Merriam-Webster's
Medical
Desk
Dictionary

Merriam-Webster's
Medical
Desk
Dictionary

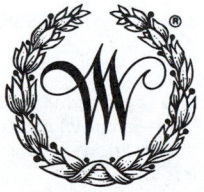

MERRIAM-WEBSTER, INCORPORATED, *Publishers*
Springfield, Massachusetts, U.S.A.

A GENUINE MERRIAM-WEBSTER

The name *Webster* alone is no guarantee of excellence. It is used by a number of publishers and may serve mainly to mislead an unwary buyer.

Merriam-Webster™ is the name you should look for when you consider the purchase of dictionaries or other fine reference books. It carries the reputation of a company that has been publishing since 1831 and is your assurance of quality and authority.

Library of Congress Cataloging in Publication Data

Merriam-Webster's medical desk dictionary
      p. cm.
   ISBN: 1-4180-0057-4 (hardcover)
   ISBN: 1-4180-0056-6 (softcover)
   1. Medicine—Dictionaries.   I. Merriam-Webster, Inc.

R121.M564 2002
610'.3—dc21   2001058656

Made in the United States of America

345678910XXX09080706

Contents

Preface

Merriam-Webster's Medical Desk Dictionary introduces a new concept in medical dictionaries. It combines a medical word list selected and defined on the basis of citational evidence with a number of features expected in a Merriam-Webster® desk dictionary such as pronunciations, end-of-line division points, functional labels, common derivatives, and irregular inflected forms. It includes British terms and spelling variants and is a record of medical English as it is used both in the United States and in international technical and general literature.

The 2005 copyrighted revision of this dictionary is a major updating including the addition of more than 500 new words and senses.

One of the most difficult challenges faced by the editors of this dictionary has been to keep both the number of vocabulary entries and the defining vocabulary within manageable limits. Without constraints on both elements, any dictionary can quickly expand to many times its intended size. If the number of entries is controlled but the defining vocabulary is not, the definitions may contain numerous words that are not entered in the dictionary itself or in a readily available, standard, general dictionary of English.

This challenge was met in two important ways. First, the number of vocabulary entries was controlled through a critical review of the medically relevant citations drawn from the more than 15,700,000 citations in the Merriam-Webster offices. A corpus of the most recent citations, consisting of more than 80 million words, is available for full-text search and retrieval. The database is continuously updated as new citational evidence becomes available.

Second, the defining vocabulary was controlled by a rigorous cross-reference process which ensured that every word used in a definition was entered in this book or in Merriam-Webster's Collegiate Dictionary. Whenever a cross-reference editor found a word in a definition that was not entered in the Collegiate Dictionary, the definer had to enter that word in this dictionary or rewrite the definition without the word.

This dictionary includes a number of other noteworthy features. First, the dictionary contains thousands of illustrations of words used in context, including hundreds of actual quotations from respected medical writers and publications. Second, there are more than one thousand short biographical sketches, each of which is placed after an entry word derived from the person's name. Third, this dictionary includes an innovative cross-reference feature: words occurring only as part of compound terms are entered at their own place in alphabetical sequence with a cross-reference to the compound terms themselves. Thus, *herpetiformis* has a cross-reference to *dermatitis herpetiformis,* and *longus* is followed by a list of 11 compound terms of which it is a part. These cross-reference entries and lists may help the reader unfamiliar with medical terminology to find the place of definition of compound terms. Fourth, the 2005 update of this dictionary implements the taxonomic nomenclature of the viruses down to the species level according to the most recent report of the International Committee on Taxonomy of Viruses (ICTV) available at the time of editing. The ICTV is part of the Virology Division of the International Union of Microbiological Societies.

The front matter of this book includes three important sections. The Explanatory Notes describe the conventions, devices, and techniques that one will find used throughout this book. All users of the dictionary are urged to read this section through and then to consult it for special information as they need to. The Explanatory Notes are followed by an informative and entertaining essay on the history and etymology of medical English by John H. Dirckx, M.D. The third section of the front matter is a gathering of entries for prefixes, suffixes, and combining forms that are commonly encountered in medical writing.

The back matter contains two sections that dictionary users have long found helpful. The first is a listing of Signs and Symbols that cannot readily be alphabetized. The second is a Handbook of Style in which various stylistic conventions (such as those of punctuation and capitalization) are summarized and exemplified. The Handbook of Style concludes with a comparative review of the styles used in preparing a bibliographic list of references for a scientific article, monograph, or book.

In this dictionary, those entries known to be trademarks or service marks are so labeled and are treated in accordance with a formula approved by the United States Trademark Association. No entry in this dictionary, however, should be regarded as affecting the validity of any trademark or service mark.

Merriam-Webster's Medical Desk Dictionary is designed to serve as an interface between the language of doctor and the language of patient, between sports medicine and the sports page, between the technical taxonomic names and the common names of plants, animals, and microorganisms, and between the old and the new in medical terminology. The user of this dictionary will find, for example, that the *abs, delts, glutes, lats, pecs,* and *quads* of the physical fitness enthusiast are the *abdominal muscles, deltoids, glutei, latissimi dorsi, pectorales,* and *quadriceps muscles* of the formal anatomist. Both medicine and science sometimes give the impression that the latest technical terminology has no antecedents. There may be no clue on the medical page of the reader's daily newspaper that the bacteria referred to as *Gardnerella* and *Helicobacter* were formerly classified as *Haemophilus* and *Campylobacter.* Medical writers may neglect to mention that the *auditory tube* and the *uterine tubes* of formal anatomy are widely known as the *eustachian tube* and *fallopian tubes.* All of these words are entered and defined in this dictionary with mention of synonyms or former terminology where appropriate.

It is the intent of the editors that this dictionary serve the purposes of all those who seek information about medical English as it is currently spoken and written, whether in the context of a clinical setting, in correctly rendered spoken and written text, or from the perspective of medical lexicography as an art and science.

Merriam-Webster's Medical Desk Dictionary is the result of a collective effort by the staff of Merriam-Webster, Incorporated. Stephen J. Perrault and Peter D. Haraty assisted the editor in preparing definitions for the original 1986 copyright, and Joan I. Narmontas assisted in defining and updating entries for the 1996, 2002, and 2005 revisions. Christopher C. Connor assisted in defining tasks for the 2005 update. For the 2002 and 2005 updates, Joshua S. Guenter, Ph.D., was responsible for pronunciations, building on the previous work of John K. Bollard, Ph.D., David B. Justice, Ph.D., and Brian M. Sietsema, Ph.D. All of the biographical paragraphs were written by Michael G.

Belanger. Jocelyn White Franklin prepared the Handbook of Style in the back matter. Cross-reference work for the updates was performed by Donna L. Rickerby, building on the previous work of Eileen M. Haraty. The manuscript for the 1986 copyright was copyedited principally by Robert D. Copeland, and the 1996, 2002, and 2005 revisions were copyedited by Madeline L. Novak. Other specialized editorial assistance was provided by Georgette B. Boucher, Susan L. Brady, Daniel B. Brandon, Jennifer N. Cislo, Robert D. Copeland, Kathleen M. Doherty, Carol A. Fugiel, Michael D. Roundy, Maria A. Sansalone, Adrienne M. Scholz, and Emily A. Vezina. Thomas F. Pitoniak, Ph.D., managed production for the 2005 update. Madeline L. Novak coordinated all editorial operations. Frederick C. Mish, Ph.D., Editor in Chief, contributed advice at several stages in the development of the book and John M. Morse, President and Publisher, made major contributions to the design and scheduling of the original and updated versions.

Roger W. Pease, Jr., Ph.D.
Editor

Explanatory Notes

Entries

Main Entries

A boldface letter or a combination of such letters, including punctuation marks and diacritics where needed, that is set flush with the left-hand margin of each column of type is a main entry or entry word. The main entry may consist of letters set solid, of letters joined by a hyphen, or of letters separated by one or more spaces:

al·ler·gy . . . *n*

¹an·ti–in·flam·ma·to·ry . . . *adj*

blood vessel *n*

non–A, non–B hepatitis . . . *n*

The material in lightface type that follows each main entry explains and justifies its inclusion in the dictionary.

Variation in the styling of compound words in English is frequent and widespread. It is often completely acceptable to choose freely among open, hyphenated, and closed alternatives. To save space for other information, this dictionary usually limits itself to a single styling for a compound. When a compound is widely used and one styling predominates, that styling is shown. When a compound is uncommon or when the evidence indicates that two or three stylings are approximately equal in frequency, the styling shown is based on the treatment of parallel compounds.

Order of Main Entries

The main entries follow one another in alphabetical order letter by letter without regard to intervening spaces or hyphens: *elastic stocking* follows *elasticity* and *right-handed* follows *right hand*. Words that often begin with the abbreviation *St.* in common usage have the abbreviation spelled out: *Saint Anthony's fire, Saint Vitus' dance*.

Full words come before parts of words made up of the same letters. Solid words come first and are followed by hyphenated compounds and then by open compounds. Lowercase entries come before entries that begin with a capital letter:

meta . . . *adj*

meta- . . . *prefix*

work·up . . . *n*

work up . . . *vt*

tri·chi·na . . . *n*

Trichina *n*

Entries containing an Arabic numeral within or at the end of the word are alphabetized as if the number were spelled out: *glucose phosphate* comes after *glucose-1=phosphate* and before *glucose-6-phosphate,* while *LD50* is between *LD* and *LDH*. Some chemical terms are preceded by one or more Arabic numerals or by a chemical prefix abbreviated to a Roman or Greek letter or by a combination of the two usually set off by a hyphen. In general, the numerical or abbreviated prefix is ignored in determining the word's alphabetical place: *N=allylnormorphine* is entered in the letter *a*, *5-hydroxytryptamine* in the letter *h*, and *β₂-microglobulin* in the letter *m*. However, if the prefix is spelled out, it is used in alphabetizing the word: *beta globulin* is entered in the letter *b*, and *levo-dihydroxyphenylalanine* in the letter *l*. In a few cases, entries have been made at more than one place to assist the reader in finding the place of definition, especially when the prefix has variants: *gamma=aminobutyric acid,* defined in the letter *g*, is often written with a Greek letter as *γ-aminobutyric acid,* and an entry has been made in the letter *a* to direct the reader to the place of definition.

If the names of two chemical substances differ only in their prefixes, the terms are alphabetized first by the main part of the word and then in relation to each other according to the prefix: *L-PAM* immediately precedes *2-PAM* in the letter *p*.

Guide Words

A pair of guide words is printed at the top of each page. The entries that fall alphabetically between the guide words are found on that page.

It is important to remember that alphabetical order rather than position of an entry on the page determines the selection of guide words. The first guide word is the alphabetically first entry on the page. The second guide word is usually the alphabetically last entry on the page:

alkalotic • alloantigen

The entry need not be a main entry. Another boldface word—a variant, an inflected form, or a defined or undefined run-on—may be selected as a guide word. For this reason the last main entry on a page is not always the last entry alphabetically:

cesarean section • challenging

All guide words must themselves be in alphabetical order from page to page throughout the dictionary; thus, the alphabetically last entry on a page is not used if it follows alphabetically the first guide word on the next page.

Homographs

When main entries are spelled alike, they are called homographs and are distinguished by superscript numerals preceding each word:

[1]**an·orex·ic** ... *adj*

[2]**anorexic** *n*

[1]**mi·crom·e·ter** ... *n*

[2]**mi·cro·me·ter** ... *n*

Although homographs are spelled alike, they may differ in pronunciation, derivation, or functional classification (as part of speech). The order of homographs is usually historical: the one first used in English is entered first. In this dictionary abbreviations and symbols are listed last in a series of homographs and are not given superscripts. Abbreviations appear before symbols when both are present.

End-of-Line Division

The centered dots within entry words indicate division points at which a hyphen may be put at the end of a line of print or writing. Centered dots are not shown after a single initial letter or before a single terminal letter because printers seldom cut off a single letter:

abort ... *vi*

body ... *n*

Nor are they shown at second and succeeding homographs unless these differ among themselves in division or pronunciation:

[1]**mu·tant** ... *adj*

[2]**mutant** *n*

[1]**pre·cip·i·tate** \pri-'sip-ə-ˌtāt\ *vb*

[2]**pre·cip·i·tate** \pri-'sip-ət-ət, -ə-ˌtāt\ *n*

There are acceptable alternative end-of-line divisions just as there are acceptable variant spellings and pronunciations. No more than one division is, however, shown for an entry in this dictionary.

Many words have two or more common pronunciation variants, and the same end-of-line division is not always appropriate for each of them. The division *du·o·de·num,* for example, best fits the variant \ˌd(y)ü-ə-'dē-nəm\ whereas the division *du·od·e·num* best fits the variant \d(y)ù-'äd-ən-əm\. In instances like this, the division falling farther to the left is used, regardless of the order of the pronunciations:

du·o·de·num \ˌd(y)ü-ə-'dē-nəm, d(y)ù-'äd-ən-əm\

A double hyphen at the end of a line in this dictionary stands for a hyphen that belongs at that point in a hyphenated word and that is retained when the word is written as a unit on one line:

Bac·te·roi·des \-'rȯid-(ˌ)ēz\ *n* **1** *cap* : a genus of gram= negative anaerobic bacteria that belong to ...

Variants

When a main entry is followed by the word *or* and another spelling, the two spellings are equal variants:

ten·di·ni·tis *or* ten·don·itis

If two variants joined by *or* are out of alphabetical order, they remain equal variants. The one printed first is, however, slightly more common than the second:

se·ro·log·i·cal ... *or* se·ro·log·ic

When another spelling is joined to the main entry by the word *also,* the spelling after *also* is a secondary variant and occurs less frequently than the first:

lip·id ... *also* lip·ide

If there are two secondary variants, the second is joined to the first by *or.* Once the word *also* is used to signal a secondary variant, all following variants are joined by *or* (except as discussed in the next paragraph):

[1]**ce·sar·e·an** *or* cae·sar·e·an *also* ce·sar·i·an *or* cae·sar·i·an

If one variant has an italic label *Brit* (for "British") or *chiefly Brit,* the label applies to all of the variants given after it. If the *Brit* label is preceded by *also,* the variants appearing before the label are preferred in British as well as in U.S. usage to those following the label. If a variant after the first one following a *Brit* or *chiefly Brit* label is preceded by *also,* it and succeeding variants are secondary British variants:

ster·il·ize *also Brit* ster·il·ise ... *vt* -ized *also Brit* -ised; -iz·ing *also Brit* -is·ing

hem·ag·glu·ti·nin ... *also* he·mo·ag·glu·ti·nin ... *or chiefly Brit* haem·ag·glu·ti·nin *also* hae·mo·ag·glu·ti·nin *n*

A variant whose own alphabetical place is at some distance from the main entry is also entered at its own place with a cross-reference to the main entry. Such variants at consecutive or nearly consecutive entries are listed together, and if there are five or more they are usually collected in a table:

tendonitis *var of* TENDINITIS

procaryote, procaryotic *var of* PROKARYOTE, PROKARYOTIC

Each boldface word in the list below is a variant of the word to its right in small capitals.

desamidate	DEAMIDATE	desamidization	DEAMIDIZATION
desamida- tion	DEAMIDATION	desamidize	DEAMIDIZE
		desaminase	DEAMINASE

Run-on Entries

A main entry may be followed by one or more derivatives or by a homograph with a different functional label. These are run-on entries. Each is introduced by a lightface dash and each has a functional label. They are not defined, however, since their meanings can readily be derived from the meaning of the root word:

healthy ... *adj* ... — **health·i·ly** ... *adv* — **health·i·ness** ... *n*

drift ... *n* ... — **drift** *vi*

A main entry may be followed by one or more phrases containing the entry word. These are also run-on entries. Each is introduced by a lightface dash but there is no functional label. They are, however, defined since their meanings are more than the sum of the meanings of their elements:

breath ... *n* ... — **out of breath** : ...

run ... *vi* ... — **run a fever** *or* **run a temperature** : ...

Variants are shown, where appropriate, at run-on entries:

par·a·sit·ize *also Brit* par·a·sit·ise ... *vt* ... — **par·a·sit·iza·tion** *also Brit* par·a·sit·isa·tion ... *n*

A run-on entry is an independent entry with respect to function and status. Labels at the main entry do not apply unless they are repeated.

Pronunciation

The matter between a pair of reversed virgules \ \ following the entry word indicates the pronunciation. The symbols used are listed in the chart printed on the page facing the first page of the dictionary proper. An abbreviated list appears at the bottom of the second column of each right-hand page of the vocabulary.

Syllables

A hyphen is used in the pronunciation to show syllabic division. These hyphens sometimes coincide with the centered dots in the entry word that indicate end-of-line division; sometimes they do not:

ab·scess \'ab-ˌses\

met·ric \'me-trik\

Stress

A high-set mark \'\ indicates primary (strongest) stress or accent; a low-set mark \ˌ\ indicates secondary (medium) stress or accent:

ear·ache \'i(ə)r-ˌāk\

The stress mark stands at the beginning of the syllable that receives the stress.

Variant Pronunciations

The presence of variant pronunciations indicates that not all educated speakers pronounce words the same way. A second- or third-place variant is not to be regarded as less acceptable than the pronunciation that is given first. It may, in fact, be used by as many educated speakers as the first variant, but the requirements of the printed page are such that one must precede the other:

oral \'ōr-əl, 'òr-, 'är-\

um·bi·li·cus \ˌəm-'bil-i-kəs, ˌəm-bə-'lī-\

A variant that is appreciably less common is preceded by the word *also*:

se·nile \'sēn-ˌīl *also* 'sen-\

Sometimes a geographical label precedes a variant:

meth·ane \'meth-ˌān, *Brit usu* 'mē-ˌthān\

Parentheses in Pronunciations

Symbols enclosed by parentheses represent elements that are present in the pronunciation of some speakers but are absent from the pronunciation of other speakers, elements that are present in some but absent from other utterances of the same speaker, or elements whose presence or absence is uncertain:

neu·ral \'n(y)ùr-əl\

re·sponse \ri-'spän(t)s\

Partial and Absent Pronunciations

When a main entry has less than a full pronunciation, the missing part is to be supplied from a pronunciation in a preceding entry or within the same pair of reversed virgules:

psy·cho·sur·gery \-'sərj-(ə-)rē\

vit·i·li·go \ˌvit-əl-'ī-(ˌ)gō *also* -'ē-\

The pronunciation of the first two syllables of *psycho-surgery* is found at the main entry *psychosurgeon:*

psy·cho·sur·geon \ˌsī-kō-'sər-jən\

The hyphens before and after \'ē\ in the pronunciation of *vitiligo* indicate that both the first and the last parts of the pronunciation are to be taken from the immediately preceding pronunciation.

When a variation of stress is involved, a partial pronunciation may be terminated at the stress mark which stands at the beginning of a syllable not shown:

li·gate \'lī-ˌgāt, lī-'\

In general, no pronunciation is indicated for open compounds consisting of two or more English words that have own-place entry:

lateral collateral ligament n

A pronunciation is shown, however, for any unentered element of an open compound:

Meiss·ner's corpuscle \'mīs-nərz-\

Only the first entry in a sequence of numbered homographs is given a pronunciation if their pronunciations are the same:

¹**sig·moid** \'sig-ˌmòid\ *adj*

²**sigmoid** n

The pronunciation of unpronounced derivatives run on at a main entry is a combination of the pronunciation at the main entry and the pronunciation of the suffix or final element.

Abbreviations, Acronyms, and Symbols

Pronunciations are not usually shown for entries with the functional labels *abbr* or *symbol* since they are usually spoken by saying the individual letters in sequence or by giving the expansion. The pronunciation is given only if there is an unusual and unexpected way of saying the abbreviation or symbol:

ICU *abbr* intensive care unit

Al *symbol* aluminum

CABG \'kab-ij\ *abbr* coronary artery bypass graft

Acronyms (as *DNA* and *HEPA*) and compounds (as *ACE inhibitor*) consisting of an acronym and a word element which have one of the traditional parts of speech labels (usually *n, adj, adv,* or *vb* in this book) are given a pronunciation even when the word is spoken by pronouncing the letters in sequence:

DNA \ˌdē-ˌen-'ā\ *n*

HEPA \'hep-ə\ *adj*

ACE inhibitor \'ās-, ˌā-(ˌ)sē-'ē-\ *n*

Functional Labels

An italic label indicating a part of speech or some other functional classification follows the pronunciation or, if no pronunciation is given, the main entry. Of the eight traditional parts of speech, five appear in this dictionary as follows:

> **con·ta·gious** ... *adj*
>
> **op·ti·cal·ly** ... *adv*
>
> **phy·si·cian** ... *n*
>
> **per** ... *prep*
>
> **pre·scribe** ... *vb*

If a verb is both transitive and intransitive, the labels *vt* and *vi* introduce the subdivisions:

> **op·er·ate** ... *vb* ... *vi* ... ∼ *vt*

A boldface swung dash ∼ is used to stand for the main entry (as *operate*) and separate the subdivisions of the verb. If there are no subdivisions, the label *vt* or *vi* takes the place of *vb:*

> **med·i·cate** ... *vt*
>
> ²**faint** *vi*

Other italic labels used to indicate functional classifications, both in the main vocabulary section and in the section of the front matter containing the combining forms, include:

> **tid** *abbr*
>
> **pleur-** *or* **pleuro-** *comb form*
>
> **-poi·e·sis** ... *n comb form*
>
> **-poi·et·ic** ... *adj comb form*
>
> **dys-** *prefix*
>
> **-lyt·ic** ... *adj suffix*
>
> **-i·a·sis** ... *n suffix*
>
> **Rolf·ing** ... *service mark*
>
> **Ca** *symbol*
>
> **Val·ium** ... *trademark*
>
> **sig·na** ... *vb imper*

Two functional labels are sometimes combined:

> **calm·ative** ... *n or adj*
>
> **cold tur·key** ... *n* ... — **cold turkey** *adv or vt*

Inflected Forms

The inflected forms recorded in this dictionary include the plurals of nouns; the past tense, the past participle when it differs from the past tense, and the present participle of verbs; and the comparative and superlative forms of adjectives and adverbs. When these inflected forms are created in a manner considered regular in English (as by adding *-s* or *-es* to nouns, *-ed* and *-ing* to verbs, and *-er* and *-est* to adjectives and adverbs) and when it seems that there is nothing about the formation to give the dictionary user doubts, the inflected form is not shown in order to save space for information more likely to be sought.

If the inflected form is created in an irregular way or if the dictionary user is likely to have doubts about it (even if it is formed regularly), the inflected form is shown in boldface either in full or, especially when the word has three or more syllables, cut back to a convenient and easily recognizable point.

The inflected forms of nouns, verbs, adjectives, and adverbs are shown in this dictionary when suffixation brings about a change in final *y* to *i*, when the word ends in *-ey*, when there are variant inflected forms, and when the dictionary user might have doubts about the spelling of the inflected form:

> **thirsty** ... *adj* **thirst·i·er; -est**
>
> ²**atrophy** ... *vb* **-phied; -phy·ing**
>
> **kid·ney** ... *n, pl* **kidneys**
>
> **sar·co·ma** ... *n, pl* **-mas** *also* **-ma·ta**
>
> ¹**burn** ... *vb* **burned** ... *or* **burnt** ...; **burn·ing**
>
> **sta·tus** ... *n, pl* **sta·tus·es**

A plural is also shown for a noun when it ends in a consonant plus *o* or in a double *oo*, and when its plural is identical with the singular. Many nouns in medical English have highly irregular plurals modeled after their language of origin. Sometimes more than one element of a compound term is pluralized:

> **ego** ... *n, pl* **egos**
>
> **HMO** ... *n, pl* **HMOs**
>
> ²**tattoo** *n, pl* **tattoos**
>
> ¹**pu·bes** ... *n, pl* **pubes**
>
> **en·ceph·a·li·tis** ... *n, pl* **-lit·i·des**
>
> **cor pul·mo·na·le** ... *n, pl* **cor·dia pul·mo·na·lia**

Nouns that are plural in form and that are regularly used with a plural verb are labeled *n pl*. Nouns that are plural in form but are not always construed as plural are appropriately labeled:

> **in·nards** ... *n pl*
>
> **rick·ets** ... *n pl but sing in constr*
>
> **smelling salts** *n pl but sing or pl in constr*

A noun that is singular in construction takes a singular verb when it is used as a subject; a noun that is plural in construction takes a plural verb when it is used as a subject.

The inflected forms of verbs, adjectives, and adverbs are also shown whenever suffixation brings about a doubling of a final consonant, elision of a final *e*, or a radical change in the base word itself. The principal parts of a verb are shown when a final *-c* changes to *-ck* in suffixation:

> ²**scar** *vb* **scarred; scar·ring**
>
> **hot** ... *adj* **hot·ter; hot·test**
>
> **op·er·ate** ... *vb* **-at·ed; -at·ing**
>
> **sane** ... *adj* **san·er; san·est**
>
> ¹**break** ... *vb* **broke** ...; **bro·ken** ...; **break·ing**
>
> ¹**ill** ... *adj* **worse** ...; **worst**
>
> ²**panic** *vb* **pan·icked** ...; **pan·ick·ing**

Regularly inflected forms are shown when it is desirable to indicate the pronunciation of one of the inflected forms:

²**blister** *vb* **blis·tered; blis·ter·ing** \-t(ə-)riŋ\

Inflected forms may be shown at run-on entries and may be cut back like inflected forms of main entries:

¹**scab** ... *n* ... — **scab·by** ... *adj* **scab·bi·er; -est**
rem·e·dy ... *n* ... — **remedy** *vt* **-died; -dy·ing**

Capitalization

Most entries in this dictionary begin with a lowercase letter, indicating that the word is not ordinarily capitalized. A few entries have an italic label *often cap*, indicating that the word is as likely to begin with a capital letter as not and is equally acceptable either way. Some entries begin with an uppercase letter, which indicates that the word is usually capitalized:

pan·cre·as ... *n*

braille ... *n, often cap*

Gol·gi ... *adj*

The capitalization of entries that are open or hyphenated compounds is similarly indicated by the form of the entry or by an italic label:

heart attack *n*

¹**neo–Freud·ian** ... *adj, often cap N*

Agent Orange ... *n*

Many acronyms are written entirely or partly in capitals, and this fact is shown by the form of the entry or by an italic label:

UTI ... *n*

cgs *adj, often cap C&G&S*

A word that is capitalized in some senses and lowercase in others shows variations from the form of the main entry by the use of italic labels at the appropriate senses:

strep·to·coc·cus ... *n* 1 *cap*

pill ... *n* ... 2 *often cap*

Attributive Nouns

The italicized label *often attrib* placed after the functional label *n* indicates that the noun is often used as an adjective equivalent in attributive position before another noun:

blood ... *n, often attrib*

hos·pi·tal ... *n, often attrib*

Examples of the attributive use of these nouns are *blood circulation* and *hospital ward*.

While any noun may occasionally be used in attribution, the label *often attrib* is limited to those having broad attributive use. This label is not used when an adjective homograph (as *serum*) is entered. When it is desired to show that a compound term is frequently used in attribution, a usage note follows the definition together with a verbal illustration indicating whether or not a hyphen is typically used:

spin echo *n* ... — usu. used attributively ⟨*spin-echo* magnetic resonance imaging of the cervical spine⟩ ...

Etymology

Etymologies showing the origin of particular words are given in this dictionary only for some abbreviations and acronyms and for all eponyms.

If an entry for an abbreviation is followed by the expansion from which it is derived, no etymology is given. However, if the abbreviation is derived from a phrase in a foreign language or in English that is not mentioned elsewhere in the entry, that phrase and its language of origin (if other than English) is given in square brackets following the functional label:

IFN *abbr* interferon

bid *abbr* [Latin *bis in die*] twice a day

Words derived from the names of persons are called eponyms. Eponymous entries in this dictionary are followed by a short biographical sketch of the person or a brief account of the legendary, mythical, or fictional figure from whose name the term is derived:

Pas·teur effect ... *n* ...
Pas·teur \pȧs-tœr\, **Louis (1822–1895),** French chemist and bacteriologist. Pasteur made contributions that rank with the greatest in modern science. His achievements include ...

Doubtful dates are followed by a question mark, and approximate dates are preceded by *ca* (circa). In some instances only the years of principal activity are given, preceded by the abbreviation *fl* (flourished):

sap·phic ... *adj or n* ...
Sap·pho ... (*fl ca* 610 BC–*ca* 580 BC), Greek lyric poet.

If a series of main entries is derived from the name of one person, the paragraph usually follows the first entry. The dictionary user who turns, for example, to *pasteurella, pasteurellosis, pasteurization, pasteurize,* or *Pasteur treatment* and seeks biographical information is expected to glance back to the first entry in the sequence, *Pasteur effect.*

If an eponym is compounded from the names of two or more individuals, several sketches may follow a single entry either as separate paragraphs (as at *Watson⸗Crick*) or incorporated into a single paragraph (as at *Guillain-Barré syndrome*).

If an eponymous entry is defined by a synonymous cross-reference to the entry where a biographical paragraph appears, no other cross-reference is made. However, if the definition of an eponymous entry contains no clue as to the location of the paragraph, the name of the individual is given following the entry and a directional cross-reference is made to the appropriate entry:

gland of Bartholin *n* : BARTHOLIN'S GLAND

gland of Bow·man ... *n* : any of the tubular and often branched glands occurring beneath the olfactory epithelium of the nose ...
W. Bowman — see BOWMAN'S CAPSULE

A paragraph on C. T. Bartholin can be found at *Bartholin's gland* and one on William Bowman at *Bowman's capsule.*

Usage

Usage Labels

Three types of status labels are used in this dictionary—temporal, regional, and stylistic—to signal that a word or a sense of a word is restricted in usage.

The temporal label *obs* for "obsolete" means that there is no evidence of use since 1755:

eryn·go ... *n* ... *obs*

The temporal label *archaic* means that a word or sense once in common use is found only rarely today:

em·bryo ... *n* ... **1** *archaic*

The labels *obs* and *archaic* are comments on the word being defined. When a thing, as distinguished from the word used to designate it, is obsolete or outmoded with respect to some use or application or is part of a discredited theory or concept, appropriate orientation is usually given in the definition:

black bile *n* : the one of the four humors of ancient and medieval physiology that was believed to be secreted by the kidneys and spleen and to cause melancholy

A word or sense limited in use to a specific region of the English-speaking world has an appropriate label. The adverb *chiefly* precedes a label when the word has some currency outside a specified region, and a double label is used to indicate currency in each of two specific regions:

red bug ... *n, Southern & Midland*

ap·pen·di·cec·to·my ... *n* ... *Brit*

enzootic ataxia *n, chiefly Austral*

The stylistic label *slang* is used with words or senses that are especially appropriate in contexts of extreme informality, that usually have a currency not limited to a particular region or area of interest, and that are composed typically of shortened forms or extravagant or facetious figures of speech. Words with the label *slang* are entered if they have been or in the opinion of the editors are likely to be encountered in communicating with patients especially in emergencies. A few words from the huge informal argot of medicine are entered with the label *med slang* because they have appeared in general context or have been the subject of discussion in medical journals:

ben·ny ... *n* ... *slang*

go·mer ... *n, med slang*

Subject orientation is generally given in the definition; however, a guide phrase is sometimes used to indicate a specific application of a word or sense:

¹drug ... *n* **1** ... **b** *according to the Food, Drug, and Cosmetic Act*

erupt ... *vi* **1** *of a tooth*

Illustrations of Usage

Definitions are sometimes followed by verbal illustrations that show a typical use of the word in context. These illustrations are enclosed in angle brackets, and the word being illustrated is usually replaced by a lightface swung dash. The swung dash stands for the boldface entry word, and it may be followed by an italicized suffix:

¹med·i·cal ... *adj* ... **2** ... ⟨a ∼ emergency⟩

ab·sorb ... *vt* **1** ... ⟨surgical sutures which can be ∼*ed* by the body⟩

The swung dash is not used when the form of the boldface entry word is changed in suffixation, and it is not used for open compounds:

ab·nor·mal·i·ty ... *n* ... **2** ... ⟨brain-wave *abnormalities*⟩

tie off ... *vt* ... ⟨*tie off* a bleeding vessel⟩

Illustrative quotations are also used to show words in typical contexts:

peri·tu·bu·lar ... *adj* ... ⟨∼ fibroblasts of the renal cortex —Deborah R. Bosman *et al*⟩

hos·pi·tal·ize ... *vt* ... ⟨the child was *hospitalized* at once for diagnosis and treatment —*Jour. Amer. Med. Assoc.*⟩

Usage Notes

Definitions are sometimes followed by usage notes that give supplementary information about such matters as idiom, syntax, semantic relationship, and status. For trademarks and service marks, a usage note is used in place of a definition. A usage note is introduced by a lightface dash:

pill ... *n* ... **2** ... : ... — usu. used with *the*

¹purge ... *vb* ... *vt* ... **2** : ... — used of a liquid

bug ... *n* **1 a** : ... — not used technically

hs *abbr* ... — used esp. in writing prescriptions

Pro·zac ... *trademark* — used for a preparation of the hydrochloride of fluoxetine

Sometimes a usage note calls attention to one or more terms with the same denotation as the main entry or to an abbreviation for it:

lep·ro·sy ... *n* ... : a chronic disease caused by infection with an acid-fast bacillus of the genus *Mycobacterium* (*M. leprae*) ... — called also *hansenosis, Hansen's disease, lepra*

blood pressure *n* : pressure exerted by the blood upon the ... — abbr. *BP*

The called-also terms are shown in italic type. If the called-also term falls alphabetically more than one entry away from the principal entry, it is entered in alphabetical sequence with the sole definition being a synonymous cross-reference to the entry where it appears in the usage note:

han·sen·osis ... *n* ... : LEPROSY

Hansen's disease *n* : LEPROSY

lep·ra ... *n* : LEPROSY

Two or more usage notes are separated by a semicolon:

parathyroid hormone *n* : a hormone of the parathyroid gland that ... — abbr. *PTH;* called also *parathormone*

Sense Division

A boldface colon is used in this dictionary to introduce a definition:

pul·mo·nary ... *adj* : relating to, functioning like, associated with, or carried on by the lungs

It is also used to separate two or more definitions of a single sense:

¹quack ... *n* : a pretender to medical skill : an ignorant or dishonest practitioner

Boldface Arabic numerals separate the senses of a word that has more than one sense:

nerve ... *n* **1** : any of the filamentous bands of nervous tissue that connect parts of the nervous system with the other organs ... **2 nerves** *pl* : a state or condition of nervous agitation or irritability **3** : the sensitive pulp of a tooth

Boldface lowercase letters separate the subsenses of a word:

¹dose ... *n* **1 a** : the measured quantity of a therapeutic agent to be taken at one time **b** : the quantity of radiation administered or absorbed **2** : a gonorrheal infection

Lightface numerals in parentheses indicate a further division of subsenses:

ra·di·a·tion ... *n* ... **2 a** : ... **b** (1) : the process of emitting radiant energy ... (2) : the combined processes of emission, transmission, and absorption of radiant energy

A lightface colon following a definition and immediately preceding two or more subsenses indicates that the subsenses are subsumed by the preceding definition:

mac·u·la ... *n* ... **2** : an anatomical structure having the form of a spot differentiated from surrounding tissues: as **a** : MACULA ACUSTICA **b** : MACULA LUTEA

extensor ret·i·nac·u·lum ... *n* **1** : either of two fibrous bands of fascia crossing the front of the ankle: **a** : a lower band ... **b** : an upper band ...

The word *as* may or may not follow the lightface colon. Its presence (as at *macula*) indicates that the following subsenses are typical or significant examples. Its absence (as at *extensor retinaculum*) indicates that the subsenses which follow are exhaustive.

Sometimes a particular semantic relationship between senses is suggested by the use of one of four italic sense dividers: *esp, specif, also,* or *broadly.* The sense divider *esp* (for *especially*) is used to introduce the most common meaning subsumed in the more general preceding definition. The sense divider *specif* (for *specifically*) is used to introduce a common but highly restricted meaning subsumed in the more general preceding definition. The sense divider *also* is used to introduce a meaning that is closely related to but may be considered less important than the preceding sense. The sense divider *broadly* is used to introduce an extended or wider meaning of the preceding definition.

The order of senses within an entry is historical: the sense known to have been first used in English is entered first. This is not to be taken to mean, however, that each sense of a multisense word developed from the immediately preceding sense. It is altogether possible that sense 1 of a word has given rise to sense 2 and sense 2 to sense 3, but frequently sense 2 and sense 3 may have arisen independently of one another from sense 1.

Information coming between the entry word and the first definition of a multisense word applies to all senses and subsenses. Information applicable only to some senses or subsenses is given between the appropriate boldface numeral or letter and the symbolic colon:

bur ... *n* **1** *usu* burr

trep·o·ne·ma ... *n* **1** *cap* ... **2** *pl* **-ma·ta** ... *or* **-mas**

Names of Plants, Animals & Microorganisms

The most familiar names of living and formerly living things are the common or vernacular names (as *mosquito, poison ivy,* or *Epstein-Barr virus*) that are determined by popular usage.

In contrast, the scientific names of biological classification are governed by four highly prescriptive, internationally recognized codes of nomenclature for zoology, botany, bacteriology, and virology. These systems of names classify each kind of organism into a hierarchy of groups—taxa—with each kind of organism having one—and only one—correct name and belonging to one—and only one—taxon at each level of classification in the hierarchy.

The taxonomic names of biological nomenclature are used in this dictionary in the definitions of the common names of plants, animals, and microorganisms and in the definitions of diseases and products relating to specific plants, animals, and microorganisms when those organisms do not have entries of their own. In general, the species names of organisms do not have their own entries, but the names of genera, families, and higher taxa may. Taxonomic names that are not given own-place entry will appear only within parentheses when used in a definition. If a name is used in a definition and is not inside parentheses, there is an entry for it at its own alphabetical place:

dust mite *n* : any of various mites (esp. family Pyroglyphidae) implicated in human allergic reactions ...

Rocky Moun·tain spotted fever ... *n* : an acute bacterial disease ... that is caused by a bacterium of the genus *Rickettsia* (*R. rickettsii*) usu. transmitted by ixodid ticks and esp. by the American dog tick and Rocky Mountain wood tick

sand·fly fever ... *n* : a virus disease ... caused by either of two bunyaviruses of the genus *Phlebovirus* transmitted by the bite of a sand fly of the genus *Phlebotomus* (esp. *P. papatasii*) ...

The use of Pyroglyphidae inside parentheses indicates that this family does not have own-place entry in the A to Z vocabulary section of this dictionary. The use of *Rickettsia, Phlebovirus,* and *Phlebotomus* outside of parentheses indicates that definitions of these genera are entered at their own places. The scientific names of the *American dog tick* and *Rocky Mountain wood tick* will be found at the entries for these organisms.

Many common names are derived directly from the names of taxa, and especially genera, with little or no modification. The genus name (as *Acarus* or *Chlamydia* or *Lentivirus*) is capitalized and italicized but is never pluralized. In contrast, the common or vernacular name (as acarus or chlamydia or lentivirus) is not usually capitalized or italicized but does take a plural (as acari or chlamydiae or lentiviruses). In many cases both the systematic taxonomic name and the common name derived from it are entered in this dictionary:

> **giar·dia** ... *n* **1** *cap* : a genus of flagellate protozoans inhabiting the intestines of various mammals and including one (*G. lamblia* syn. *Lamblia intestinalis*) that is associated with diarrhea in humans **2** : any flagellate of the genus *Giardia*
>
> **ephed·ra** ... *n* **1 a** *cap* : a large genus of jointed nearly leafless shrubs (family Gnetaceae) of dry or desert regions that have the leaves reduced to scales at the nodes and include some (esp. *E. sinica*) that are a source of ephedrine ... **b** : any plant of the genus *Ephedra* ...
>
> **mor·bil·li·vi·rus** ... *n* **1** *cap* : a genus of single-stranded RNA viruses of the family *Paramyxoviridae* that includes the causative agents of measles, canine distemper, and rinderpest **2** : any of the genus *Morbillivirus* of paramyxoviruses

The entries defining the names of plants, animals, and microorganisms are usually oriented to a taxon higher in the systematic hierarchy by including in the definition either a systematic name of higher rank (as *Chlamydiaceae* at *chlamydia*), a common name (as *poxvirus* at *orthopoxvirus*, or a technical adjective (as *digenetic* at *Schistosomatoidea*):

> **chla·myd·ia** ... *n* **1** *cap* : the type genus of the family Chlamydiaceae comprising coccoid to spherical gram-negative intracellular parasitic bacteria ...
>
> **or·tho·pox·vi·rus** ... *n* **1** *cap* : a genus of poxviruses that are brick-shaped ... and that include the vaccina virus and the causative agents of cowpox, monkeypox, mousepox, and smallpox
>
> **Schis·to·so·ma·toi·dea** ... *n pl* : a superfamily of digenetic trematodes that lack a metacercaria ...

When a common name or technical adjective is used for orientation to a higher taxon, the name of the higher taxon will usually be found in the definition of the common name or technical adjective. For example, the definition of *poxvirus* includes the name of the family *Poxviridae,* and the definition of *digenetic* contains the name of the higher taxon Digenea.

Linnaean Nomenclature of Plants, Animals, and Bacteria

The nomenclatural codes for botany, zoology, and bacteriology follow the binomial nomenclature of Carolus Linnaeus, who employed a New Latin vocabulary for the names of organisms and the names of ranks in the hierarchy of classification.

The fundamental taxon is the genus. It includes a group of closely related kinds of plants (as the genus *Digitalis,* which contains the foxgloves), a group of closely related kinds of animals (as the genus *Canis,* which includes coyotes, jackals, wolves, and domesticated dogs), or a group of closely related kinds of bacteria (as the genus *Streptococcus,* which includes numerous pathogens of humans and domesticated animals). The genus name is an italicized and capitalized singular noun.

The unique name of each kind of organism or species in the Linnaean system is the binomial or species name which consists of two parts: a genus name and an italicized lowercase word—the specific epithet—denoting the species. The name for a variety or subspecies—the trinomial, variety name, or subspecies name—adds a similar varietal or subspecific epithet. The head louse (*Pediculus humanus capitis*) is a subspecies of the species (*Pediculus humanus*) to which the body louse belongs.

The genus name in a binomial may be abbreviated to its initial letter if it has previously been spelled out in full within the same text. In this dictionary, a genus name will be found abbreviated before a specific epithet when the genus is spelled out in full earlier within the same sense or within a group of senses that fall under a single boldface sense number:

> **scar·let fever** ... *n* : an acute contagious febrile disease caused by Group A bacteria of the genus *Streptococcus* (esp. various strains of *S. pyogenes*) and characterized ...

In Linnaean nomenclature, the names of taxa higher than the genus (as family, order, and class) are capitalized plural nouns that are often used with singular verbs and are not abbreviated in normal use. They are not italicized.

Sometimes two or more different New Latin names can be found used in current literature for the same organism or group. This may happen, for example, when old monographs and field guides are kept in print after name changes occur or when there are legitimate differences of opinion about the validity of the names. To help the reader in recognizing an organism or group in such cases, alternative names are shown as synonyms in this dictionary:

> **Bedsonia** *n, syn of* CHLAMYDIA
>
> **plague** ... *n* ... **2** : a virulent contagious febrile disease that is caused by a bacterium of the genus *Yersinia* (*Y. pestis* syn. *Pasteurella pestis*) ...

Virus Nomenclature

The system of naming viruses evolved in a series of reports by a committee of the International Union of Microbiological Societies. The report published in 2000 with the title *Virus Taxonomy: Seventh Report of the International Committee on Taxonomy of Viruses (7th Rept. of the ICTV)* is the one followed in this dictionary. The code of nomenclature developed there is independent of the three Linnaean systems governing the taxonomy of plants, animals, and bacteria and differs in the way names are constructed and written.

Except as noted below, the names for species, genera, and families of viruses used in this dictionary are those that are recognized by the International Committee on Taxonomy of Viruses. Such names appear in italics and are preceded by the name of the taxon ("species," "genus," or "family") in roman before the italicized name.

The name of a species consists of an italicized phrase in which the first word is capitalized, other words are lowercase unless derived from a proper name, and the last word is *virus*. The name of a genus is usually a single capitalized word ending in -*virus*. The name of a family is a single capitalized word ending in -*viridae*:

> **small·pox** ... *n* : an acute contagious febrile disease of humans that is caused by a poxvirus of the genus *Orthopoxvirus* (species *Variola virus*) ...

pox·vi·rus ... *n* : any of the family *Poxviridae* of brick‑shaped or ovoid double-stranded DNA viruses

Unlike the Linnaean codes, virus nomenclature does not have in place a protocol for handling synonyms, names that were once in good standing but have been replaced by others. Several names (as family Myxoviridae and family Papovaviridae) that were once in good standing are not found in any of the indices of the *7th Rept. of the ICTV*. At best a word or two of explanation is offered in the articles on the taxa replacing them. In order to provide continuity, entries for some defunct taxa are retained in this dictionary when their names are still in common use:

Pa·po·va·vi·ri·dae ... *n pl* : a former family of double‑stranded DNA viruses that included the polyomaviruses and the papillomaviruses before they were placed in their own families

The names of the two families to which the viruses included in the former family Papovaviridae are now assigned can be found at the definitions of polyomavirus and *papillomavirus*.

Cross-Reference

Four different kinds of cross-references are used in this dictionary: directional, synonymous, cognate, and inflectional. In each instance the cross-reference is readily recognized by the lightface small capitals in which it is printed.

A cross-reference usually following a lightface dash and beginning with *see* or *compare* is a directional cross‑reference. It directs the dictionary user to look elsewhere for further information. A *compare* cross‑reference is regularly appended to a definition; a *see* cross-reference may stand alone:

car·ri·er ... *n*   **1 a** ... compare RESERVOIR 2, VECTOR 2

iron ... *n*   **1** ... — symbol *Fe*; see ELEMENT table

mammary artery — see INTERNAL THORACIC ARTERY

A *see* cross-reference may be used to indicate the place of definition of an entry containing one or more Arabic numerals or abbreviated chemical prefixes that might cause doubt. Examples of chemical names are given above at "Order of Main Entries." The entry below follows the entry for the abbreviation *GP:*

G₁ phase, G₂ phase — see entries alphabetized as G ONE PHASE, G TWO PHASE

A *see* cross-reference may appear after the definition of the name of a generic drug to refer the reader to one or more trademarks used for preparations of the drug:

flu·ox·e·tine ... *n* ... — see PROZAC

hy·dro·co·done ... *n* ... — see HYCODAN, VICODIN

A cross-reference immediately following a boldface colon is a synonymous cross-reference. It may stand alone as the only definitional matter, it may follow an analytical definition, or it may be one of two synonymous cross-references separated by a comma:

serum hepatitis *n* : HEPATITIS B

sys·tem·a·tist ... *n* : a classifying scientist : TAXONOMIST

ad·i·po·sis ... *n* ... **1** : ADIPOSITY, OBESITY

A synonymous cross-reference indicates that a definition at the entry cross-referred to can be substituted as a definition for the entry or the sense or subsense in which the cross-reference appears.

A cross-reference following an italic *var of* is a cognate cross-reference:

anchylostomiasis *var of* ANCYLOSTOMIASIS

manoeuvre *chiefly Brit var of* MANEUVER

A cross-reference following an italic label that identifies an entry as an inflected form is an inflectional cross‑reference. Inflectional cross-references appear only when the inflected form falls alphabetically at some distance from the main entry:

corpora *pl of* CORPUS

broke *past of* BREAK

When guidance seems needed as to which one of several homographs or which sense of a multisense word is being referred to, a superscript numeral may precede the cross-reference or a sense number may follow it or both:

ossa *pl of* ¹OS

lateral cuneiform bone *n* : CUNEIFORM BONE 1c

Combining Forms, Prefixes & Suffixes

Combining forms, prefixes, and suffixes of medical importance are listed in a separate section in the front matter beginning at page 27a. However, a few of chemical significance (as **d-** and **orth-** *or* **ortho-**) are entered in alphabetical sequence in the dictionary because of the frequency with which they are prefixed to the names of chemical substances, often in abbreviated form and set off by a hyphen.

Abbreviations & Symbols

Abbreviations and symbols for chemical elements are included as main entries in the vocabulary:

RQ *abbr* respiratory quotient

Li *symbol* lithium

Abbreviations are usually entered without periods and have been normalized to one form of capitalization. In practice, however, there is considerable variation, and stylings other than those given in this dictionary are often acceptable.

The more common abbreviations and the symbols of chemical elements also appear after the definition at the entries for the terms they represent:

respiratory quotient *n* : ... — abbr. *RQ*

Symbols that are not capable of being alphabetized are included in a separate section of the back matter headed "Signs and Symbols."

Abbreviations Used in This Book

abbr	abbreviation	*D.C.*	District of Columbia	*N.Y.*	New York
AD	anno Domini	*Dept*	Department	*obs*	obsolete
adj	adjective	*Dr.*	Doctor	*occas*	occasionally
adv	adverb	*Encyc*	Encyclopedia	*orig*	originally
Amer	American	*esp*	especially	*part*	participle
Assoc	Association	*et al*	and others	*pl*	plural
attrib	attributive	*etc*	et cetera	*prep*	preposition
Austral	Australian	*F*	Fahrenheit	*pres*	present
AV	Authorized Version	*fl*	flourished	*prob*	probably
b	born	*g*	gram	*Rev*	Review
BC	before Christ	*imper*	imperative	*sing*	singular
Biog	Biography	*Jour*	Journal	*So*	South
Biol	Biological	*Ky*	Kentucky	*SoAfr*	South African
Bk	Book	*Lk*	Luke	*specif*	specifically
Brit	British	*Mag*	Magazine	*spp*	species (pl)
Bull	Bulletin	*Mass*	Massachusetts	*St.*	Saint
C	Celsius	*Med*	Medical, Medicine	*syn*	synonym
ca	circa	*ml*	milliliter	*Univ*	University
Canad	Canadian	*mm*	millimeter	*U.S.*	United States
cap	capitalized	*Mt.*	Mount	*usu*	usually
cc	cubic centimeter	*n*	noun	*v*	versus
Chem	Chemical	*NewEng*	New England	*var*	variant
Coll	College	*NewZeal*	New Zealand	*vb*	verb
comb	combining	*nm*	nanometer	*vi*	verb intransitive
constr	construction	*No*	North	*vt*	verb transitive
d	died	*n pl*	noun plural	*Yr*	Year

The History and Etymology of Medical English

John H. Dirckx, M.D.

The language of modern medicine, a vigorous, versatile idiom of vast range and formidable intricacy, expands constantly to meet the needs of a complex and rapidly evolving discipline. Medical English in its broadest sense includes not only the official nomenclatures of the basic medical sciences (such as anatomy, biochemistry, pathology, and immunology) and the clinical specialties (such as pediatrics, dermatology, thoracic surgery, and psychiatry) but also a large body of less formal expressions, a sort of trade jargon used by physicians and their professional associates in speech, correspondence, and record-keeping.

Despite the decrees of official boards and committees, medical language tends to grow and change in much the same ways as the vernacular. New terms and expressions appear as if by spontaneous generation to meet new needs, and established words readily acquire new meanings. No firm distinction can be drawn between formal terminology and argot, or between current and obsolescent nomenclature, for expressions that began as informal or shorthand terms may achieve formal status because of their aptness and usefulness, while others whose inaccuracy or inappropriateness have become obvious may survive for decades in speech and even in textbooks.

The parallel between medical English and the common speech also holds true in other ways. Just as no single person can possibly know and use all the words recorded in an unabridged dictionary, no single physician knows and uses all the terms in a medical dictionary. Purists within the profession often object to certain pronunciations and uses of technical terms, but the majority of physicians go on remorselessly pronouncing and using them in ways that seem natural and useful and, as always, it is the standard of usage that finally determines what is correct and what a word really means.

Since pronunciation, spelling, and even meaning depend on usage rather than etymology, it has often been said that the least important thing about a word is its history. And yet, to trace the history of medical terminology is to trace the history of medicine itself, for every stage of that history has left its mark on the working vocabulary of the modern physician. Each new discovery in anatomy, physiology, pathology, and pharmacology has called forth a new name, and a great many of these names, no matter how haphazardly and irregularly coined, no matter how unsuitable in the light of later discoveries, have remained in use. An etymological survey of this rich lexical medley we call medical English, where terms used by Hippocrates jostle others made up yesterday, where we find words from classical languages adapted, often ingeniously and sometimes violently, to modern concepts, and where the names of celebrated persons, mythic figures, and remote places lend human interest and a spice of the exotic, should claim the attention of anyone having a professional or avocational concern with medicine or one of its allied fields.

For convenience, medical terms currently used by speakers of English may be grouped in eight classes: 1) terms borrowed from everyday English; 2) Greek and Latin terms preserved from ancient and medieval medicine; 3) modern coinages, chiefly from classical language elements; 4) terms based on proper names; 5) borrowings from modern foreign languages; 6) trade names; 7) argot and figurative formations; and 8) abbreviations.

Since maintaining health is ultimately each person's own responsibility, professional practitioners of medicine have never held an exclusive right to treat diseases, much less to name and discuss them. Physicians have been borrowing "medical" words from lay English as long as the language has existed.

The history of English falls naturally into three stages. During the Old English or Anglo-Saxon period (A.D. 450–1150), a group of Germanic dialects carried into Britain from northwestern Europe by invading continental tribes including Saxons, Angles, and Jutes gradually diffused and coalesced, receiving important additions from the Old Norse of Scandinavian pirates and marauders and the Latin of Christian missionaries and lesser ones from the languages of foreign traders and the conquered Celts. As Middle English (1150–1500) evolved, most of the inflectional endings of its nouns, adjectives, and verbs weakened and were gradually lost, and it assimilated a vast number of French words brought into Britain after the Norman Conquest (1066). Modern English differs from later Middle English in many of its vowel sounds, in the stabilization of its spelling after the invention of printing, and in its increasing richness in loan words and new formations.

Many modern terms used by both physicians and laity for parts or regions of the body (*arm, back, breast, hand, head, neck*), internal organs and tissues (*heart, liver, lung, blood, bone, fat*), and common symptoms and diseases (*ache, itch, measles, sore, wart, wound*) derive from Anglo-Saxon origins. *Leg, scalp, skin,* and *skull,* also dating from the earliest period of English, can be traced to Old Norse. We find most of these words in the works of Geoffrey Chaucer (ca 1342–1400), the first important figure in English literary history, and in addition others that entered Middle English via Norman French from medical Latin (*canker, jaundice*) and Greek (*cholera, melancholy*). *Migraine, plague,* and *pleurisy,* also adapted by French from classical words, appear in other Middle English authors.

Though all of these structures, symptoms, and ailments have formal names in the technical language of medicine, physicians generally prefer to use the common English words. They do not, however, always use them in the same way as the laity. For example, medicine has found it expedient to narrow and fix the meanings of some words taken over from lay speech. The anatomist limits the sense of *arm* to the part of the upper extremity between the shoulder and the elbow, and of *leg* to the part of the lower extremity between the knee and the ankle. To the microbiologist and the specialist in infectious diseases, *plague* means a specific communicable disease, not just any epidemic. To the cardiologist, *heart failure* denotes a group of sharply defined clinical syndromes, not just any breakdown of heart function. Similarly, *chill, depression, joint, migraine, shock, stillborn, strain,* and *tenderness* all have more restricted meanings in medical English than in lay speech.

In discussing human anatomy, physicians use some words, such as *flank* and *loin,* that the general populace applies only to animals, and others, such as *belly* and *gut,* that many of the laity regard as impolite. On the other hand, physicians find it best to avoid certain common words of shifting or dubious meaning and to substitute others (usually borrowed from classical languages or fabricated from classical material) whose meaning can be arbitrarily limited. For example, *hip* may be undesirably vague when the context fails to indicate whether the reference is to the thigh, the pelvis, the joint between them, the entire bodily region around this joint, or, euphemistically, the buttock. A patient may complain of dizziness, but the physician cannot be content with a term whose range of meanings includes such disparate symptoms as vertigo, disequilibrium, sleepiness, and nausea.

Physicians have been accused of adopting and clinging to an abstruse terminology based on dead languages in order to keep their patients in ignorance or even to conceal their own ignorance. But apart from cases of ambiguity as with *dizziness* and *hip,* or of brand-new concepts for which the common speech can supply no suitable names, the medical profession is only too ready to borrow or modify plain English expressions. Medical English includes a great many lively and even poetic compounds and phrases built of native material, some of them involving metaphor or hyperbole: *bamboo spine, the bends, clubfoot, frozen shoulder, hammertoe, harelip, knock-knee, mallet finger, saddle block, strawberry mark,* and *wandering pacemaker.*

The enormous stock of Greek words and word elements in the medical vocabulary, a source of difficulties for physicians and laity alike, owes its origin to the fact that Western medicine, insofar as we have written records of it, began with Hippocrates in the Periclean Age of Greece. It can be said with equal truth that Western civilization itself took shape in the same era, when the world and everything in it, from the phenomena of nature to human relations and institutions, first came under the scrutiny of that soaring analytic spirit, tempered by profound wisdom, that found its most perfect expression in Socrates. The presence in modern English of such words borrowed or derived from Greek as *astronomy, character, criticism, democracy, dialogue, emphasis, idea, paragraph, problem, system, theme, theory,* and *thesis* attests to the enduring influence of ancient Greek thought on modern culture. The philosophers Plato and Aristotle, the dramatists Sophocles and Euripides, and the historians Herodotus and Thucydides were all roughly contemporary with Hippocrates.

Revered as the Father of Medicine, Hippocrates (ca 460–ca 370 B.C.) was the guiding spirit if not the founder of the world's first school of scientific medicine on the Greek island of Kos, the site of a famous temple to Aesculapius, god of healing. Tradition assigns to Hippocrates the role of separating medicine from religion by teaching that diseases have organic causes and must be combated by physical measures. He also worked out a primitive system of physiology and pathology based on the physics of Empedocles and the numerology of Pythagoras, and established the ethical directives for physicians embodied in the celebrated Hippocratic oath (which, however, is thought to be by a later hand).

The Corpus Hippocraticum, one of the wonders of ancient learning, is a collection of medical works covering a remarkable range of topics including medical history, geographic medicine, dietetics, prognosis, surgery, and orthopedics. Although no modern scholar believes that all these works are by the same author, a substantial number of them seem to show the same fertile, inquiring, incisive mind at work, and it is through these that Hippocrates has exerted so powerful an influence on all subsequent medical theory and practice. The oldest Greek medical terms in current use appear in the Hippocratic writings themselves, among them *anthrax, asthma, bronchus, condyloma, dyspnea, dysthymia, erythema, erysipelas, orthopnea,* and *tenesmus.*

These words were not, of course, invented by Hippocrates (*asthma* appears in the *Iliad*) but borrowed by him from the common speech and adapted to serve the needs of the fledgling science. The modern physician uses all of these terms, generally with more specific meanings than did Hippocrates, and sometimes with radically different ones. The principal reason for the survival of these words from a classical language is that for centuries after Hippocrates, Greek medicine was virtually the only medicine worthy of the name in the Western world, just as Greek philosophy and science dominated Western thought until long after the beginning of the Christian era. Aristotle (384–322 B.C.), remembered chiefly as a philosopher and the formulator of the system of logic still most widely accepted today, was also a brilliant anatomist and physiologist, and a few of our medical Greek words (*alopecia, aorta, epiglottis, nystagmus, pancreas*) made early appearances in his works.

Centuries before Hippocrates, the priests of Egypt learned something about anatomy and pathology through the exercise of their duties as embalmers of the dead. Egyptian medicine, as revealed to us by tantalizingly sparse remnants of ancient writings on papyrus, seems to have been, like Greek medicine before Hippocrates, a branch of religion. There is evidence that early Egyptian science and mathematics influenced the development of these disciplines in Greece, and that, long before Alexander the Great conquered Egypt and annexed it to the Hellenic world, some Egyptian medical lore had reached Greece. A few medical terms that we customarily derive from Greek ultimately had Egyptian origins: *ammonia*, from an ancient term for ammonium chloride, of which large natural deposits were found near a shrine of the Egyptian deity Ammon (Amen) in Libya; *gum* 'vegetable exudation' from Egyptian *qmy.t* via Greek *kommi; stibium*, the chemical name for the element antimony and the basis for its international symbol, Sb, from Egyptian *stm* by way of Greek *stimmi*.

Long after Rome in its turn conquered Greece and absorbed the best of Hellenic learning and culture, most physicians in Rome and the provinces were Greek slaves or freedmen or Greek-speaking immigrants from the Near East or North Africa. Hence the lore of the craft continued to be passed on in the language of Hippocrates. Aretaeus of Cappadocia, who practiced and wrote in the first century after Christ, discussed *asphyxia* and apparently invented the term *diabetes*. His contemporary, the medical botanist Dioscorides, used the terms *eczema, kerion*, and *trachoma*. Galen (A.D. 129–199), a native of Pergamum in Asia Minor, moved to Rome early in his career, devoted many years to the study and practice of medicine, and became court physician to the emperor Marcus Aurelius. His voluminous writings in Greek on anatomy, physiology, pathology, and therapeutics have earned him second place in medicine's pantheon. Among words that first appear in his writings may be mentioned *allantois, atheroma, coccyx, epididymis*, and *peritoneum*.

In discussing parts of the body or common diseases a medical writer may find lay terms sufficient, but to write about new concepts or discoveries the writer must either invent new words or use old ones in new ways. From the dawn of medical history, writers on anatomy and pathology have yielded to the natural impulse to create metaphors to name new things. Thus the bone at the lower end of the spine was called *coccyx*, Greek for 'cuckoo', because of its beaklike shape, and the opening from the stomach into the small intestine became the *pylorus* 'gatekeeper'. Loss of hair was termed *alopecia* because it suggested the appearance of a fox (*alopex*) with mange, and a person with an abnormally ravenous appetite was said to have *bulimia* 'the hunger of an ox'. Perhaps none of these words was the invention of a physician, but they all appear in early Greek medical writings, setting a precedent for subsequent medical word-making in all Western languages down to the present day.

With the collapse of the Byzantine Empire, the Greek language went into eclipse as a medium of scientific and technical communication. Even the masterpieces of Greek drama, philosophy, and history dropped out of sight, to be rediscovered centuries later in the Renaissance. Meanwhile Latin, the language of republican and imperial Rome and its western provinces, flourished as both a widespread vernacular and a literary language. While the popular speech was evolving into regional dialects that would in time become Italian, Spanish, Catalan, Portuguese, French, Provençal, and Rumanian, the classical language, enshrined in the prose of Cicero and the verses of the Augustan poets, survived with changes as the international language of learning, science, jurisprudence, and the Church.

The first Roman writer on medicine, Aulus Cornelius Celsus, who lived in the first century after Christ, was probably not a physician. His eight books *De Medicina (On Medicine)*, perhaps translated or adapted from a Greek work, review the whole subject of medical theory and practice in lucid, even elegant Latin. The immense historical value of Celsus's writings lies partly in his nomenclature, for besides recording numerous Greek medical terms for which Latin offered no suitable equivalents (*aphthae, ascites, cremaster, lagophthalmos, mydriasis, opisthotonos, staphyloma, tetanus*), he also gives the earliest medical applications of many Latin words still in use today (*angina, caries, delirium, fistula, impetigo, mucus, radius, scabies, tabes, tibia, varus, verruca, vertebra, virus*).

Celsus's contemporary, Pliny the Elder (A.D. ca 23–79), an indefatigable if somewhat incautious student of the natural sciences (he died while observing at close range an eruption of Vesuvius), was also a prolific writer. He devoted several books of his monumental *Naturalis Historia (Natural History)* to medical topics, and recorded for the first time the medical uses of such Latin terms as *acetabulum, pruritus*, and *tinea*. Whereas Celsus's rigorously scientific work remained virtually lost from about the fifth century to the fifteenth, when its rediscovery stirred the medical world to its foundations, Pliny's compendium of myth and misinformation became one of the nonfiction best sellers of antiquity, and by the Middle Ages it was firmly established as a popular encyclopedia.

During the centuries following the decline of classical culture, the progress of medicine, as of all the arts and sciences, slowed nearly to a halt. Scientific investigation languished; education consisted largely in the uncritical memorization of ancient lore. In medicine the teachings of Galen, known through Latin translations and commentaries, maintained an unchallenged supremacy for more than a thousand years. But gradual though it was, the development of medical knowledge during the Dark Ages led to a slow accretion of technical Latin terms representing modifications of and additions to the lexical legacy of the ancients.

In the ninth century, when European letters and science were at their lowest ebb, Islamic scholars began a revival of Western learning, translating Aristotle, Galen, and other Greek authors into Syriac and Arabic and subjecting their teachings to searching analysis and impartial verification. The Persian physicians Rhazes, Haly Abbas, and Avicenna, the Arabians Averroës and Albucasis, and the Jew Maimonides performed important original research and made valuable contributions to medical literature. Traces of their influence linger in many terms of Arabic and Persian origin referring to anatomy, chemistry, and pharmacy that made their way into medical English by way of medieval Latin: *alcohol, alkali, benzoin, bezoar, camphor, nuchal, retina, safranin, saphenous, soda*, and *sugar*.

With the resurgence of intellectual activity in the Renaissance, vigorous and original thinkers arose all over Europe to overthrow the hallowed errors of ancient authorities. In medicine, the earliest revolution came in anatomy with the painstaking dissections and detailed drawings of Leonardo and Vesalius, who dared to show where Galen had gone wrong. Fallopius, Servetus, Sylvius, and many others followed their lead. Increasingly minute descriptions of the human body called for an ever more elaborate nomenclature. The printing, in 1502, of the *Onomasticon (Word-book)* of Julius Pollux (second century A.D.), a sort of dictionary that happened to include a section on anatomic terms, enabled anatomists to drop most of the Arabic names for parts of the body then commonly found in textbooks and reintroduce such classical Greek terms as *amnion, atlas, axis, canthus, gastrocnemius, tragus,* and *trochanter*.

But the system of anatomic nomenclature that had been largely codified by the end of the sixteenth century, while including a substantial body of Greek terms, was chiefly Latin. Once again metaphor played an extensive role in the choice of terms. Anatomists named body parts after plants (*glans* 'acorn', *uvula* 'little grape'), animals (*cochlea* 'snail', *vermis* 'worm'), architectural elements (*tectum* 'roof', *vestibulum* 'entrance hall'), household implements (*clavicula* 'little key', *malleus* 'hammer'), articles of clothing (*tunica* 'tunic', *zona* 'belt'), topographic features (*fossa* 'ditch', *fovea* 'pit'), and even other body parts (*capitellum* 'little head', *ventriculus* 'little belly'). By contrast, scores of other Latin anatomic terms, including many that we still use, seem almost painfully literal (*extensor pollicis longus* 'long extender of the thumb', *foramen magnum* 'big hole'). The investigation of the fine structure of the body and of disease-causing microorganisms, made possible by the invention of the simple and compound microscopes, demanded a new stock of terms, and again many of those adopted were descriptive figures (*bacillus* 'little stick', *glomerulus* 'little ball of yarn', *nucleus* 'kernel').

Medicine in the modern sense came into being only with the commencement of the scientific era. Physiology, pathology, pharmacology, and surgery, formulated on an increasingly rational basis, required increasingly rigorous and systematized language. As long as Latin was understood by all educated persons, medical textbooks and monographs continued to be written in that language and lectures to be delivered in it. New medical terms were Latin in form if not always in lexical origin. The modern vocabulary of medicine contains, besides many words known to Celsus, other terms borrowed from Latin at a much later date, such as *angina pectoris, cor bovinum, fetor hepaticus, molluscum contagiosum, placenta previa, rubeola, torticollis,* and *vaccinia*.

In the days when a doctor's prescription was a kind of recipe calling for several ingredients, prescriptions were written in an elaborate, ritualized, grammatically debased form of Latin. This pharmaceutical Latin flourished until about the middle of the twentieth century, and many abbreviations based on it are still in use today (*b.i.d., bis in die* 'twice a day'; *p.c., post cibos* 'after meals'; *p.r.n., pro re nata* 'as the occasion arises').

Although not directly connected with medicine, the system of classificatory naming of all living things devised by the Swedish naturalist Linnaeus (1707–1778) plays an important role in medical communication.

Linnaean nomenclature, fundamentally Latin with a substantial admixture of Greek stems and proper nouns, includes terms for disease-causing bacteria and fungi as well as more complex organisms of medical importance.

It is one thing for medicine to borrow a classical Greek or Latin word such as *typhus* or *scabies* and assign it a specific technical meaning, and another to combine classical stems and affixes to make entirely new words like *hypercholesterolemia* and *proprioception*. Most new medical terms formed from classical elements during the past hundred years have been of the latter kind, which we may call coinages for want of a more distinctive label.

Coinage entails two kindred processes, derivation (or affixation) and compounding. Derivation here refers to the attachment of one or more prefixes or suffixes to a word or stem, as when the prefix *endo-* 'within' and the suffix *-itis* 'inflammation of' are added to the base word *metra* 'uterus' to form *endometritis* 'inflammation of the uterine lining'. Compounding is the joining of two or more adjective, noun, or verb stems, as when the English stems derived from Greek *megas* 'large', *karyon* 'nut, nucleus', and *kytos* 'vessel, cell' are combined to form *megakaryocyte* 'a bone marrow cell with a large, irregular nucleus'. Derivation is exemplified by English *outlandish* and *unfriendly*, compounding by *headache* and *windpipe*.

The combining form of a classical word consists of its stem plus, if needed, a linking vowel, usually *o* but sometimes *i* with Latin words. Thus *brady-*, as in *bradycardia*, is from Greek *bradys* 'slow'; *cortico-*, as in *corticothalamic*, from Latin *cortex, corticis* 'bark'; *hemat-* or *hemato-*, as in *hematopoiesis*, from Greek *haima, haimatos* 'blood'; *femoro-*, as in *femoropopliteal*, from Latin *femur, femoris* 'thigh'; *gastr-* or *gastro-*, as in *gastroesophageal*, from Greek *gaster, gastros* 'stomach'; *my-* or *myo-*, as in *myoneural*, from Greek *mys, myos* 'mouse, muscle'; *ov-* or *ovi-* or *ovo-*, as in *oviduct*, from Latin *ovum, ovi* 'egg'. The linking vowel is generally omitted before a following vowel: *gastritis, hematemesis, hematuria*. The final element of a classical coinage may be anglicized (*colostomy, dermatome* with silent final *e*, *fibroblast, herniorrhaphy*) or not (*hemochromatosis, keratoconus, polyhydramnios, asystole* with *e* pronounced).

Although in earlier times makers of new terms followed classical precedents more diligently and accurately than now, medical coinages have never adhered strictly to any rule, not even that of self-consistency. Medical language has not hesitated to shorten stems, drop awkward syllables, or use unorthodox forms of juncture. The meanings of some stems have wavered between two extremes (*carcinogenic* 'causing cancer' but *nephrogenic* 'arising in the kidney') or even gone in entirely new directions under the influence of analogy. The suffix *-itis*, in classical Greek merely a means of turning a noun into an adjective (as with English *-en* in *golden*), took on its special meaning 'inflammation of' because it often appeared in Greek phrases such as *nephritis nosos* 'kidney disease'. Even as early as the time of Hippocrates, it was customary to shorten a phrase of this kind by omitting the noun. Similarly, the Greek suffix *-ma* that was a means of forming a noun from a verb stem (as in *drama* and *diploma*) fused with the linking vowel -o- appeared in English as the combining form -oma with the medical sense of 'tumor, neoplasm' because it figured in a number of ancient terms, such as sarcoma and condyloma denoting abnormal growths.

For centuries, classical scholars thought it unscholarly to join Greek and Latin material in the same word. Since most of the living medical prefixes and suffixes, including the ubiquitous and indispensable -itis and -oma, were of Greek pedigree, matching Greek stems were dredged up from the depths of oblivion for combination with them, even when synonyms of Latin derivation were already in general use. Thus, although the common adjectives oral, mammary, and renal embody the Latin words for 'mouth', 'breast', and 'kidney' respectively, the corresponding Greek stems appear in stomatitis, mastectomy, and nephrosis. Now that objections to Greek-Latin hybrids have largely died out, many such words (appendicitis, hypertension, radiology) thrive without the stigma of scholarly reproach. Indeed, compounds of Greek with French (culdoscopy, goitrogenic), English (antibody, hemiblock), German (antiscorbutic, kernicterus), and Arabic (alcoholism, alkalosis) now find universal acceptance. Meanwhile the medical lexicon remains rich beyond its needs in Greek stems and in Greek-Latin synonym pairs such as hypodermic/subcutaneous, scaphoid/navicular, and xiphoid/ensiform.

The hundreds of classical stems and affixes in daily use virtually invite further coinages, and in fact physicians produce nonce words and ad hoc formations from this material at a rate that defies the lexicographer to keep pace. Each new word may become the basis of a whole dynasty of derivative or analogical formations. Nouns, equipped with appropriate suffixes, readily change into verbs and adjectives, and vice versa. Many terms arise by back-formation, the process of creating an imaginary precursor or a shortened unconventional word from an existing form, such as to diagnose from diagnosis, to perfuse from perfusion, and precordium from precordial.

At all periods of history, proper nouns denoting persons and places have been incorporated into adjectives, verbs, other nouns, and phrases, as in Jeffersonian, Americanize, Marxism, and Halley's comet. Eponymy, the derivation of words from personal names, has added to the medical vocabulary such diverse expressions as Addison's disease, chagoma, cushingoid, descemetocele, facies Hippocratica, galenical, and parkinsonism. Besides terms like these honoring distinguished physicians, others stand as monuments to important patients: bacitracin, an antibiotic named for Margaret Tracy, from whose tissues it was first isolated; Carrión's disease (bartonellosis), named for Daniel A. Carrión, a Peruvian student who inoculated himself experimentally with the disease and died of it; Hartnup disease, a heredofamilial metabolic disorder named for an English family of which several members were so affected; HeLa cells, a line of cultured human malignant cells named for Henrietta Lacks, from whose cervical carcinoma they are all descended; Legionnaires' disease, pneumonitis due to a bacterium of the genus Legionella, the disease and the genus both named for the American Legion, at whose convention in 1976 the first recognized outbreak occurred.

Names of prominent figures in myth, legend, and popular fiction have also found their way into the physician's lexicon. Atropine, a drug extracted from belladonna and various related plants of the genus Atropa and used as an antispasmodic for smooth muscle, is named, in allusion to its lethal properties, for Atropos, one of the three Fates, who was reputed to cut off each person's thread of life at the moment appointed for death. Morphine, a narcotic extracted from the juice of the poppy, is named for Morpheus, the god of sleep. Satyriasis, abnormal sexual excitability in the male, refers to the Satyrs, mythic sylvan deities with a leaning toward lechery. Pickwickian syndrome, extreme obesity with hypoventilation, refers to Joe the fat boy in Dickens's Pickwick Papers.

Most of the medical terms that incorporate geographic allusions are names of infectious diseases or their causative agents and refer to sites where these diseases are specially prevalent or endemic or where they were first identified or studied. In some of these terms, the names preserve their original form, as in Lyme disease, a tick-borne spirochetal infection named for a town in Connecticut, and Norwalk virus, which causes outbreaks of diarrhea in school children and is named after a city in Ohio. For other terms the geographic origins are not so evident: coxsackievirus, any of a group of human viruses causing various acute febrile syndromes, named for Coxsackie, New York; maduromycosis, a fungal skin disease, named after the city of Madura, India; tularemia, an infection of rodents sometimes transmitted to humans, first identified in Tulare County, California.

These terms based on proper nouns impart an element of novelty as well as a liberal dimension to what might otherwise be a depressingly prosaic assemblage of dry lexical bones gathered from the graveyard of dead languages. In a similar way, terms borrowed from modern foreign languages lend a cosmopolitan flavor to medical speech and writing. There are logical reasons why speakers of English customarily use foreign words for certain diseases, symptoms, or drugs. During the nineteenth century, the teachings and writings of Continental medical authorities played an essential part in the education of British and American physicians. Up until World War I, Americans flocked to Paris and Vienna for specialty training, and brought back French and German words and phrases for which no English equivalents seemed quite right. Numerous French words continue in use today in clinical medicine (ballottement 'shaking', bruit 'noise', grand mal 'big disease', petit mal 'little disease'), surgery (bougie 'dilator', curette 'scraper', débridement 'unbridling, cutting loose', rongeur 'gnawer'), and obstetrics (cerclage 'encirclement', cul de sac 'bottom of the bag', fourchette 'little fork', souffle 'blowing'). The suffix -ase, used to form the names of enzymes, first appeared in diastase, a French respelling of Greek diastasis 'separation'. The sugar suffix -ose dates from French glucose, based on Greek gleukos 'sweet wine'. The phrase milieu intérieur, applied in French by Claude Bernard in the 1850s to his concept of internal physical and chemical equilibrium, is used in English today to designate the same concept.

German words also abound in medical English. Mittelschmerz 'middle pain' (that is, pain midway between menses) is a well-established term for the pain of ovulation. *Spinnbarkeit* 'stretchability' refers to the consistency of cervical mucus under the influence of estrogen. *Magenstrasse* 'stomach street' picturesquely designates a portion of the stomach whose longitudinal folds seem designed to channel food toward the intestine. A number of German terms have been retained in English for findings first reported by German or Austrian scientists: *mast* 'stuffed' *cell* in histology, *gestalt* 'shape' in psychiatry, *anlage* 'foundation' in embryology, *quellung* 'swelling' in microbiology. The term *eyeground* for the retina and associated structures as examined with the ophthalmoscope probably owes its origin to German *Augenhintergrund*. *Antibody* is a translation, or at least a partial translation, of *Antikörper*, and *sitz bath* bears the same relation to *Sitzbad*. The adjective *German* in *German measles*, a synonym for *rubella*, probably came into use in the sense of 'false' or 'illusory', but may allude to the German term *Rötheln*, by which the disease was widely known in the nineteenth and early twentieth centuries.

Most of the Spanish and Portuguese loans in medical use denote diseases endemic in tropical colonies established by Spain and Portugal in the Old and New Worlds, or drugs derived from plants first found in those regions. Spanish *espundia* (apparently an alteration of *esponja* 'sponge') and *pinta* 'splotch of paint' are names for tropical infections based on their appearance, and Portuguese *albino* 'little white one' was first applied to the occasional African slave without skin pigment. Spanish *curare* and Portuguese *ipecacuanha* are derived from South American Indian words, Portuguese *ainhum* from an African word. Other medical terms of African origin are *kwashiorkor* and *tsetse*.

Among Italian words in modern medical English, *pellagra* and *malaria* denote diseases once endemic in Italy. *Influenza* and *petechia* are also Italian in origin. *Kala-azar* is Hindi for 'black disease', and *beriberi* means 'extreme weakness' in Sinhalese. *Tsutsugamushi* 'dangerous bug' *disease* and *sodoku* 'rat venom' are from Japanese.

Trade names inevitably figure in workaday medical parlance, as they do in the speech of the general public. Nearly all drugs in common use and many dressing materials, instruments, and appliances bear trade names that are simpler, more euphonious, and more distinctive than their generic names. The trade name of an especially successful product may become a generic term for all similar products despite the efforts of the manufacturer to assert its legal rights in the name. *Aspirin*, *lanolin*, and *milk of magnesia* were once trade names; *Band-Aid*, *Vaseline*, and (in Canada) *Aspirin* still are. When Jokichi Takamine isolated the hormone of the adrenal medulla in 1901 he called it *Adrenalin* and patented both name and product. This created difficulties for the compilers of the *United States Pharmacopeia*, since regulations forbade the inclusion of trade names. The term *epinephrine*, the Greek equivalent of *Adrenalin*, which had been suggested in 1897 by John Jacob Abel, was therefore substituted in the *U.S. Pharmacopeia*, but meanwhile *adrenaline* (with final *e*) had slipped into the *British Pharmacopoeia*. Nowadays *epinephrine* and *adrenaline* are generally used interchangeably for both the natural hormone and the drug, although Parke-Davis holds the rights to *Adrenalin* as a trademark for a preparation of epinephrine used as a drug.

Physicians would not be human if they never playfully made up unconventional expressions or indulged in humorous distortions of technical terminology. What motives lie behind the creation of medical argot—the natural relish for a secret group language, the poetic impulse gone astray, a spirit of rebellion against regimentation of language and thought, or a craving for comic relief—need not concern us here. As mentioned earlier, no sharp distinction can be drawn between formal terminology and medical argot. Clearly *retinitis pigmentosa* and *antihemophilic factor* belong to formal language; just as clearly *red-hot belly* in the sense of 'an abdomen showing signs of acute inflammation' and *electric lights and watermelons* as a jocular variation on *electrolyte and water balance* do not. Between these extremes lie a large number of expressions that, without being perfectly orthodox in formation or altogether serious in tone, hover on the verge of respectability, and occasionally achieve it. Since this dictionary is based on a bank of citations from printed sources, it includes only such examples of medical slang as find their way at least occasionally into published literature.

Many terms now ratified by long use began as figures of speech, euphemisms, or experiments in onomatopoeia. An unconscious anthropomorphism has influenced the physician's way of talking about disease-causing microorganisms, which are described as *fastidious, resistant*, or *sensitive*, and about neoplasms, which may be *benign, invasive*, or *malignant*. Many expressions in daily use seem based on the notion that medical practice is a warfare waged against disease. The physician plans an *aggressive* clinical *strategy*, choosing *weapons* from his *arsenal* (or *armamentarium*) to augment the patient's *defenses* against *attacking* organisms or *foreign* substances.

Despite the nature of their calling, physicians are not much less squeamish than others about naming and discussing certain body parts and functions, nor less ready to substitute euphemisms for cruder and more explicit terms. Some expressions still in use, such as *stool* for *feces* and *void* for *urinate*, were already well established in lay speech by the end of the Middle English period. During the Victorian era, medical language copied the extreme prudishness of demotic English: childbirth was disguised as *confinement* and a leg masqueraded as a *limb*. Modern medicine continues to sugarcoat its less palatable pills, calling one kind of abortion a *menstrual extraction* and substituting *chemical dependency* for *drug addiction*. Even *disease, infirmity*, and *invalid* are somewhat euphemistic in tone, hinting at illness by denying wellness.

Onomatopoeia is the creation of a word whose very pronunciation seems to echo the thing named, as in the case of *screech, squawk*, and *whisper*. Any discussion of medical onomatopoeia must ignore the lines dividing languages and epochs, for the process has undoubtedly been at work since the origin of speech. In fact, at one time linguists were ready to trace all words to this source. Although that theory is no longer held, onomatopoeia still provides the most reasonable explanation for certain recurring associations between sound and sense, such as the relations between [sn] and the nose (*sneeze, sniffle, snore*) and between [gl] and swallowing (*deglutition, gullet, singultus*). Greek *borboryg-*

mus, bruxism, and *rhonchus,* Latin *crepitus, murmur,* and *stertor,* and English *croup, hiccup,* and *wheeze* are also plainly onomatopoetic in origin. Less evidently so, because of phonetic refinements, are *eructation, rale,* and *sternutation.*

The more frequently a medical word or phrase is used, the more likely it is to undergo some kind of shortening in both speech and writing. Spoken shortenings on the order of "CA" for *cancer* and "scope" for *bronchoscope* do not often achieve formal status, but the list of written abbreviations that have become standard grows steadily longer. The most common type of written abbreviation is the initialism, consisting of the initials of the words in a phrase or of the key elements in a compound term: *BUN, blood urea nitrogen; ECG, electrocardiogram; HMO, health maintenance organization.*

When, instead of saying the letters separately, one customarily pronounces such an abbreviation as a word (*AIDS, acquired immune deficiency syndrome; CABG,* pronounced "cabbage," *coronary artery bypass graft*) it is often called an acronym. An acronym may be treated as an ordinary word and combined with stems or affixes, as in *vipoma* 'a neoplasm that secretes VIP (vasoactive intestinal polypeptide)'. Other kinds of shortening to which medical terms are subject include telescoping of phrases (*arbovirus, arthropod-borne virus*) and omission of one or more words from a phrase (*steroid* for *adrenal cortical steroid*).

Not all shorthand expressions are abbreviations in the strict sense; sometimes letters or numbers are chosen arbitrarily to designate the members of a group or series. Thus the letters *A, B, C,* and so on, as used to designate the vitamins, are not abbreviations of more elaborate names (though, as an exception, *vitamin K* refers to Danish *koagulation*). Nor are the letters *P, Q, R, S,* and *T,* as applied to the electrocardiogram (as in *P wave, QRS complex,* and *QT interval*), abbreviations for words beginning with those letters. Greek letters as well as Arabic and Roman numerals figure in many medical terms: *alpha-fetoprotein, beta-hemolysis, gamma-aminobutyric acid, factor V, HLA-B27 antigen.*

These, then, are the ways in which nearly all of the words, phrases, and expressions in this dictionary have come into being. We often forget that words are first of all combinations of sounds, and only later marks on paper. The pronunciation of a word *is* that word, no matter what it means, how it is used, or how we choose to spell it. The pronunciation of medical terms by speakers of English tends to parallel the somewhat unruly practice of the general language. Classical precedents are largely ignored in the pronunciation of Greek and Latin words, particularly as to vowel sounds and syllable stress. Words and proper names borrowed from foreign languages fare little better, and the reproduction of French phonology is usually essayed with more zeal than accuracy. Moreover, an attempt at French pronunciation is often forced on words (*chalazion, raphe, tamponade, troche*) not actually borrowed from that language.

Although medical English may give a superficial impression of order and system, it does not possess these qualities in much higher degree than the common

speech. In fact, the ceaseless proliferation and endless semantic fusion and differentiation of medical terms have created a variety of problems. The presence in the medical lexicon of four or more names for many anatomic structures, many diseases, and many diagnostic and therepeutic procedures makes it awkward to maintain consistency in medical record-keeping, gathering statistics, billing for medical services, and assigning health insurance benefits, not to mention difficulties in medical and paramedical education and publishing.

Several official and quasi-official groups have sought, with varying degrees of success, to establish and even enforce standard nomenclatures for their spheres of interest and influence. Many of these groups have international memberships, hold periodic congresses at which experts agree (or disagree) on changes in terminology, and publish official lists, indexes, atlases, or keys of approved terms. The editors of this dictionary continuously monitor such attempts to write prescriptions for the use of medical language, but entries are made in the vocabulary section only when there is proof of compliance as evidenced by citations for actual use in the general and medical literature.

Some systems of naming and classification pertain to the basic sciences, and thus have a broader relevance than their connection with medicine. The Linnaean classification of all living things, including disease-causing organisms, has been mentioned already. Linnaeus's *Systema Naturae* survives in the official nomenclatures, consistently expanded and revised, of botany, zoology, microbiology, and now virology. The *Nomina Anatomica (NA)* is an official body of anatomic, histologic, and embryologic nomenclature, entirely in Latin, that is revised every five years by an International Congress of Anatomists. The International Union of Pure and Applied Chemistry (IUPAC) has established rules for the naming of chemical substances, old and new.

In spite of such attempts at standardization, medical language as a whole does not match the regularity of chemical and taxonomic nomenclature but it is no less precise and consistent than, for example, the technical vocabularies of banking, geology, aeronautics, and law, nor less useful and convenient for those who speak and write it daily in their professional work.

There is a recent and growing trend in some official nomenclatures to assign numeric equivalents to certain specialized medical terms. The Nomenclature Committee of the International Union of Biochemistry and Molecular Biology publishes recommendations on the nomenclature and classification of enymes, in which each is assigned a unique number. Thus 1.1.1.27. stands for lactate dehydrogenase. The *International System for Human Gene Nomenclature (ISGN)* standardizes the notation used to distinguish genes (including onco-genes, which transmit a tendency to develop certain cancers) and their positions (loci) on chromosomes. One form of early-onset breast cancer is induced by the BRCA1 oncogene, located at position 17q21 (band 1 in region 2 on the long arm of human chromosome 17).

The *ICD (International Classification of Diseases)* is an adaptation, endorsed by the U.S. Department of Health and Human Services, of the World Health Organization's *Manual of the International Statistical Classification of Diseases, Injuries and Causes of Death. ICD* provides an elaborate classification of diseases, injuries, and inherited disorders, in which each condition is accompanied by a numeric or alphanumeric code. Simple acute appendicitis is designated as 540.9, Kaposi's sarcoma as M9140/3, and death by capital punishment as E978. In recent years *ICD* has been updated annually, and extensively revised at longer intervals.

Closely coordinated with *ICD*, and partly derived from it, is the *Diagnostic and Statistical Manual of Mental Disorders (DSM)*, first published in 1952 by the American Psychiatric Association. The *DSM* classifies, names, and supplies diagnostic criteria for each mental disorder. Code numbers are those of *ICD*.

Although *ICD* contains a section of diagnostic and therapeutic procedures, a more elaborate classification is published by the Americal Medical Association as the *Physician's Current Procedural Terminology (CPT)*, with its own set of five-digit numeric codes. The *CPT* code number for an appendectomy, for example, is 44950.

One might sum up the history of medical English by saying that it has grown and evolved as an integral part of the common language, choosing and even manufacturing its vocabulary to suit the special needs of medical practitioners, investigators, teachers, and writers, but generally clinging to the phonetic, semantic, and syntactic habits of plain English. The individual histories of medical words may be both fascinating and instructive, but they do not necessarily help in determining correct meanings or current spellings. Indeed, the entry of a term into the medical vocabulary is not the end of its history but only the beginning.

The meaning we accept nowadays for a word may be but the latest of many it has borne. In the Greek of Hippocrates, *aorta* refers to the lower respiratory tract and *bronchus* means the throat, gullet, or windpipe indifferently, as does *stomachos* in Homer. In classical Latin, *vulva* means 'uterus' and *uterus* generally means 'belly'. We retain the term *influenza* for a group of specific viral syndromes although we no longer attribute them to the malign influence (for that is the purport of the term) of the heavenly bodies. We preserve terms alluding to Hippocratic pathophysiology, such as *cholera, chyme, crisis, dyscrasia, humoral, hypochondria*, and *melancholia*, although the concepts for which these terms stand were rejected as invalid early in the nineteenth century. These words remain in use because over the years they have lost their original meanings and acquired others. Cholera is now a specific bacterial infection, and a blood dyscrasia is a disturbance in the formation of blood cells, both notions that would have baffled Hippocrates.

These hardy survivors illustrate the point, often overlooked and sometimes vigorously contested, that the meaning or definition of a word depends on association and analogy, not necessarily on its history or etymology. The portal vein got its name from the *porta* or gate of the liver, a cleft on the underside of the organ where this vein enters. For centuries the portal vein was believed to be the only blood vessel in the body that both begins and ends in capillaries. For this reason the term *portal* lost its earlier associations and came to mean 'beginning and ending in capillaries'. When a similar arrangement was finally discovered in the pituitary gland, the vessels there were called the *pituitary portal system*. Because the sense of *colic* (Greek *kolikos*) has shifted from the literal one of 'pertaining to the colon' to 'any intermittent, cramping pain in the lower trunk', we can speak without incongruity of *renal colic* 'the pain caused by a stone in a kidney or ureter'.

The definitions assigned to terms such as *abortion, acupuncture, chiropractic, holistic medicine, macrobiotic diet*, and *wellness* by advocates of these disciplines or practices may differ radically from the definitions of their opponents, and these again from those of disinterested observers. Our language both reflects and shapes our ways of perceiving, dividing, and classifying reality. As modern medical thought becomes less empirical and superstitious, more coherent and linear, so does modern medical language. The words may sound the same, look the same on paper, but their connotations shift with the passing years, responding to shifts in theory, doctrine, and point of view.

The quest for the exact meaning of a medical term is more than just an academic exercise. Words are our most effective means of recording and transmitting information, and almost our only way of dealing with complex and abstract subjects. The precision and perspicuity with which words are used determine the efficacy of educational and informational endeavors and the validity of written records. On the meaning of a single word in a hospital chart may hinge thousands of dollars in insurance benefits, millions in litigation settlements, even the life of the patient. In this light the importance of an accurate, up-to-date dictionary of medical English with definitions based on current usage citations can hardly be exaggerated.

A living language is a dynamic process, not a static product, and no dictionary of it can ever be definitive. The editors of this dictionary have not set out to assign meanings to words arbitrarily, much less to fix them unalterably, but only to record the meanings that the words presently convey in actual use. Drawing on the full lexicographic resources of Merriam-Webster, Incorporated, the editors have produced a current word list that includes new formations and omits terms no longer used, and have supplied current definitions as reflected in recently published material. The result is a uniquely authoritative and up-to-date reference work for professional, student, and layperson.

Prefixes, Suffixes, and Combining Forms

This list gathers together and defines prefixes, suffixes, and combining forms that are commonly encountered in medical writing. The functional labels used in this list include *comb form*, for "combining form," *prefix*, and *suffix*. In addition, a suffix or terminal combining form that always produces words belonging to one part of speech is further identified by addition of a part-of-speech label.

> **nas-** *or* **naso-** *also* **nasi-** *comb form*
> **pre-** *prefix*
> **-itic** *adj suffix*
> **-ite** *n suffix*
> **-blast** *n comb form*

a- \('\)ā *also* (')a *or* (')ä\ *or* **an-** \(')an\ *prefix* : not : without ⟨*a*sexual⟩ — *a-* before consonants other than *h* and sometimes even before *h*, *an-* before vowels and usu. before *h* ⟨*a*chromatic⟩ ⟨*an*astigmatic⟩ ⟨*an*hydrous⟩

ab- *prefix* : from : away : off ⟨*ab*oral⟩

abdomin- *or* **abdomino-** *comb form* **1** : abdomen ⟨*abdomino*plasty⟩ **2** : abdominal and ⟨*abdomino*perineal⟩

acanth- *or* **acantho-** *comb form* **1** : spine : prickle : projection ⟨*acantho*cyte⟩ **2** : prickle cell layer ⟨*acanth*oma⟩

acar- *or* **acari-** *or* **acaro-** *comb form* : mite ⟨*acar*iasis⟩ ⟨*acar*icide⟩

achromat- *or* **achromato-** *comb form* : uncolored except for shades of black, gray, and white ⟨*achromat*opsia⟩

acr- *or* **acro-** *comb form* **1** : top : peak : summit ⟨*acro*cephaly⟩ **2** : height ⟨*acro*phobia⟩ **3** : extremity of the body ⟨*acro*cyanosis⟩

acromio- *comb form* **1** : acromion ⟨*acromio*plasty⟩ **2** : acromial and ⟨*acromio*clavicular⟩

actin- *or* **actini-** *or* **actino-** *comb form* **1** : of, utilizing, or caused by actinic radiation (as X-rays) ⟨*actino*therapy⟩ **2** : actinomycete ⟨*actino*phage⟩

acu- *comb form* **1** : performed with or as if with a needle ⟨*acu*puncture⟩ **2** : applied to selected areas of the body (as in acupuncture) ⟨*acu*pressure⟩

-a·cu·sis \ə-'kyü-səs\ *n comb form* : hearing ⟨dipl*acusis*⟩ ⟨hyper*acusis*⟩

aden- *or* **adeno-** *comb form* : gland : glandular ⟨*aden*itis⟩ ⟨*adeno*fibroma⟩

adip- *or* **adipo-** *comb form* : fat : fatty tissue ⟨*adip*ic acid⟩ ⟨*adipo*cyte⟩

adren- *or* **adreno-** *comb form* **1 a** : adrenal glands ⟨*adreno*cortical⟩ **b** : adrenal and ⟨*adreno*genital⟩ **2** : adrenaline ⟨*adren*ergic⟩

-aemia *chiefly Brit var of* -EMIA

aer- *or* **aero-** *comb form* **1** : air : atmosphere ⟨*aer*ate⟩ ⟨*aero*bic⟩ **2** : gas ⟨*aero*sol⟩ **3** : aviation ⟨*aero*medicine⟩

aesthesio- *chiefly Brit var of* ESTHESIO-

aetio- *chiefly Brit var of* ETIO-

-a·gogue \ə-ˌgäg\ *n comb form* : substance that promotes the secretion or expulsion of ⟨chol*agogue*⟩ ⟨emmen*agogue*⟩

alg- *or* **algo-** *comb form* : pain ⟨*algo*lagnia⟩

-al·gia \'al-j(ē-)ə\ *n comb form* : pain ⟨neur*algia*⟩

ali- *comb form* : wing or winglike part ⟨*ali*sphenoid⟩

all- *or* **allo-** *comb form* **1** : other : different : atypical ⟨*aller*gy⟩ ⟨*allo*some⟩ **2** *allo-* : isomeric form or variety of (a specified chemical compound) ⟨*allo*purinol⟩

allelo- *comb form* : alternative ⟨*allelo*morph⟩

alveol- *or* **alveolo-** *comb form* **1** : alveolus ⟨*alveol*ectomy⟩ **2** : alveolar and ⟨*alveolo*nasal⟩

ambi- *prefix* : both ⟨*ambi*valence⟩ ⟨*ambi*sexuality⟩

ambly- *or* **amblyo-** *comb form* : connected with amblyopia ⟨*amblyo*scope⟩

amnio- *comb form* : amnion ⟨*amnio*centesis⟩

amphi- *or* **amph-** *prefix* : on both sides : of both kinds : both ⟨*amphi*mixis⟩

amygdal- *or* **amygdalo-** *comb form* **1** : almond ⟨*amygdal*in⟩ **2** : amygdala ⟨*amygdal*ectomy⟩ ⟨*amygdalo*tomy⟩

amyl- *or* **amylo-** *comb form* : starch ⟨*amyl*ase⟩ ⟨*amylo*pectin⟩

an- *var of* A-

ana- *or* **an-** *prefix* : up : upward ⟨*ana*bolism⟩

andr- *or* **andro-** *comb form* **1** : male ⟨*andro*gen⟩ **2** : male and ⟨*andro*gynous⟩

angi- *or* **angio-** *comb form* **1** : blood or lymph vessel ⟨*angio*ma⟩ ⟨*angio*genesis⟩ **2** : blood vessels and ⟨*angio*cardiography⟩

-an·gi·um \'an-jē-əm\ *n comb form, pl* **-an·gia** \-jē-ə\ : vessel : receptacle ⟨mes*angium*⟩

anhydr- *or* **anhydro-** *comb form* : lacking water ⟨*anhydre*mia⟩

\ə\ **abut** \ᵊ\ **kitten** \ər\ **further** \a\ **ash** \ā\ **ace** \ä\ **cot, cart** \aú\ **out** \ch\ **chin** \e\ **bet** \ē\ **easy** \g\ **go** \i\ **hit** \ī\ **ice** \j\ **job** \ŋ\ **sing** \ō\ **go** \ò\ **law** \òi\ **boy** \th\ **thin** \t͟h\ **the** \ü\ **loot** \ú\ **foot** \y\ **yet** \zh\ **vision** *See also* Pronunciation Symbols page

anis- *or* **aniso-** *comb form* : unequal ⟨*anis*eikonia⟩ ⟨*anis*ocytosis⟩

ankyl- *or* **ankylo-** *also* **anchyl-** *or* **anchylo-** *comb form* : stiffness : immobility ⟨*ankyl*osis⟩

¹ano- *prefix* : upward ⟨*ano*opsia⟩

²ano- *comb form* **1** : anus ⟨*ano*scope⟩ **2** : anus and ⟨*ano*rectal⟩

ante- *prefix* **1** : anterior : forward ⟨*ante*cornu⟩ **2 a** : prior to : earlier than ⟨*ante*partum⟩ **b** : in front of ⟨*ante*brachium⟩

antero- *comb form* : anterior and : extending from front to ⟨*antero*lateral⟩ ⟨*antero*posterior⟩

-an·them \'an(t)-thəm\ *or* **-an·the·ma** \-thə-mə\ *n comb form,* *pl* **-anthems** *or* **-an·them·a·ta** \ˌan-'them-ət-ə\ : eruption : rash ⟨en*anthem*⟩ ⟨ex*anthema*⟩

anthrac- *or* **anthraco-** *comb form* : carbon : coal ⟨*anthrac*osis⟩ ⟨*anthraco*silicosis⟩

anthrop- *or* **anthropo-** *comb form* : human being ⟨*anthropo*philic⟩

anti- *or* **ant-** *or* **anth-** *prefix* **1** : opposing in effect or activity : inhibiting ⟨*ant*acid⟩ ⟨*anth*elmintic⟩ ⟨*anti*histamine⟩ **2** : serving to prevent, cure, or alleviate ⟨*anti*anxiety⟩

antr- *or* **antro-** *comb form* : antrum ⟨*antro*stomy⟩

aort- *or* **aorto-** *comb form* **1** : aorta ⟨*aort*itis⟩ **2** : aortic and ⟨*aorto*coronary⟩

apic- *or* **apici-** *or* **apico-** *comb form* : apex : tip esp. of an organ ⟨*apic*ectomy⟩

apo- *or* **ap-** *or* **aph-** *prefix* **1** : from : away from : free from ⟨*apo*chromatic⟩ **2** : formed from : related to ⟨*apo*morphine⟩

append- *or* **appendo-** *or* **appendic-** *or* **appendico-** *comb form* : vermiform appendix ⟨*append*ectomy⟩ ⟨*appendic*itis⟩

arachn- *or* **arachno-** *comb form* : spider ⟨*arachno*dactyly⟩

arch- *or* **archi-** *prefix* : primitive : original : primary ⟨*arch*enteron⟩

argent- *or* **argenti-** *or* **argento-** *comb form* : silver ⟨*argento*philic⟩

argyr- *or* **argyro-** *comb form* : silver ⟨*argyr*ia⟩

-ar·i·um \'er-ē-əm\ *n suffix, pl* **-ar·i·ums** *or* **-ar·ia** \-ē-ə\ : thing or place belonging to or connected with ⟨sanit*arium*⟩

ars- *comb form* : arsenic ⟨*ars*ine⟩ ⟨*ars*phenamine⟩

arteri- *or* **arterio-** *comb form* **1** : artery ⟨*arterio*graphy⟩ **2** : arterial and ⟨*arterio*venous⟩

arthr- *or* **arthro-** *comb form* : joint ⟨*arthr*algia⟩ ⟨*arthro*pathy⟩

-ase \ˌās, ˌāz\ *n suffix* : enzyme ⟨prote*ase*⟩ ⟨ure*ase*⟩

asthen- *or* **astheno-** *comb form* : weak ⟨*asthen*opia⟩

astr- *or* **astro-** *comb form* **1** : star : star-shaped ⟨*astro*cyte⟩ **2** : astrocyte ⟨*astro*blastoma⟩ ⟨*astro*glia⟩

astragal- *or* **astragalo-** *comb form* : astragalus ⟨*astragal*ectomy⟩

atel- *or* **atelo-** *comb form* : defective ⟨*atel*ectasis⟩

athero- *comb form* : atheroma ⟨*athero*genic⟩

atlant- *or* **atlanto-** *comb form* **1** : atlas ⟨*atlant*al⟩ **2** : atlantal and ⟨*atlanto*occipital⟩

atri- *or* **atrio-** *comb form* **1** : atrium ⟨*atri*al⟩ **2** : atrial and ⟨*atrio*ventricular⟩

audio- *comb form* **1** : hearing ⟨*audio*logy⟩ **2** : sound ⟨*audio*genic⟩

aur- *or* **auri-** *comb form* : ear ⟨*aur*al⟩

auriculo- *comb form* : of or belonging to an auricle of the heart and ⟨*auriculo*ventricular⟩

aut- *or* **auto-** *comb form* : self : same one ⟨*aut*ism⟩ **a** : of, by, affecting, from, or for the same individual ⟨*auto*graft⟩ ⟨*auto*transfusion⟩ ⟨*auto*vaccination⟩ **b** : arising or produced within the individual and acting toward or directed toward or against the individual or the individual's own body, tissues, or molecules ⟨*auto*immunity⟩ ⟨*auto*suggestion⟩ ⟨*auto*erotism⟩

ax- *or* **axo-** *comb form* : axon ⟨*axo*dendritic⟩

az- *or* **azo-** *comb form* : containing nitrogen or the azo group ⟨*azo*protein⟩

azot- *or* **azoto-** *comb form* : nitrogen : nitrogenous substance ⟨*azot*uria⟩

azygo- *comb form* : azygos ⟨*azygo*graphy⟩

bacill- *or* **bacilli-** *or* **bacillo-** *comb form* : bacillus ⟨*bacill*osis⟩

bacter- *or* **bacteri-** *or* **bacterio-** *comb form* : bacteria : bacterial ⟨*bacteri*olysis⟩

balan- *or* **balano-** *comb form* : glans penis ⟨*balan*itis⟩ ⟨*balano*posthitis⟩

balne- *or* **balneo-** *comb form* : bath : bathing ⟨*balneo*therapy⟩

bar- *or* **baro-** *comb form* : weight : pressure ⟨*bar*iatrics⟩ ⟨*baro*trauma⟩

basi- *also* **baso-** *comb form* **1** : of or belonging to the base or lower part of ⟨*basi*cranial⟩ **2** : chemical base ⟨*baso*philic⟩

benz- *or* **benzo-** *comb form* **1** : related to benzene or benzoic acid ⟨*benzo*ate⟩ **2** : containing a benzene ring fused on one side to one side of another ring ⟨*benz*imidazole⟩

¹bi- *prefix* **1 a** : two ⟨*bi*lateral⟩ **b** : into two parts ⟨*bi*furcate⟩ **2** : twice : doubly : on both sides ⟨*bi*convex⟩ **3** : between, involving, or affecting two (specified) symmetrical parts ⟨*bi*labial⟩ **4 a** : containing one (specified) constituent in double the proportion of the other constituent or in double the ordinary proportion ⟨*bi*carbonate⟩ **b** : DI- ⟨*bi*phenyl⟩

²bi- *or* **bio-** *comb form* : life : living organisms or tissue ⟨*bio*chemistry⟩ ⟨*bio*luminescence⟩

bili- *comb form* **1** : bile ⟨*bili*ary⟩ **2** : derived from bile ⟨*bili*rubin⟩

bin- *comb form* : two : two by two : two at a time ⟨*bin*aural⟩

-bi·o·sis \ˌ(ˌ)bī-'ō-səs, bē-\ *n comb form, pl* **-bi·o·ses** \-ˌsēz\ : mode of life ⟨para*biosis*⟩ ⟨sym*biosis*⟩

-bi·ot·ic \bī-'ät-ik\ *adj comb form* **1** : relating to life ⟨anti*biotic*⟩ **2** : having a (specified) mode of life ⟨necro*biotic*⟩

blast- *or* **blasto-** *comb form* : bud : budding : germ ⟨*blasto*disc⟩ ⟨*blast*ula⟩

-blast \ˌblast\ *n comb form* : formative unit esp. of living matter : germ : cell layer ⟨epi*blast*⟩

-blas·tic \'blas-tik\ *adj comb form* : sprouting or germinating (in a specified way) ⟨hemocyto*blastic*⟩ : having (such or so many) sprouts, buds, or germ layers ⟨meso*blastic*⟩

blephar- *or* **blepharo-** *comb form* **1** : eyelid ⟨*blepharo*spasm⟩ **2** : cilium : flagellum ⟨*blepharo*plast⟩

brachi- *or* **brachio-** *comb form* **1** : arm ⟨*brachio*radialis⟩ **2** : brachial and ⟨*brachio*cephalic artery⟩

brachy- *comb form* : short ⟨*brachy*cephalic⟩ ⟨*brachy*dactylous⟩

brady- *comb form* : slow ⟨*brady*cardia⟩

brom- *or* **bromo-** *comb form* **1** : bromine ⟨*brom*ide⟩ **2** *now usu bromo-* : containing bromine in place of hydrogen — in names of organic compounds ⟨*bromo*uracil⟩

bronch- *or* **broncho-** *comb form* : bronchial tube : bronchial ⟨*bronch*itis⟩

bronchi- *or* **bronchio-** *comb form* : bronchial tubes ⟨*bronchi*ectasis⟩

bucco- *comb form* : buccal and ⟨*bucco*lingual⟩

bulb- *or* **bulbo-** *comb form* **1** : bulb ⟨*bulb*ar⟩ **2** : bulbar and ⟨*bulbo*spinal⟩ ⟨*bulbo*urethral gland⟩

-bu·lia *also* **-bou·lia** \'b(y)ü-lē-ə\ *n comb form* : condition of having (such) will ⟨a*bulia*⟩

-bulic *adj comb form* : of, relating to, or characterized by a (specified) state of will ⟨a*bulic*⟩

-caine \ˌkān\ *n comb form* : synthetic alkaloid anesthetic ⟨pro*caine*⟩ ⟨lido*caine*⟩

calcaneo- *comb form* : calcaneal and ⟨*calcaneo*cuboid⟩

calori- *comb form* : heat ⟨*calori*genic⟩ ⟨*calori*meter⟩

-cap·nia \'kap-nē-ə\ *n comb form* : carbon dioxide in the blood ⟨hyper*capnia*⟩ ⟨hypo*capnia*⟩

capsul- *or* **capsuli-** *or* **capsulo-** *comb form* : capsule ⟨*capsul*itis⟩ ⟨*capsul*ectomy⟩

carcin- *or* **carcino-** *comb form* : tumor : cancer ⟨*carcino*genic⟩

cardi- *or* **cardio-** *comb form* : heart : cardiac : cardiac and ⟨*cardio*gram⟩ ⟨*cardio*vascular⟩

-car·dia \'kärd-ē-ə\ *n comb form* : heart action or location (of a specified type) ⟨dextro*cardia*⟩ ⟨tachy*cardia*⟩

-car·di·um \'kärd-ē-əm\ *n comb form, pl* **-car·dia** \-ē-ə\ : heart ⟨epi*cardium*⟩

cario- *comb form* : caries ⟨*cario*genic⟩ ⟨*cario*static⟩

carp- *or* **carpo-** *comb form* **1** : carpus ⟨*carp*ectomy⟩ **2** : carpal and ⟨*carpo*metacarpal⟩

cary- *or* **caryo-** *var of* KARY-

cata- *or* **cat-** *or* **cath-** *prefix* : down ⟨*cat*amnesis⟩ ⟨*cata*plexy⟩

cec- *or* **ceci-** *or* **ceco-** *comb form* : cecum ⟨*cec*itis⟩ ⟨*ceco*stomy⟩

¹-cele \ˌsēl\ *n comb form* : tumor : hernia ⟨cysto*cele*⟩

²-cele *var of* -COELE

celi- *or* **celio-** *comb form* : belly : abdomen ⟨*celio*scopy⟩ ⟨*celi*otomy⟩

cephal- *or* **cephalo-** *comb form* **1** : head ⟨*cephal*ad⟩ ⟨*cepha*lometry⟩ **2** : cephalic and ⟨*cephalo*pelvic disproportion⟩

-ceph·a·lus \'sef-ə-ləs, *Brit also* 'kef-\ *n comb form, pl* **-ceph·a·li** \-ˌlī\ : cephalic abnormality (of a specified type) ⟨hydro*cephalus*⟩ ⟨micro*cephalus*⟩

cerebell- *or* **cerebelli-** *or* **cerebello-** *comb form* : cerebellum ⟨*cerebell*itis⟩

cerebr- *or* **cerebro-** *comb form* **1** : brain : cerebrum ⟨*cere*bration⟩ **2** : cerebral and ⟨*cerebro*spinal⟩

cervic- *or* **cervici-** *or* **cervico-** *comb form* **1** : neck : cervix of an organ ⟨*cervic*itis⟩ **2** : cervical and ⟨*cervico*thoracic⟩ ⟨*cervico*vaginal⟩

cheil- *or* **cheilo-** *also* **chil-** *or* **chilo-** *comb form* : lip ⟨*cheil*itis⟩ ⟨*cheilo*plasty⟩

chem- *or* **chemo-** *also* **chemi-** *comb form* : chemical : chemistry ⟨*chemo*therapy⟩

chir- *or* **chiro-** *also* **cheir-** *or* **cheiro-** *comb form* : hand ⟨*chiro*practic⟩

chlor- *or* **chloro-** *comb form* **1** : green ⟨*chlor*ine⟩ ⟨*chlor*osis⟩ **2** : chlorine : containing or caused by chlorine ⟨*chlor*acne⟩ ⟨*chlor*dane⟩

chol- *or* **chole-** *or* **cholo-** *comb form* : bile : gall ⟨*chol*ate⟩ ⟨*chole*lith⟩ ⟨*chol*orrhea⟩

chondr- *or* **chondri-** *or* **chondro-** *comb form* : cartilage ⟨*chondr*al⟩ ⟨*chondro*cranium⟩

chromat- *or* **chromato-** *comb form* **1** : color ⟨*chromat*id⟩ **2** : chromatin ⟨*chromat*olysis⟩

chyl- *or* **chyli-** *or* **chylo-** *comb form* : chyle ⟨*chyl*uria⟩ ⟨*chylo*thorax⟩

-chy·lia \'kī-lē-ə\ *n comb form* : condition of having (such) chyle ⟨a*chylia*⟩

cin- *or* **cino-** *var of* KIN-

cirs- *or* **cirso-** *comb form* : swollen vein : varix ⟨*cirs*oid⟩

cleid- *or* **cleido-** *comb form* **1** : clavicle ⟨*cleido*tomy⟩ **2** : clavicular : clavicular and ⟨*cleido*cranial dyostasis⟩

clinico- *comb form* : clinical : clinical and ⟨*clinico*pathologic⟩

clitorid- *or* **clitorido-** *comb form* : clitoris ⟨*clitorid*ectomy⟩

-coc·cus \'käk-əs\ *n comb form, pl* **-coc·ci** \'käk-ˌsī *also* 'käk-ˌī, *sometimes* 'käk-(ˌ)(s)ē\ : berry-shaped organism ⟨gono*coccus*⟩ ⟨Micro*coccus*⟩

coccyg- *or* **coccygo-** *comb form* : coccyx ⟨*coccyg*ectomy⟩

-coele *or* **-coel** *also* **-cele** \ˌsēl\ *n comb form* : cavity : chamber : ventricle ⟨blasto*coel*⟩

col- *or* **coli-** *or* **colo-** *comb form* **1** : colon ⟨*col*itis⟩ ⟨*colo*stomy⟩ **2** : colon bacillus ⟨*coli*form⟩

colp- *or* **colpo-** *comb form* : vagina ⟨*colp*itis⟩ ⟨*colpo*scope⟩

-col·pos \'käl-ˌpäs\ *n comb form* : vaginal disorder (of a specified type) ⟨hydrometro*colpos*⟩

condyl- *or* **condylo-** *comb form* : joint : condyle ⟨*condyl*ectomy⟩ ⟨*condyl*oid⟩

copr- *or* **copro-** *comb form* **1** : dung : feces ⟨*copro*lith⟩ **2** : obscenity ⟨*copro*lalia⟩

coraco- *comb form* : coracoid and ⟨*coraco*humeral⟩

corne- *or* **corneo-** *comb form* : cornea : corneal and ⟨*corneo*scleral⟩

cortico- *comb form* **1** : cortex ⟨*cortico*tropic⟩ **2** : cortical and ⟨*cortico*spinal⟩

cost- *or* **costi-** *or* **costo-** *comb form* : rib : costal and ⟨*costo*chondral⟩

cox- *or* **coxo-** *comb form* : hip : thigh : of the hip and ⟨*coxo*femoral⟩

crani- *or* **cranio-** *comb form* **1** : cranium ⟨*cranio*metry⟩ **2** : cranial and ⟨*cranio*sacral⟩

-cra·nia \'krā-nē-ə\ *n comb form* : condition of the skull or head ⟨hemi*crania*⟩

crico- *comb form* **1** : cricoid cartilage and ⟨*crico*thyroid⟩ **2** : of the cricoid cartilage and ⟨*crico*pharyngeal⟩

-crotic *adj comb form* : having (such) a heartbeat or pulse ⟨di*crotic*⟩

-cro·tism \krə-ˌtiz-əm\ *n comb form* : condition of having (such) a heartbeat or pulse ⟨di*crotism*⟩

cry- *or* **cryo-** *comb form* : cold : freezing ⟨*cryo*gen⟩ ⟨*cryo*surgery⟩

crypt- *or* **crypto-** *comb form* : hidden : covered ⟨*crypto*genic⟩

culdo- *comb form* : pouch of Douglas ⟨*culdo*scopy⟩

cyan- *or* **cyano-** *comb form* **1** : blue ⟨*cyan*osis⟩ **2** : cyanide ⟨*cyano*genetic⟩

cycl- *or* **cyclo-** *comb form* **1** : ciliary body (of the eye) ⟨*cycl*itis⟩ ⟨*cyclo*dialysis⟩ **2** : containing a ring of atoms — in names of organic compounds ⟨*cyclo*hexane⟩

cyst- *or* **cysti-** *or* **cysto-** *comb form* **1** : bladder ⟨*cyst*itis⟩ ⟨*cysto*plasty⟩ **2** : cyst ⟨*cysto*gastrostomy⟩

-cyst \ˌsist\ *n comb form* : bladder : sac ⟨blasto*cyst*⟩

cyt- *or* **cyto-** *comb form* **1** : cell ⟨*cyto*logy⟩ **2** : cytoplasm ⟨*cyto*kinesis⟩

-cyte \ˌsīt\ *n comb form* : cell ⟨leuko*cyte*⟩

dacry- *or* **dacryo-** *comb form* : lacrimal ⟨*dacryo*cyst⟩

dactyl- *or* **dactylo-** *comb form* : finger : toe : digit ⟨*dactylo*logy⟩

-dac·tyl·ia \ˌdak-'til-ē-ə\ *n comb form* : -DACTYLY ⟨a*dactylia*⟩

-dac·tyl·ism \'dak-tə-ˌliz-əm\ *n comb form* : -DACTYLY ⟨oligo*dactylism*⟩

-dac·ty·lous \'dak-tə-ləs\ *adj comb form* : having (such or so many) fingers or toes ⟨brachy*dactylous*⟩

-dac·ty·ly \'dak-tə-lē\ *n comb form, pl* **-lies** : condition of having (such or so many) fingers or toes ⟨poly*dactyly*⟩ ⟨syn*dactyly*⟩

dent- *or* **denti-** *or* **dento-** *comb form* **1** : tooth ⟨*dent*al⟩ **2** : dental and ⟨*dento*facial⟩

derm- *or* **derma-** *or* **dermo-** *comb form* : skin ⟨*derm*al⟩ ⟨*dermo*pathy⟩

-derm \ˌdərm\ *n comb form* : skin : covering ⟨ecto*derm*⟩

-der·ma \'dər-mə\ *n comb form, pl* **-dermas** *or* **-der·ma·ta** \-mət-ə\ : skin or skin ailment of a (specified) type ⟨sclero*derma*⟩

dermat- *or* **dermato-** *comb form* : skin ⟨*dermat*itis⟩ ⟨*dermato*logy⟩

-der·ma·tous \'dər-mət-əs\ *adj comb form* : having a (specified) type of skin ⟨sclero*dermatous*⟩

-der·mia \'dər-mē-ə\ *n comb form* : skin or skin ailment of a (specified) type ⟨kerato*dermia*⟩

-der·mis \'dər-məs\ *n comb form* : layer of skin or tissue ⟨epi*dermis*⟩

-de·sis \də-səs\ *n comb form, pl* **-de·ses** \-ˌsēz\ : binding or fixation ⟨arthro*desis*⟩

desm- *or* **desmo-** *comb form* : connective tissue ⟨*desmo*cranium⟩ ⟨*desmo*cyte⟩

dextr- *or* **dextro-** *comb form* **1** : right : on or toward the right ⟨*dextro*cardia⟩ **2** *usu* **dextro-** : dextrorotatory ⟨*dextro*amphetamine⟩

di- *comb form* **1** : twice : twofold : double ⟨*di*phasic⟩ ⟨*di*zygotic⟩ **2** : containing two atoms, radicals, or groups ⟨*di*oxide⟩

\ə\ abut \ᵊ\ kitten \ər\ further \a\ ash \ā\ ace \ä\ cot, cart \au̇\ out \ch\ chin \e\ bet \ē\ easy \g\ go \i\ hit \ī\ ice \j\ job \ŋ\ sing \ō\ go \ȯ\ law \ȯi\ boy \th\ thin \t͟h\ the \ü\ loot \u̇\ foot \y\ yet \zh\ vision *See also* Pronunciation Symbols page

dipl- *or* **diplo-** *comb form* : double : twofold ⟨*diplo*coccus⟩ ⟨*dipl*opia⟩

disc- *or* **disci-** *or* **disco-** *also* **disk-** *or* **disko-** *comb form* : disk ⟨*disci*form⟩

disto- *also* **dist-** *or* **disti-** *comb form* : distal ⟨*disto*buccal⟩

dolicho- *comb form* : long ⟨*dolicho*cephalic⟩

dorso- *or* **dorsi-** *also* **dors-** *comb form* **1** : dorsal ⟨*dorsi*flexion⟩ **2** : dorsal and ⟨*dorso*lateral⟩

duoden- *or* **duodeno-** *comb form* **1** : duodenum ⟨*duoden*itis⟩ **2** : duodenal and ⟨*duodeno*jejunal⟩

-dy·nam·ia \dī-'nam-ē-ə, də-, -'nām-\ *comb form* : strength : condition of having (such) strength ⟨a*dynamia*⟩

dys- *prefix* **1** : abnormal ⟨*dys*chromia⟩ **2** : difficult ⟨*dys*pnea⟩ — compare EU- 1a **3** : impaired ⟨*dys*function⟩

e- *prefix* : missing : absent ⟨*e*dentulous⟩

ec- *prefix* : out of : outside of : outside ⟨*ec*crine⟩

ecto- *also* **ect-** *comb form* : outside : external ⟨*ecto*derm⟩ ⟨*ecto*cornea⟩ — compare END- 1, EXO- 1

-ec·to·my \'ek-tə-mē\ *n comb form, pl* **-ec·to·mies** : surgical removal ⟨gast*rectomy*⟩ ⟨append*ectomy*⟩

ectro- *comb form* : congenitally absent — usu. indicating absence of a particular limb or part ⟨*ectro*dactyly⟩

-ei *pl of* -EUS

elast- *or* **elasto-** *comb form* : elasticity ⟨*elast*osis⟩

embol- *or* **embolo-** *comb form* **1** : embolus ⟨*embol*ectomy⟩ **2** : interpolation ⟨*embolo*lalia⟩

embry- *or* **embryo-** *comb form* : embryo ⟨*embry*oma⟩ ⟨*embryo*genesis⟩

embryon- *or* **embryoni-** *comb form* : embryo ⟨*embryon*ic⟩

-emia \'ē-mē-ə\ *also* **-he·mia** \'hē-\ *or chiefly Brit* **-ae·mia** \'ē-mē-ə\ *also* **-hae·mia** \'hē-\ *n comb form* **1** : condition of having (such) blood ⟨leuk*emia*⟩ ⟨septic*emia*⟩ **2** : condition of having (a specified thing) in the blood ⟨chol*emia*⟩ ⟨ure*mia*⟩

encephal- *or* **encephalo-** *comb form* **1** : brain ⟨*encephal*itis⟩ ⟨*encephalo*cele⟩ **2** : of, relating to, or affecting the brain and ⟨*encephalo*myelitis⟩

-en·ce·pha·lia \-(ˌ)en-sə-'fāl-yə\ *n comb form* : condition of having (such) a brain ⟨an*encephalia*⟩

-en·ceph·a·lus \in-'sef-ə-ləs\ *n comb form, pl* **-en·ceph·a·li** \-ˌlī, -ˌlē\ **1** : fetus having (such) a brain ⟨ini*encephalus*⟩ **2** : condition of having (such) a brain ⟨hydr*encephalus*⟩

-en·ceph·a·ly \in-'sef-ə-lē\ *n comb form, pl* **-en·ceph·a·lies** \in-'sef-ə-lēz\ : condition of having (such) a brain ⟨micr*encephaly*⟩

end- *or* **endo-** *comb form* **1** : within : inside ⟨*end*aural⟩ ⟨*endo*skeleton⟩ — compare ECTO-, EXO- 1 **2** : taking in ⟨*endo*thermic⟩

endotheli- *or* **endothelio-** *comb form* : endothelium ⟨*endo*thelioma⟩

ent- *or* **ento-** *comb form* : inner : within ⟨*ent*optic⟩

enter- *or* **entero-** *comb form* **1** : intestine ⟨*enter*itis⟩ **2** : intestinal and ⟨*entero*hepatic⟩

ependym- *or* **ependymo-** *comb form* : ependyma ⟨*ependym*itis⟩

epi- *or* **ep-** *prefix* : upon ⟨*epi*bulbar⟩ : besides ⟨*epi*phenomenon⟩ : attached to ⟨*epi*didymis⟩ : outer ⟨*epi*blast⟩ : after ⟨*epi*genesis⟩

epiderm- *or* **epidermo-** *comb form* : epidermis ⟨*epiderm*itis⟩ ⟨*epidermo*lysis⟩

epididym- *or* **epididymo-** *comb form* **1** : epididymis ⟨*epididym*ectomy⟩ **2** : epididymis and ⟨*epididymo*-orchitis⟩

epilept- *or* **epilepti-** *or* **epilepto-** *comb form* : epilepsy ⟨*epilept*oid⟩ ⟨*epilepti*form⟩ ⟨*epilepto*genic⟩

episio- *comb form* **1** : vulva ⟨*episio*tomy⟩ **2** : vulva and ⟨*episio*perineorrhaphy⟩

epithel- *or* **epitheli-** *or* **epithelio-** *comb form* : epithelium ⟨*epitheli*oma⟩

erg- *or* **ergo-** *comb form* : work ⟨*ergo*meter⟩

-er·gic \(ˌ)ər-jik\ *adj comb form* **1** : allergic ⟨hyper*ergic*⟩ **2** : exhibiting or stimulating activity esp. of (such) a neurotransmitter substance ⟨adren*ergic*⟩ ⟨dopamin*ergic*⟩

ergo- *comb form* : ergot ⟨*ergo*sterol⟩

eroto- *comb form* : sexual desire ⟨*eroto*mania⟩

erythr- *or* **erythro-** *comb form* **1** : red ⟨*erythro*cyte⟩ **2** : erythrocyte ⟨*erythr*oid⟩

eso- *prefix* : inner ⟨*eso*tropia⟩

esophag- *or* **esophago-** *or chiefly Brit* **oesophag-** *or* **oesophago-** *comb form* **1** : esophagus ⟨*esophag*ectomy⟩ ⟨*esophago*plasty⟩ **2** : esophagus and ⟨*esophago*gastrectomy⟩

esthesio- *or chiefly Brit* **aesthesio-** *comb form* : sensation ⟨*esthesio*metry⟩

estr- *or* **estro-** *or chiefly Brit* **oestr-** *or* **oestro-** *comb form* : estrus ⟨*estro*gen⟩

ethmo- *comb form* : ethmoid and ⟨*ethmo*maxillary⟩

etio- *or chiefly Brit* **aetio-** *comb form* **1** : cause ⟨*etio*logic⟩ ⟨*etio*pathogenesis⟩ **2** : formed by chemical degradation of a (specified) compound ⟨*etio*porphyrin⟩

eu- *comb form* **1 a** : well : easily ⟨*eu*plastic⟩ — compare DYS- 2 **b** : good : normal ⟨*eu*thyroid⟩ **2** : true ⟨*eu*globulin⟩

-e·us \ē-əs\ *n comb form, pl* **-ei** \ē-ˌī\ *also* **-e·us·es** \ē-ə-səz\ : muscle that constitutes, has the form of, or joins a (specified) part, thing, or structure ⟨glut*eus*⟩ ⟨rhomboid*eus*⟩ ⟨iliococcyg*eus*⟩

exo- *or* **ex-** *comb form* **1** : outside : outer ⟨*exo*enzyme⟩ ⟨*exo*skeleton⟩ — compare ECTO-, END- 1 **2** : turning out ⟨*exo*thermic⟩

extra- *prefix* : outside : beyond ⟨*extra*uterine⟩

extro- *prefix* : outside : outward ⟨*extro*vert⟩ — compare INTRO-

-fa·cient \'fā-shənt\ *adj comb form* : making : causing ⟨aborti*facient*⟩ ⟨rube*facient*⟩

facio- *comb form* : facial and ⟨*facio*scapulohumeral⟩

femoro- *comb form* : femoral and ⟨*femoro*popliteal⟩

feto- *or* **feti-** *or chiefly Brit* **foeto-** *or* **foeti-** *comb form* : fetus ⟨*feti*cide⟩ ⟨*feto*metry⟩

fibr- *or* **fibro-** *comb form* **1** : fiber : fibrous tissue ⟨*fibro*genesis⟩ **2** : fibrous and ⟨*fibro*elastic⟩

fili- *or* **filo-** *comb form* : thread ⟨*fili*form⟩

fluor- *or* **fluoro-** *comb form* **1** : fluorine ⟨*fluor*osis⟩ **2** *also* **fluori-** : fluorescence ⟨*fluoro*scope⟩

fore- *comb form* **1** : occurring earlier : occurring beforehand ⟨*fore*play⟩ **2 a** : situated at the front : in front ⟨*fore*leg⟩ **b** : front part of (something specified) ⟨*fore*arm⟩ ⟨*fore*brain⟩

-form \ˌform\ *adj comb form* : in the form or shape of : resembling ⟨chorei*form*⟩ ⟨epilepti*form*⟩

fronto- *comb form* : frontal bone and ⟨*fronto*parietal⟩

-fuge \ˌfyüj\ *n comb form* : one that drives away ⟨febri*fuge*⟩ ⟨vermi*fuge*⟩

fungi- *comb form* : fungus ⟨*fungi*cide⟩

fusi- *comb form* : spindle ⟨*fusi*form⟩

galact- *or* **galacto-** *comb form* **1** : milk ⟨*galacto*poiesis⟩ **2** : related to galactose ⟨*galacto*lipid⟩

gamet- *or* **gameto-** *comb form* : gamete ⟨*gamet*ic⟩ ⟨*gameto*genesis⟩

-gam·ic \'gam-ik\ *adj comb form* : -GAMOUS ⟨mono*gamic*⟩

-g·a·mous \gə-məs\ *adj comb form* **1** : characterized by having or practicing (such) a marriage or (such or so many) marriages ⟨mono*gamous*⟩ **2** : having (such) gametes or reproductive organs or (such) a mode of fertilization ⟨heterog*amous*⟩

-g·a·my \gə-mē\ *n comb form, pl* **-g·a·mies** **1** : marriage ⟨mono*gamy*⟩ **2** : possession of (such) gametes or reproductive organs or (such) a mode of fertilization ⟨hetero*gamy*⟩

gangli- *or* **ganglio-** *comb form* : ganglion ⟨*ganli*oma⟩ ⟨*ganglio*neuroma⟩

gastr- *or* **gastro-** *also* **gastri-** *comb form* **1** : belly : stomach ⟨*gastr*itis⟩ **2** : gastric and ⟨*gastro*intestinal⟩

gen- *or* **geno-** *comb form* **1** : race : ethnic group ⟨*geno*cide⟩ **2** : genus : kind ⟨*geno*type⟩ **3** : gene ⟨*geno*me⟩

-gen \jən, jen\ *also* **-gene** \ˌjēn\ *n comb form* **1** : producer

⟨aller*gen*⟩ ⟨carcino*gen*⟩ **2** : one that is (so) produced ⟨phos*gene*⟩

-ge·net·ic \jə-ˈnet-ik\ *adj comb form* : -GENIC ⟨psychogenet*ic*⟩

-gen·ic \ˈjen-ik *sometimes* ˈjē-nik\ *adj comb form* **1** : producing : forming ⟨carcino*genic*⟩ **2** : produced by : formed from ⟨nephro*genic*⟩

genito- *comb form* : genital and ⟨*genito*urinary⟩

-g·e·nous \jə-nəs\ *adj comb form* **1** : producing : yielding ⟨ero*genous*⟩ **2** : produced by : arising or originating in ⟨neuro*genous*⟩ ⟨endo*genous*⟩

-g·e·ny \jə-nē\ *n comb form, pl* **-g·e·nies** : generation : production ⟨embryo*geny*⟩ ⟨lyso*geny*⟩

geront- *or* **geronto-** *comb form* : aged one : old age ⟨*geront*ology⟩

-geu·sia \ˈgü-zē-ə, ˈjü-, -sē-ə, -zhə\ *n comb form* : a (specified) condition of the sense of taste ⟨a*geusia*⟩ ⟨dys*geusia*⟩

gingiv- *or* **gingivo-** *comb form* **1** : gum : gums ⟨*gingiv*itis⟩ **2** : gums and ⟨*gingivo*stomatitis⟩

gli- *or* **glio-** *comb form* **1** : gliomatous ⟨*glio*blastoma⟩ **2** : glial ⟨*gli*oma⟩

-g·lia \glē-ə\ *n comb form* : glia made up of a (specified) kind or size of element ⟨micro*glia*⟩ ⟨oligodendro*glia*⟩

glomerul- *or* **glomerulo-** *comb form* : glomerulus of the kidney ⟨*glomerul*itis⟩ ⟨*glomerulo*nephritis⟩

gloss- *or* **glosso-** *comb form* **1** : tongue ⟨*gloss*itis⟩ ⟨*gloss*opathy⟩ **2** : language ⟨*glosso*lalia⟩

-glos·sia \ˈglä-sē-ə, ˈglȯ\ *n comb form* : condition of having (such) a tongue ⟨micro*glossia*⟩

gluc- *or* **gluco-** *comb form* : glucose ⟨*gluco*kinase⟩ ⟨*gluco*neogenesis⟩

glyc- *or* **glyco-** *comb form* **1** : carbohydrate and esp. sugar ⟨*glyc*uresis⟩ ⟨*glyco*protein⟩ **2** : glycine ⟨*glyc*yl⟩

glycer- *or* **glycero-** *comb form* **1** : glycerol ⟨*glycer*yl⟩ **2** : related to glycerol or glyceric acid ⟨*glycer*aldehyde⟩

-g·na·thous *adj comb form* : having (such) a jaw ⟨opisthog*nathous*⟩

-g·no·sia \g-ˈnō-zhə\ *n comb form* : -GNOSIS ⟨a*gnosia*⟩ ⟨prosopa*gnosia*⟩

-g·no·sis \g-ˈnō-səs\ *n comb form, pl* **-g·no·ses** \-ˌsēz\ : knowledge : cognition : recognition ⟨stereo*gnosis*⟩

-g·nos·tic \g-ˈnäs-tik\ *adj comb form* : characterized by or relating to (such) knowledge ⟨pharmaco*gnostic*⟩

-g·no·sy \g-nə-sē\ *n comb form, pl* **-g·no·sies** : -GNOSIS ⟨pharmaco*gnosy*⟩

gon- *or* **gono-** *comb form* : sexual : generative : semen : seed ⟨*gono*duct⟩

goni- *or* **gonio-** *comb form* : corner : angle ⟨*gonio*meter⟩

-g·o·ny \gə-nē\ *n comb form, pl* **-g·o·nies** : manner of generation or reproduction ⟨schizo*gony*⟩

-gram \ˌgram\ *n comb form* : drawing : writing : record ⟨cardio*gram*⟩

granul- *or* **granuli-** *or* **granulo-** *comb form* **1** : granular ⟨*granulo*cyte⟩ **2** : granulocyte ⟨*granulo*blast⟩

-graph \ˌgraf\ *n comb form* **1** : something written ⟨mono*graph*⟩ **2** : instrument for making or transmitting records ⟨electrocardio*graph*⟩

-graph·ia \ˈgra-fē-ə\ *n comb form* : writing characteristic of a (specified) usu. psychological abnormality ⟨dys*graphia*⟩ ⟨dermo*graphia*⟩

grapho- *comb form* : writing ⟨*grapho*logy⟩

gynec- *or* **gyneco-** *or chiefly Brit* **gynaec-** *or* **gynaeco-** *comb form* : woman ⟨*gyneco*id⟩ ⟨*gyneco*logy⟩

haem- *or* **haemo-** *chiefly Brit var of* HEM-

haema- *chiefly Brit var of* HEMA-

haemat- *or* **haemato-** *chiefly Brit var of* HEMAT-

-haemia *chiefly Brit var of* -EMIA

hapt- *or* **hapto-** *comb form* : contact : touch : combination ⟨*hapt*ic⟩ ⟨*hapto*globin⟩

heli- *or* **helio-** *comb form* : sun ⟨*helio*therapy⟩

helic- *or* **helico-** *comb form* : helix : spiral ⟨*helic*al⟩ ⟨*helico*trema⟩

helminth- *or* **helmintho-** *comb form* : helminth ⟨*helminth*iasis⟩ ⟨*helmintho*logy⟩

hem- *or* **hemo-** *or chiefly Brit* **haem-** *or* **haemo-** *comb form* : blood ⟨*hem*al⟩ ⟨*hem*angioma⟩ ⟨*hemo*philia⟩

hema- *or chiefly Brit* **haema-** *comb form* : HEM- ⟨*hema*cytometer⟩

hemat- *or* **hemato-** *or chiefly Brit* **haemat-** *or* **haemato-** *comb form* : HEM- ⟨*hemat*emesis⟩ ⟨*hemato*genous⟩

hemi- *prefix* : half ⟨*hemi*block⟩ ⟨*hemi*pelvectomy⟩

-hemia *var of* -EMIA

hemo- *var of* HEM-

hepat- *or* **hepato-** *comb form* **1** : liver ⟨*hepat*itis⟩ ⟨*hepato*toxic⟩ **2** : hepatic and ⟨*hepato*biliary⟩

heredo- *comb form* : hereditary ⟨*heredo*familial⟩

hernio- *comb form* : hernia ⟨*hernio*rrhaphy⟩ ⟨*hernio*tomy⟩

herpet- *or* **herpeto-** *comb form* **1** : reptile or reptiles ⟨*herpe*tophobia⟩ **2** : herpes ⟨*herpet*iform⟩

heter- *or* **hetero-** *comb form* : other than usual : other : different ⟨*hetero*graft⟩

hidr- *or* **hidro-** *comb form* : sweat glands ⟨*hidr*adenitis⟩

hist- *or* **histo-** *comb form* : tissue ⟨*hist*amine⟩ ⟨*histo*physiology⟩

histi- *or* **histio-** *comb form* : tissue ⟨*histio*cyte⟩

hol- *or* **holo-** *comb form* **1** : complete : total ⟨*holo*enzyme⟩ **2** : completely : totally ⟨*holo*endemic⟩

hom- *or* **homo-** *comb form* **1** : one and the same : similar : alike ⟨*homo*zygous⟩ **2** : derived from the same species ⟨*homo*graft⟩ **3** : homosexual ⟨*homo*phobia⟩

home- *or* **homeo-** *also* **homoi-** *or* **homoio-** *or chiefly Brit* **homoe-** *or* **homoeo-** *comb form* : like : similar ⟨*homeo*stasis⟩ ⟨*homoio*thermy⟩

hy- *or* **hyo-** *comb form* **1** : of, relating to, or connecting with the hyoid bone ⟨*hyo*glossus⟩ **2** : hyoid and ⟨*hyo*thyroid⟩

hyal- *or* **hyalo-** *comb form* : glass : glassy : hyaline ⟨*hyal*uronic acid⟩ ⟨*hyalo*gen⟩

hydr- *or* **hydro-** *comb form* **1** : water ⟨*hydro*therapy⟩ **2 a** : liquid : fluid ⟨*hydro*kinetics⟩ **b** : fluid accumulation ⟨*hydro*cephalus⟩ ⟨*hydro*nephrosis⟩

hymen- *or* **hymeno-** *comb form* : hymen : membrane ⟨*hymen*ectomy⟩ ⟨*hymeno*tomy⟩

hyper- *prefix* **1** : excessively ⟨*hyper*sensitive⟩ **2** : excessive ⟨*hyper*emia⟩ ⟨*hyper*tension⟩

hypn- *or* **hypno-** *comb form* **1** : sleep ⟨*hypn*agogic⟩ **2** : hypnotism ⟨*hypno*anesthesia⟩

hypo- *or* **hyp-** *prefix* **1** : under : beneath : down ⟨*hypo*blast⟩ ⟨*hypo*dermic⟩ **2** : less than normal or normally ⟨*hyp*esthesia⟩ ⟨*hypo*tension⟩

hypothalamico- *or* **hypothalamo-** *comb form* **1** : hypothalamus ⟨*hypothalamo*tomy⟩ **2** : hypothalamic and ⟨*hypothalamico*-hypophyseal⟩

hyps- *or* **hypsi-** *or* **hypso-** *comb form* : high ⟨*hypsi*cranic⟩

hyster- *or* **hystero-** *comb form* **1** : womb ⟨*hystero*tomy⟩ **2** : hysteria ⟨*hystero*genic⟩

-i·a·sis \ˈī-ə-səs\ *n suffix, pl* **-i·a·ses** \-ˌsēz\ : disease having characteristics of or produced by (something specified) ⟨amebi*asis*⟩ ⟨ancylostomi*asis*⟩ ⟨onchocerci*asis*⟩

-i·at·ric \ē-ˈa-trik\ *also* **-i·at·ri·cal** \-tri-kəl\ *adj comb form* : of or relating to (such) medical treatment or healing ⟨pedi*atric*⟩

-i·at·rics \ē-ˈa-triks\ *n pl comb form but sing or pl in constr* : medical treatment ⟨pedi*atrics*⟩

-i·a·trist \ˈī-ə-trəst, *in a few words* ē-ˈa-trəst\ *n comb form* : physician : healer ⟨psychi*atrist*⟩ ⟨podi*atrist*⟩

iatro- *comb form* **1** : physician : medicine : healing ⟨*iatro*genic⟩ **2 a** : physician and ⟨*iatro*chemist⟩ **b** : medicine or healing and ⟨*iatro*physics⟩

\ə\ **abut** \ˈə\ **kitten** \ər\ **further** \a\ **ash** \ā\ **ace** \ä\ **cot, cart**
\au̇\ **out** \ch\ **chin** \e\ **bet** \ē\ **easy** \g\ **go** \i\ **hit** \ī\ **ice** \j\ **job**
\ŋ\ **sing** \ō\ **go** \ȯ\ **law** \ȯi\ **boy** \th\ **thin** \t͟h\ **the** \ü\ **loot**
\u̇\ **foot** \y\ **yet** \zh\ **vision** *See also* Pronunciation Symbols page

-i·a·try \\'ī-ə-trē, *in a few words* ē-ˌa-trē\ *n comb form, pl* **-i·a·tries** : medical treatment : healing ⟨podi*atry*⟩ ⟨psychi*atry*⟩

ichthy- *or* **ichthyo-** *comb form* : fish ⟨*ichthyo*sarcotoxism⟩

-ics \iks\ *n pl suffix but sing or pl in constr* **1** *usu sing in constr* : study : knowledge : skill : practice ⟨opt*ics*⟩ ⟨orthoped*ics*⟩ **2** *usu pl in constr* : characteristic actions or activities ⟨hyster*ics*⟩ **3** *usu pl in constr* : characteristic qualities, operations, or phenomena ⟨acoust*ics*⟩ ⟨phonet*ics*⟩

icter- *or* **ictero-** *comb form* **1** : jaundice ⟨*icter*oid⟩ **2** : jaundice and ⟨*ictero*anemia⟩

¹-id \əd, (ˌ)id\ *also* **-ide** \īd\ *n suffix* : skin rash caused by (something specified) ⟨bacter*id*⟩ ⟨syphil*id*⟩

²-id *n suffix* **1** : structural element of a lower molar or premolar ⟨protocon*id*⟩ **2** : structure, body, or particle of a (specified) kind ⟨chromat*id*⟩

-i·da \əd-ə\ *n pl suffix* : animals that are or have the form of — in names of higher taxa (as orders and classes) ⟨Arachni*da*⟩ — **-i·dan** \əd-ən, əd-ᵊn\ *n or adj suffix*

-i·dae \ə-ˌdē\ *n pl suffix* : members of the family of — in names of zoological families ⟨Homin*idae*⟩ ⟨Ixod*idae*⟩

idio- *comb form* **1** : one's own : personal : separate : distinct ⟨*idio*type⟩ ⟨*idio*syncrasy⟩ **2** : self-produced : arising within ⟨*idio*pathic⟩ ⟨*idio*ventricular⟩

-i·dro·sis \i-'drō-səs\ *n comb form, pl* **-i·dro·ses** \-ˌsēz\ : a specified form of sweating ⟨chrom*idrosis*⟩

ile- *also* **ileo-** *comb form* **1** : ileum ⟨*ile*itis⟩ **2** : ileal and ⟨*ile*ocecal⟩

ilio- *comb form* : iliac and ⟨*ilio*inguinal⟩

immuno- *comb form* **1** : physiological immunity ⟨*immuno*logy⟩ **2** : immunologic ⟨*immuno*chemistry⟩ : immunologically ⟨*immuno*compromised⟩ : immunology and ⟨*immuno*genetics⟩

¹in- *or* **il-** *or* **im-** *or* **ir-** *prefix* : not — usu. *il-* before *l* ⟨*il*legitimate⟩; *im-* before *b, m,* or *p* ⟨*im*balance⟩ ⟨*im*mobile⟩ ⟨*im*palpable⟩; *ir-* before *r* ⟨*ir*reducible⟩; and *in-* before other sounds ⟨*in*operable⟩

²in- *or* **il-** *or* **im-** *or* **ir-** *prefix* : in : within : into : toward : on ⟨*ir*radiation⟩ — usu. *il-* before *l; im-* before *b, m,* or *p; ir-* before *r;* and *in-* before other sounds

-in \ən, ᵊn, ˌin\ *n suffix* **1 a** : neutral chemical compound ⟨insul*in*⟩ **b** : enzyme ⟨pancreat*in*⟩ **c** : antibiotic ⟨penicill*in*⟩ **2** : pharmaceutical product ⟨niac*in*⟩

infero- *comb form* : below and ⟨*infero*medial⟩

infra- *prefix* **1** : below ⟨*infra*human⟩ ⟨*infra*hyoid⟩ **2** : within ⟨*infra*specific⟩ **3** : below in a scale or series ⟨*infra*red⟩

ino- *comb form* : fiber : fibrous ⟨*ino*tropic⟩

inter- *comb form* : between : among ⟨*inter*cellular⟩ ⟨*inter*costal⟩

in·tra- \ˌin-trə, -(ˌ)trä\ *prefix* **1 a** : within ⟨*intra*cerebellar⟩ **b** : during ⟨*intra*natal⟩ **c** : between layers of ⟨*intra*dermal⟩ **2** : INTRO- ⟨an *intra*muscular injection⟩

intro- *prefix* **1** : in : into ⟨*intro*jection⟩ **2** : inward : within ⟨*intro*vert⟩ — compare EXTRO-

ir- *var of* IN-

irid- *or* **irido-** *comb form* **1** : iris of the eye ⟨*irid*ectomy⟩ **2** : iris and ⟨*irido*cyclitis⟩

is- *or* **iso-** *comb form* **1** : equal : homogeneous : uniform ⟨*iso*caloric⟩ ⟨*iso*morph⟩ **2** : for or from different individuals of the same species ⟨*iso*agglutinin⟩

ischi- *or* **ischio-** *comb form* **1** : ischium ⟨*ischi*ectomy⟩ **2** : ischial and ⟨*ischio*rectal⟩

-ism \ˌiz-əm\ *n suffix* **1** : act, practice, or process ⟨hypnot*ism*⟩ **2 a** : state, condition, or property ⟨heterothall*ism*⟩ **b** : abnormal state or condition resulting from excess of a (specified) thing or marked by resemblance to a (specified) person or thing ⟨alcohol*ism*⟩ ⟨morphin*ism*⟩ ⟨mongol*ism*⟩

-ite \ˌīt\ *n suffix* **1** : substance produced through some (specified) process ⟨anabol*ite*⟩ ⟨catabol*ite*⟩ **2** : segment or constituent part of a body or of a bodily part ⟨som*ite*⟩ ⟨dendr*ite*⟩

-it·ic \'it-ik\ *adj suffix* : of, resembling, or marked by — in adjectives formed from nouns usu. ending in *-ite* ⟨dendr*itic*⟩ and *-itis* ⟨bronch*itic*⟩

-i·tis \'īt-əs *also but not shown at individual entries* 'ēt-\ *n suffix, pl* **-i·tis·es** *also* **-it·i·des** \'it-ə-ˌdēz\ *or* **-i·tes** \'īt-(ˌ)ēz, 'ēt-\ : disease usu. inflammatory of a (specified) part or organ : inflammation of ⟨laryng*itis*⟩ ⟨appendic*itis*⟩ ⟨bronch*itis*⟩

jejun- *or* **jejuno-** *comb form* **1** : jejunum ⟨*jejun*itis⟩ **2** : jejunum and ⟨*jejuno*ileitis⟩

juxta- *comb form* : situated near ⟨*juxta*glomerular⟩

kary- *or* **karyo-** *also* **cary-** *or* **caryo-** *comb form* : nucleus of a cell ⟨*karyo*kinesis⟩ ⟨*karyo*type⟩

kerat- *or* **kerato-** *comb form* : cornea ⟨*kerat*itis⟩

kin- *or* **kine-** *or* **kino-** *or* **cin-** *or* **cino-** *comb form* : motion : action ⟨*kin*esthesia⟩

kinesi- *or* **kinesio-** *comb form* : movement ⟨*kinesio*logy⟩

-ki·ne·sia \kə-'nē-zhə, kī-, -zhē-ə\ *n comb form* : movement : motion ⟨hyper*kinesia*⟩

kinet- *or* **kineto-** *comb form* : movement : motion ⟨*kineto*cardiogram⟩

klept- *or* **klepto-** *comb form* : stealing : theft ⟨*klepto*mania⟩

labio- *comb form* : labial and ⟨*labio*lingual⟩

lact- *or* **lacti-** *or* **lacto-** *comb form* **1** : milk ⟨*lacto*genesis⟩ **2 a** : lactic acid ⟨*lact*ate⟩ **b** : lactose ⟨*lact*ase⟩

laev- *or* **laevo-** *Brit var of* LEV-

-lag·nia \'lag-nē-ə\ *comb form* : sexual excitement ⟨klepto*lagnia*⟩ ⟨uro*lagnia*⟩

-la·lia \'lā-lē-ə\ *n comb form* : speech disorder (of a specified type) ⟨echo*lalia*⟩

lamin- *or* **lamini-** *or* **lamino-** *comb form* : lamina ⟨*lamin*itis⟩ ⟨*lamino*graph⟩

laryng- *or* **laryngo-** *comb form* **1** : larynx ⟨*laryng*itis⟩ **2 a** : laryngeal ⟨*laryngo*spasm⟩ **b** : laryngeal and ⟨*laryngo*pharyngeal⟩

lecith- *or* **lecitho-** *comb form* : yolk of an egg ⟨*lecith*al⟩ ⟨*lecitho*in⟩

leio- *or* **lio-** *comb form* : smooth ⟨*leio*myoma⟩

-lep·sy \ˌlep-sē\ *also* **-lep·sia** \'lep-sē-ə\ *or* **-lep·sis** \'lep-səs\ *n comb form, pl* **-lep·sies** *also* **-lep·sias** *or* **-lep·ses** \'lep-ˌsēz\ : taking : seizure ⟨epi*lepsy*⟩ ⟨narco*lepsy*⟩

lept- *or* **lepto-** *comb form* : small : weak : thin : fine ⟨*lepto*rrhine⟩ ⟨*lepto*tene⟩

leuk- *or* **leuko-** *or chiefly Brit* **leuc-** *or* **leuco-** *comb form* **1** : white : colorless : weakly colored ⟨*leuko*cyte⟩ ⟨*leukor*rhea⟩ **2** : leukocyte ⟨*leuk*emia⟩ **3** : white matter of the brain ⟨*leuko*encephalitis⟩

leukocyt- *or* **leukocyto-** *or chiefly Brit* **leucocyt-** *or* **leucocyto-** *comb form* : leukocyte ⟨*leukocyto*sis⟩

lev- *or* **levo-** *or Brit* **laev-** *or* **laevo-** *comb form* **1** : left : on the left side : to the left ⟨*levo*cardia⟩ **2** : levorotatory ⟨*levu*lose⟩

-lex·ia \'lek-sē-ə\ *n comb form* : reading of (such) a kind or with (such) an impairment ⟨dys*lexia*⟩

lingu- *or* **lingui-** *or* **linguo-** *comb form* : tongue ⟨*lingui*form⟩

lip- *or* **lipo-** *comb form* : fat : fatty tissue : fatty ⟨*lip*oid⟩ ⟨*lipo*protein⟩

liss- *or* **lisso-** *comb form* : smooth ⟨*liss*encephaly⟩

lith- *or* **litho-** *comb form* : calculus ⟨*lith*iasis⟩ ⟨*litho*tripsy⟩

-lith \ˌlith\ *n comb form* : calculus ⟨uro*lith*⟩

lob- *or* **lobi-** *or* **lobo-** *comb form* : lobe ⟨*lob*ectomy⟩ ⟨*lobo*tomy⟩

log- *or* **logo-** *comb form* : word : thought : speech : discourse ⟨*logo*rrhea⟩

-l·o·gy \l-ə-jē\ *n comb form, pl* **-l·o·gies** : doctrine : theory : science ⟨physio*logy*⟩

lumb- *or* **lumbo-** *comb form* : lumbar and ⟨*lumbo*sacral⟩

lumi- *comb form* : formed by irradiation ⟨*lumi*rhodopsin⟩

lute- *or* **luteo-** *comb form* : corpus luteum ⟨*lute*al⟩ ⟨*luteo*lysis⟩

lymph- *or* **lympho-** *comb form* : lymph : lymphatic tissue ⟨*lymph*edema⟩ ⟨*lympho*granuloma⟩

lymphangi- *or* **lymphangio-** *comb form* : lymphatic vessels ⟨*lymphangio*graphy⟩

lys- *or* **lysi-** *or* **lyso-** *comb form* : lysis ⟨*lys*in⟩ ⟨*lyso*lecithin⟩

-ly·sis \l-ə-səs, ˈlī-səs\ *n comb form, pl* **-l·y·ses** \l-ə-ˌsēz\ 1 : decomposition ⟨auto*lysis*⟩ 2 : disintegration : breaking down ⟨auto*lysis*⟩ 3 a : relief or reduction ⟨neuro*lysis*⟩ b : detachment ⟨epidermo*lysis*⟩

-lyte \ˌlīt\ *n comb form* : substance capable of undergoing (such) decomposition ⟨electro*lyte*⟩

-lyt·ic \ˈlit-ik\ *adj suffix* : of, relating to, or effecting (such) decomposition ⟨hydro*lytic*⟩

macr- *or* **macro-** *comb form* : large ⟨*macro*molecule⟩ ⟨*macrocyte*⟩

macul- *or* **maculo-** *comb form* : macule : macular and ⟨*maculo*papular⟩

mal- *comb form* 1 : bad ⟨*mal*practice⟩ 2 a : abnormal ⟨*mal*formation⟩ b : abnormally ⟨*mal*formed⟩ 3 a : inadequate ⟨*mal*adjustment⟩ b : inadequately ⟨*mal*nourished⟩

malac- *or* **malaco-** *comb form* : soft ⟨*malaco*plakia⟩

malari- *or* **malario-** *comb form* : malaria ⟨*malario*logy⟩

mamm- *or* **mamma-** *or* **mammi-** *or* **mammo-** *comb form* : breast ⟨*mamm*ectomy⟩ ⟨*mammo*gram⟩

mandibul- *or* **mandibuli-** *or* **mandibulo-** *comb form* : mandibular and ⟨*mandibulo*facial dysostosis⟩

mast- *or* **masto-** *comb form* : breast : nipple : mammary gland ⟨*mast*itis⟩

-mas·tia \ˈmas-tē-ə\ *n comb form* : condition of having (such or so many) breasts or mammary glands ⟨gyneco*mastia*⟩ ⟨macro*mastia*⟩

maxill- *or* **maxilli-** *or* **maxillo-** *comb form* 1 : maxilla ⟨*maxill*ectomy⟩ 2 : maxillary and ⟨*maxillo*facial⟩

maz- *or* **mazo-** *comb form* : breast ⟨*mazo*plasia⟩

meat- *or* **meato-** *comb form* : meatus ⟨*meato*plasty⟩

medi- *or* **medio-** *comb form* : middle ⟨*medio*lateral⟩

medico- *comb form* : medical : medical and ⟨*medico*legal⟩

mega- *or* **meg-** *comb form* 1 : great : large ⟨*mega*colon⟩ ⟨*mega*dose⟩ 2 : million : multiplied by one million ⟨*mega*curie⟩

megal- *or* **megalo-** *comb form* 1 : large ⟨*megalo*cyte⟩ : abnormally large ⟨*megalo*cephaly⟩ 2 : grandiose ⟨*megalo*mania⟩

-meg·a·ly \ˈmeg-ə-lē\ *n comb form, pl* **-meg·a·lies** : abnormal enlargement (of a specified part) ⟨hepato*megaly*⟩ ⟨spleno*megaly*⟩

melan- *or* **melano-** *comb form* 1 : black : dark ⟨*melan*in⟩ ⟨*melan*oma⟩ 2 : melanin ⟨*melano*genesis⟩

-me·lia \ˈmē-lē-ə\ *n comb form* : condition of the limbs ⟨micro*melia*⟩ ⟨hemi*melia*⟩

-melus \mə-ləs\ *n comb form, pl* **-meli** \-ˌlī\ : one having a (specified) abnormality of the limbs ⟨phoco*melus*⟩

membran- *or* **membrani-** *or* **membrano-** *comb form* : membrane ⟨*membrano*proliferative glomerulonephritis⟩

men- *or* **meno-** *comb form* : menstruation ⟨*meno*pause⟩ ⟨*meno*rrhagia⟩

mening- *or* **meningo-** *also* **meningi-** *comb form* 1 : meninges ⟨*meningo*coccus⟩ ⟨*mening*itis⟩ 2 : meninges and ⟨*meningo*encephalitis⟩

¹mer- *or* **mero-** *comb form* : thigh ⟨*mer*algia⟩

²mer- *or* **mero-** *comb form* : part : partial ⟨*mero*blastic⟩

-mere \ˌmir\ *n comb form* : part : segment ⟨blasto*mere*⟩ ⟨centro*mere*⟩

mes- *or* **meso-** *comb form* 1 a : mid : in the middle ⟨*meso*cardia⟩ ⟨*meso*derm⟩ b : mesentery or membrane supporting a (specified) part ⟨*meso*cecum⟩ ⟨*meso*colon⟩ 2 : intermediate (as in size or type) ⟨*meso*morph⟩

mesio- *comb form* : mesial and ⟨*mesio*distal⟩ ⟨*mesio*buccal⟩

meta- *or* **met-** *prefix* 1 : occurring later than or in succession to : after ⟨*met*estrus⟩ 2 : situated behind or beyond ⟨*met*encephalon⟩ ⟨*meta*carpus⟩ 3 : change in : transformation of ⟨*meta*plasia⟩

metall- *or* **metallo-** *comb form* : containing a metal atom or ion in the molecule ⟨*metallo*porphyrin⟩

-me·ter \mət-ər *sometimes* ˌmēt-\ *n comb form* : instrument or means for measuring ⟨calori*meter*⟩

meth- *or* **metho-** *comb form* : methyl ⟨*meth*amphetamine⟩

metr- *or* **metro-** *comb form* : uterus ⟨*metr*itis⟩

-me·tra \ˈmē-trə\ *n comb form* : a (specified) condition of the uterus ⟨hemato*metra*⟩

-met·ric \ˈme-trik\ *or* **-met·ri·cal** \ˈme-tri-kəl\ *adj comb form* 1 : of, employing, or obtained by (such) a meter ⟨calori*metric*⟩ 2 : of or relating to (such) an art, process, or science of measuring ⟨psycho*metric*⟩

-me·tri·um \ˈmē-trē-əm\ *n comb form, pl* **-me·tria** : part or layer of the uterus ⟨endo*metrium*⟩

-metry \mə-trē\ *n comb form, pl* **-metries** : art, process, or science of measuring (something specified) ⟨audio*metry*⟩

micr- *or* **micro-** *comb form* 1 a : small : minute ⟨*micro*aneurysm⟩ b : used for or involving minute quantities or variations ⟨*micro*analysis⟩ 2 a : using microscopy ⟨*micro*dissection⟩ : used in microscopy ⟨*micro*needle⟩ b : revealed by or having its structure discernible only by microscopical examination ⟨*micro*organism⟩ 3 : abnormally small ⟨*micro*cyte⟩

milli- *comb form* : thousandth — used esp. in terms belonging to the metric system ⟨*milli*rad⟩

mis- *prefix* : badly : wrongly ⟨*mis*diagnose⟩

mit- *or* **mito-** *comb form* 1 : thread ⟨*mito*chondrion⟩ 2 : mitosis ⟨*mito*genesis⟩

-m·ne·sia \m-ˈnē-zhə\ *n comb form* : a (specified) type or condition of memory ⟨par*amnesia*⟩

mon- *or* **mono-** *comb form* 1 : one : single ⟨*mono*filament⟩ 2 : affecting a single part ⟨*mono*plegia⟩

morph- *or* **morpho-** *comb form* : form : shape : structure : type ⟨*morpho*logy⟩

-morph \ˌmȯrf\ *n comb form* : one having (such) a form ⟨ecto*morph*⟩ ⟨iso*morph*⟩

-mor·phic \ˈmȯr-fik\ *adj comb form* : having (such) a form ⟨endo*morphic*⟩

-mor·phism \ˈmȯr-ˌfiz-əm\ *n comb form* : quality or state of having (such) a form ⟨poly*morphism*⟩

-mor·phous \ˈmȯr-fəs\ *adj comb form* : having (such) a form ⟨poly*morphous*⟩

-mor·phy \ˌmȯr-fē\ *n comb form, pl* **-mor·phies** : quality or state of having (such) a form ⟨homo*morphy*⟩ ⟨meso*morphy*⟩

moto- *comb form* : motion : motor ⟨*moto*neuron⟩

muc- *or* **muci-** *or* **muco-** *comb form* 1 : mucus ⟨*muc*in⟩ ⟨muco*protein*⟩ 2 : mucous and ⟨*muco*purulent⟩

multi- *comb form* 1 a : many : multiple : much ⟨*multi*neuronal⟩ b : consisting of, containing, or having more than two ⟨*multi*nucleate⟩ c : more than one ⟨*multi*parous⟩ 2 : affecting many parts ⟨*multi*glandular⟩

muscul- *or* **musculo-** *comb form* 1 : muscle ⟨*muscul*ar⟩ 2 : muscular and ⟨*musculo*skeletal⟩

my- *or* **myo-** *comb form* 1 a : muscle ⟨*my*asthenia⟩ ⟨*myo*globin⟩ b : muscular and ⟨*myo*neural⟩ 2 : myoma and ⟨*myo*fibroma⟩

myc- *or* **myco-** *comb form* : fungus ⟨*myc*elium⟩ ⟨*myco*logy⟩ ⟨*myc*osis⟩

-my·ces \ˈmī-ˌsēz\ *n comb form* : fungus — used esp. in taxonomic names of fungi and certain bacteria resembling fungi and in their corresponding vernacular names ⟨Blasto*myces*⟩ ⟨strepto*myces*⟩

mycet- *or* **myceto-** *comb form* : fungus ⟨*myceto*ma⟩

-my·cete \ˈmī-ˌsēt, ˌmī-ˈsēt\ *n comb form* : fungus ⟨actino*mycete*⟩

-my·cin \ˈmīs-ᵊn\ *n comb form* : substance obtained from a fungus ⟨erythro*mycin*⟩

myel- *or* **myelo-** *comb form* : marrow: as a : bone marrow ⟨*myelo*cyte⟩ b : spinal cord ⟨*myelo*dysplasia⟩

-my·e·lia \ˌmī-ˈē-lē-ə\ *n comb form* : a (specified) condition of the spinal cord ⟨hemato*myelia*⟩ ⟨syringo*myelia*⟩

myl- *or* **mylo-** *comb form* : molar ⟨*mylo*hyoid⟩

myo- *var of* MY-

---

myom- or **myomo-** comb form : myoma ⟨myomectomy⟩

myring- or **myringo-** comb form : tympanic membrane ⟨myringotomy⟩

myx- or **myxo-** comb form **1** : mucus ⟨myxocyte⟩ ⟨myxoma⟩ **2** : myxoma ⟨myxosarcoma⟩

nan- or **nano-** comb form : dwarf ⟨nanocephalic⟩ ⟨nanosomia⟩

nano- comb form : one billionth (10⁻⁹) part of ⟨nanosecond⟩

narc- or **narco-** comb form **1** : numbness : stupor ⟨narcose⟩ **2** : narcosis : narcotic ⟨narcohypnosis⟩ ⟨narcoanesthesia⟩ **3** : deep sleep ⟨narcolepsy⟩

nas- or **naso-** also **nasi-** comb form **1** : nose : nasal ⟨nasoscope⟩ ⟨nasosinusitis⟩ **2** : nasal and ⟨nasolabial⟩

ne- or **neo-** comb form **1 a** : new : recent ⟨neonatal⟩ **b** : chemically new — used for compounds isomeric with or otherwise related to an indicated compound ⟨neostigmine⟩ **2** : new and abnormal ⟨neoplasm⟩

necr- or **necro-** comb form **1 a** : those that are dead : the dead : corpses ⟨necrophilia⟩ **b** : one that is dead : corpse ⟨necropsy⟩ **2** : death : conversion to dead tissue : atrophy ⟨necrosis⟩

nemat- or **nemato-** comb form **1** : thread ⟨nematocyst⟩ **2** : nematode ⟨nematology⟩

nephr- or **nephro-** comb form : kidney ⟨nephrectomy⟩ ⟨nephrology⟩

-neph·ros \'nef-rəs, 'nef-ˌräs\ n comb form, pl **-neph·roi** \'nef-ˌrȯi\ : kidney ⟨pronephros⟩

nerv- or **nervi-** or **nervo-** comb form : NEUR- ⟨nervine⟩

neur- or **neuro-** comb form **1** : nerve ⟨neural⟩ ⟨neurology⟩ **2** : neural : neural and ⟨neuromuscular⟩

neutro- comb form **1** : neutral ⟨neutrophil⟩ **2** : neutrophil ⟨neutropenia⟩

nicotin- or **nicotino-** comb form **1** : nicotine ⟨nicotinic⟩ **2** : nicotinic acid ⟨nicotinamide⟩

noci- comb form : pain ⟨nociceptor⟩

-n·o·my \n-ə-mē\ n comb form, pl **-n·o·mies** : system of laws or sum of knowledge regarding a (specified) field ⟨taxonomy⟩

non- prefix : not : reverse of : absence of ⟨nonallergic⟩

norm- or **normo-** comb form : normal ⟨normergic⟩ ⟨normoblast⟩ ⟨normotension⟩

nos- or **noso-** comb form : disease ⟨nosology⟩

not- or **noto-** comb form : back : back part ⟨notochord⟩

nucle- or **nucleo-** comb form **1** : nucleus ⟨nucleon⟩ ⟨nucleoplasm⟩ **2** : nucleic acid ⟨nucleoprotein⟩

nucleol- or **nucleolo-** comb form : nucleolus ⟨nucleolar⟩

nymph- or **nympho-** also **nymphi-** comb form : nymph : nymphae ⟨nymphomania⟩

o- or **oo-** comb form : egg : ovum ⟨oocyte⟩

occipit- or **occipito-** comb form : occipital and ⟨occipitotemporal⟩

occlus- or **occluso-** : occlusion ⟨occlusal⟩

ocul- or **oculo-** comb form **1** : eye ⟨oculomotor⟩ **2** : ocular and ⟨oculocutaneous⟩

odont- or **odonto-** comb form : tooth ⟨odontitis⟩ ⟨odontoblast⟩

-o·dont \ə-ˌdänt\ adj comb form : having teeth of a (specified) nature ⟨mesodont⟩ ⟨heterodont⟩

-o·don·tia \ə-ˌdän-ch(ē-)ə\ n comb form : form, condition, or mode of treatment of the teeth ⟨orthodontia⟩

-o·dyn·ia \ə-ˈdin-ē-ə\ n comb form : pain ⟨anodynia⟩ ⟨pleurodynia⟩

oesophag- or **oesophago-** chiefly Brit var of ESOPHAG-

oestr- or **oestro-** chiefly Brit var of ESTR-

¹-ol \ˌȯl, ˌōl\ n suffix : chemical compound (as an alcohol or phenol) containing hydroxyl ⟨glycerol⟩

²-ol n comb form : hydrocarbon chemically related to benzene ⟨xylol⟩ — not used in systematic chemical nomenclature

ole- or **oleo-** also **olei-** comb form : oil ⟨olein⟩

olig- or **oligo-** comb form **1** : few ⟨oligopeptide⟩ **2** : deficiency : insufficiency ⟨oliguria⟩ ⟨oligochromemia⟩

-o·ma \'ō-mə\ n suffix, pl **-o·mas** \-məz\ also **-o·ma·ta** \-mət-ə\ : tumor ⟨adenoma⟩ ⟨fibroma⟩

oment- or **omento-** comb form : omentum ⟨omentectomy⟩ ⟨omentopexy⟩

omphal- or **omphalo-** comb form **1** : umbilicus ⟨omphalitis⟩ **2** : umbilical and ⟨omphalomesenteric⟩

onco- or **oncho-** comb form **1** : tumor ⟨oncology⟩ **2** : bulk : mass ⟨oncometer⟩

-one \ˌōn, 'ōn\ n suffix : ketone or related or analogous compound or class of compounds ⟨lactone⟩ ⟨quinone⟩

ont- or **onto-** comb form : organism ⟨ontogeny⟩

-ont \ˌänt\ n comb form : cell : organism ⟨schizont⟩

onych- or **onycho-** comb form : nail of the finger or toe ⟨onychauxis⟩ ⟨onychodystrophy⟩

-o·nych·ia \ə-ˈnik-ē-ə\ n comb form : condition of the nails of the fingers or toes ⟨leukonychia⟩

-o·nych·i·um \ə-ˈnik-ē-əm\ n comb form : fingernail : toenail : region of the fingernail or toenail ⟨eponychium⟩ ⟨hyponychium⟩

oo- var of O-

oophor- or **oophoro-** comb form : ovary ⟨oophorectomy⟩

ophthalm- or **ophthalmo-** comb form : eye ⟨ophthalmology⟩ : eyeball ⟨ophthalmitis⟩

-oph·thal·mia \ˌäf-ˈthal-mē-ə, ˌäp-ˈthal-mē-ə\ n comb form : condition of having (such) eyes ⟨microphthalmia⟩

-o·pia \'ō-pē-ə\ n comb form **1** : condition of having (such) vision ⟨diplopia⟩ **2** : condition of having (such) a visual defect ⟨hyperopia⟩

opisth- or **opistho-** comb form : dorsal : posterior ⟨opisthocranion⟩ ⟨opisthotonos⟩

-op·sia \ˈäp-sē-ə\ n comb form, pl **-opsias** : vision of a (specified) kind or condition ⟨hemianopsia⟩

opson- or **opsono-** comb form : opsonin ⟨opsonic⟩ ⟨opsonization⟩

-op·sy \ˌäp-sē, əp-\ n comb form, pl **-op·sies** : examination ⟨biopsy⟩ ⟨necropsy⟩

opto- comb form **1** : vision ⟨optometry⟩ **2** : optic : optic and ⟨optokinetic⟩

-or·chi·dism \'ȯr-kə-ˌdiz-əm\ also **-or·chism** \'ȯr-ˌkiz-əm\ n comb form : a (specified) form or condition of the testes ⟨cryptorchidism⟩

-o·rex·ia \ə-ˈrek-sē-ə, ə-ˈrek-shə\ n comb form : appetite ⟨anorexia⟩

organ- or **organo-** comb form **1** : organ ⟨organelle⟩ ⟨organogenesis⟩ **2** : organic ⟨organomercury⟩

ori- comb form : mouth ⟨orifice⟩

oro- comb form **1** : mouth ⟨oropharynx⟩ **2** : oral and ⟨orofacial⟩ ⟨oronasal⟩

orth- or **ortho-** comb form **1** : straight : upright : vertical ⟨orthograde⟩ **2** : perpendicular ⟨orthorhombic⟩ **3** : correct : corrective ⟨orthodontia⟩

-ose \ˌōs\ n suffix **1** : carbohydrate; esp : sugar ⟨fructose⟩ ⟨pentose⟩ **2** : primary hydrolysis product ⟨proteose⟩

-o·side \ə-ˌsīd\ n suffix : glycoside or similar compound ⟨ganglioside⟩

-o·sis \'ō-səs\ n suffix, pl **-o·ses** \'ō-ˌsēz\ or **-o·sis·es** **1 a** : action : process : condition ⟨hypnosis⟩ **b** : abnormal or diseased condition ⟨leukosis⟩ **2** : increase : formation ⟨leukocytosis⟩

osm- or **osmo-** comb form : odor : smell ⟨osmics⟩ ⟨osmophore⟩

osmo- comb form : osmosis : osmotic ⟨osmoregulation⟩

osse- or **osseo-** comb form : bone ⟨ossein⟩

ossi- comb form : bone ⟨ossify⟩

oste- or **osteo-** comb form : bone ⟨osteal⟩ ⟨osteomyelitis⟩

osteochondr- or **osteochondro-** comb form : bone and cartilage ⟨osteochondropathy⟩

-os·to·sis \ˌäs-ˈtō-səs\ n comb form, pl **-os·to·ses** \-ˌsēz\ or **-os·to·sis·es** : ossification of a (specified) part or to a (specified) degree ⟨hyperostosis⟩

ot- or **oto-** comb form **1** : ear ⟨otitis⟩ **2** : ear and ⟨otolaryngology⟩

¹**-ot·ic** \\'ät-ik\\ *adj suffix* **1 a** : of, relating to, or characterized by a (specified) action, process, or condition ⟨symbi*otic*⟩ **b** : having an abnormal or diseased condition of a (specified) kind ⟨epizo*otic*⟩ **2** : showing an increase or a formation of ⟨leukocyt*otic*⟩

²**-otic** \\'ōt-ik\\ *adj comb form* : having (such) a relationship to the ear ⟨peri*otic*⟩

ov- or **ovi-** or **ovo-** *comb form* : egg ⟨*ovi*form⟩ : ovum ⟨*ovi*duct⟩ ⟨*ovo*cyte⟩ ⟨*ovo*genesis⟩

ovari- or **ovario-** also **ovar-** *comb form* **1** : ovary ⟨*ovari*ectomy⟩ ⟨*ovario*tomy⟩ **2** : ovary and ⟨*ovario*hysterectomy⟩

oxy- *comb form* **1** : sharp : pointed : acute ⟨*oxy*cephaly⟩ **2** : quick ⟨*oxy*tocic⟩ **3** : acid ⟨*oxy*ntic⟩

pachy- *comb form* : thick ⟨*pachy*tene⟩

paed- or **paedo-** *chiefly Brit var of* ²PED-

-pa·gus \\pə-gəs\\ *n comb form, pl* **-pa·gi** \\pə-,jī, -,gī\\ : congenitally united twins with a (specified) type of fixation ⟨crani*opagus*⟩

palato- *comb form* **1** : palate : of the palate ⟨*palato*gram⟩ ⟨*palato*plasty⟩ **2** : palatal and ⟨*palato*maxillary⟩

pale- or **paleo-** or *chiefly Brit* **palae-** or **palaeo-** *comb form* : early : old ⟨*paleo*pathology⟩

pali- *comb form* : pathological state characterized by repetition of a (specified) act ⟨*pali*lalia⟩

pan- *comb form* **1** : all : completely ⟨*pan*agglutinable⟩ **2** : whole : general ⟨*pan*carditis⟩ ⟨*pan*leukopenia⟩

pancreat- or **pancreato-** *comb form* **1** : pancreas : pancreatic ⟨*pancreat*ectomy⟩ ⟨*pancreat*in⟩ **2** : pancreas and ⟨*pancreato*duodenectomy⟩

pancreatico- *comb form* : pancreatic : pancreatic and ⟨*pancreatico*duodenal⟩

papill- or **papillo-** *comb form* **1** : papilla ⟨*papill*iform⟩ ⟨*papill*itis⟩ **2** : papillary ⟨*papill*edema⟩ ⟨*papill*oma⟩

papulo- *comb form* : characterized by papules and ⟨*papulo*pustular⟩ ⟨*papulo*vesicular⟩

para- or **par-** *prefix* **1** : beside : alongside of : beyond : aside from ⟨*para*thyroid⟩ ⟨*par*enteral⟩ **2 a** : faulty : abnormal ⟨*par*esthesia⟩ **b** : associated in a subsidiary or accessory capacity ⟨*para*medical⟩ **c** : closely resembling : almost ⟨*para*typhoid⟩

parasit- or **parasito-** *also* **parasiti-** *comb form* : parasite ⟨*parasit*emia⟩ ⟨*parasiti*cide⟩

parieto- *comb form* : parietal and ⟨*parieto*temporal⟩

-p·a·rous \\p-(ə-)rəs\\ *adj comb form* : giving birth to : producing ⟨bi*parous*⟩

parthen- or **partheno-** *comb form* : virgin : without fertilization ⟨*parthen*ogenesis⟩

parv- or **parvi-** *also* **parvo-** *comb form* : small ⟨*parvo*virus⟩

path- or **patho-** *comb form* **1** : pathological ⟨*patho*biology⟩ **2** : pathological state : disease ⟨*patho*gen⟩ ⟨*path*ergy⟩

-path \\,path\\ *n comb form* **1** : practitioner of a (specified) system of medicine that emphasizes one aspect of disease or its treatment ⟨naturo*path*⟩ **2** : one affected with a disorder (of such a part or system) ⟨psycho*path*⟩

-path·ia \\'path-ē-ə\\ *n comb form* : -PATHY 2 ⟨hyper*pathia*⟩

-path·ic \\'path-ik\\ *adj comb form* **1** : feeling or affected in a (specified) way ⟨tele*pathic*⟩ **2** : affected by disease of a (specified) part or kind ⟨myo*pathic*⟩ **3** : relating to therapy based on a (specified) unitary theory of disease or its treatment ⟨homeo*pathic*⟩

-pa·thy \\pə-thē\\ *n comb form, pl* **-pa·thies** **1** : feeling ⟨apa*thy*⟩ ⟨tele*pathy*⟩ **2** : disease of a (specified) part or kind ⟨idio*pathy*⟩ ⟨myo*pathy*⟩ **3** : therapy or system of therapy based on a (specified) unitary theory of disease or its treatment ⟨homeo*pathy*⟩

¹**ped-** or **pedi-** or **pedo-** *comb form* : foot : feet ⟨*pedi*cure⟩

²**ped-** or **pedo-** or *chiefly Brit* **paed-** or **paedo-** *comb form* : child : children ⟨*pedi*atrics⟩

-pel·ic \\'pel-ik\\ *adj comb form* : having (such) a pelvis ⟨dolicho*pellic*⟩

pelv- or **pelvi-** or **pelvo-** *comb form* : pelvis ⟨*pelv*ic⟩ ⟨*pelv*imetry⟩

-pe·nia \\'pē-nē-ə\\ *n comb form* : deficiency of ⟨erythro*penia*⟩ ⟨eosino*penia*⟩

-pep·sia \\'pep-shə, 'pep-sē-ə\\ *n comb form* : digestion ⟨dys*pepsia*⟩

pept- or **pepto-** *comb form* : protein fragment or derivative ⟨*pept*ide⟩

peri- *prefix* **1** : near : around ⟨*peri*menopausal⟩ **2** : enclosing : surrounding ⟨*peri*neurium⟩

pericardi- or **pericardio-** or **pericardo-** *comb form* **1** : pericardium ⟨*pericardi*ectomy⟩ **2** : pericardial and ⟨*pericardio*phrenic artery⟩

perineo- *comb form* : perineum ⟨*perineo*tomy⟩

periost- or **perioste-** or **periosteo-** *comb form* : periosteum ⟨*periost*itis⟩

periton- or **peritone-** or **peritoneo-** *comb form* **1** : peritoneum ⟨*periton*itis⟩ **2** : peritoneal and ⟨*peritoneo*venous shunt⟩

-pexy \\,pek-sē\\ *n comb form, pl* **-pex·ies** : fixation : making fast ⟨gastro*pexy*⟩

phac- or **phaco-** or **phak-** or **phako-** *comb form* : lens ⟨*phaco*emulsification⟩

phag- or **phago-** *comb form* **1** : eating : feeding ⟨*phag*edena⟩ **2** : phagocyte ⟨*phago*lysis⟩

-phage \\,fāj *also* ,fàzh\\ *n comb form* : one that eats ⟨bacterio*phage*⟩

-pha·gia \\'fā-j(ē-)ə\\ *n comb form* : -PHAGY ⟨dys*phagia*⟩

-pha·gous \\fə-gəs\\ *adj comb form* : feeding esp. on a (specified) kind of food ⟨hemato*phagous*⟩

-ph·a·gy \\f-ə-jē\\ *n comb form, pl* **-ph·a·gies** : eating : eating of a (specified) type or substance ⟨geo*phagy*⟩

phak- or **phako-** *var of* PHAC-

phall- or **phallo-** *comb form* : penis ⟨*phallo*plasty⟩

pharmaco- *comb form* : medicine : drug ⟨*pharmaco*logy⟩ ⟨*pharmaco*therapy⟩

pharyng- or **pharyngo-** *comb form* **1** : pharynx ⟨*pharyng*itis⟩ **2** : pharyngeal and ⟨*pharyngo*esophageal⟩

-pha·sia \\'fā-zh(ē-)ə\\ *also* **-pha·sy** \\fə-sē\\ *n comb form, pl* **-pha·sias** *also* **-pha·sies** : speech disorder (of a specified type esp. relating to the symbolic use of language) ⟨dys*phasia*⟩

-phe·mia \\'fē-mē-ə\\ *n comb form* : speech disorder (of a specified type esp. relating to the articulation or fluency of speech sounds) ⟨a*phemia*⟩

¹**-phil** \\,fil\\ or **-phile** \\,fīl\\ *n comb form* : lover : one having an affinity for or a strong attraction to ⟨acido*phil*⟩

²**-phil** or **-phile** *adj comb form* : loving : having a fondness or affinity for ⟨hemo*phile*⟩

-phil·ia \\'fil-ē-ə\\ *n comb form* **1** : tendency toward ⟨hemo*philia*⟩ **2** : abnormal appetite or liking for ⟨necro*philia*⟩

-phil·i·ac \\'fil-ē-,ak\\ *n comb form* **1** : one having a tendency toward ⟨hemo*philiac*⟩ **2** : one having an abnormal appetite or liking for ⟨copro*philiac*⟩

-phil·ic \\'fil-ik\\ *adj comb form* : having an affinity for : loving ⟨acido*philic*⟩

-ph·i·lous \\f-(ə-)ləs\\ *adj comb form* : loving : having an affinity for ⟨erythro*philous*⟩

phleb- or **phlebo-** *comb form* : vein ⟨*phleb*itis⟩ ⟨*phlebo*sclerosis⟩

-phobe \\,fōb\\ *n comb form* : one fearing or averse to (something specified) ⟨chromo*phobe*⟩

-pho·bia \\'fō-bē-ə\\ *n comb form* **1** : abnormal fear of ⟨acro*phobia*⟩ **2** : intolerance or aversion for ⟨photo*phobia*⟩

-pho·bic \\'fō-bik\\ or **-ph·o·bous** \\f-ə-bəs\\ *adj comb form* **1** : having an aversion for or fear of ⟨agora*phobic*⟩ **2** : lacking affinity for ⟨hydro*phobic*⟩

phon- or **phono-** *comb form* : sound : voice : speech : tone ⟨*phon*ation⟩

-pho·nia or **-pho·ny** *n comb form, pl* **-pho·nias** or **-pho·nies**

\\ə\\ abut \\ᵊ\\ kitten \\ər\\ further \\a\\ ash \\ā\\ ace \\ä\\ cot, cart \\aú\\ out \\ch\\ chin \\e\\ bet \\ē\\ easy \\g\\ go \\i\\ hit \\ī\\ ice \\j\\ job \\ŋ\\ sing \\ō\\ go \\ò\\ law \\òi\\ boy \\th\\ thin \\t͟h\\ the \\ü\\ loot \\ú\\ foot \\y\\ yet \\zh\\ vision   *See also* Pronunciation Symbols page

: speech disorder (of a specified type esp. relating to phonation) ⟨dys*phonia*⟩

-pho·re·sis \fə-'rē-səs\ *n comb form, pl* **-pho·re·ses** \-₁sēz\ : transmission ⟨electro*phoresis*⟩

-pho·ria \'fōr-ē-ə, 'fȯr-\ *n comb form* : bearing : state : tendency ⟨eu*phoria*⟩ ⟨hetero*phoria*⟩

-phor·ic \'fȯr-ik\ *adj comb form* : having (such) a bearing or tendency ⟨thanato*phoric*⟩

phos- *comb form* : light ⟨*phos*phene⟩

phosph- *or* **phospho-** *comb form* : phosphoric acid : phosphate ⟨*phospho*lipid⟩

phosphor- *or* **phosphoro-** *comb form* : phosphoric acid ⟨*phosphoro*lysis⟩

phot- *or* **photo-** *comb form* : light : radiant energy ⟨*photo*dermatitis⟩

phra·sia \'frā-zh(ē-)ə, 'frā-zē-ə\ *n comb form* : speech disorder (of a specified type) ⟨embolo*phrasia*⟩ ⟨para*phrasia*⟩

phren- *or* **phreno-** *comb form* **1** : mind ⟨*phren*ology⟩ **2** : diaphragm ⟨*phren*ic⟩

phreni- *comb form* : phrenic nerve ⟨*phreni*cotomy⟩

-phre·nia \'frē-nē-ə *also* 'fren-ē-ə\ *n comb form* : disordered condition of mental functions ⟨hebe*phrenia*⟩

phthisio- *comb form* : phthisis ⟨*phthisio*therapy⟩

phyl- *or* **phylo-** *comb form* : tribe : race : phylum ⟨*phylo*geny⟩

physi- *or* **physio-** *comb form* **1** : physical ⟨*physio*therapy⟩ : physical and ⟨*physio*psychic⟩ **2** : physiological ⟨*physio*psychology⟩ : physiological and ⟨*physio*pathologic⟩

phyt- *or* **phyto-** *comb form* : plant ⟨*phyto*toxin⟩

-phyte \₁fīt\ *n comb form* **1** : plant having a (specified) characteristic or habitat ⟨sapro*phyte*⟩ **2** : pathological growth ⟨osteo*phyte*⟩

pico- *comb form* **1** : one trillionth (10⁻¹²) part of ⟨*pico*gram⟩ **2** : very small ⟨*pico*rnavirus⟩

pil- *or* **pili-** *or* **pilo-** *comb form* : hair ⟨*pilo*motor⟩

-pla·sia \'plā-zh(ē-)ə\ *or* **-pla·sy** \₁plā-sē, -plə-sē\ *n comb form, pl* **-pla·sias** *or* **-pla·sies** : development : formation ⟨dys*plasia*⟩ ⟨hetero*plasia*⟩

plasm- *or* **plasmo-** *comb form* : plasma ⟨*plasm*apheresis⟩

-plasm \₁plaz-əm\ *n comb form* : formative or formed material (as of a cell or tissue) ⟨cyto*plasm*⟩ ⟨endo*plasm*⟩

-plast \₁plast\ *n comb form* : organized particle or granule : cell ⟨chloro*plast*⟩

-plas·tic \'plas-tik\ *adj comb form* **1** : developing : forming ⟨thrombo*plastic*⟩ **2** : of or relating to (something designated by a term ending in *-plasia, -plasm,* or *-plasty*) ⟨neo*plastic*⟩

-plas·ty \₁plas-tē\ *n comb form, pl* **-plas·ties** : plastic surgery ⟨osteo*plasty*⟩

-plasy *var of* -PLASIA

platy- *also* **plat-** *comb form* : flat : broad ⟨*platy*pelloid⟩

-ple·gia \'plē-j(ē-)ə\ *n comb form* : paralysis ⟨di*plegia*⟩

pleur- *or* **pleuro-** *comb form* **1** : pleura ⟨*pleuro*pneumonia⟩ **2** : pleura and ⟨*pleuro*peritoneal⟩

-ploid \₁plȯid\ *adj comb form* : having or being a chromosome number that bears (such) a relationship to or is (so many) times the basic chromosome number characteristic of a given plant or animal group ⟨poly*ploid*⟩

-pnea *or chiefly Brit* **-pnoea** \(p)-nē-ə\ *n comb form* : breath : breathing ⟨hyper*pnea*⟩ ⟨ap*nea*⟩

pneum- *or* **pneumo-** *comb form* **1** : air : gas ⟨*pneumo*thorax⟩ **2** : lung ⟨*pneumo*coniosis⟩ : pulmonary and ⟨*pneumo*gastric nerve⟩ **3** : respiration ⟨*pneumo*graph⟩ **4** : pneumonia ⟨*pneumo*coccus⟩

pneumat- *or* **pneumato-** *comb form* **1** : air : vapor : gas ⟨*pneumato*sis⟩ **2** : respiration ⟨*pneumato*graph⟩

pneumon- *or* **pneumono-** *comb form* : lung ⟨*pneumono*ctomy⟩ ⟨*pneumono*centesis⟩

-pnoea *chiefly Brit var of* -PNEA

pod- *or* **podo-** *comb form* **1** : foot ⟨*pod*iatry⟩ **2** : hoof ⟨*podo*dermatitis⟩

-poi·e·sis \(₁)pȯi-'ē-səs\ *n comb form, pl* **-poi·e·ses** \-'ē-₁sēz\ : production : formation ⟨lympho*poiesis*⟩

-poi·et·ic \(₁)pȯi-'et-ik\ *adj comb form* : productive : formative ⟨lympho*poietic*⟩

poli- *or* **polio-** *comb form* : of or relating to the gray matter of the brain or spinal cord ⟨*polio*myelitis⟩

poly- *comb form* **1** : many : several : much : MULTI- ⟨*poly*arthritis⟩ **2** : excessive : abnormal : HYPER- ⟨*poly*dactyly⟩

-pore \₁pōr\ *n comb form* : opening ⟨blasto*pore*⟩

post- *prefix* **1** : after : later than ⟨*post*operative⟩ ⟨*post*coronary⟩ **2** : behind : posterior to ⟨*post*canine⟩

postero- *comb form* : posterior and ⟨*postero*anterior⟩ ⟨*postero*lateral⟩

-prax·ia \'prak-sē-ə\ *n comb form* : performance of movements ⟨a*praxia*⟩

-prax·is \'prak-səs\ *n comb form, pl* **-prax·is·es** *also* **-prax·es** \'prak-₁sēz\ : therapeutic treatment usu. by a (specified) system or agency ⟨chiro*praxis*⟩

pre- *prefix* **1** : earlier than : prior to : before ⟨*pre*natal⟩ ⟨*pre*cancerous⟩ **2** : in front of : before ⟨*pre*anal⟩ ⟨*pre*axial⟩ ⟨*pre*molar⟩

presby- *or* **presbyo-** *comb form* : old age ⟨*presby*opia⟩ ⟨*presby*ophrenia⟩

pro- *prefix* **1 a** : PRE- 1 ⟨*pro*chondral⟩ **b** : rudimentary : immature : PROT- 1 ⟨*pro*erythrocyte⟩ **c** : being a precursor of ⟨*pro*insulin⟩ **2** : front : anterior ⟨*pro*nephros⟩ **3** : projecting ⟨*pro*gnathous⟩

proct- *or* **procto-** *comb form* **1 a** : rectum ⟨*procto*scope⟩ **b** : rectum and ⟨*procto*sigmoidectomy⟩ **2** : anus and rectum ⟨*procto*logy⟩

pros- *prefix* : in front ⟨*pros*encephalon⟩

prosop- *or* **prosopo-** *comb form* : face ⟨*prosop*agnosia⟩

prostat- *or* **prostato-** *comb form* : prostate gland ⟨*prostat*ectomy⟩ ⟨*prostat*itis⟩

prot- *or* **proto-** *comb form* **1** : beginning : giving rise to ⟨*proto*oncogene⟩ **2** : principal ⟨*proto*cone⟩

prote- *or* **proteo-** *comb form* : protein ⟨*proteo*lysis⟩

pseud- *or* **pseudo-** *comb form* : false : spurious ⟨*pseud*arthrosis⟩ ⟨*pseudo*tumor⟩

psych- *or* **psycho-** *comb form* **1** : mind : mental processes and activities ⟨*psycho*dynamic⟩ ⟨*psycho*logy⟩ **2** : psychological methods ⟨*psycho*analysis⟩ ⟨*psycho*therapy⟩ **3** : brain ⟨*psycho*surgery⟩ **4** : mental and ⟨*psycho*somatic⟩

pteryg- *or* **pterygo-** *comb form* : pterygoid and ⟨*pterygo*maxillary⟩

ptyal- *or* **ptyalo-** *comb form* : saliva ⟨*ptyal*ism⟩

-p·ty·sis \p-tə-səs\ *n comb form, pl* **-pty·ses** \p-tə-₁sēz\ : spewing : expectoration ⟨hemo*ptysis*⟩ ⟨plasmo*ptysis*⟩

pulmon- *also* **pulmoni-** *or* **pulmono-** *comb form* : lung ⟨*pulmon*ectomy⟩

pupillo- *comb form* : pupil ⟨*pupillo*meter⟩

py- *or* **pyo-** *comb form* : pus ⟨*py*emia⟩ ⟨*pyo*rrhea⟩

pyel- *or* **pyelo-** *comb form* : renal pelvis ⟨*pyelo*graphy⟩

pykn- *or* **pykno-** *also* **pycn-** *or* **pycno-** *comb form* **1** : close : compact : dense : bulky ⟨*pykn*ic⟩ **2** : marked by short stature or shortness of digits ⟨*pykno*dysostosis⟩

pyl- *or* **pyle-** *or* **pylo-** *comb form* : portal vein ⟨*pyle*phlebitis⟩

pylor- *or* **pyloro-** *comb form* : pylorus ⟨*pyloro*plasty⟩

pyo- *var of* PY-

pyr- *or* **pyro-** *comb form* **1** : fire : heat ⟨*pyro*mania⟩ **2** : fever ⟨*pyro*gen⟩

pyret- *or* **pyreto-** *comb form* : fever ⟨*pyreto*therapy⟩

quin- *or* **quino-** *comb form* **1** : quina : cinchona bark ⟨*qui*nine⟩ ⟨*quino*line⟩ **2** : quinoline ⟨*quin*ethazone⟩

rachi- *or* **rachio-** *comb form* : spine ⟨*rachi*schisis⟩

radi- *or* **radio-** *comb form* **1** : radiant energy : radiation ⟨*radio*active⟩ ⟨*radio*paque⟩ **2** : radioactive ⟨*radio*element⟩ **3** : radium : X-rays ⟨*radio*therapy⟩ **4** : radioactive isotopes esp. as produced artificially ⟨*radio*carbon⟩

rect- *or* **recto-** *comb form* **1** : rectum ⟨*rect*al⟩ **2** : rectal and ⟨*recto*vaginal⟩

reni- *or* **reno-** *comb form* **1** : kidney ⟨*reni*form⟩ **2** : renal and ⟨*reno*vascular⟩

reticul- *or* **reticulo-** *comb form* : reticulum ⟨*reticulo*cyte⟩

retin- *or* **retino-** *comb form* : retina ⟨*retin*itis⟩ ⟨*retino*scopy⟩

retro- *prefix* **1** : backward : back ⟨*retro*flexion⟩ **2** : situated behind ⟨*retro*lental⟩ ⟨*retro*pubic⟩

rhabd- *or* **rhabdo-** *comb form* : rodlike structure ⟨*rhabdo*virus⟩

rheo- *comb form* : flow : current ⟨*rheo*stat⟩

rhin- *or* **rhino-** *comb form* **1 a** : nose ⟨*rhin*itis⟩ ⟨*rhino*logy⟩ **b** : nose and ⟨*rhino*laryngology⟩ ⟨*rhino*pharyngitis⟩ **2 a** : nasal ⟨*rhino*lith⟩ **b** : nasal and ⟨*rhino*pharyngeal⟩

rhod- *or* **rhodo-** *comb form* : rose : red ⟨*rhodo*psin⟩

rib- *or* **ribo-** *comb form* : related to ribose ⟨*ribo*flavin⟩

-r·rha·chis \r-ə-kəs\ *n comb form* : spine ⟨hemato*rrhachis*⟩

-r·rha·gia \ˈrā-j(ē-)ə, ˈrā-zhə, ˈräj-ə, ˈräzh-\ *n comb form* : abnormal or excessive discharge or flow ⟨metro*rrhagia*⟩ — **-r·rha·gic** \ˈra-jik\ *adj comb form*

-r·rha·phy \r-ə-fē\ *n comb form, pl* **-r·rha·phies** : suture : sewing ⟨cardio*rrhaphy*⟩ ⟨nephro*rrhaphy*⟩

-r·rhea *or chiefly Brit* **-r·rhoea** \ˈrē-ə\ *n comb form* : flow : discharge ⟨logo*rrhea*⟩ ⟨leuko*rrhea*⟩

-r·rhex·is \ˈrek-səs\ *n comb form, pl* **-r·rhex·es** \ˈrek-ˌsēz\ **1** : rupture ⟨hystero*rrhexis*⟩ **2** : splitting ⟨onycho*rrhexis*⟩

-r·rhoea *chiefly Brit var of* -RRHEA

sacchar- *or* **sacchari-** *or* **saccharo-** *comb form* : sugar ⟨*sacchar*ide⟩

sacr- *or* **sacro-** *comb form* **1** : sacrum ⟨*sacr*al⟩ **2** : sacral and ⟨*sacro*iliac⟩

salicyl- *or* **salicylo-** *comb form* : related to salicylic acid ⟨*salicyl*amide⟩

salping- *or* **salpingo-** *comb form* **1** : fallopian tube ⟨*salpingo*plasty⟩ **2** : eustachian tube ⟨*salpingo*pharyngeus⟩

sanguino- *comb form* : blood ⟨*sanguino*purulent⟩

sapr- *or* **sapro-** *comb form* **1** : rotten : putrid ⟨*sapr*emia⟩ **2** : dead or decaying organic matter ⟨*sapro*phyte⟩

sarc- *or* **sarco-** *comb form* **1** : flesh ⟨*sarc*oid⟩ **2** : striated muscle ⟨*sarco*lemma⟩

scaph- *or* **scapho-** *comb form* : scaphoid ⟨*scapho*cephaly⟩

scapul- *or* **scapulo-** *comb form* **1** : scapula ⟨*scapulo*pexy⟩ **2** : scapular and ⟨*scapulo*humeral⟩

scat- *or* **scato-** *comb form* : excrement ⟨*scat*oma⟩ ⟨*scato*logy⟩

-schi·sis \skə-səs\ *n comb form, pl* **-schi·ses** \skə-ˌsēz\ *also* **-schi·sis·es** : breaking up of attachments or adhesions : fissure ⟨gastro*schisis*⟩ ⟨cranio*schisis*⟩

schisto- *comb form* : cleft : divided ⟨*schisto*cyte⟩

schiz- *or* **schizo-** *comb form* **1** : characterized by or involving cleavage ⟨*schizo*gony⟩ **2** : schizophrenia ⟨*schizo*id⟩

scler- *or* **sclero-** *comb form* **1** : hard ⟨*sclero*derma⟩ **2** : sclera ⟨*scler*itis⟩

-scope \ˌskōp\ *n comb form* : means (as an instrument) for viewing or observing ⟨micro*scope*⟩ ⟨laparo*scope*⟩

-scop·ic \ˈskäp-ik\ *adj comb form* : viewing or observing ⟨laparo*scopic*⟩

-s·co·py \s-kə-pē\ *n comb form, pl* **-s·co·pies** : viewing : observation ⟨radio*scopy*⟩ ⟨laparo*scopy*⟩

scroful- *or* **scrofulo-** *comb form* : scrofula ⟨*scrofulo*derma⟩

scrot- *or* **scroti-** *or* **scroto-** *comb form* : scrotum ⟨*scroto*plasty⟩

sebi- *or* **sebo-** *comb form* : fat : grease : sebum ⟨*sebo*rrhea⟩

secret- *or* **secreto-** *comb form* : secretion ⟨*secret*in⟩

-sect \ˌsekt\ *vb comb form* : cut : divide ⟨hemi*sect*⟩ ⟨tran*sect*⟩

sensori- *also* **senso-** *comb form* : sensory : sensory and ⟨*sensori*motor⟩

sept- *or* **septo-** *also* **septi-** *comb form* : septum ⟨*sept*al⟩ ⟨*septo*plasty⟩

sero- *comb form* **1** : serum ⟨*sero*logy⟩ ⟨*sero*diagnosis⟩ **2** : serous and ⟨*sero*purulent⟩

sial- *or* **sialo-** *comb form* : saliva ⟨*sialo*lith⟩ ⟨*sialo*rrhea⟩

sider- *or* **sidero-** *comb form* : iron ⟨*sidero*penia⟩

silic- *or* **silico-** *comb form* **1** : relating to or containing silicon or its compounds ⟨*silic*one⟩ **2** : silicosis and ⟨*silico*tuberculosis⟩

sino- *also* **sinu-** *comb form* : relating to a sinus or sinuses and ⟨*sino*atrial node⟩

skelet- *or* **skeleto-** *comb form* **1** : skeleton ⟨*skelet*al⟩ **2** : skeletal and ⟨*skeleto*muscular⟩

socio- *comb form* **1** : society : social ⟨*socio*path⟩ **2** : social and ⟨*socio*psychological⟩

somat- *or* **somato-** *comb form* **1** : body ⟨*somato*genic⟩ ⟨*somato*logy⟩ **2** : somatic and ⟨*somato*psychic⟩

-some \ˌsōm\ *n comb form* **1** : body ⟨chromo*some*⟩ **2** : chromosome ⟨mono*some*⟩

-so·mia \ˈsō-mē-ə\ *n comb form* : condition of having (such) a body ⟨micro*somia*⟩

-som·ic \ˈsō-mik\ *adj comb form* : having or being a chromosome complement of which one or more but not all chromosomes or genomes exhibit (such) a degree of reduplication ⟨mono*somic*⟩

somnambul- *comb form* : sleep in which motor acts are performed ⟨somnambul*ist*⟩

somni- *comb form* : sleep ⟨*somni*facient⟩

son- *or* **sono-** *comb form* : sound ⟨*sono*gram⟩

sperm- *or* **spermo-** *or* **sperma-** *or* **spermi-** *comb form* : seed : germ : sperm ⟨*spermi*cidal⟩

spermat- *or* **spermato-** *comb form* : seed : spermatozoon ⟨*spermat*id⟩ ⟨*spermato*cyte⟩

-sper·mia \ˈspər-mē-ə\ *n comb form* : condition of having or producing (such) sperm ⟨a*spermia*⟩

-sper·mic \ˈspər-mik\ *adj comb form* : being the product of (such) a number of spermatozoa : resulting from (such) a multiple fertilization ⟨poly*spermic*⟩

-sper·my \ˈspər-mē\ *n comb form, pl* **-sper·mies** : state of exhibiting or resulting from (such) a fertilization ⟨poly*spermy*⟩

sphen- *or* **spheno-** *comb form* : sphenoid and ⟨*spheno*palatine⟩

spher- *or* **sphero-** *comb form* : spherical ⟨*sphero*cyte⟩

sphingo- *comb form* : sphingomyelin ⟨*sphingo*sine⟩

sphygmo- *comb form* : pulse ⟨*sphygmo*gram⟩

spin- *or* **spini-** *or* **spino-** *comb form* **1** : spinal column : spinal cord ⟨*spino*tectal tract⟩ **2** : of, relating to, or involving the spinal cord and ⟨*spino*thalamic⟩

spiro- *comb form* : respiration ⟨*spiro*meter⟩

splanchno- *comb form* : viscera ⟨*splanchno*logy⟩

splen- *or* **spleno-** *comb form* : spleen ⟨*splen*ectomy⟩ ⟨*spleno*megaly⟩

spondyl- *or* **spondylo-** *comb form* : vertebra : vertebrae ⟨*spondyl*arthritis⟩ ⟨*spondylo*pathy⟩

spongi- *or* **spongio-** *comb form* : spongy ⟨*spongio*blast⟩

spor- *or* **spori-** *or* **sporo-** *comb form* : seed : spore ⟨*sporo*cyst⟩ ⟨*spori*cidal⟩

staphyl- *or* **staphylo-** *comb form* **1** : uvula ⟨*staphyl*ectomy⟩ **2** : staphylococcal ⟨*staphylo*coagulase⟩

-stat \ˌstat\ *n comb form* : agent causing inhibition of growth without destruction ⟨bacterio*stat*⟩

stato- *comb form* : balance : equilibrium ⟨*stato*lith⟩

steat- *or* **steato-** *comb form* : fat ⟨*steat*oma⟩

stere- *or* **stereo-** *comb form* **1** : stereoscopic ⟨*stereo*psis⟩ **2** : having or dealing with three dimensions of space ⟨*stereo*taxic⟩

stern- *or* **sterno-** *comb form* **1** : breast : sternum : breastbone ⟨*sterno*tomy⟩ **2** : sternal and ⟨*sterno*costal⟩

stomat- *or* **stomato-** *comb form* : mouth ⟨*stomat*itis⟩ ⟨*stomato*logy⟩

-sto·mia \ˈstō-mē-ə\ *n comb form* : mouth exhibiting (such) a condition ⟨xero*stomia*⟩

\ə\ **abut** \ᵊ\ **kitten** \ər\ **further** \a\ **ash** \ā\ **ace** \ä\ **cot, cart**
\aú\ **out** \ch\ **chin** \e\ **bet** \ē\ **easy** \g\ **go** \i\ **hit** \ī\ **ice** \j\ **job**
\ŋ\ **sing** \ō\ **go** \ó\ **law** \ói\ **boy** \th\ **thin** \th̲\ **the** \ü\ **loot**
\ú\ **foot** \y\ **yet** \zh\ **vision**   *See also* Pronunciation Symbols page

-s·to·my \s-tə-mē\ *n comb form, pl* **-s·to·mies** : surgical operation establishing a usu. permanent opening into (such) a part ⟨entero*stomy*⟩

strepto- *comb form* **1** : twisted : twisted chain ⟨*strepto*coccus⟩ **2** : streptococcus ⟨*strepto*kinase⟩

styl- *or* **stylo-** *comb form* : styloid process ⟨*stylo*glossus⟩

-style \ˌstīl\ *n comb form* : animal part resembling a pillar ⟨zygo*style*⟩

sub- *prefix* **1** : under : beneath : below ⟨*sub*aponeurotic⟩ **2** : subordinate portion of : subdivision of ⟨*sub*species⟩ **3** : less than completely or perfectly ⟨*sub*normal⟩

sulf- *or* **sulfo-** *or chiefly Brit* **sulph-** *or* **sulpho-** *comb form* : sulfur : containing sulfur ⟨*sulf*arsphenamine⟩

super- *prefix* **1** : greater than normal : excessive ⟨*super*ovulation⟩ **2** : situated or placed above, on, or at the top of ⟨*super*ciliary⟩; *specif* : situated on the dorsal side of

supero- *comb form* : situated above ⟨*supero*lateral⟩

supra- *prefix* **1** : SUPER- 2 ⟨*supra*orbital⟩ **2** : transcending ⟨*supra*molecular⟩

sympath- *or* **sympatho-** *comb form* : sympathetic nerve : sympathetic nervous system ⟨*sympatho*lytic⟩

sympathetico- *comb form* : SYMPATH- ⟨*sympathetico*mimetic⟩

sympathico- *comb form* : SYMPATH- ⟨*sympathico*tonia⟩

syn- *or* **sym-** *prefix* **1** : with : along with : together ⟨*sym*biosis⟩ **2** : at the same time ⟨*syn*esthesia⟩

syndesm- *or* **syndesmo-** *comb form* **1** : ligament ⟨*syndesmo*sis⟩ **2** : connection : contact ⟨*syndesmo*chorial⟩

syphil- *or* **syphilo-** *comb form* : syphilis ⟨*syphilo*ma⟩

syring- *or* **syringo-** *comb form* : tube : fistula ⟨*syringo*bulbia⟩

tabo- *comb form* : progressive wasting : tabes ⟨*tabo*paresis⟩

tachy- *comb form* : rapid : accelerated ⟨*tachy*cardia⟩

taen- *or* **taeni-** *also* **ten-** *or* **teni-** *comb form* : tapeworm ⟨*taen*iasis⟩

talo- *comb form* : astragalar and ⟨*talo*tibial⟩

tarso- *comb form* **1** : tarsus ⟨*tarso*metatarsal⟩ **2** : tarsal plate ⟨*tarso*rrhaphy⟩

tel- *or* **telo-** *also* **tele-** *comb form* : end ⟨*tel*angiectasia⟩

temporo- *comb form* : temporal and ⟨*temporo*mandibular⟩

ten- *or* **teni-** *var of* TAEN-

¹-tene \ˌtēn\ *adj comb form* : having (such or so many) chromosomal filaments ⟨poly*tene*⟩ ⟨pachy*tene*⟩

²-tene *n comb form* : stage of meiotic prophase characterized by (such) chromosomal filaments ⟨diplo*tene*⟩ ⟨pachy*tene*⟩

teno- *comb form* : tendon ⟨*teno*synovitis⟩

terat- *or* **terato-** *comb form* : developmental malformation ⟨*terato*genic⟩

thalam- *or* **thalamo-** *comb form* **1** : thalamus ⟨*thalamo*tomy⟩ **2** : thalamic and ⟨*thalamo*cortical⟩

thanat- *or* **thanato-** *comb form* : death ⟨*thanato*logy⟩

therm- *or* **thermo-** *comb form* : heat ⟨*thermo*receptor⟩

-ther·mia \ˈthər-mē-ə\ *or* **-ther·my** \ˌthər-mē\ *n comb form, pl* **-ther·mias** *or* **-ther·mies** : state of heat : generation of heat ⟨dia*thermy*⟩ ⟨hypo*thermia*⟩

thi- *or* **thio-** *comb form* : containing sulfur ⟨*thia*mine⟩ ⟨*thio*pental⟩

thorac- *or* **thoraci-** *or* **thoraco-** *comb form* **1** : chest : thorax ⟨*thoraco*plasty⟩ **2** : thoracic and ⟨*thoraco*lumbar⟩

-thrix \(ˌ)thriks\ *n comb form, pl* **-tri·ches** \trə-ˌkēz\ *or* **-thrixes** : pathological condition of having (such) hair ⟨lepo*thrix*⟩ ⟨monile*thrix*⟩

thromb- *or* **thrombo-** *comb form* **1** : blood clot : clotting of blood ⟨*thromb*in⟩ ⟨*thrombo*plastic⟩ **2** : marked by or associated with thrombosis ⟨*thrombo*angiitis⟩

thym- *or* **thymo-** *comb form* : thymus ⟨*thym*ic⟩ ⟨*thymo*cyte⟩

-thy·mia \ˈthī-mē-ə\ *n comb form* : condition of mind and will ⟨cyclo*thymia*⟩ ⟨dys*thymia*⟩

thyr- *or* **thyro-** *comb form* **1** : thyroid ⟨*thyro*globulin⟩ **2** : thyroid and ⟨*thyro*arytenoid⟩

tibio- *comb form* : tibial and ⟨*tibio*femoral⟩

-tome \ˌtōm\ *n comb form* **1** : part : segment ⟨myo*tome*⟩ **2** : cutting instrument ⟨micro*tome*⟩

-t·o·my \t-ə-mē\ *n comb form, pl* **-t·o·mies** : incision : section ⟨laparo*tomy*⟩

-to·nia \ˈtō-nē-ə\ *n comb form* : condition or degree of tonus ⟨myo*tonia*⟩

tono- *comb form* **1** : tone ⟨*tono*topic⟩ **2** : pressure ⟨*tono*meter⟩

tonsill- *or* **tonsillo-** *comb form* : tonsil ⟨*tonsill*ectomy⟩ ⟨*tonsillo*tome⟩

-to·ny \ˌtō-nē, tⁿn-ē\ *n comb form, pl* **-to·nies** : -TONIA ⟨hyper*tony*⟩

top- *or* **topo-** *comb form* : local ⟨*top*ectomy⟩ ⟨*topo*gnosia⟩

tox- *or* **toxi-** *or* **toxo-** *comb form* **1** : toxic : poisonous ⟨*tox*in⟩ **2** : toxin : poison ⟨*toxi*genic⟩

toxic- *or* **toxico-** *comb form* : poison ⟨*toxico*logy⟩ ⟨*toxic*osis⟩

trache- *or* **tracheo-** *comb form* **1** : trachea ⟨*tracheo*scopy⟩ **2** : tracheal and ⟨*tracheo*bronchial⟩

trachel- *or* **trachelo-** *comb form* **1** : neck ⟨*trachelo*mastoid muscle⟩ **2** : uterine cervix ⟨*trachelo*plasty⟩

trans- *prefix* **1** : through ⟨*trans*cutaneous⟩ **2** : so or such as to change or transfer ⟨*trans*amination⟩

traumat- *or* **traumato-** *comb form* : wound : trauma ⟨*trauma*tism⟩

-tre·ma \ˈtrē-mə\ *n comb form, pl* **-tremas** *or* **-tre·ma·ta** \ˈtrē-mət-ə\ : hole : orifice : opening ⟨helico*trema*⟩

trich- *or* **tricho-** *comb form* : hair : filament ⟨*tricho*mycosis⟩

-triches *pl of* -THRIX

-trich·ia \ˈtrik-ē-ə\ *n comb form* : condition of having (such) hair ⟨oligo*trichia*⟩ ⟨hypo*trichia*⟩

troph- *or* **tropho-** *comb form* : nutritive ⟨*tropho*plasm⟩

-tro·phic \ˈtrō-fik\ *adj comb form* **1** : of, relating to, or characterized by (such) nutrition or growth ⟨hyper*trophic*⟩ **2** : -TROPIC ⟨lipo*trophic*⟩

-tro·phy \trə-fē\ *n comb form, pl* **-tro·phies** : nutrition : nurture : growth ⟨hypo*trophy*⟩

-tro·pia \ˈtrō-pē-ə\ *n comb form* : condition of (such) a deviation in the line of vision ⟨eso*tropia*⟩ ⟨hyper*tropia*⟩

-tro·pic \ˈtrō-pik\ *adj comb form* **1** : turning, changing, or tending to turn or change in a (specified) manner or in response to a (specified) stimulus ⟨geo*tropic*⟩ **2** : attracted to or acting upon (something specified) ⟨neuro*tropic*⟩

-tro·pin \ˈtrō-pən\ *or* **-tro·phin** \-fən\ *n comb form* : hormone ⟨gonado*tropin*⟩ ⟨somato*tropin*⟩

trypan- *or* **trypano-** *comb form* : trypanosome ⟨*trypano*cidal⟩

tubercul- *or* **tuberculo-** *comb form* **1** : tubercle ⟨*tubercul*ar⟩ **2** : tubercle bacillus ⟨*tubercul*in⟩ **3** : tuberculosis ⟨*tubercu*loid⟩

ulcero- *comb form* **1** : ulcer ⟨*ulcero*genic⟩ **2** : ulcerous and ⟨*ulcero*glandular⟩

ultra- *prefix* **1** : beyond in space : on the other side ⟨*ultra*violet⟩ **2** : beyond the range or limits of : transcending ⟨*ultra*microscopic⟩

ur- *or* **uro-** *comb form* **1** : urine ⟨*ur*ic⟩ **2** : urinary tract ⟨*uro*logy⟩ **3** : urinary and ⟨*uro*genital⟩ **4** : urea ⟨*ur*acil⟩

uran- *or* **urano-** *comb form* : palate ⟨*urano*plasty⟩

ure- *or* **ureo-** *comb form* : urea ⟨*ure*ase⟩

uretero- *comb form* **1** : ureter ⟨*uretero*graphy⟩ **2** : ureteral and ⟨*uretero*ileal⟩

urethr- *or* **urethro-** *comb form* : urethra ⟨*urethr*itis⟩ ⟨*urethro*scope⟩

-uria \ˈ(y)ùr-ē-ə\ *n comb form* **1** : presence of (a specified substance) in urine ⟨albumin*uria*⟩ **2** : condition of having (such) urine ⟨poly*uria*⟩; *esp* : abnormal or diseased condition marked by the presence of (a specified substance) ⟨py*uria*⟩

uric- *or* **urico-** *comb form* : uric acid ⟨*urico*lysis⟩

urin- *or* **urino-** *comb form* : UR- ⟨*urin*ary⟩ ⟨*urino*genital⟩

uro- *var of* UR-

uter- *or* **utero-** *comb form* **1** : uterus ⟨*uter*ectomy⟩ **2** : uterine and ⟨*utero*placental⟩

vag- *or* **vago-** *comb form* : vagus nerve ⟨*vago*tomy⟩ ⟨*vago*tonia⟩

vagin- *also* **vagini-** *comb form* : vagina ⟨*vagin*ectomy⟩

-va·lent \\'vā-lənt\\ *adj comb form* : having (so many) chromosomal strands or homologous chromosomes ⟨univa*lent*⟩

valvul- *or* **valvulo-** *comb form* : small valve : fold ⟨*valvul*itis⟩ ⟨*valvulo*tome⟩

varic- *or* **varico-** *comb form* : varix ⟨*varic*osis⟩ ⟨*varico*cele⟩

vas- *or* **vaso-** *comb form* **1** : vessel: as **a** : blood vessel ⟨*vaso*motor⟩ **b** : vas deferens ⟨*vas*ectomy⟩ **2** : vascular and ⟨*va*sovagal⟩

vascul- *or* **vasculo-** *comb form* : vessel; *esp* : blood vessel ⟨*vasculo*toxic⟩

ven- *or* **veni-** *or* **veno-** *comb form* : vein ⟨*veni*puncture⟩ ⟨*veno*stasis⟩

ventr- *or* **ventri-** *or* **ventro-** *comb form* **1** : abdomen ⟨*ven*tral⟩ **2** : ventral and ⟨*ventro*medial⟩

vermi- *comb form* : worm ⟨*vermi*cide⟩ ⟨*vermi*form⟩

vesico- *comb form* : of or relating to the urinary bladder and ⟨*vesico*urethral⟩

vesicul- *or* **vesiculo-** *comb form* **1** : vesicle ⟨*vesicul*ectomy⟩ **2** : vesicular and ⟨*vesiculo*bullous⟩

viscer- *or* **visceri-** *or* **viscero-** *comb form* : visceral : viscera ⟨*viscero*tropic⟩

vitell- *or* **vitello-** *comb form* : yolk : vitellus ⟨*vitello*genesis⟩

vivi- *comb form* : alive : living ⟨*vivi*section⟩

vulv- *or* **vulvo-** *comb form* **1** : vulva ⟨*vulv*itis⟩ **2** : vulvar and ⟨*vulvo*vaginal⟩

xanth- *or* **xantho-** *comb form* : yellow ⟨*xanth*oma⟩

xen- *or* **xeno-** *comb form* **1** : strange : foreign ⟨*xeno*biotic⟩ **2** : HETER- ⟨*xeno*graft⟩

xer- *or* **xero-** *comb form* : dry : arid ⟨*xero*derma⟩

xiph- *or* **xiphi-** *or* **xipho-** *comb form* **1** : sword-shaped ⟨*xiphi*sternum⟩ **2** : xiphoid and ⟨*xipho*costal⟩

zo- *or* **zoo-** *comb form* : animal ⟨*zoo*nosis⟩

-zo·ic \\'zō-ik\\ *adj comb form* : having a (specified) animal mode of existence ⟨holo*zoic*⟩ ⟨sapro*zoic*⟩

-zo·on \\'zō-,än, -ən\\ *n comb form* : animal ⟨spermato*zoon*⟩

zyg- *or* **zygo-** *comb form* **1** : pair ⟨*zyg*apophysis⟩ **2** : union : fusion ⟨*zygo*genesis⟩

zygomatico- *comb form* : zygomatic and ⟨*zygomatico*facial⟩

-zy·gous \\'zī-gəs\\ *adj comb form* : having (such) a zygotic constitution ⟨hetero*zygous*⟩

zym- *or* **zymo-** *comb form* : enzyme ⟨*zymo*gen⟩

-zyme \\,zīm\\ *n comb form* : enzyme ⟨lyso*zyme*⟩

Pronunciation Symbols

ə .... banana, collide, abut

ˈə, ˌə .... humdrum, abut

ə .... immediately preceding \l\, \n\, \m\, \ŋ\, as in battle, mitten, eaten, and sometimes open\ˈōp-ᵊm\, lock and key \-ᵊŋ-\; immediately following \l\, \m\, \r\, as often in French table, prisme, titre

ər .... further, merger, bird

ˈər- }
ˈə-r } .... as in two different pronunciations of hurry \ˈhər-ē, ˈhə-rē\

a .... mat, map, mad, gag, snap, patch

ā .... day, fade, date, aorta, drape, cape

ä .... bother, cot, and, with most American speakers, father, cart

ȧ .... father as pronounced by speakers who do not rhyme it with bother; French patte

au̇ .... now, loud, out

b .... baby, rib

ch .... chin, nature \ˈnā-chər\ (actually, this sound is \t\ + \sh\)

d .... did, adder

e .... bet, bed, peck

ˈē, ˌē .... beat, nosebleed, evenly, easy

ē .... easy, mealy

f .... fifty, cuff

g .... go, big, gift

h .... hat, ahead

hw .... whale as pronounced by those who do not have the same pronunciation for both whale and wail

i .... tip, banish, active

ī .... site, side, buy, tripe (actually, this sound is \ä\ + \i\, or \ȧ\ + \i\)

j .... job, gem, edge, join, judge (actually, this sound is \d\ + \zh\)

k .... kin, cook, ache

ḵ .... German ich, Buch; one pronunciation of loch

l .... lily, pool

m .... murmur, dim, nymph

n .... no, own

n .... indicates that a preceding vowel or diphthong is pronounced with the nasal passages open, as in French un bon vin blanc \œⁿ-bōⁿ-vaⁿ-bläⁿ\

ŋ .... sing \ˈsiŋ\, singer \ˈsiŋ-ər\, finger \ˈfiŋ-gər\, ink \ˈiŋk\

ō .... bone, know, beau

ȯ .... saw, all, gnaw, caught

œ .... French boeuf, German Hölle

œ̄ .... French feu, German Höhle

ȯi .... coin, destroy

p .... pepper, lip

r .... red, car, rarity

s .... source, less

sh .... as in shy, mission, machine, special (actually, this is a single sound, not two); with a hyphen between, two sounds as in grasshopper \ˈgras-ˌhäp-ər\

t .... tie, attack, late, later, latter

th .... as in thin, ether (actually, this is a single sound, not two); with a hyphen between, two sounds as in knighthood \ˈnīt-ˌhu̇d\

t̲h̲ .... then, either, this (actually, this is a single sound, not two)

ü .... rule, youth, union \ˈyün-yən\, few \ˈfyü\

u̇ .... pull, wood, book, curable \ˈkyu̇r-ə-bəl\, fury \ˈfyu̇(ə)r-ē\

ue .... German füllen, hübsch

ue̅ .... French rue, German fühlen

v .... vivid, give

w .... we, away; in some words having final \(ˌ)ō\, \(ˌ)yü\, or \(ˌ)ü\ a variant \ə-w\ occurs before vowels, as in \ˈfäl-ə-wiŋ\, covered by the variant \ə(-w)\ or \yə(-w)\ at the entry word

y .... yard, young, cue \ˈkyü\, mute \ˈmyüt\, union \ˈyün-yən\

y .... indicates that during the articulation of the sound represented by the preceding character the front of the tongue has substantially the position it has for the articulation of the first sound of yard, as in French digne \dēnʸ\

z .... zone, raise

zh .... as in vision, azure \ˈazhər\ (actually, this is a single sound, not two); with a hyphen between, two sounds as in hogshead \ˈhȯgz-ˌhed, ˈhägz-\

\ .... slant line used in pairs to mark the beginning and end of a transcription: \ˈpen\

ˈ .... mark preceding a syllable with primary (strongest) stress: \ˈpen-mən-ˌship\

ˌ .... mark preceding a syllable with secondary (medium) stress: \ˈpen-mən-ˌship\

- .... mark of syllable division

( ) .... indicate that what is symbolized between is present in some utterances but not in others: factory \ˈfak-t(ə-)rē\

A Dictionary of Medical English

A

a *abbr* **1** about **2** absent **3** absolute **4** absorbency; absorbent **5** accommodation **6** acetum **7** acid; acidity **8** actin **9** active; activity **10** allergist; allergy **11** alpha **12** anode **13** answer **14** ante **15** anterior **16** aqua **17** area **18** artery **19** asymmetric; asymmetry

A \'ā\ *n* : the one of the four ABO blood groups characterized by the presence of antigens designated by the letter A and by the presence of antibodies against the antigens present in the B blood group

A *abbr* **1** adenine **2** ampere

Å *symbol* angstrom

āā *also* **aa** *abbr* [Latin *ana*] of each — used at the end of a list of two or more substances in a prescription to indicate that equal quantities of each are to be taken

AA *abbr* **1** achievement age **2** Alcoholics Anonymous

AAF *abbr* ascorbic acid factor

AAL *abbr* anterior axillary line

AAMA *abbr* American Association of Medical Assistants

AAMT *abbr* American Association for Medical Transcription

A&P *abbr* **1** anterior and posterior **2** auscultation and percussion

A&W *abbr* alive and well

ab \'ab\ *n* : ABDOMINAL — usu. used in pl. ⟨highly developed ∼*s*⟩ ⟨∼ exercises⟩

ab *abbr* **1** abort; abortion **2** about

AB \'ā-'bē\ *n* : the one of the four ABO blood groups characterized by the presence of antigens designated by the letters A and B and by the absence of antibodies against these antigens

AB *abbr* **1** aid to blind **2** [Latin *artium baccalaureus*] bachelor of arts

abac·te·ri·al \ˌā-(ˌ)bak-'tir-ē-əl\ *adj* : not caused by or characterized by the presence of bacteria ⟨∼ prostatitis⟩

A band *n* : one of the cross striations in striated muscle that contain myosin filaments and appear dark under the light microscope and light in polarized light

aba·sia \ə-'bā-zh(ē-)ə\ *n* : inability to walk caused by a defect in muscular coordination — compare ASTASIA — **aba·sic** \ə-'bā-sik, -zik\ *adj*

Ab·be condenser \'ab-ə-, 'ab-ē-\ *n* : an adjustable substage lens used as a condenser for a compound microscope

Abbe, Ernst Karl (1840–1905), German physicist. Abbe was a professor of physics and mathematics, a director of astronomical and meteorological observatories, and a research director at an optical works. He made a great number of improvements in the design of the microscope. He introduced the apochromatic lens system in 1868, and his condenser for compound microscopes in 1870, and an oil immersion lens in 1878.

Ab·be–Est·lan·der operation \-'āst-ˌlän-dər-, -'est-ˌlan-\ *n* : the grafting of a flap of tissue from one lip of the oral cavity to the other lip to correct a defect using a pedicle with an arterial supply

Abbe, Robert (1851–1928), American surgeon. Abbe is known for his pioneer work in the use of radium to treat cancer, for the use of X-rays to detect kidney stones, and

for the use of catgut rings to support the intestines during operations for intestinal anastomosis. One of the foremost surgeons of his day, he specialized in plastic surgery for a time.

Estlander, Jakob August (1831–1881), Finnish surgeon. In 1879 Estlander published an article recommending that chronic empyema be treated by resecting one or more ribs in order to allow obliteration of the cavity.

ABC *abbr* atomic, biological, and chemical

ab·cix·i·mab \ˌab-'sik-si-mab, -sē-\ *n* : a powerful anticlotting drug that inhibits platelet aggregation by binding to a glycoprotein receptor on human platelets and that consists of the Fab fragment from a chimeric monoclonal antibody prepared from humans and mice — see REOPRO

abd *abbr* abdomen; abdominal

Ab·der·hal·den reaction \'äp-dər-ˌhäl-dən-\ *n* : the occurrence in body fluids of proteolytic enzymes specific for foreign proteins introduced into the body parenterally

Abderhalden, Emil (1877–1950), Swiss physiologist. Abderhalden is most noteworthy for his investigations in biochemistry. He produced more than 1,000 publications, writing on such subjects as enzymes, hormones, amino acids, proteins, and nutrition. In 1909 he discovered that upon the entry of a foreign protein into the blood, the bodily reaction is a defensive fermentation that causes disintegration of the protein. His name was given to the reaction. In 1912 he developed a serological test for pregnancy based on this reaction. The test proved to be unreliable, however, and was superseded in 1928 by the Aschheim-Zondek test.

abdom *abbr* abdomen; abdominal

ab·do·men \'ab-də-mən, -ˌdō-; əb-'dō-mən, ab-\ *n* **1 a** : the part of the body between the thorax and the pelvis with the exception of the back — called also *belly* **b** : the cavity of this part of the trunk lined by the peritoneum, enclosed by the body walls, the diaphragm, and the pelvic floor, and containing the visceral organs (as the stomach, intestines, and liver) **c** : the portion of this cavity between the diaphragm and the brim of the pelvis — compare PELVIC CAVITY **2** : the posterior often elongated region of the body behind the thorax in arthropods

¹ab·dom·i·nal \ab-'däm-ən-°l\ *adj* **1** : of, belonging to, or affecting the abdomen ⟨∼ organs⟩ ⟨∼ pain⟩ ⟨∼ surgery⟩ **2** : performed by entry through the abdominal wall ⟨an ∼ hysterectomy⟩ — **ab·dom·i·nal·ly** \-ē-\ *adv*

²abdominal *n* : an abdominal muscle (as an oblique or a rectus abdominis) esp. of the anterolateral region — usu. used in pl.

abdominal aorta *n* : the portion of the aorta between the diaphragm and the bifurcation into the right and left common iliac arteries

abdominal cavity *n* : ABDOMEN 1b

abdominal hernia *n* : any of various hernias (as an inguinal

---

\ə\ abut \ᵊ\ kitten \ər\ further \a\ ash \ā\ ace \ä\ cot, cart \aů\ out \ch\ chin \e\ bet \ē\ easy \g\ go \i\ hit \ī\ ice \j\ job \ŋ\ sing \ō\ go \ó\ law \ói\ boy \th\ thin \t̲h̲\ the \ü\ loot \ů\ foot \y\ yet \zh\ vision *See also* Pronunciation Symbols page

hernia, umbilical hernia, or spigelian hernia) in which an anatomical part (as a section of the intestine) protrudes through an opening, tear, or weakness in the abdominal wall musculature

abdominal reflex *n* : contraction of the muscles of the abdominal wall in response to stimulation of the overlying skin

abdominal region *n* : any of the nine areas into which the abdomen is divided by four imaginary planes of which two are vertical passing through the middle of the inguinal ligament on each side and two are horizontal passing respectively through the junction of the ninth rib and costal cartilage and through the top of the iliac crest — see EPIGASTRIC 2b, HYPOCHONDRIAC 2b, HYPOGASTRIC 1, ILIAC 2, LUMBAR 2, UMBILICAL 2

abdominal ring *n* : INGUINAL RING

abdominis — see OBLIQUUS EXTERNUS ABDOMINIS, OBLIQUUS INTERNUS ABDOMINIS, RECTUS ABDOMINIS, TRANSVERSUS ABDOMINIS

ab·dom·i·no·pel·vic \(ˌ)ab-ˌdäm-ə-nō-'pel-vik, əb-\ *adj* : relating to or being the abdominal and pelvic cavities of the body

ab·dom·i·no·per·i·ne·al \-ˌper-ə-'nē-əl\ *adj* : relating to the abdominal and perineal regions

abdominoperineal resection *n* : resection of a part of the lower bowel together with adjacent lymph nodes through abdominal and perineal incisions

ab·dom·i·no·plas·ty \(ˌ)ab-'däm-ə-nō-ˌplas-tē\ *n, pl* -ties : cosmetic surgery of the abdomen that typically involves removal of excess skin and fat and tightening of the abdominal muscles — called also *tummy tuck*

ab·dom·i·nous \ab-'däm-ə-nəs, əb-\ *adj* : having a large belly

ab·duce \ab-'d(y)üs\ *vt* **ab·duced; ab·duc·ing** : ABDUCT

ab·du·cens \ab-'d(y)ü-ˌsenz\ *n, pl* **ab·du·cen·tes** \ˌab-d(y)ü-'sent-(ˌ)ēz\ : ABDUCENS NERVE

abducens nerve *n* : either of the sixth pair of cranial nerves which are motor nerves, arise beneath the floor of the fourth ventricle, and supply the lateral rectus muscle of each eye — called also *abducent nerve, sixth cranial nerve*

ab·du·cent \ab-'d(y)üs-ᵊnt\ *adj* : serving to abduct ⟨an ∼ muscle⟩ — compare ADDUCENT

abducent nerve *n* : ABDUCENS NERVE

ab·duct \ab-'dəkt, əb- *also* 'ab-ˌ\ *vt* : to draw away (as a limb) from a position near or parallel to the median axis of the body ⟨the peroneus longus extends, ∼s, and everts the foot —C. R. Bardeen⟩; *also* : to move (similar parts) apart ⟨∼ adjoining fingers⟩ — **ab·duc·tion** \ab-'dək-shən, əb-\ *n*

ab·duc·tor \ab-'dək-tər\ *n, pl* **ab·duc·to·res** \ˌab-ˌdək-'tōr-(ˌ)ēz, -'tȯr-\ *or* **abductors** : a muscle that draws a part away from the median line of the body or from the axis of an extremity

abductor dig·i·ti min·i·mi \-ˌdij-ət-(ˌ)ē-'min-ə-(ˌ)mē\ *n* **1** : a muscle of the hand that abducts the little finger and flexes the phalanx nearest the hand **2** : a muscle of the foot that abducts the little toe

abductor hal·lu·cis \-'hal-(y)ə-səs, -'hal-ə-kəs\ *n* : a muscle of the foot that abducts the big toe

abductor pol·li·cis brev·is \-ˌpäl-ə-səs-'brev-əs, -ə-kəs-\ *n* : a thin flat muscle of the hand that abducts the thumb at right angles to the plane of the palm

abductor pollicis lon·gus \-'lȯŋ-gəs\ *n* : a muscle of the forearm that abducts the thumb and wrist

Abegg's rule \'ä-ˌbegz-, -ˌbeks-\ *n* : a rule in chemistry: for a given chemical element (as sulfur) the sum of the absolute value of its negative valence of maximum absolute value (as –2 for sulfur in H_2S) and its positive valence of maximum value (as +6 for sulfur in H_2SO_4) is often equal to 8

Abegg, Richard Wilhelm Heinrich (1869–1910), Danish chemist. Abegg's major contribution to science was his work on chemical valence. His hypothesis that eight electrons in the outer shell of an atom gives the most stable configuration has been shown to be true of the second principal shell. With chemist Guido Bodländer he proposed a theory of valence based on electrical affinities. Abegg also investigated the freezing points of dilute solutions.

ab·em·bry·on·ic \ˌab-ˌem-brē-'än-ik\ *adj* : remote from the embryo proper

aberrans — see DUCTULUS ABERRANS, VAS ABERRANS OF HALLER

ab·er·rant \a-'ber-ənt, ə-; 'ab-ə-rənt, -ˌe(ə)r-ənt\ *adj* **1** : straying from the right or normal way ⟨∼ behavior⟩ **2** : deviating from the usual or natural type : ATYPICAL ⟨∼ salivary tissue⟩

ab·er·ra·tion \ˌab-ə-'rā-shən\ *n* **1** : failure of a mirror, refracting surface, or lens to produce exact point-to-point correspondence between an object and its image **2** : unsoundness or disorder of the mind **3** : an aberrant organ or individual — **ab·er·ra·tion·al** \-shnəl, -shən-əl\ *adj*

abey·ance \ə-'bā-ən(t)s\ *n* : temporary inactivity or suspension (as of function or a symptom)

ABFP *abbr* American Board of Family Practice

ab·frac·tion \ab-'frak-shən\ *n* : a mechanism that is postulated to explain loss of tooth enamel and dentin in cervical areas of teeth exposed to similar amounts of brushing, general erosion, or abrasion compared to unaffected teeth but to considerably more contact in the crown area and that is held to involve flexure of the cervical hard tissue associated with crown contacts and eventual fatigue and loss or cracking of the hard tissue involved; *also* : a lesion produced by this

ab·i·ence \'ab-ē-ən(t)s\ *n* : a tendency to withdraw from a stimulus object or situation — compare ADIENCE

ab·i·ent \'ab-ē-ənt\ *adj* : characterized by avoidance or withdrawal ⟨an ∼ response⟩ — compare ADIENT

abi·es \'ā-bē-ˌēz, 'ab-ē-\ *n* **1** *cap* : a genus (family Pinaceae) of north temperate evergreen trees that comprise the true firs (as the balsam fir), are characterized by flattish leaves, smooth circular leaf scars, and erect cones, and are valued for their wood **2** *pl* **abies** : any tree of the genus *Abies* : FIR

abio·gen·e·sis \ˌā-ˌbī-ō-'jen-ə-səs\ *n* : the supposed spontaneous origination of living organisms directly from lifeless matter — called also *spontaneous generation;* compare BIOGENESIS — **abi·og·e·nist** \ˌā-(ˌ)bī-'äj-ə-nəst\ *or* **abio·gen·e·sist** \-ˌbī-ō-'jen-ə-səst\ *n*

abio·gen·ic \ˌā-ˌbī-ō-'jen-ik\ *adj* : not produced by the action of living organisms — **abio·gen·i·cal·ly** \-i-k(ə-)lē\ *adv*

abi·o·log·i·cal \ˌā-ˌbī-ə-'läj-i-kəl\ *adj* : not biological; *esp* : not involving or produced by organisms ⟨∼ synthesis of amino acids⟩ — **abi·o·log·i·cal·ly** \-i-k(ə-)lē\ *adv*

abi·ot·ic \ˌā-(ˌ)bī-'ät-ik\ *adj* : not biotic : ABIOLOGICAL ⟨the ∼ environment⟩ — **abi·ot·i·cal·ly** \-i-k(ə-)le\ *adv*

abi·ot·ro·phy \ˌā-(ˌ)bī-'ä-trə-fē\ *n, pl* **-phies** : degeneration or loss of function or vitality in an organism or in cells or tissues not due to any apparent injury ⟨senile dementia and related *abiotrophies* —David Bowen⟩ — **abio·tro·phic** \ˌā-ˌbī-ō-'trō-fik, -'träf-ik\ *adj*

ab·lac·ta·tion \ˌab-ˌlak-'tā-shən\ *n* : the act of weaning

ablas·te·mic \ˌā-ˌblas-'tē-mik, -'tem-ik\ *adj* : not germinal : incapable of blastema formation

ablas·tin \ə-'blas-tən, ā-\ *n* : an antibody in the blood of infected animals that inhibits the reproduction of the infecting organism

ab·late \a-'blāt\ *vt* **ab·lat·ed; ab·lat·ing** : to remove or destroy esp. by cutting or abrading ⟨∼ diseased tissue⟩

ab·la·tion \a-'blā-shən\ *n* : the process of ablating; *esp* : surgical removal

ab·la·tio pla·cen·tae \a-ˌblā-sh(ē-)ō-plə-'sent-(ˌ)ē\ *n* : ABRUPTIO PLACENTAE

ab·la·tive \a-'blā-tiv, ə-\ *adj* : relating to or involving surgical ablation ⟨∼ treatment⟩ ⟨∼ techniques⟩

abled \'ā-bəld\ *adj* : capable of unimpaired function ⟨the senior citizens, those less ∼ in some way —Richard Hair⟩ — compare DIFFERENTLY ABLED

ab·lu·tion \ə-'blü-shən, a-'blü-\ *n* : the washing of one's body or part of it — **ab·lu·tion·ary** \-shə-ˌner-ē\ *adj*

ABMT *abbr* autologous bone marrow transplant

¹**ab·nor·mal** \(ˈ)ab-'nȯr-məl\ *adj* : deviating from the normal, average, or expected ⟨∼ development⟩ ⟨results of the Pap smear were ∼⟩ ⟨∼ actions departing from accepted standards of social behavior⟩ — **ab·nor·mal·ly** \-mə-lē\ *adv*

²abnormal *n* : an abnormal person

ab·nor·mal·i·ty \ˌab-nər-ˈmal-ət-ē, -(ˌ)nȯr-\ *n, pl* **-ties** **1** : the quality or state of being abnormal **2** : something abnormal ⟨brain-wave *abnormalities*⟩

abnormal psychology *n* : a branch of psychology concerned with mental and emotional disorders (as neuroses, psychoses, and mental retardation) and with certain incompletely understood normal phenomena (as dreams and hypnosis)

ABO blood group \ˌā-(ˌ)bē-ˈō-\ *n* : one of the four blood groups A, B, AB, or O comprising the ABO system

ab·oma·si·tis \ˌab-(ˌ)ō-mə-ˈsīt-əs\ *n* : inflammation of the abomasum

ab·oma·sum \ˌab-ō-ˈmā-səm\ *n, pl* **-sa** \-sə\ : the fourth compartment of the ruminant stomach that follows the omasum and has a true digestive function — compare RUMEN, RETICULUM — **ab·oma·sal** \-səl\ *adj*

ab·orad \(ˈ)a-ˈbōr-ˌad, -ˈbȯr-\ *adv* : away from the mouth

ab·oral \(ˈ)a-ˈbōr-əl, -ˈbȯr-\ *adj* : situated opposite to or away from the mouth — **ab·oral·ly** \-ə-lē\ *adv*

abort \ə-ˈbȯ(ə)rt\ *vi* : to bring forth premature or stillborn offspring ⟨the patient ~ed spontaneously⟩ — compare MISCARRY ~ *vt* **1 a** : to induce the abortion of or give birth to prematurely **b** : to terminate the pregnancy of before term **2** : to stop in the early stages ⟨~ a disease⟩ — **abort·er** *n*

abor·ti·cide \ə-ˈbȯrt-ə-ˌsīd\ *n* **1** : the act of destroying a fetus within the uterus **2** : an agent that destroys the fetus and causes abortion

¹abor·ti·fa·cient \ə-ˌbȯrt-ə-ˈfā-shənt\ *adj* : inducing abortion

²abortifacient *n* : an agent (as a drug) that induces abortion

abor·tion \ə-ˈbȯr-shən\ *n* **1** : the termination of a pregnancy after, accompanied by, resulting in, or closely followed by the death of the embryo or fetus: **a** : spontaneous expulsion of a human fetus during the first 12 weeks of gestation — compare MISCARRIAGE **b** : induced expulsion of a human fetus **c** : expulsion of a fetus of a domestic animal often due to infection at any time before completion of pregnancy — see CONTAGIOUS ABORTION, TRICHOMONIASIS b, VIBRIONIC ABORTION **2** : arrest of development of an organ so that it remains imperfect or is absorbed **3** : the arrest of a disease in its earliest stage ⟨~ of a cold⟩

abor·tion·ist \-sh(ə-)nəst\ *n* : one who induces abortion

abortion pill *n* : a drug taken orally to induce abortion esp. early in pregnancy; *esp* : RU-486

abor·tive \ə-ˈbȯrt-iv\ *adj* **1** : imperfectly formed or developed : RUDIMENTARY **2 a** : ABORTIFACIENT **b** : cutting short ⟨~ treatment of pneumonia⟩ **c** : failing to develop completely or typically ⟨an ~ case of poliomyelitis⟩

abor·tus \ə-ˈbȯrt-əs\ *n* : an aborted fetus; *specif* : a human fetus less than 12 weeks old or weighing at birth less than 17 ounces

ABO system \ˌā-(ˌ)bē-ˈō-\ *n* : the basic system of antigens of human blood behaving in heredity as an allelic unit to produce any of the ABO blood groups

aboulia, aboulic *var of* ABULIA, ABULIC

abra·chia \(ˈ)ā-ˈbrak-ē-ə, -ˈbrāk-\ *n* : congenital lack of arms

abrad·ant \ə-ˈbrād-ᵊnt\ *n* : ABRASIVE — **abradant** *adj*

abrade \ə-ˈbrād\ *vt* **abrad·ed; abrad·ing** : to irritate or roughen by rubbing : CHAFE

abra·sion \ə-ˈbrā-zhən\ *n* **1** : wearing, grinding, or rubbing away by friction **2 a** : the rubbing or scraping of the surface layer of cells or tissue from an area of the skin or mucous membrane; *also* : a place so abraded **b** : the mechanical wearing away of the tooth surfaces by chewing

¹abra·sive \ə-ˈbrā-siv, -ziv\ *adj* : tending to abrade ⟨an ~ substance⟩ — **abra·sive·ness** *n*

²abrasive *n* : a substance (as emery or pumice) used for abrading, smoothing, or polishing — called also *abradant*

ab·re·ac·tion \ˌab-rē-ˈak-shən\ *n* : the expression and emotional discharge of unconscious material (as a repressed idea or emotion) by verbalization esp. in the presence of a therapist — compare CATHARSIS 2 — **ab·re·act** \-ˈakt\ *vb*

ab·re·ac·tive \-ˈak-tiv\ *adj* : relating to or capable of producing abreaction ⟨~ technique⟩

abro·sia \(ˈ)ā-ˈbrō-zhə\ *n* : abstinence from food

ab·rup·tion \ə-ˈbrəp-shən, ə-\ *n* : a sudden breaking off : detachment of portions from a mass ⟨placental ~⟩

ab·rup·tio pla·cen·tae \ə-ˌbrəp-shē-ˌō-plə-ˈsent-(ˌ)ē, -tē-ˌō-\ *n, pl* **abruptio pla·cen·ta·rum** \-ˌplas-ᵊn-ˈtar-əm, -ˈtär-\ *or* **ab·rup·ti·o·nes placentarum** \-shē-ˌō-(ˌ)nēz-, -tē-ˌō-ˌnäs-\ : premature detachment of the placenta from the wall of the uterus — called also *ablatio placentae*

Abrus \ˈā-brəs, ˈä-\ *n* : a genus of leguminous tropical vines having purplish flowers and flat pods — see ROSARY PEA 1

abs \ˈabz\ *pl of* AB

abs *abbr* **1** absent **2** absolute

ab·scess \ˈab-ˌses\ *n, pl* **ab·scess·es** \ˈab-səs-ˌēz, -ˌses-, -əz\ : a localized collection of pus surrounded by inflamed tissue — **ab·scessed** \-ˌsest\ *adj*

ab·scis·sion \ab-ˈsizh-ən\ *n* : the act or process of cutting off : ABLATION

ab·sco·pal \ab-ˈskō-pəl\ *adj* : relating to or being an effect on a nonirradiated part of the body that results from irradiation of another part

ab·sence seizure \ˈab-sən(t)s-\ *n* : a nonconvulsive generalized seizure that is marked by the transient impairment or loss of consciousness usu. with a blank stare, that begins and ends abruptly and is usu. unremembered afterward, and that is seen chiefly in mild types of epilepsy — called also *absence, petit mal*

ab·sinthe *also* **ab·sinth** \ˈab-(ˌ)sin(t)th\ *n* **1** : WORMWOOD **2** : a green liqueur flavored with wormwood or a substitute, anise, and other aromatics

ab·sin·thin \ab-ˈsin(t)-thən, ˈab-ˌ\ *n* : a bitter white crystalline compound $C_{15}H_{20}O_4$ constituting the bitter principle of wormwood

ab·sin·thism \ˈab-sən-ˌthiz-əm, -ˌsin-\ *n* : a diseased condition resulting from habitual excessive use of absinthe that contains oils of wormwood — **ab·sin·this·mic** \ˌab-sən-ˈthiz-mik\ *adj*

ab·sin·thi·um \ab-ˈsin(t)-thē-əm\ *n, pl* **-thi·um** **1** : WORMWOOD **2 a** : the dried leaves and flowering tops of a common wormwood (*Artemisia absinthium*) once used as a bitter tonic and stomachic **b** : oil of wormwood used as an ingredient of absinthe

ab·sin·thol \ˈab-sən-ˌthȯl, -ˌsin-, -ˌthōl\ *n* : THUJONE

ab·so·lute \ˌab-sə-ˈlüt\ *adj* **1** : pure or relatively free from mixture ⟨~ methanol⟩ **2** : relating to, measured on, or being a temperature scale based on absolute zero ⟨~ temperature⟩

absolute alcohol *n* : DEHYDRATED ALCOHOL

absolute humidity *n* : the amount of water vapor present in a unit volume of air — compare RELATIVE HUMIDITY

absolute refractory period *n* : the period immediately following the firing of a nerve fiber when it cannot be stimulated no matter how great a stimulus is applied — called also *absolute refractory phase;* compare RELATIVE REFRACTORY PERIOD

absolute zero *n* : a theoretical temperature characterized by complete absence of heat and equivalent to exactly −273.15°C or −459.67°F

ab·sorb \əb-ˈsȯ(ə)rb, -ˈzȯ(ə)rb\ *vt* **1** : to take up esp. by capillary, osmotic, solvent, or chemical action ⟨surgical sutures which can be ~ed by the body⟩ ⟨the blood in the lungs ~s oxygen⟩ **2** : to transform (radiant energy) into a different form usu. with a resulting rise in temperature ⟨chlorophyll reflects green light and ~s the other colors of light⟩ — **ab·sorb·able** \əb-ˈsȯr-bə-bəl, -ˈzȯr-\ *adj* — **ab·sorb·er** *n*

ab·sor·bance \əb-ˈsȯr-bən(t)s, -ˈzȯr-\ *n* : the ability of a solution or a layer of a substance to absorb radiation that is expressed mathematically as the negative common logarithm of the transmittance of the substance or solution — called also *optical density*

\ə\ abut \ᵊ\ kitten \ər\ further \a\ ash \ā\ ace \ä\ cot, cart
\au̇\ out \ch\ chin \e\ bet \ē\ easy \g\ go \i\ hit \ī\ ice \j\ job
\ŋ\ sing \ō\ go \ȯ\ law \ȯi\ boy \th\ thin \th\ the \ü\ loot
\u̇\ foot \y\ yet \zh\ vision   *See also* Pronunciation Symbols page

¹ab·sor·be·fa·cient \əb-ˌsȯr-bə-ˈfā-shənt, -ˌzȯr-\ *adj* : causing or promoting absorption

²absorbefacient *n* : an agent causing or promoting absorption

ab·sor·ben·cy \əb-ˈsȯr-bən-sē, -ˈzȯr-\ *n, pl* **-cies** **1** : the quality or state of being absorbent **2** *or* **ab·sor·ban·cy** \-bən-sē\ : ABSORBANCE

ab·sor·bent *also* **ab·sor·bant** \-bənt\ *adj* : able to absorb ⟨∼ gauze⟩ — **absorbent** *also* **absorbant** *n*

absorbent cotton *n* : cotton made absorbent by chemically freeing it from its fatty matter

ab·sorp·ti·om·e·ter \əb-ˌsȯrp-shē-ˈäm-ət-ər, -ˌzȯrp-, -tē-ˈäm-\ *n* **1** : an instrument for measuring the reduction of pressure in a gas as it is absorbed by a liquid to determine the absorption rate **2** : a colorimeter for transparent fluids usu. employing photoelectric means of comparison — **ab·sorp·ti·o·met·ric** \-shē-ō-ˈme-trik, -tē-\ *adj*

ab·sorp·ti·om·e·try \-ˈäm-ə-trē\ *n, pl* **-tries** : the use of an absorptiometer to determine the amount of radiation absorbed (as by living tissue) — see DUAL ENERGY X-RAY ABSORPTIOMETRY, DUAL PHOTON ABSORPTIOMETRY, SINGLE PHOTON ABSORPTIOMETRY

ab·sorp·tion \əb-ˈsȯrp-shən, -ˈzȯrp-\ *n* **1** : the process of absorbing or of being absorbed ⟨∼ of nourishment in the small intestine⟩ — compare ADSORPTION **2** : interception of radiant energy or sound waves

absorption coefficient *n* : the fraction of incident radiant energy which is absorbed per unit thickness, per unit mass, or per atom of an absorber — called also *coefficient of absorption*

absorption spectrum *n* : an electromagnetic spectrum in which a decrease in intensity of radiation at specific wavelengths or ranges of wavelengths characteristic of an absorbing substance (as chlorophyll) is manifested esp. as a pattern of dark lines or bands — compare EMISSION SPECTRUM

ab·sorp·tive \əb-ˈsȯrp-tiv, -ˈzȯrp-\ *adj* : relating to or functioning in absorption ⟨the ∼ surface of the small intestine⟩

ab·sorp·tiv·i·ty \əb-ˌsȯrp-ˈtiv-ət-ē, -ˌzȯrp-\ *n, pl* **-ties** : the property of a body that determines the fraction of incident radiation absorbed by the body

ab·stain \əb-ˈstān, ab-\ *vi* : to refrain deliberately and often with an effort of self-denial from an action or practice (as consumption of a food or a drug or indulgence in sexual intercourse) — **ab·stain·er** *n*

¹ab·ster·gent \əb-ˈstər-jənt, ab-\ *adj* : having a cleansing or detergent effect

²abstergent *n* : a substance used in cleansing : DETERGENT

ab·sti·nence \ˈab-stə-nən(t)s\ *n* **1** : voluntary forbearance esp. from sexual intercourse or from eating some foods **2** : habitual abstaining from intoxicating beverages — **ab·sti·nent** \-nənt\ *adj*

¹ab·stract \ˈab-ˌstrakt\ *n* **1** : a written summary of the key points esp. of a scientific paper **2** : a pharmaceutical preparation made by mixing a powdered solid extract of a vegetable substance with lactose in such proportions that one part of the final product represents two parts of the original drug from which the extract was made

²ab·stract \ˈab-ˌstrakt, ab-ˈ\ *vt* : to make an abstract of — **ab·strac·tor** *or* **ab·stract·er** \-tər\ *n*

abt *abbr* about

abu·lia *or* **abou·lia** \ā-ˈb(y)ü-lē-ə, ə-\ *n* : abnormal lack of ability to act or to make decisions that is characteristic of certain psychotic and neurotic conditions — **abu·lic** *also* **abou·lic** \-lik\ *adj*

¹abuse \ə-ˈbyüs\ *n* **1** : improper or excessive use or treatment ⟨drug ∼⟩ ⟨long-term ∼ of tranquilizers⟩ **2** : physical maltreatment: as **a** : the act of violating sexually : RAPE **b** *under some statutes* : rape or indecent assault not amounting to rape

²abuse \ə-ˈbyüz\ *vt* **abused; abus·ing** **1** : to use excessively ⟨∼ alcohol⟩; *also* : to use without medical justification ⟨*abusing* painkillers⟩ **2** : to treat so as to injure or damage ⟨∼ a child⟩ **3 a** : MASTURBATE **b** : to subject to abuse and

esp. to rape or indecent assault — **abus·able** \-ˈbyü-zə-bəl\ *adj* — **abus·er** *n*

abut·ment \ə-ˈbət-mənt\ *n* : a tooth to which a prosthetic appliance (as a denture) is attached for support

ac *abbr* **1** acute **2** [Latin *ante cibum*] before meals — used in writing prescriptions

Ac *symbol* actinium

AC *abbr* alternating current

aca·cia \ə-ˈkā-shə\ *n* **1** *cap* : a genus of woody leguminous plants of warm regions having pinnate leaves and white or yellow flower clusters — see CATECHU **2** : any of the genus *Acacia* of leguminous plants **3** : GUM ARABIC

acal·cu·lia \ˌā-ˌkal-ˈkyü-lē-ə\ *n* : lack or loss of the ability to perform simple arithmetic tasks

acal·cu·lous \ˌā-ˈkal-kyə-ləs\ *adj* : not affected with, caused by, or associated with gallstones ⟨∼ cholecystitis⟩

acanth·amoe·ba \ə-ˌkanth-ə-ˈmē-bə\ *n* **1** *cap* : a genus of free-living amebas (family Acanthamoebidae of the order Amoebida) found esp. in soil and freshwater either in the form of feeding and asexually replicating trophozoites or dormant double-walled cysts and including several (as *A. culbertsoni* and *A. castellanii*) which are pathogenic in humans causing infections of the skin, respiratory tract, eye (as keratitis esp. in contact lens wearers), and brain (as meningoencephalitis esp. in immunocompromised individuals) **2** : any of the genus *Acanthamoeba* of amebas

acan·thi·on \ə-ˈkan(t)-thē-ən, -thē-ˌän\ *n* : a point at the base of the anterior nasal spine

Acan·tho·ceph·a·la \ə-ˌkan(t)-thə-ˈsef-ə-lə\ *n pl* : a group of elongated parasitic intestinal worms with a hooked proboscis that as adults lack a digestive tract and absorb food through the body wall, and that are usu. classified as a separate phylum related to the phylum Platyhelminthes

acan·tho·ceph·a·lan \-lən\ *n* : any of the phylum Acanthocephala of unsegmented parasitic worms — called also *spiny-headed worm* — **acanthocephalan** *adj*

Acan·tho·chei·lo·ne·ma \-ˌkī-lə-ˈnē-mə\ *n* : a common genus of tropical filarial worms parasitic in humans and monkeys

acan·tho·cyte \ə-ˈkan(t)-thə-ˌsīt\ *n* : an abnormal red blood cell having variously shaped protoplasmic projections

acan·thoid \ə-ˈkan(t)-ˌthȯid\ *adj* : shaped like a spine

ac·an·thol·y·sis \ˌak-ˌan-ˈthäl-ə-səs, ˌā-ˌkan-, ˌak-ən-\ *n, pl* **-y·ses** \-ˌsēz\ : atrophy of the stratum spinosum of the epidermis

ac·an·tho·ma \-ˈthō-mə\ *n, pl* **-mas** *also* **-ma·ta** \-mət-ə\ : a tumor originating in the skin and developing through excessive growth of skin cells esp. of the stratum spinosum

ac·an·tho·sis \-ˈthō-səs\ *n, pl* **-tho·ses** \-ˌsēz\ : a benign overgrowth of the stratum spinosum of the skin — **ac·an·thot·ic** \-ˈthät-ik\ *adj*

acanthosis ni·gri·cans \-ˈnig-rə-ˌkanz, -ˈnī-grə-\ *n* : a skin disease characterized by gray-black warty patches usu. situated in the axilla or groin or on elbows or knees and sometimes associated with cancer of abdominal viscera

acap·nia \ə-ˈkap-nē-ə, (ˈ)ā-\ *n* : a condition of carbon dioxide deficiency in blood and tissues — **acap·ni·al** \-əl\ *adj*

Ac·a·pul·co gold \ˌak-ə-ˌpúl-(ˌ)kō-, ˌäk-\ *n* : marijuana grown in Mexico that is held to be very potent

acar·dius \(ˈ)ā-ˈkärd-ē-əs\ *n* : one of a pair of twin fetuses that is formed without a heart and that is usu. joined to the other fetus on which it depends for its circulation

acari *pl of* ACARUS

Ac·a·ri \ˈak-ə-ˌrī, -ˌrē\ *n pl* : a cosmopolitan and very large order of the class Arachnida comprising the mites and ticks most of which lack distinct demarcation into cephalothorax and abdomen and have no book lungs, many of which are parasites of plants, animals, or humans, and some of which are vectors of important diseases

ac·a·ri·a·sis \ˌak-ə-ˈrī-ə-səs\ *n, pl* **-a·ses** \-ˌsēz\ : infestation with or disease caused by mites — called also *acarinosis*

acar·i·cid·al \ə-ˌkar-ə-ˈsīd-ᵊl\ *adj* : having a lethal effect on mites ⟨an ∼ compound⟩

A
B

acar·i·cide \ə-'kar-ə-ˌsīd\ *n* : a pesticide that kills mites and ticks

ac·a·rid \'ak-ə-rəd\ *n* : any of the order Acari of arachnids; *esp* : any of the family Acaridae of mites — **acarid** *adj*

Acar·i·dae \ə-'kar-ə-ˌdē\ *n pl* : a large and widely distributed family of mites that feed on organic substances (as preserved meats, hides, seeds, and grains) and are sometimes responsible for dermatitis in persons exposed to repeated contacts with infested products — see GROCER'S ITCH

Ac·a·ri·na \ˌak-ə-'rī-nə, -'rē-\ *n pl, syn of* ACARI

ac·a·rine \'ak-ə-ˌrīn, -ˌrēn, -rən\ *adj* : of, relating to, or caused by mites or ticks ⟨∼ dermatitis⟩ — **acarine** *n*

ac·a·ri·no·sis \ˌak-ə-rə-'nō-səs\ *n, pl* **-no·ses** \-ˌsēz\ : ACARIASIS

ac·aro·der·ma·ti·tis \ˌak-ə-(ˌ)rō-ˌdər-mə-'tīt-əs\ *n* : dermatitis caused by mites

ac·a·rol·o·gy \ˌak-ə-'räl-ə-jē\ *n, pl* **-gies** : a branch of zoology that is concerned with the study of mites and ticks — **ac·a·rol·o·gist** \-jəst\ *n*

ac·a·ro·pho·bia \ˌak-ə-rō-'fō-bē-ə, -ə-rə-\ *n* **1** : an abnormal dread of skin infestation with small crawling organisms **2** : a delusion that the skin is infested with small crawling organisms

ac·a·rus \'ak-ə-rəs\ *n* **1** *cap* : a genus of arachnids including a number of small mites and formerly including all mites and ticks **2** *pl* **ac·a·ri** \-ˌrī, -ˌrē\ : MITE; *esp* : one of the genus *Acarus* or formerly included in this genus

acathisia *var of* AKATHISIA

acau·dal \(')ā-'kȯd-ᵊl\ *or* **acau·date** \-'kȯ-ˌdāt\ *adj* : having no tail

acc *abbr* **1** acceleration **2** according

ac·cel·er·ate \ik-'sel-ə-ˌrāt\ *vb* **-at·ed; -at·ing** *vt* : to cause to move faster or speed up ⟨*accelerated* speech and motor activity in manic patients⟩; *also* : to cause to undergo acceleration ∼ *vi* : to move faster : gain speed

ac·cel·er·a·tion \ik-ˌsel-ə-'rā-shən, (ˌ)ak-\ *n* **1** : the act or process of accelerating : the state of being accelerated **2** : change of velocity; *also* : the rate of this change **3** : advancement in mental growth or achievement beyond the average for one's age

acceleration of gravity *n* : the acceleration of a body in free fall under the influence of the earth's gravity expressed as the rate of increase of velocity per unit of time with the value 980.665 centimeters per second per second — abbr. **g**

ac·cel·er·a·tive \ik-'sel-ə-ˌrāt-iv, ak-\ *adj* : ACCELERATORY

ac·cel·er·a·tor \ik-'sel-ə-ˌrāt-ər, ak-\ *n* : one that accelerates: as **a** : a muscle or nerve that speeds the performance of an action ⟨a cardiac ∼⟩ **b** : a substance that speeds a chemical reaction **c** : an apparatus for imparting high velocities to charged particles (as electrons)

accelerator globulin *n* : FACTOR V

accelerator nerve *n* : a nerve whose impulses increase the rate of the heart

ac·cel·er·a·to·ry \ik-'sel-ə-rə-ˌtōr-ē, ak-, -ˌtȯr-\ *adj* : relating to or tending to cause acceleration ⟨∼ forces⟩

ac·cel·er·in \ik-'sel-ə-ˌrin, ak-\ *n* : the activated form of factor V

ac·cel·er·om·e·ter \ik-ˌsel-ə-'räm-ət-ər, ak-\ *n* : an instrument for measuring acceleration or for detecting and measuring vibrations

ac·cep·tor \ik-'sep-tər, ak-\ *n* : an atom, molecule, or subatomic particle capable of receiving another entity (as an electron) esp. to form a compound — compare DONOR 2

ac·ces·so·ri·us \ˌak-sə-'sōr-ē-əs, -'sȯr-\ *n, pl* **-so·rii** \-ē-ˌī, -ē-ˌē\ **1** : a muscle reinforcing the action of another **2** : ACCESSORY NERVE

¹ac·ces·so·ry \ik-'ses-(ə-)rē, ak-\ *adj* **1** : aiding, contributing, or associated in a secondary way: as **a** : being or functioning as a vitamin ⟨∼ food substances⟩ **b** : associated in position or function with something (as an organ or lesion) usu. of more importance ⟨the testis and ∼ male ducts and glands —B. T. Scheer⟩ **2** : SUPERNUMERARY ⟨∼ spleens⟩

²accessory *n, pl* **-ries** : ACCESSORY NERVE

accessory hemiazygos vein *n* : a vein that drains the upper left side of the thoracic wall, descends along the left side of the spinal column, and empties into the azygos or hemiazygos veins near the middle of the thorax

accessory nerve *n* : either of a pair of motor nerves that are the 11th cranial nerves, arise from the medulla and the upper part of the spinal cord, and supply chiefly the pharynx and muscles of the upper chest, back, and shoulders — called also *accessorius, accessory, spinal accessory nerve*

accessory olivary nucleus *n* : any of several small masses or layers of gray matter that are situated adjacent to the inferior olive and of which there are typically two on each side: **a** : one situated on each side dorsal to the inferior olive — called also *dorsal accessory olivary nucleus* **b** : one situated on each side medial to the inferior olive — called also *medial accessory olivary nucleus*

accessory pancreatic duct *n* : a duct of the pancreas that branches from the chief pancreatic duct and opens into the duodenum above it — called also *duct of Santorini*

ac·ci·dent \'ak-səd-ənt, -sə-ˌdent; 'aks-dənt\ *n* **1** : an unfortunate event resulting from carelessness, unawareness, ignorance, or a combination of causes **2** : an unexpected bodily event of medical importance esp. when injurious ⟨a cerebrovascular ∼⟩ **3** : an unexpected happening causing loss or injury which is not due to any fault or misconduct on the part of the person injured but for which legal relief may be sought — **ac·ci·den·tal** \ˌak-sə-'dent-ᵊl\ *adj* — **ac·ci·den·tal·ly** \-'dent-lē, -ᵊl-ē\ *also* **ac·ci·dent·ly** \-'dent-lē\ *adv*

accidental death *n* : death by accidental means usu. sudden and violent; *also* : death occurring as the unforeseen and chance result of an intended act

accidental injury *n* : injury occurring as the unforeseen and chance result of a voluntary act

accident–prone *adj* **1** : having a greater than average number of accidents **2** : having personality traits that predispose to accidents ⟨∼ individuals⟩

ac·cli·mate \'ak-lə-ˌmāt; ə-'klī-mət, -ˌmāt\ *vb* **-mat·ed; -mat·ing** : ACCLIMATIZE

ac·cli·ma·tion \ˌak-lə-'mā-shən, -ˌlī-\ *n* : acclimatization esp. by physiological adjustment of an organism to environmental change

ac·cli·ma·tize *or Brit* **ac·cli·ma·tise** \ə-'klī-mə-ˌtīz\ *vb* **-tized** *or Brit* **-tised; -tiz·ing** *or Brit* **-tis·ing** *vt* : to adapt to a new temperature, altitude, climate, environment, or situation ∼ *vi* : to become acclimatized — **ac·cli·ma·ti·za·tion** *or Brit* **ac·cli·ma·ti·sa·tion** \ə-ˌklī-mət-ə-'zā-shən\ *n*

ac·com·mo·date \ə-'käm-ə-ˌdāt\ *vi* **-dat·ed; -dat·ing** : to adapt oneself; *also* : to undergo visual accommodation — **ac·com·mo·da·tive** \-ˌdāt-iv\ *adj*

ac·com·mo·da·tion \ə-ˌkäm-ə-'dā-shən\ *n* : an adaptation or adjustment esp. of a bodily part (as an organ): as **a** : the automatic adjustment of the eye for seeing at different distances effected chiefly by changes in the convexity of the crystalline lens **b** : the range over which such adjustment is possible

ac·couche·ment \ˌa-ˌküsh-'mäⁿ, ə-'küsh-ˌ\ *n* : the time or act of giving birth

accouchement for·cé \-(ˌ)fȯr-'sā\ *n, pl* **ac·couche·ments for·cés** \-'mäⁿ(z)-, -ˌmäⁿ(z)-\ : artificially forced and hastened delivery

ac·cou·cheur \ˌa-ˌkü-'shər\ *n* : one that assists at a birth; *esp* : OBSTETRICIAN

ac·cou·cheuse \ˌa-ˌkü-'shə(r)z, -'shüz\ *n* : MIDWIFE

ac·cre·tio cor·dis \ə-ˌkrē-sh(ē)ō-'kȯrd-əs\ *n* : adhesive pericarditis in which there are adhesions extending from the pericardium to the mediastinum, pleurae, diaphragm, and chest wall

ac·cre·tion \ə-'krē-shən\ *n* : the process of growth or enlargement; *esp* : increase by external addition or accumula-

---

\ə\ **abut** \ᵊ\ **kitten** \ər\ **further** \a\ **ash** \ā\ **ace** \ä\ **cot, cart** \au̇\ **out** \ch\ **chin** \e\ **bet** \ē\ **easy** \g\ **go** \i\ **hit** \ī\ **ice** \j\ **job** \ŋ\ **sing** \ō\ **go** \ȯ\ **law** \ȯi\ **boy** \th\ **thin** \t̲h̲\ **the** \ü\ **loot** \u̇\ **foot** \y\ **yet** \zh\ **vision** *See also* Pronunciation Symbols page

tion (as by adhesion of external parts or particles) — compare APPOSITION 1, INTUSSUSCEPTION 2 — **ac·cre·tion·ary** \-shə-ˌner-ē\ *adj*

accumbens — see NUCLEUS ACCUMBENS

Ac·cu·pril \'a-kyü-ˌpril\ *trademark* — used for a preparation of the hydrochloride of quinapril

Ac·cu·tane \'a-kyù-ˌtān\ *trademark* — used for a preparation of isotretinoin

Ace \'ās\ *trademark* — used for a bandage with elastic properties

ACE inhibitor \'ās-, ˌā-(ˌ)sē-'ē-\ *n* : any of a group of antihypertensive drugs (as captopril) that relax arteries and promote renal excretion of salt and water by inhibiting the activity of an angiotensin converting enzyme

acel·lu·lar \(')ā-'sel-yə-lər\ *adj* **1** : containing no cells ⟨∼ vaccines⟩ **2** : not divided into cells : consisting of a single complex cell — used esp. of protozoans and ciliates

acen·tric \(')ā-'sen-trik\ *adj* : lacking a centromere ⟨∼ chromosomes⟩

ace·pha·lia \(')ā-sə-'fāl-yə, -'fā-lē-ə\ *n* : absence of a head

aceph·a·lo·cyst \(')ā-'sef-ə-lō-ˌsist, ə-'sef-\ *n* : a hydatid that has not developed a head

aceph·a·lous \(')ā-'sef-ə-ləs, ə-'sef-\ *adj* : lacking a head or having the head reduced

aceph·a·lus \(')ā-'sef-ə-ləs, ə-'sef-\ *n, pl* **-li** \-ˌlī, -ˌlē\ : a headless fetus

ac·er·o·la \ˌas-ə-'rō-lə\ *n* : a West Indian shrub (genus *Malpighia*) with mildly acid cherrylike fruits rich in vitamin C

acer·vu·lus \ə-'sər-vyə-ləs\ *n, pl* **-vu·li** \-ˌlī, -ˌlē\ : BRAIN SAND

acervulus ce·re·bri \-sə-'rē-ˌbrī, -'ser-ə-ˌbrī, -ˌbrē\ *n* : BRAIN SAND

aces·cent \ə-'ses-ʰnt, a-'ses-\ *adj* : slightly sour ⟨an ∼ flavor⟩

aces·o·dyne \ə-'ses-ə-ˌdīn\ *adj* : mitigating or relieving pain : ANODYNE

ace·sul·fame–K \'ā-sē-ˌsəl-ˌfām-'kā\ *n* : a white crystalline powder C₄H₄KNO₄S that is a cyclic organic potassium salt, has a sweetness much more intense that sucrose, and is used as a noncaloric sweetener in foods and beverages — called also *acesulfame potassium*

aceta *pl of* ACETUM

acetabular notch \-'näch\ *n* : a notch in the rim of the acetabulum through which blood vessels and nerves pass

ac·e·tab·u·lo·plas·ty \ˌas-ə-'tab-yə-(ˌ)lō-ˌplas-tē\ *n, pl* **-ties** : plastic surgery on the acetabulum intended to restore its normal state (as by repairing or enlarging its cavity)

ac·e·tab·u·lum \-'tab-yə-ləm\ *n, pl* **-lums** *or* **-la** \-lə\ **1** : the cup-shaped socket in the hip bone **2** : a sucker of an invertebrate (as a trematode or leech) — **ac·e·tab·u·lar** \-lər\ *adj*

ac·e·tal \'as-ə-ˌtal\ *n* : any of various compounds characterized by the group C(OR)₂ and obtained esp. by heating aldehydes or ketones with alcohols

ac·et·al·de·hyde \ˌas-ə-'tal-də-ˌhīd\ *n* : a colorless volatile water-soluble liquid aldehyde C₂H₄O used chiefly in organic synthesis that can cause irritation to mucous membranes

acet·amide \ə-'set-ə-ˌmīd, ˌas-ət-'am-ˌīd\ *n* : a white crystalline amide C₂H₅NO of acetic acid used esp. as a solvent and in organic synthesis

acet·amin·o·phen \ə-ˌsēt-ə-'min-ə-fən, ˌas-ət-\ *n* : a crystalline compound C₈H₉NO₂ that is a hydroxy derivative of acetanilide and is used in chemical synthesis and in medicine instead of aspirin to relieve pain and fever — called also *paracetamol;* see LIQUIPRIN, PANADOL, TYLENOL

ac·et·an·i·lide *or* **ac·et·an·i·lid** \ˌas-ə-'tan-ʰl-ˌīd, -ʰl-əd\ *n* : a white crystalline compound C₈H₉NO that is derived from aniline and acetic acid and is used esp. to relieve pain or fever — called also *phenylacetamide*

ac·et·ar·sone \ˌas-ət-'är-ˌsōn\ *also* **ac·et·ar·sol** \-ˌsól, -ˌsōl\ *n* : a white powder C₈H₁₀AsNO₅ used in the treatment of trichomonal vaginitis and Vincent's angina and in some countries in the treatment of amebiasis

ac·e·tate \'as-ə-ˌtāt\ *n* : a salt or ester of acetic acid

ac·et·azol·amide \ˌas-ət-ə-'zōl-ə-ˌmīd, -'zäl-, -məd\ *n* : a diuretic drug C₄H₆N₄O₃S₂ used esp. to treat glaucoma, control epileptic seizures, prevent or treat altitude sickness, and

treat edema associated with congestive heart failure

ace·te·nyl \ə-'sēt-ə-ˌnil, -'sēt-ʰn-əl\ *n* : ETHINYL

ace·tic \ə-'sēt-ik\ *adj* : of, relating to, or producing acetic acid or vinegar

acetic acid *n* : a colorless pungent liquid acid C₂H₄O₂ that is the chief acid of vinegar and that is used esp. in synthesis (as of plastics) and occas. in medicine as an astringent and styptic

acetic anhydride *n* : a colorless liquid (CH₃CO)₂O with a pungent odor and lacrimatory and vesicant action that is used esp. in making acetyl derivatives (as aspirin)

ace·ti·fy \ə-'sēt-ə-ˌfī, -'set-\ *vt* **-fied; -fy·ing** : to turn into acetic acid or vinegar — **ace·ti·fi·ca·tion** \-ˌsēt-ə-fə-'kā-shən, -ˌset-\ *n* — **ace·ti·fi·er** \-'sēt-ə-ˌfī(-ə)r, -'set-\ *n*

acetimeter *var of* ACETOMETER

ac·e·tin \'as-ət-ən\ *n* : any of three liquid acetates formed when glycerol and acetic acid are heated together: **a** : one C₃H₅(OH)₂C₂H₃O₂ containing only one acetate group that is used chiefly in the manufacture of explosives — called also *monoacetin* **b** : one C₃H₅(OH)(C₂H₃O₂)₂ containing two acetate groups that is used chiefly as a plasticizer and solvent — called also *diacetin* **c** : one C₃H₅(C₂H₃O₂)₃ containing three acetate groups that is used chiefly as a plasticizer and solvent and as a fixative in perfumes — called also *triacetin*

ace·to·ac·e·tate \ˌas-ə-tō-'as-ə-ˌtāt, ə-'sēt-ō-\ *n* : a salt or ester of acetoacetic acid

ace·to·ac·e·tic acid \ˌas-ə-(ˌ)tō-ə-ˌsēt-ik-, ə-ˌsēt-ō-\ *n* : an unstable acid C₄H₆O₃ that is one of the ketone bodies found in abnormal amounts in the blood and urine in certain conditions of impaired metabolism (as in starvation and diabetes mellitus) — called also *diacetic acid*

ace·to·bac·ter \ə-'sēt-ō-ˌbak-tər\ *n* **1** *cap* : a genus of aerobic ellipsoidal to rod-shaped bacteria (family Pseudomonadaceae) that grow in the presence of alcohol, secure energy by oxidizing organic compounds to organic acids (as alcohol to acetic acid), and are important esp. in the production of vinegar **2** : a bacterium of the genus *Acetobacter*

ace·to·hex·amide \ˌas-ə-tō-'hek-sə-ˌməd, ə-'sēt-ō-, -ˌmīd\ *n* : a sulfonylurea drug C₁₅H₂₀N₂O₄S used in the oral treatment of some of the milder forms of diabetes in adults to lower the level of glucose in the blood

acet·o·in \ə-'set-ō-wən\ *n* : a colorless liquid hydroxy ketone C₄H₈O₂ formed from various carbohydrates by fermentation — called also *acetylmethylcarbinol*

ac·e·tol·y·sis \ˌas-ə-'täl-ə-səs\ *n, pl* **-y·ses** \ə-ˌsēz\ **1** : a chemical reaction analogous to hydrolysis in which acetic acid plays a role similar to that of water **2** : simultaneous acetylation and hydrolysis

ace·to·me·roc·tol \ˌas-ə-(ˌ)tō-mə-'räk-ˌtòl, ə-ˌsēt-ō-, -ˌtōl\ *n* : a white crystalline mercury derivative C₁₆H₂₄HgO₃ of phenol used in solution as a topical antiseptic

ac·e·tom·e·ter \ˌas-ə-'täm-ət-ər\ *also* **ace·to·tim·e·ter** \-'tim-\ *n* : an instrument for estimating the amount of acetic acid in a solution (as vinegar)

ace·to·mor·phine \ˌas-ə-tō-'mór-ˌfēn, ə-ˌsēt-ō-\ *n* : HEROIN

ace·to·naph·thone \-'nap-ˌthōn, -'naf-\ *n* : either of two isomeric colorless crystalline ketones C₁₀H₇COCH₃

ac·e·tone \'as-ə-ˌtōn\ *n* : a volatile fragrant flammable liquid ketone C₃H₆O used chiefly as a solvent and in organic synthesis and found in abnormal quantities in diabetic urine — called also *propanone* — **ac·e·ton·ic** \ˌas-ə-'tän-ik\ *adj*

acetone body *n* : KETONE BODY

ac·e·ton·emia *or chiefly Brit* **ac·e·ton·ae·mia** \ˌas-ə-tō-'nē-mē-ə\ *n* : KETOSIS 2; *also* : KETONEMIA 1 — **ac·e·ton·emic** *or chiefly Brit* **ac·e·ton·ae·mic** \-'nē-mik\ *adj*

ac·e·to·nide \ˌas-ə-'tō-ˌnīd\ *n* : a cyclic acetal formed esp. by reaction of acetone with both hydroxyl groups of a diol — see FLUOCINOLONE ACETONIDE

ace·to·ni·trile \ˌas-ə-tō-'nī-trəl, ə-'sēt-ō-, -ˌtrēl\ *n* : the colorless liquid nitrile CH₃CN of acetic acid usu. made by dehydration of acetamide and used chiefly in organic synthesis and as a solvent — called also *methyl cyanide*

ac·e·ton·uria \ˌas-ə-tō-'n(y)ùr-ē-ə\ *n* : KETONURIA

ace·to·phe·net·i·din \ˌas-ə-(ˌ)tō-fə-'net-əd-ən, ə-ˌsēt-ō-\ *also*

ac·et·phe·net·i·din \,as-ət-fə-\ *n* : PHENACETIN

ace·to·phe·none \,as-ə-tō-fə-'nōn, ə-'sēt-ō-\ *n* : a colorless liquid ketone $CH_3COC_6H_5$ formerly used as a hypnotic but now used chiefly in perfumery — called also *hypnone*

ace·to·sol·u·ble \-'säl-yə-bəl\ *adj* : soluble in acetic acid

ace·tous \ə-'sēt-əs, 'as-ət-əs\ *adj* : relating to or producing vinegar ⟨∼ fermentation⟩

ac·e·tract \'as-ə-,trakt\ *n* : a powdered preparation made by extracting a vegetable drug with an alcoholic menstruum containing 5 to 10 percent acetic acid ⟨∼ of nux vomica⟩

ace·tum \ə-'sēt-əm\ *n, pl* **ace·ta** \-'sēt-ə\ **1** : VINEGAR **2** : a liquid preparation made by extracting a vegetable drug with dilute acetic acid

ace·tyl \ə-'sēt-ºl, 'as-ət-; 'as-ə-,tēl\ *n* : the radical CH_3CO of acetic acid

acet·y·lase \ə-'set-ºl-,ās\ *n* : any of a class of enzymes that accelerate the synthesis of acetic acid esters (as acetylcholine)

acet·y·late \ə-'set-ºl-,āt\ *vt* **-lat·ed; -lat·ing** : to introduce the acetyl radical into (a compound) — **acet·y·la·tion** \-,set-ºl-'ā-shən\ *n* — **acet·y·la·tive** \-'set-ºl-,āt-iv\ *adj*

ace·tyl·cho·line \ə-,set-ºl-'kō-,lēn, -,sēt-; ,as-ə-,tēl\ *n* : a neurotransmitter $C_7H_{17}NO_3$ released at autonomic synapses and neuromuscular junctions, active in the transmission of nerve impulses, and formed enzymatically in the tissues from choline — **ace·tyl·cho·lin·ic** \-kō-'lin-ik\ *adj*

ace·tyl·cho·lin·es·ter·ase \-,kō-lə-'nes-tə-,rās, -,rāz\ *n* : an enzyme that occurs esp. in some nerve endings and in the blood and promotes the hydrolysis of acetylcholine

acetyl CoA \-,kō-'ā\ *n* : ACETYL COENZYME A

acetyl coenzyme A *n* : a compound $C_{25}H_{38}N_7O_{17}P_3S$ formed as an intermediate in metabolism and active as a coenzyme in biological acetylations

ace·tyl·cys·te·ine \ə-,sēt-ºl-'sis-tə-,ēn, ,as-ə-,tēl-, ,as-ət-ºl-\ *n* : a mucolytic agent $C_5H_9NO_3S$ used esp. to reduce the viscosity of abnormally viscid respiratory tract secretions — see MUCOMYST

acet·y·lene \ə-'set-ºl-ən, -ºl-,ēn\ *n* : a colorless gaseous hydrocarbon $HC \equiv CH$ made esp. by the action of water on calcium carbide and used chiefly in organic synthesis and as a fuel (as in welding and soldering) — called also *ethyne* — **acet·y·le·nic** \ə-,set-ºl-'ē-nik, -'en-ik\ *adj*

ace·tyl·meth·yl·car·bi·nol \ə-,sēt-ºl-,meth-əl-'kär-bə-,nól, ,as-ə-,tēl-, ,as-ət-ºl-, -,nōl\ *n* : ACETOIN

ace·tyl·phen·yl·hy·dra·zine \-,fen-ºl-'hī-drə-,zēn, -,fēn-\ *n* : a white crystalline compound $C_8H_{10}ON_2$ less toxic than phenylhydrazine and used in the symptomatic treatment of polycythemia

ace·tyl·sa·lic·y·late \ə-,sēt-ºl-sə-'lis-ə-,lāt\ *n* : a salt or ester of acetylsalicylic acid

ace·tyl·sal·i·cyl·ic acid \ə-'sēt-ºl-,sal-ə-,sil-ik-\ *n* : ASPIRIN 1

ace·tyl·trans·fer·ase \-'tran(t)s-fər-,ās, -,āz\ *n* : any of several enzymes that catalyze the transfer of acetyl groups — called also *transacetylase*

AcG *abbr* [accelerator globulin] factor V

Ac–glob·u·lin \'ā-,sē-,gläb-yə-lən, 'ak-,gläb-\ *n* : FACTOR V

ACh *abbr* acetylcholine

acha·la·sia \,ā-kə-'lā-zh(ē-)ə\ *n* : failure of a ring of muscle (as a sphincter) to relax ⟨∼ of the esophagus⟩ ⟨∼ of the anal sphincter⟩ — compare CARDIOSPASM

¹ache \'āk\ *vi* **ached; ach·ing** : to suffer a usu. dull persistent pain

²ache *n* **1** : a usu. dull persistent pain **2** : a condition marked by aching

AChE *abbr* acetylcholinesterase

achieve·ment age \ə-'chēv-mənt-\ *n* : the level of an individual's educational achievement as measured by a standardized test and expressed as the age (as 8 years 6 months) for which the test score would be the average score — called also *educational age;* compare CHRONOLOGICAL AGE

achievement test *n* : a standardized test for measuring the skill or knowledge attained by an individual in one or more fields of work or study — compare INTELLIGENCE TEST

Achil·lea \,ak-ə-'lē-ə, ə-'kil-ē-ə\ *n* : a large genus of temperate composite herbs of the northern hemisphere that have divided leaves and small heads of disk and ray flowers, are a source of achilleine, and include one (*A. millefolium*) formerly widely used as a medicinal herb

achil·le·ine *or chiefly Brit* **achil·le·in** \ak-ə-'lē-ən, ə-'kil-ē-, -,ēn\ *n* : a brownish red bitter alkaloid $C_{20}H_{38}N_2O_{15}$ found in plants of the genus *Achillea*

Achil·les reflex \ə-'kil-ēz-\ *n* : ANKLE JERK

Achilles tendon *n* : the strong tendon joining the muscles in the calf of the leg to the bone of the heel — called also *tendon of Achilles;* compare HAMSTRING

Achilles, Greek mythological character. One of the most illustrious of warriors, Achilles was the offspring of a sea nymph who sought to achieve immortality for her son by dipping him in the river Styx in Hades. Holding Achilles by the heel, she left this one area unprotected. Later, in the Trojan War, he was fatally wounded when an arrow struck the very spot where he was vulnerable. Since classical times, the heel and Achilles have been commonly associated.

achi·ral \,ā-'kī-rəl\ *adj* : of or relating to a molecule that is superimposable on its mirror image : not chiral

achlor·hy·dria \,ā-,klōr-'hī-drē-ə, -,klór-\ *n* : absence of hydrochloric acid from the gastric juice — compare HYPERCHLORHYDRIA, HYPOCHLORHYDRIA — **achlor·hy·dric** \-'hī-drik\ *adj*

acho·lia \(')ā-'kō-lē-ə, -'kä-\ *n* : deficiency or absence of bile

achol·ic \(')ā-'käl-ik\ *or* **acho·lous** \(')ā-'kō-ləs, -'käl-əs; 'ak-ə-ləs\ *adj* : exhibiting deficiency of bile ⟨∼ stools⟩

achol·uria \,ā-kō-'l(y)úr-ē-ə, -kä-\ *n* : absence of bile pigment from the urine — **achol·uric** \-'l(y)úr-ik\ *adj*

achon·dro·pla·sia \,ā-,kän-drə-'plā-zh(ē-)ə\ *n* : a genetic disorder disturbing normal growth of cartilage, resulting in a form of dwarfism characterized by a usu. normal torso and shortened limbs, and usu. inherited as an autosomal dominant — compare ATELIOSIS

¹achon·dro·plas·tic \-'plas-tik\ *adj* : relating to or affected with achondroplasia

²achondroplastic *n* : one affected with achondroplasia

Acho·ri·on \ə-'kōr-ē-,än, -'kór-\ *n, syn of* TRICHOPHYTON

achroa·cyte \(')ā-'krō-ə-,sīt\ *n* : a colorless cell; *specif* : LYMPHOCYTE

achroma *var of* ACHROMIA

achro·ma·cyte \(')ā-'krō-mə-,sīt\ *n* : a decolorized red blood cell

achro·ma·sia \,ā-krō-'mā-zh(ē-)ə, ,ak-rō-\ *n* **1** : ACHROMIA **2** *of cells or tissues* : loss of the usual reaction to stains

ach·ro·mat \'ak-rə-,mat\ *n* : ACHROMATIC LENS

ach·ro·mat·ic \,ak-rə-'mat-ik\ *adj* **1** : refracting light without dispersing it into its constituent colors : giving images practically free from extraneous colors ⟨an ∼ telescope⟩ **2** : not readily colored by the usual staining agents **3** : possessing or involving no hue : being or involving only black, gray, or white ⟨∼ visual sensations⟩ ⟨∼ light stimuli⟩ — **ach·ro·mat·i·cal·ly** \-i-k(ə-)lē\ *adv*

achromatic figure *n* : the mitotic spindle and associated cell structures that do not stain with the usual cytochemical dyes — compare CHROMATIC FIGURE

achromatic lens *n* : a compound lens made by combining lenses of different glasses (as flint glass and crown glass) with different focal powers so that the light emerging from the lens forms an image almost free from unwanted colors

achro·ma·tin \(')ā-'krō-mət-ən\ *n* : the part of the cell nucleus that is not readily colored by basic stains — compare CHROMATIN

achro·ma·tism \(')ā-'krō-mə-,tiz-əm, a-\ *n* : the quality or state of being achromatic

achro·ma·tize *or Brit* **achro·ma·tise** \(')ā-'krō-mə-,tīz\ *vt* **-tized** *or Brit* **-tised; -tiz·ing** *or Brit* **-tis·ing** : to make achromatic ⟨∼ a lens⟩

---

achro·mato·cyte \ˌā-krō-'mat-ə-ˌsīt, ˌak-rō-; (')ā-'krō-mət-, ak-'rō-\ *n* : ACHROMACYTE

achro·ma·tol·y·sis \ˌā-krō-mə-'täl-ə-səs, ˌak-ˌrō-\ *n, pl* **-y·ses** \-ˌsēz\ : disorganization of the achromatic part of a cell

achro·ma·top·sia \ˌā-krō-mə-'täp-sē-ə\ *n* : a visual defect marked by total color blindness in which the colors of the spectrum are seen as tones of white-gray-black

achro·mia \(')ā-'krō-mē-ə\ *also* **achro·ma** \-mə\ *n* : absence of normal pigmentation esp. in red blood cells and skin — **achro·mic** \(')ā-'krō-mik\ *adj*

Achro·mo·bac·ter \(')ā-'krō-mə-ˌbak-tər\ *n, syn of* ALCALIG-ENES

achro·mo·trich·ia \ˌā-ˌkrō-mə-'trik-ē-ə\ *n* : absence of pigment in the hair

achy \'ā-kē\ *adj* **ach·i·er; ach·i·est** : affected with aches — **ach·i·ness** *n*

achy·lia \(')ā-'kī-lē-ə\ *n* : ACHYLIA GASTRICA — **achy·lous** \(')ā-'kī-ləs\ *adj*

achylia gas·tri·ca \-'gas-trik-ə\ *n* **1** : partial or complete absence of gastric juice **2** : ACHLORHYDRIA

acic·u·lar \ə-'sik-yə-lər\ *adj* : shaped like a needle ⟨~ crystals⟩

¹ac·id \'as-əd\ *adj* **1** : sour, sharp, or biting to the taste **2 a** : of, relating to, or being an acid; *also* : having the reactions or characteristics of an acid ⟨an ~ solution⟩ **b** *of salts and esters* : derived by partial exchange of replaceable hydrogen ⟨~ sodium carbonate NaHCO₃⟩ **c** : marked by or resulting from an abnormally high concentration of acid ⟨~ indigestion⟩ — not used technically

²acid *n* **1** : a sour substance; *specif* : any of various typically water-soluble and sour compounds that in solution are capable of reacting with a base to form a salt, that redden litmus, that have a pH less than 7, and that are hydrogen-containing molecules or ions able to give up a proton to a base or are substances able to accept an unshared pair of electrons from a base **2** : LSD

acid–base balance \ˌas-əd-ˌbās-\ *n* : the state of equilibrium between proton donors and proton acceptors in the buffering system of the blood that is maintained at approximately pH 7.35 to 7.45 under normal conditions in arterial blood

acid deposition *n* : deposition of acidity in the environment by acid precipitation or by acid-containing or acid=producing gases and particles

acid dye *n* : any of a large class of dyes that contain acidic groups usu. in the form of sodium or potassium salts, that are soluble in water, and that are used esp. in aqueous or alcoholic solution for staining cytoplasm and various acidophilic structures of cells and tissues

ac·i·de·mia *or chiefly Brit* **ac·i·dae·mia** \ˌas-ə-'dē-mē-ə\ *n* : a condition in which the hydrogen-ion concentration in the blood is increased

acid–fast \'as-əd-ˌfast\ *adj* : not easily decolorized by acids (as when stained) — used esp. of bacteria and tissues

acid fuchsin *also* **acid fuchsine** *n* : an acid dye used chiefly in histology as a general cytoplasmic stain and for demonstration of special elements (as mitochondria) — called also *acid magenta*

acid·ic \ə-'sid-ik, a-\ *adj* **1** : acid-forming **2** : ACID

acid·i·fy \-ə-ˌfī\ *vb* **-fied; -fy·ing** *vt* **1** : to make acid **2** : to convert into an acid ~ *vi* : to become acid — **acid·i·fi·able** \ə-ˌsid-ə-'fī-ə-bəl, a-\ *adj* — **acid·i·fi·ca·tion** \-fə-'kā-shən\ *n* — **acid·i·fi·er** \ə-'sid-ə-ˌfī(-ə)r, a-\ *n*

ac·i·dim·e·ter \ˌas-ə-'dim-ət-ər\ *n* : an apparatus for measuring the strength or the amount of acid present in a mixture or solution — **acid·i·met·ric** \ə-ˌsid-ə-'me-trik\ *adj* — **ac·i·dim·e·try** \ˌas-ə-'dim-ə-trē\ *n, pl* **-tries**

acid·i·ty \ə-'sid-ət-ē, a-\ *n, pl* **-ties 1** : the quality, state, or degree of being sour or chemically acid ⟨the ~ of lemon juice⟩ **2** : the quality or state of being excessively or abnormally acid : HYPERACIDITY

acid magenta *n* : ACID FUCHSIN

acid maltase deficiency *n* : POMPE'S DISEASE

acid·o·gen·ic \ə-ˌsid-ə-'jen-ik, ˌas-əd-ō-\ *adj* : acid-forming ⟨~ bacteria⟩

¹acid·o·phil \ə-'sid-ə-ˌfil, a-\ *also* **acid·o·phile** \-ˌfīl\ *adj* : ACID-OPHILIC 1

²acidophil *also* **acidophile** : a substance, tissue, or organism that stains readily with acid stains — called also *oxyphile*

acid·o·phil·ia \ə-ˌsid-ə-'fil-ē-ə, ˌas-ə-dō-\ *n* : EOSINOPHILIA

acid·o·phil·ic \-'fil-ik\ *adj* **1** : staining readily with acid stains : ACIDOPHIL ⟨~ white blood cells⟩ **2** : preferring or thriving in a relatively acid environment ⟨~ bacteria⟩

ac·i·doph·i·lus \ˌas-ə-'däf-(ə-)ləs\ *n* : a lactobacillus (*Lactobacillus acidophilus*) that is added esp. to dairy products (as yogurt and milk) or prepared as a dietary supplement, is part of the normal intestinal and vaginal flora, and is used therapeutically esp. to promote intestinal health; *also* : a preparation containing such bacteria

ac·i·do·sis \ˌas-ə-'dō-səs\ *n, pl* **-do·ses** \-ˌsēz\ : an abnormal condition of reduced alkalinity of the blood and tissues that is marked by sickly sweet breath, headache, nausea and vomiting, and visual disturbances and is usu. a result of excessive acid production — compare ALKALOSIS, KETOSIS 1 — **ac·i·dot·ic** \-'dät-ik\ *adj*

acid phosphatase *n* : a phosphatase (as the phosphomonoesterase from the prostate gland) optimally active in acid medium

acid precipitation *n* : precipitation (as rain or snow) having increased acidity caused by environmental factors (as atmospheric pollutants)

acid rain *n* : acid precipitation esp. in the form of rain

acid snow *n* : acid precipitation in the form of snow

acid·u·late \ə-'sij-ə-ˌlāt\ *vt* **-lat·ed; -lat·ing** : to make acid or slightly acid — **acid·u·la·tion** \-ˌsij-ə-'lā-shən\ *n*

acid·u·lous \ə-'sij-ə-ləs\ *adj* : somewhat acid to the taste

ac·id·uria \ˌas-ə-'d(y)ùr-ē-ə\ *n* : the condition of having acid in the urine esp. in abnormal amounts — see AMINOACIDURIA

ac·id·uric \ˌas-ə-'d(y)ùr-ik\ *adj* : tolerating a highly acid environment; *also* : ACIDOPHILIC 2

ac·id·yl \'as-ə-ˌdil, -ˌdēl\ *n* : ACYL

ac·i·nar \'as-ə-nər, -ˌnär\ *adj* : of, relating to, or comprising an acinus ⟨pancreatic ~ cells⟩

acin·ic \ə-'sin-ik\ *adj* : ACINAR ⟨~ carcinoma⟩

ac·i·nose \'as-ə-ˌnōs\ *adj* : ACINOUS ⟨an ~ gland⟩

ac·i·nous \'as-ə-nəs, ə-'sī-nəs\ *adj* : consisting of or containing acini

ac·i·nus \'as-ə-nəs, ə-'sī-\ *n, pl* **aci·ni** \-ˌnī\ : any of the small sacs or alveoli that terminate the ducts of some exocrine glands and are lined with secretory cells

Acip·Hex \'as-ə-ˌfeks\ *trademark* — used for a preparation of the sodium salt of rabeprazole

ack·ee *var of* AKEE

ACL \ˌā-(ˌ)sē-'el\ *n* : ANTERIOR CRUCIATE LIGAMENT

ac·la·sis \'ak-lə-səs\ *n, pl* **ac·la·ses** \-ˌsēz\ : continuity of structure (as in hereditary deforming chondrodysplasia) between normal and pathological tissue

aclas·tic \ə-'klas-tik, (')ā-\ *adj* : incapable of refracting light

ACLS *abbr* advanced cardiac life support

ac·me \'ak-mē\ *n* : the highest or most critical point or stage (as of growth or development)

ac·mes·the·sia *or chiefly Brit* **ac·maes·the·sia** \ˌak-ˌmes-'thēzh(ē-)ə\ *n* : cutaneous sensation of a sharp point but without pain

acnae vulgares *pl of* ACNE VULGARIS

ac·ne \'ak-nē\ *n* : a disorder of the skin caused by inflammation of the skin glands and hair follicles; *specif* : a form found chiefly in adolescents and marked by pimples esp. on the face — **ac·ned** \-nēd\ *adj*

ac·ne·form \'ak-nē-ˌfòrm\ *or* **ac·ne·i·form** \'ak-nē-ə-ˌfòrm, ak-'nē-\ *adj* : resembling acne ⟨an ~ eruption on the skin⟩

ac·ne·gen·ic \ˌak-ni-'jen-ik\ *adj* : producing or increasing the severity of acne ⟨the ~ effect of some hormones⟩

ac·ne ro·sa·cea \ˌak-nē-rō-'zā-sh(ē-)ə\ *n, pl* **ac·nae ro·sa·ce·ae** \ˌak-nē-rō-'zā-shē-ˌē\ : ROSACEA

acne ur·ti·ca·ta \-ˌərt-ə-'kāt-ə\ *n* : an acneform eruption of the skin characterized by itching papular wheals

acne vul·gar·is \-ˌvəl-'gar-əs, -'ger-\ *n, pl* **acnae vul·gar·es** \-'gar-ˌēz, -'ger-\ : a chronic acne involving mainly the face, chest, and shoulders that is common in adolescent humans and various domestic animals and is characterized by the intermittent formation of discrete papular or pustular lesions often resulting in considerable scarring

ac·ni·tis \ak-'nīt-əs\ *n* : the formation of papulonecrotic tuberculids esp. on the face

ACNM *abbr* American College of Nurse-Midwives

Ac·o·can·thera \ˌak-ō-'kan(t)-thə-rə\ *n* : a genus of white-flowered African shrubs or trees (family Apocynaceae) most of which are very poisonous

acoe·lo·mate \('ā-'sē-lə-ˌmāt\ *n* : an invertebrate lacking a coelom; *esp* : one belonging to the group comprising the flatworms and nemerteans (class Nemertea or Nemertinea) and characterized by bilateral symmetry and a digestive cavity that is the only internal cavity — **acoelomate** *adj*

ac·o·ine \'ak-ə-ˌwēn, -wən\ *n* : a white crystalline derivative $C_{23}H_{26}ClN_3O_3$ of guanidine used as a local anesthetic

acon·i·tase \ə-'kän-ə-ˌtās\ *n* : an enzyme occurring in many animal and plant tissues that accelerates the conversion of citric acid first into aconitic acid and then into isocitric acid

ac·o·nite \'ak-ə-ˌnīt\ *n* **1** : MONKSHOOD **2** : the dried tuberous root of a monkshood (*Aconitum napellus*) formerly used as a cardiac and respiratory sedative

ac·o·nit·ic acid \ˌak-ə-ˌnit-ik-\ *n* : a white crystalline acid $C_3H_3(COOH)_3$ that occurs in aconite, sugarcane, and beet roots and is obtained as a by-product in sugar manufacture or by dehydration of citric acid by sulfuric acid

acon·i·tine \ə-'kän-ə-ˌtēn, -tən\ *n* : a white crystalline intensely poisonous alkaloid $C_{34}H_{47}NO_{11}$ from the root and leaves of monkshood

Ac·o·ni·tum \ˌak-ə-'nīt-əm\ *n* : a genus of poisonous herbs (family Ranunculaceae) found in temperate regions and having palmately divided leaves and very irregular blue, purple, or yellow flowers — see MONKSHOOD, WOLFSBANE

acou·me·ter \ə-'kü-mət-ər, 'ak-ü-ˌmēt-ər\ *n* : AUDIOMETER

acous·ma \ə-'küz-mə\ *n, pl* **-mas** *or* **-ma·ta** \-mət-ə\ : an auditory hallucination of a simple nonverbal character (as a buzzing or ringing)

acous·tic \ə-'kü-stik\ *or* **acous·ti·cal** \-sti-kəl\ *adj* : of or relating to the sense or organs of hearing, to sound, or to the science of sounds ⟨∼ apparatus of the ear⟩ ⟨∼ energy⟩: as **a** : deadening or absorbing sound ⟨∼ tile⟩ **b** : operated by or utilizing sound waves — **acous·ti·cal·ly** \-k(ə-)lē\ *adv*

acoustic meatus *n* : AUDITORY CANAL

acoustic microscope *n* : a microscope in which ultrasound is used to scan a sample and then is converted to an electric signal from which an image is reconstructed on a video screen — **acoustic microscopy** *n*

acoustic nerve *n* : AUDITORY NERVE

acoustic neuroma *n* : a nonmalignant usu. slow-growing tumor involving the Schwann cells of a vestibular nerve that may cause deafness, tinnitus, and disturbance of the sense of balance and may be life threatening if not treated

acous·tics \ə-'kü-stiks\ *n pl but sing or pl in constr* : a science that deals with the production, control, transmission, reception, and effects of sound

acoustic tubercle *n* : a pear-shaped prominence on the inferior cerebellar peduncle including the dorsal nucleus of the cochlear nerve

ACP *abbr* American College of Physicians

ac·quain·tance rape \ə-'kwānt-ᵊn(t)s-\ *n* : rape committed by someone known to the victim

ac·quire \ə-'kwī(ə)r\ *vt* **ac·quired; ac·quir·ing** : to come to have as a new or additional characteristic, trait, or ability (as by sustained effort, by mutation, or through environmental forces) ⟨a cognitive system . . . that is *acquired* in early childhood —Noam Chomsky⟩ ⟨bacteria that ∼ tolerance to antibiotics⟩ ⟨insects that ∼ resistance to insecticides⟩

ac·quired *adj* **1** : arising in response to the action of the environment on the organism (as in the use or disuse of an organ) ⟨∼ characteristics⟩ — compare GENETIC 2, HEREDITARY **2** : developed after birth ⟨∼ heart murmurs⟩ —

compare CONGENITAL 2, FAMILIAL, HEREDITARY

acquired immune deficiency syndrome *n* : AIDS

acquired immunity *n* : immunity that develops after exposure to a suitable agent (as by an attack of a disease or by injection of antigens) — compare ACTIVE IMMUNITY, NATURAL IMMUNITY, PASSIVE IMMUNITY

acquisita — see EPIDERMOLYSIS BULLOSA ACQUISITA

acquired immunodeficiency syndrome *n* : AIDS

ac·ral \'ak-rəl\ *adj* : of or belonging to the extremities of peripheral body parts ⟨∼ cyanosis⟩

acra·nia \(')ā-'krā-nē-ə\ *n* : congenital partial or total absence of the skull

Acrania *n pl, in some classifications* : a division of the phylum or subkingdom Chordata comprising the hemichordates, tunicates, and lancelets and including all the chordates without true heads and anterior brains — compare VERTEBRATA

Ac·re·mo·ni·um \ˌak-ri-'mō-nē-əm\ *n* : a genus of imperfect fungi with conidia held together by a slimy secretion in more or less spherical heads at the ends of fertile branches

ac·rid \'ak-rəd\ *adj* : irritatingly sharp and harsh or unpleasantly pungent in taste or odor — **ac·rid·ly** *adv*

ac·ri·dine \'ak-rə-ˌdēn\ *n* : a colorless crystalline compound $C_{13}H_9N$ occurring in coal tar and important as the parent compound of dyes and pharmaceuticals

acridine orange *n* : a basic orange dye structurally related to acridine and used esp. to stain nucleic acids

ac·ri·fla·vine \ˌak-rə-'flā-ˌvēn, -vən\ *n* : a yellow acridine dye $C_{14}H_{14}N_3Cl$ obtained by methylation of proflavine as red crystals or usu. in admixture with proflavine as a deep orange powder and used often in the form of its reddish brown hydrochloride as an antiseptic esp. for wounds

ac·ro·blast \'ak-rə-ˌblast\ *n* : a derivative of the Golgi apparatus that gives rise in spermatogenesis to the acrosome

ac·ro·cen·tric \ˌak-rō-'sen-trik\ *adj* : having the centromere situated so that one chromosomal arm is much shorter than the other — compare METACENTRIC, TELOCENTRIC — **acrocentric** *n*

ac·ro·ceph·a·lo·syn·dac·ty·ly \-ˌsef-ə-(ˌ)lō-sin-'dak-tə-lē\ *n, pl* **-lies** : a congenital syndrome characterized by a peaked head and webbed or fused fingers and toes

ac·ro·ceph·a·ly \ˌak-rə-'sef-ə-lē\ *also* **ac·ro·ce·pha·lia** \ˌak-rō-sə-'fāl-yə\ *n, pl* **-lies** *also* **-lias** : OXYCEPHALY — **ac·ro·ce·phal·ic** \ˌak-rō-sə-'fal-ik\ *adj*

ac·ro·chor·don \ˌak-rə-'kór-ˌdän\ *n* : SKIN TAG

ac·ro·cy·a·no·sis \ˌak-rō-ˌsī-ə-'nō-səs\ *n, pl* **-no·ses** \-ˌsēz\ : blueness or pallor of the extremities usu. associated with pain and numbness and caused by vasomotor disturbances (as in Raynaud's disease); *specif* : a disorder of the arterioles of the exposed parts of the hands and feet involving abnormal contraction of the arteriolar walls intensified by exposure to cold and resulting in bluish mottled skin, chilling, and sweating of the affected parts — **ac·ro·cy·a·not·ic** \-'nät-ik\ *adj*

ac·ro·der·ma·ti·tis \ˌak-rō-ˌdər-mə-'tīt-əs\ *n* : inflammation of the skin of the extremities

acrodermatitis chron·i·ca atroph·i·cans \-ˌkrän-i-kə-ə-'träf-i-ˌkanz\ *n* : a skin condition of the extremities that is a late manifestation of Lyme disease esp. when untreated and is characterized by erythematous and edematous lesions which tend to become atrophic giving the skin the appearance of wrinkled tissue paper

acrodermatitis en·tero·path·i·ca \-ˌent-ə-rō-'path-i-kə\ *n* : a severe human skin and gastrointestinal disease inherited as a recessive autosomal trait that is characterized by the symptoms of zinc deficiency and clears up when zinc is added to the diet

ac·ro·dyn·ia \ˌak-rō-'din-ē-ə\ *n* : a disease of infants and young children that is an allergic reaction to mercury, is

---

\ə\ **abut** \ᵊ\ **kitten** \ər\ **further** \a\ **ash** \ā\ **ace** \ä\ **cot, cart**
\aú\ **out** \ch\ **chin** \e\ **bet** \ē\ **easy** \g\ **go** \i\ **hit** \ī\ **ice** \j\ **job**
\ŋ\ **sing** \ō\ **go** \ò\ **law** \òi\ **boy** \th\ **thin** \t͟h\ **the** \ü\ **loot**
\ú\ **foot** \y\ **yet** \zh\ **vision** *See also* Pronunciation Symbols page

characterized by dusky pink discoloration of hands and feet with local swelling and intense itching, and is accompanied by insomnia, irritability, and sensitivity to light — called also *erythredema, pink disease, Swift's disease* — **ac·ro·dyn·ic** \-ˈdin-ik\ *adj*

ac·ro·ge·ria \-ˈjer-ē-ə, -ˈjir-\ *n* : looseness and wrinkling of the skin of the hands and feet that is caused by loss of subcutaneous fat and collagen and gives the appearance of premature aging

ac·ro·ker·a·to·sis \-ˌker-ə-ˈtō-səs\ *n, pl* **-to·ses** \-ˌsēz\ : hyperkeratosis of the hands and feet

acro·le·in \ə-ˈkrō-lē-ən\ *n* : a toxic colorless liquid aldehyde C_3H_4O with acrid odor and irritating vapors that polymerizes readily into resins and is used chiefly in organic synthesis (as of methionine) — called also *acrylaldehyde*

[1]ac·ro·me·gal·ic \ˌak-rō-mə-ˈgal-ik\ *adj* : exhibiting acromegaly

[2]acromegalic *n* : one affected with acromegaly

ac·ro·meg·a·loid \ˌak-rō-ˈmeg-ə-ˌlóid\ *adj* : resembling acromegaly ⟨∼ features⟩

ac·ro·meg·a·ly \ˌak-rō-ˈmeg-ə-lē\ *n, pl* **-lies** : a disorder that is caused by chronic overproduction of growth hormone by the pituitary gland and is characterized by a gradual and permanent enlargement of the flat bones (as the lower jaw) and of the hands and feet, abdominal organs, nose, lips, and tongue and that develops after ossification is complete — compare GIGANTISM

acro·mi·al \ə-ˈkrō-mē-əl\ *adj* : of, relating to, or situated near the acromion ⟨an ∼ branch of an artery⟩

acromial process *n* : ACROMION

ac·ro·mi·cria \ˌak-rō-ˈmik-rē-ə, -ˈmīk-\ *n* : abnormal smallness of the extremities

acro·mio·cla·vic·u·lar \ə-ˌkrō-mē-(ˌ)ō-klə-ˈvik-yə-lər\ *adj* : relating to, being, or affecting the joint connecting the acromion and the clavicle ⟨∼ arthritis⟩

acro·mi·on \ə-ˈkrō-mē-ˌän, -ən\ *n* : the outer end of the spine of the scapula that protects the glenoid cavity, forms the outer angle of the shoulder, and articulates with the clavicle — called also *acromial process, acromion process*

acro·mi·on·ec·to·my \ə-ˌkrō-mē-ˌän-ˈek-tə-mē, -mē-ə-ˈnek-\ *n, pl* **-mies** : partial or total surgical excision of the acromion

acromion process *n* : ACROMION

ac·ro·mio·plas·ty \ə-ˌkrō-mē-ō-ˈplas-tē\ *n, pl* **-ties** : excision of the anterior hook of the acromion for the relief of pressure on the rotator cuff produced during movement of the joint between the glenoid cavity and the humerus

acro·pa·chy \ˈak-rō-ˌpak-ē, ə-ˈkräp-ə-kē\ *n, pl* **-pa·chies** : OSTEOARTHROPATHY

ac·ro·par·es·the·sia *or chiefly Brit* **ac·ro·par·aes·the·sia** \ˌak-rō-ˌpar-əs-ˈthē-zh(ē-)ə\ *n* : a condition of burning, tingling, or pricking sensations or numbness in the extremities present on awaking and of unknown cause or produced by compression of nerves during sleep

acrop·a·thy \ə-ˈkräp-ə-thē\ *n, pl* **-thies** : a disease affecting the extremities

ac·ro·phobe \ˈak-rə-ˌfōb\ *n* : an individual affected with acrophobia

ac·ro·pho·bia \ˌak-rə-ˈfō-bē-ə\ *n* : abnormal or pathological dread of being in a high place : fear of heights — **ac·ro·pho·bic** \-bik\ *adj*

ac·ro·sclero·der·ma \ˌak-rō-ˌskler-ə-ˈdər-mə\ *n* : scleroderma affecting the extremities, face, and chest

ac·ro·scle·ro·sis \ˌak-rō-sklə-ˈrō-səs\ *n, pl* **-ro·ses** \-ˌsēz\ : ACROSCLERODERMA

ac·ro·some \ˈak-rə-ˌsōm\ *n* : an anterior prolongation of a spermatozoon that releases egg-penetrating enzymes — **ac·ro·so·mal** \ˌak-rə-ˈsō-məl\ *adj*

ac·ryl·al·de·hyde \ˌak-rə-ˈlal-də-ˌhīd\ *n* : ACROLEIN

ac·ry·late \ˈak-rə-ˌlāt\ *n* **1** : a salt or ester of acrylic acid **2** : ACRYLIC RESIN

[1]acryl·ic \ə-ˈkril-ik\ *adj* : of or relating to acrylic acid or its derivatives ⟨∼ polymers⟩

[2]acrylic *n* : ACRYLIC RESIN

acrylic acid *n* : a synthetic unsaturated liquid acid $C_3H_4O_2$ that polymerizes readily to form useful products (as water=soluble thickening agents)

acrylic resin *n* : a glassy acrylic thermoplastic made by polymerizing acrylic or methacrylic acid or a derivative of either and used for cast and molded parts (as of medical prostheses and dental appliances) or as coatings and adhesives

ac·ry·lo·ni·trile \ˌak-rə-lō-ˈnī-trəl, -ˌtrēl\ *n* : a colorless volatile flammable liquid nitrile C_3H_3N used chiefly in organic synthesis and for polymerization

ACS *abbr* antireticular cytotoxic serum

ACSW *abbr* Academy of Certified Social Workers

[1]act \ˈakt\ *n* **1** : a motor performance leading to a definite result **2** : a dealing with objects (as by moving, perceiving, or desiring them)

[2]act *vi* **1** : to perform an act : BEHAVE **2** : to produce an effect ⟨wait for a medicine to ∼⟩

act *abbr* active

Ac·taea \ak-ˈtē-ə\ *n* : a small genus of white-flowered herbs of the buttercup family (Ranunculaceae) comprising the baneberries and having acrid poisonous berries

ACTH \ˌā-ˌsē-(ˌ)tē-ˈāch\ *n* : a protein hormone of the anterior lobe of the pituitary gland that stimulates the adrenal cortex — called also *adrenocorticotropic hormone*

ac·tin \ˈak-tən\ *n* : a protein found esp. in microfilaments (as those comprising myofibrils) and active in muscular contraction, cellular movement, and maintenance of cell shape — see F-ACTIN, G-ACTIN

ac·tin·ic \ak-ˈtin-ik\ *adj* : of, relating to, resulting from, or exhibiting chemical changes produced by radiant energy esp. in the visible and ultraviolet parts of the spectrum ⟨∼ injury and carcinogenesis —*Jour. Amer. Med. Assoc.*⟩ ⟨∼ keratosis⟩ — **ac·tin·i·cal·ly** \-i-k(ə-)lē\ *adv*

actinic rays *n pl* : radiation (as in the violet and ultraviolet parts of the spectrum) having marked photochemical action

ac·ti·nism \ˈak-tə-ˌniz-əm\ *n* : the actinic property of radiant energy

ac·tin·i·um \ak-ˈtin-ē-əm\ *n* : a radioactive trivalent metallic element that resembles lanthanum in chemical properties and that is found esp. in pitchblende — symbol *Ac*; see ELEMENT table

ac·ti·no·bac·il·lo·sis \ˌak-tə-(ˌ)nō-ˌbas-ə-ˈlō-səs, ak-ˌtin-ō-\ *n, pl* **-lo·ses** \-ˌsēz\ : a disease that affects domestic animals (as cattle and swine) and sometimes humans, resembles actinomycosis, and is caused by a bacterium of the genus *Actinobacillus* (*A. lignieresii*) — see WOODEN TONGUE

ac·ti·no·ba·cil·lus \-bə-ˈsil-əs\ *n* **1** *cap* : a genus of aerobic gram-negative parasitic bacteria of the family Pasteurellaceae forming filaments resembling streptobacilli — see ACTINOBACILLOSIS **2** *pl* **-li** \-ˌī\ : a bacterium of the genus *Actinobacillus*

ac·ti·no·chem·is·try \-ˈkem-ə-strē\ *n, pl* **-tries** : chemistry in its relations to actinism : PHOTOCHEMISTRY

ac·ti·no·der·ma·ti·tis \-ˌdər-mə-ˈtīt-əs\ *n, pl* **-ti·tis·es** *or* **-tit·i·des** \-ˈtit-ə-ˌdēz\ : dermatitis resulting from exposure to sunlight, X-rays, or radiation from radium

ac·ti·no·graph \ak-ˈtin-ə-ˌgraf\ *n* : an instrument for determining the intensity of direct solar radiation

ac·ti·nol·o·gy \ˌak-tə-ˈnäl-ə-jē\ *n, pl* **-gies** : a science that deals with actinism and photochemical effects

ac·ti·nom·e·ter \ˌak-tə-ˈnäm-ət-ər\ *n* : any of various instruments for measuring the intensity of incident radiation; *esp* : one in which the intensity of radiation is measured by the speed of a photochemical reaction — **ac·ti·no·met·ric** \-nō-ˈme-trik\ *adj* — **ac·ti·nom·e·try** \-ˈnäm-ə-trē\ *n, pl* **-tries**

ac·ti·no·my·ces \ˌak-tə-(ˌ)nō-ˈmī-ˌsēz, ak-ˌtin-ō-\ *n* **1** *cap* : a genus of filamentous or rod-shaped gram-positive bacteria of the family Actinomycetaceae that includes usu. commensal and sometimes pathogenic forms inhabiting mucosal surfaces esp. of the oral cavity — compare ACTINOMYCOSIS **2** *pl* **actinomyces** : a bacterium of the genus *Actinomyces* — **ac·ti·no·my·ce·tal** \-ˌmī-ˈsēt-ᵊl\ *adj*

Ac·ti·no·my·ce·ta·ce·ae \-ˌmī-sə-ˈtā-sē-ˌē\ *n pl* : a family of filamentous or rod-shaped bacteria of the order Actinomy-cetales that are often branched, sometimes produce conidia, and sometimes form a mycelium that readily breaks up into bacillary elements

Ac·ti·no·my·ce·ta·les \-ˌmī-sə-'tā-(ˌ)lēz\ *n pl* : an order of fil-amentous or rod-shaped bacteria tending strongly to the de-velopment of branches and true mycelium and lacking pho-tosynthetic pigment — see MYCOBACTERIACEAE, STREPTO-MYCETACEAE

ac·ti·no·my·cete \-'mī-ˌsēt, -mī-'sēt\ *n* : a bacterium (as an actinomyces or a streptomyces) of the order Actinomyceta-les — see ACTINOMYCOSIS — **ac·ti·no·my·ce·tous** \-mī-'sēt-əs\ *adj*

ac·ti·no·my·ce·tin \-ˌmī-'sēt-ᵊn\ *n* : a bacteriolytic fluid sub-stance that is obtained from a soil bacterium of the genus *Streptomyces* (*S. albus*) and that lyses various bacteria (as liv-ing streptococci or heat-killed colon bacilli)

ac·ti·no·my·cin \-'mīs-ᵊn\ *n* : any of various red or yellow=red mostly toxic polypeptide antibiotics isolated from soil bacteria (esp. *Streptomyces antibioticus*); *specif* : one used to inhibit DNA or RNA synthesis

actinomycin D *n* : DACTINOMYCIN

ac·ti·no·my·co·ma \-ˌmī-'kō-mə\ *n, pl* **-mas** *or* **-ma·ta** \-mət-ə\ : the characteristic granulomatous lesion of actinomyco-sis

ac·ti·no·my·co·sis \ˌak-tə-nō-ˌmī-'kō-səs\ *n, pl* **-co·ses** \-ˌsēz\ : infection with or disease caused by actinomyces; *esp* : a chronic disease of cattle, swine, and humans characterized by hard granulomatous masses usu. in the mouth and jaws — see ACTINOMYCOMA — **ac·ti·no·my·cot·ic** \-'kät-ik\ *adj*

ac·ti·non \'ak-tə-ˌnän\ *n* : a gaseous radioactive isotope of ra-don that has a half-life of about four seconds

ac·tin·o·phage \ak-'tin-ə-ˌfāj\ *n* : a bacteriophage that devel-ops in and lyses an actinomycete

ac·ti·no·phy·to·sis \ˌak-tə-(ˌ)nō-ˌfī-'tō-səs, ak-ˌtin-ō-\ *n, pl* **-to·ses** \-ˌsēz\ : STREPTOTRICHOSIS

ac·ti·no·spec·ta·cin \ˌak-tə-(ˌ)nō-'spek-tə-sən, ak-ˌtin-ō-\ *n* : SPECTINOMYCIN

ac·ti·no·ther·a·py \-'ther-ə-pē\ *n, pl* **-pies** : application for therapeutic purposes of the chemically active rays of the electromagnetic spectrum (as ultraviolet light or X-rays)

ac·tion \'ak-shən\ *n* **1** : the process of exerting a force or bringing about an effect that results from the inherent ca-pacity of an agent ⟨protein synthesis is an expression of gene ~⟩ ⟨insecticidal ~⟩ **2** : a function or the performance of a function of the body (as defecation) or of one of its parts ⟨the normal baby has three or four ~s of the bowel in 24 hours —Morris Fishbein⟩ ⟨heart ~⟩ **3** : an act of will **4 actions** *pl* : BEHAVIOR ⟨aggressive ~s⟩

action potential *n* : a momentary reversal in the potential difference across a plasma membrane (as of a nerve cell or muscle fiber) that occurs when a cell has been activated by a stimulus — called also *spike potential;* compare RESTING PO-TENTIAL; see AFTERPOTENTIAL, GENERATOR POTENTIAL, PREPOTENTIAL

ac·ti·vat·ed charcoal \'ak-tə-ˌvā-təd-\ *n* : a highly adsorbent fine black odorless tasteless powdered charcoal used in med-icine esp. as an antidote in many forms of poisoning and as an antiflatulent

ac·ti·va·tion energy \ˌak-tə-'vā-shən-\ *n* : the minimum amount of energy required to convert a normal stable mole-cule into a reactive molecule — called also *energy of activa-tion*

ac·ti·va·tor \'ak-tə-ˌvāt-ər\ *n* **1** : a substance (as a chloride ion) that increases the activity of an enzyme — compare CO-ENZYME **2** : a substance given off by developing tissue that stimulates differentiation of adjacent tissue; *also* : a struc-ture giving off such a stimulant

ac·tive \'ak-tiv\ *adj* **1** : capable of acting or reacting esp. in some specific way ⟨an ~ enzyme⟩ ⟨~ nitrogen⟩ **2** : tend-ing to progress or to cause degeneration ⟨~ tuberculosis⟩ **3** : exhibiting optical activity **4** : requiring the expenditure of energy ⟨~ calcium ion uptake⟩ — **ac·tive·ly** *adv*

active immunity *n* : usu. long-lasting immunity that is ac-

quired through production of antibodies within the organ-ism in response to the presence of antigens — compare AC-QUIRED IMMUNITY, NATURAL IMMUNITY, PASSIVE IMMUNI-TY

active site *n* : a region esp. of a biologically active protein (as an enzyme) where catalytic activity takes place and whose shape permits the binding only of a specific reactant mole-cule

active transport *n* : movement of a chemical substance by the expenditure of energy against a gradient in concentra-tion or electrical potential across a plasma membrane

ac·tiv·i·ty \ak-'tiv-ət-ē\ *n, pl* **-ties** **1** : natural or normal function: as **a** : a process (as digestion) that an organism carries on or participates in by virtue of being alive **b** : a similar process actually or potentially involving mental func-tion; *specif* : an educational procedure designed to stimulate learning by firsthand experience **2** : the characteristic of acting chemically or of promoting a chemical reaction ⟨the ~ of a catalyst⟩

ac·to·my·o·sin \ˌak-tə-'mī-ə-sən\ *n* : a viscous contractile complex of actin and myosin concerned together with ATP in muscular contraction

Ac·tos \'ak-ˌtōz\ *trademark* — used for a preparation of the hydrochloride of pioglitazone

act out \(')akt-'aút\ *vt* : to express (as an impulse or a fantasy) directly in overt behavior without modification to comply with social norms ⟨*act out* an adolescent fantasy⟩ ~ *vi* : to behave badly or in a socially unacceptable often self=defeating manner esp. as a means of venting painful emo-tions (as fear or frustration)

ac·tu·al cautery \'ak-ch(ə-w)əl-, 'aksh-wəl-\ *n* : an agent (as a hot iron, electrocautery, or moxa) used to destroy tissue by heat — called also *thermocautery;* compare POTENTIAL CAU-TERY

actual neurosis *n* : a neurosis characterized by hypochon-driacal complaints or somatic manifestations held by Freud to be caused by sexual disturbances — compare PSYCHO-NEUROSIS

Ac·u·ar·ia \ˌak-yə-'war-ē-ə\ *n* : a genus of spiruroid nema-todes including destructive parasites found in the gizzard walls of gallinaceous birds and having intermediate stages in insects (as grasshoppers) or crustaceans

acu·ity \ə-'kyü-ət-ē\ *n, pl* **-ities** : keenness of sense perception ⟨~ of hearing⟩ — see VISUAL ACUITY

acu·le·ate \ə-'kyü-lē-ət\ *adj* : having a sting ⟨~ insects⟩

acuminata — see VERRUCA ACUMINATA

acu·mi·nate \ə-'kyü-mə-nət\ *adj* : tapering to a slender point

acuminatum — see CONDYLOMA ACUMINATUM

acu·pres·sure \'ak-(y)ə-ˌpresh-ər\ *n* : the application of pres-sure (as with the thumbs or fingertips) to the same discrete points on the body stimulated in acupuncture that is used for its therapeutic effects (as the relief of tension or pain) — see SHIATSU — **acu·pres·sur·ist** \-ˌpresh-ə-rəst\ *n*

acu·punc·ture \-ˌpəŋ(k)-chər\ *n* : an orig. Chinese practice of inserting fine needles through the skin at specific points esp. to cure disease or relieve pain (as in surgery)

acu·punc·tur·ist \-ˌpəŋ(k)-chə-rəst\ *n* : a person who spe-cializes in treatment by the use of acupuncture

acu·sec·tor \'ak-yü-ˌsek-tər, -ˌtó(ə)r\ *n* : RADIO KNIFE

acustica — see MACULA ACUSTICA

acuta — see PITYRIASIS LICHENOIDES ET VARIOLIFORMIS ACUTA

acute \ə-'kyüt\ *adj* **1** : sensing or perceiving accurately, clearly, effectively, or sensitively ⟨~ vision⟩ **2 a** : charac-terized by sharpness or severity ⟨~ pain⟩ ⟨an ~ infection⟩ **b** (1) : having a sudden onset, sharp rise, and short course ⟨an ~ disease⟩ ⟨an ~ inflammation⟩ — compare CHRONIC 2a (2) : ACUTE CARE ⟨an ~ hospital⟩ **c** : lasting a short time ⟨~ experiments⟩ — **acute·ly** *adv* — **acute·ness** *n*

\ə\ **abut** \ᵊ\ **kitten** \ər\ **further** \a\ **ash** \ā\ **ace** \ä\ **cot, cart** \aú\ **out** \ch\ **chin** \e\ **bet** \ē\ **easy** \g\ **go** \i\ **hit** \ī\ **ice** \j\ **job** \ŋ\ **sing** \ō\ **go** \ó\ **law** \ói\ **boy** \th\ **thin** \t͟h\ **the** \ü\ **loot** \ú\ **foot** \y\ **yet** \zh\ **vision** *See also* Pronunciation Symbols page

acute abdomen *n* : an acute internal abdominal condition requiring immediate operation

acute care *adj* : providing or concerned with short-term medical care esp. for serious acute disease or trauma ⟨*acute care* hospitals⟩ ⟨an *acute care* nursing unit⟩ — compare CHRONIC CARE, INTENSIVE CARE — **acute care** *n*

acute disseminated encephalomyelitis *n* : an acute disease of the brain and spinal cord with variable symptoms that is thought to be an allergic or immune response following infectious disease or vaccination

acute febrile neutrophilic dermatosis *n* : SWEET'S SYNDROME

acute lymphoblastic leukemia *n* : lymphocytic leukemia that is marked by an abnormal increase in the number of lymphoblasts, that is characterized by rapid onset and progression of symptoms which include fever, anemia, pallor, fatigue, appetite loss, bleeding, thrombocytopenia, granulocytopenia, bone and joint pain, and enlargement of the lymph nodes, liver, and spleen, and that occurs chiefly during childhood — abbr. *ALL;* compare CHRONIC LYMPHOCYTIC LEUKEMIA

acute lymphocytic leukemia *n* : ACUTE LYMPHOBLASTIC LEUKEMIA — abbr. *ALL*

acute myelogenous leukemia *n* : myelogenous leukemia that is marked by an abnormal increase in the number of myeloblasts esp. in bone marrow and blood, that is characterized by symptoms similar to those of acute lymphoblastic leukemia, and that may occur either in childhood or adulthood — abbr. *AML;* called also *acute myeloblastic leukemia, acute myelocytic leukemia, acute myeloid leukemia;* see ACUTE NONLYMPHOCYTIC LEUKEMIA; compare CHRONIC MYELOGENOUS LEUKEMIA

acute necrotizing ulcerative gingivitis *n* : a progressive painful disease of the mouth that is marked esp. by dirty gray ulceration of the mucous membranes, spontaneous hemorrhaging of the gums, and a foul odor to the breath and that is associated with the presence of large numbers of Vincent's organisms — called also *fusospirochetosis, necrotizing ulcerative gingivitis, trench mouth, Vincent's infection*

acute nonlymphocytic leukemia *n* : any of several forms of myelogenous leukemia marked by an abnormal increase in the number of immature white blood cells (as monoblasts, myeloblasts, or promyelocytes) that are not of the same lineage as B cells and T cells and occur esp. in the blood and bone marrow; *esp* : ACUTE MYELOGENOUS LEUKEMIA

acute respiratory distress syndrome *n* : ADULT RESPIRATORY DISTRESS SYNDROME

acute yellow atrophy *n* : a severe usu. fatal disorder in which the liver degenerates and is reduced in size as a result of toxic chemicals, infection, or other agents

acy·a·not·ic \ˌā-ˌsī-ə-ˈnät-ik\ *adj* : characterized by the absence of cyanosis ⟨~ patients⟩ ⟨~ heart disease⟩

acy·clic \(ˈ)ā-ˈsī-klik, -ˈsik-lik\ *adj* 1 : not occurring in periods or cycles ⟨~ gonadotropin secretion⟩ 2 : having an open-chain structure; *esp* : ALIPHATIC ⟨an ~ compound⟩

acy·clo·vir \ā-ˈsī-klō-ˌvir\ *n* : a cyclic nucleoside $C_8H_{11}N_5O_3$ used esp. to treat shingles, genital herpes, and chicken pox — see ZOVIRAX

ac·yl \ˈas-əl, -ēl; ˈā-səl\ *n* : a radical derived usu. from an organic acid by removal of the hydroxyl from all acid groups

ac·yl·al \ˈas-əl-ˌlal, ˈā-sə-\ *n* : an acid derivative of an aldehyde or a ketone containing the group $>C(OOCR)_2$ or $>C(OR)OOCR$

ac·yl·ase \-ˌlās, -ˌlāz\ *n* : any of several enzymes that hydrolyze acylated amino acids

¹**ac·yl·ate** \-ˌlāt\ *vt* **-at·ed; -at·ing** : to introduce an acyl group into — **ac·y·la·tion** \ˌas-ə-ˈlā-shən, ˌā-sə-\ *n*

²**ac·yl·ate** \ˈas-ə-ˌlāt, ˈā-sə-lət\ *n* : a salt or ester of an organic acid ⟨titanium ~s⟩

acys·tic \(ˈ)ā-ˈsis-tik\ *adj* : not enclosed in a bladder ⟨~ tapeworm larvae⟩

AD *abbr* 1 Alzheimer's disease 2 average deviation

ADA *abbr* 1 adenosine deaminase 2 American Dietetic Association

adac·tyl·ia \ˌā-ˌdak-ˈtil-ē-ə\ *n* : congenital lack of fingers or toes

adac·ty·lous \(ˈ)ā-ˈdak-tə-ləs\ *adj* : being without fingers or toes

Ad·a·lat \ˈad-ə-ˌlat\ *trademark* — used for a preparation of nifedipine

ad·a·man·tine \ˌad-ə-ˈman-ˌtēn, -ˌtīn, -ˈmant-ᵊn\ *adj* : characterized by extreme hardness or luster

ad·a·man·ti·no·ma \ˌad-ə-ˌmant-ᵊn-ˈō-mə\ *n, pl* **-mas** *also* **-ma·ta** \-ˌmət-ə\ : AMELOBLASTOMA — **ad·a·man·ti·no·ma·tous** \ˌad-ə-ˌmant-ᵊn-ˈäm-ət-əs, -ˈōm-\ *adj*

ad·a·man·to·blast \ˌad-ə-ˈmant-ə-ˌblast\ *n* : AMELOBLAST

ad·a·man·to·blas·to·ma \ˌad-ə-ˌmant-ə-ˌblа-ˈstō-mə\ *n, pl* **-mas** *also* **-ma·ta** \-ˌmət-ə\ : AMELOBLASTOMA

Ad·am's ap·ple \ˌad-əm-ˈzap-əl\ *n* : the projection in the front of the neck that is formed by the thyroid cartilage and is particularly prominent in males

Adam, biblical character. According to the Bible, Adam was the first man, the husband of Eve, and later the father of Cain and Abel. Adam and Eve lived in the garden of Eden until they ate a forbidden fruit, traditionally held to be an apple. As a punishment they were expelled from Eden. Adam lived a total of 930 years. The term *Adam's apple* arose through a misinterpretation of the Hebrew for "protuberance on man" used to denote this anatomical part. The late Hebrew word for protuberance is very similar to the word for apple, and Adam in Hebrew can refer to "man" in general as well as the biblical figure. Thus the expression was misinterpreted, perhaps owing to the association of Adam with apples.

ad·ams·ite \ˈad-əm-ˌzīt\ *n* : a yellow crystalline arsenical $C_{12}H_9AsCIN$ used as a respiratory irritant in some forms of tear gas — called also *diphenylaminechlorarsine*

Adams, Roger (1889–1971), American chemist. One of the foremost organic chemists of his day, Adams is remembered for determining the chemical composition of several natural substances. He analyzed chaulmoogra oil, the toxic cottonseed pigment gossypol, marijuana, and many alkaloids. He was the first American chemist to produce butacaine and procaine. He also worked in stereochemistry and with platinum catalysts and on the synthesis of medicinal compounds. He developed the poisonous gas adamsite for the U.S. Army during World War I, but the war ended before it could be used.

Adams–Stokes attack *n* : STOKES-ADAMS SYNDROME

R. Adams — see STOKES-ADAMS SYNDROME

J. Stokes — see CHEYNE-STOKES RESPIRATION

Adams–Stokes disease *n* : STOKES-ADAMS SYNDROME

Adams–Stokes syndrome *n* : STOKES-ADAMS SYNDROME

Ad·an·so·nia \ˌad-ᵊn-ˈsō-nē-ə, ˌad-ˌan-, -nyə\ *n* : a genus of trees (family Bombacaceae) having palmately divided leaves, white pendent flowers, and capsular fruits — see BAOBAB

Adan·son \à-däⁿ-sōⁿ, ˈad-ᵊn-sən\, **Michel (1727–1806),** French naturalist. Adanson played a major, although unrecognized, role in introducing modern statistical methods into systematic botany. In 1763–64 he published *Familles des plantes* in which he proposed a system of plant classification and nomenclature based on many characters instead of a few selected ones. Although the system enjoyed a period of usage, it was superseded by the Linnaean system.

adapt \ə-ˈdapt\ *vt* : to make fit (as for a specific or new use or situation) often by modification ⟨~ed himself to the new position⟩ ~ *vi* : to become adapted : undergo adaptation

ad·ap·ta·tion \ˌad-əp-ˈtā-shən, -ˌap-\ *n* 1 : the act or process of adapting : the state of being adapted ⟨his ingenious ~ of the electric cautery knife to . . . surgery —George Blumer⟩ 2 : adjustment to environmental conditions: as **a** : adjustment of a sense organ to the intensity or quality of stimulation **b** : modification of an organism or its parts that makes it more fit for existence under the conditions of its environment — compare ADJUSTMENT 1b — **ad·ap·ta·tion·al** \-shnəl, -shən-ᵊl\ *adj* — **ad·ap·ta·tion·al·ly** \-ē\ *adv*

adapt·er *also* **adap·tor** \ə-ˈdap-tər\ *n* 1 : one that adapts 2

a : a device for connecting two parts (as of different diameters) of an apparatus **b** : an attachment for adapting apparatus for uses not orig. intended

adapter RNA *or* **adaptor RNA** *n* : TRANSFER RNA

adap·tive \ə-'dap-tiv\ *adj* : capable of, suited to, or contributing to adaptation ⟨∼ traits that enhance survival —*Science News*⟩ — **adap·tive·ly** *adv* — **adap·tive·ness** *n*

adaptive radiation *n* : evolutionary diversification of a generalized ancestral form with production of a number of adaptively specialized forms

ad·ap·tom·e·ter \ad-ˌap-'täm-ət-ər\ *n* : a device for determining the efficiency of dark adaptation in the human eye — **ad·ap·tom·e·try** \-'täm-ə-trē\ *n, pl* **-tries**

ADC *abbr* aid to dependent children

add *abbr* adduction; adductor

ADD *abbr* attention deficit disorder

ad·der \'ad-ər\ *n* **1** : the common venomous European viper of the genus *Vipera* (*V. berus*); *broadly* : a terrestrial viper of the family Viperidae **2** : any of several No. American snakes (as the hognose snakes) that are harmless but are popularly believed to be venomous

¹ad·dict \ə-'dikt\ *vt* : to cause (a person) to become physiologically dependent upon a substance

²ad·dict \'ad-(ˌ)ikt\ *n* : one who is addicted to a substance

ad·dic·tion \ə-'dik-shən\ *n* : compulsive physiological need for and use of a habit-forming substance (as heroin, nicotine, or alcohol) characterized by tolerance and by well-defined physiological symptoms upon withdrawal; *broadly* : persistent compulsive use of a substance known by the user to be physically, psychologically, or socially harmful — compare HABITUATION

ad·dic·tive \ə-'dik-tiv\ *adj* : causing or characterized by addiction ⟨∼ drugs⟩

Ad·dis count \'ad-ə-ˌskaůnt\ *n* : a technique for the quantitative determination of cells, casts, and protein in a 12-hour urine sample used in the diagnosis and treatment of kidney disease

Addis, Thomas (1881–1949), American physician. Addis is most notable for his work in pathology and in particular for the study of kidney function. In 1925 he presented his method for counting cells in urinary sediments. The resultant figure is used to diagnose pathological conditions in the kidney and is now known as the Addis count. He is also known for his test, first reported in 1922, for determining the specific gravity of the urine. Addis's other areas of research included blood coagulation, hemophilia, plasma, and glycosuria.

Ad·di·so·ni·an \ˌad-ə-'sō-nē-ən, -nyən\ *adj* : of, relating to, or affected with Addison's disease ⟨∼ crisis⟩ ⟨∼ patient⟩

Addison, Thomas (1793–1860), English physician. Regarded as the father of modern endocrinology, Addison inaugurated the study of internal secretion and the endocrine glands. With John Morgan, he wrote the first book in English on the action of poisons in the living body, and he was the first to use static electricity in the treatment of spasmodic diseases. In 1849 he published a preliminary description of adrenocortical insufficiency. In an 1855 monograph he gave a full, classic description of this syndrome and an equally classic description of pernicious anemia. Shortly afterward, the French physician Armand Trousseau named these two diseases Addison's disease and addisonian anemia. Addison also produced original and significant works on tuberculosis, pneumonia, and skin disease.

addisonian anemia *n, often cap 1st A* : PERNICIOUS ANEMIA

Ad·di·son's anemia \'ad-ə-sənz-\ *n* : PERNICIOUS ANEMIA

Addison's disease *n* : a destructive disease marked by deficient adrenocortical secretion and characterized by extreme weakness, loss of weight, low blood pressure, gastrointestinal disturbances, and brownish pigmentation of the skin and mucous membranes

¹ad·di·tive \'ad-ət-iv\ *adj* : having or relating to a value or effect that is the sum of individual values or effects: as **a** : relating to the sum of the pharmacological responses produced by the concurrent administration of two or more

drugs capable of producing the same kind of effect **b** : having a genetic effect that is the sum of the individual effects — **ad·di·tive·ly** *adv* — **ad·di·tiv·i·ty** \ˌad-ə-'tiv-ət-ē\ *n, pl* **-ties**

²additive *n* : a substance added to another in relatively small amounts to effect a desired change in properties; *esp* : an agent added to a foodstuff to improve color, flavor, texture, or keeping qualities

ad·du·cent \ə-'d(y)üs-ᵊnt, a-\ *adj* : serving to adduct ⟨an ∼ muscle⟩ — compare ABDUCENT

¹ad·duct \ə-'dəkt, a-\ *vt* : to draw (as a limb) toward or past the median axis of the body; *also* : to bring together (similar parts) ⟨∼ the fingers⟩ — **ad·duc·tive** \-'dək-tiv\ *adj*

²ad·duct \'ad-ˌəkt\ *n* : a chemical addition product

ad·duc·tion \ə-'dək-shən, a-\ *n* : the action of adducting : the state of being adducted

ad·duc·tor \-'dək-tər\ *n* **1** : any of three powerful triangular muscles that contribute to the adduction of the human thigh: **a** : one arising from the superior ramus of the pubis and inserted into the middle third of the linea aspera — called also *adductor longus* **b** : one arising from the inferior ramus of the pubis and inserted into the iliopectineal line and the upper part of the linea aspera — called also *adductor brevis* **c** : one arising from the inferior ramus of the pubis and the ischium and inserted behind the first two into the linea aspera — called also *adductor magnus* **2** : any of several muscles other than the adductors of the thigh that draw a part toward the median line of the body or toward the axis of an extremity

adductor brev·is \-'brev-əs\ *n* : ADDUCTOR 1b

adductor hal·lu·cis \-'hal-(y)ə-səs, -'hal-ə-kəs\ *n* : a muscle of the foot that adducts and flexes the big toe and helps to support the arch of the foot — called also *adductor hallucis muscle*

adductor lon·gus \-'lòn-gəs\ *n* : ADDUCTOR 1a

adductor mag·nus \-'mag-nəs\ *n* : ADDUCTOR 1c

adductor pol·li·cis \-'päl-ə-səs, -ə-kəs\ *n* : a muscle of the hand with two heads that adducts the thumb by bringing it toward the palm — called also *adductor pollicis muscle*

adductor tubercle *n* : a tubercle on the proximal part of the medial epicondyle of the femur that is the site of insertion of the adductor magnus

ad·e·nase \'ad-ᵊn-ˌās, -ˌāz\ *n* : an enzyme found esp. in animal tissue (as liver) that hydrolyzes adenine to hypoxanthine and ammonia

aden·drit·ic \ˌā-den-'drit-ik\ *adj* : lacking dendrites ⟨∼ melanocytes⟩

aden·i·form \ə-'den-ə-ˌfórm, -'dēn-\ *adj* : resembling a gland

ad·e·nine \'ad-ᵊn-ˌēn\ *n* : a purine base $C_5H_5N_5$ that codes hereditary information in the genetic code in DNA and RNA — compare CYTOSINE, GUANINE, THYMINE, URACIL

adenine arabinoside *n* : VIDARABINE

ad·e·ni·tis \ˌad-ᵊn-'īt-əs\ *n* : inflammation of a gland; *esp* : LYMPHADENITIS

ad·e·no·ac·an·tho·ma \ˌad-ᵊn-(ˌ)ō-ˌak-ˌan-'thō-mə\ *n, pl* **-mas** *also* **-ma·ta** \-mət-ə\ : an adenocarcinoma with epithelial cells differentiated and proliferated into squamous cells

ad·e·no·car·ci·no·ma \-ˌkärs-ᵊn-'ō-mə\ *n, pl* **-mas** *also* **-ma·ta** \-mət-ə\ : a malignant tumor originating in glandular epithelium — **ad·e·no·car·ci·no·ma·tous** \-mət-əs\ *adj*

ad·e·no·cys·to·ma \-sis-'tō-mə\ *n, pl* **-mas** *also* **-ma·ta** \-mət-ə\ : an adenoma with a tendency to cyst formation

ad·e·no·fi·bro·ma \-ˌfī-'brō-mə\ *n, pl* **-mas** *also* **-ma·ta** \-mət-ə\ : a benign tumor of glandular and fibrous tissue

ad·e·no·hy·poph·y·sis \-hī-'päf-ə-səs, *n, pl* **-y·ses** \-ə-ˌsēz\ : the anterior part of the pituitary gland that is derived from the embryonic pharynx and is primarily glandular in nature — called also *anterior lobe;* compare NEUROHYPOPHYSIS —

\ə\ **abut** \ᵊ\ **kitten** \ər\ **further** \a\ **ash** \ā\ **ace** \ä\ **cot, cart** \aů\ **out** \ch\ **chin** \e\ **bet** \ē\ **easy** \g\ **go** \i\ **hit** \ī\ **ice** \j\ **job** \ŋ\ **sing** \ō\ **go** \ò\ **law** \ói\ **boy** \th\ **thin** \th̲\ **the** \ü\ **loot** \ů\ **foot** \y\ **yet** \zh\ **vision** *See also* Pronunciation Symbols page

ad·e·no·hy·poph·y·se·al \-(ˌ)hī-ˌpäf-ə-ˈsē-əl\ *or* ad·e·no·hy·po·phys·i·al \-ˌhī-pə-ˈfiz-ē-əl\ *adj*

¹ad·e·noid \ˈad-ᵊn-ˌóid, ˈad-ˌnóid\ *adj* **1** : of, like, or relating to glands or glandular tissue; *esp* : like or belonging to lymphoid tissue **2** : of or relating to the adenoids ⟨in the ~ region of the pharynx⟩ **3 a** : of, relating to, or affected with abnormally enlarged adenoids ⟨a severe ~ condition⟩ ⟨an ~ patient⟩ **b** : characteristic of one affected with abnormally enlarged adenoids ⟨~ facies⟩

²adenoid *n* **1** : an abnormally enlarged mass of lymphoid tissue at the back of the pharynx characteristically obstructing the nasal and ear passages and inducing mouth breathing, nasality, postnasal discharge, and dullness of facial expression — usu. used in pl. **2** : PHARYNGEAL TONSIL

ad·e·noi·dal \ˌad-ᵊn-ˈóid-ᵊl\ *adj* : exhibiting the characteristics (as snoring, mouth breathing, and voice nasality) of one affected with abnormally enlarged adenoids : ADENOID — not usu. used technically

ad·e·noid·ec·to·my \ˌad-ᵊn-ˌói-ˈdek-tə-mē\ *n, pl* **-mies** : surgical removal of the adenoids

ad·e·noid·ism \ˈad-ᵊn-ˌói-ˌdiz-əm\ *n* : a group of symptoms (as an adenoid facies) associated with the presence of enlarged adenoids

ad·e·noid·itis \ˌad-ᵊn-ˌói-ˈdīt-əs\ *n* : inflammation of the adenoids

ad·e·no·lym·pho·cele \ˌad-ᵊn-(ˌ)ō-ˈlim(p)-fə-ˌsēl\ *n* : dilation of lymph nodes or vessels caused by an obstruction

ad·e·no·lym·pho·ma \-lim-ˈfō-mə\ *n, pl* **-mas** *also* **-ma·ta** \-mət-ə\ : a tumor of the salivary glands characterized by transformation into and proliferation of squamous tissue and increase of ectopic lymphoid tissue

ad·e·no·ma \ˌad-ᵊn-ˈō-mə\ *n, pl* **-mas** *also* **-ma·ta** \-mət-ə\ : a benign tumor of a glandular structure or of glandular origin — ad·e·no·ma·tous \-mət-əs\ *adj*

ad·e·no·ma·toid \ˌad-ᵊn-ˈō-mə-ˌtóid\ *adj* : relating to or resembling an adenoma ⟨~ tumors of the fallopian tube⟩

ad·e·no·ma·to·sis \ˌad-ᵊn-ˌō-mə-ˈtō-səs\ *n, pl* **-to·ses** \-ˌsēz\ : a condition marked by multiple growths consisting of glandular tissue

ad·e·no·mere \ˈad-ᵊn-(ˌ)ō-ˌmi(ə)r\ *n* : the part of a developing gland destined to become responsible for its functioning

ad·e·no·my·o·ma \ˌad-ᵊn-(ˌ)ō-ˌmī-ˈō-mə\ *n, pl* **-mas** *also* **-ma·ta** \-mət-ə\ : a benign tumor composed of muscular and glandular elements

ad·e·no·my·o·sis \-ˌmī-ˈō-səs\ *n, pl* **-o·ses** \-ˌsēz\ : endometriosis esp. when the endometrial tissue invades the myometrium

ad·e·no·neu·ral \-ˈn(y)ùr-əl\ *adj* : of or relating to a gland and nerve ⟨~ junction⟩

ad·e·nop·a·thy \ˌad-ᵊn-ˈäp-ə-thē, ˌad-ə-ˈnäp-\ *n, pl* **-thies** : any disease or enlargement involving glandular tissue; *esp* : one involving lymph nodes ⟨cervical ~⟩

aden·o·sine \ə-ˈden-ə-ˌsēn, -sən\ *n* : a nucleoside $C_{10}H_{13}N_5O_4$ that is a constituent of RNA yielding adenine and ribose on hydrolysis

adenosine deaminase *n* : an enzyme which catalyzes the conversion of adenosine to inosine and whose deficiency causes a form of severe combined immunodeficiency disease as a result of the accumulation of toxic metabolites which inhibit DNA synthesis — abbr. *ADA*

adenosine diphosphate *n* : ADP

adenosine mo·no·phos·phate \-ˌmän-ə-ˈfäs-ˌfāt, -ˌmō-nə-\ *n* : AMP

adenosine phosphate *n* : any of three phosphates of adenosine: **a** : AMP **b** : ADP **c** : ATP

adenosine 3′,5′–monophosphate \-ˌthrē-ˌfīv-\ *n* : CYCLIC AMP

adenosine tri·phos·pha·tase \-trī-ˈfäs-fə-ˌtās, -ˌtāz\ *n* : ATPASE

adenosine tri·phos·phate \-trī-ˈfäs-ˌfāt\ *n* : ATP

ad·e·no·sis \ˌad-ᵊn-ˈō-səs\ *n, pl* **-no·ses** \-ˌsēz\ : a disease of glandular tissue; *esp* : one involving abnormal proliferation or occurrence of glandular tissue ⟨vaginal ~⟩

S–aden·o·syl·me·thi·o·nine *also* aden·o·syl·me·thi·o·nine \(ˌ)es-)ə-ˌden-ə-ˌsil-mə-ˈthī-ə-ˌnēn, (ˌes-)ˌad-ᵊn-ə-ˌsil-\ *n* : the active sulfonium form of methionine $C_{15}H_{22}N_6O_5S$ that acts as a methyl group donor in various biochemical transmethylation reactions (as the formation of epinephrine or creatine), that is formed when methionine reacts with ATP, and that is an intermediate in the formation of homocysteine — see SAME

ad·e·no·tome \ˈad-ᵊn-(ˌ)ō-ˌtōm\ *n* : an instrument for the surgical excision of the adenoids

ad·e·not·o·my \ˌad-ᵊn-ˈät-ə-mē\ *n, pl* **-mies** : the operation of dissecting, incising, or removing a gland and esp. the adenoids

Ad·e·no·vi·ri·dae \ˌad-ᵊn-ō-ˈvir-ə-ˌdē\ *n pl* : a family of double-stranded DNA viruses shaped like a 20-sided polyhedron, orig. identified in human adenoid tissue, causing infections (as pharyngoconjunctival fever) of the respiratory system, conjunctiva, and gastrointestinal tract, and including some capable of inducing malignant tumors in experimental animals

ad·e·no·vi·rus \ˌad-ᵊn-ō-ˈvī-rəs\ *n* : any of the family *Adenoviridae* of double-stranded DNA viruses — ad·e·no·vi·ral \-rəl\ *adj*

ad·e·nyl \ˈad-ᵊn-il\ *n* : a monovalent radical $C_5H_4N_5$ derived from adenine

ade·nyl·ate cyclase \ə-ˌden-ᵊl-ət-, ˌad-ᵊn-(ˌ)il-, -ˌāt-\ *n* : an enzyme that catalyzes the formation of cyclic AMP from ATP

ad·e·nyl cyclase \ˌad-ᵊn-il-\ *n* : ADENYLATE CYCLASE

ad·e·nyl·ic acid \ˌad-ᵊn-il-ik-\ *n* : AMP

ad·eps \ˈad-ˌeps\ *n, pl* ad·i·pes \ˈad-ə-ˌpēz\ : purified internal abdominal fat of the hog used in pharmacy in the preparation of ointments — called also *lard*

adeps la·nae \-ˈlä-(ˌ)nē, -ˈlä-ˌnī\ *n, pl* adipes lanae : LANOLIN

ADH *abbr* antidiuretic hormone

ADHD *abbr* attention-deficit/hyperactivity disorder

ad·here \ad-ˈhi(ə)r, əd-\ *vb* ad·hered; ad·her·ing *vi* **1** : to hold fast or stick by or as if by gluing, suction, grasping, or fusing ⟨a gauze bandage *adhering* to the wound⟩ **2** : to become joined (as in pathological adhesion) ⟨the lung sometimes ~s to the pleura⟩ ~ *vt* : to cause to stick fast — ad·her·ence \-ˈhir-ən(t)s\ *n*

ad·he·sion \ad-ˈhē-zhən, əd-\ *n* **1** : the action or state of adhering; *specif* : a sticking together of substances (as of glue and wood or of parts united by growth) **2 a** : the abnormal union of surfaces normally separate by the formation of new fibrous tissue resulting from an inflammatory process; *also* : the newly formed uniting tissue ⟨pleural ~s⟩ **b** : the union of wound edges esp. by first intention **3** : the molecular attraction exerted between the surfaces of bodies in contact — compare COHESION 2 — ad·he·sion·al \-ˈhēzh-nəl, -ˈhē-zhən-ᵊl\ *adj*

¹ad·he·sive \-ˈhē-siv, -ziv\ *adj* **1 a** : tending to adhere or cause adherence ⟨~ resins⟩ **b** : prepared for adhering ⟨an ~ bandage⟩ **2** : characterized by adhesions ⟨~ inflammation⟩ — ad·he·sive·ly *adv*

²adhesive *n* **1** : an adhesive substance; *esp* : a substance (as glue, starch, paste, or mucilage) that bonds two materials together by adhering to the surface of each **2** : ADHESIVE TAPE

adhesive capsulitis *n* : FROZEN SHOULDER

adhesive pericarditis *n* : pericarditis in which adhesions form between the two layers of pericardium — see ACCRETIO CORDIS, CONCRETIO CORDIS

adhesive tape *n* : tape coated on one side with an adhesive mixture; *esp* : one used for covering wounds

adi·a·do·ko·ki·ne·sis *or* adi·a·do·cho·ki·ne·sis \ˌad-ē-ˌad-ə-ˌkō-kə-ˈnē-səs, ə-ˌdī-ə-ˌdō-(ˌ)kō-, -kī-ˈnē-\ *n, pl* **-ne·ses** \-ˌsēz\ : inability to make movements exhibiting a rapid change of motion (as in quickly rotating the wrist one way and then the other) due to cerebellar dysfunction — compare DYSDIADOCHOKINESIA

Ad·i·an·tum \ˌad-ē-ˈant-əm\ *n* : a genus of ferns (family Polypodiaceae) with delicate palmately branched fronds comprising the maidenhair ferns and including two No.

American forms (*A. pedatum* and the Venushair *A. capillus-veneris*) that have been used in the preparation of expectorants and demulcents

ad·i·ence \'ad-ē-ən(t)s\ *n* : a tendency to approach or accept a stimulus object or situation — compare ABIENCE

ad·i·ent \-ənt\ *adj* : characterized by adience ⟨∼ behavior⟩ — compare ABIENT

Ad·ie's syndrome \'ā-dēz-\ *or* **Ad·ie syn·drome** \-dē-\ *n* : a neurologic syndrome that affects esp. women between 20 and 40 and is characterized by an abnormally dilated pupil, absent or diminished light reflexes of the eye, abnormal accommodation, and lack of ankle-jerk and knee-jerk reflexes

Adie \'ā-dē\, **William John (1886–1935),** British neurologist. Adie was on the staff at Charing Cross Hospital, Royal London Ophthalmic Hospital, and London's National Hospital for Nervous Diseases. He described the neurological disorder now known as Adie's syndrome in 1931. He is also remembered for his description of a kind of idiopathic narcolepsy and for the chapters on diseases of the nervous system that he contributed to medical textbooks.

Adin·i·da \ə-'din-ə-də\ *n pl* : a suborder of primitive flagellate protozoans of the order Dinoflagellata having two flagella but lacking a transverse groove — **adin·i·dan** \-dən\ *adj or n*

adipes *pl of* ADEPS

adipes lanae *pl of* ADEPS LANAE

ad·i·phen·ine \ˌad-i-'fen-ˌēn\ *n* : an antispasmodic drug administered in the form of its hydrochloride $C_{20}H_{25}NO_2 \cdot HCl$ — see TRASENTINE

adip·ic acid \ə-'dip-ik-\ *n* : a white crystalline dicarboxylic acid $C_6H_{10}O_4$ formed by oxidation of various fats and also made synthetically for use esp. in the manufacture of nylon

ad·i·po·cere \'ad-ə-pə-ˌsi(ə)r\ *n* : a waxy or unctuous brownish substance consisting chiefly of fatty acids and calcium soaps produced by chemical changes affecting dead body fat and muscle long buried or immersed in moisture — **ad·i·poc·er·ous** \ˌad-ə-'päs-(ə-)rəs, -pə-'sir-əs\ *adj*

ad·i·po·cyte \'ad-ə-pə-ˌsīt\ *n* : FAT CELL

ad·i·po·gen·e·sis \ˌad-ə-pō-'jen-ə-səs\ *n, pl* **-e·ses** \-ˌsēz\ : the formation of fat or fatty tissue

ad·i·po·ge·net·ic \ˌad-ə-(ˌ)pō-jə-'net-ik\ *adj* : fat-producing

ad·i·pose \'ad-ə-ˌpōs\ *adj* : of or relating to fat; *broadly* : FAT

adipose tissue *n* : connective tissue in which fat is stored and which has the cells distended by droplets of fat

ad·i·po·sis \ˌad-ə-'pō-səs\ *n, pl* **-po·ses** \-ˌsēz\ **1** : ADIPOSITY, OBESITY **2** : the condition of fatty infiltration or degeneration of single organs (as the heart or liver)

adiposis do·lo·ro·sa \-ˌdō-lə-'rō-sə, -zə\ *n* : a condition of generalized obesity characterized by pain in the abnormal deposits of fat

ad·i·pos·i·ty \ˌad-ə-'päs-ət-ē\ *n, pl* **-ties** : the quality or state of being fat : OBESITY

ad·i·po·so·gen·i·tal dystrophy \ˌad-ə-ˌpō-sō-ˌjen-ət-°l-\ *n* : a combination of obesity, retarded development of the sex glands, and changes in secondary sex characteristics that results from impaired function or disease of the pituitary gland and hypothalamus — called also *Fröhlich's syndrome*

adiposus — see PANNICULUS ADIPOSUS

adip·sia \ā-'dip-sē-ə, ə-\ *n* : loss of thirst; *also* : abnormal and esp. prolonged abstinence from the intake of fluids

ad·i·tus \'ad-ət-əs\ *n, pl* **aditus** *or* **ad·i·tus·es** : a passage or opening for entrance

adj *abbr* adjunct

¹ad·junct \'aj-ˌəŋ(k)t\ *n* **1** : a person associated with or assisting another in some duty or service **2** : ADJUVANT b ⟨drugs used as short-term ∼s in weight-loss programs⟩

²adjunct *adj* **1** : added or joined as an accompanying object or circumstance **2** : attached in a subordinate or temporary capacity to a staff ⟨an ∼ psychiatrist⟩

ad·junc·tive \ə-'jəŋ(k)-tiv, a-\ *adj* : involving the medical use of an adjunct ⟨∼ therapy⟩ — **ad·junc·tive·ly** *adv*

ad·just \ə-'jəst\ *vt* : to bring about orientation or adaptation of (oneself) ∼ *vi* **1** : to adapt oneself (as to climate, food, or new working hours) **2** : to achieve mental and behavioral

balance between one's own needs and the demands of others — **ad·just·abil·i·ty** \-ˌjəs-tə-'bil-ət-ē\ *n, pl* **-ties** — **ad·just·able** \-'jəs-tə-bəl\ *adj* — **ad·jus·tive** \-'jəs-tiv\ *adj*

ad·just·ed *adj* : having achieved an often specified and usu. harmonious relationship with the environment or with other individuals ⟨a happy, ∼ed schoolchild⟩

ad·just·ment \ə-'jəs(t)-mənt\ *n* **1** : the act or process of adjusting: as **a** : the process of modifying one's behavior in changed circumstances or an altered environment in order to fulfill psychological, physiological, and social needs **b** : a functional and often transitory alteration by which an organism adapts to its immediate environment — compare ADAPTATION 2b **2** : a means (as a mechanism) by which things are adjusted one to another ⟨∼s for brightness⟩ — **ad·just·men·tal** \ə-ˌjəs(t)-'ment-°l, ˌaj-ˌəs(t)-\ *adj*

adjustment disorder *n* : any of a group of psychological disorders characterized by emotional or behavioral symptoms that occur in response to a specific stressor (as divorce or unemployment) and are either excessive or impair social or occupational functioning and relationships

¹ad·ju·vant \'aj-ə-vənt\ *adj* **1** : serving to aid or contribute **2** : assisting in the prevention, amelioration, or cure of disease ⟨∼ chemotherapy following surgery⟩

²adjuvant *n* : one that helps or facilitates: as **a** : an ingredient (as in a prescription or solution) that facilitates or modifies the action of the principal ingredient ⟨the beneficial activity of the spray is enhanced by ∼s⟩ **b** : something (as a drug or method) that enhances the effectiveness of a medical treatment ⟨used chemotherapy as an ∼ to surgery⟩ **c** : a substance enhancing the immune response to an antigen

ADL *abbr* activities of daily living

Ad·le·ri·an \ad-'lir-ē-ən, äd-\ *adj* : of, relating to, or being a theory and technique of psychotherapy emphasizing the importance of feelings of inferiority, a will to power, and overcompensation in neurotic processes

Ad·ler \'äd-lər\, **Alfred (1870–1937),** Austrian psychiatrist. Along with Sigmund Freud and Carl Jung, Adler is considered one of the founders of modern psychiatry. At one time a close associate of Freud, Adler broke with Freud esp. over the emphasis placed on sex as an underlying cause of neurosis. In 1907 he advanced his theory that physical defects may affect the psyche, producing feelings of inferiority and attempts at psychological compensation which, if unsuccessful, may lead to neurosis. The concept of the inferiority complex has grown out of Adler's work.

ad-lib \(')ad-'lib\ *adj* : made or done spontaneously : not controlled by a schedule ⟨∼ feeding of animals⟩

ad lib \(')ad-'lib\ *adv* : without restraint or imposed limit : as much or as often as is wanted ⟨the animals were given water *ad lib* —*Science*⟩ — often used in writing prescriptions

ad li·bi·tum \(')ad-'lib-ət-əm\ *adv* : AD LIB

adm *abbr* **1** administration; administrator **2** admission; admit

ad·max·il·lary \(')ad-'mak-sə-ˌler-ē\ *adj* : near or connected with the maxilla

ad·mi·nic·u·lum lin·e·ae al·bae \ˌad-mə-ˌnik-yə-ləm-ˌlin-ē-ˌē-'al-ˌbē, -ē-ˌī-, -ˌbī\ *n* : the deeper attachment of the inferior end of the linea alba that spreads out into a triangular sheet and attaches posteriorly to the crest of the pubis

ad·min·is·ter \əd-'min-ə-stər\ *vt* **ad·min·is·tered; ad·min·is·ter·ing** \-st(ə-)riŋ\ : to give (as medicine) remedially ⟨the antibiotic may be ∼ed orally or by injection⟩

ad·min·is·tra·tion \əd-ˌmin-ə-'strā-shən, (ˌ)ad-\ *n* **1** : the act of giving medication ⟨∼ of a dose of antitoxin —Morris Fishbein⟩ **2** : the direction of the execution of something ⟨∼ of a quarantine law —V. G. Heiser⟩

ad·mit \əd-'mit, ad-\ *vt* **ad·mit·ted; ad·mit·ting** : to accept into a hospital as an inpatient ⟨he was *admitted* last night for chest pains⟩

\ə\ **abut** \ᵊ\ **kitten** \ər\ **further** \a\ **ash** \ā\ **ace** \ä\ **cot, cart** \aů\ **out** \ch\ **chin** \e\ **bet** \ē\ **easy** \g\ **go** \i\ **hit** \ī\ **ice** \j\ **job** \ŋ\ **sing** \ō\ **go** \ò\ **law** \òi\ **boy** \th\ **thin** \th̲\ **the** \ü\ **loot** \ů\ **foot** \y\ **yet** \zh\ **vision** *See also* Pronunciation Symbols page

ad·nexa \ad-'nek-sə\ *n pl* : conjoined, subordinate, or associated anatomic parts ⟨the uterine ∼ include the ovaries and fallopian tubes⟩ — **ad·nex·al** \-səl\ *adj*

ad·nex·i·tis \ad-,nek-'sīt-əs\ *n* : inflammation of adnexa (as of the uterus)

ad·o·les·cence \ad-ᵊl-'es-ᵊn(t)s\ *n* **1** : the state or process of growing up **2** : the period of life from puberty to maturity terminating legally at the age of majority

¹**ad·o·les·cent** \-ᵊnt\ *n* : one that is in the state of adolescence

²**adolescent** *adj* : of, relating to, or being in adolescence — **ad·o·les·cent·ly** *adv*

ado·nis \ə-'dän-əs, -'dō-nəs\ *n* **1** *cap* : a small genus of herbs of the buttercup family (Ranunculaceae) having alternate finely dissected leaves and solitary red or yellow flowers **2** : the herbage of a plant of the genus *Adonis* (*A. vernalis*) formerly used like digitalis to treat dropsy

Adonis, Greek mythological character. Adonis was a beautiful youth much loved by the goddess Aphrodite. While hunting he was attacked and killed by a wild boar. The grieving Aphrodite caused a red-flowered plant to spring forth from his shed blood. Linnaeus named the genus *Adonis* after the mythological character.

adon·i·tol \ə-'dän-ə-,tȯl, -,tōl\ *n* : a crystalline pentose alcohol $C_5H_{12}O_5$ occurring naturally in a plant (*Adonis vernalis*) and obtainable by reduction of ribose — called also *ribitol*

adop·tive immunotherapy \ə-'däp-tiv-\ *n* : treatment esp. for cancer in which lymphocytes are removed from a patient, cultured with interleukin-2 to induce their transformation into lymphokine-activated killer cells, and returned to the patient's body along with interleukin-2

ad·oral \(,)ad-'ȯr-əl, -'ȯr-, -'är-\ *adj* : situated near the mouth

ADP \,ā-,dē-'pē, ā-'dē-,pē\ *n* : a nucleotide $C_{10}H_{15}N_5O_{10}P_2$ composed of adenosine and two phosphate groups that is formed in living cells as an intermediate between ATP and AMP and that is reversibly converted to ATP for the storing of energy by the addition of a high-energy phosphate group — called also *adenosine diphosphate*

¹**ad·re·nal** \ə-'drēn-ᵊl\ *adj* : of, relating to, or derived from the adrenal glands or their secretion — **ad·re·nal·ly** \-ᵊl-ē\ *adv*

²**adrenal** *n* : ADRENAL GLAND

ad·re·nal·ec·to·mized \ə-,drēn-ᵊl-'ek-tə-,mīzd, -,dren-\ *adj* : having had the adrenal glands surgically removed

ad·re·nal·ec·to·my \-tə-mē\ *n, pl* **-mies** : surgical removal of one or both adrenal glands

adrenal gland *n* : either of a pair of complex endocrine organs near the anterior medial border of the kidney consisting of a mesodermal cortex that produces glucocorticoid, mineralocorticoid, and androgenic hormones and an ectodermal medulla that produces epinephrine and norepinephrine — called also *adrenal, suprarenal gland*

Adren·a·lin \ə-'dren-ᵊl-ən\ *trademark* — used for a preparation of levorotatory epinephrine

adren·a·line \ə-'dren-ᵊl-ən\ *n* : EPINEPHRINE — recognized by the *British Pharmaceutical Codex* as the preferred name for epinephrine in Great Britain

adren·a·lin·emia *or chiefly Brit* **adren·a·lin·ae·mia** \ə-,dren-ᵊl-ə-'nē-mē-ə\ *n* : the presence of abnormal amounts of epinephrine in the blood

adren·a·lone \ə-'dren-ᵊl-,ōn\ *n* : a sympathomimetic amine $C_9H_{11}NO_3$ with both alpha- and beta-adrenergic activity

ad·ren·ar·che \,ad-rə-'när-kē\ *n* : an increase in the production of androgens by the adrenal cortex that usu. occurs during the eighth or ninth year of life

adren·er·gen \ə-'dren-ər-jən\ *n* : a drug having a physiological action resembling that of adrenaline

ad·ren·er·gic \,ad-rə-'nər-jik\ *adj* **1** : liberating or activated by adrenaline or a substance like adrenaline ⟨∼ nerve fibers⟩ — compare CHOLINERGIC 1, NORADRENERGIC **2** : resembling adrenaline esp. in physiological action ⟨∼ drugs⟩ — **ad·ren·er·gi·cal·ly** \-ji-k(ə-)lē\ *adv*

ad·re·no·chrome \ə-'drē-nə-,krōm\ *n* : a red-colored mixture of quinones derived from epinephrine by oxidation and yielding a product like melanin on further oxidation

ad·re·no·cor·ti·cal \ə-,drē-nō-'kȯrt-i-kəl\ *adj* : of, relating to, or derived from the cortex of the adrenal glands ⟨∼ hormone deficiency⟩

ad·re·no·cor·ti·coid \-,kȯid\ *n* : a hormone secreted by the adrenal cortex — **adrenocorticoid** *adj*

ad·re·no·cor·ti·co·mi·met·ic \-,kȯrt-i-(,)kō-mə-'met-ik, -mī-\ *adj* : simulating the action of hormones of the adrenal cortex in physiological effect

ad·re·no·cor·ti·co·ste·roid \-'sti(ə)r-,ȯid, -'ste(ə)r-\ *n* : a steroid (as cortisone or cortisol) obtained from, resembling, or having physiological effects like those of hormones of the adrenal cortex

ad·re·no·cor·ti·co·tro·pic \-'trō-pik, -'träp-ik\ *also* **ad·re·no·cor·ti·co·tro·phic** \-'trō-fik, -'träf-ik\ *adj* : acting on or stimulating the adrenal cortex ⟨∼ activity⟩

adrenocorticotropic hormone *or* **adrenocorticotrophic hormone** *n* : ACTH

ad·re·no·cor·ti·co·tro·pin \-'trō-pən\ *also* **ad·re·no·cor·ti·co·tro·phin** \-'trō-fən\ *n* : ACTH

adre·no·gen·i·tal syndrome \ə-,drē-nō-,jen-ət-ᵊl-, -,dren-ō-\ *n* : CUSHING'S SYNDROME

adre·no·glo·mer·u·lo·tro·pin \-glä-,mer-(y)ə-lō-'trō-pən, -glə-\ *n* : a substance that is thought to be secreted by the brain or pineal gland and is reported to stimulate aldosterone secretion by the adrenal glands

adre·no·leu·ko·dys·tro·phy *or chiefly Brit* **adre·no·leu·co·dys·tro·phy** \-,lü-kō-'dis-trə-fē\ *n, pl* **-phies** : a rare demyelinating disease of the central nervous system that is inherited as an X-linked recessive trait chiefly affecting males in childhood and that is characterized by progressive blindness, deafness, tonic spasms, and mental deterioration — abbr. *ALD;* called also *encephalitis periaxialis diffusa, Schilder's disease, Schilder's encephalitis*

adre·no·lyt·ic \ə-,drēn-ᵊl-'it-ik, -,dren-\ *adj* : blocking the release or action of adrenaline at nerve endings

adre·no·med·ul·lary \ə-,drē-nō-'med-ᵊl-,er-ē, -,dren-ō-, -'mej-ə-,ler-; -mə-'dəl-ə-rē\ *adj* : relating to or derived from the medulla of the adrenal glands ⟨∼ extracts⟩

adre·no·pause \ə-'drē-nə-,pȯz, -'dren-ə-\ *n* : a stage of life supposed to be characterized by reduction or cessation of production of hormones by the adrenal glands

adre·no·re·cep·tor \ə-,drē-nō-ri-'sep-tər, -,dren-ō-\ *n* : an adrenergic receptor

adre·no·ste·rone \ə-,drē-nō-stə-'rōn, -,dren-ō-; ,ad-rə-'näs-tə-,\ *n* : a crystalline steroid $C_{19}N_{24}O_3$ obtained from the adrenal cortex and having androgenic activity

adre·no–sym·pa·thet·ic \ə-,drē-nō-,sim-pə-'thet-ik, -,dren-ō-\ *adj* **1** : of or relating to the adrenergic portion of the autonomic nervous system **2** : of or involving interaction of the sympathetic nervous system and the adrenal gland

adre·no·tro·pic \-'trō-pik, -'träp-ik\ *or* **adre·no·tro·phic** \-'trō-fik, -'träf-ik\ *adj* : ADRENOCORTICOTROPIC

Adria·my·cin \,ā-drē-ə-'mīs-ᵊn, ,ad-rē-\ *trademark* — used for a preparation of the hydrochloride of doxorubicin

ad·sorb \ad-'sȯ(ə)rb, -'zȯ(ə)rb\ *vt* : to take up and hold by adsorption ∼ *vi* : to become adsorbed — **ad·sorb·abil·i·ty** \-,sȯr-bə-'bil-ət-ē, -,zȯr-\ *n, pl* **-ties** — **ad·sorb·able** \-'sȯr-bə-bəl, -'zȯr-\ *adj*

ad·sor·bate \ad-'sȯr-bət, -'zȯr-, -,bāt\ *n* : an adsorbed substance

¹**ad·sor·bent** \-bənt\ *adj* : having the capacity or tendency to adsorb

²**adsorbent** *n* : a usu. solid substance that adsorbs another substance

ad·sorp·tion \ad-'sȯrp-shən, -'zȯrp-\ *n* : the adhesion in an extremely thin layer of molecules (as of gases, solutes, or liquids) to the surfaces of solid bodies or liquids with which they are in contact — compare ABSORPTION — **ad·sorp·tive** \-'sȯrp-tiv, -'zȯrp-\ *adj*

¹**adult** \ə-'dəlt, 'ad-,əlt\ *adj* : fully developed and mature

²**adult** *n* **1** : one that has arrived at full development or maturity esp. in size, strength, or intellectual capacity **2** : a human male or female after a specific age (as 18 or 21)

adul·ter·ant \ə-'dəl-t(ə-)rənt\ *n* : an adulterating substance or agent — **adulterant** *adj*

adul·ter·ate \ə-'dəl-tə-ˌrāt\ *vt* **-at·ed; -at·ing** : to corrupt, debase, or make impure by the addition of a foreign or inferior substance; *esp* : to prepare for sale by replacing more valuable with less valuable or inert ingredients — **adul·ter·a·tor** \-ˌrāt-ər\ *n*

adul·ter·a·tion \ə-ˌdəl-tə-'rā-shən\ *n* **1** : the process of adulterating : the condition of being adulterated **2** : an adulterated product

adult·hood \ə-'dəlt-ˌhùd\ *n* : the state or time of being an adult

adult–onset diabetes *n* : TYPE 2 DIABETES

adult respiratory distress syndrome *n* : respiratory failure in adults or children that results from diffuse injury to the endothelium of the lung (as in sepsis, chest trauma, massive blood transfusion, aspiration of the gastric contents, or pneumonia) and is characterized by pulmonary edema with an abnormally high amount of protein in the edematous fluid and by difficult rapid breathing and hypoxemia — *abbr. ARDS*; called also *acute respiratory distress syndrome*

adult T–cell leukemia *n* : a serious syndrome that is characterized by high counts of malignant T cells, hepatosplenomegaly, lymphadenopathy, skin lesions, and hypercalcemia and that is associated with the retrovirus HTLV-I — called also *adult T-cell leukemia/lymphoma*

Ad·vair Dis·kus \'ad-ˌver-'dis-kəs\ *trademark* — used for a preparation of fluticasone propionate and a salt of salmeterol

ad·vance di·rec·tive \əd-'van(t)s-də-'rek-tiv, -dī-\ *n* : a legal document (as a living will) signed by a living competent person in order to provide guidance for medical and health-care decisions (as the termination of life support and organ donation) in the event that the person becomes incompetent to make such decisions

ad·vance·ment \əd-'van(t)-smənt\ *n* : detachment of a muscle or tendon from its insertion and reattachment (as in the surgical correction of strabismus) at a more advanced point from its insertion ⟨flexor tendon ∼⟩

advancement flap *n* : a flap of tissue stretched and sutured in place to cover a defect at a nearby position

ad·ven·ti·tia \ˌad-vən-'tish-(ē-)ə, -ˌ(ˌ)ven-\ *n* : the outer layer that makes up a tubular organ or structure and esp. a blood vessel, is composed of collagenous and elastic fibers, and is not covered with peritoneum — called also *tunica adventitia, tunica externa*

ad·ven·ti·tial \-əl\ *adj* : of or relating to an adventitia

ad·ven·ti·tious \-əs\ *adj* **1 a** : arising sporadically or in other than the usual location ⟨an ∼ part in embryonic development⟩ **b** : occurring spontaneously or accidentally in a country or region to which it is not native ⟨an ∼ insect⟩ **2** : ADVENTITIAL **3** : not congenital ⟨∼ deafness⟩ — **ad·ven·ti·tious·ly** *adv*

adventitious cyst *n* : a cyst formed about a foreign object in the body

Ad·vil \'ad-(ˌ)vil\ *trademark* — used for a preparation of ibuprofen

ady·na·mia \ˌā-dī-'nam-ē-ə, ˌad-ə-, -'nām-\ *n* : asthenia caused by disease

ady·nam·ic \ˌā-(ˌ)dī-'nam-ik, ˌad-ə-'nam-\ *adj* : characterized by or causing a loss of strength or function ⟨∼ fevers such as typhoid⟩ ⟨∼ ileus⟩

ae *or* **aet** *or* **aetat** *abbr* [Latin *aetatis*] of age; aged

ae·des \ā-'ē-(ˌ)dēz\ *n* **1** *cap* : a large cosmopolitan genus of mosquitoes that includes vectors of some diseases (as yellow fever and dengue) **2** *pl* **aedes** : any mosquito of the genus *Aedes* — **ae·dine** \-ˌdīn, -ˌdēn\ *adj*

aegophony *chiefly Brit var of* EGOPHONY

aelurophobe, aelurophobia *var of* AILUROPHOBE, AILUROPHOBIA

aer·ate \'a(-ə)r-ˌāt, 'e(-ə)r-\ *vt* **aer·at·ed; aer·at·ing** **1** : to supply (the blood) with oxygen by respiration **2** : to supply or impregnate (as a liquid) with air **3** *Brit* : CARBONATE 2 — **aer·a·tion** \ˌa(-ə)r-'ā-shən, ˌe(-ə)r-\ *n*

aer·a·tor \'a(-ə)r-ˌāt-ər, 'e(-ə)r-\ *n* : one that aerates; *esp* : an apparatus for aerating something (as sewage)

aer·if·er·ous \ˌa(-ə)r-'if-(ə-)rəs, ˌe(-ə)r-\ *adj* : containing or conveying air

aero·al·ler·gen \ˌar-ō-'al-ər-jən, ˌer-ō-\ *n* : an allergen carried in the air

Aero·bac·ter \'ar-ō-ˌbak-tər, 'er-\ *n* : a taxonomically invalid genus of aerobic gram-negative bacteria of the family Enterobacteriaceae whose species are now assigned to the genera *Enterobacter* and *Klebsiella*

aer·obe \'a(-ə)r-ˌōb, 'e(-ə)r-\ *n* : an organism (as a bacterium) that lives only in the presence of oxygen

aer·o·bic \ˌa(-ə)r-'ō-bik, ˌe(-ə)r-\ *adj* **1** : living, active, or occurring only in the presence of oxygen ⟨∼ respiration⟩ **2** : of, relating to, or induced by aerobes **3 a** : of, relating to, or being activity which increases the body's demand for oxygen thereby resulting in a marked temporary increase in respiration and heart rate ⟨∼ exercise⟩ **b** : relating to, resulting from, or used in aerobics or aerobic activity ⟨∼ shoes⟩ — **aer·o·bi·cal·ly** \-bi-k(ə-)lē\ *adv*

aer·o·bics \-biks\ *n pl* **1** *sing or pl in constr* : a system of physical conditioning involving exercises (as running, walking, swimming, or calisthenics) strenuously performed so as to cause marked temporary increase in respiration and heart rate **2** : aerobic exercises

aero·bi·ol·o·gy \ˌar-ō-bī-'äl-ə-jē, ˌer-\ *n, pl* **-gies** : the science dealing with the occurrence, transportation, and effects of airborne materials or microorganisms (as viruses, pollen, or pollutants) — **aero·bi·o·log·i·cal** \-ˌbī-ə-'läj-i-kəl\ *adj* — **aero·bi·o·log·i·cal·ly** \-k(ə-)lē\ *adv*

aero·bi·o·scope \-'bī-ə-ˌskōp\ *n* : an apparatus used to collect air for determination of its bacterial count

aero·bi·o·sis \ˌar-ō-bī-'ō-səs, ˌer-, -bē-\ *n, pl* **-o·ses** \-ˌsēz\ : life in the presence of air or oxygen — **aero·bi·ot·ic** \-'ät-ik\ *adj* — **aero·bi·ot·i·cal·ly** \-i-k(ə-)lē\ *adv*

aero·cele \'a(-ə)r-ō-ˌsēl, 'e(-ə)r-\ *n* : a cavity or pouch swollen with gas (as air) ⟨an intracranial ∼⟩

aer·odon·tal·gia \ˌar-ō-dän-'tal-j(ē-)ə, ˌer-\ *n* : toothache resulting from atmospheric decompression (as in high-altitude flying or confinement in decompression chambers) — **aer·odon·tal·gic** \-jik\ *adj*

aer·odon·tia \ˌar-ō-'dän-ch(ē-)ə, ˌer-\ *n* : the branch of dentistry associated with dental problems arising in connection with flying

aero·dy·nam·ics \-dī-'nam-iks\ *n pl but sing or pl in constr* : a branch of dynamics that deals with the motion of air and other gaseous fluids and with the forces acting on bodies in motion relative to such fluids — **aero·dy·nam·ic** \-ik\ *also* **aero·dy·nam·i·cal** \-i-kəl\ *adj* — **aero·dy·nam·i·cal·ly** \-i-k(ə-)lē\ *adv* — **aero·dy·nam·i·cist** \-'nam-ə-səst\ *n*

aero·em·bo·lism \-'em-bə-ˌliz-əm\ *n* **1** : a gaseous embolism **2** : decompression sickness caused by rapid ascent to high altitudes and resulting exposure to rapidly lowered air pressure — called also *aeroemphysema, air bends*

aero·em·phy·se·ma \ˌar-ō-ˌem(p)-fə-'zē-mə, ˌer-, -'sē-\ *n* : AEROEMBOLISM 2

aero·gel \'a(-ə)r-ō-ˌjel, 'e(-ə)r-\ *n* : a highly porous solid formed by replacement of liquid in a gel with a gas so that there is little shrinkage

ae·rog·e·nous \ˌa(-ə)r-'äj-ə-nəs, ˌe(-ə)r-\ *adj* : transmitted by or involving transmission by air ⟨the ∼ route of infection —*Veterinary Record*⟩ — **ae·rog·e·nous·ly** *adv*

aero·med·i·cal \ˌar-ō-'med-i-kəl, ˌer-\ *adj* **1** : of or relating to aeromedicine **2** : relating to or involving air transportation to a medical facility

aero·med·i·cine \ˌar-ō-'med-ə-sən, ˌer-, *Brit usu* ˌer-ō-'med-sən\ *n* : a branch of medicine that deals with the diseases and disturbances arising from flying and the associated physiological and psychological problems

aer·om·e·ter \ˌa(-ə)r-'äm-ət-ər, ˌe(-ə)r-\ *n* : an instrument for ascertaining the weight or density of air or other gases

---

\ə\ abut \ᵊ\ kitten \ər\ further \a\ ash \ā\ ace \ä\ cot, cart \aù\ out \ch\ chin \e\ bet \ē\ easy \g\ go \i\ hit \ī\ ice \j\ job \ŋ\ sing \ō\ go \ò\ law \òi\ boy \th\ thin \t̲h̲\ the \ü\ loot \ù\ foot \y\ yet \zh\ vision *See also* Pronunciation Symbols page

aero·neu·ro·sis \ˌar-ō-n(y)ù-ˈrō-səs, ˌer-\ *n, pl* **-ro·ses** \-ˌsēz\ : a functional nervous disorder of flight personnel that is caused by emotional stress and characterized by physical symptoms (as restlessness, abdominal pains, and diarrhea)

aero–oti·tis \ˌar-ō-ō-ˈtīt-əs, ˌer-\ *n* : AERO-OTITIS MEDIA

aero–otitis me·dia \-ˈmēd-ē-ə\ *n* : the traumatic inflammation of the middle ear resulting from differences between atmospheric pressure and pressure in the middle ear and occurring in high-altitude flyers, caisson or tunnel workers, and deep-sea divers

aero·pause \ˈar-ō-ˌpȯz, ˈer-\ *n* : the level above the earth's surface where the atmosphere becomes too thin to support aircraft and human life

aero·pha·gia \ˌar-ō-ˈfā-j(ē-)ə, ˌer-\ *also* **aer·oph·a·gy** \ˌa(-ə)r-ˈäf-ə-jē, ˌe(-ə)r-\ *n, pl* **-gias** *also* **-gies** : the swallowing of air esp. in hysteria

aero·pho·bia \ˌar-ō-ˈfō-bē-ə, ˌer-\ *n* : abnormal or excessive fear of drafts or of fresh air — **aero·pho·bic** \-bik\ *adj*

aero·plank·ton \ˌar-ō-ˈplaŋ(k)-tən, ˌer-, -ˌtän\ *n* : small airborne organisms (as flying insects)

aero·scope \ˈa(-ə)r-ō-ˌskōp, ˈe(-ə)r-\ *n* : an apparatus for collecting small particles and organisms suspended in the air

aero·si·nus·itis \ˌar-ō-ˌsī-n(y)ə-ˈsīt-əs, ˌer-\ *n* : the traumatic inflammation of the nasal sinuses resulting from the difference between atmospheric pressure and the pressure within the sinus cavities and occurring in high-altitude flyers, caisson or tunnel workers, and deep-sea divers

aero·sol \ˈar-ə-ˌsäl, ˈer-, -ˌsȯl\ *n* **1** : a suspension of fine solid or liquid particles in gas ⟨smoke, fog, and mist are ~*s*⟩ **2** : a substance (as an insecticide or medicine) dispensed from a pressurized container as an aerosol; *also* : the container for this

aero·sol·iza·tion \ˌar-ə-ˌsäl-ə-ˈzā-shən, ˌer-, -ˌsȯl-\ *n* : dispersal (as of a medicine) in the form of an aerosol ⟨~ of penicillin⟩

aero·sol·ize \ˈar-ə-ˌsäl-ˌīz, ˈer-, -ˌsȯl-\ *vt* **-ized; -iz·ing** : to disperse (as a medicine, bactericide, or insecticide) as an aerosol ⟨*aerosolized* pentamidine, which is sprayed directly into the lungs —C. C. Mann⟩ — **aero·sol·iz·er** *n*

aero·space medicine \ˈar-ō-ˌspās-, ˈer-\ *n* : a medical specialty concerned with the health and medical problems of flight personnel both in the earth's atmosphere and in space

aero·tax·is \ˌar-ō-ˈtak-səs, ˌer-\ *n* : a taxis in which air or oxygen is the directive factor

aero·ther·a·peu·tics \ˌar-ō-ˌther-ə-ˈpyüt-iks, ˌer-\ *n pl but sing in constr* : the treatment of disease by varying pressure or composition of air breathed by the patient

aero·ther·a·py \ˌar-ō-ˈther-ə-pē, ˌer-\ *n, pl* **-pies** : AEROTHERAPEUTICS

aer·oti·tis \ˌar-ō-ˈtīt-əs, ˌer-\ *n* : AERO-OTITIS MEDIA

aero·to·nom·e·ter \ˌar-ōt-ə²n-ˈäm-ət-ər, ˌer-\ *n* : an instrument for determining the partial pressures of gases in the blood

aer·ot·ro·pism \ˌa(-ə)r-ˈä-trə-ˌpiz-əm, ˌe(-ə)r-\ *n* : response (as by bacteria) to changes in oxygen tension

Aes·cu·la·pi·an \ˌes-kyə-ˈlā-pē-ən\ *adj* : of or relating to Aesculapius or the healing art : MEDICAL

Aesculapius — see STAFF OF AESCULAPIUS

Aes·cu·la·pi·an staff \ˌes-kyə-ˈlā-pē-ən-\ *n* : STAFF OF AESCULAPIUS

Aes·cu·la·pi·us \-pē-əs\ *n* : PHYSICIAN

Aesculapius — see STAFF OF AESCULAPIUS

aesculetin, aesculin *var of* ESCULETIN, ESCULIN

aesthesia, aesthesiometer, aesthesiometry, aesthesio·physiology *chiefly Brit var of* ESTHESIA, ESTHESIOMETER, ESTHESIOMETRY, ESTHESIOPHYSIOLOGY

aestival, aestivate, aestivation *var of* ESTIVAL, ESTIVATE, ESTIVATION

aet, aetat *var of* AE

Each boldface word in the list below is a chiefly British variant of the word to its right in small capitals.

aetiologic	ETIOLOGIC	**aetiologically**	ETIOLOGICALLY
aetiological	ETIOLOGIC	**aetiology**	ETIOLOGY

aetiopatho·genesis	ETIOPATHO·GENESIS	**aetioporphy·rin**	ETIOPORPHY·RIN

AF *abbr* **1** atrial fibrillation **2** audio frequency

AFB *abbr* acid-fast bacillus

afe·brile \(ˈ)ā-ˈfeb-ˌrīl *also* -ˈfēb-\ *adj* : free from fever : not marked by fever

¹af·fect \ˈaf-ˌekt\ *n* : the conscious subjective aspect of an emotion considered apart from bodily changes — compare FEELING 3

²af·fect \ə-ˈfekt, a-\ *vt* : to produce an effect upon; *esp* : to produce a material influence upon or alteration in ⟨paralysis ~*ed* his limbs⟩

¹af·fec·tion \ə-ˈfek-shən\ *n* **1** : a moderate feeling or emotion **2** : the feeling aspect (as in pleasure or displeasure) of consciousness

²affection *n* **1** : the action of affecting : the state of being affected **2 a** : a bodily condition **b** : DISEASE, MALADY ⟨a pulmonary ~⟩

af·fec·tive \a-ˈfek-tiv\ *adj* : relating to, arising from, or influencing feelings or emotions : EMOTIONAL ⟨~ symptoms⟩ — **af·fec·tive·ly** *adv* — **af·fec·tiv·i·ty** \ˌaf-ˌek-ˈtiv-ət-ē\ *n, pl* **-ties**

affective disorder *n* : MOOD DISORDER

¹af·fer·ent \ˈaf-ə-rənt, -ˌer-ənt\ *adj* : bearing or conducting inward; *specif* : conveying impulses toward the central nervous system — compare EFFERENT — **af·fer·ent·ly** *adv*

²afferent *n* : an afferent anatomical part (as a nerve) ⟨the effect on the hypothalamus of ~*s* from the stomach⟩

af·fin·i·ty \ə-ˈfin-ət-ē\ *n, pl* **-ties** **1** : an attractive force between substances or particles that causes them to enter into and remain in chemical combination **2** : a relation between biological groups involving resemblance in structural plan and indicating a common origin

affinity chromatography *n* : chromatography in which a macromolecule (as a protein) is isolated and purified by passing it in solution through a column that has been treated with a substance having a ligand for which the macromolecule has an affinity that causes it to be retained on the column

af·flux \ˈaf-ˌləks\ *n* : a flowing esp. of a bodily fluid to or toward a bodily part ⟨an ~ of blood to the head⟩

afi·brin·o·gen·emia *or chiefly Brit* **afi·brin·o·gen·ae·mia** \ˌā-(ˌ)fī-ˌbrin-ə-jə-ˈnē-mē-ə\ *n* : an abnormality of blood clotting caused by usu. congenital absence of fibrinogen in the blood and marked by a tendency to prolonged bleeding

Afip·ia \ə-ˈfip-ē-ə\ *n* : a genus of gram-negative bacilli including one (*A. felis*) associated with some cases of cat scratch disease

af·la·tox·in \ˌaf-lə-ˈtäk-sən\ *n* : any of several carcinogenic mycotoxins that are produced esp. in stored agricultural crops (as peanuts) by molds (as *Aspergillus flavus*)

AFM *abbr* atomic force microscope; atomic force microscopy

AFP *abbr* alpha-fetoprotein

Af·ri·can horse sickness \ˌaf-ri-kən-\ *n* : a serious and commonly fatal disease of horses and sometimes other mammals including rarely humans that is caused by a reovirus of the genus *Orbivirus* (serotypes of species *African horse sickness virus*), that is endemic in parts of central and southern Africa, that is characterized by fever, edematous swellings, and internal hemorrhage, and that is transmitted by biting flies of the genus *Culicoides* — called also *horsesickness*

Af·ri·can·ized bee \ˌaf-ri-kə-ˌnīzd-\ *n* : a honeybee that originated in Brazil as an accidental hybrid between an aggressive African subspecies (*Apis mellifera scutellata*) and previously established European honeybees and has spread to Mexico and the southernmost U.S. by breeding with local bees producing populations retaining most of the African bee's traits — called also *Africanized honeybee, killer bee*

African sleeping sickness *n* : SLEEPING SICKNESS 1

African swine fever *n* : an acute highly contagious usu. fatal febrile disease that affects only swine (family Suidae), that resembles but is more severe than hog cholera, that is indigenous to Africa where wild swine (as the warthog and bushpig) act as natural reservoirs, that has spread to and caused epidemics in the western hemisphere, and that is caused by a double-stranded DNA virus (species *African swine fever virus* of the genus *Asfivirus,* family *Asfarviridae*) having a capsid with icosahedral symmetry — called also *swine fever*

African trypanosomiasis *n* : any of several trypanosomiases caused by African trypanosomes; *esp* : SLEEPING SICKNESS 1

af·ter·birth \'af-tər-ˌbərth\ *n* : the placenta and fetal membranes that are expelled after delivery — called also *secundines*

af·ter·brain \-ˌbrān\ *n* : the posterior subdivision of the hindbrain : MYELENCEPHALON

af·ter·care \-ˌke(ə)r, -ˌka(ə)r\ *n* : the care, treatment, help, or supervision given to persons discharged from an institution (as a hospital or prison)

af·ter·cat·a·ract \-ˌkat-ə-ˌrakt\ *n* : an opacity of the lens capsule that occurs following an operation for cataract

af·ter·damp \-ˌdamp\ *n* : a toxic gas mixture remaining after an explosion of firedamp in mines and consisting principally of carbon dioxide, carbon monoxide, and nitrogen

af·ter·dis·charge \-(ˌ)dis(h)-ˌchärj\ *n* : discharge of neural impulses (as by a ganglion cell) after termination of the initiating stimulus

af·ter·ef·fect \'af-tə-ri-ˌfekt\ *n* **1** : an effect that follows its cause after an interval ⟨the ∼s of surgery⟩ **2** : a secondary result esp. in the action of a drug coming on after the subsidence of the first effect

af·ter·im·age \-ˌrim-ij\ *n* : a usu. visual sensation occurring after stimulation by its external cause has ceased — called also *aftersensation, aftervision*

af·ter·load \'af-tər-ˌlōd\ *n* : the force against which a ventricle contracts that is contributed to by the vascular resistance esp. of the arteries and by the physical characteristics (as mass and viscosity) of the blood

af·ter·pain \-ˌpān\ *n* **1** : pain that follows its cause only after a distinct interval ⟨the ∼ of a tooth extraction⟩ **2 after-pains** *pl* : pains that follow the termination of labor and are associated with contraction of the uterus toward its nonpregnant size

af·ter·po·ten·tial \-pə-ˌten-chəl\ *n* : the sequence of electrical events that follows the action potential of nerve activity and that usu. takes the form of a negative followed by a positive potential with both being of much smaller amplitude than the action potential — compare PREPOTENTIAL

af·ter·sen·sa·tion \-sen-ˌsā-shən, sən-\ *n* : a sensation occurring after stimulation by its external cause has ceased; *esp* : AFTERIMAGE

af·ter·taste \-ˌtāst\ *n* : persistence of a sensation (as of flavor or an emotion) after the stimulating agent or experience has gone

af·ter·vi·sion \-ˌvizh-ən\ *n* : AFTERIMAGE

af·to·sa \af-'tō-sə, -zə\ *n* : FOOT-AND-MOUTH DISEASE

Ag *symbol* [Latin *argentum*] silver

aga·lac·tia \ˌā-gə-'lak-sh(ē-)ə, -tē-ə\ *n* : the failure of the secretion of milk from any cause other than the normal ending of the lactation period — **aga·lac·tic** \-tik\ *adj*

aga·mete \(ˌ)ā-'gam-ˌēt, 'a-gə-ˌmēt, ˌā-gə-'mēt\ *n* : an asexual reproductive cell (as a spore or a merozoite)

agam·ic \(ˌ)ā-'gam-ik\ *adj* : ASEXUAL, PARTHENOGENETIC — **agam·i·cal·ly** \-i-k(ə-)lē\ *adv*

agam·ma·glob·u·lin·emia *or chiefly Brit* **agam·ma·glob·u·lin·ae·mia** \(ˌ)ā-gam-ə-ˌgläb-yə-lə-'nē-mē-ə\ *n* : a pathological condition in which the body forms few or no gamma globulins or antibodies — compare DYSGAMMAGLOBULINEMIA

aga·mog·o·ny \ˌā-gə-'mäg-ə-nē, ˌag-ə-\ *n, pl* **-nies** : asexual reproduction; *specif* : SCHIZOGONY

Aga·mo·mer·mis \(ˌ)ā-gam-ə-'mər-məs, ˌag-ə-mō-\ *n* : a genus of nematode worms (family Mermithidae) that are normally free-living as adults and parasites of insects as larvae but may accidentally parasitize humans

agam·ont \(ˌ)ā-'gam-ˌänt\ *n* : SCHIZONT

agan·gli·on·ic \(ˌ)ā-ˌgaŋ-glē-'än-ik\ *adj* : lacking ganglia

agar \'äg-ər\ *n* **1** : a gelatinous colloidal extractive of a red alga (as of the genera *Gelidium, Gracilaria,* and *Eucheuma*) used esp. in culture media or as a gelling and stabilizing agent in foods **2** : a culture medium containing agar

agar–agar \ˌäg-ər-'äg-ər\ *n* : AGAR

aga·ric \'ag-ə-rik, ə-'gar-ik\ *n* **1** : the dried fruit body of a mushroom (*Fomes officinalis* syn. *Polyporus officinalis*) formerly used in the treatment of excessive perspiration (as in the night sweats of tuberculosis) — called also *larch agaric* **2** : a fungus of the family Agaricaceae and esp. of the genus *Agaricus*

Agar·i·ca·ce·ae \ə-ˌgar-ə-'kā-sē-ˌē\ *n pl* : a large family of fungi (order Agaricales) that contains the genera *Agaricus* and *Amanita* and includes many familiar mushrooms with the sporophore usu. consisting of a central stalk and a cap like an umbrella on the lower surface of which are numerous lamellae bearing the hymenium

agar·i·cin \ə-'gar-ə-sən\ *n* : an impure form of the active principle of medicinal agaric

Agar·i·cus \-ə-kəs\ *n* : a genus that is the type of the family Agaricaceae, comprises fungi with gills and brown spores, and includes several (as the meadow mushroom) that are edible

aga·rose \'ag-ə-ˌrōs, 'äg-, -ˌrōz\ *n* : a polysaccharide obtained from agar that is used esp. as a supporting medium in gel electrophoresis

agas·tric \(ˌ)ā-'gas-trik\ *adj* : lacking a stomach or distinct digestive canal ⟨the tapeworm is ∼⟩

aga·ve \ə-'gäv-ē\ *n* **1** *cap* : a genus of plants (family Agavaceae) that are native to tropical America and to the southwestern U.S., have spiny-margined leaves in basal rosettes and tall spikes of flowers, and include some that are cultivated for their fiber or sap or for ornament **2** : a plant (as the century plant) of the genus *Agave*

¹age \'āj\ *n* **1 a** : the part of life from birth to a given time ⟨a child 10 years of ∼⟩ **b** : the time or part of life at which some particular event, qualification, or capacity arises, occurs, or is lost ⟨of reproductive ∼⟩ ⟨∼ of onset⟩ — see MIDDLE AGE **c** : an advanced stage of life **2** : an individual's development measured in terms of the years requisite for like development of an average individual ⟨a child of 7 with a mental ∼ of 10⟩ — see BINET AGE, MENTAL AGE

²age *vb* **aged; ag·ing** *or* **age·ing** *vi* : to become old : show the effects or the characteristics of increasing age ∼ *vt* : to cause to become old

agen·e·sis \(ˌ)ā-'jen-ə-səs\ *n, pl* **-e·ses** \-ˌsēz\ : lack or failure of development (as of a body part)

agen·i·tal·ism \(ˌ)ā-'jen-ət-ᵊl-ˌiz-əm\ *n* : an abnormal condition associated with lack of or incompletely developed sex organs and caused by deficient secretion of sex hormones

age·nize \'ā-jə-ˌnīz\ *vt* **-nized; -niz·ing** : to treat (flour) with nitrogen trichloride

agent \'ā-jənt\ *n* **1** : something that produces or is capable of producing an effect **2** : a chemically, physically, or biologically active principle — see OXIDIZING AGENT, REDUCING AGENT

Agent Orange \-'är-inj, -'är(-ə)nj, -'ȯr-inj, -'ȯr(-ə)nj\ *n* : an herbicide widely used as a defoliant in the Vietnam War that is composed of 2,4-D and 2,4,5-T and contains dioxin as a contaminant

age of con·sent \-kən-'sent\ *n* : the age at which one is legally competent to give consent esp. to marriage or to sexual intercourse

age–related macular degeneration *n* : macular degeneration that affects the elderly in either a slowly progressing form marked esp. by the accumulation of yellow deposits in and thinning of the macula lutea or in a rapidly progressing

---

\ə\ **abut** \ᵊ\ **kitten** \ər\ **further** \a\ **ash** \ā\ **ace** \ä\ **cot, cart**
\aů\ **out** \ch\ **chin** \e\ **bet** \ē\ **easy** \g\ **go** \i\ **hit** \ī\ **ice** \j\ **job**
\ŋ\ **sing** \ō\ **go** \ȯ\ **law** \ȯi\ **boy** \th\ **thin** \t̲h̲\ **the** \ü\ **loot**
\ů\ **foot** \y\ **yet** \zh\ **vision** *See also* Pronunciation Symbols page

form marked by scarring produced by bleeding and fluid leakage below the macula lutea

age spots *n pl* : benign flat spots evenly colored with darker pigment that occur on sun-exposed skin (as of the hands) esp. of persons aged 50 and over — called also *lentigo senilis, liver spots*

ageu·sia \ə-ˈgyü-zē-ə, (ˈ)ā-, -ˈjü-, -sē-\ *n* : the absence or impairment of the sense of taste — **ageu·sic** \-zik, -sik\ *adj*

ag·ger \ˈaj-ər\ *n* : an anatomical prominence

¹**ag·glom·er·ate** \ə-ˈgläm-ə-ˌrāt\ *vt* **-at·ed; -at·ing** : to gather into a ball, mass, or cluster — **ag·glom·er·a·tion** \ə-ˌgläm-ə-ˈrā-shən\ *n*

²**ag·glom·er·ate** \-rət\ *n* : a jumbled mass or collection ⟨probably a virus or ∼s of a virus —E. A. Steinhaus⟩

agglut *abbr* agglutination

ag·glu·ti·na·bil·i·ty \ə-ˌglüt-ᵊn-ə-ˈbil-ət-ē\ *n, pl* **-ties** : capacity (as of red blood cells) to be agglutinated — **ag·glu·ti·na·ble** \-ˈglüt-ᵊn-ə-bəl\ *adj*

¹**ag·glu·ti·nant** \ə-ˈglüt-ᵊn-ənt\ *adj* : causing or tending to cause adhesion

²**agglutinant** *n* : an agglutinating substance

¹**ag·glu·ti·nate** \-ᵊn-ˌāt\ *vb* **-nat·ed; -nat·ing** *vt* : to cause to undergo agglutination ∼ *vi* : to undergo agglutination

²**ag·glu·ti·nate** \-ᵊn-ət, -ᵊn-ˌāt\ *n* : a clump of agglutinated material (as blood cells or bacteria)

ag·glu·ti·na·tion \ə-ˌglüt-ᵊn-ˈā-shən\ *n* : a reaction in which particles (as red blood cells or bacteria) suspended in a liquid collect into clumps and which occurs esp. as a serological response to a specific antibody

agglutination test *n* : any of several tests based on the ability of a specific serum to cause agglutination of a suitable system and used in the diagnosis of infections, the identification of microorganisms, and in blood typing — compare WIDAL TEST

ag·glu·ti·na·tive \ə-ˈglüt-ᵊn-ˌāt-iv, -ət-\ *adj* : causing or produced by agglutination ⟨∼ proteins⟩

ag·glu·ti·nin \ə-ˈglüt-ᵊn-ən\ *n* : a substance (as an antibody) producing agglutination

ag·glu·ti·no·gen \ə-ˈglüt-ᵊn-ə-jən\ *n* : an antigen whose presence results in the formation of an agglutinin — **ag·glu·ti·no·gen·ic** \-ˌglüt-ᵊn-ə-ˈjen-ik\ *adj*

ag·glu·ti·no·scope \ə-ˈglüt-ᵊn-ə-ˌskōp\ *n* : an instrument used to facilitate visual observation of agglutination (as in a test tube)

ag·gra·vate \ˈag-rə-ˌvāt\ *vt* **-vat·ed; -vat·ing** **1** : to make worse, more serious, or more severe ⟨movement may ∼ the pain⟩ **2** : to produce inflammation in : IRRITATE ⟨surgery ∼ed the nerve⟩

¹**ag·gre·gate** \ˈag-ri-gət\ *adj* : formed by the collection of units or particles into a body, mass, or amount

²**ag·gre·gate** \-ˌgāt\ *vt* **-gat·ed; -gat·ing** : to collect or gather into a mass or whole ⟨*aggregated* human albumin⟩

³**ag·gre·gate** \-gət\ *n* : a mass or body of units or parts somewhat loosely associated with one another

ag·gres·sin \ə-ˈgres-ᵊn\ *n* : a hypothetical substance held to contribute to the virulence of pathogenic bacteria by paralyzing the host defensive mechanisms (as the white blood cells) and held to be produced by the bacteria in the body of the host

ag·gres·sion \ə-ˈgresh-ən\ *n* : hostile, injurious, or destructive behavior or outlook esp. when caused by frustration

ag·gres·sive \ə-ˈgres-iv\ *adj* **1** : tending toward or exhibiting aggression ⟨∼ behavior⟩ **2** : growing, developing, or spreading rapidly ⟨∼ bone tumors⟩ **3** : more severe, intensive, or comprehensive than usual esp. in dosage or extent ⟨∼ chemotherapy⟩ ⟨∼ surgical intervention⟩ — compare CONSERVATIVE — **ag·gres·sive·ly** *adv* — **ag·gres·sive·ness** *n* — **ag·gres·siv·i·ty** \ˌag-ˌre-ˈsiv-ət-ē\ *n, pl* **-ties**

ag·gres·sor \ə-ˈgres-ər\ *n* : one who exhibits aggression

aging *pres part of* AGE

agitans — see PARALYSIS AGITANS

agitated depression *n* : a psychotic state characterized by restlessness, overactivity, anxiety, and despair but not accompanied by gross disorganization or deterioration

ag·i·ta·tion \ˌaj-ə-ˈtā-shən\ *n* : a state of excessive psychomotor activity accompanied by increased tension and irritability — **ag·i·tat·ed** \ˈaj-ə-ˌtāt-əd\ *adj*

ag·i·to·pha·sia \ˌaj-ət-ō-ˈfā-zh(ē-)ə\ *n* : extremely rapid speech marked by deletion and distortion of sounds, syllables, and words

aglo·mer·u·lar \ˌā-glə-ˈmer-(y)ə-lər, -glō-\ *adj* : lacking glomeruli

aglu·con \ag-ˈlü-ˌkän\ *or* **aglu·cone** \-ˌkōn\ *n* : AGLYCONE; *esp* : one combined with glucose in a glucoside

agly·cone \-ˈlī-ˌkōn\ *also* **agly·con** \-ˌkän\ *n* : an organic compound (as a phenol or alcohol) combined with the sugar portion of a glycoside

ag·ma·tine \ˈag-mə-ˌtēn\ *n* : a base $C_5H_{14}N_4$ formed from arginine in putrefaction

ag·mi·nate \ˈag-mə-nət, -ˌnāt\ *or* **ag·mi·nat·ed** \-ˌnāt-əd\ *adj* : grouped together ⟨*agminated* glands⟩

ag·nail \ˈag-ˌnāl\ *n* : a sore or inflammation about a fingernail or toenail; *also* : HANGNAIL

ag·na·thia \ag-ˈnā-thē-ə, (ˈ)ā-ˈnā-, -ˈnath-ē-\ *n* : the congenital complete or partial absence of one or both jaws

ag·na·thus \-ˈnā-thəs\ *n* : an individual and esp. a fetus affected with agnathia

ag·no·gen·ic \ˌag-nō-ˈjen-ik\ *adj* : of unknown cause ⟨∼ metaplasia⟩

ag·no·sia \ag-ˈnō-zhə, -shə\ *n* : loss or diminution of the ability to recognize familiar objects or stimuli usu. as a result of brain damage — see VISUAL AGNOSIA

ag·nos·te·rol \ag-ˈnäs-tə-ˌròl, -ˌrōl\ *n* : a crystalline tetracyclic triterpenoid alcohol $C_{30}H_{47}OH$ obtained from wool fat

ag·o·nal \ˈag-ən-ᵊl\ *adj* : of, relating to, or associated with agony and esp. the death agony ⟨chemical changes in the blood during the ∼ state —*Jour. Amer. Med. Assoc.*⟩

ag·o·nist \ˈag-ə-nəst\ *n* **1** : a muscle that on contracting is automatically checked and controlled by the opposing simultaneous contraction of another muscle — called also *agonist muscle, prime mover;* compare ANTAGONIST a, SYNERGIST 2 **2** : a chemical substance (as a drug) capable of combining with a receptor on a cell and initiating the same reaction or activity typically produced by the binding of an endogenous substance ⟨binding of adrenergic ∼s⟩ — compare ANTAGONIST b

ag·o·nis·tic \ˌag-ə-ˈnis-tik\ *adj* : of, relating to, or being aggressive or defensive social interaction (as fighting, fleeing, or submitting) between individuals usu. of the same species ⟨∼ behavior⟩

agonist muscle *n* : AGONIST 1

ag·o·ny \ˈag-ə-nē\ *n, pl* **-nies** **1** : intense pain of mind or body **2** : the struggle that precedes death

ag·o·ra·pho·bia \ˌag(-ə)-rə-ˈfō-bē-ə\ *n* : abnormal fear of being helpless in a situation from which escape may be difficult or embarrassing that is characterized initially often by panic or anticipatory anxiety and finally by avoidance of open or public places

¹**ag·o·ra·pho·bic** \-ˈfō-bik\ *adj* : of, relating to, or affected with agoraphobia ⟨∼ attacks⟩ ⟨an ∼ patient⟩

²**agoraphobic** *or* **ag·o·ra·phobe** \ˈag(-ə)-rə-ˌfōb\ *also* **ag·o·ra·pho·bi·ac** \ˌag(-ə)-rə-ˈfō-bē-ˌak\ *n* : a person affected with agoraphobia

agou·ti \ə-ˈgüt-ē\ *n* **1** : a rodent of the genus *Dasyprocta* (esp. *D. leporina*) **2** : a grizzled color of fur resulting from the barring of each hair in several alternate dark and light bands

agram·ma·tism \(ˈ)ā-ˈgram-ə-ˌtiz-əm\ *n* : the pathological inability to use words in grammatical sequence

agran·u·lo·cyte \(ˈ)ā-ˈgran-yə-lō-ˌsīt\ *n* : a white blood cell without cytoplasmic granules — compare GRANULOCYTE

agran·u·lo·cyt·ic angina \ā-ˌgran-yə-lō-ˌsit-ik-\ *n* : AGRANULOCYTOSIS

agran·u·lo·cy·to·sis \ˌā-ˌgran-yə-lō-ˌsī-ˈtō-səs\ *n, pl* **-to·ses** \-ˌsēz\ : an acute febrile condition marked by severe depression of the granulocyte-producing bone marrow and by prostration, chills, swollen neck, and sore throat sometimes with local ulceration and believed to be basically a response to the side effects of certain drugs of the coal-tar series (as aminopyrine) — called also *agranulocytic angina, granulocytopenia*

agraph·ia \(ˈ)ā-ˈgraf-ē-ə\ *n* : the pathological loss of the ability to write — **agraph·ic** \-ˈgraf-ik\ *adj*

Ag·ro·py·ron \ˌag-rō-ˈpī-ˌrän\ *n* : a widely distributed genus of chiefly perennial grasses that includes quack grass

Ag·ry·lin \ˈag-rə-lin\ *trademark* — used for a preparation of the hydrochloride of anagrelide

agryp·nia \ə-ˈgrip-nē-ə, a-\ *n* : INSOMNIA

agt *abbr* agent

ague \ˈā-(ˌ)gyü\ *n* 1 : a fever (as malaria) marked by paroxysms of chills, fever, and sweating that recur at regular intervals 2 : a fit of shivering : CHILL

AHA \ˌā-(ˌ)āch-ˈā\ *n* : ALPHA HYDROXY ACID

AHA *abbr* 1 American Heart Association 2 American Hospital Association

AHF *abbr* 1 antihemophilic factor 2 [*anti*hemophilic *fac*tor] factor VIII

AHG *abbr* antihemophilic globulin

AI *abbr* artificial insemination

AICD *abbr* automatic implantable cardioverter defibrillator

aich·mo·pho·bia \ˌāk-mə-ˈfō-bē-ə, -mō-\ *n* : a morbid fear of sharp or pointed objects (as a needle or a pointing finger)

aid \ˈād\ *n* 1 : the act of helping or treating; *also* : the help or treatment given ⟨in need of immediate medical ∼⟩ 2 : an assisting person or group ⟨a laboratory ∼⟩ — compare AIDE 3 : something by which assistance is given : an assisting device ⟨a visual ∼⟩; *esp* : HEARING AID

AID *abbr* artificial insemination by donor

aide \ˈād\ *n* : a person who acts as an assistant ⟨volunteer ∼s⟩ ⟨psychiatric ∼s⟩ — see NURSE'S AIDE

aid·man \ˈād-ˌman\ *n, pl* **aid·men** \-ˌmen\ : an army medical corpsman attached to a field unit

AIDS \ˈādz\ *n* : a disease of the human immune system that is characterized cytologically esp. by a reduction in the numbers of CD4-bearing helper T cells to 20 percent or less of normal thereby rendering the subject highly vulnerable to life-threatening conditions (as Pneumocystis carinii pneumonia) and to some that become life threatening (as Kaposi's sarcoma) and that is caused by infection with HIV commonly transmitted in infected blood esp. during illicit intravenous drug use and in bodily secretions (as semen) during sexual intercourse — called also *acquired immune deficiency syndrome, acquired immunodeficiency syndrome*

AIDS–related complex *n* : a group of symptoms (as fever, weight loss, and lymphadenopathy) that is associated with the presence of antibodies to HIV and is followed by the development of AIDS in a certain proportion of cases — abbr. *ARC*

aid station *n* : a station for giving emergency medical treatment; *specif* : a medical installation near the front lines where wounded receive emergency treatment

AIDS virus *n* : HIV

AIH *abbr* artificial insemination by husband

ail \ˈā(ə)l\ *vt* : to affect with an unnamed disease or physical or emotional pain or discomfort — used only of unspecified causes ⟨what ∼s the patient⟩ ∼ *vi* : to become affected with pain or discomfort ⟨was ∼*ing* from a cold⟩

ai·lan·thus \ā-ˈlan(t)-thəs, ī-\ *n* 1 *cap* : a small genus of chiefly tropical Asian trees and shrubs (family Simaroubaceae) with bitter bark, pinnate leaves, and terminal panicles of ill-scented greenish flowers; *esp* : TREE OF HEAVEN 2 : a tree of the genus *Ailanthus*

ail·ment \ˈā(ə)l-mənt\ *n* : a bodily disorder or chronic disease

ai·lu·ro·phobe \ī-ˈlur-ə-ˌfōb, ā-\ *or* **ae·lu·ro·phobe** \ē-\ *n* : a person who hates or fears cats

ai·lu·ro·pho·bia *or* **ae·lu·ro·pho·bia** \-ˌlur-ə-ˈfō-bē-ə\ *n* : abnormal fear of cats

ai·nhum \ī-ˈnyüm, -ˈnyüⁿ\ *n* : a tropical disease of unknown cause that results in increasing fibrous constriction and ultimately in spontaneous amputation of the toes and esp. the little toes

air \ˈa(ə)r, ˈe(ə)r\ *n* : a mixture of invisible odorless tasteless sound-transmitting gases that is composed by volume chiefly of 78 percent nitrogen, 21 percent oxygen, 0.9 percent argon, 0.03 percent carbon dioxide, varying amounts of water vapor, and minute amounts of rare gases (as helium), that surrounds the earth with half its mass within four miles of the earth's surface, that has a pressure at sea level of about 14.7 pounds per square inch, and that has a density of 1.293 grams per liter at 0°C and 760 mm pressure

air bends *n pl* : AEROEMBOLISM 2

air·borne \-ˌbōrn\ *adj* : carried or transported by the air ⟨∼ allergens⟩ ⟨∼ bacteria⟩

Air·bra·sive \ˈa(ə)r-ˌbrā-siv, ˈe(ə)r-, -ziv\ *trademark* — used for an apparatus designed to abrade surfaces by means of a jet of gas carrying abrasive powder under pressure

Air·cast \ˈa(ə)r-ˌkast, ˈe(ə)r-\ *trademark* — used for a pneumatic brace

air cell *n* : a cavity or receptacle for air; *esp* : ALVEOLUS b

air embolism *n* : obstruction of the circulation by air that has gained entrance to veins usu. through wounds — compare AEROEMBOLISM

air hunger *n* : deep labored breathing at an increased or decreased rate (as in acidosis)

air sac *n* : ALVEOLUS b

air·sick \ˈa(ə)r-ˌsik, ˈe(ə)r-\ *adj* : affected with motion sickness associated with flying — **air·sick·ness** *n*

air sinus *n* : an air-containing cavity (as a paranasal sinus and esp. a maxillary sinus) in bone

air·way \-ˌwā\ *n* : a passageway for air into or out of the lungs; *specif* : a device passed into the trachea by way of the mouth or nose or through an incision to maintain a clear respiratory passageway (as during anesthesia, convulsions, or in obstructive laryngitis) — see UPPER AIRWAY

AJ *abbr* ankle jerk

aj·o·wan oil \ˈaj-ə-ˌwän-\ *n* : an almost colorless essential oil containing thymol that is obtained from the fruit of a plant (*Carum copticum*) and is used in pharmaceuticals

AK *abbr* above knee

akar·y·ote \(ˈ)ā-ˈkar-ē-ˌōt\ *n* : a cell lacking a nucleus

aka·thi·sia *also* **aca·thi·sia** \ˌā-ka-ˈthizh-(ē-)ə, ˌa-, -ˈthēzh-\ *n* : a condition characterized by uncontrollable motor restlessness

akee *or* **ack·ee** \ˈak-ē, a-ˈkē\ *n* : the fruit of a tree (*Blighia sapida* of the family Sapindaceae) native to tropical West Africa but grown in the Caribbean area, Florida, and Hawaii for its white or yellowish fleshy aril which is edible when ripe but is poisonous when immature or overripe and that has a toxic pink raphe attaching the aril to the seed; *also* : the tree

aki·ne·sia \ˌā-kī-ˈnē-zh(ē-)ə\ *n* : loss or impairment of voluntary activity (as of a muscle)

aki·ne·sis \ˌā-kə-ˈnē-səs, -kī-\ *n, pl* **aki·ne·ses** \-ˌsēz\ : AKINESIA

aki·net·ic \-ˈnet-ik\ *adj* : of, relating to, or affected by akinesia ⟨an ∼ and myoclonic seizure⟩

Al *symbol* aluminum

ala \ˈā-lə\ *n, pl* **alae** \-ˌlē\ : a wing or a winglike anatomic process or part; *esp* : ALA NASI

Ala *abbr* alanine; alanyl

ALA *abbr* aminolevulinic acid

alaeque — see LEVATOR LABII SUPERIORIS ALAEQUE NASI

ala·lia \(ˈ)ā-ˈlā-lē-ə, ə-, -ˈlal-ē-\ *n* : MUTISM, APHASIA

ala na·si \-ˈnā-ˌsī, -ˌzī\ *n, pl* **alae na·si** \-ˌsī, -ˌzī\ : the expanded outer wall of cartilage on each side of the nose

al·a·nine \ˈal-ə-ˌnēn\ *n* : a simple nonessential crystalline amino acid $C_3H_7NO_2$ formed esp. by the hydrolysis of proteins — abbr. *Ala*

alanine aminotransferase *n* : an enzyme which promotes transfer of an amino group from glutamic acid to pyruvic acid and which when present in abnormally high levels in the blood is a diagnostic indication of liver disease — abbr. *ALT;* called also *glutamic pyruvic transaminase*

\ə\ **abut** \ˈ\ **kitten** \ər\ **further** \a\ **ash** \ā\ **ace** \ä\ **cot, cart**
\aú\ **out** \ch\ **chin** \e\ **bet** \ē\ **easy** \g\ **go** \i\ **hit** \ī\ **ice** \j\ **job**
\ŋ\ **sing** \ō\ **go** \ó\ **law** \ói\ **boy** \th\ **thin** \t͟h\ **the** \ü\ **loot**
\ú\ **foot** \y\ **yet** \zh\ **vision** *See also* Pronunciation Symbols page

al·a·nyl \'al-ə-ˌnil\ *n* : the amino acid radical or residue H₂NCHCH₃CO– of alanine — abbr. *Ala*

alar \'ā-lər\ *adj* : of or resembling a wing or wings

alar cartilage *n* : one of the pair of lower lateral cartilages of the nose

alar ligament *n* **1** : either of a pair of strong rounded fibrous cords of which one arises on each side of the cranial part of the odontoid process, passes obliquely and laterally upward, and inserts on the medial side of a condyle of the occipital bone — called also *check ligament;* see APICAL LIGAMENT OF THE DENS **2** : either of two folds of the synovial membrane of the knee that resemble fringes

alarm reaction \ə-'lärm-\ *n* : the initial reaction of an organism (as increased hormonal activity) to stress

alas·trim \'al-ə-ˌstrim, ˌal-ə-'; ə-'las-trəm\ *n* : VARIOLA MINOR

alb *abbr* albumin

al·ba \'al-bə\ *n* : the white matter of the brain and spinal cord

alba — see CERA ALBA, LINEA ALBA, MATERIA ALBA, PHLEGMASIA ALBA DOLENS, PNEUMONIA ALBA

albae — see ADMINICULUM LINEAE ALBAE

al·bas·pi·din \al-'bas-pə-(ˌ)dēn\ *n* : a white crystalline compound C₂₅H₃₂O₈ extracted from aspidium that has anthelmintic properties

al·be·do \al-'bēd-(ˌ)ō\ *n, pl* **-dos** : the fraction of incident light or electromagnetic radiation that is reflected by a surface or body (as the moon or the skin)

Al·bers–Schön·berg disease \'al-bərz-'shərn-ˌbərg-, -'shōn-\ *n* : OSTEOPETROSIS a

Albers–Schönberg \'äl-ˌbers-'shœn-ˌberk\, **Heinrich Ernst (1865–1921),** German roentgenologist. Albers-Schönberg was the first specialist in the field of roentgenology (now called radiology). He held the post of professor of roentgenology and founded an institute of roentgenology in Germany. He is credited with discovering that X-rays can cause damage to the reproductive organs. In 1903 he introduced a device consisting of a moving grid of lead strips used for producing sharper X-ray images by eliminating the oblique rays that pass through them before reaching the film. He described osteopetrosis, now also known as Albers-Schönberg disease, in a paper in a journal published in 1903–04.

albicans — see CORPUS ALBICANS

albicantes — see LINEAE ALBICANTES

al·bi·nism \'al-bə-ˌniz-əm, al-'bī-\ *n* : the condition of an albino — **al·bi·nis·tic** \ˌal-bə-'nis-tik\ *adj*

al·bi·no \al-'bī-(ˌ)nō\ *n, pl* **-nos** : an organism exhibiting deficient pigmentation; *esp* : a human being who is congenitally deficient in pigment and usu. has a milky or translucent skin, white or colorless hair, and eyes with pink or blue iris and deep-red pupil — compare MELANO — **al·bin·ic** \-'bin-ik\ *adj*

al·bi·no·ism \al-'bī-nə-ˌwiz-əm\ *n* : ALBINISM

al·bi·not·ic \ˌal-bə-'nät-ik\ *adj* **1** : of, relating to, or affected with albinism **2** : tending toward albinism

al·bo·ci·ne·re·ous \ˌal-(ˌ)bō-sə-'nir-ē-əs\ *adj* : composed of white and gray matter

al·bu·gin·ea \ˌal-b(y)ə-'jin-ē-ə\ *n, pl* **al·bu·gin·e·ae** \-ē-ˌī, -ˌē\ : TUNICA ALBUGINEA

album — see PRONTOSIL ALBUM

al·bu·men \al-'byü-mən; 'al-ˌbyü-, -byə-\ *n* **1** : the white of an egg **2** : ALBUMIN

al·bu·min \al-'byü-mən; 'al-ˌbyü-, -byə-\ *n* : any of numerous simple heat-coagulable water-soluble proteins that occur in blood plasma or serum, muscle, the whites of eggs, milk, and other animal substances and in many plant tissues and fluid

al·bu·mi·nate \al-'byü-mə-ˌnāt, -nət\ *n* : a compound derived from an albumin (as by the action of acids or alkalies or by combination with another substance)

¹al·bu·min·oid \-mə-ˌnȯid\ *adj* : resembling albumin

²albuminoid *n* **1** : PROTEIN 1 **2** : SCLEROPROTEIN

al·bu·mi·nom·e·ter \al-ˌbyü-mə-'näm-ət-ər\ *n* : an instrument usu. consisting of a graduated tube for determining the presence and amount of protein (esp. albumin) in a liquid (as urine)

al·bu·mi·nose \al-'byü-mə-ˌnōs, -ˌnōz\ *n* : ALBUMOSE

al·bu·min·ous \al-'byü-mə-nəs\ *adj* : relating to, containing, or having the properties of albumen or albumin

al·bu·min·uria \al-ˌbyü-mə-'n(y)ùr-ē-ə\ *n* : the presence of albumin in the urine that is usu. a symptom of disease of the kidneys but sometimes a response to other diseases or physiological disturbances of benign nature — **al·bu·min·uric** \-'n(y)ùr-ik\ *adj*

al·bu·mose \'al-byə-ˌmōs, al-'byü-, -ˌmōz\ *n* : any of various products of enzymatic protein hydrolysis

al·bu·mos·uria \ˌal-ˌbyü-mōs-'yùr-ē-ə\ *n* : the presence of proteoses in the urine

al·bu·te·rol \al-'byü-tə-ˌrȯl, -ˌrōl\ *n* : a beta-agonist bronchodilator that is administered in the form of its sulfate (C₁₃H₂₁NO₃)₂·H₂SO₄ as an inhalational aerosol or as a tablet to treat bronchospasm associated esp. with asthma and chronic obstructive pulmonary disease — called also *salbutamol;* see COMBIVENT, PROVENTIL, VENTOLIN

alc *abbr* alcohol

al·ca·lig·e·nes \ˌal-kə-'lij-ə-ˌnēz\ *n* **1** *cap* : a genus of gram-negative motile bacteria that do not ferment carbohydrates and are aerobes or facultative anaerobes, commonly occur in water and soil, and include some (as *A. faecalis*) that are found in the intestines of vertebrates including humans and are usu. harmless but have been associated with opportunistic infections **2** *pl* **alcaligenes** : an organism of the genus *Alcaligenes*

alcapton, alcaptonuria, alcaptonuric *var of* ALKAPTON, ALKAPTONURIA, ALKAPTONURIC

al·che·my \'al-kə-mē\ *n, pl* **-mies** : the medieval chemical science and speculative philosophy whose aims were the transmutation of the base metals into gold, the discovery of a universal cure for diseases, and the discovery of a means of indefinitely prolonging life — **al·che·mist** \-məst\ *n* — **al·che·mis·tic** \ˌal-kə-'mis-tik\ *or* **al·che·mis·ti·cal** \-ti-kəl\ *adj*

Al·cock's canal \'al-ˌkäks-,ȯl-\ *n* : a fascial compartment on the lateral wall of the ischiorectal fossa containing the pudendal arteries, veins, and nerves

Alcock, Benjamin (b 1801), British anatomist. In 1836 Alcock published an article on iliac arteries in which he described the canal that now bears his name.

al·co·gel \'al-kə-ˌjel\ *n* : a gel formed by the coagulation of an alcosol

al·co·hol \'al-kə-ˌhȯl\ *n* **1 a** : ethanol esp. when considered as the intoxicating agent in fermented and distilled liquors **b** : drink (as whiskey or beer) containing ethanol **c** : a mixture of ethanol and water that is usu. 95 percent ethanol **2** : any of various compounds that are analogous to ethanol in constitution and that are hydroxyl derivatives of hydrocarbons

al·co·hol·ate \'al-kə-ˌhȯl-ˌāt, -ˌhäl-, ˌal-kə-'\ *n* : a crystallizable compound of a substance with alcohol in which the alcohol plays a part analogous to that of water of crystallization

¹al·co·hol·ic \ˌal-kə-'hȯl-ik, -'häl-\ *adj* **1 a** : of, relating to, or caused by alcohol ⟨∼ hepatitis⟩ **b** : containing alcohol **2** : affected with alcoholism — **al·co·hol·i·cal·ly** \-i-k(ə-)lē\ *adv*

²alcoholic *n* : one affected with alcoholism

alcoholic fermentation *n* : a process in which some sugars (as glucose) are converted into alcohol and carbon dioxide by the action of various yeasts, molds, or bacteria on carbohydrate materials (as dough or sugar solutions) some of which do not themselves undergo fermentation but can be hydrolyzed into fermentable substances (as in the production of alcohol and alcoholic beverages)

al·co·hol·ism \'al-kə-ˌhȯ-ˌliz-əm, -kə-hə-\ *n* **1** : continued excessive or compulsive use of alcoholic drinks **2 a** : poisoning by alcohol **b** : a chronic progressive potentially fatal psychological and nutritional disorder associated with excessive and usu. compulsive drinking of ethanol and characterized by frequent intoxication leading to dependence on or addiction to the substance, impairment of the ability to work and socialize, destructive behaviors (as drunken driving), tissue damage (as cirrhosis of the liver), and severe withdrawal symptoms upon detoxification

al·co·hol·ist \-ˌhȯl-əst\ *n* : ALCOHOLIC

al·co·hol·ize *also Brit* **al·co·hol·ise** \'al-kə-ˌhȯ-ˌlīz\ *vt* **-ized** *also Brit* **-ised; -iz·ing** *also Brit* **-is·ing   1 a** : to treat or saturate with alcohol   **b** : to subject to the influence of alcohol   **2** : to convert into alcohol — **al·co·hol·iza·tion** *also Brit* **al·co·hol·isa·tion** \ˌal-kə-ˌhȯl-ə-'zā-shən, -ˌhäl-\ *n*

al·co·hol·om·e·ter \ˌal-kə-ˌhȯ-'läm-ət-ər\ *n* : a device for determining the alcoholic strength of liquids — **al·co·hol·om·e·try** \-'läm-ə-trē\ *n, pl* **-tries**

al·co·hol·ophil·ia \ˌal-kə-ˌhȯl-ə-'fil-ē-ə, -ˌhäl-\ *n* : an abnormal desire for alcohol

al·co·hol·y·sis \-'häl-ə-səs, -'hȯl-\ *n, pl* **-y·ses** \-ˌsēz\ : a chemical reaction analogous to hydrolysis in which an alcohol plays a role similar to that of water ⟨∼ of oils and fats⟩

al·co·sol \'al-kə-ˌsȯl, -ˌsōl\ *n* : a sol in which the liquid is alcohol

ALD *abbr* adrenoleukodystrophy

al·de·hyde \'al-də-ˌhīd\ *n* : ACETALDEHYDE; *broadly* : any of various highly reactive compounds typified by acetaldehyde and characterized by the group CHO — **al·de·hy·dic** \ˌal-də-'hīd-ik\ *adj*

al·der buckthorn \'ȯl-dər-\ *n* : a common European tree of the genus *Rhamnus* (*R. frangula*) with a bark that has medicinal properties — see FRANGULA

al·di·carb \'al-də-ˌkärb\ *n* : a persistent highly toxic agricultural carbamate pesticide $C_7H_{14}N_2O_2S$ used against insects, mites, and nematodes

al·do·bi·uron·ic acid \ˌal-(ˌ)dō-ˌbī-yə-ˌrän-ik-\ *n* : an acidic disaccharide in which one of the two sugar constituents is a uronic acid joined as a glycoside to a hexose or pentose unit

al·do·hex·ose \ˌal-dō-'hek-ˌsōs, -ˌsōz\ *n* : an aldehydic hexose (as glucose or mannose)

al·dol \'al-ˌdȯl, -ˌdōl\ *n* : a colorless beta-hydroxy aldehyde $C_4H_8O_2$; *broadly* : any of various similar aldehydes

al·dol·ase \'al-də-ˌlās, -ˌlāz\ *n* : a crystalline enzyme that occurs widely in living systems and catalyzes reversibly the cleavage of a fructose ester into triose sugars

al·don·ic acid \(ˌ)al-ˌdän-ik-\ *n* : any of a class of acids (as gluconic acid) formed from aldoses (as glucose) by oxidizing the aldehyde group to a carboxyl group

al·dose \'al-ˌdōs, -ˌdōz\ *n* : a sugar containing one aldehyde group per molecule

al·do·side \'al-də-ˌsīd\ *n* : any glycoside derived from an aldose

al·do·ste·rone \al-'däs-tə-ˌrōn; ˌal-dō-'sti(ə)r-ˌōn, -stə-'rōn\ *n* : a steroid hormone $C_{21}H_{28}O_5$ of the adrenal cortex that functions in the regulation of the salt and water balance of the body

al·do·ste·ron·ism \-ˌrō-ˌniz-əm, -'rō-\ *n* : a condition that is characterized by excessive secretion of aldosterone and typically by loss of body potassium, muscular weakness, and elevated blood pressure — called also *hyperaldosteronism*

al·dox·ime \al-'däk-ˌsēm\ *n* : an oxime of an aldehyde

al·drin \'al-drən, 'ȯl-\ *n* : an exceedingly poisonous cyclodiene insecticide $C_{12}H_8Cl_6$

K. Alder — see DIELDRIN

alec·i·thal \(')ā-'les-ə-thəl\ *adj, of an egg* : ISOLECITHAL

alem·bic \ə-'lem-bik\ *n* : an apparatus formerly used in distillation

alem·mal \(')ā-'lem-əl\ *adj* : being without neurilemma

alen·dro·nate \ə-'len-drə-ˌnāt\ *n* : a hydrated bisphosphonate sodium salt $C_4H_{12}NNaO_7P_2 \cdot 3H_2O$ used to inhibit bone resorption esp. in the treatment of osteoporosis in postmenopausal women and Paget's disease of bone — called also *alendronate sodium;* see FOSAMAX

Al·e·tris \'al-ə-trəs\ *n* : a small genus of bitter-rooted herbs (family Liliaceae) found in eastern No. America and Asia and including one (*A. farinosa*) used esp. formerly to treat a variety of ailments

aleu·ke·mia *or chiefly Brit* **aleu·kae·mia** \ˌā-lü-'kē-mē-ə\ *n* : leukemia in which the circulating white blood cells are normal or decreased in number; *esp* : ALEUKEMIC LEUKEMIA

aleu·ke·mic *or chiefly Brit* **aleu·kae·mic** \-'kē-mik\ *adj* : not marked by increase in circulating white blood cells

aleukemic leukemia *n* : leukemia resulting from changes in the tissues forming white blood cells and characterized by a normal or decreased number of white blood cells in the circulating blood — called also *aleukemic myelosis*

al·eu·rone \'al-yə-ˌrōn\ *n* : protein matter in the form of minute granules or grains occurring in seeds in endosperm or in a special peripheral layer — **al·eu·ron·ic** \ˌal-yə-'rän-ik\ *adj*

Aleve \ə-'lēv\ *trademark* — used for a preparation of the sodium salt of naproxen

Al·ex·an·der technique \ˌal-ig-'zan-dər\ *n, often cap T* : a technique for positioning and moving the body that is believed to reduce tension

Alexander, Frederick Matthias (1869–1955), Australian elocutionist. By the 1890s Alexander had established himself as a professional reciter or elocutionist, touring the Australian outback in a one-man variety show that included the declaiming of Shakespeare. Episodes of crippling hoarseness became increasingly frequent until he was forced to quit and seek a solution to the problem. His discovery that he tended to pull his head back, thereby depressing the larynx, during the act of declaiming led him to develop his technique for a stress-reducing alignment of the head, neck, and back. In addition to greater ease in his public speaking, he noticed an improvement in his overall health and well-being. He devoted the rest of his life to the teaching and propagation of his technique. A course for training teachers in the Alexander technique was established in London in 1931.

Al·ex·an·dri·an senna \ˌal-ig-ˌzan-drē-ən-, ˌel-\ *n* : senna obtained from a cassia (*Cassia acutifolia*) esp. in northern Africa

alex·ia \ə-'lek-sē-ə\ *n* : aphasia characterized by loss of ability to read — **alex·ic** \-'lek-sik\ *adj*

alex·in \ə-'lek-sən\ *also* **alex·ine** \-sən, -ˌsēn\ *n* : COMPLEMENT 3 — **al·ex·in·ic** \ˌal-ˌek-'sin-ik\ *adj*

alex·i·thy·mia \ə-ˌleks-i-'thī-mē-ə\ *n* : inability to express one's feelings

alfa — see INTERFERON ALFA

ALG *abbr* antilymphocyte globulin; antilymphocytic globulin

al·ga \'al-gə\ *n, pl* **al·gae** \'al-(ˌ)jē\ *also* **algas** : a plant or plantlike organism of any of several phyla, divisions, or classes of chiefly aquatic usu. chlorophyll-containing nonvascular organisms of polyphyletic origin that usu. include the green, yellow-green, brown, and red algae in the eukaryotes and esp. formerly included the cyanobacteria in the prokaryotes — **al·gal** \-gəl\ *adj*

al·ge·do·nic \ˌal-jə-'dän-ik\ *adj* : characterized by or relating to pain esp. as associated with pleasure

al·ge·sia \al-'jē-zē-ə, -'jē-zhə\ *n* : sensitivity to pain — **al·ge·sic** \-'jē-zik, -sik\ *adj*

al·ge·sim·e·ter \ˌal-jə-'sim-ət-ər\ *n* : an instrument used in determining acuteness of pain perception — **al·ge·sim·e·try** \-'sim-ə-trē\ *n, pl* **-tries**

al·get·ic \al-'jet-ik\ *adj* : relating to or causing pain

al·gi·cide *or* **al·gae·cide** \'al-jə-ˌsīd\ *n* : an agent used to kill algae — **al·gi·cid·al** \ˌal-jə-'sīd-ᵊl\ *adj*

al·gid \'al-jəd\ *adj* : marked by prostration, cold and clammy skin, and low blood pressure — used chiefly of a severe form of malaria

al·gin \'al-jən\ *n* : any of various colloidal substances derived from marine brown algae and esp. giant kelp: as   **a** : ALGINIC ACID   **b** : a soluble salt of alginic acid used esp. as a stabilizing, emulsifying, or thickening agent in foods (as ice cream), pharmaceuticals, and cosmetics and as a base for dental-impression materials — called also *sodium alginate*

\ə\ **abut** \ᵊ\ **kitten** \ər\ **further** \a\ **ash** \ā\ **ace** \ä\ **cot, cart** \au̇\ **out** \ch\ **chin** \e\ **bet** \ē\ **easy** \g\ **go** \i\ **hit** \ī\ **ice** \j\ **job** \ŋ\ **sing** \ō\ **go** \ȯ\ **law** \ȯi\ **boy** \th\ **thin** \t͟h\ **the** \ü\ **loot** \u̇\ **foot** \y\ **yet** \zh\ **vision**   See also Pronunciation Symbols page

al·gi·nate \'al-jə-ˌnāt\ *n* : a salt of alginic acid

al·gin·ic acid \(ˌ)al-ˌjin-ik-\ *n* : an insoluble colloidal acid $(C_6H_8O_6)_n$ that in the form of its salts is a constituent of the cell walls of brown algae and is used in making dental preparations and in preparing pharmaceuticals

al·glu·ce·rase \al-'glü-sə-ˌrās\ *n* : modified human glucocerebrosidase administered for enzyme replacement therapy in the treatment of Gaucher's disease — see CEREDASE

¹al·go·gen·ic \al-gō-'jen-ik\ *adj* : producing pain

²algogenic *adj* : reducing body temperature

al·go·lag·nia \ˌal-gō-'lag-nē-ə\ *n* : a perversion (as masochism or sadism) in which pleasure and esp. sexual gratification is obtained by inflicting or suffering pain — **al·go·lag·nic** \-nik\ *adj*

al·go·lag·ni·ac \-nē-ˌak\ *n* : one who practices algolagnia

al·go·lag·nist \-nəst\ *n* : ALGOLAGNIAC

al·gol·o·gist \al-'gäl-ə-jəst\ *n* : PHYCOLOGIST

al·gol·o·gy \al-'gäl-ə-jē\ *n, pl* **-gies** : PHYCOLOGY — **al·go·log·i·cal** \ˌal-gə-'läj-i-kəl\ *adj*

al·gom·e·ter \al-'gäm-ət-ər\ *n* : an instrument for measuring the smallest pressure upon the skin that will arouse a sensation of pain

al·gom·e·try \-ə-trē\ *n, pl* **-tries** : the measurement of pain sensitivity (as by an algometer)

al·go·phil·ia \ˌal-gō-'fil-ē-ə\ *n* : a morbid pleasure in the pain either of oneself or of others

al·goph·i·list \al-'gäf-ə-ləst\ *n* : one who is subject to algophilia

al·go·pho·bia \ˌal-gə-'fō-bē-ə\ *n* : morbid fear of pain

al·gor \'al-ˌgȯ(ə)r\ *n* : a sensation of coldness : CHILL

al·gor mor·tis \-'mȯrt-əs\ *n* : the gradual cooling of the body following death

al·i·cy·clic \ˌal-ə-'sī-klik, -'sik-lik\ *adj* : of, relating to, or being an organic compound that contains a ring but is not aromatic — compare ALIPHATIC

alien·ate \'ā-lē-ə-ˌnāt, 'āl-yə-\ *vt* **-at·ed; -at·ing** : to make unfriendly, hostile, or indifferent where attachment formerly existed

alien·ation \ˌā-lē-ə-'nā-shən, ˌāl-yə-\ *n* **1** : a withdrawing or separation of a person or a person's affections from an object or position of former attachment ⟨~ . . . from the values of one's society and family —S. L. Halleck⟩ **2** : MENTAL ALIENATION

alien·ist \'ā-lē-ə-nəst, 'āl-yə-\ *n* : PSYCHIATRIST; *esp* : one specializing in the legal aspects of psychiatry

ali·es·ter·ase \ˌal-ē-'es-tə-ˌrās, 'al-ē-ˌ, -ˌrāz\ *n* : an esterase that promotes the hydrolysis of ester links esp. in aliphatic esters of low molecular weight

ali·form \'ā-lə-ˌfȯrm, 'al-ə-\ *adj* : having winglike extensions : wing-shaped

al·i·ment \'al-ə-mənt\ *n* : a food or nutrient substance

al·i·men·ta·ry \ˌal-ə-'ment-ə-rē, -'men-trē\ *adj* : of, concerned with, or relating to nourishment or to the function of nutrition : NUTRITIVE ⟨~ processes of the body⟩

alimentary canal *n* : the tubular passage that extends from mouth to anus, functions in digestion and absorption of food and elimination of residual waste, and includes the mouth, pharynx, esophagus, stomach, small intestine, and large intestine

alimentary system *n* : the organ system devoted to the ingestion, digestion, and assimilation of food and the discharge of residual wastes and consisting of the alimentary canal and those glands or parts of complex glands that secrete digestive enzymes

al·i·men·ta·tion \ˌal-ə-mən-'tā-shən, -ˌmen-\ *n* : the act or process of affording nutriment or nourishment ⟨intravenous ~⟩

al·i·men·to·ther·a·py \ˌal-ə-ˌmen-tō-'ther-ə-pē\ *n, pl* **-pies** : the treatment of disease by dietetic methods

ali·na·sal \ˌā-lə-'nā-zəl, 'ā-lə-ˌ, ˌal-ə-', 'al-ə-ˌ\ *adj* : relating to the nasal alae

al·i·phat·ic \ˌal-ə-'fat-ik\ *adj* : of, relating to, or being an organic compound (as an alkane or alkene) having an open-chain structure — compare ALICYCLIC, AROMATIC 2

¹al·i·quot \'al-ə-ˌkwät\ *adj* : being an equal fractional part (as of a solution)

²aliquot *n* : an aliquot part ⟨remove 50 ml ~s at ten minute intervals⟩

³aliquot *vt* : to divide (as a solution) into equal parts

¹ali·sphe·noid \ˌā-ləs-'fē-ˌnȯid, ˌal-əs-\ *adj* : belonging or relating to or forming the wings of the sphenoid or the pair of bones that fuse with other sphenoidal elements to form the greater wings of the sphenoid in the adult

²alisphenoid *n* : an alisphenoid bone; *esp* : GREATER WING

alive \ə-'līv\ *adj* : having life : not dead or inanimate

aliz·a·rin \ə-'liz-ə-rən\ *also* **aliz·a·rine** \-rən, -ˌrēn\ *n* **1** : an orange or red crystalline compound $C_{14}H_8O_4$ formerly prepared from madder and now made synthetically from anthraquinone that was formerly used in dyeing but is now used more in making red pigments **2** : any of a group of dyes that are similar to alizarin in dyeing properties or derivation

alk *abbr* alkaline

al·ka·le·mia *or chiefly Brit* **al·ka·lae·mia** \ˌal-kə-'lē-mē-ə\ *n* : a condition in which the hydrogen ion concentration in the blood is decreased

al·ka·les·cence \ˌal-kə-'les-ᵊn(t)s\ *n* : the property or degree of being alkaline : ALKALINITY — **al·ka·les·cent** \-ᵊnt\ *adj*

al·ka·li \'al-kə-ˌlī\ *n, pl* **-lies** *or* **-lis** : a substance (as a hydroxide or carbonate of an alkali metal) having marked basic properties — compare BASE

alkali disease *n* : SELENOSIS

al·ka·li·fy \al-'kal-ə-ˌfī, 'al-kə-lə-\ *vb* **-fied; -fy·ing** *vt* : to convert or change into an alkali : make alkaline ~ *vi* : to become alkaline

alkali metal *n* : any of the univalent mostly basic metals of group I of the periodic table comprising lithium, sodium, potassium, rubidium, cesium, and francium

al·ka·lim·e·ter \ˌal-kə-'lim-ət-ər\ *n* : an apparatus for measuring the strength or the amount of alkali in a mixture or solution — **al·ka·lim·e·try** \-'lim-ə-trē\ *n, pl* **-tries**

al·ka·line \'al-kə-lən, -ˌlīn\ *adj* : of, relating to, containing, or having the properties of an alkali or alkali metal : BASIC; *esp, of a solution* : having a pH of more than 7 — **al·ka·lin·i·ty** \ˌal-kə-'lin-ət-ē\ *n, pl* **-ties**

alkaline earth *n* **1** : an oxide of an alkaline earth metal **2** : ALKALINE EARTH METAL

alkaline earth metal *n* : any of the bivalent strongly basic metals of group II of the periodic table comprising beryllium, magnesium, calcium, strontium, barium, and radium

alkaline phosphatase *n* : any of the phosphatases (as phosphomonoesterase from blood plasma or milk) optimally active in alkaline medium and occurring in esp. high concentrations in bone, the liver, the kidneys, and the placenta

al·ka·lin·ize *also Brit* **al·ka·lin·ise** \'al-kə-lə-ˌnīz\ *vt* **-ized** *also Brit* **-ised; -iz·ing** *also Brit* **-is·ing** : to make alkaline ⟨alkalinized the urine with a drug⟩ — **al·ka·lin·iza·tion** *also Brit* **al·ka·lin·isa·tion** \ˌal-kə-ˌlin-ə-'zā-shən, -lə-nə-\ *n*

alkali reserve *n* : the concentration of one or more basic ions or substances in a fluid medium that buffer its pH by neutralizing acid; *esp* : the concentration of bicarbonate in the blood

al·ka·lize *also Brit* **al·ka·lise** \'al-kə-ˌlīz\ *vt* **-lized** *also Brit* **-lised; -liz·ing** *also Brit* **-lis·ing** : ALKALINIZE — **al·ka·li·za·tion** *also Brit* **al·ka·li·sa·tion** \ˌal-kə-lə-'zā-shən\ *n*

al·ka·liz·er *also Brit* **al·ka·lis·er** \'al-kə-ˌlī-zər\ *n* : an alkalinizing agent

al·ka·loid \'al-kə-ˌlȯid\ *n* : any of numerous usu. colorless, complex, and bitter organic bases (as morphine or caffeine) containing nitrogen and usu. oxygen that occur esp. in seed plants and are typically physiologically active — **al·ka·loi·dal** \ˌal-kə-'lȯid-ᵊl\ *adj*

al·ka·lom·e·try \ˌal-kə-'läm-ə-trē\ *n, pl* **-tries** **1** : the quantitative determination of alkaloids **2** : the administration of alkaloids according to an exact system of dosage

al·ka·lo·sis \ˌal-kə-'lō-səs\ *n, pl* **-lo·ses** \-ˌsēz\ : an abnormal condition of increased alkalinity of the blood and tissues — compare ACIDOSIS, KETOSIS

al·ka·lot·ic \ˌal-kə-ˈlät-ik\ *adj* : marked by the presence of or tendency toward alkalosis ⟨an ∼ state⟩

al·kane \ˈal-ˌkān\ *n* : any of a series of saturated aliphatic hydrocarbons C_nH_{2n+2} (as methane) — called also *paraffin*

al·ka·net \ˈal-kə-ˌnet\ *n* **1** : a European plant (*Alkanna tinctoria*) of the borage family; *also* : its root **2** : a red dyestuff prepared from the root

al·kan·nin \al-ˈkan-ən\ *n* : a red crystalline coloring matter $C_{16}H_{16}O_5$ obtained from alkanet and used chiefly in coloring beverages and fatty and oily pharmaceutical and cosmetic preparations

al·kap·ton *or* **al·cap·ton** \al-ˈkap-ˌtän, -tən\ *n* : HOMOGENTISIC ACID

al·kap·ton·uria *or* **al·cap·ton·uria** \(ˌ)al-ˌkap-tə-ˈn(y)ùrē-ə\ *n* : a rare recessive metabolic anomaly in humans marked by inability to complete the degradation of tyrosine and phenylalanine resulting in the presence of alkapton in the urine

¹**al·kap·ton·uric** *or* **al·cap·ton·uric** \-ˈn(y)ùr-ik\ *n* : one affected with alkaptonuria

²**alkaptonuric** *or* **alcaptonuric** *adj* : of, relating to, or affected with alkaptonuria

al·ka·ver·vir \ˌal-kə-ˈvər-ˌvi(ə)r, al-ˈkav-ə(r)-\ *n* : a preparation containing ester alkaloids obtained from a hellebore (*Veratrum viride*) and used in treating hypertension

al·kene \ˈal-ˌkēn\ *n* : any of numerous unsaturated hydrocarbons having one double bond; *specif* : any of a series of aliphatic hydrocarbons C_nH_{2n} (as ethylene)

alk·oxy \ˈal-ˌkäk-sē\ *adj* : of, relating to, or containing a monovalent radical composed of an alkyl group united with oxygen

alky *abbr* alkalinity

¹**al·kyl** \ˈal-kəl\ *adj* : of, relating to, or being an alkyl ⟨∼ mercurials attack the brain cells —L. J. Goldwater⟩

²**alkyl** *n* **1** : a monovalent aliphatic radical C_nH_{2n+1} (as methyl); *broadly* : a monovalent aliphatic, aromatic-aliphatic, or alicyclic hydrocarbon radical **2** : a compound of one or more alkyl groups with a metal

al·kyl·amine \ˈal-kə-lə-ˌmēn, ˌal-kə-lə-ˈmēn, -ˈlam-ən, -ˈlam-ˌēn\ *n* : an amine (as methylamine) containing one or more alkyl groups

al·kyl·ate \ˈal-kə-ˌlāt\ *vt* **-at·ed; -at·ing** : to introduce one or more alkyl groups into (a compound) — **al·kyl·ation** \ˌal-kə-ˈlā-shən\ *n*

alkylating agent *n* : a substance that causes replacement of hydrogen by an alkyl group esp. in a biologically important molecule; *specif* : one with mutagenic activity that inhibits cell division and growth and is used to treat some cancers

ALL *abbr* acute lymphoblastic leukemia, acute lymphocytic leukemia

al·lan·to·cho·ri·on \ə-ˌlan-(ˌ)tō-ˈkōr-ē-ˌän, -ˈkòr-\ *n* : an embryonic membrane consisting of a fused allantois and chorion

al·lan·to·ic \ˌal-ən-ˈtō-ik, ˌal-ˌan-\ *adj* : relating to, contained in, or characterized by an allantois

allantoic vesicle *n* : the cavity of the allantois

¹**al·lan·toid** \ə-ˈlan-ˌtòid, -tə-wəd\ *adj* : of or relating to the allantois

²**allantoid** *n* : ALLANTOIS

al·lan·to·in \ə-ˈlan-tə-wən\ *n* : a crystalline oxidation product $C_4H_6N_4O_3$ of uric acid used to promote healing of local wounds and infections

al·lan·to·is \ə-ˈlant-ə-wəs\ *n, pl* **al·lan·to·ides** \ˌal-ən-ˈtō-ə-ˌdēz, ˌal-ˌan-\ : a vascular fetal membrane of reptiles, birds, or mammals that is formed as a pouch from the hindgut and that in placental mammals is intimately associated with the chorion in formation of the placenta

Al·le·gra \ə-ˈleg-rə, -ˈlā-grə\ *trademark* — used for a preparation of the hydrochloride of fexofenadine

al·lele \ə-ˈlē(ə)l\ *n* **1** : any of the alternative forms of a gene that may occur at a given locus **2** : either of a pair of alternative Mendelian characters (as ability versus inability to taste the chemical phenylthiocarbamide) — **al·le·lic** \-ˈlē-lik, -ˈlel-ik\ *adj* — **al·lel·ism** \-ˈlē(ə)l-ˌiz-əm, -ˈlel-ˌiz-\ *n*

al·le·lo·ca·tal·y·sis \ə-ˌlel-(ˌ)ō-kə-ˈtal-ə-səs, -lē-(ˌ)lō-\ *n, pl* **-y-**

ses \-ˌsēz\ : the mutually stimulating effect on the rate of growth and reproduction of two or more microorganisms in a volume of medium as compared to the rate of a single microorganism in a like volume of the same medium — **al·le·lo·cat·a·lyst** \-ˈkat-ᵊl-əst\ *n* — **al·le·lo·cat·a·lyt·ic** \-ˌkat-ᵊl-ˈit-ik\ *adj*

al·le·lo·morph \ə-ˈlel-ə-ˌmòrf, -ˈlē-lə-\ *n* : ALLELE — **al·le·lo·mor·phic** \ə-ˌlel-ə-ˈmòr-fik, -ˌlē-lə-\ *adj* — **al·le·lo·mor·phism** \ə-ˈlel-ə-ˌmòr-ˌfiz-əm, -ˈlē-lə-\ *n*

al·ler·gen \ˈal-ər-jən\ *n* : a substance that induces allergy ⟨inhaled ∼s⟩ ⟨a suspected food ∼⟩

al·ler·gen·ic \ˌal-ər-ˈjen-ik\ *adj* : having the capacity to induce allergy ⟨∼ plants⟩ — **al·ler·ge·nic·i·ty** \-jə-ˈnis-ət-ē\ *n, pl* **-ties**

al·ler·gic \ə-ˈlər-jik\ *adj* **1** : of, relating to, or characterized by allergy ⟨an ∼ reaction⟩ ⟨∼ diseases⟩ **2** : affected with allergy : subject to an allergic reaction ⟨he is ∼ to pollen⟩

allergic encephalomyelitis *n* : encephalomyelitis produced by an allergic response following the introduction of an antigenic substance into the body

allergic rhinitis *n* : rhinitis caused by exposure to an allergen; *esp* : HAY FEVER

al·ler·gin \ˈal-ər-jən\ *n* : ALLERGEN

al·ler·gist \-jəst\ *n* : a specialist in allergy

al·ler·gi·za·tion \ˌal-ər-jə-ˈzā-shən\ *n* : the process of becoming sensitive to an allergen

al·ler·gol·o·gy \ˌal-ər-ˈgäl-ə-jē\ *n, pl* **-gies** : a branch of medicine concerned with allergy

al·ler·gy \ˈal-ər-jē\ *n, pl* **-gies** **1** : altered bodily reactivity (as hypersensitivity) to an antigen in response to a first exposure ⟨his bee-venom ∼ may render a second sting fatal⟩ **2** : exaggerated or pathological reaction (as by sneezing, respiratory embarrassment, itching, or skin rashes) to substances, situations, or physical states that are without comparable effect on the average individual **3** : medical practice concerned with allergies

al·le·thrin \ˈal-ə-thrən\ *n* : a light yellow viscous oily synthetic insecticide $C_{19}H_{26}O_3$ used esp. in household aerosols

al·le·vi·ate \ə-ˈlē-vē-ˌāt\ *vt* **-at·ed; -at·ing** : to make (as symptoms) less severe or more bearable ⟨a lotion to ∼ itching⟩ — **al·le·vi·a·tion** \-ˌlē-vē-ˈā-shən\ *n*

al·le·vi·a·tive \ə-ˈlē-vē-ˌāt-iv\ *adj* : tending to alleviate : PALLIATIVE ⟨a medicine that is ∼ but not curative⟩

al·li·cin \ˈal-ə-sən\ *n* : a liquid compound $C_6H_{10}OS_2$ with a garlic odor and antibacterial properties formed from alliin by enzymatic action

al·li·ga·tion \ˌal-ə-ˈgā-shən\ *n* : a process or rule for the solution of problems concerning the compounding or mixing of ingredients differing in price or quality: **a** : one applied when a definite mixture is required — called also *alligation alternate* **b** : one applied when the price or quality of the mixture is to be determined — called also *alligation medial*

al·li·in \ˈal-ē-ən\ *n* : a crystalline amino acid $C_6H_{11}NO_3S$ occurring in garlic oil

al·li·um \ˈal-ē-əm\ *n* **1** *cap* : a genus of bulbous herbs (as an onion, garlic, or leek) of the lily family distinguished by a characteristic odor, sheathing, mostly basal leaves, and clusters of usu. white, blue, purple, pink, or red flowers **2 a** : a plant of the genus *Allium* **b** : the bulb of garlic formerly used in medicine esp. as an expectorant and rubefacient

al·lo·an·ti·body \ˌal-ō-ˈant-i-ˌbäd-ē\ *n, pl* **-bod·ies** : an antibody produced following introduction of an alloantigen into the system of an individual of a species lacking that particular antigen — called also *isoantibody*

al·lo·an·ti·gen \ˌal-ō-ˈant-ə-jən\ *n* : a genetically determined antigen present in some but not all individuals of a species (as those of a particular blood group) and capable of inducing the production of an alloantibody by individuals which

\ə\ abut \ᵊ\ kitten \ər\ further \a\ ash \ā\ ace \ä\ cot, cart
\aù\ out \ch\ chin \e\ bet \ē\ easy \g\ go \i\ hit \ī\ ice \j\ job
\ŋ\ sing \ō\ go \ò\ law \òi\ boy \th\ thin \t̲h̲\ the \ü\ loot
\ù\ foot \y\ yet \zh\ vision *See also* Pronunciation Symbols page

lack it — called also *isoantigen* — **al·lo·an·ti·gen·ic** \-₁ant-ə-'jen-ik\ *adj*

al·lo·bar·bi·tal \₁al-ə-'bär-bə-₁tol\ *n* : a white crystalline barbiturate $C_{10}H_{12}N_2O_3$ used as a sedative and hypnotic — called also *diallylbarbituric acid*

al·lo·bar·bi·tone \-₁tōn\ *n, chiefly Brit* : ALLOBARBITAL

al·lo·chi·ria *also* **al·lo·chei·ria** \₁al-ə-'kir-ē-ə\ *n* : a condition associated with a central nervous lesion in which sensation is referred to a locus on the side of the body opposite to the place on which the skin is stimulated

al·lo·cor·tex \-'kor-₁teks\ *n* : ARCHIPALLIUM

Al·lo·der·ma·nys·sus \-₁dər-mə-'nis-əs\ *n* : a genus of bloodsucking mites parasitic on rodents including one (*A. sanguineus*) implicated as a vector of rickettsialpox in humans

al·lo·dyn·ia \₁al-ə-'din-ē-ə\ *n* : pain resulting from a stimulus (as a light touch of the skin) which would not normally provoke pain; *also* : a condition marked by allodynia

al·lo·er·o·tism \₁al-ō-'er-ə-₁tiz-əm\ *also* **al·lo·erot·i·cism** \-i-'rät-ə-₁siz-əm\ *n* : sexual feeling or activity directed toward another person — called also *heteroerotism;* compare AUTOEROTISM — **al·lo·erot·ic** \-i-'rät-ik\ *adj*

al·lo·ge·ne·ic \₁al-ō-jə-'nē-ik\ *also* **al·lo·gen·ic** \-'jen-ik\ *adj* : involving, derived from, or being individuals of the same species that are sufficiently unlike genetically to interact antigenically ⟨~ skin grafts⟩ — compare SYNGENEIC, XENOGENEIC

al·lo·graft \'al-ə-₁graft\ *n* : a homograft between allogeneic individuals — **allograft** *vt*

al·lo·im·mune \₁al-ō-i-'myün\ *adj* : of, relating to, or characterized by isoimmunization ⟨~ reactivity⟩

al·lo·iso·leu·cine \₁al-ō-₁ī-sə-'lü-₁sēn\ *n* : either of two stereoisomers of isoleucine of which one is present in bodily fluids of individuals affected with maple syrup urine disease

al·lom·e·try \ə-'läm-ə-trē\ *n, pl* **-tries** : relative growth of a part in relation to an entire organism or to a standard; *also* : the measure and study of such growth — **al·lo·met·ric** \₁al-ə-'me-trik\ *adj*

al·lo·morph \'al-ə-₁morf\ *n* 1 : any of two or more distinct crystalline forms of the same substance 2 : a pseudomorph that has undergone change or substitution of material — **al·lo·mor·phic** \₁al-ə-'mor-fik\ *adj* — **al·lo·mor·phism** \'al-ə-₁mor-₁fiz-əm\ *n*

al·lo·path \'al-ə-₁path\ *n* : one who practices allopathy

al·lop·a·thy \ə-'läp-ə-thē, a-\ *n, pl* **-thies** 1 : a system of medical practice that aims to combat disease by use of remedies (as drugs or surgery) producing effects different from or incompatible with those produced by the disease being treated — compare HOMEOPATHY 2 : a system of medical practice making use of all measures that have proved of value in treatment of disease — **al·lo·path·ic** \₁al-ə-'path-ik\ *adj* — **al·lo·path·i·cal·ly** \-i-k(ə-)lē\ *adv*

al·lo·phen·ic \₁al-ə-'fen-ik\ *adj* : produced from a mosaic cellular mass composed of cells integrated from two or more genetically different embryos

al·lo·poly·ploid \₁al-ō-'päl-i-₁ploid\ *n* : an individual or strain whose chromosomes are composed of more than two genomes each of which has been derived more or less complete but possibly modified from one of two or more species — compare AUTOPOLYPLOID — **allopolyploid** *adj* — **al·lo·poly·ploi·dy** \-₁ploid-ē\ *n, pl* **-dies**

al·lo·psy·chic \₁al-ō-'sī-kik\ *adj* : related mentally to the outside world ⟨~ adjustment⟩ — compare AUTOPSYCHIC

al·lo·pu·ri·nol \₁al-ō-'pyur-ə-₁nol, -₁nōl\ *n* : a drug $C_5H_4N_4O$ used to promote excretion of uric acid esp. in the treatment of gout

all–or–none \₁o-lər-'nən\ *adj* : marked either by complete operation or effect or by none at all ⟨~ response of a nerve cell⟩

all–or–none law *n* : a principle in physiology: in any single nerve or muscle fiber the response to a stimulus above threshold level is maximal and independent of the intensity of the stimulus

all–or–noth·ing \-'nəth-iŋ\ *adj* : ALL-OR-NONE

al·lose \'al-₁ōs\ *n* : a synthetic sugar $C_6H_{12}O_6$ stereoisomeric with glucose and epimeric with altrose

al·lo·some \'al-ə-₁sōm\ *n* : an atypical chromosome; *esp* : SEX CHROMOSOME — compare AUTOSOME

al·lo·ste·ric \₁al-ō-'ster-ik, -'sti(ə)r-\ *adj* : of, relating to, or being a change in the shape and activity of a protein (as an enzyme) that results from combination with another substance at a point other than the chemically active site — **al·lo·ste·ri·cal·ly** \-i-k(ə-)lē\ *adv* — **al·lo·ste·ry** \'al-ō-₁ster-ē, -₁sti(ə)r-\ *n, pl* **-ries**

al·lo·te·tra·ploid \₁al-ō-'te-trə-₁ploid\ *n* : AMPHIDIPLOID — **al·lo·te·tra·ploi·dy** \-₁ploid-ē\ *n, pl* **-dies**

al·lo·trans·plant \₁al-ō-tran(t)s-'plant\ *vt* : to transplant between genetically different individuals — **al·lo·trans·plant** \-'tran(t)s-₁\ *n* — **al·lo·trans·plan·ta·tion** \-₁tran(t)s-₁plan-'tā-shən\ *n*

al·lo·trope \'al-ə-₁trōp\ *n* : a form showing allotropy

al·lo·tro·phic \₁al-ə-'träf-ik, -'trō-fik, 'al-ə-₁\ *adj* 1 : having an altered and esp. a lowered nutritive value ⟨~ foods⟩ 2 : HETEROTROPHIC

al·lot·ro·py \ə-'lä-trə-pē\ *n, pl* **-pies** : the existence of a substance and esp. an element in two or more different forms (as of crystals) in the same phase — **al·lo·trop·ic** \₁al-ə-'träp-ik\ *adj* — **al·lo·trop·i·cal·ly** \-i-k(ə-)lē\ *adv*

al·lo·type \'al-ə-₁tīp\ *n* : an alloantigen that is part of a plasma protein (as an antibody) — compare IDIOTYPE, ISOTYPE — **al·lo·typ·ic** \₁al-ə-'tip-ik\ *adj* — **al·lo·typ·i·cal·ly** \-i-k(ə-)lē\ *adv* — **al·lo·typy** \'al-ə-₁tī-pē\ *n, pl* **-typ·ies**

al·lox·an \ə-'läk-sən\ *n* : a crystalline compound $C_4H_2N_2O_4$ causing diabetes mellitus when injected into experimental animals; *also* : one of its similarly acting derivatives — called also *mesoxalylurea*

al·lox·azine \ə-'läk-sə-₁zēn\ *n* : either of two acidic compounds $C_{10}H_6N_4O_2$ containing a pyrimidine ring: **a** : a grayish green powder obtained by reaction of alloxan with the ortho form of phenylenediamine **b** : ISOALLOXAZINE

al·loy \'al-₁oi, ə-'loi\ *n* 1 : the degree of mixture with base metals 2 : a substance composed of two or more metals or of a metal and a nonmetal intimately united usu. by being fused together and dissolving in each other when molten; *also* : the state of union of the components — **al·loy** \ə-'loi, 'al-₁oi\ *vt*

al·lo·zyme \'al-ə-₁zīm\ *n* : any of the variants of an enzyme that are determined by alleles at a single genetic locus — **al·lo·zy·mic** \₁al-ə-'zī-mik\ *adj*

all·spice \'ol-₁spīs\ *n* : the berry of a West Indian tree of the genus *Pimenta* (*P. dioica*) of the myrtle family; *also* : the allspice tree

allspice oil *n* : PIMENTA OIL

all–trans \'ol-₁tranz\ *adj* : characterized by a trans arrangement of chemical groups at every double bond or ring in a molecule

all–trans–retinoic acid *n* : TRETINOIN

al·lyl \'al-əl\ *n, often attrib* : an unsaturated monovalent radical C_3H_5 compounds of which are found in the oils of garlic and mustard — **al·lyl·ic** \ə-'lil-ik, a-\ *adj*

al·lyl·amine \₁al-ə-lə-₁mēn, ₁al-ə-'lam-₁ēn, ə-'lil-ə-₁mēn\ *n* : a pungent strongly basic liquid C_3H_7N used in the synthesis of some pharmaceuticals (as mercurial diuretics)

allyl iso·thio·cy·a·nate \-₁ī-sō-₁thī-ə-'sī-ə-₁nāt, -nət\ *n* : a colorless pungent irritating liquid ester C_4H_5NS that is the chief constituent of mustard oil used in medicine and is used as a flavoring agent and as a medical counterirritant — called also *allyl mustard oil*

N–**al·lyl·nor·mor·phine** \₁en-₁al-əl-₁nor-'mor-₁fēn\ *n* : NALORPHINE

al·lyl·thio·urea \₁al-əl-₁thī-ō-'yur-ē-ə\ *n* : a white crystalline compound $C_4H_8N_2S$ used esp. formerly to promote absorption of scar tissue — called also *thiosinamine*

al·mond \'äm-ənd, 'am-; 'äl-mənd, 'al-\ *n* 1 : a small tree (*Prunus amygdalus*) of the rose family with flowers and young fruit resembling those of the peach 2 : the drupaceous fruit of the almond; *esp* : its ellipsoidal edible kernel used as a nut — compare AMYGDALIN

almond oil *n* **1 a :** a colorless or pale yellow bland and nearly odorless nondrying fatty oil expressed from sweet or bitter almonds and used as an emollient in pharmaceuticals and cosmetics — called also *expressed almond oil, sweet almond oil* **b :** a colorless to yellow essential oil owing its characteristic odor and flavor to benzaldehyde and its toxicity to hydrocyanic acid that is obtained from bitter almonds and is used in medicine as an emollient and after removal of the hydrocyanic acid as a flavoring agent — called also *bitter almond oil* **2 :** any of several essential oils very similar in properties and uses to bitter almond oil and obtained from amygdalin-containing kernels (as of the peach or apricot) other than almonds — called also *bitter almond oil*

al·mon·er \'äm-ə-nər, 'al-mə-\ *n, Brit* : a social-service worker in a hospital

al·oe \'al-(₁)ō\ *n* **1** *cap* : a large genus of succulent chiefly southern African plants of the lily family with basal leaves and spicate flowers **2** : a plant of the genus *Aloe* **3** : the dried juice of the leaves of various aloes used esp. formerly as a purgative and tonic — usu. used in pl. but sing. in constr. **4 :** ALOE VERA 2

al·oe–em·o·din \₁al-ō-'em-ə-dən\ *n* : an orange-yellow crystalline cathartic compound $C_{15}H_{10}O_5$ obtained from aloes, rhubarb, and senna leaves

alo·et·ic \₁al-ō-'et-ik\ *adj* : using, consisting of, containing, or belonging to aloes ⟨∼ medicines⟩

aloe vera \-'ver-ə, -'vir-\ *n* **1 :** a plant of the genus *Aloe* (*A. barbadensis* syn. *A. vera*) whose leaves furnish a gelatinous emollient extract used esp. in cosmetics and skin creams **2** : an extract of the aloe vera plant; *also* : a preparation composed predominantly of such an extract

alo·gia \(')ā-'lō-j(ē-)ə\ *n* : inability to speak esp. when caused by a brain lesion

al·o·in \'al-ə-wən\ *n* : a bitter yellow crystalline cathartic obtained from the aloe and containing one or more glycosides (as barbaloin)

al·o·pe·cia \₁al-ə-'pē-sh(ē-)ə\ *n* : loss of hair, wool, or feathers : BALDNESS — **al·o·pe·cic** \-'pē-sik\ *adj*

alopecia ar·e·a·ta \-₁ar-ē-'āt-ə, -'ät-\ *n* : sudden loss of hair esp. of the scalp or face in circumscribed patches with little or no inflammation

¹al·pha \'al-fə\ *n* **1 :** the 1st letter of the Greek alphabet — symbol A or α **2 :** ALPHA PARTICLE **3 :** ALPHA WAVE

²alpha *or* α- *adj* **1 :** of or relating to one of two or more closely related chemical substances ⟨the *alpha* chain of hemoglobin⟩ ⟨α-yohimbine⟩ — used somewhat arbitrarily to specify ordinal relationship or a particular physical form, esp. one that is allotropic, isomeric, stereoisomeric, or sometimes polymeric (as in α-D-glucose) **2 :** closest in position in the structure of an organic molecule to a particular group or atom; *also* : occurring at or having a structure characterized by such a position ⟨α-substitution⟩

al·pha–ad·ren·er·gic \'al-fə-₁ad-rə-'nər-jik\ *adj* : of, relating to, or being an alpha-receptor ⟨∼ blocking action⟩

al·pha–ad·re·no·cep·tor \-ə-'drē-nə-₁sep-tər\ *also* **al·pha–ad·re·no·re·cep·tor** \-ri-₁sep-tər\ *n* : ALPHA-RECEPTOR

al·pha–ami·no acid *or* α-**ami·no acid** \-ə-₁mē-nō-\ *n* : any of the more than 20 amino acids that have an amino group in the alpha position with most having the general formula $RCH(NH_2)COOH$, that are synthesized in plant and animal tissues, that are considered the building blocks of proteins from which they can be obtained by hydrolysis, and that play an important role in metabolism, growth, maintenance, and repair of tissue — see ESSENTIAL AMINO ACID, NONESSENTIAL AMINO ACID

al·pha–block·er \-₁bläk-ər\ *n* : any of a group of drugs (as phenoxybenzamine and phentolamine) that combine with and block the activity of an alpha-receptor and that are used esp. to treat hypertension — compare BETA-BLOCKER

alpha cell *n* : an acidophilic glandular cell (as of the pancreas or the adenohypophysis) — compare BETA CELL

alpha–fetoprotein *or* α-**fetoprotein** *or chiefly Brit* **alpha–foetoprotein** *or* α-**foetoprotein** *n* : a fetal blood protein present abnormally in adults with some forms of cancer (as of

the liver) and normally in the amniotic fluid of pregnant women but with very low levels tending to be associated with Down syndrome in the fetus and very high levels with neural tube defects (as spina bifida) in which the tube remains open

alpha globulin *n* : any of several globulins of plasma or serum that have at alkaline pH the greatest electrophoretic mobility next to albumin — compare BETA GLOBULIN, GAMMA GLOBULIN

al·pha–he·lix *or* α-**he·lix** \₁al-fə-'hē-liks\ *n* : the coiled structural arrangement of many proteins consisting of a single chain of amino acids stabilized by hydrogen bonds — compare BETA-SHEET, DOUBLE HELIX — **al·pha–he·li·cal** \-'hel-i-kəl, -'hē-li-\ *adj*

alpha hemolysis *n* : a greenish discoloration and partial hemolysis of the red blood cells immediately surrounding colonies of some streptococci on blood agar plates — compare BETA HEMOLYSIS

alpha hydroxy acid *n* : any of various carboxylic acids with a hydroxyl group attached at the alpha position; *specif* : one (as glycolic acid, malic acid, or lactic acid) that occurs in natural products (as fruits, sugarcane, or yogurt) and is used in cosmetics for its exfoliating effect on the surface layer of the skin — called also *AHA*

al·pha–hy·poph·amine *also* α-**hypophamine** \₁al-fə-hī-'päf-ə-₁mēn, -mən\ *n* : OXYTOCIN 1

alpha interferon *n* : an interferon produced by various white blood cells that inhibits viral replication, suppresses cell proliferation, and regulates immune response and that is used in a form obtained from recombinant DNA to treat hairy cell leukemia, AIDS-related Kaposi's sarcoma, condylomata acuminata, and certain chronic hepatitides — called also *interferon alpha;* compare BETA INTERFERON, GAMMA INTERFERON

al·pha–ke·to·glu·ta·rate *or* α-**ketoglutarate** \₁al-fə-₁kēt-ō-glü-'tä-₁rāt, -'glüt-ə-₁rāt\ *n* : a ketoglutarate of alpha-ketoglutaric acid

al·pha–ke·to·glu·tar·ic acid *or* α-**ketoglutaric acid** \-₁kēt-ō-glü-₁tar-ik-\ *n* : the alpha keto isomer of ketoglutaric acid formed in various metabolic processes (as the Krebs cycle)

alpha–lipoprotein *or* α-**lipoprotein** *n* : HDL

al·pha–naph·thol \al-fə-'naf-₁thȯl, -'nap-, -₁thōl\ *n* : NAPHTHOL a

al·pha–naph·thyl·thio·urea *also* α-**naph·thyl·thio·urea** \-₁naf-thəl-₁thī-ə-yu̇-'rē-ə, -'nap-\ *n* : ANTU

al·pha–1–an·ti·tryp·sin \-₁wən-₁ant-i-'trip-sən, -₁an-₁tī-\ *n* : a trypsin-inhibiting serum protein which inhibits the digestive action of elastase on the tissues of the lungs and whose deficiency is associated with the development of emphysema

alpha particle *n* : a positively charged nuclear particle identical with the nucleus of a helium atom that consists of two protons and two neutrons and is ejected at high speed in certain radioactive transformations — called also *alpha, alpha ray*

alpha radiation *n* : a stream of alpha particles

alpha ray *n* : ALPHA PARTICLE

al·pha–re·cep·tor \'al-fə-ri-₁sep-tər\ *n* : any of a group of receptors that are present on cell surfaces of some effector organs and tissues innervated by the sympathetic nervous system and that mediate certain physiological responses (as vasoconstriction, relaxation of intestinal muscle, and contraction of most smooth muscle) when bound by specific adrenergic agents — compare BETA-RECEPTOR

alpha rhythm *n* : ALPHA WAVE

al·pha–to·coph·er·ol \₁al-fə-tō-'käf-ə-₁rȯl, -₁rōl\ *n* : a tocopherol $C_{29}H_{50}O_2$ with high vitamin E potency

Al·pha·vi·rus \'al-fə-₁vī-rəs\ *n* : a genus of single-stranded RNA viruses of the family *Togaviridae* that are transmitted

---

\ə\ abut \ᵊ\ kitten \ər\ further \a\ ash \ā\ ace \ä\ cot, cart
\au̇\ out \ch\ chin \e\ bet \ē\ easy \g\ go \i\ hit \ī\ ice \j\ job
\ŋ\ sing \ō\ go \ȯ\ law \ȯi\ boy \th\ thin \th\ the \ü\ loot
\u̇\ foot \y\ yet \zh\ vision   *See also* Pronunciation Symbols page

by arthropods and esp. mosquitoes and that include the Mayaro virus, Semliki Forest virus, Sindbis virus, and the causative agents of chikungunya and equine encephalomyelitis

alpha wave *n* : an electrical rhythm of the brain with a frequency of 8 to 13 cycles per second that is often associated with a state of wakeful relaxation — called also *alpha*

Al·port syndrome \'al-ˌpȯrt-\ *n* : a usu. X-linked inherited disorder that is typically more severe in males, is characterized esp. by hematuria, hearing loss, abnormalities of the eye, and progressive renal failure, and is caused by defective or absent collagen normally present in basement membranes

  Alport, Arthur Cecil (1880–1959), British physician. Born in South Africa and trained in Edinburgh, Scotland, Alport served with the Royal Army Medical Corps in South West Africa and the Balkans during World War I. After the war he worked as a specialist in tropical medicine for the Ministry of Pensions in London. Beginning in 1922 he served as assistant director of a newly established medical unit at St. Mary's Hospital. In 1927 he reported on three generations of a family with combinations of progressive hereditary nephritis and deafness, noting that hematuria was the most common presenting symptom. In 1937 he went to Cairo to take the post of professor of medicine at King Faud I Hospital, but he later returned to his old hospital in London. The eponym *Alport syndrome* was coined in his honor in 1961.

al·praz·o·lam \al-'praz-ə-ˌlam\ *n* : a benzodiazepine tranquilizer $C_{17}H_{13}ClN_4$ used esp. in the treatment of mild to moderate anxiety — see XANAX

al·pren·o·lol \al-'pren-ə-ˌlȯl, -ˌlōl\ *n* : a beta-adrenergic blocking agent $C_{15}H_{23}NO_2$ that has been used as the hydrochloride in the treatment of cardiac arrhythmias

al·pros·ta·dil \al-'präs-tə-dil\ *n* : a vasodilating prostaglandin $C_{20}H_{34}O_5$ used esp. to treat erectile dysfunction — called also *prostaglandin E₁*

ALS *abbr* **1** amyotrophic lateral sclerosis **2** antilymphocyte serum; antilymphocytic serum

al·ser·ox·y·lon \ˌal-sə-'räk-sə-ˌlän\ *n* : a complex extract from a rauwolfia (*Rauwolfia serpentina*) of the Indian subcontinent, Myanmar, Thailand, and Java that has a physiological action resembling but milder than that of reserpine

Al·sto·nia \ȯl-'stō-nē-ə\ *n* : a genus of trees or shrubs (family Apocynaceae) found in tropical Asia, Australia, and Polynesia having white funnel-shaped flowers and including several (esp. *A. constricta*) whose bark has been used medicinally for its antiperiodic and antipyretic properties (as in the treatment of malaria)

  Alston \'ȯl-stən\, **Charles (1683–1760),** British physician and botanist. Alston was a lecturer in botany and materia medica at the University of Edinburgh. He was noted for being a staunch opponent of the Linnaean system of classification. The genus *Alstonia* was named in his honor in 1810.

al·sto·nine \'ȯl-stə-ˌnēn\ *n* : an alkaloid $C_{21}H_{20}N_2O_4$ found in the bark of a tree of the genus *Alstonia* (*A. constricta*)

alt *abbr* **1** alternate **2** altitude

ALT *abbr* alanine aminotransferase

Al·tace \'al-ˌtās\ *trademark* — used for a preparation of ramipril

al·te·plase \'al-tə-ˌplās\ *n* : TISSUE PLASMINOGEN ACTIVATOR

al·ter \'ȯl-tər\ *vt* **al·tered; al·ter·ing** \-t(ə-)riŋ\ : CASTRATE 1, SPAY

al·ter·ant \'ȯl-tə-rənt\ *n* : ALTERATIVE

¹al·ter·ative \'ȯl-tə-ˌrāt-iv, -rət-\ *n* : a drug used empirically to alter favorably the course of an ailment

²alterative *adj* : causing alteration

altered state of consciousness *n* : any of various states of awareness (as dreaming sleep, a drug-induced hallucinogenic state, or a trance) that deviate from and are usu. clearly demarcated from ordinary waking consciousness

alternans — see PULSUS ALTERNANS

Al·ter·nar·ia \ˌȯl-tər-'nar-ē-ə\ *n* : a genus of imperfect fungi (family Dematiaceae) producing chains of dark conidia tapering at the upper end and arranged like bricks

al·ter·nate host \'ȯl-tər-nət-, *chiefly Brit* ȯl-'tər-\ *n* : INTERMEDIATE HOST 1

al·ter·nat·ing personality \ˌȯl-tər-ˌnāt-iŋ- *also* ˌal-\ *n* : MULTIPLE PERSONALITY DISORDER

alternating psychosis *n* : BIPOLAR DISORDER

al·ter·na·tion of generations \ˌȯl-tər-'nā-shən *also* ˌal-\ *n* : the occurrence of two or more forms differently produced in the life cycle of a plant or animal usu. involving the regular alternation of a sexual with an asexual generation but not infrequently consisting of alternation of a dioecious generation with one or more parthenogenetic generations

al·ter·na·tive \ȯl-'tər-nət-iv, al-\ *adj* : of, relating to, or based on alternative medicine ⟨∼ therapies⟩

alternative medicine *n* : any of various systems of healing or treating disease (as homeopathy, chiropractic, naturopathy, Ayurveda, or faith healing) that are not included in the traditional curricula taught in medical schools of the U.S. and Britain

al·thaea \al-'thē-ə\ *n* **1** *cap* : a genus of Old World herbs of the mallow family that have terminal spikelike clusters of showy flowers and include the hollyhock and marshmallow **2** *or* **al·thea** : the dried root of the marshmallow deprived of its brown corky layer and small roots and used as a demulcent and emollient — called also *marshmallow root*

al·ti·tude sickness \ˌal-tə-ˌt(y)üd-\ *n* : the effects (as nosebleed, nausea, or headache) of oxygen deficiency in the blood and tissues developed at high altitudes with reduced atmospheric pressure

Alt·mann's granules \'ȯlt-mənz-, 'ält-ˌmänz-\ *n pl* : minute granules in protoplasm once regarded as its ultimate formative units but now physically equated with mitochondria

  Altmann, Richard (1852–1900), German histologist. Around 1890 Altmann advanced his theory that the fundamental units of protoplasm are granular particles whose existence he inferred from particles observed at the limits of resolution of the light microscope. They subsequently became identified with his name. The particles now are thought to be cellular organelles known as mitochondria whose morphology and cellular function have been worked out with the aid of the much greater resolving power of the electron microscope.

al·tri·gen·der·ism \ˌal-trə-'jen-də-ˌriz-əm\ *n* : the state or period of development in which one becomes socially interested in or attracted to members of the opposite sex

al·trose \'al-ˌtrōs, -ˌtrōz\ *n* : a synthetic syrupy sugar $C_6H_{12}O_6$ stereoisomeric with glucose and epimeric with allose

al·um \'al-əm\ *n* **1** : either of two colorless or white crystalline double sulfates of aluminum used in medicine internally as emetics and locally as astringents and styptics: **a** : one $KAl(SO_4)_2 \cdot 12H_2O$ that is a sulfate of aluminum and potassium — called also *potassium alum* **b** : one consisting of an ammonium aluminum sulfate $NH_4Al(SO_4)_2 \cdot 12H_2O$ — called also *ammonia alum, ammonium alum* **2** : any of various double salts isomorphous with potassium aluminum sulfate

alu·men \ə-'lü-mən\ *n, pl* **alumens** *or* **alu·mi·na** \-mə-nə\ : ALUM

alu·mi·na \ə-'lü-mə-nə\ *n* : an oxide of aluminum Al_2O_3 that occurs native as corundum and in hydrated forms (as in bauxite) and is used in antacids — called also *aluminum oxide*

al·u·min·i·um \ˌal-yə-'min-ē-əm\ *n, chiefly Brit* : ALUMINUM

alu·mi·num \ə-'lü-mə-nəm\ *n, often attrib* : a bluish silver-white malleable ductile light trivalent metallic element that has good electrical and thermal conductivity, high reflectivity, and resistance to oxidation and is the most abundant metal in the earth's crust where it always occurs in combination — symbol *Al;* see ELEMENT table

aluminum chloride *n* : a deliquescent compound $AlCl_3$ or Al_2Cl_3 that is used as a topical astringent and antiseptic on the skin, in some deodorants to control sweating, and in the anhydrous form as a catalyst — see MUCICARMINE

aluminum hydroxide *n* : any of several white gelatinous or crystalline hydrates $Al_2O_3 \cdot nH_2O$ of alumina; *esp* : one $Al_2O_3 \cdot 3H_2O$ or $Al(OH)_3$ used in medicine as an antacid

aluminum oxide *n* : ALUMINA

aluminum sulfate *n* : a colorless salt Al$_2$(SO$_4$)$_3$ that is a powerful astringent and is used as a local antiperspirant and in water purification

Al·u·pent \'a-lü-ˌpent\ *trademark* — used for a preparation of the sulfate of metaproterenol

alv *abbr* alveolar

alvei *pl of* ALVEUS

al·ve·o·lar \al-'vē-ə-lər\ *adj* **1** : of, relating to, resembling, or having alveoli **2** : of, relating to, or constituting the part of the jaws where the teeth arise, the air cells of the lungs, or glands with secretory cells about a central space

alveolar arch *n* : the arch of the upper or lower jaw formed by the alveolar processes

alveolar artery *n* : any of several arteries supplying the teeth; *esp* : POSTERIOR SUPERIOR ALVEOLAR ARTERY — compare INFERIOR ALVEOLAR ARTERY

alveolar canals *n pl* : the canals in the jawbones for the passage of the dental nerves and associated vessels

alveolar ducts *n pl* : the somewhat enlarged terminal sections of the bronchioles that branch into the terminal alveoli

alveolar index *n* : GNATHIC INDEX

alveolaris — see PYORRHEA ALVEOLARIS

alveolar nerve — see INFERIOR ALVEOLAR NERVE, SUPERIOR ALVEOLAR NERVE

alveolar point *n* : PROSTHION

alveolar process *n* : the bony ridge or raised thickened border on each side of the upper or lower jaw that contains the sockets of the teeth — called also *alveolar ridge*

alveolar vein — see INFERIOR ALVEOLAR VEIN, POSTERIOR SUPERIOR ALVEOLAR VEIN

al·ve·o·late \al-'vē-ə-lət\ *adj* : pitted like a honeycomb — **al·ve·o·la·tion** \(ˌ)al-ˌvē-ə-'lā-shən\ *n*

al·ve·o·lec·to·my \al-ˌvē-ə-'lek-tə-mē, ˌal-vē-\ *n, pl* **-mies** : surgical excision of a portion of an alveolar process usu. as an aid in fitting dentures

al·ve·o·li·tis \ˌal-ˌvē-ə-'līt-əs, ˌal-vē-\ *n* : inflammation of one or more alveoli esp. of the lung

al·ve·o·lo·con·dyl·e·an \al-ˌvē-ə-ˌlō-kän-'dil-ē-ən, -ˌkän-də-'lē-ən\ *adj* : of or relating to the plane which passes through the occipital condyles and the alveolar point

al·ve·o·lo·na·sal \al-ˌvē-ə-lō-'nā-zəl, ˌal-vē-\ *adj* : of or relating to the alveolar point and the nasion

al·ve·o·lo·plas·ty \al-'vē-ə-(ˌ)lō-ˌplas-tē\ *or* **al·veo·plas·ty** \'al-vē-ō-\ *n, pl* **-ties** : surgical shaping of the dental alveoli and alveolar processes esp. after extraction of several teeth or in preparation for dentures

al·ve·o·lus \al-'vē-ə-ləs\ *n, pl* **-li** \-ˌlī, -(ˌ)lē\ : a small cavity or pit: as **a** : a socket in the jaw for a tooth **b** : any of the small thin-walled air-containing compartments of the lung that are typically arranged in saclike clusters into which an alveolar duct terminates and from which respiratory gases are exchanged with the pulmonary capillaries **c** : an acinus of a compound gland **d** : any of the pits in the wall of the stomach into which the glands open

al·ve·us \'al-vē-əs\ *n, pl* **al·vei** \-vē-ˌī, -ˌē\ : a thin layer of medullary nerve fibers on the ventricular surface of the hippocampus

Alz·hei·mer's disease \'älts-ˌhī-mərz-, 'ȯlts-, 'alts-, 'alz-\ *also* **Alzheimer disease** \-mər\ *n* : a degenerative brain disease of unknown cause that is the most common form of dementia, that usu. starts in late middle age or in old age as a memory loss for recent events spreading to memories for more distant events and progressing over the course of five to ten years to a profound intellectual decline characterized by dementia and personal helplessness, and that is marked histologically by the degeneration of brain neurons esp. in the cerebral cortex and by the presence of neurofibrillary tangles and plaques containing beta-amyloid — abbr. *AD;* called also *Alzheimer's;* compare PRESENILE DEMENTIA

Alzheimer, Alois (1864–1915), German neurologist. Alzheimer was noted for his work in the pathology of the nervous system. The majority of his medical contributions centered on neurohistology. Alzheimer published papers on topics that include acute alcoholic delirium, schizophrenia, epilepsy, syphilitic meningomyelitis and encephalitis, gliosis, Huntington's disease, and hysterical bulbar paralysis. In 1894 he published a noteworthy description of arteriosclerotic atrophy of the brain. With Franz Nissl he produced *Histologic and Histopathologic Studies of the Cerebral Cortex* (1904–08), a six-volume encyclopedia that described normal and abnormal structures in the central nervous system. In 1907 he published his classic description of presenile dementia. The disease was later named in his honor by the German psychiatrist Emil Kraepelin.

Am *symbol* americium

AM *abbr* **1** [Latin *ante meridiem*] before noon **2** [Medieval Latin *Artium Magister*] master of arts

AMA *abbr* **1** against medical advice **2** American Medical Association

amaas \'äm-ˌäs\ *n* : VARIOLA MINOR

am·a·cri·nal \ˌam-ə-'krīn-əl, ˌā-ma-'\ *or* **am·a·crine** \'am-ə-ˌkrīn, (ˈ)ā-'mak-ˌrīn\ *adj* : of, relating to, or being an amacrine cell

amacrine cell *n* : a unipolar nerve cell found in the retina, in the olfactory bulb, and in close connection with the Purkinje cells of the cerebellum

amal·gam \ə-'mal-gəm\ *n* : an alloy of mercury with another metal that is solid or liquid at room temperature according to the proportion of mercury present and is used esp. in making tooth cements

amal·gam·ate \ə-'mal-gə-ˌmāt\ *vt* **-at·ed; -at·ing** : to unite in or as if in an amalgam; *esp* : to merge into a single body — **amal·gam·ation** \ə-ˌmal-gə-'mā-shən\ *n* — **amal·gam·ator** \-'mal-gə-ˌmāt-ər\ *n*

am·an·din \'äm-ən-dən, 'am-; ə-'man-\ *n* : the typical protein of sweet almonds and peach kernels with the properties of a globulin

am·a·ni·ta \ˌam-ə-'nīt-ə, -'nēt-\ *n* **1** *cap* : a genus of widely distributed white-spored basidiomycetous fungi (family Amanitaceae) that includes some deadly poisonous forms (as the death cap) **2** : a fungus of the genus *Amanita*

am·a·ni·tin \-'nit-ᵊn, -'nēt-\ *n* : a highly toxic cyclic peptide produced by the death cap that selectively inhibits mammalian RNA polymerase

aman·ta·dine \ə-'mant-ə-ˌdēn\ *n* : a drug administered orally esp. in the form of its hydrochloride C$_{10}$H$_{17}$N·HCl to prevent infection (as by the virus causing influenza A) by interfering with virus penetration into host cells and in the treatment of Parkinson's disease — see SYMMETREL

am·a·ranth \'am-ə-ˌran(t)th\ *n* **1** : any plant of the genus *Amaranthus* **2** : a red acid azo dye C$_{20}$H$_{11}$N$_2$Na$_3$O$_{10}$S$_3$ that is used chiefly in coloring foods, beverages, and pharmaceutical preparations and in dyeing wool and silk

Am·a·ran·thus \ˌam-ə-'ran(t)-thəs\ *n* : a large genus of coarse herbs (family Amaranthaceae, the amaranth family) including some which produce pollen that is an important hay fever allergen

amarga — see CASCARA AMARGA

am·a·roid \'am-ə-ˌroid\ *n* : any bitter vegetable extractive of definite chemical composition other than an alkaloid or glucoside

amas·tia \(ˈ)ā-'mas-tē-ə\ *n* : the absence or underdevelopment of the mammary glands

ama·tho·pho·bia \ˌam-ə-thə-'fō-bē-ə\ *n* : fear of dust

am·au·ro·sis \ˌam-ȯ-'rō-səs\ *n, pl* **-ro·ses** \-ˌsēz\ : partial or complete loss of sight occurring esp. without an externally perceptible change in the eye — **am·au·rot·ic** \-'rät-ik\ *adj*

amaurosis fu·gax \-'f(y)ü-ˌgaks\ *n* : temporary partial or complete loss of sight esp. from the effects of excessive acceleration (as in flight)

amaurotic family idiocy *n* : AMAUROTIC IDIOCY

\ə\ abut \ᵊ\ kitten \ər\ further \a\ ash \ā\ ace \ä\ cot, cart
\au̇\ out \ch\ chin \e\ bet \ē\ easy \g\ go \i\ hit \ī\ ice \j\ job
\ŋ\ sing \ō\ go \ȯ\ law \ȯi\ boy \th\ thin \t͟h\ the \ü\ loot
\u̇\ foot \y\ yet \zh\ vision   *See also* Pronunciation Symbols page

amaurotic idiocy *n* : any of several recessive genetic conditions characterized by the accumulation of lipid-containing cells in the viscera and nervous system, mental retardation, and impaired vision or blindness; *esp* : TAY-SACHS DISEASE

amax·o·pho·bia \ə-ˌmak-sə-ˈfō-bē-ə\ *n* : fear of being in or riding in a vehicle

amb *abbr* **1** ambulance **2** ambulatory

am·ber \ˈam-bər\ *n* : a hard yellowish to brownish translucent fossil resin that takes a fine polish and is used chiefly in making ornamental objects (as beads) — **amber** *adj*

am·ber·gris \ˈam-bər-ˌgris, -ˌgrē(s)\ *n* : a waxy substance found floating in or on the shores of tropical waters, believed to originate in the intestines of the sperm whale, and used in perfumery as a fixative

am·bi·dex·ter·i·ty \ˌam-bi-(ˌ)dek-ˈster-ət-ē\ *n, pl* **-ties** : the quality or state of being ambidextrous

am·bi·dex·trous \ˌam-bi-ˈdek-strəs\ *adj* : using both hands with equal ease — **am·bi·dex·trous·ly** *adv*

Am·bi·en \ˈam-bē-ˌen\ *trademark* — used for a preparation of the tartrate of zolpidem

am·bi·ent \ˈam-bē-ənt\ *adj* : surrounding on all sides ⟨the ~ environment⟩ ⟨~ air pollution⟩

ambiguus — see NUCLEUS AMBIGUUS

am·bi·lat·er·al \ˌam-bi-ˈlat-ə-rəl, -ˈla-trəl\ *adj* : relating to or affecting both sides : BILATERAL — **am·bi·lat·er·al·i·ty** \-ˌlat-ə-ˈral-ət-ē\ *n, pl* **-ties** — **am·bi·lat·er·al·ly** \-ˈlat-ə-rə-lē, -ˈla-trə-lē\ *adv*

am·bi·o·pia \ˌam-bē-ˈō-pē-ə\ *n* : DIPLOPIA

am·bi·sex·u·al \ˌam-bi-ˈseksh-(ə-)wəl, -ˈsek-shəl\ *adj* : BISEXUAL ⟨an ~ fantasy⟩ ⟨~ embryos⟩ — **ambisexual** *n* — **am·bi·sex·u·al·i·ty** \-ˌsek-shə-ˈwal-ət-ē\ *n, pl* **-ties**

am·bi·tend·en·cy \ˈam-bi-ˌten-dən-sē\ *n, pl* **-cies** : a tendency to act in opposite ways or directions : the presence of opposing behavioral drives

am·biv·a·lence \am-ˈbiv-ə-lən(t)s\ *n* : simultaneous and contradictory attitudes or feelings (as attraction and repulsion) toward an object, person, or action ⟨~ which is expressed in behavior by alternating obedience and rebellion —G. S. Blum⟩ — **am·biv·a·lent** \-lənt\ *adj* — **am·biv·a·lent·ly** *adv*

am·biv·a·len·cy \-lən-sē\ *n, pl* **-cies** : AMBIVALENCE

am·bi·ver·sion \ˌam-bi-ˈvər-zhən, -shən\ *n* : the personality configuration of an ambivert — **am·bi·ver·sive** \-ˈvər-siv, -ziv\ *adj*

am·bi·vert \ˈam-bi-ˌvərt\ *n* : a person having characteristics of both extrovert and introvert

Am·bly·om·ma \ˌam-blē-ˈäm-ə\ *n* : a genus of ixodid ticks including the lone star tick (*A. americanum*) of the southern U.S. and the African bont tick (*A. hebraeum*)

am·bly·ope \ˈam-blē-ˌōp\ *n* : an individual affected with amblyopia

am·bly·opia \ˌam-blē-ˈō-pē-ə\ *n* : dimness of sight esp. in one eye without apparent change in the eye structures — called also *lazy eye, lazy-eye blindness* — **am·bly·opic** \-ˈō-pik, -ˈäp-ik\ *adj*

am·bly·o·scope \ˈam-blē-ə-ˌskōp\ *n* : an instrument for training amblyopic eyes to function properly

am·bo·cep·tor \ˈam-bō-ˌsep-tər\ *n* : an antibody that lyses an antigen (as a bacterium) in combination with complement

am·bon \ˈam-ˌbän\ *also* **am·bo** \-ˌbō\ *n, pl* **ambo·nes** \am-ˈbō-(ˌ)nēz\ : the fibrocartilaginous ring around an articular cavity

am·bos \ˈam-ˌbäs\ *n* : INCUS

Am·bro·sia \am-ˈbrō-zh(ē-)ə\ *n* : a genus of mostly American composite herbs that includes the ragweeds

Am·bu \ˈam-ˌbü\ *trademark* — used for an artificial respiration device consisting of a bag that is squeezed by hand

am·bu·lance \ˈam-b(y)ə-lən(t)s *also* -ˌlan(t)s\ *n* : a vehicle equipped for transporting the injured or sick

am·bu·lant \ˈam-byə-lənt\ *adj* : walking or in a walking position; *specif* : AMBULATORY ⟨an ~ patient⟩

am·bu·late \-ˌlāt\ *vi* **-lat·ed; -lat·ing** : to move from place to place ⟨the patient was allowed to ~ in her room⟩ — **am·bu·la·tion** \ˌam-byə-ˈlā-shən\ *n*

am·bu·la·to·ry \ˈam-byə-lə-ˌtōr-ē, -ˌtȯr-\ *adj* **1** : of, relating to, or adapted to walking ⟨~ exercise⟩ **2 a** : able to walk about and not bedridden ⟨an ~ patient⟩ **b** : performed on or involving an ambulatory patient or an outpatient ⟨an ~ electrocardiogram⟩ ⟨~ medical care⟩ — **am·bu·la·to·ri·ly** \ˌam-byə-lə-ˈtōr-ə-lē, -ˈtȯr-\ *adv*

AMD *abbr* age-related macular degeneration

ame·ba *or chiefly Brit* **amoe·ba** \ə-ˈmē-bə\ *n, pl* **-bas** *or* **-bae** \-(ˌ)bē\ : a protozoan of the genus *Amoeba*; *broadly* : an ameboid protozoan (as a naked rhizopod) — **ame·bic** *or chiefly Brit* **amoe·bic** \-bik\ *adj*

am·e·bi·a·sis *or chiefly Brit* **am·oe·bi·a·sis** \ˌam-i-ˈbī-ə-səs\ *n, pl* **-a·ses** \-ˌsēz\ : infection with or disease caused by amebas (esp. *Entamoeba histolytica*)

amebic abscess *n* : a specific purulent invasive lesion commonly of the liver caused by parasitic amebas (esp. *Entamoeba histolytica*)

amebic dysentery *n* : acute human intestinal amebiasis caused by a common ameba of the genus *Entamoeba* (*E. histolytica*) and marked by dysentery, abdominal pain, and erosion of the intestinal wall

ame·bi·cide *also* **ame·ba·cide** *or chiefly Brit* **amoe·bi·cide** *also* **amoe·ba·cide** \ə-ˈmē-bə-ˌsīd\ *n* : a substance used to kill or capable of killing amebas and esp. parasitic amebas — **ame·bi·cid·al** *also* **ame·ba·cid·al** *or chiefly Brit* **amoe·bi·cid·al** *also* **amoe·ba·cid·al** \ə-ˌmē-bə-ˈsīd-ᵊl\ *adj*

ame·bi·form *or chiefly Brit* **amoe·bi·form** \ə-ˈmē-bə-ˌfȯrm\ *adj* : AMEBOID

ame·bo·cyte *or chiefly Brit* **amoe·bo·cyte** \ə-ˈmē-bə-ˌsīt\ *n* : a cell (as a phagocyte) having ameboid form or movements

ame·boid *or chiefly Brit* **amoe·boid** \ə-ˈmē-ˌbȯid\ *adj* : resembling an ameba specif. in moving or changing shape by means of protoplasmic flow ⟨~ movement of monocytes⟩

ame·bu·la *or chiefly Brit* **amoe·bu·la** \ə-ˈmē-byə-lə\ *n, pl* **-las** *or* **-lae** \-(ˌ)lē\ **1** : a small ameba **2** : any of various small cells or organisms (as in some stages of myxomycetes or gregarines) resembling an ameba in form

amei·o·sis \ˌā-ˌmī-ˈō-səs\ *n, pl* **-o·ses** \-ˌsēz\ : suppression of one of the meiotic divisions (as in parthenogenesis) resulting in nonreduction of chromosomes

amei·ot·ic \ˌā-ˌmī-ˈät-ik\ *adj* : lacking meiosis

amel·a·not·ic \ˌā-ˌmēl-ə-ˈnät-ik\ *adj* : containing little or no melanin ⟨~ melanocytes⟩ ⟨~ malignant melanoma⟩

ameli *pl of* AMELUS

ame·lia \ə-ˈmē-lē-ə, (ˌ)ā-\ *n* : congenital absence of one or more limbs

am·e·lo·blast \ˈam-ə-lō-ˌblast\ *n* : any of a group of columnar epithelial cells that produce and deposit enamel on the surface of a developing vertebrate tooth — **am·e·lo·blas·tic** \ˌam-ə-lō-ˈblas-tik\ *adj*

am·e·lo·blas·to·ma \ˌam-ə-lō-bla-ˈstō-mə\ *n, pl* **-mas** *also* **-ma·ta** \-ˌmət-ə\ : a tumor of the jaw derived from remnants of the embryonic rudiment of tooth enamel — called also *adamantinoma*

am·e·lo·den·tin·al \-ˈden-ˌtēn-ᵊl, -den-ˈtēn-\ *adj* : of or relating to enamel and dentin ⟨the ~ junction of a tooth⟩

am·e·lo·gen·e·sis \-ˈjen-ə-səs\ *n, pl* **-e·ses** \-ˌsēz\ : the process of forming tooth enamel

amelogenesis im·per·fec·ta \-ˌim-(ˌ)pər-ˈfek-tə\ *n* : faulty development of tooth enamel that is genetically determined

am·e·lus \ˈam-ə-ləs, (ˈ)ā-ˈmel-əs\ *n, pl* **am·e·li** \-ˌlī, -ˌlē; -ˌī, -ˌē\ : a limbless fetus

amen·or·rhea *or chiefly Brit* **amen·or·rhoea** \ˌā-ˌmen-ə-ˈrē-ə, ˌäm-ˌen-\ *n* : abnormal absence or suppression of menstruation — see PRIMARY AMENORRHEA, SECONDARY AMENORRHEA — **amen·or·rhe·ic** *or chiefly Brit* **amen·or·rhoe·ic** \-ˈrē-ik\ *adj*

amen·tia \(ˈ)ā-ˈmen-ch(ē-)ə, (ˈ)ä-\ *n* : MENTAL RETARDATION; *specif* : a condition of lack of development of intellectual capacity

Amer·i·can cockroach \ə-ˈmer-i-kən-\ *n* : a cockroach of the genus *Periplaneta* (*P. americana*) that is a common domestic pest infesting ships or buildings (as homes, warehouses, or bakeries) in the northern hemisphere

American dog tick *n* : a common No. American ixodid tick of the genus *Dermacentor* (*D. variabilis*) esp. of dogs and humans that is an important vector of Rocky Mountain spotted fever and tularemia — called also *dog tick*

American hellebore *n* : a false hellebore (*Veratrum viride*) of the eastern U.S.; *also* : its roots and rhizome

American storax *n* : STORAX 2

American trypanosomiasis *n* : CHAGAS' DISEASE

am·er·i·ci·um \ˌam-ə-ˈris(h)-ē-əm\ *n* : a radioactive metallic element produced by bombardment of plutonium with high= energy neutrons — symbol *Am*; see ELEMENT table

Ames test \ˈāmz-\ *n* : a test for identifying potential carcinogens by studying the frequency with which they cause histidine-producing genetic mutants in bacterial colonies of the genus *Salmonella* (*S. typhimurium*) initially lacking the ability to synthesize histidine

> **Ames, Bruce Nathan** (*b* 1928), American biochemist. In 1976 Ames devised his test for carcinogenesis of a substance.

ameth·o·caine \ə-ˈmeth-ə-ˌkān\ *n* : TETRACAINE

am·e·thop·ter·in \ˌam-ə-ˈthäp-tə-rən\ *n* : METHOTREXATE

am·e·trope \ˈam-ə-ˌtrōp\ *n* : an ametropic individual

am·e·tro·pia \ˌam-ə-ˈtrō-pē-ə\ *n* : an abnormal refractive eye condition (as myopia, hyperopia, or astigmatism) in which images fail to focus upon the retina — **am·e·tro·pic** \-ˈtrō-pik, -ˈträp-ik\ *adj*

AMI *abbr* acute myocardial infarction

am·i·an·thoid \ˌam-ē-ˈan-ˌthóid\ *adj* : resembling fine silky asbestos

am·i·dase \ˈam-ə-ˌdās, -ˌdāz\ *n* : an enzyme that hydrolyzes acid amides usu. with the liberation of ammonia

am·ide \ˈam-ˌīd, -əd\ *n* : an organic compound derived from ammonia or an amine by replacement of an atom of hydrogen with an acyl group — compare IMIDE — **amid·ic** \ə-ˈmid-ik, a-\ *adj*

am·i·dine \ˈam-ə-dēn, -dən\ *n* : any of various strong monobasic compounds containing an amino and an imino group attached to the same carbon atom and having the general formula $RC(=NH)NH_2$

ami·do \ə-ˈmēd-(ˌ)ō, ˈam-ə-ˌdō\ *adj* : relating to or containing an organic amide group — often used in combination

am·i·done \ˈam-ə-ˌdōn\ *n* : METHADONE

ami·do·py·rine \ə-ˌmēd-ō-ˈpī-ˌrēn, ˌam-ə-(ˌ)dō-, -rən\ *n* : AMINOPYRINE

am·i·dox·ime \ˌam-ə-ˈdäk-ˌsēm, -səm\ *n* : the oxime of an amide having the general formula $RC(=NOH)NH_2$

amil·o·ride \ə-ˈmil-ə-ˌrīd\ *n* : a diuretic $C_6H_8ClN_7O$ that promotes sodium excretion and potassium retention

amim·ia \(ˈ)ā-ˈmim-ē-ə\ *n* **1** : loss or impairment of the power of communicating thought by gestures, due to cerebral disease or injury **2** : loss of the power to give facial expression to emotion (as in a smile) because of paralysis of the facial muscles

¹am·i·nate \ˈam-ə-ˌnāt\ *n* : a compound with an amine

²aminate *vt* **-nat·ed; -nat·ing** : to introduce the amino group into : convert into an amine — **am·i·na·tion** \ˌam-ə-ˈnā-shən\ *n*

amin·azine \ə-ˈmēn-ə-ˌzēn\ *or* **amin·azin** \-ˌzēn, -zən\ *n* : CHLORPROMAZINE

amine \ə-ˈmēn, ˈam-ˌēn\ *n* : any of a class of organic compounds derived from ammonia by replacement of one, two, or three hydrogen atoms with alkyl groups — see PRIMARY AMINE, SECONDARY AMINE, TERTIARY AMINE

ami·no \ə-ˈmē-(ˌ)nō\ *adj* : relating to, being, or containing an amine group — often used in combination

ami·no·ace·tic acid \ə-ˌmē-(ˌ)nō-ə-ˌsēt-ik-\ *n* : GLYCINE

amino acid *n* : an amphoteric organic acid containing the amino group NH_2; *esp* : ALPHA-AMINO ACID

ami·no·ac·i·de·mia *or chiefly Brit* **ami·no·ac·i·dae·mia** \ə-ˌmē-nō-ˌas-ə-ˈdē-mē-ə\ *n* : a condition in which the concentration of amino acids in the blood is abnormally increased

ami·no·ac·id·uria \-ˌas-ə-ˈd(y)ùr-ē-ə\ *n* : a condition in which one or more amino acids are excreted in excessive amounts

ami·no·ac·yl \-ˈas-əl, -ēl; -ˈā-səl\ *n* : an acyl radical derived from an amino acid

ami·no·ac·yl·ate \-ˈas-ə-ˌlāt, -ˈā-sə-\ *vt* **-at·ed; -at·ing** : to introduce an aminoacyl into ⟨enzymes which ∼ transfer RNA⟩ — **ami·no·ac·yl·a·tion** \-ˌas-ə-ˈlā-shən, -ˌā-sə-\ *n*

aminoacyl–tRNA *n* : a transfer RNA formed by the enzymatic action of aminoacyl-tRNA synthetase

aminoacyl–tRNA synthetase *n* : any of a class of amino= acid-specific enzymes that catalyze an ATP-driven reaction producing an ester linkage between a carboxyl group of an amino acid and a hydroxyl group of its corresponding transfer RNA to form aminoacyl-tRNA during the early stage of protein synthesis — called also *aminoacyl-transfer RNA synthetase*

ami·no·ben·zo·ate \-ˈben-zə-ˌwāt\ *n* : a salt or ester of an aminobenzoic acid and esp. of para-aminobenzoic acid

ami·no·ben·zo·ic acid \ə-ˌmē-nō-ben-ˌzō-ik-\ *n* : any of three crystalline derivatives $C_7H_7NO_2$ of benzoic acid: as **a** : PARA-AMINOBENZOIC ACID **b** : ANTHRANILIC ACID

γ–aminobutyric acid *var of* GAMMA-AMINOBUTYRIC ACID

ami·no·glu·teth·i·mide \-glü-ˈteth-ə-ˌmīd\ *n* : a glutethimide derivative $C_{13}H_{16}N_2O_2$ used esp. as an anticonvulsant

ami·no·gly·co·side \-ˈglī-kə-ˌsīd\ *n* : any of a group of antibiotics (as streptomycin and neomycin) that inhibit bacterial protein synthesis and are active esp. against gram-negative bacteria

am·i·nol·y·sis \ˌam-ə-ˈnäl-ə-səs\ *n, pl* **-y·ses** \-ˌsēz\ **1** : ammonolysis or any analogous decomposition in which an amine takes the place of ammonia **2** : hydrolytic deamination (as the conversion of an amino acid into a hydroxy acid) — **ami·no·lyt·ic** \ə-ˌmē-nə-ˈlit-ik\ *adj*

amino nitrogen *n* : the nitrogen atom of an amino group

ami·no·pep·ti·dase \ə-ˌmē-nō-ˈpep-tə-ˌdās, -ˌdāz\ *n* : an enzyme (as one found in the duodenum) that hydrolyzes peptides by acting on the peptide bond next to a terminal amino acid containing a free amino group

am·i·noph·er·ase \ˌam-ə-ˈnäf-ə-ˌrās, -ˌrāz\ *n* : TRANSAMINASE

am·i·noph·yl·line \ˌam-ə-ˈnäf-ə-lən\ *n* : a theophylline derivative $C_{16}H_{24}N_{10}O_4$ used esp. to stimulate the heart in congestive heart failure and to dilate the air passages in respiratory disorders — called also *theophylline ethylenediamine*

β–ami·no·pro·pio·ni·trile \ˌbāt-ə-ə-ˌmē-nō-ˌprō-pē-ō-ˈnī-trəl, -ˌtrīl\ *n* : a potent lathyrogen $C_3H_6N_2$

am·i·nop·ter·in \ˌam-ə-ˈnäp-tə-rən\ *n* : a derivative $C_{19}H_{20}$-N_8O_5 of glutamic acid that is a folic acid antagonist and has been used as a rodenticide and antileukemic agent

ami·no·py·rine \ə-ˌmē-nō-ˈpī(ə)r-ˌēn\ *n* : a white crystalline compound $C_{13}H_{17}N_3O$ formerly used to relieve pain and fever but now largely abandoned for this purpose because of the occurrence of fatal agranulocytosis as a side effect in some users

ami·no·sal·i·cyl·ic acid \ə-ˌmē-nō-ˌsal-ə-ˌsil-ik-\ *n* : any of four isomeric derivatives $C_7H_7O_3N$ of salicylic acid that have a single amino group; *esp* : PARA-AMINOSALICYLIC ACID

ami·no·thi·a·zole \ə-ˌmē-nō-ˈthī-ə-ˌzōl\ *n* : a light yellow crystalline heterocyclic amine $C_3H_4N_2S$ that has been used as a thyroid inhibitor in the treatment of hyperthyroidism

ami·no·trans·fer·ase \-ˈtran(t)s-fə-ˌrās, -ˌrāz\ *n* : TRANSAMINASE

ami·o·da·rone \ə-ˈmē-ō-də-ˌrōn\ *n* : an antiarrhythmic drug administered in the form of its hydrochloride $C_{25}H_{29}I_2NO_3$·HCl and used to treat life-threatening ventricular arrhythmias

ami·to·sis \ˌā-mī-ˈtō-səs\ *n, pl* **-to·ses** \-ˌsēz\ : cell division by simple cleavage of the nucleus and division of the cytoplasm without spindle formation or appearance of chromosomes — called also *direct cell division* — **ami·tot·ic** \-ˈtät-ik\ *adj* — **ami·tot·i·cal·ly** \-i-k(ə-)lē\ *adv*

\ə\ abut \ᵊ\ kitten \ər\ further \a\ ash \ā\ ace \ä\ cot, cart
\aù\ out \ch\ chin \e\ bet \ē\ easy \g\ go \i\ hit \ī\ ice \j\ job
\ŋ\ sing \ō\ go \ò\ law \òi\ boy \th\ thin \t͟h\ the \ü\ loot
\ù\ foot \y\ yet \zh\ vision *See also* Pronunciation Symbols page

am·i·trip·ty·line \,am-ə-'trip-tə-ˌlēn\ *n* : a tricyclic antidepressant drug that is administered in the form of its hydrochloride $C_{20}H_{23}N \cdot HCl$ and has been used to treat migraine headaches and neuropathic pain as well as depression

AML *abbr* acute myeloblastic leukemia; acute myelocytic leukemia; acute myelogenous leukemia; acute myeloid leukemia

am·lo·di·pine \am-'lō-də-ˌpēn\ *n* : a calcium channel blocker administered in the form of its besylate $C_{20}H_{25}ClN_2O_5 \cdot C_6H_5SO_3H$ in the treatment of hypertension and angina pectoris — see LOTREL, NORVASC

am·me·ter \'am-ˌēt-ər\ *n* : an instrument for measuring electric current in amperes — compare MILLIAMMETER

am·mo·nia \ə-'mō-nyə\ *n* **1** : a pungent colorless gaseous alkaline compound of nitrogen and hydrogen NH_3 that is very soluble in water and can easily be condensed to a liquid by cold and pressure **2** : AMMONIA WATER

ammonia alum *n* : ALUM 1b

am·mo·ni·ac \ə-'mō-nē-ˌak\ *n* : the aromatic gum resin of a Persian herb (*Dorema ammoniacum*) of the carrot family used as an expectorant and stimulant and in plasters

ammoniac — see SAL AMMONIAC

am·mo·ni·a·cal \,am-ə-'nī-ə-kəl\ *also* **am·mo·ni·ac** \ə-'mō-nē-ˌak\ *adj* : of, relating to, containing, or having the properties of ammonia

am·mo·ni·ate \ə-'mō-nē-ˌāt\ *vt* **-at·ed; -at·ing** **1** : to combine or impregnate with ammonia or an ammonium compound **2** : to subject to ammonification — **am·mo·ni·a·tion** \-ˌmō-nē-'ā-shən\ *n*

ammonia water *n* : a water solution of ammonia — called also *spirit of hartshorn*

am·mo·ni·fi·ca·tion \ə-ˌmän-ə-fə-'kā-shən, -ˌmō-nə-\ *n* **1** : the act or process of ammoniating **2** : decomposition with production of ammonia or ammonium compounds esp. by the action of bacteria on nitrogenous organic matter — **am·mo·ni·fy** \-ˌfī\ *vb* **-fied; -fy·ing**

am·mo·ni·um \ə-'mō-nē-əm\ *n* : an ion NH_4^+ derived from ammonia by combination with a hydrogen ion and known in organic compounds (as quaternary ammonium compounds) and in compounds (as salts) that resemble in properties the compounds of the alkali metals

ammonium alum *n* : ALUM 1b

ammonium carbonate *n* : a carbonate of ammonium; *specif* : the commercial mixture of the bicarbonate and carbamate used esp. in smelling salts

ammonium chloride *n* : a white crystalline volatile salt NH_4Cl that is used in dry cells and as an expectorant — called also *sal ammoniac*

ammonium hydroxide *n* : a weakly basic compound NH_4OH that is formed when ammonia dissolves in water and that exists only in solution

ammonium nitrate *n* : a colorless crystalline salt NH_4NO_3 used in explosives and fertilizers and in veterinary medicine as an expectorant and urinary acidifier

ammonium sulfate *n* : a colorless crystalline salt $(NH_4)_2SO_4$ used as a fertilizer and in medicine as a local analgesic

am·mo·nol·y·sis \,am-ə-'näl-ə-səs\ *n, pl* **-y·ses** \-ˌsēz\ : a chemical reaction similar to hydrolysis in which ammonia reacts with another compound usu. to form an amine ⟨the ∼ of organic esters yields acid amides⟩ — **am·mo·no·lyt·ic** \ə-ˌmō-nə-'lit-ik, ˌam-ə-, ˌmän-ə-; ˌam-ə-(ˌ)nō-\ *adj*

am·ne·sia \am-'nē-zhə\ *n* **1** : loss of memory sometimes including the memory of personal identity due to brain injury, shock, fatigue, repression, or illness or sometimes induced by anesthesia ⟨a period of ∼ after the wreck⟩ **2** : a gap in one's memory ⟨an ∼ concerning her high-school years⟩

am·ne·si·ac \-z(h)ē-ˌak\ *also* **am·ne·sic** \-zik, -sik\ *n* : a person affected with amnesia

am·ne·sic \am-'nē-zik, -sik\ *also* **am·ne·si·ac** \-z(h)ē-ˌāk\ *adj* : of or relating to amnesia : affected with or caused by amnesia ⟨an ∼ patient⟩ ⟨an ∼ trauma⟩

am·nes·tic \am-'nes-tik\ *adj* : AMNESIC; *also* : causing amnesia ⟨electroconvulsive shock as an ∼ agent⟩

amnii — see LIQUOR AMNII

am·nio \'am-nē-ō\ *n* : AMNIOCENTESIS

am·nio·cen·te·sis \,am-nē-ō-(ˌ)sen-'tē-səs\ *n, pl* **-te·ses** \-ˌsēz\ : the surgical insertion of a hollow needle through the abdominal wall and into the uterus of a pregnant female to obtain amniotic fluid esp. to examine the fetal chromosomes for an abnormality and for the determination of sex

am·nio·gen·e·sis \,am-nē-(ˌ)ō-'jen-ə-səs\ *n, pl* **-e·ses** \-ˌsēz\ : amnion formation

am·ni·og·ra·phy \,am-nē-'äg-rə-fē\ *n, pl* **-phies** : radiographic visualization of the outlines of the uterine cavity, placenta, and fetus after injection of a radiopaque substance into the amnion

am·ni·on \'am-nē-ˌän, -ən\ *n, pl* **amnions** *or* **am·nia** \-nē-ə\ : a thin membrane forming a closed sac about the embryos and fetuses of reptiles, birds, and mammals and containing the amniotic fluid — called also *amniotic sac*

am·nio·scope \'am-nē-ə-ˌskōp\ *n* : an endoscope for observation of the amnion and its contents

am·ni·os·co·py \,am-nē-'äs-kə-pē\ *n, pl* **-pies** : visual observation of the amnion and its contents by means of an endoscope

Am·ni·o·ta \,am-nē-'ōt-ə\ *n pl* : the group of vertebrates that are characterized by embryonic and fetal development with an amnion and include birds, reptiles, and mammals — **am·ni·ote** \'am-nē-ˌōt\ *adj or n*

am·ni·ot·ic \,am-nē-'ät-ik\ *adj* **1** : of or relating to the amnion **2** : characterized by the development of an amnion

amniotic band *n* : strands of amniotic tissue that are formed by premature rupture of the amnion and that become entangled esp. in the extremities of the developing fetus often limiting growth and resulting in various physical abnormalities (as limb or digit distortion or amputation)

amniotic band syndrome *n* : the highly variable group of physical abnormalities that can result from the formation of amniotic bands

amniotic cavity *n* : the fluid-filled space between the amnion and the fetus

amniotic fluid *n* : the serous fluid in which the embryo and fetus is suspended within the amnion

amniotic fold *n* : any of the folds that consist of ectoderm and the outer layer of mesoderm, that arise from the extraembryonic blastoderm first at the head, then at the tail, and finally on each side, and that form the amnion and much of the chorion

amniotic sac *n* : AMNION

am·ni·ot·o·my \,am-nē-'ät-ə-mē\ *n, pl* **-mies** : intentional rupture of the fetal membranes to induce or facilitate labor

amo·bar·bi·tal \,am-ə-'bär-bə-ˌtōl\ *n* : a barbiturate $C_{11}H_{18}N_2O_3$ used as a hypnotic and sedative; *also* : its sodium salt — called also *amylobarbitone;* see AMYTAL, TUINAL

amo·di·a·quine \,am-ə-'dī-ə-ˌkwin, -ˌkwēn\ *or* **amo·di·a·quin** \-ˌkwin\ *n* : a compound derived from quinoline and used in the form of its dihydrochloride $C_{20}H_{22}ClN_3O \cdot 2HCl \cdot 2H_2O$ as an antimalarial

Each boldface word in the list below is a chiefly British variant of the word to its right in small capitals.

amoeba	AMEBA	amoebicide	AMEBICIDE
amoebacidal	AMEBICIDAL	amoebiform	AMEBIFORM
amoebacide	AMEBICIDE	amoebocyte	AMEBOCYTE
amoebiasis	AMEBIASIS	amoeboid	AMEBOID
amoebic	AMEBIC	amoebula	AMEBULA
amoebicidal	AMEBICIDAL		

Amoe·ba \ə-'mē-bə\ *n* : a large genus of naked rhizopod protozoans that have lobed and never anastomosing pseudopodia and are widely distributed in fresh and salt water and moist terrestrial environments

Amoe·bo·tae·nia \ə-ˌmē-(ˌ)bō-'tē-nē-ə\ *n* : a genus of tapeworms (family Dilepididae) parasitic in the intestines of poultry

amok \ə-'mək, -'mäk\ *also* **amuck** \-'mək\ *n* : an episode of sudden mass assault against people or objects usu. by a single individual following a period of brooding that has traditionally been regarded as occurring esp. in Malaysian culture but is now increasingly viewed as psychopathological behavior occurring worldwide in numerous countries and cultures — **amok** *also* **amuck** *adj or adv*

amor·phin·ism \(')ā-'mòr-ˌfē-ˌniz-əm, -fə-\ *n* : the condition caused by depriving an addict of morphine

amor·phous \ə-'mòr-fəs\ *adj* **1** : having no apparent shape or organization **2** : having no real or apparent crystalline form

amor·phus \ə-'mòr-fəs\ *n, pl* **amor·phi** \-ˌfī, -ˌfē\ *or* **amor·phus·es** : a fetus without head, heart, or limbs

amox·a·pine \ə-'mäk-sə-ˌpēn\ *n* : a tricyclic antidepressant drug $C_{17}H_{16}ClN_3O$

amox·i·cil·lin *or Brit* **amox·y·cil·lin** \ə-ˌmäk-sē-'sil-ən\ *n* : a semisynthetic penicillin $C_{16}H_{19}N_3O_5S$ derived from ampicillin — see AMOXIL, AUGMENTIN, LAROTID

Amox·il \ə-'mäk-sil\ *trademark* — used for a preparation of amoxicillin

amp *abbr* **1** amperage **2** ampere **3** ampule **4** amputation

AMP \ˌā-ˌem-'pē\ *n* : a nucleotide $C_{10}H_{12}N_5O_3H_2PO_4$ that is composed of adenosine and one phosphate group and is reversibly convertible to ADP and ATP in metabolic reactions — called also *adenosine monophosphate;* compare CYCLIC AMP

am·per·age \'am-p(ə-)rij, -ˌpi(ə)r-ij\ *n* : the strength of a current of electricity expressed in amperes

am·pere \'am-ˌpi(ə)r *also* -ˌpe(ə)r\ *n* **1** : the practical mks unit of electric current that is equivalent to a flow of one coulomb per second or to the steady current produced by one volt applied across a resistance of one ohm **2** : the base unit of electric current in the International System of Units that is equal to a constant current which when maintained in two straight parallel conductors of infinite length and negligible circular sections one meter apart in a vacuum produces between the conductors a force equal to 2×10^{-7} newton per meter of length

Am·père \äⁿ-per\, **André Marie** (1775–1836), French physicist. Ampère is credited with founding, naming, and developing the science of electrodynamics. He was the formulator of two laws in electromagnetism relating magnetic fields to electric currents. The first person to develop techniques for measuring electricity, he invented an instrument that was a forerunner of the galvanometer. In 1881 at the suggestion of Sir Charles Bright, an international congress on electricity adopted *ampere* as a term for the standard unit of electric current.

am·phet·amine \am-'fet-ə-ˌmēn, -mən\ *n* : a racemic sympathomimetic amine $C_9H_{13}N$ or one of its derivatives (as dextroamphetamine or methamphetamine) frequently abused as a stimulant of the central nervous system but used clinically esp. in the form of its sulfate $C_9H_{13}N·H_2SO_4$ to treat attention deficit disorder and narcolepsy and formerly as a short-term appetite suppressant — see BENZEDRINE

am·phi·ar·thro·di·al \ˌam-fē-(ˌ)är-'thrōd-ē-əl\ *adj* : characterized by amphiarthrosis

am·phi·ar·thro·sis \-'thrō-səs\ *n, pl* **-thro·ses** \-ˌsēz\ : a slightly movable articulation (as a symphysis or a syndesmosis)

am·phi·as·ter \'am-fē-ˌas-tər\ *n* : the achromatic figure of mitotic cell division esp. in animal cells in which two asters are connected by a spindle — **am·phi·as·tral** \ˌam-fē-'as-trəl\ *adj*

Am·phib·ia \am-'fib-ē-ə\ *n pl* **1** : a class of subphylum Vertebrata comprising forms (as the frogs, toads, newts, and salamanders) that are intermediate in many respects between fishes and reptiles, are cold-blooded with nucleated red blood cells and a 3-chambered heart, and that have gilled aquatic larvae and air-breathing adults **2** : the members of the class Amphibia — **am·phib·i·an** \-ē-ən\ *n or adj*

am·phi·blas·tic \ˌam(p)-fə-'blas-tik\ *adj* : characterized by complete but unequal segmentation — used of telolecithal eggs

am·phi·bole \'am(p)-fə-ˌbōl\ *n* : any of a group of complex silicate minerals with like crystal structures that contain calcium, sodium, magnesium, aluminum, and iron ions or a combination of them — see CROCIDOLITE

am·phi·bol·ic \ˌam(p)-fə-'bäl-ik\ *adj* : having an uncertain or irregular outcome — used of stages in fevers or the critical period of disease when prognosis is uncertain ⟨the ∼ period is popularly known as the crisis —G. F. Boddie⟩

am·phi·cen·tric \-'sen-trik\ *adj* : converging at both ends — used of a plexus of blood vessels having one afferent and one efferent trunk

am·phi·cra·nia \-'krā-nē-ə\ *n* : pain affecting both sides of the head — compare HEMICRANIA

am·phi·dip·loid \ˌam(p)-fi-'dip-ˌlòid\ *n* : an interspecific hybrid having a complete diploid chromsome set from each parent form — **amphidiploid** *adj* — **am·phi·dip·loi·dy** \-ˌlòid-ē\ *n, pl* **-dies**

am·phi·mic·tic \ˌam(p)-fi-'mik-tik\ *adj* : capable of interbreeding freely and of producing fertile offspring — **am·phi·mic·ti·cal·ly** \-ti-k(ə-)lē\ *adv*

am·phi·mix·is \-'mik-səs\ *n, pl* **-mix·es** \-ˌsēz\ **1** : the union of gametes in sexual reproduction **2** : the combining of pregenital, anal, and urethral eroticism in the development of genital sexuality

am·phi·ox·us \ˌam(p)-fē-'äk-səs\ *n, pl* **-oxi** \-ˌsī, -ˌsē\ *or* **-ox·us·es** : a lancelet of the genus *Branchiostoma; broadly* : LANCELET

Amphioxus *n, syn of* BRANCHIOSTOMA

am·phi·path·ic \ˌam-fə-'path-ik\ *adj* : AMPHIPHILIC — **am·phi·path** \'am-fə-ˌpath\ *n*

am·phi·phil·ic \ˌam-fə-'fil-ik\ *adj* : of, relating to, consisting of, or being one or more molecules (as of a glycolipid or sphingolipid) in a biological membrane having a polar water-soluble terminal group attached to a water-insoluble hydrocarbon chain — **am·phi·phile** \'am-fə-ˌfīl\ *n*

am·phi·ploid \'am(p)-fi-ˌplòid\ *adj, of an interspecific hybrid* : having at least one complete diploid set of chromosomes derived from each ancestral species — **amphiploid** *n* — **am·phi·ploi·dy** \-ˌplòid-ē\ *n, pl* **-dies**

Am·phi·sto·ma·ta \ˌam(p)-fi-'stō-mət-ə\ *n pl, in some classifications* : a suborder of the subclass Digenea comprising digenetic trematodes somewhat conical in form with a highly developed posterior acetabulum — compare GASTRODISCOIDES, PARAMPHISTOMUM, WATSONIUS

am·phi·stome \'am(p)-fi-ˌstōm\ *n* : any of the suborder Amphistomata of digenetic trematodes — **amphistome** *adj*

am·phit·ri·chous \am-'fi-trə-kəs\ *adj* : having flagella at both ends

am·pho·lyte \'am(p)-fə-ˌlīt\ *n* : an amphoteric electrolyte — **am·pho·lyt·ic** \ˌam(p)-fə-'lit-ik\ *adj*

am·pho·phil \'am(p)-fə-ˌfil\ *n* : an amphophilic cell

am·pho·phil·ic \ˌam(p)-fə-'fil-ik\ *also* **am·pho·phil** \'am(p)-fə-ˌfil\ *or* **am·phoph·i·lous** \am-'fäf-ə-ləs\ *adj* : staining with both acid and basic dyes : NEUTROPHIL ⟨∼ cytoplasm⟩

am·phor·ic \am-'fòr-ik\ *adj* : resembling the sound made by blowing across the mouth of an empty bottle ⟨∼ breathing⟩ ⟨∼ sounds⟩ — **am·pho·ric·i·ty** \ˌam-fə-'ris-ət-ē\ *n, pl* **-ties**

am·pho·ter·ic \ˌam(p)-fə-'ter-ik\ *adj* : partly one and partly the other; *specif* : capable of reacting chemically either as an acid or as a base — **am·pho·ter·ism** \-'ter-ˌiz-əm\ *n*

am·pho·ter·i·cin \ˌam(p)-fə-'ter-ə-sən\ *n* : either of two polyenic antifungal substances obtained from a soil bacterium of the genus *Streptomyces* (*S. nodosus*); *esp* : AMPHOTERICIN B

amphotericin B *n* : the amphotericin that is clinically useful against deep-seated and systemic fungal infections

am·pi·cil·lin \ˌam-pə-'sil-ən\ *n* : a penicillin $C_{16}H_{19}N_3O_4S$ that is effective against gram-negative and gram-positive bacteria and is used in anhydrous forms, as the trihydrate, or as the sodium salt to treat various infections of the urinary, respiratory, and intestinal tracts — see PENBRITIN

am·plex·us \am-'plek-səs\ *n* : the mating embrace of a frog or toad during which eggs are shed into the water and there fertilized

---

\ə\ abut \ᵊ\ kitten \ər\ further \a\ ash \ā\ ace \ä\ cot, cart \aù\ out \ch\ chin \e\ bet \ē\ easy \g\ go \i\ hit \ī\ ice \j\ job \ŋ\ sing \ō\ go \ò\ law \òi\ boy \th\ thin \t͟h\ the \ü\ loot \ù\ foot \y\ yet \zh\ vision *See also* Pronunciation Symbols page

am·pli·fi·ca·tion \ˌam-plə-fə-'kā-shən\ *n* **1** : an act, example, or product of amplifying **2** : a usu. massive replication of genetic material and esp. of a gene or DNA sequence (as in a polymerase chain reaction)

am·pli·fi·er \'am-plə-ˌfī(ə)r\ *n* : one that amplifies; *specif* : an electronic device (as in a computer or sound-reproducing system) for amplifying voltage, current, or power

am·pli·fy \-ˌfī\ *vt* **-fied; -fy·ing** **1** : to make larger or greater (as in amount or intensity) **2** : to increase the strength or amount of; *esp* : to make louder **3** : to cause (a gene or DNA sequence) to undergo amplification

am·pli·tude \'am-plə-ˌt(y)üd\ *n* **1** : the extent or range of a quality, property, process, or phenomenon: as **a** : the extent of a vibratory movement (as of a pendulum) measured from the mean position to an extreme **b** : the maximum departure of the value of an alternating current or wave from the average value

amplitude of accommodation *n* : the difference between the refracting power of the eye when adjusted for vision at the far point and when adjusted for vision at the near point

am·pule *or* **am·poule** *also* **am·pul** \'am-ˌpyü(ə)l, -ˌpül\ *n* **1** : a hermetically sealed small bulbous glass vessel that is used to hold a solution for esp. hypodermic injection **2** : a vial resembling an ampule

am·pul·la \am-'pu̇l-ə, 'am-ˌpyü-lə\ *n, pl* **-lae** \-ˌlē\ : a saccular anatomic swelling or pouch: as **a** : the dilatation containing a patch of sensory epithelium at one end of each semicircular canal of the ear **b** : one of the dilatations of the lactiferous tubules of the mammary glands that serve as reservoirs for milk **c** (1) : the middle portion of the fallopian tube (2) : the distal dilatation of a vas deferens near the opening of the duct leading from the seminal vesicle **d** : a terminal dilatation of the rectum just before it joins the anal canal

ampulla of Va·ter \-'fät-ər\ *n* : a trumpet-mouthed dilatation of the duodenal wall at the opening of the fused pancreatic and common bile ducts — called also *papilla of Vater*

Vater, Abraham (1684–1751), German anatomist. Vater was a professor of anatomy and botany and later of pathology and therapeutics at Wittenberg. In 1710 he first noted the ampulla that has been named after him, but he did not publish a description of it until 1720. In 1717 he described the terminal capsules of certain sensory nerve fibers. They were later described by the Italian anatomist Filippo Pacini in 1840. Now these corpuscles are more commonly identified with Pacini than with Vater.

ampullaris — see CRISTA AMPULLARIS

am·pul·la·ry \am-'pu̇l-ə-rē\ *also* **am·pul·lar** \-'pu̇l-ər\ *adj* : resembling or relating to an ampulla

am·pul·lu·la \am-'pu̇l-yə-lə, -'pəl-\ *n, pl* **-lae** \-ˌlē\ : a minute ampulla (as of the lymphatics or laceals)

am·pu·tate \'am-pyə-ˌtāt\ *vt* **-tat·ed; -tat·ing** : to cut (as a limb) from the body — **am·pu·ta·tion** \ˌam-pyə-'tā-shən\ *n*

amputation neuroma *n* : NEUROMA 2

am·pu·tee \ˌam-pyə-'tē\ *n* : one that has had a limb amputated

amt *abbr* amount

amuck *var of* AMOK

amu·sia \(')ā-'myü-zē-ə, -zhə\ *n* **1** : a condition marked by inability to produce music — called also *motor amusia* **2** : a condition marked by inability to comprehend music — compare APHASIA

amy·e·lia \ˌā-(ˌ)mī-'ē-lē-ə, ˌam-(ˌ)ī-, -'el-ē-ə\ *n* : congenital absence of the spinal cord

amy·e·lin·ic \ˌā-ˌmī-ə-'lin-ik\ *adj* : UNMYELINATED

amyg·da·la \ə-'mig-də-lə\ *n, pl* **-lae** \-ˌlē, -ˌlī\ : the one of the four basal ganglia in each cerebral hemisphere that is part of the limbic system and consists of an almond-shaped mass of gray matter in the roof of the lateral ventricle — called also *amygdaloid body, amygdaloid nucleus*

amyg·da·lase \-də-ˌlās, -ˌlāz\ *n* : an enzyme found in the bitter almond that contributes to the hydrolysis of amygdalin to hydrocyanic acid

amyg·da·lec·to·my \ə-ˌmig-də-'lek-tə-mē\ *n, pl* **-mies** : surgical removal of the amygdala — **amyg·da·lec·to·mized** \-tə-ˌmīzd\ *adj*

amyg·da·lin \ə-'mig-də-lən\ *n* : a white crystalline cyanogenetic glucoside $C_{20}H_{27}NO_{11}$ found esp. in the seeds of the apricot, peach, and bitter almond

amyg·da·line \-lən, -ˌlīn\ *adj* **1** : of, relating to, or resembling an almond **2** : of or relating to a tonsil

amyg·da·loid \-ˌlȯid\ *adj* **1** : almond-shaped **2** : of, relating to, or affecting an amygdala ⟨∼ lesions⟩

amygdaloid body *n* : AMYGDALA

amygdaloid nucleus *n* : AMYGDALA

amyg·da·lot·o·my \ə-ˌmig-də-'lät-ə-mē\ *n, pl* **-mies** : destruction of part of the amygdala of the brain (as for the control of epilepsy) by surgical incision

am·yl \'am-əl\ *n* : a univalent hydrocarbon radical C_5H_{11} that occurs in various isomeric forms and is derived from pentane — called also *pentyl*

am·y·la·ceous \ˌam-ə-'lā-shəs\ *adj* : of, relating to, or having the characteristics of starch : STARCHY

amyl acetate *n* : a colorless liquid acetate $C_7H_{14}O_2$ of amyl alcohol that has a pleasant fruity odor and is used as a solvent and in the manufacture of artificial fruit essences

amyl alcohol *n* : any of eight isomeric alcohols $C_5H_{12}O$ used esp. as solvents and in making esters; *also* : either of two commercially produced mixtures of amyl alcohols used esp. as solvents

am·y·lase \'am-ə-ˌlās, -ˌlāz\ *n* : any of a group of enzymes (as amylopsin) that catalyze the hydrolysis of starch and glycogen or their intermediate hydrolysis products

am·y·lene \-ˌlēn\ *n* : any of several low-boiling alkenes (as pentene) with the formula C_5H_{10} that have anesthetic properties but are unsafe to use because of their toxicity and flammability

amyl nitrite *n* : a pale yellow pungent flammable liquid ester $C_5H_{11}NO_2$ of commercial amyl alcohol and nitrous acid that is used chiefly in medicine as a vasodilator esp. in treating angina pectoris and illicitly as an aphrodisiac — called also *isoamyl nitrite;* compare POPPER

am·y·lo·bar·bi·tone \ˌam-ə-lō-'bär-bə-ˌtōn\ *n, Brit* : AMOBARBITAL

am·y·lo·dex·trin \-'dek-strən\ *n* : an intermediate product of the hydrolysis of starch that is soluble in water and gives a blue color with iodine

am·y·loid \'am-ə-ˌlȯid\ *n* **1** : a nonnitrogenous starchy food **2** : a waxy translucent substance consisting primarily of protein that is deposited in some animal organs and tissue under abnormal conditions (as in Alzheimer's disease) — see BETA-AMYLOID — **amyloid** *adj*

amyloid be·ta–pro·tein *also* **amyloid β–pro·tein** \-ˌbāt-ə-'prō-ˌtēn, *chiefly Brit* -ˌbē-tə-\ *n* : BETA-AMYLOID

amyloid degeneration *n* : AMYLOIDOSIS

am·y·loid·o·sis \ˌam-ə-ˌlȯi-'dō-səs\ *n, pl* **-o·ses** \-ˌsēz\ : a disorder characterized by the deposition of amyloid in organs or tissues of the animal body — see PARAMYLOIDOSIS

amyloid precursor protein *n* : a transmembrane protein from which beta-amyloid is derived by proteolytic cleavage by secretases — abbr. APP

am·y·lo·lyt·ic \ˌam-ə-lō-'lit-ik\ *adj* : characterized by or capable of the enzymatic splitting of starch into soluble products ⟨∼ enzymes⟩ ⟨∼ activity⟩ — **am·y·lol·y·sis** \ˌam-ə-'läl-ə-səs\ *n, pl* **-y·ses** \-ˌsēz\

am·y·lo·pec·tin \ˌam-ə-lō-'pek-tən\ *n* : a component of starch that has a high molecular weight and branched structure and does not tend to gel in aqueous solutions

am·y·lo·plast \'am-ə-lō-ˌplast\ *n* : a colorless starch-forming plastid

am·y·lop·sin \ˌam-ə-'läp-sən\ *n* : the amylase of the pancreatic juice

am·y·lose \'am-ə-ˌlōs, -ˌlōz\ *n* **1** : any of various polysaccharides (as starch or cellulose) **2** : a component of starch characterized by its straight chains of glucose units and by the tendency of its aqueous solutions to set to a stiff gel **3** : any of various compounds $(C_6H_{10}O_5)_x$ obtained by the hydrolysis of starch

am·y·lum \-ləm\ *n* : STARCH

amyo·stat·ic \ˌā-ˌmī-ə-ˈstat-ik\ *adj* : characterized by muscular tremors that interfere with standing

amyo·to·nia \ˌā-ˌmī-ə-ˈtō-nē-ə\ *n* : deficiency of muscle tone

amyotonia con·gen·i·ta \-kən-ˈjen-ət-ə\ *n* : a congenital disease of infants characterized by flaccidity of the skeletal muscles resulting in an inability to move freely or maintain upright posture

amyo·tro·phia \ˌā-ˌmī-ə-ˈtrō-fē-ə\ *or* **amy·ot·ro·phy** \-ˌmī-ˈä-trə-fē\ *n, pl* **-phi·as** *or* **-phies** : atrophy of a muscle

amyo·tro·phic \-ˈträf-ik, -ˈtrō-fik\ *adj* : relating to or marked by amyotrophia

amyotrophic lateral sclerosis *n* : a rare fatal progressive degenerative disease that affects pyramidal motor neurons, usu. begins in middle age, and is characterized esp. by increasing and spreading muscular weakness — abbr. *ALS;* called also *Lou Gehrig's disease*

Am·y·tal \ˈam-ə-ˌtȯl\ *trademark* — used for a preparation of amobarbital

ana \ˈan-ə\ *adv* : of each an equal quantity — used in writing prescriptions

ANA *abbr* **1** American Nurses Association **2** antinuclear antibodies; antinuclear antibody

an·a·bae·na \ˌan-ə-ˈbē-nə\ *n* **1** *cap* : a genus of freshwater cyanobacteria (family Nostocaceae) having cells in beadlike filaments and often contaminating reservoirs **2** : a cyanobacterium of the genus *Anabaena*

anab·a·sine \ə-ˈnab-ə-ˌsēn, -sən\ *n* : an insecticidal liquid alkaloid $C_{10}H_{14}N_2$ related to nicotine and found in tobacco and in a nearly leafless Asian subshrub (*Anabasis aphylla*) of the goosefoot family (Chenopodiaceae)

ana·bi·o·sis \ˌan-ə-bī-ˈō-səs, -bē-\ *n, pl* **-o·ses** \-ˌsēz\ : a state of suspended animation induced in some organisms by desiccation — **ana·bi·ot·ic** \-ˈät-ik\ *adj*

anabolic steroid *n* : any of a group of usu. synthetic hormones that are derivatives of testosterone, are used medically esp. to promote tissue growth, and are sometimes abused by athletes to increase the size and strength of their muscles and improve endurance

anab·o·lism \ə-ˈnab-ə-ˌliz-əm\ *n* : the constructive part of metabolism concerned esp. with macromolecular synthesis — compare CATABOLISM — **an·a·bol·ic** \ˌan-ə-ˈbäl-ik\ *adj*

anab·o·lite \-ˌlīt\ *also* **anab·o·lin** \-lən\ *n* : a product of an anabolic process

an·acid·i·ty \ˌan-ə-ˈsid-ət-ē\ *n, pl* **-ties** : ACHLORHYDRIA

an·a·clit·ic \ˌan-ə-ˈklit-ik\ *adj* : of, relating to, or characterized by the direction of love toward an object (as the mother) that satisfies nonsexual needs (as hunger)

anaclitic depression *n* : impaired development of an infant resulting from separation from its mother

anac·ro·tism \ə-ˈnak-rə-ˌtiz-əm\ *n* : an abnormality of the blood circulation characterized by a secondary notch in the ascending part of a sphygmographic tracing of the pulse — **an·a·crot·ic** \ˌan-ə-ˈkrät-ik\ *adj*

ana·cul·ture \ˈan-ə-ˌkəl-chər\ *n* : a mixed bacterial culture; *esp* : one used in the preparation of autogenous vaccines

anaemia, anaemic, anaemically *chiefly Brit var of* ANEMIA, ANEMIC, ANEMICALLY

an·aer·obe \ˈan-ə-ˌrōb; (ˈ)an-ˈa(-ə)r-ˌōb, -ˈe(-ə)r-\ *n* : an anaerobic organism

an·aer·o·bic \ˌan-ə-ˈrō-bik; ˌan-ˌa(-ə)r-ˈō-, -ˌe(-ə)r-\ *adj* **1 a** : living, active, or occurring in the absence of free oxygen ⟨during heavy exercise ~ respiration occurs, pyruvic acid acts as a hydrogen acceptor, and lactic acid builds up in the tissues⟩ **b** : of, relating to, or being activity in which the body incurs an oxygen debt ⟨~ sports⟩ ⟨an ~ workout⟩ **2** : relating to or induced by anaerobes — **an·aer·o·bi·cal·ly** \-bi-k(ə-)lē\ *adv*

an·aero·bi·o·sis \ˌan-ə-rō-(ˌ)bī-ˈō-səs, -bē-; ˌan-ˌa(-ə)r-ō-, -ˌe(-ə)r-\ *n, pl* **-o·ses** \-ˌsēz\ : life in the absence of air or free oxygen

Each boldface word in the following list is a chiefly British variant of the word to its right in small capitals.

anaesthesia	ANESTHESIA
anaesthesiologist	ANESTHESIOLOGIST
anaesthesiology	ANESTHESIOLOGY
anaesthetic	ANESTHETIC
anaesthetically	ANESTHETICALLY
anaesthetisation	ANESTHETIZATION
anaesthetise	ANESTHETIZE
anaesthetist	ANESTHETIST
anaesthetization	ANESTHETIZATION
anaesthetize	ANESTHETIZE

an·a·gen \ˈan-ə-ˌjen\ *n* : the active phase of the hair growth cycle preceding telogen

anag·re·lide \ə-ˈnag-rə-ˌlīd\ *n* : a phosphodiesterase inhibitor administered esp. in the form of its hydrochloride $C_{10}H_7Cl_2N_3O \cdot HCl$ to treat thrombocytosis because of its antiplatelet activity — see AGRYLIN

anal \ˈān-ᵊl\ *adj* **1** : of, relating to, or situated near the anus **2 a** : of, relating to, or characterized by the stage of psychosexual development in psychoanalytic theory during which the child is concerned esp. with its feces **b** : of, relating to, or characterized by personality traits (as parsimony, meticulousness, and ill humor) considered typical of fixation at the anal stage of development — compare GENITAL 3, ORAL 3, PHALLIC 2 — **anal·ly** \-ᵊl-ē\ *adv*

anal *abbr* **1** analysis **2** analytic **3** analyze

anal canal *n* : the terminal section of the rectum

¹an·a·lep·tic \ˌan-ə-ˈlep-tik\ *adj* : of, relating to, or acting as an analeptic

²analeptic *n* : a restorative agent; *esp* : a drug that acts as a stimulant on the central nervous system

anal eroticism *n* : the experiencing of pleasurable sensations or sexual excitement associated with or symbolic of stimulation of the anus — called also *anal erotism* — **anal erotic** *adj*

an·al·ge·sia \ˌan-ᵊl-ˈjē-zhə, -z(h)ē-ə\ *n* : insensibility to pain without loss of consciousness

¹an·al·ge·sic \-ˈjē-zik, -sik\ *adj* : relating to, characterized by, or producing analgesia

²analgesic *n* : an agent for producing analgesia

an·al·get·ic \-ˈjet-ik\ *n or adj* : ANALGESIC

anal·i·ty \ā-ˈnal-ət-ē\ *n, pl* **-ties** : an anal psychological state, stage, or quality

an·al·ler·gic \ˌan-ə-ˈlər-jik, ˌan-ᵊl-ˈər-\ *adj* : not allergic ⟨~ persons⟩

anal·o·gous \ə-ˈnal-ə-gəs\ *adj* : having similar function but a different structure and origin ⟨~ organs⟩

an·a·logue *or* **an·a·log** \ˈan-ᵊl-ˌȯg, -ˌäg\ *n* **1** : something that is analogous or similar to something else **2** : an organ similar in function to an organ of another animal or plant but different in structure and origin **3** *usu analog* : a chemical compound that is structurally similar to another but differs slightly in composition (as in the replacement of one atom by an atom of a different element or in the presence of a particular functional group)

anal·o·gy \ə-ˈnal-ə-jē\ *n, pl* **-gies** : functional similarity between anatomical parts without similarity of structure and origin — compare HOMOLOGY 1

anal–re·ten·tive \ˈān-ᵊl-ri-ˈten-tiv\ *adj* : characterized by personality traits (as frugality and obstinacy) held to be psychological sequelae of toilet training — compare ANAL 2b — **anal retentiveness** *n*

anal retentive *n* : an anal-retentive individual

anal sadism *n* : the cluster of personality traits (as aggressiveness, negativism, destructiveness, and outwardly directed rage) typical of the anal stage of development — **anal–sa·dis·tic** \ˌān-ᵊl-sə-ˈdis-tik *also* -sā- *or* -sa-\ *adj*

anal sphincter *n* : either of two sphincters controlling the closing of the anus: **a** : an outer sphincter of striated muscle extending from the coccyx to the central tendinous part of the perineum and surrounding the anus immediately beneath the skin — called also *external anal sphincter, sphincter ani externus* **b** : an inner sphincter formed by thickening of

\ə\ abut \ᵊ\ kitten \ər\ further \a\ ash \ā\ ace \ä\ cot, cart \au̇\ out \ch\ chin \e\ bet \ē\ easy \g\ go \i\ hit \ī\ ice \j\ job \ŋ\ sing \ō\ go \ȯ\ law \ȯi\ boy \th\ thin \t̲h̲\ the \ü\ loot \u̇\ foot \y\ yet \zh\ vision *See also* Pronunciation Symbols page

the circular smooth muscle of the rectum — called also *internal anal sphincter, sphincter ani internus*

anal verge \-'vərj\ *n* : the distal margin of the anal canal comprising the muscular rim of the anus

anal·y·sand \ə-'nal-ə-ˌsand\ *n* : one who is undergoing psychoanalysis

analyse, analyser *Brit var of* ANALYZE, ANALYZER

anal·y·sis \ə-'nal-ə-səs\ *n, pl* **-y·ses** \-ˌsēz\ **1** : separation of a whole into its component parts **2 a** : the identification or separation of ingredients of a substance **b** : a statement of the constituents of a mixture **3** : PSYCHOANALYSIS

analysis of variance *n* : analysis of variation in an experimental outcome and esp. of a statistical variance in order to determine the contributions of given factors or variables to the variance

an·a·lyst \'an-ᵊl-əst\ *n* **1** : a person who analyzes or who is skilled in analysis **2** : PSYCHOANALYST

an·a·lyte \'an-ᵊl-ˌīt\ *n* : a chemical substance that is the subject of a chemical analysis

an·a·lyt·ic \ˌan-ᵊl-'it-ik\ *or* **an·a·lyt·i·cal** \-i-kəl\ *adj* **1** : of or relating to analysis; *esp* : separating something into component parts or constituent elements **2** : PSYCHOANALYTIC — **an·a·lyt·i·cal·ly** \-i-k(ə-)lē\ *adv*

analytic psychology *n* : a modification of psychoanalysis due to C. G. Jung that adds to the concept of the personal unconscious a racial or collective unconscious and advocates that psychotherapy be conducted in terms of the patient's present-day conflicts and maladjustments

an·a·lyze *or Brit* **an·a·lyse** \'an-ᵊl-ˌīz\ *vt* **-lyzed** *or Brit* **-lysed**; **-lyz·ing** *or Brit* **-lys·ing** **1** : to study or determine the nature and relationship of the parts of by analysis; *esp* : to examine by chemical analysis **2** : PSYCHOANALYZE

an·a·lyz·er *or Brit* **an·a·lys·er** \-ər\ *n* : the part of a polariscope that receives the light after polarization and exhibits the properties of light — compare POLARIZER

an·am·ne·sis \ˌan-ˌam-'nē-səs\ *n, pl* **-ne·ses** \-ˌsēz\ **1** : a recalling to mind **2** : a preliminary case history of a medical or psychiatric patient

an·am·nes·tic \-'nes-tik\ *adj* **1** : of or relating to an anamnesis **2** : of or relating to a second rapid increased production of antibodies in response to an immunogenic substance after serum antibodies from a first response can no longer be detected in the blood

an·am·ni·on·ic \ˌan-ˌam-nē-'än-ik\ *adj* : not developing an amnion

An·am·ni·o·ta \-nē-'ōt-ə\ *n pl* : a group of vertebrates that develop no amnion and that include the cyclostomes, fishes, and amphibians — **an·am·ni·ote** \an-'am-nē-ˌōt\ *adj or n*

ana·mor·pho·sis \ˌan-ə-'mȯr-fə-səs\ *n, pl* **-pho·ses** \-ˌsēz\ : a gradually ascending progression or change of form from one type to another in the evolution of a group of animals or plants

an·an·a·sta·sia \ˌan-ˌan-ə-'stā-zh(ē-)ə\ *n* : a hysterical condition characterized by inability to stand up

anan·da·mide \ə-'nan-də-ˌmīd\ *n* : a derivative of arachidonic acid that occurs naturally in the brain and in some foods (as chocolate) and that binds to the same brain receptors as the cannabinoids (as THC)

an·an·kas·tic *or* **an·an·cas·tic** \ˌan-(ˌ)an-'kas-tik\ *adj* : of, relating to, or arising from compulsion esp. in an obsessive or compulsive neurosis ⟨an ∼ reaction⟩

anaph·a·lan·ti·a·sis \ˌan-ˌaf-ə-ˌlan-'tī-ə-səs, ə-ˌnaf-\ *n* : hair loss from the eyebrows

ana·phase \'an-ə-ˌfāz\ *n* : the stage of mitosis and meiosis in which the chromosomes move toward the poles of the spindle — **ana·pha·sic** \ˌan-ə-'fā-zik\ *adj*

anaph·o·ret·ic \ˌan-ˌaf-ə-'ret-ik, ə-ˌnaf-\ *adj* : causing or characterized by diminished activity of the sweat glands ⟨∼ deodorants⟩

an·aph·ro·di·sia \ˌan-ˌaf-rə-'dē-zh(ē-)ə, -'dizh-(ē-)ə\ *n* : absence or impairment of sexual desire

¹an·aph·ro·dis·i·ac \-'dē-zē-ˌak, -'diz-ē-\ *adj* : of, relating to, or causing anaphrodisia

²anaphrodisiac *n* : an anaphrodisiac agent

ana·phy·lac·tic \ˌan-ə-fə-'lak-tik\ *adj* : of, relating to, affected by, or causing anaphylaxis or anaphylactic shock — **ana·phy·lac·ti·cal·ly** \-ti-k(ə-)lē\ *adv*

anaphylactic shock *n* : an often severe and sometimes fatal systemic reaction in a susceptible individual upon a second exposure to a specific antigen (as wasp venom or penicillin) after previous sensitization that is characterized esp. by respiratory symptoms, fainting, itching, and hives

ana·phy·lac·to·gen \-tə-jən\ *n* : any substance capable of producing a condition of anaphylaxis — **an·a·phy·lac·to·gen·ic** \-ˌlak-tə-'jen-ik\ *adj*

ana·phy·lac·toid \-'lak-ˌtȯid\ *adj* : resembling anaphylaxis or anaphylactic shock

an·a·phyl·a·tox·in \ˌan-ə-ˌfil-ə-'täk-sən\ *n* : a toxic substance postulated to be formed in blood serum treated with some bacterial polysaccharides in order to explain the anaphylaxis that results when the treated and modified serum is injected into experimental animals

ana·phy·lax·is \ˌan-ə-fə-'lak-səs\ *n, pl* **-lax·es** \-ˌsēz\ **1** : hypersensitivity (as to foreign proteins or drugs) resulting from sensitization following prior contact with the causative agent **2** : ANAPHYLACTIC SHOCK

an·a·pla·sia \ˌan-ə-'plā-zh(ē-)ə\ *n* : reversion of cells to a more primitive or undifferentiated form

an·a·plas·ma \ˌan-ə-'plaz-mə\ *n* **1** *cap* : a genus of bacteria of the family Anaplasmataceae that are found in the red blood cells of ruminants, resemble small masses of chromatin without cytoplasm, are transmitted by biting arthropods, and cause anaplasmosis **2** *pl* **-ma·ta** \-mət-ə\ *or* **-mas** : any bacterium of the genus *Anaplasma*

An·a·plas·ma·ta·ce·ae \ˌan-ə-ˌplaz-mə-'tā-sē-ˌē\ *n pl* : a family of obligately parasitic bacteria of the order Rickettsiales that are enclosed in a membrane, have an internal structure resembling that of members of the related family Rickettsiaceae, occur in short chains or in irregular groups in red blood cells or free in the blood of various vertebrates, and are classified in several genera including the genus *Anaplasma*

an·a·plas·mo·sis \-ˌplaz-'mō-səs\ *n, pl* **-mo·ses** \-ˌsēz\ : a tick-borne disease of cattle, sheep, and deer caused by a bacterium of the genus *Anaplasma* (*A. marginale*) and characterized esp. by anemia and by jaundice — called also *gall sickness, galziekte*

an·a·plas·tic \ˌan-ə-'plas-tik\ *adj* : characterized by, composed of, or being cells which have reverted to a relatively undifferentiated state ⟨∼ carcinomas⟩

an·a·plas·tol·o·gy \-ˌplas-'täl-ə-jē\ *n, pl* **-gies** : a branch of medical technology concerned with the preparation and fitting of prosthetic devices (as artificial eyes and surgical implants) to individual specifications and with the study of the materials from which they are fabricated — **an·a·plas·tol·o·gist** \-ə-jest\ *n*

an·a·rith·mia \ˌan-ə-'rith-mē-ə, -'rith-\ *n* : loss of the ability to count (as resulting from a brain lesion)

an·ar·thria \an-'är-thrē-ə\ *n* : inability to articulate remembered words as a result of a brain lesion — compare APHASIA

an·a·sar·ca \ˌan-ə-'sär-kə\ *n* : generalized edema with accumulation of serum in the connective tissue — **an·a·sar·cous** \-kəs\ *adj*

an·a·stal·sis \ˌan-ə-'stȯl-səs, -'stäl-, -'stal-\ *n, pl* **-stal·ses** \-ˌsēz\ : ANTIPERISTALSIS

an·a·state \'an-ə-ˌstāt\ *n* : ANABOLITE

an·astig·mat \a-'nas-tig-ˌmat, ˌan-ə-'stig-\ *n* : an anastigmatic lens

an·astig·mat·ic \ˌan-ə-(ˌ)stig-'mat-ik, ˌan-ˌas-tig-\ *adj* : not astigmatic — used esp. of lenses that are able to form approximately point images of object points

anas·to·mose \ə-'nas-tə-ˌmōz, -ˌmōs\ *vb* **-mosed; -mos·ing** *vt* : to connect or join by anastomosis ∼ *vi* : to communicate by anastomosis

anas·to·mo·sis \ə-ˌnas-tə-'mō-səs, ˌan-əs-\ *n, pl* **-mo·ses** \-ˌsēz\ **1 a** : a communication between or coalescence of blood vessels **b** : the surgical union of parts and esp. hollow tubular parts ⟨∼ of the ureter and colon is surgically practicable⟩ **2** : a product of anastomosis; *esp* : a network (as of channels or branches) produced by anastomosis — **anas·to·mot·ic** \-'mät-ik\ *adj*

an·as·tral \(')an-'as-trəl\ *adj* : lacking asters — used of achromatic figures

anat *abbr* anatomic; anatomical; anatomy

an·a·tom·ic \ˌan-ə-'täm-ik\ *or* **an·a·tom·i·cal** \-i-kəl\ *adj* **1** : of or relating to anatomy ⟨*anatomical* knowledge⟩ **2** : STRUCTURAL 1 ⟨an ∼ obstruction⟩ — **an·a·tom·i·cal·ly** \-i-k(ə-)lē\ *adv*

Anatomica — see BASLE NOMINA ANATOMICA, NOMINA ANATOMICA

anatomical dead space *n* : the dead space in that portion of the respiratory system which is external to the alveoli and includes the air-conveying ducts from the nostrils to the terminal bronchioles — compare PHYSIOLOGICAL DEAD SPACE

anatomical position *n* : the normal position of the human body when active

an·a·tom·i·co·path·o·log·ic \ˌan-ə-ˌtäm-ə-(ˌ)kō-ˌpath-ə-'läj-ik\ *or* **an·a·tom·i·co·path·o·log·i·cal** \-i-kəl\ *adj* : of or relating to anatomy and pathology or to pathological anatomy

anat·o·mist \ə-'nat-ə-məst\ *n* : a specialist in anatomy

anat·o·mize *or Brit* **anat·o·mise** \-ˌmīz\ *vt* **-mized** *or Brit* **-mised; -miz·ing** *or Brit* **-mis·ing** : to cut in pieces in order to display or examine the structure and use of the parts : DISSECT

anat·o·my \ə-'nat-ə-mē\ *n, pl* **-mies** **1** : a branch of morphology that deals with the structure of organisms — compare PHYSIOLOGY 1 **2** : a treatise on anatomic science or art **3** : the art of separating the parts of an organism in order to ascertain their position, relations, structure, and function : DISSECTION **4** : structural makeup esp. of an organism or any of its parts

ana·tox·in \ˌan-ə-'täk-sən\ *n* : TOXOID

an·au·dia \an-'ȯd-ē-ə, ən-\ *n* : loss of voice : APHONIA

an·au·tog·e·nous \ˌan-ȯ-'täj-ə-nəs\ *adj* : requiring a meal esp. of blood to produce eggs ⟨∼ mosquitoes⟩

an·chor \'aŋ-kər\ *vt* **an·chored; an·chor·ing** \-k(ə-)riŋ\ : to relate psychologically to a point or frame of reference (as to a person, a situation, an object, or a conceptual scheme)

an·chor·age \'aŋ-k(ə-)rij\ *n* **1** : the act of securing or fastening firmly **2** : something (as a tooth) that provides a secure hold ⟨∼ for a dental plate⟩ **3** : a point or frame of psychological reference

anchylose, anchylosis, anchylotic *var of* ANKYLOSE, ANKYLOSIS, ANKYLOTIC

anchylostomiasis *var of* ANCYLOSTOMIASIS

¹an·cil·lary \'an(t)-sə-ˌler-ē, *esp Brit* an-'sil-ə-rē\ *adj* : being auxiliary or supplementary ⟨use of a drug as ∼ to surgical treatment⟩ ⟨∼ staff⟩ ⟨∼ diagnostic services⟩

²ancillary *n, pl* **-lar·ies** **1** *Brit* : one who assists or is supplementary to another person **2** : a supplemental diagnostic or therapeutic medical service (as magnetic resonance imaging or radiotherapy)

an·co·nal \(')aŋ-'kōn-ᵊl\ *also* **an·co·ne·al** \-'kō-nē-əl\ *adj* : of, relating to, or belonging to the elbow ⟨∼ pain⟩

an·co·ne·us \aŋ-'kō-nē-əs\ *n, pl* **-nei** \-nē-ˌī\ : a small triangular extensor muscle that is superficially situated behind and below the elbow and that extends the forearm — called also *anconeus muscle*

An·cy·los·to·ma \ˌaŋ-ki-'läs-tə-mə, ˌan(t)-sə-\ *n* : the type genus of the family Ancylostomatidae comprising hookworms that have buccal teeth resembling hooks and are intestinal parasites of mammals including humans — compare NECATOR

An·cy·lo·sto·mat·i·dae \ˌaŋ-kə-ˌlō-(ˌ)stō-'mat-ə-ˌdē, ˌan(t)-sə-, -ˌläs-tə-\ *n pl* : a family of nematodes containing the hookworms

an·cy·lo·stome \aŋ-'kil-ə-ˌstōm, an-'sil-\ *or* **an·kyl·o·stome** \-'kil-\ *n* : any of the genus *Ancylostoma* of hookworms

an·cy·lo·sto·mi·a·sis \ˌaŋ-ki-lō-stə-'mī-ə-səs, ˌan(t)-sə-\ *or* **an·ky·lo·sto·mi·a·sis** \-kī-lō-\ *also* **an·chy·lo·sto·mi·a·sis** \-kī-lō-\ *n, pl* **-a·ses** \-ˌsēz\ : infestation with or disease

caused by hookworms; *esp* : a lethargic anemic state due to blood loss through the feeding of hookworms in the small intestine — called also *hookworm disease*

ancyroid *var of* ANKYROID

an·dro \'an-drō\ *n* : ANDROSTENEDIONE

an·dro·gam·one \ˌan-drə-'gam-ˌōn\ *n* : a gamone in a male cell

an·dro·gen \'an-drə-jən\ *n* : a male sex hormone (as testosterone) — **an·dro·gen·ic** \ˌan-drə-'jen-ik\ *adj*

an·dro·gen·e·sis \ˌan-drə-'jen-ə-səs\ *n, pl* **-e·ses** \-ˌsēz\ : development in which the embryo contains only paternal chromosomes due to failure of the egg nucleus to participate in fertilization — compare GYNOGENESIS — **an·dro·ge·net·ic** \-jə-'net-ik\ *adj*

androgenetic alopecia *n* : hereditary androgen-dependent hair loss that is associated with the shrinkage of hair follicles and the shortening of the anagen phase of hair growth and that is typically characterized by moderate to severe hair loss on the temples and crown in men and diffuse thinning on the crown in women — see MALE-PATTERN BALDNESS

an·drog·e·nize *or Brit* **an·drog·e·nise** \an-'draj-ə-ˌnīz\ *vt* **-nized** *or Brit* **-nised; -niz·ing** *or Brit* **-nis·ing** : to treat or influence with male sex hormone esp. in excessive amounts ⟨neonatally *androgenized* female rats⟩

an·dro·gyne \'an-drə-ˌjīn\ *n* : HERMAPHRODITE 1

an·drog·y·nism \an-'draj-ə-ˌniz-əm\ *n* : the quality or state of being androgynous : HERMAPHRODITISM

an·drog·y·nous \an-'draj-ə-nəs\ *adj* : having the characteristics or nature of both male and female — **an·drog·y·ny** \-nē\ *n, pl* **-nies**

an·droid \'an-ˌdrȯid\ *adj* **1** *of the pelvis* : having the angular form and narrow outlet typical of the human male ⟨a disproportionate number of difficult labors occur in women with ∼ pelvises⟩ — compare ANTHROPOID, GYNECOID, PLATYPELLOID **2** : relating to or characterized by the distribution of body fat chiefly in the abdominal region ⟨∼ obesity⟩ — compare GYNECOID

an·drol·o·gist \an-'dral-ə-jəst\ *n* : a specialist in andrology

an·drol·o·gy \-jē\ *n, pl* **-gies** : a branch of medicine concerned with male diseases and esp. with those affecting the male reproductive system

Andromachi — see THERIACA ANDROMACHI

an·drom·e·da \an-'dram-əd-ə\ *n* **1** *cap* : a small genus of low evergreen boreal or arctic shrubs of the heath family (Ericaceae) having drooping white or pinkish flowers in terminal umbels and including several that are sources of andromedotoxin **2** : any plant of the genus *Andromeda*

an·drom·e·do·tox·in \an-ˌdram-əd-(ˌ)ō-'täk-sən\ *n* : a toxic compound $C_{31}H_{50}O_{10}$ found in various plants (as members of the genus *Andromeda*) of the heath family (Ericaceae) that lowers the blood pressure of animals when taken in small doses

an·dro·mi·met·ic \ˌan-drō-mə-'met-ik, -mī-\ *adj* : simulating the effect of androgen

an·dro·pause \'an-drə-ˌpȯz\ *n* : a gradual and highly variable decline in the production of androgenic hormones and esp. testosterone in the human male together with its associated effects that is held to occur during and after middle age but is often difficult to discriminate from the effects of confounding factors (as chronic illness, stress, or medication use) that can depress testosterone levels — called also *male climacteric, male menopause, viropause*

an·dro·pho·bia \ˌan-drə-'fō-bē-ə\ *n* : an abnormal dread of men : repugnance to the male sex — **an·dro·pho·bic** \-'fō-bik\ *adj*

an·dro·stane \'an-drə-ˌstān\ *n* : a crystalline saturated steroid hydrocarbon $C_{19}H_{32}$ obtainable from androsterone by reduction

---

\ə\ abut \ᵊ\ kitten \ər\ further \a\ ash \ā\ ace \ä\ cot, cart
\au̇\ out \ch\ chin \e\ bet \ē\ easy \g\ go \i\ hit \ī\ ice \j\ job
\ŋ\ sing \ō\ go \ȯ\ law \ȯi\ boy \th\ thin \th\ the \ü\ loot
\u̇\ foot \y\ yet \zh\ vision *See also* Pronunciation Symbols page

an·dro·stene·di·one \ˌan-drə-ˌsten-'dī-ˌōn, -'sten-dē-ˌōn\ *n* : a steroid sex hormone $C_{19}H_{26}O_2$ that is secreted by the testes, ovaries, and adrenal cortex and is a precursor of testosterone and estrogen

an·dros·ter·one \an-'dräs-tə-ˌrōn\ *n* : an androgenic hormone that is a hydroxy ketone $C_{19}H_{30}O_2$ found in human urine

Anec·tine \ə-'nek-tən\ *trademark* — used for a preparation of succinylcholine

an·elec·trot·o·nus \ˌan-əl-ˌek-'trät-ᵊn-əs\ *n* : the decreased irritability of a nerve in the region of a positive electrode or anode on the passage of a current of electricity through it — compare CATELECTROTONUS — **an·elec·tro·ton·ic** \-ˌek-trə-'tän-ik\ *adj*

ane·mia *or chiefly Brit* **anae·mia** \ə-'nē-mē-ə\ *n* 1 : a condition in which the blood is deficient in red blood cells, in hemoglobin, or in total volume — see APLASTIC ANEMIA, HYPERCHROMIC ANEMIA, HYPOCHROMIC ANEMIA, MEGALOBLASTIC ANEMIA, MICROCYTIC ANEMIA, PERNICIOUS ANEMIA, SICKLE-CELL ANEMIA; compare OLIGOCYTHEMIA 2 : ISCHEMIA — **ane·mic** *or chiefly Brit* **anae·mic** \ə-'nē-mik\ *adj* — **ane·mi·cal·ly** *or chiefly Brit* **anae·mi·cal·ly** \-mi-k(ə-)lē\ *adv*

anem·o·ne \ə-'nem-ə-nē\ *n* 1 *cap* : a genus of herbs of the buttercup family (Ranunculaceae) widely distributed in temperate and subarctic regions that have lobed or divided leaves and showy flowers and that include some (as a pasqueflower) used medicinally esp. formerly 2 : a plant or flower of the genus *Anemone*

anem·o·nin \ə-'nem-ə-nən\ *n* : an acrid poisonous compound containing two lactone groups and obtained esp. from some plants of the genus *Anemone* and a related genus (*Ranunculus*) containing the buttercups

an·en·ce·pha·lia \ˌan-ˌen-sə-'fāl-yə\ *n* : ANENCEPHALY

¹**an·en·ce·phal·ic** \ˌan-ˌen-(ˌ)en(t)-sə-'fal-ik\ *adj* : of, relating to, or affected with anencephaly ⟨an ~ fetus⟩

²**anencephalic** *n* : an anencephalic fetus or newborn

an·en·ceph·a·lus \ˌan-(ˌ)en-'sef-ə-ləs\ *n, pl* **-li** \-ˌlī\ : ANENCEPHALY

an·en·ceph·a·ly \ˌan-(ˌ)en-'sef-ə-lē\ *n, pl* **-lies** : congenital absence of all or a major part of the brain

an·en·ter·ous \(')an-'ent-ə-rəs\ *adj* : having no stomach or intestine

aneph·ric \(')a-'nef-rik, (')ā-\ *adj* : being without functioning kidneys ⟨~ patients on dialysis⟩

an·er·gy \'an-(ˌ)ər-jē\ *n, pl* **-gies** : a condition in which the body fails to react to an injected allergen or antigen (as tuberculin) — **an·er·gic** \-jik\ *adj*

an·er·oid \'an-ə-ˌrȯid\ *adj* : containing no liquid or actuated without the use of liquid ⟨an ~ manometer⟩

aneroid barometer *n* : a barometer in which the action of atmospheric pressure in bending a metallic surface is made to move a pointer

an·es·the·sia *or chiefly Brit* **an·aes·the·sia** \ˌan-əs-'thē-zhə\ *n* 1 : loss of sensation esp. to touch usu. resulting from a lesion in the nervous system or from some other abnormality 2 : loss of sensation and usu. of consciousness without loss of vital functions artificially produced by the administration of one or more agents that block the passage of pain impulses along nerve pathways to the brain

an·es·the·si·ol·o·gist *or chiefly Brit* **an·aes·the·si·ol·o·gist** \ˌan-əs-ˌthē-zē-'äl-ə-jəst\ *n* : ANESTHETIST; *specif* : a physician specializing in anesthesiology

an·es·the·si·ol·o·gy *or chiefly Brit* **an·aes·the·si·ol·o·gy** \-jē\ *n, pl* **-gies** : a branch of medical science dealing with anesthesia and anesthetics

¹**an·es·thet·ic** *or chiefly Brit* **an·aes·thet·ic** \ˌan-əs-'thet-ik\ *adj* 1 : capable of producing anesthesia ⟨~ agents⟩ 2 : of, relating to, or caused by anesthesia ⟨an ~ effect⟩ ⟨~ symptoms⟩ — **an·es·thet·i·cal·ly** *or chiefly Brit* **an·aes·thet·i·cal·ly** \-i-k(ə-)lē\ *adv*

²**anesthetic** *or chiefly Brit* **anaesthetic** *n* : a substance that produces anesthesia

anes·the·tist *or chiefly Brit* **anaes·the·tist** \ə-'nes-thət-əst, Brit -'nēs-\ *n* : one trained to administer anesthetics — compare ANESTHESIOLOGIST

anes·the·tize *or chiefly Brit* **anaes·the·tize** *also* **anaes·the·tise** \-thə-ˌtīz\ *vt* **-tized** *or chiefly Brit* **-tized** *also* **-tised; -tiz·ing** *or chiefly Brit* **-tiz·ing** *also* **-tis·ing** : to subject to anesthesia — **anes·the·ti·za·tion** *or chiefly Brit* **anaes·the·ti·za·tion** *also* **anaes·the·ti·sa·tion** \ə-ˌnes-thət-ə-'zā-shən, Brit -ˌnēs-\ *n*

an·es·trous *or chiefly Brit* **an·oes·trous** \(')an-'es-trəs, Brit -'ēs-\ *adj* 1 : not exhibiting estrus 2 : of or relating to anestrus

an·es·trus *or chiefly Brit* **an·oes·trus** \-trəs\ *n* : the period of sexual quiescence between two periods of sexual activity in cyclically breeding mammals — compare ESTRUS

an·e·thole \'an-ə-ˌthōl\ *n* : an ether $C_{10}H_{12}O$ obtained esp. from the oils of anise and fennel in the form of soft shining scales and used in flavoring and in cosmetics

ane·thum \ə-'nē-thəm\ *n* 1 *cap* : a small genus of Asian herbs of the family Umbelliferae with dissected foliage and yellow flowers that includes dill and fennel 2 *pl* **-tha** \-thə\ *or* **-thums** : the dried ripe fruit of a dill (*Anethum graveolens*) that is used in medicine as a carminative and stomachic

an·eu·ploid \'an-yù-ˌplȯid\ *adj* : having or being a chromosome number that is not an exact multiple of the usu. haploid number — compare EUPLOID — **aneuploid** *n* — **an·eu·ploi·dy** \-ˌplȯid-ē\ *n, pl* **-dies**

an·eu·rine \'an-yə-ˌrēn, (')ā-'nyù(ə)r-ˌēn\ *also* **an·eu·rin** \-rən, -ən\ *n* : THIAMINE

aneu·ro·gen·ic \ˌan-ə-(n)yùr-ə-'jen-ik\ *adj, of embryonic parts* : developing without the normal neural component ⟨a grafted limb bud is ~⟩

an·eu·rysm *also* **an·eu·rism** \'an-yə-ˌriz-əm\ *n* : an abnormal blood-filled dilatation of a blood vessel and esp. an artery resulting from disease of the vessel wall — **an·eu·rys·mal** *also* **an·eu·ris·mal** \ˌan-yə-'riz-məl\ *adj* — **an·eu·rys·mal·ly** \-ē\ *adv*

ANF *abbr* atrial natriuretic factor

angel dust \'ān-jəl-ˌdəst\ *n* : PHENCYCLIDINE

an·gel·i·ca \an-'jel-i-kə\ *n* 1 *cap* : a genus of usu. white-flowered herbs of the family Umbelliferae native to the northern hemisphere and New Zealand 2 : any plant of the genus *Angelica*; *esp* : a biennial or perennial herb (*A. archangelica*) having young stems that are candied and roots and seeds that yield a flavoring oil — see ANGELICA ROOT

an·gel·ic acid \(ˌ)an-ˌjel-ik-\ *n* : an unsaturated crystalline acid $C_5H_8O_2$ that occurs as an ester esp. in angelica root and together with tiglic acid in oil from the common European chamomile (*Anthemis nobilis*)

angelica root *n* : the dried rhizome and roots of any of several plants of the genus *Angelica* (esp. *A. archangelica*) formerly used esp. as a carminative and emmenagogue

An·gel·man syndrome \'an-jəl-mən-, 'än-\ *also* **An·gel·man's syndrome** \-mənz-\ *n* : a genetic disorder characterized by severe mental retardation, seizures, ataxic gait, jerky movements, lack of speech, microencephaly, and frequent smiling and laughter

  Angelman, Harry (1915–1996), British pediatrician. Angelman began his career in pediatrics at Booth Hall Children's Hospital in Manchester, England. After serving with the Royal Medical Corps in India during World War II, he became a resident at the Royal Liverpool Children's Hospital. In 1950 he became a consultant pediatrician to a group of hospitals in Warrington. It was there in the early 1960s that he examined three children who seemed to be affected with the same genetic disorder. In the 1980s the Angelman Syndrome Foundation was established in the U.S. His description of the disorder was published in 1965, and the name *Angelman syndrome* subsequently came to be used.

an·gen·e·sis \an-'jen-ə-səs\ *n, pl* **-e·ses** \-ˌsēz\ : regeneration esp. of tissues

an·gi·i·tis \ˌan-jē-'īt-əs\ *n, pl* **-it·i·des** \-'īt-ə-ˌdēz\ : VASCULITIS

an·gi·na \an-ˈjī-nə, ˈan-jə-\ *n* : a disease marked by spasmodic attacks of intense suffocative pain: as **a** : a severe inflammatory or ulcerated condition of the mouth or throat ⟨diphtheritic ∼⟩ — see LUDWIG'S ANGINA, VINCENT'S ANGINA **b** : ANGINA PECTORIS — **an·gi·nal** \an-ˈjīn-ᵊl, ˈan-jən-\ *adj*

angina pec·to·ris \-ˈpek-t(ə-)rəs\ *n* : a disease marked by brief paroxysmal attacks of chest pain precipitated by deficient oxygenation of the heart muscles — see UNSTABLE ANGINA; compare CORONARY INSUFFICIENCY, HEART ATTACK, HEART FAILURE 1

an·gi·noid \ˈan-jə-ˌnȯid, an-ˈjī-\ *adj* : resembling angina

an·gi·nose \ˈan-jə-ˌnōs, an-ˈjī-\ *or* **an·gi·nous** \(ˈ)an-ˈjī-nəs, ˈan-jə-\ *adj* : relating to angina or angina pectoris

an·gio·blast \ˈan-jē-ə-ˌblast\ *n* **1** : one of the extraembryonic mesenchyme cells that differentiate into the endothelium of the embryonic blood vessels **2** : the mesenchymal tissue that gives rise to embryonic blood cells and blood vessels — **an·gio·blas·tic** \ˌan-jē-ə-ˈblas-tik\ *adj*

an·gio·car·dio·gram \ˌan-jē-ō-ˈkärd-ē-ə-ˌgram\ *n* : a radiograph of the heart and its blood vessels prepared by angiocardiography

an·gio·car·di·og·ra·phy \-ˌkärd-ē-ˈäg-rə-fē\ *n, pl* **-phies** : the radiographic visualization of the heart and its blood vessels after injection of a radiopaque substance — **an·gio·car·dio·graph·ic** \-ē-ə-ˈgraf-ik\ *adj*

an·gio·cho·li·tis \ˌan-jē-ə-kō-ˈlīt-əs\ *n* : CHOLANGITIS

an·gio·cyst \ˈan-jē-ə-ˌsist\ *n* : a pouch of mesothelial tissue having blood-forming properties

an·gio·ede·ma *or Brit* **an·gio—oe·de·ma** \ˌan-jē-ō-i-ˈdē-mə\ *n, pl* **-mas** *also* **-ma·ta** \-mət-ə\ : an allergic skin disease characterized by patches of circumscribed swelling involving the skin and its subcutaneous layers, the mucous membranes, and sometimes the viscera — called also *angioneurotic edema, giant urticaria, Quincke's disease, Quincke's edema*

an·gio·gen·e·sis \-ˈjen-ə-səs\ *n, pl* **-e·ses** \-ˌsēz\ : the formation and differentiation of blood vessels — **an·gio·gen·ic** \-ˈjen-ik\ *adj*

an·gio·gram \ˈan-jē-ə-ˌgram\ *n* **1** : a radiograph made by angiography **2** : ANGIOGRAPHY

an·gi·og·ra·pher \ˌan-jē-ˈäg-rə-fər\ *n* : a physician or a certified X-ray technician who prepares or interprets angiograms

an·gi·og·ra·phy \-fē\ *n, pl* **-phies** : the radiographic visualization of the blood vessels after injection of a radiopaque substance — **an·gio·graph·ic** \ˌan-jē-ə-ˈgraf-ik\ *adj* — **an·gio·graph·i·cal·ly** \-i-k(ə-)lē\ *adv*

an·gi·oid \ˈan-jē-ˌȯid\ *adj* : resembling a blood vessel or lymphatic

an·gio·ker·a·to·ma \ˌan-jē-ō-ˌker-ə-ˈtō-mə\ *n, pl* **-mas** *also* **-ma·ta** \-mət-ə\ : a skin disease characterized by small warty elevations or telangiectasias and epidermal thickening

an·gi·ol·o·gy \ˌan-jē-ˈäl-ə-jē\ *n, pl* **-gies** : the study of blood vessels and lymphatics

an·gi·o·ma \ˌan-jē-ˈō-mə\ *n, pl* **-mas** *also* **-ma·ta** \-mət-ə\ : a tumor (as a hemangioma or lymphangioma) composed chiefly of blood vessels or lymphatic vessels — **an·gi·o·ma·tous** \-mət-əs\ *adj*

an·gi·o·ma·to·sis \ˌan-jē-ō-ˌmə-ə-ˈtō-səs\ *n, pl* **-to·ses** \-ˌsēz\ : a condition characterized by the formation of multiple angiomas

an·gio·neu·rot·ic edema \-n(y)ù-ˌrät-ik-\ *n* : ANGIOEDEMA

angio—oedema *Brit var of* ANGIOEDEMA

an·gi·op·a·thy \ˌan-jē-ˈäp-ə-thē\ *n, pl* **-thies** : a disease of the blood or lymph vessels

an·gio·plas·ty \ˈan-jē-ə-ˌplas-tē\ *n, pl* **-ties** : surgical repair or recanalization of a blood vessel; *esp* : BALLOON ANGIOPLASTY

an·gio·sar·co·ma \ˌan-jē-ō-sär-ˈkō-mə\ *n, pl* **-mas** *also* **-ma·ta** \-mət-ə\ : a rare malignant vascular tumor (as of the liver or breast)

an·gio·sco·to·ma \-skə-ˈtō-mə\ *n, pl* **-mas** *or* **-ma·ta** \-mət-ə\ : a blind spot or defect in the visual field produced by dilated retinal vessels that is esp. prevalent in persons long exposed to high altitudes

an·gio·sco·tom·e·try \-skō-ˈtäm-ə-trē\ *n, pl* **-tries** : the charting of scotomas and esp. angioscotomas

an·gio·spasm \ˈan-jē-ō-ˌspaz-əm\ *n* : spasmodic contraction of the blood vessels with increase in blood pressure — **an·gio·spas·tic** \ˌan-jē-ō-ˈspas-tik\ *adj*

an·gio·sperm \ˈan-jē-ə-ˌspərm\ *n* : any of a class (Angiospermae) of vascular plants (as orchids or roses) that have the seeds in a closed ovary and include the monocotyledons and dicotyledons — compare GYMNOSPERM — **an·gio·sper·mous** \ˌan-jē-ə-ˈspər-məs\ *adj*

an·gi·os·to·my \ˌan-jē-ˈäs-tə-mē\ *n, pl* **-mies** : the surgical establishment of an opening into a blood vessel esp. through a cannula

an·gio·ten·sin \ˌan-jē-ō-ˈten(t)-sən\ *n* **1** : either of two forms of a kinin of which one has marked physiological activity and the other is its physiologically inactive precursor; *esp* : ANGIOTENSIN II **2** : a synthetic amide derivative of angiotensin II used to treat some forms of hypotension

an·gio·ten·sin·ase \ˌan-jē-ō-ˈten(t)-sə-ˌnās, -ˌnāz\ *n* : any of several enzymes in the blood that hydrolyze angiotensin — called also *hypertensinase*

angiotensin con·vert·ing enzyme \-kən-ˌvərt-iŋ-\ *n* : a proteolytic enzyme that converts angiotensin I to angiotensin II — see ACE INHIBITOR

angiotensin converting enzyme inhibitor *n* : ACE INHIBITOR

an·gio·ten·sin·o·gen \-ten(t)-ˈsin-ə-jən\ *n* : a serum globulin formed by the liver that is cleaved by renin to produce angiotensin I — called also *hypertensinogen*

angiotensin I \-ˈwən\ *n* : the physiologically inactive form of angiotensin that is composed of 10 amino acid residues and is a precursor of angiotensin II

angiotensin II \-ˈtü\ *n* : a protein with vasoconstrictive activity that is composed of eight amino acid residues and is the physiologically active form of angiotensin

an·gio·ton·ic \ˌan-jē-ō-ˈtän-ik\ *adj* : inducing or involving increased tonus in the wall of a blood vessel ⟨an ∼ substance⟩ ⟨∼ spasm⟩

an·gio·to·nin \-ˈtō-nən\ *n* : ANGIOTENSIN

an·gle \ˈaŋ-gəl\ *n* **1** : a corner whether constituting a projecting part or a partially enclosed space **2 a** : the figure formed by two lines extending from the same point **b** : a measure of an angle or of the amount of turning necessary to bring one line or plane into coincidence with or parallel to another — **an·gled** \-gəld\ *adj*

an·gle·ber·ry \ˈaŋ-gəl-ˌber-ē\ *n, pl* **-ries** : a papilloma or warty growth of the skin or mucous membranes of cattle and sometimes horses often occurring in great numbers

angle–closure glaucoma *n* : glaucoma in which the drainage channel for the aqueous humor composed of the attachment at the edge of the iris and the junction of the sclera and cornea is blocked by the iris — called also *closed-angle glaucoma, narrow-angle glaucoma;* compare OPEN-ANGLE GLAUCOMA

angle of depression *n* : the angle formed by the line of sight and the horizontal plane for an object below the horizontal

angle of elevation *n* : the angle formed by the line of sight and the horizontal plane for an object above the horizontal

angle of incidence *n* : the angle that a line (as a ray of light) falling on a surface or interface makes with the normal drawn at the point of incidence

angle of reflection *n* : the angle between a reflected ray and the normal drawn at the point of incidence to a reflecting surface

angle of refraction *n* : the angle between a refracted ray and the normal drawn at the point of incidence to the interface at which refraction occurs

angle of the jaw *n* : GONIAL ANGLE

angle of the mandible *n* : GONIAL ANGLE

\ə\ **abut** \ᵊ\ **kitten** \ər\ **further** \a\ **ash** \ā\ **ace** \ä\ **cot, cart**
\aù\ **out** \ch\ **chin** \e\ **bet** \ē\ **easy** \g\ **go** \i\ **hit** \ī\ **ice** \j\ **job**
\ŋ\ **sing** \ō\ **go** \ȯ\ **law** \ȯi\ **boy** \th\ **thin** \t̲h̲\ **the** \ü\ **loot**
\ù\ **foot** \y\ **yet** \zh\ **vision** *See also* Pronunciation Symbols page

an·gos·tu·ra bark \ˌaŋ-gə-'st(y)ùr-ə-\ *n* : the aromatic bitter bark of either of two So. American trees (*Galipea officinalis* and *Cusparia trifoliata*) of the rue family used esp. formerly as a tonic and antipyretic — called also *angostura*

ang·strom \'aŋ-strəm *also* 'ȯŋ-\ *n* : a unit of length equal to one ten-billionth of a meter

Ångström, Anders Jonas (1814–1874), Swedish astronomer and physicist. One of the early formulators of the science of modern spectroscopy, Ångström wrote extensively on terrestrial magnetism, the conduction of heat, and especially spectroscopy. He published a monumental map of the normal solar spectrum that expressed the length of light waves in units of one ten-millionth of a millimeter, a unit of length now known as the angstrom. He discovered that hydrogen is present in the sun's atmosphere, and he was the first to examine the spectrum of the aurora borealis.

angstrom unit *n* : ANGSTROM

An·guil·lu·la \aŋ-'gwil-yə-lə\ *n, syn of* TURBATRIX

an·gu·lar \'aŋ-gyə-lər\ *adj* **1 a** : having an angle or angles   **b** : forming an angle or corner : sharp-cornered   **2** : measured by an angle ⟨~ distance⟩   **3** : relating to or having a chemical structure in which a component ring or group is attached at an angle and not in a straight line ⟨an ~ methyl group⟩   **4** : relating to or situated near an anatomical angle ⟨the ~ head of the levator labii superioris⟩; *specif* : relating to or situated near the inner angle of the eye — **an·gu·lar·i·ty** \ˌaŋ-gyə-'lar-ə-tē\ *n, pl* **-ties** — **an·gu·lar·ly** *adv*

angular aperture *n* : the angle subtended at the principal focus of an optical system (as a microscope) by the diameter of its entrance for light

angular artery *n* : the terminal part of the facial artery that passes up alongside the nose to the inner angle of the orbit

angular gyrus *n* : the cerebral gyrus of the posterior part of the external surface of the parietal lobe that arches over the posterior end of the sulcus between the superior and middle gyri of the temporal lobe — called also *angular convolution*

angularis — see INCISURA ANGULARIS

angular vein *n* : a vein that comprises the first part of the facial vein and runs obliquely down at the side of the upper part of the nose

an·gu·la·tion \ˌaŋ-gyə-'lā-shən\ *n* **1** : the action of making angular   **2** : an angular position, formation or shape; *esp* : an abnormal bend or curve in an organ — **an·gu·late** \'aŋ-gyə-ˌlāt\ *vb* **-lat·ed; -lat·ing**

anguli — see LEVATOR ANGULI ORIS

an·gu·lus \'aŋ-gyə-ləs\ *n, pl* **an·gu·li** \-ˌlī, -ˌlē\ : an anatomical angle; *also* : an angular part or relationship

an·he·do·nia \ˌan-hē-'dō-nē-ə\ *n* : a psychological condition characterized by inability to experience pleasure in acts which normally produce it — compare ANALGESIA — **an·he·don·ic** \-'dän-ik\ *adj*

an·hi·dro·sis *also* **an·hy·dro·sis** \ˌan-hi-'drō-səs, -hī-\ *or* **an·idro·sis** \ˌan-i-'\ *n, pl* **-dro·ses** \-ˌsēz\ : abnormal deficiency or absence of sweating

¹an·hi·drot·ic *also* **an·hy·drot·ic** *or* **an·idrot·ic** \-'drät-ik\ *adj* : tending to check sweating

²anhidrotic *also* **anhydrotic** *or* **anidrotic** *n* : an anhidrotic agent

anhyd *abbr* anhydrous

an·hy·drase \an-'hī-ˌdrās, -ˌdrāz\ *n* : an enzyme (as carbonic anhydrase) promoting a specific dehydration reaction and the reverse hydration reaction

an·hy·drate \-ˌdrāt\ *vt* **-drat·ed; -drat·ing** : DEHYDRATE; *esp* : to dehydrate quickly in food processing — **an·hy·dra·tion** \ˌan-(ˌ)hī-'drā-shən\ *n*

an·hy·dre·mia *or chiefly Brit* **an·hy·drae·mia** \ˌan-(ˌ)hī-'drē-mē-ə\ *n* : an abnormal reduction of water in the blood — **an·hy·dre·mic** *or chiefly Brit* **an·hy·drae·mic** \-mik\ *adj*

an·hy·dride \(')an-'hī-ˌdrīd\ *n* : a compound derived from another (as an acid) by removal of the elements of water

an·hy·dro·hy·droxy·pro·ges·ter·one \ˌan-ˌhī-drō-ˌhī-ˌdräk-sē-prō-'jes-tə-ˌrōn\ *n* : ETHISTERONE

anhydrosis, anhydrotic *var of* ANHIDROSIS, ANHIDROTIC

an·hy·drous \(')an-'hī-drəs\ *adj* : free from water and esp.

water that is chemically combined in a crystalline substance ⟨~ ammonia⟩

ani *pl of* ANUS

ani — see LEVATOR ANI, PRURITUS ANI, SPHINCTER ANI EXTERNUS, SPHINCTER ANI INTERNUS

an·ic·ter·ic \ˌan-(ˌ)ik-'ter-ik\ *adj* : not accompanied or characterized by jaundice ⟨~ hepatitis⟩

anidrosis, anidrotic *var of* ANHIDROSIS, ANHIDROTIC

anile \'an-ˌīl, 'ā-ˌnīl\ *adj* : SENILE — **anil·i·ty** \a-'nil-ət-ē, ā-, ə-\ *n, pl* **-ties**

an·i·lide \'an-ᵊl-əd, -ˌīd\ *n* : an amide (as acetanilide) in which hydrogen of the amido group is replaced by phenyl : an acyl derivative of aniline

an·i·line \'an-ᵊl-ən\ *n* : an oily liquid poisonous amine $C_6H_5NH_2$ obtained esp. by the reduction of nitrobenzene and used chiefly in organic synthesis (as of dyes and pharmaceuticals) — **aniline** *adj*

aniline blue *n* : one of the soluble blue dyes used as a biological dye

aniline dye *n* : a dye made by the use of aniline or one chemically related to such a dye; *broadly* : a synthetic organic dye

ani·lin·gus \ˌā-ni-'liŋ-gəs\ *or* **ani·linc·tus** \-'liŋ(k)-təs\ *n* : erotic stimulation achieved by contact between mouth and anus

an·i·lin·ism \'an-ᵊl-ə-ˌniz-əm\ *n* : poisoning from fumes inhaled in the manufacture of aniline

an·i·ma \'an-ə-mə\ *n* **1** : an individual's true inner self that in the analytic psychology of C. G. Jung reflects archetypal ideals of conduct; *also* : an inner feminine part of the male personality — compare ANIMUS, PERSONA   **2** *in old pharmacy* **a** : the active ingredient of an animal or vegetable drug   **b** : a dried plant juice or an aqueous extract

¹an·i·mal \'an-ə-məl\ *n* **1** : any of a kingdom (Animalia) of living things including many-celled organisms and often many of the single-celled ones (as protozoans) that typically differ from plants in having cells without cellulose walls, in lacking chlorophyll and the capacity for photosynthesis, in requiring more complex food materials (as proteins), in being organized to a greater degree of complexity, and in having the capacity for spontaneous movement and rapid motor response to stimulation   **2 a** : one of the lower animals as distinguished from human beings   **b** : MAMMAL; *broadly* : VERTEBRATE

²animal *adj* **1** : of, relating to, or derived from animals   **2** : of or relating to the animal pole of an egg or to the part from which ectoderm normally develops

an·i·mal·cule \ˌan-ə-'mal-(ˌ)kyü(ə)l\ *also* **an·i·mal·cu·lum** \-'mal-kyə-ləm\ *n, pl* **-cules** *also* **-cu·la** \-kyə-lə\ : a minute usu. microscopic organism

animal heat *n* : BODY HEAT

animal kingdom *n* : a basic group of natural objects that includes all living and extinct animals — compare MINERAL KINGDOM, PLANT KINGDOM

animal magnetism *n* : a spiritlike force alleged by the Austrian physician Franz Anton Mesmer (1734–1815) to reside within himself and to be active in his use of therapeutic hypnosis — see MESMERISM

animal model *n* : an animal sufficiently like humans in its anatomy, physiology, or response to a pathogen to be used in medical research in order to obtain results that can be extrapolated to human medicine; *also* : a pathological or physiological condition that occurs in such an animal and is similar (as in its pathology or physiology) to a human condition ⟨experimental allergic encephalomyelitis is a useful *animal model* in the study of multiple sclerosis in humans⟩

animal pole *n* : the point on the surface of an egg that is diametrically opposite to the vegetal pole and usu. marks the most active part of the protoplasm or the part containing least yolk

animal protein factor *n* : vitamin B_{12} or a concentrate containing this vitamin and usu. antibiotics that is obtained esp. in the fermentation production of vitamin B_{12} and chlortetracycline and is used as a supplement in some animal and poultry feeds

animal psychology *n* : a branch of psychology concerned with the behavior of animals other than humans

animal starch *n* : GLYCOGEN

an·i·mate \'an-ə-mət\ *adj* **1** : possessing or characterized by life **2** : of or relating to animal life as opposed to plant life

an·i·mat·ed \-ˌmāt-əd\ *adj* **1** : endowed with life or the qualities of life **2** : full of movement and activity

an·i·ma·tion \ˌan-ə-'mā-shən\ *n* : the state of being animate or animated — see SUSPENDED ANIMATION

an·i·mat·ism \'an-ə-mə-ˌtiz-əm\ *n* : attribution of consciousness and personality but not of individual spirit to such natural phenomena as thunderstorms and earthquakes and to such objects as plants and stones — compare ANIMISM — **an·i·ma·tis·tic** \ˌan-ə-mə-'tis-tik\ *adj*

an·i·mism \'an-ə-ˌmiz-əm\ *n* **1** : a doctrine that the vital principle of organic development is immaterial spirit **2** : attribution of conscious life to nature or natural objects — **an·i·mist** \-məst\ *n* — **an·i·mis·tic** \ˌan-ə-'mis-tik\ *adj*

an·i·mus \'an-ə-məs\ *n* : an inner masculine part of the female personality in the analytic psychology of C. G. Jung — compare ANIMA 1

an·ion \'an-ˌī-ən\ *n* : the ion in an electrolyzed solution that migrates to the anode; *broadly* : a negatively charged ion

an·ion·ic \ˌan-(ˌ)ī-'än-ik\ *adj* **1** : of or relating to anions **2** : characterized by an active and esp. surface-active anion — **an·ion·i·cal·ly** \-i-k(ə-)lē\ *adv*

an·ion·ot·ro·py \ˌan-ˌī-ə-'nä-trə-pē\ *n, pl* **-pies** : tautomerism involving migration of an anion (as chloride, hydroxyl, or acetate) of which the best-known type is allylic rearrangement — compare CATIONOTROPY, PROTOTROPY — **an·ion·o·tro·pic** \-nə-'träp-ik, -'trō-pik\ *adj*

an·irid·ia \ˌan-ī-'rid-ē-ə\ *n* : congenital or traumatically induced absence or defect of the iris

an·i·sa·ki·a·sis \ˌan-ə-sə-'kī-ə-sis\ *n* : intestinal infection caused by the larvae of a nematode (family Anisakidae and esp. *Anisakis marina*) and usu. contracted by eating raw fish (as in sushi)

an·ise \'an-əs\ *n* : an herb (*Pimpinella anisum*) of the family Umbelliferae having carminative and aromatic seeds; *also* : ANISEED

ani·seed *also* **an·ise·seed** \'an-ə(s)-ˌsēd\ *n* : the seed of anise often used as a flavoring in liqueurs and in cooking

aniseed oil *n* : ANISE OIL

an·is·ei·ko·nia \ˌan-ˌī-ˌsī-'kō-nē-ə\ *n* : a defect of binocular vision in which the two retinal images of an object differ in size — **an·is·ei·kon·ic** \-'kän-ik\ *adj*

anise oil *n* **1** : a colorless or pale yellow essential oil obtained from the dried fruits of anise and used as a flavoring agent and as a carminative **2** : STAR ANISE OIL

an·iso·co·ria \ˌan-ˌī-sō-'kōr-ē-ə\ *n* : inequality in the size of the pupils of the eyes

an·iso·cy·to·sis \-ˌsī-'tō-səs\ *n, pl* **-to·ses** \-ˌsēz\ : variation in size of cells and esp. of the red blood cells (as in pernicious anemia) — **an·iso·cy·tot·ic** \-'tät-ik\ *adj*

an·isog·a·mous \ˌan-(ˌ)ī-'säg-ə-məs\ *also* **an·iso·gam·ic** \-ˌī-sə-'gam-ik\ *adj* : characterized by fusion of heterogamous gametes or of individuals that usu. differ chiefly in size ⟨~ reproduction⟩ — **an·isog·a·my** \-(ˌ)ī-'säg-ə-mē\ *n, pl* **-mies**

an·iso·me·tro·pia \ˌan-ˌī-sə-mə-'trō-pē-ə\ *n* : unequal refractive power in the two eyes — **an·iso·me·tro·pic** \-'träp-ik, -'trō-pik\ *adj*

an·iso·trop·ic \(ˌ)an-ˌī-sə-'träp-ik\ *adj* : exhibiting properties with different values when measured in different directions : not isotropic ⟨an ~ crystal⟩ — **an·isot·ro·pism** \-ˌī-'sä-trə-ˌpiz-əm\ *n* — **an·isot·ro·py** \-pē\ *n, pl* **-pies**

an·i·so·ylat·ed plasminogen–streptokinase activator complex \ˌan-ə-'sō-i-ˌlāt-əd-\ *n* : ANISTREPLASE

an·i·strep·lase \ˌan-i-'strep-(ˌ)lās, ˌan-(ˌ)ī-; ə-'nis-trə-ˌplās\ *n* : a thrombolytic complex of plasminogen and streptokinase used esp. to treat heart attack and to lyse thrombi in coronary arteries — called also *APSAC*

an·kle \'aŋ-kəl\ *n* **1 a** : the joint between the foot and the leg that constitutes in humans a ginglymus joint between the tibia and fibula above and the talus below — called also *an-*

kle joint **b** : the region of the ankle joint **2** : the joint between the cannon bone and pastern (as in the horse)

an·kle·bone \'aŋ-kəl-ˌbōn\ *n* : TALUS 1

ankle jerk *n* : a reflex downward movement of the foot produced by a spasmodic contraction of the muscles of the calf in response to sudden extension of the leg or the striking of the Achilles' tendon above the heel — called also *Achilles reflex*

ankle joint *n* : ANKLE 1a

an·ky·lose *also* **an·chy·lose** \'aŋ-ki-ˌlōs, -ˌlōz\ *vb* **-losed; -losing** *vt* : to unite or stiffen by ankylosis ⟨a joint *ankylosed* by surgery⟩ ~ *vi* : to undergo ankylosis

ankylosing spondylitis *n* : rheumatoid arthritis of the spine — called also *Marie-Strümpell disease, rheumatoid spondylitis*

an·ky·lo·sis *also* **an·chy·lo·sis** \ˌaŋ-ki-'lō-səs\ *n, pl* **-lo·ses** \-ˌsēz\ : stiffness or fixation of a joint by disease or surgery — **an·ky·lot·ic** *also* **an·chy·lot·ic** \-'lät-ik\ *adj*

An·ky·lo·sto·ma \ˌaŋ-ki-'läs-tə-mə\ *n, syn of* ANCYLOSTOMA

ankylostome, ankylostomiasis *var of* ANCYLOSTOME, ANCYLOSTOMIASIS

an·ky·roid \aŋ-'kī-ˌróid, 'aŋ-kə-\ *also* **an·cy·roid** \an-'sī-', 'an-sə-\ *adj* : shaped like a hook

an·la·ge \'än-ˌläg-ə\ *n, pl* **-gen** \-ən\ *also* **-ges** \-əz\ : the foundation of a subsequent development; *esp* : PRIMORDIUM

an·nat·to \ə-'nät-(ˌ)ō, -'nat-\ *n* : a yellowish red dyestuff made from the pulp around the seeds of a tropical tree (*Bixa orellana* of the family Bixaceae) and used esp. for coloring oils, butter, and cheese

an·neal \ə-'nē(ə)l\ *vt* **1** : to heat and then cool (as steel or glass) usu. for softening and making less brittle **2** : to heat and then cool (double-stranded nucleic acid) in order to separate strands and induce combination at lower temperatures esp. with complementary strands ~ *vi* : to be capable of combining with complementary nucleic acid by a process of heating and cooling ⟨some bacterial nucleic acid ~s well with eukaryotic DNA⟩

an·nec·tant *or chiefly Brit* **an·nec·tent** \ə-'nek-tənt, a-\ *adj* **1** : serving to connect or join **2** : intergrading between populations or taxonomic groups

An·nel·i·da \ə-'nel-ə-də, a-\ *n pl* : a phylum of coelomate and usu. elongated segmented invertebrates (as earthworms, various marine worms, and leeches) — **an·ne·lid** \'an-ᵊl-əd\ *n or adj* — **an·nel·i·dan** \ə-'nel-əd-ən, a-\ *adj or n*

an·nu·lar \'an-yə-lər\ *adj* : of, relating to, or forming a ring ⟨the ~ diaphragm of a microscope⟩

annulare — see GRANULOMA ANNULARE

annular ligament *n* : a ringlike ligament or band of fibrous tissue encircling a part: **a** : any of the transverse bands holding in place the extensor and flexor tendons of the wrist and ankle **b** : a strong band of fibers surrounding the head of the radius and retaining it in the radial notch of the ulna — called also *orbicular ligament* **c** : any of several strengthening bands of the tendon sheaths of the digits **d** : a ring attaching the base of the stapes to the oval window

an·nu·lus \'an-yə-ləs\ *n, pl* **-li** \-ˌlī\ *also* **-lus·es** : a ringlike part, structure, or marking; *esp* : any of various ringlike anatomical parts (as the inguinal ring)

annulus fi·bro·sus \-fī-'brō-səs, -fi-\ *also* **an·u·lus fi·bro·sus** \'an-yə-ləs-\ *n* : a ring of fibrous or fibrocartilaginous tissue (as of an intervertebral disk or surrounding an orifice of the heart)

ano·ci·as·so·ci·a·tion \ə-ˌnō-sē-ə-ˌsō-sē-'ā-shən, a-, -ˌsō-shē-\ *n* : a method of preventing shock and exhaustion incident to surgical operations by preventing communication between the area of operation and the nervous system esp. by means of a local anesthetic or sharp dissection

ano·ci·a·tion \ə-ˌnō-sē-'ā-shən, a-\ *n* : ANOCIASSOCIATION

\ə\ abut \ᵊ\ kitten \ər\ further \a\ ash \ā\ ace \ä\ cot, cart
\aù\ out \ch\ chin \e\ bet \ē\ easy \g\ go \i\ hit \ī\ ice \j\ job
\ŋ\ sing \ō\ go \ò\ law \òi\ boy \th\ thin \th\ the \ü\ loot
\ú\ foot \y\ yet \zh\ vision *See also* Pronunciation Symbols page

an·od·al \a-ˈnōd-ᵊl\ *adj* : of, relating to, or attracted to an anode : ANODIC ⟨∼ potentials⟩ — used esp. in the life sciences — **an·od·al·ly** \-ē\ *adv*

an·ode \ˈan-ˌōd\ *n* **1** : the electrode of an electrochemical cell at which oxidation occurs: as **a** : the positive terminal of an electrolytic cell **b** : the negative terminal of a storage battery that is delivering current **2** : the electron-collecting electrode of an electron tube — compare CATHODE

an·od·ic \a-ˈnäd-ik\ *adj* : of, at, or relating to an anode — **an·od·i·cal·ly** \-i-k(ə-)lē\ *adv*

an·odon·tia \ˌan-ō-ˈdän-ch(ē-)ə\ *n* : an esp. congenital absence of teeth

¹an·o·dyne \ˈan-ə-ˌdīn\ *adj* : serving to ease pain

²anodyne *n* : a drug that allays pain

an·o·dy·nia \ˌan-ə-ˈdin-ē-ə, -ˈdīn-\ *n* : absence of pain

an·o·dy·nous \an-ˈäd-ᵊn-əs, ˌan-ə-ˈdī-nəs\ *adj* : ANODYNE

an·o·e·sis \-ˈwē-səs\ *n, pl* **-e·ses** \-ˌsēz\ : consciousness that is pure passive receptiveness without understanding or intellectual organization of the materials presented — **an·o·et·ic** \-ˈwet-ik\ *adj*

anoestrous, anoestrus *chiefly Brit var of* ANESTROUS, ANESTRUS

ano·gen·i·tal \ˌā-nō-ˈjen-ə-tᵊl\ *adj* : of, relating to, or involving the genital organs and the anus ⟨∼ infections⟩

anom·a·lo·scope \ə-ˈnäm-ə-lə-ˌskōp\ *n* : an optical device designed to test color vision by matching a yellow light which may be varied in intensity with a combination of red and green lights of constant intensity

anom·a·lous \ə-ˈnäm-ə-ləs\ *adj* : deviating from normal ⟨∼ development⟩ ⟨∼ pulmonary venous drainage —*Physicians' Current Procedural Terminology*⟩; *specif* : having abnormal vision with respect to a particular color but not color-blind ⟨she was almost red ∼ —*Nature*⟩

anom·a·ly \ə-ˈnäm-ə-lē\ *n, pl* **-lies** : a deviation from normal esp. of a bodily part ⟨the infants demonstrated congenital *anomalies*⟩ ⟨personality *anomalies*⟩

an·o·mer \ˈan-ə-mər\ *n* : a cyclic stereoisomer of a carbohydrate with isomerism involving only the arrangement of atoms or groups at the aldehyde or ketone position — **an·o·mer·ic** \ˌan-ə-ˈmer-ik\ *adj*

ano·mia \ə-ˈnäm-ē-ə, -ˈnō-mē-\ *n* : ANOMIC APHASIA

ano·mic \ə-ˈnäm-ik, ā-, -ˈnō-mik\ *adj* : relating to or characterized by anomie

anomic aphasia *n* : loss of the power to use or understand words denoting objects

an·o·mie *also* **an·o·my** \ˈan-ə-mē\ *n* : social instability resulting from a breakdown of standards and values; *also* : personal unrest, alienation, and anxiety that comes from a lack of purpose or ideals

an·onych·ia \ˌan-ə-ˈnik-ē-ə\ *n* : congenital absence of the nails

anon·y·ma \ə-ˈnän-ə-mə, a-\ *n, pl* **-mae** \-ˌmē, -ˌmī\ *or* **-mas** : BRACHIOCEPHALIC ARTERY

ano·op·sia \ˌan-ō-ˈäp-sē-ə\ *or* **an·op·sia** \ə-ˈnäp-, a-, -ˈnōp-\ *n* : upward strabismus

anoph·e·les \ə-ˈnäf-ə-ˌlēz\ *n* **1** *cap* : a genus of mosquitoes that includes all mosquitoes that transmit malaria to humans **2** : any mosquito of the genus *Anopheles* — **anopheles** *adj* — **anoph·e·line** \-ˌlīn\ *adj or n*

anoph·e·li·cide \ə-ˈnäf-ə-lə-ˌsīd\ *n* : an agent that destroys anopheles mosquitoes

anoph·e·lism \-ə-ˌliz-əm\ *n* : infestation of a locality with anopheles mosquitoes

an·oph·thal·mia \ˌan-əf-ˈthal-mē-ə, -əp-, -äf-, -äp-\ *n* : congenital absence of the eyes — **an·oph·thal·mic** \-ˈthal-mik\ *adj*

an·oph·thal·mos \-ˈthal-məs\ *n* **1** : ANOPHTHALMIA **2** : an individual born without eyes

an·opia \ə-ˈnō-pē-ə, a-\ *n* : a defect of vision; *esp* : HEMIANOPSIA

ano·plas·ty \ˈā-nə-ˌplas-tē, ˈan-ə-\ *n, pl* **-ties** : plastic surgery on the anus (as for stricture)

An·op·lo·ceph·a·la \ˌan-ə-(ˌ)plō-ˈsef-ə-lə\ *n* : a genus of taenioid tapeworms including some parasites of horses

An·op·lo·ce·phal·i·dae \-se-ˈfal-ə-ˌdē\ *n pl* : a family of taenioid tapeworms with unarmed scolices that live as adults in the intestines of various herbivores and pass their larval stages in some free-living mites — **an·op·lo·ceph·a·lid** \-ˈsef-ə-ləd\ *adj*

An·o·plu·ra \ˌan-ə-ˈplùr-ə\ *n pl* : an order of insects comprising the sucking lice and in some classifications the bird lice

anopsia *var of* ANOOPSIA

an·or·chid·ism \ə-ˈnór-kə-ˌdiz-əm, a-\ *n* : congenital absence of one or both testes

ano·rec·tal \ˌā-nō-ˈrek-tᵊl, ˌan-ə-\ *adj* : of, relating to, or involving both the anus and rectum ⟨∼ surgery⟩

¹an·o·rec·tic \ˌan-ə-ˈrek-tik\ *also* **an·o·ret·ic** \-ˈret-ik\ *adj* **1 a** : lacking appetite **b** : ANOREXIC 2 **2** : causing loss of appetite ⟨∼ drugs⟩

²anorectic *also* **anoretic** *n* **1** : an anorectic agent **2** : ANOREXIC

an·orex·ia \ˌan-ə-ˈrek-sē-ə, -ˈrek-shə\ *n* **1** : loss of appetite esp. when prolonged **2** : ANOREXIA NERVOSA

anorexia ner·vo·sa \-(ˌ)nər-ˈvō-sə, -zə\ *n* : a serious eating disorder primarily of young women in their teens and early twenties that is characterized esp. by a pathological fear of weight gain leading to faulty eating patterns, malnutrition, and usu. excessive weight loss

¹an·orex·i·ant \ˌan-ə-ˈrek-sē-ənt, -ˈrek-shənt\ *n* : a drug that suppresses appetite

²anorexiant *adj* : ANORECTIC 2

¹an·orex·ic \-ˈrek-sik\ *adj* **1** : ANORECTIC 1a, 2 **2** : affected with anorexia nervosa

²anorexic *n* : a person affected with anorexia nervosa

an·orex·i·gen·ic \-ˌrek-sə-ˈjen-ik\ *adj* : ANORECTIC 2

an·or·gan·ic \ˌan-ór-ˈgan-ik\ *adj* : INORGANIC

an·or·gas·mia \ˌā-nór-ˈgaz-mē-ə\ *n* : sexual dysfunction characterized by failure to achieve orgasm — **an·or·gas·mic** \-mik\ *adj*

an·or·tho·pia \ˌan-(ˌ)ór-ˈthō-pē-ə\ *n* : distorted vision in which straight lines appear bent or curved

ano·scope \ˈā-nə-ˌskōp\ *n* : an instrument for facilitating visual examination of the anal canal

ano·sco·py \ā-ˈnäs-kə-pē, ə-\ *n, pl* **-pies** : visual examination of the anal canal with an anoscope — **ano·scop·ic** \ˌā-nə-ˈskäp-ik\ *adj*

an·os·mat·ic \ˌan-(ˌ)äz-ˈmat-ik, ˌan-əz-\ *adj* : lacking the sense of smell

an·os·mia \a-ˈnäz-mē-ə\ *n* : loss or impairment of the sense of smell — **an·os·mic** \-mik\ *adj*

an·os·phre·sia \ˌan-əs-ˈfrē-zh(ē-)ə, ˌan-(ˌ)äs-\ *also* **an·os·phra·sia** \-ˈfrā-\ *n* : ANOSMIA

an·otia \an-ˈō-sh(ē-)ə\ *n* : congenital absence of the ears

ano·vag·i·nal \ˌā-nō-ˈvaj-ən-ᵊl\ *adj* : connecting the anal canal and the vagina ⟨an ∼ fistula⟩

¹an·ovu·lant \a-ˈnäv-yə-lənt, -ˈnōv-\ *adj* : ANOVULATORY 2 ⟨∼ pills⟩

²anovulant *n* : a drug that suppresses ovulation

an·ovu·lar \-lər\ *adj* : not accompanied by ovulation : ANOVULATORY ⟨∼ menstruation⟩

an·ovu·la·tion \ˌan-ˌäv-yə-ˈlā-shən, -ˌōv-\ *n* : failure or absence of ovulation

an·ovu·la·to·ry \(ˈ)an-ˈäv-yə-lə-ˌtōr-ē, -ˈōv-, -ˌtór-\ *adj* **1** : not involving or associated with ovulation ⟨∼ bleeding⟩ **2** : suppressing ovulation ⟨∼ drugs⟩

an·ox·emia *or chiefly Brit* **an·ox·ae·mia** \ˌan-äk-ˈsē-mē-ə\ *n* : a condition of subnormal oxygenation of the arterial blood — **an·ox·emic** *or chiefly Brit* **an·ox·ae·mic** \-mik\ *adj*

an·ox·ia \ə-ˈnäk-sē-ə, a-\ *n* : hypoxia esp. of such severity as to result in permanent damage — **an·ox·ic** \-sik\ *adj*

ANP *abbr* atrial natriuretic peptide

ans *abbr* answer

ANS *abbr* autonomic nervous system

an·sa \ˈan-sə\ *n, pl* **an·sae** \-ˌsē\ : a loop-shaped anatomical structure

ansa cer·vi·ca·lis \-ˌsər-və-ˈkal-əs, -ˈkā-ləs\ *n* : a nerve loop from the upper cervical nerves that accompanies the hypoglossal nerve and innervates the infrahyoid muscles

ansa hy·po·glos·si \-ˌhī-pə-ˈgläs-ˌī, -ˈglòs-, -ˌ(ˌ)ē\ *n* : ANSA CERVICALIS

An·said \ˈan-sed\ *trademark* — used for a preparation of flurbiprofen

ansa sub·cla·via \ˈan-sə-ˌsəb-ˈklā-vē-ə\ *n* : a nerve loop of sympathetic fibers passing around the subclavian artery

anserina — see CUTIS ANSERINA

anserinus — see PES ANSERINUS

an·si·form \ˈan(t)-sə-ˌfò(ə)rm\ *adj* : having a shape like a loop ⟨an ∼ lobule⟩

Ant·a·buse \ˈant-ə-ˌbyüs\ *trademark* — used for a preparation of disulfiram

¹ant·ac·id \(ˈ)ant-ˈas-əd\ *also* **an·ti·ac·id** \ˌant-ē-ˈas-əd, ˌan-ˌtī-\ *adj* : tending to counteract acidity

²antacid *also* **antiacid** *n* : an agent (as an alkali or absorbent) that counteracts or neutralizes acidity

an·tag·o·nism \an-ˈtag-ə-ˌniz-əm\ *n* : opposition in physiological action: **a** : contrariety in the effect of contraction of muscles (as the extensors and flexors of a part) **b** : interaction of two or more substances such that the action of any one of them on living cells or tissues is lessened (as by interference with the uptake or by an opposing physiological reaction) — compare SYNERGISM

an·tag·o·nist \-nəst\ *n* : an agent that acts in physiological opposition ⟨contact between a tooth and its ∼ in the opposing jaw⟩: as **a** : a muscle that contracts with and limits the action of an agonist with which it is paired — called also *antagonistic muscle;* compare AGONIST 1, SYNERGIST 2 **b** : a chemical that acts within the body to reduce the physiological activity of another chemical substance (as an opiate); *esp* : one that opposes the action on the nervous system of a drug or a substance occurring naturally in the body by combining with and blocking its nervous receptor — compare AGONIST 2

an·tag·o·nis·tic \(ˌ)an-ˌtag-ə-ˈnis-tik\ *adj* **1** : characterized by or resulting from antagonism ⟨∼ antibiotics⟩ **2** : relating to or being muscles that are antagonists ⟨skeletal muscles arranged in ∼ pairs⟩ — **an·tag·o·nis·ti·cal·ly** \-ti-k(ə-)lē\ *adv*

antagonistic muscle *n* : ANTAGONIST a

an·tag·o·nize *also Brit* **an·tag·o·nise** \an-ˈtag-ə-ˌnīz\ *vt* **-nized** *also Brit* **-nised; -niz·ing** *also Brit* **-nis·ing** : to act in antagonism to : COUNTERACT ⟨these effects are *antagonized* by atropine —Ernest Bueding & Harry Most⟩

an·te·bra·chi·al \ˌant-i-ˈbrā-kē-əl\ *or* **an·ti·bra·chi·al** \ˌant-ē-, ˌan-ˌti-\ *adj* : relating to the antebrachium

an·te·bra·chi·um *or* **an·ti·bra·chi·um** \-ˈbrā-kē-əm\ *n, pl* **-chia** \-kē-ə\ : the part of the arm or forelimb between the brachium and the carpus : FOREARM

antecardium *var of* ANTICARDIUM

an·te·cor·nu \ˈant-i-ˌkòr-(ˌ)n(y)ü\ *n, pl* **-nua** \-n(y)ə-wə\ : the anterior cornu of either lateral ventricle of the brain

an·te·cu·bi·tal \ˌant-i-ˈkyü-bət-ᵊl\ *adj* : of or relating to the inner or front surface of the forearm ⟨the ∼ area⟩

antecubital fossa *n* : a triangular cavity of the elbow that contains a tendon of the biceps, the median nerve, and the brachial artery

an·te·flex·ion \ˌant-i-ˈflek-shən\ *n* : a displacement forward of an organ (as the uterus) so that its axis is bent upon itself

an·te·grade \ˈant-i-ˌgrād\ *adj* : ANTEROGRADE 2

an·te·mor·tem \-ˈmòrt-əm\ *adj* : preceding death

an·te·na·tal \-ˈnāt-ᵊl\ *adj* **1** : PRENATAL ⟨∼ diagnosis of birth defects⟩ **2** *Brit* : concerned with the care and treatment of the unborn child and of pregnant women ⟨∼ clinics⟩ — **an·te·na·tal·ly** \-ē\ *adv*

an·te·par·tum \-ˈpärt-əm\ *adj* : relating to the period before parturition : before childbirth ⟨∼ infection⟩ ⟨∼ care⟩

an·te·ri·or \an-ˈtir-ē-ər\ *adj* **1** : relating to or situated near or toward the head or toward the part in headless animals most nearly corresponding to the head **2** : situated toward the front of the body : VENTRAL — used in human anatomy because of the upright posture of humans — **an·te·ri·or·ly** *adv*

anterior cerebral artery *n* : CEREBRAL ARTERY a

anterior chamber *n* : a space in the eye bounded in front by the cornea and in back by the iris and middle part of the lens — compare POSTERIOR CHAMBER

anterior choroid artery *or* **anterior choroidal artery** *n* : CHOROID ARTERY

anterior column *n* : VENTRAL HORN

anterior commissure *n* : a band of nerve fibers crossing from one side of the brain to the other just anterior to the third ventricle

anterior communicating artery *n* : COMMUNICATING ARTERY a

anterior corticospinal tract *n* : VENTRAL CORTICOSPINAL TRACT

anterior cranial fossa *n* : CRANIAL FOSSA c

anterior cruciate ligament *n* : a cruciate ligament of each knee that is attached in front to the more medial aspect of the tibia, that passes upward, backward, and laterally through the middle of the knee crossing the posterior cruciate ligament to attach to the femur, that functions to prevent hyperextension of the knee and to keep the tibia from sliding forward in relation to the femur, and that is subject to sports injury esp. by tearing — called also *ACL*

anterior crural nerve *n* : FEMORAL NERVE

anterior facial vein *n* : FACIAL VEIN

anterior fontanel *or* **anterior fontanelle** *n* : the fontanel occurring at the meeting point of the coronal and sagittal sutures

anterior fossa *n* : CRANIAL FOSSA c

anterior funiculus *n* : a longitudinal division on each side of the spinal cord comprising white matter between the anterior median fissure and the ventral root — called also *ventral funiculus;* compare LATERAL FUNICULUS, POSTERIOR FUNICULUS

anterior gray column *n* : VENTRAL HORN

anterior horn *n* **1** : VENTRAL HORN **2** : the cornu of the lateral ventricle of each cerebral hemisphere that curves outward and forward into the frontal lobe — compare INFERIOR HORN, POSTERIOR HORN 2

anterior humeral circumflex artery *n* : an artery that branches from the axillary artery in the shoulder, curves around the front of the humerus, is distributed or gives off branches distributed esp. to the shoulder joint, head of the humerus, biceps brachii, and deltoid muscle, and anastomoses with the posterior humeral circumflex artery — compare POSTERIOR HUMERAL CIRCUMFLEX ARTERY

anterior inferior cerebellar artery *n* : an artery that arises from the basilar artery either alone or by a common trunk with the internal auditory artery, divides into branches distributed to the anterior parts of the inferior surface of the cerebellum, and gives off a branch that anastomoses with the posterior inferior cerebellar artery

anterior inferior iliac spine *n* : a projection on the anterior margin of the ilium that is situated below the anterior superior iliac spine and is separated from it by a notch — called also *anterior inferior spine*

anterior intercostal artery *n* : INTERCOSTAL ARTERY a

an·te·ri·or·i·ty \(ˌ)an-ˌtir-ē-ˈòr-ət-ē\ *n, pl* **-ties** : the quality or state of being anterior

anterior jugular vein *n* : JUGULAR VEIN c

anterior lingual gland *n* : either of two mucus-secreting glands of the tip of the tongue of which one is located on each side of the frenulum on the underside of the tongue

anterior lobe *n* : ADENOHYPOPHYSIS

anterior median fissure *n* : a groove along the anterior midline of the spinal cord that incompletely divides it into symmetrical halves — called also *ventral median fissure*

anterior nasal spine *n* : the nasal spine that is formed by the union of processes of the two premaxillae and projects upward between the anterior nares

---

\ə\ **abut** \ᵊ\ **kitten** \ər\ **further** \a\ **ash** \ā\ **ace** \ä\ **cot, cart** \aù\ **out** \ch\ **chin** \e\ **bet** \ē\ **easy** \g\ **go** \i\ **hit** \ī\ **ice** \j\ **job** \ŋ\ **sing** \ō\ **go** \ò\ **law** \òi\ **boy** \th\ **thin** \t͟h\ **the** \ü\ **loot** \ù\ **foot** \y\ **yet** \zh\ **vision** *See also* Pronunciation Symbols page

anterior pillar of the fauces *n* : PALATOGLOSSAL ARCH
anterior root *n* : VENTRAL ROOT
anterior sacrococcygeal muscle *n* : SACROCOCCYGEUS VENTRALIS
anterior scalene *n* : SCALENUS a
anterior spinal artery *n* : SPINAL ARTERY a
anterior spinocerebellar tract *n* : SPINOCEREBELLAR TRACT b
anterior spinothalamic tract *n* : SPINOTHALAMIC TRACT a
anterior superior iliac spine *n* : a projection at the anterior end of the iliac crest — called also *anterior superior spine*
anterior synechia *n* : SYNECHIA a
anterior temporal artery *n* : TEMPORAL ARTERY 3a
anterior tibial artery *n* : TIBIAL ARTERY b
anterior tibial nerve *n* : DEEP PERONEAL NERVE
anterior tibial vein *n* : TIBIAL VEIN b
anterior triangle *n* : a triangular region that is a landmark in the neck, has its apex at the sternum pointing downward, and is bounded in front by the anterior midline of the neck, behind by the anterior margin of the sternocleidomastoid muscle, and above by the inferior margin of the lower jaw — compare POSTERIOR TRIANGLE
anterior ulnar recurrent artery *n* : ULNAR RECURRENT ARTERY a
an·tero·grade \'ant-ə-(ˌ)rō-ˌgrād\ *adj* **1** : effective for a period immediately following a shock or seizure; *specif* : effective for and in effect during the period from the time of seizure to the present ⟨prolonged retrograde and ∼ amnesia —*Jour. Amer. Med. Assoc.*⟩ **2** : occurring or performed in the normal or forward direction of conduction or flow: as **a** : occurring along nerve cell processes away from the cell body ⟨∼ axonal transport⟩ **b** : occurring in the normal direction or path of blood circulation ⟨restoration of ∼ flow in an occluded coronary artery⟩ — compare RETROGRADE 3
an·tero·in·fe·ri·or \ˌant-ə-(ˌ)rō-in-'fir-ē-ər\ *adj* : located in front and below ⟨the patella is at the ∼ aspect of the femur —L. L. Langley⟩ — **an·tero·in·fe·ri·or·ly** *adv*
an·tero·lat·er·al \-'lat-ə-rəl, -'la-trəl\ *adj* : situated or occurring in front and to the side — **an·tero·lat·er·al·ly** \-ē\ *adv*
an·tero·me·di·al \-'mēd-ē-əl\ *adj* : located in front and toward the middle
an·tero·pos·te·ri·or \-pō-'stir-ē-ər, -pä-\ *adj* : concerned with or extending along a direction or axis from front to back or from anterior to posterior — **an·tero·pos·te·ri·or·ly** *adv*
an·tero·su·pe·ri·or \-sù-'pir-ē-ər\ *adj* : located in front and above — **an·tero·su·pe·ri·or·ly** *adv*
an·te·ver·sion \ˌant-i-'vər-zhən, -shən\ *n* : a condition of being anteverted — used esp. of the uterus
an·te·vert \'ant-i-ˌvərt, ˌant-i-'\ *vt* : to displace (a body organ) so that the whole axis is directed farther forward than normal
anthelix *var of* ANTIHELIX
¹an·thel·min·tic \ˌant-ˌhel-'min-tik, ˌan-ˌthel-\ *also* **an·thel·min·thic** \-'min-thik\ *adj* : expelling or destroying parasitic worms (as tapeworms) of the intestine
²anthelmintic *also* **anthelminthic** *n* : an anthelmintic drug
an·tho·cy·a·nin \ˌan(t)-thə-'sī-ə-nən\ *also* **an·tho·cy·an** \-'sī-ən, -ˌan\ *n* : any of various soluble glycoside pigments producing blue to red coloring in flowers and plants
an·thra·cene \'an(t)-thrə-ˌsēn\ *n* : a crystalline cyclic hydrocarbon $C_{14}H_{10}$ obtained from coal-tar distillation
an·thra·coid \'an(t)-thrə-ˌkòid\ *adj* : resembling anthrax
an·thra·co·sil·i·co·sis \ˌan(t)-thrə-(ˌ)kō-ˌsil-ə-'kō-səs\ *also* **an·thra·sil·i·co·sis** \ˌan(t)-thrə-\ *n, pl* **-co·ses** \-ˌsēz\ : massive fibrosis of the lungs resulting from inhalation of carbon and quartz dusts and marked by shortness of breath
an·thra·co·sis \ˌan(t)-thrə-'kō-səs\ *n, pl* **-co·ses** \-ˌsēz\ : a benign deposition of coal dust within the lungs from inhalation of sooty air — **an·thra·cot·ic** \-'kät-ik\ *adj*
an·thra·cy·cline \ˌan(t)-thrə-'sī-ˌklēn\ *n* : any of a class of antineoplastic drugs (as doxorubicin) derived from an actinomycete of the genus *Streptomyces* (esp. *S. peucetius*)

an·thra·lin \'an(t)-thrə-lən\ *n* : a yellowish brown crystalline compound $C_{14}H_{10}O_3$ used in the treatment of skin diseases (as psoriasis) — called also *dithranol*
an·thra·ni·late \an-'thran-ᵊl-ˌāt, ˌan(t)-thrə-'nil-ˌāt\ *n* : a salt or ester of anthranilic acid
an·thra·nil·ic acid \ˌan(t)-thrə-ˌnil-ik-\ *n* : the ortho-substituted aminobenzoic acid $NH_2C_6H_4COOH$ used as an intermediate in the manufacture of dyes (as indigo), pharmaceuticals, and perfumes
an·thra·qui·none \ˌan(t)-thrə-kwin-'ōn, -'kwin-ˌōn\ *n* : a yellow crystalline ketone $C_{14}H_8O_2$ often derived from anthracene and used esp. in the manufacture of dyes
anthrasilicosis *var of* ANTHRACOSILICOSIS
an·thrax \'an-ˌthraks\ *n, pl* **-thra·ces** \-thrə-ˌsēz\ : an infectious disease of warm-blooded animals (as cattle and sheep) caused by a spore-forming bacterium (*Bacillus anthracis*), transmissible to humans esp. by the handling of infected products (as hair), and characterized by external ulcerating nodules or by lesions in the lungs
an·throne \'an-ˌthrōn, an-'\ *n* : a pale yellow alkali-insoluble crystalline ketone $C_{14}H_{10}O$ used in sulfuric-acid solution as a colorimetric reagent for determination of carbohydrates (as sugar in body fluids)
an·thro·po·gen·e·sis \ˌan(t)-thrə-pə-'jen-ə-səs\ *n, pl* **-e·ses** \-ˌsēz\ : the origin and development of humans — **an·thro·po·ge·net·ic** \-(ˌ)pō-jə-'net-ik\ *adj*
an·thro·po·gen·ic \-pə-'jen-ik\ *adj* : of, relating to, or resulting from the influence of human beings on nature ⟨∼ sources of pollution⟩
an·thro·pog·o·ny \ˌan(t)-thrə-'päg-ə-nē\ *n, pl* **-nies** : ANTHROPOGENESIS
an·thro·pog·ra·phy \-'päg-rə-fē\ *n, pl* **-phies** : a branch of anthropology dealing with the distribution of humans as distinguished by physical character, language, institutions, and customs
¹an·thro·poid \'an(t)-thrə-ˌpòid\ *adj* **1** : resembling humans — used esp. of apes of the family Pongidae **2** *of the pelvis* : having a relatively great anteroposterior dimension — compare ANDROID, GYNECOID, PLATYPELLOID
²anthropoid *n* : APE 2
anthropoid ape *n* : APE 2
An·thro·poi·dea \ˌan(t)-thrə-'pòid-ē-ə\ *n pl* : the suborder of Primates including the monkeys, apes, and humans — **an·thro·poi·de·an** *adj*
an·thro·pol·o·gy \ˌan(t)-thrə-'päl-ə-jē\ *n, pl* **-gies** : the science of humans; *esp* : the study of humans in relation to distribution, origin, classification, and relationship of races, physical character, environmental and social relations, and culture — **an·thro·po·log·i·cal** \-pə-'läj-i-kəl\ *adj* — **an·thro·po·log·i·cal·ly** \-i-k(ə-)lē\ *adv* — **an·thro·pol·o·gist** \ˌan(t)-thrə-'päl-ə-jəst\ *n*
an·thro·pom·e·ter \ˌan(t)-thrə-'päm-ət-ər\ *n* : an instrument used for making anthropometric measurements and consisting of four hollow graduated tubes that fit into one another to form a rigid rod
an·thro·pom·e·try \-'päm-ə-trē\ *n, pl* **-tries** : the study of human body measurements esp. on a comparative basis — **an·thro·po·met·ric** \-pə-'me-trik\ *adj*
an·thro·po·mor·phism \ˌan(t)-thrə-pə-'mòr-ˌfiz-əm\ *n* : an interpretation of what is not human or personal in terms of human or personal characteristics — compare THERIOMORPHISM — **an·thro·po·mor·phic** \-fik\ *adj* — **an·thro·po·mor·phi·cal·ly** \-i-k(ə-)lē\ *adv*
an·thro·poph·a·gous \ˌan(t)-thrə-'päf-ə-gəs\ *adj* : feeding on human flesh
an·thro·poph·a·gy \-ə-jē\ *n, pl* **-gies** : CANNIBALISM 1
an·thro·po·phil·ic \ˌan(t)-thrə-(ˌ)pō-'fil-ik\ *also* **an·thro·poph·i·lous** \-'päf-ə-ləs\ *adj* : attracted to humans esp. as a source of food ⟨∼ mosquitoes⟩; *also* : indicating relative attraction to humans ⟨∼ indices of certain forest insects⟩
an·thro·po·pho·bia \-(ˌ)pō-'fō-bē-ə\ *n* : a pathological fear of people or human companionship
an·ti·abor·tion \ˌant-ē-ə-'bòr-shən, ˌan-ˌtī-\ *adj* : opposed to abortion and esp. to the legalization of abortion ⟨an ∼ bill⟩

an·ti·abor·tion·ist \-sh(ə-)nəst\ *n* : a person who is opposed to abortion and esp. to the legalization of abortion — called also *prolifer, right-to-lifer*

antiacid *var of* ANTACID

an·ti–ac·ne \-'ak-nē\ *adj* : alleviating the symptoms of acne ⟨an ∼ ointment⟩

an·ti·ag·gres·sin \ant-ē-ə-'gres-ən, an-ti-\ *n* : an antibody that acts against an aggressin

an·ti·ag·gres·sion \-ə-'gresh-ən\ *adj* : tending to prevent aggressive behavior ⟨∼ drugs⟩

an·ti·ag·ing \-'āj-iŋ\ *adj* : used or tending to prevent or lessen the effects of aging ⟨∼ skin creams⟩

an·ti–AIDS \-'ādz\ *adj* : used to treat or delay the development of AIDS ⟨the ∼ drug AZT⟩

¹**an·ti·al·ler·gic** \-ə-'lər-jik\ *also* **an·ti·al·ler·gen·ic** \-,al-ər-'jen-ik\ *adj* : tending to relieve or control allergic symptoms

²**antiallergic** *also* **antiallergenic** *n* : an antiallergic agent

an·ti·an·a·phy·lax·is \-,an-ə-fə-'lak-səs\ *n, pl* **-lax·es** \-,sēz\ **1** : a condition in which an anaphylactic reaction is not obtained because of the presence of free antibodies in the blood **2** : the state of desensitization to an antigen

an·ti·an·dro·gen \-'an-drə-jən\ *n* : a substance that tends to inhibit the production, activity, or effects of a male sex hormone — **an·ti·an·dro·gen·ic** \-,an-drə-'jen-ik\ *adj*

an·ti·ane·mic *or chiefly Brit* **an·ti·anae·mic** \-ə-'nē-mik\ *adj* : effective in or relating to the prevention or correction of anemia

antianemic factor *n* : a substance having antianemic activity; *esp* : VITAMIN B₁₂ — called also *antianemic principle*

an·ti·an·gi·nal \-an-'jīn-ᵊl, -'an-jən-ᵊl\ *adj* : used or tending to prevent or relieve angina pectoris ⟨∼ drugs⟩

an·ti·an·gio·gen·e·sis \-,an-jē-ō-'jen-ə-səs\ *n, pl* **-e·ses** \-,sēz\ : the prevention or inhibition of angiogenesis — **an·ti·an·gio·gen·ic** \-'jen-ik\ *adj*

an·ti·an·ti·body \ant-ē-'ant-i-,bäd-ē, ,an-,tī-\ *n, pl* **-bod·ies** : an antibody with specific immunologic activity against another antibody

an·ti·anx·i·ety \-(,)aŋ-'zī-ət-ē\ *adj* : tending to prevent or relieve anxiety ⟨∼ drugs⟩

¹**an·ti·ar·rhyth·mic** \-(,)ā-'rith-mik\ *adj* : counteracting or preventing cardiac arrhythmia ⟨an ∼ agent⟩

²**antiarrhythmic** *n* : an antiarrhythmic agent

¹**an·ti·ar·thrit·ic** \-är-'thrit-ik\ *or* **an·ti·ar·thri·tis** \-'thrīt-əs\ *adj* : tending to relieve or prevent arthritic symptoms

²**antiarthritic** *n* : an antiarthritic agent

an·ti–asth·ma \-'az-mə\ *or* **an·ti·asth·mat·ic** \-az-'mat-ik, *Brit* -as-\ *adj* : used to relieve the symptoms of asthma ⟨∼ drugs⟩

antiasthmatic *n* : an anti-asthma drug

¹**an·ti·bac·te·ri·al** \ant-i-bak-'tir-ē-əl, ,an-,tī-\ *adj* : directed or effective against bacteria

²**antibacterial** *n* : an antibacterial agent

an·ti·bi·o·sis \ant-i-bī-'ät-ik, ,an-,tī-; ,ant-i-bē-\ *n, pl* **-o·ses** \-,sēz\ : antagonistic association between organisms to the detriment of one of them or between one organism and a metabolic product of another

¹**an·ti·bi·ot·ic** \-bī-'ät-ik, -bē-\ *adj* **1** : tending to prevent, inhibit, or destroy life **2** : of or relating to antibiotics or to antibiosis — **an·ti·bi·ot·i·cal·ly** \-i-k(ə-)lē\ *adv*

²**antibiotic** *n* : a substance produced by or a semisynthetic substance derived from a microorganism and able in dilute solution to inhibit or kill another microorganism

an·ti·body \'ant-i-,bäd-ē\ *n, pl* **-bod·ies** : any of a large number of proteins of high molecular weight that are produced normally by specialized B cells after stimulation by an antigen and act specifically against the antigen in an immune response, that are produced abnormally by some cancer cells, and that typically consist of four subunits including two heavy chains and two light chains — called also *immunoglobulin*

antibrachial, antibrachium *var of* ANTEBRACHIAL, ANTEBRACHIUM

an·ti·can·cer \ant-i-'kan(t)-sər, ,an-,tī-\ *adj* : used or effective against cancer ⟨∼ drugs⟩ ⟨∼ activity⟩

an·ti·car·cin·o·gen \-kär-'sin-ə-jən, -'kärs-ᵊn-ə-,jen\ *n* : an anticarcinogenic agent

¹**an·ti·car·ci·no·gen·ic** \-,kärs-ᵊn-ō-'jen-ik\ *adj* : tending to inhibit or prevent the activity of a carcinogen or the development of carcinoma ⟨an ∼ substance⟩

²**anticarcinogenic** *n* : ANTICARCINOGEN

an·ti·car·dio·lip·in antibody \-,kärd-ē-ō-'lip-ən-\ *n* : an antibody that is directed against phospholipids and esp. cardiolipin and is associated with increased risk for recurring arterial and venous thromboses — called also *anticardiolipin*

an·ti·car·di·um \-'kär-dē-əm\ *or* **an·te·car·di·um** \,ant-i-\ *n, pl* **-dia** \-dē-ə\ : the pit of the stomach : EPIGASTRIUM

an·ti·car·ies \,ant-i-'ka(ə)r-ēz, ,an-,tī-, -'ke(ə)r-\ *adj* : tending to inhibit the formation of caries ⟨∼ effects⟩

an·ti·car·io·gen·ic \-,kar-ē-ō-'jen-ik, -,ker-\ *adj* : ANTICARIES

an·ti·cat·a·lyst \-'kat-ᵊl-əst\ *n* **1** : NEGATIVE CATALYST **2** : a catalytic poison

an·ti·ca·thex·is \-kə-'thek-səs, -ka-\ *n, pl* **-thex·es** \-,sēz\ : the transfer of mental or emotional energy from an impulse to one of an opposite kind ⟨fear of suffocation may be expressed by way of ∼ in the words "free to breathe"⟩

an·ti·cath·ode \-'kath-,ōd\ *n* : TARGET 2a

an·ti·choice \-'chȯis\ *adj* : ANTIABORTION — **an·ti·choic·er** \-ər\ *n*

an·ti·cho·les·ter·ol \-kə-'les-tə-,rȯl, -,rōl\ *adj* : tending to reduce the level of cholesterol in the blood ⟨∼ drugs⟩

¹**an·ti·cho·lin·er·gic** \-,kō-lə-'nər-jik\ *adj* : opposing or blocking the physiological action of acetylcholine

²**anticholinergic** *n* : a drug having an anticholinergic action

an·ti·cho·lin·es·ter·ase \-'nes-tə-,rās, -,rāz\ *n* : any substance (as neostigmine) that inhibits a cholinesterase by combination with it

an·tic·i·pate \an-'tis-ə-,pāt\ *vb* **-pat·ed; -pat·ing** *vt* : to give advance thought to ∼ *vi* : to come before the expected time — used esp. of medical symptoms

an·tic·i·pa·tion \(,)an-,tis-ə-'pā-shən\ *n* **1** : occurrence (as of a disease or symptom) before the normal or expected time **2** : mental attitude that influences a later response

an·ti·clot·ting \,ant-i-'klät-iŋ, ,an-,tī-\ *adj* : inhibiting the clotting of blood ⟨∼ factors⟩

an·tic·ne·mi·on \,an-tik-'nē-mē-,än, -ən\ *n* : the front of the leg : SHIN

¹**an·ti·co·ag·u·lant** \,ant-i-kō-'ag-yə-lənt, ,an-,tī-\ *adj* : of, relating to, or utilizing anticoagulants ⟨∼ therapy⟩

²**anticoagulant** *n* : a substance (as a drug) that hinders coagulation and esp. coagulation of the blood : BLOOD THINNER

an·ti·co·ag·u·la·tion \-kō-,ag-yə-'lā-shən\ *n* : the process of hindering the clotting of blood esp. by treatment with an anticoagulant — **an·ti·co·ag·u·late** \-kō-'ag-yə-,lāt\ *vt* **-lat·ed; -lat·ing** — **an·ti·co·ag·u·la·to·ry** \-yə-lə-,tōr-ē\ *adj*

an·ti·co·ag·u·la·tive \-'ag-yə-,lāt-iv\ *adj* : ANTICOAGULANT ⟨∼ activity⟩

an·ti·co·ag·u·lin \-yə-lən\ *n* : a substance (as one in the saliva of blood-sucking insects or in snake venom) that retards clotting of vertebrate blood

an·ti·co·don \,ant-i-'kō-,dän\ *n* : a triplet of nucleotide bases in transfer RNA that identifies the amino acid carried and binds to a complementary codon in messenger RNA during protein synthesis at a ribosome

an·ti·com·ple·ment \-'käm-plə-mənt\ *n* : a substance that interferes with the activity of complement

an·ti·com·ple·men·ta·ry \-,käm-plə-'ment-ə-rē, -'men-trē\ *adj* : having the capacity to remove or inactivate complement nonspecifically ⟨the ∼ protein in cobra venom⟩

¹**an·ti·con·vul·sant** \-kən-'vəl-sənt\ *also* **an·ti·con·vul·sive** \-siv\ *n* : an anticonvulsant drug

²**anticonvulsant** *also* **anticonvulsive** *adj* : used or tending to control or prevent convulsions (as in epilepsy)

\ə\ **abut** \ᵊ\ **kitten** \ər\ **further** \a\ **ash** \ā\ **ace** \ä\ **cot, cart** \au̇\ **out** \ch\ **chin** \e\ **bet** \ē\ **easy** \g\ **go** \i\ **hit** \ī\ **ice** \j\ **job** \ŋ\ **sing** \ō\ **go** \ȯ\ **law** \ȯi\ **boy** \th\ **thin** \th̲\ **the** \ü\ **loot** \u̇\ **foot** \y\ **yet** \zh\ **vision** *See also* Pronunciation Symbols page

an·ti·cus \an-'tī-kəs\ *adj* : ANTERIOR

anticus — see BRACHIALIS ANTICUS, SCALENUS ANTICUS, SCALENUS ANTICUS SYNDROME, TIBIALIS ANTICUS

an·ti·dan·druff \-'dan-drəf\ *adj* : tending to remove or prevent dandruff ⟨an ∼ shampoo⟩

¹**an·ti·de·pres·sant** \ant-i-di-'pres-ᵊnt, ˌan-ˌtī-\ *also* **an·ti·de·pres·sive** \-'pres-iv\ *adj* : used or tending to relieve or prevent psychic depression

²**antidepressant** *also* **antidepressive** *n* : an antidepressant drug — called also *energizer, psychic energizer, psychostimulant;* compare TRICYCLIC ANTIDEPRESSANT

¹**an·ti·di·a·bet·ic** \-ˌdī-ə-'bet-ik\ *n* : an antidiabetic drug

²**antidiabetic** *adj* : tending to relieve diabetes ⟨∼ drugs⟩

¹**an·ti·di·ar·rhe·al** *or chiefly Brit* **an·ti·di·ar·rhoe·al** \-ˌdī-ə-'rē-əl\ *adj* : tending to prevent or relieve diarrhea

²**antidiarrheal** *or chiefly Brit* **antidiarrhoeal** *n* : an antidiarrheal agent

an·ti·di·ure·sis \-ˌdī-(y)ə-'rē-səs\ *n, pl* **-ure·ses** \-ˌsēz\ : reduction in or suppression of the excretion of urine

¹**an·ti·di·uret·ic** \-'ret-ik\ *adj* : tending to oppose or check excretion of urine

²**antidiuretic** *n* : an antidiuretic substance

antidiuretic hormone *n* : VASOPRESSIN

an·ti·dot·al \ant-i-'dōt-ᵊl\ *adj* : of, relating to, or acting as an antidote — **an·ti·dot·al·ly** \-ᵊl-ē\ *adv*

an·ti·dote \'ant-i-ˌdōt\ *n* : a remedy that counteracts the effects of poison

an·ti·dro·mic \ant-i-'dräm-ik, -'drōm-\ *adj* **1** : proceeding or conducting in a direction opposite to the usual one — used esp. of a nerve impulse or fiber ⟨∼ action potentials⟩ **2** : characterized by antidromic conduction ⟨∼ tachycardia in which impulses travel from the ventricle to the atrium via the atrioventricular node⟩ — **an·ti·dro·mi·cal·ly** \-i-k(ə-)lē\ *adv*

an·ti·drug \ˌan-ˌtī-'drəg, ˌant-i\ *adj* **1** : counteracting the effect of a drug **2** : acting against or opposing illicit drugs or their use ⟨∼ activist⟩ ⟨∼ program⟩

¹**an·ti·dys·en·ter·ic** \ant-i-ˌdis-ᵊn-'ter-ik, ˌan-ˌtī-\ *adj* : tending to relieve or prevent dysentery

²**antidysenteric** *n* : an antidysenteric agent

¹**an·ti·emet·ic** \ant-ē-ə-'met-ik, ˌan-ˌtī-\ *adj* : used or tending to prevent or check vomiting ⟨∼ drugs⟩

²**antiemetic** *n* : an antiemetic agent

an·ti·en·zyme \-'en-ˌzīm\ *n* : an inhibitor of enzyme action; *esp* : one produced by living cells

¹**an·ti·ep·i·lep·tic** \-ˌep-ə-'lep-tik\ *adj* : tending to suppress or prevent epilepsy ⟨∼ treatment⟩

²**antiepileptic** *n* : an antiepileptic drug

an·ti·es·tro·gen *or chiefly Brit* **an·ti·oes·tro·gen** \-'es-trə-jən, *Brit* -'ēs-\ *n* : a substance that inhibits the physiological action of an estrogen — **an·ti·es·tro·gen·ic** *or chiefly Brit* **an·ti·oes·tro·gen·ic** \-ˌes-trə-'jen-ik, *Brit* -ˌēs-\ *adj*

an·ti·fer·til·i·ty \ant-i-(ˌ)fər-'til-ət-ē, ˌan-ˌtī-\ *adj* : having the capacity or tending to reduce or destroy fertility : CONTRACEPTIVE ⟨∼ agents⟩ ⟨∼ properties of a new drug⟩

an·ti·fi·bril·la·to·ry \-'fib-rə-lə-ˌtōr-ē, -'fīb-, -ˌtȯr-\ *adj* : tending to suppress or prevent cardiac fibrillation

an·ti·fi·bri·no·ly·sin \-ˌfī-brən-ᵊl-'īs-ᵊn\ *n* : an antibody that acts specifically against fibrinolysins of hemolytic streptococci and that is used chiefly in some diagnostic tests — called also *antistreptokinase*

an·ti·fi·bri·no·ly·sis \-'ī-səs\ *n, pl* **-ly·ses** \-ˌsēz\ : the action of an antifibrinolysin in opposing streptococcal fibrinolysis — **an·ti·fi·bri·no·lyt·ic** \-'lit-ik\ *adj*

¹**an·ti·flat·u·lent** \-'flach-ə-lənt\ *adj* : preventing or relieving flatulence

²**antiflatulent** *n* : an antiflatulent agent

an·ti·flu \-'flü\ *adj* : used to prevent infection by the orthomyxoviruses causing influenza ⟨an ∼ drug⟩

an·ti·flu·o·ri·da·tion·ist \-ˌflur-ə-'dāsh-(ə-)nəst\ *n* : a person who is vigorously opposed to the fluoridation of public water supplies

¹**an·ti·fun·gal** \ˌant-i-'fəŋ-gəl, ˌan-ˌtī-\ *adj* : destroying fungi or inhibiting their growth : FUNGICIDAL, FUNGISTATIC ⟨∼ drugs⟩ ⟨∼ activity⟩ ⟨∼ therapy⟩

²**antifungal** *n* : an antifungal agent

an·ti·gen \'ant-i-jən\ *n* : any substance (as an immunogen or a hapten) foreign to the body that evokes an immune response either alone or after forming a complex with a larger molecule (as a protein) and that is capable of binding with a product (as an antibody or T cell) of the immune response — **an·ti·gen·ic** \ˌant-i-'jen-ik\ *adj* — **an·ti·gen·i·cal·ly** \-i-k(ə-)lē\ *adv*

an·ti·gen·emia *or chiefly Brit* **an·ti·gen·ae·mia** \ˌant-i-jə-'nē-mē-ə\ *n* : the condition of having an antigen in the blood

antigenic determinant *n* : EPITOPE

an·ti·gen·ic·i·ty \-'nis-ət-ē\ *n, pl* **-ties** : the capacity to act as an antigen ⟨a vaccine with reduced ∼⟩

antigen–presenting cell *n* : any of various cells (as a macrophage or a B cell) that take up and process an antigen into a form that when displayed at the cell surface in combination with a molecule of the major histocompatibility complex is recognized by and serves to activate a specific helper T cell

an·ti·glob·u·lin \ˌant-i-'gläb-yə-lən, ˌan-ˌtī-\ *n* : an antibody that combines with and precipitates globulin

an·ti·go·nad·o·trop·ic \-ˌgō-ˌnad-ə-'träp-ik\ *adj* : tending to inhibit the physiological activity of gonadotropic hormones

an·ti·go·nad·o·tro·pin \-'trō-pən\ *n* : an antigonadotropic substance

an·ti–G suit \ˌan-ˌtī-'jē-\ *n* : G SUIT

an·ti·he·lix \-'hē-liks\ *also* **ant·he·lix** \(')ant-\ *n, pl* **-li·ces** \-'hel-ə-ˌsēz, -'hē-lə-\ *or* **-lix·es** \-'hē-lik-səz\ : the curved elevation of cartilage within or in front of the helix

an·ti·he·mo·phil·ic factor *or chiefly Brit* **an·ti·hae·mo·phil·ic factor** \-ˌhē-mə-ˌfil-ik-\ *n* : FACTOR VIII

antihemophilic globulin *or chiefly Brit* **antihaemophilic globulin** *n* : FACTOR VIII

an·ti·hem·or·rhag·ic *or chiefly Brit* **an·ti·haem·or·rhag·ic** \-ˌhem-ə-'raj-ik\ *adj* : tending to prevent or arrest hemorrhage

an·ti·her·pes \-'hər-(ˌ)pēz\ *adj* : acting against a herpesvirus or the symptoms caused by infection with it ⟨the ∼ drug acyclovir⟩ ⟨∼ antibodies⟩

an·ti·hi·drot·ic \-hid-'rät-ik, -hī-'drät-\ *adj* : tending to reduce or prevent sweat secretion

¹**an·ti·his·ta·mine** \ant-i-'his-tə-ˌmēn, ˌan-ˌtī-, -mən\ *adj* : tending to block or counteract the physiological action of histamine ⟨human blood lacks ∼ activity⟩

²**antihistamine** *n* : any of various compounds that oppose the actions of histamine and are used esp. for treating allergic reactions (as hay fever), cold symptoms, and motion sickness

an·ti·his·ta·min·ic \-ˌhis-tə-'min-ik\ *adj or n* : ANTIHISTAMINE

an·ti·hor·mone \-'hȯr-ˌmōn\ *n* **1** : a fraction of blood globulin that is capable of rendering ineffective a protein‐containing heterologous hormone when the latter is administered over a period of time and that is now generally considered to be a true antibody formed in response to the presence of foreign protein **2** : a substance (as tamoxifen) that blocks the action or inhibits the production of a hormone

an·ti·hu·man \ˌant-i-'hyü-mən, ˌan-ˌtī-, -'yü-\ *adj* : reacting strongly with human antigens ⟨∼ antibodies⟩

an·ti·hy·per·lip·id·emic *or chiefly Brit* **an·ti·hy·per·lip·id·ae·mic** \-ˌhī-pər-ˌlip-əd-'ē-mik\ *adj* : acting to prevent or counteract the accumulation of lipids in the blood ⟨an ∼ drug⟩

¹**an·ti·hy·per·ten·sive** \-ˌhī-pər-'ten(t)-siv\ *also* **an·ti·hy·per·ten·sion** \-'hī-pər-ˌten-chən\ *adj* : used or effective against high blood pressure ⟨∼ drugs⟩

²**antihypertensive** *n* : an antihypertensive agent (as a drug)

an·ti·id·io·type \ˌan-ˌtī-'id-ē-ə-ˌtīp\ *n* : an antibody that treats another antibody as an antigen and suppresses its immunoreactivity — **an·ti·id·io·typ·ic** \-ˌid-ē-ə-'tip-ik\ *adj*

¹**an·ti·im·mu·no·glob·u·lin** \ˌant-ē-ˌim-yə-nō-'gläb-yə-lən, ˌan-ˌtī-, -ˌim-yü-nō-\ *adj* : acting against specific antibodies ⟨∼ antibodies⟩ ⟨∼ sera⟩

²**anti–immunoglobulin** *n* : an anti-immunoglobulin agent

¹an·ti–in·fec·tive \-in-'fek-tiv\ *adj* : used against or tending to counteract or prevent infection ⟨~ agents⟩

²anti–infective *n* : an anti-infective agent

¹an·ti–in·flam·ma·to·ry \-in-'flam-ə-ˌtōr-ē, -ˌtór-\ *adj* : counteracting inflammation

²anti–inflammatory *n, pl* **-ries** : an anti-inflammatory agent (as a drug)

¹an·ti–in·su·lin \-'in(t)-s(ə-)lən\ *adj* : tending to counteract the physiological action of insulin

²anti–insulin *n* : an anti-insulin substance

an·ti·ke·to·gen·e·sis \ˌant-i-ˌkēt-ō-'jen-ə-səs, ˌan-ˌtī-\ *n, pl* **-e·ses** \-ˌsēz\ : the prevention or suppression of ketosis

an·ti·ke·to·gen·ic \-'jen-ik\ *adj* : tending to prevent or counteract ketosis

an·ti·leu·ke·mic \-lü-'kē-mik\ *also* **an·ti·leu·ke·mia** \-mē-ə\ *or chiefly Brit* **an·ti·leu·kae·mic** *also* **an·ti·leu·kae·mia** *adj* : counteracting the effects of leukemia

anti–lewisite — see DIMERCAPROL

an·ti·lu·et·ic \-lü-'et-ik\ *n* : ANTISYPHILITIC

an·ti·lym·pho·cyte globulin \-ˌlim(p)-fə-ˌsīt-\ *n* : serum globulin containing antibodies against lymphocytes that is used similarly to antilymphocyte serum

antilymphocyte serum *n* : a serum containing antibodies against lymphocytes that is used for suppressing graft rejection caused by lymphocyte-controlled immune responses in organ or tissue transplant recipients

an·ti·lym·pho·cyt·ic globulin \-ˌlim(p)-fə-ˌsit-ik-\ *n* : ANTILYMPHOCYTE GLOBULIN

antilymphocytic serum *n* : ANTILYMPHOCYTE SERUM

an·ti·ly·sin \-'līs-ᵊn\ *n* : a substance that is antagonistic to a lysin and protects cells from its attack

an·ti·ly·sis \-'lī-səs\ *n, pl* **-ly·ses** \-ˌsēz\ : the action of an antilysin — **an·ti·lyt·ic** \-'lit-ik\ *adj*

¹an·ti·ma·lar·i·al \-mə-'ler-ē-əl\ *or* **an·ti·ma·lar·ia** \-ē-ə\ *adj* : serving to prevent, check, or cure malaria

²antimalarial *n* : an antimalarial drug

an·ti·man·ic \-'man-ik\ *adj* : counteracting or preventing mania and esp. mania associated with bipolar disorder

an·ti·mere \'ant-i-ˌmi(ə)r\ *n* : either of a pair of opposite corresponding symmetrical bodily parts (as the halves of a bilaterally symmetrical animal)

an·ti·me·tab·o·lite \ˌant-i-mə-'tab-ə-ˌlīt, ˌan-ˌtī-\ *n* : a substance (as a sulfa drug) that replaces or inhibits the utilization of a metabolite

¹an·ti·mi·cro·bi·al \ˌant-i-mī-ˌkrō-bē-əl\ *also* **an·ti·mi·cro·bic** \-'krō-bik\ *adj* : destroying or inhibiting the growth of microorganisms and esp. pathogenic microorganisms

²antimicrobial *also* **antimicrobic** *n* : an antimicrobial substance

¹an·ti·mi·tot·ic \ˌant-i-mī-'tät-ik, ˌan-ˌtī-\ *adj* : inhibiting or disrupting mitosis ⟨~ agents⟩ ⟨~ activity⟩

²antimitotic *n* : an antimitotic substance

¹an·ti·mo·ni·al \ˌant-ə-'mō-nē-əl\ *adj* : of, relating to, or containing antimony

²antimonial *n* : an antimonial substance or preparation

an·ti·mo·nide \'ant-ə-mə-ˌnīd, -nəd\ *n* : a binary compound of antimony with a more positive element

an·ti·mo·ny \'ant-ə-ˌmō-nē\ *n, pl* **-nies** : a trivalent and pentavalent metalloid element that is commonly metallic silvery white, crystalline, and brittle and is used esp. in alloys and semiconductors and in medicine as a constituent of various antiprotozoal agents (as tartar emetic) — symbol *Sb*; see ELEMENT table

an·ti·mo·nyl \'ant-ə-mə-ˌnil, -ˌnēl\ *n* : a monovalent radical SbO composed of antimony and oxygen held to exist in the molecules of tartar emetic and some basic salts of antimony

antimonyltartrate — see POTASSIUM ANTIMONYLTARTRATE

antimony potassium tartrate *n* : TARTAR EMETIC

an·ti·mus·ca·rin·ic \ˌant-i-ˌməs-kə-'rin-ik\ *adj* : inhibiting muscarinic physiological effects ⟨an ~ agent⟩

an·ti·mu·ta·gen·ic \ˌant-i-ˌmyüt-ə-'jen-ik, ˌan-ˌtī-\ *adj* : reducing the rate of mutation ⟨~ substances⟩

an·ti·my·cin A \ˌant-i-ˌmīs-ᵊn-'ā\ *n* : a crystalline antibiotic

$C_{28}H_{40}N_2O_9$ used esp. as a fungicide, insecticide, and miticide — called also *antimycin*

an·ti·my·cot·ic \ˌant-i-mī-'kät-ik, ˌan-ˌtī-\ *adj or n* : ANTIFUNGAL

an·ti·nau·sea \-'nó-zē-ə, -sē-; -'nó-zhə, -shə\ *also* **an·ti·nau·se·ant** \-'nó-zē-ənt, -zhē-, -sē-, -shē-\ *adj* : preventing or counteracting nausea ⟨~ drugs⟩

an·ti·nau·se·ant \-'nó-zē-ənt, -zhē-, -sē-, -shē-\ *n* : an anti-nausea agent

¹an·ti·neo·plas·tic \-ˌnē-ə-'plas-tik\ *adj* : inhibiting or preventing the growth and spread of neoplasms or malignant cells ⟨treated with a regimen of ~ drugs⟩

²antineoplastic *n* : an antineoplastic agent

an·ti·neu·rit·ic \-n(y)ù-'rit-ik\ *adj* : preventing or relieving neuritis ⟨an ~ vitamin⟩

an·tin·i·on \an-'tin-ē-ən, -ˌän\ *n* : the most forward projecting part of the forehead that is between the eyebrows and opposite to the inion

an·ti·no·ci·cep·tive \ˌant-i-ˌnō-si-'sep-tiv, ˌan-ˌtī-\ *adj* : ANALGESIC

an·ti·nu·cle·ar \-'n(y)ü-klē-ər\ *adj* : being antibodies or autoantibodies that react with components and esp. DNA of cell nuclei and that tend to occur frequently in connective tissue diseases (as systemic lupus erythematosus, rheumatoid arthritis, and Sjögrens syndrome)

antioestrogen, antioestrogenic *chiefly Brit var of* ANTIESTROGEN, ANTIESTROGENIC

an·ti·on·co·gene \-'äŋ-kō-ˌjēn\ *n* : TUMOR SUPPRESSOR GENE

an·ti·ox·i·dant \ˌant-ē-'äk-səd-ənt, ˌan-ˌtī-\ *n* : any of various substances (as beta-carotene, vitamin C, and alpha-tocopherol) that inhibit oxidation or reactions promoted by oxygen and peroxides and that include many held to protect the living body from the deleterious effects of free radicals — **antioxidant** *adj*

an·ti·par·al·lel \ˌant-i-'par-ə-ˌlel, ˌan-ˌtī-, -ləl\ *adj* : parallel but oppositely directed or oriented ⟨two ~ chains of nucleotides comprise DNA⟩

an·ti·par·a·sit·ic \ˌant-i-ˌpar-ə-'sit-ik, ˌan-ˌtī-\ *adj* : acting against parasites ⟨~ drugs⟩

an·ti·par·kin·so·nian \-ˌpär-kən-'sō-nē-ən, -nyən\ *also* **an·ti·par·kin·son** \-'pär-kən-sən\ *adj* : tending to relieve parkinsonism ⟨~ drugs⟩

an·ti·pa·thet·ic \ˌant-i-pə-'thet-ik\ *adj* **1** : having a natural opposition to something ⟨an immune response which can be both ~ to the tumour . . . and protective —*Nature*⟩ **2** : inducing or characterized by antipathy

an·tip·a·thy \an-'tip-ə-thē\ *n, pl* **-thies** **1** : settled aversion or dislike **2** : an object of aversion — **an·ti·path·ic** \ˌant-i-'path-ik\ *adj*

¹an·ti·pe·ri·od·ic \ˌant-i-ˌpir-ē-'äd-ik, ˌan-ˌtī-\ *adj* : preventing periodic returns of disease

²antiperiodic *n* : an antiperiodic agent

an·ti·peri·stal·sis \-ˌper-ə-'stól-səs, -'stäl-, -'stal-\ *n, pl* **-stal·ses** \-ˌsēz\ : reversed peristalsis

an·ti·peri·stal·tic \-tik\ *adj* **1** : opposed to or checking peristaltic motion **2** : relating to antiperistalsis

an·ti·per·spi·rant \ˌant-i-'pər-sp(ə-)rənt, ˌan-ˌtī-\ *n* : a cosmetic preparation used to check excessive perspiration

an·ti·phlo·gis·tic \-flə-'jis-tik\ *adj or n* : ANTI-INFLAMMATORY

an·ti·phos·pho·lip·id \-ˌfäs-fō-'lip-əd\ *adj* : relating to, being, or associated with antibodies (as anticardiolipin antibodies) that act against phospholipids and increase the risk of venous and arterial thromboses and thrombocytopenia ⟨~ syndrome⟩

an·ti·plas·min \-'plaz-mən\ *n* : a substance (as an antifibrinolysin) that inhibits the action of plasmin

---

\ə\ **abut** \ᵊ\ **kitten** \ər\ **further** \a\ **ash** \ā\ **ace** \ä\ **cot, cart**
\aú\ **out** \ch\ **chin** \e\ **bet** \ē\ **easy** \g\ **go** \i\ **hit** \ī\ **ice** \j\ **job**
\ŋ\ **sing** \ō\ **go** \ó\ **law** \ói\ **boy** \th\ **thin** \th\ **the** \ü\ **loot**
\ù\ **foot** \y\ **yet** \zh\ **vision** *See also* Pronunciation Symbols page

an·ti·plas·tic \-'plas-tik\ *adj* : preventing or checking the process of healing or granulation

an·ti·plate·let \-'plāt-lət\ *adj* : acting against or destroying blood platelets ⟨∼ drugs⟩

an·ti·pneu·mo·coc·cal \-ₙn(y)ü-mə-'käk-əl\ *or* **an·ti·pneu·mo·coc·cic** \-'käk-(ₙ)sik\ *or* **an·ti·pneu·mo·coc·cus** \-'käk-əs\ *adj* : destroying or inhibiting pneumococci

an·ti·pode \'ant-ə-ₙpōd\ *n, pl* **an·tip·o·des** \an-'tip-ə-ₙdēz\ **1** : the exact opposite **2** : ENANTIOMER

an·ti·pol·lu·tion \ₙant-i-pə-'lü-shən, ₙan-ₙtī-\ *adj* : designed to prevent, reduce, or eliminate pollution ⟨∼ laws⟩ — **antipol·lution** *n* — **an·ti·pol·lu·tion·ist** \-sh(ə-)nəst\ *n*

an·ti·pro·lif·er·a·tive \-prə-'lif-ə-ₙrāt-iv, -rət-iv\ *adj* : used or tending to inhibit cell growth ⟨∼ effects on tumor cells⟩

an·ti·pro·te·ase \-'prōt-ē-ₙās, -ₙāz\ *n* : a substance that inhibits the enzymatic activity of a protease

an·ti·pro·throm·bin \-(ₙ)prō-'thräm-bən\ *n* : a substance that interferes with the conversion of prothrombin to thrombin — compare ANTITHROMBIN, HEPARIN

¹an·ti·pro·to·zo·al \-ₙprōt-ə-'zō-əl\ *adj* : tending to destroy or inhibit the growth of protozoans

²antiprotozoal *n* : an antiprotozoal agent

¹an·ti·pru·rit·ic \-prü-'rit-ik\ *adj* : tending to check or relieve itching ⟨∼ effects⟩

²antipruritic *n* : an antipruritic agent

an·ti·pseu·do·mo·nal \-ₙsüd-ə-'mōn-ᵊl, -sü-'däm-ən-ᵊl\ *adj* : tending to destroy bacteria of the genus *Pseudomonas* ⟨∼ activity⟩

¹an·ti·psy·chot·ic \ₙant-i-sī-'kät-ik, -ₙan-ₙtī-\ *adj* : of, being, or involving the use of an antipsychotic ⟨∼ drugs⟩

²antipsychotic *n* : any of the powerful tranquilizers (as the phenothiazines or butyrophenones) used esp. to treat psychosis and believed to act by blocking dopamine nervous receptors — called also *neuroleptic*

an·ti·py·re·sis \-ₙpī-'rē-səs\ *n, pl* **-re·ses** \-ₙsēz\ : treatment of fever by use of antipyretics

¹an·ti·py·ret·ic \-pī-'ret-ik\ *n* : an antipyretic agent — called also *febrifuge*

²antipyretic *adj* : preventing, removing, or allaying fever

an·ti·py·rine \-'pī(ə)r-ₙēn\ *also* **an·ti·py·rin** \-ən\ *n* : an analgesic and antipyretic C₁₁H₁₂N₂O formerly widely used but now largely replaced in oral use by less toxic drugs (as aspirin) — called also *phenazone*

¹an·ti·ra·chit·ic \-rə-'kit-ik\ *adj* : used or tending to prevent the development of rickets ⟨an ∼ vitamin⟩

²antirachitic *n* : an antirachitic agent

an·ti·re·jec·tion \-ri-'jek-shən\ *adj* : used or tending to prevent organ or tissue transplant rejection ⟨∼ drugs⟩

an·ti·ren·nin \ₙant-i-'ren-ən, ₙan-ₙtī-\ *n* : an antibody that inhibits the coagulating activity of rennin on milk

an·ti·re·sorp·tive \-(')rē-'sȯrp-tiv, -'zȯrp-\ *adj* : tending to slow or block the resorption of bone ⟨∼ therapies for osteoporosis may include the use of bisphosphonates or selective estrogen receptor modulators⟩ ⟨an ∼ agent⟩

an·ti·re·tic·u·lar cytotoxic serum \-rə-'tik-yə-lər-\ *n* : a serum prepared from blood of horses inoculated with cells of normal human spleen and bone marrow and claimed to have restorative and regenerative effects on certain reticular tissues in humans

¹an·ti·ret·ro·vi·ral \-'re-trō-ₙvī-rəl\ *adj* : acting, used, or effective against retroviruses ⟨∼ drugs⟩ ⟨∼ therapy⟩

²antiretroviral *n* : an antiretroviral drug

¹an·ti·rheu·mat·ic \-rù-'mat-ik\ *adj* : alleviating or preventing rheumatism ⟨∼ therapy⟩

²antirheumatic *n* : an antirheumatic agent

an·ti·ri·cin \-'rīs-ᵊn, -'ris-\ *n* : an antitoxin antagonistic to ricin

an·ti·schis·to·so·mal \-ₙshis-tə-'sō-məl\ *adj* : tending to destroy or inhibit the development and reproduction of schistosomes

an·ti·schizo·phren·ic \-ₙskit-sə-'fren-ik\ *adj* : tending to relieve or suppress the symptoms of schizophrenia

¹an·ti·scor·bu·tic \-skȯr-'byüt-ik\ *adj* : counteracting scurvy ⟨the ∼ vitamin is vitamin C⟩

²antiscorbutic *n* : a remedy for scurvy

an·ti·se·cre·tory \-'sē-krə-ₙtȯr-ē, *esp Brit* -si-'krēt-ə-rē\ *adj* : tending to inhibit secretion ⟨∼ effects⟩

an·ti·sei·zure \-'sē-zhər\ *adj* : preventing or counteracting seizures ⟨∼ drugs⟩

an·ti·sense \'an-ₙtī-ₙsens, 'an-ti-\ *adj* : having a sequence complementary to a segment of genetic material; *specif* : of, being, relating to, or possessing a sequence of DNA or RNA that is complementary to and pairs with a specific messenger RNA blocking it from being translated into protein and serving to inhibit gene function ⟨∼ RNA⟩ ⟨∼ drug therapy to inhibit malignant cell proliferation⟩ ⟨∼ research⟩ — compare MISSENSE, NONSENSE

an·ti·sep·sis \ₙant-ə-'sep-səs\ *n, pl* **-sep·ses** \-ₙsēz\ : the inhibiting of the growth and multiplication of microorganisms by antiseptic means

¹an·ti·sep·tic \ₙant-ə-'sep-tik\ *adj* **1 a** : opposing sepsis, putrefaction, or decay; *esp* : preventing or arresting the growth of microorganisms (as on living tissue) **b** : acting or protecting like an antiseptic **2** : relating to or characterized by the use of antiseptics **3** : free of living microorganisms : scrupulously clean : ASEPTIC — **an·ti·sep·ti·cal·ly** \-ti-k(ə-)lē\ *adv*

²antiseptic *n* : a substance (as hydrogen peroxide) that checks the growth or action of microorganisms esp. in or on living tissue; *also* : GERMICIDE

an·ti·sep·ti·cize *or chiefly Brit* **an·ti·sep·ti·cise** \-'sep-tə-ₙsīz\ *vt* **-cized** *or chiefly Brit* **-cised; -ciz·ing** *or chiefly Brit* **-cis·ing** : to make antiseptic

an·ti·se·rum \'ant-i-ₙsir-əm, 'an-ₙtī-, -ₙser-\ *n* : a serum containing antibodies — called also *immune serum*

an·ti·sex \ₙan-tī-'seks\ *or* **an·ti·sex·u·al** \-'seksh-(ə-)wəl\ *adj* : antagonistic toward sex; *esp* : tending to reduce or eliminate the sex drive or sexual activity

an·ti·si·al·a·go·gic \ₙant-i-ₙsī-ₙal-ə-'gäj-ik, ₙan-tī-, -'gōj-\ *adj* : tending to inhibit the flow of saliva

an·ti·si·der·ic \-sə-'der-ik\ *n* : a pharmaceutical agent that counteracts the physiological action of iron

an·ti·so·cial \-'sō-shəl\ *adj* : hostile or harmful to organized society: as **a** : being or marked by behavior deviating sharply from the social norm **b** : of, relating to, or characterized by an antisocial personality, the antisocial personality disorder, or behavior typical of either

antisocial personality *n* : a personality exhibiting traits typical of the antisocial personality disorder and often considered as predisposed toward criminality — called also *psychopathic personality*

antisocial personality disorder *n* : a personality disorder that is characterized by antisocial behavior exhibiting pervasive disregard for and violation of the rights, feelings, and safety of others starting in childhood or the early teenage years and continuing into adulthood, that is often marked by a lack of remorse for having hurt, mistreated, or stolen from others, and that in practice is often difficult to diagnose because it is confounded with disorders in which drug addiction or substance abuse is a factor — called also *psychopathic personality disorder*

¹an·ti·spas·mod·ic \-spaz-'mäd-ik\ *n* : an antispasmodic agent

²antispasmodic *adj* : capable of preventing or relieving spasms or convulsions

an·ti·sperm \-'spərm\ *adj* : destroying or inactivating sperm

an·ti·strep·to·coc·cal \-ₙstrep-tə-'käk-əl\ *or* **an·ti·strep·to·coc·cic** \-'käk-(s)ik\ *adj* : tending to destroy or inhibit the growth and reproduction of streptococci ⟨∼ antibodies⟩

an·ti·strep·to·ki·nase \-ₙstrep-tō-'kī-ₙnās, -ₙnāz\ *n* : ANTIFIBRINOLYSIN

an·ti·strep·to·ly·sin \-ₙstrep-tə-'līs-ᵊn\ *n* : an antibody against a streptolysin produced by an individual injected with a streptolysin-forming streptococcus

¹an·ti·syph·i·lit·ic \-ₙsif-ə-'lit-ik\ *adj* : effective against syphilis ⟨∼ treatment⟩

²antisyphilitic *n* : an antisyphilitic agent

an·ti·the·nar \ₙant-i-'thē-nər, ₙan-ₙtī-, an-'tith-ə-, -ₙnär\ *adj* **1**

A
B

: situated opposite to the palm or sole   **2** : HYPOTHENAR EMINENCE

an·ti·throm·bic \ˌant-i-ˈthräm-bik, ˌan-ˌtī-\ *adj* : of or resembling that of an antithrombin 〈~ activity〉

an·ti·throm·bin \-ˈthräm-bən\ *n* : any of a group of substances in blood that inhibit blood clotting by inactivating thrombin — compare ANTIPROTHROMBIN, HEPARIN

an·ti·throm·bo·plas·tin \-ˌthräm-bə-ˈplas-tən\ *n* : an anticoagulant substance that counteracts the effects of thromboplastin

¹an·ti·throm·bot·ic \-thräm-ˈbät-ik\ *adj* : used against or tending to prevent thrombosis 〈~ agents〉 〈~ therapy〉

²antithrombotic *n* : an antithrombotic agent

an·ti·thy·roid \-ˈthī-ˌroid\ *adj* : able to counteract excessive thyroid activity 〈~ drugs〉

an·ti·tox·ic \-ˈtäk-sik\ *adj* **1** : counteracting toxins 〈~ versus antibacterial immunity〉   **2** : being or containing antitoxins 〈~ serum〉

an·ti·tox·in \ˌant-i-ˈtäk-sən\ *n* : an antibody that is capable of neutralizing the specific toxin (as a specific causative agent of disease) that stimulated its production in the body and is produced in animals for medical purposes by injection of a toxin or toxoid with the resulting serum being used to counteract the toxin in other individuals; *also* : an antiserum containing antitoxins

an·ti·tox·i·no·gen·ic \-ˌtäk-sə-nə-ˈjen-ik, -ˈtäk-ˌsin-ə-\ *adj* : stimulating the production of antitoxin

an·ti·trag·i·cus \ˌant-i-ˈtraj-ə-kəs\ *n, pl* **-i·ci** \-ə-ˌsī, -ˌsē\ : a small muscle arising from the outer part of the antitragus and inserted into the antihelix

an·ti·tra·gus \-ˈtrā-gəs\ *n, pl* **-gi** \-ˌjī, -ˌgī\ : a prominence on the lower posterior portion of the concha of the external ear opposite the tragus

an·ti·try·pano·som·al \-trip-ˌan-ə-ˈsō-məl\ *or* **an·ti·try·pano·some** \-trip-ˈan-ə-ˌsōm\ *adj* : TRYPANOCIDAL

an·ti·tryp·sin \ˌant-i-ˈtrip-sən, ˈan-ˌtī-\ *n* : a substance that inhibits the action of trypsin — see ALPHA-1-ANTITRYPSIN — **an·ti·tryp·tic** \-ˈtrip-tik\ *adj*

an·ti·tu·ber·cu·lous \ˌant-i-t(y)ù-ˈbər-kyə-ləs, ˌan-ˌtī-\ *or* **an·ti·tu·ber·cu·lo·sis** \-ˌbər-kyə-ˈlō-səs\ *also* **an·ti·tu·ber·cu·lar** \-ˈbər-kyə-lər\ *adj* : used or effective against tuberculosis 〈~ drugs〉 〈~ activity〉

an·ti·tu·mor \ˈant-i-ˌt(y)ü-mər, ˈan-ˌtī-\ *also* **an·ti·tu·mor·al** \-mə-rəl\ *or chiefly Brit* **an·ti·tu·mour** *also* **an·ti·tu·mour·al** *adj* : preventing or inhibiting the formation or growth of tumors : ANTICANCER 〈~ agents〉 〈~ activity〉

¹an·ti·tus·sive \ˌant-i-ˈtəs-iv, ˌan-ˌtī-\ *adj* : tending or having the power to act as a cough suppressant 〈~ action〉

²antitussive *n* : a cough suppressant

an·ti·ty·phoid \-ˈtī-ˌfoid, -tī-ˈfoid\ *adj* : tending to prevent or cure typhoid

an·ti·ul·cer \-ˈəl-sər\ *adj* : tending to prevent or heal ulcers 〈~ drugs〉

an·ti·ven·in \-ˈven-ən\ *n* : an antitoxin to a venom; *also* : an antiserum containing such an antitoxin

An·ti·vert \ˈant-i-ˌvərt, ˈan-ˌtī-\ *trademark* — used for a preparation of the hydrochloride of meclizine

¹an·ti·vi·ral \-ˈvī-rəl\ *also* **an·ti·vi·rus** \-rəs\ *adj* : acting, effective, or directed against viruses 〈~ drugs〉

²antiviral *n* : an antiviral agent and esp. a drug

an·ti·vi·ta·min \ˈant-i-ˌvīt-ə-mən, ˈan-ˌtī-, *Brit usu* -ˌvit-\ *n* : a substance that makes a vitamin metabolically ineffective

an·ti·vivi·sec·tion \ˌant-i-ˌviv-ə-ˈsek-shən, ˌan-ˌtī-, -ˈviv-ə-\ *n, often attrib* : opposition to animal experimentation and esp. vivisection 〈the ~ movement〉 — **an·ti·vivi·sec·tion·ist** \-ˌviv-ə-ˈsek-sh(ə-)nəst\ *n*

an·ti·xe·roph·thal·mic \-ˌzir-äf-ˈthal-mik, -äp-\ *adj* : preventing or curing xerophthalmia 〈vitamin A is the ~ vitamin〉

an·ti·zy·mot·ic \-zī-ˈmät-ik\ *n* : a substance that inhibits enzymatic action

An·ton's syndrome \ˈan-ˌtänz-\ *n* : a disorder marked by psychological denial and rationalization of clinically evident loss of vision

An·ton \ˈän-ˌtōn\, **Gabriel (1858–1933),** German neuropsychiatrist. Anton first described the syndrome that bears his name in an article published in 1899.

antra *pl of* ANTRUM

an·tral \ˈan-trəl\ *adj* : of or relating to an antrum 〈the ~ part of the stomach〉

an·trec·to·my \an-ˈtrek-tə-mē\ *n, pl* **-mies** : excision of an antrum (as of the stomach or mastoid)

an·trorse \ˈan-ˌtró(ə)rs\ *adj* : directed forward or upward — **an·trorse·ly** *adv*

an·tro·scope \ˈan-trə-ˌskōp\ *n* : an instrument for illuminating and examining an antrum (as the maxillary sinus)

an·tros·to·my \an-ˈträs-tə-mē\ *n, pl* **-mies** : the operation of opening an antrum (as for drainage); *also* : the opening made in such an operation

an·trot·o·my \-ˈträt-ə-mē\ *n, pl* **-mies** : incision of an antrum; *also* : ANTROSTOMY

an·trum \ˈan-trəm\ *n, pl* **an·tra** \-trə\ : a cavity within a bone (as the maxilla) or hollow organ (as the stomach)

antrum of High·more \-ˈhī-ˌmō(ə)r, -ˌmó(ə)r\ *n* : MAXILLARY SINUS

   Highmore, Nathaniel (1613–1685), British surgeon. Highmore is remembered for his studies in anatomy. In 1651 he published a treatise on human anatomy that was noteworthy for its sound treatment of the circulation of the blood. This treatise also contains his description of the air cavity of the maxilla, now known as the maxillary sinus or antrum of Highmore. The cavity had been discovered previously and had actually been illustrated by Leonardo da Vinci. Highmore is also known for his description of the incomplete partition that divides the scrotum into two sacs each containing a testis.

ANTU \ˈan-ˌtü\ *n* : a chemical $C_{11}H_{10}N_2S$ produced as a gray powder for use as a rat poison — called also *alpha-naphthylthiourea*

anu·cle·ate \(ˈ)ā-ˈn(y)ü-klē-ət\ *also* **anu·cle·at·ed** \-klē-ˌāt-əd\ *adj* : lacking a cell nucleus

anulus fibrosus *var of* ANNULUS FIBROSUS

an·u·re·sis \ˌan-(y)ə-ˈrē-səs\ *n, pl* **-re·ses** \-ˌsēz\ : retention of urine in the urinary bladder : failure or inability to void urine — **an·u·ret·ic** \-ˈret-ik\ *adj*

an·uria \ə-ˈn(y)ùr-ē-ə, a-\ *n* : absence of or defective urine excretion — **an·uric** \-ˈn(y)ùr-ik\ *adj*

anus \ˈā-nəs\ *n, pl* **anus·es** *or* **ani** \ˈā-(ˌ)nī\ : the posterior opening of the alimentary canal

an·vil \ˈan-vəl\ *n* : INCUS

anx·i·ety \aŋ-ˈzī-ət-ē\ *n, pl* **-eties** **1 a** : a painful or apprehensive uneasiness of mind usu. over an impending or anticipated ill   **b** : a cause of anxiety   **2** : an abnormal and overwhelming sense of apprehension and fear often marked by physiological signs (as sweating, tension, and increased pulse), by doubt concerning the reality and nature of the threat, and by self-doubt about one's capacity to cope with it

anxiety disorder *n* : any of various disorders (as panic disorder, obsessive-compulsive disorder, a phobia, or generalized anxiety disorder) in which anxiety is a predominant feature — called also *anxiety neurosis, anxiety state*

anxiety equivalent *n* : an intense somatic symptom (as palpitation of the heart) that replaces fear in an attack of anxiety

anxiety hysteria *n* : an anxiety disorder and esp. a phobia when the mental aspects of anxiety are emphasized over any accompanying physical symptoms (as heart palpitations and breathlessness) — used esp. in early Freudian psychiatry

anxiety neurosis *n* : ANXIETY DISORDER

anxiety reaction *n* : reaction to a feared situation or object in which various manifestations of anxiety (as shortness of breath, abdominal pain, increased heart rate, or irritability) are prominent

\ə\ abut \ᵊ\ kitten \ər\ further \a\ ash \ā\ ace \ä\ cot, cart
\aù\ out \ch\ chin \e\ bet \ē\ easy \g\ go \i\ hit \ī\ ice \j\ job
\ŋ\ sing \ō\ go \ó\ law \ói\ boy \th\ thin \ṯh\ the \ü\ loot
\ù\ foot \y\ yet \zh\ vision   *See also* Pronunciation Symbols page

¹**anx·io·lyt·ic** \ˌaŋ-zē-ō-ˈlit-ik, ˌaŋ(k)-sē-\ *n* : a drug that relieves anxiety

²**anxiolytic** *adj* : relieving anxiety

anx·ious \ˈaŋ(k)-shəs\ *adj* **1** : characterized by extreme uneasiness of mind or brooding fear about some contingency ⟨~ students⟩ **2** : characterized by, resulting from, or causing anxiety ⟨an ~ time in the hospital waiting room⟩

AOB *abbr* alcohol on breath

aor·ta \ā-ˈȯrt-ə\ *n, pl* **-tas** *or* **-tae** \-ē\ : the large arterial trunk that carries blood from the heart to be distributed by branch arteries through the body

aor·tic \ā-ˈȯrt-ik\ *also* **aor·tal** \-ˈȯrt-ᵊl\ *adj* : of, relating to, or affecting an aorta ⟨the ~ media⟩ ⟨an ~ aneurysm⟩

aortic arch *n* **1** : one of the arterial branches in vertebrate embryos that exist in a series of pairs with one on each side of the embryo, that connect the ventral arterial system lying anterior to the heart to the dorsal arterial system above the alimentary tract, and that persist in adult fishes but are reduced or much modified in the adult of higher forms **2** : ARCH OF THE AORTA

aortic dissection *n* : a pathological splitting of the aortic media

aortic hiatus *n* : an opening in the diaphragm through which the aorta passes

aortic incompetence *n* : AORTIC REGURGITATION

aortic insufficiency *n* : AORTIC REGURGITATION

aortic murmur *n* : a heart murmur originating at the aortic valve

aor·ti·co·pul·mo·nary \ā-ˌȯrt-ə-kō-ˈpůl-mə-ˌner-ē, -ˈpəl-\ *adj* : relating to or joining the aorta and the pulmonary artery ⟨an ~ anastomosis⟩

aor·ti·co·re·nal \-ˈrēn-ᵊl\ *adj* : relating to or situated near the aorta and the kidney

aortic regurgitation *n* : leakage of blood from the aorta back into the left ventricle during diastole because of failure of an aortic valve to close properly — called also *aortic incompetence, aortic insufficiency, Corrigan's disease*

aortic sinus *n* : SINUS OF VALSALVA

aortic stenosis *n* : a condition usu. the result of disease in which the aorta and esp. its orifice is abnormally narrow

aortic valve *n* : the semilunar valve separating the aorta from the left ventricle that prevents blood from flowing back into the left ventricle

aor·ti·tis \ˌā-ȯr-ˈtīt-əs\ *n* : inflammation of the aorta

aor·to·cor·o·nary \ˌā-ȯrt-ə-ˈkȯr-ə-ˌner-ē, -ˈkär-\ *adj* : of, relating to, or joining the aorta and the coronary arteries ⟨~ bypass surgery⟩

aor·to·fem·o·ral \-ˈfem(-ə)-rəl\ *adj* : of, relating to, or joining the abdominal aorta and the femoral arteries ⟨an ~ bypass graft⟩

aor·to·gram \ā-ˈȯrt-ə-ˌgram\ *n* : an X-ray picture of the aorta made by arteriography

aor·tog·ra·phy \ˌā-ȯr-ˈtäg-rə-fē\ *n, pl* **-phies** : arteriography of the aorta — **aor·to·graph·ic** \(ˌ)ā-ȯrt-ə-ˈgraf-ik\ *adj*

aor·to·il·i·ac \ˌā-ȯrt-ō-ˈil-ē-ˌak\ *adj* : of, relating to, or joining the abdominal aorta and the iliac arteries ⟨an ~ bypass graft⟩

aor·to·pul·mo·nary win·dow \ˌā-ȯrt-ō-ˈpůl-mə-ˌner-ē-ˈwin-(ˌ)dō, -ˌpəl-\ *n* : a congenital circulatory defect in which there is direct communication between the aorta and the pulmonary artery — called also *aortopulmonary fenestration*

aor·to·sub·cla·vi·an \-ˌsəb-ˈklā-vē-ən\ *adj* : relating to or joining the aorta and the subclavian arteries ⟨~ bypass graft —*Physicians' Current Procedural Terminology*⟩

AOTA *abbr* American Occupational Therapy Association

ap *abbr* apothecaries

AP *abbr* **1** action potential **2** alkaline phosphatase **3** anterior pituitary **4** anteroposterior **5** aortic pressure

APAP *abbr* [N-*acetyl*-*para*-*amino*phenol] acetaminophen — used esp. when combined with a prescription drug ⟨hydrocodone/*APAP*⟩

apar·a·lyt·ic \ˌā-ˌpar-ə-ˈlit-ik\ *adj* : not characterized by paralysis ⟨benign ~ illness —Harry Hoogstraal⟩

ap·a·thet·ic \ˌap-ə-ˈthet-ik\ *adj* : having or showing little or no feeling or emotion — **ap·a·thet·i·cal·ly** \-i-k(ə-)lē\ *adv*

ap·a·thy \ˈap-ə-thē\ *n, pl* **-thies** : lack of feeling or emotion

ap·a·tite \ˈap-ə-ˌtīt\ *n* : any of a group of calcium phosphate minerals occurring variously as hexagonal crystals, as granular masses, or in fine-grained masses as the chief constituent of bones and teeth and of phosphate rock; *esp* : calcium phosphate fluoride Ca₅F(PO₄)₃

APC *abbr* aspirin, phenacetin, and caffeine

APD *abbr* **1** auditory processing disorder **2** automated peritoneal dialysis

ape \ˈāp\ *n* **1** : MONKEY; *esp* : one of the larger tailless or short-tailed Old World forms **2** : any of the large tailless semierect primates (as the chimpanzee, gorilla, orangutan, or gibbon) that comprise two primate families (Pongidae and Hylobatidae) — called also *anthropoid, anthropoid ape*

¹**ape·ri·ent** \ə-ˈpir-ē-ənt\ *adj* : gently causing the bowels to move : LAXATIVE

²**aperient** *n* : an aperient agent

ape·ri·od·ic \ˌā-pir-ē-ˈäd-ik\ *adj* **1** : of irregular occurrence **2** : not having periodic vibrations : not oscillatory

aperi·stal·sis \ˌā-per-ə-ˈstȯl-səs, -ˈstäl-, -ˈstal-\ *n, pl* **-stal·ses** \-ˌsēz\ : absence of peristalsis

¹**aper·i·tive** \ə-ˈper-ət-iv\ *adj* **1** : APERIENT **2** : stimulating the appetite

²**aperitive** *n* : APERIENT

ap·er·tom·e·ter \ˌap-ər-ˈtäm-ət-ər\ *n* : an instrument for measuring the numerical aperture of objectives (as those of a microscope)

ap·er·tu·ra \ˌap-ə(r)-ˈchù(ə)r-ə, -ˈt(y)ù(ə)r-\ *n, pl* **-tu·rae** \-ˌī, -ˌē\ : an anatomical opening or aperture

ap·er·ture \ˈap-ə(r)-ˌchù(ə)r, -chər, -ˌt(y)ù(ə)r\ *n* **1** : an opening or open space **2** : the diameter of the stop in an optical system that determines the diameter of the bundle of rays traversing the instrument

apex \ˈā-ˌpeks\ *n, pl* **apex·es** *or* **api·ces** \ˈā-pə-ˌsēz\ : a narrowed or pointed end of an anatomical structure: as **a** : the narrow somewhat conical upper part of a lung extending into the root **b** : the lower pointed end of the heart situated in humans opposite the space between the cartilages of the fifth and sixth ribs on the left side **c** : the extremity of the root of a tooth

apex·car·di·og·ra·phy \ˌā-ˌpek-ˌskärd-ē-ˈäg-rə-fē\ *n, pl* **-phies** : a procedure for measuring the beat in the apex region of the heart by recording movements in the nearby wall of the chest

APF *abbr* animal protein factor

Ap·gar score \ˈap-ˌgär-ˈskō(ə)r, -ˈskȯ(ə)r\ *n* : an index used to evaluate the condition of a newborn infant based on a rating of 0, 1, or 2 for each of the five characteristics of color, heart rate, response to stimulation of the sole of the foot, muscle tone, and respiration with 10 being a perfect score

Apgar, Virginia (1909–1974), American physician. Apgar began her medical career as an anesthesiologist and was for many years an attending anesthesiologist. As a result of her duties in the hospital delivery room, she developed a concern for the lack of immediate medical attention given the newborn. To rectify the situation she developed the Apgar score as a simple, quick test to determine the need for emergency treatment. The test soon became a standard procedure in hospitals all over the world. Turning to the study of congenital anomalies, Apgar became an authority on teratology and proper prenatal care.

apha·gia \ā-ˈfā-j(ē-)ə, a-\ *n* : loss of the ability to swallow

apha·kia \ə-ˈfā-kē-ə, a-\ *n* : absence of the crystalline lens of the eye; *also* : the resulting anomalous state of refraction

¹**apha·kic** \ə-ˈfā-kik, a-\ *adj* : of, relating to, or affected with aphakia ⟨the ~ eye⟩

²**aphakic** *n* : an individual who has had the lens of an eye removed

apha·sia \ə-ˈfā-zh(ē-)ə\ *n* : loss or impairment of the power to use or comprehend words usu. resulting from brain damage — see MOTOR APHASIA; compare AMUSIA, ANARTHRIA

¹apha·sic \ə-ˈfā-zik\ *adj* : of, relating to, or affected with aphasia

²aphasic *or* **apha·si·ac** \ə-ˈfā-z(h)ē-ˌak\ *n* : an individual affected with aphasia

apha·si·ol·o·gy \ə-ˌfā-z(h)ē-ˈäl-ə-jē\ *n, pl* **-gies** : the study of aphasia including its linguistic, psychological, and neurological aspects — **apha·si·ol·o·gist** \-jəst\ *n*

Aphas·mid·ia \ˌā-ˌfaz-ˈmid-ē-ə\ *n pl* : a subclass of Nematoda comprising worms in which the sensory organs are often bristlelike, phasmids are lacking or greatly reduced, the lateral cervical papillae are absent, and the sensory depressions situated laterally at the anterior end are usu. modified — compare PHASMIDIA

aphe·mia \ə-ˈfē-mē-ə\ *n* : MOTOR APHASIA

aphe·re·sis \ˌa-fə-ˈrē-səs\ *n, pl* **-re·ses** \-ˌsēz\ : withdrawal of blood from a donor's body, removal of one or more components (as plasma, blood platelets, or white blood cells) from the blood, and transfusion of the remaining blood back into the donor — called also *pheresis;* see PLATELETPHERESIS; compare PLASMAPHERESIS

apho·nia \(ˈ)ā-ˈfō-nē-ə\ *n* : loss of voice and of all but whispered speech — **apho·nic** \-ˈfän-ik, -ˈfō-nik\ *adj*

aphos·pho·ro·sis \ˌā-ˌfäs-fə-ˈrō-səs\ *n, pl* **-ro·ses** \-ˌsēz\ : a deficiency disease esp. of domestic cattle caused by inadequate intake of dietary phosphorus and marked by lameness, scouring, and loss of appetite

aphra·sia \ə-ˈfrā-zh(ē-)ə, a-\ *n* **1** : an inability to utter words in intelligible order **2** : pathological refusal to speak — **aphra·sic** \-zik\ *adj*

aph·ro·di·sia \ˌaf-rə-ˈdē-zh(ē-)ə, -ˈdizh-(ē-)ə\ *n* : sexual desire esp. when violent

Aph·ro·di·te \ˌaf-rə-ˈdīt-ē\, Greek mythological character. Aphrodite was the ancient Greek goddess of sexual love, fertility, and beauty. In Greek mythology Aphrodite was renowned for her mortal lovers, who included Adonis and Anchises. By the latter, she became the mother of Aeneas. Aphrodite was identified by the Romans with Venus.

¹aph·ro·di·si·ac \ˌaf-rə-ˈdē-zē-ˌak, -ˈdiz-ē-\ *also* **aph·ro·di·sia·cal** \ˌaf-rəd-ə-ˈzī-ə-kəl, -ˈsī-\ *adj* : exciting sexual desire

²aphrodisiac *n* : an aphrodisiac agent

aph·tha \ˈaf-thə, ˈap-thə\ *also* **ap·tha** \ˈap-\ *n, pl* **aph·thae** *also* **ap·thae** \-ˌthē\ **1** : a speck, flake, or blister on the mucous membranes (as in the mouth or gastrointestinal tract or on the lips) characteristic of some diseases (as thrush) **2** : one of the vesicles filled with clear serous fluid that occur in the mouth, on the udder, and in the spaces between the digits of cloven-footed animals in some diseases — usu. used in pl. **3** : a disease (as foot-and-mouth disease) characterized by aphthae — **aph·thic** \-thik\ *adj*

aph·thoid \ˈaf-ˌthȯid, ˈap-\ *adj* : having the characteristics of aphthae; *specif* : resembling thrush

aph·thon·gia \af-ˈthän-j(ē-)ə\ *n* : aphasia due to spasm of the tongue

aph·tho·sis \af-ˈthō-səs\ *n, pl* **-tho·ses** \-ˌsēz\ : a condition characterized by the formation of aphthae

aph·thous \ˈaf-thəs, ˈap-\ *adj* : of, relating to, or characterized by aphthae ⟨~ lesions⟩

aphthous fever *n* : FOOT-AND-MOUTH DISEASE

aphthous stomatitis *n* : a very common disorder of the oral mucosa that is characterized by the formation of canker sores on movable mucous membranes and that has a multiple etiology but is not caused by the virus causing herpes simplex

api·cal \ˈā-pi-kəl *also* ˈap-i-\ *adj* : of, relating to, or situated at an apex — **api·cal·ly** \-k(ə-)lē\ *adv*

apical foramen *n* : the opening of the pulp canal in the root of a tooth

apical ligament of the dens *n* : a fibrous cord between the two alar ligaments that extends from the tip of the dens to the anterior margin of the foramen magnum — called also *apical dental ligament*

apic·ec·to·my \ˌā-pə-ˈsek-tə-mē\ *n, pl* **-mies** : surgical removal of an anatomical apex (as of the root of a tooth or of the petrous portion of the temporal bone)

apices *pl of* APEX

api·ci·tis \ˌā-pə-ˈsīt-əs, ˌap-ə-\ *n, pl* **-ci·tes** \-ˈsī-ˌtēz\ : inflammation of an anatomical apex (as of a lung, the root of a tooth, or the petrous portion of the temporal bone)

api·co·ec·to·my \ˌā-pi-(ˌ)kō-ˈek-tə-mē, ˌap-i-\ *n, pl* **-mies** : excision of the root tip of a tooth

api·col·y·sis \ˌap-i-ˈkäl-ə-səs\ *n, pl* **-y·ses** \-ˌsēz\ : collapse of the apex of a lung induced by surgical means in order to obliterate its cavity esp. in the treatment of pulmonary tuberculosis

Api·um \ˈā-pē-əm, ˈap-ē-\ *n* : a genus of Eurasian herbs of the carrot family that includes celery

apla·cen·tal \ˌā-plə-ˈsent-ᵊl\ *adj* : having or developing no placenta

ap·la·nat·ic \ˌap-lə-ˈnat-ik, ˌā-plə-\ *adj* : free from or corrected for spherical aberration ⟨an ~ lens⟩ — **ap·la·nat·i·cal·ly** \-i-k(ə-)lē\ *adv*

aplan·a·tism \ā-ˈplan-ə-ˌtiz-əm, ˈap-lə-ˌnat-ˌiz-\ *n* : freedom from spherical aberration

apla·sia \(ˈ)ā-ˈplā-zh(ē)ə, ə-\ *n* : incomplete or faulty development of an organ or part

aplas·tic \(ˈ)ā-ˈplas-tik\ *adj* **1** : not exhibiting growth or change in structure **2** : of, relating to, or exhibiting aplasia

aplastic anemia *n* : anemia that is characterized by defective function of the blood-forming organs (as the bone marrow) and is caused by toxic agents (as chemicals or X-rays) or is idiopathic in origin — called also *hypoplastic anemia*

ap·nea *or chiefly Brit* **ap·noea** \ˈap-nē-ə, ap-ˈnē-\ *n* **1** : transient cessation of respiration whether normal (as in hibernating animals) or abnormal (as that caused by certain drugs) — see SLEEP APNEA **2** : ASPHYXIA — **ap·ne·ic** *or chiefly Brit* **ap·noe·ic** \ap-ˈnē-ik\ *adj*

ap·neu·sis \ap-ˈn(y)ü-səs\ *n, pl* **ap·neu·ses** \-ˌsēz\ : sustained tonic contraction of the respiratory muscles resulting in prolonged inspiration

ap·neus·tic \-ˈn(y)ü-stik\ *adj* : relating to, concerned with, or exhibiting apneusis ⟨the ~ area in the lower pons —S. W. Jacob & C. A. Francone⟩

apo \ˈa-ˌpō\ *n* : APOLIPOPROTEIN ⟨~s A-I and B were assayed⟩

apo·car·ter·e·sis \ˌap-ə-ˌkärt-ə-ˈrē-səs\ *n, pl* **-e·ses** \-ˌsēz\ : commission of suicide by starvation

apo·chro·mat·ic \ˌap-ə-krō-ˈmat-ik\ *adj* : free of chromatic and spherical aberration ⟨an ~ lens⟩

apo·crine \ˈap-ə-krən, -ˌkrīn, -ˌkrēn\ *adj* : producing a fluid secretion by pinching off one end of the secreting cells which then reform and repeat the process ⟨~ glands⟩; *also* : produced by an apocrine gland — compare ECCRINE, HOLOCRINE, MEROCRINE

Apoc·y·num \ə-ˈpäs-ə-nəm\ *n* : a genus of chiefly American perennial herbs of the dogbane family (Apocynaceae) with opposite leaves and small white or pink flowers comprising the dogbanes of which several (esp. *A. androsaemifolium* and *A. cannabium*) are the source of substances with physiological activity resembling digitalis — see INDIAN HEMP 1

ap·o·dal \ˈap-əd-ᵊl\ *or* **ap·o·dous** \-əd-əs\ *adj* : having no feet

apo·en·zyme \ˌap-ō-ˈen-ˌzīm\ *n* : a protein that forms an active enzyme system by combination with a coenzyme and determines the specificity of this system for a substrate

ap·o·fer·ri·tin \ˌap-ə-ˈfer-ət-ən\ *n* : a colorless crystalline protein capable of storing iron in bodily cells esp. of the liver by combining with iron to form ferritin

apo·lar \(ˈ)ā-ˈpō-lər\ *adj* : having no poles ⟨polar and ~ binding sites in a protein⟩

apo·li·po·pro·tein \ˌap-ə-ˌlī-pō-ˈprō-ˌtēn, -ˌlip-ō-, -ˈprōt-ē-ən\ *n* : any of the proteins that combine with a lipid to form a lipoprotein and that are now grouped into four classes designated *A, B, C,* and *E* and formerly into a fifth class *D* now

---

\ə\ **abut** \ᵊ\ **kitten** \ər\ **further** \a\ **ash** \ā\ **ace** \ä\ **cot, cart** \au̇\ **out** \ch\ **chin** \e\ **bet** \ē\ **easy** \g\ **go** \i\ **hit** \ī\ **ice** \j\ **job** \ŋ\ **sing** \ō\ **go** \ȯ\ **law** \ȯi\ **boy** \th\ **thin** \th\ **the** \ü\ **loot** \u̇\ **foot** \y\ **yet** \zh\ **vision** *See also* Pronunciation Symbols page

considered part of *A* — often followed by the letter designating the class or by the letter and a number expressed in Roman or Arabic numerals to indicate a specific member of the class ⟨∼ *B* is a major component of LDL⟩

apo·mor·phine \ap-ə-ˈmȯr-ˌfēn\ *n* : a crystalline morphine derivative $C_{17}H_{17}NO_2$ that is a dopamine agonist and is administered as the hydrochloride for its powerful emetic action

apo·neu·ro·sis \ˌap-ə-n(y)u̇-ˈrō-səs\ *n, pl* **-ro·ses** \-ˌsēz\ : any of the broad flat sheets of dense fibrous collagenous connective tissue that cover, invest, and form the terminations and attachments of various muscles — **apo·neu·rot·ic** \-ˈrät-ik\ *adj*

aponeurotica — see GALEA APONEUROTICA

apo·nia \(ˈ)ā-ˈpō-nē-ə, (ˈ)ä-, -nyə\ *n* : freedom from pain

apoph·y·sis \ə-ˈpäf-ə-səs\ *n, pl* **-y·ses** \-ˌsēz\ : an expanded or projecting part esp. of an organism — **apoph·y·se·al** \-ˌpäf-ə-ˈsē-əl\ *adj*

apoph·y·si·tis \ə-ˌpäf-ə-ˈsīt-əs\ *n* : inflammation of an apophysis

ap·o·plec·tic \ˌap-ə-ˈplek-tik\ *adj* **1** : of, relating to, or causing stroke **2** : affected with, inclined to, or showing symptoms of stroke — **ap·o·plec·ti·cal·ly** \-ti-k(ə-)lē\ *adv*

ap·o·plec·ti·form \-ˈplek-tə-ˌfȯrm\ *adj* : resembling stroke ⟨∼ seizures⟩

ap·o·plexy \ˈap-ə-ˌplek-sē\ *n, pl* **-plex·ies** **1** : STROKE **2** : copious hemorrhage into a cavity or into the substance of an organ ⟨abdominal ∼⟩ ⟨adrenal ∼⟩

apo·pro·tein \ˌap-ə-ˈprō-ˌtēn, -ˈprōt-ē-ən\ *n* : a protein that combines with a prosthetic group to form a conjugated protein

apop·to·sis \ˌap-ə(p)-ˈtō-sis, -äp-, -ō-; ˌā-ˌpäp-\ *n* : a genetically determined process of cell self-destruction that is marked by the fragmentation of nuclear DNA, is activated either by the presence of a stimulus or by the removal of a stimulus or suppressing agent, is a normal physiological process eliminating DNA-damaged, superfluous, or unwanted cells (as immune cells targeted against the self in the development of self-tolerance or larval cells in amphibians undergoing metamorphosis), and when halted (as by genetic mutation) may result in uncontrolled cell growth and tumor formation — called also *programmed cell death* — **apop·tot·ic** \-ˈtät-ik\ *adj*

apoth·e·car·ies' measure \ə-ˈpäth-ə-ˌker-ēz-\ *n* : a system of liquid units of measure used in compounding medical prescriptions that include the gallon, pint, fluid ounce, fluid dram, and minim

apothecaries' weight *n* : a system of weights used chiefly by pharmacists in compounding medical prescriptions that include the pound of 12 ounces, the dram of 60 grains, and the scruple

apoth·e·cary \ə-ˈpäth-ə-ˌker-ē\ *n, pl* **-car·ies** **1** : a person who prepares and sells drugs or compounds for medicinal purposes : DRUGGIST, PHARMACIST **2** : PHARMACY 2a

ap·ox·e·sis \ˌap-äk-ˈsē-səs\ *n* : the removal of deposits from the root surfaces of teeth by a scraper

ap·o·zem \ˈap-ə-ˌzem\ *or* **apoz·e·ma** \ə-ˈpäz-ə-mə\ *n* : a pharmaceutical decoction

apo·zy·mase \ˌap-ə-ˈzī-ˌmās, -ˌmāz\ *n* : the protein portion of a zymase

app *abbr* appendix

APP *abbr* amyloid precursor protein

ap·pa·ra·tus \ˌap-ə-ˈrat-əs, -ˈrät-\ *n, pl* **-tus·es** *or* **-tus** : a group of anatomical and cytological parts having a common function ⟨the respiratory ∼⟩ — see GOLGI APPARATUS

ap·par·ent \ə-ˈpar-ənt, -ˈper-\ *adj* **1** : clear or manifest to the senses ⟨no ∼ cause for the condition⟩ **2** : manifest to the senses or mind as real or true on the basis of evidence that may or may not be valid upon deeper investigation ⟨the ∼ stimulating action of a sedative drug may actually result from its depressant effect —D. W. Maurer & V. H. Vogel⟩

apparent motion *n* : an optical illusion in which stationary objects viewed in quick succession or in relation to moving objects appear to be in motion — called also *apparent movement;* see PHI PHENOMENON

ap·pear·ance \ə-ˈpir-ən(t)s\ *n* **1** : the action or process of becoming evident to the senses ⟨the sudden ∼ of a rash on the body⟩ **2** : the outward or visible aspect of something ⟨a tumor with a spongy ∼⟩ — **ap·pear** \ə-ˈpi(ə)r\ *vi*

ap·pend·age \ə-ˈpen-dij\ *n* : a subordinate or derivative body part; *esp* : a limb or analogous part (as a seta)

ap·pen·dec·to·my \ˌap-ən-ˈdek-tə-mē\ *n, pl* **-mies** : surgical removal of the vermiform appendix

ap·pen·di·ceal \ə-ˌpen-də-ˈsē-əl\ *also* **ap·pen·di·cal** \ə-ˈpen-di-kəl\ *or* **ap·pen·di·cial** \ˌap-ən-ˈdish-əl\ *adj* : of, relating to, or involving the vermiform appendix ⟨∼ inflammation⟩

ap·pen·di·cec·to·my \ə-ˌpen-də-ˈsek-tə-mē\ *n, pl* **-mies** *Brit* : APPENDECTOMY

ap·pen·di·ces epi·ploi·cae \ə-ˌpen-də-ˌsēz-ˌep-i-ˈplȯi-sē\ *n pl* : small peritoneal pouches filled with fat that are situated along the large intestine

ap·pen·di·ci·tis \ə-ˌpen-də-ˈsīt-əs\ *n* : inflammation of the vermiform appendix — called also *epityphlitis*

ap·pen·di·cos·to·my \ə-ˌpen-də-ˈkäs-tə-mē\ *n, pl* **-to·mies** : the surgical operation of opening the vermiform appendix to irrigate the large intestine

ap·pen·dic·u·lar \ˌap-ən-ˈdik-yə-lər\ *adj* : of or relating to an appendage: **a** : of or relating to a limb or limbs ⟨the ∼ skeleton⟩ **b** : APPENDICEAL

ap·pen·dix \ə-ˈpen-diks\ *n, pl* **-dix·es** *or* **-di·ces** \-də-ˌsēz\ : a bodily outgrowth or process; *specif* : VERMIFORM APPENDIX

ap·per·ceive \ˌap-ər-ˈsēv\ *vt* **-ceived; -ceiv·ing** : to have apperception of

ap·per·cep·tion \-ˈsep-shən\ *n* : mental perception; *esp* : the process of understanding something perceived in terms of previous experience — compare ASSIMILATION 3 — **ap·per·cep·tive** \-ˈsep-tiv\ *adj*

ap·per·son·a·tion \(ˌ)a-ˌpərs-ᵊn-ˈā-shən, ə-\ *n* : the incorporation of characteristics of external objects or persons through a process of identification with them

ap·pe·stat \ˈap-ə-ˌstat\ *n* : the neural center in the brain that regulates appetite and is thought to be in the hypothalamus

ap·pe·tite \ˈap-ə-ˌtīt\ *n* : any of the instinctive desires necessary to keep up organic life; *esp* : the desire to eat — **ap·pe·ti·tive** \-ˌtīt-iv\ *adj*

ap·pe·ti·tion \ˌap-ə-ˈtish-ən\ *n* : a longing for or seeking after something

appl *abbr* applied

ap·pla·nate \ˈap-lə-ˌnāt, (ˈ)a-ˈplā-ˌnāt\ *adj* : flattened or horizontally expanded

ap·pla·na·tion \ˌap-lə-ˈnā-shən\ *n* : abnormal flattening of a convex surface (as of the cornea of the eye)

applanation tonometer *n* : an ophthalmologic instrument used to determine pressure within the eye by measuring the force necessary to flatten an area of the cornea with a small disk

ap·ple \ˈap-əl\ *n* : the fleshy usu. rounded and red, yellow, or green edible pome fruit of a tree (genus *Malus*) of the rose family; *also* : an apple tree

ap·pli·ance \ə-ˈplī-ən(t)s\ *n* : an instrument or device designed for a particular use ⟨prosthetic ∼s⟩ ⟨an orthodontic ∼ used to move misaligned teeth into proper occlusion⟩

ap·pli·ca·tion \ˌap-lə-ˈkā-shən\ *n* **1** : an act of applying ⟨the ∼ of a dressing to a wound⟩ **2** : a medicated or protective layer or material ⟨an oily ∼ for dry skin⟩

ap·pli·ca·tor \ˈap-lə-ˌkāt-ər\ *n* : one that applies; *specif* : a device for applying a substance (as medicine)

ap·plied \ə-ˈplīd\ *adj* : put to practical use; *esp* : applying general principles to solve definite problems ⟨∼ sciences⟩ ⟨∼ psychology⟩

ap·ply \ə-ˈplī\ *vt* **ap·plied; ap·ply·ing** : to lay or spread on ⟨∼ antiseptic to a cut⟩

ap·pos·able \ə-ˈpō-zə-bəl\ *adj* : OPPOSABLE — **ap·pos·abil·i·ty** \-ˌpō-zə-ˈbil-ət-ē\ *n, pl* **-ties**

ap·po·si·tion \ˌap-ə-ˈzish-ən\ *n* **1** : the placing of things in juxtaposition or proximity; *specif* : deposition of successive layers upon those already present (as in cell walls) — compare ACCRETION, INTUSSUSCEPTION 2 **2** : the state of being in juxtaposition or proximity (as in the drawing together of cut edges of tissue in healing) — **ap·pose** \ə-'pōz\ vt **apposed; ap·pos·ing — ap·po·si·tion·al** \ˌap-ə-'zish-nəl, -ən-ᵊl\ adj

ap·proach \ə-'prōch\ n : the surgical procedure by which access is gained to a bodily part

approach–approach conflict n : psychological conflict that results when a choice must be made between two desirable alternatives — compare APPROACH-AVOIDANCE CONFLICT, AVOIDANCE-AVOIDANCE CONFLICT

approach–avoidance conflict n : psychological conflict that results when a goal is both desirable and undesirable — called also *approach-avoidance;* compare APPROACH= APPROACH CONFLICT, AVOIDANCE-AVOIDANCE CONFLICT

approx abbr approximate; approximately

ap·prox·i·mal \ə-'präk-sə-məl\ adj : CONTIGUOUS ⟨∼ surfaces of teeth⟩

¹**ap·prox·i·mate** \ə-'präk-sə-mət\ adj : located close together

²**ap·prox·i·mate** \-ˌmāt\ vt **-mat·ed; -mat·ing** : to bring together ⟨∼ cut edges of tissue⟩ — **ap·prox·i·ma·tion** \ə-ˌpräk-sə-'mā-shən\ n

appt abbr appointment

aprax·ia \(')ā-'prak-sē-ə\ n : loss or impairment of the ability to execute complex coordinated movements without muscular or sensory impairment — compare EUPRAXIA — **aprac·tic** \-'prak-tik\ or **aprax·ic** \-'prak-sik\ adj

apri·cot–ker·nel oil \'ap-rə-ˌkät-ˌkərn-ᵊl-, 'ā-prə-\ n : PERSIC OIL a

aproc·tous \(')ā-'präk-təs\ adj : lacking an anal orifice

apron \'ā-prən, -pərn\ n, often attrib **1** : a garment usu. of cloth or plastic usu. tied around the waist and used esp. to protect clothing **2** : an anatomical structure that resembles an apron; esp : HOTTENTOT APRON

apros·ex·ia \ˌā-prä-'sek-sē-ə\ n : abnormal inability to sustain attention

apro·so·pus \ā-'prō-sə-pəs\ n : a teratological fetus lacking all or part of the face

apro·ti·nin \ā-'prōt-ə-nin\ n : a polypeptide used for its protease-inhibiting properties esp. in the treatment of pancreatitis — see TRASYLOL

APSAC \'ap-ˌsak\ n : ANISTREPLASE

ap·sel·a·phe·sia \ˌap-ˌsel-ə-'fē-zē-ə, -zhə\ n : loss or impairment of the sense of touch

aptha var of APHTHA

ap·ti·tude \'ap-tə-ˌt(y)üd\ n : a natural or acquired capacity or ability; esp : a tendency, capacity, or inclination to learn or understand

aptitude test n : a standardized test designed to predict an individual's ability to learn certain skills — compare INTELLIGENCE TEST

apty·a·lism \ā-'tī-ə-ˌliz-əm\ n : absence of or deficiency in secretion of saliva

ap·y·rase \'ap-ə-ˌrās, -ˌrāz\ n : any of several enzymes that hydrolyze ATP with the liberation of phosphate and energy

apy·ret·ic \ˌā-ˌpī-'ret-ik, ˌap-ə-'ret-\ adj : being without fever : AFEBRILE

apy·rex·ia \ˌā-pī-'rek-sē-ə, ˌap-ə-'\ also **apy·rexy** \(ˌ)ā-'pī-ˌrek-sē, 'ap-ə-\ n, pl **-rex·ias** also **-rex·ies** : absence or intermission of fever — **apy·rex·i·al** \ˌā-pī-'rek-sē-əl, ˌap-ə-\ adj

aq abbr aqua; aqueous

AQ abbr accomplishment quotient; achievement quotient

aqua \'ak-wə, 'äk-\ n, pl **aquae** \'ak-(ˌ)wē, 'äk-ˌwī\ or **aquas** : WATER; esp : an aqueous solution

aqua pu·ra \ˌak-wə-'pyür-ə, ˌäk-\ n : pure water

aqua re·gia \-'rē-j(ē-)ə\ n : a mixture of nitric and hydrochloric acids that dissolves gold or platinum — called also *nitrohydrochloric acid*

aquat·ic \ə-'kwät-ik, -'kwat-\ adj : growing or living in or frequenting water ⟨∼ mosquito larvae⟩

aqua vi·tae \ˌak-wə-'vīt-ē, ˌäk-\ n : a strong alcoholic liquor

aq·ue·duct \'ak-wə-ˌdəkt\ n : a canal or passage in a part or organ

aqueduct of Fallopius n : FACIAL CANAL

G. Fallopio — see FALLOPIAN

aqueduct of Syl·vi·us \-'sil-vē-əs\ n : a channel connecting the third and fourth ventricles of the brain — called also *cerebral aqueduct, sylvian aqueduct*

Du·bois \d(y)üb-'wä\ (*Latin* **Jacques Jacobus Sylvius**) **(1478–1555),** French anatomist. The teacher of Andreas Vesalius and later his steadfast opponent, Dubois attempted to reconcile the best of classical teachings, principally those of Galen, with contemporary observations. Confident that Galen was omniscient in all matters medical, Dubois published in 1555 a systematic account of anatomy based on Galen's writings. He presented a relatively modern method of numbering branches of vessels, structures, and relationships. One of the structures described therein was the channel connecting the third and fourth ventricles of the brain; although his description was not original, the passage became known as the aqueduct of Sylvius, after his latinized professional name.

¹**aque·ous** \'ā-kwē-əs, 'ak-wē-\ adj **1 a** : of, relating to, or resembling water ⟨an ∼ vapor⟩ **b** : made from, with, or by water ⟨an ∼ solution⟩ **2** : of or relating to the aqueous humor

²**aqueous** n : AQUEOUS HUMOR

aqueous flare n : FLARE 3

aqueous humor n : a transparent fluid occupying the space between the crystalline lens and the cornea of the eye

aquos·i·ty \ə-'kwäs-ət-ē, ā-\ n, pl **-ties** : the quality or state of being moist or wet

Ar symbol argon

ara–A \ˌar-ə-'ā\ n : VIDARABINE

ar·a·ban \'ar-ə-ˌban\ n : a pentosan yielding arabinose on hydrolysis

arabic — see GUM ARABIC

arab·i·nose \ə-'rab-ə-ˌnōs, -ˌnōz\ n : a white crystalline aldose sugar $C_5H_{10}O_5$ occurring esp. in vegetable gums

ara·bi·no·side \ˌar-ə-'bin-ə-ˌsīd, ə-'rab-ə-nō-ˌsīd\ n : a glycoside that yields arabinose on hydrolysis

arab·i·tol \ə-'rab-ə-ˌtȯl, -ˌtōl\ n : a sweet crystalline alcohol $C_5H_7(OH)_5$ obtained by the reduction of arabinose

ar·a·chid·ic acid \ˌar-ə-ˌkid-ik-\ n : a white crystalline saturated fatty acid $C_{20}H_{40}O_2$ found in the form of esters esp. in vegetable fats and oils (as peanut oil)

ara·chid·o·nate \ˌar-ə-'kid-ᵊn-ˌāt\ n : a salt or ester of arachidonic acid

ar·a·chi·don·ic acid \ˌar-ə-kə-ˌdän-ik-\ n : a liquid unsaturated fatty acid $C_{20}H_{32}O_2$ that occurs in most animal fats, is a precursor of prostaglandins, and is considered essential in animal nutrition

ar·a·chis oil \'ar-ə-kəs-\ n : PEANUT OIL

Arach·ni·da \ə-'rak-nəd-ə\ n pl : a large class of arthropods that are mostly air-breathing by means of trachea or book lungs, that include the spiders and scorpions, mites, and ticks, and that have a segmented body divided into two regions of which the anterior bears four pairs of legs but no antennae — **arach·nid** \-nəd\ adj or n

arach·nid·ism \-nə-ˌdiz-əm\ n : poisoning caused by the bite or sting of an arachnid (as a spider, tick, or scorpion); esp : a syndrome marked by extreme pain and muscular rigidity due to the bite of a black widow spider

ar·ach·ni·tis \ˌar-ˌak-'nīt-əs\ n : ARACHNOIDITIS

arach·no·dac·ty·ly \ə-ˌrak-nō-'dak-tə-lē\ n, pl **-lies** : a hereditary condition characterized esp. by excessive length of the fingers and toes — see CONGENITAL CONTRACTURAL ARACHNODACTYLY

¹**arach·noid** \ə-'rak-ˌnȯid\ n : a thin membrane of the brain and spinal cord that lies between the dura mater and the pia mater

\ə\ abut \ᵊ\ kitten \ər\ further \a\ ash \ā\ ace \ä\ cot, cart
\aú\ out \ch\ chin \e\ bet \ē\ easy \g\ go \i\ hit \ī\ ice \j\ job
\ŋ\ sing \ō\ go \ȯ\ law \ȯi\ boy \th\ thin \th\ the \ü\ loot
\ú\ foot \y\ yet \zh\ vision *See also* Pronunciation Symbols page

²**arachnoid** also **arach·noi·dal** \ə-ˌrak-ˈnȯid-ᵊl\ adj : of or relating to the arachnoid ⟨the ~ membrane⟩

arach·noi·dea \ə-ˌrak-ˈnȯid-ē-ə\ n : ARACHNOID

arachnoid granulation n : any of the small whitish processes that are enlarged villi of the arachnoid membrane of the brain which protrude into the superior sagittal sinus and into depressions in the neighboring bone — called also *arachnoid villus, pacchionian body*

arach·noid·ism \ə-ˈrak-ˌnȯid-ˌiz-əm\ n : ARACHNIDISM

arach·noid·itis \ə-ˌrak-ˌnȯid-ˈīt-əs\ n : inflammation of the arachnoid membrane

arachnoid villus n : ARACHNOID GRANULATION

arach·no·ly·sin \ə-ˌrak-nō-ˈlīs-ᵊn\ n : a hemolysin secreted by some spiders

arach·no·pho·bia \ə-ˌrak-nə-ˈfō-bē-ə\ n : pathological fear or loathing of spiders

¹**arach·no·pho·bic** \-bik\ adj : of, relating to, or affected with arachnophobia

²**arach·no·pho·bic** or **arach·no·phobe** \ə-ˈrak-nə-ˌfōb\ n : an individual affected with arachnophobia

ara·lia \ə-ˈrā-lē-ə, -lyə\ n 1 cap : a large genus (family Araliaceae) of widely distributed often aromatic herbs, shrubs, and trees with compound leaves and umbellate flowers that includes some with medicinal properties 2 : a plant of the genus *Aralia* 3 : the dried rhizome and roots of the American spikenard (*Aralia racemosa*) used as a diaphoretic and aromatic

ar·a·ro·ba \ˌar-ə-ˈrō-bə\ n : GOA POWDER

ar·bor \ˈär-bər\ n : a branching anatomical structure resembling a tree

ar·bo·res·cent \ˌär-bə-ˈres-ᵊnt\ adj : resembling a tree in growth, structure, or appearance

ar·bo·ri·za·tion or Brit **ar·bo·ri·sa·tion** \ˌär-bə-rə-ˈzā-shən\ n : a treelike figure or arrangement of branching parts; esp : a treelike part or process (as a dendrite) of a nerve cell ⟨the terminal ~ of an axon⟩

ar·bo·rize or Brit **ar·bo·rise** \ˈär-bə-ˌrīz\ vi **-rized** or Brit **-rised**; **-riz·ing** or Brit **-ris·ing** : to branch freely and repeatedly ⟨the nerve fibers *arborized*⟩

ar·bo·vi·rol·o·gist \ˌär-bə-ˌvī-ˈräl-ə-jəst\ n : a specialist in arbovirology

ar·bo·vi·rol·o·gy \ˌär-bə-ˌvī-ˈräl-ə-jē\ n, pl **-gies** : a branch of virology that deals with the arboviruses

ar·bo·vi·rus \-ˈvī-rəs\ n : any of various RNA viruses (as an arenavirus, bunyavirus, or flavivirus) transmitted principally by arthropods and including the causative agents of encephalitis, yellow fever, and dengue — **ar·bo·vi·ral** \-rəl\ adj

ar·bu·tin \är-ˈbyüt-ᵊn, ˈär-byət-ən\ n : a crystalline glucoside $C_{12}H_{16}O_7$ found in the leaves of various plants (as the bearberry) of the heath family (Ericaceae) and sometimes used as a urinary antiseptic

Ar·bu·tus \är-ˈbyüt-əs\ n : a genus of shrubs and trees of the heath family (Ericaceae) having white or pink flowers and scarlet berries and including some from which arbutin is obtained

arc \ˈärk\ n 1 : an arched or curved anatomical part, distance, or pathway — see REFLEX ARC 2 : a sustained luminous discharge of electricity across a gap in a circuit or between electrodes

ARC abbr 1 AIDS-related complex 2 American Red Cross

ar·cade \är-ˈkād\ n 1 : an anatomical structure comprising a series of arches 2 : DENTAL ARCH

arch \ˈärch\ n 1 : an anatomical structure that resembles an arch in form or function: as **a** : either of two vaulted portions of the bony structure of the foot that impart elasticity to it: (1) : a longitudinal arch supported posteriorly by the basal tuberosity of the calcaneus and anteriorly by the heads of the metatarsal bones (2) : a transverse arch consisting of the metatarsals and first row of tarsals and resulting from elevation of the central anterior portion of the median longitudinal arch **b** : ARCH OF THE AORTA 2 : a fingerprint in which all the ridges run from side to side and make no backward turn

ar·cha·ic \är-ˈkā-ik\ adj 1 : typical of a previously dominant

evolutionary stage ⟨~ features of a fossil skull⟩ 2 : having the characteristics of primitive humans and their animal forebears esp. as represented in the unconscious and appearing in behavior as manifestations of the unconscious

arch·en·ter·on \är-ˈkent-ə-ˌrän, -rən\ n, pl **-tera** \-ə-rə\ : the cavity of the gastrula of an embryo forming a primitive gut — called also *gastrocoel*

ar·che·spo·ri·um \ˌär-ki-ˈspȯr-ē-əm, -ˈspȯr-\ n, pl **-spo·ria** \-ē-ə\ : the cell or group of cells from which spore mother cells develop — **ar·che·spo·ri·al** \ˌär-ki-ˈspȯr-ē-əl, -ˈspȯr-\ adj

ar·che·type \ˈär-ki-ˌtīp\ n **1 a** : a primitive generalized plan of structure deduced from the characters of a natural group of plants or animals and assumed to be the characteristic of the ancestor from which they are all descended **b** : the original ancestor of a group of plants or animals **2** : an inherited idea or mode of thought in the psychology of C. G. Jung that is derived from the experience of the race and is present in the unconscious of the individual — **ar·che·typ·al** \ˌär-ki-ˈtī-pəl\ adj

ar·chi·a·ter \ˈär-kē-ˌāt-ər, ˌär-kē-ˈ\ n : a chief physician orig. of the court of a Hellenistic king or a Roman emperor

ar·chi·carp \ˈär-kē-ˌkärp\ n : the female sex organ in ascomycetous fungi

ar·chil \ˈär-chəl\ also **or·chil** \ˈȯr-\ n 1 : a violet dye obtained from lichens (genera *Rocella* and *Lecanora*) — see CUDBEAR 2 : a lichen that yields archil

ar·chi·pal·li·um \ˌär-ki-ˈpal-ē-əm\ n : the olfactory part of the cerebral cortex comprising the hippocampus and part of the parahippocampal gyrus — compare NEOPALLIUM

ar·chi·tec·ton·ics \-tek-ˈtän-iks\ n pl but sing or pl in constr : the structural arrangement or makeup of an anatomical part or system ⟨the ~ of nuclei in the cerebellum⟩ — **ar·chi·tec·ton·ic** \-ik\ adj

ar·chi·tec·ture \ˈär-kə-ˌtek-chər\ n : the basic structural form esp. of a bodily part or of a large molecule ⟨the ~ and function of the cerebral cortex⟩ ⟨the complex molecular ~ of muscle cells —Carolyn Cohen⟩ — **ar·chi·tec·tur·al** \ˌär-kə-ˈtek-chə-rəl, -ˈtek-shrəl\ adj — **ar·chi·tec·tur·al·ly** \-ē\ adv

arch of Cor·ti \-ˈkȯrt-ē\ n : any of the series of arches composing the tunnel of Corti — compare ORGAN OF CORTI

A. Corti — see ORGAN OF CORTI

arch of the aorta n : the curved transverse part of the aorta that connects the ascending aorta with the descending aorta — called also *aortic arch*

arch of the fauces n : PILLAR OF THE FAUCES

ar·ci·form \ˈär-sə-ˌfȯrm\ adj : having the form of an arch ⟨lesions of tinea corporis in ~ configurations⟩

arc·to·staph·y·los \ˌärk-(ˌ)tō-ˈstaf-ə-ləs, -ˌläs\ n 1 cap : a genus of chiefly No. American woody plants of the heath family (Ericaceae) with alternate evergreen leaves, nodding flowers, and fruits that are drupes 2 : a plant (as the bearberry) of the genus *Arctostaphylos*

ar·cu·a·le \ˌär-kyə-ˈwā-(ˌ)lē\ n, pl **-lia** \-lē-ə\ : any of the primitive cartilages or structural elements of which a typical vertebra is formed

ar·cu·ate \ˈär-kyə-wət, -ˌwāt\ adj : curved like a bow ⟨~ fibers in the brain⟩

arcuate artery n : any of the branches of the interlobar arteries of the kidney that form arches over the base of the pyramids

arcuate ligament — see LATERAL ARCUATE LIGAMENT, MEDIAL ARCUATE LIGAMENT, MEDIAN ARCUATE LIGAMENT

arcuate nucleus n : any of several cellular masses in the thalamus, hypothalamus, or medulla oblongata

arcuate popliteal ligament n : a triangular ligamentous band in the posterior part of the knee that passes medially downward from the lateral condyle of the femur to the area between the condyles of the tibia and to the head of the fibula — compare OBLIQUE POPLITEAL LIGAMENT

arcuate vein n : any of the veins of the kidney that accompany the arcuate arteries, drain blood from the interlobular veins, and empty into the interlobar veins

ar·cu·a·tion \ˌär-kyə-ˈwā-shən\ *n* : an arching or curving

ar·cus \ˈär-kəs\ *n, pl* **arcus** : an anatomical arch

arcus se·nil·is \-sə-ˈnil-əs\ *n* : a whitish ring-shaped or bow-shaped deposit in the cornea that frequently occurs in old age

ARD *abbr* acute respiratory disease

ar·dor uri·nae \ˈär-ˌdȯr-yù-ˈrī-nē, -dər-, -yə-, -ˌnī\ *n* : a scalding sensation during urination

ARDS *abbr* acute respiratory distress syndrome; adult respiratory distress syndrome

ar·ea \ˈar-ē-ə, ˈer-\ *n* : a part of the cerebral cortex having a particular function — see ASSOCIATION AREA, MOTOR AREA, SENSORY AREA

area opa·ca \-ō-ˈpā-kə\ *n* : the peripheral opaque area that surrounds the area pellucida of a vertebrate embryo (as of a bird) formed by discoidal cleavage

area pel·lu·ci·da \-pə-ˈlü-səd-ə\ *n* : the pellucid central area that immediately surrounds a vertebrate embryo (as of a bird) formed by discoidal cleavage

area pla·cen·ta·lis \-ˌplas-ən-ˈtā-ləs\ *n* : the part of the trophoblast in early placental vertebrate embryos that lies in immediate contact with the uterine mucosa

area po·stre·ma \-pō-ˈstrē-mə, -päs-ˈtrē-\ *n* : a tongue-shaped structure in the caudal region of the fourth ventricle of the brain

areata — see ALOPECIA AREATA

area vas·cu·lo·sa \-ˌvas-kyə-ˈlō-sə\ *n* : the inner portion of the area opaca in which blood and blood-vessel formation is initiated

are·ca \ə-ˈrē-kə, ˈar-ə-kə\ *n* **1** *cap* : a small genus of pinnate-leaved palms of tropical Asia having thick-rinded fruits and including the betel palm **2** : a palm of the genus *Areca* or of any of several related genera; *esp* : BETEL PALM

arec·o·line \ə-ˈrek-ə-ˌlēn\ *n* : a toxic parasympathomimetic alkaloid C₈H₁₃NO₂ that is used as a veterinary anthelmintic and occurs naturally in betel nuts

are·flex·ia \ˌā-ri-ˈflek-sē-ə\ *n* : absence of reflexes — **are·flex·ic** \-ˈflek-sik\ *adj*

are·gen·er·a·tive \ˌā-ri-ˈjen-ə-ˌrāt-iv, -ˈjen-(ə)rət-\ *adj* : relating to or being aplastic anemia

ar·e·na·ceous \ˌar-ə-ˈnā-shəs\ *adj* : resembling, made of, or containing sand or sandy particles

ar·e·na·tion \ˌar-ə-ˈnā-shən\ *n* : the therapeutic application of sand to the body

Are·na·vi·ri·dae \ˌar-ə-nə-ˈvir-ə-ˌdē, ə-ˌrē-\ *n pl* : a family of single-stranded RNA viruses that have a grainy appearance due to the presence of ribosomes in the virion and that are usu. transmitted to humans by infected wild rodents through contamination of food and personal items or by inhalation of the airborne virus

are·na·vi·rus \ˌar-ə-nə-ˈvī-rəs, ə-ˌrē-\ *n* **1** *cap* : a genus of the family *Arenaviridae* that includes the Machupo virus, the Junin virus, and the causative agents of lymphocytic choriomeningitis and Lassa fever **2** : any of the family *Arenaviridae* of single-stranded RNA viruses

are·o·la \ə-ˈrē-ə-lə\ *n, pl* **-lae** \-ˌlē\ *or* **-las** : a small area between things or about something: as **a** : the colored ring around the nipple or around a vesicle or pustule **b** : the portion of the iris that borders the pupil of the eye

are·o·lar \-lər\ *adj* **1** : of, relating to, or like an areola **2** : of, relating to, or consisting of areolar tissue

areolar tissue *n* : fibrous connective tissue having the fibers loosely arranged in a net or meshwork

are·o·late \-lət, -ˌlāt\ *adj* : divided into or marked by areolae ⟨∼ colonies of bacteria⟩ — **are·o·la·tion** \ˌə-ˌrē-ə-ˈlā-shən\ *n*

ar·e·om·e·ter \ˌar-ē-ˈäm-ət-ər\ *n* : HYDROMETER — **ar·e·o·met·ric** \-ē-ə-ˈme-trik\ *or* **ar·e·o·met·ri·cal** \-tri-kəl\ *adj* — **ar·e·o·met·ri·cal·ly** \-k(ə-)lē\ *adv*

Arg *abbr* arginine; arginyl

Ar·gas \ˈär-gəs, -ˌgas\ *n* : a genus of ticks of the family Argasidae including the fowl ticks (as *A. persicus*)

Ar·gas·i·dae \är-ˈgas-ə-ˌdē\ *n pl* : a family of ticks of the superfamily Ixodoidea that comprises the soft ticks and includes a number of medically and economically important ticks all of which lack a scutum and exhibit no marked sexual dimorphism — see ARGAS, ORNITHODOROS — **ar·gas·id** \-əd\ *adj*

ar·gen·taf·fin \är-ˈjent-ə-fən\ *or* **ar·gen·taf·fine** \-fən, -ˌfēn\ *adj* **1 a** : depositing reduced silver from ammoniated silver hydroxide solutions — used of certain cell granules containing phenols or polyamines **b** : of, relating to, or being argentaffin cells **2** : ARGYROPHILIC — **ar·gen·taf·fin·i·ty** \-ˌjent-ə-ˈfin-ət-ē\ *n, pl* **-ties**

argentaffin cell *or* **argentaffine cell** *n* : any of various specialized epithelial cells of the gastrointestinal tract that stain readily with silver salts

ar·gen·taf·fin·o·ma \är-ˌjent-ə-fə-ˈnō-mə\ *n, pl* **-mas** *also* **-ma·ta** \-mət-ə\ : CARCINOID

ar·gen·tic \är-ˈjent-ik\ *adj* : of, relating to, or containing silver esp. when bivalent

ar·gen·to·phil·ic \är-ˌjent-ə-ˈfil-ik\ *also* **ar·gen·to·phil** \-ˈjent-ə-ˌfil\ *or* **ar·gen·to·phile** \-ˌfīl\ *adj* : ARGYROPHILIC

ar·gen·tous \är-ˈjent-əs\ *adj* : of, relating to, or containing silver esp. when monovalent

ar·gi·nase \ˈär-jə-ˌnās, -ˌnāz\ *n* : a crystalline enzyme that converts naturally occurring arginine into ornithine and urea

ar·gi·nine \ˈär-jə-ˌnēn\ *n* : a crystalline basic amino acid C₆H₁₄N₄O₂ derived from guanidine — abbr. *Arg*

arginine vasopressin *n* : vasopressin in which the eighth amino acid residue in its polypeptide chain is an arginine residue (as in most mammals including humans) rather than a lysine residue (as in pigs) — abbr. *AVP*

ar·gi·nyl \ˈär-jə-ˌnil\ *n* : the amino acid radical or residue (NH₂)₂CNHCH₂CH(NH₂)CO– of arginine — abbr. *Arg*

ar·gon \ˈär-ˌgän\ *n* : a colorless odorless inert gaseous element found in the air and in volcanic gases and used esp. in lasers and electric bulbs — symbol *Ar*; see ELEMENT table

Ar·gyll Rob·ert·son pupil \är-ˌgīl-ˈräb-ərt-sən-\ *n* : a pupil characteristic of neurosyphilis that fails to react to light but still reacts in accommodation to distance

Robertson, Douglas Argyll (1837–1909), British ophthalmologist. The leading ophthalmologist in Scotland, Robertson specialized in the physiology and diseases of the eye. He published more than fifty medical papers on such topics as etiology of glaucoma, retinitis pigmentosa, and hydrophthalmos. In 1869 he produced his most significant contribution, an article concerned with accommodation in miosis associated with spinal diseases. Robertson was also a popular teacher, and the naming of the condition in his honor gave rise to the quip that it was "far better to be an Argyll Robertson pupil than to have one."

ar·gyr·ia \är-ˈjir-ē-ə\ *n* : permanent dark discoloration of skin caused by overuse of medicinal silver preparations

Ar·gy·rol \ˈär-jə-ˌrȯl, -ˌrōl\ *trademark* — used for a silver-protein compound whose aqueous solution is used as a local antiseptic esp. for mucous membranes

ar·gyr·o·phil·ia \ˌär-jə-(ˌ)rō-ˈfil-ē-ə, -rə-\ *n* : the property of being argyrophilic

ar·gyr·o·phil·ic \ˌär-jə-(ˌ)rō-ˈfil-ik, -rə-\ *also* **ar·gyr·o·phil** \ˈär-jə-(ˌ)rō-ˌfil, -rə-\ *or* **ar·gyr·o·phile** \-ˌfīl\ *adj* : having an affinity for silver — used of certain cells, structures, or tissues that selectively reduce silver salts to metallic silver ⟨∼ cytoplasmic inclusions⟩

ar·gy·ro·sis \ˌär-jə-ˈrō-səs\ *n, pl* **-ro·ses** \-ˈrō-ˌsēz\ : ARGYRIA

ari·bo·fla·vin·osis \ˌā-ˌrī-bə-ˌflā-və-ˈnō-səs\ *n, pl* **-oses** \-ˌsēz\ : a deficiency disease due to inadequate intake of riboflavin and characterized by sores on the mouth — called also *hyporiboflavinosis*

Ar·i·cept \ˈar-ə-ˌsept, ˈer-\ *trademark* — used for a preparation of the hydrochloride of donepezil

Aris·to·lo·chia \(ˌ)a-ˌris-tə-ˈlō-kē-ə\ *n* : a large genus (the type of the family Aristolochiaceae) of mostly tropical herbs or woody vines with pungent aromatic rootstocks and very irregular flowers that includes several that have been used medicinally (as Texas snakeroot and Virginia snakeroot)

arith·mo·ma·nia \ə-ˌrith-mō-ˈmā-nē-ə, -nyə\ *n* : a morbid compulsion to count objects

arm \ˈärm\ *n* **1 a** : a human upper limb **b** : the part of the human upper limb between the shoulder and the wrist; *also* : BRACHIUM **2 a** : the forelimb of a vertebrate other than a human being **b** : a limb of an invertebrate animal **c** : any of the usu. two parts of a chromosome lateral to the centromere

ar·ma·men·tar·i·um \ˌär-mə-ˌmen-ˈter-ē-əm, -mən-\ *n, pl* **-tar·ia** \-ē-ə\ : the equipment, pharmaceuticals, and methods used in medicine

armed \ˈärmd\ *adj* **1** : having an arm or arms esp. of a specified kind or number — usu. used in combination ⟨long=*armed*⟩ ⟨two-*armed*⟩ **2** : having a spiny rostellum ⟨a tapeworm ∼ with numerous hammer-shaped hooks⟩

arm·pit \ˈärm-ˌpit\ *n* : the hollow beneath the junction of the arm and shoulder : AXILLA

Ar·neth index \ˈär-ˌnet-\ *n* : an age classification of blood granulocytes and esp. neutrophils that is based on the number of lobes of the nucleus with increasing lobulation regarded as indicative of increasing age — see SHIFT TO THE LEFT, SHIFT TO THE RIGHT; compare SCHILLING INDEX

  Arneth, Joseph (1873–1955), German physician. Arneth specialized in hematology and wrote several studies of diseases of the blood. He introduced the Arneth index in 1904 and advocated its use as a valuable aid in determining the reaction of bone marrow to infectious agents.

ar·ni·ca \ˈär-ni-kə\ *n* **1** *cap* : a large genus of composite herbs having flower heads that are discoid or have bright yellow rays **b** : a plant of the genus *Arnica* **2 a** : the dried flower head of any of several herbs of the genus *Arnica* (esp. *A. montana*) used for stimulant and local irritant effect esp. in the form of a liniment for bruises, sprains, and swellings **b** : a tincture made from arnica

aro·ma·tase \ə-ˈrō-mə-ˌtās, -ˌtāz\ *n* : an enzyme or complex of enzymes that promotes the conversion of an androgen (as testosterone) into estrogens (as estradiol)

aro·ma·ther·a·py \ə-ˌrō-mə-ˈther-ə-pē\ *n, pl* **-pies** : massage of the body and esp. of the face with a preparation of fragrant essential oils extracted from herbs, flowers, and fruits; *broadly* : the use of aroma to enhance a feeling of well-being — **aro·ma·ther·a·pist** \-pəst\ *n*

¹aro·mat·ic \ˌar-ə-ˈmat-ik\ *adj* **1** : of, relating to, or having a smell or odor **2** *of an organic compound* : characterized by increased chemical stability resulting from the delocalization of electrons in a ring system (as benzene) containing usu. multiple conjugated double bonds — compare ALICYCLIC, ALIPHATIC

²aromatic *n* **1** : an aromatic plant, drug, or medicine **2** : an aromatic organic compound

aromatic ammonia spirit *n* : a solution of ammonia and ammonium carbonate in alcohol and distilled water perfumed with the oils of lemon, lavender, and nutmeg and used as a stimulant, carminative, and antacid — called also *aromatic spirit of ammonia*

aromatic bitters *n pl* : bitters that contain aromatic oils but little tannin

aromatic spirit of ammonia *n* : AROMATIC AMMONIA SPIRIT

aro·ma·tize *or Brit* **aro·ma·tise** \ə-ˈrō-mə-ˌtīz\ *vt* **-tized** *or Brit* **-tised; -tiz·ing** *or Brit* **-tis·ing** **1** : to make aromatic : FLAVOR **2** : to convert into one or more aromatic compounds — **aro·ma·ti·za·tion** \-ˌrō-mət-ə-ˈzā-shən\ *n*

arous·al \ə-ˈrau̇-zəl\ *n* : the act of arousing : state of being aroused ⟨sexual ∼⟩; *specif* : responsiveness to stimuli ⟨altered states of consciousness . . . associated with relaxation or low ∼ —Paul Bakan⟩

arouse \ə-ˈrau̇z\ *vt* **aroused; arous·ing** **1** : to rouse or stimulate to action or to physiological readiness for activity ⟨became sexually *aroused*⟩ **2** : to give rise to ⟨a response *aroused* by a stimulus⟩

ar·rec·tor \ə-ˈrek-tər, a-\ *n, pl* **ar·rec·to·res** \ˌar-ˌek-ˈtōr-(ˌ)ēz\ *or* **ar·rec·tors** : ERECTOR

arrector pi·li muscle \-ˈpī-ˌlī-, -ˈpil-ē-\ *n* : one of the small fan-shaped smooth muscles associated with the base of each hair that contract when the body surface is chilled and erect the hairs, compress an oil gland above each muscle, and produce the appearance of goose bumps — called also *erector pili muscle, pilomotor muscle*

¹ar·rest \ə-ˈrest\ *vt* : to bring to a standstill or state of inactivity ⟨∼ed tuberculosis⟩ ⟨∼ed labor⟩ ∼ *vi* : to undergo cardiac arrest ⟨the . . . patient has ∼ed while being transported to surgery —Wayne Fields⟩ — **ar·rest·ment** *n*

²arrest *n* : the condition of being stopped ⟨developmental ∼⟩ — see CARDIAC ARREST; compare CURE 1, REMISSION

ar·rhe·no·blas·to·ma \ə-ˌrē-nō-bla-ˈstō-mə, ə-ˌrē-nō-\ *n, pl* **-mas** *also* **-ma·ta** \-mət-ə\ : a sometimes malignant tumor of the ovary that by the secretion of male hormone induces development of secondary male characteristics — compare GYNANDROBLASTOMA

ar·rhe·not·o·ky \ˌar-ə-ˈnät-ə-kē\ *n, pl* **-kies** : parthenogenesis in which only males are produced — compare DEUTEROTOKY, THELYTOKY

ar·rhyth·mia \ā-ˈrith-mē-ə\ *n* : an alteration in rhythm of the heartbeat either in time or force

ar·rhyth·mic \-mik\ *adj* **1** : lacking rhythm or regularity ⟨∼ locomotor activity⟩ **2** : of, relating to, characterized by, or resulting from arrhythmia ⟨∼ risk⟩ ⟨∼ death⟩

ar·row·root \ˈar-ō-ˌrüt, ˈar-ə-, -ˌru̇t\ *n* **1 a** : any plant of the genus *Maranta*; *esp* : one (*M. arundinacea*) whose roots yield an easily digested edible starch **b** : any of several plants (as of the genera *Zamia* and *Curcuma*) that yield a similar starch **2** : starch yielded by an arrowroot

ARRT *abbr* **1** American registered respiratory therapist **2** American Registry of Radiologic Technologists

ar·sa·nil·ic acid \ˌärs-ᵊn-ˌil-ik-\ *n* : any of the poisonous crystalline isomeric acids $NH_2C_6H_4AsO(OH)_2$; *esp* : the para isomer analogous to sulfanilic acid used in making organic arsenical drugs

ar·se·nate \ˈärs-nət, -ᵊn-ət, -ᵊn-ˌāt\ *n* : a salt or ester of an arsenic acid

¹ar·se·nic \ˈärs-nik, -ᵊn-ik\ *n* **1** : a trivalent and pentavalent solid poisonous element that is commonly metallic steel=gray, crystalline, and brittle — symbol *As*; see ELEMENT table **2** : ARSENIC TRIOXIDE

²ar·sen·ic \är-ˈsen-ik\ *adj* : of, relating to, or containing arsenic esp. with a valence of five

ar·sen·ic acid \är-ˌsen-ik-\ *n* : any of three arsenic-containing acids that are analogous to the phosphoric acids

¹ar·sen·i·cal \är-ˈsen-i-kəl\ *adj* : of, relating to, containing, or caused by arsenic ⟨an ∼ drug⟩ ⟨∼ poisoning⟩

²arsenical *n* : a compound or preparation containing arsenic

ar·sen·i·cal·ism \-kə-ˌliz-əm\ *n* : chronic arsenic poisoning

ar·se·nic trioxide \ˌärs-nik-, -ᵊn-ik-\ *n* : a poisonous trioxide As_2O_3 or As_4O_6 of arsenic that was formerly used in medicine and dentistry but has been abandoned for therapeutic purposes and is now used esp. as an insecticide and weed killer — called also *arsenic, arsenious acid, arsenious oxide, white arsenic*

ar·se·nide \ˈärs-ᵊn-ˌīd\ *n* : a binary compound of arsenic with a more positive element

ar·se·ni·ous \är-ˈsē-nē-əs\ *also* **ar·se·nous** \ˈärs-nəs, -ᵊn-əs\ *adj* : of, relating to, or containing arsenic esp. when trivalent

arsenious acid *n* : ARSENIC TRIOXIDE; *also* : any of several acids derived from arsenic trioxide

arsenious oxide *n* : ARSENIC TRIOXIDE

ar·se·nite \ˈärs-ə-ˌnīt\ *n* : a salt or ester of an arsenious acid

ar·se·ni·um \är-ˈsē-nē-əm\ *n* : ARSENIC

ar·se·niu·ret·ted *or* **ar·se·niu·ret·ed** \är-ˈsen-yə-ˌret-əd, -ˈsen-\ *adj* : combined with arsenic ⟨∼ hydrogen⟩

ar·se·no·ther·a·py \ˌärs-nō-ˈther-ə-pē, ˌärs-ᵊn-ō-, är-ˌsen-ō-\ *n, pl* **-pies** : treatment of disease with any form of arsenic

arsenous *var of* ARSENIOUS

ar·sen·ox·ide \ˌärs-ᵊn-ˈäk-ˌsīd\ *n* : an active metabolic product of an arsenical (as arsphenamine) that is the base of oxophenarsine

ar·sine \är-ˈsēn, ˈär-ˌ\ *n* : a colorless flammable extremely poisonous gas AsH₃ with an odor like garlic; *also* : a derivative of arsine

ar·so·ni·um \är-ˈsō-nē-əm\ *n* : a monovalent arsenic-containing radical AsH₄ analogous to the ammonium radical NH₄

ars·phen·a·mine \ärs-ˈfen-ə-ˌmēn, -mən\ *n* : a light-yellow toxic hygroscopic powder C₁₂Cl₂H₁₄As₂N₂O₂·2H₂O formerly used in the treatment esp. of syphilis and yaws — called also *salvarsan, six-o-six*

ART *abbr* accredited record technician

artefact, artefactual *chiefly Brit var of* ARTIFACT, ARTIFACTUAL

ar·te·mis·ia \ˌärt-ə-ˈmizh(-ē)-ə, -ˈmē-zh(ē)-ə, -ˈmiz-ē-ə\ *n* **1** *cap* : a genus of composite shrubs and herbs (as the sagebrushes and santonicas) that have strongly scented foliage and small rayless flower heads **2** : any plant of the genus *Artemisia*

   Ar·te·mis \ˈärt-ə-məs\, Greek mythological character. Artemis was the Greek goddess of the hunt, wild animals, and the forest. She was identified with the Roman goddess Diana. Artemis was also worshiped as a goddess of chastity and childbirth. The genus *Artemisia* of composite plants was named after her, and a plant of this genus was formerly used to promote menstruation.

ar·te·mis·i·nin \ˌärt-ə-ˈmis-ᵊn-ən\ *n* : an antimalarial drug C₁₅H₂₂O₅ that is a peroxide derivative of sesquiterpene and is obtained from the leaves of a Chinese artemisia (*Artemisia annua*) or made synthetically

ar·te·re·nol \ˌärt-ə-ˈrē-ˌnȯl, -ˌnōl\ *n* : NOREPINEPHRINE

ar·te·ria \är-ˈtir-ē-ə\ *n, pl* **-ri·ae** \-ē-ˌē\ : ARTERY

ar·te·ri·al \är-ˈtir-ē-əl\ *adj* **1** : of or relating to an artery **2** : relating to or being the bright red blood present in most arteries that has been oxygenated in lungs or gills — compare VENOUS 3 — **ar·te·ri·al·ly** \-ē-ə-lē\ *adv*

ar·te·ri·al·ize *also Brit* **ar·te·ri·al·ise** \är-ˈtir-ē-ə-ˌlīz\ *vt* **-ized** *also Brit* **-ised; -iz·ing** *also Brit* **-is·ing** : to transform (venous blood) into arterial blood by oxygenation — **ar·te·ri·al·iza·tion** \-ˌtir-ē-ə-lə-ˈzā-shən\ *n*

ar·te·rio·cap·il·lary \är-ˌtir-ē-ō-ˈkap-ə-ˌler-ē, *Brit usu* -kə-ˈpil-ə-rē\ *adj* : relating to, situated in, or affecting the arteries and capillaries ⟨∼ obliteration⟩

ar·te·rio·gram \är-ˈtir-ē-ə-ˌgram\ *n* : a radiograph of an artery made by arteriography

ar·te·ri·og·ra·phy \är-ˌtir-ē-ˈäg-rə-fē\ *n, pl* **-phies** : the radiographic visualization of an artery after injection of a radiopaque substance — **ar·te·rio·graph·ic** \-ē-ə-ˈgraf-ik\ *adj* — **ar·te·rio·graph·i·cal·ly** \-i-k(ə-)lē\ *adv*

ar·te·ri·o·la \är-ˌtir-ē-ˈō-lə\ *n, pl* **-lae** \-ˌlē\ : ARTERIOLE

ar·te·ri·ole \är-ˈtir-ē-ˌōl\ *n* : any of the small terminal twigs of an artery that ends in capillaries — **ar·te·ri·o·lar** \-ˌtir-ē-ˈō-ˌlär, -lər\ *adj*

ar·te·rio·li·tis \är-ˌtir-ē-ō-ˈlīt-əs\ *n* : inflammation of the arterioles

ar·te·rio·lo·ne·cro·sis \är-ˌtir-ē-ˌō-(ˌ)lō-nə-ˈkrō-səs, -ē-ə-ˌlō-, -ne-\ *n, pl* **-cro·ses** \-ˌsēz\ : necrosis of the arterioles

ar·te·rio·lop·a·thy \-ē-ə-ˈläp-ə-thē\ *n, pl* **-thies** : disease of the arterioles

ar·te·rio·lo·scle·ro·sis \är-ˌtir-ē-ˌō-(ˌ)lō-sklə-ˈrō-səs, -ē-ə-ˌlō-\ *n, pl* **-ro·ses** \-ˌsēz\ : thickening of the intima of arterioles (as of the kidney in hypertension) by hyaline and fatty deposits that reduce the lumen and obstruct blood flow

ar·te·rio·lu·mi·nal \är-ˌtir-ē-ō-ˈlü-mən-ᵊl\ *adj* : relating to or being the small vessels that branch from the arterioles of the heart and empty directly into its lumen

ar·te·rio·mes·en·ter·ic \-ˌmez-ᵊn-ˈter-ik, -ˌmes-\ *adj* : relating to or involving the arteries and mesentery

ar·te·ri·op·a·thy \är-ˌtir-ē-ˈäp-ə-thē\ *n, pl* **-thies** : a disease of the arteries

ar·te·ri·or·rha·phy \är-ˌtir-ē-ˈȯr-ə-fē\ *n, pl* **-phies** : a surgical operation of suturing an artery

ar·te·rio·scle·ro·sis \är-ˌtir-ē-ō-sklə-ˈrō-səs\ *n, pl* **-ro·ses** \-ˌsēz\ : a chronic disease characterized by abnormal thickening and hardening of the arterial walls with resulting loss of elasticity — compare ATHEROSCLEROSIS

arteriosclerosis ob·lit·e·rans \-ä-ˈblit-ə-ˌranz\ *n* : chronic arteriosclerosis marked by occlusion of arteries and esp. those supplying the extremities

¹**ar·te·rio·scle·rot·ic** \-ˈrät-ik\ *adj* : of, relating to, or affected with arteriosclerosis

²**arteriosclerotic** *n* : an arteriosclerotic individual

arteriosi — see CONUS ARTERIOSUS

ar·te·rio·si·nu·soi·dal \är-ˌtir-ē-ō-ˌsī-n(y)ə-ˈsȯid-ᵊl\ *adj* : relating to or being the vessels that connect the arterioles and sinusoids of the heart

ar·te·rio·spasm \är-ˈtir-ē-ō-ˌspaz-əm\ *n* : spasm of an artery — **ar·te·rio·spas·tic** \-ˌtir-ē-ō-ˈspas-tik\ *adj*

arteriosum — see LIGAMENTUM ARTERIOSUM

arteriosus — see CONUS ARTERIOSUS, DUCTUS ARTERIOSUS, PATENT DUCTUS ARTERIOSUS, TRUNCUS ARTERIOSUS

ar·te·ri·ot·o·my \är-ˌtir-ē-ˈät-ə-mē\ *n, pl* **-mies** : the surgical incision of an artery

ar·te·rio·ve·nous \är-ˌtir-ē-ō-ˈvē-nəs\ *adj* : of, relating to, or connecting the arteries and veins ⟨∼ anastomoses⟩

ar·ter·i·tis \ˌärt-ə-ˈrīt-əs\ *n, pl* **-te·rit·i·des** \-ˈrit-ə-ˌdēz\ : arterial inflammation — see GIANT CELL ARTERITIS — **ar·ter·it·ic** \-ˈrit-ik\ *adj*

ar·tery \ˈärt-ə-rē\ *n, pl* **-ter·ies** : any of the tubular branching muscular- and elastic-walled vessels that carry blood from the heart through the body

ar·thral \ˈär-thrəl\ *adj* : of or relating to a joint

ar·thral·gia \är-ˈthral-j(ē-)ə\ *n* : pain in one or more joints — **ar·thral·gic** \-jik\ *adj*

ar·threc·to·my \är-ˈthrek-tə-mē\ *n, pl* **-mies** : surgical excision of a joint

¹**ar·thrit·ic** \är-ˈthrit-ik\ *adj* : of, relating to, or affected with arthritis — **ar·thrit·i·cal·ly** \-i-k(ə-)lē\ *adv*

²**arthritic** *n* : a person affected with arthritis

ar·thri·tis \är-ˈthrīt-əs\ *n, pl* **-thrit·i·des** \-ˈthrit-ə-ˌdēz\ : inflammation of joints due to infectious, metabolic, or constitutional causes; *also* : a specific arthritic condition (as gouty arthritis or psoriatic arthritis)

arthritis de·for·mans \-dē-ˈfȯr-ˌmanz\ *n* : a chronic arthritis marked by deformation of affected joints

ar·thro·cen·te·sis \ˌär-(ˌ)thrō-sen-ˈtē-səs\ *n, pl* **-te·ses** \-ˌsēz\ : surgical puncture of a joint (as for the withdrawal of fluid)

ar·thro·co·nid·i·um \ˌär-(ˌ)thrō-kə-ˈnid-ē-əm\ *n, pl* **-ia** \-ē-ə\ : one of the small conidia borne in chains by various fungi (as of the genera *Coccidioides* and *Trichosporon*) — called also *arthrospore*

ar·throd·e·sis \är-ˈthräd-ə-səs\ *n, pl* **-e·ses** \-ˌsēz\ : the surgical immobilization of a joint so that the bones grow solidly together : artificial ankylosis

ar·thro·dia \är-ˈthrōd-ē-ə\ *n, pl* **-di·ae** \-ē-ˌē\ : GLIDING JOINT — **ar·thro·di·al** \-ē-əl\ *adj* — **ar·throd·ic** \-ˈthräd-ik\ *adj*

ar·thro·dys·pla·sia \ˌär-(ˌ)thrō-dis-ˈplā-zh(ē-)ə, -zē-ə\ *n* : abnormal development of a joint

ar·throg·e·nous \är-ˈthräj-ə-nəs\ *adj* : developing vegetative resting cells (as arthrospores) that function as spores ⟨∼ fungi⟩

ar·thro·gram \ˈär-thrə-ˌgram, -thrō-\ *n* : a radiograph of a joint made by arthrography

ar·throg·ra·phy \är-ˈthräg-rə-fē\ *n, pl* **-phies** : the radiographic visualization of a joint (as the hip or shoulder) after the injection of a radiopaque substance — **ar·thro·graph·ic** \ˌär-thrə-ˈgraf-ik\ *adj*

ar·thro·gry·po·sis \ˌär-(ˌ)thrō-gri-ˈpō-səs\ *n* **1** : congenital fixation of a joint in an extended or flexed position **2** : any

---

\ə\ **abut** \ᵊ\ **kitten** \ər\ **further** \a\ **ash** \ā\ **ace** \ä\ **cot, cart**
\aù\ **out** \ch\ **chin** \e\ **bet** \ē\ **easy** \g\ **go** \i\ **hit** \ī\ **ice** \j\ **job**
\ŋ\ **sing** \ō\ **go** \ȯ\ **law** \ȯi\ **boy** \th\ **thin** \t̲h̲\ **the** \ü\ **loot**
\ù\ **foot** \y\ **yet** \zh\ **vision** *See also* Pronunciation Symbols page

of a group of congenital conditions characterized by reduced mobility of multiple joints due to contractures causing fixation of the joints in extension or flexion

arthrogryposis mul·ti·plex con·gen·i·ta \-'məl-tə-ˌpleks-kən-'jen-ət-ə\ *n* : ARTHROGRYPOSIS 2

ar·throl·o·gy \är-'thräl-ə-jē\ *n, pl* **-gies** : a science concerned with the study of joints

ar·throl·y·sis \är-'thräl-ə-səs\ *n, pl* **-y·ses** \-ˌsēz\ : surgical restoration of mobility to an ankylosed joint

ar·throm·e·ter \är-'thräm-ət-ər\ *n* : an instrument for measuring the range of movement of a joint

arthropathica — see PSORIASIS ARTHROPATHICA

ar·throp·a·thy \är-'thräp-ə-thē\ *n, pl* **-thies** : a disease of a joint

ar·thro·plas·ty \'är-thrə-ˌplas-tē\ *n, pl* **-ties** : plastic surgery of a joint (as the hip or knee) : the operative formation or restoration of a joint

Ar·throp·o·da \är-'thräp-əd-ə\ *n pl* : a phylum of invertebrate animals (as insects, arachnids, and crustaceans) having a segmented body and jointed appendages, usu. a shell of chitin molted at intervals, and an anterior brain dorsal to the alimentary canal and connected with a ventral chain of ganglia — **ar·thro·pod** \'är-thrə-ˌpäd\ *adj or n* — **ar·throp·o·dan** \är-'thräp-əd-ən\ *adj*

ar·thro·scope \'är-thrə-ˌskōp\ *n* : an endoscope that is inserted through an incision near a joint (as the knee) and is used for the visual examination, diagnosis, and treatment of the interior of a joint

ar·thros·co·py \är-'thräs-kə-pē\ *n, pl* **-pies** : examination of a joint with an arthroscope; *also* : joint surgery using an arthroscope — **ar·thro·scop·ic** \ˌär-thrə-'skäp-ik\ *adj*

ar·thro·sis \är-'thrō-səs\ *n, pl* **-thro·ses** \-ˌsēz\ **1** : an articulation or line of juncture between bones **2** : a degenerative disease of a joint

ar·thro·spore \'är-thrə-ˌspō(ə)r, -ˌspȯ(ə)r\ *n* : ARTHROCONIDIUM

ar·throt·o·my \är-'thrät-ə-mē\ *n, pl* **-mies** : incision into a joint

Ar·thus reaction \'är-thəs-, är-'tüēs-\ *n* : a reaction that follows injection of an antigen into an animal in which hypersensitivity has been previously established and that involves infiltrations, edema, sterile abscesses, and in severe cases gangrene — called also *Arthus phenomenon*

Ar·thus \är-tüēs\, **Nicolas Maurice (1862–1945),** French bacteriologist and physiologist. Arthus was primarily concerned with venoms and antivenins and with coagulability and anticoagulants. In 1890 he published an article on coagulation that demonstrated for the first time the essential role of calcium in blood coagulation. In 1903, in an article reporting a study involving repeated injections of horse serum into rabbits, he reported discovery of the phenomenon of local anaphylaxis, a phenomenon that has since become identified with his name.

ar·tic·u·lar \är-'tik-yə-lər\ *adj* : of or relating to a joint

articular capsule *n* : JOINT CAPSULE

articular cartilage *n* : cartilage that covers the articular surfaces of bones

articular disk *n* : a cartilage (as the meniscus of the temporomandibular joint) interposed between two articular surfaces and partially or completely separating the joint cavity into two compartments

articular lamella *n* : the layer of compact bone to which the articular cartilage is attached

articular process *n* : either of two processes on each side of a vertebra that articulate with adjoining vertebrae: **a** : one on each side of the neural arch that projects upward and articulates with an inferior articular process of the next more cranial vertebra — called also *superior articular process* **b** : one on each side of the neural arch that projects downward and articulates with a superior articular process of the next more caudal vertebra — called also *inferior articular process*

¹ar·tic·u·late \är-'tik-yə-lət\ *adj* : consisting of segments united by joints : JOINTED ⟨∼ animals⟩

²ar·tic·u·late \-ˌlāt\ *vb* **-lat·ed; -lat·ing** *vt* **1** : to utter distinct-

ly **2** : to unite by means of a joint **3** : to arrange (artificial teeth) on an articulator ∼ *vi* **1** : to utter articulate sounds **2** : to become united or connected by or as if by a joint ⟨bones that ∼ with each other⟩

ar·tic·u·la·tion \(ˌ)är-ˌtik-yə-'lā-shən\ *n* **1** : the action or manner in which the parts come together at a joint ⟨a sketch showing the ∼ of the limbs⟩ **2 a** : a joint between bones or cartilages in the vertebrate skeleton that is immovable when the bones are directly united, slightly movable when they are united by an intervening substance, or more or less freely movable when the articular surfaces are covered with smooth cartilage and surrounded by a joint capsule — see AMPHIARTHROSIS, DIARTHROSIS, SYNARTHROSIS **b** : a movable joint between rigid parts of any animal (as between the segments of an insect appendage) **3 a** : the act or manner of articulating **b** : an articulated utterance or sound **4 a** (1) : the act of properly arranging artificial teeth (2) : an arrangement of artificial teeth — see OCCLUSION 2a

ar·tic·u·la·tor \är-'tik-yə-ˌlāt-ər\ *n* : one that articulates; *specif* : an apparatus used in dentistry for obtaining correct articulation of artificial teeth

ar·tic·u·la·to·ry \är-'tik-yə-lə-ˌtōr-ē, -ˌtȯr-\ *adj* : of or relating to articulation ⟨paralysis of the ∼ muscles —Josephine Semmes⟩

articulo — see IN ARTICULO MORTIS

ar·ti·fact *or chiefly Brit* **ar·te·fact** \'ärt-ə-ˌfakt\ *n* **1** : a product of artificial character due to extraneous (as human) agency; *specif* : a product or formation in a microscopic preparation of a fixed tissue or cell that is caused by manipulation or reagents and is not indicative of actual structural relationships **2** : an electrocardiographic and electroencephalographic wave that arises from sources other than the heart or brain — **ar·ti·fac·tu·al** *or chiefly Brit* **ar·te·fac·tu·al** \ˌärt-ə-'fak-chə-(-wə)l, -'faksh-wəl\ *adj*

ar·ti·fi·cial \ˌärt-ə-'fish-əl\ *adj* **1** : humanly contrived often on a natural model ⟨an ∼ limb⟩ **2** : based on differential morphological characters not necessarily indicative of natural relationships ⟨an ∼ key for identification of a group of organisms⟩ — **ar·ti·fi·cial·ly** \-'fish-(ə-)lē\ *adv*

artificial insemination *n* : introduction of semen into part of the female reproductive tract (as the cervical opening, uterus, or fallopian tube) by other than natural means

artificial kidney *n* : an apparatus designed to do the work of the kidney during temporary stoppage of kidney function — called also *hemodialyzer*

artificial respiration *n* : the process of restoring or initiating breathing by forcing air into and out of the lungs to establish the rhythm of inspiration and expiration — see BACK PRESSURE-ARM LIFT METHOD, MOUTH-TO-MOUTH

Ar·tio·dac·ty·la \ˌärt-ē-ō-'dak-tə-lə\ *n pl* : an order of hoofed mammals (as the sheep, goat, pig, camel, or ox) with an even number of functional toes on each foot — compare PERISSODACTYLA — **ar·tio·dac·tyl** \-'dak-tᵊl\ *n or adj* — **ar·tio·dac·ty·lous** \-tə-ləs\ *adj*

ary·ep·i·glot·tic \ˌar-ē-ˌep-ə-'glät-ik\ *adj* : relating to or linking the arytenoid cartilage and the epiglottis ⟨∼ folds⟩

ar·yl \'ar-əl\ *n* : a radical (as phenyl) derived from an aromatic hydrocarbon by the removal of one hydrogen atom

ary·te·no·ep·i·glot·tic \ˌar-ə-ˌtē-(ˌ)nō-ˌep-ə-'glät-ik, ə-'rit-ᵊn-(ˌ)ō-\ *or* **ary·te·no·ep·i·glot·tid·e·an** \-ˌep-ə-glä-'tid-ē-ən\ *adj* : ARYEPIGLOTTIC

¹ary·te·noid \ˌar-ə-'tē-ˌnȯid, ə-'rit-ᵊn-ˌȯid\ *adj* **1** : relating to or being either of two small cartilages to which the vocal cords are attached and which are situated at the upper back part of the larynx **2** : relating to or being either of a pair of small muscles or an unpaired muscle of the larynx

²arytenoid *n* : an arytenoid cartilage or muscle

ary·te·noi·dec·to·my \ˌar-ə-ˌtē-ˌnȯi-'dek-tə-mē, ə-'rit-ᵊn-ˌȯi-\ *n, pl* **-mies** : surgical excision of an arytenoid cartilage

ary·te·noi·do·pexy \ˌar-ət-ə-'nȯid-ə-ˌpek-sē, ə-ˌrit-ᵊn-'ȯid-ə-\ *n, pl* **-pex·ies** : surgical fixation of arytenoid muscles or cartilages

as *abbr* astigmatism

As *symbol* arsenic

AS *abbr* **1** aortic stenosis **2** arteriosclerosis

ASA *abbr* [*a*cetyl*s*alicylic *a*cid] aspirin

asa·fet·i·da *or* **asa·foet·i·da** \ˌas-ə-ˈfit-əd-ē, -ˈfet-əd-ə\ *n* : the fetid gum resin of the root of several Asian plants of the genus *Ferula* (esp. *F. assafoetida, F. foetida,* or *F. narthex*) that was formerly used in medicine esp. as an antispasmodic and in folk medicine as a general prophylactic against disease

ASAP *abbr* as soon as possible

as·a·rum \ˈas-ə-rəm\ *n* **1** *cap* : a genus of herbs (family Aristolochiaceae) that are native to temperate regions of the northern hemisphere, have pungent aromatic roots and dull-colored flowers, and include the wild ginger **2** : the dried rhizome and roots of wild ginger used as aromatic bitters and as a flavoring agent

as·bes·tos \as-ˈbes-təs, az-\ *n* : any of several minerals that readily separate into long flexible fibers, that have been implicated as causes of certain cancers, and that have been used esp. formerly as fireproof insulating materials

as·bes·to·sis \ˌas-ˌbes-ˈtō-səs, ˌaz-\ *n, pl* **-to·ses** \-ˌsēz\ : a pneumoconiosis due to asbestos particles that is marked by fibrosis and scarring of lung tissue

as·ca·ri·a·sis \ˌas-kə-ˈrī-ə-səs\ *n, pl* **-a·ses** \-ˌsēz\ : infestation with or disease caused by ascarids

as·car·i·cid·al \ə-ˌskar-ə-ˈsīd-ᵊl\ *adj* : capable of destroying ascarids

as·car·i·cide \ə-ˈskar-ə-ˌsīd\ *n* : an agent destructive of ascarids

as·ca·rid \ˈas-kə-rəd\ *n* : a nematode worm of the family Ascaridae — **ascarid** *adj*

As·car·i·dae \ə-ˈskar-ə-ˌdē\ *n pl* : a family of large nematode worms (superfamily Ascaridoidea) that are usu. parasitic in the intestines of vertebrates, have three well-developed lips and a simple cylindrical esophagus, and include the common roundworm (*Ascaris lumbricoides*) parasitic in the human intestine — see ASCARIDIA, ASCARIS

As·ca·rid·ia \ˌas-kə-ˈrid-ē-ə\ *n* : a genus of nematode worms of the family Ascaridae that include an important intestinal parasite (*A. galli*) of some domestic fowl and esp. the chicken and that are distinguished from other ascarids by the presence of a preanal sucker

as·car·i·di·a·sis \ə-ˌskar-ə-ˈdī-ə-səs\ *n, pl* **-a·ses** : ASCARIASIS

as·car·i·do·sis \ə-ˌskar-ə-ˈdō-səs\ *n, pl* **-do·ses** \-ˌsēz\ : ASCARIASIS

as·ca·ris \ˈas-kə-rəs\ *n* **1** *cap* : a genus of Ascaridae comprising nematode worms with a 3-lipped mouth, resembling earthworms in size and superficial appearance, and including one (*A. lumbricoides*) parasitic in the human intestine **2** *pl* **as·car·i·des** \ə-ˈskar-ə-ˌdēz\ : ASCARID

As·ca·rops \ˈas-kə-ˌräps\ *n* : a genus of nematode worms (family Spiruridae) including a common reddish stomach worm (*A. strongylina*) of wild and domestic swine

as·cend \ə-ˈsend\ *vi* : to move upward: as **a** : to conduct nerve impulses toward or to the brain ⟨nerve fibers that ∼ to a nucleus of the brain⟩ ⟨∼ing and descending tracts⟩ **b** : to affect the extremities and esp. the lower limbs first and then the central nervous system ⟨∼ing paralysis⟩

ascending aorta *n* : the part of the aorta from its origin to the beginning of the arch

ascending colon *n* : the part of the large intestine that extends from the cecum to the bend on the right side below the liver — compare DESCENDING COLON, TRANSVERSE COLON

ascending lumbar vein *n* : a longitudinal vein on each side that connects the lumbar veins and is frequently the origin of the azygos vein on the right side and of the hemiazygos vein on the left

ascending palatine artery *n* : PALATINE ARTERY 1a

Asc·hel·min·thes \ˌask-(ˌ)hel-ˈmin-ˌthēz\ *n pl, in some classifications* : a phylum of pseudocoelomate animals including the major taxa Rotifera, Gastrotricha, Kinorhyncha, Nematoda, Nematomorpha, and sometimes the Acanthocephala all of which are sometimes regarded as independent phyla

Asch·heim–Zon·dek test \ˈäsh-(ˌ)hīm-ˈzän-dik-, -ˌtsän-\ *n* : a test formerly used esp. to determine human pregnancy in its early stages on the basis of the effect of a subcutaneous injection of the patient's urine on the ovaries of an immature female mouse

Asch·heim \ˈäsh-(ˌ)hīm\, **Selmor Samuel (1878–1965),** and **Zon·dek** \ˈtsón-ˌdek\, **Bernhard (1891–1966),** German obstetrician-gynecologists. In 1927 Aschheim and Zondek demonstrated that gonadotropic hormones are produced by the anterior lobe of the pituitary gland. They also isolated a gonadotropin now known as human chorionic gonadotropin in the urine of pregnant women. These discoveries led to the development in 1928 of their test for pregnancy. Zondek was also the author of a major work on the hormones of the ovary and the anterior pituitary.

Asch·off body \ˈä-ˌshóf-\ *n* : one of the tiny lumps in heart muscle that are typical of rheumatic heart disease and consist of swollen collagen, cells, and fibrils; *also* : one of the similar but larger lumps found under the skin esp. in rheumatic fever or polyarthritis — called also *Aschoff nodule*

Aschoff, Karl Albert Ludwig (1866–1942), German pathologist. One of the foremost pathologists of his time, Aschoff undertook noteworthy investigations into cholelithiasis, thrombosis, scurvy, and appendicitis. He also made a classic histopathologic study of myocarditis, and in 1904 in an article on myocarditis associated with acute rheumatic fever he presented his classic description of the inflammatory nodule (now known as the Aschoff body or nodule) that is characteristic of this rheumatic condition. Aschoff is also known for his later work on phagocytic cells, which he grouped into the reticuloendothelial system.

asci *pl of* ASCUS

as·ci·tes \ə-ˈsīt-ēz\ *n, pl* **ascites** : abnormal accumulation of serous fluid in the spaces between tissues and organs in the cavity of the abdomen — called also *hydroperitoneum* — **as·cit·ic** \-ˈsit-ik\ *adj*

as·cle·pi·as \ə-ˈsklē-pē-əs, a-\ *n* **1** *cap* : a genus (family Asclepiadaceae) of perennial herbs found chiefly in No. America with flowers having a corona of five concave hoods each of which bears a slender horn — see BUTTERFLY WEED, MILKWEED **2** : any plant of the genus *Asclepias* **3** : the dried root of the butterfly weed formerly used as a diaphoretic and expectorant — called also *pleurisy root*

Aesculapius — see STAFF OF AESCULAPIUS

as·co·carp \ˈas-kə-ˌkärp\ *n* : the mature fruiting body of an ascomycetous fungus; *broadly* : such a body with its enclosed asci, spores, and paraphyses — **as·co·carp·ic** \ˌas-kə-ˈkär-pik\ *adj*

as·co·go·ni·um \ˌas-kə-ˈgō-nē-əm\ *n, pl* **-nia** \-nē-ə\ : the fertile basal often one-celled portion of an archicarp; *broadly* : ARCHICARP

as·co·my·cete \ˌas-kō-ˈmī-sə-(ˌ)tē, as-ˈkō-mi-ˌsēt\ *n* : any of a group of higher fungi (as yeasts and molds) with spores formed in asci that are variously considered to form a class (Ascomycetes), a subdivision (Ascomycotina), or a division (Ascomycota) — **as·co·my·ce·tous** \ˌas-kō-ˈmī-sēt-əs, ˌas-(ˌ)kō-mi-ˈsēt-əs\ *adj*

As·co·my·ce·tes \ˌas-kō-ˌmī-ˈsēt-ˌēz\ *n pl* : a large class of higher fungi comprising the ascomycetes when they are considered a class

As·co·my·co·ta \ˌas-kō-ˌmī-ˈkō-tə\ *n pl* : a division of higher fungi comprising the ascomycetes when they are considered a division

As·co·my·co·ti·na \ˌas-kō-ˌmī-kō-ˈtī-nə\ *n pl* : a subdivision of higher fungi comprising the ascomycetes when they are considered a subdivision

ascor·bate \ə-ˈskór-ˌbāt, -bət\ *n* : a salt of ascorbic acid

ascor·bic acid \ə-ˌskór-bik-\ *n* : VITAMIN C

as·co·spore \ˈas-kə-ˌspō(ə)r, -ˌspó(ə)r\ *n* : one of the spores contained in an ascus — **as·co·spor·ic** \ˌas-kə-ˈspór-ik, -ˈspór-\ *adj*

\ə\ **abut** \ᵊ\ kitten \ər\ **further** \a\ **ash** \ā\ **ace** \ä\ **cot, cart** \aú\ **out** \ch\ **chin** \e\ bet \ē\ **easy** \g\ **go** \i\ **hit** \ī\ **ice** \j\ **job** \ŋ\ **sing** \ō\ **go** \ó\ **law** \ói\ **boy** \th\ **thin** \t͟h\ **the** \ü\ **loot** \ú\ **foot** \y\ **yet** \zh\ **vision** *See also* Pronunciation Symbols page

as·co·spo·rog·e·nous \ˌas-ˌkō-spə-ˈräj-ə-nəs\ *adj* : having the capacity to form ascospores ⟨∼ yeasts⟩

ASCP *abbr* American Society of Clinical Pathologists

as·cus \ˈas-kəs\ *n, pl* **as·ci** \ˈas-ˌ(k)ī, -ˌkē\ : the membranous oval or tubular sporangium of an ascomycete

ASCVD *abbr* arteriosclerotic cardiovascular disease

asep·sis \(ˈ)ā-ˈsep-səs, ə-\ *n, pl* **asep·ses** \-ˌsēz\   **1** : the condition of being aseptic   **2** : the methods of producing or maintaining an aseptic condition

asep·tic \-ˈsep-tik\ *adj*   **1** : preventing infection ⟨∼ techniques⟩   **2** : free or freed from pathogenic microorganisms ⟨an ∼ operating room⟩ — **asep·ti·cal·ly** \-ti-k(ə-)lē\ *adv*

asex·u·al \(ˈ)ā-ˈseksh-(ə-)wəl, -ˈsek-shəl\ *adj*   **1** : lacking sex or functional sexual organs   **2** : produced without sexual action or differentiation ⟨∼ spores⟩ — **asex·u·al·i·ty** \ˌā-ˌsek-shə-ˈwal-ət-ē\ *n, pl* **-ties** — **asex·u·al·ly** \-ˈseksh-(ə-)wə-lē, -(ə-)lē\ *adv*

asexual generation *n* : a generation that reproduces only by asexual processes — used of organisms exhibiting alternation of generations

asex·u·al·i·za·tion *also Brit* **asex·u·al·i·sa·tion** \(ˈ)ā-ˌseksh-(ə-)wə-lə-ˈzā-shən, -ˌsek-shə-lə-\ *n* : the process of destroying the capacity for reproduction esp. by surgical means : STERILIZATION, CASTRATION

asexual reproduction *n* : reproduction (as cell division, spore formation, fission, or budding) without union of individuals or gametes

ash \ˈash\ *n, often attrib*   **1** : the solid residue left when combustible material is thoroughly burned or is oxidized by chemical means   **2 ashes** *pl* : the remains of the dead human body after cremation or disintegration

ASHD *abbr* arteriosclerotic heart disease

Asian flu \ˌā-zhən-, -shən-\ *n* : influenza that is caused by a subtype (H2N2) of the orthomyxovirus causing influenza A and that was responsible for about 70,000 deaths in the U.S. in the influenza pandemic of 1957–1958 — called also *Asian influenza;* compare HONG KONG FLU, SPANISH FLU

Asian tiger mosquito *n* : a black-and-white striped Asian mosquito of the genus *Aedes* (*A. albopictus*) that transmits the causative viruses of several diseases (as dengue and Japanese B encephalitis) in Asia and that has been introduced into the U.S. — called also *tiger mosquito*

Asi·at·ic cholera \ˌā-z(h)ē-ˌat-ik-\ *n* : cholera of Asian origin that is produced by virulent strains of the causative vibrio (*Vibrio cholerae*)

¹asleep \ə-ˈslēp\ *adj*   **1** : being in a state of sleep   **2** : lacking sensation : NUMB

²asleep *adv* : into a state of sleep

Asn *abbr* asparagine; asparaginyl

aso·cial \(ˈ)ā-ˈsō-shəl\ *adj* : not social: as   **a** : rejecting or lacking the capacity for social interaction ⟨an ∼ or reclusive attitude —A. T. Weaver⟩   **b** : ANTISOCIAL ⟨some type of ∼ act such as truancy, shoplifting, property damage, boisterousness —Edward Press & James Sterling⟩

Asp *abbr* aspartic acid; aspartyl

as·pa·rag·i·nase \ˌas-pə-ˈraj-ə-ˌnās, -ˌnāz\ *n* : an enzyme that hydrolyzes asparagine to aspartic acid and ammonia

L–asparaginase — see entry alphabetized in the letter *l*

as·par·a·gine \ə-ˈspar-ə-ˌjēn\ *n* : a white crystalline amino acid $C_4H_8N_2O_3$ that is an amide of aspartic acid — abbr. *Asn*

as·par·ag·i·nyl \ˌas-pə-ˈraj-ə-nəl, -ˌnēl\ *n* : the amino acid radical or residue $H_2NCOCH_2CH(NH_2)CO-$ of asparagine — abbr. *Asn*

as·par·a·gus \ə-ˈspar-ə-gəs\ *n*   **1** *cap* : a genus of Old World perennial herbs of the lily family (Liliaceae) having erect much-branched stems, minute scalelike leaves, and narrow filiform branchlets that function as leaves   **2 a** : any plant of the genus *Asparagus*; *esp* : a plant (*A. officinalis*) widely cultivated for its tender edible young shoots   **b** : the root of cultivated asparagus formerly used as a diuretic

as·par·tame \ˈas-pər-ˌtām, ə-ˈspär-\ *n* : a crystalline dipeptide ester $C_{14}H_{18}N_2O_5$ that is synthesized from the amino acids phenylalanine and aspartic acid and is used as a low-calorie sweetener — see NUTRASWEET

as·par·tase \ə-ˈspär-ˌtās, -ˌtāz\ *n* : an enzyme that occurs in various bacteria, yeasts, and higher plants and that catalyzes the conversion reaction of aspartic acid to fumaric acid by the removal of ammonia and also the reverse reaction of the addition of ammonia to fumaric acid

as·par·tate \-ˌtāt\ *n* : a salt or ester of aspartic acid

aspartate aminotransferase *n* : an enzyme that promotes transfer of an amino group from glutamic acid to oxaloacetic acid and that when present in abnormally high levels in the blood is a diagnostic indication of heart attack or liver disease — called also *aspartate transaminase, glutamic= oxaloacetic transaminase*

aspartate transaminase *n* : ASPARTATE AMINOTRANSFERASE

as·par·tic acid \ə-ˌspärt-ik-\ *n* : a crystalline amino acid $C_4H_7NO_4$ that is obtained from many proteins by hydrolysis — abbr. *Asp*

as·par·to·ki·nase \ə-ˌspärt-ō-ˈkī-ˌnās, -ˌnāz\ *n* : an enzyme that catalyzes the phosphorylation of aspartic acid by ATP

as·par·tyl \ə-ˈspärt-ᵊl, as-ˈpär-ˌtēl\ *n* : the amino acid radical or residue $-OCCH_2CH(NH_2)CO-$ of aspartic acid — abbr. *Asp*

aspe·cif·ic \(ˈ)ā-spi-ˈsif-ik\ *adj* : not specific ⟨∼ binding limits the anticoagulant effect of unfractionated heparin —Giancarlo Agnelli⟩

as·pect \ˈas-ˌpekt\ *n*   **1** : the part of an object (as an organ) in a particular position ⟨the medial ∼s of the knees —R. H. Nyquist⟩   **2** : a particular status or phase in which something appears or may be regarded ⟨the medicolegal ∼s of pregnancy —*Bull. of Meharry Med. Coll.*⟩

aspera — see LINEA ASPERA

As·per·ger's syndrome \ˈäs-ˌpər-gərz-\ *also* **As·per·ger syndrome** \-gər\ *n* : a developmental disorder characterized by impaired social and occupational skills, by normal language and cognitive development, and by restricted, repetitive, and stereotyped patterns of behavior, interests, and activities often with above average performance in a narrow field against a general background of deficient functioning — called also *Asperger's disorder*

As·per·ger \ˈäs-ˌper-gər\, **Hans,** 20th-century Austrian psychiatrist. Asperger first described the syndrome that bears his name in an article published in 1944.

as·per·gil·lin \ˌas-pər-ˈjil-ən\ *n*   **1** : an amorphous black pigment found in the spores of various fungi of the genus *Aspergillus*   **2** : an antibacterial substance isolated from two molds of the genus *Aspergillus* (*A. flavus* and *A. fumigatus*) and reported to possess activity against both gram-positive and gram-negative bacteria

as·per·gil·lo·sis \ˌas-pər-(ˌ)jil-ˈō-səs\ *n, pl* **-lo·ses** \-ˌsēz\ : infection with or disease caused (as in poultry) by molds of the genus *Aspergillus*

as·per·gil·lus \-ˈjil-əs\ *n*   **1** *cap* : a genus of ascomycetous fungi with branched radiate sporophores including many common molds   **2** *pl* **-gil·li** \-ˈjil-ˌī, -(ˌ)ē\ : any fungus of the genus *Aspergillus*

asper·ma·tism \(ˈ)ā-ˈspər-mə-ˌtiz-əm\ *n* : ASPERMIA

asper·mia \-ˈspər-mē-ə\ *n* : inability to produce or ejaculate semen — compare AZOOSPERMIA — **asper·mic** \-mik\ *adj*

aspher·ic \(ˈ)ā-ˈsfi(ə)r-ik, -ˈsfer-\ *or* **aspher·i·cal** \-i-kəl\ *adj* : departing slightly from the spherical form esp. in order to correct for spherical aberration ⟨an ∼ lens⟩

as·phyx·ia \as-ˈfik-sē-ə, əs-\ *n* : a lack of oxygen or excess of carbon dioxide in the body that is usu. caused by interruption of breathing and that causes unconsciousness — compare SUFFOCATION — **as·phyx·i·al** \-sē-əl\ *adj*

as·phyx·i·ant \-sē-ənt\ *n* : an agent (as a gas) capable of causing asphyxia

as·phyx·i·ate \-sē-ˌāt\ *vb* **-at·ed; -at·ing** *vt* : to cause asphyxia in; *also* : to kill or make unconscious through inadequate oxygen, presence of noxious agents, or other obstruction to normal breathing ∼ *vi* : to become asphyxiated — **as·phyx·i·a·tion** \-ˌfik-sē-ˈā-shən\ *n* — **as·phyx·i·a·tor** \-ˈfik-sē-ˌāt-ər\ *n*

as·pid·i·nol \a-'spid-³n-₁ol, -₁ol\ *n* : a yellow crystalline compound C₁₂H₁₆O₄ found in the rhizome of the male fern

as·pid·i·um \as-'pid-ē-əm, əs-\ *n, pl* **-ia** \-ē-ə\ : a drug consisting of the rhizome and stipes esp. of the male fern used as the oleoresinous extract for the expulsion of tapeworms

as·pi·do·sper·ma \₁as-pə-(₁)dō-'spər-mə\ *n* **1** *cap* : a genus of tropical American trees or rarely shrubs of the dogbane family that includes the white quebracho **2** : the dried bark of the quebracho (*Aspidosperma quebracho*) used as a respiratory sedative in dyspnea and in asthma — called also *quebracho bark*

as·pi·do·sper·mine \-'spər-₁mēn, -mən\ *n* : a bitter crystalline alkaloid C₂₂H₃₀N₂O₂ that is obtained from quebracho bark and was formerly used in the form of its sulfate as a respiratory stimulant and antispasmodic and as an antipyretic in typhoid fever

¹as·pi·rate \'as-pə-₁rāt\ *vt* **-rat·ed; -rat·ing** **1** : to draw by suction **2** : to remove (as blood) by aspiration ⟨the portal vein is exposed and blood is *aspirated* with a 50-ml. syringe —*Biol. Abstracts*⟩ **3** : INHALE ⟨*aspirated* material into the respiratory tract —*Anesthesia Digest*⟩

²as·pi·rate \'as-p(ə-)rət\ *n* : material removed by aspiration

as·pi·ra·tion \₁as-pə-'rā-shən\ *n* : a drawing of something in, out, up, or through by or as if by suction: as **a** : the act of breathing and esp. of breathing in **b** : the withdrawal of fluid or friable tissue from the body **c** : the taking of foreign matter into the lungs with the respiratory current — **as·pi·ra·tion·al** \-shnəl, -shən-³l\ *adj*

as·pi·ra·tor \'as-pə-₁rāt-ər\ *n* : an apparatus for producing suction or moving or collecting materials by suction; *esp* : a hollow tubular instrument connected with a partial vacuum and used to remove fluid or tissue or foreign bodies from the body

as·pi·rin \'as-p(ə-)rən\ *n, pl* **aspirin** *or* **aspirins** **1** : a white crystalline derivative C₉H₈O₄ of salicylic acid used for relief of pain and fever **2** : a tablet of aspirin

aspo·rog·e·nous \(')ā-spə-'räj-ə-nəs, -spó-\ *also* **aspo·ro·gen·ic** \-₁spör-ə-'jen-ik, -₁spór-\ *adj* : not spore-bearing : not producing spores ⟨~ yeasts⟩

aspor·ous \(')ā-'spōr-əs, -'spór-\ *adj* : not having true spores

aspor·u·late \(')ā-'spōr-(y)ə-lət, -'spór-\ *adj* : not sporulating

as·sas·sin bug \ə-'sas-³n-\ *n* : any bug of the family Reduviidae — compare CONENOSE

¹as·say \'as-₁ā, a-'sā\ *n* **1** : examination and determination as to characteristics (as weight, measure, or quality) **2** : analysis (as of a drug) to determine the presence, absence, or quantity of one or more components — compare BIOASSAY **3** : a substance to be assayed; *also* : the tabulated result of assaying

²as·say \a-'sā, 'as-₁ā\ *vt* : to analyze (an impure substance or mixture) for one or more specific components ⟨the sample was ~*ed* for drug content⟩

as·sim·i·la·ble \ə-'sim-ə-lə-bəl\ *adj* : capable of being assimilated

¹as·sim·i·late \ə-'sim-ə-₁lāt\ *vb* **-lat·ed; -lat·ing** *vt* **1** : to take in and utilize as nourishment : absorb into the system **2** : to absorb into the cultural tradition of a population or group ⟨the community *assimilated* many immigrants⟩ ~ *vi* **1** : to become absorbed or incorporated into the system ⟨some foods ~ more readily than others⟩ **2** : to become culturally assimilated

²as·sim·i·late \-lət, -₁lāt\ *n* : something that is assimilated

as·sim·i·la·tion \ə-₁sim-ə-'lā-shən\ *n* **1 a** : an act, process, or instance of assimilating **b** : the state of being assimilated **2** : the incorporation or conversion of nutrients into protoplasm that in animals follows digestion and absorption and in higher plants involves both photosynthesis and root absorption **3** : the process of receiving new facts or of responding to new situations in conformity with what is already available to consciousness — compare APPERCEPTION

as·sim·i·la·tive \ə-'sim-ə-₁lāt-iv, -lət-\ *adj* : of, relating to, or causing assimilation

as·sim·i·la·to·ry \-lə-₁tōr-ē, -₁tór-\ *adj* : ASSIMILATIVE

¹as·sist \ə-'sist\ *vt* : to give usu. supplementary support or aid

to ⟨~ the patient up the stairs⟩ ⟨~ respiration mechanically⟩ ~ *vi* : to give support or aid

²assist *n* : an act or procedure that provides assistance ⟨external pressure circulatory ~ employs compression of the lower extremities —P. W. Wright⟩

as·sist·ed living \ə-₁sis-təd-\ *n* : a system of housing and limited care that is designed for senior citizens who need some assistance with day-to-day activities but are not sufficiently incapacitated to require care in a nursing home and that usu. includes private quarters, meals, personal assistance, housekeeping aid, monitoring of medications, and nurses' visits ⟨an *assisted living* facility⟩

assisted suicide *n* : suicide by an individual facilitated by means or information (as a gun or indication of the lethal dosage of a drug) provided by someone else aware of the individual's intent; *esp* : PHYSICIAN-ASSISTED SUICIDE

as·sist·ive \ə-'sis-tiv\ *adj* : providing aid or assistance; *specif* : designed or intended to assist disabled persons ⟨walked with an ~ device⟩ ⟨~ technology for disabled persons⟩

assn *abbr* association

¹as·so·ci·ate \ə-'sō-s(h)ē-₁āt\ *vb* **-at·ed; -at·ing** *vt* **1** : to join or connect (things) together **2** : to bring together in a relationship ⟨infectious disease *associated* with a rise in body temperature⟩ ~ *vi* **1** : to combine or join with other parts ⟨fibrils of the sensory neurons ~ with motor neurons —S. J. Jacob & C. A. Francone⟩ **2** : to engage in free association ⟨the patient *associated* freely about his childhood⟩

²as·so·ci·ate \ə-'sō-s(h)ē-ət, -shət, -s(h)ē-₁āt\ *adj* : ranking immediately below the senior or chief position ⟨~ clinical professor of medicine⟩ ⟨~ medical examiner⟩

³as·so·ci·ate *like²*\ *n* **1** : a research worker or teacher affiliated with a professional organization or institution and ranking below a professor or full member ⟨a research ~ in pathology⟩ **2** *often cap* : a degree conferred esp. by a junior college ⟨an *Associate* in Technical Arts degree in nursing —*Skagit Valley Coll. Catalog*⟩

as·so·ci·a·tion \ə-₁sō-sē-'ā-shən, -shē-\ *n* **1** : the act of associating **2** : something linked in memory or imagination with a thing or person **3** : the process of forming mental connections or bonds between sensations, ideas, or memories **4** : the aggregation of chemical species to form (as with hydrogen bonds) loosely bound chemical complexes — compare POLYMERIZATION 1 — **as·so·ci·a·tion·al** \-shnəl, -shən-³l\ *adj*

association area *n* : an area of the cerebral cortex considered to function in linking and coordinating the sensory and motor areas

association fiber *n* : a nerve fiber connecting different parts of the brain; *esp* : any of the fibers connecting different areas within the cortex of each cerebral hemisphere — compare PROJECTION FIBER

as·so·ci·a·tion·ism \ə-₁sō-sē-'ā-shə-₁niz-əm, -₁sō-shē-\ *n* : a reductionist school of psychology that holds that the content of consciousness can be explained by the association and reassociation of irreducible sensory and perceptual elements — **as·so·ci·a·tion·is·tic** \-₁ā-shə-'nis-tik\ *adj*

as·so·ci·a·tion·ist \-nəst\ *n* : an adherent of associationism

association neuron *n* : INTERNEURON

as·so·cia·tive \ə-'sō-s(h)ē-₁āt-iv, -shət-iv\ *adj* **1** : of or relating to association esp. of ideas or images ⟨an ~ symbol⟩ **2 a** : dependent on or characterized by association ⟨an ~ reaction⟩ **b** : acquired by a process of learning ⟨an ~ reflex⟩

associative learning *n* : a learning process in which discrete ideas and percepts which are experienced together become linked to one another — compare PAIRED-ASSOCIATE LEARNING

associative neuron *n* : INTERNEURON

as·sor·ta·tive \ə-'sort-ət-iv\ *adj* : being nonrandom mating based on like or unlike characteristics

---

\ə\ **abut** \³\ **kitten** \ər\ **further** \a\ **ash** \ā\ **ace** \ä\ **cot, cart**
\aù\ **out** \ch\ **chin** \e\ **bet** \ē\ **easy** \g\ **go** \i\ **hit** \ī\ **ice** \j\ **job**
\ŋ\ **sing** \ō\ **go** \ò\ **law** \òi\ **boy** \th\ **thin** \th̲\ **the** \ü\ **loot**
\ù\ **foot** \y\ **yet** \zh\ **vision**   *See also* Pronunciation Symbols page

assortment — see INDEPENDENT ASSORTMENT

asst *abbr* assistant

AST *abbr* aspartate transaminase

asta·sia \ə-'stā-zh(ē-)ə\ *n* : muscular incoordination in standing — compare ABASIA

asta·sia–aba·sia \ə-'stā-zh(ē-)ə-ab-'ā-zhə, -əb-\ *n* : inability to stand and walk resulting from muscular incoordination

astat·ic \ə-'stat-ik\ *adj* : of or relating to astasia ⟨childhood ~ seizures⟩

as·ta·tine \'as-tə-ˌtēn\ *n* : a radioactive halogen element discovered by bombarding bismuth with helium nuclei and also formed by radioactive decay — symbol *At;* called also *ekaiodine;* see ELEMENT table

as·tem·i·zole \a-'stem-ə-ˌzōl, ə-, -ˌzól\ *n* : an antihistamine $C_{28}H_{31}FN_4O$ now withdrawn from use because of its link to ventricular arrythmias and cardiac arrest — see HISMANAL

as·ter \'as-tər\ *n* : a system of gelated cytoplasmic rays arranged radially about a centriole at either end of the mitotic or meiotic spindle — called also *cytaster*

astere·og·no·sis \(ˌ)ā-ˌster-ē-äg-'nō-səs, -ˌstir-\ *n, pl* **-no·ses** \-ˌsēz\ : loss of the ability to recognize the shapes of objects by handling them

as·te·ri·on \a-'tir-ē-ˌän, -ən\ *n, pl* **-ria** \-ē-ə\ : the point behind the ear where the parietal, temporal, and occipital bones meet — **as·te·ri·on·ic** \(ˌ)as-ˌtir-ē-'än-ik\ *adj*

as·te·rix·is \ˌas-tə-'rik-sis\ *n* : a motor disorder characterized by jerking movements (as of the outstretched hands) and associated with various encephalopathies due esp. to faulty metabolism

aster·nal \(ˌ)ā-'stərn-əl\ *adj* : not sternal: **a** : unattached to the sternum ⟨the floating ribs are ~⟩ **b** : having no sternum

as·ter·oid \'as-tə-ˌróid\ *adj* : resembling a star

as·the·nia \as-'thē-nē-ə\ *n* : lack or loss of strength : DEBILITY

as·then·ic \as-'then-ik\ *adj* **1** : of, relating to, or exhibiting asthenia : DEBILITATED **2** : characterized by slender build and slight muscular development : ECTOMORPHIC

as·the·no·pia \ˌas-thə-'nō-pē-ə\ *n* : weakness or rapid fatigue of the eyes often accompanied by pain and headache — **as·the·no·pic** \-'näp-ik, -'nō-pik\ *adj*

asth·ma \'az-mə\ *n* : a chronic lung disorder that is marked by recurring episodes of airway obstruction (as from bronchospasm) manifested by labored breathing accompanied esp. by wheezing and coughing and by a sense of constriction in the chest, and that is triggered by hyperreactivity to various stimuli (as allergens or rapid change in air temperature)

¹asth·mat·ic \az-'mat-ik, *Brit* as-\ *adj* : of, relating to, or affected with asthma ⟨an ~ attack⟩ — **asth·mat·i·cal·ly** \-i-k(ə-)lē\ *adv*

²asthmatic *n* : a person affected with asthma

asthmaticus — see STATUS ASTHMATICUS

asth·mo·gen·ic \ˌaz-mə-'jen-ik\ *adj* : causing asthmatic attacks

¹as·tig·mat·ic \ˌas-tig-'mat-ik\ *adj* : affected with, relating to, or correcting astigmatism

²astigmatic *n* : a person affected with astigmatism

astig·ma·tism \ə-'stig-mə-ˌtiz-əm\ *n* **1** : a defect of an optical system (as a lens) causing rays from a point to fail to meet in a focal point resulting in a blurred and imperfect image **2** : a defect of vision due to astigmatism of the refractive system of the eye and esp. to corneal irregularity — compare EMMETROPIA, MYOPIA

astig·mia \-mē-ə\ *n* : ASTIGMATISM

as·tig·mom·e·ter \ˌas-(ˌ)tig-'mäm-ət-ər\ *or* **as·tig·ma·tom·e·ter** \ə-ˌstig-mə-'täm-\ *n* : an apparatus for measuring the degree of astigmatism

as tol *abbr* as tolerated

asto·ma·tous \(ˌ)ā-'stäm-ət-əs, -'stōm-\ *adj* : having no mouth; *esp* : lacking a cytostome ⟨~ ciliates⟩

as·trag·a·lar \ə-'strag-ə-lər\ *adj* : of or relating to the astragalus

astrag·a·lec·to·my \ə-ˌstrag-ə-'lek-tə-mē\ *n, pl* **-mies** : surgical removal of the astragalus

as·trag·a·lus \ə-'strag-ə-ləs\ *n, pl* **-li** \-ˌlī, -ˌlē\ : one of the proximal bones of the tarsus of the higher vertebrates — see TALUS 1

as·tral \'as-trəl\ *adj* : of or relating to a mitotic or meiotic aster

astral ray *n* : one of the thin fibrils that make up the mitotic or meiotic aster

¹as·trin·gent \ə-'strin-jənt\ *adj* : having the property of causing contraction of soft organic tissues ⟨~ cosmetic lotions⟩: **a** : tending to shrink mucous membranes or raw or exposed tissues : checking discharge (as of serum or mucus) : STYPTIC **b** : tending to pucker the tissues of the mouth ⟨~ fruits⟩ — **as·trin·gen·cy** \-jən-sē\ *n, pl* **-cies**

²astringent *n* : an astringent agent or substance

as·tro·bi·ol·o·gist \ˌas-trō-bī-'äl-ə-jəst\ *n* : EXOBIOLOGIST

as·tro·bi·ol·o·gy \-(ˌ)bī-ə-jē\ *n, pl* **-gies** : EXOBIOLOGY

as·tro·blast \'as-trə-ˌblast\ *n* : a primordial astrocyte — **as·tro·blas·tic** \ˌas-trə-'blas-tik\ *adj*

as·tro·blas·to·ma \ˌas-trə-(ˌ)blas-'tō-mə\ *n, pl* **-mas** *also* **-ma·ta** \-mət-ə\ : an astrocytoma of moderate malignancy

as·tro·cyte \'as-trə-ˌsīt\ *n* : a star-shaped cell; *esp* : any comparatively large much-branched glial cell — **as·tro·cyt·ic** \ˌas-trə-'sit-ik\ *adj*

as·tro·cy·to·ma \ˌas-trə-sī-'tō-mə\ *n, pl* **-mas** *also* **-ma·ta** \-mət-ə\ : a nerve-tissue tumor composed of astrocytes

as·tro·glia \as-'träg-lē-ə, ˌas-trə-'glī-ə\ *n* : glial tissue composed of astrocytes — **as·tro·gli·al** \-əl\ *adj*

as·tro·sphere \'as-trə-ˌsfi(ə)r\ *n* : an aster exclusive of the centrosome

asyl·la·bia \ˌā-sə-'lā-bē-ə\ *n* : aphasia in which the patient can recognize letters but cannot form their sounds into syllables

asy·lum \ə-'sī-ləm\ *n* : an institution for the relief or care of the destitute or sick and esp. the insane

asym·bo·lia \ˌā-sim-(ˌ)bō-lē-ə\ *n* : loss of the power to understand previously familiar symbols and signs usu. in consequence of a brain lesion

asym·met·ri·cal \ˌā-sə-'me-tri-kəl\ *or* **asym·met·ric** \-trik\ *adj* **1** : not symmetrical **2** *usu* asymmetric, *of a carbon atom* : bonded to four different atoms or groups — **asym·met·ri·cal·ly** \-tri-k(ə-)lē\ *adv*

asym·me·try \(ˌ)ā-'sim-ə-trē\ *n, pl* **-tries** **1** : lack or absence of symmetry: as **a** : lack of proportion between the parts of a thing; *esp* : want of bilateral symmetry ⟨~ in the development of the two sides of the brain⟩ **b** : lack of coordination of two parts acting in connection with one another ⟨~ of convergence of the eyes⟩ **2** : lack of symmetry in spatial arrangement of atoms and groups in a molecule

asymp·tom·at·ic \ˌā-ˌsim(p)-tə-'mat-ik\ *adj* : presenting no symptoms of disease ⟨~ amebiasis⟩ — **asymp·tom·at·i·cal·ly** \-i-k(ə-)lē\ *adv*

asyn·ap·sis \ˌā-sə-'nap-səs\ *n, pl* **-ap·ses** \-ˌsēz\ : failure of pairing of homologous chromosomes in meiosis

asyn·clit·ism \(ˌ)ā-'sin-klə-ˌtiz-əm, -'siŋ-\ *n* : presentation of the fetal head during childbirth with the axis oriented obliquely to the axial planes of the pelvis

asy·ner·gia \ˌā-sə-'nər-j(ē-)ə\ *or* **asyn·er·gy** \(ˌ)ā-'sin-ər-jē\ *n, pl* **-gi·as** *or* **-gies** : lack of coordination (as of muscles) ⟨~ results in jerkiness, overaction and imperfect muscle control —C. H. Best & N. B. Taylor⟩ — **asy·ner·gic** \ˌā-sə-'nər-jik\ *adj*

asys·to·le \(ˌ)ā-'sis-tə-(ˌ)lē\ *n* : a condition of weakening or cessation of systole — **asys·tol·ic** \ˌā-sis-'täl-ik\ *adj* — **asys·to·lism** \(ˌ)ā-'sis-tə-ˌliz-əm\ *n*

asys·to·lia \ˌā-sis-'tō-lē-ə\ *n* : ASYSTOLE

at *abbr* airtight

At *symbol* astatine

Ata·brine \'at-ə-brən\ *n* : a preparation of quinacrine — formerly a U.S. registered trademark

atac·tic \(ˌ)ā-'tak-tik\ *adj* : lacking regularity or coordination; *specif* : characterized by ataxia

¹**at·a·rac·tic** \ˌat-ə-'rak-tik\ *or* **at·a·rax·ic** \-'rak-sik\ *adj* : tending to tranquilize ⟨~ drugs⟩

²**ataractic** *or* **ataraxic** *n* : TRANQUILIZER

at·a·rax·ia \ˌat-ə-'rak-sē-ə\ *or* **at·a·raxy** \'at-ə-ˌrak-sē\ *n, pl* **-rax·ias** *or* **-rax·ies** : calmness untroubled by mental or emotional disquiet

at·a·vism \'at-ə-ˌviz-əm\ *n* **1** : recurrence in an organism of a trait or character typical of an ancestral form and usu. due to genetic recombination **2** : an individual or character manifesting atavism : THROWBACK — **at·a·vis·tic** \ˌat-ə-'vis-tik\ *adj* — **at·a·vis·ti·cal·ly** \-ti-k(ə-)lē\ *adv*

atax·apha·sia \ə-ˌtak-sə-'fā-zh(ē-)ə\ *or* **ataxi·apha·sia** \ə-ˌtak-sē-ə-'fā-\ *n* : aphasia marked by inability to order words into sentences

atax·ia \ə-'tak-sē-ə, (')ā-\ *n* : an inability to coordinate voluntary muscular movements that is symptomatic of some nervous disorders — **atax·ic** \-sik\ *adj*

atax·ia·gram \ə-'tak-sē-ə-ˌgram\ *n* : a record obtained with an ataxiameter

atax·ia·graph \ə-'tak-sē-ə-ˌgraf\ *n* : ATAXIAMETER

atax·i·am·e·ter \ə-ˌtak-sē-'am-ət-ər\ *n* : an instrument for measuring involuntary tremor and unsteadiness (as the swaying of the whole body in the erect posture)

ataxic cerebral palsy *n* : cerebral palsy marked by hypotonic muscles and poor coordination and balance

ate *past of* EAT

at·el·ec·ta·sis \ˌat-ᵊl-'ek-tə-səs\ *n, pl* **-ta·ses** \-ˌsēz\ : collapse of the expanded lung; *also* : defective expansion of the pulmonary alveoli at birth — **at·el·ec·tat·ic** \-ek-'tat-ik\ *adj*

ate·li·o·sis *or chiefly Brit* **ate·lei·o·sis** \ə-ˌtel-ē-'ō-səs, -ˌtē-lē-\ *n, pl* **-o·ses** \-ˌsēz\ : incomplete development; *esp* : dwarfism associated with anterior pituitary deficiencies and marked by essentially normal intelligence and proportions though often retarded sexual development — compare ACHONDROPLASIA

¹**ate·li·ot·ic** *or chiefly Brit* **ate·lei·ot·ic** \-'ät-ik\ *adj* : of, relating to, or affected with ateliosis

²**ateliotic** *or chiefly Brit* **ateleiotic** *n* : an individual affected with ateliosis

at·e·lo·my·elia \ˌat-ᵊl-(ˌ)ō-mī-'ē-lē-ə\ *n* : defective development of the spinal cord

aten·o·lol \ə-'ten-ə-ˌlȯl, -ˌlōl\ *n* : a beta-blocker $C_{14}H_{22}N_2O_3$ used in the treatment of hypertension — see TENORMIN

ath·er·ec·to·my \ˌath-ə-'rek-tə-mē\ *n, pl* **-mies** : surgical removal of atheromatous plaque from within a blood vessel by threading a catheter with a rotating cutting blade through blood vessels to the point of the lesion and using the blade to shave away the plaque

ather·mic \(')ā-'thər-mik\ *adj* : not accompanied by fever or a rise in temperature ⟨~ effects on living tissue⟩

ath·ero·gen·e·sis \ˌath-ə-rō-'jen-ə-səs\ *n, pl* **-e·ses** \-ˌsēz\ : the formation of atheroma

ath·ero·gen·ic \-'jen-ik\ *adj* : relating to or causing atherogenesis ⟨~ diets⟩ — **ath·ero·ge·nic·i·ty** \-jə-'nis-ə-tē\ *n, pl* **-ties**

ath·er·o·ma \ˌath-ə-'rō-mə\ *n, pl* **-mas** *also* **-ma·ta** \-mət-ə\ **1** : fatty degeneration of the inner coat of the arteries **2** : an abnormal fatty deposit in an artery — **ath·er·o·ma·tous** \-'rō-mət-əs\ *adj*

ath·er·o·ma·to·sis \ˌath-ə-rō-mə-'tō-səs\ *n, pl* **-to·ses** \-ˌsēz\ : a disease characterized by atheromatous degeneration of the arteries

ath·ero·scle·ro·sis \ˌath-ə-rō-sklə-'rō-səs\ *n, pl* **-ro·ses** \-ˌsēz\ : an arteriosclerosis characterized by atheromatous deposits in and fibrosis of the inner layer of the arteries — **ath·ero·scle·rot·ic** \-sklə-'rät-ik\ *adj* — **ath·ero·scle·rot·i·cal·ly** \-i-k(ə-)lē\ *adv*

¹**ath·e·toid** \'ath-ə-ˌtȯid\ *adj* : exhibiting or characteristic of athetosis ⟨~ children⟩ ⟨~ movements⟩

²**athetoid** *n* : an athetoid individual

athetoid cerebral palsy *n* : cerebral palsy marked by involuntary uncontrolled writhing movements — called also *dyskinetic cerebral palsy*

ath·e·to·sis \ˌath-ə-'tō-səs\ *n, pl* **-to·ses** \-ˌsēz\ : a nervous dis-

order that is marked by continual slow movements esp. of the extremities and usu. due to a brain lesion

ath·e·tot·ic \ˌath-ə-'tät-ik\ *or* **ath·e·to·sic** \-'tō-sik\ *adj* : relating to athetosis : ATHETOID

ath·lete's foot \ˌath-ˌlēts-\ *n* : ringworm of the feet — called also *tinea pedis*

ath·let·ic \ath-'let-ik\ *adj* : characterized by heavy frame, large chest, and powerful muscular development : MESOMORPHIC

athletic supporter *n* : a supporter for the genitals worn by boys and men participating in sports or strenuous activities — called also *jockstrap;* see CUP 3a(1)

athrep·sia \ə-'threp-sē-ə, ā-\ *n* : MARASMUS — **athrep·tic** \ə-'threp-tik, (')ā-\ *adj*

ath·ro·cyte \'ath-rə-ˌsīt\ *n* : a cell capable of athrocytosis — **ath·ro·cyt·ic** \ˌath-rə-'sit-ik\ *adj*

ath·ro·cy·to·sis \ˌath-rə-sī-'tō-səs\ *n, pl* **-to·ses** \-ˌsēz\ : the capacity of some cells (as of the proximal convoluted tubule of the kidney) to pick up foreign material and store it in granular form in the cytoplasm

athy·mic \(')ā-'thī-mik\ *adj* : lacking a thymus

athy·re·o·sis \ˌā-ˌthī-rē-'ō-səs\ *n, pl* **-o·ses** \-ˌsēz\ : an abnormal condition caused by absence or functional deficiency of the thyroid gland — **athy·re·ot·ic** \-'ät-ik\ *adj*

At·i·van \'at-i-ˌvan\ *trademark* — used for a preparation of lorazepam

At·kins diet \'at-kənz-\ *n* : a weight loss program that emphasizes a diet low in carbohydrates along with little restriction on protein, fat, or total caloric intake

Atkins, Robert Coleman (1930–2003), American cardiologist and nutritionist. In 1972 he published *Dr. Atkins' Diet Revolution,* the first of seven best-selling diet books. His controversial system of weight loss was based upon an extremely low intake of carbohydrates that induces ketosis and forces the body to burn stored fat. He operated the Atkins Center for Complementary Medicine, and in 1999 established a foundation to support research on ways in which a low-carbohydrate diet can prevent or treat a variety of illnesses. Despite varying medical opinions on the efficacy and health effects of his method of weight loss, it gained popularity and prompted a demand for low-carbohydrate foods.

at·lan·tad \ət-'lan-ˌtad, at-\ *adv* : toward the atlas

at·lan·tal \-'lant-ᵊl\ *adj* **1** : of or relating to the atlas **2** : ANTERIOR 1, CEPHALIC

at·lan·to·ax·i·al \ət-ˌlant-ō-'ak-sē-əl, at-\ *adj* : relating to or being anatomical structures that connect the atlas and the axis

at·lan·to·oc·cip·i·tal \-ˌäk-'sip-ət-ᵊl\ *adj* : relating to or being structures (as a joint or ligament) joining the atlas and the occipital bone

at·las \'at-ləs\ *n* : the first vertebra of the neck

Atlas, Greek mythological character. In Greek legend Atlas was a Titan who took part in the revolt against the gods. As a punishment he was condemned to hold the heavens aloft forever. Atlas was usually represented as a human figure bearing the heavens or the celestial globe upon his shoulders.

ATLS *trademark* — used for an instruction course for assessing patient condition in the case of trauma

atm *abbr* atmosphere; atmospheric

at·mol·y·sis \ət-'mäl-ə-səs, at-\ *n, pl* **-y·ses** \-ˌsēz\ : the act or process of separating mingled gases of unequal diffusibility by transmission through porous substances

at·mom·e·ter \at-'mäm-ət-ər\ *n* : an instrument for measuring the evaporating capacity of the air

at·mo·sphere \'at-mə-ˌsfi(ə)r\ *n* **1** : the whole mass of air surrounding the earth **2** : the air of a locality **3** : a unit of pressure equal to the pressure of the air at sea level or to

---

101,325 pascals or to approximately 14.7 pounds per square inch — **at·mo·spher·ic** \ˌat-mə-ˈsfi(ə)r-ik, -ˈsfer-\ *adj*

atmospheric pressure *n* : the pressure exerted in every direction at any given point by the weight of the atmosphere

at·om \ˈat-əm\ *n* : the smallest particle of an element that can exist either alone or in combination — **atom·ic** \ə-ˈtäm-ik\ *adj* — **atom·i·cal·ly** \-i-k(ə-)lē\ *adv*

atomic cock·tail \-ˈkäk-ˌtāl\ *n* : a radioactive substance (as iodide of sodium) dissolved in water and administered orally to patients with cancer

atomic energy *n* : energy that can be liberated by changes in the nucleus of an atom (as by fission of a heavy nucleus or fusion of light nuclei into heavier ones with accompanying loss of mass)

atomic force microscope *n* : an instrument used for mapping the atomic-scale topography of a surface by means of the repulsive electronic forces between the surface and the tip of a microscopic probe moving above the surface — abbr. *AFM*

atomic force microscopy *n* : the art or process of using an atomic force microscope — abbr. *AFM*

atomic heat *n* : the heat capacity per gram-atomic weight of any element : the specific heat in calories per degree per gram multiplied by the atomic weight — compare MOLECULAR HEAT

atomic hypothesis *n* : ATOMIC THEORY 1

atomic mass *n* : the mass of an atom usu. expressed in atomic mass units; *also* : ATOMIC WEIGHT — compare MASS NUMBER

atomic mass unit *n* : a unit of mass for expressing masses of atoms, molecules, or nuclear particles equal to $\frac{1}{12}$ the mass of a single atom of the most abundant carbon isotope ^{12}C — called also *dalton*

atomic num·ber \-ˈnəm-bər\ *n* : an experimentally determined number characteristic of a chemical element that represents the number of protons in the nucleus which in a neutral atom equals the number of electrons outside the nucleus and that determines the place of the element in the periodic table — see ELEMENT table

atomic theory *n* **1** : a theory of the nature of matter: all material substances are composed of minute particles or atoms of a comparatively small number of kinds and all the atoms of the same kind are uniform in size, weight, and other properties — called also *atomic hypothesis* **2** : any of several theories of the structure of the atom; *esp* : one based on experimentation and theoretical considerations holding that the atom is composed essentially of a small positively charged comparatively heavy nucleus surrounded by a comparatively large arrangement of electrons

atomic weight *n* : the mass of one atom of an element; *specif* : the average mass of an atom of an element as it occurs in nature that is expressed in atomic mass units — see ELEMENT table

at·om·ism \ˈat-ə-ˌmiz-əm\ *n* **1** : a doctrine that the universe is composed of simple indivisible minute particles **2** : a psychological doctrine that perceptions, thoughts, and all mental processes are built up by the combination of simple elements

at·om·is·tic \ˌat-ə-ˈmis-tik\ *adj* **1** : of or relating to atoms or atomism **2** : considering the primary concern of psychology to be the content of consciousness or the succession of ideas or mental experiences rather than the integrated conscious self

at·om·ize *or Brit* **at·om·ise** \ˈat-ə-ˌmīz\ *vt* **-ized** *or Brit* **-ised**; **-iz·ing** *or Brit* **-is·ing** : to convert to minute particles or to a fine spray ⟨an *atomized* medicated powder⟩ — **at·om·iza·tion** *or Brit* **at·om·isa·tion** \ˌat-ə-mə-ˈzā-shən\ *n*

at·om·iz·er *or Brit* **at·om·is·er** \ˈat-ə-ˌmī-zər\ *n* : an instrument for atomizing usu. a perfume, disinfectant, or medicament

aton·ic \(ˈ)ā-ˈtän-ik, (ˈ)a-\ *adj* : characterized by atony ⟨an ∼ bladder⟩

ato·nic·i·ty \ˌā-tō-ˈnis-ət-ē, ˌat-ə-ˈnis-\ *n, pl* **-ties** : lack of normal tension or tonus ⟨intestinal ∼ as a cause of constipation⟩

at·o·ny \ˈat-ᵊn-ē\ *or* **ato·nia** \(ˈ)ā-ˈtō-nē-ə\ *n, pl* **-nies** *or* **-ni·as** : lack of physiological tone esp. of a contractile organ

ato·pen \ˈat-ə-pən, -ˌpen\ *n* : an agent inducing atopic allergy

ato·pog·no·sis \ˌā-ˌtäp-äg-ˈnō-səs, -ˌtōp-\ *n, pl* **-no·ses** \-ˌsēz\ : absence or loss of the power of topognosia

at·o·py \ˈat-ə-pē\ *n, pl* **-pies** : a prob. hereditary allergy characterized by symptoms (as asthma, hay fever, or hives) produced upon exposure esp. by inhalation to the exciting environmental antigen — **atop·ic** \(ˈ)ā-ˈtäp-ik, -ˈtō-pik\ *adj*

ator·va·stat·in \ə-ˌtȯr-və-ˈstat-ᵊn, -ˈtȯr-və-ˌstat-\ *n* : a statin that is administered orally (as in hypercholesterolemia) in the form of its hydrated calcium salt $(C_{33}H_{34}FN_2O_5)_2Ca\cdot 3H_2O$ to lower lipid levels in the blood — see LIPITOR

atox·ic \(ˈ)ā-ˈtäk-sik\ *adj* : not toxic ⟨∼ antibiotics⟩

ATP \ˌā-ˌtē-ˈpē, ā-ˈtē-ˌpē\ *n* : a phosphorylated nucleotide $C_{10}H_{16}N_5O_{13}P_3$ composed of adenosine and three phosphate groups that supplies energy for many biochemical cellular processes by undergoing enzymatic hydrolysis esp. to ADP — called also *adenosine triphosphate*

ATPase \ˌā-ˌtē-ˈpē-ˌās, -ˌāz\ *n* : an enzyme that hydrolyzes ATP; *esp* : one that hydrolyzes ATP to ADP and inorganic phosphate — called also *adenosine triphosphatase*

atre·sia \ə-ˈtrē-zhə\ *n* **1** : absence or closure of a natural passage of the body ⟨∼ of the small intestine⟩ **2** : absence or disappearance of an anatomical part (as an ovarian follicle) by degeneration

atre·sic \-zik, -sik\ *adj* : ATRETIC

atret·ic \ə-ˈtret-ik\ *adj* : of, relating to, or marked by atresia ⟨∼ follicles⟩

atria *pl of* ATRIUM

atri·al \ˈā-trē-əl\ *adj* : of, relating to, or affecting an atrium ⟨∼ electrical activity⟩ ⟨∼ disorders⟩

atrial fibrillation *n* : very rapid uncoordinated contractions of the atria of the heart resulting in a lack of synchronism between heartbeat and pulse beat — called also *auricular fibrillation*

atrial flutter *n* : an irregularity of the heartbeat in which the contractions of the atrium exceed in number those of the ventricle — called also *auricular flutter*

atrial natriuretic factor *n* : ATRIAL NATRIURETIC PEPTIDE — abbr. *ANF*

atrial natriuretic peptide *n* : a peptide hormone secreted by myocytes of the cardiac atria that in pharmacological doses promotes salt and water excretion and lowers blood pressure — abbr. *ANP*

atrial septum *n* : INTERATRIAL SEPTUM

atrich·ia \ā-ˈtrik-ē-ə, ə-\ *n* : congenital or acquired baldness : ALOPECIA

atri·chous \ˈa-trə-kəs, (ˈ)ā-ˈtrik-əs\ *adj* : having no flagellum

atrio·ven·tric·u·lar \ˌā-trē-(ˌ)ō-ven-ˈtrik-yə-lər\ *adj* **1** : of, relating to, or situated between an atrium and ventricle **2** : of, involving, or being the atrioventricular node

atrioventricular bundle *n* : BUNDLE OF HIS

atrioventricular canal *n* : the canal joining the atrium and ventricle in the tubular embryonic heart

atrioventricular node *n* : a small mass of tissue that is situated in the wall of the right atrium adjacent to the septum between the atria, passes impulses received from the sinoatrial node to the ventricles by way of the bundle of His, and in some pathological states replaces the sinoatrial node as pacemaker of the heart

atrioventricular valve *n* : a valve between an atrium and ventricle of the heart : AURICULOVENTRICULAR VALVE: **a** : MITRAL VALVE **b** : TRICUSPID VALVE

atri·um \ˈā-trē-əm\ *n, pl* **atria** \-trē-ə\ *also* **atri·ums** : an anatomical cavity or passage; *esp* : a chamber of the heart that receives blood from the veins and forces it into a ventricle or ventricles

At·ro·pa \ˈa-trə-pə\ *n* : a genus of Eurasian and African herbs (as belladonna) of the family Solanaceae that have entire leaves, a usu. bell-shaped calyx and corolla, and a fruit that is a berry and that are a source of medicinal alkaloids (as atropine and scopolamine)

At·ro·pos \'a-trə-ˌpäs, -pəs\, Greek mythological character. The three Fates of Greek mythology were pictured as old women who spun out every person's destiny as if it were a thread. Clotho spun the thread, Lachesis measured it out, and Atropos cut it off. Belladonna was the first plant to be named in the genus *Atropa*. As the plant is highly poisonous, the genus was appropriately named after the goddess who cut the thread of life.

atro·phic \(ˈ)ā-ˈtrō-fik, ə-, -ˈträf-ik\ *adj* : relating to or characterized by atrophy ⟨an ∼ jaw⟩

atrophicans — see ACRODERMATITIS CHRONICA ATROPHICANS

atrophic arthritis *n* : RHEUMATOID ARTHRITIS

atrophic rhinitis *n* **1** : a chronic disease of swine that is characterized by purulent inflammation of the nasal mucosa, atrophy of the nasal conchae, and abnormal swelling and distortion of the face **2** : OZENA

atrophicus — see LICHEN SCLEROSUS ET ATROPHICUS

atrophic vaginitis *n* : inflammation of the vagina with thinning of the epithelial lining that occurs following menopause and is due to a deficiency of estrogen

¹**at·ro·phy** \'a-trə-fē\ *n, pl* **-phies** : decrease in size or wasting away of a body part or tissue; *also* : arrested development or loss of a part or organ incidental to the normal development or life of an animal or plant

²**atrophy** \'a-trə-fē, -ˌfī\ *vb* **-phied; -phy·ing** *vi* : to undergo atrophy ⟨the inactive muscles *atrophied*⟩ ∼ *vt* : to cause to undergo atrophy ⟨disuse *atrophied* the arm⟩

at·ro·pine \'a-trə-ˌpēn\ *n* : a racemic mixture of hyoscyamine usu. obtained from belladonna and related plants of the family Solanaceae and used esp. in the form of its hydrated sulfate $(C_{17}H_{23}NO_3)_2 \cdot H_2SO_4 \cdot H_2O$ for its anticholinergic effects (as relief of smooth muscle spasms or dilation of the pupil of the eye)

at·ro·pin·ism \-ˌpē-ˌniz-əm\ *n* : poisoning by atropine

at·ro·pin·iza·tion *also Brit* **at·ro·pin·isa·tion** \ˌa-trə-ˌpē-nə-ˈzā-shən\ *n* : the physiological condition of being under the influence of atropine — **at·ro·pin·ize** *also Brit* **at·ro·pin·ise** \'a-trə-pə-ˌnīz\ *vt* **-ized** *also Brit* **-ised; -iz·ing** *also Brit* **-is·ing**

at·ro·scine \'a-trə-ˌsēn, -sən\ *n* : racemic scopolamine

at·tach·ment \ə-ˈtach-mənt\ *n* : the physical connection by which one thing is attached to another ⟨sever the ∼s of a muscle to a bone⟩ — **at·tach** \ə-ˈtach\ *vb*

¹**at·tack** \ə-ˈtak\ *vt* : to begin to affect or to act on injuriously ⟨tumors ∼ed the kidneys⟩ ⟨∼ed by a fever⟩

²**attack** *n* : a fit of sickness; *esp* : an active episode of a chronic or recurrent disease

at·tar \'at-ər, 'a-ˌtär\ *n* : a fragrant essential oil; *esp* : ATTAR OF ROSES

attar of roses *n* : a fragrant essential oil obtained by distillation from petals esp. of damask rose and with geraniol and citronellol as its principal odorous constituents

at·tempt·er \ə-ˈtem(p)-tər\ *n* : one who attempts suicide

at·tend \ə-ˈtend\ *vt* : to visit or stay with professionally as a physician or nurse — **at·tend·er** *n*

at·ten·dance \ə-ˈten-dən(t)s\ *n* : service at a hospital ⟨a physician in ∼⟩

at·ten·dant \ə-ˈten-dənt\ *n* : a person who attends another to perform a service ⟨ward ∼s⟩

¹**at·tend·ing** \ə-ˈtend-in\ *adj* : serving as a physician or surgeon on the staff of a hospital, regularly visiting and treating patients, and often supervising students, fellows, and the house staff ⟨the final responsibility for adequate records rests upon the shoulders of the ∼ staff —*Jour. Amer. Med. Assoc.*⟩

²**attending** *n* : an attending physician or surgeon ⟨making decisions to operate with the consent of an ∼ —Don Gold⟩

at·ten·tion \ə-ˈten-chən\ *n* **1** : the act or state of attending : the application of the mind to any object of sense or thought **2 a** : an organismic condition of selective awareness or perceptual receptivity; *specif* : the complex of neuromuscular adjustments that permit maximum excitability or

responsiveness to a given class of stimuli **b** : the process of focusing consciousness to produce greater vividness and clarity of certain of its contents relative to others — **at·ten·tion·al** \-ˈtench-nəl, -ˈten-chən-ᵊl\ *adj*

attention deficit disorder *n* : a syndrome of disordered learning and disruptive behavior that is not caused by any serious underlying physical or mental disorder and that has several subtypes characterized primarily by symptoms of inattentiveness or primarily by symptoms of hyperactivity and impulsive behavior (as in speaking out of turn) or by the significant expression of all three — abbr. *ADD;* called also *minimal brain dysfunction*

attention–deficit/hyperactivity disorder *n* : ATTENTION DEFICIT DISORDER

at·ten·u·ate \ə-ˈten-yə-ˌwāt\ *vt* **-at·ed; -at·ing** : to reduce the severity of (a disease) or virulence or vitality of (a pathogenic agent) ⟨a procedure to ∼ severe diabetes⟩ ⟨*attenuated* bacilli⟩

at·ten·u·a·tion \ə-ˌten-yə-ˈwā-shən\ *n* : a decrease in the pathogenicity or vitality of a microorganism or in the severity of a disease

at·tic \'at-ik\ *n* : the small upper space of the middle ear — called also *epitympanic recess*

at·ti·co·mas·toid \ˌat-ə-kō-ˈmas-ˌtòid\ *adj* : of or relating to the attic and the mastoid

at·ti·co·to·my \ˌat-ə-ˈkät-ə-mē\ *n, pl* **-mies** : surgical incision of the tympanic attic

at·ti·tude \'at-ə-ˌt(y)üd\ *n* **1** : the arrangement of the parts of the body : POSTURE **2 a** : a mental position with regard to a fact or state **b** : a feeling or emotion toward a fact or state **3** : an organismic state of readiness to respond in a characteristic way to a stimulus (as an object, concept, or situation)

at·ti·tu·di·nal \ˌat-ə-ˈt(y)üd-nəl, -ᵊn-əl\ *adj* : relating to, based on, or expressive of personal attitudes or feelings ⟨∼ responses of college students⟩

at·trac·tion \ə-ˈtrak-shən\ *n* : a force acting mutually between particles of matter, tending to draw them together, and resisting their separation — **at·tract** \ə-ˈtrakt\ *vt*

at·tri·tion \ə-ˈtrish-ən\ *n* : the act of rubbing together; *also* : the act of wearing or grinding down by friction ⟨∼ of teeth⟩ — **at·tri·tion·al** \-ˈtrish-nəl, -ˈtrish-ən-ᵊl\ *adj*

at wt *abbr* atomic weight

atyp·ia \(ˈ)ā-ˈtip-ē-ə\ *n* : ATYPISM

atyp·i·cal \(ˈ)ā-ˈtip-i-kəl\ *adj* : not typical : not like the usual or normal type — **atyp·i·cal·ly** \(ˈ)ā-ˈtip-i-k(ə-)lē\ *adv*

atypical pneumonia *n* : PRIMARY ATYPICAL PNEUMONIA

atyp·ism \(ˈ)ā-ˈtī-ˌpiz-əm\ *n* : the condition of being uncharacteristic or lacking uniformity ⟨cellular ∼⟩

au *abbr* **1** angstrom unit **2** antitoxin unit

Au *symbol* [L *aurum*] gold

au·di·al \'òd-ē-əl\ *adj* : of, relating to, or affecting the sense of hearing : AURAL

au·di·ble \'òd-ə-bəl\ *adj* : heard or capable of being heard — **au·di·bil·i·ty** \ˌòd-ə-ˈbil-ət-ē\ *n, pl* **-ties** — **au·di·bly** \'òd-ə-blē\ *adv*

¹**au·dile** \'ò-ˌdīl\ *n* : a person whose mental imagery is auditory rather than visual or motor — compare MOTILE, TACTILE, VISUALIZER

²**audile** *adj* **1** : of or relating to hearing : AUDITORY **2** : of, relating to, or being an audile

au·dio frequency \'òd-ē-(ˌ)ō-\ *n* : the frequency of an audible sound wave usu. in the range between 15 and 20,000 hertz

au·dio·gen·ic \ˌòd-ē-ō-ˈjen-ik\ *adj* : produced by frequencies corresponding to sound waves — used esp. of epileptoid responses ⟨∼ seizures⟩

au·dio·gram \'òd-ē-ō-ˌgram\ *n* : a graphic representation of

\ə\ abut \ᵊ\ kitten \ər\ further \a\ ash \ā\ ace \ä\ cot, cart
\aù\ out \ch\ chin \e\ bet \ē\ easy \g\ go \i\ hit \ī\ ice \j\ job
\ŋ\ sing \ō\ go \ò\ law \òi\ boy \th\ thin \th\ the \ü\ loot
\ù\ foot \y\ yet \zh\ vision *See also* Pronunciation Symbols page

the relation of vibration frequency and the minimum sound intensity for hearing

au·di·ol·o·gist \ˌȯd-ē-ˈäl-ə-jəst\ *n* : a specialist in audiology

au·di·ol·o·gy \ˌȯd-ē-ˈäl-ə-jē\ *n, pl* **-gies** : a branch of science dealing with hearing; *specif* : therapy of individuals having impaired hearing — **au·di·o·log·i·cal** \-ē-ə-ˈläj-i-kəl\ *also* **au·di·o·log·ic** \-ē-ə-ˈläj-ik\ *adj*

au·di·om·e·ter \ˌȯd-ē-ˈäm-ət-ər\ *n* : an instrument used in measuring the acuity of hearing — called also *acoumeter*

au·di·om·e·try \ˌȯd-ē-ˈäm-ə-trē\ *n, pl* **-tries** : the testing and measurement of hearing acuity for variations in sound intensity and pitch and for tonal purity — **au·dio·met·ric** \ˌȯd-ē-ō-ˈme-trik\ *adj* — **au·di·om·e·trist** \ˌȯd-ē-ˈäm-ə-trəst\ *n*

au·dio·vi·su·al \ˌȯd-ē-(ˌ)ō-ˈvizh-(ə)-wəl, -ˈvizh-əl\ *adj* : of, relating to, or involving both hearing and sight

au·di·tion \ȯ-ˈdish-ən\ *n* **1** : the power or sense of hearing **2** : the act of hearing

¹au·di·to·ry \ˈȯd-ə-ˌtōr-ē, -ˌtȯr-\ *adj* **1** : of or relating to hearing **2** : attained, experienced, or produced through or as if through hearing ⟨∼ images⟩ ⟨∼ hallucinations⟩ **3** : marked by great susceptibility to impressions and reactions produced by acoustic stimuli ⟨an ∼ individual⟩

²auditory *n, pl* **-ries** : AUDITORY NERVE

auditory aphasia *n* : inability to understand spoken words

auditory area *n* : a sensory area in the temporal cortex associated with the organ of hearing — called also *auditory center, auditory cortex*

auditory canal *n* : either of two passages of the ear — called also *acoustic meatus, auditory meatus;* see EXTERNAL AUDITORY CANAL, INTERNAL AUDITORY CANAL

auditory cell *n* : a hair cell of the organ of Corti

auditory center *n* : AUDITORY AREA

auditory cortex *n* : AUDITORY AREA

auditory meatus *n* : AUDITORY CANAL

auditory nerve *n* : either of the eighth pair of cranial nerves connecting the inner ear with the brain, transmitting impulses concerned with hearing and balance, and composed of the cochlear nerve and the vestibular nerve — called also *acoustic nerve, auditory, eighth cranial nerve, vestibulocochlear nerve*

auditory pit *n* : the indentation of thickened surface ectoderm that forms the embryonic ear — called also *otic pit*

auditory placode *n* : either of the anterior lateral areas of ectoderm that invaginate and sink beneath the body surface to form the inner ear structures of vertebrate embryos — called also *otic placode*

auditory point *n* : the lowest part of the notch between the incurved rim of the outer ear and the tragus

auditory processing disorder *n* : CENTRAL AUDITORY PROCESSING DISORDER

auditory tube *n* : EUSTACHIAN TUBE

auditory vesicle *n* : the saccular invagination of ectoderm from which the vertebrate inner ear develops — called also *otic vesicle*

Auer·bach's plexus \ˈau̇(-ə)r-ˌbäks-, -ˌbäks-\ *n* : MYENTERIC PLEXUS

Auer·bach \ˈau̇(-ə)r-ˌbäk, -ˌbäk\, **Leopold (1828–1897),** German anatomist. Auerbach made important contributions to microscopic anatomy. His published works numbered almost fifty and included papers on the neuropsychiatric functions of lower animals, the unicellularity of amebas, the anatomy of the lymphatic and capillary vessels, and fertilization of the egg. In 1862 he published his description of a plexus of autonomic nerve fibers in the intestines of vertebrates. Shortly afterward he presented his description of the ganglion cells situated in the plexus. The plexus is now commonly called the myenteric plexus but is sometimes known by Auerbach's name.

aug·ment \ˈȯg-ˌment, ˈȯg-ˌment\ *vt* : to increase in size, amount, degree, or severity ⟨diabetes mellitus is ∼ed by hyperthyroidism —C. H. Thienes⟩

aug·men·ta·tion \ˌȯg-mən-ˈtā-shən, -ˌmen-\ *n* **1** : the act, action, or process of augmenting **2** : something that augments

Aug·men·tin \ȯg-ˈment-ᵊn\ *trademark* — used for a preparation of amoxicillin and the potassium salt of clavulanic acid

au·la \ˈau̇-lə, ˈȯ-\ *n, pl* **au·las** *or* **au·lae** \-ˌlī, -ˌlē\ : the anterior part of the third ventricle of the brain leading to the lateral ventricles

au·ra \ˈȯr-ə\ *n, pl* **auras** *also* **au·rae** \-ē\ : a subjective sensation (as of voices or colored lights or crawling and numbness) experienced before an attack of some nervous disorders (as epilepsy or migraine)

au·ral \ˈȯr-əl\ *adj* : of or relating to the ear or to the sense of hearing — **au·ral·ly** \-ə-lē\ *adv*

Au·reo·my·cin \ˌȯr-ē-ō-ˈmīs-ᵊn\ *trademark* — used for a preparation of the hydrochloride of chlortetracycline

au·ric \ˈȯr-ik\ *adj* : of, relating to, or derived from gold

au·ri·cle \ˈȯr-i-kəl\ *n* **1 a** : PINNA   **b** : an atrium of the heart **2** : an angular or ear-shaped anatomical lobe or process (as an auricular appendage of the heart)

au·ric·u·la \ȯ-ˈrik-yə-lə\ *n, pl* **-lae** \-ˌlē\ : AURICLE; *esp* : AURICULAR APPENDAGE

au·ric·u·lar \ȯ-ˈrik-yə-lər\ *adj* **1** : of, relating to, or using the ear or the sense of hearing **2** : understood or recognized by the sense of hearing **3** : of or relating to an auricle or auricular appendage ⟨∼ fibrillation⟩

auricular appendage *n* : an ear-shaped pouch projecting from each atrium of the heart — called also *auricular appendix*

auricular artery — see POSTERIOR AURICULAR ARTERY

auricular fibrillation *n* : ATRIAL FIBRILLATION

auricular flutter *n* : ATRIAL FLUTTER

au·ric·u·lar·is \ȯ-ˌrik-yə-ˈlar-əs, -ˈlär-\ *n, pl* **-lar·es** \-ˌēz\ : any of three muscles attached to the cartilage of the external ear that assist in moving the scalp and in some individuals the external ear itself and that consist of one that is anterior, one superior, and one posterior in position — called also respectively *auricularis anterior, auricularis superior, auricularis posterior*

auricular point *n* : the center of the external auditory canal

auricular tubercle of Darwin *n* : DARWIN'S TUBERCLE

auricular vein — see POSTERIOR AURICULAR VEIN

au·ric·u·late \ȯ-ˈrik-yə-lət\ *adj* : having ears or auricles

au·ric·u·lo·in·fra·or·bit·al plane \ȯ-ˌrik-yə-(ˌ)lō-ˌin-frə-ˌȯr-bət-ᵊl-, -(ˌ)frä-\ *n* : the plane that passes through the auricular points and the lowest points of the orbits

au·ric·u·lo·tem·po·ral nerve \-ˌtem-p(ə-)rəl-\ *n* : the branch of the mandibular nerve that supplies sensory fibers to the skin of the external ear and temporal region and autonomic fibers from the otic ganglion to the parotid gland

au·ric·u·lo·ven·tric·u·lar \ȯ-ˌrik-yə-(ˌ)lō-ven-ˈtrik-yə-lər, -vən-\ *adj* : ATRIOVENTRICULAR

auriculoventricular valve *n* : ATRIOVENTRICULAR VALVE

au·rin \ˈȯr-ən\ *n* : a poisonous red dye $C_{19}H_{14}O_3$ used chiefly as an indicator and dye intermediate — called also *rosolic acid*

au·rist \ˈȯr-əst\ *n* : an ear specialist

au·ro·ther·a·py \ˌȯr-ō-ˈther-ə-pē, ˈȯr-ō-ˌ\ *n, pl* **-pies** : CHRYSOTHERAPY

au·ro·thio·glu·cose \ˌȯr-ō-ˌthī-ō-ˈglü-ˌkōs, -ˌkōz\ *n* : GOLD THIOGLUCOSE

aurothiosulfate — see SODIUM AUROTHIOSULFATE

au·ru·lent \ˈȯr-(y)ə-lənt\ *adj* : golden in color

au·rum \ˈȯr-əm, ˈau̇r-\ *n* : GOLD

au·rum po·ta·bi·le \ˌau̇-rəm-pə-ˈtäb-ə-lē, ˌȯr-, -ˈtab-\ *n* : a formerly used cordial or medicine consisting of some volatile oil in which minute particles of gold were suspended

aus·cul·tate \ˈȯ-skəl-ˌtāt\ *vt* **-tat·ed; -tat·ing** : to examine by auscultation — **aus·cul·ta·to·ry** \ȯ-ˈskəl-tə-ˌtōr-ē, -ˌtȯr-\ *adj*

aus·cul·ta·tion \ˌȯ-skəl-ˈtā-shən\ *n* : the act of listening to sounds arising within organs (as the lungs or heart) as an aid to diagnosis and treatment

aus·cul·ta·tor \ˈȯ-skəl-ˌtāt-ər\ *n* : a person who performs auscultation

Aus·tra·lia antigen \ȯ-ˈstrāl-yə-, ä-, ə-\ *also* **Aus·tra·lian antigen** \-yən-\ *n* : HEPATITIS B SURFACE ANTIGEN

au·ta·coid \ˈȯt-ə-ˌkȯid\ *n* : a physiologically active substance (as a serotonin, bradykinin, or angiotensin) produced by and acting within the body

autecious var of AUTOECIOUS

au·tism \'ȯ-ˌtiz-əm\ n : a developmental disorder that appears by age three and that is variable in expression but is recognized and diagnosed by impairment of the ability to form normal social relationships, by impairment of the ability to communicate with others, and by stereotyped behavior patterns esp. as exhibited by a preoccupation with repetitive activities of restricted focus rather than with flexible and imaginative ones

¹**au·tis·tic** \ȯ-'tis-tik\ adj : of, relating to, or marked by autism ⟨∼ behavior⟩ ⟨∼ children⟩

²**autistic** n : an individual affected with autism

au·to·ac·ti·va·tion \ˌȯt-ō-ˌak-tə-'vā-shən\ n : AUTOCATALYSIS

au·to·ag·glu·ti·na·tion \ˌȯt-ō-ə-ˌglüt-ᵊn-'ā-shən\ n : agglutination of red blood cells by cold agglutinins in an individual's own serum usu. at lower than body temperature

au·to·ag·glu·ti·nin \-ə-'glüt-ᵊn-ən\ n : an antibody that agglutinates the red blood cells of the individual producing it — compare COLD AGGLUTININ

au·to·anal·y·sis \-ə-'nal-ə-səs\ n, pl -y·ses \-ˌsēz\ 1 : self-treatment by psychoanalysis 2 : automatic chemical analysis

Au·to·an·a·lyz·er \'ȯt-ō-ˌan-ᵊl-ˌī-zər\ trademark — used for an instrument designed for automatic chemical analysis (as of blood glucose level)

au·to·an·ti·body \ˌȯt-(ˌ)ō-'ant-i-ˌbäd-ē\ n, pl -bod·ies : an antibody active against a tissue constituent of the individual producing it

au·to·an·ti·gen \ˌȯt-(ˌ)ō-'ant-i-ˌjen\ n : an antigen that is a normal bodily constituent and against which the immune system produces autoantibodies — **au·to·an·ti·gen·ic** \-ˌant-i-'jen-ik\ adj

au·to·as·phyx·i·a·tion \-as-ˌfik-sē-'ā-shən\ n : asphyxiation of an organism by the products of its own metabolism

au·to·ca·tal·y·sis \ˌȯt-ō-kə-'tal-ə-səs\ n, pl -y·ses \-ˌsēz\ : catalysis of a reaction by one of its products — called also autoactivation — **au·to·cat·a·lyt·ic** \-ˌkat-ᵊl-'it-ik\ adj — **au·to·cat·a·lyt·i·cal·ly** \-i-k(ə-)lē\ adv

au·toch·tho·nous \(')ȯ-'täk-thə-nəs\ adj 1 a : indigenous or endemic to a region ⟨∼ malaria⟩ b : contracted in the area where reported ⟨∼ cases of malaria in the U.S.⟩ 2 : originated in that part of the body where present — used chiefly of pathological conditions — **au·toch·tho·nous·ly** \-lē\ adv

au·to·clav·able \'ȯt-ə-ˌklā-və-bəl, ˌȯt-ə-'\ adj : able to withstand the action of an autoclave — **au·to·clav·abil·i·ty** \ˌȯt-ə-ˌklā-və-'bil-ət-ē\ n, pl -ties

¹**au·to·clave** \'ȯt-ō-ˌklāv\ n : an apparatus (as for sterilizing) using superheated steam under pressure

²**autoclave** vt -claved; -clav·ing : to treat in an autoclave

au·to·crine \-krin\ adj : of, relating to, promoted by, or being a substance secreted by a cell and acting on surface receptors of the same cell ⟨∼ stimulation of T cell growth⟩ ⟨∼ growth of some breast cancers —M. E. Lippman⟩ — compare PARACRINE

au·to·cy·tol·y·sis \ˌȯt-ō-sī-'täl-ə-səs\ n, pl -y·ses \-ˌsēz\ : autolysis of cells

au·to·di·ges·tion \-dī-'jes(h)-chən, -də-\ n : AUTOLYSIS

au·toe·cious also **au·te·cious** \ȯ-'tē-shəs\ adj : passing through all life stages on the same host ⟨∼ rusts⟩ — **au·toe·cism** \-'tē-ˌsiz-əm\ n

au·to·er·o·tism \ˌȯt-ō-'er-ə-ˌtiz-əm\ or **au·to·erot·i·cism** \-i-'rät-ə-ˌsiz-əm\ n 1 : sexual gratification obtained solely through stimulation by oneself of one's own body — compare ALLOEROTISM 2 : sexual feeling arising without known external stimulation — **au·to·erot·ic** \-i-'rät-ik\ adj — **au·to·erot·i·cal·ly** \-i-k(ə-)lē\ adv

au·tog·a·my \ȯ-'täg-ə-mē\ n, pl -mies : SELF-FERTILIZATION; esp : conjugation of two sister cells or sister nuclei of protozoans or fungi — **au·tog·a·mous** \-məs\ adj

au·to·gen·ic \ˌȯt-ə-'jen-ik\ adj 1 : AUTOGENOUS 2 : of or relating to any of several relaxation techniques that actively

involve the patient (as by self-hypnosis, meditation, or biofeedback) in attempts to control physiological variables (as body temperature and blood pressure) ⟨∼ training⟩

au·to·gen·i·tal \-'jen-ə-tᵊl\ adj : of or relating to one's own genital organs ⟨∼ stimulation⟩

au·tog·e·nous \ȯ-'täj-ə-nəs\ adj 1 : produced independently of external influence or aid : ENDOGENOUS 2 : orginating or derived from sources within the same individual ⟨an ∼ graft⟩ ⟨∼ vaccine⟩ 3 : not requiring a meal of blood to produce eggs ⟨∼ mosquitoes⟩ — **au·tog·e·nous·ly** adv — **au·tog·e·ny** \ȯ-'täj-ə-nē\ n, pl -nies

au·tog·no·sis \ˌȯt-əg-'nō-səs\ n, pl -no·ses \-ˌsēz\ : an understanding of one's own psychodynamics

au·to·graft \'ȯt-ō-ˌgraft\ n : a tissue or organ that is transplanted from one part to another part of the same body — **autograft** vt

au·to·he·mo·ly·sin or chiefly Brit **au·to·hae·mo·ly·sin** \ˌȯt-ō-ˌhē-mə-'līs-ᵊn\ n : a hemolysin that acts on the red blood cells of the individual in whose blood it is found

au·to·he·mo·ly·sis or chiefly Brit **au·to·hae·mo·ly·sis** \-hi-'mäl-ə-səs, -ˌhē-mə-'lī-səs\ n, pl -ly·ses \-ˌsēz\ : hemolysis of red blood cells by factors in the serum of the person from whom the blood is taken

au·to·he·mo·ther·a·py or chiefly Brit **au·to·hae·mo·ther·a·py** \-ˌhē-mō-'ther-ə-pē\ n, pl -pies : treatment of disease by modification (as by irradiation) of the patient's own blood or by its introduction (as by intramuscular injection) outside the bloodstream

au·to·hyp·no·sis \ˌȯt-ō-hip-'nō-səs\ n, pl -no·ses \-ˌsēz\ : self-induced and usu. automatic hypnosis — **au·to·hyp·not·ic** \-'nät-ik\ adj

au·to·im·mune \-im-'yün\ adj : of, relating to, or caused by antibodies or T cells that attack molecules, cells, or tissues of the organism producing them ⟨∼ diseases⟩

au·to·im·mu·ni·ty \ˌȯt-ō-im-'yü-nət-ē\ n, pl -ties : a condition in which the body produces an immune response against its own tissue constituents

au·to·im·mu·ni·za·tion or Brit **au·to·im·mu·ni·sa·tion** \-ˌim-yə-nə-'zā-shən also -im-ˌyü-nə-\ n : production by the body of an immune response against its own tissue constituents

au·to·im·mu·nize or Brit **au·to·im·mu·nise** \-'im-yə-ˌnīz\ vt -nized or Brit -nised; -niz·ing or Brit -nis·ing : to induce autoimmunity in

au·to·in·fec·tion \-in-'fek-shən\ n : reinfection with larvae produced by parasitic worms already in the body — compare HYPERINFECTION

au·to·in·oc·u·la·ble \ˌȯt-ō-in-'äk-yə-lə-bəl\ adj : capable of being transmitted by inoculation from one part of the body to another ⟨certain kinds of warts are ∼⟩

au·to·in·oc·u·la·tion \-in-ˌäk-yə-'lā-shən\ n 1 : inoculation with vaccine prepared from material from one's own body 2 : spread of infection from one part to other parts of the same body

au·to·in·tox·i·ca·tion \-in-ˌtäk-sə-'kā-shən\ n : poisoning by toxic substances produced within the body

au·to·ki·ne·sis \ˌȯt-ō-kə-'nē-səs, -kī-\ n, pl -ne·ses \-ˌsēz\ : spontaneous or voluntary movement — **au·to·ki·net·ic** \-'net-ik\ adj

au·tol·o·gous \ȯ-'täl-ə-gəs\ adj 1 : derived from the same individual ⟨∼ grafts⟩ ⟨incubated lymphoid cells with ∼ tumor cells⟩ — compare HETEROLOGOUS 1, HOMOLOGOUS 2a 2 : involving one individual as both donor and recipient (as of blood) ⟨∼ transfusion⟩ ⟨∼ bone marrow transplants⟩

au·tol·y·sate \ȯ-'täl-ə-ˌsāt, -ˌzāt\ also **au·tol·y·zate** \-ˌzāt\ n : a product of autolysis

au·tol·y·sin \-ə-sən\ n : a substance that produces autolysis

au·tol·y·sis \-ə-səs\ n, pl -y·ses \-ə-ˌsēz\ : breakdown of all or part of a cell or tissue by self-produced enzymes — called

---

\ə\ abut \ᵊ\ kitten \ər\ further \a\ ash \ā\ ace \ä\ cot, cart
\aù\ out \ch\ chin \e\ bet \ē\ easy \g\ go \i\ hit \ī\ ice \j\ job
\ŋ\ sing \ō\ go \ȯ\ law \ȯi\ boy \th\ thin \t͟h\ the \ü\ loot
\ù\ foot \y\ yet \zh\ vision   See also Pronunciation Symbols page

also *self-digestion* — **au·to·lyt·ic** \ˌȯt-ᵊl-ˈit-ik\ *adj*
au·to·lyze *or Brit* **au·to·lyse** \ˈȯt-ᵊl-ˌīz\ *vb* **-lyzed** *or Brit* **-lysed; -lyz·ing** *or Brit* **-lys·ing** *vi* : to undergo autolysis ~ *vt* : to subject to autolysis
au·to·ma·nip·u·la·tion \ˌȯt-ō-mə-ˌnip-yə-ˈlā-shən\ *n* : physical stimulation of the genital organs by oneself — **au·to·ma·nip·u·la·tive** \-ˈnip-yə-ˌlāt-iv\ *adj*
au·tom·a·tism \ȯ-ˈtäm-ə-ˌtiz-əm\ *n* **1** : an automatic action; *esp* : any action performed without the doer's intention or awareness **2** : the power or fact of moving or functioning without conscious control either independently of external stimulation (as in the beating of the heart) or more or less directly under the influence of external stimuli (as in the dilating or contracting of the pupil of the eye)
au·to·mat·o·graph \ˌȯt-ə-ˈmat-ə-ˌgraf\ *n* : AUTOSCOPE
au·to·mix·is \ˌȯt-ə-ˈmik-səs\ *n, pl* **-mix·es** \-ˌsēz\ : parthenogenesis in which the chromosomes of a haploid gamete divide without nuclear division resulting in formation of a diploid nucleus
au·to·mne·sia \ˌȯt-əm-ˈnē-zhə, ˌȯt-ō-ˈnē-\ *n* : memory of earlier experience without any apparent associative condition
au·to·nom·ic \ˌȯt-ə-ˈnäm-ik\ *adj* **1 a** : acting or occurring involuntarily ⟨~ reflexes⟩ **b** : relating to, affecting, or controlled by the autonomic nervous system ⟨~ ganglia⟩ ⟨~ dysfunction⟩ **2** : having an effect upon tissue supplied by the autonomic nervous system ⟨~ drugs⟩ — **au·to·nom·i·cal·ly** \-i-k(ə)lē\ *adv*
autonomic nervous system *n* : a part of the vertebrate nervous system that innervates smooth and cardiac muscle and glandular tissues and governs involuntary actions (as secretion, vasoconstriction, or peristalsis) and that consists of the sympathetic nervous system and the parasympathetic nervous system — called also *vegetative nervous system;* compare CENTRAL NERVOUS SYSTEM, PERIPHERAL NERVOUS SYSTEM
au·ton·o·mous \ȯ-ˈtän-ə-məs\ *adj* **1** : of, relating to, or marked by autonomy **2 a** : not forming a part (as does an embryo or seed) in the developmental sequence of an organism **b** : responding, reacting, or developing independently of the whole ⟨a tumor is an ~ growth⟩ **3** : under control of the autonomic nervous system — **au·ton·o·mous·ly** *adv*
au·ton·o·my \-mē\ *n, pl* **-mies** **1** : the quality or state of being independent, free, and self-directing **2** : independence from the organism as a whole in the capacity of a part for growth, reactivity, or responsiveness
auto–oxidation *var of* AUTOXIDATION
au·toph·a·gy \ȯ-ˈtäf-ə-jē\ *n, pl* **-gies** : digestion of cellular constituents by enzymes of the same cell — **au·toph·a·gic** \-jik\ *adj*
au·to·pho·bia \ˌȯt-ə-ˈfō-bē-ə\ *n* : morbid fear of solitude
au·to·plas·tic \ˌȯt-ō-ˈplas-tik\ *adj* : of, relating to, or involving autoplasty ⟨an ~ graft⟩ — **au·to·plas·ti·cal·ly** \-ti-k(ə)lē\ *adv*
au·to·plas·ty \ˈȯt-ə-ˌplas-tē\ *n, pl* **-ties** : the repairing of lesions with tissue from the same body
au·to·poly·ploid \ˌȯt-ō-ˈpäl-i-ˌplȯid\ *n* : an individual or strain whose chromosome complement consists of more than two complete copies of the genome of a single ancestral species — compare ALLOPOLYPLOID — **autopolyploid** *adj* — **au·to·poly·ploi·dy** \-ˌplȯid-ē\ *n, pl* **-dies**
au·to·pro·throm·bin \ˌȯt-ō-prō-ˈthräm-bən\ *n* : any of several blood factors formed in the conversion of prothrombin to thrombin: as **a** : FACTOR VII **b** : FACTOR IX
autoprothrombin I \-ˈwən\ *n* : FACTOR VII
autoprothrombin II \-ˈtü\ *n* : FACTOR IX
¹**au·top·sy** \ˈȯ-ˌtäp-sē, ˈȯt-əp-\ *n, pl* **-sies** : an examination of the body after death usu. with such dissection as will expose the vital organs for determining the cause of death or the character and extent of changes produced by disease — called also *necropsy, postmortem, postmortem examination*
²**autopsy** *vt* **-sied; -sy·ing** : to perform an autopsy on
au·to·psy·chic \ˈȯt-ə-ˌsī-kik\ *adj* : of or relating to awareness of one's own mind and personality — compare ALLOPSYCHIC

au·to·ra·dio·gram \ˌȯt-ō-ˈrād-ē-ə-ˌgram\ *n* : AUTORADIOGRAPH
¹**au·to·ra·dio·graph** \-ˌgraf\ *n* : an image produced on a photographic film or plate by the radiations from a radioactive substance in an object which is in close contact with the emulsion — called also *radioautogram, radioautograph*
²**autoradiograph** *vt* : to subject to autoradiography
au·to·ra·dio·graph·ic \-ˌrād-ē-ə-ˈgraf-ik\ *adj* : of or relating to autoradiographs or to autoradiography
au·to·ra·di·og·ra·phy \-ˌrād-ē-ˈäg-rə-fē\ *n, pl* **-phies** : the process of making autoradiographs
au·to·re·ac·tive \ˌȯt-ō-rē-ˈak-tiv\ *adj* : produced by an organism and acting against its own cells or tissues ⟨~ T cells⟩
au·to·reg·u·la·tion \ˌȯt-ō-ˌreg-yə-ˈlā-shən\ *n* : the maintenance of relative constancy of a physiological process by a bodily part or system under varying conditions; *esp* : the maintenance of a constant supply of blood to an organ in spite of varying arterial pressure ⟨the influence of vasoactive agents on ~ of renal flow *—Science*⟩ — **au·to·reg·u·late** \-ˈreg-yə-ˌlāt\ *vb* **-lat·ed; -lat·ing** — **au·to·reg·u·la·to·ry** \-ˈreg-yə-lə-ˌtōr-ē, -ˌtȯr-\ *adj*
au·to·scope \ˈȯt-ə-ˌskōp\ *n* : a device for recording or magnifying small involuntary movements of the body
au·tos·co·py \ȯ-ˈtäs-kə-pē\ *n, pl* **-pies** : visual hallucination of an image of one's body
au·to·sen·si·ti·za·tion *or Brit* **au·to·sen·si·ti·sa·tion** \ˌȯt-ō-ˌsen(t)-sət-ə-ˈzā-shən, -ˌsen(t)-stə-ˈzā-\ *n* : AUTOIMMUNIZATION
au·to·se·rum \ˈȯt-ō-ˌsir-əm\ *n* : a serum used to treat the same patient from which it was taken
au·to·sex·ing \ˈȯt-ō-ˌsek-siŋ\ *adj* : exhibiting different characters in the two sexes at birth or hatching ⟨~ poultry⟩
au·to·site \-ˌsīt\ *n* : the larger part of a double fetus that is usu. capable of independent existence and nourishes both itself and the parasitic twin — compare OMPHALOSITE
au·to·some \ˈȯt-ə-ˌsōm\ *n* : a chromosome other than a sex chromosome — called also *nonsex chromosome;* compare ALLOSOME — **au·to·so·mal** \ˌȯt-ə-ˈsō-məl\ *adj* — **au·to·so·mal·ly** \-mə-lē\ *adv*
au·to·sug·gest·ibil·i·ty \ˌȯt-ō-sə(g)-ˌjes-tə-ˈbil-ət-ē\ *n, pl* **-ties** : the quality or state of being subject to autosuggestion — **au·to·sug·gest·i·ble** \-ˈjes-tə-bəl\ *adj*
au·to·sug·ges·tion \-sə(g)-ˈjes(h)-chən\ *n* : an influencing of one's own attitudes, behavior, or physical condition by mental processes other than conscious thought : SELF-HYPNOSIS — compare HETEROSUGGESTION — **au·to·sug·gest** \-sə(g)-ˈjest\ *vt*
au·to·ther·a·py \ˈȯt-ō-ˌther-ə-pē, ˌȯt-ō-ˈ\ *n, pl* **-pies** : SELF-TREATMENT
au·tot·o·my \ȯ-ˈtät-ə-mē\ *n, pl* **-mies** : reflex separation of a part from the body esp. in an invertebrate
au·to·top·ag·no·sia \ˌȯt-ō-ˌtäp-ig-ˈnō-zhə\ *n* : loss of the power to recognize or orient a bodily part due to a brain lesion
au·to·tox·emia *or chiefly Brit* **au·to·tox·ae·mia** \-täk-ˈsē-mē-ə\ *n* : AUTOINTOXICATION
autotoxicus — see HORROR AUTOTOXICUS
au·to·tox·in \ˈȯt-ə-ˌtäk-sən, ˌȯt-ə-ˈ\ *n* : any toxin produced within the body
au·to·trans·form·er \ˌȯt-ō-tran(t)s-ˈfȯr-mər\ *n* : a transformer in which the primary and secondary coils have part or all of their turns in common
au·to·trans·fuse \-tran(t)s-ˈfyüz\ *vt* **-fused; -fus·ing** : to subject to autotransfusion
au·to·trans·fu·sion \-tran(t)s-ˈfyü-zhən\ *n* : return of autologous blood to the patient's own circulatory system
au·to·trans·plant \-ˈtran(t)s-ˌplant\ *n* : AUTOGRAFT — **au·to·trans·plant** \-tran(t)s-ˈ\ *vt*
au·to·trans·plan·ta·tion \-ˌtran(t)s-ˌplan-ˈtā-shən\ *n* : the action of autotransplanting : the condition of being autotransplanted
au·to·troph \ˈȯt-ə-ˌtrōf, -ˌträf\ *n* : an autotrophic organism
au·to·tro·phic \ˌȯt-ə-ˈtrō-fik\ *adj* **1** : needing only carbon

dioxide or carbonates as a source of carbon and a simple inorganic nitrogen compound for metabolic synthesis **2** : not requiring a specified exogenous factor for normal metabolism — **au·to·tro·phi·cal·ly** \-fi-k(ə-)lē\ *adv*

au·to·tro·phy \'ȯt-ə-ˌtrō-fē, ȯ-'tä-trə-fē\ *n, pl* **-phies** : the condition of being autotrophic; *also* : the process by which an autotrophic organism obtains energy from carbon dioxide or carbonates and inorganic substances

au·to·vac·ci·na·tion \'ȯt-ō-ˌvak-sə-ˌnā-shən\ *n* : vaccination of an individual by material from the individual's own body or with a vaccine prepared from such material

au·tox·i·da·tion \ȯ-ˌtäk-sə-'dā-shən\ *also* **au·to–ox·i·da·tion** \ˌȯt-ō-ˌäk-sə-'dā-shən\ *n* : oxidation by direct combination with oxygen (as in air) at ordinary temperatures ⟨the rancidity of fats and oils is caused by ∼⟩

au·tumn cro·cus \ˌȯt-əm-'krō-kəs\ *n* : an autumn-blooming herb (*Colchicum autumnale*) of the lily family (Liliaceae) that is the source of medicinal colchicum

aux *abbr* auxiliary

aux·an·o·gram \ȯg-'zan-ə-ˌgram, ȯk-'san-\ *n* : a plate culture (as of bacteria) in which variable conditions are provided for growth in order to determine the effects of a particular condition or agent on the growth of a test organism

aux·a·nog·ra·phy \ˌȯg-zə-'näg-rə-fē, ˌȯk-sə-\ *n, pl* **-phies** : the study of growth-promoting or growth-inhibiting agents by means of auxanograms — **aux·an·o·graph·ic** \ȯg-ˌzan-ə-'graf-ik, ȯk-ˌsan-\ *adj* — **aux·an·o·graph·i·cal·ly** \-i-k(ə-)lē\ *adv*

aux·e·sis \ȯg-'zē-səs, ȯk-'sē-\ *n, pl* **-e·ses** \-ˌsēz\ : GROWTH; *specif* : increase of cell size without cell division — **aux·et·ic** \-'zet-ik, -'set-\ *adj*

¹aux·il·ia·ry \ȯg-'zil-yə-rē, -'zil-(ə-)rē\ *adj* : serving to supplement or assist ⟨∼ springs in a dental appliance⟩

²auxiliary *n* **1** : one who assists or serves another person esp. in dentistry **2** : an organization that assists (as by donations or volunteer services) the work esp. of a hospital

aux·in \'ȯk-sən\ *n* : an organic substance that is able in low concentrations to promote elongation of plant shoots and usu. to control other specific growth effects; *broadly* : PLANT HORMONE

auxo·chrome \'ȯk-sə-ˌkrōm\ *n* : a salt-forming group (as hydroxyl or amino) that when introduced into a chromogen produces a dye — **auxo·chrom·ic** \ˌȯk-sə-'krō-mik\ *adj*

auxo·cyte \'ȯk-sə-ˌsīt\ *n* : a gamete-forming cell (as an oocyte) or spore-forming cell during its growth period

auxo·drome \-ˌdrōm\ *n* : a plotted curve indicating the relative development of a child at any given age

auxo·troph \-ˌtrōf, -ˌträf\ *n* : an auxotrophic strain or individual

auxo·tro·phic \ˌȯk-sə-'trō-fik\ *adj* : requiring a specific growth substance beyond the minimum required for normal metabolism and reproduction of the parental or wild-type strain ⟨∼ bacterial mutants⟩ — compare PROTOTROPHIC

aux·ot·ro·phy \ȯk-'sä-trə-fē\ *n, pl* **-phies** : the condition of being auxotrophic

av *abbr* **1** average **2** avoirdupois

AV *abbr* **1** arteriovenous **2** atrioventricular

aval·vu·lar \(')ā-'val-vyə-lər\ *adj* **1** : lacking valves **2** : not affecting valves

Avan·dia \ä-ˌvan-'dē-ə\ *trademark* — used for a preparation of the maleate of rosiglitazone

avas·cu·lar \(')ā-'vas-kyə-lər\ *adj* : having few or no blood vessels ⟨the lens is a very ∼ structure⟩ ⟨∼ necrosis⟩

avas·cu·lar·i·ty \-ˌvas-kyə-'lar-ət-ē\ *n, pl* **-ties** : the condition of having few or no blood vessels ⟨cartilage ∼⟩

avascular necrosis *n* : necrosis of bone tissue due to impaired or disrupted blood supply (as that caused by traumatic injury or disease) and marked by severe pain in the affected region and by weakened bone that may flatten and collapse — called also *osteonecrosis*

avdp *abbr* avoirdupois

Ave·na \ə-'vē-nə\ *n* : a genus of widely distributed grasses (family Gramineae) with deeply furrowed grains that include the commonly cultivated oat (*A. sativa*)

ave·nin \ə-'vē-nən, 'av-ə-nən\ *or* **ave·nine** \-ˌnēn\ *n* : the glutelin of oats

Aven·tyl \'av-ən-ˌtil\ *trademark* — used for a preparation of nortriptyline

aver·sion \ə-'vər-zhən, -shən\ *n* **1** : a feeling of repugnance toward something with a desire to avoid or turn from it **2** : a tendency to extinguish a behavior or to avoid a thing or situation and esp. a usu. pleasurable one because it is or has been associated with a noxious stimulus ⟨conditioning of food ∼s by drug injection⟩

aversion therapy *n* : therapy intended to suppress an undesirable habit or behavior (as smoking or overeating) by associating the habit or behavior with a noxious or punishing stimulus (as an electric shock)

aver·sive \ə-'vər-siv, -ziv\ *adj* : tending to avoid or causing avoidance of a noxious or punishing stimulus ⟨behavior modification by ∼ conditioning⟩ — **aver·sive·ly** *adv* — **aver·sive·ness** *n*

Aves \'ā-ˌvēz\ *n pl* : a class of Vertebrata that includes all fossil and recent birds

avi·an \'ā-vē-ən\ *adj* : of, relating to, or derived from birds

avian encephalomyelitis *n* : a usu. fatal infection of young chickens caused by a picornavirus (genus *Hepatovirus*) and characterized by ataxic gait and weakening of the legs and by tremor esp. of the head and neck — called also *epidemic tremor*

avian influenza *n* : a highly variable mild to fulminant influenza typically of domestic and wild birds that is characterized usu. by respiratory symptoms but sometimes by gastrointestinal, integumentary, and urogenital symptoms and that is caused by strains (as H5N1) of the orthomyxovirus causing influenza A which do not normally infect humans but which may mutate and be transmitted to other vertebrates (as humans) causing epidemics — called also *bird flu, fowl plague*

avi·an·ize *or Brit* **avi·an·ise** \'ā-vē-ə-ˌnīz\ *vt* **-ized** *or Brit* **-ised; -iz·ing** *or Brit* **-is·ing** : to modify or attenuate (as a virus) by repeated culture in a developing chick embryo

avian leukosis *n* : any of a group of diseases (as lymphoid leukosis) of poultry that are caused by strains of a retrovirus (species *Avian leukosis virus* of the genus *Alpharetrovirus*), that involve disturbed blood formation, and that are distinguished individually by special manifestations (as paralysis, tumor formation, leukemia, and eye damage) — called also *avian leukosis complex*

avian tuberculosis *n* : tuberculosis of birds usu. caused by a bacterium of the genus *Mycobacterium* (*M. avium*); *also* : infection of mammals (as swine) by the same bacterium

avi·din \'av-əd-ən\ *n* : a protein found in white of egg that inactivates biotin by combining with it

avir·u·lent \(')ā-'vir-(y)ə-lənt\ *adj* : not virulent ⟨an ∼ tubercle bacillus⟩ — compare NONPATHOGENIC

avis — see CALCAR AVIS

avi·ta·min·osis \ˌā-ˌvīt-ə-mə-'nō-səs, *Brit also* ˌā-vi-ˌtam-ə-\ *n, pl* **-o·ses** \-ˌsēz\ : disease (as pellagra) resulting from a deficiency of one or more vitamins — called also *hypovitaminosis* — **avi·ta·min·ot·ic** \-mə-'nät-ik\ *adj*

avium — see CALCAR AVIS, MYCOBACTERIUM AVIUM COMPLEX, MYCOBACTERIUM AVIUM-INTRACELLULARE COMPLEX

A–V node *or* **AV node** \'ā-'vē-\ *n* : ATRIOVENTRICULAR NODE

Avo·ga·dro's law \ˌav-ə-ˌgäd-(ˌ)rōz-, ˌäv-, -ˌgad-\ *n* : a law in chemistry: equal volumes of all gases at the same temperature and pressure contain equal numbers of molecules — called also *Avogadro's hypothesis*

 Avo·ga·dro \ˌav-ə-'gäd-(ˌ)rō, ˌäv-\, **Count Amedea (1776–1856),** Italian physicist and chemist. Avogadro is considered one of the founders of physical chemistry. In 1811, he made

---

\ə\ **abut** \ᵊ\ **kitten** \ər\ **further** \a\ **ash** \ā\ **ace** \ä\ **cot, cart**
\au̇\ **out** \ch\ **chin** \e\ **bet** \ē\ **easy** \g\ **go** \i\ **hit** \ī\ **ice** \j\ **job**
\ŋ\ **sing** \ō\ **go** \ȯ\ **law** \ȯi\ **boy** \th\ **thin** \t͟h\ **the** \ü\ **loot**
\u̇\ **foot** \y\ **yet** \zh\ **vision** *See also* Pronunciation Symbols page

his outstanding scientific contribution: his hypothesis, now accepted as a scientific law, that equal volumes of gases at the same temperature and pressure contain the same number of molecules. This hypothesis was a landmark in 19th-century chemistry and is one of the basic concepts of modern chemistry.

Avogadro's number *or* **Avogadro number** \-₁gäd-(₁)rō-, -₁gad-\ *n* : the number 6.023×10^{23} indicating the number of atoms or molecules in a mole of any substance — compare AVOGADRO'S LAW

avoid·ance \ə-'void-ᵊn(t)s\ *n, often attrib* : the act or practice of keeping away from or withdrawing from something undesirable ⟨reinforced by escape or ∼ of electric shock —E. S. Katkin & E. N. Murray⟩ ⟨∼ learning⟩; *esp* : an anticipatory response undertaken to avoid a noxious stimulus ⟨conditioned ∼ in mice⟩

avoidance–avoidance conflict *n* : psychological conflict that results when a choice must be made between two undesirable alternatives — compare APPROACH-APPROACH CONFLICT, APPROACH-AVOIDANCE CONFLICT

avoid·ant \ə-'void-ᵊnt\ *adj* : characterized by turning away or by withdrawal or defensive behavior ⟨the ∼ detached schizophrenic patient —Norman Cameron⟩ ⟨an ∼ personality⟩

av·oir·du·pois \₁av-ərd-ə-'poiz, -'pwä\ *adj* : expressed in avoirdupois weight ⟨∼ units⟩ ⟨5 ounces ∼⟩ ⟨2 ∼ ounces⟩

avoirdupois pound *n* : POUND b

avoirdupois weight *n* : a system of weights based on a pound of 16 ounces and an ounce of 437.5 grains (28.350 grams) and in general use in the U.S. except for precious metals, gems, and drugs

AVP *abbr* arginine vasopressin

avulse \ə-'vəls\ *vt* **avulsed; avuls·ing** : to separate by avulsion ⟨an *avulsed* ligament⟩

avul·sion \ə-'vəl-shən\ *n* : a tearing away of a body part accidentally or surgically ⟨∼ of the fingernail⟩

avulsion fracture *n* : the detachment of a bone fragment that results from the pulling away of a ligament, tendon, or joint capsule from its point of attachment on a bone — called also *sprain fracture*

ax *abbr* axis

axe·nic \(')ā-'zen-ik, -'zēn-\ *adj* : free from other living organisms ⟨an ∼ culture of bacteria⟩ — **axe·ni·cal·ly** \-i-k(ə-)lē\ *adv*

axes *pl of* AXIS

ax·i·al \'ak-sē-əl\ *adj* **1** : of, relating to, or having the characteristics of an axis **2 a** : situated around, in the direction of, on, or along an axis **b** : extending in a direction essentially perpendicular to the plane of a cyclic structure (as of cyclohexane) ⟨∼ hydrogens⟩ — compare EQUATORIAL

axial skeleton *n* : the skeleton of the trunk and head

Ax·id \'ak-sid\ *trademark* — used for a preparation of nizatidine

ax·ile \'ak-₁sīl\ *adj* : relating to or situated in an axis

ax·il·la \ag-'zil-ə, ak-'sil-\ *n, pl* **-lae** \-(₁)ē, -₁ī\ *or* **-las** : the cavity beneath the junction of the arm or anterior appendage and shoulder or pectoral girdle containing the axillary artery and vein, a part of the brachial plexus of nerves, many lymph nodes, and fat and areolar tissue; *esp* : ARMPIT

ax·il·lary \'ak-sə-₁ler-ē\ *adj* : of, relating to, or located near the axilla ⟨∼ lymph nodes⟩ ⟨∼ temperature⟩

axillary artery *n* : the part of the main artery of the arm that lies in the axilla and that is continuous with the subclavian artery above and the brachial artery below

axillary fossa *n* : AXILLA

axillary gland *n* : AXILLARY NODE

axillary nerve *n* : a large nerve arising from the posterior cord of the brachial plexus and supplying the deltoid and teres minor muscles and the skin of the shoulder

axillary node *n* : any of the lymph nodes of the axilla — called also *axillary gland*

axillary vein *n* : the large vein passing through the axilla continuous with the basilic vein below and the subclavian vein above

ax·is \'ak-səs\ *n, pl* **ax·es** \-₁sēz\ **1 a** : a straight line about which a body or a geometric figure rotates or may be thought of as rotating **b** : a straight line with respect to which a body, organ, or figure is symmetrical **2 a** : the second vertebra of the neck of the higher vertebrates that is prolonged anteriorly within the foramen of the first vertebra and united with the dens which serves as a pivot for the atlas and head to turn upon — called also *epistropheus* **b** : any of various central, fundamental, or axial parts ⟨the cerebrospinal ∼⟩ ⟨the skeletal ∼⟩ **c** : AXILLA

axis cylinder *n* : AXON; *esp* : the axon of a myelinated neuron

axo·ax·o·nal \₁ak-sō-'ak-sən-ᵊl, -ak-'sän-, -'sōn-\ *or* **axo·ax·on·ic** \-ak-'sän-ik\ *adj* : relating to or being a synapse between an axon of one neuron and an axon of another

axo·den·drit·ic \₁ak-sō-den-'drit-ik\ *adj* : relating to or being a nerve synapse between an axon of one neuron and a dendrite of another

axo·lem·ma \'ak-sə-₁lem-ə\ *n* : the plasma membrane of an axon

ax·om·e·ter \ak-'säm-ət-ər\ *n* : an instrument used to locate the position of optical axes; *esp* : one used to adjust a pair of spectacles properly with respect to the axes of the eyes

ax·on \'ak-₁sän\ *also* **ax·one** \-₁sōn\ *n* : a usu. long and single nerve-cell process that usu. conducts impulses away from the cell body — **ax·o·nal** \'ak-sən-ᵊl; ak-'sän-, -'sōn-\ *adj*

ax·o·neme \'ak-sə-₁nēm\ *n* : the fibrillar bundle of a flagellum or cilium that usu. consists of nine pairs of microtubules in a ring around a single central pair — **ax·o·ne·mal** \₁ak-sə-'nē-məl\ *adj*

axon hillock *n* : the prominence on a nerve-cell body from which an axon arises

ax·on·ot·me·sis \₁ak-sə-nət-'mē-səs\ *n, pl* **-tme·ses** \-'mē-₁sēz\ : axonal nerve damage (as from compression or crushing) that does not completely sever the surrounding endoneurial sheath so that regeneration can take place

axo·plasm \'ak-sə-₁plaz-əm\ *n* : the protoplasm of an axon — **axo·plas·mic** \₁ak-sə-'plaz-mik\ *adj*

axo·so·mat·ic \₁ak-sō-sō-'mat-ik\ *adj* : relating to or being a nerve synapse between the cell body of one neuron and an axon of another

axo·style \'ak-sō-₁stīl\ *n* : an axial rod present in many parasitic flagellates that is variously regarded as locomotor or supporting in function

ax·ot·o·my \ak-'sät-ə-mē\ *n, pl* **-mies** : the cutting or severing of a neuron's axon — **ax·ot·o·mized** \-mīzd\ *adj*

Ayer·za's disease \ə-'yər-zəz-\ *n* : a complex of symptoms marked esp. by cyanosis, dyspnea, polycythemia, and sclerosis of the pulmonary artery

Ayerza, Abel (1861–1918), Argentinean physician. Ayerza was a professor of clinical medicine at the National University of Buenos Aires. In 1901 he studied a case in which cyanosis and sclerosis of the pulmonary vessels appeared during autopsy. He reported his findings only in a lecture. A student, Francisco C. Arrillaga, incorporated the observations in a 1912 thesis and published a full description of the disease in 1925.

Ay·ur·ve·da \₁ī-yər-'vād-ə, -'ved-\ *n* : a form of alternative medicine that is the traditional system of medicine of India, that preceded and evolved independently of Western medicine, and that seeks to treat and integrate body, mind, and spirit using a comprehensive holistic approach esp. by emphasizing diet, herbal remedies, exercise, meditation, breathing, and physical therapy — **Ay·ur·ve·dic** \-ik\ *adj* — **Ay·ur·ve·dist** \-əst\ *n*

Ayurvedic medicine *n* : AYURVEDA

Az *abbr* [French *azote*] nitrogen

5–aza·cy·ti·dine \'fīv-₁az-ə-'sit-ə-₁dēn, -'sīt-\ *or* **azacytidine** *n* : an antineoplastic cytidine analog $C_8H_{12}N_4O_5$ that has been used experimentally in the treatment of some leukemias and cancers

aza·se·rine \₁az-ə-'ser-₁ēn, -'si(ə)r-, -ən\ *n* : an antibiotic $C_5H_7N_3O_4$ that has been used to inhibit the growth of some tumors without significant clinical success

aza·thi·o·prine \ˌaz-ə-'thī-ə-ˌprēn\ *n* : a purine antimetabolite $C_9H_7N_7O_2S$ that is used esp. as an immunosuppressant — see IMURAN

azeo·trope \ā-'zē-ə-ˌtrōp\ *n* : a liquid mixture that is characterized by a constant minimum or maximum boiling point which is lower or higher than that of any of the components and that distills without change in composition — **azeo·tro·pic** \ˌzē-ə-'trō-pik, -'träp-ik\ *adj*

azide \'ā-ˌzīd, 'az-ˌīd\ *n* : a compound containing the group N_3 combined with an element or radical

az·i·do \'a-zə-(ˌ)dō\ *adj* : relating to or containing the monovalent group N_3 — often used in combination

az·i·do·thy·mi·dine \ˌaz-i-dō-'thī-mə-ˌdēn\ *n* : AZT

azine \'ā-ˌzēn, 'az-ˌēn\ *n* **1** : any of numerous organic compounds with a nitrogenous 6-membered ring **2** : a compound of the general formula RCH=NN=CHR or R_2C=NN=CR_2 formed by the action of hydrazine on aldehydes or ketones

azin·phos·meth·yl \ˌāz-²n-fäs-'meth-əl, ˌaz-\ *n* : an organophosphorus pesticide $C_{10}H_{12}N_3O_3PS_2$ used against insects and mites

azith·ro·my·cin \ə-ˌzith-rō-'mīs-²n\ *n* : a semisynthetic macrolide antibiotic $C_{38}H_{72}N_2O_{12}$ that is derived from erythromycin and is used esp. as an antibacterial agent — see ZITHROMAX

Az·ma·cort \'az-mə-ˌkȯrt\ *trademark* — used for a preparation of the acetonide of triamcinolone

azo \'ā-(ˌ)zō, 'az-(ˌ)ō\ *adj* : relating to or containing the bivalent group N=N united at both ends to carbon

azo dye *n* : any of numerous dyes containing azo groups

azole \'ā-ˌzōl, 'az-ˌōl\ *n* : any of numerous compounds characterized by a 5-membered ring containing at least one atom of nitrogen

azo·lit·min \ˌaz-ō-'lit-mən, ˌāz-\ *n* : a dark red nitrogenous coloring matter obtained from litmus and used as an acid-base indicator

azo·osper·mia \ˌā-zō-ə-'spər-mē-ə, ə-ˌzō-\ *n* : absence of spermatozoa from the seminal fluid — compare ASPERMIA — **azo·osper·mic** \-'spər-mik\ *adj*

azo·pro·tein \ˌā-zō-'prō-ˌtēn, -'prōt-ē-ən\ *n* : any of various compounds made by coupling a protein (as serum albumin) with a diazotized amine (as histamine or sulfanilamide), and sometimes used as synthetic antigens

azo·sul·fa·mide *or chiefly Brit* **azo·sul·pha·mide** \ˌā-zō-'səl-fə-ˌmīd\ *n* : a dark red crystalline azo compound $C_{18}H_{14}N_4Na_2O_{10}S_3$ of the sulfa class having antibacterial effect similar to that of sulfanilamide — called also *prontosil soluble*

azo·te·mia *or chiefly Brit* **azo·tae·mia** \ˌā-zō-'tē-mē-ə\ *n* : an excess of urea and other nitrogenous wastes in the blood as a result of kidney insufficiency — compare UREMIA — **azo·te·mic** *or chiefly Brit* **azo·tae·mic** \-'tē-mik\ *adj*

az·oth \'az-ˌȯth\ *n* **1** : mercury regarded by alchemists as the first principle of metals **2** : the universal remedy of Paracelsus

azo·to·bac·ter \ā-'zōt-ə-ˌbak-tər\ *n* **1** *cap* : a genus of large rod-shaped or spherical bacteria occurring in soil and sewage and fixing atmospheric nitrogen **2** : any bacterium of the genus *Azotobacter*

azo·tom·e·ter \ˌā-zō-'täm-ət-ər\ *n* : NITROMETER

azo·tor·rhea *or chiefly Brit* **azo·tor·rhoea** \ˌā-zōt-ə-'rē-ə\ *n* : excessive discharge of nitrogenous substances in the feces or urine

azo·tu·ria \ˌā-zō-'t(y)ùr-ē-ə\ *n* : an abnormal condition of horses characterized by an excesss of urea or other nitrogenous substances in the urine and by muscle damage esp. to the hindquarters

AZT \ˌā-(ˌ)zē-'tē\ *n* : an antiviral drug $C_{10}H_{13}N_5O_4$ that inhibits replication of some retroviruses (as HIV) and is used to treat AIDS — called also *azidothymidine, ZDV, zidovudine;* see RETROVIR

az·tre·o·nam \ˌaz-'trē-ō-ˌnam, 'az-trē-\ *n* : a synthetic monobactam antibiotic $C_{13}H_{17}N_5O_8S_2$ used esp. against gram-negative bacteria

azure \'azh-ər\ *n* : any of several dyes used as biological stains

azy·gog·ra·phy \ˌā-zī-'gäg-rə-fē\ *n, pl* **-phies** : radiographic visualization of the azygos system of veins after injection of a radiopaque medium

¹azy·gos \ā-'zī-gəs\ *n* : an azygos anatomical part

²azy·gos *also* **azy·gous** \(')ā-'zī-gəs\ *adj* : not being one of a pair ⟨the ∼ muscle of the uvula⟩ ⟨the ∼ system of veins⟩

azygos vein *n* : any of a system of three veins which drain the thoracic wall and much of the abdominal wall and which form a collateral circulation when either the inferior or superior vena cava is obstructed; *esp* : a vein that receives blood from the right half of the thoracic and abdominal walls, ascends along the right side of the spinal column, and empties into the superior vena cava — compare ACCESSORY HEMIAZYGOS VEIN, HEMIAZYGOS VEIN

B

b *abbr* **1** bacillus **2** barometric **3** bath **4** Baumé scale **5** behavior **6** bel **7** bicuspid **8** born **9** brother

B \'bē\ *n* : the one of the four ABO blood groups characterized by the presence of antigens designated by the letter B and by the presence of antibodies against the antigens present in the A blood group

B *symbol* boron

BA *abbr* bronchial asthma

Ba *symbol* barium

Bab·cock test \'bab-ˌkäk-\ *n* : a test for determining the fat content of milk and milk products

　Babcock, Stephen Moulton (1843–1931), American agricultural chemist. During his career Babcock provided agriculture with a number of inventions and procedures, the Babcock test being the foremost. The introduction of this test, devised in 1890, discouraged the watering down of milk, resulted in a scale for milk prices based on quality, and provided a new impetus for the improvement of dairy herds. Babcock also invented an improved viscometer, which is used for measuring the viscosity of milk and other liquids, and did research on the nutritional value of various feeds, thereby providing groundwork for the discovery of vitamin A.

Ba·bes–Ernst granule \'bäb-ˌesh-'ərn(t)st-\ *n* : a metachromatic granule in protoplasm — called also *Babes-Ernst body*

　Babès, Victor (1854–1926), Romanian bacteriologist. In 1888 Babès made two important discoveries. With the German pathologist Paul Ernst he discovered and described the metachromatic granules seen in the protoplasm of bacteria. These granules stain deeply with aniline dyes and are now known as Babes-Ernst granules or bodies. He also discovered a group of small protozoan parasites that invade the blood of various animals and are now placed in the genus *Babesia*, named after him.

　Ernst, Paul (1859–1937), German pathologist. Director of the pathological institute at Heidelberg, Ernst specialized in the pathology of cells and the nervous system. In

\ə\ **abut** \ˈ\ **kitten** \ər\ **further** \a\ **ash** \ā\ **ace** \ä\ **cot, cart** \aù\ **out** \ch\ **chin** \e\ **bet** \ē\ **easy** \g\ **go** \i\ **hit** \ī\ **ice** \j\ **job** \ŋ\ **sing** \ō\ **go** \ò\ **law** \òi\ **boy** \th\ **thin** \th\ **the** \ü\ **loot** \ù\ **foot** \y\ **yet** \zh\ **vision** *See also* Pronunciation Symbols page

1889 in an article he again described the Babes-Ernst granules.

ba·be·sia \bə-'bē-zh(ē-)ə\ *n* **1** *cap* : the type genus of the family Babesiidae **2** : any of the sporozoans of the genus *Babesia* or sometimes the family Babesiidae that are parasitic in mammalian red blood cells (as in Texas fever) and are transmitted by the bite of a tick — called also *piroplasm*

V. **Babès** — see BABES-ERNST GRANULE

babe·si·a·sis \ˌbab-ə-'sī-ə-səs\ *n, pl* **-a·ses** \-ˌsēz\ : BABESIOSIS

Ba·be·si·i·dae \ˌbab-ə-'zī-ə-ˌdē, -'zē-\ *n pl* : a family of the order Haemosporidia comprising minute protozoan parasites of mammalian red blood cells that are transmitted from host to host by the bite of a tick intermediate host and cause some destructive diseases of domestic animals — see BABESIA

ba·be·si·o·sis \bə-ˌbē-zē-'ō-səs\ *n, pl* **-o·ses** \-ˌsēz\ : infection with or disease caused by babesias — called also *babesiasis*

Ba·bin·ski reflex \bə-ˌbin-skē-\ *also* **Ba·bin·ski's reflex** \-skēz-\ *n* : a reflex movement in which when the sole is tickled the great toe turns upward instead of downward and which is normal in infancy but indicates damage to the central nervous system (as in the pyramidal tracts) when occurring later in life — called also *Babinski, Babinski sign, Babinski's sign;* compare PLANTAR REFLEX

Babinski, Joseph–François–Felix (1857–1932), French neurologist. One of the leading neurologists of his time, Babinski published more than 200 papers, making many important contributions to clinical neurology. In 1896 he made his most famous contribution, his original description of the plantar reflex. He is also known for his critical analysis of cerebellar physiology and symptomatology. He introduced the concept of asynergia and described adiadokokinesis, the inability to perform rapid alternating movements.

ba·by \'bā-bē\ *n, pl* **babies** **1** : an extremely young child; *esp* : INFANT **2** : an extremely young animal — **baby** *adj* — **ba·by·hood** \-bē-ˌhůd\ *n* — **ba·by·ish** \-ish\ *adj*

baby oil *n* : a usu. fragrant mineral oil that is used esp. to moisturize and cleanse the skin; *also* : any of various oils used similarly

baby talk *n* **1** : the syntactically imperfect speech or phonetically modified forms used by small children learning to talk **2** : the consciously imperfect or altered speech often used by adults in speaking to small children

baby tooth *n* : MILK TOOTH

bac·cate \'bak-ˌāt\ *adj* : pulpy throughout like a berry

Bac·il·la·ce·ae \ˌbas-ə-'lā-sē-ˌē\ *n pl* : a family including the genera *Bacillus* and *Clostridium* and comprising typically rod-shaped usu. gram-positive bacteria of the order Eubacteriales that produce endospores

ba·cil·la·ry \'bas-ə-ˌler-ē, bə-'sil-ə-rē\ *also* **ba·cil·lar** \bə-'sil-ər, 'bas-ə-lər\ *adj* **1** : shaped like a rod; *also* : consisting of small rods **2** : of, relating to, or caused by bacilli ⟨∼ meningitis⟩

bacillary angiomatosis *n* : a disease esp. of the skin that occurs in immunocompromised individuals, that is characterized by reddish elevated lesions often surrounded by a scaly ring, that may spread to produce a more widespread systemic disorder, and that is caused by either of two bacteria of the genus *Bartonella* (*B. henselae* and *B. quintana*) — called also *epithelioid angiomatosis*

ba·cille Calmette–Guérin \ba-'sēl-, bä-\ *n* : BACILLUS CALMETTE-GUÉRIN

bac·il·le·mia *or chiefly Brit* **bac·il·lae·mia** \ˌbas-ə-'lē-mē-ə\ *n* : BACTEREMIA

ba·cil·li·form \bə-'sil-ə-ˌfȯrm\ *adj* : shaped like a rod : BACILLARY

bac·il·lo·sis \ˌbas-ə-'lō-səs\ *n, pl* **-lo·ses** \-ˌsēz\ : infection with bacilli

bac·il·lu·ria \ˌbas-ə-'lůr-ē-ə, -əl-'yůr-\ *n* : the passage of bacilli with the urine — **bac·il·lu·ric** \-'lůr-ik, -'yůr-\ *adj*

ba·cil·lus \bə-'sil-əs\ *n, pl* **-li** \-ˌī *also* -ē\ **1 a** *cap* : a genus of rod-shaped gram-positive endospore-producing usu. aerobic bacteria of the family Bacillaceae that include many saprophytes and some parasites (as *B. anthracis* of anthrax)

b : any bacterium of the genus *Bacillus*; *broadly* : a straight rod-shaped bacterium **2** : BACTERIUM; *esp* : a disease-producing bacterium

bacillus Cal·mette–Gué·rin \-ˌkal-'met-(ˌ)gā-'ran, -'ran\ *n* : an attenuated strain of tubercle bacillus developed by repeated culture on a medium containing bile and used in preparation of tuberculosis vaccines — called also *bacille Calmette-Guérin;* compare BCG VACCINE

Cal·mette \kȧl-met\, **Albert Léon Charles (1863–1933),** French bacteriologist, and **Gué·rin** \gā-ran\, **Camille (1872–1961),** French veterinarian. A pupil of Louis Pasteur, Calmette founded in 1891 the Pasteur Institute in Saigon, in what is now Vietnam, where he discovered an antivenin snake venom serum. In 1908 his discovery that virulent bovine tubercle bacilli became less virulent after being cultured on a medium containing bile led to his development in 1927 with Camille Guérin of a tuberculosis vaccine from a strain of tubercle bacillus now known as bacillus Calmette-Guérin. The acronym of the name of the bacillus forms part of the name of their discovery, BCG vaccine, which is widely used in the vaccination of children against tuberculosis.

bac·i·tra·cin \ˌbas-ə-'trās-ᵊn\ *n* : a polypeptide antibiotic isolated from a bacillus (*Bacillus subtilis* or *B. licheniformis*) and usu. used topically esp. against gram-positive bacteria

Tra·cy \'trā-sē\, **Margaret,** American hospital patient. The antibiotic bacitracin was first identified in 1945 in wound drainage from Margaret Tracy.

back \'bak\ *n* **1 a** : the rear part of the human body esp. from the neck to the end of the spine **b** : the corresponding part of a lower animal (as a quadruped) **c** : SPINAL COLUMN **2** : the part of the upper surface of the tongue behind the front and lying opposite the soft palate when the tongue is at rest

back·ache \'bak-ˌāk\ *n* : a pain in the lower back

back·board \-ˌbȯrd\ *n* : a stiff board on which an injured person and esp. one with neck or spinal injuries is placed and immobilized in order to prevent further injury during transport

back·bone \-'bōn, -ˌbōn\ *n* **1** : SPINAL COLUMN, SPINE **2** : the longest chain of atoms or groups of atoms in a usu. long molecule (as a polymer or protein)

¹back·cross \'bak-ˌkrȯs\ *vt* : to cross (a first-generation hybrid) with one of the parental types

²backcross *n* : a mating that involves backcrossing; *also* : an individual produced by backcrossing

back·ing \'bak-iŋ\ *n* : the metal portion of a dental crown, bridge, or similar structure to which a porcelain or plastic tooth facing is attached

back mutation *n* : mutation of a previously mutated gene to its former condition

back pressure–arm lift method *n* : artificial respiration in which the operator kneels at the head of the prone victim, compresses the chest manually by pressure on the back, and then pulls up the elbows thereby expanding the lungs — called also *Holger Nielsen method*

back·rest \'bak-ˌrest\ *n* : a rest for the back

back·side \-ˌsīd\ *n* : BUTTOCKS — often used in pl.

bac·lo·fen \'bak-lō-ˌfen\ *n* : a gamma-aminobutyric acid analog $C_{10}H_{12}ClNO_2$ used as a relaxant of skeletal muscle esp. in treating spasticity (as in multiple sclerosis)

bact *abbr* **1** bacteria; bacterial **2** bacteriological; bacteriology **3** bacterium

bac·ter·emia *or chiefly Brit* **bac·ter·ae·mia** \ˌbak-tə-'rē-mē-ə\ *n* : the usu. transient presence of bacteria in the blood — **bac·ter·emic** *or chiefly Brit* **bac·ter·ae·mic** \-mik\ *adj*

¹bacteria *pl of* BACTERIUM

²bac·te·ria \bak-'tir-ē-ə\ *n* **1** : BACTERIUM — not usu. used technically ⟨caused by a ∼ borne by certain tiny ticks —*Wall Street Jour.*⟩ ⟨a single ∼—there are roughly 200 in each cough—apparently can infect a person —Cheryl Clark⟩ **2** *pl, cap* : a domain in the system of classification dividing all organisms into three major domains of life that includes the prokaryotes that are bacteria but not those that are archaebacteria or archaea — compare EUBACTERIA

Bac·te·ri·a·ce·ae \\(ˌ)bak-ˌtir-ē-ˈā-sē-ˌē\ *n pl* **1** *in some classi-fications* : a large family of rod-shaped usu. gram-negative bacteria of the order Eubacteriales that produce no spores and have a complex metabolism utilizing amino acids and generally carbohydrates **2** *in former classifications* : a family comprising all simple cylindrical bacteria lacking a sheath and including the family Bacteriaceae, the genus *Bacillus,* and a number of other groups

bac·te·ri·al \bak-ˈtir-ē-əl\ *adj* : of, relating to, or caused by bacteria ⟨a ∼ chromosome⟩ ⟨∼ infection⟩ ⟨∼ endocardi-tis⟩ — **bac·te·ri·al·ly** \-ə-lē\ *adv*

bacterial vag·i·no·sis \-ˌvaj-ə-ˈnō-səs\ *n* : vaginitis that is marked by a grayish vaginal discharge usu. of foul odor and that is associated with the presence of a bacterium esp. of the genus *Gardnerella* (*G. vaginalis* syn. *Haemophilus vaginalis*) — abbr. *BV;* called also *nonspecific vaginitis*

bacterial virus *n* : BACTERIOPHAGE

bac·te·ri·cid·al \bak-ˌtir-ə-ˈsīd-ᵊl\ *also* **bac·te·ri·o·cid·al** \-ˌtir-ē-ə-ˈsīd-\ *adj* : destroying bacteria — **bac·te·ri·cid·al·ly** \-ᵊl-ē\ *adv* — **bac·te·ri·cide** \-ˈtir-ə-ˌsīd\ *n*

bac·te·ri·cid·in \bak-ˌtir-ə-ˈsīd-ᵊn\ *or* **bac·te·ri·o·cid·in** \-ˌtir-ē-ə-ˈsīd-\ *n* : a bactericidal antibody

bac·ter·id \ˈbak-tə-rəd, -ˌrid\ *n* : a skin eruption associated with bacterial infection — compare ²ID

bac·ter·in \ˈbak-tə-rən\ *n* : a suspension of killed or attenuat-ed bacteria for use as a vaccine

bac·te·rio·chlo·ro·phyll \bak-ˌtir-ē-ō-ˈklōr-ə-ˌfil, -ˈklȯr-, -fəl\ *n* : a pyrrole derivative in photosynthetic bacteria relat-ed to the chlorophyll of higher plants

bac·te·ri·o·cin \bak-ˈtir-ē-ə-sən\ *n* : an antibiotic (as colicin) produced by bacteria

bac·te·ri·o·gen·ic \bak-ˌtir-ē-ə-ˈjen-ik\ *also* **bac·te·ri·og·e·nous** \-ē-ˈäj-ə-nəs\ *adj* : caused by bacteria

bac·te·ri·ol·o·gist \(ˌ)bak-ˌtir-ē-ˈäl-ə-jəst\ *n* : a specialist in bacteriology

bac·te·ri·ol·o·gy \(ˌ)bak-ˌtir-ē-ˈäl-ə-jē\ *n, pl* **-gies** **1** : a sci-ence that deals with bacteria and their relations to medicine, industry, and agriculture **2** : bacterial life and phenomena — **bac·te·ri·o·log·ic** \bak-ˌtir-ē-ə-ˈläj-ik\ *or* **bac·te·ri·o·log·i·cal** \-ˈläj-i-kəl\ *adj* — **bac·te·ri·o·log·i·cal·ly** \-i-k(ə-)lē\ *adv*

bac·te·ri·o·ly·sin \bak-ˌtir-ē-ə-ˈlīs-ᵊn\ *n* : an antibody that acts to destroy a bacterium

bac·te·ri·ol·y·sis \(ˌ)bak-ˌtir-ē-ˈäl-ə-səs\ *n, pl* **-y·ses** \-ˌsēz\ : destruction or dissolution of bacterial cells — **bac·te·ri·o·lyt·ic** \bak-ˌtir-ē-ə-ˈlit-ik\ *adj*

bac·te·ri·o·phage \bak-ˈtir-ē-ə-ˌfāj, -ˌfäzh\ *n* : a virus that in-fects bacteria — called also *phage* — **bac·te·ri·oph·a·gy** \(ˌ)bak-ˌtir-ē-ˈäf-ə-jē\ *n, pl* **-gies**

bacteriophage lambda *n* : PHAGE LAMBDA

bac·te·ri·o·pro·tein \bak-ˌtir-ē-ō-ˈprō-ˌtēn, -ˈprōt-ē-ən\ *n* : a protein present in bacteria

bac·te·ri·o·rho·dop·sin \bak-ˌtir-ē-ō-rō-ˈdäp-sən\ *n* : a purple-pigmented protein that is found in the outer mem-brane of a bacterium (*Halobacterium salinarium* syn. *H. ha-lobium*) and that converts light energy into chemical energy in the synthesis of ATP

bac·te·ri·o·sta·sis \bak-ˌtir-ē-ō-ˈstā-səs\ *n, pl* **-sta·ses** \-ˌsēz\ : inhibition of the growth of bacteria without destruction

bac·te·ri·o·stat \-ˈtir-ē-ō-ˌstat\ *also* **bac·te·ri·o·stat·ic** \-ˌtir-ē-ō-ˈstat-ik\ *n* : an agent that causes bacteriostasis

bac·te·ri·o·stat·ic \-ˌtir-ē-ō-ˈstat-ik\ *adj* : causing bacterio-stasis ⟨a ∼ agent⟩ — **bac·te·ri·o·stat·i·cal·ly** \-i-k(ə-)lē\ *adv*

bac·te·ri·o·ther·a·py \bak-ˌtir-ē-ō-ˈther-ə-pē\ *n, pl* **-pies** : the treatment of disease by the use of bacteria or their products — **bac·te·ri·o·ther·a·peu·tic** \-ˌther-ə-ˈpyüt-ik\ *adj*

bac·te·ri·o·tox·in \-ˈtäk-sən\ *n* : a specific substance that de-stroys or inhibits bacteria growth

bac·te·ri·o·tro·pic \-ˈträp-ik, -ˈtrōp-\ *adj* : directed toward bacteria or affecting them in a specific way

bac·te·ri·um \bak-ˈtir-ē-əm\ *n, pl* **-ria** \-ē-ə\ : any of a do-main (Bacteria) of prokaryotic round, spiral, or rod-shaped single-celled microorganisms that may lack cell walls or are gram-positive or gram-negative if they have cell walls, that are often aggregated into colonies or motile by means of fla-

gella, that typically live in soil, water, organic matter, or the bodies of plants and animals, that are usu. autotrophic, sap-rophytic, or parasitic in nutrition, and that are noted for their biochemical effects and pathogenicity; *broadly* : PRO-KARYOTE

bac·te·ri·uria \bak-ˌtir-ē-ˈ(y)ùr-ē-ə\ *n* : the presence of bac-teria in the urine — **bac·te·ri·uric** \-ˈ(y)ùr-ik\ *adj*

bac·te·rize *or Brit* **bac·te·rise** \ˈbak-tə-ˌrīz\ *vt* **-rized** *or Brit* **-rised; -riz·ing** *or Brit* **-ris·ing** : to subject to bacterial action — **bac·te·ri·za·tion** *or Brit* **bac·te·ri·sa·tion** \ˌbak-tə-rə-ˈzā-shən\ *n*

Bac·te·roi·da·ce·ae \ˌbak-tə-ˌrȯi-ˈdā-sē-ˌē\ *n pl* : a family of extremely varied gram-negative bacteria (order Eubacteria-les) that usu. live in the alimentary canal or on mucous sur-faces of warm-blooded animals and are sometimes associat-ed with acute infective processes — see BACTEROIDES

Bac·te·roi·des \-ˈrȯid-(ˌ)ēz\ *n* **1** *cap* : a genus of gram=negative anaerobic bacteria that belong to the family Bacte-roidaceae, that have rounded ends, produce no endospores and no pigment, and that occur usu. in the normal intestinal flora **2** *pl* **-roides** : a bacterium of the genus *Bacteroides* or of a closely related genus

Bac·trim \ˈbak-trim\ *trademark* — used for a preparation of sulfamethoxazole and trimethoprim

Bac·tro·ban \ˈbak-trō-ˌban\ *trademark* — used for a prepa-ration of mupirocin

bac·u·lum \ˈbak-yə-ləm\ *n, pl* **-lums** \-ləmz\ *or* **-la** \-lə\ : a slender bone reinforcing the penis in many mammals

bad cholesterol \ˈbad-\ *n* : LDL

BaE *or* **BAE** *abbr* barium enema

¹bag \ˈbag\ *n* : a pouched or pendulous bodily part or organ: as **a** : UDDER **b** : a pendulous outpouching of flabby skin ⟨an aging face with ∼s below the eyes⟩

²bag *vt* **bagged; bag·ging** : to ventilate the lungs of (a patient) using a hand-squeezed bag attached to a face mask

ba·gasse \bə-ˈgas\ *n* : plant residue (as of sugarcane or grapes) left after a product (as juice) has been extracted

bagasse disease *n* : BAGASSOSIS

bag·as·so·sis \ˌbag-ə-ˈsō-səs\ *n, pl* **-so·ses** \-ˌsēz\ : an indus-trial disease characterized by cough, difficult breathing, chills, fever, and prolonged weakness and caused by the in-halation of the dust of bagasse

bag of waters *n* : the double-walled fluid-filled sac that en-closes and protects the fetus in the mother's womb and that breaks releasing its fluid during the birth process — see WA-TER BAG

Bain·bridge reflex \ˈbān-(ˌ)brij-\ *n* : a homeostatic reflex mechanism that causes acceleration of heartbeat following the stimulation of local muscle spindles when blood pressure in the venae cavae and right atrium is increased

Bainbridge, Francis Arthur (1874–1921), British physiol-ogist. In 1914 in an article on cardiac reflexes Bainbridge described a reflex action that is produced by inhibition of tone of the vagus nerve and excitation of the cardiac accel-erator nerves. The reflex has since been known by his name.

Ba·ker's cyst \ˈbā-kərz-\ *n* : a swelling behind the knee that is composed of a membrane-lined sac filled with synovial fluid and is associated with certain joint disorders (as arthri-tis)

Baker, William Morrant (1839–1896), British physician. Baker spent most of his career at London's St. Bartholo-mew's Hospital, serving as lecturer in anatomy and physiol-ogy and rising to the rank of full surgeon. He also served as examiner in surgery at St. Bart's and at the universities of London and Durham. In 1877 he published the first of two reports on synovial cysts of the knee joint. His 1885 follow=up report added six new cases and extended the affected sites to other major joints. Baker's other major contribution

\ə\ abut \ᵊ\ kitten \ər\ further \a\ ash \ā\ ace \ä\ cot, cart \aù\ out \ch\ chin \e\ bet \ē\ easy \g\ go \i\ hit \ī\ ice \j\ job \ŋ\ sing \ō\ go \ò\ law \òi\ boy \th\ thin \t̲h̲\ the \ü\ loot \ù\ foot \y\ yet \zh\ vision   *See also* Pronunciation Symbols page

was an original description, published in 1873, of a kind of infective dermatitis now known as erysipeloid.

bak·er's itch \ˌbā-kərz-\ *n* : GROCER'S ITCH

baker's yeast *n* : a yeast (as *Saccharomyces cerevisiae*) used or suitable for use as leaven

bak·ing soda \'bā-kiŋ-\ *n* : SODIUM BICARBONATE

bal *abbr* balance

BAL \ˌbē-(ˌ)ā-'el\ *n* : DIMERCAPROL

bal·ance \'bal-ən(t)s\ *n* **1** : an instrument for weighing **2** : mental and emotional steadiness **3 a** : the relation in physiology between the intake of a particular nutrient and its excretion — used with *positive* when the nutrient is in excess of the bodily metabolic requirement and with *negative* when dietary inadequacy and withdrawal of bodily reserves is present; see NITROGEN BALANCE, WATER BALANCE **b** : the maintenance (as in laboratory cultures) of a population at about the same condition and level

bal·anced \-ən(t)st\ *adj* **1** : having the physiologically active elements mutually counteracting ⟨a ∼ solution⟩ **2** *of a diet or ration* : furnishing all needed nutrients in the amount, form, and proportions needed to support healthy growth and productivity

ba·lan·ic \bə-'lan-ik\ *adj* : of or relating to the glans of the penis or of the clitoris

bal·a·ni·tis \ˌbal-ə-'nīt-əs\ *n* : inflammation of the glans penis

bal·a·no·pos·thi·tis \ˌbal-ə-(ˌ)nō-päs-'thīt-əs\ *n* : inflammation of the glans penis and of the foreskin

bal·a·no·pre·pu·tial \ˌbal-ə-(ˌ)nō-prē-'pyü-shəl\ *adj* : relating to or situated near the glans penis and the foreskin

bal·an·ti·di·a·sis \ˌbal-ən-tə-'dī-ə-səs, bə-ˌlan-\ *also* **bal·an·tid·i·o·sis** \ˌbal-ən-ˌtid-ē-'ō-səs\ *n, pl* **-a·ses** *also* **-o·ses** \-ˌsēz\ : infection with or disease caused by protozoans of the genus *Balantidium*

bal·an·tid·i·um \ˌbal-ən-'tid-ē-əm\ *n* **1** *cap* : a genus of large parasitic ciliate protozoans (order Heterotricha) including one (*B. coli*) that infests the intestines of some mammals and esp. swine and may cause a chronic ulcerative dysentery in humans **2** *pl* **-ia** \-ē-ə\ : a protozoan of the genus *Balantidium* — **bal·an·tid·i·al** \-ē-əl\ *or* **bal·an·tid·ic** \-'tid-ik\ *adj*

bald \'bȯld\ *adj* : lacking all or a significant part of the hair on the head or sometimes on other parts of the body — **bald** *vi*

bald·ness *n* : the state of being bald — see MALE-PATTERN BALDNESS

Bal·kan frame \'bȯl-kən-\ *n* : a frame employed in the treatment of fractured bones of the leg or arm that provides overhead weights and pulleys for suspension, traction, and continuous extension of the splinted fractured limb

¹ball \'bȯl\ *n* : a round or roundish body or mass: as **a** : a roundish protuberant part of the body: as **(1)** : the rounded eminence by which the base of the thumb is continuous with the palm of the hand **(2)** : the rounded broad part of the sole of the human foot between toes and arch and on which the main weight of the body first rests in normal walking **(3)** : the padded rounded underside of a human finger or toe near the tip **b** : EYEBALL **c** *often vulgar* : TESTIS **d** : a large pill (as one used in veterinary medicine) : BOLUS

²ball *vt* : to give a medicinal ball to (as a horse)

ball–and–socket joint *n* : an articulation (as the hip joint) in which the rounded head of one bone fits into a cuplike cavity of the other and admits movement in any direction — called also *enarthrosis*

ball·ing iron \'bȯl-iŋ-\ *n* : a long metal instrument with a cup-shaped depression at one end for placing solid medicine in the posterior part of the mouth of a horse or ox so that it will have to be swallowed whole — called also *balling gun*

bal·lism \'bal-ˌiz-əm\ *or* **bal·lis·mus** \bə-'liz-məs\ *n, pl* **-lisms** *or* **-lis·mus·es** : the abnormal swinging jerking movements sometimes seen in chorea

bal·lis·to·car·dio·gram \bə-'lis-tō-'kärd-ē-ə-ˌgram\ *n* : the record made by a ballistocardiograph

bal·lis·to·car·dio·graph \-ˌgraf\ *n* : a device for measuring the amount of blood passing through the heart in a specified time by recording the recoil movements of the body that re-

sult from contraction of the heart muscle in ejecting blood from the ventricles — **bal·lis·to·car·dio·graph·ic** \-ˌkärd-ē-ə-'graf-ik\ *adj* — **bal·lis·to·car·di·og·ra·phy** \-ē-'äg-rə-fē\ *n, pl* **-phies**

¹bal·loon \bə-'lün\ *n* : a nonporous bag of tough light material that can be inflated (as in a bodily cavity) with air or gas ⟨gastroesophageal tamponade by introduction of a ∼ into the stomach⟩

²balloon *vt* : to inflate or distend like a balloon ∼ *vi* : to swell or puff out

balloon angioplasty *n* : dilation of an obstructed atherosclerotic artery by the passage of a balloon catheter through the vessel to the area of disease where inflation of the catheter's tip compresses the plaque against the vessel wall

balloon catheter *n* : a catheter that has two lumens and an inflatable tip which can be expanded by the passage of gas, water, or a radiopaque medium through one of the lumens and that is used esp. to measure blood pressure in a blood vessel or to expand a partly closed or obstructed bodily passage or tube (as a coronary artery) — called also *balloon=tipped catheter;* see PERCUTANEOUS TRANSLUMINAL ANGIOPLASTY; compare SWAN-GANZ CATHETER

bal·lot·ta·ble \bə-'lät-ə-bəl\ *adj* : identifiable by ballottement

bal·lotte·ment \bə-'lät-mənt\ *n* : a sharp upward pushing against the uterine wall with a finger inserted into the vagina for diagnosing pregnancy by feeling the return impact of the displaced fetus; *also* : a similar procedure for detecting a floating kidney

balm \'bä(l)m, *NewEng also* 'bȧm\ *n* **1** : a balsamic resin; *esp* : one from small tropical evergreen trees (genus *Commiphora* of the family Burseraceae) **2** : an aromatic preparation (as a healing ointment) **3** : a soothing restorative agency

balm of Gil·e·ad \-'gil-ē-əd\ *n* **1** : a small evergreen African and Asian tree (*Commiphora meccanensis* of the family Burseraceae) with aromatic leaves **2** : a fragrant oleoresin from the balm of Gilead — called also *Mecca balsam*

bal·ne·ol·o·gy \ˌbal-nē-'äl-ə-jē\ *n, pl* **-gies** : the science of the therapeutic use of baths

bal·neo·ther·a·peu·tics \ˌbal-nē-ō-ˌther-ə-'pyüt-iks\ *n pl but sing or pl in constr* : BALNEOTHERAPY

bal·neo·ther·a·py \-'ther-ə-pē\ *n, pl* **-pies** : the treatment of disease by baths

bal·sam \'bȯl-səm\ *n* **1 a** : an aromatic and usu. oily and resinous substance flowing from various plants; *esp* : any of several resinous substances containing benzoic or cinnamic acid and used esp. in medicine **b** : a preparation containing resinous substances and having a balsamic odor **2** : a balsam-yielding tree **3** : BALM 3 — **bal·sam·ic** \bȯl-'sam-ik\ *adj*

balsam fir *n* : a resinous American evergreen tree (*Abies balsamea*) that is widely used for pulpwood and as a Christmas tree and that is the source of Canada balsam

balsam of Pe·ru \-pə-'rü\ *n* : a leguminous balsam from a tropical American tree (*Myroxylon pereirae*) used esp. as an irritant and to promote wound healing — called also *Peru balsam, Peruvian balsam*

balsam of To·lu \-tə-'lü\ *n* : a balsam from a tropical American leguminous tree (*Myroxylon balsamum*) used esp. as an expectorant and as a flavoring for cough syrups — called also *tolu, tolu balsam*

bam·boo spine \(ˌ)bam-'bü-\ *n* : a spinal column in the advanced stage of ankylosing spondylitis esp. as observed in an X-ray with ossified layers at the margins of the vertebrae giving the whole an appearance of a stick of bamboo

ba·nal \bə-'nal, ba-, -'näl; bā-'nal; 'bān-ᵊl\ *adj* : of a common or ordinary kind ⟨∼ skin organisms⟩ ⟨a ∼ inflammation⟩

ba·nana oil \bə-'nan-ə-ˌȯi(ə)l\ *n* : AMYL ACETATE

Ban·croft·i·an filariasis \'ban-ˌkrȯf-tē-ən-, 'baŋ-\ *or* **Ban·croft's filariasis** \-ˌkrȯf(t)s-\ *n* : filariasis caused by a slender white filaria of the genus *Wuchereria* (*W. bancrofti*) that is transmitted in larval form by mosquitoes, lives in lymph vessels and lymphoid tissues periodically shedding larvae into the peripheral bloodstream, and often causes elephantiasis by blocking lymphatic drainage

Ban·croft \'ban-ˌkròft, 'baṇ-\, **Joseph (1836–1894),** British physician. In 1877 Bancroft discovered a species of nematode parasite (*Wuchereria bancrofti*) and announced his discovery the following year in an article on filarial disease.

band \'band\ *n* **1** : a thin flat encircling strip esp. for binding: as **a** : a strip of cloth used to protect a newborn baby's navel — called also *bellyband* **b** : a thin flat strip of metal that encircles a tooth ⟨orthodontic ∼s⟩ **2** : a strip separated by some characteristic color or texture or considered apart from what is adjacent: as **a** : a stripe, streak, or other elongated mark on an animal; *esp* : one transverse to the long axis of the body **b** : a line or streak of differentiated cells **c** : one of the alternating dark and light segments of skeletal muscle fibers **d** : BAND FORM **e** : a strip of abnormal tissue either congenital or acquired; *esp* : a strip of connective tissue that causes obstruction of the bowel

¹ban·dage \'ban-dij\ *n* : a strip of fabric used to cover a wound, hold a dressing in place, immobilize an injured part, or apply pressure — see CAPELINE, ESMARCH BANDAGE, PRESSURE BANDAGE, SPICA, VELPEAU BANDAGE

²bandage *vb* **ban·daged; ban·dag·ing** *vt* : to bind, dress, or cover with a bandage ⟨∼ a wound⟩ ⟨∼ a sprained ankle⟩ ∼ *vi* : to apply a bandage — **ban·dag·er** *n*

Band–Aid \'ban-ˌdād\ *trademark* — used for a small adhesive strip with a gauze pad for covering minor wounds

band form *n* : a young neutrophil in the stage of development following a metamyelocyte and having an elongated nucleus that has not yet become lobed as in a mature neutrophil — called also *band cell, stab cell*

band keratopathy *n* : calcium deposition in Bowman's membrane and the stroma of the cornea that appears as an opaque gray streak and occurs in hypercalcemia and various chronic inflammatory conditions of the eye

ban·dy \'ban-dē\ *adj* **1** *of legs* : bowed outward at or below the knee **2** : BOWLEGGED

ban·dy–leg \-ˌleg, -ˌlāg\ *n* : BOWLEG — **ban·dy–leg·ged** \-ˌleg-əd, -ˌlāg-, *Brit usu* -ˌlegd\ *adj*

bane \'bān\ *n* : POISON — see HENBANE

bane·ber·ry \'bān-ˌber-ē, *Brit often & US sometimes* -b(ə-)rē\ *n, pl* **-ber·ries 1** : the acid poisonous berry of any plant of the genus *Actaea* **2** : a plant of the genus *Actaea*

bang *var of* BHANG

Bang's disease \'baṇz-\ *n* : BRUCELLOSIS; *specif* : contagious abortion of cattle caused by a bacterium of the genus *Brucella* (*B. abortus*) — called also *Bang's*

Bang, Bernhard Lauritz Frederik (1848–1932), Danish veterinarian. In 1897 Bang discovered that a bacterium (*Brucella abortus*) caused contagious abortion in cattle and one form of undulant fever in human beings. He also made important contributions to the control of bovine tuberculosis and to the research on smallpox vaccination and bacillary disease in animals.

bank \'baṇk\ *n* : a place where something is held available ⟨data ∼⟩; *esp* : a depot for the collection and storage of a biological product of human origin for medical use ⟨a sperm ∼⟩ ⟨an eye ∼⟩ — see BLOOD BANK

bant \'bant\ *vi* : to practice banting : DIET

ban·ting \'bant-iṇ\ *n, often cap* : a method of dieting for obesity by avoiding sweets and carbohydrates

Banting, William (1797–1878), British undertaker and coffin maker. A well-known obese Londoner, Banting increased in weight as his years increased in number. Finally, when he was 66, his bodily size reached the point where it was almost literally unbearable. After trying various remedies, all fruitless, he consulted William Harvey, who devised for him a high-protein, low-carbohydrate diet. The diet was a splendid success. Eager to spread the good word, Banting in 1863 published the pamphlet *A Letter on Corpulence,* in which he described the wonder diet. Soon "to bant" became a familiar phrase in British households, and *banting* immortalized a reduced man.

Ban·ti's disease \ˌbänt-ēz-\ *n* : a disorder characterized by

congestion and great enlargement of the spleen usu. accompanied by anemia, leukopenia, and cirrhosis of the liver — called also *Banti's syndrome*

Banti, Guido (1852–1925), Italian physician. Banti was one of the most eminent Italian pathologists of the early 20th century. In addition, he was a capable clinician, histologist, and bacteriologist. As an anatomist he added to the knowledge of aphasia, and as a bacteriologist studied the pathogenesis of infectious diseases caused by bacteria. His most important medical contributions were in the study of the pathology of the spleen and of leukemia. In 1894 he described the spleen disorder that is now known as Banti's disease or Banti's syndrome. In 1913 he composed a basic definition of leukemia that still stands.

bao·bab \'baù-ˌbab, 'bā-ə-ˌbab\ *n* : a broad-trunked Old World tropical tree (*Adansonia digitata*) of the silk-cotton family (Bombacaceae) with an edible acid fruit resembling a gourd, leaves and bark formerly used medicinally, and bark that is used in making paper, cloth, and rope

¹bar \'bär\ *n, often attrib* **1 a** : a piece of metal that connects parts of a removable partial denture **b** : the part of the wall of a horse's hoof that is bent inward toward the frog at the heel on each side and that extends toward the center of the sole **2** : a straight stripe, band, or line much longer than it is wide: as **a** : a transverse ridge on the roof of a horse's mouth — usu. used in pl. **b** : the space in front of the molar teeth of a horse in which the bit is placed

²bar *vt* **barred; bar·ring** : to cut free and ligate (a vein in a horse's leg) above and below the site of a projected operative procedure

³bar *n* : a unit of pressure equal to 100,000 pascals or to one million dynes per square centimeter or to 0.9869 atmosphere

bar *abbr* barometer; barometric

bar·ag·no·sis \ˌbar-ˌag-'nō-səs, bar-'ag-ˌ\ *n, pl* **-no·ses** \-ˌsēz\ : loss of barognosis

Bá·rá·ny chair \bə-'rän-(y)ē-ˌcha(ə)r, -ˌche(ə)r\ *n* : a chair used esp. for demonstrating the effects of circular motion (as on airplane pilots)

Bá·rá·ny \'bá-ˌränʸ\, Robert (1876–1936), Austrian otologist. Bárány's major field of investigation was equilibrium in humans. His investigations into the relationship between the vestibular apparatus of the inner ear and the nervous system prepared the way for the creation of a new field of medicine, otoneurology. Studying the rotatory reaction of the vestibular system, he was able to define the sensation of dizziness in terms of such objective signs as definite eye movements and muscular reactions. In 1906 he devised two tests to measure vestibular function. The first was a caloric test that produced nystagmus by the injection of warm or cold water into the external auditory canal. The second test involved the use of a rotating chair to produce nystagmus. The chair used to administer the test is now known as the Bárány chair. In 1914, Bárány was awarded the Nobel Prize for Physiology or Medicine.

barb \'bärb\ *n, slang* : BARBITURATE

barbae — see SYCOSIS BARBAE, TINEA BARBAE

barb·al·o·in \bär-'bal-ə-wən\ *n* : a yellow crystalline compound $C_{20}H_{18}O_9$ isolated from aloin

bar·ber·ry \'bär-ˌber-ē, *Brit often & US sometimes* -b(ə-)rē\ *n, pl* **-ries 1** : any shrub of the genus *Berberis* **2 a** : an evergreen shrub of the genus *Mahonia* (esp. *M. aquifolium*) **b** : BERBERIS 2

bar·ber's itch \ˌbär-bər-'zich\ *n* : ringworm of the face and neck — called also *tinea barbae*

barber's pole worm \'bär-bərz-ˌpōl-\ *also* **bar·ber pole worm** \-bər\ *n* : a nematode stomach worm of the genus *Haemonchus* (*H. contortus*) that occurs typically in the abomasum of ruminants (as sheep) and rarely in humans

bar·bi·tal \'bär-bə-ˌtòl, -ˌtal\ *n* : a crystalline barbiturate

---

$C_8H_{12}N_2O_3$ formerly used as a sedative and hypnotic often in the form of its soluble sodium salt — see VERONAL

bar·bi·tone \'bär-bə-ˌtōn\ *n, Brit* : BARBITAL

bar·bi·tu·rate \bär-'bich-ə-rət, -ˌrāt; ˌbär-bə-'t(y)ùr-ət, -'t(y)ú(ə)r-ˌāt\ *n* **1** : a salt or ester of barbituric acid **2** : any of various derivatives of barbituric acid (as phenobarbital) that are used esp. as sedatives, hypnotics, and antispasmodics and are often addictive

bar·bi·tu·ric acid \ˌbär-bə-ˌt(y)ùr-ik-\ *n* : a synthetic crystalline acid $C_4H_4N_2O_3$ that is a derivative of pyrimidine; *also* : any of its acid derivatives of which some are used as hypnotics

bar·bi·tur·ism \bär-'bich-ə-ˌriz-əm, 'bär-bə-chə-\ *n* : a condition characterized by deleterious effects on the mind or body by excess use of barbiturates

bar·bo·ne \bär-'bō-nē\ *n* : pasteurellosis of the domestic buffalo — called also *barbone disease*

bar·bo·tage \ˌbär-bə-'täzh\ *n* : the production of spinal anesthesia by repeated injection and removal of fluid

bare·foot doctor \ˌba(ə)r-ˌfüt-, ˌbe(ə)r-\ *n* : an auxiliary medical worker trained to provide health care in rural areas of China

bar·ia·tri·cian \ˌbar-ē-ə-'trish-ən\ *n* : a specialist in bariatrics

bar·iat·rics \ˌbar-ē-'a-triks\ *n pl but sing in constr* : a branch of medicine that deals with the treatment of obesity — **bar·iat·ric** \-'trik\ *adj*

bar·ic \'bar-ik\ *adj* : of or relating to barium

ba·ril·la \bə-'rēl-yə, -'rē-(y)ə\ *n* **1** : an Algerian plant (*Halogeton souda*) formerly burned as a source of sodium carbonate **2** : an impure sodium carbonate made from the ashes of barillas and formerly used esp. in making soap and glass

bar·i·to·sis \ˌbar-ə-'tō-səs\ *n, pl* **-to·ses** \-ˌsēz\ : pneumoconiosis caused by inhalation of dust composed of barium or its compounds

bar·i·um \'bar-ē-əm, 'ber-\ *n* **1** : a silver-white malleable toxic bivalent metallic element of the alkaline-earth group that occurs only in combination — symbol *Ba*; see ELEMENT table **2** : BARIUM SULFATE

barium chloride *n* : a water-soluble toxic salt $BaCl_2 \cdot 2H_2O$ used as a reagent in analysis and as a cardiac stimulant

barium enema *n* : a suspension of barium sulfate injected into the lower bowel to render it radiopaque, usu. followed by injection of air to inflate the bowel and increase definition, and used in the radiographic diagnosis of intestinal lesions

barium meal *n* : a solution of barium sulfate that is swallowed by a patient to facilitate fluoroscopic or radiographic diagnosis

barium sulfate *n* : a colorless crystalline insoluble salt $BaSO_4$ occurring in nature as barite and used medically chiefly as a radiopaque substance

barium ti·tan·ate \-'tīt-ˌ²n-ˌāt\ *n* : a white crystalline compound $BaTiO_3$ used in hearing aids, phonograph pickups, and ceramic transducers

bark \'bärk\ *n* **1** : the tough exterior covering of a woody root or stem **2** : CINCHONA 3

bar·ley \'bär-lē\ *n* : a cereal grass (genus *Hordeum*, esp. *H. vulgare*) having the flowers in dense spikes with long awns; *also* : its seed used in malt beverages and in breakfast foods and stock feeds

Bar·low's disease \'bär-ˌlōz-\ *n* : INFANTILE SCURVY

Barlow, Sir Thomas (1845–1945), British physician. Barlow is noteworthy for his research and discoveries in children's diseases. In 1883 he described infantile scurvy, now known as Barlow's disease. He was the first to distinguish infantile scurvy from rickets, and tuberculosis from simple meningitis.

Barlow's syndrome *n* : MITRAL VALVE PROLAPSE

Barlow, John Brereton (b 1924), South African cardiologist. Barlow first described mitral valve prolapse in an article on late systolic murmurs that was published in 1963.

barn \'bärn\ *n* : a unit of area equal to 10^{-24} square centimeters that is used in nuclear physics for measuring cross section

bar·og·no·sis \ˌbar-ˌäg-'nō-səs, ˌbar-əg-\ *n, pl* **-no·ses** \-ˌsēz\ : the perception of weight by the cutaneous and muscle senses

baro·gram \'bar-ə-ˌgram\ *n* : a barographic tracing

baro·graph \-ˌgraf\ *n* : a self-registering barometer — **baro·graph·ic** \ˌbar-ə-'graf-ik\ *adj*

baro·phil·ic \ˌbar-ə-'fil-ik\ *adj* : thriving under high environmental pressures — used of deep-sea organisms

baro·re·cep·tor \ˌbar-ō-ri-'sep-tər\ *also* **baro·cep·tor** \-ō-'sep-\ *n* : a sensory nerve ending esp. in the walls of large arteries (as the carotid sinus and arch of the aorta) that is sensitive to changes in blood pressure — called also *pressoreceptor*

baro·re·flex \'bar-ō-ˌrē-ˌfleks\ *n* : the reflex mechanism by which baroreceptors regulate blood pressure that includes transmission of nerve impulses from the baroreceptors to the medulla in response to a change in blood pressure and that produces vasodilation and a decrease in heart rate when blood pressure increases and vasoconstriction and an increase in heart rate when blood pressure decreases — called also *baroreceptor reflex*

baro·scope \'bar-ə-ˌskōp\ *n* : an apparatus for showing that the loss of weight of an object in air equals the weight of the air displaced by it

Ba·ros·ma \bə-'räz-mə\ *n* : a genus of southern African strong-scented evergreen shrubs (family Rutaceae) from some of which buchu is obtained

baro·tac·tic \'bar-ō-ˌtak-tik\ *adj* : of, relating to, or being a barotaxis

baro·tax·is \ˌbar-ō-'tak-səs\ *n, pl* **-tax·es** \-ˌsēz\ : a taxis in which pressure is the orienting stimulus

baro·trau·ma \-'trau̇-mə, -'trò-\ *n, pl* **-mas** *also* **-ma·ta** \-mət-ə\ : injury of a part or organ as a result of changes in barometric pressure; *esp* : AERO-OTITIS MEDIA

Barr body \'bär-\ *n* : a densely staining inactivated condensed X chromosome that is present in each somatic cell of most female mammals and is used as a test of genetic femaleness (as in a fetus or an athlete) — called also *sex chromatin*

Barr, Murray Llewellyn (1908–1995), Canadian anatomist. A professor of microanatomy, Barr specialized in cytological research, especially as it applies to genetically determined anomalies of sex determination and development, cancer, and mental disease. His most notable work dealt with sex chromatin, now known as the Barr body. In 1949 he noted that females had in the nuclei of their nerve cells a mass of chromatin that males did not. Further study revealed that this sex difference in the nuclei of resting cells is found in most mammals.

bar·rel chest \'bar-əl-\ *n* : the enlarged chest with a rounded cross section and fixed horizontal position of the ribs that occurs in chronic pulmonary emphysema

bar·ren \'bar-ən\ *adj* : incapable of producing offspring — used esp. of females or matings — **bar·ren·ness** \-ən-nəs\ *n*

Bar·rett's esophagus \'bar-its-, 'ber-\ *n* : metaplasia of the lower esophagus that is characterized by replacement of squamous epithelium with columnar epithelium, occurs esp. as a result of chronic gastroesophageal reflux, and is associated with an increased risk for esophageal carcinoma — called also *Barrett's epithelium*

Barrett, Norman Rupert (1903–1979), British surgeon. Barrett's numerous positions included those of surgeon at King Edward VII Sanatorium, Midhurst, and at London's St. Thomas's and Brompton Hospitals; lecturer in surgery at the University of London; and examiner in surgery at the universities of Cambridge, Oxford, Birmingham, London, and Khartoum. He also served as editor of *Thorax* and contributed to several surgery textbooks.

bar·ri·er \'bar-ē-ər\ *n* **1** : a material object or set of objects that separates, demarcates, or serves as a barricade — see BLOOD-BRAIN BARRIER, PLACENTAL BARRIER **2** : a factor that tends to restrict the free movement, mingling, or interbreeding of individuals or populations ⟨behavioral and geographic ∼s to hybridization⟩

bar·tho·lin·itis \bär-ˌtō-lə-ˈnīt-əs\ *n, pl* **-lin·ites** \-ˈnī-ˌtēz\ : inflammation of the Bartholin's glands

Bar·tho·lin's gland \ˌbärt-ᵊl-ənz-, ˌbär-thə-lənz-\ *n* : either of two oval racemose glands lying one to each side of the lower part of the vagina and secreting a lubricating mucus — called also *gland of Bartholin, greater vestibular gland;* compare COWPER'S GLAND

Bar·tho·lin \bär-ˈtŭl-in\, **Caspar Thomèson (1655–1738),** Danish anatomist. Belonging to a family that produced three generations of eminent anatomists, Bartholin made a number of significant contributions to anatomy. In 1675 he first described the glands in the female reproductive tract that are homologous to Cowper's glands in the male and that now honor his name.

bar·ton·el·la \ˌbärt-ᵊn-ˈel-ə\ *n* **1** *cap* : a genus of gram-negative bacteria that is the type genus of the family Bartonellaceae and includes one (*B. bacilliformis*) causing bartonellosis transmitted by sand flies and another (*B. henselae* syn. *Rochalimaea henselae*) causing cat scratch disease **2** : any bacterium of the genus *Bartonella*

Bar·ton \ˈbär-ˌtōn\, **Alberto L. (1874–1950),** Peruvian physician. In 1909 Barton published an article on elements found in the red blood cells of patients with Oroya fever. In this article he identified the blood parasite (*Bartonella bacilliformis*) that is the causative agent of Oroya fever and verruga peruana. The organism is now placed in the genus *Bartonella*, which was named after him in 1915.

Bar·ton·el·la·ce·ae \ˌbärt-ᵊn-ˌel-ˈla-sē-ˌē\ *n pl* : a family of bacteria of the order Rickettsiales that invade blood and tissue cells of humans and other vertebrates and are often transmitted by bloodsucking arthropods

bar·ton·el·lo·sis \-ˌel-ˈō-səs\ *n, pl* **-lo·ses** \-ˌsēz\ : a disease or infection caused by bacteria of the genus *Bartonella; specif* : a disease of mammals including humans that occurs in So. America, is characterized by severe anemia and high fever followed by an eruption like warts on the skin, and is caused by a bacterium of the genus *Bartonella* (*B. bacilliformis*) that invades the red blood cells and is transmitted by sand flies (genus *Phlebotomus*) — called also *Carrión's disease;* see OROYA FEVER, VERRUGA PERUANA

Bart·ter's syndrome \ˈbärt-ərz-\ *n* : a kidney disorder that usu. first appears during childhood and is characterized esp. by hypokalemia, aldosteronism, hyperreninemia, and juxtaglomerular cell hyperplasia

Bartter, Frederic Crosby (1914–1983), American physiologist. Bartter's numerous medical positions included those of chief of the clinical endocrinology branch of the National Heart Institute; professor of pediatrics at Howard University and of medicine at Georgetown University, both in Washington, D.C.; associate chief of staff for research at Audie Murphy Veterans Hospital and professor of medicine at the University of Texas Health Science Center, both in San Antonio. In the course of his career he contributed over 300 articles on endocrinology and physiology. His areas of research included the physiology of the adrenal and parathyroid glands, especially the production of aldosterone. Besides describing the syndrome that now bears his name, he also described a syndrome marked by inappropriate antidiuretic hormone production, and he defined the biochemical basis of Cushing's syndrome.

bar·ye \ˈbar-ē\ *n* : the cgs unit of pressure equal to 0.1 pascal or to one dyne per square centimeter

ba·ry·ta \bə-ˈrīt-ə\ *n* : any of several compounds of barium

ba·sad \ˈbā-ˌsad\ *adv* : toward the base

ba·sal \ˈbā-səl, -zəl\ *adj* **1** : relating to, situated at, or forming the base **2** : of, relating to, or essential for maintaining the fundamental vital activities of an organism (as respiration, heartbeat, or excretion) ⟨a ~ diet⟩ — see BASAL METABOLISM **3** : serving as or serving to induce an initial comatose or unconscious state that forms a basis for further anesthetization ⟨~ narcosis⟩ ⟨a ~ anesthetic⟩ — **ba·sal·ly** \-ē\ *adv*

basal body *n* : a minute distinctively staining cell organelle found at the base of a flagellum or cilium and resembling a centriole in structure — called also *basal granule, kinetosome*

basal cell *n* : one of the innermost cells of the deeper epidermis of the skin

basal–cell carcinoma *n* : a skin cancer derived from and preserving the form of the basal cells of the skin

basale — see STRATUM BASALE

basal ganglion *n* : any of four deeply placed masses of gray matter within each cerebral hemisphere comprising the caudate nucleus, the lentiform nucleus, the amygdala, and the claustrum — usu. used in pl.; called also *basal nucleus*

basal granule *n* : BASAL BODY

basalia — see STRATUM BASALE

ba·sa·lis \bā-ˈsā-ləs\ *n, pl* **-les** \-ˌlēz\ : the basal part of the endometrium that is not shed during menstruation — see DECIDUA BASALIS

basal lamina *n* **1** : the part of the gray matter of the embryonic neural tube from which the motor nerve roots arise **2** : a thin extracellular layer composed chiefly of collagen, proteoglycans, and glycoproteins (as laminin and fibronectin) that lies adjacent to the basal surface of epithelial cells or surrounds individual muscle, fat, and Schwann cells and that separates these cells from underlying or surrounding connective tissue or adjacent cells — compare RETICULAR LAMINA

basal length *n* : the distance from gnathion to basion

basal metabolic rate *n* : the rate at which heat is given off by an organism at complete rest

basal metabolism *n* : the turnover of energy in a fasting and resting organism using energy solely to maintain vital cellular activity, respiration, and circulation as measured by the basal metabolic rate

basal nucleus *n* : BASAL GANGLION

basal plate *n* : an underlying structure: as **a** : the ventral portion of the neural tube **b** : the part of the decidua of a placental mammal that is intimately fused with the placenta

base \ˈbās\ *n, pl* **bas·es** \ˈbā-səz\ **1** : that portion of a bodily organ or part by which it is attached to another more central structure of the organism ⟨the ~ of the thumb⟩ **2 a** : the usu. inactive ingredient of a preparation serving as the vehicle for the active medicinal preparation ⟨the fatty ~ of an ointment⟩ **b** : the chief active ingredient of a preparation — called also *basis* **3 a** : any of various typically water-soluble and bitter tasting compounds that in solution have a pH greater than 7, are capable of reacting with an acid to form a salt, and are molecules or ions able to take up a proton from an acid or are substances able to give up an unshared pair of electrons to an acid — compare ALKALI **b** : any of the five purine or pyrimidine bases of DNA and RNA that include cytosine, guanine, adenine, thymine, and uracil **4** : FREEBASE — **based** \ˈbāst\ *adj*

Ba·se·dow's disease \ˈbäz-ə-ˌdōz-\ *n* : GRAVES' DISEASE

Basedow, Karl Adolph von (1799–1854), German physician. Basedow practiced general medicine, surgery, and ophthalmology, but he is best known for his study of Graves' disease. The English physician Caleb H. Parry first mentioned the disease in 1815, and in 1835 the first full description was given by the Irish physician Robert L. Graves. However, the 1840 description by Basedow is considered to be classic. His description presented the three classic symptoms: goiter, exophthalmos, and tachycardia.

base·line \ˈbā-ˌslīn\ *n* : a set of critical observations or data used for comparison or a control

base·ment membrane \ˌbā-smənt-\ *n* **1** : a thin extracellular supporting layer that separates a layer of epithelial cells from the underlying lamina propria and is composed of the basal lamina and reticular lamina **2** : BASAL LAMINA

¹base pair \-ˈpa(ə)r, -ˈpe(ə)r\ *n* : one of the pairs of nucleotide

\ə\ abut \ᵊ\ kitten \ər\ further \a\ ash \ā\ ace \ä\ cot, cart
\aů\ out \ch\ chin \e\ bet \ē\ easy \g\ go \i\ hit \ī\ ice \j\ job
\ŋ\ sing \ō\ go \ȯ\ law \ȯi\ boy \th\ thin \t̲h̲\ the \ü\ loot
\ů\ foot \y\ yet \zh\ vision *See also* Pronunciation Symbols page

bases on complementary strands of nucleic acid that consist of a purine on one strand joined to a pyrimidine on the other strand by hydrogen bonds holding together the two strands much like the rungs of a ladder and that include adenine linked to thymine in DNA or to uracil in RNA and guanine linked to cytosine in both DNA and RNA

²**base pair** *vi* : to participate in formation of a base pair ⟨adenine *base pairs* with thymine⟩

base pair·ing \-'pa(ə)r-iŋ, -'pe(ə)r-\ *n* : the pairing of purine and pyrimidine bases cross-linked by hydrogen bonds in two complementary strands of DNA

base·plate \'bās-ˌplāt\ *n* **1** : the portion of an artificial denture in contact with the jaw **2** : the sheet of plastic material used in the making of trial denture plates

base unit *n* : one of a set of simple units in a system of measurement that is based on a natural phenomenon or established standard and from which other units may be derived — see INTERNATIONAL SYSTEM OF UNITS

basi–bregmatic height *var of* BASION-BREGMA HEIGHT

ba·sic \'bā-sik *also* -zik\ *adj* **1** : of, relating to, or forming the base or essence **2 a** : of, relating to, containing, or having the character of a base **b** : having an alkaline reaction

basic dye *n* : any of various chiefly synthetic dyes that react as bases, produce clear brilliant colors, and are used esp. as histological stains

ba·si·chro·ma·tin \ˌbā-sē-'krō-mət-ən\ *n* : chromatin which stains readily with basic dyes — compare OXYCHROMATIN

ba·sic·i·ty \bā-'sis-ət-ē\ *n, pl* **-ties** : the quality, state, or degree of being a base

ba·si·cra·ni·al \ˌbā-si-'krā-nē-əl\ *adj* : of or relating to the base of the skull

basic stain *n* : a basic dye used as a stain

ba·sid·io·my·cete \bə-ˌsid-ē-ō-'mī-ˌsēt, -ˌmī-'sēt\ *n* : any of a group of higher fungi that have septate hyphae and spores borne on a basidium produced directly from the mycelium or as an outgrowth of a spore, that include rusts, smuts, and numerous edible forms (as many mushrooms), and that are variously considered to comprise a class (Basidiomycetes), a subdivision (Basidiomycotina), or a division (Basidiomycota) — **ba·sid·io·my·ce·tous** \-mī-'sēt-əs\ *adj*

Ba·sid·io·my·ce·tes \-mī-'sēt-ˌēz\ *n pl* : a class of higher fungi comprising the basidiomycetes when they are considered a class

Ba·sid·io·my·co·ta \-(ˌ)mī-'kōt-ə\ *n pl* : a division of higher fungi comprising the basidiomycetes when they are considered a division

Ba·sid·io·my·co·ti·na \-ˌmī-kō-'tē-nə\ *n pl* : a subdivision of higher fungi comprising the basidiomycetes when they are considered a subdivision

ba·sid·io·spore \bə-'sid-ē-ə-ˌspō(ə)r, -ˌspȯ(ə)r\ *n* : a spore produced by a basidium

ba·sid·i·um \bə-'sid-ē-əm\ *n, pl* **-ia** \-ē-ə\ : a structure on a basidiomycete in which karyogamy occurs followed by meiosis to form usu. four basidiospores

ba·si·fa·cial \ˌbā-si-'fā-shəl\ *adj* : of or relating to the lower part of the face

¹**ba·si·hy·al** \-'hī(-ə)l\ *adj* : of, relating to, or being a median element or bone at the ventral point of the hyoid arch that in humans forms the body of the hyoid bone

²**basihyal** *n* : a basihyal bone

ba·si·hy·oid \-'hī-ˌȯid\ *adj or n* : BASIHYAL

bas·i·lar \'baz-(ə-)lər, 'bas- *also* 'bāz- *or* 'bās-\ *adj* : of, relating to, or situated at the base ⟨∼ fractures of the skull⟩

basilar artery *n* : an unpaired artery that is formed by the union of the two vertebral arteries, runs forward within the skull just under the pons, divides into the two posterior cerebral arteries, and supplies the pons, cerebellum, posterior part of the cerebrum, and the inner ear

basilar groove *n* : the depression in the upper surface of the basilar process on which the medulla rests

basilar index *n* : the ratio of the distance between the basion and the alveolar point to the total length of the skull multiplied by 100

basilar membrane *n* : a membrane that extends from the margin of the bony shelf of the cochlea to the outer wall and that supports the organ of Corti

basilar meningitis *n* : a usu. tuberculous inflammation of the meninges at the base of the brain

basilar plate *n* : PARACHORDAL PLATE

basilar process *n* : an anterior median projection of the occipital bone in front of the foramen magnum articulating in front with the body of the sphenoid by the basilar suture

ba·sil·ic vein \bə-'sil-ik-\ *n* : a vein of the upper arm lying along the inner border of the biceps muscle, draining the whole limb, and opening into the axillary vein

ba·sin \'bās-ᵊn\ *n* **1** : an open usu. circular vessel with sloping or curving sides used typically for holding water for washing **2** : the quantity contained in a basin

¹**ba·si·oc·cip·i·tal** \ˌbā-sē-äk-'sip-ət-ᵊl\ *adj* : relating to or being a bone in the base of the cranium immediately in front of the foramen magnum that is represented in humans by the basilar process of the occipital bone

²**basioccipital** *n* : the basioccipital bone

ba·si·on \'bā-sē-ˌän, -zē-\ *n* : the midpoint of the anterior margin of the foramen magnum

basion–bregma height *or* **ba·si–bregmatic height** \ˌbā-si-\ *n* : the distance between the basion and bregma

basion–prosthion line *n* : a line from the basion to the prosthion

ba·sip·e·tal \bā-'sip-ət-ᵊl, -'zip-\ *adj* : proceeding from the apex toward the base or from above downward — **ba·sip·e·tal·ly** \-ᵊl-ē\ *adv*

ba·sis \'bā-səs\ *n, pl* **ba·ses** \-ˌsēz\ **1** : any of various anatomical parts that function as a foundation **2** : BASE 2b

¹**ba·si·sphe·noid** \ˌbā-səs-'fē-ˌnȯid\ *also* **ba·si·sphe·noi·dal** \-səs-fi-'nȯid-ᵊl\ *adj* : relating to or being the part of the base of the cranium that lies between the basioccipital and the presphenoid bones and that usu. ossifies separately and becomes a part of the sphenoid bone only in the adult

²**basisphenoid** *n* : the basisphenoid bone

ba·si·ver·te·bral \ˌbā-si-(ˌ)vər-'tē-brəl, -'vərt-ə-\ *adj* : of or relating to the centrum of a vertebra

bas·ket cell \'bas-kət-\ *n* : any of the cells in the molecular layer of the cerebellum whose axons pass inward and end in a basketlike network around the Purkinje cells

Basle Nomina Anatomica \'bä-zəl-\ *n* : the anatomical nomenclature adopted at the 1895 meeting of the German Anatomical Society at Basel, Switzerland, and superseded by the Nomina Anatomica adopted at the Sixth International Congress of Anatomists in 1955 — abbr. *BNA*

baso *abbr* basophil

ba·so·cyte \'bā-sə-ˌsīt, -zə-\ *n* : BASOPHIL

ba·so·phil \'bā-sə-ˌfil, -zə-\ *or* **ba·so·phile** \-ˌfīl\ *n* : a basophilic substance or structure; *esp* : a white blood cell with basophilic granules that is similar in function to a mast cell

ba·so·phil·ia \ˌbā-sə-'fil-ē-ə, -zə-\ *n* **1** : tendency to stain with basic dyes **2** : an abnormal condition in which some tissue element has increased basophilia

ba·so·phil·ic \-'fil-ik\ *also* **ba·so·phil** \'bā-sə-ˌfil, -zə-\ *or* **ba·so·phile** \-ˌfīl\ *adj* : staining readily with or being a basic stain

basophilism — see PITUITARY BASOPHILISM

bas·so·rin \'bas-ə-rən, 'bäs-\ *n* : a substance that is a constituent of some gums (as tragacanth) and is insoluble in water but swells to form a gel — compare TRAGACANTHIN

bast fiber \'bast-\ *n* : a strong woody fiber obtained chiefly from the phloem of plants and used esp. in cordage, matting, and fabrics — called also *bast*

bat \'bat\ *n* : any of an order (Chiroptera) of nocturnal placental flying mammals with forelimbs modified to form wings

¹**bath** \'bath, 'bȧth\ *n, pl* **baths** \'bathz, 'baths, 'bȧthz, 'bȧths\ **1** : a washing or soaking (as in water) of all or part of the body — see MUD BATH, SITZ BATH **2 a** : water used for bathing **b** (1) : a medium for regulating the temperature of something placed in or on it (2) : a vessel containing this

medium **3** : a place resorted to esp. for medical treatment by bathing : SPA — usu. used in pl.

²**bath** *vt, Brit* : to give a bath to ~ *vi, Brit* : to take a bath

¹**bathe** \ˈbāth\ *vb* **bathed; bath·ing** *vt* **1** : to wash in a liquid (as water) **2** : to apply water or a liquid medicament to ⟨~ the eye with warm water⟩ ~ *vi* : to take a bath

²**bathe** *n, Brit* : the act or action of bathing : BATH

bath·mo·trop·ic \ˌbath-mə-ˈträp-ik\ *adj* : modifying the degree of excitability of the cardiac musculature — used esp. of the action of the cardiac nerves

bath·mot·ro·pism \bath-ˈmä-trə-ˌpiz-əm\ *n* : the state of being bathmotropic

bath·tub \ˈbath-ˌtəb, ˈbȧth-\ *n* : a usu. fixed tub for bathing

ba·tracho·tox·in \bə-ˌtrak-ə-ˈtäk-sən, ˌba-trə-kō-\ *n* : a very powerful steroid venom $C_{31}H_{42}N_2O_6$ extracted from the skin of a So. American frog (*Phyllobates aurotaenia*)

Bat·ten disease \ˈbat-ⁿn-\ *n* : a fatal lipofuscinosis that is inherited as an autosomal recessive trait, has an onset between five and eight or nine years of age, and is marked by early symptoms which progress to blindness, paralysis, and dementia

Batten, Frederick Eustace (1865–1918), British neurologist and pediatrician. In London, Batten held posts at the Hospital for Sick Children and at the National Hospital for the Paralysed and Epileptic. His research centered on the histology of disorders of the nervous system. In 1902 he published the first description of a fatal form of lipofuscinosis that is often known as *Batten disease*. Additional descriptions of the disease were separately published by the German neurologists Heinrich Vogt in 1905 and Walter Spielmeyer in 1908. Batten is also remembered for his 1903 description of a benign form of congenital muscular dystrophy. The author of more than 100 medical papers, he published a book on acute poliomyelitis in 1916.

bat·tered child syndrome \ˌbat-ərd-\ *n* : the complex of physical injuries (as fractures, hematomas, and contusions) that results from gross abuse (as by a parent) of a young child — compare SHAKEN BABY SYNDROME

battered wom·an syndrome \-ˈwu̇-mən-, -ˈwō-, -ˈwə-\ *also* **battered wom·an's syndrome** \-mənz-\ *n* : the highly variable symptom complex of physical and psychological injuries exhibited by a woman repeatedly abused esp. physically by her mate — called also *battered wife syndrome, battered women's syndrome*

bat·tery \ˈbat-ə-rē, ˈba-trē\ *n, pl* **-ter·ies** **1 a** : a combination of apparatus for producing a single electrical effect **b** : a group of two or more cells connected together to furnish electric current; *also* : a single cell that furnishes electric current **2** : a group or series of tests; *esp* : a group of intelligence or personality tests given to a subject as an aid in psychological analysis

bat·tle fatigue \ˈbat-ⁿl-\ *n* : COMBAT FATIGUE — **bat·tle-fa·tigued** *adj*

bat·yl alcohol \ˌbat-ⁿl-\ *n* : a colorless crystalline alcohol $C_{21}H_{44}O_3$ obtained esp. from many shark-liver oils and ray-liver oils and from the yellow marrow of cattle bones

Bau·hin's valve \ˈbō-ˌanz-, bō-ˈaⁿz-\ *n* : ILEOCECAL VALVE

Bau·hin \bō-aⁿ\, **Gaspard** *or* **Caspar (1560–1624),** Swiss anatomist and botanist. Bauhin served for almost all of his career on the medical faculty at the University of Basel. There he taught both anatomy and botany and as a teacher of anatomy exerted a wide influence. Bauhin first became aware of the ileocecal valve in 1579, in the course of a private dissection, and he published an early account of the valve in 1588.

Bau·mé *also* **Bau·me** *or* **Beau·mé** \bō-ˈmā, ˈbō-(ˌ)mā\ *adj* : being, measured according to, or calibrated in accordance with a Baumé scale ⟨a *Baumé* hydrometer⟩

Bau·mé \bō-mā\, **Antoine (1728–1804),** French chemist. Baumé operated a pharmacy and dispensary and designed industrial and laboratory apparatus. In 1768 he designed a hydrometer with a scale having two fixed points (the density of distilled water and that of a salt solution of known concentration), thus enabling the production of properly

calibrated instruments. The scale has been named after him, and his name serves as an adjective indicating relationship to or use of the scale.

Baumé scale *n* : either of two hydrometer scales that indicate specific gravity in arbitrarily defined but constant degrees: **a** : one for liquids lighter than water on which specific gravity S at 60°F (15.6°C) is related to the Baumé reading n in degrees by $S = 140 \div (130 + n)$ **b** : one for liquids heavier than water on which specific gravity S at 60°F (15.6°C) is related to the Baumé reading n in degrees by $S = 145 \div (145 - n)$

bay·ber·ry \ˈbā-ˌber-ē, *Brit often & US sometimes* -b(ə-)rē\ *n, pl* **-ries** **1** : a West Indian tree of the genus *Pimenta* (*P. racemosa*) of the myrtle family yielding a yellow aromatic oil **2 a** : any of several wax myrtles; *esp* : a hardy shrub (*Myrica pensylvanica*) of coastal eastern No. America bearing dense clusters of small globular nuts covered with grayish white wax **b** : the fruit of a bayberry

BBB *abbr* **1** blood-brain barrier **2** bundle branch block

BBT *abbr* basal body temperature

BC *abbr* board-certified

B cell *n* : any of the lymphocytes that have antigen-binding antibody molecules on the surface, that comprise the antibody-secreting plasma cells when mature, and that in mammals differentiate in the bone marrow — called also *B lymphocyte;* compare T CELL

BCG *abbr* **1** bacillus Calmette-Guérin **2** ballistocardiogram **3** bromocresol green

BCG vaccine \ˌbē-(ˌ)sē-ˈjē-\ *n* : a vaccine prepared from a living attenuated strain of tubercle bacilli and used to vaccinate human beings against tuberculosis

A. L. C. Calmette and **C. Guérin** — see BACILLUS CALMETTE-GUÉRIN

BCLS *abbr* basic cardiac life support

BCNU \ˌbē-ˌsē-ˌen-ˈyü\ *n* : a nitrosourea $C_5H_9Cl_2N_3O_2$ used as an antineoplastic drug — called also *carmustine*

B complex *n* : VITAMIN B COMPLEX

b.d. *abbr* [Latin *bis die*] twice a day — used in writing prescriptions

bdel·li·um \ˈdel-ē-əm\ *n* : a gum resin similar to myrrh obtained from various trees (genus *Commiphora*) of the East Indies and Africa

bdel·lo·vi·brio \ˌdel-ō-ˈvib-rē-ˌō\ *n, pl* **-brios** **1** *cap* : a genus of bacteria that are parasitic on other bacteria **2** : any bacterium of the genus *Bdellovibrio*

B–DNA \ˌbē-ˌdē-ˌen-ˈā\ *n* : the right-handed typical form of double helix DNA in which the chains twist up and to the right around the front of the axis of the helix and that has usu. ten base pairs in each helical turn and two grooves on the external surface — compare Z-DNA

Bé *abbr* Baumé

Be *symbol* beryllium

BE *abbr* **1** barium enema **2** below elbow **3** board-eligible

bead·ed lizard \ˌbēd-əd-\ *n* : a large yellow and black venomous lizard (*Heloderma horridum*) of Mexico that is related to the Gila monster

beaded ribs *n pl* : ribs with the beading that is characteristic of rickets

bead·ing \ˈbēd-iŋ\ *n* : the beadlike nodules occurring in rickets at the junction of the ribs with their cartilages — called also *rachitic rosary, rosary*

bea·ker \ˈbē-kər\ *n* : a deep widemouthed thin-walled vessel usu. with a lip for pouring that is used esp. in science laboratories

beam \ˈbēm\ *n* **1** : a ray or shaft of light **2** : a collection of nearly parallel rays (as X-rays) or a stream of particles (as electrons)

bear \\'ba(ə)r, 'be(ə)r\\ *vt* **bore** \\'bō(ə)r, 'bȯ(ə)r\\; **borne** \\'bō(ə)rn, 'bȯ(ə)rn\\ *also* **born** \\'bȯ(ə)rn\\; **bear·ing** : to give birth to

bear·ber·ry \\-ˌber-ē, *Brit often & US sometimes* -b(ə-)rē\\ *n, pl* **-ries** : a trailing evergreen plant (*Arctostaphylos uva-ursi*) of the heath family (Ericaceae) with astringent foliage and red berries — see UVAURSI

beard \\'bi(ə)rd\\ *n* : the hair that grows on a man's face often excluding the mustache — **beard·ed** \\-əd\\ *adj*

bear down \\(')ba(ə)r-'daůn, (')be(ə)r-\\ *vi* : to contract the abdominal muscles and the diaphragm during childbirth

bear·ing *n* : an object, surface, or point that supports

¹beat \\'bēt\\ *vi* **beat**; **beat·en** \\'bēt-ᵊn\\ *or* **beat**; **beat·ing** : PULSATE, THROB

²beat *n* : a single stroke or pulsation (as of the heart) ⟨ectopic ∼s⟩ — see EXTRASYSTOLE

Beaumé *var of* BAUMÉ

Beau's lines \\'bōz-\\ *n pl* : transverse grooves or ridges on the nail plate that are temporary and usu. occur after a severe illness

Beau \\bō\\, **Joseph–Honoré–Simon (1806–1865),** French physician. Beau successively served on the staffs of St. Antoine's and Cochin Hospitals. He is credited with being one of the first to apply physiological concepts to the study of pathology and with observing that functional disorders often precede anatomical disorders. His areas of research included epilepsy, dyspepsia, hysteria, and disorders of the heart and lungs. He is remembered for his descriptions of asystole, in 1836, and Beau's lines, in 1846.

be·bee·rine \\bə-'bi(ə)r-ˌēn, -ən; 'beb-(ē-)ə-ˌrēn\\ *n* : a crystalline alkaloid $C_{36}H_{38}N_3O_6$ known in two optically different forms; *esp* : the dextrorotatory form

Bechterew's nucleus *var of* BEKHTEREV'S NUCLEUS

Beck Depression Inventory \\'bek-\\ *n* : a standardized psychiatric questionnaire in which the subject rates each statement on a sliding scale and that is used in the diagnosis of depression

Beck, Aaron Temkin (b 1921), American psychiatrist. Beck held the concurrent positions of professor of psychiatry at the University of Pennsylvania, section chief at Philadelphia General Hospital, and consultant to Philadelphia's Veterans Administration Hospital. His areas of research included depression, suicide, cognitive aspects of psychopathology, cognitive therapy, and anxiety and panic disorders. He developed his depression inventory in the 1970s as a diagnostic and therapeutic tool for the treatment of childhood mood disorders. It uses a total of eighteen criteria for depressive illness.

Beck·er muscular dystrophy \\'bek-ər-\\ *or* **Beck·er's muscular dystrophy** \\-ərz-\\ *n* : a less severe form of Duchenne muscular dystrophy with later onset and slower progression of the disease that is inherited as an X-linked recessive trait and is characterized by dystrophin of deficient or abnormal molecular weight

Becker, P. E., 20th-century German human geneticist. Becker spent the earlier part of his career as a lecturer at the psychiatric and neurological clinic at the University of Freiberg. He went on to hold the post of Professor of Human Genetics at the University of Göttingen. He wrote numerous books and articles on human genetics, especially concerning hereditary myopathies and in particular myotonia. He was the first to recognize a benign X-linked recessive form of muscular dystrophy, publishing his first report in 1955.

Beck·with–Wie·de·mann syndrome \\'bek-wəth-'wēd-ə-mən-, -ˌman-\\ *n* : an inherited disease that is characterized by macroglossia, umbilical hernia, hypoglycemia, abnormal enlargement of the viscera, and increased risk of Wilms' tumor and rhabdomyosarcoma

Beckwith, John Bruce (b 1933), American pathologist. Beckwith held positions as professor of pathology and pediatrics at the University of Washington's Medical School and chairman of the department of pathology at Children's Hospital in Denver. His areas of research included sudden death during infancy and pathogenesis of tumors in children. He described the syndrome which now bears his name as well as Wiedemann's in an article published independently of Wiedemann in 1964.

Wie·de·mann \\'vē-də-ˌmän\\, **Hans Rudolf (b 1915),** German pediatrician. In the course of his career Wiedemann served as director of children's clinics in Bonn, Krefeld, and Kiel and on the medical faculty at the universities of Bonn and Kiel. He published several articles on congenital malformations, including the first report on the effects of thalidomide, and on hereditary diseases of the skeleton and nervous system. In 1964 he published an independent description of the syndrome that now bears his name as well as Beckwith's.

bec·lo·meth·a·sone \\ˌbek-lə-'meth-ə-ˌzōn, -ˌsōn\\ *n* : a steroid anti-inflammatory drug administered in the form of its dipropionate $C_{28}H_{37}ClO_7$ as an oral inhalant to treat asthma and as a nasal spray to treat rhinitis — see BECONASE

Bec·on·ase \\'bek-ə-ˌnās, -ˌnāz\\ *trademark* — used for a preparation of the dipropionate of beclomethasone

Bec·que·rel ray \\(ˌ)bek-ˌrel-, ˌbek-ə-\\ *n* : a ray emitted by a radioactive substance — used before radioactive emissions were classified as alpha and beta particles and gamma-ray photons

Becque·rel \\bek-rel\\, **Antoine–Henri (1852–1908),** French physicist. The father of modern atomic and nuclear physics, Becquerel is most notable for his discovery of radioactivity. In 1896 he demonstrated that uranium salts are radioactive and emit rays. For a time the rays were called Becquerel rays. His observations led Pierre and Marie Curie to their discovery of radium. Becquerel also undertook research into light polarization, magnetism, and the passage of light through crystals. He was awarded the Nobel Prize for Physics in 1903.

bed \\'bed\\ *n* **1 a** : a piece of furniture on or in which one may lie and sleep — see HOSPITAL BED **b** : the equipment and services needed to care for one hospitalized patient **2** : a layer of specialized or altered tissue esp. when separating dissimilar structures — see NAIL BED, VASCULAR BED

bed·bound \\'bed-ˌbaůnd\\ *adj* : confined to bed : BEDRIDDEN

bed·bug \\'bed-ˌbəg\\ *n* : a wingless bloodsucking bug (*Cimex lectularius*) sometimes infesting houses and esp. beds and feeding on human blood — called also *chinch*

bed·fast \\'bed-ˌfast\\ *adj* : BEDRIDDEN

bed·lam \\'bed-ləm\\ *n* **1** *obs* : MADMAN, LUNATIC **2** *often cap* : a lunatic asylum

bed·lam·ite \\-lə-ˌmīt\\ *n* : MADMAN, LUNATIC — **bedlamite** *adj*

bed·pan \\'bed-ˌpan\\ *n* : a shallow vessel used by a bedridden person for urination or defecation

bed rest *n* : confinement of a sick person to bed

bed·rid·den \\'bed-ˌrid-ᵊn\\ *also* **bed·rid** \\-ˌrid\\ *adj* : confined to bed (as by illness)

¹bed·side \\'bed-ˌsīd\\ *n* : a place beside a bed esp. of a bedridden person

²bedside *adj* **1** : of, relating to, or conducted at the bedside of a bedridden patient ⟨a ∼ diagnosis⟩ **2** : suitable for a bedridden person ⟨∼ reading⟩

bedside manner *n* : the manner that a physician assumes toward patients

bed·so·nia \\bed-'sō-nē-ə\\ *n, pl* **-ni·ae** \\-nē-ˌē, -ˌī\\ : CHLAMYDIA 2a

Bed·son \\'bed-sᵊn\\, **Sir Samuel Phillips (1886–1969),** English bacteriologist. Bedson undertook important original research on blood platelets and their relationships with various hemorrhagic states. He concentrated upon the study of filterable viruses. In 1930 Bedson, George T. Western, and Samuel L. Simpson reported their discovery that the causative agent of psittacosis is filterable. A former name for the group of microorganisms that includes this causative agent honors Bedson. In other research on viruses he made significant serological investigations into primary atypical and viral pneumonias and the use of penicillin in treating those infections.

Bedsonia *n, syn of* CHLAMYDIA

bed·sore \'bed-ˌsō(ə)r, -ˌso(ə)r\ *n* : an ulceration of tissue deprived of adequate blood supply by prolonged pressure — called also *decubitus, decubitus ulcer, pressure sore;* compare PRESSURE POINT 1

bed·wet·ting \-ˌwet-iŋ\ *n* : enuresis esp. when occurring in bed during sleep — **bed·wet·ter** \-ˌwet-ər\ *n*

bee \'bē\ *n* : HONEYBEE; *broadly* : any of numerous hymenopteran insects (superfamily Apoidea) that differ from the related wasps esp. in the heavier hairier body and in having sucking as well as chewing mouthparts, that feed on pollen and nectar, and that store both and often also honey — see AFRICANIZED BEE

beef \'bēf\ *n, pl* **beefs** \'bēfs\ *or* **beeves** \'bēvz\ : the flesh of an adult domestic bovine (as a steer or cow) used as food

beef measles *n pl but sing or pl in constr* : the infestation of beef muscle by cysticerci of the beef tapeworm which make oval white vesicles giving a measly appearance to beef

beef tapeworm *n* : an unarmed tapeworm of the genus *Taenia* (*T. saginata*) that infests the human intestine as an adult, has a cysticercus larva that develops in cattle, and is contracted through ingestion of the larva in raw or rare beef

Beer's law \ˌbā(ə)rz-, ˌbe(ə)rz-\ *n* : a statement in physics usu. made in either of two mathematically equivalent ways: (1) the transmittance of a chemical solution is an exponential function of the product of the concentration of the solution and the distance light travels through it (2) the absorbance of a chemical solution is directly proportional to the product of its concentration and the distance light travels through it

Beer \'bā(ə)r\, **August (1825–1863)**, German physicist. Beer is known primarily for his research on optics and his discovery of the law of absorption of light that bears his name. In 1854 he published *Introduction to Higher Optics.*

bees·wax \'bēz-ˌwaks\ *n* **1** : WAX 1 **2 a** : YELLOW WAX **b** : WHITE WAX

be·have \bi-'hāv\ *vb* **be·haved; be·hav·ing** *vt* : to bear or conduct (oneself) in a particular way ∼ *vi* : to act, function, or react in a particular way

be·hav·ior *or chiefly Brit* **be·hav·iour** \bi-'hā-vyər\ *n* **1** : the manner of conducting oneself **2 a** : anything that an organism does involving action and response to stimulation **b** : the response of an individual, group, or species to its environment — **be·hav·ior·al** *or chiefly Brit* **be·hav·iour·al** \-vyə-rəl\ *adj* — **be·hav·ior·al·ly** *or chiefly Brit* **be·hav·iour·al·ly** \-rə-lē\ *adv*

behavioral science *n* : a science (as psychology, sociology, or anthropology) that deals with human action and seeks to generalize about human behavior in society — **behavioral scientist** *n*

be·hav·ior·ism *or chiefly Brit* **be·hav·iour·ism** \bi-'hā-vyə-ˌriz-əm\ *n* : a school of psychology that takes the objective evidence of behavior (as measured responses to stimuli) as the only concern of its research and the only basis of its theory without reference to conscious experience — compare COGNITIVE PSYCHOLOGY — **be·hav·ior·is·tic** *or chiefly Brit* **be·hav·iour·is·tic** \-ˌhā-vyə-'ris-tik\ *adj*

¹be·hav·ior·ist *or chiefly Brit* **be·hav·iour·ist** \-rəst\ *n* : a person who advocates or practices behaviorism

²behaviorist *adj* : of or relating to behaviorism ⟨∼ psychology⟩

behavior modification *also* **behavioral modification** *n* : psychotherapy that is concerned with the treatment (as by desensitization or aversion therapy) of observable behaviors rather than underlying psychological processes and that applies learning principles to substitute desirable responses and behavior patterns for undesirable ones (as phobias or obsessions) — called also *behavior therapy;* compare COGNITIVE THERAPY

behavior therapist *or* **behavioral therapist** *n* : a specialist in behavior modification

behavior therapy *or* **behavioral therapy** *n* : BEHAVIOR MODIFICATION

Beh·cet's syndrome \'bā-sɒts-\ *n* : a group of symptoms of

unknown etiology that occur esp. in young men and include esp. ulcerative lesions of the mouth and genitalia and inflammation of the eye (as uveitis and iridocyclitis) — called also *Behcet's disease*

Beh·çet \be-'chet\, **Hulusi (1889–1948)**, Turkish dermatologist. Behçet published his original description of Behcet's syndrome in 1937.

bej·el \'bej-əl\ *n* : a disease that is chiefly endemic in children in northern Africa and Asia Minor, is marked by bone and skin lesions, and is caused by a spirochete of the genus *Treponema* very similar to the causative agent of syphilis

Bekh·te·rev's nucleus *or* **Bech·te·rew's nucleus** \'bek-tə-ˌrefs-, -ˌrevz-\ *n* : SUPERIOR VESTIBULAR NUCLEUS

Bekh·te·rev \'byāk-tər-yəf\, **Vladimir Mikhailovich (1857–1927)**, Russian neuropathologist. A pioneer in clinical research on mental diseases, Bekhterev founded the psychoneurological institute in St. Petersburg. The author of more than 800 publications, Bekhterev published several original descriptions that include papers on ankylosing spondylitis in 1892 and on the superior vestibular nucleus (Bekhterev's nucleus) in 1908. In 1910 he published a major work, *Objective Psychology,* in which he applied the Pavlovian principles of the conditioned reflex to psychological problems. This study influenced the development of behaviorism in the U.S.

bel \'bel\ *n* : ten decibels — abbr. *b*

Bell \'bel\, **Alexander Graham (1847–1922)**, American inventor. Bell began his career in the fields of speech and acoustics. Training teachers of the deaf, he and his father developed "visible speech," a system of symbolic representations of the physical process of speech. His investigations into the application of electricity to the production and analysis of sound resulted in the invention of a multiplexing telegraph system. Further experimentation in telegraphy led to work on a method of electrically transmitting actual voice sounds, and in 1876 his work culminated in the invention of the telephone. Later inventions included a telephonic device using the modulation of a light beam, an audiometer, an improved phonograph, and an electrical induction device for the detection of metallic objects in the body. Throughout his life he remained deeply interested in the teaching of speech to the deaf.

¹belch \'belch\ *vi* : to expel gas suddenly from the stomach through the mouth ∼ *vt* : to expel (gas) from the stomach suddenly : ERUCT

²belch *n* : an act or instance of belching : ERUCTATION

bel·em·noid \'bel-əm-ˌnȯid, bə-'lem-\ *adj* : shaped like a dart

bel·la·don·na \ˌbel-ə-'dän-ə\ *n* **1** : an Old World poisonous plant of the genus *Atropa* (*A. belladonna*) having purple or green flowers, glossy black berries, and a root and leaves that yield atropine — called also *deadly nightshade* **2** : a medicinal preparation (as atropine) extracted from the belladonna plant and containing anticholinergic alkaloids

bell jar \'bel-ˌjär\ *n* : a bell-shaped usu. glass vessel designed to cover objects or to contain gases or a vacuum

Bell-Ma·gen·die law \'bel-ˌmà-zhaⁿ-'dē-\ *n* : BELL'S LAW

Bell, Sir Charles (1774–1842), British anatomist. Bell was the leading anatomist of his time as well as an eminent surgeon. In 1802 he published a series of engravings showing the anatomy of the brain and the nervous system. In 1811 he published one of the most seminal works in all of neurology, *Idea of a New Anatomy of the Brain.* In 1830, he produced an expanded work, *The Nervous System of the Human Body.* In these books he distinguished between sensory nerves and motor nerves and announced his finding that the anterior roots of the spinal nerves are motor in function, while the posterior roots are sensory. First presented in 1811, this statement is alternately known as Bell's law or

\ə\ **abut** \ᵊ\ **kitten** \ər\ **further** \a\ **ash** \ā\ **ace** \ä\ **cot, cart**
\au̇\ **out** \ch\ **chin** \e\ **bet** \ē\ **easy** \g\ **go** \i\ **hit** \ī\ **ice** \j\ **job**
\ŋ\ **sing** \ō\ **go** \ȯ\ **law** \ȯi\ **boy** \th\ **thin** \th̲\ **the** \ü\ **loot**
\u̇\ **foot** \y\ **yet** \zh\ **vision** *See also* Pronunciation Symbols page

as the Bell-Magendie law, due to the fact that François Magendie later elaborated on it. One of the classic descriptions in Bell's *Nervous System of the Human Body* is his detailed account of the facial nerve, which he had originally described in 1821. He also described the facial paralysis resulting from a lesion of this nerve. The paralysis is now known as Bell's palsy.

Ma·gen·die \mȧ-zhaⁿ-dē\, **François (1783–1855),** French physiologist. An experimental physiologist, Magendie is remembered for his pioneering investigations into the effects of drugs on various parts of the body. His researches led to the scientific application of such compounds as strychnine and morphine into medical practice. In 1821 he founded the first journal devoted to experimental physiology. The following year he confirmed and elaborated upon Bell's law. He was the first to actually prove the functional difference of the spinal nerves. Magendie was also one of the first to observe anaphylaxis, discovering in 1839 that rabbits tolerating a single injection of egg albumin often died following a second injection.

bel·lows \'bel-(ˌ)ōz, -əz\ *n pl but sing or pl in constr* : LUNGS

Bell's law \'belz-\ *n* : a statement in physiology: the roots of the spinal nerves coming from the ventral portion of the spinal cord are motor in function and those coming from the dorsal portion are sensory — called also *Bell-Magendie law*

Bell's palsy *n* : paralysis of the facial nerve producing distortion on one side of the face

bel·ly \'bel-ē\ *n, pl* **bellies 1 a** : ABDOMEN 1a **b** : the undersurface of an animal's body **c** : WOMB, UTERUS **d** : the stomach and its adjuncts **2** : the enlarged fleshy body of a muscle

bel·ly·ache \'bel-ē-ˌāk\ *n* : pain in the abdomen and esp. in the stomach : STOMACHACHE

bel·ly·band \'bel-ē-ˌband\ *n* : a band around or across the belly; *esp* : BAND 1a

belly but·ton \-ˌbət-ᵊn\ *n* : the human navel

be·me·gride \'bem-ə-ˌgrīd, 'bē-mə-\ *n* : an analeptic drug $C_{18}H_{13}NO_2$ used esp. to counteract the effects of barbiturates

Ben·a·dryl \'ben-ə-ˌdril\ *trademark* — used for a preparation of the hydrochloride of diphenhydramine

ben·a·ze·pril \bən-'ā-zə-pril\ *n* : an ACE inhibitor administered orally in the form of its hydrochloride $C_{24}H_{28}N_2O_5$·HCl for the treatment of hypertension — see LOTENSIN, LOTREL

Bence–Jones protein \ˌben(t)s-ˌjōnz-\ *n* : a polypeptide composed of one or two antibody light chains that is found esp. in the urine of persons affected with multiple myeloma

  Bence–Jones, Henry (1814–1873), British physician. In 1848 Bence-Jones published an article announcing his discovery of a special protein (now known as Bence-Jones protein) in the urine of patients suffering from softening of the bones. The first physician to note the occurrence of xanthine in urine, Bence-Jones was also a recognized authority on diseases of the stomach and kidneys.

Ben·der Gestalt test \'ben-dər-\ *n* : a drawing test in which the subject copies geometric figures and which is used esp. to assess organic brain damage and degree of maturation of the nervous system

  Bender, Lauretta (1897–1987), American psychiatrist. In 1935 Bender published *Visual Motor Gestalt and Its Clinical Use.* She developed the psychological test that is associated with her name. Much of her career was devoted to child neurology, psychiatry, and psychology.

bends \'ben(d)z\ *n pl but sing or pl in constr* : the painful manifestations (as joint pain) of decompression sickness; *also* : DECOMPRESSION SICKNESS — usu. used with *the* ⟨a case of the ∼⟩

Ben·e·dict's solution \'ben-ə-ˌdik(t)(s)-\ *n* : a blue solution that contains sodium carbonate, sodium citrate, and copper sulfate $CuSO_4$ and is used to test for reducing sugars in Benedict's test

  Ben·e·dict \'ben-ə-ˌdikt\, **Stanley Rossiter (1884–1936),** American chemist. Benedict's major contribution was in

analytical biochemistry. His precise techniques for analyzing such biological materials as blood and urine made possible new discoveries in the body's chemistry. He explored the significance of his findings both to normal metabolism and to the diagnosis and treatment of disease. In 1909 Benedict presented a new method for the detection of reducing sugars. It is an improvement and modification of the classical test for sugar in the urine using Fehling's solution.

Ben·e·dict's test \-ˌdik(t)s-\ *n* : a test for the presence of a reducing sugar (as in urine) by heating the solution to be tested with Benedict's solution which yields a red, yellow, or orange precipitate upon warming with a reducing sugar (as glucose or maltose)

bengal — see ROSE BENGAL

Ben–Gay \ˌben-'gā\ *trademark* — used for a preparation of methyl salicylate and menthol

be·nign \bi-'nīn\ *adj* **1** : of a mild type or character that does not threaten health or life ⟨∼ malaria⟩ ⟨a ∼ tumor⟩ — compare MALIGNANT 1 **2** : having a good prognosis : responding favorably to treatment ⟨a ∼ psychosis⟩

benign intracranial hypertension *n* : PSEUDOTUMOR CEREBRI

be·nig·ni·ty \bi-'nig-nət-ē\ *n, pl* **-ties** : the quality or state of being benign ⟨determine the ∼ or malignancy of a tumor⟩

benign prostatic hyperplasia *n* : adenomatous hyperplasia of the periurethral part of the prostate gland that occurs esp. in men over 50 years old and that tends to obstruct urination by constricting the urethra — abbr. *BPH;* called also *benign prostatic hypertrophy*

ben·ne *or* **bene** \'ben-ē\ *n* : SESAME

benne oil *n* : SESAME OIL

ben·ny \'ben-ē\ *n, pl* **bennies** *slang* : a tablet of amphetamine taken as a stimulant

ben·ton·ite \'bent-ᵊn-ˌīt\ *n* : an absorptive and colloidal clay used in pharmacy esp. to stabilize suspensions — **ben·ton·it·ic** \ˌbent-ᵊn-'it-ik\ *adj*

benz·al·de·hyde \ben-'zal-də-ˌhīd\ *n* : a colorless nontoxic aromatic liquid C_6H_5CHO found in essential oils (as in peach kernels) and used in flavoring and perfumery, in pharmaceuticals, and in synthesis of dyes

benz·al·ko·ni·um chloride \ˌben-zal-ˌkō-nē-əm-\ *n* : a white or yellowish white mixture of chloride salts obtained as a bitter aromatic powder or gelatinous pieces that is used as an antiseptic and germicide — see ZEPHIRAN

benz·an·thra·cene \ben-'zan(t)-thrə-ˌsēn\ *n* : a crystalline feebly carcinogenic cyclic hydrocarbon $C_{18}H_{12}$ that is found in small amounts in coal tar

ben·za·thine penicillin G \'ben-zə-ˌthēn-, -thən-\ *n* : PENICILLIN G BENZATHINE

Ben·ze·drine \'ben-zə-ˌdrēn\ *n* : a preparation of the sulfate of amphetamine $(C_9H_{13}N)_2 \cdot H_2SO_4$ formerly used in medicine — formerly a U.S. registered trademark

ben·zene \'ben-ˌzēn, ben-'\ *n* : a colorless volatile flammable toxic liquid aromatic hydrocarbon C_6H_6 used in organic synthesis, as a solvent, and as a motor fuel — called also *benzol* — **ben·ze·noid** \'ben-zə-ˌnȯid\ *adj*

benzene hexa·chlo·ride \-ˌhek-sə-'klō(ə)r-ˌīd, -'klō(ə)r-\ *n* : any of several stereoisomeric chlorine derivatives $C_6H_6Cl_6$ of cyclohexane in which the chlorine atoms are all attached to different carbon atoms : BHC; *esp* : GAMMA BENZENE HEXACHLORIDE — see LINDANE

benzene ring *n* : a plane symmetrical ring of six carbon atoms which is characteristic of benzene and related aromatic compounds and in which the electrons forming three conjugated double bonds are distributed over the entire ring

ben·zene·sul·fo·nate *or chiefly Brit* **ben·zene·sul·pho·nate** \ˌben-ˌzēn-'səl-fə-ˌnāt\ *n* : BESYLATE

ben·zene·sul·fon·ic acid *or chiefly Brit* **ben·zene·sul·phon·ic acid** \ˌben-ˌzēn-ˌsəl-ˌfän-ik-, -ˌfän-\ *n* : a colorless crystalline acid $C_6H_5SO_3H$ made by sulfonating benzene and used in organic synthesis, in the form of its besylate in pharmacology, and in the form of derivatives as detergents

ben·zes·trol \ben-'zes-ˌtrȯl, -ˌtrōl\ *n* : a crystalline estrogenic diphenol $C_{20}H_{26}O_2$

ben·zi·dine \\'ben-zə-ˌdēn\ *n* : a crystalline base $C_{12}H_{12}N_2$ used esp. in making dyes and in a test for blood

benzidine test *n* : a test for blood (as in feces) based on its production of a blue color in a solution of benzidine, sodium peroxide, and glacial acetic acid

benzilate — see QUINUCLIDINYL BENZILATE

benz·imid·azole \\ˌben-ˌzim-ə-ˈdaz-ˌōl, ˌben-zə-ˈmid-ə-ˌzōl\ *n* : a crystalline base $C_7H_6N_2$ used esp. to inhibit the growth of various viruses, parasitic worms, and fungi; *also* : one of its derivatives

ben·zine \\'ben-ˌzēn, ben-'\ *n* : any of various volatile flammable petroleum distillates used esp. as solvents or as motor fuels

ben·zo·[a]·py·rene \\ˌben-zō-ˌā-ˈpī(ə)r-ˌēn, -zō-ˌal-fə-, -pī-ˈrēn\ *also* **3,4–benz·py·rene** \\-benz-ˈpī(ə)r-ˌēn, -ˌbenz-pī-ˈrēn\ *n* : the yellow crystalline highly carcinogenic isomer of the benzopyrene mixture that is formed esp. in the burning of cigarettes, coal, and gasoline

ben·zo·ate \\'ben-zə-ˌwāt\ *n* : a salt or ester of benzoic acid

benzoate of soda *n* : SODIUM BENZOATE

ben·zo·caine \\'ben-zə-ˌkān\ *n* : a white crystalline ester $C_9H_{11}NO_2$ used as a local anesthetic — called also *ethyl aminobenzoate*

ben·zo·di·az·e·pine \\ˌben-zō-dī-ˈaz-ə-ˌpēn\ *n* : any of a group of aromatic lipophilic amines (as diazepam and chlordiazepoxide) used esp. as tranquilizers

ben·zo·ic acid \\ben-ˌzō-ik-\ *n* : a white crystalline acid $C_6H_6O_2$ found naturally (as in benzoin or in cranberries) or made synthetically and used esp. as a preservative of foods, in medicine, and in organic synthesis

ben·zo·in \\'ben-zə-wən, -ˌwēn; -ˌzóin\ *n* **1** : a hard fragrant yellowish balsamic resin from trees (genus *Styrax* of the family Styracaceae) of southeastern Asia used esp. as an expectorant and topically to relieve skin irritations **2** : a white crystalline hydroxy ketone $C_{14}H_{12}O_2$ made from benzaldehyde **3** : a tree yielding benzoin

ben·zol \\'ben-ˌzól, -ˌzōl\ *n* : BENZENE; *also* : a mixture of benzene and other aromatic hydrocarbons

ben·zol·ism \\'ben-zə-ˌliz-əm\ *n* : poisoning by benzene

ben·zo·mor·phan \\ˌben-zō-ˈmór-ˌfan\ *n* : any of a group of synthetic compounds including some potent analgesics (as phenazocine or pentazocine)

ben·zo·phe·none \\ˌben-zō-fi-ˈnōn, -ˈfē-ˌnōn\ *n* : a colorless crystalline ketone $C_{13}H_{10}O$ used chiefly in perfumery and sunscreens; *also* : a derivative of benzophenone

ben·zo·py·rene \\ˌben-zō-ˈpī(ə)r-ˌēn, -pī-ˈrēn\ *or* **benz·py·rene** \\benz-ˈpī(ə)r-ˌēn, ˌbenz-pī-ˈrēn\ *n* : a mixture of two isomeric hydrocarbons $C_{20}H_{12}$ of which one is highly carcinogenic — see BENZO[A]PYRENE

ben·zo·qui·none \\ˌben-zō-kwin-ˈōn, -ˈkwin-ˌ\ *n* : QUINONE 1

ben·zo·sul·fi·mide *or chiefly Brit* **ben·zo·sul·phi·mide** \\ˌben-zō-ˈsəl-fə-ˌmīd\ *n* : SACCHARIN

ben·zo·yl \\'ben-zə-ˌwil, -ˌzóil\ *n* : the radical C_6H_5CO of benzoic acid

benzoyl peroxide *n* : a white crystalline flammable compound $C_{14}H_{10}O_4$ used in bleaching and in medicine esp. in the treatment of acne

benz·pyr·in·i·um bromide \\ˌbenz-pə-ˈrin-ē-əm-\ *n* : a cholinergic drug $C_{15}H_{17}BrN_2O_2$ that has actions and uses similar to those of neostigmine and has been used esp. to relieve postoperative urinary retention — called also *benzpyrinium*

benz·tro·pine \\benz-ˈtrō-ˌpēn, -pən\ *n* : a parasympatholytic drug administered in the form of its mesylate $C_{21}H_{25}NO\cdot CH_4O_3S$ esp. in the treatment of Parkinson's disease

ben·zyl \\'ben-ˌzēl, -zəl\ *n* : a monovalent radical $C_6H_5CH_2$ derived from toluene

benzyl benzoate *n* : a colorless oily ester $C_{14}H_{12}O_2$ used in medicine formerly as an antispasmodic and now in the form of a lotion as a scabicide and in perfumery as a fixative and solvent

ben·zyl·pen·i·cil·lin \\'ben-ˌzēl-(ˌ)pen-ə-ˈsil-ən, -zəl-\ *n* : PENICILLIN G

ber·ba·mine \\'bər-bə-ˌmēn, -mən\ *n* : a crystalline alkaloid $C_{37}H_{40}N_2O_6$ found esp. in barberry

ber·ber·ine \\'bər-bə-ˌrēn\ *n* : a bitter crystalline yellow alkaloid $C_{20}H_{19}NO_5$ obtained from the roots of various plants (as barberry) and used as a tonic and antiperiodic

ber·ber·is \\'bər-bə-rəs\ *n* **1** *cap* : a large genus of shrubs (family Berberidaceae) that usu. have prickly stems, yellow flowers, and red or blackish berries — compare MAHONIA **2** : the dried rhizome and roots of some barberries of the genus *Mahonia* (esp. *M. aquifolium*) that contain a number of alkaloids (as berberine and berbamine)

beri·beri \\ˌber-ē-ˈber-ē\ *n* : a deficiency disease marked by inflammatory or degenerative changes of the nerves, digestive system, and heart and caused by a lack of or inability to assimilate thiamine — called also *kakke*

berke·li·um \\'bər-klē-əm\ *n* : a radioactive metallic element produced by bombarding americium 241 with helium ions — symbol *Bk*; see ELEMENT table

ber·lock dermatitis \\'bər-ˌläk-\ *n* : a brownish discoloration of the skin that develops on exposure to sunlight after the use of perfume containing certain essential oils

Ber·noul·li effect \\bər-ˌnü-lē-, ber-ˌnü-ē-, ˌber-ˌnü-ˌ(y)ē-\ *n* : the change in pressure observed in a fluid stream in accordance with Bernoulli's principle

Ber·noul·li \\bər-ˈnü-lē, ber-ˈnü-ē, ˌber-ˈnü-ˌ(y)ē\, **Daniel (1700–1782),** Swiss mathematician and physicist. Bernoulli came from an illustrious family that produced eight outstanding mathematicians in three generations. In 1724 he demonstrated his own mathematical ability by producing a treatise on differential equations and the physics of flowing water. In 1738 he published his great work, *Hydrodynamica*. The work examined the basic properties of fluid flow, particularly density, pressure, and velocity. Bernoulli stated the fundamental relationships between these properties, set forth the principle now known as Bernoulli's principle, and established the basis for the kinetic theory of gases and heat. A scientist of catholic interests, he did research on such diverse subjects as astronomy, the properties of vibrating and rotating bodies, gravity, magnetism, tides and ocean currents, and probability theory.

Ber·noul·li's principle \\-lēz-, -ēz-, -ˌ(y)ēz-\ *also* **Bernoulli principle** *n* : a principle in hydrodynamics: the pressure in a stream of fluid is reduced as the speed of flow is increased

ber·serk \\bə(r)-ˈsərk, ˌbər-, -ˈzərk, ˈbər-ˌ\ *adj* : marked by crazed or frenzied behavior suggestive of sudden mental imbalance — usu. used in the phrase *go berserk* — **berserk** *adv*

Ber·tin's column \\ber-ˌtaⁿz-\ *n* : RENAL COLUMN

Ber·tin \\ber-taⁿ\, **Exupère Joseph (1712–1781),** French anatomist. Bertin is known primarily for his study of the kidneys. He wrote classic descriptions of the renal columns, which are also known as the columns of Bertin, and of the nasal conchae. He also studied blood circulation in the fetus, the anatomy of the lacrimal system, and the organs of speech.

be·ryl·li·o·sis \\bə-ˌril-ē-ˈō-səs\ *also* **ber·yl·lo·sis** \\ˌber-ə-ˈlō-\ *n, pl* **-li·o·ses** \\-ˌsēz\ *or* **-lo·ses** \\-ˌsēz\ : poisoning resulting from exposure to fumes and dusts of beryllium compounds or alloys and occurring chiefly as an acute pneumonitis or as a granulomatosis involving esp. the lungs

be·ryl·li·um \\bə-ˈril-ē-əm\ *n* : a steel-gray light strong brittle toxic bivalent metallic element used chiefly as a hardening agent in alloys — symbol *Be*; see ELEMENT table

bes·ti·al·i·ty \\ˌbes-chē-ˈal-ət-ē, ˌbēs-\ *n, pl* **-ties** : sexual relations between a human being and a lower animal

bes·yl·ate \\'bes-ə-ˌlāt\ *n* : a salt or ester of a benzenesulfonic acid — called also *benzenesulfonate*

¹be·ta \\'bāt-ə, *chiefly Brit* 'bē-tə\ *n* **1** : the second letter of the Greek alphabet — symbol B or β **2** : BETA PARTICLE **3** : BETA WAVE

²beta *or* **β-** *adj* **1** : of or relating to one of two or more closely related chemical substances ⟨the *beta* chain of hemoglobin⟩

\ə\ abut \ᵊ\ kitten \ər\ further \a\ ash \ā\ ace \ä\ cot, cart
\aú\ out \ch\ chin \e\ bet \ē\ easy \g\ go \i\ hit \ī\ ice \j\ job
\ŋ\ sing \ō\ go \ó\ law \ói\ boy \th\ thin \th\ the \ü\ loot
\ú\ foot \y\ yet \zh\ vision *See also* Pronunciation Symbols page

⟨β-yohimbine⟩ — used somewhat arbitrarily to specify ordinal relationship or a particular physical form and esp. one that is allotropic, isomeric, stereoisomeric, or sometimes polymeric (as in β-D-glucose) **2** : second in position in the structure of an organic molecule from a particular group or atom; *also* : occurring at or having a structure characterized by such a position ⟨∼ substitution⟩ **3** : producing a zone of decolorization when grown on blood media — used of some hemolytic streptococci or of the hemolysis they cause

be·ta–ad·ren·er·gic \-ٍ,ad-rə-'nər-jik\ *adj* : of, relating to, or being a beta-receptor ⟨a ∼ blocking agent⟩

beta–adrenergic receptor *n* : BETA-RECEPTOR

be·ta–adre·no·cep·tor \-ə-'drē-nə-ٍsep-tər\ *also* **be·ta–adre·no·re·cep·tor** \-ri-ٍsep-tər\ *n* : BETA-RECEPTOR

be·ta–ag·o·nist \-'ag-ə-nəst\ *n* : any of various drugs (as albuterol or terbutaline) that combine with and activate a beta-receptor

be·ta–am·y·loid *also* β–**amyloid** \-'am-ə-ٍloid\ *n* : an amyloid that is derived from amyloid precursor protein and is the primary component of plaques characteristic of Alzheimer's disease — called also *amyloid beta-protein, beta=amyloid protein*

be·ta–block·ade \-blä-'kād\ *n* : blockade of beta-receptor activity

be·ta–block·er \-'bläk-ər\ *n* : any of a group of drugs (as propranolol) that combine with and block the activity of a beta-receptor to decrease the heart rate and force of contractions and lower high blood pressure and that are used esp. to treat hypertension, angina pectoris, and ventricular and supraventricular arrhythmias — compare ALPHA=BLOCKER

be·ta–block·ing \-'bläk-iŋ\ *adj* : blocking or relating to the blocking of beta-receptor activity ⟨∼ drugs⟩ ⟨the ∼ activity of atenolol⟩

be·ta–car·o·tene *or* β–**carotene** \-'kar-ə-ٍtēn\ *n* : an isomer of carotene that is found in dark green and dark yellow vegetables and fruits

beta cell *n* : any of various secretory cells distinguished by their basophilic staining characters: as **a** : a pituitary basophil **b** : an insulin-secreting cell of the islets of Langerhans — compare ALPHA CELL

Be·ta·dine \'bāt-ə-ٍdīn, *chiefly Brit* 'bē-tə-\ *trademark* — used for a preparation of povidone-iodine

be·ta–en·dor·phin *or* β–**endorphin** \ٍbāt-ə-en-'dȯr-fən, *chiefly Brit* ٍbē-tə-\ *n* : an endorphin of the pituitary gland with much greater analgesic potency than morphine that occurs free and as the terminal sequence of 31 amino acids in the polypeptide chain of beta-lipotropin

beta globin *also* β–**glo·bin** \-'glō-bən\ *n* : the chain of hemoglobin that is designated beta and that when deficient or defective causes various anemias (as beta-thalassemia or sickle=cell anemia)

beta globulin *n* : any of several globulins of plasma or serum that have at alkaline pH electrophoretic mobilities intermediate between those of the alpha globulins and gamma globulins

beta–glucan *n* : any of several polysaccharides consisting of glucose units and including one found in endosperm cell walls of cereal grains (as barley and oats)

beta hemolysis *n* : a sharply defined clear colorless zone of hemolysis surrounding colonies of certain streptococci on blood agar plates — compare ALPHA HEMOLYSIS

be·ta–he·mo·lyt·ic *or chiefly Brit* **be·ta–hae·mo·lyt·ic** \ٍbāt-ə-ٍhē-mə-'lit-ik, *chiefly Brit* ٍbē-tə-\ *adj* : capable of causing beta hemolysis ⟨∼ streptococci⟩

be·ta–hy·poph·amine *also* β–**hypophamine** \-hī-'päf-ə-ٍmēn, -mən\ *n* : VASOPRESSIN

be·ta·ine \'bēt-ə-ٍēn\ *n* : a sweet crystalline quaternary ammonium salt $C_5H_{11}NO_2$ that was first isolated in beet juice and is used to treat homocystinuria and is also used in the form of its hydrochloride $C_5H_{11}NO_2 \cdot HCl$ as a source of hydrochloric acid esp. to treat hypochlorhydria

beta interferon *n* : an interferon that is produced esp. by fibroblasts, possesses antiviral activity, and is used in a form obtained from recombinant DNA esp. in the treatment of multiple sclerosis marked by recurrent attacks alternating with periods of remission — compare ALPHA INTERFERON, GAMMA INTERFERON

be·ta–lac·tam *or* β–**lactam** \ٍbāt-ə-'lak-ٍtam, *chiefly Brit* ٍbē-tə-\ *n* : any of a large class of natural and semisynthetic antibiotics (as the penicillins and cephalosporins) with a lactam ring

be·ta–lac·ta·mase *or* β–**lactamase** \-'lak-tə-ٍmās, -ٍmāz\ *n* : an enzyme found esp. in staphylococcal bacteria that inactivates penicillins by hydrolyzing them — called also *penicillinase*

beta–lipoprotein *or* β–**lipoprotein** *n* : LDL

be·ta–li·po·tro·pin \-ٍlip-ə-'trō-pən, -ٍlī-pə-\ *n* : a lipotropin of the adenohypophysis of the pituitary gland that contains beta-endorphin as the terminal sequence of 31 amino acids in its polypeptide chain

be·ta·meth·a·sone \-'meth-ə-ٍzōn, -ٍsōn\ *n* : a potent glucocorticoid $C_{22}H_{29}FO_5$ that is isomeric with dexamethasone and has potent anti-inflammatory activity

be·ta–naph·thol \-'naf-ٍthȯl, -'nap-, -ٍthȯl\ *n* : NAPHTHOL b

be·ta–ox·i·da·tion \'bāt-ə-ٍäk-sə-'dā-shən, *chiefly Brit* 'bē-tə-\ *n* : stepwise catabolism of fatty acids in which two-carbon fragments are successively removed from the carboxyl end of the chain

beta particle *n* : a high-speed electron; *specif* : one emitted during radioactive decay of an atomic nucleus

be·ta–pleat·ed sheet \-'plēt-əd-\ *n* : BETA SHEET

beta ray *n* **1** : BETA PARTICLE **2** : a stream of beta particles

be·ta–re·cep·tor \-ri-ٍsep-tər\ *n* : any of a group of receptors that are present on cell surfaces of some effector organs and tissues innervated by the sympathetic nervous system and that mediate certain physiological responses (as vasodilation, relaxation of bronchial and uterine smooth muscle, and increased heart rate) when bound by specific adrenergic agents — called also *beta-adrenergic receptor, beta=adrenoceptor;* compare ALPHA-RECEPTOR

beta rhythm *n* : BETA WAVE

be·ta–sheet \-ٍshēt\ *n* : the structural arrangement of many proteins in which two or more short regions of the polypeptide chain align adjacently and are stabilized by hydrogen bonds into sheets with a pleated or accordionlike appearance — called also *beta-pleated sheet;* compare ALPHA=HELIX

be·ta–thal·as·se·mia *or* β–**thalassemia** *or Brit* **be·ta–thal·as·sae·mia** *or* β–**thalassaemia** \-ٍthal-ə-'sē-mē-ə\ *n* : thalassemia in which the hemoglobin chain designated beta is affected and which comprises Cooley's anemia in the homozygous condition and thalassemia minor in the heterozygous condition

beta wave *n* : an electrical rhythm of the brain with a frequency of 13 to 30 cycles per second that is associated with normal conscious waking experience — called also *beta*

be·tel \'bēt-ᵊl\ *n* : a climbing pepper (*Piper betle*) of southeastern Asia whose leaves are chewed together with betel nut and mineral lime as a stimulant masticatory

betel nut *n* : the astringent seed of the betel palm that is a source of arecoline

betel palm *n* : a pinnate-leaved palm of the genus *Areca* (*A. catechu*) of Asia that has an orange-colored drupe with an outer fibrous husk

be·tha·ne·chol \bə-'thā-nə-ٍkȯl, -'than-ə-, -ٍkōl\ *n* : a parasympathomimetic agent administered in the form of its chloride $C_7H_{17}ClN_2O_2$ and used esp. to treat gastric and urinary retention — see URECHOLINE

Bet·u·la \'bech-ə-lə\ *n* : a genus of trees and shrubs (family Betulaceae) of arctic and temperate regions of the northern hemisphere comprising the birches and including one (*B. lenta*) which is the source of birch oil

betula oil *n* : BIRCH OIL

be·tween·brain \bi-'twēn-ٍbrān\ *n* : DIENCEPHALON

Betz cell \'bets-\ *n* : a very large pyramidal nerve cell of the motor area of the cerebral cortex

Betz, Vladimir Aleksandrovich (1834–1894), Russian

anatomist. In 1874 Betz discovered and described the giant pyramidal cells of the motor area of the cerebral cortex.

Bex·tra \'bek-strə\ *trademark* — used for a preparation of valdecoxib

be·zoar \'bē-ˌzō(ə)r, -ˌzò(ə)r\ *n* : any of various calculi found in the gastrointestinal organs esp. of ruminants — called also *bezoar stone*

BFP *abbr* biologic false-positive

BGH *abbr* bovine growth hormone

Bh *symbol* bohrium

BH *abbr* bill of health

BHA \ˌbē-ˌāch-'ā\ *n* : a phenolic antioxidant $C_{11}H_{16}O_2$ used esp. to preserve fats and oils in food — called also *butylated hydroxyanisole*

bhang *also* **bang** \'bäŋ, 'bóŋ, 'baŋ\ *n* **1 a** : HEMP 1 **b** : the leaves and flowering tops of uncultivated hemp : CANNABIS — compare MARIJUANA **2** : an intoxicant product obtained from bhang — compare HASHISH

BHC \ˌbē-(ˌ)āch-'sē\ *n* **1** : BENZENE HEXACHLORIDE **2** : LINDANE

BHT \ˌbē-ˌāch-'tē\ *n* : a phenolic antioxidant $C_{15}H_{24}O$ used esp. to preserve fats and oils in food, cosmetics, and pharmaceuticals — called also *butylated hydroxytoluene*

Bi *symbol* bismuth

bi·ace·tyl \ˌbī-ə-'sēt-əl, (ˌ)bī-'as-ət-əl\ *n* : DIACETYL

bi·ar·tic·u·lar \ˌbī-(ˌ)är-'tik-yə-lər\ *adj* : of or relating to two joints

bi·au·ric·u·lar \-ò-'rik-yə-lər\ *adj* : of or relating to the two auditory openings

bib·lio·clast \'bib-lē-ə-ˌklast, -lē-ō-\ *n* : a destroyer or mutilator of books

bib·lio·klep·to·ma·nia \ˌbib-lē-ō-ˌklep-tə-'mā-nē-ə, -nyə\ *n* : kleptomania involving a morbid tendency to steal books

bib·lio·ma·nia \ˌbib-lē-ə-'mā-nē-ə, -nyə\ *n* : extreme preoccupation with collecting books

bib·lio·ma·ni·ac \-'mā-nē-ə,ˌak\ *n* : one affected with bibliomania

bib·lio·ther·a·pist \-'ther-ə-pəst\ *n* : one who practices bibliotherapy

bib·lio·ther·a·py \-'ther-ə-pē\ *n, pl* **-pies** : the use of selected reading materials as therapeutic adjuvants in medicine and in psychiatry; *also* : guidance in the solution of personal problems through directed reading — **bib·lio·ther·a·peu·tic** \-ther-ə-'pyüt-ik\ *adj*

bib·u·lous \'bib-yə-ləs\ *adj* : highly absorbent ⟨~ paper⟩

bi·cam·er·al \(ˌ)bī-'kam-(ə-)rəl\ *adj* : having two chambers

bi·cap·su·lar \(ˌ)bī-'kap-sə-lər\ *adj* : having two capsules or a 2-celled capsule

bi·carb \'bī-ˌkärb, bī-'\ *n* : SODIUM BICARBONATE

bi·car·bon·ate \(ˌ)bī-'kär-bə-ˌnāt, -nət\ *n* : an acid carbonate

bicarbonate of soda *n* : SODIUM BICARBONATE

bi·cau·dal \(ˌ)bī-'kòd-əl\ *also* **bi·cau·date** \-'kò-ˌdāt\ *adj* : having or terminating in two tails

bi·cel·lu·lar \-'sel-yə-lər\ *adj* : having or composed of two cells

bi·ceps \'bī-ˌseps\ *n, pl* **biceps** *also* **bi·ceps·es** : a muscle having two heads: as **a** : the large flexor muscle of the front of the upper arm **b** : the large flexor muscle of the back of the upper leg

biceps bra·chii \-'brā-kē-ˌē, -ˌī\ *n* : BICEPS a

biceps fe·mo·ris \-'fē-mə-rəs, -'fem-ə-\ *n* : BICEPS b

biceps flex·or cu·bi·ti \-'flek-ˌsòr-'kyü-bə-ˌtī, -bət-ē\ *n* : BICEPS a

bi·chlo·ride \(ˌ)bī-'klō(ə)r-ˌīd, -'klò(ə)r-\ *n* : MERCURIC CHLORIDE

bichloride of mercury *n* : MERCURIC CHLORIDE

bi·chro·mate \(ˌ)bī-'krō-ˌmāt, 'bī-krō-\ *n* : a dichromate esp. of sodium or potassium — **bi·chro·mat·ed** \-ˌmāt-əd\ *adj*

bi·cil·i·ate \(ˌ)bī-'sil-ē-ət, -ē-ˌāt\ *or* **bi·cil·i·at·ed** \-ē-ˌāt-əd\ *adj* : having two cilia

bi·cip·i·tal \(ˌ)bī-'sip-ət-əl\ *adj* **1** *of muscles* : having two heads or origins **2** : of or relating to a biceps muscle

bicipital aponeurosis *n* : an aponeurosis that is given off as a broad medial expansion of the tendon of the biceps brachii at the elbow and that descends medially over the brachial artery to fuse with the deep fascia covering the origins of the flexor muscles of the forearm — called also *lacertus fibrosus*

bicipital groove *n* : a furrow on the upper part of the humerus occupied by the long head of the biceps — called also *intertubercular groove*

bicipital tuberosity *n* : the rough eminence which is on the anterior inner aspect of the neck of the radius and into which the tendon of the biceps is inserted

bi·con·cave \ˌbī-(ˌ)kän-'kāv, (ˌ)bī-'kän-ˌ\ *adj* : concave on both sides ⟨~ vertebrae⟩ ⟨a ~ lens⟩ — **bi·con·cav·i·ty** \ˌbī-(ˌ)kän-'kav-ət-ē\ *n, pl* **-ties**

bi·con·vex \ˌbī-(ˌ)kän-'veks, (ˌ)bī-'kän-ˌ, ˌbī-kən-'\ *adj* : convex on both sides ⟨a ~ lens⟩ — **bi·con·vex·i·ty** \ˌbī-kən-'vek-sət-ē, -(ˌ)kän-\ *n, pl* **-ties**

bi·cor·nu·ate \(ˌ)bī-'kòrn-yə-ˌwāt, -wət\ *or* **bi·cor·nate** \-'kòr-ˌnāt, -nət\ *adj* : having two horns or horn-shaped processes ⟨a ~ uterus⟩

bi·cu·cul·line \bī-'kùk-yə-ˌlēn, -lən\ *n* : a convulsant alkaloid $C_{20}H_{17}NO_6$ obtained from plants (family Fumariaceae) and having the capacity to antagonize the action of gamma-aminobutyric acid in the central nervous system

¹bi·cus·pid \(ˌ)bī-'kəs-pəd\ *adj* : having or ending in two points ⟨~ teeth⟩

²bicuspid *n* : either of the two double-pointed teeth that in humans are situated between the canines and the molars on each side of each jaw : PREMOLAR 1

bicuspid valve *n* : MITRAL VALVE

bi·cy·clic \(ˌ)bī-'sī-klik, -'sik-lik\ *adj* : containing two usu. fused rings in the structure of the molecule

bid *abbr* [Latin *bis in die*] twice a day — used in writing prescriptions

bi·det \bi-'dā\ *n* : a bathroom fixture about the height of the seat of a chair used esp. for bathing the external genitals and the posterior parts of the body

bi·di·rec·tion·al \ˌbī-də-'rek-shnəl, -dī-, -shən-əl\ *adj* : involving, moving, or taking place in two usu. opposite directions ⟨~ flow of materials in axons⟩ ⟨~ replication of DNA⟩ — **bi·di·rec·tion·al·ly** \-ē\ *adv*

Bie·brich scarlet \'bē-ˌbrik-'skär-lət, -ˌbrik-\ *n* : an acid azo dye that is used as a biological stain for cytoplasm

bi·fid \'bī-ˌfid, -fəd\ *adj* : divided into two equal lobes or parts by a median cleft ⟨repair of a ~ digit⟩

bifida — see SPINA BIFIDA, SPINA BIFIDA OCCULTA

bi·fla·gel·late \(ˌ)bī-'flaj-ə-lət, -ˌlāt; ˌbī-flə-'jel-ət\ *adj* : having two flagella

¹bi·fo·cal \(ˌ)bī-'fō-kəl\ *adj* **1** : having two focal lengths **2** : having one part that corrects for near vision and one for distant vision ⟨a ~ eyeglass lens⟩

²bifocal *n* **1** : a bifocal glass or lens **2 bifocals** *pl* : eyeglasses with bifocal lenses

bi·func·tion·al \ˌbī-'fəŋk-shən-əl\ *adj* : having two functions ⟨~ reagents⟩ ⟨~ neurons⟩

bi·fur·cate \'bī-(ˌ)fər-ˌkāt, bī-'fər-\ *vi* **-cat·ed; -cat·ing** : to divide into two branches or parts — **bi·fur·cate** \(ˌ)bī-'fər-kət, -ˌkāt; 'bī-(ˌ)fər-ˌkāt\ *or* **bi·fur·cat·ed** \-ˌkāt-əd\ *adj* — **bi·fur·ca·tion** \ˌbī-(ˌ)fər-'kā-shən\ *n*

bi·gem·i·ny \bī-'jem-ə-nē\ *n, pl* **-nies** : the state of having a pulse characterized by two beats close together with a pause following each pair of beats — **bi·gem·i·nal** \-ən-əl\ *adj*

bi·ge·ner·ic \ˌbī-jə-'ner-ik\ *adj* : of, relating to, or involving two genera ⟨a ~ hybrid⟩

big·head \'big-ˌhed\ *n* : any of several diseases of animals: as **a** : equine osteoporosis **b** : an acute photosensitization of sheep and goats that follows the ingestion of various plants — compare FAGOPYRISM

big toe \ˌbig-\ *n* : the innermost and largest digit of the foot — called also *great toe*

bi·gua·nide \(ˌ)bī-'gwän-ˌīd, -əd\ *n* : any of a group of

\ə\ abut \ᵊ\ kitten \ər\ further \a\ ash \ā\ ace \ä\ cot, cart
\aù\ out \ch\ chin \e\ bet \ē\ easy \g\ go \i\ hit \ī\ ice \j\ job
\ŋ\ sing \ō\ go \ò\ law \òi\ boy \th\ thin \th\ the \ü\ loot
\ù\ foot \y\ yet \zh\ vision *See also* Pronunciation Symbols page

hypoglycemia-inducing drugs (as metformin) used esp. in the treatment of diabetes — see PROGUANIL

bi·ki·ni incision \bə-'kē-nē-\ *n* : PFANNENSTIEL'S INCISION

bi·la·bi·al \(')bī-'lā-bē-əl\ *adj* : of or relating to both lips

bi·lat·er·al \(')bī-'lat-ə-rəl, -'la-trəl\ *adj* **1** : of, relating to, or affecting the right and left sides of the body or the right and left members of paired organs 〈~ nephrectomy〉 〈~ tumors of the adrenal glands〉 **2** : having bilateral symmetry — **bi·lat·er·al·ism** \-,iz-əm\ *n* — **bi·lat·er·al·i·ty** \(')bī-,lat-ə-'ral-ət-ē, -,la-'tral-\ *n, pl* **-ties** — **bi·lat·er·al·ly** \(')bī-'lat-ə-rə-lē, -'la-trə-lē\ *adv*

bilateral symmetry *n* : symmetry in which similar anatomical parts are arranged on opposite sides of a median axis so that one and only one plane can divide the individual into essentially identical halves

bi·lay·er \'bī-,lā-ər, -,le(-ə)r\ *n* : a film or membrane with two molecular layers 〈a ~ of phospholipid molecules〉 — **bilayer** *adj*

bile \'bī(ə)l\ *n* **1** : a yellow or greenish viscid alkaline fluid secreted by the liver and passed into the duodenum where it aids esp. in the emulsification and absorption of fats — called also *fel* **2** : either of two humors associated in old physiology with irascibility and melancholy

bile acid *n* : any of several steroid acids (as cholic acid) that occur in bile usu. in the form of sodium salts conjugated with glycine or taurine

bile duct *n* : a duct by which bile passes from the liver or gallbladder to the duodenum

bile fluke *n* : CHINESE LIVER FLUKE

bile pigment *n* : any of several coloring matters (as bilirubin or biliverdin) in bile

bile salt *n* **1** : a salt of bile acid **2 bile salts** *pl* : a dry mixture of the salts of the gall of the ox used as a liver stimulant and as a laxative — called also *ox bile extract, oxgall*

bile vessel *n* : any of numerous fine channels within the liver that conduct bile

bil·har·zia \bil-'här-zē-ə, -'härt-sē-\ *n* **1** : SCHISTOSOME **2** : SCHISTOSOMIASIS — **bil·har·zi·al** \-zē-əl, -sē-\ *adj*

Bil·harz \'bil-,härts\, **Theodor Maximillian (1825–1862)**, German anatomist and helminthologist. Bilharz became a professor of anatomy in Cairo. While there in 1851 he described the disease schistosomiasis in a letter. In 1852 he discovered that the causative parasite was a hitherto unknown trematode, and he published a description the following year. Heinrich Meckel von Hemsbach created the genus *Bilharzia* in 1856 to contain the trematode discovered by Bilharz. The genus was subsequently suppressed by international agreement, and all three trematodes causing schistosomiasis are now placed in the genus *Schistosoma*. However, the term bilharzia (written without an initial capital letter and without italics) denoting the disease or its causative agent and the term bilharziasis denoting the disease are derived from the genus and continue to honor Bilharz's contributions to tropical parasitology.

Bilharzia *n, syn of* SCHISTOSOMA

bil·har·zi·a·sis \,bil-,här-'zī-ə-səs, -,härt-'sī-\ *n, pl* **-a·ses** \-,sēz\ : SCHISTOSOMIASIS

bili *abbr* bilirubin

bil·i·ary \'bil-ē-,er-ē\ *adj* **1** : of, relating to, or conveying bile 〈~ stasis〉 **2** : affecting the bile-conveying structures 〈~ disorders〉

biliary atresia *n* : absence or underdevelopment of the bile ducts and esp. the extrahepatic bile ducts

biliary calculus *n* : GALLSTONE

biliary cirrhosis *n* : cirrhosis of the liver due to inflammation or obstruction of the bile ducts resulting in the accumulation of bile in and functional impairment of the liver

biliary duct *n* : BILE DUCT

biliary dyskinesia *n* : pain or discomfort in the epigastric region resulting from spasm esp. of the sphincter of Oddi following cholecystectomy

biliary fever *n* : piroplasmosis esp. of dogs and horses

biliary tree *n* : the bile ducts and gallbladder

bili·cy·a·nin \,bil-ə-'sī-ə-nən\ *n* : a blue pigment found in gallstones and formed by oxidation of biliverdin or bilirubin

bil·i·fi·ca·tion \,bil-ə-fə-'kā-shən, ,bī-lə-\ *n* : formation and excretion of bile

bili·fus·cin \,bil-ə-'fəs-ən\ *n* : a brown pigment found in human gallstones and in old bile and formed by oxidation of biliverdin

bil·ious \'bil-yəs\ *adj* **1** : of or relating to bile **2** : marked by or affected with disordered liver function and esp. excessive secretion of bile — **bil·ious·ness** *n*

bil·i·ru·bin \,bil-i-'rü-bən, 'bil-i-,\ *n* : a reddish yellow pigment $C_{33}H_{36}N_4O_6$ that occurs esp. in bile and blood and causes jaundice if accumulated in excess

bil·i·ru·bi·ne·mia *or chiefly Brit* **bil·i·ru·bi·nae·mia** \,bil-i-,rü-bə-'nē-mē-ə\ *n* : HYPERBILIRUBINEMIA

bil·i·ru·bi·nu·ria \-'n(y)ùr-ē-ə\ *n* : excretion of bilirubin in the urine

bil·i·ver·din \,bil-i-'vərd-ᵊn, 'bil-i-,\ *n* : a green pigment $C_{33}H_{34}N_4O_6$ that occurs in bile and is an intermediate in the degradation of hemoglobin heme groups to bilirubin

bill of health \,bil-əv-\ *n* : a duly authenticated certificate of the state of health of a ship's company and of a port with regard to infectious diseases that is given to the ship's master at the time of leaving the port

bi·lo·bate \(')bī-'lō-,bāt\ *adj* : divided into two lobes

bi·lobed \(')bī-'lōbd\ *adj* : divided into two lobes 〈a ~ nucleus〉 〈a ~ organ〉

bi·lob·u·lar \(')bī-'läb-yə-lər\ *adj* : having or divided into two lobules

bi·loc·u·lar \-'läk-yə-lər\ *or* **bi·loc·u·late** \-lət\ *adj* : divided into two cells or compartments

Bil·tri·cide \'bil-trə-,sīd\ *trademark* — used for a preparation of praziquantel

bi·man·u·al \(')bī-'man-yə(-wə)l\ *adj* : done with or requiring the use of both hands 〈a ~ pelvic examination〉 — **bi·man·u·al·ly** \-ē\ *adv*

bi·mas·toid \-'mas-,tòid\ *adj* : of, relating to, or joining the two mastoid processes

bi·mo·lec·u·lar \,bī-mə-'lek-yə-lər\ *adj* **1** : relating to or formed from two molecules **2** : being two molecules thick — **bi·mo·lec·u·lar·ly** *adv*

bi·na·ry \'bī-nə-rē, -,ner-ē\ *adj* **1** : compounded or consisting of or marked by two things or parts **2 a** : composed of two chemical elements, an element and a radical that acts as an element, or two such radicals **b** : utilizing two harmless ingredients that upon combining form a lethal substance (as a gas)

binary fission *n* : reproduction of a cell by division into two approximately equal parts — compare MULTIPLE FISSION

bin·au·ral \(')bī-'nòr-əl, (')bin-'ôr-\ *adj* : of, relating to, or involving two or both ears — **bin·au·ral·ly** \-ə-lē\ *adv*

¹bind \'bīnd\ *vb* **bound** \'baùnd\; **bind·ing** *vt* **1** : to wrap up (an injury) with a cloth : BANDAGE 〈~ing up the gash with clean gauze〉 **2** : to take up and hold usu. by chemical forces : combine with 〈cellulose ~s water〉 **3** : to make costive : CONSTIPATE ~ *vi* **1 a** : to form a cohesive mass **b** : to combine or be taken up esp. by chemical action 〈antibody ~s to a specific antigen〉 **2** : to hamper free movement

²bind *n* **1** : something that binds : the act of binding : the state of being bound — see DOUBLE BIND

bind·er \'bīn-dər\ *n* **1** : a broad bandage applied (as about the chest or abdomen) for support 〈a breast ~〉 〈an obstetrical ~〉 **2** : a substance (as glucose or acacia) used in pharmacy to hold together the ingredients of a compressed tablet

Bi·net age \bē-'nā-, bi-\ *n* : mental age as determined by the Binet-Simon scale

Bi·net \bē-nā\, **Alfred (1857–1911)**, French psychologist, and **Si·mon** \sē-mōⁿ\, **Théodore (1873–1961)**, French physician. Binet was the founder of French experimental psychology. His major contribution to psychology was his introduction of new ways of measuring intelligence. In 1905 Binet and Théodore Simon developed for the French Ministry of Education the first test for measuring intelligence.

A
B

Originally the test was designed for detecting mentally retarded children. The test now honors the names of both men, although the mental age of a person, as determined by the test, is called simply the Binet age. Revised in 1908, the Binet-Simon scale was widely administered and much imitated.

Bi·net–Si·mon scale \bi-ˌnā-sē-ˈmōⁿ-\ n : an intelligence test consisting orig. of tasks graded from the level of the average 3-year-old to that of the average 12-year-old but later extended in range — called also *Binet-Simon test, Binet test;* see STANFORD-BINET TEST

binge \ˈbinj\ vi **binged; binge·ing** or **bing·ing** : to eat compulsively or greedily esp. as a symptom of bulimia ⟨a self-destructive pattern of smoking, starving, and ∼*ing* —Carol Tavris⟩ — **bing·er** \-ər\ n

binge eating n : uncontrolled compulsive eating esp. as a symptom of bulimia or binge eating disorder

binge eating disorder n : an eating disorder characterized by recurring episodes of binge eating accompanied by a sense of lack of control and often negative feelings about oneself but without intervening periods of compensatory behavior (as self-induced vomiting, purging by laxatives, fasting, or prolonged exercise)

bin·io·dide \(ˈ)bī-ˈnī-ə-ˌdīd, (ˈ)bin-ˈī-\ n : DIIODIDE

¹**bin·oc·u·lar** \bī-ˈnäk-yə-lər, bə-\ adj : of, relating to, using, or adapted to the use of both eyes ⟨∼ vision⟩ ⟨a ∼ microscope⟩ — **bin·oc·u·lar·ly** \bī-ˈnäk-yə-lər-lē, bə-\ adv

²**bin·oc·u·lar** \bə-ˈnäk-yə-lər, bī-\ n : a binocular optical instrument

bi·no·mi·al \bī-ˈnō-mē-əl\ n : a biological species name consisting of two terms — **binomial** adj

binomial nomenclature n : a system of nomenclature in which each species of animal or plant receives a name of two terms of which the first identifies the genus to which it belongs and the second the species itself

bin·ovu·lar \(ˈ)bī-ˈnäv-yə-lər, -ˈnōv-\ adj : BIOVULAR

bi·nu·cle·ate \(ˈ)bī-ˈn(y)ü-klē-ət\ also **bi·nu·cle·at·ed** \-klē-ˌāt-əd\ adj : having two nuclei ⟨∼ lymphocytes⟩ ⟨∼ cysts⟩

bi·nu·cle·o·late \(ˈ)bī-ˈn(y)ü-klē-ə-ˌlāt, -lət\ adj : having two nucleoli

bio·ac·cu·mu·la·tion \ˌbī-ō-ə-ˌkyü-myə-ˈlā-shən\ n : the accumulation of a substance (as a pesticide) in a living organism — **bio·ac·cu·mu·late** \-ə-ˈkyü-m(y)ə-ˌlāt\ vb **-lated; -lating** — **bio·ac·cu·mu·la·tive** \-ˌlāt-iv, -lət-\ adj

bio·acous·tic \-ə-ˈküs-tik\ adj : of or relating to the relation between living things and sound

bio·ac·ous·ti·cian \-ˌak-ˌü-ˈstish-ən, -ə-ˌkü-\ n : an expert in bioacoustics

bio·acous·tics \-ə-ˈküs-tiks\ n pl but sing in constr : a branch of science that deals with the relation between living things and sound

bio·ac·tive \-ˈak-tiv\ adj : having an effect on a living organism ⟨∼ molecules⟩ ⟨∼ pharmaceuticals and pesticides⟩ — **bio·ac·tiv·i·ty** \-ak-ˈtiv-ət-ē\ n, pl **-ties**

bio·as·say \-ˈas-ˌā, -a-ˈsā\ n : determination of the relative strength of a substance (as a drug) by comparing its effect on a test organism with that of a standard preparation — **bio·as·say** \-a-ˈsā, -ˈas-ˌā\ vt

bio·as·tro·nau·tics \-ˌas-trə-ˈnot-iks, -ˈnät-\ n pl but sing or pl in constr : the medical and biological aspect of astronautics

bio·au·tog·ra·phy \-ò-ˈtäg-rə-fē\ n, pl **-phies** : the identification or comparison of organic compounds separated by chromatography by means of their effect on living organisms and esp. microorganisms — **bio·au·to·graph** \-ˈòt-ə-ˌgraf\ n — **bio·au·to·graph·ic** \-ˌòt-ə-ˈgraf-ik\ adj

bio·avail·abil·i·ty \-ə-ˌvā-lə-ˈbil-ət-ē\ n, pl **-ties** : the degree and rate at which a substance (as a drug) is absorbed into a living system or is made available at the site of physiological activity — **bio·avail·able** \-ˈvā-lə-bəl\ adj

bio·be·hav·ior·al \-bi-ˈhā-vyə-rəl\ adj : of, relating to, or involving the interaction of behavior and biological processes ⟨a ∼ approach to health⟩

bio·cat·a·lyst \-ˈkat-ᵊl-əst\ n : ENZYME

bio·chem·i·cal \-ˈkem-i-kəl\ adj **1** : of or relating to bio-

chemistry **2** : characterized by, produced by, or involving chemical reactions in living organisms ⟨∼ derangements⟩ — **biochemical** n — **bio·chem·i·cal·ly** \-k(ə-)lē\ adv

biochemical oxygen de·mand \-di-ˌmand\ n : the oxygen used in meeting the metabolic needs of aerobic microorganisms in water rich in organic matter (as water polluted with sewage) — called also *biological oxygen demand, oxygen demand*

bio·chem·ist \-ˈkem-əst\ n : a chemist specializing in biochemistry

bio·chem·is·try \-ˈkem-ə-strē\ n, pl **-tries 1** : chemistry that deals with the chemical compounds and processes occurring in organisms **2** : the chemical characteristics and reactions of a particular living system or biological substance ⟨a change in the patient's ∼ accompanied her psychological depression⟩

bio·chem·or·phol·o·gy \-ˌkem-(ˌ)òr-ˈfäl-ə-jē\ n, pl **-gies** : the study of the relationship between the chemical structure of a compound and its biological action

bio·chip \ˈbī-ō-ˌchip\ n : MICROARRAY

bio·cide \ˈbī-ə-ˌsīd\ n : a substance (as DDT) that is destructive to many different organisms — **bio·cid·al** \ˌbī-ə-ˈsīd-ᵊl\ adj

bio·clean \ˈbī-ō-ˌklēn\ adj : free or almost free of harmful or potentially harmful organisms (as bacteria) ⟨a ∼ room⟩

bio·cli·mat·ic \ˌbī-ō-klī-ˈmat-ik\ adj : of, relating to, or concerned with the relations of climate and living matter

bio·cli·mat·ics \-iks\ n pl but sing or pl in constr : BIOCLIMATOLOGY

bio·cli·ma·tol·o·gy \-ˌklī-mə-ˈtäl-ə-jē\ n, pl **-gies** : a branch of knowledge concerned with the direct and indirect impact of climate or sometimes other geophysical factors on living matter

bio·col·loid \-ˈkäl-ˌòid\ n : a colloid or colloidal mixture of plant or animal origin — **bio·col·loi·dal** \-(ˌ)ō-kə-ˈlòid-ᵊl, -kä-\ adj

bio·com·pat·i·bil·i·ty \-kəm-ˌpat-ə-ˈbil-ət-ē\ n, pl **-ties** : the condition of being compatible with living tissue or a living system by not being toxic or injurious and not causing immunological rejection — **bio·com·pat·i·ble** \-kəm-ˈpat-ə-bəl\ adj

bi·o·cy·tin \-ˈsīt-ᵊn\ n : a colorless crystalline peptide $C_{16}H_{28}N_4O_4S$ occurring naturally (as in yeast) and yielding biotin and lysine on hydrolysis

bio·de·grad·able \-di-ˈgrād-ə-bəl\ adj : capable of being broken down esp. into innocuous products by the action of living things (as microorganisms) — **bio·de·grad·abil·i·ty** \-ˌgrād-ə-ˈbil-ət-ē\ n, pl **-ties** — **bio·deg·ra·da·tion** \-ˌdeg-rə-ˈdā-shən\ n — **bio·de·grade** \-di-ˈgrād\ vb **-grad·ed; -grad·ing**

bio·dy·nam·ics \-dī-ˈnam-iks\ n pl but sing or pl in constr **1** : the dynamic relationships existing between organisms, their physiology, and their environment ⟨the ∼ of human beings in space⟩ **2** : the study of the biodynamics of an organism or group of organisms — **bio·dy·nam·ic** \-ik\ adj

bio·elec·tri·cal \-i-ˈlek-tri-kəl\ or **bio·elec·tric** \-trik\ adj : of or relating to electric phenomena in living organisms ⟨human cortical ∼ activity⟩ — **bio·elec·tric·i·ty** \-ˌlek-ˈtris-ət-ē, -ˈtris-tē\ n, pl **-ties**

bio·elec·tro·gen·e·sis \-i-ˌlek-trə-ˈjen-ə-səs\ n, pl **-e·ses** \-ˌsēz\ : the production of electricity by living organisms

bio·elec·tron·ics \-i-(ˌ)lek-ˈträn-iks\ n pl but sing in constr **1** : a branch of science that deals with electronic control of physiological function esp. as applied in medicine to compensate for defects of the nervous system **2** : a branch of science that deals with the role of electron transfer in biological processes — **bio·elec·tron·ic** \-ik\ adj

bio·en·er·get·ics \-ˌen-ər-ˈjet-iks\ n pl but sing in constr **1**

\ə\ **abut** \ᵊ\ **kitten** \ər\ **further** \a\ **ash** \ā\ **ace** \ä\ **cot, cart**
\aù\ **out** \ch\ **chin** \e\ **bet** \ē\ **easy** \g\ **go** \i\ **hit** \ī\ **ice** \j\ **job**
\ŋ\ **sing** \ō\ **go** \ò\ **law** \òi\ **boy** \th\ **thin** \th̲\ **the** \ü\ **loot**
\ù\ **foot** \y\ **yet** \zh\ **vision** *See also* Pronunciation Symbols page

: the biology of energy transformations and energy exchanges within and between living things and their environments **2** : a system of therapy that combines breathing and body exercises, psychological therapy, and the free expression of impulses and emotions and that is held to increase well=being by releasing blocked physical and psychic energy — **bio·en·er·get·ic** \-ik\ *adj*

¹**bio·en·gi·neer** \-ˌen-jə-'ni(ə)r\ *n* : a person specializing in bioengineering

²**bioengineer** *vt* : to modify or produce by bioengineering ⟨~ed insulin⟩

bio·en·gi·neer·ing \-ˌen-jə-'ni(ə)r-iŋ\ *n* : biological or medical application of engineering principles (as the theory of control systems in models of the nervous system) or engineering equipment (as in the construction of artificial organs); *broadly* : BIOTECHNOLOGY

bio·en·vi·ron·men·tal \-in-ˌvī-rə-'ment-ᵊl, -ˌvī-(ə)r(n)-\ *adj* : of, relating to, affecting, or utilizing living things, their environment, and the interactions between them ⟨~ effects of pollution⟩ ⟨~ pest control⟩

bio·equiv·a·lence \-i-'kwiv-(ə)-lən(t)s\ *n* : the property wherein two drugs with identical active ingredients (as a brand-name drug and its generic equivalent) or two different dosage forms (as tablet and oral suspension) of the same drug possess similar bioavailability and produce the same effect at the site of physiological activity — **bio·equiv·a·lent** \-lənt\ *adj*

bio·equiv·a·len·cy \-lən(t)-sē\ *n, pl* **-cies** : BIOEQUIVALENCE

bio·eth·i·cist \-'eth-ə-səst\ *n* : an expert in bioethics

bio·eth·ics \-'eth-iks\ *n pl but usu sing in constr* : the discipline dealing with the ethical implications of biological research and applications esp. in medicine — **bio·eth·ic** \-'eth-ik\ *n* — **bio·eth·i·cal** \-'eth-i-kəl\ *adj*

bio·feed·back \-'fēd-ˌbak\ *n* : the technique of making unconscious or involuntary bodily processes (as heartbeat or brain waves) perceptible to the senses (as by the use of an oscilloscope) in order to manipulate them by conscious mental control

bio·film \'bī-ō-ˌfilm\ *n* : a thin usu. resistant layer of microorganisms (as bacteria) that form on and coat various surfaces (as of catheters or water pipes)

bio·fla·vo·noid \ˌbī-ō-'flā-və-ˌnȯid\ *n* : any of various biologically active flavonoids (as hesperidin and quercetin) derived from plants and found esp. in fruits and vegetables (as grapes, citrus fruits, and peppers)

bio·gen·e·sis \-'jen-ə-səs\ *n, pl* **-e·ses** \-ˌsēz\ **1** : the development of life from preexisting life — compare ABIOGENESIS **2** : a supposed tendency for stages in the evolutionary history of a race to briefly recur during the development and differentiation of an individual of that race **3** : the synthesis of chemical compounds or structures in the living organism — compare BIOSYNTHESIS — **bio·ge·net·ic** \-jə-'net-ik\ *adj*

biogenetic law *n* : a theory of development much disputed in biology: an organism passes through successive stages resembling the series of ancestral types from which it has descended so that the ontogeny of the individual is a recapitulation of the phylogeny of the group

bio·gen·ic \-'jen-ik\ *adj* : produced by living organisms ⟨~ amine metabolism in depressed patients —D. L. Murphy⟩

bio·geo·chem·is·try \-ˌjē-ō-'kem-ə-strē\ *n, pl* **-tries** : a science that deals with the relation of earth chemicals to plant and animal life in an area — **bio·geo·chem·i·cal** \-'kem-i-kəl\ *adj*

bio·ge·og·ra·pher \-jē-'äg-rə-fər\ *n* : a specialist in biogeography

bio·ge·og·ra·phy \-jē-'äg-rə-fē\ *n, pl* **-phies** : a branch of biology that deals with the geographical distribution of animals and plants — **bio·geo·graph·ic** \-ˌjē-ə-'graf-ik\ *or* **bio·geo·graph·i·cal** \-i-kəl\ *adj*

bio·haz·ard \'bī-ō-ˌhaz-ərd, -'haz-\ *n* : a biological agent or condition (as an infectious organism or insecure laboratory procedures) that constitutes a hazard to humans or the environment; *also* : a hazard posed by such an agent or condition — **bio·haz·ard·ous** \-'haz-ərd-əs\ *adj*

bio·in·for·mat·ics \ˌbī-ō-ˌin-fər-'ma-tiks\ *n pl but sing in constr* : the collection, classification, storage, and analysis of biochemical and biological information using computers esp. as applied in molecular genetics and genomics — **bio·in·for·mat·ic** \-tik\ *adj*

bio·in·or·gan·ic \-ˌin-ȯr-'gan-ik\ *adj* : of, relating to, or concerned with the application of inorganic chemistry and its techniques (as nuclear magnetic resonance) to the study of biological processes and substances (as metalloproteins) in which inorganic substances are important constituents or play important roles

bio·in·stru·men·ta·tion \'bī-ō-ˌin-strə-mən-'tā-shən, -ˌmen-\ *n* : the development and use of instruments for recording and transmitting physiological data (as from astronauts in flight); *also* : the instruments themselves

biol *abbr* biologic; biological; biologist; biology

bi·o·log·ic \ˌbī-ə-'läj-ik\ *or* **bi·o·log·i·cal** \-i-kəl\ *n* : a biological product (as a globulin, serum, vaccine, antitoxin, or antigen) used in the prevention or treatment of disease

biological *also* **biologic** *adj* **1** : of or relating to biology or to life and living processes **2** : used in or produced by applied biology **3** : related by direct genetic relationship rather than by adoption or marriage ⟨an adoptee who searched for years for her ~ parents⟩ — **bi·o·log·i·cal·ly** \-i-k(ə-)lē\ *adv*

biological clock *n* : an inherent timing mechanism in a living system (as a cell) that is inferred to exist in order to explain various cyclical behaviors and physiological processes

biological control *n* : reduction in numbers or elimination of pest organisms by interference with their ecology (as by the introduction of parasites or diseases)

biological half–life *or* **biologic half–life** *n* : the time that a living body requires to eliminate one half the quantity of an administered substance (as a radioisotope) through its normal channels of elimination

biological oxygen de·mand \-di-ˌmand\ *n* : BIOCHEMICAL OXYGEN DEMAND

biological war·fare \-'wȯr-ˌfa(ə)r, -ˌfe(ə)r\ *n* : warfare involving the use of biological weapons; *also* : warfare involving the use of herbicides

biological weap·on \-'wep-ən\ *n* : a harmful biological agent (as a pathogenic microorganism or a neurotoxin) used as a weapon to cause death or disease usu. on a large scale

biologic false–positive *n* : a positive serological reaction for syphilis given by blood of a person who does not have syphilis

bi·ol·o·gist \bī-'äl-ə-jəst\ *n* : a specialist in biology

bi·ol·o·gy \-jē\ *n, pl* **-gies** **1** : a branch of science that deals with living organisms and vital processes **2 a** : the plant and animal life of a region or environment **b** : the laws and phenomena relating to an organism or group **3** : a treatise on biology

bio·lu·mi·nes·cence \ˌbī-ō-ˌlü-mə-'nes-ᵊn(t)s\ *n* : the emission of light from living organisms; *also* : the light so produced — **bio·lu·mi·nes·cent** \-ᵊnt\ *adj*

bi·ol·y·sis \bī-'äl-ə-səs\ *n, pl* **-y·ses** \-ˌsēz\ : decomposition by living organisms of sewage and other complex materials — **bi·o·lyt·ic** \ˌbī-ə-'lit-ik\ *adj*

bio·mark·er \'bī-ō-ˌmär-kər\ *n* : a distinctive biological or biologically derived indicator (as a biochemical metabolite in the body) of a process, event, or condition (as aging, disease, or exposure to a toxic substance) ⟨age-related ~s of disease and degenerative change —Janet Raloff⟩

bio·mass \-ˌmas\ *n* : the amount of living matter (as in a unit area or volume of habitat)

bio·ma·te·ri·al \ˌbī-ō-mə-'tir-ē-əl\ *n* : a natural or synthetic material (as a polymer or metal) that is suitable for introduction into living tissue esp. as part of a medical device (as an artificial heart valve or joint)

bio·math·e·ma·ti·cian \-ˌmath-(ə-)mə-'tish-ən\ *n* : a specialist in biomathematics

bio·math·e·mat·ics \-ˌmath-ə-'mat-iks\ *n pl but usu sing in constr* : the principles of mathematics that are of special use in biology and medicine — **bio·math·e·mat·i·cal** \-i-kəl\ *adj*

bio·me·chan·ics \-mi-'kan-iks\ *n pl but sing or pl in constr*

: the mechanical bases of biological, esp. muscular, activity; *also* : the study of the principles and relations involved — **bio·me·chan·i·cal** \-i-kəl\ *adj*

bio·med·i·cal \-'med-i-kəl\ *adj* **1** : of or relating to biomedicine **2** : of, relating to, or involving biological, medical, and physical science — **bio·med·i·cal·ly** \-k(ə-)lē\ *adv*

biomedical engineering *n* : BIOENGINEERING — **biomedical engineer** *n*

bio·med·i·cine \-'med-ə-sən, *Brit usu* -'med-sən\ *n* : medicine based on the application of the principles of the natural sciences and esp. biology and biochemistry; *also* : a branch of medical science concerned esp. with the capacity of human beings to survive and function in abnormally stressful environments and with the protective modification of such environments

bio·mem·brane \-'mem-ˌbrān\ *n* : a membrane either on the surface or interior of a cell that is composed of protein and lipid esp. in sheets only a few molecules thick and that limits the diffusion and transport of materials

bi·om·e·ter \bī-'äm-ət-ər\ *n* : a device for measuring carbon dioxide given off by living matter

bio·me·tri·cian \ˌbī-ō-me-'trish-ən\ *n* : a specialist in biometry

bio·met·rics \-'me-triks\ *n pl but sing or pl in constr* : BIOMETRY

bi·om·e·try \bī-'äm-ə-trē\ *n, pl* **-tries** : the statistical analysis of biological observations and phenomena — **bio·met·ric** \ˌbī-ō-'me-trik\ *or* **bio·met·ri·cal** \-tri-kəl\ *adj*

bio·mi·cro·scope \ˌbī-ō-'mī-krə-ˌskōp\ *n* : a low-power binocular microscope placed horizontally and used with a slit lamp for detailed examination of the anterior part of the eye

bio·mi·cros·co·py \-mī-'kräs-kə-pē\ *n, pl* **-pies** : the microscopic examination and study of living cells and tissues; *specif* : examination of the living eye with the biomicroscope

bio·mol·e·cule \-'mäl-i-ˌkyü(ə)l\ *n* : an organic molecule and esp. a macromolecule (as a protein or nucleic acid) in living organisms — **bio·mo·lec·u·lar** \-mə-'lek-yə-lər\ *adj*

bi·on·ic \bī-'än-ik\ *adj* **1** : of or relating to bionics **2 a** : having normal biological capability or performance enhanced by or as if by electronic or electromechanical devices **b** : comprising or made up of artificial body parts that enhance or substitute for a natural biological capability ⟨a ~ heart⟩

bi·on·ics \bī-'än-iks\ *n pl but sing or pl in constr* : a science concerned with the application of data about the functioning of biological systems to the solution of engineering problems

bi·o·nom·ics \ˌbī-ə-'näm-iks\ *n pl but sing or pl in constr* : ECOLOGY 1, 2 — **bi·o·nom·ic** \-ik\ *or* **bi·o·nom·i·cal** \-i-kəl\ *adj* — **bi·o·nom·i·cal·ly** \-i-k(ə-)lē\ *adv*

bio·or·gan·ic \ˌbī-ō-ȯr-'gan-ik\ *adj* : of, relating to, or concerned with the organic chemistry of biologically significant substances ⟨a ~ chemist⟩

¹bio·phar·ma·ceu·ti·cal \ˌbī-ō-ˌfär-mə-'süt-i-kəl\ *adj* : of or relating to biopharmaceutics or biopharmaceuticals

²biopharmaceutical *n* : a pharmaceutical produced by biotechnology and esp. by genetic engineering

bio·phar·ma·ceu·tics \-iks\ *n pl but sing in constr* : the study of the relationships between the physical and chemical properties, dosage, and form of administration of a drug and its activity in the living body

bi·o·phore \'bī-ə-ˌfō(ə)r, -ˌfȯ(ə)r\ *n* : the ultimate supramolecular vital unit in August Weismann's theory of life processes that is conceived as the basic building block of living structures — see DETERMINANT 1a

bio·pho·tom·e·ter \ˌbī-ō-fō-'täm-ət-ər\ *n* : an instrument for measuring the rate and efficiency of dark adaptation of the eye used esp. in detecting vitamin A deficiency

bio·phys·i·cist \-'fiz-(ə-)səst\ *n* : a specialist in biophysics

bio·phys·ics \-'fiz-iks\ *n* : a branch of science concerned with the application of physical principles and methods to biological problems — **bio·phys·i·cal** \-i-kəl\ *adj*

bio·phys·i·og·ra·phy \-ˌfiz-ē-'äg-rə-fē\ *n, pl* **-phies** : descriptive zoology and botany

bio·plast \'bī-ō-ˌplast\ *n* **1** : ALTMANN'S GRANULES **2** : a functional unit of living protoplasm : CELL

bio·poly·mer \ˌbī-ō-'päl-ə-mər\ *n* : a polymeric substance (as a protein or polysaccharide) formed in a biological system

bio·pros·the·sis \-präs-'thē-səs, -'präs-thə-\ *n, pl* **-the·ses** \-ˌsēz\ : a prosthesis (as a porcine heart valve) consisting of an animal part or containing animal tissue — **bio·pros·thet·ic** \-präs-'thet-ik\ *adj*

¹bi·op·sy \'bī-ˌäp-sē\ *n, pl* **-sies** : the removal and examination of tissue, cells, or fluids from the living body

²biopsy *vt* **-sied; -sy·ing** : to perform a biopsy on ⟨the intestinal polyps were removed and *biopsied*⟩

bio·psy·chol·o·gy \ˌbī-ō-sī-'käl-ə-jē\ *n, pl* **-gies** : psychology as related to biology or as a part of the vital processes — **bio·psy·chol·o·gist** \-sī-'käl-ə-jəst\ *n*

bio·psy·cho·so·cial \-ˌsī-kō-'sō-shəl\ *adj* : of, relating to, or concerned with the biological, psychological, and social aspects in contrast to the strictly biomedical aspects of disease

bi·or·bit·al \(')bī-'ȯr-bət-ᵊl\ *adj* : of or relating to the two orbits; *specif* : relating to a measure taken between the outer borders of the bony orbits on the skull or between the outer corners of the eyes on the living body

bio·re·ac·tor \ˌbī-ō-rē-'ak-tər\ *n* : a device or apparatus in which living organisms and esp. bacteria synthesize useful substances (as interferon) or break down harmful ones (as in sewage)

bio·re·search \-ri-'sərch, -'rē-ˌ\ *n* : research in biology

bio·rhythm \'bī-ō-ˌrith-əm\ *n* : an innately determined rhythmic biological process or function (as sleep behavior); *also* : an innate rhythmic determiner of such a process or function — **bio·rhyth·mic** \ˌbī-ō-'rith-mik\ *adj* — **bio·rhyth·mic·i·ty** \-rith-'mis-ət-ē\ *n, pl* **-ties**

bi·os \'bī-ˌäs\ *n* : a mixture of vitamins of the B complex essential for the optimum growth of some yeasts

bio·safe·ty \'bī-ō-ˌsāf-tē\ *n, pl* **-ties** : safety with respect to the effects of biological research on humans and the environment

bio·sat·el·lite \ˌbī-ō-'sat-ᵊl-ˌīt\ *n* : an artificial satellite for carrying a living human being, animal, or plant

bio·sci·ence \'bī-ō-ˌsī-ən(t)s\ *n* : BIOLOGY; *also* : LIFE SCIENCE — **bio·sci·en·tif·ic** \ˌbī-ō-ˌsī-ən-'tif-ik\ *adj* — **bio·sci·en·tist** \'bī-ō-ˌsī-ənt-əst\ *n*

bi·ose \'bī-ˌōs\ *n* : DISACCHARIDE

bio·sen·sor \'bī-ō-ˌsen-ˌsȯ(ə)r, -ˌsen(t)-sər\ *n* : a device that is sensitive to a physical or chemical stimulus (as heat or an ion) and transmits information about a life process

bio·sphere \'bī-ə-ˌsfi(ə)r\ *n* **1** : the part of the world in which life can exist **2** : living beings together with their environment

bio·stat·is·ti·cian \ˌbī-ō-ˌstat-ə-'stish-ən\ *n* : an expert in biostatistics

bio·sta·tis·tics \-stə-'tis-tiks\ *n pl but sing in constr* : statistical processes and methods applied to the analysis of biological phenomena

bio·syn·the·sis \-'sin(t)-thə-səs\ *n, pl* **-the·ses** \-ˌsēz\ : production of a chemical compound by a living organism — **bio·syn·thet·ic** \-sin-'thet-ik\ *adj* — **bio·syn·thet·i·cal·ly** \-i-k(ə-)lē\ *adv*

bio·syn·the·size *also Brit* **bio·syn·the·sise** \-'sin(t)-thə-ˌsīz\ *vt* **-sized** *also Brit* **-sised; -siz·ing** *also Brit* **-sis·ing** : to produce by biosynthesis

bio·tech \'bī-ō-ˌtek\ *n* : BIOTECHNOLOGY 1

bio·tech·ni·cal \ˌbī-ō-'tek-ni-kəl\ *adj* : of or relating to biotechnology

bio·tech·nol·o·gy \-tek-'näl-ə-jē\ *n, pl* **-gies** **1** : applied biological science (as bioengineering or recombinant DNA technology) **2** : ERGONOMICS — **bio·tech·no·log·i·cal** \-ˌtek-nə-'läj-i-kəl\ *adj* — **bio·tech·no·log·i·cal·ly** \-k(ə-)lē\ *adv* — **bio·tech·nol·o·gist** \-tek-'näl-ə-jəst\ *n*

\ə\ abut \ᵊ\ kitten \ər\ further \a\ ash \ā\ ace \ä\ cot, cart \aú\ out \ch\ chin \e\ bet \ē\ easy \g\ go \i\ hit \ī\ ice \j\ job \ŋ\ sing \ō\ go \ȯ\ law \ȯi\ boy \th\ thin \t̲h̲\ the \ü\ loot \ú\ foot \y\ yet \zh\ vision *See also* Pronunciation Symbols page

bio·te·lem·e·try \-tə-'lem-ə-trē\ *n, pl* **-tries** : remote detection and measurement of a human or animal condition, activity, or function (as heartbeat or body temperature) — **bio·tel·e·met·ric** \-ˌtel-ə-'me-trik\ *adj*

bio·ter·ror \-'ter-ər\ *n, often attrib* : BIOTERRORISM ⟨a ∼ attack⟩

bio·ter·ror·ism \-'ter-ər-ˌiz-əm\ *n* : terrorism involving the use of biological weapons — **bio·ter·ror·ist** \-ər-əst\ *adj or n*

bi·ot·ic \bī-'ät-ik\ *adj* : of or relating to life; *esp* : caused or produced by living beings

bi·o·tin \'bī-ət-ən\ *n* : a colorless crystalline growth vitamin $C_{10}H_{16}N_2O_3S$ of the vitamin B complex found esp. in yeast, liver, and egg yolk — called also *vitamin H*

bio·tox·in \'bī-ō-ˌtäk-sən\ *n* : a toxic substance of biological origin

bio·trans·for·ma·tion \'bī-ō-ˌtran(t)s-fər-'mā-shən, -ˌfor-\ *n* : the transformation of chemical compounds in a living system

bio·type \-ˌtīp\ *n* : the organisms sharing a specified genotype; *also* : the genotype shared or its distinguishing peculiarity

bi·ovu·lar \(')bī-'äv-yə-lər, -'ōv-\ *adj, of fraternal twins* : derived from two ova

bio·war·fare \ˌbī-ō-'wor-ˌfar\ *n* : BIOLOGICAL WARFARE

bio·weap·on \'bī-ō-ˌwep-ən\ *n* : BIOLOGICAL WEAPON

bi·pa·ren·tal \ˌbī-pə-'rent-əl\ *adj* : of, relating to, involving, or derived from two parents ⟨∼ reproduction⟩ — **bi·pa·ren·tal·ly** \-əl-ē\ *adv*

bi·pa·ri·etal \ˌbī-pə-'rī-ət-əl\ *adj* : of or relating to the parietal bones; *specif* : being a measurement between the most distant opposite points of the two parietal bones

bip·a·rous \'bip-ə-rəs\ *adj* : bringing forth two young at a birth

bi·par·tite \(')bī-'pär-ˌtīt\ *adj* : divided into two parts

bi·ped \'bī-ˌped\ *n* : a two-footed animal — **biped** *or* **bi·ped·al** \(')bī-'ped-əl\ *adj*

bi·pen·nate \(')bī-'pen-ˌāt\ *adj* : BIPENNIFORM

bi·pen·ni·form \-'pen-i-ˌfo(ə)rm\ *adj* : resembling a feather barbed on both sides — used of muscles

bi·per·i·den \bī-'per-ə-dən\ *n* : a white crystalline muscle relaxant $C_{21}H_{29}NO$ used esp. to reduce the symptoms (as tremors, akinesia, and muscle rigidity) associated with Parkinson's disease

bi·phas·ic \(')bī-'fā-zik\ *adj* : having two phases ⟨a ∼ life cycle⟩ ⟨a ∼ immune response⟩ ⟨a ∼ stimulatory effect⟩

bi·phe·nyl \(')bī-'fen-əl, -'fēn-\ *n* : a white crystalline hydrocarbon $C_6H_5C_6H_5$ — called also *diphenyl*

bi·po·lar \(')bī-'pō-lər\ *adj* **1** : having or involving the use of two poles ⟨∼ encephalograph leads⟩ **2** *of a neuron* : having an efferent and an afferent process **3** : being, characteristic of, or affected with a bipolar disorder ⟨∼ depression⟩ ⟨∼ affectively ill patients⟩ — compare UNIPOLAR 2

bipolar disorder *n* : any of several mood disorders characterized usu. by alternating episodes of depression and mania or by episodes of depression alternating with mild nonpsychotic excitement — called also *bipolar affective disorder, bipolar illness, manic depression, manic-depressive psychosis;* compare MAJOR DEPRESSIVE DISORDER

bi·po·ten·ti·al·i·ty \ˌbī-pə-ˌten-chē-'al-ət-ē\ *n, pl* **-ties** : capacity to function as or develop into male or female

bi·ra·mous \(')bī-'rā-məs\ *adj* : having two branches

birch oil \'bərch-\ *n* : an essential oil that consists chiefly of methyl salicylate and is obtained from the bark and twigs of the sweet birch (*Betula lenta*) — called also *betula oil, sweet-birch oil;* compare OIL OF WINTERGREEN

bird flu \'bərd-\ *n* : AVIAN INFLUENZA

bird louse *n* : BITING LOUSE

bi·re·frac·tive \ˌbī-ri-'frak-tiv\ *adj* : having or characterized by birefringence : BIREFRINGENT

bi·re·frin·gence \ˌbī-ri-'frin-jən(t)s\ *n* : the refraction of light in an anisotropic material in two slightly different directions to form two rays — **bi·re·frin·gent** \-jənt\ *adj*

bi·ro·ta·tion \ˌbī-rō-'tā-shən\ *n* : MUTAROTATION

¹birth \'bərth\ *n* **1** : the emergence of a new individual from the body of its parent **2** : the act or process of bringing forth young from the womb

²birth *vt* : to give birth to ⟨allowed to ∼ her child in her own way —Nancy Robinson⟩ ∼ *vi* : to bring forth or be brought forth as a child or young ⟨contend that ∼*ing* is a natural process, rather than a medical procedure —Kit Miniclier⟩ ⟨the baby ∼*ed* breech —Jayne Anne Phillips⟩

³birth *adj* : BIOLOGICAL 3 ⟨spent years searching for his ∼ parents⟩

birth canal *n* : the channel formed by the cervix, vagina, and vulva through which the fetus passes during birth

birth cer·tif·i·cate \-(ˌ)sər-'tif-i-kət\ *n* : a copy of an official record of a person's date and place of birth and parentage

birth control *n* **1** : control of the number of children born esp. by preventing or lessening the frequency of conception : CONTRACEPTION **2** : contraceptive devices or preparations

birth control pill *n* : any of various preparations that usu. contain a combination of a progestogen (as norethindrone) and an estrogen (as ethinyl estradiol) but sometimes only a progestogen, are taken orally esp. on a daily basis, and act as contraceptives typically preventing ovulation by suppressing secretion of gonadotropins (as luteinizing hormone) — called also *oral contraceptive, oral contraceptive pill*

birth defect *n* : a physical or biochemical defect (as cleft palate, phenylketonuria, or Down syndrome) that is present at birth and may be inherited or environmentally induced

birth·ing center \ˌbər-thiŋ-\ *n* : a facility usu. staffed by nurse-midwives that provides a less institutionalized setting than a hospital for women who wish to deliver by natural childbirth

birthing room *n* : a comfortably furnished hospital room where both labor and delivery take place and in which the baby usu. remains during the hospital stay

birth·mark \'bərth-ˌmärk\ *n* : an unusual mark or blemish on the skin at birth : NEVUS — **birthmark** *vt*

birth pang *n* : one of the regularly recurrent pains that are characteristic of childbirth — usu. used in pl.

birth·rate \'bər-ˌthrāt\ *n* : the ratio between births and individuals in a specified population and time often expressed as number of live births per hundred or per thousand population per year — called also *natality*

birth·root \'bər-ˌthrüt, -ˌthrut\ *n* : any of several trilliums with astringent roots used in folk medicine

birth trauma *n* : the physical injury or emotional shock sustained by an infant in the process of birth

bis·a·co·dyl \ˌbis-ə-'kō-(ˌ)dil\ *n* : a white crystalline laxative $C_{22}H_{19}NO_4$ administered orally or as a suppository

bis·cuit \'bis-kət\ *n* : porcelain after the first firing and before glazing

¹bi·sex·u·al \(')bī-'seksh-(ə-)wəl, -'sek-shəl\ *adj* **1 a** : possessing characters of both sexes : HERMAPHRODITIC **b** : of, relating to, or characterized by a tendency to direct sexual desire toward individuals of both sexes **2** : of, relating to, or involving two sexes — **bi·sex·u·al·i·ty** \ˌbī-ˌsek-shə-'wal-ət-ē\ *n, pl* **-ties** — **bi·sex·u·al·ly** \(')bī-'seksh-(ə-)wə-lē, -(ə-)lē\ *adv*

²bisexual *n* : a bisexual individual

bis·hy·droxy·cou·ma·rin \ˌbis-(ˌ)hī-ˌdräk-sē-'kü-mə-rən\ *n* : DICUMAROL

Bis·marck brown \'biz-ˌmärk-\ *n* : a brown basic diazo dye that is used as a biological stain

Bis·marck–Schön·hau·sen \'bis-ˌmärk-shœn-'hau-zən\, **Otto Edward Leopold von (1815–1898)**, German chancellor. The dye Bismarck brown was named in his honor.

bis·muth \'biz-məth\ *n* : a heavy brittle grayish white chiefly trivalent metallic element that is chemically like arsenic and antimony and that is used in alloys and pharmaceuticals — symbol *Bi;* see ELEMENT table — **bis·mu·thic** \biz-'məth-ik, -'myü-thik\ *adj*

bismuth sub·car·bon·ate \-ˌsəb-'kär-bə-ˌnāt, -nət\ *n* : a white or pale yellowish white powder that is a basic salt of varying composition obtained by reaction of a carbonate with a bismuth salt and used chiefly in treating gastrointestinal disorders, topically as a protective in lotions and ointments, and in cosmetics

bismuth subnitrate *n* : a white bismuth-containing powder $Bi_5O(OH)_9(NO_3)_4$ used in medicine similarly to bismuth subcarbonate

bismuth sub·sa·lic·y·late \-ˌsəb-sə-ˈlis-ə-ˌlāt\ *n* : an antidiarrheal drug $C_7H_5BiO_4$ also used to relieve heartburn, indigestion, and nausea — see PEPTO-BISMOL

bis·phos·pho·nate \(ˌ)bī-ˈfäs-fə-ˌnāt\ *n* : any of a group of carbon-substituted analogs (as etidronate) of pyrophosphate that are potent inhibitors of osteoclast-mediated bone resorption

bis·tou·ry \ˈbis-tə-rē\ *n, pl* **-ries** : a small slender straight or curved surgical knife with a sharp or blunt point

bi·sul·fate *or chiefly Brit* **bi·sul·phate** \(ˈ)bī-ˈsəl-ˌfāt\ *n* : an acid sulfate

bi·sul·fide *or chiefly Brit* **bi·sul·phide** \-ˌfīd\ *n* : DISULFIDE

bi·sul·fite *or chiefly Brit* **bi·sul·phite** \-ˌfīt\ *n* : an acid sulfite

bi·tar·trate \(ˈ)bī-ˈtär-ˌtrāt\ *n* : an acid tartrate

bitch \ˈbich\ *n* : the female of the dog or some other carnivorous mammals

¹**bite** \ˈbīt\ *vb* **bit** \ˈbit\; **bit·ten** \ˈbit-ᵊn\ *also* **bit**; **bit·ing** \ˈbīt-iŋ\ *vt* **1** : to seize esp. with teeth or jaws so as to enter, grip, or wound **2** : to wound, pierce, or sting esp. with a fang or a proboscis ∼ *vi* : to bite or have the habit of biting something

²**bite** *n* **1** : the act or manner of biting; *esp* : OCCLUSION 2a **2** : a wound made by biting

bite block *n* : a device used chiefly in dentistry for recording the spatial relation of the jaws esp. in respect to the occlusion of the teeth

bi·tem·po·ral \(ˈ)bī-ˈtem-p(ə-)rəl\ *adj* : relating to, involving, or joining the two temporal bones or the areas that they occupy

bite plane *n* : a removable dental appliance used to cover the occlusal surfaces of the teeth so that they cannot be brought into contact

bite plate *n* : a removable usu. plastic dental appliance used in orthodontics and prosthodontics to assist in therapy or diagnosis: as **a** : a U-shaped device worn in the upper or lower jaw and used esp. to reposition the jaw or prevent bruxism by covering the occlusal surfaces of the teeth so that they cannot be brought into contact **b** : RETAINER 2

bite·wing \ˈbīt-ˌwin\ *n* : dental X-ray film designed to show the crowns of the upper and lower teeth simultaneously

biting fly *n* : a dipteran fly (as a mosquito, midge, or horsefly) having mouthparts adapted for piercing and biting

biting louse *n* : any of numerous wingless insects of the order Mallophaga that are mostly parasitic on birds but sometimes on mammals, have mouths adapted to biting instead of sucking, and feed on feathers, hair, or skin of the host often causing injury — called also *bird louse*

biting midge *n* : any of a large family (Ceratopogonidae) of tiny long-legged dipteran flies that have piercing mouthparts, attack birds and various mammals including humans, and include various vectors of filarial worms

Bi·tot's spots \bē-ˈtōz-\ *n* : shiny pearly spots of triangular shape occurring on the conjunctiva in severe vitamin A deficiency esp. in children

    Bi·tot \bē-tō\, **Pierre A. (1822–1888)**, French physician. Bitot's description of the spots now known as Bitot's spots was first published in 1863.

bi·tro·chan·ter·ic \ˌbī-ˌtrō-kən-ˈter-ik\ *adj* : of, relating to, or between the two trochanters or trochanter points

bit·ter \ˈbit-ər\ *adj* : being or inducing the one of the four basic taste sensations that is peculiarly acrid, astringent, or disagreeable and suggestive of an infusion of hops — compare SALT 2, SOUR, SWEET — **bit·ter·ness** *n*

bitter almond *n* : an almond with a bitter taste that contains amygdalin; *also* : a tree (*Prunus dulcis amara*) of the rose family (Rosaceae) producing bitter almonds

bitter almond oil *n* **1** : ALMOND OIL 1b, 2 **2** : BENZALDEHYDE

bitter orange oil *n* : ORANGE OIL b

bitter principle *n* : any of various neutral substances of strong bitter taste (as aloin) extracted from plants

bit·ters \ˈbit-ərz\ *n pl* : a usu. alcoholic solution of bitter and often aromatic plant products used esp. in preparing mixed drinks or as a mild tonic

bitter salts *n pl* : EPSOM SALTS

bit·ter·sweet \ˈbit-ər-ˌswēt, ˌbit-ər-ˈ\ *n* : a sprawling poisonous weedy nightshade (*Solanum dulcamara*) with purple flowers and oval reddish orange berries that is the source of dulcamara

bi·uret \ˈbī-yə-ˈret, ˈbī-yə-ˌ\ *n* : a white crystalline compound $N_3H_5C_2O_2$ formed by heating urea

biuret reaction *n* : a reaction that is shown by biuret, proteins, and most peptides on treatment in alkaline solution with copper sulfate and that results in a violet color

biuret test *n* : a test esp. for proteins using the biuret reaction

bi·va·lence \(ˈ)bī-ˈvā-lən(t)s\ *n* : BIVALENCY

bi·va·len·cy \(ˈ)bī-ˈvā-lən-sē\ *n, pl* **-cies** : the quality or state of being bivalent

¹**bi·va·lent** \(ˈ)bī-ˈvā-lənt\ *adj* **1 a** : DIVALENT **b** : having two combining sites ⟨a ∼ antibody capable of binding to two molecules of an antigen⟩ **2** : associated in pairs in synapsis **3** : conferring immunity to two diseases or two serotypes ⟨a ∼ vaccine protecting against hepatitis A and hepatitis B⟩

²**bivalent** *n* : a pair of synaptic chromosomes

¹**bi·valve** \ˈbī-ˌvalv\ *also* **bi·valved** \-ˌvalvd\ *adj* : having or consisting of two corresponding movable pieces suggesting the shells of mollusks ⟨a ∼ speculum⟩ ⟨a ∼ cast⟩

²**bivalve** *vt* **bi·valved; bi·valv·ing** : to split (a cast) along one or two sides (as to relieve pressure)

bi·ven·ter \(ˈ)bī-ˈvent-ər\ *n* : a muscle with two bellies

bi·ven·tral \-ˈven-trəl\ *adj* : having two bellies : DIGASTRIC

bix·in \ˈbik-sən\ *n* : a red-brown carotenoid acid ester $C_{25}H_{30}O_4$ constituting the chief coloring matter of annatto and used similarly

¹**bi·zy·go·mat·ic** \ˌbī-ˌzī-gə-ˈmat-ik\ *adj* : of or relating to the two cheekbones; *specif* : relating to a measure of facial width taken between the most lateral points on the external surfaces of the zygomatic arches

²**bizygomatic** *n* : the bizygomatic width of the face

BJ *abbr* biceps jerk

Bk *symbol* berkelium

BK *abbr* below knee

black–and–blue \ˌblak-ən-ˈblü\ *adj* : darkly discolored from blood effused by bruising

black bile *n* : the one of the four humors of ancient and medieval physiology that was believed to be secreted by the kidneys and spleen and to cause melancholy

black cohosh *n* : a perennial herb of the genus *Cimicifuga* (*C. racemosa*) whose rhizome and roots are the source of cimicifuga — called also *black snakeroot, bugbane*

black cohosh root *n* : CIMICIFUGA 2

black damp *n* : a nonexplosive mine gas that is a mixture containing carbon dioxide and is incapable of supporting life or flame — compare FIREDAMP

black death *n, often cap B&D* **1** : PLAGUE 2 **2** : a severe epidemic of plague and esp. bubonic plague that occurred in Asia and Europe in the 14th century

black disease *n* : a fatal toxemia of sheep associated with simultaneous infection by liver flukes (*Fasciola hepatica*) and an anaerobic toxin-producing clostridium (*Clostridium novyi*) and characterized by liver necrosis and subcutaneous hemorrhage — compare BLACKLEG, BRAXY, LIVER ROT, MALIGNANT EDEMA

black eye *n* : a discoloration of the skin around the eye from bruising

black·fly \ˈblak-ˌflī\ *n, pl* **-flies** : any of a family (Simuliidae) and esp. genus *Simulium* of bloodsucking dipteran flies

---

\ə\ **abut** \ᵊ\ **kitten** \ər\ **further** \a\ **ash** \ā\ **ace** \ä\ **cot, cart**
\aů\ **out** \ch\ **chin** \e\ **bet** \ē\ **easy** \g\ **go** \i\ **hit** \ī\ **ice** \j\ **job**
\ŋ\ **sing** \ō\ **go** \ȯ\ **law** \ȯi\ **boy** \th\ **thin** \t͟h\ **the** \ü\ **loot**
\ů\ **foot** \y\ **yet** \zh\ **vision** *See also* Pronunciation Symbols page

black hairy tongue *n* : BLACKTONGUE 1

black·head \'blak-,hed\ *n* 1 : a small plug of sebum blocking the duct of a sebaceous gland esp. on the face — compare MILIUM 2 : a destructive disease of turkeys and related birds caused by a protozoan of the genus *Histomonas* (*H. meleagridis*) that invades the intestinal ceca and liver — called also *enterohepatitis, histomoniasis, infectious enterohepatitis*

black hellebore *n* 1 : a European hellebore of the genus *Helleborus* (*H. niger*) having white or purplish roselike flowers produced in winter and a highly purgative root — called also *Christmas rose* 2 : the root of black hellebore

black henbane *n* : HENBANE

black·leg \'blak-,leg, -,lāg\ *n* : an enzootic usu. fatal toxemia esp. of young cattle caused by toxins produced by an anaerobic soil bacterium of the genus *Clostridium* (*C. chauvoei* syn. *C. feseri*) — called also *black quarter, quarter evil, quarter ill, symptomatic anthrax;* compare BLACK DISEASE, MALIGNANT EDEMA

black–legged tick \'blak-'legd-, -'lāgd-; -'leg-əd-, -'lā-gəd-\ *n* : either of two ixodid ticks: **a** : DEER TICK **b** : a tick (*Ixodes pacificus*) of the western U.S. and British Columbia that is the vector of several diseases (as Lyme disease)

black lung *n* : pneumoconiosis caused by habitual inhalation of coal dust — called also *black lung disease;* compare SILICOSIS

black mustard *n* 1 : a yellow-flowered annual Eurasian herb (*Brassica nigra*) that is a source of table mustard 2 : the dried ripe seed of black mustard or a relative (*Brassica juncea*) that was formerly much used in medicine as a rubefacient and emetic

black–necked cobra \,blak-,nekt-\ *n* : a venomous and aggressive African elapid snake (*Naja nigricollis*) that rarely bites but discharges by spitting a venom that is harmless to the intact skin but may cause blindness if it enters the eyes — called also *spitting cobra*

black·out \'blak-,aut\ *n* : a transient dulling or loss of vision, consciousness, or memory ⟨an alcoholic ∼⟩ — compare GRAYOUT, REDOUT

black out \(')blak-'aut\ *vi* : to undergo a temporary loss of vision, consciousness, or memory (as from temporary impairment of cerebral circulation, retinal anoxia, a traumatic emotional blow, or an alcoholic binge) — compare GRAY OUT, RED OUT ∼ *vt* : to cause to black out

black pepper *n* : a condiment that consists of the fruit of an East Indian plant of the genus *Piper* (*P. nigrum*) ground with the black husk still on

black quarter *n* : BLACKLEG

black rat *n* : a rat of the genus *Rattus* (*R. rattus*) that infests houses and has been the chief vector of bubonic plague

black snake·root \-'snā-,krüt, -,krüt\ *n* : BLACK COHOSH

black spot *n* : a spotting of frozen meat caused by an imperfect fungus of the genus *Cladosporium* (*C. herbarum*)

black·tongue \'blak-,təŋ\ *n* 1 : a dark furry or hairy discoloration of the tongue 2 : a disease of dogs that is caused by a deficient diet and that is identical with pellagra in humans

black vomit *n* 1 : vomit consisting of dark-colored matter 2 : a condition characterized by black vomit; *esp* : YELLOW FEVER

black·wa·ter \'blak-,wòt-ər, -,wät-\ *n* : any of several diseases (as blackwater fever or Texas fever) characterized by dark-colored urine

blackwater fever *n* : a rare febrile complication of repeated malarial attacks that is marked by destruction of blood cells with hemoglobinuria and extensive kidney damage

black wid·ow \-'wid-,ō\ *n* : a venomous New World spider of the genus *Latrodectus* (*L. mactans*) the female of which is black with an hourglass-shaped red mark on the underside of the abdomen

blad·der \'blad-ər\ *n* 1 : a membranous sac in animals that serves as the receptacle of a liquid or contains gas; *esp* : URINARY BLADDER 2 : a vesicle or pouch forming part of an animal body ⟨the ∼ of a tapeworm larva⟩

bladder worm *n* : CYSTICERCUS

blade \'blād\ *n* 1 : a broad flat body part (as the shoulder blade) 2 : the flat portion of the tongue immediately behind the tip; *also* : this portion together with the tip 3 : a flat working and esp. cutting part of an implement (as a scalpel)

blain \'blān\ *n* : an inflammatory swelling or sore

Bla·lock–Taus·sig operation \'blā-,läk-'tau-sig-\ *n* : surgical correction of the tetralogy of Fallot — called also *blue= baby operation*

> **Blalock, Alfred (1899–1964),** and **Taussig, Helen B. (1898–1986),** American physicians. Blalock and Taussig were on the staff of Johns Hopkins Hospital. Based upon Taussig's theory that the cause of cyanosis in infants was a functional lack of oxygen, Blalock (a surgeon) developed an operation in which the pulmonary artery and a healthy systemic artery were spliced to bypass any constriction or blockage, thereby giving the lungs sufficient blood for oxygenation. The Blalock-Taussig operation was first performed in 1944; it marked the beginning of modern heart surgery.

¹blast \'blast\ *n* 1 : an explosion or violent detonation 2 : the violent effect produced in the vicinity of an explosion that consists of a wave of increased atmospheric pressure followed by a wave of decreased atmospheric pressure — **blast** *vb*

²blast *n* : BLAST CELL

blast cell *n* : an immature cell; *esp* : a usu. large blood cell precursor that is in the earliest stage of development in which it is recognizably committed to development along a particular cell lineage

blast crisis *n* : the terminal stage of chronic myelogenous leukemia that is characterized by a marked increase in the proportion of blast cells, by fever and pain in the bones, and by increased severity of anemia, thrombocytopenia, and splenomegaly — called also *blastic crisis*

blas·te·ma \bla-'stē-mə\ *n, pl* **-mas** *also* **-ma·ta** \-mət-ə\ : a mass of living substance capable of growth and differentiation — **blas·te·mat·ic** \,blas-tə-'mat-ik\ *or* **blas·te·mic** \bla-'stē-mik, -'stem-ik\ *adj*

blas·tic crisis \'blas-tik-\ *n* : BLAST CRISIS

blas·to·coel *or* **blas·to·coele** \'blas-tə-,sēl\ *n* : the cavity of a blastula — called also *segmentation cavity* — **blas·to·coe·lic** \,blas-tə-'sē-lik\ *adj*

blas·to·cyst \'blas-tə-,sist\ *n* : the modified blastula of a placental mammal

blas·to·cyte \-,sīt\ *n* : an undifferentiated embryonic cell

blas·to·derm \-,dərm\ *n* : a blastodisc after completion of cleavage and formation of the blastocoel — called also *discoblastula*

blas·to·derm·ic vesicle \,blas-tə-,dər-mik-\ *n* : BLASTOCYST

blas·to·disc *or* **blas·to·disk** \'blas-tə-,disk\ *n* : the embryo= forming portion of an egg with discoidal cleavage usu. appearing as a small disc on the upper surface of the yolk mass

blas·to·gen·e·sis \,blas-tə-'jen-ə-səs\ *n, pl* **-e·ses** \-,sēz\ : the transformation of lymphocytes into larger cells capable of undergoing mitosis — **blas·to·gen·ic** \-'jen-ik\ *adj*

blas·to·mere \'blas-tə-,mi(ə)r\ *n* : a cell produced during cleavage of a fertilized egg — called also *cleavage cell* — **blas·to·mer·ic** \,blas-tə-'mi(ə)r-ik, -'mer-\ *adj*

Blas·to·my·ces \,blas-tə-'mī-,sēz\ *n* : a genus of yeastlike fungi that contains the causative agent (*B. dermatitidis*) of North American blastomycosis and that formerly included the causative agent (*Paracoccidioides brasiliensis* syn. *B. brasiliensis*) of South American blastomycosis

Blas·to·my·ce·tes \-mī-'sēt-,ēz\ *n pl, in some classifications* : a class of pathogenic imperfect fungi that typically grow like yeasts by budding but sometimes form a mycelium and conidia on artificial media — **blas·to·my·cete** \-'mī-,sēt, -mī-'sēt\ *n*

blas·to·my·ce·tic \-,mī-'sēt-ik\ *adj* 1 *also* **blas·to·my·ce·tous** \-'sēt-əs\ : of or relating to the class Blastomycetes ⟨∼ fungi⟩ 2 : of, relating to, or caused by blastomycetes ⟨∼ dermatitis⟩

blas·to·my·cin \-'mīs-ᵊn\ *n* : a preparation of growth products of the causative agent (*Blastomyces dermatitidis*) of North American blastomycosis that is used esp. to test for this disease

blas·to·my·co·sis \-ˌmī-'kō-səs\ *n, pl* **-co·ses** \-ˌsēz\ : either of two infectious diseases caused by yeastlike fungi — see BLASTOMYCES, NORTH AMERICAN BLASTOMYCOSIS, SOUTH AMERICAN BLASTOMYCOSIS — **blas·to·my·cot·ic** \-'kät-ik\ *adj*

blas·to·neu·ro·pore \ˌblas-tō-'n(y)u̇r-ō-ˌpō(ə)r, -ˌpȯ(ə)r\ *n* : a temporary opening formed by the union of the blastopore and neuropore in some embryos

blas·toph·tho·ria \ˌblas-təf-'thȯr-ē-ə, -'thȯr-\ *n* : degeneration of the germ cells believed to be due to chronic poisoning (as by alcohol) or to disease — **blas·toph·tho·ric** \-'thȯr-ik, -'thȯr-\ *adj*

blas·to·pore \'blas-tə-ˌpō(ə)r, -ˌpȯ(ə)r\ *n* : the opening of the archenteron — **blas·to·por·al** \ˌblas-tə-'pōr-əl, -'pȯr-\ *or* **blas·to·por·ic** \-'pōr-ik, -'pȯr-\ *adj*

blas·to·sphere \'blas-təs-ˌfi(ə)r\ *n* : BLASTULA; *esp* : BLASTOCYST — **blas·to·spher·ic** \ˌblas-təs-'fi(ə)r-ik, -'fer-\ *adj*

blas·to·spore \'blas-tə-ˌspō(ə)r, -ˌspȯ(ə)r\ *n* : a fungal spore that is produced by budding and that acts as a resting spore or (as in yeasts) gives rise to another spore or a hypha

blas·tot·o·my \blas-'tät-ə-mē\ *n, pl* **-mies** : separation of cleavage cells during early stages of embryonic development

blas·tu·la \'blas-chə-lə\ *n, pl* **-las** *or* **-lae** \-ˌlē\ : an early metazoan embryo typically having the form of a hollow fluid-filled rounded cavity bounded by a single layer of cells — compare GASTRULA, MORULA — **blas·tu·lar** \-lər\ *adj* — **blas·tu·la·tion** \ˌblas-chə-'lā-shən\ *n*

Blat·ta \'blat-ə\ *n* : a genus (family Blattidae) of cockroaches that includes the oriental cockroach

Blat·tel·la \blə-'tel-ə\ *n* : a genus of cockroaches that includes the German cockroach

Blaud's pill \'blōdz-, 'blȯ(d)z-\ *n* : a pill consisting essentially of ferrous carbonate used in the treatment of anemia

Blaud \blō\, **Pierre (1774–1858),** French physician. In 1832 Blaud published an article on chlorosis in which he introduced the pill that now bears his name.

blaze \'blāz\ *n* : a white or gray streak in the hair of the head

bld *abbr* blood

bleach·ing powder \ˌblē-chiŋ-\ *n* : a white powder consisting chiefly of calcium hydroxide, calcium chloride, and calcium hypochlorite used as a bleach, disinfectant, or deodorant — called also *chloride of lime, chlorinated lime*

¹blear \'bli(ə)r\ *vt* : to make (the eyes) sore or watery

²blear *adj* : dim with water or tears — **blear–eyed** \-'īd\ *adj*

bleary \'bli(ə)r-ē\ *adj, of the eyes or vision* : dull or dimmed esp. from fatigue or sleep

bleb \'bleb\ *n* **1** : a small blister — compare BULLA 2 **2** : something resembling a bleb; *esp* : a vesicular outpocketing of a plasma or nuclear membrane — **bleb·by** \'bleb-ē\ *adj*

¹bleed \'blēd\ *vb* **bled** \'bled\; **bleed·ing** *vi* **1** : to emit or lose blood ⟨hemophiliacs often ∼ severely from the slightest scratch⟩ **2** : to escape by oozing or flowing (as from a wound) ∼ *vt* : to remove or draw blood from

²bleed *n* : the escape of blood from vessels : HEMORRHAGE ⟨a massive gastrointestinal ∼⟩

bleed·er \'blēd-ər\ *n* **1** : one that draws blood; *esp* : a person who draws blood for medical reasons : BLOODLETTER **2** : HEMOPHILIAC **3** : a large blood vessel (as one cut during surgery) that is losing blood **4** : a horse that has experienced exercise-induced pulmonary hemorrhage

bleed·ing \-iŋ\ *n* : an act, instance, or result of being bled or the process by which something is bled: as **a** : the escape of blood from vessels : HEMORRHAGE **b** : the operation of bleeding a person medically : PHLEBOTOMY

bleeding time *n* : a period of time of usu. about two and a half minutes during which a small wound (as a pinprick) continues to bleed

blem·ish \'blem-ish\ *n* : a mark of physical deformity or injury: as **a** : any small mark on the skin (as a pimple or birthmark) ⟨∼es symptomatic of acne⟩ **b** : a defect of an animal (as a horse) that detracts from its appearance but does not interfere with its usefulness

blend·ing inheritance \'blend-iŋ-\ *n* : the expression in offspring of phenotypic characters (as pink flower color from red and white parental plants) intermediate between those of the parents; *also* : inheritance in a now discarded theory in which the genetic material of offspring was held to be a uniform blend of that of the parents — compare MENDELIAN INHERITANCE, QUANTITATIVE INHERITANCE

blen·noid \'blen-ˌȯid\ *adj* : resembling mucus : MUCOID

blen·nor·rha·gia \ˌblen-ə-'rā-j(ē-)ə\ *n* **1** : BLENNORRHEA **2** : GONORRHEA

blennorrhagica — see KERATOSIS BLENNORRHAGICA

blennorrhagicum — see KERATODERMA BLENNORRHAGICUM

blen·nor·rhea *or chiefly Brit* **blen·nor·rhoea** \ˌblen-ə-'rē-ə\ *n* : an excessive secretion and discharge of mucus — **blen·nor·rhe·al** *or chiefly Brit* **blen·nor·rhoe·al** \-'rē-əl\ *adj*

bleo·my·cin \ˌblē-ə-'mīs-ᵊn\ *n* : a mixture of glycoprotein antibiotics derived from a streptomyces (*Streptomyces verticillus*) and used in the form of the sulfates as an antineoplastic agent

bleph·a·ral \'blef-ə-rəl\ *adj* : of or relating to the eyelids

bleph·a·rism \-ˌriz-əm\ *n* : spasm of the eyelids

bleph·a·ri·tis \ˌblef-ə-'rīt-əs\ *n, pl* **-rit·i·des** \-'rit-ə-ˌdēz\ : inflammation of the eyelids and esp. of their margins

bleph·a·ro·con·junc·ti·vi·tis \ˌblef-ə-(ˌ)rō-kən-ˌjəŋ(k)-tə-'vīt-əs\ *n* : inflammation of the eyelid and conjunctiva

bleph·a·ro·plast \'blef-ə-rō-ˌplast\ *n* : a basal body esp. of a flagellated cell

bleph·a·ro·plas·ty \-ˌplas-tē\ *n, pl* **-ties** : plastic surgery on an eyelid esp. to remove fatty or excess tissue

bleph·a·rop·to·sis \ˌblef-ə-rəp-'tō-səs\ *n, pl* **-to·ses** \-ˌsēz\ : a drooping or abnormal relaxation of the upper eyelid

bleph·a·ro·spasm \'blef-ə-rō-ˌspaz-əm, -rə-\ *n* : spasmodic winking from involuntary contraction of the orbicularis oculi muscle of the eyelids

bleph·a·ro·stat \-ˌstat\ *n* : an instrument for holding the eyelids apart (as during an operation)

bleph·a·rot·o·my \ˌblef-ə-'rät-ə-mē\ *n, pl* **-mies** : surgical incision of an eyelid

blew *past of* BLOW

blight \'blīt\ *n, Austral* : an inflammation of the eye in which the eyelids discharge a thick mucous substance that often seals them up for days and minute granular pustules develop inside the lid — called also *sandy blight*

¹blind \'blīnd\ *adj* **1 a** : lacking or deficient in sight; *esp* : having less than ¹/₁₀ of normal vision in the more efficient eye when refractive defects are fully corrected by lenses **b** : of or relating to sightless persons ⟨∼ care⟩ **2 a** : made or done without sight of certain objects or knowledge of certain facts that could serve for guidance or cause bias ⟨a ∼ taste test⟩ ⟨a ∼ clinical trial⟩ — see DOUBLE-BLIND, SINGLE-BLIND **b** : having no knowledge of information that may cause bias during the course of an experiment or test ⟨researchers ∼ to whether the investigational drug is administered⟩ **3** : having but one opening or outlet ⟨the cecum is a ∼ pouch⟩ — **blind·ly** \'blīn-(d)lē\ *adv* — **blind·ness** \'blīn(d)-nəs\ *n*

²blind *vt* : to make blind

blind gut *n* : a digestive cavity open at only one end; *esp* : the cecum of the large intestine

blind side *n* : the side on which one who is blind in one eye cannot see

blind spot *n* : the small circular area in the retina where the optic nerve enters the eye that is devoid of rods and cones and is insensitive to light — called also *optic disk*

\ə\ **abut** \ᵊ\ **kitten** \ər\ **further** \a\ **ash** \ā\ **ace** \ä\ **cot, cart**
\au̇\ **out** \ch\ **chin** \e\ **bet** \ē\ **easy** \g\ **go** \i\ **hit** \ī\ **ice** \j\ **job**
\ŋ\ **sing** \ō\ **go** \ȯ\ **law** \ȯi\ **boy** \th\ **thin** \th̲\ **the** \ü\ **loot**
\u̇\ **foot** \y\ **yet** \zh\ **vision** *See also* Pronunciation Symbols page

blind stag·gers \-'stag-ərz\ *n pl but sing or pl in constr* : a severe form of selenosis characterized esp. by impairment of vision, an unsteady gait, and a tendency of the affected animal to stand with the forehead pressing against an immovable obstacle; *also* : a similar condition not caused by selenium poisoning

¹blink \'bliŋk\ *vi* : to close and open the eyes involuntarily (as when struggling against drowsiness or when dazzled) ~ *vt* **1** : to close and open (the eye) involuntarily **2** : to remove (as tears) from the eye by blinking

²blink *n* : a usu. involuntary shutting and opening of the eye

¹blis·ter \'blis-tər\ *n* **1** : a fluid-filled elevation of the epidermis — compare WATER BLISTER **2** : an agent that causes blistering — **blis·tery** \-t(ə-)rē\ *adj*

²blister *vb* **blis·tered; blis·ter·ing** \-t(ə-)riŋ\ *vi* : to become affected with blisters ~ *vt* : to raise a blister on

blister beetle *n* : any of various beetles (as the Spanish fly) that are used medicinally dried and powdered to raise blisters on the skin; *broadly* : any of numerous soft-bodied beetles (family Meloidae)

blister gas *n* : VESICANT

¹bloat \'blōt\ *vt* : to make turgid: **a** : to produce edema in **b** : to cause or result in accumulation of gas in the digestive tract of ⟨cucumbers sometimes ~ me⟩ **c** : to cause abdominal distension in ~ *vi* : to become turgid

²bloat *n* **1** : a digestive disturbance of ruminant animals and esp. cattle marked by accumulation of gas in one or more stomach compartments **2** : a condition of large dogs marked by distension and usu. life-threatening rotation of the stomach

¹block \'bläk\ *n, often attrib* **1** : interruption of normal physiological function of a tissue or organ ⟨respiratory ~ due to carbon monoxide⟩; *esp* : HEART BLOCK **2 a** : BLOCK ANESTHESIA **b** : NERVE BLOCK 1 **3** : interruption of a train of thought by competing thoughts or psychological suppression

²block *vt* **1** : to prevent normal functioning of (a bodily element) ⟨~ a nerve with novocaine⟩ **2** : to obstruct the effect of ⟨a carboxyl group ~ed by esterification⟩ ~ *vi* : to experience or exhibit psychological blocking or blockage — **block·er** \-ər\ *n*

¹block·ade \blä-'kād\ *n* **1 a** : interruption of normal physiological function (as transmission of nerve impulses) of a cellular receptor, tissue, or organ **b** : inhibition of a physiologically active substance (as a hormone) **2** : the process of reducing the phagocytic capabilities of the reticuloendothelial system by loading it with harmless material (as India ink or lampblack) which engages its cells in phagocytosis and prevents them from reacting to new antigenic material — compare BLOCKING ANTIBODY

²blockade *vt* **block·ad·ed; block·ad·ing** : to subject to blockade

block·age \'bläk-ij\ *n* : the action of blocking or the state of being blocked: as **a** : BLOCKADE 2 **b** : internal resistance to understanding a communicated idea, to learning new material, or to adopting a new mode of response because of existing habitual ways of thinking, perceiving, and acting — compare BLOCKING

block anesthesia *n* : local anesthesia (as by injection) produced by interruption of the flow of impulses along a nerve trunk — compare REGIONAL ANESTHESIA

block·er \'bläk-ər\ *n* : one that blocks — see ALPHA‐BLOCKER, BETA-BLOCKER, CALCIUM CHANNEL BLOCKER

block·ing \'bläk-iŋ\ *n* : interruption of a trend of associative thought by the arousal of an opposing trend or through the welling up into consciousness of a complex of unpleasant ideas — compare BLOCKAGE b

blocking antibody *n* : an antibody that combines with an antigen without visible reaction but prevents another antibody from later combining with or producing its usual effect on that antigen — called also *incomplete antibody*

blood \'bləd\ *n, often attrib* **1** : the fluid that circulates in the heart, arteries, capillaries, and veins of a vertebrate animal carrying nourishment and oxygen to and bringing away waste products from all parts of the body **2** : a fluid of an invertebrate comparable to blood **3** : blood regarded in medieval physiology as one of the four humors and believed to be the seat of the emotions **4** : descent from parents of recognized breed or pedigree

blood bank *n* : a place for storage of or an institution storing blood or plasma; *also* : blood so stored — **blood bank·er** \-ˌbaŋ-kər\ *n*

blood bank·ing \-ˌbaŋ-kiŋ\ *n* : the activity of administering or working in a blood bank

blood–borne \-ˌbȯrn\ *adj* : carried or transmitted by the blood ⟨a ~ disease⟩ ⟨~ pathogens⟩

blood–brain barrier *n* : a naturally occurring barrier created by the modification of brain capillaries (as by reduction in fenestration and formation of tight cell-to-cell contacts) that prevents many substances from leaving the blood and crossing the capillary walls into the brain tissues — abbr. *BBB*

blood cell *n* : a cell or platelet normally present in blood — see RED BLOOD CELL, WHITE BLOOD CELL

blood clot *n* : CLOT

blood count *n* : the determination of the blood cells in a definite volume of blood; *also* : the number of cells so determined — see COMPLETE BLOOD COUNT, DIFFERENTIAL BLOOD COUNT

blood doping *n* : a technique for temporarily improving athletic performance in which oxygen-carrying red blood cells previously withdrawn from an athlete are injected back just before an event — called also *blood packing*

blood dust *n* : HEMOCONIA

blood fluke *n* : SCHISTOSOME

blood gas *n* : dissolved carbon dioxide and oxygen in blood typically expressed in terms of partial pressure; *also* : a test of usu. arterial blood to measure the partial pressures and concentrations of carbon dioxide and oxygen along with the pH and bicarbonate level

blood group *n* : one of the classes (as A, B, AB, or O) into which individual vertebrates and esp. human beings or their blood can be separated on the basis of the presence or absence of specific antigens in the blood — called also *blood type*

blood group·ing \-ˈgrüp-iŋ\ *n* : BLOOD TYPING

blood heat *n* : a temperature approximating that of the human body

blood island *n* : any of the reddish areas in the extraembryonic mesoblast of developing vertebrate eggs where blood cells and vessels are forming — called also *blood islet*

blood·less \'bləd-ləs\ *adj* : free from or lacking blood ⟨a ~ surgical field⟩ — **blood·less·ly** *adv*

blood·let·ter \'bləd-ˌlet-ər\ *n* : a practitioner of phlebotomy

blood·let·ting \-ˌlet-iŋ\ *n* : PHLEBOTOMY

blood·mo·bile \-mō-ˌbēl\ *n* : a motor vehicle staffed and equipped for collecting blood from donors

blood packing *n* : BLOOD DOPING

blood plasma *n* : the pale yellow fluid portion of whole blood that consists of water and its dissolved constituents including proteins (as albumin, fibrinogen, and globulins), electrolytes (as sodium and chloride), sugars (as glucose), lipids (as cholesterol and triglycerides), metabolic waste products (as urea), amino acids, hormones, and vitamins — compare SERUM a(1)

blood platelet *n* : PLATELET

blood poisoning *n* : SEPTICEMIA

blood pressure *n* : pressure exerted by the blood upon the walls of the blood vessels and esp. arteries, usu. measured on the radial artery by means of a sphygmomanometer, and expressed in millimeters of mercury either as a fraction having as numerator the maximum pressure that follows systole of the left ventricle of the heart and as denominator the minimum pressure that accompanies cardiac diastole or as a whole number representing the first value only ⟨a *blood pressure* of ¹²⁰⁄₈₀⟩ ⟨a *blood pressure* of 120⟩ — abbr. *BP*

blood·root \-ˌrüt, -ˌrút\ *n* : an herb (*Sanguinaria canadensis*) of the poppy family that has red sap and has a rootstock and roots used as an emetic and expectorant

blood serum *n* : SERUM a(1)

blood·shot \'bləd-ˌshät\ *adj, of an eye* : inflamed to redness

blood·stain \-ˌstān\ *n* : a discoloration caused by blood

blood·stained \-ˌstānd\ *adj* : stained with blood

blood·stream \-ˌstrēm\ *n* : the flowing blood in a circulatory system

blood·suck·er \-ˌsək-ər\ *n* : an animal that sucks blood; *esp* : LEECH — **blood·suck·ing** \-iŋ\ *adj*

blood sugar *n* : the glucose in the blood; *also* : its concentration (as in milligrams per 100 milliliters)

blood test *n* : a test of the blood (as a serological test for syphilis)

blood thin·ner \-ˌthin-ər\ *n* : a drug used to prevent the formation of blood clots by hindering coagulation of the blood

blood type *n* : BLOOD GROUP

blood typing *n* : the action or process of determining an individual's blood group — called also *blood grouping*

blood vessel *n* : any of the vessels through which blood circulates in the body

blood·worm \'bləd-ˌwərm\ *n* : any of several comparatively large bloodsucking nematode worms of the genus *Strongylus* that are parasitic in the large intestine of horses and have larvae which wander in the viscera and sometimes lodge in the intestinal blood vessels causing colic or more rarely a fatal aneurysm — called also *palisade worm, red worm*

bloody \'bləd-ē\ *adj* **blood·i·er; -est** **1 a** : containing or made up of blood **b** : of or contained in the blood **2 a** : smeared or stained with blood **b** : dripping blood : BLEEDING ⟨a ∼ nose⟩ — **blood·i·ly** \'bləd-ᵊl-ē\ *adv* — **blood·i·ness** \'bləd-ē-nəs\ *n*

bloody flux *n* **1** : diarrhea in which blood is mixed with the intestinal discharge **2** : SWINE DYSENTERY

blot \'blät\ *n* : a nitrocellulose sheet that contains spots of immobilized macromolecules (as of DNA, RNA, or protein) or their fragments and that is used to identify specific components of the spots by applying a suitable molecular probe (as a complementary nucleic acid or a radiolabeled antibody) — see NORTHERN BLOT, SOUTHERN BLOT, WESTERN BLOT — **blot** *vt*

blotch \'bläch\ *n* : a discolored patch on the skin ⟨the face and neck were covered with large reddish ∼es⟩ — **blotch** *vt* — **blotchy** \-ē\ *adj*

¹blow \'blō\ *vt* **blew** \'blü\; **blown** \'blōn\; **blow·ing** **1** : to free (the nose) of mucus and debris by forcible exhalation **2** *of blowflies and flesh flies* : to deposit eggs or larvae on or in

²blow *n* **1** : the act of some insects of depositing eggs or larvae; *also* : a larva so deposited (as in a wound) — used chiefly of blowflies and flesh flies **2** : forcible ejection of air from the body (as in freeing the nose of mucus and debris)

blow·fish \-ˌfish\ *n* : PUFFER

blow·fly \-ˌflī\ *n, pl* **-flies** : any dipteran fly (as a bluebottle or a screwworm) of the family Calliphoridae

blow·pipe \'blō-ˌpīp\ *n* : a tubular instrument used in anatomy and zoology for revealing or cleaning a bodily cavity by forcing air into it

BLS *abbr* basic life support

blub·ber finger \'bləb-ər-\ *n* : SEAL FINGER

¹blue \'blü\ *adj* **blu·er; blu·est** : of the color blue

²blue *n* **1** : a color whose hue is that of the clear sky or that of the portion of the color spectrum lying between green and violet **2** : a pigment or dye that colors blue — see PRUSSIAN BLUE

blue asbestos *n* : CROCIDOLITE

blue baby *n* : an infant with a bluish tint usu. from a congenital heart defect marked by mingling of venous and arterial blood

blue–baby operation *n* : BLALOCK-TAUSSIG OPERATION

blue bag *n* : gangrenous mastitis of sheep

blue·bot·tle \'blü-ˌbät-ᵊl\ *n* : any of several blowflies (genus *Calliphora*) that have an iridescent blue body or abdomen and make a loud buzzing noise in flight

blue cohosh *n* : a tall herb (*Caulophyllum thalictroides* of the

family Berberidaceae) of eastern No. America and Asia having large blue berrylike fruits and a thick knotty rootstock that was formerly used as an antispasmodic and emmenagogue

blue comb \-ˈkōm\ *n* : an acute infectious disease of domestic turkeys that is caused by a coronavirus (genus *Coronavirus*) and is characterized by lack of appetite, weight loss, and wet droppings — called also *blue comb disease, mud fever*

blue flag \-ˈflag\ *n* **1** : either of two common blue-flowered irises (*Iris versicolor* and *I. virginica*) of the eastern and central U.S. with rhizomes formerly used medicinally as a cathartic and emetic **2** : the dried rhizome of a blue flag — called also *blue flag root*

blue–green alga \'blü-ˈgrēn-\ *n* : CYANOBACTERIUM

blue heav·en \-ˈhev-ən\ *n, slang* : amobarbital or its sodium derivative in a blue tablet or capsule

blue mold *n* : any of various fungi of the genus *Penicillium* that produce blue or blue-green surface growths

blue nevus *n* : a small blue or bluish black spot on the skin that is sharply circumscribed, rounded, and flat or slightly raised and is usu. benign but often mistaken for a melanoma

blue–ringed octopus \-ˈriŋd-ˈäk-tə-pəs, -ˌpüs\ *n* : a venomous octopus (*Hapalochlaena maculosa* syn. *Octopus maculosa*) of the Indo-Pacific region that is esp. common along the southern coast of Australia, is capable of inflicting a fatal bite due to the injection of tetrodotoxin, and undergoes skin color changes when aroused displaying brilliant blue rings

blues \'blüz\ *n pl but sing or pl in constr* : low spirits : MELANCHOLY — **blue** \'blü\ *adj*

blue spot *n* : MONGOLIAN SPOT

blue–tongue \'blü-ˌtəŋ\ *n* : a noncontagious virus disease esp. of sheep that is caused by a reovirus of the genus *Orbivirus* (species *Bluetongue virus*) transmitted by biting flies of the genus *Culicoides* and that is characterized by hyperemia and cyanosis and by swelling and sloughing of the mucous membranes esp. about the mouth and tongue — called also *soremuzzle*

blunt dissection \'blənt-\ *n* : surgical separation of tissue layers by means of an instrument without a cutting edge or by the fingers

blunt trauma *n* : a usu. serious injury caused by a blunt object or collision with a blunt surface (as in a vehicle accident or fall from a building) ⟨the patient died of *blunt trauma* to the head⟩ — called also *blunt force trauma*

blush \'bləsh\ *vi* : to become red in the face esp. from shame, modesty, or confusion — **blush** *n*

B lym·pho·cyte \'bē-ˈlim(p)-fə-ˌsīt\ *n* : B CELL

BM *abbr* **1** Bachelor of Medicine **2** basal metabolism **3** bowel movement

BMD *abbr* bone mineral density

BMI *abbr* body mass index

BMR *abbr* basal metabolic rate

BMT *abbr* bone marrow transplant; bone marrow transplantation

BNA *abbr* Basle Nomina Anatomica

BO *abbr* body odor

board \'bō(ə)rd, 'bò(ə)rd\ *n* **1** : a group of persons having supervisory, managerial, investigatory, or advisory powers ⟨medical licensing ∼s⟩ ⟨a ∼ of health⟩ **2** : an examination given by an examining board — often used in pl. ⟨passed his medical ∼s⟩

board–certified *adj* : being a physician who has graduated from medical school, completed residency, trained under supervision in a specialty, and passed a qualifying exam given by a medical specialty board — abbr. *BC*

board–el·i·gi·ble \-ˈel-ə-jə-bəl\ *adj* : being a physician who has graduated from medical school, completed residency,

---

\ə\ abut \ᵊ\ kitten \ər\ further \a\ ash \ā\ ace \ä\ cot, cart
\aů\ out \ch\ chin \e\ bet \ē\ easy \g\ go \i\ hit \ī\ ice \j\ job
\ŋ\ sing \ō\ go \ò\ law \òi\ boy \th\ thin \t̲h̲\ the \ü\ loot
\ů\ foot \y\ yet \zh\ vision *See also* Pronunciation Symbols page

trained under supervision in a specialty, and is eligible to take a qualifying exam given by a medical specialty board — abbr. *BE*

BOD *abbr* biochemical oxygen demand; biological oxygen demand

Bo·dan·sky unit \bə-'dan(t)-skē-, -'dän(t)-\ *n* : a unit based on the activity of phosphatase toward sodium beta-glycerophosphate that is used as a measure of phosphatase concentration (as in the blood) esp. in the diagnosis of various pathological conditions and that for the blood has a normal value averaging about 7 for children and 4 for adults

  Bodansky, Aaron (1887–1960), American biochemist. Bodansky published reports on determining the phosphatase concentration in blood in 1932 and 1933.

bodi·ly \'bäd-ᵊl-ē\ *adj* : of or relating to the body ⟨∼ organs⟩

Bo·do \'bō-(ˌ)dō\ *n* : a genus of minute usu. ovoid biflagellate kinetoplastid protozoans (family Bodonidae) that are common in stagnant water, dung, and sewage and include numerous intestinal commensals of vertebrates

body \'bäd-ē\ *n, pl* **bod·ies 1 a :** the organized physical substance of an animal or plant either living or dead: as (1) : the material part or nature of a human being (2) : a dead organism : CORPSE **b :** a human being **2 a :** the main part of a plant or animal body esp. as distinguished from limbs and head : TRUNK **b :** the main part of an organ (as the uterus) **3 :** a kind or form of matter : a material substance — see KETONE BODY

body bag *n* : a large zippered bag (as of rubber or vinyl) in which a human corpse is placed esp. for transportation

body build \-ˌbild\ *n* : the distinctive physical makeup of a human being

body cavity *n* : a cavity within an animal body; *specif* : COELOM

body clock \-'kläk\ *n* : the internal mechanisms that schedule bodily functions and activities — not usu. used technically

body dysmorphia *n* : BODY DYSMORPHIC DISORDER

body dysmorphic disorder *n* : pathological preoccupation with an imagined or slight physical defect of one's body to the point of causing significant stress or behavioral impairment in several areas (as work and personal relationships)

body heat *n* : heat produced in the body of a living animal by metabolic and physical activity — called also *animal heat*

body image *n* : a subjective picture of one's own physical appearance established both by self-observation and by noting the reactions of others

body louse *n* : a louse feeding primarily on the body; *esp* : a sucking louse of the genus *Pediculus* (*P. humanus humanus*) feeding on the human body and living in clothing — called also *cootie*

body mass index *n* : a measure of body fat that is the ratio of the weight of the body in kilograms to the square of its height in meters ⟨a *body mass index* in adults of 25 to 29.9 is considered an indication of overweight, and 30 or more an indication of obesity⟩ — abbr. *BMI;* called also *Quetelet index*

body odor *n* : an unpleasant odor from a perspiring or unclean person

body ringworm *n* : TINEA CORPORIS

body snatch·er \-'snach-ər\ *n* : one esp. in former times who illegally removed usu. recently interred corpses from graves for medical dissection or for sale for this purpose

body stalk *n* : the mesodermal cord that contains the umbilical vessels and that connects a fetus with its chorion

body wall *n* : the external surface of the animal body consisting of ectoderm and mesoderm and enclosing the body cavity

body·work \-ˌwərk\ *n* : therapeutic touching or manipulation of the body by using specialized techniques

Boeck's disease \'beks-, 'bərks-\ *n* : SARCOIDOSIS

  Boeck \'bœk\, **Caesar Peter Moeller (1845–1917),** Norwegian dermatologist. Boeck is known primarily for his description in 1899 of sarcoidosis or lupus pernio. The condition had been described previously and in 1917 was more fully described by Jorgen Nilsen Schaumann, but Boeck's description is known for its treatment of the cutaneous lesions and their histologic structure.

Boeck's sarcoid *n* : SARCOIDOSIS

Bohr effect \'bō(ə)r-, 'bȯ(ə)r-\ *n* : the decrease in oxygen affinity of a respiratory pigment (as hemoglobin or hemocyanin) in response to decreased blood pH resulting from increased carbon dioxide concentration

  Bohr, Christian (1855–1911), Danish physiologist. Bohr is known for two contributions to medical science: an 1891 study of the exchange of gases in respiration and the discovery that the affinity of blood for oxygen depends on carbon dioxide pressure. This discovery was reported in 1904 and is now known as the Bohr effect.

bohr·i·um \'bōr-ē-əm, 'bȯr-\ *n* : a short-lived radioactive element that is artificially produced — symbol *Bh*; see ELEMENT table

Bohr theory *n* : a theory in early quantum physics: an atom consists of a positively charged nucleus about which revolves one or more electrons of quantized energy

  Bohr, Niels Henrik David (1885–1962), Danish physicist. Bohr was the foremost influence on and major contributor to the development of quantum theory in the first half of the 20th century. In 1913 he postulated the theory that bears his name and that laid the groundwork for modern atomic physics. During World War II he worked in Britain and the U.S. on atomic bomb projects. Bohr was awarded the Nobel Prize for Physics in 1922.

boil \'bȯi(ə)l\ *n* : a localized swelling and inflammation of the skin resulting from usu. bacterial infection of a hair follicle and adjacent tissue, having a hard central core, and forming pus — called also *furuncle*

boil·ing point \'bȯi-liŋ-ˌpȯint\ *n* : the temperature at which a liquid boils

Bol·ling·er body \'bäl-iŋ-ər-\ *n* : one of the inclusion bodies that occur in epithelial cells of birds affected with fowl pox

  Bollinger, Otto (1843–1909), German pathologist. Bollinger is considered to be one of the founders of comparative pathology and made important contributions to both human and veterinary medicine. In 1870 he published the first description of botryomycosis. In 1876 he discovered actinomycosis in cattle, publishing a description the following year. The inclusion bodies characteristic of fowl pox are called Bollinger bodies in his honor.

bo·lom·e·ter \bō-'läm-ət-ər\ *n* : a very sensitive thermometer used in the detection and measurement of feeble thermal radiation and esp. adapted to the study of infrared spectra — **bo·lo·met·ric** \ˌbō-lə-'me-trik\ *adj* — **bo·lo·met·ri·cal·ly** \-tri-k(ə-)lē\ *adv*

bo·lus \'bō-ləs\ *n, pl* **bo·lus·es 1 :** a rounded mass: as **a :** a large pill **b :** a soft mass of chewed food **2 a :** a dose of a substance (as a drug) given intravenously **b :** a large dose of a substance given by injection for the purpose of rapidly achieving the needed therapeutic concentration in the bloodstream ⟨the patient receives a ∼ dose to reach the minimum effective analgesic concentration —J. F. Camp⟩ ⟨subcutaneous injection of a premeal ∼ of fast-acting insulin⟩

bomb calorimeter \'bäm-\ *n* : a calorimeter used to determine the heat of combustion of a substance in a chamber consisting of a strong steel shell

bombé — see IRIS BOMBÉ

bom·be·sin \'bäm-bə-sin\ *n* : a polypeptide that is found in the brain and gastrointestinal tract and has been shown experimentally to cause the secretion of various substances (as gastrin and cholecystokinin) and to inhibit intestinal motility

bomb fly *n* : the adult of the northern cattle grub

bond \'bänd\ *n* : an attractive force that holds together atoms, ions, or groups of atoms in a molecule or crystal — usu. represented in formulas by a line — **bond** *vb*

bond·ing *n* **1 :** the formation of a close relationship (as between a mother and child or between a person and an animal) esp. through frequent or constant association — see MALE BONDING **2 :** a dental technique in which a material and esp. plastic or porcelain is attached to a tooth surface to correct minor defects (as chipped or discolored teeth) esp. for cosmetic purposes

bone \'bōn\ *n, often attrib* **1** : one of the hard parts of the skeleton of a vertebrate ⟨a shoulder ∼⟩ ⟨the ∼s of the arm⟩ **2** : any of various hard animal substances or structures (as baleen or ivory) akin to or resembling bone **3** : the hard largely calcareous connective tissue of which the adult skeleton of most vertebrates is chiefly composed ⟨cancellous ∼⟩ ⟨compact ∼⟩ — compare CARTILAGE 1

bone·let \-lət\ *n* : a small bone : OSSICLE

bone marrow *n* : a soft highly vascular modified connective tissue that occupies the cavities and cancellous part of most bones and occurs in two forms: **a** : a whitish or yellowish bone marrow consisting chiefly of fat cells and predominating in the cavities of the long bones — called also *yellow marrow* **b** : a reddish bone marrow containing little fat, being the chief seat of red blood cell and blood granulocyte formation, and occurring in the normal adult only in cancellous tissue esp. in certain flat bones — called also *red marrow*

bone·set·ter \-ˌset-ər\ *n* : a person who sets broken or dislocated bones usu. without being a licensed physician

bo·no·bo \bə-'nō-bō; 'bä-nə-bō, -nō-\ *n* : a rare anthropoid ape of the genus *Pan* (*P. paniscus*) that has a more slender build and longer limbs than the related common chimpanzee (*P. troglodytes*) — called also *pygmy chimpanzee*

bont tick \'bänt-\ *n* : a southern African tick of the genus *Amblyomma* (*A. hebraeum*) that attacks livestock, birds, and sometimes humans and transmits heartwater of sheep, goats, and cattle; *broadly* : any African tick of the genus *Amblyomma*

bony *also* **bon·ey** \'bō-nē\ *adj* **bon·i·er; -est** : consisting of or resembling bone ⟨∼ prominences of the skull⟩

bony labyrinth *n* : the cavity in the petrous portion of the temporal bone that contains the membranous labyrinth of the inner ear — called also *osseous labyrinth*

book lung \'bůk-\ *n* : a saccular breathing organ in many arachnids containing thin folds of membrane arranged like the leaves of a book

Bo·oph·i·lus \bō-'äf-ə-ləs\ *n* : a genus of ticks some of which are pests esp. of cattle and are vectors of disease — see CATTLE TICK

boost·er \'bü-stər\ *n* : a substance that increases the effectiveness of a medicament; *esp* : BOOSTER SHOT

booster shot *n* : a supplementary dose of an immunizing agent — called also *booster, booster dose*

bo·rac·ic acid \bə-ˌras-ik-\ *n* : BORIC ACID

bo·rate \'bō(ə)r-ˌāt, 'bȯ(ə)r-\ *n* : a salt or ester of a boric acid

bo·rat·ed \-ˌāt-əd\ *adj* : mixed or impregnated with borax or boric acid

bo·rax \'bō(ə)r-ˌaks, 'bȯ(ə)r-, -əks\ *n* : a white crystalline compound that consists of a hydrated sodium borate $Na_2B_4O_7 \cdot 10H_2O$, that occurs as a mineral or is prepared from other minerals, and that is used esp. as a flux, cleansing agent, and water softener and as a preservative

bor·bo·ryg·mus \ˌbȯr-bə-'rig-məs\ *n, pl* **-mi** \-ˌmī\ : a rumbling sound made by the movement of gas in the intestine — **bor·bo·ryg·mic** \-mik\ *adj*

bor·der \'bȯrd-ər\ *n* : an outer part or edge — see BRUSH BORDER

bor·der·line \-ˌlīn\ *adj* **1** : being in an intermediate position or state : not fully classifiable as one thing or its opposite; *esp* : not quite up to what is usual, standard, or expected ⟨∼ intelligence⟩ **2** : exhibiting typical but not altogether conclusive symptoms ⟨a ∼ diabetic⟩ **3** : of, relating to, being, or exhibiting a behavior pattern typical or suggestive of borderline personality disorder ⟨a ∼ patient⟩ ⟨∼ behavior⟩

borderline personality disorder *n* : a disordered behavior pattern with onset by early adulthood that is characterized by multiple types of psychological instability and impulsiveness, often involves fear of abandonment and a risk of suicide, and may ameliorate with age

Bor·de·tel·la \ˌbȯrd-ə-'tel-ə\ *n* : a genus of bacteria comprising very short gram-negative strictly aerobic coccuslike bacilli and including the causative agent (*B. pertussis*) of whooping cough

J.–J.–B.–V. Bordet — see BORDET-GENGOU

Bor·det–Gen·gou \bȯr-'dä-zhäⁿ-'gü\ *adj* : of, relating to, or for use in connection with the Bordet-Gengou bacillus ⟨*Bordet-Gengou* media⟩

Bor·det \bȯr-dā\, **Jules–Jean–Baptiste–Vincent (1870– 1961)**, Belgian bacteriologist, and **Gen·gou** \zhaⁿ-gü\, **Octave (1875–1957)**, French bacteriologist. Bordet was an outstanding immunologist. His discovery of the role of antibodies and complement in immunity was a development vital to the modern diagnosis and treatment of many dangerous contagious diseases. His research on the destruction of bacteria and foreign red corpuscles in blood serum is generally held to constitute the beginnings of serology. In 1901 he and Gengou published the first of their reports on complement fixation. This reaction is the basis of many tests for infection, including the Wassermann test for syphilis and reactions for gonococcus infection, glanders, and hydatid disease. In 1906 they discovered the causative agent of whooping cough, now known as the Bordet-Gengou bacillus. Bordet was awarded the Nobel Prize for Physiology or Medicine in 1919.

Bordet–Gengou bacillus *n* : a small ovoid bacillus of the genus *Bordetella* (*B. pertussis*) that is the causative agent of whooping cough

¹bore *past of* BEAR

²bore \'bō(ə)r, 'bȯ(ə)r\ *n* **1** : the long usu. cylindrical hollow part of something (as a tube or artery) **2** : the internal diameter of a tube (as a hypodermic needle, catheter, or sound) ⟨a small-*bore* catheter⟩

bo·ric \'bōr-ik, 'bȯr-\ *adj* : of or containing boron

boric acid *n* : a white crystalline acid H_3BO_3 obtained from its salts and used esp. as a weak antiseptic — called also *boracic acid, orthoboric acid*

borne *past part of* BEAR

bor·ne·ol \'bȯr-nē-ˌȯl, -ˌōl\ *n* : a crystalline cyclic alcohol $C_{10}H_{17}OH$ that occurs in two enantiomeric forms, is found in essential oils, and is used esp. in perfumery

Born·holm disease \'bȯrn-ˌhōlm-\ *n* : EPIDEMIC PLEURODYNIA

bo·ron \'bō(ə)r-ˌän, 'bȯ(ə)r-\ *n* : a trivalent metalloid element found in nature only in combination and used in metallurgy and in composite structural materials — symbol *B*; see ELEMENT table — **bo·ron·ic** \bȯr-'än-ik, bōr-\ *adj*

Bor·rel body \bə-'rel-, bȯr-'el-\ *n* : one of the particles making up a Bollinger body

Bor·rel \bȯr-el\, **Amédée (1867–1936)**, French bacteriologist. With Albert L. Calmette, Borrel developed in 1895 a vaccine for use against bubonic plague. In 1898 he diagnosed sheep pox. He also investigated cancer, cell division in tumors, the action of glycogen on tumors, tuberculosis, and bacteriophages.

bor·re·lia \bə-'rel-ē-ə, -'rē-lē-\ *n* **1** *cap* : a genus of small flexible spirochetes of the family Spirochaetaceae that are parasites of humans and warm-blooded animals and include the causative agents of septicemia in chickens (*B. recurrentis*), relapsing fever in Africa (*B. duttoni*), and Lyme disease in the U.S. (*B. burgdorferi*) **2** : a spirochete of the genus *Borrelia*

bor·re·lia·cid·al \bə-ˌrel-ē-ə-'sīd-ᵊl, -ˌrē-lē-\ *adj* : destroying spirochetes of the genus *Borrelia* and esp. the causative agent (*B. burgdorferi*) of Lyme disease ⟨∼ antibodies⟩

bor·rel·i·o·sis \bə-ˌrel-ē-'ō-səs, -ˌrē-l-\ *n, pl* **-o·ses** \-ˌsēz\ : infection with or disease caused by a spirochete of the genus *Borrelia*; *specif* : LYME DISEASE

boss \'bäs, 'bȯs\ *n* : a protuberant part or body ⟨a ∼ on an animal's horn⟩

\ə\ abut \ᵊ\ kitten \ər\ further \a\ ash \ā\ ace \ä\ cot, cart \au̇\ out \ch\ chin \e\ bet \ē\ easy \g\ go \i\ hit \ī\ ice \j\ job \ŋ\ sing \ō\ go \ȯ\ law \ȯi\ boy \th\ thin \t͟h\ the \ü\ loot \u̇\ foot \y\ yet \zh\ vision *See also* Pronunciation Symbols page

bos·se·lat·ed \'bäs-ə-ˌlāt-əd, 'bòs-\ *adj* : marked or covered with small bosses ⟨a ~ tumor⟩

boss·ing \'bäs-iŋ, 'bòs-\ *n* : a boss or a swelling resembling a boss

bot *also* **bott** \'bät\ *n* : the larva of a botfly; *esp* : one infesting the horse

bot *abbr* **1** botanical; botanist; botany **2** bottle

¹bo·tan·i·cal \bə-'tan-i-kəl\ *adj* **1** : of or relating to plants or botany **2** : derived from plants — **bo·tan·i·cal·ly** \-k(ə-)lē\ *adv*

²botanical *n* : a vegetable drug esp. in the crude state

bot·a·nist \'bät-ᵊn-əst, 'bät-nəst\ *n* : a specialist in botany or in a branch of botany

bot·a·ny \'bät-ᵊn-ē, 'bät-nē\ *n, pl* **-nies 1** : a branch of biology dealing with plant life **2 a** : plant life **b** : the properties and life phenomena exhibited by a plant, plant type, or plant group **3** : a botanical treatise or study; *esp* : a particular system of botany

botch \'bäch\ *n* : an inflammatory sore

bot·fly \'bät-ˌflī\ *n, pl* **-flies** : any of various stout dipteran flies of the family Oestridae that have larvae parasitic in cavities or tissues of various mammals including humans

bo·thrid·i·um \bō-'thrid-ē-əm\ *n, pl* **-ia** \-ē-ə\ *or* **-i·ums** : one of the outgrowths from the head of tapeworms esp. of the order Tetraphyllidea that act as holdfasts

Both·rio·ceph·a·lus \ˌbäth-rē-ō-'sef-ə-ləs\ *n* : a genus of tapeworms of the order Pseudophyllidea with two bothria that is sometimes considered to include the common fish tapeworm of humans — compare DIPHYLLOBOTHRIUM

both·ri·um \'bäth-rē-əm\ *n, pl* **-ria** \-rē-ə\ *or* **-riums** : a slit, groove, or depression esp. on the holdfast of a pseudophyllidean tapeworm

Bo·tox \'bō-ˌtäks\ *trademark* — used for a preparation of botulinum toxin type A

bot·ry·oid \'bä-trē-ˌòid\ *adj* : having the form of a bunch of grapes

botryoides — see SARCOMA BOTRYOIDES

bot·ry·o·my·co·ma \ˌbä-trē-(ˌ)ō-mī-'kō-mə\ *n, pl* **-mas** *or* **-ma·ta** \-mət-ə\ : one of the vascular granulomatous masses occurring in botryomycosis

bot·ry·o·my·co·sis \-'kō-səs\ *n, pl* **-co·ses** \-ˌsēz\ : a bacterial infection of domestic animals and humans marked by the formation of usu. superficial vascular granulomatous masses, associated esp. with wounds, and sometimes followed by metastatic visceral tumors — **bot·ry·o·my·cot·ic** \-'kät-ik\ *adj*

bot·tle \'bät-ᵊl\ *n, often attrib* **1** : a rigid or semirigid container typically of glass or plastic having a comparatively narrow neck or mouth and usu. no handle — see WASH BOTTLE **2** : liquid food usu. consisting of milk and supplements that is fed from a bottle (as to an infant) in place of mother's milk

bottle baby *n* : a baby fed chiefly or wholly on the bottle as contrasted with a baby that is chiefly or wholly breast-fed

bot·tle-feed \'bät-ᵊl-ˌfēd\ *vt* **-fed; -feed·ing** : to feed (an infant) from a bottle rather than by breast-feeding

bottle jaw *n* : a pendulous edematous condition of the tissues under the lower jaw in cattle and sheep resulting from infestation with bloodsucking gastrointestinal parasites (as of the genus *Haemonchus*)

bot·u·lin \'bäch-ə-lən\ *n* : BOTULINUM TOXIN

bot·u·li·num \ˌbäch-ə-'lī-nəm\ *also* **bot·u·li·nus** \-nəs\ *n* : a spore-forming bacterium of the genus *Clostridium* (*C. botulinum*) that secretes botulinum toxin — **bot·u·li·nal** \-'līn-ᵊl\ *adj*

botulinum toxin *also* **botulinus toxin** *n* : a very powerful bacterial neurotoxin that acts primarily on the parasympathetic nervous system, is produced by botulinum, blocks release of acetylcholine at the neuromuscular junction, and causes botulism — often used with one of the letters *A* to *G* to designate one of seven distinct types; called also *botulin*

botulinum toxin type A *n* : a purified botulinum toxin of high molecular weight that is used by injection esp. to treat strabismus, blepharospasm, spasmodic torticollis, and severe axillary hyperhidrosis and in cosmetic dermatology and plastic surgery to minimize wrinkles — see BOTOX

bot·u·lism \'bäch-ə-ˌliz-əm\ *n* : acute food poisoning caused by botulinum toxin produced in food by a bacterium of the genus *Clostridium* (*C. botulinum*) and characterized by muscle weakness and paralysis, disturbances of vision, swallowing, and speech, and a high mortality rate — see BOTULINUM TOXIN, LIMBERNECK

Bou·chard's node \bü-'shärz-\ *n* : a bony enlargement of the middle joint of a finger that is commonly associated with osteoarthritis — compare HEBERDEN'S NODE

Bouchard, Charles Jacques (1837–1915), French pathologist. For most of his career Bouchard was associated with the Faculty of Medicine at the University of Paris, being head of its clinic from 1868 and a member of the faculty from 1869. He became known for his research in urosepsis as well as for his work on diseases resulting from malnutrition. Bouchard is also remembered for his pioneering use of X-rays to diagnose bone diseases, fractures, and dislocations. In 1884 he made the connection between osteoarthritis and bony enlargements of the middle joints of the fingers.

bou·gie \'bü-ˌzhē, -ˌjē\ *n* **1** : a tapering cylindrical instrument for introduction into a tubular passage of the body **2** : SUPPOSITORY

bou·gi·nage *or* **bou·gie·nage** \ˌbü-zhē-'näzh\ *n* : the dilation of a tubular cavity (as a constricted esophagus) with a bougie

bouil·lon \'bü(l)-ˌyän, 'bù(l)-; 'bùl-yən; 'bü-ˌyōⁿ\ *n* : a clear seasoned soup made usu. from lean beef

Bou·in's fluid \(')bü-'anz-, 'bwaⁿz-\ *n* : a fixing and preserving solution consisting of picric acid, formaldehyde, and glacial acetic acid — called also *Bouin, Bouin's solution*

Bouin \bwaⁿ, (')bü-'an\, Pol André (1870–1962), French histologist. In collaboration with Paul Ancel for thirty years, Bouin undertook research on the physiology of reproduction that laid the groundwork for the development of reproductive endocrinology. Among other things, the pair successfully demonstrated that the testis has a dual function and that the Leydig cells of the testis control the secondary sex characteristics in the male. Bouin's fluid was introduced in 1897.

boulimia *var of* BULIMIA

bound \'baùnd\ *adj* **1** : made costive : CONSTIPATED **2** : held in chemical or physical combination ⟨~ water in a molecule⟩

bour·tree \'bù(ə)r-(ˌ)trē, 'bò(ə)r-\ *n, Brit* : a large Eurasian black-fruited elderberry (*Sambucus nigra*) formerly valued as a source of dyestuffs and of several folk remedies

bou·ton \bü-'tōⁿ\ *n* : a terminal club-shaped enlargement of a nerve fiber at a synapse with another neuron — called also *end foot*

bou·ton·neuse fever \ˌbü-tò-'nœz-\ *n* : a disease of the Mediterranean area that is characterized by headache, pain in muscles and joints, and an eruption over the body and is caused by a tick-borne rickettsia (*Rickettsia conorii*) — called also *fièvre boutonneuse, Marseilles fever;* see TICK-BITE FEVER, TICK TYPHUS

Bo·vic·o·la \bō-'vik-ə-lə\ *n* : a genus of biting lice (order Mallophaga) including several that infest the hair of domestic mammals

bo·vine \'bō-ˌvīn, -ˌvēn\ *n* : an ox (genus *Bos*) or a closely related animal — **bovine** *adj*

bovine mastitis *n* : inflammation of the udder of a cow resulting from injury or more commonly from bacterial infection — see SUMMER MASTITIS

bovine spongiform encephalopathy *n* : a fatal spongiform encephalopathy of cattle affecting the nervous system, resembling or identical with scrapie of sheep and goats, and prob. caused by a prion transmitted by infected tissue in food — abbr. *BSE;* called also *mad cow disease*

bovine viral diarrhea *n* : an infectious disease of cattle that is characterized by fever, diarrhea, loss of appetite, dehydration, excessive salivation, and ulceration of the gastrointestinal tract, that is caused by two flaviviruses of the genus *Pestivirus* (species *Bovine viral diarrhea virus 1* and species *Bovine viral diarrhea virus 2*), and that tends to occur in herds with high morbidity but low mortality — called also *bovine virus diarrhea, mucosal disease*

bovinum — see COR BOVINUM

bow \'bō\ *n* : a frame for the lenses of eyeglasses; *also* : the curved sidepiece of the frame passing over the ear

bow·el \'baú(-ə)l\ *n* : INTESTINE, GUT; *also* : one of the divisions of the intestines — usu. used in pl. except in medical use ⟨move your ~*s*⟩ ⟨surgery of the involved ~⟩

bowel worm *n* : a common strongylid nematode worm of the genus *Chabertia* (*C. ovina*) infesting the colon of sheep and feeding on blood and tissue — called also *large-mouthed bowel worm*

bow·en·oid papulosis \'bō-ə-ˌnóid-\ *n* : a condition that is usu. associated with a genetic variant of the human papillomavirus and is characterized by pigmented papules in the anogenital area which are histologically similar to those of Bowen's disease but usu. follow a benign course

J. T. Bowen — see BOWEN'S DISEASE

Bow·en's disease \'bō-ənz-\ *n* : a precancerous lesion of the skin or mucous membranes characterized by small solid elevations covered by thickened horny tissue

   Bowen, John Templeton (1857–1941), American dermatologist. In 1912 Bowen published the first description of the dermatosis which now bears his name.

bow·leg \'bō-ˌleg, -ˌlāg, 'bō-\ *n* : a leg bowed outward at or below the knee — called also *genu varum*

bow-legged \'bō-'leg(-ə)d, -'lāg(-ə)d\ *adj* : having bowlegs

Bow·man's capsule \ˌbō-mənz-\ *n* : a thin membranous double-walled capsule surrounding the glomerulus of a vertebrate nephron through which glomerular filtrate passes to the proximal convoluted tubule — called also *capsule of Bowman, glomerular capsule*; see RENAL CORPUSCLE

   Bowman, Sir William (1816–1892), British ophthalmologist, anatomist, and physiologist. Bowman was the foremost ophthalmic surgeon of 19th-century Britain. He is known in particular for his studies of the anatomy and physiology of the eye; the structure now known as Bowman's membrane was described by him in 1847. Bowman is equally notable for his studies of the kidney and urinary secretion; his original description of Bowman's capsule was published in 1842. In addition to these achievements, he discovered and described striated muscle in 1840.

Bowman's gland *n* : GLAND OF BOWMAN

Bowman's membrane *n* : the thin outer layer of the substantia propria of the cornea immediately underlying the epithelium

box·ing \'bäk-siŋ\ *n* : construction of the base of a dental cast by building up the walls of an impression while preserving important landmarks

Boyle's law \ˌbói(ə)lz-\ *n* : a statement in physics: the volume of a gas at constant temperature varies inversely with the pressure exerted on it

   Boyle, Robert (1627–1691), British physicist. Considered one of the fathers of modern chemistry, Boyle is known especially for his pioneering experiments on the properties of gases. In 1662 he published his findings stating the relation concerning the compression and expansion of a gas at constant temperature (Boyle's law). Boyle also wrote the first English treatise on electricity and espoused the theory that matter is corpuscular in composition. This theory was an important forerunner of modern chemical theory.

bp *abbr* base pair

BP *abbr* **1** blood pressure **2** boiling point **3** British Pharmacopoeia

BPH *abbr* benign prostatic hyperplasia; benign prostatic hypertrophy

BPharm \'bē-'färm\ *n* : bachelor of pharmacy

Br *symbol* bromine

¹**brace** \'brās\ *n* **1** : an appliance that gives support to moving able parts (as a joint or a fractured bone), to weak muscles (as in paralysis), or to strained ligaments (as of the lower back) **2 braces** *pl* : an orthodontic appliance usu. of metallic wire that is used esp. to exert pressure to straighten misaligned teeth and that is not removable by the patient

²**brace** *vt* **braced; brac·ing** : to furnish or support with a brace

bra·chi·al \'brā-kē-əl\ *adj* : of or relating to the arm or a process like an arm

brachial artery *n* : the chief artery of the upper arm that is a direct continuation of the axillary artery and divides into the radial and ulnar arteries just below the elbow — see DEEP BRACHIAL ARTERY

bra·chi·alis \ˌbrā-kē-'al-əs, -'āl-, -'äl-\ *n* : a flexor that lies in front of the lower part of the humerus whence it arises and is inserted into the ulna

brachialis an·ti·cus \-an-'tī-kəs\ *n* : BRACHIALIS

brachial plexus *n* : a complex network of nerves that is formed chiefly by the lower four cervical nerves and the first thoracic nerve, lies partly within the axilla, and supplies nerves to the chest, shoulder, and arm

brachial vein *n* : one of a pair of veins accompanying the brachial artery and uniting with each other and with the basilic vein to form the axillary vein

brachii — see BICEPS BRACHII, TRICEPS BRACHII

bra·chio·ce·phal·ic artery \ˌbrā-kē-(ˌ)ō-sə-ˌfal-ik-\ *n* : a short artery that arises from the arch of the aorta and divides into the carotid and subclavian arteries of the right side — called also *brachiocephalic trunk, innominate artery*

brachiocephalicus — see TRUNCUS BRACHIOCEPHALICUS

brachiocephalic vein *n* : either of two large veins that occur one on each side of the neck, receive blood from the head and neck, are formed by the union of the internal jugular and the subclavian veins, and unite to form the superior vena cava — called also *innominate vein*

bra·chio·ra·di·alis \ˌbrā-kē-ō-ˌrād-ē-'al-əs, -'āl-, -'äl-\ *n, pl* **-ales** \-'al-ˌēz, -'āl-, -'äl-\ : a flexor of the radial side of the forearm arising from the lateral supracondylar ridge of the humerus and inserted into the styloid process of the radius

bra·chi·um \'brā-kē-əm\ *n, pl* **-chia** \-kē-ə\ : the upper segment of the arm or forelimb extending from the shoulder to the elbow

brachium con·junc·ti·vum \-ˌkän-(ˌ)jəŋ(k)-'tī-vəm\ *n* : CEREBELLAR PEDUNCLE a

brachium pon·tis \-'pänt-əs\ *n* : CEREBELLAR PEDUNCLE b

brachy·ce·phal·ic \ˌbrak-i-sə-'fal-ik\ *adj* : short-headed or broad-headed with a cephalic index of over 80 — **brachy·ceph·a·ly** \-'sef-ə-lē\ *n, pl* **-lies**

brachy·dac·ty·lous \ˌbrak-i-'dak-tə-ləs\ *adj* : having abnormally short digits — **brachy·dac·ty·ly** \-lē\ *n, pl* **-lies**

brachy·dont \'brak-i-ˌdänt\ *also* **brachy·odont** \'brak-ē-ō-ˌdänt\ *adj* **1** *of teeth* : having short crowns, well-developed roots, and only narrow canals in the roots (as in humans) — compare HYPSODONT **2** : having brachydont teeth

brachy·fa·cial \ˌbrak-i-'fā-shəl\ *adj* : having a short or broad face

brachy·mor·phic \-'mór-fik\ *adj* : ENDOMORPHIC, PYKNIC

brachy·ther·a·py \-'ther-ə-pē\ *n, pl* **-pies** : radiotherapy in which the source of radiation is placed (as by implantation) in or close to the area being treated

brachy·uran·ic \-yúr-'an-ik\ *adj* : having a short or narrow alveolar arch with a palatal index of 115 or above — **brachy·ur·a·ny** \-'yúr-ə-nē\ *n, pl* **-nies**

Brad·ford frame \'brad-fərd-\ *n* : a rectangular metal frame fitted with adjustable straps of canvas or webbing and used to support a patient with disease or fractures of the spine, hip, or pelvis

   Bradford, Edward Hickling (1848–1926), American orthopedist. The inventor of the Bradford frame, Bradford

---

\ə\ **abut** \ᵊ\ **kitten** \ər\ **further** \a\ **ash** \ā\ **ace** \ä\ **cot, cart**
\aú\ **out** \ch\ **chin** \e\ **bet** \ē\ **easy** \g\ **go** \i\ **hit** \ī\ **ice** \j\ **job**
\ŋ\ **sing** \ō\ **go** \ó\ **law** \ói\ **boy** \th\ **thin** \t̲h̲\ **the** \ü\ **loot**
\ú\ **foot** \y\ **yet** \zh\ **vision**   *See also* Pronunciation Symbols page

described the frame in a treatise on orthopedic surgery published in 1890. Originally designed for handling children with tuberculosis of the spine, the frame was later modified for use in other orthopedic conditions.

brad·sot \'brad-sət\ *n* : BRAXY 1

bra·dy·car·dia \ˌbräd-i-'kärd-ē-ə *also* ˌbrad-\ *n* : relatively slow heart action whether physiological or pathological — compare TACHYCARDIA

bra·dy·crot·ic \-'krät-ik\ *adj* : marked by or inducing slowness of pulse ⟨∼ and stress-relieving action of reserpine —*Jour. Amer. Med. Assoc.*⟩

bra·dy·ki·ne·sia \-kī-'nē-zh(ē-)ə, -kə-, -zē-ə\ *n* : extreme slowness of movements and reflexes (as in catatonic schizophrenia or in weightless spaceflight)

bra·dy·ki·nin \-'kī-nən\ *n* : a kinin that is formed locally in injured tissue, acts in vasodilation of small arterioles, is considered to play a part in inflammatory processes, and is composed of a chain of nine amino acid residues — see KALLIDIN

bra·dy·lex·ia \-'lek-sē-ə\ *n* : abnormally slow performance in reading

bra·dy·pha·sia \-'fā-zh(ē-)ə\ *n* : abnormal slowness of speech

bra·dy·phra·sia \-'frā-zh(ē-)ə\ *n* : BRADYPHASIA

bra·dy·phre·nia \-'frē-nē-ə\ *n* : a condition characterized by slowness of mental processes

bra·dy·pnea *or chiefly Brit* **bra·dy·pnoea** \ˌbräd-ə(p)-'nē-ə *also* ˌbrad-\ *n* : abnormally slow breathing

bra·dy·rhyth·mia \ˌbräd-i-'rith-mē-ə *also* ˌbrad-\ *n* : BRADYCARDIA

braille \'brā(ə)l\ *n, often cap* : a system of writing for the blind that uses characters made up of raised dots — **braille** *vt* **brailled; braill·ing**

Braille \bràY\, **Louis (1809–1852)**, French inventor and teacher. Braille was blind and while at a school for the blind in Paris met Charles Barbier. Barbier had devised a system of writing for the blind in which simple messages coded in dots were embossed on cardboard. In 1824 Braille started work on adapting this system, developing a system in which a six-dot code represented letters and characters. He published treatises on his system in 1829 and 1837.

braille·writ·er \-ˌrīt-ər\ *n, often cap* : a machine for writing braille

brain \'brān\ *n* **1** : the portion of the vertebrate central nervous system enclosed in the skull and continuous with the spinal cord through the foramen magnum that is composed of neurons and supporting and nutritive structures (as glia) and that integrates sensory information from inside and outside the body in controlling autonomic function (as heartbeat and respiration), in coordinating and directing correlated motor responses, and in the process of learning — see FOREBRAIN, HINDBRAIN, MIDBRAIN **2** : a nervous center in invertebrates comparable in position and function to the vertebrate brain

brain attack *n* : STROKE

brain·case \-ˌkās\ *n* : the part of the skull that encloses the brain — see CRANIUM

brain death *n* : final cessation of activity in the central nervous system esp. as indicated by a flat electroencephalogram for a predetermined length of time — **brain–dead** *adj*

brain hormone *n* : any of various hormones (as serotonin and melatonin) produced in or acting on the vertebrate brain or central nervous system — not usu. used technically

brain·pan \'brān-ˌpan\ *n* : BRAINCASE

brain sand \-ˌsand\ *n* : small grains of calcareous matter in the brain (as in the pineal gland) that occur esp. in association with aging — called also *acervulus, acervulus cerebri*

brain stem \-ˌstem\ *n* : the part of the brain composed of the midbrain, pons, and medulla oblongata and connecting the spinal cord with the forebrain and cerebrum

brain vesicle *n* : any of the divisions into which the developing embryonic brain of vertebrates is marked off by incomplete transverse constrictions

brain·wash·ing \'brān-ˌwȯsh-iŋ, -ˌwäsh-\ *n* : a forcible indoctrination to induce someone to give up basic political, social, or religious beliefs and attitudes and to accept contrasting regimented ideas — **brain·wash** *vt* — **brainwash** *n* — **brain·wash·er** *n*

brain wave *n* **1** : rhythmic fluctuations of voltage between parts of the brain resulting in the flow of an electric current **2** : a current produced by brain waves — compare ALPHA WAVE, BETA WAVE

bran \'bran\ *n* : the edible broken seed coats of cereal grain separated from the flour or meal by sifting or bolting

branch \'branch\ *n* **1** : something that extends from or enters into a main body or source ⟨a ∼ of an artery⟩ **2** : an area of knowledge that may be considered apart from related areas ⟨pathology is a ∼ of medicine⟩ — **branch** *vi* — **branched** \'brancht\ *adj*

branched chain *n* : an open chain of atoms having one or more side chains

bran·chia \'braŋ-kē-ə\ *n, pl* **-chi·ae** \-kē-ˌē, -ˌī\ : ²GILL 1

bran·chi·al \-kē-əl\ *adj* : of or relating to the gills or to parts of the body derived from the embryonic branchial arches and clefts

branchial arch *n* : one of a series of bony or cartilaginous arches that develop in the walls of the mouth cavity and pharynx of a vertebrate embryo, consist typically of a curved segmented bar or rod on each side meeting the contralateral bar or rod at the ventral end, and correspond to the gill arches of fishes and amphibians — called also *pharyngeal arch, visceral arch*

branchial cleft *n* : one of the open or potentially open clefts that occur on each side of the neck region of a vertebrate embryo between the branchial arches, are formed by the meeting of an external furrow in the ectoderm with a pharyngeal pouch, may or may not extend through from the exterior to the cavity of the mouth and pharynx, and correspond to the gill slits of fishes and amphibians — called also *pharyngeal cleft, pharyngeal slit, visceral cleft*

bran·chi·og·e·nous \ˌbraŋ-kē-'äj-ə-nəs\ *adj* : arising from or formed by the branchial clefts or arches

bran·chi·oma \ˌbraŋ-kē-'ō-mə\ *n, pl* **-omas** *or* **-oma·ta** \-mət-ə\ : a tumor and esp. a carcinoma affecting branchial tissues

bran·chio·mere \'braŋ-kē-ə-ˌmi(ə)r\ *n* : a branchial segment; *esp* : one of the metameres indicated by the branchial arches and clefts of the embryo of air-breathing vertebrates — **bran·chio·mer·ic** \ˌbraŋ-kē-ə-'mer-ik\ *adj*

bran·chi·om·er·ism \ˌbraŋ-kē-'äm-ə-ˌriz-əm\ *n* : segmentation into branchiomeres

Bran·chi·os·to·ma \ˌbraŋ-kē-'äs-tə-mə\ *n* : a genus of lancelets (family Branchiostomidae) with paired gonads and symmetrical metapleura — compare AMPHIOXUS

bran·dy \'bran-dē\ *n, pl* **brandies** : an alcoholic liquor distilled from wine or fermented fruit juice (as of apples)

brash \'brash\ *n* **1** : an attack of illness; *esp* : a short severe illness **2** : WATER BRASH

brava — see PAREIRA BRAVA

brawny \'brȯ-nē\ *adj* **brawn·i·er; -est** : being swollen and hard ⟨a ∼ infected foot⟩

Brax·ton–Hicks contractions \ˌbrak-stən-'hiks-\ *n pl* : relatively painless nonrhythmic contractions of the uterus that occur during pregnancy with increasing frequency over time but are not associated with labor

Hicks, John Braxton (1823–1897), British gynecologist. In 1871 Hicks presented evidence before the Obstetrical Society that contractions of the uterus appear early in pregnancy and persist through delivery. A year later he published his findings on these contractions, which now bear his name.

braxy \'brak-sē\ *n, pl* **brax·ies** **1** : a malignant edema of sheep that involves gastrointestinal invasion by a spore-forming bacterium of the genus *Clostridium* (*C. septicum*), produces an enterotoxemia characterized by staggering, convulsions, coma, and death, and is common in Iceland, Scotland, and Norway — compare BLACK DISEASE **2** : a sheep dead from natural causes and esp. from disease; *also* : mutton from such a carcass

bra·yera \brə-'yer-ə, 'brā-ə-rə\ *n* : the dried pistillate flowers of an ornamental Ethiopian tree (*Hagenia abyssinica*) sometimes used as an anthelmintic

BRCA \ˌbē-(ˌ)är-(ˌ)sē-'ā\ *n* : either of two tumor supressor genes that in mutated form tend to be associated with an increased risk of certain cancers and esp. breast and ovarian cancers

bread mold \'bred-\ *n* : any of various molds found esp. on bread; *esp* : one of the genus *Rhizopus* (*R. nigricans*)

breadth–height index \'bretth-'hīt-\ *n* : the ratio of the maximum breadth of the head or skull to its maximum height multiplied by 100

¹break \'brāk\ *vb* **broke** \'brōk\; **bro·ken** \'brō-kən\; **break·ing** *vt* **1 a** : to snap into pieces : FRACTURE ⟨~ a bone⟩ **b** : to fracture the bone of (a bodily part) ⟨the blow *broke* her arm⟩ **c** : to dislocate or dislocate and fracture a bone of (the neck or back) **2 a** : to cause an open wound in : RUPTURE ⟨~ the skin⟩ **b** : to rupture the surface of and permit flowing out or effusing ⟨~ an artery⟩ ⟨he *broke* several veins during his seizure⟩ ~ *vi* **1** : to fail in health or strength — often used with *down* ⟨he *broke* down under the strain⟩ **2** : to suffer complete or marked loss of resistance, composure, resolution, morale, or command of a situation — often used with *down* ⟨the prisoner *broke* down under interrogation and told the whole story⟩

²break *n* **1 a** : an act or action of breaking : FRACTURE **b** : the act of opening a gap in an electrical circuit **2 a** : a condition produced by breaking ⟨the ~ in her leg⟩ **b** : a gap in an otherwise continuous electric circuit **3** : the occurrence of a disease in a person or esp. in a domestic animal supposed to be immune to or to have been completely isolated from exposure to that disease

break·bone fever \ˌbrāk-ˌbōn-\ *n* : DENGUE

¹break·down \'brāk-ˌdaun\ *n* : the action or result of breaking down: as **a** : a failure to function **b** : a physical, mental, or nervous collapse **c** : the process of decomposing ⟨~ of food during digestion⟩

²breakdown *adj* : obtained or resulting from disintegration or decomposition of a substance ⟨a ~ product of purine⟩

break down \(ˈ)brāk-'daun\ *vt* : to separate (as a chemical compound) into simpler substances : DECOMPOSE ~ *vi* **1** : to stop functioning because of breakage or wear **2** : to undergo decomposition

breaking point *n* : the point at which a person gives way under stress

break out \(ˈ)brā-'kaut\ *vi* **1** : to be affected with a skin eruption and esp. one indicative of the presence of a particular disease ⟨*breaking out* with measles⟩ **2** *of a disease* : to manifest itself by skin eruptions **3** : to become covered with ⟨*break out* in a sweat⟩

break·through bleeding \ˌbrāk-ˌthrü-\ *n* : an abnormal flow of blood from the uterus that occurs between menstrual periods esp. due to irregular sloughing of the endometrium in women on contraceptive hormones

breast \'brest\ *n* **1** : either of the pair of mammary glands extending from the front of the chest in pubescent and adult females of humans and some other mammals; *also* : either of the analogous but rudimentary organs of the male chest esp. when enlarged **2** : the fore or ventral part of the body between the neck and the abdomen

breast·bone \'bres(t)-'bōn, -ˌbōn\ *n* : STERNUM

breast–feed \'brest-ˌfēd\ *vt* : to feed (a baby) from a mother's breast rather than from a bottle

breast lift *n* : plastic surgery to elevate and often reshape a sagging breast — called also *mastopexy*

breath \'breth\ *n* **1 a** : the faculty of breathing ⟨recovering her ~ after the race⟩ **b** : an act or an instance of breathing or inhaling **2 a** : air inhaled and exhaled in breathing ⟨bad ~⟩ **b** : something (as moisture on a cold surface) produced by breath or breathing — **out of breath** : breathing very rapidly (as from strenuous exercise)

Breath·a·ly·zer \'breth-ə-ˌlī-zər\ *trademark* — used for a device consisting of a small tube of chemically sensitized crystals connected to a balloon that is used to determine the alcohol content of a breath sample

breathe \'brēth\ *vb* **breathed; breath·ing** *vi* **1** : to draw air into and expel it from the lungs : RESPIRE; *broadly* : to take in oxygen and give out carbon dioxide through natural processes **2** : to inhale and exhale freely ~ *vt* : to inhale and exhale ⟨*breathing* fresh air⟩

breath·er \'brē-thər\ *n* : one that breathes usu. in a specified way — see MOUTH BREATHER

breathing tube *n* : ENDOTRACHEAL TUBE

breath·less \'breth-ləs\ *adj* **1** : panting or gasping for breath **2** : suffering from dyspnea

¹breech \'brēch\ *n* **1** : the hind end of the body : BUTTOCKS **2** : BREECH PRESENTATION; *also* : a fetus that is presented at the uterine cervix buttocks or legs first

²breech *adv* : in the manner of a breech delivery or breech presentation ⟨her children were born ~ —Laura Cunningham⟩ ⟨the baby birthed ~ —Jayne Anne Phillips⟩

breech delivery *n* : delivery of a fetus by breech presentation — called also *breech birth*

breech presentation *n* : presentation of the fetus in which the buttocks or legs are the first parts to appear at the uterine cervix

¹breed \'brēd\ *vb* **bred** \'bred\; **breed·ing** *vt* **1** : to produce (offspring) by hatching or gestation **2** : to propagate (plants or animals) sexually and usu. under controlled conditions **3 a** : MATE **b** : to mate with : INSEMINATE **c** : IMPREGNATE **1** ~ *vi* **1 a** : to produce offspring by sexual union **b** : COPULATE, MATE **2** : to propagate animals or plants

²breed *n* : a group of animals or plants presumably related by descent from common ancestors and visibly similar in most characters; *esp* : such a group differentiated from the wild type under domestication

breed·er \'brē-dər\ *n* : one that breeds: as **a** : an animal or plant kept for propagation **b** : one engaged in the breeding of a specified organism

breg·ma \'breg-mə\ *n, pl* **-ma·ta** \-mət-ə\ : the point of junction of the coronal and sagittal sutures of the skull — **breg·mat·ic** \breg-'mat-ik\ *adj*

brei \'brī\ *n* : a finely and uniformly divided tissue suspension used esp. in metabolic experimentation

bre·tyl·i·um \brə-'til-ē-əm\ *n* : an antiarrhythmic drug administered in the form of its tosylate $C_{18}H_{24}BrNO_3S$ in the treatment of ventricular fibrillation and tachycardia and formerly used as an antihypertensive

brevia — see VASA BREVIA

brevis — see ABDUCTOR POLLICIS BREVIS, ADDUCTOR BREVIS, EXTENSOR CARPI RADIALIS BREVIS, EXTENSOR DIGITORUM BREVIS, EXTENSOR HALLUCIS BREVIS, EXTENSOR POLLICIS BREVIS, FLEXOR DIGITI MINIMI BREVIS, FLEXOR DIGITORUM BREVIS, FLEXOR HALLUCIS BREVIS, FLEXOR POLLICIS BREVIS, PALMARIS BREVIS, PERONEUS BREVIS

brew·er's yeast \'brü-ərz-\ *n* : the dried pulverized cells of a yeast of the genus *Saccharomyces* (*S. cerevisiae*) used in brewing and esp. as a source of B-complex vitamins

BRI *abbr* building-related illness

bridge \'brij\ *n* **1 a** : the upper bony part of the nose **b** : the curved part of a pair of glasses that rests upon this part of the nose **2 a** : PONS **b** : a strand of protoplasm extending between two cells **c** : a partial denture held in place by anchorage to adjacent teeth **d** : a connection (as an atom or group of atoms) that joins two different parts of a molecule (as opposite sides of a ring) **e** : an area of physical continuity between two chromatids persisting during the later phases of mitosis and constituting a possible source of somatic genetic change

bridge·work \-ˌwərk\ *n* : dental bridges; *also* : prosthodontics concerned with their construction

---

\ə\ abut \ᵊ\ kitten \ər\ **further** \a\ **ash** \ā\ **ace** \ä\ **cot, cart**
\au̇\ **out** \ch\ **chin** \e\ **bet** \ē\ **easy** \g\ **go** \i\ **hit** \ī\ **ice** \j\ **job**
\ŋ\ **sing** \ō\ **go** \ȯ\ **law** \ȯi\ **boy** \th\ **thin** \t͟h\ **the** \ü\ **loot**
\u̇\ **foot** \y\ **yet** \zh\ **vision** *See also* Pronunciation Symbols page

bri·dle \'brīd-ºl\ *n* : FRENULUM

bright·ness \'brīt-nəs\ *n* : the one of the three psychological dimensions of color perception by which visual stimuli are ordered continuously from light to dark and which is correlated with light intensity — compare HUE, SATURATION 4a

Bright's disease \'brīts-\ *n* : any of several kidney diseases marked esp. by albumin in the urine

   Bright, Richard (1789–1858), British internist and pathologist. One of the foremost physicians of his day, Bright was particularly interested in diseases of the pancreas, duodenum, liver, and especially the kidneys. In 1827 he published an important work on kidney disease describing the association between diseased kidneys, dropsy, and albuminous urine. His name is associated with a group of diseases characterized by urine of this type.

bril·liant green \'bril-yənt-\ *n, often cap B&G* : a basic triphenylmethane dye used in culture media and in triple dye

Brill's disease \'brilz-\ *n* : an acute infectious disease milder than epidemic typhus but caused by the same rickettsia

   Brill, Nathan Edwin (1860–1925), American physician. In 1910, after studying 221 cases, Brill published the first description of the disease now known as Brill's disease.

brim·stone \'brim-ˌstōn\ *n* : SULFUR

Bri·nell hardness \brə-ˌnel-\ *n* : the hardness of a metal or alloy measured by hydraulically pressing a hard ball under a standard load into the specimen

   Brinell, Johan August (1849–1925), Swedish engineer. After studying the internal composition of steel during cooling and heating, Brinell devised his hardness test, which was first displayed in 1900 at the Paris Exposition.

Brinell hardness number *n* : a number expressing Brinell hardness and denoting the load applied in testing in kilograms divided by the spherical area of indentation produced in the specimen in square millimeters

bring up \(ˈ)briŋ-ˈəp\ *vt* : VOMIT

bris·ket \'bris-kət\ *n* : the breast or lower chest of a quadruped animal

bris·tle \'bris-əl\ *n* : a short stiff coarse hair or filament

Brit·ish an·ti·lew·is·ite \'brit-ish-ˌant-ē-ˈlü-ə-ˌsīt, -ˌan-ˌtī-\ *n* : DIMERCAPROL

   W. L. Lewis — see LEWISITE

British thermal unit *n* : the quantity of heat required to raise the temperature of one pound of water one degree Fahrenheit at a specified temperature (as 39°F) — abbr. *Btu*

brit·tle \'brit-ºl\ *adj* : affected with or being a form of type 1 diabetes characterized by large and unpredictable fluctuations in blood glucose level ⟨∼ diabetes⟩ ⟨a ∼ diabetic⟩

¹**broach** \'brōch\ *n* : a fine tapered flexible instrument used in dentistry to remove dental pulp and to dress a root canal

²**broach** *vt* : to open (a vein) to draw blood

broad bean \'brȯd-ˌbēn\ *n* : the large flat edible seed of an Old World upright vetch (*Vicia faba*); *also* : this plant widely grown for its seeds and as fodder — called also *fava bean;* see FAVISM

broad ligament *n* : either of the two lateral ligaments of the uterus composed of a double sheet of peritoneum, passing from the sides of the uterus to the side walls of the pelvis, giving passage between the two layers of each ligament to the uterine tubes, blood vessels, and the epoophoron and paroophoron, and bearing the ovary suspended from the dorsal surface

broad–spectrum *adj* : effective against a wide range of organisms (as insects or bacteria) ⟨∼ antibiotics⟩ — compare NARROW-SPECTRUM

Bro·ca's aphasia \(ˌ)brō-ˌkäz-, ˌbrō-kəz-\ *n* : MOTOR APHASIA

   Bro·ca \brȯ-kä\, **Pierre–Paul (1824–1880)**, French surgeon and anthropologist. One of the great French anthropologists, Broca founded modern craniometry and made extensive comparative studies of the craniums and brains of the races of humankind. In 1861 he announced his discovery that the center of articulate speech is usually in the third left frontal convolution of the brain—an area now most commonly known as Broca's area. His discovery furnished

the first anatomical proof of localization of brain function. He associated loss of the power of speech with brain lesions, a condition that is now commonly termed motor aphasia or Broca's aphasia.

Broca's area *n* : a brain center associated with the motor control of speech and usu. located in the left but sometimes in the right inferior frontal gyrus — called also *Broca's convolution, Broca's gyrus, convolution of Broca*

Broca scale *n* : a color chart for rating skin color

Broca's point *n* : the midpoint of the external auditory canal

Brod·mann area \'bräd-mən-\ *or* **Brod·mann's area** \-mənz-\ *n* : one of the several structurally distinguishable and presumably functionally distinct regions into which the cortex of each cerebral hemisphere can be divided

   Brod·mann \'brȯt-ˌmän, 'bräd-mən\, **Korbinian (1868–1918)**, German neurologist. Brodmann was a pioneer in the study of the comparative cellular structure of the mammalian cortex. In 1909 he published a book that remains the only comprehensive work on the subject. The occipital and preoccipital areas (now known as the Brodmann areas) of the cerebral cortex were first described by him in 1908.

broke *past of* BREAK

bro·ken \'brō-kən\ *adj* : having undergone or been subjected to fracture ⟨a ∼ leg⟩

broken wind *n* : HEAVES 1

bro·ken–wind·ed \-'wind-əd\ *adj* : affected with heaves

bromacetone *var of* BROMOACETONE

¹**bro·mate** \'brō-ˌmāt\ *n* : a salt of bromic acid

²**bromate** *vt* **bro·mat·ed; bro·mat·ing** : to treat with a bromate; *broadly* : BROMINATE

bro·me·lain *also* **bro·me·lin** \'brō-mə-lən\ *n* : a protease obtained from the juice of the pineapple

brom·hi·dro·sis \ˌbrō-mə-'drō-səs *also* ˌbrōm-hə-\ *also* **bro·mi·dro·sis** \ˌbrō-mə-\ *n, pl* **-dro·ses** \-ˌsēz\ : foul-smelling sweat

bro·mic acid \'brō-mik-\ *n* : an unstable strongly oxidizing acid $HBrO_3$ known only in solution or in the form of its salts

bro·mide \'brō-ˌmīd\ *n* **1** : a binary compound of bromine with another element or a radical including some (as potassium bromide) used as sedatives **2** : a dose of bromide taken usu. as a sedative

bro·mi·nate \'brō-mə-ˌnāt\ *vt* **-nat·ed; -nat·ing** : to treat or cause to combine with bromine or a compound of bromine — **bro·mi·na·tion** \ˌbrō-mə-'nā-shən\ *n*

bro·mine \'brō-ˌmēn\ *n* : a nonmetallic halogen element that is isolated as a deep red corrosive toxic fuming liquid of disagreeable odor — symbol *Br*; see ELEMENT table

bro·min·ism \'brō-mə-ˌniz-əm\ *n* : BROMISM

bro·mism \'brō-ˌmiz-əm\ *n* : an abnormal state due to excessive or prolonged use of bromides

bro·mo \'brō-(ˌ)mō\ *n, pl* **bromos** : a dose of a proprietary effervescent mixture used as a headache remedy, sedative, and antacid; *also* : such a proprietary product

bro·mo·ac·e·tone \ˌbrō-mō-'as-ə-ˌtōn\ *also* **brom·ac·e·tone** \(ˈ)brō-'mas-ə-ˌtōn\ *n* : a colorless lacrimatory not very stable liquid compound C_3H_5OBr

bro·mo·ben·zyl cyanide \ˌbrō-mō-ˌben-ˌzēl-, -ˌzəl-\ *also* **brom·ben·zyl cyanide** \ˌbrōm-ˌben-\ *n* : a light-yellow oily lacrimatory compound C_8H_6BrN having an odor of sour fruit

bro·mo·cre·sol green \ˌbrō-mō-ˌkrē-ˌsȯl-, -ˌsȯl-\ *also* **brom·cre·sol green** \ˌbrōm-ˌkrē-\ *n* : a brominated acid dye that is obtained as a yellowish crystalline powder and is used as an acid-base indicator

bro·mo·crip·tine \ˌbrō-mō-'krip-ˌtēn\ *n* : a polypeptide alkaloid $C_{32}H_{40}BrN_5O_5$ that is a derivative of ergot and mimics the activity of dopamine in selectively inhibiting prolactin secretion

bro·mo·de·oxy·ur·i·dine \ˌbrō-mō-ˌdē-ˌäk-sē-'yùr-ə-ˌdēn, -dən\ *or* **5–bro·mo·de·oxy·ur·i·dine** \'fīv-\ *n* : a mutagenic analog $C_9H_{11}O_5NBr$ of thymidine that induces chromosomal breakage esp. in heterochromatic regions and has been used to selectively destroy actively dividing cells — abbr. *BUdR*

bro·mo·der·ma \'brō-mə-,dər-mə\ *n* : a skin eruption caused in susceptible persons by the use of bromides

bro·mo·phe·nol blue \,brō-mō-,fē-,nōl-, -,nól-, -fi-\ *also* **brom·phe·nol blue** \(,)brōm-\ *n* : a dye $C_{19}H_{10}Br_4O_5S$ obtained as pinkish crystals and used as an acid-base indicator

bro·mo·ura·cil \,brō-mō-'yùr-ə-,sil, -səl\ *n* : a mutagenic uracil derivative $C_4H_3N_2O_2Br$ that is an analog of thymine and pairs readily with adenine and sometimes with guanine during bacterial or bacteriophage DNA synthesis

brom·phen·ir·a·mine \,brōm-fen-'ir-ə-,mēn, -fən-\ *n* : an H_1 antagonist of histamine administered in the form of its maleate $C_{16}H_{19}BrN_2·C_4H_4O_4$ esp. to treat allergies and the common cold

bronchi *pl of* BRONCHUS

bron·chi·al \'brän-kē-əl\ *adj* : of or relating to the bronchi or their ramifications in the lungs — **bron·chi·al·ly** \-ə-lē\ *adv*

bronchial artery *n* : any branch of the descending aorta or first intercostal artery that accompanies the bronchi

bronchial asthma *n* : asthma resulting from spasmodic contraction of bronchial muscles

bronchial gland *n* : any of the lymphatic glands situated at the bifurcation of the trachea and along the bronchi

bronchial pneumonia *n* : BRONCHOPNEUMONIA

bronchial tree *n* : the bronchi together with their branches

bronchial tube *n* : a primary bronchus; *also* : any of its branches

bronchial vein *n* : any vein accompanying the bronchi and their branches and emptying into the azygos and superior intercostal veins

bron·chi·ec·ta·sis \,brän-kē-'ek-tə-səs\ *also* **bron·chi·ec·ta·sia** \-ek-'tā-zh(ē-)ə\ *n, pl* **-ta·ses** \-,sēz\ *also* **-ta·sias** \-zh(ē-)əz\ : a chronic inflammatory or degenerative condition of one or more bronchi or bronchioles marked by dilatation and loss of elasticity of the walls — **bron·chi·ec·tat·ic** \-ek-'tat-ik\ *adj*

bron·chio·gen·ic \,brän-kē-ō-'jen-ik\ *adj* : BRONCHOGENIC

bron·chi·ole \'brän-kē-,ōl\ *n* : a minute thin-walled branch of a bronchus — **bron·chi·o·lar** \,brän-kē-'ō-lər\ *adj*

bron·chi·ol·ec·ta·sis \,brän-kē-ō-'lek-tə-səs\ *n, pl* **-ta·ses** \-,sēz\ : dilatation of the bronchioles

bron·chi·ol·itis \-ō-'līt-əs\ *n* : inflammation of the bronchioles

bronchiolitis ob·lit·er·ans \-ə-'blit-ə-,ranz\ *n* : a pathological process producing obstruction of the bronchioles due to inflammation and fibrosis and occurring as a complication of various lung conditions (as some forms of pneumonia) or physiological insults (as inhalation of a toxic substance)

bron·chi·o·lus \brän-'kī-ə-ləs\ *n, pl* **-o·li** \-,lī\ : BRONCHIOLE

bron·chi·tis \brän-'kīt-əs, bräŋ-\ *n* : acute or chronic inflammation of the bronchial tubes; *also* : a disease marked by this — **bron·chit·ic** \-'kit-ik\ *adj*

bron·chi·um \'brän-kē-əm\ *n, pl* **bron·chia** \-kē-ə\ : a branch of a bronchus; *esp* : one joining a primary bronchus to its bronchioles

bron·cho·al·ve·o·lar \,brän-kō-al-'vē-ə-lər\ *adj* : of, relating to, or involving the bronchioles and alveoli of the lungs ⟨~ lavage as a diagnostic technique⟩

bron·cho·con·stric·tion \,brän-kō-kən-'strik-shən\ *n* : constriction of the bronchial air passages — **bron·cho·con·stric·tive** \-tiv\ *adj*

[1]**bron·cho·con·stric·tor** \-'strik-tər\ *adj* : causing or involving bronchoconstriction ⟨~ effects⟩ ⟨~ responses⟩

[2]**bronchoconstrictor** *n* : a drug or natural substance in the body causing bronchoconstriction

bron·cho·di·la·ta·tion \,brän-kō-,dil-ə-'tā-shən, -,dī-lə-\ *n* : BRONCHODILATION

bron·cho·di·la·tion \-dī-'lā-shən\ *n* : expansion of the bronchial air passages

[1]**bron·cho·di·la·tor** \-dī-'lāt-ər, -'dī,lāt-\ *also* **bron·cho·di·la·to·ry** \-dī-'lāt-ə-rē\ *adj* : relating to or causing expansion of the bronchial air passages ⟨~ activity⟩ ⟨~ drugs⟩

[2]**bronchodilator** *n* : a drug that relaxes bronchial muscle resulting in expansion of the bronchial air passages

bron·cho·gen·ic \,brän-kə-'jen-ik\ *adj* : of, relating to, or arising in or by way of the air passages of the lungs ⟨~ carcinoma⟩

bron·cho·gram \'brän-kə-,gram, -kō-\ *n* : a radiograph of the bronchial tree after injection of a radiopaque substance

bron·chog·ra·phy \brän-'käg-rə-fē, bräŋ-\ *n, pl* **-phies** : the radiographic visualization of the bronchi and their branches after injection of a radiopaque substance — **bron·cho·graph·ic** \,brän-kə-'graf-ik\ *adj*

bron·cho·li·thi·a·sis \,brän-kō-(,)kō-lə-'thī-ə-səs\ *n, pl* **-a·ses** \-,sēz\ : a condition in which concretions are present in a bronchus

bron·cho·mo·ni·li·a·sis \-,mō-nə-'lī-ə-səs, -,män-ə-\ *n, pl* **-a·ses** \-,sēz\ : infection of the bronchi with fungi of the genus *Candida*

bron·cho·mo·tor \'brän-kō-,mōt-ər\ *adj* : relating to or affecting contraction or dilation of the bronchial air passages ⟨~ activity⟩

bron·cho·my·co·sis \,brän-kō-mī-'kō-səs\ *n, pl* **-co·ses** \-,sēz\ : any bronchial disease caused by a fungus (as of the genus *Candida*)

bron·choph·o·ny \brän-'käf-ə-nē\ *n, pl* **-nies** : the sound of the voice heard through the stethoscope over a healthy bronchus and over other portions of the chest in cases of consolidation of the lung tissue — compare PECTORILOQUY

bron·cho·plas·ty \'brän-kə-,plas-tē\ *n, pl* **-ties** : surgical repair of a bronchial defect

bron·cho·pleu·ral \,brän-kō-'plùr-əl\ *adj* : joining a bronchus and the pleural cavity ⟨a ~ fistula⟩

bron·cho·pneu·mo·nia \,brän-(,)kō-n(y)ù-'mō-nyə\ *n* : pneumonia involving many relatively small areas of lung tissue — called also *bronchial pneumonia, lobular pneumonia* — **bron·cho·pneu·mon·ic** \-'män-ik\ *adj*

bron·cho·pul·mo·nary \,brän-kō-'pùl-mə-,ner-ē, -'pəl-\ *adj* : of, relating to, or affecting the bronchi and the lungs ⟨~ disease⟩ ⟨~ tissue⟩

bronchopulmonary dysplasia *n* : a chronic lung condition that is caused by tissue damage to the lungs, is marked by inflammation, exudate, scarring, fibrosis, and emphysema, and usu. occurs in immature infants who have received mechanical ventilation and supplemental oxygen as treatment for respiratory distress syndrome

bron·chor·rhea *or chiefly Brit* **bron·chor·rhoea** \,brän-kə-'rē-ə\ *n* : the excessive discharge of mucus from the air passages of the lung

bron·cho·scope \'brän-kə-,skōp\ *n* : a usu. flexible endoscope for inspecting and passing instruments into the bronchi (as to obtain tissue for biopsy)

bron·cho·scop·ic \,brän-kə-'skäp-ik\ *adj* : of, relating to, or performed by bronchoscopy or the use of a bronchoscope ⟨a ~ biopsy⟩

bron·chos·co·pist \brän-'käs-kə-pəst, bräŋ-\ *n* : a physician trained in the use of the bronchoscope or in the performance of bronchoscopy

bron·chos·co·py \brän-'käs-kə-pē, bräŋ-\ *n, pl* **-pies** : the use of a bronchoscope in the examination or treatment of the bronchi

bron·cho·spasm \'brän-kə-,spaz-əm\ *n* : constriction of the air passages of the lung (as in asthma) by spasmodic contraction of the bronchial muscles — **bron·cho·spas·tic** \,brän-kə-'spas-tik\ *adj*

bron·cho·spi·rom·e·try \,brän-kō-spī-'räm-ə-trē\ *n, pl* **-tries** : independent measurement of the vital capacity of each lung by means of a spirometer in direct continuity with one of the primary bronchi — **bron·cho·spi·rom·e·ter** \-'räm-ət-ər\ *n* — **bron·cho·spi·ro·met·ric** \-,spī-rə-'me-trik\ *adj*

bron·cho·ste·no·sis \,brän-kō-stə-'nō-səs\ *n, pl* **-no·ses** \-,sēz\ : stenosis of a bronchus

bron·chus \'brän-kəs\ *n, pl* **bron·chi** \'brän-,kī, -,kē\ : either of the two primary divisions of the trachea that lead respectively into the right and the left lung; *broadly* : BRONCHIAL TUBE

bron·to·pho·bia \ˌbränt-ə-'fō-bē-ə\ *n* : abnormal fear of thunder

¹brood \'brüd\ *n* : the young of an animal or a family of young; *esp* : the young (as of a bird or insect) hatched or cared for at one time

²brood *vt* **1 a** : to sit on or incubate (eggs) **b** : to produce by or as if by incubation **2** : to think anxiously or gloomily about ∼ *vi* **1** *of a bird* : to brood eggs or young **2 a** : to dwell gloomily on a subject **b** : to be in a state of depression

broom \'brüm, 'brùm\ *n* : any of various leguminous shrubs (esp. genera *Cytisus* and *Genista*) with long slender branches, upright growth, small leaves, and usu. showy yellow flowers; *esp* : SCOTCH BROOM — see BROOM TOP

broom top *n* : the almost leafless branches of the Scotch broom (*Cytisus scoparius*) that contain the alkaloid sparteine; *esp* : these tops prepared for pharmaceutical use — usu. used in pl.

broth \'bròth\ *n, pl* **broths** \'bròths, 'bròthz\ **1** : liquid in which meat or sometimes vegetable food has been cooked **2** : a fluid culture medium

brow \'braú\ *n* **1** : EYEBROW **2** : either of the lateral prominences of the forehead **3** : FOREHEAD

brown adipose tissue *n* : BROWN FAT

brown alga *n* : any of a major taxonomic group (Phaeophyta) of variable mostly marine algae (as a laminaria) with chlorophyll masked by brown pigment — see ALGIN, LAMINARIN

brown dog tick *n* : a widely distributed reddish brown tick of the genus *Rhipicephalus* (*R. sanguineus*) that occurs on dogs and other mammals and on some birds and that transmits canine babesiosis and possibly other diseases

brown fat *n* : a mammalian heat-producing tissue occurring esp. in human fetuses and newborn infants and in hibernating animals — called also *brown adipose tissue*

Brown·ian motion \ˌbraú-nē-ən-\ *n* : a random movement of microscopic particles suspended in liquids or gases resulting from the impact of molecules of the fluid surrounding the particles — called also *Brownian movement*

Brown \'braún\, **Robert (1773–1858)**, British botanist. Brown was one of the leading botanists of his day. In 1801 he accompanied a surveying expedition to and around Australia, acting as the company's naturalist. In 1805 he returned to Great Britain with about 3,900 species of plants, and in 1810 he published a great work on the flora of Australia. In the field of botany he is also known for his substantial contributions to plant morphology, embryology, and geography, for improving plant classification and making a fundamental distinction between gymnosperms and angiosperms, for establishing and defining new families and genera, and for describing and naming the nucleus of a plant cell. He published his observations on Brownian motion in 1831.

brown lung disease *n* : BYSSINOSIS — called also *brown lung*

brown rat *n* : a common domestic rat of the genus *Rattus* (*R. norvegicus*) that has been introduced worldwide — called also *Norway rat*

brown recluse spider *n* : a venomous spider of the genus *Loxosceles* (*L. reclusa*) introduced esp. into the southern and central U.S. that produces a dangerous cytotoxin which can cause necrotic lesions — called also *brown recluse*

brown snake *n* : any of several Australian venomous elapid snakes esp. of the genus *Demansia*; *esp* : a widely distributed brownish or blackish snake (*D. textilis*)

brow·ridge \'braú-ˌrij\ *n* : SUPERCILIARY RIDGE

BRP *abbr* bathroom privileges

bru·cel·la \brü-'sel-ə\ *n* **1** *cap* : a genus of nonmotile capsulated bacteria of the family Brucellaceae that cause disease in humans and domestic animals **2** *pl* **-cel·lae** \-'sel-(ˌ)ē\ *or* **-cel·las** : any bacterium of the genus *Brucella*

Bruce \'brüs\, **Sir David (1855–1931)**, British bacteriologist. While on the island of Malta in 1886, Bruce discovered the bacterial cause of undulant or Malta fever; he reported his findings the following year. He called the causal organism *Micrococcus melitensis* but in 1920 the genus was renamed *Brucella* in his honor. Also, the disease caused by bacteria of this genus is now usually known as brucellosis. Bruce later did extensive research on trypanosomiasis. In 1894 he investigated nagana in Zululand, and in 1903 he started his investigation of sleeping sickness in Uganda.

Bru·cel·la·ce·ae \ˌbrü-sə-'lā-sē-ˌē\ *n pl* : a family of small gram-negative coccoid to rod-shaped bacteria of the order Eubacteriales that are obligate parasites chiefly of warmᵇblooded vertebrates and that include a number of serious pathogens — see BRUCELLA

bru·cel·lin \brü-'sel-ən\ *n* : a cell-free polysaccharideᵇcontaining culture filtrate of brucellae used in skin tests to detect the presence of brucella infections

bru·cel·lo·sis \ˌbrü-sə-'lō-səs\ *n, pl* **-lo·ses** \-ˌsēz\ : a disease caused by bacteria of the genus *Brucella*: **a** : a disease of humans of sudden or insidious onset and long duration caused by any of four organisms (*Brucella melitensis* of goats, *B. suis* of hogs and rarely cattle, *B. abortus* of cattle and rarely hogs, and *B. canis* of dogs), characterized by great weakness, extreme exhaustion on slight effort, night sweats, chills, remittent fever, and generalized aches and pains, and acquired through direct contact with infected animals or animal products or from the consumption of milk, dairy products, or meat from infected animals — called also *Malta fever, undulant fever* **b** : CONTAGIOUS ABORTION

bru·cine \'brü-ˌsēn\ *n* : a poisonous alkaloid $C_{23}H_{26}N_2O_4$ found with strychnine esp. in nux vomica

Bruce \'brüs\, **James (1730–1794)**, British explorer. Bruce is famous primarily for his journey in 1768–1773 to the source of the Blue Nile in Ethiopia. In the course of his travels he encountered a new tree (*Brucea antidysenterica*) and introduced the seeds to Great Britain. In 1779 the genus containing this tree was named in his honor. In 1819 a new alkaloid was isolated from a sample of bark erroneously thought to be from this tree. The alkaloid was called brucine after the botanist although it was later discovered that the bark was actually from the nux vomica.

Brud·zin·ski sign \brü-'jin-skē-, brüd-'zin-\ *or* **Brud·zin·ski's sign** \-skē(z)-\ *n* : any of several symptoms of meningeal irritation occurring esp. in meningitis: as **a** : flexion of the lower limbs induced by passive flexion of the head on the chest **b** : flexion of one lower limb following passive flexion of the other

Brudzinski, Josef (1874–1917), Polish physician. Brudzinski described in 1908 a sign of meningitis in which the passive flexion of one lower limb results in a contralateral reflex in the other. In 1909 he described another sign of meningitis: a bending of the neck results in flexure movements of the ankle, knee, and hip.

¹bruise \'brüz\ *vb* **bruised; bruis·ing** *vt* **1** : to inflict a bruise on : CONTUSE **2** : WOUND, INJURE; *esp* : to inflict psychological hurt on ∼ *vi* : to undergo bruising ⟨she ∼s easily⟩

²bruise *n* **1** : an injury transmitted through unbroken skin to underlying tissue causing rupture of small blood vessels and escape of blood into the tissue with resulting discoloration : CONTUSION **2** : an injury esp. to the feelings

bruit \'brü-ē\ *n* : any of several generally abnormal sounds heard on auscultation ⟨an audible ∼ produced by an artery⟩

Brun·ner's gland \'brùn-ərz-\ *n* : any of the compound racemose glands in the submucous layer of the duodenum that secrete alkaline mucus and a potent proteolytic enzyme — called also *duodenal gland, gland of Brunner*

Brunner, Johann Conrad (1653–1727), Swiss anatomist. Brunner is known for his work on the pancreas and duodenum. In 1683 he made pioneering experimental excisions of the spleen and pancreas in dogs and noted the resultant extreme thirst and polyuria. In 1672 he discovered the glands of the duodenum that bear his name and published a report on them in 1688. He believed that the glands secreted a

A
B

juice similar to that of the pancreas and that they played a chief role in intestinal digestion.

Brunn's membrane \\'brünz-\ *n* : the part of the nasal mucous membrane that serves as an organ of smell

Brunn, Albert von (1849–1895), German anatomist. Brunn described the membrane that bears his name in *Senseorgans,* a posthumous work published in 1897.

brush border \\,brəsh-\ *n* : a stria of microvilli on the plasma membrane of an epithelial cell (as in a kidney tubule) that is specialized for absorption

brux·ism \\'brək-,siz-əm\ *n* : the habit of unconsciously gritting or grinding the teeth esp. in situations of stress or during sleep

bruxo·ma·nia \\,brək-sō-'mā-nē-ə, -nyə\ *n* : BRUXISM

bry·o·nia \\brī-'ō-nē-ə\ *n* **1** *cap* : a small genus of perennial Old World tendril-bearing vines (family Cucurbitaceae) with red or black fruit — see BRYONY **2** : the dried root of a bryony (*Bryonia alba* or *B. dioica*) used as a cathartic

bry·o·ny \\'brī-ə-nē\ *n, pl* **-nies** : any plant of the genus *Bryonia*

BS *abbr* **1** bowel sounds **2** breath sounds

BSE *abbr* bovine spongiform encephalopathy

BSN *abbr* bachelor of science in nursing

BST *abbr* blood serological test

BT *abbr* **1** bedtime **2** brain tumor

Btu *abbr* British thermal unit

bub·ble boy disease \\'bəb-əl-'bȯi-\ *n* : SEVERE COMBINED IMMUNODEFICIENCY

bu·bo \\'b(y)ü-(,)bō\ *n, pl* **buboes** : an inflammatory swelling of a lymph node esp. in the groin — **bu·bon·ic** \\b(y)ü-'bän-ik\ *adj*

bubonic plague *n* : plague caused by a bacterium of the genus *Yersinia* (*Y. pestis* syn. *Pasteurella pestis*) and characterized esp. by the formation of buboes — compare PNEUMONIC PLAGUE

bu·bon·o·cele \\b(y)ü-'bän-ə-,sēl\ *n* : an inguinal hernia; *esp* : a hernia in which the hernial pouch descends only as far as the groin and forms a swelling there like a bubo

bu·bon·u·lus \\b(y)ü-'bän-(y)ə-ləs\ *n, pl* **-li** \\-(,)lē, -,lī\ : a nodule or abscess formed in lymphangitis affecting the dorsal aspect of the penis

buc·ca \\'bək-ə\ *n, pl* **buc·cae** \\-(,)ē\ : CHEEK 1

buc·cal \\'bək-əl\ *adj* **1** : of, relating to, near, involving, or supplying a cheek ⟨the ~ surface of a tooth⟩ ⟨the ~ branch of the facial nerve⟩ **2** : of, relating to, involving, or lying in the mouth ⟨the ~ cavity⟩ — **buc·cal·ly** \\-ə-lē\ *adv*

buccal gland *n* : any of the small racemose mucous glands in the mucous membrane lining the cheeks

buc·ci·na·tor \\'bək-sə-,nāt-ər\ *n* : a thin broad muscle forming the wall of the cheek and serving to compress the cheek against the teeth and to retract the angle of the mouth — called also *buccinator muscle*

buc·co·lin·gual \\,bək-ō-'liŋ-g(yə-)wəl\ *adj* **1** : relating to or affecting the cheek and the tongue **2** : of or relating to the buccal and lingual aspects of a tooth ⟨the ~ width of a molar⟩ — **buc·co·lin·gual·ly** \\-g(yə-)wə-lē\ *adv*

buc·co·pha·ryn·geal \\-,far-ən-'jē-əl, -fə-'rin-j(ē-)əl\ *adj* : relating to or near the cheek and the pharynx ⟨the ~ fascia of the buccinator⟩

buccopharyngeal membrane *n* : a membrane in an early embryo composed of ectoderm and endoderm and separating the head end of the gut from the stomodeum — called also *oral membrane, oral plate, pharyngeal membrane*

Büch·ner funnel \\'bük-nər-\ *n* : a cylindrical often porcelain filtering funnel that has a perforated plate on which the filter paper is placed and that is used usu. with a vacuum

Büch·ner \\'buɛk-nər\, **Ernst,** German chemist. Büchner introduced his funnel in 1888.

bu·chu \\'b(y)ü-(,)k(y)ü\ *n* **1** : the dried leaves of various plants (genera *Barosma* and *Diosma* of the family Rutaceae) used as a diuretic and diaphoretic **2** : a plant that supplies buchu

buck·thorn \\'bək-,thȯ(ə)rn\ *n* : a shrub or tree of the genus *Rhamnus* sometimes having thorny branches and often containing purgative principles in bark or sap and producing fruits sometimes used as a source of yellow and green dyes or pigments — see CASCARA BUCKTHORN

buck·tooth \\-'tüth\ *n, pl* **buck·teeth** : a large projecting front tooth — **buck–toothed** \\-'tütht\ *adj*

¹bud \\'bəd\ *n* **1 a** : an asexual reproductive structure **b** : a primordium having potentialities for growth and development into a definitive structure ⟨an embryonic limb ~⟩ ⟨a horn ~⟩ **2** : an anatomical structure (as a tactile corpuscle) resembling a bud

²bud *vi* **bud·ded; bud·ding** : to reproduce asexually esp. by the pinching off of a small part of the parent

bu·des·o·nide \\,byü-'des-ō-,nīd\ *n* : an anti-inflammatory glucocorticoid $C_{25}H_{34}O_6$ used to treat both allergic and non-allergic rhinitis

BUdR *abbr* bromodeoxyuridine

Buer·ger's disease \\'bər-gərz-, 'bùr-\ *n* : thromboangiitis of the small arteries and veins of the extremities and esp. the feet resulting in occlusion, ischemia, and gangrene — called also *thromboangiitis obliterans*

Buerger, Leo (1879–1943), American pathologist. In 1908 Buerger published an article on thromboangiitis obliterans. He presented the first clear description of this disease and distinguished it from endarteritis obliterans.

bu·fa·gin \\'byü-fə-jən\ *n* : a toxic steroid $C_{24}H_{34}O_5$ obtained from the poisonous secretion of a skin gland on the back of the neck of a large toad (*Bufo marinus*) that resembles digitalis in physiological activity; *also* : any of several similar substances from secretions of other toads — compare BUFOTOXIN

¹buff·er \\'bəf-ər\ *n* **1** : a substance or mixture of substances (as bicarbonates and some proteins in biological fluids) that in solution tends to stabilize the hydrogen-ion concentration by neutralizing within limits both acids and bases **2** : BUFFER SOLUTION

²buffer *vt* : to treat (as a solution or its acidity) with a buffer; *also* : to prepare (aspirin) with an antacid

buffer solution *n* : a solution that usu. contains on the one hand either a weak acid (as carbonic acid) together with one of the salts of this acid or with at least one acid salt of a weak acid or on the other hand a weak base (as ammonia) together with one of the salts of the base and that by its resistance to changes in hydrogen-ion concentration on the addition of acid or base is useful in many chemical, biological, and technical processes

buffy coat \\'bəf-ē-\ *n* : the superficial layer of yellowish or buff coagulated plasma from which the red corpuscles have settled out in slowly coagulated blood

bu·fo \\'b(y)ü-(,)fō\ *n* **1** *cap* : a large genus (family Bufonidae) of toads that contains the common toads of America and Europe and is represented on all the continents except Australia **2** : any toad of the genus *Bufo*

bu·fo·gen·in \\,byü-fə-'jen-ən, byü-'fäj-ə-nən\ *n* : BUFAGIN

bu·fo·ta·lin \\,byü-fə-'tal-ən, -'tä-lən\ *n* : a toxic steroid $C_{26}H_{36}O_6$ obtained esp. from the skin glands of the common toad of Europe (*Bufo vulgaris*) — see BUFOTOXIN

bu·fo·ten·ine \\,byü-fə-'ten-,ēn, -ən\ *or* **bu·fo·ten·in** \\-ən\ *n* : a toxic hallucinogenic alkaloid $C_{12}H_{16}N_2O$ that is obtained esp. from poisonous secretions of toads and from some mushrooms and has hypertensive and vasoconstrictor activity

bu·fo·tox·in \\-'täk-sən\ *n* : a toxic steroid $C_{40}H_{60}N_4O_{10}$ obtained from the skin glands of the common toad of Europe (*Bufo vulgaris*) that resembles digitalis in physiological activity and yields bufotalin on hydrolysis; *also* : any of several similar steroids from the secretions of other toads — compare BUFAGIN

bug \\'bəg\ *n* **1 a** : an insect or other creeping or crawling invertebrate animal (as a spider) — not used technically **b**

\ə\ abut \ʰ\ kitten \ər\ further \a\ ash \ā\ ace \ä\ cot, cart
\aù\ out \ch\ chin \e\ bet \ē\ easy \g\ go \i\ hit \ī\ ice \j\ job
\ŋ\ sing \ō\ go \ȯ\ law \ȯi\ boy \th\ thin \t̲h̲\ the \ü\ loot
\ù\ foot \y\ yet \zh\ vision *See also* Pronunciation Symbols page

: any of various insects commonly considered esp. obnoxious: as (1) : BEDBUG (2) : COCKROACH (3) : HEAD LOUSE **c** : any of the order Hemiptera and esp. of its suborder Heteroptera of insects that have sucking mouthparts, forewings thickened at the base, and that lack a pupal stage between the immature stages and the adult — called also *true bug* **2 a** : a disease-producing microorganism and esp. a germ **b** : a disease caused by such microorganisms; *esp* : any of various respiratory conditions (as influenza or grippe) of virus origin

bug·bane \ˈbəg-ˌbān\ *n* : a plant of the genus *Cimicifuga*; *esp* : BLACK COHOSH

bug·gery \ˈbəg-ə-rē\ *n, pl* **-ger·ies** : SODOMY

bu·gle·weed \ˈbyü-gəl-ˌwēd\ *n* : any mint of the genus *Lycopus*; *esp* : a mildly narcotic and astringent herb (*L. virginicus*) of the eastern half of the U.S.

building–related illness \ˈbil-diŋ-ri-ˌlāt-əd-\ *n* : a clinically diagnosable disease or condition (as Legionnaires' disease or an allergic reaction) caused by a microorganism or substance demonstrably present in a building — abbr. *BRI*; compare SICK BUILDING SYNDROME

bulb \ˈbəlb\ *n* **1** : a rounded dilation or expansion of something cylindrical ⟨the ∼ of a thermometer⟩; *esp* : a rounded or pear-shaped enlargement on a small base ⟨the ∼ of an eyedropper⟩ **2** : a rounded part: as **a** : a rounded enlargement of one end of a part — see BULB OF THE PENIS, BULB OF THE VESTIBULE, END BULB, HAIR BULB, OLFACTORY BULB **b** : MEDULLA OBLONGATA; *broadly* : the hindbrain exclusive of the cerebellum **c** : a thick-walled muscular enlargement of the pharynx of certain nematode worms

bul·bar \ˈbəl-bər, -ˌbär\ *adj* : of or relating to a bulb; *specif* : involving the medulla oblongata

bulbar paralysis *n* : destruction of nerve centers of the medulla oblongata and paralysis of the parts innervated from the medulla with interruption of their functions (as swallowing or speech)

bulbi *pl of* BULBUS

bulbi — see PHTHISIS BULBI

bul·bo·cap·nine \ˌbəl-bō-ˈkap-ˌnēn, -nən\ *n* : a crystalline alkaloid $C_{19}H_{19}NO_4$ that induces catalepsy and that is obtained from the roots of plants of the genus *Corydalis* and from squirrel corn

bul·bo·cav·er·no·sus \ˌbəl-(ˌ)bō-ˌkav-ər-ˈnō-səs\ *n, pl* **-no·si** \-ˌsī\ : a muscle that in the male surrounds and compresses the bulb of the penis and the bulbar portion of the urethra and in the female divides into lateral halves that extend from immediately behind the clitoris along either side of the vagina to the central tendon of the perineum and serve to compress the vagina — see SPHINCTER VAGINAE

bul·bo·cav·er·nous \-ˈkav-ər-nəs\ *adj* : of, relating to, or located near the bulb of the penis

bulb of the penis *n* : the proximal expanded part of the corpus cavernosum of the male urethra

bulb of the vestibule *n* : a structure in the female vulva that is homologous to the bulb of the penis and the adjoining corpus spongiosum in the male and that consists of an elongated mass of erectile tissue on each side of the vaginal opening united anteriorly to the contralateral mass by a narrow median band passing along the lower surface of the clitoris

bul·bo·spi·nal \ˌbəl-bō-ˈspīn-ᵊl\ *adj* : of, relating to, or interconnecting the medulla oblongata and the spinal cord ⟨∼ nerve fibers⟩

bul·bo·spon·gi·o·sus muscle \ˌbəl-(ˌ)bō-ˌspən-jē-ˈō-səs-\ *n* : BULBOCAVERNOSUS

bul·bo·ure·thral \-yù-ˈrē-thrəl\ *adj* : of or relating to the bulb of the penis and the urethra

bulbourethral gland *n* : COWPER'S GLAND

bul·bous \ˈbəl-bəs\ *adj* : resembling a bulb esp. in roundness or the gross enlargement of a part ⟨the ∼ expansion at the base of a hair⟩

bul·bus \ˈbəl-bəs\ *n, pl* **bul·bi** \-ˌbī, -ˌbē\ : a bulb-shaped anatomical part

bu·lim·a·rex·ia \bü-ˌlim-ə-ˈrek-sē-ə, byü-, -ˌlē-mə-\ *n* : BULIMIA 2 — **bu·lim·a·rex·ic** \-sik\ *n or adj*

bu·lim·ia \byü-ˈlim-ē-ə, bü-, -ˈlē-mē-\ *also* **bou·lim·ia** \bü-\ *n* **1** : an abnormal and constant craving for food — called also *hyperorexia* **2** : a serious eating disorder that occurs chiefly in females, is characterized by compulsive overeating usu. followed by self-induced vomiting or laxative or diuretic abuse, and is often accompanied by guilt and depression

bulimia ner·vo·sa \-(ˌ)nər-ˈvō-sə, -zə\ *n* : BULIMIA 2

¹bu·lim·ic \-ˈlim-ik, -ˈlē-mik\ *adj* : of, relating to, or affected with bulimia ⟨∼ patients⟩

²bulimic *n* : an individual affected with bulimia

bulk \ˈbəlk\ *n* : material (as indigestible fibrous residues of food) that forms a mass in the intestine; *esp* : FIBER 2

bul·la \ˈbùl-ə\ *n, pl* **bul·lae** \ˈbùl-ˌē, -ˌī\ **1** : a hollow thin-walled rounded bony prominence **2** : a large vesicle or blister — compare BLEB

bul·late \ˈbùl-ˌāt\ *adj* : like or having a bulla

bull neck *n* : a thick short powerful neck — **bull·necked** \ˈbùl-ˈnekt\ *adj*

bull·nose \ˈbùl-ˌnōz\ *n* : a necrobacillosis arising in facial wounds of swine and characterized by swelling of the face, nose, and mouth and sloughing of the tissues

bullosa — see EPIDERMOLYSIS BULLOSA

bul·lous \ˈbùl-əs\ *adj* : resembling or characterized by bullae : VESICULAR ⟨∼ lesions⟩

bullous pemphigoid *n* : a chronic skin disease affecting esp. elderly individuals that is characterized by the formation of numerous hard blisters over a widespread area

bu·met·a·nide \byü-ˈmet-ə-ˌnīd\ *n* : a powerful diuretic $C_{17}H_{20}N_2O_5S$ used in the treatment of edema — see BUMEX

Bu·mex \ˈbyü-ˌmeks\ *trademark* — used for a preparation of bumetanide

BUN \ˌbē-ˌyü-ˈen\ *n* : the concentration of nitrogen in the form of urea in the blood

bun·dle \ˈbən-dᵊl\ *n* : a small band of mostly parallel fibers (as of nerve or muscle) : FASCICULUS, TRACT

bundle branch *n* : either of the parts of the bundle of His passing respectively to the right and left ventricles

bundle branch block *n* : heart block due to a lesion in one of the bundle branches

bundle of His \-ˈhis\ *n* : a slender bundle of modified cardiac muscle that passes from the atrioventricular node in the right atrium to the right and left ventricles by way of the septum and that maintains the normal sequence of the heartbeat by conducting the wave of excitation from the right atrium to the ventricles — called also *atrioventricular bundle, His bundle*

His, Wilhelm (1863–1934), German physician. A pioneer cardiologist, His was one of the first to recognize that the heartbeat originates in nodes of modified heart muscle. In 1893 he described the atrioventricular bundle, which is now often known as the bundle of His. He is also remembered for his description of trench fever in 1916, when it was a major medical problem.

bun·ga·ro·tox·in \ˈbəŋ-gə-rō-ˌtäk-sən\ *n* : a potent polypeptide neurotoxin that is obtained from krait venom and yields three electrophoretic fractions of which the one designated α is used esp. to label acetylcholine receptors at neuromuscular junctions because it binds irreversibly to them and blocks their activity — often used with one of the Greek prefixes α-, β-, or γ- to indicate the electrophoretic fractions

Bun·ga·rus \ˈbəŋ-ˌgä-rəs\ *n* : a genus of extremely venomous Asian snakes that include the kraits and are related to the cobras but have shorter fangs and are without a dilatable hood

bun·ion \ˈbən-yən\ *n* : an inflamed swelling of the small fluid-filled sac on the first joint of the big toe accompanied by enlargement and protrusion of the joint — compare HALLUX VALGUS

bun·ion·ec·to·my \ˌbən-yə-ˈnek-tə-mē\ *n, pl* **-mies** : surgical excision of a bunion

bu·no·dont \ˈbyü-nə-ˌdänt\ *adj* : having tubercles on the crown of the molar teeth — compare LOPHODONT

Bu·nos·to·mum \byü-ˈnäs-tə-məm\ *n* : a genus of nematode worms including the hookworms of sheep and cattle

Bun·sen burn·er \\'bən(t)-sən-ˌbər-nər\ *n* : a gas burner consisting typically of a straight tube with small holes at the bottom where air enters and mixes with the gas to produce an intensely hot blue flame

Bun·sen \\'bün-zən\, **Robert Wilhelm (1811–1899)**, German chemist. Bunsen is credited with a number of discoveries and inventions. In 1834 he discovered that freshly precipitated, hydrated ferric oxide is an antidote for arsenic poisoning. The most famous of his inventions, the Bunsen burner, was actually a minor refinement of inventions by Aimé Argand and Michael Faraday. Bunsen introduced his version in 1855.

Bun·ya·vi·ri·dae \ˌbən-yə-'vir-ə-ˌdē\ *n pl* : a family of single-stranded RNA viruses that are spherical to pleomorphic in shape with projections of glycoprotein embedded in a surface bilayer of lipid, that are usu. transmitted by the bite of an arthropod (as a mosquito) or in the bodily secretions of rodents, that infect vertebrates and arthropods, and that include the hantaviruses and the causative agents of Nairobi sheep disease, Rift Valley fever, sandfly fever, and some forms of encephalitis (as La Crosse encephalitis) and hemorrhagic fever — see PHLEBOVIRUS

bun·ya·vi·rus \\'bən-yə-ˌvī-rəs\ *n* **1** *cap* : a genus of numerous single-stranded RNA viruses (as the La Crosse virus) of the family *Bunyaviridae* that are usu. transmitted by mosquitoes or ticks **2** : any of the family *Bunyaviridae* of single-stranded RNA viruses

buph·thal·mos \b(y)üf-'thal-məs, ˌbəf-, -ˌmäs\ *also* **buph·thal·mia** \-mē-ə\ *n, pl* **-mos·es** *also* **-mias** : marked enlargement of the eye that is usu. congenital and attended by symptoms of glaucoma

bu·piv·a·caine \byü-'piv-ə-ˌkān\ *n* : a local anesthetic $C_{18}H_{28}N_2O$ that is like lidocaine in its action but is longer acting

bu·pre·nor·phine \ˌbyü-prə-'nor-ˌfēn, -fən\ *n* : a semisynthetic narcotic analgesic that is derived from thebaine and is administered in the form of its hydrochloride $C_{29}H_{41}NO_4 \cdot$ HCl intravenously or intramuscularly to treat moderate to severe pain and sublingually to treat opioid dependence

bu·pro·pi·on \byü-'prō-pē-ˌän, -ən\ *n* : a drug administered in the form of its hydrochloride $C_{13}H_{18}ClNO \cdot HCl$ as an antidepressant and as an aid to stop smoking usu. without the side effects of depressed libido and weight gain — see WELLBUTRIN, ZYBAN

bur \\'bər\ *n* **1** *usu* **burr** : a small surgical cutting tool (as for making an opening in bone) **2** : a bit used on a dental drill

bur·den \\'bərd-ᵊn\ *n* : LOAD 3 ⟨worm ∼⟩ ⟨cancer ∼⟩

bur·dock \\'bər-ˌdäk\ *n* : any of a genus (*Arctium*) of coarse composite herbs bearing globular flower heads with prickly bracts and including one (*A. lappa*) that is the source of lappa

bu·rette *or* **bu·ret** \byù-'ret\ *n* : a graduated glass tube with a small aperture and stopcock for delivering measured quantities of liquid or for measuring the liquid or gas received or discharged

Bur·kitt's lymphoma \ˌbər-kəts-\ *also* **Burkitt lymphoma** \-kət-\ *n* : a malignant lymphoma that affects primarily the upper and lower jaws, orbit, retroperitoneal tissues situated near the pancreas, kidneys, ovaries, testes, thyroid, adrenal glands, heart, and pleura, that occurs esp. in children of central Africa, and that is associated with Epstein-Barr virus

Burkitt, Denis Parsons (1911–1993), British surgeon. In 1957 while in Uganda, Burkitt identified for the first time the cancer that now bears his name. In 1970 he published a monograph entitled *Burkitt's Lymphoma*.

Burkitt's tumor *also* **Burkitt tumor** *n* : BURKITT'S LYMPHOMA

¹burn \\'bərn\ *vb* **burned** \\'bərnd, 'bərnt\ *or* **burnt** \\'bərnt\; **burn·ing** *vi* **1** : to produce or undergo discomfort or pain ⟨iodine ∼s so⟩ ⟨ears ∼ing from the cold⟩ **2** : to receive sunburn ⟨she ∼s easily⟩ ∼ *vt* : to injure or damage by exposure to fire, heat, or radiation ⟨∼ed his hand⟩

²burn *n* **1** : bodily injury resulting from exposure to heat, caustics, electricity, or some radiations, marked by varying degrees of skin destruction and hyperemia often with the formation of watery blisters and in severe cases by charring of the tissues, and classified according to the extent and degree of the injury — see FIRST-DEGREE BURN, SECOND-DEGREE BURN, THIRD-DEGREE BURN **2** : an abrasion having the appearance of a burn ⟨friction ∼s⟩ ⟨cold ∼⟩ **3** : a burning sensation ⟨the ∼ of iodine applied to a cut⟩

burn center *also* **burns center** *n* : a specialized facility usu. affiliated with a hospital that provides advanced care and treatment for patients with severe burn

burn·er \\'bər-nər\ *n* : STINGER 2

¹burn·ing \\'bər-niŋ\ *adj* **1** : affecting with or as if with heat ⟨a ∼ fever⟩ **2** : resembling that produced by a burn ⟨a ∼ sensation on the tongue⟩

²burning *n* : a sensation of being on fire or excessively heated ⟨gastric ∼⟩

burning mouth syndrome *n* : a chronic burning sensation of the oral mucous membranes esp. of the tongue that is typically accompanied by dryness of the mouth and disturbances in taste, that chiefly affects postmenopausal women, and that is of unknown cause

burn·out \\'bərn-ˌaùt\ *n* **1 a** : exhaustion of physical or emotional strength usu. as a result of prolonged stress or frustration **b** : a person affected with burnout **2** : a person showing the effects of drug abuse

Bu·row's solution \\'bü-(ˌ)rō(z)-\ *n* : a solution of the acetate of aluminum used as an antiseptic and astringent

Burow, Karl August von (1809–1874), German military surgeon and anatomist. In 1857 Burow introduced his solution which was originally compounded from alum and lead acetate. He is also known for his description of certain veins of the kidneys in 1835.

¹burp \\'bərp\ *n* : BELCH

²burp *vi* : BELCH ∼ *vt* : to help (a baby) expel gas from the stomach esp. by patting or rubbing the back

burr *var of* BUR

bur·row \\'bər-(ˌ)ō, 'bə-(ˌ)rō\ *n* : a passage or gallery formed in or under the skin by the wandering of a parasite (as the mite of scabies or a foreign hookworm) — **burrow** *vb*

bur·sa \\'bər-sə\ *n, pl* **bur·sas** \-səz\ *or* **bur·sae** \-ˌsē, -ˌsī\ : a bodily pouch or sac: as **a** : a small serous sac between a tendon and a bone **b** : BURSA OF FABRICIUS — **bur·sal** \-səl\ *adj*

bursa cop·u·la·trix \-ˌkäp-yə-'lā-triks\ *n* : a thin fan or bell-shaped expansion of the cuticle of the tail of many male nematode worms that functions as a copulatory structure

bursa of Fa·bri·cius \-fə-'brish(-ē)-əs\ *n* : a blind glandular sac that opens into the cloaca of birds and functions in B cell production

Fabricius, Johann Christian (1745–1808), Danish entomologist. Fabricius was one of the outstanding entomologists of his time. A student of Carolus Linnaeus, he is known for his extensive taxonomic research that led to his classifying insects according to the structure of their mouthparts and not of their wings. His entomological classification was first published in 1775 followed by another work a year later. Eventually he named and described about 10,000 insects. He is also remembered for his views on evolution. He held that new species and varieties could arise through hybridization and by environmental influences on structure and function.

bur·sec·to·my \(ˌ)bər-'sek-tə-mē\ *n, pl* **-mies** : excision of a bursa (as the bursa of Fabricius of a chicken) — **bur·sec·to·mize** \-ˌmīz\ *vt* **-mized; -miz·ing**

bur·si·tis \(ˌ)bər-'sīt-əs\ *n* : inflammation of a bursa (as of the shoulder or elbow)

bush·mas·ter \\'bùsh-ˌmas-tər\ *n* : a tropical American pit viper (*Lachesis mutus*) that is the largest New World venomous snake — called also *surucucu*

\ə\ abut \ᵊ\ kitten \ər\ further \a\ ash \ā\ ace \ä\ cot, cart \aù\ out \ch\ chin \e\ bet \ē\ easy \g\ go \i\ hit \ī\ ice \j\ job \ŋ\ sing \ō\ go \ò\ law \òi\ boy \th\ thin \t͟h\ the \ü\ loot \ù\ foot \y\ yet \zh\ vision *See also* Pronunciation Symbols page

Bu·Spar \\'byü-ˌspär\ *trademark* — used for a preparation of the hydrochloride of buspirone

bu·spi·rone \byü-'spī-ˌrōn\ *n* : a mild antianxiety tranquilizer that is administered in the form of its hydrochloride $C_{21}H_{31}N_5O_2 \cdot HCl$ and does not induce significant tolerance or psychological dependence — see BUSPAR

bu·sul·fan \byü-'səl-fən\ *n* : an antineoplastic agent $C_6H_{14}O_6S_2$ used in the treatment of chronic myelogenous leukemia — see MYLERAN

bu·ta·bar·bi·tal \ˌbyüt-ə-'bär-bə-ˌtȯl\ *n* : a synthetic barbiturate used esp. in the form of its sodium salt $C_{10}H_{15}N_2NaO_3$ as a sedative and hypnotic

bu·ta·caine \'byüt-ə-ˌkān, ˌbyüt-ə-'\ *n* : a local anesthetic that is an ester of para-aminobenzoic acid and is applied in the form of its white crystalline sulfate $(C_{18}H_{30}N_2O_2)_2 \cdot H_2SO_4$ to mucous membranes

bu·tane \'byü-ˌtān\ *n* : either of two isomeric flammable gaseous alkanes C_4H_{10} obtained usu. from petroleum or natural gas and used as fuels

bu·ta·nol \'byüt-ᵊn-ˌȯl, -ˌōl\ *n* : either of two butyl alcohols $C_4H_{10}O$ derived from normal butane

Bu·ta·zol·i·din \ˌbyüt-ə-'zäl-əd-ən\ *n* : a preparation of phenylbutazone — formerly a U.S. registered trademark

bute \'byüt\ *n* : PHENYLBUTAZONE

bu·tene \'byü-ˌtēn\ *n* : either of two butylenes having a straight-chain structure

bu·te·nyl \'byüt-ᵊn-əl\ *n* : any of three monovalent radicals C_4H_7 derived from a butene by removal of one hydrogen atom — see CROTYL

bu·to·py·ro·nox·yl \ˌbyüt-ə-ˌpī-rə-'näk-səl\ *n* : a yellow to reddish brown liquid $C_{12}H_{18}O_4$ used as an insect repellent — see INDALONE

bu·tor·pha·nol \ˌbyüt-'ȯr-fə-ˌnȯl\ *n* : a synthetic analgesic and antitussive opioid drug administered in the form of its tartrate $C_{21}H_{29}NO_2 \cdot C_4H_6O_6$ as a nasal spray or by injection esp. for the relief of pain — see STADOL

butoxide — see PIPERONYL BUTOXIDE

but·ter \'bət-ər\ *n* **1** : a solid emulsion of fat globules, air, and water made by churning milk or cream and used as food **2** : a buttery substance; *esp* : any of various fatty oils remaining nearly solid at ordinary temperatures

but·ter·fat \-ˌfat\ *n* : the natural fat of milk and chief constituent of butter consisting essentially of a mixture of glycerides (as butyrin, olein, and palmitin)

¹but·ter·fly \-ˌflī\ *n, pl* **-flies** **1** *pl* : a feeling of hollowness or queasiness caused esp. by emotional or nervous tension or anxious anticipation **2** : a bandage with wing-shaped extensions

²butterfly *adj* : being, relating to, or affecting the area of the face including both cheeks connected by a band across the nose ⟨the typical ∼ lesion of lupus erythematosus⟩

butterfly needle *n* : a short needle that has plastic tabs on either side which aid esp. in manipulating and stabilizing the needle during insertion

butterfly weed \-ˌwēd\ *n* : an orange-flowered milkweed of the genus *Asclepias* (*A. tuberosa*) of eastern No. America that is a source of asclepias — called also *pleurisy root*

but·ter·milk \'bət-ər-ˌmilk\ *n* **1** : the liquid left after butter has been churned from milk or cream **2** : cultured milk made by the addition of suitable bacteria to sweet milk

but·tock \'bət-ək\ *n* **1** : the back of a hip that forms one of the fleshy parts on which a person sits **2 buttocks** *pl* : the seat of the body; *also* : the corresponding part of a quadruped — RUMP

but·ton \'bət-ᵊn\ *n* : something that resembles a small knob or disk: as **a** : the terminal segment of a rattlesnake's rattle **b** : COTYLEDON 1

bu·tyl \'byüt-ᵊl\ *n* : any of four isomeric monovalent radicals C_4H_9 derived from butanes

butyl alcohol *n* : any of four flammable alcohols C_4H_9OH (as butanol) derived from butanes and used in organic synthesis and as solvents

bu·tyl·at·ed hy·droxy·an·i·sole \ˌbyüt-ᵊl-ˌāt-əd-hī-ˌdräk-sē-'an-ə-ˌsōl\ *n* : BHA

butylated hy·droxy·tol·u·ene \-hī-ˌdräk-sē-'täl-yə-ˌwēn\ *n* : BHT

bu·tyl·ene \'byüt-ᵊl-ˌēn\ *n* : any of three isomeric hydrocarbons C_4H_8 of the ethylene series obtained usu. by cracking petroleum

butyl nitrite *n* : a colorless pungent liquid $C_4H_9NO_2$ inhaled by drug users for its stimulating effects which are similar to those of amyl nitrite — called also *isobutyl nitrite*

bu·ty·rate \'byüt-ə-ˌrāt\ *n* : a salt or ester of butyric acid

bu·tyr·ic \byü-'tir-ik\ *adj* : relating to or producing butyric acid ⟨∼ fermentation⟩

butyric acid *n* : either of two isomeric fatty acids $C_4H_8O_2$: **a** : a normal acid of unpleasant odor found in rancid butter and in perspiration **b** : ISOBUTYRIC ACID

bu·tyr·in \'byüt-ə-rən\ *n* : any of the three liquid glycerides of butyric acid; *esp* : TRIBUTYRIN

bu·ty·ro·phe·none \ˌbyüt-ə-(ˌ)rō-fə-'nōn\ *n* : any of a class of antipsychotic drugs (as haloperidol) used esp. in the treatment of schizophrenia

bu·tyr·yl \'byüt-ə-rəl\ *n* : the radical C_4H_7O- of normal butyric acid

BV *abbr* bacterial vaginosis

B vitamin *n* : any vitamin of the vitamin B complex

BW *abbr* **1** blood Wassermann **2** body weight

Bx *abbr* [by analogy with *Rx*] biopsy

by·pass \'bī-ˌpas\ *n* : a surgically established shunt ⟨cardiopulmonary ∼ of blood from the right atrium to the aorta⟩; *also* : a surgical procedure for the establishment of a shunt — see CORONARY BYPASS, GASTRIC BYPASS, JEJUNOILEAL BYPASS — **bypass** *vt*

bys·si·no·sis \ˌbis-ə-'nō-səs\ *n, pl* **-no·ses** \-ˌsēz\ : an occupational respiratory disease associated with inhalation of cotton, flax, or hemp dust and characterized initially by chest tightness, shortness of breath, and cough, and eventually by irreversible lung disease — called also *brown lung, brown lung disease, mill fever*

BZ \'bē-'zē\ *n* : a war gas $C_{21}H_{23}NO_3$ that when breathed produces incapacitating physical and mental effects — called also *quinuclidinyl benzilate*

C

c *abbr* **1** calorie **2** canine **3** cathode **4** centimeter **5** clonus **6** closure **7** cobalt **8** coefficient **9** contact **10** contraction **11** coulomb **12** curie **13** cylinder **14** *or* **c̄** [Latin *cum*] with — used in writing prescriptions

C *abbr* **1** Celsius **2** centigrade **3** cervical — used esp. with a number from 1 to 7 to indicate a vertebra or segment of the spinal cord **4** cocaine **5** complement **6** congius **7** cytosine

C *symbol* carbon

Ca *symbol* calcium

CA *abbr* **1** cancer **2** carcinoma **3** cardiac arrest **4** certified acupuncturist **5** chronological age

CABG \'kab-ij\ *abbr* coronary artery bypass graft

Cab·ot's ring \'kab-əts-\ *or* **Cab·ot ring** \-ət-\ *n* : a ringlike body present in many immature red blood cells that stains with nuclear dyes and may represent remains of the nuclear membrane

> **Cabot, Richard Clarke (1868–1939),** American physician. Cabot is known for his pioneering work in medical social service. His most outstanding contribution to medical knowledge was a 1914 article on heart disease that for the first time gave proper emphasis to its etiologic diagnosis. 1903 was the year in which he described the ringlike bodies (Cabot's rings) found in the red blood corpuscles in severe cases of anemia.

CAC *abbr* cardiac accelerator center

ca·cao \kə-'kaú, kə-'kā-(ˌ)ō\ *n, pl* **cacaos** **1** : the dried partly fermented fatty seeds of a So. American evergreen tree (*Theobroma cacao* of the family Sterculiaceae) that are used in making cocoa, chocolate, and cocoa butter — called also *cacao bean, cocoa bean* **2** : a tree having small yellowish flowers followed by fleshy pods with many seeds that bear cacao — called also *chocolate tree*

cacao butter *var of* COCOA BUTTER

ca·chec·tic \kə-'kek-tik, ka-\ *adj* : relating to or affected by cachexia

ca·chet \ka-'shā\ *n* : a medicinal preparation for swallowing consisting of a case usu. of rice-flour paste containing an unpleasant-tasting medicine — called also *wafer, wafer capsule*

ca·chex·ia \kə-'kek-sē-ə, ka-\ *also* **ca·chexy** \kə-'kek-sē, ka-; 'kak-ˌek-\ *n, pl* **-chex·ias** *also* **-chex·ies** : general physical wasting and malnutrition usu. associated with chronic disease

caco·de·mo·nia \ˌkak-ə-dē-'mō-nē-ə\ *or* **caco·de·mo·no·ma·nia** \-ˌdē-mə-nō-'mā-nē-ə\ *n* : insanity in which the patient has the delusion of being possessed by an evil spirit

cac·o·dyl \'kak-ə-ˌdil\ *n* : an arsenical radical As(CH₃)₂ whose compounds have a vile smell and are usu. poisonous

cac·o·dyl·ate \ˌkak-ə-'dil-ˌāt\ *n* : a salt of cacodylic acid

cac·o·dyl·ic acid \ˌkak-ə-ˌdil-ik-\ *n* : a toxic crystalline compound of arsenic C₂H₇AsO₂ used esp. as an herbicide

ca·cos·mia \kə-'käs-mē-ə, ka-, -'käz-\ *n* : a hallucination of a disagreeable odor

CAD *abbr* coronary artery disease

ca·dav·er \kə-'dav-ər\ *n, pl* **-ers** *also* **-era** \-ə-rə\ : a dead body; *specif* : one intended for use in medical education or research — **ca·dav·er·ic** \-(ə-)rik\ *adj*

ca·dav·er·ine \kə-'dav-ə-ˌrēn\ *n* : a syrupy colorless poisonous ptomaine C₅H₁₄N₂ formed by decarboxylation of lysine esp. in putrefaction of flesh

ca·dav·er·ous \kə-'dav-(ə-)rəs\ *adj* **1** : of or relating to a corpse **2** *of a complexion* : being pallid or livid like a corpse

cade \'kād\ *n* : PRICKLY JUNIPER

cade oil *n* : JUNIPER TAR

caderas — see MAL DE CADERAS

cad·mi·um \'kad-mē-əm\ *n* : a bluish white malleable ductile toxic bivalent metallic element used esp. in protective platings and in bearing metals — symbol *Cd*; see ELEMENT table

cadmium sulfide *n* : a yellow-brown poisonous salt CdS used esp. in electronic parts, in photoelectric cells, and in the treatment of seborrheic dermatitis of the scalp

ca·du·ceus \kə-'d(y)ü-sē-əs, -shəs\ *n, pl* **-cei** \-sē-ˌī\ : a medical insignia bearing a representation of a staff with two entwined snakes and two wings at the top: **a** : one of the symbols of a physician — compare STAFF OF AESCULAPIUS **b** : the emblem of a medical corps or a department of the armed services (as of the U.S. Army)

Each boldface word in the list below is a chiefly British variant of the word to its right in small capitals.

caecal	CECAL	caecostomy	CECOSTOMY
caecally	CECALLY	caecotomy	CECOTOMY
caecectomy	CECECTOMY	caecum	CECUM
caecitis	CECITIS	caenogenetic	CENOGENETIC
caecopexy	CECOPEXY		

Cae·no·rhab·di·tis \ˌsē-nō-rab-'dīt-əs\ *n* : a genus of nematodes (order Rhabditida) that includes a small typically hermaphroditic soil nematode (*C. elegans*) which has a transparent body and is extensively studied in laboratories esp. in relation to genetics, animal development, and neurobiology

caeruleus — see MORBUS CAERULEUS

Cae·sal·pin·ia \ˌsez-ˌal-'pin-ē-ə, ˌsē-ˌzal-\ *n* : a genus of usu. small spiny tropical trees of the family Leguminosae that have small whitish-green, yellow, or reddish flowers in showy racemes and that include the divi-divi

caesarean *also* **caesarian** *var of* CESAREAN

caesium *chiefly Brit var of* CESIUM

ca·fé au lait spot \ka-ˌfā-ō-'lā-\ *n* : any of the medium brown spots usu. on the trunk, pelvis, and creases of the elbow and knees that are often numerous in neurofibromatosis — usu. used in pl.

caf·fe·ic acid \(ˌ)ka-ˌfē-ik-\ *n* : a yellow crystalline acid C₉H₈O₄ obtained by hydrolysis of chlorogenic acid

caf·feine \ka-'fēn, 'ka-ˌ; 'kaf-ē-ən\ *n* : a bitter alkaloid C₈H₁₀N₄O₂ found esp. in coffee, tea, and kola nuts and used medicinally as a stimulant and diuretic — **caf·fein·ic** \ka-'fē-nik, ˌkaf-ē-'in-ik\ *adj*

caf·fein·ism \-ˌiz-əm\ *n* : a morbid condition caused by caffeine (as from excessive consumption of coffee)

cage \'kāj\ *n* : an arrangement of atoms or molecules so bonded as to enclose a space in which another atom or ion (as of a metal) can reside

ca·hin·ca root \kə-'hiŋ-kə-\ *also* **ca·in·ca root** \kə-'iŋ-kə-\ *n* **1** : the root of a tropical American shrub (*Chiococca alba*) used medicinally as a purgative and diuretic **2** : the root of a So. American shrub (*Chiococca anguifuga*) used as an antidote for snake poison

CAI *abbr* confused artificial insemination

cais·son disease \'kā-ˌsän-, -'kās-ᵊn-; *Brit often* kə-'sün-\ *n* : DECOMPRESSION SICKNESS

caj·e·put *also* **caj·u·put** \'kaj-ə-pət, -ˌpút\ *n* : an Australian and southeast Asian tree (*Melaleuca quinquenervia* syn. *M. leucadendron*) of the myrtle family (Myrtaceae) that yields a pungent medicinal oil and has been introduced into Florida — called also *paperbark*

cajeput oil *or* **cajuput oil** *n* : a pungent essential oil obtained from plants of the genus *Melaleuca* and esp. cajeput and used chiefly as a local application in skin disease and as a stimulating expectorant

---

\ə\ **abut** \ᵊ\ **kitten** \ər\ **further** \a\ **ash** \ā\ **ace** \ä\ **cot, cart**
\aú\ **out** \ch\ **chin** \e\ **bet** \ē\ **easy** \g\ **go** \i\ **hit** \ī\ **ice** \j\ **job**
\ŋ\ **sing** \ō\ **go** \ò\ **law** \òi\ **boy** \th\ **thin** \t̲h̲\ **the** \ü\ **loot**
\ú\ **foot** \y\ **yet** \zh\ **vision**   *See also* Pronunciation Symbols page

C
D

caj·e·put·ol *or* **caj·u·put·ol** \'kaj-ə-pə-ˌtȯl, -ˌtōl\ *n* : EUCALYPTOL

caked breast \'kākt-\ *n* : a localized hardening in one or more segments of a lactating breast caused by accumulation of blood in dilated veins and milk in obstructed ducts

cal *abbr* small calorie

Cal *abbr* large calorie

Cal·a·bar bean \'kal-ə-ˌbär-\ *n* : the dark brown poisonous seed of a tropical African woody vine of the genus *Physostigma* (*P. venenosum*) that is used as a source of physostigmine

Calabar swelling *n* : a transient subcutaneous swelling marking the migratory course through the tissues of the adult filarial eye worm of the genus *Loa* (*L. loa*) — compare LOAIASIS

cal·a·mine \'kal-ə-ˌmīn, -mən\ *n* : a mixture of zinc oxide or zinc carbonate with a small amount of ferric oxide that is used in lotions, liniments, and ointments

cal·a·mus \'kal-ə-məs\ *n, pl* **-mi** \-ˌmī, -ˌmē\ **1** : SWEET FLAG **2** : the aromatic peeled and dried rhizome of the sweet flag that is the source of a carcinogenic essential oil

Cal·an \'kal-ˌän, -ən\ *trademark* — used for a preparation of the hydrochloride of verapamil

cal·ca·ne·al \kal-'kā-nē-əl\ *also* **cal·ca·ne·an** \-ən\ *adj* **1** : relating to the heel **2** : relating to the calcaneus

calcaneal tendon *n* : ACHILLES TENDON

cal·ca·neo·cu·boid \(ˌ)kal-ˌkā-nē-ō-'kyü-ˌbȯid\ *adj* : of or relating to the calcaneus and the cuboid bone ⟨~ articulations⟩

calcaneocuboid ligament *n* : either of two ligaments of the tarsus connecting the calcaneus and the cuboid

calcaneonavicular — see PLANTAR CALCANEONAVICULAR LIGAMENT

cal·ca·ne·um \kal-'kā-nē-əm\ *n, pl* **-nea** \-nē-ə\ : CALCANEUS

cal·ca·ne·us \-nē-əs\ *n, pl* **-nei** \-nē-ˌī\ : a tarsal bone that in humans is the large bone of the heel — called also *heel bone, os calcis*

cal·car \'kal-ˌkär\ *n, pl* **cal·car·ia** \kal-'kar-ē-ə, -'ker-\ : a spurred anatomical prominence

calcar avis \-'ā-vəs, -'ä-\ *n, pl* **calcaria avi·um** \-vē-əm\ : a curved ridge on the medial wall of the posterior horn of each lateral ventricle of the brain opposite the calcarine sulcus

cal·car·e·ous \kal-'kar-ē-əs, -'ker-\ *adj* **1** : resembling calcite or calcium carbonate esp. in hardness **2** : consisting of or containing calcium carbonate; *also* : containing calcium

cal·ca·rine \'kal-kə-ˌrīn\ *adj* : belonging to or situated near the calcar avis

calcarine sulcus *n* : a sulcus in the mesial surface of the occipital lobe of the cerebrum — called also *calcarine fissure*

calces *pl of* CALX

cal·cic \'kal-sik\ *adj* : derived from or containing calcium or lime : rich in calcium

cal·ci·co·sis \ˌkal-sə-'kō-səs\ *n, pl* **-co·ses** \-ˌsēz\ : pneumoconiosis caused by inhalation of limestone dust

cal·cif·er·ol \kal-'sif-ə-ˌrȯl, -ˌrōl\ *n* : an alcohol $C_{28}H_{43}OH$ usu. prepared by irradiation of ergosterol and used as a dietary supplement in nutrition and medicinally esp. in the control of rickets — called also *ergocalciferol, viosterol, vitamin D, vitamin D₂; see* DRISDOL

cal·cif·er·ous \kal-'sif-(ə-)rəs\ *adj* : producing or containing calcium carbonate

cal·cif·ic \kal-'sif-ik\ *adj* : involving or caused by calcification ⟨~ lesions⟩ ⟨~ periarthritis⟩

cal·ci·fi·ca·tion \ˌkal-sə-fə-'kā-shən\ *n* **1** : impregnation with calcareous matter: as **a** : deposition of calcium salts within the matrix of cartilage often as the preliminary step in the formation of bone — compare OSSIFICATION 1a **b** : abnormal deposition of calcium salts within tissue **2** : a calcified structure or part

cal·ci·fy \'kal-sə-ˌfī\ *vb* **-fied; -fy·ing** *vt* : to make calcareous by deposit of calcium salts ~ *vi* : to become calcareous

cal·cim·e·ter \kal-'sim-ət-ər\ *n* : an instrument to measure the calcium in body fluids

cal·ci·na·tion \ˌkal-sə-'nā-shən\ *n* : the act or process of calcining : the state of being calcined

¹cal·cine \kal-'sīn\ *vb* **cal·cined; cal·cin·ing** *vt* : to heat (as inorganic materials) to a high temperature but without fusing in order to drive off volatile matter or to effect changes (as oxidation or pulverization) ~ *vi* : to undergo calcination

²cal·cine \'kal-ˌsīn\ *n* : a product (as a metal oxide) of calcination or roasting

cal·ci·no·sis \ˌkal-sə-'nō-səs\ *n, pl* **-no·ses** \-ˌsēz\ : the abnormal deposition of calcium salts in a part or tissue of the body

cal·ci·phy·lax·is \ˌkal-sə-fə-'lak-səs\ *n, pl* **-lax·es** \-ˌsēz\ : an adaptive response that follows systemic sensitization by a calcifying factor (as a vitamin D) and a challenge (as with a metallic salt) and that involves local inflammation and sclerosis with calcium deposition — **cal·ci·phy·lac·tic** \-'lak-tik\ *adj* — **cal·ci·phy·lac·ti·cal·ly** \-ti-k(ə-)lē\ *adv*

calcis — see OS CALCIS

cal·cite \'kal-ˌsīt\ *n* : a mineral $CaCO_3$ consisting of calcium carbonate crystallized in hexagonal form and including common limestone, chalk, and marble — **cal·cit·ic** \kal-'sit-ik\ *adj*

cal·ci·to·nin \ˌkal-sə-'tō-nən\ *n* : a polypeptide hormone esp. from the thyroid gland that tends to lower the level of calcium in the blood plasma — called also *thyrocalcitonin*

cal·ci·tri·ol \ˌkal-sə-'trī-ˌȯl, -ˌōl\ *n* : a physiologically active metabolic derivative $C_{27}H_{44}O_3$ of cholecalciferol that is synthesized in the liver and kidney and stimulates the intestinal absorption of calcium — called also *1,25-dihydroxycholecalciferol*

cal·ci·um \'kal-sē-əm\ *n, often attrib* : a silver-white bivalent metallic element that is an alkaline earth metal, occurs only in combination, and is an essential constituent of most plants and animals — symbol *Ca*; see ELEMENT table

calcium blocker *n* : CALCIUM CHANNEL BLOCKER

calcium carbonate *n* : a calcium salt $CaCO_3$ that is found in limestone, chalk, marble, plant ashes, bones, and many shells, that is obtained also as a white precipitate by passing carbon dioxide into a suspension of calcium hydroxide in water, and that is used in dentifrices and in pharmaceuticals as an antacid and to supplement bodily calcium stores

calcium channel blocker *n* : any of a class of drugs (as verapamil) that prevent or slow the influx of calcium ions into smooth muscle cells esp. of the heart and that are used esp. to treat some forms of angina pectoris and some cardiac arrhythmias — called also *calcium blocker*

calcium chloride *n* : a salt $CaCl_2$ used in medicine as a source of calcium and as a diuretic

calcium gluconate *n* : a white crystalline or granular powdery salt $C_{12}H_{22}CaO_{14}$ used to supplement bodily calcium stores

calcium hydroxide *n* : a strong alkali $Ca(OH)_2$ commonly sold in water solution or as an ingredient of bleaching powder — see LIMEWATER, SODA LIME

calcium hypochlorite *n* : a chlorine-containing white powder $CaCl_2O_2$ used esp. as a bleaching agent, disinfectant, bactericide, and fungicide

calcium lactate *n* : a white almost tasteless crystalline salt $C_6H_{10}CaO_6·5H_2O$ used chiefly in medicine as a source of calcium and in foods (as in baking powder)

calcium levulinate *n* : a white powdery salt $C_{10}H_{14}CaO_6·H_2O$ used in medicine as a source of calcium

calcium oxalate *n* : a colorless crystalline salt $CaC_2O_4·H_2O$ that is noted for its insolubility and is sometimes excreted in urine or retained in the form of urinary calculi

calcium pantothenate *n* : a white powdery salt $C_{18}H_{32}CaN_2O_{10}$ made synthetically and used as a source of pantothenic acid

calcium phosphate *n* : any of various phosphates of calcium: as **a** : the phosphate $CaHPO_4$ used in pharmaceutical preparations and animal feeds **b** : a naturally occurring phosphate of calcium $Ca_5(F,Cl,OH,½CO_3)(PO_4)_3$ that contains other elements or radicals and is the chief constituent of bones and teeth

calcium–phosphorus ratio *n* : the proportional relation existing between calcium and phosphorus in the form of phosphate in body fluids and bone that in humans is normally about 2.2 to 1

calcium propionate *n* : a mold-inhibiting calcium salt $C_6H_{10}CaO_4$ used chiefly as a food preservative (as in bread)

calcium stearate *n* : a white powder consisting essentially of calcium salts of stearic acid and palmitic acid and used as a conditioning agent in food and pharmaceuticals

calcium sulfate *n* : a white calcium salt $CaSO_4$ used esp. as a diluent in tablets and in hydrated form as plaster of paris

calcium sulfite *n* : a white calcium salt $CaSO_3$ prepared as a powder and used esp. as a disinfectant and preservative

cal·co·sphe·rite \ˌkal-kō-ˈsfi(ə)r-ˌīt\ *n* : a granular or laminated deposit of calcium salts in the body

cal·cu·lo·sis \ˌkal-kyə-ˈlō-səs\ *n, pl* **-lo·ses** \-ˌsēz\ : the formation of or the condition of having a calculus or calculi

cal·cu·lous \ˈkal-kyə-ləs\ *adj* : caused or characterized by a calculus or calculi

cal·cu·lus \-ləs\ *n, pl* **-li** \-ˌlī, -ˌlē\ *also* **-lus·es** **1** : a concretion usu. of mineral salts around organic material found esp. in hollow organs or ducts **2** : a concretion on teeth : TARTAR

Cald·well–Luc operation \ˈkōld-ˌwel-ˈlük-, ˈkäld-, -ˈlüek-\ *n* : a surgical procedure used esp. for clearing a blocked or infected maxillary sinus that involves entering the sinus through the mouth by way of an incision into the canine fossa above a canine tooth, cleaning the sinus, and creating a new and enlarged opening for drainage through the nose

Caldwell, George Walter (1866–1946), American surgeon. Caldwell was a pioneer in nasal surgery and is credited with devising a number of surgical procedures. In 1893 he described an operative procedure for the treatment of severe disorders of the maxillary sinus in which an auxiliary opening is provided in the anterior wall through the canine fossa. His procedure became widely used in the treatment of maxillary sinus empyema. Several of his papers described diseases of the nasal sinuses.

Luc \lüek\, **Henri (1855–1925),** French laryngologist. Luc is credited with devising several surgical procedures involving the sinuses and with developing various surgical instruments. His description of what is now known as the Caldwell-Luc operation was published in 1889, predating Caldwell's by four years.

¹cal·e·fa·cient \ˌkal-ə-ˈfā-shənt\ *adj* : making warm

²calefacient *n* : a calefacient agent

ca·len·du·la \kə-ˈlen-jə-lə\ *n* **1** *cap* : a small genus of yellow-rayed composite herbs of temperate regions **2** : any plant of the genus *Calendula* **3** : the dried florets of plants of the genus *Calendula* (esp. *C. officinalis*) sometimes used as a mild aromatic and diaphoretic

ca·len·du·lin \-lən\ *n* : a yellowish pigment that is the physiologically active substance in calendula

calf \ˈkaf, ˈkáf\ *n, pl* **calves** \ˈkavz, ˈkávz\ : the fleshy back part of the leg below the knee

calf bone *n* : FIBULA

calf diphtheria *n* : an infectious disease of the mouth and pharynx of calves and young cattle associated with the presence of large numbers of a bacterium of the genus *Fusobacterium* (*F. necrophorum*) and commonly passing into pneumonia or generalized septicemia if untreated

cal·i·ber *or chiefly Brit* **cal·i·bre** \ˈkal-ə-bər, *Brit also* kə-ˈlē-\ *n* : the diameter of a round or cylindrical body; *esp* : the internal diameter of a hollow cylinder

cal·i·brate \ˈkal-ə-ˌbrāt\ *vt* **-brat·ed; -brat·ing** **1** : to ascertain the caliber of (as a thermometer tube) **2** : to determine, rectify, or mark the graduations of (as a thermometer tube) **3** : to standardize (as a measuring instrument) by determining the deviation from a standard so as to ascertain the proper correction factors — **cal·i·bra·tion** \ˌkal-ə-ˈbrā-shən\ *n* — **cal·i·bra·tor** \ˈkal-ə-ˌbrāt-ər\ *n*

caliceal *var of* CALYCEAL

calices *pl of* CALIX

Cal·i·ci·vi·ri·dae \kə-ˌlis-ə-ˈvir-ə-ˌdē, -ˌlē-sē-, -ˌlē-chē-\ *n pl* : a family of single-stranded RNA viruses with icosahedral symmetry that have numerous cup-shaped depressions on the surface but no lipoprotein envelope forming the outer layer of the virion and that include the Norwalk virus and the causative viruses of hepatitis E and vesicular exanthema

cal·i·ci·vi·rus \kə-ˈlis-ə-ˌvī-rəs, -ˈlē-sē-, -ˈlē-chē-\ *n* : any of the family *Caliciviridae* of single-stranded RNA viruses

cal·i·for·ni·um \ˌkal-ə-ˈfȯr-nē-əm\ *n* : an artificially prepared radioactive element discovered by bombarding an isotope of curium with alpha particles — symbol *Cf*; see ELEMENT table

¹cal·i·per *or chiefly Brit* **cal·li·per** \ˈkal-ə-pər\ *n* **1** : any of various measuring instruments having two usu. adjustable arms, legs, or jaws used to measure thickness, diameter, and distance between surfaces — usu. used in pl. ⟨a pair of ∼s⟩ **2** : CALIPER SPLINT

²caliper *or chiefly Brit* **calliper** *vt* **-pered; -per·ing** \-p(ə-)riŋ\ : to measure by or as if by calipers

caliper splint *n* : a support for the leg consisting of two metal rods extending between a foot plate and a padded thigh band and worn so that the weight is borne mainly by the hip bone — called also *caliper*

cal·i·saya bark \ˌkal-ə-ˌsī-ə-\ *n* : cinchona bark obtained from either of two cinchonas (*Cinchona calisaya* and *C. ledgeriana*) or from a hybrid of either of these with other cinchonas — called also *yellow cinchona*

cal·is·then·ic *or Brit* **cal·lis·then·ic** \ˌkal-əs-ˈthen-ik\ *adj* : of or relating to calisthenics

cal·is·then·ics *or Brit* **cal·lis·then·ics** \-iks\ *n pl but sing or pl in constr* **1** : systematic rhythmic bodily exercises performed usu. without apparatus **2** *usu sing in constr* : the art or practice of calisthenics

calix *var of* CALYX

call·ing \ˈkȯ-liŋ\ *n* : the characteristic cry of a female cat in heat; *also* : the period of heat

calliper *chiefly Brit var of* CALIPER

Cal·liph·o·ra \kə-ˈlif-(ə-)rə\ *n* : a genus of the family Calliphoridae that includes large bluebottle flies — **cal·liph·o·rine** \-ˈlif-ə-ˌrīn\ *adj*

Cal·li·phor·i·dae \ˌkal-ə-ˈfȯr-ə-ˌdē\ *n pl* : a family of large usu. hairy metallic blue or green flies comprising the blowflies (as a bluebottle) and a few related forms with parasitic larvae — **cal·liph·o·rid** \kə-ˈlif-ə-rəd\ *adj or n*

callisthenic, callisthenics *Brit var of* CALISTHENIC, CALISTHENICS

Cal·li·tro·ga \ˌkal-ə-ˈtrō-gə\ *n, syn* COCHLIOMYIA

cal·lo·sal \kə-ˈlō-səl, ka-\ *adj* : of, relating to, or adjoining the corpus callosum

cal·lose \ˈkal-ˌōs, -ˌōz\ *n* : a carbohydrate component of plant cell walls

cal·los·i·ty \ka-ˈläs-ət-ē, kə-\ *n, pl* **-ties** : the quality or state of being callous; *esp* : marked or abnormal hardness and thickness (as of the skin)

callosum — see CORPUS CALLOSUM

cal·lous \ˈkal-əs\ *adj* **1** : being hardened and thickened **2** : having calluses

cal·loused *or* **cal·lused** \ˈkal-əst\ *adj* : CALLOUS 2 ⟨∼ hands⟩

cal·lus \ˈkal-əs\ *n* **1** : a thickening of or a hard thickened area on skin **2** : a mass of exudate and connective tissue that forms around a break in a bone and is converted into bone in the healing of the break

calm·ant \ˈkäm-ənt, ˈkälm-\ *n* : SEDATIVE

calm·ative \ˈkäm-ət-iv, ˈkäl-mət-\ *n or adj* : SEDATIVE

cal·mod·u·lin \ˌkal-ˈmäj-ə-lən\ *n* : a calcium-binding protein that mediates cellular metabolic processes (as muscle-fiber contraction) by regulating the activity of specific calcium-dependent enzymes

cal·o·mel \ˈkal-ə-məl, -ˌmel\ *n* : a white tasteless compound Hg_2Cl_2 used esp. as a fungicide and insecticide and formerly in medicine as a purgative — called also *mercurous chloride*

\ə\ abut \ˈə\ kitten \ər\ further \a\ ash \ā\ ace \ä\ cot, cart
\aù\ out \ch\ chin \e\ bet \ē\ easy \g\ go \i\ hit \ī\ ice \j\ job
\ŋ\ sing \ō\ go \ȯ\ law \ȯi\ boy \th\ thin \t̲h̲\ the \ü\ loot
\ù\ foot \y\ yet \zh\ vision *See also* Pronunciation Symbols page

cal·or \ˈkal-ˌȯ(ə)r\ *n* : bodily heat that is a sign of inflammation

ca·lor·ic \kə-ˈlȯr-ik, -ˈlȯr-, -ˈlär-; ˈkal-ə-rik\ *adj* **1** : of or relating to heat **2** : of or relating to calories — **ca·lo·ri·cal·ly** \kə-ˈlȯr-i-k(ə-)lē, -ˈlȯr-, -ˈlär-\ *adv*

cal·o·rie *also* **cal·o·ry** \ˈkal-(ə-)rē\ *n, pl* **-ries** **1 a** : the amount of heat required at a pressure of one atmosphere to raise the temperature of one gram of water one degree Celsius that is equal to about 4.19 joules — abbr. *cal;* called also *gram calorie, small calorie* **b** : the amount of heat required to raise the temperature of one kilogram of water one degree Celsius that is equal to 1000 gram calories or 3.968 Btu — abbr. *Cal;* called also *kilocalorie, kilogram calorie, large calorie* **2 a** : a unit equivalent to the large calorie expressing heat-producing or energy-producing value in food when oxidized in the body **b** : an amount of food having an energy‑producing value of one large calorie

cal·o·ri·fa·cient \kə-ˌlȯr-ə-ˈfā-shənt, -ˌlȯr-, -ˌlär-; ˌkal-ə-rə-ˈfā-\ *adj* : heat-producing — usu. used of foods

cal·o·rif·ic \ˌkal-ə-ˈrif-ik\ *adj* **1** : CALORIC **2** : of or relating to the production of heat

cal·o·ri·gen·ic \kə-ˌlȯr-ə-ˈjen-ik, -ˌlȯr-, -ˌlär-; ˌkal-ə-rə-\ *adj* : generating heat or energy ⟨∼ foodstuffs⟩

cal·o·rim·e·ter \ˌkal-ə-ˈrim-ət-ər\ *n* : any of several apparatuses for measuring quantities of absorbed or evolved heat or for determining specific heats — see BOMB CALORIMETER, OXYCALORIMETER — **ca·lo·ri·met·ric** \ˌkal-ə-rə-ˈme-trik; kə-ˌlȯr-ə-, -ˌlȯr-, -ˌlär-\ *adj* — **ca·lo·ri·met·ri·cal·ly** \-tri-k(ə-)lē\ *adv* — **cal·o·rim·e·try** \ˌkal-ə-ˈrim-ə-trē\ *n, pl* **-tries**

ca·lum·ba \kə-ˈləm-bə\ *or* **co·lom·bo** \-(ˌ)bō\ *n* : the root of an African plant (*Jatrorrhiza palmata* of the family Menispermaceae) that contains columbin and is used as a tonic — called also *calumba root, colombo root*

cal·va \ˈkal-və\ *n, pl* **calvas** *or* **cal·vae** \-ˌvē, -ˌvī\ : the upper part of the human cranium

cal·var·ia \kal-ˈvar-ē-ə\ *n, pl* **-i·ae** \-ē-ˌē, -ē-ˌī\ : CALVARIUM

cal·var·i·um \-ē-əm\ *n, pl* **-ia** \-ē-ə\ : an incomplete skull; *esp* : the portion of a skull including the braincase and excluding the lower jaw or lower jaw and facial portion — **cal·var·i·al** \-ē-əl\ *adj*

calves *pl of* CALF

cal·vi·ti·es \kal-ˈvish-ē-ˌēz, -ˈvish-(ˌ)ēz\ *n, pl* **calvities** : the condition of being bald : BALDNESS

¹calx \ˈkalks\ *n, pl* **calx·es** *or* **cal·ces** \ˈkal-ˌsēz\ : the crumbly residue left when a metal or mineral has been subjected to calcination or combustion; *esp* : ¹LIME

²calx *n, pl* **calces** : HEEL

ca·ly·ce·al *or* **ca·li·ce·al** \ˌkal-ə-ˈsē-əl, ˌkā-lə-\ *adj* : of or relating to a calyx

calyces *pl of* CALYX

ca·ly·cine \ˈkā-lə-ˌsīn, ˈkal-ə-\ *also* **ca·lyc·i·nal** \kə-ˈlis-ᵊn-əl\ *adj* : relating to or resembling a calyx

cal·y·cle \ˈkal-i-kəl\ *n* : CALYCULUS

ca·lyc·u·lus \kə-ˈlik-yə-ləs\ *n, pl* **-li** \-ˌlī, -ˌlē\ : a small cup‑shaped structure (as a taste bud)

Ca·lym·ma·to·bac·te·ri·um \kə-ˌlim-ət-ō-bak-ˈtir-ē-əm\ *n* : a genus of pleomorphic nonmotile rod bacteria of the family Brucellaceae including only the causative agent (*C. granulomatis*) of granuloma inguinale — see DONOVAN BODY

ca·lyx *also* **ca·lix** \ˈkā-liks *also* ˈkal-iks\ *n, pl* **ca·lyx·es** *or* **ca·ly·ces** \ˈkā-lə-ˌsēz *also* ˈkal-ə-\ *also* **ca·li·ces** : a cuplike division of the renal pelvis surrounding one or more renal papillae

CAM *abbr* complementary and alternative medicine

cam·bo·gia \kam-ˈbō-jə\ *n* : GAMBOGE

cam·era lu·ci·da \ˌkam-(ə-)rə-ˈlü-səd-ə\ *n* : an instrument that by means of a prism or mirrors and often a microscope causes a virtual image of an object to appear as if projected upon a plane surface so that an outline may be traced

cam·i·sole \ˈkam-ə-ˌsōl\ *n* : a long-sleeved straitjacket

camomile *var of* CHAMOMILE

camomile oil *var of* CHAMOMILE OIL

cAMP *abbr* cyclic AMP

cam·phene \ˈkam-ˌfēn\ *n* : any of several terpenes related to camphor; *esp* : a colorless crystalline terpene $C_{10}H_{16}$ found in three optically different forms in several essential oils, made synthetically from pinene, and used in insecticides

cam·phor \ˈkam(p)-fər\ *n* : a tough gummy volatile aromatic crystalline compound $C_{10}H_{16}O$ obtained esp. from the wood and bark of the camphor tree and used topically as a liniment and mild analgesic, as a plasticizer, and as an insect repellent; *also* : any of several similar compounds (as some terpene alcohols and ketones) — **cam·phor·ic** \kam-ˈfȯr-ik, -ˈfär-\ *adj*

cam·pho·ra·ceous \ˌkam(p)-fə-ˈrā-shəs\ *adj* : being or having the properties of camphor ⟨a ∼ odor⟩

cam·phor·at·ed \ˈkam(p)-fə-ˌrāt-əd\ *adj* : impregnated or treated with camphor ⟨paregoric is a ∼ tincture of opium⟩

camphorated oil *n* : a solution of about 20 percent camphor in cottonseed oil used as a counterirritant — called also *camphor liniment*

camphoric acid *n* : a white crystalline acid $C_{10}H_{16}O_2$ existing in three optically different forms; *esp* : the dextrorotatory form obtained by the oxidation of dextrorotatory camphor and used in pharmaceuticals

camphor liniment *n* : CAMPHORATED OIL

camphor oil *n* : an essential oil obtained by distilling the wood and other parts of the camphor tree

camphor tree *n* : a large Asian evergreen tree of the genus *Cinnamomum* (*C. camphora*) that is grown in warm areas and has smooth branches and shining lanceolate leaves and from which camphor is obtained

cam·pim·e·ter \kam-ˈpim-ət-ər\ *n* : an instrument for testing indirect or peripheral visual perception of form and color — **cam·pim·e·try** \-ə-trē\ *n, pl* **-tries**

camp·to·cor·mia \ˌkam(p)-tə-ˈkȯr-mē-ə\ *n* : a condition marked by forward bending of the trunk that is sometimes accompanied by lumbar pain

camp·to·dac·ty·ly \ˌkam(p)-tə-ˈdak-tə-lē\ *n, pl* **-lies** : permanent flexion of one or more finger joints

camp·to·the·cin \ˌkamp-tə-ˈthē-sən\ *n* : an alkaloid $C_{20}H_{16}N_2O_4$ from the wood of a Chinese tree (*Camptotheca acuminata* of the family Nyssaceae) that has shown some antileukemic and anticancer activity in animal studies; *also* : a semisynthetic or synthetic derivative of this

cam·py·lo·bac·ter \ˈkam-pə-lō-ˌbak-tər\ *n* **1** *cap* : a genus of slender spirally curved rod bacteria of the family Spirillaceae that are gram-negative, microaerophilic, and motile with a characteristic motion resembling a corkscrew, that do not form spores, and that include forms formerly included in the genus *Spirillum* or *Vibrio* of which some are pathogenic for domestic animals or humans — see HELICOBACTER **2** : any bacterium of the genus *Campylobacter*

Canada balsam \ˌkan-əd-ə-\ *n* : an oleoresin exuded by the balsam fir and used as a transparent cement esp. in microscopy for mounting specimens and in optical instruments — called also *Canada turpentine*

can·a·dine \ˈkan-ə-ˌdēn, -əd-ən\ *n* : a crystalline alkaloid $C_{20}H_{21}NO_4$ found in the root of the goldenseal

ca·nal \kə-ˈnal\ *n* : a tubular anatomical passage or channel : DUCT — see ALIMENTARY CANAL, HAVERSIAN CANAL, INGUINAL CANAL

can·a·lic·u·lar \ˌkan-ᵊl-ˈik-yə-lər\ *adj* : relating to, resembling, or provided with a canaliculus

can·a·lic·u·lus \-yə-ləs\ *n, pl* **-li** \-ˌlī, -ˌlē\ : a minute canal in a bodily structure: as **a** : one of the hairlike channels ramifying a haversian system in bone and linking the lacunae with one another and with the haversian canal **b** : one of the narrow spaces between cells in the anastomosing cords of cells that make up a liver lobule

ca·na·lis \kə-ˈnal-əs, -ˈnäl-\ *n, pl* **ca·na·les** \-ˈnal-(ˌ)ēz, -ˈnäl-(ˌ)ās\ : CANAL

ca·na·li·za·tion *or Brit* **ca·na·li·sa·tion** \ˌkan-ᵊl-ə-ˈzā-shən\ *n* **1** : surgical formation of holes or canals for drainage without tubes **2** : natural formation of new channels in tissue (as formation of new blood vessels through a blood clot) **3** : establishment of new pathways in the central nervous system by repeated passage of nerve impulses **4** : the developmental buffering and homeostatic processes by which a particular kind of organism forms a relatively constant phenotype although individuals may have a variety of genotypes and environmental conditions may vary

can·a·lize *or Brit* **can·a·lise** \'kan-ᵊl-ˌīz\ *vb* **-lized** *or Brit* **-lised; -liz·ing** *or Brit* **-lis·ing** *vt* : to drain (a wound) by forming channels without the use of tubes ∼ *vi* : to develop new channels (as new capillaries in a blood clot)

canal of Schlemm \-'shlem\ *n* : a circular canal lying in the substance of the sclerocorneal junction of the eye and draining the aqueous humor from the anterior chamber into the veins draining the eyeball — called also *Schlemm's canal, sinus venosus sclerae*

Schlemm, Friedrich S. (1795–1858), German anatomist. Schlemm described the canal of Schlemm in 1830. His description was not the first, for the canal had been noted as early as 1778.

Can·a·va·lia \ˌkan-ə-'vā-lē-ə, -'vāl-yə\ *n* : a small genus of tropical twining herbs of the family Leguminosae that have long tough pods with large seeds and include the jack bean

ca·na·val·in \ˌkan-ə-'val-ən, kə-'nav-ə-lən\ *n* : a globulin found in the jack bean

Can·a·van disease \'kan-ə-ˌvan-\ *also* **Can·a·van's disease** \-ˌvanz-\ *n* : a rare usu. fatal demyelinating disease of infancy that is characterized by spongy degeneration of the brain caused by an enzyme deficiency inherited as an autosomal recessive trait and that typically affects individuals of eastern European Jewish ancestry

Canavan, Myrtelle May (1879–1953), American pathologist. Canavan served as a pathologist for Boston State Hospital and the Massachusetts Department of Mental Health. She also held positions on the faculty of Boston medical schools. Her areas of research included chronic manganese poisoning, enostosis, the pathology of the mentally retarded, and the mental health of the offspring of schizophrenics. She described Canavan disease in 1931.

ca·na·van·ine \ˌkan-ə-'van-ˌēn, -'vän-; kə-'nav-ə-ˌnēn\ *n* : an amino acid $C_5H_{12}O_3N_4$ occurring esp. in the jack bean that is an inhibitor of protein synthesis

canc *abbr* canceled

can·cel·late \kan-'sel-ət, 'kan(t)-sə-ˌlāt\ *or* **can·cel·lat·ed** \'kan(t)-sə-ˌlāt-əd\ *adj* : CANCELLOUS

can·cel·li \kan-'sel-ˌī, -(ˌ)ē\ *n pl* **1** : the intersecting osseous plates and bars of which cancellous bone is composed **2** : the interstices between the plates and bars of cancellous bone

can·cel·lous \kan-'sel-əs, 'kan(t)-sə-ləs\ *adj* : having a porous structure made up of intersecting plates and bars that form small cavities or cells ⟨∼ bone⟩ — compare COMPACT

can·cer \'kan(t)-sər\ *n* **1** : a malignant tumor of potentially unlimited growth that expands locally by invasion and systemically by metastasis **2** : an abnormal state marked by a cancer — **can·cer·ous** \'kan(t)s-(ə-)rəs\ *adj*

can·cer·ate \-sə-ˌrāt\ *vi* **-at·ed; -at·ing** : to become cancerous : develop into a cancer

cancer eye *n* : a malignant squamous cell epithelioma of cattle that originates in the mucous membranes of the eye, that is common in regions of intense sunlight and chiefly affects animals with white or light-colored skin about the eyes but prob. has a multiple etiology, and that ultimately destroys the eye and adjacent bony structures

can·cer–eyed \'kan(t)-sər-'īd\ *adj* : affected with cancer eye

can·cer·i·ci·dal *or* **can·cer·o·ci·dal** \ˌkan(t)-sə-rə-'sīd-ᵊl\ *adj* : destructive of cancer cells

can·cer·iza·tion *or Brit* **can·cer·isa·tion** \ˌkan(t)-sə-rə-'zā-shən\ *n* : transformation into cancer or from a normal to a cancerous state ⟨∼ of a wart⟩ ⟨epithelial ∼⟩

can·cer·o·gen·ic \ˌkan(t)-sə-rə-'jen-ik, -rō-\ *or* **can·cer·i·gen·ic** \-sə-rə-\ *adj* : CARCINOGENIC

can·cer·ol·o·gy \ˌkan(t)-sə-'räl-ə-jē\ *n, pl* **-gies** : the study of cancer — compare ONCOLOGY — **can·cer·ol·o·gist** \-'räl-ə-jəst\ *n*

can·cer·o·lyt·ic \ˌkan(t)-sə-rə-'lit-ik\ *adj* : CARCINOLYTIC

can·cer·pho·bia \ˌkan(t)-sər-'fō-bē-ə\ *or* **can·cer·o·pho·bia** \-sər-ō-'fō-\ *n* : an abnormal dread of cancer

¹can·croid \'kaŋ-ˌkröid\ *adj* : resembling a cancer ⟨a ∼ tumor⟩

²cancroid *n* : a skin cancer of low or moderate malignancy

can·crum oris \ˌkaŋ-krəm-'ōr-əs, -'ór-, -'är-\ *n, pl* **can·cra oris** \-krə-\ : noma of the oral tissues — called also *gangrenous stomatitis*

can·de·la \kan-'dē-lə, -'del-ə\ *n* : the base unit of luminous intensity in the International System of Units that is equal to the luminous intensity in a given direction of a source which emits monochromatic radiation of frequency 540×10^{12} hertz and has a radiant intensity in that direction of $\frac{1}{683}$ watt per unit solid angle — abbr. *cd;* called also *candle*

can·di·cin \ˌkan-də-'sid-ᵊn\ *n* : an antibiotic obtained from a streptomyces (*Streptomyces griseus*) and active against some fungi of the genus *Candida*

can·di·da \'kan-dəd-ə\ *n* **1** *cap* : a genus of parasitic fungi that resemble yeasts, produce small amounts of mycelium, occur esp. in the mouth, vagina, and intestinal tract where they are usu. benign but can become pathogenic, and have been grouped with the imperfect fungi but are now often placed with the ascomycetes **2** : any fungus of the genus *Candida*; *esp* : one (*C. albicans*) causing thrush — **can·di·dal** \-dəd-ᵊl\ *adj*

can·di·di·a·sis \ˌkan-də-'dī-ə-səs\ *n, pl* **-a·ses** \-ˌsēz\ : infection with or disease caused by a fungus of the genus *Candida* — called also *monilia, moniliasis*

can·dle \'kan-dᵊl\ *n* **1** : a medicated candle or lozenge used for fumigation **2** : CANDELA

can·dle–foot \-'fút\ *n* : FOOTCANDLE

can·dy strip·er \'kan-dē-ˌstrī-pər\ *n* : a volunteer nurse's aide

ca·nic·o·la fever \kə-ˌnik-ə-lə-\ *n* : an acute disease in humans and dogs characterized by gastroenteritis and mild jaundice and caused by a spirochete of the genus *Leptospira* (*L. canicola*)

Can·i·dae \'kan-ə-ˌdē\ *n pl* : a cosmopolitan family of carnivorous mammals that includes the wolves, jackals, foxes, coyote, and the domestic dog — **can·id** \'kan-əd\ *n*

¹ca·nine \'kā-ˌnīn, *Brit also* 'kan-ˌīn\ *n* **1** : a conical pointed tooth; *esp* : one situated between the lateral incisor and the first premolar **2** : any member of the family Canidae : DOG

²canine *adj* : of or relating to dogs or to the family Canidae

canine distemper *n* : DISTEMPER a

canine fossa *n* : a depression external to and somewhat above the prominence on the surface of the superior maxillary bone caused by the socket of the canine tooth

ca·ni·ni·form \(ˈ)kā-'nī-nə-ˌfórm, kə-\ *adj* : having the form of a typical canine tooth

ca·ni·nus \kā-'nī-nəs, kə-\ *n, pl* **ca·ni·ni** \-'nī-ˌnī\ : LEVATOR ANGULI ORIS

Ca·nis \'kā-nəs, 'kan-\ *n* : the type genus of the family Canidae that includes the domestic dog, the wolves and jackals, and sometimes in older classifications the foxes

ca·ni·ti·es \kə-'nish-ē-ˌēz\ *n* : grayness or whiteness of the hair

can·ker \'kaŋ-kər\ *n* **1 a** (1) : an erosive or spreading sore (2) *obs* : GANGRENE **b** : CANKER SORE **2 a** : a chronic inflammation of the ear in dogs, cats, or rabbits; *esp* : a localized form of mange **b** : a chronic and progressive inflammation of the deep horn-producing tissues of the frog and sole of the hooves of horses resulting in softening and destruction of the horny layers

can·kered \-kərd\ *adj* : affected with canker ⟨a ∼ mouth⟩

\ə\ **abut** \ᵊ\ **kitten** \ər\ **further** \a\ **ash** \ā\ **ace** \ä\ **cot, cart**
\aú\ **out** \ch\ **chin** \e\ **bet** \ē\ **easy** \g\ **go** \i\ **hit** \ī\ **ice** \j\ **job**
\ŋ\ **sing** \ō\ **go** \ó\ **law** \ói\ **boy** \th\ **thin** \th̲\ **the** \ü\ **loot**
\ú\ **foot** \y\ **yet** \zh\ **vision** *See also* Pronunciation Symbols page

canker sore *n* : a small painful ulcer esp. of the mouth; *esp* : a painful shallow ulceration of the oral mucous membranes that has a grayish-white base surrounded by a reddish inflamed area and is characteristic of aphthous stomatitis — compare COLD SORE

can·na·bi·di·ol \ˌkan-ə-bə-ˈdī-ˌȯl, kə-ˈnab-ə-, -ˌȯl\ *n* : a crystalline diphenol $C_{21}H_{28}(OH)_2$ obtained from the hemp plant that is physiologically inactive but is rearranged by acids into THC

can·na·bi·noid \ˈkan-ə-bə-ˌnȯid, kə-ˈnab-ə-\ *n* : any of various chemical constituents (as THC) of cannabis or marijuana

can·na·bi·nol \ˈkan-ə-bə-ˌnȯl, kə-ˈnab-ə-, -ˌnōl\ *n* : a physiologically inactive crystalline cannabinoid $C_{21}H_{26}O_2$

can·na·bis \ˈkan-ə-bəs\ *n* **1 a** *cap* : a genus of annual herbs (family Moraceae) that have leaves with three to seven elongate leaflets and pistillate flowers in spikes along the leafy erect stems and that include the hemp (*C. sativa*) **b** : HEMP 1 **2** : any of the preparations (as marijuana or hashish) or chemicals (as THC) that are derived from the hemp and are psychoactive

cannabis in·di·ca \-ˈin-di-kə\ *n*, *pl* **can·na·bes in·di·cae** \ˈkan-ə-ˌbēz-ˈin-də-ˌsē, -ˌbäs-ˈin-di-ˌkī\ : cannabis of a variety obtained in India

can·na·bism \ˈkan-ə-ˌbiz-əm\ *n* **1** : habituation to the use of cannabis **2** : chronic poisoning from excessive smoking or chewing of cannabis

can·ni·bal \ˈkan-ə-bəl\ *n* : one that eats the flesh of its own kind — **cannibal** *adj*

can·ni·bal·ism \-bə-ˌliz-əm\ *n* **1** : the usu. ritualistic eating of human flesh by a human being **2** : the eating of the flesh or the eggs of any animal by its own kind **3** : the pecking and tearing of the live flesh of its own members in a domestic poultry flock — compare PECKING ORDER **4** : oral sadism

can·non \ˈkan-ən\ *n* : the part of the leg in which the cannon bone is found

cannon bone *n* : a bone in hoofed mammals that supports the leg from the hock joint to the fetlock

can·nu·la *also* **can·u·la** \ˈkan-yə-lə\ *n*, *pl* **-las** *or* **-lae** \-ˌlē, -ˌlī\ : a small tube for insertion into a body cavity, duct, or vessel

can·nu·lar \ˈkan-yə-lər\ *adj* : TUBULAR

can·nu·late \-ˌlāt\ *vt* **-lat·ed; -lat·ing** : to insert a cannula into — **can·nu·la·tion** \ˌkan-yə-ˈlā-shən\ *n*

can·nu·lize \ˈkan-yə-ˌlīz\ *vt* **-lized; -liz·ing** : CANNULATE — **can·nu·li·za·tion** \ˌkan-yə-lə-ˈzā-shən\ *n*

ca·no·la \kə-ˈnō-lə\ *n* **1** : a rape plant (*Brassica napus* of the mustard family) of an improved variety with seeds that are low in erucic acid and are the source of canola oil **2** : CANOLA OIL

canola oil *n* : an edible vegetable oil obtained from the seeds of canola that is high in monounsaturated fatty acids

cant \ˈkant\ *n* : an oblique or slanting surface

can·thal \ˈkan(t)-thəl\ *adj* : belonging to a canthus

can·thar·i·dal \kan-ˈthar-əd-ᵊl\ *adj* : relating to or containing cantharides ⟨a ~ plaster⟩

can·thar·i·date \-ə-ˌdāt\ *vt* **-dat·ed; -dat·ing** : to treat or impregnate with cantharides

can·thar·i·din \kan-ˈthar-əd-ən\ *n* : a bitter crystalline compound $C_{10}H_{12}O_4$ that is the active blister-producing ingredient of cantharides

can·thar·i·dism \-ə-ˌdiz-əm\ *n* : poisoning due to misuse of cantharides

can·tha·ris \ˈkan(t)-thə-rəs\ *n*, *pl* **can·thar·i·des** \kan-ˈthar-ə-ˌdēz\ **1** : SPANISH FLY 1 **2** *cantharides pl but sing or pl in constr* : a preparation of dried beetles and esp. Spanish flies that contains cantharidin and is used in medicine as a blister-producing agent and formerly as an aphrodisiac — called also *Spanish fly*

Can·tha·ris \ˈkan(t)-thə-rəs\ *n*, *syn of* LYTTA

can·tha·xan·thin \ˌkan-thə-ˈzan-ˌthin\ *n* : a carotenoid $C_{40}H_{52}O_2$ used esp. as a color additive for food

can·thus \ˈkan(t)-thəs\ *n*, *pl* **can·thi** \ˈkan-ˌthī, -ˌthē\ : either of the angles formed by the meeting of the upper and lower eyelids

canula *var of* CANNULA

caou·tchouc \ˈkaù-ˌchúk, -ˌchük, -ˌchü\ *n* : RUBBER 1

¹cap \ˈkap\ *n, often attrib* **1** : a natural cover or top: as **a** : PILEUS **b** : PATELLA, KNEECAP **2** : something that serves as a cover or protection esp. for a tip, knob, or end (as of a tooth) **3** *Brit* : CERVICAL CAP **4** : a cluster of molecules or chemical groups bound to one end or a region of a cell, virus, or molecule ⟨the cell surface receptors were redistributed into ~s⟩

²cap *vb* **capped; cap·ping** *vt* **1** : to invest (a student nurse) with a cap as an indication of completion of a probationary period of study **2** : to cover (a diseased or exposed part of a tooth) with a protective substance **3** : to form a chemical cap on ⟨the *capped* end of a messenger RNA⟩ ~ *vi* : to form or produce a chemical cap

cap *abbr* **1** capacity **2** capsule

ca·pac·i·tance \kə-ˈpas-ət-ən(t)s\ *n* **1 a** : the property of an electric nonconductor that permits the storage of energy as a result of the separation of charge occurring when opposite surfaces of the nonconductor are maintained at a difference of potential **b** : the measure of this property equal to the ratio of the charge on either surface to the potential difference between the surfaces **2** : a part of a circuit or network that possesses capacitance

ca·pac·i·tate \-ə-ˌtāt\ *vt* **-tat·ed; -tat·ing** : to cause (sperm) to undergo capacitation

ca·pac·i·ta·tion \kə-ˌpas-ə-ˈtā-shən\ *n* : the change undergone by sperm in the female reproductive tract that enables them to penetrate and fertilize an egg

ca·pac·i·tor \kə-ˈpas-ət-ər\ *n* : a device giving capacitance and usu. consisting of conducting plates or foils separated by thin layers of dielectric (as air or mica) with the plates on opposite sides of the dielectric layers oppositely charged by a source of voltage and the electrical energy of the charged system stored in the polarized dielectric

ca·pac·i·ty \kə-ˈpas-ət-ē, -ˈpas-tē\ *n*, *pl* **-ties** **1 a** : the ability to hold, receive, store, or accommodate **b** : a measure of content : the measured ability to contain : VOLUME ⟨a beaker with a ~ of one liter⟩ — see VITAL CAPACITY **c** (1) : CAPACITANCE (2) : the quantity of electricity that a battery can deliver under specified conditions **2** : legal qualification, competency, power, or fitness **3 a** : power to grasp and analyze ideas and cope with problems **b** : blended power, strength, and ability ⟨encourage physical activity to the limit of the child's ~ —Morris Fishbein⟩

CAPD *abbr* **1** central auditory processing disorder **2** continuous ambulatory peritoneal dialysis

cap·e·line \ˈkap-ə-ˌlēn, -lən\ *n* : a cup-shaped bandage for the head, the shoulder, or the stump of an amputated limb

cap·il·lar·ia \ˌkap-ə-ˈlar-ē-ə\ *n* **1** *cap* : a genus of slender white nematode worms of the family Trichuridae that includes serious pathogens of the alimentary tract of fowls and some tissue and organ parasites of mammals including one (*C. hepatica*) which is common in rodents and occas. invades the human liver sometimes with fatal results **2** : a nematode worm of the genus *Capillaria* — **cap·il·lar·id** \-ˈlar-əd, kə-ˈpil-ə-rəd\ *n*

ca·pil·la·ri·a·sis \kə-ˌpil-ə-ˈrī-ə-səs\ *also* **cap·il·lar·i·o·sis** \ˌkap-ə-ˌler-ē-ˈō-səs\ *n*, *pl* **-a·ses** \-ə-ˌsēz\ *also* **-o·ses** \-ˈō-ˌsēz\ : infestation with or disease caused by nematode worms of the genus *Capillaria*

cap·il·lar·i·ty \ˌkap-ə-ˈlar-ət-ē\ *n*, *pl* **-ties** : the action by which the surface of a liquid where it is in contact with a solid (as in a capillary tube) is elevated or depressed depending on the relative attraction of the molecules of the liquid for each other and for those of the solid

cap·il·lar·o·scope \ˌkap-ə-ˈlar-ə-ˌskōp\ *n* : a microscope that permits visual examination of the living capillaries in nail beds, skin, and conjunctiva

cap·il·la·ros·co·py \ˌkap-ə-lə-ˈräs-kə-pē\ *also* **cap·il·lar·i·os-**

co·py \-ˌler-ē-ˈäs-\ *n, pl* **-pies** : diagnostic examination of capillaries, esp. of the nail beds, with a microscope

¹**cap·il·lary** \ˈkap-ə-ˌler-ē, *Brit usu* kə-ˈpil-ə-rē\ *adj* **1 a** : resembling a hair esp. in slender elongated form **b** : having a very small bore ⟨a ∼ tube⟩ **2** : involving, held by, or resulting from surface tension **3** : of or relating to capillaries or capillarity

²**capillary** *n, pl* **-lar·ies** : a capillary tube; *esp* : any of the smallest blood vessels connecting arterioles with venules and forming networks throughout the body

capillary attraction *n* : the force of adhesion between a solid and a liquid in capillarity

capillary bed *n* : the whole system of capillaries of a body, part, or organ

ca·pil·li·cul·ture \kə-ˈpil-ə-ˌkəl-chər\ *n* : treatment to cure or prevent baldness

ca·pil·lus \kə-ˈpil-əs\ *n, pl* **ca·pil·li** \-ˈpil-ˌī, -(ˌ)ē\ : a hair esp. of the head

capita *pl of* CAPUT

capita succedanea *pl of* CAPUT SUCCEDANEUM

¹**cap·i·tate** \ˈkap-ə-ˌtāt\ *adj* : abruptly enlarged and globular

²**capitate** *n* : the largest bone of the wrist that is situated between the hamate and the trapezoid in the distal row of carpal bones and that articulates with the third metacarpal

cap·i·tat·ed \ˈkap-ə-ˌtāt-əd\ *adj* : of, relating to, participating in, or being a health-care system in which a medical provider is given a set fee per patient (as by an HMO) regardless of treatment required

cap·i·ta·tion \ˌkap-ə-ˈtā-shən\ *n* **1** : a fixed per capita payment made periodically to a medical service provider (as a physician) by a managed care group (as an HMO) in return for medical care provided to enrolled individuals **2** : a capitated health-care system

cap·i·ta·tum \ˌkap-ə-ˈtāt-əm, -ˈtät-\ *n, pl* **cap·i·ta·ta** \-ˈtāt-ə, -ˈtät-\ : CAPITATE

cap·i·tel·lum \ˌkap-ə-ˈtel-əm\ *n, pl* **-tel·la** \-ˈtel-ə\ : a knoblike protuberance esp. at the end of a bone (as the humerus)

capitis — see LONGISSIMUS CAPITIS, LONGUS CAPITIS, OBLIQUUS CAPITIS INFERIOR, OBLIQUUS CAPITIS SUPERIOR, PEDICULOSIS CAPITIS, RECTUS CAPITIS POSTERIOR MAJOR, RECTUS CAPITIS POSTERIOR MINOR, SEMISPINALIS CAPITIS, SPINALIS CAPITIS, SPLENIUS CAPITIS, TINEA CAPITIS

ca·pit·u·lar \kə-ˈpich-ə-lər, -ˌlär\ *adj* : of or relating to a capitulum

ca·pit·u·lum \-ə-ləm\ *n, pl* **-la** \-lə\ : a rounded protuberance of an anatomical part: as **a** : the knob at the end of a bone or cartilage **b** : the beak of a tick composed of the mouthparts and palpi

Cap·lets \ˈka-pləts\ *trademark* — used for capsule-shaped medicinal tablets

cap·no·gram \ˈkap-nō-ˌgram\ *n* : the waveform tracing produced by a capnograph

cap·no·graph \ˈkap-nō-ˌgraf\ *n* : a monitoring device that measures the concentration of carbon dioxide in exhaled air and displays a numerical readout and waveform tracing — compare CAPNOMETER — **cap·no·graph·ic** \ˌkap-nō-ˈgraf-ik\ *adj* — **cap·nog·ra·phy** \kap-ˈnäg-rə-fē\ *n*

cap·nom·e·ter \kap-ˈnäm-ə-tər\ *n* : a monitoring device that measures and numerically displays the concentration of carbon dioxide in exhaled air — compare CAPNOGRAPH — **cap·nom·e·try** \-trē\ *n*

ca·pon \ˈkā-ˌpän, -pən\ *n* : a castrated male chicken

ca·pon·iza·tion *or Brit* **ca·pon·isa·tion** \ˌkā-pə-nə-ˈzā-shən\ *n* : castration esp. of a fowl — **ca·pon·ize** *or Brit* **ca·pon·ise** \ˈkā-pə-ˌnīz, -ˌpän-ˌīz\ *vt* **-ized** *or Brit* **-ised; -iz·ing** *or Brit* **-is·ing**

Cap·o·ten \ˈkap-ō-ˌten\ *trademark* — used for a preparation of captopril

cap·rate \ˈkap-ˌrāt\ *n* : a salt or ester of capric acid

cap·re·o·my·cin \ˌkap-rē-ō-ˈmīs-ᵊn\ *n* : an antibiotic obtained from a bacterium of the genus *Streptomyces* (*S. capreolus*) that is used to treat tuberculosis

cap·ric acid \ˌkap-rik-\ *n* : a fatty acid $C_{10}H_{20}O_2$ found in fats and oils and used in flavors and perfumes — called also *decanoic acid*

cap·rin \ˈkap-rən\ *n* : a caprate of glycerol found esp. in butter

cap·ro·ate \ˈkap-rə-ˌwāt\ *n* : a salt or ester of caproic acid

ca·pro·ic acid \kə-ˌprō-ik-\ *n* : a liquid fatty acid $C_6H_{12}O_2$ that is found as a glycerol ester in fats and oils or made synthetically and used in pharmaceuticals and flavors — called also *hexanoic acid*

cap·ro·in \ˈkap-rə-wən\ *n* : a caproate of glycerol found esp. in butter

cap·ro·yl \ˈkap-rə-ˌwil, -ˌwēl\ *n* : the group $C_5H_{11}CO-$ of caproic acid

cap·ry·late \ˈkap-rə-ˌlāt\ *n* : a salt or ester of caprylic acid — called also *octanoate;* see SODIUM CAPRYLATE

ca·pryl·ic acid \kə-ˌpril-ik-\ *n* : a fatty acid $C_8H_{16}O_2$ of rancid odor occurring in fats and oils and used in perfumes — called also *octanoic acid*

cap·sa·icin \kap-ˈsā-ə-sən\ *n* : a colorless irritant phenolic amide $C_{18}H_{27}NO_3$ found in various capsicums that gives hot peppers their hotness and that is used in topical creams for its analgesic properties

cap·si·cum \ˈkap-si-kəm\ *n* **1** *cap* : a genus of tropical herbs and shrubs of the nightshade family (Solanaceae) widely cultivated for their many-seeded usu. fleshy-walled berries **2** : any plant of the genus *Capsicum* — called also *pepper* **3** : the dried ripe fruit of some capsicums (as *C. frutescens*) used as a gastric and intestinal stimulant

cap·sid \ˈkap-səd\ *n* : the protein shell of a virus particle that surrounds its nucleic acid — **cap·sid·al** \-səd-ᵊl\ *adj*

cap·so·mer \ˈkap-sə-mər\ *or* **cap·so·mere** \ˈkap-sə-ˌmi(ə)r\ *n* : one of the subunits making up a viral capsid

cap·su·la \ˈkap-sə-lə\ *n, pl* **cap·su·lae** \-ˌlē, -ˌlī\ : CAPSULE

cap·su·lar \ˈkap-sə-lər\ *adj* : of, relating to, affecting, or resembling a capsule ⟨a ∼ contracture⟩

capsular contracture *n* : contracture involving a capsule or capsule-shaped structure; *specif* : shrinking and tightening of the mass of scar tissue around a breast implant that occurs esp. with some silicone implants and may result in pain and in unnatural firmness and distortion of the breast

capsularis — see DECIDUA CAPSULARIS

capsular ligament *n* : JOINT CAPSULE

cap·su·lat·ed \-ˌlāt-əd\ *also* **cap·su·late** \-ˌlāt, -lət\ *adj* : enclosed in a capsule ⟨a ∼ staphylococcus⟩

cap·su·la·tion \ˌkap-sə-ˈlā-shən\ *n* : enclosure in a capsule

cap·sule \ˈkap-səl, -(ˌ)sül\ *n* **1 a** : a membrane or saclike structure enclosing a part or organ ⟨the ∼ of the kidney⟩ **b** : either of two layers or laminae of white matter in the cerebrum: (1) : a layer that consists largely of fibers passing to and from the cerebral cortex and that lies internal to the lentiform nucleus — called also *internal capsule* (2) : one that lies between the lentiform nucleus and the claustrum — called also *external capsule* **2** : a shell usu. of gelatin for packaging something (as a drug or vitamins); *also* : a usu. medicinal or nutritional preparation for oral use consisting of the shell and its contents **3** : a viscous or gelatinous often polysaccharide envelope surrounding certain microscopic organisms (as the pneumococcus)

cap·su·lec·to·my \ˌkap-sə-ˈlek-tə-mē\ *n, pl* **-mies** : excision of a capsule (as of a joint, kidney, or lens)

capsule of Bow·man \-ˈbō-mən\ *n* : BOWMAN'S CAPSULE

capsule of Glis·son \-ˈglis-ᵊn\ *n* : GLISSON'S CAPSULE

capsule of Te·non \-tə-ˈnōⁿ\ *n* : TENON'S CAPSULE

cap·su·li·tis \ˌkap-sə-ˈlīt-əs\ *n* : inflammation of a capsule (as that of the crystalline lens)

cap·su·lor·rha·phy \ˌkap-sə-ˈlȯr-ə-fē\ *n, pl* **-phies** : suture of a cut or wounded capsule (as of the knee joint)

\ə\ **abut** \ᵊ\ **kitten** \ər\ **further** \a\ **ash** \ā\ **ace** \ä\ **cot, cart**
\aů\ **out** \ch\ **chin** \e\ **bet** \ē\ **easy** \g\ **go** \i\ **hit** \ī\ **ice** \j\ **job**
\ŋ\ **sing** \ō\ **go** \ȯ\ **law** \ȯi\ **boy** \th\ **thin** \t̲h̲\ **the** \ü\ **loot**
\ů\ **foot** \y\ **yet** \zh\ **vision** *See also* Pronunciation Symbols page

cap·su·lot·o·my \-'lät-ə-mē\ *n, pl* **-mies** : incision of a capsule esp. of the crystalline lens (as in a cataract operation)

cap·to·pril \'kap-tə-ˌpril\ *n* : an antihypertensive drug $C_9H_{15}NO_3S$ that is an ACE inhibitor — see CAPOTEN

ca·put \'käp-ˌut, -ət; 'kap-ət\ *n, pl* **ca·pi·ta** \'käp-ə-ˌtä, 'kap-ət-ə\ **1** : a knoblike protuberance (as of a bone or muscle) **2** : CAPUT SUCCEDANEUM

caput suc·ce·da·ne·um \-ˌsək-sə-'dā-nē-əm\ *n, pl* **capita suc·ce·da·nea** \-nē-ə\ : an edematous swelling formed under the presenting part of the scalp of a newborn infant as a result of trauma sustained during delivery

Car·a·fate \'kar-ə-ˌfāt\ *trademark* — used for a preparation of sucralfate

car·a·mel \'kar-ə-məl, -ˌmel; 'kär-məl\ *n* : an amorphous brittle brown and somewhat bitter substance obtained by heating sugar and used as a coloring and flavoring agent

ca·ra·te \kə-'rät-ē\ *n* : PINTA

car·a·way \'kar-ə-ˌwā\ *n* **1** : a biennial usu. white-flowered aromatic herb (*Carum carvi*) of the carrot family (Umbelliferae) with pungent fruits **2** : the fruit of caraway that is used in cookery and confectionery and is the source of caraway oil — called also *caraway seed*

caraway oil *n* : an essential oil obtained from caraway seeds and used in pharmaceuticals and as a flavoring agent in foods and liqueurs

caraway seed *n* : CARAWAY 2

carb \'kärb\ *or* **car·bo** \'kär-ˌbō\ *n* : CARBOHYDRATE; *also* : a high-carbohydrate food — usu. used in pl.

car·ba·chol \'kär-bə-ˌkȯl, -ˌkōl\ *n* : a synthetic parasympathomimetic drug $C_6H_{15}ClN_2O_2$ that is used in veterinary medicine and topically to treat glaucoma

car·ba·mate \'kär-bə-ˌmāt, kär-'bam-ˌāt\ *n* : a salt or ester of carbamic acid — see URETHANE

car·ba·maz·e·pine \ˌkär-bə-'maz-ə-ˌpēn\ *n* : a tricyclic anticonvulsant and analgesic $C_{15}H_{12}N_2O$ used in the treatment of trigeminal neuralgia and epilepsy — see TEGRETOL

car·bam·ic acid \(ˌ)kär-ˌbam-ik-\ *n* : an acid CH_3NO_2 known in the form of salts and esters

carb·amide \'kär-bə-ˌmīd, kär-'bam-əd\ *n* : UREA

carb·ami·no \ˌkär-bə-'mē-(ˌ)nō\ *adj* : relating to any of various carbamic acid derivatives formed by reaction of carbon dioxide with an amino acid or a protein (as hemoglobin)

carb·ami·no·he·mo·glo·bin *or chiefly Brit* **carb·ami·no·hae·mo·glo·bin** \ˌkärb-ə-ˌmē-(ˌ)nō-'hē-mə-ˌglō-bən\ *n* : CARBHEMOGLOBIN

car·ba·myl \'kär-bə-ˌmil\ *or* **car·bam·o·yl** \kär-'bam-ə-ˌwil\ *n* : the radical NH_2CO- of carbamic acid

carb·an·ion \kär-'ban-ˌī-ən, -ˌī-ˌän\ *n* : an organic ion carrying a negative charge on a carbon atom

car·bar·sone \kär-'bär-ˌsōn\ *n* : a white powder $C_7H_9N_2O_4As$ used esp. in treating intestinal amebiasis

car·ba·ryl \'kär-bə-ˌril\ *n* : a carbamate insecticide effective against numerous crop, forage, and forest pests — see SEVIN

car·ba·zole \'kär-bə-ˌzōl\ *n* : a crystalline slightly basic cyclic compound $C_{12}H_9N$ found in anthracene and used in making dyes and in testing for carbohydrates (as sugars)

car·ben·i·cil·lin \ˌkär-ben-ə-'sil-ən\ *n* : a broad-spectrum semisynthetic penicillin $C_{17}H_{18}N_2O_6S$ that is used esp. against gram-negative bacteria (as pseudomonas)

carb·he·mo·glo·bin \(ˈ)kärb-'hē-mə-ˌglō-bən\ *or* **car·bo·hemo·glo·bin** \ˌkär-(ˌ)bō-\ *or chiefly Brit* **carb·hae·mo·glo·bin** *or* **car·bo·hae·mo·glo·bin** *n* : a compound of hemoglobin with carbon dioxide

car·bide \'kär-ˌbīd\ *n* : a binary compound of carbon with a more electropositive element

car·bi·do·pa \ˌkär-bə-'dō-pə\ *n* : a drug $C_{10}H_{14}N_2O_4 \cdot H_2O$ that inhibits decarboxylation of L-dopa in tissues outside the brain and that is administered with L-dopa in the treatment of Parkinson's disease to increase the amount of L-dopa available for transport to the brain

car·bi·nol \'kär-bə-ˌnȯl, -ˌnōl\ *n* : METHANOL; *also* : an alcohol derived from it

¹car·bo \'kär-ˌbō\ *n* : CHARCOAL

²carbo *var of* CARB

car·bo·ben·zoxy \ˌkär-(ˌ)bō-ˌben-'zäk-sē\ *or* **car·bo·ben·zy·loxy** \-ˌben-zə-'läk-sē\ *adj* : relating to or containing the group $-COOCH_2C_6H_5$ ⟨∼ synthesis of peptides⟩

car·bo·cy·clic \ˌkär-bō-'sī-klik, -'sik-lik\ *adj* : being or having an organic ring composed of carbon atoms

carbohaemoglobin *chiefly Brit var of* CARBHEMOGLOBIN

carbohemoglobin *var of* CARBHEMOGLOBIN

car·bo·hy·drase \ˌkär-bō-'hī-ˌdrās, -bə-, -ˌdrāz\ *n* : any of a group of enzymes (as amylase) that promote hydrolysis or synthesis of a carbohydrate (as a disaccharide)

car·bo·hy·drate \-ˌdrāt, -drət\ *n* : any of various neutral compounds of carbon, hydrogen, and oxygen (as sugars, starches, and celluloses) most of which are formed by green plants and which constitute a major class of animal foods

car·bo·late \'kär-bə-ˌlāt\ *n* : a salt of carbolic acid

car·bo·lat·ed \-ˌlāt-əd\ *adj* : PHENOLATED

car·bol·fuch·sin \ˌkär-(ˌ)bäl-'fyük-sən, -(ˌ)bȯl-\ *n* : a mixture of an aqueous solution of phenol and an alcoholic solution of fuchsin used as a stain in microscopy esp. in staining bacteria

carbolfuchsin paint \-'pānt\ *n* : a solution containing boric acid, phenol, resorcinol, and fuchsin in acetone, alcohol, and water that is applied externally in the treatment of fungal infections of the skin — called also *Castellani's paint*

car·bol·ic \kär-'bäl-ik\ *n* : PHENOL 1

carbolic acid *n* : PHENOL 1

car·bo·li·gase \ˌkär-bō-'lī-ˌgās, -ˌgāz\ *n* : an enzyme that catalyzes the combination of carbon atoms in some metabolic reactions

car·bo·line \'kär-bə-ˌlēn\ *n* : any of various isomers that have the formula $C_{11}H_8N_2$ and are structurally related to indole and pyridine

car·bo·lized *or Brit* **car·bo·lised** \-ˌlīzd\ *adj* : PHENOLATED

car·bo–load \'kär-ˌbō-ˌlōd\ *vi* : to consume a large amount of carbohydrates through food intake usu. in order to improve performance in an upcoming athletic event (as a marathon)

car·bo·my·cin \ˌkär-bə-'mīs-ᵊn\ *n* : a colorless crystalline basic macrolide antibiotic $C_{42}H_{67}NO_{16}$ produced by a bacterium of the genus *Streptomyces* (*S. halstedii*) and active esp. in inhibiting the growth of gram-positive bacteria — see MAGNAMYCIN

car·bon \'kär-bən\ *n, often attrib* : a nonmetallic element found native (as in diamonds and graphite) or as a constituent of coal, petroleum, asphalt, limestone, and organic compounds or obtained artificially (as in activated charcoal) — symbol *C*; see ELEMENT table

¹car·bon·ate \'kär-bə-ˌnāt, -nət\ *n* : a salt or ester of carbonic acid

²car·bon·ate \-ˌnāt\ *vt* **-at·ed; -at·ing** **1** : to convert into a carbonate **2** : to impregnate with carbon dioxide — **car·bon·ation** \ˌkär-bə-'nā-shən\ *n*

carbon bisulfide *n* : CARBON DISULFIDE

carbon cycle *n* : the cycle of carbon in living beings in which carbon dioxide is fixed by photosynthesis to form organic nutrients and is ultimately restored to the inorganic state by respiration and protoplasmic decay

carbon dioxide *n* : a heavy colorless gas CO_2 that does not support combustion, dissolves in water to form carbonic acid, is formed esp. in animal respiration and in the decay or combustion of animal and vegetable matter, is absorbed from the air by plants in photosynthesis, and is used in the carbonation of beverages

carbon disulfide *n* : a colorless flammable poisonous liquid CS_2 used as a solvent for rubber and as an insect fumigant — called also *carbon bisulfide*

carbon 14 \-(ˈ)fōr(t)-'tēn, -(ˈ)fȯr(t)-\ *n* : a heavy radioactive isotope of carbon of mass number 14 used esp. in tracer studies and in dating archaeological and geological materials

car·bon·ic \kär-'bän-ik\ *adj* : of, relating to, or derived from carbon, carbonic acid, or carbon dioxide

carbonic acid *n* : a weak dibasic acid H_2CO_3 known only in solution that reacts with bases to form carbonates

carbonic acid gas *n* : CARBON DIOXIDE

car·bon·ic an·hy·drase \-an-'hī-₁drās, -₁drāz\ *n* : a zinc-containing enzyme that occurs in living tissues (as red blood cells) and aids carbon-dioxide transport from the tissues and its release from the blood in the lungs by catalyzing the reversible hydration of carbon dioxide to carbonic acid

car·bo·ni·um ion \kär-'bō-nē-əm-\ *n* : an organic ion that contains a positively charged carbon atom

car·bon·ize *or Brit* **car·bon·ise** \'kär-bə-₁nīz\ *vb* **-ized** *or Brit* **-ised; -iz·ing** *or Brit* **-is·ing** *vt* : to convert into carbon or a carbonic residue ∼ *vi* : to become carbonized or charred — **car·bon·iza·tion** *or Brit* **car·bon·isa·tion** \₁kär-bə-nə-'zā-shən\ *n*

carbon monoxide *n* : a colorless odorless very toxic gas CO that burns to carbon dioxide with a blue flame and is formed as a product of the incomplete combustion of carbon

carbon tetrachloride *n* : a colorless nonflammable toxic carcinogenic liquid CCl_4 that has an odor resembling that of chloroform and is used as a solvent and a refrigerant — called also *tetrachloromethane*

car·bon·yl \'kär-bə-₁nil, -₁nēl\ *n* : an organic functional group CO occurring in aldehydes, ketones, carboxylic acids, esters, and their derivatives

car·bon·yl·he·mo·glo·bin *or chiefly Brit* **car·bon·yl·hae·mo·glo·bin** \-'hē-mə-₁glō-bən\ *n* : CARBOXYHEMOGLOBIN

car·bo·plat·in \'kär-bō-₁plat-ᵊn\ *n* : a platinum-containing antineoplastic drug $C_6H_{12}N_2O_4Pt$ that is an analog of cisplatin with somewhat reduced toxicity and that is used in the treatment of various cancers (as of the ovary or lung)

car·boxy·he·mo·glo·bin *or chiefly Brit* **car·boxy·hae·mo·glo·bin** \(₁)kär-₁bäk-sē-'hē-mə-₁glō-bən\ *n* : a very stable combination of hemoglobin and carbon monoxide formed in the blood when carbon monoxide is inhaled with resulting loss of ability of the blood to combine with oxygen

car·box·yl \kär-'bäk-səl\ *n* : a monovalent group –COOH typical of organic acids — called also *carboxyl group* — **car·box·yl·ic** \₁kär-(₁)bäk-'sil-ik\ *adj*

car·box·yl·ase \kär-'bäk-sə-₁lās, -₁lāz\ *n* : an enzyme that catalyzes decarboxylation or carboxylation

¹car·box·yl·ate \-₁lāt\ *vt* **-at·ed; -at·ing** : to introduce carboxyl or carbon dioxide into (a compound) with formation of a carboxylic acid — **car·box·yl·ation** \(₁)kär-₁bäk-sə-'lā-shən\ *n*

²car·box·yl·ate \-₁lāt, -lət\ *n* : a salt or ester of a carboxylic acid

carboxyl group *n* : CARBOXYL

carboxylic acid *n* : an organic acid (as an acetic acid) containing one or more carboxyl groups

car·boxy·meth·yl·cel·lu·lose \(₁)kär-₁bäk-sē-₁meth-əl-'sel-yə-₁lōs, -₁lōz\ *n* : an acid ether derivative of cellulose that in the form of its sodium salt is used as a thickening, emulsifying, and stabilizing agent and as a bulk laxative in medicine

car·boxy·pep·ti·dase \-'pep-tə-₁dās, -₁dāz\ *n* : an enzyme that hydrolyzes peptides and esp. polypeptides by splitting off sequentially the amino acids at the end of the peptide chain which contain free carboxyl groups

car·bro·mal \kär-'brō-məl\ *n* : a white crystalline compound $C_7H_{13}BrN_2O_2$ used as a sedative and hypnotic

car·bun·cle \'kär-₁bəŋ-kəl\ *n* : a painful local purulent inflammation of the skin and deeper tissues with multiple openings for the discharge of pus and usu. necrosis and sloughing of dead tissue — **car·bun·cu·lar** \kär-'bəŋ-kyə-lər\ *adj*

car·bun·cu·lo·sis \kär-₁bəŋ-kyə-'lō-səs\ *n, pl* **-lo·ses** \-₁sēz\ : a condition marked by the formation of many carbuncles simultaneously or in rapid succession

car·byl·amine \₁kär-₁bil-ə-'mēn, -'bil-ə-₁mēn\ *n* : ISOCYANIDE

car·cass \'kär-kəs\ *n* : a dead body : CORPSE; *esp* : the dressed body of a meat animal

car·ce·ag \'kär-sē-₁ag\ *n* : babesiosis of the sheep

car·ci·no·em·bry·on·ic antigen \₁kärs-ᵊn-ō-₁em-brē-₁än-ik-\ *n* : a glycoprotein present in fetal gut tissues during the first two trimesters of pregnancy and in peripheral blood of patients with some forms of cancer (as of the digestive system or the breast) — abbr. *CEA*

car·cin·o·gen \kär-'sin-ə-jən, 'kärs-ᵊn-ə-₁jen\ *n* : a substance or agent causing cancer

car·ci·no·gen·e·sis \₁kärs-ᵊn-ō-'jen-ə-səs\ *n, pl* **-e·ses** \-₁sēz\ : the production of cancer

car·ci·no·gen·ic \₁kärs-ᵊn-ō-'jen-ik\ *adj* : producing or tending to produce cancer ⟨the ∼ action of certain chemicals —*Jour. Amer. Med. Assoc.*⟩ — **car·ci·no·gen·i·cal·ly** \-i-k(ə-)lē\ *adv* — **car·ci·no·ge·nic·i·ty** \-jə-'nis-ət-ē\ *n, pl* **-ties**

car·ci·noid \'kärs-ᵊn-₁óid\ *n* : a benign or malignant tumor arising esp. from the mucosa of the gastrointestinal tract (as in the stomach or appendix)

carcinoid syndrome *n* : a syndrome that is caused by vasoactive substances secreted by carcinoid tumors and is characterized by flushing, cyanosis, abdominal cramps, diarrhea, and valvular heart disease

car·ci·no·lyt·ic \₁kärs-ᵊn-ō-'lit-ik\ *adj* : destructive to cancer cells

car·ci·no·ma \₁kärs-ᵊn-'ō-mə\ *n, pl* **-mas** *also* **-ma·ta** \-mət-ə\ : a malignant tumor of epithelial origin — compare SARCOMA — **car·ci·no·ma·tous** \-'ō-mət-əs\ *adj*

carcinoma in situ *n* : carcinoma in the stage of development when the cancer cells are still within their site of origin (as the mouth or uterine cervix) — abbr. *CIS*

car·ci·no·ma·toid \₁kärs-ᵊn-'äm-ə-₁tóid, -'ō-mə-\ *adj* : resembling a carcinoma

car·ci·no·ma·to·sis \-₁ō-mə-'tō-səs\ *n, pl* **-to·ses** \-₁sēz\ : a condition in which multiple carcinomas develop simultaneously usu. after dissemination from a primary source

car·ci·no·sar·co·ma \'kärs-ᵊn-ō-(₁)sär-'kō-mə\ *n, pl* **-mas** *also* **-ma·ta** \-mət-ə\ : a malignant tumor combining elements of carcinoma and sarcoma

car·ci·no·sis \₁kärs-ᵊn-'ō-səs\ *n, pl* **-no·ses** \-₁sēz\ : dissemination of carcinomatous growths in the body : CARCINOMATOSIS

car·da·mom \'kärd-ə-məm, -₁mäm\ *n* : the aromatic capsular fruit of an Indian herb (*Elettaria cardamomum*) of the ginger family with seeds used as a spice and in medicine; *also* : this plant

cardamom oil *n* : a colorless or pale-yellow essential oil with a camphoraceous odor and pungent taste distilled from cardamom seeds and used in pharmaceutical preparations and as a flavoring for foods

car·dia \'kärd-ē-ə\ *n, pl* **car·di·ae** \-ē-₁ē\ *or* **cardias** **1** : the opening of the esophagus into the stomach **2** : the part of the stomach adjoining the cardia

¹car·di·ac \'kärd-ē-₁ak\ *adj* **1 a** : of, relating to, situated near, or acting on the heart **b** : of or relating to the cardia of the stomach **2** : of, relating to, or affected with heart disease

²cardiac *n* : an individual with heart disease

cardiac arrest *n* : abrupt temporary or permanent cessation of the heartbeat (as from ventricular fibrillation or asystole) — called also *sudden cardiac arrest*

cardiac asthma *n* : asthma due to heart disease (as heart failure) that occurs in paroxysms usu. at night and is characterized by difficult wheezing respiration, pallor, and anxiety — called also *paroxysmal dyspnea*

cardiac cycle *n* : the complete sequence of events in the heart from the beginning of one beat to the beginning of the following beat : a complete heartbeat including systole and diastole

cardiac failure *n* : HEART FAILURE

cardiac gland *n* : any of the branched tubular mucus-secreting glands of the cardia of the stomach; *also* : one of the similar glands of the esophagus

cardiac impulse *n* : the wave of cardiac excitation passing

\ə\ **abut** \ᵊ\ **kitten** \ər\ **further** \a\ **ash** \ā\ **ace** \ä\ **cot, cart**
\aú\ **out** \ch\ **chin** \e\ **bet** \ē\ **easy** \g\ **go** \i\ **hit** \ī\ **ice** \j\ **job**
\ŋ\ **sing** \ō\ **go** \ó\ **law** \ói\ **boy** \th\ **thin** \th̲\ **the** \ü\ **loot**
\ú\ **foot** \y\ **yet** \zh\ **vision** *See also* Pronunciation Symbols page

from the sinoatrial node to the atrioventricular node and along the bundle of His and initiating the cardiac cycle; *broadly* : HEARTBEAT

cardiac muscle *n* : the principal muscle tissue of the vertebrate heart that is made up of elongated striated muscle fibers each of which consists of a single cell that has an intrinsic rhythm of contraction and relaxation even when isolated, is joined physically at its often branched ends to other such cells by intercalated disks, and in intact myocardial tissue is synchronized to function in contraction esp. by electrical signals of extrinsic origin passing through gap junctions in the intercalated disks — compare SMOOTH MUSCLE, STRIATED MUSCLE

cardiac nerve *n* : any of the three nerves connecting the cervical ganglia of the sympathetic nervous system with the cardiac plexus: **a** : one arising esp. from the inferior cervical ganglion or the stellate ganglion — called also *inferior cardiac nerve* **b** : one arising esp. from the middle cervical ganglion — called also *middle cardiac nerve* **c** : one arising esp. from the superior cervical ganglion — called also *superior cardiac nerve*

cardiac neurosis *n* : NEUROCIRCULATORY ASTHENIA

cardiac orifice *n* : CARDIA 1

cardiac out·put \-ˈaut-ˌput\ *n* : the volume of blood ejected from the left side of the heart in one minute — called also *minute volume*

cardiac plexus *n* : a nerve plexus of the autonomic nervous system supplying the heart and neighboring structures and situated near the heart and the arch and ascending part of the aorta

cardiac reserve *n* : the difference between the rate at which a heart pumps blood at a particular time and its maximum capacity for pumping blood

cardiac sphincter *n* : the somewhat thickened muscular ring surrounding the opening between the esophagus and the stomach

cardiac tamponade *n* : mechanical compression of the heart by large amounts of fluid or blood within the pericardial space that limits the normal range of motion and function of the heart

cardiac valve *n* : HEART VALVE

cardiac vein *n* : any of the veins returning the blood from the tissues of the heart that open into the right atrium either directly or through the coronary sinus: as **a** : one that begins at the apex of the lower part of the heart, ascends in the sulcus between the ventricles in front, and curves around the heart to the left to join the coronary sinus in back — called also *great cardiac vein* **b** : one that begins at the apex of the lower part of the heart and ascends along the sulcus between the ventricles in back to join the right extremity of the coronary sinus — called also *middle cardiac vein* **c** : a vein that drains blood from the back of the atrium and ventricle on the right side of the heart, passes along the coronary sulcus, and empties into the coronary sinus near its opening into the right atrium — called also *small cardiac vein*

cardiae *pl of* CARDIA

car·di·al·gia \ˌkärd-ē-ˈal-j(ē-)ə\ *n* **1** : HEARTBURN **2** : pain in the heart

car·di·ec·to·my \ˌkärd-ē-ˈek-tə-mē\ *n, pl* **-mies** : excision of the cardiac portion of the stomach

car·di·nal vein \ˌkärd-nəl-, -ᵊn-əl-\ *n* : any of four longitudinal veins of the vertebrate embryo running anteriorly and posteriorly along each side of the spinal column with the pair on each side meeting at and discharging blood to the heart through the corresponding duct of Cuvier — called also *cardinal sinus, Cuvierian vein*

¹car·dio \ˈkärd-ē-(ˌ)ō\ *adj* : CARDIOVASCULAR 2 ⟨~ exercises⟩ ⟨worked out on ~ machines⟩

²cardio *n* : cardiovascular exercise ⟨30 minutes of ~ daily⟩

car·dio·ac·cel·er·a·tor \ˌkärd-ē-(ˌ)ō-ik-ˈsel-ə-ˌrāt-ər, -ak-\ *also* **car·dio·ac·cel·er·a·to·ry** \-ˈsel-ə-rə-ˌtōr-ē, -ˌtòr-\ *adj* : speeding up the action of the heart — **car·dio·ac·cel·er·a·tion** \-ˌsel-ə-ˈrā-shən\ *n*

car·dio·ac·tive \-ˈak-tiv\ *adj* : having an influence on the heart ⟨~ drugs⟩ — **car·dio·ac·tiv·i·ty** \-ak-ˈtiv-ət-ē\ *n, pl* **-ties**

car·dio·cir·cu·la·to·ry \-ˈsər-kyə-lə-ˌtōr-ē, -ˌtòr-\ *adj* : of or relating to the heart and circulatory system ⟨temporary ~ assist⟩

car·dio·dy·nam·ics \-dī-ˈnam-iks\ *n pl but sing or pl in constr* : the dynamics of the heart's action in pumping blood — **car·dio·dy·nam·ic** \-ik\ *adj*

car·dio·gen·ic \-ˈjen-ik\ *adj* : originating in the heart or caused by a cardiac condition ⟨~ pulmonary edema⟩

cardiogenic plate *n* : an area of splanchnic mesoderm anterior to the head process of the early mammalian embryo that subsequently gives rise to the heart

cardiogenic shock *n* : shock resulting from failure of the heart to pump an adequate amount of blood as a result of heart disease and esp. heart attack

car·dio·gram \ˈkärd-ē-ə-ˌgram\ *n* : the curve or tracing made by a cardiograph

car·dio·graph \-ˌgraf\ *n* : an instrument that registers graphically movements of the heart — **car·di·og·ra·pher** \ˌkärd-ē-ˈäg-rə-fər\ *n* — **car·dio·graph·ic** \ˌkärd-ē-ə-ˈgraf-ik\ *adj* — **car·di·og·ra·phy** \ˌkärd-ē-ˈäg-rə-fē\ *n, pl* **-phies**

car·dio·in·hib·i·to·ry \ˌkärd-ē-(ˌ)ō-in-ˈhib-ə-ˌtōr-ē, -ˌtòr-\ *adj* : interfering with or slowing the normal sequence of events in the cardiac cycle ⟨the ~ center of the medulla⟩

car·dio·lip·in \ˌkärd-ē-ō-ˈlip-ən\ *n* : a phospholipid obtained esp. from beef heart and used in combination with lecithin and cholesterol as an antigen in diagnostic blood tests for syphilis

car·di·ol·o·gy \ˌkärd-ē-ˈäl-ə-jē\ *n, pl* **-gies** : the study of the heart and its action and diseases — **car·di·o·log·i·cal** \-ē-ə-ˈläj-i-kəl\ *adj* — **car·di·ol·o·gist** \-ē-ˈäl-ə-jəst\ *n*

car·di·o·meg·a·ly \ˌkärd-ē-ō-ˈmeg-ə-lē\ *n, pl* **-lies** : enlargement of the heart

car·di·om·e·ter \ˌkärd-ē-ˈäm-ət-ər\ *n* : an instrument used in measuring the force of the heart's action — **car·di·o·met·ric** \-ē-ə-ˈme-trik\ *adj* — **car·di·om·e·try** \-ē-ˈäm-ə-trē\ *n, pl* **-tries**

car·di·o·my·op·a·thy \ˈkärd-ē-ō-(ˌ)mī-ˈäp-ə-thē\ *n, pl* **-thies** : any structural or functional disease of heart muscle that is marked esp. by hypertrophy of cardiac muscle, by enlargement of the heart, by rigidity and loss of flexibility of the heart walls, or by narrowing of the ventricles but is not due to a congenital developmental defect, to coronary atherosclerosis, to valve dysfunction, or to hypertension

car·dio·path \ˈkärd-ē-ə-ˌpath\ *n* : CARDIAC

car·di·op·a·thy \ˌkärd-ē-ˈäp-ə-thē\ *n, pl* **-thies** : any disease of the heart

car·dio·pho·bia \ˌkärd-ē-ə-ˈfō-bē-ə\ *n* : abnormal fear of heart disease

car·dio·plas·ty \ˈkärd-ē-ō-ˌplas-tē\ *n, pl* **-ties** : plastic surgery performed on the gastric cardiac sphincter

car·dio·ple·gia \ˌkärd-ē-ō-ˈplē-j(ē-)ə\ *n* : temporary cardiac arrest induced (as by drugs) during heart surgery — **car·dio·ple·gic** \-jik\ *adj*

car·dio·pro·tec·tive \-prə-ˈtek-tiv\ *adj* : serving to protect the heart ⟨~ effects of ACE inhibitors⟩ ⟨a ~ agent⟩

car·dio·pul·mo·nary \ˌkärd-ē-ō-ˈpul-mə-ˌner-ē, -ˈpəl-\ *adj* : of or relating to the heart and lungs ⟨the ~ system⟩ ⟨a ~ bypass that diverts blood from the entrance to the right atrium through an oxygenator directly to the aorta⟩

cardiopulmonary resuscitation *n* : a procedure designed to restore normal breathing after cardiac arrest that includes the clearance of air passages to the lungs, the mouth-to-mouth method of artificial respiration, and heart massage by the exertion of pressure on the chest — abbr. *CPR*

car·dio·re·nal \-ˈrēn-ᵊl\ *adj* : of or relating to the heart and the kidneys ⟨~ disorders⟩

car·dio·res·pi·ra·to·ry \ˌkärd-ē-ō-ˈres-p(ə-)rə-ˌtōr-ē, -ri-ˈspī-rə-, -ˌtòr-\ *adj* : of or relating to the heart and the respiratory system : CARDIOPULMONARY ⟨~ ailments⟩ ⟨~ responses⟩

car·di·or·rha·phy \ˌkärd-ē-'ȯr-ə-fē\ *n, pl* **-phies** : a surgical operation of suturing the heart muscle (as in the repair of a stab wound)

car·dio·scle·ro·sis \ˌkärd-ē-(ˌ)ō-sklə-'rō-səs\ *n, pl* **-ro·ses** \-ˌsēz\ : induration of the heart caused by formation of fibrous tissue in the cardiac muscle

car·dio·scope \'kärd-ē-ə-ˌskōp\ *n* **1** : an instrument that permits direct visual inspection of the interior of the heart **2** : an instrument that permits continuous electrocardiographic observation of the heart's action during an operation **3** : an instrument equipped with a screen on which tracings of the heart's action and sounds can be shown

car·dio·spasm \-ˌspaz-əm\ *n* : failure of the cardiac sphincter to relax during swallowing with resultant esophageal obstruction — compare ACHALASIA — **car·dio·spas·tic** \ˌkärd-ē-ō-'spas-tik\ *adj*

car·dio·ta·chom·e·ter \ˌkärd-ē-(ˌ)ō-ta-'käm-ət-ər, -tə-'käm-\ *n* : a device for prolonged graphic recording of the heartbeat — **car·dio·tacho·met·ric** \-ˌtak-ə-'me-trik\ *adj* — **car·dio·ta·chom·e·try** \-ta-'käm-ə-trē, -tə-'käm-\ *n, pl* **-tries**

car·dio·tho·ra·cic \-thə-'ras-ik\ *adj* : relating to, involving, or specializing in the heart and chest ⟨∼ surgery⟩

car·di·ot·o·my \ˌkärd-ē-'ät-ə-mē\ *n, pl* **-mies** **1** : surgical incision of the heart **2** : surgical incision of the stomach cardia

¹**car·dio·ton·ic** \ˌkärd-ē-ō-'tän-ik\ *adj* : tending to increase the tonus of heart muscle ⟨∼ steroids⟩

²**cardiotonic** *n* : a cardiotonic substance

car·dio·tox·ic \-'täk-sik\ *adj* : having a toxic effect on the heart — **car·dio·tox·ic·i·ty** \-täk-'sis-ət-ē\ *n, pl* **-ties**

¹**car·dio·vas·cu·lar** \-'vas-kyə-lər\ *adj* **1** : of, relating to, or involving the heart and blood vessels ⟨∼ disease⟩ **2** : used, designed, or performed to cause a temporary increase in heart rate (as to improve heart function and reduce the risk of heart disease) ⟨a ∼ workout⟩ ⟨treadmills, stationary bicycles, and other ∼ equipment⟩

²**cardiovascular** *n* : a substance (as a drug) that affects the heart or blood vessels

car·dio·ver·sion \-'vər-zhən *also* -shən\ *n* : application of an electric shock in order to restore normal heartbeat

car·dio·vert \'kärd-ē-ō-ˌvərt\ *vt* : to subject to cardioversion ⟨∼ed the patient to sinus rhythm⟩

car·dio·ver·ter \'kärd-ē-ō-ˌvərt-ər\ *n* : a device for the administration of an electric shock in cardioversion

car·di·tis \kär-'dīt-əs\ *n, pl* **car·dit·i·des** \-'dit-ə-ˌdēz\ : inflammation of the heart muscle : MYOCARDITIS

Car·di·zem \'kär-də-ˌzem, -zəm\ *trademark* — used for a preparation of the hydrochloride of diltiazem

Car·du·ra \ˌkär-'dúr-ə\ *trademark* — used for a preparation of doxazosin

care \'ka(ə)r, 'ke(ə)r\ *n* : responsibility for or attention to health, well-being, and safety — see ACUTE CARE, HEALTH CARE, INTENSIVE CARE, PRIMARY CARE, TERTIARY CARE — **care** *vi* **cared; car·ing**

care·giv·er \-ˌgiv-ər\ *n* : a person who provides direct care (as for children, elderly people, or the chronically ill) ⟨parents and other ∼s⟩ — **care·giv·ing** \-iŋ\ *n*

Car·i·ca \'kar-i-kə\ *n* : a genus (the type of the family Caricaceae) of chiefly tropical American trees that includes the papaya

car·ies \'ka(ə)r-ēz, 'ke(ə)r-\ *n, pl* **caries** : a progressive destruction of bone or tooth; *esp* : tooth decay

ca·ri·na \kə-'rī-nə, -'rē-\ *n, pl* **carinas** *or* **ca·ri·nae** \-'rī-ˌnē, -'rē-ˌnī\ : any of various keel-shaped anatomical structures, ridges, or processes: as **a** : a ridge on the lower surface of the fornix of the brain **b** : the ventral distal part of the vagina

car·i·nate \'kar-ə-ˌnāt, -nət\ *adj* : having or shaped like a keel or carina

carinii — see PNEUMOCYSTIS CARINII PNEUMONIA

car·io·gen·ic \ˌkar-ē-ō-'jen-ik\ *adj* : producing or promoting the development of tooth decay ⟨∼ foods⟩ ⟨∼ bacteria⟩

car·io·stat·ic \-'stat-ik\ *adj* : tending to inhibit the formation of dental caries ⟨the ∼ action of fluorides⟩

car·i·ous \'kar-ē-əs, 'ker-\ *adj* : affected with caries ⟨∼ teeth⟩

ca·ri·so·pro·dol \kə-ˌrī-sə-'prō-ˌdȯl, -zə-, -ˌdōl\ *n* : a drug $C_{12}H_{24}N_2O_4$ related to meprobamate that is used to relax muscle and relieve pain

carm·al·um \kär-'mal-əm\ *n* : a stain composed of carminic acid, alum, and water for use in microscopy

¹**car·mi·na·tive** \kär-'min-ət-iv, 'kär-mə-ˌnāt-\ *adj* : expelling gas from the stomach or intestines so as to relieve flatulence or abdominal pain or distension

²**carminative** *n* : a carminative agent

car·mine \'kär-mən, -ˌmīn\ *n* : a vivid red lake consisting essentially of an aluminum salt of carminic acid made from cochineal and used as a biological stain and as coloring in foods, drugs, and cosmetics; *also* : any of various coloring matters (as indigo carmine) other than carmine

car·min·ic acid \kär-ˌmin-ik-\ *n* : a red crystalline anthraquinone dye $C_{22}H_{20}O_{13}$ best known as the essential coloring matter of cochineal and used chiefly as a biological stain

car·mus·tine \'kär-mə-ˌstēn\ *n* : BCNU

car·ni·fi·ca·tion \ˌkär-nə-fə-'kā-shən\ *n* : the process by which lung tissue becomes converted into fibrous tissue as a result of unresolved pneumonia

car·ni·tine \'kär-nə-ˌtēn\ *n* : a quaternary ammonium compound $C_7H_{15}NO_3$ that is present esp. in vertebrate muscle, is involved in the transfer of fatty acids across mitochondrial membranes, and in humans is obtained from food (as meat or milk) or is synthesized from a lysine derivative

car·niv·o·ra \kär-'niv-ə-rə\ *n pl* **1** *cap* : an order of eutherian mammals that are mostly carnivorous and have teeth adapted for flesh eating **2** : carnivorous animals; *esp* : members of the order Carnivora — **car·ni·vore** \'kär-nə-ˌvō(ə)r, -ˌvȯ(ə)r\ *n*

car·niv·o·rous \kär-'niv-(ə-)rəs\ *adj* **1** : subsisting or feeding on animal tissues **2** : of or relating to the carnivores — **car·niv·o·rous·ly** *adv* — **car·niv·o·rous·ness** *n*

car·no·sine \'kär-nə-ˌsēn, -sən\ *n* : a colorless crystalline dipeptide $C_9H_{14}N_4O_3$ occurring in the muscles of most mammals

carnosus — see PANNICULUS CARNOSUS

car·ob \'kar-əb\ *n* **1** : a Mediterranean evergreen leguminous tree (*Ceratonia siliqua*) with racemose red flowers **2** : a carob pod; *also* : its sweet pulp

carob flour *n* : a powder extracted from the fruit of the carob tree and used in the pharmaceutical, textile, and food industries as a thickener, stabilizer, and sizing agent

car·o·tene \'kar-ə-ˌtēn\ *n* : any of several orange or red crystalline hydrocarbon pigments (as $C_{40}H_{56}$) that occur in the chromoplasts of plants and in the fatty tissues of plant-eating animals and are convertible to vitamin A — see BETA= CAROTENE

car·o·ten·emia *also* **car·o·tin·emia** *or chiefly Brit* **car·o·ten·ae·mia** *also* **car·o·tin·ae·mia** \ˌkar-ət-ə-'nē-mē-ə, -ət-ᵊn-'ē-\ *n* : the presence in the circulating blood of carotene which may cause a yellowing of the skin resembling jaundice

ca·rot·en·oid *also* **ca·rot·in·oid** \kə-'rät-ᵊn-ˌȯid\ *n* : any of various usu. yellow to red pigments (as carotenes) found widely in plants and animals and characterized chemically by a long aliphatic polyene chain composed of eight isoprene units — **carotenoid** *adj*

caroticum — see GLOMUS CAROTICUM

ca·rot·id \kə-'rät-əd\ *adj* : of, situated near, or involving a carotid artery ⟨∼ arteriography⟩

carotid artery *n* : either of the two main arteries that supply blood to the head of which the left in humans arises from the arch of the aorta and the right by bifurcation of the brachiocephalic artery with each passing along the corresponding anterolateral aspect of the neck and dividing opposite the upper border of the thyroid cartilage into an external branch

\ə\ abut \ᵊ\ kitten \ər\ further \a\ ash \ā\ ace \ä\ cot, cart \aú\ out \ch\ chin \e\ bet \ē\ easy \g\ go \i\ hit \ī\ ice \j\ job \ŋ\ sing \ō\ go \ȯ\ law \ȯi\ boy \th\ thin \t̲h̲\ the \ü\ loot \ú\ foot \y\ yet \zh\ vision *See also* Pronunciation Symbols page

supplying the face, tongue, and external parts of the head and an internal branch supplying the brain, eye, and other internal parts of the head — called also *carotid;* see COMMON CAROTID ARTERY, EXTERNAL CAROTID ARTERY, INTERNAL CAROTID ARTERY

carotid body *n* : a small body of vascular tissue that adjoins the carotid sinus, functions as a chemoreceptor sensitive to change in the oxygen content of blood, and mediates reflex changes in respiratory activity — called also *carotid gland, glomus caroticum*

carotid canal *n* : the canal by which the internal carotid artery enters the skull — called also *carotid foramen*

carotid gland *n* : CAROTID BODY

carotid plexus *n* : a network of nerves of the sympathetic nervous system surrounding the internal carotid artery

carotid sinus *n* : a small but richly innervated arterial enlargement that is located near the point in the neck where the common carotid artery divides into the internal and the external carotid arteries and that functions in the regulation of heart rate and blood pressure

carotid triangle *n* : SUPERIOR CAROTID TRIANGLE

carotinaemia *chiefly Brit var of* CAROTENEMIA

carotinemia *var of* CAROTENEMIA

carotinoid *var of* CAROTENOID

car·pa·ine \'kär-pə-ˌēn\ *n* : a crystalline alkaloid $C_{14}H_{25}NO_2$ obtained esp. from the leaves, fruit, and seeds of the papaya

¹car·pal \'kär-pəl\ *adj* : relating to the carpus

²carpal *n* : a carpal element : CARPALE

car·pa·le \kär-'pal-(ˌ)ē, -'pāl-, -'päl-\ *n, pl* **-lia** \-ē-ə\ : a carpal bone; *esp* : one of the distal series articulating with the metacarpals

carpal tunnel *n* : a passage between the flexor retinaculum of the hand and the carpal bones that is sometimes a site of compression of the median nerve

carpal tunnel syndrome *n* : a condition caused by compression of the median nerve in the carpal tunnel and characterized esp. by weakness, pain, and disturbances of sensation in the hand and fingers — abbr. *CTS*

car·pec·to·my \kär-'pek-tə-mē\ *n, pl* **-mies** : excision of a carpal bone

car·phol·o·gy \kär-'fäl-ə-jē\ *also* **car·pho·lo·gia** \ˌkär-fə-'lō-j(ē-)ə\ *n, pl* **-gies** *also* **-gias** : an aimless semiconscious plucking at the bedclothes observed in conditions of exhaustion or stupor or in high fevers — called also *floccillation*

carpi — see EXTENSOR CARPI RADIALIS BREVIS, EXTENSOR CARPI RADIALIS LONGUS, EXTENSOR CARPI ULNARIS, FLEXOR CARPI RADIALIS, FLEXOR CARPI ULNARIS

car·pi·tis \kär-'pīt-əs\ *n* : arthritis of the carpal joint in domestic animals

car·po·meta·car·pal \ˌkär-pō-'met-ə-ˌkär-pəl\ *adj* : relating to, situated between, or joining a carpus and metacarpus ⟨a ∼ joint⟩ ⟨a ∼ ligament⟩

car·po·ped·al spasm \ˌkär-pə-ˌped-ᵊl-, -ˌpēd-ᵊl\ *n* : a spasmodic contraction of the muscles of the hands and feet or esp. of the wrists and ankles in disorders such as alkalosis and tetany

car·pus \'kär-pəs\ *n, pl* **car·pi** \-ˌpī, -ˌpē\ **1** : WRIST **2** : the group of bones supporting the wrist comprising in humans a proximal row which contains the scaphoid, lunate, triquetrum, and pisiform that articulate with the radius and a distal row which contains the trapezium, trapezoid, capitate, and hamate that articulate with the metacarpals

car·ra·geen *also* **car·ra·gheen** \'kar-ə-ˌgēn\ *n* **1** : IRISH MOSS 2 **2** : CARRAGEENAN

car·ra·geen·an *or* **car·ra·geen·in** \ˌkar-ə-'gē-nən\ *n* : a colloid extracted from various red algae and esp. Irish moss and used esp. as a suspending agent (as in foods) and as a clarifying agent (as for beverages) and in controlling crystal growth in frozen confections

car·riage \'kar-ij\ *n* : the condition of harboring a pathogen within the body ⟨immunization against hepatitis B reduced the rate of HBV ∼⟩ ⟨asymptomatic ∼ of the pneumococcus in the nasopharynx⟩

car·ri·er \'kar-ē-ər\ *n* **1 a** : a person, animal, or plant that harbors and transmits the causative agent of an infectious disease; *esp* : one who carries the causative agent systemically but is asymptomatic or immune to it ⟨a ∼ of typhoid fever⟩ — compare RESERVOIR 2, VECTOR 2 **b** : an individual possessing a specified gene and capable of transmitting it to offspring but not expressing or only weakly expressing its phenotype; *esp* : one that is heterozygous for a recessive factor **2** : a usu. inactive substance used in association with an active substance esp. for aiding in the application of the active substance: as **a** : a support for a catalyst **b** : a vehicle serving esp. as a diluent (as for an insecticide or a drug) **3** : a substance (as a catalyst) by whose agency some element or group is transferred from one compound to another

Car·ri·ón's disease \ˌkar-ē-'ōnz-\ *n* : BARTONELLOSIS

Car·ri·ón \ˌkär-ē-'ōn\, **Daniel A. (1850–1885),** Peruvian medical student. Carrión allowed himself to be inoculated with the blood of a patient suffering from verruga peruana. He died with the symptoms of Oroya fever, thereby proving the association between the two. Bartonellosis was named Carrión's disease in his honor by the Peruvian physician Ernesto Odriozola.

car·ron oil \'kar-ən-\ *n* : a lotion of equal parts of linseed oil and limewater formerly applied to burns and scalds — called also *lime liniment*

car·rot \'kar-ət\ *n* : a biennial plant of the genus *Daucus* (*D. carota*) that bears seeds which have been used esp. as a diuretic and stimulant and that in cultivated varieties has a yellow or orange-red tapering root which is used as a vegetable; *also* : its root

car·ry \'kar-ē\ *vt* **car·ried; car·ry·ing 1** : to harbor (a pathogen) within the body ⟨many are unaware they ∼ the virus and could be infecting others —Donald MacGillis⟩ **2** : to possess a specified gene ⟨women who ∼ genes that increase the risk of breast cancer —Liz Szabo⟩; *specif* : to possess one copy of a specified recessive gene and be capable of transmitting it to offspring ⟨screening tests to see whether parents ∼ genes for cystic fibrosis, Tay-Sachs disease or other defects —Lisa Greene⟩

car·sick \'kär-ˌsik\ *adj* : affected with motion sickness esp. in an automobile — **car sickness** *n*

car·tha·mus \'kär-thə-məs\ *n* : SAFFLOWER 2

car·ti·lage \'kärt-ᵊl-ij, 'kärt-lij\ *n* **1** : a usu. translucent somewhat elastic tissue that composes most of the skeleton of vertebrate embryos and except for a small number of structures (as some joints, respiratory passages, and the external ear) is replaced by bone during ossification in the higher vertebrates **2** : a part or structure composed of cartilage

cartilage bone *n* : a bone formed by ossification of cartilage — compare MEMBRANE BONE

cartilage of Ja·cob·son \-'jā-kəb-sən, -kəp-\ *n* : VOMERONASAL CARTILAGE

cartilage of San·to·ri·ni \-ˌsant-ə-'rē-nē\ *n* : CORNICULATE CARTILAGE

G. D. Santorini — see DUCT OF SANTORINI

cartilage of Wris·berg \-'riz-ˌbərg, -'vris-ˌberk\ *n* : CUNEIFORM CARTILAGE

Wris·berg \'vris-ˌberk\, **Heinrich August (1739–1808),** German anatomist. A professor of anatomy, Wrisberg published a number of works containing original anatomical descriptions. In 1764 he published a work on embryonic anatomy in which he gave clear descriptions of the cuneiform cartilages of the larynx (cartilages of Wrisberg), a ganglion of the superficial cardiac plexus (Wrisberg's ganglion), the lateral meniscus of the knee, and the fibers connecting the motor and the sensory roots of the trigeminal nerve. In 1777 he produced a treatise on the anatomy of the nervous system that contained classic descriptions of the nervus intermedius of the facial nerve, and a nerve supplying the medial side of the upper arm. Each of these is sometimes called the nerve of Wrisberg.

car·ti·lag·i·noid \ˌkärt-ᵊl-'aj-ə-ˌnȯid\ *adj* : resembling cartilage

car·ti·lag·i·nous \-nəs\ *adj* : composed of, relating to, or resembling cartilage

Car·um \'kar-əm\ *n* : a large genus of biennial aromatic herbs (family Umbelliferae) that have white or yellow flowers in compound umbels and include caraway

car·un·cle \'kar-əŋ-kəl, kə-'rəŋ-\ *n* : a small fleshy growth; *specif* : a reddish growth situated at the urethral meatus in women and causing pain and bleeding — see LACRIMAL CARUNCLE

ca·run·cu·la \kə-'rəŋ-kyə-lə\ *n, pl* **-lae** \-ˌlē, -ˌlī\ : CARUNCLE

car·va·crol \'kär-və-ˌkról, -ˌkról\ *n* : a liquid phenol $C_{10}H_{14}O$ found in essential oils of various mints (as thyme) and used as a fungicide and disinfectant

ca·san·thra·nol \kə-'san(t)-thrə-ˌnòl\ *n* : a cathartic mixture of glycosides extracted from cascara sagrada — see PERICOLACE

cas·cade \(ˌ)kas-'kād\ *n* : a molecular, biochemical, or physiological process occurring in a succession of stages each of which is closely related to or depends on the output of the previous stage ⟨a ∼ of enzymatic reactions⟩ ⟨the ∼ of events comprising the immune response⟩

cas·cara \kas-'kar-ə, -'kär-; 'kas-kə-rə\ *n* **1** : CASCARA BUCKTHORN **2** : CASCARA SAGRADA

cascara amar·ga \-ə-'mär-gə\ *n* : the dried bark of a tropical American tree (*Picramnia antidesma*) formerly used in the treatment of syphilis and skin diseases — called also *Honduras bark*

cascara buckthorn *n* : a buckthorn of the genus *Rhamnus* (*R. purshiana*) of the Pacific coast of the U.S. yielding cascara sagrada — called also *cascara, coffeeberry*

cascara sa·gra·da \-sə-'gräd-ə\ *n* : the dried bark of cascara buckthorn used as a mild laxative — called also *cascara, chittam bark*

cas·ca·ril·la \ˌkas-kə-'ril-ə, -'rē-ə\ *n* **1** : the aromatic bark of a West Indian shrub (*Croton eluteria*) used for making incense and as a tonic — called also *cascarilla bark* **2** : the shrub that yields cascarilla bark

case \'kās\ *n* **1** : the circumstances and situation of a particular person or group **2 a** : an instance of disease or injury ⟨10 ∼s of pneumonia⟩ **b** : PATIENT 1

ca·se·ase \'kā-sē-ˌās, -ˌāz\ *n* : an enzyme that is formed by some bacteria, that decomposes casein, and that is used in ripening cheese

ca·se·ate \'kā-sē-ˌāt\ *vi* **-at·ed; -at·ing** : to undergo caseation

ca·se·ation \ˌkā-sē-'ā-shən\ *n* : necrosis with conversion of damaged tissue into a soft cheesy substance

case·book \'kās-ˌbúk\ *n* : a book containing medical records of illustrative cases that is used for reference and instruction

case history *n* : a record of an individual's personal or family history and environment for use in analysis or instructive illustration

casei — see LACTOBACILLUS CASEI FACTOR

ca·sein \'kā-ˌsēn, ka-'\ *n* : any of several phosphoproteins of milk: as **a** : one that occurs as a colloidal suspension in milk — called also *caseinogen* **b** : one that is produced when milk is curdled by rennet, is the chief constituent of cheese, and is used in making plastics — called also *paracasein*

ca·sein·ate \kā-'sē-ˌnāt, 'kā-sē-ə-ˌnāt\ *n* : a compound of casein with a metal (as calcium or sodium)

ca·sein·o·gen \kā-'sē-nə-jən, ˌkā-sē-'in-ə-jən\ *n* : CASEIN a

case·load \'kās-ˌlōd\ *n* : the number of cases handled (as by a clinic) in a particular period

case man·ag·er \-'man-ij-ər\ *n* : a person (as a social worker or nurse) who assists in the planning, coordination, monitoring, and evaluation of medical services for a patient with emphasis on quality of care, continuity of services, and cost-effectiveness; *also* : CASEWORKER — **case man·age·ment** \-mənt\ *n*

caseosa — see VERNIX CASEOSA

ca·se·ous \'kā-sē-əs\ *adj* : marked by caseation

caseous lymphadenitis *n* : a chronic infectious disease of sheep and goats characterized by caseation of the lymph glands and occas. of parts of the lungs, liver, spleen, and kidneys that is caused by a bacterium of the genus *Corynebacterium* (*C. pseudotuberculosis*) — called also *pseudotuberculosis*

case·work \'kā-ˌswərk\ *n* : social work involving direct consideration of the problems, needs, and adjustments of the individual case (as a person or family in need of financial or psychiatric aid) — **case·work·er** \-ˌswər-kər\ *n*

cas·sette *also* **ca·sette** \kə-'set, ka-\ *n* **1** : a lightproof magazine for holding film or plates for use in a camera; *specif* : one for holding the intensifying screens and film in X-ray photography **2** : a small plastic cartridge containing magnetic tape with the tape on one reel passing to the other

cas·sia \'kash-ə, *esp 2* 'kas-ē-ə\ *n* **1** : any of the coarser varieties of cinnamon bark — see CHINESE CINNAMON **2** *cap* : a genus of leguminous herbs, shrubs, and trees that are native to warm regions and have pinnate leaves and nearly regular flowers — see SENNA **3** : CASSIA FISTULA

cassia bark *n* : CHINESE CINNAMON 1

cassia fis·tu·la \-'fis(h)-chə-lə\ *n* : the dried pods of a tree of the genus *Cassia* (*C. fistula*) the sweet pulp of which is a mild laxative

cassia oil *n* : CINNAMON OIL

¹cast \'kast\ *vt* **cast; cast·ing** **1** : to give a shape to (a substance) by pouring in liquid or plastic form into a mold and letting harden without pressure **2** : to form by casting

²cast *n* **1** : a slight strabismus **2 a** : something that is formed by casting in a mold or form; *esp* : an impression taken from an object by using a liquid or plastic substance **b** : a rigid casing (as of fiberglass or of gauze impregnated with plaster of paris) used for immobilizing a usu. diseased or broken part **3** : a mass of plastic matter formed in cavities of diseased organs (as the kidneys) and discharged from the body

Cas·ta·nea \ka-'stā-nē-ə\ *n* : a small genus of rough-barked trees or shrubs (family Fagaceae) native to temperate regions that includes the chestnut of eastern No. America

Cas·tel·la·ni's paint \ˌkas-tə-ˌlän-ēz-'pānt\ *n* : CARBOL-FUCHSIN PAINT

Cas·tel·la·ni \ˌkas-tə-'län-ē\, **Aldo (1878–1971),** Italian physician. Castellani was a specialist in tropical diseases. His numerous contributions to tropical medicine include the discovery in 1903 of a species of trypanosome (*Trypanosoma gambiense*) in the spinal fluid of patients suffering from sleeping sickness, the discovery in 1905 that yaws is caused by a spirochete (*Treponema pertenue*), and the isolation of new strains of fungi causing dermatoses.

cas·tile soap \(ˌ)kas-ˌtēl-\ *n* : a fine hard bland soap made from olive oil and sodium hydroxide; *also* : any of various similar soaps

cast·ing *n* **1** : the act or process of making casts or impressions or of shaping in a mold **2** : something cast in a mold

cas·tor bean \'kas-tər-\ *n* : the very poisonous seed of the castor-oil plant; *also* : CASTOR-OIL PLANT

castor–bean tick *n* : a widely distributed tick of the genus *Ixodes* (*I. ricinus*) that is a vector of piroplasmosis and various virus diseases of domestic animals

castor oil *n* : a pale viscous fatty oil from castor beans used esp. as a cathartic or lubricant

castor–oil plant *n* : a tropical Old World herb of the genus *Ricinus* (*R. communis*) widely grown as an ornamental or for its oil-rich castor beans that are a source of castor oil

¹cas·trate \'kas-ˌtrāt\ *vt* **cas·trat·ed; cas·trat·ing** **1 a** : to deprive of the testes : GELD **b** : to deprive of the ovaries : SPAY **2** : to render impotent or deprive of vitality esp. by psychological means ⟨uses these ideas . . . as an instrument to ∼ and destroy him —Harold Clurman⟩ — **cas·trat·er** *or* **cas·tra·tor** \-ər\ *n* — **cas·tra·tion** \kas-'trā-shən\ *n*

²castrate *n* : a castrated individual

castration complex *n* : a child's fear or delusion of genital

\ə\ **abut** \ᵊ\ **kitten** \ər\ **further** \a\ **ash** \ā\ **ace** \ä\ **cot, cart**
\aú\ **out** \ch\ **chin** \e\ **bet** \ē\ **easy** \g\ **go** \i\ **hit** \ī\ **ice** \j\ **job**
\ŋ\ **sing** \ō\ **go** \ò\ **law** \ói\ **boy** \th\ **thin** \th̲\ **the** \ü\ **loot**
\ú\ **foot** \y\ **yet** \zh\ **vision** *See also* Pronunciation Symbols page

injury at the hands of the parent of the same sex as punishment for unconscious guilt over oedipal strivings; *broadly* : the often unconscious fear or feeling of bodily injury or loss of power at the hands of authority

ca·su·al·ty \\'kazh-əl-tē, 'kazh-(ə-)wəl-\\ *n, pl* **-ties** **1** : a serious or fatal accident **2** : a military person lost through death, wounds, injury, sickness, internment, or capture or through being missing in action **3 a** : injury or death from accident **b** : one injured or killed (as by accident)

ca·su·is·tic \\ˌkazh-ə-'wis-tik\\ *adj* : of or based on the study of actual cases or case histories ⟨a ∼ approach⟩

cat \\'kat\\ *n, often attrib* **1** : a carnivorous mammal (*Felis catus*) long domesticated and kept as a pet or for catching rats and mice **2** : any of a family (Felidae) of mammals including the domestic cat, lion, tiger, leopard, jaguar, cougar, wildcat, lynx, and cheetah

CAT *abbr* computed axial tomography; computerized axial tomography

cata·bi·o·sis \\ˌkat-ə-bī-'ō-səs, -bē-\\ *n, pl* **-o·ses** \\-ˌsēz\\ : the degenerative biological changes accompanying cellular senescence — **cata·bi·ot·ic** \\-'ät-ik\\ *adj*

cat·a·bol·ic *also* **kat·a·bol·ic** \\ˌkat-ə-'bäl-ik\\ *adj* : of or relating to catabolism — **cat·a·bol·i·cal·ly** \\-i-k(ə-)lē\\ *adv*

ca·tab·o·lism *also* **ka·tab·o·lism** \\kə-'tab-ə-ˌliz-əm\\ *n* : destructive metabolism involving the release of energy and resulting in the breakdown of complex materials within the organism — compare ANABOLISM

ca·tab·o·lite \\-ˌlīt\\ *n* : a product of catabolism

ca·tab·o·lize *or Brit* **ca·tab·o·lise** \\-ˌlīz\\ *vb* **-lized** *or Brit* **-lised; -liz·ing** *or Brit* **-lis·ing** *vt* : to subject to catabolism ∼ *vi* : to undergo catabolism

cata·crot·ic \\ˌkat-ə-'krät-ik\\ *adj* : relating to, being, or characterized by a pulse tracing in which the descending part of the curve is marked by secondary peaks due to two or more expansions of the artery in the same beat

cata·di·op·tric \\ˌkat-ə-dī-'äp-trik\\ *adj* : belonging to, produced by, or involving both the reflection and the refraction of light ⟨∼ prisms⟩

cat·a·lase \\'kat-əl-ˌās, -ˌāz\\ *n* : a red crystalline enzyme that consists of a protein complex with hematin groups and catalyzes the decomposition of hydrogen peroxide into water and oxygen — **cat·a·lat·ic** \\ˌkat-əl-'at-ik\\ *adj*

cat·a·lep·sy \\'kat-əl-ˌep-sē\\ *n, pl* **-sies** : a condition of suspended animation and loss of voluntary motion associated with hysteria and schizophrenia in humans and with organic nervous disease in animals and characterized by a trancelike state of consciousness and a posture in which the limbs hold any position they are placed in — compare WAXY FLEXIBILITY

¹cat·a·lep·tic \\ˌkat-əl-'ep-tik\\ *adj* : of, having the characteristics of, or affected with catalepsy ⟨a ∼ state⟩ ⟨a ∼ person⟩ — **cat·a·lep·ti·cal·ly** \\-ti-k(ə-)lē\\ *adv*

²cataleptic *n* : one affected with catalepsy

cat·a·lep·toid \\ˌkat-əl-'ep-ˌtȯid\\ *adj* : resembling catalepsy

cat·a·lo·gia \\ˌkat-əl-'ō-j(ē-)ə\\ *n* : VERBIGERATION

ca·tal·y·sis \\kə-'tal-ə-səs\\ *n, pl* **-y·ses** \\-ˌsēz\\ : a change and esp. increase in the rate of a chemical reaction induced by a catalyst

cat·a·lyst \\'kat-əl-əst\\ *n* : a substance (as an enzyme) that enables a chemical reaction to proceed under different conditions (as at a lower temperature) than otherwise possible

cat·a·lyt·ic \\ˌkat-əl-'it-ik\\ *adj* : causing, involving, or relating to catalysis ⟨a ∼ reaction⟩ — **cat·a·lyt·i·cal·ly** \\-'it-i-k(ə-)lē\\ *adv*

cat·a·lyze *or Brit* **cat·a·lyse** \\'kat-əl-ˌīz\\ *vt* **-lyzed** *or Brit* **-lysed; -lyz·ing** *or Brit* **-lys·ing** : to bring about the catalysis of (a chemical reaction) — **cat·a·lyz·er** *or Brit* **cat·a·lys·er** *n*

cata·me·nia \\ˌkat-ə-'mē-nē-ə\\ *n pl* : MENSES — **cata·me·ni·al** \\-nē-əl\\ *adj*

cat·a·mite \\'kat-ə-ˌmīt\\ *n* : a boy kept by a pederast — called also *pathic*

Cat·a·mi·tus \\ˌkat-ə-'mīt-əs, -'mēt-\\ (*Greek* **Gan·y·mede** \\'gan-i-ˌmēd\\), Greek mythological character. Ganymede was an attractive Trojan boy who was abducted to Olympus

to become the cupbearer of Zeus and later his homosexual lover.

cat·am·ne·sis \\ˌkat-ˌam-'nē-səs\\ *n, pl* **-ne·ses** \\-ˌsēz\\ : the follow-up medical history of a patient — **cat·am·nes·tic** \\-'nes-tik\\ *adj*

cata·pha·sia \\ˌkat-ə-'fā-zh(ē-)ə\\ *n* : VERBIGERATION

cat·a·pho·re·sis \\ˌkat-ə-fə-'rē-səs\\ *n, pl* **-re·ses** \\-ˌsēz\\ : ELECTROPHORESIS — **cat·a·pho·ret·ic** \\-'ret-ik\\ *adj* — **cat·a·pho·ret·i·cal·ly** \\-i-k(ə-)lē\\ *adv*

cat·a·pla·sia \\ˌkat-ə-'plā-zh(ē-)ə\\ *n* : reversion of cells or tissues to a more embryonic condition — **cat·a·plas·tic** \\-'plas-tik\\ *adj*

cat·a·plasm \\'kat-ə-ˌplaz-əm\\ *n* : POULTICE

cat·a·plec·tic \\ˌkat-ə-'plek-tik\\ *adj* : of, relating to, or affected with cataplexy

cat·a·plexy \\'kat-ə-ˌplek-sē\\ *n, pl* **-plex·ies** \\-sēz\\ : a sudden loss of muscle control with retention of clear consciousness that follows a strong emotional stimulus (as elation, surprise, or anger) and is a characteristic symptom of narcolepsy

cat·a·ract \\'kat-ə-ˌrakt\\ *n* : a clouding of the lens of the eye or its surrounding transparent membrane that obstructs the passage of light

cat·a·ract·ous \\'kat-ə-ˌrak-təs\\ *adj* : of, relating to, or affected with an eye cataract

ca·tar·ia \\kə-'tar-ē-ə\\ *n* **1** : CATNIP **2** : the dried leaves and flowering tops of catnip formerly used in medicine (as in the treatment of infantile colic) — called also *catnip*

ca·tarrh \\kə-'tär\\ *n* : inflammation of a mucous membrane in humans or animals; *esp* : one chronically affecting the human nose and air passages — **ca·tarrh·al** \\-əl\\ *adj* — **ca·tarrh·al·ly** \\-ə-lē\\ *adv*

catarrhal fever *n* : MALIGNANT CATARRHAL FEVER

Cat·ar·rhi·na \\ˌkat-ə-'rī-nə\\ *n pl, in many classifications* : a division of Anthropoidea comprising the Old World monkeys, higher apes, and humans — **cat·ar·rhine** *also* **cat·a·rhine** \\'kat-ə-ˌrīn\\ *adj or n*

cata·state \\'kat-ə-ˌstāt\\ *n* : CATABOLITE — **cata·stat·ic** \\ˌkat-ə-'stat-ik\\ *adj*

ca·tas·tro·phe \\kə-'tas-trə-fē\\ *n* : death (as from an inexplicable cause) before, during, or after an operation

cat·a·stroph·ic \\ˌkat-ə-'sträf-ik\\ *adj* **1** : of, relating to, resembling, or resulting in catastrophe **2** *of an illness* : financially ruinous

cata·to·nia \\ˌkat-ə-'tō-nē-ə\\ *n* : a marked psychomotor disturbance that may involve stupor or mutism, negativism, rigidity, purposeless excitement, echolalia, echopraxia, and inappropriate or bizarre posturing and is associated with various medical conditions (as schizophrenia and mood disorders)

¹cata·ton·ic \\ˌkat-ə-'tän-ik\\ *adj* : of, relating to, marked by, or affected with catatonia ⟨∼ schizophrenia⟩ ⟨∼ rigidity⟩ ⟨∼ patients⟩ — **cata·ton·i·cal·ly** \\-i-k(ə-)lē\\ *adv*

²catatonic *n* : a catatonic individual

cat·bite fever \\ˌkat-ˌbīt-\\ *n* : RAT-BITE FEVER

catch·ment area \\'kach-mənt-\\ *n* : the geographical area served by an institution

cat cry syndrome \\-ˌkrī-\\ *n* : CRI DU CHAT SYNDROME

cat distemper *n* : PANLEUKOPENIA

cat·e·chin \\'kat-ə-ˌkin\\ *n* : a crystalline compound $C_{15}H_{14}O_6$ that is related chemically to the flavones, is found in catechu, and is used in dyeing and tanning; *also* : a derivative of this compound

cat·e·chol \\'kat-ə-ˌkȯl, -ˌkōl\\ *n* **1** : CATECHIN **2** : PYROCATECHOL

cat·e·chol·amine \\ˌkat-ə-'kō-lə-ˌmēn, -'kȯ-\\ *n* : any of various amines (as epinephrine, norepinephrine, and dopamine) that contain a dihydroxy benzene ring, that are derived from tyrosine, and that function as hormones or neurotransmitters or both

cat·e·chol·amin·er·gic \\-ˌkō-lə-mē-'nər-jik\\ *adj* : involving, liberating, or mediated by catecholamine ⟨∼ neurons in the brain⟩ ⟨∼ transmission in the nervous system⟩

cat·e·chu \\'kat-ə-ˌchü, -ˌshü\\ *n* : any of several dry, earthy, or resinous astringent substances obtained from tropical plants of Asia: as   **a** : an extract of the heartwood of an East Indian acacia (*Acacia catechu*) that was formerly used in medicine   **b** : GAMBIER

cat·elec·trot·o·nus \ˌkat-i-ˌlek-ˈträt-ᵊn-əs\ *n* : the local depolarization and increased irritability of a nerve in the region of the negative electrode or cathode on the passage of a current of electricity through it — compare ANELECTROTONUS

cat·e·noid \ˈkat-ə-ˌnȯid\ *adj* : FILIFORM — used esp. of the colonies of some protozoans

ca·ten·u·late \kə-ˈten-yə-lət\ *adj* : shaped like a chain ⟨∼ colonies of bacteria⟩

cat fever *n*   **1** : a respiratory infection accompanied by fever — used esp. in the U.S. Navy   **2** : PANLEUKOPENIA

cat flea \ˈkat-ˌflē\ *n* : a common often pestiferous flea of the genus *Ctenocephalides* (*C. felis*) that breeds chiefly on cats, dogs, and rats

cat·gut \-ˌgət\ *n* : a tough cord made usu. from sheep intestines and used esp. for sutures in closing wounds

cath \ˈkath\ *vt* : to insert a catheter into : subject to catheterization

cath *abbr*   **1** cathartic   **2** catheter; catheterization   **3** cathode

Catha \ˈkath-ə\ *n* : a genus of African evergreen shrubs (family Celastraceae) that have thick leaves, white flowers, and a seed with a white aril at the base and that include the khat

ca·thar·sis *also* **ka·thar·sis** \kə-ˈthär-səs\ *n, pl* **ca·thar·ses** *also* **ka·thar·ses** \-ˌsēz\   **1** : PURGATION   **2** : elimination of a complex by bringing it to consciousness and affording it expression — compare ABREACTION

¹**ca·thar·tic** \kə-ˈthärt-ik\ *adj* : of, relating to, or producing catharsis

²**cathartic** *n* : a cathartic medicine : PURGATIVE

ca·thect \kə-ˈthekt, ka-\ *vt* : to invest with mental or emotional energy

ca·thec·tic \kə-ˈthek-tik, ka-\ *adj* : of, relating to, or invested with mental or emotional energy

ca·thep·sin \kə-ˈthep-sən\ *n* : any of several intracellular proteases of animal tissue that aid in autolysis in some diseased conditions and after death

cath·e·ter \ˈkath-ət-ər, ˈkath-tər\ *n* : a tubular medical device for insertion into canals, vessels, passageways, or body cavities for diagnostic or therapeutic purposes (as to permit injection or withdrawal of fluids or to keep a passage open)

catheter fever *n* : fever ascribed to the passage of a urethral catheter and associated with infection of the bladder

cath·e·ter·iza·tion *or Brit* **cath·e·ter·isa·tion** \ˌkath-ət-ə-rə-ˈzā-shən, ˌkath-tə-rə-\ *n* : the use of or insertion of a catheter (as in or into the bladder, trachea, or heart) — **cath·e·ter·ize** *or Brit* **cath·e·ter·ise** \ˈkath-ət-ə-ˌrīz, ˈkath-tə-\ *vt* **-ized** *or Brit* **-ised; -iz·ing** *or Brit* **-is·ing**

cath·e·ter·ized *or Brit* **cath·e·ter·ised** *adj* : obtained by catheterization ⟨∼ urine specimens⟩

ca·thex·is \kə-ˈthek-səs, ka-\ *n, pl* **ca·thex·es** \-ˌsēz\   **1** : investment of mental or emotional energy in a person, object, or idea   **2** : libidinal energy that is either invested or being invested

cath·od·al \ˈkath-ˌōd-ᵊl\ *adj* : of, relating to, or attracted to a cathode : CATHODIC ⟨∼ potentials⟩ ⟨∼ hemoglobins⟩ — used esp. in the life sciences — **cath·od·al·ly** \-ē\ *adv*

cath·ode \ˈkath-ˌōd\ *n*   **1** : the electrode of an electrochemical cell at which reduction occurs: as   **a** : the negative terminal of an electrolytic cell   **b** : the positive terminal of a storage battery that is delivering current   **2** : the electron-emitting electrode of an electron tube — compare ANODE

cathode-ray oscilloscope *n* : OSCILLOSCOPE

cathode-ray tube *n* : a vacuum tube in which a beam of electrons is projected on a fluorescent screen to produce a luminous spot

cath·od·ic \ka-ˈthōd-ik\ *adj* : of, at, or relating to a cathode — **cath·od·i·cal·ly** \-i-k(ə-)lē\ *adv*

ca·thol·i·con \kə-ˈthäl-ə-ˌkän\ *n* : something that is a cure-all or panacea

cat·ion \ˈkat-ˌī-ən\ *n* : the ion in an electrolyzed solution that migrates to the cathode; *broadly* : a positively charged ion

cat·ion·ic \ˌkat-(ˌ)ī-ˈän-ik\ *adj*   **1** : of or relating to cations   **2**

: characterized by an active and esp. surface-active cation ⟨a ∼ dye⟩ — **cat·ion·i·cal·ly** \-i-k(ə-)lē\ *adv*

cat·ion·ot·ro·py \ˌkat-ˌī-ə-ˈnä-trə-pē\ *n, pl* **-pies** : tautomerism (as prototropy) involving migration of a cation — compare ANIONOTROPY

cat louse *n* : a biting louse (*Felicola subrostratus*) of the family Trichodectidae common on cats esp. in warm regions

cat·mint \ˈkat-ˌmint\ *n* : CATNIP 1

cat·nip \-ˌnip\ *also* **cat·nep** \-ˌnep, -nəp\ *n*   **1** : a strong-scented mint (*Nepeta cataria*) that has small pale flowers in terminal spikes and contains a substance attractive to cats — called also *cataria, catmint*   **2** : CATARIA 2

ca·top·tric \kə-ˈtäp-trik\ *adj* : being or using a mirror to focus light — **ca·top·tri·cal·ly** \-tri-k(ə-)lē\ *adv*

cat plague *n* : PANLEUKOPENIA

CAT scan \ˈkat-ˈskan, ˌsē-ˌā-ˈtē-\ *n* : a sectional view of the body constructed by computed tomography — called also *CT scan*

CAT scan·ner \-ˈskan-ər\ *n* : a medical instrument consisting of integrated X-ray and computing equipment and used for computed tomography — called also *CT scanner*

CAT scanning *n* : the action or process of making a CAT scan with a CAT scanner — called also *CT scanning*

cat scratch disease *n* : an illness that is characterized by chills, slight fever, and swelling of the lymph glands and is caused by a gram-negative bacterium of the genus *Bartonella* (*B. henselae* syn. *Rochalimaea henselae*) transmitted esp. by a cat scratch — called also *cat scratch fever*

cat tapeworm *n* : a common tapeworm of the genus *Taenia* (*T. taeniaeformis* or *T. crassicollis*) of cats who ingest cysticercus-infected livers of various rodents

cat·tery \ˈkat-ə-rē\ *n, pl* **-ter·ies** : a place for the breeding, raising, or care of cats

cattle fly \ˈkat-ᵊl-ˌflī\ *n* : HORN FLY

cattle grub \-ˌgrəb\ *n* : either of two warble flies of the genus *Hypoderma* esp. in the larval stage: **a** : COMMON CATTLE GRUB   **b** : NORTHERN CATTLE GRUB

cattle louse *n* : a louse infesting cattle — see LONG-NOSED CATTLE LOUSE, SHORT-NOSED CATTLE LOUSE

cattle plague *n* : RINDERPEST

cattle tick *n* : either of two ixodid ticks of the genus *Boophilus* (*B. annulatus* and *B. microplus*) that infest cattle and transmit the protozoan which causes Texas fever

cattle–tick fever *n* : TEXAS FEVER

cat typhoid *n* : PANLEUKOPENIA

Cau·ca·sian \kȯ-ˈkā-zhən, -ˈkazh-ən\ *adj*   **1** : of or relating to the white race of humankind as classified according to physical features   **2** : of or relating to the white race as defined by law specif. as composed of persons of European, No. African, or southwest Asian ancestry — **Caucasian** *n*

cau·da \ˈkaȯd-ə, ˈkȯd-\ *n, pl* **cau·dae** \ˈkaȯ-ˌdī, ˈkȯ-ˌdē\ : a taillike appendage : TAIL

cau·dad \ˈkȯ-ˌdad\ *adv* : toward the tail or posterior end

cauda equi·na \-ek-ˈwē-nə, -ē-ˈkwī-nə\ *n, pl* **caudae equi·nae** \-ek-ˈwē-ˌnī, -ē-ˈkwī-ˌnē\ : the roots of the upper sacral nerves that extend beyond the termination of the spinal cord at the first lumbar vertebra in the form of a bundle of filaments within the vertebral canal resembling a horse's tail

cau·da he·li·cis \-ˈhel-ə-kəs, -ə-səs\ *n, pl* **caudae helicis** : the lower posterior part of the helix of the external ear

cau·dal \ˈkȯd-ᵊl\ *adj*   **1** : of, relating to, or being a tail   **2** : situated in or directed toward the hind part of the body — **cau·dal·ly** \-ᵊl-ē\ *adv*

caudal anesthesia *n* : loss of pain sensation below the navel produced by injection of an anesthetic into the caudal portion of the vertebral canal — called also *caudal analgesia*

caudal artery *n* : the portion of the dorsal aorta of a vertebrate that passes into the tail

cau·date lobe \ˌkȯ-ˌdāt-\ *n* : a lobe of the liver bounded on

---

\ə\ abut \ᵊ\ kitten \ər\ further \a\ ash \ā\ ace \ä\ cot, cart \aȯ\ out \ch\ chin \e\ bet \ē\ easy \g\ go \i\ hit \ī\ ice \j\ job \ŋ\ sing \ō\ go \ȯ\ law \ȯi\ boy \th\ thin \t͟h\ the \ü\ loot \ȯ\ foot \y\ yet \zh\ vision   *See also* Pronunciation Symbols page

the right by the inferior vena cava, on the left by the fissure of the ductus venosus, and connected with the right lobe by a narrow prolongation — called also *spigelian lobe*

caudate nucleus *n* : the one of the four basal ganglia in each cerebral hemisphere that comprises a mass of gray matter in the corpus striatum, forms part of the floor of the lateral ventricle, and is separated from the lentiform nucleus by the internal capsule — called also *caudate*

cau·da·to·len·tic·u·lar \kȯ-ˌdāt-ō-len-ˈtik-yə-lər\ *adj* : relating to the caudate and lentiform nuclei of the corpus striatum

caul \ˈkȯl\ *n* **1** : GREATER OMENTUM **2** : the inner embryonic membrane of higher vertebrates esp. when covering the head at birth

cau·li·flow·er ear \ˌkȯ-li-ˌflaủ-(ə)r-, ˌkäl-i-\ *n* : an ear deformed from injury and excessive growth of reparative tissue

cauliflower excrescence *n* : a wartlike growth of tissue that is usu. a condyloma but sometimes a stage of cancer and resembles a cauliflower — called also *cauliflower growth*

cau·sal·gia \kȯ-ˈzal-j(ē-)ə, -ˈsal-\ *n* : a constant usu. burning pain resulting from injury to a peripheral nerve — **cau·sal·gic** \-jik\ *adj*

¹caus·tic \ˈkȯ-stik\ *adj* : capable of destroying or eating away organic tissue and esp. animal tissue by chemical action ⟨silver nitrate and sulfuric acid are ∼ agents⟩ — **caus·ti·cal·ly** \-sti-k(ə-)lē\ *adv* — **caus·tic·i·ty** \kȯ-ˈstis-ət-ē\ *n, pl* **-ties**

²caustic *n* : a caustic agent: as **a** : a substance that burns or destroys organic tissue by chemical action : ESCHAROTIC **b** : SODIUM HYDROXIDE

caustic potash *n* : POTASSIUM HYDROXIDE

caustic soda *n* : SODIUM HYDROXIDE

cau·ter \ˈkȯt-ər\ *n* : an iron for cauterizing : CAUTERY

cau·ter·ant \ˈkȯt-ə-rənt\ *n* : a cauterizing substance

cau·ter·ize *or Brit* **cau·ter·ise** \ˈkȯt-ə-ˌrīz\ *vt* **-ized** *or Brit* **-ised; -iz·ing** *or Brit* **-is·ing** : to sear with a cautery or caustic — **cau·ter·iza·tion** *or Brit* **cau·ter·isa·tion** \ˌkȯt-ə-rə-ˈzā-shən\ *n*

cau·tery \ˈkȯt-ə-rē\ *n, pl* **-ter·ies** **1** : the act or effect of cauterizing : CAUTERIZATION **2** : an agent (as a hot iron or caustic) used to burn, sear, or destroy tissue

cav *abbr* cavity

¹ca·va \ˈkäv-ə, ˈkā-və\ *n, pl* **ca·vae** \ˈkäv-ˌē, -ˌī; ˈkā-ˌvē\ : VENA CAVA — **ca·val** \-vəl\ *adj*

²cava *pl of* CAVUM

cav·ern \ˈkav-ərn\ *n* : a cavity (as in the lung) caused by disease

cav·er·no·ma \ˌkav-ər-ˈnō-mə\ *n, pl* **-mas** *also* **-ma·ta** \-mət-ə\ : a cavernous vascular tumor or angioma

cav·er·nos·to·my \-ˈnäs-tə-mē\ *n, pl* **-mies** : incision and drainage of a tuberculous cavity

cavernosum — see CORPUS CAVERNOSUM

cav·ern·ous \ˈkav-ər-nəs\ *adj* **1** : having caverns or cavities **2** *of tissue* : composed largely of vascular sinuses and capable of dilating with blood to bring about the erection of a body part

cavernous plexus *n* : a nerve plexus of the sympathetic nervous system that lies below and internal to the carotid artery at each side of the sella turcica

cavernous respiration *n* : a peculiar blowing respiratory sound heard over abnormal lung cavities

cavernous sinus *n* : either of a pair of large venous sinuses situated in a groove at the side of the body of the sphenoid bone in the cranial cavity and opening behind into the petrosal sinuses

Ca·via \ˈkā-vē-ə\ *n* : a genus of rodents that contains the guinea pig

cav·i·tary \ˈkav-ə-ˌter-ē\ *adj* : of, relating to, or characterized by bodily cavitation ⟨∼ tuberculosis⟩ ⟨∼ lesions⟩

cav·i·ta·tion \ˌkav-ə-ˈtā-shən\ *n* **1** : the process of cavitating; *esp* : the formation of cavities in an organ or tissue esp. in disease **2** : a cavity formed by cavitation — **cav·i·tate** \ˈkav-ə-ˌtāt\ *vb* **-tat·ed; -tat·ing**

cav·i·ty \ˈkav-ət-ē\ *n, pl* **-ties** **1** : an unfilled space within a mass — see PELVIC CAVITY **2** : an area of decay in a tooth : CARIES

cav·og·ra·phy \kav-ˈäg-rə-fē\ *n, pl* **-phies** : angiography of the vena cava

ca·vo·sur·face \ˈkā-vō-ˌsər-fəs, ˌkav-ō-\ *adj* : of or relating to the wall of a cavity and the natural surface of a tooth

ca·vum \ˈkäv-əm, ˈkā-vəm\ *n, pl* **ca·va** \ˈkäv-ə, ˈkā-və\ : an anatomical recess or hollow: as **a** : the lower part of the concha of the ear adjoining the origin of the helix **b** : the nasal cavity

cavus — see PES CAVUS

ca·vy \ˈkā-vē\ *n, pl* **ca·vies** : any of several short-tailed So. American rodents (family Caviidae); *esp* : GUINEA PIG

cb *abbr* centibar

Cb *symbol* columbium

CB *abbr* [Latin *Chirurgiae Baccalaureus*] bachelor of surgery

CBC *abbr* complete blood count

CBD *abbr* **1** closed bladder drainage **2** common bile duct

CBF *abbr* cerebral blood flow

CBR *abbr* **1** chemical, bacteriological, and radiological **2** chemical, biological, and radiological

CBW *abbr* chemical and biological warfare

cc *abbr* cubic centimeter

CC *abbr* **1** chief complaint **2** commission certified **3** critical condition **4** current complaint

CCI *abbr* chronic coronary insufficiency

CCK *abbr* cholecystokinin

CCT *abbr* chocolate-coated tablet

CCU *abbr* **1** cardiac care unit **2** coronary care unit **3** critical care unit

cd *abbr* candela

Cd *symbol* cadmium

CD *abbr* **1** cluster of differentiation — used with an integer to denote any of numerous antigenic proteins found chiefly on the surface of leukocytes (as T cells or B cells); see CD4, CD8 **2** communicable disease **3** constant drainage **4** contagious disease **5** convulsive disorder **6** curative dose

CDC *abbr* **1** calculated date of confinement **2** Centers for Disease Control

CD8 \ˌsē-(ˌ)dē-ˈāt\ *n, often attrib* : a glycoprotein found esp. on the surface of cytotoxic T cells that usu. functions to facilitate recognition by cytotoxic T cell receptors of antigens complexed with molecules of a class that are found on the surface of most nucleated cells and are the product of genes of the major histocompatibility complex

CD4 \-ˈfōr, -ˈfȯr\ *n, often attrib* : a large glycoprotein that is found esp. on the surface of helper T cells, that is the receptor for HIV, and that usu. functions to facilitate recognition by helper T cell receptors of antigens complexed with molecules of a class that are found on the surface of antigen=presenting cells (as B cells and macrophages) and are the product of genes of the major histocompatibility complex

cDNA \ˌsē-ˌdē-ˌen-ˌā\ *n* : a DNA that is complementary to a given RNA which serves as a template for synthesis of the DNA in the presence of reverse transcriptase — called also *complementary DNA*

Ce *symbol* cerium

CE *abbr* cardiac enlargement

CEA *abbr* carcinoembryonic antigen

ce·cal *or chiefly Brit* **cae·cal** \ˈsē-kəl\ *adj* : of or like a cecum — **ce·cal·ly** *or chiefly Brit* **cae·cal·ly** \-kə-lē\ *adv*

cecal worm *n* : a worm parasitizing the cecum; *specif* : a nematode worm of the genus *Heterakis* (*H. gallinae*) that infests gallinaceous birds and serves as an intermediate host and transmitter of the protozoan causing blackhead

ce·cec·to·my *or chiefly Brit* **cae·cec·to·my** \sē-ˈsek-tə-mē\ *n, pl* **-mies** : surgical excision of all or part of the cecum

ce·ci·tis *or chiefly Brit* **cae·ci·tis** \sē-ˈsīt-əs\ *n* : inflammation of the cecum

Ce·clor \ˈsē-ˌklȯr, -ˌklör\ *trademark* — used for a preparation of cefaclor

C
D

ce·co·pexy or chiefly Brit **cae·co·pexy** \'sē-kə-ˌpek-sē\ n, pl **-pex·ies** : a surgical operation to fix the cecum to the abdominal wall

ce·cos·to·my or chiefly Brit **cae·cos·to·my** \sē-'käs-tə-mē\ n, pl **-mies** : the surgical formation of an opening into the cecum to serve as an artificial anus

ce·cot·o·my or chiefly Brit **cae·cot·o·my** \sē-'kät-ə-mē\ n, pl **-mies** : incision of the cecum

ce·cum or chiefly Brit **cae·cum** \'sē-kəm\ n, pl **ce·ca** or chiefly Brit **cae·ca** \-kə\ : a cavity open at one end (as the blind end of a duct); esp : the blind pouch at the beginning of the large intestine into which the ileum opens from one side and which is continuous with the colon

ce·dar·wood oil \'sēd-ər-ˌwùd-\ n : an essential oil obtained from the heartwood of cedars and used in soaps and perfumes and with immersion lenses in microscopy — called also cedar oil

cef·a·clor \'sef-ə-klȯr, -klōr\ n : a semisynthetic cephalosporin antibiotic $C_{15}H_{14}ClN_3O_4S\cdot H_2O$ that is administered orally to treat a wide range of bacterial infections of the skin and the respiratory and urinary tracts — see CECLOR

ce·faz·o·lin \si-'faz-ə-lən\ n : a semisynthetic cephalosporin antibiotic that is administered parenterally in the form of its sodium salt $C_{14}H_{13}N_8NaO_4S_3$

cef·ix·ime \ˌsef-'iks-ˌēm\ n : a semisynthetic cephalosporin antibiotic $C_{16}H_{15}N_5O_7S_2$ that is administered orally and is effective esp. against gram-negative bacteria and streptococci

cef·o·tax·ime \ˌsef-ə-'tak-ˌsēm\ n : a semisynthetic cephalosporin antibiotic that is administered parenterally in the form of its sodium salt $C_{16}H_{16}N_5NaO_7S_2$

ce·fox·i·tin \si-'fäk-sət-ən\ n : a semisynthetic cephamycin antibiotic that is administered parenterally in the form of its sodium salt $C_{16}H_{16}N_3NaO_7S_2$

cef·taz·i·dime \sef-'taz-ə-ˌdēm\ n : a semisynthetic cephalosporin antibiotic that is administered parenterally in the form of its hydrate $C_{22}H_{22}N_6O_7S_2\cdot 5H_2O$

Cef·tin \'sef-tin\ trademark — used for a preparation of an ester of cefuroxime

cef·tri·ax·one \ˌsef-ˌtrī-'ak-ˌsōn\ n : a semisynthetic cephalosporin antibiotic that is administered parenterally in the form of its hydrated disodium salt $C_{18}H_{16}N_8Na_2O_7S_3\cdot 3\frac{1}{2}H_2O$

ce·fur·ox·ime \si-'fyùr-ə-ˌzēm\ n : a semisynthetic cephalosporin antibiotic that is administered parenterally in the form of its sodium salt $C_{16}H_{15}N_4NaO_8S$ or orally as an ester derivative $C_{20}H_{22}N_4O_{10}S$ — see CEFTIN

Cel abbr Celsius

cel·an·dine \'sel-ən-ˌdīn, -ˌdēn\ n : a yellow-flowered biennial Eurasian herb (Chelidonium majus) of the poppy family naturalized in the eastern U.S. that has been used medicinally esp. as a diuretic — see CHELIDONIUM 2

ce·la·tion \si-'lā-shən\ n : concealment of pregnancy or childbirth

Cel·e·brex \'sel-ə-ˌbreks\ trademark — used for a preparation of celecoxib

cel·e·cox·ib \ˌsel-ə-'käk-sib\ n : an NSAID $C_{17}H_{14}F_3N_3O_2S$ that is a COX-2 inhibitor administered orally esp. to relieve the pain and inflammation of osteoarthritis and rheumatoid arthritis — see CELEBREX

Ce·lex·a \sə-'lek-sə\ trademark — used for a preparation of the hydrobromide of citalopram

¹ce·li·ac or chiefly Brit **coe·li·ac** \'sē-lē-ˌak\ adj 1 : of or relating to the abdominal cavity 2 : belonging to or prescribed for celiac disease ⟨the ∼ syndrome⟩ ⟨a ∼ diet⟩

²celiac or chiefly Brit **coeliac** n : a celiac part (as a nerve)

celiac artery n : a short thick artery arising from the aorta just below the diaphragm and dividing almost immediately into the gastric, hepatic, and splenic arteries — called also celiac axis, truncus celiacus

celiac disease n : a chronic hereditary intestinal disorder in which an inability to absorb the gliadin portion of gluten results in the gliadin triggering an immune response that damages the intestinal mucosa — called also celiac sprue, gluten‑sensitive enteropathy, nontropical sprue, sprue

celiac ganglion n : either of a pair of collateral sympathetic

ganglia that are the largest of the autonomic nervous system and lie one on each side of the celiac artery near the adrenal gland on the same side

celiac plexus n : a nerve plexus that is situated in the abdomen behind the stomach and in front of the aorta and the crura of the diaphragm, surrounds the celiac artery and the root of the superior mesenteric artery, contains several ganglia of which the most important are the celiac ganglia, and distributes nerve fibers to all the abdominal viscera — called also solar plexus

celiac sprue n : CELIAC DISEASE

celiacus — see TRUNCUS CELIACUS

ce·li·os·co·py or chiefly Brit **coe·li·os·co·py** \ˌsē-lē-'äs-kə-pē\ n, pl **-pies** : examination of the abdominal cavity by surgical insertion of an endoscope through the abdominal wall

ce·li·ot·o·my or chiefly Brit **coe·li·ot·o·my** \ˌsē-lē-'ät-ə-mē\ n, pl **-mies** : surgical incision of the abdomen

cell \'sel\ n 1 : a small compartment or bounded space 2 : a small usu. microscopic mass of protoplasm bounded externally by a semipermeable membrane, usu. including one or more nuclei and various nonliving products, capable alone or interacting with other cells of performing all the fundamental functions of life, and forming the smallest structural unit of living matter capable of functioning independently

cell body n : the nucleus-containing central part of a neuron exclusive of its axons and dendrites that is the major structural element of the gray matter of the brain and spinal cord, the ganglia, and the retina — called also perikaryon, soma

cell count n : a count of cells esp. of the blood or other body fluid in a standard volume (as a cubic millimeter)

cell cycle n : the complete series of events from one cell division to the next — see G₁ PHASE, G₂ PHASE, M PHASE, S PHASE

cell division n : the process by which cells multiply involving both nuclear and cytoplasmic division — compare MEIOSIS, MITOSIS

celled \'seld\ adj : having (such or so many) cells — used in combination ⟨single-celled organisms⟩

cel·lif·u·gal \(')sel-'if-(y)ə-gəl\ or **cel·lu·lif·u·gal** \ˌsel-yə-'lif-\ adj : conducting or conducted away from a cell body — used chiefly of nerve-cell processes and nerve impulses

cel·lip·e·tal \(')sel-'ip-ət-əl\ or **cel·lu·lip·e·tal** \ˌsel-yə-'lip-\ adj : conducting or conducted toward a cell body — used chiefly of nerve-cell processes and nerve impulses

cell line n : a cell culture selected for uniformity from a cell population derived from a usu. homogeneous tissue source (as an organ) ⟨a newly established cell line derived from human endometrial carcinoma —Biol. Abstracts⟩

cell-me·di·at·ed \'sel-ˌmēd-ē-ˌāt-əd\ adj : relating to or being the part of immunity or the immune response that is mediated primarily by T cells and esp. cytotoxic T cells rather than by antibodies secreted by B cells ⟨∼ immunity⟩ ⟨∼ reactions⟩ — compare HUMORAL 2

cell membrane n 1 : a membrane of a cell; esp : PLASMA MEMBRANE 2 : CELL WALL

cel·lo·bi·ose \ˌsel-ə-'bī-ˌōs, -ˌōz\ n : a faintly sweet disaccharide $C_{12}H_{22}O_{11}$ obtained by partial hydrolysis of cellulose — called also cellose

cell of Clau·di·us \-'klaùd-ē-əs, -'klȯd-\ n : one of the low cuboidal cells covering the outermost part of the basilar membrane of the organ of Corti

Clau·di·us \'klaùd-ē-ùs\, **Friedrich Matthias (1822–1869)**, Austrian anatomist. Claudius studied the hearing organs of land and marine mammals. In 1852 he described those cells in the organ of Corti which are now known as the cells of Claudius.

cell of Cor·ti \-'kȯrt-ē\ n : a hair cell in the organ of Corti

A. Corti — see ORGAN OF CORTI

\ə\ abut \ᵊ\ kitten \ər\ further \a\ ash \ā\ ace \ä\ cot, cart \aù\ out \ch\ chin \e\ bet \ē\ easy \g\ go \i\ hit \ī\ ice \j\ job \ŋ\ sing \ō\ go \ȯ\ law \ȯi\ boy \th\ thin \t̲h̲\ the \ü\ loot \ù\ foot \y\ yet \zh\ vision   See also Pronunciation Symbols page

cell of Dei·ters \-ˈdīt-ərz, -ərs\ *n* : one of the modified supporting cells prolonged into a process ending in a terminal plate that are placed among and alternate with the outer hair cells of the organ of Corti — called also *Deiters' cell*

Dei·ters \ˈdīt-ərs\, **Otto Friedrich Karl (1834–1863)**, German anatomist. A student of Rudolf Virchow, Deiters made several significant contributions to the study of the anatomy of the nervous system and the inner ear. In 1865 his magnum opus on the brain and spinal marrow in mammals was posthumously published. It contained his descriptions of the structures now called the cells of Deiters and Deiters' nucleus.

cell of Hen·sen \-ˈhen(t)-sən\ *n* : one of the supporting columnar cells between the outer hair cells and the cells of Claudius in the organ of Corti

Hensen, Viktor (1835–1924), German physiologist and marine biologist. Hensen did basic research on the physiology of hearing and sight in humans and in lower animals as well. In 1863 he studied the morphology of the human cochlea and described the cells now known as the cells of Hensen. He also discovered that the fibers of the cochlear basilar membrane are resonant corpuscles capable of vibrating. In his examination of human sight he studied the dispersion of cones in the center of the retina. In the lower animals he investigated the organs of hearing in grasshoppers, decapods, and various fishes. His companion interest in marine biology led to an investigation of plankton (he was the first to use the term *plankton*) as well as of fishes.

cell of Ley·dig \-ˈlīd-ig\ *n* : LEYDIG CELL

cel·loi·din \se-ˈlȯid-ᵊn\ *n* : a purified pyroxylin used chiefly in microscopy

cel·lose \ˈsel-(ˌ)ōs, -(ˌ)ōz\ *n* : CELLOBIOSE

cell plate *n* : a disk formed in the phragmoplast of a dividing plant cell that eventually forms the middle lamella of the wall between the daughter cells

cell sap \-ˈsap\ *n*   **1** : the liquid contents of a plant cell vacuole   **2** : CYTOSOL

cell theory *n* : a theory in biology that includes one or both of the statements that the cell is the fundamental structural and functional unit of living matter and that the organism is composed of autonomous cells with its properties being the sum of those of its cells

cel·lu·la \ˈsel-yə-lə\ *n, pl* **cel·lu·lae** \-ˌlē\ : a small cell : CELLULE

cel·lu·lar \ˈsel-yə-lər\ *adj*   **1** : of, relating to, or consisting of cells   **2** : CELL-MEDIATED ⟨∼ immunity⟩ — **cel·lu·lar·i·ty** \ˌsel-yə-ˈlar-ət-ē\ *n, pl* **-ties**

cellular respiration *n* : any of various energy-yielding oxidative reactions in living matter that typically involve transfer of oxygen and production of carbon dioxide and water as end products

cel·lu·lase \ˈsel-yə-ˌlās, -ˌlāz\ *n* : an enzyme that hydrolyzes cellulose

cel·lule \ˈsel-(ˌ)yü(ə)l\ *n* : a small cell

cellulifugal *var of* CELLIFUGAL

cel·lu·lin \ˈsel-yə-lən\ *n* : a carbohydrate resembling cellulose that is chiefly of animal origin but is also found in some fungi

cellulipetal *var of* CELLIPETAL

cel·lu·lite \ˈsel-yə-ˌlīt, -ˌlēt\ *n* : deposits of subcutaneous fat within fibrous connective tissue (as in the thighs, hips, and buttocks) that give a puckered and dimpled appearance to the skin surface

cel·lu·li·tis \ˌsel-yə-ˈlīt-əs\ *n* : diffuse and esp. subcutaneous inflammation of connective tissue

cel·lu·lo·lyt·ic \ˌsel-yə-lō-ˈlit-ik\ *adj* : hydrolyzing or having the capacity to hydrolyze cellulose ⟨∼ bacteria⟩

cel·lu·los·an \ˌsel-yə-ˈlōs-ᵊn, -ˌlō-ˈsan\ *n* : any of several carbohydrates (as xylan and mannan) occurring in close association with cellulose in cell walls

cel·lu·lose \ˈsel-yə-ˌlōs, -ˌlōz\ *n* : a polysaccharide $(C_6H_{10}O_5)_x$ of glucose units that constitutes the chief part of the cell walls of plants, occurs naturally in such fibrous products as cotton and kapok, and is the raw material of many manufactured goods (as paper, rayon, and cellophane)

cellulose acetate phthalate *n* : a derivative of cellulose used as a coating for enteric tablets

cellulose nitrate *n* : any of several esters of nitric acid formed by the action of nitric acid on cellulose (as paper, linen, or cotton) and used for making explosives, plastics, and varnishes — called also *nitrocellulose;* see GUNCOTTON, PYROXYLIN

¹cel·lu·los·ic \ˌsel-yə-ˈlō-sik, -zik\ *adj* : of, relating to, or made from cellulose ⟨∼ fibers⟩

²cellulosic *n* : a substance made from cellulose or a derivative of cellulose

cell wall *n* : the usu. rigid nonliving permeable wall that surrounds the plasma membrane and encloses and supports the cells of most plants, bacteria, fungi, and algae

Cel·sius \ˈsel-sē-əs, -shəs\ *adj* : relating to or having a scale for measuring temperature on which the interval between the triple point and the boiling point of water is divided into 99.99 degrees with 0.01° being the triple point and 100.00° the boiling point — abbr. *C*; compare CENTIGRADE

Celsius, Anders (1701–1744), Swedish astronomer. Celsius's major contribution was his thermometer scale. Although not the first thermometer with a 100-degree scale, his scale, described in 1742, used the freezing and boiling points of water as its two fixed points, with 0° for the boiling point and 100° for the freezing point. Five years later the system was reversed so that 0° represented the freezing point and 100° represented the boiling point and then it gradually gained acceptance. Since about 1800 *Celsius* has been used as an adjective to designate a thermometer based on the revised scale and more recently to indicate the scale itself.

ce·ment \si-ˈment\ *n*   **1** : CEMENTUM   **2** : a plastic composition made esp. of zinc or silica for filling dental cavities

ce·men·ta·tion \ˌsē-ˌmen-ˈtā-shən\ *n* : the act or process of attaching (as a dental restoration to a natural tooth) by means of cement

ce·ment·i·cle \si-ˈment-i-kəl\ *n* : a calcified body formed in the periodontal membrane of a tooth

ce·ment·i·fi·ca·tion \si-ˌment-ə-fə-ˈkā-shən\ *n* : the process by which cementum of a tooth is formed

ce·ment·ite \si-ˈment-ˌīt\ *n* : a hard brittle iron carbide Fe_3C in steel, cast iron, and iron-carbon alloys

ce·ment·o·blast \si-ˈment-ə-ˌblast\ *n* : one of the specialized osteoblasts of the dental sac that produce cementum

ce·men·to·enam·el \si-ˌment-ō-i-ˈnam-əl\ *adj* : of, relating to, or joining the cementum and enamel of a tooth

ce·men·to·ma \ˌsē-ˌmen-ˈtō-mə\ *n, pl* **-mas** *also* **-ma·ta** \-mət-ə\ : a tumor resembling cementum in structure

ce·men·tum \si-ˈment-əm\ *n* : a specialized external bony layer covering the dentin of the part of a tooth normally within the gum — called also *cement;* compare DENTIN, ENAMEL

cen *abbr* central

cen·es·the·sia *or chiefly Brit* **coen·aes·the·sia** \ˌsē-nəs-ˈthē-zhə\ *n* : the general feeling of inhabiting one's body that arises from multiple stimuli from various bodily organs — **cen·es·thet·ic** *or chiefly Brit* **coen·aes·thet·ic** \-ˈthet-ik\ *adj*

ce·no·ge·net·ic *or* **coe·no·ge·net·ic** *or chiefly Brit* **cae·no·ge·net·ic** \ˌsē-nə-jə-ˈnet-ik, ˌsen-ə-\ *adj* : relating to or being a specialized adaptive character (as the amnion or chorion surrounding the embryo of higher vertebrates) that is not represented in primitive ancestral forms

cen·sor \ˈsen(t)-sər\ *n* : a hypothetical psychic agency that represses unacceptable notions before they reach consciousness — **cen·so·ri·al** \sen-ˈsōr-ē-əl, -ˈsȯr-\ *adj*

cen·sor·ship \ˈsen(t)-sər-ˌship\ *n* : exclusion from consciousness by the psychic censor

cen·ter *or chiefly Brit* **cen·tre** \ˈsent-ər\ *n* : a group of nerve cells having a common function ⟨the brain stem's respiratory ∼⟩ — called also *nerve center*

center of ossification *n* : a point within a developing bone at which ossification begins within the preexistent cartilaginous matrix

cen·te·sis \sen-'tē-səs\ *n, pl* **cen·te·ses** \-ˌsēz\ : surgical puncture (as of a tumor or membrane) — usu. used in compounds ⟨para*centesis*⟩ ⟨thora*centesis*⟩

cen·ti·bar \'sent-ə-ˌbär\ *n* : a unit of atmospheric pressure equal to ¹⁄₁₀₀ bar — abbr. *cb*

cen·ti·grade \'sent-ə-ˌgrād, 'sänt-\ *adj* : relating to, conforming to, or having a thermometer scale on which the interval between the freezing and boiling points of water is divided into 100 degrees with 0° representing the freezing point and 100° the boiling point ⟨10° ∼⟩ — abbr. *C*; compare CELSIUS

cen·ti·gram *or chiefly Brit* **cen·ti·gramme** \-ˌgram\ *n* : a unit of mass and weight equal to ¹⁄₁₀₀ gram

cen·ti·li·ter *or chiefly Brit* **cen·ti·li·tre** \'sent-i-ˌlēt-ər, 'sänt-\ *n* : a unit of liquid capacity equal to ¹⁄₁₀₀ liter

cen·ti·me·ter *or chiefly Brit* **cen·ti·me·tre** \'sent-ə-ˌmēt-ər, 'sänt-\ *n* : a unit of length equal to ¹⁄₁₀₀ meter

centimeter–gram–second *or chiefly Brit* **centimetre–gram–second** *also* **centimetre–gramme–second** *adj* : CGS

cen·ti·mor·gan \'sen-tə-ˌmȯr-gən\ *n* : a genetic unit equivalent to ¹⁄₁₀₀ of a morgan

cen·ti·nor·mal \'sent-ə-ˌnȯr-məl\ *adj, of a chemical solution* : having ¹⁄₁₀₀ of normal strength

cen·ti·pede \'sent-ə-ˌpēd\ *n* : any member of the class Chilopoda of long flattened many-segmented predaceous arthropods with each segment bearing one pair of legs of which the foremost pair is modified into poison fangs

cen·ti·poise \'sent-ə-ˌpȯiz\ *n* : a unit of viscosity equal to ¹⁄₁₀₀ poise

cen·ti·stoke \'sent-ə-ˌstōk\ *n* : a unit of kinematic viscosity equal to ¹⁄₁₀₀ stoke

centra *pl of* CENTRUM

¹cen·trad \'sen-ˌtrad\ *adv or adj* : toward the center (as of the body) ⟨∼ to the epidermis⟩

²centrad *n* : a unit of angular measure equal to ¹⁄₁₀₀ of a radian or about 0.57 degrees

cen·tral \'sen-trəl\ *adj* **1** : of or concerning the centrum of a vertebra **2 a** : of, relating to, or comprising the brain and spinal cord **b** : originating within the central nervous system : caused by factors originating in the central nervous system ⟨∼ precocious puberty⟩ **3** : affecting or involving the trunk of the body and esp. the abdomen ⟨∼ adiposity⟩ — **cen·tral·ly** \-trə-lē\ *adv*

central artery *n* : a branch of the ophthalmic artery or the lacrimal artery that enters the substance of the optic nerve and supplies the retina

central artery of the retina *n* : a branch of the ophthalmic artery that passes to the retina in the middle of the optic nerve and branches to form the arterioles of the retina — called also *central retinal artery*

central auditory processing disorder *n* : a disorder that is marked by a deficit in the way the brain receives, differentiates, analyzes, and interprets auditory information (as speech) and that is not attributable to impairments in peripheral hearing or intellect

central body *n* : CENTROSOME 2

central canal *n* : a minute canal running through the gray matter of the whole length of the spinal cord and continuous anteriorly with the ventricles of the brain

central deafness *n* : hearing loss or impairment resulting from defects in the central nervous system (as in the auditory area) rather than in the ear itself or the auditory nerve — compare CONDUCTION DEAFNESS, NERVE DEAFNESS

central diabetes insipidus *n* : diabetes insipidus caused by insufficient production of vasopressin and resulting from damage (as from injury, infection or disease) to the pituitary gland or hypothalamus

central dogma *n* : a theory in genetics and molecular biology subject to several exceptions that genetic information is coded in self-replicating DNA and undergoes unidirectional transfer to messenger RNAs in transcription which act as templates for protein synthesis in translation

centralis — see FOVEA CENTRALIS

central line *n* : an IV line that is inserted into a large vein (as the superior vena cava) typically in the neck or near the heart for therapeutic or diagnostic purposes (as to administer medicines or fluids or withdraw blood)

central lobe *n* : INSULA

central nervous system *n* : the part of the nervous system which in vertebrates consists of the brain and spinal cord, to which sensory impulses are transmitted and from which motor impulses pass out, and which supervises and coordinates the activity of the entire nervous system — compare AUTONOMIC NERVOUS SYSTEM, PERIPHERAL NERVOUS SYSTEM

central pain *n* : pain resulting from a lesion in the brain or spinal cord

central pontine myelinolysis *n* : disintegration of the myelin sheaths in the pons that is associated with malnutrition and esp. with alcoholism

central retinal artery *n* : CENTRAL ARTERY OF THE RETINA

central retinal vein *n* : CENTRAL VEIN OF THE RETINA

central sulcus *n* : the sulcus separating the frontal lobe of the cerebral cortex from the parietal lobe — called also *fissure of Rolando, Rolandic fissure*

central tendon *n* : a 3-lobed aponeurosis located near the central portion of the diaphragm caudal to the pericardium and composed of intersecting planes of collagenous fibers

central vein *n* : any of the veins in the lobules of the liver that occur one in each lobule running from the apex to the base, receive blood from the sinusoids, and empty into the sublobular veins — called also *intralobular vein*

central vein of the retina *n* : a vein that is formed by union of the veins draining the retina, passes with the central artery of the retina in the optic nerve, and empties into the superior ophthalmic vein — called also *central retinal vein*

central venous pressure *n* : the venous pressure of the right atrium of the heart obtained by inserting a catheter into the median cubital vein and advancing it to the right atrium through the superior vena cava — abbr. *CVP*

centre *chiefly Brit var of* CENTER

cen·tric \'sen-trik\ *adj* **1** : of or relating to a nerve center **2** : of, relating to, or having a centromere **3** *of dental occlusion* : involving spatial relationships such that all teeth of both jaws meet in a normal manner and forces exerted by the lower on the upper jaw are perfectly distributed in the dental arch

cen·trif·u·gal \sen-'trif-yə-gəl, -'trif-i-gəl\ *adj* : passing outward (as from a nerve center to a muscle or gland) : EFFERENT — **cen·trif·u·gal·ly** \-gə-lē\ *adv*

cen·trif·u·gal·ize *or Brit* **cen·trif·u·gal·ise** \-gə-ˌlīz\ *vt* **-ized** *or Brit* **-ised; -iz·ing** *or Brit* **-is·ing** : CENTRIFUGE — **cen·trif·u·gal·iza·tion** *or Brit* **cen·trif·u·gal·isa·tion** \-ˌtrif-yə-gə-lə-'zā-shən\ *n*

cen·trif·u·ga·tion \ˌsen-trə-fyu̇-'gā-shən\ *n* : the process of centrifuging

¹cen·tri·fuge \'sen-trə-ˌfyüj\ *n* : a machine using centrifugal force for separating substances of different densities, for removing moisture, or for simulating gravitational effects

²centrifuge *vt* **-fuged; -fug·ing** : to subject to centrifugal action esp. in a centrifuge

cen·tri·lob·u·lar \ˌsen-trə-'läb-yə-lər\ *adj* : relating to or affecting the center of a lobule ⟨∼ necrosis in the liver⟩; *also* : affecting the central parts of the lobules containing clusters of branching functional and anatomical units of the lung ⟨∼ emphysema⟩

cen·tri·ole \'sen-trē-ˌōl\ *n* : one of a pair of cellular organelles that occur esp. in animals, are adjacent to the nucleus, function in the formation of the spindle apparatus during cell division, and consist of a cylinder with nine microtubules arranged peripherally in a circle

\ə\ **abut** \ᵊ\ **kitten** \ər\ **further** \a\ **ash** \ā\ **ace** \ä\ **cot, cart** \au̇\ **out** \ch\ **chin** \e\ **bet** \ē\ **easy** \g\ **go** \i\ **hit** \ī\ **ice** \j\ **job** \ŋ\ **sing** \ō\ **go** \ȯ\ **law** \ȯi\ **boy** \th\ **thin** \t̲h̲\ **the** \ü\ **loot** \u̇\ **foot** \y\ **yet** \zh\ **vision** *See also* Pronunciation Symbols page

cen·trip·e·tal \sen-'trip-ət-ᵊl\ *adj* : passing inward (as from a sense organ to the brain or spinal cord) : AFFERENT — **cen·trip·e·tal·ly** \-ᵊl-ē\ *adv*

cen·tro·lec·i·thal \ˌsen-trō-'les-ə-thəl\ *adj, of an egg* : having the yolk massed centrally and surrounded by a thin layer of clear cytoplasm — compare ISOLECITHAL, TELOLECITHAL

cen·tro·mere \'sen-trə-ˌmi(ə)r\ *n* : the point or region on a chromosome to which the spindle attaches during mitosis and meiosis — called also *kinetochore* — **cen·tro·mer·ic** \ˌsen-trə-'mi(ə)r-ik, -'mer-\ *adj*

cen·tro·some \'sen-trə-ˌsōm\ *n* **1** : CENTRIOLE **2** : the centriole-containing region of clear cytoplasm adjacent to the cell nucleus — **cen·tro·so·mic** \ˌsen-trə-'sō-mik\ *adj*

cen·tro·sphere \'sen-trə-ˌsfi(ə)r\ *n* : the differentiated layer of cytoplasm surrounding the centriole within the centrosome

cen·trum \'sen-trəm\ *n, pl* **centrums** *or* **cen·tra** \-trə\ **1** : the center esp. of an anatomical part **2** : the body of a vertebra ventral to the neural arch

Cen·tru·roi·des \ˌsen-trə-'rȯi-(ˌ)dēz\ *n* : a genus of scorpions containing the only U.S. forms dangerous to humans

ce·pha·eline \se-'fā-ə-ˌlēn, -lən\ *n* : a colorless crystalline alkaloid $C_{28}H_{38}N_2O_4$ extracted from ipecac root

Cepha·elis \ˌsef-ə-'ē-ləs\ *n* : a large genus of tropical shrubs and trees (family Rubiaceae) that have small tubular flowers crowded into dense heads and that include ipecac

ceph·a·lad \'sef-ə-ˌlad\ *adv* : toward the head or anterior end of the body

ceph·a·lal·gia \ˌsef-ə-'lal-j(ē-)ə\ *n* : HEADACHE

ceph·a·lex·in \ˌsef-ə-'lek-sən\ *n* : a semisynthetic cephalosporin $C_{16}H_{17}N_3O_4S$ with a spectrum of antibiotic activity similar to the penicillins that is often administered in the form of its hydrochloride $C_{16}H_{17}N_3O_4S \cdot HCl$

ce·phal·gia \se-'fal-jə, -jē-ə\ *n* : HEADACHE

ceph·al·he·ma·to·ma *or chiefly Brit* **ce·phal·hae·ma·to·ma** \ˌsef-əl-ˌhē-mə-'tō-mə\ *n, pl* **-mas** *also* **-ma·ta** \-'mät-ə\ : a usu. benign swelling formed from a hemorrhage beneath the periosteum of the skull and occurring esp. over one or both of the parietal bones in newborn infants as a result of trauma sustained during delivery

ce·phal·ic \sə-'fal-ik\ *adj* **1** : of or relating to the head **2** : directed toward or situated on or in or near the head — **ce·phal·i·cal·ly** \-i-k(ə-)lē\ *adv*

cephalic flexure *n* : the middle of the three anterior flexures of an embryo in which the front part of the brain bends downward in an angle of 90 degrees — called also *cranial flexure*

cephalic index *n* : the ratio multiplied by 100 of the maximum breadth of the head to its maximum length — compare CRANIAL INDEX

cephalic vein *n* : any of various superficial veins of the arm; *specif* : a large vein of the upper arm lying along the outer edge of the biceps muscle and emptying into the axillary vein

ceph·a·lin \'kef-ə-lən, 'sef-\ *also* **keph·a·lin** \'kef-\ *n* : PHOSPHATIDYLETHANOLAMINE

ceph·a·li·za·tion *or Brit* **ceph·a·li·sa·tion** \ˌsef-ə-lə-'zā-shən\ *n* : an evolutionary tendency to specialization of the body with concentration of sensory and neural organs in an anterior head

ceph·a·lo·cau·dal \ˌsef-ə-lō-'kȯd-ᵊl\ *adj* : proceeding or occurring in the long axis of the body esp. in the direction from head to tail — **ceph·a·lo·cau·dal·ly** \-ᵊl-ē\ *adv*

Ceph·a·lo·chor·da \-'kȯrd-ə\ *n pl, syn of* CEPHALOCHORDATA

Ceph·a·lo·chor·da·ta \-ˌkȯr-'dät-ə, -'dāt-ə\ *n pl* : a subphylum or other major taxon of the phylum Chordata comprising the lancelets and characterized by extension of the notochord to the anterior as well as to the posterior end of the body

ceph·a·lo·gram \'sef-ə-lə-ˌgram\ *n* : a radiograph of the head esp. for orthodontic purposes

ceph·a·lom·e·ter \ˌsef-ə-'läm-ət-ər\ *n* : an instrument for measuring the head

ceph·a·lom·e·try \ˌsef-ə-'läm-ə-trē\ *n, pl* **-tries** : the science

of measuring the head in living individuals (as to assess craniofacial growth and development) — **ceph·a·lo·met·ric** \-lō-'me-trik\ *adj*

ceph·a·lo·pel·vic disproportion \ˌsef-ə-lō-ˌpel-vik-\ *n* : a condition in which a maternal pelvis is small in relation to the size of the fetal head

Ceph·a·lop·o·da \ˌsef-ə-'läp-əd-ə\ *n pl* : a class of mollusks including the squids, cuttlefishes, and octopuses that have a tubular siphon under the head, a group of muscular arms around the front of the head which are usu. furnished with suckers, highly developed eyes, and usu. a bag of inky fluid which can be ejected for defense or concealment — **ceph·a·lo·pod** \'sef-ə-lə-ˌpäd\ *adj or n* — **ceph·a·lop·o·dan** \ˌsef-ə-'läp-əd-ən\ *adj or n*

ceph·a·lor·i·dine \ˌsef-ə-'lȯr-ə-ˌdēn, -'lär-\ *n* : a semisynthetic broad-spectrum antibiotic $C_{19}H_{17}N_3O_4S_2$ derived from a cephalosporin

ceph·a·lo·spo·rin \ˌsef-ə-lə-'spȯr-ən, -'spȯr-\ *n* : any of several beta-lactam antibiotics produced by an imperfect fungus of the genus *Acremonium* or made semisynthetically

Ceph·a·lo·spo·ri·um \-'spōr-ē-əm, -'spȯr-\ *n, syn of* ACREMONIUM

ceph·a·lo·thin \'sef-ə-lə-(ˌ)thin\ *n* : a semisynthetic broad= spectrum antibiotic $C_{16}H_{15}N_2NaO_6S_2$ that is an analog of a cephalosporin and is effective against penicillin-resistant staphylococci

ceph·a·lo·tho·ra·cop·a·gus \ˌsef-ə-ˌlō-ˌthȯr-ə-'käp-ə-gəs, -ˌthȯr-\ *n, pl* **-a·gi** \-ˌgī, -ˌgē\ : teratological twin fetuses joined at the head, neck, and thorax

ceph·a·lo·tho·rax \ˌsef-ə-lə-'thō(ə)r-ˌaks, -'thȯ(ə)r-\ *n* : the united head and thorax of an arachnid or higher crustacean

cepha·my·cin \ˌsef-ə-'mīs-ᵊn\ *n* : any of several beta-lactam antibiotics that are produced by various bacteria of the genus *Streptomyces* and are related to the cephalosporins

CER *abbr* conditioned emotional response

ce·ra al·ba \ˌsir-ə-'al-bə\ *n* : WHITE WAX

ce·ra·ceous \sə-'rā-shəs\ *adj* : resembling wax

ce·ra fla·va \ˌsir-ə-'fläv-ə, -'flā-və\ *n* : YELLOW WAX

cer·amide \'sir-ə-ˌmīd\ *n* : any of a group of amido sphingolipids formed by linking a fatty acid to sphingosine and found widely in small amounts in plant and animal tissue

cer·amide·tri·hexo·si·dase \ˌsir-ə-ˌmīd-ˌtrī-ˌhek-sə-'sī-ˌdās, -ˌdāz\ *n* : an enzyme that breaks down ceramidetrihexoside and is deficient in individuals affected with Fabry's disease

cer·amide·tri·hexo·side \-(ˌ)trī-'hek-sə-ˌsīd\ *n* : a lipid that accumulates in body tissues of individuals affected with Fabry's disease

ce·rate \'si(ə)r-ˌāt\ *n* : an unctuous preparation for external use consisting of wax or resin mixed with oil, lard, and medicinal ingredients

cer·a·to·hy·al \ˌser-ə-(ˌ)tō-'hī-əl\ *or* **cer·a·to·hy·oid** \-'hī-ˌȯid\ *n* : the smaller inner projection of the two lateral projections on each side of the human hyoid bone — called also *lesser cornu;* compare THYROHYAL

Cer·a·to·phyl·lus \ˌser-ə-(ˌ)tō-'fil-əs\ *n* : a genus of fleas formerly coextensive with the family Dolichopsyllidae but now restricted to some parasites of the bird

cer·car·ia \(ˌ)sər-'kar-ē-ə, -'ker-\ *n, pl* **-i·ae** \-ē-ˌē\ : a usu. tadpole-shaped larval trematode worm that develops in a molluscan host from a redia — **cer·car·i·al** \-ē-əl\ *adj*

cer·clage \ser-'kläzh, (ˌ)sər-\ *n* : any of several procedures for increasing tissue resistance in a functionally incompetent uterine cervix that usu. involve reinforcement with an inert substance esp. in the form of sutures near the internal opening

Cer·com·o·nas \(ˌ)sər-'käm-ə-nəs\ *n* : a genus of commensal or coprophilous flagellated protozoans of the order Kinetoplastida having two flagella

Cer·co·pi·the·ci·dae \ˌsȯr-kō-pə-'thē-sə-ˌdē, -'thē-kə-\ *n pl* : a family of primates that includes all the Old World monkeys except the anthropoid apes and is coextensive with a superfamily (Cercopithecoidea) — **cer·co·pith·e·coid** \-'pith-ə-ˌkȯid, -pə-'thē-\ *adj or n*

Cer·co·pi·the·cus \-pə-'thē-kəs, -'pith-\ *n* : a genus of the family Cercopithecidae that includes slender long-tailed African monkeys comprising the guenons and related forms with cheek pouches and ischial callosities

cer·cus \'sər-kəs\ *n, pl* **cer·ci** \'sər-ˌsī, -ˌkī\ : either of a pair of simple or segmented appendages at the posterior end of various arthropods

cere \'si(ə)r\ *vt* **cered; cer·ing** : to wrap in or as if in a cerecloth

ce·rea flex·i·bil·i·tas \ˌsir-ē-ə-ˌflek-sə-'bil-ə-ˌtas, -ˌtäs\ *n* : the capacity (as in catalepsy) to maintain the limbs or other bodily parts in whatever position they have been placed

¹ce·re·al \'sir-ē-əl\ *adj* : relating to grain or to the plants that produce it; *also* : made of grain

²cereal *n* **1** : a plant (as a grass) yielding farinaceous grain suitable for food; *also* : its grain **2** : a prepared foodstuff of grain

cerebella *pl of* CEREBELLUM

cer·e·bel·lar \ˌser-ə-'bel-ər\ *adj* **1** : of, relating to, or affecting the cerebellum ⟨∼ neurons⟩ ⟨∼ dysfunction⟩ **2** : caused by disease of the cerebellum ⟨∼ ataxia⟩

cerebellar artery *n* : any of several branches of the basilar and vertebral arteries that supply the cerebellum — see ANTERIOR INFERIOR CEREBELLAR ARTERY, POSTERIOR INFERIOR CEREBELLAR ARTERY, SUPERIOR CEREBELLAR ARTERY

cerebellar peduncle *n* : any of three large bands of nerve fibers that join each hemisphere of the cerebellum with the parts of the brain below and in front: **a** : one connecting the cerebellum with the midbrain — called also *brachium conjunctivum, pedunculus cerebellaris superior, superior cerebellar peduncle* **b** : one connecting the cerebellum with the pons — called also *brachium pontis, middle cerebellar peduncle, middle peduncle, pedunculus cerebellaris medius* **c** : one that connects the cerebellum with the medulla oblongata and the spinal cord — called also *inferior cerebellar peduncle, pedunculus cerebellaris inferior, restiform body*

cerebelli — see FALX CEREBELLI, TENTORIUM CEREBELLI

cer·e·bel·li·tis \ˌser-ə-bə-'līt-əs, -be-\ *n* : inflammation of the cerebellum

cer·e·bel·lo·pon·tine angle \ˌser-ə-ˌbel-ō-ˌpän-ˌtēn-, -ˌtīn-\ *n* : a region of the brain at the junction of the pons and cerebellum that is a frequent site of tumor formation

cer·e·bel·lo·ru·bral \ˌser-ə-ˌbel-ō-'rü-brəl\ *adj* : of or relating to the cerebellum and red nucleus

cer·e·bel·lum \ˌser-ə-'bel-əm\ *n, pl* **-bellums** *or* **-bel·la** \-'bel-ə\ : a large dorsally projecting part of the brain concerned esp. with the coordination of muscles and the maintenance of bodily equilibrium, situated between the brain stem and the back of the cerebrum and formed in humans of two lateral lobes and a median lobe

cerebra *pl of* CEREBRUM

ce·re·bral \sə-'rē-brəl, 'ser-ə-\ *adj* **1** : of or relating to the brain or the intellect **2** : of, relating to, affecting, or being the cerebrum ⟨∼ blood flow⟩ ⟨∼ toxoplasmosis⟩

cerebral accident *n* : STROKE

cerebral apophysis *n* : PINEAL GLAND

cerebral aqueduct *n* : AQUEDUCT OF SYLVIUS

cerebral artery *n* : any of the arteries supplying the cerebral cortex: **a** : an artery that arises from the internal carotid artery, forms the anterior portion of the circle of Willis where it is linked to the artery on the opposite side by the anterior communicating artery, and passes on to supply the medial surfaces of the cerebrum — called also *anterior cerebral artery* **b** : an artery that arises from the internal carotid artery, passes along the lateral fissure, and supplies the lateral surfaces of the cerebral cortex — called also *middle cerebral artery* **c** : an artery that arises by the terminal forking of the basilar artery where it forms the posterior portion of the circle of Willis and passes on to supply the lower surfaces of the temporal and occipital lobes — called also *posterior cerebral artery*

cerebral cortex *n* : the convoluted surface layer of gray mat-

ter of the cerebrum that functions chiefly in coordination of sensory and motor information — called also *pallium;* see NEOCORTEX

cerebral dominance *n* : dominance in development and functioning of one of the cerebral hemispheres

cerebral edema *n* : the accumulation of fluid in and resultant swelling of the brain that may be caused by trauma, a tumor, lack of oxygen at high altitudes, or exposure to toxic substances

cerebral hemisphere *n* : either of the two hollow convoluted lateral halves of the cerebrum

cerebral hemorrhage *n* : the bleeding into the tissue of the brain and esp. of the cerebrum from a ruptured blood vessel

cerebral palsy *n* : a disability resulting from damage to the brain before, during, or shortly after birth and outwardly manifested by muscular incoordination and speech disturbances — see ATAXIC CEREBRAL PALSY, ATHETOID CEREBRAL PALSY, SPASTIC CEREBRAL PALSY — **cerebral palsied** *adj*

cerebral peduncle *n* : either of two large bundles of nerve fibers passing from the pons forward and outward to form the main connection between the cerebral hemispheres and the spinal cord

cerebral vein *n* : any of various veins that drain the surface and inner tissues of the cerebral hemispheres — see GALEN'S VEIN, GREAT CEREBRAL VEIN

cer·e·brate \'ser-ə-ˌbrāt\ *vi* **-brat·ed; -brat·ing** : to use the mind — **cer·e·bra·tion** \ˌser-ə-'brā-shən\ *n*

cerebri — see ACERVULUS CEREBRI, CRURA CEREBRI, FALX CEREBRI, HYPOPHYSIS CEREBRI, PSEUDOTUMOR CEREBRI

cere·bri·form \sə-'rē-brə-ˌförm, 'ser-ə-brə-\ *adj* : like the brain in form or structure : CONVOLUTED ⟨a fleshy . . . lesion with an irregular ∼ surface —J. A. Shields *et al*⟩

cer·e·brip·e·tal \ˌser-ə-'brip-ət-ᵊl\ *adj, of nerve fibers or impulses* : AFFERENT

cer·e·broid \'ser-ə-ˌbroid\ *adj* : resembling or analogous to the cerebrum or brain

cer·e·bron·ic acid \ˌser-ə-ˌbrän-ik-\ *n* : a hydroxy fatty acid obtained from phrenosin by hydrolysis

cer·e·brose \'ser-ə-ˌbrōs, -ˌbrōz\ *n* : GALACTOSE

ce·re·bro·side \sə-'rē-brə-ˌsīd, 'ser-ə-brə-\ *n* : any of various lipids composed of ceramide and a monosaccharide and found esp. in the myelin sheath of nerves

ce·re·bro·spi·nal \sə-ˌrē-brō-'spīn-ᵊl, ˌser-ə-brō-\ *adj* : of or relating to the brain and spinal cord or to these together with the cranial and spinal nerves that innervate voluntary muscles

cerebrospinal fever *n* : CEREBROSPINAL MENINGITIS

cerebrospinal fluid *n* : a liquid that is comparable to serum but contains less dissolved material, that is secreted from the blood into the lateral ventricles of the brain by the choroid plexus, circulates through the ventricles to the spaces between the meninges about the brain and spinal cord, and is resorbed into the blood through the subarachnoid sinuses, and that serves chiefly to maintain uniform pressure within the brain and spinal cord — called also *spinal fluid;* compare LYMPH

cerebrospinal meningitis *n* : inflammation of the meninges of both brain and spinal cord; *specif* : an infectious often epidemic and fatal meningitis caused by the meningococcus — called also *cerebrospinal fever*

ce·re·bro·to·nia \sə-ˌrē-brə-'tō-nē-ə, ˌser-ə-brə-\ *n* : a pattern of temperament that is marked by predominance of intellectual over social or physical factors and by exhibition of sensitivity, introversion, and shyness — compare SOMATOTONIA, VISCEROTONIA

ce·re·bro·vas·cu·lar \sə-ˌrē-brō-'vas-kyə-lər, ˌser-ə-brō-\ *adj* : of or involving the cerebrum and the blood vessels supplying it ⟨∼ disease⟩

\ə\ **abut** \ᵊ\ **kitten** \ər\ **further** \a\ **ash** \ā\ **ace** \ä\ **cot, cart**
\aů\ **out** \ch\ **chin** \e\ **bet** \ē\ **easy** \g\ **go** \i\ **hit** \ī\ **ice** \j\ **job**
\ŋ\ **sing** \ō\ **go** \ȯ\ **law** \ȯi\ **boy** \th\ **thin** \t̲h̲\ **the** \ü\ **loot**
\ů\ **foot** \y\ **yet** \zh\ **vision**   *See also* Pronunciation Symbols page

cerebrovascular accident *n* : STROKE

ce·re·brum \sə-'rē-brəm, 'ser-ə-brəm\ *n, pl* **-brums** *or* **-bra** \-brə\ **1** : BRAIN 1 **2** : an enlarged anterior or upper part of the brain; *esp* : the expanded anterior portion of the brain that in higher mammals overlies the rest of the brain, consists of cerebral hemispheres and connecting structures, and is considered to be the seat of conscious mental processes : TELENCEPHALON

cere·cloth \'si(ə)r-ˌklȯth\ *n* : cloth treated with melted wax or gummy matter and formerly used esp. for wrapping a dead body

Cer·e·dase \'ser-ə-ˌdās\ *trademark* — used for a preparation of alglucerase

cere·ment \'ser-ə-mənt, 'si(ə)r-mənt\ *n* : a shroud for the dead; *esp* : CERECLOTH — usu. used in pl.

Ce·ren·kov *also* **Che·ren·kov** \chər-'(y)eŋ-kəf\ *adj* **1** : of, relating to, or being Cerenkov radiation or the process that produces such radiation ⟨the ∼ effect⟩ **2** : being a device that makes use of Cerenkov radiation ⟨a ∼ counter⟩

Cherenkov, Pavel Alekseevich (1904–1990), Russian physicist. Cherenkov first discovered Cerenkov radiation in 1934. Later research by Igor Y. Tamm and Ilya M. Frank led to a definite explanation of the phenomenon. Discovery of Cerenkov radiation led to studies in cosmic rays and high-energy subatomic particles. Cherenkov, Frank, and Tamm were awarded the Nobel Prize for Physics in 1958.

Cerenkov radiation *also* **Cherenkov radiation** *n* : light produced by charged particles (as electrons) traversing a transparent medium at a speed greater than that of light in the same medium — called also *Cerenkov light*

cer·e·sin \'ser-ə-sən\ *n* : a white or yellow hard brittle wax made by purifying ozokerite and used as a substitute for beeswax

ce·ri·um \'sir-ē-əm\ *n* : a malleable ductile metallic element that is the most abundant of the rare-earth group — symbol *Ce*; see ELEMENT table

cerium oxalate *n* : a mixture of the oxalates of cerium metals formerly used to allay gastric irritation

ce·roid \'sir-ˌȯid\ *n* : a yellow to brown pigment found esp. in the liver in cirrhosis

ce·ro·tic acid \sə-ˌrōt-ik-, -ˌrät-\ *n* : a solid fatty acid $C_{26}H_{52}O_2$ occurring in waxes (as beeswax) and some fats

cert *abbr* certificate; certification; certified; certify

cer·ti·fi·ca·tion \ˌsərt-ə-fə-'kā-shən\ *n* : the act of certifying : the state of being certified ⟨psychiatrists with subspecialty board ∼ in geriatrics —Gary Kennedy⟩

certified milk *n* : pasteurized or unpasteurized milk produced in dairies which operate under the rules and regulations of an authorized medical milk commission

cer·ti·fy \'sərt-ə-ˌfī\ *vb* **-fied; -fy·ing** *vt* **1** : to attest authoritatively; *esp* : to attest officially to the insanity of **2** : to designate as having met the requirements to practice medicine or a particular medical specialty ∼ *vi* : to attest by a certificate ⟨five year program leading to examination by the American Board which *certifies* in that specialty —*Bull. of Meharry Med. Coll.*⟩ — **cer·ti·fi·able** \ˌsər-tə-'fī-ə-bəl\ *adj* — **cer·ti·fi·ably** \-blē\ *adv*

cerulea — see PHLEGMASIA CERULEA DOLENS

ce·ru·lo·plas·min \sə-ˌrü-lō-'plaz-mən\ *n* : a blue copper-binding serum oxidase that is deficient in Wilson's disease and that may catalyze the conversion of ferrous iron in tissues to ferric iron

ce·ru·men \sə-'rü-mən\ *n* : EARWAX

ce·ru·mi·nous \sə-'rü-mə-nəs\ *also* **ce·ru·mi·nal** \-nᵊl\ *adj* : relating to or secreting earwax

ceruminous gland *n* : one of the modified sweat glands of the ear that produce earwax

ce·ruse \sə-'rüs, 'si(ə)r-ˌüs\ *n* **1** : white lead as a pigment **2** : a cosmetic containing white lead

cerv *abbr* cervical

cer·vi·cal \'sər-vi-kəl, *Brit usu* sər-'vī-kəl\ *adj* : of or relating to a neck or cervix ⟨∼ cancer⟩

cervical canal *n* : the passage through the cervix uteri

cervical cap *n* : a usu. rubber or plastic contraceptive device in the form of a thimble-shaped molded cap that fits snugly over the uterine cervix and blocks sperm from entering the uterus — called also *Dutch cap*

cervical flexure *n* : a ventral bend in the neural tube of the vertebrate embryo marking the point of transition from brain to spinal cord

cervical ganglion *n* : any of three sympathetic ganglia on each side of the neck: **a** : a ganglion at the top of the sympathetic chain that lies between the internal carotid artery and the second and third cervical vertebrae and that sends postganglionic fibers to the heart, larynx, and pharynx, and to the head — called also *superior cervical ganglion* **b** : a ganglion at the level of the carotid cartilage that is the smallest of the cervical ganglia, that varies in its presence or absence, size, form, and position, and that sends fibers to the fifth and sixth cervical nerves — called also *middle cervical ganglion;* see THYROID GANGLION **c** : a ganglion that is located between the base of the transverse process of the seventh cervical vertebra and the fifth rib and is usu. partly or completely fused with the first thoracic ganglion to form the stellate ganglion — called also *inferior cervical ganglion*

cervicalis — see ANSA CERVICALIS

cervical nerve *n* : one of the spinal nerves of the cervical region of which there are eight on each side in most mammals including humans

cervical plexus *n* : a plexus formed by the anterior divisions of the four upper cervical nerves

cervical plug *n* : a mass of tenacious secretion by glands of the uterine cervix present during pregnancy and tending to close the uterine orifice

cervical rib *n* : a supernumerary rib sometimes found in the neck above the usual first rib

cervical vertebra *n* : any of the seven vertebrae of the neck

cer·vi·cec·to·my \ˌsər-və-'sek-tə-mē\ *n, pl* **-mies** : surgical excision of the uterine cervix — called also *trachelectomy*

cervicis — see ILIOCOSTALIS CERVICIS, LONGISSIMUS CERVICIS, SEMISPINALIS CERVICIS, SPINALIS CERVICIS, SPLENIUS CERVICIS, TRANSVERSALIS CERVICIS

cer·vi·ci·tis \ˌsər-və-'sīt-əs\ *n* : inflammation of the uterine cervix

cer·vi·co·fa·cial \ˌsər-və-(ˌ)kō-'fā-shəl\ *adj* : of, relating to, or affecting the neck and face ⟨∼ actinomycosis⟩

cervicofacial nerve *n* : a branch of the facial nerve supplying the lower part of the face and upper part of the neck

cer·vi·co·tho·rac·ic \ˌsər-vi-(ˌ)kō-thə-'ras-ik, -thȯ-\ *adj* : of or relating to the neck and thorax ⟨∼ sympathectomy⟩

cer·vi·co·vag·i·nal \-'vaj-ən-ᵊl\ *adj* : of or relating to the uterine cervix and the vagina ⟨∼ flora⟩ ⟨∼ carcinoma⟩

cer·vix \'sər-viks\ *n, pl* **cer·vi·ces** \-və-ˌsēz, ˌsər-'vī-(ˌ)sēz\ *or* **cervixes** **1** : NECK 1a; *esp* : the back part of the neck **2** : a constricted portion of an organ or part: as **a** : the narrow lower or outer end of the uterus **b** : the constricted cementoenamel junction on a tooth

cervix cor·nu \-'kȯr-ˌn(y)ü\ *n* : CERVIX 2b

cervix ute·ri \-'yüt-ə-ˌrī\ *n* : CERVIX 2a

ce·ryl alcohol \'sir-əl-\ *n* : a white crystalline alcohol $C_{26}H_{53}OH$ occurring as an ester in waxes (as beeswax)

CES *abbr* central excitatory state

¹ce·sar·e·an *or* **cae·sar·e·an** *also* **ce·sar·i·an** *or* **cae·sar·i·an** \si-'zar-ē-ən, -'zer-\ *adj* : of, relating to, or being a cesarean section ⟨a ∼ birth⟩

²cesarean *or* **caesarean** *also* **cesarian** *or* **caesarian** *n* : CESAREAN SECTION

Cae·sar \'sē-zər\, **Gaius Julius (100–44 BC),** Roman general and statesman. Caesar's connection with the cesarean section is unclear. It is thought by some that the operation was named after Caesar himself because of the popular, although probably erroneous, belief that he was born by this means. On the other hand, it is argued that the general's family, the Julii, acquired the cognomen Caesar (from Latin *caedere*, to cut) because the operation was once performed on a forebear. It is also thought that cesarean section may derive from *lex Caesaria,* the name, under the Caesars, for the law that ordered the operation be performed on women

C
D

dying in late pregnancy or in childbirth.

cesarean section *n* : surgical incision of the walls of the abdomen and uterus for delivery of offspring

ce·si·um *or chiefly Brit* **cae·si·um** \'sē-zē-əm\ *n* : a silver=white soft ductile element of the alkali metal group that is the most electropositive element known and that is used esp. in photoelectric cells — symbol *Cs*; see ELEMENT table

Ces·to·da \ses-'tōd-ə\ *n pl* : a class of the phylum Platyhelminthes comprising the tapeworms and including dorsoventrally flattened parasitic usu. segmented flatworms without cilia that lack a digestive tract and typically consist of a differentiated scolex and a chain of proglottides each including a set of reproductive organs

Ces·to·dar·ia \ses-tə-'dar-ē-ə\ *n* : a subclass of the class Cestoda comprising unsegmented intestinal parasites of sharks, rays, and primitive bony fish — **ces·to·dar·ian** \-ē-ən\ *n*

ces·tode \'ses-ˌtōd\ *n* : TAPEWORM — **cestode** *adj*

ces·to·di·a·sis \ˌses-tə-'dī-ə-səs\ *n, pl* **-a·ses** \-ˌsēz\ : infestation with tapeworms

Ces·toi·dea \ses-'tȯid-ē-ə\ *n pl, syn of* CESTODA

ce·ta·ce·um \si-'tā-s(h)ē-əm, -shəm\ *n* : SPERMACETI

ce·tir·i·zine \se-'tir-ə-ˌzēn\ *n* : an H₁ antagonist administered orally in the form of its dihydrochloride C₂₁H₂₅ClN₂O₃·2HCl to treat allergic rhinitis and chronic hives — see ZYRTEC

Ce·trar·ia \si-'trar-ē-ə\ *n* : a genus of foliose lichens (family Parmeliaceae) chiefly of northern latitudes that includes Iceland moss

cet·ri·mide \'se-trə-ˌmīd\ *n* : a mixture of bromides of ammonium used esp. as a detergent and antiseptic

ce·tyl \'sēt-ᵊl\ *n* : a monovalent chemical group C₁₆H₃₃ found in compounds that occur in waxes (as beeswax and spermaceti)

cetyl alcohol *n* : a waxy crystalline alcohol C₁₆H₃₄O obtained by the saponification of spermaceti or the hydrogenation of palmitic acid and used esp. in pharmaceutical and cosmetic preparations and in making detergents

ce·tyl·py·ri·din·i·um chloride \ˌsēt-ᵊl-ˌpī-rə-ˌdin-ē-əm-\ *n* : a white powder consisting of a hydrated quaternary ammonium salt C₂₁H₃₈ClN·H₂O and used as a cationic detergent and antiseptic

cev·a·dil·la \ˌscv-ə-'dil-ə, -'dē-(y)ə\ *n* : SABADILLA

cev·a·dine \'sev-ə-ˌdēn, -dən\ *n* : a poisonous crystalline alkaloid C₃₂H₄₉NO₉ found esp. in sabadilla seeds — called also *crystalline veratrine*

ce·vi·tam·ic acid \ˌsē-(ˌ)vī-ˌtam-ik-\ *n* : VITAMIN C

cf *abbr* [Latin *confer*] compare

Cf *symbol* californium

CF *abbr* **1** complement fixation **2** cystic fibrosis

CFS *abbr* chronic fatigue syndrome

CFT *abbr* complement fixation test

CG *abbr* chorionic gonadotropin

C gene \'sē-\ *n* : a gene that codes genetic information for the constant region of an immunoglobulin — compare V GENE

cgs *adj, often cap C&G&S* : of, relating to, or being a system of units based on the centimeter as the unit of length, the gram as the unit of mass, and the second defined as 1/86,400 of a mean solar day as the unit of time ⟨∼ units⟩

ch *abbr* **1** child **2** chronic

Cha·ber·tia \shə-'bert-ē-ə, -'bərt-\ *n* : a genus of nematode worms of the family Strongylidae including one (*C. ovina*) that infests the colon esp. of sheep and causes a bloody diarrhea

    Cha·bert \shà-ber\, **Philibert (1737–1814)**, French veterinarian. Chabert is remembered for his classic descriptions of glanders in 1779 and anthrax in 1780.

¹**chafe** \'chāf\ *vt* **chafed; chaf·ing** : to irritate or make sore by or as if by rubbing

²**chafe** *n* : injury caused by friction

Cha·gas' disease \'shäg-əs-(əz-)\ *n* : a tropical American disease that is caused by a protozoan of the genus *Trypanosoma* (*T. cruzi*) transmitted by reduviid bugs esp. of the genus *Triatoma,* that has an acute form primarily affecting children and marked by chagoma, fever, edema, enlargement of the spleen, liver, and lymph nodes, and sometimes by myocardi-tis, and that also has a chronic form which may or may not follow an acute episode, progresses over time, and is marked esp. by cardiac and gastrointestinal complications (as myocarditis, ventricular hypertrophy, megacolon, or megaesophagus)

    Chagas, Carlos Ribeiro Justiniano (1879–1934), Brazilian physician. Early in his career Chagas undertook a malaria control campaign that used pyrethrum to disinfect households and that proved to be the first successful campaign against malaria in the history of Brazil. During 1909 and 1910 Chagas discovered and described the disease named after him. He discovered that it is caused by a species of trypanosome transmitted by bloodsucking reduviid bugs and that it is manifested by fever and edema and later by cardiac disturbances. He also described its epidemiology and some of its pathogenic hosts.

cha·go·ma \shə-'gō-mə\ *n, pl* **-mas** *or* **-ma·ta** \-mət-ə\ : a swelling resembling a tumor that appears at the site of infection in Chagas' disease

chain \'chān\ *n, often attrib* **1** : a series of things (as bacteria) linked, connected, or associated together **2** : a number of atoms or chemical groups united like links in a chain

κ–chain *var of* KAPPA CHAIN

chain reaction *n* : a self-sustaining chemical or nuclear reaction yielding energy or products that cause further reactions of the same kind

chain reflex *n* : a series of responses each serving as a stimulus that evokes the next response

chair·bound \'cha(ə)r-ˌbaùnd, 'che(ə)r-\ *adj* : confined (as by illness or incapacity) to sitting in a chair

chair·side \'cha(ə)r-ˌsīd, 'che(ə)r-\ *adj* : relating to, performed in the vicinity of, or assisting in the work done on a patient in a dentist's chair ⟨a dental ∼ assistant⟩

chair time *n* : the time that a dental patient spends in the dentist's chair

cha·la·sia \kə-'lā-zhə, ka-\ *n* : the relaxation of a ring of muscle (as the cardiac sphincter of the esophagus) surrounding a bodily opening

cha·la·za \kə-'lā-zə, -'laz-ə\ *n, pl* **-zae** \-ˌzē\ *or* **-zas** : either of a pair of spiral bands in the white of a bird's egg that extend from the yolk and attach to opposite ends of the lining membrane

cha·la·zi·on \kə-'lā-zē-ən, -ˌän\ *n, pl* **-zia** \-zē-ə\ : a small circumscribed tumor of the eyelid formed by retention of secretions of the meibomian gland and sometimes accompanied by inflammation

chal·i·co·sis \ˌkal-i-'kō-səs\ *n, pl* **-co·ses** \-ˌsēz\ : a pulmonary disorder occurring among stonecutters that is caused by inhalation of stone dust

chalk \'chȯk\ *n* : a soft white, gray, or buff limestone composed chiefly of the shells of foraminifers and sometimes used medicinally as a source of calcium carbonate — called also *creta;* see PRECIPITATED CHALK, PREPARED CHALK — **chalky** \'chȯ-kē\ *adj*

chalk·stone \'chȯk-ˌstōn\ *n* : a concretion resembling chalk that is composed mainly of urate of sodium and found esp. in and about the small joints of persons suffering from gout : TOPHUS

¹**chal·lenge** \'chal-ənj\ *vt* **chal·lenged; chal·leng·ing** : to administer a physiological and esp. an immunologic challenge to (an organism or cell)

²**challenge** *n* : the process of provoking or testing physiological activity by exposure to a specific substance; *esp* : a test of immunity by exposure to an antigen after immunization against it

chal·lenged *adj* : having a physical or mental disability or deficiency ⟨skiing programs for physically ∼ athletes —Craig Hansell⟩

\ə\ abut \ᵊ\ kitten \ər\ further \a\ ash \ā\ ace \ä\ cot, cart
\aù\ out \ch\ chin \e\ bet \ē\ easy \g\ go \i\ hit \ī\ ice \j\ job
\ŋ\ sing \ō\ go \ȯ\ law \ȯi\ boy \th\ thin \th\ the \ü\ loot
\ù\ foot \y\ yet \zh\ vision *See also* Pronunciation Symbols page

cha·lone \'kā-ˌlōn, 'kal-ˌōn\ n : a substance (as a glycoprotein) that inhibits mitosis in the specific tissue which secretes it

¹**cha·ly·be·ate** \kə-'lib-ē-ət, -'lē-bē-\ adj : impregnated with salts of iron; also : having a taste due to iron ⟨∼ water⟩

²**chalybeate** n : a chalybeate liquid or medicine

cham·ber \'chām-bər\ n : an enclosed space within the body of an animal — see ANTERIOR CHAMBER, POSTERIOR CHAMBER

Cham·ber·land filter \'chām-bər-lən(d)-, shäⁿ-ber-läⁿ-\ n : a candle-shaped porcelain filter used chiefly to filter out microorganisms (as from culture media)

Cham·ber·land \shäⁿ-ber-läⁿ\, **Charles–Édouard (1851–1908)**, French bacteriologist. A close associate of Louis Pasteur, Chamberland devised a number of major techniques and apparatuses for the study of bacteriology. He discovered that certain spores need twenty minutes boiling at 115°C in order to be killed. His experiments in sterilization led to his development of the autoclave, an apparatus that revolutionized sterilization. His invention of the heated porcelain filter that bears his name later helped in the discovery of microbial exotoxins and filterable viruses. The filter's ability to purify drinking water was another enduring benefit. During his career Chamberland participated in Pasteur's experiments and discoveries, eventually having responsibility over the preparation of vaccines.

chamber pot n : a bedroom vessel for urination and defecation

cham·o·mile or **cam·o·mile** \'kam-ə-ˌmīl, -ˌmēl\ n   **1 a** : a composite herb (*Chamaemelum nobile* syn. *Anthemis nobilis*) of Europe and No. Africa having strong-scented foliage and flower heads that contain a bitter principle used as an antispasmodic or a diaphoretic   **b** : any of several related composite plants (genera *Anthemis* and *Matricaria*); esp : a Eurasian herb of the genus *Matricaria* (*M. recutita* syn. *M. chamomilla*) naturalized in No. America and having foliage and flower heads that contain the bitter principle found in chamomile (*C. nobile*)   **2** : the dried flower heads of either of two chamomiles (*Chamaemelum nobile* and *Matricaria recutita*) used as aromatic bitters

chamomile oil or **camomile oil** n : a blue aromatic essential oil obtained from the flower heads of either of two chamomiles (*Anthemis nobilis* or *Matricaria chamomilla*)

chan·cre \'shaŋ-kər\ n : a primary sore or ulcer at the site of entry of a pathogen (as in tularemia); esp : the initial lesion of syphilis — **chan·crous** \-k(ə-)rəs\ adj

chan·cri·form \'shaŋ-krə-ˌfórm\ adj : resembling a chancre

chan·croid \'shaŋ-ˌkróid\ n : a venereal disease caused by a hemophilic bacterium of the genus *Haemophilus* (*H. ducreyi*) and characterized by chancres that differ from those of syphilis in lacking firm indurated margins — called also *soft chancre;* see DUCREY'S BACILLUS — **chan·croi·dal** \shaŋ-'króid-ᵊl\ adj

change of life \ˌchān-jəv-'līf\ n   **1** : MENOPAUSE 1a(2)   **2** : ANDROPAUSE

chan·nel \'chan-ᵊl\ n   **1** : a usu. tubular enclosed passage   **2 a** : a passage created in a selectively permeable membrane by a conformational change in membrane proteins — see ION CHANNEL   **b** : a protein or cluster of proteins that functions as a channel — see CALCIUM CHANNEL BLOCKER

chao·tro·pic \ˌkā-ə-'trōp-ik, -'träp-\ adj : disrupting the structure of water, macromolecules, or a living system so as to promote activities (as change in protein conformation in solution or migration through a chromatographic medium) inhibited by such structure

¹**chap** \'chap\ vb **chapped; chap·ping** vi : to crack or open in slits ⟨the hands and lips often ∼ in winter⟩ ∼ vt : to cause to open in slits or cracks ⟨*chapped* lips⟩

²**chap** n : a crack in or a sore roughening of the skin caused by exposure to wind or cold

chap·er·one \'shap-ə-ˌrōn\ n : any of a class of proteins (as heat shock proteins) that facilitate the proper folding of proteins by binding to and stabilizing unfolded or partially folded proteins — called also *chaperone protein, molecular chaperone*

Chap Stick \'chap-ˌstik\ *trademark* — used for a lip balm in stick form

char·ac·ter \'kar-ik-tər\ n   **1** : one of the attributes or features that make up and distinguish the individual   **2** : the detectable expression of the action of a gene or group of genes   **3** : the complex of mental and ethical traits marking and often individualizing a person, group, or nation

¹**char·ac·ter·is·tic** \ˌkar-ik-tə-'ris-tik\ adj : serving to reveal and distinguish the individual character — **char·ac·ter·is·ti·cal·ly** \-ti-k(ə-)lē\ adv

²**characteristic** n : a distinguishing trait, quality, or property

char·ac·ter·olog·i·cal \ˌkar-ik-t(ə-)rə-'läj-i-kəl\ adj : of, relating to, or based on character or the study of character including its development and its differences in different individuals — **char·ac·ter·olog·i·cal·ly** \-'läj-i-k(ə-)lē\ adv

char·ac·ter·ol·o·gy \-tə-'räl-ə-jē\ n, pl **-gies** : the study of character including its development and its differences in different individuals — **char·ac·ter·ol·o·gist** \-jəst\ n

cha·ras \'chär-əs\ n : HASHISH

char·bon \'shär-bən, -ˌbän; shär-bōⁿ\ n : ANTHRAX

char·coal \'chär-ˌkōl\ n : a dark or black porous carbon prepared from vegetable or animal substances (as from wood by charring in a kiln from which air is excluded) — see ACTIVATED CHARCOAL

Char·cot–Ley·den crystals \ˌshär-ˌkō-'lī-dᵊn-\ n pl : minute colorless crystals that occur in various pathological discharges and esp. in the sputum following an asthmatic attack and that are thought to be formed by the disintegration of eosinophils

Char·cot \shár-kō\, **Jean–Martin (1825–1893)**, French neurologist. One of the fathers of modern neurology, Charcot created the greatest neurological clinic of his time. An eminent clinician and pathologist as well as a neurologist, he practiced the method which correlates the moribund patient's symptoms with the lesions discovered during the autopsy. He was the first to describe the disintegration of ligaments and joint surfaces, the condition now known as Charcot's joint or Charcot's disease, caused by tabes dorsalis. He did pioneering work on the determination of the brain centers responsible for specific nervous functions. He demonstrated the clear relationship between psychology and physiology, and his work on hysteria and hypnosis stimulated Sigmund Freud, one of his students, to pursue the psychological origins of neurosis.

Leyden, Ernst Viktor von (1832–1910), German physician. Leyden was a professor of medicine at the University of Berlin and a renowned neurologist. In 1869 he described the crystals found in the sputum of bronchial asthma patients. The crystals had already been described by Charcot in 1853, and consequently they are associated with the names of both men.

Char·cot–Ma·rie–Tooth disease \ˌ(ˌ)shär-ˌkō-mə-ˌrē-'tüth-\ n : PERONEAL MUSCULAR ATROPHY

P. Marie — see MARIE-STRÜMPELL DISEASE

Tooth, Howard Henry (1856–1925), British physician. Tooth enjoyed a varied career as a consulting physician to a British hospital for the paralyzed and epileptic, as an examiner in medicine at Cambridge and Durham universities, and as physician to British troops in Malta. In 1886 he published a description of peroneal muscular atrophy. In that same year an independent description of the disease was published jointly by Jean-Martin Charcot and Pierre Marie.

Char·cot's joint \(ˌ)shär-ˌkōz-\ or **Char·cot joint** \-ˌkō-\ n : a destructive condition affecting one or more joints, occurring in diseases of the spinal cord, and ultimately resulting in a flail joint — called also *Charcot's disease*

¹**charge** \'chärj\ vt **charged; charg·ing** : to give an electric charge to

²**charge** n   **1** : a plaster or ointment used on a domestic animal   **2** : a definite quantity of electricity; esp : an excess or deficiency of electrons in a body   **3** : CATHEXIS 2

C
D

charge nurse *n* : a nurse who is in charge of a health-care unit (as a hospital ward, emergency room, or nursing home)

char·la·tan \'shär-lət-ən\ *n* : QUACK

Charles' law *also* **Charles's law** \ˌchärl(-z)z-\ *n* : a statement in physics: the volume of a given mass of gas at a constant pressure varies directly as its absolute temperature

   Charles \shärl\, **Jacques–Alexandre–César (1746–1823),** French physicist and inventor. Charles discovered the law that bears his name about 1787. He was a pioneer in the field of ballooning who conceived the idea of using hydrogen as the medium of displacement and in 1783 participated in the first hydrogen balloon flight.

char·ley horse \'chär-lē-ˌhȯrs\ *n* : a muscular pain, cramping, or stiffness esp. of the quadriceps that results from a strain or bruise

chart \'chärt\ *n* **1** : a sheet giving information esp. in tabular form; *esp* : a record of medical information for a patient **2** : GRAPH **3** : a sheet of paper ruled and graduated for use in a recording instrument — **chart** *vt*

char·ta \'kärt-ə\ *n, pl* **char·tae** \-ˌē\ **1** : a strip of paper impregnated or coated with a medicinal substance and used for external application **2** : a paper folded to contain a medicinal powder

char·tu·la \'kär-chə-lə\ *n, pl* **char·tu·lae** \-ˌlē\ : a folded paper containing a single dose of a medicinal powder

Chas·tek paralysis \ˌchas-ˌtek-\ *n* : a fatal paralytic vitamin deficiency of foxes and minks that are bred in captivity and fed raw fish and that is caused by enzymatic inactivation of thiamine by thiaminase present in the fish

   Chas·tek \'chas-ˌtek\, **John Simeon (1886–1954),** American breeder of fur-bearing animals. In 1932 in Glencoe, Minnesota, a new disease of foxes was recognized for the first time on Chastek's farm. R. G. Green and C. A. Evans studied the pathology of the disease and in 1940 published an article in which they reported that the paralysis was due to a deficiency of thiamine caused by the presence of raw fish in the diet.

chaul·moo·gra \chȯl-'mü-grə\ *n* : any of several East Indian trees (family Flacourtiaceae) that yield chaulmoogra oil

chaulmoogra oil *n* : any of several fats and oils expressed from the seeds of chaulmoogras and used esp. formerly in the treatment of skin diseases and leprosy

chaul·moo·grate \chȯl-'mü-grət, -ˌgrāt\ *n* : a salt or ester of chaulmoogric acid

chaul·moo·gric acid \(ˌ)chȯl-ˌmü-grik-\ *n* : a crystalline unsaturated acid $C_{18}H_{32}O_2$ found as an ester esp. in chaulmoogra oil

ChB *abbr* [Latin *Chirugiae Baccalaureus*] Bachelor of Surgery

CHD *abbr* **1** childhood disease **2** coronary heart disease

ChE *abbr* cholinesterase

check·bite \'chek-ˌbīt\ *n* **1 a** : an act of biting into a sheet of material (as wax) to record the relation between the opposing surfaces of upper and lower teeth **b** : the record obtained **2** : the material for checkbites

check ligament \'chek-\ *n* **1** : ALAR LIGAMENT 1 **2** : either of two expansions of the sheaths of rectus muscles of the eye each of which prob. restrains the activity of the muscle with which it is associated: **a** : an expansion of the sheath of the lateral rectus that is attached to the lacrimal bone — called also *lateral check ligament* **b** : an expansion of the sheath of the medial rectus that is attached to the zygomatic bone — called also *medial check ligament*

check·up \'chek-ˌəp\ *n* : EXAMINATION; *esp* : a general physical examination

Che·diak–Hi·ga·shi syndrome \shäd-ˌyäk-hē-ˌgäsh-ē-\ *n* : a genetic disorder inherited as an autosomal recessive and characterized by partial albinism, abnormal granules in the white blood cells, and marked susceptibility to bacterial infections

   Che·diak \shäd-yäk\, **Moises (*fl* 1952),** French physician, and **Hi·ga·shi** \hē-gäsh-ē\, **Ototaka (*fl* 1954),** Japanese physician. Chediak and Higashi independently of each other discovered the genetic disorder that bears their names.

cheek \'chēk\ *n* **1** : the fleshy side of the face below the eye and above and to the side of the mouth; *broadly* : the lateral aspect of the head **2** : BUTTOCK 1

cheek·bone \'chēk-ˌbōn, -ˌbōn\ *n* : the prominence below the eye that is formed by the zygomatic bone; *also* : ZYGOMATIC BONE

cheek tooth *n* : any of the molar or premolar teeth

cheese fly \'chēz-\ *n* : a dipteran fly of the genus *Piophila (P. casei)* that is the adult form of the cheese skipper

cheese skip·per \-ˌskip-ər\ *n* : the cheese fly larva that lives in cheese and cured meats and is a cause of intestinal myiasis

cheesy \'chē-zē\ *adj* **chees·i·er; -est** : resembling cheese in consistency ⟨∼ lesions⟩ ⟨a ∼ discharge⟩

cheil·ec·tro·pi·on *also* **chil·ec·tro·pi·on** \ˌkī-ˌlek-'trō-pē-ˌän, -ən\ *n* : an abnormal turning outward of one or both lips

chei·li·tis *or* **chi·li·tis** \kī-'līt-əs\ *n* : inflammation of the lip

chei·lo·plas·ty \'kī-lō-ˌplas-tē\ *n, pl* **-ties** : plastic surgery to repair lip defects — **chei·lo·plas·tic** \ˌkī-lō-'plas-tik\ *adj*

chei·los·chi·sis \kī-'läs-kə-səs\ *n, pl* **-chi·ses** \-ˌsēz\ : CLEFT LIP

chei·lo·sis \kī-'lō-səs\ *n, pl* **-lo·ses** \-ˌsēz\ : an abnormal condition of the lips characterized by scaling of the surface and by the formation of fissures in the corners of the mouth

chei·ro·kin·es·thet·ic *or chiefly Brit* **chei·ro·kin·aes·thet·ic** \ˌkī-rō-ˌkin-əs-'thet-ik, -ˌkī-nəs-; *Brit usu* -ˌkī-nēs-\ *adj* : relating to or concerned with the subjective perception of hand movements (as in writing) ⟨∼ centers of the brain⟩

chei·rol·o·gy *or* **chi·rol·o·gy** \kī-'räl-ə-jē\ *n, pl* **-gies** : the study of the hand

chei·ro·pom·pho·lyx \ˌkī-rō-'päm(p)-fə-ˌliks\ *n* : a skin disease characterized by itching vesicles or blebs occurring in groups on the hands or feet

chei·ro·scope \'kī-rə-ˌskōp\ *n* : an apparatus that is used to present an image to one eye which must be drawn in a space visible only to the other eye and that serves to improve binocular vision and coordination of hand and eye

¹che·late \'kē-ˌlāt\ *adj* : of, relating to, or having the ring structure typical of a chelate

²chelate *vb* **che·lat·ed; che·lat·ing** *vt* : to combine with (a metal) so as to form a chelate ring ∼ *vi* : to react so as to form a chelate ring — **che·lat·able** \-ˌlāt-ə-bəl\ *adj* — **che·la·tion** \kē-'lā-shən\ *n*

³chelate *n* : a compound having a ring structure that usu. contains a metal ion held by coordinate bonds

che·lat·ing agent \'kē-ˌlā-tiŋ-\ *n* : CHELATOR

chelation therapy *n* : the use of a chelator (as EDTA) to bind with a metal (as lead or iron) in the body to form a chelate so that the metal loses its toxic effect or physiological activity

che·la·tor \'kē-ˌlāt-ər\ *n* : any of various compounds that combine with metals to form chelates and that include some used medically in the treatment of metal poisoning (as by lead)

che·lic·era \ki-'lis-ə-rə\ *n, pl* **-er·ae** \-ˌrē\ : one of the anterior pair of appendages of an arachnid often specialized as fangs — **che·lic·er·al** \-ə-rəl\ *adj*

chel·i·do·ni·um \ˌkel-ə-'dō-nē-əm\ *n* **1** *cap* : a genus of yellow-flowered herbs of the poppy family (Papaveraceae) that have yellowish acrid juice and include the celandine **2** : a preparation of celandine (*Chelidonium majus*) used esp. formerly as a diuretic

cheloid *var of* KELOID

che·lo·ni·an \ki-'lō-nē-ən\ *n* : TURTLE — **chelonian** *adj*

chem *abbr* chemical; chemist; chemistry

¹chem·i·cal \'kem-i-kəl\ *adj* **1** : of, relating to, used in, or produced by chemistry **2 a** : acting or operated or produced by chemicals **b** : detectable by chemical means — **chem·i·cal·ly** \-i-k(ə-)lē\ *adv*

\ə\ abut \ᵊ\ kitten \ər\ further \a\ ash \ā\ ace \ä\ cot, cart \aú\ out \ch\ chin \e\ bet \ē\ easy \g\ go \i\ hit \ī\ ice \j\ job \ŋ\ sing \ō\ go \ȯ\ law \ȯi\ boy \th\ thin \t̲h̲\ the \ü\ loot \ú\ foot \y\ yet \zh\ vision *See also* Pronunciation Symbols page

²**chemical** *n* **1** : a substance (as an element or chemical compound) obtained by a chemical process or used for producing a chemical effect **2** : DRUG 2

chemical dependence *n* : addiction to or dependence on drugs — **chemically dependent** *adj*

chemical dependency *n* : CHEMICAL DEPENDENCE

chemical peel *n* : a cosmetic procedure for the removal of facial blemishes and wrinkles involving the application of a caustic chemical and esp. an acid (as trichloroacetic acid) to the skin

chemical pneumonia *n* : an acute generalized inflammation of the lungs caused by the inhalation of irritating gases or soluble dusts

chemical sense *n* : a nervous mechanism for the physiological reception of and response to chemical stimulation; *specif* : the central nervous process (as in smelling and tasting) initiated by excitation of special receptors sensitive to chemical substances in solution — compare CHEMORECEPTOR

chemical shift *n* : the characteristic displacement of the magnetic resonance frequency of a sample nucleus from that of a reference nucleus that provides the basis for generating and interpreting nuclear magnetic resonance and magnetic resonance imaging data

chemical toilet *n* : a toilet rendering waste matter innocuous by chemical decomposition and employed where running water is not available

chemical warfare *n* : tactical warfare using incendiary mixtures, smokes, or irritant, burning, poisonous, or asphyxiating gases

che·mi·lu·mi·nes·cence \ˌkem-i-ˌlü-mə-'nes-ᵊn(t)s, ˌkē-mi-\ *n* : luminescence (as bioluminescence) due to chemical reaction usu. at low temperatures — **che·mi·lu·mi·nes·cent** \-'nes-ᵊnt\ *adj*

chemi·os·mot·ic \ˌkem-ē-äz-'mät-ik\ *adj* : relating to or being a hypothesis that seeks to explain the mechanism of ATP formation in oxidative phosphorylation by mitochondria and chloroplasts without recourse to the formation of high-energy intermediates by postulating the formation of an energy gradient of hydrogen ions across the organelle membranes that results in the reversible movement of hydrogen ions to the outside and is generated by electron transport or the activity of electron carriers

che·mi·sorp·tion \ˌkem-i-'sorp-shən, ˌkē-mi-, -'zorp-\ *n* : the usu. irreversible process of the atoms in a surface (as of a solid) forming chemical bonds with molecules that come in contact with them 〈~ of gaseous nitrogen on iron catalysts〉 — **che·mi·sorb** \'kem-i-ˌsö(ə)rb, 'kē-mi-, -'zö(ə)rb\ *vt*

chem·ist \'kem-əst\ *n* **1** : one trained in chemistry **2** *Brit* : PHARMACIST

chem·is·try \'kem-ə-strē\ *n, pl* **-tries** **1** : a science that deals with the composition, structure, and properties of substances and of the transformations that they undergo **2 a** : the composition and chemical properties of a substance 〈the ~ of hemoglobin〉 **b** : chemical processes and phenomena (as of an organism) 〈blood ~〉

chemist's shop *n, Brit* : a place where medicines are sold

chemo \'kē-ˌmō\ *n* : CHEMOTHERAPY

che·mo·at·trac·tant \ˌkē-mō-ə-'trak-tənt *also* ˌkem-ō-\ *n* : a chemical agent that induces movement of chemotactic cells in the direction of its highest concentration

che·mo·au·to·troph \-'ot-ə-ˌtrof\ *n* : an organism having a chemoautotrophic method of nutrition

che·mo·au·to·tro·phic \-ˌot-ə-'trō-fik\ *adj* : being autotrophic and oxidizing some inorganic compound as a source of energy 〈~ bacteria〉 — **che·mo·au·tot·ro·phy** \-ȯ-'tä-trə-fē\ *n, pl* **-phies**

chemoceptor *var of* CHEMORECEPTOR

che·mo·dec·to·ma \-'dek-tə-mə\ *n, pl* **-mas** *also* **-ma·ta** \-mət-ə\ : a tumor that affects tissue (as of the carotid body) populated with chemoreceptors

che·mo·dif·fer·en·ti·a·tion \-ˌdif-ə-ˌren-chē-'ā-shən\ *n* : differentiation at the molecular level assumed to precede morphological differentiation in embryogenesis

che·mo·kine \-'kīn\ *n* : any of a group of chemotactic cytok-

ines that are produced by various cells (as at sites of inflammation), that are thought to provide directional cues for the movement of white blood cells (as T cells, monocytes, and neutrophils), and that include some playing a role in HIV infection because the cell surface receptors to which they bind are also used by specific strains of HIV for entry into cells

che·mo·ki·ne·sis \-kə-'nē-səs, -kī-\ *n, pl* **-ne·ses** \-ˌsēz\ : increased activity of free-moving organisms produced by a chemical agency — **che·mo·ki·net·ic** \-kə-'net-ik, -kī-\ *adj*

che·mo·nu·cle·ol·y·sis \-ˌn(y)ü-klē-'äl-ə-səs\ *n, pl* **-y·ses** \-ˌsēz\ : treatment of a slipped disk by the injection of chymopapain to dissolve the displaced nucleus pulposus

che·mo·pal·li·dec·to·my \-ˌpal-ə-'dek-tə-mē\ *n, pl* **-mies** : destruction of the globus pallidus by the injection of a chemical agent (as ethyl alcohol) esp. for the relief of parkinsonian tremors

che·mo·pre·ven·tion \-pri-'ven-chən\ *n* : the use of chemical agents to prevent the development of cancer — **che·mo·pre·ven·tive** \-'ven-tiv\ *adj*

che·mo·pro·phy·lax·is \-ˌprō-fə-'lak-səs *also* -ˌpräf-ə-\ *n, pl* **-lax·es** \-ˌsēz\ : the prevention of infectious disease by the use of chemical agents — **che·mo·pro·phy·lac·tic** \-'lak-tik\ *adj*

che·mo·ra·di·a·tion \-ˌrād-ē-'ā-shən\ *n* : CHEMORADIOTHERAPY

che·mo·ra·dio·ther·a·py \-ˌrād-ē-ō-'ther-ə-pē\ *n* : treatment that combines chemotherapy and radiotherapy 〈~ for advanced esophageal cancer〉 — called also *chemoradiation*

che·mo·re·cep·tion \-ri-'sep-shən\ *n* : the physiological reception of chemical stimuli — **che·mo·re·cep·tive** \-'sep-tiv\ *adj*

che·mo·re·cep·tor \-ri-'sep-tər\ *also* **che·mo·cep·tor** \'kē-mō-ˌsep-tər *also* 'kem-ō-\ *n* : a sense organ (as a taste bud) responding to chemical stimuli

¹**che·mo·re·flex** \ˌkē-mō-'rē-ˌfleks *also* ˌkem-ō-\ *n* : a physiological reflex initiated by a chemical stimulus or in a chemoreceptor

²**chemoreflex** *adj* : of, relating to, or dependent on a chemoreflex

che·mo·re·sis·tance \-ri-'zis-tən(t)s\ *n* : the quality or state of being resistant to a chemical (as a drug) 〈~ in a series of lung adenocarcinoma samples —J. C. Willey *et al*〉 — **che·mo·re·sis·tant** \-tənt\ *adj*

che·mo·sen·si·tiv·i·ty \-ˌsen(t)-sə-'tiv-ət-ē\ *n, pl* **-ties** : susceptibility (as of a disease-causing bacterium or a cancer cell) to the action of a chemical agent (as a therapeutic drug) — **che·mo·sen·si·tive** \-'sen(t)-sət-iv, -'sen(t)-stiv\ *adj*

chemosensitivity test·ing \-'tes-tiŋ\ *n* : the comparative testing of a variety of drugs for their effect on a sample of biopsied tissue or a cultured disease-causing microorganism taken from a patient to determine which drugs will provide the most effective therapy

che·mo·sen·so·ry \-'sen(t)s-(ə-)rē\ *adj* : of, relating to, or functioning in the sensory reception of chemical stimuli 〈~ hairs〉 〈insect ~ behavior〉

che·mo·sis \kə-'mō-səs\ *n, pl* **-mo·ses** \-ˌsēz\ : swelling of the conjunctival tissue around the cornea

chem·os·mo·sis \ˌkē-ˌmäz-'mō-səs, -ˌmäs-; ˌkem-ˌäz-, -ˌäs-\ *n, pl* **-mo·ses** \-ˌsēz\ : chemical action taking place through an intervening membrane — **chem·os·mot·ic** \-'mät-ik\ *adj*

che·mo·stat \'kē-mə-ˌstat, 'kem-ə-\ *n* : a device in which bacteria are kept uniformly suspended in a culture medium that is constantly renewed and maintained chemically unaltered by a continuous flow of new medium through it and which is used esp. in quantitative studies of mutation rates

che·mo·ster·il·ant \ˌkē-mō-'ster-ə-lənt *also* ˌkem-ō-\ *n* : a substance that produces irreversible sterility (as of an insect) without marked alteration of mating habits or life expectancy — **che·mo·ster·il·iza·tion** *or Brit* **che·mo·ster·il·isa·tion** \-ˌster-ə-lə-'zā-shən\ *n* — **che·mo·ster·il·ize** *or Brit* **che·mo·ster·il·ise** \-'ster-ə-ˌlīz\ *vb* **-ized** *or Brit* **-ised; -iz·ing** *or Brit* **-is·ing**

che·mo·sur·gery \-'sərj-(ə-)rē\ *n, pl* **-ger·ies** : removal by chemical means of diseased or unwanted tissue — **che·mo·sur·gi·cal** \-'sər-ji-kəl\ *adj*

che·mo·syn·the·sis \-'sin(t)-thə-səs\ *n, pl* **-the·ses** : synthesis of organic compounds (as in living cells) by energy derived from chemical reactions — **che·mo·syn·thet·ic** \-sin-'thet-ik\ *adj*

chemosynthetic bacteria *n pl* : bacteria that obtain energy required for metabolic processes from exothermic oxidation of inorganic or simple organic compounds without the aid of light

che·mo·tac·tic \-'tak-tik\ *adj* : involving, inducing, or exhibiting chemotaxis — **che·mo·tac·ti·cal·ly** \-ti-k(ə-)lē\ *adv*

che·mo·tax·is \-'tak-səs\ *n, pl* **-tax·es** \-ˌsēz\ : orientation or movement of an organism or cell in relation to chemical agents

che·mo·ther·a·peu·sis \-ˌther-ə-'pyü-səs\ *n, pl* **-peu·ses** \-ˌsēz\ : CHEMOTHERAPY

che·mo·ther·a·peu·tant \-ˌther-ə-'pyüt-ᵊnt\ *n* : a chemotherapeutic agent

¹**che·mo·ther·a·peu·tic** \-ˌther-ə-'pyüt-ik\ *also* **che·mo·ther·a·peu·ti·cal** \-i-kəl\ *adj* : of, relating to, or used in chemotherapy — **che·mo·ther·a·peu·ti·cal·ly** \-i-k(ə-)lē\ *adv*

²**chemotherapeutic** *or* **chemotherapeutical** *n* : an agent used in chemotherapy

chemotherapeutic index *n* : the ratio of the maximum tolerated dose of a chemical agent used in chemotherapy to its minimum effective dose

che·mo·ther·a·peu·tics \-iks\ *n pl but sing or pl in constr* : CHEMOTHERAPY

che·mo·ther·a·pist \-'ther-ə-pəst\ *n* : a specialist in chemotherapy

che·mo·ther·a·py \-'ther-ə-pē\ *n, pl* **-pies** : the use of chemical agents in the treatment or control of disease or mental disorder

che·mot·ic \ki-'mät-ik\ *adj* : marked by or affected with chemosis ⟨∼ reactions⟩ ⟨∼ and hyperemic conjunctivas⟩

che·mot·ro·pism \ki-'mä-trə-ˌpiz-əm, ke-\ *n* : orientation of cells or organisms in relation to chemical stimuli — **che·mo·tro·pic** \ˌkē-mə-'trō-pik\ *adj* — **che·mo·tro·pi·cal·ly** \-pi-k(ə-)lē\ *adv*

che·no·de·ox·y·cho·lic acid \ˌkē-(ˌ)nō-ˌdē-ˌäk-si-ˌkō-lik-, -ˌkäl-ik-\ *or* **che·no·des·ox·y·cho·lic acid** \-ˌdez-ˌäk-\ *n* : a bile acid $C_{24}H_{40}O_4$ that is usu. found conjugated with glycine or taurine in various vertebrates (as hens, geese, hogs, and bears) including humans, that facilitates fat absorption and cholesterol excretion, and that is used to dissolve gallstones which are not calcified — called also *chenodiol*

che·no·di·ol \ˌkē-nō-'dī-ˌȯl, -ˌōl\ *n* : CHENODEOXYCHOLIC ACID

Che·no·po·di·um \ˌkē-nō-'pōd-ē-əm\ *n* : a large genus (the type of the family Chenopodiaceae) of glabrous herbs that include the goosefoots (as Mexican tea) and occur in temperate regions of the world

chenopodium oil *n* : a colorless or pale yellow toxic essential oil of unpleasant odor and taste obtained from Mexican tea plants and formerly used as an anthelmintic

Cherenkov, Cherenkov radiation *var of* CERENKOV, CERENKOV RADIATION

cher·ry \'cher-ē\ *n, pl* **cherries** **1** : any of numerous trees and shrubs (genus *Prunus*) of the rose family that bear pale yellow to deep red or blackish smooth-skinned drupes enclosing a smooth seed and that belong to any of several varieties including some cultivated for their fruits or ornamental flowers **2** : the fruit of a cherry

cher·ub·ism \'cher-(y)ə-ˌbiz-əm\ *n* : a hereditary condition characterized by swelling of the jawbones and esp. in young children by a characteristic facies marked by protuberant cheeks and upturned eyes

chest \'chest\ *n* **1** : MEDICINE CHEST **2** : the part of the body enclosed by the ribs and sternum

chest·nut \'ches-(ˌ)nət\ *n* **1 a** : a tree or shrub of the genus *Castanea* (*C. dentata*) that is found in eastern No. America and the leaf of which was formerly used to prepare an infusion for the treatment of whooping cough **b** : the edible nut of a chestnut **2** : a callosity on the inner side of the leg of the horse

chesty \'ches-tē\ *adj* : of, relating to, or affected with disease of the chest — not used technically

Cheyne–Stokes respiration \ˌchān(-ē)-ˌstōks-\ *n* : cyclic breathing marked by a gradual increase in the rapidity of respiration followed by a gradual decrease and total cessation for from 5 to 50 seconds and found esp. in advanced kidney and heart disease, asthma, and increased intracranial pressure — called also *Cheyne-Stokes breathing*

Cheyne, John (1777–1836), British physician. One of the founding fathers of modern medicine in Ireland, Cheyne published reports on a number of medical subjects, including stroke, epidemic fevers, dysentery, melena, jaundice of the newborn, incipient phthisis, and fatal erethism of the stomach. In 1808 he produced an original description of acute hydrocephalus. In 1818 he published his original observations on a kind of breathing irregularity which was to become known as Cheyne-Stokes respiration.

Stokes, William (1804–1878), British physician. Stokes produced more than 140 books and articles, covering such medical topics as intestinal disorders, mediastinal tumors, hydrocephalus, cerebrospinal meningitis, cancer of the mouth, and sarcoma of the scrotum. His most important works were concerned with diseases of the chest, heart, and aorta. His book *Diseases of the Chest* (1837) was the first treatise on the subject in modern medicine. His 1846 description of heart block, described previously by Giovanni Morgagni and later by Robert Adams, was a classic, detailed description that was based on case histories from several sources. In 1854 Stokes used Cheyne's observations on respiration as a point of departure and wrote an extended description of the condition now known as Cheyne-Stokes respiration.

CHF *abbr* congestive heart failure

chg *abbr* change

Chi·ari–From·mel syndrome \kē-'är-ē-'frȯm-əl-, -'främ-\ *n* : a condition usu. occurring postpartum and characterized by amenorrhea, galactorrhea, obesity, and atrophy of the uterus and ovaries

Chiari, Johann Baptist (1817–1854), German surgeon. Chiari is remembered for his contributions to obstetrics and especially gynecology. A member of the staff of the first maternity clinic in Vienna, he later held the post of professor of obstetrics in Prague. With two colleagues he produced a work on clinical obstetrics and gynecology which was published in 1855 after Chiari's death. In the large section he wrote on diseases of the uterus, Chiari made his early observations on atrophy of the uterus.

From·mel \'frȯm-əl\, **Richard Julius Ernst (1854–1912)**, German gynecologist. Frommel in 1882 published his description of atrophy of the uterus due to prolonged lactation. Because of Chiari's earlier contribution, the disorder is now known as the Chiari-Frommel syndrome.

chi·asm \'kī-ˌaz-əm, 'kē-\ *n* : CHIASMA 1

chi·as·ma \kī-'az-mə, kē-\ *n, pl* **-ma·ta** \-mət-ə\ **1** : an anatomical intersection or decussation — see OPTIC CHIASMA **2** : a cross-shaped configuration of paired chromatids visible in the diplotene of meiotic prophase and considered the cytological equivalent of genetic crossing-over — **chi·as·mat·ic** \ˌkī-əz-'mat-ik, ˌkē-\ *adj*

chiasmatic groove *n* : a narrow transverse groove that lies near the front of the superior surface of the body of the sphenoid bone, is continuous with the optic foramen, and houses the optic chiasma — called also *optic groove*

chick·en cholera \'chik-ən-\ *n* : FOWL CHOLERA

\ə\ **abut** \ᵊ\ **kitten** \ər\ **further** \a\ **ash** \ā\ **ace** \ä\ **cot, cart** \aȯ\ **out** \ch\ **chin** \e\ **bet** \ē\ **easy** \g\ **go** \i\ **hit** \ī\ **ice** \j\ **job** \ŋ\ **sing** \ō\ **go** \ȯ\ **law** \ȯi\ **boy** \th\ **thin** \th̲\ **the** \ü\ **loot** \u̇\ **foot** \y\ **yet** \zh\ **vision** *See also* Pronunciation Symbols page

chick·en mite \\,chik-ən-\ *n* : a small mite of the genus *Dermanyssus* (*D. gallinae*) that infests poultry esp. in warm regions — called also *poultry mite*

chicken pox *n* : an acute contagious disease esp. of children that is marked by low-grade fever and formation of vesicles and that is caused by a herpesvirus of the genus *Varicellovirus* (species *Human herpesvirus 3*) — called also *varicella;* see SHINGLES

chicken tick *n* : FOWL TICK

chief cell \\,chēf-\ *n* **1** : one of the cells that line the lumen of the fundic glands of the stomach: **a** : a small cell with granular cytoplasm that secretes pepsin **b** : a larger cell with hyaline cytoplasm and a mucoid secretion — compare PARIETAL CELL **2** : one of the secretory cells of the parathyroid glands

chig·ger \'chig-ər, 'jig-\ *n* **1** : CHIGOE 1 **2** : a 6-legged mite larva of the family Trombiculidae that sucks the blood of vertebrates and causes intense irritation

chi·goe \'chig-(,)ō, 'chē-(,)gō\ *n* **1** : a tropical flea belonging to the genus *Tunga* (*T. penetrans*) of which the fertile female causes great discomfort by burrowing under the skin — called also *chigger, sand flea* **2** : CHIGGER 2

chi kung *also* **ch'i kung** \'chē-'kuŋ\ *n, often cap C&K* : QIGONG

chik·un·gun·ya \,chik-ən-'gún-yə, ,chik-úŋ-\ *n* : a febrile disease that resembles dengue, occurs esp. in parts of Africa, India, and southeastern Asia, and is caused by a togavirus of the genus *Alphavirus* (species *Chikungunya virus*) transmitted by mosquitoes esp. of the genus *Aedes* — called also *chikungunya fever*

chil·blain \'chil-,blān\ *n* : an inflammatory swelling or sore caused by exposure (as of the feet or hands) to cold — called also *pernio*

child \'chī(ə)ld\ *n, pl* **chil·dren** \'chil-drən, -dərn\ **1** : an unborn or recently born person **2** : a young person esp. between infancy and youth — **with child** : PREGNANT

child·bear·ing \'chīl(d)-,bar-iŋ, -,ber-\ *n* : the act of bringing forth children — **childbearing** *adj*

child·bed \-,bed\ *n* : the condition of a woman in childbirth

childbed fever *n* : PUERPERAL FEVER

child·birth \'chīl(d)-,bərth\ *n* : PARTURITION

child guidance *n* : the clinical study and treatment of the personality and behavior problems of esp. maladjusted and delinquent children by a staff of specialists usu. comprising a physician or psychiatrist, a clinical psychologist, and a psychiatric social worker

child·hood \'chīld-,húd\ *n* : the state or period of being a child

child psychiatry *n* : psychiatry applied to the treatment of children

child psychology *n* : the study of the psychological characteristics of infants and children and the application of general psychological principles to infancy and childhood

children *pl of* CHILD

chilectropion *var of* CHEILECTROPION

Chile saltpeter \'chil-ē-\ *n* : sodium nitrate esp. occurring naturally (as in caliche) — called also *Chile niter*

chilitis *var of* CHEILITIS

¹chill \'chil\ *n* **1** : a sensation of cold accompanied by shivering **2** : a disagreeable sensation of coldness

²chill *vi* **1 a** : to become cold **b** : to shiver or quake with or as if with cold **2** : to become affected with a chill ~ *vt* : to make cold or chilly

chill factor *n* : WINDCHILL

Chi·lo·mas·tix \,kī-lō-'mas-tiks\ *n* : a genus of pear-shaped protozoans of the subphylum Mastigophora possessing three flagella and usu. occurring commensally in the intestines of various vertebrates and including one (*C. mesnili*) that occurs as a nonpathogenic parasite in the cecum and colon of humans

Chi·lop·o·da \kī-'läp-əd-ə\ *n pl* : a class of arthropods comprising the centipedes — **chi·lop·o·dan** \-əd-ən\ *adj or n*

chi·me·ra *or* **chi·mae·ra** \kī-'mir-ə, kə-\ *n* : an individual, organ, or part consisting of tissues of diverse genetic constitution

    Chimera, Greek mythological character. The Chimera was a fire-breathing she-monster made up of the front parts of a lion, the middle parts of a goat, and the tail of a snake.

chi·me·ric \kī-'mir-ik, kə-, -'mer-\ *adj* : relating to, derived from, or being a genetic chimera or its genetic material ⟨a ~ cat⟩ ⟨~ genes⟩

chi·me·rism \kī-'mi(ə)r-,iz-əm, kə-; 'kī-mə-,riz-\ *n* : the state of being a genetic chimera

chim·pan·zee \,chim-,pan-'zē, ,shim-, -pən-; chim-'pan-zē, shim-\ *n* : an anthropoid ape of the genus *Pan* (*P. troglodytes*) found in equatorial Africa that is smaller and more arboreal than the gorilla — see BONOBO

chi·myl alcohol \'kī-məl-\ *n* : a crystalline alcohol $C_{19}H_{40}O_3$ obtained esp. from fish-liver oils and the yellow marrow of cattle bones

chin \'chin\ *n* : the lower portion of the face lying below the lower lip and including the prominence of the lower jaw — called also *mentum* — **chin·less** \-ləs\ *adj*

Chi·na white \'chī-nə-'(h)wīt\ *n, often cap W* **1** : a pure potent form of heroin originating in southeastern Asia **2** : an illicit analog of the analgesic fentanyl that resembles heroin in its physical appearance and physiological effects

chin·bone \'chin-'bōn, -,bōn\ *n* : JAW 1b; *esp* : the median anterior part of the bone of the human lower jaw

chinch \'chinch\ *n* : BEDBUG

Chi·nese cinnamon \,chī-,nēz-, -,nēs-\ *n* **1** : the bark of a Chinese tree of the genus *Cinnamomum* (*C. cassia*) that is the source of cinnamon oil — called also *cassia bark* **2** : the tree that yields Chinese cinnamon

Chinese liver fluke *n* : a common and destructive Asian liver fluke of the genus *Clonorchis* (*C. sinensis*) that has a complex life cycle involving a mollusk and a fish as intermediate hosts and that esp. in eastern and southeastern Asia is a serious human parasite invading the liver following the consumption of raw infected fish and causing clonorchiasis

Chinese res·tau·rant syndrome \-'res-t(ə-)rənt-, -tə-,ränt-, -,tränt-, -tərnt-\ *n* : a group of symptoms (as numbness of the neck, arms, and back with headache, dizziness, and palpitations) that is held to affect susceptible persons eating food and esp. Chinese food heavily seasoned with monosodium glutamate

Chinese rhubarb *n* : a rhubarb of the genus *Rheum* (*R. officinale*) from whose rhizome and roots medicinal rhubarb is obtained

chin fly *n* : THROAT BOTFLY

chi·ni·o·fon \kə-'nī-ə-,fän\ *n* : a yellow powder composed of a sulfonic acid $C_9H_6INO_4S$ derived from quinoline, the sodium salt of this acid, and sodium bicarbonate and used in the treatment of amebiasis

chi·on·ablep·sia \,kī-,än-ə-'blep-sē-ə\ *n* : SNOW BLINDNESS

chip–blow·er \'chip-,blō-(ə)r\ *n* : a dental instrument typically consisting of a rubber bulb with a long metal tube that is used to blow drilling debris from a cavity being prepared for filling

chi·ral \'kī-rəl\ *adj* : of or relating to a molecule that is nonsuperimposable on its mirror image — **chi·ral·i·ty** \kī-'ral-ət-ē\ *n, pl* **-ties**

chiral center *n* : an atom esp. in an organic molecule that has four different atoms or groups attached to it

chi·rop·o·dy \kə-'räp-əd-ē, shə- *also* kī-\ *n, pl* **-dies** : PODIATRY — **chi·ro·po·di·al** \,kī-rə-'pōd-ē-əl\ *adj* — **chi·rop·o·dist** \kə-'räp-əd-əst, shə- *also* kī-\ *n*

chi·ro·prac·tic \'kī-rə-,prak-tik\ *n* : a system of therapy which holds that disease results from a lack of normal nerve function and which employs manipulation and specific adjustment of body structures (as the spinal column) — **chiropractic** *adj* — **chi·ro·prac·tor** \-tər\ *n*

chi·ro·prax·is \'kī-rə-,prak-səs, ,kī-rə-'\ *n, pl* **-prax·es** \-,sēz\ : CHIROPRACTIC

Chi·rop·tera \kī-'räp-tə-rə\ *n pl* : an order of eutherian

C
D

mammals modified for true flight comprising the recent and extinct bats — **chi·rop·ter** \kī-'räp-tər\ n — **chi·rop·ter·an** \(')kī-'räp-tə-rən\ adj or n

chi·rur·geon \kī-'rər-jən\ n, archaic : SURGEON

chi·rur·gi·cal \kī-'rər-ji-kəl\ adj, archaic : of or relating to surgery : SURGICAL

chis·el \'chiz-əl\ n : a metal tool with a cutting edge at the end of a blade; esp : one used in dentistry (as for cutting or shaping enamel)

chi·tin \'kīt-ᵊn\ n : a horny polysaccharide that forms part of the hard outer integument esp. of insects, arachnids, and crustaceans — **chi·tin·ous** \'kīt-ᵊn-əs, 'kīt-nəs\ adj

chi·to·bi·ose \,kīt-ə-'bī-(,)ōs, -(,)ōz\ n : a disaccharide obtained from chitin by hydrolysis

chit·tam bark \'chit-əm-,bärk\ n : CASCARA SAGRADA

chl abbr chloroform

chla·myd·ia \klə-'mid-ē-ə\ n **1** cap : the type genus of the family Chlamydiaceae comprising coccoid to spherical gram-negative intracellular parasitic bacteria and including one (C. trachomatis) that causes or is associated with various diseases of the eye and genitourinary tract including trachoma, lymphogranuloma venereum, cervicitis, and some forms of nongonococcal urethritis **2** pl **-i·ae** \-ē-,ē, -ī\ also **-ias a** : a bacterium of the genus Chlamydia **b** : an infection or disease caused by chlamydiae — **chla·myd·ial** \-ē-əl\ adj

Chla·myd·i·a·ce·ae \,klə-,mid-ē-'ā-sē-,ē\ n pl : a family of bacteria (order Chlamydiales) that are related to members of the order Rickettsiales, that are obligate parasites in the cells of warm-blooded vertebrates, and that include the causative agents of trachoma, lymphogranuloma venereum, and psittacosis

chla·mydo·spore \klə-'mid-ə-,spō(ə)r, -,spò(ə)r\ n : a thick-walled usu. resting fungal spore

chlo·as·ma \klō-'az-mə\ n, pl **-ma·ta** \-mət-ə\ : irregular brownish or blackish spots esp. on the face that occur sometimes in pregnancy and in disorders of or functional changes in the uterus and ovaries

chloracetic acid var of CHLOROACETIC ACID

chloracetophenone var of CHLOROACETOPHENONE

chlor·ac·ne \(')klōr-'ak-nē, (')klòr-\ n : a skin eruption resembling acne and resulting from exposure to chlorine or its compounds

chlo·ral \'klōr-əl, 'klòr-\ n **1** : a pungent colorless oily aldehyde C_2HCl_3O used in making DDT and chloral hydrate **2** : CHLORAL HYDRATE

chlo·ral·form·amide \,klōr-əl-'fòr-mə-,mīd, -məd; -,fòr-'mam-,īd, -əd; ,klòr-\ n : a colorless crystalline compound $C_3H_4Cl_3NO_2$ used as a hypnotic

chloral hydrate n : a bitter white crystalline drug $C_2H_3Cl_3O_2$ used as a hypnotic and sedative or in knockout drops

chlo·ral·ose \'klōr-ə-,lōs, 'klòr-, -,lōz\ n : a bitter crystalline compound $C_8H_{11}Cl_3O_6$ used esp. to anesthetize animals — **chlo·ral·osed** \-,lōst, -,lōzd\ adj

chlo·ram·bu·cil \klōr-'am-byə-,sil, klòr-\ n : an anticancer drug $C_{14}H_{19}Cl_2NO_2$ that is a derivative of nitrogen mustard and is used esp. to treat leukemias, multiple myeloma, some lymphomas, and Hodgkin's disease

chlo·ra·mine \'klōr-ə-,mēn, 'klòr-\ n **1** : any of three compounds formed by the reaction of dilute hypochlorous acid with ammonia; esp : a colorless oily bactericidal compound NH_2Cl having an ammoniacal odor **2** : any of various organic compounds containing nitrogen and chlorine esp. when the chlorine is attached to the nitrogen atom (as in the groups –NHCl and –NCl₂); esp : CHLORAMINE-T

chloramine–B \-'bē\ n : a white crystalline compound $C_6H_5ClNNaO_2S·2H_2O$ used as an antiseptic

chloramine–T \-'tē\ n : a white or faintly yellow crystalline compound $C_7H_7ClNNaO_2S·3H_2O$ used as an antiseptic (as in treating wounds) — compare DICHLORAMINE-T

chlor·am·phen·i·col \,klōr-,am-'fen-i-,kòl, ,klòr-, -,kōl\ n : a broad-spectrum antibiotic $C_{11}H_{12}Cl_2N_2O_5$ isolated from cul-

tures of a soil actinomycete of the genus Streptomyces (S. venezuelae) or prepared synthetically — see CHLOROMYCETIN

chlor·ane·mia or chiefly Brit **chlor·anae·mia** \,klōr-ə-'nē-mē-ə, ,klòr-\ n **1** : CHLOROSIS — **chlor·ane·mic** or chiefly Brit **chlor·anae·mic** \-'nē-mik\ adj

chlo·rate \'klō(ə)r-,āt, 'klò(ə)r-\ n : a salt containing the anion ClO_3^- ⟨∼ of potassium⟩

chlor·bu·tol \'klòr-byə-,tòl\ n, chiefly Brit : CHLOROBUTANOL

chlor·cy·cli·zine \klōr-'sī-klə-,zēn\ n : a cyclic antihistamine administered in the form of its hydrochloride $C_{18}H_{21}-ClN_2·HCl$

chlor·dane \'klò(ə)r-,dān\ also **chlor·dan** \-,dan\ n : a highly chlorinated viscous volatile liquid insecticide $C_{10}H_6Cl_8$

chlor·di·az·epox·ide \,klōr-dī-,az-ə-'päk-,sīd, ,klòr-\ n : a benzodiazepine that is structurally and pharmacologically related to diazepam and is used in the form of its hydrochloride $C_{16}H_{14}ClN_3O·HCl$ esp. as a tranquilizer and to treat the withdrawal symptoms of alcoholism — see LIBRIUM

chlo·rel·la \klə-'rel-ə\ n **1** cap : a genus of unicellular green algae potentially a source of high-grade protein and B-complex vitamins **2** : any alga of the genus Chlorella

chlo·rel·lin \-'rel-ən\ n : a substance obtained from algae esp. of the genus Chlorella that inhibits bacterial growth

chlor·e·mia or chiefly Brit **chlor·ae·mia** \klōr-'ē-mē-ə, klòr-\ n **1** : CHLOROSIS **2** : excess of chlorides in the blood

chlor·hex·i·dine \klōr-'hek-sə-,dīn, klòr-, -,dēn\ n : an antibacterial compound $C_{22}H_{30}Cl_2N_{10}$ that is a biguanide derivative used as a local antiseptic (as in mouthwash) and disinfectant esp. in the form of its hydrochloride, gluconate, or acetate

chlo·ric \'klōr-ik, 'klòr-\ adj : relating to or obtained from chlorine esp. with a valence of five ⟨a radiolabeled ∼ anion⟩

chloric acid n : a strong acid $HClO_3$ like nitric acid in oxidizing properties but far less stable that is obtained from its salts (as the chlorate of sodium) as a colorless aqueous solution

chlo·ride \'klō(ə)r-,īd, 'klò(ə)r-\ n **1** : a compound of chlorine with another element or radical; esp : a salt or ester of hydrochloric acid — called also muriate **2** : a monovalent anion consisting at one atom of chlorine

chloride of lime n : BLEACHING POWDER

chloride shift \-'shift\ n : the passage of chloride ions from the blood plasma into the red blood cells when carbon dioxide enters the plasma from the tissues and their return to the plasma when the carbon dioxide is discharged in the lungs that is a major factor both in maintenance of blood pH and in transport of carbon dioxide

chlo·ri·nate \'klōr-ə-,nāt, 'klòr-\ vt **-nat·ed; -nat·ing** : to treat or cause to combine with chlorine or a chlorine compound — **chlo·ri·na·tion** \,klōr-ə-'nā-shən, ,klòr-\ n

chlorinated lime n : BLEACHING POWDER

chlo·rine \'klō(ə)r-,ēn, 'klò(ə)r-, -ən\ n : a halogen element that is isolated as a heavy greenish yellow gas of pungent odor and is used esp. as a bleach, oxidizing agent, and disinfectant in water purification — symbol Cl; see ELEMENT table

chlo·rite \-,īt\ n : a salt containing the anion ClO_2^-

chlor·mer·o·drin \klōr-'mer-ə-drən, klòr-\ n : a mercurial compound $C_5H_{11}ClHgN_2O_2$ formerly used esp. as a diuretic

chlo·ro·ace·tic acid \,klōr-ō-ə-,sēt-ik-\ also **chlor·ace·tic acid** \,klōr-ə-\ n : MONOCHLOROACETIC ACID

chlo·ro·ace·to·phe·none \,klōr-ō-,as-ət-(,)ō-fə-'nōn, ,klòr-, -ō-ə-,sēt-\ or **chlor·ace·to·phe·none** \,klōr-,as-, ,klòr-ə-,sēt-, ,klòr-\ n : a chlorine derivative of acetophenone; esp : the alpha derivative C_8H_7ClO used esp. in solution as a tear gas — abbr. CN

chlo·ro·ane·mia or chiefly Brit **chlo·ro·anae·mia** \,klōr-ō-ə-'nē-mē-ə, ,klòr-\ n : CHLOROSIS

---

chlo·ro·az·o·din \\ˌklōr-ō-ˈaz-əd-ən, ˌklȯr-\ *n* : a yellow crystalline compound $C_2H_4Cl_2N_6$ used in solution as a surgical antiseptic

chlo·ro·bu·ta·nol \-ˈbyüt-³n-ˌȯl, -ˌōl\ *n* : a white crystalline alcohol $C_4H_7Cl_3O$ with an odor and taste like camphor that is used as a local anesthetic, sedative, and preservative (as for hypodermic solutions)

chlo·ro·cre·sol \-ˈkrē-ˌsȯl, -ˌsōl\ *n* : any of several chlorine derivatives of the cresols; *esp* : the para derivative C_7H_7ClO used as an antiseptic and preservative

chlo·ro·cru·o·rin \-ˈkrü-ə-rən\ *n* : a green iron-containing respiratory pigment related chemically to hemoglobin and found in the blood of some marine polychaete worms

¹chlo·ro·form \ˈklȯr-ə-ˌfȯrm, ˈklȯr-\ *n* : a colorless volatile heavy toxic liquid $CHCl_3$ with an ether odor used esp. as a solvent — called also *trichloromethane*

²chloroform *vt* : to treat with chloroform esp. so as to produce anesthesia or death

chlo·ro·gen·ic acid \ˌklȯr-ə-ˌjen-ik-, ˌklȯr-\ *n* : a crystalline acid $C_{16}H_{18}O_9$ occurring in various plant parts (as potatoes or coffee beans)

chlo·ro·gua·nide \ˌklōr-o-ˈgwän-ˌīd, ˌklȯr-, -əd\ *also* **chlor·gua·nide** \(ˈ)klȯr-ˈgwän-, (ˈ)klȯr-\ *n* : PROGUANIL

chlo·ro·leu·ke·mia *or chiefly Brit* **chlo·ro·leu·kae·mia** \-lü-ˈkē-mē-ə\ *n* : CHLOROMA

chlo·ro·ma \klə-ˈrō-mə\ *n, pl* **-mas** *also* **-ma·ta** \-mət-ə\ : a leukemic condition marked by the formation of usu. green-colored tumors composed of myeloid tissue; *also* : one of these tumors — **chlo·rom·a·tous** \-ˈräm-ət-əs\ *adj*

chlo·ro·meth·ane \ˌklōr-ō-ˈmeth-ˌān, ˌklȯr-\ *n* : METHYL CHLORIDE

chlo·rom·e·try \klōr-ˈäm-ə-trē, klȯr-\ *n, pl* **-tries** : the quantitative measurement of chlorine

Chlo·ro·my·ce·tin \ˌklōr-ō-mī-ˈsēt-³n, ˌklȯr-\ *trademark* — used for chloramphenicol

chlo·ro·per·cha \ˌklōr-ə-ˈpər-chə, ˌklȯr-\ *n* : a solution of gutta-percha in chloroform used esp. in dentistry (as for filling a root canal)

chlo·ro·phe·nol \ˌklōr-ō-ˈfē-ˌnōl, -ˌnȯl, ˌklȯr-, -fi-ˈ-\ *also* **chlor·phe·nol** \(ˈ)klȯr-, (ˈ)klȯr-\ *n* : any of three derivatives C_6H_5ClO of phenol containing a single chlorine atom per molecule; *esp* : the para derivative that is used as a topical antiseptic

chlo·ro·phen·o·thane \ˌklōr-ō-ˈfen-ə-ˌthān, ˌklȯr-\ *n* : DDT

chlo·ro·phyll \ˈklōr-ə-ˌfil, ˈklȯr-, -fəl\ *n* **1** : the green photosynthetic coloring matter of plants found in chloroplasts and made up chiefly of a blue-black ester $C_{55}H_{72}MgN_4O_5$ and a dark green ester $C_{55}H_{70}MgN_4O_6$ — called also respectively *chlorophyll a, chlorophyll b* **2** : a waxy green chlorophyll-containing substance extracted from green plants and used as a coloring agent or deodorant — **chlo·ro·phyl·lous** \ˌklōr-ə-ˈfil-əs, ˌklȯr-\ *also* **chlo·ro·phyl·lose** \-ˈfil-ˌōs, -(ˌ)fil-ˈ\ *adj*

chlo·ro·pia \klōr-ˈō-pē-ə, klȯr-\ *n* : CHLOROPSIA

chlo·ro·pic·rin \ˌklōr-ə-ˈpik-rən, ˌklȯr-\ *n* : a heavy colorless liquid CCl_3NO_2 that causes tears and vomiting and is used esp. as a soil fumigant — called also *nitrochloroform*

Chlo·rop·i·dae \klōr-ˈäp-ə-ˌdē, klȯr-; klə-ˈräp-\ *n pl* : a family of small nearly hairless flies with broad heads and short antennae including some which are irritating though nonbiting pests about the eyes of humans and various animals and are sometimes implicated in the transmission of diseases (as yaws) — see HIPPELATES, SIPHUNCULINA

chlo·ro·plast \ˈklōr-ə-ˌplast, ˈklȯr-\ *n* : a plastid that contains chlorophyll and is the site of photosynthesis and starch formation — **chlo·ro·plas·tic** \ˌklōr-ə-ˈplas-tik, ˌklȯr-\ *adj*

chlo·ro·pro·caine \ˌklōr-ō-ˈprō-ˌkān, ˌklȯr-\ *n* : a local anesthetic administered by injection in the form of its hydrochloride $C_{13}H_{19}ClN_2O_2 \cdot HCl$ — see NESACAINE

chlo·rop·sia \klōr-ˈäp-sē-ə, klȯr-; klə-ˈräp-\ *n* : a visual defect in which all objects appear green

chlo·ro·quine \ˈklōr-ə-ˌkwēn, ˈklȯr-\ *n* : an antimalarial drug administered in the form of its diphosphate $C_{18}H_{26}-ClN_3 \cdot 2H_3PO_4$ or hydrochloride $C_{18}H_{26}ClN_3 \cdot HCl$

chlo·ro·sis \klə-ˈrō-səs\ *n, pl* **-ro·ses** \-ˌsēz\ : an iron-

deficiency anemia esp. of adolescent girls that may impart a greenish tint to the skin — called also *greensickness* — **chlo·rot·ic** \-ˈrät-ik\ *adj*

chlo·ro·then \ˈklȯr-ə-ˌthen, ˈklȯr-\ *n* : an antihistamine usu. administered in the form of its citrate $C_{14}H_{19}Cl_2N_3S \cdot C_6H_8O_7$

chlo·ro·thi·a·zide \ˌklōr-ə-ˈthī-ə-ˌzīd, ˌklȯr-\ *n* : a thiazide diuretic $C_7H_6ClN_3O_4S_2$ that is taken orally or is administered in the form of its sodium salt $C_7H_5ClN_3NaO_4S_2$ by intravenous injection esp. in the treatment of edema and hypertension — see DIURIL

chlo·ro·thy·mol \-ˈthī-ˌmȯl, -ˌmōl\ *n* : any of several chlorine derivatives of thymol; *esp* : the para derivative $C_{10}H_{13}ClO$ used as a germicide (as in mouthwashes)

chlo·ro·tri·an·i·sene \-ˌtrī-ˈan-ə-ˌsēn\ *n* : a synthetic estrogen $C_{23}H_{21}ClO_3$ that is administered orally in the treatment of menopause-related conditions (as atrophic vaginitis and kraurosis vulvae), abnormal estrogen deficiency (as in hypogonadism), or in the palliative treatment of some prostate cancers

chlo·rous \ˈklȯr-əs, ˈklȯr-\ *adj* : relating to or obtained from chlorine esp. with a valence of three

chlorous acid *n* : a strongly oxidizing acid $HClO_2$ known only in solution and in the form of its salts (as the chlorite of sodium)

chlo·ro·xy·le·nol \ˌklōr-ō-ˈzī-lə-ˌnȯl, ˌklȯr-, -ˌnōl\ *n* : any of several chlorine derivatives of the xylenols; *esp* : the para derivative C_8H_9ClO used as an antiseptic and germicide

chlor·phen·e·sin carbamate \(ˌ)klȯr-fen-ə-sin-, (ˌ)klȯr-\ *n* : a white crystalline powdery drug $C_{10}H_{12}ClNO_4$ used to relax skeletal muscle

chlor·phen·ir·amine \-fen-ˈir-ə-ˌmēn, -mən, -fən-\ *n* : an antihistamine that is usu. administered in the form of its maleate $C_{16}H_{19}ClN_2 \cdot C_4H_4O_4$

chlorphenol *var of* CHLOROPHENOL

chlor·prom·a·zine \klȯr-ˈpräm-ə-ˌzēn, klȯr-\ *n* : a phenothiazine derivative that has antipsychotic, sedative, and antiemetic properties and is used in the form of its hydrochloride $C_{17}H_{19}ClN_2S \cdot HCl$ esp. to manage the symptoms of psychotic disorders (as schizophrenia) — see LARGACTIL, THORAZINE

chlor·prop·amide \-ˈpräp-ə-ˌmīd, -ˈprōp-\ *n* : a sulfonylurea drug $C_{10}H_{13}ClN_2O_3S$ used orally to reduce blood sugar in the treatment of mild diabetes

chlor·pyr·i·fos \-ˈpir-ə-fäs, -ˈpī-rə-\ *n* : a toxic crystalline organophosphate pesticide $C_9H_{11}Cl_3NO_3PS$ that inhibits acetylcholinesterase and is used to control insect pests and ticks

chlor·tet·ra·cy·cline \ˌklȯr-ˌte-trə-ˈsī-ˌklēn, ˌklȯr-\ *n* : a yellow crystalline broad-spectrum antibiotic $C_{22}H_{23}ClN_2O_8$ produced by a soil actinomycete of the genus *Streptomyces* (*S. aureofaciens*) and sometimes used in animal feeds to stimulate growth — see AUREOMYCIN

chlor·thal·i·done \klȯr-ˈthal-ə-ˌdōn, klȯr-\ *n* : a sulfonamide $C_{14}H_{11}ClN_2O_4S$ that is a long-acting diuretic used in the treatment of hypertension and in the treatment of edema associated esp. with congestive heart failure, renal dysfunction, cirrhosis of the liver, or corticosteroid and estrogen therapy — see HYGROTON

CHO *abbr* carbohydrate

cho·a·na \ˈkō-ə-nə\ *n, pl* **-nae** \-ˌnē\ : either of the pair of posterior apertures of the nasal cavity that open into the nasopharynx — called also *posterior naris* — **cho·a·nal** \-nəl\ *adj*

Cho·a·no·tae·nia \ˌkō-ə-(ˌ)nō-ˈtē-nē-ə\ *n* : a genus of taenioid tapeworms including a number of intestinal parasites of birds of which one (*C. infundibulum*) is an important pest of chickens and turkeys

chocolate tree *n* : CACAO 2

¹choke \ˈchōk\ *vb* **choked; chok·ing** *vt* : to keep from breathing in a normal way by compressing or obstructing the trachea or by poisoning or adulterating available air ~ *vi* : to have the trachea blocked entirely or partly

²choke *n* **1** : the act of choking **2 chokes** *pl* : decompression sickness when marked by suffocation — used with *the*

choked disk *n* : PAPILLEDEMA

chol *abbr* cholesterol

cholaemia, cholaemic *chiefly Brit var of* CHOLEMIA, CHOLE-MIC

cho·la·gog·ic \ˌkäl-ə-ˈgäj-ik, ˌkōl-\ *adj* : being a cholagogue : inducing a flow of bile

cho·la·gogue \ˈkäl-ə-ˌgäg, ˈkōl-\ *n* : an agent that promotes an increased flow of bile

cho·lane \ˈkō-ˌlān\ *n* : a crystalline steroid hydrocarbon $C_{24}H_{42}$ from which the bile acids are derived

chol·an·gio·car·ci·no·ma \kə-ˌlan-jē-ə-ˌkärs-ᵊn-ˈō-mə\ *n* : a usu. slow-growing malignant tumor of the bile duct that arises from biliary epithelium and is typically an adenocarcinoma

chol·an·gio·gram \kə-ˈlan-jē-ə-ˌgram, kō-\ *n* : a radiograph of the bile ducts made after the ingestion or injection of a radiopaque substance

chol·an·gi·og·ra·phy \kə-ˌlan-jē-ˈäg-rə-fē, (ˌ)kō-\ *n, pl* **-phies** : radiographic visualization of the bile ducts after ingestion or injection of a radiopaque substance — **chol·an·gio·graph·ic** \-jē-ə-ˈgraf-ik\ *adj*

chol·an·gi·ole \kə-ˈlan-jē-ˌōl, kō-\ *n* : a bile canaliculus

chol·an·gio·li·tis \kə-ˌlan-jē-ə-ˈlīt-əs, (ˌ)kō-\ *n, pl* **-lit·i·des** \-ˈlit-ə-ˌdēz\ : inflammation of bile capillaries — **chol·an·gi·o·lit·ic** \-ˈlit-ik\ *adj*

chol·an·gi·o·ma \kə-ˌlan-jē-ˈō-mə, (ˌ)kō-\ *n, pl* **-mas** *also* **-ma·ta** \-mət-ə\ : a tumor of a bile duct

cholangiopancreatography — see ENDOSCOPIC RETROGRADE CHOLANGIOPANCREATOGRAPHY

chol·an·gi·tis \ˌkō-ˌlan-ˈjīt-əs\ *n, pl* **-git·i·des** \-ˈjit-ə-ˌdēz\ : inflammation of one or more bile ducts — called also *angiocholitis*

cho·lan·ic acid \(ˌ)kō-ˌlan-ik-\ *n* : a colorless crystalline acid $C_{23}H_{39}COOH$ some of whose hydroxy and keto derivatives constitute the bile acids

chol·ano·poi·e·sis \kə-ˌlan-ō-ˌpȯi-ˈē-səs, (ˌ)kō-\ *n, pl* **-e·ses** \-ˌsēz\ : synthesis of cholic acid, its derivatives, or bile by the liver

chol·an·threne \kō-ˈlan-ˌthrēn\ *n* : a pale yellow crystalline polycyclic carcinogenic hydrocarbon $C_{20}H_{14}$ — compare METHYLCHOLANTHRENE

cho·late \ˈkō-ˌlāt\ *n* : a salt or ester of cholic acid

cho·le·cal·cif·er·ol \ˌkō-lə-(ˌ)kal-ˈsif-ə-ˌrȯl, -ˌrōl\ *n* : a sterol $C_{27}H_{43}OH$ that is a natural form of vitamin D found esp. in fish, egg yolks, and fish-liver oils and is formed in the skin on exposure to sunlight or ultraviolet rays — called also *vitamin D, vitamin D_3*

cho·le·chro·mo·poi·e·sis \ˌkō-lə-ˌkrō-mō-ˌpȯi-ˈē-səs\ *n, pl* **-e·ses** \-ˌsēz\ : formation of bile pigments by the liver

cho·le·cyst \ˈkō-lə-ˌsist, ˈkäl-\ *n* : GALLBLADDER — **cho·le·cys·tic** \ˌkō-lə-ˈsis-tik, ˌkäl-ə-\ *adj*

cho·le·cys·ta·gogue \ˌkō-lə-ˈsist-ə-ˌgäg, ˌkäl-ə-\ *n* : an agent (as cholecystokinin) that causes the gallbladder to discharge bile

cho·le·cys·tec·to·mized \-(ˌ)sis-ˈtek-tə-ˌmīzd\ *adj* : having had the gallbladder removed

cho·le·cys·tec·to·my \ˌkō-lə-(ˌ)sis-ˈtek-tə-mē\ *n, pl* **-mies** : surgical excision of the gallbladder

cho·le·cys·ten·ter·os·to·my \-ˌtent-ə-ˈräs-tə-mē\ *or* **cho·le·cys·to·en·ter·os·to·my** \-ˌsis-tō-ˌent-\ *n, pl* **-mies** : surgical union of and creation of a passage between the gallbladder and the intestine

cho·le·cys·ti·tis \-(ˌ)sis-ˈtīt-əs\ *n, pl* **-tit·i·des** \-ˈtit-ə-ˌdēz\ : inflammation of the gallbladder

cho·le·cys·to·gram \-ˈsis-tə-ˌgram\ *n* : a radiograph of the gallbladder made after ingestion or injection of a radiopaque substance

cho·le·cys·tog·ra·phy \-(ˌ)sis-ˈtäg-rə-fē\ *n, pl* **-phies** : the radiographic visualization of the gallbladder after ingestion or injection of a radiopaque substance — **cho·le·cys·to·graph·ic** \-ˌsis-tə-ˈgraf-ik\ *adj*

¹cho·le·cys·to·ki·net·ic \-ˌsis-tə-kə-ˈnet-ik, -kī-\ *adj* : tending to cause the gallbladder to contract and discharge bile

²cholecystokinetic *n* : CHOLECYSTAGOGUE

cho·le·cys·to·ki·nin \-ˌsis-tə-ˈkī-nən\ *n* : a hormone secreted esp. by the duodenal mucosa that regulates the emptying of the gallbladder and secretion of enzymes by the pancreas and that has been found in the brain — called also *cholecystokinin-pancreozymin, pancreozymin*

cho·le·cys·tor·rha·phy \-(ˌ)sis-ˈtȯr-ə-fē\ *n, pl* **-phies** : repair of the gallbladder by suturing

cho·le·cys·tos·to·my \ˌkō-lə-(ˌ)sis-ˈtäs-tə-mē\ *n, pl* **-mies** : surgical incision of the gallbladder usu. to effect drainage

cho·le·cys·tot·o·my \-ˈtät-ə-mē\ *n, pl* **-mies** : surgical incision of the gallbladder esp. for exploration or to remove a gallstone

cho·le·doch·al \ˈkō-lə-ˌdäk-əl, kə-ˈled-ə-kəl\ *adj* : relating to, being, or occurring in the common bile duct ⟨a ∼ cyst⟩

cho·le·do·chi·tis \kə-ˌled-ə-ˈkīt-əs, ˌkō-lə-də-\ *n* : inflammation of the common bile duct

cho·led·o·cho·du·o·de·nos·to·my \kə-ˌled-ə-(ˌ)kō-ˌd(y)ü-ə-də-ˈnäs-tə-mē, -d(y)ü-ˌäd-ᵊn-ˈäs-\ *n, pl* **-mies** : surgical creation of a passage uniting the common bile duct and the duodenum

cho·led·o·cho·je·ju·nos·to·my \-ji-(ˌ)jü-ˈnäs-tə-mē\ *n, pl* **-mies** : surgical creation of a passage uniting the common bile duct and the jejunum

cho·led·o·cho·li·thi·a·sis \-lith-ˈī-ə-səs\ *n, pl* **-a·ses** \-ˌsēz\ : a condition marked by presence of calculi in the gallbladder and common bile duct

cho·led·o·cho·li·thot·o·my \-lith-ˈät-ə-mē\ *n, pl* **-mies** : surgical incision of the common bile duct for removal of a gallstone

cho·led·o·chor·ra·phy \kə-ˌled-ə-ˈkȯr-ə-fē, -ˈkȯr-\ *n, pl* **-ra·phies** : surgical union of the separated ends of the common bile duct by suturing

cho·led·o·chos·to·my \-ˈkäs-tə-mē\ *n, pl* **-mies** : surgical incision of the common bile duct usu. to effect drainage

cho·led·o·chot·o·my \-ˈkät-ə-mē\ *n, pl* **-mies** : surgical incision of the common bile duct

cho·led·o·chus \kə-ˈled-ə-kəs\ *n, pl* **-o·chi** \-ˌkī, -ˌkē\ : COMMON BILE DUCT

cho·le·glo·bin \ˈkō-lə-ˌglō-bən, ˈkäl-ə-\ *n* : a green pigment that occurs in bile, is a combination of globin and a ferric salt of biliverdin, and is formed by breakdown of hemoglobin

cho·le·ic acid \kə-ˌlē-ik-, kō-\ *n* : DEOXYCHOLIC ACID; *also* : a molecular compound of this acid (as with a fatty acid or a hydrocarbon)

cho·le·lith \ˈkō-li-ˌlith, ˈkäl-i-\ *n* : GALLSTONE

cho·le·li·thi·a·sis \ˌkō-li-lith-ˈī-ə-səs\ *n, pl* **-a·ses** \-ˌsēz\ : production of gallstones; *also* : the resulting abnormal condition

cho·le·mia *or chiefly Brit* **cho·lae·mia** \kō-ˈlē-mē-ə\ *n* : the presence of excess bile in the blood usu. indicative of liver disease — **cho·le·mic** *or chiefly Brit* **cho·lae·mic** \-mik\ *adj*

cho·le·poi·e·sis \ˌkō-lə-ˌpȯi-ˈē-səs, ˌkäl-ə-\ *n, pl* **-e·ses** \-ˈē-ˌsēz\ : production of bile — compare CHOLERESIS — **cho·le·poi·et·ic** \-ˌpȯi-ˈet-ik\ *adj*

chol·era \ˈkäl-ə-rə\ *n* : any of several diseases of humans and domestic animals usu. marked by severe gastrointestinal symptoms: as **a** : an acute diarrheal disease caused by an enterotoxin produced by various strains of a comma-shaped gram-negative bacterium of the genus *Vibrio* (*V. cholerae* syn. *V. comma*) when it is present in large numbers in the proximal part of the human small intestine — see ASIATIC CHOLERA **b** : FOWL CHOLERA **c** : HOG CHOLERA — **chol·e·ra·ic** \ˌkäl-ə-ˈrā-ik\ *adj*

chol·era in·fan·tum \ˌkäl-ə-rə-in-ˈfant-əm\ *n* : an acute noncontagious intestinal disturbance of infants formerly common in congested areas of high humidity and temperature but now rare

cholera mor·bus \-ˈmȯr-bəs\ *n* : a gastrointestinal disturbance characterized by abdominal pain, diarrhea, and sometimes vomiting — not used technically

---

\ə\ **abut** \ᵊ\ **kitten** \ər\ **further** \a\ **ash** \ā\ **ace** \ä\ **cot, cart** \au̇\ **out** \ch\ **chin** \e\ **bet** \ē\ **easy** \g\ **go** \i\ **hit** \ī\ **ice** \j\ **job** \ŋ\ **sing** \ō\ **go** \ȯ\ **law** \ȯi\ **boy** \th\ **thin** \t͟h\ **the** \ü\ **loot** \u̇\ **foot** \y\ **yet** \zh\ **vision** *See also* Pronunciation Symbols page

cholera vib·rio \-'vib-rē-ˌō\ *n* : the bacterium of the genus *Vibrio* (*V. cholerae* syn. *V. comma*) that causes cholera

cho·le·re·sis \ˌkō-lə-'rē-səs, ˌkäl-ə-\ *n, pl* **-re·ses** \-ˌsēz\ : the flow of bile from the liver esp. when increased above a previous or normal level — compare CHOLAGOGUE, CHOLEPOIESIS, HYDROCHOLERESIS

¹**cho·le·ret·ic** \ˌkō-lə-'ret-ik, ˌkäl-ə-\ *adj* : promoting bile secretion by the liver ⟨∼ action of bile salts⟩

²**choleretic** *n* : a choleretic agent

cho·ler·ic \'käl-ə-rik, kə-'ler-ik\ *adj* : easily moved to often unreasonable or excessive anger : hot-tempered

chol·er·i·form \'käl-(ə-)rə-ˌform\ *adj* : resembling cholera

chol·er·oid \'käl-ə-ˌroid\ *adj* : resembling cholera

cho·le·scin·ti·gram \ˌkō-lə-'sin-tə-ˌgram\ *n* : a picture produced by cholescintigraphy

cho·le·scin·tig·ra·phy \-sin-'tig-rə-fē\ *n, pl* **-phies** : scintigraphy of the biliary system

cho·les·tane \kə-'les-ˌtān\ *n* : a crystalline saturated steroid hydrocarbon $C_{27}H_{48}$ obtained from cholesterol by reduction

cho·les·ta·nol \-'les-tə-ˌnol, -ˌnōl\ *n* : a monohydroxy alcohol $C_{27}H_{47}OH$ derived from cholestane

cho·le·sta·sis \ˌkō-lə-'stā-səs, ˌkäl-ə-\ *n, pl* **-sta·ses** \-'stā-ˌsēz\ : a checking or failure of bile flow — **cho·le·stat·ic** \ˌkō-lə-'stat-ik, ˌkäl-ə-\ *adj*

cho·les·te·a·to·ma \kə-ˌles-tē-ə-'tō-mə, ˌkō-lə-ˌstē-, ˌkäl-ə-\ *n, pl* **-mas** *also* **-ma·ta** \-mət-ə\ **1** : an epidermoid cyst usu. in the brain arising from aberrant embryonic rests and appearing as a compact shiny flaky mass — called also *pearly tumor* **2** : a tumor usu. growing in a confined space (as the middle ear or mastoid) and frequently constituting a sequel to chronic otitis media — **cho·les·te·a·to·ma·tous** \-mət-əs\ *adj*

cho·les·ter·ic \kə-'les-tə-rik; ˌkō-lə-'ster-ik, ˌkäl-ə-\ *adj* : of, relating to, or resembling cholesterol or its derivatives

cho·les·ter·in \kə-'les-tə-rən\ *n* : CHOLESTEROL

cho·les·ter·ol \kə-'les-tə-ˌrōl, -ˌrol\ *n* : a steroid alcohol $C_{27}H_{45}OH$ present in animal cells and body fluids that regulates membrane fluidity, functions as a precursor molecule in various metabolic pathways, and as a constituent of LDL may cause arteriosclerosis

cho·les·ter·ol·emia \kə-ˌles-tə-rə-'lē-mē-ə\ *also* **cho·les·ter·emia** \-tə-'rē-mē-ə\ *or chiefly Brit* **cho·les·ter·ol·ae·mia** *also* **cho·les·ter·ae·mia** *n* : the presence of cholesterol in the blood

cho·les·ter·ol·osis \kə-ˌles-tə-rə-'lō-səs\ *n, pl* **-oses** \-ˌsēz\ : CHOLESTEROSIS

cho·les·ter·o·sis \kə-ˌles-tə-'rō-səs\ *n, pl* **-o·ses** \-ˌsēz\ : abnormal deposition of cholesterol (as in blood vessels or the gallbladder)

cho·le·styr·amine \kō-'les-tir-ə-ˌmēn\ *n* : a strongly basic ion exchange resin that forms insoluble complexes with bile acids and has been used to lower cholesterol levels in hypercholesterolemic patients

cho·lic acid \ˌkō-lik-\ *n* : a crystalline bile acid $C_{24}H_{40}O_5$

cho·line \'kō-ˌlēn\ *n* : a basic compound $C_5H_{15}NO_2$ that is found in various foods (as egg yolk and legumes) or is synthesized in the liver and that is a component of lecithin, is a precursor of acetylcholine, and is essential to liver function

choline acetyltransferase *n* : an enzyme that catalyzes the synthesis of acetylcholine from acetyl coenzyme A and choline

cho·lin·er·gic \ˌkō-lə-'nər-jik\ *adj* **1** *of autonomic nerve fibers* : liberating, activated by, or involving acetylcholine — compare ADRENERGIC 1, NORADRENERGIC **2** : resembling acetylcholine esp. in physiological action ⟨a ∼ drug⟩ — **cho·lin·er·gi·cal·ly** \-ji-k(ə-)lē\ *adv*

cho·lin·es·ter·ase \ˌkō-lə-'nes-tə-ˌrās, -ˌrāz\ *n* **1** : ACETYLCHOLINESTERASE **2** : an enzyme that hydrolyzes choline esters and that is found esp. in blood plasma — called also *pseudocholinesterase*

¹**cho·li·no·lyt·ic** \ˌkō-lə-nō-'lit-ik\ *adj* : interfering with the action of acetylcholine or cholinergic agents

²**cholinolytic** *n* : a cholinolytic substance

¹**cho·li·no·mi·met·ic** \ˌkō-lə-nō-mə-'met-ik, ˌkäl-ə-, -mī-\ *adj* : resembling acetylcholine or simulating its physiologic action

²**cholinomimetic** *n* : a cholinomimetic substance

cho·li·no·re·cep·tor \-ri-'sep-tər\ *n* : a receptor for acetylcholine in a postsynaptic membrane

cho·lor·rhea *or chiefly Brit* **cho·lor·rhoea** \ˌkäl-ə-'rē-ə, ˌkō-lə-\ *n* : excessive secretion of bile

chol·uria \kō-'l(y)ùr-ē-ə, kə-\ *n* : presence of bile in urine

chon·dral \'kän-drəl\ *adj* : of or relating to cartilage

chondri *pl of* CHONDRUS

Chon·drich·thy·es \kän-'drik-thē-ˌēz\ *n pl* : a class comprising cartilaginous fishes with well-developed jaws and including the sharks, skates, rays, chimeras, and extinct related forms — compare CYCLOSTOMATA

chon·dri·fi·ca·tion \ˌkän-drə-fə-'kā-shən\ *n* : formation of or conversion into cartilage

chon·dri·fy \'kän-drə-ˌfī\ *vb* **-fied; -fy·ing** *vt* : to convert into cartilage ∼ *vi* : to become converted into cartilage

chon·drin \'kän-drən\ *n* : a horny substance obtainable from cartilage and similar to and often associated with gelatin — compare CHONDROMUCOID

chon·drio·some \'kän-drē-ə-ˌsōm\ *n* : MITOCHONDRION — **chon·drio·som·al** \ˌkän-drē-ə-'sōm-əl\ *adj*

chon·dri·tis \kän-'drīt-əs\ *n* : inflammation of cartilage

chon·dro·blast \'kän-drə-ˌblast, -drō-\ *n* : a cell that produces cartilage — **chon·dro·blas·tic** \ˌkän-drə-'blas-tik, -drō-\ *adj*

chon·dro·clast \'kän-drə-ˌklast, -drō-\ *n* : a cell that absorbs cartilage — compare OSTEOCLAST 1

chon·dro·cos·tal \ˌkän-drə-'käs-t³l, -drō-\ *adj* : of or relating to the costal cartilages and the ribs

chon·dro·cra·ni·um \ˌkän-drə-'krā-nē-əm, -drō-\ *n, pl* **-nia** : the embryonic cartilaginous cranium; *also* : the part of the adult skull derived therefrom — compare OSTEOCRANIUM

chon·dro·cyte \'kän-drə-ˌsīt, -drō-\ *n* : a cartilage cell

chon·dro·dys·pla·sia \ˌkän-drə-dis-'plāzh(-ē)-ə, -drō-\ *n* : a hereditary skeletal disorder characterized by the formation of exostoses at the epiphyses and resulting in arrested development and deformity — called also *dyschondroplasia*

chon·dro·dys·tro·phia \-dis-'trō-fē-ə\ *n* : ACHONDROPLASIA

chon·dro·dys·tro·phy \-'dis-trə-fē\ *n, pl* **-phies** : ACHONDROPLASIA — **chon·dro·dys·tro·phic** \-dis-'trō-fik\ *adj*

chon·dro·gen·e·sis \-'jen-ə-səs\ *n, pl* **-e·ses** \-ˌsēz\ : the development of cartilage — **chon·dro·ge·net·ic** \-jə-'net-ik\ *adj*

chon·dro·gen·ic \-'jen-ik\ *adj* : relating to or characterized by chondrogenesis : CHONDROGENETIC ⟨∼ activity⟩

chon·dro·glos·sus \ˌkän-drə-'gläs-əs, -drō-\ *n, pl* **-glos·si** \-'gläs-ˌī, -ē\ : a muscle arising from the lesser cornu of the hyoid bone and blending with the intrinsic muscles of the tongue

chon·droid \'kän-ˌdroid\ *adj* : resembling cartilage ⟨innervation of ∼ tissue⟩

chon·droi·tin \kän-'droit-³n, -'drō-ət-ən\ *n* : any of several glycosaminoglycans occurring in sulfated form in variou̓s tissues (as cartilage and tendons)

chondroitin sulfate *n* : any of several sulfated forms of chondroitin found in various tissues (as cartilage, adult bone, and tendons)

chon·droi·tin·sul·fu·ric acid \kän-ˌdroit-³n-ˌsəl-ˌfyùr-ik-, -ˌdrō-ət-ən-\ *n* : CHONDROITIN SULFATE

chon·drol·o·gy \kän-'dräl-ə-jē\ *n, pl* **-gies** : a branch of anatomy concerned with cartilage

chon·dro·ma \kän-'drō-mə\ *n, pl* **-mas** *also* **-ma·ta** \-mət-ə\ : a benign tumor containing the structural elements of cartilage — compare CHONDROSARCOMA — **chon·dro·ma·tous** \(')kän-'dräm-ət-əs, -'drōm-\ *adj*

chon·dro·ma·la·cia \ˌkän-drō-mə-'lā-sh(ē-)ə\ *n* : abnormal softness of cartilage

chondromalacia patellae *n* : pain over the front of the knee with softening of the articular cartilage of the patella — compare RUNNER'S KNEE

chon·dro·mu·coid \-'myü-ˌkȯid\ *n* : a white amorphous substance obtainable from the matrix of cartilage and consisting of a protein that resembles gelatin and is combined with chondroitin sulfate — compare CHONDRIN

chon·dro–os·teo·dys·tro·phy \-ˌäs-tē-ō-'dis-trə-fē\ *n, pl* **-phies** : any of several mucopolysaccharidoses (as Hurler's syndrome) characterized esp. by disorders of bone and cartilage

chon·dro·pha·ryn·ge·us \-fə-'rin-jē-əs, -ˌfar-ən-'jē-əs\ *n, pl* **-gei** \-jē-ˌī, -'jē-ˌī\ : the muscle arising from the lesser cornu of the hyoid bone and forming part of the middle constrictor of the pharynx

chon·dro·phyte \'kän-drō-ˌfīt\ *n* : an outgrowth or spur of cartilage

chon·dro·pro·tein \ˌkän-drō-'prō-ˌtēn, -'prōt-ē-ən\ *n* : any of various glycoproteins (as chondromucoid) that yield on hydrolysis chondroitin sulfate and a protein

chon·dro·sa·mine \kän-'drō-sə-ˌmēn, -mən\ *n* : an amino sugar $C_6H_{13}NO_5$ obtained from chondroitin sulfate and related compounds

chon·dro·sar·co·ma \ˌkän-drō-sär-'kō-mə\ *n, pl* **-mas** *also* **-ma·ta** \-mət-ə\ : a sarcoma containing cartilage cells rarely arising as a primary tumor but more frequently developing as a secondary growth by malignant degeneration of a chondroma

chon·dro·ster·nal \ˌkän-drō-'stərn-ᵊl\ *adj* : of or relating to the costal cartilages and sternum

chon·drot·o·my \kän-'drät-ə-mē\ *n, pl* **-mies** : the cutting or dissection of cartilage

chon·dro·xi·phoid \ˌkän-drō-'zī-ˌfȯid, -'zif-ˌȯid\ *adj* : connecting a costal cartilage and the xiphoid process

chon·drus \'kän-drəs\ *n* **1** *cap* : a small genus of red algae (family Gigartinaceae) having rather coarse branching fronds **2** *pl* **chon·dri** \-ˌdrī\ : IRISH MOSS 1

Cho·part's joint \(')shō-'pärz-\ *n* : the tarsal joint that comprises the talonavicular and calcaneocuboid articulations

    Cho·part \shō-pár\, **François (1743–1795),** French surgeon. Chopart was a notable instructor of medicine and eventually became a professor of surgery. In 1792 he devised a method for amputating the forepart of the foot at the joint between the two rows of bones in the tarsus in cases involving diabetic gangrene. The joint was named in his honor by one of his students.

chord \'kȯrd\ *n* : CORD 2

chor·da \'kȯr-də\ *n, pl* **chor·dae** \-ˌdē\ : CORD 2; *specif* : NOTOCHORD

chord·al \'kȯrd-ᵊl\ *adj* : of or relating to an anatomical cord (as the notochord or spinal cord) — used chiefly in combination ⟨peri*chordal*⟩ — **chord·al·ly** \-ē\ *adv*

chor·da·meso·derm \ˌkȯrd-ə-'mez-ə-ˌdərm *also* -'mes-\ *n* : the portion of the embryonic mesoderm that forms notochord and related structures and induces the formation of neural structures — **chor·da·meso·der·mal** \-ˌmez-ə-'dər-məl, -ˌmes-\ *adj*

Chor·da·ta \kȯr-'dät-ə, -'dāt-ə\ *n pl* : a phylum comprising animals having at least at some stage of development a more or less well-developed notochord, a dorsally situated central nervous system, and gill clefts in the walls of the pharynx and including the vertebrates, lancelets, and tunicates — **chor·date** \'kȯ(ə)r-ˌdāt, 'kȯrd-ət\ *n or adj*

chorda ten·din·ea \-ˌten-'din-ē-ə\ *n, pl* **chordae ten·din·e·ae** \-ē-ˌē\ : any of the delicate tendinous cords that are attached to the edges of the atrioventricular valves of the heart and to the papillary muscles and serve to prevent the valves from being pushed into the atrium during the ventricular contraction

chorda tym·pa·ni \-'tim-pə-ˌnī\ *n* : a branch of the facial nerve that traverses the middle ear cavity and the infratemporal fossa and supplies autonomic fibers to the sublingual and submandibular glands and sensory fibers to the anterior part of the tongue

chor·dee \'kȯr-ˌdē, -ˌdā, ˌkȯr-'\ *n* : painful erection of the penis often with a downward curvature that may be present in a congenital condition (as hypospadias) or accompany gonorrhea

chor·di·tis \kȯr-'dīt-əs\ *n* : inflammation of a cord or cords (as the vocal or spermatic cords)

chor·do·ma \kȯr-'dō-mə\ *n, pl* **-mas** *also* **-ma·ta** \-mət-ə\ : a malignant tumor that is derived from remnants of the embryonic notochord and occurs along the spine attacking esp. the bones at the base of the skull or near the coccyx

chordotomy *var of* CORDOTOMY

cho·rea \kə-'rē-ə\ *n* : any of various nervous disorders of infectious or organic origin marked by spasmodic movements of the limbs and facial muscles and by incoordination — called also *Saint Vitus' dance;* see HUNTINGTON'S DISEASE, SYDENHAM'S CHOREA — **cho·re·at·ic** \ˌkōr-ē-'at-ik, ˌkȯr-\ *adj* — **cho·re·ic** \kə-'rē-ik\ *adj*

cho·re·i·form \kə-'rē-ə-ˌfȯrm\ *adj* : resembling chorea ⟨∼ convulsions⟩

cho·reo·ath·e·toid \ˌkōr-ē-(ˌ)ō-'ath-ə-ˌtȯid, ˌkȯr-\ *or* **cho·reo·ath·e·tot·ic** \-ˌath-ə-'tät-ik\ *adj* : resembling or characteristic of choreoathetosis ⟨∼ movements⟩

cho·reo·ath·e·to·sis \-ˌath-ə-'tō-səs\ *n, pl* **-to·ses** \-ˌsēz\ : a nervous disturbance marked by the involuntary purposeless and uncontrollable movements characteristic of chorea and athetosis

cho·re·oid \'kōr-ē-ˌȯid, 'kȯr-\ *adj* : CHOREIFORM

cho·ri·al·lan·to·is \ˌkōr-ē-ō-ə-'lant-ə-wəs, ˌkȯr-\ *n, pl* **-to·ides** \-ō-ˌal-ən-'tō-ə-ˌdēz, -ō-ˌal-ˌan-\ : a vascular fetal membrane composed of the fused chorion and adjacent wall of the allantois that in the hen's egg is used as a living culture medium for viruses and for tissues — called also *chorioallantoic membrane* — **cho·rio·al·lan·to·ic** \-ˌal-ən-'tō-ik\ *adj*

cho·rio·am·ni·o·ni·tis \-ˌam-nē-ō-'nīt-əs\ *n* : inflammation of the fetal membranes

cho·rio·an·gi·o·ma \-ˌan-jē-'ō-mə\ *n, pl* **-mas** *also* **-ma·ta** \-mət-ə\ : a benign vascular tumor of the chorion

cho·rio·cap·il·lar·is \-ˌkap-ə-'lar-əs\ *n* : the inner of the two vascular layers of the choroid of the eye that is composed largely of capillaries

cho·rio·car·ci·no·ma \-ˌkärs-ᵊn-'ō-mə\ *n, pl* **-mas** *also* **-ma·ta** \-mət-ə\ : a malignant tumor derived from trophoblastic tissue consisting of syncytiotrophoblasts and cytotrophoblasts that develops typically in the uterus following pregnancy, miscarriage, or abortion esp. when associated with a hydatidiform mole or rarely in the testes or ovaries chiefly as a component of a mixed germ-cell tumor

cho·rio·ep·i·the·li·o·ma \-ˌep-ə-ˌthē-lē-'ō-mə\ *n, pl* **-mas** *also* **-ma·ta** \-mət-ə\ : CHORIOCARCINOMA — **cho·rio·ep·i·the·li·o·ma·tous** \-mət-əs\ *adj*

chorioid, chorioiditis *var of* CHOROID, CHOROIDITIS

cho·ri·o·ma \ˌkōr-ē-'ō-mə, ˌkȯr-\ *n, pl* **-mas** *or* **-ma·ta** \-mət-ə\ : a tumor (as a choriocarcinoma) formed of chorionic tissue

cho·rio·men·in·gi·tis \ˌkōr-ē-(ˌ)ō-ˌmen-ən-'jīt-əs, ˌkȯr-\ *n, pl* **-git·i·des** \-'jit-ə-ˌdēz\ : cerebral meningitis; *specif* : LYMPHOCYTIC CHORIOMENINGITIS

cho·ri·on \'kōr-ē-ˌän, 'kȯr-\ *n* : the highly vascular outer embryonic membrane that is associated with the allantois in the formation of the placenta

cho·ri·on·ep·i·the·li·o·ma \ˌkōr-ē-ˌän-ˌep-ə-ˌthē-lē-'ō-mə, ˌkȯr-\ *n, pl* **-mas** *also* **-ma·ta** \-mət-ə\ : CHORIOCARCINOMA

chorion fron·do·sum \-frən-'dō-səm\ *n* : the part of the chorion that has persistent villi and that with the decidua basalis forms the placenta — see CHORIONIC VILLUS SAMPLING

cho·ri·on·ic \ˌkōr-ē-'än-ik, ˌkȯr-\ *adj* **1** : of, relating to, or being part of the chorion ⟨∼ villi⟩ **2** : secreted or produced by chorionic or a related tissue (as in the placenta or a choriocarcinoma) ⟨human ∼ gonadotropin⟩

---

chorionic somatomammotropin *n* : PLACENTAL LACTOGEN

chorionic villus sampling *also* **chorionic villi sampling** *n* : biopsy of the chorion frondosum through the abdominal wall or by way of the vagina and uterine cervix at 10 to 12 weeks of gestation to obtain fetal cells for the prenatal diagnosis of chromosomal abnormalities — abbr. *CVS*

Cho·ri·op·tes \ˌkȯr-ē-ˈäp-ˌtēz, ˌkȯr-\ *n* : a genus of small parasitic mites infesting domestic animals and causing chorioptic mange — **cho·ri·op·tic** \-ˈäp-tik\ *adj*

chorioptic mange *n* : mange caused by mites of the genus *Chorioptes* that usu. attack only the surface of the skin esp. about the feet and lower legs or in cattle at the base of the tail — compare DEMODECTIC MANGE, SARCOPTIC MANGE

cho·rio·ret·i·nal \ˌkȯr-ē-ō-ˈret-ᵊn-əl, -ˈret-nəl\ *adj* : of, relating to, or affecting the choroid and the retina of the eye ⟨∼ burns⟩ ⟨∼ lesions⟩

cho·rio·ret·i·ni·tis \-ˌret-ᵊn-ˈīt-əs\ *also* **cho·roi·do·ret·i·ni·tis** \kə-ˌrȯid-ō-\ *n, pl* **-nit·i·des** \-ˈit-ə-ˌdēz\ : inflammation of the retina and choroid of the eye

cho·roid \ˈkō(ə)r-ˌȯid, ˈkȯ(ə)r-\ *also* **cho·ri·oid** \ˈkȯr-ē-ˌȯid, ˈkȯr-\ *n* : a vascular membrane containing large branched pigment cells that lies between the retina and the sclera of the eye — called also *choroid coat* — **choroid** *or* **cho·roi·dal** \kə-ˈrȯid-ᵊl\ *adj*

choroid artery *or* **choroidal artery** *n* : an artery that arises from the internal carotid artery and supplies the choroid plexus of the lateral ventricle of the brain and adjacent structures — called also *anterior choroid artery*

choroid coat *n* : CHOROID

choroidea — see TELA CHOROIDEA

cho·roi·de·re·mia *or chiefly Brit* **cho·roi·de·rae·mia** \ˌkȯr-ˌȯid-ə-ˈrē-mē-ə, ˈkȯr-\ *n* : progressive degeneration of the choroid that is an X-linked trait chiefly affecting males and that is characterized by night blindness, constriction of the visual field, and eventual blindness

cho·roid·itis \ˌkȯr-ˌȯi-ˈdīt-əs, ˌkȯr-\ *or* **cho·ri·oid·itis** \ˌkȯr-ē-ȯi-, ˌkȯr-\ *n* : inflammation of the choroid of the eye

cho·roi·do·iri·tis \kə-ˌrȯid-ō-ī-ˈrīt-əs\ *n* : inflammation of the choroid and the iris of the eye

cho·roid·op·a·thy \ˌkȯr-ˌȯi-ˈdäp-ə-thē, ˌkȯr-\ *n, pl* **-thies** : a diseased condition affecting the choroid of the eye

choroidoretinitis *var of* CHORIORETINITIS

choroid plexus *n* : a highly vascular portion of the pia mater that projects into the ventricles of the brain and is thought to secrete the cerebrospinal fluid

chr *abbr* chronic

Christ·mas disease \ˈkris-məs-\ *n* : a hereditary sex-linked hemorrhagic disease involving absence of a coagulation factor in the blood and failure of the clotting mechanism — called also *hemophilia B;* compare HEMOPHILIA

Christmas, Stephen, British child patient. Christmas was the youngest of seven patients in a study at an Oxford, England, hospital undertaken by Rosemary Biggs and her associates of a newly discovered condition resembling hemophilia. Christmas was the first patient examined in detail, and the disease was named after him. In 1952, Biggs and her associates published their first article on Christmas disease.

Christmas factor *n* : FACTOR IX

Christmas rose *n* : BLACK HELLEBORE 1

chromaesthesia *chiefly Brit var of* CHROMESTHESIA

chro·maf·fin \ˈkrō-mə-fən\ *adj* : staining deeply with chromium salts ⟨∼ cells of the adrenal medulla⟩

chro·maf·fi·no·ma \ˌkrō-mə-fə-ˈnō-mə, krō-ˌmaf-ə-\ *n, pl* **-mas** *also* **-ma·ta** \-mət-ə\ : a tumor containing chromaffin cells; *esp* : PHEOCHROMOCYTOMA

chro·man \ˈkrō-ˌman\ *n* : a bicyclic heterocyclic compound $C_9H_{10}O$ that is the parent nucleus of the tocopherols

chro·ma·phil \ˈkrō-mə-ˌfil\ *adj* : CHROMAFFIN ⟨∼ tissue⟩

chro·mate \ˈkrō-ˌmāt\ *n* : a salt of chromic acid

chro·mat·ic \krō-ˈmat-ik\ *adj* **1** : of, relating to, or characterized by color or color phenomena or sensations ⟨∼ perception⟩ ⟨∼ stimuli⟩ **2** : capable of being colored by staining agents ⟨∼ substances⟩

chromatic aberration *n* : aberration caused by differences in the refraction of light at different frequencies

chromatic figure *n* : the mitotic or meiotic chromosomes — compare ACHROMATIC FIGURE

chro·ma·tic·i·ty \ˌkrō-mə-ˈtis-ət-ē\ *n, pl* **-ties** : the quality of color characterized by its dominant or complementary wavelength and purity taken together

chromatic vision *n* **1** : normal color vision in which the colors of the spectrum are distinguished and evaluated **2** : CHROMATOPSIA

chro·ma·tid \ˈkrō-mə-təd\ *n* : one of the usu. paired and parallel strands of a duplicated chromosome joined by a single centromere — see CHROMONEMA

chro·ma·tin \ˈkrō-mət-ən\ *n* : a complex of a nucleic acid with basic proteins (as histone) in eukaryotic cells that is usu. dispersed in the interphase nucleus and condensed into chromosomes in mitosis and meiosis — **chro·ma·tin·ic** \ˌkrō-mə-ˈtin-ik\ *adj*

chro·ma·tism \ˈkrō-mə-ˌtiz-əm\ *n* **1** : CHROMATIC ABERRATION **2** : CHROMESTHESIA

chro·mato·gram \krō-ˈmat-ə-ˌgram, krə-\ *n* **1** : the pattern formed on the adsorbent medium by the layers of components separated by chromatography **2** : a time-based graphic record (as of concentration of eluted materials) of a chromatographic separation

chro·mato·graph \krō-ˈmat-ə-ˌgraf, krə-\ *n* : an instrument for performing chromatographic separations and producing chromatograms — **chromatograph** *vb* — **chro·ma·tog·ra·pher** \ˌkrō-mə-ˈtäg-rə-fər\ *n*

chro·ma·tog·ra·phy \ˌkrō-mə-ˈtäg-rə-fē\ *n, pl* **-phies** : a process in which a chemical mixture carried by a liquid or gas is separated into components as a result of differential distribution of the solutes as they flow around or over a stationary liquid or solid phase — see AFFINITY CHROMATOGRAPHY, COCHROMATOGRAPHY, COLUMN CHROMATOGRAPHY, ELECTROCHROMATOGRAPHY, GAS CHROMATOGRAPHY, GAS-LIQUID CHROMATOGRAPHY, GEL FILTRATION, HIGH= PERFORMANCE LIQUID CHROMATOGRAPHY, ION= EXCHANGE CHROMATOGRAPHY, LIQUID CHROMATOGRAPHY, PAPER CHROMATOGRAPHY, PARTITION CHROMATOGRAPHY, RADIOCHROMATOGRAPHY, THIN-LAYER CHROMATOGRAPHY — **chro·mato·graph·ic** \ˌkrō-ˌmat-ə-ˈgraf-ik, krə-\ *adj* — **chro·mato·graph·i·cal·ly** \-i-k(ə-)lē\ *adv*

chro·ma·toid \ˈkrō-mə-ˌtȯid\ *adj* : resembling chromatin esp. in affinity for stains ⟨∼ granules⟩

chro·ma·tol·y·sis \ˌkrō-mə-ˈtäl-ə-səs\ *n, pl* **-y·ses** \-ˌsēz\ : the dissolution and breaking up of chromophil material (as chromatin) of a cell and esp. a neuron — **chro·mato·lyt·ic** \ˌkrō-ˌmat-ᵊl-ˈit-ik, krə-\ *adj*

chro·ma·tom·e·ter \ˌkrō-mə-ˈtäm-ət-ər\ *n* **1** : a color diagram or chart so arranged as to serve as a scale of colors **2** : an instrument for measuring color perception

chromatophil, chromatophile *var of* CHROMOPHIL

chro·mato·phil·ia \ˌkrō-ˌmat-ə-ˈfil-ē-ə, ˌkrō-mət-ə-\ *also* **chro·moph·i·ly** \krō-ˈmäf-ə-lē\ *n, pl* **-ias** *also* **-lies** : the quality or state of being chromophil

chro·ma·to·pho·ral \ˌkrō-mə-ˈtäf-(ə-)rəl, krə-ˌmat-ə-ˈfōr-əl, -ˈfȯr-\ *adj* : of or belonging to a chromatophore

chro·mato·phore \krō-ˈmat-ə-ˌfō(ə)r, krə-, -ˌfȯ(ə)r\ *n* **1** : a pigment-bearing cell esp. in the skin **2** : the organelle of photosynthesis in photosynthetic bacteria (as the cyanobacteria) : CHROMOPLAST, CHLOROPLAST — **chro·mato·phor·ic** \-ˌmat-ə-ˈfōr-ik, -ˈfȯr-\ *adj*

chro·ma·top·sia \ˌkrō-mə-ˈtäp-sē-ə\ *n* : a disturbance of vision which is sometimes caused by drugs and in which colorless objects appear colored

chro·ma·to·sis \ˌkrō-mə-ˈtō-səs\ *n, pl* **-to·ses** \-ˌsēz\ : PIGMENTATION; *specif* : deposit of pigment in a normally unpigmented area or excessive pigmentation in a normally pigmented site

chrome \ˈkrōm\ *n* **1** : CHROMIUM **2** : a chromium pigment

chrom·es·the·sia *or chiefly Brit* **chrom·aes·the·sia** \ˌkrō-mes-ˈthē-zh(ē-)ə\ *n* : synesthesia in which color is perceived in response to stimuli (as words or numbers) that contain no element of color — called also *chromatism, color hearing*

chrome yellow *n* : a yellow pigment consisting essentially of neutral lead chromate PbCrO₄

chromhidrosis *var of* CHROMIDROSIS

chro·mic \\'krō-mik\\ *adj* : of, relating to, or derived from chromium esp. with a valence of three

chromic acid *n* : an acid H_2CrO_4 analogous to sulfuric acid but known only in solution and esp. in the form of its salts (as lead chromate) most of which are yellow and are toxic causing ulcers on the skin or mucous membranes

chro·mi·cize \\'krō-mə-ˌsīz\\ *vt* **-cized; -ciz·ing** : to treat (catgut) with a compound of chromium

chromidial substance *n* : NISSL SUBSTANCE

chro·mid·i·um \\krə-'mid-ē-əm, krō-\\ *n, pl* **-ia** \\-ē-ə\\ : a chromatin or chromatinlike granule in the cytoplasm of a cell; *esp* : one of nuclear origin — **chro·mid·i·al** \\krə-'mid-ē-əl, krō-\\ *adj*

chro·mi·dro·sis \\ˌkrō-mə-'drō-səs\\ *also* **chrom·hi·dro·sis** \\ˌkrōm-(h)ə-\\ *n, pl* **-dro·ses** \\-ˌsēz\\ : secretion of colored sweat

chro·mi·um \\'krō-mē-əm\\ *n* : a blue-white metallic element found naturally only in combination and used esp. in alloys and in electroplating — symbol *Cr*; see ELEMENT table

chromium picolinate *n* : a biologically active chromium salt $C_{18}H_{12}CrN_3O_6$ containing three picolinic acid ligands that is used as a dietary supplement

chro·mo·bac·te·ri·um \\ˌkrō-mō-bak-'tir-ē-əm\\ *n* **1** *cap* : a genus of aerobic gram-negative saprophytic soil and water bacteria (family Rhizobiaceae) producing a violet pigment **2** *pl* **-ria** \\-ē-ə\\ : a bacterium of the genus *Chromobacterium*

chro·mo·blast \\'krō-mə-ˌblast\\ *n* : an anatomical cell that develops into a pigment cell

chro·mo·blas·to·my·co·sis \\ˌkrō-mə-ˌblas-tə-ˌmī-'kō-səs\\ *n, pl* **-co·ses** \\-ˌsēz\\ : a skin disease that is caused by any of several pigmented fungi esp. of the genera *Phialophora, Cladosporium,* and *Fonsecaea* and is marked by the formation of warty colored nodules usu. on the legs — called also *chromomycosis*

chro·mo·cen·ter \\'krō-mə-ˌsent-ər\\ *n* : a densely staining nuclear body associated with the chromatin of some cells — **chro·mo·cen·tric** \\ˌkrō-mə-'sen-trik\\ *adj*

chro·mo·cyte \\'krō-mə-ˌsīt\\ *n* : a pigmented anatomical cell — called also *color cell*

chro·mo·gen \\'krō-mə-jən\\ *n* **1 a** : a precursor of a biochemical pigment **b** : a compound not itself a dye but containing a chromophore and so capable of becoming one **2** : a pigment-producing microorganism ⟨many bacteria are ∼s⟩ — **chro·mo·gen·ic** \\ˌkrō-mə-'jen-ik\\ *adj*

chro·mo·gen·e·sis \\ˌkrō-mə-'jen-ə-səs\\ *n, pl* **-e·ses** \\-ˌsēz\\ : color production (as by the metabolic activities of bacteria and fungi)

chro·mo·isom·er·ism \\ˌkrō-(ˌ)mō-ī-'säm-ə-ˌriz-əm\\ *n* : isomerism in which the isomers are of different colors — used esp. of cases in which the isomers are tautomeric

chro·mo·li·poid \\ˌkrō-mə-'lī-ˌpȯid, -'lip-ˌȯid\\ *n* : LIPOCHROME

¹chro·mo·mere \\'krō-mə-ˌmi(ə)r\\ *n* : the highly refractile portion of a blood platelet — compare HYALOMERE

²chromomere *n* : one of the small bead-shaped and heavily staining concentrations of chromatin that are linearly arranged along the chromosome — **chro·mo·mer·ic** \\ˌkrō-mə-'mer-ik, -'mi(ə)r-\\ *adj*

chro·mom·e·ter \\krō-'mäm-ət-ər, krō-\\ *n* : an apparatus for comparing the color of a substance with a standard esp. to determine the degree of purity or percentage of a constituent : COLORIMETER

chro·mo·my·co·sis \\ˌkrō-mə-ˌmī-'kō-səs\\ *n, pl* **-co·ses** \\-ˌsēz\\ : CHROMOBLASTOMYCOSIS

chro·mone \\'krō-ˌmōn\\ *n* : a colorless crystalline cyclic ketone $C_9H_6O_2$; *also* : a derivative (as flavone) of this ketone

chro·mo·ne·ma \\ˌkrō-mə-'nē-mə\\ *n, pl* **-ne·ma·ta** \\-'nē-mət-ə\\ : the coiled filamentous core of a chromatid — **chro·mo-**

ne·mat·ic \\-ni-'mat-ik\\ *or* **chro·mo·ne·mal** \\-'nē-məl\\ *or* **chro·mo·ne·ma·tal** \\-'nē-mət-²l, -'nem-ət-\\ *adj*

¹chro·mo·phil \\'krō-mə-ˌfil\\ *also* **chro·mo·phil·ic** \\ˌkrō-mə-'fil-ik\\ *or* **chro·mo·phile** \\'krō-mə-ˌfī(ə)l\\ *or* **chro·mato·phil** \\krō-'mat-ə-ˌfil\\ *or* **chro·mato·phile** \\-ˌfī(ə)l\\ *adj* **1** : staining readily with dyes **2** : CHROMAFFIN

²chromophil *or* **chromophile** *or* **chro·mato·phil** *or* **chro·mato·phile** *n* : a chromophil cell or substance

chromophily *var of* CHROMATOPHILIA

¹chro·mo·phobe \\'krō-mə-ˌfōb\\ *also* **chro·mo·pho·bic** \\ˌkrō-mə-'fō-bik\\ *adj* : not readily absorbing stains : difficult to stain ⟨∼ tumors⟩ — **chro·mo·pho·by** \\'krō-mə-ˌfō-bē, krō-'mäf-ə-bē\\ *n, pl* **-bies**

²chromophobe *n* : a chromophobe cell esp. of the pituitary gland

chro·mo·phore \\'krō-mə-ˌfō(ə)r, -ˌfȯ(ə)r\\ *n* : a chemical group (as an azo group) that absorbs light at a specific frequency and so imparts color to a molecule; *also* : a colored chemical compound — **chro·mo·phor·ic** \\ˌkrō-mə-'fōr-ik, -'fär-\\ *adj*

chro·moph·o·rous \\(')krō-'mäf-(ə-)rəs\\ *adj* : containing pigment as an integral part of the protoplasm

chro·mo·phy·to·sis \\ˌkrō-mə-ˌfī-'tō-səs\\ *n, pl* **-to·ses** \\-ˌsēz\\ : TINEA VERSICOLOR

chro·mo·plast \\'krō-mə-ˌplast\\ *n* : a colored plastid usu. containing red or yellow pigment (as carotene)

chro·mo·pro·tein \\ˌkrō-mə-'prō-ˌtēn, -'prōt-ē-ən\\ *n* : any of various proteins (as hemoglobins, carotenoids, or flavoproteins) having a pigment as a prosthetic group

chro·mos·co·py \\krō-'mäs-kə-pē\\ *n, pl* **-pies** : diagnosis of gastric or renal function by the administration of dyes and subsequent examination of the stomach contents or the urine

chro·mo·some \\'krō-mə-ˌsōm, -ˌzōm\\ *n* : any of the usu. linear bodies of the cell nucleus of eukaryotic organisms, the usu. circular bodies of prokaryotic organisms (as bacteria), or esp. in some schools of molecular biology the genomes of DNA viruses (as bacteriophages) that take up basophilic stains and contain most or all of the genes of the organism ⟨both the ∼s of cells and those of viruses can duplicate only in the complex environment of a living cell —J. D. Watson⟩ ⟨an episome, an element that may exist as a free circular plasmid, or that may become integrated into the bacterial ∼ as a linear sequence —Benjamin Lewin⟩ — **chro·mo·som·al** \\ˌkrō-mə-'sō-məl, -'zō-\\ *adj* — **chro·mo·som·al·ly** \\-mə-lē\\ *adv*

chromosome complement *n* : the entire group of chromosomes in a nucleus

chromosome number *n* : the usu. constant number of chromosomes characteristic of a particular kind of animal or plant

chro·mo·ther·a·py \\ˌkrō-mō-'ther-ə-pē\\ *n, pl* **-pies** : treatment of disease by colored lights

chro·mo·trich·i·al \\-'trik-ē-əl\\ *adj* : concerned with or modifying hair color

chron·ax·ie *or* **chron·axy** \\'krōn-ˌak-sē, 'krän-\\ *also* **chron·ax·ia** \\krō-'nak-sē-ə, krə-, krän-'ak-\\ *n, pl* **-ax·ies** *also* **-ax·ias** : the minimum time required for excitation of a structure (as a nerve cell) by a constant electric current of twice the threshold voltage — compare RHEOBASE

chro·nax·im·e·ter \\ˌkrō-ˌnak-'sim-ət-ər, ˌkrän-ˌak-\\ *n* : a device for measuring chronaxie

chro·nax·im·e·try \\ˌkrō-ˌnak-'sim-ə-trē, ˌkrän-ˌak-\\ *n, pl* **-tries** : the measurement of chronaxie — **chro·nax·i·met·ric** \\ˌkrō-ˌnak-sə-'me-trik\\ *adj* — **chro·nax·i·met·ri·cal·ly** \\-tri-k(ə-)lē\\ *adv*

¹chron·ic \\'krän-ik\\ *also* **chron·i·cal** \\-i-kəl\\ *adj* **1 a** : marked by long duration, by frequent recurrence over a long time, and often by slowly progressing seriousness : not acute ⟨∼

\\ə\\ **abut** \\ᵊ\\ **kitten** \\ər\\ **further** \\a\\ **ash** \\ā\\ **ace** \\ä\\ **cot, cart** \\au̇\\ **out** \\ch\\ **chin** \\e\\ **bet** \\ē\\ **easy** \\g\\ **go** \\i\\ **hit** \\ī\\ **ice** \\j\\ **job** \\ŋ\\ **sing** \\ō\\ **go** \\ȯ\\ **law** \\ȯi\\ **boy** \\th\\ **thin** \\t̲h̲\\ **the** \\ü\\ **loot** \\u̇\\ **foot** \\y\\ **yet** \\zh\\ **vision** *See also* Pronunciation Symbols page

indigestion⟩ ⟨her hallucinations became ∼⟩ **b** : suffering from a disease or ailment of long duration or frequent recurrence ⟨a ∼ arthritic⟩ ⟨∼ sufferers from asthma⟩ **2 a** : having a slow progressive course of indefinite duration — used esp. of degenerative invasive diseases, some infections, psychoses, and inflammations ⟨∼ heart disease⟩ ⟨∼ arthritis⟩ ⟨∼ tuberculosis⟩; compare ACUTE 2b(1) **b** : infected with a disease-causing agent (as a virus) and remaining infectious over a long period of time but not necessarily expressing symptoms ⟨∼ carriers may remain healthy but still transmit the virus causing hepatitis B⟩ — **chron·i·cal·ly** \-i-k(ə-)lē\ *adv* — **chro·nic·i·ty** \krä-'nis-ət-ē, krō-\ *n, pl* **-ties**

²**chronic** *n* : one that suffers from a chronic disease

chronica — see ACRODERMATITIS CHRONICA ATROPHICANS

chronic alcoholism *n* : ALCOHOLISM 2b

chronic care *adj* : providing or concerned with long-term medical care lasting usu. more than 90 days esp. for individuals with chronic physical or mental impairment ⟨*chronic care* hospitals⟩ ⟨a *chronic care* nurse⟩ — compare ACUTE CARE, INTENSIVE CARE — **chronic care** *n*

chronic fatigue syndrome *n* : a disorder of uncertain cause that is characterized by persistent profound fatigue usu. accompanied by impairment in short-term memory or concentration, sore throat, tender lymph nodes, muscle or joint pain, and headache unrelated to any preexisting medical condition and that typically has an onset at about 30 years of age — abbr. *CFS;* called also *myalgic encephalomyelitis*

chronic granulocytic leukemia *n* : CHRONIC MYELOGENOUS LEUKEMIA

chronic granulomatous disease *n* : either of two diseases that are inherited as X-linked and autosomal traits, are characterized by recurrent infections which lead to granuloma formation at infection sites (as the skin or lungs), and result from a defect in the ability of white blood cells to destroy bacteria and fungi

chronic lymphocytic leukemia *n* : lymphocytic leukemia that is marked by an abnormal increase in the number of mature lymphocytes and esp. B cells, that is characterized by slow onset and progression of symptoms which include anemia, pallor, fatigue, appetite loss, granulocytopenia, thrombocytopenia, hypogammaglobulinemia, and enlargement of the lymph nodes, liver, and spleen, and that occurs esp. in older adults — abbr. *CLL;* compare ACUTE LYMPHOCYTIC LEUKEMIA

chronic myelogenous leukemia *n* : myelogenous leukemia that is marked by an abnormal increase in mature and immature granulocytes (as neutrophils, eosinophils, and myelocytes) esp. in bone marrow and blood, that is characterized by fatigue, weakness, loss of appetite, spleen and liver enlargement, anemia, thrombocytopenia, and ultimately a dangerous increase in blast cells and esp. myeloblasts and lymphoblasts, that occurs esp. in adults, and that is associated with the presence of the Philadelphia chromosome — abbr. *CML;* called also *chronic myelocytic leukemia, chronic myeloid leukemia, chronic granulocytic leukemia;* compare ACUTE MYELOGENOUS LEUKEMIA

chronic obstructive pulmonary disease *n* : pulmonary disease (as emphysema or chronic bronchitis) that is characterized by chronic typically irreversible airway obstruction resulting in a slowed rate of exhalation — abbr. *COPD*

chronicum — see ERYTHEMA CHRONICUM MIGRANS

chronicus — see LICHEN SIMPLEX CHRONICUS

chro·no·bi·ol·o·gist \ˌkrän-ə-bī-'äl-ə-jəst, ˌkrō-nə-\ *n* : a specialist in chronobiology

chro·no·bi·ol·o·gy \ˌkrän-ə-bī-'äl-ə-jē, ˌkrō-nə-\ *n, pl* **-gies** : the study of biological rhythms — **chro·no·bi·o·log·ic** \-ˌbī-ə-'läj-ik\ *or* **chro·no·bi·o·log·i·cal** \-i-kəl\ *adj*

chro·no·graph \'krän-ə-ˌgraf, 'krō-nə-\ *n* : an instrument for measuring and recording time intervals: as **a** : an instrument having a revolving drum on which a stylus makes marks **b** : a watch incorporating the functions of a stopwatch — **chro·no·graph·ic** \ˌkrän-ə-'graf-ik, ˌkrō-nə-\ *adj* — **chro·nog·ra·phy** \krə-'näg-rə-fē\ *n*

chro·no·log·i·cal age \ˌkrän-ºl-ˌäj-i-kəl-, ˌkrōn-\ *n* : the age of a person as measured from birth to a given date — compare ACHIEVEMENT AGE

chro·nom·e·ter \krə-'näm-ət-ər\ *n* : an instrument for measuring time; *esp* : one designed to keep time with great accuracy

chro·no·met·ric \ˌkrän-ə-'me-trik, ˌkrō-nə-\ *also* **chro·no·met·ri·cal** \-tri-kəl\ *adj* : of or relating to a chronometer or chronometry

chro·nom·e·try \krə-'näm-ə-trē\ *n, pl* **-tries** : the science of measuring time esp. by periods or intervals

chro·no·pho·to·graph \ˌkrän-ə-'fōt-ə-ˌgraf, ˌkrō-nə-\ *n* : a photograph or a series of photographs of a moving object taken to record and exhibit successive phases of the object's motion — **chro·no·pho·to·graph·ic** \-ˌfōt-ə-'graf-ik\ *adj* — **chro·no·pho·tog·ra·phy** \-fə-'täg-rə-fē\ *n*

chro·no·ther·a·peu·tics \-ˌther-ə-'pyüt-iks\ *n pl but sing in constr* : CHRONOTHERAPY 2 — **chro·no·ther·a·peu·tic** \-'pyüt-ik\ *adj*

chro·no·ther·a·py \ˌkrän-ə-'ther-ə-pē, ˌkrō-nə-\ *n, pl* **-pies** **1** : treatment of a sleep disorder (as insomnia) by changing sleeping and waking times in an attempt to reset the patient's biological clock **2** : the administration of medication in coordination with the body's circadian rhythms to maximize effectiveness and minimize side effects

chro·no·trop·ic \-'träp-ik\ *adj* : influencing the rate esp. of the heartbeat ⟨the ∼ effects of epinephrine⟩

chro·not·ro·pism \krə-'nä-trə-ˌpiz-əm\ *n* : interference with the rate of the heartbeat

chrys·a·ro·bin \ˌkris-ə-'rō-bən\ *n* : a brownish to orange-yellow powder obtained esp. from Goa powder and used to treat skin diseases (as psoriasis)

chry·si·a·sis \krə-'sī-ə-səs\ *n, pl* **-a·ses** \-ˌsēz\ : an ash-gray or mauve pigmentation of the skin due to deposition of gold in the tissues following parenteral administration of gold preparations

Chrys·o·my·ia \ˌkris-ə-'mī-(y)ə\ *n* : a genus of blowflies including the Old World screwworms

chrys·o·phan·ic acid \ˌkris-ə-ˌfan-ik-\ *n* : a yellow crystalline phenol $C_{15}H_{10}O_4$ occurring esp. in rhubarb and senna leaves

Chrys·ops \'kris-ˌäps\ *n* : a large widely distributed genus of small horseflies (family Tabanidae) of which the American deerflies are pests of humans and animals and in certain areas transmit tularemia while the African mango flies are vectors of the eye worm (*Loa loa*)

chryso·ther·a·py \ˌkris-ə-'ther-ə-pē\ *n, pl* **-pies** : treatment (as of arthritis) by injection of gold salts — called also *aurotherapy*

Churg–Strauss syndrome \'chərg-'straus-\ *n* : granulomatosis that typically affects the lungs but may involve other organs or tissues (as the skin or kidneys), is accompanied by vasculitis, eosinophilia, and asthma, and is sometimes considered to be a variant form of polyarteritis nodosa

Churg, Jacob (*b* 1910), and **Strauss, Lotte (1913–1985),** American pathologists. Churg and Strauss spent virtually the whole of their medical careers at Mount Sinai Hospital and Medical School in New York City. Churg's areas of research included vascular diseases, renal structure and diseases, and pneumoconioses. Strauss specialized in pediatric pathology. They described the syndrome that bears their names in articles published in 1951.

Chvos·tek's sign \(kə-)ˌvos-ˌtek(s)-\ *or* **Chvos·tek sign** \(kə-)ˌvos-ˌtek-\ *n* : a twitch of the facial muscles following gentle tapping over the facial nerve in front of the ear that indicates hyperirritability of the facial nerve

Chvos·tek \'kvos-ˌtek\, **Franz (1835–1884),** Austrian surgeon. Chvostek was a military doctor and professor at a military medical school in Vienna. In 1876 he published an article in which he announced his discovery that in a patient with tetany, tapping the optic nerve in front of the ear produces a spasm of the cheek muscles. This sign of tetany now bears his name.

chyl·an·gi·o·ma \ˌkī-ˌlan-jē-'ō-mə\ *n, pl* **-mas** *also* **-ma·ta** \-mət-ə\ : a tumor composed of intestinal lymph vessels containing chyle

chyle \'kī(ə)l\ *n* : lymph that is milky from emulsified fats, characteristically present in the lacteals, and most apparent during intestinal absorption of fats

chyli — see CISTERNA CHYLI

chy·lif·er·ous \(ˈ)kī-'lif-(ə-)rəs\ *adj* : transmitting or conveying chyle ⟨∼ vessels⟩

chy·li·fi·ca·tion \ˌkī-lə-fə-'kā-shən, ˌkil-ə-\ *n* : the formation of chyle

chy·li·form \'kī-lə-ˌfȯrm\ *adj* : resembling chyle ⟨∼ fluid⟩

chy·lo·cele \'kī-lə-ˌsēl\ *n* : an effusion of chyle in the tunica vaginalis of the testis

chy·lo·mi·cron \ˌkī-lō-'mī-ˌkrän\ *n* : a lipoprotein rich in triglyceride and common in the blood during fat digestion and assimilation

chy·lo·mi·cro·ne·mia *or chiefly Brit* **chy·lo·mi·cro·nae·mia** \-ˌmī-krə-'nē-mē-ə\ *n* : an excessive number of chylomicrons in the blood ⟨postprandial ∼⟩

chy·lo·peri·to·ne·um \-ˌper-ət-ᵊn-'ē-əm\ *n, pl* **-ne·ums** *or* **-nea** \-'ē-ə\ : the presence of chyle in the peritoneal cavity

chy·lo·pneu·mo·tho·rax \-ˌn(y)ü-mə-'thō(ə)r-ˌaks, -'thȯ(ə)r-\ *n, pl* **-rax·es** *or* **-ra·ces** \-'thōr-ə-ˌsēz, -'thȯr-\ : the presence of air and chyle in the pleural cavity

chy·lo·poi·e·sis \-poi-'ē-səs\ *n, pl* **-e·ses** \-ˌsēz\ : CHYLIFICATION — **chy·lo·poi·et·ic** \-'et-ik\ *adj*

chy·lo·sis \kī-'lō-səs\ *n, pl* **-lo·ses** \-ˌsēz\ : CHYLIFICATION

chy·lo·tho·rax \-'thō(ə)r-ˌaks, -'thȯ(ə)r-\ *n, pl* **-rax·es** *or* **-ra·ces** \-'thōr-ə-ˌsēz, -'thȯr-\ : an effusion of chyle or chylous fluid into the thoracic cavity

chy·lous \'kī-ləs\ *adj* : consisting of or like chyle ⟨∼ ascites⟩

chy·lu·ria \kī-'l(y)ùr-ē-ə\ *n* : the presence of chyle in the urine as a result of organic disease (as of the kidney) or of mechanical lymphatic esp. parasitic obstruction

chyme \'kīm\ *n* : the semifluid mass of partly digested food expelled by the stomach into the duodenum — **chy·mous** \'kī-məs\ *adj*

chy·mi·fi·ca·tion \ˌkī-mə-fə-'kā-shən, ˌkim-ə-\ *n* : the conversion of food into chyme by the digestive action of gastric juice

chy·mo·pa·pa·in \ˌkī-mō-pə-'pā-ən, -'pī-ən\ *n* : a proteolytic enzyme from the latex of the papaya that is used in meat tenderizer and has been used medically in chemonucleolysis

chy·mo·sin \'kī-mə-sən\ *n* : RENNIN

chy·mo·tryp·sin \ˌkī-mō-'trip-sən\ *n* : a protease that hydrolyzes peptide bonds and is formed in the intestine from chymotrypsinogen — compare TRYPSIN

chy·mo·tryp·sin·o·gen \-ˌtrip-'sin-ə-jən\ *n* : a zymogen that is secreted by the pancreas and is converted by trypsin to chymotrypsin

chy·mo·tryp·tic \ˌkī-mō-'trip-tik\ *adj* : of, relating to, produced by, or performed with chymotrypsin ⟨∼ peptide mapping⟩

CI *abbr* chemotherapeutic index

Ci·al·is \sē-'al-əs\ *trademark* — used for a preparation of tadalafil

cic·a·tri·cial \ˌsik-ə-'trish-əl\ *adj* : relating to or having the character of a cicatrix ⟨excision of a ∼ lesion⟩

ci·ca·trix \'sik-ə-ˌtriks, sə-'kā-triks\ *n, pl* **ci·ca·tri·ces** \ˌsik-ə-'trī-(ˌ)sēz, sə-'kā-trə-ˌsēz\ : a scar resulting from formation and contraction of fibrous tissue in a flesh wound

cic·a·tri·zant *or Brit* **cic·a·tri·sant** \ˌsik-ə-'trīz-ᵊnt\ *adj* : promoting the healing of a wound or the formation of a cicatrix

cic·a·tri·za·tion *or Brit* **cic·a·tri·sa·tion** \ˌsik-ə-trə-'zā-shən\ *n* : scar formation at the site of a healing wound

cic·a·trize *or Brit* **cic·a·trise** \'sik-ə-ˌtrīz\ *vb* **-trized** *or Brit* **-trised; -triz·ing** *or Brit* **-tris·ing** *vt* **1** : to induce the formation of a scar in **2** : SCAR ∼ *vi* : to heal by forming a scar

CICU *abbr* coronary intensive care unit

Ci·cu·ta \sə-'kyüt-ə\ *n* : a small genus of perennial herbs of the family Umbelliferae that have tuberous deadly poisonous roots and twice or thrice pinnate or ternate leaves — see SPOTTED COWBANE, WATER HEMLOCK

cic·u·tox·in \ˌsik-yə-'täk-sən, 'sik-yə-ˌ\ *n* : an amorphous poisonous principle $C_{19}H_{26}O_3$ in water hemlock, spotted cowbane, and related plants of the genus *Cicuta*

cigarette drain *n* : a cigarette-shaped gauze wick enclosed in rubber dam tissue or rubber tubing for draining wounds — called also *Penrose drain*

ci·gua·tera \ˌsē-gwə-'ter-ə, ˌsig-\ *n* : poisoning caused by the ingestion of various normally edible tropical fish in whose flesh a toxic substance (as one produced by some dinoflagellates) has accumulated

ci·gua·tox·in \'sē-gwə-ˌtäk-sən, 'sig-wə-\ *n* : a potent heat‑stable neurotoxin that is produced by a marine dinoflagellate (*Gambierdiscus toxicus*) and causes ciguatera poisoning in those who eat fish (as barracuda or amberjack) in which toxic levels of it have become concentrated; *also* : any of several related neurotoxins causing ciguatera

cilia *pl of* CILIUM

ciliaris — see ORBICULUS CILIARIS, ZONULA CILIARIS

cil·i·ary \'sil-ē-ˌer-ē\ *adj* **1** : of or relating to cilia ⟨∼ movement⟩ **2** : of, relating to, or being the annular suspension of the lens of the eye ⟨a ∼ arteriole⟩ ⟨∼ spasm⟩

ciliary artery *n* : any of several arteries that arise from the ophthalmic artery or its branches and supply various parts of the eye — see LONG POSTERIOR CILIARY ARTERY, SHORT POSTERIOR CILIARY ARTERY

ciliary body *n* : an annular structure on the inner surface of the anterior wall of the eyeball composed largely of the ciliary muscle and bearing the ciliary processes

ciliary ganglion *n* : a small autonomic ganglion on the nasociliary branch of the ophthalmic nerve receiving preganglionic fibers from the oculomotor nerve and sending postganglionic fibers to the ciliary muscle and to the sphincter pupillae — called also *lenticular ganglion*

ciliary muscle *n* : a circular band of smooth muscle fibers situated in the ciliary body and serving as the chief agent in accommodation when it contracts by drawing the ciliary processes centripetally and relaxing the suspensory ligament of the lens so that the lens is permitted to become more convex

ciliary nerve — see LONG CILIARY NERVE, SHORT CILIARY NERVE

ciliary process *n* : any of the vascular folds on the inner surface of the ciliary body that give attachment to the suspensory ligament of the lens

ciliary ring *n* : ORBICULUS CILIARIS

ciliary zonule *n* : ZONULE OF ZINN

Cil·i·a·ta \ˌsil-ē-'āt-ə\ *n pl, in some classifications* : a large class of chiefly free-living protozoans that feed on complex organic matter, have cilia or cirri throughout the vegetative stages of the life cycle, and usu. have nuclei of two kinds

cil·i·ate \'sil-ē-ət, -ē-ˌāt\ *n* : any of the phylum Ciliophora of ciliate protozoans

cil·i·at·ed \'sil-ē-ˌāt-əd\ *or* **ciliate** *adj* : provided with cilia ⟨*ciliated* epithelium⟩ ⟨the *ciliate* protozoans⟩ — **cil·i·ate·ly** *adv* — **cil·i·a·tion** \ˌsil-ē-'ā-shən\ *n*

Cil·i·oph·o·ra \ˌsil-ē-'äf-(ə-)rə\ *n pl* : a phylum of protozoans that possess cilia during some phase of the life cycle and usu. have nuclei of two kinds — compare SARCOMASTIGOPHORA — **cil·i·oph·o·ran** \-'äf-(ə-)rən\ *adj or n*

cil·io·ret·i·nal \ˌsil-ē-ō-'ret-ᵊn-əl, -'ret-nəl\ *adj* : of, relating to, or supplying the part of the eye including the ciliary body and the retina ⟨a ∼ arteriole⟩

cil·i·um \'sil-ē-əm\ *n, pl* **cil·ia** \-ē-ə\ **1** : EYELASH **2** : a minute short hairlike process often forming part of a fringe; *esp* : one of a cell that is capable of lashing movement and serves esp. in free unicellular organisms to produce locomotion or in higher forms a current of fluid

ci·met·i·dine \sī-'met-ə-ˌdēn\ *n* : an H₂ antagonist $C_{10}H_{16}N_6S$ that like histamine contains the ring structure of imidazole

\ə\ **abut** \ᵊ\ **kitten** \ər\ **further** \a\ **ash** \ā\ **ace** \ä\ **cot, cart** \aù\ **out** \ch\ **chin** \e\ **bet** \ē\ **easy** \g\ **go** \i\ **hit** \ī\ **ice** \j\ **job** \ŋ\ **sing** \ō\ **go** \ȯ\ **law** \ȯi\ **boy** \th\ **thin** \th\ **the** \ü\ **loot** \ù\ **foot** \y\ **yet** \zh\ **vision** *See also* Pronunciation Symbols page

and is used to inhibit gastric acid secretion in conditions in which such secretion produces duodenal or gastric ulcers or erosive lesions (as in serious cases of gastroesophageal reflux disease) — see TAGAMET

ci·mex \'sī-ˌmeks\ *n* **1** *pl* **ci·mi·ces** \'sī-mə-ˌsēz, 'sim-ə-\ : BEDBUG **2** *cap* : the type genus of the family Cimicidae comprising the common bedbug and a few related insects

Ci·mic·i·dae \sī-'mis-ə-ˌdē, sə-\ *n pl* : a small family of flat-bodied wingless bloodsucking bugs of the order Hemiptera including the bedbug and some pests of birds and bats

cim·i·cif·u·ga \ˌsim-ə-'sif-yə-gə\ *n* **1 a** *cap* : a small genus of perennial herbs (family Ranunculaceae) having white flowers in long racemes — see BLACK COHOSH **b** : a plant of the genus *Cimicifuga* **2** : the dried rhizome and roots of black cohosh (*Cimicifuga racemosa*) that were formerly used as a sedative and alterative in the treatment of rheumatism and chorea — called also *black cohosh root*

cim·i·cif·u·gin \-yə-jən\ *n* : a resinoid prepared from the roots and rhizome of black cohosh (*Cimicifuga racemosa*) that has been used as a nerve tonic and antispasmodic

cin·cho·caine \'siŋ-kə-ˌkān, 'sin-\ *n, chiefly Brit* : DIBUCAINE

cin·cho·na \siŋ-'kō-nə, sin-'chō-\ *n* **1** *cap* : a large genus of So. American trees and shrubs of the madder family **2** : a tree of the genus *Cinchona* **3** : the dried bark of any of several trees of the genus *Cinchona* (esp. *C. ledgeriana* and *C. succirubra* or their hybrids) containing alkaloids (as quinine, cinchonine, quinidine, and cinchonidine) and being used esp. formerly as a specific in malaria, an antipyretic in other fevers, and a tonic and stomachic — called also *cinchona bark, Jesuits' bark, Peruvian bark*

Chin·chón \chin-'chōn\, **Countess of (Doña Francisca Henriquez de Ribera),** vicereine. According to a legend first given out in 1663 and supposedly based on a now-lost letter, Countess Chinchón, the wife of the viceroy of Peru, fell ill with malaria. The governor of a neighboring province quickly provided a remedy in the form of a certain tree bark. The countess experienced a seemingly miraculous recovery, and word of the bark's extraordinary powers quickly spread. The name of the countess henceforth became associated with the bark. While the story is apocryphal, Linnaeus perpetuated the name of the countess, albeit in misspelled form, by designating the genus of that tree *Cinchona* in her honor.

cin·chon·amine \siŋ-'kō-nə-ˌmēn, sin-'chō-, -mən\ *n* : a white crystalline alkaloid $C_{19}H_{24}N_2O$ obtained from some So. American shrubs (genus *Remijia*) of the madder family that has been used as a substitute for and is more toxic than quinine

¹**cin·chon·ic** \siŋ-'kän-ik, sin-'chän-\ *adj* : belonging to or obtained from cinchona

²**cinchonic** *n* : a constituent or preparation of cinchona used in medicine

cin·cho·ni·dine \-'kän-ə-ˌdēn, -'kō-nə-, -'chō-nə-\ *n* : a bitter crystalline alkaloid $C_{19}H_{22}N_2O$ stereoisomeric with cinchonine that is found in cinchona bark and used like quinine

cin·cho·nine \'siŋ-kə-ˌnēn, 'sin-chə-\ *n* : a bitter white crystalline alkaloid $C_{19}H_{22}N_2O$ found esp. in cinchona bark and used like quinine

cin·cho·nism \'siŋ-kə-ˌniz-əm, 'sin-chə-\ *n* : a disorder due to excessive or prolonged use of cinchona or its alkaloids and marked by temporary deafness, ringing in the ears, headache, dizziness, and rash

cin·cho·nize *or Brit* **cin·cho·nise** \-ˌnīz\ *vt* **-nized** *or Brit* **-nised; -niz·ing** *or Brit* **-nis·ing** : to treat (as a malarial patient) with cinchona or one of its alkaloids (as quinine)

cin·cho·phen \-ˌfen, -fən\ *n* : a bitter white crystalline compound $C_{16}H_{11}NO_2$ made synthetically that is used for treating gout and rheumatism but is damaging to the liver

cine·an·gio·car·di·og·ra·phy \ˌsin-ē-ˌan-jē-ō-ˌkärd-ē-'äg-rə-fē\ *n, pl* **-phies** : motion-picture photography of a fluoroscopic screen recording passage of a contrasting medium through the chambers of the heart and large blood vessels — **cine·an·gio·car·dio·graph·ic** \-ˌkärd-ē-ō-'graf-ik\ *adj*

cine·an·gi·og·ra·phy \-ˌan-jē-'äg-rə-fē\ *n, pl* **-phies** : motion-

picture photography of a fluorescent screen recording passage of a contrasting medium through the blood vessels — **cine·an·gio·graph·ic** \-jē-ə-'graf-ik\ *adj*

cine·flu·o·rog·ra·phy \-ˌflu̇-(ə)r-'äg-rə-fē\ *n, pl* **-phies** : the process of making motion pictures of images of objects by means of X-rays with the aid of a fluorescent screen (as for revealing the motions of organs in the body) — compare CINERADIOGRAPHY — **cine·flu·o·ro·graph·ic** \-ˌflu̇(-ə)r-ə-'graf-ik\ *adj*

cinematics *var of* KINEMATICS

cin·e·mat·o·graph \ˌsin-ə-'mat-ə-ˌgraf\ *n* : a visual record obtained by cinematography ⟨∼s of the spontaneously fibrillating auricle —*Jour. Amer. Med. Assoc.*⟩

cin·e·ma·tog·ra·phy \ˌsin-ə-mə-'täg-rə-fē\ *n, pl* **-phies** : the art or science of motion-picture photography ⟨X-ray fluoroscopic ∼⟩ — **cin·e·mat·o·graph·ic** \-ˌmat-ə-'graf-ik\ *adj* — **cin·e·mat·o·graph·i·cal·ly** \-i-k(ə)lē\ *adv*

cin·e·ole \'sin-ē-ˌōl\ *n* : EUCALYPTOL

cine·pho·to·mi·cro·graph \ˌsin-ē-ˌfōt-ə-'mī-krə-ˌgraf\ *n* : a motion picture made by cinephotomicrography

cine·pho·to·mi·crog·ra·phy \-mī-'kräg-rə-fē\ *n, pl* **-phies** : MICROCINEMATOGRAPHY

cin·e·plas·ty \'sin-ə-ˌplas-tē\ *also* **ki·ne·plas·ty** \'kin-ə-, 'kī-nə-\ *n, pl* **-ties** **1** : surgical fitting of a lever to a muscle in an amputation stump to facilitate the operation of an artificial hand **2** : surgical isolation of a loop of muscle of chest or arm, covering it with skin, and attaching to it a prosthetic device to be operated by contraction of the muscle in the loop — **cin·e·plas·tic** \ˌsin-ə-'plas-tik\ *also* **ki·ne·plas·tic** \ˌkin-ə-, ˌkī-nə-\ *adj*

cine·ra·di·og·ra·phy \ˌsin-ē-ˌrād-ē-'äg-rə-fē\ *n, pl* **-phies** : the process of making radiographs of moving objects (as the heart or joints) in sufficiently rapid sequence so that the radiographs or copies made from them may be projected as motion pictures — compare CINEFLUOROGRAPHY — **cine·ra·dio·graph·ic** \-ˌrād-ē-ō-'graf-ik\ *adj*

ci·ne·rea \sə-'nir-ē-ə\ *n* : the gray matter of nerve tissue

cinereum — see TUBER CINEREUM

cine·roent·gen·og·ra·phy \ˌsin-ē-ˌrent-gən-'äg-rə-fē\ *n, pl* **-phies** : CINERADIOGRAPHY

cin·gu·late gyrus \ˌsiŋ-gyə-lət-, -ˌlāt-\ *n* : a medial gyrus of each cerebral hemisphere that partly surrounds the corpus callosum

cin·gu·lec·to·my \ˌsiŋ-gyə-'lek-tə-mē\ *n, pl* **-mies** : CINGULOTOMY

cin·gu·lot·o·my \ˌsiŋ-gyə-'lät-ə-mē\ *n, pl* **-mies** : surgical destruction of all or part (as the cingulum) of the cingulate gyrus

cin·gu·lum \'siŋ-gyə-ləm\ *n, pl* **cin·gu·la** \-lə\ **1** : a ridge about the base of the crown of a tooth **2** : a tract of association fibers lying within the cingulate gyrus and connecting the callosal and hippocampal convolutions of the brain

cin·na·bar \'sin-ə-ˌbär\ *n* **1** : native red sulfide of mercury HgS that is the only important ore of mercury **2** : artificial red sulfide of mercury used esp. as a pigment

cin·na·mal·de·hyde \ˌsin-ə-'mal-də-ˌhīd\ *n* : an aromatic oily aldehyde C_9H_8O occurring as the chief constituent of cinnamon-bark oil and cinnamon oil and used as a flavor

cin·na·mate \'sin-ə-ˌmāt, sə-'nam-ət\ *n* : a salt or ester of cinnamic acid

cin·na·mene \'sin-ə-ˌmēn\ *n* : STYRENE

cin·nam·ic \sə-'nam-ik\ *adj* : obtained or derived from cinnamon oil or cinnamic acid ⟨∼ aldehyde⟩

cinnamic acid *n* : a white crystalline odorless acid $C_9H_8O_2$ found esp. in cinnamon oil and storax

Cin·na·mo·mum \ˌsin-ə-'mō-məm\ *n* : a large genus of Asian and Australian aromatic trees and shrubs of the laurel family (Lauraceae) that have small flowers in panicles and include the camphor tree, cinnamon, and Chinese cinnamon

cin·na·mon \'sin-ə-mən\ *n, often attrib* **1** : any of several Asian trees of the genus *Cinnamomum* **2 a** : the highly aromatic bark of a cinnamon that yields cinnamaldehyde and other aromatic products in the form of cinnamon oil — see

CHINESE CINNAMON b : an aromatic spice prepared from the dried inner bark of a cinnamon (esp. *C. zeylanicum*)

cinnamon–bark oil *n* : a light-yellow essential oil obtained from the bark of a Sri Lankan tree of the genus *Cinnamomum* (*C. zeylanicum*) and used in medicine, flavoring, and perfumery — called also *cinnamon oil*

cinnamon oil *n* : an oil obtained from a tree or shrub of the genus *Cinnamomum*: as **a** : CINNAMON-BARK OIL **b** : a yellowish or brownish essential oil obtained from the leaves and young twigs of a cinnamon tree (*Cinnamomum cassia*) and used chiefly as a flavoring — called also *cassia oil*

cinnamon water *n* : a saturated solution of cinnamon oil in distilled water used as a vehicle for some drugs

Cip·ro \'sip-rō\ *trademark* — used for a preparation of ciprofloxacin

cip·ro·flox·a·cin \ˌsip-rə-'fläk-sə-sən, -rō-\ *n* : a fluoroquinolone $C_{17}H_{18}FN_3O_3$ that is often administered in the form of its hydrochloride $C_{17}H_{18}FN_3O_3 \cdot HCl$ and is effective esp. against gram-negative bacteria — see CIPRO

cir·ca·di·an \(ˌ)sər-'kad-ē-ən, -'kād-; ˌsər-kə-'dī-ən, -'dē-\ *adj* : being, having, characterized by, or occurring in approximately 24-hour periods or cycles (as of biological activity or function) ⟨~ periodicity⟩ ⟨~ rhythms in behavior or physiological activity⟩ — compare INFRADIAN, ULTRADIAN

circ·an·nu·al \(')sər-'kan-yə(-wə)l\ *adj* : having, characterized by, or occurring in approximately yearly periods or cycles (as of biological activity or function) ⟨~ rhythmicity⟩

cir·ci·nate \'sər-sᵊn-ˌāt\ *adj, of lesions* : having a sharply circumscribed and somewhat circular margin ⟨scaly ~ dermatophytids⟩

čir·cle \'sər-kəl\ *n* **1 a** : a closed plane curve every point of which is equidistant from a fixed point within the curve **b** : the plane surface bounded by such a curve **2** : something (as an anatomical part) in the form of a circle or section of a circle ⟨an arterial ~⟩ — see CIRCLE OF WILLIS

circle of Wil·lis \-'wil-əs\ *n* : a complete ring of arteries at the base of the brain that is formed by the cerebral and communicating arteries and is a site of aneurysms

Willis, Thomas (1621–1675), British physician. One of the major figures of English medicine in the 17th century, Willis was a founder of the Royal Society. With all his notable achievements, he is known especially for his extensive study of the nervous system. In 1664 he produced *Cerebri Anatome* ("Anatomy of the Brain"), the most complete and accurate description of the nervous system up to that time. This work contained his description of the circular anastomosis of arteries at the base of the brain that is now known as the circle of Willis. His description was not the first but it was the first complete one and was accompanied by an equally complete illustration.

circling disease *n* : listeriosis of sheep or cattle

cir·cuit \'sər-kət\ *n* : the complete path of an electric current including usu. the source of electric energy

cir·cuit·ry \'sər-kə-trē\ *n* **1 a** : the detailed plan or arrangement of an electric circuit **b** : the components of an electric circuit **2** : the network of interconnected neurons in the nervous system and esp. the brain; *also* : the neuronal pathways of the brain along which electrical and chemical signals travel

cir·cu·lar \'sər-kyə-lər\ *adj* : MANIC-DEPRESSIVE; *esp* : BIPOLAR 3 ⟨the exalted phase of the mental ~ state —Havelock Ellis⟩

circular dichroism *n* **1** : the property (as of an optically active medium) of unequal absorption of right and left plane-polarized light so that the emergent light is elliptically polarized **2** : a spectroscopic technique that makes use of circular dichroism

circulares — see PLICAE CIRCULARES

circular polarization *n* : polarization in which the mutually perpendicular components of a transverse wave radiation have equal amplitudes but differ in phase by 90 degrees — **circularly polarized** *adj*

circular sinus *n* : a circular venous channel around the pituitary gland formed by the cavernous and intercavernous sinuses

cir·cu·late \'sər-kyə-ˌlāt\ *vi* **-lat·ed; -lat·ing** : to flow or be propelled naturally through a closed system of channels (as blood vessels) ⟨blood ~s through the body⟩

circulating nurse *n* : a registered nurse who makes preparations for an operation and continually monitors the patient and staff during its course, who works in the operating room outside the sterile field in which the operation takes place, and who records the progress of the operation, accounts for the instruments, and handles specimens

cir·cu·la·tion \ˌsər-kyə-'lā-shən\ *n* : the movement of blood through the vessels of the body that is induced by the pumping action of the heart and serves to distribute nutrients and oxygen to and remove waste products from all parts of the body — see PULMONARY CIRCULATION, SYSTEMIC CIRCULATION

cir·cu·la·to·ry \'sər-kyə-lə-ˌtōr-ē, -ˌtȯr-\ *adj* : of or relating to circulation or the circulatory system ⟨~ failure⟩

circulatory system *n* : the system of blood, blood vessels, lymphatics, and heart concerned with the circulation of the blood and lymph

cir·cu·lin \'sər-kyə-lən\ *n* : an antibiotic consisting of a mixture of polypeptides related to polymyxin that is obtained from a soil bacterium of the genus *Bacillus* (*B. circulans*) and is active esp. against gram-negative bacteria (as colon bacilli)

cir·cu·lus \-ləs\ *n, pl* **-li** \-ˌlī\ : an anatomical circle or ring esp. of veins or arteries

cir·cum·cise \'sər-kəm-ˌsīz\ *vt* **-cised; -cis·ing** : to cut off the prepuce of (a male) or the clitoris of (a female) — **cir·cum·cis·er** *n*

cir·cum·ci·sion \ˌsər-kəm-'sizh-ən\ *n* **1** : the act of circumcising: **a** : the cutting off of the foreskin of males that is practiced as a religious rite by Jews and Muslims and as a sanitary measure in modern surgery **b** : FEMALE GENITAL MUTILATION **2** : the condition of being circumcised

cir·cum·cor·ne·al injection \ˌsir-kəm-ˌkȯr-nē-əl-\ *n* : enlargement of the ciliary and conjunctival blood vessels near the margin of the cornea with reduction in size peripherally

cir·cum·duc·tion \ˌsər-kəm-'dək-shən\ *n* : movement of a limb or extremity so that the distal end describes a circle while the proximal end remains fixed — **cir·cum·duct** \-'dəkt\ *vt*

cir·cum·flex \'sər-kəm-ˌfleks\ *adj, of nerves and blood vessels* : bending around

circumflex artery *n* : any of several paired curving arteries: as **a** : either of two arteries that branch from the deep femoral artery or from the femoral artery itself: (1) : LATERAL FEMORAL CIRCUMFLEX ARTERY (2) : MEDIAL FEMORAL CIRCUMFLEX ARTERY **b** : either of two branches of the axillary artery that wind around the neck of the humerus: (1) : ANTERIOR HUMERAL CIRCUMFLEX ARTERY (2) : POSTERIOR HUMERAL CIRCUMFLEX ARTERY **c** : CIRCUMFLEX ILIAC ARTERY **d** : a branch of the subscapular artery supplying the muscles of the shoulder

circumflex iliac artery *n* : either of two arteries arching anteriorly near the inguinal ligament: **a** : an artery lying internal to the iliac crest and arising from the external iliac artery **b** : a more superficially located artery that is a branch of the femoral artery

circumflex nerve *n* : AXILLARY NERVE

cir·cum·len·tal \ˌsər-kəm-'lent-ᵊl, 'sər-kəm-ˌ\ *adj* : situated around the lens of the eye

cir·cum·nu·cle·ar \-'n(y)ü-klē-ər\ *n* : situated around a nucleus (as of a cell)

cir·cum·oral \-'ōr-əl, -'ȯr-, -'är-\ *adj* : surrounding the mouth ⟨~ pallor⟩

\ə\ **abut** \ᵊ\ **kitten** \ər\ **further** \a\ **ash** \ā\ **ace** \ä\ **cot, cart** \au̇\ **out** \ch\ **chin** \e\ **bet** \ē\ **easy** \g\ **go** \i\ **hit** \ī\ **ice** \j\ **job** \ŋ\ **sing** \ō\ **go** \ȯ\ **law** \ȯi\ **boy** \th\ **thin** \th\ **the** \ü\ **loot** \u̇\ **foot** \y\ **yet** \zh\ **vision** *See also* Pronunciation Symbols page

C
D

cir·cum·scribed \'sər-kəm-ˌskrībd\ *adj* : confined to a limited area ⟨a ~ neurosis⟩ ⟨~ loss of hair⟩

cir·cum·stan·ti·al·i·ty \ˌsər-kəm-ˌstan-chē-ˈal-ət-ē\ *n, pl* **-ties** : a conversational pattern (as in some manic states) exhibiting excessive attention to irrelevant and digressive details

cir·cum·val·late \ˌsər-kəm-ˈval-ˌāt, -ˈval-ət\ *adj* : enclosed by a ridge of tissue

circumvallate papilla *n* : any of approximately 12 large papillae near the back of the tongue each of which is surrounded with a marginal sulcus and supplied with taste buds responsive esp. to bitter flavors — called also *vallate papilla*

circumvallate placenta *n* : a placenta with a dense ring around the periphery produced by excessive growth of the surrounding tissue of the uterus

cir·rho·gen·ic \ˌsir-ə-ˈje-nik\ *adj* : tending to cause cirrhosis of the liver ⟨a ~ diet⟩ ⟨chronic ~ hepatitis⟩

cir·rhog·e·nous \sə-ˈräg-ə-nəs\ *adj* : CIRRHOGENIC

cir·rho·sis \sə-ˈrō-səs\ *n, pl* **-rho·ses** \-ˌsēz\ : widespread disruption of normal liver structure by fibrosis and the formation of regenerative nodules that is caused by any of various chronic progressive conditions affecting the liver (as long-term alcohol abuse or hepatitis) — see BILIARY CIRRHOSIS

¹**cir·rhot·ic** \sə-ˈrät-ik\ *adj* : of, relating to, caused by, or affected with cirrhosis ⟨~ degeneration⟩ ⟨a ~ liver⟩

²**cirrhotic** *n* : an individual affected with cirrhosis

cir·rus \'sir-əs\ *n, pl* **cir·ri** \'si(ə)r-ˌī\ : a slender usu. flexible animal appendage: as **a** : a fused group of cilia functioning like a limb on some protozoans **b** : the male copulatory organ of some worms

cir·soid \'sər-ˌsȯid\ *adj* : resembling a dilated tortuous vein ⟨a ~ aneurysm of the scalp⟩

cis \'sis\ *adj* **1** : characterized by having certain atoms or groups of atoms on the same side of the longitudinal axis of a double bond or of the plane of a ring in a molecule **2** : relating to or being an arrangement of two very closely linked genes in the heterozygous condition in which both mutant alleles are on one chromosome and both wild-type alleles are on the homologous chromosome — compare TRANS 2

CIS *abbr* carcinoma in situ

cis·plat·in \'sis-ˌplat-ᵊn\ *n* : a platinum-containing antineoplastic drug $Cl_2H_6N_2Pt$ that functions as an alkylating agent, produces crosslinks in DNA between and within strands, and is used esp. as a palliative therapy in testicular and ovarian tumors and in advanced bladder cancer — see PLATINOL

cis–platinum \-ˈplat-ᵊn-əm\ *n* : CISPLATIN

cis·tern \'sis-tərn\ *n* : a fluid-containing sac or cavity in an organism

cis·ter·na \sis-ˈtər-nə\ *n, pl* **-nae** \-ˌnē\ : CISTERN: as **a** : CISTERNA MAGNA **b** : CISTERNA CHYLI **c** : one of the interconnected flattened vesicles or tubules comprising the endoplasmic reticulum

cisterna chy·li \-ˈkī-ˌlī\ *n, pl* **cisternae chyli** : a dilated lymph channel usu. opposite the first and second lumbar vertebrae and marking the beginning of the thoracic duct

cis·ter·nal \sis-ˈtərn-ᵊl\ *adj* : of or relating to a cisterna and esp. the cisterna magna ⟨~ puncture⟩ — **cis·ter·nal·ly** \-ē\ *adv*

cisterna mag·na \-ˈmag-nə\ *n, pl* **cisternae mag·nae** \-ˌnē\ : a large subarachnoid space between the caudal part of the cerebellum and the medulla oblongata

cis·ter·nog·ra·phy \ˌsis-(ˌ)tər-ˈnäg-rə-fē\ *n, pl* **-phies** : radiographic visualization of the subarachnoid spaces containing cerebrospinal fluid following injection of an opaque contrast medium

cis·tron \'sis-ˌträn\ *n* : a segment of DNA that is equivalent to a gene and that specifies a single functional unit (as a protein or enzyme) — **cis·tron·ic** \sis-ˈträn-ik\ *adj*

ci·tal·o·pram \sī-ˈtal-ə-ˌpram, si-\ *n* : an antidepressant drug that is administered orally in the form of its hydrobromide $C_{20}H_{21}FN_2O \cdot HBr$ and functions as an SSRI — see CELEXA

Ci·tel·lus \sī-ˈtel-əs\ *n* : a genus of rodents (family Sciuridae) including the typical ground squirrels

cit·ral \'si-ˌtral\ *n* : an unsaturated liquid isomeric aldehyde $C_{10}H_{16}O$ of many essential oils that has a strong lemon odor and is used esp. in perfumery and as a flavoring

cit·rate \'si-ˌtrāt\ *n* : a salt or ester of citric acid

cit·rat·ed \'si-ˌtrāt-əd\ *adj* : treated with a citrate esp. of sodium or potassium to prevent coagulation ⟨~ blood⟩

citrate synthase *n* : an enzyme that catalyzes condensation of acetyl coenzyme A with oxaloacetate to form citric acid in the Krebs cycle — called also *citrogenase*

cit·ric acid \ˌsi-trik-\ *n* : a sour organic acid $C_6H_8O_7$ occurring in cellular metabolism, obtained esp. from lemon and lime juices or by fermentation of sugars, and used as a flavoring

citric acid cycle *n* : KREBS CYCLE

cit·rin \'si-trən\ *n* : a crystalline water-soluble flavonoid concentrate that was orig. prepared from lemons and is used as a source of bioflavonoids

ci·tri·nin \si-ˈtrī-nən\ *n* : a toxic antibiotic $C_{13}H_{14}O_5$ that is produced esp. by two molds of the genus *Penicillium* (*P. citrinum*) and the genus *Aspergillus* (*A. niveus*) and is effective against some gram-positive bacteria

cit·rog·e·nase \sə-ˈträj-ə-ˈnās, -ˌnāz\ *n* : CITRATE SYNTHASE

cit·ro·nel·la \ˌsi-trə-ˈnel-ə\ *n* **1** : CITRONELLA OIL **2** : a fragrant grass (*Cymbopogon nardus*) of southern Asia that yields citronella oil

cit·ro·nel·lal \-ˈnel-ˌal\ *n* : an aldehyde $C_{10}H_{18}O$ with a lemony odor that is obtained esp. from citronella oil and that is used in perfumery and as an insect repellent

citronella oil *n* : a yellowish essential oil with a lemony odor obtained from either of two grasses and used esp. as an insect repellent: **a** : an oil from citronella grass containing chiefly geraniol **b** : an oil from a related grass (*Cymbopogon winterianus*) containing citronellal, citronellol, and geraniol

cit·ro·nel·lol \-ˈnel-ˌȯl, -ˌōl\ *n* : an unsaturated liquid alcohol $C_{10}H_{20}O$ with a roselike odor that is found in two optically active forms in many essential oils (as rose oil) and is used in perfumery and soaps

ci·trov·o·rum factor \sə-ˈträv-ə-rəm-\ *n* : LEUCOVORIN

cit·rul·lin \si-ˈtrəl-ən, ˈsi-trəl-\ *n* : a purgative yellow resinous preparation of the colocynth

cit·rul·line \'si-trə-ˌlēn; si-ˈtrəl-ˌēn, -ən\ *n* : a crystalline amino acid $C_6H_{13}N_3O_3$ formed esp. as an intermediate in the conversion of ornithine to arginine in the living system

cit·rul·lin·emia *or chiefly Brit* **cit·rul·lin·aemia** \ˌsi-trə-lə-ˈnē-mē-ə, si-ˌtrəl-ə-ˈnē-\ *n* : an inherited disorder of amino acid metabolism accompanied by excess amounts of citrulline in the blood, urine, and cerebrospinal fluid and by ammonia intoxication

cit·rus \'si-trəs\ *n, often attrib* **1** *cap* : a genus of often thorny trees and shrubs of the rue family (Rutaceae) grown in warm regions for their edible fruit (as the orange, lemon, lime, or mandarin) with firm usu. thick rind and pulpy flesh **2** *pl* **citruses** *or* **citrus** : any plant or fruit of the genus *Citrus* or a related genus

civ·et \'siv-ət\ *n* **1** : CIVET CAT **2** : a thick yellowish musky-odored substance found in a pouch near the sexual organs of the civet cat and used in perfume

civet cat *n* : any of several carnivorous mammals (family Viverridae); *esp* : a long-bodied short-legged African animal (*Civettictis civetta*) that produces most of the civet of commerce

civ·e·tone \'siv-ə-ˌtōn\ *n* : a crystalline ketone $C_{17}H_{30}O$ that constitutes the characteristic odorous constituent of civet and that is used in perfumes

CJD *abbr* Creutzfeldt-Jakob disease

CK *abbr* creatine kinase

cl *abbr* **1** centiliter **2** clavicle **3** clinic **4** closure

Cl *abbr* chloride

Cl *symbol* chlorine

CL *abbr* **1** chest and left arm **2** corpus luteum **3** critical list

CLA *abbr* certified laboratory assistant

Clad·o·spo·ri·um \ˌklad-ə-ˈspȯr-ē-əm, -ˈspȯr-\ *n* : a genus of imperfect fungi having conidia borne on branched conidiophores and the conidia with usu. one or in age two or three septa and including some economically important species — see BLACK SPOT

clair·au·di·ence \kla(ə)r-ˈȯd-ē-ən(t)s, kle(ə)r-, -ˈäd-\ *n* : the power or faculty of hearing something not present to the ear but regarded as having objective reality — **clair·au·di·ent** \-ənt\ *adj*

clair·voy·ance \kla(ə)r-ˈvȯi-ən(t)s, kle(ə)r-\ *n* : the power or faculty of discerning objects or matters not present to the senses — called also *cryptesthesia*

¹**clair·voy·ant** \-ənt\ *adj* : of or relating to clairvoyance

²**clairvoyant** *n* : one having the power of clairvoyance

clam·my \ˈklam-ē\ *adj* **clam·mi·er; -est** : being moist and sticky ⟨a patient in shock may be cold and ∼ —*Emergency Medicine*⟩ ⟨∼ sweating⟩

¹**clamp** \ˈklamp\ *n* : any of various instruments or appliances having parts brought together for holding or compressing something; *esp* : an instrument used to hold, compress, or crush vessels and hollow organs and to aid in surgical excision of parts ⟨an arterial ∼⟩

²**clamp** *vt* : to fasten with or as if with a clamp ⟨the descending thoracic aorta was ∼ed —W. A. Banks *et al*⟩

clang association \ˈklaŋ-\ *n* : word association (as in a psychological test) based on sound rather than meaning

clap \ˈklap\ *n* : GONORRHEA — often used with *the*

cla·rif·i·cant \klə-ˈrif-ə-kənt\ *n* : a substance that clears a liquid of turbidity

clar·i·fy \ˈklar-ə-ˌfī\ *vb* **-fied; -fy·ing** *vt* : to make (as a liquid) clear or pure usu. by freeing from suspended matter ⟨∼ sewage⟩ ∼ *vi* : to become clear — **clar·i·fi·ca·tion** \ˌklar-ə-fə-ˈkā-shən\ *n* — **clar·i·fi·er** \ˈklar-ə-ˌfī-(ə)r\ *n*

Clar·i·nex \ˈklar-ə-ˌneks\ *trademark* — used for a preparation of desloratadine

cla·rith·ro·my·cin \klə-ˌrith-rə-ˈmīs-ᵊn\ *n* : a semisynthetic macrolide antibiotic $C_{38}H_{69}NO_{13}$ used esp. in the treatment of various respiratory tract infections

Clar·i·tin \ˈklar-ə-ˌtin\ *trademark* — used for a preparation of loratadine

Clarke's column \ˈklärks-\ *n* : NUCLEUS DORSALIS

Clarke, Jacob Augustus Lockhart (1817–1880), British anatomist. Clarke devoted himself to research in microscopic anatomy. His most significant work was on the brain and spinal cord. In 1851 he published his description of the column of nerve cells that now bears his name. He is also known for his original description of syringomyelia, reported in 1867.

clas·mato·cyte \klaz-ˈmat-ə-ˌsīt\ *n* : MACROPHAGE — **clas·mato·cyt·ic** \(ˌ)klaz-ˌmat-ə-ˈsit-ik\ *adj*

clas·ma·to·sis \ˌklaz-mə-ˈtō-səs\ *n, pl* **-to·ses** \-ˌsēz\ : fragmentation esp. of cells

clasp \ˈklasp\ *n* : a device designed to encircle a tooth to hold a denture in place

class \ˈklas\ *n, often attrib* : a group, set, or kind marked by common attributes or a common attribute; *esp* : a major category in biological taxonomy ranking above the order and below the phylum or division ⟨the ∼ Mammalia⟩

clas·sic \ˈklas-ik\ *or* **clas·si·cal** \-i-kəl\ *adj* : standard or recognized esp. because of great frequency or consistency of occurrence ⟨the ∼ triad of urethritis, conjunctivitis, and arthritis signaling Reiter's syndrome —*Emergency Medicine*⟩

classical conditioning *n* : conditioning in which the conditioned stimulus (as the sound of a bell) is paired with and precedes the unconditioned stimulus (as the sight of food) until the conditioned stimulus alone is sufficient to elicit the response (as salivation in a dog) — compare OPERANT CONDITIONING

clas·si·fi·ca·tion \ˌklas-(ə)fə-ˈkā-shən\ *n* **1** : the act or process of classifying **2** : systematic arrangement of animals and plants in groups or categories according to established criteria; *specif* : TAXONOMY 2

clas·si·fy \ˈklas-ə-ˌfī\ *vt* **-fied; -fy·ing** : to arrange in classes that have systematic relations usu. founded on common properties ⟨how would you ∼ these animals⟩

clas·tic \ˈklas-tik\ *adj* : capable of being taken apart — used of anatomical models made of detachable pieces

¹**clath·rate** \ˈklath-ˌrāt\ *adj* : relating to or being a compound formed by the inclusion of molecules of one kind in cavities of the crystal lattice of another

²**clathrate** *n* : a clathrate compound

clath·rin \ˈklath-rin\ *n* : the major component protein of a cagelike polyhedral molecular arrangement that forms on the cytoplasmic side of a cell's plasma membrane and coats the endocytotic vesicles which bud off from the membrane

clau·di·ca·tion \ˌklȯd-ə-ˈkā-shən\ *n* **1** : the quality or state of being lame **2** : INTERMITTENT CLAUDICATION

claus·tro·phil·ia \ˌklȯ-strə-ˈfil-ē-ə\ *n* : an abnormal desire for confinement in an enclosed space

claus·tro·phobe \ˈklȯ-strə-ˌfōb\ *n* : one affected with claustrophobia

claus·tro·pho·bia \ˌklȯ-strə-ˈfō-bē-ə\ *n* : abnormal dread of being in closed or narrow spaces

¹**claus·tro·pho·bic** \ˌklȯ-strə-ˈfō-bik\ *adj* **1** : suffering from or inclined to claustrophobia **2** : inducing or suggesting claustrophobia — **claus·tro·pho·bi·cal·ly** \-bi-k(ə-)lē\ *adv*

²**claustrophobic** *n* : CLAUSTROPHOBE

claus·trum \ˈklȯ-strəm, ˈklau̇-\ *n, pl* **claus·tra** \-strə\ : the one of the four basal ganglia in each cerebral hemisphere that consists of a thin lamina of gray matter between the lentiform nucleus and the insula

cla·va \ˈklā-və, ˈkläv-ə\ *n, pl* **cla·vae** \ˈklā-vē, ˈkläv-ˌī\ : a clublike structure: as **a** : the fruiting body of some fungi **b** : a slight bulbous enlargement that forms part of the wall of the fourth ventricle of the brain and is the seat of a nucleus contributing axons to the lemniscus — **cla·val** \ˈklā-vəl, ˈkläv-əl\ *adj*

clav·a·cin \ˈklav-ə-sən, ˈkläv-\ *n* : PATULIN

cla·vate \ˈklā-ˌvāt\ *adj* : gradually thickening toward the distal end

clavi *pl of* CLAVUS

Clav·i·ceps \ˈklav-ə-ˌseps\ *n* : a genus of ascomycetous fungi (family Hypocreaceae) parasitic upon the ovaries of various grasses and forming characteristic sclerotia from which arise the ascus-bearing heads

clav·i·cle \ˈklav-i-kəl\ *n* : a bone of the pectoral girdle that links the scapula and sternum, is situated just above the first rib on either side of the neck, and has the form of a narrow elongated S — called also *collarbone* — **cla·vic·u·lar** \kla-ˈvik-yə-lər, klə-\ *adj*

cla·vic·u·la \klə-ˈvik-yə-lə, kla-\ *n, pl* **-u·lae** \-ˌlē, -ˌlī\ : CLAVICLE

clavicular notch *n* : a notch on each side of the upper part of the manubrium that is the site of articulation with a clavicle

cla·vic·u·lec·to·my \kla-ˌvik-yə-ˈlek-tə-mē, klə-\ *n, pl* **-mies** : surgical removal of all or part of a clavicle

clav·i·form \ˈklav-ə-ˌfȯrm\ *adj* : shaped like a club

clav·i·for·min \ˌklav-i-ˈfȯr-mən, ˌkläv-\ *n* : PATULIN

clav·u·la·nate \ˈklav-yə-lə-ˌnāt\ *n* : a salt of clavulanic acid

clav·u·lan·ic acid \ˌklav-yə-ˌlan-ik-\ *n* : a beta-lactam antibiotic $C_8H_9NO_5$ produced by a bacterium of the genus *Streptomyces* (*S. clavuligerus*) that is a beta-lactamase inhibitor and is usu. used in the form of its clavulanate salt of potassium esp. in combination with amoxicillin — see AUGMENTIN

cla·vus \ˈklā-vəs, ˈkläv-əs\ *n, pl* **cla·vi** \ˈklā-ˌvī, ˈkläv-ˌē\ : CORN

claw \ˈklȯ\ *n* : a sharp usu. slender and curved nail on the toe of an animal — **clawed** \ˈklȯd\ *adj*

claw foot *n* : a deformity of the foot characterized by an exaggerated curvature of the longitudinal arch

claw hand *n* : a deformity of the hand characterized by extreme extension of the wrist and the first phalanges and extreme flexion of the other phalanges

---

\ə\ **abut** \ᵊ\ **kitten** \ər\ **further** \a\ **ash** \ā\ **ace** \ä\ **cot, cart** \au̇\ **out** \ch\ **chin** \e\ **bet** \ē\ **easy** \g\ **go** \i\ **hit** \ī\ **ice** \j\ **job** \ŋ\ **sing** \ō\ **go** \ȯ\ **law** \ȯi\ **boy** \th\ **thin** \th̲\ **the** \ü\ **loot** \u̇\ **foot** \y\ **yet** \zh\ **vision** *See also* Pronunciation Symbols page

claw toe *n* : HAMMERTOE

Clay·ton gas \\'klāt-ᵊn-\ *n* : a poisonous gas mixture used on ships for exterminating vermin

Clayton, T. A., 19th-century British chemist who invented the apparatus for generating the gas known as Clayton gas.

¹**clean** \\'klēn\ *adj* **1 a** : free from dirt or pollution **b** : free from disease or infectious agents ⟨a pullorum-*clean* flock⟩ ⟨keep installations ∼ of TB infection⟩ **2** : free from smudges or anything that tends to obscure ⟨a ∼ set of fingerprints⟩ **3** *of a horse's leg* : free from curbs or bunches below the hock **4** : free from drug addiction

²**clean** *vt* **1** : to brush (the teeth) with a cleanser (as a dentifrice) **2** : to perform dental prophylaxis on (the teeth)

clean bill of health *n* : a bill of health certifying absence of infectious disease

cleanse \\'klenz\ *vt* **cleansed; cleans·ing** : to make clean

cleans·er \\'klen-zər\ *n* : a preparation including a cleaning agent for cleansing the skin, the teeth, or glass surfaces

¹**clear** \\'kli(ə)r\ *adj* **1** *of the skin or complexion* : good in texture and color and without blemish or discoloration **b** *of an animal coat* : of uniform shade without spotting **2** : free from abnormal sounds on auscultation

²**clear** *vt* **1** : to render (a specimen for microscopic examination) transparent by the use of an agent (as an essential oil) that modifies the index of refraction **2** : to rid (the throat) of phlegm or of something that makes the voice indistinct or husky

clear·ance \\'klir-ən(t)s\ *n* : the volume of blood or plasma that could be freed of a specified constituent in a specified time (usu. one minute) by excretion of the constituent into the urine through the kidneys — called also *renal clearance*

clearing agent *n* : any substance used to clear a specimen or preparation for microscopic examination

cleav·age \\'klē-vij\ *n* **1** : the series of synchronized mitotic cell divisions of the fertilized egg that results in the formation of the blastomeres and changes the single-celled zygote into a multicellular embryo; *also* : one of these cell divisions **2** : the splitting of a molecule into simpler molecules

cleavage cell *n* : BLASTOMERE

cleave \\'klēv\ *vt* **cleaved; cleav·ing** : to subject to chemical cleavage ⟨a protein *cleaved* by an enzyme⟩

cleft \\'kleft\ *n* **1** : a usu. abnormal fissure or opening esp. when resulting from failure of parts to fuse during embryonic development **2** : a usu. V-shaped indented formation : a hollow between ridges or protuberances ⟨the anal ∼ of the human body⟩ **3** : the hollow space between the two branches of the frog or the frog and bars or between the bulbs of the heel of a horse's hoof **4** : a crack on the bend of the pastern of a horse **5** : a division of the cleft foot of an animal **6** : SYNAPTIC CLEFT

cleft lip *n* : a birth defect characterized by one or more clefts in the upper lip resulting from failure of the embryonic parts of the lip to unite — called also *cheiloschisis, harelip*

cleft palate *n* : congenital fissure of the roof of the mouth produced by failure of the two maxillae to unite during embryonic development and often associated with cleft lip — called also *palatoschisis*

clei·do·cra·ni·al dysostosis \\ˌklī-dō-ˈkrā-nē-əl-\ *n* : a rare condition inherited as an autosomal dominant and characterized esp. by partial or complete absence of the clavicles, defective ossification of the skull, and faulty occlusion due to missing, misplaced, or supernumerary teeth

clei·do·ic \\klī-ˈdō-ik\ *adj, of an egg* : enclosed in a relatively impervious shell which reduces free exchange with the environment ⟨the eggs of birds are ∼⟩

clei·dot·o·my \\klī-ˈdät-ə-mē\ *n, pl* **-o·mies** : surgical division of the clavicles to effect delivery of a fetus with broad shoulders

cleis·to·the·ci·um \\ˌklīs-tə-ˈthē-sē-əm\ *n, pl* **-cia** \-sē-ə\ : a closed spore-bearing structure in some ascomycetous fungi from which the asci and spores are released only by decay or disintegration — **cleis·to·the·ci·al** \-sē-əl\ *adj*

clem·as·tine \\'klem-ə-ˌstēn\ *n* : an antihistamine administered in the form of its fumarate $C_{21}H_{26}ClNO \cdot C_4H_4O_4$

cle·oid \\'klē-ˌóid\ *n* : a dental excavator with a claw-shaped working point

clerk \\'klərk\ *n* : a third- or fourth-year medical student undergoing clinical training in a clerkship — **clerk** *vi*

clerk·ship \-ˌship\ *n* : a course of clinical medical training in a specialty (as pediatrics, internal medicine, or psychiatry) that usu. lasts a minimum of several weeks and takes place during the third or fourth year of medical school ⟨third-year medical study involves ∼s in five areas, of which surgery is among the most arduous —*N.Y. Times Mag.*⟩

click \\'klik\ *n* : a short sharp sound heard in auscultation and associated with various abnormalities of the heart

¹**cli·mac·ter·ic** \\klī-ˈmak-t(ə-)rik, ˌklī-ˌmak-ˈter-ik\ *adj* : constituting or characterized by the climacteric ⟨the ∼ state⟩

²**climacteric** *n* **1** : MENOPAUSE 1a(2) **2** : ANDROPAUSE

cli·mac·te·ri·um \\ˌklī-ˌmak-ˈtir-ē-əm\ *n, pl* **-ria** \-ē-ə\ : the bodily and psychic changes accompanying the transition from middle life to old age; *specif* : menopause and the bodily and mental changes that accompany it

cli·mac·tic \\klī-ˈmak-tik\ *adj* : of, relating to, or constituting a climax

cli·ma·tol·o·gy \\ˌklī-mə-ˈtäl-ə-jē\ *n, pl* **-gies** : the science that deals with climates and their phenomena — **cli·ma·to·log·i·cal** \\ˌklī-mət-ᵊl-ˈäj-i-kəl\ *adj* — **cli·ma·to·log·i·cal·ly** \-k(ə-)lē\ *adv* — **cli·ma·tol·o·gist** \\ˌklī-mə-ˈtäl-ə-jəst\ *n*

cli·ma·to·ther·a·py \\ˌklī-mət-ō-ˈther-ə-pē\ *n, pl* **-pies** : treatment of disease by means of residence in a suitable climate

cli·max \\'klī-ˌmaks\ *n* **1** : the highest or most intense point **2** : ORGASM **3 a** : MENOPAUSE 1a(2) **b** : ANDROPAUSE

clin *abbr* clinical

clin·da·my·cin \\ˌklin-də-ˈmīs-ᵊn\ *n* : an antibiotic $C_{18}H_{33}$-ClN_2O_5S derived from and used similarly to lincomycin

clin·ic \\'klin-ik\ *n* **1 a** : a session or class of medical instruction in a hospital held at the bedside of patients serving as case studies **b** : a group of selected patients presented with discussion before doctors (as at a convention) for purposes of instruction **2 a** : an institution connected with a hospital or medical school where diagnosis and treatment are made available to outpatients **b** : a form of group practice in which several physicians (as specialists) work in cooperative association

clin·i·cal \\'klin-i-kəl\ *adj* **1** : of, relating to, or conducted in or as if in a clinic: **a** : involving or concerned with the direct observation and treatment of living patients ⟨engaged in full-time ∼ practice⟩ ⟨∼ professor of obstetrics and gynecology⟩ **b** : of, relating to, based on, or characterized by observable and diagnosable symptoms of disease ⟨the ∼ picture on admission was that of mild depression in an extremely rigid personality —*Occupational Therapy & Rehabilitation*⟩ ⟨three of these six foods were actually the cause of symptoms, and upon their elimination, ∼ cure was effected —*Jour. of Pediatrics*⟩ **c** : applying objective or standardized methods (as interviews and personality or intelligence tests) to the description, evaluation, and modification of human behavior ⟨∼ psychology⟩ **2** *of a sacrament* : administered on a sickbed or deathbed ⟨∼ baptism⟩ — **clin·i·cal·ly** \-k(ə-)lē\ *adv*

clinical crown *n* : the part of a tooth that projects above the gums

clinical depression *n* : depression of sufficient severity to be brought to the attention of a physician and to require treatment; *specif* : MAJOR DEPRESSIVE DISORDER

clinical thermometer *n* : a thermometer for measuring body temperature that has a constriction in the tube above the bulb preventing movement of the column of liquid downward once it has reached its maximum temperature so that it continues to indicate the maximum temperature until the liquid is shaken back down into the bulb — called also *fever thermometer*

clinical trial *n* : a scientifically controlled study of the safety and effectiveness of a therapeutic agent (as a drug or vaccine) using consenting human subjects

cli·ni·cian \\klin-ˈish-ən\ *n* : an individual qualified in the clinical practice of medicine, psychiatry, or psychology as distinguished from one specializing in laboratory or research techniques or in theory

clin·i·co·path·o·log·ic \'klin-i-(,)kō-,path-ə-'läj-ik\ *or* **clin·i·co·path·o·log·i·cal** \-'läj-i-kəl\ *adj* : relating to or concerned both with the signs and symptoms directly observable by the physician and with the results of laboratory examination ⟨a ~ study of the patient⟩ — **clin·i·co·path·o·log·i·cal·ly** \-i-k(ə-)lē\ *adv*

cli·no·dac·ty·ly \,klī-nō-'dak-tə-lē\ *n, pl* **-ty·lies** : a deformity of the hand marked by deviation or deflection of the fingers

cli·noid process \'klī-,nóid-\ *n* : any of several processes of the sphenoid bone

clip \'klip\ *n* : a device used to arrest bleeding from vessels or tissues during operations

clit·i·on \'klit-ē-,än\ *n, pl* **clit·ia** \-ē-ə\ : the median point of the anterior margin of the clivus

clit·o·ri·dec·to·my \,klit-ə-rə-'dek-tə-mē\ *also* **clit·o·rec·to·my** \-'rek-tə-mē\ *n, pl* **-mies** : excision of all or part of the clitoris

clitoridis — see GLANS CLITORIDIS, PREPUTIUM CLITORIDIS

clit·o·ris \'klit-ə-rəs, kli-'tór-əs\ *n, pl* **clit·o·ri·des** \kli-'tór-ə-,dēz\ : a small erectile organ at the anterior or ventral part of the vulva homologous to the penis — **clit·o·ral** \'klit-ə-rəl\ *also* **clit·or·ic** \kli-'tór-ik, -'tär-\ *adj*

cli·vus \'klī-vəs\ *n, pl* **cli·vi** \-,vī\ : the smooth sloping surface on the upper posterior part of the body of the sphenoid bone supporting the pons and the basilar artery

CLL *abbr* chronic lymphocytic leukemia

clo·aca \klō-'ā-kə\ *n, pl* **-acae** \-,kē, -,sē\ **1 a** : the common chamber into which the intestinal, urinary, and generative canals discharge esp. in monotreme mammals, birds, reptiles, amphibians, and elasmobranch fishes **b** : the terminal part of the embryonic hindgut of a mammal before it divides into rectum, bladder, and genital precursors **2** : a passage in a bone leading to a cavity containing a sequestrum — **clo·acal** \-'ā-kəl\ *adj*

cloacal membrane *n* : a plate of fused embryonic ectoderm and endoderm closing the fetal anus

clo·a·ci·tis \,klō-ə-'sīt-əs\ *n* : a chronic inflammatory process of the cloaca of the domestic chicken that is of undetermined cause but is apparently transmitted by copulation — called also *vent gleet*

clo·be·ta·sol \klō-'bāt-ə-,sól\ *n* : a potent synthetic corticosteroid that is used topically in the form of its propionate $C_{25}H_{32}ClFO_5$ esp. to treat inflammatory skin conditions

clock \'kläk\ *n* : BIOLOGICAL CLOCK

clo·faz·i·mine \klō-'faz-ə-,mēn, -mən\ *n* : a reddish brown powdered dye $C_{27}H_{22}Cl_2N_4$ that is a derivative of phenazine used esp. to treat lepromatous leprosy and to treat tuberculosis in AIDS patients caused by bacteria of the Mycobacterium avium complex

clo·fi·brate \klō-'fīb-,rāt, -'fib-\ *n* : a synthetic drug $C_{12}H_{15}ClO_3$ used esp. to lower abnormally high concentrations of fats and cholesterol in the blood

Clo·mid \'klō-mid\ *trademark* — used for a preparation of the citrate of clomiphene

clo·mi·phene \'kläm-ə-,fēn, 'klōm-\ *n* : a synthetic drug used in the form of its citrate $C_{26}H_{28}ClNO \cdot C_6H_8O_7$ to induce ovulation — see CLOMID

clo·mip·ra·mine \klō-'mip-rə-,mēn\ *n* : a tricyclic antidepressant used in the form of its hydrochloride $C_{19}H_{23}ClN_2 \cdot HCl$ to treat obsessive-compulsive disorder

clo·naz·e·pam \(,)klō-'naz-ə-,pam\ *n* : a benzodiazepine $C_{15}H_{10}ClN_3O_3$ used esp. as an anticonvulsant in the treatment of epilepsy

¹clone \'klōn\ *n* **1** : the aggregate of the asexually produced progeny of an individual; *also* : a group of replicas of all or part of a macromolecule (as DNA or an antibody) **2** : an individual grown from a single somatic cell of its parent and genetically identical to it — **clon·al** \'klōn-⁹l\ *adj* — **clon·al·ly** \-⁹l-ē\ *adv*

²clone *vb* **cloned; clon·ing** *vt* : to propagate a clone from

⟨frogs have been successfully *cloned* by transplanting nuclei from body cells to enucleated eggs⟩ ~ *vi* : to produce a clone

clon·ic \'klän-ik\ *adj* : exhibiting, relating to, or involving clonus ⟨~ contraction⟩ ⟨~ spasm⟩ — **clo·nic·i·ty** \klō-'nis-ət-ē, klä-\ *n, pl* **-ties**

clon·i·co·ton·ic \,klän-i-kō-'tän-ik\ *adj* : being both clonic and tonic ⟨~ convulsions⟩

clo·ni·dine \'klän-ə-,dēn, 'klōn-, -,dīn\ *n* : an antihypertensive drug used in the form of its hydrochloride $C_9H_9Cl_2N_3 \cdot HCl$ esp. to treat essential hypertension, to prevent migraine headache, and to diminish opiate withdrawal symptoms

clo·nism \'klō-,niz-əm, 'klän-,iz-\ *n* : the condition of being affected with clonus

clo·nor·chi·a·sis \,klō-nór-'kī-ə-səs\ *also* **clo·nor·chi·o·sis** \-(,)nór-kē-'ō-səs\ *n, pl* **-a·ses** \-,sēz\ *also* **-o·ses** \-,sēz\ : infestation with or disease caused by the Chinese liver fluke (*Clonorchis sinensis*) that invades bile ducts of the liver after ingestion in uncooked fish and when present in numbers causes severe systemic reactions including edema, liver enlargement, and diarrhea

Clo·nor·chis \klō-'nór-kəs\ *n* : a genus of trematode worms of the family Opisthorchiidae that includes the Chinese liver fluke (*C. sinensis*)

clo·nus \'klō-nəs\ *n* : a series of alternating contractions and partial relaxations of a muscle that in some nervous diseases occurs in the form of convulsive spasms involving complex groups of muscles and is believed to result from alteration of the normal pattern of motor neuron discharge — compare TONUS 2

clo·pid·o·grel \klō-'pid-ə-,grel\ *n* : an antithrombotic agent that is administered in the form of its bisulfate $C_{16}H_{16}ClNO_2S \cdot H_2SO_4$ and inhibits ADP-induced aggregation of platelets — see PLAVIX

clor·az·e·pate \,klór-'az-ə-,pāt, ,klór-\ *n* : a benzodiazepine dipotassium salt $C_{16}H_{10}ClKN_2O_3 \cdot KOH$ administered orally to treat anxiety, partial seizures, and acute alcohol withdrawal — called also *clorazepate dipotassium;* see TRANXENE

closed \'klōzd\ *adj* **1** : being a complete self-contained system with nothing transferred in or out ⟨a ~ thermodynamic system⟩ **2** : covered by unbroken skin ⟨a ~ fracture⟩ **3** : not discharging pathogenic organisms to the outside ⟨a case of ~ tuberculosis⟩ — compare OPEN 2

closed–angle glaucoma *n* : ANGLE-CLOSURE GLAUCOMA

closed reduction *n* : the reduction of a displaced part (as a fractured bone) by manipulation without incision — compare OPEN REDUCTION

clos·trid·i·um \kläs-'trid-ē-əm\ *n* **1** *cap* : a genus of saprophytic rod-shaped or spindle-shaped usu. gram-positive bacteria of the family Bacillaceae that are anaerobic or require very little free oxygen and are nearly cosmopolitan in soil, water, sewage, and animal and human intestines, that are very active biochemically comprising numerous fermenters of carbohydrates with vigorous production of acid and gas, many nitrogen-fixers, and others which rapidly putrefy proteins, and that include important pathogens — see BLACKLEG, BOTULISM, GAS GANGRENE, TETANUS BACILLUS **2** *pl* **clos·trid·ia** \-ē-ə\ **a** : any bacterium of the genus *Clostridium* **b** : a spindle-shaped or ovoid bacterial cell; *esp* : one swollen at the center by an endospore — **clos·trid·i·al** \-ē-əl\ *adj*

clo·sure \'klō-zhər\ *n* **1 a** : an act of closing up or condition of being closed up ⟨~ of the eyelids⟩ ⟨early ~ of fontanels and sutures —W. A. D. Anderson⟩ **b** : a drawing together of edges or parts to form a united integument ⟨wound ~ by

---

\ə\ **abut** \⁹\ **kitten** \ər\ **further** \a\ **ash** \ā\ **ace** \ä\ **cot, cart** \aú\ **out** \ch\ **chin** \e\ **bet** \ē\ **easy** \g\ **go** \i\ **hit** \ī\ **ice** \j\ **job** \ŋ\ **sing** \ō\ **go** \ó\ **law** \ói\ **boy** \th\ **thin** \th\ **the** \ü\ **loot** \ú\ **foot** \y\ **yet** \zh\ **vision** *See also* Pronunciation Symbols page

suture immediately after laceration⟩ **2** : a cap, lid, or stopper for sealing a container (as a serum vial) **3** : the perception of incomplete figures or situations as though complete by ignoring the missing parts or by compensating for them by projection based on past experience **4** : an often comforting or satisfying sense of finality ⟨therapy brought ~ to the victim's family⟩

¹**clot** \'klät\ *n* : a coagulated mass produced by clotting of blood

²**clot** *vb* **clot·ted; clot·ting** *vi* : to undergo a sequence of complex chemical and physical reactions that results in conversion of fluid blood into a coagulum and that involves shedding of blood, release of thromboplastin from blood platelets and injured tissues, inactivation of heparin by thromboplastin permitting calcium ions of the plasma to convert prothrombin to thrombin, interaction of thrombin with fibrinogen to form an insoluble fibrin network in which blood cells and plasma are trapped, and contraction of the network to squeeze out excess fluid : COAGULATE ~ *vt* : to cause to form into or as if into a clot

clot–bust·er \'klät-ˌbəs-tər\ *n* : a drug (as streptokinase or tissue plasminogen activator) used to dissolve blood clots — **clot–bust·ing** \-tiŋ\ *adj*

clot retraction *n* : the process by which a blood clot becomes smaller and draws the edges of a broken blood vessel together and which involves the shortening of fibrin threads and the squeezing out of excess serum

clo·tri·ma·zole \klō-'trī-mə-ˌzōl, -ˌzȯl\ *n* : an antifungal agent $C_{22}H_{17}ClN_2$ used to treat candida infections, tinea, and ringworm — see LOTRIMIN

clot·ting factor \'klät-iŋ-\ *n* : any of several plasma components (as fibrinogen, prothrombin, and thromboplastin) that are involved in the clotting of blood — see FACTOR VIII, PLASMA THROMBOPLASTIN ANTECEDENT, TRANSGLUTAMINASE; compare FACTOR V, FACTOR VII, FACTOR IX, FACTOR X, FACTOR XII, FACTOR XIII

clove \'klōv\ *n* **1 a** : the pungent fragrant aromatic reddish brown dried flower bud of a tropical evergreen tree (*Syzygium aromaticum*) of the myrtle family (Myrtaceae) that yields clove oil **b** : a spice consisting of whole or ground cloves — usu. used in pl. **2** : the tree that is the source of cloves and is prob. native to the Moluccas but is now widely cultivated in the tropics

clo·ven foot \ˌklō-vən-\ *n* : a foot (as of a sheep) divided into two parts at its distal extremity — **clo·ven–foot·ed** \-'fut-əd\ *adj*

cloven hoof *n* : CLOVEN FOOT — **clo·ven–hoofed** \-'huft, -'huft, -'huvd, -'huvd\ *adj*

clove oil *n* : a colorless to pale yellow essential oil that is obtained from cloves, is a source of eugenol, has a powerful germicidal action, and is used topically to relieve toothache

clover disease *n* : an acute photosensitization of white or light-skinned animals feeding on leguminous plants and esp. clovers — called also *trifoliosis*

clo·ver·leaf skull \'klō-vər-ˌlēf-\ *n* : a birth defect in which some or all of the usu. separate bones of the skull have grown together resulting in a 3-lobed skull with associated deformities of the features and skeleton — called also *kleeblattschädel*

clown·ism \'klau̇-ˌniz-əm\ *n* : an abnormal emotional display accompanied by grotesque actions (as in hystero-epilepsy)

clox·a·cil·lin \ˌkläk-sə-'sil-ən\ *n* : a semisynthetic oral penicillin $C_{19}H_{17}ClN_3NaO_5S$ effective esp. against staphylococci which secrete beta-lactamase — see TEGOPEN

clo·za·pine \'klō-zə-ˌpēn\ *n* : an antipsychotic drug $C_{18}H_{19}ClN_4$ with serious side effects (as seizures and agranulocytosis) that is used in the management of schizophrenia — see CLOZARIL

Clo·za·ril \'klō-zə-ril\ *trademark* — used for a preparation of clozapine

clubbed \'kləbd\ *adj* **1** : having a bulbous enlargement of the tip with convex overhanging nail ⟨a ~ finger⟩ **2** : affected with clubfoot

club·bing \'kləb-iŋ\ *n* : the condition of being clubbed ⟨~ of the fingers and toes⟩

club·foot \'kləb-ˌfut\ *n, pl* **club·feet** \-ˌfēt\ **1** : any of numerous congenital deformities of the foot in which it is twisted out of position or shape — called also *talipes;* compare TALIPES EQUINOVARUS, TALIPES EQUINUS, TALIPES VALGUS, TALIPES VARUS **2** : a foot affected with clubfoot — **club·foot·ed** \-'fut-əd\ *adj*

club fungus \'kləb-\ *n* : any of a family (Clavariaceae) of basidiomycetes with a simple or branched often club-shaped sporophore

club·hand \-ˌhand\ *n* **1** : a congenital deformity in which the hand is short and distorted **2** : a hand affected with club-hand

club moss *n* : any of an order (Lycopodiales) of primitive vascular plants including several (genus *Lycopodium*) whose spores are used as a dusting powder and to coat pills

¹**clump** \'kləmp\ *n* : a clustered mass of particles (as bacteria or blood cells) — compare AGGLUTINATION

²**clump** *vi* : to form clumps ~ *vt* : to arrange in or cause to form clumps ⟨the serum ~s the bacteria⟩

clu·pe·ine \'klü-pē-ən, -ˌēn\ *also* **clu·pe·in** \-ən\ *n* : a protamine contained in the spermatozoa of the herring

clus·ter \'kləs-tər\ *n* : a larger than expected number of cases of disease (as leukemia) occurring in a particular locality, group of people, or period of time

cluster headache *n* : a headache that is characterized by severe unilateral pain in the eye or temple, affects primarily men, and tends to recur in a series of attacks — called also *histamine cephalalgia, histamine cephalgia, Horton's syndrome*

clut·ter·ing \'klət-ə-riŋ\ *n* : a speech defect in which phonetic units are dropped, condensed, or otherwise distorted as a result of overly rapid agitated utterance

Clut·ton's joints \ˌklət-ᵊnz-\ *n pl* : symmetrical hydrarthrosis esp. of the knees or elbows that occurs in congenital syphilis

Clutton, Henry Hugh (1850–1909), British surgeon. Clutton's major area of interest concerned diseases of the bones and joints. In 1886 he published his single major paper, describing a malady of the knee that occurs in children who have congenital syphilis. The condition has since become known as Clutton's joints.

cly·sis \'klī-səs\ *n, pl* **cly·ses** \-ˌsēz\ : the introduction of large amounts of fluid into the body usu. by parenteral injection to replace that lost (as from hemorrhage or in dysentery or burns), to provide nutrients, or to maintain blood pressure — see HYPODERMOCLYSIS, PHLEBOCLYSIS, PROCTOCLYSIS

clys·ma \'kliz-mə\ *n, pl* **-ma·ta** \-mət-ə\ : ENEMA

clys·ter \'klis-tər\ *n* : ENEMA

cm *abbr* centimeter

Cm *symbol* curium

CM *abbr* **1** [Latin *Chirurgiae Magister*] Master of Surgery **2** circular muscle

CMA *abbr* certified medical assistant

CMHC *abbr* Community Mental Health Center

CML *abbr* chronic myelocytic leukemia; chronic myelogenous leukemia; chronic myeloid leukemia

CMV *abbr* cytomegalovirus

CN *abbr* chloroacetophenone

CNA *abbr* certified nurse's aide

cne·mi·al \'nē-mē-əl\ *adj* : relating to the shin or shinbone

cne·mis \'nē-məs\ *n, pl* **cnem·i·des** \'nem-ə-ˌdēz\ : SHIN, TIBIA

Cni·dar·ia \nī-'dar-ē-ə\ *n pl* : a phylum of more or less radially symmetrical invertebrate animals that lack a true body cavity, possess tentacles studded with nematocysts, and include the hydroids, jellyfishes, sea anemones, and corals — **cni·dar·i·an** \-ē-ən\ *n* : COELENTERATE — **cnidarian** *adj*

cni·do·blast \'nid-ə-ˌblast\ *n* : a cell of a coelenterate that develops a nematocyst or develops into a nematocyst

CNM *abbr* certified nurse-midwife

CNP *abbr* continuous negative pressure

CNS *abbr* central nervous system

Co *abbr* coenzyme

Co *symbol* cobalt

CO *abbr* cardiac output

c/o *abbr* complains of

co·ac·er·vate \kō-'as-ər-ˌvāt\ *n* : an aggregate of colloidal droplets held together by electrostatic attractive forces — **co·ac·er·va·tion** \(ˌ)kō-ˌas-ər-'vā-shən\ *n*

co·adapt·ed \ˌkō-ə-'dap-təd\ *adj* : mutually adapted esp. by natural selection ⟨∼ gene complexes⟩ — **co·ad·ap·ta·tion** \ˌkō-ˌad-ˌap-'tā-shən, -əp-\ *n*

co·ad·min·is·tra·tion \ˌkō-əd-ˌmin-ə-'strā-shən, -(ˌ)ad-\ *n* : the administration of two or more drugs together — **co·ad·min·is·ter** \-'min-ə-stər\ *vt*

coag *abbr* coagulate; coagulation

coag time *abbr* coagulation time

coagula *pl of* COAGULUM

co·ag·u·lant \kō-'ag-yə-lənt\ *n* : something that produces coagulation

co·ag·u·lase \kō-'ag-yə-ˌlās, -ˌlāz\ *n* : any of several enzymes that cause coagulation (as of blood)

¹**co·ag·u·late** \kō-'ag-yə-ˌlāt\ *vb* **-lat·ed; -lat·ing** *vt* **1** : to cause to become viscous or thickened into a coherent mass : CLOT ⟨blood platelets that ∼ blood —Sonni Efron⟩ ⟨rennin ∼s milk⟩ **2** : to subject to coagulation ⟨high-frequency radio waves used to cut and ∼ tissue —Alan Goldstein⟩ ∼ *vi* : to become coagulated : undergo coagulation — **co·ag·u·la·bil·i·ty** \kō-ˌag-yə-lə-'bil-ət-ē\ *n* — **co·ag·u·la·ble** \-'ag-yə-lə-bəl\ *adj*

²**co·ag·u·late** \-lət, -ˌlāt\ *n* : COAGULUM

co·ag·u·la·tion \kō-ˌag-yə-'lā-shən\ *n* **1 a** : a change to a viscous, jellylike, or solid state; *esp* : a change from a liquid to a thickened curdlike state not by evaporation but by chemical reaction ⟨the spontaneous ∼ of freshly drawn blood⟩ ⟨the ∼ of milk by rennin⟩ **b** : the process by which such change of state takes place consisting of the alteration of a soluble substance (as a protein) into an insoluble form or of the flocculation or separation of colloidal or suspended matter **2** : a substance or body formed by coagulation : COAGULUM **3** : disruption of tissue by physical means (as by application of an electric current) so that denaturation and clumping of protein occur ⟨diathermic ∼ of tissues during surgery to seal bleeding blood vessels⟩ — see ELECTROCOAGULATION, PHOTOCOAGULATION

coagulation time *n* : the time required by shed blood to clot that is a measure of the normality of the blood

co·ag·u·la·tor \kō-'ag-yə-ˌlāt-ər\ *n* : an agent that causes coagulation — **co·ag·u·la·to·ry** \-lə-ˌtōr-ē, -ˌtòr-\ *adj*

co·ag·u·lin \kō-'ag-yə-lən\ *n* **1** : PRECIPITIN **2 a** : a postulated tissue constituent able to induce conversion of fibrinogen to fibrin in the absence of prothrombin or thrombin **b** : THROMBOPLASTIN

co·ag·u·lom·e·ter \kō-ˌag-yə-'läm-ət-ər\ *n* : an apparatus for measuring the time required for a sample of fluid (as blood) to coagulate

co·ag·u·lop·a·thy \-'läp-ə-thē\ *n, pl* **-thies** : a disease or condition affecting the blood's ability to coagulate

co·ag·u·lum \kō-'ag-yə-ləm\ *n, pl* **-u·la** \-lə\ *or* **-u·lums** : a coagulated mass or substance : CLOT

co·alesce \ˌkō-ə-'les\ *vi* **co·alesced; co·alesc·ing** : to grow together — **co·ales·cence** \-'les-ᵊn(t)s\ *n*

coal tar \'kōl-\ *n* : tar obtained by distillation of bituminous coal and used in the treatment of some skin diseases by direct local application to the skin

co·apt \kō-'apt\ *vt* : to close or fasten together : cause to adhere ⟨the margins of the wound were then closely ∼ed with sutures —*Biol. Abstracts*⟩

co·ap·ta·tion \(ˌ)kō-ˌap-'tā-shən\ *n* : the adaptation or adjustment of parts to each other : the joining or fitting together (as of the ends of a broken bone or the edges of a wound)

co·arct \kō-'ärkt\ *vt* : to cause (the aorta) to become narrow or (the heart) to constrict

co·arc·ta·tion \(ˌ)kō-ˌärk-'tā-shən\ *n* : a stricture or narrowing esp. of a canal or vessel (as the aorta)

coarse \'kō(ə)rs, 'kò(ə)rs\ *adj* **1** : visible to the naked eye or by means of a compound microscope ⟨∼ particles⟩ **2** *of a tremor* : of wide excursion ⟨a ∼ tremor of the extremities⟩ **3** : harsh, raucous, or rough in tone — used of some sounds heard in auscultation in pathological states of the chest ⟨∼ rales⟩

coat \'kōt\ *n* **1** : the external growth on an animal **2** : a layer of one substance covering or lining another; *esp* : one covering or lining an organ ⟨the ∼ of the eyeball⟩

coat·ed \-əd\ *adj, of the tongue* : covered with a yellowish white deposit of desquamated cells, bacteria, and debris usu. as an accompaniment of digestive disorder

Coats's disease \'kōts-, 'kōt-səz-\ *n* : a chronic inflammatory disease of the eye that is characterized by white or yellow areas around the optic disk due to edematous accumulation under the retina and that leads to destruction of the macula and to blindness

> **Coats, George (1876–1915),** British ophthalmologist. In 1908 Coats published the first description of the inflammatory condition of the eye that results from hemorrhage under the retina and is now known by his name.

co·bal·a·min \kō-'bal-ə-mən\ *also* **co·bal·a·mine** \-ˌmēn\ *n* : VITAMIN B₁₂

co·balt \'kō-ˌbòlt\ *n* : a tough lustrous silver-white magnetic metallic element that is related to and occurs with iron and nickel and is used esp. in alloys — symbol *Co*; see ELEMENT table

co·bal·tic \kō-'bòl-tik\ *adj* : of, relating to, or containing cobalt esp. with a valence of three

co·bal·tous \kō-'bòl-təs\ *adj* : of, relating to, or containing cobalt esp. with a valence of two

cobalt 60 \-'sik-stē\ *n* : a heavy radioactive isotope of cobalt having the mass number 60 produced in nuclear reactors and used as a source of gamma rays esp. in place of radium (as in the treatment of cancer and in radiography) — called also *radiocobalt*

co·bra \'kō-brə\ *n* **1** : any of several very venomous Asian and African elapid snakes of the genera *Naja* and *Ophiophagus* that when excited expand the skin of the neck into a broad hood by movement of the anterior ribs — see INDIAN COBRA, KING COBRA **2** : either of two African snakes that spit their venom from a distance: **a** : BLACK-NECKED COBRA **b** : RINGHALS **3** : MAMBA

COC *abbr* cathodal opening contraction

co·ca \'kō-kə\ *n* **1** : any of several So. American shrubs (genus *Erythroxylon* of the family Erythroxylaceae); *esp* : one (*E. coca*) that is the primary source of cocaine **2** : dried leaves of a coca (as *Erythroxylon coca*) containing alkaloids including cocaine

co·caine \kō-'kān, 'kō-ˌ\ *n* : a bitter crystalline alkaloid C₁₇H₂₁NO₄ obtained from coca leaves that is used medically esp. in the form of its hydrochloride C₁₇H₂₁NO₄·HCl as a topical anesthetic and illicitly for its euphoric effects and that may result in a compulsive psychological need

co·cain·ism \kō-'kā-ˌniz-əm\ *n* : habituation to cocaine

co·cain·ize *or Brit* **co·cain·ise** \kō-'kā-ˌnīz\ *vt* **-ized** *or Brit* **-ised; -iz·ing** *or Brit* **-is·ing** : to treat or anesthetize with cocaine — **co·cain·iza·tion** *or Brit* **co·cain·isa·tion** \-ˌkā-nə-'zā-shən\ *n*

co·car·box·yl·ase \ˌkō-kär-'bäk-sə-ˌlās, -ˌlāz\ *n* : a coenzyme C₁₂H₁₉ClN₄O₇P₂S·H₂O that is important in metabolic reactions (as decarboxylation in the Krebs cycle) — called also *thiamine pyrophosphate*

co·car·cin·o·gen \ˌkō-kär-'sin-ə-jən, kō-'kärs-ᵊn-ə-ˌjen\ *n* : an agent that aggravates the carcinogenic effects of another substance — **co·car·cin·o·gen·ic** \ˌkō-ˌkärs-ᵊn-ō-'jen-ik\ *adj*

coc·cal \'käk-əl\ *adj* : of or relating to a coccus

cocci *pl of* COCCUS

---

coc·cid·ia \käk-'sid-ē-ə\ *n pl* **1** *cap* : a large order of schizo-gonic telosporidian sporozoans typically parasites of the di-gestive epithelium of vertebrates and higher invertebrates and including several forms of great economic importance — see CRYPTOSPORIDIUM, EIMERIA, HAEMOGREGARINA, ISOSPORA **2** : sporozoans of the order Coccidia — **coc·cid·i·al** \(')käk-'sid-ē-əl\ *adj*

coc·cid·i·an \-ē-ən\ *n* : any sporozoan of the order Coccidia — **coccidian** *adj*

coc·cid·i·oi·dal \(ˌ)käk-ˌsid-ē-'oid-əl\ *adj* : belonging to, re-sembling, or caused by fungi of the genus *Coccidioides* ⟨∼ infection⟩

Coc·cid·i·oi·des \-'oid-ˌēz\ *n* : a genus of imperfect fungi having a septate mycelium and endospores and including one (*C. immitis*) causing coccidioidomycosis

coc·cid·i·oi·din \-'oid-ᵊn, -'oi-ˌdin\ *n* : an antigen derived from a fungus of the genus *Coccidioides* (*C. immitis*) while in its mycelial phase and used to detect skin sensitivity to and, by inference, infection with this organism — compare SPHERULIN

coc·cid·i·oi·do·my·co·sis \-ˌoid-ō-(ˌ)mī-'kō-səs\ *n, pl* **-co·ses** \-ˌsēz\ : a disease of humans and domestic animals caused by a fungus of the genus *Coccidioides* (*C. immitis*) and marked esp. by fever and localized pulmonary symptoms — called also *San Joaquin fever, San Joaquin valley fever, valley fever*

coc·cid·io·my·co·sis \(ˌ)käk-ˌsid-ē-ō-(ˌ)mī-'kō-səs\ *n, pl* **-co·ses** \-ˌsēz\ : COCCIDIOIDOMYCOSIS

coc·cid·i·o·sis \(ˌ)käk-ˌsid-ē-'ō-səs\ *n, pl* **-o·ses** \-ˌsēz\ : infes-tation with or disease caused by coccidia

coc·cid·io·stat \(')käk-'sid-ē-ō-ˌstat\ *n* : a chemical agent added to animal feed (as for poultry) that serves to retard the life cycle or reduce the population of pathogenic coccidia to the point that disease is minimized and the host develops im-munity

coc·co·ba·cil·la·ry \ˌkäk-(ˌ)ō-'bas-ə-ˌler-ē, -bə-'sil-ə-rē\ *adj* : of, relating to, or being a coccobacillus ⟨∼ organisms⟩

coc·co·ba·cil·lus \-bə-'sil-əs\ *n, pl* **-li** \-ˌī *also* -ē\ : a very short bacillus esp. of the genus *Pasteurella*

Coccobacillus *n, syn of* PASTEURELLA

coc·co·gen·ic \ˌkäk-ō-'jen-ik\ *also* **coc·ci·gen·ic** \ˌkäk-sə-'jen-\ *adj* : caused by a coccus ⟨∼ disease⟩

coc·coid \'käk-ˌoid\ *adj* : of, related to, or resembling a coc-cus — **coccoid** *n*

coc·cu·lus \'käk-yə-ləs\ *n, pl* **cocculus** : the very poisonous bean-shaped berry of a woody vine (*Anamirta cocculus*) of the East Indies that yields picrotoxin

cocculus in·di·cus \-'in-də-kəs\ *n* : COCCULUS

coc·cus \'käk-əs\ *n, pl* **coc·ci** \'käk-ˌ(s)ī *also* -(ˌ)(s)ē\ **1** : a spherical bacterium **2** : COCHINEAL

coc·cy·dyn·ia \ˌkäk-sə-'din-ē-ə\ *n* : COCCYGODYNIA

coc·cy·geal \käk-'sij-(ē-)əl\ *adj* : of, relating to, or affecting the coccyx ⟨a ∼ fracture⟩

coccygeal body *n* : GLOMUS COCCYGEUM

coccygeal ganglion *n* : a small ganglion anterior to the coc-cyx at the caudal junction of the two gangliated cords of the sympathetic nervous system

coccygeal gland *n* : GLOMUS COCCYGEUM

coccygeal nerve *n* : either of the 31st or lowest pair of spinal nerves

coc·cy·gec·to·my \ˌkäk-sə-'jek-tə-mē\ *n, pl* **-mies** : the surgi-cal removal of the coccyx

coccygeum — see GLOMUS COCCYGEUM

coc·cy·ge·us \käk-'sij-ē-əs\ *n, pl* **coc·cyg·ei** \-jē-ˌī\ : a muscle arising from the ischium and sacrospinous ligament and in-serted into the coccyx and sacrum — called also *coccygeus muscle, ischiococcygeus*

coc·cy·go·dyn·ia \ˌkäk-sə-(ˌ)gō-'din-ē-ə\ *n* : pain in the coc-cyx and adjacent regions

coc·cyx \'käk-siks\ *n, pl* **coc·cy·ges** \'käk-sə-ˌjēz\ *also* **coc-cyx·es** \'käk-sik-səz\ : a small bone that articulates with the sacrum and that usu. consists of four fused vertebrae which form the terminus of the spinal column

co·chi·neal \'käch-ə-ˌnēl, 'kō-chə-\ *n* : a red dye consisting of the dried bodies of female cochineal insects used esp. as a bi-ological stain and as an indicator

cochineal insect *n* : a small bright red cactus-feeding scale insect (*Dactylopius coccus*) the females of which are the source of cochineal

co·chle·a \'kō-klē-ə, 'käk-lē-ə\ *n, pl* **co·chle·as** *or* **co·chle·ae** \'kō-klē-ˌē, 'käk-lē-ˌē, -ˌī\ : a division of the bony labyrinth of the inner ear coiled into the form of a snail shell and consist-ing of a spiral canal in the petrous part of the temporal bone in which lies a smaller membranous spiral passage that com-municates with the saccule at the base of the spiral, ends blindly near its apex, and contains the organ of Corti — **co·chle·ar** \'kō-klē-ər, 'käk-lē-ər\ *adj*

cochlear canal *n* : SCALA MEDIA

cochlear duct *n* : SCALA MEDIA

co·chle·ar·i·form \-'ar-ə-ˌfȯrm\ *adj* : shaped like a spoon

cochlear implant *n* : an electrical prosthetic device that en-ables individuals with sensorineural hearing loss to recognize some sounds and that consists of an external microphone and speech processor that receive and convert sound waves into electrical signals which are transmitted to one or more electrodes implanted in the cochlea where they stimulate the auditory nerve — **cochlear implantation** *n*

cochlearis — see DUCTUS COCHLEARIS

cochlear microphonic *n* : an electrical potential arising in the cochlea when the mechanical energy of a sound stimulus is transformed to electrical energy as the action potential of the transmitting nerve — called also *microphonic*

cochlear nerve *n* : a branch of the auditory nerve that arises in the spiral ganglion of the cochlea and conducts sensory stimuli from the organ of hearing to the brain — called also *cochlear, cochlear branch, cochlear division*

cochlear nucleus *n* : the nucleus of the cochlear nerve situ-ated in the caudal part of the pons and consisting of dorsal and ventral parts which are continuous and lie on the dorsal and lateral aspects of the inferior cerebellar peduncle

co·chle·ate \'kō-klē-ət, -ˌāt, 'käk-lē-\ *adj* : having the form of a snail shell

co·chleo·ves·tib·u·lar \ˌkō-klē-(ˌ)ō-ve-'stib-yə-lər, ˌkäk-lē-\ *adj* : relating to or affecting the cochlea and vestibule of the ear ⟨∼ disorders⟩

Coch·lio·my·ia \ˌkäk-lē-ə-'mī-(y)ə\ *n* : a genus of No. Amer-ican blowflies of the family Calliphoridae that includes the screwworms (*C. hominivorax* and *C. macellaria*)

co·chro·ma·tog·ra·phy \ˌkō-ˌkrō-mə-'täg-rə-fē\ *n, pl* **-phies** : chromatography of two or more samples together; *esp* : identification of an unknown substance by chromato-graphic comparison with a known substance — **co·chro·mato·graph** \ˌkō-ˌkrō-'mat-ə-ˌgraf, -krə-\ *vb*

co·cil·la·na \ˌkō-sə-'lan-ə, -'län-ə *also* -'lā-nə\ *n* : the dried bark of a So. American tree (*Guarea rusbyi*) used as an ex-pectorant

Cock·ayne syndrome \kä-'kān-\ *n* : a rare disease that is in-herited as an autosomal recessive trait, is marked esp. by growth and developmental failure, photosensitivity, and pre-mature aging, and that is either present at birth or has an on-set during infancy or childhood — called also *Cockayne's syndrome*

Cockayne, Edward Alfred (1880–1956), British physician. After service in Russia with the British Royal Navy during World War I, Cockayne became outpatient physician at Middlesex Hospital as well as at the Hospital for Sick Chil-dren, both in London. In 1934 he rose to the position of full professor at the Hospital for Sick Children and remained there for the rest of his career. His major interests were en-docrinology and rare genetic diseases in children. In 1934 he published the monograph *Inherited Abnormalities of the Skin and its Appendages,* the first book to be exclusively concerned with genodermatoses. Cockayne syndrome was first described in 1936, in an article on a form of dwarfism marked by retinal atrophy and deafness.

cock·eye \'käk-ˌī, -'ī\ *n* : a squinting eye

cock·eyed \'käk-'īd\ *adj* : having a cockeye

cock·roach \'käk-ˌrōch\ *n* : any of an order or suborder (Blattodea syn. Blattalia) of chiefly nocturnal insects including some that are domestic pests — see BLATTA, BLATTELLA, PERIPLANETA

cock·tail \'käk-ˌtāl\ *n* : a mixture of agents usu. in solution that is taken or used esp. for medical treatment or diagnosis ⟨a potent ∼ of antiretroviral drugs —Zia Jaffrey⟩ ⟨chemotherapy ∼s to treat cancer —J. L. Swerdlow⟩

COCl *abbr* cathodal opening clonus

co·coa \'kō-(ˌ)kō\ *n* **1** : CACAO 2 **2 a** : powdered ground roasted cacao beans from which a portion of the fat has been removed **b** : a beverage prepared by heating powdered cocoa with water or milk

cocoa bean *n* : CACAO 1

cocoa butter *or* **cacao butter** *n* : a pale vegetable fat obtained from cacao beans that is used in the manufacture of chocolate candy, in cosmetics as an emollient, and in pharmacy for making suppositories — called also *theobroma oil*

co·con·scious \(')kō-'kän-chəs\ *n* : mental processes outside the main stream of consciousness but sometimes available to it — **coconscious** *adj*

co·con·scious·ness *n* : COCONSCIOUS

co·co·nut \'kō-kə-(ˌ)nət\ *n* **1** : the fruit of the coconut palm having an outer fibrous husk with a nut containing thick edible meat and coconut milk **2** : the edible meat of the coconut

coconut oil *n* : a nearly colorless fatty oil or white semisolid fat extracted from fresh coconuts and used esp. in making soaps and food products

coc·to·sta·ble \ˌkäk-tə-'stā-bəl\ *adj* : unaltered by heating to the temperature of boiling water

co·cul·ti·va·tion \ˌkō-ˌkəl-tə-'vā-shən\ *n* : cultivation of two types of cell or tissue in the same medium — **co·cul·ti·vate** \-'kəl-tə-ˌvāt\ *vt* **-vat·ed; -vat·ing**

cod \'käd\ *n, pl* **cod** *also* **cods** : any of various bottom-dwelling fishes (family Gadidae, the cod family) that usu. occur in cold marine waters and often have barbels and three dorsal fins: as **a** : one (*Gadus morhua*) of the No. Atlantic that is an important food fish **b** : one (*Gadus macrocephalus*) of the Pacific Ocean

co·da·mine \'kōd-ə-ˌmēn, -mən\ *n* : a crystalline alkaloid $C_{20}H_{25}NO_4$ found in the aqueous extract of opium

¹code \'kōd\ *n* **1** : GENETIC CODE **2** : CODE BLUE

²code *vb* **cod·ed; cod·ing** *vt* : to specify the genetic code for ⟨an amino acid *coded* by a nucleotide sequence⟩ ∼ *vi* **1** : to specify the genetic code ⟨the DNA sequence of the gene that ∼s for that protein —Gina B. Kolata⟩ **2** : to experience cardiac arrest or respiratory failure ⟨the patient *coded* a second time⟩

code blue *n, often cap C&B* : a declaration of or a state of medical emergency and call for medical personnel and equipment to attempt to resuscitate a patient esp. when in cardiac arrest or respiratory distress or failure ⟨summoned by emergency *Code Blues,* doctors had brought her back to life more than once —Bill Bryan⟩; *also* : the attempt to resuscitate the patient

co·de·car·box·yl·ase \ˌkō-ˌdē-kär-'bäk-sə-ˌlās, -ˌlāz\ *n* : the coenzyme $C_8H_{10}NO_6P$ of various amino acid decarboxylases and transaminases

co·deine \'kō-ˌdēn, 'kōd-ē-ən\ *n* : a morphine derivative that is found in opium, is weaker in action than morphine, and is used esp. in the form of its sulfate $(C_{18}H_{21}NO_3)_2 \cdot H_2SO_4$ or phosphate $C_{18}H_{21}NO_3 \cdot H_3PO_4$ esp. as an analgesic and an antitussive

co·de·pen·dence \ˌkō-di-'pen-dən(t)s\ *n* : CODEPENDENCY

co·de·pen·den·cy \-dən-sē\ *n, pl* **-cies** : a psychological condition or a relationship in which a person is controlled or manipulated by another who is affected with a pathological condition (as an addiction to alcohol or heroin); *broadly* : dependence on the needs of or control by another

¹co·de·pen·dent \-dənt\ *n* : a codependent person

²codependent *adj* : participating in or exhibiting codependency ⟨a ∼ relationship⟩ ⟨a ∼ and abusive spouse⟩

co·dex \'kō-ˌdeks\ *n, pl* **co·di·ces** \'kōd-ə-ˌsēz, 'käd-\ : an official or standard collection of drug formulas and descriptions ⟨a ∼ similar to the British Pharmaceutical Codex⟩

cod–liver oil *n* : a pale yellow fatty oil obtained from the liver of the cod (*Gadus morhua*) and related fishes and used in medicine (as in the prophylaxis of rickets) chiefly as a source of vitamins A and D — compare FISH-LIVER OIL

co·dom·i·nant \(')kō-'däm-ə-nənt\ *adj* : being fully expressed in the heterozygous condition ⟨the alleles controlling blood groups A and B are ∼ since an individual with both alleles belongs to blood group AB⟩ — **codominant** *n*

co·don \'kō-ˌdän\ *n* : a specific sequence of three consecutive nucleotides that is part of the genetic code and that specifies a particular amino acid in a protein or starts or stops protein synthesis — called also *triplet*

coeff *or* **coef** *abbr* coefficient

co·ef·fi·cient \ˌkō-ə-'fish-ənt\ *n* : a number that serves as a measure of some property (as of a substance) or characteristic (as of a device or process) and that is commonly used as a factor in computations ⟨the ∼ of expansion of a metal⟩ — see ABSORPTION COEFFICIENT

coefficient of absorption *n* : ABSORPTION COEFFICIENT

coefficient of inbreeding *n* : a measure of the degree of inbreeding in a population expressed as the expected proportion of homozygous loci in an individual at which both alleles can be traced back to the same ancestor — called also *inbreeding coefficient*

coefficient of viscosity *n* : VISCOSITY 2

co·elec·tro·pho·re·sis \ˌkō-i-ˌlek-trə-fə-'rē-səs\ *n* : electrophoresis of two substances together

Coe·len·ter·a·ta \si-ˌlent-ə-'rät-ə\ *n pl, syn of* CNIDARIA

coe·len·ter·ate \si-'lent-ə-ˌrāt, -rət\ *n* : any invertebrate animal of the phylum Cnidaria — called also *cnidarian* — **coelenterate** *adj*

coeliac, coelioscopy, coeliotomy *chiefly Brit var of* CELIAC, CELIOSCOPY, CELIOTOMY

coe·lom \'sē-ləm\ *n, pl* **coeloms** *or* **coe·lo·ma·ta** \si-'lō-mət-ə\ : the usu. epithelium-lined body cavity of metazoans above the lower worms that forms a large space when well developed between the digestive tract and the body wall — **coe·lo·mate** \'sē-lə-ˌmāt\ *adj or n* — **coe·lo·mic** \si-'läm-ik, -'lō-mik\ *adj*

coenaesthesia, coenaesthetic *chiefly Brit var of* CENESTHESIA, CENESTHETIC

coe·no·cyte \'sē-nə-ˌsīt\ *n* **1 a** : a multinucleate mass of protoplasm resulting from repeated nuclear division unaccompanied by cell fission **b** : an organism consisting of such a structure **2** : SYNCYTIUM 1 — **coe·no·cyt·ic** \ˌsē-nə-'sit-ik\ *adj*

coenogenetic *var of* CENOGENETIC

coe·nu·ri·a·sis \ˌsēn-yə-'rī-ə-səs\ *n, pl* **-a·ses** \-ˌsēz\ : COENUROSIS

coe·nu·ro·sis \ˌsēn-yə-'rō-səs, ˌsen-\ *n, pl* **-ro·ses** \-ˌsēz\ : infestation with or disease caused by coenuri (as gid of sheep)

coe·nu·rus \sə-'n(y)ùr-əs, sē-\ *n, pl* **-nu·ri** \-'n(y)ù(ə)r-ˌī\ : a complex tapeworm larva growing interstitially in vertebrate tissues and consisting of a large fluid-filled sac from the inner wall of which numerous scolices develop — see GID, MULTICEPS

co·en·zyme \(')kō-'en-ˌzīm\ *n* : a thermostable nonprotein compound that forms the active portion of an enzyme system after combination with an apoenzyme — compare ACTIVATOR 1 — **co·en·zy·mat·ic** \(ˌ)kō-ˌen-zə-'mat-ik, -(ˌ)zī-\ *adj* — **co·en·zy·mat·i·cal·ly** \-i-k(ə)lē\ *adv*

coenzyme A *n* : a coenzyme $C_{21}H_{36}N_7O_{16}P_3S$ that occurs in all living cells and is essential to the metabolism of carbohydrates, fats, and some amino acids

coenzyme Q *n* : UBIQUINONE

coenzyme Q10 *n* : a ubiquinone $C_{59}H_{90}O_4$ of humans and

---

\ə\ abut \ᵊ\ kitten \ər\ further \a\ ash \ā\ ace \ä\ cot, cart
\aù\ out \ch\ chin \e\ bet \ē\ easy \g\ go \i\ hit \ī\ ice \j\ job
\ŋ\ sing \ō\ go \ò\ law \òi\ boy \th\ thin \t͟h\ the \ü\ loot
\ù\ foot \y\ yet \zh\ vision   *See also* Pronunciation Symbols page

C
D

most other mammals that has a side chain with ten isoprenoid units and possesses antioxidant properties

coeruleus, coerulei — see LOCUS COERULEUS

co·fac·tor \'kō-ˌfak-tər\ *n* **1** : a substance that acts with another substance to bring about certain effects; *esp* : COEN-
ZYME **2** : something (as a diet or virus) that acts with or aids
another factor in causing disease

cof·fee·ber·ry \'kȯ-fē-ˌber-ē, 'käf-ē-\ *n* : CASCARA BUCK-
THORN

cof·fin bone \'kȯ-fən-\ *n* : the bone enclosed within the hoof
of the horse — called also *pedal bone*

cogener *var of* CONGENER

Cog·gins test \'käg-ənz-\ *n* : a serological immunodiffusion
test for the diagnosis of equine infectious anemia esp. in
horses by the presence of antibodies to the causative retrovirus — called also *Coggins* — **Coggins test** *vt*

    Coggins, Leroy (*b* 1932), American veterinary virologist.
Coggins held successive positions as professor of veterinary
virology at Cornell and North Carolina State Universities.
In addition to his research on equine infections anemia, his
areas of research included equine influenza and the viruses
of variola, hog cholera, bovine viral diarrhea, and African
swine fever. He introduced the Coggins test in 1970.

Cog·nex \'käg-ˌneks\ *trademark* — used for a preparation of
tacrine

cog·ni·tion \käg-'nish-ən\ *n* **1** : cognitive mental processes
2 : a conscious intellectual act ⟨conflict between ∼*s*⟩

cog·ni·tive \'käg-nət-iv\ *adj* : of, relating to, or being conscious intellectual activity (as thinking, reasoning, remembering, imagining, or learning words) ⟨the ∼ elements of
perception —C. H. Hamburg⟩ — **cog·ni·tive·ly** *adv*

cognitive behavioral therapy *also* **cognitive behavior
therapy** *n* : COGNITIVE THERAPY

cognitive dissonance *n* : psychological conflict resulting
from simultaneously held incongruous beliefs and attitudes
(as a fondness for smoking and a belief that it is harmful)

cognitive psychology *n* : a branch of psychology concerned
with mental processes (as perception, thinking, learning, and
memory) esp. with respect to the internal events occurring
between sensory stimulation and the overt expression of behavior — compare BEHAVIORISM — **cognitive psychologist**
n

cognitive science *n* : an interdisciplinary science that draws
on many fields (as psychology, artificial intelligence, linguis-
tics, and philosophy) in developing theories about human
perception, thinking, and learning — **cognitive scientist** *n*

cognitive therapy *n* : psychotherapy esp. for depression that
emphasizes the substitution of desirable patterns of thinking
for maladaptive or faulty ones — compare BEHAVIOR MODI-
FICATION — **cognitive therapist** *n*

COH *abbr* carbohydrate

co·he·sion \kō-'hē-zhən\ *n* **1** : the act or process of sticking
together tightly **2** : the molecular attraction by which the
particles of a body are united throughout the mass — compare ADHESION 3

co·he·sive \kō-'hē-siv, -ziv\ *adj* : exhibiting or producing cohesion — **co·he·sive·ly** *adv* — **co·he·sive·ness** *n*

Cohn·heim's area \'kōn-ˌhīmz-\ *n* : one of the polygonal areas seen in transverse sections of a striated muscle fiber representing a bundle of cut ends of fibrils surrounded by sarcoplasm

    Cohnheim, Julius Friedrich (1839–1884), German pathol-
ogist. A pupil of Rudolf Virchon at Berlin's Pathological Institute, Cohnheim made pioneering investigations into the
causes of inflammation. In 1867 he found that inflammation is the result of the passage of white blood cells into the
tissues through capillary walls and that pus consists mainly
of disintegrated white blood cells. After witnessing Robert
Koch demonstrate that the anthrax bacillus is infectious,
Cohnheim himself successfully induced tuberculosis in a
rabbit and thus paved the way for Koch's discovery of the
tubercle bacillus. Cohnheim also developed the now standard procedure of freezing tissue before cutting it into thin
slices for microscopic examination. In 1865 he described

the arrangements seen in the transverse sections of muscle
fiber; these patterns are now known as Cohnheim's areas.

co·ho·ba \kō-'hō-bə\ *n* : a narcotic snuff made from the
seeds of a tropical American tree (*Piptadenia peregrina*)

co·ho·ba·tion \ˌkō-ə-'bā-shən, ˌkō-(h)ō-'bā-\ *n* : repeated distillation usu. by subjecting a distillate to a new act of distillation — **co·ho·bate** \'kō-ə-ˌbāt, 'kō-(h)ō-, kə-'hō-\ *vt*
-**bat·ed;**
-**bat·ing**

co·hort \'kō-ˌhȯ(ə)rt\ *n* : a group of individuals having a statistical factor (as age or risk) in common ⟨the population
consisted of two ∼*s*: 204 clearly exposed and 163 not exposed —R. R. Suskind *et al*⟩

co·hosh \'kō-ˌhäsh\ *n* : any of several American medicinal or
poisonous plants: as **a** : BLACK COHOSH **b** : BLUE COHOSH

co·in·fec·tion \ˌkō-in-'fek-shən\ *n* : concurrent infection of a
cell or organism with two microorganisms ⟨pneumonia
caused by ∼ with an orthomyxovirus and a streptococcus⟩
— **co·in·fect** \-'fekt\ *vt*

coin lesion \'kȯin-\ *n* : a round well-circumscribed nodule in
a lung that is seen in an X-ray photograph as a shadow the
size and shape of a coin

coital exanthema *n* : EQUINE COITAL EXANTHEMA

co·ition \kō-'ish-ən\ *n* : COITUS — **co·ition·al** \-'ish-nəl, -ən-
ᵊl\ *adj*

co·itus \'kō-ət-əs, kō-'ēt-\ *n* : physical union of male and female genitalia accompanied by rhythmic movements : SEX-
UAL INTERCOURSE 1 — compare ORGASM — **co·ital** \-ət-ᵊl,
-'ēt-\ *adj* — **co·ital·ly** \-ᵊl-ē\ *adv*

coitus in·ter·rup·tus \-ˌint-ə-'rəp-təs\ *n* : coitus in which the
penis is withdrawn prior to ejaculation to prevent the deposit
of sperm in the vagina

coitus res·er·va·tus \-ˌrez-ər-'vāt-əs\ *n* : prolonged coitus in
which ejaculation of sperm is deliberately withheld — called
also *karezza*

col *abbr* **1** colony **2** color

cola *pl of* COLON

co·la·mine \'kō-lə-ˌmēn, kō-'lam-ən\ *n* : ethanolamine esp. as
a component of certain phosphatides (as cephalin)

cola nut, cola tree *var of* KOLA NUT, KOLA TREE

col·chi·cine \'käl-chə-ˌsēn, 'käl-kə-\ *n* : a poisonous alkaloid
$C_{22}H_{25}NO_6$ that inhibits mitosis, is extracted from the corms
or seeds of the autumn crocus, and is used in the treatment
of gout and acute attacks of gouty arthritis

col·chi·cum \-kəm\ *n* **1** *cap* : a genus of chiefly fall⸗
blooming Old World corm-producing herbs (family Liliaceae) that produce flowers resembling crocuses **2** : a bulb,
flower, or plant (as the autumn crocus) of the genus *Colchicum* **3** : the dried corm or dried ripe seeds of the autumn
crocus containing the alkaloid colchicine, possessing an
emetic, diuretic, and cathartic action, and used to treat gout
— called also *colchicum root*

¹cold \'kōld\ *adj* **1 a** : having or being a temperature that is
noticeably lower than body temperature and esp. that is un-
comfortable for humans ⟨a ∼ drafty room⟩ **b** : having a
relatively low temperature or one that is lower than normal
or expected ⟨the bath water has gotten ∼⟩ **c** : receptive to
the sensation of coldness : stimulated by cold ⟨a ∼ spot is a
typical receptor in higher vertebrates⟩ **2** : marked by the
loss of normal body heat ⟨∼ hands⟩ **3** : DEAD **4** : exhibiting little or no radioactivity — **cold·ness** \'kōl(d)-nəs\ *n*

²cold *n* **1** : bodily sensation produced by loss or lack of heat
2 : a bodily disorder popularly associated with chilling: **a** *in
humans* : COMMON COLD **b** *in domestic animals* : CORYZA

COLD *abbr* chronic obstructive lung disease

cold abscess *n* : a chronic abscess of slow formation and
with little evidence of inflammation

cold agglutinin *n* : any of several agglutinins sometimes present in the blood (as that of many patients with primary
atypical pneumonia) that at low temperatures agglutinate
compatible as well as incompatible red blood cells, including
the patient's own — called also *cold hemagglutinin;* compare
AUTOAGGLUTININ

cold–blood·ed \'kōl(d)-'bləd-əd\ *adj* : having a body temperature not internally regulated but approximating that of the environment : POIKILOTHERMIC ⟨∼ amphibians and reptiles⟩ — **cold–blood·ed·ness** *n*

cold cream *n* : a soothing and cleansing cosmetic basically consisting of a perfumed emulsion of a bland vegetable oil or heavy mineral oil

cold pack *n* : a sheet or blanket wrung out of cold water, wrapped around the patient's body, and covered with dry blankets — compare HOT PACK

cold sore *n* : a vesicular lesion that typically occurs in or around the mouth, that initially causes pain, burning, or itching before bursting and crusting over, and that is caused by a herpes simplex virus which remains dormant in the body and may be reactivated by a variety of factors (as stress, fever, or sunburn) — called also *fever blister;* compare CANKER SORE

cold sweat *n* : perspiration accompanied by feelings of chill or cold and usu. induced or accompanied by dread, fear, or shock

cold tur·key \-'tər-kē\ *n* : abrupt complete cessation of the use of an addictive drug; *also* : the symptoms experienced by one undergoing withdrawal from a drug — **cold turkey** *adv or vt*

col·ec·to·my \kə-'lek-tə-mē, kō-\ *n, pl* **-mies** : excision of a portion or all of the colon

co·le·op·te·ra \ˌkō-lē-'äp-tə-rə\ *n pl* **1** *cap* : the largest order of insects comprising the beetles and weevils and being distinguished by a pair of forewings that are usu. hard and rigid, are never used for flight, and serve as a protective covering for the delicate flight wings and the upper surface of the abdomen **2** : insects that are beetles — **co·le·op·te·ran** \-rən\ *n or adj* — **co·le·op·te·rist** \-rəst\ *n* — **co·le·op·te·rous** \-rəs\ *adj*

co·les·ti·pol \kə-'les-tə-ˌpȯl\ *n* : a strongly basic ion exchange resin with an affinity for bile acids that is used in the form of its hydrochloride to treat hypercholesterolemia and disorders associated with the accumulation of bile acids

co·li \'kō-ˌlī\ *adj* : of or relating to bacteria normally inhabiting the intestine or colon and esp. to species of the genus *Escherichia* (as *E. coli*) — **coli** *n*

coli — see MELANOSIS COLI, TAENIA COLI, VALVULA COLI

co·li·ba·cil·la·ry \ˌkō-lə-'bas-ə-ˌler-ē, -bə-'sil-ə-rē\ *adj* : of, relating to, or caused by the colon bacillus ⟨∼ infection⟩

co·li·ba·cil·lo·sis \-ˌbas-ə-'lō-səs\ *n, pl* **-lo·ses** \-ˌsēz\ : infection with or disease caused by colon bacilli (esp. *E. coli*)

coli bacillus *n* : COLON BACILLUS

¹col·ic \'käl-ik\ *n* **1** : an attack of acute abdominal pain localized in a hollow organ or part (as the small intestine, ureter, or bile duct) and often caused by spasm, obstruction, or twisting **2** : a condition marked by recurrent episodes of prolonged and uncontrollable crying and irritability in an otherwise healthy infant that is of unknown cause and usu. subsides after three to four months of age

²colic *adj* : of or relating to colic : COLICKY ⟨∼ crying⟩

³co·lic \'kō-lik, 'käl-ik\ *adj* : of or relating to the colon ⟨∼ lymph nodes⟩

col·i·ca \'käl-i-kə\ *n* : COLIC 1

colica dex·tra \-'dek-strə\ *n* : COLIC ARTERY a

colica me·dia \-'mēd-ē-ə\ *n* : COLIC ARTERY b

colic artery *n* : any of three arteries that branch from the mesenteric arteries and supply the large intestine: **a** : a branch of the superior mesenteric artery serving the ascending colon — called also *colica dextra, right colic artery* **b** : a branch of the superior mesenteric artery serving the transverse colon — called also *colica media, middle colic artery* **c** : a branch of the inferior mesenteric artery supplying the descending colon — called also *colica sinistra, left colic artery*

colica sin·is·tra \-'sin-ə-strə\ *n* : COLIC ARTERY c

co·li·cin \'kō-lə-sən\ *also* **co·li·cine** \-ˌsēn\ *n* : any of various antibacterial proteins that are produced by some strains of intestinal bacteria (as *E. coli*) having a specific plasmid and that often act to inhibit macromolecular synthesis in related strains

co·li·ci·no·ge·nic \ˌkō-lə-sən-ə-'jen-ik, ˌkäl-ə-, -ˌsēn-\ *adj* **1** : producing or having the capacity to produce colicins ⟨∼ bacteria⟩ **2** : conferring the capacity to produce colicins ⟨∼ genetic material⟩ — **co·li·ci·no·ge·nic·i·ty** \-jə-'nis-ət-ē\ *n, pl* **-ties**

co·li·ci·nog·e·ny \ˌkō-lə-sə-'näj-ə-nē, ˌkäl-ə-\ *n, pl* **-nies** : the capacity to produce colicins

col·icky \'käl-i-kē\ *adj* **1** : relating to or associated with colic ⟨∼ pain⟩ **2** : suffering from colic ⟨∼ babies⟩

co·li·form \'kō-lə-ˌfȯrm, 'käl-ə-\ *adj* : of, relating to, or being gram-negative rod-shaped bacteria (as *E. coli*) normally present in the intestine ⟨monitored ∼ levels in drinking water⟩ — **coliform** *n*

co·lin·ear \(')kō-'lin-ē-ər\ *adj* : having corresponding parts arranged in the same linear order ⟨good evidence . . . that the gene and its polypeptide product are ∼ —J. D. Watson⟩ — **co·lin·ear·i·ty** \(ˌ)kō-ˌlin-ē-'ar-ət-ē\ *n, pl* **-ties**

co·li·phage \'kō-lə-ˌfāj, -ˌfäzh\ *n* : a bacteriophage active against colon bacilli

co·lis·tin \kə-'lis-tən, kō-\ *n* : a polymyxin produced by a bacterium of the genus *Bacillus* (*B. polymyxa* var. *colistinus*) and used against some gram-negative pathogens esp. of the genera *Pseudomonas, Escherichia, Klebsiella,* and *Shigella*

co·li·tis \kō-'līt-əs, kə-\ *n* : inflammation of the colon — see ULCERATIVE COLITIS

coll *abbr* **1** collect; collection **2** colloidal **3** collyrium

colla *pl of* COLLUM

col·la·gen \'käl-ə-jən\ *n* : an insoluble fibrous protein of vertebrates that is the chief constituent of the fibrils of connective tissue (as in skin and tendons) and of the organic substance of bones and yields gelatin and glue on prolonged heating with water — **col·la·gen·ic** \ˌkäl-ə-'jen-ik\ *adj* — **col·lag·e·nous** \kə-'laj-ə-nəs\ *adj*

col·la·ge·nase \kə-'laj-ə-ˌnās, 'käl-ə-jə-, -ˌnāz\ *n* : any of a group of proteolytic enzymes that decompose collagen and gelatin

collagen disease *n* : CONNECTIVE TISSUE DISEASE

col·la·gen·o·lyt·ic \ˌkäl-ə-jən-ə-'lit-ik, -ˌjen-\ *adj* : relating to or having the capacity to break down collagen ⟨∼ activity⟩ ⟨∼ enzymes⟩

col·la·ge·no·sis \ˌkäl-ə-jə-'nō-səs\ *n, pl* **-no·ses** \-ˌsēz\ : CONNECTIVE TISSUE DISEASE

collagen vascular disease *n* : CONNECTIVE TISSUE DISEASE

¹col·lapse \kə-'laps\ *vb* **col·lapsed; col·laps·ing** *vi* **1** : to fall or shrink together abruptly and completely : fall into a jumbled or flattened mass through the force of external pressure ⟨a blood vessel that *collapsed*⟩ **2** : to break down in vital energy, stamina, or self-control through exhaustion or disease; *esp* : to fall helpless or unconscious ∼ *vt* : to cause to collapse ⟨*collapsing* an infected lung⟩ — **col·laps·ibil·i·ty** \-ˌlap-sə-'bil-ət-ē\ *n* — **col·laps·ible** \-'lap-sə-bəl\ *adj*

²collapse *n* **1** : a breakdown in vital energy, strength, or stamina : complete sudden enervation ⟨the daughter's mental ∼ through mounting frustration —Leslie Rees⟩ **2** : a state of extreme prostration and physical depression resulting from circulatory failure, great loss of body fluids, or heart disease and occurring terminally in diseases such as cholera, typhoid fever, and pneumonia **3** : an airless state of a lung of spontaneous origin or induced surgically — see ATELECTASIS **4** : an abnormal falling together of the walls of an organ ⟨∼ of blood vessels⟩

col·lar \'käl-ər\ *n* : a band (as of cotton) worn around the neck for therapeutic purposes (as protection, support, or retention of body heat)

col·lar·bone \'käl-ər-ˌbōn, ˌkäl-ər-'\ *n* : CLAVICLE

¹col·lat·er·al \kə-'lat-ə-rəl, -'la-trəl\ *adj* **1** : relating to or being branches of a bodily part ⟨∼ sprouting of nerves⟩ **2** : relating to or being part of the collateral circulation ⟨∼ circulatory vessels⟩ ⟨∼ blood flow⟩

\ə\ abut \ᵊ\ kitten \ər\ further \a\ ash \ā\ ace \ä\ cot, cart
\au̇\ out \ch\ chin \e\ bet \ē\ easy \g\ go \i\ hit \ī\ ice \j\ job
\ŋ\ sing \ō\ go \ȯ\ law \ȯi\ boy \th\ thin \t̲h̲\ the \ü\ loot
\u̇\ foot \y\ yet \zh\ vision *See also* Pronunciation Symbols page

²**collateral** n **1** : a branch esp. of a blood vessel, nerve, or the axon of a nerve cell ⟨excitation of axon ∼s⟩ **2** : a bodily part (as a ligament) that is lateral in position

collateral circulation n : circulation of blood established through enlargement of minor vessels and anastomosis of vessels with those of adjacent parts when a major vein or artery is functionally impaired (as by obstruction); also : the modified vessels through which such circulation occurs

collateral ganglion n : any of several autonomic ganglia (as the celiac ganglion) not in the sympathetic chain — called also prevertebral ganglion

collateral ligament n : any of various ligaments on one or the other side of a hinge joint (as the knee, elbow, or the joints between the phalanges of the toes and fingers): as **a** : LATERAL COLLATERAL LIGAMENT **b** : MEDIAL COLLATERAL LIGAMENT

collateral sulcus n : a sulcus of the tentorial surface of the cerebrum lying below and external to the calcarine sulcus and causing an elevation on the floor of the lateral ventricle between the hippocampi — called also collateral fissure

col·lec·ting tubule \kə-ˈlek-tiŋ-\ n : a nonsecretory tubule that receives urine from several nephrons and discharges it into the pelvis of the kidney — called also collecting duct

col·lec·tive unconscious \kə-ˈlek-tiv-\ n : the genetically determined part of the unconscious that esp. in the psychoanalytic theory of C. G. Jung occurs in all the members of a people or race

Col·les' fracture \ˈkäl-əs-, ˈkäl-ˌēz-\ n : a fracture of the lower end of the radius with backward displacement of the lower fragment and radial deviation of the hand at the wrist that produces a characteristic deformity — compare SMITH FRACTURE

> **Col·les** \ˈkäl-əs\, **Abraham (1773–1843),** British surgeon. Colles' enduring contributions are his anatomical description of the fascia of the perineum in 1811, his description of a fracture at the distal end of the radius (Colles' fracture) in 1814, and his clinical observations in 1837 on the contagion of syphilis.

col·lic·u·lus \kə-ˈlik-yə-ləs\ n, pl **-u·li** \-ˌlī, -lē\ : an anatomical prominence; esp : any of the four prominences constituting the corpora quadrigemina — see INFERIOR COLLICULUS, SUPERIOR COLLICULUS

col·li·ga·tive \ˈkäl-ə-ˌgāt-iv\ adj : depending on the number of particles (as molecules) and not on the nature of the particles ⟨pressure is a ∼ property⟩

col·li·mate \ˈkäl-ə-ˌmāt\ vt **-mat·ed; -mat·ing** : to make (as rays of light) parallel — **col·li·ma·tion** \ˌkäl-ə-ˈmā-shən\ n

col·li·ma·tor \ˈkäl-ə-ˌmāt-ər\ n : a device for obtaining a beam of radiation (as X-rays) of limited cross section

col·li·qua·tion \ˌkäl-i-ˈkwā-zhən, -shən\ n : the breakdown and liquefaction of tissue

col·liq·ua·tive \ˈkäl-i-ˌkwät-iv, kə-ˈlik-wət-iv\ adj : producing or characterized by colliquation ⟨∼ necrobiosis⟩

col·lo·di·on \kə-ˈlōd-ē-ən\ n : a viscous solution of pyroxylin used esp. as a coating for wounds or for photographic films

col·loid \ˈkäl-ˌoid\ n **1** : a gelatinous or mucinous substance found in tissues in disease or normally (as in the thyroid) **2 a** : a substance consisting of particles that are dispersed throughout another substance and are too small for resolution with an ordinary light microscope but are incapable of passing through a semipermeable membrane **b** : a mixture (as smoke) consisting of a colloid together with the medium in which it is dispersed — **col·loi·dal** \kə-ˈloid-ᵊl, kä-\ adj — **col·loi·dal·ly** \-ᵊl-ē\ adv

col·loi·do·cla·sia \ˌkäl-ˌoid-ə-ˈklā-zh(ē-)ə, kə-ˌloid-\ n : disequilibrium of the colloid system of the body that is associated with anaphylactic shock and thought to be caused by the presence of undigested colloids in the blood — **col·loi·do·clas·tic** \-ˈklas-tik\ adj

col·lum \ˈkäl-əm\ n, pl **col·la** \-ə\ : an anatomical neck or neckline part or process

col·lu·nar·i·um \ˌkäl-ə-ˈnar-ē-əm\ n, pl **-nar·ia** \-ē-ə\ : a medicated solution for instillation into the nostrils as a wash or spray or as drops

col·lu·to·ri·um \ˌkäl-ə-ˈtōr-ē-əm, -ˈtor-\ n, pl **-to·ria** \-ē-ə\ : MOUTHWASH

col·lyr·i·um \kə-ˈlir-ē-əm\ n, pl **-ia** \-ē-ə\ or **-i·ums** : an eye lotion : EYEWASH

col·o·bo·ma \ˌkäl-ə-ˈbō-mə\ n, pl **-mas** also **-ma·ta** \-mət-ə\ : a fissure of the eye usu. of congenital origin — **col·o·bo·ma·tous** \-mət-əs\ adj

co·lo·co·lic \ˌkäl-ə-ˈkäl-ik, ˌkō-lə-, -ˈkō-lik\ adj : relating to two parts of the colon

col·o·cynth \ˈkäl-ə-ˌsin(t)th\ n : a Mediterranean and African herbaceous vine (Citrullus colocynthis) related to the watermelon; also : its spongy fruit from which a powerful cathartic is prepared

colombo var of CALUMBA

co·lom·bo root \kə-ˈläm-(ˌ)bō-ˈrüt, -ˈrut\ n : CALUMBA

co·lon \ˈkō-lən\ n, pl **colons** or **co·la** \-lə\ : the part of the large intestine that extends from the cecum to the rectum

colon bacillus n : any of several bacilli esp. of the genus Escherichia that are normally commensal in vertebrate intestines; esp : E. COLI

¹**co·lon·ic** \kō-ˈlän-ik, kə-\ adj : of or relating to the colon

²**colonic** n : ENEMA 1 — see HIGH COLONIC

colonic irrigation n : ENEMA 1

col·o·nize \ˈkäl-ə-ˌnīz\ vb **-nized; -niz·ing** vt **1** : to establish a colony in or on ⟨the parasitic roundworms . . . have succeeded in colonizing a great variety of hosts —W. H. Dowdeswell⟩ **2** : to isolate in supervised groups ∼ vi, of microorganisms : to become established in a habitat (as a host or a wound) ⟨these bacteria in turn ∼ in other parts of the body —R. A. Runnells⟩ — **co·lo·ni·za·tion** \ˌkäl-ə-nə-ˈzā-shən\ n

co·lon·o·scope \kō-ˈlän-ə-ˌskōp\ n : a flexible endoscope for inspecting and passing instruments into the colon (as to obtain tissue for biopsy)

co·lo·nos·co·py \ˌkō-lə-ˈnäs-kə-pē, ˌkäl-ə-\ n, pl **-pies** : endoscopic examination of the colon ⟨transabdominal ∼ with a sigmoidoscope via colotomy⟩ — **co·lon·o·scop·ic** \kō-ˌlän-ə-ˈskäp-ik\ adj

col·o·ny \ˈkäl-ə-nē\ n, pl **-nies** : a circumscribed mass of microorganisms usu. growing in or on a solid medium

col·o·ny–stim·u·lat·ing factor \-ˌstim-yə-ˌlāt-iŋ-\ n : any of several glycoproteins that promote the differentiation of stem cells esp. into blood granulocytes and macrophages and that stimulate their proliferation into colonies in culture — see GRANULOCYTE COLONY-STIMULATING FACTOR, GRANULOCYTE-MACROPHAGE COLONY-STIMULATING FACTOR, INTERLEUKIN-3, MACROPHAGE COLONY-STIMULATING FACTOR

col·o·pexy \ˈkäl-ə-ˌpek-sē\ n, pl **-pex·ies** : the operation of suturing the sigmoid colon to the abdominal wall

co·lo·pho·ny \kə-ˈläf-ə-nē, ˈkäl-ə-ˌfō-\ n, pl **-nies** : ROSIN

co·lo·proc·tos·to·my \ˌkō-lə-ˌpräk-ˈtäs-tə-mē, ˌkäl-ə-\ n, pl **-mies** : surgical formation of an artificial passage between the colon and the rectum

col·or or chiefly Brit **col·our** \ˈkəl-ər\ n **1 a** : a phenomenon of light (as red, brown, pink, or gray) or visual perception that enables one to differentiate otherwise identical objects **b** : the aspect of objects and light sources that may be described in terms of hue, lightness, and saturation for objects and hue, brightness, and saturation for light sources **c** : a hue as contrasted with black, white, or gray **2** : complexion tint; esp : the tint characteristic of good health — **color** or chiefly Brit **colour** adj

Col·o·ra·do tick fever \ˌkäl-ə-ˈrad-(ˌ)ō-, -ˈräd-\ n : a mild disease of the western U.S. and western Canada that is characterized by intermittent fever, malaise, headaches, myalgia, and the absence of a rash and is caused by a reovirus (species Colorado tick fever virus of the genus Coltivirus) transmitted by the Rocky Mountain wood tick

col·or–blind \-ˌblīnd\ adj : affected with partial or total inability to distinguish one or more chromatic colors — **color blindness** n

color cell n : CHROMOCYTE

co·lo·rec·tal \ˌkō-lə-ˈrek-tᵊl, ˌkäl-ə-\ *adj* : relating to or affecting the colon and the rectum ⟨∼ cancer⟩

color filter *n* : FILTER 3b

color hearing *n* : CHROMESTHESIA

col·or·im·e·ter \ˌkəl-ə-ˈrim-ət-ər\ *n* : any of various instruments used to objectively determine the color of a solution — **col·or·i·met·ric** \ˌkəl-ə-rə-ˈme-trik\ *adj* — **col·or·i·met·ri·cal·ly** \-tri-k(ə-)lē\ *adv* — **col·or·im·e·try** \ˌkəl-ə-ˈrim-ə-trē\ *n, pl* **-tries**

color index *n* : a figure that represents the ratio of the amount of hemoglobin to the number of red cells in a given volume of blood and that is a measure of the normality of the hemoglobin content of the individual cells

color vision *n* : perception of and ability to distinguish colors

co·los·to·mize \kə-ˈläs-tə-ˌmīz\ *vt* **-mized; -miz·ing** : to perform a colostomy on

co·los·to·my \kə-ˈläs-tə-mē\ *n, pl* **-mies** : surgical formation of an artificial anus by connecting the colon to an opening in the abdominal wall — compare COLOTOMY

colostomy bag *n* : a container kept constantly in position to receive feces discharged through the opening created by a colostomy

colostomy belt *n* : a belt or girdle designed to hold a colostomy bag securely against the opening created by a colostomy

co·los·trum \kə-ˈläs-trəm\ *n* : milk secreted for a few days after parturition and characterized by high protein and antibody content — **co·los·tral** \-trəl\ *adj*

colostrum corpuscle *n* : a cell in the colostrum that contains fat globules and is thought to be a degenerated phagocytic cell of the mammary gland

co·lot·o·my \kə-ˈlät-ə-mē\ *n, pl* **-mies** : surgical incision of the colon — compare COLOSTOMY

colour *chiefly Brit var of* COLOR

col·pec·to·my \käl-ˈpek-tə-mē\ *n, pl* **-mies** : partial or complete surgical excision of the vagina — called also *vaginectomy*

col·peu·ryn·ter \ˌkäl-pyə-ˈrint-ər\ *n* : an inflatable bag used to dilate the vagina or cervical canal

col·peu·ry·sis \käl-ˈpyùr-ə-səs\ *n* : dilation of the vagina (as by a colpeurynter)

col·pi·tis \käl-ˈpīt-əs\ *n* : VAGINITIS

col·po·cen·te·sis \ˌkäl-(ˌ)pō-sen-ˈtē-səs\ *n, pl* **-te·ses** \-ˌsēz\ : surgical puncture of the vagina

col·po·clei·sis \ˌkäl-pō-ˈklī-səs\ *n, pl* **-clei·ses** \-ˌsēz\ : the suturing of posterior and anterior walls of the vagina to prevent uterine prolapse

col·po·per·i·ne·or·rha·phy \ˌkäl-pō-ˌper-ə-(ˌ)nē-ˈòr-ə-fē\ *n, pl* **-phies** : the suturing of an injury to the vagina and the perineum

col·po·pexy \ˈkäl-pə-ˌpek-sē\ *n, pl* **-pex·ies** : fixation of the vagina by suturing it to the adjacent abdominal wall

col·po·plas·ty \ˈkäl-pə-ˌplas-tē\ *n, pl* **-ties** : VAGINOPLASTY

col·por·rha·phy \käl-ˈpòr-ə-fē\ *n, pl* **-phies** : surgical repair of the vaginal wall

col·po·scope \ˈkäl-pə-ˌskōp\ *n* : a magnifying instrument designed to facilitate visual inspection of the vagina and cervix — **col·po·scop·ic** \ˌkäl-pə-ˈskäp-ik\ *adj* — **col·po·scop·i·cal·ly** \-i-k(ə-)lē\ *adv* — **col·pos·co·py** \käl-ˈpäs-kə-pē\ *n, pl* **-pies**

col·po·stat \ˈkäl-pə-ˌstat\ *n* : a medical appliance or instrument (as a radium applicator) designed to facilitate vaginal treatment

col·pot·o·my \käl-ˈpät-ə-mē\ *n, pl* **-mies** : surgical incision of the vagina

colts·foot \ˈkōlts-ˌfùt\ *n, pl* **coltsfoots** **1** : a perennial yellow-flowered composite herb (*Tussilago farfara*) native to Europe but now nearly cosmopolitan that has leaves which are the source of farfara **2** : FARFARA

Co·lu·bri·dae \kə-ˈl(y)ü-brə-ˌdē\ *n pl* : a large cosmopolitan family of nonvenomous terrestrial, arboreal, or sometimes aquatic snakes — **col·u·brid** \ˈkäl-(y)ə-ˌbrəd\ *n or adj*

col·u·brine \ˈkäl-(y)ə-ˌbrīn\ *adj* : of or relating to snakes of the family Colubridae : COLUBRID

co·lum·bin \kə-ˈləm-bən\ *n* : a bitter crystalline constituent of calumba

co·lum·bi·um \kə-ˈləm-bē-əm\ *n* : NIOBIUM

col·u·mel·la \ˌkäl-(y)ə-ˈmel-ə\ *n, pl* **-mel·lae** \-ˈmel-(ˌ)ē\ *also* -ˌī\ **1** : any of various anatomical parts likened to a column: **a** : the bony central axis of the cochlea **b** : the lower part of the nasal septum **2** : the central sterile portion of the sporangium in various fungi (*Mucor* and related genera) — **col·u·mel·lar** \-ər\ *adj* — **col·u·mel·late** \-ˌāt, -ət\ *adj*

col·umn \ˈkäl-əm\ *n* : a longitudinal subdivision of the spinal cord that resembles a column or pillar: as **a** : any of the principal longitudinal subdivisions of gray matter or white matter in each lateral half of the spinal cord — see DORSAL HORN, GRAY COLUMN, LATERAL COLUMN 1, VENTRAL HORN; compare FUNICULUS a **b** : any of a number of smaller bundles of spinal nerve fibers : FASCICULUS

co·lum·na \kə-ˈləm-nə\ *n, pl* **-nae** \-ˌnē, -ˌnī\ *also* **-nas** : an anatomical structure that suggests a column in form — usu. used in combination

co·lum·nar \kə-ˈləm-nər\ *adj* : of, relating to, being, or composed of tall narrow somewhat cylindrical or prismatic epithelial cells ⟨∼ epithelium⟩ ⟨∼ tissue⟩

column chromatography *n* : chromatography in which the substances to be separated are introduced onto the top of a column packed with an adsorbent (as silica gel or alumina), pass through the column at different rates that depend on the affinity of each substance for the adsorbent and for the solvent or solvent mixture, and are usu. collected in solution as they pass from the column at different times — compare GAS CHROMATOGRAPHY, PAPER CHROMATOGRAPHY, THIN-LAYER CHROMATOGRAPHY

column of Ber·tin \-ber-ˈtaⁿ\ *n* : RENAL COLUMN

E. J. Bertin — see BERTIN'S COLUMN

column of Bur·dach \-ˈbər-dək, -ˈbùr-, -ˌdäk\ *n* : FASCICULUS CUNEATUS

Bur·dach \ˈbùr-däk\, **Karl Friedrich (1776–1847),** German anatomist. Burdach was a specialist in the anatomy and physiology of the nervous system, particularly the brain and spinal cord. He also delved into embryology, making studies of embryonic brains. His significant contributions to neuroanatomy were his descriptions of many of the fiber bundles of the brain and spinal cord. In 1806 he gave the first complete description of the fasciculus cuneatus, sometimes known as Burdach's column. In addition he wrote a physiology textbook.

co·ma \ˈkō-mə\ *n* : a state of profound unconsciousness caused by disease, injury, or poison

co·ma·tose \ˈkō-mə-ˌtōs, ˈkäm-ə-\ *adj* : of, resembling, or affected with coma ⟨a ∼ patient⟩ ⟨a ∼ condition⟩

com·bat fatigue \ˈkäm-ˌbat-\ *n* : post-traumatic stress disorder occurring under wartime conditions (as combat) that cause intense stress — called also *battle fatigue, shell shock, war neurosis*

combination therapy *n* : the use of two or more therapies and esp. drugs to treat a disease or condition ⟨a *combination therapy* for asthma using a beta-agonist and corticosteroid⟩

com·bi·na·to·ri·al chemistry \ˌkäm-bə-nə-ˈtòr-ē-əl-, kəm-ˌbī-nə-, -ˈtòr-\ *n* : a branch of applied chemistry concerned with the rapid synthesis and screening of large numbers of different but related chemical compounds generated from a mixture of known building blocks in order to recover new substances optimally suited for a specific function ⟨using *combinatorial chemistry* to develop new pharmaceuticals and catalysts⟩

com·bine \kəm-ˈbīn\ *vb* **com·bined; com·bin·ing** *vt* : to cause to unite into a chemical compound ∼ *vi* : to unite to form a chemical compound — **com·bi·na·tion** \ˌkäm-bə-ˈnā-shən\ *n*

\ə\ **abut** \ᵊ\ **kitten** \ər\ **further** \a\ **ash** \ā\ **ace** \ä\ **cot, cart** \aù\ **out** \ch\ **chin** \e\ **bet** \ē\ **easy** \g\ **go** \i\ **hit** \ī\ **ice** \j\ **job** \ŋ\ **sing** \ō\ **go** \ò\ **law** \òi\ **boy** \th\ **thin** \t̲h̲\ **the** \ü\ **loot** \ù\ **foot** \y\ **yet** \zh\ **vision** *See also* Pronunciation Symbols page

Com·bi·vent \\'käm-bə-ˌvent\\ *trademark* — used for a preparation of ipratropium bromide and the sulfate of albuterol

com·bus·ti·ble \\kəm-'bəs-tə-bəl\\ *adj* : capable of combustion ⟨~ anesthetics⟩

com·bus·tion \\kəm-'bəs-chən\\ *n* : a usu. very rapid chemical process (as oxidation) that produces heat and usu. light; *also* : a slower oxidation (as in the body)

com·e·do \\'käm-ə-ˌdō\\ *n, pl* **com·e·do·nes** \\ˌkäm-ə-'dō-(ˌ)nēz\\ : BLACKHEAD 1

com·e·do·car·ci·no·ma \\ˌkäm-ə-ˌdō-ˌkärs-ᵊn-'ō-mə\\ *n, pl* **-mas** *also* **-ma·ta** \\-mət-ə\\ : breast cancer that arises in the larger ducts and is characterized by slow growth, late metastasis, and the accumulation of solid plugs of atypical and degenerating cells in the ducts

com·e·do·gen·ic \\ˌkäm-əd-ə-'jen-ik\\ *adj* : tending to clog pores esp. by the formation of blackheads ⟨a ~ cosmetic⟩

come to \\'kəm-'tü\\ *vi* : to recover consciousness

comitans — see VENA COMITANS

com·ma bacillus \\'käm-ə-\\ *n* : CHOLERA VIBRIO

com·men·sal \\kə-'men(t)-səl\\ *adj* : of, relating to, or living in a state of commensalism — **commensal** *n* — **com·men·sal·ly** \\-sə-lē\\ *adv*

com·men·sal·ism \\-sə-ˌliz-əm\\ *n* : a relation between two kinds of organisms in which one obtains food or other benefits from the other without damaging or benefiting it

com·mi·nute \\'käm-ə-ˌn(y)üt\\ *vt* **-nut·ed; -nut·ing** : to reduce to minute particles ⟨prolonged trituration to ~ a therapeutic agent⟩ — **com·mi·nu·tion** \\ˌkäm-ə-'n(y)ü-shən\\ *n*

com·mi·nut·ed *adj* : being a fracture in which the bone is splintered or crushed into numerous pieces ⟨a ~ elbow fracture⟩

com·mis·su·ra \\ˌkäm-ə-'shùr-ə\\ *n, pl* **-rae** \\-ˌrē\\ : COMMISSURE

com·mis·sure \\'käm-ə-ˌshù(ə)r\\ *n* **1** : a point or line of union or junction between two anatomical parts (as the lips at their angles or adjacent heart valves) **2** : a connecting band of nerve tissue in the brain or spinal cord — see ANTERIOR COMMISSURE, CORPUS CALLOSUM, GRAY COMMISSURE, HABENULAR COMMISSURE, HIPPOCAMPAL COMMISSURE, POSTERIOR COMMISSURE; compare MASSA INTERMEDIA — **com·mis·su·ral** \\ˌkäm-ə-'shùr-əl\\ *adj*

com·mis·sur·ot·o·my \\ˌkäm-ə-ˌshù(ə)r-'ät-ə-mē, -shə-'rät-\\ *n, pl* **-mies** : the operation of cutting through a band of muscle or nerve fibers; *specif* : separation of the flaps of a mitral valve to relieve mitral stenosis : VALVULOTOMY

com·mit \\kə-'mit\\ *vt* **com·mit·ted; com·mit·ting** : to place in a prison or mental institution ⟨a patient *committed* by the court to a state hospital⟩ — **com·mit·ta·ble** \\-'mit-ə-bəl\\ *adj*

com·mit·ment \\kə-'mit-mənt\\ *n* : a consignment to a penal or mental institution

com·mon \\'käm-ən\\ *adj* : formed of or dividing into two or more branches ⟨the ~ facial vein⟩ ⟨~ iliac vessels⟩

common bile duct *n* : the duct formed by the union of the hepatic and cystic ducts and opening into the duodenum — called also *ductus choledochus*

common cardinal vein *n* : DUCT OF CUVIER

common carotid artery *n* : the part of either carotid artery between its point of origin and its division into the internal and external carotid arteries — called also *common carotid*

common cattle grub *n* : a cattle grub of the genus *Hypoderma* (*H. lineatum*) which is found throughout the U.S. and whose larva is particularly destructive to cattle

common cold *n* : an acute contagious disease of the upper respiratory tract that is marked by inflammation of the mucous membranes of the nose, throat, eyes, and eustachian tubes with a watery then purulent discharge and is caused by any of several viruses (as a rhinovirus or an adenovirus)

common iliac artery *n* : ILIAC ARTERY 1

common iliac vein *n* : ILIAC VEIN a

common interosseous artery *n* : a short thick artery that arises from the ulnar artery near the proximal end of the radius on the dorsal side of the interosseous membrane and that divides into anterior and posterior branches which pass down the forearm toward the wrist

common peroneal nerve *n* : the smaller of the branches into which the sciatic nerve divides passing obliquely outward and downward from the popliteal space and to the neck of the fibula where it divides into the deep peroneal nerve and the superficial peroneal nerve that supply certain muscles and skin areas of the leg and foot — called also *lateral popliteal nerve, peroneal nerve*

common salt *n* : SALT 1a

com·mo·tio \\kə-'mō-sh(ē-)ō\\ *n* : CONCUSSION

com·mo·tio cor·dis \\kə-'mō-shē-ō-'kòrd-əs\\ *n* : concussion of the heart that is caused by a blow to the chest over the region of the heart by a blunt object (as a baseball, hockey puck, or fist) which does not penetrate the body and that usu. results in ventricular fibrillation leading to sudden cardiac death if treatment by defibrillation is not immediately given

com·mu·ni·ca·ble \\kə-'myü-ni-kə-bəl\\ *adj* : capable of being transmitted from person to person, animal to animal, animal to human, or human to animal : TRANSMISSIBLE — **com·mu·ni·ca·bil·i·ty** \\-ˌmyü-ni-kə-'bil-ət-ē\\ *n, pl* **-ties**

communicable disease *n* : an infectious disease transmissible (as from person to person) by direct contact with an affected individual or the individual's discharges or by indirect means (as by a vector) — compare CONTAGIOUS DISEASE

communicans — see GRAY RAMUS COMMUNICANS, RAMUS COMMUNICANS, WHITE RAMUS COMMUNICANS

communicantes — see RAMUS COMMUNICANS

com·mu·ni·cate \\kə-'myü-nə-ˌkāt\\ *vt* **-cat·ed; -cat·ing** : to cause to pass from one to another ⟨some diseases are easily *communicated*⟩

communicating artery *n* : any of three arteries in the brain that form parts of the circle of Willis: **a** : one connecting the anterior cerebral arteries — called also *anterior communicating artery* **b** : either of two arteries that occur one on each side of the circle of Willis and connect an internal carotid artery with a posterior cerebral artery — called also *posterior communicating artery*

com·mu·ni·ca·tion \\kə-ˌmyü-nə-'kā-shən\\ *n* **1** : the act or process of transmitting information (as about ideas, attitudes, emotions, or objective behavior) ⟨nonverbal interpersonal ~⟩ ⟨emotional ~ between parent and child —G. S. Blum⟩: **a** : exchange of information between individuals through a common system of signs, symbols, or behavior ⟨pictorial representation is a usable channel of ~ between humans and the chimpanzee⟩ ⟨the function of pheromones in insect ~⟩ **b** : personal rapport ⟨a lack of ~ between young and old persons⟩ **2** : information communicated **3** : a connection between bodily parts ⟨an artificial ~ between the esophagus and the stomach⟩

communis — see EXTENSOR DIGITORUM COMMUNIS

com·mu·ni·ty \\kə-'myü-nət-ē\\ *n, pl* **-ties** : a unified body of individuals: as **a** : the people with common interests living in a particular area; *broadly* : the area itself ⟨the problems of a large ~⟩ **b** : an interacting population of various kinds of individuals (as species) in a common location **c** : a group of people with a common characteristic or interest living together within a larger society ⟨a ~ of retired persons⟩

co·mor·bid \\(ˌ)kō-'mòr-bəd\\ *adj* : existing simultaneously with and usu. independently of another medical condition ⟨laparoscopic surgery for symptomatic gallstones may be contraindicated by ~ cardiopulmonary disease⟩

co·mor·bid·i·ty \\-mòr-'bid-ə-tē\\ *n, pl* **-ties** : a comorbid condition ⟨diabetes patients tend to present with a long list of *comorbidities* —Fred Gebhart⟩; *also* : the occurrence of comorbid conditions : occurrence as a comorbid condition ⟨the hallmark of depression in older people is its ~ with medical illness —*U.S. Dept. of Health & Human Services*⟩

comp *abbr* **1** comparative; compare **2** composition **3** compound

com·pact \\kəm-'pakt, käm-', 'käm-ˌ\\ *adj* : having a dense structure without small cavities or cells ⟨~ bone⟩ — compare CANCELLOUS

com·pac·ta \\kəm-'pak-tə\\ *n* : the part of a bone made up of compact bone (as the shaft wall of a long bone)

C
D

compacta — see PARS COMPACTA

compactum — see STRATUM COMPACTUM

com·par·a·tive \kəm-ˈpar-ət-iv\ *adj* : characterized by the systematic comparison of phenomena and esp. of likenesses and dissimilarities ⟨∼ anatomy⟩ ⟨the study of blood types by ∼ analysis⟩

comparative psychology *n* : the study of the relationships between species differences and behavior esp. in reference to genetics and evolution

com·par·a·tor \kəm-ˈpar-ət-ər\ *n* **1** : an apparatus used for determining concentration of dissolved substances (as hydrogen ions) in solution by color comparison with known standards **2** : an instrument, device, or set of charts (as for use in chemical analysis and medical diagnosis) for the determination and specification of colors by direct comparison with a standardized system of colors

com·part·men·tal·iza·tion *or Brit* **com·part·men·tal·isa·tion** \kəm-ˌpärt-ˌment-ᵊl-ə-ˈzā-shən\ *n* : isolation or splitting off of part of the personality or mind with lack of communication and consistency between the parts — **com·part·men·tal·ize** *or Brit* **com·part·men·tal·ise** \-ˈment-ᵊl-ˌīz\ *vt* **-ized** *or Brit* **-ised; -iz·ing** *or Brit* **-is·ing**

com·part·men·tal syndrome \kəm-ˌpärt-ˈment-ᵊl-, -ˌkäm-\ *n* : COMPARTMENT SYNDROME

com·part·men·ta·tion \kəm-ˌpärt-mən-ˈtā-shən, -ˌmen-\ *n* : intracellular partitioning of cellular substances and metabolic activities by membranes

com·part·ment syndrome \kəm-ˈpärt-mənt-\ *n* : a painful condition resulting from the expansion or overgrowth of enclosed tissue (as of a leg muscle) within its anatomical enclosure (as a muscular sheath) producing pressure that interferes with circulation and adversely affects the function and health of the tissue itself — called also *compartmental syndrome*

com·pat·i·ble \kəm-ˈpat-ə-bəl\ *adj* **1** : capable of existing together in a satisfactory relationship (as marriage) **2** : capable of being used in transfusion or grafting without immunological reaction (as agglutination or tissue rejection) ⟨treatment of hemophilia by transfusion of ∼ blood⟩ **3** *of medications* : capable of being administered jointly without interacting to produce deleterious effects or impairing their respective actions — **com·pat·i·bil·i·ty** \-ˌpat-ə-ˈbil-ət-ē\ *n, pl* **-ties**

Com·pa·zine \ˈkäm-pə-ˌzēn\ *trademark* — used for a preparation of prochlorperazine

com·pen·sate \ˈkäm-pən-ˌsāt, -ˌpen-\ *vb* **-sat·ed; -sat·ing** *vt* : to subject to or remedy by physiological compensation ⟨*compensated* hypertensive patients⟩ ∼ *vi* : to undergo or engage in psychic or physiological compensation ⟨his aggression was an attempt to ∼ for inherent passivity⟩

com·pen·sat·ed *adj* : buffered so that there is no change in the pH of the blood ⟨∼ acidosis⟩ ⟨∼ alkalosis⟩ — compare UNCOMPENSATED

com·pen·sa·tion \ˌkäm-pən-ˈsā-shən, -ˌpen-\ *n* **1** : correction of an organic defect by excessive development or by increased functioning of another organ or unimpaired parts of the same organ ⟨cardiac ∼⟩ — see DECOMPENSATION **2** : a psychological mechanism by which feelings of inferiority, frustration, or failure in one field are counterbalanced by achievement in another

com·pen·sa·to·ry \kəm-ˈpen(t)-sə-ˌtōr-ē, -ˌtȯr-\ *adj* : making up for a loss; *esp* : serving as psychic or physiological compensation ⟨∼ enlargement of the heart⟩ ⟨to overcome this feeling of inferiority by developing such ∼ mechanisms as intelligent aggression or shrewdness —Edward Sapir⟩

com·pe·tence \ˈkäm-pət-ən(t)s\ *n* : the quality or state of being functionally adequate ⟨drugs that improve the ∼ of a failing heart⟩: as **a** : the properties of an embryonic field that enable it to respond in a characteristic manner to an organizer **b** : readiness of bacteria to undergo genetic transformation

com·pe·ten·cy \-ən-sē\ *n, pl* **-cies** : COMPETENCE

com·pe·tent \ˈkäm-pət-ənt\ *adj* : having the capacity to func-

tion or develop in a particular way; *specif* : having the capacity to respond (as by producing an antibody) to an antigenic determinant ⟨immunologically ∼ cells⟩

com·pet·i·tive \kəm-ˈpet-ət-iv\ *adj* : depending for effectiveness on the relative concentration of two or more substances ⟨∼ inhibition of an enzyme⟩ ⟨∼ protein binding⟩ — **com·pet·i·tive·ly** *adv*

com·plain \kəm-ˈplān\ *vi* : to speak of one's illness or symptoms ⟨the patient visited the office ∼*ing* of weight loss⟩

com·plaint \kəm-ˈplānt\ *n* : a bodily ailment or disease ⟨bloating and other digestive ∼s —Christine Gorman⟩

com·ple·ment \ˈkäm-plə-mənt\ *n* **1** : a group or set (as of chromosomes or DNA) that is typical of the complete organism or one of its parts — see CHROMOSOME COMPLEMENT **2** : a complementary color **3** : the thermolabile group of proteins in normal blood serum and plasma that in combination with antibodies causes the destruction esp. of particulate antigens (as bacteria and foreign blood corpuscles)

com·ple·men·tar·i·ty \ˌkäm-plə-(ˌ)men-ˈtar-ət-ē, -mən-\ *n, pl* **-ties** : correspondence in reverse of part of one molecule to part of another: as **a** : the arrangement of chemical groups and electric charges that enables a combining group of an antibody to combine with a specific determinant group of an antigen or hapten **b** : the correspondence between strands or nucleotides of DNA or sometimes RNA that permits their precise pairing ⟨evolution of the contemporary genetic code involving purine-pyrimidine ∼ —Struther Arnott & P. J. Bond⟩

com·ple·men·ta·ry \ˌkäm-plə-ˈment-ə-rē, -ˈmen-trē\ *adj* **1** : relating to or constituting one of a pair of contrasting colors that produce a neutral color when combined in suitable proportions **2** : characterized by molecular complementarity; *esp* : characterized by the capacity for precise pairing of purine and pyrimidine bases between strands of DNA and sometimes RNA such that the structure of one strand determines the other — **com·ple·men·ta·ri·ly** \-ˈmen-trə-lē, -(ˌ)men-ˈter-ə-lē, -ˈment-ə-rə-lē\ *adv* — **com·ple·men·ta·ri·ness** \-ˈment-ə-rē-nəs, -ˈmen-trē-\ *n*

complementary DNA *n* : CDNA

complementary medicine *n* : any of the practices (as acupuncture) of alternative medicine accepted and utilized by mainstream medical practitioners; *also* : ALTERNATIVE MEDICINE

com·ple·men·ta·tion \ˌkäm-plə-(ˌ)men-ˈtā-shən, -mən-\ *n* **1** : the formation of neutral colors from complementary colors **2** : production of normal phenotype in an individual heterozygous for two closely related mutations with one on each homologous chromosome and at a slightly different position

complement fixation *n* : the process of binding serum complement to the product formed by the union of an antibody and the antigen for which it is specific that occurs when complement is added to a mixture (in proper proportion) of such an antibody and antigen

complement–fixation test *n* : a diagnostic test for the presence of a particular antibody in the serum of a patient that involves inactivation of the complement in the serum, addition of measured amounts of the antigen for which the antibody is specific and of foreign complement, and detection of the presence or absence of complement fixation by the addition of a suitable indicator system — compare WASSERMANN TEST

com·plete \kəm-ˈplēt\ *adj* **1** *of insect metamorphosis* : characterized by the occurrence of a pupal stage between the motile immature stages and the adult — compare INCOMPLETE 1 **2** *of a bone fracture* : characterized by a break passing entirely across the bone — compare INCOMPLETE 2

\ə\ **abut** \ᵊ\ **kitten** \ər\ **further** \a\ **ash** \ā\ **ace** \ä\ **cot, cart**
\au̇\ **out** \ch\ **chin** \e\ **bet** \ē\ **easy** \g\ **go** \i\ **hit** \ī\ **ice** \j\ **job**
\ŋ\ **sing** \ō\ **go** \ȯ\ **law** \ȯi\ **boy** \th\ **thin** \t̲h̲\ **the** \ü\ **loot**
\u̇\ **foot** \y\ **yet** \zh\ **vision** *See also* Pronunciation Symbols page

complete blood count *n* : a blood count that includes separate counts for red and white blood cells — called also *complete blood cell count;* compare DIFFERENTIAL BLOOD COUNT

com·ple·tion test \kəm-'plē-shən-\ *n* : an intelligence test requiring that the test taker complete a whole (as a sentence or picture) from which certain parts have been omitted

¹**com·plex** \käm-'pleks, kəm-', 'käm-ˌ\ *adj* **1** : having many varied interrelated parts, patterns, or elements and consequently hard to understand ⟨~ behavior⟩ ⟨a ~ personality⟩ ⟨~ plants and animals⟩ **2** : formed by the union of simpler chemical substances ⟨~ proteins⟩

²**com·plex** \'käm-ˌpleks\ *n* **1** : a group of repressed memories, desires, and ideas that exert a dominant influence on the personality and behavior ⟨a guilt ~⟩ — see CASTRATION COMPLEX, ELECTRA COMPLEX, INFERIORITY COMPLEX, OEDIPUS COMPLEX, PERSECUTION COMPLEX, SUPERIORITY COMPLEX **2** : a group of chromosomes arranged or behaving in a particular way — see GENE COMPLEX **3** : a chemical association of two or more species (as ions or molecules) joined usu. by weak electrostatic bonds rather than by covalent bonds **4** : the sum of the factors (as symptoms and lesions) characterizing a disease ⟨primary tuberculous ~⟩

³**com·plex** \käm-'pleks, kəm-', 'käm-ˌ\ *vt* **1** : to form into a complex ⟨RNA ~ed with protein⟩ **2** : CHELATE ~ *vi* : to form a complex ⟨hormones which must ~ with specific receptors⟩

complex carbohydrate *n* : a polysaccharide (as starch or cellulose) consisting of usu. hundreds or thousands of monosaccharide units; *also* : a food (as rice or pasta) composed primarily of such polysaccharides

com·plex·ion \kəm-'plek-shən\ *n* **1** : the combination of the hot, cold, moist, and dry qualities held in medieval physiology to determine the quality of a body **2** : the hue or appearance of the skin and esp. of the face ⟨a dark ~⟩ — **com·plex·ioned** \-shənd\ *adj*

com·plex·us \kəm-'plek-səs, käm-\ *n* : SEMISPINALIS CAPITIS — called also *complexus muscle*

com·pli·ance \kəm-'plī-ən(t)s\ *n* **1** : the ability or process of yielding to changes in pressure without disruption of structure or function ⟨a study of pulmonary ~⟩ ⟨the tone of colonic muscle as judged by ~ of the gut wall —S. C. Truelove⟩ **2** : the process of complying with a regimen of treatment ⟨simplified drug regimens may encourage better ~⟩

com·pli·cate \'käm-plə-ˌkāt\ *vt* **-cat·ed; -cat·ing** : to cause to be more complex or severe ⟨a virus disease *complicated* by bacterial infection⟩

com·pli·cat·ed *adj, of a bone fracture* : characterized by injury to nearby parts

com·pli·ca·tion \ˌkäm-plə-'kā-shən\ *n* : a secondary disease or condition that develops in the course of a primary disease or condition and arises either as a result of it or from independent causes

com·po·nent \kəm-'pō-nənt, 'käm-ˌ, käm-'\ *n* : a constituent part ⟨the exocrine and endocrine ~s of the pancreas⟩

com·pos men·tis \ˌkäm-pə-'sment-əs\ *adj* : of sound mind, memory, and understanding

¹**com·pound** \käm-'paúnd, kəm-', 'käm-ˌ\ *vt* : to form by combining parts ⟨~ a medicine⟩

²**com·pound** \'käm-ˌpaúnd, käm-', kəm-'\ *adj* : composed of or resulting from union of separate elements, ingredients, or parts ⟨a ~ substance⟩ ⟨~ glands⟩

³**com·pound** \'käm-ˌpaúnd\ *n* : something formed by a union of elements or parts; *specif* : a distinct substance formed by chemical union of two or more ingredients in definite proportion by weight

com·pound benzoin tincture \(ˌ)käm-ˌpaúnd-, kəm-\ *n* : FRIAR'S BALSAM

compound fracture *n* : a bone fracture resulting in an open wound through which bone fragments usu. protrude — compare SIMPLE FRACTURE

compound microscope *n* : a microscope consisting of an objective and an eyepiece mounted in a telescoping tube

¹**com·press** \kəm-'pres\ *vt* **1** : to press or squeeze together ⟨a

ligament in the wrist was ~ing a nerve⟩ **2** : to reduce in size or volume as if by squeezing ⟨~ air⟩

²**com·press** \'käm-ˌpres\ *n* **1** : a covering consisting usu. of a folded cloth that is applied and held firmly by the aid of a bandage over a wound dressing to prevent oozing **2** : a folded wet or dry cloth applied firmly to a part (as to allay inflammation)

com·pressed air \kəm-ˌprest-'a(ə)r, käm-, -'e(ə)r\ *n* : air under pressure greater than that of the atmosphere

compressed–air disease *n* : DECOMPRESSION SICKNESS

compressed–air illness *n* : DECOMPRESSION SICKNESS

com·pres·sion \kəm-'presh-ən\ *n* : the act, process, or result of compressing esp. when involving a compressing force on a bodily part ⟨~ of an artery by forceps⟩ ⟨~ of the brain by the bones of a depressed fracture⟩

compression fracture *n* : fracture (as of a vertebra) caused by compression of one bone against another

com·pres·sor \-'pres-ər\ *n* : one that compresses: as **a** : a muscle that compresses a part **b** : a machine that compresses gases

¹**com·pro·mise** \'käm-prə-ˌmīz\ *vt* **-mised; -mis·ing** : to cause the impairment of ⟨certain chemical agents may ~ placental function⟩ ⟨a *compromised* immune system⟩

²**compromise** *n* : the condition of having been compromised : IMPAIRMENT ⟨cardiovascular ~⟩ ⟨patients at risk for airway ~ —David Jaffe *et al*⟩

Comp·ton effect \'käm(p)-tən-\ *n* : the loss of energy and concomitant increase in wavelength of a usu. high-energy photon (as of X-rays or gamma rays) that occurs upon collision of the photon with an electron

Compton, Arthur Holly (1892–1962), American physicist. Compton is generally regarded as one of the great figures in modern physics. A leader in the development of nuclear energy and investigations on cosmic rays, he discovered the effect that now bears his name in 1923. This discovery helped to establish that electromagnetic radiation has a dual nature, as a wave and as a particle. While at the University of Chicago, he was from 1942 to 1945 the director of the project that developed the first self-sustaining atomic chain reaction. He discovered the variation in the intensity of cosmic rays with the latitude and altitude of the observer and a method for the production of plutonium in quantity. In 1927 he was awarded, along with Charles T. R. Wilson, the Nobel Prize for Physics for his discovery of the Compton effect.

Compton scattering *n* : the scattering of a high-energy photon with loss of energy that occurs in the Compton effect

com·pul·sion \kəm-'pəl-shən\ *n* : an irresistible persistent impulse to perform an act (as excessive hand washing); *also* : the act itself — compare OBSESSION, PHOBIA

¹**com·pul·sive** \-'pəl-siv\ *adj* : of, relating to, caused by, or suggestive of psychological compulsion or obsession ⟨repetitive and ~ behavior⟩ ⟨a ~ gambler⟩ — **com·pul·sive·ly** *adv* — **com·pul·sive·ness** *n* — **com·pul·siv·i·ty** \kəm-ˌpəl-'siv-ət-ē, ˌkäm-\ *n, pl* **-ties**

²**compulsive** *n* : one who is subject to a psychological compulsion

com·put·ed axial tomography \kəm-ˌpyüt-əd-\ *n* : COMPUTED TOMOGRAPHY — abbr. *CAT*

computed tomographic *adj* : using, produced by, or obtained by computed tomography ⟨a *computed tomographic* scan of the abdomen⟩ ⟨*computed tomographic* findings⟩

computed tomography *n* : radiography in which a three-dimensional image of a body structure is constructed by computer from a series of plane cross-sectional images made along an axis — abbr. *CT*

com·pu·ter·ized axial tomography \kəm-ˌpyüt-ə-ˌrīzd-\ *n* : COMPUTED TOMOGRAPHY — abbr. *CAT*

computerized tomography *n* : COMPUTED TOMOGRAPHY — abbr. *CT*

con·al·bu·min \ˌkän-al-'byü-mən, 'kän-al-ˌ\ *n* : a protein of the white of an egg that is obtained from the filtrate from the crystallization of ovalbumin and that combines with iron salts to form a red iron-protein complex

C
D

co·nar·i·um \kō-'nar-ē-əm\ *n, pl* **co·nar·ia** \-ē-ə\ : PINEAL GLAND

co·na·tion \kō-'nā-shən\ *n* : an inclination (as an instinct, a drive, a wish, or a craving) to act purposefully : IMPULSE 2 — **co·na·tive** \'kō-nət-iv, -ₙnāt-; 'kän-ət-\ *adj*

conc *abbr* concentrated; concentration

con·ca·nav·a·lin \ₙkän-kə-'nav-ə-lən\ *n* : either of two crystalline globulins occurring esp. in the seeds of the jack bean; *esp* : one that is a potent hemagglutinin

con·cat·e·nate \kän-'kat-ə-nət, kən-\ *adj* : linked together

Con·ca·to's disease \kän-ₙkät-(ₙ)ōz-, kōn-, kən-\ *n* : POLYSEROSITIS

Con·ca·to \kōn-'kät-(ₙ)ō, kän-\, **Luigi Maria (1825–1882)**, Italian physician. In 1881 Concato published a classic description of the inflammation of the serous membranes that is now known as Concato's disease.

con·cave \kän-'kāv, 'kän-ₙ\ *adj* : hollowed or rounded inward like the inside of a bowl

con·cav·i·ty \kän-'kav-ət-ē\ *n, pl* **-ties** **1** : a concave surface or space **2** : the quality or state of being concave

con·ca·vo—concave \kän-ₙkā-(ₙ)vō-\ *adj* : concave on both sides

concavo—convex *adj* : concave on one side and convex on the other

con·ceive \kən-'sēv\ *vb* **con·ceived; con·ceiv·ing** *vt* : to become pregnant with (young) ~ *vi* : to become pregnant

¹con·cen·trate \'kän(t)-sən-ₙtrāt, -ₙsen-\ *vb* **-trat·ed; -trat·ing** *vt* **1 a** : to bring or direct toward a common center or objective : FOCUS **b** : to accumulate (a toxic substance) in bodily tissues ⟨fish ~ mercury⟩ **2** : to make less dilute ⟨~ syrup⟩ ~ *vi* : to fix one's powers, efforts, or attention on one thing ⟨~ on a problem⟩ — **con·cen·tra·tor** \-ₙtrāt-ər\ *n*

²concentrate *n* : something prepared by concentration; *esp* : a food reduced in bulk by elimination of fluid ⟨orange juice ~⟩

con·cen·tra·tion \ₙkän(t)-sən-'trā-shən, -ₙsen-\ *n* **1** : the act or action of concentrating: as **a** : a directing of the attention or of the mental faculties toward a single object **b** : an increasing of strength (as of a solute or a gas in a mixture) or a purifying by partial or total removal of diluents, solvents, admixed gases, extraneous material, or waste (as by evaporation or diffusion) **2** : a crude active principle of a vegetable esp. for pharmaceutical use in the form of a powder or resin **3** : the relative content of a component (as dissolved or dispersed material) of a solution, mixture, or dispersion that may be expressed in percentage by weight or by volume, in parts per million, or in grams per liter

con·cen·tric \kən-'sen-trik, (ˈ)kän-\ *adj* : having a common center ⟨~ circles⟩ — **con·cen·tri·cal·ly** \-tri-k(ə-)lē\ *adv*

con·cept \'kän-ₙsept\ *n* **1** : something conceived in the mind **2** : an abstract or generic idea generalized from particular instances

con·cep·tion \kən-'sep-shən\ *n* **1 a** : the process of becoming pregnant involving fertilization or implantation or both **b** : EMBRYO, FETUS **2 a** : the capacity, function, or process of forming or understanding ideas or abstractions or their symbols **b** : a general idea

con·cep·tive \kən-'sep-tiv\ *adj* : capable of or relating to conceiving ⟨problems either of sexual inadequacy or ~ inadequacy —W. H. Masters & V. E. Johnson⟩

con·cep·tu·al \kən-'sep-chə(-wə)l, kän-, -'sepsh-wəl\ *adj* : of, relating to, or consisting of concepts — **con·cep·tu·al·ly** *adv*

con·cep·tus \kən-'sep-təs\ *n, pl* **-tus·es** *also* **-ti** \-ₙtī\ : a fertilized egg, embryo, or fetus

Con·cer·ta \kän-'sert-ə\ *trademark* — used for a preparation of the hydrochloride of methylphenidate

conch \'käŋk, 'känch, 'kóŋk\ *n, pl* **conchs** \'käŋks, 'kóŋks\ *or* **conch·es** \'kän-chəz\ : CONCHA 1

con·cha \'käŋ-kə *also* 'kóŋ-\ *n, pl* **con·chae** \-ₙkē, -ₙkī\ **1** : the largest and deepest concavity of the external ear **2** : NASAL CONCHA — **con·chal** \-kəl\ *adj*

con·cor·dant \kən-'kórd-ᵊnt\ *adj, of twins* : similar with respect to one or more particular characters — compare DISCORDANT — **con·cor·dance** \-ᵊn(t)s\ *n*

con·cre·ment \'käŋ-krə-mənt, 'kän-\ *n* : CONCRETION

con·cres·cence \kän-'kres-ᵊn(t)s, kän-\ *n* : a growing together : COALESCENCE; *esp* : convergence and fusion of the lateral lips of the blastopore to form the primordium of an embryo

con·cre·tio cor·dis \ₙkän-'krēt-ē-ō-'kórd-əs\ *n* : adhesive pericarditis with the space between the layers of the pericardium mostly or completely obliterated by dense scar tissue

con·cre·tion \kän-'krē-shən, kən-\ *n* : a hard usu. inorganic mass (as a bezoar or tophus) formed in a living body

con·cuss \kən-'kəs\ *vt* : to affect with concussion

con·cus·sion \kən-'kəsh-ən\ *n* **1** : a hard blow or collision **2** : a condition resulting from the stunning, damaging, or shattering effects of a hard blow; *esp* : a jarring injury of the brain resulting in disturbance of cerebral function and sometimes marked by permanent damage — **con·cus·sive** \-'kəs-iv\ *adj*

cond *abbr* condition

con·den·sa·tion \ₙkän-den-'sā-shən, -dən-\ *n* **1** : the act or process of condensing: as **a** : a chemical reaction involving union between molecules often with elimination of a simple molecule (as water) to form a new more complex compound of often greater molecular weight **b** : the conversion of a substance (as water) from the vapor state to a denser liquid or solid state usu. initiated by a reduction in temperature of the vapor **2** : representation of several apparently discrete ideas by a single symbol esp. in dreams **3** : an abnormal hardening of an organ or tissue ⟨connective tissue ~s⟩

con·dense \kən-'den(t)s\ *vb* **con·densed; con·dens·ing** *vt* : to make denser or more compact; *esp* : to subject to condensation ~ *vi* **1** : to undergo condensation **2** : to become visibly dense or more compact ⟨the chromosomes ~ during prophase⟩ — **con·dens·able** \-'den(t)s-sə-bəl\ *adj*

condensed *adj* : reduced to a more compact or dense form ⟨~ metaphase chromosomes⟩ ⟨~ heterochromatin⟩

condensed milk *n* : evaporated milk with sugar added

con·dens·er \kən-'den(t)s-sər\ *n* **1 a** : a lens or mirror used to concentrate light on an object **b** : an apparatus in which gas or vapor is condensed **2** : CAPACITOR

con·di·ment \'kän-də-mənt\ *n* : something used to enhance the flavor of food; *esp* : a pungent seasoning — **con·di·men·tal** \ₙkän-də-'ment-ᵊl\ *adj*

¹con·di·tion \kən-'dish-ən\ *n* **1** : something essential to the appearance or occurrence of something else; *esp* : an environmental requirement ⟨available oxygen is an essential ~ for animal life⟩ **2 a** : a usu. defective state of health ⟨a serious heart ~⟩ **b** : a state of physical fitness ⟨exercising to get into ~⟩

²condition *vt* **con·di·tioned; con·di·tion·ing** \-'dish-(ə-)niŋ\ : to cause to undergo a change so that an act or response previously associated with one stimulus becomes associated with another — **con·di·tion·able** \-(-ə-)nə-bəl\ *adj*

con·di·tion·al \kən-'dish-nəl, -ən-ᵊl\ *adj* **1 a** : CONDITIONED ⟨~ reflex⟩ ⟨~ response⟩ **b** : eliciting a conditional response ⟨a ~ stimulus⟩ **2** : permitting survival only under special growth or environmental conditions ⟨~ lethal mutations⟩ — **con·di·tion·al·ly** \-'dish-nə-lē, -ən-ᵊl-ē\ *adv*

con·di·tioned *adj* : determined or established by conditioning

con·dom \'kän-dəm *also* 'kən-\ *n* **1** : a sheath commonly of rubber worn over the penis (as to prevent conception or venereal infection during coitus) — called also *sheath* **2** : a device that is designed to be inserted into the vagina before coitus and that resembles in form and function the condom used by males

cond ref *abbr* conditioned reflex

cond resp *abbr* conditioned response

con·duct \kən-'dəkt *also* 'kän-ₙdəkt\ *vt* : to act as a medium

---

\ə\ abut \ᵊ\ kitten \ər\ further \a\ ash \ā\ ace \ä\ cot, cart
\aù\ out \ch\ chin \e\ bet \ē\ easy \g\ go \i\ hit \ī\ ice \j\ job
\ŋ\ sing \ō\ go \ó\ law \ói\ boy \th\ thin \t̲h̲\ the \ü\ loot
\ù\ foot \y\ yet \zh\ vision   *See also* Pronunciation Symbols page

for conveying ~ *vi* : to have the quality of transmitting something (as light, heat, sound, or electricity)

con·duc·tance \kən-'dək-tən(t)s\ *n* **1** : the power, readiness, or capacity to conduct something ⟨neural ~⟩ ⟨changes in membrane ~ to ions⟩ **2** : the readiness with which a conductor transmits an electric current expressed as the reciprocal of electrical resistance

con·duc·tion \kən-'dək-shən\ *n* **1 a** : transmission through or by means of a conductor; *also* : the transfer of heat through matter by communication of kinetic energy from particle to particle with no net displacement of the particles **b** : CONDUCTIVITY **2** : the transmission of excitation through living tissue and esp. nervous tissue ⟨~ of impulses to the brain⟩

conduction deafness *n* : hearing loss or impairment resulting from interference with the transmission of sound waves to the organ of Corti — called also *conductive deafness, transmission deafness;* compare CENTRAL DEAFNESS, NERVE DEAFNESS

con·duc·tive \-'dək-tiv\ *adj* **1** : having conductivity : relating to conduction (as of electricity) **2** : caused by failure in the mechanisms for sound transmission in the external or middle ear ⟨~ hearing loss⟩

conductive deafness *n* : CONDUCTION DEAFNESS

con·duc·tiv·i·ty \ˌkän-ˌdək-'tiv-ət-ē, kən-\ *n, pl* **-ties** : the quality or power of conducting or transmitting: as **a** : the reciprocal of electrical resistivity **b** : the quality of living matter responsible for the transmission of and progressive reaction to stimuli

con·duc·to·met·ric *also* **con·duc·ti·met·ric** \kən-ˌdək-tə-'me-trik\ *adj* **1** : of or relating to the measurement of conductivity **2** : being or relating to titration based on determination of changes in the electrical conductivity of the solution

con·duc·tor \kən-'dək-tər\ *n* **1 a** : a material or object that permits an electric current to flow easily **b** : a material capable of transmitting another form of energy (as heat or sound) **2** : a bodily part (as a nerve fiber) that transmits excitation

con·du·ran·gin \ˌkän-də-'raŋ-(g)ən, -'ran-jən\ *n* : a bitter poisonous yellowish glucoside obtained from condurango

con·du·ran·go \-'raŋ-(ˌ)gō\ *n* : the dried bark of a So. American vine (*Marsdenia cundurango*) used as an alterative and stomachic — see CONDURANGIN

con·dy·lar \'kän-də-lər\ *adj* : of or relating to a condyle

con·dy·lar·thro·sis \ˌkän-də-lär-'thrō-səs\ *n, pl* **-thro·ses** \-ˌsēz\ : articulation by means of a condyle (as that between the head and spinal column involving the occipital condyles and the atlas)

con·dyle \'kän-ˌdīl *also* -d°l\ *n* : an articular prominence of a bone — used chiefly of such as occur in pairs resembling a pair of knuckles (as those of the occipital bone for articulation with the atlas, those at the distal end of the humerus and femur, and those of the lower jaw); see LATERAL CONDYLE, MEDIAL CONDYLE

con·dy·lec·to·my \ˌkän-dī-'lek-tə-mē, -d°l-'ek-\ *n, pl* **-mies** : surgical removal of a condyle

con·dy·li·on \kən-'dil-ē-ən, kän-\ *n* : the lateral tip of the condyle of the lower jaw

con·dy·loid \'kän-də-ˌloid\ *adj* : shaped like or situated near a condyle : relating to a condyle

condyloid foramen *n* : a foramen in front of each condyle of the occipital bone

condyloid joint *n* : an articulation (as that between the metacarpals of the hand and the first phalanx of the fingers) in which an ovoid head is received into an elliptical cavity permitting all movements except axial rotation

condyloid process *n* : the rounded process by which the ramus of the mandible articulates with the temporal bone

con·dy·lo·ma \ˌkän-də-'lō-mə\ *n, pl* **-ma·ta** \-mət-ə\ *also* **-mas** : GENITAL WART — **con·dy·lo·ma·tous** \-mət-əs\ *adj*

condyloma acu·mi·na·tum \-ə-ˌkyü-mə-'nāt-əm\ *n, pl* **condylomata acu·mi·na·ta** \-'nāt-ə\ : GENITAL WART

condyloma la·tum \-'lā-təm\ *n, pl* **condylomata la·ta** \-tə\

: a highly infectious flattened often hypertrophic papule of secondary syphilis that forms in moist areas of skin and at mucocutaneous junctions

cone \'kōn\ *n* **1** : a solid having a circular base and sides that slope evenly to a point **2 a** : any of the conical photosensitive receptor cells of the vertebrate retina that function in color vision — compare ROD **b** : any of a family (Conidae) of numerous somewhat conical tropical gastropod mollusks that include a few highly poisonous forms — see CONUS **3** : a cusp of a tooth esp. in the upper jaw

cone·nose \'kōn-ˌnōz\ *n* : any of various large bloodsucking reduviid bugs esp. of the genus *Triatoma* including some capable of inflicting painful bites — called also *kissing bug;* compare ASSASSIN BUG

conf *abbr* conference

con·fab·u·la·tion \kən-ˌfab-yə-'lā-shən, ˌkän-\ *n* : a filling in of gaps in memory by unconstrained fabrication (as in Korsakoff's psychosis) — **con·fab·u·late** \kən-'fab-yə-ˌlāt\ *vi* **-lat·ed; -lat·ing** — **con·fab·u·la·to·ry** \-yə-lə-ˌtōr-ē, -ˌtȯr-\ *adj*

con·fec·tio \kən-'fek-shē-ˌō, -'fek-tē-\ *n, pl* **-ti·o·nes** \-ˌfek-shē-'ō-ˌnēz, -ˌfek-tē-'ō-ˌnäs\ : CONFECTION

con·fec·tion \kən-'fek-shən\ *n* : a medicinal preparation usu. made with sugar, syrup, or honey — called also *electuary*

con·fig·u·ra·tion \kən-ˌfig-(y)ə-'rā-shən, ˌkän-\ *n* **1 a** : relative arrangement of parts or elements **b** : the stable structural makeup of a chemical compound esp. with reference to the space relations of the constituent atoms **2** : GESTALT ⟨personality ~⟩ — **con·fig·u·ra·tion·al** \-shnəl, -shən-°l\ *adj* — **con·fig·u·ra·tion·al·ly** \-ē\ *adv* — **con·fig·u·ra·tive** \-'fig-(y)ə-rət-iv\ *adj*

con·fine \kən-'fīn\ *vt* **con·fined; con·fin·ing** : to keep from leaving accustomed quarters (as one's room or bed) under pressure of infirmity, childbirth, or detention

con·fined \kən-'fīnd\ *adj* : undergoing childbirth

con·fine·ment \kən-'fīn-mənt\ *n* : an act of confining : the state of being confined; *esp* : LYING-IN

con·flict \'kän-ˌflikt\ *n* : mental struggle resulting from incompatible or opposing needs, drives, wishes, or external or internal demands — **con·flict·ful** \'kän-ˌflikt-fəl\ *adj* — **con·flict·less** \'kän-ˌflikt-tləs\ *adj* — **con·flic·tu·al** \kän-'flik-ch(ə-w)əl, kən-\ *adj*

con·flict·ed \kən-'flik-təd\ *adj* : having or experiencing emotional conflict ⟨working women were much more ~ about working than full-time mothers were about staying home —*People*⟩

con·flu·ence of sinuses \'kän-ˌflü-ən(t)s-, kən-'flü-\ *n* : the junction of several of the sinuses of the dura mater in the internal occipital region — called also *confluence of the sinuses, torcular Herophili*

con·flu·ens si·nu·um \(ˌ)kän-ˌflü-ən(t)(s)-'sīn-yə-wəm\ *n* : CONFLUENCE OF SINUSES

con·flu·ent \'kän-ˌflü-ənt, kən-\ *adj* **1** : flowing or coming together; *also* : run together ⟨~ pustules⟩ **2** : characterized by confluent lesions ⟨~ smallpox⟩ — compare DISCRETE

con·fo·cal \(ˈ)kän-'fō-kəl\ *adj* : having the same foci ⟨~ lenses⟩ — **con·fo·cal·ly** \-kə-lē\ *adv*

con·for·ma·tion \ˌkän-(ˌ)fȯr-'mā-shən, -fər-\ *n* : any of the spatial arrangements of a molecule that can be obtained by rotation of the atoms about a single bond — **con·for·ma·tion·al** \-shnəl, -shən-°l\ *adj* — **con·for·ma·tion·al·ly** \-ē\ *adv*

con·form·er \kən-'fȯr-mər\ *n* : a mold (as of plastic) used to prevent collapse or closing of a cavity, vessel, or opening during surgical repair

con·fused \kən-'fyüzd\ *adj* : affected with mental confusion

con·fu·sion \kən-'fyü-zhən\ *n* : disturbance of consciousness characterized by inability to engage in orderly thought or by lack of power to distinguish, choose, or act decisively — **con·fu·sion·al** \-zhnəl, -zhən-°l\ *adj*

cong *abbr* **1** congenital **2** congius

con·geal \kən-'jē(ə)l\ *vt* **1** : to change from a fluid to a solid state by or as if by cold **2** : to make viscid or curdled : CO-AGULATE ~ *vi* : to become congealed

con·ge·la·tion \ˌkän-jə-ˈlā-shən\ *n* : the process or result of congealing and esp. freezing

con·ge·ner \ˈkän-jə-nər, kən-ˈjē-\ *also* **co·ge·ner** \ˈkō-ˌjē-nər, kō-ˈ\ *n* **1** : a member of the same taxonomic genus as another plant or animal **2** : a chemical substance related to another ⟨tetracycline and its ~s⟩ — **con·ge·ner·ic** \ˌkän-jə-ˈner-ik\ *adj*

congenita — see AMYOTONIA CONGENITA, ARTHROGRYPOSIS MULTIPLEX CONGENITA, MYOTONIA CONGENITA, OSTEOGENESIS IMPERFECTA CONGENITA

con·gen·i·tal \kän-ˈjen-ə-tᵊl\ *adj* **1** : existing at or dating from birth ⟨~ deafness⟩ **2** : acquired during development in the uterus and not through heredity ⟨~ syphilis⟩ — compare ACQUIRED 2, FAMILIAL, HEREDITARY — **con·gen·i·tal·ly** \-tᵊl-ē\ *adv*

congenital con·trac·tur·al arachnodactyly \-kən-ˈtrak-chə-rəl-, -kän-\ *n* : a disorder that is similar to or a variant of Marfan syndrome, is inherited as a dominant autosomal trait, and is characterized esp. by arachnodactyly, joint contracture, and scoliosis

congenital megacolon *n* : HIRSCHSPRUNG'S DISEASE

con·gest·ed \kən-ˈjes-təd\ *adj* : containing an excessive accumulation esp. of blood or mucus ⟨~ mucous membranes⟩ ⟨~ lungs⟩

con·ges·tion \kən-ˈjes(h)-chən\ *n* : an excessive accumulation esp. of blood or mucus ⟨vascular ~⟩ ⟨nasal ~⟩

con·ges·tive \-ˈjes-tiv\ *adj* : having to do with congestion

congestive heart failure *n* : heart failure in which the heart is unable to maintain adequate circulation of blood in the tissues of the body or to pump out the venous blood returned to it by the venous circulation — compare CORONARY FAILURE

con·gi·us \ˈkän-jē-əs\ *n, pl* **con·gii** \-jē-ˌī\ : GALLON — abbr. *cong* or *C*

con·glo·bate \kän-ˈglō-ˌbāt, kən-\ *vt* **-bat·ed; -bat·ing** : to form into a round compact mass — **con·glo·bate** \-bət, -ˌbāt\ *adj* — **con·glo·ba·tion** \ˌkän-(ˌ)glō-ˈbā-shən\ *n*

¹**con·glom·er·ate** \kən-ˈgläm-(ə-)rət\ *adj* : made up of parts from various sources or of various kinds

²**con·glom·er·ate** \-ə-ˌrāt\ *vb* **-at·ed; -at·ing** *vt* : to gather (something) into a mass or coherent whole ~ *vi* : to gather into a mass or coherent whole — **con·glom·er·a·tive** \-ˈgläm-(ə-)rət-iv, -ə-ˌrāt-\ *adj*

³**con·glom·er·ate** \-(ə-)rət\ *n* : a composite mass or mixture

con·glom·er·a·tion \kən-ˌgläm-ə-ˈrā-shən, ˌkän-\ *n* **1** : the act of conglomerating : the state of being conglomerated **2** : something conglomerated : a mixed coherent mass

con·glu·tin \kən-ˈglüt-ᵊn, ˈkän-ˌ\ *n* : a protein found esp. in almonds and in seeds from some plants (as peas or beans) of the family Leguminosae

con·glu·ti·nate \kən-ˈglüt-ᵊn-ˌāt, kän-\ *vb* **-nat·ed; -nat·ing** *vt* : to unite by or as if by a glutinous substance ~ *vi* : to become conglutinated ⟨blood platelets ~ in blood clotting⟩

con·glu·ti·na·tion \kən-ˌglüt-ᵊn-ˈā-shən, ˌkän-\ *n* : the act or action of conglutinating or the consequent quality or state of being conglutinated: as **a** : the union or establishment of continuity of parts — now used only of abnormal adhesion of contiguous surfaces **b** (1) : a reaction of agglutination and lysis brought about by addition of bovine serum to antibody-treated cells (2) : agglutination brought about by serum albumin or plasma proteins when added to cells coated with blocking antibody

con·glu·ti·nin \kən-ˈglüt-ᵊn-ən, (ˈ)kän-\ *n* : a heat-stable protein of bovine serum that combines with red blood cells which have been treated with antibody and that causes rapid strong agglutination followed by lysis

Congo red \ˌkäŋ-(ˌ)gō-ˈred\ *n* : an azo dye $C_{32}H_{22}N_6Na_2O_6S_2$ that is red in alkaline and blue in acid solution and that is used in a number of diagnostic tests and esp. for the detection of amyloidosis since the injected dye tends to be retained by abnormal amyloid deposits

con·gress \ˈkäŋ-grəs *also* -rəs, *Brit usu* ˈkäŋ-ˌgres\ *n* : COITUS

con·hy·drine \kän-ˈhī-drən, -ˌdrēn\ *n* : a poisonous crystalline alkaloid $C_8H_{17}NO$ occurring in poison hemlock

coni *pl of* CONUS

con·i·cal \ˈkän-i-kəl\ *or* **con·ic** \ˈkän-ik\ *adj* : resembling a cone esp. in shape — **con·i·cal·ly** \-k(ə-)lē\ *adv*

co·nid·i·al \kə-ˈnid-ē-əl\ *adj* : of or relating to conidia

co·nid·io·phore \kə-ˈnid-ē-ə-ˌfō(ə)r, -ˌfȯ(ə)r\ *n* : a structure that bears conidia; *specif* : a specialized hyphal branch that produces successive conidia usu. by abstriction — **co·nid·i·oph·o·rous** \-ˌnid-ē-ˈäf-(ə-)rəs\ *adj*

co·nid·io·spore \-ˌspō(ə)r, -ˌspȯ(ə)r\ *n* : CONIDIUM

co·nid·i·um \kə-ˈnid-ē-əm\ *n, pl* **-ia** \-ē-ə\ : an asexual spore produced on a conidiophore

co·ni·ine \ˈkō-nē-ˌēn\ *n* : a poisonous alkaloid $C_8H_{17}N$ found in poison hemlock (*Conium maculatum*)

co·ni·um \kō-ˈnī-əm, ˈkō-nē-\ *n* **1** *a cap*) : a genus of poisonous herbs (family Umbelliferae) that have spotted stems, large divided leaves and white flowers and that include the poison hemlock **b** : a plant of the genus *Conium* **2** : the dried full-grown but unripe fruit of the poison hemlock containing coniine and its methyl derivative and used as a narcotic and sedative

con·iza·tion \ˌkō-nə-ˈzā-shən, ˌkän-ə-\ *n* : the electrosurgical excision of a cone of tissue from a diseased uterine cervix

con·joined \kən-ˈjȯind, kän-\ *adj* : of, relating to, or being conjoined twins ⟨~ twinning⟩ ⟨~ twin neonates⟩

conjoined twins *n pl* : twins that are physically united at some part or parts of their bodies at the time of birth

con·ju·gal \ˈkän-ji-gəl, kən-ˈjü-\ *adj* : of or relating to the married state or to married persons and their relations ⟨~ happiness⟩ — **con·ju·gal·ly** \-gə-lē\ *adv*

conjugal rights *n pl* : the sexual rights or privileges implied by and involved in the marriage relationship : the right of sexual intercourse between husband and wife

con·ju·gant \ˈkän-ji-gənt\ *n* : either of a pair of conjugating gametes or organisms

con·ju·gase \ˈkän-jə-ˌgās, -ˌgāz\ *n* : any of a group of enzymes found in blood or in certain organs (as kidney and pancreas) and in some vegetables (as potatoes) that bring about the breakdown of conjugates of pteroylglutamic acid

con·ju·ga·ta \ˌkän-jə-ˈgät-ə\ *n, pl* **-ga·tae** \-ˈgät-ˌē\ : CONJUGATE DIAMETER

¹**con·ju·gate** \ˈkän-ji-gət, -jə-ˌgāt\ *adj* **1** : functioning or operating simultaneously as if joined ⟨~ eye movements⟩ **2** *of an acid or base* : related by the difference of a proton ⟨the acid NH_4^+ and the base NH_3 are ~ to each other⟩ — **con·ju·gate·ly** *adv*

²**con·ju·gate** \-jə-ˌgāt\ *vb* **-gat·ed; -gat·ing** *vt* : to unite (as with the elimination of water) so that the product is easily broken down (as by hydrolysis) into the original compounds ⟨benzoic acid is *conjugated* with glycine to hippuric acid in the body⟩ ~ *vi* **1** : to pair and fuse in conjugation **2** : to pair in synapsis

³**conjugate** \-ji-gət, -jə-ˌgāt\ *n* : a chemical compound formed by the union of two compounds or united with another compound

con·ju·gat·ed \ˈkän-jə-ˌgāt-əd\ *adj* : formed by the union of two compounds or united with another compound ⟨some enzymes are ~⟩ ⟨~ bile acids⟩

conjugated estrogen *n* : a mixture of estrogens and esp. of estrone and equilin for oral administration in the form of the sodium salts of their sulfate esters — usu. used in pl. but sing. or pl. in constr. ⟨*conjugated estrogens* is a mixture —*U.S. Pharmacopeia XXII/National Formulary XVII*, 22d Ed.⟩; see PREMARIN, PREMPRO

conjugate diameter *n* : the anteroposterior diameter of the human pelvis measured from the sacral promontory to the pubic symphysis — called also *conjugata, true conjugate*

\ə\ **abut** \ᵊ\ **kitten** \ər\ **further** \a\ **ash** \ā\ **ace** \ä\ **cot, cart** \au̇\ **out** \ch\ **chin** \e\ **bet** \ē\ **easy** \g\ **go** \i\ **hit** \ī\ **ice** \j\ **job** \ŋ\ **sing** \ō\ **go** \ȯ\ **law** \ȯi\ **boy** \th\ **thin** \t͟h\ **the** \ü\ **loot** \u̇\ **foot** \y\ **yet** \zh\ **vision** *See also* Pronunciation Symbols page

conjugated protein *n* : a compound of a protein with a non-protein ⟨hemoglobin is a *conjugated protein* of heme and globin⟩

conjugate vaccine *n* : a vaccine containing bacterial capsular polysaccharide joined to a protein to enhance immunogenicity; *esp* : one that is used to immunize infants and children against invasive disease caused by Hib bacteria and that contains the Hib capsular polysaccharide polyribosylribitol phosphate bound to diphtheria or tetanus toxoid or to an outer membrane protein of the meningococcus

con·ju·ga·tion \ˌkän-jə-ˈgā-shən\ *n*   **1** : the act of conjugating : the state of being conjugated   **2 a** : fusion of usu. similar gametes with ultimate union of their nuclei that occurs in most fungi and in some algae (as green algae)   **b** : temporary cytoplasmic union with exchange of nuclear material that is the usual sexual process in ciliated protozoans   **c** : the one-way transfer of DNA between bacteria in cellular contact — **con·ju·ga·tion·al** \-shnəl, -shən-ᵊl\ *adj*

con·junc·ti·va \ˌkän-ˌjəŋ(k)-ˈtī-və, kən-\ *n, pl* **-vas** *or* **-vae** \-(ˌ)vē\ : the mucous membrane that lines the inner surface of the eyelids and is continued over the forepart of the eyeball — **con·junc·ti·val** \-vəl\ *adj*

con·junc·ti·vi·tis \kən-ˌjəŋ(k)-ti-ˈvīt-əs\ *n* : inflammation of the conjunctiva

con·junc·tivo·plas·ty \kən-ˈjəŋ(k)-ti-(ˌ)vō-ˌplas-tē\ *n, pl* **-plas·ties** : plastic repair of a defect in the conjunctiva

con·junc·tivo·rhi·nos·to·my \kən-ˌjəŋ(k)-ti-(ˌ)vō-ˌrī-ˈnäs-tə-mē\ *n, pl* **-to·mies** : surgical creation of a passage through the conjunctiva to the nasal cavity

con·nate \kä-ˈnāt, ˈkän-ˌāt\ *adj* : firmly united ⟨~ bones⟩ — **con·nate·ly** *adv*

con·nec·tive tissue \kə-ˌnek-tiv-\ *n* : a tissue of mesodermal origin that consists of various cells (as fibroblasts and macrophages) and interlacing protein fibers (as of collagen) embedded in a chiefly carbohydrate ground substance, that supports, ensheathes, and binds together other tissues, and that includes loose and dense forms (as adipose tissue, tendons, ligaments, and aponeuroses) and specialized forms (as cartilage and bone)

connective tissue disease *n* : any of various diseases or abnormal states (as rheumatoid arthritis, systemic lupus erythematosus, polyarteritis nodosa, rheumatic fever, and dermatomyositis) characterized by inflammatory or degenerative changes in connective tissue — called also *collagen disease, collagenolysis, collagen vascular disease*

con·nec·tor \kə-ˈnek-tər\ *n* : something that connects; *esp* : a part of a partial denture which joins its components

connector neuron *n* : INTERNEURON

conniventes — see VALVULAE CONNIVENTES

Conn's syndrome \ˈkänz-\ *n* : PRIMARY ALDOSTERONISM
> **Conn, Jerome W. (1907–1994),** American physician. Conn had a long and distinguished career as a member of the medical faculty at the university hospital in Ann Arbor, Michigan. For many years he also served as director of the hospital's division of metabolism and endocrinology. He received numerous awards for his contributions to endocrinology. Conn also undertook studies in human nutrition, metabolic disorders, and normal human metabolism.

¹co·noid \ˈkō-ˌnȯid\ *or* **co·noi·dal** \kō-ˈnȯid-ᵊl\ *adj* : shaped like or nearly like a cone

²conoid *n* : a cone-shaped structure; *esp* : a hollow organelle shaped like a truncated cone that occurs at the anterior end of the organism in some developmental stages of some sporozoans (as of the genus *Sarcocystis*)

conoid ligament *n* : the posterior fasciculus of the coraco-clavicular ligament connecting the conoid tubercle and the base of the coracoid

conoid tubercle *n* : a prominence on the underside of the clavicle that forms one attachment of the conoid ligament

con·qui·nine \ˈkän-kwə-ˌnēn, ˈkän-\ *n* : QUINIDINE

con·san·guine \kän-ˈsaŋ-gwən, kən-\ *adj* : CONSANGUINEOUS

con·san·guin·e·ous \ˌkän-ˌsan-ˈgwin-ē-əs, -ˌsaŋ-\ *adj* : of the same blood or origin; *specif* : relating to or involving persons (as first cousins) that are relatively closely related ⟨~ marriages⟩ — **con·san·guin·i·ty** \-ˈgwin-ət-ē\ *n, pl* **-ties**

con·science \ˈkän-chən(t)s\ *n* : the part of the superego in psychoanalysis that transmits commands and admonitions to the ego

¹con·scious \ˈkän-chəs\ *adj*   **1** : capable of or marked by thought, will, design, or perception : relating to, being, or being part of consciousness ⟨the ~ mind⟩ ⟨~ and unconscious processes⟩   **2** : having mental faculties undulled by sleep, faintness, or stupor ⟨became ~ after the anesthesia wore off⟩ — **con·scious·ly** \-lē\ *adv*

²conscious *n* : CONSCIOUSNESS 3

con·scious·ness \ˈkän-chə-snəs\ *n*   **1** : the totality in psychology of sensations, perceptions, ideas, attitudes, and feelings of which an individual or a group is aware at any given time or within a given time span ⟨altered states of ~, such as sleep, dreaming and hypnosis —Bob Gaines⟩   **2** : waking life (as that to which one returns after sleep, trance, or fever) in which one's normal mental powers are present ⟨the ether wore off and the patient regained ~⟩   **3** : the upper part of mental life of which the person is aware as contrasted with unconscious processes

conscious sedation *n* : an induced state of sedation characterized by a minimally depressed consciousness such that the patient is able to continuously and independently maintain a patent airway, retain protective reflexes, and remain responsive to verbal commands and physical stimulation — compare DEEP SEDATION

con·sen·su·al \kən-ˈsench-(ə-)wəl, -ˈsen-chəl\ *adj*   **1** : existing or made by mutual consent ⟨~ sexual behavior⟩   **2** : relating to or being the constrictive pupillary response of an eye that is covered when the other eye is exposed to light — **con·sen·su·al·ly** \-ē\ *adv*

conservation of energy *n* : a principle in physics: the total energy of an isolated system remains constant irrespective of whatever internal changes may take place with energy disappearing in one form reappearing in another — called also *first law of thermodynamics, law of conservation of energy*

conservation of mass *n* : a principle in classical physics: the total mass of any material system is neither increased nor diminished by reactions between the parts — called also *conservation of matter, law of conservation of matter*

con·ser·va·tive \kən-ˈsər-vət-iv\ *adj* : not extreme or drastic; *esp* : designed to preserve parts or restore or preserve function ⟨~ treatment of prostate cancer by watchful waiting or hormonal therapy in contrast to radical prostatectomy⟩ — compare AGGRESSIVE 3, RADICAL — **con·ser·va·tive·ly** *adv*

¹con·serve \ˈkän-ˌsərv\ *n* : an obsolete medicinal preparation made by mixing undried vegetable drugs with sufficient powdered sugar to form a soft mass — compare CONFECTION

²con·serve \kən-ˈsərv\ *vt* **con·served; con·serv·ing** : to maintain (a quantity) constant during a process of chemical, physical, or evolutionary change ⟨a DNA sequence that has been *conserved*⟩

con·sol·i·da·tion \kən-ˌsäl-ə-ˈdā-shən\ *n* : the process by which an infected lung passes from an aerated collapsible condition to one of airless solid consistency through the accumulation of exudate in the alveoli and adjoining ducts ⟨pneumonic ~⟩; *also* : tissue that has undergone consolidation ⟨areas of ~⟩

con·so·lute \ˈkän(t)-sə-ˌlüt\ *adj* : miscible in all proportions : mutually soluble — used of two or more liquids

con·spe·cif·ic \ˌkän(t)-spi-ˈsif-ik\ *adj* : of the same species — **conspecific** *n*

const *abbr* constant

¹con·stant \ˈkän(t)-stənt\ *adj* : remaining unchanged — **con·stant·ly** *adv*

²constant *n* : something invariable or unchanging; *esp* : a number that has a fixed value in a given situation or universally or that is characteristic of some substance or instrument

constant region *n* : the part of the polypeptide chain of a light or heavy chain of an antibody that ends in a free carboxyl group –COOH and that is relatively constant in its sequence of amino acid residues from one antibody to another — called also *constant domain;* compare VARIABLE REGION

con·stel·la·tion \ˌkän(t)-stə-'lā-shən\ *n* : a set of ideas, conditions, symptoms, or traits that fall into or appear to fall into a pattern: as **a** : a group of stimulus conditions or factors affecting personality and behavior development ⟨the way in which family ∼ and handling of punishment influenced this particular boy —S. B. Sarason⟩ **b** : a group of behavioral or personality traits

con·sti·pate \'kän(t)-stə-ˌpāt\ *vt* **-pat·ed; -pat·ing** : to make costive : cause constipation in

constipated *adj* : affected with constipation

con·sti·pa·tion \ˌkän(t)-stə-'pā-shən\ *n* : abnormally delayed or infrequent passage of dry hardened feces

con·sti·tu·tion \ˌkän(t)-stə-'t(y)ü-shən\ *n* **1** : the physical makeup of the individual comprising inherited qualities modified by environment **2** : the structure of a compound as determined by the kind, number, and arrangement of atoms in its molecule — **con·sti·tu·tion·al** \-shnəl, -shən-ᵊl\ *adj*

con·sti·tu·tion·al \-shnəl, -shən-ᵊl\ *n* : a walk taken for one's health

con·sti·tu·tive \'kän(t)-stə-ˌt(y)üt-iv, kən-'stich-ət-iv\ *adj* **1 a** : of, relating to, or being an enzyme or protein produced in relatively constant amounts in all cells of an organism without regard to cell environmental conditions (as the concentration of a substrate) — compare INDUCIBLE a **b** : controlling production of or coding genetic information for a constitutive enzyme or protein ⟨∼ genes⟩ ⟨∼ mutations⟩ **2** : being chromatin of a chromosomal region that is condensed into heterochromatin in all cells of an organism rather than just some — **con·sti·tu·tive·ly** *adv*

con·strict \kən-'strikt\ *vt* **1** : to make narrow or draw together ⟨∼ the pupil of the eye⟩ **2** : to subject (as a body part) to compression ⟨∼ a nerve⟩ ∼ *vi* : to become constricted — **con·stric·tive** \-'strik-tiv\ *adj*

con·stric·tion \-'strik-shən\ *n* **1** : an act or product of constricting **2** : the quality or state of being constricted **3** : something that constricts

con·stric·tor \-'strik-tər\ *n* : a muscle that contracts a cavity or orifice or compresses an organ — see INFERIOR CONSTRICTOR, MIDDLE CONSTRICTOR, SUPERIOR CONSTRICTOR

constrictor pha·ryn·gis inferior \-fə-'rin-jəs-\ *n* : INFERIOR CONSTRICTOR

constrictor pharyngis me·di·us \-'mēd-ē-əs\ *n* : MIDDLE CONSTRICTOR

constrictor pharyngis superior *n* : SUPERIOR CONSTRICTOR

con·struct \'kän-ˌstrəkt\ *n* : something constructed esp. by mental synthesis ⟨form a ∼ of a physical object by mentally assembling and integrating sense-data⟩

con·sult \kən-'səlt\ *vt* : to ask the advice or opinion of ⟨∼ a doctor⟩

con·sul·tant \kən-'səlt-ᵊnt\ *n* : one (as a physician, surgeon, or psychologist) called in for professional advice or services

con·sul·ta·tion \ˌkän(t)-səl-'tā-shən\ *n* : a deliberation between physicians on a case or its treatment

con·sul·ta·tive \kən-'səl-tət-iv, 'kän(t)-səl-ˌtāt-iv\ *adj* : of, relating to, or intended for consultation ⟨neurologic services are typically ∼ —*Physicians' Current Procedural Terminology*⟩

con·sult·ing \kən-'səl-tiŋ\ *adj* : serving as a consultant ⟨a ∼ physician⟩ ⟨a ∼ psychologist⟩

con·sum·ma·to·ry \kən-'səm-ə-ˌtōr-ē, -ˌtȯr-\ *adj* : of, relating to, or being a response or act (as eating or copulating) that terminates a period of usu. goal-directed behavior

con·sump·tion \kən-'səm(p)-shən\ *n* **1** : a progressive wasting away of the body esp. from pulmonary tuberculosis **2** : TUBERCULOSIS

¹con·sump·tive \-'səm(p)-tiv\ *adj* : of, relating to, or affected with consumption ⟨a ∼ cough⟩ ⟨a ∼ child⟩ — **con·sump·tive·ly** *adv*

²consumptive *n* : an individual affected with consumption

cont *abbr* **1** containing **2** contents **3** continue; continued

¹con·tact \'kän-ˌtakt\ *n* **1** : union or junction of body surfaces ⟨sexual ∼⟩ **2 a** : the junction of two electrical conductors through which a current passes **b** : a special part that has been made for such a junction **3** : direct experience through the senses ⟨loss of ∼ with reality⟩ **4** : CONTACT LENS

²contact *adj* : caused or transmitted by direct or indirect contact (as with an allergen or a contagious disease) ⟨a ∼ allergy⟩

contact inhibition *n* : cessation of cellular undulating movements upon contact with other cells with accompanying cessation of cell growth and division

con·tact lens \'kän-ˌtakt-\ *n* : a thin lens designed to fit over the cornea and usu. worn to correct defects in vision

con·ta·gion \kən-'tā-jən\ *n* **1** : the transmission of a disease by direct or indirect contact **2** : CONTAGIOUS DISEASE **3** : a disease-producing agent (as a virus)

contagiosa — see IMPETIGO CONTAGIOSA, MOLLUSCUM CONTAGIOSUM

contagiosum — see MOLLUSCUM CONTAGIOSUM

con·ta·gious \-jəs\ *adj* **1** : communicable by contact ⟨tuberculosis in the ∼ stage⟩ — compare INFECTIOUS 2 **2** : bearing contagion ⟨many persons . . . are ∼ long before they are aware of the presence of their disease —*Jour. Amer. Med. Assoc.*⟩ **3** : used for contagious diseases ⟨a ∼ ward⟩ — **con·ta·gious·ly** *adv* — **con·ta·gious·ness** *n*

contagious abortion *n* **1** : brucellosis in domestic animals characterized by abortion: **a** : brucellosis affecting esp. cattle that is caused by a brucella (*Brucella abortus*), that is contracted by ingestion, by copulation, or possibly by wound infection, and that is characterized by proliferation of the causative organism in the fetal membranes inducing abortion, subsequent invasion of the regional lymph nodes and udder with the formation of chronic foci of infection, and sometimes reinvasion of the uterus when pregnancy is reestablished **b** : any brucellosis of swine or goats having a somewhat similar course to bovine brucellosis but usu. caused by different brucellae **2** : any of several contagious or infectious diseases of domestic animals marked by abortion (as vibrionic abortion of sheep or an acute salmonellosis of the mare) — called also *infectious abortion*

contagious disease *n* : an infectious disease communicable by contact with one who has it, with a bodily discharge of such a patient, or with an object touched by such a patient or by bodily discharges — compare COMMUNICABLE DISEASE

con·ta·gium \kən-'tā-j(ē-)əm\ *n, pl* **-gia** \-j(ē-)ə\ : a virus or living organism capable of causing a communicable disease

con·tam·i·nant \kən-'tam-ə-nənt\ *n* : something that contaminates

con·tam·i·nate \kən-'tam-ə-ˌnāt\ *vt* **-nat·ed; -nat·ing 1** : to soil, stain, or infect by contact or association ⟨bacteria *contaminated* the wound⟩ **2** : to make inferior or impure by admixture ⟨air *contaminated* by sulfur dioxide⟩ — **con·tam·i·na·tive** \-ˌnāt-iv\ *adj* — **con·tam·i·na·tor** \-ˌnāt-ər\ *n*

con·tam·i·na·tion \kən-ˌtam-ə-'nā-shən\ *n* **1** : a process of contaminating : a state of being contaminated **2** : something that contaminates

con·tent \'kän-ˌtent\ *n* **1** : something contained — usu. used in pl. ⟨the stomach ∼s⟩ **2** : the subject matter or symbolic significance of something — see LATENT CONTENT, MANIFEST CONTENT **3** : the amount of specified material contained ⟨the sulfur ∼ of a sample⟩

con·tig·u·ous \kən-'tig-yə-wəs\ *adj* : being in actual contact : touching along a boundary or at a point — **con·ti·gu·ity** \ˌkänt-ə-'gyü-ət-ē\ *n, pl* **-it·ies** — **con·tig·u·ous·ly** *adv*

\ə\ abut \ᵊ\ kitten \ər\ further \a\ ash \ā\ ace \ä\ cot, cart
\aù\ out \ch\ chin \e\ bet \ē\ easy \g\ go \i\ hit \ī\ ice \j\ job
\ŋ\ sing \ō\ go \ȯ\ law \ȯi\ boy \th\ thin \th̲\ the \ü\ loot
\ù\ foot \y\ yet \zh\ vision   *See also* Pronunciation Symbols page

con·ti·nence \'känt-ᵊn-ən(t)s\ *n* **1** : self-restraint in refraining from sexual intercourse **2** : the ability to retain a bodily discharge voluntarily ⟨fecal ∼⟩

con·ti·nent \'känt-ᵊn-ənt\ *adj* : exercising continence — **con·ti·nent·ly** *adv*

con·ti·nu·ity \ˌkänt-ᵊn-'(y)ü-ət-ē\ *n, pl* **-it·ies** : uninterrupted connection, succession, or union

con·tin·u·ous \kən-'tin-yə-wəs\ *adj* : marked by uninterrupted extension in space, time, or sequence : continuing without intermission or recurring regularly after minute interruptions ⟨∼ vitamin injections⟩ — **con·tin·u·ous·ly** *adv*

continuous phase *n* : DISPERSION MEDIUM

continuous positive airway pressure *n* : a technique of assisting breathing by maintaining the air pressure in the lungs and air passages constant and above atmospheric pressure throughout the breathing cycle — abbr. *CPAP*; compare POSITIVE END-EXPIRATORY PRESSURE

¹con·tour \'kän-ˌtü(ə)r\ *n* : an outline esp. of a curving or irregular figure; *also* : the line representing this outline

²contour *vt* : to shape the contour of ⟨∼ a gingiva in gingivoplasty⟩

con·tra·cep·tion \ˌkän-trə-'sep-shən\ *n* : deliberate prevention of conception or impregnation — **con·tra·cep·tive** \-'sep-tiv\ *adj or n*

contraceptive pill *n* : BIRTH CONTROL PILL

con·tract \kən-'trakt *also* 'kän-ˌtrakt\ *vt* **1** : to become affected with ⟨∼ pneumonia⟩ **2** : to reduce to smaller size by or as if by squeezing or drawing together ⟨treatment . . . inhibits spindle formation and ∼s chromosomes —Ernst Mayr⟩ **3** *of a muscle or muscle fiber* : to cause to undergo contraction; *esp* : to cause to shorten and thicken ∼ *vi* **1** : to draw together so as to become diminished in size **2** *of a muscle or muscle fiber* : to undergo contraction; *esp* : to shorten and thicken — **con·tract·ibil·i·ty** \kən-ˌtrak-tə-'bil-ət-ē, ˌkän-\ *n, pl* **-ties** — **con·tract·ible** \kən-'trak-tə-bəl, 'kän-ˌ\ *adj*

contracted pelvis *n* : a pelvis that is abnormally small in one or more principal diameters and that consequently interferes with normal parturition

con·trac·tile \kən-'trak-tᵊl, -ˌtīl\ *adj* : having or concerned with the power or property of contracting ⟨∼ proteins of muscle fibrils⟩

contractile vacuole *n* : a vacuole in a unicellular organism that contracts regularly to discharge fluid from the body

con·trac·til·i·ty \ˌkän-ˌtrak-'til-ət-ē\ *n, pl* **-ties** : the capability or quality of shrinking or contracting; *esp* : the power of muscle fibers of shortening into a more compact form

con·trac·tion \kən-'trak-shən\ *n* **1** : the action or process of contracting : the state of being contracted ⟨∼ of hepatitis⟩ ⟨lung expansion and ∼ in breathing —P. G. Donohue⟩ **2** : the action of a functioning muscle or muscle fiber in which force is generated accompanied esp. by shortening and thickening of the muscle or muscle fiber or sometimes by its lengthening ⟨isometric ∼⟩ ⟨isotonic ∼⟩; *esp* : the shortening and thickening of a functioning muscle or muscle fiber **3** : one of usu. a series of rhythmic tightening actions of the uterine muscles (as during menstruation or labor)

con·trac·tor \'kän-ˌtrak-tər, kən-'\ *n* : something (as a muscle) that contracts or shortens

con·trac·ture \kən-'trak-chər\ *n* : a permanent shortening (as of muscle, tendon, or scar tissue) producing deformity or distortion — see DUPUYTREN'S CONTRACTURE

con·tra·in·di·cate \ˌkän-trə-'in-də-ˌkāt\ *vt* **-cat·ed; -cat·ing** : to make (a treatment or procedure) inadvisable

con·tra·in·di·ca·tion \-ˌin-də-'kā-shən\ *n* : something (as a symptom or condition) that makes a particular treatment or procedure inadvisable

con·tra·lat·er·al \-'lat-ə-rəl, -'la-trəl\ *adj* : occurring on, affecting, or acting in conjunction with a part on the opposite side of the body ⟨the motor cortex controls ∼ muscles⟩ — compare IPSILATERAL

con·trast bath \'kän-ˌtrast-\ *n* : a therapeutic immersion of a part of the body (as an extremity) alternately in hot and cold water

contrast medium *n* : a substance (as a solution of iodine or suspension of barium sulfate) comparatively opaque to X-rays that is introduced into the body (as by injection or swallowing) to contrast an internal part (as the gastrointestinal tract, kidneys, or blood vessels) with its surrounding tissue in radiographic visualization — called also *contrast agent, contrast material*

con·tre·coup \'kōn-trə-ˌkü, 'kän-\ *n* : injury (as when the brain strikes the skull) occurring on the side of an organ opposite to the side on which a blow or impact is received — compare COUP

con·trec·ta·tion \ˌkän-(ˌ)trek-'tā-shən\ *n* : the initial stage of the sexual act concerned with manual contact and tumescence

¹con·trol \kən-'trōl\ *vb* **con·trolled; con·trol·ling** *vt* **1** : to incorporate suitable controls in ⟨a *controlled* experiment⟩ **2** : to reduce the incidence or severity of esp. to innocuous levels ⟨∼ an insect population⟩ ⟨a vaccine for *controlling* outbreaks of cholera⟩ ∼ *vi* : to incorporate controls in an experiment or study — used with *for* ⟨failure to ∼ for the difference in the rate of smoking between the two groups —Howard Bauchner *et al*⟩

²control *n* **1** : an act or instance of controlling something ⟨∼ of acute intermittent porphyria⟩ **2** : one that is used in controlling something: as **a** : an experiment in which the subjects are treated as in a parallel experiment except for omission of the procedure or agent under test and which is used as a standard of comparison in judging experimental effects — called also *control experiment* **b** : one (as an organism, culture, or group) that is part of a control

con·trolled \kən-'trōld\ *adj* : regulated by law with regard to possession and use ⟨∼ drugs⟩

controlled hypotension *n* : low blood pressure induced and maintained to reduce blood loss or to provide a bloodless field during surgery

con·tu·sion \kən-'t(y)ü-zhən\ *n* : injury to tissue usu. without laceration : BRUISE 1 — **con·tuse** \-'t(y)üz\ *vt* **con·tused; con·tus·ing**

co·nus \'kō-nəs\ *n* **1** *cap* : a very large genus (the type of the family Conidae) of tropical marine snails comprising the cones and including many harmless forms and a few chiefly in the southwest Pacific that are highly dangerous because they are capable of biting with the radula and injecting a paralytic venom that has been known to cause death in humans **2** *pl* **co·ni** \-ˌnī, -(ˌ)nē\ : CONUS ARTERIOSUS

co·nus ar·te·ri·o·sus \'kō-nə-sär-ˌtir-ē-'ō-səs\ *n, pl* **co·ni ar·te·ri·o·si** \-ˌnī-är-ˌtir-ē-'ō-ˌsī, -(ˌ)nē-\ : a conical prolongation of the right ventricle from which the pulmonary arteries emerge — called also *conus*

conus med·ul·lar·is \-ˌmed-ᵊl-'er-əs, -ˌmej-ə-'ler-\ *n* : a tapering lower part of the spinal cord at the level of the first lumbar segment

conv *abbr* convalescent

con·va·lesce \ˌkän-və-'les\ *vi* **-lesced; -lesc·ing** : to recover health and strength gradually after sickness or weakness

con·va·les·cence \-'les-ᵊn(t)s\ *n* **1** : gradual recovery of health and strength after disease ⟨a patient well advanced in ∼⟩ **2** : the time between the subsidence of a disease and complete restoration to health ⟨quiet and rest during ∼⟩

¹con·va·les·cent \-'les-ᵊnt\ *adj* **1** : recovering from sickness or debility : partially restored to health or strength ⟨∼ patients⟩ **2** : of, for, or relating to convalescence or convalescents ⟨∼ stages⟩ ⟨a ∼ ward⟩ — **con·va·les·cent·ly** *adv*

²convalescent *n* : one recovering from sickness

convalescent home *n* : an institution for the care of convalescing patients

con·val·la·mar·in \kən-ˌval-ə-'mar-ən, ˌkän-və-'lam-ə-rən\ *n* : a bitter poisonous glycoside extracted from the dried rhizome and roots of the lily of the valley

con·val·lar·ia \ˌkän-və-'lar-ē-ə\ *n* **1** *cap* : a genus of plants of the lily family (Liliaceae) that includes the lily of the valley (*C. majalis*) **2** : the dried rhizome and roots of the lily of the valley that contain several cardioactive glycosides

con·val·lar·in \ˌkän-və-ˈlar-ən, kən-ˈval-ə-rən\ *n* : a poisonous glycoside extracted from the dried rhizome, roots, and flowers of the lily of the valley

con·val·la·tox·in \ˌkän-ˌval-ə-ˈtäk-sən, -vəl-\ *n* : a glycoside $C_{29}H_{42}O_{10}$ obtained esp. from the dried rhizome, roots, and flowers of the lily of the valley that acts on the heart and that on hydrolysis yields strophanthidin and rhamnose

con·vec·tion \kən-ˈvek-shən\ *n* **1** : the circulatory motion that occurs in a fluid at a nonuniform temperature owing to the variation of its density and the action of gravity **2** : the transfer of heat by convection in a fluid — **con·vec·tion·al** \-shnəl, -shən-ᵊl\ *adj* — **con·vec·tive** \-ˈvek-tiv\ *adj*

con·ver·gence \kən-ˈvər-jən(t)s\ *n* **1** : an embryonic movement that involves streaming of material from the dorsal and lateral surfaces of the gastrula toward the blastopore and concurrent shifting of lateral materials toward the middorsal line and that is a process fundamental to the establishment of the germ layers **2** : independent development of similar characters (as of body structure in whales and fishes) by animals or plants of different groups that is often associated with similarity of habits or environment **3** : movement of the two eyes so coordinated that the images of a single point fall on corresponding points of the two retinas **4** : overlapping synaptic innervation of a single cell by more than one nerve fiber — compare DIVERGENCE 2 — **con·verge** \-ˈvərj\ *vb* **con·verged; con·verg·ing** — **con·ver·gent** \-ˈvər-jənt\ *adj*

convergent think·ing \-ˈthiŋk-iŋ\ *n* : thinking (as in answering a multiple-choice question) that weighs alternatives within an existing construct or model in solving a problem or answering a question to find one best solution and that is measured by IQ tests — compare DIVERGENT THINKING — **convergent think·er** \-ər\ *n*

con·ver·sion \kən-ˈvər-zhən, -shən\ *n* **1** : the transformation of an unconscious mental conflict into a symbolically equivalent bodily symptom **2** : GENE CONVERSION

conversion disorder *n* : a psychoneurosis in which bodily symptoms (as paralysis of the limbs) appear without physical basis — called also *conversion hysteria, conversion reaction*

con·vex \kän-ˈveks; ˈkän-ˌ, kən-ˈ\ *adj* : curved or rounded like the exterior of a sphere or circle ⟨~ lenses are used to correct for farsightedness⟩ — **con·vex·i·ty** \kən-ˈvek-sət-ē, kän-\ *n, pl* **-ties**

con·vexo–concave \kən-ˌvek-(ˌ)sō-, kän-\ *adj* **1** : CONCAVO-CONVEX **2** : having the convex side of greater curvature than the concave

convexo–convex *adj* : BICONVEX

con·vo·lute \ˈkän-və-ˌlüt\ *adj* : rolled or wound together with one part upon another

con·vo·lut·ed \-ˌlü-təd\ *adj* : folded in curved or tortuous windings; *specif* : having convolutions ⟨the highly ~ human cerebral cortex⟩

convoluted tubule *n* **1** : PROXIMAL CONVOLUTED TUBULE **2** : DISTAL CONVOLUTED TUBULE

con·vo·lu·tion \ˌkän-və-ˈlü-shən\ *n* : any of the irregular ridges on the surface of the brain and esp. of the cerebrum — called also *gyrus;* compare SULCUS — **con·vo·lu·tion·al** \-shnəl, -shən-ᵊl\ *adj*

convolution of Broca *n* : BROCA'S AREA

con·vol·vu·lin \kən-ˈväl-vyə-lən, -ˈvȯl-\ *n* : an ether-insoluble glucosidic constituent of true jalap resin

con·vol·vu·lus \-ˈväl-vyə-ləs, also -ˈväv-yə-, -ˈvȯv-yə-\ *n* **1** *cap* : a genus of erect trailing or twining herbs and shrubs (family Convolvulaceae) chiefly of temperate regions **2** *pl* **-lus·es** *or* **-li** \-ˌlī, -ˌlē\ : a plant of the genus *Convolvulus*

¹con·vul·sant \kən-ˈvəl-sənt\ *adj* : causing convulsions : CONVULSIVE 1

²convulsant *n* : an agent and esp. a drug that produces convulsions

con·vulse \kən-ˈvəls\ *vb* **con·vulsed; con·vuls·ing** *vt* : to shake or agitate violently; *esp* : to shake or cause to shake with or as if with irregular spasms ⟨was *convulsed* with pain⟩ ~ *vi* : to become affected with convulsions ⟨some children will inevitably ~ when fever reaches a high point —H. R. Litchfield & L. H. Dembo⟩

con·vul·sion \kən-ˈvəl-shən\ *n* : an abnormal violent and involuntary contraction or series of contractions of the muscles — often used in pl. ⟨a patient suffering from ~s⟩

con·vul·sive \kən-ˈvəl-siv\ *adj* **1** : constituting or producing a convulsion ⟨~ disorders⟩ **2** : caused by or affected with convulsions ⟨~ motions⟩ ⟨a ~ patient⟩ — **con·vul·sive·ly** *adv*

convulsive therapy *n* : SHOCK THERAPY

Coo·ley's anemia \ˌkü-lēz-\ *n* : a severe thalassemic anemia that is associated with the presence of microcytes, enlargement of the liver and spleen, increase in the erythroid bone marrow, and jaundice and that occurs esp. in children of Mediterranean parents — called also *thalassemia major*

Cooley, Thomas Benton (1871–1945), American pediatrician. Cooley was one of the first modern pediatricians and a founder of the American Academy of Pediatrics. Interested in the etiology of childhood diseases, he focused his research on hematology and the anemias. His most important contribution was the identification of the familial anemia that bears his name. In 1927 Cooley, E. R. Witwer, and O. P. Lee described this anemia, frequently called thalassemia, that at first was thought to occur only in children of Mediterranean stock.

Coo·lidge tube \ˈkü-lij-\ *n* : a vacuum tube for the generation of X-rays in which the cathode consists of a spiral filament of incandescent tungsten and the target serves as the anode and consists of massive tungsten and in which the temperature of the cathode determines the intensity of the X-rays while the applied voltage determines wavelength

Coolidge, William David (1873–1975), American engineer and physicist. In 1913 Coolidge invented an X-ray tube (now known as the Coolidge tube) that was the prototype of the modern X-ray tube.

Coo·mas·sie blue \kü-ˌmas-ē-ˈblü, -ˌmäs-\ *n* : a bright blue acid dye used as a biological stain esp. for proteins in gel electrophoresis

Coombs test \ˈkümz-\ *n* : an agglutination test used to detect proteins and esp. antibodies on the surface of red blood cells

Coombs, Robert Royston Amos (b 1921), British immunologist. Coombs, along with A. E. Mourant and R. R. Race, devised in 1945 the test now known as the Coombs test.

Coo·pe·ria \kü-ˈpir-ē-ə\ *n* : a genus of small reddish brown nematode worms (family Trichostrongylidae) including several species infesting the small intestine of sheep, goats, and cattle and sometimes held responsible for marked catarrhal inflammation, anemia, and diarrhea — **coop·er·id** \ˈküp-ə-rəd\ *n*

Cur·tice \ˈkərt-əs\, **Cooper (1856–1939),** American veterinarian. Throughout his career Curtice worked on the eradication of various diseases in sheep, cattle, and poultry. He specialized in parasitology, investigating ticks and worms in particular. The genus *Cooperia* of nematode worms is derived from his first name.

Coo·per's ligament \ˌkü-pərz-, ˌkup-ərz-\ *n* : a strong ligamentous band extending upward and backward from the base of Gimbernat's ligament along the iliopectineal line to which it is attached — called also *ligament of Cooper*

Coo·per \ˈkü-pər, *US also* ˈkup-ər\, **Sir Astley Paston (1768–1841),** British surgeon. The foremost surgeon of his day, Cooper is known in part for his pioneering treatments for aneurysm. In 1808 he ligated the common carotid artery and the external iliac arteries and in 1817 he ligated the abdominal continuation of the descending aorta. In 1829 he published a work on the anatomy and diseases of the breast

\ə\ **abut** \ᵊ\ **kitten** \ər\ **further** \a\ **ash** \ā\ **ace** \ä\ **cot, cart**
\aù\ **out** \ch\ **chin** \e\ **bet** \ē\ **easy** \g\ **go** \i\ **hit** \ī\ **ice** \j\ **job**
\ŋ\ **sing** \ō\ **go** \ȯ\ **law** \ȯi\ **boy** \th\ **thin** \th̲\ **the** \ü\ **loot**
\ù\ **foot** \y\ **yet** \zh\ **vision** *See also* Pronunciation Symbols page

in which he described those ligaments which are the connective tissue attachments of the mammary gland to the overlying skin. The ligaments have since been named in his honor.

coord *abbr* coordination

co·or·di·nate \kō-'ȯrd-ᵊn-ˌāt\ *vb* **-nat·ed; -nat·ing** *vt* : to bring into a common action, movement, or condition ⟨∼ muscular movements⟩ ∼ *vi* : to function together in a concerted way

co·or·di·nate bond \-ᵊn-ət-\ *n* : a covalent bond that consists of a pair of electrons supplied by only one of the two atoms it joins

co·or·di·nat·ed \-ᵊn-ˌāt-əd\ *adj* : able to use more than one set of muscle movements to a single end ⟨a well-*coordinated* athlete⟩

co·or·di·na·tion \(ˌ)kō-ˌȯrd-ᵊn-'ā-shən\ *n* **1** : the act or action of coordinating **2** : the harmonious functioning of parts (as muscle and nerves) for most effective results

coordination compound *n* : a compound or ion with a central usu. metallic atom or ion combined by coordinate bonds with a definite number of surrounding ions, groups, or molecules — called also *coordination complex*

co·os·si·fy \kō-'äs-ə-ˌfī\ *vi* **-fied; -fy·ing** : to grow together by ossification (as of bones or parts of a bone) : ANKYLOSE — **co·os·si·fi·ca·tion** \(ˌ)kō-ˌäs-ə-fə-'kā-shən\ *n*

coo·tie \'küt-ē\ *n* : BODY LOUSE

co·pai·ba \kō-'pī-bə, -'pā-; ˌkō-pə-'ē-bə\ *n* : an oleoresin obtained from several pinnate-leaved So. American leguminous trees (genus *Copaifera*) that has a stimulant action on mucous membranes; *also* : one of these trees

co–pay \'kō-ˌpā\ *n* : CO-PAYMENT

co–pay·ment \(ˈ)kō-'pā-mənt\ *n* : a relatively small fixed fee required by a health insurer (as an HMO) to be paid by the patient at the time of each office visit, outpatient service, or filling of a prescription

COPD *abbr* chronic obstructive pulmonary disease

cope \'kōp\ *vi* **coped; cop·ing** : to deal with and attempt to overcome problems and difficulties — usu. used with *with* ⟨teachers *coping* with violence in schools⟩

COPE *abbr* chronic obstructive pulmonary emphysema

Co·pep·o·da \kō-'pep-ə-də\ *n pl* : a subclass of Crustacea comprising minute aquatic forms abundant in both fresh and salt waters and including one order (Eucopepoda) whose members are chiefly free-living and important as fish food and another order (Branchiura) whose members are parasitic on the skin and gills of fish — **co·pe·pod** \'kō-pə-ˌpäd\ *n or adj*

cop·i·o·pia \ˌkäp-ē-'ō-pē-ə\ *n* : ASTHENOPIA

co·pol·y·mer \(ˈ)kō-'päl-ə-mər\ *n* : a product of copolymerization — called also *heteropolymer* — **co·pol·y·mer·ic** \ˌkō-ˌpäl-ə-'mer-ik\ *adj*

co·po·ly·mer·iza·tion *or Brit* **co·po·ly·mer·isa·tion** \ˌkō-pə-ˌlim-ə-rə-'zā-shən, ˌkō-ˌpäl-ə-mə-\ *n* : the polymerization of two substances (as two different monomers) together — **co·po·ly·mer·ize** *or Brit* **co·po·ly·mer·ise** \ˌkō-pə-'lim-ə-ˌrīz, ˌkō-'päl-ə-mə-\ *vb* **-ized** *or Brit* **-ised; -iz·ing** *or Brit* **-is·ing**

cop·per \'käp-ər\ *n, often attrib* : a common reddish metallic element that is ductile and malleable and one of the best conductors of heat and electricity — symbol *Cu*; see ELEMENT table — **cop·pery** \'käp-(ə-)rē\ *adj*

cop·per·as \'käp-(ə-)rəs\ *n* : a green hydrated ferrous sulfate $FeSO_4 \cdot 7H_2O$ used esp. in making inks and pigments — used esp. of commercial grades not to be used internally

cop·per·head \'käp-ər-ˌhed\ *n* **1** : a pit viper (*Agkistrodon contortrix*) widely distributed in upland areas of the eastern and central U.S. that typically attains a length of three feet (0.9 meter), is coppery brown above with dark transverse blotches, and is capable of inflicting a very painful but rarely fatal bite **2** : a very venomous but sluggish Australian elapid snake of the genus *Denisonia* (*D. superba*)

copper sulfate *n* : the sulfate of bivalent copper that is best known as the blue crystalline hydrate $CuSO_4 \cdot 5H_2O$, is used as an algicide and fungicide, and has been used medicinally

in solution as an emetic but is not now recommended for such use because of its potential toxicity — called also *cupric sulfate*

cop·ro·an·ti·body \ˌkäp-rō-'ant-i-ˌbäd-ē\ *n, pl* **-bod·ies** : an antibody whose presence in the intestinal tract can be demonstrated by examination of an extract of the feces

cop·ro·lag·nia \ˌkäp-rə-'lag-nē-ə\ *n* : sexual excitement produced by contact with feces — **cop·ro·lag·nist** \-nəst\ *n*

cop·ro·la·lia \-'lā-lē-ə\ *n* **1** : obsessive or uncontrollable use of obscene language **2** : the use of obscene (as scatological) language as sexual gratification — **cop·ro·la·lic** \-'lal-ik\ *adj*

cop·ro·lith \'käp-rə-ˌlith\ *n* : a mass of hard fecal matter in the intestine

cop·ro·pha·gia \ˌkäp-rə-'fā-j(ē-)ə\ *n* : COPROPHAGY

co·proph·a·gy \kə-'präf-ə-jē\ *n, pl* **-gies** : the eating of excrement that is normal behavior among many esp. young animals but in humans is a symptom of some forms of insanity — **co·proph·a·gist** \-jəst\ *n* — **co·proph·a·gous** \-ə-gəs\ *or* **cop·ro·phag·ic** \ˌkäp-rə-'faj-ik\ *adj*

cop·ro·phil·ia \ˌkäp-rə-'fil-ē-ə\ *n* : marked interest in excrement; *esp* : the use of feces or filth for sexual excitement — **cop·ro·phil·i·ac** \-ē-ˌak\ *n*

cop·ro·phil·ic \ˌkäp-rə-'fil-ik\ *adj* **1** : relating to coprophilia **2** : COPROPHILOUS

cop·roph·i·lous \kä-'präf-ə-ləs\ *adj* : growing or living on dung ⟨∼ fungi⟩

cop·ro·por·phy·rin \ˌkäp-rə-'pȯr-fə-rən\ *n* : any of four isomeric porphyrins $C_{36}H_{38}N_4O_8$ of which types I and III are found in feces and urine esp. in certain pathological conditions and also in yeast

co·pros·ta·nol \kə-'präs-tə-ˌnȯl, -ˌnōl\ *n* : a crystalline sterol $C_{27}H_{47}OH$ formed by bacterial reduction of cholesterol in the intestines and present in feces

co·pros·ter·ol \-tə-ˌrȯl, -ˌrōl\ *n* : COPROSTANOL

cop·ro·zo·ic \ˌkäp-rə-'zō-ik\ *adj* : living in feces ⟨∼ protozoans⟩ — **cop·ro·zo·on** \-'zō-ˌän\ *n, pl* **-zoa** \-zō-ə\

cop·u·la \'käp-yə-lə\ *n, pl* **copulas** *also* **cop·u·lae** \-ˌlē\ **1** : a connecting anatomical structure **2** : sexual union : COPULATION

cop·u·late \'käp-yə-ˌlāt\ *vi* **-lat·ed; -lat·ing 1** : to engage in sexual intercourse **2** *of gametes* : to fuse permanently — compare CONJUGATE 1 — **cop·u·la·tion** \ˌkäp-yə-'lā-shən\ *n* — **cop·u·la·to·ry** \'käp-yə-lə-ˌtȯr-ē, -ˌtȯr-\ *adj*

copulatrix — see BURSA COPULATRIX

co·quille \kō-'kil, -'kēl\ *n* : an oval glass of curved surface and uniform thickness used in eyeglasses — called also *coquille lens*

cor *abbr* corrected

CoR *abbr* Congo red

cor·a·cid·i·um \ˌkȯr-ə-'sid-ē-əm\ *n, pl* **-cid·ia** \-dē-ə\ : the oncosphere of a tapeworm at about the time of hatching while still surrounded by the embryophore

cor·a·co·acro·mi·al \ˌkȯr-ə-(ˌ)kō-ə-'krō-mē-əl\ *adj* : relating to or connecting the acromion and the coracoid process

cor·a·co·bra·chi·a·lis \ˌkȯr-ə-(ˌ)kō-brā-kē-'ā-ləs\ *n, pl* **-a·les** \-ˌlēz\ : a muscle extending between the coracoid process and the middle of the medial surface of the humerus — called also *coracobrachialis muscle*

cor·a·co·cla·vic·u·lar ligament \-klə-ˌvik-yə-lər-, -klə-\ *n* : a ligament that joins the clavicle and the coracoid process of the scapula — see CONOID LIGAMENT

cor·a·co·hu·mer·al \-'hyüm-(ə-)rəl\ *adj* : relating to or connecting the coracoid process and the humerus

¹cor·a·coid \'kȯr-ə-ˌkȯid, 'kär-\ *adj* : of, relating to, or being a process of the scapula in most mammals or a well-developed cartilage bone of many lower vertebrates that extends from the scapula to or toward the sternum — see PECTORAL GIRDLE

²coracoid *n* : a coracoid bone or process

coracoid process *n* : a process of the scapula in most mammals representing the remnant of the coracoid bone of lower vertebrates that has become fused with the scapula and in humans is situated on its superior border and serves for the attachment of various muscles

coral snake \'kȯr-əl-, 'kär-\ *n* : any of several venomous chiefly tropical New World elapid snakes of the genus *Micrurus* that are brilliantly banded in red, black, and yellow or white and include two (*M. fulvius* and *M. euryxanthus*) ranging northward into the southern U.S.

cor·bo·vi·num \'kȯr-bō-'vī-nəm\ *n* : a greatly enlarged heart

cord \'kȯ(ə)rd\ *n* **1** : a long slender flexible material usu. consisting of several strands (as of thread or yarn) woven or twisted together **2** : a slender flexible anatomical structure (as a nerve) — see SPERMATIC CORD, SPINAL CORD, UMBILICAL CORD, VOCAL CORD 1

cor·date \'kȯ(ə)r-ˌdāt\ *adj* : shaped like a heart — **cor·date·ly** *adv*

cord blood *n* : blood from the umbilical cord of a fetus or newborn

cor·dec·to·my \kȯr-'dek-tə-mē\ *n, pl* **-mies** : surgical removal of one or more vocal cords

cor·dial \'kȯr-jəl\ *n* : an invigorating and stimulating medicine, food, or drink

cordia pulmonalia *pl of* COR PULMONALE

cor·di·form \'kȯrd-ə-ˌfȯrm\ *adj* : shaped like a heart ⟨a ~ bothridium of a tapeworm⟩

cordiform tendon *n* : the central tendon of the diaphragm

cordis — see ACCRETIO CORDIS, COMMOTIO CORDIS, CONCRETIO CORDIS, MORBUS CORDIS, VENAE CORDIS MINIMAE

cor·do·cen·te·sis \ˌkȯr-dō-(ˌ)sen-'tē-səs\ *n* : the withdrawal of a sample of fetal blood from the umbilical cord by transabdominal insertion of a needle guided by ultrasound

cor·dot·o·my *or* **chor·dot·o·my** \kȯr-'dät-ə-mē\ *n, pl* **-mies** : surgical division of a tract of the spinal cord for relief of severe intractable pain

core \'kō(ə)r, 'kȯ(ə)r\ *n* : the central part of a body, mass, or part

core biopsy *n* : a biopsy in which a cylindrical sample of tissue is obtained (as from a kidney or breast) by a hollow needle — compare FINE NEEDLE ASPIRATION, WEDGE BIOPSY

co·re·ly·sis \ˌkōr-ə-'lī-səs, ˌkȯr-; kȯ-'rel-ə-səs, kō-\ *n, pl* **-ly·ses** \-ˌsēz\ : the operation of breaking loose adhesions formed between the iris and adjacent parts

co·re·pres·sor \ˌkō-ri-'pres-ər\ *n* : a small molecule that activates a particular genetic repressor by combining with it

core protein *n* : any of various proteins that play a major structural or functional role in a large molecular complex of which they are part: as **a** : an inner coat of protein that surrounds the genetic material of some viruses **b** : a protein forming part of a proteoglycan and to which glycosaminoglycans attach

core temperature *n* : the temperature deep within a living body (as in the viscera)

co·ri·a·myr·tin \ˌkōr-ē-ə-'mərt-ᵊn, ˌkȯr-\ *n* : a bitter poisonous crystalline compound $C_{15}H_{18}O_5$ found in an Old World dye plant (*Coriaria myrtifolia* of the family Coriariaceae)

co·ri·an·der \'kōr-ē-ˌan-dər, ˌkȯr-ē-', 'kȯr-, ˌkȯr-\ *n* **1** : an Old World herb (*Coriandrum sativum*) of the carrot family (Umbelliferae) with aromatic fruits **2** : the ripened dried fruit of coriander used as a flavoring — called also *coriander seed*

Co·ri cycle \'kōr-ē-, 'kȯr-\ *n* : the cycle in carbohydrate metabolism consisting of the conversion of glycogen to lactic acid in muscle, diffusion of the lactic acid into the bloodstream which carries it to the liver where it is converted into glycogen, and the breakdown of liver glycogen to glucose which is transported to muscle by the bloodstream and reconverted into glycogen

Cori, Carl Ferdinand (1896–1984) and **Gerty Theresa (1896–1957)**, American biochemists. In 1936 the Coris discovered the activated intermediate glucose-1-phosphate that is often called the Cori ester. In 1942 they isolated and purified the enzyme responsible for catalyzing the conversion of glycogen to glucose-1-phosphate. In 1943 they achieved the test-tube synthesis of glycogen. Proof of the glucose-glycogen interconversion allowed them to formulate what is now known as the Cori cycle. Their discoveries led to a new understanding of hormonal influence on the

interconversion of sugar and starches in the animal organism. In 1947, the Coris were awarded the Nobel Prize for Physiology or Medicine.

Cori ester *n* : GLUCOSE-1-PHOSPHATE

co·ri·um \'kōr-ē-əm, 'kȯr-\ *n, pl* **co·ria** \-ē-ə\ : DERMIS

corm \'kȯ(ə)rm\ *n* : a rounded thick modified underground stem base bearing membranous or scaly leaves and buds and acting as a vegetative reproductive structure

corn \'kȯ(ə)rn\ *n* : a local hardening and thickening of epidermis (as on a toe)

cor·nea \'kȯr-nē-ə\ *n* : the transparent part of the coat of the eyeball that covers the iris and pupil and admits light to the interior — **cor·ne·al** \-əl\ *adj*

cor·ne·itis \ˌkȯr-nē-'īt-əs\ *n* : KERATITIS

cor·neo·scler·al \ˌkȯr-nē-ə-'skler-əl\ *adj* : of, relating to, or affecting both the cornea and the sclera ⟨the ~ junction⟩

cor·ne·ous \'kȯr-nē-əs\ *adj* : of a texture resembling horn

cor·ner \'kȯ(r)-nər\ *n* : CORNER TOOTH

corner tooth *n* : one of the third or outer pair of incisor teeth of each jaw of a horse — compare DIVIDER, NIPPER 2

cor·ne·um \'kȯr-nē-əm\ *n, pl* **cor·nea** \-ē-ə\ : STRATUM CORNEUM

cor·nic·u·late cartilage \kȯr-ˌnik-yə-lət-\ *n* : either of two small nodules of yellow elastic cartilage articulating with the apex of the arytenoid — called also *cartilage of Santorini*

cor·nic·u·lum \kȯr-'nik-yə-ləm\ *n, pl* **-u·la** \-lə\ : a small horn-shaped part or process

cor·ni·fi·ca·tion \ˌkȯr-nə-fə-'kā-shən\ *n* **1** : conversion into horn or a horny substance or tissue **2** : the histological and cytological changes that occur in the vaginal epithelium esp. of a rodent in response to stimulation by an estrogen and that have been used as a bioassay for estrogenicity of chemicals (as pesticides) in the environment

cor·ni·fy \'kȯr-nə-fī\ *vi* **-fied; -fy·ing** : to become converted or changed into horn or horny substance or tissue ⟨*cornified* layers of epithelial cells⟩

corn oil *n* : a yellow fatty oil obtained from the germ of Indian corn kernels that is used in medicine as a solvent and as a vehicle for injections — called also *maize oil*

cor·nu \'kȯr-(ˌ)n(y)ü\ *n, pl* **cor·nua** \-n(y)ə-wə\ : a horn-shaped anatomical structure (as either of the lateral divisions of a bicornuate uterus, one of the lateral processes of the hyoid bone, or one of the gray columns of the spinal cord) — **cor·nu·al** \-n(y)ə-wəl\ *adj*

cor·nus \'kȯr-nəs\ *n* **1** *cap* : a genus of shrubs and small trees (family Cornaceae) usu. having very hard wood and perfect flowers with a 2-celled ovary and comprising the dogwoods **2** : the dried bark of the root of the flowering dogwood (*Cornus florida*) containing a bitter principle sometimes used as a mild astringent and stomachic

corny \'kȯr-nē\ *adj* **corn·i·er; -est** : relating to or having corns on the feet

co·ro·na \kə-'rō-nə\ *n* : the upper portion of a bodily part (as a tooth or the skull)

co·ro·nal \'kȯr-ən-ᵊl, 'kär-; kə-'rōn-\ *adj* **1** : of, relating to, or being a corona **2** : lying in the direction of the coronal suture **3** : of or relating to the frontal plane that passes through the long axis of the body

cor·o·nale \ˌkȯr-ə-'nal-(ˌ)ē, -'nāl-, -'näl-\ *n* : the point of the coronal suture marking the greatest diameter of the frontal bone

coronal suture *n* : a suture extending across the skull between the parietal and frontal bones — called also *frontoparietal suture*

co·ro·na ra·di·a·ta \kə-'rō-nə-ˌrād-ē-'āt-ə, -'ät-\ *n, pl* **co·ro·nae ra·di·a·tae** \-(ˌ)nē-ˌrād-ē-'āt-(ˌ)ē, -'ät-\ **1** : the zone of small follicular cells immediately surrounding the ovum in

\ə\ abut \ᵊ\ kitten \ər\ further \a\ ash \ā\ ace \ä\ cot, cart \au̇\ out \ch\ chin \e\ bet \ē\ easy \g\ go \i\ hit \ī\ ice \j\ job \ŋ\ sing \ō\ go \ȯ\ law \ȯi\ boy \th\ thin \t͟h\ the \ü\ loot \u̇\ foot \y\ yet \zh\ vision *See also* Pronunciation Symbols page

the graafian follicle and accompanying the ovum on its discharge from the follicle   2 : a large mass of myelinated nerve fibers radiating from the internal capsule to the cerebral cortex

¹cor·o·nary \'kȯr-ə-ˌner-ē, 'kär-\ adj   1 : resembling a crown or circlet : encircling another part   2 a : of, relating to, affecting, or being the coronary arteries or veins of the heart ⟨a ∼ bypass⟩; broadly : of or relating to the heart   b : of, relating to, or affected with coronary artery disease ⟨a ∼ care unit⟩ ⟨a diet for the young ∼ male⟩

²coronary n, pl -nar·ies   1 a : CORONARY ARTERY   b : CORONARY VEIN   2 : CORONARY THROMBOSIS; broadly : HEART ATTACK

coronary artery n : either of two arteries that arise one from the left and one from the right side of the aorta immediately above the semilunar valves and supply the tissues of the heart itself

coronary artery bypass n : CORONARY BYPASS

coronary artery disease n : a condition and esp. one caused by atherosclerosis that reduces the blood flow through the coronary arteries to the heart muscle and typically results in chest pain or heart damage — called also coronary disease, coronary heart disease

coronary band n : a thickened band of extremely vascular tissue that lies at the upper border of the wall of the hoof of the horse and related animals and that plays an important part in the secretion of the horny walls — called also coronary cushion

coronary bypass n : a surgical bypass operation performed to shunt blood around an obstruction in a coronary artery that usu. involves grafting one end of a segment of vein (as of the saphenous vein) removed from another part of the body into the aorta and the other end into the coronary artery beyond the obstructed area to allow for increased blood flow — called also coronary artery bypass

coronary disease n : CORONARY ARTERY DISEASE

coronary failure n : heart failure in which the heart muscle is deprived of the blood necessary to meet its functional needs as a result of narrowing or blocking of one or more of the coronary arteries — compare CONGESTIVE HEART FAILURE

coronary heart disease n : CORONARY ARTERY DISEASE

coronary insufficiency n : cardiac insufficiency of relatively mild degree — compare ANGINA PECTORIS, HEART ATTACK, HEART FAILURE 1

coronary ligament n   1 : the folds of peritoneum connecting the posterior surface of the liver and the diaphragm   2 : a part of the joint capsule of the knee connecting each meniscus with the margin of the head of the tibia

coronary occlusion n : the partial or complete blocking (as by a thrombus, by spasm, or by sclerosis) of a coronary artery

coronary plexus n : one of two nerve plexuses that are extensions of the cardiac plexus along the coronary arteries

coronary sclerosis n : sclerosis of the coronary arteries of the heart

coronary sinus n : a venous channel that is derived from the sinus venosus, is continuous with the largest of the cardiac veins, receives most of the blood from the walls of the heart, and empties into the right atrium

coronary sulcus n : a depression surrounding the heart at the atrioventricular junction and giving passage to coronary arteries, coronary veins, and the coronary sinus

coronary thrombosis n : the blocking of a coronary artery of the heart by a thrombus

coronary valve n : the fold of endocardium at the opening of the coronary sinus into the right atrium — called also valve of Thebesius

coronary vein n   1 a : any of several veins that drain the tissues of the heart and empty into the coronary sinus   b : CARDIAC VEIN — not used technically   2 : a vein draining the lesser curvature of the stomach and emptying into the portal vein

Co·ro·na·vi·ri·dae \kə-ˌrō-nə-'vir-ə-ˌdē\ n pl : a family of single-stranded RNA viruses that are surrounded by a lipoprotein envelope with large club-shaped projections and that infect birds and many mammals including humans but with each species of virus usu. having a restricted range of hosts

co·ro·na·vi·rus \kə-'rō-nə-ˌvī-rəs\ n   1 cap : a genus of single-stranded RNA viruses of the family Coronaviridae that includes the causative agents of blue comb, feline infectious peritonitis, and SARS   2 : any virus of the family Coronaviridae; esp : one of the genus Coronavirus

cor·o·ner \'kȯr-ə-nər, 'kär-\ n : a usu. elected public officer who is typically not required to have specific medical qualifications and whose principal duty is to inquire by an inquest into the cause of any death which there is reason to suppose is not due to natural causes — see MEDICAL EXAMINER 1

cor·o·net \ˌkȯr-ə-'net, ˌkär-\ n : the lower part of a horse's pastern where the horn terminates in skin

co·ro·ni·on \kə-'rō-nē-ˌän, -ən\ n, pl -nia \-nē-ə\ : the tip of the coronoid process of the mandible

cor·o·ni·tis \ˌkȯr-ə-'nīt-əs\ n : inflammation of the coronary band of animals

cor·o·noid \'kȯr-ə-ˌnȯid\ adj : of, relating to, or indicating the coronoid process or coronoid fossa ⟨∼ teeth⟩

cor·o·noid·ec·to·my \ˌkȯr-ə-ˌnȯi-'dek-tə-mē\ n, pl -mies : surgical removal of the mandibular coronoid process

coronoid fossa n : a depression of the humerus into which the coronoid process fits when the arm is flexed — compare OLECRANON FOSSA

coronoid process n   1 : the anterior process of the superior border of the ramus of the mandible   2 : a flared process of the lower anterior part of the upper articular surface of the ulna fitting into the coronoid fossa when the arm is flexed

corpora pl of CORPUS

cor·po·ral \'kȯr-p(ə-)rəl\ adj : of, relating to, or affecting the body ⟨∼ punishment⟩

cor·po·ra quad·ri·gem·i·na \ˌkȯr-p(ə-)rə-ˌkwäd-rə-'jem-ə-nə\ n pl : two pairs of colliculi on the dorsal surface of the midbrain composed of white matter externally and gray matter within, the superior pair containing correlation centers for optic reflexes and the inferior pair containing correlation centers for auditory reflexes

cor·po·re·al \kȯr-'pōr-ē-əl, -'pȯr-\ adj : having, consisting of, or relating to a physical material body

corporis — see PEDICULOSIS CORPORIS, TINEA CORPORIS

corpse \'kȯ(ə)rps\ n : a dead body esp. of a human being

corps·man \'kō(ə)r(z)-mən, 'kȯ(ə)r(z)-\ n, pl corps·men \-mən\ : a military enlisted person trained to give first aid and minor medical treatment

cor·pu·lence \'kȯr-pyə-lən(t)s\ n : the state of being excessively fat

cor·pu·len·cy \-lən-sē\ n, pl -cies : CORPULENCE

cor·pu·lent \-lənt\ adj : having a large bulky body : OBESE — cor·pu·lent·ly adv

cor pul·mo·na·le \ˌkȯr-ˌpúl-mə-'näl-ē, -ˌpəl-, -'nal-\ n, pl cor·dia pul·mo·na·lia \'kȯrd-ē-ə-ˌpúl-mə-'näl-ē-ə, -ˌpəl-, -'nal-\ : disease of the heart characterized by hypertrophy and dilatation of the right ventricle and secondary to disease of the lungs or their blood vessels

cor·pus \'kȯr-pəs\ n, pl cor·po·ra \-p(ə-)rə\   1 : the human or animal body esp. when dead   2 : the main part or body of a bodily structure or organ ⟨the ∼ of the jaw⟩ — see CORPUS UTERI

corpus al·bi·cans \-'al-bə-ˌkanz\ n, pl corpora al·bi·can·tia \-ˌal-bə-'kan-chē-ə\   1 : MAMMILLARY BODY   2 : the white fibrous scar that remains in the ovary after resorption of the corpus luteum and replaces a discharged graafian follicle

corpus cal·lo·sum \-ka-'lō-səm\ n, pl corpora cal·lo·sa \-sə\ : the great band of commissural fibers uniting the cerebral hemispheres

corpus ca·ver·no·sum \-ˌkav-ər-'nō-səm\ n, pl corpora ca·ver·no·sa \-sə\ : a mass of erectile tissue with large interspaces capable of being distended with blood; esp : one of those that form the bulk of the body of the penis or of the clitoris

cor·pus·cle \'kȯr-(ˌ)pəs-əl\ n   1 : a living cell; esp : one (as a red or white blood cell or a cell in cartilage or bone) not aggregated into continuous tissues **2** : any of various small circumscribed multicellular bodies — usu. used with a qualifying term ⟨Malpighian ~*s*⟩ — **cor·pus·cu·lar** \kȯr-ˈpəs-kyə-lər\ *adj*

corpuscle of Herbst \-ˈhe(ə)rpst\ *n* : any of several tactile organs that are found in birds and are related to Pacinian corpuscles

   Herbst, Ernst Friedrich Gustav H. (1803–1893), German anatomist. Herbst spent his career teaching at the university at Göttingen. He also published numerous articles on subjects that included the air capacity of the lungs, the treatment of hydrogen cyanide poisoning, Asiatic cholera, and the lymphatic system. In 1848 he published an article on Pacinian corpuscles in which he described the tactile organs that now honor his name.

corpuscle of Krause *n* : KRAUSE'S CORPUSCLE

corpuscle of Meissner *n* : MEISSNER'S CORPUSCLE

corpus de·lic·ti \-di-ˈlik-ˌtī, -(ˌ)tē\ *n, pl* **corpora delicti 1** : the substantial and fundamental fact (as, in murder, actual death and its occurrence as a result of criminal agency) necessary to prove the commission of a crime **2** : the material substance (as the body of the victim of a murder) upon which a crime has been committed

corpus he·mor·rhag·i·cum *or chiefly Brit* **corpus hae·mor·rhag·i·cum** \-ˌhem-ə-ˈraj-i-kəm\ *n* : a ruptured graafian follicle containing a blood clot that is absorbed as the cells lining the follicle form the corpus luteum

corpus lu·te·um \-ˈlüt-ē-əm, -lü-ˈtē-əm\ *n, pl* **corpora lu·tea** \-ə\ : a yellowish mass of progesterone-secreting endocrine tissue that consists of pale secretory cells derived from granulosa cells, that forms immediately after ovulation from the ruptured graafian follicle in the mammalian ovary, and that regresses rather quickly if the ovum is not fertilized but persists throughout the ensuing pregnancy if it is fertilized

corpus spon·gi·o·sum \-ˌspən-jē-ˈō-səm, -ˌspän-\ *n* : the median longitudinal column of erectile tissue of the penis that contains the urethra and is ventral to the two corpora cavernosa

corpus stri·a·tum \-ˌstrī-ˈāt-əm\ *n, pl* **corpora stri·a·ta** \-ˈāt-ə\ : cither of a pair of masses of nerve tissue which lie beneath and external to the anterior cornua of the lateral ventricles of the brain and form part of their floor and each of which contains a caudate nucleus and a lentiform nucleus separated by sheets of white matter to give the mass a striated appearance in section

corpus uteri \-ˈyüt-ə-ˌrī\ *n* : the main body of the uterus above the constriction behind the cervix and below the openings of the fallopian tubes

cor·rect \kə-ˈrekt\ *vt* : to alter or adjust so as to bring to some standard or required condition ⟨~ a lens for spherical aberration⟩ — **cor·rect·able** \-ˈrek-tə-bəl\ *adj*

cor·rec·tion \kə-ˈrek-shən\ *n* : the action or an instance of correcting or neutralizing a harmful or undesirable condition ⟨~ of acidity⟩ ⟨~ of visual defects with glasses⟩

¹**cor·rec·tive** \kə-ˈrek-tiv\ *adj* : intended to correct ⟨~ lenses⟩ ⟨~ surgery⟩ — **cor·rec·tive·ly** *adv*

²**corrective** *n* : a medication that removes undesirable or unpleasant side effects of other medication ⟨phenobarbital acts as a ~ in overcoming the insomnia produced by ephedrine⟩

cor·re·spond·ing points \ˌkȯr-ə-ˌspän-diŋ-\ *n pl* : points on the retinas of the two eyes which when simultaneously stimulated normally produce a single visual impression

Cor·ri·gan's disease \ˌkȯr-i-gənz-\ *n* : AORTIC REGURGITATION

   Corrigan, Sir Dominic John (1802–1880), British pathologist. Corrigan produced more than 100 communications on a great variety of maladies. His more important writings include his identification in 1829 of the peculiar expanding pulsation of an aneurysm of the aortic arch, his description in 1838 of cirrhosis of the lungs, and his 1854 article that reported in cases of chronic copper poisoning the appearance of a purple line along the gums. In 1832 he published a description of aortic regurgitation. Although Corrigan's description was not original, this disease became identified with him when a French physician, Armand Trousseau, termed it "maladie de Corrigan." The pulse associated with aortic regurgitation or Corrigan's disease subsequently became identified with him also. The alternate term, *water=hammer pulse,* was introduced in 1852 by G. H. Barlow.

Corrigan's pulse *or* **Corrigan pulse** *n* : a pulse characterized by a sharp rise to full expansion followed by immediate collapse that is seen in aortic insufficiency — called also *water-hammer pulse*

cor·ri·gent \ˈkȯr-ə-jənt\ *n* : a substance added to a medicine to modify its action or counteract a disagreeable effect

cor·rode \kə-ˈrōd\ *vb* **cor·rod·ed; cor·rod·ing** *vt* : to eat away by degrees as if by gnawing; *esp* : to wear away gradually usu. by chemical action ~ *vi* : to undergo corrosion

cor·ro·sion \kə-ˈrō-zhən\ *n* **1** : the action, process, or effect of corroding ⟨arterial ~ that characterizes arteriosclerosis —*Jour. Amer. Med. Assoc.*⟩ **2** : a study specimen of an organ or other structure prepared by injection of hollow parts (as blood vessels) with a plastic and subsequent removal of the surrounding tissue by corrosion

¹**cor·ro·sive** \-ˈrō-siv, -ziv\ *adj* : tending or having the power to corrode ⟨~ acids⟩ ⟨a ~ gas⟩ — **cor·ro·sive·ness** *n*

²**corrosive** *n* : a substance that corrodes : CAUSTIC

corrosive sublimate *n* : MERCURIC CHLORIDE

cor·ru·ga·tor \ˈkȯr-ə-ˌgāt-ər\ *n* : a muscle that contracts the skin into wrinkles; *esp* : one that draws the eyebrows together and wrinkles the brow in frowning

cort *abbr* cortex; cortical

cor·tex \ˈkȯr-ˌteks\ *n, pl* **cor·ti·ces** \ˈkȯrt-ə-ˌsēz\ *or* **cor·tex·es 1 a** : the outer or superficial part of an organ or body structure (as the kidney, adrenal gland, or a hair); *esp* : CEREBRAL CORTEX **b** : the outer part of some organisms (as paramecia) **2 a** : a plant bark or rind (as cinchona) used medicinally **b** : the peel of any of several fruits — used esp. in the writing of medical prescriptions

cor·tex·one \ˈkȯr-ˌtek-ˌsōn\ *n* : DESOXYCORTICOSTERONE

cor·ti·cal \ˈkȯrt-i-kəl\ *adj* **1** : of, relating to, or consisting of cortex ⟨~ tissue⟩ **2** : involving or resulting from the action or condition of the cerebral cortex ⟨~ blindness⟩ — **cor·ti·cal·ly** \-k(ə-)lē\ *adv*

cor·ti·cate \ˈkȯrt-ə-ˌkāt, -kət\ *adj* : covered with bark or with a cortex or specially developed external investment

cor·ti·cif·u·gal \ˌkȯrt-ə-ˈsif-yə-gəl, -ˈsif-i-gəl\ *adj* : originating within and passing away from the cortex ⟨a ~ nerve fiber⟩

cor·ti·cip·e·tal \-ˈsip-ət-ᵊl\ *adj* : originating without and passing to or toward the cerebral cortex ⟨a ~ nerve fiber⟩

cor·ti·co·ad·re·nal \ˌkȯr-ti-kō-ə-ˈdrēn-ᵊl\ *adj* : of or relating to the cortex of the adrenal gland ⟨~ hormones⟩ ⟨~ insufficiency⟩

cor·ti·co·af·fer·ent \ˌkȯrt-i-kō-ˈaf-ə-rənt, -ˌer-ənt\ *adj* : CORTICIPETAL

cor·ti·co·bul·bar \-ˈbəl-bər, -ˌbär\ *adj* : relating to or connecting the cerebral cortex and the medulla oblongata

cor·ti·co·ef·fer·ent \-ˈef-ə-rənt; -ˈef-ˌer-ənt, -ˌē-ˌfer-\ *adj* : CORTICIFUGAL

cor·ti·coid \ˈkȯrt-i-ˌkȯid\ *n* : CORTICOSTEROID — **corticoid** *adj*

cor·ti·co·pe·dun·cu·lar \ˌkȯrt-i-kō-pi-ˈdəŋ-kyə-lər\ *adj* : of or relating to the cerebral cortex and peduncles

cor·ti·co·pon·tine \-ˈpän-ˌtīn\ *adj* : relating to or connecting the cerebral cortex and the pons

cor·ti·co·pon·to·cer·e·bel·lar \-ˌpän-tō-ˌser-ə-ˈbel-ər\ *adj* : of, relating to, or being a tract of nerve fibers or a path for nervous impulses that passes from the cerebral cortex through the internal capsule to the pons to the white matter and cortex of the cerebellum

---

\ə\ **abut** \ᵊ\ **kitten** \ər\ **further** \a\ **ash** \ā\ **ace** \ä\ **cot, cart**
\aú\ **out** \ch\ **chin** \e\ **bet** \ē\ **easy** \g\ **go** \i\ **hit** \ī\ **ice** \j\ **job**
\ŋ\ **sing** \ō\ **go** \ȯ\ **law** \ȯi\ **boy** \th\ **thin** \t͟h\ **the** \ü\ **loot**
\ù\ **foot** \y\ **yet** \zh\ **vision**   *See also* Pronunciation Symbols page

cor·ti·co·ru·bral tract \-'rü-brəl-\ *n* : a conducting path of the brain extending from the cortex of the frontal lobe to the red nucleus

cor·ti·co·spi·nal \-'spīn-ᵊl\ *adj* : of or relating to the cerebral cortex and spinal cord or to the corticospinal tract ⟨∼ neurons⟩

corticospinal tract *n* : any of four columns of motor fibers of which two run on each side of the spinal cord and which are continuations of the pyramids of the medulla oblongata : PYRAMIDAL TRACT: **a** : LATERAL CORTICOSPINAL TRACT **b** : VENTRAL CORTICOSPINAL TRACT

cor·ti·co·ste·roid \ˌkȯrt-i-kō-'sti(ə)r-ˌȯid *also* -'ste(ə)r-\ *n* : any of various adrenal-cortex steroids (as corticosterone, cortisone, and aldosterone) that are divided on the basis of their major biological activity into glucocorticoids and mineralocorticoids

cor·ti·co·ste·rone \ˌkȯrt-ə-'käs-tə-ˌrōn, -i-kō-stə-'; ˌkȯrt-i-kō-'sti(ə)r-ˌōn, -'ste(ə)r-\ *n* : a colorless crystalline corticosteroid $C_{21}H_{30}O_4$ of the adrenal cortex that is important in protein and carbohydrate metabolism

cor·ti·co·tha·lam·ic \ˌkȯrt-i-kō-thə-'lam-ik\ *adj* : of or relating to the cerebral cortex and the thalamus

cor·ti·co·tro·pic \-'trō-pik\ *also* **cor·ti·co·tro·phic** \-fik\ *adj* : influencing or stimulating the adrenal cortex ⟨∼ activity of synthetic human ACTH⟩

cor·ti·co·tro·pin \-pən\ *also* **cor·ti·co·tro·phin** \-fən\ *n* : ACTH; *also* : a preparation of ACTH that is used esp. in the treatment of rheumatoid arthritis and rheumatic fever

corticotropin–releasing factor *also* **corticotrophin–releasing factor** *n* : a substance secreted by the median eminence of the hypothalamus that regulates the release of ACTH by the anterior lobe of the pituitary gland — abbr. *CRF*

corticotropin–releasing hormone *also* **corticotrophin–releasing hormone** *n* : CORTICOTROPIN-RELEASING FACTOR

cor·tin \'kȯrt-ᵊn\ *n* **1** : the active principle of the adrenal cortex now known to consist of several hormones **2** : an aqueous hormone-containing extract of the adrenal cortex

Cor·ti's ganglion \'kȯrt-ēz-, 'kȯr-ˌtēz-\ *n* : SPIRAL GANGLION

A. Corti — see ORGAN OF CORTI

cor·ti·sol \'kȯrt-ə-ˌsȯl, -ˌzȯl, -ˌsōl, -ˌzōl\ *n* : a glucocorticoid $C_{21}H_{30}O_5$ produced by the adrenal cortex upon stimulation by ACTH that mediates various metabolic processes (as gluconeogenesis), has anti-inflammatory and immunosupressive properties, and whose levels in the blood may become elevated in response to physical or psychological stress — called also *hydrocortisone*

cor·ti·sone \-ˌsōn, -ˌzōn\ *n* : a glucocorticoid $C_{21}H_{28}O_5$ that is produced naturally in small amounts by the adrenal cortex and is administered in the form of its synthetic acetate $C_{23}H_{30}O_6$ esp. as replacement therapy for deficient adrenocortical secretion and as an anti-inflammatory agent (as for rheumatoid arthritis) — compare 11-DEHYDROCORTICOSTERONE

co·run·dum \kə-'rən-dəm\ *n* : a very hard mineral Al_2O_3 that consists of alumina occurring in massive form and as variously colored crystals which include the ruby and sapphire

co·ryd·a·lis \kə-'rid-ᵊl-əs\ *n* **1 a** *cap* : a large genus of herbs (family Fumariaceae) that are native to southern Africa and temperate regions of the northern hemisphere and have a several-seeded capsular fruit — see BULBOCAPNINE, CRYPTOPINE **b** : any plant of the genus *Corydalis* **2** : the dried tubers of squirrel corn and Dutchman's-breeches containing the alkaloid bulbocapnine and formerly used as a tonic

Cor·y·ne·bac·te·ri·a·ce·ae \ˌkȯr-ə-(ˌ)nē-bak-ˌtir-ē-'ā-sē-ˌē\ *n pl, in some former classifications* : a family of chiefly gram≠ positive and nonmotile pleomorphic rod-shaped bacteria comprising important parasites as well as saprophytes of soil and dairy products and including a number of diverse genera (as *Corynebacterium, Erysipelothrix,* and *Listeria*)

cor·y·ne·bac·te·ri·um \-'tir-ē-əm\ *n* **1** *cap* : a large genus of usu. gram-positive nonmotile bacteria that do not produce spores, occur as irregular or branching rods often banded

with metachromatic granules, and include a number of important animal and plant pathogens — see DIPHTHERIA 2 *pl* **-ria** \-ē-ə\ : any bacterium of the genus *Corynebacterium*

co·ryne·form \kə-'rin-ə-ˌfȯrm\ *adj* : being or resembling bacteria of the genus *Corynebacterium* ⟨∼ soil isolates⟩

co·ry·za \kə-'rī-zə\ *n* : an acute inflammatory contagious disease involving the upper respiratory tract: **a** : COMMON COLD **b** : any of several diseases of domestic animals characterized by inflammation of and discharge from the mucous membranes of the upper respiratory tract, sinuses, and eyes; *esp* : INFECTIOUS CORYZA — **co·ry·zal** \-zəl\ *adj*

cos·me·ceu·ti·cal \ˌkäz-mə-'süt-i-kəl\ *n* : a preparation (as of benzoyl peroxide or retinol) that possesses both cosmetic and pharmaceutical properties

cos·me·sis \käz-'mē-səs\ *n, pl* **-me·ses** \-ˌsēz\ **1** : preservation, restoration, or enhancement of physical appearance ⟨café au lait macules themselves require treatment only if ∼ is requested —D. L. Stulberg *et al*⟩ ⟨the improved hip replacement resulted in a quicker recovery and better ∼⟩ **2** : the outer aesthetic covering (as of silicone) of a limb prosthesis

¹**cos·met·ic** \käz-'met-ik\ *n* : a cosmetic preparation for external use

²**cosmetic** *adj* **1** : of, relating to, or making for beauty esp. of the complexion ⟨∼ salves⟩ **2** : correcting defects esp. of the face ⟨∼ surgery⟩ — **cos·met·i·cal·ly** \-i-k(ə-)lē\ *adv*

cos·me·ti·cian \ˌkäz-mə-'tish-ən\ *n* : a person who is professionally trained in the use of cosmetics

cos·me·tol·o·gist \-'täl-ə-jəst\ *n* : a person who gives beauty treatments (as to skin and hair)

cos·me·tol·o·gy \-jē\ *n, pl* **-gies** : the cosmetic treatment of the skin, hair, and nails

cos·mid \'käz-məd\ *n* : a plasmid into which a short nucleotide sequence of a bacteriophage has been inserted to create a vector capable of cloning large fragments of DNA

cos·ta \'käs-tə\ *n, pl* **cos·tae** \-(ˌ)tē, -ˌtī\ : RIB

cos·tal \'käs-tᵊl\ *adj* : of, relating to, involving, or situated near a rib ⟨∼ fractures caused by violent coughing⟩

costal breathing *n* : inspiration and expiration produced chiefly by movements of the ribs

costal cartilage *n* : any of the cartilages that connect the distal ends of the ribs with the sternum and by their elasticity permit movement of the chest in respiration

costal process *n* : the ventral or anterior root of the transverse process of a cervical vertebra

costarum — see LEVATORES COSTARUM

cos·tec·to·my \käs-'tek-tə-mē\ *n, pl* **-mies** : surgical removal of all or part of a rib

cos·tive \'käs-tiv, 'kȯs-\ *adj* **1** : affected with constipation **2** : causing constipation — **cos·tive·ness** *n*

cos·to·cen·tral \ˌkäs-tə-'sen-trəl, -tō-\ *adj* : relating to or joining a rib and a vertebral centrum ⟨∼ articulations⟩

cos·to·cer·vi·cal trunk \-'sər-və-kəl-\ *n* : a branch of the subclavian artery that divides to supply the first or first two intercostal spaces and the deep structures of the neck — see INTERCOSTAL ARTERY b

cos·to·chon·dral \-'kän-drəl\ *adj* : relating to or joining a rib and costal cartilage ⟨a ∼ junction⟩

cos·to·chon·dri·tis \-kän-'drīt-əs\ *n* : TIETZE'S SYNDROME

cos·to·cla·vic·u·lar \-klə-'vik-yə-lər, -klä-\ *adj* : of or relating to a ligament connecting the costal cartilage of the first rib with the clavicle

cos·to·cor·a·coid \-'kȯr-ə-ˌkȯid\ *adj* : relating to or joining the ribs and the coracoid process

costocoracoid membrane *n* : a strong fascia that ensheathes and extends between the subclavius and pectoralis minor muscles and protects the axillary vessels and nerves

cos·to·di·a·phrag·mat·ic \ˌkäs-tə-dī-ə-frə(g)-'mat-ik, ˌkäs-tō-, -ˌfrag-\ *adj* : relating to or involving the ribs and diaphragm ⟨the ∼ movement in inspiration⟩

cos·to·phren·ic \ˌkäs-tō-'fren-ik, -tə-\ *adj* : of or relating to the ribs and the diaphragm

cos·to·tome \'käs-tə-ˌtōm\ *n* : a surgical instrument for cutting the ribs and opening the thoracic cavity

cos·to·trans·verse \ˌkäs-tə-tran(t)s-ˈvərs, -tō-, -tranz-, -ˈtran(t)s-ˌ, -ˈtranz-ˌ\ *adj* : relating to or connecting a rib and the transverse process of a vertebra ⟨a ~ joint⟩

cos·to·trans·ver·sec·to·my \-ˌtran(t)s-(ˌ)vər-ˈsek-tə-mē, -ˌtranz-\ *n, pl* **-mies** : surgical excision of part of a rib and the transverse process of the adjoining vertebra

cos·to·ver·te·bral \-(ˌ)vər-ˈtē-brəl *also* -ˈvərt-ə-\ *adj* : of or relating to a rib and its adjoining vertebra ⟨~ approach in an operation for herniated intervertebral disk⟩ ⟨~ pain⟩

cos·to·xi·phoid \-ˈzī-ˌfȯid, -ˈzif-ˌȯid\ *adj* : relating to or connecting a costal cartilage and the xiphoid process

¹cot \ˈkät\ *n* : a protective cover for a finger — called also *fingerstall*

²cot *n* : a wheeled stretcher for hospital, mortuary, or ambulance service

COTA *abbr* certified occupational therapy assistant

co·tar·nine \kō-ˈtär-ˌnēn, -nən\ *n* : a crystalline alkaloid that is obtained by the oxidation of narcotine and has been used chiefly in the form of its chloride $C_{12}H_{14}ClNO_3$ to check bleeding esp. from small blood vessels

cot death *n, chiefly Brit* : SUDDEN INFANT DEATH SYNDROME

co·throm·bo·plas·tin \(ˌ)kō-ˌthräm-bō-ˈplas-tən\ *n* : FACTOR VII

co·tin·ine \ˈkōt-ᵊn-ˌēn, -ˌīn\ *n* : an alkaloid $C_{10}H_{12}N_2O$ that is the principal metabolite of nicotine and is widely used as an indicator of recent exposure to nicotine

co·trans·duc·tion \ˌkō-ˌtran(t)s-ˈdək-shən\ *n* : transduction involving two or more genetic loci carried by a single bacteriophage

co–tri·mox·a·zole \ˌkō-ˌtrī-ˈmäk-sə-ˌzōl\ *n* : a bactericidal combination of trimethoprim and sulfamethoxazole in the ratio of one to five used esp. for chronic urinary tract infections

cot·ton \ˈkät-ᵊn\ *n, often attrib* **1** : a soft usu. white fibrous substance composed of the hairs surrounding the seeds of various erect freely branching tropical plants (genus *Gossypium*) of the mallow family and used extensively in making threads, yarns, and fabrics (as in surgical dressings) **2** : a plant producing this cotton

cot·ton·mouth \ˈkät-ᵊn-ˌmau̇th\ *n* : WATER MOCCASIN

cottonmouth moccasin *n* : WATER MOCCASIN

cot·ton·seed oil \ˈkät-ᵊn-ˌsēd-\ *n* : a fatty oil that is obtained from cottonseed, is pale yellow after refining, contains principally glycerides of linoleic, oleic, and palmitic acids, and is used chiefly in salad and cooking oils and after hydrogenation in shortenings and margarine

cotton–wool *n, Brit* : ABSORBENT COTTON

cot·y·le·don \ˌkät-ᵊl-ˈēd-ᵊn\ *n* **1** : a lobule of a mammalian placenta **2** : the first leaf or one of the first pair or whorl of leaves developed by the embryo of a seed plant or of some lower plants (as ferns) — **cot·y·le·don·ary** \-ˈēd-ᵊn-ˌer-ē\ *adj*

cot·y·loid \ˈkät-ᵊl-ˌȯid\ *adj* : of or relating to an acetabulum

¹couch \ˈkau̇ch\ *vt* : to treat (a cataract or a person who has a cataract) by displacing the lens of the eye into the vitreous body

²couch *n* : an article of furniture used (as by a patient undergoing psychoanalysis) for sitting or reclining — **on the couch** : receiving psychiatric treatment

couch grass *n* : QUACK GRASS

¹cough \ˈkȯf\ *vi* : to expel air from the lungs suddenly with an explosive noise usu. in a series of efforts ~ *vt* : to expel by coughing — often used with *up* ⟨~ up mucus⟩

²cough *n* **1** : an ailment manifesting itself by frequent coughing ⟨he has a bad ~⟩ **2** : an explosive expulsion of air from the lungs acting as a protective mechanism to clear the air passages or as a symptom of pulmonary disturbance

cough drop *n* : a lozenge or troche used to relieve coughing

cough syrup *n* : any of various sweet usu. medicated liquids used to relieve coughing

cou·lomb \ˈkü-ˌläm, -ˌlōm, kü-ˈ\ *n* : the practical mks unit of electric charge equal to the quantity of electricity transferred by a current of one ampere in one second

Cou·lomb \kü-lōⁿ\, **Charles–Augustin de (1736–1806),**

French physicist. A pioneer in electrical theory, Coulomb is known for his formulation of the law (now identified with him) in physics regarding the force between two electrical charges. He also established that the attraction and repulsion of unlike and like magnetic poles varies inversely as the square of the distance between them. In the course of his career Coulomb did research on friction as applied to machinery, on windmills, and on the elasticity of metal and silk fibers. The electrical unit of measure was named in his honor in 1881 by the Paris Congress on electricity.

Cou·ma·din \ˈkü-mə-dən\ *trademark* — used for a preparation of warfarin

cou·ma·phos \ˈkü-mə-ˌfäs\ *n* : an organophosphorus systemic insecticide $C_{14}H_{16}ClO_5PS$ administered esp. to cattle and poultry as a feed additive

cou·ma·rin \ˈkü-mə-rən\ *n* : a toxic white crystalline lactone $C_9H_6O_2$ with an odor of new-mown hay found in plants or made synthetically and used esp. in perfumery and as the parent compound in various anticoagulant agents (as warfarin); *also* : a derivative of this compound

¹coun·sel \ˈkau̇n(t)-səl\ *n* : advice given esp. as a result of consultation

²counsel *vt* **-seled** *or* **-selled; -sel·ing** *or* **-sel·ling** \-s(ə-)liŋ\ : to advise esp. seriously and formally after consultation

coun·sel·ee \ˌkau̇n(t)-sə-ˈlē\ *n* : one who is being counseled

coun·sel·ing *n* : professional guidance of the individual by utilizing psychological methods esp. in collecting case history data, using various techniques of the personal interview, and testing interests and aptitudes

coun·sel·or *or* **coun·sel·lor** \ˈkau̇n(t)-s(ə-)lər\ *n* : a person engaged in counseling

¹count \ˈkau̇nt\ *vt* : to indicate or name by units or groups so as to find the total number of units involved

²count *n* **1 a** : the action or process of counting **b** : a total obtained by counting **2** : the total number of individual things in a given unit or sample (as of blood) obtained by counting all or a subsample of them — see ADDIS COUNT, BLOOD COUNT, CELL COUNT, RED BLOOD COUNT, WHITE COUNT

¹count·er \ˈkau̇nt-ər\ *n* : a level surface over which transactions are conducted or food is served or on which goods are displayed or work is conducted ⟨a lunch ~⟩ — **over the counter** : without a prescription ⟨drugs available *over the counter*⟩

²counter *n* : one that counts; *esp* : a device for indicating a number or amount — see GEIGER COUNTER

coun·ter·act \ˌkau̇nt-ə-ˈrakt\ *vt* : to make ineffective or restrain or neutralize the usu. ill effects of by an opposite force ⟨vitamin K ~s the effects of warfarin⟩ — **coun·ter·ac·tion** \-ˈrak-shən\ *n*

coun·ter·con·di·tion·ing \ˌkau̇nt-ər-kən-ˈdish-(ə-)niŋ\ *n* : conditioning in order to replace an undesirable response (as fear) to a stimulus (as an engagement in public speaking) by a favorable one

¹coun·ter·cur·rent \ˈkau̇nt-ər-ˌkər-ənt, -ˌkə-rənt\ *n* : a current flowing in a direction opposite that of another current

²countercurrent \ˌkau̇nt-ər-ˈ\ *adj* **1** : flowing in an opposite direction **2** : involving flow of materials in opposite directions ⟨~ dialysis⟩ ⟨the ~ system of the kidney⟩

coun·ter·elec·tro·pho·re·sis \ˌkau̇nt-ər-i-ˌlek-trə-fə-ˈrē-səs\ *n, pl* **-re·ses** \-ˌsēz\ : an electrophoretic method of testing blood esp. for hepatitis antigens

coun·ter·im·mu·no·elec·tro·pho·re·sis \ˌkau̇nt-ər-ˌim-yə-nō-i-ˌlek-trō-fə-ˈrē-səs\ *n, pl* **-re·ses** : COUNTERELECTROPHORESIS

coun·ter·ir·ri·tant \-ˈir-ə-tənt\ *n* : an agent applied locally to produce superficial inflammation with the object of reducing inflammation in deeper adjacent structures — **counterirritant** *adj*

\ə\ **abut** \ᵊ\ **kitten** \ər\ **further** \a\ **ash** \ā\ **ace** \ä\ **cot, cart** \au̇\ **out** \ch\ **chin** \e\ **bet** \ē\ **easy** \g\ **go** \i\ **hit** \ī\ **ice** \j\ **job** \ŋ\ **sing** \ō\ **go** \ȯ\ **law** \ȯi\ **boy** \th\ **thin** \t̲h̲\ **the** \ü\ **loot** \u̇\ **foot** \y\ **yet** \zh\ **vision** *See also* Pronunciation Symbols page

coun·ter·ir·ri·ta·tion \-ˌir-ə-ˈtā-shən\ n : the reaction produced by treatment with a counterirritant; *also* : the treatment itself

coun·ter·open·ing \ˈkau̇n-tər-ˌōp-(ə-)niŋ\ n : an aperture on the opposite side or in a different place; *specif* : a surgical opening made opposite another to facilitate drainage (as of an abscess)

coun·ter·pho·bic \-ˌfō-bik\ adj : relating to or characterized by a preference for or the seeking out of a situation that is feared ⟨∼ reaction patterns⟩

coun·ter·pul·sa·tion \-ˌpəl-ˌsā-shən\ n : a technique for reducing the workload on the heart by lowering systemic blood pressure just before or during expulsion of blood from the ventricle and by raising blood pressure during diastole — see INTRA-AORTIC BALLOON COUNTERPULSATION

coun·ter·punc·ture \-ˌpən(k)-chər\ n : a surgical counteropening

coun·ter·shock \-ˌshäk\ n : a therapeutic shock of electricity applied to a heart for the purpose of altering a disturbed rhythm (as in chronic atrial fibrillation) ⟨delivering a life‑saving ∼ within seconds of an arrhythmic episode —John Maurice⟩

¹**coun·ter·stain** \-ˌstān\ n : a stain used to color parts of a microscopy specimen not affected by another stain; *esp* : a cytoplasmic stain used to contrast with or enhance a nuclear stain

²**counterstain** vt : to stain (a tissue or microscopy specimen) with an additional usu. contrasting color

coun·ter·trac·tion \ˈkau̇nt-ər-ˌtrak-shən\ n : a traction opposed to another traction used in reducing fractures

coun·ter·trans·fer·ence \ˌkau̇nt-ər-tran(t)s-ˈfər-ən(t)s, -ˈtran(t)s-(ˌ)\ n 1 : psychological transference esp. by a psychotherapist during the course of treatment; *esp* : the psychotherapist's reactions to the patient's transference 2 : the complex of feelings of a psychotherapist toward the patient

coup \ˈkü\ n : injury occurring on the side of an organ (as the brain) on which a blow or impact is received — compare CONTRECOUP

cou·pling \ˈkəp-liŋ, -ə-liŋ\ n 1 : the joint together with its supporting structures between the last lumbar vertebra and the sacrum that joins the hindquarters of a quadruped to the trunk; *broadly* : the part of the body or the conformation and proportionate length of the part of the body that joins the hindquarters to the forequarters 2 : the tendency of linked traits to be inherited together in offspring of a double heterozygote when both dominant genes occur on one chromosome and both recessive genes occur on the homologous chromosome — compare REPULSION 3 : BIGEMINY

course \ˈkō(ə)rs, ˈkȯ(ə)rs\ n 1 : the series of events or stages comprising a natural process ⟨the ∼ of a disease⟩ 2 : a series of doses or medications administered over a designated period ⟨a ∼ of three doses daily for five days⟩

cours·es \ˈkōr-səz, ˈkȯr-\ n pl : MENSES

court plaster \ˈkō(ə)rt-, ˈkȯ(ə)rt-\ n : an adhesive plaster esp. of silk coated with isinglass and glycerin

cou·vade \kü-ˈväd\ n : a custom in some cultures in which when a child is born the father takes to bed as if bearing the child and submits himself to fasting, purification, or taboos

Cou·ve·laire uterus \ˌkü-və-ˈle(ə)r-\ n : a pregnant uterus in which the placenta has detached prematurely with extravasation of blood into the uterine musculature

Cou·ve·laire \kü̇v(-ə)-ler\, **Alexandre (1873–1948),** French obstetrician. A leading specialist in obstetrics and gynecology, Couvelaire did original research on the anatomy of the pregnant uterus, uterine hemorrhages, and the pathology of newborn infants. In 1912 he published a work on the condition affecting the pregnant uterus that has been named after him.

co·va·lence \(ˈ)kō-ˈvā-lən(t)s\ n : valence characterized by the sharing of electrons — **co·va·lent** \-lənt\ adj — **co·va·lent·ly** adv

co·va·len·cy \-lən-sē\ n, pl **-cies** : COVALENCE

covalent bond n : a chemical bond formed between atoms by the sharing of electrons

cov·er glass \ˈkəv-ər-ˌglas\ n : a piece of very thin glass used to cover material on a glass microscope slide

cov·er·slip \ˈkəv-ər-ˌslip\ n : COVER GLASS

cowbane — see SPOTTED COWBANE

Cow·dria \ˈkau̇-drē-ə\ n : a genus of small pleomorphic intracellular rickettsial bacteria known chiefly from ticks but including the causative organism (*C. ruminantium*) of heartwater of ruminants

Cow·dry \ˈkau̇-drē\, **Edmund Vincent (1888–1975),** American anatomist. Cowdry's areas of research included the pathology of virus diseases, rickettsial diseases, malaria, yellow fever, and east coast fever. In 1924 he discovered the causative organism (*Cowdria ruminantium*) of heartwater.

cow·hage *also* **cow·age** \ˈkau̇-ij\ n : a tropical leguminous woody vine (*Mucuna pruriens*) with crooked pods covered with barbed hairs that cause intense itching; *also* : these hairs formerly used as a vermifuge

cow hock \ˈkau̇-ˌhäk\ n : a hock of a horse or dog that turns or bends inward like that of a cow so that the shanks of the hind legs are very close — **cow–hocked** \-ˌhäkt\ adj

Cow·per's gland \ˌkau̇-pərz-, ˌkü-pərz-, ˌku̇p-ərz-\ n : either of two small glands of which one lies on each side of the male urethra below the prostate gland and discharges a secretion into the semen — called also *bulbourethral gland, gland of Cowper;* compare BARTHOLIN'S GLAND

Cow·per \ˈkau̇-pər, ˈkü-pər, ˈku̇p-ər\, **William (1666–1709),** British anatomist. In 1702 Cowper described the bulbourethral glands. The glands had been described previously, in 1684 by the French surgeon Jean Méry, but Cowper's description was so excellent that ever since they have been more commonly known as Cowper's glands.

cow·pox \ˈkau̇-ˌpäks\ n : a mild eruptive disease of the cow that is caused by a poxvirus of the genus *Orthopoxvirus* (species *Cowpox virus*) and that when communicated to humans protects against smallpox — called also *variola vaccinia*

cox \ˈkäks\ n : CYCLOOXYGENASE

coxa \ˈkäk-sə\ n, pl **cox·ae** \-ˌsē, -ˌsī\ : HIP JOINT, ¹HIP

cox·al·gia \käk-ˈsal-j(ē-)ə\ n : pain in the hip

coxa vara \ˌkäk-sə-ˈvar-ə\ n : a deformed hip joint in which the neck of the femur is bent downward

Cox·i·el·la \ˌkäk-sē-ˈel-ə\ n : a genus of small pleomorphic rickettsial bacteria occurring intercellularly in ticks and intracellularly in the cytoplasm of vertebrates and including the causative organism (*C. burnetii*) of Q fever

Cox \ˈkäks\, **Herald Rea (b 1907),** American bacteriologist. Cox's areas of research include neurotropic virus diseases, rickettsial diseases, virus infections, and vaccines. In 1937 Frank MacFarlane Burnet, an Australian physician, reported his discovery with Mavis Freeman of the causative organism of Q fever. At about the same time Cox isolated this causative agent. The genus *Coxiella* of bacteria created to contain the rickettsial agent (*Coxiella burnetii*) was named after Cox and the species after Burnet.

cox·i·tis \käk-ˈsīt-əs\ n, pl **cox·it·i·des** \-ˈsit-ə-ˌdēz\ : inflammation of the hip joint

coxo·fem·o·ral \ˌkäk-sō-ˈfem-(ə-)rəl\ adj : of or relating to the hip and thigh

COX–1 \ˈkäks-ˈwən\ n : the isoform of cyclooxygenase that is expressed in most tissues of the body and is not involved in producing the pain and inflammation of arthritis

cox·sack·ie·vi·rus \(ˈ)käk-ˌsak-ē-ˈvī-rəs\ n : any of numerous serotypes of three picornaviruses of the genus *Enterovirus* (species *Human enterovirus A, Human enterovirus B,* and *Human enterovirus C*) associated with human diseases (as meningitis or herpangina) — see EPIDEMIC PLEURODYNIA

COX–2 \ˈkäks-ˈtü\ n 1 : the isoform of cyclooxygenase that is expressed esp. in the brain and kidneys and at sites of inflammation 2 : COX-2 INHIBITOR

COX–2 inhibitor n : any of a class of drugs (as celecoxib) that selectively block the isoform COX-2 but not the isoform COX-1 of cyclooxygenase and that are intended to relieve the pain and inflammation of arthritis while minimizing gastrointestinal side effects — called also *COX-2 blocker*

Co·zaar \'kō-ˌzär\ *trademark* — used for a preparation of the potassium salt of losartan

CP *abbr* **1** capillary pressure **2** cerebral palsy **3** chemically pure **4** compare **5** constant pressure **6** cor pulmonale

CPAP \'sē-ˌpap\ *abbr* continuous positive airway pressure

CPB *abbr* competitive protein binding

CPC *abbr* chronic passive congestion

cpd *abbr* compound

CPE *abbr* cytopathogenic effects

C–pep·tide \'sē-'pep-ˌtīd\ *n* : a protein fragment 35 amino acid residues long produced by enzymatic cleavage of proinsulin in the formation of insulin

CPI *abbr* constitutional psychopathic inferiority

CPK *abbr* creatine phosphokinase

CPM *abbr* counts per minute

CPR *abbr* cardiopulmonary resuscitation

CPV *abbr* canine parvovirus

CPZ *abbr* chlorpromazine

Cr *abbr* creatinine

Cr *symbol* chromium

CR *abbr* **1** cardiorespiratory **2** chest and right arm **3** clot retraction **4** conditioned reflex; conditioned response

crab \'krab\ *n* **1** : any of a tribe (Brachyura) of chiefly marine crustaceans with a short broad usu. flattened carapace, a small abdomen that curls forward beneath the body, short antennae, and the anterior pair of limbs modified as grasping pincers **2** **crabs** *pl* : infestation with crab lice

crab louse *n, pl* **crab lice** : a sucking louse of the genus *Pthirus* (*P. pubis*) infesting the pubic region of the human body

crack \'krak\ *n, often attrib* : a potent form of cocaine that is obtained by treating the hydrochloride of cocaine with sodium bicarbonate to create small chips used illicitly usu. for smoking

crack baby *n* : an infant born physiologically addicted to crack as a result of continued exposure to the drug in the mother's womb

cra·dle \'krād-ᵊl\ *n* **1** : a bed or cot for a baby usu. on rockers or pivots **2 a** : a frame to keep the bedclothes from contact with an injured part of the body **b** : a frame placed on the neck of an animal to keep it from biting an injury or sore

cradle cap *n* : a seborrheic condition in infants that usu. affects the scalp and is characterized by greasy gray or dark brown adherent scaly crusts

¹**cramp** \'kramp\ *n* **1** : a painful involuntary spasmodic contraction of a muscle ⟨a ∼ in the leg⟩ **2** : a temporary paralysis of muscles from overuse — see WRITER'S CRAMP **3 a** : sharp abdominal pain — usu. used in pl. **b** : persistent and often intense though dull lower abdominal pain associated with dysmenorrhea — usu. used in pl.

²**cramp** *vt* : to affect with or as if with a cramp or cramps ⟨gout ∼ing his limbs⟩ ∼ *vi* : to suffer from cramps

cra·ni·ad \'krā-nē-ˌad\ *adv* : toward the head or anterior end ⟨the artery extends ∼⟩

cra·ni·al \'krā-nē-əl\ *adj* **1** : of or relating to the skull or cranium **2** : CEPHALIC ⟨the ∼ end of the spinal column⟩ — **cra·ni·al·ly** \-ə-lē\ *adv*

cranial arteritis *n* : GIANT CELL ARTERITIS

cranial capacity *n* : the cubic capacity of the braincase estimated for the living by a formula based on head measurements and determined for the skull by filling the cranial cavity with particulate material (as mustard seed or small shot) and measuring the volume of the latter

cranial flexure *n* : CEPHALIC FLEXURE

cranial fossa *n* : any of the three large depressions in the posterior, middle, and anterior aspects of the floor of the cranial cavity: **a** : the posterior one that is the largest and deepest of the three and lodges the cerebrum, pons, and medulla oblongata — called also *posterior cranial fossa, posterior fossa* **b** : the middle one that lodges the temporal lobes laterally and the hypothalamus medially — called also *middle cranial fossa, middle fossa* **c** : the anterior one that lodges the frontal lobes — called also *anterior cranial fossa, anterior fossa*

cra·ni·al·gia \ˌkrā-nē-'al-j(ē-)ə\ *n* : pain occurring within the skull : HEADACHE

cranial index *n* : the ratio multiplied by 100 of the maximum breadth of the bare skull to its maximum length from front to back — compare CEPHALIC INDEX

cranial nerve *n* : any of the 12 paired nerves that arise from the lower surface of the brain with one of each pair on each side and pass through openings in the skull to the periphery of the body — see ABDUCENS NERVE, ACCESSORY NERVE, AUDITORY NERVE, FACIAL NERVE, GLOSSOPHARYNGEAL NERVE, HYPOGLOSSAL NERVE, OCULOMOTOR NERVE, OLFACTORY NERVE, OPTIC NERVE, TRIGEMINAL NERVE, TROCHLEAR NERVE, VAGUS NERVE

Cra·ni·a·ta \ˌkrā-nē-'āt-ə\ *n pl, syn of* VERTEBRATA

cra·ni·ate \'krā-nē-ət, -ˌāt\ *adj* **1** : VERTEBRATE **2** : having a cranium — **craniate** *n*

cra·ni·ec·to·my \ˌkrā-nē-'ek-tə-mē\ *n, pl* **-mies** : the surgical removal of a portion of the skull

cra·nio·ce·re·bral \ˌkrā-nē-ō-sə-'rē-brəl, -'ser-ə-\ *adj* : involving both cranium and brain ⟨∼ injury⟩

cra·nio·cla·sis \ˌkrā-nē-ō-'klas-əs, -nē-'äk-lə-səs\ *n, pl* **-cla·ses** \-'klas-ˌēz, -lə-ˌsēz\ : the crushing of the fetal head during a difficult delivery

cra·nio·fa·cial \ˌkrā-nē-ō-'fā-shəl\ *adj* : of, relating to, or involving both the cranium and the face ⟨∼ abnormalities⟩

craniofacial dysostosis *n* : CROUZON SYNDROME

craniofacial index *n* : the ratio of the breadth of the cranium to the breadth of the face

cra·nio·fe·nes·tria \-fə-'nes-trē-ə\ *n* : a congenital bony defect of the skull characterized by areas in which no bone forms

cra·nio·graph \'krā-nē-ə-ˌgraf\ *n* : an instrument used for the accurate depiction of a skull in outline

cra·ni·ol·o·gy \ˌkrā-nē-'äl-ə-jē\ *n, pl* **-gies** : a science dealing with variations in size, shape, and proportions of skulls among the human races

cra·ni·om·e·ter \ˌkrā-nē-'äm-ət-ər\ *n* : an instrument for measuring skulls

cra·ni·om·e·try \-'äm-ə-trē\ *n, pl* **-tries** : a science dealing with cranial measurement — **cra·nio·met·ric** \ˌkrā-nē-ō-'me-trik\ *or* **cra·nio·met·ri·cal** \-tri-kəl\ *adj*

cra·ni·op·a·gus \ˌkrā-nē-'äp-ə-gəs\ *n, pl* **-a·gi** \-ə-ˌjē, -ˌjī\ : a pair of twins joined at the heads

cra·ni·op·a·thy \ˌkrā-nē-'äp-ə-thē\ *n, pl* **-thies** : a disease of the skull bones

cra·nio·pha·ryn·geal \ˌkrā-nē-ō-ˌfar-ən-'jē-əl, -fə-'rin-j(ē-)əl\ *adj* : relating to or connecting the cavity of the skull and the pharynx ⟨the ∼ canal connecting the hypophyseal diverticulum with buccal ectoderm in the fetus⟩

cra·nio·pha·ryn·gi·o·ma \-ˌfar-ən-jē-'ō-mə, -fə-ˌrin-jē-'ō-mə\ *n, pl* **-mas** *also* **-ma·ta** \-'mət-ə\ : a tumor of the brain near the pituitary gland that develops esp. in children or young adults from epithelium derived from the embryonic craniopharyngeal canal and that is often associated with increased intracranial pressure

cra·nio·phore \'krā-nē-ə-ˌfō(ə)r\ *n* : a device for holding skulls in position (as for taking measurements)

cra·nio·plas·ty \-ˌplas-tē\ *n, pl* **-ties** : the surgical correction of skull defects

cra·nio·ra·chis·chi·sis \ˌkrā-nē-(ˌ)ō-rə-'kis-kə-səs\ *n, pl* **-chi·ses** \-ˌsēz\ : a congenital fissure of the skull and spine

cra·nio·sa·cral \ˌkrā-nē-ō-'sak-rəl, -'sā-krəl\ *adj* **1** : of or relating to the cranium and the sacrum **2** : PARASYMPATHETIC ⟨the ∼ division of the autonomic nervous system⟩

cra·ni·os·chi·sis \ˌkrā-nē-'äs-kə-səs\ *n, pl* **-chi·ses** \-ˌsēz\ : a congenital fissure of the skull

cra·ni·os·co·pist \ˌkrā-nē-'äs-kə-ˌpist\ *n* : a specialist in cranioscopy

\ə\ **abut** \ᵊ\ **kitten** \ər\ **further** \a\ **ash** \ā\ **ace** \ä\ **cot, cart** \aú\ **out** \ch\ **chin** \e\ **bet** \ē\ **easy** \g\ **go** \i\ **hit** \ī\ **ice** \j\ **job** \ŋ\ **sing** \ō\ **go** \ó\ **law** \ói\ **boy** \th\ **thin** \th̲\ **the** \ü\ **loot** \ú\ **foot** \y\ **yet** \zh\ **vision** *See also* Pronunciation Symbols page

cra·ni·os·co·py \-'äs-kə-pē\ *n, pl* **-pies** : observations on or examination of the human skull — **cra·nio·scop·ic** \ˌkrā-nē-ə-'skäp-ik\ *adj*

cra·nio·ste·no·sis \ˌkrā-nē-(ˌ)ō-stə-'nō-səs\ *n, pl* **-no·ses** \-ˌsēz\ : malformation of the skull caused by premature closure of the cranial sutures

cra·nio·syn·os·to·sis \-ˌsin-ˌäs-'tō-səs\ *n, pl* **-to·ses** \-ˌsēz\ *or* **-to·sis·es** : premature fusion of the sutures of the skull

cra·nio·ta·bes \ˌkrā-nē-ə-'tā-(ˌ)bēz\ *n, pl* **craniotabes** : a thinning and softening of the infantile skull in spots usu. due to rickets or syphilis

cra·nio·tome \'krā-nē-ə-ˌtōm\ *n* : an instrument used in performing craniotomy

cra·ni·ot·o·my \ˌkrā-nē-ə-'ät-ə-mē\ *n, pl* **-mies** **1** : the operation of cutting or crushing the fetal head to effect delivery 〈fetal *craniotomies* . . . performed to save the life of the mother —R. E. Frisch〉 **2** : surgical opening of the skull

cra·ni·um \'krā-nē-əm\ *n, pl* **-ni·ums** *or* **-nia** \-nē-ə\ : SKULL; *specif* : BRAINCASE

crank \'kraŋk\ *n* : CRYSTAL 2

crap·u·lous \'krap-yə-ləs\ *adj* **1** : marked by intemperance esp. in eating or drinking **2** : sick from excessive indulgence in liquor

cra·ter \'krāt-ər\ *n* : an eroded lesion of a wall or surface 〈ulcer ~s〉

cra·ter·iza·tion \ˌkrāt-ər-ə-'zā-shən\ *n* : surgical excision of a crater-shaped piece of bone

craw–craw \'krȯ-ˌkrȯ\ *n* : an itching skin disease produced by the larvae of the filarial worm causing onchocerciasis migrating in the subcutaneous tissues; *broadly* : ONCHOCERCIASIS

craze \'krāz\ *vb* **crazed; craz·ing** *vt* : to make insane or as if insane 〈*crazed* by pain and fear〉 ~ *vi* : to become insane

craz·ing \'krāz-iŋ\ *n* : the formation of minute cracks (as in acrylic resin teeth) usu. attributed to shrinkage or to moisture

cra·zy \'krā-zē\ *adj* **craz·i·er; -est** : MAD 1, INSANE — **cra·zi·ly** \-zə-lē\ *adv* — **cra·zi·ness** \-zē-nəs\ *n*

crazy bone *n* : FUNNY BONE

crazy chick disease \-'chik-\ *n* : a disease of the nervous system of young chickens caused by inadequate intake of vitamin E and marked by severe muscular incoordination, tremors, and encephalomalacia followed by paralysis and by renal congestion and failure — called also *crazy chick*

CRD *abbr* chronic respiratory disease

C–re·ac·tive protein \ˌsē-rē-ˌak-tiv-\ *n* : a protein produced by the liver that is normally present in trace amounts in the blood serum but is elevated during episodes of acute inflammation (as those associated with neoplastic disease, chronic infection, or coronary artery disease)

cream \'krēm\ *n* **1** : the yellowish part of milk containing from 18 to about 40 percent butterfat **2** : something having the consistency of cream; *esp* : a usu. emulsified medicinal or cosmetic preparation — **creamy** \'krē-mē\ *adj*

¹**crease** \'krēs\ *n* : a line or mark made by or as if by folding a pliable substance (as the skin)

²**crease** *vb* **creased; creas·ing** *vt* : to make a crease in or on 〈aging had *creased* her face〉 ~ *vi* : to become creased

cre·atine \'krē-ə-ˌtēn, -ət-ᵊn\ *n* : a white crystalline nitrogenous substance $C_4H_9N_3O_2$ found esp. in vertebrate muscle either free or as phosphocreatine

creatine kinase *n* : any of three isoenzymes found esp. in vertebrate skeletal and myocardial muscle and the brain that catalyze the transfer of a high-energy phosphate group from phosphocreatine to ADP with the formation of ATP and creatine and typically occur in elevated levels in the blood following injury to brain or muscle tissue

creatine phosphate *n* : PHOSPHOCREATINE

creatine phosphokinase *n* : CREATINE KINASE

cre·at·i·nine \krē-'at-ᵊn-ˌēn, -ᵊn-ən\ *n* : a white crystalline strongly basic compound $C_4H_7N_3O$ formed from creatine and found esp. in muscle, blood, and urine

cre·atin·uria \ˌkrē-ə-tə-'n(y)ùr-ē-ə, -ət-ᵊn-'(y)ùr-\ *n* : the presence of creatine in urine; *esp* : an increased or abnormal amount in the urine 〈marked ~ may accompany some endocrine disorders〉

crèche \'kresh, 'krāsh\ *n* **1** : DAY NURSERY **2** : a foundling hospital

creep·er \'krē-pər\ *n* **1** : a genetic anomaly of the domestic fowl marked by shortening and thickening of the long bones in the heterozygote and completely lethal when homozygous **2** : CREEPER FOWL

creeper fowl *n* : an individual fowl exhibiting creeper

creep·ing eruption \'krē-piŋ-\ *n* : a human skin disorder that is characterized by a red line of eruption which fades at one end as it progresses at the other and that is usu. caused by insect or worm larvae and esp. those of the dog hookworm burrowing in the deeper layers of the skin — called also *larval migrans, larva migrans*

creeps \'krēps\ *n pl* : a deficiency disease esp. of sheep and cattle associated with an abnormal calcium-phosphorus ratio in the diet and characterized by progressive anemia, painful softening of the bones, and a stiff slow gait

cre·mains \kri-'mānz\ *n pl* : the ashes of a cremated human body

cre·mas·ter \krē-'mas-tər, krə-\ *n* : a thin muscle consisting of loops of fibers derived from the internal oblique muscle and descending upon the spermatic cord to surround and suspend the testicle — called also *cremaster muscle* — **cre·mas·ter·ic** \ˌkrē-mə-'ster-ik\ *adj*

cre·mate \'krē-ˌmāt, kri-'\ *vt* **cre·mat·ed; cre·mat·ing** : to reduce (as a dead body) to ashes by burning — **cre·ma·tion** \kri-'mā-shən\ *n*

cre·ma·to·ri·um \ˌkrē-mə-'tōr-ē-əm, ˌkrem-ə-, -'tòr-\ *n, pl* **-ri·ums** *or* **-ria** \-ē-ə\ : CREMATORY

cre·ma·to·ry \'krē-mə-ˌtōr-ē, 'krem-ə-, -ˌtòr-\ *n, pl* **-ries** : a furnace for cremating; *also* : an establishment containing such a furnace — **crematory** *adj*

crème \'krem, 'krēm\ *n, pl* **crèmes** \'krem(z), 'krēmz\ : CREAM 2

cre·nat·ed \'krē-ˌnāt-əd\ *also* **cre·nate** \-ˌnāt\ *adj* : having the margin or surface cut into rounded scallops 〈~ red blood cells〉

cre·na·tion \kri-'nā-shən\ *n* : shrinkage of red blood cells resulting in crenated margins

cren·o·cyte \'kren-ə-ˌsīt, 'krē-nə-\ *n* : a red blood cell with notched serrated edges (as that resulting from crenation)

cre·oph·a·gy \krē-'äf-ə-jē\ *n, pl* **-gies** : the use of flesh as food

cre·o·sote \'krē-ə-ˌsōt\ *n* **1** : a clear or yellowish flammable oily liquid mixture of phenolic compounds obtained by the distillation of wood tar esp. from beech wood and used esp. as a disinfectant and as an expectorant in chronic bronchitis **2** : a brownish oily liquid consisting chiefly of aromatic hydrocarbons obtained by distillation of coal tar and used esp. as a wood preservative

cre·o·sote oil \'krē-ə-ˌsōt-\ *n* **1** : the part of the wood-tar distillate from which creosote is obtained by refining **2** : CREOSOTE 2

crep·i·tant \'krep-ət-ənt\ *adj* : having or making a crackling sound

crepitant rale *n* : a peculiar crackling sound audible with inspiration in pneumonia and other lung diseases

crep·i·tate \'krep-ə-ˌtāt\ *vi* **-tat·ed; -tat·ing** : to produce or experience crepitation

crep·i·ta·tion \ˌkrep-ə-'tā-shən\ *n* : a grating or crackling sound or sensation (as that produced by the fractured ends of a bone moving against each other or as that in tissues affected with gas gangrene) 〈~ in the arthritic knee〉

crep·i·tus \'krep-ət-əs\ *n, pl* **crepitus** : CREPITATION

cre·pus·cu·lar \kri-'pəs-kyə-lər\ *adj* **1** : of, relating to, or resembling twilight 〈~ depths of personality —William James〉 **2** : active in the twilight 〈~ animals〉

cres·cent \'kres-ᵊnt\ *n* **1** : a crescent-shaped anatomical structure or section **2** : the gametocyte of the falciparum malaria parasite that is shaped like a crescent and constitutes a distinguishing character of malignant tertian malaria

crescent of Gian·nuz·zi *or* **crescent of Gia·nuz·zi** \-jə-'nüt-sē\ *n* : DEMILUNE

G. Giannuzzi — see DEMILUNE OF GIANNUZZI

cre·sol \'krē-ˌsȯl, -ˌsōl\ *n* **1** : any of three poisonous colorless crystalline or liquid isomeric phenols C_7H_8O that are used as disinfectants, in making phenolic resins and plasticizers, and in organic synthesis — see METACRESOL, ORTHOCRESOL, PARACRESOL **2** : a mixture of cresol isomers — called also *tricresol*

crest \'krest\ *n* **1** : a showy tuft or process on the head of an animal esp. a bird **2** : a process or prominence on a part of an animal body: as **a** : the upper curve or ridge of the neck of a quadruped (as a horse); *also* : the mane borne on such a crest **b** : a ridge esp. on a bone ⟨the ∼ of the tibia⟩ — see FRONTAL CREST, OCCIPITAL CREST

cre·syl \'kres-əl, 'krē-ˌsil\ *n* : TOLYL

cre·syl·ic \kri-'sil-ik\ *adj* : of or relating to cresol or creosote

cresyl vi·o·let \-'vī(-ə)-lət\ *n* : an oxazine dye used as a biological stain esp. in histology

cre·ta \'krēt-ə\ *n* : CHALK

cre·tin \'krēt-ᵊn\ *n, often offensive* : one affected with cretinism — **cre·tin·ous** \-ᵊn-əs\ *adj*

cre·tin·ism \-ᵊn-ˌiz-əm\ *n* : a usu. congenital abnormal condition marked by physical stunting and mental retardation and caused by severe thyroid deficiency — called also *infantile myxedema*

cre·tin·oid \-ᵊn-ˌȯid\ *adj* : resembling or suggestive of cretinism

Creutz·feldt–Ja·kob disease *also* **Creutz·feld–Ja·kob disease** \ˌkrȯits-ˌfelt-ˌyä-(ˌ)kōb-\ *n* : a rare progressive fatal spongiform encephalopathy now usu. considered to be caused by a prion and marked by the development of porous brain tissue, premature dementia in middle age, and gradual loss of muscular coordination — abbr. *CJD*; called also *Jakob-Creutzfeldt disease*; see VARIANT CREUTZFELDT-JAKOB DISEASE

Creutz·feldt \'krȯits-ˌfelt\, **Hans Gerhard (1885–1964)**, and **Ja·kob** \'yä-ˌkōp\, **Alfons Maria (1884–1931)**, German psychiatrists. Creutzfeldt published his description of the disease now known as Creutzfeldt-Jakob disease in 1920. A year later in the same neurological journal Jakob offered his description. Although Creutzfeldt's description is the original one, Jakob's is the better known of the two, so the disease is named in honor of both men.

crev·ice \'krev-əs\ *n* : a narrow fissure or cleft ⟨an ulcerated periodontal ∼⟩ — see GINGIVAL CREVICE

cre·vic·u·lar \krə-'vik-yə-lər\ *adj* : of, relating to, or involving a crevice and esp. the gingival crevice ⟨gingival ∼ fluid⟩

CRF *abbr* corticotropin-releasing factor

CRH *abbr* corticotropin-releasing hormone

crib \'krib\ *n* **1** : a manger for feeding animals **2 a** : a stall for a stabled animal **b** : a small child's bedstead with high enclosing usu. slatted sides

crib·bing \'krib-iŋ\ *n* : a vice of horses characterized by gnawing (as at a manger) while slobbering and salivating

crib biting *n* : CRIBBING

crib death *n* : SUDDEN INFANT DEATH SYNDROME

crib·rate \'kri-ˌbrāt, -brət\ *adj* : resembling a sieve — **crib·rate·ly** *adv*

cri·bra·tion \krə-'brā-shən\ *n* : the act or an instance of sifting (as drugs)

crib·ri·form \'krib-rə-ˌfȯrm\ *adj* : pierced with small holes

cribriform fascia *n* : the perforated fascia covering the saphenous opening in the fascia lata of the thigh and giving passage to various blood and lymph vessels

cribriform plate *n* **1** : the horizontal plate of the ethmoid bone perforated with numerous foramina for the passage of the olfactory nerve filaments from the nasal cavity — called also *lamina cribrosa* **2** : LAMINA DURA

cribrosa — see LAMINA CRIBROSA

Cri·ce·ti·dae \krī-'sēt-ə-ˌdē, krə-, -'set-\ *n pl* : a family of small rodents that includes the hamsters, voles, lemmings, gerbils, and New World rats and mice and is often grouped with the murids — **cri·ce·tid** \-'sēt-əd, -'set-\ *adj or n*

Cri·ce·tu·lus \-'sēt-ᵊl-əs, -'set-\ *n* : a large genus of small short-tailed Asian hamsters that resemble the New World white-footed mice

Cri·ce·tus \-'sēt-əs, -'set-\ *n* : the type genus of Cricetidae that includes the common hamster (*C. cricetus*) of Europe and Russia and in some classifications the golden hamster (*Mesocricetus auratus* syn. *C. cricetus*) and related forms

¹crick \'krik\ *n* : a painful spasmodic condition of muscles (as of the neck or back)

²crick *vt* : to cause a crick in (as the neck)

cri·co·ar·y·te·noid \ˌkrī-kō-ˌar-ə-'tē-ˌnȯid, -kō-ə-'rit-ᵊn-ˌȯid\ *n* **1** : a muscle of the larynx that arises from the upper margin of the arch of the cricoid cartilage, inserts into the front of the process of the arytenoid cartilage, and helps to narrow the opening of the vocal cords — called also *lateral cricoarytenoid* **2** : a muscle of the larynx that arises from the posterior surface of the lamina of the cricoid cartilage, inserts into the posterior of the process of the arytenoid cartilage, and widens the opening of the vocal cords — called also *posterior cricoarytenoid*

cri·coid cartilage \'krī-ˌkȯid-\ *n* : a cartilage of the larynx which articulates with the lower cornua of the thyroid cartilage and with which the arytenoid cartilages articulate — called also *cricoid*

cri·coid·ec·to·my \ˌkrī-ˌkȯid-'ek-tə-mē\ *n, pl* **-mies** : surgical excision of the cricoid cartilage

cri·co·pha·ryn·geal \ˌkrī-kō-ˌfar-ən-'jē-əl, -fə-'rin-j(ē-)əl\ *adj* : of or relating to the cricoid cartilage and the pharynx

¹cri·co·thy·roid \-'thī-ˌrȯid\ *adj* : relating to or connecting the cricoid cartilage and the thyroid cartilage

²cricothyroid *n* : a triangular muscle of the larynx that is attached to the cricoid and thyroid cartilages and is the principal tensor of the vocal cords — called also *cricothyroid muscle*

cri·co·thy·roi·de·us \ˌkrī-kō-thī-'rȯid-ē-əs\ *n, pl* **-dei** \-ē-ˌī\ : CRICOTHYROID

cricothyroid membrane *n* : a membrane of yellow elastic tissue that is attached below to the cricoid cartilage, in front to the thyroid cartilage, and in back to the arytenoid cartilages and that forms the vocal ligaments with its thickened upper margins

cri·co·thy·roi·dot·o·my \-ˌthī-ˌrȯi-'dät-ə-mē\ *n, pl* **-mies** : CRICOTHYROTOMY

cri·co·thy·rot·o·my \-'rät-ə-mē\ *n, pl* **-mies** : tracheotomy by incision through the skin and cricothyroid membrane esp. as an emergency procedure for relief of an obstructed airway

cri du chat syndrome \ˌkrē-dü-'shä-, -də-\ *n* : an inherited condition characterized by a mewing cry, mental retardation, physical anomalies, and the absence of part of a chromosome — called also *cat cry syndrome*

crim·i·nol·o·gy \ˌkrim-ə-'näl-ə-jē\ *n, pl* **-gies** : the scientific study of crime as a social phenomenon, of criminals, and of penal treatment — **crim·i·no·log·i·cal** \-ən-ᵊl-'äj-i-kəl\ *adj* — **crim·i·no·log·i·cal·ly** \-k(ə)lē\ *adv* — **crim·i·nol·o·gist** \ˌkrim-ə-'näl-ə-jəst\ *n*

¹crip·ple \'krip-əl\ *n, sometimes offensive* : a lame or partly disabled individual

²cripple *adj* : being a cripple : LAME

³cripple *vt* **crip·pled; crip·pling** \-(ə)liŋ\ : to deprive of the use of a limb and esp. a leg ⟨*crippled* by arthritis⟩

crip·pler \-(ə)lər\ *n* : a disease that results in crippling ⟨polio was once a major ∼ of children⟩

cri·sis \'krī-səs\ *n, pl* **cri·ses** \-ˌsēz\ **1** : the turning point for better or worse in an acute disease or fever; *esp* : a sudden turn for the better (as sudden abatement in severity of symptoms or abrupt drop in temperature) — compare LYSIS 1 **2**

\ə\ abut \ᵊ\ kitten \ər\ further \a\ ash \ā\ ace \ä\ cot, cart
\aú\ out \ch\ chin \e\ bet \ē\ easy \g\ go \i\ hit \ī\ ice \j\ job
\ŋ\ sing \ō\ go \ȯ\ law \ȯi\ boy \th\ thin \th\ the \ü\ loot
\ú\ foot \y\ yet \zh\ vision   *See also* Pronunciation Symbols page

: a paroxysmal attack of pain, distress, or disordered function ⟨tabetic ∼⟩ ⟨cardiac ∼⟩   **3** : an emotionally significant event or radical change of status in a person's life   **4 : a** psychological or social condition characterized by unusual instability caused by excessive stress and either endangering or felt to endanger the continuity of an individual or group; *esp* : such a social condition requiring the transformation of cultural patterns and values

crisis center *n* : a facility run usu. by nonprofessionals who counsel those who telephone for help in a personal crisis

cris·ta \'kris-tə\ *n, pl* **cris·tae** \-ˌtē, -ˌtī\   **1** : one of the areas of specialized sensory epithelium in the ampullae of the semicircular canals of the ear serving as end organs for the labyrinthine sense — called also *crista ampullaris*   **2** : a membranous spiral fold running the length of the body of certain spirochetes   **3** : an elevation of the surface of a bone for the attachment of a muscle or tendon   **4** : any of the inwardly projecting folds of the inner membrane of a mitochondrion

crista am·pul·lar·is \-ˌam-p(y)ü-'lar-əs\ *n* : CRISTA 1

crista gal·li \-'gal-ē, -'gȯ-lē\ *n* : an upright process on the anterior portion of the cribriform plate to which the anterior part of the falx cerebri is attached

crit *abbr* critical

cri·thid·ia \krə-'thid-ē-ə\ *n*   **1** *cap* : a genus of flagellates of the family Trypanosomatidae that are exclusively parasites of invertebrates esp. in the digestive tract of insects and that occur typically as elongated forms morphologically like trypanosomes but pass through developmental stages all in a single host in which they are indistinguishable from typical leptomonas and leishmanias   **2 a** : any flagellate of the genus *Crithidia*   **b** : any flagellate of the family Trypanosomatidae when exhibiting a typical form of a crithidia

cri·thid·i·al \-ē-əl\ *adj* : of, like, or relating to crithidias : CRITHIDIFORM

cri·thid·i·form \-də-ˌfȯrm\ *adj* : resembling a crithidia in structure

crit·i·cal \'krit-i-kəl\ *adj*   **1 a** : relating to, indicating, or being the stage of a disease at which an abrupt change for better or worse may be anticipated with reasonable certainty ⟨the ∼ phase of a fever⟩   **b** : being or relating to an illness or condition involving danger of death ⟨∼ care⟩ ⟨a ∼ head injury⟩   **2 a** : of sufficient size to sustain a chain reaction — used of a mass of fissionable material   **b** : sustaining a chain reaction — used of a nuclear reactor — **crit·i·cal·ly** \-k(ə-)lē\ *adv*

Crix·i·van \'krik-sə-ˌvan\ *trademark* — used for a preparation of the sulfate of indinavir

CRNA *abbr* certified registered nurse anesthetist

CRO *abbr* cathode-ray oscilloscope

cro·ci·do·lite \ˌkrō-'sī-də-ˌlīt, -'sid-ə-\ *n* : a purplish blue to greenish mineral of the amphibole group that causes asbestosis and cancer in the form of mesotheliomas — called also *blue asbestos*

crock \'kräk\ *n, slang* : a complaining medical patient whose illness is largely imaginary or psychosomatic

cro·cus \'krō-kəs\ *n, pl* **cro·cus·es**   **1** *pl also* **crocus** or **cro·ci** \-ˌkē, -ˌkī, -ˌsī\ : any of a large genus (*Crocus*) of perennial herbs of the iris family (Iridaceae)   **2** : SAFFRON 1

Crohn's disease \'krōnz-\ *also* **Crohn disease** \'krōn-\ *n* : chronic ileitis that typically involves the distal portion of the ileum, often spreads to the colon, and is characterized by diarrhea, cramping, and loss of appetite and weight with local abscesses and scarring — called also *regional enteritis, regional ileitis*

    Crohn, Burrill Bernard (1884–1983), American physician. Crohn spent his career studying diseases of the intestines. In 1932 he published an article on regional ileitis. Since then that disease has also been known as Crohn's disease.

cromoglycate — see SODIUM CROMOGLYCATE

cro·mo·lyn sodium \ˌkrō-mə-lən-\ *n* : a drug $C_{23}H_{14}Na_2O_{11}$ that inhibits the release of histamine from mast cells and is used usu. as an inhalant to prevent the onset of bronchial asthma attacks — called also *cromolyn, disodium cromoglycate, sodium cromoglycate;* see INTAL

crop \'kräp\ *n* : a pouched enlargement of the gullet of many birds that serves as a receptacle for food and for its preliminary maceration

¹cross \'krȯs\ *n*   **1** : a device composed of an upright bar traversed by a horizontal one   **2 a** : an act of crossing dissimilar individuals   **b** : a crossbred individual or kind

²cross *vt* : to cause (an animal or plant) to interbreed with one of a different kind : HYBRIDIZE ⟨the ∼*ing* of two cattle breeds⟩ ∼ *vi* : INTERBREED, HYBRIDIZE

³cross *adj* : CROSSBRED, HYBRID

cross·abil·i·ty \ˌkrȯ-sə-'bil-ət-ē\ *n, pl* **-ties** : the ability of different species or varieties to cross with each other

cross·able \'krȯ-sə-bəl\ *adj* : capable of being crossed

cross agglutination *n* : agglutination of cells of one species by serum of an animal immunized against another usu. closely related species — called also *paragglutination*

cross·bred \'krȯs-'bred\ *adj* : produced by crossbreeding : HYBRID — **cross·bred** \-ˌbred\ *n*

¹cross·breed \'krȯs-ˌbrēd, -'brēd\ *vb* **-bred** \-ˌbred, -'bred\ **-breed·ing** *vt* : HYBRIDIZE, CROSS; *esp* : to cross (two varieties or breeds) within the same species ∼ *vi* : to engage in or undergo crossing or hybridization

²cross·breed \-ˌbrēd\ *n* : HYBRID

cross·bridge \'krȯs-ˌbrij\ *n* : the globular head of a myosin molecule that projects from a myosin filament in muscle and in the sliding filament hypothesis of muscle contraction is held to attach temporarily to an adjacent actin filament and draw it into the A band of a sarcomere between the myosin filaments

crossed \'krȯst\ *adj* : forming a decussation ⟨a ∼ tract of nerve fibers⟩

crossed pyramidal tract *n* : LATERAL CORTICOSPINAL TRACT

cross–eye \'krȯ-ˌsī\ *n*   **1** : strabismus in which the eye turns inward toward the nose — called also *esotropia;* compare WALLEYE 2a   **2 cross–eyes** \-ˌsīz\ *pl* : eyes affected with cross-eye ⟨the treatment of *cross-eyes*⟩ — **cross–eyed** \-ˌsīd\ *adj*

cross–fer·tile \'krȯs-'fərt-ᵊl\ *adj* : fertile in a cross or capable of cross-fertilization

cross–fer·til·iza·tion *or Brit* **cross–fer·til·isa·tion** \-ˌfərt-ᵊl-ə-'zā-shən\ *n* : fertilization in which the gametes are produced by separate individuals or sometimes by individuals of different kinds

cross–fer·til·ize *or Brit* **cross–fer·til·ise** \-'fərt-ᵊl-ˌīz\ *vb* **-ized** *or Brit* **-ised; -iz·ing** *or Brit* **-is·ing** *vt* : to accomplish cross-fertilization of ∼ *vi* : to undergo cross-fertilization

cross–fir·ing \'krȯs-'fi(ə)r-iŋ\ *n* : a method of radiation therapy in which the rays are directed from different points to meet at the same point in the patient

cross·ing–over \ˌkrȯ-siŋ-'ō-vər\ *n* : an interchange of genes or segments between homologous chromosomes

cross–link \'krȯ-ˌsliŋk\ *n* : a crosswise connecting part (as an atom or group) that connects parallel chains in a complex chemical molecule (as a protein) — **cross–link** *vb*

cross–link·age \'krȯ-'sliŋ-kij\ *n* : the process of forming cross-links; *also* : CROSS-LINK

cross·match·ing \'krȯ-'smach-iŋ\ *or* **cross·match** \-'smach\ *n* : the testing of the compatibility of the bloods of a transfusion donor and a recipient by mixing the serum of each with the red cells of the other to determine the absence of agglutination reactions — **crossmatch** *vt*

¹cross·over \'krȯ-ˌsō-vər\ *n*   **1** : an instance or product of genetic crossing-over   **2** : a crossover interchange in an experiment

²crossover *adj* : involving or using interchange of the control group and the experimental group during the course of an experiment ⟨a double-blind ∼ study⟩

cross–re·ac·tion \ˌkrȯs-rē-'ak-shən\ *n* : reaction of one antigen with antibodies developed against another antigen — **cross–re·act** \-'akt\ *vi*

cross–re·ac·tive \-rē-'ak-tiv\ *adj* : capable of undergoing cross-reaction ⟨∼ antigens⟩ ⟨∼ antibodies⟩ — **cross–re·ac·tiv·i·ty** \-(ˌ)rē-ˌak-ˈtiv-ət-ē\ *n, pl* **-ties**

cross section *n* : a cutting or piece of something cut off at right angles to an axis; *also* : a representation of such a cutting — **cross–sec·tion·al** \ˌkrò(s)-ˈsek-shnəl, -shən-ᵊl\ *adj*

cross–ster·ile \ˈkròs-ˈ(s)ter-əl\ *adj* : mutually sterile — **cross–ste·ril·i·ty** \ˌkròs-(s)tə-ˈril-ət-ē\ *n, pl* **-ties**

cross–tol·er·ance \ˈkrò-ˈstäl(-ə)-rən(t)s\ *n* : tolerance or resistance to a drug that develops through continued use of another drug with similar pharmacological action

cro·ta·lar·ia \ˌkrō-tə-ˈlar-ē-ə, ˌkrä-\ *n* **1** *cap* : a large genus of usu. tropical and subtropical plants of the family Leguminosae with yellow flowers and inflated pods including some containing toxic alkaloids esp. in the seeds that are poisonous to farm animals and humans **2** : any plant of the genus *Crotalaria* — called also *rattlebox*

cro·ta·lar·i·o·sis \ˌkròt-ᵊl-ˌar-ē-ˈō-səs, ˌkrät-\ *n, pl* **-o·ses** \-ˌsēz\ : CROTALISM

¹cro·ta·lid \ˈkròt-ᵊl-əd, -id\ *adj* **1** : of or belonging to the family Crotalidae ⟨∼ snakes⟩ **2** : typical of a pit viper ⟨∼ venom⟩

²crotalid *n* : a crotalid snake

Cro·tal·i·dae \krō-ˈtal-ə-ˌdē\ *n pl* : a family of venomous snakes sometimes regarded as a subfamily (Crotalinae) of the family Viperidae comprising the pit vipers

cro·ta·lin \ˈkròt-ᵊl-ən, ˈkrät-\ *n* : rattlesnake venom

cro·ta·line \-ᵊl-ˌīn, -ᵊl-ən\ *adj* : CROTALID ⟨∼ snakes⟩

cro·ta·lism \-ᵊl-ˌiz-əm\ *n* : the poisoning or poisoned condition of animals caused by eating a leguminous plant (*Crotalaria sagittalis*) or other plants of the same genus in the field or as hay — called also *crotalariosis;* compare WALKABOUT DISEASE

Cro·ta·lus \-ᵊl-əs\ *n* : the type genus of the family Crotalidae that includes many of the rattlesnakes

cro·taph·i·on \krō-ˈtaf-ē-ˌän\ *n* : a point at the tip of the greater wing of the sphenoid

crotch \ˈkräch\ *n* : an angle formed by the parting of two legs, branches, or members

cro·tin \ˈkròt-ᵊn\ *n* : a mixture of poisonous proteins found in the seeds of a small Asian tree (*Croton tiglium*) related to the spurges

cro·ton \ˈkròt-ᵊn\ *n* **1** *cap* : a genus of herbs and shrubs of the spurge family **2** : an herb or shrub of the genus *Croton*: as **a** : one (*C. eluteria*) of the Bahamas yielding cascarilla bark **b** : an Asian plant (*C. tiglium*) yielding croton oil

Cro·ton bug \ˈkròt-ᵊn-\ *n* : GERMAN COCKROACH

cro·ton·ic acid \(ˌ)krō-ˌtän-ik-\ *n* : an unsaturated aliphatic acid $C_4H_6O_2$ that occurs in croton oil

croton oil \ˈkròt-ᵊn-\ *n* : a viscid acrid fixed oil from an Asian plant of the genus *Croton* (*C. tiglium*) that was formerly used as a drastic cathartic but is now used esp. in pharmacological experiments as an irritant

cro·ton·o·yl \ˈkròt-ᵊn-ə-ˌwil, -ˌwēl\ *n* : the monovalent group $CH_3CH=CHCO-$ of crotonic acid

cro·to·nyl \ˈkròt-ᵊn-ˌil, -ˌēl\ *n* **1** : CROTONOYL **2** : CROTYL

cro·tyl \ˈkròt-ᵊl, ˈkrō-ˌtil\ *n* : the butenyl group $CH_3CH=CHCH_2-$

croup \ˈkrüp\ *n* : inflammation, edema, and subsequent obstruction of the larynx, trachea, and bronchi esp. of infants and young children that is typically caused by a virus and is marked by episodes of difficult breathing and hoarse metallic cough — **croup·ous** \ˈkrü-pəs\ *adj* — **croupy** \-pē\ *adj* **croup·i·er; -est**

Crou·zon's disease \ˌkrü-ˈzänz-\ *also* **Crouzon disease** \-ˈzän-\ *n* : CROUZON SYNDROME

Crouzon syndrome *also* **Crouzon's syndrome** *n* : an inherited disorder that is controlled by an autosomal dominant gene and that is characterized by malformation of the skull due to premature ossification and closure of the sutures and by widely spaced eyes, abnormal protrusion of the eyeballs, a beaked nose, and underdevelopment of the maxilla with protrusion of the mandible — called also *craniofacial dysostosis*

Crou·zon \krü-zōᵐ\, **Octave (1874–1938),** French neurolo-

gist. In 1906 Crouzon was appointed chief of the clinic and laboratory at the Hôtel de Dieu in Paris. Two years later he joined the staff of Salpêtrière Hospital's school of nursing. In 1937 he ascended to the chairmanship of medical-social welfare at the Paris Faculty. His researches in hereditary diseases encompassed neurological disorders, cerebellar ataxia, and chronic rheumatism. He also studied familial encephalitis, hysteria, epilepsy, and post-traumatic disorders of the nervous system. His studies in familial bone diseases resulted in his original description in 1912 of craniofacial dysostosis, the disorder that now bears his name.

¹crown \ˈkraún\ *n* **1** : the topmost part of the skull or head **2** : the part of a tooth external to the gum or an artificial substitute for this

²crown *vt* : to put an artificial crown on (a tooth) ∼ *vi, in childbirth* : to appear at the vaginal opening — used of the first part (as the crown of the head) of the infant to appear ⟨an anesthetic was given when the head ∼*ed*⟩

crow's–foot \ˈkrōz-ˌfùt\ *n, pl* **crow's–feet** \-ˌfēt\ : any of the wrinkles around the outer corners of the eyes — usu. used in pl.

CrP *abbr* creatine phosphate

CRP *abbr* C-reactive protein

CRT \ˌsē-(ˌ)är-ˈtē\ *n, pl* **CRTs** *or* **CRT's** : CATHODE-RAY TUBE; *also* : a display device incorporating a cathode-ray tube

CRT *abbr* complex reaction time

CRTT *abbr* certified respiratory therapy technician

cru·ci·ate \ˈkrü-shē-ˌāt\ *adj* : shaped like a cross ⟨a ∼ bandage⟩ ⟨a ∼ incision⟩

cruciate ligament *n* : any of several more or less cross-shaped ligaments: as **a** : either of two ligaments in the knee joint which cross each other from femur to tibia: (1) : ANTERIOR CRUCIATE LIGAMENT (2) : POSTERIOR CRUCIATE LIGAMENT **b** : a complex ligament made up of the transverse ligament of the atlas and vertical fibrocartilage extending from the dens to the border of the foramen magnum

cru·ci·ble \ˈkrü-sə-bəl\ *n* : a vessel of a very refractory material (as porcelain) used for melting and calcining a substance that requires a high degree of heat

crude protein \ˈkrüd-\ *n* : the approximate amount of protein in foods that is calculated from the determined nitrogen content by multiplying by a factor (as 6.25 for many foods and 5.7 for wheat) derived from the average percentage of nitrogen in the food proteins and that may contain an appreciable error if the nitrogen is derived from nonprotein material or from a protein of unusual composition

crura *pl of* CRUS

cru·ra ce·re·bri \ˌkrù(ə)r-ə-ˈser-ə-ˌbrī, -ˈker-ə-ˌbrē\ *n pl* : CRUS 2c

crura for·ni·cis \-ˈfòr-nə-ˌsis, -ə-ˌkis\ *n pl* : CRUS 2e

cru·ral \ˈkrù(ə)r-əl\ *adj* : of or relating to the thigh or leg; *specif* : FEMORAL ⟨∼ artery⟩ ⟨∼ nerve⟩

crural arch *n* : INGUINAL LIGAMENT

crural septum *n* : a thin fascia that normally closes the femoral ring and prevents descent of abdominal viscera into the femoral canal

cruris — see TINEA CRURIS

crus \ˈkrüs, ˈkrəs\ *n, pl* **cru·ra** \ˈkrü(ə)r-ə\ **1** : the part of the hind limb between the femur or thigh and the ankle or tarsus : SHANK **2** : any of various anatomical parts likened to a leg or to a pair of legs: as **a** : either of the diverging proximal ends of the corpora cavernosa **b** : the tendinous attachments of the diaphragm to the bodies of the lumbar vertebrae forming the sides of the aortic opening — often used in pl. **c** *crura pl* : the peduncles of the cerebrum — called also *crura cerebri* **d** *crura pl* : the peduncles of the cerebellum **e**

\ə\ **abut** \ᵊ\ **kitten** \ər\ **further** \a\ **ash** \ā\ **ace** \ä\ **cot, cart** \aù\ **out** \ch\ **chin** \e\ **bet** \ē\ **easy** \g\ **go** \i\ **hit** \ī\ **ice** \j\ **job** \ŋ\ **sing** \ō\ **go** \ò\ **law** \òi\ **boy** \th\ **thin** \th̶\ **the** \ü\ **loot** \ù\ **foot** \y\ **yet** \zh\ **vision** *See also* Pronunciation Symbols page

C
D

crura pl : the posterior pillars of the fornix — called also *crura fornicis* **f** (1) : a long bony process of the incus that articulates with the stapes; *also* : a shorter one projecting from the body of the incus perpendicular to this   (2) : either of the two bony processes forming the sides of the arch of the stapes

crush syndrome \\'krəsh-\ *n* : the physical responses to severe crushing injury of muscle tissue involving esp. shock and partial or complete renal failure; *also* : the renal failure associated with such responses

crust \\'krəst\ *n* **1** : SCAB 2 **2** : an encrusting deposit of serum, cellular debris, and bacteria present over or about lesions in some skin diseases (as impetigo or eczema) — **crust** *vb*

crus·ta \\'krəs-tə\ *n, pl* **crus·tae** \-ˌtē, -ˌtī\ : the lower or ventral of the two parts into which the substantia nigra divides the cerebral peduncles

crus·ta·cea \ˌkrəs-'tā-sh(ē-)ə\ *n pl* **1** *cap* : a large class of mostly aquatic arthropods that have a chitinous or calcareous and chitinous exoskeleton, a pair of often much modified appendages on each segment, and two pairs of antennae and that include the lobsters, shrimps, crabs, wood lice, water fleas, and barnacles **2** : arthropods of the class Crustacea — **crus·ta·cean** \-shən\ *adj or n*

¹**crutch** \\'krəch\ *n* **1** : a support typically fitting under the armpit for use as an aid in walking **2** : the crotch esp. of an animal

²**crutch** *vt* : to support on crutches

cry·mo·ther·a·py \ˌkrī-mō-'ther-ə-pē\ *n, pl* **-pies** : CRYOTHERAPY

cryo·bi·ol·o·gist \ˌkrī-ō-bī-'äl-ə-jəst\ *n* : a specialist in cryobiology

cryo·bi·ol·o·gy \ˌkrī-ō-bī-'äl-ə-jē\ *n, pl* **-gies** : the study of the effects of extremely low temperature on biological systems (as cells or organisms) — **cryo·bi·o·log·i·cal** \-ˌbī-ə-'läj-i-kəl\ *adj*

cryo·cau·tery \-'kȯt-ə-rē\ *n, pl* **-ter·ies** : destruction of tissue by use of extreme cold

cryo·ex·trac·tion \-ik-'strak-shən\ *n* : extraction of a cataract through use of a cryoprobe whose refrigerated tip adheres to and freezes tissue of the lens permitting its removal

cryo·ex·trac·tor \-ik-'strak-tər, -'ek-ˌ\ *n* : a cryoprobe used for removal of cataracts

cryo·fi·brin·o·gen \-fī-'brin-ə-jən\ *n* : fibrinogen that precipitates upon cooling to 4°C and redissolves at 37°C

cryo·gen \\'krī-ə-jən\ *n* : a substance for obtaining low temperatures — called also *cryogenic*

cryo·gen·ic \ˌkrī-ə-'jen-ik\ *adj* **1 a** : of or relating to the production of very low temperatures **b** : being or relating to very low temperatures **2** : requiring or involving the use of a cryogenic temperature ⟨∼ surgery⟩ ⟨∼ arterial thrombolysis⟩ — **cryo·gen·i·cal·ly** \-i-k(ə)lē\ *adv*

cryo·gen·ics \-iks\ *n pl but sing or pl in constr* : a branch of physics that deals with the production and effects of very low temperatures

cryo·glob·u·lin \ˌkrī-ō-'gläb-yə-lən\ *n* : any of several proteins similar to gamma globulins (as in molecular weight) that precipitate usu. in the cold from blood serum esp. in pathological conditions (as multiple myeloma) and that redissolve on warming

cryo·glob·u·lin·emia *or chiefly Brit* **cryo·glob·u·lin·aemia** \-ˌgläb-yə-lə-'nē-mē-ə\ *n* : the condition of having abnormal quantities of cryoglobulins in the blood

cry·om·e·ter \krī-'äm-ət-ər\ *n* : an instrument for the measurement of low temperature

cry·on·ics \krī-'än-iks\ *n pl but usu sing in constr* : the practice of freezing the body of a person who has died from a disease in hopes of restoring life at some future time when a cure for the disease has been developed — **cry·on·ic** \-ik\ *adj*

cryo·pexy \\'krī-ə-ˌpek-sē\ *n, pl* **-pex·ies** : cryosurgery for fixation of the retina in retinal detachment or for repair of a retinal tear or hole

cryo·phil·ic \ˌkrī-ə-'fil-ik\ *adj* : thriving at low temperatures

cryo·pre·cip·i·tate \ˌkrī-ō-prə-'sip-ət-ət, -'sip-ə-ˌtāt\ *n* : a precipitate (as factor VIII) that is formed by cooling a solution (as blood plasma) — **cryo·pre·cip·i·ta·tion** \-ˌsip-ə-'tā-shən\ *n*

cryo·pres·er·va·tion \-ˌprez-ər-'vā-shən\ *n* : preservation (as of sperm or eggs) by subjection to extremely low temperatures — **cryo·pre·serve** \-pri-'zərv\ *vt* **-served; -serv·ing**

cryo·probe \\'krī-ə-ˌprōb\ *n* : a blunt chilled instrument used to freeze tissues in cryosurgery

cryo·pro·tec·tive \ˌkrī-ō-prə-'tek-tiv\ *adj* : serving to protect against the deleterious effects of subjection to freezing temperatures ⟨a ∼ agent⟩ — **cryo·pro·tec·tant** \-tənt\ *n or adj*

cryo·pro·tein \ˌkrī-ə-'prō-ˌtēn, -'prōt-ē-ən\ *n* : a protein (as cryoglobulin) in the blood that can be precipitated by cooling and redissolved by warming

cryo·scope \\'krī-ə-ˌskōp\ *n* : an instrument for determining freezing points

cry·os·co·py \krī-'äs-kə-pē\ *n, pl* **-pies** : the determination of the lowered freezing points produced in liquid by dissolved substances in order to find the molecular weights of solutes and various properties of solutions — **cryo·scop·ic** \ˌkrī-ə-'skäp-ik\ *adj*

cryo·stat \\'krī-ə-ˌstat\ *n* : an apparatus for maintaining a constant low temperature esp. below 0°C (as by means of liquid helium); *esp* : one containing a microtome for obtaining sections of frozen tissue — **cryo·stat·ic** \ˌkrī-ə-'stat-ik\ *adj*

cryo·sur·geon \ˌkrī-ō-'sər-jən\ *n* : a surgeon who is a specialist in cryosurgery

cryo·sur·gery \ˌkrī-ō-'sərj-(ə-)rē\ *n, pl* **-ger·ies** : surgery in which diseased or abnormal tissue (as a tumor or wart) is destroyed or removed by freezing (as by the use of liquid nitrogen) — **cryo·sur·gi·cal** \-ji-kəl\ *adj*

cryo·ther·a·py \-'ther-ə-pē\ *n, pl* **-pies** : the therapeutic use of cold; *esp* : CRYOSURGERY

crypt \\'kript\ *n* **1** : an anatomical pit, depression, or invagination ⟨a developing tooth in its bony ∼⟩ — see TONSILLAR CRYPT **2** : a simple tubular gland (as a crypt of Lieberkühn)

crypt·ec·to·my \krip-'tek-tə-mē\ *n, pl* **-mies** : surgical removal or destruction of a crypt

crypt·es·the·sia *or chiefly Brit* **crypt·aes·the·sia** \ˌkrip-tes-'thē-zh(ē-)ə\ *n* : CLAIRVOYANCE — **crypt·es·thet·ic** *or chiefly Brit* **crypt·aes·thet·ic** \-tes-'thet-ik, -tis-\ *adj*

cryp·tic \\'krip-tik\ *adj* **1** : serving to conceal ⟨∼ coloration in animals⟩ **2** : not recognized ⟨a ∼ infection⟩ ⟨∼ cases of lead poisoning⟩ — **cryp·ti·cal·ly** \-ti-k(ə-)lē\ *adv*

cryp·ti·tis \krip-'tīt-əs\ *n* : inflammation of a crypt (as an anal crypt)

cryp·to·bi·o·sis \ˌkrip-(ˌ)tō-ˌbī-'ō-səs, -(ˌ)bē-\ *n, pl* **-o·ses** \-ˌsēz\ : the reversible cessation of metabolism under extreme environmental conditions (as low temperature)

cryp·to·coc·co·sis \ˌkrip-tə-(ˌ)kä-'kō-səs\ *n, pl* **-co·ses** \-(ˌ)sēz\ : an infectious disease that is caused by a fungus of the genus *Cryptococcus* (*C. neoformans*) and is characterized by the production of nodular lesions or abscesses in subcutaneous tissues, joints, and esp. the lungs, brain, and meninges and often by pneumonia or meningitis — called also *torulosis*

cryp·to·coc·cus \-'käk-əs\ *n* **1** *cap* : a genus of budding imperfect fungi that resemble yeasts and include a number of saprophytes and a few serious pathogens **2** *pl* **-coc·ci** \-'käk-ˌ(s)ī, -ˌ(s)ē\ : any fungus of the genus *Cryptococcus* — **cryp·to·coc·cal** \-'käk-əl\ *adj*

cryp·to·crys·tal·line \ˌkrip-tō-'kris-tə-lən\ *adj* : having a crystalline structure so fine that no distinct particles are recognizable under the microscope

crypt of Lie·ber·kühn \-'lē-bər-ˌk(y)ün, -ˌkēn\ *n* : any of the tubular glands of the intestinal mucous membrane — called also *gland of Lieberkühn, intestinal gland, Lieberkühn's gland*

Lie·ber·kühn \\'lē-bər-ˌkēn\, **Johannes Nathanael (1711–1756),** German anatomist. In 1745 Lieberkühn described for the first time the structure and function of the glands, now known as the crypts of Lieberkühn, attached to the villi of the intestines. He went on to explore the circulatory

C

D

vessels of animals, devising special microscopes to view in greater detail the intricacies of fluid motion within the living animal. One of the instruments which he devised was a microscope with a silver speculum that used sunlight and projected the image on a screen.

crypt of Mor·ga·gni \-mȯr-'gän-yē\ *n* : any of the pouched cavities of the rectal mucosa immediately above the anorectal junction, intervening between vertical folds of the rectal mucosa

Morgagni, Giovanni Battista (1682–1771), Italian anatomist and pathologist. Often called the "father of pathology," Morgagni is considered to be the founder of modern pathological anatomy. He was the first to demonstrate the necessity for basing diagnosis, prognosis, and treatment on knowledge of anatomical conditions. In 1761 he published *De Sedibus et Causis Morborum* (The Seats and Causes of Diseases), a monumental work that established him as one of the greatest figures in the history of medicine.

cryp·to·gam \'krip-tə-ˌgam\ *n* : a plant or plantlike organism (as a fern, moss, alga, or fungus) reproducing by spores and not producing flowers or seed — **cryp·to·gam·ic** \ˌkrip-tə-'gam-ik\ *or* **cryp·tog·a·mous** \krip-'täg-ə-məs\ *adj*

Cryp·to·ga·mia \ˌkrip-tə-'gam-ē-ə, -'gäm-\ *n, in former classifications* : a class or subkingdom including all cryptogams — compare PHANEROGAMIA

cryp·to·ge·net·ic \ˌkrip-tō-jə-'net-ik\ *adj* : CRYPTOGENIC

cryp·to·gen·ic \ˌkrip-tə-'jen-ik\ *adj* : of obscure or unknown origin ⟨∼ epilepsy⟩ — compare PHANEROGENIC

cryp·tom·ne·sia \ˌkrip-ˌtäm-'nē-zhə\ *n* : the appearance in consciousness of memory images which are not recognized as such but which appear as original creations — **cryp·tom·ne·sic** \-'nē-zik, -sik\ *adj*

cryp·to·pine \'krip-tə-ˌpēn, -pən\ *n* : a colorless crystalline alkaloid $C_{21}H_{23}NO_5$ obtained from opium and plants of the genus *Corydalis*

[1]crypt·or·chid \krip-'tȯr-kəd\ *adj* : affected with cryptorchidism — compare MONORCHID

[2]cryptorchid *n* : a cryptorchid individual

crypt·or·chi·dism \-kə-ˌdiz-əm\ *also* **crypt·or·chism** \-ˌkiz-əm\ *n* : a condition in which one or both testes fail to descend normally — compare MONORCHIDISM

cryp·to·spo·rid·i·o·sis \ˌkrip-tō-spȯr-ˌid-ē-'ō-səs\ *n, pl* **-o·ses** \-ˌsēz\ : infection with or disease caused by cryptosporidia

cryp·to·spo·rid·i·um \ˌkrip-tō-spȯr-'id-ē-əm\ *n* **1** *cap* : a genus of protozoans of the order Coccidia that are parasitic in the gut of many vertebrates including humans and that sometimes cause diarrhea esp. in individuals who are immunocompromised (as in AIDS) **2** *pl* **-rid·ia** \-ē-ə\ : any protozoan of the genus *Cryptosporidium*

cryp·to·xan·thin \ˌkrip-tə-'zan(t)-thən\ *n* : a red crystalline carotenoid alcohol $C_{40}H_{55}OH$ that occurs in many plants (as yellow corn and papaya), in blood serum, and in some animal products (as butter and egg yolk) and that is a precursor of vitamin A

cryp·to·xan·thol \-'zan-ˌthȯl\ *n* : CRYPTOXANTHIN

cryp·to·zo·ite \-'zō-ˌīt\ *n* : a malaria parasite that develops in tissue cells and gives rise to the forms that invade blood cells — compare METACRYPTOZOITE

cryp·to·zy·gous \ˌkrip-tə-'zī-gəs, (')krip-'täz-ə-gəs\ *adj* : having a wide skull and a narrow face so that the zygomatic arches are concealed when the skull is viewed from above — **cryp·to·zy·gy** \'krip-tə-ˌzī-gē, krip-'täz-ə-gē, -jē\ *n, pl* **-gies**

cryst *abbr* crystalline; crystallized

crys·tal \'kris-t°l\ *n* **1** : a body that is formed by the solidification of a chemical element, a compound, or a mixture and has a regularly repeating internal arrangement of its atoms and often external plane faces **2** : ICE 2; *broadly* : methamphetamine in any form when used illicitly — **crystal** *adj*

crys·tal·lin \'kris-tə-lən\ *n* : either of two globulins in the crystalline lens

crystallina — see MILIARIA CRYSTALLINA

crys·tal·line \'kris-tə-lən *also* -ˌlīn, -ˌlēn\ *adj* **1** : composed of or resembling crystals **2 a** : formed by crystallization : having regular arrangement of the atoms in a space lattice

— see AMORPHOUS 2 **b** : having the internal structure though not necessarily the external form of a crystal ⟨granite is only ∼, while quartz crystal is perfectly crystallized⟩ — **crys·tal·lin·i·ty** \ˌkris-tə-'lin-ət-ē\ *n, pl* **-ties**

crystalline lens *n* : the lens of the eye

crystalline veratrine *n* : CEVADINE

crys·tal·li·za·tion *also Brit* **crys·tal·li·sa·tion** \ˌkris-tə-lə-'zā-shən\ *n* : the process of crystallizing; *also* : a form resulting from this

crys·tal·lize *also* **crys·tal·ize** *also Brit* **crys·tal·lise** *or* **crys·tal·ise** \'kris-tə-ˌlīz\ *vb* **-lized** *also* **-ized** *also Brit* **-lised** *or* **-ised**; **-liz·ing** *also* **-iz·ing** *also Brit* **-lis·ing** *or* **-is·ing** *vt* : to cause to form crystals or assume crystalline form; *esp* : to cause to form perfect or large crystals ∼ *vi* : to become crystallized — often used with *out* ⟨the solid *crystallized* out⟩ — **crys·tal·liz·able** \-ˌlī-zə-bəl\ *adj*

crys·tal·lo·gram \'kris-tə-lō-ˌgram, kri-'stal-ə-\ *n* : a photographic record of crystal structure obtained by the use of X-rays

crys·tal·log·ra·phy \ˌkris-tə-'läg-rə-fē\ *n, pl* **-phies** : a science that deals with the forms and structures of crystals — see X-RAY CRYSTALLOGRAPHY — **crys·tal·log·ra·pher** \-fər\ *n* — **crys·tal·lo·graph·ic** \-lə-'graf-ik\ *adj* — **crys·tal·lo·graph·i·cal·ly** \-ik(ə-)lē\ *adv*

crys·tal·loid \'kris-tə-ˌlȯid\ *n* **1** : a substance that forms a true solution and is capable of being crystallized **2** : a particle of protein that has the properties of crystal and is found esp. in oily seeds — **crystalloid** *or* **crys·tal·loi·dal** \ˌkris-tə-'lȯid-°l\ *adj*

crys·tal·lu·ria \ˌkris-tə-'l(y)ùr-ē-ə\ *n* : the presence of crystals in the urine indicating renal irritation (as that caused by sulfa drugs)

crystal meth *n* : ICE 2 — called also *crystal methamphetamine*

crystal violet *n* : a triphenylmethane dye found in gentian violet — called also *methylrosaniline chloride*

cs *abbr* **1** case **2** cesarean section **3** conditioned stimulus **4** consciousness **5** corticosteroid **6** current strength

Cs *symbol* cesium

CS \ˌsē-'es\ *n* : a potent lacrimatory and nausea-producing gas $C_{10}H_5ClN_2$ used in riot control and chemical warfare

C–sec·tion \'sē-ˌsek-shən\ *n* : CESAREAN SECTION

CSF \ˌsē-(ˌ)es-'ef\ *n* : COLONY-STIMULATING FACTOR

CSF *abbr* cerebrospinal fluid

CSM *abbr* cerebrospinal meningitis

CT *abbr* **1** circulation time **2** coated tablet **3** compressed tablet **4** computed tomography; computerized tomography

CTa *abbr* catamenia

CTC *abbr* chlortetracycline

CTD *abbr* cumulative trauma disorder

Cteno·ce·phal·i·des \ˌten-ō-sə-'fal-ə-ˌdēz\ *n* : a genus of fleas of the family Pulicidae including the dog flea (*C. canis*) and cat flea (*C. felis*)

CTL \ˌsē-(ˌ)tē-'el\ *n* : CYTOTOXIC T LYMPHOCYTE

ctr *abbr* center

CTS *abbr* carpal tunnel syndrome

CT scan \(')sē-'tē-\ *n* : CAT SCAN

CT scanner *n* : CAT SCANNER

CT scanning *n* : CAT SCANNING

cu *abbr* cubic

Cu *symbol* copper

CU *abbr* clinical unit

cu·beb \'kyü-ˌbeb\ *n* : the dried unripe berry of a tropical shrub (*Piper cubeba*) of the pepper family that was formerly used medicinally when powdered for its effect on mucous membranes esp. as a urinary antiseptic and to treat chronic bronchitis

[1]cu·bi·tal \'kyü-bət-°l\ *adj* : of or relating to a cubitus ⟨∼ nerve⟩

²**cubital** *n* : CUBITUS

cubiti — see BICEPS FLEXOR CUBITI

cu·bi·tus \'kyü-bət-əs\ *n, pl* **cu·bi·ti** \-bə-ˌtī\ **1** : FOREARM, ANTEBRACHIUM **2** : ULNA

cubitus valgus *n* : a condition of the arm in which the forearm deviates away from the midline of the body when extended

cubitus varus *n* : a condition of the arm in which the forearm deviates toward the midline of the body when extended

¹**cu·boid** \'kyü-ˌbȯid\ *adj* **1** : relating to or being the cuboid ⟨the ~ bone⟩ **2** : shaped approximately like a cube

²**cuboid** *n* : the outermost bone in the distal row of tarsal bones of the foot that supports the fourth and fifth metatarsals

cu·boi·dal \kyü-'bȯid-ᵊl\ *adj* **1** : CUBOID 2 **2** : composed of nearly cubical elements ⟨~ epithelium⟩

CUC *abbr* chronic ulcerative colitis

cu·cum·ber \'kyü-(ˌ)kəm-bər\ *n* : the fruit of a vine (*Cucumis sativus*) of the gourd family that is cultivated as a garden vegetable and that has diuretic seeds; *also* : this vine

cud \'kəd, 'ku̇d\ *n* : food brought up into the mouth by a ruminating animal from its first stomach to be chewed again

cud·bear \'kəd-ˌba(ə)r, -ˌbe(ə)r\ *n* : a reddish coloring matter from lichens that is sometimes considered a form of archil and is used in coloring pharmaceutical preparations

> **Gor·don** \'gȯrd-ᵊn\, **Cuthbert**, British chemist. Sometime in the 18th century Gordon first patented the dye now known as cudbear, the name being derived from his first name.

cue \'kyü\ *n* : a minor stimulus acting as an indication of the nature of the perceived object or situation ⟨foreshortened lines in the picture are ~s to depth perception⟩

cuff \'kəf\ *n* **1** : an inflatable band that is wrapped around an extremity to control the flow of blood through the part when recording blood pressure with a sphygmomanometer **2** : an anatomical structure shaped like a cuff; *esp* : ROTATOR CUFF ⟨repair of complete shoulder ~ avulsion —*Physicians' Current Procedural Terminology*⟩

cuffed \'kəft\ *adj* : provided with an often inflatable encircling part ⟨used a ~ endotracheal tube to provide an air supply while preventing aspiration of foreign material⟩

cui·rass \kwi-'ras, kyü-\ *n* **1** : a plaster cast for the trunk and neck **2** : a respirator that covers the chest or the chest and abdomen and provides artificial respiration by means of an electric pump

cul–de–sac \'kəl-di-ˌsak, 'ku̇l-; ˌkəl-di-', ˌku̇l-\ *n, pl* **culs–de–sac** \'kəl(z)-, 'ku̇l(z)-, ˌkəl(z)-, ˌku̇l(z)-\ *also* **cul–de–sacs** \-ˌsaks, -'saks\ **1** : a blind diverticulum or pouch; *also* : the closed end of such a pouch **2** : POUCH OF DOUGLAS

cul–de–sac of Douglas *n* : POUCH OF DOUGLAS

cul·do·cen·te·sis \ˌkəl-dō-ˌsen-'tē-səs, ˌku̇l-\ *n, pl* **-te·ses** \-ˌsēz\ : removal of material from the pouch of Douglas by means of puncture of the vaginal wall

cul·dos·co·py \ˌkəl-'däs-kə-pē, ˌku̇l-\ *n, pl* **-pies** : a technique for endoscopic visualization and minor operative procedures on the female pelvic organs in which the instrument is introduced through a puncture in the wall of the pouch of Douglas — **cul·do·scop·ic** \ˌkəl-də-'skäp-ik, ˌku̇l-\ *adj*

cul·dot·o·my \ˌkəl-'dät-ə-mē, ˌku̇l-\ *n, pl* **-mies** : surgical incision of the pouch of Douglas

cu·lex \'kyü-ˌleks\ *n* **1** *cap* : a large cosmopolitan genus of mosquitoes that includes the common house mosquito (*C. pipiens*) of Europe and No. America, a widespread tropical mosquito (*C. quinquefasciatus* syn. *C. fatigans*) which transmits some filarial worms parasitic in humans, and other mosquitoes which have been implicated as vectors of virus encephalitides and possibly of other human and animal diseases **2** : a mosquito of the genus *Culex* — **cu·li·cine** \'kyü-lə-ˌsīn\ *adj or n*

Cu·lic·i·dae \kyü-'lis-ə-ˌdē\ *n pl* : a family of slender long-legged dipteran flies having the body and appendages partly covered with hairs or scales and the mouthparts adapted for piercing and sucking, comprising the mosquitoes, and having active aquatic larvae known as wrigglers

cu·li·cide \'kyü-lə-ˌsīd\ *n* : an insecticide that destroys mosquitoes

Cu·li·coi·des \ˌkyü-lə-'kȯid-ˌēz\ *n* : a genus of bloodsucking midges (family Ceratopogonidae) of which some are intermediate hosts of filarial parasites

cul·men \'kəl-mən\ *n* : a lobe of the cerebellum lying in the superior vermis just in front of the primary fissure

cult *abbr* culture

cul·ti·vate \'kəl-tə-ˌvāt\ *vt* **-vat·ed; -vat·ing** : CULTURE 1 ⟨viruses *cultivated* in brain tissue⟩

cul·ti·va·tion \ˌkəl-tə-'vā-shən\ *n* : CULTURE 2

cultural anthropology *n* : anthropology that deals with human culture esp. with respect to social structure, language, law, politics, religion, magic, art, and technology — compare PHYSICAL ANTHROPOLOGY — **cultural anthropologist** *n*

¹**cul·ture** \'kəl-chər\ *n* **1 a** : the integrated pattern of human behavior that includes thought, speech, action, and artifacts and depends upon the human capacity for learning and transmitting knowledge to succeeding generations **b** : the customary beliefs, social forms, and material traits of a racial, religious, or social group **2 a** : the act or process of growing living material (as bacteria or viruses) in prepared nutrient media **b** : a product of cultivation in nutrient media — **cul·tur·al** \'kəlch-(ə-)rəl\ *adj* — **cul·tur·al·ly** \-rə-lē\ *adv*

²**culture** *vt* **cul·tured; cul·tur·ing** \'kəlch-(ə-)riŋ\ **1** : to grow (as microorganisms or tissues) in a prepared medium **2** : to start a culture from ⟨~ soil⟩; *also* : to make a culture of ⟨~ milk⟩

culture shock *n* : a sense of confusion and uncertainty sometimes with feelings of anxiety that may affect people exposed to an alien culture or environment without adequate preparation

Cul·ver's physic \'kəl-vərz-\ *n* : CULVER'S ROOT

> **Culver**, American physician. Culver's root or physic is commonly supposed to have been named after a Dr. Culver, who presumably used the herb for medicinal purposes. The doctor has never been specifically identified. All that is known for certain is that by 1716 Culver's root was common enough for Cotton Mather to mention it in his writings, noting that it was "Famous for the cure of Consumptions."

Culver's root *n* **1** : a tall perennial herb (*Veronicastrum virginicum*) common in eastern No. America **2** : the rhizome and roots of Culver's root used as a cathartic — called also *leptandra*

cu·mu·la·tive \'kyü-myə-lət-iv, -ˌlāt-\ *adj* : increasing in effect by successive doses (as of a drug or poison) ⟨~ poisoning by organochlorine pesticides —Jack Clincy⟩ — **cu·mu·la·tive·ly** *adv*

cumulative trauma disorder *n* : REPETITIVE STRAIN INJURY — abbr. *CTD*

cu·mu·lus \'kyü-myə-ləs\ *n, pl* **cu·mu·li** \-ˌlī, -ˌlē\ : the projecting mass of granulosa cells that bears the developing ovum in a graafian follicle — called also *discus proligerus*

cumulus ooph·o·rus \-ō-'äf-ə-rəs\ *n* : CUMULUS

cu·ne·ate \'kyü-nē-ˌāt, -ət\ *adj* : narrowly triangular with the acute angle toward the base

cuneate fasciculus *n, pl* **cuneate fasciculi** : FASCICULUS CUNEATUS

cuneate lobe *n* : CUNEUS

cuneate nucleus *n* : NUCLEUS CUNEATUS

cuneatus — see FASCICULUS CUNEATUS, NUCLEUS CUNEATUS

cunei *pl of* CUNEUS

¹**cu·ne·i·form** \kyü-'nē-ə-ˌfȯrm, 'kyü-n(ē-)ə-\ *adj* **1** : of, relating to, or being a cuneiform bone or cartilage **2** *of a human skull* : wedge-shaped as viewed from above

²**cuneiform** *n* : a cuneiform bone or cartilage

cuneiform bone *n* **1** : any of three small bones of the tarsus situated between the navicular and the first three metatarsals: **a** : one on the medial side of the foot that is just proximal to the first metatarsal bone and is the largest of the three bones — called also *medial cuneiform, medial cunei-form bone* **b** : one that is situated between the other two bones proximal to the second metatarsal bone and is the smallest of the three bones — called also *intermediate cuneiform, intermediate cuneiform bone* **c** : one that is situated proximal to the third metatarsal bone and that lies between the intermediate cuneiform bone and the cuboid — called also *lateral cuneiform, lateral cuneiform bone* **2** : TRIQUE-TRAL BONE

cuneiform cartilage *n* : either of a pair of rods of yellow elastic cartilage of which each lies on one side of the larynx in an aryepiglottic fold just below the arytenoid cartilage — called also *cartilage of Wrisberg*

cu·ne·us \'kyü-nē-əs\ *n, pl* **cu·nei** \-nē-ˌī\ : a convolution of the mesial surface of the occipital lobe of the brain above the calcarine sulcus that forms a part of the visual area

cu·nic·u·lus \kyü-'nik-(y)ə-ləs\ *n, pl* **cu·nic·u·li** \-ˌlī, -ˌlē\ : the burrow of an itch mite in the skin

cun·ni·lin·gus \ˌkən-i-'liŋ-gəs\ *also* **cun·ni·linc·tus** \-'liŋ(k)-təs\ *n* : oral stimulation of the vulva or clitoris — **cun·ni·lin·guism** \-'liŋ-gə-ˌwiz-əm\ *n*

cun·nus \'kən-əs\ *n, pl* **cun·ni** \-ˌnī, -(ˌ)nē\ : the female external genitals : VULVA

¹**cup** \'kəp\ *n* **1** : a usu. open bowl-shaped drinking vessel often having a handle and a stem and base and sometimes a lid **2** : a drinking vessel and its contents : the beverage or food contained in a cup ⟨a second ~ of coffee⟩ **3** : something resembling a cup ⟨invagination of the blastula to form a multilayered cellular ~⟩: as **a** (1) : an athletic supporter reinforced for providing extra protection to the wearer in certain strenuous sports (as boxing, hockey, or football) (2) : either of the two parts of a brassiere that are shaped like and fit over the breasts **b** : a small bell-shaped glass formerly used in cupping **c** : a cap of metal shaped like the femoral head and used in plastic reconstruction of the hip joint

²**cup** *vb* **cupped; cup·ping** *vt* : to treat by cupping ~ *vi* : to undergo or perform cupping

cup·ping *n* **1** : a technique formerly employed for drawing blood to the surface of the body by application of a glass vessel from which air had been evacuated by heat to form a partial vacuum **2** : a concave depression in a body organ; *also* : the formation of such a depression

cu·pre·ine \'k(y)ü-prē-ˌēn, -prē-ən\ *n* : a crystalline alkaloid $C_{19}H_{22}N_2O_2$ that occurs esp. in cinchona bark and is closely related to quinine

cu·pric \'k(y)ü-prik\ *adj* : of, relating to, or containing copper with a valence of two

cupric sulfate *n* : COPPER SULFATE

cu·pu·la \'kyü-p(y)ə-lə\ *n, pl* **cu·pu·lae** \-ˌlē\ **1** : the bony apex of the cochlea **2** : the peak of the pleural sac covering the apex of the lung

cur *abbr* **1** curative **2** current

cur·able \'kyur-ə-bəl\ *adj* : capable of being cured — **cur·abil·i·ty** *n, pl* **-ties**

cu·ra·re *also* **cu·ra·ri** \k(y)ù-'rär-ē\ *n* : a dried aqueous extract esp. of a vine (as *Strychnos toxifera* of the family Loganiaceae or *Chondodendron tomentosum* of the family Menispermaceae) that produces muscle relaxation and is used in arrow poisons by So. American Indians — compare TUBOCURARINE

cu·ra·ri·form \k(y)ü-'rär-ə-ˌfòrm\ *adj* : producing or characterized by the muscular relaxation typical of curare ⟨~ drugs⟩

cu·ra·rine \-'rär-ən, -ˌēn\ *n* : any of several alkaloids from curare

cu·ra·rize *or Brit* **cu·ra·rise** \-'rär-ˌīz\ *vt* **-rized** *or Brit* **-rised; -riz·ing** *or Brit* **-ris·ing** : to treat with curare — **cu·ra·ri·za·tion** *or Brit* **cu·ra·ri·sa·tion** \-ˌrär-ə-'zā-shən\ *n*

cu·ra·tive \'kyur-ət-iv\ *adj* : relating to or used in the cure of diseases — **curative** *n* — **cu·ra·tive·ly** *adv*

curb \'kərb\ *n* : a swelling on the back of the hind leg of a horse just behind the lowest part of the hock joint that is due to strain or rupture of the ligament and generally causes lameness

cur·cu·ma \'kər-kyə-mə\ *n* : TURMERIC 2

curd \'kərd\ *n* : the thick casein-rich part of coagulated milk — **curdy** \-ē\ *adj*

¹**cure** \'kyù(ə)r\ *n* **1** : recovery from a disease ⟨his ~ was complete⟩; *also* : remission of signs or symptoms of a disease esp. during a prolonged period of observation ⟨a clinical ~⟩ ⟨5-year ~ of cancer⟩ — compare ARREST **2** : a drug, treatment, regimen, or other agency that cures a disease ⟨quinine is a ~ for malaria⟩ **3** : a course or period of treatment; *esp* : one designed to interrupt an addiction or compulsive habit or to improve general health ⟨take a ~ for alcoholism⟩ ⟨an annual ~ at a spa⟩ **4** : SPA **5** *maritime law* : the medical care awarded a person in the merchant marine who is injured or taken sick in the course of duty

²**cure** *vb* **cured; cur·ing** *vt* : HEAL : **a** : to restore to health, soundness, or normality ⟨*curing* her patients rapidly by new procedures⟩ **b** : to bring about recovery from ⟨antibiotics ~ many formerly intractable infections⟩ ~ *vi* **1** : to effect a cure ⟨careful living ~*s* more often than it kills⟩ **2** : to take a cure (as in a sanatorium or at a spa) — **cur·er** *n*

cu·ret·tage \ˌkyur-ə-'täzh\ *n* : a surgical scraping or cleaning by means of a curette

¹**cu·rette** *also* **cu·ret** \kyù-'ret\ *n* : a surgical instrument that has a scoop, loop, or ring at its tip and is used in performing curettage

²**curette** *also* **curet** *vt* **cu·rett·ed; cu·rett·ing** : to perform curettage on — **cu·rette·ment** \kyü-'ret-mənt\ *n*

cu·rie \'kyu(ə)r-(ˌ)ē, kyù-'rē\ *n* **1** : a unit quantity of any radioactive nuclide in which 3.7×10^{10} disintegrations occur per second **2** : a unit of radioactivity equal to 3.7×10^{10} disintegrations per second

Cu·rie \kūē-rē\, **Pierre (1859–1906)** and **Marie Słodowska (1867–1934),** French chemists and physicists. The Curies were two of the most important and influential figures in modern physics. Their major joint contributions include the discovery, with Henri Becquerel, of radioactivity, and the discovery and isolation of radium and polonium in 1898. In 1910 the first International Congress of Radiology honored the husband and wife team by establishing *curie* as a term for a unit of measurement for radioactivity. The element curium was named in honor of the Curies in 1944 by its discoverers, a team of scientists at the University of Chicago. The Curies were awarded the Nobel Prize for Physics in 1903, and Marie Curie was awarded the Nobel Prize for Chemistry in 1911.

cu·rine \'kyù-ˌrēn\ *n* : a crystalline alkaloid $C_{36}H_{38}N_2O_6$ that is structurally very similar to tubocurarine and is obtained from the same tropical vine : levorotatory bebeerine

cu·ri·um \'kyùr-ē-əm\ *n* : a metallic radioactive element produced artificially — symbol *Cm*; see ELEMENT table

Cur·ling's ulcer \'kər-liŋz-\ *n* : acute gastroduodenal ulceration following severe skin burns

Curling, Thomas Blizard (1811–1888), British surgeon. Curling is noteworthy for writing two historically important descriptions. In 1850 he published what is thought to be the first accurate clinical picture of cretinism. In 1849 he had examined two cases in which there was a complete absence of thyroid tissue. In 1842 he published his finding that acute ulceration of the duodenum could result from severe skin burns. In 1866 in a follow-up report he described finding burn cases with acute perforated ulcers.

cur·rent \'kər-ənt, 'kə-rənt\ *n* **1** : the part of a fluid body (as air or water) moving continuously in a certain direction **2** : a flow of electric charge; *also* : the rate of such flow

cur·va·ture \'kər-və-ˌchù(ə)r, -chər, -ˌt(y)ù(ə)r\ *n* **1** : an abnormal curving (as of the spine) — see KYPHOSIS, SCOLIOSIS **2** : a curved surface of an organ (as the stomach) — see GREATER CURVATURE, LESSER CURVATURE

\ə\ abut \ˈ\ kitten \ər\ further \a\ ash \ā\ ace \ä\ cot, cart \aù\ out \ch\ chin \e\ bet \ē\ easy \g\ go \i\ hit \ī\ ice \j\ job \ŋ\ sing \ō\ go \ò\ law \òi\ boy \th\ thin \t̲h̲\ the \ü\ loot \ù\ foot \y\ yet \zh\ vision *See also* Pronunciation Symbols page

cush·ing·oid \\'kush-iŋ-ˌöid\ *adj, often cap* : resembling Cushing's disease esp. in facies or habitus ⟨developed ∼ features after receiving ACTH⟩

Cush·ing's disease \ˌkush-iŋz-\ *n* : Cushing's syndrome esp. when caused by excessive production of ACTH by the pituitary gland

Cushing, Harvey Williams (1869–1939), American neurosurgeon. Cushing first gained a reputation by publishing an important work on the pituitary gland in 1912. In 1930 he gave the first description of the condition named in his honor. Throughout his career he wrote numerous monographs on the surgery of the brain and worked on the classification of brain tumors. He also contributed to studies of blood pressure in surgery and developed the method of operating with local anesthesia.

Cushing's syndrome *n* : an abnormal bodily condition that is caused by excess corticosteroids and esp. cortisol usu. from adrenal or pituitary hyperfunction and that is characterized by a variety of signs and symptoms including esp. a change in appearance marked by moon facies with plethora, obesity, easy bruising, slow wound healing, and hypokalemia — called also *adrenogenital syndrome*

cush·ion \\'kush-ən\ *n* **1** : a bodily part resembling a pad **2** : a medical procedure or drug that eases discomfort without necessarily affecting the basic condition of the patient

cusp \\'kəsp\ *n* **1** : a point on the grinding surface of a tooth **2** : a fold or flap of a cardiac valve — **cus·pal** \\'kəs-pəl\ *adj*

cus·pid \\'kəs-pəd\ *n* : a canine tooth

cus·pi·date \\'kəs-pə-ˌdāt\ *adj* : having a cusp : terminating in a point ⟨∼ molars⟩

cus·to·di·al \ˌkəs-'tōd-ē-əl\ *adj* **1** : relating to, providing, or being protective care or services for basic needs ⟨nursing and ∼ care⟩ **2** : having sole or primary custody of a child ⟨the ∼ parent⟩

¹cut \\'kət\ *vb* **cut; cut·ting** *vt* **1 a** : to penetrate with or as if with an edged instrument **b** : to cut or operate on in surgery: as **(1)** : to subject (a domestic animal) to castration **(2)** : to perform lithotomy on **c** : to experience the emergence of (a tooth) through the gum **2** : to subject to trimming or paring ⟨∼ one's nails⟩ ∼ *vi* **1** : to function as or in the manner of an edged tool ⟨a knife that ∼s well⟩ **2** : to cut in surgery : OPERATE

²cut *n* **1** : a product of cutting: as **a** : an opening made with an edged instrument **b** : a wound made by something sharp **2** : a stroke or blow with the edge of a sharp implement (as a knife)

cu·ta·ne·ous \kyù-'tā-nē-əs\ *adj* : of, relating to, or affecting the skin ⟨a ∼ infection⟩ ⟨four ∼ nerves arise from the cervical plexus⟩ — **cu·ta·ne·ous·ly** *adv*

cutaneous T–cell lymphoma *n* : any of several lymphomas (as mycosis fungoides or Sezary syndrome) that are marked by clusters of malignant helper T cells in the epidermis causing skin lesions and eruptions which typically progress to tumors and may spread to lymph nodes and internal organs

cut·down \\'kət-ˌdaùn\ *n* : incision of a superficial blood vessel (as a vein) to facilitate insertion of a catheter (as for administration of fluids)

Cu·te·re·bra \ˌkyüt-ə-'rē-brə, kyù-'ter-ə-brə\ *n* : the type genus of the family Cuterebridae comprising large usu. dark-colored botflies with larvae that form tumors under the skin of rodents, cats, and other small mammals

Cu·te·reb·ri·dae \ˌkyüt-ə-'reb-rə-ˌdē\ *n pl* : a family of chiefly New World botflies that occur under the skin or sometimes in the throat or nasal sinuses of various mammals and that include a botfly (*Dermatobia hominis*) that normally parasitizes humans — see CUTEREBRA — **cu·te·re·brid** \ˌkyüt-ə-'rē-brəd, kyù-'ter-ə-brəd\ *n*

cu·te·re·brine \ˌkyüt-ə-'rē-brən, (')kyù-'ter-ə-brən, -ˌbrīn\ *adj* : of or relating to the genus *Cuterebra* or the family Cuterebridae

cutes anserinae *pl of* CUTIS ANSERINA

cutes verae *pl of* CUTIS VERA

cu·ti·cle \\'kyüt-i-kəl\ *n* **1** : an outer covering layer: as **a** : the outermost layer of integument composed of epidermis

b : the outermost membranous layer of a hair consisting of cornified epithelial cells **2** : dead or horny epidermis (as that surrounding the base and sides of a fingernail or toenail) — **cu·tic·u·lar** \kyù-'tik-yə-lər\ *adj*

cu·tic·u·lar·iza·tion *or Brit* **cu·tic·u·lar·isa·tion** \kyù-ˌtik-yə-lə-rə-'zā-shən\ *n* : the state of being or process of becoming cuticularized ⟨gradual ∼ of the vaginal mucosa⟩

cu·tic·u·lar·ized *or Brit* **cu·tic·u·lar·ised** \-'tik-yə-lə-ˌrīzd\ *adj* : covered with or altered into cuticle ⟨∼ cells⟩

cu·ti·re·ac·tion \ˌkyüt-i-rē-'ak-shən, 'kyüt-ə-rē-\ *n* : a local inflammatory reaction of the skin that occurs in certain infectious diseases following the application to or injection into the skin of a preparation of organisms producing the disease

cu·tis \\'kyüt-əs\ *n, pl* **cu·tes** \\'kyü-ˌtēz\ *or* **cu·tis·es** : DERMIS

cutis an·se·ri·na \ˌ-an(t)-sə-'rī-nə\ *n, pl* **cutes an·se·ri·nae** \-'rī-ˌnē\ : GOOSE BUMPS

cutis ve·ra \-'vi(ə)r-ə\ *n, pl* **cutes ve·rae** \-'vi(ə)r-ˌē\ : DERMIS

cu·vette \kyü-'vet\ *n* : a small often transparent laboratory vessel (as a tube)

Cu·vie·ri·an vein \(')kyü-'vi(ə)r-ē-ən-, ˌkyü-vē-'i(ə)r-\ *n* : CARDINAL VEIN

Cu·vier \\'k(y)ü-vē-ˌā, kūē-vyā\, **Georges** (*orig.* **Jean–Léopold–Nicolas–Frédéric) (1769–1832),** French naturalist. One of the great French naturalists of the early 19th century, Cuvier is credited with essentially founding the studies of comparative anatomy and paleontology. In 1817 he published his magnum opus, *Le Règne animal,* his classification of the animal kingdom in which he divided all animals into vertebrate, molluscan, articulate, and radiate types. Around 1800 in one of his lessons on comparative anatomy he described the common cardinal veins that now honor his name.

CV *abbr* cardiovascular

CVA *abbr* cerebrovascular accident

CVD *abbr* cardiovascular disease

CVP *abbr* central venous pressure

CVR *abbr* **1** cardiovascular renal **2** cardiovascular respiratory **3** cerebrovascular resistance

CVS *abbr* chorionic villus sampling

CW *abbr* crutch walking

Cy *abbr* cyanogen

cy·an·ic \sī-'an-ik\ *adj* : relating to or containing cyanogen

cy·a·nide \\'sī-ə-ˌnīd, -nəd\ *n* : any of several compounds (as potassium cyanide) that contain the radical CN having a chemical valence of one, react with and inactivate respiratory enzymes, and are rapidly lethal producing drowsiness, tachycardia, coma, and finally death

cy·a·no·ac·ry·late \ˌsī-ə-nō-'ak-rə-ˌlāt, sī-ˌan-ō-\ *n* : any of several liquid acrylate monomers that readily polymerize as anions and are used as adhesives in industry and in medicine on living tissue to close wounds in surgery

cy·a·no·bac·te·ri·um \-bak-'tir-ē-əm\ *n, pl* **-ria** \-ē-ə\ : any of a major group (Cyanobacteria) of photosynthetic bacteria that produce molecular oxygen and use water as an electron-donating substrate in photosynthesis — called also *blue-green alga*

cy·a·no·co·bal·a·min \-kō-'bal-ə-mən\ *also* **cy·a·no·co·bal·a·mine** \-ˌmēn\ *n* : VITAMIN B_{12}

cy·ano·gen \sī-'an-ə-jən\ *n* **1** : a monovalent group –CN present in cyanides **2** : a colorless flammable poisonous gas $(CN)_2$

cy·a·no·ge·net·ic \ˌsī-ə-nō-jə-'net-ik, sī-ˌan-ō-\ *or* **cy·a·no·gen·ic** \-'jen-ik\ *adj* : capable of producing cyanide (as hydrogen cyanide) ⟨a ∼ plant that is dangerous to livestock⟩ — **cy·a·no·gen·e·sis** \-'jen-ə-səs\ *n, pl* **-e·ses** \-ˌsēz\

cy·a·no·met·he·mo·glo·bin \ˌsī-ə-nō-(')met-'hē-mə-ˌglō-bən\ *or* **cy·an·met·he·mo·glo·bin** \ˌsī-ˌan-(')met-, ˌsī-ən-\ *or chiefly Brit* **cy·a·no·met·hae·mo·glo·bin** *or* **cy·an·met·hae·mo·glo·bin** *n* : a bright red crystalline compound formed by the action of hydrogen cyanide on methemoglobin in the cold or on oxyhemoglobin at body temperature

cy·ano·phile \sī-'an-ə-ˌfīl\ *also* **cy·ano·phil** \-ˌfil\ *n* : a cyanophilous tissue element

C

D

cy·a·noph·i·lous \ˌsī-ə-ˈnäf-ə-ləs\ *also* **cy·a·no·phil·ic** \ˌsī-ə-nō-ˈfil-ik\ *adj* : having an affinity for blue or green dyes ⟨∼ tissues⟩

cy·a·nosed \ˈsī-ə-ˌnōst, -ˌnōzd\ *adj* : affected with cyanosis

cy·a·no·sis \ˌsī-ə-ˈnō-səs\ *n, pl* **-no·ses** \-ˌsēz\ : a bluish or purplish discoloration (as of skin) due to deficient oxygenation of the blood — **cy·a·not·ic** \-ˈnät-ik\ *adj*

cy·an·urate \ˌsī-ə-ˈn(y)ù(ə)r-ˌāt, -ˈn(y)ùr-ət\ *n* : a salt or ester of cyanuric acid; *esp* : one that is used to disinfect water

cy·an·uric acid \ˌsī-ə-ˌn(y)ùr-ik-\ *n* : a crystalline weak acid $C_3H_3N_3O_3$ used esp. in swimming pools to protect the available chlorine from dissipation by sunlight

cy·ber·net·i·cian \ˌsī-(ˌ)bər-nə-ˈtish-ən\ *n* : a specialist in cybernetics

cy·ber·net·i·cist \ˌsī-bər-ˈnet-ə-səst\ *n* : CYBERNETICIAN

cy·ber·net·ics \ˌsī-bər-ˈnet-iks\ *n pl but sing or pl in constr* : the science of communication and control theory that is concerned esp. with the comparative study of automatic control systems (as the nervous system and brain and mechanical-electrical communication systems) — **cy·ber·net·ic** \-ik\ *also* **cy·ber·net·i·cal** \-i-kəl\ *adj* — **cy·ber·net·i·cal·ly** \-i-k(ə-)lē\ *adv*

cy·borg \ˈsī-ˌbò(ə)rg\ *n* : a bionic human

cy·ca·sin \ˈsī-kə-sən\ *n* : a glucoside $C_8H_{16}N_2O_7$ that occurs in cycads and results in toxic and carcinogenic effects when introduced into mammals

cy·cla·mate \ˈsī-klə-ˌmāt, -mət\ *n* : an artificially prepared salt of sodium or calcium used esp. formerly as a sweetener but now largely discontinued because of the possibly harmful effects of its metabolic breakdown product cyclohexylamine

cy·cla·min \ˈsī-klə-mən, ˈsik-lə-\ *n* : a white amorphous saponin constituting the active principle of the root of a cyclamen (*Cyclamen europaeum*) and formerly used as an emetic and purgative

cy·clan·de·late \ˌsī-ˈklan-dᵊl-ˌāt\ *n* : an antispasmodic drug $C_{17}H_{24}O_3$ used esp. as a vasodilator in the treatment of diseased arteries

cy·clase \ˈsī-ˌklās, -ˌklāz\ *n* : an enzyme (as adenyl cyclase) that catalyzes cyclization of a compound

cy·claz·o·cine \sī-ˈklaz-ə-ˌsēn, -sən\ *n* : an analgesic drug $C_{18}H_{25}NO$ that inhibits the effect of morphine and related addictive drugs and is used in the treatment of drug addiction

¹cy·cle \ˈsī-kəl\ *n* **1** : a recurring series of events: as **a** (1) : a series of stages through which an organism tends to pass once in a fixed order ⟨the common ∼ of birth, growth, senescence and death —T. C. Schneirla & Gerard Piel⟩; *also* : a series of stages through which a population of organisms tends to pass more or less in synchrony ⟨the mosquito-hatching ∼⟩ — see LIFE CYCLE (2) : a series of physiological, biochemical, or psychological stages that recur in the same individual — see CARDIAC CYCLE, MENSTRUAL CYCLE; KREBS CYCLE **b** : one complete performance of a vibration, electric oscillation, current alternation, or other periodic process **c** : a series of ecological stages through which a substance tends to pass and which usu. but not always leads back to the starting point ⟨the ∼ of nitrogen in the living world⟩ **2** : RING 2 — **cy·clic** \ˈsī-klik *also* ˈsik-lik\ *or* **cy·cli·cal** \ˈsī-kli-kəl, ˈsik-li-\ *adj* — **cy·cli·cal·ly** \-k(ə-)lē\ *also* **cy·clic·ly** \ˈsī-kli-klē, ˈsik-li-\ *adv*

²cycle *vi* **cycled; cycling** : to undergo the estrous cycle ⟨the mare has begun *cycling*⟩

cy·clec·to·my \sī-ˈklek-tə-mē, sik-ˈlek-\ *n, pl* **-mies** : surgical removal of part of the ciliary muscle or body

cyclic adenosine monophosphate *n* : CYCLIC AMP

cyclic AMP *n* : a cyclic mononucleotide of adenosine that is formed from ATP and is responsible for the intracellular mediation of hormonal effects on various cellular processes (as lipid metabolism, membrane transport, and cell proliferation) — abbr. *cAMP;* called also *adenosine 3',5'-monophosphate*

cyclic GMP \-ˌjē-ˌem-ˈpē\ *n* : a cyclic mononucleotide of guanosine that acts similarly to cyclic AMP as a second mes-

senger in response to hormones — called also *cyclic guanosine monophosphate, guanosine 3',5'-monophosphate*

cyclic guanosine monophosphate *n* : CYCLIC GMP

cy·clic·i·ty \sī-ˈklis-ət-ē, sik-ˈlis-\ *n, pl* **-ties** : the quality or state of being cyclic ⟨estrous ∼⟩

cyclicly *var of* CYCLICALLY

cy·clin \ˈsī-klən, ˈsik-lən\ *n* : any of a group of proteins active in controlling the cell cycle and in initiating DNA synthesis

cy·cli·tis \sə-ˈklīt-əs, sī-\ *n* : inflammation of the ciliary body

cy·cli·tol \ˈsī-klə-ˌtòl, ˈsik-lə-ˌtōl\ *n* : an alicyclic polyhydroxy compound (as inositol)

cy·cli·za·tion *or Brit* **cy·cli·sa·tion** \ˌsīk-(ə-)lə-ˈzā-shən, ˌsik-\ *n* : formation of one or more rings in a chemical compound

cy·clize *or Brit* **cy·clise** \ˈsīk-(ə-)ˌlīz, ˈsik-\ *vb* **cy·clized** *or Brit* **cy·clised; cy·cliz·ing** *or Brit* **cy·clis·ing** *vt* : to subject to cyclization ∼ *vi* : to undergo cyclization

cy·cli·zine \ˈsīk-lə-ˌzēn\ *n* : an antiemetic drug used esp. in the form of its hydrochloride $C_{18}H_{22}N_2$·HCl in the treatment of motion sickness — see MAREZINE

cy·clo·bar·bi·tal \ˌsī-klō-ˈbär-bə-ˌtòl, ˌsik-lō-\ *n* : a white crystalline compound $C_{12}H_{16}N_2O_3$ used as a sedative and hypnotic

cy·clo·ben·za·prine \-ˈben-zə-ˌprēn, -prən\ *n* : a skeletal muscle relaxant administered in the form of its hydrochloride $C_{20}H_{21}N$·HCl to relieve muscle spasms and pain

cy·clo·di·al·y·sis \-dī-ˈal-ə-səs\ *n, pl* **-y·ses** \-ˌsēz\ : surgical detachment of the ciliary body from the sclera to reduce tension in the eyeball in some cases of glaucoma

cy·clo·dia·ther·my \-ˈdī-ə-ˌthər-mē\ *n, pl* **-mies** : partial or complete destruction of the ciliary body by diathermy to relieve some conditions (as glaucoma) characterized by increased tension within the eyeball

cy·clo·di·ene \-ˈdī-ˌēn, -dī-ˈ\ *n* : an organic insecticide (as aldrin, dieldrin, or chlordane) with a chlorinated methylene group forming a bridge across a 6-membered carbon ring

Cy·clo·gyl \ˈsī-klō-ˌjil\ *trademark* — used for a preparation of the hydrochloride of cyclopentolate

cy·clo·hex·ane \ˌsī-klō-ˈhek-ˌsān, ˌsik-lō-\ *n* : a pungent saturated cyclic hydrocarbon C_6H_{12} found in petroleum or made synthetically and used chiefly as a solvent and in organic synthesis

cy·clo·hex·i·mide \-ˈhek-sə-ˌmīd, -məd\ *n* : an agricultural fungicide $C_{15}H_{23}NO_4$ that is obtained from a soil bacterium of the genus *Streptomyces* (*S. griseus*)

cy·clo·hex·yl·a·mine \-hek-ˈsil-ə-ˌmēn\ *n* : a colorless liquid amine $C_6H_{11}NH_2$ of cyclohexane that is believed to be harmful as a metabolic breakdown product of cyclamate

¹cy·cloid \ˈsī-ˌklòid\ *n* : a cycloid individual

²cycloid *adj* : relating to, having, or being a personality characterized by alternating high and low moods — compare CYCLOTHYMIC

cy·clo·oxy·gen·ase \ˌsī-klō-ˈäk-si-jə-ˌnās, -äk-ˈsij-ə-, -ˌnāz\ *n* : an enzyme that catalyzes the conversion of arachidonic acid to prostaglandins, that is inactivated by aspirin and other NSAIDs, and that has two isoforms of which one is involved in the cascade of events producing the pain and inflammation of arthritis and the other is not — see COX-1, COX-2

cy·clo·pen·to·late \ˌsī-klō-ˈpen-tə-ˌlāt, ˌsik-lō-\ *n* : an anticholinergic drug used esp. in the form of its hydrochloride $C_{17}H_{25}NO_3$·HCl to dilate the pupil of the eye for ophthalmologic examination — see CYCLOGYL

cyclopes *pl of* CYCLOPS

cy·clo·pho·ria \-ˈfōr-ē-ə, -ˈfòr-\ *n* : a form of heterophoria in which the vertical axis of the eye rotates to the right or left due to weakness of the oblique muscles — **cy·clo·phor·ic** \-ˈfòr-ik, -ˈfär-\ *adj*

\ə\ **abut** \ᵊ\ **kitten** \ər\ **further** \a\ **ash** \ā\ **ace** \ä\ **cot, cart** \aů\ **out** \ch\ **chin** \e\ **bet** \ē\ **easy** \g\ **go** \i\ **hit** \ī\ **ice** \j\ **job** \ŋ\ **sing** \ō\ **go** \ò\ **law** \òi\ **boy** \th\ **thin** \t̲h̲\ **the** \ü\ **loot** \ů\ **foot** \y\ **yet** \zh\ **vision** *See also* Pronunciation Symbols page

cy·clo·phos·pha·mide \-ˈfäs-fə-ˌmīd\ *n* : an immunosuppressive and antineoplastic drug $C_7H_{15}Cl_2N_2O_2P$ used to treat lymphomas and some leukemias — see CYTOXAN

cy·clo·phre·nia \-ˈfrē-nē-ə\ *n* : BIPOLAR DISORDER

Cy·clo·phyl·lid·ea \-fə-ˈlid-ē-ə\ *n pl* : an order of the subclass Cestoda that consists of tapeworms with four suckers on the scolex and the vitellaria condensed into a mass adjacent to the ovary and that includes most of the medically and economically important tapeworms of the higher vertebrates — **cy·clo·phyl·lid·e·an** \-ē-ən\ *adj or n*

cy·clo·pia \sī-ˈklō-pē-ə\ *also* **cy·clo·py** \ˈsī-klə-pē\ *n, pl* **-pias** *also* **-pies** : a developmental anomaly characterized by the presence of a single median eye

cy·clo·ple·gia \ˌsī-klō-ˈplē-j(ē-)ə, ˌsik-lō-\ *n* : paralysis of the ciliary muscle of the eye

¹**cy·clo·ple·gic** \-ˈplē-jik\ *adj* : producing, involving, or characterized by cycloplegia ⟨~ agents⟩ ⟨~ refraction⟩

²**cycloplegic** *n* : a cycloplegic agent

cy·clo·pro·pane \-ˈprō-ˌpān\ *n* : a flammable gaseous saturated cyclic hydrocarbon C_3H_6 sometimes used as a general anesthetic

cy·clops \ˈsī-ˌkläps\ *n* **1** *pl* **cy·clo·pes** \sī-ˈklō-(ˌ)pēz\ : an individual or fetus abnormal in having a single eye or the usual two orbits fused **2** *cap* : a genus of minute free-swimming copepods that have a large median eye, a pear-shaped body tapering posteriorly, and long antennules used in swimming, that are widely distributed and abundant in fresh waters, that are important elements in certain aquatic food chains, and that directly affect humans as intermediate hosts of certain parasitic worms — see GUINEA WORM **3** *pl* **cyclops** : a copepod water flea of the genus *Cyclops*

cyclopy *var of* CYCLOPIA

cy·clo·ser·ine \ˌsī-klō-ˈse(ə)r-ˌēn, ˌsik-lō-\ *n* : a broad‑spectrum antibiotic $C_3H_6N_2O_2$ produced by an actinomycete of the genus *Streptomyces* (*S. orchidaceus*) and used esp. in the treatment of tuberculosis

cy·clo·sis \sī-ˈklō-səs\ *n, pl* **-ses** \-ˌsēz\ : the streaming of protoplasm within a cell

Cy·clo·spora \ˌsī-klō-ˈspòr-ə\ *n* : a genus of coccidian protozoans that produce an oocyst containing two sporocysts with each sporocyst containing two sporozoites and that include one (*C. cayetanensis*) causing diarrhea in humans

cy·clo·spo·ri·a·sis \-spə-ˈrī-ə-səs\ *n, pl* **-a·ses** \-ˌsēz\ : infection with or disease caused by a coccidian protozoan of the genus *Cyclospora*

cy·clo·spor·in \ˌsī-klə-ˈspòr-ᵊn\ *n* : any of a group of polypeptides obtained as metabolites from various imperfect fungi (as *Tolypocladium inflatum* syn. *Trichoderma polysporum*); *esp* : CYCLOSPORINE

cyclosporin A *n* : CYCLOSPORINE

cy·clo·spor·ine \ˌsī-klə-ˈspòr-ᵊn, -ˌēn\ *n* : a cyclosporin $C_{62}H_{111}N_{11}O_{12}$ used as an immunosuppressive drug esp. to prevent rejection of transplanted organs

Cy·clo·sto·ma·ta \ˌsī-klō-ˈstō-mət-ə, ˌsik-lō-, -ˈstäm-ət-ə\ *n pl* : a class or other taxon of primitive vertebrates that have a large jawless sucking mouth, no limbs or paired fins, a wholly cartilaginous skeleton with persistent notochord, and 6 to 14 pairs of gill pouches and that include the lampreys and the hagfishes — compare CHONDRICHTHYES

cy·clo·stome \ˈsī-klə-ˌstōm, ˈsik-lə-\ *n* : any vertebrate of the major taxonomic group Cyclostomata

Cy·clos·to·mi \sī-ˈkläs-tə-ˌmī\ *n pl, syn of* CYCLOSTOMATA

cy·clo·thyme \ˈsī-klə-ˌthīm\ *n* : a cyclothymic individual

cy·clo·thy·mia \ˌsī-klə-ˈthī-mē-ə\ *n* : a cyclothymic mood disorder

¹**cy·clo·thy·mic** \-ˈthī-mik\ *adj* : relating to, having, or being a mood disorder characterized by alternating short episodes of depression and hypomania in a form less severe than that of bipolar disorder — compare CYCLOID

²**cyclothymic** *n* : a cyclothymic individual

cy·clo·tome \ˈsī-klə-ˌtōm\ *n* : a knife used in cyclotomy

cy·clot·o·my \sī-ˈklät-ə-mē\ *n, pl* **-mies** : incision or division of the ciliary body

cy·clo·tron \ˈsī-klə-ˌträn\ *n* : an accelerator in which charged particles (as protons, deuterons, or ions) are propelled by an alternating electric field in a constant magnetic field

cy·clo·tro·pia \ˌsī-klə-ˈtrō-pē-ə\ *n* : squint in which the eye rolls outward or inward around its front-to-back axis : rotational strabismus

Cy·do·nia \sī-ˈdō-nē-ə\ *n* : a monotypic genus of small Asian trees (family Rosaceae) that includes the quince (*C. oblonga*)

cy·e·sis \sī-ˈē-səs\ *n, pl* **cy·e·ses** \-ˌsēz\ : PREGNANCY ⟨full‑term abdominal ~ —*Jour. Amer. Med. Assoc.*⟩

cyl *abbr* cylinder; cylindrical

¹**cyl·in·droid** \ˈsil-ən-ˌdrȯid, sə-ˈlin-\ *n* : a spurious or mucous urinary cast that resembles a hyaline cast but has one tapered, stringy, twisted end

²**cylindroid** *adj* : shaped somewhat like a cylinder ⟨the esophagus is more or less ~ —J. T. Lucker⟩

cyl·in·dro·ma \ˌsil-ən-ˈdrō-mə\ *n, pl* **-mas** *also* **-ma·ta** \-mət-ə\ : a tumor characterized by cylindrical masses consisting of epithelial cells and hyalinized stroma: **a** : a malignant tumor esp. of the respiratory tract or salivary glands **b** : a benign tumor of the skin and esp. the scalp

cyl·in·dru·ria \ˌsil-ən-ˈdrúr-ē-ə\ *n* : the presence of casts in the urine

cy·ma·rin \ˈsī-mə-rən, ˈsim-ə- *also* sə-ˈmar-ən\ *n* : a cardiac glycoside $C_{30}H_{44}O_9$ occurring esp. in plants of the genus *Apocynum*

cy·ma·rose \ˈsī-mə-(ˌ)rōs, ˈsim-ə- *also* -(ˌ)rōz\ *n* : a sugar $C_7H_{14}O_4$ occurring as a constituent of some cardiac glycosides (as cymarin)

cym·ba \ˈsim-bə\ *n, pl* **cym·bae** \-(ˌ)bē, -ˌbī\ : the upper part of the concha of the ear

cym·bo·ce·phal·ic \ˌsim-bō-sə-ˈfal-ik\ *adj, of a head or skull* : having a prolonged receding forehead and a projecting occiput — **cym·bo·ceph·a·ly** \-ˈsef-ə-lē\ *n, pl* **-lies**

cy·no·mol·gus monkey \ˌsī-nə-ˌmäl-gəs-\ *n* : a macaque (*Macaca fascicularis* syn. *M. cynomolgus*) of southeastern Asia, Borneo, and the Philippines that is often used in medical research

cy·no·pho·bia \-ˈfō-bē-ə\ *n* : a morbid fear of dogs

Cy·pri·ni·dae \sə-ˈprin-ə-ˌdē, -ˈprīn-\ *n pl* : a large family (order Ostariophysi) of freshwater fishes that includes the carps, barbels, tenches, breams, goldfishes, chubs, dace, shiners, and most of the freshwater minnows — **cyp·ri·nid** \ˈsip-rə-nəd\ *n or adj*

cy·pro·hep·ta·dine \ˌsī-prō-ˈhep-tə-ˌdēn\ *n* : a drug $C_{21}H_{21}N$ that acts antagonistically to histamine and serotonin and is used esp. in the treatment of asthma

cy·prot·er·one \sī-ˈprät-ə-ˌrōn\ *n* : a synthetic steroid used in the form of its acetate $C_{24}H_{29}ClO_4$ to inhibit androgenic secretions (as testosterone)

cyr·tom·e·ter \sər-ˈtäm-ət-ər\ *n* : an instrument used for delineating or measuring the dimensions of curved surfaces esp. of the chest and head

Cys *abbr* cysteine; cysteinyl

cyst \ˈsist\ *n* **1** : a closed sac having a distinct membrane and developing abnormally in a body cavity or structure **2** : a body resembling a cyst: as **a** : a capsule formed about a minute organism going into a resting or spore stage; *also* : this capsule with its contents **b** : a resistant cover about a parasite produced by the parasite or the host — compare HYDATID 2a

cyst·ad·e·no·ma \ˌsis-ˌtad-ᵊn-ˈō-mə\ *n, pl* **-mas** *also* **-ma·ta** \-mət-ə\ : an adenoma marked by a cystic structure — **cyst·ad·e·no·ma·tous** \-mət-əs\ *adj*

cys·ta·mine \ˈsis-tə-ˌmēn\ *n* : a cystine derivative $C_4H_{12}N_2S_2$

cys·ta·thi·o·nine \ˌsis-tə-ˈthī-ə-ˌnēn\ *n* : a sulfur-containing amino acid $C_7H_{14}N_2O_4S$ formed as an intermediate in the conversion of methionine to cysteine

cys·te·amine \sis-ˈtē-ə-mən\ *n* : a cysteine derivative used in the form of its bitartrate $C_2H_7NS·C_4H_6O_6$ to treat cystinosis and esp. formerly as an antidote for acetaminophen overdose

cys·tec·to·my \sis-ˈtek-tə-mē\ *n, pl* **-mies** **1** : the surgical excision of a cyst ⟨ovarian ~⟩ **2** : the removal of all or a portion of the urinary bladder

cys·te·ic acid \'sis-tē-ik-\ *n* : a crystalline amino acid $C_3H_7NO_5S$ formed by oxidation of cysteine or cystine and yielding taurine on decarboxylation

cys·teine \'sis-tə-ˌēn\ *n* : a sulfur-containing amino acid $C_3H_7NO_2S$ occurring in many proteins and glutathione and readily oxidizable to cystine — abbr. *Cys*

cys·tei·nyl \'sis-tē-ˌnil, sis-'tē-ə-\ *n* : the amino acid radical or residue $HSCH_2CH(NH_2)CO-$ of cysteine — abbr. *Cys*

cys·tic \'sis-tik\ *adj* **1** : relating to, composed of, or containing cysts ⟨~ tissue⟩ ⟨a ~ tumor⟩ **2** : of or relating to the urinary bladder or the gallbladder **3** : enclosed in a cyst ⟨a ~ worm larva⟩

cystica — see OSTEITIS FIBROSA CYSTICA, OSTEITIS FIBROSA CYSTICA GENERALISTA

cystic duct *n* : the duct from the gallbladder that unites with the hepatic duct to form the common bile duct

cys·ti·cer·ci·a·sis \ˌsis-tə-sər-'sī-ə-səs\ *n, pl* **-a·ses** \-ˌsēz\ : CYSTICERCOSIS

cys·ti·cer·coid \-'sər-ˌkȯid\ *n* : a tapeworm larva having an invaginated scolex and solid hind part

cys·ti·cer·co·sis \-(ˌ)sər-'kō-səs\ *n, pl* **-co·ses** \-ˌsēz\ : infestation with or disease caused by cysticerci

cys·ti·cer·cus \-'sər-kəs\ *n, pl* **-cer·ci** \-'sər-ˌsī, -ˌkī\ : a tapeworm larva that consists of a fluid-filled sac containing an invaginated scolex, is situated in the tissues of an intermediate host, and is capable of developing into an adult tapeworm when eaten by a suitable definitive host — called also *bladder worm, measle* — **cys·ti·cer·cal** \-'sər-kəl\ *adj*

cystic fibrosis *n* : a hereditary disease prevalent esp. in Caucasian populations that appears usu. in early childhood, is inherited as an autosomal recessive monogenic trait, involves functional disorder of the exocrine glands, and is marked esp. by faulty digestion due to a deficiency of pancreatic enzymes, by difficulty in breathing due to mucus accumulation in airways, and by excessive loss of salt in the sweat — called also *fibrocystic disease of the pancreas, mucoviscidosis*

cys·ti·cid·al \ˌsis-tə-'sīd-ᵊl\ *adj* : killing or tending to kill an encysted stage of an organism ⟨a ~ agent such as chlorine⟩

cys·tig·er·ous \(')sis-'tij-(ə-)rəs\ *adj* : containing or producing cysts ⟨~ tissue⟩

cys·tine \'sis-ˌtēn\ *n* : an amino acid $C_6H_{12}N_2O_4S_2$ that is a dimer of cysteine, is widespread in proteins (as keratins), and is a major metabolic sulfur source

cys·ti·no·sis \ˌsis-tə-'nō-səs\ *n, pl* **-no·ses** \-ˌsēz\ : a recessive autosomally inherited disease characterized esp. by cystinuria and deposits of cystine throughout the body — **cys·ti·not·ic** \-'nät-ik\ *adj*

cys·tin·uria \ˌsis-tə-'n(y)ùr-ē-ə\ *n* : a metabolic defect characterized by excretion of excessive amounts of cystine in the urine and sometimes by the formation of stones in the urinary tract and inherited as an autosomal recessive trait — **cys·tin·uric** \-'n(y)ùr-ik\ *adj*

cys·ti·tis \sis-'tīt-əs\ *n, pl* **cys·tit·i·des** \-'tit-ə-ˌdēz\ : inflammation of the urinary bladder — **cys·tit·ic** \(')sis-'tit-ik\ *adj*

cys·to·cele \'sis-tə-ˌsēl\ *n* : hernia of a bladder and esp. the urinary bladder : vesical hernia

cys·to·cer·cous \ˌsis-tə-'sər-kəs\ *adj, of a cercaria* : having a space in the tail into which the body can be retracted

cys·to·gas·tros·to·my \ˌsis-tō-(ˌ)gas-'träs-tə-mē\ *n, pl* **-mies** : creation of a surgical opening between the stomach and a nearby cyst for drainage

cys·to·gram \'sis-tə-ˌgram\ *n* : a radiograph made by cystography

cys·tog·ra·phy \sis-'täg-rə-fē\ *n, pl* **-phies** : X-ray photography of the urinary bladder after injection of a contrast medium — **cys·to·graph·ic** \-tə-'graf-ik\ *adj*

¹cys·toid \'sis-ˌtȯid\ *adj* : resembling a bladder

²cystoid *n* : a cystoid structure; *specif* : a mass resembling a cyst but lacking a membrane — called also *pseudocyst*

cys·to·je·ju·nos·to·my \ˌsis-tō-ji-jü-'näs-tə-mē\ *n, pl* **-mies** : surgical creation of a passage from the jejunum to a nearby cyst for drainage

cys·to·lith \'sis-tə-ˌlith\ *n* : a urinary calculus — **cys·to·lith·ic** \ˌsis-tə-'lith-ik\ *adj*

cys·to·li·thi·a·sis \ˌsis-tō-lith-'ī-ə-səs\ *n, pl* **-a·ses** \-ˌsēz\ : the presence of calculi in the urinary bladder

cys·to·li·thot·o·my \-lith-'ät-ə-mē\ *n, pl* **-mies** : surgical removal of a calculus from the urinary bladder

cys·to·ma \sis-'tō-mə\ *n, pl* **-mas** *also* **-ma·ta** \-mət-ə\ : a tumor containing cysts — **cys·to·ma·tous** \sis-'täm-ət-əs, -'tōm-\ *adj*

cys·tom·e·ter \sis-'täm-ət-ər\ *n* : an instrument designed to measure pressure within the urinary bladder in relation to its capacity — **cys·to·met·ric** \ˌsis-tə-'me-trik\ *adj* — **cys·tom·e·try** \sis-'täm-ə-trē\ *n, pl* **-tries**

cys·to·met·ro·gram \ˌsis-tə-'me-trə-ˌgram, -'mē-\ *n* : a graphic recording of a cystometric measurement

cys·to·me·trog·ra·phy \-mə-'träg-rə-fē\ *n, pl* **-phies** : the process of making a cystometrogram

cys·to·plas·ty \'sis-tə-ˌplas-tē\ *n, pl* **-ties** : plastic surgery on the urinary bladder

cys·to·py·eli·tis \ˌsis-tə-ˌpī-ə-'līt-əs\ *n* : inflammation of the urinary bladder and of the pelvis of one or both kidneys

cys·to·py·elog·ra·phy \-ˌpī-ə-'läg-rə-fē\ *n, pl* **-phies** : radiography of the urinary bladder, the ureter, and the renal pelvis after injection of these organs with a contrast medium

cys·to·py·elo·ne·phri·tis \-ˌpī-(ə-)lō-ni-'frīt-əs\ *n, pl* **-ne·phrit·i·des** \-'frit-ə-ˌdēz\ *also* **-ne·phri·tis·es** \-'frīt-ə-səz\ : inflammation of the urinary bladder and of the cortex and pelvis of one or both kidneys

cys·tor·rha·phy \sis-'tōr-ə-fē, -'tȯr-\ *n, pl* **-phies** : suture of a wound, injury, or rupture in the urinary bladder

cys·to·sar·co·ma phyl·lodes \ˌsis-tō-sär-ˌkō-mə-'fī-ˌlōdz\ *n* : a slow-growing tumor of the breast that resembles a fibroadenoma

¹cys·to·scope \'sis-tə-ˌskōp\ *n* : a rigid endoscope for inspecting and passing instruments into the urethra and bladder — **cys·to·scop·ic** \ˌsis-tə-'skäp-ik\ *adj* — **cys·tos·co·pist** \sis-'täs-kə-pəst\ *n*

²cystoscope *vt* **-scoped; -scop·ing** : to examine (as a patient) with a cystoscope

cys·tos·co·py \sis-'täs-kə-pē\ *n, pl* **-pies** : the use of a cystoscope to examine the bladder

cys·tos·to·my \sis-'täs-tə-mē\ *n, pl* **-mies** : formation of an opening into the urinary bladder by surgical incision

cys·to·tome \'sis-tə-ˌtōm\ *n* **1** : an instrument used for cystotomy **2** : an instrument used in opening the capsule of the lens in cataract operations

cys·tot·o·my \sis-'tät-ə-mē\ *n, pl* **-mies** : surgical incision of the urinary bladder

cys·to·ure·ter·itis \ˌsis-tō-ˌyùr-ət-ə-'rīt-əs\ *n* : combined inflammation of the urinary bladder and ureters

cys·to·ure·thro·cele \ˌsis-tō-yù-'rē-thrə-ˌsēl\ *n* : herniation of the neck of the female bladder and associated urethra into the vagina

cys·to·ure·thro·gram \-yù-'rē-thrə-ˌgram\ *n* : an X-ray photograph of the urinary bladder and urethra made after injection of these organs with a contrast medium

cys·to·ure·throg·ra·phy \-ˌyùr-i-'thräg-rə-fē\ *n, pl* **-phies** : radiography for the purpose of preparing a cystourethrogram — **cys·to·ure·thro·graph·ic** \-yù-ˌrē-thrə-'graf-ik\ *adj*

cys·to·ure·thro·scope \ˌsis-tō-yù-'rē-thrə-ˌskōp\ *n* : an endoscope used for the visual examination of the posterior urethra and bladder — **cys·to·ure·thros·co·py** \-ˌyùr-i-'thräs-kə-pē\ *n, pl* **-pies**

cyst·ous \'sis-təs\ *adj* : CYSTIC

cyt·ar·a·bine \sīt-'ar-ə-ˌbēn\ *n* : CYTOSINE ARABINOSIDE

cy·tase \'sīt-ˌās, -ˌāz\ *n* : any of several enzymes found in the seeds of various plants (as cereals) that have the power of making soluble the material of cell walls by hydrolyzing mannan, galactan, xylan, and araban

cyt·as·ter \'sīt-ˌas-tər\ *n* : ASTER

\ə\ abut \ᵊ\ kitten \ər\ further \a\ ash \ā\ ace \ä\ cot, cart \aù\ out \ch\ chin \e\ bet \ē\ easy \g\ go \i\ hit \ī\ ice \j\ job \ŋ\ sing \ō\ go \ȯ\ law \ȯi\ boy \th\ thin \th\ the \ü\ loot \ù\ foot \y\ yet \zh\ vision *See also* Pronunciation Symbols page

cy·ti·dine \\'sit-ə-ˌdēn, 'sīt-\\ *n* : a nucleoside containing cytosine

cy·ti·dyl·ic acid \\ˌsit-ə-ˌdil-ik-, ˌsīt-\\ *n* : a nucleotide containing cytosine

cyt·i·sine \\'sit-ə-ˌsēn, -sən\\ *n* : a bitter crystalline very poisonous alkaloid $C_{11}H_{14}N_2O$ found in many plants of the family Leguminosae and formerly used as a cathartic and diuretic — called also *sophorine*

cy·to·ar·chi·tec·ton·ics \\ˌsīt-ō-ˌär-kə-(ˌ)tek-'tän-iks\\ *n pl but sing or pl in constr* : CYTOARCHITECTURE — **cy·to·ar·chi·tec·ton·ic** \\-ik\\ *adj*

cy·to·ar·chi·tec·ture \\ˌsīt-ō-'är-kə-ˌtek-chər\\ *n* : the cellular makeup of a bodily tissue or structure — **cy·to·ar·chi·tec·tur·al** \\ˌär-kə-'tek-chə-rəl, -shrəl\\ *adj* — **cy·to·ar·chi·tec·tur·al·ly** \\-ē\\ *adv*

cy·to·blast \\'sīt-ə-ˌblast\\ *n* : NUCLEUS 1

cy·to·cha·la·sin \\ˌsīt-ō-kə-'lā-sən\\ *n* : any of a group of metabolites isolated from fungi (esp. *Helminthosporium dematioideum*) that inhibit various cell processes

cy·to·chem·is·try \\-'kem-ə-strē\\ *n, pl* **-tries** 1 : microscopical biochemistry 2 : the chemistry of cells — **cy·to·chem·i·cal** \\-'kem-i-kəl\\ *adj* — **cy·to·chem·i·cal·ly** \\-i-k(ə-)lē\\ *adv* — **cy·to·chem·ist** \\-'kem-əst\\ *n*

cy·to·chrome \\'sīt-ə-ˌkrōm\\ *n* : any of several intracellular hemoprotein respiratory pigments that are enzymes functioning in electron transport as carriers of electrons

cytochrome c *n, often italicized 3d c* : the most abundant and stable of the cytochromes

cytochrome oxidase *n* : an iron-porphyrin enzyme important in cellular respiration because of its ability to catalyze the oxidation of reduced cytochrome c in the presence of oxygen

cy·to·cid·al \\ˌsīt-ə-'sīd-ᵊl\\ *adj* : killing or tending to kill individual cells ⟨∼ RNA viruses⟩

cy·to·clas·tic \\ˌsīt-ə-'klas-tik\\ *adj* : tending to destroy cells

cy·to·di·ag·no·sis \\ˌsīt-ō-ˌdī-ig-'nō-səs, -əg-\\ *n, pl* **-no·ses** \\-ˌsēz\\ : diagnosis based upon the examination of cells found in the tissues or fluids of the body — **cy·to·di·ag·nos·tic** \\-'näs-tik\\ *adj*

cy·to·di·er·e·sis \\ˌsīt-ō-dī-'er-ə-səs\\ *n, pl* **-e·ses** \\-ˌsēz\\ : CYTOKINESIS

cy·to·dif·fer·en·ti·a·tion \\ˌsīt-ō-ˌdif-ə-ˌren-chē-'ā-shən\\ *n* : the development of specialized cells (as muscle, blood, or nerve cells) from undifferentiated precursors

cy·to·gene \\'sīt-ə-ˌjēn\\ *n* : a self-replicating cytoplasmic gene or determinant (as those of certain plant plastids) — compare PLASMAGENE

cy·to·gen·e·sis \\ˌsīt-ə-'jen-ə-səs\\ *n, pl* **-e·ses** \\-ˌsēz\\ : cell formation and development

cy·to·ge·net·i·cist \\ˌsīt-ō-jə-'net-ə-səst\\ *n* : a person who specializes in cytogenetics

cy·to·ge·net·ics \\-jə-'net-iks\\ *n pl but sing or pl in constr* : a branch of biology that deals with the study of heredity and variation by the methods of both cytology and genetics — **cy·to·ge·net·ic** \\-jə-'net-ik\\ *or* **cy·to·ge·net·i·cal** \\-i-kəl\\ *adj* — **cy·to·ge·net·i·cal·ly** \\-i-k(ə-)lē\\ *adv*

cy·to·gen·ic \\ˌsīt-ə-'jen-ik\\ *or* **cy·tog·e·nous** \\sī-'täj-ə-nəs\\ *adj* : producing cells

cy·toid body \\ˌsī-ˌtoid-\\ *n* : one of the white globular masses resembling cells that are found in the retina in some abnormal conditions

cy·to·kine \\'sīt-ə-ˌkīn\\ *n* : any of a class of immunoregulatory proteins (as interleukin, tumor necrosis factor, and interferon) that are secreted by cells esp. of the immune system

cy·to·ki·ne·sis \\ˌsīt-ō-kə-'nē-səs, -kī-\\ *n, pl* **-ne·ses** \\-ˌsēz\\ 1 : the cytoplasmic changes accompanying mitosis 2 : cleavage of the cytoplasm into daughter cells following nuclear division — compare KARYOKINESIS — **cy·to·ki·net·ic** \\-'net-ik\\ *adj*

cy·to·ki·nin \\ˌsīt-ə-'kī-nən\\ *n* : any of various plant growth substances that are usu. derivatives of adenine

cytol *abbr* cytological; cytology

cy·tol·o·gy \\sī-'täl-ə-jē\\ *n, pl* **-gies** 1 : a branch of biology dealing with the structure, function, multiplication, patholo-gy, and life history of cells 2 : the cytological aspects of a process or structure — **cy·to·log·i·cal** \\ˌsīt-ᵊl-'äj-i-kəl\\ *or* **cy·to·log·ic** \\-'äj-ik\\ *adj* — **cy·to·log·i·cal·ly** \\-i-k(ə-)lē\\ *adv* — **cy·tol·o·gist** \\sī-'täl-ə-jəst\\ *n*

cy·to·ly·sin \\ˌsīt-ᵊl-'īs-ᵊn\\ *n* : a substance (as an antibody that lyses bacteria) producing cytolysis

cy·tol·y·sis \\sī-'täl-ə-səs\\ *n, pl* **-y·ses** \\-ˌsēz\\ : the usu. pathological dissolution or disintegration of cells — **cy·to·lyt·ic** \\ˌsīt-ᵊl-'it-ik\\ *adj*

cytolytic T cell *n* : CYTOTOXIC T CELL

cytolytic T lymphocyte *n* : CYTOTOXIC T CELL

cy·to·me·gal·ic \\ˌsīt-ō-mi-'gal-ik\\ *adj* : characterized by or causing the formation of enlarged cells

cytomegalic inclusion disease *n* : a severe disease esp. of newborns that is caused by the cytomegalovirus and usu. affects the salivary glands, brain, kidneys, liver, and lungs — called also *inclusion disease*

cy·to·meg·a·lo·vi·rus \\ˌsīt-ə-ˌmeg-ə-lō-'vī-rəs\\ *n* : a herpesvirus (species *Human herpesvirus 5* of the genus *Cytomegalovirus*) that causes cellular enlargement and formation of eosinophilic inclusion bodies esp. in the nucleus and that acts as an opportunistic infectious agent in immunosuppressed conditions (as AIDS)

cy·to·mem·brane \\ˌsīt-ō-'mem-ˌbrān\\ *n* : one of the cellular membranes including those of the plasma membrane, endoplasmic reticulum, nuclear envelope, and Golgi apparatus; *specif* : UNIT MEMBRANE

cy·tom·e·ter \\sī-'täm-ət-ər\\ *n* : an apparatus for counting and measuring cells

cy·tom·e·try \\sī-'täm-ə-trē\\ *n, pl* **-tries** : a technical specialty concerned with the counting of cells and esp. blood cells — see FLOW CYTOMETRY — **cy·to·met·ric** \\ˌsīt-ə-'me-trik\\ *adj*

cy·to·mor·phol·o·gy \\ˌsīt-ə-mòr-'fäl-ə-jē\\ *n, pl* **-gies** : the morphology of cells — **cy·to·mor·pho·log·i·cal** \\-ˌmòr-fə-'läj-i-kəl\\ *adj*

cy·to·mor·pho·sis \\ˌsīt-ō-'mòr-fə-səs *also* -mòr-'fō-\\ *n, pl* **-pho·ses** \\-ˌsēz\\ : the series of developmental changes undergone by a cell during its life

cy·ton \\'sī-ˌtän\\ *n* : CELL; *esp* : NEURON

cy·to·path·ic \\ˌsīt-ə-'path-ik\\ *adj* : of, relating to, characterized by, or producing pathological changes in cells ⟨∼ agents⟩

cy·to·patho·gen·ic \\-ˌpath-ə-'jen-ik\\ *adj* : pathological for or destructive to cells — **cy·to·patho·ge·nic·i·ty** \\-jə-'nis-ət-ē\\ *n, pl* **-ties**

cy·to·pa·thol·o·gy \\-pə-'thäl-ə-jē, -pa-\\ *n, pl* **-gies** : a branch of pathology that deals with manifestations of disease at the cellular level — **cy·to·patho·log·ic** \\-ˌpath-ə-'läj-ik\\ *also* **cy·to·patho·log·i·cal** \\-i-kəl\\ *adj* — **cy·to·patho·log·i·cal·ly** \\-i-k(ə-)lē\\ *adv* — **cy·to·pa·thol·o·gist** \\-pə-'thäl-ə-jəst, -pa-\\ *n*

cy·to·pem·phis \\ˌsīt-ə-'pem(p)-fəs\\ *n* : CYTOPEMPSIS

cy·to·pemp·sis \\-'pem(p)-səs\\ *n* : transportation of a substance into a cell and through the cytoplasm in a vesicle followed by its release to the exterior without utilization by the cell

cy·to·pe·nia \\-'pē-nē-ə\\ *n* : a deficiency of cellular elements of the blood; *esp* : deficiency of a specific element (as granulocytes in granulocytopenia) — **cy·to·pe·nic** \\-'pē-nik\\ *adj*

cy·to·phag·ic \\-'faj-ik\\ *adj* : of, relating to, or involving phagocytosis ⟨a ∼ test⟩

cy·to·phar·ynx \\-'far-iŋ(k)s\\ *n* : a channel leading from the surface into the protoplasm of some unicellular organisms and functioning in ciliates as a gullet

cy·to·phil·ic \\ˌsīt-ə-'fil-ik\\ *adj* : having an affinity for cells

cy·to·pho·tom·e·ter \\ˌsīt-ō-fō-'täm-ət-ər\\ *n* : a photometer for use in cytophotometry

cy·to·pho·tom·e·try \\-(ˌ)fō-'täm-ə-trē\\ *n, pl* **-tries** : photometry applied to the study of the cell or its constituents — **cy·to·pho·to·met·ric** \\-ˌfōt-ə-'me-trik\\ *adj* — **cy·to·pho·to·met·ri·cal·ly** \\-tri-k(ə-)lē\\ *adv*

cy·to·phys·i·ol·o·gy \\-ˌfiz-ē-'äl-ə-jē\\ *n, pl* **-gies** : the physiology of cells — **cy·to·phys·i·o·log·i·cal** \\-ē-ə-'läj-i-kəl\\ *adj* — **cy·to·phys·i·o·log·i·cal·ly** \\-i-k(ə-)lē\\ *adv*

C
D

cy·to·pi·pette \ˌsīt-ō-pī-'pet\ *n* : a pipette with a bulb that contains a fluid which is released into the vagina and then sucked back with a sample of cells for a vaginal smear

cy·to·plasm \'sīt-ə-ˌplaz-əm\ *n* : the organized complex of inorganic and organic substances external to the nuclear membrane of a cell and including the cytosol and membrane-bound organelles (as mitochondria or chloroplasts) — **cy·to·plas·mic** \ˌsīt-ə-'plaz-mik\ *adj* — **cy·to·plas·mi·cal·ly** \-mi-k(ə-)lē\ *adv*

cy·to·poi·e·sis \ˌsīt-ə-ˌpȯi-'ē-səs\ *n, pl* **-e·ses** \-ˌsēz\ : production of cells

cy·to·ryc·tes *or* **cy·tor·rhyc·tes** \-'rik-ˌtēz\ *n, pl* **cytoryctes** *or* **cytorrhyctes** : any of various inclusion bodies (as the Guarnieri bodies) orig. considered a genus of protozoans

cy·to·sine \'sīt-ə-ˌsēn\ *n* : a pyrimidine base C₄H₅N₃O that codes genetic information in the polynucleotide chain of DNA or RNA — compare ADENINE, GUANINE, THYMINE, URACIL

cytosine arabinoside *n* : a cytotoxic antineoplastic agent C₉H₁₃N₃O₅ that is a synthetic isomer of the naturally occurring nucleoside of cytosine and arabinose and is used esp. in the treatment of acute myelogenous leukemia in adults

cy·to·skel·e·ton \ˌsīt-ō-'skel-ət-ᵊn\ *n* : the network of protein filaments and microtubules in the cytoplasm that controls cell shape, maintains intracellular organization, and is involved in cell movement — **cy·to·skel·e·tal** \-ᵊl\ *adj*

cy·to·sol \'sīt-ə-ˌsäl, -ˌsȯl\ *n* : the fluid portion of the cytoplasm exclusive of organelles and membranes — called also *hyaloplasm, ground substance* — **cy·to·sol·ic** \ˌsīt-ə-'säl-ik, -'sȯl-\ *adj*

cy·to·some \'sīt-ə-ˌsōm\ *n* : the cytoplasmic portion of the cell

cy·to·spec·tro·pho·tom·e·try \ˌsīt-ə-ˌspek-trō-fō-'täm-ə-trē\ *n, pl* **-tries** : the application of spectrophotometry to the study of cells and esp. to the quantitative estimation of their constituents (as DNA)

¹**cy·to·stat·ic** \ˌsīt-ə-'stat-ik\ *adj* : tending to retard cellular activity and multiplication ⟨∼ treatment of tumor cells⟩ — **cy·to·stat·i·cal·ly** \-i-k(ə-)lē\ *adv*

²**cytostatic** *n* : a cytostatic agent

cy·to·stome \'sīt-ə-ˌstōm\ *n* : the mouth of a unicellular organism

cy·to·tax·on·o·my \ˌsīt-ō-(ˌ)tak-'sän-ə-mē\ *n, pl* **-mies** **1** : study of the relationships and classification of organisms using both classical systematic techniques and comparative studies of chromosomes **2** : the nuclear cytologic makeup of a kind of organism — **cy·to·tax·o·nom·ic** \-ˌtak-sə-'näm-ik\ *also* **cy·to·tax·o·nom·i·cal** \-i-kəl\ *adj* — **cy·to·tax·o·nom·i·cal·ly** \-i-k(ə-)lē\ *adv*

cy·to·tech \'sīt-ə-ˌtek\ *n* : CYTOTECHNOLOGIST

cy·to·tech·ni·cian \ˌsīt-ə-(ˌ)tek-'nish-ən\ *n* : CYTOTECHNOLOGIST

cy·to·tech·nol·o·gist \-'näl-ə-jəst\ *n* : a medical technician trained in cytotechnology

cy·to·tech·nol·o·gy \-'näl-ə-jē\ *n, pl* **-gies** : a specialty in medical technology concerned with the identification of cells and cellular abnormalities (as in cancer)

cy·to·tox·ic \ˌsīt-ə-'täk-sik\ *adj* : toxic to cells ⟨∼ lymphocytes⟩ ⟨∼ drugs⟩ — **cy·to·tox·ic·i·ty** \-(ˌ)täk-'sis-ət-ē\ *n, pl* **-ties**

cytotoxic T cell *n* : a T cell that usu. bears CD8 molecular markers on its surface and that functions in cell-mediated immunity by destroying a cell (as a virus-infected cell) having a specific antigenic molecule on its surface — called also *CTL, cytolytic T cell, cytolytic T lymphocyte, killer T cell, killer T lymphocyte;* compare HELPER T CELL, SUPPRESSOR T CELL

cytotoxic T lymphocyte *n* : CYTOTOXIC T CELL

cy·to·tox·in \ˌsīt-ə-'täk-sən\ *n* : a substance (as a toxin or antibody) having a toxic effect on cells

cy·to·tro·pho·blast \ˌsīt-ə-'trō-fə-ˌblast\ *n* : the inner cellular layer of the trophoblast of an embryonic placental mammal that gives rise to the plasmodial syncytiotrophoblast covering the placental villi — called also *Langhans' layer, layer of Langhans* — **cy·to·tro·pho·blas·tic** \-ˌtrō-fə-'blas-tik\ *adj*

cy·to·tro·pic \ˌsīt-ə-'trō-pik, -'träp-ik\ *adj* : attracted to cells ⟨a ∼ virus⟩

Cy·tox·an \sī-'täk-sən\ *trademark* — used for a preparation of cyclophosphamide

cy·to·zo·ic \ˌsīt-ə-'zō-ik\ *adj* : parasitic within a cell — used esp. of protozoans

cy·to·zo·on \-'zō-ˌän\ *n, pl* **-zoa** \-'zō-ə\ : a cytozoic animal

cy·to·zyme \'sīt-ə-ˌzīm\ *n* : THROMBOPLASTIN

D

d *abbr* **1** dalton **2** date **3** daughter **4** day **5** dead **6** deceased **7** deciduous **8** degree **9** density **10** developed **11** deviation **12** dexter **13** diameter **14** died **15** diopter **16** disease **17** divorced **18** dorsal **19** dose **20** duration

D *symbol* deuterium

d- \ˌdē, 'dē\ *prefix* **1** : dextrorotatory — usu. printed in italic ⟨*d*-tartaric acid⟩ **2** : having a similar configuration at a selected carbon atom to the configuration of dextrorotatory glyceraldehyde — usu. printed as a small capital ⟨D-fructose⟩

2,4–D — see entry alphabetized as TWO,FOUR-D

da *abbr* **1** daughter **2** day

DA *abbr* delayed action

da·boia \də-'bȯi-ə\ *n* **1** *also* **da·boya** : RUSSELL'S VIPER **2** *cap, in some classifications* : a genus of vipers that includes only Russell's viper

da·car·ba·zine \də-'kär-bə-ˌzēn\ *n* : an antineoplastic agent C₆H₁₀N₆O used to treat esp. metastatic malignant melanoma, tumors of adult soft tissue, and Hodgkin's disease

dacrya *pl of* DACRYON 9

dac·ryo·ad·e·nec·to·my \ˌdak-rē-(ˌ)ō-ˌad-ᵊn-'ek-tə-mē\ *n, pl* **-mies** : excision of a lacrimal gland

dac·ryo·cyst \'dak-rē-ə-ˌsist\ *n* : LACRIMAL SAC

dac·ryo·cys·tec·to·my \ˌdak-rē-(ˌ)ō-sis-'tek-tə-mē\ *n, pl* **-mies** : excision of a lacrimal sac

dac·ryo·cys·ti·tis \-sis-'tīt-əs\ *n* : inflammation of the lacrimal sac

dac·ryo·cys·to·blen·no·rhea *or chiefly Brit* **dac·ryo·cys·to·blen·no·rhoea** \-ˌsis-tə-ˌblen-ə-'rē-ə\ *n* : chronic dacryocystitis with constriction of the lacrimal duct and consequent decomposition of tears

dac·ryo·cys·tog·ra·phy \-sis-'täg-rə-fē\ *n, pl* **-phies** : radiographic visualization of the lacrimal sacs and associated structures after injection of a contrast medium

dac·ryo·cys·to·rhi·nos·to·my \-ˌsis-tə-ˌrī-'näs-tə-mē\ *n, pl* **-mies** : surgical creation of a passage for drainage between the lacrimal sac and the nasal cavity

dac·ryo·cys·tos·to·my \-sis-'täs-tə-mē\ *n, pl* **-mies** : an operation on a lacrimal sac to form a new opening (as for drainage)

dac·ryo·cys·tot·o·my \-sis-'tät-ə-mē\ *n, pl* **-mies** : incision (as for drainage) of a lacrimal sac

\ə\ abut \ᵊ\ kitten \ər\ further \a\ ash \ā\ ace \ä\ cot, cart \au̇\ out \ch\ chin \e\ bet \ē\ easy \g\ go \i\ hit \ī\ ice \j\ job \ŋ\ sing \ō\ go \ȯ\ law \ȯi\ boy \th\ thin \t͟h\ the \ü\ loot \u̇\ foot \y\ yet \zh\ vision *See also* Pronunciation Symbols page

dac·ryo·lith \'dak-rē-ə-ˌlith\ *n* : a concretion formed in a lacrimal passage

dac·ryo·li·thi·a·sis \ˌdak-rē-(ˌ)ō-li-'thī-ə-səs\ *n, pl* **-a·ses** \-ˌsēz\ : the formation of dacryoliths; *also* : a condition in which dacryoliths are present

dac·ry·on \'dak-rē-ˌän\ *n, pl* **dac·rya** \-rē-ə\ : the point of junction of the anterior border of the lacrimal bone with the frontal bone

dac·ryo·ste·no·sis \ˌdak-rē-(ˌ)ō-sti-'nō-səs\ *n, pl* **-no·ses** \-ˌsēz\ : a narrowing of the lacrimal duct

dac·ti·no·my·cin \ˌdak-tə-nō-'mīs-ᵊn\ *n* : a toxic antineoplastic drug $C_{62}H_{86}N_{12}O_{16}$ of the actinomycin group — called also *actinomycin D*

dac·tyl \'dak-tᵊl\ *n* : a finger or toe

dac·tyl·i·on \dak-'til-ē-ˌän\ *n* : the tip of the middle finger

dac·ty·log·ra·phy \ˌdak-tə-'läg-rə-fē\ *n, pl* **-phies** : the scientific study of fingerprints as a means of identification — **dac·ty·log·ra·pher** \-rə-fər\ *n*

dac·ty·lol·o·gy \ˌdak-tə-'läl-ə-jē\ *n, pl* **-gies** : FINGER SPELLING

dac·ty·los·co·py \-'läs-kə-pē\ *n, pl* **-pies** : identification by comparison of fingerprints; *also* : classification of fingerprints — **dac·tyl·o·scop·ic** \ˌdak-tə-lə-'skäp-ik\ *adj* — **dac·ty·los·co·pist** \-'läs-kə-pəst\ *n*

dac·ty·lo·sym·phy·sis \ˌdak-tə-lō-'sim(p)-fə-səs\ *n, pl* **-phy·ses** \-ˌsēz\ : SYNDACTYLY

dag·ga \'dag-ə, 'däg-ə\ *n* **1** *chiefly SoAfr* : MARIJUANA **2** : either of two relatively nontoxic So. African herbs (*Leonotis leonurus* and *L. orata*) smoked like tobacco

DAH *abbr* disordered action of the heart

dahll·ite \'däl-ˌīt\ *n* : a complex naturally occurring derivative of apatite that is closely related to the inorganic constituents of bones, dental enamel, and dentin

    Dahll \'däl\, **Tellef (1825–1893),** Norwegian mineralogist and geologist. Dahll was employed as a geologist by private mining concerns and for a time was a surveyor of mines. He also helped to edit geological maps of Norway and other parts of northern Scandinavia. In 1888, the mineral dahllite was named after him and his brother Johann, also a mineralogist.

daid·zein \'dād-ˌzīn, -ˌzēn\ *n* : an isoflavone $C_{15}H_{10}O_4$ found chiefly in legumes and esp. soybeans

Dal·mane \'dal-ˌmān\ *trademark* — used for a preparation of the hydrochloride of flurazepam

dal·ton \'dȯlt-ᵊn\ *n* : a unit of mass for expressing masses of atoms, molecules, or nuclear particles equal to ¹⁄₁₂ of the atomic mass of the most abundant carbon isotope ^{12}C : ATOMIC MASS UNIT — used chiefly in biochemistry; abbr. *d*

    Dalton, John (1766–1844), British chemist and physicist. One of the fathers of modern physical science, Dalton formulated the atomic theory of matter, a theory that established chemistry as a true science. He determined the relative weights of atoms and developed the laws of definite and multiple proportions. He formulated several laws relating to gases, including Dalton's law or the law of partial pressures. His wide interests included meteorology, in which he made valuable observations on the aurora borealis, trade winds, and rain. In 1794 he systematically described and explained the form of color blindness known as Daltonism. He himself was color-blind.

Dal·ton·ism \-ᵊn-ˌiz-əm\ *n* : red-green color blindness occurring as a recessive sex-linked genetic trait; *broadly* : any form of color blindness

Dalton's law *n* : LAW OF PARTIAL PRESSURES

¹dam \'dam\ *n* : a female parent — used esp. of a domestic animal

²dam *n* : RUBBER DAM — see DENTAL DAM

dam *abbr* dekameter

dam·ar *or* **dam·mar** \'dam-ər\ *n* : any of various resins obtained chiefly in Malaysia and Indonesia from several timber trees (as genera *Shorea* and *Vatica* of the family Dipterocarpaceae and genus *Canarium* of the family Burseraceae) and used as a mounting medium in microscopy and in varnishes and inks

damp \'damp\ *n* : a noxious or stifling gas or vapor; *esp* : one occurring in coal mines — usu. used in pl.; see BLACK DAMP, FIREDAMP

da·na·zol \'dä-nə-ˌzōl, 'dan-ə-, -ˌzȯl\ *n* : a synthetic androgenic derivative $C_{22}H_{27}NO_2$ of ethisterone that suppresses gonadotropin secretion by the adenohypophysis and is used esp. in the treatment of endometriosis

D&C \'dē-ən(d)-'sē\ *n* : DILATION AND CURETTAGE

D&E \'dē-ən(d)-'ē\ *n* : DILATION AND EVACUATION

dan·de·li·on \'dan-dᵊl-ˌī-ən\ *n* : any plant of the genus *Taraxacum*; *esp* : an herb (*T. officinale*) sometimes grown as a potherb and nearly cosmopolitan as a weed

dan·der \'dan-dər\ *n* : DANDRUFF; *specif* : minute scales from hair, feathers, or skin that may act as allergens

dan·druff \'dan-drəf\ *n* : scaly white or grayish flakes of dead skin cells esp. of the scalp; *also* : the condition marked by excessive shedding of such flakes and usu. accompanied by itching — **dan·druffy** \-ē\ *adj*

D&X \'dē-ən(d)-'eks\ *n* : DILATION AND EXTRACTION

dan·dy fever \'dan-dē-\ *n* : DENGUE

Dane particle \'dān-\ *n* : a spherical particle found in the serum in hepatitis B that is the virion of the causative double-stranded DNA virus

    Dane, David Maurice Surrey (1923–1998), British pathologist. A group of British scientists, led by Dane, discovered the Dane particle in 1970. By 1974 the viral identity of the particle had been confirmed by scientists.

Da·nysz phenomenon \'dän-ish-\ *n* : the exhibition of residual toxicity by a mixture of toxin and antitoxin in which the toxin has been added in several increments to an amount of antitoxin sufficient to completely neutralize it if it had been added as a single increment — called also *Danysz effect*

    Danysz, Jean (1860–1928), Polish-French pathologist. Danysz reported on the Danysz phenomenon in an 1899 article on toxins and antitoxins. He is also known for two other achievements: the isolation in 1900 of the bacterium (*Salmonella typhimurium*) that is the most frequent cause of human food poisoning, and the first use of radium in treating malignant diseases in 1903.

daph·ne \'daf-(ˌ)nē\ *n* **1** *cap* : a genus of Eurasian shrubs (family Thymelaeaceae) that have often fragrant flowers without petals and that include the mezereon **2** : a plant of the genus *Daphne*

daph·nin \'daf-nən\ *n* : a bitter crystalline glucoside $C_{15}H_{16}O_9$ occurring esp. in plants of the genus *Daphne* (as *D. mezereum*)

dap·pen dish \'dap-ən-\ *n* : a small heavy 10-sided piece of glass each end of which is ground into a small cup for mixing dental medicaments or fillings — called also *dappen glass*

dap·sone \'dap-ˌsōn, -ˌzōn\ *n* : an antimicrobial agent $C_{12}H_{12}N_2O_2S$ used esp. to treat leprosy and dermatitis herpetiformis — called also *diaminodiphenyl sulfone*

Da·rier's disease \dar-'yāz-, där-\ *n* : a genetically determined skin condition characterized by patches of keratotic papules — called also *keratosis follicularis*

    Da·rier \där-yā\, **Jean Ferdinand (1856–1938),** French dermatologist. Darier is known for classic descriptions of three conditions affecting the skin: the hereditary dermatosis now known as Darier's disease (1889), acanthosis nigricans (1893), and the skin eruptions associated with tuberculosis (1896).

dark adaptation \ˌdärk-\ *n* : the phenomena including dilation of the pupil, increase in retinal sensitivity, shift of the region of maximum luminosity toward the blue, and regeneration of rhodopsin by which the eye adapts to conditions of reduced illumination — compare LIGHT ADAPTATION — **dark–adapt·ed** \'därk-ə-ˌdap-təd\ *adj*

dark field *n* : the dark area that serves as the background for objects viewed in an ultramicroscope — **dark–field** *adj*

dark–field microscope *n* : ULTRAMICROSCOPE — **dark–field microscopy** *n*

darm·stadt·i·um \ˌdärm-'stat-ē-əm\ *n* : a short-lived radioactive element produced artificially — symbol *Ds*; see ELEMENT table

D'Ar·son·val current \'där-sᵊn-ˌvȯl-, -ˌval-\ *n* : a high-frequency oscillating current of low voltage and high amperage used in diathermy

Ar·son·val \är-sōⁿ-vál\, **Jacques–Arsène d'** (1851–1940), French biophysicist. D'Arsonval did pioneering work in electrotherapy. In 1892 he introduced the use of high-frequency currents to treat diseases of the skin and mucous membranes. The current is now known as the D'Arsonval current.

dar·tos \'där-ˌtäs, 'därt-əs\ *n* : a thin layer of vascular contractile tissue that contains smooth muscle fibers but no fat and is situated beneath the skin of the scrotum or beneath that of the labia majora

Dar·vo·cet–N \'där-vō-ˌset-'en\ *trademark* — used for a preparation of the napsylate of propoxyphene in combination with acetaminophen

Dar·von \'där-ˌvän\ *trademark* — used for a preparation of the hydrochloride of propoxyphene

Dar·win·ian \där-'win-ē-ən\ *adj* : of or relating to Charles Darwin, his theories esp. of evolution, or his followers — **Darwinian** *n*

Dar·win \'där-wən\, **Charles Robert** (1809–1882), British naturalist. Darwin is celebrated for his documentation of the theory of evolution and the development of the principle of natural selection. In 1831 he began a five-year voyage around the world, making stopovers in So. America where he gained critical insight into the variation between populations of animals on the various islands and the mainland which played an important role in the development of his ideas on evolution. In 1859 he published *On the Origin of Species by Means of Natural Selection*. This landmark work brought about a revolution in biology and firmly established the study of evolution as part of the science of biology. *The Descent of Man*, 1871, was a follow-up work that contained his related theory of sexual selection. Darwin was not the first to question the immutability of species in nature or to conceive the notion of evolution, but he added to the theorizing of Lamarck and others the concept of natural selection and voluminous documentary evidence.

Dar·win·ism \'där-wə-ˌniz-əm\ *n* : a theory of the origin and perpetuation of new species of animals and plants that offspring of a given organism vary, that natural selection favors the survival of some of these variations over others, that new species have arisen and may continue to arise by these processes, and that widely divergent groups of plants and animals have arisen from the same ancestors; *broadly* : a theory of biological evolution — **Dar·win·ist** \-wə-nəst\ *n or adj*

Darwin's tubercle *n* : the slight projection occas. present on the edge of the external human ear and assumed by some scientists to represent the pointed part of the ear of quadrupeds — called also *auricular tubercle of Darwin*

Das·y·proc·ta \ˌdas-ə-'präk-tə\ *n* : a genus (the type of the family Dasyproctidae) of rodents comprising the agoutis and having relatively long legs

DAT *abbr* delayed action tablet

da·ta \'dāt-ə, 'dat-, 'dät-\ *n pl but sing or pl in constr* : factual information (as measurements or statistics) used as a basis for reasoning, discussion, or calculation ⟨the ∼ is plentiful and easily available —H. A. Gleason, Jr.⟩ ⟨comprehensive ∼ on the incidence of Lyme disease⟩

date rape \'dāt-\ *n* : rape committed by the victim's date; *broadly* : ACQUAINTANCE RAPE

date rape drug *n* : a drug (as GHB or flunitrazepam) administered surreptitiously (as in a drink) to induce an unconscious or sedated state in a potential date rape victim

da·tu·ra \də-'t(y)ùr-ə\ *n* **1** *cap* : a genus of widely distributed strong-scented herbs, shrubs, or trees of the family Solanaceae including some used as sources of medicinal alkaloids (as stramonium from jimsonweed) or in folk rites or illicitly for their poisonous, narcotic, or hallucinogenic properties **2** : any plant or flower of the genus *Datura*

dau *abbr* daughter

Dau·ben·ton's plane \'dō-bən-ˌtōⁿz-, dō-bäⁿ-tōⁿz-\ *n* : a plane that passes through the opisthion and the orbitalia on a skull

Dau·ben·ton \dō-bäⁿ-tōⁿ\, **Louis–Jean–Marie** (1716–1800), French naturalist. Daubenton was a pioneer in the fields of comparative anatomy and paleontology. His major contribution to anatomy was his share of a massive multi-volume work on natural history by fellow naturalist Georges Buffon (1707–1788). He described Daubenton's plane around 1751.

Dau·cus \'dȯ-kəs\ *n* : a genus of chiefly Old World herbs (family Umbelliferae) that have compound umbels of mostly white flowers and prickly fruit and include the carrot and wild carrot

¹daugh·ter \'dȯt-ər\ *n* **1 a** : a human female having the relation of child to a parent **b** : a female offspring of an animal **2** : an atomic species that is the product of the radioactive decay of a given element ⟨radon is the ∼ of radium⟩

²daughter *adj* **1** : having the characteristics or relationship of a daughter **2** : belonging to the first generation of offspring, organelles, or molecules produced by reproduction, division, or replication ⟨a ∼ cell⟩ ⟨∼ chromosomes⟩

dau·no·my·cin \ˌdȯ-nə-'mīs-ᵊn, ˌdaù-\ *n* : DAUNORUBICIN

dau·no·ru·bi·cin \-'rü-bə-sən\ *n* : an antibiotic that is a nitrogenous glycoside and is used in the form of its hydrochloride $C_{27}H_{29}NO_{10} \cdot HCl$ esp. in the treatment of some leukemias

dawn phenomenon \'dȯn-\ *n* : a rise in the level of glucose in the blood plasma that occurs in early morning before breakfast and that may progress to hyperglycemia in diabetics and esp. in those affected with type 1 diabetes — compare SOMOGYI EFFECT

day·dream \'dā-ˌdrēm\ *n* : a visionary creation of the imagination experienced while awake; *esp* : a gratifying reverie usu. of wish fulfillment — **daydream** *vi* — **day·dream·er** *n*

day·mare \'dā-ˌma(ə)r, -ˌme(ə)r\ *n* : a nightmarish fantasy experienced while awake

day nursery *n* : a public center for the care and education of young children

Day·pro \'dā-prō\ *trademark* — used for a preparation of oxaprozin

day re·lease \-ri-'lēs\ *n, Brit* : a program in hospitals, prisons, and jails in which patients or prisoners are permitted to spend part of the day outside their institution of confinement studying, training, or working

Db *symbol* dubnium

DBCP \ˌdē-(ˌ)bē-(ˌ)sē-'pē\ *n* : a halocarbon compound $C_3H_5Br_2Cl$ used as an agricultural pesticide that is a suspected carcinogen and cause of sterility in human males — called also *dibromochloropropane*

dbl *abbr* double

DBP *abbr* diastolic blood pressure

DC *abbr* **1** Dental Corps **2** diagnostic center **3** direct current **4** doctor of chiropractic

DCc *abbr* double concave

DCIS *abbr* ductal carcinoma in situ

DCR *abbr* direct critical response

DD *abbr* developmentally disabled

DDAVP \ˌdē-(ˌ)dē-(ˌ)ā-(ˌ)vē-'pē\ *trademark* — used for a preparation of the acetate of desmopressin

ddC \ˌdē-(ˌ)dē-'sē\ *n, often all cap* : a synthetic nucleoside analog $C_9H_{13}N_3O_3$ that inhibits replication of retroviruses and is used in the treatment of advanced HIV infection — called also *dideoxycytidine, zalcitabine*

DDD \ˌdē-(ˌ)dē-'dē\ *n* : an insecticide $C_{14}H_{10}Cl_4$ closely related chemically and similar in properties to DDT

DDE \-'ē\ *n* : a persistent organochlorine $C_{15}H_8Cl_4$ that is produced by the metabolic breakdown of DDT

ddI \-'ī\ *n, often all cap* : a synthetic nucleoside analog

\ə\ **abut** \ᵊ\ **kitten** \ər\ **further** \a\ **ash** \ā\ **ace** \ä\ **cot, cart**
\au̇\ **out** \ch\ **chin** \e\ **bet** \ē\ **easy** \g\ **go** \i\ **hit** \ī\ **ice** \j\ **job**
\ŋ\ **sing** \ō\ **go** \ȯ\ **law** \ȯi\ **boy** \th\ **thin** \th̲\ **the** \ü\ **loot**
\u̇\ **foot** \y\ **yet** \zh\ **vision** *See also* Pronunciation Symbols page

$C_{10}H_{12}N_4O_3$ having properties and uses similar to those of ddC — called also *didanosine, dideoxyinosine;* see VIDEX

DDS *abbr* doctor of dental science; doctor of dental surgery

DDT \ˌdē-ˌdē-ˈtē\ *n* : a colorless odorless water-insoluble crystalline insecticide $C_{14}H_9Cl_5$ that tends to accumulate in ecosystems and has toxic effects on many vertebrates — called also *chlorophenothane, dicophane*

DDVP \ˌdē-ˌdē-vē-ˈpē\ *n* : DICHLORVOS

de·acid·i·fy \ˌdē-ə-ˈsid-ə-ˌfī\ *vt* **-fied; -fy·ing** : to remove acid from : reduce the acidity of (as by neutralization) — **de·acid·i·fi·ca·tion** \-ˌsid-ə-fə-ˈkā-shən\ *n*

de·ac·ti·vate \(ˈ)dē-ˈak-tə-ˌvāt\ *vt* **-vat·ed; -vat·ing** **1** : to make inactive or ineffective **2** : to deprive of chemical activity ⟨∼ an enzyme⟩ — **de·ac·ti·va·tion** \-ˌak-tə-ˈvā-shən\ *n*

¹dead \ˈded\ *adj* **1** : deprived of life : having died ⟨∼ of scarlet fever⟩ **2** : lacking power to move, feel, or respond : NUMB

²dead *n, pl* **dead** : one that is dead — usu. used collectively

dead·ly \ˈded-lē\ *adj* **dead·li·er; -est** : likely to cause or capable of causing death ⟨a ∼ disease⟩ ⟨a ∼ poison⟩ ⟨a ∼ instrument⟩ — **dead·li·ness** \-nəs\ *n*

deadly nightshade *n* : BELLADONNA 1

dead space *n* **1** : space in the respiratory system in which air does not undergo significant gaseous exchange — see ANATOMICAL DEAD SPACE, PHYSIOLOGICAL DEAD SPACE **2** : a space (as that in the chest following excision of a lung) left in the body as the result of a surgical procedure

deaf \ˈdef\ *adj* : lacking or deficient in the sense of hearing — **deaf·ness** *n*

deaf–aid \ˈdef-ˌād\ *n, chiefly Brit* : HEARING AID

deaf·en \ˈdef-ən\ *vb* **deaf·ened; deaf·en·ing** \-(ə-)niŋ\ *vt* : to make deaf ∼ *vi* : to cause deafness or stun one with noise — **deaf·en·ing·ly** \-(ə-)niŋ-lē\ *adv*

de·af·fer·en·ta·tion \ˌdē-ˌaf-ə-ˌren-ˈtā-shən\ *n* : the freeing of a motor nerve from sensory components by severing the dorsal root central to the dorsal ganglion

¹deaf–mute \ˈdef-ˈmyüt\ *adj, often offensive* : lacking the sense of hearing and the ability to speak — **deaf–mute·ness** *n, sometimes offensive* — **deaf–mut·ism** \-ˈmyüt-ˌiz-əm\ *n, sometimes offensive*

²deaf–mute *n, often offensive* : a deaf person who cannot speak

de·am·i·dase \(ˈ)dē-ˈam-ə-ˌdās, -ˌdāz\ *n* : an enzyme which hydrolyzes amides with the removal of the amido group

de·am·i·date \-ˌdāt\ *or* **des·am·i·date** \(ˈ)des-\ *vt* **-dat·ed; -dat·ing** : to remove the amido group from (a compound) — **de·am·i·da·tion** \ˌdē-ˌam-ə-ˈdā-shən\ *or* **des·am·i·da·tion** \ˌdes-\ *n*

de·am·i·di·za·tion \ˌdē-ˌam-əd-ə-ˈzā-shən\ *also* **des·am·i·di·za·tion** \ˌdes-\ *n* : the process of deamidizing : DEAMIDATION

de·am·i·dize \(ˈ)dē-ˈam-ə-ˌdīz\ *also* **des·am·i·dize** \(ˈ)des-\ *vt* **-dized; -diz·ing** : DEAMIDATE

de·am·i·nase \(ˈ)dē-ˈam-ə-ˌnās, -ˌnāz\ *also* **des·am·i·nase** \(ˈ)des-\ *n* : an enzyme that hydrolyzes amino compounds (as amino acids) with removal of the amino group

de·am·i·nate \-ˌnāt\ *vt* **-nat·ed; -nat·ing** : to remove the amino group from (a compound) — **de·am·i·na·tion** \(ˌ)dē-ˌam-ə-ˈnā-shən\ *n*

de·am·i·nize \(ˈ)dē-ˈam-ə-ˌnīz\ *vt* **-nized; -niz·ing** : DEAMINATE — **de·am·i·ni·za·tion** \ˌdē-ˌam-ə-nə-ˈzā-shən\ *n*

de·a·nol \ˈdē-ə-ˌnȯl\ *n* : DMAE

death \ˈdeth\ *n* **1** : the irreversible cessation of all vital functions esp. as indicated by permanent stoppage of the heart, respiration, and brain activity : the end of life — see BRAIN DEATH **2** : the cause or occasion of loss of life ⟨drinking was the ∼ of him⟩ **3** : the state of being dead ⟨in ∼ as in life⟩

death·bed \ˈdeth-ˌbed\ *n* **1** : the bed in which a person dies **2** : the last hours of life — **on one's deathbed** : near the point of death

death cap *n* : a very poisonous mushroom of the genus *Amanita* (*A. phalloides*) of deciduous woods of No. America and Europe that varies in color from pure white to olive or yellow and has a prominent volva at the base — called also *death cup;* see THIOCTIC ACID

death instinct *n* : an innate and unconscious tendency toward self-destruction postulated in psychoanalytic theory to explain aggressive and destructive behavior not satisfactorily explained by the pleasure principle — called also *Thanatos;* compare EROS

death point *n* : a limit (as of degree of heat or cold) beyond which an organism or living protoplasm cannot survive

death rate *n* : the ratio of deaths to number of individuals in a population usu. expressed as number of deaths per hundred or per thousand population for a given time

death rattle *n* : a rattling or gurgling sound produced by air passing through mucus in the lungs and air passages of a dying person

death wish *n* : the conscious or unconscious desire for the death of another or of oneself — called also *destrudo*

de·bil·i·tate \di-ˈbil-ə-ˌtāt\ *vt* **-tat·ed; -tat·ing** : to impair the strength of ⟨a body *debilitated* by disease⟩ — **de·bil·i·ta·tion** \-ˌbil-ə-ˈtā-shən\ *n*

de·bil·i·ty \di-ˈbil-ət-ē\ *n, pl* **-ties** : the quality or state of being weak, feeble, or infirm; *esp* : physical weakness

de·bride \di-ˈbrēd, dā-\ *vt* **de·brid·ed; de·brid·ing** : to cleanse by debridement

de·bride·ment \di-ˈbrēd-mənt, dā-, -ˌmänt, -ˌmäⁿ\ *n* : the usu. surgical removal of lacerated, devitalized, or contaminated tissue

de·bris \də-ˈbrē, dā-ˈ, ˈdā-ˌ, *Brit usu* ˈdeb-(ˌ)rē\ *n, pl* **debris** : organic waste from dead or damaged tissue ⟨a wound obscured by blood and ∼ —*Emergency Medicine*⟩

de·bris·o·quin \di-ˈbris-ō-ˌkwin\ *or* **de·bris·o·quine** \-ˌkwīn\ *n* : an antihypertensive drug used esp. in the form of its sulfate $(C_{10}H_{13}N_3)_2 \cdot H_2SO_4$

de·bulk \(ˌ)dē-ˈbəlk *also* -ˈbulk\ *vt* : to remove all or most of the substance of (a tumor or lesion) ⟨surgical ∼*ing* of hepatic tumor masses —*Scientific Amer. Medicine Bull.*⟩

dec *abbr* **1** deceased **2** decompose

Dec·a·dron \ˈdek-ə-ˌdrän\ *trademark* — used for a preparation of dexamethasone

decagram, decaliter, decameter *var of* DEKAGRAM, DEKALITER, DEKAMETER

decagramme, decalitre, decametre *chiefly Brit var of* DEKAGRAM, DEKALITER, DEKAMETER

de·cal·ci·fi·ca·tion \(ˌ)dē-ˌkal-sə-fə-ˈkā-shən\ *n* : the removal or loss of calcium or calcium compounds (as from bones or soil) — **de·cal·ci·fy** \(ˈ)dē-ˈkal-sə-ˌfī\ *vt* **-fied; -fy·ing**

deca·me·tho·ni·um \ˌdek-ə-mə-ˈthō-nē-əm\ *n* : a synthetic ion used esp. in the form of its bromide $C_{16}H_{38}Br_2N_2$ or iodide $C_{16}H_{38}I_2N_2$ as a skeletal muscle relaxant

dec·ane \ˈdek-ˌān\ *n* : any of several isomeric liquid alkanes $C_{10}H_{22}$

dec·a·noate \ˌdek-ə-ˈnō-ˌāt\ *n* : CAPRATE

dec·a·no·ic acid \ˌdek-ə-ˌnō-ik-\ *n* : CAPRIC ACID

de·cant \di-ˈkant\ *vt* : to draw off (a liquid) without disturbing the sediment or the lower liquid layers — **de·can·ta·tion** \ˌdē-ˌkan-ˈtā-shən\ *n*

deca·pep·tide \ˌdek-ə-ˈpep-ˌtīd\ *n* : a polypeptide (as angiotensin I) that consists of a chain of 10 amino acids

¹de·cap·i·tate \di-ˈkap-ə-ˌtāt\ *vt* **-tat·ed; -tat·ing** : to cut off the head of — **de·cap·i·ta·tion** \-ˌkap-ə-ˈtā-shən\ *n*

²de·cap·i·tate \-ə-ˌtāt, -ət-ət\ *adj* : relating to or being a decapitated experimental animal

de·cap·su·late \ˌdē-ˈkap-sə-ˌlāt\ *vt* **-lat·ed; -lat·ing** : to remove the capsule from ⟨∼ a kidney⟩ — **de·cap·su·la·tion** \ˌdē-ˌkap-sə-ˈlā-shən\ *n*

de·car·box·yl·ase \ˌdē-kär-ˈbäk-sə-ˌlās, -ˌlāz\ *n* : any of a group of enzymes that accelerate decarboxylation esp. of amino acids

de·car·box·yl·ate \-sə-ˌlāt\ *vt* **-at·ed; -at·ing** : to remove carboxyl from — **de·car·box·yl·a·tion** \-ˌbäk-sə-ˈlā-shən\ *n*

¹de·cay \di-ˈkā\ *vi* : to undergo decomposition ∼ *vt* : to destroy by decomposition

C
D

²**decay** *n* **1 a :** ROT 1; *specif* : aerobic decomposition of proteins chiefly by bacteria **b :** the product of decay **2 a :** spontaneous decrease in the number of radioactive atoms in radioactive material **b :** spontaneous disintegration (as of an atom or a nuclear particle)

decay constant *n* : the constant ratio of the number of radioactive atoms disintegrating in any specified short unit interval of time to the total number of atoms of the same kind still intact at the beginning of that interval — called also *disintegration constant*

decd *abbr* deceased

de·cease \di-'sēs\ *n* : departure from life : DEATH — **decease** *vi* **de·ceased; de·ceas·ing**

¹**de·ceased** \-'sēst\ *adj* : no longer living; *esp* : recently dead — used of persons

²**deceased** *n, pl* **deceased** : a dead person ⟨the will of the ∼⟩

de·ce·dent \di-'sēd-³nt\ *n* : a deceased person — used chiefly in law

de·cel·er·ate \(')dē-'sel-ə-ˌrāt\ *vb* **-at·ed; -at·ing** *vt* : to reduce the speed of : slow down ∼ *vi* : to move at decreasing speed — **de·cel·er·a·tion** \(ˌ)dē-ˌsel-ə-'rā-shən\ *n*

de·cer·e·brate \(')dē-'ser-ə-brət, -ˌbrāt; ˌdē-sə-'rē-brət\ *adj* **1 :** having the cerebrum removed or made inactive ⟨∼ rats⟩ **2 :** characteristic of decerebration ⟨∼ rigidity⟩

de·cer·e·bra·tion \(ˌ)dē-ˌser-ə-'brā-shən\ *n* : loss of cerebral function (as from disease, trauma, or surgical cutting of the brain stem); *also* : removal of the cerebrum (as by surgery) — **de·cer·e·brate** \(')dē-'ser-ə-ˌbrāt\ *vt* **-brat·ed; -brat·ing**

de·chlo·ri·nate \(')dē-'klōr-ə-ˌnāt, -'klȯr-\ *vt* **-nat·ed; -nat·ing** : to remove chlorine from ⟨∼ water⟩ — **de·chlo·ri·na·tion** \(ˌ)dē-ˌklōr-ə-'nā-shən, -ˌklȯr-\ *n*

deci·bel \'des-ə-bəl, -ˌbel\ *n* **1 a :** a unit for expressing the ratio of two amounts of electric or acoustic signal power equal to 10 times the common logarithm of this ratio **b :** a unit for expressing the ratio of the magnitudes of two electric voltages or currents or analogous acoustic quantities equal to 20 times the common logarithm of the voltage or current ratio **2 :** a unit for expressing the relative intensity of sounds on a scale from zero for the average least perceptible sound to about 130 for the average pain level

de·cid·ua \di-'sij-ə-wə\ *n, pl* **-uae** \-ˌwē\ **1 :** the part of the mucous membrane lining the uterus that in higher placental mammals undergoes special modifications in preparation for and during pregnancy and is cast off at parturition, being made up in the human of a part lining the uterus, a part enveloping the embryo, and a part participating with the chorion in the formation of the placenta — see DECIDUA BASALIS, DECIDUA CAPSULARIS, DECIDUA PARIETALIS **2 :** the mucous membrane of the uterus cast off in the ordinary process of menstruation — **de·cid·u·al** \-ə-wəl\ *adj*

decidua ba·sa·lis \-bə-'sā-ləs\ *n* : the part of the endometrium in the pregnant human female that participates with the chorion in the formation of the placenta

decidua cap·su·lar·is \-ˌkap-sə-'lar-əs\ *n* : the part of the decidua in the pregnant human female that envelops the embryo

decidua pa·ri·etal·is \-pə-ˌrī-ə-'tal-əs\ *n* : the part of the decidua in the pregnant human female lining the uterus

decidua pla·cen·tal·is \-ˌplā-sən-'tal-əs, -sen-\ *n* : DECIDUA BASALIS

decidua re·flexa \-ri-'flek-sə\ *n* : DECIDUA CAPSULARIS

decidua ser·o·ti·na \-ˌser-ə-'tē-nə, -'tī-\ *n* : DECIDUA BASALIS

de·cid·u·ate \di-'sij-ə-wət\ *adj* : having the fetal and maternal tissues firmly interlocked so that a layer of maternal tissue is torn away at parturition and forms a part of the afterbirth

decidua ve·ra \-'vir-ə, -'ver-\ *n* : DECIDUA PARIETALIS

de·cid·u·itis \di-ˌsij-ə-'wīt-əs\ *n* : inflammation of the decidua

de·cid·u·oma \-'wō-mə\ *n, pl* **-ma·ta** \-ˌmət-ə\ *also* **-mas** **1 :** a mass of tissue formed in the uterus following pregnancy that contains remnants of chorionic or decidual tissue **2 :** decidual tissue induced in the uterus (as by trauma) in the absence of pregnancy

de·cid·u·o·sis \-'wō-səs\ *n, pl* **-o·ses** \-ˌsēz\ : the occurrence of decidual tissue in an ectopic site (as the cervix or vagina)

de·cid·u·ous \di-'sij-ə-wəs\ *adj* **1 :** falling off or shed at a certain stage in the life cycle **2 :** having deciduous parts ⟨a ∼ dentition⟩

deciduous tooth *n* : MILK TOOTH

deci·gram *also Brit* **deci·gramme** \'des-ə-ˌgram\ *n* : a metric unit of mass and weight equal to ¹⁄₁₀ gram

deci·li·ter *or chiefly Brit* **deci·li·tre** \'des-ə-ˌlēt-ər\ *n* : a metric unit of capacity equal to ¹⁄₁₀ liter

deci·me·ter *or chiefly Brit* **deci·me·tre** \'des-ə-ˌmēt-ər\ *n* : a metric unit of length equal to ¹⁄₁₀ meter

deci·nor·mal \ˌdes-ə-'nȯr-məl\ *adj, of a chemical solution* : having one tenth of the normal strength

de·clar·a·tive \di-'klar-ət-iv, -'kler-\ *adj* : being or comprising memory characterized by the conscious recall of facts and events — compare PROCEDURAL

de·claw \(ˌ)dē-'klȯ\ *vt* : to remove the claws of (a cat) usu. with the nail matrix and all or part of the last bone of the toe

¹**de·cline** \di-'klīn\ *vi* **de·clined; de·clin·ing** : to tend toward an impaired state or a weaker condition

²**decline** *n* **1 :** the process of declining; *esp* : a gradual physical or mental sinking and wasting away **2 :** the period during which the end of life is approaching **3 :** a wasting disease; *esp* : pulmonary tuberculosis

de·clive \di-'klīv\ *n* : a part of the monticulus of the cerebellum that is dorsal to the culmen

de·clot \(')dē-'klät\ *vt* **de·clot·ted; de·clot·ting** : to remove blood clots from ⟨the serum histidine concentration in casual samples, properly *declotted* and stored —D. A. Gerber⟩

de·coct \di-'käkt\ *vt* **1 :** to prepare by boiling : extract the flavor or active principle of by boiling **2 :** to steep in hot water

de·coc·tion \-'käk-shən\ *n* **1 :** the act or process of boiling usu. in water so as to extract the flavor or active principle — compare INFUSION 1b(1) **2 a :** an extract or liquid preparation obtained by decocting **b :** a liquid preparation made by boiling a medicinal plant with water usu. in the proportion of 5 parts of the drug to 100 parts of water

de·coc·tum \-'käk-təm\ *n, pl* **de·coc·ta** \-tə\ : DECOCTION 2b

¹**de·col·or·ant** *or Brit* **de·col·our·ant** \(')dē-'kəl-ər-ənt, -ə-rənt\ *n* : a substance that removes color

²**decolorant** *or Brit* **decolourant** *adj* : capable of removing color

de·col·or·a·tion *or Brit* **de·col·our·a·tion** \ˌdē-ˌkəl-ə-'rā-shən\ *n* : the process of decolorizing

de·col·or·ize *or Brit* **de·col·our·ise** \(')dē-'kəl-ə-ˌrīz\ *vt* **-or·ized** *or Brit* **-our·ized** *also* **-our·ised; -or·iz·ing** *or Brit* **-our·iz·ing** *also* **-our·is·ing** : to remove color from ⟨∼ vinegar by adsorption of impurities on activated charcoal⟩ — **de·col·or·iza·tion** *or Brit* **de·col·our·iza·tion** *also* **de·col·our·isa·tion** \(')dē-ˌkəl-ə-rə-'zā-shən\ *n* — **de·col·or·iz·er** *or Brit* **de·col·our·iz·er** *also* **de·col·our·is·er** \(')dē-'kəl-ə-ˌrī-zər\ *n*

de·com·pen·sate \(')dē-'käm-pən-ˌsāt, -ˌpen-\ *vi* **-sat·ed; -sat·ing** : to undergo decompensation — **de·com·pen·sa·to·ry** \ˌdē-kəm-'pen(t)-sə-ˌtōr-ē, -ˌtȯr-\ *adj*

de·com·pen·sa·tion \(ˌ)dē-ˌkäm-pən-'sā-shən, -pen-\ *n* : loss of physiological compensation or psychological balance; *esp* : inability of the heart to maintain adequate circulation

de·com·pose \ˌdē-kəm-'pōz\ *vb* **-posed; -pos·ing** *vt* : to separate into constituent parts or elements or into simpler compounds ⟨∼ water by electrolysis⟩ ∼ *vi* : to undergo chemical breakdown : DECAY, ROT ⟨fruit ∼s⟩ — **de·com·pos·abil·i·ty** \-ˌpō-zə-'bil-ət-ē\ *n, pl* **-ties** — **de·com·pos·able** \-'pō-zə-bəl\ *adj*

de·com·pos·er \ˌdē-kəm-'pō-zər\ *n* : any of various organisms (as many bacteria and fungi) that return constituents of

\ə\ abut \ᵊ\ kitten \ər\ further \a\ ash \ā\ ace \ä\ cot, cart
\au̇\ out \ch\ chin \e\ bet \ē\ easy \g\ go \i\ hit \ī\ ice \j\ job
\ŋ\ sing \ō\ go \ȯ\ law \ȯi\ boy \th\ thin \th\ the \ü\ loot
\u̇\ foot \y\ yet \zh\ vision   *See also* Pronunciation Symbols page

organic substances to ecological cycles by feeding on and breaking down dead protoplasm

de·com·po·si·tion \(ˌ)dē-ˌkäm-pə-ˈzish-ən\ *n* : the act or process of decomposing : the state of being decomposed: **a** : the separation or resolution (as of a substance) into constituent parts or elements or into simpler compounds ⟨∼ of mercuric oxide into mercury and oxygen⟩ **b** : organic decay ⟨the ∼ of a dead body⟩

de·com·press \ˌdē-kəm-ˈpres\ *vt* : to release from pressure or compression

de·com·pres·sion \-ˈpresh-ən\ *n* : the act or process of releasing from pressure or compression: as **a** : reduction of pressure: (1) : the decrease of ambient air pressure experienced in an air lock on return to atmospheric pressure after a period of breathing compressed air (as in a diving bell or caisson) or experienced in ascent to a great altitude without a pressure suit or pressurized cabin (2) : the decrease of water pressure experienced by a diver when ascending rapidly **b** : an operation or technique used to relieve pressure upon an organ (as in fractures of the skull or spine) or within a hollow organ (as in intestinal obstruction)

decompression chamber *n* **1** : a chamber in which excessive pressure can be reduced gradually to atmospheric pressure **2** : a chamber in which an individual can be gradually subjected to decreased atmospheric pressure (as in simulating conditions at high altitudes)

decompression sickness *n* : a sometimes fatal disorder that is marked by neuralgic pains and paralysis, distress in breathing, and often collapse and that is caused by the release of gas bubbles (as of nitrogen) in tissue upon too rapid decrease in air pressure after a stay in a compressed atmosphere — called also *bends, caisson disease, decompression illness, decompression syndrome*; see AEROEMBOLISM

de·com·pres·sive \ˌdē-kəm-ˈpres-iv\ *adj* : tending to relieve or reduce pressure

de·con·di·tion \ˌdē-kən-ˈdish-ən\ *vt* **1** : to cause to lose physical fitness ⟨inactivity ∼s a bedridden person⟩ **2** : to cause extinction of (a conditioned response)

de·con·di·tion·ing \-ˈdish-(ə-)niŋ\ *n* : a decrease in the responsiveness of heart muscle that sometimes occurs after long periods of weightlessness and may be marked by decrease in blood volume and pooling of the blood in the legs upon return to normal conditions

¹de·con·ges·tant \ˌdē-kən-ˈjes-tənt\ *n* : an agent that relieves congestion (as of mucous membranes)

²decongestant *adj* : relieving or tending to relieve congestion ⟨nasal ∼ action⟩

de·con·ges·tion \-ˈjes(h)-chən\ *n* : the process of relieving congestion — **de·con·gest** \-ˈjest\ *vt* — **de·con·ges·tive** \-ˈjes-tiv\ *adj*

de·con·tam·i·nate \ˌdē-kən-ˈtam-ə-ˌnāt\ *vt* **-nat·ed; -nat·ing** : to rid of contamination (as radioactive material) — **de·con·tam·i·na·tion** \-ˌtam-ə-ˈnā-shən\ *n*

¹de·cor·ti·cate \(ˈ)dē-ˈkȯrt-ə-ˌkāt\ *vt* **-cat·ed; -cat·ing** : to remove all or part of the cortex from (as the brain)

²de·cor·ti·cate \-ˌkāt, -kət\ *adj* : lacking a cortex and esp. the cerebral cortex ⟨experiments with ∼ cats⟩

de·cor·ti·ca·tion \(ˌ)dē-ˌkȯrt-i-ˈkā-shən\ *n* : the surgical removal of the cortex of an organ, an enveloping membrane, or a constrictive fibrinous covering ⟨the ∼ of a lung⟩

de·crep·i·tate \di-ˈkrep-ə-ˌtāt\ *vb* **-tat·ed; -tat·ing** *vt* : to roast or calcine (as salt) so as to cause crackling or until crackling stops ∼ *vi* : to become decrepitated — **de·crep·i·ta·tion** \-ˌkrep-ə-ˈtā-shən\ *n*

de·cu·bi·tal \di-ˈkyü-bət-ᵊl\ *adj* **1** : relating to or resulting from lying down ⟨a ∼ sore⟩ **2** : relating to or resembling a decubitus

de·cu·bi·tus \-bət-əs\ *n, pl* **-bi·ti** \-bət-ˌī, -ˌē\ **1** : a position assumed in lying down ⟨the dorsal ∼⟩ **2 a** : ULCER **b** : BEDSORE **3** : prolonged lying down (as in bed)

decubitus ulcer *n* : BEDSORE

de·cus·sate \ˈdek-ə-ˌsāt, di-ˈkəs-ˌāt\ *vb* **-sat·ed; -sat·ing** : to intersect in the form of an X

de·cus·sa·tio \ˌdē-(ˌ)kə-ˈsā-sh(ē-)ō\ *n, pl* **-sa·ti·o·nes** \-ˌsā-shē-ˈō-ˌnēz\ : DECUSSATION

de·cus·sa·tion \ˌdē-(ˌ)kə-ˈsā-shən\ *n* **1** : the action of intersecting or crossing (as of nerve fibers) esp. in the form of an X — see DECUSSATION OF PYRAMIDS **2 a** : a band of nerve fibers that connects unlike centers on opposite sides of the nervous system **b** : a crossed tract of nerve fibers passing between centers on opposite sides of the central nervous system : COMMISSURE

decussation of pyramids *n* : the crossing of the fibers of the corticospinal tracts from one side of the central nervous system to the other near the junction of the medulla and the spinal cord — called also *pyramidal decussation*

de·dif·fer·en·ti·ate \(ˈ)dē-ˌdif-ə-ˈren-chē-ˌāt\ *vi* **-at·ed; -at·ing** : to undergo dedifferentiation

de·dif·fer·en·ti·a·tion \-ˌren-chē-ˈā-shən\ *n* : reversion of specialized structures (as cells) to a more generalized or primitive condition often as a preliminary to major physiological or structural change

deep \ˈdēp\ *adj* **1 a** : extending well inward from an outer surface ⟨a ∼ gash⟩ **b** (1) : not located superficially within the body or one of its parts ⟨∼ pressure receptors in muscles⟩ (2) : resulting from or involving stimulation of deep structures ⟨∼ pain⟩ ⟨∼ reflexes⟩ **2** : being below the level of the conscious ⟨∼ neuroses⟩ — **deep·ly** *adv*

deep brachial artery *n* : the largest branch of the brachial artery in the upper part of the arm — called also *profunda artery*

deep cervical vein *n* : a tributary of the vertebral vein that drains blood esp. from the deeper parts of the back of the neck

deep epigastric artery *n* : EPIGASTRIC ARTERY b

deep external pudendal artery *n* : EXTERNAL PUDENDAL ARTERY b

deep facial vein *n* : a tributary of the facial vein that drains part of the pterygoid plexus and neighboring structures

deep fascia *n* : a firm fascia that ensheathes and binds together muscles and other internal structures — compare SUPERFICIAL FASCIA

deep femoral artery *n* : the large deep branch of the femoral artery formed where it divides about two inches (five centimeters) below the inguinal ligament — called also *profunda artery, profunda femoris, profunda femoris artery*

deep inguinal ring *n* : the internal opening of the inguinal canal — called also *internal inguinal ring*; compare SUPERFICIAL INGUINAL RING, INGUINAL RING

deep lingual artery *n* : the terminal part of the lingual artery supplying the tip of the tongue — called also *ranine artery*

deep palmar arch *n* : PALMAR ARCH a

deep peroneal nerve *n* : a nerve that arises as a branch of the common peroneal nerve where it forks between the fibula and the peroneus longus and that innervates or gives off branches innervating the muscles of the anterior part of the leg, the extensor digitorum brevis of the foot, and the skin between the big toe and the second toe — called also *anterior tibial nerve*; compare SUPERFICIAL PERONEAL NERVE

deep petrosal nerve *n* : a sympathetic nerve that originates in the carotid plexus, passes through the cartilage of the Eustachian tube, joins with the greater petrosal nerve at the entrance of the pterygoid canal to form the Vidian nerve, and as part of this nerve passes through the pterygopalatine ganglion without forming synapses to be distributed to the mucous membranes of the nasal cavity and palate

deep sedation *n* : an induced state of sedation characterized by depressed consciousness such that the patient is unable to continuously and independently maintain a patent airway and experiences a partial loss of protective reflexes and ability to respond to verbal commands or physical stimulation — compare CONSCIOUS SEDATION

deep temporal artery *n* : TEMPORAL ARTERY 1

deep temporal nerve *n* : either of two motor branches of the mandibular nerve on each side of the body that are distributed to the temporalis

C
D

deep temporal vein *n* : TEMPORAL VEIN b

deep vein thrombosis *n* : a condition marked by the formation of a thrombus within a deep vein (as of the leg or pelvis) that may be asymptomatic or be accompanied by symptoms (as swelling and pain) and that is potentially life threatening if dislodgment of the thrombus results in pulmonary embolism — abbr. *DVT*

deer·fly \'di(ə)r-ˌflī\ *n, pl* **-flies** : any of numerous small horseflies esp. of the genus *Chrysops* that include important vectors of tularemia

deerfly fever *n* : TULAREMIA

deer tick \'di(ə)r-\ *n* : a tick of the genus *Ixodes* (*I. scapularis* syn. *I. dammini*) that transmits the bacterium causing Lyme disease

deet \'dēt\ *n, often all cap* : a colorless oily liquid insect and tick repellent $C_{12}H_{17}NO$

def *abbr* **1** defecation **2** deficient **3** definite

de·fat \(ˈ)dē-ˈfat\ *vt* **de·fat·ted; de·fat·ting** : to remove fat from

def·e·cate *or chiefly Brit* **def·ae·cate** \'def-i-ˌkāt\ *vb* **-cat·ed; -cat·ing** *vt* : to discharge from the anus ∼ *vi* : to discharge feces from the bowels

def·e·ca·tion *or chiefly Brit* **def·ae·ca·tion** \ˌdef-i-ˈkā-shən\ *n* : discharge of feces

de·fect \'dē-ˌfekt, di-ˈ\ *n* : a lack or deficiency of something necessary for adequacy in form or function ⟨a hearing ∼⟩

¹de·fec·tive \di-ˈfek-tiv\ *adj* : falling below the norm in structure or in mental or physical function ⟨∼ eyesight⟩ — **de·fec·tive·ness** \-nəs\ *n*

²defective *n* : one that is subnormal physically or mentally

de·fem·i·nize *or Brit* **de·fem·i·nise** \(ˈ)dē-ˈfem-ə-ˌnīz\ *vt* **-nized** *or Brit* **-nised; -niz·ing** *or Brit* **-nis·ing** : to divest of feminine qualities or physical characteristics : MASCULINIZE — **de·fem·i·ni·za·tion** *or Brit* **de·fem·i·ni·sa·tion** \-ˌfem-ə-nə-ˈzā-shən\ *n*

de·fense *or chiefly Brit* **de·fence** \di-ˈfen(t)s\ *n* : a means or method of protecting the physical or functional integrity of body or mind ⟨ability to concentrate urine may be interpreted as a renal ∼ of body volume fluid —Jack Metcoff⟩

defense mechanism *n* **1** : an often unconscious mental process (as repression, projection, or sublimation) that makes possible compromise solutions to personal problems **2** : a defensive reaction by an organism

de·fen·sin \di-ˈfen(t)-sən\ *n* : any of a class of peptides that are found in neutrophils and have antimicrobial and cytotoxic properties

de·fen·sive \di-ˈfen(t)-siv, 'dē-ˌ\ *adj* **1** : serving to defend or protect (as the ego) ⟨face-saving is a common ∼ reaction —*Psychology Today*⟩ **2** : devoted to resisting or preventing aggression or attack ⟨∼ behavior⟩ — **de·fen·sive·ly** *adv* — **de·fen·sive·ness** *n*

defensive medicine *n* : the practice of ordering medical tests, procedures, or consultations of doubtful clinical value in order to protect the prescribing physician from malpractice suits

deferens — see DUCTUS DEFERENS, VAS DEFERENS

def·er·ent \'def-ə-rənt, -ˌer-ənt\ *adj* : of, relating to, or supplying the vas deferens ⟨∼ arteries⟩

def·er·en·tial \ˌdef-ə-ˈren-chəl\ *adj* : DEFERENT

de·fer·ox·amine \ˌdē-fə-ˈräk-sə-ˌmēn\ *n* : a chelator that is used in the form of its mesylate $C_{25}H_{48}N_6O_8 \cdot CH_4O_3S$ as an antidote to iron poisoning or overload

de·fer·ves·cence \ˌdē-(ˌ)fər-ˈves-ᵊn(t)s, ˌdef-ər-\ *n* : the subsidence of a fever — **de·fer·vesce** \-ˈves\ *vi* **-vesced; -vesc·ing**

de·fi·bril·la·tion \(ˌ)dē-ˌfib-rə-ˈlā-shən, -ˌfīb-\ *n* : restoration (as by an electric shock) of the rhythm of a fibrillating heart — **de·fi·bril·late** \(ˈ)dē-ˈfib-rə-ˌlāt, -ˈfīb-\ *vt* **-lat·ed; -lat·ing**

de·fi·bril·la·tor \(ˈ)dē-ˈfib-rə-ˌlāt-ər, -ˈfīb-\ *n* : an electronic device used to defibrillate a heart by applying an electric shock to it

de·fi·brin·ate \(ˈ)dē-ˈfib-rə-ˌnāt, -ˈfīb-\ *vt* **-at·ed; -at·ing** : to remove fibrin from (blood) — **de·fi·brin·ation** \(ˌ)dē-ˌfib-rə-ˈnā-shən, -ˌfīb-\ *n*

de·fi·cien·cy \di-ˈfish-ən-sē\ *n, pl* **-cies** **1** : a shortage of substances (as vitamins) necessary to health **2** : DELETION

deficiency anemia *n* : NUTRITIONAL ANEMIA

deficiency disease *n* : a disease (as scurvy) caused by a lack of essential dietary elements and esp. a vitamin or mineral

¹de·fi·cient \di-ˈfish-ənt\ *adj* **1** : lacking in some necessary quality or element ⟨a ∼ diet⟩ **2** : not up to a normal standard or complement ⟨∼ strength⟩ **3** : having, relating to, or characterized by a genetic deletion

²deficient *n* : one that is deficient ⟨a mental ∼⟩

de·fi·cit \'def-(ə)-sət, *Brit also* di-ˈfis-ət, 'dē-fə-sət\ *n* : a deficiency of a substance ⟨a potassium ∼⟩; *also* : a lack or impairment of a functional capacity ⟨cognitive ∼s⟩

de·fined \di-ˈfīnd\ *adj, of a culture medium* : consisting wholly of chemically identified substances in precisely determined proportions

def·i·ni·tion \ˌdef-ə-ˈnish-ən\ *n* : the action or the power of making definite and clear ⟨the ∼ of a microscope lens⟩

de·fin·i·tive \di-ˈfin-ət-iv\ *adj* : fully differentiated or developed ⟨a ∼ organ⟩

definitive host *n* : the host in which the sexual reproduction of a parasite takes place — compare INTERMEDIATE HOST 1

de·flec·tion \di-ˈflek-shən\ *n* **1** : a turning aside or deviation from a straight line **2** : the departure of an indicator or pointer from the zero reading on the scale of an instrument — **de·flect** \di-ˈflekt\ *vb*

de·flo·ra·tion \ˌdef-lə-ˈrā-shən, ˌdē-flə-\ *n* : rupture of the hymen — **de·flo·rate** \'def-lə-ˌrāt, 'dē-flə-, 'dē-flə-\ *vt* **-rat·ed; -rat·ing**

de·flo·res·cence \ˌdef-lə-ˈres-ᵊn(t)s; ˌdē-ˌflōr-ˈes-, -ˌflȯr-\ *n* : the fading or disappearance of the eruption in an exanthematous disease

de·flu·vi·um \dē-ˈflü-vē-əm\ *n* : the pathological loss of a part (as hair or nails)

de·fo·cus \(ˈ)dē-ˈfō-kəs\ *vt* **de·fo·cused; de·fo·cus·ing** : to cause to be out of focus ⟨∼ed her eye⟩ ⟨a ∼ed image⟩

deformans — see ARTHRITIS DEFORMANS, DYSTONIA MUSCULORUM DEFORMANS, OSTEITIS DEFORMANS, OSTEODYSTROPHIA DEFORMANS

de·formed \di-ˈfȯ(ə)rmd, dē-\ *adj* : misshapen esp. in body or limbs

de·for·mi·ty \di-ˈfȯr-mət-ē\ *n, pl* **-ties** **1** : the state of being deformed **2** : a physical blemish or distortion ⟨*deformities* caused by thalidomide⟩

deg *abbr* **1** degeneration **2** degree

de·gen·er·a·cy \di-ˈjen-(ə-)rə-sē\ *n, pl* **-cies** **1** : the state of being degenerate **2** : the process of becoming degenerate **3** : sexual perversion **4** : the coding of an amino acid by more than one codon of the genetic code

¹de·gen·er·ate \di-ˈjen-(ə-)rət\ *adj* **1 a** : having declined (as in nature, character, structure, or function) from an ancestral or former state; *esp* : having deteriorated progressively (as in the process of evolution) esp. through loss of structure and function **b** : having sunk to a lower and usu. corrupt and vicious state **2** : having more than one codon representing an amino acid; *also* : being such a codon

²de·gen·er·ate \di-ˈjen-ə-ˌrāt\ *vi* **-at·ed; -at·ing** **1** : to sink into a low intellectual or moral state **2** : to pass from a higher to a lower type or condition: as **a** : to gradually deteriorate so that normal function or structure is impaired or lost ⟨the retina *degenerated*⟩ **b** : to decline from the standards of a species, race, or breed **3** : to evolve or develop into a less autonomous or less functionally active form ⟨*degenerated* into dependent parasites⟩

³de·gen·er·ate \di-ˈjen-(ə-)rət\ *n* : one that is degenerate: as **a** : one degraded from the normal moral standard **b** : a sexual pervert

de·gen·er·a·tion \di-ˌjen-ə-ˈrā-shən, ˌdē-\ *n* **1** : intellectual or moral decline tending toward dissolution of character or integrity : a progressive worsening of personal adjustment

\ə\ **abut** \ᵊ\ **kitten** \ər\ **further** \a\ **ash** \ā\ **ace** \ä\ **cot, cart**
\au̇\ **out** \ch\ **chin** \e\ **bet** \ē\ **easy** \g\ **go** \i\ **hit** \ī\ **ice** \j\ **job**
\ŋ\ **sing** \ō\ **go** \ȯ\ **law** \ȯi\ **boy** \th\ **thin** \t̲h̲\ **the** \ü\ **loot**
\u̇\ **foot** \y\ **yet** \zh\ **vision** *See also* Pronunciation Symbols page

2 a : progressive deterioration of physical characters from a level representing the norm of earlier generations or forms : regression of the morphology of a group or kind of organism toward a simpler less highly organized state ⟨parasitism leads to ∼⟩ **b** : deterioration of a tissue or an organ in which its vitality is diminished or its structure impaired; *esp* : deterioration in which specialized cells are replaced by less specialized cells (as in fibrosis or in malignancies) or in which cells are functionally impaired (as by deposition of abnormal matter in the tissue)

de·gen·er·a·tive \di-'jen-ə-ˌrāt-iv, -'jen-(ə-)rət-\ *adj* : of, relating to, involving, or tending to cause degeneration ⟨∼ conditions of the nervous system —Morris Fishbein⟩ ⟨∼ changes⟩ ⟨a ∼ muscle disorder⟩

degenerative arthritis *n* : OSTEOARTHRITIS

degenerative disease *n* : a disease (as arteriosclerosis, diabetes mellitus, or osteoarthritis) characterized by progressive degenerative changes in tissue

degenerative joint disease *n* : OSTEOARTHRITIS

de·germ \(')dē-'jərm\ *vt* : to remove germs from (as the skin) — **de·germ·ation** \(')dē-ˌjər-'mā-shən\ *n*

de·glu·ti·tion \ˌdē-glü-'tish-ən, ˌdeg-lü-\ *n* : the act, power, or process of swallowing

de·glu·ti·to·ry \di-'glüt-ə-ˌtōr-ē, -ˌtòr-\ *adj* : serving for or aiding in swallowing

de·grad·able \di-'grād-ə-bəl\ *adj* : capable of being chemically degraded ⟨∼ detergents⟩ — **de·grad·abil·i·ty** \-ˌgrād-ə-'bil-ət-ē\ *n, pl* **-ties**

deg·ra·da·tion \ˌdeg-rə-'dā-shən\ *n* : change of a chemical compound to a less complex compound — **deg·ra·da·tive** \'deg-rə-ˌdāt-iv\ *adj*

de·grade \di-'grād\ *vt* **de·grad·ed; de·grad·ing** : to reduce the complexity of (a chemical compound) by splitting off one or more groups or larger components : DECOMPOSE ⟨cellulose is *degraded* by the action of some bacteria⟩ ∼ *vi* : to undergo chemical degradation

de·gran·u·la·tion \(ˌ)dē-ˌgran-yə-'lā-shən\ *n* : the process of losing granules; *specif* : the process by which cytoplasmic granules (as of mast cells) release their contents — **de·gran·u·late** \-'gran-yə-ˌlāt\ *vi* **-lat·ed; -lat·ing**

de·gree \di-'grē\ *n* **1** : a measure of damage to tissue caused by injury or disease — see FIRST-DEGREE BURN, SECOND= DEGREE BURN, THIRD-DEGREE BURN **2 a** : a title conferred on students by a college, university, or professional school on completion of a unified program of study **b** : an academic title conferred honorarily **3** : one of the divisions or intervals marked on a scale of a measuring instrument; *specif* : any of various units for measuring temperature **4** : a 360th part of the circumference of a circle — **de·greed** \-'grēd\ *adj*

de·gus·ta·tion \ˌdē-ˌgəs-'tā-shən, di-\ *n* : the action or an instance of tasting or savoring — **de·gust** \di-'gəst\ *vt*

de·hisce \di-'his\ *vi* **de·hisced; de·hisc·ing** : to undergo dehiscence

de·his·cence \di-'his-ᵊn(t)s\ *n* : the parting of the sutured lips of a surgical wound ⟨wound ∼ resulting from infection⟩

de·hu·mid·i·fy \ˌdē-hyü-'mid-ə-ˌfī, ˌdē-yü-\ *vt* **-fied; -fy·ing** : to remove moisture from (as air) — **de·hu·mid·i·fi·ca·tion** \-ˌmid-ə-fə-'kā-shən\ *n* — **de·hu·mid·i·fi·er** \-'mid-ə-ˌfī-(ə)r\ *n*

de·hy·drant \(')dē-'hī-drənt\ *n* : a dehydrating substance

de·hy·drase \(')dē-'hī-ˌdrās, -ˌdrāz\ *n* **1** : DEHYDRATASE **2** : DEHYDROGENASE

de·hy·dra·tase \(')dē-'hī-drə-ˌtās, -ˌtāz\ *n* : an enzyme that catalyzes the removal of oxygen and hydrogen from metabolites in the proportion in which they form water

de·hy·drate \(')dē-'hī-ˌdrāt\ *vb* **-drat·ed; -drat·ing** *vt* **1** : to remove bound water or hydrogen and oxygen from (a chemical compound) in the proportion in which they form water **2** : to remove water from (as foods) ∼ *vi* : to lose water or body fluids — **de·hy·dra·tor** \-ˌdrāt-ər\ *n*

dehydrated alcohol *n* : ethanol for pharmaceutical use that at 15.56°C contains not less than 99.2 percent ethanol by weight or 99.5 percent by volume and has a specific gravity of not more than 0.7964 — called also *absolute alcohol*

de·hy·dra·tion \ˌdē-hī-'drā-shən\ *n* : the process of dehydrating; *esp* : an abnormal depletion of body fluids

de·hy·dro·ace·tic acid \(ˌ)dē-ˌhī-drō-ə-ˌsēt-ik-\ *n* : a crystalline acid $C_8H_8O_4$ related to pyrone and used as a fungicide, bactericide, and plasticizer

de·hy·dro·ascor·bic acid \-ə-ˌskòr-bik-\ *n* : a crystalline oxidation product $C_6H_6O_6$ of vitamin C that occurs at times in some foodstuffs (as fruits, vegetables, and milk) and can be reduced to vitamin C

de·hy·dro·chlo·ri·nase \(ˌ)dē-ˌhī-drə-'klōr-ə-ˌnās, -'klòr-, -ˌnāz\ *n* : an enzyme that dehydrochlorinates a chlorinated hydrocarbon (as DDT) and is found esp. in some DDT resistant insects

de·hy·dro·chlo·ri·na·tion \-ˌklōr-ə-'nā-shən, -ˌklòr-\ *n* : the process of removing hydrogen and chlorine or hydrogen chloride from a compound — **de·hy·dro·chlo·ri·nate** \-'klōr-ə-ˌnāt, -'klòr-\ *vt* **-nat·ed; -nat·ing**

de·hy·dro·cho·late \-'kō-ˌlāt\ *n* : a salt of dehydrocholic acid

7–de·hy·dro·cho·les·ter·ol \'sev-ən-(ˌ)dē-ˌhī-drō-kə-'les-tə-ˌrōl, -ˌròl\ *n* : a crystalline steroid alcohol $C_{27}H_{43}OH$ that occurs (as in the skin) chiefly in higher animals and humans and that yields vitamin D_3 on irradiation with ultraviolet light

24–dehydrocholesterol \ˌtwen-tē-'fōr-, ˌtwən-, -'fòr-\ *n* : DESMOSTEROL

de·hy·dro·cho·lic acid \(ˌ)dē-ˌhī-drə-ˌkō-lik-\ *n* : a colorless crystalline acid $C_{24}H_{34}O_5$ made by the oxidation of cholic acid and used often in the form of its sodium salt $C_{24}H_{33}NaO_5$ esp. as a laxative and choleretic

11–de·hy·dro·cor·ti·co·ste·rone \i-'lev-ən-(ˌ)dē-ˌhī-drō-ˌkòrt-ə-'käs-tə-ˌrōn, -i-(ˌ)kō-stə-'; -ˌkòrt-i-kō-'sti(ə)r-ˌōn\ *n* : a steroid $C_{21}H_{28}O_4$ extracted from the adrenal cortex and also made synthetically — compare CORTISONE

de·hy·dro·epi·an·dros·ter·one \(ˌ)dē-ˌhī-drō-ˌep-ē-an-'dräs-tə-ˌrōn\ *n* : an androgenic ketosteroid $C_{19}H_{28}O_2$ secreted by the adrenal cortex that is an intermediate in the biosynthesis of testosterone — abbr. *DHA, DHEA*

de·hy·dro·ge·nase \ˌdē-(ˌ)hī-'drāj-ə-ˌnās, (')dē-'hī-drə-jə-, -ˌnāz\ *n* : an enzyme that accelerates the removal of hydrogen from metabolites and its transfer to other substances — see SUCCINATE DEHYDROGENASE

de·hy·dro·ge·nate \ˌdē-(ˌ)hī-'drāj-ə-ˌnāt, (')dē-'hī-drə-jə-\ *vt* **-nat·ed; -nat·ing** : to remove hydrogen from — **de·hy·dro·ge·na·tion** \ˌdē-(ˌ)hī-ˌdräj-ə-'nā-shən, (ˌ)dē-ˌhī-drə-jə-\ *n*

de·hy·dro·ge·nize *or Brit* **de·hy·dro·ge·nise** \(')dē-'hī-drə-jə-ˌnīz\ *vt* **-nized** *or Brit* **-nised; -niz·ing** *or Brit* **-nis·ing** : DEHYDROGENATE

de·hy·dro·iso·an·dros·ter·one \(ˌ)dē-ˌhī-drō-ˌī-sō-an-'dräs-tə-ˌrōn\ *n* : DEHYDROEPIANDROSTERONE

de·hyp·no·tize *or Brit* **de·hyp·no·tise** \(')dē-'hip-nə-ˌtīz\ *vt* **-tized** *or Brit* **-tised; -tiz·ing** *or Brit* **-tis·ing** : to remove from hypnosis

de·in·sti·tu·tion·al·iza·tion \(ˌ)dē-ˌin(t)-stə-ˌt(y)üsh-nə-lə-'zā-shən, -ˌt(y)ü-shən-ᵊl-ə-'zā-\ *n* : the release of institutionalized individuals from institutional care (as in a psychiatric hospital) to care in the community — **de·in·sti·tu·tion·al·ize** \-'t(y)üsh-nə-ˌlīz, -'t(y)ü-shən-ᵊl-ˌīz\ *vt* **-ized; -iz·ing**

de·io·din·ation \(ˌ)dē-ˌī-ə-də-'nā-shən\ *n* : the removal of iodine from a compound (as a thyroid hormone)

de·ion·ize *or Brit* **de·ion·ise** \(')dē-'ī-ə-ˌnīz\ *vt* **-ized** *or Brit* **-ised; -iz·ing** *or Brit* **-is·ing** : to remove ions from ⟨∼ water by ion exchange⟩ — **de·ion·iza·tion** \(ˌ)dē-ˌī-ə-nə-'zā-shən\ *n* — **de·ion·iz·er** \(')dē-'ī-ə-ˌnī-zər\ *n*

Dei·ters' cell \'dīt-ərz-, 'dīt-ər-səz-\ *n* **1** : CELL OF DEITERS **2** : an astrocyte of the glia

Deiters' nucleus *n* : LATERAL VESTIBULAR NUCLEUS

dé·jà vu \ˌdā-ˌzhä-'v(y)ü, dā-zhà-vœ̅\ *n* : PARAMNESIA b

de·jec·ta \di-'jek-tə\ *n pl* : FECES, EXCREMENT

de·ject·ed \di-'jek-təd\ *adj* : cast down in spirits : DEPRESSED

de·jec·tion \-'jek-shən\ *n* **1** : lowness of spirits : DEPRESSION, MELANCHOLY **2 a** : the act or process of defecating **b** : FECES, EXCREMENT

deka·gram *or* **deca·gram** *or chiefly Brit* **deca·gramme** \'dek-ə-ˌgram\ *n* : a metric unit of mass and weight equal to 10 grams

deka·li·ter *or* **deca·li·ter** *or chiefly Brit* **deca·li·tre** \-ˌlēt-ər\ *n* : a metric unit of capacity equal to 10 liters

deka·me·ter *or* **deca·me·ter** *or chiefly Brit* **deca·me·tre** \-ˌmēt-ər\ *n* : a metric unit of length equal to 10 meters

del *abbr* delusion

de·lam·i·nate \(ˈ)dē-ˈlam-ə-ˌnāt\ *vi* **-nat·ed; -nat·ing** : to undergo delamination

de·lam·i·na·tion \(ˌ)dē-ˌlam-ə-ˈnā-shən\ *n* **1** : separation into constituent layers **2** : gastrulation in which the endoderm is split off as a layer from the inner surface of the blastoderm and the archenteron is represented by the space between this endoderm and the yolk mass

de·layed hypersensitivity \di-ˈlād-\ *n* : hypersensitivity (as in a tuberculin test) which is mediated by T cells and in which the typical symptoms of inflammation and induration appear in an individual previously exposed to an antigen after an interval of 12 to 48 hours following a subsequent exposure (as by injection of the antigen under the skin)

delayed–stress disorder *n* : POST-TRAUMATIC STRESS DISORDER

delayed–stress syndrome *n* : POST-TRAUMATIC STRESS DISORDER

de·lead \(ˈ)dē-ˈled\ *vt* : to remove lead from ⟨~ a chemical⟩

del·e·te·ri·ous \ˌdel-ə-ˈtir-ē-əs\ *adj* : harmful often in a subtle or an unexpected way ⟨the ~ effects of radiation and chemotherapy on the marrow —Christine Gorman⟩ ⟨~ genes⟩

de·le·tion \di-ˈlē-shən\ *n* **1** : the absence of a section of genetic material from a gene or chromosome **2** : the mutational process that results in a deletion

delicti — see CORPUS DELICTI

de·lin·quen·cy \di-ˈliŋ-kwən-sē, -ˈlin-\ *n, pl* **-cies** : conduct that is out of accord with accepted behavior or the law; *esp* : JUVENILE DELINQUENCY

¹de·lin·quent \-kwənt\ *n* : a transgressor against duty or the law esp. in a degree not constituting crime; *specif* : JUVENILE DELINQUENT

²delinquent *adj* **1** : offending by neglect or violation of duty or of law **2** : of, relating to, or characteristic of delinquents : marked by delinquency — **de·lin·quent·ly** *adv*

del·i·ques·cence \ˌdel-i-ˈkwes-ᵊn(t)s\ *n* : the action or process of dissolving or becoming liquid esp. by a deliquescent substance; *also* : the resultant state or the liquid produced — **del·i·quesce** \-ˈkwes\ *vi* **-quesced; -quesc·ing**

del·i·ques·cent \-ᵊnt\ *adj* : tending to melt or dissolve; *esp* : tending to undergo gradual dissolution and liquefaction by the attraction and absorption of moisture from the air

¹de·lir·i·ant \di-ˈlir-ē-ənt\ *adj* : producing or tending to produce delirium

²deliriant *n* : a deliriant agent

de·lir·i·ous \di-ˈlir-ē-əs\ *adj* **1** : of, relating to, or characteristic of delirium **2** : affected with or marked by delirium — **de·lir·i·ous·ly** *adv*

de·lir·i·um \di-ˈlir-ē-əm\ *n* : a mental disturbance characterized by confusion, disordered speech, and hallucinations

delirium tre·mens \-ˈtrē-mənz, -ˈtrem-ənz\ *n* : a violent delirium with tremors that is induced by excessive and prolonged use of alcoholic liquors — called also *d.t.'s*

de·liv·er \di-ˈliv-ər\ *vb* **de·liv·ered; de·liv·er·ing** \-(ə-)riŋ\ *vt* **1 a** : to assist (a parturient female) in giving birth ⟨she was ~ed of a fine boy⟩ **b** : to aid in the birth of ⟨sometimes it is necessary to ~ a child with forceps⟩ **2** : to give birth to ⟨she ~ed a pair of healthy twins after a short labor⟩ ~ *vi* : to give birth to offspring ⟨patients that repeatedly ~ prematurely present special problems⟩

de·liv·ery \di-ˈliv-(ə-)rē\ *n, pl* **-er·ies 1** : the act of giving birth : the expulsion or extraction of a fetus and its membranes : PARTURITION **2** : the procedure of assisting birth of the fetus and expulsion of the placenta by manual, instrumental, or surgical means

delivery room *n* : a hospital room esp. equipped for the delivery of pregnant women

de·lo·mor·phous \ˌdē-lō-ˈmȯr-fəs\ *or* **de·lo·mor·phic** \-fik\ *adj* : having a definite or fixed form ⟨the parietal cells of the cardiac glands are ~⟩

de·louse \(ˈ)dē-ˈlaús, -ˈlaúz\ *vt* **de·loused; de·lous·ing** : to remove lice from

del·phi·nine \'del-fə-ˌnēn, -nən\ *n* : a poisonous crystalline alkaloid $C_{33}H_{45}NO_9$ obtained esp. from seeds of the stavesacre

del·phin·i·um \del-ˈfin-ē-əm\ *n* **1** *cap* : a large genus of the buttercup family (Ranunculaceae) that comprises chiefly perennial herbs with divided leaves and flowers in showy spikes and includes several esp. of the western U.S. that are toxic to grazing animals and esp. cattle — see LARKSPUR, STAVESACRE **2** : any plant of the genus *Delphinium*

delt \'delt\ *n* : DELTOID — usu. used in pl.

¹del·ta \'del-tə\ *n* **1** : the fourth letter of the Greek alphabet — symbol Δ or δ **2** : any of various things felt to resemble a capital Δ; *esp* : the triangular terminus of a pattern in a fingerprint formed either by bifurcation of a ridge or by divergence of two ridges that are parallel beyond it **3** : DELTA WAVE

²delta *or* **δ-** *adj* **1** : of or relating to one of four or more closely related chemical substances ⟨the ~ chain of fetal hemoglobin⟩ ⟨δ-yohimbine⟩ — used somewhat arbitrarily to specify ordinal relationship or a particular physical form and esp. one that is allotropic, isomeric, or stereoisomeric (as in δ-benzene hexachloride) **2** : fourth in position in the structure of an organic molecule from a particular group or atom; *also* : having a structure characterized by such a position ⟨δ-hydroxy acids⟩ ⟨δ-lactones⟩

delta agent *n* : HEPATITIS D VIRUS

delta hepatitis *n* : HEPATITIS D

del·ta–9–tet·ra·hy·dro·can·nab·i·nol *or* **Δ⁹–tetrahydrocannabinol** \ˈdel-tə-ˈnīn-ˌte-trə-ˌhī-drə-kə-ˈnab-ə-ˌnȯl, -ˌnōl\ *n* : THC a

del·ta–9–THC *or* **Δ⁹–THC** \-ˌtē-āch-ˈsē\ *n* : THC a

delta virus *n* : HEPATITIS D VIRUS

delta wave *n* : a high amplitude electrical rhythm of the brain with a frequency of less than 6 hertz that occurs esp. in deep sleep, in infancy, and in many diseased conditions of the brain — called also *delta, delta rhythm*

¹del·toid \'del-ˌtȯid\ *n* : a large triangular muscle that covers the shoulder joint, serves to raise the arm laterally, arises from the upper anterior part of the outer third of the clavicle and from the acromion and spine of the scapula, and is inserted into the outer side of the middle of the shaft of the humerus — called also *deltoid muscle;* see DELTOID TUBEROSITY

²deltoid *adj* : relating to, associated with, or supplying the deltoid ⟨the ~ branch of the thoracoacromial artery⟩

del·toi·de·us \del-ˈtȯid-ē-əs\ *n, pl* **-dei** \-ē-ˌē, -ˌī\ : DELTOID

deltoid ligament *n* : a strong radiating ligament of the inner aspect of the ankle that binds the base of the tibia to the bones of the foot

deltoid tuberosity *n* : a rough triangular bump on the outer side of the middle of the humerus that is the site of insertion of the deltoid

delts \'delts\ *pl of* DELT

de·lude \di-ˈlüd\ *vt* **de·lud·ed; de·lud·ing** : to mislead the mind or judgment of

de·lu·sion \di-ˈlü-zhən\ *n* **1 a** : the act of deluding : the state of being deluded **b** : an abnormal mental state characterized by the occurrence of psychotic delusions **2** : a false belief regarding the self or persons or objects outside the self that persists despite the facts and occurs in some psychotic states — compare HALLUCINATION 1, ILLUSION 2a

de·lu·sion·al \di-ˈlüzh-nəl, -ˈlü-zhən-ᵊl\ *adj* : relating to, based on, or affected by delusions ⟨a ~ patient⟩

delusion of reference *n* : IDEA OF REFERENCE

\ə\ **abut** \ᵊ\ **kitten** \ər\ **further** \a\ **ash** \ā\ **ace** \ä\ **cot, cart**
\aú\ **out** \ch\ **chin** \e\ **bet** \ē\ **easy** \g\ **go** \i\ **hit** \ī\ **ice** \j\ **job**
\ŋ\ **sing** \ō\ **go** \ȯ\ **law** \ȯi\ **boy** \th\ **thin** \t̲h̲\ **the** \ü\ **loot**
\ú\ **foot** \y\ **yet** \zh\ **vision** *See also* Pronunciation Symbols page

C
D

De·man·sia \di-'man(t)-sē-ə\ *n* : a genus of snakes of the family Elapidae comprising the venomous Australian brown snake and related forms

van Die·men \vän-'dē-mən\, **Anthony (1593–1645)**, Dutch colonial administrator. Van Diemen was governor-general of the Dutch East Indies from 1636. During his tenure he greatly extended Dutch commerce and influence in the area under his control. In 1842 the genus *Demansia* was named in his honor by the British naturalist John Edward Gray (1800–1875).

de·mar·cate \di-'mär-ˌkāt, 'dē-ˌ\ *vt* **-cat·ed; -cat·ing 1** : to mark or determine the limits of **2** : to set apart clearly or distinctly as if by definite limits or boundaries — **de·mar·ca·tion** *also* **de·mar·ka·tion** \ˌdē-ˌmär-'kā-shən\ *n*

demarcation potential *n* : INJURY POTENTIAL

de·mas·cu·lin·ize *also Brit* **de·mas·cu·lin·ise** \(ˌ)dē-'mas-kyə-lə-ˌnīz, di-\ *vt* **-ized** *also Brit* **-ised; -iz·ing** *also Brit* **-is·ing** : to remove the masculine character or qualities of — **de·mas·cu·lin·iza·tion** *also Brit* **de·mas·cu·lin·isa·tion** \-ˌmas-kyə-lə-nə-'zā-shən, -ˌnī-'\ *n*

dem·e·car·i·um \ˌdem-i-'kar-ē-əm, -'ker-\ *n* : a long-acting cholinesterase-inhibiting quaternary ammonium compound that is a derivative of neostigmine and is used as the bromide $C_{32}H_{52}Br_2N_4O_4$ in an ophthalmic solution esp. in the treatment of glaucoma and esotropia

de·mec·lo·cy·cline \ˌdem-ə-klō-'sī-ˌklēn\ *n* : a broad-spectrum tetracycline antibiotic produced by an actinomycete of the genus *Streptomyces* (*S. aureofaciens*) and used esp. in the form of its hydrochloride $C_{21}H_{21}ClN_2O_8 \cdot HCl$

de·ment·ed \di-'ment-əd\ *adj* **1** : MAD, INSANE **2** : suffering from or exhibiting cognitive dementia — **de·ment·ed·ly** *adv* — **de·ment·ed·ness** *n*

de·men·tia \di-'men-chə\ *n* : a usu. progressive condition (as Alzheimer's disease) marked by the development of multiple cognitive deficits (as memory impairment, aphasia, and inability to plan and initiate complex behavior) — **de·men·tial** \-chəl\ *adj*

dementia par·a·lyt·i·ca \-ˌpar-ə-'lit-i-kə\ *n, pl* **de·men·ti·ae par·a·lyt·i·cae** \di-'men-chē-ˌē-ˌpar-ə-'lit-i-ˌsē\ : GENERAL PARESIS

dementia prae·cox \-'prē-ˌkäks\ *n* : SCHIZOPHRENIA

dementia pu·gi·lis·ti·ca \-ˌpyü-jə-'lis-tə-kə\ *n* : a syndrome affecting boxers that is caused by cumulative cerebral injuries and is characterized by impaired cognitive processes (as thinking and remembering, impaired and often slurred speech, and slow poorly coordinated movements esp. of the legs

de·ment·ing \di-'ment-iŋ\ *adj* : causing or characterized by dementia ⟨memory loss, confusion and disorientation . . . are common symptoms of ∼ illness —Abigail Van Buren⟩

Dem·er·ol \'dem-ə-ˌról, -ˌrōl\ *trademark* — used for meperidine

de·meth·yl·a·tion \(ˌ)dē-ˌme-thə-'lā-shən\ *n* : the process of removing a methyl group from a chemical compound — **de·meth·yl·ate** \(')dē-'me-thə-ˌlāt\ *vt* **-at·ed; -at·ing**

demi·lune \'dem-ē-ˌlün\ *n* : one of the small crescentic groups of granular deeply staining zymogen-secreting cells lying between the clearer mucus-producing cells and the basement membrane in the alveoli of mixed salivary glands — called also *crescent of Giannuzzi*

demilune of Gian·nuz·zi *also* **demilune of Gia·nuz·zi** \-jä-'nüt-sē\ *n* : DEMILUNE

Giannuzzi, Giuseppe (1839–1876), Italian anatomist. Giannuzzi undertook significant research into several areas of anatomy and physiology. He is best known for his discovery of the demilunes or crescents which are now identified with both him and Heidenhain.

demilune of Hei·den·hain \-'hīd-ᵊn-ˌhīn\ *n* : DEMILUNE

Heidenhain, Rudolf Peter Heinrich (1834–1897), German histologist and physiologist. Heidenhain studied glandular secretions in the salivary glands, pancreas, breast, and stomach. He formulated a law of glandular secretion, which states that secretion always involves a change in the structure of the gland. He considered all secretory phenomena to be intracellular processes. Heidenhain is also known for his descriptions of the columnar cells of the uriniferous tubules (1861), of certain large border cells of the gastric glands (1870), and the crescentic cells or demilunes of the mucous glands.

de·min·er·al·iza·tion *also Brit* **de·min·er·al·isa·tion** \(ˌ)dē-ˌmin-(ə-)rə-lə-'zā-shən\ *n* **1** : loss of minerals (as salts of calcium) from the body esp. in disease **2** : the process of removing mineral matter or salts (as from water) — **de·min·er·al·ize** *also Brit* **de·min·er·al·ise** \(ˌ)dē-'min-(ə-)rə-ˌlīz\ *vt* **-ized** *also Brit* **-ised; -iz·ing** *also Brit* **-is·ing**

dem·o·dec·tic \ˌdem-ə-'dek-tik\ *adj* **1** : of or relating to the genus *Demodex* **2** : caused by mites of the genus *Demodex*

demodectic mange *n* : mange caused by mites of the genus *Demodex* that burrow in the hair follicles esp. of dogs causing pustule formation and spreading bald patches — compare CHORIOPTIC MANGE, SARCOPTIC MANGE

de·mo·dex \'dem-ə-ˌdeks, 'dēm-\ *n* **1** *cap* : a genus (coextensive with a family Demodicidae) of minute elongated cylindrical mites with the legs greatly reduced that live in the hair follicles esp. about the face of humans and various furred mammals and in the latter often cause demodectic mange **2** : any mite of the genus *Demodex* : FOLLICLE MITE

dem·o·di·co·sis \ˌdem-ō-də-'kō-səs\ *n, pl* **-co·ses** \-ˌsēz\ : DEMODECTIC MANGE

de·mo·graph·ic \ˌdē-mə-'graf-ik, ˌdem-ə-\ *adj* **1** : of or relating to demography **2** : relating to the dynamic balance of a population esp. with regard to density and capacity for expansion or decline — **de·mo·graph·i·cal·ly** \-i-k(ə-)lē\ *adv*

de·mog·ra·phy \di-'mäg-rə-fē\ *n, pl* **-phies** : the statistical study of human populations esp. with reference to size and density, distribution, and vital statistics — **de·mog·ra·pher** \-fər\ *n*

de·mon·o·ma·nia \ˌdē-mə-nə-'mā-nē-ə, -nyə\ *n* : a delusion of being possessed by evil spirits

dem·on·strate \'dem-ən-ˌstrāt\ *vb* **-strat·ed; -strat·ing** *vt* **1** : to show clearly ⟨*demonstrated* the artery arteriographically⟩ **2** : to prove or make clear by reasoning or evidence ∼ *vi* : to make a demonstration

dem·on·stra·tion \ˌdem-ən-'strā-shən\ *n* : an act, process, or means of demonstrating to the intelligence; *esp* : a proof by experiment ⟨a ∼ of the neutralization of an acid by a base⟩

dem·on·stra·tor \'dem-ən-ˌstrāt-ər\ *n* : a teacher or teacher's assistant who demonstrates principles or theories studied (as by dissection, experiment, or chemical preparation)

¹de·mul·cent \di-'məl-sᵊnt\ *adj* : tending to soothe or soften ⟨∼ expectorants which give a protective coating to the throat —*Therapeutic Notes*⟩

²demulcent *n* : a usu. mucilaginous or oily substance (as tragacanth) capable of soothing or protecting an abraded mucous membrane

de·my·elin·at·ing \(')dē-'mī-ə-lə-ˌnāt-iŋ\ *adj* : causing or characterized by the loss or destruction of myelin ⟨∼ diseases⟩ ⟨a ∼ agent⟩

de·my·eli·na·tion \(ˌ)dē-ˌmī-ə-lə-'nā-shən\ *n* : the state resulting from the loss or destruction of myelin; *also* : the process of such loss or destruction

de·my·elin·iza·tion *or Brit* **de·my·elin·isa·tion** \-lə-nə-'zā-shən\ *n* : DEMYELINATION

de·na·tur·ant \(')dē-'nāch-(ə-)rənt\ *n* : a denaturing agent

de·na·tur·ation \(ˌ)dē-ˌnā-chə-'rā-shən\ *n* : the process of denaturing

de·na·ture \(')dē-'nā-chər\ *vb* **de·na·tured; de·na·tur·ing** \-'nāch-(ə-)riŋ\ *vt* : to deprive of natural qualities: as **a** : to make (alcohol) unfit for drinking (as by adding an obnoxious substance) without impairing usefulness for other purposes **b** : to modify the molecular structure of (as a protein or DNA) esp. by heat, acid, alkali, or ultraviolet radiation so as to destroy or diminish some of the original properties and esp. the specific biological activity ∼ *vi* : to become denatured

den·dri·form \'den-drə-ˌform\ *adj* : resembling a tree in structure

den·drite \'den-ˌdrīt\ *n* : any of the usu. branching protoplasmic processes that conduct impulses toward the body of a nerve cell — **den·drit·ic** \den-'drit-ik\ *adj*

dendritic cell *n* : any of various antigen-presenting cells with long irregular processes

den·dro·den·drit·ic \ˌden-drō-ˌden-'drit-ik\ *adj* : relating to or being a nerve synapse between a dendrite of one cell and a dendrite of another

den·droid \'den-ˌdrȯid\ *adj* : resembling a tree in form or in pattern of growth ⟨∼ colonies of algae⟩

den·dron \'den-drən, -ˌdrän\ *n, pl* **dendrons** *also* **den·dra** \-drə\ : DENDRITE

de·ner·vate \'dē-(ˌ)nər-ˌvāt\ *vt* **-vat·ed; -vat·ing** : to deprive of a nerve supply (as by cutting a nerve) — **de·ner·va·tion** \ˌdē-(ˌ)nər-'vā-shən\ *n*

den·gue \'deŋ-gē, -ˌgā\ *n* : an acute infectious disease that is characterized by headache, severe joint pain, and a rash and that is caused by a single-stranded RNA virus of the genus *Flavivirus* (species *Dengue virus*) transmitted by mosquitoes of the genus *Aedes* — called also *breakbone fever, dandy fever, dengue fever*

dengue hemorrhagic fever *n* : dengue marked by hemorrhagic symptoms (as hemorrhagic lesions of the skin, thrombocytopenia, and reduction in the fluid part of the blood) — called also *hemorrhagic dengue*

de·ni·al \di-'nī(-ə)l\ *n* : a psychological defense mechanism in which confrontation with a personal problem or with reality is avoided by denying the existence of the problem or reality

den·i·da·tion \ˌden-ə-'dā-shən\ *n* : the sloughing of the endometrium of the uterus esp. during menstruation

Den·i·so·nia \ˌden-ə-'sō-nē-ə, -nyə\ *n* : a genus of venomous Australian snakes of the family Elapidae including the copperhead (*D. superba*)

> **Den·i·son** \'den-ə-sən\, **Sir William Thomas (1804–1871),** Australian statesman. Denison was governor of New South Wales from 1854 to 1861. In his spare time he was an avid conchologist. In 1860 he appointed as a curator of the Australian Museum Johann Ludwig Gerard Krefft (1830–1881). Krefft was an all-around zoologist but specialized in snakes. His published works include some 200 articles and a book-length work on the snakes of Australia. One of the species described was the Australian copperhead, which he named *Denisonia superba* after his benefactor.

de·ni·tri·fi·ca·tion \(ˌ)dē-ˌnī-trə-fə-'kā-shən\ *n* : the loss or removal of nitrogen or nitrogen compounds; *specif* : reduction of nitrates or nitrites commonly by bacteria (as in soil) that usu. results in the escape of nitrogen into the air — **de·ni·tri·fy** \(')dē-'nī-trə-ˌfī\ *vt* **-fied; -fy·ing**

de·ni·tri·fi·er \(')dē-'nī-trə-ˌfī(-ə)r\ *n* : a denitrifying agent (as a denitrifying bacterium)

denitrifying bacteria *n pl* : various bacteria (as *Thiobacillus denitrificans* and *Paracoccus denitrificans*) that bring about denitrification — used esp. of forms that reduce nitrates to nitrites or nitrites to nitrogen gas (as many common putrefactive organisms of manure and soil)

de·ni·trog·e·nate \(ˌ)dē-ˌnī-'träj-ə-ˌnāt\ *vt* **-nat·ed; -nat·ing** : to reduce the stored nitrogen in the body by forced breathing of pure oxygen for a period of time esp. as a measure designed to prevent development of decompression sickness — **de·ni·trog·e·na·tion** \-ˌträj-ə-'nā-shən\ *n*

dens \'denz\ *n, pl* **den·tes** \'den-ˌtēz\ : a toothlike process that projects from the anterior end of the centrum of the axis in the spinal column, serves as a pivot on which the atlas rotates, and is morphologically the centrum of the atlas though detached from that vertebra and more or less perfectly united with the next one behind — called also *odontoid process*

densa — see MACULA DENSA

den·sim·e·ter \'den-'sim-ət-ər\ *n* : an instrument for determining mass density or specific gravity — **den·si·met·ric** \ˌden(t)-sə-'me-trik\ *adj*

den·si·tom·e·ter \ˌden(t)-sə-'täm-ət-ər\ *n* : an instrument for determining optical, photographic, or mass density ⟨diag-

nose osteoporosis using an X-ray bone ∼⟩ — **den·si·to·met·ric** \ˌden(t)-sət-ə-'me-trik\ *adj* — **den·si·tom·e·try** \ˌden(t)-sə-'täm-ə-trē\ *n, pl* **-tries**

den·si·ty \'den(t)-sət-ē, -stē\ *n, pl* **-ties 1** : the quantity per unit volume, unit area, or unit length: as **a** : the mass of a substance per unit volume **b** : the distribution of a quantity (as mass, electricity, or energy) per unit usu. of space **c** : the average number of individuals or units per space unit ⟨a population ∼ of 500 per square mile⟩ **2 a** : the degree of opacity of a translucent medium **b** : ABSORBANCE

dent *abbr* dental; dentist; dentistry

den·tal \'dent-ᵊl\ *adj* **1** : relating to, specializing in, or used in dentistry ⟨∼ surgery⟩ ⟨∼ students⟩ **2** : relating to or used on the teeth ⟨∼ paste⟩ — **den·tal·ly** \-ē\ *adv*

dental arch *n* : the curve of the row of teeth in each jaw — called also *arcade*

dental artery *n* : any of the several small arteries (as the inferior alveolar artery) derived from the maxillary artery that supply the teeth and adjacent parts

dental dam *n* : a rubber dam used in dentistry

dental en·gine \-'en-jən\ *n* : a dentist's drilling machine for rotating drills, burs, or other instruments at high speed

dental floss *n* : a waxed thread used to clean between the teeth

dental formula *n* : an abridged expression for the number and kind of teeth of mammals in which the kind of teeth are represented by *i* (incisor), *c* (canine), *pm* (premolar) or *b* (bicuspid), and *m* (molar) and the number in each jaw is written like a fraction with the figures above the horizontal line showing the number in the upper jaw and those below the number in the lower jaw and with a dash separating the figures representing the teeth on each side of the jaw ⟨the *dental formula* of a human adult is

$$i\ \frac{2-2}{2-2},\ c\ \frac{1-1}{1-1},\ b\ or\ pm\ \frac{2-2}{2-2},\ m\ \frac{3-3}{3-3} = 32⟩$$

dental hygienist *n* : a person who assists a dentist esp. in cleaning teeth

dental index *n* : a measure of the relative size of teeth that is obtained by finding the distance from the anterior surface of the first premolar tooth to the posterior surface of the last molar, dividing by the distance from the nasion to the basion, and multiplying by 100

dental lamina *n* : a linear zone of epithelial cells of the covering of each embryonic jaw that grows down into the developing gums and gives rise to the enamel organs of the teeth — called also *dental ridge*

dental nerve — see INFERIOR ALVEOLAR NERVE

dental papilla *n* : the mass of mesenchyme that occupies the cavity of each enamel organ and gives rise to the dentin and the pulp of the tooth

dental plate *n* : DENTURE 2

dental pulp *n* : the highly vascular sensitive tissue occupying the central cavity of a tooth

dental sac *n* : the mesenchymal investment of the developing tooth and enamel organ that differentiates into cementoblasts about the dentin and forms a connective tissue sheath about the enamel organ

dental surgeon *n* : DENTIST; *esp* : one engaging in oral surgery

dental technician *n* : a technician who makes dental appliances

den·tate \'den-ˌtāt\ *adj* : having teeth or pointed conical projections

dentate gyrus *n* : a narrow strip of cortex associated with the hippocampal sulcus that continues forward to the uncus

dentate ligament *n* : DENTICULATE LIGAMENT

dentate nucleus *n* : a large laminar nucleus of gray matter forming an incomplete capsule within the white matter of each cerebellar hemisphere

---

C
D

dentes pl of DENS
den·ti·cle \'dent-i-kəl\ n : PULP STONE
den·tic·u·late \den-'tik-yə-lət\ or **den·tic·u·lat·ed** \-ˌlāt-əd\ adj : finely dentate or serrate
denticulate ligament n : a band of fibrous pia mater extending along the spinal cord on each side between the dorsal and ventral roots — called also *dentate ligament*
den·ti·frice \'dent-ə-frəs\ n : a powder, paste, or liquid for cleaning the teeth
den·tig·er·ous \den-'tij-ə-rəs\ adj : bearing teeth or structures resembling teeth
dentigerous cyst n : an epithelial cyst containing fluid and one or more imperfect teeth usu. thought to result from defects in the enamel-forming structures
den·tin \'dent-°n\ or **den·tine** \'den-ˌtēn, den-'tēn\ n : a calcareous material similar to bone but harder and denser that composes the principal mass of a tooth, is formed by the odontoblasts of the surface of the dental papilla, and consists of a matrix containing minute parallel tubules which open into the pulp cavity and during life contain processes of the cells of the pulp — compare CEMENTUM, ENAMEL — **den·tin·al** \'dent-°n-əl; 'den-ˌtēn-°l, den-'\ adj
dentinal tubule n : one of the minute parallel tubules of the dentin of a tooth that communicate with the dental pulp
den·tino·blast \den-'tē-nə-ˌblast\ n : a mesenchymal cell that forms dentin
den·tino·enam·el \den-ˌtē-nō-i-'nam-əl\ adj : relating to or connecting the dentin and enamel of a tooth
den·tino·gen·e·sis \den-ˌtē-nə-'jen-ə-səs\ n, pl **-e·ses** \-ˌsēz\ : the formation of dentin
dentinogenesis im·per·fec·ta \-ˌim-pər-'fek-tə\ n : a disorder of tooth development inherited as an autosomal dominant and characterized by relatively soft enamel in both the primary and permanent teeth that makes the teeth abnormally vulnerable to fracture, abrasion, and wear
den·tino·gen·ic \ˌdent-°n-ō-'jen-ik\ adj : forming dentin
den·ti·noid \den-'tē-ˌnòid\ n : the immature still uncalcified matrix of dentin
den·ti·no·ma \ˌdent-°n-'ō-mə\ n, pl **-mas** also **-ma·ta** \-mət-ə\ : an odontoma containing dentin
den·tist \'dent-əst\ n : a licensed practitioner who is skilled in the prevention, diagnosis, and treatment of diseases, injuries, and malformations of the teeth, jaws, and mouth and who makes and inserts false teeth
den·tist·ry \'dent-ə-strē\ n, pl **-ries** : the art or profession of a dentist
den·ti·tion \den-'tish-ən\ n **1** : the development and cutting of teeth **2** : the character of a set of teeth esp. with regard to their number, kind, and arrangement **3** : TEETH
den·to·al·ve·o·lar \ˌdent-ō-al-'vē-ə-lər\ adj : of, relating to, or involving the teeth and their sockets ⟨~ structures⟩
den·to·fa·cial \ˌdent-ə-'fā-shəl\ adj : of or relating to the dentition and face
den·to·gin·gi·val \-'jin-jə-vəl\ adj : of, relating to, or connecting the teeth and the gums ⟨the ~ junction⟩
den·toid \'den-ˌtòid\ adj : resembling a tooth : ODONTOID
den·tu·lous \'den-chə-ləs\ adj : having teeth
den·ture \'den-chər\ n **1** : a set of teeth **2** : an artificial replacement for one or more teeth; esp : a set of false teeth — called also *dental plate*
den·tur·ism \'den-chə-ˌriz-əm\ n : the practice or profession of a denturist
den·tur·ist \-rəst\ n : a dental technician who makes, fits, and repairs dentures directly for the public
de·nu·da·tion \ˌdē-n(y)ü-'dā-shən, ˌden-yù-\ n : the act or process of removing surface layers (as of skin) or an outer covering (as of myelin); also : the condition that results from this — **de·nude** \di-'n(y)üd\ vt **de·nud·ed; de·nud·ing**
¹de·odor·ant \dē-'ōd-ə-rənt\ adj : destroying or masking offensive odors
²deodorant n : any of various preparations or solutions (as a soap or disinfectant) that destroy or mask unpleasant odors; esp : a cosmetic that neutralizes perspiration odors
de·odor·ize or Brit **de·odor·ise** \dē-'ōd-ə-ˌrīz\ vt **-ized** or Brit

-ised; -iz·ing or Brit **-is·ing** : to eliminate or prevent the offensive odor of — **de·odor·iza·tion** or Brit **de·odor·isa·tion** \-ˌōd-ə-rə-'zā-shən\ n — **de·odor·iz·er** or Brit **de·odor·is·er** n
de·on·tol·o·gy \ˌdē-ˌän-'täl-ə-jē\ n, pl **-gies** : the theory or study of moral obligation — **de·on·to·log·i·cal** \ˌdē-ˌänt-°l-'äj-i-kəl\ adj — **de·on·tol·o·gist** \ˌdē-ˌän-'täl-ə-jəst\ n
de·ox·i·da·tion \(ˌ)dē-ˌäk-sə-'dā-shən\ n : the process of deoxidizing; also : the state of being deoxidized
de·ox·i·dize or Brit **de·ox·i·dise** \(')dē-'äk-sə-ˌdīz\ vt **-dized** or Brit **-dised; -diz·ing** or Brit **-dis·ing** : to remove oxygen from — **de·ox·i·diz·er** or Brit **de·ox·i·dis·er** \-ˌdī-zər\ n
de·oxy \(ˌ)dē-'äk-sē\ also **des·oxy** \(ˌ)des-\ adj : containing less oxygen per molecule than the compound from which it is derived ⟨~ sugars⟩ — usu. used in combination ⟨*deoxy*ribonucleic acid⟩ ⟨*desoxy*corticosterone⟩
de·oxy·cho·late \(ˌ)dē-ˌäk-sē-'kō-ˌlāt\ also **des·oxy·cho·late** \ˌdes-\ n : a salt or ester of deoxycholic acid
de·oxy·cho·lic acid \(ˌ)dē-ˌäk-sē-ˌkō-lik-\ or **des·oxy·cho·lic acid** \ˌdes-\ n : a crystalline acid $C_{24}H_{40}O_4$ found esp. in bile and used as a choleretic and digestant and in the synthesis of adrenocortical hormones (as cortisone)
deoxycorticosterone var of DESOXYCORTICOSTERONE
deoxycortone chiefly Brit var of DESOXYCORTONE
de·oxy·cy·ti·dine \(ˌ)dē-ˌäk-sē-'sit-ə-ˌdēn, -'sīt-\ n : a nucleoside consisting of cytosine combined with deoxyribose that occurs esp. as a component of DNA
de·ox·y·gen·ate \(ˌ)dē-'äk-si-jə-ˌnāt, ˌdē-äk-'sij-ə-\ vt **-at·ed; -at·ing** : to remove oxygen from — **de·ox·y·gen·ation** \(ˌ)dē-ˌäk-si-jə-'nā-shən, ˌdē-äk-ˌsij-ə-\ n
de·ox·y·gen·at·ed adj : having the hemoglobin in the reduced state
de·oxy·ri·bo·nu·cle·ase \(')dē-'äk-si-ˌrī-bō-'n(y)ü-klē-ˌās, -ˌāz\ also **des·oxy·ri·bo·nu·cle·ase** \(')des-\ n : an enzyme that hydrolyzes DNA to nucleotides — called also *DNase*
de·oxy·ri·bo·nu·cle·ic acid \(')dē-'äk-si-ˌrī-bō-n(y)ü-ˌklē-ik-, -ˌklā-\ also **des·oxy·ri·bo·nu·cle·ic acid** \(')des-\ n : DNA
de·oxy·ri·bo·nu·cleo·pro·tein \(ˌ)dē-ˌäk-sē-ˌrī-bō-ˌn(y)ü-klē-ō-'prō-ˌtēn, -'prōt-ē-ən\ also **des·oxy·ri·bo·nu·cleo·pro·tein** \ˌdes-\ n : a nucleoprotein that yields DNA on hydrolysis
de·oxy·ri·bo·nu·cle·o·tide also **des·oxy·ri·bo·nu·cle·o·tide** \-'n(y)ü-klē-ə-ˌtīd\ n : a nucleotide that contains deoxyribose and is a constituent of DNA
de·oxy·ri·bose \(ˌ)dē-ˌäk-si-'rī-ˌbōs, -ˌbōz\ also **des·oxy·ri·bose** \ˌdes-\ n : a pentose sugar $C_5H_{10}O_4$ that is a structural element of DNA
Dep·a·kene \'dep-ə-ˌkēn\ trademark — used for a preparation of valproic acid
De·pa·kote \'dep-ə-ˌkōt\ trademark — used for a preparation of divalproex sodium
de·pan·cre·atize \(')dē-'paŋ-krē-ə-ˌtīz, -'pan-\ vt **-atized; -atiz·ing** : to deprive of the pancreas and thereby induce inability to utilize glucose and impair the digestion of fats
de·pen·dence \di-'pen-dən(t)s\ n **1** : the quality or state of being dependent upon or unduly subject to the influence of another **2 a** : drug addiction **b** : HABITUATION 2b
de·pen·den·cy \-dən-sē\ n, pl **-cies** : DEPENDENCE
¹de·pen·dent \di-'pen-dənt\ adj **1** : unable to exist, sustain oneself, or act appropriately or normally without the assistance or direction of another **2** : affected with a drug dependence **3** : affecting the lower part of the body and esp. the legs ⟨~ edema⟩ — **de·pen·dent·ly** adv
²dependent also **dependant** n : one that is dependent (as on drugs or a person)
dependent drainage n : the process of draining from a higher to a lower place under the influence of gravity ⟨gauze wicks are inserted in the wound to facilitate *dependent drainage* —D. N. Gerding et al⟩
dependent lividity n : a purplish color assumed by the lowest-lying parts of a recently dead body due to the downward flow and pooling of blood under the influence of gravity

de·per·son·al·iza·tion *or Brit* **de·per·son·al·isa·tion** \(ˌ)dē-ˌpər-snə-lə-ˈzā-shən, -ˌpərs-ᵊn-ə-lə-\ *n* : the act or process of causing or the state resulting from loss of the sense of personal identity; *esp* : a psychopathological syndrome characterized by loss of identity and feelings of unreality or strangeness about one's own behavior — **de·per·son·al·ize** *or Brit* **de·per·son·al·ise** \(ˈ)dē-ˈpər-snə-ˌlīz, -ˈpərs-ᵊn-ə-\ *vt* **-ized** *or Brit* **-ised; -iz·ing** *or Brit* **-is·ing**

de·phos·phor·y·la·tion \(ˌ)dē-ˌfäs-ˌfȯr-ə-ˈlā-shən\ *n* : the process of removing phosphate groups from an organic compound (as ATP) by hydrolysis; *also* : the resulting state — **de·phos·phor·y·late** \(ˈ)dē-fäs-ˈfȯr-ə-ˌlāt\ *vt* **-lat·ed; -lat·ing**

de·pig·men·ta·tion \(ˌ)dē-ˌpig-mən-ˈtā-shən, -ˌmen-\ *n* : loss of normal pigmentation

de·pig·ment·ed \(ˈ)dē-ˈpig-mənt-əd, -ˌment-\ *adj* : having undergone depigmentation : deprived of pigment ⟨~ skin⟩

de·pig·ment·ing \-iŋ\ *adj* : causing or used to produce depigmentation ⟨a ~ agent⟩

dep·i·la·tion \ˌdep-ə-ˈlā-shən\ *n* : the removal of hair, wool, or bristles by chemical or mechanical methods — **dep·i·late** \ˈdep-ə-ˌlāt\ *vt* **-lat·ed; -lat·ing**

¹de·pil·a·to·ry \di-ˈpil-ə-ˌtōr-ē, -ˌtȯr-\ *adj* : having the power to remove hair

²depilatory *n* : a cosmetic for the temporary removal of undesired hair

de·plete \di-ˈplēt\ *vt* **de·plet·ed; de·plet·ing** : to empty (as the blood vessels) of a principal substance ⟨a body *depleted* by excessive blood loss⟩ ⟨tissues *depleted* of vitamins⟩

de·ple·tion \di-ˈplē-shən\ *n* : the act or process of depleting or the state of being depleted: as **a** : the reduction or loss of blood, body fluids, chemical constituents, or stored materials from the body (as by hemorrhage or malnutrition) **b** : a debilitated state caused by excessive loss of body fluids or other constituents

de·po·lar·iza·tion *or Brit* **de·po·lar·isa·tion** \(ˌ)dē-ˌpō-lə-rə-ˈzā-shən\ *n* : loss of polarization; *esp* : loss of the difference in charge between the inside and outside of the plasma membrane of a muscle or nerve cell due to a change in permeability and migration of sodium ions to the interior

de·po·lar·ize *or Brit* **de·po·lar·ise** \(ˈ)dē-ˈpō-lə-ˌrīz\ *vt* **-ized** *or Brit* **-ised; -iz·ing** *or Brit* **-is·ing** : to subject (as a plasma membrane) to depolarization — **de·po·lar·iz·er** *or Brit* **de·po·lar·is·er** \-ˌrī-zər\ *n*

de·po·lym·er·ase \ˌdē-pə-ˈlim-ə-ˌrās, -ˌrāz; -ˈpäl-ə-mə-ˌrās, -ˌrāz\ *n* : any of various enzymes (as nucleases) that bring about depolymerization

de·po·ly·mer·ize *or Brit* **de·po·ly·mer·ise** \(ˈ)dē-pə-ˈlim-ə-ˌrīz, -ˈpäl-ə-mə-\ *vb* **-ized** *or Brit* **-ised; -iz·ing** *or Brit* **-is·ing** *vt* : to decompose (macromolecules) into relatively simple compounds (as monomers) ⟨*depolymerized* nucleic acids⟩ ~ *vi* : to undergo decomposition into simpler compounds — **de·po·ly·mer·iza·tion** *or Brit* **de·po·ly·mer·isa·tion** \ˌdē-pə-ˌlim-ə-rə-ˈzā-shən, (ˌ)dē-ˌpäl-ə-mə-rə-\ *n*

Depo–Pro·vera \ˈdep-ō-prō-ˈver-ə\ *trademark* — used for an aqueous suspension of medroxyprogesterone acetate

¹de·pos·it \di-ˈpäz-ət\ *vt* **de·pos·it·ed** \-ˈpäz-ət-əd, -ˈpäz-təd\; **de·pos·it·ing** \-ˈpäz-ət-iŋ, -ˈpäz-tiŋ\ : to lay down or foster the accumulation of as a deposit ⟨crystals are ~*ed* in the articular cartilage, the synovium, and the capsule —*Med. Radiography & Photography*⟩

²deposit *n* : matter laid down or accumulated esp. in a living organism by a normal or abnormal process ⟨removal of calcium ~*s* in his knees by arthroscopic surgery⟩

de·po·si·tion \ˌdep-ə-ˈzi-shən, ˌdē-pə-\ *n* **1** : a process of depositing something ⟨the ~ and clearance of a metabolic product⟩ **2** : something deposited : DEPOSIT ⟨beta-amyloid ~*s* in Alzheimer's disease⟩

¹de·pot \ˈdep-(ˌ)ō, ˈdēp-\ *n* : a bodily location where a substance is stored usu. for later utilization ⟨fat ~*s* as a source of energy⟩

²depot *adj* : being in storage ⟨~ fat⟩; *also* : acting over a prolonged period ⟨~ insulin⟩

depr *abbr* depression

dep·re·nyl \ˈdep-rə-ˌnil\ *n* : an optically active compound $C_{13}H_{17}N$ that is a monoamine oxidase inhibitor; *esp* : SELEGILINE

de·press \di-ˈpres\ *vt* **1** : to diminish the activity, strength, or yield of ⟨able to ~ irritability of the heart muscle by the use of such a drug as procaine⟩ **2** : to lower in spirit or mood

¹de·pres·sant \-ᵊnt\ *adj* : tending to depress; *esp* : lowering or tending to lower functional or vital activity ⟨a drug with a ~ effect on heart rate⟩

²depressant *n* : one that depresses; *specif* : an agent that reduces bodily functional activity or an instinctive desire (as appetite) ⟨a ~ of intestinal spasm⟩

de·pressed \di-ˈprest\ *adj* **1** : low in spirits; *specif* : affected by psychological depression ⟨a severely ~ patient⟩ **2 a** : having the central part lower than the margin ⟨a ~ pustule⟩ **b** : dorsoventrally flattened ⟨the tapeworm is a ~ animal —R. A. Wardle & J. A. McLeod⟩

depressed fracture *n* : a fracture esp. of the skull in which the fragment is depressed below the normal surface

de·pres·sion \di-ˈpresh-ən\ *n* **1** : a displacement downward or inward ⟨~ of the jaw⟩ **2** : an act of depressing or a state of being depressed: as **a** (1) : a state of feeling sad (2) : a psychoneurotic or psychotic disorder marked esp. by sadness, inactivity, difficulty with thinking and concentration, a significant increase or decrease in appetite and time spent sleeping, feelings of dejection and hopelessness, and sometimes suicidal thoughts or an attempt to commit suicide **b** : a reduction in functional activity, amount, quality, or force ⟨~ of autonomic function⟩ ⟨~ of red blood cells⟩

¹de·pres·sive \di-ˈpres-iv\ *adj* **1** : tending to depress **2** : of, relating to, marked by, or affected by psychological depression ⟨the patient was paranoid and ~⟩ ⟨~ symptoms⟩

²depressive *n* : one who is affected with or prone to psychological depression

depressive disorder *n* : any of several mood disorders and esp. dysthymia and major depressive disorder that are characterized by prolonged or recurring symptoms of psychological depression without manic episodes — see MAJOR DEPRESSIVE DISORDER

de·pres·sor \di-ˈpres-ər\ *n* : one that depresses: as **a** : a muscle that draws down a part — compare LEVATOR **b** : a device for pressing a part down or aside — see TONGUE DEPRESSOR **c** : a nerve or nerve fiber that decreases the activity or the tone of the organ or part it innervates

depressor nerve *n* : a nerve whose stimulation tends to decrease the activity or tone of the part or organ that it innervates

depressor sep·ti \-ˈsep-ˌtī\ *n* : a small muscle of each side of the upper lip that is inserted into the nasal septum and wing of the nose on each side and constricts the nasal opening by drawing the wing downward

de·pri·va·tion \ˌdep-rə-ˈvā-shən, ˌdē-prī-\ *n* : the act or process of removing or the condition resulting from removal of something normally present and usu. essential for mental or physical well-being ⟨his nervous system may have been affected by early oxygen —Jack Fincher⟩ ⟨sleep ~⟩

de·prive \di-ˈprīv\ *vt* **de·prived; de·priv·ing** : to take something away from and esp. something that is usu. considered essential for mental or physical well-being ⟨a child *deprived* of emotional support⟩ ⟨tissue *deprived* of oxygen⟩

de·pro·gram *or chiefly Brit* **de·pro·gramme** \(ˌ)dē-ˈprō-ˌgram, -grəm\ *vt* **-grammed** *also* **-gramed; -gramming** *also* **-graming** : to dissuade or try to dissuade from strongly held convictions (as of a religious nature) or a firmly established or innate behavior pattern ⟨the necessity of countering propaganda and *deprogramming* the indoctrinated —Toni Cade Bambara⟩

de·pro·tein·ate \(ˈ)dē-ˈprō-ˌtē-ˌnāt, -ˈprōt-ē-ə-ˌnāt\ *vt* **-at·ed;**

-at·ing : DEPROTEINIZE — **de·pro·tein·ation** \(ˌ)dē-ˌprō-ˌtē-'nā-shən, -ˌprōt-ē-ə-\ n

de·pro·tein·iza·tion or chiefly Brit **de·pro·tein·isa·tion** \(ˌ)dē-ˌprō-ˌtē-nə-'zā-shən, -ˌprōt-ē-ə-nə-\ n : the process of removing protein

de·pro·tein·ize or Brit **de·pro·tein·ise** \(')dē-'prō-ˌtē-ˌnīz, -'prōt-ē-ə-ˌnīz\ vt **-ized** or Brit **-ised; -iz·ing** or Brit **-is·ing** : to subject to deproteinization ⟨deproteinized blood⟩

depth \'depth\ n, pl **depths** \'depth, 'dep(t)s\ **1** : the distance between upper and lower or between dorsal and ventral points of a body **2** : the quality of a state of consciousness, a bodily state, or a physiological function of being intense or complete ⟨the ∼ of anesthesia⟩ ⟨the ∼ of respiration⟩

depth perception n : the ability to judge the distance of objects and the spatial relationship of objects at different distances

depth psychology n : PSYCHOANALYSIS; also : psychology concerned esp. with the unconscious mind

dep·u·ra·tion \ˌdep-yə-'rā-shən\ n : purification of impurities or heterogeneous matter ⟨∼ of shellfish from polluted waters⟩ — **dep·u·rate** \'dep-yə-ˌrāt\ vt **-rat·ed; -rat·ing**

de·Quer·vain's disease \də-(ˌ)kər-'vaⁿz-\ n : inflammation of tendons and their sheaths at the styloid process of the radius that often causes pain in the thumb side of the wrist

Quer·vain \ker-vaⁿ\, **Fritz de (1868–1940),** Swiss physician. The author of a major text on surgery, Quervain was known for his work on the pathology and surgery of the thyroid. He worked also on the prevention of goiter. He described the inflammatory process now known as deQuervain's disease in 1895.

de·range·ment \di-'rānj-mənt\ n **1** : a disturbance of normal bodily functioning or operation ⟨∼s in the secretion of adaptive hormones —Hans Selye⟩ **2** : INSANITY — **de·range** \di-'rānj\ vt **de·ranged; de·rang·ing**

de·re·al·iza·tion or Brit **de·re·al·isa·tion** \(ˌ)dē-ˌrē-ə-lə-'zā-shən, -ˌrī-ə-\ n : a feeling of altered reality that occurs often in schizophrenia and in some drug reactions

de·re·ism \'dē-rē-ˌiz-əm, 'dā-rā-; dē-'rē-iz-əm, dā-'rā-\ n : thinking directed away from reality and not following ordinary rules of logic — **de·re·is·tic** \ˌdē-(ˌ)rē-'is-tik, ˌdā-(ˌ)rā-\ adj — **de·re·is·ti·cal·ly** \-ti-k(ə-)lē\ adv

de·re·press \ˌdē-ri-'pres\ vt : to activate (a gene or enzyme) by releasing from a blocked state — **de·re·pres·sion** \-'presh-ən\ n

¹de·riv·a·tive \di-'riv-ət-iv\ adj **1** : formed by derivation **2** : made up of or marked by derived elements

²derivative n **1** : something that is obtained from, grows out of, or results from an earlier or more fundamental state or condition **2 a** : a chemical substance related structurally to another substance and theoretically derivable from it **b** : a substance that can be made from another substance

de·rive \di-'rīv\ vb **de·rived; de·riv·ing** vt : to take, receive, or obtain, esp. from a specified source; specif : to obtain (a chemical substance) actually or theoretically from a parent substance ∼ vi : to have or take origin — **der·i·va·tion** \ˌder-ə-'vā-shən\ n

derm abbr dermatologist; dermatology

der·ma \'dər-mə\ n : DERMIS

derm·abra·sion \ˌdər-mə-'brā-zhən\ n : surgical removal of skin blemishes or imperfections (as scars or tattoos) by abrasion (as with sandpaper or wire brushes)

Der·ma·cen·tor \'dər-mə-ˌsent-ər\ n : a large widely distributed genus of ornate ticks of the family Ixodidae including a number that attack humans and other mammals and several that are vectors of important diseases (as Rocky Mountain spotted fever)

der·mal \'dər-məl\ adj **1** : of or relating to skin and esp. to the dermis : CUTANEOUS **2** : EPIDERMAL

Der·ma·nys·si·dae \ˌdər-mə-'nis-ə-ˌdē\ n pl : a family of parasitic mites having the chelicerae adapted for piercing — **der·ma·nys·sid** \-'nis-əd\ adj

Der·ma·nys·sus \-'nis-əs\ n : the type genus of the family Dermanyssidae comprising a number of blood-sucking mites that are parasitic on birds — see CHICKEN MITE

der·ma·ti·tis \ˌdər-mə-'tīt-əs\ n, pl **-ti·tis·es** or **-tit·i·des** \-'tit-ə-ˌdēz\ : inflammation of the skin — called also dermitis — **der·ma·tit·ic** \-'tit-ik\ adj

dermatitis her·pe·ti·for·mis \-ˌhər-pə-tə-'fór-məs\ n : chronic dermatitis characterized by eruption of itching papules, vesicles, and lesions resembling hives typically in clusters

Der·ma·to·bia \ˌdər-mə-'tō-bē-ə\ n : a genus of botflies including one (D. hominis) whose larvae live under the skin of domestic mammals and sometimes of humans in tropical America

der·ma·to·fi·bro·ma \ˌdər-mət-ō-fī-'brō-mə\ n, pl **-mas** also **-ma·ta** \-mət-ə\ : a benign chiefly fibroblastic nodule of the skin found esp. on the extremities of adults

der·ma·to·fi·bro·sar·co·ma \-ˌfī-brō-sär-'kō-mə\ n, pl **-mas** also **-ma·ta** \-mət-ə\ : a fibrosarcoma affecting the skin

dermatofibrosarcoma pro·tu·ber·ans \-prō-'t(y)ü-bə-ˌranz\ n : a dermal fibroblastic tumor composed of firm nodular masses that usu. do not metastasize

der·ma·to·glyph·ics \ˌdər-mət-ə-'glif-iks\ n pl but sing or pl in constr **1** : skin patterns; esp : patterns of the specialized skin of the inferior surfaces of the hands and feet **2** : the science of the study of skin patterns — **der·ma·to·glyph·ic** \-ik\ adj

der·ma·to·graph·ia \-'graf-ē-ə\ n : DERMOGRAPHISM

der·ma·to·graph·ism \-'graf-ˌiz-əm\ n : DERMOGRAPHISM

der·ma·tog·ra·phy \ˌdər-mə-'täg-rə-fē\ n, pl **-phies** : anatomical description of the skin

der·ma·to·his·tol·o·gy \ˌdər-mət-ō-his-'täl-ə-jē\ n, pl **-gies** : histology of the skin — **der·ma·to·his·to·log·ic** \-ˌhis-tə-'läj-ik\ adj

der·ma·toid \'dər-mə-ˌtóid\ adj : resembling skin

der·ma·to·log·ic \ˌdər-mət-ᵊl-'äj-ik\ or **der·ma·to·log·i·cal** \-i-kəl\ adj : of or relating to dermatology

der·ma·to·log·i·cal \-i-kəl\ n : a medicinal agent for application to the skin

der·ma·tol·o·gy \ˌdər-mə-'täl-ə-jē\ n, pl **-gies** : a branch of science dealing with the skin, its structure, functions, and diseases — **der·ma·tol·o·gist** \-mə-'täl-ə-jəst\ n

der·ma·tome \'dər-mə-ˌtōm\ n **1** : an instrument for cutting skin for use in grafting **2** : the lateral wall of a somite from which the dermis is produced — **der·ma·to·mal** \ˌdər-mə-'tō-məl\ or **der·ma·to·mic** \-mik\ adj

der·ma·to·mere \'dər-mət-ə-ˌmi(ə)r, (ˌ)dər-'mat-ə-\ n : DERMATOME 2

der·ma·to·my·co·sis \ˌdər-mət-ō-ˌmī-'kō-səs, (ˌ)dər-ˌmat-\ n, pl **-co·ses** \-ˌsēz\ : a disease (as ringworm) of the skin caused by infection with a fungus — called also epidermomycosis

der·ma·to·my·o·si·tis \-ˌmī-ə-'sīt-əs\ n, pl **-si·tis·es** or **-sit·i·des** \-'sit-ə-ˌdēz\ : polymyositis that is accompanied by involvement of the skin and that is typically marked by reddish erythematous eruptions esp. on the face, neck, upper trunk and distal half of the limbs, by periorbital edema, by violet-colored erythema of the eyelids and region over the upper eyelids, and sometimes by cutaneous vasculitis or subcutaneous calcification

der·ma·to·path·ia \-'path-ē-ə\ n : DERMOPATHY — **der·ma·to·path·ic** \-'path-ik\ adj

der·ma·to·pa·thol·o·gy \-pə-'thäl-ə-jē, -pa-\ n, pl **-gies** : pathology of the skin — **der·ma·to·pa·thol·o·gist** \-jəst\ n

der·ma·top·a·thy \ˌdər-mə-'täp-ə-thē\ n, pl **-thies** : DERMOPATHY

Der·ma·toph·a·goi·des \ˌdər-mə-ˌtäf-ə-'gói-(ˌ)dēz\ n : a genus of mites (family Pyroglyphidae) including several that scavenge shed flakes of human skin and dander and cause allergy — see HOUSE-DUST MITE

der·ma·to·phyte \(ˌ)dər-'mat-ə-ˌfīt, 'dər-mət-ə-\ n : a fungus parasitic upon the skin or skin derivatives (as hair or nails) — compare DERMATOMYCOSIS — **der·ma·to·phyt·ic** \(ˌ)dər-ˌmat-ə-'fit-ik, ˌdər-mət-\ adj

der·ma·to·phy·tid \(ˌ)dər-ˌmat-ə-'fit-əd, ˌdər-mət-\ n : a skin eruption associated with a fungus infection; esp : one considered to be due to allergic reaction

der·ma·to·phy·to·sis \-fī-'tō-səs\ *n, pl* **-to·ses** \-ˌsēz\ : a disease (as athlete's foot) of the skin or skin derivatives that is caused by a dermatophyte

der·ma·to·plas·ty \(ˌ)dər-'mat-ə-ˌplas-tē, 'dər-mət-\ *n, pl* **-ties** : plastic surgery of the skin

der·ma·to·scle·ro·sis \ˌdər-mət-ō-sklə-'rō-səs\ *n, pl* **-ro·ses** \-ˌsēz\ : SCLERODERMA

der·ma·to·sis \ˌdər-mə-'tō-səs\ *n, pl* **-to·ses** \-ˌsēz\ : a disease of the skin

der·ma·to·ther·a·py \(ˌ)dər-ˌmat-ə-'ther-ə-pē, ˌdər-mət-\ *n, pl* **-pies** : the treatment of skin diseases

der·ma·to·zoo·no·sis \-ˌzō-ə-'nō-səs\ *n, pl* **-no·ses** \-ˌsēz\ : skin disease caused by animal parasites of the skin

der·mic \'dər-mik\ *adj* : DERMAL

der·mis \'dər-məs\ *n* : the sensitive vascular inner mesodermic layer of the skin — called also *corium, cutis, cutis vera, derma*

der·mi·tis \(ˌ)dər-'mīt-əs\ *n* : DERMATITIS

der·mo·graph·ia \ˌdər-mə-'graf-ē-ə\ *n* : DERMOGRAPHISM

der·mog·ra·phism \(ˌ)dər-'mäg-rə-ˌfiz-əm\ *n* : a condition in which pressure or friction on the skin gives rise to a transient raised usu. reddish mark so that a line traced on the skin becomes visible — called also *dermatographia, dermatographism* — **der·mo·graph·ic** \ˌdər-mə-'graf-ik\ *adj*

der·moid \'dər-ˌmóid\ *also* **der·moi·dal** \(ˌ)dər-'móid-ᵊl\ *adj* **1** : made up of cutaneous elements and esp. ectodermal derivatives ⟨a ∼ tumor⟩ **2** : resembling skin

dermoid cyst *n* : a cystic tumor often of the ovary that contains skin and skin derivatives (as hair or teeth) — called also *dermoid*

der·mom·e·ter \(ˌ)dər-'mäm-ət-ər\ *n* : an instrument used to measure the electrical resistance of the skin

der·mo·ne·crot·ic \ˌdər-mō-ni-'krät-ik\ *adj* : relating to or causing necrosis of the skin ⟨a ∼ toxin⟩ ⟨∼ effects⟩

der·mop·a·thy \(ˌ)dər-'mäp-ə-thē\ *n, pl* **-thies** : a disease of the skin — called also *dermatopathia, dermatopathy*

der·mo·tro·pic \ˌdər-mə-'trō-pik, -'träp-ik\ *adj* : attracted to, localizing in, or entering by way of the skin ⟨∼ viruses⟩ — compare NEUROTROPIC, PANTROPIC

der·ren·ga·de·ra \(ˌ)der-ˌeŋ-gə-'der-ə\ *n* : MAL DE CADERAS

DES \ˌdē-(ˌ)ē-'es\ *n* : DIETHYLSTILBESTROL

de·salt \(ˈ)dē-'sólt\ *vt* : to remove salt from

Each boldface word in the list below is a variant of the word to its right in small capitals.

desamidate	DEAMIDATE	**desamidize**	DEAMIDIZE
desamidation	DEAMIDATION	**desaminase**	DEAMINASE
desamidization	DEAMIDIZATION		

de·sat·u·rate \(ˌ)dē-'sach-ə-ˌrāt\ *vb* **-rat·ed; -rat·ing** *vt* : to cause to become unsaturated ⟨∼ carbon chains⟩ ∼ *vi* : to become unsaturated — **de·sat·u·ra·tion** \(ˌ)dē-ˌsach-ə-'rā-shən\ *n*

des·ce·met·o·cele \ˌdes-ə-'met-ə-ˌsēl\ *n* : protrusion of Descemet's membrane through the cornea

Des·ce·met's membrane \ˌdes-(ə-)'māz-\ *n* : a transparent highly elastic apparently structureless membrane that covers the inner surface of the cornea and is lined with endothelium — called also *membrana of Descemet, posterior elastic lamina*

    Des·ce·met \des-mā\, **Jean (1732–1810),** French physician. Descemet's areas of study ranged from treatment of gout and measles to the anatomy of the eye and skin. Around 1759 he published a complete description of the membrane now known as Descemet's membrane, which had been first described in 1729 by a British ophthalmologist, Benedict Duddell.

de·scend \di-'send\ *vi* : to pass from a higher place or level to a lower one ⟨normally the testicle ∼s into the scrotum between the seventh and ninth month in utero —*Therapeutic Notes*⟩

de·scend·ing \'dē-ˌsen-diŋ, di-'\ *adj* **1** : moving or directed downward ⟨∼ infection from the kidney —*Therapeutic Notes*⟩ **2** : being a nerve, nerve fiber, or nerve tract that carries nerve impulses in a direction away from the central nervous system : EFFERENT, MOTOR ⟨the ∼ branch of a nerve⟩

descending aorta *n* : the part of the aorta from the arch to its bifurcation into the two common iliac arteries that passes downward in the thoracic and abdominal cavities

descending colon *n* : the part of the large intestine on the left side that extends from the bend below the spleen to the sigmoid colon — compare ASCENDING COLON, TRANSVERSE COLON

de·scen·sus \di-'sen(t)-səs\ *n* : the process of descending or prolapsing ⟨∼ of the uterus⟩

de·scent \di-'sent\ *n* **1** : the act or process of descending from a higher to a lower location ⟨∼ of the testes into the scrotum⟩ **2 a** : derivation from an ancestor **b** : the fact or process of originating by generation from an ancestral stock (as a species or genus) **3** : a former method of distillation in which the material was heated in a vessel having its outlet underneath so that the vapors produced were forced to descend

de·sen·si·tize *also Brit* **de·sen·si·tise** \(ˈ)dē-'sen(t)-sə-ˌtīz\ *vt* **-tized** *also Brit* **-tised; -tiz·ing** *also Brit* **-tis·ing** : to make less sensitive : reduce sensitivity in ⟨∼ a nerve with a local anesthetic⟩: as **a** : to make (a sensitized or hypersensitive individual) insensitive or nonreactive to a sensitizing agent **b** : to extinguish an emotional response (as of fear, anxiety, or guilt) to stimuli which formerly induced it : make emotionally insensitive ⟨evidence that violence on television ∼s children to actual violence —Stephanie Harrington⟩ **c** : to decrease a response (as of a cell receptor) progressively following prolonged exposure to a stimulus ⟨formation of cAMP was reduced significantly in *desensitized* cells and remained low in the continuous presence of agonist —S. M. Nilius *et al*⟩ — **de·sen·si·ti·za·tion** *also Brit* **de·sen·si·ti·sa·tion** \(ˌ)dē-ˌsen-sət-ə-'zā-shən, -ˌsen-stə-'zā-\ *n*

de·sen·si·tiz·er *also Brit* **de·sen·si·tis·er** \(ˈ)dē-'sen(t)-sə-ˌtī-zər\ *n* : a desensitizing agent; *esp* : a drug that reduces sensitivity to pain ⟨a dentin ∼⟩

de·ser·pi·dine \di-'sər-pə-ˌdēn\ *n* : an alkaloid $C_{32}H_{38}N_2O_8$ obtained from a plant of the genus *Rauwolfia* (*R. canescens*) that is structurally related to reserpine, blocks adrenergic neurons, and is used esp. as an antihypertensive and sometimes as a tranquilizer

des·ert sore \'dez-ərt-\ *n* : an ulcer of unknown cause affecting chiefly the extremities and occurring in desert regions of the tropics

de·sex \(ˈ)dē-'seks\ *vt* : CASTRATE 1, SPAY

de·sex·u·al·ize *or Brit* **de·sex·u·al·ise** \(ˈ)dē-'seksh-(ə-)wə-ˌlīz, -'sek-shə-ˌlīz\ *vt* **-ized** *or Brit* **-ised; -iz·ing** *or Brit* **-is·ing** **1** : to deprive of sexual characters or power **2** : to divest of sexual quality — **de·sex·u·al·iza·tion** *or Brit* **de·sex·u·al·isa·tion** \(ˌ)dē-ˌseksh-(ə-)wə-lə-'zā-shən, -ˌsek-shə-lə-\ *n*

¹des·ic·cant \'des-i-kənt\ *adj* : tending to dry or desiccate

²desiccant *n* : a drying agent (as calcium chloride)

des·ic·cate \'des-i-ˌkāt\ *vb* **-cat·ed; -cat·ing** *vt* **1** : to dry up or cause to dry up : deprive or exhaust of moisture; *esp* : to dry thoroughly ⟨uses radio frequencies of 100,000 Hz to 10,000,000 Hz to cut, coagulate, and ∼ tissue —Bettyann Hutchisson *et al*⟩ **2** : to preserve a food by drying : DEHYDRATE ⟨*desiccated* coconut⟩ ∼ *vi* : to become dried up : undergo a desiccating process

des·ic·ca·tion \ˌdes-i-'kā-shən\ *n* : the act or process of desiccating or the state of being or becoming desiccated; *esp* : a complete or nearly complete deprivation of moisture (as by vaporization or by evaporation) or of water not chemically combined : DEHYDRATION ⟨from the long-wave diathermy machine two distinct currents are obtained which produce ∼ and electrocoagulation respectively —W. H. Schmidt⟩

de·sic·ca·tive \'des-i-ˌkāt-iv, di-'sik-ət-\ *adj* : drying up or tending to dry up ⟨intense ∼ characteristics⟩

des·ic·ca·tor \'des-i-ˌkāt-ər\ *n* **1** : a container (as a glass jar) fitted with an airtight cover and containing at the bottom a

---

desiccating agent (as calcium chloride) **2** : a machine or apparatus for desiccating food usu. by the aid of heat and sometimes in a vacuum

de·sign \di-'zīn\ n : a plan or protocol for carrying out or accomplishing something (esp. a scientific experiment); *also* : the process of preparing this — **design** *vt*

de·sign·er drug \di-,zī-nər-\ n **1** : a synthetic version of a controlled substance (as heroin) that is produced with a slightly altered molecular structure to avoid classification as an illicit drug **2** : a synthetic drug created (as by genetic engineering) to treat a particular medical condition esp. by producing a specific effect on the body's biochemistry

de·si·pra·mine \,dez-ə-'pram-ən, də-'zip-rə-,mēn\ n : a tricyclic antidepressant administered in the form of its hydrochloride $C_{18}H_{22}N_2 \cdot HCl$ esp. in the treatment of endogenous depressions (as a bipolar disorder) — see NORPRAMIN, PERTOFRANE

des·lo·rat·a·dine \,dez-lə-'rat-ə-,dēn, -,dīn\ n : a long-acting H_1 antagonist $C_{19}H_{19}ClN_2$ that is used to treat seasonal and perennial allergic rhinitis and chronic hives — see CLARINEX

des·meth·yl·imip·ra·mine \,des-,meth-əl-im-'ip-rə-,mēn\ n : DESIPRAMINE

des·mo·cra·ni·um \,dez-mə-'krā-nē-əm, ,des-, -mō-\ n, pl **-ni·ums** or **-nia** \-nē-ə\ : the earliest mesenchymal precursor of the chondrocranium

des·mo·cyte \'dez-mə-,sīt, ,des-, -mō-\ n : any of certain elongated interstitial cells (as a fibroblast)

Des·mo·dus \dez-'mōd-əs\ n : a monotypic genus of a subfamily (Desmodontinae of the family Phyllostomidae) containing a common So. American vampire bat (*D. rotundus*)

des·moid \'dez-,moid\ n : a dense benign connective-tissue tumor

des·mo·lase \'dez-mə-,lās, -,lāz\ n : an enzyme (as aldolase) capable of breaking or forming a carbon-to-carbon bond in a molecule and playing a role in respiration and fermentation

des·mo·pla·sia \,dez-mə-'plā-zh(ē-)ə, ,des-, -mō-\ n : formation of fibrous connective tissue by proliferation of fibroblasts

des·mo·plas·tic \-'plas-tik\ adj : characterized by the formation of fibrous tissue 〈a ~ fibroma〉 〈~ malignant melanomas〉

des·mo·pres·sin \,des-mō-'pres-°n\ n : a synthetic hormone that is administered in the form of its hydrated acetate salt $C_{46}H_{64}N_{14}O_{12}S_2 \cdot C_2H_4O_2 \cdot 3H_2O$ and is used for its antidiuretic effect in treating diabetes insipidus due to injury to the neurohypophyseal system and nocturnal enuresis and for its effect of increasing certain clotting factors in treating some bleeding disorders — see DDAVP

des·mo·some \'dez-mə-,sōm\ n : a specialized local thickening of the plasma membrane of an epithelial cell that serves to anchor contiguous cells together — **des·mo·som·al** \-,sō-məl\ adj

des·mos·ter·ol \dez-'mäs-tə-,rȯl, -,rōl\ n : a precursor $C_{27}H_{43}OH$ of cholesterol that tends to accumulate in blood serum when cholesterol synthesis is inhibited — called also *24-dehydrocholesterol*

des·mot·ro·pism \dez-'mä-trə-,piz-əm\ n : tautomerism in which both tautomeric forms have been isolated

des·mot·ro·py \-trə-pē\ n, pl **-pies** : DESMOTROPISM

deso·ges·trel \des-ə-'jes-tril\ n : a synthetic progestogen $C_{22}H_{30}O$ used in birth control pills in combination with ethinyl estradiol

deso·mor·phine \,dez-ə-'mȯr-,fēn\ n : a synthetic morphine derivative $C_{17}H_{21}NO_2$ used as an analgesic

de·sorb \(')dē-'sȯ(ə)rb, -'zȯ(ə)rb\ vt : to remove (a sorbed substance) by the reverse of adsorption or absorption

de·sorp·tion \-'sȯrp-shən, -'zȯrp-\ n : the process of desorbing

Each boldface word in the list below is a variant of the word to its right in small capitals.

desoxy	DEOXY
desoxycholate	DEOXYCHOLATE
desoxycholic acid	DEOXYCHOLIC ACID
desoxyribonuclease	DEOXYRIBONUCLEASE
desoxyribonucleic acid	DEOXYRIBONUCLEIC ACID
desoxyribonucleoprotein	DEOXYRIBONUCLEOPROTEIN
desoxyribonucleotide	DEOXYRIBONUCLEOTIDE
desoxyribose	DEOXYRIBOSE

des·oxy·cor·ti·co·ste·rone \(,)dez-,äk-si-,kȯrt-i-'käs-tə-,rōn, -i-,kō-stə-'rōn\ or **des·oxy·cor·ti·co·ste·rone** \(,)dē-\ n : a steroid hormone $C_{21}H_{30}O_3$ of the adrenal cortex

des·oxy·cor·tone \(,)dez-,äk-si-'kȯr-,tōn\ or chiefly Brit **de·oxy·cor·tone** \(,)dē-\ n : DESOXYCORTICOSTERONE

de·spe·ci·ate \(')dē-'spē-s(h)ē-,āt\ vt **-at·ed; -at·ing** : to remove the characteristic antigenicity of (a foreign protein) by chemical or other treatment — **de·spe·ci·a·tion** \(,)dē-,spē-s(h)ē-'ā-shən\ n

des·qua·mate \'des-kwə-,māt\ vi **-mat·ed; -mat·ing** : to peel off in the form of scales : scale off 〈*desquamated* epithelial cells〉 — **des·qua·ma·tion** \,des-kwə-'mā-shən\ n

des·qua·ma·tive \'des-kwə-,māt-iv, di-'skwam-ət-\ adj : attended by or causing desquamation 〈~ interstitial pneumonia〉

des·qua·ma·to·ry \'des-kwə-mə-,tōr-ē, di-'skwam-ə-, -,tȯr-\ adj : characterized by or used for desquamation

de·stain \(')dē-'stān\ vt : to selectively remove stain from (a specimen for microscopic study)

des·thio·bi·o·tin \des-,thī-ō-'bī-ət-ən\ n : a crystalline acid $C_{10}H_{18}N_2O_3$ obtained from biotin by removal of sulfur and held to be a precursor of biotin in some organisms (as many yeasts and bacteria)

de·stroy·ing an·gel \di-,strȯi(-i)ŋ-'ān-jəl\ n : any of several very poisonous pure white mushrooms of the genus *Amanita* (as *A. verna, A. virosa*, or *A. ocreata*); *also* : a death cap (*A. phalloides*) whether white or colored

de·stru·do \di-'strü-(,)dō\ n : DEATH WISH

de·syn·chro·ni·za·tion also Brit **de·syn·chro·ni·sa·tion** \(,)dē-,siŋ-krə-nə-'zā-shən, -,sin-\ n : the process or result of getting out of synchronization 〈electrocortical ~ and autonomic arousal —Jackson Beatty〉 — **de·syn·chro·nize** also Brit **de·syn·chro·nise** \(')dē-'siŋ-krə-,nīz, -'sin-\ vt **-nized** also Brit **-nised; -niz·ing** also Brit **-nis·ing**

de·syn·chro·nized sleep n : REM SLEEP

de·tached retina \di-'tacht-\ n : RETINAL DETACHMENT

de·tach·ment of the retina \di-'tach-mənt-\ n : RETINAL DETACHMENT

de·tail·er \di-'tā-lər, 'dē-,tā-\ n : DETAIL MAN

de·tail man \di-'tā(ə)l-, 'dē-,tāl-\ n : a representative of a drug manufacturer who introduces new products and esp. drugs to medical and pharmaceutical professionals (as physicians or pharmacists)

de·tec·tor \di-'tek-tər\ n : one that detects; *esp* : a device for detecting the presence of electromagnetic waves or of radioactivity

¹**de·ter·gent** \di-'tər-jənt\ adj : having a cleansing action

²**detergent** n : a cleansing agent: as **a** : SOAP 1 **b** : any of numerous synthetic water-soluble or liquid organic preparations that are chemically different from soaps but are able to emulsify oils, hold dirt in suspension, and act as wetting agents

de·te·ri·o·rate \di-'tir-ē-ə-,rāt\ vi **-rat·ed; -rat·ing** : to become impaired in quality, functioning, or condition : DEGENERATE 〈her health *deteriorated*〉 〈*deteriorating* vision〉

de·te·ri·o·ra·tion \di-,tir-ē-ə-'rā-shən\ n : the action or process of deteriorating : the state of having deteriorated 〈personality ~〉 〈neurological ~〉

de·ter·mi·nant \di-'tərm-(ə-)nənt\ n **1 a** : a hypothetical aggregate of biophores conceived as comparable to the gene of more recent biological theory **b** : GENE **2** : EPITOPE

de·ter·mi·nate \di-'tərm-(ə-)nət\ adj : relating to, being, or undergoing determinate cleavage 〈a ~ egg〉

determinate cleavage n : cleavage of an egg in which each division irreversibly separates portions of the zygote with specific potencies for further development — compare INDETERMINATE CLEAVAGE

de·ter·mi·na·tion \di-,tər-mə-'nā-shən\ n **1** : a fixing or finding of the position, magnitude, quantity, value, or character of something: as **a** : the act, process, or result of an accurate measurement **b** : an identification of the taxonomic position of a plant or animal **2** : the fixation of the destiny of undifferentiated embryonic tissue — compare DIFFERENTIATION 2b

de·ter·mine \di-ˈtər-mən\ vt **de·ter·mined; de·ter·min·ing** \-ˈtərm-(ə-)niŋ\ **1 a** : to obtain definite information about with regard to quantity, character, magnitude, or location ⟨~ the ionic concentration⟩ ⟨~ the creatinine in blood serum⟩ **b** : to discover the taxonomic position or the generic and specific names of **2** : to bring about the determination of ⟨~ the fate of a cell⟩

de·ter·min·er \-ˈtərm-(ə-)nər\ n : GENE

de·ter·min·ism \di-ˈtər-mə-ˌniz-əm\ n **1** : a theory or doctrine that acts of the will, occurrences in nature, or social or psychological phenomena are causally determined by preceding events or natural laws ⟨explained behavior by the combination of an environmental and a genetic ~⟩ **2** : the quality or state of being determined — **de·ter·min·is·tic** \-ˌtər-mə-ˈnis-tik\ also **de·ter·min·ist** \-ˈtərm-(ə-)nəst\ adj — **de·ter·min·is·ti·cal·ly** \-ˌtər-mə-ˈnis-ti-k(ə-)lē\ adv

de·ter·min·ist \di-ˈtərm-(ə-)nəst\ n : an adherent of determinism

de·ter·rence \di-ˈtər-ən(t)s, -ˈter-; -ˈtə-rən(t)s; dē-\ n : the inhibition of criminal behavior by fear esp. of punishment

¹de·ter·sive \di-ˈtər-siv, -ziv\ adj : relating to or having detergent or cleansing activity ⟨a ~ agent⟩

²detersive n : a cleansing agent : DETERGENT

de·tick \(ˈ)dē-ˈtik\ vt : to remove ticks from ⟨~ dogs⟩

detn abbr detention

de·tor·sion \(ˈ)dē-ˈtȯr-shən\ n : the removal of torsion; specif : correction of abnormal twist (as of the intestine)

¹de·tox \(ˈ)dē-ˈtäks\ n **1** often attrib : detoxification from an intoxicating or addictive substance ⟨began performing ultra rapid ~es —Carol Ann Campbell & Fredrick Kunkle⟩ ⟨a ~ program⟩ ⟨a ~ clinic⟩ **2** : a detox program or facility ⟨spent five days in ~ at a local hospital —Karl Ross⟩

²detox vt : DETOXIFY 2

de·tox·i·cant \(ˈ)dē-ˈtäk-si-kənt\ n : a detoxicating agent

de·tox·i·cate \(ˈ)dē-ˈtäk-sə-ˌkāt\ vt **-cat·ed; -cat·ing** : DETOXIFY — **de·tox·i·ca·tion** \(ˌ)dē-ˌtäk-sə-ˈkā-shən\ n

de·tox·i·fi·er \(ˈ)dē-ˈtäk-sə-ˌfī-ər\ n : DETOXICANT

de·tox·i·fy \(ˈ)dē-ˈtäk-sə-ˌfī\ vb **-fied; -fy·ing** vt **1 a** : to remove a poison or toxin or the effect of such from **b** : to render (a harmful substance) harmless **2** : to free (as a drug user or an alcoholic) from an intoxicating or an addictive substance in the body or from dependence on or addiction to such a substance ⟨the clinic started ~ing him by gradually lowering his dosage —J. M. Markham⟩ ~ vi : to become free of addiction to a drug or alcohol — **de·tox·i·fi·ca·tion** \(ˌ)dē-ˌtäk-sə-fə-ˈkā-shən\ n

de·tri·tion \di-ˈtrish-ən\ n : a wearing off or away

de·tri·tus \di-ˈtrīt-əs\ n, pl **de·tri·tus** \-ˈtrīt-əs, -ˈtrī-ˌtüs\ : loose material resulting from disintegration (as of tissue)

de·tru·sor \di-ˈtrü-zər, -sər\ n : the outer largely longitudinally arranged musculature of the bladder wall — called also detrusor muscle

detrusor uri·nae \-yə-ˈrī-(ˌ)nē\ n : the external longitudinal musculature of the urinary bladder

de·tu·ba·tion \ˌdē-t(y)ü-ˈbā-shən\ n : EXTUBATION

de·tu·mes·cence \ˌdē-t(y)ü-ˈmes-ᵊn(t)s\ n : subsidence or diminution of swelling or erection — **de·tu·mes·cent** \-ᵊnt\ adj

deu·ter·anom·a·lous \ˌd(y)üt-ə-rə-ˈnäm-ə-ləs\ adj : exhibiting partial loss of green color vision so that an increased intensity of this color is required in a mixture of red and green to match a given yellow

deu·ter·anom·a·ly \-ə-lē\ n, pl **-lies** : the condition of being deuteranomalous — compare PROTANOMALY, TRICHROMATISM 2

deu·ter·an·ope \ˈd(y)üt-ə-rə-ˌnōp\ n : an individual affected with deuteranopia

deu·ter·an·opia \ˌd(y)üt-ə-rə-ˈnō-pē-ə\ n : color blindness marked by usu. complete loss of ability to distinguish colors — **deu·ter·an·opic** \-ˈnō-pik, -ˈnäp-ik\ adj

deu·ter·ate \ˈd(y)üt-ə-ˌrāt\ vt **-at·ed; -at·ing** : to introduce deuterium into (a compound)

deu·te·ri·um \d(y)ü-ˈtir-ē-əm\ n : an isotope of hydrogen that has one proton and one neutron in its nucleus and that has twice the mass of ordinary hydrogen — called also heavy hydrogen

deuterium oxide n : HEAVY WATER

deu·ter·o·my·cete \ˌd(y)üt-ə-rə-ˈmī-ˌsēt\ n : IMPERFECT FUNGUS — **deu·ter·o·my·ce·tous** \-ˌmī-ˈsēt-əs\ adj

Deu·ter·o·my·ce·tes \-ˌmī-ˈsēt-ēz\ n pl : a class of fungi comprising the imperfect fungi when they are considered a class

Deu·ter·o·my·co·ta \-ˌmī-ˈkōt-ə\ n pl : a division of fungi comprising the imperfect fungi when they are considered a division

Deu·ter·o·my·co·ti·na \-ˌmī-kə-ˈtī-nə\ n pl : a subdivision of fungi comprising the imperfect fungi when they are considered a subdivision

deu·ter·on \ˈd(y)üt-ə-ˌrän\ n : a deuterium nucleus

deu·ter·ot·o·kous \ˌd(y)üt-ə-ˈrät-ə-kəs\ adj : exhibiting deuterotoky : producing both male and female offspring parthenogenetically

deu·ter·ot·o·ky \-ˈrät-ə-kē\ n, pl **-kies** : the parthenogenetic production of both males and females — compare ARRHENOTOKY, THELYTOKY

deu·tom·er·ite \d(y)ü-ˈtäm-ə-ˌrīt\ n : the posterior segment of the trophozoite of some gregarines

deu·to·plasm \ˈd(y)üt-ə-ˌplaz-əm\ n : the nutritive inclusions of protoplasm; esp : the yolk reserves of an egg — **deu·to·plas·mic** \ˌd(y)üt-ə-ˈplaz-mik\ adj

deu·to·plas·mol·y·sis \ˌd(y)üt-(ˌ)ō-plaz-ˈmäl-ə-səs\ n, pl **-y·ses** \-ˌsēz\ : elimination of part of the yolk content of an egg following fertilization or during cleavage

deux — see FOLIE À DEUX

de·vas·cu·lar·iza·tion or Brit **de·vas·cu·lar·isa·tion** \(ˌ)dē-ˌvas-kyə-lə-rə-ˈzā-shən\ n : loss of the blood supply to a bodily part due to destruction or obstruction of blood vessels — **de·vas·cu·lar·ized** or Brit **de·vas·cu·lar·ised** \-ˈvas-kyə-lə-ˌrīzd\ adj

devel abbr development

de·vel·op \di-ˈvel-əp\ vt **1 a** : to make active or promote the growth of ⟨~ed their muscles by weight lifting⟩ **b** : to cause to grow and differentiate along lines natural to its kind ⟨the zygote is gradually ~ed into the adult plant or animal⟩ **2** : to become infected or affected by ⟨~ed pneumonia⟩ ~ vi **1** : to go through a process of natural growth, differentiation, or evolution by successive stages ⟨the fever ~s normally⟩ ⟨the embryo ~s into a well-formed human being⟩ **2** : to acquire secondary sex characteristics ⟨she is ~ing rapidly for a girl of 12⟩

de·vel·op·ment \di-ˈvel-əp-mənt\ n **1** : the action or process of developing: as **a** : the process of growth and differentiation by which the potentialities of a zygote, spore, or embryo are realized **b** : the gradual advance through evolutionary stages : EVOLUTION **2** : the state of being developed ⟨the great muscular ~ of weight lifters⟩ — **de·vel·op·men·tal** \-ˌvel-əp-ˈment-ᵊl\ adj — **de·vel·op·men·tal·ly** \-ē\ adv

developmental anatomy n : the anatomy of the embryo or fetus

developmentally disabled adj : having a physical or mental disability (as mental retardation) that becomes apparent in childhood and prevents, impedes, or limits normal development including the ability to learn or to care for oneself — abbr. DD — **developmental disability** n

developmental quo·tient \-ˈkwō-shənt\ n : a number expressing the development of a child determined by dividing

C

D

the age of the group into which test scores place the child by the child's chronological age and multiplying by 100 — abbr. *DQ*

de·vi·ance \'dē-vē-ən(t)s\ *n* : deviant quality, state, or behavior

¹de·vi·ant \-ənt\ *adj* : deviating esp. from some accepted norm : characterized by deviation (as from a standard of conduct) ⟨socially ∼ behavior⟩

²deviant *n* : something that deviates from a norm; *esp* : a person who differs markedly (as in social adjustment or sexual behavior) from what is considered normal for a group

¹de·vi·ate \'dē-vē-ət, -vē-ˌāt\ *adj* : characterized by or given to significant departure from the behavioral norms of a particular society

²deviate *n* : one that deviates from a norm; *esp* : a person who differs markedly from a group norm

de·vi·at·ed septum \ˌdē-vē-ˌāt-əd-\ *n* : deviation of the nasal septum from its normal position that results from a developmental abnormality or trauma and may be asymptomatic or cause nasal obstruction and predispose to sinusitis and nosebleed

de·vi·a·tion \ˌdē-vē-'ā-shən\ *n* : an act or instance of diverging from an established way or in a new direction: as **a** : evolutionary differentiation involving interpolation of new stages in the ancestral pattern of morphogenesis **b** : noticeable or marked departure from accepted norms of behavior

de·vice \di-'vīs\ *n* : a piece of equipment or a mechanism designed to serve a special purpose or perform a special function

dev·il's–grip \'dev-əlz-'grip\ *n, pl* **devil's–grips 1** : a malformation of sheep that consists of an indentation near the withers and down behind the shoulder as if a string had been put round that part of the sheep and tightened **2** : EPIDEMIC PLEURODYNIA

de·vi·tal·iza·tion *or Brit* **de·vi·tal·isa·tion** \(ˌ)dē-ˌvīt-ᵊl-ə-'zā-shən\ *n* **1** : an act of devitalizing; *esp* : destruction and usu. removal of the pulp from a tooth **2** : the condition of being devitalized

de·vi·tal·ize *or Brit* **de·vi·tal·ise** \(')dē-'vīt-ᵊl-ˌīz\ *vt* **-ized** *or Brit* **-ised; -iz·ing** *or Brit* **-is·ing** : to deprive of life or vitality: as **a** : to refine (as foodstuffs) to the point that essential or desirable constituents are lost **b** : to subject (a tooth or its pulp) to devitalization

de·vi·ta·min·ize \(')dē-'vīt-ə-mə-ˌnīz\ *or Brit* **de·vit·a·min·ise** \(')dē-'vit-\ *vt* **-ized** *or Brit* **-ised; -iz·ing** *or Brit* **-is·ing** : to deprive (as food) of vitamins esp. by cooking or hulling

dew·claw \'d(y)ü-ˌklo\ *n* : a vestigial digit not reaching to the ground on the foot of a mammal; *also* : a claw or hoof terminating such a digit — **dew·clawed** \-ˌklod\ *adj*

dew·lap \'d(y)ü-ˌlap\ *n* : loose skin hanging under the neck esp. of a bovine animal — **dew·lapped** \-ˌlapt\ *adj*

de·worm \(')dē-'wərm\ *vt* : to rid (as a dog) of worms : WORM

de·worm·er \(')dē-'wər-mər\ *n* : WORMER

dex \'deks\ *n* : the sulfate of dextroamphetamine

DEXA *abbr* dual energy X-ray absorptiometry

dexa·meth·a·sone \ˌdek-sə-'meth-ə-ˌsōn, -ˌzōn\ *n* : a synthetic glucocorticoid $C_{22}H_{29}FO_5$ also used in the form of its acetate $C_{24}H_{31}FO_6$ or sodium phosphate $C_{22}H_{28}FNa_2O_8P$ esp. as an anti-inflammatory and antiallergic agent — see DECADRON

dex·am·phet·amine \ˌdek-sam-'fet-ə-ˌmēn, -mən\ *n, chiefly Brit* : DEXTROAMPHETAMINE

Dex·e·drine \'dek-sə-ˌdrēn, -drən\ *trademark* — used for a preparation of the sulfate of dextroamphetamine

dex·fen·flur·a·mine \ˌdeks-'fen-flùr-ə-ˌmēn\ *n* : the dextrorotatory form of fenfluramine formerly used in the form of its hydrochloride to treat obesity but no longer used due to its association with heart disease affecting the heart valves — see FEN-PHEN

dex·ies \'dek-sēz\ *n pl, slang* : tablets or capsules of the sulfate of dextroamphetamine

dex·ter \'dek-stər\ *adj* : relating to or situated on the right ⟨the ∼ wing of a fowl⟩ — **dexter** *adv*

dex·ter·i·ty \dek-'ster-ət-ē\ *n, pl* **-ties 1** : readiness and grace in physical activity; *esp* : skill and ease in using the hands **2** : mental skill or quickness

dex·ter·ous *also* **dex·trous** \'dek-st(ə-)rəs\ *adj* **1** : skillful and competent with the hands **2** : mentally adroit and skillful — **dex·ter·ous·ly** *adv* — **dex·ter·ous·ness** *n*

dextra — see COLICA DEXTRA

dex·trad \'dek-ˌstrad\ *adv* : toward the right side : DEXTRALLY

¹dex·tral \'dek-strəl\ *adj* : of or relating to the right; *esp* : RIGHT-HANDED — **dex·tral·ly** \-strə-lē\ *adv*

²dextral *n* : a person exhibiting dominance of the right hand and eye

dex·tral·i·ty \dek-'stral-ət-ē\ *n, pl* **-ties** : the quality or state of having the right side or some parts (as the hand or eye) different from and usu. more efficient than the left or corresponding parts; *also* : RIGHT-HANDEDNESS

dex·tran \'dek-ˌstran, -strən\ *n* : any of numerous biopolymers $(C_6H_{10}O_5)_n$ of variable molecular weight that are produced esp. by the fermentation of sucrose by bacteria of the genus *Leuconostoc* (as *L. mesenteroides*), are found in dental plaque, and are used esp. after suitable chemical modification as blood plasma substitutes, as packing materials in chromatography, and as pharmaceutical agents — compare LEVAN

dex·tran·ase \-strə-ˌnās, -ˌnāz\ *n* : a hydrolase that prevents tooth decay by breaking down dextran and eliminating plaque

dex·trin \'dek-strən\ *also* **dex·trine** \-ˌstrēn, -strən\ *n* : any of various soluble gummy polysaccharides $(C_6H_{10}O_5)_n$ obtained from starch by the action of heat, acids, or enzymes and used as adhesives, as sizes for paper and textiles, as thickening agents (as in syrups), and in beer

dex·trino·gen·ic \ˌdek-strə-nō-'jen-ik\ *adj* : producing dextrins ⟨∼ activity⟩ — compare SACCHAROGENIC

dex·tro \'dek-(ˌ)strō\ *adj* : DEXTROROTATORY

dex·tro·am·phet·amine \ˌdek-(ˌ)strō-am-'fet-ə-ˌmēn, -mən\ *n* : a drug consisting of dextrorotatory amphetamine that is usu. administered in the form of its sulfate $(C_9H_{13}N)_2 \cdot H_2SO_4$, is a strong stimulant of the central nervous system, is a common drug of abuse, and is used medicinally esp. in the treatment of narcolepsy and attention deficit disorder — called also *dexamphetamine;* see DEXEDRINE

dex·tro·car·dia \ˌdek-strō-'kär-dē-ə\ *n* : an abnormal condition in which the heart is situated on the right side and the great blood vessels of the right and left sides are reversed — **dex·tro·car·di·al** \-dē-əl\ *adj*

dex·tro·car·dio·gram \ˌdek-strō-'kärd-ē-ə-ˌgram\ *n* : the part of an electrocardiogram recording activity of the right side of the heart — compare LEVOCARDIOGRAM

dex·troc·u·lar \(')dek-'sträk-yə-lər\ *adj* : using the right eye habitually or more effectively than the left — **dex·troc·u·lar·i·ty** \ˌdek-ˌsträk-yə-'lar-ət-ē\ *n, pl* **-ties**

dex·tro·me·thor·phan \ˌdek-strō-mi-'thòr-ˌfan\ *n* : a nonaddictive cough suppressant that is widely used esp. in the form of its hydrobromide $C_{18}H_{25}NO \cdot HBr$ in over-the-counter cough and cold preparations and is a codeine analog of levorphanol lacking the analgesic properties of codeine and producing little or no depression of the central nervous system

dex·tro·po·si·tion \ˌdek-strō-pə-'zish-ən\ *n* : displacement to the right — used chiefly of the aorta

dex·tro·pro·poxy·phene \ˌdek-strə-prō-'päk-sə-ˌfēn\ *n* : PROPOXYPHENE

dex·tro·ro·ta·tion \ˌdek-strə-rō-'tā-shən\ *n* : right-handed or clockwise rotation — used of the plane of polarization of light

dex·tro·ro·ta·to·ry \-'rōt-ə-ˌtōr-ē, -ˌtòr-\ *also* **dex·tro·ro·ta·ry** \-'rōt-ə-rē\ *adj* : turning clockwise or toward the right; *esp* : rotating the plane of polarization of light toward the right ⟨∼ crystals⟩ — compare LEVOROTATORY

dex·trose \'dek-ˌstrōs, -ˌstrōz\ *n* : dextrorotatory glucose — called also *grape sugar*

dex·tro·si·nis·tral \ˌdek-strə-ˈsin-əs-trəl, -sə-ˈnis-\ *adj* **1** : extending from the right toward the left **2** : naturally left-handed but trained to use the right hand in writing — **dex·tro·si·nis·tral·ly** \-ē\ *adv*

dextrous *var of* DEXTEROUS

dex·tro·ver·sion \ˈdek-strə-ˌvər-zhən, -shən\ *n* : movement or turning (as of the eyes) to the right

d4T \ˌdē-ˌfȯr-ˈtē\ *n* : a synthetic antiretroviral nucleoside $C_{10}H_{12}N_2O_4$ that is an analog of thymidine and is administered orally in the treatment of HIV infection — called also *stavudine*

DFP \ˌdē-ˌef-ˈpē\ *n* : ISOFLUROPHATE

dg *abbr* decigram

DHA *abbr* **1** dehydroepiandrosterone **2** dihydroxyacetone **3** docosahexaenoic acid

DHEA *abbr* dehydroepiandrosterone

dho·bie itch \ˈdō-bē-\ *n* : ringworm attacking moist parts of the body (as the groin)

DHPG \ˈdē-ˌāch-ˈpē-ˈjē\ *n* : GANCICLOVIR

DHT *abbr* dihydrotestosterone

DI *abbr* diabetes insipidus

dia *abbr* **1** diameter **2** diathermy

Di·a·βe·ta \ˌdī-ə-ˈbā-tə\ *trademark* — used for a preparation of glyburide

di·a·be·tes \ˌdī-ə-ˈbēt-ēz, -ˈbēt-əs\ *n, pl* **diabetes** : any of various abnormal conditions characterized by the secretion and excretion of excessive amounts of urine; *esp* : DIABETES MELLITUS

diabetes in·sip·i·dus \-in-ˈsip-əd-əs\ *n* : a disorder that is caused by insufficient secretion of vasopressin by the pituitary gland or by a failure of the kidneys to respond to circulating vasopressin and that is characterized by intense thirst and by the excretion of large amounts of urine — see CENTRAL DIABETES INSIPIDUS, NEPHROGENIC DIABETES INSIPIDUS

diabetes mel·li·tus \-ˈmel-ət-əs\ *n* : a variable disorder of carbohydrate metabolism caused by a combination of hereditary and environmental factors and usu. characterized by inadequate secretion or utilization of insulin, by excessive urine production, by excessive amounts of sugar in the blood and urine, and by thirst, hunger, and loss of weight — see TYPE 1 DIABETES, TYPE 2 DIABETES

¹**di·a·bet·ic** \ˌdī-ə-ˈbet-ik\ *adj* **1** : of or relating to diabetes or diabetics **2** : affected with diabetes **3** : occurring in or caused by diabetes ⟨a ∼ coma⟩ **4** : suitable for diabetics ⟨∼ food⟩

²**diabetic** *n* : a person affected with diabetes

diabeticorum — see NECROBIOSIS LIPOIDICA DIABETICORUM

di·a·be·to·gen·ic \ˌdī-ə-ˌbēt-ə-ˈjen-ik\ *adj* : producing diabetes ⟨∼ drugs⟩ ⟨a ∼ diet⟩

di·a·be·tol·o·gist \ˌdī-ə-bə-ˈtäl-ə-jəst\ *n* : a specialist in diabetes

di·ac·e·tate \(ˈ)dī-ˈas-ə-ˌtāt\ *n* **1** : an acid derivative (as a salt or ester) containing two acetate groups **2** : ACETOACETATE

di·ac·e·tic acid \ˌdī-ə-ˌsēt-ik-\ *n* : ACETOACETIC ACID

di·ac·e·tin \dī-ˈas-ət-ən\ *n* : ACETIN b

¹**di·ac·e·tyl** \ˌdī-ə-ˈsēt-ᵊl, dī-ˈas-ət-ᵊl\ *adj* : containing two acetyl groups

²**diacetyl** *n* : a greenish yellow liquid compound $(CH_3CO)_2$ that has an odor like that of quinone, that is chiefly responsible for the odor of butter and contributes to the aroma of coffee and tobacco, and that is used as a flavoring agent in foods (as margarine) — called also *biacetyl*

di·ac·e·tyl·mor·phine \-ˈmȯr-ˌfēn\ *n* : HEROIN

¹**di·ac·id** \(ˈ)dī-ˈas-əd\ *or* **di·acid·ic** \ˌdī-ə-ˈsid-ik\ *adj* **1** : able to react with two molecules of a monobasic acid or one of a dibasic acid to form a salt or ester — used esp. of bases **2** : containing two replaceable hydrogen atoms — used esp. of acid salts

²**diacid** *n* : an acid with two acid hydrogen atoms

diad *var of* DYAD

dia·der·mal \ˌdī-ə-ˈdər-məl\ *or* **dia·der·mat·ic** \-dər-ˈmat-ik\ *or* **dia·der·mic** \-ˈdər-mik\ *adj* : acting through the skin ⟨a ∼ allergy⟩ ⟨a ∼ ointment⟩

di·a·do·cho·ki·ne·sia *or* **di·a·do·ko·ki·ne·sia** \ˌdī-ˌad-ə-ˌkō-kə-ˈnē-zh(ē-)ə, ˌdī-ə-ˌdō-(ˌ)kō-, -kī-ˈnē-\ *n* : the normal power of alternating diametrically opposite muscular actions (as flexion and extension of a limb) — **di·a·do·cho·ki·net·ic** *or* **di·a·do·ko·ki·net·ic** \-kə-ˈnet-ik, -kī-ˈnet-\ *adj*

di·a·do·cho·ki·ne·sis \-kə-ˈnē-səs, -kī-\ *n, pl* **-ne·ses** \-ˌsēz\ : DIADOCHOKINESIA

di·ag·nose \ˈdī-ig-ˌnōs, -ˌnōz, ˌdī-ig-ˈ, -əg-\ *vb* **-nosed; -nos·ing** *vt* **1** : to recognize (as a disease) by signs and symptoms **2** : to diagnose a disease or condition in ⟨*diagnosed* the patient⟩ ∼ *vi* : to make a diagnosis — **di·ag·nos·able** *also* **di·ag·nose·able** \ˌdī-ig-ˈnō-sə-bəl, -əg-, -zə-\ *adj*

di·ag·no·sis \ˌdī-ig-ˈnō-səs, -əg-\ *n, pl* **-no·ses** \-ˌsēz\ **1 a** : the art or act of identifying a disease from its signs and symptoms **b** : the decision reached by diagnosis ⟨a ∼ of pneumonia⟩ **2** : a concise technical description of a taxon

diagnosis related group *n* : DRG

¹**di·ag·nos·tic** \-ˈnäs-tik\ *also* **di·ag·nos·ti·cal** \-ti-kəl\ *adj* **1** : of, relating to, or used in diagnosis **2** : using the methods of or yielding a diagnosis ⟨a ∼ service⟩ ⟨∼ properties⟩ — **di·ag·nos·ti·cal·ly** \-ti-k(ə-)lē\ *adv*

²**diagnostic** *n* : the art or practice of diagnosis — often used in pl.

di·ag·nos·ti·cian \-(ˌ)näs-ˈtish-ən\ *n* : a specialist in medical diagnostics

dia·ki·ne·sis \ˌdī-ə-kə-ˈnē-səs, -(ˌ)kī-\ *n, pl* **-ne·ses** \-ˌsēz\ : the final stage of the meiotic prophase marked by contraction of the bivalents — **dia·ki·net·ic** \-ˈnet-ik\ *adj*

Dia·lis·ter \ˌdī-ə-ˈlis-tər\ *n* : a genus of minute gram-negative parasitic strictly anaerobic bacteria of the family Bacteroidaceae that grow only in fresh sterile tissue or ascitic fluid and comprise cells occurring singly, in pairs, or in short chains

di·al·lel \ˈdī-ə-ˌlel\ *adj* : relating to or being the crossing of each of several individuals with two or more others in order to determine the relative genetic contribution of each parent to specific characters in the offspring

di·al·lyl \(ˈ)dī-ˈal-əl\ *adj* : containing two allyl groups

di·al·lyl·bar·bi·tu·ric acid \(ˌ)dī-ˌal-əl-ˌbär-bə-ˌt(y)ùr-ik-\ *n* : ALLOBARBITAL

di·al·y·sance \dī-ˈal-ə-sən(t)s\ *n* : blood volume in milliliters per unit time cleared of a substance by dialysis (as by an artificial kidney)

di·al·y·sate \dī-ˈal-ə-ˌzāt, -ˌsāt\ *also* **di·al·y·zate** \-ˌzāt\ *n* **1** : the material that passes through the membrane in dialysis — called also *diffusate* **2** : the liquid into which material passes by way of the membrane in dialysis — called also *diffusate*

di·al·y·sis \dī-ˈal-ə-səs\ *n, pl* **-y·ses** \-ˌsēz\ **1** : the separation of substances in solution by means of their unequal diffusion through semipermeable membranes; *esp* : such a separation of colloids from soluble substances **2** : either of two medical procedures to remove wastes or toxins from the blood and adjust fluid and electrolyte imbalances by utilizing rates at which substances diffuse through a semipermeable membrane: **a** : the process of removing blood from an artery (as of a kidney patient), purifying it by dialysis, adding vital substances, and returning it to a vein — called also *hemodialysis* **b** : a procedure performed in the peritoneal cavity in which the peritoneum acts as the semipermeable membrane — called also *peritoneal dialysis* — **di·a·lyt·ic** \ˌdī-ə-ˈlit-ik\ *adj*

dialysis dementia *n* : a neurological syndrome that occurs in some long-term dialysis patients, is associated with aluminum deposits in bone and the brain from aluminum-containing compounds in the dialysis fluid or in antacids

\ə\ abut \ᵊ\ kitten \ər\ further \a\ ash \ā\ ace \ä\ cot, cart \aù\ out \ch\ chin \e\ bet \ē\ easy \g\ go \i\ hit \ī\ ice \j\ job \ŋ\ sing \ō\ go \ȯ\ law \ȯi\ boy \th\ thin \th̲\ the \ü\ loot \ù\ foot \y\ yet \zh\ vision *See also* Pronunciation Symbols page

prescribed to control phosphorus balance, and is characterized by progressive dementia, dyspraxia, facial grimaces, and myoclonic seizures

di·a·lyz·able *or Brit* **di·a·lys·able** \'dī-ə-ˌlī-zə-bəl\ *adj* : capable of being dialyzed or of dialyzing; *esp* : capable of diffusing through a dialyzing membrane — **di·a·lyz·abil·i·ty** *or Brit* **di·a·lys·abil·i·ty** \ˌdī-ə-ˌlī-zə-ˈbil-ət-ē\ *n, pl* **-ties**

di·a·lyze *or Brit* **di·a·lyse** \'dī-ə-ˌlīz\ *vb* **-lyzed** *or Brit* **-lysed**; **-lyz·ing** *or Brit* **-lys·ing** *vt* : to subject to dialysis : separate or obtain by dialysis ~ *vi* : to undergo dialysis : diffuse through a suitable membrane

di·a·lyz·er *or Brit* **di·a·lys·er** \-ˌlī-zər\ *n* : an apparatus in which dialysis is carried out consisting essentially of one or more containers for liquids separated into compartments by membranes

diam *abbr* diameter

di·am·e·ter \dī-ˈam-ət-ər\ *n* **1** : a unit of magnification for an optical instrument equal to the number of times the linear dimensions of an object are apparently increased ⟨a microscope magnifying 60 ~*s*⟩ **2** : one of the maximal breadths of a part of the body ⟨the transverse ~ of the inlet of the pelvis⟩

di·amide \'dī-ə-ˌmīd, dī-ˈam-əd\ *n* : a compound containing two amido groups

di·am·i·dine \(ˈ)dī-ˈam-ə-ˌdēn, -dən\ *n* : any of a group of compounds (as pentamidine and stilbamidine) containing two of the groups –C(=NH)NH₂

di·amine \'dī-ə-ˌmēn, dī-ˈam-ən\ *n* : a compound containing two amino groups

diamine oxidase *n* : HISTAMINASE

di·ami·no \ˌdī-ə-ˈmē-(ˌ)nō\ *adj* : relating to or containing two amino or substituted amino groups

di·ami·no·di·phe·nyl sulfone *or chiefly Brit* **di·ami·no·di·phe·nyl sulphone** \ˌdī-ə-ˌmē-(ˌ)nō-ˌdī-ˌfen-ᵊl-, -ˌfēn-\ *n* : DAPSONE

di·a·mond·back rattlesnake \'dī-(ə-)mən(d)-ˌbak-\ *n* : either of two large and deadly rattlesnakes of the genus *Crotalus* (*C. adamanteus* of the southeastern U.S. and *C. atrox* of the south central and southwestern U.S. and Mexico) — called also *diamondback, diamondback rattler*

dia·mor·phine \ˌdī-ə-ˈmȯr-ˌfēn\ *n* : HEROIN

dia·pause \'dī-ə-ˌpȯz\ *n* : a period of physiologically enforced dormancy between periods of activity

dia·paus·ing \-ˌpȯ-ziŋ\ *adj* : undergoing diapause

di·a·pe·de·sis \ˌdī-ə-pə-ˈdē-səs\ *n, pl* **-de·ses** \-ˌsēz\ : the passage of blood cells through capillary walls into the tissues — called also *emigration* — **di·a·pe·det·ic** \-ˈdet-ik\ *adj*

¹di·a·per \'dī-(ə-)pər\ *n* : a basic garment esp. for infants consisting of a folded cloth or other absorbent material drawn up between the legs and fastened about the waist

²diaper *vt* **di·a·pered**; **di·a·per·ing** \-p(ə-)riŋ\ : to put on or change the diaper of (an infant)

diaper rash *n* : skin irritation of the diaper-covered area and usu. the buttocks of an infant esp. from exposure to feces and urinary ammonia

di·aph·a·nom·e·ter \dī-ˌaf-ə-ˈnäm-ət-ər\ *n* : an instrument for measuring transparency (as of air or liquids) — **di·aph·a·no·met·ric** \-nə-ˈme-trik\ *adj*

di·aph·a·no·scope \dī-ˈaf-ə-nō-ˌskōp\ *n* : a device for examining the accessory nasal sinuses of domestic animals — **di·aph·a·nos·co·py** \-ˈnäs-kə-pē\ *n, pl* **-pies**

di·aph·o·rase \dī-ˈaf-ə-ˌrās, -ˌrāz\ *n* : a flavoprotein enzyme capable of oxidizing the reduced form of NAD

di·a·pho·re·sis \ˌdī-ə-fə-ˈrē-səs, (ˌ)dī-ˌaf-ə-\ *n, pl* **-re·ses** \-ˌsēz\ : PERSPIRATION; *esp* : profuse perspiration artificially induced

¹di·a·pho·ret·ic \-ˈret-ik\ *adj* **1** : having the power to increase sweating **2** : perspiring profusely : covered with sweat : SWEATY

²diaphoretic *n* : an agent capable of inducing sweating

di·a·phragm \'dī-ə-ˌfram\ *n* **1** : a body partition of muscle and connective tissue; *specif* : the partition separating the chest and abdominal cavities in mammals — see PELVIC DIAPHRAGM, UROGENITAL DIAPHRAGM **2** : a device that limits

the aperture of a lens or optical system **3** : a molded cap usu. of thin rubber fitted over the uterine cervix to act as a mechanical contraceptive barrier

di·a·phrag·ma sel·lae \ˌdī-ə-ˈfrag-mə-ˈsel-ˌī, -ˌē\ *n* : a small horizontal fold of the dura mater that roofs over the sella turcica and is pierced by a small opening for the infundibulum

di·a·phrag·mat·ic \ˌdī-ə-frə(g)-ˈmat-ik, -ˌfrag-\ *adj* : of, involving, or resembling a diaphragm ⟨~ hernia⟩

di·a·phys·e·al \ˌdī-ˌaf-ə-ˈsē-əl, -ˈzē-\ *or* **di·a·phys·i·al** \ˌdī-ə-ˈfiz-ē-əl\ *adj* : of, relating to, or involving a diaphysis

di·a·phy·sec·to·my \ˌdī-ə-fə-ˈzek-tə-mē, -ˈsek-\ *n, pl* **-mies** : surgical excision of all or part of a diaphysis (as of the clavicle, femur, or fibula)

di·aph·y·sis \dī-ˈaf-ə-səs\ *n, pl* **-y·ses** \-ˌsēz\ : the shaft of a long bone — compare EPIPHYSIS 1

di·apoph·y·sis \ˌdī-ə-ˈpäf-ə-səs\ *n, pl* **-y·ses** \-ˌsēz\ : a transverse process of a vertebra that is an outgrowth of the neural arch on the dorsal side; *esp* : one of the dorsal pair of such processes when two or more pairs are present

Di·ap·to·mus \dī-ˈap-tə-məs\ *n* : a genus (the type of the family Diaptomidae) of widely distributed freshwater copepods including some which serve as intermediate hosts for the fish tapeworm of humans — **di·ap·to·mid** \-məd\ *n*

di·ar·rhea *or chiefly Brit* **di·ar·rhoea** \ˌdī-ə-ˈrē-ə\ *n* : abnormally frequent intestinal evacuations with more or less fluid stools

di·ar·rhe·al *or chiefly Brit* **di·ar·rhoe·al** \-ˈrē-əl\ *adj* : DIARRHEIC

di·ar·rhe·ic *or chiefly Brit* **di·ar·rhoe·ic** \-ˈrē-ik\ *adj* : of or relating to diarrhea

di·ar·rhet·ic *or chiefly Brit* **di·ar·rhoet·ic** \-ˈret-ik\ *adj* : DIARRHEIC

di·ar·thro·di·al \ˌdī-ˌär-ˈthrōd-ē-əl\ *adj* : of, relating to, or exhibiting diarthrosis

di·ar·thro·sis \ˌdī-ˌär-ˈthrō-səs\ *n, pl* **-thro·ses** \-ˌsēz\ **1** : articulation that permits free movement **2** : a freely movable joint — called also *synovial joint*

di·ar·tic·u·lar \ˌdī-ˌär-ˈtik-yə-lər\ *adj* : of or involving two joints

di·as·chi·sis \dī-ˈas-kə-səs\ *n, pl* **-chi·ses** \-ˌsēz\ : the breaking up of a pattern of brain activity by a localized injury that temporarily throws the whole activity out of function though destroying only part of a structure

di·a·scope \'dī-ə-ˌskōp\ *n* : a plate of glass pressed against the skin so as to expel the blood from a part and show anatomical changes — **di·a·scop·ic** \ˌdī-ə-ˈskäp-ik\ *adj* — **di·as·co·py** \dī-ˈas-kə-pē\ *n, pl* **-pies**

di·a·stase \'dī-ə-ˌstās, -ˌstāz\ *n* **1** : AMYLASE; *esp* : a mixture of amylases from malt **2** : ENZYME

di·a·sta·sic \ˌdī-ə-ˈstā-sik, -zik\ *adj* : DIASTATIC

di·as·ta·sis \dī-ˈas-tə-səs\ *n, pl* **-ta·ses** \-ˌsēz\ **1** : an abnormal separation of parts normally joined together **2** : the rest phase of cardiac diastole occurring between filling of the ventricle and the start of atrial contraction

di·a·stat·ic \ˌdī-ə-ˈstat-ik\ *adj* : relating to or having the properties of diastase; *esp* : converting starch into sugar

di·a·ste·ma \ˌdī-ə-ˈstē-mə\ *n, pl* **-mas** *or* **-ma·ta** \-mət-ə\ : a space between teeth in a jaw — **di·a·ste·mat·ic** \-sti-ˈmat-ik\ *adj*

di·a·ste·ma·to·my·e·lia \ˌdī-ə-ˌstē-mət-ō-mī-ˈē-lē-ə, -ˌstem-ət-\ *n* : congenital division of all or part of the spinal cord

di·as·ter \(ˈ)dī-ˈas-tər\ *n* : a stage in mitotic cell division in which the divided and separated chromosomes group themselves near the poles of the spindle preparatory to forming new nuclei

di·a·ste·reo·mer \ˌdī-ə-ˈster-ē-ō-(ˌ)mər, -ˈstir-\ *or* **di·a·ste·reo·iso·mer** \-ˌster-ē-ō-ˈī-sə-mər, -ˌstir-\ *n* : an isomer that is a stereoisomer of a compound having two or more chiral centers and that is not a mirror image of another stereoisomer of the same compound — **di·a·ste·reo·mer·ic** \-ˌster-ē-ō-ˈmer-ik, -ˌstir-\ *or* **di·a·ste·reo·iso·mer·ic** \-ˌī-sə-ˈmer-ik\ *adj* — **di·a·ste·reo·isom·er·ism** \-ˌī-ˈsäm-ə-ˌriz-əm\ *n*

di·as·to·le \dī-'as-tə-(ˌ)lē\ *n* **1** : the passive rhythmical expansion or dilation of the cavities of the heart during which they fill with blood — compare SYSTOLE **2** : the rhythmical expansion of a pulsating vacuole (as of an ameba) — **di·a·stol·ic** \ˌdī-ə-'stäl-ik\ *adj*

diastolic blood pressure *n* : the lowest arterial blood pressure of a cardiac cycle occurring during diastole of the heart — called also *diastolic pressure;* compare SYSTOLIC BLOOD PRESSURE

di·a·stroph·ic dwarfism \ˌdī-ə-'sträf-ik-\ *n* : an inherited dysplasia affecting bones and joints and characterized esp. by clubfoot, deformities of the digits of the hand, malformed pinnae, and cleft palate

dia·ther·mal \ˌdī-ə-'thər-məl\ *adj* : DIATHERMIC

dia·ther·mic \-mik\ *adj* : of or relating to diathermy ⟨~ treatment⟩

dia·ther·mo·co·ag·u·la·tion \ˌdī-ə-ˌthər-mə-kō-ˌag-yə-'lā-shən\ *n* : ELECTROCOAGULATION

dia·ther·my \'dī-ə-ˌthər-mē\ *n, pl* **-mies** : the generation of heat in tissue by electric currents for medical or surgical purposes — called also *endothermy;* see ELECTROCOAGULATION, SHORTWAVE DIATHERMY

di·ath·e·sis \dī-'ath-ə-səs\ *n, pl* **-e·ses** \-ˌsēz\ : a constitutional predisposition toward a particular state or condition and esp. one that is abnormal or diseased — **di·a·thet·ic** \ˌdī-ə-'thet-ik\ *adj*

di·a·tom \'dī-ə-ˌtäm\ *n* : any of a class (Bacillariophyceae) of minute planktonic unicellular or colonial algae with silicified skeletons that form diatomite

di·a·to·ma·ceous \ˌdī-ət-ə-'mā-shəs, (ˌ)dī-ˌat-\ *adj* : consisting of or abounding in diatoms or their siliceous remains

diatomaceous earth *n* : DIATOMITE

di·atom·ic \ˌdī-ə-'täm-ik\ *adj* : consisting of two atoms : having two atoms in the molecule

di·at·o·mite \dī-'at-ə-ˌmīt\ *n* : a light friable siliceous material derived chiefly from diatom remains and used esp. as a filter — called also *diatomaceous earth*

dia·tri·zo·ate \ˌdī-ə-ˌtrī-'zō-ˌāt\ *n* : either of two salts of the acid $C_{11}H_9I_3N_2O_4$ administered in solution as a radiopaque medium for various forms of radiographic diagnosis — see HYPAQUE

di·az·e·pam \dī-'az-ə-ˌpam\ *n* : a synthetic tranquilizer $C_{16}H_{13}ClN_2O$ used esp. to relieve anxiety and tension and as a muscle relaxant — see VALIUM

di·a·zine \'dī-ə-ˌzēn, dī-'az-ⁿn\ *n* : any of three heterocyclic aromatic compounds $C_4H_4N_2$ that consist of a six-membered ring and differ in the proximity of the nitrogen atoms to each other

Di·az·i·non \dī-'az-ə-ˌnän\ *trademark* — used for an organophosphate insecticide $C_{12}H_{21}N_2O_3PS$ that is a cholinesterase inhibitor dangerous to humans if ingested

di·azo \dī-'az-(ˌ)ō\ *adj* **1** : relating to or containing the group N_2 composed of two nitrogen atoms united to a single carbon atom of an organic radical **2** : relating to or containing diazonium

di·azo·ben·zene·sul·fon·ic acid *or chiefly Brit* **di·azo·ben·zene·sul·phon·ic acid** \ˌdī-ˌaz-(ˌ)ō-ˌben-ˌzēn-ˌsəl-'fän-ik-\ *n* : a white or reddish crystalline acid derivative $C_6H_4N_2O_3S$ of sulfanilic acid that is used as the reagent in the diazo reaction

di·a·zo·ni·um \ˌdī-ə-'zō-nē-əm\ *n* : the monovalent cation N_2^+ that is composed of two nitrogen atoms united to carbon in an organic radical and that usu. exists in salts used in the manufacture of azo dyes

diazo reaction *n* : a reaction in which a diazo compound is made or used; *specif* : a reaction in various diseases (as typhoid fever) consisting of a red discoloration of the urine on addition of diazobenzenesulfonic acid

di·az·o·tize *or Brit* **di·az·o·tise** \dī-'az-ə-ˌtīz\ *vt* **-tized** *or Brit* **-tised; -tiz·ing** *or Brit* **-tis·ing** : to convert (a compound) into a diazo compound (as a diazonium salt) — **di·az·o·ti·za·tion** *or Brit* **di·az·o·ti·sa·tion** \-ˌaz-ət-ə-'zā-shən\ *n*

di·az·ox·ide \ˌdī-ˌaz-'äk-ˌsīd\ *n* : a drug $C_8H_7ClN_2O_2S$ used in the treatment of hypoglycemia and in the emergency treatment of hypertension

di·ba·sic \(')dī-'bā-sik\ *adj* **1** : having two replaceable hydrogen atoms — used of acids **2** : containing two atoms of a monovalent metal

dibasic sodium phosphate *n* : SODIUM PHOSPHATE 2

di·benz·an·thra·cene *or* **1,2:5,6–di·benz·an·thra·cene** \(ˌwən-ˌtü-ˌfīv-ˌsiks-)dī-ˌben-'zan(t)-thrə-ˌsēn\ *n* : an orange-brown crystalline actively carcinogenic cyclic hydrocarbon $C_{22}H_{14}$ found in trace amounts in coal tar

di·ben·zo·fu·ran \ˌdī-ˌben-zō-'fyu̇-ˌran, -fyə-'ran\ *n* : a highly toxic chemical compound $C_{12}H_8O$ that is used in chemical synthesis and as an insecticide and is a hazardous pollutant in its chlorinated form

Di·both·rio·ceph·a·lus \(ˌ)dī-ˌbäth-rē-ō-'sef-ə-ləs\ *n, syn of* DIPHYLLOBOTHRIUM

di·bro·mide \(')dī-'brō-ˌmīd\ *n* : an organic compound containing two atoms of bromine

di·bro·mo·chlo·ro·pro·pane \(ˌ)dī-ˌbrō-mō-ˌklōr-ō-'prō-ˌpān, -ˌklȯr-\ *n* : DBCP

di·bu·caine \dī-'byü-ˌkān, 'dī-ˌ\ *n* : a local anesthetic $C_{20}H_{29}N_3O_2$ that is used for temporary relief of pain and itching esp. from burns, sunburn, insect bites, or hemorrhoids — called also *cinchocaine*

dibucaine number *n* : a number expressing the percentage by which cholinesterase activity in a serum sample is inhibited by dibucaine

di·bu·tyl \(')dī-'byüt-ⁿl\ *adj* : containing two butyl groups in the molecule

dibutyl phthal·ate \-'thal-ˌāt\ *n* : a colorless oily ester $C_{16}H_{22}O_4$ used chiefly as a solvent, plasticizer, pesticide, and repellent (as for chiggers and mites)

di·car·box·yl·ic \ˌdī-ˌkär-ˌbäk-'sil-ik\ *adj* : containing two carboxyl groups in the molecule

dicaryon, dicaryotic *var of* DIKARYON, DIKARYOTIC

di·cen·tric \(')dī-'sen-trik\ *adj* : having two centromeres ⟨a ~ chromosome⟩ — **dicentric** *n*

di·ceph·a·lus \(')dī-'sef-ə-ləs\ *n, pl* **-a·li** \-ˌlī\ : a teratological fetus having two distinct heads

di·chlo·ra·mine–T \ˌdī-ˌklōr-ə-ˌmēn-'tē, -ˌklȯr-\ *n* : a yellow crystalline compound $C_7H_7Cl_2NO_2S$ used esp. formerly as an antiseptic — compare CHLORAMINE-T

di·chlor·eth·yl sulfide \(ˌ)dī-ˌklōr-ˌeth-əl-, -ˌklȯr-\ *also* **di·chlo·ro·eth·yl sulfide** \-ˌklōr-ō-ˌeth-, -ˌklȯr-\ *n* : MUSTARD GAS

di·chlo·ride \(')dī-'klō(ə)r-ˌīd, -'klȯ(ə)r-\ *n* : a compound containing two atoms of chlorine

di·chlo·ro·ben·zene \(ˌ)dī-ˌklōr-ə-'ben-ˌzēn, -ˌklȯr-, -(ˌ)ben-'\ *n* : any of three isomeric benzene derivatives $C_6H_4Cl_2$ (as paradichlorobenzene) that differ in the relative placements of the two chlorine atoms

p–dichlorobenzene *var of* PARADICHLOROBENZENE

di·chlo·ro·di·flu·o·ro·meth·ane \-ˌdī-ˌflu̇r-ə-'meth-ˌān\ *n* : a nontoxic nonflammable gas CCl_2F_2 used as a refrigerant and as a propellant

di·chlo·ro·meth·ane \-'meth-ˌān\ *n* : METHYLENE CHLORIDE

di·chlo·ro·phen·ar·sine \-fen-'är-ˌsēn, -ˌär-'sēn\ *n* : an arsenical formerly used in the form of its white powdery hydrochloride $C_6H_6AsCl_2NO \cdot HCl$ in the treatment of syphilis

2,4–di·chlo·ro·phen·oxy·ace·tic acid *also* **di·chlo·ro·phen·oxy·ace·tic acid** \(ˌtü-ˌfȯr-)dī-ˌklōr-ō-(ˌ)fen-ˌäk-sē-ə-ˌsēt-ik-, (ˌtü-ˌfȯr-), -ˌklȯr-\ *n* : 2,4-D

di·chlor·vos \(')dī-'klō(ə)r-ˌväs, -'klȯ(ə)r-, -vəs\ *n* : an organophosphorus insecticide and anthelmintic $C_4H_7Cl_2O_4P$ used esp. in veterinary medicine — called also *DDVP*

di·cho·ri·al \(')dī-'kōr-ē-əl, -'kȯr-\ *adj* : having two chorions and two placentas — used esp. of human fraternal twins

---

\ə\ **abut** \ᵊ\ **kitten** \ər\ **further** \a\ **ash** \ā\ **ace** \ä\ **cot, cart**
\au̇\ **out** \ch\ **chin** \e\ **bet** \ē\ **easy** \g\ **go** \i\ **hit** \ī\ **ice** \j\ **job**
\ŋ\ **sing** \ō\ **go** \ȯ\ **law** \ȯi\ **boy** \th\ **thin** \t͟h\ **the** \ü\ **loot**
\u̇\ **foot** \y\ **yet** \zh\ **vision** *See also* Pronunciation Symbols page

di·cho·ri·on·ic \ˌdī-ˌkōr-ē-'än-ik, -ˌkȯr-\ *adj* : DICHORIAL

dich·ot·ic \(')dī-'kōt-ik\ *adj* : relating to or involving the presentation of a stimulus to one ear that differs in some respect (as pitch, loudness, frequency, or energy) from a stimulus presented to the other ear ⟨∼ listening⟩ — **dich·oti·cal·ly** \-i-k(ə-)lē\ *adv*

di·chot·o·mous \dī-'kät-ə-məs *also* də-\ *adj* : dividing into two parts ⟨∼ branching⟩ — **di·chot·o·mous·ly** *adv*

dichotomous key *n* : a key for the identification of organisms based on a series of choices between alternative characters

di·chot·o·my \dī-'kät-ə-mē *also* də-\ *n, pl* **-mies** : a division or forking into branches; *esp* : repeated bifurcation

di·chro·ic \dī-'krō-ik\ *adj* **1** : having the property of dichroism ⟨a ∼ crystal⟩ **2** : DICHROMATIC

di·chro·ism \'dī-(ˌ)krō-ˌiz-əm\ *n* : the property of some crystals and solutions of absorbing one of two plane-polarized components of transmitted light more strongly than the other; *also* : the property of exhibiting different colors by reflected or transmitted light — compare CIRCULAR DICHROISM 1

di·chro·mat \'dī-krō-ˌmat, (')dī-'\ *n* : one affected with dichromatism

di·chro·mate \(')dī-'krō-ˌmāt, 'dī-krō-\ *n* : a usu. orange to red chromium salt containing the anion $Cr_2O_7{}^{2-}$ ⟨∼ of potassium⟩

di·chro·mat·ic \ˌdī-krō-'mat-ik\ *adj* **1** : having or exhibiting two colors **2** : of, relating to, or exhibiting dichromatism

di·chro·ma·tism \dī-'krō-mə-ˌtiz-əm\ *n* **1** : the state or condition of being dichromatic **2** : partial color blindness in which only two colors are perceptible

di·chro·ma·top·sia \(ˌ)dī-ˌkrō-mə-'täp-sē-ə\ *n* : DICHROMATISM 2

Dick test \'dik-\ *n* : a test to determine susceptibility or immunity to scarlet fever by an injection of scarlet fever toxin

Dick, George Frederick (1881–1967) and **Gladys Henry (1881–1963),** American physicians. In 1923 the Dicks isolated the hemolytic streptococcus that causes scarlet fever. They also developed the toxin used for immunization and a method for preventing the disease—a toxin-antitoxin injection. The Dick test was developed in 1924.

di·clo·fe·nac \dī-'klō-fə-ˌnak\ *n* : a nonsteroidal antiinflammatory drug used in the form of its sodium salt $C_{14}H_{10}Cl_2NNaO_2$ or potassium salt $C_{14}H_{10}Cl_2KNaO_2$ esp. to treat the symptoms of rheumatoid arthritis, osteoarthritis, and ankylosing spondylitis — see VOLTAREN

di·clox·a·cil·lin \(ˌ)dī-ˌkläk-sə-'sil-ən\ *n* : a semisynthetic penicillin used in the form of its hydrated sodium salt $C_{19}H_{16}Cl_2N_3NaO_5S \cdot H_2O$ esp. against beta-lactamase producing staphylococci

di·co·phane \'dī-kə-ˌfān\ *n* : DDT

di·cou·ma·rin \(')dī-'kü-mə-rən\ *n* : DICUMAROL

dicoumarol *var of* DICUMAROL

Di·cro·coe·li·i·dae \ˌdī-krə-sə-'lī-ə-ˌdē\ *n pl* : a family of small to medium-sized flattened or more or less cylindrical digenetic trematode worms that as adults parasitize the biliary ducts or occas. other viscera of vertebrates

Di·cro·coe·li·um \ˌdī-krə-'sē-lē-əm\ *n* : a widely distributed genus that is the type of the family Dicrocoeliidae and that includes small lanceolate digenetic trematodes infesting the livers of ruminants or occas. other mammals including humans — see LANCET FLUKE

di·crot·ic \(')dī-'krät-ik\ *adj* **1** *of the pulse* : having a double beat (as in certain febrile states in which the heart is overactive and the arterial walls are lacking in tone) — compare MONOCROTIC **2** : being or relating to the second part of the arterial pulse occurring during diastole of the heart or of an arterial pressure recording made during the same period — **di·cro·tism** \'dī-krə-ˌtiz-əm\ *n*

dicrotic notch *n* : a secondary upstroke in the descending part of a pulse tracing corresponding to the transient increase in aortic pressure upon closure of the aortic valve — called also *dicrotic wave*

Dic·ty·o·cau·lus \ˌdik-tē-ə-'kȯ-ləs\ *n* : a genus of small slender lungworms of the family Metastrongylidae infesting mammals (as ruminants) and often causing severe bronchial symptoms or even pneumonia in young animals

dic·tyo·ki·ne·sis \ˌdik-tē-ō-kī-'nē-səs\ *n, pl* **-ne·ses** \-ˌsēz\ : fission of the Golgi apparatus as a normal reproductive process

dic·tyo·some \'dik-tē-ə-ˌsōm\ *n* : any of the membranous or vesicular structures making up the Golgi apparatus

di·cu·ma·rol *also* **di·cou·ma·rol** \dī-'k(y)ü-mə-ˌról, -ˌról\ *n* : a crystalline compound $C_{19}H_{12}O_6$ that acts similarly to warfarin and is used esp. in preventing and treating thromboembolic disease

di·cy·clic \(')dī-'sī-klik, -'sik-lik\ *adj* : BICYCLIC

di·cy·clo·mine \(')dī-'sī-klə-ˌmēn, -'sik-lə-\ *n* : an anticholinergic drug used in the form of its hydrochloride $C_{19}H_{35}NO_2 \cdot HCl$ for its antispasmodic effect on smooth muscle in gastrointestinal functional disorders

di·dac·tic \dī-'dak-tik, də-\ *adj* : involving lecture and textbook instruction rather than demonstration and laboratory study

di·dan·o·sine \dī-'dan-ə-ˌsēn\ *n* : DDI

di·del·phia \(')dī-'del-fē-ə\ *n* : the condition of having a double uterus — **di·del·phic** \-fik\ *adj*

Di·del·phis \dī-'del-fəs\ *n* : a genus of marsupials (family Didelphidae) that includes the common opossum (*D. virginiana*) of the eastern U.S. and a few related tropical forms

di·de·oxy·cy·ti·dine \ˌdī-(ˌ)dē-ˌäk-sē-'sīt-ə-ˌdēn, -'sīt-\ *n* : DDC

di·de·oxy·ino·sine \-'in-ə-ˌsēn, -'ī-nə-, -sən\ *n* : DDI

¹die \'dī\ *vi* **died; dy·ing** \'dī-iŋ\ **1** : to suffer total and irreversible loss of the bodily attributes and functions that constitute life **2** : to suffer or face the pains of death

²die *n, pl* **dies** \'dīz\ : any of various tools or devices for imparting a desired shape, form, or finish to a material or for impressing an object or material

diel·drin \'dē(ə)l-drən\ *n* : a white crystalline persistent chlorinated hydrocarbon insecticide $C_{12}H_8Cl_6O$

Diels \'dē(ə)ls\, **Otto Paul Hermann (1876–1954),** and **Alder** \'òl-dər\, **Kurt (1902–1958),** German chemists. Diels and Alder made an important contribution to organic chemistry with their development of a method for synthesizing a ring of six carbon atoms. This is now known as the Diels-Alder reaction, from which aldrin and dieldrin are derived. In 1928 Diels and Alder published their first paper on the subject. The insecticides aldrin and dieldrin were first prepared by the method which is now widely used in the synthesis of organic compounds. Diels and Alder were awarded the Nobel Prize for Chemistry in 1950.

di·elec·tric \ˌdī-i-'lek-trik\ *n* : a nonconductor of direct electric current — **dielectric** *adj*

di·en·ceph·a·lon \ˌdī-ən-'sef-ə-ˌlän, ˌdī-(ˌ)en-, -lən\ *n* : the posterior subdivision of the forebrain — called also *betweenbrain, interbrain* — **di·en·ce·phal·ic** \-sə-'fal-ik\ *adj*

die·ner \'dē-nər\ *n* : a laboratory helper esp. in a medical school

di·en·es·trol \ˌdī-ə-'nes-ˌtról, -ˌtról\ *or chiefly Brit* **di·en·oes·trol** \ˌdī-ə-'nēs-\ *n* : a white crystalline estrogenic compound $C_{18}H_{18}O_2$ structurally related to diethylstilbestrol and used topically to treat atrophic vaginitis and kraurosis vulvae

Di·ent·amoe·ba \ˌdī-ˌent-ə-'mē-bə\ *n* : a genus of amebic protozoans parasitic in the intestines of humans and monkeys that include one (*D. fragilis*) known to cause abdominal pain, anorexia, and loose stools in humans

di·es·ter \'dī-ˌes-tər\ *n* : a compound containing two ester groups

di·es·trus \(')dī-'es-trəs\ *also* **di·es·trum** \-trəm\ *or chiefly Brit* **di·oes·trus** *also* **di·oes·trum** \-'ēs-\ *n* : a period of sexual quiescence that intervenes between two periods of estrus — **di·es·trous** \-trəs\ *also* **di·es·tru·al** \-trə-wəl\ *or chiefly Brit* **di·oes·trous** *also* **di·oes·tru·al** *adj*

¹di·et \'dī-ət\ *n* **1** : food and drink regularly provided or consumed **2** : habitual nourishment **3** : the kind and amount of food prescribed for a person or animal for a special reason **4** : a regimen of eating and drinking sparingly so as to reduce one's weight ⟨going on a ∼⟩

C
D

²**diet** *vt* **1** : to cause to take food **2** : to cause to eat and drink sparingly or according to prescribed rules ∼ *vi* : to eat sparingly or according to prescribed rules

³**diet** *adj* : reduced in calories ⟨a ∼ soft drink⟩

¹**di·etary** \ˈdī-ə-ˌter-ē\ *n*, *pl* **di·etar·ies** : the kinds and amounts of food available to or eaten by an individual, group, or population

²**dietary** *adj* : of or relating to a diet or to the rules of a diet ⟨a ∼ disease⟩ ⟨∼ habits⟩ — **di·etari·ly** \ˌdī-ə-ˈter-ə-lē\ *adv*

dietary fiber *n* : FIBER 2

Dietary Reference Intake *n* : a set of guidelines for the daily intake of nutrients (as vitamins, protein, and fats) and other food components (as fiber) that include recommended daily allowances, adequate daily intake values for nutrients having undetermined recommended daily allowances, and tolerable upper level values of daily intake — abbr. *DRI*

dietary supplement *n* : a product taken orally that contains one or more ingredients that are intended to supplement one's diet and are not considered food; *specif, according to the Dietary Supplements Health and Education Act* : a product other than tobacco that is taken by mouth, that contains one or more vitamins, minerals, herbs or other botanicals, amino acids, substances supplementing the diet by increasing the daily dietary intake, or a concentrate, constituent, metabolite, extract, or combination of these, that is not represented as a food or as constituting a meal or the sole item of the diet, and that contains as part of its labeling the words *dietary supplement*

di·et·er \ˈdī-ət-ər\ *n* : one that diets; *esp* : a person that consumes a reduced allowance of food in order to lose weight

di·etet·ic \ˌdī-ə-ˈtet-ik\ *adj* **1** : of or relating to diet **2** : adapted (as by the elimination of salt or sugar) for use in special diets — **di·etet·i·cal·ly** \-i-k(ə-)lē\ *adv*

di·etet·ics \-ˈtet-iks\ *n pl but sing or pl in constr* : the science or art of applying the principles of nutrition to feeding

di·eth·yl \(ˈ)dī-ˈeth-əl\ *adj* : containing two ethyl groups in a molecule

diethylamide — see LYSERGIC ACID DIETHYLAMIDE

di·eth·yl·amine \(ˌ)dī-ˌeth-ə-lə-ˈmēn, -ˈlam-ˌēn\ *n* : a colorless flammable volatile liquid base $(C_2H_5)_2NH$ having a fishy odor and used chiefly in organic synthesis

di·eth·yl·car·bam·azine \ˌdī-ˌeth-əl-kär-ˈbam-ə-ˌzēn, -zən\ *n* : an anthelmintic derived from piperazine and administered in the form of its crystalline citrate $C_{10}H_{21}N_3O \cdot C_6H_8O_7$ esp. to control filariasis in humans and large roundworms in dogs and cats

di·eth·yl·ene glycol \ˌeth-ə-ˌlēn-\ *n* : a sweet toxic syrupy compound $C_4H_{10}O_3$ used chiefly as a solvent, humectant, and plasticizer and in the production of polyester resins

di·eth·yl ether \(ˌ)dī-ˌeth-əl-\ *n* : ETHER 2a

di·eth·yl·pro·pi·on \(ˌ)dī-ˌeth-əl-ˈprō-pē-ˌän\ *n* : a sympathomimetic amine related structurally to amphetamine and used esp. in the form of its hydrochloride $C_{13}H_{19}NO \cdot HCl$ as an appetite suppressant to promote weight loss — see TENUATE

di·eth·yl·stil·bes·trol \-stil-ˈbes-ˌtrol, -ˌtrōl\ *or chiefly Brit* **di·eth·yl·stil·boes·trol** \-ˈbēs-\ *n* : a colorless crystalline synthetic compound $C_{18}H_{20}O_2$ used as a potent estrogen but contraindicated in pregnancy for its tendency to cause cancer or birth defects in offspring — called also *DES, stilbestrol*

di·eti·tian *or* **di·eti·cian** \ˌdī-ə-ˈtish-ən\ *n* : a specialist in dietetics

Die·tl's crisis \ˈdēt-ᵊlz-\ *n* : an attack of violent pain in the kidney region accompanied by chills, nausea, vomiting, and collapse that is caused by the formation of kinks in the ureter and is usu. associated with a floating kidney

　Die·tl \ˈdēt-ᵊl\, **Josef (1804–1878)**, Polish physician. Dietl was a leading proponent of a school of medicine advocating that physicians can only diagnose and describe diseases, not cure them. His single medical contribution was his description of Dietl's crisis.

di·e·to·ther·a·py \ˌdī-ət-ō-ˈther-ə-pē\ *n*, *pl* **-pies** : a branch of dietetics concerned with therapeutic uses of food and diet

diet pill *n* : a pill and esp. one containing amphetamine pre-

scribed esp. formerly to promote weight loss by increasing metabolism or depressing appetite

dif·fer·en·tia \ˌdif-ə-ˈren-ch(ē-)ə\ *n*, *pl* **-ti·ae** \-chē-ˌē, -chē-ˌī\ : the element, feature, or factor that distinguishes one entity, state, or class from another; *esp* : a characteristic trait distinguishing a species from other species of the same genus

dif·fer·en·tial \ˌdif-ə-ˈren-chəl\ *adj* **1** : of, relating to, or constituting a difference ⟨∼ birth rates in different economic levels⟩ **2** : making a distinction between individuals or classes ⟨∼ cell counts⟩ ⟨∼ staining⟩ — **dif·fer·en·tial·ly** \-ˈrench-(ə-)lē\ *adv*

differential blood count *n* : a blood count which includes separate counts for each kind of white blood cell — compare COMPLETE BLOOD COUNT, WHITE COUNT

differential cell count *n* : a count of cells that includes a separate count for each type of cell; *esp* : DIFFERENTIAL BLOOD COUNT

differential diagnosis *n* : the distinguishing of a disease or condition from others presenting similar symptoms

dif·fer·en·ti·ate \ˌdif-ə-ˈren-chē-ˌāt\ *vb* **-at·ed; -at·ing** *vt* **1** : to constitute a difference that distinguishes ⟨the history of the injury also ∼s these two fractures —J. S. Keene *et al*⟩ **2** : to cause differentiation of in the course of development **3** : to discriminate or give expression to a specific difference that distinguishes ⟨quickly learned to ∼ sharp pain from dull pain⟩ **4** : to cause differentiation in (a specimen for microscopic examination) by staining ∼ *vi* **1** : to recognize or express a difference ⟨∼ between humans and the rest of the primates⟩ **2** : to undergo differentiation ⟨when a B cell matures, it ∼s into a plasma cell that secretes antibodies —R. C. Gallo⟩

dif·fer·en·ti·a·tion \-ˌren-chē-ˈā-shən\ *n* **1 a** : the act of describing a thing by giving its differentia **b** : the enhancement of microscopically visible differences between tissue or cell parts by partial selective decolorization or removal of excess stain (as in regressive staining) **c** : the development of a discriminating conditioned response with a positive response to one stimulus and absence of the response on the application of similar but discriminably different stimuli **2 a** : modification of different parts of the body for performance of particular functions; *also* : specialization of parts or organs in the course of evolution **b** : the sum of the developmental processes whereby apparently unspecialized cells, tissues, and structures attain their adult form and function — compare DETERMINATION 2

dif·fer·ent·ly abled \ˈdif-ərnt-lē-ˈā-bəld, ˈdif-(ə-)rənt-\ *adj* : DISABLED, CHALLENGED

dif·flu·ent \ˈdif-ˌlü-ənt, -lə-wənt\ *adj* : characterized by mushiness or deliquescence ⟨in typhoid fever the parenchyma of the spleen becomes ∼⟩

dif·fract \dif-ˈrakt\ *vt* : to cause to undergo diffraction

dif·frac·tion \dif-ˈrak-shən\ *n* : a modification which light undergoes in passing by the edges of opaque bodies or through narrow slits or in being reflected from ruled surfaces and in which the rays appear to be deflected and to produce fringes of parallel light and dark or colored bands; *also* : a similar modification of other waves (as sound waves)

diffraction grating *n* : GRATING

diffraction pattern *n* : an often photographic pattern produced by diffraction (as of light or X-rays)

diffusa — see ENCEPHALITIS PERIAXIALIS DIFFUSA

dif·fu·sate \di-ˈfyü-ˌzāt\ *n* : DIALYSATE

¹**dif·fuse** \dif-ˈyüs\ *adj* : not concentrated or localized ⟨∼ sclerosis⟩

²**dif·fuse** \dif-ˈyüz\ *vb* **dif·fused; dif·fus·ing** *vt* **1** : to subject (as a light beam) to diffusion **2** : to break up and distribute (incident light) by reflection (as from a rough surface) ∼ *vi* : to undergo diffusion

---

\ə\ abut \ᵊ\ kitten \ər\ further \a\ ash \ā\ ace \ä\ cot, cart
\au̇\ out \ch\ chin \e\ bet \ē\ easy \g\ go \i\ hit \ī\ ice \j\ job
\ŋ\ sing \ō\ go \ȯ\ law \ȯi\ boy \th\ thin \t̠h\ the \ü\ loot
\u̇\ foot \y\ yet \zh\ vision　*See also* Pronunciation Symbols page

dif·fus·ible \dif-'yü-zə-bəl\ *adj* : capable of diffusing or of being diffused — **dif·fus·ibil·i·ty** \-,yü-zə-'bil-ət-ē\ *n, pl* **-ties**

dif·fu·sion \dif-'yü-zhən\ *n* **1** : the process whereby particles of liquids, gases, or solids intermingle as the result of their spontaneous movement caused by thermal agitation and in dissolved substances move from a region of higher to one of lower concentration **2 a** : reflection of light by a rough reflecting surface **b** : transmission of light through a translucent material — **dif·fu·sion·al** \-'yüzh-nəl, -ən-ºl\ *adj*

Di·flu·can \dī-'flük-,än, -ºn\ *trademark* — used for a preparation of fluconazole

di·flu·ni·sal \(,)dī-'flü-nə-,sal\ *n* : a nonsteroidal anti‑ inflammatory drug $C_{13}H_8F_2O_3$ related to aspirin that is used to relieve mild to moderately severe pain — see DOLOBID

di·gal·lic acid \(,)dī-,gal-ik-\ *n* : TANNIC ACID 1

di·ga·met·ic \,dī-gə-'met-ik\ *adj* : forming two kinds of germ cells

di·gas·tric \(')dī-'gas-trik\ *adj* **1** : having two bellies separated by a median tendon **2** : of or relating to a digastric muscle

digastric muscle *n* : either of a pair of muscles having two bellies separated by a median tendon that extend from the anterior inferior margin of the mandible to the temporal bone and serve to depress the lower jaw and raise the hyoid bone esp. during swallowing — called also *digastric*

di·gas·tri·cus \-tri-kəs\ *n* : DIGASTRIC MUSCLE

Di·ge·nea \dī-'jē-nē-ə\ *n pl* : a subclass, suborder, or other taxon of trematode worms which have a complex life cycle involving alternation of sexual reproduction as an internal parasite of a vertebrate with asexual reproduction in a mollusk and often including developmental stages in still other hosts and which include a number of parasites (as the Chinese liver fluke) of humans — compare MONOGENEA — **di·ge·ne·an** \-ən\ *adj or n*

di·gen·e·sis \(')dī-'jen-ə-səs\ *n, pl* **-e·ses** \-,sēz\ : successive reproduction by sexual and asexual methods

di·ge·net·ic \,dī-jə-'net-ik\ *adj* **1** : of or relating to digenesis **2** : of or relating to the taxon Digenea of trematode worms

Di·George syndrome \də-'jörj-\ *also* **Di·George's syn·drome** \-'jör-jəz\ *n* : a rare congenital disease that is characterized esp. by absent or underdeveloped thymus and parathyroid glands, heart defects, immunodeficiency, hypocalcemia, and characteristic facial features (as wide-set eyes, small jaws, and low-set ears) and is typically caused by a deletion on the chromosome numbered 22

Di George, Angelo Mario (b 1921), American endocrinologist and pediatrician. A professor of pediatrics at Temple University's School of Medicine, Di George served as chief of endocrine and metabolic services at St. Christopher's Hospital for Children in Philadelphia. He also held the positions of assistant chief of pediatrics at Philadelphia General Hospital from 1956 to 1966 and lecturer at the U.S. Naval Hospital in Philadelphia from 1967 to 1980. His principal areas of research were disorders of growth, pubertal development, thyroid dysfunction, and hypocalcemia. DiGeorge syndrome was first reported in 1965.

¹di·gest \'dī-,jest\ *n* : a product of digestion

²di·gest \dī-'jest, də-\ *vt* **1** : to convert (food) into absorbable form **2 a** : to soften, decompose, or break down by heat and moisture or chemicals **b** : to extract soluble ingredients from by warming with a liquid ∼ *vi* **1** : to digest food **2** : to become digested

di·ges·ta \dī-'jes-tə, də-\ *n pl* : something undergoing digestion (as food in the stomach)

di·ges·tant \-'jes-tənt\ *n* : a substance (as an enzyme) that digests or aids in digestion — compare DIGESTIVE 1

di·gest·er \-'jes-tər\ *n* **1** : one that digests **2** : a medicine or an article of food that aids digestion **3** *also* **di·ges·tor** : a vessel or apparatus for digesting

di·gest·ibil·i·ty \-,jes-tə-'bil-ət-ē\ *n, pl* **-ties 1** : the fitness of something for digestion **2** : the percentage of a foodstuff taken into the digestive tract that is absorbed into the body

di·gest·ible \-'jes-tə-bəl\ *adj* : capable of being digested

di·ges·tion \dī-'jes(h)-chən, də-\ *n* : the action, process, or power of digesting; *esp* : the process of making food absorbable by mechanically and enzymatically breaking it down into simpler chemical compounds in the alimentary canal

¹di·ges·tive \-'jes-tiv\ *n* **1** : something that aids digestion esp. of food — compare DIGESTANT **2** : a substance which promotes suppuration

²digestive *adj* **1** : relating to or functioning in digestion ⟨∼ processes⟩ **2** : having the power to cause or promote digestion ⟨∼ enzymes⟩ — **di·ges·tive·ly** *adv* — **di·ges·tive·ness** *n*

digestive gland *n* : a gland secreting digestive enzymes

digestive system *n* : the bodily system concerned with the ingestion, digestion, and absorption of food : ALIMENTARY SYSTEM

dig·i·lan·id \,dij-ə-'lan-əd\ *or* **dig·i·lan·ide** \-,īd, -əd\ *n* : LANATOSIDE

digilanid A *or* **digilanide A** *n* : LANATOSIDE a

digilanid B *or* **digilanide B** *n* : LANATOSIDE b

digilanid C *or* **digilanide C** *n* : LANATOSIDE c

dig·it \'dij-ət\ *n* : any of the divisions (as a finger or toe) in which the limbs of amphibians and all higher vertebrates including humans terminate, which are typically five in number but may be reduced (as in the horse), and which typically have a series of phalanges bearing a nail, claw, or hoof at the tip

dig·i·tal \'dij-ət-ºl\ *adj* **1** : of, relating to, or supplying one or more fingers or toes ⟨a ∼ branch of an artery⟩ **2** : done with a finger ⟨a ∼ rectal examination⟩ — **dig·i·tal·ly** \-ē\ *adv*

dig·i·tal·in \,dij-ə-'tal-ən *also* -'tāl-\ *n* **1** : a white crystalline steroid glycoside $C_{36}H_{56}O_{14}$ obtained from seeds of the common European foxglove (*Digitalis purpurea*) **2** : a mixture of the glycosides of digitalis leaves or seeds

dig·i·tal·is \-əs\ *n* **1 a** *cap* : a genus of Eurasian herbs of the snapdragon family (Scrophulariaceae) that have alternate leaves and racemes of showy bell-shaped flowers and comprise the foxgloves **b** : FOXGLOVE **2** : the dried leaf of the common European foxglove (*Digitalis purpurea*) that contains physiologically active glycosides, that is a powerful cardiotonic acting to increase the force of myocardial contraction, to slow the conduction rate of nerve impulses through the atrioventricular node, and to promote diuresis, and that is used in standardized powdered form esp. in the treatment of congestive heart failure and in the management of atrial fibrillation, atrial flutter, and paroxysmal tachycardia of the atria; *broadly* : any of various glycosides (as digoxin or digitoxin) that are constituents of digitalis or are derived from a related foxglove (*D. lanata*)

dig·i·ta·li·za·tion *also Brit* **dig·i·ta·li·sa·tion** \,dij-ət-ºl-ə-'zā-shən\ *n* : the administration of digitalis (as in heart disease) until the desired physiological adjustment is attained; *also* : the bodily state so produced

dig·i·ta·lize *also Brit* **dig·i·ta·lise** \'dij-ət-ºl-,īz\ *vt* **-lized** *also Brit* **-lised; -liz·ing** *also Brit* **-lis·ing** : to subject to digitalization

digital nerve *n* **1** : any of several branches of the median nerve and the ulnar nerve supplying the fingers and thumb **2** : any of several branches of the medial plantar nerve supplying the toes

dig·i·tal·ose \,dij-ə-'tal-,ōs *also* -'tāl-, -,ōz\ *n* : a sugar $C_7H_{14}O_5$ obtained esp. from digitalin by hydrolysis

dig·i·tate \'dij-ə-,tāt\ *adj* : having digits

dig·i·ta·tion \,dij-ə-'tā-shən\ *n* : a process that resembles a finger

Dig·i·tek \'dij-ə-,tek\ *trademark* — used for a preparation of digoxin

digiti — see ABDUCTOR DIGITI MINIMI, EXTENSOR DIGITI MINIMI, EXTENSOR DIGITI QUINTI PROPRIUS, FLEXOR DIGITI MINIMI BREVIS, OPPONENS DIGITI MINIMI

dig·i·ti·grade \'dij-ət-ə-,grād\ *adj* : walking or adapted for walking on the digits with the posterior of the foot more or less raised ⟨cats and dogs are ∼ mammals⟩ — compare PLANTIGRADE — **digitigrade** *n*

dig·i·to·nin \ˌdij-ə-'tō-nən\ *n* : a steroid saponin $C_{56}H_{92}O_{29}$ occurring in the leaves and seeds of foxglove

dig·i·to·plan·tar \ˌdij-ət-ə-'plant-ər, -'plan-ˌtär\ *adj* : of or relating to the toes and the plantar surface of the foot

digitorum — see EXTENSOR DIGITORUM BREVIS, EXTENSOR DIGITORUM COMMUNIS, EXTENSOR DIGITORUM LONGUS, FLEXOR DIGITORUM BREVIS, FLEXOR DIGITORUM LONGUS, FLEXOR DIGITORUM PROFUNDUS, FLEXOR DIGITORUM SUPERFICIALIS

dig·i·toxi·gen·in \ˌdij-ə-ˌtäk-sə-'jen-ən\ *n* : a steroid lactone $C_{23}H_{34}O_4$ obtained esp. by hydrolysis of digitoxin

dig·i·tox·in \ˌdij-ə-'täk-sən\ *n* : a poisonous glycoside $C_{41}H_{64}O_{13}$ that is the most active constituent of digitalis; *also* : a mixture of digitalis glycosides consisting chiefly of digitoxin

dig·i·tox·ose \-'täk-ˌsōs *also* -ˌsōz\ *n* : a sugar $C_6H_{12}O_4$ obtained by the hydrolysis of several glycosides of digitalis (as digitoxin or gitoxin)

di·glos·sia \dī-'gläs-ē-ə\ *n* : the condition of having the tongue bifid

di·glyc·er·ide \dī-'glis-ə-ˌrīd\ *n* : an ester of glycerol that contains two ester groups and involves one or two acids

di·gox·in \dij-'äk-sən, dig-\ *n* : a poisonous cardiotonic glycoside $C_{41}H_{64}O_{14}$ obtained from the leaves of a foxglove (*Digitalis lanata*) and used similarly to digitalis — see DIGITEK, LANOXIN

di·hy·brid \(ˌ)dī-'hī-brəd\ *adj* : of, relating to, involving, or being an individual or strain that is heterozygous at two genetic loci — **dihybrid** *n*

di·hy·drate \('')dī-'hī-ˌdrāt\ *n* : a hydrate containing two molecules of water

di·hy·drat·ed \-ˌdrāt-əd\ *adj* : combined with two molecules of water

di·hy·dro \-(ˌ)drō\ *adj* : combined with two atoms of hydrogen ⟨cortisol is a ~ derivative of cortisone⟩ — often used in combination

dihydrochalcone — see NEOHESPERIDIN DIHYDROCHALCONE

di·hy·dro·chlo·ride \(ˌ)dī-ˌhī-drə-'klō(ə)r-ˌīd, -'klȯ(ə)r-\ *n* : a hydrochloride containing two molecules of hydrochloric acid ⟨quinine ~ $C_{20}H_{24}N_2O_2 \cdot 2HCl$⟩

di·hy·dro·co·de·inone \-kō-'dē-ə-ˌnōn\ *n* : HYDROCODONE

di·hy·dro·er·go·cor·nine \-ˌhī-drō-ˌər-gō-'kȯr-ˌnēn, -nən\ *n* : a hydrogenated derivative $C_{31}H_{41}N_5O_5$ of an ergot alkaloid from ergot that is used in the treatment of peripheral vascular diseases and hypertension

di·hy·dro·er·got·a·mine \-ˌər-'gät-ə-ˌmēn\ *n* : a hydrogenated derivative of ergotamine that is used in the form of its mesylate $C_{33}H_{37}N_5O_5 \cdot CH_4O_3S$ in the treatment of migraine

di·hy·dro·fo·late reductase \-'fō-ˌlāt-\ *n* : an enzyme that catalyzes the reduction of a folate having one of its rings with two double bonds and two attached hydrogen atoms into the dihydro form differing only in having one double bond and four hydrogen atoms in the same ring, that is essential for DNA and protein synthesis, and that is targeted by some anticancer drugs (as methotrexate) in order to inhibit its positive effect on tumor cell growth and reproduction

dihydrogen — see SODIUM DIHYDROGEN PHOSPHATE

di·hy·dro·mor·phi·none \(ˌ)dī-ˌhī-drō-'mȯr-fə-ˌnōn\ *n* : HYDROMORPHONE

di·hy·dro·strep·to·my·cin \-ˌstrep-tə-'mīs-ᵊn\ *n* : a toxic antibiotic $C_{21}H_{41}N_7O_{12}$ formerly used in the treatment of tuberculosis, tularemia, and infections caused by gram-negative organisms but abandoned because of its tendency to impair hearing

di·hy·dro·tachy·ste·rol \-ˌtak-i-'ster-ˌȯl, -'stir-, -ˌōl\ *n* : a crystalline alcohol $C_{28}H_{45}OH$ used in the treatment of hypocalcemia (as in hypoparathyroidism)

di·hy·dro·tes·tos·ter·one \-te-'stäs-tə-ˌrōn\ *n* : a biologically active metabolite $C_{19}H_{30}O_2$ of testosterone having similar androgenic activity and produced in various tissues (as of the skin and prostate) — abbr. *DHT*

di·hy·dro·the·elin \-'thē-ə-lən\ *n* : ESTRADIOL

di·hy·droxy \ˌdī-hī-'dräk-sē\ *adj* : containing two hydroxyl groups in a molecule — often used in combination

di·hy·droxy·ac·e·tone \ˌdī-hī-ˌdräk-sē-'as-ə-ˌtōn\ *n* : a glyceraldehyde isomer $C_3H_6O_3$ that is used esp. to stain the skin to simulate a tan

1,25-di·hy·droxy·cho·le·cal·cif·er·ol \-ˌwən-ˌtwen-tē-ˌfīv-ˌdī-hī-ˌdräk-sē-ˌkō-lə-(ˌ)kal-'sif-ə-ˌrȯl, -ˌrōl\ *n* : CALCITRIOL

di·hy·droxy·phe·nyl·al·a·nine \ˌdī-hī-ˌdräk-sē-ˌfen-ᵊl-'al-ə-ˌnēn, -ˌfēn-\ *n* **1** *or* 3,4-**dihydroxyphenylalanine** \ˌthrē-ˌfȯr-\ : DOPA **2** *or* L-**3,4-dihydroxyphenylalanine** \'el-\ *or* L-**dihydroxyphenylalanine** : L-DOPA

di·io·dide \(')dī-'ī-ə-ˌdīd\ *n* : a compound containing two atoms of iodine combined with an element or radical

di·io·do·hy·droxy·quin \ˌdī-ˌī-ə-ˌdō-hī-'dräk-si-kwən\ *n* : IODOQUINOL

di·io·do·hy·droxy·quin·o·line \-hī-ˌdräk-si-'kwin-ᵊl-ˌēn\ *n* : IODOQUINOL

di·io·do·ty·ro·sine \-'tī-rə-ˌsēn\ *n* : an iodinated tyrosine $C_9H_9I_2NO_3$ that is produced in the thyroid gland from monoiodotyrosine and that combines with monoiodotyrosine to form triiodothyronine — called also *iodogorgoic acid*

di·iso·pro·pyl \ˌdī-ˌī-sə-'prō-pəl\ *adj* : containing two isopropyl groups in a molecule

diisopropyl fluorophosphate *n* : ISOFLUROPHATE

di·kary·on *also* **di·cary·on** \(')dī-'kar-ē-ˌän, -ən\ *n* **1** : a pair of associated but unfused haploid nuclei of a fungus cell capable of participating in repeated cell division as separate entities prior to their ultimate fusion **2** : a cell having or a mycelium made up of cells each having a dikaryon — compare HOMOKARYON

di·kary·o·tic *also* **di·cary·o·tic** \ˌdī-ˌkar-ē-'ät-ik\ *adj* : characterized by the presence of two nuclei in each cell

di·ke·tone \(')dī-'kē-ˌtōn\ *n* : a chemical compound containing two ketone groups

di·ke·to·pi·per·a·zine \(ˌ)dī-ˌkēt-ō-pī-'per-ə-ˌzēn\ *n* **1** : a compound $C_4H_6N_2O_2$ that is obtainable from two molecules of glycine by dehydration and may be regarded as a cyclic dipeptide **2** : any of various cyclic compounds formed similarly to diketopiperazine from alpha-amino acids other than glycine or obtained by partial hydrolysis of proteins

dil *abbr* dilute

di·lac·er·a·tion \(ˌ)dī-ˌlas-ə-'rā-shən\ *n* : injury (as partial fracture) to a developing tooth that results in a curve in the long axis as development continues — **di·lac·er·at·ed** \-'las-ə-ˌrā-təd\ *adj*

Di·lan·tin \dī-'lant-ᵊn, də-\ *trademark* — used for a preparation of phenytoin

dilat *abbr* dilatation

di·la·ta·tion \ˌdil-ə-'tā-shən, ˌdī-lə-\ *n* **1** : the condition of being stretched beyond normal dimensions esp. as a result of overwork or disease or of abnormal relaxation ⟨~ of the heart⟩ ⟨~ of the stomach⟩ **2** : DILATION 2

di·la·ta·tor \'dil-ə-ˌtāt-ər, 'dī-lə-\ *n* : DILATOR b

di·late \dī-'lāt, 'dī-\ *vb* **di·lat·ed; di·lat·ing** *vt* : to enlarge, stretch, or cause to expand ⟨~ his pupils with atropine⟩ ⟨the drug ~s peripheral arteries⟩ ~ *vi* : to become expanded or swollen ⟨the cervix was *dilating*⟩ ⟨the pupils *dilated*⟩

di·la·tion \dī-'lā-shən\ *n* **1** : the state of being dilated : DILATATION **2** : the action of stretching or enlarging an organ or part of the body ⟨cervical ~⟩ ⟨~ of the pupil with atropine⟩

dilation and curettage *n* : a medical procedure in which the uterine cervix is dilated and a curette is inserted into the uterus to scrape away the endometrium (as for the diagnosis or treatment of abnormal bleeding or for surgical abortion during the early part of the second trimester of pregnancy) — called also *D&C*

dilation and evacuation *n* : a surgical abortion that is typically performed midway during the second trimester of

---

\ə\ **abut** \ᵊ\ **kitten** \ər\ **further** \a\ **ash** \ā\ **ace** \ä\ **cot, cart** \aů\ **out** \ch\ **chin** \e\ **bet** \ē\ **easy** \g\ **go** \i\ **hit** \ī\ **ice** \j\ **job** \ŋ\ **sing** \ō\ **go** \ȯ\ **law** \ȯi\ **boy** \th\ **thin** \th̲\ **the** \ü\ **loot** \ů\ **foot** \y\ **yet** \zh\ **vision** *See also* Pronunciation Symbols page

pregnancy and in which the uterine cervix is dilated and fetal tissue is removed using surgical instruments (as a forceps and curette) and suction — called also *D&E*

dilation and extraction *n* : a surgical abortion that is typically performed during the third trimester or later part of the second trimester of pregnancy and in which the uterine cervix is dilated and death of the fetus is induced after it has passed partway through the birth canal — called also *D&X, partial-birth abortion*

di·la·tom·e·ter \ˌdil-ə-ˈtäm-ət-ər, ˌdīl-\ *n* : an instrument for measuring thermal dilatation or expansion esp. in determining coefficients of expansion of liquids or solids — **di·la·to·met·ric** \ˌdil-ət-ə-ˈme-trik\ *adj* — **di·la·to·met·ri·cal·ly** \-tri-k(ə-)lē\ *adv* — **di·la·tom·e·try** \ˌdil-ə-ˈtäm-ə-trē, ˌdīl-\ *n, pl* **-tries**

di·la·tor \(ˈ)dī-ˈlāt-ər, də-\ *n* : one that dilates: as **a** : an instrument for expanding a tube, duct, or cavity ⟨a urethral ∼⟩ — called also *divulsor* **b** : a muscle that dilates a part **c** : a drug (as a vasodilator) causing dilation

Di·lau·did \(ˌ)dī-ˈlȯ-did\ *trademark* — used for a preparation of hydromorphone

dil·do \ˈdil-(ˌ)dō\ *n, pl* **dildos** *also* **dildoes** : an object resembling a penis used for sexual stimulation

dill \ˈdil\ *n* : any of several plants of the family Umbelliferae; *esp* : a European herb (*Anethum graveolens*) with aromatic seeds and foliage that are used in flavoring foods and esp. pickles

dill oil *n* : either of two essential oils derived from the common dill: **a** : a colorless or pale yellow oil having a sweetish acrid taste that is obtained from the dried ripe fruits of the dill and is used as an aromatic carminative and as a flavoring agent **b** : a similar oil obtained from the whole dill plant and used as a flavoring agent

dill·seed oil \ˈdil-ˌsēd-\ *n* : DILL OIL a

dill·weed oil \-ˌwēd-\ *n* : DILL OIL b

dil·ti·a·zem \dil-ˈtī-ə-(ˌ)zem\ *n* : a calcium channel blocker used esp. in the form of its hydrochloride $C_{22}H_{26}N_2O_4S \cdot HCl$ as a coronary vasodilator — see CARDIZEM

¹dil·u·ent \ˈdil-yə-wənt\ *n* : a diluting agent (as the vehicle in a medicinal preparation)

²diluent *adj* : making thinner or less concentrated by admixture : DILUTING

¹di·lute \dī-ˈlüt, də-\ *vt* **di·lut·ed; di·lut·ing** : to make thinner or more liquid by admixture — **di·lut·er** *also* **di·lu·tor** \-ər\ *n*

²dilute *adj* : of relatively low strength or concentration ⟨a ∼ solution⟩

di·lu·tion \dī-ˈlü-shən, də-\ *n* **1** : the action of diluting : the state of being diluted **2** : something (as a solution) that is diluted

dim *abbr* diminished

di·men·hy·dri·nate \ˌdī-ˌmen-ˈhī-drə-ˌnāt\ *n* : a crystalline antihistamine $C_{24}H_{28}ClN_5O_3$ used esp. to prevent nausea (as in motion sickness)

di·men·sion \də-ˈmen-chən *also* dī-\ *n* : measure in one direction; *specif* : one of three or four coordinates determining a position in space or space and time

di·mer \ˈdī-mər\ *n* : a compound formed by the union of two radicals or two molecules of a simpler compound; *specif* : a polymer formed from two molecules of a monomer — **di·mer·ic** \(ˈ)dī-ˈmer-ik\ *adj* — **di·mer·iza·tion** *or Brit* **di·mer·isa·tion** \ˌdī-mə-rə-ˈzā-shən\ *n* — **di·mer·ize** *or Brit* **di·mer·ise** \ˈdī-mə-ˌrīz\ *vt* **-ized** *or Brit* **-ised; -iz·ing** *or Brit* **-is·ing**

di·mer·cap·rol \ˌdī-(ˌ)mər-ˈkap-ˌrȯl, -ˌrōl\ *n* : a colorless viscous oily compound $C_3H_8OS_2$ with an offensive odor developed as an antidote to lewisite and used in treating arsenic, mercury, and gold poisoning — called also *BAL, British anti-lewisite*

di·meth·yl \(ˈ)dī-ˈmeth-əl\ *adj* : containing two methyl groups in a molecule — often used in combination

di·meth·yl·ami·no·eth·a·nol \(ˈ)dī-ˌmeth-ə-lə-ˌmē-nō-ˈeth-ə-ˌnȯl, -ˌnōl\ *n* : DMAE

di·meth·yl·benz·an·thra·cene \-ben-ˈzan(t)-thrə-ˌsēn\ *also* **7,12–di·meth·yl·benz·[a]·an·thra·cene** \ˌsev-ən-ˌtwelv-(ˌ)dī-

ˌmeth-əl-ben-ˈzan(t)-thrə-ˌsēn\ *n* : a carcinogenic polycyclic aromatic hydrocarbon $C_{20}H_{16}$ widely used in experimental research on carcinogenesis using animal models (as mice or rats) — abbr. *DMBA*

di·meth·yl·ni·tros·amine \(ˌ)dī-ˌmeth-əl-(ˌ)nī-ˈtrō-sə-ˌmēn\ *n* : a carcinogenic nitrosamine $C_2H_6N_2O$ that occurs esp. in tobacco smoke — called also *nitrosodimethylamine*

di·meth·yl phthalate \(ˌ)dī-ˌmeth-əl-\ *n* : a colorless liquid ester $C_{10}H_{10}O_4$ used chiefly as a plasticizer and insect repellent

di·meth·yl·poly·si·lox·ane \-ˌpäl-ē-sə-ˈläk-ˌsān, -sī-\ *n* : a polymer of silicone used esp. in pharmaceutical and cosmetic preparations — see SIMETHICONE

dimethyl sulfate *n* : a carcinogenic sulfate $(CH_3)_2SO_4$ containing two methyl groups that is esp. irritating to the respiratory tract

dimethyl sulfoxide *n* : an anti-inflammatory agent $(CH_3)_2SO$ used in the treatment of interstitial cystitis — called also *DMSO*

di·meth·yl·tryp·ta·mine \-ˈtrip-tə-ˌmēn\ *n* : a naturally occurring or easily synthesized hallucinogenic drug $C_{12}H_{16}N_2$ that is chemically similar to but shorter acting than psilocybin — called also *DMT*

di·meth·yl·tu·bo·cu·ra·rine \-ˌt(y)ü-bō-kyù-ˈrär-ən, -ˌēn\ *n* : a derivative of tubocurarine; *esp* : METOCURINE IODIDE

di·mor·phic \(ˈ)dī-ˈmȯr-fik\ *adj* **1** : DIMORPHOUS 1 **2** : occurring in two distinct forms

di·mor·phism \-ˌfiz-əm\ *n* : the condition or property of being dimorphic or dimorphous: as **a** (1) : the existence of two different forms (as of color or size) of a species esp. in the same population (2) : the existence of an organ in two different forms **b** : crystallization of a chemical compound in two different forms

di·mor·phous \(ˈ)dī-ˈmȯr-fəs\ *adj* **1** : crystallizing in two different forms **2** : DIMORPHIC 2

¹dim·ple \ˈdim-pəl\ *n* : a slight natural indentation or hollow in the surface of some part of the human body (as on a cheek or the chin)

²dimple *vb* **dim·pled; dim·pling** \-p(ə-)liŋ\ *vt* : to mark with dimples ∼ *vi* : to exhibit or form dimples

di·ner·ic \(ˈ)dī-ˈner-ik, də-\ *adj* : of or relating to the interface between two mutually immiscible liquids (as oil and water) contained in the same vessel

dinitrate — see ISOSORBIDE DINITRATE

di·ni·tro·ben·zene \ˌdī-ˌnī-trō-ˈben-ˌzēn, -ben-ˈ\ *n* : any of three isomeric toxic derivatives $C_6H_4(NO_2)_2$ of benzene

di·ni·tro–o–cre·sol \ˌdī-ˌnī-trō-ˌō-ˈkrē-ˌsȯl, -ˌsōl\ *also* **di·ni·tro–or·tho–cre·sol** \-ˌȯr-thō-\ *n* : a yellow crystalline compound $C_7H_6N_2O_5$ used esp. as an insecticide and herbicide — called also *DNOC*

di·ni·tro·phe·nol \-ˈfē-ˌnȯl, -fi-ˈ\ *n* : any of six isomeric crystalline compounds $C_6H_4N_2O_5$ some of whose derivatives are pesticides; *esp* : a highly toxic compound that increases fat metabolism and was formerly used in weight control

Di·no·flag·el·la·ta \ˌdī-nō-ˌflaj-ə-ˈlät-ə, -ˈlāt-\ *n pl* : an order of chiefly marine usu. solitary phytoflagellates that are typically enclosed in a cellulose envelope, that have one transverse flagellum running in a groove about the body, one posterior flagellum extending out from a similar median groove, usu. a single nucleus, and yellow, brown, or occas. green chromoplasts, and that include luminescent forms, important elements of marine food chains, and the flagellates of the genera *Gonyaulax* and *Gymnodinium* that cause red tide

di·no·fla·gel·late \ˌdī-nō-ˈflaj-ə-lət, -ˌlāt, -flə-ˈjel-ət\ *n* : any of the order Dinoflagellata of phytoflagellates

di·nu·cle·o·tide \(ˌ)dī-ˈn(y)ü-klē-ə-ˌtīd\ *n* : a nucleotide consisting of two units each composed of a phosphate, a pentose, and a purine or pyrimidine base

Di·oc·to·phy·ma \(ˌ)dī-ˌäk-tə-ˈfī-mə\ *n* : a genus of nematode worms including a single species (*D. renale*) which is a destructive parasite of the kidney of dogs, minks, and sometimes humans

Di·oc·to·phy·me \-ˈfī-(ˌ)mē\ *n, syn of* DIOCTOPHYMA

di·o·done \ˈdī-ə-ˌdōn\ *n* : IODOPYRACET

dioestrous, dioestrual, dioestrum, dioestrus *chiefly Brit var of* DIESTROUS, DIESTRUAL, DIESTRUM, DIESTRUS

di·ol \'dī-ˌȯl, -ˌōl\ *n* : a compound containing two hydroxyl groups

di·op·ter *or chiefly Brit* **di·op·tre** \dī-'äp-tər, 'dī-ˌäp-\ *n* : a unit of measurement of the refractive power of a lens equal to the reciprocal of the focal length in meters

di·op·tom·e·ter \ˌdī-ˌäp-'täm-ət-ər\ *n* : an instrument used in measuring the accommodation and refraction of the eye — **di·op·tom·e·try** \-'täm-ə-trē\ *n, pl* **-tries**

di·op·tric \(')dī-'äp-trik\ *also* **di·op·tri·cal** \-tri-kəl\ *adj* **1** : producing or serving in refraction of a beam of light : REFRACTIVE; *specif* : assisting vision by refracting and focusing light ⟨the ∼ power of a lens⟩ **2** : produced by means of refraction ⟨∼ images⟩ — **di·op·tri·cal·ly** \-tri-k(ə-)lē\ *adv*

di·op·trics \dī-'äp-triks\ *n pl but sing in constr* **1** : a branch of optics dealing with the refraction of light esp. by lenses **2** : refractive optics esp. of a lens or system of lenses ⟨correction of refractive error of the peripheral ∼ of the eye —Anne Lamont *et al*⟩

di·ose \'dī-ˌōs, -ˌōz\ *n* : a monosaccharide (as glycolaldehyde) that contains two carbon atoms

di·os·gen·in \ˌdī-ˌäz-'jen-ən, -'äz-jə-nən\ *n* : a crystalline steroid sapogenin $C_{27}H_{42}O_3$ obtained esp. from yams (genus *Dioscorea*) and used as a starting material for the synthesis of steroid hormones (as cortisone and progesterone)

Di·os·py·ros \dī-'äs-pə-ˌrōs\ *n* : a genus of trees and shrubs of the ebony family (Ebenaceae) with hard fine wood, oblong leaves, and small bell-shaped flowers that includes an American persimmon (*D. virginiana*) whose bark has been used as an astringent

di·otic \(')dī-'ät-ik\ *adj* : affecting or relating to the two ears : BINAURAL

Di·o·van \'dī-ə-ˌvan\ *trademark* — used for a preparation of valsartan

di·ovu·lar \-'äv-yə-lər, -'ōv-\ *adj* : BIOVULAR

di·ox·ane \dī-'äk-ˌsān\ *also* **di·ox·an** \-sən, -ˌsan\ *n* : a flammable toxic liquid $C_4H_8O_2$ used esp. as a solvent and as a clearing agent for histological preparations

di·ox·ide \(')dī-'äk-ˌsīd\ *n* : an oxide (as carbon dioxide) containing two atoms of oxygen in a molecule

di·ox·in \(')dī-'äk-sən\ *n* : any of several persistent toxic heterocyclic hydrocarbons that occur esp. as by-products of various industrial processes (as pesticide manufacture and paper milling) and waste incineration; *esp* : TCDD — see AGENT ORANGE

di·oxy·ben·zone \(ˌ)dī-ˌäk-sē-'ben-ˌzōn, -ben-'\ *n* : a sunscreen $C_{14}H_{12}O_4$ that absorbs throughout the ultraviolet spectrum and is used for protection against sunburn and in drug-induced light-sensitive states

¹dip \'dip\ *vt* **dipped; dip·ping** : to immerse (as a sheep or hog) in an antiseptic or parasiticidal solution

²dip *n* **1** : a liquid preparation of an insecticide or parasiticide which is applied to animals by immersing them in it — see SHEEP-DIP **2** : a vat or tank in which dip is used

DIP *abbr* distal interphalangeal

di·pen·tene \(')dī-'pen-ˌtēn\ *n* : a liquid terpene hydrocarbon $C_{10}H_{16}$ that is found in many essential oils, is a constituent of terebene, and is used chiefly as a solvent and dispersing agent (as for resins and varnishes) — compare LIMONENE

di·pep·ti·dase \dī-'pep-tə-ˌdās, -ˌdāz\ *n* : any of various enzymes that hydrolyze dipeptides but not polypeptides

di·pep·tide \(')dī-'pep-ˌtīd\ *n* : a peptide that yields two molecules of amino acid on hydrolysis

Di·pet·a·lo·ne·ma \(ˌ)dī-ˌpet-ᵊl-ō-'nē-mə\ *n* : a genus of tropical filarial worms whose adults occur in connective tissue and skin of primates including humans and whose microfilariae occur in their blood

Di·pet·a·lo·ne·mat·i·dae \-nə-'mat-ə-ˌdē\ *n pl* : a family of filarial worms distinguished by possession of slender larvae with no anterior spines and including most filarial worms parasitic in humans and domestic animals

diph *abbr* diphtheria

di·pha·sic \(')dī-'fā-zik\ *adj* : having two phases: as **a** : ex-

hibiting a stage of stimulation followed by a stage of depression or vice versa ⟨the ∼ action of certain drugs⟩ **b** : relating to or being a record of a nerve impulse that is negative and positive ⟨a ∼ action potential⟩ — compare MONOPHASIC 1, POLYPHASIC 1

di·phen·an \dī-'fen-ən\ *n* : a crystalline ester $C_{14}H_{13}NO_2$ administered in the treatment of pinworms

di·phen·hy·dra·mine \ˌdī-fen-'hī-drə-ˌmēn\ *n* : an antihistamine used esp. in the form of its hydrochloride $C_{17}H_{21}NO \cdot HCl$ to treat allergy symptoms and motion sickness and to induce sleep — see BENADRYL

di·phe·nol \(')dī-'fen-ˌȯl, -'fēn-, -ˌōl\ *n* : a chemical compound (as pyrocatechol or resorcinol) containing two phenolic hydroxyl groups

di·phen·oxy·late \ˌdī-ˌfen-'äk-sə-ˌlāt\ *n* : an antidiarrheal agent chemically related to meperidine and administered in the form of its hydrochloride $C_{30}H_{32}N_2O_2 \cdot HCl$ in combination with the sulfate of atropine — see LOMOTIL

di·phe·nyl \(')dī-'fen-ᵊl, -'fēn-\ *n* : BIPHENYL

di·phe·nyl·amine \(ˌ)dī-ˌfen-ᵊl-ə-'mēn, -ˌfēn-, -ᵊl-'am-ən\ *n* : a crystalline pleasant-smelling compound $(C_6H_5)_2NH$ that has been used in veterinary medicine, in the manufacture of dyes, and in stabilizing explosives

di·phe·nyl·amine·chlor·ar·sine \-ˌklȯr-'är-ˌsēn, -ˌklȯr-, -sən\ *n* : ADAMSITE

di·phe·nyl·chlo·ro·ar·sine \-ˌklȯr-ō-'är-ˌsēn, -ˌklȯr-, -sən\ *also* **di·phe·nyl·chlor·ar·sine** \-ˌklȯr-'är-, -ˌklȯr-\ *n* : a colorless crystalline arsenical $(C_6H_5)_2AsCl$ used during World War I esp. by the Germans for producing a toxic smoke causing sneezing and vomiting

di·phe·nyl·hy·dan·to·in \-hī-'dant-ə-wən\ *n* : PHENYTOIN

di·phos·gene \(')dī-'fäz-ˌjēn\ *n* : a liquid compound $C_2Cl_4O_2$ used as a poison gas in World War I

di·phos·phate \(')dī-'fäs-ˌfāt\ *n* : a phosphate containing two phosphate groups

diphosphoglucose — see URIDINE DIPHOSPHOGLUCOSE

2,3–di·phos·pho·glyc·er·ate *also* **di·phos·pho·glyc·er·ate** \(ˌtü-ˌthrē-)ˌdī-ˌfäs-fō-'glis-ə-ˌrāt\ *n* : an isomeric ester of diphosphoglyceric acid that occurs in human red blood cells and facilitates release of oxygen by decreasing the oxygen affinity of hemoglobin

di·phos·pho·gly·cer·ic acid *or* **1,3–di·phos·pho·gly·cer·ic acid** \(ˌwən-ˌthrē-)(')dī-ˌfäs-fō-glis-ˌer-ik-\ *n* : a diphosphate $C_3H_8O_9P_2$ of glyceric acid that is an important intermediate in photosynthesis and in glycolysis and fermentation

di·phos·pho·pyr·i·dine nucleotide \-ˌpir-ə-ˌdēn-\ *n* : NAD

diph·the·ria \dif-'thir-ē-ə, dip-\ *n* : an acute febrile contagious disease typically marked by the formation of a false membrane esp. in the throat and caused by a bacterium of the genus *Corynebacterium* (*C. diphtheriae*) which produces a toxin causing inflammation of the heart and nervous system — **diph·the·ri·al** \-ē-əl\ *adj*

¹diph·the·ric \-'ther-ik, -'thir-\ *adj* : DIPHTHERITIC

²diphtheric *n* : one suffering from diphtheria

diph·the·rit·ic \ˌdif-thə-'rit-ik, ˌdip-\ *adj* : relating to, produced in, or affected with diphtheria ⟨a ∼ membrane⟩ ⟨a ∼ child⟩; *also* : resembling diphtheria esp. in the formation of a false membrane ⟨∼ dysentery⟩

¹diph·the·roid \'dif-thə-ˌrȯid\ *adj* : resembling diphtheria

²diphtheroid *n* : a bacterium (esp. genus *Corynebacterium*) that resembles the bacterium of diphtheria but does not produce diphtheria toxin

di·phy·let·ic \ˌdī-fī-'let-ik\ *adj* : derived from two lines of evolutionary descent ⟨∼ dinosaurs⟩

di·phyl·lo·both·ri·a·sis \(ˌ)dī-ˌfil-ō-bäth-'rī-ə-səs\ *n, pl* **-a·ses** \-ˌsēz\ : infestation with or disease caused by the fish tapeworm (*Diphyllobothrium latum*)

Di·phyl·lo·both·ri·i·dae \-'rī-ə-ˌdē\ *n pl* : a family of tapeworms that belong to the order Pseudophyllidea and have a

---

\ə\ abut \ᵊ\ kitten \ər\ further \a\ ash \ā\ ace \ä\ cot, cart
\au̇\ out \ch\ chin \e\ bet \ē\ easy \g\ go \i\ hit \ī\ ice \j\ job
\ŋ\ sing \ō\ go \ȯ\ law \ȯi\ boy \th\ thin \t͟h\ the \ü\ loot
\u̇\ foot \y\ yet \zh\ vision *See also* Pronunciation Symbols page

C
D

complex life history with more than one intermediate host and the scolex of the adult usu. grooved and lacking suckers or hooks

Di·phyl·lo·both·ri·um \-'bäth-rē-əm\ *n* : a large genus of tapeworms that is the type genus of the family Diphyllobothriidae and that comprises a number of parasites of fish-eating birds and mammals including the common fish tapeworm (*D. latum*) of humans — compare BOTHRIOCEPHALUS

¹di·phy·odont \(')dī-'fī-ə-ˌdänt\ *adj* : marked by the successive development of deciduous and permanent sets of teeth ⟨humans are ~ mammals⟩ ⟨a ~ dentition⟩ — compare MONOPHYODONT, POLYPHYODONT

²diphyodont *n* : a diphyodont animal

dip·la·cu·sis \ˌdip-lə-'kyü-səs\ *n, pl* **-cu·ses** \-ˌsēz\ : the hearing of a single tone as if it were two tones of different pitch

di·ple·gia \dī-'plē-j(ē-)ə\ *n* : paralysis of corresponding parts (as the legs) on both sides of the body

dip·lo·ba·cil·lus \ˌdip-lō-bə-'sil-əs\ *n, pl* **-cil·li** \-ˌī *also* -ē\ : any of certain small aerobic gram-negative rod-shaped bacilli that are related to the genus *Haemophilus* and are parasitic on mucous membranes — **dip·lo·ba·cil·la·ry** \-'bas-ə-ˌler-ē, -bə-'sil-ə-rē\ *adj*

dip·lo·blas·tic \-'blas-tik\ *adj* : having two germ layers — used of an embryo that lacks a true mesoderm

dip·lo·car·dia \-'kärd-ē-ə\ *n* : a cardiac condition in which the right and left halves of the heart are separated by a fissure

dip·lo·car·di·ac \-'kärd-ē-ə-ˌak\ *adj* : having the heart completely divided so that one side is systemic and the other is pulmonary

dip·lo·coc·cus \-'käk-əs\ *n* : any of various encapsulated bacteria (as the pneumococcus) that usu. occur in pairs and that were formerly grouped in a single taxon (genus *Diplococcus*) but are now all assigned to other genera — **dip·lo·coc·cal** \-əl\ *adj*

dip·loe \'dip-lə-ˌwē\ *n* : cancellous bony tissue between the external and internal layers of the skull

dip·lo·et·ic \ˌdip-lə-'wet-ik\ *adj* : DIPLOIC

di·plo·ic \də-'plō-ik, dī-\ *adj* : of or relating to the diploe

diploic vein *n* : any of several veins situated in channels in the diploe

¹dip·loid \'dip-ˌlòid\ *adj* : having the basic chromosome number doubled — **dip·loi·dy** \-ˌlòid-ē\ *n, pl* **-dies**

²diploid *n* : a single cell, individual, or generation characterized by the diploid chromosome number

dip·lo·kary·on \ˌdip-lō-'kar-ē-ˌän\ *n* : a nucleus possessing twice the diploid number of chromosomes : a tetraploid nucleus — **dip·lo·kary·ot·ic** \-ˌkar-ē-'ät-ik\ *adj*

dip·lo·mate \'dip-lə-ˌmāt\ *n* : one who holds a diploma; *esp* : a physician qualified to practice in a medical specialty by advanced training and experience in the specialty followed by passing an intensive examination by a national board of senior specialists

dip·lo·my·elia \ˌdip-lō-mī-'ē-lē-ə\ *n* : duplication of the spinal cord

dip·lo·ne·ma \ˌdip-lə-'nē-mə\ *n* : the chromosomes of the diplotene stage of meiotic prophase

dip·lo·neu·ral \-'n(y)ùr-əl\ *adj* : supplied by two different nerves

dip·lont \'dip-ˌlänt\ *n* : an organism with somatic cells having the diploid chromosome number — compare HAPLONT — **dip·lon·tic** \dip-'länt-ik\ *adj*

dip·lo·phase \'dip-lə-ˌfāz\ *n* : a diploid phase in a life cycle

dip·lo·pia \dip-'lō-pē-ə\ *n* : a disorder of vision in which two images of a single object are seen (as from unequal action of the eye muscles) — called also *double vision* — **dip·lo·pic** \-'lō-pik, -'läp-ik\ *adj*

dip·lo·sis \dip-'lō-səs\ *n, pl* **dip·lo·ses** \-ˌsēz\ : restoration of the somatic chromosome number by fusion of two gametes in fertilization

dip·lo·some \'dip-lə-ˌsōm\ *n* : a double centriole

dip·lo·tene \'dip-lə-ˌtēn\ *n* : a stage of meiotic prophase

which follows the pachytene and during which the paired homologous chromosomes begin to separate and chiasmata become visible — **diplotene** *adj*

di·po·lar \'dī-ˌpō-lər, -'pō-\ *adj* : of, relating to, or having a dipole

di·pole \'dī-ˌpōl\ *n* **1** : a pair of equal and opposite electric charges or magnetic poles of opposite sign separated by a small distance **2** : a body or system (as a molecule) having such charges

di·po·tas·sium \ˌdī-pə-'tas-ē-əm\ *adj* : containing two atoms of potassium in a molecule

di·pro·pi·o·nate \(ˌ)dī-'prō-pē-ə-ˌnāt\ *n* : an ester containing two propionate groups

di·pro·so·pus \ˌdī-prə-'sō-pəs\ *n* : a fetus with two faces

dip·so·ma·nia \ˌdip-sə-'mā-nē-ə, -nyə\ *n* : an uncontrollable craving for alcoholic liquors — **dip·so·ma·ni·ac** \-nē-ˌak\ *n* — **dip·so·ma·ni·a·cal** \ˌdip-sō-mə-'nī-ə-kəl\ *adj*

dip·stick \'dip-ˌstik\ *n* : a chemically sensitive strip of paper used to identify one or more constituents (as glucose or protein) of urine by immersion

Dip·tera \'dip-t(ə-)rə\ *n pl* : a large order of winged or rarely wingless insects (as the housefly, mosquitoes, midges, and gnats) that have the anterior wings usu. functional and the posterior wings reduced to small club-shaped structures functioning as sensory flight stabilizers and that have a segmented larva often without a head, eyes, or legs

dip·ter·an \'dip-tə-rən\ *n* : any insect of the order Diptera — **dipteran** *adj* — **dip·ter·ous** \-rəs\ *adj*

Dip·ter·yx \'dip-tə-(ˌ)riks\ *n* : a small genus of tropical American trees of the family Leguminosae having opposite pinnate leaves and including several whose seeds are a source of coumarin — see TONKA BEAN

dipus — see SYMPUS DIPUS

di·py·gus \(')dī-'pī-gəs, 'dip-ə-gəs\ *n, pl* **di·py·gi** \-ˌgī\ : a teratological fetus with a double pelvis, genitals, and extremities

di·py·li·di·a·sis \ˌdī-ˌpī-lə-'dī-ə-səs, *pl* **-a·ses** \-ˌsēz\ : infestation with the dog tapeworm (*Dipylidium caninum*)

Di·py·lid·i·um \ˌdī-ˌpī-'lid-ē-əm, -pə-\ *n* : a genus of taenioid tapeworms including the common dog tapeworm (*D. caninum*) that is a cosmopolitan parasite of dogs, cats, and other carnivores and occas. infests humans

di·pyr·i·dam·ole \(')dī-ˌpir-ə-'dam-ˌōl, -ˌōl\ *n* : a drug $C_{24}H_{40}N_8O_4$ used as a coronary vasodilator — see PERSANTINE

di·rect cell division \də-'rekt-, dī-\ *n* : AMITOSIS

direct current *n* : an electric current flowing in one direction only and substantially constant in value — abbr. *DC*

di·rec·tive \də-'rek-tiv, dī-\ *adj* : of or relating to psychotherapy in which the therapist introduces information, content, or attitudes not previously expressed by the client

di·rec·tor \də-'rek-tər, dī-\ *n* : an instrument grooved to guide and limit the motion of a surgical knife

direct pyramidal tract *n* : VENTRAL CORTICOSPINAL TRACT

di·rhin·ic \(')dī-'rin-ik, -'rīn-\ *adj* : affecting both nostrils alike

Di·ro·fi·lar·ia \ˌdī-(ˌ)rō-fə-'lar-ē-ə\ *n* : a genus of filarial worms of the superfamily Filarioidea that includes the heartworm (*D. immitis*) — **di·ro·fi·lar·i·al** \-ē-əl\ *adj*

di·ro·fil·a·ri·a·sis \-ˌfil-ə-'rī-ə-səs\ *n, pl* **-a·ses** \-ˌsēz\ : infestation with filarial worms of the genus *Dirofilaria* and esp. with the heartworm (*D. immitis*)

dirty \'dərt-ē\ *adj* **dirt·i·er; -est** : contaminated with infecting organisms ⟨~ wounds⟩

dis *abbr* **1** disabled **2** disease

dis·abil·i·ty \ˌdis-ə-'bil-ət-ē\ *n, pl* **-ties** **1** : the condition of being disabled **2** : inability to pursue an occupation because of physical or mental impairment

dis·able \dis-'ā-bəl, diz-\ *vt* **dis·abled; dis·abling** \-b(ə-)liŋ\ : to deprive of a mental or physical capacity

dis·abled *adj* : incapacitated by illness, injury, or wounds; *broadly* : physically or mentally impaired

disabled list \-ˌlist\ *n* : a list of athletes unable to play because of injury or illness

dis·able·ment \-mənt\ *n* : the act of becoming disabled to the extent that full wages cannot be earned; *also* : the state of being so disabled

di·sac·cha·ri·dase \(ˈ)dī-ˈsak-ə-rə-ˌdās, -ˌdāz\ *n* : an enzyme (as maltase or lactase) that hydrolyzes disaccharides

di·sac·cha·ride \(ˈ)dī-ˈsak-ə-ˌrīd\ *n* : any of a class of sugars (as sucrose) that on hydrolysis yields two monosaccharide molecules — called also *biose, double sugar*

dis·ag·gre·gate \(ˈ)dis-ˈag-ri-ˌgāt\ *vb* **-gat·ed; -gat·ing** *vt* : to separate into component parts ⟨∼ polyribosomes⟩ ∼ *vi* : to break up or apart ⟨the molecules of a gel ∼ to form a sol⟩ — **dis·ag·gre·ga·tion** \(ˌ)dis-ˌag-ri-ˈgā-shən\ *n*

dis·ar·tic·u·la·tion \ˌdis-är-ˌtik-yə-ˈlā-shən\ *n* : separation or amputation of a body part at a joint ⟨∼ of the shoulder⟩ — **dis·ar·tic·u·late** \-ˈtik-yə-ˌlāt\ *vb* **-lat·ed; -lat·ing**

dis·as·sim·i·late \ˌdis-ə-ˈsim-ə-ˌlāt\ *vt* **-lat·ed; -lat·ing** : to subject to catabolism — **dis·as·sim·i·la·tion** \-ˌsim-ə-ˈlā-shən\ *n* — **dis·as·sim·i·la·tive** \-ˈsim-ə-ˌlāt-iv\ *adj*

dis·azo \dis-ˈaz-ō\ *adj* : containing two azo groups in a molecule ⟨∼ dyes⟩

disc, discectomy *var of* DISK, DISKECTOMY

disch *abbr* discharge; discharged

¹**dis·charge** \dis(h)-ˈchärj, ˈdis(h)-ˌ\ *vb* **dis·charged; dis·charg·ing** *vt* **1** : to release from confinement, custody, or care ⟨∼ a patient from the hospital⟩ **2 a** : to give outlet to or emit ⟨a boil *discharging* pus⟩ **b** : to release or give expression to (a pent-up emotion or a repressed impulse) ⟨*discharged* his anxiety by working out with a punching bag⟩ ∼ *vi* : to pour forth fluid or other contents

²**dis·charge** \ˈdis(h)-ˌchärj, dis(h)-ˈ\ *n* **1** : the act of relieving of something ⟨∼ of a repressed impulse⟩ **2** : release from confinement, custody, or care ⟨returned to work the day after ∼ from the hospital⟩ **3** : something that is emitted or evacuated ⟨a purulent ∼ from a wound⟩ ⟨a thick white vaginal ∼⟩

disci *pl of* DISCUS

dis·ci·form \ˈdis-(k)ə-ˌfȯrm\ *adj* : round or oval in shape

dis·cis·sion \də-ˈsish-ən, -ˈsizh-\ *n* : an incision (as in treating cataract) of the capsule of the lens of the eye

dis·clos·ing \dis-ˈklō-ziŋ\ *adj* : being or using an agent (as a tablet or liquid) that contains a usu. red dye that adheres to and stains dental plaque

dis·co·blas·tic \ˌdis-kō-ˈblas-tik\ *adj* : MEROBLASTIC

dis·co·blas·tu·la \-ˈblas-chə-lə\ *n, pl* **-las** *or* **-lae** \-(ˌ)lē, -ˌlī\ : BLASTODERM

dis·co·gas·tru·la \-ˈgas-trə-lə\ *n, pl* **-las** *or* **-lae** \-(ˌ)lē, -ˌlī\ : a gastrula derived from a blastoderm

discogram, discography *var of* DISKOGRAM, DISKOGRAPHY

¹**dis·coid** \ˈdis-ˌkȯid\ *adj* **1** : resembling a disk : being flat and circular ⟨the red blood cell is a biconcave ∼ body⟩ **2** : characterized by macules ⟨∼ lupus erythematosus⟩

²**discoid** *n* : an instrument with a disk-shaped blade used in dentistry for carving

dis·coi·dal \dis-ˈkȯid-ᵊl\ *adj* : of, resembling, or producing a disk; *esp* : having the villi restricted to one or more disklike areas

discoidal cleavage *n* : meroblastic cleavage in which a disk of cells is produced at the animal pole of the zygote (as in bird eggs)

dis·con·tin·u·ous phase \ˌdis-kən-ˈtin-yə-wəs-\ *n* : DISPERSED PHASE

dis·cop·a·thy \dis-ˈkäp-ə-thē\ *n, pl* **-thies** : any disease affecting an intervertebral disk

dis·co·pla·cen·ta \ˌdis-kō-plə-ˈsent-ə\ *n* : a discoidal placenta

dis·cor·dant \dis-ˈkȯrd-ᵊnt\ *adj, of twins* : dissimilar with respect to one or more particular characters — compare CONCORDANT — **dis·cor·dance** \-ᵊn(t)s\ *n*

dis·crete \dis-ˈkrēt, ˈdis-ˌ\ *adj* : characterized by distinct unconnected lesions ⟨∼ smallpox⟩ — compare CONFLUENT 2

dis·crim·i·na·bil·i·ty \dis-ˌkrim-ə-nə-ˈbil-ət-ē\ *n, pl* **-ties 1** : the quality of being distinguishable ⟨the ∼ of two stimuli⟩ **2** : the ability to distinguish between different stimuli ⟨loss of ∼ for blue-yellow differences⟩ — **dis·crim·i·na·ble** \-ˈkrim-ə-nə-bəl\ *adj*

dis·crim·i·nate \dis-ˈkrim-ə-ˌnāt\ *vb* **-nat·ed; -nat·ing** *vt* : to respond selectively to (a stimulus) ∼ *vi* : to respond selectively ⟨the capacity of organisms to ∼ —J. A. Swets⟩

dis·crim·i·na·tion \dis-ˌkrim-ə-ˈnā-shən\ *n* : the process by which two stimuli differing in some aspect are responded to differently ⟩ DIFFERENTIATION

dis·cus \ˈdis-kəs\ *n, pl* **dis·ci** \-ˌkī, -kē\ : any of various rounded and flattened anatomical structures

discus pro·lig·er·us \-prō-ˈlij-(ə-)rəs\ *n* : CUMULUS

dis·ease \diz-ˈēz\ *n* : an impairment of the normal state of the living animal or plant body or one of its parts that interrupts or modifies the performance of the vital functions, is typically manifested by distinguishing signs and symptoms, and is a response to environmental factors (as malnutrition, industrial hazards, or climate), to specific infective agents (as worms, bacteria, or viruses), to inherent defects of the organism (as genetic anomalies), or to combinations of these factors : SICKNESS, ILLNESS — called also *morbus;* compare HEALTH 1 — **dis·eased** \-ˈēzd\ *adj*

dis·equi·lib·ri·um \(ˌ)dis-ˌē-kwə-ˈlib-rē-əm, -ˌek-wə-\ *n, pl* **-ri·ums** *or* **-ria** \-rē-ə\ : loss or lack of equilibrium ⟨ionic ∼ in a resting nerve cell⟩ ⟨emotional ∼⟩

disfunction *var of* DYSFUNCTION

disgenic *var of* DYSGENIC

dis·ha·bit·u·a·tion \ˌdis-hə-ˌbich-ə-ˈwā-shən\ *n* : restoration to full strength of a response that has become weakened by habituation — **dis·ha·bit·u·ate** \-ˈbich-ə-ˌwāt\ *vb* **-at·ed; -at·ing**

dis·har·mo·ny \(ˈ)dis-ˈhär-mə-nē\ *n, pl* **-nies** : lack of harmony — see OCCLUSAL DISHARMONY

dish–face deformity \ˈdish-ˌfās-\ *n* : a condition in which the face appears somewhat concave because of underdevelopment of the nasal and maxillary regions

dish·pan hands \ˈdish-ˌpan-\ *n pl but sing or pl in constr* : a condition of dryness, redness, and scaling of the hands that results typically from repeated exposure to, sensitivity to, or overuse of cleaning materials (as detergents) used in housework

dis·in·fect \ˌdis-ᵊn-ˈfekt\ *vt* : to free from infection esp. by destroying harmful microorganisms — **dis·in·fec·tion** \-ˈfek-shən\ *n*

¹**dis·in·fec·tant** \-ˈfek-tənt\ *n* : an agent that frees from infection; *esp* : a chemical that destroys vegetative forms of harmful microorganisms (as bacteria and fungi) esp. on inanimate objects but that may be less effective in destroying spores

²**disinfectant** *adj* : serving or tending to disinfect : suitable for use in disinfecting

dis·in·fest \ˌdis-ᵊn-ˈfest\ *vt* : to rid of small animal pests (as insects) — **dis·in·fes·ta·tion** \(ˌ)dis-ˌin-ˌfes-ˈtā-shən\ *n*

dis·in·fes·tant \ˌdis-ᵊn-ˈfes-tənt\ *n* : a disinfesting agent

dis·in·hib·it \ˌdis-in-ˈhib-ət\ *vt* : to cause the loss or reduction of an inhibition ⟨∼ a reflex⟩ ⟨∼ violent tendencies⟩ — **dis·in·hi·bi·tion** \-ˌin-(h)ə-ˈbish-ən\ *n*

dis·in·hib·i·to·ry \-in-ˈhib-ə-ˌtōr-ē, -ˌtȯr-\ *adj* : tending to overcome psychological inhibition ⟨∼ drugs⟩

dis·in·sec·tion \ˌdis-ᵊn-ˈsek-shən\ *n* : DISINSECTIZATION

dis·in·sect·iza·tion *or Brit* **dis·in·sect·isa·tion** \ˌdis-(ˌ)in-ˌsek-tə-ˈzā-shən\ *n* : removal of insects (as from an aircraft)

dis·in·ser·tion \-(ˌ)in-ˈsər-shən\ *n* **1** : rupture of a tendon at its point of attachment to a bone **2** : peripheral separation of the retina from its attachment at the ora serrata

dis·in·te·grate \(ˈ)dis-ˈint-ə-ˌgrāt\ *vb* **-grat·ed; -grat·ing** *vt* : to break or decompose into constituent elements, parts, or small particles ∼ *vi* **1** : to break or separate into constituent elements or parts **2** : to undergo a change in composition ⟨an atomic nucleus that ∼s because of radioactivity⟩ — **dis·in·te·gra·tion** \(ˌ)dis-ˌint-ə-ˈgrā-shən\ *n*

disintegration constant *n* : DECAY CONSTANT

dis·in·te·gra·tor \(ˈ)dis-ˈint-ə-ˌgrāt-ər\ *n* : one that causes the

C
D

\ə\ abut \ᵊ\ kitten \ər\ further \a\ ash \ā\ ace \ä\ cot, cart
\aů\ out \ch\ chin \e\ bet \ē\ easy \g\ go \i\ hit \ī\ ice \j\ job
\ŋ\ sing \ō\ go \ȯ\ law \ȯi\ boy \th\ thin \t̲h̲\ the \ü\ loot
\ů\ foot \y\ yet \zh\ vision   *See also* Pronunciation Symbols page

disintegration of something; *specif* : a substance used in tablet formulations to cause the tablet to break up on contact with moisture and exert its medicinal action promptly

dis·in·ter \ˌdis-ᵊn-ˈtər\ *vt* : to take out of the grave or tomb — **dis·in·ter·ment** \-mənt\ *n*

dis·in·tox·i·cate \ˌdis-ᵊn-ˈtäk-sə-ˌkāt\ *vt* **-cat·ed; -cat·ing** : DETOXIFY 2 — **dis·in·tox·i·ca·tion** \-ˌtäk-sə-ˈkā-shən\ *n*

dis·junc·tion \dis-ˈjəŋ(k)-shən\ *n* : the separation of chromosomes or chromatids during anaphase of mitosis or meiosis

disk *or* **disc** \ˈdisk\ *n* : any of various rounded or flattened anatomical structures: as **a** : a mammalian blood cell **b** : BLIND SPOT **c** : INTERVERTEBRAL DISK — see SLIPPED DISK

disk·ec·to·my *also* **disc·ec·to·my** \dis-ˈkek-tə-mē\ *n, pl* **-mies** : surgical removal of an intervertebral disk

disk·o·gram *also* **disc·o·gram** \ˈdis-kə-ˌgram\ *n* : a radiograph of an intervertebral disk made after injection of a radiopaque substance

dis·kog·ra·phy *also* **dis·cog·ra·phy** \dis-ˈkäg-rə-fē\ *n, pl* **-phies** : the process of making a diskogram

dis·lo·cate \ˈdis-lō-ˌkāt, -lə-; (ˈ)dis-ˈlō-ˌkāt\ *vt* **-cat·ed; -cat·ing** : to put (a body part) out of order by displacing a bone from its normal connections with another bone ⟨he *dislocated* his shoulder⟩; *also* : to displace (a bone) from normal connections with another bone ⟨the humerus was *dislocated* in the fall⟩

dis·lo·ca·tion \ˌdis-(ˌ)lō-ˈkā-shən, -lə-\ *n* : displacement of one or more bones at a joint : LUXATION

dis·mem·ber \(ˈ)dis-ˈmem-bər\ *vt* **dis·mem·bered; dis·mem·ber·ing** \-b(ə-)riŋ\ : to cut off or disjoin the limbs, members, or parts of — **dis·mem·ber·ment** \-bər-mənt\ *n*

dismutase — see SUPEROXIDE DISMUTASE

dis·mu·ta·tion \ˌdis-myü-ˈtā-shən\ *n* : a process of simultaneous oxidation and reduction — used esp. of compounds taking part in biological processes

di·so·di·um \(ˈ)dī-ˈsōd-ē-əm\ *adj* : containing two atoms of sodium in a molecule

disodium cromoglycate *n* : CROMOLYN SODIUM

disodium ed·e·tate \-ˈed-ə-ˌtāt\ *n* : a hydrated disodium salt $C_{10}H_{14}N_2Na_2O_8 \cdot 2H_2O$ of EDTA that has an affinity for calcium and is used to treat hypercalcemia and pathological calcification

di·so·mic \(ˈ)dī-ˈsō-mik\ *adj* : having one or more chromosomes present in twice the normal number but not having the entire genome doubled — **di·so·my** \-mē\ *n, pl* **-mies**

di·so·mus \-məs\ *n, pl* **di·so·mi** \-ˌmī\ *or* **di·so·mus·es** : a 2-bodied teratological fetus

di·so·pyr·a·mide \ˌdī-(ˌ)sō-ˈpi(ə)r-ə-ˌmīd\ *n* : a cardiac depressant administered in the form of its phosphate $C_{21}H_{29}N_3O \cdot H_3PO_4$ in the treatment of life-threatening ventricular arrhythmias

¹dis·or·der \(ˈ)dis-ˈȯrd-ər, (ˈ)diz-\ *vt* **dis·or·dered; dis·or·der·ing** \-ˈȯrd-(ə-)riŋ\ : to disturb the regular or normal functions of

²disorder *n* : an abnormal physical or mental condition : AILMENT ⟨an intestinal ∼⟩ ⟨a nervous ∼⟩

dis·or·dered *adj* **1** : not functioning in a normal orderly healthy way ⟨∼ bodily functions⟩ **2** : mentally unbalanced ⟨a ∼ patient⟩ ⟨a ∼ mind⟩

dis·or·ga·ni·za·tion *or Brit* **dis·or·ga·ni·sa·tion** \(ˌ)dis-ˌȯrg-(ə-)nə-ˈzā-shən\ *n* : psychopathological inconsistency in personality, mental functions, or overt behavior ⟨psychotic ∼⟩ ⟨psychomotor ∼⟩ — **dis·or·ga·nize** *or Brit* **dis·or·ga·nise** \(ˈ)dis-ˈȯr-gə-ˌnīz\ *vt* **-nized** *or Brit* **-nised; -niz·ing** *or Brit* **-nis·ing**

dis·ori·ent \(ˈ)dis-ˈōr-ē-ˌent, -ˈȯr-\ *vt* : to produce a state of disorientation in : DISORIENTATE ⟨the next day the patient was ∼*ed* but not comatose —*Jour. Amer. Med. Assoc.*⟩

dis·ori·en·ta·tion \(ˌ)dis-ˌōr-ē-ən-ˈtā-shən, -ˌȯr-, -ˌen-\ *n* : a usu. transient state of confusion esp. as to time, place, or identity often as a result of disease or drugs — **dis·ori·en·tate** \(ˈ)dis-ˈōr-ē-ən-ˌtāt, -ˈȯr-, -ˌen-\ *vt* **-tat·ed; -tat·ing**

disp *abbr* dispensary

dis·pa·rate \dis-ˈpar-ət, ˈdis-p(ə-)rət\ *adj* : indicating or stimulating dissimilar points on the retina of each eye

dis·par·i·ty \dis-ˈpar-ət-ē\ *n, pl* **-ties** : the state of being different or dissimilar (as in the sensory information received) — see RETINAL DISPARITY

dis·pen·sa·ry \dis-ˈpen(t)s-(ə-)rē\ *n, pl* **-ries** : a place where medicine or medical or dental treatment is dispensed

dis·pen·sa·tion \ˌdis-pən-ˈsā-shən, -ˌpen-\ *n* : the act of dispensing ⟨the ∼ of medicines⟩

dis·pen·sa·to·ry \dis-ˈpen(t)s-ə-ˌtōr-ē, -ˌtȯr-\ *n, pl* **-ries** **1** : a book or medicinal formulary containing a systematic description of the drugs and preparations used in medicine — compare PHARMACOPOEIA 1 **2** : DISPENSARY

dis·pense \dis-ˈpen(t)s\ *vt* **dis·pensed; dis·pens·ing** **1** : to put up (a prescription or medicine) **2** : to prepare and distribute (medication)

dispensing optician *n, Brit* : a person qualified and licensed to fit and supply eyeglasses

di·sper·my \ˈdī-ˌspər-mē\ *n, pl* **-mies** : the entrance of two spermatozoa into one egg — compare MONOSPERMY, POLYSPERMY

dis·pers·al \dis-ˈpər-səl\ *n* : the act or result of dispersing; *specif* : the process or result of the spreading of organisms from one place to another

dis·perse \dis-ˈpərs\ *vb* **dis·persed; dis·pers·ing** *vt* : to spread or distribute from a fixed or constant source: as **a** : to subject (as light) to dispersion **b** : to distribute (as fine particles) more or less evenly throughout a medium ∼ *vi* : to become dispersed

dispersed phase *or* **disperse phase** *n* : the phase in a two-phase system that consists of finely divided particles (as colloidal particles), droplets, or bubbles of one substance distributed through another substance — called also *discontinuous phase, internal phase*

disperse system *n* : DISPERSION 3b, COLLOID 2b

dis·per·sion \dis-ˈpər-zhən, -shən\ *n* **1** : the act or process of dispersing : the state of being dispersed **2** : the separation of light into colors by refraction or diffraction with formation of a spectrum; *also* : the separation of radiation into components in accordance with some varying characteristic (as energy) **3 a** : a dispersed substance **b** : a system consisting of a dispersed substance and the medium in which it is dispersed : COLLOID 2b — called also *disperse system*

dispersion medium *n* : the liquid, gaseous, or solid phase in a two-phase system in which the particles of the dispersed phase are distributed — called also *continuous phase, external phase*

dis·per·si·ty \dis-ˈpər-sət-ē\ *n, pl* **-ties** : the state or the degree of chemical dispersion

dis·per·sive \-ˈpər-siv, -ziv\ *adj* **1** : of or relating to dispersion ⟨a ∼ medium⟩ ⟨the ∼ power of a lens⟩ **2** : tending to disperse — **dis·per·sive·ness** *n*

dis·per·soid \-ˌsȯid\ *n* : finely divided particles of one substance dispersed in another

dis·place \(ˈ)dis-ˈplās\ *vt* **-placed; -plac·ing** **1 a** : to remove from the usual or proper place ⟨in heterotopia the gray portions of the cord are *displaced* so that patches of gray matter are scattered among the bundles of white fibers —R. L. Cecil *et al*⟩ **b** : to shift (an emotion or behavior) from a maladaptive or unacceptable object or form of outlet to a more adaptive or acceptable one ⟨∼ punishable behavior by directing it towards things that cannot punish —B. F. Skinner⟩ **2** : to set free from chemical combination by taking the place of ⟨zinc ∼*s* the hydrogen of dilute acids⟩ **3** : to subject to percolation

dis·place·ment \-ˈplā-smənt\ *n* **1 a** : the act or process of removing something from its usual or proper place or the state resulting from this : DISLOCATION ⟨the ∼ of a knee joint⟩ **b** : PERCOLATION 3 **2** : the quantity in which or the degree to which something is displaced **3 a** : the redirection of an emotion or impulse from its original object (as an idea or person) to something that is more acceptable **b** : SUBLIMATION 2 **c** : the substitution of another form of behavior for what is usual or expected esp. when the usual response is nonadaptive — called also *displacement activity, displacement behavior*

dis·pro·por·tion \ˌdis-prə-ˈpȯr-shən, -ˈpȯr-\ *n* : absence of symmetry or the proper dimensional relationship ⟨a ∼ between the large head and the average-size body⟩ — see CEPHALOPELVIC DISPROPORTION

dis·rup·tion \dis-ˈrəp-shən\ *n* : the act or process of breaking apart or rupturing ⟨bandaged her leg tightly to prevent ∼ of the partly healed wound⟩ — **dis·rupt** \dis-ˈrəpt\ *vt*

dis·rup·tive \dis-ˈrəp-tiv\ *adj* : characterized by psychologically disorganized behavior ⟨a confused, incoherent, and ∼ patient in the manic phase⟩

dissd *abbr* dissolved

dissecans — see OSTEOCHONDRITIS DISSECANS

dis·sect \dis-ˈekt; dī-ˈsekt, ˈdī-ˌ\ *vt* : to cut so as to separate into pieces or to expose the several parts of (as an animal or a cadaver) for scientific examination; *specif* : to separate or follow along natural lines of cleavage (as through connective tissue) ⟨∼ out the regional lymph nodes⟩ ⟨a ∼*ing* aneurysm⟩ ∼ *vi* : to make a medical dissection — **dis·sec·tor** \-ər\ *n*

dissecting microscope *n* : a low-magnification stereomicroscope used esp. for examining or dissecting biological specimens

dis·sec·tion \dis-ˈek-shən; dī-ˈsek-, ˈdī-ˌ\ *n* **1** : the act or process of dissecting or separating: as **a** : the surgical removal along natural lines of cleavage of tissues which are or might become diseased **b** : the digital separation of tissues (as in heart-valve operations) — compare FINGER FRACTURE **c** : a pathological splitting or separation of tissue — see AORTIC DISSECTION **2 a** : something (as a part or the whole of an animal) that has been dissected **b** : an anatomical specimen prepared in this way

dis·sem·i·nat·ed \dis-ˈem-ə-ˌnāt-əd\ *adj* : widely dispersed in a tissue, organ, or the entire body ⟨∼ cutaneous leishmaniasis⟩ ⟨∼ gonococcal disease⟩ — **dis·sem·i·na·tion** \-ˌem-ə-ˈnā-shən\ *n*

dis·sep·i·ment \dis-ˈep-ə-mənt\ *n* : a dividing tissue : SEPTUM

dis·sim·i·la·tion \(ˌ)dis-ˌim-ə-ˈlā-shən\ *n* : CATABOLISM — **dis·sim·i·late** \(ˈ)dis-ˈim-ə-ˌlāt\ *vt* -lat·ed; -lat·ing — **dis·sim·i·la·tive** \-ˌlāt-iv\ *adj* — **dis·sim·i·la·to·ry** \-lə-ˌtōr-ē, -ˌtȯr-\ *adj*

¹dis·so·ciant \dis-ˈō-s(h)ē-ənt, -ˈō-shənt\ *adj, of microorganisms* : MUTANT

²dissociant *n* : a dissociant strain or individual

dis·so·ci·ate \(ˈ)dis-ˈō-s(h)ē-ˌāt\ *vb* -at·ed; -at·ing *vt* : to subject to chemical dissociation ∼ *vi* **1** : to undergo dissociation **2** : to mutate esp. reversibly

dis·so·ci·at·ed *adj* **1** : giving evidence of or marked by psychological dissociation ⟨a ∼ personality⟩ **2** : formed by dissociation ⟨∼ pneumococci⟩

dis·so·ci·a·tion \(ˌ)dis-ˌō-sē-ˈā-shən, -shē-\ *n* **1** : the act or process of dissociating : the state of being dissociated: as **a** : the process by which a chemical combination breaks up into simpler constituents; *esp* : one that results from the action of energy (as heat) on a gas or of a solvent on a dissolved substance **b** : the separation of whole segments of the personality (as in multiple personality disorder) or of discrete mental processes (as in the schizophrenias) from the mainstream of consciousness or of behavior with loss of integrated awareness and autonomous functioning of the separated segments or parts **2** : the process by which some biological stocks (as of certain bacteria) differentiate into two or more distinct and relatively permanent strains; *also* : such a strain

dissociation constant *n* : a constant that depends upon the equilibrium between the dissociated and undissociated forms of a chemical combination; *esp* : IONIZATION CONSTANT — symbol *K*

dis·so·cia·tive \(ˈ)dis-ˈō-s(h)ē-ˌāt-iv, -shət-iv\ *adj* : of, relating to, or tending to produce dissociation ⟨a ∼ chemical reaction⟩ ⟨hypnosis theoretically induces a ∼ state in the subject so that he or she is not aware of all that is occurring in consciousness —Rita L. Atkinson *et al*⟩

dissociative identity disorder *n* : MULTIPLE PERSONALITY DISORDER

dis·so·lu·tion \ˌdis-ə-ˈlü-shən\ *n* : the act or process of dissolving: as **a** : separation into component parts **b** : DEATH 1 ⟨grew convinced of his friend's approaching ∼ —Elinor Wylie⟩ **c** : LIQUEFACTION **d** : SOLUTION 1a

dis·solve \diz-ˈälv, -ˈȯlv\ *vb* **dis·solved; dis·solv·ing** *vt* **1** : to cause to pass into solution ⟨∼ sugar in water⟩ **2** : to cause to melt or liquefy ∼ *vi* **1** : to become fluid **2** : to pass into solution — **dis·solv·able** \-ˈäl-və-bəl, -ˈȯl-\ *adj* — **dis·solv·er** *n*

dis·sol·vent \diz-ˈäl-vənt, -ˈȯl-\ *adj* : SOLVENT — **dissolvent** *n*

dis·so·nance \ˈdis-ə-nən(t)s\ *n* : inconsistency between the beliefs one holds or between one's actions and one's beliefs — see COGNITIVE DISSONANCE

dis·tad \ˈdis-ˌtad\ *adv* : toward or near the distal part or end

dis·tal \ˈdis-tᵊl\ *adj* **1** : situated away from the point of attachment or origin or a central point: as **a** : located away from the center of the body ⟨the ∼ end of a bone⟩ — compare PROXIMAL 1a **b** : located away from the mesial plane of the body — compare MESIAL 2 **c** : of, relating to, or being the surface of a tooth that is next to the following tooth counting from the middle of the front of the upper or lower jaw or that faces the back of the mouth in the case of the last tooth on each side — compare MESIAL 3, PROXIMAL 1b **2** : physical or social rather than sensory — compare PROXIMAL 2 — **dis·tal·ly** \-ē\ *adv*

distal convoluted tubule *n* : the convoluted portion of the nephron lying between the loop of Henle and the nonsecretory part of the nephron and concerned esp. with the concentration of urine — called also *convoluted tubule, distal tubule*

distalis — see PARS DISTALIS

distal radioulnar joint *n* : a pivot joint between the lower end of the ulna and the ulnar notch on the lower end of the radius that permits rotation of the distal end of the radius around the longitudinal axis of the ulna — called also *inferior radioulnar joint*

dis·tem·per \dis-ˈtem-pər\ *n* : a disordered or abnormal bodily state esp. of quadruped mammals: as **a** : a highly contagious virus disease esp. of dogs that is marked by fever, leukopenia, and respiratory, gastrointestinal, and neurological symptoms and that is caused by a paramyxovirus of the genus *Morbillivirus* (species *Canine distemper virus*) — called also *canine distemper* **b** : STRANGLES **c** : PANLEUKOPENIA **d** : a severe frequently fatal infectious nasopharyngeal inflammation of rabbits

dis·tem·per·oid \dis-ˈtem-pə-ˌrȯid\ *adj* : resembling distemper; *specif* : of, relating to, or being an attenuated canine distemper virus used to develop immunity to natural distemper infection

dis·tend \dis-ˈtend\ *vt* : to enlarge or stretch out (as from internal pressure) ⟨∼*ed* veins⟩ ∼ *vi* : to become expanded

dis·ten·si·ble \-ˈten(t)-sə-bəl\ *adj* : capable of being distended, extended, or dilated ⟨∼ blood vessels⟩ — **dis·ten·si·bil·i·ty** \-ˌten(t)-sə-ˈbil-ət-ē\ *n, pl* **-ties**

dis·ten·sile \dis-ˈten(t)-səl *also* -ˈten-ˌsīl\ *adj* **1** : DISTENSIBLE **2** : causing distension

dis·ten·sion *or* **dis·ten·tion** \dis-ˈten-chən\ *n* : the act of distending or the state of being distended esp. unduly or abnormally ⟨no noticeable ∼ of the abdomen —Benjamin Spock⟩

dis·till *also* **dis·til** \dis-ˈtil\ *vb* **dis·tilled; dis·till·ing** *vt* **1** : to subject to or transform by distillation **2** : to obtain by or as if by distillation **3** : to obtain an extract from (as a plant) by infusion and distillation ⟨making medicines by ∼*ing* herbs⟩ ∼ *vi* **1** : to undergo distillation **2** : to condense or drop from a still after distillation

C
D

\ə\ abut \ᵊ\ kitten \ər\ **fur**ther \a\ ash \ā\ ace \ä\ cot, cart
\au̇\ out \ch\ chin \e\ bet \ē\ easy \g\ go \i\ hit \ī\ ice \j\ job
\ŋ\ sing \ō\ go \ȯ\ law \ȯi\ boy \th\ thin \t͟h\ the \ü\ loot
\u̇\ foot \y\ yet \zh\ vision *See also* Pronunciation Symbols page

dis·til·late \'dis-tə-ˌlāt, -lət; dis-'til-ət\ *n* : a liquid product condensed from vapor during distillation

dis·til·la·tion \ˌdis-tə-'lā-shən\ *n* **1** : a process that consists of driving gas or vapor from liquids or solids by heating and condensing to liquid products and that is used esp. for purification, fractionation, or the formation of new substances **2** : something distilled

dis·to·buc·cal \ˌdis-tō-'bək-əl\ *adj* : relating to or located on the distal and buccal surfaces of a molar or premolar ⟨the ∼ cusp of the first molar⟩ — **dis·to·buc·cal·ly** \-ə-lē\ *adv*

dis·to·clu·sion \-'klü-zhən\ *n* : malposition of a lower tooth or teeth distal to the upper when the jaws are closed

dis·to·lin·gual \-'liŋ-g(ə-)wəl\ *adj* : relating to or situated on the distal and lingual surfaces of a tooth ⟨the ∼ cusp⟩

Dis·to·ma \'dis-tə-mə\ *n, syn of* FASCIOLA

Dis·to·ma·ta \dī-'stō-mət-ə\ *n pl, in some classifications* : a large suborder of the order Prosostomata comprising flukes with oral and ventral suckers and with the reproductive organs mostly posterior to the ventral sucker — **dis·to·mate** \-ˌmāt, -mət\ *adj* — **di·stome** \'dī-ˌstōm\ *adj or n*

dis·to·ma·to·sis \ˌdī-ˌstō-mə-'tō-səs\ *n, pl* **-to·ses** \-ˌsēz\ : infestation with or disease (as liver rot) caused by digenetic trematode worms

dis·to·mi·a·sis \ˌdī-stō-'mī-ə-səs\ *n, pl* **-a·ses** \-ˌsēz\ : DISTOMATOSIS

Dis·to·mum \'dis-tə-məm\ *n, syn of* FASCIOLA

dis·tor·tion \dis-'tòr-shən\ *n* **1** : the censorship of unacceptable unconscious impulses so that they are unrecognizable to the ego in the manifest content of a dream **2** : a lack of correspondence of size or intensity in an image resulting from defects in an optical system

dis·to·ver·sion \'dis-tō-ˌvər-zhən, -shən\ *n* : tipping of a tooth so that the crown projects in a distal direction

dis·tract·i·bil·i·ty \dis-ˌtrak-tə-'bil-ət-ē\ *n, pl* **-ties** : a condition in which the attention of the mind is easily distracted by small and irrelevant stimuli — **dis·tract·ible** \-'trak-tə-bəl\ *adj*

dis·trac·tion \dis-'trak-shən\ *n* **1 a** : diversion of the attention **b** : mental derangement **2** : excessive separation (as from improper traction) of fracture fragments — **dis·tract** \dis-'trakt\ *vt*

dis·tress \dis-'tres\ *n* : pain or suffering affecting the body, a bodily part, or the mind ⟨gastric ∼⟩ ⟨respiratory ∼⟩

dis·tri·bu·tion \ˌdis-trə-'byü-shən\ *n* : the pattern of branching and termination of a ramifying anatomical structure (as a nerve or artery)

distribution coefficient *n* : PARTITION COEFFICIENT

dis·trict nurse \ˌdis-trikt-\ *n, Brit* : a qualified nurse who is employed by a local authority to visit and treat patients in their own homes — compare VISITING NURSE

dis·tur·bance \dis-'tər-bən(t)s\ *n* : the state of being emotionally disturbed

dis·turbed \dis-'tərbd\ *adj* **1** : showing symptoms of emotional illness or mental disorder ⟨∼ children⟩ ⟨∼ behavior⟩ **2** : designed for or occupied by disturbed patients ⟨∼ wards⟩

di·sul·fide *or chiefly Brit* **di·sul·phide** \(')dī-'səl-ˌfīd\ *n* **1** : a compound containing two atoms of sulfur combined with an element or radical **2** : an organic compound containing the bivalent group SS composed of two sulfur atoms

di·sul·fi·ram *or chiefly Brit* **di·sul·phi·ram** \dī-'səl-fə-ˌram\ *n* : a compound $C_{10}H_{20}N_2S_4$ that causes a severe physiological reaction to alcohol and is used esp. in the treatment of alcoholism — called also *tetraethylthiuram disulfide;* see ANTABUSE

di·ter·pene \(')dī-'tər-ˌpēn\ *n* : any of a class of terpenes $C_{20}H_{32}$ containing twice as many atoms in a molecule as monoterpenes; *also* : a derivative of such a terpene

di·thio \(')dī-'thī-(ˌ)ō\ *adj* : relating to or containing two atoms of sulfur usu. in place of two oxygen atoms ⟨∼ acids⟩

di·thio·thre·i·tol \(ˌ)dī-ˌthī-ō-'thrē-ə-ˌtòl, -ˌtōl\ *n* : a reducing agent $C_4H_{10}O_2S_2$ used esp. in biochemical reactions to sever bonds (as in a protein) composed of disulfide groups

di·thra·nol \'dī-thrə-ˌnòl, 'dith-rə-, -ˌnōl\ *n, chiefly Brit* : ANTHRALIN

di·ure·sis \ˌdī-(y)ə-'rē-səs\ *n, pl* **di·ure·ses** \-ˌsēz\ : an increased excretion of urine

[1]di·uret·ic \ˌdī-(y)ə-'ret-ik\ *adj* : tending to increase the excretion of urine — **di·uret·i·cal·ly** \-i-k(ə-)lē\ *adv*

[2]diuretic *n* : an agent that increases the excretion of urine

Di·ur·il \'dī-yùr-il\ *trademark* — used for a preparation of chlorothiazide

di·ur·nal \dī-'ərn-ᵊl\ *adj* **1** : having a daily cycle ⟨∼ rhythms⟩ **2 a** : of, relating to, or occurring in the daytime ⟨∼ activity⟩ **b** : chiefly active during the daytime ⟨∼ mosquitoes⟩ — **di·ur·nal·ly** \-ᵊl-ē\ *adv*

div *abbr* **1** divide; division **2** divorced

di·va·lent \(')dī-'vā-lənt\ *adj* : having a chemical valence of two ⟨∼ calcium⟩; *also* : bonded to two other atoms or groups ⟨a ∼ methylene group⟩

di·val·pro·ex sodium \ˌdī-ˌval-prō-eks-, -ˌval-'prō-\ *n* : a coordination compound of valproate and valproic acid that is used esp. to treat manic episodes of bipolar disorder and absence seizures of epilepsy — called also *divalproex;* see DEPAKOTE

di·ver·gence \də-'vər-jən(t)s, dī-\ *n* **1 a** : a drawing apart **b** : the acquisition of dissimilar characters by related organisms under the influence of unlike environments **2** : dissemination of the effect of activity of a single nerve cell through multiple synaptic connections — compare CONVERGENCE 4 — **di·verge** \-'vərj\ *vb* **di·verged; di·verg·ing** — **di·ver·gent** \-'vər-jənt\ *adj*

divergent think·ing \-'thiŋk-iŋ\ *n* : creative thinking that may follow many lines of thought and tends to generate new and original solutions to problems — compare CONVERGENT THINKING — **divergent think·er** \-ər\ *n*

diverging lens *n* : a lens that causes divergence of rays : a concave lens — called also *negative lens*

div·er's palsy \ˌdī-vərz-\ *n* : DECOMPRESSION SICKNESS

diver's paralysis *n* : DECOMPRESSION SICKNESS

diverticula *pl of* DIVERTICULUM

di·ver·tic·u·lar \ˌdī-vər-'tik-yə-lər\ *adj* : consisting of or resembling a diverticulum

diverticular disease *n* : a disorder characterized by diverticulosis or diverticulitis

di·ver·tic·u·lec·to·my \ˌdī-vər-ˌtik-yə-'lek-tə-mē\ *n, pl* **-mies** : the surgical removal of a diverticulum

di·ver·tic·u·li·tis \-'līt-əs\ *n* : inflammation or infection of a diverticulum of the colon that is marked by abdominal pain or tenderness often accompanied by fever, chills, and cramping

di·ver·ti·cu·lop·exy \-'läp-ək-sē\ *n, pl* **-ex·ies** : surgical obliteration or fixation of a diverticulum

di·ver·tic·u·lo·sis \-'lō-səs\ *n, pl* **-lo·ses** \-ˌsēz\ : an intestinal condition characterized by the presence of diverticula in the colon that is typically symptomless but may be marked by symptoms (as bleeding or constipation)

di·ver·tic·u·lum \ˌdī-vər-'tik-yə-ləm\ *n, pl* **-la** \-lə\ **1** : an abnormal pouch or sac opening from a hollow organ (as the colon or bladder) **2** : a blind tube or sac branching off from a cavity or canal of the body ⟨the liver is an anterior ∼ of the intestine—Gordon Alexander⟩

di·vide \də-'vīd\ *vb* **di·vid·ed; di·vid·ing** *vt* : to separate into two or more parts ⟨∼ a nerve surgically⟩ ∼ *vi* : to undergo replication, multiplication, fission, or separation into parts ⟨actively *dividing* cells⟩

di·vid·er \də-'vīd-ər\ *n* : the second incisor tooth of a horse situated between the center and corner incisors on each side — compare NIPPER 2

di·vi–di·vi \ˌdē-vē-'dē-vē, ˌdiv-ē-'div-ē\ *n* **1** : a small leguminous tropical American tree of the genus *Caesalpinia* (*C. coriaria*) with twisted astringent pods that contain a large proportion of tannin **2** : the pods of the divi-divi

di·vi·sion \də-'vizh-ən\ *n* **1** : the act or process of dividing : the state of being divided — see CELL DIVISION **2** : a

C
D

group of organisms forming part of a larger group; *specif* : a primary category of the plant kingdom — **di·vi·sion·al** \-'vizh-nəl, -'vizh-ən-°l\ *adj*

di·vul·sion \dī-'vəl-shən\ *n* : a tearing apart — **di·vulse** \-'vəls\ *vt* **di·vulsed; di·vuls·ing**

di·vul·sor \-'vəl-sər\ *n* : DILATOR a

di·zy·got·ic \ˌdī-zī-'gät-ik\ *also* **di·zy·gous** \(')dī-'zī-gəs\ *adj, of twins* : FRATERNAL

diz·zi·ness \'diz-ē-nəs\ *n* : the condition of being dizzy; *esp* : a sensation of unsteadiness accompanied by a feeling of movement within the head — compare VERTIGO 1

diz·zy \'diz-ē\ *adj* **diz·zi·er; -est** 1 : having a whirling sensation in the head with a tendency to fall 2 : mentally confused — **diz·zi·ly** \'diz-ə-lē\ *adv*

DJD *abbr* degenerative joint disease

dkg *abbr* dekagram

dkl *abbr* dekaliter

dkm *abbr* dekameter

dl *abbr* deciliter

dl- *prefix* 1 *also* **d,l-** : consisting of equal amounts of the dextrorotatory and levorotatory forms of a specified compound — usu. printed in italic ⟨*dl*-tartaric acid⟩; compare RACEMIC 2 : consisting of equal amounts of the D- and L- forms of a specified compound — usu. printed as small capitals ⟨DL⸗fructose⟩; compare RACEMIC

DL *abbr* danger list

DLE *abbr* disseminated lupus erythematosus

dm *abbr* decimeter

DM *abbr* 1 diabetes mellitus 2 diastolic murmur 3 [Latin *dystrophia myotonica*] myotonic dystrophy

DMAE \ˌdē-ˌem-ˌā-'ē\ *n* : a choline analog $C_4H_{11}NO$ formerly investigated for use in medicine (as in the treatment of tardive dyskinesia) but now used esp. as a dietary supplement and skin toner — called also *deanol, dimethylaminoethanol*

DMBA *abbr* dimethylbenzanthracene

DMD *abbr* 1 [Latin *dentariae medicinae doctor*] doctor of dental medicine 2 Duchenne muscular dystrophy; Duchenne's muscular dystrophy

DMF *abbr* decayed, missing, and filled teeth

DMSO \ˌdē-ˌem-ˌes-'ō\ *n* : DIMETHYL SULFOXIDE

DMT \ˌdē-(ˌ)em-'tē\ *n* : DIMETHYLTRYPTAMINE

DNA \ˌdē-ˌen-'ā\ *n* : any of various nucleic acids that are usu. the molecular basis of heredity, are constructed of a double helix held together by hydrogen bonds between purine and pyrimidine bases which project inward from two chains containing alternate links of deoxyribose and phosphate, and that in eukaryotes are localized chiefly in cell nuclei — called also *deoxyribonucleic acid;* see RECOMBINANT DNA

DNA chip \-'chip\ *n* : DNA MICROARRAY

DNA fingerprint *n* : the base-pair pattern in an individual's DNA obtained by DNA fingerprinting — called also *genetic fingerprint*

DNA fingerprinting *n* : a technique used esp. for identification (as for forensic purposes) by extracting and identifying the base-pair pattern of an individual's DNA — called also *DNA typing, genetic fingerprinting*

DNA methylation *n* : the enzymatically controlled methylation of a nucleotide base (as cytosine in eukaryotes) in a molecule of DNA that plays a role in suppressing gene expression

DNA methyltransferase *n* : a methyltransferase that promotes the covalent addition of a methyl group to a specific nucleotide base in a molecule of DNA

DNA microarray *n* : a microarray of immobilized single⸗stranded DNA fragments of known nucleotide sequence that is used esp. in the identification and sequencing of DNA samples and in the analysis of gene expression (as in a cell or tissue)

DNA polymerase *n* : any of several polymerases that promote replication or repair of DNA usu. using single-stranded DNA as a template

DNAR *abbr* do not attempt resuscitation

DN·ase \(')dē-'en-ˌās, -ˌāz\ *also* **DNA·ase** \(ˌ)dē-ˌen-'ā-ˌās, -ˌāz\ *n* : DEOXYRIBONUCLEASE

DNA typing *n* : DNA FINGERPRINTING

DNA virus *n* : a virus whose genome consists of DNA

DNOC \ˌdē-ˌen-ˌō-'sē\ *n* : DINITRO-O-CRESOL

DNR *abbr* do not resuscitate

DO *abbr* 1 doctor of optometry 2 doctor of osteopathy

DOA *abbr* dead on arrival

DOB *abbr* date of birth

Do·bell's solution \(')dō-'belz\ *n* : an aqueous solution of sodium borate, sodium bicarbonate, glycerin, and phenol used as a spray for the nose and throat

    Do·bell \dō-'bel\, **Horace Benge (1828–1917),** British physician. Dobell devoted much of his career to originating and establishing in Britain the system of hydropathic treatment.

do·bu·ta·mine \dō-'byüt-ə-ˌmēn\ *n* : a strongly inotropic catecholamine administered intravenously in the form of its hydrochloride $C_{18}H_{23}NO_3 \cdot HCl$ esp. to increase cardiac output and lower wedge pressure in heart failure and after cardiopulmonary bypass surgery

doc \'däk\ *n* : DOCTOR — used chiefly as a familiar term of address

doc *abbr* document

do·ce·tax·el \ˌdō-sə-'tak-səl\ *n* : a semisynthetic antineoplastic drug $C_{43}H_{53}NO_{14} \cdot 3H_2O$ derived from the needles of a yew tree (*Taxus baccata*) of Europe — see TAXOTERE

doc·i·ma·sia \ˌdäs-ə-'mā-zh(ē-)ə\ *n* : determination as to whether a dead infant was stillborn by placing the body in water in which it sinks unless the infant has expanded the lungs in respiration

doc·i·ma·sy \'däs-ə-mə-sē\ *n, pl* **-sies** : DOCIMASIA

¹**dock** \'däk\ *n* : any plant of the genus *Rumex*

²**dock** *vi* : to combine with a molecular receptor ⟨the AIDS virus ~ed on the T cell receptor⟩

do·co·sa·hex·a·e·no·ic acid \ˌdō-kō-sə-ˌhek-sə-ˌē-ˌnō-ik-\ *n* : an omega-3 fatty acid $C_{22}H_{32}O_2$ found esp. in fish of cold waters — abbr. *DHA*

¹**doc·tor** \'däk-tər\ *n* 1 a : a person who has earned one of the highest academic degrees (as a PhD) conferred by a university b : a person awarded an honorary doctorate by a college or university 2 : a person skilled or specializing in healing arts; *esp* : one (as a physician, dentist, or veterinarian) who holds an advanced degree and is licensed to practice

²**doctor** *vb* **doc·tored; doc·tor·ing** \-t(ə-)riŋ\ *vt* 1 : to give medical treatment to 2 : CASTRATE 1, SPAY ⟨have your pet cat ~ed⟩ ~ *vi* : to practice medicine

doc·trine of signatures \'däk-trən-\ *n* : a theory in old natural philosophy: the outward appearance of a body signalizes its special properties (as of magic or healing virtue) and there is a relationship between the outward qualities of a medicinal object and the diseases against which it is effective

doc·u·sate \'däk-yü-ˌsāt\ *n* : any of several laxative salts and esp. the sodium salt $C_{20}H_{37}NaO_7S$ used to soften stools — see PERI-COLACE

do·dec·a·no·ic acid \(ˌ)dō-ˌdek-ə-ˌnō-ik-, ˌdō-dək-\ *n* : LAURIC ACID

do·de·cyl \'dōd-ə-ˌsil\ *n* : an alkyl radical $C_{12}H_{25}$; *esp* : the normal radical $CH_3(CH_2)_{10}CH_2-$ — see SODIUM DODECYL SULFATE

DOE *abbr* dyspnea on exertion

dog \'dȯg\ *n, often attrib* : a highly variable carnivorous domesticated mammal of the genus *Canis* (*C. familiaris*) closely related to the common wolf (*Canis lupus*); *broadly* : any member of the family Canidae

dog·bane \'dȯg-ˌbān\ *n* : any plant of the genus *Apocynum*

dog·fish \-ˌfish\ *n* : any of various small sharks (as of the families Squalidae, Carcharhinidae, and Scyliorhinidae) that often appear in schools near shore, prey chiefly on fish and invertebrates, and are a valuable food source

dog flea *n* : a flea of the genus *Ctenocephalides* (*C. canis*) that feeds chiefly on dogs and cats

---

\ə\ abut \°\ kitten \ər\ further \a\ ash \ā\ ace \ä\ cot, cart \au̇\ out \ch\ chin \e\ bet \ē\ easy \g\ go \i\ hit \ī\ ice \j\ job \ŋ\ sing \ō\ go \ȯ\ law \ȯi\ boy \th\ thin \t̲h̲\ the \ü\ loot \u̇\ foot \y\ yet \zh\ vision *See also* Pronunciation Symbols page

dog tapeworm *n* : a tapeworm of the genus *Dipylidium* (*D. caninum*) occurring in dogs and cats and sometimes in humans — called also *double-pored tapeworm*

dog tick *n* : any of several ticks infesting dogs and commonly other animals: as **a** : AMERICAN DOG TICK **b** : an Australian tick of the genus *Ixodes* (*I. holocyclus*) that chiefly infests native marsupials and that may cause respiratory paralysis in dogs or humans by its bite

dog·wood \'dȯ-ˌgwu̇d\ *n* : any tree or shrub of the genus *Cornus*

dol \'dōl\ *n* : a unit for the measurement of pain intensity usu. taken as one tenth of the range of increasing sensation from that produced by the least perceptible stimulus to that at which further increase in stimulation causes no further increase in sensation

dolens — see PHLEGMASIA ALBA DOLENS, PHLEGMASIA CERULEA DOLENS

dol·i·cho·ceph·al \ˌdäl-i-kō-'sef-əl\ *n, pl* **-ceph·als** *also* **-ceph·a·li** \-ə-ˌlī\ : a dolichocephalic person

dol·i·cho·ce·phal·ic \-sə-'fal-ik\ *adj* : having a relatively long head with a cephalic index of less than 75 — **dol·i·cho·ceph·a·ly** \-'sef-ə-lē\ *n, pl* **-lies**

dol·i·cho·co·lon \-'kō-lən\ *n* : an abnormally long colon

dol·i·cho·cra·ni·al \-'krā-nē-əl\ *adj* : having a relatively long head with a cranial index of less than 75 — **dol·i·cho·cra·ny** \'däl-i-kō-ˌkrā-nē\ *n, pl* **-nies**

dol·i·cho·cra·nic \-'krā-nik\ *adj* : DOLICHOCRANIAL

dol·i·cho·fa·cial \-'fā-shəl\ *adj* : LEPTOPROSOPIC

dol·i·cho·hi·er·ic \-'hī-'er-ik\ *adj* : having a relatively long narrow sacrum with a sacral index of less than 100 — compare PLATYHIERIC, SUBPLATYHIERIC

dol·i·cho·mor·phic \-'mȯr-fik\ *adj* : having a light build with relatively long body members (as the head and neck)

dol·i·cho·pel·lic \-'pel-ik\ *adj* : having a pelvis relatively long dorsoventrally with a pelvic index of 95 or more — **dol·i·cho·pel·ly** \'däl-i-kō-ˌpel-ē\ *n, pl* **-lies**

Dol·i·cho·psyl·li·dae \ˌdäl-i-kō-'sil-ə-ˌdē, -ˌkäp-'sil-\ *n pl* : a family of fleas chiefly of temperate zones including many that attack rodents and act as vectors of plague among rodents — see CERATOPHYLLUS

dol·i·chu·ran·ic \ˌdäl-i-kyu̇-'ran-ik\ *adj* : having a maxillo= alveolar index of less than 110

Do·lo·bid \'dō-lə-ˌbid\ *trademark* — used for a preparation of diflunisal

do·lor *or chiefly Brit* **do·lour** \'dō-lər, 'däl-ər\ *n* **1** *obs* : physical pain — used in old medicine as one of five cardinal symptoms of inflammation **2** : mental suffering or anguish

do·lor·if·ic \ˌdō-lə-'rif-ik, ˌdäl-ə-\ *adj* : causing pain or grief

do·lo·rim·e·try \ˌdō-lə-'rim-ə-trē, ˌdäl-ə-\ *n, pl* **-tries** : a method of measuring intensity of pain perception in degrees ranging from unpleasant to unbearable by using heat applied to the skin as a gauge — **do·lo·ri·met·ric** \ˌdō-lə-rə-'me-trik, ˌdäl-ə-\ *adj* — **do·lo·ri·met·ri·cal·ly** \-tri-k(ə-)lē\ *adv*

do·lo·rol·o·gy \ˌdō-lə-'räl-ə-jē, ˌdäl-ə-\ *n, pl* **-gies** : a medical specialty concerned with the study and treatment of pain

dolorosa — see ADIPOSIS DOLOROSA

do·lor·ous \'dō-lə-rəs, 'däl-ə-\ *adj* **1** : causing, characterized by, or affected with physical pain ⟨∼ sensations⟩ **2** : causing, marked by, or expressive of misery or grief — **do·lor·ous·ly** *adv*

DOM \ˌdē-(ˌ)ō-'em\ *n* : STP

do·main \dō-'mān, də-\ *n* **1** : any of the three-dimensional subunits of a protein that together make up its tertiary structure, that are formed by folding its linear peptide chain, and that are variously considered to be the basic units of protein structure, function, and evolution ⟨immunoglobulin light chains have two ∼s and heavy chains have four or five ∼s, depending on class —*Jour. Amer. Med. Assoc.*⟩ **2** : the highest taxonomic category in biological classification ranking above the kingdom

dome \'dōm\ *n* : a rounded-arch element in the wave tracing in an electroencephalogram ⟨the spike and ∼ pattern characteristic of absence seizures⟩

do·mi·cil·i·ary \ˌdäm-ə-'sil-ē-ˌer-ē, ˌdō-mə-\ *adj* **1** : provided or attended in the home rather than in an institution ⟨∼ midwifery⟩ **2** : providing, constituting, or provided by an institution for chronically ill or permanently disabled persons requiring minimal medical attention ⟨∼ care⟩

dom·i·nance \'däm-(ə)-nən(t)s\ *n* : the fact or state of being dominant: as **a** : the relative position of an individual in a social hierarchy — compare PECKING ORDER **b** : the property of one of a pair of alleles or traits that suppresses expression of the other in the heterozygous condition **c** : functional asymmetry between a pair of bodily structures (as the right and left hands)

¹dom·i·nant \-nənt\ *adj* **1** : exerting forcefulness or having dominance in a social hierarchy **2** : being the one of a pair of bodily structures that is the more effective or predominant in action ⟨the ∼ eye⟩ **3** : of, relating to, or exerting genetic dominance — **dom·i·nant·ly** *adv*

²dominant *n* **1** : a dominant genetic character or factor **2** : a dominant individual in a social hierarchy

dom·i·na·tor \-ˌnāt-ər\ *n* : a brightness receptor in the retina of the eye that is supposedly a group of cones linked to the terminals of a single nerve fiber

do·mo·ic acid \də-'mō-ik-\ *n* : a neurotoxic analog $C_{15}H_{21}NO_6$ of glutamic acid that is produced by some diatoms (esp. genus *Pseudonitzschia*) and has caused poisoning in vertebrates (as whales, birds, and humans) that have consumed diatom-contaminated fish or shellfish

DOMS *abbr* delayed onset muscle soreness

do·nee \dō-'nē\ *n* : a recipient of biological material (as blood or a graft)

don·ep·e·zil \ˌdän-'ep-ə-zil\ *n* : a reversible acetylcholinesterase inhibitor used as the hydrochloride $C_{24}H_{29}NO_3$·HCl in the palliative treatment of mild to moderate dementia of the type occurring in Alzheimer's disease — see ARICEPT

Don Juan \('̇)dän-'(̇h)wän, *Brit usu* dän-'jü-ən\ *n, pl* **Don Juans** : a man who pursues women promiscuously

  Don Juan, legendary character. In Spanish legend Don Juan de Tenorio is a Seville nobleman who is infamous for his seduction of women. After one such episode he kills the conquest's father. Afterwards he visits the slain man's tomb, over which an effigy has been erected. Don Juan mockingly invites the statue to supper. The invitation is accepted, and the statue drags Don Juan to hell. Don Juan is now generally regarded as a symbol of libertinism.

Don Juan·ism \-'(h)wän-ˌiz-əm, -'jü-ə-ˌniz-əm\ *n, pl* **Don Juanisms** : male sexual promiscuity : SATYRIASIS

Don·nan equilibrium \'dän-ən-\ *n* : the ionic equilibrium reached in a solution of an electrolyte whose ions are diffusible through a semipermeable membrane but are distributed unequally on the two sides of the membrane because of the presence of a nondiffusible colloidal ion (as a protein ion) on one side of the membrane

  Donnan, Frederick George (1870–1956), British chemist. A university professor for most of his career, Donnan made important contributions as a colloid chemist. Apart from the theory of membrane equilibrium named after him, he did research during World War I on chemical warfare and nitrogen products. He did early research on synthetic ammonia and nitric acid and helped in the development of mustard gas.

do·nor \'dō-nər, -ˌnȯ(ə)r\ *n* **1** : one used as a source of biological material (as blood or an organ) **2** : a compound capable of giving up a part (as an atom, chemical group, or elementary particle) for combination with an acceptor

Don·o·van body \'dän-ə-vən-, 'dən-\ *n* : an encapsulated gram-negative bacterium of the genus *Calymmatobacterium* (*C. granulomatis*) that is the causative agent of granuloma inguinale and is characterized by one or two opposite polar chromatin masses — compare LEISHMAN-DONOVAN BODY

  C. Donovan — see LEISHMAN-DONOVAN BODY

Don·o·va·nia \ˌdän-ə-'vā-nē-ə, ˌdən-, -nyə\ *n, syn of* CALYMMATOBACTERIUM

  C. Donovan — see LEISHMAN-DONOVAN BODY

do·pa \'dō-pə, -(ˌ)pä\ *n* : an amino acid $C_9H_{11}NO_4$ that in the

C
D

levorotatory form is found in the broad bean and is used in the treatment of Parkinson's disease — called also *dihydroxyphenylalanine*

L–dopa — see entry alphabetized in the letter *l*

do·pa·mine \'dō-pə-ˌmēn\ *n* : a monoamine $C_8H_{11}NO_2$ that is a decarboxylated form of dopamine and occurs esp. as a neurotransmitter in the brain and as an intermediate in the biosynthesis of epinephrine — see INTROPIN

do·pa·mi·ner·gic \ˌdō-pə-ˌmē-'nər-jik\ *adj* : liberating, activated by, or involving dopamine or related substances ⟨the mesolimbic ∼ pathway⟩ ⟨∼ activity⟩ ⟨∼ neurons⟩

¹dope \'dōp\ *n* **1 a** : a preparation of an illicit, habit-forming, or narcotic drug (as opium, heroin, or marijuana) **b** : a preparation given to a racehorse to help or hinder its performance **2** : a narcotic addict

²dope *vb* **doped; dop·ing** *vt* : to give a narcotic to ∼ *vi* : to take dope

dop·er \'dō-pər\ *n* : a habitual or frequent user of drugs

Dopp·ler \'däp-lər\ *adj* **1** : of, relating to, or utilizing a shift in frequency in accordance with the Doppler effect **2** : of, relating to, using, or produced by Doppler ultrasound ⟨a ∼ examination⟩ ⟨∼ images⟩

Doppler, Christian Johann (1803–1853), Austrian physicist and mathematician. Doppler first described the Doppler effect in 1842. It is used in astronomical measurements and in radar and modern navigation. He also investigated the colors in double stars and the effect of rotation of objects on the properties of light and sound waves.

Doppler echocardiography *n* : Doppler ultrasound used to measure cardiovascular blood flow velocity for diagnostic purposes (as for evaluating valve function)

Doppler effect *n* : a change in the frequency with which waves (as sound, light, or radio waves) from a given source reach an observer when the source and the observer are in motion with respect to each other so that the frequency increases or decreases according to the speed at which the distance is decreasing or increasing — compare SHIFT a

Doppler ultrasound *n* : ultrasound that utilizes the Doppler effect to measure movement or flow in the body and esp. blood flow — called also *Doppler ultrasonography*

do·ra·pho·bia \ˌdōr-ə-'fō-bē-ə, ˌdȯr-\ *n* : a dread of touching the skin or fur of an animal

dorsa *pl of* DORSUM

dor·sad \'dȯ(ə)r-ˌsad\ *adv* : toward the back : DORSALLY

¹dor·sal \'dȯr-səl\ *adj* **1 a** : being or located near, on, or toward the upper surface of an animal (as a quadruped) opposite the lower or ventral surface **b** : being or located near, on, or toward the back or posterior part of the human body **2** *chiefly Brit* : THORACIC — **dor·sal·ly** \-sə-lē\ *adv*

²dorsal *n* : a dorsally located part; *esp* : a thoracic vertebra

dorsal accessory olivary nucleus *n* : ACCESSORY OLIVARY NUCLEUS a

dorsal carpal ligament *n* : a broad flat ligament at the back of the wrist serving to hold in place the tendons of the extensor muscles

dorsal horn *n* : a longitudinal subdivision of gray matter in the dorsal part of each lateral half of the spinal cord that receives terminals from some afferent fibers of the dorsal roots of the spinal nerves — called also *dorsal column, posterior column, posterior gray column, posterior horn;* compare LATERAL COLUMN 1, VENTRAL HORN

dorsal interosseus *n* **1** : any of four small muscles of the hand each of which arises by two heads from the dorsal aspect of two adjacent metacarpals, extends along the interval between them to insert into the base of the proximal phalanx of the thumb side of the index finger, the little-finger or thumb side of the middle finger, or the little-finger side of the fourth finger, and acts to draw the fingers away from the long axis of the middle finger, flex the fingers at the metacarpophalangeal joints, and extend their distal two phalanges **2** : any of four small muscles of the foot each of which arises by two heads from the dorsal aspects of the adjacent sides of two metatarsals, extends along the interval between them to insert into the base of the first phalanx of the medial side of

the second toe or the lateral side of the second, third, or fourth toe, and acts to draw the toes away from the long axis of the second toe, flex their proximal phalanges, and extend the distal phalanges

dorsal interosseous muscle *n* : DORSAL INTEROSSEUS

dor·sa·lis \dȯr-'sal-əs, -'sāl-, -'säl-\ *n, pl* **dor·sa·les** \-'sal-(ˌ)ēz, -'sāl-; -'säl-ˌās\ : any of several arteries situated in and supplying the back of the parts with which they are associated — see INTEROSSEUS DORSALIS, NUCLEUS DORSALIS, SACROCOCCYGEUS DORSALIS, TABES DORSALIS

dorsalis pe·dis \-'ped-əs, -'pēd-\ *n* : an artery of the upper surface of the foot that is a direct continuation of the anterior tibial artery — called also *dorsalis pedis artery*

dorsal lip *n* : the margin of the fold of blastula wall that delineates the dorsal limit of the blastopore, constitutes the primary organizer, and forms the point of origin of chordamesoderm

dorsal mesogastrium *n* : MESOGASTRIUM 2

dorsal root *n* : the one of the two roots of a spinal nerve that passes posteriorly to the spinal cord separating the posterior and lateral funiculi and that consists of sensory fibers — called also *posterior root;* compare VENTRAL ROOT

dorsal root ganglion *n* : SPINAL GANGLION

dorsal spinocerebellar tract *n* : SPINOCEREBELLAR TRACT a

dorsal vertebra *n* : THORACIC VERTEBRA

dorsi — see ILIOCOSTALIS DORSI, LATISSIMUS DORSI, LONGISSIMUS DORSI

dor·si·duct \'dȯr-sə-ˌdəkt\ *vt* : to turn or draw toward the back

dor·si·flex \-ˌfleks\ *vi* : to flex in a dorsal direction ⟨the toe will ∼⟩ ∼ *vt* : to cause to flex in a dorsal direction ⟨various central lesions both ∼ and supinate the foot⟩

dor·si·flex·ion \ˌdȯr-sə-'flek-shən\ *n* : flexion in a dorsal direction; *esp* : flexion of the foot in an upward direction — compare PLANTAR FLEXION

dor·si·flex·or \'dȯr-sə-ˌflek-sər\ *n* : a muscle causing flexion in a dorsal direction

dor·si·spi·nal \ˌdȯr-sə-'spīn-əl\ *adj* : of or relating to the back and spine

dor·so·lat·er·al \ˌdȯr-sō-'lat-ə-rəl, -'la-trəl\ *adj* : of, relating to, or involving both the back and the sides ⟨lesions of the ∼ hypothalamus⟩ — **dor·so·lat·er·al·ly** \-ē\ *adv*

dorsolateral tract *n* : a slender column of white matter between the dorsal gray column and the periphery of the spinal cord — called also *Lissauer's tract, tract of Lissauer*

dor·so·lum·bar \ˌdȯr-sō-'ləm-bər, -ˌbär\ *adj* : of or involving structures in the region occupied by the dorsal and lumbar vertebrae ⟨∼ myelitis⟩ ⟨a ∼ laminectomy⟩

dorsolumbar nerve *n* : a small nerve connecting the last thoracic nerve with the lumbar plexus

dor·so·me·di·al \-'mēd-ē-əl\ *adj* : located toward the back and near the midline

dor·so·ven·tral \-'ven-trəl\ *adj* : relating to, involving, or extending along the axis joining the dorsal and ventral sides ⟨∼ compression⟩ — **dor·so·ven·tral·i·ty** \-ven-'tral-ət-ē\ *n, pl* **-ties** — **dor·so·ven·tral·ly** \-'ven-trə-lē\ *adv*

dor·sum \'dȯr-səm\ *n, pl* **dor·sa** \-sə\ **1** : the upper surface of an appendage or part **2** : BACK 1a, b; *esp* : the entire dorsal surface of an animal

dos *abbr* dosage

dos·age \'dō-sij\ *n* **1 a** : the addition of an ingredient or the application of an agent in a measured dose **b** : the presence and relative representation or strength of a factor or agent (as a gene) **2 a** : DOSE 1 **b** (1) : the giving of a dose (2) : regulation or determination of doses

dosage compensation *n* : the genetic mechanism by which the same effect on the phenotype is produced by a pair of identical sex-linked genes in the sex (as the human female)

\ə\ **abut** \ᵊ\ **kitten** \ər\ **further** \a\ **ash** \ā\ **ace** \ä\ **cot, cart** \aů\ **out** \ch\ **chin** \e\ **bet** \ē\ **easy** \g\ **go** \i\ **hit** \ī\ **ice** \j\ **job** \ŋ\ **sing** \ō\ **go** \ȯ\ **law** \ȯi\ **boy** \th\ **thin** \t̲h̲\ **the** \ü\ **loot** \ů\ **foot** \y\ **yet** \zh\ **vision** *See also* Pronunciation Symbols page

having the two sex chromosomes of the same type as by a single gene in the sex (as the human male) having the two sex chromosomes of different types or having only one sex chromosome (as in the males of some insects)

¹**dose** \'dōs\ *n* **1 a :** the measured quantity of a therapeutic agent to be taken at one time **b :** the quantity of radiation administered or absorbed **2 :** a gonorrheal infection

²**dose** *vb* **dosed; dos·ing** *vt* **1 :** to divide (as a medicine) into doses **2 :** to give a dose to; *esp* **:** to give medicine to **3 :** to treat with an application or agent ∼ *vi* **:** to take medicine ⟨he is forever *dosing* but he gets worse⟩

dose–response *adj* **:** of, relating to, or graphing the pattern of physiological response to varied dosage (as of a drug or radiation) in which there is typically little or no effect at very low dosages and a toxic or unchanging effect at high dosages with the maximum increase in effect somewhere between the extremes ⟨nicotine was rated as highly euphoric, with ∼ curves similar to those of cocaine, amphetamines and morphine —Sandra Blakeslee⟩

do·sim·e·ter \dō-'sim-ət-ər\ *also* **dose·me·ter** \'dō-ˌsmēt-ər\ *n* **:** a device for measuring doses of radiations (as X-rays) — **do·si·met·ric** \ˌdō-sə-'me-trik\ *adj* — **do·sim·e·try** \dō-'sim-ə-trē\ *n, pl* **-tries**

dot \'dät\ *n* **:** a small spot or speck — see MAURER'S DOTS, SCHUFFNER'S DOTS

dot·age \'dōt-ij\ *n* **:** a state or period of senile decay marked by decline of mental poise and alertness

dot·ard \'dōt-ərd\ *n* **:** a person in his or her dotage

dou·ble bind \'dəb-əl-'bīnd\ *n* **:** a psychological predicament in which a person receives from a single source conflicting messages that allow no appropriate response to be made

dou·ble–blind \ˌdəb-əl-'blīnd\ *adj* **:** of, relating to, or being an experimental procedure in which neither the subjects nor the experimenters know which subjects are in the test and control groups during the actual course of the experiments — compare OPEN-LABEL, SINGLE-BLIND

double bond *n* **:** a chemical bond in which two pairs of electrons are shared by two atoms in a molecule and which is usu. represented in chemical formulas by two lines (as in the formula for ethylene $H_2C=CH_2$) — compare TRIPLE BOND; see UNSATURATED b

double chin *n* **:** a fleshy or fatty fold under the chin — **dou·ble–chinned** \-'chind\ *adj*

double decomposition *n* **:** a chemical reaction between two compounds in which part of the first compound becomes united with part of the second and the remainder of the first compound becomes united with the remainder of the second (as in AB + CD → AD + BC) — called also *metathesis*

double helix *n* **:** a helix or spiral consisting of two strands in the surface of a cylinder that coil around its axis; *esp* **:** the structural arrangement of DNA in space that consists of paired polynucleotide strands stabilized by cross-links between purine and pyrimidine bases — compare ALPHA= HELIX, WATSON-CRICK MODEL — **dou·ble–he·li·cal** \-'hel-i-kəl, -'hē-li-\ *adj*

dou·ble–joint·ed \ˌdəb-əl-'joint-əd\ *adj* **:** having a joint that permits an exceptional degree of freedom of motion of the parts joined ⟨a ∼ athlete highly susceptible to injury⟩

double pneumonia *n* **:** pneumonia affecting both lungs

dou·ble–pored tapeworm \'dəb-əl-ˌpō(ə)rd-, -ˌpo(ə)rd-\ *n* **:** DOG TAPEWORM

double sugar *n* **:** DISACCHARIDE

dou·blet \'dəb-lət\ *n* **1 :** something consisting of two identical or similar parts: as **a :** a lens consisting of two components **b :** a spectrum line having two close components **2 :** a set of two identical or similar things; *esp* **:** one of nine pairs of microtubules found in cilia and flagella

double vision *n* **:** DIPLOPIA

¹**douche** \'düsh\ *n* **1 a :** a jet or current of liquid (as a cleansing solution) directed against or into a bodily part or cavity (as the vagina) **b :** an act of cleansing with a douche **2 :** a device for giving douches

²**douche** *vb* **douched; douch·ing** *vt* **:** to administer or apply a douche to ∼ *vi* **:** to take a douche

Doug·las bag \'dəg-ləs-ˌbag\ *n* **:** an inflatable bag used to collect expired air for the determination of oxygen consumption and basal metabolic rate

Douglas, Claude Gordon (1882–1963), British physiologist. From his laboratory at Oxford, Douglas contributed significantly to the knowledge of human respiratory function. In 1911 he introduced the large airtight bag known as the Douglas bag for use in collecting expired respiratory gases.

Douglas's cul–de–sac \'dəg-lə-səz-\ *n* **:** POUCH OF DOUG-LAS

Douglas's pouch *n* **:** POUCH OF DOUGLAS

dou·la \'dü-lə\ *n* **:** a woman experienced in childbirth who provides advice, information, emotional support, and physical comfort to a mother before, during, and just after childbirth

douloureux — see TIC DOULOUREUX

dou·rine \'dü(ə)r-ˌēn, 'dü-ˌrēn\ *n* **:** a contagious disease esp. of horses and asses that is caused by a member of the genus *Trypanosoma* (*T. equiperdum*) transmitted during copulation and that commonly assumes a chronic course marked by inflammation of the genitals, subcutaneous edematous plaques, low-grade fever, progressive paralysis, emaciation, and death

Do·ver's powder \'dō-vərz-\ *n* **:** a powder of ipecac and opium that is now compounded in the U.S. with lactose and in England with potassium sulfate and that is used as an anodyne and diaphoretic

Do·ver \'dō-vər\, **Thomas (1660–1742),** British physician. A pupil of the eminent physician Thomas Sydenham, Dover made the unique choice of combining a medical career with that of a buccaneer. Constantly at odds with the medical establishment, he published in 1732 a volume of his nostrums, almost all of them worthless or worse, the exception being his sole legacy—Dover's powder.

dow·a·ger's hump \'daù-i-jərz-\ *n* **:** an abnormal outward curvature of the upper back with round shoulders and stooped posture caused esp. by bone loss and anterior compression of the vertebrae in osteoporosis

down·er \'daù-nər\ *n* **:** a depressant drug; *esp* **:** BARBITURATE

down·growth \'daù-nˌgrōth\ *n* **:** the growing downward of a structure; *also* **:** the product of such growth

down·reg·u·la·tion \ˌdaù-nˌreg-yə-'lā-shən\ *n* **:** the process of reducing or suppressing a response to a stimulus; *specif* **:** reduction in a cellular response to a molecule (as insulin) due to a decrease in the number of receptors on the cell surface — **down·reg·u·late** \-'reg-yə-ˌlāt\ *vb* **-lat·ed; -lat·ing**

Down's \'daùnz\ *also* **Down** \'daùn\ *n, often attrib* **:** DOWN SYNDROME ⟨a *Down's* patient⟩ ⟨a *Down* baby⟩

down·stream \'daù-n-'strēm\ *adv or adj* **:** in the same direction along a molecule of DNA or RNA as that in which transcription and translation take place and toward the end having a hydroxyl group attached to the position labeled 3′ in the terminal nucleotide ⟨a nucleotide sequence located ∼ from the regulatory gene⟩ ⟨effects on the expression of ∼ genes⟩ — compare UPSTREAM

Down syndrome *or* **Down's syndrome** *n* **:** a congenital condition characterized by moderate to severe mental retardation, slanting eyes, a broad short skull, broad hands with short fingers, and by trisomy of the human chromosome numbered 21 — called also *trisomy 21*

Down \'daùn\, **John Langdon Haydon (1828–1896),** British physician. Down published in 1866 a treatise on the degeneration of race as a result of marriages of consanguinity. He classified individuals exhibiting mental retardation according to the supposed physiognomic features of various races including the American Indian, Caucasian, Ethiopian, and Mongolian. Although his classification is invalid, one kind of moderate to severe mental retardation was known until recently as mongolism and is now called Down syndrome or Down's syndrome.

dox·a·zo·sin \däk-'sā-zō-sin\ *n* **:** a quinazoline alpha= blocker administered in the form of its mesylate

C
D

$C_{23}H_{25}N_5O_5 \cdot CH_4O_3S$ to relieve urethral obstruction in benign prostatic hyperplasia and to treat hypertension — see CARDURA

dox·e·pin \'däk-sə-ˌpin, -pən\ *n* : a tricyclic antidepressant administered in the form of its hydrochloride $C_{19}H_{21}NO \cdot HCl$ — see SINEQUAN

doxo·ru·bi·cin \ˌdäk-sə-'rü-bə-sən\ *n* : an anthracycline antibiotic with broad antineoplastic activity that is obtained from a bacterium of the genus *Streptomyces* (*S. peucetius*) and is administered in the form of its hydrochloride $C_{27}H_{29}NO_{11} \cdot HCl$ — see ADRIAMYCIN

doxy·cy·cline \ˌdäk-sə-'sī-ˌklēn\ *n* : a broad-spectrum tetracycline antibiotic $C_{22}H_{24}N_2O_8$ with potent antibacterial activity that is often taken by travelers as a prophylactic against diarrhea — see VIBRAMYCIN

dox·yl·amine \däk-'sil-ə-ˌmēn, -mən\ *n* : an antihistamine derived from pyridine and usu. administered in the form of its succinate $C_{17}H_{22}N_2O \cdot C_4H_6O_4$

doz *abbr* dozen

DP *abbr* **1** doctor of pharmacy **2** doctor of podiatry

DPA *abbr* diphenylamine

DPH *abbr* **1** department of public health **2** doctor of public health

D phase \'dē-ˌfāz\ *n* : M PHASE

DPM *abbr* doctor of podiatric medicine

DPN \ˌdē-ˌ(ˌ)pē-'en\ *n* : NAD

DPT *abbr* diphtheria-pertussis-tetanus (vaccine)

DQ *abbr* developmental quotient

dr *abbr* **1** dram **2** dressing

Dr *abbr* doctor

DR *abbr* delivery room

drachm *var of* DRAM

drac·on·ti·a·sis \ˌdrak-ˌän-'tī-ə-səs\ *n, pl* **-a·ses** \-ˌsēz\ : DRACUNCULIASIS

dra·cun·cu·li·a·sis \drə-ˌkən-kyə-'lī-ə-səs\ *n, pl* **-a·ses** \-ˌsēz\ : infestation with or disease caused by the guinea worm that has been eradicated in many regions but not in Africa — called also *guinea worm disease*

dra·cun·cu·lo·sis \-'lō-səs\ *n, pl* **-lo·ses** \-ˌsēz\ : DRACUNCULIASIS

Dra·cun·cu·lus \drə-'kən-kyə-ləs\ *n* : a genus (the type of the family Dracunculidae) of greatly elongated nematode worms including the guinea worm

draft *or chiefly Brit* **draught** \'draft, 'dråft\ *n* **1** : a portion (as of medicine) poured out or mixed for drinking : DOSE **2** : a current of air in a closed-in space — **drafty** *or chiefly Brit* **draughty** \'draf-tē, 'dråf-\ *adj*

dra·gée \dra-'zhā\ *n* : a sugar-coated medicated confection

¹drain \'drān\ *vt* **1 a** : to draw off (liquid) gradually or completely ⟨∼ pus from an abscess⟩ **b** : to exhaust physically or emotionally **2** : to carry away or give passage to a bodily fluid or a discharge from ⟨∼ an abscess⟩ ⟨the eustachian tube ∼s the middle ear —H. G. Armstrong⟩ ∼ *vi* : to flow off gradually ⟨blood ∼*ing* from a wound⟩

²drain *n* : a tube or cylinder usu. of absorbent material for drainage of a wound — see CIGARETTE DRAIN

drain·age \'drā-nij\ *n* **1** : the act or process of drawing off fluids from a cavity or wound by means of suction or gravity **2** : a process of releasing internal conflicts or pent-up feelings (as hostility or guilt)

Draize test \'drāz-\ *n* : a test that is used as a criterion for harmfulness of chemicals to the human eye and that involves dropping the test substance into one eye of rabbits without anesthesia with the other eye used as a control — called also *Draize eye test*

Draize, John Henry (1900–1992), American pharmacologist. Draize spent the better part of his career as a pharmacologist with the U.S. government's Food and Drug Administration. His areas of research included skin pharmacology, the toxicity and pharmacology of drugs, and the testing of cosmetics. He introduced the Draize test for cosmetics in 1944.

dram *also* **drachm** \'dram\ *n* **1** : either of two units of weight: **a** : an avoirdupois unit equal to 1.772 grams or

27.344 grains **b** : a unit of apothecaries' weight equal to 3.888 grams or 60 grains **2** : FLUID DRAM

Dram·amine \'dram-ə-ˌmēn *also* -mən\ *trademark* — used for a preparation of dimenhydrinate

dra·ma·ti·za·tion *or Brit* **dra·ma·ti·sa·tion** \ˌdram-ət-ə-'zā-shən, ˌdräm-\ *n* : the transformation which in psychoanalytic theory the underlying dream thoughts undergo into dramatic and pictorial form before they can take part in the actual dream

drank *past and past part of* DRINK

¹drape \'drāp\ *vt* **draped; drap·ing** : to shroud or enclose with surgical drapes

²drape *n* : a sterile covering used in an operating room — usu. used in pl.

¹dras·tic \'dras-tik\ *adj* : acting rapidly or violently — used chiefly of purgatives — **dras·ti·cal·ly** \-ti-k(ə-)lē\ *adv*

²drastic *n* : a powerful medicinal agent; *esp* : a strong purgative

draught, draughty *chiefly Brit var of* DRAFT, DRAFTY

draw \'drȯ\ *vb* **drew** \'drü\ **drawn** \'drȯn\ **draw·ing** *vt* **1** : to cause to move toward or localize in a surface ⟨using a poultice to ∼ inflammation to a head⟩; *esp* : to cause (an unwanted element) to depart (as from the body or a lesion) ⟨this will help ∼ the poison⟩ **2** : INHALE ⟨she *drew* a deep breath⟩ **3** : to remove the viscera of : EVISCERATE ∼ *vi* **1** : to cause local congestion : induce blood or other body fluid to localize at a particular point : be effective as a blistering agent or counterirritant — used of a poultice and comparable means of medication **2** *of a lesion* : to become localized — used in the phrase *draw to a head*

draw·sheet \'drȯ-ˌshēt\ *n* : a narrow sheet used chiefly in hospitals and stretched across the bed lengthwise often over a rubber sheet underneath the patient's trunk

DRE *abbr* digital rectal exam; digital rectal examination

¹dream \'drēm\ *n, often attrib* : a series of thoughts, images, or emotions occurring during sleep and esp. during REM sleep — compare DAYDREAM

²dream \'drēm\ *vb* **dreamed** \'drem(p)t, 'drēmd\ *or* **dreamt** \'drem(p)t\; **dream·ing** \'drē-miŋ\ *vi* **1** : to have a dream **2** : to indulge in daydreams or fantasies ∼ *vt* : to have a dream of — **dream·er** \'drē-mər\ *n*

dream·work \'drēm-ˌwərk\ *n* : the process of concealing the latent content of dreams from the conscious mind

¹drench \'drench\ *n* : a poisonous or medicinal drink; *specif* : a large dose of medicine mixed with liquid and put down the throat of an animal

²drench *vt* : to administer a drench to (an animal)

drep·a·no·cyte \'drep-ə-nə-ˌsīt\ *n* : SICKLE CELL 1 — **drep·a·no·cyt·ic** \ˌdrep-ə-nə-'sit-ik\ *adj*

drep·a·no·cy·to·sis \ˌdrep-ə-(ˌ)nō-ˌsī-'tō-səs\ *n, pl* **-to·ses** \-ˌsēz\ **1** : SICKLE-CELL ANEMIA **2** : SICKLE-CELL TRAIT

dress \'dres\ *vb* : to apply dressings or medicaments to

dress·er \'dres-ər\ *n* : a person who serves as a doctor's assistant esp. in the dressing of lesions

dress·ing \-iŋ\ *n* : a covering (as of ointment or gauze) applied to a lesion

Dress·ler's syndrome \'dres-lərz-\ *n* : pericarditis after heart attack that is often recurrent and may be accompanied by fever, pericardial and pleural effusions, pleurisy, lung infiltrates, and joint pain

Dressler, William (1890–1969), American cardiologist. Born in Poland, Dressler served as associate chief of a hospital devoted to cardiac care in Vienna from 1924 to 1938. In that year he emigrated to the U.S., becoming chief of the cardiac clinic at Maimonides Hospital in Brooklyn, N.Y., the following year. While there, he published *Clinical Cardiology* (1942) and, with Hugo Roesler, *Atlas of Clinical Cardiology* (1948). In 1955 he described for the first time recurrent pericarditis following heart attack.

\ə\ abut \ᵊ\ kitten \ər\ further \a\ ash \ā\ ace \ä\ cot, cart
\au̇\ out \ch\ chin \e\ bet \ē\ easy \g\ go \i\ hit \ī\ ice \j\ job
\ŋ\ sing \ō\ go \ȯ\ law \ȯi\ boy \th\ thin \th̲\ the \ü\ loot
\u̇\ foot \y\ yet \zh\ vision *See also* Pronunciation Symbols page

drew *past of* DRAW

DRG \'dē-'är-'jē\ *n* : any of the payment categories that are used to classify patients and esp. Medicare patients for the purpose of reimbursing hospitals for each case in a given category with a fixed fee regardless of the actual costs incurred and that are based esp. on the principal diagnosis, surgical procedure used, age of patient, and expected length of stay in the hospital — called also *diagnosis related group*

DRI *abbr* Dietary Reference Intake

dried *past and past part of* DRY

drier *comparative of* DRY

driest *superlative of* DRY

drift \'drift\ *n* 1 : movement of a tooth in the dental arch 2 : GENETIC DRIFT — **drift** *vi*

¹**drill** \'dril\ *vt* : to make a hole in with a drill ⟨the dentist ∼ed the tooth for a filling⟩ ∼ *vi* : to make a hole with a drill ⟨painless dental ∼ing⟩

²**drill** *n* : an instrument with an edged or pointed end for making holes in hard substances (as bones or teeth) by revolving

¹**drink** \'driŋk\ *vb* **drank** \'draŋk\; **drunk** \'drəŋk\ *or* **drank**; **drink·ing** *vt* : SWALLOW, IMBIBE ⟨∼ liquid⟩ ∼ *vi* 1 : to take liquid into the mouth for swallowing 2 : to partake of alcoholic beverages esp. habitually; *specif* : to indulge in alcoholic beverages with disagreeable effect

²**drink** *n* 1 : liquid suitable for swallowing esp. to quench thirst or to provide nourishment or refreshment 2 : alcoholic liquor 3 : a draft or portion of liquid (as water or a prepared beverage) taken or to be taken by an individual at one time

Drink·er respirator \'driŋ-kər-\ *n* : IRON LUNG

Drinker, Philip (1894–1972), American industrial hygienist. Drinker introduced the Drinker respirator, or iron lung, in 1929. He also invented a small chamber for maintaining respiration in newborn babies. During his career he studied industrial hygiene, the control of air pollution, and toxicology.

¹**drip** \'drip\ *vb* **dripped; drip·ping** *vt* : to let fall in drops ∼ *vi* 1 : to let fall drops of moisture or liquid 2 : to fall in drops

²**drip** *n* 1 a : a falling in drops — see POSTNASAL DRIP b : liquid that falls, overflows, or is extruded in drops 2 : a device for the administration of a fluid at a slow rate esp. into a vein ⟨was hooked up to an intravenous ∼⟩; *also* : a material so administered ⟨a glucose ∼⟩ — see GRAVITY DRIP

Dris·dol \'dris-,dȯl, -,dōl\ *trademark* — used for a preparation of calciferol

drive \'drīv\ *n* 1 : an urgent, basic, or instinctual need : a motivating physiological condition of the organism ⟨a sexual ∼⟩ 2 : an impelling culturally acquired concern, interest, or longing ⟨a ∼ for perfection⟩

dro·mo·ma·nia \,dräm-ə-'mā-nē-ə, ,drōm-\ *n* : an exaggerated desire to wander

dro·mo·trop·ic \-'träp-ik\ *adj* : affecting the conductivity of cardiac muscle — used of the influence of cardiac nerves

dro·nab·i·nol \,drō-'nab-ə-nȯl\ *n* : a synthetic delta-9-tetrahydrocannabinol that is used to control nausea caused by chemotherapy and to stimulate appetite in cases of AIDS-induced anorexia — see MARINOL

drool \'drül\ *vi* 1 : to secrete saliva in anticipation of food 2 : to let saliva or some other substance flow from the mouth ⟨side effects included drowsiness and ∼ing⟩ — **drool** *n*

¹**drop** \'dräp\ *n* 1 a : the quantity of fluid that falls in one spherical mass b **drops** *pl* : a dose of medicine measured by drops ⟨eye ∼s for dilating the pupil of the eye⟩ 2 : the smallest practical unit of liquid measure that varies in size according to the specific gravity and viscosity of the liquid and to the conditions under which it is formed — compare MINIM

²**drop** *vb* **dropped; drop·ping** *vi* : to fall in drops ∼ *vt* 1 *of an animal* : to give birth to ⟨lambs *dropped* in June⟩ 2 : to take (a drug) orally ⟨∼ acid⟩

dro·per·i·dol \drō-'per-ə-,dȯl\ *n* : a butyrophenone tranquilizer $C_{22}H_{22}FN_3O_2$ used as a premedication for surgery, as an antiemetic in cancer chemotherapy, and as an antipsychotic in severely disturbed psychotic states

drop foot *n* : FOOT DROP

drop·let \'dräp-lət\ *n* : a tiny drop (as of a liquid)

droplet infection *n* : infection transmitted by airborne droplets of saliva or sputum containing infectious organisms

drop·per \'dräp-ər\ *n* : a short glass tube fitted with a rubber bulb and used to measure liquids by drops — called also *eyedropper, medicine dropper* — **drop·per·ful** \-,fu̇l\ *n*

drop·si·cal \'dräp-si-kəl\ *adj* : relating to or affected with edema

drop·sy \'dräp-sē\ *n, pl* **drop·sies** : EDEMA

dro·soph·i·la \drō-'säf-ə-lə, drə-\ *n* 1 *cap* : a genus of small dipteran flies that include many (as *D. melanogaster*) extensively used in genetic research 2 : any fly of the genus *Drosophila*

drown \'draún\ *vb* **drowned** \'draúnd\ **drown·ing** \'draú-niŋ\ *vi* 1 : to suffocate in water or some other liquid 2 : to suffocate because of excess of body fluid that interferes with the passage of oxygen from the lungs to the body tissues (as in pulmonary edema) ∼ *vt* : to suffocate by submersion esp. in water ⟨∼ed three kittens⟩

drowsy \'draú-zē\ *adj* **drows·i·er; -est** : ready to fall asleep : SLEEPY — **drows·i·ly** \-zə-lē\ *adv* — **drows·i·ness** \-zē-nəs\ *n*

DrPH *abbr* doctor of public health

¹**drug** \'drəg\ *n* 1 a : a substance used as a medication or in the preparation of medication b *according to the Food, Drug, and Cosmetic Act* (1) : a substance recognized in an official pharmacopoeia or formulary (2) : a substance intended for use in the diagnosis, cure, mitigation, treatment, or prevention of disease (3) : a substance other than food intended to affect the structure or function of the body (4) : a substance intended for use as a component of a medicine but not a device or a component, part, or accessory of a device 2 : something and often an illicit substance that causes addiction, habituation, or a marked change in consciousness

²**drug** *vb* **drugged; drug·ging** *vt* 1 : to affect with a drug; *esp* : to stupefy by a narcotic drug 2 : to administer a drug to ∼ *vi* : to take drugs for narcotic effect

drug–fast \'drəg-,fast\ *adj* : resistant to the action of a drug

drug·gie *also* **drug·gy** \'drəg-ē\ *n, pl* **druggies** : a person who habitually uses drugs

drug·gist \'drəg-əst\ *n* : an individual who sells or dispenses drugs and medicines: as a : PHARMACIST b : a person who owns or manages a drugstore

drug·mak·er \'drəg-,mā-kər\ *n* : one that manufactures pharmaceuticals

drug·store \-,stō(ə)r, -,stȯ(ə)r\ *n* : a retail store where medicines and miscellaneous articles (as food, cosmetics, and film) are sold — called also *pharmacy*

drum \'drəm\ *n* : TYMPANIC MEMBRANE

drum·head \-,hed\ *n* : TYMPANIC MEMBRANE

drum·stick \-,stik\ *n* : a small projection from the cell nucleus that occurs in a small percentage of the polymorphonuclear leukocytes in the normal human female

¹**drunk** *past part of* DRINK

²**drunk** \'drəŋk\ *adj* 1 : having the faculties impaired by alcohol 2 : of, relating to, or caused by intoxication : DRUNKEN ⟨convicted of ∼ driving —*Time*⟩

³**drunk** *n* 1 : a period of drinking to intoxication or of being intoxicated 2 : one who is drunk; *esp* : DRUNKARD

drunk·ard \'drəŋ-kərd\ *n* : one suffering from or subject to acute or chronic alcoholism : one who habitually becomes drunk

drunk·en \'drəŋ-kən\ *adj* 1 : DRUNK 1 ⟨a ∼ driver⟩ 2 a : given to habitual excessive use of alcohol b : of, relating to, or characterized by intoxication ⟨∼ parties⟩ c : resulting from or as if from intoxication ⟨a ∼ stupor⟩ — **drunk·en·ly** *adv* — **drunk·en·ness** \-kən-nəs\ *n*

drunk·o·me·ter \,drəŋ-'käm-ət-ər, 'drəŋ-kə-,mēt-\ *n* : a device for measuring alcohol content of the blood by chemical analysis of the breath

druse \'drüz, 'drü-zə\ *n, pl* **dru·sen** \'drü-zən\ : one of the small yellowish deposits of cellular debris that accumulate between the pigmented epithelial layer of the retina and the

C

D

inner collagenous layer of the choroid, that are typically associated with aging, and that may be a sign of certain pathological conditions (as age-related macular degeneration)

¹dry \\'drī\\ *adj* **dri·er** \\'drī-(-ə)r\\; **dri·est** \\'drī-əst\\ **1** : marked by the absence or scantiness of secretions, effusions, or other forms of moisture **2** *of a cough* : not accompanied by the raising of mucus or phlegm

²dry *vb* **dried; dry·ing** *vt* : to make dry ~ *vi* : to become dry

dry eye *n* : a condition associated with inadequate tear production and marked by redness of the conjunctiva, by itching and burning of the eye, and usu. by filaments of desquamated epithelial cells adhering to the cornea — called also *keratoconjunctivitis sicca*

dry eye syndrome *n* : DRY EYE

dry gangrene *n* : gangrene that develops in the presence of arterial obstruction, is sharply localized, and is characterized by dryness of the dead tissue which is sharply demarcated from adjacent tissue by a line of inflammation

dry lab *n* : a laboratory for making computer simulations or for data analysis esp. by computers (as in bioinformatics) — called also *dry laboratory;* compare WET LAB

dry labor *n* : childbirth characterized by premature escape of the amniotic fluid

dry measure *n* : a series of units of capacity for dry commodities

dry mouth *n* : XEROSTOMIA

dry–nurse \\(')drī-'nərs\\ *vt* **dry–nursed; dry–nurs·ing** : to act as dry nurse to

dry nurse *n* : a nurse who takes care of but does not breastfeed another woman's baby

dry–out \\'drī-,au̇t\\ *adj* : providing detoxification treatment ⟨checked into a ~ clinic⟩

dry out \\(')drī-'au̇t\\ *vt* : to subject to withdrawal from the use of alcohol or drugs : DETOXIFY **2** ~ *vi* : to undergo an extended period of withdrawal from alcohol or drug use esp. at a special clinic : DETOXIFY

dry pleurisy *n* : pleurisy in which the exudation is mainly fibrinous

dry socket *n* : a tooth socket in which after tooth extraction a blood clot fails to form or disintegrates without undergoing organization; *also* : a condition that is marked by the occurrence of such a socket or sockets and that is usu. accompanied by neuralgic pain but without suppuration

Ds *symbol* darmstadtium

DSC *abbr* doctor of surgical chiropody

DSD *abbr* dry sterile dressing

DSW *abbr* **1** doctor of social welfare **2** doctor of social work

d.t. \\(')dē-'tē\\ *n, often cap D&T, chiefly Brit* : D.T.'S

DT *abbr* **1** distance test **2** duration of tetany

DTN *abbr* diphtheria toxin normal

DTP *abbr* diphtheria-tetanus-pertussis (vaccine)

d.t.'s \\(')dē-'tēz\\ *n pl, often cap D&T* : DELIRIUM TREMENS

DU *abbr* diagnosis undetermined

du·al energy X–ray absorptiometry \\'d(y)ü-əl-\\ *n* : absorptiometry in which the density or mass of a material (as bone or fat) is measured by comparing the amounts of absorption by the material of x-radiation of two different energies generated by an X-ray tube and which is used esp. for determining bone mineral content — abbr. *DEXA, DXA*

du·al·ism \\'d(y)ü-ə-,liz-əm\\ *n* **1** : a theory that considers reality to consist of two irreducible elements or modes (as mind and matter) **2** : a theory in hematology holding that the blood cells arise from two kinds of stem cells one of which yields lymphatic elements and the other myeloid elements — **du·al·ist** \\-ə-ləst\\ *n* — **du·al·is·tic** \\,d(y)ü-ə-'lis-tik\\ *adj*

dual photon absorptiometry *n* : absorptiometry that functions and is used similarly to dual energy X-ray absorptiometry but that utilizes X-rays generated by a radioscope

DUB *abbr* dysfunctional uterine bleeding

dub·ni·um \\'düb-nē-əm, 'dəb-\\ *n* : a short-lived radioactive element that is artificially produced — symbol *Db*; see ELEMENT table

Du·boi·sia \\d(y)ü-'bȯi-zē-ə\\ *n* : a genus of white-flowered Australian shrubs or small trees of the family Solanaceae that yield alkaloids having an action similar to atropine

Du·bois \\d(y)üb-'wä, dūē-bwä\\, **François Noel Alexandre (1752–1824),** French botanist. Dubois was a prolific writer of botanical works, none of which have proved to be of lasting significance. The genus *Duboisia* was named in his honor in 1810 by the British botanist Robert Brown (1773–1858).

Du·chenne \\dü-'shen, də-\\ *also* **Du·chenne's** \\-'shenz\\ *adj* : relating to or being Duchenne muscular dystrophy

Du·chenne \\dūē-shen\\, **Guillaume–Benjamin–Amand (1806–1875),** French neurologist. Duchenne is widely recognized as the founder of electrotherapy. Dedicating his career to the study of disorders associated with nerves and muscles, he used, as early as 1830, faradic currents in treating patients. He built his own machine for electrical stimulation of nerves and muscles. In 1855 he published a volume concerning the electrophysiology of the muscular system. He is also known for his classic descriptions of a number of medical disorders involving atrophy of muscles or paralysis.

Duchenne dystrophy *also* **Duchenne's dystrophy** *n* : DUCHENNE MUSCULAR DYSTROPHY

Duchenne muscular dystrophy *also* **Duchenne's muscular dystrophy** *n* : a severe progressive form of muscular dystrophy of males that appears in early childhood, affects the muscles of the legs before those of the arms and the proximal muscles of the limbs before the distal ones, is inherited as an X-linked recessive trait, is characterized by complete absence of the protein dystrophin, and usu. has a fatal outcome by age 20 — abbr. *DMD*; see BECKER MUSCULAR DYSTROPHY

duck \\'dək\\ *n, pl* **ducks** *or* **duck** : any of various swimming birds (family Anatidae, the duck family) in which the neck and legs are short, the feet typically webbed, the bill often broad and flat, and the sexes usu. different from each other in plumage

duck sickness *n* : a highly destructive form of botulism affecting esp. wild ducks in areas of the western U.S. in which drought has caused decay of aquatic vegetation thereby permitting excessive multiplication of a form of botulinum bacterium (*Clostridium botulinum* type C) and spreading of its characteristic toxin in feeding areas — called also *duck disease*

Du·crey's bacillus \\dü-'krāz-\\ *n* : a gram-negative bacillus of the genus *Haemophilus* (*H. ducreyi*) that is the causative agent of chancroid

Du·crey \\dü-'krā\\, **Augusto (1860–1940),** Italian dermatologist. Ducrey published in 1889 an announcement of his discovery of the organism which causes chancroid and now bears his name.

duct \\'dəkt\\ *n* : a bodily tube or vessel esp. when carrying the secretion of a gland

duc·tal \\'dək-t³l\\ *adj* : of or belonging to a duct : made up of ducts ⟨the biliary ~ system⟩

ductal carcinoma in situ *n* : any of a histologically variable group of precancerous growths or early carcinomas of the lactiferous ducts that have the potential of becoming invasive and spreading to other tissues — abbr. *DCIS*

duc·tile \\'dək-t³l, -,tīl\\ *adj* : capable of being drawn out or hammered thin ⟨~ metal⟩ — **duc·til·i·ty** \\,dək-'til-ət-ē\\ *n, pl* **-ties**

duc·tion \\'dək-shən\\ *n* : a turning or rotational movement of the eye

duct·less \\'dək-tləs\\ *adj* : being without a duct

ductless gland *n* : ENDOCRINE GLAND

duct of Bar·tho·lin \\-'bärt-³l-ən, -'bär-thə-lən, -bär-'tül-in\\ *n* : a relatively large duct draining the sublingual gland and opening into Wharton's duct or near it

---

\\ə\\ **abut** \\³\\ **kitten** \\ər\\ **further** \\a\\ **ash** \\ā\\ **ace** \\ä\\ **cot, cart**
\\au̇\\ **out** \\ch\\ **chin** \\e\\ **bet** \\ē\\ **easy** \\g\\ **go** \\i\\ **hit** \\ī\\ **ice** \\j\\ **job**
\\ŋ\\ **sing** \\ō\\ **go** \\ȯ\\ **law** \\ȯi\\ **boy** \\th\\ **thin** \\th\\ **the** \\ü\\ **loot**
\\u̇\\ **foot** \\y\\ **yet** \\zh\\ **vision** *See also* Pronunciation Symbols page

C. T. Bartholin — see BARTHOLIN'S GLAND

duct of Bel·li·ni \-be-'lē-nē\ *n* : any of the large excretory ducts of the uriniferous tubules of the kidney that open on the free surface of the papillae

Bellini, Lorenzo (1643–1704), Italian anatomist and physiologist. Bellini is important as one of the founders of Italian iatrophysics. He pioneered in the use of physical laws to explain the function of the human body. For three decades he served as professor of theoretical medicine and then of anatomy at the University of Pisa, Italy. In 1662 he published his first paper, an important study of the structure and function of the kidneys. Rejecting Galen's characterization of the kidneys as a mass of undifferentiated material, he uncovered a complicated structure composed of fibers, open spaces, and densely packed tubules. In his paper he described the renal excretory ducts that are now associated with his name. In 1665, in another classic essay, he recognized the papillae of the tongue as the organs of taste. Bellini was also among the first to recognize the value of urinalysis as an aid to diagnosis.

duct of Cu·vier \-'k(y)ü-vē-ˌā, -kūēv-'yā\ *n* : either of a pair of large transverse venous sinuses that conduct blood from the cardinal veins to the sinus venosus of the vertebrate embryo — called also *common cardinal vein*

G. Cuvier — see CUVIERIAN VEIN

duct of Gart·ner \-'gart-nər\ *n* : GARTNER'S DUCT

duct of Ri·vi·nus \-rə-'vē-nəs\ *n* : any of several small inconstant efferent ducts of the sublingual gland

Rivinus, Augustus Quirinus (1652–1723), German anatomist and botanist. Rivinus described the excretory ducts of the sublingual glands in an article on dyspepsia published in 1678. In 1701 he made a list of the recognized drugs of the time. He classified certain drugs as useless or undesirable and tried to remove from the materia medica of his time such substances as feces and urine. In the field of botanical taxonomy he is remembered for his attempts to classify plants more systematically. He was one of the first botanists to use a binomial nomenclature.

duct of San·to·ri·ni \-ˌsant-ə-'rē-nē, -ˌsänt-\ *n* : ACCESSORY PANCREATIC DUCT

Santorini, Giovanni Domenico (1681–1737), Italian anatomist. A professor of anatomy and medicine at Venice, Santorini published major works on anatomy in 1705 and 1724. In the latter work he wrote classic descriptions of the accessory pancreatic duct and of the small nodule at the tip of each arytenoid cartilage. He also treated such anatomical features as the facial muscles and the ampullae of Vater. He was one of the most skillful dissectors of his time, and his works on anatomy are noted for their lucid descriptions and precise graphic illustrations.

duct of Wir·sung \-'vir-(ˌ)zùŋ, -zəŋ\ *n* : PANCREATIC DUCT a

Wirsung, Johann Georg (1600–1643), German anatomist. A professor of anatomy at Padua, Italy, Wirsung discovered and drew an illustration of the excretory duct of the pancreas in 1642. The following year he published a formal description. Shortly thereafter, he was assassinated in a dispute over his claims of discovery.

duct·ule \'dək-(ˌ)t(y)ü(ə)l\ *n* : a small duct

duc·tu·li ef·fe·ren·tes \'dək-t(y)ə-ˌlī-ˌef-ə-'ren-(ˌ)tēz, -(ˌ)lē-\ *n pl* : a group of ducts that convey sperm from the testis to the epididymis

duc·tu·lus \'dək-t(y)ə-ləs\ *n, pl* **-li** \-ˌlī, -(ˌ)lē\ : DUCTULE

ductulus ab·er·rans \-'ab-ə-ˌranz\ *n, pl* **ductuli ab·er·ran·tes** \-ˌab-ə-'ran-ˌtēz\ : VAS ABERRANS OF HALLER — called also *ductulus aberrans inferior*

duc·tus \'dək-təs\ *n, pl* **ductus** : DUCT

ductus ar·te·ri·o·sus \-är-ˌtir-ē-'ō-səs\ *n* : a short broad vessel in the fetus that connects the pulmonary artery with the aorta and conducts most of the blood directly from the right ventricle to the aorta bypassing the lungs

ductus cho·le·do·chus \-kə-'led-ə-kəs\ *n* : COMMON BILE DUCT

ductus co·chle·ar·is \-ˌkō-klē-'ar-əs, -ˌkäk-lē-\ *n* : SCALA MEDIA

ductus de·fer·ens \-'def-ə-ˌrenz, -rənz\ *n, pl* **ductus de·fer·en·tes** \-ˌdef-ə-'ren-tēz\ : VAS DEFERENS

ductus ejac·u·la·to·ri·us \-i-ˌjak-yə-lə-'tōr-ē-əs, -'tòr-\ *n* : EJACULATORY DUCT

ductus en·do·lym·phat·i·cus \-ˌen-dō-lim-'fat-i-kəs\ *n* : a tubular process of the membranous labyrinth of the ear that ends blindly but has its base in communication with both the utricle and the saccule

ductus re·uni·ens \-rē-'(y)ü-nē-ˌenz\ *n* : a passage in the ear that connects the cochlea and the saccule

ductus ve·no·sus \-vi-'nō-səs\ *n* : a vein passing through the liver and connecting the left umbilical vein with the inferior vena cava of the fetus, losing its circulatory function after birth, and persisting as the ligamentum venosum of the liver

due \'d(y)ü\ *adj* : expected to be born in the normal course of events ⟨the baby is ~ in November⟩; *also* : expected to give birth ⟨she's ~ this month⟩

Duf·fy \'dəf-ē\ *adj* : relating to, characteristic of, or being a system of blood groups determined by the presence or absence of any of several antigens in red blood cells ⟨~ blood group system⟩ ⟨~ antigens⟩ ⟨~ blood typing⟩

Duffy, Richard (1906–1956), British hemophiliac. In 1949 Duffy was given a blood transfusion after having developed a large hematoma on his chest. When he developed a reaction to the transfusion, the research unit at London's Postgraduate Medical School compared samples of his blood with donor blood and discovered the existence of a new blood group system. In 1950 the researchers, Marie Cutbush, Patrick L. Mollison, and Dorothy M. Parkin, reported their discovery in a letter to *Nature* and named the blood group system in honor of the patient.

Dührs·sen's incisions \'düer-sənz-\ *n pl* : a set of three incisions in the cervix of the uterus to facilitate delivery if dilation is inadequate

Dührs·sen \'düer-sən\, **Alfred (1862–1933),** German obstetrician-gynecologist. Dührssen is regarded as one of the founders of modern surgical gynecology. In 1893 he developed a technique for facilitating labor by making incisions in the cervix which are now known as Dührssen's incisions. In 1895 he introduced a new variation of the cesarean section in which the surgery was performed via the vaginal canal. A full description of the operation was published in 1898. He also did research on abdominal cancer.

dul·ca·ma·ra \ˌdəl-kə-'mär-ə, -'mar-\ *n* **1** : BITTERSWEET **2** : the dried stems of bittersweet of the genus *Solanum* (*S. dulcamara*) formerly used as a diuretic and sedative

dul·ci·tol \'dəl-sə-ˌtól, -ˌtōl\ *n* : GALACTITOL

dull \'dəl\ *adj* **1** : mentally slow or stupid **2** : slow in perception or sensibility **3** : lacking sharpness of edge or point ⟨a ~ scalpel⟩ **4** : lacking in force, intensity, or acuteness ⟨a ~ pain⟩ — **dull** *vb* — **dull·ness** *or* **dul·ness** \'dəl-nəs\ *n* — **dul·ly** \'dəl-ē\ *adv*

Du·long and Pe·tit's law \'d(y)ü-ˌlòŋ-ən-pə-'tēz-, d(y)ü-'\ *n* : a law in physics and chemistry: the specific heats of most solid elements multiplied by their atomic weights are nearly the same averaging a little over six calories per degree Celsius per gram-atomic weight

Du·long \düe-lōⁿ\, **Pierre–Louis (1785–1838),** and **Pe·tit** \p(ə-)tē\, **Alexis–Thérèse (1791–1820),** French physicists. Dulong and Petit collaborated on important studies of temperature measurement and heat transfer. In 1815 they made the first accurate comparison between air and mercury thermometers. Two years later they showed that Newton's law of cooling is true only for small differences in temperature. In 1819 they demonstrated that the heat produced in the compression of a gas is proportional to the work done. In that same year they formulated the law concerning specific heats that now bears their names.

dumb \'dəm\ *adj* **1** : lacking the human power of speech ⟨~ animals⟩ **2** *of a person, often offensive* : lacking the ability to speak — **dumb·ly** \'dəm-lē\ *adv* — **dumb·ness** *n*

dumb rabies *n* : PARALYTIC RABIES

dum·dum fever \ˌdəm-ˌdəm-\ *n* : KALA-AZAR

C
D

dum·mi·ness \'dəm-ē-nəs\ *n* : the condition of being a dummy — used esp. of a horse

¹dum·my \'dəm-ē\ *n, pl* **dummies** **1** : a horse lacking the ability to respond to ordinary stimuli because of cerebral damage esp. following encephalomyelitis **2** : PONTIC **3** : PLACEBO

²dummy *adj* : being a placebo ⟨those who unknowingly receive a ∼ pill instead of the real thing —Nicholas Wade⟩

dump·ing syndrome \'dəm-piŋ-\ *n* : a condition characterized by weakness, dizziness, flushing and warmth, nausea, and palpitation immediately or shortly after eating and produced by abnormally rapid emptying of the stomach esp. in individuals who have had part of the stomach removed

duodena *pl of* DUODENUM

du·o·de·nal gland \ˌd(y)ü-ə-ˈdēn-ᵊl-, d(y)ü-ˈäd-ᵊn-əl-\ *n* : BRUNNER'S GLAND

duodenal tube *n* : a long flexible rubber tube that can be passed through the esophagus and stomach into the duodenum

duodenal ulcer *n* : a peptic ulcer situated in the duodenum

du·o·de·nec·to·my \d(y)ü-ˌäd-ᵊn-ˈek-tə-mē\ *n, pl* **-mies** : excision of all or part of the duodenum

du·o·de·ni·tis \d(y)ü-ˌäd-ᵊn-ˈīt-əs\ *n* : inflammation of the duodenum

du·o·de·no·cho·led·o·chot·o·my \d(y)ü-ˌäd-ᵊn-ō-kə-ˌled-ə-ˈkät-ə-mē\ *n, pl* **-mies** : choledochotomy performed by approach through the duodenum by incision

du·o·de·nog·ra·phy \d(y)ü-ˌäd-ᵊn-ˈäg-rə-fē\ *n, pl* **-phies** : radiographic visualization of the duodenum with a contrast medium

du·o·de·no·je·ju·nal \d(y)ü-ˌäd-ᵊn-ō-ji-ˈjün-ᵊl\ *adj* : of, relating to, or joining the duodenum and the jejunum ⟨the ∼ junction⟩

du·o·de·no·je·ju·nos·to·my \-ji-jü-ˈnäs-tə-mē\ *n, pl* **-mies** : a surgical operation that joins part of the duodenum and the jejunum with creation of an artificial opening between them

du·o·de·not·o·my \d(y)ü-ˌäd-ᵊn-ˈät-ə-mē\ *n, pl* **-mies** : incision of the duodenum

du·o·de·num \ˌd(y)ü-ə-ˈdē-nəm, d(y)ü-ˈäd-ᵊn-əm\ *n, pl* **-de·na** \-ˈdē-nə, -ᵊn-ə\ *or* **-de·nums** : the first, shortest, and widest part of the small intestine that in humans is about 10 inches (25 centimeters) long and that extends from the pylorus to the undersurface of the liver where it descends for a variable distance and receives the bile and pancreatic ducts and then bends to the left and finally upward to join the jejunum near the second lumbar vertebra — **du·o·de·nal** \-ˈdēn-ᵊl, -ᵊn-əl\ *adj*

dup *abbr* duplicate

du·plex \'d(y)ü-ˌpleks\ *n* : a molecule having two complementary polynucleotide strands of DNA or of DNA and RNA — **duplex** *adj*

du·pli·cate \'d(y)ü-pli-ˌkāt\ *vi* **-cat·ed; -cat·ing** : to become duplicate : REPLICATE ⟨DNA in chromosomes ∼s⟩

du·pli·ca·tion \ˌd(y)ü-pli-ˈkā-shən\ *n* **1** : the act or process of duplicating : the quality or state of being duplicated **2** : a part of a chromosome in which the genetic material is repeated; *also* : the process of forming a duplication

du·pli·ca·ture \'d(y)ü-pli-kə-ˌchů(ə)r, -chər; -ˌkā-chər\ *n* : a doubling or fold esp. of a membrane

Du·puy·tren's contracture \də-ˌpwē-ˈtraⁿz-, -ˈpwē-trənz-\ *n* : a condition marked by fibrosis with shortening and thickening of the palmar aponeurosis resulting in flexion contracture of the fingers into the palm of the hand

Du·puy·tren \də-pwē-traⁿ\, **Guillaume (1777–1835),** French surgeon. Dupuytren was the leading French surgeon of his day. His greatest achievements were in surgical pathology, and they include: the first excision of the lower jaw (1812), a successful ligation of the external iliac artery (1815), the first successful treatment of aneurysm by compression (1818), a successful ligation of the subclavian artery (1819), surgical treatment of wryneck (1822), the development of an operation for the creation of an artificial anus (1828), and a classification of burns into four divisions

(1832). The contracture that bears his name was described in 1831.

dura — see LAMINA DURA

du·ral \'d(y)ůr-əl\ *adj* : of or relating to the dura mater

dural sinus *n* : SINUS OF THE DURA MATER

du·ra ma·ter \'d(y)ůr-ə-ˌmāt-ər, -ˌmät-\ *n* : the tough fibrous membrane lined with endothelium on the inner surface that envelops the brain and spinal cord external to the arachnoid and pia mater, that in the cranium closely lines the bone, does not dip down between the convolutions, and contains numerous blood vessels and venous sinuses, and that in the spinal cord is separated from the bone by a considerable space and contains no venous sinuses — called also *dura*

dust cell \'dəst-ˌ\ *n* : a pulmonary macrophage that takes up and eliminates foreign particles introduced into the lung alveoli with inspired air

dust·ing powder \'dəst-iŋ-\ *n* : a powder used on the skin or on wounds esp. for allaying irritation or absorbing moisture

dust mite *n* : any of various mites (esp. family Pyroglyphidae) implicated in human allergic reactions to dust; *esp* : HOUSE-DUST MITE

Dutch cap \ˌdəch-ˈkap\ *n* : CERVICAL CAP

Dutch·man's–breech·es \ˌdəch-mənz-ˈbrich-əz\ *n pl but sing or pl in constr* : a delicate spring-flowering herb (*Dicentra cucullaria* of the family Fumariaceae) that occurs in the eastern U.S. and has tubers that are a source of corydalis

du·ty of care \'d(y)üt-ē-əv-ˈke(ə)r, -ˈka(ə)r\ *n* : a duty to use care toward others that would be exercised by an ordinarily resonable and prudent person in order to protect them from unnecessary risk of harm ⟨in a typical medical malpractice lawsuit, the plaintiff has the burden of proof to show that the physician had a legal *duty of care* to the patient, that the physician breached that duty, and that the breach caused injury to the plaintiff —L. F. Sparr *et al*⟩

DV *abbr* **1** daily value **2** dilute volume

DVM *abbr* doctor of veterinary medicine

DVT *abbr* deep vein thrombosis

DW *abbr* distilled water

¹dwarf \'dwȯ(ə)rf\ *n, pl* **dwarfs** \'dwȯ(ə)rfs\ *also* **dwarves** \'dwȯ(ə)rvz\ *often attrib* **1** : a person of unusually small stature; *esp* : one whose bodily proportions are abnormal **2** : an animal much below normal size

²dwarf *vt* : to restrict the growth of : STUNT

dwarf·ism \'dwȯr-ˌfiz-əm\ *n* : the condition of stunted growth

dwt *abbr* [Latin *denarius* + *weight*] pennyweight

Dx *abbr* diagnosis

DXA *abbr* dual energy X-ray absorptiometry

Dy *symbol* dysprosium

dy·ad *also* **di·ad** \'dī-ˌad, -əd\ *n* **1** : two individuals (as husband and wife) maintaining a sociologically significant relationship **2** : a meiotic chromosome after separation of the two homologous members of a tetrad — **dy·ad·ic** \dī-ˈad-ik\ *adj* — **dy·ad·i·cal·ly** \-i-k(ə-)lē\ *adv*

Dy·a·zide \'dī-ə-ˌzīd\ *trademark* — used for a preparation of hydrochlorothiazide and triamterene

dy·dro·ges·ter·one \ˌdī-drō-ˈjes-tə-ˌrōn\ *n* : a synthetic progestational agent $C_{21}H_{28}O_2$ used in the diagnosis and treatment of amenorrhea, dysmenorrhea, endometriosis, and in a test for pregnancy — called also *isopregnenone*

¹dye \'dī\ *n* **1** : color from dyeing **2** : a soluble or insoluble coloring matter

²dye *vb* **dyed; dye·ing** *vt* **1** : to impart a new and often permanent color to esp. by impregnating with a dye **2** : to impart (a color) by dyeing ⟨∼*ing* blue on yellow⟩ ∼ *vi* : to take up or impart color in dyeing

dye laser *n* : a laser in which light is emitted by a fluorescent organic dye and which can be tuned to radiate at any of a wide range of frequencies

---

\ə\ abut \ᵊ\ kitten \ər\ further \a\ ash \ā\ ace \ä\ cot, cart \aů\ out \ch\ chin \e\ bet \ē\ easy \g\ go \i\ hit \ī\ ice \j\ job \ŋ\ sing \ō\ go \ȯ\ law \ȯi\ boy \th\ thin \th̲\ the \ü\ loot \ů\ foot \y\ yet \zh\ vision *See also* Pronunciation Symbols page

dying *pres part of* DIE

dy·nam·ic \dī-'nam-ik\ *adj* **1** *also* **dy·nam·i·cal** \-i-kəl\ **a** : of or relating to physical force or energy **b** : of or relating to dynamics **2** : FUNCTIONAL 1b ⟨a ~ disease⟩ **3 a** : marked by continuous usu. productive activity or change ⟨a ~ population⟩ **b** : marked by energy or forcefulness ⟨a ~ personality⟩ — **dy·nam·i·cal·ly** \-i-k(ə-)lē\ *adv*

dy·nam·ics \dī-'nam-iks\ *n pl but sing or pl in constr* **1** : a branch of mechanics that deals with forces and their relation primarily to the motion but sometimes also to the equilibrium of bodies **2** : PSYCHODYNAMICS **3** : the pattern of change or growth of an object or phenomenon ⟨personality ~⟩ ⟨population ~⟩

dy·na·mo·gen·e·sis \,dī-nə-mō-'jen-ə-səs\ *n, pl* **-e·ses** \-,sēz\ : an increase in the mental or motor activity of an already functioning bodily system that accompanies any added sensory stimulation — **dy·na·mo·gen·ic** \-'jen-ik\ *adj*

dy·na·mog·e·ny \,dī-nə-'mäj-ə-nē\ *n, pl* **-nies** : DYNAMO-GENESIS

dy·na·mom·e·ter \,dī-nə-'mäm-ət-ər\ *n* : an instrument for measuring the force of muscular contraction esp. of the hand — **dy·na·mo·met·ric** \-nə-mō-'me-trik\ *adj*

dyne \'dīn\ *n* : the unit of force in the cgs system equal to the force that would give a free mass of one gram an acceleration of one centimeter per second per second

dy·nein \'dī-,nēn, -,nē-ən\ *n* : an ATPase that cross-links adjacent microtubules and that by controlling their relative sliding motion regulates the movement of cellular organelles and structures (as the beating of cilia and flagella and the movement of chromosomes to the poles of the spindle)

dy·nor·phin \dī-'nȯr-fən\ *n* : any of a group of potent opioids found in the mammalian central nervous system that have a strong affinity for opiate receptors

dy·phyl·line \dī-'fil-,ēn\ *n* : a theophylline derivative $C_{10}H_{14}N_4O_4$ used as a diuretic and for its bronchodilator and peripheral vasodilator effects — called also *hyphylline*

dys·acou·sia \dis-ə-'kü-zh(ē-)ə\ *n* : DYSACUSIS

dys·acu·sis *also* **dysacousis** \-'kü-səs\ *n, pl* **-acu·ses** *also* **-acou·ses** \-,sēz\ : a condition in which ordinary sounds produce discomfort or pain

dys·ad·ap·ta·tion \dis-,ad-,ap-'tā-shən, -əp-\ *n* : an impaired ability of the iris and retina to adapt properly to variations in light intensities that is often indicative of vitamin A deficiency

dysaesthesia, dysaesthetic *chiefly Brit var of* DYSESTHESIA, DYSESTHETIC

dys·ar·thria \dis-'är-thrē-ə\ *n* : difficulty in articulating words due to disease of the central nervous system — compare DYSPHASIA — **dys·ar·thric** \-thrik\ *adj*

dys·ar·thro·sis \,dis-,är-'thrō-səs\ *n, pl* **-thro·ses** \-,sēz\ **1** : a condition of reduced joint motion due to deformity, dislocation, or disease **2** : DYSARTHRIA

dys·au·to·no·mia \,dis-,ȯt-ə-'nō-mē-ə\ *n* : a disorder of the autonomic nervous system that causes disturbances in all or some autonomic functions and may result from the course of a disease (as diabetes) or from injury or poisoning; *esp* : FAMILIAL DYSAUTONOMIA — **dys·au·to·nom·ic** \-'näm-ik\ *adj*

dys·ba·rism \'dis-bə-,riz-əm\ *n* : the complex of symptoms (as the bends, headache, or mental disturbance) that accompanies exposure to excessively low or rapidly changing environmental air pressure

dys·cal·cu·lia \,dis-kal-'kyü-lē-ə\ *n* : impairment of mathematical ability due to an organic condition of the brain

dys·che·zia \dis-'kē-zē-ə, -zh(ē-)ə; -'kez-ē-ə, -'kezh-(ē-)ə\ *n* : constipation associated with a defective reflex for defecation — **dys·che·zic** \-'kē-zik, -'kez-ik\ *adj*

dys·chon·dro·pla·sia \dis-,kän-drō-'plā-zh(ē-)ə\ *n* : CHON-DRODYSPLASIA

dys·chro·mia \dis-'krō-mē-ə\ *n* : abnormal pigmentation of the skin ⟨periocular ~⟩

dys·cra·sia \dis-'krā-zh(ē-)ə\ *n* : an abnormal condition of the body; *esp* : an imbalance of components of the blood

dys·di·ad·o·cho·ki·ne·sia *or* **dys·di·ad·o·ko·ki·ne·sia** \,dis-,dī-,ad-ə-,kō-kī-'nē-zh(ē-)ə\ *n* : impairment of the ability to make movements exhibiting a rapid change of motion that is caused by cerebellar dysfunction — compare ADIADOKOKI-NESIS

dys·en·do·crin·ism \dis-'en-də-krə-,niz-əm\ *n* : a disorder of endocrine function

dys·en·ter·ic \,dis-ᵊn-'ter-ik\ *adj* : of or relating to dysentery

dys·en·ter·i·form \-'ter-ə-,fȯ(ə)rm\ *adj* : resembling that of dysentery ⟨~ stools⟩ ⟨~ symptoms⟩

dys·en·tery \'dis-ᵊn-,ter-ē\ *n, pl* **-ter·ies** **1** : a disease characterized by severe diarrhea with passage of mucus and blood and usu. caused by infection **2** : DIARRHEA

dys·er·gia \di-'sər-j(ē-)ə\ *n* : lack of muscular coordination due to a defect in innervation

dys·er·gy \'dis-,ər-jē, di-'sər-\ *n, pl* **-gies** : DYSERGIA

dys·es·the·sia *or chiefly Brit* **dys·aes·the·sia** \,dis-es-'thē-zh(ē-)ə\ *n* : impairment of sensitivity esp. to touch — **dys·es·thet·ic** *or chiefly Brit* **dys·aes·thet·ic** \-'thet-ik\ *adj*

dys·func·tion *also* **dis·func·tion** \(')dis-'fəŋ(k)-shən\ *n* : impaired or abnormal functioning (as of an organ of the body) — see MINIMAL BRAIN DYSFUNCTION — **dys·func·tion·al** \-shnəl, -shən-ᵊl\ *adj* — **dys·func·tion·ing** \-shə-niŋ\ *n*

dysfunctional uterine bleeding *n* : abnormal uterine bleeding that is not associated with a physical lesion (as a tumor), inflammation, or pregnancy — abbr. *DUB*

dys·gam·ma·glob·u·li·ne·mia *or chiefly Brit* **dys·gam·ma·glob·u·li·nae·mia** \,dis-,gam-ə-,gläb-yə-lə-'nē-mē-ə\ *n* : a disorder involving abnormality in structure or frequency of gamma globulins — compare AGAMMAGLOBULINEMIA

dys·gen·e·sis \(')dis-'jen-ə-səs\ *n, pl* **-e·ses** \-,sēz\ : defective development esp. of the gonads (as in Klinefelter's syndrome or Turner's syndrome)

dys·gen·ic *also* **dis·gen·ic** \(')dis-'jen-ik\ *adj* **1** : tending to promote survival of or reproduction by less well-adapted individuals (as the weak or diseased) esp. at the expense of well-adapted individuals (as the strong or healthy) ⟨the ~ effect of war⟩ **2** : biologically defective or deficient

dys·gen·ics \-iks\ *n pl but sing in constr* : the study of the accumulation and perpetuation of defective genes and traits in a population, race, or species

dys·ger·mi·no·ma \dis-,jər-mə-'nō-mə\ *n, pl* **-mas** *also* **-ma·ta** \-mət-ə\ : a germinoma of the ovary

dys·geu·sia \(')dis-'g(y)ü-zē-ə\ *n* : dysfunction of the sense of taste

dys·gon·ic \(')dis-'gän-ik\ *adj* : growing with difficulty on artificial media — used esp. of some strains of the tubercle bacillus; compare EUGONIC

dys·graph·ia \(')dis-'graf-ē-ə\ *n* : impairment of the ability to write caused by brain damage

dys·hi·dro·sis \,dis-,hī-'drō-səs, -hə-\ *also* **dys·idro·sis** \,dis-,ī-, ,dis-ə-\ *n, pl* **-dro·ses** \-,sēz\ : POMPHOLYX

dys·kary·o·sis \dis-,kar-ē-'ō-səs\ *n, pl* **-o·ses** \-,sēz\ *or* **-o·sis·es** : abnormality esp. of exfoliated cells (as from the uterine cervix) that affects the nucleus but not the cytoplasm

dys·ker·a·to·sis \,dis-,ker-ə-'tō-səs\ *n, pl* **-to·ses** \-,sēz\ : faulty development of the epidermis with abnormal keratinization — **dys·ker·a·tot·ic** \-'tät-ik\ *adj*

dys·ki·ne·sia \,dis-kə-'nē-zh(ē-)ə, -kī-\ *n* : impairment of voluntary movements resulting in fragmented or jerky motions (as in Parkinson's disease) — see TARDIVE DYSKINESIA — **dys·ki·net·ic** \-'net-ik\ *adj*

dyskinetic cerebral palsy *n* : ATHETOID CEREBRAL PALSY

dys·la·lia \dis-'lā-lē-ə, -'lal-ē-ə\ *n* : a speech defect caused by malformation of or imperfect distribution of nerves to the organs of articulation (as the tongue)

dys·lec·tic \dis-'lek-tik\ *adj or n* : DYSLEXIC

dys·lex·ia \dis-'lek-sē-ə\ *n* : a variable often familial learning disability involving difficulties in acquiring and processing language that is typically manifested by a lack of proficiency in reading, spelling, and writing

¹dys·lex·ic \-'lek-sik\ *adj* : affected with dyslexia

²dyslexic *n* : a dyslexic person

dys·lip·id·emia *or chiefly Brit* **dys·lip·id·ae·mia** \dis-ˌlip-ə-ˈdē-mē-ə\ *n* : a condition marked by abnormal concentrations of lipids or lipoproteins in the blood — **dys·lip·id·emic** *or chiefly Brit* **dys·lip·id·ae·mic** \-mik\ *adj*

dys·lo·gia \dis-ˈlō-j(ē-)ə\ *n* : difficulty in expressing ideas through speech caused by impairment of the power of reasoning (as in certain psychoses)

dys·men·or·rhea *or chiefly Brit* **dys·men·or·rhoea** \(ˌ)dis-ˌmen-ə-ˈrē-ə\ *n* : painful menstruation — see SPASMODIC DYSMENORRHEA — **dys·men·or·rhe·ic** *or chiefly Brit* **dys·men·or·rhoe·ic** \-ˈrē-ik\ *adj*

dys·met·ria \dis-ˈme-trē-ə\ *n* : impaired ability to estimate distance in muscular action

dys·mor·phia \-ˈmȯr-fē-ə\ *n* **1** : DYSMORPHISM **2** : BODY DYSMORPHIC DISORDER — **dys·mor·phic** \-fik\ *adj*

dys·mor·phism \-ˈmȯr-ˌfiz-əm\ *n* : an anatomical malformation ⟨have facial ∼ and other structural abnormalities —R. O. Brady⟩

dys·mor·phol·o·gist \-mȯr-ˈfäl-ə-jist\ *n* : a specialist in dysmorphology

dys·mor·phol·o·gy \-ə-jē\ *n, pl* **-gies** : a branch of clinical medicine concerned with human teratology

dys·on·to·ge·net·ic \ˌdis-ˌänt-ə-jə-ˈnet-ik\ *adj* : involving abnormal cell and tissue growth and differentiation ⟨∼ mixed tumors of the vagina —*Cancer*⟩

dys·os·mia \dis-ˈäz-mē-ə, -ˈäs-\ *n* : dysfunction of the sense of smell

dys·os·to·sis \ˌdis-ˌäs-ˈtō-səs\ *n, pl* **-to·ses** \-ˌsēz\ : defective formation of bone — **dys·os·tot·ic** \-ˈtät-ik\ *adj*

dys·pa·reu·nia \ˌdis-pə-ˈrü-nē-ə, -nyə\ *n* : difficult or painful sexual intercourse

dys·pep·sia \dis-ˈpep-shə, -sē-ə\ *n* : INDIGESTION

¹dys·pep·tic \-ˈpep-tik\ *adj* : relating to or having dyspepsia — **dys·pep·ti·cal·ly** \-ti-k(ə-)lē\ *adv*

²dyspeptic *n* : a person having dyspepsia

dys·pha·gia \dis-ˈfā-j(ē-)ə\ *n* : difficulty in swallowing — **dys·phag·ic** \-ˈfaj-ik\ *adj*

dys·pha·sia \dis-ˈfā-zh(ē-)ə\ *n* : loss of or deficiency in the power to use or understand language as a result of injury to or disease of the brain — compare DYSARTHRIA

¹dys·pha·sic \-ˈfā-zik\ *adj* : relating to or affected with dysphasia

²dysphasic *n* : a dysphasic individual

dys·phe·mia \dis-ˈfē-mē-ə\ *n* : a speech disorder characterized esp. by stammering or stuttering and usu. having a psychological basis

dys·pho·nia \dis-ˈfō-nē-ə\ *n* : defective use of the voice — **dys·phon·ic** \-ˈfän-ik\ *adj*

dys·pho·ria \dis-ˈfōr-ē-ə, -ˈfȯr-\ *n* : a state of feeling unwell or unhappy — compare EUPHORIA — **dys·phor·ic** \-ˈfȯr-ik, -ˈfär-\ *adj*

dys·pi·tu·i·ta·rism \ˌdis-pə-ˈt(y)ü-ət-ə-ˌriz-əm\ *n* : any abnormal condition caused by dysfunction of the pituitary gland

dys·pla·sia \dis-ˈplā-zh(ē-)ə\ *n* **1** : variation in somatotype (as in degree of ectomorphy, endomorphy, or mesomorphy) from one part of a human body to another **2** : abnormal growth or development (as of organs or cells); *broadly* : abnormal anatomic structure due to such growth — **dys·plas·tic** \-ˈplas-tik\ *adj*

dys·pnea *or chiefly Brit* **dys·pnoea** \ˈdis(p)-nē-ə\ *n* : difficult or labored respiration — compare EUPNEA — **dys·pne·ic** *or chiefly Brit* **dys·pnoe·ic** \-nē-ik\ *adj*

dys·prax·ia \dis-ˈprak-sē-ə, -ˈprak-sh(ē-)ə\ *n* : impairment of the ability to perform coordinated movements ⟨∼s of gaze —A. G. Waltz⟩ — **dys·prax·ic** \-ˈprak-sik\ *adj*

dys·pro·si·um \dis-ˈprō-zē-əm, -zh(ē-)əm\ *n* : an element of the rare-earth group that forms highly magnetic compounds — symbol *Dy*; see ELEMENT table

dys·pro·tein·emia *or chiefly Brit* **dys·pro·tein·ae·mia** \ˌdis-ˌprōt-ⁿn-ˈē-mē-ə, -ˌprō-ˌtēn-, -ˌprōt-ē-ən-\ *n* : any abnormality of the protein content of the blood — **dys·pro·tein·emic** *or chiefly Brit* **dys·pro·tein·ae·mic** \-ˈē-mik\ *adj*

dys·ra·phism \dis-ˈrā-ˌfiz-əm, ˈdis-rə-\ *n* : incomplete fusion of parts; *esp* : defective closure of the neural tube ⟨spinal ∼⟩

dys·reg·u·la·tion \ˌdis-ˌreg-yə-ˈlā-shən, -ˌreg-ə-\ *n* : impairment of a physiological regulatory mechanism (as that governing metabolism, immune response, or organ function) — **dys·reg·u·lat·ed** \-ˈreg-yə-ˌlāt-əd, -ˈreg-ə-\ *adj*

dys·rhyth·mia \dis-ˈrith-mē-ə\ *n* **1** : an abnormal rhythm; *esp* : a disordered rhythm exhibited in a record of electrical activity of the brain or heart **2** : JET LAG — **dys·rhyth·mic** \-mik\ *adj*

dys·se·ba·cia \ˌdis-(s)ə-ˈbā-sh(ē-)ə\ *n* : a disorder of the sebaceous glands marked by reddening and accumulation of greasy flaky scales on affected areas and often indicative of a vitamin deficiency

dys·sym·bo·lia \ˌdis-ˌ(s)im-ˈbō-lē-ə\ *n* : deficiency in the ability to express thoughts in language

dys·sy·ner·gia \ˌdis-(s)ə-ˈnər-j(ē-)ə\ *n* : DYSKINESIA — **dys·sy·ner·gic** \-ˈnər-jik\ *adj*

dys·syn·er·gy \(ˈ)dis-ˈ(s)in-ər-jē\ *n, pl* **-gies** : DYSKINESIA

dys·thy·mia \dis-ˈthī-mē-ə\ *n* : a mood disorder characterized by chronic mildly depressed or irritable mood often accompanied by other symptoms (as eating and sleeping disturbances, fatigue, and poor self-esteem) — called also *dysthymic disorder*

¹dys·thy·mic \dis-ˈthī-mik\ *adj* : of, relating to, or affected with dysthymia ⟨a ∼ patient⟩

²dysthymic *n* : an individual affected with dysthymia

dysthymic disorder *n* : DYSTHYMIA

dys·to·cia \dis-ˈtō-sh(ē-)ə\ *or* **dys·to·kia** \-ˈtō-kē-ə\ *n* : slow or difficult labor or delivery — compare EUTOCIA

dys·to·nia \dis-ˈtō-nē-ə\ *n* : a state of disordered tonicity of tissues (as of muscle) — **dys·ton·ic** \-ˈtän-ik\ *adj*

dystonia mus·cu·lo·rum de·for·mans \-ˌməs-kyə-ˈlȯr-əm-di-ˈfȯr-ˌmanz\ *n* : a rare inherited neurological disorder characterized by progressive muscular spasticity causing severe involuntary contortions esp. of the trunk and limbs — called also *torsion dystonia*

dys·to·pia \dis-ˈtō-pē-ə\ *n* : malposition of an anatomical part — **dys·top·ic** \-ˈtō-pik, -ˈtäp-ik\ *adj*

dys·tro·phic \dis-ˈtrō-fik\ *adj* **1** : relating to or caused by faulty nutrition **2** : relating to or affected with a dystrophy ⟨∼ muscles⟩ **3 a** : occurring at sites of damaged or necrotic tissue ⟨∼ calcification . . . may occur despite normal serum calcium levels —Raymond Chan *et al*⟩ **b** : characterized by disordered growth ⟨fungal infection may be the cause of thickened ∼ nails⟩

dystrophica — see MYOTONIA DYSTROPHICA

dystrophic epidermolysis bullosa *n* : any of several forms of epidermolysis bullosa that are marked esp. by blister formation between the basement membrane and lamina propria often accompanied by scarring and sometimes involvement of the mucous membranes (as of the mouth or esophagus) and that are inherited as an autosomal dominant or recessive trait

dys·tro·phin \ˈdis-trə-ˌfin\ *n* : a protein of high molecular weight that is associated with a transmembrane glycoprotein complex of skeletal muscle cells and is absent in Duchenne muscular dystrophy and deficient or of abnormal molecular weight in Becker muscular dystrophy

dys·tro·phy \ˈdis-trə-fē\ *n, pl* **-phies** **1** : a condition produced by faulty nutrition ⟨waters with a high fluorine content are responsible for the dental ∼ known as mottled enamel —*Lancet*⟩ **2** : any myogenic atrophy; *esp* : MUSCULAR DYSTROPHY

dys·uria \dish-ˈ(y)ùr-ē-ə, dis-ˈyùr-\ *n* : difficult or painful discharge of urine — **dys·uric** \-ˈ(y)ùr-ik\ *adj*

\ə\ **abut** \ᵊ\ **kitten** \ər\ **further** \a\ **ash** \ā\ **ace** \ä\ **cot, cart**
\aù\ **out** \ch\ **chin** \e\ **bet** \ē\ **easy** \g\ **go** \i\ **hit** \ī\ **ice** \j\ **job**
\ŋ\ **sing** \ō\ **go** \ȯ\ **law** \ȯi\ **boy** \th\ **thin** \th̲\ **the** \ü\ **loot**
\ù\ **foot** \y\ **yet** \zh\ **vision** *See also* Pronunciation Symbols page

C
D

E

E *abbr* **1** emmetropia **2** enema **3** enzyme **4** experimenter **5** eye

ea *abbr* each

EA *abbr* educational age

EAE *abbr* experimental allergic encephalomyelitis; experimental autoimmune encephalomyelitis

ear \'i(ə)r\ *n* **1** : the characteristic vertebrate organ of hearing and equilibrium consisting in the typical mammal of a sound-collecting outer ear separated by the tympanic membrane from a sound-transmitting middle ear that in turn is separated from a sensory inner ear by membranous fenestrae **2 a** : the external ear of humans and most mammals **b** : a human earlobe ⟨had her ∼s pierced⟩ **3 a** : the sense or act of hearing **b** : acuity of hearing

ear·ache \'i(ə)r-ˌāk\ *n* : an ache or pain in the ear — called also *otalgia*

ear·drum \-ˌdrəm\ *n* : TYMPANIC MEMBRANE

eared \'i(ə)rd\ *adj* : having ears esp. of a specified kind or number ⟨a big-*eared* man⟩

ear·lobe \'i(ə)r-ˌlōb\ *n* : the pendent part of the ear esp. of humans

ear mange *n* : canker of the ear esp. in cats and dogs that is caused by mites; *esp* : OTODECTIC MANGE

ear mite *n* : any of various mites attacking the ears of mammals

ear·mold \'i(ə)r-ˌmōld\ *n* : a device of usu. acrylic, vinyl, or silicone that fits within the outer ear, is connected by way of a tube to a hearing aid worn behind the ear, and serves esp. to channel the amplified sound from the hearing aid to the ear canal

ear pick *n* : a device for removing wax or foreign bodies from the ear

ear·piece \'i(ə)r-ˌpēs\ *n* **1** : a part of an instrument (as a stethoscope or hearing aid) that is inserted into the outer opening of the ear **2** : one of the two sidepieces that support eyeglasses by passing over or behind the ears

ear·plug \-ˌpləg\ *n* : a device of pliable material for insertion into the outer opening of the ear (as to keep out water or deaden sound)

earth eating \'ərth-\ *n* : GEOPHAGY

ear tick *n* : any of several ticks infesting the ears of mammals; *esp* : SPINOSE EAR TICK

ear·wax \'i(ə)r-ˌwaks\ *n* : the yellow waxy secretion from the glands of the external ear — called also *cerumen*

ease \'ēz\ *vb* **eased; eas·ing** *vt* **1** : to free from something that pains, disquiets, or burdens ⟨*eased* and comforted the sick⟩ **2** : to take away or lessen : ALLEVIATE ⟨took an aspirin to ∼ the pain⟩ ∼ *vi* : to give freedom or relief (as from pain or discomfort) ⟨a hot bath often ∼*s* and relaxes⟩

east coast fever *n* : an acute highly fatal febrile disease of cattle esp. of eastern and southern Africa that is caused by a protozoan of the genus *Theileria* (*T. parva*) transmitted by ticks esp. of the genera *Rhipicephalus* and *Hyalomma* and is marked by intense fever, labored breathing, gastrointestinal hemorrhage, swelling of the lymph nodes, and generalized weakness and emaciation

east·ern equine encephalomyelitis \ē-stərn-\ *n* : EQUINE ENCEPHALOMYELITIS a

eat \'ēt\ *vb* **ate** \'āt, *chiefly Brit* 'et\ **eat·en** \'ēt-ᵊn\ **eat·ing** *vt* **1** : to take in through the mouth as food : ingest, chew, and swallow in turn **2** : to consume gradually : CORRODE ∼ *vi* : to take food or a meal

eating disorder *n* : any of several psychological disorders (as anorexia nervosa or bulimia) characterized by serious disturbances of eating behavior

Ea·ton agent \'ēt-ᵊn-\ *n* : a microorganism of the genus *Mycoplasma* (*M. pneumoniae*) that is the causative agent of primary atypical pneumonia

Eaton, Monroe Davis (*b* 1904), American microbiologist. Eaton worked on the isolation of the causative agent of primary atypical pneumonia; the agent is now known as the Eaton agent. He also did research on bacterial toxins, purification of diphtheria toxin, development of influenza vaccination, the immunology of malaria, the biochemistry of virus growth, and the action of viruses on cancer cells.

Eaton–Lambert syndrome *n* : LAMBERT-EATON SYNDROME

Eb·er·thel·la \ˌeb-ər-'thel-ə\ *n, in many classifications* : a genus of motile aerobic gram-negative bacteria of the family Enterobacteriaceae that produce acid but no gas on many carbohydrates, comprise a number of pathogens including the causative agent (*E. typhosa*) of typhoid fever in humans, and are sometimes placed in the genus *Salmonella* or *Bacterium*

Eberth \'ā-bərt\, **Karl Joseph (1835–1926),** German pathologist and bacteriologist. Eberth's most important work in pathology was his contribution to the understanding of thrombosis. He was one of the first pathologists to seriously undertake bacteriological investigations and one of the earliest laboratory bacteriologists. In 1879 Eberth, after studying twenty-three cases of typhoid fever, concluded that the characteristic changes found in the spleen and lymph nodes of the abdomen occurred because bacterial activity was most intense in these areas. In twelve of the cases he found rod-shaped organisms. In 1880 he reported his discovery of the typhoid bacillus. Although Eberth discovered the bacillus through histopathologic techniques, the organism was actually isolated and cultivated in 1884 by Georg Gaffky (1850–1918).

Ebo·la \i-'bō-lə, ē-; 'ē-ˌbō-\ *n* **1** : EBOLA VIRUS **2** : the hemorrhagic fever caused by the Ebola virus — called also *Ebola fever*

Ebola virus *n* : any of several single-stranded RNA viruses of the family *Filoviridae* (esp. species *Zaire Ebola virus*) of African origin that cause an often fatal hemorrhagic fever

ebri·e·ty \i-'brī-ət-ē\ *n, pl* **-ties** : INEBRIETY

eb·ul·lism \'eb-(y)ə-ˌliz-əm\ *n* : the formation of bubbles in body fluids under sharply reduced environmental pressure

eb·ur·nat·ed \'eb-ər-ˌnāt-əd, 'ē-bər-\ *adj* : hard and dense like ivory ⟨∼ cartilage⟩ ⟨∼ bone⟩

eb·ur·na·tion \ˌeb-ər-'nā-shən, ˌē-bər-\ *n* : a diseased condition in which bone or cartilage is eburnated

EBV *abbr* Epstein-Barr virus

EB virus \ˌē-'bē-\ *n* : EPSTEIN-BARR VIRUS

ecau·date \(')ē-'kȯ-ˌdāt\ *adj* : having no tail

ec·bol·ic \ek-'bäl-ik\ *n* : a drug (as an ergot alkaloid) that tends to increase uterine contractions and that is used esp. to facilitate delivery

¹ec·cen·tric \ik-'sen-trik, ek-\ *adj* : deviating from an established pattern or from accepted usage or conduct — **ec·cen·tri·cal·ly** \-tri-k(ə-)lē\ *adv*

²eccentric *n* : an eccentric individual

eccentric hypertrophy *n* : hypertrophy of the wall of a hollow organ and esp. the heart with dilatation of its cavity

ec·chon·dro·ma \ˌek-ən-'drō-mə\ *n, pl* **-ma·ta** \-mət-ə\ *also* **-mas** : a cartilaginous tumor projecting from bone or cartilage

ec·chy·mosed \'ek-ə-ˌmōzd, -ˌmōst\ *adj* : affected with ecchymosis

ec·chy·mo·sis \ˌek-ə-'mō-səs\ *n, pl* **-mo·ses** \-ˌsēz\ : the escape of blood into the tissues from ruptured blood vessels marked by a livid black-and-blue or purple spot or area; *also* : the discoloration so caused — **ec·chy·mot·ic** \-'mät-ik\ *adj*

ec·co·pro·ti·co·phor·ic \ˌek-ō-ˌprōt-ə-kō-'fȯr-ik, -ˌprät-\ *adj* : exhibiting the properties of a laxative

ec·crine \\'ek-rən, -ˌrīn, -ˌrēn\\ *adj* : of, relating to, having, or being eccrine glands — compare APOCRINE, HOLOCRINE, MEROCRINE

eccrine gland *n* : any of the rather small sweat glands that produce a fluid secretion without removing cytoplasm from the secreting cells and that are restricted to the human skin — called also *eccrine sweat gland*

ec·cri·nol·o·gy \\ˌek-rə-'näl-ə-jē\\ *n, pl* **-gies** : a branch of physiology that deals with secretion and secretory organs

ec·dy·sis \\'ek-də-səs\\ *n, pl* **ec·dy·ses** \\-də-ˌsēz\\ : the act of molting or shedding an outer cuticular layer (as in insects and crustaceans) — **ec·dys·ial** \\ek-'diz-ē-əl, -'dizh-(ē-)əl\\ *adj*

ec·dy·sone \\'ek-də-ˌsōn\\ *also* **ec·dy·son** \\-ˌsän\\ *n* : any of several arthropod hormones that in insects are produced by the prothoracic gland and that trigger molting and metamorphosis

ECF *abbr* extracellular fluid

ECG *abbr* electrocardiogram

ec·go·nine \\'ek-gə-ˌnēn, -nən\\ *n* : a crystalline alkaloid $C_9H_{15}NO_3$ obtained by hydrolysis of cocaine

Echid·noph·a·ga \\ˌek-(ˌ)id-'näf-ə-gə\\ *n* : a genus of fleas (as the sticktight flea) of the family Pulicidae of which the female remains attached to the host

ech·i·na·cea \\ˌek-i-'nā-sē-ə, -sh(ē-)ə\\ *n* : the dried rhizome, roots, or other part of any of three composite herbs (*Echinacea angustifolia*, *E. pallida*, and *E. purpurea*) that were formerly listed in the U.S. Pharmacopeia, that are now used primarily in dietary supplements and herbal remedies, and that are held to stimulate the immune system; *also* : any of these herbs — see PURPLE CONEFLOWER

echi·no·coc·co·sis \\i-ˌkī-nə-kä-'kō-səs\\ *n, pl* **-co·ses** \\-ˌsēz\\ : infestation with or disease caused by a small tapeworm of the genus *Echinococcus* (*E. granulosus*); *esp* : HYDATID DISEASE

echi·no·coc·cus \\-nə-'käk-əs\\ *n* **1** *cap* : a genus of tapeworms of the family Taeniidae that alternate a minute adult living as a harmless commensal in the intestine of dogs and other carnivores with a hydatid larva invading tissues esp. of the liver of cattle, sheep, swine, and humans, and acting as a serious often fatal pathogen **2** *pl* **-coc·ci** \\-'käk-ˌ(s)ī, -'käk-(ˌ)(s)ē\\ : any tapeworm of the genus *Echinococcus*; *also* : HYDATID 1

Echi·no·der·ma·ta \\-nə-'dər-mət-ə\\ *n pl* : a phylum of radially symmetrical coelomate marine animals consisting of the starfishes, sea urchins, and related forms — **echi·no·der·ma·tous** \\i-ˌkī-nə-'dər-mət-əs\\ *adj* — **echi·no·derm** \\i-'kī-nə-ˌdərm\\ *n*

Echi·noi·dea \\ˌek-ə-'nȯi-dē-ə\\ *n pl* : a class of motile bottom-dwelling echinoderms comprising the sea urchins and related forms — **ech·i·noid** \\'ek-ə-ˌnȯid\\ *n*

Echi·no·rhyn·chus \\i-ˌkī-nə-'riŋ-kəs\\ *n* : a genus (the type of the family Echinorhynchidae) of small cylindrical acanthocephalan worms that are parasitic in various vertebrates

echi·nu·late \\i-'kin-yə-lət, -'kīn-, -ˌlāt\\ *adj* **1** : set with small spines or prickles ⟨∼ spores⟩ **2** : having a jagged outline with pointed outgrowths ⟨an ∼ culture of bacteria⟩ — **echi·nu·la·tion** \\-ˌkin-yə-'lā-shən, -ˌkīn-\\ *n*

Echis \\'ek-əs, 'ēk-\\ *n* : a genus of vipers found in India, Arabia, and No. Africa

echo \\'ek-(ˌ)ō\\ *n, pl* **ech·oes** *also* **echos** **1** : the repetition of a sound that is caused by reflection of sound waves **2** : the sound that is due to reflection of sound waves — **echo** *vb* **ech·oed; echo·ing** \\'ek-(ˌ)ō-iŋ, 'ek-ə-wiŋ\\

echo *abbr* echocardiogram; echocardiography

echo·car·dio·gram \\ˌek-ō-'kärd-ē-ə-ˌgram\\ *n* : a visual record made by echocardiography; *also* : the procedure for producing such a record

echo·car·di·og·ra·phy \\-ˌkärd-ē-'äg-rə-fē\\ *n, pl* **-phies** : the use of ultrasound to examine and measure the structure and functioning of the heart and to diagnose abnormalities and disease — **echo·car·di·og·ra·pher** \\-fər\\ *n* — **echo·car·dio·graph·ic** \\-ē-ə-'graf-ik\\ *adj*

echo·en·ceph·a·lo·gram \\ˌek-ō-in-'sef-ə-lə-ˌgram\\ *n* : a visual record obtained by echoencephalography

echo·en·ceph·a·log·ra·phy \\-in-ˌsef-ə-'läg-rə-fē\\ *n, pl* **-phies** : the use of ultrasound to examine and measure internal structures (as the ventricles) of the skull and to diagnose abnormalities and disease — **echo·en·ceph·a·lo·graph·ic** \\-ˌsef-ə-lə-'graf-ik\\ *adj*

echo·gen·ic \\ˌek-ə-'jen-ik\\ *adj* : reflecting ultrasound waves ⟨the normal thyroid gland is uniformly ∼ —Catherine Cole-Beuglet⟩ — **echo·ge·nic·i·ty** \\-jə-'nis-ə-tē\\ *n, pl* **-ties**

echo·gram \\'ek-ō-ˌgram\\ *n* : SONOGRAM

echo·graph \\-ˌgraf\\ *n* : an instrument used for echography

echog·ra·phy \\i-'käg-rə-fē\\ *n, pl* **-phies** : ULTRASOUND 2 — **echo·graph·ic** \\ˌek-ō-'graf-ik\\ *adj* — **echo·graph·i·cal·ly** \\-i-k(ə-)lē\\ *adv*

echo·ki·ne·sis \\ˌek-ō-kə-'nē-səs, -kī-\\ *n, pl* **-ne·ses** \\-ˌsēz\\ : ECHOPRAXIA

echo·la·lia \\ˌek-ō-'lā-lē-ə\\ *n* : the often pathological repetition of what is said by other people as if echoing them — **echo·lal·ic** \\-'lal-ik\\ *adj*

echo·mim·ia \\ˌek-ō-'mim-ē-ə\\ *n* : ECHOPRAXIA

echo·prac·tic \\ˌek-ō-'prak-tik, 'ek-ō-ˌ\\ *adj* : of, relating to, or affected with echopraxia

echo·prax·ia \\ˌek-ō-'prak-sē-ə\\ *n* : pathological repetition of the actions of other people as if echoing them

echo·thi·o·phate iodide \\-ˌthī-ə-ˌfāt-\\ *n* : a long-acting anticholinesterase $C_9H_{23}INO_3PS$ used esp. to reduce intraocular pressure in the treatment of glaucoma — called also *echothiophate*

echo·vi·rus \\'ek-ō-ˌvī-rəs\\ *n* : any of numerous serotypes of a picornavirus of the genus *Enterovirus* (species *Human enterovirus B*) that are closely related to the coxsackieviruses, are found in the gastrointestinal tract, cause cytopathic changes in cells in tissue culture, and are sometimes associated with respiratory ailments and meningitis

Eck fistula \\'ek-\\ *n* : an artificial anastomosis between the portal vein and inferior vena cava by which blood from the intestinal region is diverted from the liver to flow directly to the heart

Eck, Nikolai Vladimirovich (1849–1908), Russian physiologist. Eck developed the surgical procedure that bears his name in 1877. The operation made possible the experimental study of diseases of the liver and the investigation of the role of the liver in metabolism. He was a pioneer in the surgical treatment of neoplastic disease, and he wrote on nasal and laryngeal polyps. Eck was also interested in epidemiology, sanitation, and geology.

ec·lamp·sia \\i-'klam(p)-sē-ə, e-\\ *n* : a convulsive state : an attack of convulsions: as **a** : convulsions or coma late in pregnancy in an individual affected with preeclampsia — compare TOXEMIA OF PREGNANCY **b** : a condition comparable to milk fever of cows observed in domestic animals (as dogs and cats) — **ec·lamp·tic** \\i-'klam(p)-tik, e-\\ *adj*

¹eclec·tic \\e-'klek-tik, i-\\ *adj* **1** : selecting what appears to be best in various doctrines or methods **2** : of, relating to, or practicing eclecticism — **eclec·ti·cal·ly** \\-ti-k(ə-)lē\\ *adv*

²eclectic *n* : one who uses an eclectic method or approach

eclec·ti·cism \\-'klek-tə-ˌsiz-əm\\ *n* **1** : a theory or practice (as of medicine or psychotherapy) that combines doctrines or methods (as therapeutic procedures) from diverse sources **2** : a system of medicine once popular in the U.S. that depended on plant remedies

E. coli \\ˌē-'kō-ˌlī\\ *n, pl* **E. coli** *also* **E. colis** : a straight rod-shaped gram-negative bacterium (*Escherichia coli* of the family Enterobacteriaceae) that is used in public health as an indicator of fecal pollution (as of water or food) and in medicine and genetics as a research organism and that occurs in various strains that may live as harmless inhabitants of the

---

\ə\ abut \ʲ\ kitten \ər\ further \a\ ash \ā\ ace \ä\ cot, cart
\aů\ out \ch\ chin \e\ bet \ē\ easy \g\ go \i\ hit \ī\ ice \j\ job
\ŋ\ sing \ō\ go \ȯ\ law \ȯi\ boy \th\ thin \th\ the \ü\ loot
\ů\ foot \y\ yet \zh\ vision   *See also* Pronunciation Symbols page

E
F

human lower intestine or may produce a toxin causing intestinal illness ⟨one million acid-resistant *E. coli* per gram of feces —John Schwartz⟩ ⟨this *E. coli* can survive . . . longer than all the other *E. colis* —Ed Geldreich⟩

ecol·o·gist \i-ˈkäl-ə-jəst, e-\ *n* : a person who specializes in ecology

ecol·o·gy \-jē\ *n, pl* **-gies** **1** : a branch of science concerned with the interrelationship of organisms and their environments **2** : the totality or pattern of relations between organisms and their environment **3** : HUMAN ECOLOGY — **eco·log·i·cal** \ˌē-kə-ˈläj-i-kəl, ˌek-ə-\ *also* **eco·log·ic** \-ik\ *adj* — **eco·log·i·cal·ly** \-i-k(ə-)lē\ *adv*

econ·o·my \i-ˈkän-ə-mē\ *n, pl* **-mies** **1** : the system of operation of the processes of anabolism and catabolism in living bodies ⟨the ∼ of the cell⟩ **2** : the body of an animal or plant as an organized whole ⟨disorganizing wide segments of the body ∼ —Leonard Engel⟩

eco·phys·i·ol·o·gy \ˌē-kō-ˌfiz-ē-ˈäl-ə-jē, ˌek-ō-\ *n, pl* **-gies** : the science of the interrelationships between the physiology of organisms and their environment — **eco·phys·i·o·log·i·cal** \-ē-ə-ˈläj-i-kəl\ *adj* — **eco·phys·i·ol·o·gist** \-ē-ˈäl-ə-jəst\ *n*

écor·ché \ˌā-ˌkȯr-ˈshā, ā-ˈkȯr-\ *n* : an anatomical illustration or manikin showing the muscles and bones that are visible with the skin removed

eco·sphere \ˈē-kō-ˌsfi(ə)r, ˈek-ō-\ *n* : the parts of the universe habitable by living organisms; *esp* : BIOSPHERE 1

eco·sys·tem \-ˌsis-təm\ *n* : the complex of a community and its environment functioning as an ecological unit in nature

eco·tox·i·col·o·gy \ˌē-kō-ˌtäk-si-ˈkäl-ə-jē, ˌek-ō-\ *n, pl* **-gies** : a scientific discipline combining the methods of ecology and toxicology in studying the effects of toxic substances and esp. pollutants on the environment — **eco·tox·i·co·log·i·cal** \-kə-ˈläj-i-kəl\ *adj* — **eco·tox·i·col·o·gist** \-ˈkäl-ə-jəst\ *n*

ec·pho·ria \ek-ˈfōr-ē-ə\ *n, pl* **-rias** *or* **-ri·ae** \-ē-ˌē\ : the rousing of an engram or system of engrams from a latent to an active state (as by repetition of the original stimulus or by mnemic excitation)

ec·pho·rize *or Brit* **ec·pho·rise** \ˈek-fə-ˌrīz\ *vt* **-rized** *or Brit* **-rised; -riz·ing** *or Brit* **-ris·ing** : to revive or rouse (an engram or system of engrams) from latency

écra·seur \ˌā-krä-ˈzər, ˌē-\ *n* : a surgical instrument containing a chain or wire loop that is used to encircle and sever a projecting mass of tissue (as the testicles of a horse or a pedicled tumor) by gradual tightening of the chain or loop

ec·sta·sy \ˈek-stə-sē\ *n, pl* **-sies** **1** : a trance state in which intense absorption (as in religious ideation) is accompanied by loss of sense perception and voluntary control **2** *often cap* : a synthetic amphetamine analog $C_{11}H_{15}NO_2$ used illicitly for its mood-enhancing and hallucinogenic properties — called also *MDMA, methylenedioxymethamphetamine, XTC* — **ec·stat·ic** \ek-ˈstat-ik\ *adj*

ECT *abbr* electroconvulsive therapy

ec·tad \ˈek-ˌtad\ *adv* : toward the outside — compare ENTAD

ec·tal \ˈek-tᵊl\ *adj* : situated in an exterior or outer position — compare ENTAL

ec·ta·sia \ek-ˈtā-zh(ē-)ə\ *n* : the expansion of a hollow or tubular organ

ec·ta·sis \ˈek-tə-səs\ *n, pl* **-ta·ses** \-ˌsēz\ : ECTASIA

¹ect·eth·moid \ek-ˈteth-ˌmȯid\ *n* : either of two lateral parts of the ethmoid bone that form part of the anterior wall of the orbit

²ectethmoid *adj* : lateral or external to the ethmoid bone

ec·thy·ma \ek-ˈthī-mə\ *n* **1** : a cutaneous eruption marked by large flat pustules that have a hardened base surrounded by inflammation, heal with pigmented scar formation, and occur esp. on the lower legs — **ec·thy·ma·tous** \ek-ˈthim-ət-əs, -ˈthīm-\ *adj*

ec·to·blast \ˈek-tə-ˌblast\ *n* : EPIBLAST — **ec·to·blas·tic** \ˌek-tə-ˈblas-tik\ *adj*

ec·to·car·dia \ˌek-tō-ˈkär-dē-ə\ *n* : abnormal position of the heart

ec·to·chon·dral \-ˈkän-drəl\ *adj* : on the surface of cartilage ⟨an ∼ lesion⟩ ⟨∼ bone formation⟩

ec·to·com·men·sal \-kə-ˈmen(t)-səl\ *adj* : living as a commensal on the body surface of another ⟨∼ protozoans⟩

ec·to·cor·nea \ˌek-tō-ˈkȯr-nē-ə\ *n* : the external layer of the cornea

ec·to·crine \ˈek-tə-krən, -ˌkrīn, -ˌkrēn\ *n* : a metabolite produced by an organism of one kind and utilized by one of another kind

ec·to·cyst \ˈek-tə-ˌsist\ *n* : the external layer of a hydatid cyst

ec·to·derm \ˈek-tə-ˌdərm\ *n* **1** : the outermost of the three primary germ layers of an embryo **2** : a tissue (as neural tissue) derived from ectoderm — **ec·to·der·mal** \ˌek-tə-ˈdər-məl\ *adj*

ec·to·en·zyme \ˌek-tō-ˈen-ˌzīm\ *n* : an enzyme acting outside the cell

ec·to·gen·ic \ˌek-tə-ˈjen-ik\ *adj* : ECTOGENOUS

ec·tog·e·nous \ek-ˈtäj-ə-nəs\ *adj* : capable of development apart from the host — used chiefly of pathogenic bacteria

ec·to·hor·mone \ˌek-tə-ˈhȯr-ˌmōn\ *n* : PHEROMONE — **ec·to·hor·mon·al** \-hȯr-ˈmōn-ᵊl\ *adj*

ec·to·mere \ˈek-tə-ˌmi(ə)r\ *n* : a blastomere destined to form ectoderm — **ec·to·mer·ic** \ˌek-tə-ˈmer-ik, -ˈmi(ə)r-\ *adj*

ec·to·morph \ˈek-tə-ˌmȯrf\ *n* : an ectomorphic individual

ec·to·mor·phic \ˌek-tə-ˈmȯr-fik\ *adj* **1** : of or relating to the component in W. H. Sheldon's classification of body types that measures the body's degree of slenderness, angularity, and fragility **2** : having a light body build — compare ENDOMORPHIC 2, MESOMORPHIC 2b — **ec·to·mor·phy** \ˈek-tə-ˌmȯr-fē\ *n, pl* **-phies**

ec·to·par·a·site \ˌek-tō-ˈpar-ə-ˌsīt\ *n* : a parasite that lives on the exterior of its host — compare ENDOPARASITE — **ec·to·par·a·sit·ic** \-ˌpar-ə-ˈsit-ik\ *adj*

ec·to·phyte \ˈek-tə-ˌfīt\ *n* : an ectoparasitic plant — **ec·to·phyt·ic** \ˌek-tə-ˈfit-ik\ *adj*

ec·to·pia \ek-ˈtō-pē-ə\ *n* : an abnormal congenital or acquired position of an organ or part ⟨∼ of the heart⟩

ec·top·ic \ek-ˈtäp-ik\ *adj* **1** : occurring in an abnormal position ⟨an ∼ kidney⟩ — compare ENTOPIC **2** : originating in an area of the heart other than the sinoatrial node ⟨∼ beats⟩; *also* : initiating ectopic heartbeats ⟨an ∼ pacemaker⟩ — **ec·top·i·cal·ly** \-i-k(ə-)lē\ *adv*

ectopic pregnancy *n* : gestation elsewhere than in the uterus (as in a fallopian tube or in the peritoneal cavity) — called also *ectopic gestation, extrauterine gestation, extrauterine pregnancy*

ec·to·pla·cen·ta \ˌek-tō-plə-ˈsent-ə\ *n* : TROPHOBLAST — **ec·to·pla·cen·tal** \-ˈsent-ᵊl\ *adj*

ec·to·plasm \ˈek-tə-ˌplaz-əm\ *n* : the outer relatively rigid granule-free layer of the cytoplasm usu. held to be a gel reversibly convertible to a sol — compare ENDOPLASM — **ec·to·plas·mic** \ˌek-tə-ˈplaz-mik\ *adj*

ec·to·py \ˈek-tə-pē\ *n, pl* **-pies** : ECTOPIA

ec·to·sarc \ˈek-tə-ˌsärk\ *n* : the semisolid external layer of protoplasm in some unicellular organisms (as the ameba) : ECTOPLASM — **ec·to·sar·cous** \ˌek-tə-ˈsär-kəs\ *adj*

ect·os·te·al \ek-ˈtäs-tē-əl\ *adj* : of or relating to the surface of a bone — **ect·os·te·al·ly** \-ē\ *adv*

ec·to·therm \ˈek-tə-ˌthərm\ *n* : a cold-blooded animal : POIKILOTHERM — **ec·to·ther·mic** \ˌek-tə-ˈthər-mik\ *adj*

ec·to·ther·my \-ˌthər-mē\ *n, pl* **-mies** : POIKILOTHERMISM

¹ec·to·thrix \ˈek-tə-ˌthriks\ *n* : an ectothrix fungus of the genus *Microsporum* or *Trichophyton*

²ectothrix *adj* : occurring on the surface of the hair shaft ⟨∼ fungi⟩; *also* : characterized by the presence of hyphae or arthroconidia on the surface of the hair shaft ⟨∼ tinea capitis⟩ — compare ENDOTHRIX

Ec·to·zoa \ˌek-tə-ˈzō-ə\ *n pl* : external animal parasites — often used as if a taxon

ec·tro·dac·tyl·ia \ˌek-trō-dak-ˈtil-ē-ə\ *n* : ECTRODACTYLY

ec·tro·dac·tyl·ism \-ˈdak-tə-ˌliz-əm\ *n* : ECTRODACTYLY

ec·tro·dac·ty·ly \-ˈdak-tə-lē\ *n, pl* **-lies** : congenital complete or partial absence of one or more digits — **ec·tro·dac·ty·lous** \-tə-ləs\ *adj*

ec·tro·me·lia \ˌek-trō-ˈmē-lē-ə\ *n* **1** : congenital absence or imperfection of one or more limbs **2** : MOUSEPOX — **ec·tro·me·lic** \-ˈmē-lik\ *adj*

ec·tro·pi·on \ek-ˈtrō-pē-ˌän, -pē-ən\ *n* : an abnormal turning out of a part (as an eyelid)

ec·tro·pi·um \-pē-əm\ *n* : ECTROPION

ec·ze·ma \ig-ˈzē-mə, ˈeg-zə-mə, ˈek-sə-\ *n* : an inflammatory condition of the skin characterized by redness, itching, and oozing vesicular lesions which become scaly, crusted, or hardened — **ec·zem·a·tous** \ig-ˈzem-ət-əs\ *adj*

ec·ze·ma·ti·za·tion \ig-ˌzē-mət-ə-ˈzā-shən, -ˌzem-ət-\ *n* : an eczematous skin lesion complicating a dermatitis that is not eczematous

ec·ze·ma·toid \ig-ˈzē-mə-ˌtȯid, -ˈzem-ə-\ *adj* : resembling eczema

ED *abbr* **1** effective dose **2** emergency department **3** erectile dysfunction **4** erythema dose

EDB *abbr* ethylene dibromide

ede·ma *or chiefly Brit* **oe·de·ma** \i-ˈdē-mə\ *n, pl* **-mas** *also* **-ma·ta** \-mət-ə\ : an abnormal excess accumulation of serous fluid in connective tissue or in a serous cavity — called also *dropsy*

edem·a·tous *or chiefly Brit* **oe·dem·a·tous** \-ˈdem-ət-əs\ *adj* : affected with edema ⟨an ~ patient⟩ ⟨an ~ lung⟩

Eden·ta·ta \ˌē-den-ˈtät-ə, -ˈtāt-\ *n pl* : an order of the major taxon Eutheria comprising mammals with few or no teeth and including the sloths, armadillos, and New World anteaters and formerly also the pangolins and the aardvark

¹eden·tate \(ˈ)ē-ˈden-ˌtāt\ *adj* **1** : lacking teeth **2** : being an edentate

²edentate *n* : any mammal of the order Edentata — called also *xenarthran*

eden·tu·lous \(ˈ)ē-ˈden-chə-ləs\ *adj* : TOOTHLESS

edes·tin \i-ˈdes-tən\ *n* : a crystalline globulin obtained esp. from hemp seed that contains all of the essential amino acids

edetate — see DISODIUM EDETATE

Ed·ing·er–West·phal nucleus \ˌed-iŋ-ər-ˌwest-ˌfäl-, -ˌfȯl-\ *n* : the lateral portion of the group of nerve cells lying ventral to the aqueduct of Sylvius which give rise to the autonomic fibers of the oculomotor nerve supplying the ciliary muscle and the sphincter pupillae

Ed·ing·er \ˈed-iŋ-ər\, **Ludwig (1855–1918),** German neurologist. In 1885 Edinger described for the first time a nucleus beneath the aqueduct of Sylvius that gives rise to some of the fibers of the oculomotor nerve.

West·phal \ˈwest-ˌfäl, -ˌfȯl\, **Carl Friedrich Otto (1833–1890),** German neurologist. In 1887 Westphal presented his description of the nucleus described earlier by Edinger. Since Westphal's description is more complete, he has been accorded equal credit with Edinger, and the nucleus is now usually known as the Edinger-Westphal nucleus.

EDR *abbr* electrodermal response

ed·ro·pho·ni·um \ˌed-rə-ˈfō-nē-əm\ *n* : an anticholinesterase C₁₀H₁₆ClNO used esp. to stimulate skeletal muscle and in the diagnosis of myasthenia gravis — called also *edrophonium chloride;* see TENSILON

EDTA \ˌē-ˌdē-ˌtē-ˈā\ *n* : a white crystalline acid C₁₀H₁₆N₂O₈ used in medicine as an anticoagulant and as a chelator in the treatment of lead poisoning — called also *ethylenediaminetetraacetic acid*

ed·u·ca·ble \ˈej-ə-kə-bəl\ *adj* : affected with mild mental retardation and capable of developing academic, social, and occupational skills within the capabilities of one with a mental age between 9 and 12 years — compare TRAINABLE

ed·u·ca·tion·al age \ˌej-ə-ˌkā-shnəl-, -shən-ᵊl-\ *n* : ACHIEVEMENT AGE

Edwards syndrome \ˈed-wərdz-\ *n* : TRISOMY 18

Edwards, John Hilton (*b* 1928), British geneticist. Edwards served as professor of human genetics at Birmingham University from 1969 to 1979 and at Oxford University from 1979 to 1995. He was the author of *Human Genetics* (1978) as well as numerous papers on a variety of topics in the field. His discovery of trisomy 18 in 1960 led to the association of his name with the syndrome.

EEE *abbr* eastern equine encephalomyelitis

EEG *abbr* electroencephalogram; electroencephalograph

eel·worm \ˈēl-ˌwərm\ *n* : a nematode worm; *esp* : any of various small free-living or plant-parasitic roundworms

EENT *abbr* eye, ear, nose, and throat

ef·face·ment \i-ˈfās-mənt, e-\ *n* : obliteration of the uterine cervix by shortening and softening during labor so that only the external orifice remains — **ef·face** \-ˈfās\ *vt* **ef·faced; ef·fac·ing**

ef·fect \i-ˈfekt\ *n* : something that is produced by an agent or cause ⟨obtained the same ~ with a smaller dose⟩

ef·fec·tive \i-ˈfek-tiv\ *adj* : producing a decided, decisive, claimed, or desired effect ⟨a drug judged ~ by an evaluating panel⟩ — **ef·fec·tive·ly** *adv* — **ef·fec·tive·ness** *n*

ef·fec·tor \i-ˈfek-tər, -ˌtȯ(ə)r\ *n* **1** : a bodily organ (as a gland or muscle) that becomes active in response to stimulation **2** : a molecule (as an inducer, a corepressor, or an enzyme) that activates, controls, or inactivates a process or action (as protein synthesis or the release of a second messenger)

effector cell *n* : a lymphocyte (as a T cell) that has been induced to differentiate into a form (as a cytotoxic T cell) capable of mounting a specific immune response — called also *effector lymphocyte*

ef·fem·i·na·tion \ə-ˌfem-ə-ˈnā-shən\ *n* : the taking on by a man of the mental characteristics (as passivity) traditionally associated with women

¹ef·fer·ent \ˈef-ə-rənt; ˈef-ˌer-ənt, ˈē-ˌfer-\ *adj* : conducting outward from a part or organ; *specif* : conveying nervous impulses to an effector ⟨~ neurons⟩ — compare AFFERENT — **ef·fer·ent·ly** *adv*

²efferent *n* : an efferent part (as a blood vessel or nerve fiber)

efferentes — see DUCTULI EFFERENTES

efferentia — see VASA EFFERENTIA

ef·fer·vesce \ˌef-ər-ˈves\ *vi* **-vesced; -vesc·ing** : to bubble, hiss, and foam as gas escapes — **ef·fer·ves·cence** \-ˈves-ᵊn(t)s\ *n* — **ef·fer·ves·cent** \-ᵊnt\ *adj*

Ef·fex·or \ə-ˈfek-ˌsȯr\ *trademark* — used for a preparation of the hydrochloride of venlafaxine

ef·fleu·rage \ˌef-lə-ˈräzh, -(ˌ)lü-\ *n* : a light stroking movement used in massage

ef·flo·resce \ˌef-lə-ˈres\ *vi* **-resced; -resc·ing** : to change to a powder from loss of water of crystallization

ef·flo·res·cence \ˌef-lə-ˈres-ᵊn(t)s\ *n* **1** : the process of efflorescing; *also* : the powder or crust so formed **2** : a redness of the skin or an eruption (as in a rash) — **ef·flo·res·cent** \-ᵊnt\ *adj*

ef·flu·vi·um \e-ˈflü-vē-əm\ *n, pl* **-via** \-vē-ə\ *or* **-vi·ums** : an invisible emanation; *esp* : an offensive exhalation or smell — the form *effluvia* often used with a singular verb

ef·flux \ˈef-ˌləks\ *n* **1** : something that is given off in or as if in a stream ⟨the red-blood-cell sodium ion ~⟩ **2** : the action or process of flowing or seeming to flow out ⟨the uptake and ~ of sodium ions⟩

effort syndrome \ˈef-ərt-, -ˌȯ(ə)rt-\ *n* : NEUROCIRCULATORY ASTHENIA

ef·fuse \i-ˈfyüs, e-\ *adj* : spread out flat without definite form ⟨an ~ colony of bacteria⟩

ef·fu·sion \i-ˈfyü-zhən, e-\ *n* **1 a** : the escape of a fluid from anatomical vessels by rupture or exudation **b** : the flow of a gas through an aperture whose diameter is small as compared with the distance between the molecules of the gas **2** : the fluid that escapes by extravasation — see PLEURAL EFFUSION

eges·ta \i-ˈjes-tə\ *n pl* : something egested

eges·tion \i-ˈjes(h)-chən\ *n* : the act or process of discharging undigested or waste material from a cell or organism; *specif* : DEFECATION — **egest** \i-ˈjest\ *vt* — **eges·tive** \-ˈjes-tiv\ *adj*

EGF *abbr* epidermal growth factor

\ə\ **abut** \ᵊ\ **kitten** \ər\ **further** \a\ **ash** \ā\ **ace** \ä\ **cot, cart** \aᵫ\ **out** \ch\ **chin** \e\ **bet** \ē\ **easy** \g\ **go** \i\ **hit** \ī\ **ice** \j\ **job** \ŋ\ **sing** \ō\ **go** \ȯ\ **law** \ȯi\ **boy** \th\ **thin** \t͟h\ **the** \ü\ **loot** \ᵫ\ **foot** \y\ **yet** \zh\ **vision** *See also* Pronunciation Symbols page

egg \'eg, 'āg\ *n* **1** : the hard-shelled reproductive body produced by a bird and esp. by the common domestic chicken (*Gallus gallus*) **2** : an animal reproductive body consisting of an ovum together with its nutritive and protective envelopes and having the capacity to develop into a new individual capable of independent existence **3** : OVUM

egg albumin *n* : the albumin of eggs; *esp* : OVALBUMIN

egg cell *n* : OVUM

egg·shell \'eg-ˌshel, 'āg-\ *n* : the hard exterior covering of an egg

eggshell nail *n* : a thin fingernail turning up at the outer edge seen in some diseases and nutritional disorders

egg–white injury \ˌeg-ˌ(h)wīt-, ˌāg-\ *n* : a vitamin-deficiency disease observed chiefly in animals that is induced by feeding upon an excess of raw egg white

ego \'ē-ˌ(ˌ)gō *also* 'eg-(ˌ)ō\ *n, pl* **egos** **1** : the self esp. as contrasted with another self or the world **2** : the one of the three divisions of the psyche in psychoanalytic theory that serves as the organized conscious mediator between the person and reality esp. by functioning both in the perception of and adaptation to reality — compare ¹ID, SUPEREGO

¹ego·cen·tric \ˌē-gō-'sen-trik *also* ˌeg-ō-\ *adj* **1** : limited in outlook or concern to one's own activities or needs **2** : being self-centered or selfish — **ego·cen·tri·cal·ly** \-tri-k(ə-)lē\ *adv*

²egocentric *n* : an egocentric individual

ego·cen·tric·i·ty \ˌē-gō-(ˌ)sen-'tris-ət-ē, -sən- *also* ˌeg-ō-\ *n, pl* **-ties** : the quality or state of being egocentric

ego·cen·trism \-'sen-ˌtriz-əm\ *n* **1** : EGOCENTRICITY **2** : the effort to get personal recognition esp. by socially unacceptable behavior

ego–de·fense *or chiefly Brit* **ego–de·fence** \ˌē-(ˌ)gō-di-'fen(t)s *also* ˌeg-(ˌ)ō-\ *n* : DEFENSE MECHANISM 1

ego–dys·ton·ic \-dis-'tän-ik\ *adj* : incompatible with or unacceptable to the ego — compare EGO-SYNTONIC

ego ideal *n* : the positive standards, ideals, and ambitions that according to psychoanalytic theory are assimilated from the superego

ego–in·volve·ment \-in-'välv-mənt, -'vȯlv-\ *n* : an involvement of one's self-esteem in the performance of a task or in an object — **ego–in·volve** \-'välv, -'vȯlv\ *vt* **-volved; -volving**

ego·ism \'ē-gə-ˌwiz-əm *also* 'eg-ə-\ *n* **1 a** : a doctrine that individual self-interest is the actual motive of all conscious action **b** : a doctrine that individual self-interest is the valid end of all actions **2** : excessive concern for oneself without exaggerated feelings of self-importance — compare EGOTISM — **ego·ist** \-wəst\ *n* — **ego·is·tic** \ˌē-gə-'wis-tik *also* ˌeg-ə-\ *also* **ego·is·ti·cal** \-ti-kəl\ *adj* — **ego·is·ti·cal·ly** \-ti-k(ə-)lē\ *adv*

egoistic hedonism *n* : the ethical theory that the valid aim of right conduct is one's own happiness

ego–libido *n* : libido directed toward the self — compare OBJECT LIBIDO

ego·ma·nia \ˌē-gō-'mā-nē-ə, -nyə\ *n* : the quality or state of being extremely egocentric

ego·ma·ni·ac \-nē-ˌak\ *n* : one characterized by egomania — **ego·ma·ni·a·cal** \-mə-'nī-ə-kəl\ *adj* — **ego·ma·ni·a·cal·ly** \-k(ə-)lē\ *adv*

egoph·o·ny *or chiefly Brit* **ae·goph·o·ny** \ē-'gäf-ə-nē\ *n, pl* **-nies** : a modification of the voice resembling bleating heard on auscultation of the chest in some diseases (as in pleurisy with effusion)

ego–syn·ton·ic \ˌē-gō-sin-'tän-ik *also* ˌeg-ō-\ *adj* : compatible with or acceptable to the ego — compare EGO-DYSTONIC

ego·tism \'ē-gə-ˌtiz-əm *also* 'eg-ə-\ *n* : an exaggerated sense of self-importance — compare EGOISM 2

ego·tist \-təst\ *n* : one characterized by egotism — **ego·tis·tic** \ˌē-gə-'tis-tik *also* ˌeg-ə-\ *or* **ego·tis·ti·cal** \-'tis-ti-kəl\ *adj* — **ego·tis·ti·cal·ly** \-'tis-ti-k(ə-)lē\ *adv*

Eh *symbol* standard oxidation-reduction potential

EHBF *abbr* extrahepatic blood flow

Eh·lers–Dan·los syndrome \'ā-lərz-'dan-(ˌ)läs-\ *n* : an inherited disorder of connective tissue with several clinical forms characterized esp. by extremely flexible joints, elastic skin, and excessive bruising

Eh·lers \'ā-(ˌ)lerz\, **Edvard L.** (1863–1937), Danish dermatologist. Ehlers can claim priority in recognizing Ehlers=Danlos syndrome, having reported the disorder in 1901.
Dan·los \däⁿ-lō\, **Henri–Alexandre** (1844–1912), French dermatologist. In 1908 Danlos published his own description of the syndrome to which his name and Ehlers' have become attached.

Ehr·lich·ia \er-'lik-ē-ə\ *n* : a genus of gram-negative nonmotile rickettsial bacteria that are intracellular parasites infecting the cytoplasm esp. of circulating white blood cells (as monocytes and granulocytes), that are transmitted chiefly by tick bites, and that are pathogens of animals and humans

Ehr·lich \'er-ˌlik\, **Paul** (1854–1915), German chemist and bacteriologist. Ehrlich is celebrated for his pioneering research in hematology, immunology, and chemotherapy. He held a series of research positions at several institutions, including Berlin's Charité Hospital, Robert Koch's Institute for Infectious Diseases, and Frankfurt's Royal Institute for Experimental Therapy. His contributions included the invention of a new staining technique for the tuberculosis bacillus discovered by Robert Koch. The technique proved to be vitally important for the microscopic diagnosis of tuberculosis. Ehrlich is also credited with the important discovery that oxygen consumption varies with different types of tissue and that these variations constitute a measure of the intensity of vital cell processes. Perhaps his greatest achievement was his investigation into the mechanisms of bacterial infection and immunity. He developed a method for measuring the effectiveness of sera that was adopted worldwide for the standardization of diphtheria serum. His recognition of the limitations of serum therapy led to his search for synthesized substances that can kill parasites or inhibit their growth without damaging the organism. His researches marked the birth of chemotherapy. His study of the spirochete (*Treponema pallidum*) that causes syphilis led to his discovery of salvarsan, the first effective treatment for syphilis. With Élie Metchnikoff, he was awarded the 1908 Nobel Prize for Physiology or Medicine.

ehr·lich·i·o·sis \er-ˌlik-ē-'ō-sis\ *n, pl* **-o·ses** \-ˌsēz\ : infection with or a disease caused by rickettsial bacteria of the genus *Ehrlichia*

EIA *abbr* **1** enzyme immunoassay **2** equine infectious anemia **3** exercise-induced asthma

ei·co·sa·noid \ī-'kō-sə-ˌnȯid\ *n* : any of a class of compounds (as the prostaglandins, leukotrienes, and thromboxanes) derived from polyunsaturated fatty acids (as arachidonic acid) and involved in cellular activity

ei·co·sa·pen·ta·e·no·ic acid \ˌī-kō-sə-ˌpen-tə-ē-ˌnō-ik-, -iˌnō-ik-\ *n* : an omega-3 fatty acid $C_{20}H_{30}O_2$ found esp. in fish oils — abbr. *EPA*

ei·det·ic \ī-'det-ik\ *adj* : marked by or involving extraordinarily accurate and vivid recall esp. of visual images ⟨an ∼ memory⟩ — **ei·det·i·cal·ly** \-i-k(ə-)lē\ *adv*

eighth cranial nerve \'ātth-\ *n* : AUDITORY NERVE

eighth nerve *n* : AUDITORY NERVE

Eijk·man test \'āk-mən-, 'īk-\ *n* : a test for the identification of coliform bacteria from warm-blooded animals based on the bacteria's ability to produce gas when grown in glucose media at 46°C (114.8°F)

Eijkman, Christiaan (1858–1930), Dutch physiologist. Eijkman introduced his test for coliform bacteria in a 1904 paper. His most important work, however, concerned the etiology of beriberi. While in the Dutch East Indies, he studied fowl affected with polyneuritis, a condition similar to beriberi, and discovered in 1897 that the disease was caused by a diet of polished rice. A cure was effected by restoring the discarded hulls to the diet. In 1929 Eijkman was awarded the Nobel Prize for Physiology or Medicine.

ei·ko·nom·e·ter \ˌī-kə-'näm-ət-ər\ *n* : a device to detect aniseikonia or to test stereoscopic vision

Ei·me·ria \ī-'mir-ē-ə\ *n* : a genus of coccidian protozoans that invade the visceral epithelia and esp. the intestinal wall of many vertebrates and some invertebrates and that include serious pathogens — **ei·me·ri·an** \-ē-ən\ *adj or n*

Ei·mer \ˈī-mər\, **Theodor Gustav Heinrich (1843–1898)**, German zoologist. Eimer is known largely for his opposition to the Darwinian theory of natural selection. He held that variation in organisms occurred not by chance but according to the mechanism of orthogenesis.

Ei·me·ri·idae \ˌī-mə-ˈrī-ə-ˌdē\ *n pl* : a family of protozoans of the order Coccidia that includes the genera *Eimeria* and *Isospora* of medical and veterinary importance

ein·stein \ˈīn-ˌstīn\ *n* : the radiant energy of a given frequency required to effect the complete photochemical transformation of one mole of a photosensitive substance being equal to about 0.004 erg second times the frequency in question

Ein·stein \ˈīn-ˌstīn, -ˌshtīn\, **Albert (1879–1955)**, American (German-born) physicist. Einstein is generally regarded as one of the very greatest scientists in history. His ideas and speculations have brought about the most profound revolution in scientific thought since Copernicus. In 1905 he published four great discoveries in theoretical physics: the special theory of relativity, the equivalence of mass and energy, the theory of Brownian motion, and the foundation of the photon theory of light. His famous special theory of relativity merged the traditionally absolute concepts of space and time into a space of four dimensions. In 1916 he advanced his general theory of relativity, which was substantiated by other scientists in 1919. In 1950 he introduced a merger of quantum theory with the general theory of relativity, thereby establishing one set of determinate laws for subatomic phenomena and large-scale physical phenomena. In 1952 the element einsteinium was identified by researchers at Berkeley, California, and named in his honor. Einstein was awarded the Nobel Prize for Physics in 1921.

ein·stei·ni·um \īn-ˈstī-nē-əm\ *n* : a radioactive element produced artificially — symbol *Es*; see ELEMENT table

Ei·sen·meng·er's complex \ˈī-zən-ˌmeŋ-ərz-, -sən-\ *or* **Ei·sen·meng·er complex** \-ər-\ *n* : the combination of a congenital defect in the septum between the ventricles of the heart with its early complications that include left to right blood flow through the defect, increased blood pressure in the pulmonary arteries, and hypertrophy of the right ventricle

Eisenmenger, Victor (1864–1932), German physician. Eisenmenger described Eisenmenger's complex in an article published in 1897.

Eisenmenger's syndrome *also* **Eisenmenger syndrome** *n* : the congenital septal defect of Eisenmenger's complex with its later complications that are essentially surgically irreversible and include damage to the small vessels of the lung, hypertension in the pulmonary arteries, right to left blood flow through the septal defect, marked hypertrophy of the right ventricle, and cyanosis

ejacula *pl of* EJACULUM

¹ejac·u·late \i-ˈjak-yə-ˌlāt\ *vb* **-lat·ed; -lat·ing** *vt* **1** : to eject from a living body; *specif* : to eject (semen) in orgasm ~ *vi* : to eject a fluid (as semen) — **ejac·u·la·tor** \-ˌlāt-ər\ *n*

²ejac·u·late \-lət\ *n* : the semen released by one ejaculation

ejac·u·la·tion \i-ˌjak-yə-ˈlā-shən\ *n* : the act or process of ejaculating; *specif* : the sudden or spontaneous discharging of a fluid (as semen in orgasm) from a duct — see PREMATURE EJACULATION

ejac·u·la·tio prae·cox \-ˈlā-sh(ē-)ō-ˈprē-ˌkäks\ *n* : PREMATURE EJACULATION

ejaculatorius — see DUCTUS EJACULATORIUS

ejac·u·la·to·ry \i-ˈjak-yə-lə-ˌtōr-ē, -ˌtȯr-\ *adj* : casting or throwing out; *specif* : associated with or concerned in physiological ejaculation ⟨~ vessels⟩

ejaculatory duct *n* : either of the paired ducts in the human male that are formed by the junction of the duct from the seminal vesicle with the vas deferens, pass through the prostate, and open into or close to the prostatic utricle — called also *ductus ejaculatorius*

ejac·u·lum \i-ˈjak-yə-ləm\ *n, pl* **-u·la** \-lə\ : EJACULATE

eject \i-ˈjekt\ *vt* : to force out or expel from within ⟨blood ~ed from the heart —S. F. Mason⟩ — **ejec·tion** \-ˈjek-shən\ *n*

ejec·ta \i-ˈjek-tə\ *n* : matter (as vomit) ejected from the body

ejection fraction *n* : the ratio of the volume of blood the heart empties during systole to the volume of blood in the heart at the end of diastole expressed as a percentage usu. between 50 and 80 percent

ejec·tor \i-ˈjek-tər\ *n* : something that ejects — see SALIVA EJECTOR

eka·io·dine \ˌek-ə-ˈī-ə-ˌdīn, ˌā-kə-, -əd-ən, -ə-ˌdēn\ *n* : ASTATINE

EKG \ˌē-ˌkā-ˈjē\ *n* **1** : ELECTROCARDIOGRAM **2** : ELECTROCARDIOGRAPH

elab·o·rate \i-ˈlab-ə-ˌrāt\ *vt* **-rat·ed; -rat·ing** *of a living organism* : to alter the chemical makeup of (as a foodstuff) to one more suited to bodily needs (as of assimilation or excretion); *esp* : to build up (complex organic compounds) from simple ingredients ⟨the toxin *elaborated* by the tetanus bacterium⟩

elab·o·ra·tion \i-ˌlab-ə-ˈrā-shən\ *n* **1** : the act or process of elaborating ⟨the ~ of toxic substances⟩ **2** : psychic interpretation or amplification of the content of dreams and other unconscious processes

elaeoptene *chiefly Brit var of* ELEOPTENE

el·a·id·ic acid \ˌel-ə-ˌid-ik-\ *n* : a white crystalline unsaturated acid $C_{17}H_{33}COOH$ obtained from oleic acid by isomerization

ela·i·din \ə-ˈlā-əd-ən\ *n* : a glycerol ester of elaidic acid

Elap·i·dae \ə-ˈlap-ə-ˌdē\ *n pl* : a family of venomous snakes with hollow fangs found in the warmer parts of both hemispheres and including the cobras and mambas, the coral snakes of the New World, and the majority of Australian snakes — **elap·id** \-ˈlap-əd\ *adj or n*

elas·mo·branch \i-ˈlaz-mə-ˌbraŋk\ *n, pl* **-branchs** : any fish of the class Chondrichthyes — **elasmobranch** *adj*

Elas·mo·bran·chii \i-ˌlaz-mə-ˈbraŋ-kē-ˌī\ *n pl, syn of* CHONDRICHTHYES

elas·tase \i-ˈlas-ˌtās, -ˌtāz\ *n* : an enzyme esp. of pancreatic juice that digests elastin

¹elas·tic \i-ˈlas-tik\ *adj* **1 a** *of a solid* : capable of recovering size and shape after deformation **b** *of a liquid* : capable of resisting compression **c** *of a gas* : capable of indefinite expansion **2** : capable of being easily stretched or expanded and resuming former shape — **elas·ti·cal·ly** \-ti-k(ə-)lē\ *adv*

²elastic *n* **1 a** : easily stretched rubber usu. prepared in cords, strings, or bands **b** : a band of elastic used esp. in orthodontics; *also* : one placed around a tooth at the gumline in effecting its nonsurgical removal **2 a** : an elastic fabric usu. made of yarns containing rubber **b** : something made from this fabric

elas·ti·ca \i-ˈlas-tik-ə\ *n* : either of two layers of elastic tissue present in the walls of most arteries: **a** : an inner layer between the intima and media **b** : an outer layer between the media and adventitia

elastic cartilage *n* : a yellowish flexible cartilage having the matrix infiltrated in all directions by a network of elastic fibers and occurring chiefly in the external ear, eustachian tube, and some cartilages of the larynx and epiglottis

elastic fiber *n* : a thick very elastic smooth yellowish anastomosing fiber of connective tissue that contains elastin

elas·tic·i·ty \i-ˌlas-ˈtis-ət-ē, ˌē-ˌlas-, -ˈtis-tē\ *n, pl* **-ties** : the quality or state of being elastic

elastic stocking *n* : a stocking woven or knitted with an elastic material (as rubber) and used (as in the treatment of varicose veins) to provide support for the leg

elastic tissue *n* : tissue consisting chiefly of elastic fibers that is found esp. in some ligaments and tendons

elasticum — see PSEUDOXANTHOMA ELASTICUM

\ə\ abut \ᵊ\ kitten \ər\ further \a\ ash \ā\ ace \ä\ cot, cart
\au̇\ out \ch\ chin \e\ bet \ē\ easy \g\ go \i\ hit \ī\ ice \j\ job
\ŋ\ sing \ō\ go \ȯ\ law \ȯi\ boy \th\ thin \t͟h\ the \ü\ loot
\u̇\ foot \y\ yet \zh\ vision *See also* Pronunciation Symbols page

elas·tin \i-ˈlas-tən\ *n* : a protein that is similar to collagen and is the chief constituent of elastic fibers

elas·to·lyt·ic \i-ˌlas-tə-ˈlit-ik\ *adj* : having a catalytic effect on the digestion of elastic tissue

elas·tom·e·ter \i-ˌlas-ˈtäm-ət-ər\ *n* : an instrument for measuring elasticity (as of body tissues) — **elas·tom·e·try** \i-ˌlas-ˈtäm-ə-trē\ *n, pl* **-tries**

Elas·to·plast \i-ˈlast-ə-ˌplast\ *trademark* — used for an elastic adhesive bandage used as a dressing or support (as a cast or a corset)

elas·to·sis \i-ˌlas-ˈtō-səs\ *n, pl* **-to·ses** \-ˌsēz\ : a condition marked by loss of elasticity of the skin in elderly people due to degeneration of connective tissue

ela·tion \i-ˈlā-shən\ *n* : pathological euphoria sometimes accompanied by intense pleasure — **elat·ed** \-ˈlāt-əd\ *adj*

El·a·vil \ˈel-ə-ˌvil\ *trademark* — used for a preparation of amitriptyline

el·bow \ˈel-ˌbō\ *n* **1** : the joint between the human forearm and the upper arm that supports the outer curve of the arm when bent — called also *elbow joint* **2** : a joint in the anterior limb of a lower vertebrate corresponding to the elbow

el·der \ˈel-dər\ *n* : ELDERBERRY 2

el·der·ber·ry \ˈel-də(r)-ˌber-ē\ *n, pl* **-ries** **1** : the edible black or red berrylike drupe of a tree or shrub of the genus *Sambucus* that is eaten raw or processed into preserves or wines **2** : any tree or shrub of the genus *Sambucus* including several whose flowers or fruits were once considered to have medicinal properties — see BOURTREE, SAMBUCUS 2

el·der·care \ˈel-dər-ˌka(ə)r, -ˌke(ə)r\ *n* : the care of older persons and esp. the care of an older parent by a son or daughter

elec *abbr* electric; electrical; electricity

ele·cam·pane \ˌel-i-ˌkam-ˈpān\ *n* **1** : a large coarse European composite herb of the genus *Inula* (*I. helenium*) that has yellow ray flowers, is naturalized in the U.S., and is the source of the stimulant inula **2** : INULA 1

elecampane root *n* : INULA 1

elec·tive \i-ˈlek-tiv\ *adj* : beneficial to the patient but not essential for survival ⟨an ∼ appendectomy⟩

Elec·tra complex \i-ˌlek-trə-\ *n* : the Oedipus complex when it occurs in a female

    Elec·tra \i-ˈlek-trə\, Greek mythological character. Electra was the daughter of Agamemnon and Clytemnestra and the sister of Orestes. After the murder of their father by their mother and her lover, the brother and sister conspired to murder the two lovers. The Electra complex is so named because of Electra's intense devotion to her father.

elec·tric \i-ˈlek-trik\ *or* **elec·tri·cal** \-tri-kəl\ *adj* : of, relating to, or operated by electricity — **elec·tri·cal·ly** \-tri-k(ə-)lē\ *adv*

electrical potential *or* **electric potential** *n* : the potential energy of a unit positive charge at a point in an electric field that is reckoned as the work which would be required to move the charge to its location in the electric field from an arbitrary point having zero potential (as one at infinite distance from all electric charges) and that is roughly analogous to the potential energy at a given elevation in a gravitational field

electric eel *n* : a large eel-shaped bony fish (*Electrophorus electricus* of the family Electrophoridae) of the Orinoco and Amazon basins that is capable of giving a severe shock with electricity generated by a special tract of tissue

electric field *n* : a region associated with a distribution of electric charge or a varying magnetic field in which forces due to that charge or field act upon other electric charges

electric intensity *n* : the strength of an electric field at any point as measured by the force exerted upon a unit positive charge placed at that point

elec·tric·i·ty \i-ˌlek-ˈtris-ət-ē, -ˈtris-tē\ *n, pl* **-ties** **1 a** : a fundamental entity of nature consisting of negative and positive kinds, observable in the attractions and repulsions of bodies electrified by friction and in natural phenomena (as lightning or the aurora borealis), and usu. utilized in the form of electric currents   **b** : electric current or power   **2** : a science that deals with the phenomena and laws of electricity

electric organ *n* : a specialized tract of tissue (as in the electric eel) in which electricity is generated

electric ray *n* : any of various round-bodied short-tailed rays (family Torpedinidae) of warm seas that have a pair of specialized tracts of tissue in which electricity is generated

electric shock *n* **1** : SHOCK 3   **2** : ELECTROCONVULSIVE THERAPY

electric shock therapy *n* : ELECTROCONVULSIVE THERAPY

electric shock treatment *n* : ELECTROCONVULSIVE THERAPY

elec·tro·acu·punc·ture \i-ˌlek-trō-ˈak-(y)ə-ˌpəŋ(k)-chər\ *n* : acupuncture in which a weak electric current is passed through each needle

elec·tro·anal·y·sis \-ə-ˈnal-ə-səs\ *n, pl* **-y·ses** \-ˌsēz\ : chemical analysis by electrolytic methods — **elec·tro·an·a·lyt·i·cal** \-ˌan-ᵊl-ˈit-i-kəl\ *also* **elec·tro·an·a·lyt·ic** \-ˈit-ik\ *adj*

elec·tro·an·es·the·sia *or chiefly Brit* **elec·tro·an·aes·the·sia** \-ˌan-əs-ˈthē-zhə\ *n* : anesthesia produced by means of electrical stimulation

elec·tro·bi·ol·o·gist \-ˌbī-ˈäl-ə-jəst\ *n* : a specialist in electrobiology

elec·tro·bi·ol·o·gy \-bī-ˈäl-ə-jē\ *n, pl* **-gies** : a branch of biology that deals with electrical phenomena in living organisms — **elec·tro·bi·o·log·i·cal** \-ˌbī-ə-ˈläj-i-kəl\ *adj*

elec·tro·car·dio·gram \-ˈkärd-ē-ə-ˌgram\ *n* : the tracing made by an electrocardiograph; *also* : the procedure for producing an electrocardiogram

elec·tro·car·dio·graph \-ˌgraf\ *n* : an instrument for recording the changes of electrical potential occurring during the heartbeat used esp. in diagnosing abnormalities of heart action — **elec·tro·car·dio·graph·ic** \-ˌkärd-ē-ə-ˈgraf-ik\ *adj* — **elec·tro·car·di·og·ra·phy** \-ē-ˈäg-rə-fē\ *n, pl* **-phies**

elec·tro·cau·ter·iza·tion *or Brit* **elec·tro·cau·ter·isa·tion** \-ˌkȯt-ə-rə-ˈzā-shən\ *n* : ELECTROCAUTERY 2

elec·tro·cau·tery \-ˈkȯt-ə-rē\ *n, pl* **-ter·ies** **1** : a cautery operated by an electric current   **2** : the cauterization of tissue by means of an electrocautery

elec·tro·chem·is·try \-ˈkem-ə-strē\ *n, pl* **-tries** : a science that deals with the relation of electricity to chemical changes and with the interconversion of chemical and electrical energy — **elec·tro·chem·i·cal** \-ˈkem-i-kəl\ *adj* — **elec·tro·chem·i·cal·ly** \-k(ə-)lē\ *adv* — **elec·tro·chem·ist** \-ˈkem-əst\ *n*

elec·tro·chro·ma·tog·ra·phy \-ˌkrō-mə-ˈtäg-rə-fē\ *n, pl* **-phies** : chromatography involving differential electrical migration produced by application of an electrical potential

elec·tro·co·ag·u·late \-kō-ˈag-yə-ˌlāt\ *vt* **-lat·ed; -lat·ing** : to cause the electrocoagulation of — **elec·tro·co·ag·u·la·tive** \-ˌlāt-iv\ *adj*

elec·tro·co·ag·u·la·tion \-kō-ˌag-yə-ˈlā-shən\ *n* : the surgical coagulation of tissue by diathermy — called also *diathermocoagulation*

elec·tro·co·ma \i-ˌlek-trə-ˈkō-mə\ *n* : the coma induced in electroconvulsive therapy

elec·tro·con·trac·til·i·ty \i-ˌlek-trō-ˌkän-ˌtrak-ˈtil-ət-ē, -kən-\ *n, pl* **-ties** : contractility (as of a muscle) in response to electric stimulation

elec·tro·con·vul·sive \i-ˌlek-trō-kən-ˈvəl-siv\ *adj* : of, relating to, producing, or involving a convulsive response to a shock of electricity ⟨∼ shocks⟩

electroconvulsive therapy *n* : the treatment of mental disorder and esp. depression by the application of electric current to the head of a usu. anesthetized patient that induces unconsciousness and convulsive seizures in the brain — abbr. *ECT;* called also *electric shock, electric shock therapy, electroshock therapy*

elec·tro·cor·ti·cal \-ˈkȯrt-i-kəl\ *adj* : of, relating to, or being the electrical activity occurring in the cerebral cortex

elec·tro·cor·ti·co·gram \i-ˌlek-trō-ˈkȯrt-i-kə-ˌgram\ *n* : an electroencephalogram made with the electrodes in direct contact with the brain

elec·tro·cor·ti·cog·ra·phy \-ˌkȯrt-i-ˈkäg-rə-fē\ *n, pl* **-phies**
: the process of recording electrical activity in the brain by placing electrodes in direct contact with the cerebral cortex — **elec·tro·cor·ti·co·graph·ic** \-kə-ˈgraf-ik\ *adj* — **elec·tro·cor·ti·co·graph·i·cal·ly** \-i-k(ə-)lē\ *adv*

elec·troc·u·lo·gram \i-ˌlek-ˈträk-yə-lə-ˌgram\ *n* : a recording of the moving eye

elec·tro·cute \i-ˈlek-trə-ˌkyüt\ *vt* **-cut·ed; -cut·ing** **1** : to execute (a criminal) by electricity **2** : to kill by a shock of electricity — **elec·tro·cu·tion** \-ˌlek-trə-ˈkyü-shən\ *n*

elec·trode \i-ˈlek-ˌtrōd\ *n* : a conductor used to establish electrical contact with a nonmetallic part of a circuit

elec·tro·der·mal \i-ˌlek-trō-ˈdər-məl\ *adj* : of or relating to electrical activity in or electrical properties of the skin

elec·tro·des·ic·ca·tion \i-ˌlek-trō-ˌdes-i-ˈkā-shən\ *n* : the drying of tissue by a high-frequency electric current applied with a needle-shaped electrode — called also *fulguration* — **elec·tro·des·ic·cate** \-ˈdes-i-ˌkāt\ *vt* **-cat·ed; -cat·ing**

elec·tro·di·ag·no·sis \-ˌdī-ig-ˈnō-səs\ *n, pl* **-no·ses** \-ˌsēz\ : diagnosis based on electrodiagnostic tests or procedures

elec·tro·di·ag·nos·tic \-ˌdī-ig-ˈnäs-tik\ *adj* : involving or obtained by the recording of responses to electrical stimulation or of spontaneous electrical activity (as in electromyography) for purposes of diagnosing a pathological condition ⟨∼ studies⟩ — **elec·tro·di·ag·nos·ti·cal·ly** \-ti-k(ə-)lē\ *adv*

elec·tro·di·al·y·sis \i-ˌlek-trō-dī-ˈal-ə-səs\ *n, pl* **-y·ses** \-ˌsēz\ : dialysis accelerated by an electromotive force applied to electrodes adjacent to the membranes — **elec·tro·di·a·lyt·ic** \-ˌdī-ə-ˈlit-ik\ *adj* — **elec·tro·di·a·lyze** *or Brit* **elec·tro·di·a·lyse** \-ˈdī-ə-ˌlīz\ *vt* **-lyzed** *or Brit* **-lysed; -lyz·ing** *or Brit* **-lys·ing** — **elec·tro·di·a·lyz·er** *or Brit* **elec·tro·di·a·lys·er** *n*

elec·tro·en·ceph·a·lo·gram \-in-ˈsef-ə-lə-ˌgram\ *n* : the tracing of brain waves made by an electroencephalograph

elec·tro·en·ceph·a·lo·graph \-ˌgraf\ *n* : an apparatus for detecting and recording brain waves — called also *encephalograph* — **elec·tro·en·ceph·a·lo·graph·ic** \-ˌsef-ə-lə-ˈgraf-ik\ *adj* — **elec·tro·en·ceph·a·lo·graph·i·cal·ly** \-i-k(ə-)lē\ *adv* — **elec·tro·en·ceph·a·log·ra·phy** \-ˈläg-rə-fē\ *n, pl* **-phies**

elec·tro·en·ceph·a·log·ra·pher \-in-ˌsef-ə-ˈläg-rə-fər\ *n* : a person who specializes in electroencephalography

elec·tro·en·dos·mo·sis \-ˌen-ˌdäz-ˈmō-səs, -ˌdäs-\ *n, pl* **-mo·ses** \-ˌsēz\ : ELECTROOSMOSIS — **elec·tro·en·dos·mot·ic** \-ˈmät-ik\ *adj*

elec·tro·gen·e·sis \i-ˌlek-trə-ˈjen-ə-səs\ *n, pl* **-e·ses** \-ˌsēz\ : the production of electrical activity esp. in living tissue

elec·tro·gen·ic \-ˈjen-ik\ *adj* : of or relating to the production of electrical activity in living tissue ⟨an ∼ pump causing movement of sodium ions across a membrane⟩

elec·tro·gram \i-ˈlek-trə-ˌgram\ *n* : a tracing of the electrical potentials of a tissue (as the brain or heart) made by means of electrodes placed directly in the tissue instead of on the surface of the body

elec·tro·graph·ic \i-ˌlek-trə-ˈgraf-ik\ *adj* : relating to, involving, or produced by the use of electrodes implanted directly in living tissue ⟨∼ stimulation of the brain⟩ — **elec·tro·graph·i·cal·ly** \-i-k(ə-)lē\ *adv* — **elec·trog·ra·phy** \i-ˌlek-ˈträg-rə-fē\ *n, pl* **-phies**

elec·tro·hys·tero·graph \i-ˌlek-trə-ˈhis-tə-rə-ˌgraf\ *n* : an instrument for recording electrical activity in the contracting uterine muscle during labor that is used esp. to detect abnormal labor — **elec·tro·hys·ter·og·ra·phy** \-ˌhis-tə-ˈräg-rə-fē\ *n, pl* **-phies**

elec·tro·ky·mo·graph \-ˈkī-mə-ˌgraf\ *n* : an instrument for recording graphically the motion of the heart as seen in silhouette on a fluoroscopic screen — **elec·tro·ky·mo·graph·ic** \-ˌkī-mə-ˈgraf-ik\ *adj* — **elec·tro·ky·mo·graph·i·cal·ly** \-i-k(ə-)lē\ *adv* — **elec·tro·ky·mog·ra·phy** \-kī-ˈmäg-rə-fē\ *n, pl* **-phies**

elec·trol·o·gist \i-ˌlek-ˈträl-ə-jəst\ *n* : a person who removes hair, warts, moles, and birthmarks by means of an electric current applied to the body with a needle-shaped electrode

elec·trol·y·sis \i-ˌlek-ˈträl-ə-səs\ *n, pl* **-y·ses** \-ˌsēz\ **1 a** : the producing of chemical changes by passage of an electric cur-

rent through an electrolyte **b** : subjection to this action **2** : the destruction of hair roots with an electric current

elec·tro·lyte \i-ˈlek-trə-ˌlīt\ *n* **1** : a nonmetallic electric conductor in which current is carried by the movement of ions **2 a** : a substance (as an acid, base, or salt) that when dissolved in a suitable solvent (as water) or when fused becomes an ionic conductor **b** : any of the ions (as of sodium, potassium, calcium, or bicarbonate) that in a biological fluid regulate or affect most metabolic processes (as the flow of nutrients into and waste products out of cells) — used esp. in biology and biochemistry

elec·tro·lyt·ic \i-ˌlek-trə-ˈlit-ik\ *adj* : of or relating to electrolysis or an electrolyte; *also* : involving, produced by, or used in electrolysis ⟨the anode of an ∼ cell⟩ — **elec·tro·lyt·i·cal·ly** \-i-k(ə-)lē\ *adv*

elec·tro·lyze *or Brit* **elec·tro·lyse** \i-ˈlek-trə-ˌlīz\ *vt* **-lyzed** *or Brit* **-lysed; -lyz·ing** *or Brit* **-lys·ing** : to subject to electrolysis

elec·tro·mag·net \i-ˌlek-trō-ˈmag-nət\ *n* : a core of magnetic material surrounded by a coil of wire through which an electric current is passed to magnetize the core

elec·tro·mag·net·ic \-mag-ˈnet-ik\ *adj* : of, relating to, or produced by electromagnetism — **elec·tro·mag·net·i·cal·ly** \-i-k(ə-)lē\ *adv*

electromagnetic field *n* : a field (as around a working computer or a transmitting high-voltage power line) that is made up of associated electric and magnetic components, that results from the motion of an electric charge, and that possesses a definite amount of electromagnetic energy ⟨the purported effects of *electromagnetic fields* on human health⟩

electromagnetic radiation *n* : a series of electromagnetic waves

electromagnetic spectrum *n* : the entire range of wavelengths or frequencies of electromagnetic radiation extending from gamma rays to the longest radio waves and including visible light

electromagnetic unit *n* : any of a system of electrical units based primarily on the magnetic properties of electrical currents

electromagnetic wave *n* : one of the waves that are propagated by simultaneous periodic variations of electric and magnetic field intensity and that include radio waves, infrared, visible light, ultraviolet, X-rays, and gamma rays

elec·tro·mag·ne·tism \i-ˌlek-trō-ˈmag-nə-ˌtiz-əm\ *n* **1** : magnetism developed by a current of electricity **2** : physics dealing with the relations between electricity and magnetism

elec·trom·e·ter \i-ˌlek-ˈträm-ət-ər\ *n* : any of various instruments for detecting or measuring electric-potential differences or ionizing radiations by means of the forces of attraction or repulsion between charged bodies — **elec·tro·met·ric** \-trə-ˈme-trik\ *adj*

elec·tro·mo·tive force \i-ˌlek-trō-ˈmōt-iv-, -trə-\ *n* : something that moves or tends to move electricity : the potential difference derived from an electrical source (as a cell or generator) per unit quantity of electricity passing through the source

elec·tro·myo·gram \i-ˌlek-trō-ˈmī-ə-ˌgram\ *n* : a tracing made with an electromyograph

elec·tro·myo·graph \-ˌgraf\ *n* : an instrument that converts the electrical activity associated with functioning skeletal muscle into a visual record or into sound and has been used to diagnose neuromuscular disorders and in biofeedback training — **elec·tro·myo·graph·ic** \-ˌmī-ə-ˈgraf-ik\ *adj* — **elec·tro·myo·graph·i·cal·ly** \-i-k(ə-)lē\ *adv* — **elec·tro·my·og·ra·phy** \-mī-ˈäg-rə-fē\ *n, pl* **-phies**

elec·tron \i-ˈlek-ˌträn\ *n* : an elementary particle consisting of a charge of negative electricity equal to about 1.602×10^{-19} coulomb and having a mass when at rest of about 9.109534×10^{-28} gram or about $\frac{1}{1836}$ that of a proton

elec·tro·nar·co·sis \i-ˌlek-trō-när-ˈkō-səs\ *n, pl* **-co·ses** \-ˌsēz\ : unconsciousness induced by passing a weak electric current through the brain and used in treating certain mental disorders

elec·tron–dense \i-ˈlek-ˌträn-ˈden(t)s\ *adj* : relatively impermeable to the electron beam of an electron microscope

elec·tro·neg·a·tive \i-ˌlek-trō-ˈneg-ət-iv\ *adj* **1** : charged with negative electricity **2** : having a tendency to attract electrons — **elec·tro·neg·a·tiv·i·ty** \-ˌneg-ə-ˈtiv-ət-ē\ *n, pl* **-ties**

elec·tron·ic \i-ˌlek-ˈträn-ik\ *adj* : of or relating to electrons or electronics — **elec·tron·i·cal·ly** \-i-k(ə-)lē\ *adv*

elec·tron·ics \-iks\ *n pl* **1** *sing in constr* : a branch of physics that deals with the emission, behavior, and effects of electrons (as in electron tubes and transistors) and with electronic devices **2** : electronic devices or equipment

electron micrograph *n* : a micrograph made with an electron microscope — **electron micrography** *n*

electron microscope *n* : an electron-optical instrument in which a beam of electrons is used to produce an enlarged image of a minute object — **electron microscopist** *n* — **electron microscopy** *n*

electron optics *n pl but sing in constr* : a branch of physics in which the principles of optics are applied to beams of electrons — **elec·tron–op·ti·cal** \i-ˌlek-ˌträ-ˈnäp-ti-kəl\ *adj*

electron paramagnetic resonance *n* : ELECTRON SPIN RESONANCE

electron spin resonance *n* : the resonance of unpaired electrons in a magnetic field

electron transport *n* : the sequential transfer of electrons esp. by cytochromes in cellular respiration from an oxidizable substrate to molecular oxygen by a series of oxidation≈reduction reactions

electron volt *n* : a unit of energy equal to the energy gained by an electron in passing from a point of low potential to a point one volt higher in potential : 1.60×10^{-19} joule

elec·tro·nys·tag·mog·ra·phy \i-ˌlek-trō-ˌnis-ˌtag-ˈmäg-rə-fē\ *n, pl* **-phies** : the use of electrooculography to study nystagmus — **elec·tro·nys·tag·mo·graph·ic** \-(ˌ)nis-ˌtag-mə-ˈgraf-ik\ *adj*

elec·tro·oc·u·lo·gram \i-ˌlek-trō-ˈäk-yə-lə-ˌgram\ *n* : a record of the standing voltage between the front and back of the eye that is correlated with eyeball movement (as in REM sleep) and obtained by electrodes suitably placed on the skin near the eye

elec·tro·oc·u·log·ra·phy \-ˌäk-yə-ˈläg-rə-fē\ *n, pl* **-phies** : the preparation and study of electrooculograms — **elec·tro·oc·u·lo·graph·ic** \-lə-ˈgraf-ik\ *adj*

elec·tro·os·mo·sis \i-ˌlek-trō-äz-ˈmō-səs, -äs-\ *n, pl* **-mo·ses** \-ˌsēz\ : the movement of a liquid out of or through a porous material or a biological membrane under the influence of an electric field — called also *electroendosmosis* — **elec·tro·os·mot·ic** \-ˈmät-ik\ *adj* — **elec·tro·os·mot·i·cal·ly** \-i-k(ə-)lē\ *adv*

elec·tro·phe·ro·gram \-trə-ˈfir-ə-ˌgram, -ˈfer-\ *n* : ELECTROPHORETOGRAM

elec·tro·phile \i-ˈlek-trə-ˌfīl\ *n* : an electrophilic substance (as an electron-accepting reagent)

elec·tro·phil·ic \i-ˌlek-trə-ˈfil-ik\ *adj* **1** *of an atom, ion, or molecule* : having an affinity for electrons : being an electron acceptor ⟨∼ reagents⟩ **2** : involving an electrophilic atom, ion, or molecule ⟨an ∼ reaction⟩ — **elec·tro·phil·ic·ity** \-trō-fil-ˈis-ət-ē\ *n, pl* **-ities**

elec·tro·pho·rese \i-ˌlek-trə-fə-ˈrēs, -ˈträf-ə-ˌrēs, -ˌrēz\ *vt* **-resed; -res·ing** : to subject to electrophoresis

elec·tro·pho·re·sis \-trə-fə-ˈrē-səs\ *n, pl* **-re·ses** \-ˌsēz\ : the movement of suspended particles through a fluid or gel under the action of an electromotive force applied to electrodes in contact with the suspension — called also *cataphoresis* — **elec·tro·pho·ret·ic** \-ˈret-ik\ *adj* — **elec·tro·pho·ret·i·cal·ly** \-i-k(ə-)lē\ *adv*

elec·tro·pho·reto·gram \-fə-ˈret-ə-ˌgram\ *n* : a record that consists of the separated components of a mixture (as of proteins) produced by electrophoresis in a supporting medium (as filter paper)

elec·troph·o·rus \i-ˌlek-ˈträf-ə-rəs\ *n, pl* **-ri** \-ˌrī, -ˌrē\ : a device for producing electric charges consisting of a disk that is negatively electrified by friction and a metal plate that becomes charged by induction when placed on the disk

elec·tro·phren·ic \i-ˌlek-trə-ˈfren-ik\ *adj* : relating to or induced by electrical stimulation of the phrenic nerve ⟨treatment of apnea by ∼ pacing of the sleeping patient⟩

electrophrenic respiration *n* : artificial respiration by means of an electrophrenic respirator used esp. in poliomyelitis and other conditions in which the nervous control of breathing is impaired

electrophrenic respirator *n* : a device for the regular recurrent electrical stimulation of the phrenic nerve or nerves to induce respiratory movements artificially and induce breathing

elec·tro·phys·i·ol·o·gist \i-ˌlek-trō-ˌfiz-ē-ˈäl-ə-jəst\ *n* : a specialist in electrophysiology

elec·tro·phys·i·ol·o·gy \i-ˌlek-trō-ˌfiz-ē-ˈäl-ə-jē\ *n, pl* **-gies** **1** : physiology that is concerned with the electrical aspects of physiological phenomena **2** : electrical phenomena associated with a physiological process (as the function of a body or bodily part) ⟨∼ of the eye⟩ — **elec·tro·phys·i·o·log·i·cal** \-ē-ə-ˈläj-i-kəl\ *also* **elec·tro·phys·i·o·log·ic** \-ik\ *adj* — **elec·tro·phys·i·o·log·i·cal·ly** \-i-k(ə-)lē\ *adv*

elec·tro·plexy \i-ˈlek-trə-ˌplek-sē\ *n, pl* **-plex·ies** *Brit* : ELECTROCONVULSIVE THERAPY

elec·tro·po·ra·tion \i-ˌlek-trə-pōr-ˈā-shən\ *n* : the application of an electric current to a living surface (as the skin or the plasma membrane of a cell) in order to open pores or channels through which something (as a drug or DNA) may pass — **elec·tro·po·rate** \i-ˈlek-trə-pə-ˌrāt\ *vt* **-rat·ed; -rat·ing**

elec·tro·pos·i·tive \i-ˌlek-trō-ˈpäz-ət-iv, -ˈpäz-tiv\ *adj* **1** : charged with positive electricity **2** : having a tendency to release electrons

elec·tro·py·rex·ia \-pī-ˈrek-sē-ə\ *n* : artificial fever induced by electrical means for therapeutic purposes

elec·tro·re·sec·tion \-rē-ˈsek-shən\ *n* : resection by electrosurgical means

elec·tro·ret·i·no·gram \-ˈret-ᵊn-ə-ˌgram\ *n* : a graphic record of electrical activity of the retina used esp. in the diagnosis of retinal conditions

elec·tro·ret·i·no·graph \-ˌgraf\ *n* : an instrument for recording electrical activity in the retina — **elec·tro·ret·i·no·graph·ic** \-ˌret-ᵊn-ə-ˌgraf-ik\ *adj* — **elec·tro·ret·i·nog·ra·phy** \-ᵊn-ˌäg-rə-fē\ *n, pl* **-phies**

elec·tro·scope \i-ˈlek-trə-ˌskōp\ *n* : any of various instruments for detecting the presence of an electric charge on a body, for determining whether the charge is positive or negative, or for indicating and measuring intensity of radiation

elec·tro·shock \-trō-ˌshäk\ *n* **1** : SHOCK 3 **2** : ELECTROCONVULSIVE THERAPY

electroshock therapy *n* : ELECTROCONVULSIVE THERAPY

elec·tro·sleep \i-ˈlek-trō-ˌslēp\ *n* : profound relaxation or a state of unconsciousness induced by the passage of a very low voltage electric current through the brain

elec·tro·stat·ic \i-ˌlek-trə-ˈstat-ik\ *adj* : of or relating to static electricity or electrostatics — **elec·tro·stat·i·cal·ly** \-ˈstat-i-k(ə-)lē\ *adv*

electrostatic generator *n* : VAN DE GRAFF GENERATOR

elec·tro·stat·ics \i-ˌlek-trə-ˈstat-iks\ *n pl but sing in constr* : physics that deals with phenomena due to attractions or repulsions of electric charges but not dependent upon their motion

electrostatic unit *n* : any of a system of electrical units based primarily on forces of interaction between electric charges — abbr. *esu*

elec·tro·stim·u·la·tion \i-ˌlek-trō-ˌstim-yə-ˈlā-shən\ *n* : shocks of electricity administered in nonconvulsive doses ⟨clinical cardiac ∼⟩

elec·tro·stric·tion \-'strik-shən\ *n* : deformation of a dielectric body as the result of an applied electric field — **elec·tro·stric·tive** \-'strik-tiv\ *adj*

elec·tro·sur·gery \i-ˌlek-trō-'sərj-(ə-)rē\ *n, pl* **-ger·ies** : surgery by means of diathermy — **elec·tro·sur·gi·cal** \-'sər-ji-kəl\ *adj*

elec·tro·syn·the·sis \-'sin(t)-thə-səs\ *n, pl* **-the·ses** \-ˌsēz\ : synthesis accomplished with the aid of electricity; *esp* : synthesis of an organic compound by electrolysis — **elec·tro·syn·thet·ic** \-sin-'thet-ik\ *adj* — **elec·tro·syn·thet·i·cal·ly** \-i-k(ə-)lē\ *adv*

elec·tro·tax·is \-'tak-səs\ *n, pl* **-tax·es** \-ˌsēz\ : movement in which an electric current constitutes the directive factor : GALVANOTAXIS

elec·tro·ther·a·py \-'ther-ə-pē\ *n, pl* **-pies** : treatment of disease by means of electricity (as in diathermy)

elec·tro·tome \i-'lek-trə-ˌtōm\ *n* : an electric cutting instrument used in electrosurgery

elec·tro·ton·ic \i-ˌlek-trə-'tän-ik\ *adj* **1** : of, induced by, relating to, or constituting electrotonus ⟨the ∼ condition of a nerve⟩ ⟨∼ induction of depolarization⟩ **2** : of, relating to, or being the spread of electrical activity through living tissue or cells in the absence of repeated action potentials ⟨an ∼ junction between cells⟩ — **elec·tro·ton·i·cal·ly** \-i-k(ə-)lē\ *adv*

elec·tro·to·nic·i·ty \-tō-'nis-ət-ē\ *n, pl* **-ties** : ELECTROTONUS

elec·trot·o·nus \i-ˌlek-'trät-ᵊn-əs\ *n* : the altered sensitivity of a nerve when a constant current of electricity passes through any part of it

elec·trot·ro·pism \i-lek-'trä-trə-ˌpiz-əm\ *n* : bodily orientation in relation to an electric current : GALVANOTROPISM

elec·tu·ary \i-'lek-chə-ˌwer-ē\ *n, pl* **-ar·ies** : CONFECTION; *esp* : a medicated paste prepared with a sweet (as honey), used in veterinary practice, and administered by smearing on the teeth, gums, or tongue

el·e·doi·sin \ˌel-ə-'dȯis-ᵊn\ *n* : a small protein $C_{54}H_{85}N_{13}O_{15}S$ from the salivary glands of several octopuses (genus *Eledone*) that is a powerful vasodilator and hypotensive agent

el·e·ment \'el-ə-mənt\ *n* **1** : any of the four substances air, water, fire, and earth formerly believed to compose the physical universe **2** : a constituent part: as **a** : any of more than 100 fundamental substances that consist of atoms of only one kind and that singly or in combination constitute all matter **b** : one of the distinct parts (as a lens) of a composite device (as a microscope) **c** : one of the basic constituent units (as a cell or fiber) of a tissue

el·e·men·tal \ˌel-ə-'ment-ᵊl\ *adj* : of, relating to, or being an element; *specif* : existing as an uncombined chemical element

el·e·men·ta·ry body \ˌel-ə-ˌment-ə-rē-, -ˌmen-trē-\ *n* : an infectious particle of any of several microorganisms; *esp* : a chlamydial cell of an extracellular infectious form that attaches to receptors on the membrane of the host cell and is taken up by endocytosis — compare RETICULATE BODY

elementary particle *n* **1** : any of the particles of which matter and energy are composed or which mediate the fundamental forces of nature; *esp* : one (as the photon or the electron) whose existence has not been attributed to the combination of other more fundamental entities **2** : one of the structural units of mitochondrial cristae that are observable by the electron microscope usu. as spheres or stalked spheres and are prob. the seat of fundamental energy=producing reactions

el·e·op·tene *or chiefly Brit* **el·ae·op·tene** \ˌel-ē-'äp-ˌtēn\ *n* : the liquid portion of any natural essential oil that partly solidifies in the cold — compare STEAROPTENE

el·e·phan·ti·as·ic \ˌel-ə-ˌfan-tē-'as-ik, -fən-'tī-ə-(ˌ)sik\ *adj* : affected with or characteristic of elephantiasis

el·e·phan·ti·a·sis \ˌel-ə-fən-'tī-ə-səs, -ˌfan-\ *n, pl* **-a·ses** \-ˌsēz\ : enlargement and thickening of tissues; *specif* : the enormous enlargement of a limb or the scrotum caused by obstruction of lymphatics by filarial worms of the genus *Wuchereria* (*W. bancrofti*) or a related genus (*Brugia malayi*)

CHEMICAL ELEMENTS

ELEMENT	SYMBOL	ATOMIC NUMBER	ATOMIC WEIGHT[1]
actinium	Ac	89	227.0277
aluminum	Al	13	26.98154
americium	Am	95	(243)
antimony	Sb	51	121.760
argon	Ar	18	39.948
arsenic	As	33	74.92160
astatine	At	85	(210)
barium	Ba	56	137.33
berkelium	Bk	97	(247)
beryllium	Be	4	9.012182
bismuth	Bi	83	208.98038
bohrium	Bh	107	(264)
boron	B	5	10.81
bromine	Br	35	79.904
cadmium	Cd	48	112.41
calcium	Ca	20	40.078
californium	Cf	98	(251)
carbon	C	6	12.011
cerium	Ce	58	140.116
cesium	Cs	55	132.90545
chlorine	Cl	17	35.453
chromium	Cr	24	51.996
cobalt	Co	27	58.93320
copper	Cu	29	63.546
curium	Cm	96	(247)
darmstadtium	Ds	110	(269)
dubnium	Db	105	(262)
dysprosium	Dy	66	162.50
einsteinium	Es	99	(252)
erbium	Er	68	167.259
europium	Eu	63	151.964
fermium	Fm	100	(257)
fluorine	F	9	18.998403
francium	Fr	87	(223)
gadolinium	Gd	64	157.25
gallium	Ga	31	69.723
germanium	Ge	32	72.64
gold	Au	79	196.96655
hafnium	Hf	72	178.49
hassium	Hs	108	(277)
helium	He	2	4.002602
holmium	Ho	67	164.93032
hydrogen	H	1	1.0079
indium	In	49	114.818
iodine	I	53	126.90447
iridium	Ir	77	192.217
iron	Fe	26	55.845
krypton	Kr	36	83.80
lanthanum	La	57	138.9055
lawrencium	Lr	103	(262)
lead	Pb	82	207.2
lithium	Li	3	6.941
lutetium	Lu	71	174.967
magnesium	Mg	12	24.305
manganese	Mn	25	54.93805
meitnerium	Mt	109	(268)
mendelevium	Md	101	(258)
mercury	Hg	80	200.59
molybdenum	Mo	42	95.94
neodymium	Nd	60	144.24
neon	Ne	10	20.180
neptunium	Np	93	(237)
nickel	Ni	28	58.6934

\ə\ **abut** \ᵊ\ **kitten** \ər\ **further** \a\ **ash** \ā\ **ace** \ä\ **cot, cart**
\au̇\ **out** \ch\ **chin** \e\ **bet** \ē\ **easy** \g\ **go** \i\ **hit** \ī\ **ice** \j\ **job**
\ŋ\ **sing** \ō\ **go** \ȯ\ **law** \ȯi\ **boy** \th\ **thin** \t͟h\ **the** \ü\ **loot**
\u̇\ **foot** \y\ **yet** \zh\ **vision** *See also* Pronunciation Symbols page

E
F

ELEMENT	SYMBOL	ATOMIC NUMBER	ATOMIC WEIGHT[1]
niobium	Nb	41	92.90638
nitrogen	N	7	14.0067
nobelium	No	102	(259)
osmium	Os	76	190.23
oxygen	O	8	15.9994
palladium	Pd	46	106.42
phosphorus	P	15	30.973761
platinum	Pt	78	195.078
plutonium	Pu	94	(244)
polonium	Po	84	(209)
potassium	K	19	39.0983
praseodymium	Pr	59	140.90765
promethium	Pm	61	(145)
protactinium	Pa	91	(231)
radium	Ra	88	(226)
radon	Rn	86	(222)
rhenium	Re	75	186.207
rhodium	Rh	45	102.90550
rubidium	Rb	37	85.4678
ruthenium	Ru	44	101.07
rutherfordium	Rf	104	(261)
samarium	Sm	62	150.36
scandium	Sc	21	44.95591
seaborgium	Sg	106	(266)
selenium	Se	34	78.96
silicon	Si	14	28.0855
silver	Ag	47	107.8682
sodium	Na	11	22.989770
strontium	Sr	38	87.62
sulfur	S	16	32.07
tantalum	Ta	73	180.9479
technetium	Tc	43	(98)
tellurium	Te	52	127.60
terbium	Tb	65	158.92534
thallium	Tl	81	204.3833
thorium	Th	90	232.0381
thulium	Tm	69	168.93421
tin	Sn	50	118.71
titanium	Ti	22	47.867
tungsten	W	74	183.84
uranium	U	92	(238)
vanadium	V	23	50.9415
xenon	Xe	54	131.29
ytterbium	Yb	70	173.04
yttrium	Y	39	88.90585
zinc	Zn	30	65.39
zirconium	Zr	40	91.224

[1]Weights are based on the naturally occurring isotope compositions and scaled to $^{12}C = 12$. For elements lacking stable isotopes, the mass number of the most stable nuclide is shown in parentheses.

el·e·phan·toid \,el-ə-'fan-,tȯid, 'el-ə-fən-\ *adj* : resembling, affected by, or relating to elephantiasis ⟨~ tissue⟩

el·e·vat·ed \'el-ə-,vāt-əd\ *adj* : increased esp. abnormally (as in degree or amount) ⟨~ blood pressure⟩ ⟨~ temperature⟩

el·e·va·tion \,el-ə-'vā-shən\ *n* **1** : a swelling esp. on the skin **2** : a usu. abnormal increase (as in degree or amount)

el·e·va·tor \'el-ə-,vāt-ər\ *n* **1** : a dental instrument for removing teeth or the roots of teeth which cannot be gripped with a forceps **2** : a surgical instrument for raising a depressed part (as a bone) or for separating contiguous parts

elev·enth cranial nerve \i-'lev-ən(t)th-\ *n* : ACCESSORY NERVE

elim·i·nant \i-'lim-ə-nənt\ *n* : an agent that promotes bodily elimination

elim·i·nate \-,nāt\ *vt* **-nat·ed; -nat·ing** : to expel (as waste) from the living body

elim·i·na·tion \i-,lim-ə-'nā-shən\ *n* **1** : the act of discharging or excreting waste products or foreign substances from the body **2 eliminations** *pl* : bodily discharges including urine, feces, and vomit **3** : the removal from a molecule of the constituents of a simpler molecule ⟨ethylene is formed by the ~ of water from ethanol⟩

elim·i·na·tive \i-'lim-ə-,nāt-iv\ *adj* : serving or tending to eliminate; *specif* : relating to, operating in the process of, or carrying on bodily elimination ⟨the ~ organs⟩

ELISA \ē-'lī-sə, i-, -zə\ *n* : ENZYME-LINKED IMMUNOSORBENT ASSAY

elix·ir \i-'lik-sər\ *n* : a sweetened liquid usu. containing alcohol that is used in medication either for its medicinal ingredients or as a flavoring

Eliz·a·be·than collar \i-,liz-ə-,bē-thən-\ *n* : a broad circle of stiff cardboard or other material placed about the neck of a cat or dog to prevent it from licking or biting an injured part

el·lag·ic acid \ə-,laj-ik-, e-\ *n* : a crystalline phenolic compound $C_{14}H_6O_8$ with two lactone groups that is obtained esp. from oak galls and some tannins and has hemostatic properties

el·lip·to·cyte \i-'lip-tə-,sīt\ *n* : an elliptical red blood cell — called also *ovalocyte*

el·lip·to·cy·to·sis \i-,lip-tə-,sī-'tō-səs\ *n, pl* **-to·ses** \-,sēz\ : a human hereditary trait manifested by the presence in the blood of red blood cells which are oval in shape with rounded ends — called also *ovalocytosis;* compare SICKLE-CELL TRAIT

[1]**elon·gate** \i-'lȯŋ-,gāt\ *vb* **-gat·ed; -gat·ing** *vt* : to extend the length of ~ *vi* : to grow in length

[2]**elongate** *or* **elon·gat·ed** *adj* : long in proportion to width

elon·ga·tion \(,)ē-,lȯŋ-'gā-shən\ *n* **1** : the state of being elongated or lengthened; *also* : the process of growing or increasing in length ⟨chain ~ in DNA synthesis⟩ ⟨the ~ of a muscle under tension⟩ **2** : something that is elongated

el·u·ant *or* **el·u·ent** \'el-yə-wənt\ *n* : a solvent used in eluting

el·u·ate \'el-yə-wət, -,wāt\ *n* : the washings obtained by eluting

elute \ē-'lüt\ *vt* **elut·ed; elut·ing** : to wash out or extract; *specif* : to remove (adsorbed material) from an adsorbent by means of a solvent — **elu·tion** \-'lü-shən\ *n*

elu·tri·a·tion \ē-,lü-trē-'ā-shən\ *n* **1** : the removal of substances from a mixture by washing and decanting **2** : the separation of finer lighter particles from coarser heavier particles in a mixture by means of a usu. slow upward stream of fluid so that the lighter particles are carried upward

EM *abbr* **1** electromagnetic **2** electron microscope; electron microscopy **3** emergency medicine

ema·ci·ate \i-'mā-shē-,āt\ *vb* **-at·ed; -at·ing** *vt* : to cause to lose flesh so as to become very thin ~ *vi* : to waste away physically

ema·ci·a·tion \i-,mā-s(h)ē-'ā-shən\ *n* **1** : the process of making or becoming emaciated **2** : the state of being emaciated; *esp* : a wasted condition of the body

em·a·nate \'em-ə-,nāt\ *vb* **-nat·ed; -nat·ing** *vi* : to come out from a source ~ *vt* : to give out or emit

em·a·na·tion \,em-ə-'nā-shən\ *n* **1** : the action of emanating **2 a** : something that emanates or is produced by emanation **b** : a heavy gaseous element produced by radioactive disintegration ⟨radium ~⟩

eman·ci·pa·tion \i-,man(t)-sə-'pā-shən\ *n* : gradual separation of an original homogeneous embryo into fields with different specific potentialities for development

emas·cu·late \i-'mas-kyə-,lāt\ *vt* **-lat·ed; -lat·ing** : to deprive of virility or procreative power : CASTRATE — **emas·cu·la·tion** \-,mas-kyə-'lā-shən\ *n*

emas·cu·la·tome \i-'mas-kyə-lə-,tōm\ *n* : a pair of double-hinged pincers for castrating domestic animals bloodlessly by crushing the spermatic cord through the unbroken skin

emas·cu·la·tor \-,lāt-ər\ *n* : one that emasculates; *specif* : an instrument often with a broad surface and a cutting edge used in castrating livestock

emb *abbr* embryo; embryology

Em·ba·dom·o·nas \,em-bə-'däm-ə-nəs\ *n* : a genus of small flagellates with two unequal flagella commensal in the intestines of various vertebrates including humans

em·balm \im-'bä(l)m, *NewEng also* -'bȧm\ *vt* : to treat (a dead body) so as to protect from decay — **em·balm·er** *n* — **em·balm·ment** \-'bä(l)m-mənt\ *n*

em·bar·rass \im-'bar-əs\ *vt* : to impair the activity of (a bodily function) or the function of (a bodily part) ⟨digestion ∼ed by overeating⟩

em·bar·rass·ment \im-'bar-ə-smənt\ *n* : difficulty in functioning as a result of disease ⟨cardiac ∼⟩ ⟨respiratory ∼⟩

Emb·den–Mey·er·hof pathway \'em-dən-'mī-ər-ˌhȯf-, 'emp-\ *n* : GLYCOLYSIS

Embden, Gustav Georg (1874–1933), German physiological chemist. In 1904 Embden became director of the chemistry laboratory of the medical clinic at the Frankfurt≠ Sachsenhausen municipal hospital. Eventually the clinic became an institute of the University of Frankfurt am Main. His pioneering studies in the field of physiological chemistry included research on the intermediate metabolic processes in liver tissue. He established the importance of the role of the liver in metabolism. Between 1932 and 1933 he and his assistants succeeded in tracing all of the stages of the breakdown of glycogen in the muscle to lactic acid. He is also credited with isolating several intermediate metabolic products from muscle tissue.

Meyerhof, Otto (1884–1951), German biochemist. Meyerhof held posts in physiology and physical chemistry at Kiel and other German universities. From 1929 to 1938 he headed the department of physiology at the Kaiser Wilhelm Institute for Medical Research in Heidelberg. In 1919 he demonstrated that during muscle contraction in the absence of oxygen, glycogen is converted to lactic acid. In the presence of oxygen, about one-fifth of the lactic acid is oxidized to carbon dioxide and water. The energy produced by this oxidation is then used to regenerate glycogen from the remaining lactic acid. In 1925 Meyerhof successfully extracted from muscle the group of enzymes responsible for the conversion of glycogen to lactic acid. In 1922 he and Archibald Hill shared the Nobel Prize for Physiology or Medicine for their researches into the chemistry of metabolism in muscle.

em·bed *also* **im·bed** \im-'bed\ *vt* **em·bed·ded** *also* **im·bed·ded; em·bed·ding** *also* **im·bed·ding** : to prepare (a microscopy specimen) for sectioning by infiltrating with and enclosing in a supporting substance — **em·bed·ment** \-'bed-mənt\ *n*

em·be·lia \em-'bēl-yə, -'bē-lē-ə\ *n* **1** *cap* : a large genus of Old World tropical woody vines (family Myrsinaceae) with alternate leaves and racemose flowers **2** : the dried powdered fruit of an Indian vine of the genus *Embelia* (*E. ribes*) that is used locally as a tapeworm remedy

em·bo·la·lia \ˌem-bə-'lā-lē-ə, -'lal-ē-\ *n* : EMBOLOLALIA

em·bo·lec·to·my \ˌem-bə-'lek-tə-mē\ *n, pl* **-mies** : surgical removal of an embolus

em·bo·le·mia *or chiefly Brit* **em·bo·lae·mia** \-'lē-mē-ə\ *n* : an abnormal state characterized by the presence of emboli in the blood

emboli *pl of* EMBOLUS

em·bol·ic \em-'bäl-ik, im-\ *adj* **1** : of or relating to an embolus or embolism ⟨∼ occlusion of a middle cerebral artery with cholesterol material —D. R. Gress & J. H. Eichhorn⟩ **2** : of, relating to, or produced by embory

em·bo·lism \'em-bə-ˌliz-əm\ *n* **1** : the sudden obstruction of a blood vessel by an embolus **2** : EMBOLUS

em·bo·li·za·tion *or Brit* **em·bo·li·sa·tion** \ˌem-bə-lə-'zā-shən\ *n* : the process by which or state in which a blood vessel or organ is obstructed by the lodgment of a material mass (as an embolus) ⟨pulmonary ∼⟩ ⟨∼ of a thrombus⟩; *also* : an operation in which pellets are introduced into the circulatory system in order to induce embolization in specific abnormal blood vessels

em·bo·lize *or Brit* **em·bo·lise** \'em-bə-ˌlīz\ *vb* **-lized** *or Brit* **-lised; -liz·ing** *or Brit* **-lis·ing** *vt, of an embolus* : to lodge in and obstruct (as a blood vessel or organ) ∼ *vi* : to break up into emboli or become an embolus ⟨bone marrow fragments

embolized and were swept to the lung from the site of the fracture⟩

em·bo·lo·la·lia \ˌem-bə-lō-'lā-lē-ə, -'lal-ē-\ *n* : the interpolation of meaningless sounds or words into speech

em·bo·lo·phra·sia \-'frā-zh(ē-)ə\ *n* : EMBOLOLALIA

em·bo·lo·ther·a·py \-'ther-ə-pē\ *n, pl* **-pies** : the intentional blockage of an artery with an object (as a balloon inserted by a catheter) to control or prevent hemorrhaging

em·bo·lus \'em-bə-ləs\ *n, pl* **-li** \-ˌlī\ : an abnormal particle (as an air bubble) circulating in the blood — compare THROMBUS

em·bo·ly \'em-bə-lē\ *n, pl* **-lies** : gastrula formation by simple invagination of the blastula wall

em·bra·sure \im-'brā-zhər\ *n* : the sloped valley between adjacent teeth

em·bro·cate \'em-brə-ˌkāt\ *vt* **-cat·ed; -cat·ing** : to moisten and rub (a part of the body) with lotion

em·bro·ca·tion \ˌem-brə-'kā-shən\ *n* : LINIMENT

em·bryo \'em-brē-ˌō\ *n, pl* **em·bry·os 1** *archaic* : a vertebrate at any stage of development prior to birth or hatching **2** : an animal in the early stages of growth and differentiation that are characterized by cleavage, the laying down of fundamental tissues, and the formation of primitive organs and organ systems; *esp* : the developing human individual from the time of implantation to the end of the eighth week after conception — compare FETUS

em·bryo·car·dia \ˌem-brē-ō-'kärd-ē-ə\ *n* : a symptom of heart disease in which the heart sounds resemble those of the fetal heart

em·bryo·gen·e·sis \ˌem-brē-ō-'jen-ə-səs\ *n, pl* **-e·ses** \-ˌsēz\ : the formation and development of the embryo — **em·bryo·ge·net·ic** \-jə-'net-ik\ *adj*

em·bry·og·e·ny \ˌem-brē-'äj-ə-nē\ *n, pl* **-nies** : EMBRYOGENESIS — **em·bryo·gen·ic** \-brē-ō-'jen-ik\ *adj*

em·bry·oid \'em-brē-ˌȯid\ *n* : a mass of tissue resembling an embryo — **embryoid** *adj*

embryol *abbr* embryology

em·bry·ol·o·gist \ˌem-brē-'äl-ə-jəst\ *n* : a specialist in embryology

em·bry·ol·o·gy \-jē\ *n, pl* **-gies 1** : a branch of biology dealing with embryos and their development **2** : the features and phenomena exhibited in the formation and development of an embryo — **em·bry·o·log·i·cal** \-brē-ə-'läj-i-kəl\ *also* **em·bry·o·log·ic** \-'läj-ik\ *adj* — **em·bry·o·log·i·cal·ly** \-i-k(ə-)lē\ *adv*

em·bry·o·ma \ˌem-brē-'ō-mə\ *n, pl* **-mas** *also* **-ma·ta** \-mət-ə\ : a tumor derived from embryonic structures : TERATOMA

em·bry·o·nal \em-'brī-ən-ᵊl\ *adj* : EMBRYONIC 1

embryonal carcinoma *n* : a highly malignant cancer of the testis

em·bry·o·nate \'em-brē-ə-ˌnāt\ *vi* **-nat·ed; -nat·ing** *of an egg or zygote* : to produce or differentiate into an embryo

em·bry·o·nat·ed *adj* : having an embryo

em·bry·on·ic \ˌem-brē-'än-ik\ *adj* **1** : of or relating to an embryo **2** : being in an early stage of development : INCIPIENT, RUDIMENTARY — **em·bry·on·i·cal·ly** \-i-k(ə-)lē\ *adv*

embryonic disk *n or* **embryonic disc** *n* **1 a** : BLASTODISC : BLASTODERM **2** : the part of the inner cell mass of a blastocyst from which the embryo of a placental mammal develops — called also *embryonic shield*

embryonic membrane *n* : a structure (as the amnion) that derives from the fertilized ovum but does not form a part of the embryo

em·bry·op·a·thy \ˌem-brē-'äp-ə-thē\ *n, pl* **-thies** : a developmental abnormality of an embryo or fetus esp. when caused by a disease (as German measles or mumps) in the mother

em·bryo·phore \'em-brē-ə-ˌfō(ə)r, -ˌfȯ(ə)r\ *n* : the outer cellular covering of the hexacanth embryo of a tapeworm; *broadly* : the covering and the included embryo

---

\ə\ abut \ᵊ\ kitten \ər\ further \a\ ash \ā\ ace \ä\ cot, cart \au̇\ out \ch\ chin \e\ bet \ē\ easy \g\ go \i\ hit \ī\ ice \j\ job \ŋ\ sing \ō\ go \ȯ\ law \ȯi\ boy \th\ thin \th\ the \ü\ loot \u̇\ foot \y\ yet \zh\ vision *See also* Pronunciation Symbols page

em·bry·o·tome \'em-brē-ə-ˌtōm\ *n* : an instrument used in embryotomy

em·bry·ot·o·my \ˌem-brē-'ät-ə-mē\ *n, pl* **-mies** **1** : mutilation of a fetus to facilitate removal from the uterus when natural delivery is impossible **2** : dissection of embryos for examination

em·bryo·tox·ic·i·ty \ˌem-brē-ō-ˌtäk-'sis-ət-ē\ *n, pl* **-ties** : the state of being toxic to embryos ⟨a test of the ∼ of xylene in mice and rats⟩ — **em·bryo·tox·ic** \-'täk-sik\ *adj*

em·bryo·tox·on \-'täk-ˌsän, -sən\ *n* : a congenital defect of the eye characterized by an opaque ring around the margin of the cornea

embryo transfer *n* : a procedure used esp. in animal breeding in which an embryo from a superovulated female is removed and reimplanted in the uterus of another female — called also *embryo transplant*

em·bry·o·trophe \'em-brē-ə-ˌtrōf\ *or* **em·bry·o·troph** \-ˌträf, -ˌtrȯf\ *n* : the pabulum of uterine tissue fluids and cellular debris that nourishes the embryo of a placental mammal prior to the establishment of the placental circulation — compare HEMOTROPHE, HISTOTROPHE

emer·gence \i-'mər-jən(t)s\ *n* : a recovering of consciousness (as from anesthesia)

emer·gen·cy \i-'mər-jən-sē\ *n, pl* **-cies** : an unforeseen combination of circumstances or the resulting state that calls for immediate action: as **a** : a sudden bodily alteration (as a ruptured appendix or surgical shock) such as is likely to require immediate medical attention **b** : a usu. distressing event or condition that can often be anticipated or prepared for but seldom exactly foreseen

emergency medical technician *n* : EMT

emergency medicine *n* : a medical specialty concerned with the care and treatment of acutely ill or injured patients who need immediate medical attention

emergency room *n* : a hospital room or area staffed and equipped for the reception and treatment of persons with conditions (as illness or trauma) requiring immediate medical care

emer·gent \i-'mər-jənt\ *adj* : calling for prompt or urgent action ⟨an ∼ condition in a hemophiliac⟩

emergent evolution *n* : evolution which according to some biological and philosophical theories involves the appearance of new characters and qualities (as life and consciousness) at more complex levels of organization (as the cell or organism) which cannot be predicted solely from the study of less complex levels (as the atom or molecule)

em·ery \'em-(ə-)rē\ *n, pl* **em·er·ies** *often attrib* : a dark granular mineral that consists essentially of corundum and is used for grinding and polishing; *also* : a hard abrasive powder

eme·sis \'em-ə-səs, i-'mē-\ *n, pl* **eme·ses** \-ˌsēz\ : VOMITING

¹emet·ic \i-'met-ik\ *n* : an agent that induces vomiting

²emetic *adj* : having the capacity to induce vomiting — **emet·i·cal·ly** \-i-k(ə-)lē\ *adv*

em·e·tine \'em-ə-ˌtēn\ *n* : an amorphous alkaloid $C_{29}H_{40}N_2O_4$ extracted from ipecac root and used as an emetic and expectorant

EMF *abbr* **1** electromagnetic field **2** electromotive force

EMG *abbr* electromyogram; electromyograph; electromyography

em·i·gra·tion \ˌem-ə-'grā-shən\ *n* : DIAPEDESIS

Em·i·nase \'em-i-ˌnās, -ˌnāz\ *trademark* — used for a preparation of anistreplase

em·i·nence \'em-ə-nən(t)s\ *n* : a protuberance or projection on a bodily part and esp. a bone

em·i·nen·tia \ˌem-ə-'nen-ch(ē-)ə\ *n* : EMINENCE

em·is·sary vein \'em-ə-ˌser-ē-\ *n* : any of the veins that pass through apertures in the skull and connect the venous sinuses of the dura mater with veins external to the skull

emis·sion \ē-'mish-ən\ *n* **1** : an act or instance of emitting **2 a** : something sent forth by emitting: as **(1)** : electrons discharged from a surface **(2)** : electromagnetic waves radiated by an antenna or a celestial body **(3)** : substances and esp. pollutants discharged into the air (as by a smokestack or

an automobile gasoline engine) **b** : a discharge of fluid from a living body; *esp* : EJACULATE — see NOCTURNAL EMISSION

emission spectrum *n* : an electromagnetic spectrum that derives its characteristics from the material of which the emitting source is made and from the way in which the material is excited — compare ABSORPTION SPECTRUM

emis·siv·i·ty \ˌem-ə-'siv-ət-ē, ˌē-ˌmis-'iv-\ *n, pl* **-ties** : the relative power of a surface to emit heat by radiation : the ratio of the radiant energy emitted by a surface to that emitted by a blackbody at the same temperature

em·men·a·gog·ic \i-ˌmen-ə-'gäj-ik, -ˌmēn-, -'gäg-\ *adj* : promoting menstruation

¹em·men·a·gogue \ə-'men-ə-ˌgäg, e-\ *adj* : EMMENAGOGIC

²emmenagogue *n* : an agent that promotes the menstrual discharge

em·me·trope \'em-ə-ˌtrōp\ *n* : a person having emmetropic eyes

em·me·tro·pia \ˌem-ə-'trō-pē-ə\ *n* : the normal refractive condition of the eye in which with accommodation relaxed parallel rays of light are all brought accurately to a focus upon the retina — compare ASTIGMATISM, MYOPIA — **em·me·trop·ic** \-'träp-ik, -'trōp-\ *adj*

em·o·din \'em-ə-dən\ *n* : an orange crystalline phenolic compound $C_{15}H_{10}O_5$ that is obtained from plants (as rhubarb and cascara buckthorn) and is used as a laxative

¹emol·lient \i-'mäl-yənt\ *adj* : making soft or supple; *also* : soothing esp. to the skin or mucous membrane

²emollient *n* : an emollient agent ⟨an ∼ for the hands⟩

emo·tion \i-'mō-shən\ *n* **1** : the affective aspect of consciousness **2** : a state of feeling **3** : a conscious mental reaction (as anger or fear) subjectively experienced as strong feeling usu. directed toward a specific object and typically accompanied by physiological and behavioral changes in the body — compare AFFECT — **emo·tion·al** \-shnəl, -shən-ᵊl\ *adj* — **emo·tion·al·i·ty** \-ˌmō-shə-'nal-ət-ē\ *n, pl* **-ties** — **emo·tion·al·ly** \-'mō-shnə-lē, -shən-ᵊl-ē\ *adv*

em·path·ic \em-'path-ik, im-\ *adj* : involving, characterized by, or based on empathy — **em·path·i·cal·ly** \-i-k(ə-)lē\ *adv*

em·pa·thize *or Brit* **em·pa·thise** \'em-pə-ˌthīz\ *vi* **-thized** *or Brit* **-thised; -thiz·ing** *or Brit* **-this·ing** : to experience empathy ⟨adults unable to ∼ with a child's frustrations⟩

em·pa·thy \'em-pə-thē\ *n, pl* **-thies** **1** : the imaginative projection of a subjective state into an object so that the object appears to be infused with it **2** : the action of understanding, being aware of, being sensitive to, and vicariously experiencing the feelings, thoughts, and experience of another of either the past or present without having the feelings, thoughts, and experience fully communicated in an objectively explicit manner; *also* : the capacity for empathy

em·phy·se·ma \ˌem(p)-fə-'zē-mə, -'sē-\ *n* : a condition characterized by air-filled expansions in interstitial or subcutaneous tissues; *specif* : a condition of the lung that is marked by distension and eventual rupture of the alveoli with progressive loss of pulmonary elasticity, that is accompanied by shortness of breath with or without cough, and that may lead to impairment of heart action — **em·phy·se·ma·tous** \-'zem-ət-əs, -'sem-, -'zēm-, -'sēm-\ *adj* — **em·phy·se·mic** \-'zē-mik, -'sē-\ *adj*

em·pir·ic \im-'pir-ik, em-\ *n* **1 a** : a member of an ancient sect of physicians who based their practice on experience alone disregarding all theoretical and philosophic considerations **b** : QUACK **2** : EMPIRICIST

em·pir·i·cal \-i-kəl\ *also* **em·pir·ic** \-ik\ *adj* **1** *archaic* **a** : following or used in the practice of the empirics — compare RATIONAL 2 **b** : being or befitting a quack or charlatan **2** : originating in or based on observation or experiment ⟨much medical lore had had an ∼ origin ... centuries of trial-and-error gropings after remedies —R. H. Shryock⟩ **3** : capable of being confirmed, verified, or disproved by observation or experiment ⟨∼ statements or laws⟩ — **em·pir·i·cal·ly** \-i-k(ə-)lē\ *adv*

empirical formula *n* : a chemical formula showing the simplest ratio of elements in a compound rather than the total number of atoms in the molecule ⟨CH_2O is the *empirical formula* for glucose⟩ — compare MOLECULAR FORMULA

em·pir·i·cism \im-'pir-ə-ˌsiz-əm, em-\ *n* **1 a** : a former school of medical practice based on the teachings of the empirics **b** : QUACKERY **2** : the practice of relying on observation and experiment esp. in the natural sciences

em·pir·i·cist \-səst\ *n* : one who relies on observation and experiment

em·pros·thot·o·nos \ˌem-ˌpräs-'thät-ᵊn-əs\ *n* : a tetanic spasm in which the head and feet are brought forward toward each other and the back arched

emp·ty-nest syndrome \'em(p)-tē-'nest-\ *n* : the emotional letdown often experienced by a parent whose children have grown up and moved away from home

empty sella syndrome *n* : a condition in which the subarachnoid space extends into the sella turcica causing it to become filled with cerebrospinal fluid, the pituitary gland is compressed, and the diaphragma sellae is greatly reduced but pituitary function usu. remains normal unless impaired by some other factor (as an infarction, irradiation, or a tumor)

em·py·ema \ˌem-ˌpī-'ē-mə\ *n, pl* **-ema·ta** \-mət-ə\ *also* **-emas** : the presence of pus in a bodily cavity (as the pleural cavity) — called also *pyothorax* — **em·py·emic** \-mik\ *adj*

em·py·reu·ma \ˌem-pə-'rü-mə, -ˌpī-\ *n, pl* **-ma·ta** \-mət-ə\ : the peculiar odor of the products of organic substances burned in closed vessels

em·py·reu·mat·ic \-ˌrü-'mat-ik\ *adj* : being or having an odor of burnt organic matter as a result of decomposition at high temperatures ⟨creosote and other ∼ oils⟩

EMS *abbr* **1** emergency medical service; emergency medical services **2** eosinophilia-myalgia syndrome

EMT \'ē-ˌem-'tē\ *n* : a specially trained medical technician certified to provide basic emergency services (as cardiopulmonary resuscitation) before and during transportation to a hospital — called also *emergency medical technician;* compare PARAMEDIC 2

emul *abbr* emulsion

emul·si·fi·er \i-'məl-sə-ˌfī(-ə)r\ *n* : one that emulsifies; *esp* : a surface-active agent (as a soap) promoting the formation and stabilization of an emulsion

emul·si·fy \-ˌfī\ *vt* **-fied; -fy·ing** : to disperse (as an oil) in an emulsion; *also* : to convert (two or more immiscible liquids) into an emulsion — **emul·si·fi·ca·tion** \i-ˌməl-sə-fə-'kā-shən\ *n*

emul·sin \i-'məl-sən\ *n* : any of various enzyme preparations that are obtained usu. from plants (as almonds) in the form of white amorphous powders and that contain glycosidases active on beta stereoisomers (as amygdalin or cellobiose) of the glycosides

emul·sion \i-'məl-shən\ *n* **1 a** : a system (as fat in milk) consisting of a liquid dispersed with or without an emulsifier in an immiscible liquid usu. in droplets of larger than colloidal size **b** : the state of such a system **2** : SUSPENSION 2; *esp* : a suspension of a sensitive silver salt or a mixture of halides of silver in a viscous medium (as a gelatin solution) forming a coating on photographic plates, film, or paper — **emul·sive** \-'məl-siv\ *adj*

emul·soid \i-'məl-ˌsȯid\ *n* **1** : a colloidal system consisting of a liquid dispersed in a liquid **2** : a lyophilic sol (as a gelatin solution) — **emul·soi·dal** \-ˌməl-'sȯid-ᵊl\ *adj*

emunc·to·ry \i-'məŋ(k)-t(ə-)rē\ *n, pl* **-ries** : an organ (as a kidney) or part of the body (as the skin) that carries off body wastes

en·abler \i-'nā-b(ə-)lər\ *n* : one that enables another to achieve an end; *esp* : one who enables another to persist in self-destructive behavior (as substance abuse) by providing excuses or by helping that individual avoid the consequences of such behavior

enal·a·pril \e-'nal-ə-ˌpril\ *n* : an antihypertensive drug that is an ACE inhibitor administered orally in the form of its maleate $C_{20}H_{28}N_2O_5 \cdot C_4H_4O_4$ — see VASOTEC

enal·a·pril·at \e-'nal-ə-ˌpril-ət\ *n* : the metabolically active form $C_{18}H_{24}N_2O_5 \cdot 2H_2O$ of enalapril administered intravenously — see VASOTEC

enam·el \in-'am-əl\ *n* : the intensely hard calcareous substance that forms a thin layer partly covering the teeth of many vertebrates including humans, is the hardest substance of the animal body, and consists of minute prisms secreted by ameloblasts, arranged at right angles to the surface, and bound together by a cement substance — compare CEMENTUM, DENTIN

enam·e·lo·ma \in-ˌam-ə-'lō-mə\ *n, pl* **-mas** *or* **-ma·ta** \-mət-ə\ : a benign tumor derived from the remains of the enamel organ

enamel organ *n* : an ectodermal ingrowth from the dental lamina that forms a cap with two walls separated by a reticulum of stellate cells, encloses the anterior part of the developing dental papilla and the cells of the inner enamel layer adjacent to the papilla, and differentiates into columnar ameloblasts which lay down the enamel rods of the tooth

enamel rod *n* : one of the elongated prismatic bodies making up the enamel of a tooth — called also *enamel prism*

enan·thate \i-'nan-ˌthāt\ *n* : a salt or ester of heptanoic acid — see TESTOSTERONE ENANTHATE

en·an·them \i-'nan(t)-thəm\ *or* **en·an·the·ma** \ˌen-ˌan-'thē-mə\ *n, pl* **-thems** *or* **-the·ma·ta** \-mət-ə\ : an eruption on a mucous surface — **en·an·the·ma·tous** \ˌen-ˌan-'them-ət-əs, -'thēm-\ *adj*

enan·thic acid \i-ˌnan-thik-\ *n* : HEPTANOIC ACID

en·an·tio·mer \in-'ant-ē-ə-mər\ *n* : either of a pair of chemical compounds whose molecular structures have a mirror-image relationship to each other — called also *optical antipode* — **en·an·tio·mer·ic** \-ˌant-ē-ə-'mer-ik\ *adj* — **en·an·tio·mer·i·cal·ly** \-i-k(ə-)lē\ *adv*

en·an·tio·morph \in-'ant-ē-ə-ˌmȯrf\ *n* : ENANTIOMER — **en·an·tio·mor·phic** \-ˌant-ē-ə-'mȯr-fik\ *or* **en·an·tio·mor·phous** \-fəs\ *adj* — **en·an·tio·mor·phism** \-'mȯr-ˌfiz-əm\ *n*

en·an·tio·se·lec·tive \in-ˌant-ē-ə-sə-'lek-tiv\ *adj* : relating to or being a chemical reaction in which one enantiomer of a chiral product is preferentially produced — **en·an·tio·se·lec·tive·ly** *adv*

en·an·tio·se·lec·tiv·i·ty \-sə-ˌlek-'tiv-ə-tē, -ˌsē-\ *n, pl* **-ties** : the degree to which one enantiomer of a chiral product is preferentially produced in a chemical reaction

en·ar·thro·di·al \ˌen-ˌär-'thrōd-ē-əl\ *adj* : of, relating to, or having the form of a ball-and-socket joint

en·ar·thro·sis \ˌen-ˌär-'thrō-səs\ *n, pl* **-thro·ses** \-ˌsēz\ : BALL-AND-SOCKET JOINT

en·cai·nide \en-'kā-ˌnīd\ *n* : an antiarrhythmic drug $C_{22}H_{28}N_2O_2$ withdrawn from use when it was shown to increase mortality in patients who had a recent heart attack prior to receiving the drug

en·cap·su·late \in-'kap-sə-ˌlāt\ *vb* **-lat·ed; -lat·ing** *vt* : to surround, encase, or protect in or as if in a capsule ⟨DNA has been *encapsulated* in microspheres —Paul Smaglik⟩ ∼ *vi* : to become encapsulated ⟨a bacillus that ∼*s* in the human body⟩ — **en·cap·su·la·tion** \-ˌkap-sə-'lā-shən\ *n*

en·cap·su·lat·ed *adj* : surrounded by a gelatinous or membranous envelope ⟨an ∼ drug⟩ ⟨∼ bacteria⟩

en·cap·suled \in-'kap-səld, -(ˌ)süld\ *adj* : ENCAPSULATED

en·ceinte \äⁿ(n)-'sant\ *adj* : PREGNANT

en·ce·phal·ic \ˌen(t)-sə-'fal-ik\ *adj* : of or relating to the brain; *also* : lying within the cranial cavity

en·ceph·a·li·tis \in-ˌsef-ə-'līt-əs\ *n, pl* **-lit·i·des** \-'lit-ə-ˌdēz\ : inflammation of the brain — **en·ceph·a·lit·ic** \-'lit-ik\ *adj*

encephalitis le·thar·gi·ca \-li-'thär-ji-kə, -le-\ *n* : epidemic virus encephalitis in which somnolence is marked — called also *lethargic encephalitis*

encephalitis peri·ax·i·alis dif·fu·sa \-ˌper-ē-ˌak-sē-'ā-ləs-di-'fyü-sə\ *n* : ADRENOLEUKODYSTROPHY

\ə\ abut \ᵊ\ kitten \ər\ further \a\ ash \ā\ ace \ä\ cot, cart \au̇\ out \ch\ chin \e\ bet \ē\ easy \g\ go \i\ hit \ī\ ice \j\ job \ŋ\ sing \ō\ go \ȯ\ law \ȯi\ boy \th\ thin \t͟h\ the \ü\ loot \u̇\ foot \y\ yet \zh\ vision *See also* Pronunciation Symbols page

E
F

en·ceph·a·lit·o·gen \in-ˌsef-ə-'lit-ə-jən, -ˌjen\ *n* : an encephalitogenic agent (as a virus)

en·ceph·a·lit·o·gen·ic \in-ˌsef-ə-ˌlit-ə-'jen-ik\ *adj* : tending to cause encephalitis ⟨an ∼ strain of a virus⟩

en·ceph·a·li·to·zo·on \-ˌlīt-ə-'zō-ˌän, -'zō-ən\ *n* **1** *cap* : a genus of protozoans of the order Microsporidia that infect the brain and kidneys of numerous mammals and that include one (*E. cuniculi*) infecting humans and esp. immunocompromised individuals **2** *pl* **en·ceph·a·li·to·zoa** \-'zō-ə\ : any protozoan of the genus *Encephalitozoon*

en·ceph·a·lo·cele \in-'sef-ə-lō-ˌsēl\ *n* : hernia of the brain that is either congenital or due to trauma

en·ceph·a·lo·gram \in-'sef-ə-lə-ˌgram\ *n* : an X-ray picture of the brain made by encephalography

en·ceph·a·lo·graph \-ˌgraf\ *n* **1** : ENCEPHALOGRAM **2** : ELECTROENCEPHALOGRAPH

en·ceph·a·log·ra·phy \in-ˌsef-ə-'läg-rə-fē\ *n, pl* **-phies** : radiography of the brain after the cerebrospinal fluid has been replaced by a gas (as air) — **en·ceph·a·lo·graph·ic** \-lə-'graf-ik\ *adj* — **en·ceph·a·lo·graph·i·cal·ly** \-i-k(ə-)lē\ *adv*

en·ceph·a·loid \in-'sef-ə-ˌlȯid\ *adj* : resembling the material of the brain

en·ceph·a·lo·ma·la·cia \in-ˌsef-ə-lō-mə-'lā-sh(ē-)ə\ *n* : softening of the brain due to degenerative changes in nervous tissue (as in crazy chick disease) — **en·ceph·a·lo·ma·lac·ic** \-mə-'las-ik\ *adj*

en·ceph·a·lo·men·in·gi·tis \-ˌmen-ən-'jīt-əs\ *n, pl* **-git·i·des** \-'jit-ə-ˌdēz\ : MENINGOENCEPHALITIS

en·ceph·a·lo·me·nin·go·cele \-mə-'niŋ-gə-ˌsēl, -'nin-jə-\ *n* : protrusion of both brain substance and the meninges through a fissure in the skull

en·ceph·a·lo·mere \in-'sef-ə-lə-ˌmi(ə)r\ *n* : a segment of the embryonic brain — **en·ceph·a·lo·mer·ic** \-ˌsef-ə-lə-'mer-ik\ *adj*

en·ceph·a·lo·my·eli·tis \in-ˌsef-ə-lō-ˌmī-ə-'līt-əs\ *n, pl* **-elit·i·des** \-ə-'lit-ə-ˌdēz\ : concurrent inflammation of the brain and spinal cord; *specif* : EQUINE ENCEPHALOMYELITIS — see ACUTE DISSEMINATED ENCEPHALOMYELITIS, ALLERGIC ENCEPHALOMYELITIS, AVIAN ENCEPHALOMYELITIS — **en·ceph·a·lo·my·elit·ic** \-ə-'lit-ik\ *adj*

en·ceph·a·lo·my·elop·a·thy \-ˌmī-ə-'läp-ə-thē\ *n, pl* **-thies** : any disease that affects the brain and spinal cord

en·ceph·a·lo·myo·car·di·tis \-ˌmī-ə-kär-'dīt-əs\ *n* : an acute febrile virus disease that affects numerous vertebrates including humans but is of serious clinical significance mostly in swine, that is caused by any of several strains of a picornavirus (genus *Cardiovirus*), and that in swine is characterized esp. by degeneration and inflammation of skeletal and cardiac muscle and lesions of the central nervous system

en·ceph·a·lon \in-'sef-ə-ˌlän, -lən\ *n, pl* **-la** \-lə\ : the vertebrate brain

en·ceph·a·lop·a·thy \in-ˌsef-ə-'läp-ə-thē\ *n, pl* **-thies** : a disease of the brain; *esp* : one involving alterations of brain structure — **en·ceph·a·lo·path·ic** \-lə-'path-ik\ *adj*

en·ceph·a·lo·sis \-'lō-səs\ *n, pl* **-lo·ses** \-ˌsēz\ : ENCEPHALOPATHY

en·chon·dral \(')en-'kän-drəl, (')eŋ-\ *adj* : ENDOCHONDRAL

en·chon·dro·ma \ˌen-ˌkän-'drō-mə, -ˌeŋ-\ *n, pl* **-mas** *also* **-ma·ta** \-mət-ə\ : a tumor consisting of cartilaginous tissue; *esp* : one arising where cartilage does not normally exist — **en·chon·dro·ma·tous** \-'dräm-ət-əs, -'drōm-\ *adj*

en·clave \'en-ˌklāv; 'än-ˌklāv, 'äŋ-, -ˌkläv\ *n* : something enclosed in an organ or tissue but not a continuous part of it

en·code \in-'kōd, en-\ *vt* **en·cod·ed; en·cod·ing** : to specify the genetic code for ⟨each nucleotide triplet or codon on the mRNA chain ∼s a specific amino acid —J. E. Darnell, Jr.⟩

en·co·pre·sis \ˌen-ˌkäp-'rē-səs, -kə-'prē-\ *n, pl* **-re·ses** \-ˌsēz\ : involuntary passage of feces ⟨∼ as a consequence of chronic constipation⟩ — **en·cop·ret·ic** \ˌen-ˌkäp-'ret-ik, -kə-'pret-\ *adj*

en·coun·ter group \in-'kaünt-ər, en-\ *n* : a usu. leaderless and unstructured group that seeks to develop the capacity of the individual to express feelings and to form emotional ties by unrestrained confrontation of individuals (as by physical contact, uninhibited verbalization, or nudity) — compare T-GROUP

en·crust *also* **in·crust** \in-'krəst\ *vt* : to cover, line, or overlay with a crust ∼ *vi* : to form a crust

en·crus·ta·tion \ˌ(ˌ)in-ˌkrəs-'tā-shən, ˌen-\ *var of* INCRUSTATION

en·cyst \in-'sist, en-\ *vt* : to enclose in or as if in a cyst ⟨an ∼ed tumor⟩ ∼ *vi* : to form or become enclosed in a cyst ⟨protozoans ∼ing in order to resist desiccation⟩ — **en·cyst·ment** \-'sis(t)-mənt\ *n*

en·cys·ta·tion \ˌen-ˌsis-'tā-shən\ *n* : the process of forming a cyst or becoming enclosed in a capsule

end·ame·ba *or chiefly Brit* **end·amoe·ba** \ˌen-də-'mē-bə\ *n, pl* **-bas** *or* **-bae** \-(ˌ)bē\ : any ameba of the genus *Endamoeba*

End·amoe·ba \ˌen-də-'mē-bə\ *n* : a genus of amebas including forms parasitic in the intestines of insects and in some esp. former classifications various parasites of vertebrates now usu. included in the genus *Entamoeba*

end·ar·ter·ec·to·my \ˌen-ˌdärt-ə-'rek-tə-mē\ *n, pl* **-mies** : surgical removal of the inner layer of an artery when thickened and atheromatous or occluded (as by intimal plaques)

end·ar·te·ri·al \ˌen-där-'tir-ē-əl\ *adj* : of or relating to the intima of an artery

end·ar·te·ri·tis \ˌen-ˌdärt-ə-'rīt-əs\ *also* **en·do·ar·te·ri·tis** \ˌen-dō-ˌärt-\ *n* : inflammation of the intima of one or more arteries

endarteritis ob·lit·er·ans \-ə-'blit-ə-ˌranz, -rənz\ *n* : endarteritis in which the intimal tissue proliferates and ultimately plugs the lumen of an affected artery — called also *obliterating endarteritis*

end·ar·te·ri·um \ˌen-där-'tir-ē-əm\ *n, pl* **-ria** \-ē-ə\ : the intima of an artery

end artery *n* : a terminal artery (as a coronary artery) supplying all or most of the blood to a body part without significant collateral circulation

end–au·ral \(')en-'dȯr-əl\ *adj* : performed or applied within the ear ⟨∼ surgery⟩ ⟨an ∼ dressing⟩

end·brain \'en(d)-ˌbrān\ *n* : TELENCEPHALON

end brush *n* : END PLATE

end bud *n* : TAIL BUD

end bulb *n* : a bulbous termination of a sensory nerve fiber (as in the skin or in a mucous membrane) — compare KRAUSE'S CORPUSCLE

end–di·a·stol·ic \ˌen-ˌdī-ə-'stäl-ik\ *adj* : relating to or occurring in the moment immediately preceding contraction of the heart ⟨∼ pressure⟩

¹en·dem·ic \en-'dem-ik, in-\ *adj* : restricted or peculiar to a locality or region ⟨∼ diseases⟩ ⟨an ∼ species⟩ — compare EPIDEMIC 1, SPORADIC — **en·dem·i·cal·ly** \-'dem-i-k(ə-)lē\ *adv*

²endemic *n* **1** : an endemic disease or an instance of its occurrence **2** : an endemic organism

en·de·mic·i·ty \ˌen-ˌdem-'is-ət-ē, -də-'mis-\ *n, pl* **-ties** : the quality or state of being endemic

endemic typhus *n* : MURINE TYPHUS

en·de·mism \'en-də-ˌmiz-əm\ *n* : ENDEMICITY

end·er·gon·ic \ˌen-dər-'gän-ik\ *adj* : ENDOTHERMIC 1 ⟨∼ biochemical reactions⟩ — compare EXERGONIC

en·der·mat·ic \ˌen-dər-'mat-ik\ *adj* : ENDERMIC 1

en·der·mic \en-'dər-mik\ *adj* **1** : acting through the skin or by direct application to the skin ⟨∼ ointments⟩ **2** : administered within the dermis : INTRADERMAL ⟨∼ injections⟩

end foot *n, pl* **end feet** : BOUTON

en·do·ab·dom·i·nal \ˌen-dō-ab-'däm-ən-²l, -əb-, -'däm-n²l\ *adj* : relating to or occurring in the interior of the abdomen

en·do·an·eu·rys·mor·rha·phy \ˌen-dō-ˌan-yə-ˌriz-'mȯr-ə-fē\ *n, pl* **-phies** : a surgical treatment of aneurysm that involves opening its sac and collapsing, folding, and suturing its walls so that the lumen of the blood vessel approximates normal size

endoarteritis *var of* ENDARTERITIS

en·do·bi·ot·ic \ˌen-dō-ˌbī-'ät-ik, -bē-\ *adj* : dwelling within the cells or tissues of a host ⟨∼ bacteria⟩

en·do·blast \'en-də-ˌblast\ *n* : HYPOBLAST — **en·do·blas·tic** \ˌen-də-'blas-tik\ *adj*

en·do·bron·chi·al \ˌen-dō-'brän-kē-əl\ *adj* : located within a bronchus — **en·do·bron·chi·al·ly** \-ə-lē\ *adv*

en·do·car·di·ac \-'kärd-ē-ˌak\ *adj* : ENDOCARDIAL

en·do·car·di·al \-'kärd-ē-əl\ *adj* **1** : situated within the heart **2** : of or relating to the endocardium ⟨~ biopsy⟩

endocardial fibroelastosis *n* : a condition usu. associated with congestive heart failure and enlargement of the heart that is characterized by conversion of the endocardium to fibroelastic tissue

en·do·car·di·tis \ˌen-dō-ˌkär-'dīt-əs\ *n* : inflammation of the lining of the heart and its valves

en·do·car·di·um \-'kärd-ē-əm\ *n, pl* **-dia** \-ē-ə\ : a thin serous membrane lining the cavities of the heart

en·do·cast \'en-də-ˌkast\ *n* : ENDOCRANIAL CAST

en·do·cel·lu·lar \ˌen-dō-'sel-yə-lər\ *adj* : INTRACELLULAR

en·do·cer·vi·cal \ˌen-dō-'sər-vi-kəl\ *adj* : of, relating to, or affecting the endocervix

en·do·cer·vi·ci·tis \-ˌsər-və-'sīt-əs\ *n* : inflammation of the lining of the uterine cervix

en·do·cer·vix \-'sər-viks\ *n, pl* **-vi·ces** \-və-ˌsēz\ : the epithelial and glandular lining of the uterine cervix

en·do·chon·dral \ˌen-də-'kän-drəl\ *adj* : relating to, formed by, or being ossification that takes place from centers arising in cartilage and involves deposition of lime salts in the cartilage matrix followed by secondary absorption and replacement by true bony tissue — compare INTRAMEMBRANOUS 1, PERICHONDRAL

en·do·cor·pus·cu·lar \-ˌkȯr-'pəs-kyə-lər\ *adj* : located within a red blood cell ⟨~ parasites of malaria⟩

en·do·cra·ni·al \ˌen-də-'krā-nē-əl\ *adj* : of or relating to an endocranial cast or to the cranial cavity ⟨~ volume⟩

endocranial cast *n* : a cast of the cranial cavity showing the approximate shape of the brain

¹en·do·crine \'en-də-krən, -ˌkrīn, -ˌkrēn\ *adj* **1** : secreting internally; *specif* : producing secretions that are distributed in the body by way of the bloodstream ⟨an ~ system⟩ **2** : of, relating to, affecting, or resembling an endocrine gland or secretion ⟨~ tumors⟩

²endocrine *n* **1** : HORMONE 1a **2** : ENDOCRINE GLAND

endocrine gland *n* : a gland (as the thyroid or the pituitary) that produces an endocrine secretion — called also *ductless gland, gland of internal secretion*

endocrine system *n* : the glands and parts of glands that produce endocrine secretions, help to integrate and control bodily metabolic activity, and include esp. the pituitary, thyroid, parathyroids, adrenals, islets of Langerhans, ovaries, and testes

en·do·cri·no·log·ic \ˌen-də-ˌkrin-ᵊl-'äj-ik, -ˌkrīn-, -ˌkrēn-\ *or* **en·do·cri·no·log·i·cal** \-i-kəl\ *adj* : involving or relating to the endocrine glands or secretions or to endocrinology

en·do·cri·nol·o·gy \ˌen-də-kri-'näl-ə-jē, -ˌkrī-\ *n, pl* **-gies** : a science dealing with the endocrine glands — **en·do·cri·nol·o·gist** \-jəst\ *n*

en·do·cri·nop·a·thy \-krə-'näp-ə-thē, -ˌkrī-, -ˌkrē-\ *n, pl* **-thies** : a disease marked by dysfunction of an endocrine gland — **en·do·crin·o·path·ic** \-ˌkrin-ə-'path-ik, -ˌkrīn-, -ˌkrēn-\ *adj*

en·do·cyst \'en-də-ˌsist\ *n* : the lining membrane of a hydatid cyst from which larvae are budded off

en·do·cyt·ic \ˌen-də-'sit-ik\ *adj* : of or relating to endocytosis : ENDOCYTOTIC ⟨~ vesicles⟩

en·do·cy·to·sis \-sī-'tō-səs\ *n, pl* **-to·ses** \-ˌsēz\ : incorporation of substances into a cell by phagocytosis or pinocytosis — **en·do·cy·tose** \-'sī-ˌtōs, -ˌtōz\ *vt* **-tosed; -tos·ing** — **en·do·cy·tot·ic** \-sī-'tät-ik\ *adj*

en·do·derm \'en-də-ˌdərm\ *n* : the innermost of the three primary germ layers of an embryo that is the source of the epithelium of the digestive tract and its derivatives and of the lower respiratory tract; *also* : a tissue that is derived from this germ layer — **en·do·der·mal** \ˌen-də-'dər-məl\ *adj*

end·odon·tia \ˌen-də-'dän-ch(ē-)ə\ *n* : ENDODONTICS

end·odon·tics \-'dänt-iks\ *n pl but sing in constr* : a branch of dentistry concerned with diseases of the pulp — **end·odon·tic** \-'dänt-ik\ *adj* — **end·odon·ti·cal·ly** \-'dänt-i-k(ə-)lē\ *adv*

end·odon·tist \-'dänt-əst\ *n* : a specialist in endodontics

en·do·en·zyme \ˌen-dō-'en-ˌzīm\ *n* : an enzyme that functions inside the cell — compare EXOENZYME

en·do·ep·i·the·li·al \ˌen-dō-ˌep-ə-'thē-lē-əl\ *adj* : occurring within epithelial cells ⟨~ parasites⟩

en·do·eryth·ro·cyt·ic \ˌen-dō-i-ˌrith-rə-'sit-ik\ *adj* : occurring within red blood cells — used chiefly of stages of malaria parasites

en·dog·a·my \en-'däg-ə-mē\ *n, pl* **-mies** : marriage within a specific group as required by custom or law — **en·dog·a·mous** \-məs\ *adj*

en·do·gas·tric \ˌen-dō-'gas-trik\ *adj* : of or relating to the inside of the stomach — **en·do·gas·tri·cal·ly** \-tri-k(ə-)lē\ *adv*

en·dog·e·nous \en-'däj-ə-nəs\ *also* **en·do·gen·ic** \ˌen-də-'jen-ik\ *adj* **1** : growing from or on the inside ⟨~ spores⟩ **2** : caused by factors within the body or mind or arising from internal structural or functional causes ⟨~ malnutrition⟩ ⟨~ psychic depression⟩ **3** : relating to or produced by metabolic synthesis in the body ⟨~ opioids⟩ ⟨~ amino acids⟩ — compare EXOGENOUS — **en·dog·e·nous·ly** *adv*

en·do·gna·thi·on \ˌen-də-'nā-thē-ˌän, -'nath-ē-\ *n* : the medial segment of the premaxilla situated on each side of the midline of the palate and bearing the medial incisor

En·do·li·max \-'lī-ˌmaks\ *n* : a genus of amebas that are commensal in vertebrate intestines and include one (*E. nana*) found in humans

en·do·lymph \'en-də-ˌlim(p)f\ *n* : the watery fluid in the membranous labyrinth of the ear — **en·do·lym·phat·ic** \ˌen-də-lim-'fat-ik\ *adj*

endolymphaticus — see DUCTUS ENDOLYMPHATICUS

en·do·me·ninx \ˌen-də-'mē-niŋ(k)s, -'men-iŋ(k)s\ *n, pl* **-nin·ges** \-mə-'nin-(ˌ)jēz\ : the layer of embryonic mesoderm from which the arachnoid coat and pia mater of the brain develop

en·do·me·so·derm \ˌen-dō-'mez-ə-ˌdərm, -'mēz-, -'mēs-, -'mes-\ *n* : an embryonic blastomere or cell layer not yet differentiated into mesoderm and endoderm but destined to give rise to both — called also *mesendoderm* — **en·do·me·so·der·mal** \-ˌmez-ə-'dər-məl, -ˌmēz-, -ˌmēs-, -ˌmes-\ *adj*

en·do·me·tri·al \ˌen-də-'mē-trē-əl\ *adj* : of, belonging to, or consisting of endometrium

en·do·me·tri·o·ma \-ˌmē-trē-'ō-mə\ *n, pl* **-mas** *also* **-ma·ta** \-mət-ə\ **1** : a tumor containing endometrial tissue **2** : ENDOMETRIOSIS — used chiefly of isolated foci of endometrium outside the uterus

en·do·me·tri·osis \ˌen-dō-ˌmē-trē-'ō-səs\ *n, pl* **-oses** \-ˌsēz\ : the presence and growth of functioning endometrial tissue in places other than the uterus that often results in severe pain and infertility — see ADENOMYOSIS — **en·do·me·tri·ot·ic** \-trē-'ät-ik\ *adj*

en·do·me·tri·tis \-mə-'trīt-əs\ *n* : inflammation of the endometrium

en·do·me·tri·um \-'mē-trē-əm\ *n, pl* **-tria** \-trē-ə\ : the mucous membrane lining the uterus that is composed of three layers — see STRATUM BASALE, STRATUM COMPACTUM, STRATUM SPONGIOSUM

en·do·mic·tic \ˌen-də-'mik-tik\ *adj* : of or relating to endomixis

en·do·mi·to·sis \-mī-'tō-səs\ *n, pl* **-to·ses** \-ˌsēz\ : division of chromosomes that is not followed by nuclear division and that results in an increased number of chromosomes in the cell — **en·do·mi·tot·ic** \-mī-'tät-ik\ *adj*

en·do·mix·is \-'mik-səs\ *n* : a periodic nuclear reorganization in ciliate protozoans

en·do·morph \'en-də-ˌmȯrf\ *n* : an endomorphic individual

en·do·mor·phic \ˌen-də-'mȯr-fik\ *adj* **1** : of or relating to the component in W. H. Sheldon's classification of body

---

\ə\ abut \ᵊ\ kitten \ər\ further \a\ ash \ā\ ace \ä\ cot, cart \au̇\ out \ch\ chin \e\ bet \ē\ easy \g\ go \i\ hit \ī\ ice \j\ job \ŋ\ sing \ō\ go \ȯ\ law \ȯi\ boy \th\ thin \th̲\ the \ü\ loot \u̇\ foot \y\ yet \zh\ vision *See also* Pronunciation Symbols page

types that measures the degree to which the digestive viscera are massive and the body build rounded and soft **2** : having a heavy rounded body build often with a marked tendency to become fat — compare ECTOMORPHIC 2, MESOMORPHIC 2b — **en·do·mor·phy** \'en-də-ˌmȯr-fē\ *n, pl* **-phies**

en·do·myo·car·di·al \ˌen-dō-ˌmī-ə-'kärd-ē-əl\ *adj* : of, relating to, or affecting the endocardium and the myocardium ⟨an ∼ biopsy⟩ — **en·do·myo·car·di·um** \-ē-əm\ *n, pl* **-dia** \-ē-ə\

en·do·my·si·al \ˌen-də-'miz-ē-əl, -'mizh(-ē)-əl\ *adj* : of, relating to, or affecting endomysium ⟨∼ inflammation⟩

en·do·my·si·um \-əm\ *n, pl* **-sia** \-ə\ : the delicate connective tissue surrounding the individual muscular fibers within the smallest bundles — compare EPIMYSIUM

en·do·neu·ri·um \ˌen-dō-'n(y)ùr-ē-əm\ *n, pl* **-ria** \-ē-ə\ : the delicate connective tissue network holding together the individual fibers of a nerve trunk — **en·do·neu·ri·al** \-ē-əl\ *adj*

en·do·nu·cle·ase \-'n(y)ü-klē-ˌās, -ˌāz\ *n* : an enzyme that breaks down a nucleotide chain into two or more shorter chains by cleaving the internal phosphodiester bonds — see RESTRICTION ENDONUCLEASE; compare EXONUCLEASE

en·do·nu·cleo·lyt·ic \-ˌn(y)ü-klē-ō-'lit-ik\ *adj* : cleaving a nucleotide chain into two parts at an internal point ⟨∼ nicks⟩

en·do·par·a·site \-'par-ə-ˌsīt\ *n* : a parasite that lives in the internal organs or tissues of its host — compare ECTOPARASITE — **en·do·par·a·sit·ic** \-ˌpar-ə-'sit-ik\ *adj* — **en·do·par·a·sit·ism** \-'par-ə-ˌsīt-ˌiz-əm, -sə-ˌtiz-\ *n*

en·do·pep·ti·dase \-'pep-tə-ˌdās, -ˌdāz\ *n* : any of a group of enzymes that hydrolyze peptide bonds inside the long chains of protein molecules : PROTEASE — compare EXOPEPTIDASE

en·do·peri·car·di·al \-ˌper-i-'kärd-ē-əl\ *adj* : of or involving the endocardium and pericardium ⟨∼ infection⟩

en·do·per·ox·ide \-pə-'räk-ˌsīd\ *n* : any of various biosynthetic intermediates in the formation of prostaglandins

en·do·phil·ic \ˌen-də-'fil-ik\ *adj* : ecologically associated with humans and their domestic environment ⟨mosquitoes that are ∼ vectors of malaria⟩ — compare EXOPHILIC — **en·doph·i·ly** \en-'däf-ə-lē\ *n, pl* **-lies**

en·do·phle·bi·tis \ˌen-dō-fli-'bīt-əs\ *n, pl* **-bi·tis·es** *or* **-bit·i·des** \-'bit-ə-ˌdēz\ : inflammation of the intima of a vein

en·doph·thal·mi·tis \ˌen-ˌdäf-thal-'mīt-əs\ *n* : inflammation (as from infection by a fungus of the genus *Candida*) that affects the interior of the eyeball

en·do·phyt·ic \ˌen-dō-'fit-ik\ *adj* : tending to grow inward into tissues in fingerlike projections from a superficial site of origin — used of tumors; compare EXOPHYTIC

en·do·plasm \'en-də-ˌplaz-əm\ *n* : the inner relatively fluid part of the cytoplasm — compare ECTOPLASM — **en·do·plas·mic** \ˌen-də-'plaz-mik\ *adj*

endoplasmic reticulum *n* : a system of interconnected vesicular and lamellar cytoplasmic membranes that functions esp. in the transport of materials within the cell and that is studded with ribosomes in some places — see ROUGH ENDOPLASMIC RETICULUM

en·do·poly·ploi·dy \ˌen-dō-'päl-i-ˌplȯid-ē\ *n, pl* **-dies** : a polyploid state in which the chromosomes have divided repeatedly without subsequent division of the nucleus or cell — **en·do·poly·ploid** \-ˌplȯid\ *adj*

en·do·pros·the·sis \-präs-'thē-səs\ *n, pl* **-the·ses** \-ˌsēz\ : an artificial device to replace a missing bodily part that is placed inside the body

en·do·ra·dio·sonde \-'rād-ē-ō-ˌsänd\ *n* : a microelectronic device introduced into the body to record physiological data not otherwise obtainable

end–organ *adj* : of or relating to an organ (as the liver or kidney) that is ultimately affected by a chronic or progressive disease or condition ⟨diabetic ∼ damage⟩ ⟨predictions of ∼ function and failure in severe sepsis —G. J. Slotman⟩

end organ *n* : a structure forming the peripheral terminus of a path of nerve conduction and consisting of an effector or a receptor with its associated nerve terminations

en·dor·phin \en-'dȯr-fən\ *n* : any of a group of endogenous peptides (as enkephalin and dynorphin) found esp. in the brain that bind chiefly to opiate receptors and produce some of the same pharmacological effects (as pain relief) as those of opiates; *specif* : BETA-ENDORPHIN

β**–endorphin** *var of* BETA-ENDORPHIN

en·do·sal·pinx \ˌen-dō-'sal-ˌpiŋ(k)s\ *n, pl* **-pin·ges** \-sal-'pin-ˌjēz\ : the mucous membrane lining the fallopian tube

en·do·scope \'en-də-ˌskōp\ *n* : an illuminated usu. fiber-optic flexible or rigid tubular instrument for visualizing the interior of a hollow organ or part (as the bladder or esophagus) for diagnostic or therapeutic purposes that typically has one or more channels to enable passage of instruments (as forceps or scissors) — **en·dos·co·py** \en-'däs-kə-pē\ *n, pl* **-pies**

en·do·scop·ic \ˌen-də-'skäp-ik\ *adj* : of, relating to, or performed by means of an endoscope or endoscopy — **en·do·scop·i·cal·ly** \-i-k(ə-)lē\ *adv*

endoscopic retrograde chol·an·gio·pan·cre·atog·ra·phy \-kə-ˌlan-jē-ə-ˌpan-krē-ə-'täg-rə-fē, -ˌpan-\ *n* : radiographic visualization of the pancreatic and biliary ducts by means of endoscopic injection of a contrast medium through the ampulla of Vater — called also *endoscopic cholangiopancreatography*

en·dos·co·pist \en-'däs-kə-pəst\ *n* : a person trained in the use of the endoscope

en·do·skel·e·ton \ˌen-dō-'skel-ət-ᵊn\ *n* : an internal skeleton or supporting framework in an animal — compare EXOSKELETON — **en·do·skel·e·tal** \-ət-ᵊl\ *adj*

end·os·mom·e·ter \ˌen-ˌdäs-'mäm-ət-ər, -ˌdäz-\ *n* : an instrument for measuring endosmosis — **end·os·mo·met·ric** \-mə-'me-trik\ *adj*

end·os·mo·sis \ˌen-ˌdäs-'mō-səs, -ˌdäz-\ *n, pl* **-mo·ses** \-ˌsēz\ : passage (as of a surface-active substance) through a membrane from a region of lower to a region of higher concentration — compare EXOSMOSIS — **end·os·mot·ic** \-'mät-ik\ *adj* — **end·os·mot·i·cal·ly** \-i-k(ə-)lē\ *adv*

en·do·some \'en-də-ˌsōm\ *n* **1** : a conspicuous body other than a chromatin granule that occurs within the nuclear membrane of a vesicular protozoan nucleus and is either a karyosome or a nucleolus **2** : a vesicle formed by the invagination and pinching off of the cell membrane during endocytosis

en·do·spore \-ˌspō(ə)r, -ˌspȯ(ə)r\ *n* : an asexual spore developed within the cell esp. in bacteria

en·do·spor·u·la·tion \ˌen-də-ˌspȯr-yə-'lā-shən, -ˌspȯr-\ *n* : the production of endospores

en·do·stat·in \ˌen-də-'stat-ᵊn\ *n* : a polypeptide that is a proteolytic fragment of the carboxyl terminus of a collagen found esp. in the epithelial basement membrane and that inhibits angiogenesis, tumor growth, and endothelial cell proliferation

end·os·te·al \en-'däs-tē-əl\ *adj* **1** : of or relating to the endosteum **2** : located within bone or cartilage — **end·os·te·al·ly** \-ə-lē\ *adv*

end·os·te·itis \ˌen-ˌdäs-tē-'īt-əs\ *or* **end·os·ti·tis** \-ˌdäs-'tīt-əs\ *n* : inflammation of the endosteum

end·os·te·um \en-'däs-tē-əm\ *n, pl* **-tea** \-tē-ə\ : the layer of vascular connective tissue lining the medullary cavities of bone

en·do·sym·bi·ont \ˌen-dō-'sim-ˌbī-ˌänt, -bē-\ *also* **en·do·sym·bi·ote** \-ˌōt\ *n* : a symbiotic organism living within the body of its partner

en·do·sym·bi·o·sis \ˌen-dō-ˌsim-bī-'ō-səs, -bē-\ *n, pl* **-o·ses** \-ˌsēz\ : symbiosis in which a symbiotic organism lives within the body of its partner — **en·do·sym·bi·ot·ic** \-'ät-ik\ *adj*

en·do·the·li·al \ˌen-dō-'thē-lē-əl\ *adj* : of, relating to, or produced from endothelium

en·do·the·lin \ˌen-dō-'thē-lin\ *n* : any of several polypeptides consisting of 21 amino acid residues that are produced in various cells and tissues, that play a role in regulating vasomotor activity, cell proliferation, and the production of hormones, and that have been implicated in the development of vascular disease

en·do·the·lio·cho·ri·al \-ˌthē-lē-ō-ˈkōr-ē-əl, -ˈkȯr-\ *adj* : having fetal epithelium enclosing maternal blood vessels ⟨carnivores and some insectivores have an ~ placenta⟩

en·do·the·li·o·ma \-ˌthē-lē-ˈō-mə\ *n, pl* **-mas** *also* **-ma·ta** \-mət-ə\ : a tumor developing from endothelial tissue

en·do·the·li·um \ˌen-də-ˈthē-lē-əm\ *n, pl* **-lia** \-lē-ə\ : an epithelium of mesoblastic origin composed of a single layer of thin flattened cells that lines internal body cavities (as the serous cavities or the interior of the heart)

en·do·therm \ˈen-də-ˌthərm\ *n* : a warm-blooded animal

en·do·ther·mic \ˌen-də-ˈthər-mik\ *also* **en·do·ther·mal** \-məl\ *adj* **1** : characterized by or formed with absorption of heat — compare EXOTHERMIC **2** : WARM-BLOODED

en·do·ther·my \ˈen-də-ˌthər-mē\ *n, pl* **-mies 1** : DIATHERMY **2** : physiological regulation of body temperature by metabolic means; *esp* : the property or state of being warm-blooded

¹en·do·thrix \ˈen-də-ˌthriks\ *n* : an endothrix fungus of the genus *Trichophyton* (esp. *T. tonsurans*)

²endothrix *adj* : occurring within or penetrating the hair shaft ⟨~ dermatophytes⟩; *also* : characterized by the presence of hyphae and arthroconidia within the hair shaft ⟨~ tinea capitis⟩ — compare ECTOTHRIX

en·do·tox·emia *or chiefly Brit* **en·do·tox·ae·mia** \ˌen-dō-täk-ˈsē-mē-ə\ *n* : the presence of endotoxins in the blood

en·do·tox·in \ˌen-dō-ˈtäk-sən\ *n* : a toxin of internal origin; *specif* : a poisonous substance present in bacteria (as the causative agent of typhoid fever) but separable from the cell body only on its disintegration — compare EXOTOXIN — **en·do·tox·ic** \-sik\ *adj*

en·do·tox·oid \-ˈtäk-ˌsȯid\ *n* : a toxoid derived from an endotoxin

en·do·tra·che·al \-ˈtrā-kē-əl\ *adj* **1** : placed within the trachea **2** : applied or effected through the trachea ⟨~ anesthesia⟩ ⟨~ intubation⟩

endotracheal tube *n* : a tube inserted (as through the nose or mouth) into the trachea to maintain an unobstructed passageway esp. to deliver oxygen or anesthesia to the lungs — called also *breathing tube*

end plate *n* : a complex terminal arborization of the axon of a motor neuron that contacts with a muscle fiber — called also *end brush*

end·plea·sure \(ˈ)en(d)-ˈplezh-ər, -ˈplāzh-\ *n* : pleasurable excitement that results from the release of tensions at the culmination of an act (as orgasm in sexual intercourse) — compare FOREPLEASURE

end point *n* : a point marking the completion of a process or stage of a process: as **a** : a point in a titration at which a definite effect is observed **b** : the greatest dilution (as of a virus or a vitamin) that will produce a specified effect in a biological system

end–stage \ˈend-ˌstāj\ *adj* : being or occurring in the final stages of a terminal disease or condition ⟨~ liver failure⟩

end–stage renal disease *n* : the final stage of kidney failure (as that resulting from diabetes, chronic hypertension, or glomerulonephritis) that is marked by the complete or nearly complete irreversible loss of renal function — called also *end-stage kidney disease, end-stage kidney failure, end-stage renal failure*

end–tidal \ˈend-ˌtīd-ᵊl\ *adj* : of or relating to the last portion of expired tidal air ⟨~ carbon dioxide concentrations⟩

en·e·ma \ˈen-ə-mə\ *n, pl* **enemas** *also* **ene·ma·ta** \ˌen-ə-ˈmät-ə, ˈen-ə-mə-tə\ **1** : the injection of liquid into the intestine by way of the anus (as for cleansing or examination) **2** : the liquid injected by an enema

en·er·get·ic \ˌen-ər-ˈjet-ik\ *adj* : of or relating to energy ⟨~ equation⟩

en·er·get·ics \-iks\ *n pl but sing in constr* **1** : a branch of physics that deals primarily with energy and its transformations **2** : the total energy relations and transformations of a physical, chemical, or biological system ⟨~ of muscular contraction⟩

en·er·gid \ˈen-ər-jəd, -ˌjid\ *n* : a nucleus and the body of cytoplasm with which it interacts

en·er·giz·er *or Brit* **en·er·gis·er** \-ˌjī-zər\ *n* : ANTIDEPRESSANT

en·er·gy \ˈen-ər-jē\ *n, pl* **-gies 1** : the force driving and sustaining mental activity ⟨in psychoanalytic theory the source of psychic ~ is the id⟩ **2** : the capacity for doing work

energy of activation *n* : ACTIVATION ENERGY

en·er·vate \ˈen-ər-ˌvāt\ *vt* **-vat·ed; -vat·ing 1** *obs* : to cut the nerves or tendons of **2** : to lessen the vitality or strength of ⟨heat ~s people⟩ — **en·er·va·tion** \ˌen-ər-ˈvā-shən\ *n*

en·flur·ane \en-ˈflu̇(ə)r-ˌān\ *n* : a liquid inhalational general anesthetic $C_3H_2ClF_5O$ prepared from methanol

en·gage·ment \in-ˈgāj-mənt\ *n* : the phase of parturition in which the fetal head passes into the cavity of the true pelvis

en·gi·neer \ˌen-jə-ˈni(ə)r\ *vt* : to modify or produce by genetic engineering ⟨insulin made by genetically ~ed bacteria —*Technical Survey*⟩

En·glish system \ˈiŋ-glish-, ˈin-lish-\ *n* : the foot-pound-second system of units

en·globe \in-ˈglōb\ *vt* **en·globed; en·glob·ing** : PHAGOCYTOSE — **en·globe·ment** \-mənt\ *n*

en·gorge \in-ˈgȯ(ə)rj\ *vb* **en·gorged; en·gorg·ing** *vt* : to fill with blood to the point of congestion ⟨the gastric mucosa was greatly *engorged*⟩ ~ *vi* : to suck blood to the limit of body capacity ⟨unconscious of the dog tick *engorging* on his right ankle —John Barth⟩ — **en·gorge·ment** \-mənt\ *n*

en·graft \in-ˈgraft\ *vt* : GRAFT ⟨~ed embryonic gill tissue into the back⟩ — **en·graft·ment** \-ˈgraf(t)-mənt\ *n*

en·gram *also* **en·gramme** \ˈen-ˌgram\ *n* : a hypothetical change in neural tissue postulated in order to account for persistence of memory — called also *memory trace* — **en·gram·mic** \en-ˈgram-ik\ *adj*

en·hanc·er \in-ˈhan(t)-sər, en-\ *n* : a nucleotide sequence that increases the rate of genetic transcription by increasing the activity of the nearest promoter on the same DNA molecule

en·keph·a·lin \in-ˈkef-ə-lən, -ˌ(ˌ)lin\ *n* : either of two pentapeptides with opiate and analgesic activity that occur naturally in the brain and have a marked affinity for opiate receptors: **a** : LEUCINE-ENKEPHALIN **b** : METHIONINE-ENKEPHALIN — compare ENDORPHIN

en·keph·a·lin·er·gic \-ˌkef-ə-lə-ˈnər-jik\ *adj* : liberating or activated by enkephalins ⟨~ neurons⟩

enl *abbr* enlarged

en·large \in-ˈlärj\ *vb* **en·larged; en·larg·ing** *vt* : to make larger ~ *vi* : to grow larger

en·larged *adj* : larger or greater than that formerly or normally present ⟨~ and diseased tonsils⟩

en·large·ment \in-ˈlärj-mənt\ *n* : an act or instance of enlarging : the state of being enlarged ⟨~ of the heart⟩

enol \ˈē-ˌnȯl, -ˌnōl\ *n* : an organic compound that contains a hydroxyl group bonded to a carbon atom having a double bond and that is usu. characterized by the group C=C(OH) — **eno·lic** \ē-ˈnō-lik, -ˈnäl-ik\ *adj*

eno·lase \ˈē-nə-ˌlās, -ˌlāz\ *n* : a crystalline enzyme that is found esp. in muscle and yeast and is important in the metabolism of carbohydrates

eno·lize *or Brit* **eno·lise** \-ˌlīz\ *vb* **-lized** *or Brit* **-lised; -liz·ing** *or Brit* **-lis·ing** *vt* : to convert into an enol or an enolic hydroxyl group ~ *vi* : to become enolized — **eno·liz·able** *or Brit* **eno·lis·able** \ˌē-nə-ˈlī-zə-bəl\ *adj* — **eno·li·za·tion** *or Brit* **eno·li·sa·tion** \-lə-ˈzā-shən\ *n*

en·oph·thal·mos \ˌen-ˌäf-ˈthal-məs, -ˌäp-, -ˌmäs\ *also* **en·oph·thal·mus** \-məs\ *n* : a sinking of the eyeball into the orbital cavity

en·os·to·sis \ˌen-ˌäs-ˈtō-səs\ *n, pl* **-to·ses** \-ˌsēz\ : a bony tumor arising within a bone

Eno·vid \e-ˈnō-vid\ *n* : a preparation of norethynodrel and mestranol — formerly a U.S. registered trademark

---

\ə\ abut \ᵊ\ kitten \ər\ further \a\ ash \ā\ ace \ä\ cot, cart
\au̇\ out \ch\ chin \e\ bet \ē\ easy \g\ go \i\ hit \ī\ ice \j\ job
\ŋ\ sing \ō\ go \ȯ\ law \ȯi\ boy \th\ thin \t̲h̲\ the \ü\ loot
\u̇\ foot \y\ yet \zh\ vision *See also* Pronunciation Symbols page

en·sheathe \in-'shēth\ *vt* en·sheathed; en·sheath·ing : to cover with or as if with a sheath ⟨nerve fibers *ensheathed* by myelin⟩

en·si·form \'en(t)-sə-ˌfórm\ *adj* : having sharp edges and tapering to a slender point

ensiform appendix *n* : XIPHOID PROCESS

ensiform cartilage *n* : XIPHOID PROCESS

ensiform process *n* : XIPHOID PROCESS

ENT *abbr* ear, nose, and throat

en·tad \'en-ˌtad\ *adv* : toward the inside — compare ECTAD

en·tal \'ent-ᵊl\ *adj* : situated in an interior or inner position — compare ECTAL

ent·ame·ba *or chiefly Brit* ent·amoe·ba \ˌent-ə-'mē-bə\ *n, pl* -bas *or* -bae \-(ˌ)bē\ : any ameba of the genus *Entamoeba* — ent·ame·bic *or chiefly Brit* ent·amoe·bic \-bik\ *adj*

ent·am·e·bi·a·sis *or chiefly Brit* ent·am·oe·bi·a·sis \ˌent-ˌam-i-'bī-ə-səs\ *n, pl* -a·ses \-ˌsēz\ : infection with or disease caused by an entameba

Ent·amoe·ba \ˌent-ə-'mē-bə, 'ent-ə-ˌ\ *n* : a genus of ameboid protozoans (order Amoebida) that are parasitic in the vertebrate alimentary canal and esp. in the intestines and that include the causative agent (*E. histolytica*) of amebic dysentery — see ENDAMOEBA

en·ter·al \'ent-ə-rəl\ *adj* : ENTERIC — en·ter·al·ly \-rə-lē\ *adv*

en·ter·al·gia \ˌent-ə-'ral-j(ē-)ə\ *n* : pain in the intestines : COLIC

en·ter·ec·to·my \ˌent-ə-'rek-tə-mē\ *n, pl* -mies : the surgical removal of a portion of the intestine

en·ter·ic \en-'ter-ik, in-\ *adj* 1 : of, relating to, or affecting the intestines ⟨~ diseases⟩; *broadly* : ALIMENTARY 2 : being or possessing a coating designed to pass through the stomach unaltered and to disintegrate in the intestines ⟨~ aspirin⟩

enteric fever *n* : TYPHOID FEVER; *also* : PARATYPHOID

entericus — see SUCCUS ENTERICUS

en·ter·i·tis \ˌent-ə-'rīt-əs\ *n, pl* en·ter·it·i·des \-'rit-ə-ˌdēz\ *or* en·ter·i·tis·es 1 : inflammation of the intestines and esp. of the human ileum 2 : a disease of domestic animals (as panleukopenia of cats) marked by enteritis and diarrhea

En·tero·bac·ter \'ent-ə-rō-ˌbak-tər\ *n* : a genus of aerobic gram-negative bacteria of the family Enterobacteriaceae that produce acid and gas from many sugars (as dextrose and lactose), form acetoin, are widely distributed in nature (as in feces, soil, water, and the contents of human and animal intestines), and include some that may be pathogenic

En·tero·bac·te·ri·a·ce·ae \ˌent-ə-rō-ˌbak-ˌtir-ē-'ā-sē-ˌē\ *n pl* : a large family of gram-negative straight bacterial rods of the order Eubacteriales that ferment glucose with the production of acid or acid and gas and that include the common coliform organisms and a number of serious pathogens of humans, lower animals, and plants — see EBERTHELLA, ENTEROBACTER, KLEBSIELLA, PROTEUS, SALMONELLA, SERRATIA

en·tero·bac·te·ri·ol·o·gist \ˌen-tə-rō-(ˌ)bak-ˌtir-ē-'äl-ə-jest\ *n* : a bacteriologist who specializes in bacteria of the family Enterobacteriaceae

en·tero·bac·te·ri·um \-bak-'tir-ē-əm\ *n, pl* -ria \-ē-ə\ : any bacterium of the family Enterobacteriaceae — en·tero·bac·te·ri·al \-ē-əl\ *adj*

en·tero·bi·a·sis \-'bī-ə-səs\ *n, pl* -a·ses \-ˌsēz\ : infestation with or disease caused by pinworms of the genus *Enterobius* that occurs esp. in children

En·te·ro·bi·us \ˌent-ə-'rō-bē-əs\ *n* : a genus of small nematode worms of the family Oxyuridae that includes the common pinworm (*E. vermicularis*) of the human intestine

en·ter·o·cele \'ent-ə-rō-ˌsēl\ *n* : a hernia containing a portion of the intestines

en·tero·chro·maf·fin \ˌent-ə-rō-'krō-mə-fən\ *adj* : of, relating to, or being epithelial cells of the intestinal mucosa that stain esp. with chromium salts and usu. contain serotonin

en·tero·coc·cus \-'käk-əs\ *n* 1 *cap* : a genus of gram-positive bacteria that resemble streptococci and were formerly classified with them 2 *pl* -coc·ci \-'käk-ˌ(s)ī, -'käk-

(ˌ)(s)ē\ : any bacterium of the genus *Enterococcus*; *esp* : one (*E. faecalis*) normally present in the intestine — en·tero·coc·cal \-'käk-əl\ *adj*

en·tero·coele *or* en·tero·coel \'ent-ə-rō-ˌsēl\ *n* : a coelom originating by outgrowth from the archenteron — en·tero·coe·lous \ˌent-ə-rō-'sē-ləs\ *or* en·tero·coe·lic \-lik\ *adj*

en·tero·co·li·tis \ˌent-ə-rō-kə-'līt-əs\ *n* : enteritis affecting both the large and small intestine

en·ter·o·cri·nin \-'krī-nən, -'krin-ən\ *n* : an intestinal hormone found in several animals that stimulates the digestive glands of the small intestine

en·tero·en·te·ros·to·my \ˌent-ə-rō-ˌent-ə-'räs-tə-mē\ *n, pl* -mies : surgical anastomosis of two parts of the intestine with creation of an opening between them

en·tero·gas·tric reflex \-ˌgas-trik-\ *n* : reflex inhibition of the emptying of the stomach's contents through the pylorus that occurs when the duodenum is stimulated by the presence of irritants, is overloaded, or is obstructed

en·tero·gas·trone \ˌent-ə-rō-'gas-ˌtrōn\ *n* : a hormone that is held to be produced by the duodenal mucosa and to inhibit gastric motility and secretion — compare UROGASTRONE

en·ter·og·e·nous \ˌent-ə-'räj-ə-nəs\ *adj* : originating within the intestine

en·tero·he·pat·ic \ˌent-ə-rō-hi-'pat-ik\ *adj* : of or involving the intestine and the liver ⟨~ circulation of bile salts⟩

en·tero·hep·a·ti·tis \-ˌhep-ə-'tīt-əs\ *n* : BLACKHEAD 2

en·tero·ki·nase \ˌent-ə-rō-'kī-ˌnās, -ˌnāz\ *n* : an enzyme esp. of the upper intestinal mucosa that activates trypsinogen by converting it to trypsin

en·ter·o·lith \'ent-ə-rō-ˌlith\ *n* : a calculus occurring in the intestine

en·ter·on \'ent-ə-ˌrän, -rən\ *n* : the alimentary canal or system — used esp. of the embryo

enteropathica — see ACRODERMATITIS ENTEROPATHICA

en·tero·patho·gen·ic \ˌent-ə-rō-ˌpath-ə-'jen-ik\ *adj* : tending to produce disease in the intestinal tract ⟨~ bacteria⟩ — en·tero·patho·gen \-'path-ə-jən\ *n*

en·ter·op·a·thy \ˌent-ə-'räp-ə-thē\ *n, pl* -thies : a disease of the intestinal tract

en·ter·op·to·sis \ˌent-ə-ˌräp-'tō-səs\ *n, pl* -to·ses \-ˌsēz\ : an abnormal sagging or downward displacement of the intestines — en·ter·op·tot·ic \-'tät-ik\ *adj*

en·ter·or·rha·gia \ˌent-ə-rō-'rā-j(ē-)ə\ *n* : bleeding from the intestine

en·tero·ste·no·sis \ˌent-ə-ˌrō-stə-'nō-səs\ *n, pl* -no·ses \-ˌsēz\ : stenosis of the intestine

en·ter·os·to·my \ˌent-ə-'räs-tə-mē\ *n, pl* -mies : a surgical formation of an opening into the intestine through the abdominal wall — en·ter·os·to·mal \-tə-məl\ *adj*

en·tero·tome \'ent-ə-rə-ˌtōm\ *n* : a surgical cutting instrument for opening the alimentary tract and esp. the intestine

en·te·rot·o·my \ˌent-ə-'rät-ə-mē\ *n, pl* -mies : incision into the intestines

en·tero·tox·emia *or chiefly Brit* en·tero·tox·ae·mia \ˌent-ə-rō-ˌtäk-'sē-mē-ə\ *n* : a disease (as pulpy kidney disease of lambs) attributed to absorption of a toxin from the intestine — called also *overeating disease*

en·tero·toxi·gen·ic \-ˌtäk-sə-'jen-ik\ *adj* : producing enterotoxin ⟨~ strains of E. coli⟩

en·tero·tox·in \ˌent-ə-rō-'täk-sən\ *n* : a toxic substance that is produced by microorganisms (as some staphylococci) and causes gastrointestinal symptoms (as in some forms of food poisoning or cholera)

en·tero·vi·rus \-'vī-rəs\ *n* 1 *cap* : a genus of single-stranded RNA viruses of the family *Picornaviridae* that multiply esp. in the gastrointestinal tracts of humans and swine but may infect other tissues (as nerve and muscle), that may produce clinically evident conjunctivitis, encephalitis, meningitis, myelitis, or myocarditis, and that include the poliovirus and several species including numerous serotypes named as coxsackieviruses and echoviruses 2 : any picornavirus of the genus *Enterovirus* — en·tero·vi·ral \-rəl\ *adj*

en·tero·zoa \ˌent-ə-rə-'zō-ə\ *n pl* : ENTOZOA

en·thal·py \'en-ˌthal-pē, en-'\ *n, pl* **-pies** : the sum of the internal energy of a body and the product of its volume multiplied by the pressure

en·ti·ty \'en(t)-ət-ē\ *n, pl* **-ties** : something (as a disease or condition) that has separate and distinct existence and objective or conceptual reality ⟨whether the common cold is an ∼ has been debated — *Yr. Bk. of Med.*⟩

en·to·blast \'ent-ə-ˌblast\ *n* **1** : HYPOBLAST **2** : a blastomere producing endoderm — **en·to·blas·tic** \ˌent-ə-'blas-tik\ *adj*

en·to·cone \'ent-ə-ˌkōn\ *n* : the posterointernal cusp of the talon of an upper molar tooth

en·to·co·nid \ˌent-ə-'kō-nəd\ *n* : the posterointernal cusp of the talon of a lower molar tooth

en·to·derm \'ent-ə-ˌdərm\ *n* : ENDODERM — **en·to·der·mal** \ˌent-ə-'dər-məl\ *or* **en·to·der·mic** \-mik\ *adj*

en·to·mi·on \en-'tō-mē-ˌän, -ən\ *n, pl* **-mia** \-mē-ə\ : the tip of the thickened angular part of the parietal bone that articulates with the mastoid portion of the temporal bone

en·to·mol·o·gist \ˌent-ə-'mäl-ə-jəst\ *n* : a person who is trained in or working in entomology

en·to·mol·o·gy \ˌent-ə-'mäl-ə-jē\ *n, pl* **-gies** : a branch of zoology that deals with insects — **en·to·mo·log·i·cal** \-mə-'läj-i-kəl\ *adj* — **en·to·mo·log·i·cal·ly** \-k(ə-)lē\ *adv*

en·to·mo·pho·bia \ˌent-ə-mō-'fō-bē-ə\ *n* : fear of insects

en·top·ic \(')en-'täp-ik\ *adj* : occurring in the usual place — compare ECTOPIC — **en·top·i·cal·ly** \-i-k(ə-)lē\ *adv*

ent·op·tic \(')ent-'äp-tik\ *adj* : lying or originating within the eyeball — used esp. of visual sensations due to the shadows of retinal blood vessels or of opaque particles in the vitreous body falling upon the retina

en·to·ret·i·na \ˌen-tō-'ret-ᵊn-ə, -'ret-nə\ *n* : the internal or neural portion of the retina

en·to·rhi·nal \ˌen-tə-'rī-nᵊl\ *adj* : of, relating to, or being the part of the cerebral cortex in the medial temporal lobe that serves as the main cortical input to the hippocampus

en·to·zoa \ˌent-ə-'zō-ə\ *n pl* : internal animal parasites; *esp* : the intestinal worms

en·to·zo·ic \-'zō-ik\ *adj* : living within an animal

en·trails \'en-trəlz, -ˌtrālz\ *n pl* : the bowels or viscera esp. of an animal

en·train \in-'trān\ *vt* : to determine or modify the phase or period of ⟨circadian rhythms ∼ed by a light cycle⟩ — **en·train·ment** \-'trān-mənt\ *n*

en·trap·ment \in-'trap-mənt, en-\ *n* : chronic compression of a peripheral nerve (as the median nerve or ulnar nerve) usu. between ligamentous and bony surfaces that is characterized esp. by pain, numbness, tingling, or weakness

en·tro·pi·on \en-'trō-pē-ˌän, -ən\ *n* : the inversion or turning inward of the border of the eyelid against the eyeball

en·tro·py \'en-trə-pē\ *n, pl* **-pies** : a measure of the unavailable energy in a closed thermodynamic system that is also usu. considered to be a measure of the system's disorder and that is a property of the system's state and is related to it in such a manner that a reversible change in heat in the system produces a change in the measure which varies directly with the heat change and inversely with the absolute temperature at which the change takes place; *broadly* : the degree of disorder or uncertainty in a system — **en·tro·pic** \en-'trōp-ik, -'träp-\ *adj* — **en·tro·pi·cal·ly** \-i-k(ə-)lē\ *adv*

en·ty·py \'ent-ə-pē\ *n, pl* **-pies** : a method of amnion formation in certain mammals in which the inner cell mass invaginates into the yolk sac and no amniotic folds are formed

¹enu·cle·ate \(')ē-'n(y)ü-klē-ˌāt\ *vt* **-at·ed; -at·ing** **1** : to deprive of a nucleus **2** : to remove without cutting into ⟨∼ a tumor⟩ ⟨∼ the eyeball⟩ — **enu·cle·ation** \(ˌ)ē-ˌn(y)ü-klē-'ā-shən\ *n* — **enu·cle·a·tor** \(')ē-'n(y)ü-klē-ˌāt-ər\ *n*

²enu·cle·ate \-klē-ət, -ˌāt\ *adj* : lacking a nucleus ⟨∼ cells⟩

en·ure·sis \ˌen-yù-'rē-səs\ *n, pl* **-ure·ses** \-ˌsēz\ : an involuntary discharge of urine : incontinence of urine — **en·uret·ic** \-'ret-ik\ *adj or n*

en·ve·lope \'en-və-ˌlōp, 'än-\ *n* : a natural enclosing covering (as a membrane or integument)

en·ven·om·ation \in-ˌven-ə-'mā-shən\ *n* : an act or instance of impregnating with a venom (as of a snake or spider); *also* : ENVENOMIZATION — **en·ven·om·ate** \-'ven-ə-ˌmāt\ *vt* **-at·ed; -at·ing**

en·ven·om·iza·tion *also Brit* **en·ven·om·isa·tion** \-mə-'zā-shən\ *n* : a poisoning caused by a bite or sting

en·vi·ron·ment \in-'vī-rən-mənt, -'vī(-ə)rn-\ *n* **1** : the complex of physical, chemical, and biotic factors (as climate, soil, and living things) that act upon an organism or an ecological community and ultimately determine its form and survival **2** : the aggregate of social and cultural conditions that influence the life of an individual or community — **en·vi·ron·men·tal** \-ˌvī-rən-'ment-ᵊl, -ˌvī(-ə)rn-\ *adj* — **en·vi·ron·men·tal·ly** \-ᵊl-ē\ *adv*

en·vi·ron·men·tal·ism \-ˌvī-rən-'ment-ᵊl-ˌiz-əm, -ˌvī(-ə)rn-\ *n* : a theory that views environment rather than heredity as the important factor in the development and esp. the cultural and intellectual development of an individual or group

en·vi·ron·men·tal·ist \-ᵊl-əst\ *n* **1** : an advocate of environmentalism **2** : one concerned about environmental quality esp. of the human environment with respect to the control of pollution

¹en·zo·ot·ic \ˌen-zə-'wät-ik\ *adj, of animal diseases* : peculiar to or constantly present in a locality — **en·zo·ot·i·cal·ly** \-i-k(ə-)lē\ *adv*

²enzootic *n* : an enzootic disease

enzootic ataxia *n, chiefly Austral* : SWAYBACK 3

en·zy·got·ic \ˌen-zī-'gät-ik\ *adj, of twins* : MONOZYGOTIC

en·zy·mat·ic \ˌen-zə-'mat-ik\ *also* **en·zy·mic** \en-'zī-mik\ *adj* : of, relating to, or produced by an enzyme — **en·zy·mat·i·cal·ly** \ˌen-zə-'mat-i-k(ə-)lē\ *also* **en·zy·mi·cal·ly** \en-'zī-mi-k(ə-)lē\ *adv*

en·zyme \'en-ˌzīm\ *n* : any of numerous complex proteins that are produced by living cells and catalyze specific biochemical reactions at body temperatures

enzyme immunoassay *n* : an immunoassay (as an enzyme-linked immunosorbent assay) in which an enzyme bound to an antigen or antibody functions as a label — abbr. *EIA*

enzyme–linked immunosorbent assay *n* : a quantitative in vitro test for an antibody or antigen in which the test material is adsorbed on a surface and exposed either to a complex of an enzyme linked to an antibody specific for the antigen or an enzyme linked to an anti-immunoglobulin specific for the antibody followed by reaction of the enzyme with a substrate to yield a colored product corresponding to the concentration of the test material — called also *ELISA*

en·zy·mol·o·gist \ˌen- zī-'mäl-ə-jəst\ *n* : a person who is trained in or working in enzymology

en·zy·mol·o·gy \ˌen-ˌzī-'mäl-ə-jē, -zə-\ *n, pl* **-gies** : a branch of biochemistry dealing with enzymes, their nature, activity, and significance — **en·zy·mo·log·i·cal** \ˌen-ˌzī-mə-'läj-i-kəl\ *adj*

EOG *abbr* electrooculogram

eon·ism \'ē-ə-ˌniz-əm\ *n* : TRANSVESTISM

Éon de Beau·mont \ā-ōⁿ-də-bō-mōⁿ\, **Charles (1728–1810),** French chevalier and adventurer. Although baptized as a boy, Éon was raised as a girl until he was seven. In 1755 as a secret agent for the French king, he was received at the Russian court as a woman. After several years as a special agent, he served for a time in the military as a dragoon captain. Some years later, while on a diplomatic mission in London, he was ordered by the French king to resume the dress of a woman and to retire from public life. Refusing to comply with either order, he became involved in intrigues and scandals and was the object of open and fierce betting regarding his true sex. Although he returned to France in 1777 in the guise of a man, he was again ordered by the king to dress as a woman. With the personal assistance of the queen, he was eventually presented at court in the full regalia of a woman of fashion. His last thirty-three years were

---

\ə\ abut \ᵊ\ kitten \ər\ further \a\ ash \ā\ ace \ä\ cot, cart
\aù\ out \ch\ chin \e\ bet \ē\ easy \g\ go \i\ hit \ī\ ice \j\ job
\ŋ\ sing \ō\ go \ò\ law \òi\ boy \th\ thin \t̲h̲\ the \ü\ loot
\ù\ foot \y\ yet \zh\ vision *See also* Pronunciation Symbols page

spent as a woman. A postmortem examination revealed that he had male genitalia although his features and physique were very feminine.

eos or **eosin** abbr eosinophil

eo·sin \'ē-ə-sən\ also **eo·sine** \-sən, -ˌsēn\ n **1** : a red fluorescent dye $C_{20}H_8Br_4O_5$ obtained by the action of bromine on fluorescein and used esp. in cosmetics and as a toner; also : its red to brown sodium or potassium salt used esp. as a biological stain for cytoplasmic structures **2** : any of several dyes related to eosin

eo·sin·o·cyte \ˌē-ə-'sin-ə-ˌsīt\ n : EOSINOPHIL

eo·sin·o·pe·nia \ˌē-ə-ˌsin-ə-'pē-nē-ə, -nyə\ n : an abnormal decrease in the number of eosinophils in the blood — **eo·sin·o·pe·nic** \-'pē-nik\ adj

¹eo·sin·o·phil \ˌē-ə-'sin-ə-ˌfil\ also **eo·sin·o·phile** \-ˌfīl\ adj : EOSINOPHILIC 1

²eosinophil also **eosinophile** n : a white blood cell or other granulocyte with cytoplasmic inclusions readily stained by eosin

eo·sin·o·phil·ia \-ˌsin-ə-'fil-ē-ə\ n : abnormal increase in the number of eosinophils in the blood that is characteristic of allergic states and various parasitic infections — called also acidophilia

eosinophilia–myalgia syndrome n : eosinophilia with severe myalgia and often arthralgia, rash, peripheral edema, and cough or dyspnea that occurred esp. in 1989 and 1990 in individuals who made extensive use of L-tryptophan containing a toxic contaminant — abbr. EMS; called also eosinophilia-myalgia

eo·sin·o·phil·ic \-ˌsin-ə-'fil-ik\ adj **1** : staining readily with eosin **2** : of, relating to, or characterized by eosinophilia

eosinophilic granuloma n : a disease of adolescents and young adults marked by the formation of granulomas in bone and the presence in them of macrophages and eosinophilic cells with secondary deposition of cholesterol

EPA abbr eicosapentaenoic acid

ep·ar·te·ri·al \ˌep-är-'tir-ē-əl\ adj : situated above an artery; specif : of or relating to the first branch of the right bronchus

ep·ax·i·al \(ˈ)ep-'ak-sē-əl\ also **ep·ax·on·ic** \ˌep-ˌak-'sän-ik\ adj : located above or on the dorsal side of an axis

ep·en·dy·ma \ep-'en-də-mə\ n : an epithelial membrane lining the ventricles of the brain and the canal of the spinal cord — **ep·en·dy·mal** \(ˈ)ep-'en-də-məl\ adj

ep·en·dy·mi·tis \ˌep-ˌen-də-'mīt-əs\ n, pl **-mit·i·des** \-'mit-ə-ˌdēz\ : inflammation of the ependyma

ep·en·dy·mo·ma \(ˌ)ep-ˌen-də-'mō-mə\ n, pl **-mas** also **-ma·ta** \-mət-ə\ : a glioma arising in or near the ependyma

ep·eryth·ro·zo·on \ˌep-ə-ˌrith-rə-'zō-ˌän\ n **1** cap : a genus of bacteria of the family Anaplasmataceae comprising blood parasites of vertebrates **2** pl **-zoa** \-'zō-ə\ : a bacterium of the genus Eperythrozoon

ep·eryth·ro·zo·on·o·sis \-ˌzō-ə-'nō-səs\ n, pl **-o·ses** \-ˌsēz\ : infection with or disease caused by bacteria of the genus Eperythrozoon that is esp. severe in young pigs in which it takes the form of an anemia accompanied by jaundice and is often fatal

eph·apse \'ef-ˌaps\ n : a point of contact between neurons; esp : the lateral contact between parallel fibers in a nerve or fiber tract

eph·ap·tic \(ˈ)ef-'ap-tik\ adj : relating to or being electrical conduction of a nerve impulse across an ephapse without the mediation of a neurotransmitter

ephed·ra \i-'fed-rə, 'ef-əd-rə\ n **1 a** cap : a large genus of jointed nearly leafless shrubs (family Gnetaceae) of dry or desert regions that have the leaves reduced to scales at the nodes and include some (esp. E. sinica) that are a source of ephedrine — see MA HUANG **b** : any plant of the genus Ephedra **2** : an extract of ma huang containing ephedrine and related alkaloids and used as a dietary supplement

ephed·rine \i-'fed-rən, Brit also 'ef-ə-drən\ n : a crystalline alkaloid $C_{10}H_{15}NO$ extracted from a Chinese ephedra (Ephedra sinica) or synthesized that has the physiological action of epinephrine and is usu. used in the form of its hydrochloride

$C_{10}H_{15}NO \cdot HCl$ or sulfate $(C_{10}H_{15}NO)_2 \cdot H_2SO_4$ as a bronchodilator, nasal decongestant, and vasopressor — see EPHEDRA 2, PSEUDOEPHEDRINE

ephe·lis \i-'fē-ləs\ n, pl **-li·des** \-'fē-lə-ˌdēz, -'fel-ə-\ : FRECKLE

ephem·er·al \i-'fem(-ə)-rəl, -'fēm-\ adj : lasting a very short time

ephemeral fever n : an infectious disease of cattle esp. in Africa marked by fever, muscular rigidity, conjunctivitis, and nasal discharge and usu. subsiding within two or three days — called also three-day fever

epi·an·dros·ter·one \ˌep-ē-ˌan-'dräs-tə-ˌrōn\ n : an androsterone derivative $C_{19}H_{30}O_2$ that occurs in normal human urine — called also isoandrosterone

epi·blast \'ep-ə-ˌblast\ n : the outer layer of the blastoderm : ECTODERM — **epi·blas·tic** \ˌep-ə-'blas-tik\ adj

epib·o·ly also **epib·o·le** \i-'pib-ə-lē\ n, pl **-lies** also **-les** \-lēz\ : the growing of one part about another; esp : such growth of the dorsal lip area during gastrulation — **ep·i·bol·ic** \ˌep-ə-'bäl-ik\ adj

epi·bul·bar \ˌep-i-'bəl-bər, -ˌbär\ adj : situated upon the eyeball

epi·can·thic fold \ˌep-ə-ˌkan(t)-thik-\ n : a prolongation of a fold of the skin of the upper eyelid over the inner angle or both angles of the eye

epi·can·thus \-'kan(t)-thəs\ n : EPICANTHIC FOLD

epi·car·dia \-'kärd-ē-ə\ n : the short part of the esophagus extending from the diaphragm to the stomach

epi·car·di·al \-ē-əl\ adj : of or relating to the epicardium

epi·car·di·um \-ē-əm\ n, pl **-dia** \-ē-ə\ : the visceral part of the pericardium that closely envelops the heart — called also visceral pericardium; compare PARIETAL PERICARDIUM

epi·cen·tral \-'sen-trəl\ adj : arising from the centrum of a vertebra

epi·chord·al \-'kord-ᵊl\ adj : located upon or above the notochord — used esp. of vertebrae or elements of vertebrae on the dorsal side of the notochord

epi·con·dyle \ˌep-i-'kän-ˌdīl also -dᵊl\ n : any of several prominences on the distal part of a long bone serving for the attachment of muscles and ligaments: **a** : one on the outer aspect of the distal part of the humerus or proximal to the lateral condyle of the femur — called also lateral epicondyle **b** : a larger and more prominent one on the inner aspect of the distal part of the humerus or proximal to the medial condyle of the femur — called also medial epicondyle; see EPITROCHLEA — **epi·con·dy·lar** \-də-lər\ adj

epi·con·dy·li·tis \-ˌkän-ˌdī-'līt-əs, -dᵊl-'īt-\ n : inflammation of an epicondyle or of adjacent tissues — compare TENNIS ELBOW

epi·cra·ni·al \ˌep-i-'krā-nē-əl\ adj : situated on the cranium

epicranial aponeurosis n : GALEA APONEUROTICA

epi·cra·ni·um \ˌep-i-'krā-nē-əm\ n, pl **-nia** \-nē-ə\ : the structures covering the vertebrate cranium

epi·cra·ni·us \ˌep-ə-'krā-nē-əs\ n, pl **-cra·nii** \-nē-ˌī\ : OCCIPITOFRONTALIS

¹epic·ri·sis \i-'pik-rə-səs\ n : a critical or analytical summing up esp. of a medical case history

²epi·cri·sis \'ep-i-ˌkrī-səs, ˌep-i-'\ n, pl **-cri·ses** \-ˌsēz\ : something that follows a crisis; specif : a secondary crisis

ep·i·crit·ic \ˌep-ə-'krit-ik\ adj : of, relating to, being, or mediating cutaneous sensory reception that is marked by accurate discrimination between small degrees of sensation — compare PROTOPATHIC

epi·cyte \'ep-ə-ˌsīt\ n **1** : the investing membrane of a cell **2** : an epithelial cell

¹ep·i·dem·ic \ˌep-ə-'dem-ik\ also **ep·i·dem·i·cal** \-i-kəl\ adj : affecting or tending to affect an atypically large number of individuals within a population, community, or region at the same time ⟨typhoid was ∼⟩ — compare ENDEMIC, SPORADIC **2** : of, relating to, or constituting an epidemic ⟨coronary disease . . . has hit ∼ proportions —Herbert Ratner⟩ — **ep·i·dem·i·cal·ly** \-i-k(ə-)lē\ adv

²epidemic n **1** : an outbreak of epidemic disease **2** : a natural population (as of insects) suddenly and greatly enlarged

epidemic hemorrhagic fever *n* : KOREAN HEMORRHAGIC FEVER

ep·i·de·mic·i·ty \ˌep-ə-dem-ˈis-ət-ē, ˌep-əd-ə-ˈmis-\ *n, pl* **-ties** : the quality or state of being epidemic; *specif* : the relative ability to spread from one host to others ⟨the ∼ of typhoid bacteria⟩

epidemic keratoconjunctivitis *n* : an infectious often epidemic disease that is caused by adenoviruses of the genus *Mastadenovirus* (esp. serotypes of species *Human adenovirus B* and *Human adenovirus D*) and is marked by pain, by redness and swelling of the conjunctiva, by edema of the tissues around the eye, and by tenderness of the adjacent lymph nodes

epidemic parotitis *n* : MUMPS

epidemic pleurodynia *n* : an acute epidemic form of pleurisy characterized by sudden onset with fever, headache, and acute diaphragmatic pain and caused by various coxsackieviruses (esp. serotypes of species *Human enterovirus B*) — called also *Bornholm disease, devil's-grip*

epidemic tremor *n* : AVIAN ENCEPHALOMYELITIS

epidemic typhus *n* : TYPHUS a

ep·i·de·mi·ol·o·gist \ˌep-ə-ˌdē-mē-ˈäl-ə-jəst, -ˌdem-ē-\ *n* : a specialist in epidemiology

ep·i·de·mi·ol·o·gy \-jē\ *n, pl* **-gies** **1** : a branch of medical science that deals with the incidence, distribution, and control of disease in a population **2** : the sum of the factors controlling the presence or absence of a disease or pathogen — **ep·i·de·mi·o·log·i·cal** \-ˌdē-mē-ə-ˈläj-i-kəl, -ˌdem-ē-\ *also* **ep·i·de·mi·o·log·ic** \-ik\ *adj* — **ep·i·de·mi·o·log·i·cal·ly** \-i-k(ə-)lē\ *adv*

ep·i·derm \ˈep-ə-ˌdərm\ *n* : EPIDERMIS

epi·der·mal \ˌep-ə-ˈdər-məl\ *adj* : of, relating to, or arising from the epidermis

epidermal growth factor *n* : a polypeptide hormone that stimulates cell proliferation esp. of epithelial cells by binding to receptor proteins on the cell surface — abbr. *EGF*

epidermal necrolysis *n* : TOXIC EPIDERMAL NECROLYSIS

ep·i·der·mat·ic \ˌep-ə-(ˌ)dər-ˈmat-ik\ *adj* : acting only upon the outer surface of the skin ⟨∼ ointments⟩

epi·der·mic \ˌep-ə-ˈdər-mik\ *adj* : EPIDERMAL

ep·i·der·mi·dal·iza·tion \ˌep-ə-ˌdər-məd-ᵊl-ə-ˈzā-shən\ *n* : the transformation of cuboidal cells derived from the stratum basale into flattened cells of the outer horny layer of the skin

epi·der·mis \-ˈdər-məs\ *n* **1** : the outer epithelial layer of the external integument of the animal body that is derived from the embryonic epiblast; *specif* : the outer nonsensitive and nonvascular layer of the skin of a vertebrate that overlies the dermis **2** : any of various animal integuments

epi·der·mi·tis \-(ˌ)dər-ˈmīt-əs\ *n, pl* **-mi·tis·es** *or* **-mit·i·des** \-ˈmit-ə-ˌdēz\ : inflammation of the epidermis

epi·der·mi·za·tion \-ˌdər-mə-ˈzā-shən\ *n* : EPITHELIZATION

epi·der·moid \-ˈdər-ˌmȯid\ *adj* : resembling epidermis or epidermal cells : made up of elements like those of epidermis ⟨∼ cancer of the lung⟩

epidermoid cyst *n* : a cystic tumor containing epidermal or similar tissue — called also *epidermoid;* see CHOLESTEATOMA

ep·i·der·mol·y·sis \ˌep-ə-(ˌ)dər-ˈmäl-ə-səs\ *n, pl* **-y·ses** \-ˌsēz\ : a state of detachment or loosening of the epidermis

epidermolysis bul·lo·sa \-bə-ˈlō-sə\ *n* : any of a group of inherited disorders of variable severity marked esp. by the formation of large fluid-filled blisters which develop chiefly in response to minor mechanical trauma — see DYSTROPHIC EPIDERMOLYSIS BULLOSA, EPIDERMOLYSIS BULLOSA ACQUISITA, EPIDERMOLYSIS BULLOSA SIMPLEX, JUNCTIONAL EPIDERMOLYSIS BULLOSA

epidermolysis bullosa ac·qui·si·ta \-ˌak-wə-ˈsīt-ə\ *n* : an autoimmune skin disorder similar to epidermolysis bullosa that occurs in adults and is usu. associated with another disorder (as Crohn's disease or diabetes)

epidermolysis bullosa sim·plex \-ˈsim-ˌpleks\ *n* : any of several forms of epidermolysis bullosa that are marked by blister formation within the epidermis sometimes accompa-

nied by thickening of the skin but usu. no scarring and that are chiefly inherited as an autosomal dominant trait

ep·i·der·mo·my·co·sis \-ˌdər-mō-ˌmī-ˈkō-səs\ *n, pl* **-co·ses** \-ˌsēz\ : DERMATOMYCOSIS

Ep·i·der·moph·y·ton \-(ˌ)dər-ˈmäf-ə-ˌtän\ *n* : a genus of imperfect fungi that comprises dermatophytes causing disease (as athlete's foot and tinea cruris), that now usu. includes a single species (*E. floccosum* syns. *E. inguinale* and *E. cruris*), and that is sometimes considered a synonym of *Trichophyton*

ep·i·der·moph·y·to·sis \-ˌmäf-ə-ˈtō-səs\ *n, pl* **-to·ses** \-ˌsēz\ : a disease (as athlete's foot) of the skin or nails caused by a dermatophyte

ep·i·did·y·mec·to·my \ˌep-ə-ˌdid-ə-ˈmek-tə-mē\ *n, pl* **-mies** : excision of the epididymis

ep·i·did·y·mis \ˌep-ə-ˈdid-ə-məs\ *n, pl* **-mi·des** \-mə-ˌdēz\ : a system of ductules that emerges posteriorly from the testis, holds sperm during maturation, and forms a tangled mass before uniting into a single coiled duct which comprises the highly convoluted body and tail of the system and is continuous with the vas deferens — see VASA EFFERENTIA — **ep·i·did·y·mal** \-məl\ *adj*

ep·i·did·y·mi·tis \-ˌdid-ə-ˈmīt-əs\ *n* : inflammation of the epididymis

ep·i·did·y·mo–or·chi·tis \-ˌdid-ə-ˌmō-ȯr-ˈkīt-əs\ *n* : combined inflammation of the epididymis and testis

ep·i·did·y·mo·vas·os·to·my \-vas-ˈäs-tə-mē\ *n, pl* **-mies** : surgical severing of the vas deferens with anastomosis of the distal part to the epididymis esp. to circumvent an obstruction causing sterility

¹**epi·du·ral** \ˌep-i-ˈd(y)ùr-əl\ *adj* : situated upon or administered or placed outside the dura mater ⟨∼ anesthesia⟩ ⟨an ∼ abscess⟩ — **epi·du·ral·ly** \-ə-lē\ *adv*

²**epidural** *n* : an injection of an anesthetic to produce epidural anesthesia

epidural anesthesia *n* : anesthesia produced by injection of a local anesthetic into the peridural space of the spinal cord beneath the ligamentum flavum — called also *peridural anesthesia*

epi·fol·li·cu·li·tis \ˌep-i-fə-ˌlik-yə-ˈlīt-əs\ *n* : inflammation of hair follicles

epi·gas·tric \ˌep-ə-ˈgas-trik\ *adj* **1** : lying upon or over the stomach **2 a** : of or relating to the anterior walls of the abdomen ⟨∼ veins⟩ **b** : of or relating to the abdominal region lying between the hypochondriac regions and above the umbilical region ⟨∼ distress⟩

epigastric artery *n* : any of the three arteries supplying the anterior walls of the abdomen: **a** : one that is a direct downward continuation of the internal mammary artery — called also *superior epigastric artery* **b** : one that arises from the external iliac artery near the inguinal ligament and ascends along the inner margin of the internal abdominal ring — called also *deep epigastric artery, inferior epigastric artery* **c** : one that arises from the femoral artery, passes through the saphenous opening in the fascia lata, and then ascends upon the lower part of the abdomen — called also *superficial epigastric artery*

epigastric fold *n* : a fold of peritoneum on the anterior abdominal wall covering the deep epigastric artery

epigastric plexus *n* : CELIAC PLEXUS

epi·gas·tri·um \ˌep-ə-ˈgas-trē-əm\ *n, pl* **-tria** \-trē-ə\ : the epigastric region

epi·gas·tri·us \-trē-əs\ *n* : a twin teratological fetus in which one member of the pair is underdeveloped and attached to the epigastric region of the other

epi·gen·e·sis \ˌep-ə-ˈjen-ə-səs\ *n, pl* **-e·ses** \-ˌsēz\ **1** : development involving gradual diversification and differentiation of an initially undifferentiated entity (as a zygote or spore) — compare PREFORMATION **2** : THEORY OF EPIGENESIS

epi·ge·net·ic \-jə-ˈnet-ik\ *adj* **1** : of, relating to, or produced

---

\ə\ **abut** \ᵊ\ **kitten** \ər\ **further** \a\ **ash** \ā\ **ace** \ä\ **cot, cart** \aú\ **out** \ch\ **chin** \e\ **bet** \ē\ **easy** \g\ **go** \i\ **hit** \ī\ **ice** \j\ **job** \ŋ\ **sing** \ō\ **go** \ȯ\ **law** \ȯi\ **boy** \th\ **thin** \th\ **the** \ü\ **loot** \ú\ **foot** \y\ **yet** \zh\ **vision** *See also* Pronunciation Symbols page

by epigenesis **2** : relating to, being, or involving a modification in gene expression that is independent of the DNA sequence of a gene ⟨∼ carcinogenesis⟩ ⟨∼ inheritance⟩ — **epi·ge·net·i·cal·ly** \-i-k(ə-)lē\ *adv*

epi·ge·net·ics \-iks\ *n pl but sing in constr* : the study of how genes produce their effect on the phenotype of the organism

epi·glot·tic \ˌep-ə-ˈglät-ik\ *or* **epi·glot·tal** \-ˈglät-ᵊl\ *adj* : of, relating to, or produced with the aid of the epiglottis

epi·glot·tid·e·an \ˌep-ə-glä-ˈtid-ē-ən\ *adj* : EPIGLOTTIC

epi·glot·ti·dec·to·my \-ˌglät-əd-ˈek-tə-mē\ *n, pl* **-mies** : excision of all or part of the epiglottis

epi·glot·tis \ˌep-ə-ˈglät-əs\ *n* : a thin lamella of yellow elastic cartilage that ordinarily projects upward behind the tongue and just in front of the glottis and that with the arytenoid cartilages serves to cover the glottis during the act of swallowing

ep·i·glot·ti·tis \-glät-ˈīt-əs\ *n* : inflammation of the epiglottis

epi·hy·al \ˌep-ə-ˈhī-əl\ *n* : an element of the hyoid arch that in humans is the stylohyoid ligament and in many vertebrates forms a distinct bone

epi·ker·a·to·pha·kia \ˌep-ə-ˌker-ə-tə-ˈfā-kē-ə\ *n* : the grafting of human corneal tissue to a recipient in order to correct a refractive defect (as nearsightedness, farsightedness, or astigmatism)

epil *abbr* epilepsy; epileptic

epi·la·mel·lar \ˌep-ə-lə-ˈmel-ər\ *adj* : situated outside the basement membrane

ep·i·lat·ing wax \ˈep-ə-ˌlāt-iŋ-\ *n* : a mixture of resins and waxes designed to remove cosmetically undesirable hair by being applied hot to a surface and pulled away with the embedded hairs after cooling

ep·i·la·tion \ˌep-ə-ˈlā-shən\ *n* : the loss or removal of hair

ep·i·la·tor \ˈep-ə-ˌlāt-ər\ *n* : DEPILATORY; *specif* : EPILATING WAX

ep·i·lem·ma \ˌep-ə-ˈlem-ə\ *n* : the sheath covering a terminal nerve fibril — **ep·i·lem·mal** \-ᵊl\ *adj*

ep·i·lep·sy \ˈep-ə-ˌlep-sē\ *n, pl* **-sies** : any of various disorders marked by abnormal electrical discharges in the brain and typically manifested by sudden brief episodes of altered or diminished consciousness, involuntary movements, or convulsions — see GRAND MAL, PETIT MAL; FOCAL EPILEPSY, JACKSONIAN EPILEPSY, MYOCLONIC EPILEPSY, TEMPORAL LOBE EPILEPSY

¹**ep·i·lep·tic** \ˌep-ə-ˈlep-tik\ *adj* : relating to, affected with, or having the characteristics of epilepsy — **ep·i·lep·ti·cal·ly** \-ti-k(ə-)lē\ *adv*

²**epileptic** *n* : one affected with epilepsy

epilepticus — see STATUS EPILEPTICUS

ep·i·lep·ti·form \-ˈlep-tə-ˌfòrm\ *adj* : resembling that of epilepsy ⟨an ∼ convulsion⟩

ep·i·lep·to·gen·ic \-ˌlep-tə-ˈjen-ik\ *adj* : inducing or tending to induce epilepsy ⟨an ∼ drug⟩

ep·i·lep·toid \-ˈlep-ˌtòid\ *adj* **1** : EPILEPTIFORM **2** : exhibiting symptoms resembling those of epilepsy

ep·i·loia \ˌep-ə-ˈlòi-ə\ *n* : TUBEROUS SCLEROSIS

epi·mer \ˈep-i-mər\ *n* : either of the stereoisomers of a sugar or sugar derivative that differ in the arrangement of the hydrogen atom and the hydroxyl group on the first asymmetric carbon atom of a chain — **epi·mer·ic** \ˌep-i-ˈmer-ik\ *adj*

ep·i·mere \ˈep-ə-ˌmi(ə)r\ *n* : the dorsal part of a mesodermal segment of a chordate embryo

epim·er·ite \i-ˈpim-ə-ˌrīt\ *n* : an anterior prolongation of the protomerite of many gregarines bearing organelles for attachment to the host — **epim·er·it·ic** \-ˌpim-ə-ˈrit-ik\ *adj*

epi·mor·pho·sis \ˌep-ə-ˈmòr-fə-səs\ *n, pl* **-pho·ses** \-ˌsēz\ : regeneration of a part or organism involving extensive cell proliferation followed by differentiation — compare MORPHALLAXIS

epi·myo·car·di·um \ˌep-ə-ˌmī-ə-ˈkärd-ē-əm\ *n, pl* **-dia** \-ē-ə\ : the undifferentiated splanchnic mesodermal layer of the embryonic heart that subsequently differentiates into myocardium and epicardium

epi·my·si·um \ˌep-ə-ˈmiz(h)-ē-əm\ *n, pl* **-sia** \-ē-ə\ : the external connective-tissue sheath of a muscle — compare ENDOMYSIUM

epi·neph·rine *also* **epi·neph·rin** \ˌep-ə-ˈnef-rən\ *n* : a colorless crystalline feebly basic sympathomimetic hormone $C_9H_{13}NO_3$ that is the principal blood-pressure-raising hormone secreted by the adrenal medulla, is prepared from adrenal extracts or made synthetically, and is used medicinally esp. as a heart stimulant, as a vasoconstrictor (as to treat open-angle glaucoma and life-threatening allergic reactions and to prolong the effects of local anesthetics), and as a bronchodilator — called also *adrenaline*

¹**epi·neu·ral** \ˌep-ə-ˈn(y)ùr-əl\ *adj* : arising from the neural arch of a vertebra

²**epineural** *n* : a spine or process arising from the neural arch of a vertebra

epi·neu·ri·um \ˌep-ə-ˈn(y)ùr-ē-əm\ *n* : the external connective-tissue sheath of a nerve trunk

epi·otic \ˌep-ē-ˈät-ik\ *adj* : belonging to or constituting the upper and outer element of the bony capsule of the inner ear that in humans forms a part of the temporal bone

epi·phe·nom·e·non \ˌep-i-fə-ˈnäm-ə-ˌnän, -nən\ *n* : an accidental or accessory event or process occurring in the course of a disease but not necessarily related to that disease

epiph·o·ra \i-ˈpif-ə-rə\ *n* : a watering of the eyes due to excessive secretion of tears or to obstruction of the lacrimal passages

epiph·y·se·al \i-ˌpif-ə-ˈsē-əl\ *also* **ep·i·phys·i·al** \ˌep-ə-ˈfiz-ē-əl\ *adj* : of or relating to an epiphysis

epiphyseal line *n* : the line marking the site of the epiphyseal plate

epiphyseal plate *n* : the cartilage that contains an epiphysis, unites it with the shaft, and is the site of longitudinal growth of the bone — called also *epiphyseal cartilage*

epiph·y·si·od·e·sis \i-ˌpif-ə-sē-ˈäd-ə-səs, ˌep-ə-ˌfiz-ē-\ *n, pl* **-e·ses** \-ˌsēz\ : the surgical reattachment of a separated epiphysis to the shaft of its bone

epiph·y·si·ol·y·sis \-ˈäl-ə-səs\ *n, pl* **-y·ses** \-ˌsēz\ : abnormal separation of an epiphysis from the bone shaft

epiph·y·sis \i-ˈpif-ə-səs\ *n, pl* **-y·ses** \-ˌsēz\ **1** : a part or process of a bone that ossifies separately and later becomes ankylosed to the main part of the bone; *esp* : an end of a long bone — compare DIAPHYSIS **2** : PINEAL GLAND

epiph·y·si·tis \i-ˌpif-ə-ˈsīt-əs\ *n* : inflammation of an epiphysis

epi·pi·al \ˌep-ə-ˈpī-əl\ *adj* : situated upon the pia mater

epi·plo·ec·to·my \ˌep-ə-plō-ˈek-tə-mē\ *n, pl* **-mies** : OMENTECTOMY

ep·i·plo·ic \ˌep-ə-ˈplō-ik\ *adj* : of or associated with an omentum : OMENTAL

epiploicae — see APPENDICES EPIPLOICAE

epiploic foramen *n* : the only opening between the omental bursa and the general peritoneal sac — called also *foramen of Winslow*

ep·i·plo·on \ˌep-ə-ˈplō-ˌän\ *n, pl* **-ploa** \-ˈplō-ə\ : OMENTUM; *specif* : GREATER OMENTUM

epi·pter·ic \ˌep-i(p)-ˈter-ik\ *adj* : relating to or being a small Wormian bone sometimes present in the human skull between the parietal and the greater wing of the sphenoid

epi·sclera \ˌep-ə-ˈskler-ə\ *n* : the layer of connective tissue between the conjunctiva and the sclera of the eye

epi·scler·al \-ˈskler-əl\ *adj* **1** : situated upon the sclerotic coat of the eye **2** : of or relating to the episclera

epi·scle·ri·tis \-sklə-ˈrīt-əs\ *n* : inflammation of the superficial layers of the sclera

epi·sio·per·i·ne·or·rha·phy \i-ˌpiz-ē-ō-ˌper-ə-nē-ˈòr-ə-fē, -ˌpēz-\ *n, pl* **-phies** : surgical repair of the vulva and perineum by suturing

epi·si·or·rha·phy \-ē-ˈòr-ə-fē\ *n, pl* **-phies** : surgical repair of injury to the vulva by suturing

epi·si·ot·o·my \i-ˌpiz-ē-ˈät-ə-mē, -ˌpēz-\ *n, pl* **-mies** : surgical enlargement of the vulval orifice for obstetrical purposes during parturition

ep·i·sode \ˈep-ə-ˌsōd *also* -ˌzōd\ *n* : an event that is distinctive and separate although part of a larger series; *esp* : an occurrence of a usu. recurrent pathological abnormal condition ⟨a manic ∼⟩ ⟨hypoglycemic ∼s⟩ — **ep·i·sod·ic** \,ep-ə-'säd-ik *also* -'zäd-\ *adj* — **ep·i·sod·i·cal·ly** \-i-k(ə-)lē\ *adv*

epi·some \'ep-ə-,sōm, -,zōm\ *n* : a genetic determinant (as the DNA of some bacteriophages) that can replicate either autonomously in bacterial cytoplasm or as an integral part of their chromosomes — compare PLASMID — **epi·som·al** \,ep-ə-'sō-məl, -'zō-\ *adj* — **epi·som·al·ly** \-mə-lē\ *adv*

ep·i·spa·di·as \,ep-ə-'spād-ē-əs\ *n* : a congenital defect in which the urethra opens upon the upper surface of the penis

¹**ep·i·spas·tic** \-'spas-tik\ *adj* : causing a blister or producing a serous discharge by producing inflammation

²**epispastic** *n* : VESICANT

epis·ta·sis \i-'pis-tə-səs\ *n, pl* **-ta·ses** \-,sēz\ **1 a** : suppression of a secretion or discharge **b** : a scum on the surface of urine **2** : suppression of the effect of a gene by a nonallelic gene ⟨the role of ∼ in polygenic inheritance⟩

epis·ta·sy \-tə-sē\ *n, pl* **-sies** : EPISTASIS 2

epi·stat·ic \,ep-ə-'stat-ik\ *adj* : exhibiting or produced by genetic epistasis ⟨∼ genes⟩ ⟨a trait ∼ to another trait⟩

ep·i·stax·is \,ep-ə-'stak-səs\ *n, pl* **-stax·es** \-,sēz\ : NOSEBLEED

epi·ster·nal \,ep-ə-'stərn-ᵊl\ *adj* : located on or above the sternum

ep·i·stro·phe·us \,ep-ə-'strō-fē-əs\ *n* : AXIS 2a

epi·ten·din·e·um \,ep-ə-,ten-'din-ē-əm\ *n* : white fibrous tissue covering a tendon

epith *abbr* epithelial; epithelium

epi·thal·a·mus \,ep-ə-'thal-ə-məs\ *n, pl* **-mi** \-,mī\ : a dorsal segment of the diencephalon containing the habenula and the pineal gland

ep·i·the·li·al \,ep-ə-'thē-lē-əl\ *adj* : of or relating to epithelium ⟨∼ cells⟩

ep·i·the·lio·cho·ri·al \,ep-ə-,thē-lē-ō-'kōr-ē-əl, -'kòr-\ *adj* : having maternal and fetal epithelium in contact

ep·i·the·li·oid \,ep-ə-'thē-lē-,òid\ *adj* : resembling epithelium

epithelioid angiomatosis *n* : BACILLARY ANGIOMATOSIS

ep·i·the·li·o·ma \-,thē-lē-'ō-mə\ *n, pl* **-mas** *also* **-ma·ta** \-mət-ə\ : a benign or malignant tumor derived from epithelial tissue — **ep·i·the·li·o·ma·tous** \-mət-əs\ *adj*

ep·i·the·li·um \,ep-ə-'thē-lē-əm\ *n, pl* **-lia** \-lē-ə\ : a membranous cellular tissue that covers a free surface or lines a tube or cavity of an animal body and serves esp. to enclose and protect the other parts of the body, to produce secretions and excretions, and to function in assimilation

ep·i·the·li·za·tion \,ep-ə-,thē-lə-'zā-shən\ *or* **ep·i·the·lial·iza·tion** \-,thē-lē-ə-lə-\ *or Brit* **ep·i·the·li·sa·tion** *or* **ep·i·the·lial·isa·tion** *n* : the process of becoming covered with or converted to epithelium ⟨rapid and healthy ∼ of wounds⟩

ep·i·the·lize \,ep-ə-'thē-,līz\ *or* **ep·i·the·li·al·ize** \-lē-ə-,līz\ *or Brit* **ep·i·the·lise** *or* **ep·i·the·li·al·ise** *vt* **-lized** *or Brit* **-lised; -liz·ing** *or Brit* **-lis·ing** : to cause to undergo epithelization

ep·i·them \'ep-ə-,them\ *n* : an external local application to the body (as a poultice)

ep·i·thet \'ep-ə-,thet *also* -thət\ *n* : the part of a scientific name identifying the species, variety, or other subunit within a genus — see SPECIFIC EPITHET

epi·tope \'ep-ə-,tōp\ *n* : a molecular region on the surface of an antigen capable of eliciting an immune response and of combining with the specific antibody produced by such a response — called also *determinant, antigenic determinant*

ep·i·trich·i·um \,ep-ə-'trik-ē-əm\ *n* : an outer layer of the epidermis of the fetus of many mammals beneath which the hair develops

epi·troch·lea \,ep-i-'träk-lē-ə\ *n* : the medial epicondyle at the distal end of the humerus — **epi·troch·le·ar** \-lē-ər\ *adj*

epi·tu·ber·cu·lo·sis \-t(y)ù-,bər-kyə-'lō-səs\ *n, pl* **-lo·ses** \-,sēz\ : an abnormal state of the tissues near a tuberculous lesion that is caused by the spread of products therefrom, occurs usu. in children, and is not associated with severe symptoms — **epi·tu·ber·cu·lous** \-t(y)ù-'bər-kyə-ləs\ *adj*

epi·tym·pan·ic \-tim-'pan-ik\ *adj* : situated above the tympanic membrane

epitympanic recess *n* : ATTIC

epi·tym·pa·num \-'tim-pə-nəm\ *n* : the upper portion of the middle ear — compare HYPOTYMPANUM

ep·i·typh·li·tis \,ep-ə-tə-'flīt-əs\ *n* : APPENDICITIS

Ep·i·vir \'ep-ə-,vir\ *trademark* — used for a preparation of lamivudine

epi·zoa \,ep-ə-'zō-ə\ *n pl* : ECTOZOA

epi·zo·ic \,ep-ə-'zō-ik\ *adj* : dwelling upon the body of an animal — **epi·zo·ism** \-,iz-əm\ *n* — **epi·zo·ite** \-,īt\ *n*

epi·zo·ol·o·gy \-zō-'äl-ə-jē, -zə-'wäl-\ *n, pl* **-gies** : EPIZOOTIOLOGY

epi·zo·ot·ic \,ep-ə-zə-'wät-ik\ *n* : an outbreak of disease affecting many animals of one kind at the same time; *also* : the disease itself — **epizootic** *adj* — **epi·zo·ot·i·cal·ly** \-i-k(ə-)lē\ *adv*

epizootica — see LYMPHANGITIS EPIZOOTICA

epizootic abortion *n* : CONTAGIOUS ABORTION

epizootic lymphangitis *n* : a chronic contagious inflammation that affects chiefly the superficial lymphatics and lymph nodes of horses, mules, and donkeys, that is characterized by enlargement and thickening of the vessels and softening and purulent ulceration of the nodes, and that is caused by an imperfect fungus of the genus *Histoplasma* (*H. farciminosum*) — called also *Japanese glanders, lymphangitis epizootica*

epi·zo·ot·i·ol·o·gy \,ep-ə-zə-,wät-ē-'äl-ə-jē\ *also* **epi·zo·otol·o·gy** \-,zō-ə-'täl-ə-jē\ *n, pl* **-gies** **1** : a science that deals with the character, ecology, and causes of outbreaks of animal diseases **2** : the sum of the factors controlling the occurrence of a disease or pathogen of animals — **epi·zo·oti·o·log·i·cal** \-zə-,wōt-ē-ə-'läj-i-kəl, -,wät-\ *also* **epi·zo·oti·o·log·ic** \-ik\ *adj*

EPO *abbr* erythropoietin

Ep·o·gen \'ep-ə-jən\ *trademark* — used for a preparation of erythropoietin

ep·o·nych·i·um \,ep-ə-'nik-ē-əm\ *n* **1** : the thickened layer of epidermal tissue over the developing fetal fingernail or toenail that disappears before birth except over the base of the nail where it persists as the perionychium **2** : the quick of a nail

ep·onym \'ep-ə-,nim\ *n* **1** : the person for whom something (as a disease) is or is believed to be named **2** : a name (as of a drug or a disease) based on or derived from the name of a person

epon·y·mous \i-'pän-ə-məs, e-\ *adj* : of, relating to, or named after an eponym ⟨those ∼ genetic conditions . . . such as . . . Friedreich's ataxia —R. O. Brady⟩

ep·ooph·o·ron \,ep-ō-'äf-ə-,rän, -ə-'wäf-\ *n* : a rudimentary organ homologous with the male epididymis that lies in the broad ligament of the uterus and consists of a number of small tubules which are the remains of the tubules of the mesonephros of the embryo and which open into Gartner's duct — called also *organ of Rosenmüller, parovarium*

ep·oxy \i-'päk-sē\ *adj* : containing oxygen attached to two different atoms already united in some other way; *specif* : containing a 3-membered ring consisting of one oxygen and two carbon atoms

Ep·som salt \,ep-səm-\ *n* : EPSOM SALTS

Epsom salts *n pl but sing in constr* : a bitter white crystalline salt $MgSO_4 \cdot 7H_2O$ that is a hydrated magnesium sulfate with cathartic properties — called also *bitter salts*

Ep·stein–Barr virus \,ep-,stīn-,bär-\ *n* : a herpesvirus (species *Human herpesvirus 4* of the genus *Lymphocryptovirus*) that causes infectious mononucleosis and is associated with Burkitt's lymphoma and nasopharyngeal carcinoma — abbr. *EBV;* called also *EB virus*

Ep·stein \'ep-,stīn\, **Michael Anthony** (*b* 1921), and **Barr** \'bär\, **Yvonne M.** (*b* 1932), British virologists. In 1964 Epstein and Barr isolated a herpesvirus in cultured Burkitt's

\ə\ **abut** \ᵊ\ **kitten** \ər\ **further** \a\ **ash** \ā\ **ace** \ä\ **cot, cart** \aù\ **out** \ch\ **chin** \e\ **bet** \ē\ **easy** \g\ **go** \i\ **hit** \ī\ **ice** \j\ **job** \ŋ\ **sing** \ō\ **go** \ò\ **law** \òi\ **boy** \th\ **thin** \th̶\ **the** \ü\ **loot** \ù\ **foot** \y\ **yet** \zh\ **vision** *See also* Pronunciation Symbols page

lymphoma cells. This herpesvirus, since known as the Epstein-Barr virus, is now thought to be a cause of various types of human cancers, including Burkitt's lymphoma and nasopharyngeal carcinoma. Epstein also did research on tumor cell structure and other viruses.

Ep·stein's pearls \'ep-ˌstīnz-, -ˌstēnz-\ *n pl* : temporary small white cysts that occur along the midline of the hard palate of many newborn infants

Epstein, Alois (1849–1918), Czech pediatrician. An authority on children's diseases, Epstein was director of the Children's Clinic and professor of pediatrics at Prague. He made numerous references to what are now known as Epstein's pearls in various clinical papers dealing with newborns and infants.

epu·lis \ə-'pyü-ləs\ *n, pl* **epu·li·des** \-lə-ˌdēz\ : a tumor or tumorous growth of the gum — **ep·u·loid** \'ep-yə-ˌlȯid\ *or* **ep·u·loi·dal** \ˌep-yə-'lȯid-ᵊl\ *adj*

eq *abbr* **1** equal **2** equivalent

Eq·ua·nil \'ek-wə-ˌnil\ *trademark* — used for a preparation of meprobamate

equa·tion \i-'kwā-zhən *also* -shən\ *n* : an expression representing a chemical reaction quantitatively by means of chemical symbols

equa·tion·al \i-'kwāzh-nəl, -ən-ᵊl *also* -'kwāsh-\ *adj* : dividing into two equal parts — used esp. of the mitotic cell division usu. following reduction in meiosis — **equa·tion·al·ly** \-ē\ *adv*

equa·tor \i-'kwāt-ər, 'ē-ˌ\ *n* **1** : a circle or circular band dividing the surface of a body into two usu. equal and symmetrical parts esp. at the place of greatest width ⟨the ∼ of the lens of the eye⟩ **2** : EQUATORIAL PLANE

equa·to·ri·al \ˌē-kwə-'tōr-ē-əl, ˌek-wə-, -'tȯr-\ *adj* **1** : of, located at, or relating to an equator ⟨∼ diameter⟩ **2** : extending in a direction essentially in the plane of a cyclic structure (as of cyclohexane) ⟨∼ hydrogen atoms⟩ — compare AXIAL 2b

equatorial plane *n* : the plane perpendicular to the spindle of a dividing cell and midway between the poles

equatorial plate *n* **1** : METAPHASE PLATE **2** : EQUATORIAL PLANE

equi·an·al·ge·sic \ˌē-kwi-ˌan-ᵊl-'jē-zik, ˌek-wi-, -sik\ *adj* : producing the same degree of analgesia ⟨a substance with fewer side effects than an ∼ dose of morphine⟩

equi·ca·lo·ric \ˌē-kwə-kə-'lȯr-ik, ˌek-wə-, -'lȯr-, -'lär-; -'kal-ə-rik\ *adj* : capable of yielding equal amounts of energy in the bodily economy ⟨∼ high and low protein diets⟩

Eq·ui·dae \'ek-wə-ˌdē\ *n pl* : a family of perissodactyl ungulate mammals including the horses, asses, zebras, and various extinct related mammals — see EQUUS

equi·len·in \ˌek-wə-'len-ən, ə-'kwil-ə-nən\ *n* : a weakly estrogenic steroid hormone $C_{18}H_{18}O_2$ obtained from the urine of pregnant mares

equil·i·brate \i-'kwil-ə-ˌbrāt\ *vb* **-brat·ed; -brat·ing** *vt* : to bring into or keep in equilibrium ∼ *vi* : to bring about, come to, or be in equilibrium — **equil·i·bra·tion** \-ˌkwil-ə-'brā-shən\ *n* — **equil·i·bra·to·ry** \-'kwil-ə-brə-ˌtōr-ē, -ˌtȯr-\ *adj*

equi·lib·ri·um \ˌē-kwə-'lib-rē-əm, ˌek-wə-\ *n, pl* **-ri·ums** *or* **-ria** \-rē-ə\ **1** : a state of balance between opposing forces or actions that is either static (as in a body acted on by forces whose resultant is zero) or dynamic (as in a reversible chemical reaction when the velocities in both directions are equal) **2** : a state of intellectual or emotional balance

eq·ui·lin \'ek-wə-lən\ *n* : a crystalline estrogenic hormone that is a phenolic steroid ketone $C_{18}H_{20}O_2$ and is obtained from the urine of pregnant mares

equi·mo·lar \ˌē-kwə-'mō-lər, ˌek-wə-\ *adj* **1** : of or relating to an equal number of moles ⟨an ∼ mixture of chlorine and sulfur dioxide⟩ **2** : having equal molar concentration

equi·mo·lec·u·lar \ˌē-kwə-mə-'lek-yə-lər, ˌek-wə-\ *adj* **1** : containing an equal number of molecules **2** : EQUIMOLAR 1

equina — see CAUDA EQUINA

equine \'ē-ˌkwīn, 'ek-ˌwīn\ *n* : a member of the family Equidae; *esp* : HORSE — **equine** *adj*

equine babesiosis *n* : a babesiosis that affects horses and related equines (as mules, donkeys, and zebras), is caused by two protozoans of the genus *Babesia* (*B. caballi* and *B. equi*) which parasitize red blood cells, is transmitted by ticks and esp. the tropical horse tick, and is characterized by variable clinical signs associated with destruction of red blood cells and including esp. fever, anemia, weakness, icterus, and sometimes hemoglobinuria and edema just below the skin around the head — called also *equine piroplasmosis*

equine coital exanthema *n* : a highly contagious disease of horses that is transmitted chiefly by copulation, is marked by the formation of vesicles and pustules on the mucous membranes of the genital tract, and is caused by a herpesvirus (species *Equid herpesvirus 3*) tentatively assigned to the genus *Varicellovirus* — called also *coital exanthema*

equine encephalitis *n* : EQUINE ENCEPHALOMYELITIS

equine encephalomyelitis *n* : any of three encephalomyelitides that attack chiefly equines and humans in various parts of No. and So. America and are caused by three togaviruses of the genus *Alphavirus* (species *Eastern equine encephalitis virus, Western equine encephalitis virus,* and *Venezuelan equine encephalitis virus*): **a** : one that occurs esp. in the eastern U.S. — called also *eastern equine encephalomyelitis* **b** : one that occurs esp. in the western U.S. — called also *western equine encephalomyelitis* **c** : one that occurs esp. from northern So. America to Mexico — called also *Venezuelan equine encephalitis, Venezuelan equine encephalomyelitis*

equine infectious anemia *n* : a serious sometimes fatal disease of horses that is caused by a retrovirus of the genus *Lentivirus* (species *Equine infectious anemia virus*) and is marked by intermittent fever, depression, weakness, edema, and anemia — called also *swamp fever*

equine piroplasmosis *n* : EQUINE BABESIOSIS

equinovarus — see TALIPES EQUINOVARUS

equinus — see TALIPES EQUINUS

equi·po·tent \ˌē-kwə-'pōt-ᵊnt, ˌek-wə-\ *adj* **1** : having equal effects or capacities ⟨∼ genes⟩ ⟨∼ doses of different drugs⟩ **2** *of egg protoplasm* : potentially capable of developing into any tissue

equi·po·ten·tial \-pə-'ten-chəl\ *adj* : EQUIPOTENT 2

equiv·a·lence \i-'kwiv-(ə-)lən(t)s\ *n* : the state or property of being equivalent

equiv·a·len·cy \-lən-sē\ *n, pl* **-cies** : EQUIVALENCE

¹**equiv·a·lent** \-lənt\ *adj* **1** : corresponding or virtually identical esp. in effect or function ⟨drugs that are therapeutically ∼⟩ **2** : having the same chemical combining capacity ⟨∼ quantities of two elements⟩

²**equivalent** *n* **1 a** : the relative weight of an element that has the same combining capacity as a given weight of another element : the atomic weight divided by the valence **b** : the relative weight of a radical or compound that combines with a given weight of an element, radical, or compound; *esp* : the weight of a compound that reacts with one equivalent of a given chemical element **2** : a psychopathological symptom replacing the usual one in a given disorder ⟨a twilight state may be an epileptic ∼⟩

equivalent weight *n* : EQUIVALENT 1

Eq·uus \'ek-wəs, 'ēk-\ *n* : a genus of the family Equidae that comprises the horses, asses, zebras, and related recent and extinct mammals

Er *symbol* erbium

ER *abbr* emergency room

era·sion \i-'rā-zhən, -shən\ *n* : surgical removal of diseased tissue by scraping or curetting

er·bi·um \'ər-bē-əm\ *n* : a metallic element of the rare-earth group that occurs with yttrium — symbol *Er*; see ELEMENT table

Erb's palsy \'erbz-, 'erps-\ *n* : paralysis affecting the muscles of the upper arm and shoulder that is caused by an injury during birth to the upper part of the brachial plexus

Erb, Wilhelm Heinrich (1840–1921), German neurologist.

Erb earned a reputation as an outstanding clinical neurologist and was responsible for major contributions to the understanding of neuromuscular disorders. He enjoyed a long association with the University of Heidelberg, rising to the status of professor and director of its medical clinic. His contributions included a hypothesis for the etiology of tabes dorsalis, descriptions of myotonia congenita and a juvenile form of progressive muscular atrophy, and pioneering research in electrodiagnostic studies and electrotherapy. His monographs included *Diseases of the Peripheral and Cerebrospinal Nerves* and *Handbook of Diseases of the Spinal Cord and Medulla*. He published his description of what is now known as Erb's palsy in 1874.

erect \i-ʹrekt\ *adj* **1** : standing up or out from the body ⟨~ hairs⟩ **2** : being in a state of physiological erection

erec·tile \i-ʹrek-tᵊl, -ˌtīl\ *adj* : capable of being raised to an erect position; *esp* : CAVERNOUS 2 — **erec·til·i·ty** \-ˌrek-ʹtil-ət-ē\ *n, pl* **-ties**

erectile dysfunction *n* : chronic inability to achieve or maintain an erection satisfactory for sexual intercourse : IMPOTENCE 2 — abbr. *ED*

erec·tion \i-ʹrek-shən\ *n* **1** : the state marked by firm turgid form and erect position of a previously flaccid bodily part containing cavernous tissue when that tissue becomes dilated with blood **2** : an occurrence of erection in the penis or clitoris

erec·tor \i-ʹrek-tər\ *n* : a muscle that raises or keeps a part erect — called also *arrector*

erector pi·li muscle \-ʹpī-ˌlī-, -ʹpil-ē-\ *n* : ARRECTOR PILI MUSCLE — called also *erector pili*

erector spi·nae \-ʹspē-nə, -ˌ(ˌ)nē\ *n* : SACROSPINALIS

er·e·mo·pho·bia \ˌer-ə-mō-ʹfō-bē-ə\ *n* : morbid dread of being alone

erep·sin \i-ʹrep-sən\ *n* : a proteolytic fraction obtained esp. from the intestinal juice and known to be a mixture of exopeptidases

er·e·thism \ʹer-ə-ˌthiz-əm\ *n* : abnormal irritability or responsiveness to stimulation — **ereth·ic** \ə-ʹreth-ik, er-ʹeth-\ *adj*

erg \ʹərg\ *n* : a cgs unit of work equal to the work done by a force of one dyne acting through a distance of one centimeter and equivalent to 10^{-7} joule

ERG *abbr* electroretinogram

er·ga·sia \(ˌ)ər-ʹgā-zh(ē-)ə\ *n* : integrated activity or behavior of the whole organism including both mental and physiological components

er·gas·tic \(ˌ)ər-ʹgas-tik\ *adj* : constituting the nonliving by-products (as intracellular deposits of starch or fat) of protoplasmic activity

er·gas·to·plasm \-tə-ˌplaz-əm\ *n* : ribosome-studded endoplasmic reticulum — **er·gas·to·plas·mic** \-ˌgas-tə-ʹplaz-mik\ *adj*

er·go·cal·cif·er·ol \ˌər-(ˌ)gō-kal-ʹsif-ə-ˌról, -ˌrōl\ *n* : CALCIFEROL

er·go·cor·nine \ˌər-gō-ʹkòr-ˌnēn, -nən\ *n* : a crystalline tripeptide alkaloid $C_{31}H_{39}N_5O_5$ separated from ergotoxine

er·go·cris·tine \-ʹkris-ˌtēn, -tən\ *n* : a crystalline tripeptide alkaloid $C_{35}H_{39}N_5O_5$ separated from ergotoxine

er·go·cryp·tine \-ʹkrip-ˌtēn, -tən\ *n* : an alkaloid $C_{32}H_{41}N_5O_5$ obtained from ergot

er·go·gen·ic \ˌər-gə-ʹjen-ik\ *adj* : increasing capacity for bodily or mental labor esp. by eliminating fatigue symptoms ⟨an ~ drug⟩

er·go·graph \ʹər-gə-ˌgraf\ *n* : an apparatus for measuring the work capacity of a muscle — **er·go·graph·ic** \ˌər-gə-ʹgraf-ik\ *adj*

er·go·loid mesylates \ʹər-gə-ˌlóid-\ *n pl but sing or pl in constr* : a combination of equal amounts of three ergot alkaloids used with varying success in the treatment of cognitive decline and dementia esp. in elderly patients — see HYDERGINE

er·go·ma·nia \ˌər-gə-ʹmā-nē-ə\ *n* : excessive devotion to work esp. as a symptom of mental disorder

er·go·ma·ni·ac \-nē-ˌak\ *n* : an individual affected with ergomania

er·gom·e·ter \(ˌ)ər-ʹgäm-ət-ər\ *n* : an apparatus for measuring the work performed (as by a person exercising); *also* : an exercise machine equipped with an ergometer — **er·go·met·ric** \ˌər-gə-ʹme-trik\ *adj*

er·go·met·rine \ˌər-gə-ʹme-ˌtrēn, -trən\ *n* : ERGONOVINE

er·go·nom·ics \ˌər-gə-ʹnäm-iks\ *n pl but sing or pl in constr* : an applied science concerned with the characteristics of people that need to be considered in designing things that they use in order that people and things will interact most effectively and safely — called also *human engineering, human factors engineering* — **er·go·nom·ic** \-ik\ *adj* — **er·go·nom·i·cal·ly** \-i-k(ə-)lē\ *adv*

er·gon·o·mist \(ˌ)ər-ʹgän-ə-məst\ *n* : a person trained in or working in ergonomics

er·go·no·vine \ˌər-gə-ʹnō-ˌvēn, -vən\ *n* : an alkaloid that is derived from ergot, has similar pharmacological action but reduced toxicity and a greater capacity to induce muscular contractions of the uterus, and is used esp. in the form of its maleate $C_{19}H_{23}N_3O_2 \cdot C_4H_4O_4$ to prevent or treat postpartum bleeding

er·go·phobe \ʹər-gə-ˌfōb\ *n* : one suffering from ergophobia

er·go·pho·bia \ˌər-gə-ʹfō-bē-ə\ *n* : a fear of or aversion to work

er·gos·ter·ol \(ˌ)ər-ʹgäs-tə-ˌról, -ˌrōl\ *n* : a crystalline steroid alcohol $C_{28}H_{44}O$ that occurs esp. in yeast, molds, and ergot and is converted by ultraviolet irradiation ultimately into vitamin D_2

er·got \ʹər-gət, -ˌgät\ *n* **1 a** : the black or dark purple sclerotium of fungi of the genus *Claviceps* that occurs as a club-shaped body which replaces the seed of various grasses (as rye) **b** : any fungus of the genus *Claviceps* **2** : a disease of rye and other cereals caused by fungi of the genus *Claviceps* and characterized by the presence of ergots in the seed heads — compare ERGOTISM **3 a** : the dried sclerotial bodies of an ergot fungus grown on rye and containing several ergot alkaloids **b** : ERGOT ALKALOID — **er·got·ic** \(ˌ)ər-ʹgät-ik\ *adj*

ergot alkaloid *n* : any of a group of alkaloids found in ergot or produced synthetically that include the psychedelic drug LSD as well as numerous pharmacologically useful compounds (as ergonovine and ergotamine) noted esp. for their contractile effect on smooth muscle (as of the uterus or blood vessels) — compare ERGOTISM

er·got·a·mine \(ˌ)ər-ʹgät-ə-ˌmēn\ *n* : an alkaloid that is derived from ergot and is used chiefly in the form of its tartrate $(C_{33}H_{35}N_5O_5)_2 \cdot C_4H_6O_6$ esp. in treating migraine

er·go·ther·a·py \ˌər-gō-ʹther-ə-pē\ *n, pl* **-pies** : the treatment of disease by physical work and recreation

er·go·thi·o·ne·ine \ˌər-gō-ˌthī-ʹō-nē-ˌēn, -ʹän-ē-\ *n* : a crystalline betaine $C_9H_{15}N_3O_2S$ that is found esp. in ergot and blood — called also *thioneine*

er·got·i·nine \(ˌ)ər-ʹgät-ᵊn-ˌēn, -ᵊn-ən\ *n* : a crystalline tripeptide alkaloid $C_{35}H_{39}N_5O_5$ from ergot that is relatively inactive pharmacologically

er·got·ism \ʹər-gət-ˌiz-əm\ *n* : a toxic condition produced by eating grain, grain products (as rye bread), or grasses infected with ergot fungus or by chronic excessive use of an ergot drug

er·got·ized \-ˌīzd\ *adj* : infected with ergot ⟨~ grain⟩; *also* : poisoned by ergot ⟨~ cattle⟩

er·go·tox·ine \ˌər-gə-ʹtäk-ˌsēn, -sən\ *n* **1** : a crystalline pharmacologically active alkaloid $C_{35}H_{39}N_5O_5$ from ergot that is stereoisomeric with ergotinine **2** : a mixture of isomorphous pharmacologically active alkaloids from ergot — called also *ergotoxine group*

erigens — see NERVUS ERIGENS

erig·er·on \ə-ʹrij-ə-rən, -ˌrän\ *n* **1** *cap* : a widely distributed genus of composite herbs having flower heads resembling asters **2 a** : any plant of the genus *Erigeron* **b** : the leaves and tops of plants of the genus *Erigeron* occas. and esp. formerly used as a diuretic and as a hemostatic in uterine hemorrhage **c** : ERIGERON OIL

erigeron oil *n* : a volatile oil distilled from the horseweed (*Erigeron canadensis*) and sometimes used medicinally

er·i·o·dic·ty·ol \ˌer-ē-ə-ˈdik-tē-ˌȯl, -ˌōl\ *n* : a colorless crystalline compound $C_{15}H_{12}O_6$ derived from flavanone and found esp. in the leaves of some resinous shrubs of the genus *Eriodictyon*

er·i·o·dic·ty·on \-tē-ˌän\ *n* **1 a** *cap* : a small genus of resinous shrubs (family Hydrophyllaceae) of southwestern No. America having finely reticulated leaves often woolly beneath and white or bluish flowers **b** : any plant of the genus *Eriodictyon* **2** : the dried leaves of yerba santa (*Eriodictyon californicum*) used as a flavoring in medicine esp. to disguise the taste of quinine

Er·len·mey·er flask \ˌər-lən-ˌmī(-ə)r-, ˌer-lən-\ *n* : a flat-bottomed conical flask whose shape allows the contents to be swirled without danger of spilling

Er·len·mey·er \ˈer-lən-ˌmī(-ə)r, ˈər-\, **Richard August Carl Emil (1825–1909)**, German chemist. Erlenmeyer was one of the important figures of modern organic chemistry. He produced important works in both experimental and theoretical organic chemistry. His research concentrated on the synthesis and constitution of aliphatic compounds. He discovered and synthesized isobutyric acid in 1865, synthesized guanidine in 1868, and synthesized tyrosine in 1883. He is also credited with introducing the modern structural notation for organic compounds. In 1861 he invented the flask that bears his name.

erode \i-ˈrōd\ *vt* **erod·ed; erod·ing** **1** : to eat into or away by slow destruction of substance (as by acid, infection, or cancer) ⟨acids that ~ the teeth⟩ **2** : to remove with an abrasive ⟨a dental tool that ~s the decayed area⟩

erog·e·nous \i-ˈräj-ə-nəs\ *also* **er·o·gen·ic** \ˌer-ə-ˈjen-ik\ *adj* **1** : producing sexual excitement or libidinal gratification when stimulated : sexually sensitive **2** : of, relating to, or arousing sexual feelings — **er·o·ge·ne·i·ty** \ˌer-ə-jə-ˈnē-ət-ē\ *n, pl* **-ties**

Eros \ˈe(ə)r-ˌäs, ˈi(ə)r-\ *n* : the sum of life-preserving instincts that are manifested as impulses to gratify basic needs (as sex), as sublimated impulses motivated by the same needs, and as impulses to protect and preserve the body and mind — called also *life instinct;* compare DEATH INSTINCT

Eros, Greek mythological character. Eros was the son of Aphrodite. As the Greek god of love he excited erotic love in gods and mortals with his arrows and torches.

erose \i-ˈrōs\ *adj* : having the margin irregularly notched as if gnawed ⟨an ~ edge of a bacterial colony⟩

ero·sion \i-ˈrō-zhən\ *n* **1 a** : the superficial destruction of a surface area of tissue (as mucous membrane) by inflammation, ulceration, or trauma ⟨~ of the uterine cervix⟩ **b** : progressive loss of the hard substance of a tooth **2** : an instance or product of erosion ⟨a circular ~ on the skin⟩

ero·sive \i-ˈrō-siv, -ziv\ *adj* : tending to erode or to induce or permit erosion ⟨~ lesions⟩; *also* : caused or marked by erosion ⟨~ arthritis⟩

erot·ic \i-ˈrät-ik\ *also* **erot·i·cal** \i-ˈrät-i-kəl\ *adj* **1** : of, devoted to, or tending to arouse sexual love or desire **2** : strongly marked or affected by sexual desire — **erot·i·cal·ly** \-i-k(ə-)lē\ *adv*

erot·i·ca \i-ˈrät-i-kə\ *n pl but sing or pl in constr* : literary or artistic works having an erotic theme or quality

erot·i·cism \i-ˈrät-ə-ˌsiz-əm\ *n* **1** : the arousal of or the attempt to arouse sexual feeling by means of suggestion, symbolism, or allusion (as in an art form) **2** : a state of sexual arousal or anticipation (as from stimulation of erogenous zones) **3** : insistent sexual impulse or desire

erot·i·cize *or Brit* **erot·i·cise** \-ˌsīz\ *vt* **-cized** *or Brit* **-cised; -ciz·ing** *or Brit* **-cis·ing** : to make erotic — **erot·i·ci·za·tion** *or Brit* **erot·i·ci·sa·tion** \i-ˌrät-ə-sə-ˈzā-shən\ *n*

er·o·tism \ˈer-ə-ˌtiz-əm\ *n* : EROTICISM

er·o·ti·za·tion *or Brit* **er·o·ti·sa·tion** \ˌer-ət-ə-ˈzā-shən\ *n* : the act or process of erotizing; *also* : the resulting state

er·o·tize *or Brit* **er·o·tise** \ˈer-ə-ˌtīz\ *vt* **-tized** *or Brit* **-tised; -tiz·ing** *or Brit* **-tis·ing** : to invest with erotic significance or sexual feeling

ero·to·gen·e·sis \i-ˌrōt-ə-ˈjen-ə-səs, -ˌrät-\ *n, pl* **-e·ses** \-ˌsēz\ : arousal of sexual feeling

ero·to·gen·ic \i-ˌrōt-ə-ˈjen-ik, -ˌrät-\ *adj* : EROGENOUS

er·o·tol·o·gy \ˌer-ə-ˈtäl-ə-jē\ *n, pl* **-gies** : the study and description of sexual love and lovemaking — **er·o·to·log·i·cal** \ˌer-ət-ə-ˈläj-i-kəl\ *adj*

ero·to·ma·nia \i-ˌrōt-ə-ˈmā-nē-ə, -ˌrät-\ *n* **1** : excessive sexual desire **2** : a psychological disorder marked by the delusional belief that one is the object of another person's love or sexual desire

ero·to·ma·ni·ac \-ˈmā-nē-ˌak\ *n* : one affected with erotomania

ero·to·path \i-ˈrät-ə-ˌpath, -ˈrōt-\ *n* : one affected with erotopathy

er·o·top·a·thy \ˌer-ə-ˈtäp-ə-thē\ *n, pl* **-thies** : an abnormality of sexual desire

ero·to·pho·bia \i-ˌrōt-ə-ˈfō-bē-ə, -ˌrät-\ *n* : a morbid aversion to sexual love or desire

ERPF *abbr* effective renal plasma flow

er·rat·ic \ir-ˈat-ik\ *adj* **1** : characterized by lack of consistency, regularity, or uniformity ⟨an ~ pulse⟩ **2** : deviating from what is ordinary or standard

¹er·rhine \ˈer-ˌīn\ *n* : STERNUTATOR

²errhine *adj* : STERNUTATORY

er·ror \ˈer-ər\ *n* : a deficiency or imperfection in structure or function ⟨inborn ~s of metabolism⟩

ERT *abbr* estrogen replacement therapy

eru·cic acid \i-ˌrü-sik-\ *n* : a crystalline fatty acid $C_{22}H_{42}O_2$ found in the form of glycerides esp. in rapeseed oil

eruct \i-ˈrəkt\ *vb* : BELCH

eruc·tate \i-ˈrək-ˌtāt\ *vb* **-tat·ed; -tat·ing** : BELCH

eruc·ta·tion \i-ˌrək-ˈtā-shən, ˌē-\ *n* : an act or instance of belching

erupt \i-ˈrəpt\ *vi* **1** *of a tooth* : to emerge through the gum **2** : to break out (as with a skin eruption) — **erup·tive** \-tiv\ *adj*

erup·tion \i-ˈrəp-shən\ *n* **1** : an act, process, or instance of erupting ⟨the ~ of the tooth from the gum⟩; *specif* : the breaking out of an exanthem or enanthem on the skin or mucous membrane (as in measles) **2** : something produced by an act or process of erupting: as **a** : the condition of the skin or mucous membrane caused by erupting **b** : one of the lesions (as a pustule) constituting this condition

eryn·gi·um \i-ˈrin-jē-əm\ *n* **1** *cap* : a genus of coarse bristly herbs (family Umbelliferae) that include the sea holly **2** : any plant of the genus *Eryngium*

eryn·go \i-ˈriŋ-(ˌ)gō\ *n, pl* **-goes** *or* **-gos** *obs* : candied root of the sea holly made to be used as an aphrodisiac

Erys·i·mum \i-ˈris-ə-məm\ *n* : a small genus of cruciferous herbs having small yellow flowers and slender pods

er·y·sip·e·las \ˌer-ə-ˈsip-(ə-)ləs, ˌir-\ *n* **1** : an acute febrile disease that is associated with intense often vesicular and edematous local inflammation of the skin and subcutaneous tissues and that is caused by a hemolytic streptococcus **2** : SWINE ERYSIPELAS — used esp. when the disease affects hosts other than swine

er·y·si·pel·a·tous \ˌer-ə-si-ˈpel-ət-əs, ˌir-\ *adj* **1** : of or relating to erysipelas **2** : ERYSIPELOID

¹er·y·sip·e·loid \ˌer-ə-ˈsip-(ə-)ˌlȯid, ˌir-\ *n* : an acute dermatitis resembling erysipelas that is caused by the bacterium of the genus *Erysipelothrix* (*E. rhusiopathiae*) that causes swine erysipelas, is typically marked by usu. painful reddish purple lesions esp. on the hands, and that is contracted by direct contact with infected animal flesh

²erysipeloid *adj* : resembling erysipelas

er·y·sip·e·lo·thrix \ˌer-ə-ˈsip-ə-lō-ˌthriks\ *n* **1** *cap* : a genus of gram-positive rod-shaped bacteria that form no spores, tend to produce long filaments, and are usu. considered to comprise a single species (*E. rhusiopathiae*) which is widespread in nature where nitrogenous matter is disintegrating and is the causative agent of swine erysipelas, an arthritis of lambs, and human erysipeloid **2** : a bacterium of the genus *Erysipelothrix*

er·y·the·ma \ˌer-ə-ˈthē-mə\ *n* : abnormal redness of the skin due to capillary congestion (as in inflammation)

erythema chron·i·cum mi·grans \-ˌkrän-ə-kəm-ˈmī-grənz\ *n* : ERYTHEMA MIGRANS

erythema in·fec·ti·o·sum \-in-ˌfek-shē-ˈō-səm\ *n* : FIFTH DISEASE

er·y·the·mal \ˌer-ə-ˈthē-məl\ *adj* : relating to or producing erythema ⟨∼ radiation⟩

erythema migrans *n* : a spreading annular erythematous skin lesion that is an early symptom of Lyme disease and that develops at the site of the bite of a tick (as the deer tick) infected with the causative spirochete — called also *erythema chronicum migrans*

erythema mul·ti·for·me \-ˌməl-tə-ˈfȯr-mē\ *n* : a skin disease characterized by papular or vesicular lesions and reddening or discoloration of the skin often in concentric zones about the lesions

erythema no·do·sum \-nō-ˈdō-səm\ *n* : a skin condition characterized by small tender reddened nodules under the skin (as over the shin bones) often accompanied by fever and transitory arthritic pains and commonly considered a manifestation of hypersensitivity

erythema so·la·re \-sō-ˈlar-ē\ *n* : SUNBURN

er·y·the·ma·to·gen·ic \ˌer-ə-ˌthēm-ət-ə-ˈjen-ik, -ˌthem-\ *adj* : producing erythema ⟨∼ action of certain wavelengths of light⟩

erythematosus — see LUPUS ERYTHEMATOSUS, LUPUS ERYTHEMATOSUS CELL, PEMPHIGUS ERYTHEMATOSUS, SYSTEMIC LUPUS ERYTHEMATOSUS

er·y·them·a·tous \ˌer-ə-ˈthem-ət-əs, -ˈthēm-ət-əs\ *also* **er·y·the·mic** \-ˈthē-mik\ *adj* : relating to or marked by erythema

er·y·thor·bate \ˌer-ə-ˈthȯr-ˌbāt\ *n* : a salt of erythorbic acid that is used in foods as an antioxidant

er·y·thor·bic acid \ˌer-ə-ˈthȯr-bik-\ *n* : a stereoisomer of vitamin C

er·y·thras·ma \ˌer-ə-ˈthraz-mə\ *n* : a chronic contagious dermatitis that affects warm moist areas of the body (as the armpit and groin) and is caused by a bacterium of the genus *Corynebacterium* (*C. minutissimum*)

eryth·re·de·ma *or chiefly Brit* **eryth·roe·de·ma** \i-ˌrith-rə-ˈdē-mə\ *n* : ACRODYNIA

er·y·thre·mia *or chiefly Brit* **er·y·thrae·mia** \ˌer-ə-ˈthrē-mē-ə\ *n* : POLYCYTHEMIA VERA

er·y·thrism \ˈer-ə-ˌthriz-əm\ *n* : a condition marked by exceptional prevalence of red pigmentation (as in skin or hair) — **er·y·thris·tic** \ˌer-ə-ˈthris-tik\ *also* **er·y·thris·mal** \-ˈthriz-məl\ *adj*

eryth·ri·tol \i-ˈrith-rə-ˌtȯl, -ˌtōl\ *n* : a sweet crystalline alcohol $C_4H_{10}O_4$ obtained esp. from lichens, algae, and yeast or made by reduction of erythrose — called also *erythrol*

eryth·ri·tyl tet·ra·ni·trate \i-ˈrith-rə-ˌtil-ˌte-trə-ˈnī-ˌtrāt\ *n* : a salt of erythritol with nitric acid $C_4H_{10}N_4O_{12}$ that is used esp. as a vasodilator to prevent angina pectoris — called also *erythritol tetranitrate*

eryth·ro·blast \i-ˈrith-rə-ˌblast\ *n* : a polychromatic nucleated cell of red marrow that synthesizes hemoglobin and that is an intermediate in the initial stage of red blood cell formation; *broadly* : a cell ancestral to red blood cells — compare NORMOBLAST — **eryth·ro·blas·tic** \-ˌrith-rə-ˈblas-tik\ *adj*

eryth·ro·blas·te·mia *or chiefly Brit* **eryth·ro·blas·tae·mia** \i-ˌrith-rə-ˌblas-ˈtē-mē-ə\ *n* : the presence of an abnormal number of erythroblasts in the blood

eryth·ro·blas·to·pe·nia \i-ˌrith-rə-ˌblas-tə-ˈpē-nē-ə\ *n* : a deficiency in bone marrow erythroblasts

eryth·ro·blas·to·sis \-ˌblas-ˈtō-səs\ *n, pl* **-to·ses** \-ˌsēz\ : abnormal presence of erythroblasts in the circulating blood; *esp* : ERYTHROBLASTOSIS FETALIS

erythroblastosis fe·ta·lis \-fi-ˈtal-əs\ *n* : a hemolytic disease of the fetus and newborn that is characterized by an increase

in circulating erythroblasts and by jaundice and that occurs when the system of an Rh-negative mother produces antibodies to an antigen in the blood of an Rh-positive fetus which cross the placenta and destroy fetal red blood cells — called also *hemolytic disease of the newborn, Rh disease*

erythroblastosis ne·o·na·to·rum \-ˌnē-ə-nə-ˈtōr-əm\ *n* : ERYTHROBLASTOSIS FETALIS

eryth·ro·blas·tot·ic \i-ˌrith-rə-blas-ˈtät-ik\ *adj* : of, relating to, or affected by erythroblastosis ⟨an ∼ infant⟩

eryth·ro·cyte \i-ˈrith-rə-ˌsīt\ *n* : RED BLOOD CELL — **eryth·ro·cyt·ic** \-ˌrith-rə-ˈsit-ik\ *adj*

eryth·ro·cy·the·mia *or chiefly Brit* **eryth·ro·cy·thae·mia** \i-ˌrith-rə-ˌsī-ˈthē-mē-ə\ *n* : POLYCYTHEMIA VERA

eryth·ro·cy·tom·e·ter \-sī-ˈtäm-ət-ər\ *n* : HEMACYTOMETER

eryth·ro·cy·to·pe·nia \i-ˌrith-rə-ˌsīt-ə-ˈpē-nē-ə\ *n* : deficiency of red blood cells — called also *erythropenia*

eryth·ro·cy·to·poi·e·sis \-ˌpȯi-ˈē-səs\ *n, pl* **-e·ses** \-ˈē-ˌsēz\ : ERYTHROPOIESIS

eryth·ro·cy·tor·rhex·is \-ˈrek-səs\ *n, pl* **-rhex·es** \-ˈrek-ˌsēz\ : rupture of a red blood cell

eryth·ro·cy·to·sis \i-ˌrith-rə-ˌsī-ˈtō-səs\ *n, pl* **-to·ses** \-ˈtō-ˌsēz\ : an increase in the number of circulating red blood cells esp. resulting from a known stimulus (as hypoxia) — compare POLYCYTHEMIA

eryth·ro·der·ma \-ˈdər-mə\ *n, pl* **-mas** *or* **-ma·ta** \-mət-ə\ : ERYTHEMA

eryth·ro·der·mia \-ˈdər-mē-ə\ *n* : ERYTHEMA

eryth·ro·dex·trin \-ˈdek-strən\ *also* **eryth·ro·dex·trine** \-ˌstrēn, -strən\ *n* : a dextrin that gives a red color with iodine

eryth·ro·don·tia \-ˈdän-ch(ē-)ə\ *n* : discoloration of the teeth by red or reddish brown pigmentation

eryth·ro·gen·e·sis \i-ˌrith-rə-ˈjen-ə-səs\ *n, pl* **-e·ses** \-ˌsēz\ : ERYTHROPOIESIS

eryth·ro·gen·ic \-ˈjen-ik\ *adj* **1** : producing a color sensation of redness **2** : producing red blood cells : ERYTHROPOIETIC **3** : inducing reddening of the skin ⟨∼ toxins⟩

eryth·ro·gone \i-ˈrith-rə-ˌgōn\ *n* : PROMEGALOBLAST

ery·throid \i-ˈrith-ˌrȯid, ˈer-ə-ˌthrȯid\ *adj* : relating to red blood cells or their precursors

er·y·thro·i·dine \ˌer-ə-ˈthrō-ə-ˌdēn, -əd-ᵊn\ *n* : an alkaloid $C_{16}H_{19}NO_3$ obtained from leguminous plants (genus *Erythrina*) as a mixture of stereoisomers; *esp* : the beta form of erythroidine that possesses curariform activity and acts as a depressant of the central nervous system

er·y·throl \ˈer-ə-ˌthrȯl, i-ˈrith-ˌrȯl, -ˌrōl\ *n* **1** : a liquid unsaturated dihydroxy alcohol $C_4H_8O_2$ formed by decomposition of erythritol **2** : ERYTHRITOL

eryth·ro·leu·ke·mia *or chiefly Brit* **eryth·ro·leu·kae·mia** \i-ˌrith-rə-lü-ˈkē-mē-ə\ *n* : a malignant disorder that is marked by proliferation of erythroblastic and myeloblastic tissue and in later stages by leukemia — **eryth·ro·leu·ke·mic** *or chiefly Brit* **eryth·ro·leu·kae·mic** \-mik\ *adj*

eryth·ro·leu·ko·sis *or chiefly Brit* **eryth·ro·leu·co·sis** \-lü-ˈkō-səs\ *n, pl* **-ko·ses** *or chiefly Brit* **-co·ses** \-ˌsēz\ : a leukemic disease of poultry

eryth·ro·mel·al·gia \-ˌməl-ˈal-jə\ *n* : a state of excessive dilation of the superficial blood vessels of the feet or more rarely the hands accompanied by hyperemia, increased skin temperature, and burning pain

eryth·ro·my·cin \i-ˌrith-rə-ˈmīs-ᵊn\ *n* : a broad-spectrum antibiotic $C_{37}H_{67}NO_{13}$ that is produced by a bacterium of the genus *Streptomyces* (*S. erythreus*), resembles penicillin in antibacterial activity, and is effective also against amebas, treponemata, and pinworms; *also* : a preparation of the salt (as the estolate or stearate) of erythromycin — see ILOSONE, ILOTYCIN

er·y·thron \ˈer-ə-ˌthrän\ *n* : the red blood cells and their precursors in the bone marrow

eryth·ro·pe·nia \i-ˌrith-rə-ˈpē-nē-ə\ *n* : ERYTHROCYTOPENIA

\ə\ abut \ᵊ\ kitten \ər\ further \a\ ash \ā\ ace \ä\ cot, cart \au̇\ out \ch\ chin \e\ bet \ē\ easy \g\ go \i\ hit \ī\ ice \j\ job \ŋ\ sing \ō\ go \ȯ\ law \ȯi\ boy \th\ thin \t̲h̲\ the \ü\ loot \u̇\ foot \y\ yet \zh\ vision   *See also* Pronunciation Symbols page

eryth·ro·phage \i-'rith-rə-ˌfāj\ *n* : a phagocyte that ingests red blood cells

eryth·ro·pha·gia \i-ˌrith-rə-'fāj-(ē-)ə\ *n* : ERYTHROPHAGOCYTOSIS

eryth·ro·phago·cy·to·sis \-ˌfag-ə-sə-'tō-səs, -ˌsī-\ *n, pl* **-to·ses** \-'tō-ˌsēz\ : consumption of red blood cells by macrophages and sometimes other phagocytes

er·y·throph·i·lous \ˌer-ə-'thräf-ə-ləs\ *adj* : having an affinity for red coloring matter

eryth·ro·phle·ine *or chiefly Brit* **eryth·ro·phloe·ine** \i-ˌrith-rə-'flē-ən, -'flē-ˌēn\ *n* : a white crystalline very poisonous alkaloid $C_{24}H_{39}NO_5$ extracted esp. from sassy bark

eryth·ro·pla·sia \-'plā-zh(ē-)ə\ *n* : a reddened patch with a velvety surface on the oral or genital mucosa that is considered to be a precancerous lesion

eryth·ro·poi·e·sis \i-ˌrith-rō-pȯi-'ē-səs\ *n, pl* **-e·ses** \-ˌsēz\ : the production of red blood cells (as from the bone marrow) — called also *erythrocytopoiesis, erythrogenesis* — **eryth·ro·poi·et·ic** \-'et-ik\ *adj*

erythropoietic protoporphyria *n* : a rare porphyria usu. appearing in young children and marked by excessive protoporphyrin in red blood cells, blood plasma, and feces and by skin lesions resulting from photosensitivity

eryth·ro·poi·e·tin \-'pȯi-ət-ən\ *n* : a hormonal substance that is formed esp. in the kidney and stimulates red blood cell formation — abbr. *EPO*; see EPOGEN

er·y·throp·sia \ˌer-ə-'thräp-sē-ə\ *or* **er·y·thro·pia** \ˌer-ə-'thrō-pē-ə\ *n* : a visual disturbance in which all objects appear reddish

er·y·throse \'er-ə-ˌthrōs, i-'rith-ˌrōs *also* -ˌthrōz, -ˌrōz\ *n* : a syrupy aldose sugar $C_4H_8O_4$ that is the epimer of threose

eryth·ro·sine \i-'rith-rə-sən, -ˌsēn\ *also* **eryth·ro·sin** \-sən\ *n* : a brick-red powdered xanthene dye $C_{20}H_6I_4Na_2O_5$ that is used as a biological stain and in dentistry as an agent to disclose plaque on teeth — called also *erythrosine sodium*

er·y·thro·sis \ˌer-ə-'thrō-səs\ *n, pl* **-thro·ses** \-ˌsēz\ **1** : a red or purplish color of the skin (as of the face) resulting from vascular congestion (as in polycythemia) : PLETHORA **2** : a hyperplastic condition of tissues that form red blood cells

eryth·ru·lose \i-'rith-rə-ˌlōs *also* -ˌlōz\ *n* : a syrupy ketose sugar $C_4H_8O_4$ obtained by bacterial oxidation of erythritol

Es *symbol* einsteinium

ESB *abbr* electrical stimulation of the brain

¹es·cape \is-'kāp\ *vb* **es·caped; es·cap·ing** *vi* : to avoid or find relief from something by means of an escape ∼ *vt* : to avoid or find relief from (something) by means of an escape ⟨he was unable to ∼ reality⟩

²escape *n* : an act or instance of escaping: as **a** : evasion of something undesirable ⟨find no method of ∼ from pain and suffering⟩ **b** : distraction or relief from routine or reality; *esp* : mental distraction or relief by flight into idealizing fantasy or fiction that serves to glorify the self

³escape *adj* : providing a means of escape ⟨∼ literature⟩

escape mechanism *n* : a mode of behavior or thinking adopted to evade unpleasant facts or responsibilities : DEFENSE MECHANISM 1

es·cap·ism \is-'kā-ˌpiz-əm\ *n* : habitual diversion of the mind to purely imaginative activity or entertainment as an escape from reality or routine — **es·cap·ist** \-pəst\ *adj or n*

es·char \'es-ˌkär\ *n* : a scab formed esp. after a burn

¹es·cha·rot·ic \ˌes-kə-'rät-ik\ *adj* : producing an eschar

²escharotic *n* : an escharotic agent (as a drug)

Esch·e·rich·ia \ˌesh-ə-'rik-ē-ə\ *n* : a genus of aerobic gram≈ negative rod-shaped bacteria of the family Enterobacteriaceae that form acid and gas on many carbohydrates (as dextrose and lactose) but no acetoin and that include occas. pathogenic forms (as some strains of *E. coli*) normally present in the human intestine and other forms which typically occur in soil and water

Esch·e·rich \'esh-ə-riḵ\, **Theodor (1857–1911)**, German pediatrician. A seminal figure in pediatrics, Escherich used his extensive knowledge of bacteriology, immunology, and biochemistry to greatly advance child care, especially in the areas of hygiene and nutrition. In 1886 he published a monograph in which he discussed the relationship of intestinal bacteria to the physiology of digestion in infants. Therein he gave the first description of a colon bacillus (*Escherichia coli*) now extensively used in genetic research.

es·cu·lent \'es-kyə-lənt\ *adj* : being edible — **esculent** *n*

es·cu·le·tin *or* **aes·cu·le·tin** \ˌes-kyə-'lēt-ᵊn\ *n* : a crystalline lactone $C_9H_6O_4$ obtained by hydrolysis of esculin

es·cu·lin *or* **aes·cu·lin** \'es-kyə-lən\ *n* : a glucoside $C_{15}H_{16}O_9$ from the inner bark of the horse chestnut (*Aesculus hippocastaneum*) and roots of the yellow jessamine (*Gelsemium sempervirens*) that absorbs ultraviolet rays

es·cutch·eon \is-'kəch-ən\ *n* : the configuration of adult pubic hair

es·er·ine \'es-ə-ˌrēn\ *n* : PHYSOSTIGMINE

es·er·in·ize *or Brit* **es·er·in·ise** \'es-ə-rə-ˌnīz\ *vt* **-ized** *or Brit* **-ised; -iz·ing** *or Brit* **-is·ing** : to treat with physostigmine esp. to enhance the physiological effect of acetylcholine ⟨proceeded to ∼ both eyes of a rabbit —Otto Loewi⟩

ESF *abbr* erythropoietic stimulating factor

Es·march bandage \'es-ˌmärk, 'ez-\ *or* **Es·march's bandage** \'es-ˌmärks-, 'ez-\ *n* : a tight rubber bandage for driving the blood out of a limb

Esmarch, Johannes Friedrich August von (1823–1908), German surgeon. Esmarch was a military surgeon who introduced a number of innovative measures and devices for battlefield use. The author of a widely used first-aid manual, he instituted training in first aid for civilian and military personnel. In 1869 he introduced the use of the first-aid bandage on the battlefield. Four years later during the Franco-Prussian War he developed the bandage now known as the Esmarch bandage.

es·od·ic \e-'säd-ik, -ē-\ *adj* : AFFERENT ⟨∼ nerves⟩

es·omep·ra·zole \ˌes-ō-'mep-rə-ˌzōl, -'mē-prə-, -ˌzȯl\ *n* : an isomer of omeprazole that is administered in the form of its magnesium salt $(C_{17}H_{18}N_3O_3S)_2Mg$ esp. in the treatment of erosive esophagitis, gastroesophageal reflux disease, and duodenal ulcer — see NEXIUM

esoph·a·ge·al *or chiefly Brit* **oe·soph·a·ge·al** \i-ˌsäf-ə-'jē-əl\ *adj* : of or relating to the esophagus

esophageal artery *n* : any of several arteries that arise from the front of the aorta, anastomose along the esophagus, and terminate by anastomosis with adjacent arteries

esophageal gland *n* : one of the racemose glands in the walls of the esophagus that in humans are small and serve principally to lubricate the food but in some birds secrete a milky fluid on which the young are fed

esophageal hiatus *n* : the aperture in the diaphragm that gives passage to the esophagus — see HIATAL HERNIA

esophageal plexus *n* : a nerve plexus formed by the branches of the vagus nerve which surround and supply the esophagus

esophageal speech *n* : a method of speaking which is used by individuals whose larynx has been removed and in which phonation is achieved by expelling swallowed air from the esophagus

esoph·a·gec·to·my *or chiefly Brit* **oe·soph·a·gec·to·my** \i-ˌsäf-ə-'jek-tə-mē\ *n, pl* **-mies** : excision of part of the esophagus

esophagi *pl of* ESOPHAGUS

esoph·a·gi·tis *or chiefly Brit* **oe·soph·a·gi·tis** \i-ˌsäf-ə-'jīt-əs, -'gīt-əs, (ˌ)ē-\ *n* : inflammation of the esophagus

esoph·a·go·gas·trec·to·my *or chiefly Brit* **oe·soph·a·go·gas·trec·to·my** \i-ˌsäf-ə-gō-ˌgas-'trek-tə-mē\ *n, pl* **-mies** : excision of part of the esophagus (esp. the lower third) and the stomach

esoph·a·go·gas·tric *or chiefly Brit* **oe·soph·a·go·gas·tric** \-'gas-trik\ *adj* : of, relating to, involving, or affecting the esophagus and the stomach ⟨the restoration of continuity by ∼ anastomosis —*Jour. Amer. Med. Assoc.*⟩ ⟨∼ ulcers⟩

esoph·a·go·gas·tros·co·py *or chiefly Brit* **oe·soph·a·go·gas·tros·co·py** \-ˌgas-'träs-kə-pē\ *n, pl* **-pies** : examination of the interior of the esophagus and stomach by means of an endoscope

esoph·a·go·gas·tros·to·my *or chiefly Brit* **oe·soph·a·go·gas-**

tros·to·my \-ˌgas-ˈträs-tə-mē\ *n, pl* **-mies** : the surgical formation of an artificial communication between the esophagus and the stomach

esoph·a·go·je·ju·nos·to·my *or chiefly Brit* **oe·soph·a·go·je·ju·nos·to·my** \-ˌje-jə-ˈnäs-tə-mē\ *n, pl* **-mies** : the surgical formation of an artificial communication between the esophagus and the jejunum

esoph·a·go·my·ot·o·my *or chiefly Brit* **oe·soph·a·go·my·ot·o·my** \-mī-ˈät-ə-mē\ *n, pl* **-mies** : incision through the musculature of the esophagus and esp. the distal part (as for the relief of esophageal achalasia)

esoph·a·go·plas·ty *or chiefly Brit* **oe·soph·a·go·plas·ty** \i-ˈsäf-ə-gə-ˌplas-tē\ *n, pl* **-ties** : plastic surgery for the repair or reconstruction of the esophagus

esoph·a·go·scope *or chiefly Brit* **oe·soph·a·go·scope** \-ˌskōp\ *n* : an endoscope for inspecting the interior of the esophagus

esoph·a·gos·co·pist *or chiefly Brit* **oe·soph·a·gos·co·pist** \i-ˌsäf-ə-ˈgäs-kə-pəst\ *n* : a person trained in the use of the esophagoscope

esoph·a·gos·co·py *or chiefly Brit* **oe·soph·a·gos·co·py** \i-ˌsäf-ə-ˈgäs-kə-pē\ *n, pl* **-pies** : examination of the esophagus by means of an esophagoscope — **esoph·a·go·scop·ic** *or chiefly Brit* **oe·soph·a·go·scop·ic** \i-ˌsäf-ə-gə-ˈskäp-ik\ *adj*

esophagostome, esophagostomiasis *var of* OESOPHAGOSTOME, OESOPHAGOSTOMIASIS

esoph·a·gos·to·my *or chiefly Brit* **oe·soph·a·gos·to·my** \-ˈgäs-tə-mē\ *n, pl* **-mies** : surgical creation of an artificial opening into the esophagus

esoph·a·got·o·my *or chiefly Brit* **oe·soph·a·got·o·my** \-ˈgät-ə-mē\ *n, pl* **-mies** : incision of the esophagus (as for the removal of an obstruction or the relief of esophageal achalasia)

esoph·a·gus *or chiefly Brit* **oe·soph·a·gus** \i-ˈsäf-ə-gəs\ *n, pl* **-gi** \-ˌgī -ˌjī\ : a muscular tube that in adult humans is about nine inches (23 centimeters) long and passes from the pharynx down the neck between the trachea and the spinal column and behind the left bronchus where it pierces the diaphragm slightly to the left of the middle line and joins the cardiac end of the stomach

es·o·pho·ria \ˌes-ə-ˈfōr-ē-ə, *sometimes* ˌē-sə-\ *n* : squint in which the eyes tend to turn inward toward the nose

es·o·tro·pia \ˌes-ə-ˈtrō-pē-ə, *sometimes* ˌē-sə-\ *n* : CROSS-EYE 1 — **es·o·trop·ic** \-ˈträp-ik\ *adj*

ESP \ˌē-ˌes-ˈpē\ *n* : EXTRASENSORY PERCEPTION

es·pun·dia \is-ˈpün-dē-ə, -ˈpun-\ *n* : leishmaniasis of the mouth, pharynx, and nose that is prevalent in Central and So. America

ESR *abbr* erythrocyte sedimentation rate

ESRD *abbr* end-stage renal disease

es·sence \ˈes-ᵊn(t)s\ *n* **1** : a substance considered to possess in high degree the predominant qualities of a natural product (as a plant or drug) from which it is extracted (as by distillation or infusion) **2 a** : ESSENTIAL OIL **b** : an alcoholic solution esp. of an essential oil ⟨∼ of peppermint⟩ **c** : an artificial preparation (as an alcoholic solution of one or more esters) used esp. in flavoring **d** : ELIXIR

es·sen·tial \i-ˈsen-chəl\ *adj* **1** : being, relating to, or containing an essence ⟨an ∼ odor⟩ **2** : being a substance that is not synthesized by the body in a quantity sufficient for normal health and growth and that must be obtained from the diet ⟨∼ fatty acids⟩ — compare NONESSENTIAL **3** : having no obvious or known cause : IDIOPATHIC ⟨∼ disease⟩

essential amino acid *n* : any of various alpha-amino acids that are required for normal health and growth, are either not manufactured in the body or manufactured in insufficient quantities, are usu. supplied by dietary protein, and in humans include histidine, isoleucine, leucine, lysine, methionine, phenylalanine, threonine, tryptophan, and valine

essential hypertension *n* : a common form of hypertension that occurs in the absence of any evident cause, is marked hemodynamically by elevated peripheral vascular resistance, and has multiple risk factors (as family history of hypertension, high dietary sodium intake, obesity, sedentary lifestyle,

and emotional stress) — called also *idiopathic hypertension, primary hypertension;* see MALIGNANT HYPERTENSION

essential oil *n* : any of a large class of volatile odoriferous oils of vegetable origin that give plants their characteristic odors and often other properties, that are obtained from various parts of the plants (as flowers, leaves, or bark) by steam distillation, expression, or extraction, that are usu. mixtures of compounds (as aldehydes or esters), and that are used often in the form of essences in perfumes, flavorings, and pharmaceutical preparations — called also *ethereal oil, volatile oil;* compare FATTY OIL, FIXED OIL

essential tremor *n* : a common usu. hereditary or familial disorder of movement that is characterized by uncontrolled trembling of the hands and often involuntary nodding of the head and tremulousness of the voice, that is exacerbated by anxiety and by activity, that is not associated with Parkinson's disease or any other known disease, and that responds to treatment with propranolol

EST *abbr* electroshock therapy

es·ter \ˈes-tər\ *n* : any of a class of often fragrant compounds that can be represented by the formula RCOOR′ and that are usu. formed by the reaction between an acid and an alcohol usu. with elimination of water

es·ter·ase \ˈes-tə-ˌrās, -ˌrāz\ *n* : an enzyme that accelerates the hydrolysis or synthesis of esters

es·ter·i·fy \e-ˈster-ə-ˌfī\ *vt* **-fied; -fy·ing** : to convert into an ester — **es·ter·i·fi·able** \e-ˌster-ə-ˈfī-ə-bəl\ *adj* — **es·ter·ifi·ca·tion** \-fə-ˈkā-shən\ *n*

es·ter·o·lyt·ic \ˌes-tə-rō-ˈlit-ik\ *adj* : of, relating to, carrying out, or being the splitting of an ester into its component alcohol and acid — **es·ter·ol·y·sis** \ˌes-tər-ˈäl-ə-səs\ *n, pl* **-y·ses** \-ˌsēz\

es·the·sia *or chiefly Brit* **aes·the·sia** \es-ˈthē-zh(ē-)ə\ *n* : capacity for sensation and feeling : SENSIBILITY

es·the·si·om·e·ter *or chiefly Brit* **aes·the·si·om·e·ter** \es-ˌthē-zē-ˈäm-ət-ər, -ˌthē-sē-\ *n* : an instrument for measuring sensory discrimination; *esp* : one for determining the distance by which two points pressed against the skin must be separated in order that they may be felt as separate

es·the·si·om·e·try *or chiefly Brit* **aes·the·si·om·e·try** \-ˈäm-ə-trē\ *n, pl* **-tries** : the measurement of sensory (as tactile) discrimination

es·the·sio·phys·i·ol·o·gy *or chiefly Brit* **aes·the·sio·phys·i·ol·o·gy** \es-ˌthē-zē-ō-ˌfiz-ē-ˈäl-ə-jē, -ˌthē-sē-\ *n, pl* **-gies** : the physiology of sensation and sense organs

es·thi·o·mene \es-ˈthī-ə-ˌmēn\ *n* : the chronic ulcerated state of the vulva and clitoris characteristic of lymphogranuloma in the female

es·ti·val *or* **aes·ti·val** \ˈes-tə-vəl\ *adj* : of, relating to, or occurring in the summer

es·ti·vate *or* **aes·ti·vate** \-ˌvāt\ *vi* **-vat·ed; -vat·ing** : to pass the summer in a state of torpor — compare HIBERNATE

es·ti·va·tion *or* **aes·ti·va·tion** \ˌes-tə-ˈvā-shən\ *n* : the state of one that estivates

es·to·late \ˈes-tə-ˌlāt\ *n* : the dodecyl sulfate salt of a propionate esp. of erythromycin

Es·trace \ˈes-ˌtrās\ *trademark* — used for a preparation of estradiol

Es·tra·derm \ˈes-trə-dərm\ *trademark* — used for a preparation of estradiol

es·tra·di·ol \ˌes-trə-ˈdī-ˌol, -ˌōl\ *or chiefly Brit* **oes·tra·di·ol** \ˌē-strə-ˈdī-ˌol, ē-ˈstrad-ē-ˌol, -ˌōl\ *n* : a natural estrogenic hormone that is a phenolic alcohol $C_{18}H_{24}O_2$ secreted chiefly by the ovaries, is the most potent of the naturally occurring estrogens, and is administered in its natural or semisynthetic esterified form esp. to treat menopausal symptoms — called also *dihydrotheelin;* see ESTRACE, ESTRADERM

es·tral cycle \ˈes-trəl-\ *or chiefly Brit* **oes·tral cycle** \ˈē-strəl-\ *n* : ESTROUS CYCLE

\ə\ **abut** \ᵊ\ **kitten** \ər\ **further** \a\ **ash** \ā\ **ace** \ä\ **cot, cart** \aů\ **out** \ch\ **chin** \e\ **bet** \ē\ **easy** \g\ **go** \i\ **hit** \ī\ **ice** \j\ **job** \ŋ\ **sing** \ō\ **go** \ȯ\ **law** \ȯi\ **boy** \th\ **thin** \t͟h\ **the** \ü\ **loot** \ů\ **foot** \y\ **yet** \zh\ **vision** *See also* Pronunciation Symbols page

es·trin \'es-trən\ *or chiefly Brit* **oes·trin** \'ē-strin\ *n* : an estrogenic hormone; *esp* : ESTRONE

es·trin·iza·tion \ˌes-trən-ə-'zā-shən, -ˌī-'zā-\ *or chiefly Brit* **oes·trin·iza·tion** \ˌē-strin-\ *n* **1** : the uterine and vaginal mucosal alteration characteristic of estrus **2** : treatment with estrogenic substances

es·tri·ol \'es-ˌtrī-ˌol, e-'strī-, -ˌol\ *or chiefly Brit* **oes·tri·ol** \'ē-ˌstrī-ˌol, ē-'strī-, -ˌol\ *n* : a relatively weak natural estrogenic hormone that is a glycol $C_{18}H_{24}O_3$ found in the body chiefly as a metabolite of estradiol, is the main estrogen secreted by the placenta during pregnancy, and is the estrogen typically found in the urine of pregnant women

es·tro·gen \'es-trə-jən\ *or chiefly Brit* **oes·tro·gen** \'ē-strə-jən\ *n* : any of various natural steroids (as estradiol) that are formed from androgen precursors, that are secreted chiefly by the ovaries, placenta, adipose tissue, and testes, and that stimulate the development of female secondary sex characteristics and promote the growth and maintenance of the female reproductive system; *also* : any of various synthetic or semisynthetic steroids (as ethinyl estradiol) that mimic the physiological effect of natural estrogens

es·tro·gen·ic \ˌes-trə-'jen-ik\ *or chiefly Brit* **oes·tro·gen·ic** \ˌē-strə-\ *adj* **1** : promoting estrus **2** : of, relating to, caused by, or being an estrogen — **es·tro·gen·i·cal·ly** *or chiefly Brit* **oes·tro·gen·i·cal·ly** \-i-k(ə-)lē\ *adv* — **es·tro·gen·ic·i·ty** *or chiefly Brit* **oes·tro·gen·ic·i·ty** \-jə-'nis-ət-ē\ *n, pl* **-ties**

estrogen re·place·ment therapy \-ri-'plā-smənt-\ *n* : postmenopausal administration of estrogen esp. to prevent osteoporosis and heart disease — abbr. *ERT*

es·trone \'es-ˌtrōn\ *or chiefly Brit* **oes·trone** \'ē-ˌstrōn\ *n* : a natural estrogenic hormone that is a ketone $C_{18}H_{22}O_2$ found in the body chiefly as a metabolite of estradiol, is also secreted esp. by the ovaries, and is used to treat various conditions (as ovarian failure and menopausal symptoms) relating to estrogen deficiency — see THEELIN

es·trous \'es-trəs\ *or chiefly Brit* **oes·trous** \'ē-strəs\ *adj* **1** : of, relating to, or characteristic of estrus **2** : being in heat

estrous cycle *n* : the correlated phenomena of the endocrine and generative systems of a female mammal from the beginning of one period of estrus to the beginning of the next — called also *estral cycle, estrus cycle*

es·tru·al \'es-trə-wəl\ *or chiefly Brit* **oes·tru·al** \'ē-strə-wəl\ *adj* : ESTROUS

es·tru·ate \'es-trə-ˌwāt\ *or chiefly Brit* **oes·tru·ate** \'ē-strə-\ *vi* **-at·ed; -at·ing** : to undergo estrus — **es·tru·a·tion** \ˌes-trə-'wā-shən\ *or chiefly Brit* **oes·tru·a·tion** \ˌē-strə-\ *n*

es·trus \'es-trəs\ *or* **es·trum** \-trəm\ *or chiefly Brit* **oes·trus** \'ē-strəs\ *or* **oes·trum** \'ē-strəm\ *n* **1 a** : a regularly recurrent state of sexual excitability during which the female of most mammals will accept the male and is capable of conceiving : HEAT **b** : a single occurrence of this state **2** : ESTROUS CYCLE

esu *abbr* electrostatic unit

eth·a·cryn·ic acid \ˌeth-ə-ˌkrin-ik-\ *n* : a potent synthetic diuretic $C_{13}H_{12}Cl_2O_4$ used esp. in the treatment of edema

eth·am·bu·tol \eth-'am-byù-ˌtol, -ˌtōl\ *n* : a synthetic drug used in the form of its dihydrochloride $C_{10}H_{24}N_2O_2 \cdot 2HCl$ esp. in the treatment of tuberculosis — see MYAMBUTOL

etha·mi·van \eth-'am-ə-ˌvan, ˌeth-ə-'mī-vən\ *n* : a central nervous system stimulant $C_{12}H_{17}NO_3$ related to vanillic acid and used esp. formerly as a respiratory stimulant

eth·a·nal \'eth-ə-ˌnal\ *n* : ACETALDEHYDE

eth·ane \'eth-ˌān, *Brit* 'ē-ˌthän\ *n* : a colorless odorless gaseous alkane C_2H_6 found in natural gas and used esp. as a fuel

eth·a·nol \'eth-ə-ˌnol, -ˌnōl\ *n* : a colorless volatile flammable liquid C_2H_5OH that is the intoxicating agent in liquors and is also used as a solvent — called also *ethyl alcohol, grain alcohol;* see ALCOHOL 1

eth·a·nol·amine \ˌeth-ə-'näl-ə-ˌmēn, -'nōl-\ *n* : a colorless liquid amino alcohol C_2H_7NO used esp. as a solvent for fats and oils, as soap in emulsions (as lotions or creams) when combined with fatty acids, and in gas purification — called also *monoethanolamine*

eth·chlor·vy·nol \eth-'klor-və-ˌnol, -ˌnōl\ *n* : a pungent liquid alcohol C_7H_9ClO derived from methanol and used esp. as a mild hypnotic — see PLACIDYL

eth·ene \'eth-ˌēn\ *n* : ETHYLENE 1

ether \'ē-thər\ *n* **1** : a medium that in the wave theory of light permeates all space and transmits transverse waves **2 a** : a light volatile flammable liquid $C_4H_{10}O$ used esp. formerly chiefly as an anesthetic — called also *diethyl ether, ethyl ether, ethyl oxide* **b** : any of various organic compounds characterized by an oxygen atom attached to two carbon atoms

ethe·re·al \i-'thir-ē-əl\ *adj* : relating to, containing, or resembling a chemical ether

ethereal oil *n* : ESSENTIAL OIL

ether·i·fi·ca·tion \i-ˌther-ə-fə-'kā-shən, ˌē-thər-\ *n* : the process of converting a substance (as an alcohol or phenol) into an ether — **ether·i·fy** \i-'ther-ə-ˌfī\ *vt* **-fied; -fy·ing**

ether·ize *or Brit* **ether·ise** \'ē-thə-ˌrīz\ *vt* **-ized** *or Brit* **-ised; -iz·ing** *or Brit* **-is·ing** : to treat or anesthetize with ether — **ether·iza·tion** *or Brit* **ether·isa·tion** \ˌē-thə-rə-'zā-shən\ *n*

¹**eth·i·cal** \'eth-i-kəl\ *also* **eth·ic** \-ik\ *adj* **1** : conforming to accepted professional standards of conduct **2** *of a drug* : restricted to sale only on a doctor's prescription — **eth·i·cal·ly** \'eth-i-k(ə-)lē\ *adv*

²**ethical** *n* : an ethical drug

eth·i·cist \'eth-ə-səst\ *n* : one who specializes in or is very concerned about ethics ⟨now ~s must confront the unsettling question of whether to set limits on scientific inquiry —Ricardo Sookdeo⟩

eth·ics \'eth-iks\ *n pl but sing or pl in constr* : the principles of conduct governing an individual or a group ⟨medical ~⟩

ethid·i·um bromide \e-'thid-ē-əm-\ *n* : a fluorescent mutagenic biological dye $C_{21}H_{20}BrN_3$ that is used esp. to stain nucleic acids

ethine *var of* ETHYNE

ethi·nyl *also* **ethy·nyl** \e-'thin-ᵊl, 'eth-ə-ˌnil\ *n* : a monovalent unsaturated radical $HC\equiv C-$ derived from acetylene by removal of one hydrogen atom

ethinyl estradiol *or* **ethy·nyl·es·tra·di·ol** \ˌeth-ə-nil-ˌes-trə-'dī-ˌol, -ˌol\ *or chiefly Brit* **ethi·nyl·oes·tra·di·ol** *or* **ethy·nyl·oes·tra·di·ol** \ˌeth-ə-nil-ˌē-strə-'dī-ˌol, -ē-'strad-ē-ˌol, -ˌol\ *n* : a white crystalline very potent synthetic estrogen $C_{20}H_{24}O_2$ prepared from estrone and used in combination (as with norgestrel or norethindrone) as a birth control pill or alone in the treatment of menopausal symptoms or female hypogonadism or in the palliative treatment of prostate or breast cancer — see ORTHO-NOVUM, ORTHO TRI-CYCLEN

eth·i·on·amide \ˌeth-ē-'än-ə-ˌmīd\ *n* : a compound $C_8H_{10}N_2S$ used against mycobacteria (as in tuberculosis)

ethi·o·nine \e-'thī-ə-ˌnēn\ *n* : an amino acid $C_6H_{13}NO_2S$ that is the ethyl homologue of methionine and is biologically antagonistic to methionine

ethis·ter·one \i-'this-tə-ˌrōn\ *n* : a synthetic orally effective female sex hormone $C_{21}H_{28}O_2$ administered in cases of progesterone deficiency — called also *anhydrohydroxyprogesterone, pregneninolone*

¹**eth·moid** \'eth-ˌmoid\ *or* **eth·moi·dal** \eth-'moid-ᵊl\ *adj* : of, relating to, adjoining, or being one or more bones of the walls and septum of the nasal cavity

²**ethmoid** *n* : ETHMOID BONE

ethmoidal air cells *n pl* : the cavities in the lateral masses of the ethmoid bone that are partly completed by adjoining bones and communicate with the nasal cavity — called also *ethmoidal cells*

ethmoid bone *n* : a light spongy cubical bone of the skull that is made up of thin plates and forms much of the walls of the nasal cavity and part of those of the orbits

eth·moid·ec·to·my \ˌeth-ˌmoi-'dek-tə-mē\ *n, pl* **-mies** : excision of all or some of the ethmoidal air cells or part of the ethmoid bone

eth·moid·itis \-'dīt-əs\ *n* : inflammation of the ethmoid bone or its sinuses

ethmoid sinus *also* **ethmoidal sinus** *n* : either of two sinuses each of which is situated in a lateral part of the ethmoid bone alongside the nose and consists of ethmoidal air cells

eth·mo·max·il·lary \eth-(ˌ)mō-'mak-sə-ˌler-ē, *chiefly Brit* -mak-'sil-ə-rē\ *adj* : of or relating to the ethmoid and maxillary bones

¹**eth·mo·tur·bi·nal** \eth-(ˌ)mō-'tər-bən-ᵊl\ *n* : an ethmoturbinal bone

²**ethmoturbinal** *adj* : of, relating to, or consisting of the lateral masses of the ethmoid bone that bear or consist largely of the nasal conchae in mammals

eth·nog·ra·pher \eth-'näg-rə-fər\ *n* : a specialist in ethnography

eth·nog·ra·phy \eth-'näg-rə-fē\ *n, pl* **-phies** : the study and systematic recording of human cultures; *also* : a descriptive work produced from such research — **eth·no·graph·ic** \ˌeth-nə-'graf-ik\ *or* **eth·no·graph·i·cal** \-i-kəl\ *adj* — **eth·no·graph·i·cal·ly** \-i-k(ə-)lē\ *adv*

eth·nol·o·gist \eth-'näl-ə-jəst\ *n* : a specialist in ethnology

eth·nol·o·gy \eth-'näl-ə-jē\ *n, pl* **-gies** **1** : a science that deals with the division of human beings into races and their origin, distribution, relations, and characteristics **2** : anthropology dealing chiefly with the comparative and analytical study of cultures : CULTURAL ANTHROPOLOGY — **eth·no·log·i·cal** \ˌeth-nə-'läj-i-kəl\ *also* **eth·no·log·ic** \-ik\ *adj*

eth·no·med·i·cine \ˌeth-nō-'med-ə-sən, *Brit usu* -'med-sən\ *n* : the comparative study of how different cultures view disease and how they treat or prevent it; *also* : the medical beliefs and practices of indigenous cultures — **eth·no·med·i·cal** \-'med-i-kəl\ *adj*

etho·hexa·di·ol \ˌe-(ˌ)thō-ˌhek-sə-'dī-ˌól, -'dī-ˌōl\ *n* : an odorless oily glycol $C_8H_{16}(OH)_2$ applied to the skin as an insect repellent

ethol·o·gist \ē-'thäl-ə-jəst\ *n* : a specialist in ethology

ethol·o·gy \ē-'thäl-ə-jē\ *n, pl* **-gies** : the scientific and objective study of animal behavior esp. under natural conditions — **etho·log·i·cal** \ˌē-thə-'läj-i-kəl, ˌeth-ə-\ *adj*

etho·sux·i·mide \ˌe-(ˌ)thō-'sək-sə-ˌmīd, -sə-məd\ *n* : an anticonvulsant drug $C_7H_{11}NO_2$ derived from succinic acid and used to treat epilepsy

eth·o·to·in \ˌeth-ə-'tō-ən\ *n* : an anticonvulsant drug $C_{11}H_{12}N_2O_2$ used in the treatment of epilepsy — see PEGANONE

eth·oxy \e-'thäk-sē\ *adj* : relating to or containing ethoxyl

eth·ox·yl \e-'thäk-səl\ *n* : the monovalent radical C_2H_5O composed of ethyl united with oxygen

eth·yl \'eth-əl, *Brit also* 'ē-ˌthīl\ *n* : a monovalent hydrocarbon radical C_2H_5 — **eth·yl·ic** \e-'thil-ik\ *adj*

ethyl acetate *n* : a colorless fragrant volatile flammable liquid ester $C_4H_8O_2$ used esp. as a solvent

ethyl alcohol *n* : ETHANOL

ethyl aminobenzoate *n* : BENZOCAINE

ethyl bromide *n* : a volatile liquid compound C_2H_5Br of aromatic odor that is used as an inhalation anesthetic

ethyl carbamate *n* : URETHANE 1

ethyl cellulose *n* : any of various thermoplastic substances used esp. in plastics and lacquers

ethyl chaulmoograte *n* : a pale-yellow liquid containing a mixture of the ethyl esters of the acids of chaulmoogra oil and formerly used in the treatment of leprosy

ethyl chloride *n* : a colorless pungent flammable gaseous or volatile liquid C_2H_5Cl used esp. as a topical anesthetic

eth·yl·ene \'eth-ə-ˌlēn\ *n* **1** : a colorless flammable gaseous unsaturated hydrocarbon C_2H_4 that is found in coal gas, can be produced by pyrolysis of petroleum hydrocarbons, is used in medicine as a general inhalation anesthetic, and occurs in plants functioning esp. as a natural growth regulator that promotes the ripening of fruit — called also *ethene* **2** : a divalent hydrocarbon group C_2H_4 derived from ethane — **eth·yl·enic** \ˌeth-ə-'lē-nik, -'len-ik\ *adj* — **eth·yl·eni·cal·ly** \-'lē-ni-k(ə-)lē, -'len-i-k(ə-)lē\ *adv*

ethylene bromide *n* : ETHYLENE DIBROMIDE

eth·yl·ene·di·amine \ˌeth-ə-ˌlēn-'dī-ə-ˌmēn, -dī-'am-ən\ *n* : a colorless volatile liquid base $C_2H_8N_2$ that has an ammoniacal odor and is used chiefly as a solvent, in organic synthesis, and in medicine to stabilize aminophylline when used in injections

eth·yl·ene·di·amine·tetra·ac·e·tate \ˌeth-ə-ˌlēn-ˌdī-ə-ˌmēn-ˌte-tra-'as-ə-ˌtāt, -dī-ˌam-ən-\ *n* : a salt of EDTA

eth·yl·ene·di·amine·tetra·ace·tic acid \-ə-ˌsēt-ik-\ *n* : EDTA

ethylene dibromide *n* : a colorless toxic liquid compound $C_2H_4Br_2$ that has been shown by experiments with laboratory animals to be strongly carcinogenic and that was formerly used in the U.S. as an agricultural pesticide — abbr. *EDB;* called also *ethylene bromide*

ethylene glycol *n* : a thick liquid alcohol $C_2H_6O_2$ used esp. as an antifreeze

ethylene oxide *n* : a colorless flammable toxic gaseous or liquid compound C_2H_4O used esp. in synthesis (as of ethylene glycol) and in fumigation and sterilization (as of medical instruments)

ethylene series *n* : the homologous series of unsaturated hydrocarbons C_nH_{2n} of which ethylene is the lowest member

eth·yl·es·tren·ol \ˌeth-əl-'es-trə-ˌnól, -ˌnōl\ *n* : an anabolic steroid $C_{20}H_{32}O$ having some androgenic activity — see MAXIBOLIN

ethyl ether *n* : ETHER 2a

ethyl·i·dene \e-'thil-ə-ˌdēn, 'eth-əl-\ *n* : a bivalent hydrocarbon radical >CHCH₃ isomeric with ethylene

eth·yl·mor·phine \ˌeth-əl-'mór-ˌfēn\ *n* : a synthetic toxic alkaloid that is an ethyl ether of morphine and is used esp. in the form of its hydrochloride $C_{19}H_{23}NO_3 \cdot HCl$ similarly to morphine and codeine

ethyl nitrite *n* : a pale-yellow flammable volatile liquid ester $C_2H_5NO_2$ having a pleasant odor

ethyl nitrite spirit *n* : a solution of ethyl nitrite in alcohol formerly used as a diuretic and diaphoretic

ethyl oxide *n* : ETHER 2a — used esp. of ether not intended for use in anesthesia

eth·yl·stib·amine \ˌeth-əl-'stib-ə-ˌmēn\ *n* : a drug complex containing 41 to 44 percent organic pentavalent antimony and formerly used in the treatment of leishmaniasis (as kalaazar) and filariasis — called also *neostibosan*

ethyl vanillin *n* : a white crystalline aldehyde $C_9H_{10}O_3$ that has a more intense odor and flavor than vanillin and is used as a flavoring agent

Ethyl Vi·o·let \-'vī-ə-lət\ *n* : a basic dye used esp. as a biological stain

eth·yne *also* **eth·ine** \'eth-ˌīn, e-'thīn\ *n* : ACETYLENE

eth·y·no·di·ol diacetate \ˌeth-i-nō-'dī-ˌól, -ˌól-\ *n* : a synthetic progestogen $C_{24}H_{32}O_4$ used esp. in birth control pills usu. in combination with an estrogen

ethynyl *var of* ETHINYL

ethynylestradiol *var of* ETHINYL ESTRADIOL

ethynyloestradiol *chiefly Brit var of* ETHINYL ESTRADIOL

et·i·dro·nate \ˌēt-ə-'drō-ˌnāt, ˌet-\ *n* : a white disodium bisphosphonate salt $C_2H_6Na_2O_7P_2$ that inhibits the formation, growth, and dissolution of hydroxyapatite crystals and is used esp. to treat Paget's disease of bone and to prevent or treat heterotopic ossification (as that associated with hip-replacement surgery) — called also *etidronate disodium*

etio·chol·an·ol·one \ˌēt-ē-ō-ˌkō-'lan-ə-ˌlōn *also* ˌet-\ *n* : a testosterone metabolite $C_{19}H_{30}O_2$ that occurs in urine

eti·o·late \'ēt-ē-ə-ˌlāt\ *vt* **-lat·ed; -lat·ing** : to make pale and sickly — **eti·o·la·tion** \ˌēt-ē-ə-'lā-shən\ *n*

eti·o·log·ic \ˌēt-ē-ə-'läj-ik\ *or* **eti·o·log·i·cal** \-i-kəl\ *or chiefly Brit* **ae·ti·o·log·ic** *or* **ae·ti·o·log·i·cal** *adj* **1** : of, relating to, or based on etiology ⟨~ treatment of a disease seeks to remove or correct its cause⟩ **2** : causing or contributing to the cause of a disease or condition ⟨smoking is an ~ factor in the production of arteriosclerosis —F. A. Faught⟩ — **eti·o·log·i·cal·ly** *or chiefly Brit* **ae·ti·o·log·i·cal·ly** \-i-k(ə-)lē\ *adv*

eti·ol·o·gy *or chiefly Brit* **ae·ti·ol·o·gy** \ˌēt-ē-'äl-ə-jē\ *n, pl* **-gies** **1** : the cause or causes of a disease or abnormal condition ⟨some types of cancer have a viral ~⟩ ⟨a multiple ~ in which biological, psychological, and sociocultural factors all play a role —M. E. Jackson *et al*⟩ **2 :** a branch of medical science dealing with the causes and origin of diseases

etio·patho·gen·e·sis *or chiefly Brit* **ae·tio·patho·gen·e·sis** \ˌēt-ē-ō-ˌpath-ə-ˈjen-ə-səs *also* ˌet-\ *n, pl* **-e·ses** \-ˌsēz\ **:** the cause and development of a disease or abnormal condition

etio·por·phy·rin *or chiefly Brit* **ae·tio·por·phy·rin** \-ˈpȯr-fə-rən\ *n* **:** any of four isomeric porphyrins $C_{32}H_{38}N_4$; *esp* **:** a violet crystalline pigment occurring in nature (as in petroleum and coal) and formed by degradation of chlorophyll and of heme

eto·po·side \ˌēt-ə-ˈpō-ˌsīd, ˌet-\ *n* **:** a semisynthetic podophyllotoxin derivative $C_{29}H_{32}O_{13}$ used to treat various neoplastic diseases (as carcinoma of the lungs or testicles, AIDS-related Kaposi's sarcoma, acute myelogenous leukemia, and Ewing's sarcoma)

etor·phine \ē-ˈtȯr-ˌfēn, i-\ *n* **:** a synthetic narcotic drug $C_{25}H_{33}NO_4$ related to morphine but with more potent analgesic properties

etret·i·nate \i-ˈtret-ᵊn-ˌāt\ *n* **:** a retinoid drug $C_{23}H_{30}O_3$ used esp. to treat severe recalcitrant psoriasis

Eu *symbol* europium

Eu·bac·te·ria \ˌyü-bak-ˈtir-ē-ə\ *n pl* **:** a subkingdom of prokaryotic microorganisms that is equivalent to the domain Bacteria in the three-domain classification of living things, that comprises microorganisms either lacking a cell wall, having a thick cell wall of peptidoglycan, or having a thin cell wall of peptidoglycan with an outer layer of lipoprotein, and that includes most of the familiar bacteria of medical and economic importance

eu·bac·te·ri·al \-əl\ *adj* **:** of, relating to, or being microorganisms of the subkingdom Eubacteria or the domain Bacteria

Eu·bac·te·ri·a·les \ˌyü-(ˌ)bak-ˌtir-ē-ˈā-(ˌ)lēz\ *n pl, in some former classifications* **:** an order of the class Schizomycetes comprising relatively simple nonfilamentous unbranched bacteria that show no visible sulfur or iron particles and that include spherical and rod-shaped forms

eu·bac·te·ri·um \ˌyü-bak-ˈtir-ē-əm\ *n* **1** *cap* **:** a genus of gram-positive anaerobic rod-shaped bacteria that do not form spores, that are found in the bodily cavities of animals including humans, in plant and animal products, in infections of soft tissue, and in soil, and that include some forms which may be pathogenic **2** *pl* **-ria** \-ē-ə\ **:** any microorganism of the subkingdom Eubacteria or the domain Bacteria

eu·caine \yü-ˈkān, ˈyü-ˌkān\ *n* **:** a piperidine derivative $C_{15}H_{21}NO_2$ used esp. formerly as a local anesthetic in the form of its white crystalline hydrochloride

eu·ca·lyp·tol *also* **eu·ca·lyp·tole** \ˌyü-kə-ˈlip-ˌtōl, -ˌtȯl\ *n* **:** a liquid $C_{10}H_{18}O$ with an odor of camphor that occurs in many essential oils (as of eucalyptus) and is used esp. as an expectorant and flavoring — called also *cajeputol, cineole*

eu·ca·lyp·tus \ˌyü-kə-ˈlip-təs\ *n* **1** *cap* **:** a genus of mostly Australian evergreen trees or rarely shrubs of the myrtle family that have rigid entire leaves and umbellate flowers and are widely cultivated for their gums, resins, oils, and useful woods **2** *pl* **-ti** \-ˌtī, -ˌtē\ *or* **-tus·es :** any tree or shrub of the genus *Eucalyptus* — **eucalyptus** *adj*

eucalyptus oil *n* **:** any of various essential oils obtained from the leaves of various members of the genus *Eucalyptus* (as *E. globulus*) and used in pharmaceutical preparations (as antiseptics and cough drops)

eucaryote, eucaryotic *var of* EUKARYOTE, EUKARYOTIC

euc·at·ro·pine \yü-ˈka-trə-ˌpēn\ *n* **:** a synthetic alkaloid used in the form of its white crystalline hydrochloride $C_{17}H_{25}NO_3$·HCl as a mydriatic

Eu·ces·to·da \ˌyü-ses-ˈtō-də\ *n pl, in some classifications* **:** a subclass of flatworms of the class Cestoda comprising polyzootic forms that have a scolex of varying structure and usu. distinct external segmentation and that parasitize the intestines of vertebrates

eu·chlor·hyd·ria \ˌyü-ˌklȯr-ˈhī-drē-ə\ *n* **:** the presence of the normal amount of hydrochloric acid in the gastric juice

eu·chro·ma·tin \(ˈ)yü-ˈkrō-mət-ən\ *n* **:** the genetically active portion of chromatin that is largely composed of genes — **eu·chro·mat·ic** \ˌyü-krō-ˈmat-ik\ *adj*

eu·di·om·e·ter \ˌyüd-ē-ˈäm-ət-ər\ *n* **:** an instrument for the volumetric measurement and analysis of gases — **eu·dio·met·ric** \ˌyüd-ē-ə-ˈme-trik\ *adj* — **eu·dio·met·ri·cal·ly** \-tri-k(ə-)lē\ *adv*

eu·ge·nia \yü-ˈjēn-yə, -ˈjē-nē-ə\ *n* **1** *cap* **:** a large genus of tropical trees and shrubs of the myrtle family (Myrtaceae) having aromatic leaves and including one (*E. aromatica*) that is the source of cloves **2 :** any tree of the genus *Eugenia*

Eu·gène \œ-zhen\ **(1663–1736),** Prince of Savoy. A general in the service of Austria, Eugène served brilliantly in wars against the Turks and later the French. In the Spanish War of Succession (1701–1714) he fought in a long series of campaigns and won several battles. He was one of the victors in the famous battle at Blenheim in 1704. The genus *Eugenia* was named in his honor by Carolus Linnaeus in 1753.

eu·gen·ic \yü-ˈjen-ik\ *adj* **1 :** relating to or fitted for the production of good offspring **2 :** of or relating to eugenics — **eu·gen·i·cal·ly** \-i-k(ə-)lē\ *adv*

eu·gen·i·cist \-ˈjen-ə-səst\ *n* **:** a student or advocate of eugenics

eu·gen·ics \yü-ˈjen-iks\ *n pl but sing in constr* **:** a science that deals with the improvement (as by control of human mating) of hereditary qualities of a race or breed

eu·ge·nol \ˈyü-jə-ˌnȯl, -ˌnōl\ *n* **:** a colorless aromatic liquid phenol $C_{10}H_{12}O_2$ found esp. in clove oil and used in dentistry as an analgesic

eu·gle·na \yü-ˈglē-nə\ *n* **1** *cap* **:** a genus of green freshwater flagellates of the order Euglenida often classified as algae **2 :** any member of the genus *Euglena*

Eu·gle·ni·da \yü-ˈglē-nəd-ə\ *n pl* **:** an order of protozoans of the subphylum Mastigophora comprising extremely varied flagellates that are typically green or colorless stigma-bearing solitary organisms with one or two flagella emerging anteriorly from a well-defined gullet — see EUGLENOPHYTA

eu·gle·noid \yü-ˈglē-ˌnȯid, ˈyü-glə-\ *n* **:** any flagellate of the order Euglenida — **euglenoid** *adj*

euglenoid movement *n* **:** writhing usu. nonprogressive protoplasmic movement of plastic-bodied euglenoid flagellates

Eu·gle·noph·y·ta \ˌyü-glə-ˈnäf-ət-ə\ *n pl* **:** a division of algae that is equivalent to the protozoan order Euglenida of the subphylum Mastigophora and includes mostly unicellular flagellates which are both photosynthetic and heterotrophic

eu·glob·u·lin \yü-ˈgläb-yə-lən\ *n* **:** a simple protein that does not dissolve in pure water — compare PSEUDOGLOBULIN

eu·gly·ce·mia *or chiefly Brit* **eu·gly·cae·mia** \ˌyü-glī-ˈsē-mē-ə\ *n* **:** a normal level of sugar in the blood

eu·gon·ic \(ˈ)yü-ˈgän-ik\ *adj* **:** growing readily on artificial media — used esp. of some strains of the tubercle bacillus; compare DYSGONIC

eu·kary·ote *also* **eu·cary·ote** \(ˈ)yü-ˈkar-ē-ˌōt, -ē-ət\ *n* **:** any of a domain (Eukarya) or a higher taxonomic group (Eukaryota) above the kingdom that includes organisms composed of one or more cells containing visibly evident nuclei and organelles — compare PROKARYOTE — **eu·kary·ot·ic** *also* **eu·cary·ot·ic** \-ˌkar-ē-ˈät-ik\ *adj*

Eu·my·ce·tes \ˌyü-mī-ˈsēt-ēz\ *n pl* **:** a division of fungi that includes all true fungi (as the ascomycetes and basidiomycetes) as distinguished from the slime molds — **eu·my·cete** \ˌyü-ˈmī-sēt\ *n*

eu·nuch \ˈyü-nək, -nik\ *n* **:** a man or boy deprived of the testes or external genitals — **eu·nuch·ism** \-ˌiz-əm\ *n*

¹eu·nuch·oid \ˈyü-nə-ˌkȯid\ *also* **eu·nuch·oi·dal** \-ˌkȯid-ᵊl, ˌyü-nə-ˈkȯid-ᵊl\ *adj* **:** of, relating to, or characterized by eunuchoidism **:** resembling a eunuch

²eunuchoid *n* **:** a sexually deficient individual; *esp* **:** one lacking in sexual differentiation and tending toward the intersex state

eu·nuch·oid·ism \ˈyü-nə-ˌkȯi-ˌdiz-əm\ *n* **:** a state suggestive of that of a eunuch in being marked by deficiency of sexual development, by persistence of prepubertal characteristics, and often by the presence of characteristics typical of the opposite sex

eu·on·y·mus \yü-'än-ə-məs\ *n* **1 a** *cap* : a genus (family Celastraceae) of often evergreen shrubs, small trees, or vines **b** : any member of the genus *Euonymus* **2** : the dried bark of the root of a shrub of the genus *Euonymus* (*E. atropurpureus*) used as a cathartic

eu·pa·to·rin \yü-pə-'tōr-ən\ *n* **1** : a bitter glucoside $C_{35}H_{58}NO_{10}$ occurring in boneset **2** : a resinoid prepared from boneset and formerly used as a tonic and expectorant

eu·pa·to·ri·um \-'tōr-ē-əm\ *n* **1** *cap* : a large genus of chiefly tropical composite herbs having heads of white or purplish flowers and including several (as boneset) that have been used medicinally **2** : any plant of the genus *Eupatorium*

eu·pep·sia \yü-'pep-shə, -sē-ə\ *n* : good digestion

eu·pep·tic \-'pep-tik\ *adj* : of, relating to, or having good digestion

eu·phen·ics \yü-'fen-iks\ *n pl but sing in constr* : the therapeutic techniques and procedures (as medical treatment) for amelioration of the deleterious phenotypic effects of a genetic defect esp. without altering the genetic makeup of the germ plasm of the individual — **eu·phen·ic** \-ik\ *adj*

eu·phor·bia \yü-'fȯr-bē-ə\ *n* **1** : a large genus of plants of the spurge family that have a milky juice and flowers included in an involucre which surrounds a group of several staminate flowers and a central pistillate flower and that include a number which have been used medicinally **2** : any plant of the genus *Euphorbia*; *also* : any of various other plants that belong to the spurge family

eu·pho·ria \yü-'fōr-ē-ə, -'fȯr-\ *n* : a feeling of well-being or elation; *esp* : one that is groundless, disproportionate to its cause, or inappropriate to one's life situation — compare DYSPHORIA — **eu·phor·ic** \-'fōr-ik, -'fär-\ *adj* — **eu·phor·i·cal·ly** \-i-k(ə-)lē\ *adv*

¹eu·pho·ri·ant \yü-'fōr-ē-ənt, -'fȯr-\ *n* : a drug that tends to induce euphoria

²euphoriant *adj* : tending to induce euphoria ⟨a ∼ drug⟩

eu·phor·i·gen·ic \yü-ˌfōr-ə-'jen-ik\ *adj* : tending to cause euphoria ⟨the ∼ effects of cocaine⟩

eu·plas·tic \yü-'plas-tik\ *adj* : adapted to the formation of tissue : BLASTEMATIC

eu·ploid \'yü-ˌplȯid\ *adj* : having a chromosome number that is an exact multiple of the haploid number — compare ANEUPLOID — **euploid** *n* — **eu·ploi·dy** \-ˌplȯid-ē\ *n, pl* **-dies**

eup·nea *or chiefly Brit* **eup·noea** \yüp-'nē-ə\ *n* : normal respiration — compare DYSPNEA — **eup·ne·ic** *or chiefly Brit* **eup·noe·ic** \-'nē-ik\ *adj*

eu·prax·ia \yü-'prak-sē-ə, -'prak-shə\ *n* : normally coordinated muscular performance — compare APRAXIA

eu·ro·pi·um \yü-'rō-pē-əm\ *n* : a bivalent and trivalent metallic element of the rare-earth group found in monazite sand — symbol *Eu*; see ELEMENT table

Eu·ro·ti·a·les \yü-ˌrōt-ē-'ā-lēz, -ˌrō-shē-\ *n pl* : an order of ascomycetous fungi (as the blue molds) that have a closed ascocarp with the asci scattered rather than collected into a spore-bearing layer and that include most of the human and animal dermatophytes as well as many saprobic soil or coprophilous fungi

eu·ryg·nath·ic \ˌyü-ri(g)-'nath-ik, -rē(g)-\ *also* **eu·ryg·na·thous** \yə-'rig-nə-thəs\ *adj* : having a wide jaw — **eu·ryg·na·thism** \yə-'rig-nə-ˌthiz-əm\ *n*

eu·ry·on \'yü-rē-ˌän\ *n* : either of the lateral points marking the ends of the greatest transverse diameter of the skull

eu·ry·therm \'yür-i-ˌthərm\ *n* : an organism that tolerates a wide range of temperature — **eu·ry·ther·mal** \ˌyür-i-'thər-məl\ *or* **eu·ry·ther·mic** \-mik\ *or* **eu·ry·ther·mous** \-məs\ *adj*

eu·sta·chian tonsil \yü-ˌstā-sh(ē-)ən- *also* -ˌstā-kē-ən-\ *n, often cap E* : a mass of lymphoid tissue at the pharyngeal opening of the eustachian tube

Eu·sta·chio \äü-'stäk-yō\, **Bartolomeo** (*ca* 1520–1574), Italian anatomist. Eustachio served as a professor of anatomy at a school of medicine in Rome. Between 1562 and 1563 he produced a remarkable series of treatises on the kidney, the ear, the nervous system, and the teeth. His treatise on the kidney was the first work specifically concerned with that organ. It revealed a knowledge of the kidney that exceeded previous works, and it contained the first account of the adrenal glands. The treatise on the ear contains the classic description of the Eustachian tube. Eustachio is known for an extraordinary series of 47 anatomical drawings. The set included an illustration of the sympathetic nervous system that is generally considered to be one of the best ever produced. One plate illustrated the valve in the right atrium of the fetal heart that is now known as the Eustachian valve.

eustachian tube *n, often cap E* : a bony and cartilaginous tube connecting the middle ear with the nasopharynx and equalizing air pressure on both sides of the tympanic membrane — called also *auditory tube, pharyngotympanic tube*

eustachian valve *n, often cap E* : a crescent-shaped fold of the lining membrane of the heart at the entrance of the inferior vena cava that directs the blood through the foramen ovale to the left atrium in the fetus but is rudimentary and functionless in the adult

eu·tec·tic \yü-'tek-tik\ *adj* **1** *of an alloy or solution* : having the lowest melting point possible **2** : of or relating to a eutectic alloy or solution or its melting or freezing point — **eutectic** *n*

eu·tha·na·sia \ˌyü-thə-'nā-zh(ē-)ə\ *n* : the act or practice of killing hopelessly sick or injured individuals (as persons or domestic animals) in a relatively painless way for reasons of mercy; *also* : the act or practice of allowing a hopelessly sick or injured patient to die by taking less than complete medical measures to prolong life — called also *mercy killing*

eu·tha·nize \'yü-thə-ˌnīz\ *also* **eu·than·a·tize** \yü-'than-ə-ˌtīz\ *vt* **-nized** *also* **-tized; -niz·ing** *also* **-tiz·ing** : to subject to euthanasia ⟨the dog was *euthanized* at the owner's request⟩

eu·then·ics \yü-'then-iks\ *n pl but sing or pl in constr* : a science that deals with development of human well-being by improvement of living conditions — **eu·the·nist** \yü-'then-əst, 'yü-thə-nəst\ *n*

Eu·the·ria \yü-'thir-ē-ə\ *n pl* : a major division of mammals characterized by the attachment of the developing fetus to the maternal uterus by a placenta and including all mammals living at the present time except the marsupials — **eu·the·ri·an** \-ē-ən\ *adj or n*

eu·thy·roid \(')yü-'thī-ˌrȯid\ *adj* : characterized by normal thyroid function — **eu·thy·roid·ism** \-iz-əm\ *n*

eu·to·cia \yü-'tō-sh(ē-)ə\ *n* : normal parturition — compare DYSTOCIA

evac·u·ant \i-'vak-yə-wənt\ *n* : an emetic, diuretic, or purgative agent — **evacuant** *adj*

evac·u·ate \i-'vak-yə-ˌwāt\ *vb* **-at·ed; -at·ing** *vt* **1** : to remove the contents of ⟨∼ an abscess⟩ **2** : to discharge (as urine or feces) from the body as waste : VOID ∼ *vi* : to pass urine or feces from the body — **evac·u·a·tive** \-ˌwāt-iv\ *adj*

evac·u·a·tion \i-ˌvak-yə-'wā-shən\ *n* **1** : the act or process of evacuating **2** : something evacuated or discharged

evag·i·na·tion \i-ˌvaj-ə-'nā-shən\ *n* **1** : a process of turning outward or inside out ⟨∼ of a plasma membrane⟩ **2** : a part or structure that is produced by evagination — called also *outpocketing, outpouching* — **evag·i·nate** \i-'vaj-ə-ˌnāt\ *vt* **-nat·ed; -nat·ing**

ev·a·nes·cent \ˌev-ə-'nes-ᵊnt\ *adj* : tending to disappear quickly : of relatively short duration ⟨an ∼ rash⟩

Ev·ans blue \'ev-ənz-\ *n* : a dye $C_{34}H_{24}N_6Na_4O_{14}S_4$ that on injection into the bloodstream combines with serum albumin and is used to determine blood volume colorimetrically

Evans, Herbert McLean (1882–1971), American anatomist and physiologist. Evans made classic contributions to endocrinology and vitaminology. He was one of the few scientists to study both hormones and vitamins. In 1915 he published an explanation of the physiological behavior of vital stains in the benzidine series and did research on azo

\ə\ **abut** \ᵊ\ **kitten** \ər\ **further** \a\ **ash** \ā\ **ace** \ä\ **cot, cart**
\aù\ **out** \ch\ **chin** \e\ **bet** \ē\ **easy** \g\ **go** \i\ **hit** \ī\ **ice** \j\ **job**
\ŋ\ **sing** \ō\ **go** \ȯ\ **law** \ȯi\ **boy** \th\ **thin** \th̲\ **the** \ü\ **loot**
\ù\ **foot** \y\ **yet** \zh\ **vision** *See also* Pronunciation Symbols page

dyes, and in particular the dye now called Evans blue.

evap·o·ra·tion \i-ˌvap-ə-ˈrā-shən\ *n* : the change by which any substance is converted from a liquid state into and carried off in vapor; *specif* : the conversion of a liquid into vapor in order to remove it wholly or partly from a liquid of higher boiling point or from solids dissolved in or mixed with it — **evap·o·rate** \i-ˈvap-ə-ˌrāt\ *vb* **-rat·ed; -rat·ing** — **evap·o·ra·tor** \-ˌrāt-ər\ *n*

event \i-ˈvent\ *n* : an adverse or damaging medical occurrence ⟨a heart attack or other cardiac ∼⟩

even·tra·tion \ˌē-ven-ˈtrā-shən\ *n* : protrusion of abdominal organs through the abdominal wall

ever·sion \i-ˈvər-zhən, -shən\ *n* **1** : the act of turning inside out : the state of being turned inside out ⟨∼ of the eyelid⟩ ⟨∼ of the bladder⟩ **2** : the condition (as of the foot) of being turned or rotated outward — compare INVERSION 1b — **ever·si·ble** \-ˈvər-sə-bəl\ *adj*

evert \i-ˈvərt\ *vt* : to turn outward ⟨∼ the foot⟩; *also* : to turn inside out

evir·a·tion \ˌev-ə-ˈrā-shən\ *n* : loss or deprivation of masculine qualities with assumption of feminine characteristics; *also* : a delusion in a male that he has become a woman

evis·cer·ate \i-ˈvis-ə-ˌrāt\ *vb* **-at·ed; -at·ing** *vt* **1** : to remove the viscera of **2** : to remove an organ from (a patient) or the contents of (an organ) ∼ *vi* : to protrude through a surgical incision or suffer protrusion of a part through an incision

evis·cer·a·tion \i-ˌvis-ə-ˈrā-shən\ *n* : the act or process of eviscerating

Evis·ta \ē-ˈvis-tə\ *trademark* — used for a preparation of raloxifene

evo·ca·tion \ˌē-vō-ˈkā-shən, ˌev-ə-\ *n* : INDUCTION 3b; *specif* : initiation of development of a primary embryonic axis

evo·ca·tor \ˈē-vō-ˌkāt-ər, ˈev-ə-\ *n* : the specific chemical constituent responsible for the physiological effects of an organizer

evoked potential \ē-ˈvōkt-\ *n* : an electrical response esp. in the cerebral cortex as recorded following stimulation of a peripheral sense receptor

evo·lu·tion \ˌev-ə-ˈlü-shən *also* ˌē-və-\ *n* **1** : a process of change in a certain direction ⟨tumor ∼ and progression —I. J. Fidler *et al*⟩ **2 a** : the historical development of a biological group (as a race or species) : PHYLOGENY **b** : a theory that the various types of animals and plants have their origin in other preexisting types and that the distinguishable differences are due to modifications in successive generations — **evo·lu·tion·ari·ly** \-shə-ˌner-ə-lē\ *adv* — **evo·lu·tion·ary** \-shə-ˌner-ē\ *adj*

evo·lu·tion·ist \-sh(ə-)nəst\ *n* : a student of or adherent to a theory of evolution

evolve \i-ˈvälv, -ˈvolv\ *vb* **evolved; evolv·ing** *vt* : to produce by natural evolutionary processes ∼ *vi* : to develop by or as if by evolution : undergo evolutionary change ⟨an *evolving* theory of mental functioning —S. A. Green⟩

evul·sion \i-ˈvəl-shən\ *n* : the act of extracting forcibly : EXTRACTION ⟨∼ of a tooth⟩ — **evulse** \i-ˈvəls\ *vt* **evulsed; evuls·ing**

ewe \ˈyü, ˈyō\ *n* : the female of the sheep esp. when mature; *also* : the female of various related animals

ewe–neck \-ˈnek\ *n* : a thin neck with a concave arch occurring as a defect in dogs and horses — **ewe–necked** \-ˈnekt\ *adj*

Ew·ing's sarcoma \ˈyü-iŋz-\ *n* : a malignant bone tumor esp. of a long bone or the pelvis — called also *Ewing's tumor*
  Ewing, James (1866–1943), American pathologist. Ewing was a recognized authority on the diagnosis and management of neoplastic diseases and the author of a standard text on the subject. His description of reticulum cell sarcoma was published in 1913. He described the disease now known as Ewing's sarcoma or tumor in 1921.

ex *abbr* **1** examined **2** example **3** exercise

ex·ac·er·bate \ig-ˈzas-ər-ˌbāt\ *vt* **-bat·ed; -bat·ing** : to cause (a disease or its symptoms) to become more severe ⟨her condition was *exacerbated* by lack of care⟩ — **ex·ac·er·ba·tion** \-ˌzas-ər-ˈbā-shən\ *n*

ex·act sci·ence \ig-ˈzakt-ˈsī-ən(t)s\ *n* : a science (as physics, chemistry, or astronomy) whose laws are capable of accurate quantitative expression

ex·alt \ig-ˈzolt\ *vt* : to cause (virulence) to increase ⟨virulence ∼*ed* by addition of mucin to a bacterial culture⟩; *also* : to increase the virulence of ⟨∼ a virus by repeated rapid passage through susceptible hosts⟩

ex·al·ta·tion \ˌeg-ˌzol-ˈtā-shən, ˌek-ˌsol-\ *n* **1 a** : marked or excessive intensification of a mental state or of the activity of a bodily part or function **b** : an abnormal sense of personal well-being, power, or importance : a delusional euphoria **2** : an increase in degree or intensity ⟨∼ of virulence of a virus⟩

ex·am \ig-ˈzam\ *n* : EXAMINATION

ex·am·i·na·tion \ig-ˌzam-ə-ˈnā-shən\ *n* : the act or process of inspecting or testing for evidence of disease or abnormality — see PHYSICAL EXAMINATION

ex·am·ine \ig-ˈzam-ən\ *vb* **ex·am·ined; ex·am·in·ing** \-(ə-)niŋ\ *vt* : to inspect or test for evidence of disease or abnormality ⟨the doctor *examined* the young men and found them in perfect health⟩ ∼ *vi* : to make or give an examination ⟨the doctor will ∼ at the infirmary⟩

ex·am·in·ee \ig-ˌzam-ə-ˈnē\ *n* : a person who is examined

ex·am·in·er \ig-ˈzam-(ə-)nər\ *n* : one that examines — see MEDICAL EXAMINER

ex·an·them \eg-ˈzan(t)-thəm, ˈek-ˌsan-ˌthem\ *or* **ex·an·the·ma** \ˌeg-ˌzan-ˈthē-mə\ *n, pl* **-thems** *also* **-them·a·ta** \ˌeg-ˌzan-ˈthem-ət-ə\ *or* **-themas** : an eruptive disease (as measles) or its symptomatic eruption — **ex·an·them·a·tous** \ˌeg-ˌzan-ˈthem-ət-əs\ *or* **ex·an·the·mat·ic** \-ˌzan-thə-ˈmat-ik\ *adj*

exanthema su·bi·tum *or* **exanthem subitum** \-sə-ˈbīt-əm\ *n* : ROSEOLA INFANTUM

exc *abbr* except; exception

ex·ca·vate \ˈek-skə-ˌvāt\ *vb* **-vat·ed; -vat·ing** *vt* : to form a cavity or hole in ⟨an *excavated* wisdom tooth⟩ ∼ *vi* : to make excavations or become hollowed out ⟨an area of infarction in soft tissue often tends to ∼⟩

ex·ca·va·tion \ˌek-skə-ˈvā-shən\ *n* **1** : the action or process of excavating **2** : a cavity formed by or as if by cutting, digging, or scooping

ex·ca·va·tor \ˈek-skə-ˌvāt-ər\ *n* : an instrument used to open bodily cavities (as in the teeth) or remove material from them

excavatum — see PECTUS EXCAVATUM

ex·cel·sin \ik-ˈsel-sən\ *n* : a crystalline globulin obtained from the meat of the Brazil nut

ex·ce·men·to·sis \ˌeks-si-ˌmen-ˈtō-səs\ *n, pl* **-to·ses** \-ˈtō-ˌsēz\ *or* **-to·sis·es** : abnormal outgrowth of the cementum of the root of a tooth

ex·change transfusion \iks-ˈchānj-\ *n* : simultaneous withdrawal of the recipient's blood and transfusion with the donor's blood esp. in the treatment of erythroblastosis

ex·ci·mer \ˈek-si-(ˌ)mər\ *n* **1** : an aggregate of two atoms or molecules that exists in an excited state **2** : EXCIMER LASER

excimer laser *n* : a laser that uses a compound of a halogen and a noble gas to generate radiation usu. in the ultraviolet region of the spectrum

ex·cip·i·ent \ik-ˈsip-ē-ənt\ *n* : a usu. inert substance (as gum arabic, syrup, lanolin, or starch) that forms a vehicle (as for a drug or antigen); *esp* : one that in the presence of sufficient liquid gives a medicated mixture the adhesive quality needed for the preparation of pills or tablets

ex·cise \ik-ˈsīz\ *vt* **ex·cised; ex·cis·ing** : to remove by excision : RESECT ⟨∼ a tumor⟩

ex·ci·sion \ik-ˈsizh-ən\ *n* : surgical removal or resection (as of a diseased part) — **ex·ci·sion·al** \-ˈsizh-nəl, -ᵊn-əl\ *adj*

ex·cit·able \ik-ˈsīt-ə-bəl\ *adj, of living tissue or an organism* : capable of being activated by and reacting to stimuli : exhibiting irritability ⟨the biochemistry of ∼ membranes —*Science*⟩ — **ex·cit·abil·i·ty** \-ˌsīt-ə-ˈbil-ət-ē\ *n, pl* **-ties**

¹**ex·ci·tant** \ik-ˈsīt-ᵊnt, ˈek-sət-ənt\ *adj* : tending to excite or augment ⟨∼ drugs⟩

²**excitant** *n* : an agent that arouses or augments physiological activity (as of the nervous system)

ex·ci·ta·tion \ek-ˌsī-ˈtā-shən, ˌek-sə-\ *n* : EXCITEMENT: as **a** : the disturbed or altered condition resulting from arousal of activity (as by neural or electrical stimulation) in an individual organ or tissue **b** : the arousing of such activity

ex·cit·ato·ry \ik-ˈsīt-ə-ˌtōr-ē, -ˌtȯr-\ *adj* **1** : tending to induce excitation (as of a neuron) ⟨∼ substances⟩ ⟨∼ and inhibitory pathways from the brain —W. G. Van der Kloot⟩ **2** : exhibiting, resulting from, related to, or produced by excitement or excitation ⟨an ∼ postsynaptic potential⟩

ex·cite \ik-ˈsīt\ *vt* **ex·cit·ed; ex·cit·ing 1** : to increase the activity of (as a living organism) : STIMULATE **2** : to raise (as an atomic nucleus, an atom, or a molecule) to a higher energy level

ex·cite·ment \-ˈsīt-mənt\ *n* **1** : the act of exciting **2** : the state of being excited: as **a** : aroused, augmented, or abnormal activity of an organism or functioning of an organ or part **b** : extreme motor hyperactivity (as in catatonic schizophrenia or bipolar disorder)

ex·ci·tor \-ˈsīt-ər\ *n* : an afferent nerve arousing increased action of the part that it supplies

ex·ci·to·tox·ic \ik-ˌsīt-ə-ˈtäk-sik\ *adj* : being, involving, or resulting from the action of an agent that binds to a nerve cell receptor, stimulates the cell, and damages it or causes its death ⟨∼ damage to cortical interneurons —R. C. Collins *et al*⟩ — **ex·ci·to·tox·ic·i·ty** \-ˌ)täk-ˈsis-ə-tē\ *n, pl* **-ties**

ex·ci·to·tox·in \ik-ˈsīt-ə-ˌtäk-sən\ *n* : an excitotoxic agent (as kainic acid)

ex·clu·sion \iks-ˈklü-zhən\ *n* : surgical separation of part of an organ from the rest without excision — **ex·clude** \iks-ˈklüd\ *vt* **ex·clud·ed; ex·clud·ing**

ex·coch·le·a·tion \ˌeks-ˌkäk-lē-ˈā-shən\ *n* : removal of the contents of a cavity by scraping or curetting

ex·co·ri·a·tion \(ˌ)ek-ˌskōr-ē-ˈā-shən, -ˌskȯr-\ *n* **1** : the act of abrading or wearing off the skin ⟨chafing and ∼ of the skin⟩ **2** : a raw irritated lesion (as of the skin or a mucosal surface) — **ex·co·ri·ate** \ek-ˈskōr-ē-ˌāt\ *vt* **-at·ed; -at·ing**

ex·cre·ment \ˈek-skrə-mənt\ *n* : waste matter discharged from the body; *esp* : waste (as feces) discharged from the alimentary canal — **ex·cre·men·tal** \ˌek-skrə-ˈment-ᵊl\ *adj* — **ex·cre·men·ti·tious** \-ˌmen-ˈtish-əs\ *adj*

ex·cres·cence \ik-ˈskres-ᵊn(t)s\ *n* : an outgrowth or enlargement: as **a** : a natural and normal appendage or development ⟨hair is an ∼ from the scalp⟩ **b** : an abnormal outgrowth ⟨warty ∼s in the colon⟩ — **ex·cres·cent** \ik-ˈskres-ᵊnt\ *adj*

ex·cre·ta \ik-ˈskrēt-ə\ *n pl* : waste matter eliminated or separated from an organism — compare EXCRETION 2 — **ex·cre·tal** \-ˈskrēt-ᵊl\ *adj*

ex·crete \ik-ˈskrēt\ *vt* **ex·cret·ed; ex·cret·ing** : to separate and eliminate or discharge (waste) from the blood or tissues or from the active protoplasm

ex·cret·er \-ˈskrēt-ər\ *n* : one that excretes something; *esp* : one that excretes an atypical bodily product (as a pathogenic microorganism)

ex·cre·tion \ik-ˈskrē-shən\ *n* **1** : the act or process of excreting **2 a** : something eliminated by the process of excretion that is composed chiefly of urine or sweat in mammals including humans and of comparable materials in other animals, characteristically includes products of protein degradation (as urea or uric acid), usu. differs from ordinary bodily secretions by lacking any further utility to the organism that produces it, and is distinguished from waste materials (as feces) that have merely passed into or through the alimentary canal without being incorporated into the body proper **b** : a waste product (as urine, feces, or vomit) eliminated from an animal body : EXCREMENT — not used technically

ex·cre·to·ry \ˈek-skrə-ˌtōr-ē, -ˌtȯr-\ *adj* : of, relating to, or functioning in excretion ⟨∼ ducts⟩

ex·cur·sion \ik-ˈskər-zhən\ *n* **1 a** : a movement outward and back or from a mean position or axis ⟨∼ of the femur⟩ **b** : the distance traversed **2** : one complete movement of expansion and contraction of the lungs and their membranes (as in breathing)

ex·cyst \ek(s)-ˈsist\ *vi* : to emerge from a cyst ⟨the metacercariae ∼ in the duodenum —W. A. D. Anderson⟩ — **ex·cys·ta·tion** \ˌek(s)-ˌsis-ˈtā-shən\ *n* — **ex·cyst·ment** \ˌek(s)-ˈsist-mənt\ *n*

ex·en·ter·a·tion \ig-ˌzent-ə-ˈrā-shən\ *n* **1** : EVISCERATION **2** : surgical removal of the contents of a bodily cavity (as the orbit, pelvis, or a sinus) ⟨pelvic ∼ for advanced uterine, bladder, and rectal carcinoma —*Jour. Amer. Med. Assoc.*⟩ — **ex·en·ter·ate** \ig-ˈzent-ə-ˌrāt\ *vt* **-at·ed; -at·ing**

¹**ex·er·cise** \ˈek-sər-ˌsīz\ *n* **1** : regular or repeated use of a faculty or bodily organ **2** : bodily exertion for the sake of developing and maintaining physical fitness

²**exercise** *vb* **-cised; -cis·ing** *vt* **1** : to use repeatedly in order to strengthen or develop (as a muscle) **2** : to put through exercises ∼ *vi* : to take exercise

ex·er·cis·er \ˈek-sər-ˌsī-zər\ *n* **1** : one that exercises **2** : an apparatus for use in physical exercise

Ex·er·cy·cle \ˈek-sər-ˌsī-kəl\ *trademark* — used for a stationary bicycle

ex·er·e·sis \ig-ˈzer-ə-səs\ *n, pl* **-e·ses** \-ə-ˌsēz\ : surgical removal of a part or organ (as a nerve)

ex·er·gon·ic \ˌek-(ˌ)sər-ˈgän-ik\ *adj* : EXOTHERMIC ⟨an ∼ biochemical reaction⟩ — compare ENDERGONIC

ex·er·tion·al \ig-ˈzərsh-(ə)-nəl\ *adj* : precipitated by physical exertion but usu. relieved by rest ⟨∼ rhabdomyolysis⟩

ex·flag·el·la·tion \(ˌ)eks-ˌflaj-ə-ˈlā-shən\ *n* **1** : the casting off of cilia or flagella **2** : the formation of microgametes in sporozoans (as the malaria parasite) by extrusion of nuclear material into peripheral processes resembling flagella — **ex·flag·el·late** \-ˈflaj-ə-ˌlāt\ *vi* **-lat·ed; -lat·ing**

ex·fo·li·ant \(ˌ)eks-ˈfō-lē-ənt, -ˈfōl-yənt\ *n* : a mechanical or chemical agent (as an abrasive skin wash or salicylic acid) that is applied to the skin to remove dead cells from the surface — called also *exfoliator*

ex·fo·li·ate \-ˈfō-lē-ˌāt\ *vb* **-at·ed; -at·ing** *vt* **1** : to cast off in scales or laminae **2** : to remove the surface of in scales or laminae **3** : to shed (teeth) by exfoliation ∼ *vi* **1** : to split into or give off scales, laminae, or body cells **2** : to come off in thin layers or scales : scale off

ex·fo·li·a·tion \(ˌ)eks-ˌfō-lē-ˈā-shən\ *n* : the action or process of exfoliating: as **a** : the peeling of the horny layer of the skin (as in some skin diseases) **b** : the shedding of surface components (as cells from internal body surfaces) **c** : the shedding of a superficial layer of bone or of a tooth or part of a tooth — **ex·fo·li·a·tive** \eks-ˈfō-lē-ˌāt-iv\ *adj*

exfoliative cytology *n* : the study of cells shed from body surfaces esp. for determining the presence or absence of a cancerous condition

ex·fo·li·a·tor \(ˌ)eks-ˈfō-lē-ˌāt-ər\ *n* : EXFOLIANT

ex·ha·la·tion \ˌeks-(h)ə-ˈlā-shən\ *n* **1** : the action of forcing air out of the lungs **2** : something (as the breath) that is exhaled or given off

ex·hale \eks-ˈ(h)ā(ə)l\ *vb* **ex·haled; ex·hal·ing** *vi* : to emit breath or vapor ∼ *vt* : to breathe out

ex·haust \ig-ˈzȯst\ *vt* **1 a** : to draw off or let out completely **b** : to empty by drawing off the contents; *specif* : to create a vacuum in **2 a** : to use up : consume completely **b** : to tire extremely or completely ⟨∼ed by overwork⟩ **3** : to extract completely with a solvent ⟨∼ a drug with alcohol⟩

ex·haus·tion \ig-ˈzȯs-chən\ *n* **1** : the act or process of exhausting : the state of being exhausted ⟨suffered from physical and mental ∼⟩ — see HEAT EXHAUSTION **2** : neurosis following overstrain or overexertion esp. in military combat

ex·hi·bi·tion·ism \ˌek-sə-ˈbish-ə-ˌniz-əm\ *n* **1 a** : a perversion marked by a tendency to indecent exposure **b** : an act of such exposure **2** : the act or practice of behaving so as to attract attention to oneself

ex·hi·bi·tion·ist \-ˈbish-(ə-)nəst\ *n* : one who engages in or is addicted to exhibitionism

---

\ə\ **abut** \ᵊ\ **kitten** \ər\ **further** \a\ **ash** \ā\ **ace** \ä\ **cot, cart** \au̇\ **out** \ch\ **chin** \e\ **bet** \ē\ **easy** \g\ **go** \i\ **hit** \ī\ **ice** \j\ **job** \ŋ\ **sing** \ō\ **go** \ȯ\ **law** \ȯi\ **boy** \th\ **thin** \t̲h̲\ **the** \ü\ **loot** \u̇\ **foot** \y\ **yet** \zh\ **vision** *See also* Pronunciation Symbols page

ex·hi·bi·tion·is·tic \-,bish-ə-'nis-tik\ *also* **exhibitionist** *adj* : of, relating to, or given to exhibitionism — **ex·hi·bi·tion·is·ti·cal·ly** \-ti-k(ə-)lē\ *adv*

ex·hume \igz-'(y)üm, iks-'(h)yüm\ *vt* **ex·humed; ex·hum·ing** : DISINTER ⟨the body was *exhumed* for an autopsy⟩ — **ex·hu·ma·tion** \,eks-(h)yü-'mā-shən, ,egz-(y)ü-\ *n*

ex·i·tus \'ek-sət-əs\ *n, pl* **exitus** : DEATH; *esp* : fatal termination of a disease

exo·bi·ol·o·gist \,ek-sō-bī-'äl-ə-jəst\ *n* : a specialist in exobiology — called also *astrobiologist*

exo·bi·ol·o·gy \-bī-'äl-ə-jē\ *n, pl* **-gies** : a branch of biology concerned with the search for life outside the earth and with the effects of extraterrestrial environments on living organisms — called also *astrobiology* — **exo·bi·o·log·i·cal** \-,bī-ə-'läj-i-kəl\ *adj*

exo·crine \'ek-sə-krən, -,krīn, -,krēn\ *adj* : producing, being, or relating to a secretion that is released outside its source ⟨∼ pancreatic cells⟩ ⟨∼ functions⟩ ⟨∼ insufficiency⟩

exocrine gland *n* : a gland (as a sweat gland, a salivary gland, or a kidney) that releases a secretion external to or at the surface of an organ by means of a canal or duct — called also *gland of external secretion*

exo·cri·nol·o·gy \,ek-sə-kri-'näl-ə-jē, -,krī-, -,krē-\ *n, pl* **-gies** : the study of external secretions (as pheromones) that serve an integrative function

exo·cy·clic \,ek-sō-'sī-klik, -'sik-lik\ *adj* : situated outside of a ring in a chemical structure

exo·cy·to·sis \,ek-sō-sī-'tō-səs\ *n, pl* **-to·ses** \-,sēz\ : the release of cellular substances (as secretory products) contained in cell vesicles by fusion of the vesicular membrane with the plasma membrane and subsequent release of the contents to the exterior of the cell — **exo·cy·tot·ic** \-'tät-ik\ *adj*

ex·od·ic \'ek-,säd-ik, ek-'säd-ik, eg-'zäd-ik\ *adj* : EFFERENT

ex·odon·tia \,ek-sə-'dän-ch(ē-)ə\ *n* : a branch of dentistry that deals with the extraction of teeth — **ex·odon·tist** \-'dänt-əst\ *n*

exo·en·zyme \,ek-sō-'en-,zīm\ *n* : an extracellular enzyme — compare ENDOENZYME

exo·eryth·ro·cyt·ic \,ek-sō-i-,rith-rə-'sit-ik\ *adj* : occurring outside the red blood cells — used of stages of malaria parasites

ex·og·a·my \ek-'säg-ə-mē\ *n, pl* **-mies 1** : marriage outside of a specific group esp. as required by custom or law **2** : sexual reproduction between individuals (as of a particular species) that are not closely related — **ex·og·a·mous** \ek-'säg-ə-məs\ *or* **exo·gam·ic** \,ek-sə-'gam-ik\ *adj*

exo·gas·tru·la \,ek-sō-'gas-trə-lə\ *n, pl* **-las** *or* **-lae** \-,lē, -,lī\ : an abnormal gastrula that has the presumptive endoderm increased in quantity and incapable of invagination and is therefore unable to develop further — **exo·gas·tru·la·tion** \-,gas-trə-'lā-shən\ *n*

ex·og·e·nous \ek-'säj-ə-nəs\ *also* **exo·gen·ic** \,ek-sō-'jen-ik\ *adj* **1** : growing from or on the outside ⟨∼ spores⟩ **2** : caused by factors (as food or a traumatic factor) or an agent (as a disease-producing organism) from outside the organism or system ⟨∼ obesity⟩ ⟨∼ psychic depression⟩ **3** : introduced from or produced outside the organism or system; *specif* : not synthesized within the organism or system — compare ENDOGENOUS — **ex·og·e·nous·ly** *adv*

ex·om·pha·los \ek-'säm-fə-ləs\ *n, pl* **-li** \-,lī, -lē\ : UMBILICAL HERNIA; *also* : OMPHALOCELE

ex·on \'ek-,sän\ *n* : a polynucleotide sequence in a nucleic acid that codes information for protein synthesis and that is copied and spliced together with other such sequences to form messenger RNA — compare INTRON — **ex·on·ic** \ek-'sän-ik\ *adj*

exo·nu·cle·ase \,ek-sō-'n(y)ü-klē-,ās, -,āz\ *n* : an enzyme that breaks down a nucleic acid by removing nucleotides one by one from the end of a chain — compare ENDONUCLEASE

exo·nu·cleo·lyt·ic \,ek-sō-,n(y)ü-klē-ə-'lit-ik\ *adj* : cleaving a nucleotide chain at a point adjacent to one of its ends

exo·pep·ti·dase \-'pep-tə-,dās, -,dāz\ *n* : any of a group of enzymes that hydrolyze peptide bonds formed by the terminal amino acids of peptide chains : PEPTIDASE — compare ENDOPEPTIDASE

exo·phil·ic \,ek-sə-'fil-ik\ *adj* : ecologically independent of humans and their domestic environment ⟨an ∼ species of mosquito⟩ — compare ENDOPHILIC — **ex·oph·i·ly** \ek-'säf-ə-lē\ *n, pl* **-lies**

ex·o·pho·ria \,ek-sə-'fōr-ē-ə\ *n* : latent strabismus in which the visual axes tend outward toward the temple — compare HETEROPHORIA — **ex·o·phor·ic** \,ek-sə-'fòr-ik\ *adj*

ex·oph·thal·mia \,ek-,säf-'thal-mē-ə\ *n* : EXOPHTHALMOS

exophthalmic goiter *n* : GRAVES' DISEASE

ex·oph·thal·mos *also* **ex·oph·thal·mus** \,ek-säf-'thal-məs, -səf-\ *n* : abnormal protrusion of the eyeball — **ex·oph·thal·mic** \,ek-säf-'thal-mik\ *adj*

exo·phyt·ic \,ek-sō-'fit-ik\ *adj* : tending to grow outward beyond the surface epithelium from which it originates — used of tumors; compare ENDOPHYTIC

exo·skel·e·ton \,ek-sō-'skel-ət-ᵊn\ *n* **1** : an external supportive covering of an animal (as the system of sclerites covering the body of an insect) — compare ENDOSKELETON **2** : bony or horny parts (as nails, hooves, or scales) of a vertebrate produced from epidermal tissues — **exo·skel·e·tal** \-ət-ᵊl\ *adj*

ex·os·mo·sis \,ek-(,)säs-'mō-səs, -(,)säz-\ *n, pl* **-mo·ses** \-,sēz\ : passage of material through a membrane from a region of higher to a region of lower concentration — compare ENDOSMOSIS — **ex·os·mot·ic** \-'mät-ik\ *adj*

exo·spore \'ek-sə-,spō(ə)r, -,spò(ə)r\ *n* : one of the asexual spores separated from a parent cell (as in phycomycetous fungi) by formation of a septum

ex·os·tec·to·my \,ek-(,)säs-'tek-tə-mē\ *n, pl* **-mies** : excision of an exostosis

ex·os·to·sis \,ek-(,)säs-'tō-səs\ *n, pl* **-to·ses** \-,sēz\ : a spur or bony outgrowth from a bone or the root of a tooth — **ex·os·tot·ic** \-'tät-ik\ *adj*

exo·ther·mal \,ek-sō-'thər-məl\ *adj* : EXOTHERMIC — **exo·ther·mal·ly** \-ē\ *adv*

exo·ther·mic \-'thər-mik\ *adj* : characterized by or formed with evolution of heat — compare ENDOTHERMIC — **exo·ther·mi·cal·ly** \-mi-k(ə-)lē\ *adv* — **exo·ther·mic·i·ty** \-,thər-'mis-ət-ē\ *n, pl* **-ties**

exo·tox·in \,ek-sō-'täk-sən\ *n* : a soluble poisonous substance produced during growth of a microorganism and released into the surrounding medium ⟨tetanus ∼⟩ — compare ENDOTOXIN — **exo·tox·ic** \-'täk-sik\ *adj*

exo·tro·pia \,ek-sə-'trō-pē-ə\ *n* : WALLEYE 2a

exp *abbr* **1** experiment; experimental **2** expired

ex·pand·er \ik-'span-dər\ *n* : any of several colloidal substances (as dextran) of high molecular weight used as a blood or plasma substitute for increasing the blood volume — called also *extender*

ex·pan·sion \ik-'span-chən\ *n* **1** : the act or process of expanding **2** : the quality or state of being expanded

ex·pan·sive \ik-'span(t)-siv\ *adj* : marked by or indicative of exaggerated euphoria and delusions of self-importance ⟨a patient with ∼ trends⟩ — **ex·pan·sive·ness** \-nəs\ *n*

ex·pect \ik-'spekt\ *vi* : to be pregnant : await the birth of one's child — used in progressive tenses ⟨she's ∼*ing* next month⟩

ex·pec·tan·cy \-'spek-tən-sē\ *n, pl* **-cies** : the expected amount (as of the number of years of life) based on statistical probability — see LIFE EXPECTANCY

ex·pec·tant \-tənt\ *adj* : expecting the birth of a child ⟨∼ mothers⟩

¹**ex·pec·to·rant** \ik-'spek-t(ə-)rənt\ *adj* : having the activity of an expectorant

²**expectorant** *n* : an agent that promotes the discharge or expulsion of mucus from the respiratory tract; *broadly* : ANTITUSSIVE

ex·pec·to·rate \-tə-,rāt\ *vb* **-rat·ed; -rat·ing** *vt* **1** : to eject from the throat or lungs by coughing or hawking and spitting **2** : SPIT ∼ *vi* **1** : to discharge matter from the throat or lungs by coughing or hawking and spitting **2** : SPIT

ex·pec·to·ra·tion \ik-ˌspek-tə-ˈrā-shən\ *n* **1** : the act or an instance of expectorating **2** : expectorated matter

¹ex·per·i·ment \ik-ˈsper-ə-mənt *also* -ˈspir-\ *n* **1** : a procedure carried out under controlled conditions in order to discover an unknown effect or law, to test or establish a hypothesis, or to illustrate a known law **2** : the process of testing : EXPERIMENTATION

²ex·per·i·ment \-ˌment\ *vi* : to carry out experiments — **ex·per·i·men·ta·tion** \ik-ˌsper-ə-mən-ˈtā-shən, -ˌmen- *also* -ˌspir-\ *n* — **ex·per·i·ment·er** \-ˈsper-ə-ˌment-ər *also* -ˈspir-\ *n*

ex·per·i·men·tal \ik-ˌsper-ə-ˈment-ᵊl *also* -ˌspir-\ *adj* **1** : of, relating to, or based on experience or experiment **2** : founded on or derived from experiment ⟨the heart of the ∼ method is the direct control of the thing studied —B. F. Skinner⟩ **3** *of a disease* : intentionally produced esp. in laboratory animals for the purpose of study ⟨∼ diabetes⟩ — **ex·per·i·men·tal·ly** \-ᵊl-ē\ *adv*

experimental allergic encephalomyelitis *n* : an inflammatory autoimmune disease that has been induced in laboratory animals and esp. mice by injecting them with diseased tissue from affected animals or with myelin basic protein and that because of the similarity of its pathology to multiple sclerosis in humans is used as an animal model in studying this condition — abbr. *EAE;* called also *experimental autoimmune encephalomyelitis*

ex·per·i·men·tal·ist \-ᵊl-əst\ *n* : a person conducting scientific experiments

ex·pi·ra·tion \ˌek-spə-ˈrā-shən\ *n* **1 a** (1) : the act or process of releasing air from the lungs through the nose or mouth : EXHALATION (2) : the escape of carbon dioxide from the body protoplasm (as through the blood and lungs or by diffusion) **b** *archaic* : the last emission of breath : DEATH **2** : something produced by breathing out

ex·pi·ra·to·ry \ik-ˈspī-rə-ˌtōr-ē, ek-, -ˌtȯr-; ˈek-sp(ə-)rə-\ *adj* : of, relating to, or employed in the expiration of air from the lungs ⟨∼ muscles⟩ ⟨an ∼ cough⟩

expiratory reserve volume *n* : the additional amount of air that can be expired from the lungs by determined effort after normal expiration — compare INSPIRATORY RESERVE VOLUME

ex·pire \ik-ˈspī(ə)r, *usually for vi 2 and vt* ek-\ *vb* **ex·pired; ex·pir·ing** *vi* **1** : to breathe one's last breath : DIE **2** : to emit the breath ∼ *vt* : to breathe out from or as if from the lungs ⟨the basal metabolism test ... measures the amount of carbon dioxide *expired* by the lungs —J. D. Ratcliff⟩

ex·pi·ry \ik-ˈspī(ə)r-ē, ˈek-spə-rē\ *n, pl* **-ries** **1** : exhalation of breath **2** : DEATH

¹ex·plant \(ˈ)ek-ˈsplant\ *vt* : to remove (living tissue) esp. to a medium for tissue culture — **ex·plan·ta·tion** \ˌek-ˌsplan-ˈtā-shən\ *n*

²ex·plant \ˈek-ˌsplant\ *n* : living tissue removed from an organism and placed in a medium for tissue culture

ex·plode \ik-ˈsplōd\ *vb* **ex·plod·ed; ex·plod·ing** *vt* : to cause to explode or burst noisily ⟨∼ a bomb⟩ ∼ *vi* : to undergo a rapid chemical or nuclear reaction with the production of noise, heat, and violent expansion of gases

ex·plor·ato·ry \ik-ˈsplōr-ə-ˌtōr-ē, -ˈsplȯr-, -ˌtȯr-\ *adj* : of, relating to, or being exploration ⟨∼ surgery⟩

ex·plore \ik-ˈsplō(ə)r, -ˈsplȯ(ə)r\ *vt* **ex·plored; ex·plor·ing** : to examine (as by surgery) esp. for diagnostic purposes ⟨the abdomen may need to be *explored* surgically —Donald Caslow⟩ — **ex·plo·ra·tion** \ˌek-splə-ˈrā-shən\ *n*

ex·plor·er \ik-ˈsplōr-ər, -ˈsplȯr-\ *n* : an instrument for exploring cavities esp. in teeth : PROBE 1

ex·plo·sion \ik-ˈsplō-zhən\ *n* : the act or an instance of exploding

ex·po·nen·tial \ˌek-spə-ˈnen-chəl\ *adj* : expressible or approximately expressible by an exponential function ⟨an ∼ growth rate⟩ — **ex·po·nen·tial·ly** \-ˈnench-(ə-)lē\ *adv*

ex·pose \ik-ˈspōz\ *vt* **ex·posed; ex·pos·ing** **1** : to make liable to or accessible to something (as a disease or environmental conditions) that may have a detrimental effect ⟨children ex-

posed to diphtheria⟩ **2** : to lay open to view: as **a** : to conduct (oneself) as an exhibitionist **b** : to reveal (a bodily part) esp. by dissection

ex·po·sure \ik-ˈspō-zhər\ *n* **1** : the fact or condition of being exposed: as **a** : the condition of being unprotected esp. from severe weather ⟨the hiker died of ∼ after becoming lost in the snowstorm⟩ **b** : the condition of being subject to some detrimental effect or harmful condition ⟨repeated ∼ to bronchial irritants⟩ ⟨risk ∼ to the flu⟩ ⟨benign skin discolorations caused by sun ∼ —Katie Tyndall⟩ **2** : the act or an instance of exposing — see INDECENT EXPOSURE

exposure therapy *n* : psychotherapy that involves repeated real, visualized, or simulated exposure to or confrontation with a feared situation or object or a traumatic event or memory in order to achieve habituation and that is used esp. in the treatment of post-traumatic stress disorder, anxiety disorder, or phobias

ex·press \ik-ˈspres, ek-\ *vt* **1** : to make known or exhibit by an expression **2 a** : to force out by pressure ⟨∼ milk manually or by electric pump⟩ **b** : to subject to pressure so as to extract something ⟨some pumps ∼ one breast at a time —Paula Lynn Parks⟩ **3** : to cause (a gene) to manifest its effects in the phenotype ⟨a gene selectively ∼*ed* in lung tumors⟩; *also* : to manifest or produce (a character, molecule, or effect) by a genetic process ⟨individuals with the gene ∼ symptoms of the disease⟩ ⟨differentially ∼*ed* proteins⟩

ex·pressed almond oil \ik-ˈsprest-\ *n* : ALMOND OIL 1a

ex·pres·sion \ik-ˈspresh-ən\ *n* **1 a** : something that manifests, represents, reflects, embodies, or symbolizes something else ⟨the first clinical ∼ of a disease⟩ **b** (1) : the detectable effect of a gene ⟨gene ∼ can be controlled by regulatory proteins that bind to specific sites on DNA —Mark Ptashne⟩ (2) : EXPRESSIVITY **2** : facial aspect or vocal intonation as indicative of feeling **3** : an act or product of pressing out

ex·pres·siv·i·ty \ˌek-spres-ˈiv-ət-ē\ *n, pl* **-ties** : the relative capacity of a gene to affect the phenotype of the organism of which it is a part — compare PENETRANCE

expt *abbr* experiment

exptl *abbr* experimental

ex·pul·sive \ik-ˈspəl-siv\ *adj* **1** : serving to expel ⟨∼ efforts during labor⟩ **2** : characterized by concern with the elimination of feces ⟨there are two anal phases—the earlier ∼ and the later retentive —G. S. Blum⟩ — **ex·pul·sion** \-ˈspəl-shən\ *n*

ex·qui·site \ik-ˈskwiz-ət, ek-\ *adj* : ACUTE 2a, INTENSE ⟨∼ pain⟩ — **ex·qui·site·ly** \-lē\ *adv*

ex·san·gui·na·tion \(ˌ)ek(s)-ˌsaŋ-gwə-ˈnā-shən\ *n* : the action or process of draining or losing blood — **ex·san·gui·nate** \ek(s)-ˈsaŋ-gwə-ˌnāt\ *vt* **-nat·ed; -nat·ing**

ex·san·guine \ek(s)-ˈsaŋ-gwən\ *adj* : BLOODLESS, ANEMIC — **ex·san·guin·i·ty** \ˌek(s)-ˌsaŋ-ˈgwin-ət-ē, -ˌsan-\ *n, pl* **-ties**

ex·san·gui·no·trans·fu·sion \ek(s)-ˌsaŋ-gwin-ō-ˌtrans-ˈfyü-zhən\ *n* : EXCHANGE TRANSFUSION

ex·sect \ek-ˈsekt\ *vt* : to cut out : EXCISE ⟨an ∼*ed* uterus⟩ — **ex·sec·tion** \-ˈsek-shən\ *n*

ex·sic·cate \ˈek-si-ˌkāt\ *vt* **-cat·ed; -cat·ing** : to remove moisture from : DRY ⟨*exsiccated* magnesium sulfate⟩ — **ex·sic·ca·tion** \ˌek-si-ˈkā-shən\ *n*

ex·sic·co·sis \ˌek-si-ˈkō-səs\ *n, pl* **-co·ses** \-ˌsēz\ : insufficient intake of fluids; *also* : the resulting condition of bodily dehydration

ex·stro·phy \ˈek-strə-fē\ *n, pl* **-phies** : eversion of a part or organ; *specif* : a congenital malformation of the bladder in which the normally internal mucosa of the organ lies exposed on the abdominal wall because of failure of union between the halves of the pubic symphysis and between the adjacent halves of the abdominal wall

ext *abbr* **1** external **2** extract **3** extremity

E
F

ex·tend \ik-'stend\ *vt* **1** : to straighten out (as an arm or leg) **2** : to increase the quantity or bulk of (as by adding a cheaper substance or a modifier) ⟨*~ing* ground meat with cereal⟩; *also* : ADULTERATE

extended family *n* : a family that includes in one household near relatives in addition to a nuclear family

ex·tend·er \ik-'sten-dər\ *n* **1** : a substance added to a product esp. in the capacity of a diluent, adulterant, or modifier **2** : EXPANDER

ex·ten·si·bil·i·ty \ik-,sten(t)-sə-'bil-ət-ē\ *n, pl* **-ties** : the capability of being stretched ⟨*~* of muscle⟩ — **ex·ten·si·ble** \ik-'sten(t)-sə-bəl\ *adj*

ex·ten·sion \ik-'sten-chən\ *n* **1** : the stretching of a fractured or dislocated limb so as to restore it to its natural position **2** : an unbending movement around a joint in a limb (as the knee or elbow) that increases the angle between the bones of the limb at the joint — compare FLEXION 1

ex·ten·som·e·ter \,ek-,sten-'säm-ət-ər\ *n* : an instrument for measuring minute deformations (as of a test specimen) caused by tension, compression, bending, or twisting — called also *strain gauge*

ex·ten·sor \ik-'sten(t)-sər, -,sȯ(ə)r\ *n* : a muscle serving to extend a bodily part (as a limb) — called also *extensor muscle;* compare FLEXOR

extensor car·pi ra·di·al·is brev·is \-'kär-,pī-,rā-dē-'ā-ləs-'brev-əs, -'kär-,pē-\ *n* : a short muscle on the radial side of the back of the forearm that extends and may abduct the hand

extensor carpi radialis lon·gus \-'lȯŋ-gəs\ *n* : a long muscle on the radial side of the back of the forearm that extends and abducts the hand

extensor carpi ul·nar·is \-,əl-'nar-əs\ *n* : a muscle on the ulnar side of the back of the forearm that extends and adducts the hand

extensor dig·i·ti min·i·mi \-'dij-ə-,tī-'min-ə-,mī, -'dij-ə-,tē-'min-ə-,mē\ *n* : a slender muscle on the medial side of the extensor digitorum communis that extends the little finger

extensor digiti quin·ti pro·pri·us \-'kwin-,tī-'prō-prē-əs, -'kwin-,tē-\ *n* : EXTENSOR DIGITI MINIMI

extensor dig·i·to·rum brev·is \-,dij-ə-'tōr-əm-'brev-əs\ *n* : a muscle on the dorsum of the foot that extends the toes

extensor digitorum com·mu·nis \-kə-'myün-əs, -'käm-yə-nəs\ *n* : a muscle on the back of the forearm that extends the fingers and wrist

extensor digitorum lon·gus \-'lȯŋ-gəs\ *n* : a pennate muscle on the lateral part of the front of the leg that extends the four small toes and dorsally flexes and pronates the foot

extensor hal·lu·cis brev·is \-'hal-(y)ü-səs-'brev-əs, -'hal-ə-kəs-\ *n* : the part of the extensor digitorum brevis that extends the big toe

extensor hallucis lon·gus \-'lȯŋ-gəs\ *n* : a long thin muscle situated on the shin that extends the big toe and dorsiflexes and supinates the foot

extensor in·di·cis \-'in-də-səs, -də-kəs\ *n* : a thin muscle that arises from the ulna in the more distal part of the forearm and extends the index finger

extensor indicis pro·pri·us \-'prō-prē-əs\ *n* : EXTENSOR INDICIS

extensor pol·li·cis brev·is \-'päl-ə-səs-'brev-əs, -'päl-ə-kəs-\ *n* : a muscle that arises from the dorsal surface of the radius, extends the first phalanx of the thumb, and adducts the hand

extensor pollicis lon·gus \-'lȯŋ-gəs\ *n* : a muscle that arises dorsolaterally from the middle part of the ulna, extends the second phalanx of the thumb, and abducts the hand

extensor ret·i·nac·u·lum \-,ret-ᵊn-'a-kyə-ləm\ *n* **1** : either of two fibrous bands of fascia crossing the front of the ankle: **a** : a lower band that is attached laterally to the superior aspect of the calcaneus and passes medially to divide in the shape of a Y and that passes over or both over and under the tendons of the extensor muscles at the ankle — called also *inferior extensor retinaculum* **b** : an upper band passing over and binding down the tendons of the tibialis anterior, extensor hallucis longus, extensor digitorum longus, and peroneus tertius just above the ankle joint — called also *superior ex-*

tensor retinaculum, transverse crural ligament **2** : a fibrous band of fascia crossing the back of the wrist and binding down the tendons of the extensor muscles

ex·te·ri·or \ek-'stir-ē-ər\ *adj* : being on an outside surface : situated on the outside — **ex·te·ri·or·ly** *adv*

ex·te·ri·or·ize *or Brit* **ex·te·ri·or·ise** \ek-'stir-ē-ə-,rīz\ *vt* **-ized** *or Brit* **-ised; -iz·ing** *or Brit* **-is·ing** **1** : EXTERNALIZE **2** : to bring out of the body (as for surgery) ⟨the section of perforated colon was *exteriorized*⟩ — **ex·te·ri·or·iza·tion** *or Brit* **ex·te·ri·or·isa·tion** \-,stir-ē-ə-rə-'zā-shən\ *n*

ex·tern *also* **ex·terne** \'ek-,stərn\ *n* : a nonresident doctor or medical student at a hospital — **ex·tern·ship** \-,ship\ *n*

externa — see MUSCULARIS EXTERNA, OTITIS EXTERNA, THECA EXTERNA, TUNICA EXTERNA

ex·ter·nal \ek-'stərn-ᵊl\ *adj* **1** : capable of being perceived outwardly : BODILY ⟨*~* signs of a disease⟩ **2 a** : situated at, on, or near the outside ⟨an *~* protective covering⟩ ⟨an *~* muscle⟩ **b** : directed toward the outside : having an outside object ⟨*~* perception⟩ ⟨eyesight and the other *~* senses⟩ **c** : used by applying to the outside ⟨an *~* lotion⟩ **3 a** (1) : situated near or toward the surface of the body; *also* : situated away from the mesial plane ⟨the *~* condyle of the humerus⟩ (2) : arising or acting from outside : having an outside origin ⟨*~* causes⟩ ⟨*~* stimuli⟩ **b** : of, relating to, or consisting of something outside the mind : having existence independent of the mind ⟨sensations aroused by *~* phenomena⟩ ⟨*~* reality⟩ — **ex·ter·nal·ly** \-ᵊl-ē\ *adv*

external anal sphincter *n* : ANAL SPHINCTER a

external auditory canal *n* : the auditory canal leading from the opening of the external ear to the eardrum — called also *external acoustic meatus, external auditory meatus*

external capsule *n* : CAPSULE 1b(2)

external carotid artery *n* : the outer branch of the carotid artery that supplies the face, tongue, and external parts of the head — called also *external carotid*

external ear *n* : the parts of the ear that are external to the eardrum; *also* : PINNA

external iliac artery *n* : ILIAC ARTERY 2

external iliac node *n* : any of the lymph nodes grouped around the external iliac artery and the external iliac vein — compare INTERNAL ILIAC NODE

external iliac vein *n* : ILIAC VEIN b

external inguinal ring *n* : SUPERFICIAL INGUINAL RING

external intercostal muscle *n* : INTERCOSTAL MUSCLE a — called also *external intercostal*

ex·ter·nal·ize *or Brit* **ex·ter·nal·ise** \ek-'stərn-ᵊl-,īz\ *vt* **-ized** *or Brit* **-ised; -iz·ing** *or Brit* **-is·ing** **1 a** : to transform from a mental image into an apparently real object (as in hallucinations) : attribute (a mental image) to external causation ⟨*externalizing* an obsession⟩ **b** : to invent an explanation for (an inner problem whose actual basis is known only subconsciously) by attributing to causes outside the self : RATIONALIZE, PROJECT ⟨*externalized* his failure⟩ **2** : to direct outward socially ⟨*externalized* her anger⟩ — **ex·ter·nal·iza·tion** *or Brit* **ex·ter·nal·isa·tion** \-,stərn-ᵊl-ə-'zā-shən\ *n*

external jugular vein *n* : JUGULAR VEIN b — called also *external jugular*

external malleolus *n* : MALLEOLUS a

external maxillary artery *n* : FACIAL ARTERY

external oblique *n* : OBLIQUE a(1)

external occipital crest *n* : OCCIPITAL CREST a

external occipital protuberance *n* : OCCIPITAL PROTUBERANCE a

external phase *n* : DISPERSION MEDIUM

external pterygoid muscle *n* : PTERYGOID MUSCLE a

external pudendal artery *n* : either of two branches of the femoral artery: **a** : one that is distributed to the skin of the lower abdomen, to the penis and scrotum in the male, and to one of the labia majora in the female, and that anastomoses with the internal pudendal artery — called also *superficial external pudendal artery* **b** : one that follows a deeper course, that is distributed to the medial aspect of the thigh, to the skin of the scrotum and perineum in the male, and to one of the labia majora in the female, and that anastomoses with branches of the perineal artery — called also *deep external pudendal artery*

external respiration *n* : exchange of gases between the external environment and a distributing system of the animal body (as the lungs of higher vertebrates or the tracheal tubes of insects) or between the alveoli of the lungs and the blood — compare INTERNAL RESPIRATION

external semilunar fibrocartilage *n* : MENISCUS 2a(1)

externe *var of* EXTERN

externus — see OBLIQUUS EXTERNUS, OBLIQUUS EXTERNUS ABDOMINIS, OBTURATOR EXTERNUS, SPHINCTER ANI EXTERNUS, VASTUS EXTERNUS

ex·tero·cep·tive \ˌek-stə-rō-ˈsep-tiv\ *adj* : activated by, relating to, or being stimuli received by an organism from outside ⟨∼ feedback⟩

ex·tero·cep·tor \-ˈsep-tər\ *n* : a sense receptor (as of touch, temperature, smell, vision, or hearing) excited by exteroceptive stimuli — compare INTEROCEPTOR

ex·tero·fec·tive \-ˈfek-tiv\ *adj* : of, relating to, dependent on, or constituting the part of the nervous system comprising the brain, the cranial and spinal nerves, and the spinal cord — compare INTEROFECTIVE

ex·tinct \ik-ˈstiŋ(k)t, ˈek-ˌ\ *adj* : no longer existing : lacking living representatives ⟨∼ prehistoric animals⟩

ex·tinc·tion \ik-ˈstiŋ(k)-shən\ *n* **1** : the process of becoming extinct ⟨the ∼ of a species⟩; *also* : the condition or fact of being extinct **2** : the process of eliminating or reducing a conditioned response by not reinforcing it

ex·tin·guish \ik-ˈstiŋ-(g)wish\ *vt* : to cause extinction of (a conditioned response) ⟨∼ an avoidance response⟩

ex·tir·pa·tion \ˌek-stər-ˈpā-shən\ *n* : complete excision or surgical destruction of a body part — **ex·tir·pate** \ˈek-stərˌpāt\ *vt* **-pat·ed; -pat·ing**

ex·tor·sion \ek-ˈstȯr-shən, ˈek-ˌ\ *n* : outward rotation (as of a body part) about an axis or fixed point — compare INTORSION

ex·tra·bul·bar \ˌek-strə-ˈbəl-bər\ *adj* : situated or originating outside the medulla oblongata

ex·tra·cap·su·lar \-ˈkap-sə-lər, *esp Brit* -ˈkap-syu̇-lər\ *adj* **1** : situated outside a capsule **2** *of a cataract operation* : involving removal of the front part of the capsule and the central part of the lens — compare INTRACAPSULAR 2

ex·tra·cel·lu·lar \ˌek-strə-ˈsel-yə-lər\ *adj* : situated or occurring outside a cell or the cells of the body ⟨∼ digestion⟩ ⟨∼ enzymes⟩ — **ex·tra·cel·lu·lar·ly** *adv*

ex·tra·chro·mo·som·al \-ˌkrō-mə-ˈsō-məl, -ˈzō-\ *adj* : situated or controlled by factors outside the chromosome ⟨∼ inheritance⟩ ⟨∼ DNA⟩

ex·tra·cor·po·re·al \-kȯr-ˈpōr-ē-əl, -ˈpȯr-\ *adj* : occurring or based outside the living body ⟨heart surgery employing ∼ circulation⟩ — **ex·tra·cor·po·re·al·ly** \-ē-ə-lē\ *adv*

ex·tra·cor·pus·cu·lar \-kȯr-ˈpəs-kyə-lər\ *adj* : situated outside the blood corpuscles

ex·tra·cra·ni·al \-ˈkrā-nē-əl\ *adj* : situated or occurring outside the cranium ⟨∼ arterial occlusion⟩

¹ex·tract \ik-ˈstrakt\ *vt* **1** : to pull or take out forcibly ⟨∼ed a wisdom tooth⟩ **2** : to withdraw (as the medicinally active components of a plant or animal tissue) by physical or chemical process; *also* : to treat with a solvent so as to remove a soluble substance — **ex·tract·abil·i·ty** \ik-ˌstrak-tə-ˈbil-ət-ē, (ˌ)ek-\ *n, pl* **-ties** — **ex·tract·able** *also* **ex·tract·ible** \ikˈstrak-tə-bəl, ˈek-ˌ\ *adj*

²ex·tract \ˈek-ˌstrakt\ *n* : something prepared by extracting; *esp* : a medicinally active pharmaceutical solution

ex·tract·ant \ik-ˈstrak-tənt\ *n* : a solvent (as alcohol) used in extracting

ex·trac·tion \ik-ˈstrak-shən\ *n* : the act or process of extracting something ⟨∼ of a tooth⟩

¹ex·trac·tive \ik-ˈstrak-tiv, ˈek-ˌ\ *adj* : of, relating to, or involving extraction ⟨∼ processes⟩

²extractive *n* : something extracted or extractable : EXTRACT

ex·trac·tor \ik-ˈstrak-tər, ˈek-ˌstrak-\ *n* **1** : an instrument

used in extraction (as of a tooth) **2** : an apparatus for extracting substances by means of solvents

ex·tra·cys·tic \ˌek-strə-ˈsis-tik\ *adj* : situated or originating outside a cyst or bladder

ex·tra·du·ral \-ˈd(y)u̇r-əl\ *adj* : situated or occurring outside the dura mater but within the skull ⟨an ∼ hemorrhage⟩

ex·tra·em·bry·on·ic \-ˌem-brē-ˈän-ik\ *adj* : situated outside the embryo proper; *esp* : developed from the zygote but not part of the embryo ⟨∼ membranes⟩

extraembryonic coelom *n* : the space between the chorion and amnion which in early stages is continuous with the coelom of the embryo proper

ex·tra·en·ter·ic \-en-ˈter-ik, -in-\ *adj* : situated or occurring outside the enteron ⟨∼ amebiasis⟩

ex·tra·eryth·ro·cyt·ic \ˌek-strə-iˌrith-rō-ˈsit-ik\ *adj* : EXO-ERYTHROCYTIC

ex·tra·fu·sal \-ˈfyü-zəl\ *adj* : situated outside a striated muscle spindle ⟨∼ muscle fibers⟩ — compare INTRAFUSAL

ex·tra·gen·i·tal \-ˈjen-ə-tᵊl\ *adj* : situated or originating outside the genital region or organs ⟨∼ sexual responses⟩

ex·tra·he·pat·ic \-hi-ˈpat-ik\ *adj* : situated or originating outside the liver ⟨∼ jaundice⟩ ⟨∼ tumors⟩

ex·tra·in·tes·ti·nal \-in-ˈtes-tə-nəl\ *adj* : situated or occurring outside the intestines ⟨∼ infections⟩

ex·tra·mac·u·lar \ˌek-strə-ˈmak-yə-lər\ *adj* : relating to or being the part of the retina other than the macula lutea

ex·tra·mas·toid \-ˈmas-tȯid\ *adj* : situated on or affecting the outer surface of the mastoid bone ⟨∼ infection⟩

ex·tra·med·ul·lary \-ˈmed-ᵊl-ˌer-ē, -ˈmej-ə-ˌler-ē, -mə-ˈdəl-ə-rē\ *adj* **1** : situated or occurring outside the spinal cord or the medulla oblongata **2** : located or taking place outside the bone marrow ⟨∼ hematopoiesis⟩

ex·tra·mi·to·chon·dri·al \-ˌmīt-ə-ˈkän-drē-əl\ *adj* : situated or occurring in the cell outside the mitochondria ⟨∼ synthesis of fatty acids⟩

ex·tra·mu·ral \-ˈmyu̇r-əl\ *adj* : existing or functioning outside or beyond the walls, boundaries, or precincts of an organized unit ⟨∼ medical care provided by hospital personnel⟩ — **ex·tra·mu·ral·ly** \-ə-lē\ *adv*

ex·tra·nu·cle·ar \ˌek-strə-ˈn(y)ü-klē-ər\ *adj* : situated in or affecting the parts of a cell external to the nucleus : CYTO-PLASMIC

ex·tra·oc·u·lar muscle \-ˈäk-yə-lər-\ *n* : any of six small voluntary muscles that pass between the eyeball and the orbit and control the movement of the eyeball in relation to the orbit

ex·tra·oral \-ˈȯr-əl, -ˈōr-əl, -ˈär-əl\ *adj* : situated or occurring outside the mouth ⟨an ∼ abscess⟩ ⟨an ∼ dental appliance⟩

ex·tra·peri·to·ne·al \-ˌper-ət-ᵊn-ē-əl\ *adj* : located or taking place outside the peritoneal cavity ⟨∼ surgical drainage⟩

ex·tra·pi·tu·i·tary \-pə-ˈt(y)ü-ə-ˌter-ē\ *adj* : situated or arising outside the pituitary gland

ex·tra·pla·cen·tal \-plə-ˈsent-ᵊl\ *adj* : being outside of or independent of the placenta

ex·tra·pleu·ral pneumonolysis \-ˈplu̇r-əl-\ *n* : PNEUMO-NOLYSIS a

ex·tra·pul·mo·nary \-ˈpu̇l-mə-ˌner-ē, -ˈpəl-\ *adj* : situated or occurring outside the lungs ⟨∼ tuberculosis⟩

ex·tra·pu·ni·tive \ˌek-strə-ˈpyü-nət-iv\ *adj* : tending to direct blame or punishment toward persons other than the self — compare INTROPUNITIVE

ex·tra·py·ra·mi·dal \-pə-ˈram-əd-ᵊl, -ˌpir-ə-ˈmid-ᵊl\ *adj* : situated outside of and esp. involving descending nerve tracts other than the pyramidal tracts ⟨∼ brain lesions⟩

ex·tra·re·nal \-ˈrēn-ᵊl\ *adj* : situated or occurring outside the kidneys ⟨∼ action of diuretics⟩

ex·tra·ret·i·nal \-ˈret-ᵊn-əl, -ˈret-nəl\ *adj* : situated or occurring outside the retina ⟨∼ photoreception⟩

\ə\ abut \ᵊ\ kitten \ər\ further \a\ ash \ā\ ace \ä\ cot, cart \au̇\ out \ch\ chin \e\ bet \ē\ easy \g\ go \i\ hit \ī\ ice \j\ job \ŋ\ sing \ō\ go \ȯ\ law \ȯi\ boy \th\ thin \t̲h̲\ the \ü\ loot \u̇\ foot \y\ yet \zh\ vision   *See also* Pronunciation Symbols page

E
F

ex·tra·sen·so·ry \,ek-strə-'sen)s-(ə-)rē\ *adj* : residing beyond or outside the ordinary senses

extrasensory perception *n* : perception (as in telepathy, clairvoyance, and precognition) that involves awareness of information about events external to the self not gained through the senses and not deducible from previous experience — called also *ESP*

ex·tra·so·mat·ic \,ek-strə-sō-'mat-ik\ *adj* : of, relating to, or being something that exists external to and distinct from the individual human being or the human body

ex·tra·sys·to·le \-'sis-tə-(,)lē\ *n* : a prematurely occurring beat of one of the chambers of the heart that leads to momentary arrhythmia but leaves the fundamental rhythm unchanged — called also *premature beat* — **ex·tra·sys·tol·ic** \-sis-'tāl-ik\ *adj*

ex·tra·tub·al \-'t(y)ü-bəl\ *adj* : situated outside a body duct or esp. outside the fallopian tube ⟨~ pregnancy⟩

ex·tra·uter·ine \,ek-strə-'yüt-ə-rən, -,rīn\ *adj* : situated or occurring outside the uterus

extrauterine gestation *n* : ECTOPIC PREGNANCY

extrauterine pregnancy *n* : ECTOPIC PREGNANCY

ex·tra·vag·i·nal \,ek-strə-'vaj-ən-ᵊl\ *adj* : outside an enclosing sheath (as the vagina)

¹**ex·trav·a·sate** \ik-'strav-ə-,sāt, -,zāt\ *vb* **-sat·ed; -sat·ing** *vt* : to force out or cause to escape from a proper vessel or channel ⟨*extravasated* blood⟩ ~ *vi* : to pass by infiltration or effusion from a proper vessel or channel (as a blood vessel) into surrounding tissue

²**extravasate** *n* : EXTRAVASATION 2a

ex·trav·a·sa·tion \ik-,strav-ə-'zā-shən, -'sā-\ *n* **1** : the action of extravasating **2 a** : an extravasated fluid (as blood) ⟨~s from the nose⟩ **b** : a deposit formed by extravasation

ex·tra·vas·cu·lar \,ek-strə-'vas-kyə-lər\ *adj* : not occurring or contained in body vessels ⟨~ tissue fluids⟩ ⟨~ hemolysis⟩ — **ex·tra·vas·cu·lar·ly** *adv*

ex·tra·ven·tric·u·lar \-ven-'trik-yə-lər, -vən-\ *adj* : located or taking place outside a ventricle ⟨~ lesions⟩

extraversion, extraversive, extravert, extraverted *var of* EXTROVERSION, EXTROVERSIVE, EXTROVERT, EXTROVERTED

ex·tra·vi·su·al \,ek-strə-'vizh-(ə-)wəl, -'vizh-əl\ *adj* : being beyond the limits of vision

extremis — see IN EXTREMIS

ex·trem·i·ty \ik-'strem-ət-ē\ *n, pl* **-ties 1** : the farthest or most remote part, section, or point **2** : a limb of the body; *esp* : a human hand or foot

ex·trin·sic \ek-'strin-zik, -'strin(t)-sik\ *adj* **1** : originating or due to causes or factors from or on the outside of a body, organ, or part ⟨renal tumors or cysts . . . causing ~ compression of the renal vasculature —*Scientific Amer. Medicine*⟩ **2** : originating outside a part and acting on the part as a whole — used esp. of certain muscles ⟨the ~ muscles of the tongue⟩; compare INTRINSIC 2 — **ex·trin·si·cal·ly** \-zi-k(ə-)lē, -si-\ *adv*

extrinsic factor *n* : VITAMIN B₁₂

ex·tro·ver·sion *or* **ex·tra·ver·sion** \,ek-strə-'vər-zhən, -shən\ *n* : the act, state, or habit of being predominantly concerned with and obtaining gratification from what is outside the self — compare INTROVERSION — **ex·tro·ver·sive** *or* **ex·tra·ver·sive** \-siv, -ziv\ *adj*

¹**ex·tro·vert** *also* **ex·tra·vert** \'ek-strə-,vərt\ *adj* : EXTROVERTED

²**extrovert** *also* **extravert** *n* : one whose personality is characterized by extroversion; *broadly* : a gregarious and unreserved person — compare INTROVERT

ex·tro·vert·ed *also* **ex·tra·vert·ed** \-,vərt-əd\ *adj* : marked by or suggesting extroversion; *broadly* : being a gregarious and unreserved person — compare INTROVERTED

ex·trude \ik-'strüd\ *vb* **ex·trud·ed; ex·trud·ing** *vt* : to force, press, or push out ~ *vi* : to become extruded

ex·tru·sion \ik-'strü-zhən\ *n* : the act or process of extruding ⟨~ of proteins from cells⟩

ex·tu·ba·tion \,ek-,st(y)ü-'bā-shən\ *n* : the removal of a tube esp. from the larynx after intubation — called also *detubation* — **ex·tu·bate** \ek-'st(y)ü-,bāt, 'ek-,st(y)ü-\ *vt* **-bat·ed; -bat·ing**

ex·u·ber·ant \ig-'zü-b(ə-)rənt\ *adj* : characterized by extreme proliferation ⟨~ granulation tissue⟩ ⟨remarkably ~ metastatic calcification —Sandy Muspratt⟩

ex·u·date \'ek-s(y)ù-,dāt, -shù-\ *n* : exuded matter; *esp* : the material composed of serum, fibrin, and white blood cells that escapes from blood vessels into a superficial lesion or area of inflammation

ex·u·da·tion \,ek-s(y)ù-'dā-shən, -shù-\ *n* **1** : the process of exuding **2** : EXUDATE — **ex·u·da·tive** \ig-'züd-ət-iv; 'ek-s(y)ù-,dāt-iv, -shù-\ *adj*

ex·ude \ig-'züd\ *vb* **ex·ud·ed; ex·ud·ing** *vi* **1** : to ooze out **2** : to undergo diffusion ~ *vt* : to cause to ooze or spread out in all directions

ex·u·vi·ae \ig-'zü-vē-,ē, -vē-,ī\ *n pl* : sloughed-off natural coverings of animals (as the skins of snakes)

ex·u·vi·a·tion \-,zü-vē-'ā-shən\ *n* : the process of producing exuviae

eye \'ī\ *n* **1** : an organ of sight; *esp* : a nearly spherical hollow organ that is lined with a sensitive retina, is lodged in a bony orbit in the skull, is the vertebrate organ of sight, and is normally paired **2** : all the visible structures within and surrounding the orbit and including eyelids, eyelashes, and eyebrows **3** : the faculty of seeing with eyes — **eye·less** \'ī-ləs\ *adj* — **eye·like** \-,līk\ *adj*

eye·ball \'ī-,bòl\ *n* : the more or less globular capsule of the vertebrate eye formed by the sclera and cornea together with their contained structures

eye bank *n* : a storage place for human corneas from the newly dead for transplanting to the eyes of those blind through corneal defects

eye·brow \'ī-,braù\ *n* : the ridge over the eye or hair growing on it — called also *brow*

eye chart *n* : a chart that is read at a fixed distance for purposes of testing sight; *esp* : one with rows of letters or objects of decreasing size

eye contact *n* : visual contact with another person's eyes

eye·cup \'ī-,kəp\ *n* **1** : a small oval cup with a rim curved to fit the orbit of the eye used for applying liquid remedies to the eyes **2** : OPTIC CUP

eyed \'īd\ *adj* : having an eye or eyes esp. of a specified kind or number — often used in combination ⟨a blue-*eyed* patient⟩

eyed·ness \'īd-nəs\ *n* : preference for the use of one eye instead of the other (as in using a monocular microscope)

eye doctor *n* : a specialist (as an optometrist or ophthalmologist) in the examination, treatment, or care of the eyes

eye·drop·per \'ī-,dräp-ər\ *n* : DROPPER — **eye·drop·per·ful** \-,fùl\ *n*

eye·drops \'ī-,dräps\ *n pl* : a medicated solution for the eyes that is applied in drops — **eye·drop** \-,dräp\ *adj*

eye–ear plane *n* : FRANKFORT HORIZONTAL PLANE

eye·glass \'ī-,glas\ *n* **1 a** : EYEPIECE **b** : a lens worn to aid vision; *specif* : MONOCLE **c eye·glass·es** *pl* : GLASSES, SPECTACLES **2** : EYECUP 1

eye gnat *n* : any of several small dipteran flies of the genus *Hippelates* (esp. *H. pusio*) including some that are held to be vectors of pinkeye and yaws — called also *eye fly;* compare CHLOROPIDAE, SIPHUNCULINA

eye·ground \'ī-,graùnd\ *n* : the fundus of the eye; *esp* : the retina as viewed through an ophthalmoscope

eye·hole \'ī-,hōl\ *n* : ORBIT

eye·lash \'ī-,lash\ *n* **1** : the fringe of hair edging the eyelid — usu. used in pl. **2** : a single hair of the eyelashes

eye·lid \'ī-,lid\ *n* : either of the movable lids of skin and muscle that can be closed over the eyeball — called also *palpebra*

eye·piece \'ī-,pēs\ *n* : the lens or combination of lenses at the eye end of an optical instrument — called also *ocular*

eyepiece micrometer *n* : a scale in the visual field of an eyepiece used as a measuring device — called also *ocular micrometer*

eye·sight \'ī-,sīt\ *n* : SIGHT 2

eye socket *n* : ORBIT

eye·spot \ˈī-ˌspät\ *n* **1** : a simple visual organ of pigment or pigmented cells covering a sensory termination : OCELLUS **2** : a small pigmented body of various unicellular algae

eye·strain \ˈī-ˌstrān\ *n* : weariness or a strained state of the eye

eye·tooth \ˈī-ˈtüth\ *n, pl* **eye·teeth** \-ˈtēth\ : a canine tooth of the upper jaw

eye·wash \ˈī-ˌwȯsh, -ˌwäsh\ *n* : an eye lotion

eye·wear \ˈī-ˌwa(ə)r, -ˌwe(ə)r\ *n* : corrective or protective devices (as glasses or contact lenses) for the eyes

eye·wink \ˈī-ˌwiŋk\ *n* : a wink of the eye

eye worm *n* : a parasitic worm found in the eye: as **a** : either of two slender nematode worms of the genus *Oxyspirura* (*O. mansoni* and *O. petrowi*) living beneath the nictitating membrane of the eyes of birds and esp. chickens **b** : any member of the nematode genus *Thelazia* living in the tear duct and beneath the eyelid of dogs, cats, sheep, humans, and other mammals and sometimes causing blindness **c** : an African filarial worm of the genus *Loa* (*L. loa*) that migrates through the eyeball and subcutaneous tissues of humans — compare CALABAR SWELLING

ezet·i·mibe \e-ˈzet-ə-ˌmib\ *n* : a drug $C_{24}H_{21}F_2NO_3$ that lowers the amount of cholesterol in the blood by selectively inhibiting its absorption in the intestine — see VYTORIN, ZETIA

F

f *abbr* **1** farad **2** father **3** female **4** foot **5** formula

f *symbol* **1** faraday **2** focal length **3** function

F *abbr* **1** Fahrenheit **2** French

F *symbol* fluorine

FA *abbr* fatty acid

Fab \ˈfab\ *n* : a fragment of an immunoglobulin molecule formed when the molecule is digested by papain and containing one antigen-binding site, one complete light chain, and part of one heavy chain — called also *Fab fragment*

fa·bel·la \fə-ˈbel-ə\ *n, pl* **fa·bel·lae** \-ˈbel-ˌē\ : a small fibrocartilage ossified in many animals and sometimes in humans in the tendon of the gastrocnemius muscle, behind one or both of the femoral condyles

Fab fragment *n* : FAB

Fa·bi·ana \ˌfä-bē-ˈan-ə, -ˈän-\ *n* : a genus of heathlike evergreen shrubs of the family Solanaceae of Central and So. America that include one (*F. imbricata*) whose dried leaves and twigs have been used to treat some kidney ailments

　Fa·bi·án y Fue·ro \fä-bē-ˈän-ē-ˈfwer-ō\, **Francisco (1719–1801)**, Spanish archbishop. Fabián was archbishop of Valencia, Spain. The genus *Fabiana* was named in his honor in 1794 by H. Ruiz Lopez and J. Pavon.

fab·ri·ca·tion \ˌfab-ri-ˈkā-shən\ *n* : CONFABULATION

Fa·bry's disease \ˈfäb-rēz-\ *n* : a disorder of lipid metabolism that is inherited as an X-linked recessive trait and is characterized by skin lesions esp. on the lower trunk, severe pain in the extremities, corneal opacities, and vascular disease affecting the kidneys, heart, or brain

　Fabry, Johannes (1860–1930), German dermatologist. Fabry gave the first description of the disease which bears his name in 1898.

fab·u·la·tion \ˌfab-yə-ˈlā-shən\ *n* : the act of inventing or relating false or fantastic tales

FACC *abbr* Fellow of the American College of Cardiology

FACD *abbr* Fellow of the American College of Dentists

face \ˈfās\ *n, often attrib* **1 a** : the front part of the human head including the chin, mouth, nose, cheeks, eyes, and usu. the forehead **b** : the corresponding part of the head of a lower animal **2** : SURFACE; *esp* : a front, upper, or outer surface

face bone *n* : CHEEKBONE

face·bow \ˈfās-ˌbō\ *n* : a device used in dentistry to determine the positional relationships of the maxillae to the temporomandibular joints of a patient esp. for the purpose of properly positioning dental casts on an articulator

face fly *n* : a European fly of the genus *Musca* (*M. autumnalis*) that is similar to the housefly, is widely established in No. America, and causes distress in livestock by clustering about the face

face–lift \ˈfās-ˌslift\ *n* : a plastic surgical operation for removal of facial defects (as wrinkles) typical of aging — called also *rhytidectomy* — **face–lift** *vt*

face–lifting \ˈfā-ˌslif-tiŋ\ *n* : FACE-LIFT

fac·et \ˈfas-ət\ *n* : a smooth flat or nearly flat circumscribed anatomical surface ⟨the articular ∼ of a bone⟩ — **fac·et·ed** *or* **fac·et·ted** \ˈfas-ət-əd\ *adj*

fac·et·ec·to·my \ˌfas-ət-ˈek-tə-mē\ *n, pl* **-mies** : excision of a facet esp. of a vertebra

¹fa·cial \ˈfā-shəl\ *adj* **1** : of, relating to, or affecting the face ⟨∼ neuralgia⟩ **2** : concerned with or used in improving the appearance of the face **3** : relating to or being the buccal and labial surface of a tooth — **fa·cial·ly** \-shə-lē\ *adv*

²facial *n* **1** : a treatment to improve the appearance of the face **2** : a facial part (as a nerve or artery)

facial angle *n* : the angle that is determined by the intersection of a line connecting the nasion and prosthion with the Frankfort horizontal plane and is used as a measure of prognathism

facial artery *n* : an artery that arises from the external carotid artery just superior to the lingual artery and gives off a number of branches supplying the neck and face — called also *external maxillary artery;* compare MAXILLARY ARTERY

facial bone *n* : any of the bones of the facial region of the skull that do not take part in forming the braincase and that in humans include 14 bones: two nasal bones, two maxillae of the upper jaw, two lacrimal bones, two zygomatic bones, two palatine bones, two nasal conchae, one vomer, and the mandible of the lower jaw

facial canal *n* : a passage in the petrous part of the temporal bone that extends from the internal auditory canal to the stylomastoid foramen and transmits various branches of the facial nerve — called also *aqueduct of Fallopius, fallopian aqueduct, fallopian canal*

facial colliculus *n* : a medial eminence on the floor of the fourth ventricle of the brain produced by the nucleus of the abducens nerve and the flexure of the facial nerve around it

facial index *n* : the ratio multiplied by 100 of the breadth of the face to its length

facial nerve *n* : either of the seventh pair of cranial nerves that supply motor fibers esp. to the muscles of the face and jaw and sensory and parasympathetic fibers to the tongue, palate, and fauces — called also *seventh cranial nerve, seventh nerve*

facial vein *n* : a vein that arises as the angular vein, drains the superficial structures of the face, and empties into the internal jugular vein — called also *anterior facial vein;* see DEEP FACIAL VEIN, POSTERIOR FACIAL VEIN

facial vision *n* : an awareness of obstacles independent of vision that is often considerably developed in blind persons and prob. dependent on tactile perception of reflected sound waves

\ə\ **abut** \ˈə\ **kitten** \ər\ **further** \a\ **ash** \ā\ **ace** \ä\ **cot, cart** \au̇\ **out** \ch\ **chin** \e\ **bet** \ē\ **easy** \g\ **go** \i\ **hit** \ī\ **ice** \j\ **job** \ŋ\ **sing** \ō\ **go** \ȯ\ **law** \ȯi\ **boy** \th\ **thin** \t̲h̲\ **the** \ü\ **loot** \u̇\ **foot** \y\ **yet** \zh\ **vision** *See also* Pronunciation Symbols page

fa·cies \'fā-sh(ē-,)ēz\ *n, pl* **facies** **1** : an appearance and expression of the face characteristic of a particular condition esp. when abnormal ⟨adenoid ∼⟩ — see HIPPOCRATIC FACIES, MOON FACIES **2** : an anatomical surface

facies Hip·po·crat·ica \-,hip-ə-'krat-i-kə\ *n* : HIPPOCRATIC FACIES

fa·cil·i·tate \fə-'sil-ə-,tāt\ *vt* **-tat·ed; -tat·ing** : to increase the likelihood, strength, or effectiveness of (as behavior or a response) ⟨reflexes can be *facilitated* or inhibited⟩; *also* : to lower the threshold for transmission of (an impulse)

fa·cil·i·ta·tion \fə-,sil-ə-'tā-shən\ *n* **1** : the lowering of the threshold for reflex conduction along a particular neural pathway esp. from repeated use of that pathway **2** : the increasing of the ease or intensity of a response by repeated stimulation

fa·cil·i·ta·to·ry \fə-'sil-ə-tə-,tōr-ē, -,tȯr-\ *adj* : inducing or involved in facilitation esp. of a reflex action

fa·cil·i·ty \fə-'sil-ət-ē\ *n, pl* **-ties** **1** : the quality of being easily performed **2** : ease in performance : APTITUDE **3** : something (as a hospital) that is built, installed, or established to serve a particular purpose

fac·ing \'fā-siŋ\ *n* : a front of porcelain or plastic used in dental crowns and bridgework to face the metal replacement and simulate the natural tooth

fa·cio·scap·u·lo·hu·mer·al \,fā-sh(ē)ō-,skap-yə-lō-'hyüm-(ə-)rəl\ *adj* : relating to or affecting the muscles of the face, scapula, and arm ⟨∼ muscular dystrophies⟩

FACOG *abbr* Fellow of the American College of Obstetricians and Gynecologists

FACP *abbr* Fellow of the American College of Physicians

FACR *abbr* Fellow of the American College of Radiology

FACS *abbr* Fellow of the American College of Surgeons

F–ac·tin \'ef-,ak-tən\ *n* : a fibrous actin polymerized in the form of a double helix that is produced in the presence of a metal cation (as of calcium) and ATP — compare G-ACTIN

fac·ti·tious \fak-'tish-əs\ *adj* : not produced by natural means

fac·tor \'fak-tər\ *n* **1 a** : something that actively contributes to the production of a result **b** : a substance that functions in or promotes the function of a particular physiological process or bodily system **2** : GENE — **fac·to·ri·al** \fak-'tōr-ē-əl, -'tȯr-\ *adj*

factor VIII \-'āt\ *n* : a glycoprotein clotting factor of blood plasma that is essential for blood clotting and is absent or inactive in hemophilia — called also *antihemophilic factor, thromboplastinogen*

factor XI *n* : PLASMA THROMBOPLASTIN ANTECEDENT

factor V \-'fīv\ *n* : a globulin clotting factor that occurs in inactive form in blood plasma and that in its active form is one of the factors accelerating the formation of thrombin from prothrombin in the clotting of blood — called also *accelerator globulin, labile factor, proaccelerin*

factor IX \-'nīn\ *n* : a clotting factor whose absence is associated with Christmas disease — called also *autoprothrombin II, Christmas factor*

factor VII \-'sev-ən, -'seb-ᵊm\ *n* : a clotting factor in normal blood that is formed in the kidney under the influence of vitamin K and may be deficient due to a hereditary disorder or to a vitamin K deficiency — called also *autoprothrombin I, cothromboplastin, proconvertin, stable factor*

factor X \-'ten\ *n* : a clotting factor that is converted to a proteolytic enzyme which converts prothrombin to thrombin in a reaction dependent on calcium ions and other clotting factors — called also *Stuart-Prower factor*

factor XIII \-,thər(t)-'tēn, -'thər(t)-\ *n* : a clotting factor that causes monomeric fibrin to polymerize and become stable and insoluble — called also *fibrinase;* see TRANSGLUTAMINASE

factor XII \-,twelv\ *n* : a clotting factor that facilitates blood coagulation in vivo and initiates coagulation on a firm surface (as glass) in vitro but whose deficiency tends not to promote hemorrhage — called also *Hageman factor*

facts of life \,fakt-səv-'līf\ *n pl* : the fundamental physiological processes and behavior involved in sex and reproduction

fac·ul·ta·tive \'fak-əl-,tāt-iv\ *adj* **1** : taking place under some conditions but not under others ⟨∼ parasitism⟩ **2** : exhibiting an indicated lifestyle under some environmental conditions but not under others ⟨∼ anaerobes⟩ — **fac·ul·ta·tive·ly** *adv*

fac·ul·ty \'fak-əl-tē\ *n, pl* **-ties** **1 a** : an inherent capability, power, or function ⟨the ∼ of hearing⟩ ⟨digestive ∼⟩ **b** : one of the powers of the mind formerly held by psychologists to form a basis for the explanation of all mental phenomena **2 a** : the members of a profession **b** : the teaching and administrative staff and those members of the administration having academic rank in an educational institution

FAD \,ef-(,)ā-'dē\ *n* : FLAVIN ADENINE DINUCLEOTIDE

Each boldface word in the list below is a chiefly British variant of the word to its right in small capitals.

faecal	FECAL	faecaloid	FECALOID
faecalith	FECALITH	faeces	FECES
faecally	FECALLY		

fag·o·py·rism \,fag-ō-'pī-,riz-əm\ *also* **fag·o·py·ris·mus** \-,pī-'riz-məs\ *n, pl* **-risms** *also* **-ris·mus·es** : a photosensitization esp. of swine and sheep that is due to eating large quantities of buckwheat (esp. *Fagopyrum esculentum* of the family Polygonaceae) and that appears principally on the nonpigmented parts of the skin as an intense redness and swelling with severe itching and the formation of vesicles and later sores and scabs — compare BIGHEAD b, HYPERICISM

Fah *or* **Fahr** *abbr* Fahrenheit

Fahr·en·heit \'far-ən-,hīt\ *adj* : relating or conforming to a thermometric scale on which under standard atmospheric pressure the boiling point of water is at 212 degrees above the zero of the scale, the freezing point is at 32 degrees above zero, and the zero point approximates the temperature produced by mixing equal quantities by weight of snow and common salt — abbr. *F*

Fahrenheit, Daniel Gabriel (1686–1736), German physicist. Fahrenheit devoted his career mostly to the making of precision scientific instruments. In 1709 he developed an alcohol thermometer, superseding it with a mercury thermometer in 1714. His most important achievement was his development, from the work of Olaus Roemer, of the thermometric scale that bears his name.

fail \'fā(ə)l\ *vi* **1** : to weaken or lose strength ⟨her health was ∼*ing*⟩ **2** : to stop functioning ⟨the patient's heart ∼*ed*⟩

fail·ure \'fā(ə)l-yər\ *n* : a state of inability to perform a vital function ⟨acute renal ∼⟩ ⟨respiratory ∼⟩ — see HEART FAILURE

¹**faint** \'fānt\ *adj* : weak, dizzy, and likely to faint

²**faint** *vi* : to lose consciousness because of a temporary decrease in the blood supply to the brain

³**faint** *n* : the physiological action of fainting; *also* : the resulting condition : SYNCOPE

faint·ness \-nəs\ *n* : the state or condition of being faint : partial or near loss of consciousness

faith healing \'fāth-,hē-liŋ\ *n* : a method of treating diseases by prayer and exercise of faith in God — **faith healer** *n*

fal·cate \'fal-,kāt, 'fȯl-\ *also* **fal·cat·ed** \-,kāt-əd\ *adj* : hooked or curved like a sickle

falces *pl of* FALX

fal·cial \'fal-shəl, 'fȯl-, -chəl\ *adj* : of or belonging to a falx

fal·ci·form \'fal-sə-,fȯrm, 'fȯl-\ *adj* : having the shape of a scythe or sickle

falciform ligament *n* : an anteroposterior fold of peritoneum attached to the under surface of the diaphragm and sheath of the rectus muscle and along a line on the anterior and upper surfaces of the liver extending back from the notch on the anterior margin

fal·cip·a·rum malaria \fal-'sip-ə-rəm-, fȯl-\ *n* : severe malaria caused by a parasite of the genus *Plasmodium* (*P. falciparum*) and marked by irregular recurrence of paroxysms and usu. prolonged or continuous fever — called also *malignant malaria, malignant tertian malaria, subtertian malaria;* compare VIVAX MALARIA

fal·cu·lar \'fal-kyə-lər, 'fȯl-\ *adj* **1** : shaped like a sickle **2** : belonging to or indicating a falx ⟨∼ cilia⟩

fall·en arch \'fȯ-lən-\ *n* : FLATFOOT

fall·ing sickness \'fȯ-liŋ-\ *n* : EPILEPSY

fal·lo·pi·an \fə-'lō-pē-ən\ *adj, often cap* : relating to or discovered by Fallopius

Fal·lop·pio \fäl-'lȯp-yō\ *or* **Fal·lop·pia** \-'lȯp-yä\, **Gabriele** (*Latin* **Gabriel Fal·lo·pi·us** \fə-'lō-pē-əs\) (1523–1562), Italian anatomist. A student of Andreas Vesalius and one of the great anatomists of his time, Fallopius published in 1561 *Observationes anatomicae,* a seminal work that offered a systematic description of human anatomy based on years of dissection experience. Of all the anatomical descriptions the most important were those concerning the ears, face, and genitals. He described in detail the anatomy of the middle and inner ear (including the semicircular canals), and he named the cochlea. His original description of the facial canal resulted in its subsequent eponymous designation. In his identification of the structures of the female reproductive tract he described the hymen and clitoris and gave the scientific names to the vagina and placenta. His classic (but not original) description of the human oviducts resulted in his name being associated with them.

fallopian aqueduct *n, often cap F* : FACIAL CANAL

fallopian canal *n, often cap F* : FACIAL CANAL

fallopian tube *n, often cap F* : either of the pair of tubes that carry the eggs from the ovary to the uterus — called also *uterine tube*

Fallot's tetralogy \(ˌ)fal-ˌōz-\ *n* : TETRALOGY OF FALLOT

fall·out \'fȯ-ˌlau̇t\ *n* **1** : the often radioactive particles stirred up by or resulting from a nuclear explosion and descending through the atmosphere; *also* : other polluting particles (as volcanic ash) descending likewise **2** : descent (as of fallout) through the atmosphere

false \'fȯls\ *adj* **fals·er; fals·est 1** : not corresponding to truth or reality ⟨a test for HIV which gave ∼ results⟩ **2** : artificially made ⟨∼ teeth⟩ **3** : of a kind related to or resembling another kind that is usu. designated by the unqualified vernacular ⟨∼ oats⟩ — **false·ly** *adv* — **false·ness** *n*

false hellebore *n* : any of several hellebores of the genus *Veratrum; esp* : one (*V. viride*) of the eastern U.S. with dense spikelike flower clusters and a rootstock that has been used medicinally — see AMERICAN HELLEBORE

false joint *n* : PSEUDARTHROSIS

false labor *n* : pains resembling those of normal labor but occurring at irregular intervals and without dilation of the cervix

false membrane *n* : a fibrinous deposit with enmeshed necrotic cells formed esp. in croup and diphtheria — called also *pseudomembrane*

false mo·rel \-mȯ-'rel\ *n* : any fungus of the genus *Gyromitra*

false–negative *adj* : relating to or being an individual or a test result that is erroneously classified in a negative category (as of diagnosis) because of imperfect testing methods or procedures — compare FALSE-POSITIVE — **false negative** *n*

false neurotransmitter *n* : a biological amine that can be stored in presynaptic vesicles but that has little or no effect on postsynaptic receptors when released into the synaptic cleft — called also *false transmitter*

false pelvis *n* : the upper broader portion of the pelvic cavity — called also *false pelvic cavity;* compare TRUE PELVIS

false–positive *adj* : relating to or being an individual or a test result that is erroneously classified in a positive category (as of diagnosis) because of imperfect testing methods or procedures ⟨a ∼ pregnancy test⟩ — compare FALSE‗NEGATIVE — **false positive** *n*

false pregnancy *n* : PSEUDOCYESIS, PSEUDOPREGNANCY

false rib *n* : a rib whose cartilages unite indirectly or not at all with the sternum — compare FLOATING RIB

false transmitter *n* : FALSE NEUROTRANSMITTER

false vocal cords *n pl* : the upper pair of vocal cords each of which encloses a vestibular ligament, extends from one side of the thyroid cartilage in front to the arytenoid cartilage on the same side of the larynx in back, and is not directly con-

cerned with speech production — called also *superior vocal cords, ventricular folds, vestibular folds*

fal·si·fi·ca·tion \ˌfȯl-sə-fə-'kā-shən\ *n* : a misrepresentation esp. by embellishing a true memory with false details — **fal·si·fy** \'fȯl-sə-ˌfī\ *vb* **-fied; -fy·ing**

falx \'falks, 'fȯlks\ *n, pl* **fal·ces** \'fal-ˌsēz, 'fȯl-\ : a sickle‗ shaped part or structure: as **a** : FALX CEREBRI **b** : FALX CEREBELLI

falx ce·re·bel·li \-ˌser-ə-'bel-ˌī\ *n* : the smaller of the two folds of dura mater separating the hemispheres of the brain that lies between the lateral lobes of the cerebellum

falx cer·e·bri \-'ser-ə-ˌbrī\ *n* : the larger of the two folds of dura mater separating the hemispheres of the brain that lies between the cerebral hemispheres and contains the sagittal sinuses

fam *abbr* family

FAMA *abbr* Fellow of the American Medical Association

fam·ci·clo·vir \ˌfam-'sī-klō-ˌvir\ *n* : a precursor $C_{14}H_{19}N_5O_4$ of the antiviral agent penciclovir that after oral administration is converted to penciclovir by cellular kinases and that is used esp. to treat shingles and herpes genitalis — see FAMVIR

fa·mes \'fā-ˌmēz\ *n* : HUNGER

fa·mil·ial \fə-'mil-yəl\ *adj* : tending to occur in more members of a family than expected by chance alone ⟨a ∼ disorder⟩ — compare ACQUIRED 2, CONGENITAL 2, HEREDITARY

familial adenomatous polyposis *n* : a disease of the large intestine that is marked by the formation esp. in the colon and rectum of numerous adenomatous polyps which typically become malignant if left untreated, that may be either asymptomatic or accompanied by diarrhea or bleeding, and that is inherited as an autosomal dominant trait — abbr. *FAP;* called also *familial polyposis*

familial dysautonomia *n* : a disorder of the autonomic nervous system that is inherited as an autosomal recessive trait, typically affects individuals of eastern European Jewish ancestry, and is characterized esp. by multiple sensory deficits (as of taste and pain), excessive sweating and salivation, lack of tears, difficulty in swallowing, corneal ulceration, dysarthria, orthostatic hypotension, episodic vomiting, and emotional instability

familial hypercholesterolemia *n* : a metabolic disorder that is caused by defective or absent receptors for LDLs on cell surfaces, that is marked by an increase in blood plasma LDLs and by an accumulation of LDLs in the body (as in connective tissue) resulting in xanthomas, atherosclerosis, and an increased risk of heart attack and coronary heart disease, and that is inherited as an autosomal dominant trait

familial polyposis *n* : any of several inherited diseases (as Gardner's syndrome or Peutz-Jegher's syndrome) that are characterized esp. by the formation of polyps in the gastrointestinal tract; *esp* : FAMILIAL ADENOMATOUS POLYPOSIS

fam·i·ly \'fam-(ə-)lē\ *n, pl* **-lies 1** : the basic unit in society traditionally consisting of two parents rearing their children; *also* : any of various social units differing from but regarded as equivalent to the traditional family ⟨a single-parent ∼⟩ **2** : a group of related plants or animals forming a category ranking above a genus and below an order and usu. comprising several to many genera — **family** *adj*

family doctor *n* **1** : a doctor regularly consulted by a family in time of medical need **2** : FAMILY PHYSICIAN 2

family physician *n* **1** : FAMILY DOCTOR 1 **2** : a doctor specializing in family practice

family planning \-'plan-iŋ\ *n* : planning intended to determine the number and spacing of one's children through effective methods of birth control

family practice *n* : a medical practice or specialty which provides continuing general medical care for the individual and family — abbr. *FP;* called also *family medicine*

\ə\ abut \ᵊ\ kitten \ər\ further \a\ ash \ā\ ace \ä\ cot, cart \au̇\ out \ch\ chin \e\ bet \ē\ easy \g\ go \i\ hit \ī\ ice \j\ job \ŋ\ sing \ō\ go \ȯ\ law \ȯi\ boy \th\ thin \t̲h̲\ the \ü\ loot \u̇\ foot \y\ yet \zh\ vision *See also* Pronunciation Symbols page

family practitioner *n* : FAMILY DOCTOR, FAMILY PHYSICIAN

fa·mo·ti·dine \fə-'mōt-ə-ˌdīn, -ˌdēn\ *n* : an H₂ antagonist $C_8H_{15}N_7O_2S_3$ used to inhibit gastric acid secretion esp. in the short-term treatment of gastric and duodenal ulcers and gastroesophageal reflux disease and in the treatment of disorders (as Zollinger-Ellison syndrome) involving gastric acid hypersecretion — see PEPCID

Fam·vir \'fam-ˌvir\ *trademark* — used for a preparation of famciclovir

fa·nat·i·cism \fə-'nat-ə-ˌsiz-əm\ *n* : fanatic outlook or behavior esp. as exhibited by excessive enthusiasm, unreasoning zeal, or wild and extravagant notions on some subject

Fan·co·ni's anemia \fän-'kō-nēz-, fan-\ *n* : aplastic anemia that is inherited as an autosomal recessive trait and is characterized by progressive pancytopenia, hypoplastic bone marrow, skeletal anomalies (as short stature), microcephaly, hypogonadism, and a predisposition to leukemia

Fanconi, Guido (1892–1979), Swiss pediatrician. Fanconi first described the congenital disease now known as Fanconi's anemia in 1927. He first reported on the renal dysfunction now known as Fanconi syndrome in 1931.

Fan·co·ni syndrome \-nē-\ *also* **Fanconi's syndrome** *n* : a disorder of reabsorption in the proximal convoluted tubules of the kidney characterized esp. by the presence of glucose, amino acids, and phosphates in the urine

fang \'faŋ\ *n* **1 a** : a long sharp tooth: as (1) : one by which an animal's prey is seized and held or torn (2) : one of the long hollow or grooved and often erectile teeth of a venomous snake **b** : one of a spider's chelicerae at the tip of which a poison gland opens **2** : the root of a tooth or one of the processes or prongs into which a root divides — **fanged** \'faŋd\ *adj*

fan·go \'faŋ-(ˌ)gō, 'fäŋ-\ *n* : mud and esp. a clay mud from hot springs at Battaglio, Italy, that is used in the form of hot external applications in the therapeutic treatment of certain medical conditions (as rheumatism)

Fan·nia \'fan-ē-ə\ *n* : a genus of dipteran flies (family Anthomyiidae) resembling but smaller than the common housefly and including the little housefly (*F. canicularis*) and the latrine fly (*F. scalaris*)

fan·ta·size *or Brit* **fan·ta·sise** \'fant-ə-ˌsīz\ *vb* **-sized** *or Brit* **-sised; -siz·ing** *or Brit* **-sis·ing** *vi* : to indulge in fantasy : create or develop imaginative and often fantastic views or ideas ⟨∼*s* about running away from home⟩ ∼ *vt* : to portray in the mind by fantasy ⟨likes to ∼ herself as very famous⟩

fan·tast \'fan-ˌtast\ *n* : one who indulges in fantasies and daydreaming

¹**fan·ta·sy** *also* **phan·ta·sy** \'fant-ə-sē, -zē\ *n, pl* **-sies** : the power or process of creating esp. unrealistic or improbable mental images in response to psychological need ⟨an object of ∼⟩; *also* : a mental image or a series of mental images (as a daydream) so created ⟨sexual *fantasies* of adolescence⟩

²**fantasy** *also* **phantasy** *vb* **-sied; -sy·ing** : FANTASIZE

fantom *var of* PHANTOM

FAP *abbr* familial adenomatous polyposis

FAPA *abbr* Fellow of the American Psychological Association

far·ad \'fa(ə)r-ˌad, 'far-əd\ *n* : the unit of capacitance equal to the capacitance of a capacitor between whose plates there appears a potential of one volt when it is charged by one coulomb of electricity — abbr. *f*

Far·a·day \'far-ə-ˌdā\, **Michael (1791–1867),** British physicist and chemist. Faraday ranks as one of the greatest experimental scientists of all time. In the field of electricity he demonstrated in 1821 that the force acting on a current-carrying wire in a magnetic field was circular and directed around the wire. In 1831 he discovered that an electromotive force can be induced in a circuit by varying the magnetic flux linked with the circuit, and he built an elementary electric motor and dynamo. Faraday also stated the basic laws of electrolysis and introduced the terms *anode, cathode, anion, cation,* and *electrode.*

far·a·day \'far-ə-ˌdā, -əd-ē\ *n* : the quantity of electricity transferred in electrolysis per equivalent weight of an element or ion equal to about 96,500 coulombs — symbol *f*

fa·rad·ic \fə-'rad-ik, far-'ad-\ *also* **far·a·da·ic** \far-ə-'dā-ik\ *adj* : of or relating to an asymmetric alternating current of electricity produced by an induction coil ⟨∼ muscle stimulation⟩ — compare GALVANIC

far·a·dism \'far-ə-ˌdiz-əm\ *n* : the application of a faradic current of electricity (as for therapeutic purposes)

far·a·dize *also Brit* **far·a·dise** \'far-ə-ˌdīz\ *vt* **-dized** *also Brit* **-dised; -diz·ing** *also Brit* **-dis·ing** : to treat by faradism — **far·a·di·za·tion** *also Brit* **far·a·di·sa·tion** \far-əd-ə-'zā-shən, -ˌī-'zā-\ *n* — **far·a·diz·er** *also Brit* **far·a·dis·er** \'far-ə-ˌdī-zər\ *n*

far·cy \'fär-sē\ *n, pl* **far·cies** : GLANDERS; *esp* : cutaneous glanders

far·fa·ra \'fär-fər-ə, -fə-rə\ *n* : the dried leaves of coltsfoot used in folk medicine for coughs and as a tonic

fa·ri·na \fə-'rē-nə\ *n* : a fine meal of vegetable matter (as cereal grains) used chiefly for puddings or as a breakfast cereal

far·i·na·ceous \far-ə-'nā-shəs\ *adj* **1** : containing or rich in starch **2** : having a mealy texture or surface

farm·er's lung \ˌfär-mərz-\ *n* : an acute pulmonary disorder that is characterized by sudden onset, fever, cough, expectoration, and breathlessness and that results from the inhalation of dust from moldy hay or straw

farmer's skin *n* : SAILOR'S SKIN

far·ne·sol \'fär-nə-ˌsȯl, -ˌsȯl, -ˌsōl, -ˌzȯl\ *n* : a liquid alcohol $C_{15}H_{25}OH$ that has a floral odor and that occurs in various essential oils (as citronella oil)

far point \'fär-\ *n* : the point farthest from the eye at which an object is accurately focused on the retina when the accommodation is completely relaxed, being theoretically equivalent to infinity or, for practical purposes with respect to the normal eye, equivalent to any distance greater than 20 feet (6.1 meters) — see RANGE OF ACCOMMODATION; compare NEAR POINT

¹**far·row** \'far-(ˌ)ō, -ə(-w)\ *vt* : to give birth to (a farrow) ∼ *vi, of swine* : to bring forth young — often used with *down*

²**farrow** *n* **1** : a litter of pigs **2** : an act of farrowing

³**farrow** *adj, of a cow* : not pregnant

far·sight·ed \'fär-'sīt-əd\ *adj* **1** : seeing or able to see to a great distance **2** : affected with hyperopia — **far·sight·ed·ly** *adv*

far·sight·ed·ness *n* **1** : the quality or state of being farsighted **2** : HYPEROPIA

FAS *abbr* fetal alcohol syndrome

fasc *abbr* fasciculus

fas·cia \'fash-(ē-)ə *also* 'fāsh-\ *n, pl* **-ci·ae** \-ē-ˌē\ *or* **-cias** : a sheet of connective tissue (as an aponeurosis) covering or binding together body structures; *also* : tissue occurring in such a sheet — see DEEP FASCIA, SUPERFICIAL FASCIA — **fas·cial** \-(ē-)əl\ *adj*

fasciae — see TENSOR FASCIAE LATAE

fascia la·ta \-'lät-ə, -'lāt-ə\ *n, pl* **fasciae la·tae** \-'lät-ē, -'lāt-ē\ : the deep fascia that forms a complete sheath for the thigh and has an opening in front just below the inguinal ligament for the passage of the great saphenous vein

fas·ci·cle \'fas-i-kəl\ *n* : a small bundle; *esp* : FASCICULUS — **fas·ci·cled** \-kəld\ *adj*

fas·cic·u·lar \fə-'sik-yə-lər, fa-\ *adj* : of, relating to, or consisting of fasciculi ⟨a ∼ biopsy⟩ — **fas·cic·u·lar·ly** *adv*

fasciculata — see ZONA FASCICULATA

fas·cic·u·late \-lət\ *or* **fas·cic·u·lat·ed** \-ˌlät-əd\ *adj* : FASCICULAR

fas·cic·u·la·tion \fə-ˌsik-yə-'lā-shən, fa-\ *n* : muscular twitching involving the simultaneous contraction of contiguous groups of muscle fibers

fas·cic·u·lus \fə-'sik-yə-ləs, fa-\ *n, pl* **-li** \-ˌlī\ : a slender bundle of fibers: **a** : a bundle of skeletal muscle cells bound together by fasciae and forming one of the constituent elements of a muscle **b** : a bundle of nerve fibers that follow the same course but do not necessarily have like functional connections (as in some subdivisions of the funiculi of the spinal cord) — compare TRACT 2 **c** : TRACT 2

fasciculus cu·ne·atus \-ˌkyü-nē-ˈāt-əs\ *n* : either of a pair of nerve tracts of the posterior funiculus of the spinal cord that are situated on opposite sides of the posterior median septum lateral to the fasciculus gracilis and that carry nerve fibers from the upper part of the body — called also *column of Burdach, cuneate fasciculus*

fasciculus grac·i·lis \-ˈgras-ə-ləs\ *n* : either of a pair of nerve tracts of the posterior funiculus of the spinal cord situated on opposite sides of and immediately adjacent to the posterior median septum and carrying nerve fibers from the lower part of the body — called also *gracile fasciculus*

fas·ci·ec·to·my \ˌfash-ē-ˈek-tə-mē, ˌfas-\ *n, pl* **-mies** : surgical excision of strips of fascia

fas·ci·i·tis \ˌfash-ē-ˈīt-əs, fas-\ *or* **fas·ci·tis** \fa-ˈshīt-əs, -ˈsīt-\ *n* : inflammation of a fascia

fas·ci·o·la \fə-ˈsē-ə-lə, -ˈsī-\ *n* **1** *pl* **-lae** \-ˌlē\ *or* **-las** : a narrow fascia or band of color **2** *cap* : a genus (the type of the family Fasciolidae) of digenetic trematode worms including common liver flukes of various mammals (as ruminants and humans)

fas·ci·o·lar \-lər\ *adj* : of or relating to a fasciola

fa·sci·o·li·a·sis \fə-ˌsē-ə-ˈlī-ə-səs, -ˌsī-\ *n, pl* **-a·ses** \-ˌsēz\ : infestation with or disease caused by liver flukes of the genus *Fasciola* (*F. hepatica* or *F. gigantica*)

fas·ci·o·li·cide \fə-ˈsē-ə-lə-ˌsīd, fa-\ *n* : an agent that destroys liver flukes of the genus *Fasciola* — **fas·ci·o·li·cid·al** \-ˌsē-ə-lə-ˈsīd-ᵊl\ *adj*

Fas·ci·ol·i·dae \ˌfas-ē-ˈäl-ə-dē\ *n pl* : a cosmopolitan family of digenetic trematodes chiefly infesting the livers of mammals and typically having a flattened leaf-shaped body with the ventral sucker near the anterior end — see FASCIOLA, FASCIOLOIDES, FASCIOLOPSIS

Fas·ci·o·loi·des \fə-ˌsē-ə-ˈlòid-(ˌ)ēz, -ˌsī-\ *n* : a genus of trematode worms of the family Fasciolidae including the giant liver flukes of ruminant mammals that are serious pests of livestock and game in parts of western No. America

fas·ci·o·lop·si·a·sis \-ˌläp-ˈsī-ə-səs\ *n, pl* **-a·ses** \-ˌsēz\ : infestation with or disease caused by a large intestinal fluke of the genus *Fasciolopsis* (*F. buski*)

Fas·ci·o·lop·sis \-ˈläp-səs\ *n* : a genus of trematode worms of the family Fasciolidae that includes an important intestinal parasite (*F. buski*) of humans, swine, dogs, and rabbits in much of eastern Asia

fas·ci·ot·o·my \ˌfash-ē-ˈät-ə-mē\ *n, pl* **-mies** : surgical incision of a fascia ⟨palmar ∼ for Dupuytren's contracture⟩

fasciitis *var of* FASCIITIS

¹fast \ˈfast\ *adj* **1** : firmly fixed **2 a** : having a rapid effect ⟨a ∼ medicine⟩ **b** : allowing for the rapid passage of a gas or liquid **3** : resistant to change (as from destructive action) — used chiefly of organisms and in combination with the agent resisted ⟨acid-*fast* bacteria⟩

²fast *vi* **1** : to abstain from food **2** : to eat sparingly or abstain from some foods ∼ *vt* : to deny food to ⟨the patient is ∼*ed* and given a mild hypnotic —*Lancet*⟩

³fast *n* **1** : the practice of fasting **2** : a time of fasting

fast green *n* : any of several green dyes derived from triphenylmethane that include some used as biological stains or counterstains

fas·tid·i·ous \fa-ˈstid-ē-əs, fə-\ *adj* : having complex nutritional requirements ⟨∼ microorganisms⟩ — used of bacteria that grow only in specially fortified artificial culture media

fas·tid·i·um \-ē-əm\ *n* : a strong distaste esp. for food

fas·tig·ial \fa-ˈstij-(ē-)əl\ *adj* : of or associated with the fastigium of the fourth ventricle of the brain

fastigial nucleus *n* : a nucleus lying near the midline in the roof of the fourth ventricle of the brain — called also *roof nucleus*

fas·tig·i·um \fa-ˈstij-ē-əm\ *n* **1** : the period at which the symptoms of a disease (as a febrile disease) are most pronounced **2** : the angle in the roof of the fourth ventricle of the brain

fast·ing \ˈfas-tiŋ\ *adj* : of or taken from a fasting subject ⟨∼

blood sugar levels⟩ ⟨∼ urine⟩; *also* : occurring from or caused by fasting ⟨∼ hyperglycemia⟩

fast·ness \ˈfas(t)-nəs\ *n* : resistance (as of an organism) to the action of a usu. toxic substance ⟨streptomycin ∼ developed by a strain of tubercule bacillus⟩

fast–twitch \ˈfas(t)-ˌtwich\ *adj* : of, relating to, or being muscle fiber that contracts quickly esp. during brief high= intensity physical activity requiring strength — compare SLOW-TWITCH

¹fat \ˈfat\ *adj* **fat·ter; fat·test** : notable for having an unusual amount of fat; *esp* : fleshy with superfluous flabby tissue that is not muscle : OBESE — **fat·ness** *n*

²fat *n* **1** : animal tissue consisting chiefly of cells distended with greasy or oily matter — see BROWN FAT **2 a** : oily or greasy matter making up the bulk of adipose tissue **b** : any of numerous compounds of carbon, hydrogen, and oxygen that are glycerides of fatty acids, are the chief constituents of plant and animal fat, are a major class of energy-rich food, and are soluble in organic solvents (as ether) but not in water **c** : a solid or semisolid fat as distinguished from an oil **3** : the condition of fatness : OBESITY

fa·tal \ˈfāt-ᵊl\ *adj* : causing death ⟨a ∼ diabetic coma —Havelock Ellis⟩ — **fa·tal·ly** \ˈfāt-ᵊl-ē\ *adv*

fa·tal·i·ty \fā-ˈtal-ət-ē, fə-\ *n, pl* **-ties** **1** : the quality or state of causing death or being fatal : DEADLINESS ⟨the degree of ∼ of a disease⟩ **2 a** : death resulting from a disaster ⟨a car crash causing several *fatalities*⟩ **b** : one who suffers such a death ⟨one of the *fatalities* was a small child⟩

fat cell *n* : a fat-containing cell of adipose tissue — called also *adipocyte, lipocyte*

fat de·pot \-ˈdep-(ˌ)ō *also* -ˈdēp-\ *n* : ADIPOSE TISSUE

fate \ˈfāt\ *n* : the expected result of normal development ⟨prospective ∼ of embryonic cells⟩

fat farm \ˈfat-ˌfärm\ *n* : a health spa that specializes in weight reduction

fa·ther figure \ˈfäth-ər-\ *n* : one often of particular power or influence who serves as an emotional substitute for a father

father image *n* : an idealization of one's father often projected onto someone to whom one looks for guidance and protection

fa·ti·ga·bil·i·ty *also* **fa·ti·gua·bil·i·ty** \fə-ˌtē-gə-ˈbil-ət-ē, ˌfat-i-gə-\ *n, pl* **-ties** : susceptibility to fatigue

fa·ti·ga·ble *also* **fa·ti·gua·ble** \fə-ˈtē-gə-bəl, ˈfat-i-gə-\ *adj* : susceptible to fatigue

¹fa·tigue \fə-ˈtēg\ *n* **1** : weariness or exhaustion from labor, exertion, or stress **2** : the temporary loss of power to respond induced in a sensory receptor or motor end organ by continued stimulation

²fatigue *vb* **fa·tigued; fa·tigu·ing** *vt* **1** : to weary with labor or exertion **2** : to induce a condition of fatigue in (as an effector organ) ∼ *vi* : to be affected with fatigue : become weary

fat pad \-ˌpad\ *n* : a flattened mass of fatty tissue

fat–sol·u·ble \ˈfat-ˌsäl-yə-bəl\ *adj* : soluble in fats or fat solvents ⟨the ∼ vitamins include vitamin A, vitamin D, and vitamin K⟩

fat·ty \ˈfat-ē\ *adj* **fat·ti·er; -est** **1 a** : unduly stout : CORPULENT **b** : marked by an abnormal deposit of fat ⟨a ∼ liver⟩ ⟨∼ cirrhosis⟩ **2** : derived from or chemically related to fat — **fat·ti·ness** *n*

fatty acid *n* **1** : any of numerous saturated aliphatic acids $C_nH_{2n+1}COOH$ (as lauric acid) containing a single carboxyl group and including many that occur naturally usu. in the form of esters in fats, waxes, and essential oils **2** : any of the saturated or unsaturated organic acids (as palmitic acid) that have a single carboxyl group and usu. an even number of carbon atoms and that occur naturally in the form of glycerides in fats and fatty oils

\ə\ abut \ᵊ\ kitten \ər\ further \a\ ash \ā\ ace \ä\ cot, cart \aù\ out \ch\ chin \e\ bet \ē\ easy \g\ go \i\ hit \ī\ ice \j\ job \ŋ\ sing \ō\ go \ò\ law \òi\ boy \th\ thin \t͟h\ the \ü\ loot \ù\ foot \y\ yet \zh\ vision   *See also* Pronunciation Symbols page

fatty degeneration *n* : a process of tissue degeneration marked by the deposition of fat globules in the cells — called also *steatosis*

fatty infiltration *n* : infiltration of the tissue of an organ with excess amounts of fat

fatty liver *n* **1** : an abnormal condition of the liver that is characterized by lipid accumulation in the hepatocytes to the extent that lipids account for more than five percent of liver weight and that is caused esp. by injury, malnutrition, or hepatotoxins **2** : a liver affected with fatty liver

fatty oil *n* : a fat that is liquid at ordinary temperatures and that is obtained from plants or marine animals — called also *fixed oil;* compare ESSENTIAL OIL, OIL 1, VOLATILE OIL

fau·ces \'fȯ-ˌsēz\ *n pl but sing or pl in constr* : the narrow passage from the mouth to the pharynx situated between the soft palate and the base of the tongue — called also *isthmus of the fauces* — **fau·cial** \'fȯ-shəl\ *adj*

fau·na \'fȯn-ə, 'fän-\ *n, pl* **faunas** *also* **fau·nae** \-ˌē, -ˌī\ : animal life; *esp* : the animals characteristic of a region, period, or special environment — compare FLORA 1 — **fau·nal** \-ᵊl\ *adj* — **fau·nal·ly** \-ᵊl-ē\ *adv*

fa·va bean \'fäv-ə\ *n* : BROAD BEAN

fa·ve·o·late \fə-'vē-ə-lət, -ˌlāt\ *adj* : having cavities like a honeycomb : ALVEOLATE

fa·vism \'fä-ˌviz-əm, 'fā-\ *n* : a condition esp. of males of Mediterranean descent that is marked by the development of hemolytic anemia upon consumption of broad beans or inhalation of broad bean pollen and is caused by a usu. inherited deficiency of glucose-6-phosphate

fa·vus \'fā-vəs\ *n* : a contagious skin disease of humans and many domestic animals and fowls that is caused by a fungus (as *Trichophyton schoenleinii*) — called also *honeycomb ringworm* — **fa·vic** \-vik\ *adj*

FD *abbr* focal distance

FDA *abbr* Food and Drug Administration

Fe *symbol* iron

fear \'fi(ə)r\ *n* **1** : an unpleasant often strong emotion caused by anticipation or awareness of danger and accompanied by increased autonomic activity **2** : an instance of fear — **fear** *vb*

feath·er \'feth-ər\ *n* : one of the light horny epidermal outgrowths that form the external covering of the body of birds and that consist of a shaft bearing on each side a series of barbs which bear barbules which in turn bear barbicels commonly ending in the hooked processes and interlocking with the barbules of an adjacent barb to link the barbs into a continuous vane — **feath·ered** \-ərd\ *adj*

fea·ture \'fē-chər\ *n* **1** : the structure, form, or appearance esp. of a person **2 a** : the makeup or appearance of the face or its parts **b** : a part of the face

fe·bric·u·la \fi-'brik-yə-lə\ *n* : a slight and transient fever

fe·bri·fa·cient \ˌfeb-rə-'fā-shənt, ˌfēb-\ *n* : a substance that causes fever

fe·brif·ic \fi-'brif-ik\ *adj* : producing fever

fe·brif·u·gal \fi-'brif-(y)ə-gəl, ˌfeb-rə-'fyü-gəl\ *adj* : mitigating or removing fever

feb·ri·fuge \'feb-rə-ˌfyüj\ *n or adj* : ANTIPYRETIC

fe·brile \'feb-ˌrīl *also* 'fēb-\ *adj* : FEVERISH

fe·bris \'feb-rəs, 'fäb-\ *n* : FEVER

fe·cal *or chiefly Brit* **fae·cal** \'fē-kəl\ *adj* : of, relating to, or constituting feces ⟨~ incontinence⟩ ⟨~ matter⟩ — **fe·cal·ly** *or chiefly Brit* **fae·cal·ly** \-kə-lē\ *adv*

fe·ca·lith *or chiefly Brit* **fae·ca·lith** \'fē-kə-ˌlith\ *n* : a concretion of dry compact feces formed in the intestine or vermiform appendix

fe·cal·oid *or chiefly Brit* **fae·cal·oid** \-kə-ˌlȯid\ *adj* : resembling dung

fe·ces *or chiefly Brit* **fae·ces** \'fē-(ˌ)sēz\ *n pl* : bodily waste discharged through the anus : EXCREMENT

Fech·ner's law \'fek-nərz-, 'fek-\ *n* : WEBER-FECHNER LAW

fec·u·la \'fek-yə-lə\ *n, pl* **fec·u·lae** \-ˌlē\ : a form of starch obtained from some plants (as an arrowroot)

fec·u·lent \'fek-yə-lənt\ *adj* : foul with impurities : FECAL ⟨a ~ odor of the breath⟩ — **fe·cu·lence** \-lən(t)s\ *n*

fe·cund \'fek-ənd, 'fēk-\ *adj* **1** : characterized by having produced many offspring **2** : capable of producing : not sterile or barren — **fe·cun·di·ty** \fi-'kən-dət-ē, fe-\ *n, pl* **-ties**

fe·cun·date \'fek-ən-ˌdāt, 'fēk-ən-\ *vt* **-dat·ed; -dat·ing** : IMPREGNATE — **fe·cun·da·tion** \ˌfek-ən-'dā-shən, ˌfē-kən-\ *n*

fee·ble·mind·ed \ˌfē-bəl-'mīn-dəd\ *adj* : mentally deficient — **fee·ble·mind·ed·ly** *adv* — **fee·ble·mind·ed·ness** *n*

¹feed \'fēd\ *vb* **fed** \'fed\; **feed·ing** *vt* **1 a** : to give food to **b** : to give as food **2** : to produce or provide food for ~ *vi* : to consume food : EAT

²feed *n* **1 a** : an act of eating **b** : MEAL; *esp* : a large meal **2 a** : food for livestock; *specif* : a mixture or preparation for feeding livestock **b** : the amount given at each feeding

feed·back \'fēd-ˌbak\ *n* **1** : the return to the input of part of the output of a machine, system, or process (as for producing changes in an electronic circuit that improve performance or in an automatic control device that provide self= corrective action) **2 a** : the partial reversion of the effects of a process to its source or to a preceding stage **b** : the return to a point of origin of evaluative or corrective information about an action or process ⟨patient ~ was solicited⟩; *also* : the information so transmitted

feedback inhibition *n* : inhibition of an enzyme controlling an early stage of a series of biochemical reactions by the end product when it reaches a critical concentration

fee-for-ser·vice \ˌfē-fər-'sər-vəs\ *n* : separate payment to a health-care provider for each medical service rendered to a patient — often used attributively ⟨a ~ group plan⟩

¹feel \'fē(ə)l\ *vb* **felt** \'felt\; **feel·ing** *vt* **1** : to handle or touch in order to examine, test, or explore some quality ⟨felt the compress to see if it was wet⟩ **2** : to perceive by a physical sensation coming from discrete end organs (as of the skin or muscles) ~ *vi* **1** : to receive or be able to receive a tactile sensation **2** : to search for something by using the sense of touch

²feel *n* **1** : the sense of touch **2** : SENSATION, FEELING

feel·er \'fē-lər\ *n* : one that feels; *esp* : a tactile process (as a tentacle) of an animal

feel·ing \'fē-liŋ\ *n* **1 a** : the one of the basic physical senses of which the skin contains the chief end organs and of which the sensations of touch and temperature are characteristic : TOUCH **b** : a sensation experienced through this sense **2** : an emotional state or reaction ⟨guilt ~s⟩ **3** : the overall quality of one's awareness esp. as measured along a pleasantness-unpleasantness continuum

fee split·ting \'fē-ˌsplit-iŋ\ *n* : payment by a medical specialist (as a surgeon) of a part of the specialist's fee to the physician who made the referral — **fee split·ter** \-ər\ *n*

feet *pl of* FOOT

Feh·ling's solution \'fā-liŋ(z)-\ *or* **Feh·ling solution** \-liŋ-\ *n* : a blue solution of Rochelle salt and copper sulfate used as an oxidizing agent in a test for sugars and aldehydes in which the precipitation of a red oxide of copper indicates a positive result

Fehling, Hermann von (1812–1885), German chemist. Fehling is known for his work in analytical and industrial chemistry. In 1848 he published an article on analyzing the quantity of sugar in urine in which he introduced his test for the determination of reducing sugars using a solution that he formulated.

fel \'fel\ *n* : BILE 1

fel·ba·mate \'fel-bə-ˌmāt\ *n* : an anticonvulsant drug $C_{11}H_{14}N_2O_4$ that is used to treat severe epilepsy or epilepsy that is unresponsive to other drugs

Fel·den·krais \'fel-dən-ˌkrīs\ *trademark* — used for a system of aided body movements intended to increase bodily awareness and ease tension

feld·sher \'fel(d)-shər\ *n* : a medical or surgical practitioner without full professional qualifications or status in some east European countries and esp. Russia

Fe·li·dae \'fē-lə-ˌdē\ *n pl* : a cosmopolitan family comprising lithe-bodied carnivorous mammals (as the domestic cat, lion, tiger, lynx, and cheetah) having often strikingly patterned fur, comparatively short limbs with soft pads on the feet, usu. sharp curved retractile claws, a broad and somewhat rounded head with short but powerful jaws equipped with teeth suited to grasping, tearing, and shearing through flesh, erect ears, and typically eyes with narrow or elliptical pupils and esp. adapted for seeing in dim light

fe·line \'fē-ˌlīn\ *adj* : of, relating to, or affecting cats or the family Felidae — **feline** *n*

feline distemper *n* : PANLEUKOPENIA

feline enteritis *n* : PANLEUKOPENIA

feline infectious anemia *n* : a widespread contagious disease of cats characterized by weakness, lethargy, loss of appetite, and hemolytic anemia and caused by a bacterial parasite of red blood cells belonging to the genus *Haemobartonella* (*H. felis*)

feline infectious peritonitis *n* : an almost invariably fatal infectious disease of cats caused by a single-stranded RNA virus of the genus *Coronavirus* (species *Feline coronavirus*) and characterized by fever, weight and appetite loss, and ascites with a thick yellow fluid — abbr. *FIP*

feline leukemia *n* : a disease of cats caused by the feline leukemia virus, characterized by leukemia and lymphoma, and often resulting in death

feline leukemia virus *n* : a retrovirus (species *Feline leukemia virus* of the genus *Gammaretrovirus*) that is widespread in cat populations, is usu. transmitted by direct contact, and is associated with or causes a variety of conditions and symptoms including malignant lymphoma, feline leukemia, anemia, glomerulonephritis, infertility, and immunosuppression

feline panleukopenia *n* : PANLEUKOPENIA

feline pneumonitis *n* : an infectious disease of the eyes and upper respiratory tract of cats that is caused by a bacterium of the genus *Chlamydia* (*C. psittaci*) and is characterized esp. by conjunctivitis and rhinitis

fel·late \'fel-ˌāt, fə-'lāt\ *vb* **fel·lat·ed; fel·lat·ing** *vt* : to perform fellatio on ∼ *vi* : to fellate someone

fel·la·tio \fə-'lā-shē-ˌō, fe-, -'lāt-ē-\ *also* **fel·la·tion** \-'lā-shən\ *n, pl* **-tios** *also* **-tions** : oral stimulation of the penis — **fel·la·tory** \'fel-ə-ˌtōr-ē\ *adj*

fel·la·tor \'fe-ˌlā-tər, fə-'lā-\ *n* : one who and esp. a man who performs fellatio

fel·la·trice \'fel-ə-ˌtrēs\ *n* : FELLATRIX

fel·la·trix \fe-'lā-triks\ *n, pl* **-trix·es** *or* **-tri·ces** \-trə-ˌsēz, ˌfel-ə-'trī-(ˌ)sēz\ : a woman who performs fellatio

fellea *see* VESICA FELLEA

fel·low \'fel-(ˌ)ō, -ə(-w)\ *n* : a young physician who has completed training as an intern and resident and has been granted a stipend and position allowing him or her to do further study or research in a specialty

felo–de–se \ˌfel-ōd-ə-'sā, -'sē\ *n, pl* **fe·lo·nes–de–se** \fə-ˌlō-(ˌ)nēz-də-\ *or* **felos–de–se** \ˌfel-ōz-də-\ **1** : one who commits suicide or who dies from the effects of having committed an unlawful malicious act **2** : an act of deliberate self=destruction : SUICIDE

fe·lo·di·pine \fə-'lō-də-ˌpēn, -ˌpīn\ *n* : a calcium channel blocker $C_{18}H_{19}Cl_2NO_4$ used esp. in the treatment of hypertension

fel·on *n* : WHITLOW

felt *past and past part of* FEEL

felt·work \'felt-ˌwərk\ *n* : an anatomical network (as neuropil) of fibers

Fel·ty's syndrome \'fel-tēz-\ *n* : a condition characterized by rheumatoid arthritis, neutropenia, and splenomegaly and often by weight loss, anemia, lymphadenopathy, and pigment spots on the skin

  Felty, Augustus Roi (1895–1964), American physician. Felty described the syndrome that bears his name in 1924 based on five cases including one of his own.

FeLV *abbr* feline leukemia virus

fem *abbr* **1** female **2** feminine **3** femur

¹fe·male \'fē-ˌmāl\ *n* : an individual that bears young or produces eggs as distinguished from one that produces sperm; *esp* : a woman or girl as distinguished from a man or boy

²female *adj* : of, relating to, or being the sex that bears young or produces eggs

female circumcision *n* : FEMALE GENITAL MUTILATION

female complaint *n* : any of various ill-defined disorders of the human female formerly usu. held to be associated with or attributed to the generative function

female genital mutilation *n* : clitoridectomy esp. as a cultural rite sometimes with removal of the labia that is now outlawed in some nations including the U.S. — abbr. *FGM;* called also *female circumcision*

female hormone *n* : a sex hormone (as an estrogen) primarily produced and functioning in the female

fe·male·ness \'fē-ˌmāl-nəs\ *n* : the qualities (as of form, physiology, or behavior) that distinguish an individual that produces large usu. immobile gametes from one that produces spermatozoa or spermatozoids

female pronucleus *n* : the nucleus that remains in a female gamete after the meiotic reduction division and extrusion of polar bodies and contains only one half the number of chromosomes characteristic of its species — compare MALE PRONUCLEUS

fem·i·nine \'fem-ə-nən\ *adj* **1** : FEMALE **2** : characteristic of or appropriate or peculiar to women

fem·i·nin·i·ty \ˌfem-ə-'nin-ət-ē\ *n, pl* **-ties** : the quality or nature of the female sex

fem·i·nism \'fem-ə-ˌniz-əm\ *n* : the presence of female characteristics in males

fem·i·nize *or Brit* **fem·i·nise** \'fem-ə-ˌnīz\ *vt* **-nized** *or Brit* **-nised; -niz·ing** *or Brit* **-nis·ing** : to cause (a male or castrate) to take on feminine characters (as by implantation of ovaries or administration of estrogenic substances) — **fem·i·ni·za·tion** *or Brit* **fem·i·ni·sa·tion** \ˌfem-ə-nə-'zā-shən\ *n*

femora *pl of* FEMUR

fem·o·ral \'fem-(ə-)rəl\ *adj* : of or relating to the femur or thigh

femoral artery *n* : the chief artery of the thigh that is a continuation of the external iliac artery lying in the anterior part of the thigh and is undivided until a point about two inches (5 centimeters) below the inguinal ligament where it divides into a large deep branch and a smaller superficial branch — see DEEP FEMORAL ARTERY

femoral canal *n* : the space that is situated between the femoral vein and the inner wall of the femoral sheath, is from a quarter to half an inch (6 to 13 millimeters) long, and extends from the femoral ring to the saphenous opening

femoral nerve *n* : the largest branch of the lumbar plexus that in humans comes from the second, third, and fourth lumbar nerves and supplies extensor muscles of the thigh and skin areas on the front of the thigh and medial surface of the leg and foot and that sends articular branches to the hip and knee joints — called also *anterior crural nerve*

femoral ring *n* : the oval upper opening of the femoral canal often the seat of a hernia — see CRURAL SEPTUM

femoral sheath *n* : the fascial sheath investing the femoral vessels

femoral triangle *n* : an area in the upper anterior part of the thigh bounded by the inguinal ligament, the sartorius, and the adductor longus — called also *femoral trigone, Scarpa's triangle*

femoral trigone *n* : FEMORAL TRIANGLE

femoral vein *n* : the chief vein of the thigh that is a continuation of the popliteal vein, accompanies the femoral artery in the upper part of its course, and continues above the inguinal ligament as the external iliac vein

femoris — see BICEPS FEMORIS, PROFUNDA FEMORIS, PROFUNDA FEMORIS ARTERY, QUADRATUS FEMORIS, QUADRICEPS FEMORIS, RECTUS FEMORIS

fem·o·ro·pop·li·te·al \ˌfem-ə-rō-ˌpäp-lə-'tē-əl, -päp-'lit-ē-əl\ *adj* : of, relating to, or connecting the femoral and popliteal arteries ⟨a ∼ bypass⟩

fe·mur \'fē-mər\ *n, pl* **fe·murs** *or* **fem·o·ra** \'fem-(ə-)rə\ **1**

\ə\ abut \ᵊ\ kitten \ər\ further \a\ ash \ā\ ace \ä\ cot, cart \au̇\ out \ch\ chin \e\ bet \ē\ easy \g\ go \i\ hit \ī\ ice \j\ job \ŋ\ sing \ō\ go \ȯ\ law \ȯi\ boy \th\ thin \th\ the \ü\ loot \u̇\ foot \y\ yet \zh\ vision *See also* Pronunciation Symbols page

: the proximal bone of the hind or lower limb that is the longest and largest bone in the human body, extends from the hip to the knee, articulates above with the acetabulum by a rounded head connected with the shaft of the bone by an oblique neck bearing a pair of trochanters for the attachment of muscles, and articulates with the tibia below by a pair of condyles — called also *thigh bone* **2** : the segment of an insect's leg that is third from the body

fe·nes·tra \fə-'nes-trə\ *n, pl* **-trae** \-ˌtrē, -ˌtrī\ **1** : a small anatomical opening (as in a bone): as **a** : OVAL WINDOW **b** : ROUND WINDOW **2 a** : an opening like a window cut in bone (as in the inner ear in the fenestration operation) **b** : a window cut in a surgical instrument (as an endoscope) — **fe·nes·tral** \-trəl\ *adj*

fenestra coch·le·ae \-'käk-lē-ˌē, -'kō-klē-ˌī\ *n* : ROUND WINDOW

fenestra oval·is \-ˌō-'vā-ləs\ *n* : OVAL WINDOW

fenestra ro·tun·da \-ˌrō-'tən-də\ *n* : ROUND WINDOW

fen·es·trat·ed \'fen-ə-ˌstrāt-əd\ *adj* : having one or more openings or pores ⟨∼ blood capillaries⟩ ⟨a ∼ catheter⟩

fenestrated membrane *n* : an elastic membrane of the inner coat of large arteries composed of broad elastic fibers that become fused to form a perforated sheet

fen·es·tra·tion \ˌfen-ə-'strā-shən\ *n* **1 a** : a natural or surgically created opening in a surface **b** : the presence of such openings **2** : the operation of cutting an opening in the bony labyrinth between the inner ear and tympanum to replace natural fenestrae that are not functional

fenestration operation *n* : FENESTRATION 2

fenestra ves·ti·bu·li \-ves-'tib-yə-ˌlī\ *n* : OVAL WINDOW

fen·flur·amine \ˌfen-'flur-ə-ˌmēn\ *n* : an anorectic amphetamine derivative $C_{12}H_{16}F_3N$ with little stimulant effect on the central nervous system formerly used in the form of its hydrochloride to treat obesity but no longer used due to its association with heart valve disease — see DEXFENFLURAMINE, FEN-PHEN

fen·nel \'fen-ᵊl\ *n* : a perennial European herb (*Foeniculum vulgare*) of the carrot family (Umbelliferae) introduced into No. America and cultivated for its aromatic seeds and its foliage

fennel oil *n* : a colorless or pale yellow essential oil obtained from fennel seed and used chiefly as a flavoring material

fen·o·fi·brate \ˌfen-ō-'fī-ˌbrāt\ *n* : a hypolipidemic agent $C_{20}H_{21}ClO_4$ used to treat hypercholesterolemia and hypertriglyceridemia — see TRICOR

fen·o·pro·fen \ˌfen-ə-'prō-fən\ *n* : an anti-inflammatory analgesic administered in the form of its hydrated calcium salt $C_{30}H_{26}CaO_6\cdot2H_2O$ esp. to treat arthritis

fen–phen \'fen-ˌfen\ *n* : a former diet drug combination of phentermine with either fenfluramine or dexfenfluramine — called also *phen-fen*

fen·ta·nyl \'fent-ᵊn-ˌil\ *n* : a synthetic opioid narcotic analgesic $C_{22}H_{28}N_2O$ with pharmacological action similar to morphine that is administered transdermally as a skin patch and in the form of its citrate $C_{22}H_{28}N_2O\cdot C_6H_8O_7$ is administered orally or parenterally

fenu·greek *also* **fenu·greek** \'fen-yə-ˌgrēk\ *n* : a leguminous annual Asian herb (*Trigonella foenumgraecum*) with aromatic seeds used in making curry, imitation vanilla flavoring, and some veterinary medicines

¹fer·ment \(ˌ)fər-'ment\ *vi* : to undergo fermentation ∼ *vt* : to cause to undergo fermentation — **fer·ment·able** \-ə-bəl\ *adj*

²fer·ment \'fər-ˌment *also* (ˌ)fər-'\ *n* **1 a** : a living organism (as a yeast) that causes fermentation by virtue of its enzymes **b** : ENZYME **2** : FERMENTATION

fer·men·ta·tion \ˌfər-mən-'tā-shən, -ˌmen-\ *n* **1** : a chemical change with effervescence **2** : an enzymatically controlled anaerobic breakdown of an energy-rich compound (as a carbohydrate to carbon dioxide and alcohol or to an organic acid); *broadly* : an enzymatically controlled transformation of an organic compound

fer·men·ta·tive \(ˌ)fər-'ment-ət-iv\ *adj* **1** : causing or producing a substance that causes fermentation ⟨∼ organisms⟩ **2** : of, relating to, or produced by fermentation

fer·men·ter \(ˌ)fər-'ment-ər\ *n* **1** : an organism that causes fermentation **2** *or* **fer·men·tor** : an apparatus for carrying out fermentation

fer·mi·um \'fer-mē-əm, 'fər-\ *n* : a radioactive metallic element artificially produced (as by bombardment of plutonium with neutrons) — symbol *Fm*; see ELEMENT table

fer·re·dox·in \ˌfer-ə-'däk-sən\ *n* : any of a group of iron-containing plant proteins that function as electron carriers in photosynthetic organisms and in some anaerobic bacteria

fer·ric \'fer-ik\ *adj* **1** : of, relating to, or containing iron **2** : being or containing iron usu. with a valence of three

ferric ammonium citrate *n* : a complex salt of indefinite composition that contains varying amounts of iron, that is obtained as red crystals or a brownish yellow powder or as green crystals or powder, and that was formerly used in medicine for treating iron-deficiency anemia

ferric chloride *n* : a deliquescent salt $FeCl_3$ that is used chiefly as an oxidizing agent, as a catalyst, as an etching agent in photoengraving, as a coagulant in treating industrial wastes, and in medicine in a water solution or tincture usu. as an astringent or styptic

ferric ferrocyanide *n* : PRUSSIAN BLUE 2

ferric hydroxide *n* : a hydrate $Fe_2O_3\cdot nH_2O$ of ferric oxide that is capable of acting both as a base and as a weak acid

ferric oxide *n* : the red or black oxide of iron Fe_2O_3 found in nature as hematite and as rust and also obtained synthetically and used as a pigment and for polishing

ferric pyrophosphate *n* : a green or yellowish green salt $Fe_4(P_2O_7)_3\cdot nH_2O$ that is used as a source of iron esp. when dietary intake is inadequate

fer·ri·cy·a·nide \ˌfer-ˌī-'sī-ə-ˌnīd, ˌfer-i-\ *n* **1** : the trivalent anion $Fe(CN)_6^{3-}$ **2** : a compound containing the ferricyanide anion; *esp* : the red salt $K_3Fe(CN)_6$ used in making blue pigments

fer·ri·he·mo·glo·bin *or chiefly Brit* **fer·ri·hae·mo·glo·bin** \ˌfer-ˌī-'hē-mə-ˌglō-bən, ˌfer-i-\ *n* : METHEMOGLOBIN

fer·ri·tin \'fer-ət-ən\ *n* : a crystalline iron-containing protein that functions in the storage of iron and is found esp. in the liver and spleen — compare HEMOSIDERIN

fer·ro·cy·a·nide \ˌfer-ō-'sī-ə-ˌnīd\ *n* **1** : the tetravalent anion $Fe(CN)_6^{4-}$ **2** : a compound containing the ferrocyanide anion; *esp* : the salt $K_4Fe(CN)_6$ used in making blue pigments (as Prussian blue)

fer·rous \'fer-əs\ *adj* **1** : of, relating to, or containing iron **2** : being or containing iron with a valence of two

ferrous carbonate *n* : a salt $FeCO_3$ occurring in nature or obtained synthetically as a white easily oxidizable precipitate and used in medicine in treating iron-deficiency anemia

ferrous fumarate *n* : a reddish orange to red-brown powder $C_4H_2FeO_4$ used orally in the treatment of iron-deficiency anemia

ferrous gluconate *n* : a yellowish gray or pale greenish yellow powder or granules $C_{12}H_{22}FeO_{14}$ used as a hematinic in the treatment of iron-deficiency anemia

ferrous sulfate *n* : an astringent iron salt obtained usu. in the form of its pale green crystalline hydrate $FeSO_4\cdot7H_2O$ and used in medicine chiefly for treating iron-deficiency anemia

fer·ru·gi·nous \fə-'rü-jə-nəs, fe-\ *or* **fer·ru·gin·e·ous** \ˌfer-(y)ù-'jin-ē-əs\ *adj* **1** : of, relating to, or containing iron **2** : resembling iron rust in color

fer·tile \'fərt-ᵊl, *chiefly Brit* 'fər-ˌtīl\ *adj* **1** : capable of growing or developing ⟨∼ egg⟩ **2** : developing spores or spore-bearing organs **3 a** : capable of breeding or reproducing **b** *of an estrous cycle* : marked by the production of one or more viable eggs

fer·til·i·ty \(ˌ)fər-'til-ət-ē\ *n, pl* **-ties** **1** : the quality or state of being fertile **2** : the birthrate of a population — compare MORTALITY 2b

fer·til·iza·tion *or Brit* **fer·til·isa·tion** \ˌfərt-ᵊl-ə-'zā-shən\ *n* : an act or process of making fertile: as **a** : an act or process

E

F

of fecundation, insemination, or impregnation **b** : the process of union of two gametes whereby the somatic chromosome number is restored and the development of a new individual is initiated — **fer·til·ize** or Brit **fer·til·ise** \'fərt-ᵊl-ˌīz\ vt **-ized** or Brit **-ised; -iz·ing** or Brit **-is·ing**

fertilization membrane n : a resistant membranous layer in eggs of many animals that forms following fertilization by the thickening and separation of the vitelline membrane from the cell surface and that prevents multiple fertilization

fer·til·i·zin \fər-'til-ə-zən, 'fert-ᵊl-ˌī-zən\ n : a sperm-agglutinating agent that is produced by an egg and plays a part in the preliminaries of fertilization

fer·u·la \'fer-(y)ə-lə\ n **1** cap : a genus of Old World plants of the carrot family (Umbelliferae) yielding various gum resins (as galbanum and asafetida)   **2** : a plant of the genus *Ferula*

fes·cue foot \'fes-(ˌ)kyü-\ n : a disease of the feet of cattle resembling ergotism that is associated with feeding on fescue grass (genus *Festuca*) and esp. tall fescue

¹**fes·ter** \'fes-tər\ n : a suppurating sore : PUSTULE

²**fester** vi **fes·tered; fes·ter·ing** \-t(ə-)riŋ\ : to generate pus

fes·ti·nat·ing \'fes-tə-ˌnāt-iŋ\ adj : being a walking gait (as in Parkinson's disease) characterized by involuntary acceleration — **fes·ti·na·tion** \ˌfes-tə-'nā-shən\ n

fe·tal or chiefly Brit **foe·tal** \'fēt-ᵊl\ adj : of, relating to, or being a fetus

fetal alcohol syndrome n : a highly variable group of birth defects including mental retardation, deficient growth, central nervous system dysfunction, and malformations of the skull and face that tend to occur in the offspring of women who consume large amounts of alcohol during pregnancy — abbr. *FAS*

fetal hemoglobin n : hemoglobin that consists of two alpha chains and two gamma chains and that predominates in the blood of a newborn and persists in increased proportions in some forms of anemia (as thalassemia) — called also *hemoglobin F*

fetalis — see ERYTHROBLASTOSIS FETALIS, HYDROPS FETALIS

fetal position n : a position (as of a sleeping person) in which the body lies curled up on one side with the arms and legs drawn up toward the chest and the head is bowed forward and which is assumed in some forms of psychic regression

fe·ta·tion or chiefly Brit **foe·ta·tion** \fē-'tā-shən\ n : the formation of a fetus : PREGNANCY

fe·ti·cide or chiefly Brit **foe·ti·cide** \'fēt-ə-ˌsīd\ n : the action or process of causing the death of a fetus — **fe·ti·ci·dal** or chiefly Brit **foe·ti·ci·dal** \ˌfēt-ə-'sīd-ᵊl\ adj

fet·id also **foet·id** \'fet-əd, esp Brit 'fē-tid\ adj : having a heavy offensive smell

fe·tish also **fe·tich** \'fet-ish also 'fēt-\ n : an object or bodily part whose real or fantasized presence is psychologically necessary for sexual gratification and that is an object of fixation to the extent that it may interfere with complete sexual expression

fe·tish·ism also **fe·tich·ism** \-ish-ˌiz-əm\ n : the pathological displacement of erotic interest and satisfaction to a fetish — **fe·tish·is·tic** also **fe·tich·is·tic** \ˌfet-ish-'is-tik also ˌfēt-\ adj — **fe·tish·is·ti·cal·ly** \-ti-k(ə-)lē\ adv

fet·ish·ist also **fet·ich·ist** \-ish-əst\ n : one who obtains erotic gratification by fetishism ⟨a shoe ∼ and other sex deviants⟩

fet·lock \'fet-ˌläk\ n **1 a** : a projection bearing a tuft of hair on the back of the leg above the hoof of a horse or similar animal   **b** : the tuft of hair itself   **2** : the joint of the limb at the fetlock

fe·tol·o·gist or chiefly Brit **foe·tol·o·gist** \fē-'täl-ə-jəst\ n : a specialist in fetology

fe·tol·o·gy or chiefly Brit **foe·tol·o·gy** \fē-'täl-ə-jē\ n, pl **-gies** : a branch of medical science concerned with the study and treatment of the fetus in the uterus

fe·tom·e·try or chiefly Brit **foe·tom·e·try** \fē-'täm-ə-trē\ n, pl **-tries** : measurement of a fetus (as by X-ray examination)

fe·to·pro·tein or chiefly Brit **foe·to·pro·tein** \ˌfēt-ō-'prō-ˌtēn, -'prōt-ē-ən\ n : any of several fetal antigens present in the adult in some abnormal conditions; esp : ALPHA-FETOPROTEIN

fe·tor also **foe·tor** \'fēt-ər, 'fē-ˌtȯ(ə)r\ n : a strong offensive smell

fetor he·pat·i·cus \-hi-'pat-i-kəs\ n : a characteristically disagreeable odor to the breath that is a sign of liver failure

fe·to·scope or chiefly Brit **foe·to·scope** \'fēt-ə-ˌskōp\ n **1** : an endoscope for visual examination of the pregnant uterus   **2** : a stethoscope for listening to the fetal heartbeat

fe·tos·co·py or chiefly Brit **foe·tos·co·py** \fēt-'äs-kə-pē\ n, pl **-pies** : examination of the pregnant uterus by means of a fiber-optic tube

fe·to·tox·ic \ˌfēt-ə-'täk-sik\ adj : toxic to fetuses — **fe·to·tox·ic·i·ty** \-täk-'sis-ət-ē\ n, pl **-ties**

fe·tus or chiefly Brit **foe·tus** \'fēt-əs\ n, pl **fe·tus·es** or chiefly Brit **foe·tus·es** or **foe·ti** \'fēt-ˌī\ : an unborn or unhatched vertebrate esp. after attaining the basic structural plan of its kind; specif : a developing human from usu. two months after conception to birth — compare EMBRYO

Feul·gen \'fȯil-gən\ adj : of, relating to, utilizing, or staining by the Feulgen reaction ⟨positive ∼ mitochondria⟩

Feulgen, Robert Joachim (1884–1955), German biochemist. Feulgen introduced the Feulgen reaction in 1914. This reaction, which is specific for DNA, transformed nucleic acid cytochemistry.

Feulgen reaction n : the development of a brilliant purple color by DNA in a microscopic preparation stained with a modified Schiff's reagent

¹**fe·ver** \'fē-vər\ n **1** : a rise of body temperature above the normal whether a natural response (as to infection) or artificially induced for therapeutic reasons   **2** : an abnormal bodily state characterized by increased production of heat, accelerated heart action and pulse, and systemic debility with weakness, loss of appetite, and thirst   **3** : any of various diseases of which fever is a prominent symptom — see YELLOW FEVER, TYPHOID FEVER

²**fever** vb **fe·vered; fe·ver·ing** \'fēv-(ə-)riŋ\ vt : to affect with fever ⟨the malarial plasmodia ∼ed him⟩ ∼ vi : to contract or be in a fever : be or become feverish ⟨the malaria victim ∼ed intermittently⟩

fever blister n : COLD SORE

fe·ver·ish \'fēv-(ə-)rish\ adj **1** : showing symptoms indicating fever (as increased heat and thirst or delirium) : having a fever ⟨the patient is ∼⟩; specif : abnormally hot ⟨the child's forehead felt ∼⟩   **2** : of or indicating fever ⟨a ∼ condition⟩   **3** : infected with or tending to cause fever ⟨a damp, ∼, unhealthy spot —R. L. Stevenson⟩

fever therapy n : a treatment of disease by fever induced by various artificial means

fever thermometer n : CLINICAL THERMOMETER

fex·o·fen·a·dine \ˌfek-sō-'fen-ə-ˌdēn\ n : an H₁ antagonist administered orally in the form of its hydrochloride $C_{32}H_{39}NO_4 \cdot HCl$ to relieve symptoms of seasonal allergic rhinitis — see ALLEGRA

FF abbr **1** fat free   **2** filtration fraction

FFA abbr free fatty acids

FGF abbr fibroblast growth factor

FGM abbr female genital mutilation

FHS abbr fetal heart sounds

FHT abbr fetal heart tone

fib abbr fibrillation

fi·ber or chiefly Brit **fi·bre** \'fī-bər\ n **1** : a thread or a threadlike structure or object: as   **a** : a strand of nerve tissue : AXON, DENDRITE   **b** : one of the filaments composing most of the intercellular matrix of connective tissue   **c** : one of the elongated contractile cells of muscle tissue   **2** : mostly indigestible material in food that stimulates the intestine to peristalsis — called also *bulk, dietary fiber, roughage*

\ə\ abut \ᵊ\ kitten \ər\ further \a\ ash \ā\ ace \ä\ cot, cart
\aů\ out \ch\ chin \e\ bet \ē\ easy \g\ go \i\ hit \ī\ ice \j\ job
\ŋ\ sing \ō\ go \ȯ\ law \ȯi\ boy \th\ thin \th\ the \ü\ loot
\ů\ foot \y\ yet \zh\ vision   See also Pronunciation Symbols page

fiber of Mül·ler \-'myü-lər, -'məl-ər\ *n* : any of the glial fibers that extend through the entire thickness of the retina and act as a support for the other structures — called also *Müller cell, sustentacular fiber of Müller*

   H. Müller — see MÜLLERIAN

fiber of Re·mak \-'rā-ˌmäk\ *n* : REMAK'S FIBER

fiber optics *or chiefly Brit* **fibre optics** *n pl* **1** : thin transparent fibers of glass or plastic that are enclosed by material of a lower index of refraction and that transmit light throughout their length by internal reflections; *also* : a bundle of such fibers used in an instrument (as for viewing body cavities) **2** *sing in constr* : the technique of the use of fiber optics — **fi·ber–op·tic** *or chiefly Brit* **fi·bre–op·tic** \'fī-bə-ˌräp-tik\ *adj*

fi·ber·scope *or chiefly Brit* **fi·bre·scope** \'fī-bər-ˌskōp\ *n* : a flexible endoscope that utilizes fiber optics to transmit light and is used for visual examination of inaccessible areas (as the stomach)

fiber tract *n* : TRACT 2

fibre *chiefly Brit var of* FIBER

fi·bril \'fīb-rəl, 'fib-\ *n* : a small filament or fiber: as **a** : one of the fine threads into which a striated muscle fiber can be longitudinally split **b** : NEUROFIBRIL

fi·bril·la \fī-'bril-ə, fi-; 'fī-bri-lə, 'fib-ri-lə\ *n, pl* **fi·bril·lae** \-ˌlē\ : FIBRIL

fi·bril·lar \'fib-rə-lər, 'fīb-; fī-'bril-ər, fi-\ *adj* **1** : of or like fibrils or fibers ⟨a ~ network⟩ **2** : of or exhibiting fibrillation ⟨~ twitchings⟩

fi·bril·lary \'fī-brə-ˌler-ē, 'fib-rə-; fī-'bril-ə-rē, fi-'bril-\ *adj* **1** : of or relating to fibrils or fibers ⟨~ overgrowth⟩ **2** : of, relating to, or marked by fibrillation ⟨~ chorea⟩

fi·bril·late \'fib-rə-ˌlāt, 'fīb-\ *vb* **-lat·ed; -lat·ing** *vi* : to undergo or exhibit fibrillation ~ *vt* : to cause (as the heart) to undergo fibrillation

fi·bril·la·tion \ˌfib-rə-'lā-shən, ˌfīb-\ *n* **1** : an act or process of forming fibers or fibrils **2 a** : a muscular twitching involving individual muscle fibers acting without coordination **b** : very rapid irregular contractions of the muscle fibers of the heart resulting in a lack of synchronism between heartbeat and pulse — see ATRIAL FIBRILLATION, VENTRICULAR FIBRILLATION

fi·bril·lin \'fī-brə-lin, 'fib-rə-\ *n* : a large extracellular glycoprotein of connective tissue that is a structural component of microfibrils associated esp. with elastin

fi·bril·lo·gen·e·sis \ˌfib-rə-lō-'jen-ə-səs, ˌfīb-\ *n, pl* **-e·ses** \-ˌsēz\ : the development of fibrils

fi·brin \'fī-brən\ *n* : a white insoluble fibrous protein formed from fibrinogen by the action of thrombin esp. in the clotting of blood

fi·brin·ase \-ˌās, -ˌāz\ *n* : FACTOR XIII

fibrin film \-ˌfilm\ *n* : a pliable translucent film prepared from fibrinogen and thrombin from human blood plasma and used in the surgical repair of defects

fibrin foam \-ˌfōm\ *n* : a spongy substance prepared from fibrinogen and thrombin from human blood plasma and used esp. after saturation with thrombin as an absorbable clotting agent in surgical wounds

fi·brin·o·gen \fī-'brin-ə-jən\ *n* : a plasma protein that is produced in the liver and is converted into fibrin during blood clot formation

fi·brin·o·gen·o·pe·nia \(ˌ)fī-ˌbrin-ə-ˌjen-ə-'pē-nē-ə, -nyə\ *n* : a deficiency of fibrin or fibrinogen or both in the blood

fi·bri·noid \'fib-rə-ˌnòid, 'fīb-\ *n, often attrib* : a homogeneous acidophilic refractile material that somewhat resembles fibrin and is formed in the walls of blood vessels and in connective tissue in some pathological conditions and normally in the placenta

fi·bri·no·ly·sin \ˌfī-brən-ᵊl-'īs-ᵊn\ *n* : any of several proteolytic enzymes that promote the dissolution of blood clots; *esp* : PLASMIN

fi·bri·no·ly·sis \-'ī-səs, -brə-'näl-ə-səs\ *n, pl* **-ly·ses** \-ˌsēz\ : the usu. enzymatic breakdown of fibrin — **fi·bri·no·lyt·ic** \-brən-ᵊl-'it-ik\ *adj*

fi·bri·no·pe·nia \ˌfī-brə-nō-'pē-nē-ə, -nyə\ *n* : FIBRINOGENOPENIA

fi·bri·no·pep·tide \-'pep-ˌtīd\ *n* : any of the vertebrate polypeptides that are cleaved from fibrinogen by thrombin during blood clot formation

fi·bri·no·pu·ru·lent \-'pyùr-(y)ə-lənt\ *adj* : containing, characterized by, or exuding fibrin and pus ⟨necrosis of the bowel and ~ peritonitis —*Jour. Amer. Med. Assoc.*⟩

fi·bri·nous \'fib-rə-nəs, 'fīb-\ *adj* : marked by the presence of fibrin ⟨~ pericarditis⟩ ⟨~ exudate⟩

fi·bro·ad·e·no·ma \ˌfī-(ˌ)brō-ˌad-ᵊn-'ō-mə\ *n, pl* **-mas** *also* **-ma·ta** \-mət-ə\ : adenoma with a large amount of fibrous tissue

fi·bro·are·o·lar \-ə-'rē-ə-lər\ *adj* : composed of both fibrous and areolar connective tissue

fi·bro·blast \'fīb-rə-ˌblast *also* 'fib-\ *n* : a connective-tissue cell of mesenchymal origin that secretes proteins and esp. molecular collagen from which the extracellular fibrillar matrix of connective tissue forms — **fi·bro·blas·tic** \ˌfīb-rə-'blas-tik, ˌfib-\ *adj*

fibroblast growth factor *n* : any of several protein growth factors that stimulate the proliferation esp. of endothelial cells and that promote angiogenesis — abbr. *FGF*

fi·bro·car·ti·lage \ˌfī-(ˌ)brō-'kärt-ᵊl-ij, -'kärt-lij\ *n* : cartilage in which the matrix except immediately about the cells is largely composed of fibers like those of ordinary connective tissue; *also* : a structure or part composed of such cartilage — **fi·bro·car·ti·lag·i·nous** \-ˌkärt-ᵊl-'aj-ə-nəs\ *adj*

fi·bro·cys·tic \ˌfīb-rə-'sis-tik, ˌfib-\ *adj* : characterized by the presence or development of fibrous tissue and cysts ⟨~ changes in the pancreas —*Lancet*⟩

fibrocystic disease of the pancreas *n* : CYSTIC FIBROSIS

fi·bro·cyte \'fīb-rə-ˌsīt, 'fib-\ *n* : FIBROBLAST; *specif* : a spindle-shaped cell of fibrous tissue — **fi·bro·cyt·ic** \ˌfīb-rə-'sit-ik, ˌfib-\ *adj*

fi·bro·elas·tic \ˌfī-(ˌ)brō-i-'las-tik\ *adj* : consisting of both fibrous and elastic elements ⟨~ tissue⟩

fi·bro·elas·to·sis \-ˌlas-'tō-səs\ *n, pl* **-to·ses** \-ˌsēz\ : a condition of the body or one of its organs (as the left ventricle of the heart) characterized by proliferation of fibroelastic tissue — see ENDOCARDIAL FIBROELASTOSIS

fi·bro·gen·e·sis \ˌfī-brə-'jen-ə-səs\ *n, pl* **-e·ses** \-ˌsēz\ : the development or proliferation of fibers or fibrous tissue ⟨pulmonary ~ resulting from inhalation of asbestos⟩

fi·bro·gen·ic \-'jen-ik\ *adj* : promoting the development of fibers ⟨the ~ action of silica —A. C. Heppleston⟩

¹fi·broid \'fīb-ˌroid, 'fib-\ *adj* : resembling, forming, or consisting of fibrous tissue

²fibroid *n* : a benign tumor esp. of the uterine wall that consists of fibrous and muscular tissue

fi·bro·ma \fī-'brō-mə\ *n, pl* **-mas** *also* **-ma·ta** \-mət-ə\ : a benign tumor consisting mainly of fibrous tissue — **fi·bro·ma·tous** \-mət-əs\ *adj*

fi·bro·ma·to·gen·ic \fī-ˌbrō-mət-ə-'jen-ik\ *adj* : inducing or tending to induce the development of fibromas

fi·bro·ma·toid \fī-'brō-mə-ˌtòid\ *adj* : resembling a fibroma

fi·bro·ma·to·sis \(ˌ)fī-ˌbrō-mə-'tō-səs\ *n, pl* **-to·ses** \-ˌsēz\ : a condition marked by the presence of or a tendency to develop multiple fibromas

fi·bro·my·al·gia \ˌfī-(ˌ)brō-ˌmī-'al-j(ē-)ə\ *n* : a chronic disorder characterized by widespread pain, tenderness, and stiffness of muscles and associated connective tissue structures that is typically accompanied by fatigue, headache, and sleep disturbances — called also *fibromyalgia syndrome, fibromyositis*

fi·bro·my·o·ma \-ˌmī-'ō-mə\ *n, pl* **-mas** *also* **-ma·ta** \-mət-ə\ : a mixed tumor containing both fibrous and muscle tissue — **fi·bro·my·o·ma·tous** \-mət-əs\ *adj*

fi·bro·my·o·si·tis \-ˌmī-ə-'sīt-əs\ *n* : FIBROMYALGIA

fi·bro·myx·o·ma \-mik-'sō-mə\ *n, pl* **-mas** *also* **-ma·ta** \-mət-ə\ : a myxoma containing fibrous tissue

fi·bro·nec·tin \ˌfī-brə-'nek-tən\ *n* : any of a group of glycoproteins of cell surfaces, blood plasma, and connective tissue that promote cellular adhesion and migration

fi·bro·pla·sia \ˌfī-brə-'plā-zh(ē-)ə\ *n* : the process of forming fibrous tissue (as in wound healing) — **fi·bro·plas·tic** \-'plas-tik\ *adj*

fibrosa — see OSTEITIS FIBROSA, OSTEITIS FIBROSA CYSTICA, OSTEITIS FIBROSA CYSTICA GENERALISTA, OSTEODYSTROPHIA FIBROSA, TUNICA FIBROSA

fi·bro·sar·co·ma \-sär-'kō-mə\ *n, pl* **-mas** *also* **-ma·ta** \-mət-ə\ : a sarcoma of relatively low malignancy consisting chiefly of spindle-shaped cells that tend to form collagenous fibrils

¹**fi·brose** \'fī-ˌbrōs\ *adj* : FIBROUS

²**fibrose** *vi* **-brosed; -bros·ing** : to form fibrous tissue ⟨a *fibrosed* wound⟩

fi·bro·se·rous \ˌfī-brō-'sir-əs\ *adj* : composed of a serous membrane supported by a firm layer of fibrous tissue ⟨the pericardium is a ~ sac⟩

fi·bro·sis \fī-'brō-səs\ *n, pl* **-bro·ses** \-ˌsēz\ : a condition marked by increase of interstitial fibrous tissue : fibrous degeneration

fi·bro·si·tis \ˌfī-brə-'sīt-əs\ *n* : rheumatic disorder of fibrous tissue; *esp* : FIBROMYALGIA — **fi·bro·sit·ic** \-'sit-ik\ *adj*

fibrosus — see ANNULUS FIBROSUS, LACERTUS FIBROSUS

fi·brot·ic \fī-'brät-ik\ *adj* : characterized by or affected with fibrosis ⟨the ~ liver⟩

fi·brous \'fī-brəs\ *adj* **1** : containing, consisting of, or resembling fibers ⟨collagen is a ~ protein⟩ **2** : characterized by fibrosis

fibrous ankylosis *n* : ankylosis due to the growth of fibrous tissue

fib·u·la \'fib-yə-lə\ *n, pl* **-lae** \-lē *also* -ˌlī\ *or* **-las** : the outer or postaxial and usu. the smaller of the two bones of the hind or lower limb below the knee that is the slenderest bone of the human body in proportion to its length, articulates above with the external tuberosity of the tibia and below with the talus, and has its lower end forming the external malleolus of the ankle — called also *calf bone* — **fib·u·lar** \-lər\ *adj*

fibular collateral ligament *n* : LATERAL COLLATERAL LIGAMENT

fib·u·lo·cal·ca·ne·al \ˌfib-yə-(ˌ)lō-ˌkal-'kā-nē-əl\ *adj* : belonging to the fibula and the calcaneus

fi·cin \'fīs-ᵊn\ *n* : a protease that is obtained from the latex of fig trees and is used as an anthelmintic and protein digester

Fick principle \'fik-\ *n* : a generalization in physiology which states that blood flow is proportional to the difference in concentration of a substance in the blood as it enters and leaves an organ and which is used to determine cardiac output from the difference in oxygen concentration in blood before it enters and after it leaves the lungs and from the rate at which oxygen is consumed — called also *Fick method*

Fick, Adolf Eugen (1829–1901), German physiologist. A professor of physiology, Fick was an advocate of the school of physiology that sought to determine quantitatively the fundamental capabilities of the organism's components and then explain these on the basis of general physicochemical laws of nature. Fick did research in fields of notable diversity: molecular physics, including the diffusion of water and gases, porous diffusion, endosmosis, and filtration; hydrodynamics as applied to the motion of fluids in rigid and/or elastic vessels; the origin and measurement of bioelectric phenomena; optics; the theory of heat in physics and physiology; and sound. In 1856 he published a work that is often considered to be the first textbook of biophysics. In it he stated the fundamental laws governing diffusion, one of which is now known as Fick's law. Fick made outstanding contributions in hemodynamics, and in 1870 he stated the Fick principle for the measurement of cardiac output.

Fick's law \'fiks-\ *n* : a law of chemistry and physics: the rate of diffusion of one material in another is proportional to the negative of the gradient of the concentration of the first material

FICS *abbr* Fellow of the International College of Surgeons

FID *abbr* free induction decay

field \'fē(ə)ld\ *n* **1** : an area or division of an activity ⟨a doctor eminent in her ~⟩ **2** : a complex of forces that serve as causative agents in human behavior **3 a** : a region of embryonic tissue potentially capable of a particular type of differentiation ⟨a morphogenetic ~⟩ **b** : a region or space in which a given effect (as magnetism) exists **4 a** : an area that is perceived or under observation; *esp* : the area visible through the lens of an optical instrument — see VISUAL FIELD **b** : the site of a surgical operation

field fever *n* : a European leptospirosis of humans

field hospital *n* : a military organization of medical personnel with equipment for establishing a temporary hospital in the field

field lens \-ˌlenz\ *n* : the lens in a compound eyepiece that is nearer the objective

field of force *n* : FIELD 3b

field of view \-'vyü\ *n* : FIELD 4a

field of vision *n* : VISUAL FIELD

fièvre bou·ton·neuse \'fyev-rə-ˌbü-tò-'nœz\ *n* : BOUTONNEUSE FEVER

fifth cranial nerve \'fi(f)th-, 'fift-\ *n* : TRIGEMINAL NERVE

fifth disease *n* : an acute eruptive disease esp. of children that is caused by a parvovirus (species *B19 virus* of the genus *Erythrovirus*), that is first manifested by a blotchy red rash on the cheeks followed by a maculopapular rash on the extremities, and that is usu. accompanied by fever and malaise — called also *erythema infectiosum*

fifth nerve *n* : TRIGEMINAL NERVE

fifth ventricle *n* : a cavity between the vertical lamina of the septum pellucidum that does not have a channel of communication with the other ventricles of the brain

fig \'fig\ *n* **1** : an oblong or pear-shaped fruit that is a syconium; *esp* : the edible fruit of a widely cultivated tree (*Ficus carica*) that has laxative qualities **2** : any of a genus (*Ficus*) of trees of the mulberry family that produce figs

fig *abbr* figure

fig·ure \'fig-yər, *Brit & often US* 'fig-ər\ *n* **1** : bodily shape or form esp. of a person ⟨a slender ~⟩ **2 a** : the graphic representation of a form esp. of a person **b** : a diagram or pictorial illustration of textual matter **3** : a person who is representative of or serves as a psychological substitute for someone or something else — see FATHER FIGURE

figure–ground \-'graúnd\ *adj* : relating to or being the relationships between the parts of a perceptual field which is perceived as divided into a part consisting of figures having form and standing out from the part comprising the background and being relatively formless ⟨a diagram in which ~ relationships are easily perceived as reversed⟩

fila *pl of* FILUM

fil·a·ment \'fil-ə-mənt\ *n* : a single thread or a thin flexible threadlike object, process, or appendage; *esp* : an elongated thin series of cells attached one to another or a very long thin cylindrical single cell (as of some algae, fungi, or bacteria) — **fil·a·men·tous** \ˌfil-ə-'ment-əs\ *adj*

fi·lar \'fī-lər\ *adj* : of or relating to a thread or line; *esp* : having threads across the field of view ⟨a ~ eyepiece⟩

fi·lar·ia \fə-'lar-ē-ə, -'ler-\ *n* **1** *pl* **fi·lar·i·ae** \-ē-ˌē, -ˌī\ : any of numerous slender filamentous nematodes that as adults are parasites in the blood or tissues of birds or mammals and as larvae usu. develop in biting insects (as fleas or mosquitoes) that belong to the superfamily Filarioidea, and that for the most part were once included in the genus *Filaria* but are now divided among various genera (as *Wuchereria* and *Onchocerca*) **2** *cap, in former classifications* : a genus of nematodes that included most of the filarial worms

fi·lar·i·al \-ē-əl\ *adj* : of, relating to, infested with, transmitting, or caused by filariae or related parasitic worms

fil·a·ri·a·sis *also* **fil·a·ri·o·sis** \ˌfil-ə-'rī-ə-səs\ *n, pl* **-a·ses** *also* **-o·ses** \-ˌsēz\ : infestation with or disease caused by filariae

fi·lar·i·at·ed \fə-'lar-ē-ˌāt-əd, -'ler-\ *adj* : marked by the presence of filariae ⟨a ~ person⟩

\ə\ abut \ᵊ\ kitten \ər\ **further** \a\ ash \ā\ ace \ä\ cot, cart \aú\ **out** \ch\ **chin** \e\ bet \ē\ **easy** \g\ go \i\ hit \ī\ ice \j\ **job** \ŋ\ **sing** \ō\ go \ò\ **law** \òi\ **boy** \th\ **thin** \th̲\ **the** \ü\ **loot** \ú\ **foot** \y\ **yet** \zh\ **vision** *See also* Pronunciation Symbols page

fi·lar·i·cide \fə-'lar-ə-ˌsīd, -'ler-\ *n* : an agent that is destructive to filariae — **fi·lar·i·cid·al** \-ˌlar-ə-'sīd-ᵊl, -ˌler-\ *adj*

fi·lar·i·form \-ə-ˌform\ *adj, of a larval nematode* : resembling a filaria esp. in having a slender elongated form and in possessing a delicate capillary esophagus

¹**fi·lar·i·id** \-ē-əd\ *or* **fi·lar·id** \fə-'lar-əd, 'fil-ər-əd\ *adj* : of or relating to the superfamily Filarioidea or to filariae

²**filariid** *or* **filarid** *n* : FILARIA 1

Fi·lar·i·oi·dea \fə-ˌlar-ē-'ȯid-ē-ə, -ˌler-\ *n pl* : a large superfamily of nematodes of the order Spirurida that comprises the medically important filarial worms and related forms having a slender thready body, a simple anterior end with the oral lips inconspicuous, a cylindrical esophagus lacking a bulbus, and often unequal and dissimilar copulatory spicules in the male — **fi·lar·i·oid** \fə-'lar-ē-ˌȯid, -'ler-\ *adj*

filariosis *var of* FILARIASIS

filar micrometer *n* : an instrument for accurately measuring small distances or angles that usu. consists of two parallel fine platinum wires mounted in the focal plane of a microscope or telescope with one wire being fixed and the other movable by means of a finely threaded screw

fila terminalia *pl of* FILUM TERMINALE

file \'fī(ə)l\ *n* **1** : a tool usu. of hardened steel with cutting ridges for forming or smoothing surfaces (as of a tooth) **2** : a narrow instrument for shaping fingernails with a fine rough metal or emery surface — **file** *vt* **filed; fil·ing**

fil·gras·tim \fil-'gras-təm\ *n* : a genetically engineered human granulocyte colony-stimulating factor used to decrease the incidence of infection esp. as manifested by febrile neutropenia in patients affected with nonmyeloid malignant tumors — see NEUPOGEN

fil·ial generation \'fil-ē-əl-, 'fil-yəl-\ *n* : a generation in a breeding experiment that is successive to a parental generation — compare F_1 GENERATION, F_2 GENERATION

fi·lic·ic acid \fi-ˌlis-ik-\ *n* : a phenolic anthelmintic substance that is obtained as a colorless powder from the rhizome of the common male fern

fil·i·cin \'fil-ə-sən\ *n* : FILICIC ACID; *also* : the mixture of active principles obtained from the male fern

¹**fil·i·form** \'fil-ə-ˌform, 'fī-lə-\ *adj* : shaped like a filament

²**filiform** *n* : an extremely slender bougie

filiform papilla *n* : any of numerous minute pointed papillae on the tongue

fil·i·pin \'fil-ə-pin\ *n* : an antifungal antibiotic $C_{35}H_{58}O_{11}$ produced by a bacterium of the genus *Streptomyces* (*S. filipinensis*)

fill \'fil\ *vt* **1** : to repair the cavities of (teeth) **2** : to supply as directed ⟨∼ a prescription⟩

filled milk *n* : skim milk with fat content increased by the addition of vegetable oils

fil·let \'fil-ət\ *n* : a band of anatomical fibers; *specif* : LEMNISCUS

fill·ing \'fil-iŋ\ *n* **1** : material (as gold or amalgam) used to fill a cavity in a tooth **2** : simple sporadic lymphangitis of the leg of a horse commonly due to overfeeding and insufficient exercise

film \'film\ *n* **1 a** : a thin skin or membranous covering : PELLICLE **b** : an abnormal growth on or in the eye **2 a** : an exceedingly thin layer : LAMINA **b** : a thin flexible transparent sheet of cellulose acetate or cellulose nitrate coated with a radiation-sensitive emulsion for taking photographs or making radiographs

film badge \-ˌbaj\ *n* : a small pack of sensitive photographic film worn as a badge for indicating exposure to radiation

fil·o·po·di·um \ˌfil-ə-'pō-dē-əm *also* ˌfīl-\ *also* **fil·o·pod** \'fil-ə-ˌpäd\ *n, pl* **-po·di·a** \-'pō-dē-ə\ *also* **-pods** : a long thin filamentous pseudopodium (as of a nerve cell or platelet) — **fil·o·po·di·al** \-'pō-dē-əl\ *adj*

Fi·lo·vi·ri·dae \ˌfil-ō-'vir-ə-ˌdē\ *n pl* : a family of single-stranded RNA viruses that infect vertebrates, that have a pleomorphic usu. bacilliform or filamentous shape with a helical nucleocapsid and a lipoprotein envelope with glycoprotein projections, and that include the Ebola viruses and the Marburg virus

fi·lo·vi·rus \'fī-lō-ˌvī-rəs\ *n* : any of a family *Filoviridae* of single-stranded RNA viruses

¹**fil·ter** \'fil-tər\ *n* **1** : a porous article or mass (as of paper or sand) through which a gas or liquid is passed to separate out matter in suspension **2** : an apparatus containing a filter medium **3 a** : a device or material for suppressing or minimizing waves or oscillations of certain frequencies (as of electricity, light, or sound) **b** : a transparent material (as colored glass) that absorbs light of certain wavelengths or colors selectively and is used for modifying light that reaches a sensitized photographic material — called also *color filter*

²**filter** *vb* **fil·tered; fil·ter·ing** \-t(ə-)riŋ\ *vt* **1** : to subject to the action of a filter **2** : to remove by means of a filter ∼ *vi* : to pass or move through or as if through a filter

fil·ter·able *also* **fil·tra·ble** \'fil-t(ə-)rə-bəl\ *adj* : capable of being filtered or of passing through a filter — **fil·ter·abil·i·ty** \ˌfil-t(ə-)rə-'bil-ət-ē\ *n, pl* **-ties**

filterable virus *also* **filtrable virus** *n* : any of the infectious agents that pass through a filter esp. of diatomite or unglazed porcelain with the filtrate and remain virulent and that include the viruses as presently understood and various other groups (as the mycoplasmas and rickettsiae) which were orig. considered viruses before their cellular nature was established

filter paper \-ˌpā-pər\ *n* : porous unsized paper used esp. for filtering

¹**fil·trate** \'fil-ˌtrāt\ *vb* **fil·trat·ed; fil·trat·ing** : FILTER

²**filtrate** *n* : fluid that has passed through a filter

fil·tra·tion \fil-'trā-shən\ *n* **1** : the process of filtering **2** : the process of passing through or as if through a filter; *also* : DIFFUSION ⟨the kidney produces urine by ∼⟩

fi·lum \'fī-ləm\ *n, pl* **fi·la** \-lə\ : a filamentous structure : FILAMENT

fi·lum ter·mi·na·le \'fī-ləm-ˌtər-mə-'nā-(ˌ)lē, 'fē-ləm-ˌter-mə-'näl-ˌā\ *n, pl* **fi·la ter·mi·na·lia** \'fī-lə-tər-mə-'nā-lē-ə, 'fē-lə-ˌter-mə-'näl-ē-ə\ : the slender threadlike prolongation of the spinal cord below the origin of the lumbar nerves : the last portion of the pia mater

fim·bria \'fim-brē-ə\ *n, pl* **-bri·ae** \-brē-ˌē, -ˌī\ **1** : a bordering fringe esp. at the entrance of the fallopian tubes **2** : a band of nerve fibers bordering the hippocampus and joining the fornix **3** : a pilus of a bacterium — **fim·bri·al** \-brē-əl\ *adj*

fimbriata — see PLICA FIMBRIATA

fim·bri·at·ed \'fim-brē-ˌāt-əd\ *also* **fim·bri·ate** \-ˌāt\ *adj* : having the edge or extremity fringed or bordered by slender processes ⟨the ∼ ends of the fallopian tubes⟩

fi·nas·te·ride \fə-'nas-tə-ˌrīd\ *n* : a nitrogenous steroid derivative $C_{23}H_{36}N_2O_2$ that is used esp. to treat symptoms of benign prostatic hyperplasia and to increase hair growth in male-pattern baldness and that acts by inhibiting the enzymatic conversion of testosterone to dihydrotestosterone — see PROPECIA, PROSCAR

fine \'fīn\ *adj* **fin·er; fin·est** *of bodily tremors* : of slight excursion

fine needle *n* : a long thin hollow needle with a narrow bore used esp. to obtain samples by fine needle aspiration; *also* : a solid hairlike needle used in acupuncture

fine needle aspiration *n* : the process of obtaining a sample of cells and bits of tissue for examination by applying suction through a fine needle attached to a syringe — abbr. *FNA*; compare CORE BIOPSY

fine structure *n* : microscopic structure of a biological entity or one of its parts esp. as studied in preparations for the electron microscope — **fine structural** *adj*

fin·ger \'fiŋ-gər\ *n* : any of the five terminating members of the hand : a digit of the forelimb; *esp* : one other than the thumb

fin·gered \'fiŋ-gərd\ *adj* : having fingers esp. of a specified kind or number — used in combination ⟨stubby-*fingered*⟩

finger fracture *n* : valvulotomy of the mitral commissures performed by a finger thrust through the valve — compare DISSECTION 1b

fin·ger·nail \'fiŋ-gər-ˌnāl, ˌfiŋ-gər-'nā(ə)l\ *n* : the nail of a finger

¹**fin·ger·print** \-ˌprint\ *n* **1** : the impression of a fingertip on any surface; *esp* : an ink impression of the lines on the fingertip taken for purpose of identification **2** : analytical evidence (as a spectrogram) that characterizes an object or substance; *esp* : the chromatogram or electrophoretogram obtained by cleaving a protein by enzymatic action and subjecting the resulting collection of peptides to two-dimensional chromatography or electrophoresis — compare DNA FINGERPRINTING

²**fingerprint** *vt* : to analyze (as spectrographically or chromatographically) in order to determine uniquely the identifying characteristics, origin, or constitution of ⟨each protein was ∼ed⟩ — **fin·ger·print·ing** *n*

finger spelling *n* : the representation of individual letters and numbers using standardized finger positions

fin·ger·stall \-ˌstȯl\ *n* : ¹COT

finger–stick \-ˌstik\ *adj* : relating to or being a blood test for which blood is obtained by a finger stick ⟨a ∼ test for blood sugar⟩

finger stick \-ˌstik\ *n* : an instance of pricking the skin of a finger to obtain blood from a capillary

fin·ger·tip \-ˌtip\ *n* : the tip of a finger

FIP *abbr* feline infectious peritonitis

fir \ˈfər\ *n* : any tree of the genus *Abies* — see BALSAM FIR

¹**fire** \ˈfī(ə)r\ *n, often attrib* : fever or inflammation esp. from a disease

²**fire** *vb* **fired; fir·ing** *vt* **1** : to cause to transmit a nerve impulse **2** : to sear (the leg of a horse) with a hot iron in order to convert a crippling chronic inflammation into an acute inflammation that will stimulate the natural healing responses of the body ∼ *vi* : to transmit a nerve impulse ⟨the rate at which a neuron ∼s⟩

fire ant \-ˌant\ *n* : any ant of the genus *Solenopsis*; *esp* : IMPORTED FIRE ANT

fire coral \-ˈkȯr-əl, -ˈkär-\ *n* : a colonial hydrozoan (genus *Millepora*) resembling coral and having nematocysts that inflict a painful and burning sting

fire·damp \-ˌdamp\ *n* : a combustible mine gas that consists chiefly of methane; *also* : the explosive mixture of this gas with air — compare BLACK DAMP

first aid \ˌfərst-ˈād\ *n* : emergency care or treatment given to an ill or injured person before regular medical aid can be obtained

first cranial nerve *n* : OLFACTORY NERVE

first–degree \ˈfərst-di-ˈgrē\ *adj* : of the lowest or mildest in a series of categories ⟨a ∼ laceration⟩

first–degree burn *n* : a mild burn characterized by heat, pain, and reddening of the burned surface but not exhibiting blistering or charring of tissues

first filial generation *n* : F₁ GENERATION

first generation hybrid *n* : F₁ HYBRID

first intention *n* : the healing of an incised wound by the direct union of skin edges without granulations — compare SECOND INTENTION

first law of thermodynamics *n* : CONSERVATION OF ENERGY

first–line \ˈfərst-ˈlīn\ *adj* : being the preferred, standard, or first choice ⟨∼ treatment of advanced breast cancer⟩ — compare SECOND-LINE

first messenger *n* : an extracellular substance (as the hormone epinephrine or the neurotransmitter serotonin) that binds to a cell-surface receptor and initiates intracellular activity — compare SECOND MESSENGER

first polar body *n* : POLAR BODY a

fish–liv·er oil \ˈfish-ˌliv-ər-\ *n* : a fatty oil from the livers of various fishes (as cod, halibut, or sharks) used chiefly as a source of vitamin A and formerly also of vitamin D — compare COD-LIVER OIL

fish protein concentrate *n* : a protein-rich food additive obtained as a nearly colorless and tasteless powder from ground whole fish — abbr. FPC

fish·skin disease \-ˌskin-\ *n* : ICHTHYOSIS

fish tapeworm *n* : a large tapeworm of the genus *Diphyllobothrium* (*D. latum*) that as an adult infests the human intes-tine, is sometimes associated with a peculiar macrocytic anemia resembling pernicious anemia, and goes through its early stages in copepods of the genus *Diaptomus* and intermediate stages in freshwater fishes from which it is transmitted to humans or other fish-eating mammals when raw fish is eaten

fis·sion \ˈfish-ən *also* ˈfizh-\ *n* **1** : a method of reproduction in which a living cell or body divides into two or more parts each of which grows into a whole new individual **2 a** : CLEAVAGE **2 b** : the splitting of an atomic nucleus resulting in the release of large amounts of energy — called also *nuclear fission* — **fis·sion** *vb* **fis·sioned; fis·sion·ing** \ˈfish-(ə-)niŋ *also* ˈfizh-\ — **fis·sion·al** \ˈfish-ən-əl *also* ˈfizh-\ *adj*

fis·sion·able \ˈfish-(ə-)nə-bəl, ˈfizh-\ *adj* : capable of undergoing fission and esp. atomic fission

fis·sip·a·rous \fis-ˈip-ə-rəs\ *adj* : producing new biological units or individuals by fission

Fis·sip·e·da \fis-ˈip-ə-də\ *n pl* : a suborder of the order Carnivora that includes recent land carnivores and extinct related forms — **fis·si·ped** \ˈfis-ə-ˌped\ *adj or n*

fis·su·ra \fi-ˈs(h)ů-rə, *Brit also* fi-ˈs(h)yů-rə\ *n, pl* **fis·su·rae** \-ˌrē, -ˌrī\ : FISSURE 1

fis·sur·al \ˈfish-ə-rəl, *Brit also* ˈfis(h)-yůr-əl\ *adj* : of or relating to a fissure

fis·su·ra·tion \ˌfish-ə-ˈrā-shən, *Brit also* ˌfish-yů-ˈrā-\ *n* : the state of being fissured or having fissures ⟨brain ∼⟩

fis·sure \ˈfish-ər, *Brit also* ˈfish-yůr\ *n* **1** : a natural cleft between body parts or in the substance of an organ: as **a** : any of several clefts separating the lobes of the liver **b** : any of various clefts between bones or parts of bones in the skull **c** : any of the deep clefts of the brain; *esp* : one of those located at points of elevation in the walls of the ventricles — compare SULCUS **d** : ANTERIOR MEDIAN FISSURE; *also* : POSTERIOR MEDIAN SEPTUM **2** : a break or slit in tissue usu. at the junction of skin and mucous membrane ⟨∼ of the lip⟩ **3** : a linear developmental imperfection in the enamel of a tooth — **fis·sured** \ˈfish-ərd, *Brit also* ˈfish-yůrd\ *adj*

fissure of Ro·lan·do \-rō-ˈlan-(ˌ)dō, -ˈlän-\ *n* : CENTRAL SULCUS

Rolando, Luigi (1773–1831), Italian anatomist and physiologist. Rolando did his early research on the anatomy and physiology of the nervous system in humans and animals, using comparative methods. His most important studies, however, concerned the anatomy, physiology, and embryology of the brain. He paid particular interest to the gray matter. He was the first to investigate the functions of the cerebellum. In an 1824 report on the brain he described the motor area in the cerebral cortex comprising both the precentral and the postcentral gyri. This area is now known as the Rolandic area. In 1825 he published his observations on the cerebellum. One of the features described was a fissure between the parietal and frontal lobes. This is now often called the fissure of Rolando.

fissure of Syl·vi·us \-ˈsil-vē-əs\ *n* : SYLVIAN FISSURE

fist \ˈfist\ *n* : the hand clenched with the fingers doubled into the palm and the thumb doubled inward across the fingers

fis·tu·la \ˈfis(h)-chə-lə, *Brit also* ˈfis-tyů-lə\ *n, pl* **-las** *or* **-lae** \-lē *also* -lī\ **1** : an abnormal passage that leads from an abscess or hollow organ or part to the body surface or from one hollow organ or part to another and that may be surgically created to permit passage of fluids or secretions ⟨a congenital tracheoesophageal ∼⟩ ⟨an arteriovenous ∼ was reconstructed in the right arm for dialysis —Pasteur Rasuli *et al*⟩ **2** : FISTULOUS WITHERS

fistula — see CASSIA FISTULA

fis·tu·lat·ed \-ˌlāt-əd\ *adj* : having a fistula; *esp* : having an artificial fistula ⟨study the digestive process in ∼ cows⟩

fis·tu·lec·to·my \ˌfis(h)-chə-ˈlek-tə-mē, *Brit also* ˌfist-yů-\ *n, pl* **-mies** : surgical excision of a fistula

---

\ə\ **abut** \ᵊ\ **kitten** \ər\ **further** \a\ **ash** \ā\ **ace** \ä\ **cot, cart** \aů\ **out** \ch\ **chin** \e\ **bet** \ē\ **easy** \g\ **go** \i\ **hit** \ī\ **ice** \j\ **job** \ŋ\ **sing** \ō\ **go** \ȯ\ **law** \ȯi\ **boy** \th\ **thin** \t̲h̲\ **the** \ü\ **loot** \ů\ **foot** \y\ **yet** \zh\ **vision** *See also* Pronunciation Symbols page

fis·tu·li·za·tion \-lə-ʹzā-shən, -ˌlī-\ *n* **1** : the condition of having a fistula **2** : surgical production of an artificial channel

fis·tu·lous \-ləs\ *adj* : of, relating to, or having the form or nature of a fistula

fistulous withers *n pl but usu sing in constr* : a deep-seated chronic inflammation of the withers of the horse that discharges seropurulent or bloody fluid through one or more openings and is prob. associated with infection by bacteria of the genus *Brucella* (esp. *B. abortus*)

¹**fit** \ʹfit\ *n* **1** : a sudden violent attack of a disease (as epilepsy) esp. when marked by convulsions or unconsciousness : PAROXYSM **2** : a sudden but transient attack of a physical disturbance ⟨~s of shivering⟩

²**fit** *adj* **fit·ter; fit·test** **1** : adapted to the environment so as to be capable of surviving **2** : sound physically and mentally : HEALTHY — **fit·ness** *n*

³**fit** *n* : the fact, condition, or manner of being fitted or adapted

fit·ness \ʹfit-nəs\ *n* : the capacity of an organism to survive and transmit its genotype to reproductively fertile offspring as compared to competing organisms; *also* : the contribution of an allele or genotype to the gene pool of subsequent generations as compared to that of other alleles or genotypes

¹**fix** \ʹfiks\ *vt* **1 a** : to make firm, stable, or stationary **b** : to give a permanent or final form to: as **(1)** : to change into a stable compound or available form ⟨bacteria that ~ nitrogen⟩ **(2)** : to kill, harden, and preserve for microscopic study **2** : to hold or direct steadily ⟨~es her eyes on the horizon⟩ **3 a** : RESTORE, CURE ⟨the doctor ~ed him up⟩ **b** : SPAY, CASTRATE **1** ~ *vi* : to direct the gaze or attention : FOCUS, FIXATE — often used with *on* or *upon*

²**fix** *n* : a shot of a narcotic

fix·ate \ʹfik-ˌsāt\ *vb* **fix·at·ed; fix·at·ing** *vt* **1** : to focus one's gaze on **2** : to direct (the libido) toward an infantile form of gratification ~ *vi* **1** : to focus or concentrate one's gaze or attention ⟨an infant with normal vision . . . will ~ on a light held before him —*Jour. Amer. Med. Assoc.*⟩ **2** : to undergo arrestment at a stage of development

fix·at·ed *adj* : arrested in development or adjustment; *esp* : arrested at a pregenital level of psychosexual development

fix·a·tion \fik-ʹsā-shən\ *n* **1** : the act, process, or result of fixing, fixating, or becoming fixated: as **a** : the act or an instance of focusing the eyes upon an object **b** : a persistent concentration of libidinal energies upon objects characteristic of psychosexual stages of development preceding the genital stage **c** : stereotyped behavior (as in response to frustration) **d** : an obsessive or unhealthy preoccupation or attachment **2** : the immobilization of the parts of a fractured bone esp. by the use of various metal attachments

fixation point *n* : the point in the visual field that is fixated by the two eyes in normal vision and for each eye is the point that directly stimulates the fovea of the retina

fix·a·tive \ʹfik-sət-iv\ *n* : a substance used to fix living tissue

fix·a·tor \ʹfik-ˌsā-tər\ *n* : a muscle that stabilizes or fixes a part of the body to which a muscle in the process of moving another part is attached

fixed cell *n* : a usu. large, irregular, and branching phagocytic cell existing in certain tissues (as connective tissue), lymph nodes, or spleen but sometimes becoming ameboid and moving through the tissues

fixed idea *n* : IDÉE FIXE

fixed oil *n* : a nonvolatile oil; *esp* : FATTY OIL — compare ESSENTIAL OIL

fixed virus *n* : a virus made constant in its reactions by repeated passage through a host other than the usual host

fl *abbr* fluid

FL *abbr* focal length

flab \ʹflab\ *n* : soft flabby body tissue

flab·by \ʹflab-ē\ *adj* **flab·bi·er; -est** : lacking resilience or firmness : FLACCID — **flab·bi·ness** \ʹflab-ē-nəs\ *n*

flac·cid \ʹflas-əd, ʹflak-səd\ *adj* : not firm or stiff; *also* : lacking normal or youthful firmness ⟨~ muscles⟩ — **flac·cid·i·ty** \fla(k)-ʹsid-ət-ē\ *n*, *pl* **-ties**

flaccid paralysis *n* : paralysis in which muscle tone is lacking in the affected muscles and in which tendon reflexes are decreased or absent

flagella *pl of* FLAGELLUM

fla·gel·lant \ʹflaj-ə-lənt, flə-ʹjel-ənt\ *n* : a person who responds sexually to being beaten by or to beating another flagellant person — **flagellant** *adj* — **fla·gel·lant·ism** \-ˌiz-əm\ *n*

fla·gel·lar \flə-ʹjel-ər, ʹflaj-ə-lər\ *adj* : of or relating to a flagellum

flagellar antigen *n* : H ANTIGEN

Flag·el·la·ta \ˌflaj-ə-ʹlät-ə, -ʹlāt-ə\ *n pl, syn of* MASTIGOPHORA

¹**fla·gel·late** \ʹflaj-ə-lət, -ˌlāt; flə-ʹjel-ət\ *adj* **1 a** *or* **flag·el·lat·ed** \ʹflaj-ə-ˌlāt-əd\ : having flagella **b** : shaped like a flagellum **2** : of, relating to, or caused by flagellates ⟨~ diarrhea⟩

²**flagellate** *n* : a flagellate protozoan or alga

¹**flag·el·la·tion** \ˌflaj-ə-ʹlā-shən\ *n* : the practice of a flagellant

²**flagellation** *n* : the formation or arrangement of flagella

fla·gel·li·form \flə-ʹjel-ə-ˌfȯrm\ *adj* : elongated, slender, and tapering like a flagellum ⟨~ ends of a microorganism⟩

fla·gel·lin \flə-ʹjel-ən\ *n* : a polymeric protein that is the chief constituent of bacterial flagella, that forms helical chains around the hollow core of the flagellar filament, that determines the specificity of the flagellum in eliciting an immune response by its amino acid sequence, and that within any one serogroup can vary between two antigenic states by switching between the expression of two different genes

flag·el·lo·sis \ˌflaj-ə-ʹlō-səs\ *n, pl* **-lo·ses** \-ˌsēz\ : infestation with or disease caused by flagellate protozoans

fla·gel·lum \flə-ʹjel-əm\ *n, pl* **-la** \-ə\ *also* **-lums** : a long tapering process that projects singly or in groups from a cell and is the primary organ of motion of many microorganisms

Flag·yl \ʹflag-əl\ *trademark* — used for a preparation of metronidazole

flail \ʹflā(ə)l\ *adj* : exhibiting abnormal mobility and loss of response to normal controls — used of body parts damaged by paralysis, injury, or surgery ⟨~ joint⟩

flame \ʹflām\ *vt* **flamed; flam·ing** : to cleanse or sterilize by fire

flame cell *n* : a hollow cell that has a tuft of vibratile cilia and is part of the excretory system of various lower invertebrates (as a flatworm)

flame photometer *n* : a spectrophotometer in which a spray of metallic salts in solution is vaporized in a very hot flame and subjected to quantitative analysis by measuring the intensities of the spectral lines of the metals present — **flame photometric** *adj* — **flame photometry** *n*

flammeus — see NEVUS FLAMMEUS

flank \ʹflaŋk\ *n* : the fleshy part of the side between the ribs and the hip; *broadly* : the side of a quadruped

flap \ʹflap\ *n* : a piece of tissue partly severed from its place of origin for use in surgical grafting

¹**flare** \ʹfla(ə)r, ʹfle(ə)r\ *vi* **flared; flar·ing** : to break out or intensify rapidly : become suddenly worse or more painful — often used with *up* ⟨your gallstones ~ up —W. A. Nolen⟩

²**flare** *n* **1** : a sudden outburst or worsening of a disease ⟨acute ~s in rheumatoid arthritis —*Emergency Medicine*⟩ — see FLARE-UP **2** : an area of skin flush resulting from and spreading out from a local center of vascular dilation and hyperemia ⟨urticarial ~⟩ **3** : the presence of floating particles in the fluid of the anterior chamber of the eye — called also *aqueous flare*

flare–up \-ˌəp\ *n* : a sudden increase in the symptoms of a latent or subsiding disease ⟨a ~ of malaria⟩

flash \ʹflash\ *n* : RUSH 2 — compare HOT FLASH

¹**flask** \ʹflask\ *n* : a container often somewhat narrowed toward the outlet and often fitted with a closure: as **a** : any of various usu. blown-glass vessels used for technical purposes in a laboratory **b** : a metal container in which the materials used to form a dental restoration (as a denture) are processed

²**flask** *vt* : to place (a denture) in a flask for processing

flat \ʹflat\ *adj* **flat·ter; flat·test** **1** : being or characterized by a horizontal line or tracing without peaks or depressions ⟨the EEG is ominously ∼ indicating that her brain function is gone —Don Gold⟩ **2 :** characterized by general impoverishment in the presence of emotion-evoking stimuli ⟨∼ affect often occurs in schizophrenia⟩ — **flat·ness** n

flat bone n : any of various bones (as of the skull, the jaw, the pelvis, or the rib cage) not rounded in cross section

flat·foot \-ˌfu̇t, -ˌfu̇t\ n, pl **flat·feet** \-ˌfēt, -ˌfēt\ **1 :** a condition in which the arch of the instep is flattened so that the entire sole rests upon the ground **2 :** a foot affected with flatfoot

flat–foot·ed \-ˈfu̇t-əd\ adj : affected with flatfoot; broadly : walking with a dragging or shambling gait — **flat–foot·ed·ly** adv — **flat–foot·ed·ness** n

flat plate n : a radiograph esp. of the abdomen taken with the subject lying flat

flat·u·lence \ˈflach-ə-lən(t)s\ n : the quality or state of being flatulent

flat·u·lent \-lənt\ adj **1 :** marked by or affected with gases generated in the intestine or stomach **2 :** likely to cause digestive flatulence — **flat·u·lent·ly** adv

fla·tus \ˈflāt-əs\ n : gas generated in the stomach or bowels

flat wart n : a small smooth slightly elevated wart found esp. on the face and back of the hands and that occurs chiefly in children and adolescents — called also plane wart, verruca plana

flat·worm \ˈflat-ˌwərm\ n : any worm of the phylum Platyhelminthes ; PLATYHELMINTH; esp : TURBELLARIAN

flava — see CERA FLAVA

fla·va·none \ˈflā-və-ˌnōn\ n : a colorless crystalline ketone $C_{15}H_{12}O_2$; also : any of the derivatives of this ketone many of which occur in plants often in the form of glycosides

fla·vi·an·ic acid \ˌflā-vē-ˌan-ik-, ˌflav-ē-\ n : a yellow crystalline acid $C_{10}H_6N_2O_8S$ used chiefly in precipitating arginine, tyrosine, or organic bases as insoluble salts

fla·vin \ˈflā-vən\ n : any of a class of yellow water-soluble nitrogenous pigments derived from isoalloxazine and occurring in the form of nucleotides as coenzymes of flavoproteins : PLATYHELMINTH; esp : RIBOFLAVIN

flavin adenine dinucleotide n : a coenzyme $C_{27}H_{33}N_9O_{15}P_2$ of some flavoproteins — called also FAD

fla·vine \ˈflā-ˌvēn\ n : any of a series of yellow acridine dyes (as acriflavine) often used medicinally for their antiseptic properties

flavin mononucleotide n : FMN

Fla·vi·vi·ri·dae \ˌflā-vi-ˈvir-ə-ˌdē\ n pl : a family of single=stranded RNA viruses that have a spherical virion with a capsid composed of a single protein and a lipid envelope containing two or three proteins and that include members of the genus Flavivirus transmitted by ticks and mosquitoes, the causative agents of bovine viral diarrhea and hog cholera transmitted by direct or indirect contact esp. with bodily secretions, and the causative agent of hepatitis C transmitted by contact with contaminated blood or blood products — see PESTIVIRUS

fla·vi·vi·rus \ˈflā-vi-ˌvī-rəs\ n **1** cap : a genus of the family Flaviviridae of single-stranded RNA viruses that are transmitted by arthropod vectors and esp. by ticks and mosquitoes and that include the causative agents of dengue, Japanese B encephalitis, Saint Louis encephalitis, West Nile fever, and yellow fever **2 :** any virus of the family Flaviviridae

Fla·vo·bac·te·ri·um \ˌflā-(ˌ)vō-bak-ˈtir-ē-əm, ˌflav-(ˌ)ō-\ n : a genus of nonmotile aerobic gram-negative usu. rod-shaped bacteria found esp. in soil and water including one (F. meningosepticum) that is found as a contaminant in hospitals and is associated with meningitis and septicemia esp. in newborn infants

fla·vone \ˈflā-ˌvōn\ n : a colorless crystalline ketone $C_{15}H_{10}O_2$ found in the leaves, stems, and seed capsules of many primroses; also : any of the derivatives of this ketone many of which occur as yellow plant pigments in the form of glycosides and are used as dyestuffs

¹fla·vo·noid \ˈflāv-ə-ˌnȯid, ˈflav-\ adj : of, relating to, or being a flavonoid

²flavonoid n : any of a group of aromatic compounds that have two substituted benzene rings connected by a chain of three carbon atoms and an oxygen bridge and that include many common pigments

fla·vo·nol \-ˌnȯl, -ˌnōl\ n : any of various hydroxy derivatives of flavone

fla·vo·pro·tein \ˌflāv-ō-ˈprō-ˌtēn, ˌflav-, -ˈprōt-ē-ən\ n : a dehydrogenase that contains a flavin and often a metal and plays a major role in biological oxidations

¹fla·vor or chiefly Brit **fla·vour** \ˈflā-vər\ n **1 a :** the quality of something that affects the sense of taste ⟨condiments give ∼ to food⟩ **b :** the blend of taste and smell sensations evoked by a substance in the mouth ⟨the ∼ of ripe fruit⟩ **2 :** a substance that flavors — **fla·vored** or chiefly Brit **fla·voured** \-vərd\ adj

²flavor or chiefly Brit **fla·vour** vt **fla·vored** or chiefly Brit **fla·voured; fla·vor·ing** or chiefly Brit **fla·vour·ing** \ˈflāv-(ə-)riŋ\ : to give or add flavor to

flavum — see LIGAMENTUM FLAVUM

flax·seed \ˈflak(s)-ˌsēd\ n : the small seed of flax (esp. Linum usitatissimum) used esp. as a source of oil, as a demulcent and emollient in treating inflammatory conditions of the respiratory, intestinal, and urinary passages, and as a dietary supplement — called also linseed

flea \ˈflē\ n : any of the order Siphonaptera comprising wingless bloodsucking insects that have a hard laterally compressed body and legs adapted to leaping and that feed on warm-blooded animals — see CAT FLEA, CHIGOE 1, DOG FLEA, RAT FLEA, SAND FLEA, STICKTIGHT FLEA

flea·bite \-ˌbīt\ n : the bite of a flea; also : the red spot caused by such a bite

flea–bit·ten \-ˌbit-ᵊn\ adj : bitten by or infested with fleas

flea col·lar \-ˌkäl-ər\ n : a collar for animals that contains insecticide for killing fleas

fleam \ˈflēm\ n : a sharp lancet formerly used for bloodletting

flea·seed \ˈflē-ˌsēd\ n : PSYLLIUM SEED

flea·wort \-ˌwərt, -ˌwȯ(ə)rt\ n : any of three Old World plantains of the genus Plantago (esp. P. psyllium) that are the source of psyllium seed — called also psyllium

fle·cai·nide \ˌfle-ˈkā-ˌnīd\ n : an antiarrhythmic drug administered in the form of its acetate $C_{17}H_{20}F_6N_2O_3 \cdot C_2H_4O_2$ esp. to treat serious ventricular arrhythmias

flection var of FLEXION

flesh \ˈflesh\ n : the soft parts of the body of an animal and esp. of a vertebrate; esp : the parts composed chiefly of skeletal muscle as distinguished from visceral structures, bone, and integuments — see GOOSE BUMPS, PROUD FLESH — **fleshed** \ˈflesht\ adj

flesh fly n : a dipteran fly whose maggots feed on flesh; esp : any of the family Sarcophagidae of flies some of which cause myiasis

flesh wound n : an injury involving penetration of the body musculature without damage to bones or internal organs

fleshy \ˈflesh-ē\ adj **flesh·i·er; -est** : marked by abundant flesh; esp : CORPULENT

Fletch·er·ism \ˈflech-ər-ˌiz-əm\ n : the practice of eating in small amounts and only when hungry and of chewing one's food thoroughly

Fletcher, Horace (1849–1919), American dietitian. Fletcher was plagued by obesity and indigestion most of his life. Then in 1895 he set out to find the key to good health. He developed a set of principles which he proceeded to propagate. The basic tenets were these: one should eat only when genuinely hungry and never when anxious, depressed, or otherwise preoccupied; one may eat any food that appeals to the appetite; one should chew each mouthful of food 32 times or, ideally, until the food liquefies; one should enjoy one's food.

E

F

\ə\ abut \ᵊ\ kitten \ər\ further \a\ ash \ā\ ace \ä\ cot, cart
\au̇\ out \ch\ chin \e\ bet \ē\ easy \g\ go \i\ hit \ī\ ice \j\ job
\ŋ\ sing \ō\ go \ȯ\ law \ȯi\ boy \th\ thin \th\ the \ü\ loot
\u̇\ foot \y\ yet \zh\ vision See also Pronunciation Symbols page

Fletch·er·ite \-ˌīt\ *n* : a believer in or practicer of Fletcherism

fletch·er·ize *or Brit* **fletch·er·ise** \-ˌīz\ *vt* **-ized** *or Brit* **-ised; -iz·ing** *or Brit* **-is·ing** : to reduce (food) to tiny particles esp. by prolonged chewing

flews \ˈflüz\ *n pl* : the pendulous lateral parts of a dog's upper lip

flex \ˈfleks\ *vt* **1** : to bend esp. repeatedly **2 a** : to move muscles so as to cause flexion of (a joint) ⟨stretching and ~ing his knees⟩ **b** : to move or tense (a muscle or muscles) by contraction ⟨~ed their biceps⟩

flexibilitas — see CEREA FLEXIBILITAS

flex·i·ble \ˈflek-sə-bəl\ *adj* : capable of being flexed : capable of being turned, bowed, or twisted without breaking ⟨~ bandages⟩ ⟨a ~ fiber-optic bronchoscope⟩ — **flex·i·bil·i·ty** \ˌflek-sə-ˈbil-ət-ē\ *n, pl* **-ties**

flex·ion *also* **flec·tion** \ˈflek-shən\ *n* **1** : a bending movement around a joint in a limb (as the knee or elbow) that decreases the angle between the bones of the limb at the joint — compare EXTENSION 2 **2** : a forward raising of the arm or leg by a movement at the shoulder or hip joint

flex·or \ˈflek-sər, -ˌsȯ(ə)r\ *n* : a muscle serving to bend a body part (as a limb) — called also *flexor muscle;* compare EXTENSOR

flexor car·pi ra·di·al·is \-ˈkär-ˌpī-ˌrā-dē-ˈā-ləs, -ˈkär-ˌpē-\ *n* : a superficial muscle of the palmar side of the forearm that flexes the hand and assists in abducting it

flexor carpi ul·nar·is \-ˌəl-ˈnar-əs\ *n* : a superficial muscle of the ulnar side of the forearm that flexes the hand and assists in adducting it

flexor dig·i·ti min·i·mi brev·is \-ˈdij-ə-ˌtī-ˈmin-ə-ˌmī-ˈbrev-əs, -ˈdij-ə-ˌtē-ˈmin-ə-ˌmē-\ *n* **1** : a muscle of the ulnar side of the palm of the hand that flexes the little finger **2** : a muscle of the sole of the foot that flexes the first proximal phalanx of the little toe

flexor dig·i·to·rum brevis \-ˌdij-ə-ˈtōr-əm-\ *n* : a muscle of the middle part of the sole of the foot that flexes the second phalanx of each of the four small toes

flexor digitorum lon·gus \-ˈlȯŋ-gəs\ *n* : a muscle of the tibial side of the leg that flexes the terminal phalanx of each of the four small toes

flexor digitorum pro·fund·us \-prō-ˈfən-dəs\ *n* : a deep muscle of the ulnar side of the forearm that flexes esp. the terminal phalanges of the four fingers

flexor digitorum su·per·fi·ci·al·is \-ˌsü-pər-ˌfish-ē-ˈā-ləs\ *n* : a superficial muscle of the palmar side of the forearm that flexes esp. the second phalanges of the four fingers

flexor hal·lu·cis brev·is \-ˈhal-(y)ü-səs-ˈbrev-əs, -ˈhal-ə-kəs-\ *n* : a short muscle of the sole of the foot that flexes the proximal phalanx of the big toe

flexor hallucis longus *n* : a long deep muscle of the fibular side of the leg that flexes esp. the second phalanx of the big toe

flexor muscle *n* : FLEXOR

flexor pol·li·cis brevis \-ˈpäl-ə-səs-, -ˈpäl-ə-kəs-\ *n* : a short muscle of the palm that flexes and adducts the thumb

flexor pollicis longus *n* : a muscle of the radial side of the forearm that flexes esp. the second phalanx of the thumb

flexor ret·in·ac·u·lum \-ˌret-ᵊn-ˈak-yə-ləm\ *n* **1** : a fibrous band of fascia on the medial side of the ankle that extends downward from the medial malleolus of the tibia to the calcaneus and that covers over the bony grooves containing the tendons of the flexor muscles, the posterior tibial artery and vein, and the tibial nerve as they pass into the sole of the foot **2** : a fibrous band of fascia on the palm side of the wrist and base of the hand that forms the roof of the carpal tunnel and covers the tendons of the flexor muscles and the median nerve as they pass into the hand — called also *transverse carpal ligament*

flex·u·ous \ˈfleksh-(ə-)wəs\ *adj* : lacking rigidity in structure or action ⟨~ filamentous virus particles —M. Hema *et al*⟩

flex·ure \ˈflek-shər\ *n* **1** : the quality or state of being flexed : FLEXION **2** : an anatomical turn, bend, or fold; *esp* : one of three sharp bends of the anterior part of the primary axis

of the vertebrate embryo that serve to establish the relationship of the parts of the developing brain — see CEPHALIC FLEXURE, CERVICAL FLEXURE, HEPATIC FLEXURE, PONTINE FLEXURE, SIGMOID FLEXURE, SPLENIC FLEXURE — **flex·ur·al** \-shər-əl\ *adj*

flick·er \ˈflik-ər\ *n* : the wavering or fluttering visual sensation produced by intermittent light when the interval between flashes is not small enough to produce complete fusion of the individual impressions

flicker fusion *n* : FUSION 2c(2)

flight of ideas \ˌflīt-əv-(ˌ)ī-ˈdē-əz\ *n* : a rapid shifting of ideas with only superficial associative connections between them that is expressed as a disconnected rambling from subject to subject and occurs esp. in the manic phase of bipolar disorder

flight surgeon *n* : a medical officer (as in the U.S. Air Force) qualified by additional training for specialization in the psychological and medical problems associated with flying

float·er \ˈflōt-ər\ *n* : a bit of optical debris (as a dead cell or cell fragment) in the vitreous body or lens that may be perceived as a spot before the eye; *also* : a spot in the visual field due to such debris — usu. used in pl.; compare MUSCAE VOLITANTES

float·ing \ˈflōt-iŋ\ *adj* : located out of the normal position or abnormally movable ⟨a ~ kidney⟩

floating rib *n* : any rib in the last two pairs of human ribs that have no attachment to the sternum — compare FALSE RIB

¹**floc** \ˈfläk\ *n* : a flocculent mass formed by the aggregation of a number of fine suspended particles

²**floc** *vb* **flocced** \ˈfläkt\; **floc·cing** \ˈfläk-iŋ\ *vi* : to aggregate into flocs ~ *vt* : to cause to floc

floc·cil·la·tion \ˌfläk-sə-ˈlā-shən\ *n* : CARPHOLOGY

floc·cu·lar \ˈfläk-yə-lər\ *adj* : of or relating to a flocculus

¹**floc·cu·late** \ˈfläk-yə-ˌlāt\ *vb* **-lat·ed; -lat·ing** *vt* : to cause to aggregate into a flocculent mass ⟨denature and ~ cell proteins⟩ ~ *vi* : to become flocculated — **floc·cu·la·tion** \ˌfläk-yə-ˈlā-shən\ *n*

²**floc·cu·late** \-lət, -ˌlāt\ *n* : something that has flocculated

flocculation test *n* : any of various serological tests (as the Mazzini test for syphilis) in which a positive result depends on the combination of an antigen and antibody to produce a flocculent precipitate

floc·cule \ˈfläk-(ˌ)yü(ə)l\ *n* : a small loosely aggregated bit of material suspended in or precipitated from a liquid

floc·cu·lent \-yə-lənt\ *adj* : made up of loosely aggregated particles ⟨a ~ precipitate⟩

floc·cu·lo·nod·u·lar lobe \ˌfläk-yə-(ˌ)lō-ˈnäj-ə-lər-\ *n* : the posterior lobe of the cerebellum that consists of the nodulus and paired lateral flocculi and is concerned with equilibrium

floc·cu·lus \-ləs\ *n, pl* **-li** \-ˌlī, -ˌlē\ : a small irregular lobe on the undersurface of each hemisphere of the cerebellum that is linked with the corresponding side of the nodulus by a peduncle

Flo·max \ˈflō-ˌmaks\ *trademark* — used for a preparation of the hydrochloride of tamsulosin

Flo·nase \ˈflō-ˌnās\ *trademark* — used for a preparation of fluticasone propionate administered as a nasal spray

flood \ˈfləd\ *vi* : to have an excessive menstrual flow or a uterine hemorrhage after childbirth

flood·ing \ˈfləd-iŋ\ *n* : exposure therapy in which there is prolonged confrontation with an anxiety-provoking stimulus

floor \ˈflō(ə)r, ˈflȯ(ə)r\ *n* : the lower inside surface of a hollow anatomical structure ⟨the ~ of the pelvis⟩

flo·ra \ˈflōr-ə, ˈflȯr-\ *n, pl* **floras** *also* **flo·rae** \ˈflō(ə)r-ˌē, ˈflȯ(ə)r-, -ˌī\ **1** : plant life; *esp* : the plants characteristic of a region, period, or special environment ⟨fossil ~⟩ — compare FAUNA **2** : the microorganisms (as bacteria or fungi) living in or on the body ⟨the beneficial ~ of the intestine⟩ ⟨potentially harmful skin ~⟩ — **flo·ral** \ˈflōr-əl, ˈflȯr-\ *adj*

Flor·ence flask \ˌflȯr-ən(t)s-, ˌflär-\ *n* : a round usu. flat-bottomed laboratory vessel with a long neck

flor·id \ˈflȯr-əd, ˈflär-\ *adj* : fully developed : manifesting a complete and typical clinical syndrome ⟨∼ schizophrenia⟩ ⟨∼ adolescent acne⟩ — **flor·id·ly** *adv*

¹floss \'fläs, 'flȯs\ *n* : DENTAL FLOSS

²floss *vt* : to use dental floss on (one's teeth) ⟨the correct way to ∼ your teeth⟩ ∼ *vi* : to use dental floss ⟨∼*es* daily⟩

Flo·vent \'flō-ˌvent\ *trademark* — used for a preparation of fluticasone propionate administered as an oral inhalant

¹flow \'flō\ *vi* **1** : to move with a continual change of place among the constituent particles ⟨blood ∼*s* toward the heart in veins⟩ **2** : MENSTRUATE

²flow *n* **1** : the quantity that flows in a certain time **2** : MENSTRUATION **3** : the motion characteristic of fluids

flow cytometry *n* : a technique for identifying and sorting cells and their components (as DNA) by staining with a fluorescent dye and detecting the fluorescence usu. by laser beam illumination — **flow cytometer** *n*

flow·er·ing dogwood \'flau̇(-ə)r-iŋ-\ *n* : a common spring-flowering white-bracted dogwood of the genus *Cornus* (*C. florida*) the dried bark of whose root has been used as a mild astringent and stomachic

flow·ers \'flau̇(-ə)rz\ *n pl* : a finely divided powder produced esp. by condensation or sublimation

flowers of zinc *n pl* : zinc oxide esp. as obtained as a light white powder by burning zinc for use in pharmaceutical and cosmetic preparations

flow·me·ter \'flō-ˌmēt-ər\ *n* : an instrument for measuring the velocity of flow of a fluid (as blood) in a tube or pipe

fl oz *abbr* fluid ounce

flu \'flü\ *n* **1** : INFLUENZA **2** : any of several diseases caused by bacteria or viruses and marked esp. by respiratory or intestinal symptoms — see INTESTINAL FLU — **flu·like** \-ˌlīk\ *adj*

flu·con·a·zole \flü-'kän-ə-ˌzōl\ *n* : a triazole antifungal agent $C_{13}H_{12}F_2N_6O$ used orally to treat cryptococcal meningitis and local or systemic candida infections — see DIFLUCAN

fluc·tu·ant \'flək-chə-wənt\ *adj* : movable and compressible — used of abnormal body structures (as some abscesses or tumors) ⟨the ∼ mass in his abdomen —Oliver Sacks⟩

fluc·tu·a·tion \ˌflək-chə-'wā-shən\ *n* **1** : a motion like that of waves; *esp* : the wavelike motion of a fluid collected in a natural or artificial cavity of the body observed by palpation or percussion **2 a** : a slight and nonheritable variation; *esp* : such a variation occurring in response to environmental factors **b** : recurrent and often more or less cyclic alteration (as of form, size, or color of a bodily part) — **fluc·tu·ate** \'flək-chə-ˌwāt\ *vb* **-at·ed; -at·ing**

flu·cy·to·sine \ˌflü-'sīt-ə-ˌsēn\ *n* : a white crystalline drug $C_4H_4FN_3O$ that can be synthesized from fluorouracil and is used to treat fungal infections esp. by members of the genera *Candida* and *Cryptococcus* (esp. *Cryptococcus neoformans*)

flu·dar·a·bine \flü-'dar-ə-ˌbēn\ *n* : an antineoplastic agent that is an analog of vidarabine and is administered intravenously in the form of its phosphate $C_{10}H_{13}FN_5O_7P$ esp. in the treatment of chronic lymphocytic leukemia

flu·dro·cor·ti·sone \ˌflü-drō-'kȯrt-ə-ˌsōn, -ˌzōn\ *n* : a potent mineralocorticoid drug that is derived from cortisol, possesses some glucocorticoid activity, and is administered in the form of its acetate $C_{23}H_{31}FO_6$ to treat adrenocortical insufficiency

¹flu·id \'flü-əd\ *adj* : having particles that easily move and change their relative position without a separation of the mass and that easily yield to pressure : capable of flowing

²fluid *n* : a substance (as a liquid or gas) tending to flow or conform to the outline of its container; *specif* : one in the body of an animal or plant — see CEREBROSPINAL FLUID, SEMINAL FLUID

fluid dram *or* **flu·i·dram** \'flü-ə-ˌdram\ *n* : either of two units of liquid capacity: **a** : a U.S. unit equal to ⅛ U.S. fluid ounce or 0.226 cubic inch or 3.697 milliliters **b** : a British unit equal to ⅛ British fluid ounce or 0.2167 cubic inch or 3.5516 milliliters

flu·id·ex·tract \ˌflü-ə-'dek-ˌstrakt\ *n* : an alcohol preparation of a vegetable drug containing the active constituents of one gram of the dry drug in each milliliter

flu·id·glyc·er·ate \ˌflü-əd-'glis-ə-ˌrāt\ *n* : a concentrated liquid preparation made by extracting a vegetable drug with a menstruum consisting of one volume of glycerol and three volumes of water to produce a drug strength equivalent to that of a fluidextract

flu·id·i·ty \flü-'id-ət-ē\ *n, pl* **-ties** **1** : the quality or state of being fluid **2 a** : the physical property of a substance that enables it to flow **b** : the reciprocal of viscosity

fluid ounce *n* **1** : a U.S. unit of liquid capacity equal to 1/16 pint **2** : a British unit of liquid capacity equal to 1/20 pint

flu·idram *var of* FLUID DRAM

fluke \'flük\ *n* : a flattened digenetic trematode worm; *broadly* : TREMATODE — see LIVER FLUKE

flu·nis·o·lide \flü-'nis-ə-ˌlīd\ *n* : a synthetic glucocorticoid $C_{24}H_{31}FO_6\cdot\frac{1}{2}H_2O$ administered as an oral inhalant to treat bronchial asthma and as a nasal spray to treat rhinitis

flu·ni·traz·e·pam \ˌflü-nə-'traz-ə-ˌpam, -ˌnī-\ *n* : a powerful benzodiazepine sedative and hypnotic drug $C_{16}H_{12}FN_3O_3$ that is widely prescribed for medical use in Europe, Australia, and the Republic of South Africa but is not licensed for use in the U.S. and that is a frequent illicit drug of abuse — see ROHYPNOL

flu·o·cin·o·lone ac·e·to·nide \ˌflü-ə-'sin-ᵊl-ˌōn-\ *n* : a glucocorticoid steroid $C_{24}H_{30}F_2O_6$ used esp. as an anti-inflammatory agent in the treatment of skin diseases

flu·or \'flü-ˌȯ(ə)r, 'flü-ər\ *n* : a bodily discharge ⟨make a diagnosis of pathological ∼ —*Archives of Therapeutics*⟩

flu·o·resce \flu̇-'(ə)r-'es, flȯr-, flȯr-\ *vi* **-resced; -resc·ing** : to produce, undergo, or exhibit fluorescence

flu·o·res·ce·in \-'es-ē-ən\ *n* : a yellow or red crystalline dye $C_{20}H_{12}O_5$ with a bright yellow-green fluorescence in alkaline solution that is used as the sodium salt as an aid in diagnosis (as of lesions and foreign bodies in the cornea or of brain tumors)

flu·o·res·cence \-'es-ᵊn(t)s\ *n* : luminescence that is caused by the absorption of radiation at one wavelength followed by nearly immediate reradiation usu. at a different wavelength and that ceases almost immediately when the incident radiation stops; *also* : the radiation emitted — **flu·o·res·cent** \-'es-ᵊnt\ *adj*

fluorescence microscope *n* : ULTRAVIOLET MICROSCOPE

flu·o·ri·date \'flu̇r-ə-ˌdāt, 'flȯr-, 'flȯr-\ *vt* **-dat·ed; -dat·ing** : to add a fluoride to (as drinking water) to reduce tooth decay — **flu·o·ri·da·tion** \ˌflu̇r-ə-'dā-shən, ˌflȯr-, ˌflȯr-\ *n*

flu·o·ri·da·tion·ist \-sh(ə)n-əst\ *n* : an advocate of the fluoridation of public water supplies

flu·o·ride \'flu̇(-ə)r-ˌīd\ *n* **1** : a compound of fluorine with a more electropositive element or radical **2** : the monovalent anion of fluorine — **fluoride** *adj*

flu·o·ri·dize *or Brit* **flu·o·ri·dise** \-ə-ˌdīz\ *vt* **-dized** *or Brit* **-dised; -diz·ing** *or Brit* **-dis·ing** : to treat (as the teeth) with a fluoride — **flu·o·ri·di·za·tion** *or Brit* **flu·o·ri·di·sa·tion** \ˌflu̇(-ə)r-ə-də-'zā-shən\ *n*

fluo·ri·nate \'flu̇(-ə)r-ə-ˌnāt, 'flȯr-, 'flȯr-\ *vt* **-nat·ed; -nat·ing** : to treat or cause to combine with fluorine or a compound of fluorine — **fluo·ri·na·tion** \ˌflu̇(-ə)r-ə-'nā-shən, ˌflȯr-, ˌflȯr-\ *n*

fluo·rine \'flu̇(-ə)r-ˌēn, -ən\ *n* : a nonmetallic monovalent halogen element that is normally a pale yellowish flammable irritating toxic gas — symbol *F*; see ELEMENT table

fluoroacetate — see SODIUM FLUOROACETATE

flu·o·ro·chrome \'flu̇(-ə)r-ə-ˌkrōm\ *n* : any of various fluorescent substances used in biological staining to produce fluorescence in a specimen

flu·o·rom·e·ter \ˌflu̇(-ə)r-'äm-ət-ər\ *or* **flu·o·rim·e·ter** \-'im-\ *n* : an instrument for measuring fluorescence that is used esp. to determine intensities of radiations (as X-rays) from the fluorescence they produce or from concentrations of

\ə\ abut \ᵊ\ kitten \ər\ further \a\ ash \ā\ ace \ä\ cot, cart \au̇\ out \ch\ chin \e\ bet \ē\ easy \g\ go \i\ hit \ī\ ice \j\ job \ŋ\ sing \ō\ go \ȯ\ law \ȯi\ boy \th\ thin \th\ the \ü\ loot \u̇\ foot \y\ yet \zh\ vision   *See also* Pronunciation Symbols page

substances (as uranium or vitamins of the B complex) capable of forming fluorescent compounds — **flu·o·ro·met·ric** or **flu·o·ri·met·ric** \ˌflü-(ə)r-ə-'me-trik\ adj — **flu·o·rom·e·try** or **flu·o·rim·e·try** \ˌflü-(ə)r-'äm-ə-trē\ or \-'im-\ n, pl **-tries**

flu·o·ro·phos·phate \ˌflü-(ə)r-ō-'fäs-ˌfāt\ n : a salt or ester of a fluorophosphoric acid

flu·o·ro·phos·phor·ic acid \-ˌfäs-'fȯr-ik-\ n : any of three acids made by reaction of the pentoxide of phosphorus with hydrogen fluoride; esp : an acid H_2PO_3F obtained as a colorless viscous liquid and as salts and esters some of which are nerve gases

flu·o·ro·pho·tom·e·ter \-fō-'täm-ət-ər\ n : FLUOROMETER — **flu·o·ro·pho·to·met·ric** \-ˌfōt-ə-'me-trik\ adj — **flu·o·ro·pho·tom·e·try** \-ˌfō-'täm-ə-trē\ n, pl **-tries**

flu·o·ro·quin·o·lone \-'kwin-ə-ˌlōn\ n : any of a group of fluorinated derivatives (as ciprofloxacin and levofloxacin) of quinolone that are used as antibacterial drugs

¹**flu·o·ro·scope** \'flu̇r-ə-ˌskōp\ n : an instrument used chiefly in industry and in medical diagnosis for observing the internal structure of opaque objects (as the living body) by means of the shadow cast by the object examined upon a fluorescent screen when placed between the screen and a source of X-rays — **flu·o·ro·scop·ic** \ˌflu̇r-ə-'skäp-ik\ adj — **flu·o·ro·scop·i·cal·ly** \-i-k(ə-)lē\ adv — **flu·o·ros·co·pist** \ˌflu̇(-ə)r-'äs-kə-pəst\ n — **flu·o·ros·co·py** \-pē\ n, pl **-pies**

²**fluoroscope** vt **-scoped; -scop·ing** : to examine by fluoroscopy

flu·o·ro·sis \ˌflu̇(-ə)r-'ō-səs\ n : an abnormal condition (as mottled enamel of human teeth) caused by fluorine or its compounds — **flu·o·rot·ic** \-'ät-ik\ adj

flu·o·ro·ura·cil \ˌflu̇(-ə)r-ō-'yu̇r-ə-ˌsil, -ˌsəl\ or **5–flu·o·ro·ura·cil** \'fīv-\ n : a fluorine-containing pyrimidine base $C_4H_3FN_2O_2$ used to treat some kinds of cancer

fluo·sil·i·cate \ˌflü-ə-'sil-ə-ˌkāt, -'sil-i-kət\ n : a salt of fluosilicic acid — called also *silicofluoride;* see SODIUM FLUOSILICATE

fluo·si·lic·ic acid \ˌflü-ə-sə-ˌlis-ik-\ n : an unstable corrosive poisonous acid H_2SiF_6

flu·ox·e·tine \ˌflü-'äk-sə-ˌtēn\ n : an antidepressant drug that is administered in the form of its hydrochloride $C_{17}H_{18}F_3NO·HCl$ and enhances serotonin activity — see PROZAC

flu·oxy·mes·te·rone \flə-ˌwäk-sē-'mes-tə-ˌrōn\ n : a synthetic androgen $C_{20}H_{29}FO_3$ that is administered orally and is used esp. in the treatment of testosterone deficiency in males and in the palliative treatment of breast cancer in females

flu·phen·azine \flü-'fen-ə-ˌzēn\ n : a phenothiazine tranquilizer administered esp. in the form of its dihydrochloride $C_{22}H_{26}F_3N_3OS·2HCl$ — see PROLIXIN

flur·az·e·pam \ˌflu̇r-'az-ə-ˌpam\ n : a benzodiazepine that is closely related structurally to diazepam and is used as a hypnotic in the form of its dihydrochloride $C_{21}H_{23}ClFN_3O·2HCl$ to treat insomnia and to induce periods of restful sleep — see DALMANE

flur·bip·ro·fen \flu̇r-'bip-rə-fən\ n : a nonsteroidal antiinflammatory drug $C_{15}H_{13}FO_2$ used in the symptomatic treatment of rheumatoid arthritis and osteoarthritis — see ANSAID

flur·o·thyl \'flu̇r-ə-thil\ n : a clear colorless volatile liquid convulsant $C_4H_4F_6O$ that has been used in place of electroconvulsive therapy in the treatment of mental disorder

¹**flush** \'fləsh\ n : a transitory sensation of extreme heat (as in response to some drugs or in some physiological states) ⟨menopausal ∼es⟩

²**flush** vi : to blush or become suddenly suffused with color due to vasodilation ∼ vt : to cleanse or wash out with or as if with a rush of liquid ⟨the newly sewn incision is ∼ed with saline —Don Gold⟩

flu·ta·mide \'flüt-ə-ˌmīd\ n : a nonsteroidal antiandrogen $C_{11}H_{11}F_3N_2O_3$ that is used in the treatment of prostate cancer

flu·tic·a·sone propionate \flü-'tik-ə-ˌsōn, -ˌzōn\ n : a synthetic corticosteroid $C_{25}H_{31}F_3O_5S$ administered as a nasal spray to treat allergic rhinitis, as an oral inhalant to treat and

prevent asthma, and topically as a cream or ointment to treat inflammation and pruritus of dermatoses responsive to corticosteroids — called also *fluticasone;* see ADVAIR DISKUS, FLONASE, FLOVENT

flut·ter \'flət-ər\ n : an abnormal rapid spasmodic and usu. rhythmic motion or contraction of a body part ⟨diaphragmatic ∼⟩ ⟨affected with ventricular ∼⟩ — **flutter** vi

flu·vox·a·mine \flü-'väk-sə-ˌmēn\ n : a drug that functions as an SSRI and is administered orally in the form of its maleate $C_{15}H_{21}O_2N_2F_3·C_4H_4O_4$ in the treatment of obsessive-compulsive disorder — see LUVOX

flux \'fləks\ n **1 a** : a flowing or discharge of fluid from the body esp. when excessive or abnormal: as **(1)** : DIARRHEA **(2)** : DYSENTERY **b** : the matter discharged in a flux **2** : the rate of transfer of fluid, particles, or energy across a given surface

flux density n : magnetic, electric, or radiant flux per unit area normal to the direction of the flux

fly \'flī\ n, pl **flies 1** : a winged insect — usu. used in combination ⟨emerging may*flies*⟩ ⟨a large butter*fly*⟩ **2 a** : any dipteran fly — called also *true fly, two-winged fly* **b** : a large and stout-bodied dipteran fly (as a horsefly)

fly agaric n : a poisonous mushroom of the genus *Amanita* (*A. muscaria*) that has a variably colored but typically bright-red pileus with a warty white scurf on the surface that with the related death cap is responsible for most cases of severe mushroom poisoning, that has been used as a source of poison for flypaper, and that is extensively used chiefly in northeastern Asia as an intoxicant esp. for the hallucinatory effects that it produces — called also *fly amanita, fly mushroom*

fly·belt \'flī-ˌbelt\ n : an area infested with tsetse flies

¹**fly·blow** \-ˌblō\ vt **-blew; -blown** : to deposit eggs or young larvae of a flesh fly or blowfly in

²**flyblow** n : FLY-STRIKE

fly·blown \-ˌblōn\ adj **1** : infested with flyblows **2** : covered with flyspecks

fly–strike \-ˌstrīk\ n : infestation with fly maggots — **fly-struck** \-ˌstrək\ adj

Fm symbol fermium

FMN \ˌef-ˌem-'en\ n : a yellow crystalline phosphoric ester $C_{17}H_{21}N_4O_9P$ of riboflavin that is a coenzyme of several flavoprotein enzymes — called also *flavin mononucleotide, riboflavin phosphate*

fMRI abbr functional magnetic resonance imaging

FMS abbr fibromyalgia syndrome

FNA abbr fine needle aspiration

¹**foal** \'fōl\ n : the young of an animal of the horse family; esp : one less than one year old

²**foal** vi : to give birth to a foal

foam \'fōm\ n : a light frothy mass of fine bubbles formed in or on the surface of a liquid ⟨spermicidal ∼⟩ — **foam** vb

foam cell n : a swollen vacuolate reticuloendothelial cell filled with lipid inclusions and characteristic of some conditions of disturbed lipid metabolism

foamy virus \'fō-mē\ n : any of a genus (*Spumavirus*) of non-pathogenic retroviruses that occur in mammals and are sometimes transmitted to humans from nonhuman primates — called also *spumavirus*

FOBT abbr fecal occult blood test; fecal occult blood testing

fo·cal \'fō-kəl\ adj : of, relating to, being, or having a focus — **fo·cal·ly** \-kə-lē\ adv

focal epilepsy n : epilepsy characterized by partial seizures — called also *partial epilepsy*

focal infection n : a persistent bacterial infection of some organ or region; esp : one causing symptoms elsewhere in the body

fo·cal·ize or Brit **fo·cal·ise** \'fō-kə-ˌlīz\ vb **-ized** or Brit **-ised; -iz·ing** or Brit **-is·ing** vt : to confine to a limited area ⟨the ability to ∼ a coccidioidal infection —*Jour. Amer. Med. Assoc.*⟩ ∼ vi : to become confined to a limited area ⟨pullorum disease commonly ∼s in the adult bird's ovary⟩ — **fo·cal·iza·tion** or Brit **fo·cal·isa·tion** \ˌfō-kə-lə-'zā-shən\ n

focal length \-ˌleŋ(k)th\ *n* : the distance of a focus from the surface of a lens or concave mirror — symbol *f*

focal plane *n* : a plane that is perpendicular to the axis of a lens or mirror and passes through the focus

focal point *n* : FOCUS 1a

focal seizure *n* : PARTIAL SEIZURE

fo·com·e·ter \fō-ˈkäm-ət-ər\ *also* **fo·cim·e·ter** \-ˈsim-\ *n* : an instrument for measuring either the visual or the photographic focal length of an objective or of another optical system

¹**fo·cus** \ˈfō-kəs\ *n, pl* **fo·ci** \ˈfō-ˌsī *also* -ˌkī\ *also* **fo·cus·es 1 a** : a point at which rays (as of light, heat, or sound) converge or from which they diverge or appear to diverge; *specif* : the point where the geometrical lines or their prolongations conforming to the rays diverging from or converging toward another point intersect and give rise to an image after reflection by a mirror or refraction by a lens or optical system **b** : a point of convergence of a beam of particles (as electrons) **2 a** : FOCAL LENGTH **b** : adjustment for distinct vision; *also* : the area that may be seen distinctly or resolved into a clear image **3** : a localized area of disease or the chief site of a generalized disease or infection

²**focus** *vb* **fo·cused** *also* **fo·cussed; fo·cus·ing** *also* **fo·cus·sing** *vt* **1** : to bring (as light rays) to a focus **2 a** : to adjust the focus of (as the eye or a lens) **b** : to bring (as an image) into focus ~ *vi* **1** : to come to a focus **2** : to adjust one's eye or a camera to a particular range — **fo·cus·able** \-kəs-ə-bəl\ *adj*

foenugreek *var of* FENUGREEK

Each boldface word in the list below is a chiefly British variant of the word to its right in small capitals.

foetal	FETAL	**foetometry**	FETOMETRY
foetation	FETATION	**foetoprotein**	FETOPROTEIN
foeticidal	FETICIDAL	**foetoscope**	FETOSCOPE
foeticide	FETICIDE	**foetoscopy**	FETOSCOPY
foetologist	FETOLOGIST	**foetus**	FETUS
foetology	FETOLOGY		

foeti *chiefly Brit pl of* FETUS

foetid, foetor *var of* FETID, FETOR

fog \ˈfäg, ˈfȯg\ *vt* **fogged; fog·ging** : to blur (a visual field) with lenses that prevent a sharp focus in order to relax accommodation before testing vision

foil \ˈfȯil\ *n* : very thin sheet metal (as of gold or platinum) used esp. in filling teeth

fo·la·cin \ˈfō-lə-sən\ *n* : FOLIC ACID

fo·late \ˈfō-ˌlāt\ *n* : FOLIC ACID ⟨the uptake of ~ by the mutant —*Biol. Abstracts*⟩; *also* : a salt or ester of folic acid

¹**fold** \ˈfōld\ *vi* : to become doubled or pleated

²**fold** *n* : a margin apparently formed by the doubling upon itself of a flat anatomical structure (as a membrane)

Fo·ley catheter \ˈfō-lē-\ *n* : a catheter with an inflatable balloon tip for retention in the bladder

   Foley, Frederic Eugene Basil (1891–1966), American urologist. Foley in 1937 introduced an operation for stricture at the junction of the ureter and the kidney pelvis. The operation entailed the insertion of a rubber catheter now known as the Foley catheter.

fo·li·a·ceous \ˌfō-lē-ˈā-shəs\ *adj* : resembling a leaf in form or in mode of growth

foliaceus — see PEMPHIGUS FOLIACEUS

fo·li·ate \ˈfō-lē-ət, -ˌāt\ *adj* : shaped like a leaf

foliate papilla *n* : any of the paired oval papillae of the lateral aspect of the posterior part of the tongue that are rudimentary or missing in humans but form the chief organs of taste of some other mammals (as rabbits)

fo·lic acid \ˌfō-lik-\ *n* : a crystalline vitamin $C_{19}H_{19}N_7O_6$ of the B complex that is required for normal production of red blood cells, that is used esp. in the treatment of nutritional anemias, and that occurs esp. in green leafy vegetables, liver, kidneys, dried beans, and mushrooms — called also *folacin, folate, Lactobacillus casei factor, pteroylglutamic acid, vitamin B_c, vitamin M*

fo·lie \ˌfō-ˈlē\ *n* : loss of reason : INSANITY

folie à deux \-(ˌ)ä-ˈdœ, -ˈdə\ *n, pl* **folies à deux** \ˌfō-ˈlē(z)-

(ˌ)ä-\ : the presence of the same or similar delusional ideas in two persons closely associated with one another

folie du doute \-də-ˈdüt\ *n, pl* **folies du doute** \ˌfō-lē(z)-də-\ : pathological indecisiveness esp. when extended to ordinary simple choice situations

fo·lin·ic acid \fō-ˈlin-ik-\ *n* : LEUCOVORIN

fo·li·um \ˈfō-lē-əm\ *n, pl* **fo·lia** \-lē-ə\ : one of the lamellae of the cerebellar cortex

folk medicine \ˈfōk-\ *n* : traditional medicine as practiced esp. by people isolated from modern medical services and usu. involving the use of plant-derived remedies on an empirical basis — compare HOME REMEDY

fol·li·cle \ˈfäl-i-kəl\ *n* **1** : a small anatomical cavity or deep narrow-mouthed depression; *esp* : a small simple or slightly branched gland : CRYPT **2** : a small lymph node **3** : a vesicle in the mammalian ovary that contains a developing egg surrounded by a covering of cells : OVARIAN FOLLICLE; *esp* : GRAAFIAN FOLLICLE — **fol·lic·u·lar** \fə-ˈlik-yə-lər, fä-\ *adj*

follicle mite *n* : any of several minute mites of the genus *Demodex* that are parasitic in the hair follicles

follicle–stimulating hormone *n* : a hormone from an anterior lobe of the pituitary gland that stimulates the growth of the ovum-containing follicles in the ovary and that activates sperm-forming cells — called also *follitropin*

follicularis — see KERATOSIS FOLLICULARIS

folliculi — see LIQUOR FOLLICULI, THECA FOLLICULI

fol·lic·u·lin \fə-ˈlik-yə-lən, fä-\ *n* : ESTROGEN; *esp* : ESTRONE

fol·lic·u·li·tis \fə-ˌlik-yə-ˈlīt-əs\ *n* : inflammation of one or more follicles esp. of the hair

fol·lic·u·lus \fə-ˈlik-yə-ləs\ *n, pl* **-li** \-ˌlī, -ˌlē\ : FOLLICLE

fol·li·tro·pin \ˌfäl-ə-ˈtrō-pən\ *n* : FOLLICLE-STIMULATING HORMONE

¹**fol·low–up** \ˈfäl-ə-ˌwəp, ˌfäl-\ *adj* : done, conducted, or administered in the course of following up persons esp. after institutionalization ⟨~ care for postoperative patients⟩

²**follow–up** *n* : maintenance of contact with or reexamination of a person (as a patient) at usu. prescribed intervals following diagnosis or treatment; *also* : a patient with whom such contact is maintained

follow up \ˌfäl-ə-ˈwəp\ *vt* : to maintain contact with (a person) in order to evaluate a diagnosis or to determine the effectiveness of treatment received ⟨patients who are *followed up* after their discharge⟩

¹**fo·ment** \ˈfō-ˌment\ *n* : FOMENTATION

²**fo·ment** \fō-ˈment\ *vt* : to treat with moist heat (as for easing pain)

fo·men·ta·tion \ˌfō-mən-ˈtā-shən, -ˌmen-\ *n* **1** : the application of hot moist substances to the body to ease pain **2** : the material applied in fomentation : POULTICE

fo·mite \ˈfō-ˌmīt\ *n, pl* **fo·mites** \-ˌmīts; ˈfäm-ə-ˌtēz, ˈfōm-\ : an inanimate object (as a dish, toy, book, doorknob, or clothing) that may be contaminated with infectious organisms and serve in their transmission ⟨the much maligned toilet seat is a remarkably ineffective ~ —M. F. Rein⟩ ⟨what are the most common *fomites* for rotavirus in day-care settings —*Pediatric Report's Child Health Newsletter*⟩

F₁ \ˈef-ˈwən\ *n* : F₁ GENERATION; *also* : F₁ HYBRID

F₁ generation *n* : the first generation produced by a cross and consisting of individuals heterozygous for characters in which the parents differ and are homozygous — called also *first filial generation*; compare F₂ GENERATION, P₁ GENERATION

F₁ hybrid *n* : an individual of an F₁ generation — called also *first generation hybrid*

Fon·se·caea \ˌfän-sē-ˈsē-ə\ *n* : a genus of imperfect fungi that includes two (*F. pedrosoi* and *F. compacta*) often associated with chromoblastomycosis

fon·ta·nel *or* **fon·ta·nelle** \ˌfänt-ᵊn-ˈel, ˈfänt-ᵊn-ˌ\ *n* : a membrane-covered opening in bone or between bones;

specif : any of the spaces closed by membranous structures between the uncompleted angles of the parietal bones and the neighboring bones of a fetal or young skull

food \'füd\ *n, often attrib* **1** : material consisting essentially of protein, carbohydrate, and fat used in the body of an organism to sustain growth, repair, and vital processes and to furnish energy; *also* : such material together with supplementary substances (as minerals, vitamins, and condiments) **2** : nutriment in solid form

food poisoning *n* **1** : either of two acute gastrointestinal disorders caused by bacteria or their toxic products: **a** : a rapidly developing intoxication marked by nausea, vomiting, prostration, and often severe diarrhea and caused by the presence in food of toxic products produced by bacteria (as some staphylococci) **b** : a less rapidly developing infection esp. with salmonellas that has generally similar symptoms and that results from multiplication of bacteria ingested with contaminated food **2** : a gastrointestinal disturbance occurring after consumption of food that is contaminated with chemical residues (as from sprays) or food (as some fungi) that is inherently unsuitable for human consumption

food·stuff \'füd-ˌstəf\ *n* : a substance with food value; *esp* : a specific nutrient (as a fat or protein)

food vacuole *n* : a vacuole (as in an ameba) in which ingested food is digested

foot \'fut\ *n, pl* **feet** \'fēt\ *also* **foot** **1** : the terminal part of the vertebrate leg upon which an individual stands **2** : any of various units of length based on the length of the human foot; *esp* : a unit equal to ⅓ yard or 12 inches or 30.48 centimeters — pl. *foot* used between a number and a noun ⟨a 10= *foot* pole⟩; pl. *feet* or *foot* used between a number and an adjective ⟨6 *feet* tall⟩

foot–and–mouth disease *n* : an acute contagious febrile disease esp. of cloven-hoofed animals that is caused by any of seven serotypes of a picornavirus (species *Foot-and-mouth disease virus* of the genus *Aphthovirus*) and is marked by ulcerating vesicles in the mouth, about the hooves, and on the udder and teats — called also *aftosa, aphthous fever, foot-and-mouth, hoof-and-mouth disease;* compare HAND, FOOT AND MOUTH DISEASE

foot·bath \'fut-ˌbath, -ˌbath\ *n* : a bath for cleansing, warming, soothing, or disinfecting the feet

foot·can·dle \-'kan-dᵊl\ *n* : a unit of illuminance on a surface that is everywhere one foot from a uniform point source of light of one candle and equal to one lumen per square foot

foot drop *n* : an extended position of the foot caused by paralysis of the flexor muscles of the leg — called also *drop foot*

foot·ed \'fut-əd\ *adj* : having a foot or feet esp. of a specified kind or number — often used in combination ⟨a four-*footed* animal⟩

foot·plate \-ˌplāt\ *n* : the flat oval base of the stapes

foot–pound \-'paund\ *n, pl* **foot–pounds** : a unit of work equal to the work done by a force of one pound acting through a distance of one foot in the direction of the force

foot–pound–second \ˌfut-ˌpaund-'sek-ənd\ *adj* : being or relating to a system of units based upon the foot as the unit of length, the pound as the unit of weight or mass, and the second as the unit of time — abbr. *fps*

foot·print \'fut-ˌprint\ *n* : an impression of the foot on a surface

foot·print·ing \-iŋ\ *n* : identification of the binding sites between a specific DNA and a protein by subjecting a complex of the DNA and protein to chemical digestion and comparing the resulting fragments with those obtained by digestion of the same DNA which does not have some of its cleavage sites protected by binding with the protein

foot rot *n* : a progressive inflammation of foot tissues (as between the digits) esp. of sheep or cattle; *specif* : a necrobacillosis marked by sloughing, ulceration, suppuration, and sometimes loss of the hoof

fo·ra·men \fə-'rā-mən\ *n, pl* **fo·ram·i·na** \-'ram-ə-nə\ *or* **fo·ra·mens** \-'rā-mənz\ : a small opening, perforation, or orifice : FENESTRA 1 — **fo·ram·i·nal** \fə-'ram-ən-ᵊl\ *adj*

foramen ce·cum \-'sē-kəm\ *n* : a shallow depression in the posterior dorsal midline of the tongue that is the remnant of the more cranial part of the embryonic duct from which the thyroid gland developed

foramen lac·er·um \-'las-ər-əm\ *n* : an irregular aperture on the lower surface of the skull bounded by parts of the temporal, sphenoid, and occipital bones that gives passage to the internal carotid artery

foramen mag·num \-'mag-nəm\ *n* : the opening in the skull through which the spinal cord passes to become the medulla oblongata

foramen of Lusch·ka \-'lush-kə\ *n* : either of two openings each of which is situated on one side of the fourth ventricle of the brain and communicates with the subarachnoid space
    Luschka, Hubert von (1820–1875), German anatomist. Luschka was the author of a notable textbook of human anatomy, which was published in three volumes from 1863 to 1869. In 1873 he described the anatomy and physiology of the larynx. He produced classic descriptions of the pharyngeal bursa and a small cartilaginous nodule in the anterior part of the vocal cord. He is also remembered for his classic descriptions of polyposis of the colon in 1861 and of the lateral openings in the fourth ventricle of the brain (now known as the foramina of Luschka) around 1863.

foramen of Ma·gen·die \-mə-ˌzhän-'dē\ *n* : a passage through the midline of the roof of the fourth ventricle of the brain that gives passage to the cerebrospinal fluid from the ventricles to the subarachnoid space
    F. Magendie — see BELL-MAGENDIE LAW

foramen of Mon·ro \-mən-'rō\ *n* : INTERVENTRICULAR FORAMEN
    Monro, Alexander (Secundus) (1733–1817), British anatomist. Professor of anatomy at Edinburgh, Monro was the first physician to use the stomach pump and the first to perform paracentesis. In 1783 he published observations on the anatomy and physiology of the nervous system which included a definitive description of the interventricular foramen between the lateral ventricles of the brain. He was also the author of an early, important textbook on comparative anatomy and treatises on the brain, eye, and ear.

foramen of Wins·low \-'winz-ˌlō\ *n* : EPIPLOIC FORAMEN
    Winslow, Jacob (or Jacques–Bénigne) (1669–1760), Danish anatomist. Regarded by many as the greatest European anatomist of his time, Winslow did much to condense and systematize the body of anatomical information then known. He was one of the first to study anatomy precisely and systematically. In his study of muscles he observed that muscles do not function independently, as flexors or supinators, but rather that muscles operate within a synergistic relationship. His classic descriptions of the oblique popliteal ligament and epiploic foramen were published in 1732 as part of a multivolume work on human anatomy.

foramen ova·le \-ō-'va-(ˌ)lē, -'vā-, -'vä-\ *n* **1** : an opening in the septum between the two atria of the heart that is normally present only in the fetus **2** : an oval opening in the greater wing of the sphenoid for passage of the mandibular nerve

foramen ro·tun·dum \-rō-'tən-dəm\ *n* : a circular aperture in the anterior and medial part of the greater wing of the sphenoid that gives passage to the maxillary nerve

foramen spin·o·sum \-spin-'ō-səm\ *n* : an aperture in the greater wing of the sphenoid that gives passage to the middle meningeal artery

foramina *pl of* FORAMEN

force \'fō(ə)rs, 'fo(ə)rs\ *n* : an agency or influence that if applied to a free body results chiefly in an acceleration of the body and sometimes in elastic deformation and other effects

forcé — see ACCOUCHEMENT FORCÉ

for·ceps \'fòr-səps, -ˌseps\ *n, pl* **forceps** : an instrument for grasping, holding firmly, or exerting traction upon objects esp. for delicate operations (as by surgeons, obstetricians, or dentists)

for·ci·pres·sure \'fòr-sə-ˌpresh-ər\ *n* : compression of a blood vessel with a forceps to arrest hemorrhage

For·dyce's disease \'fòr-ˌdīs-əz-\ *also* **For·dyce disease** \'fòr-ˌdīs-\ *n* : a common anomaly of the oral mucosa in

E
F

which misplaced sebaceous glands form yellowish white nodules on the lips or the lining of the mouth

Fordyce, John Addison (1858–1925), American dermatologist. Fordyce specialized in dermatology and syphilology. He was a pioneer in the modern diagnosis and treatment of syphilis. He studied the various phases of the disease, its infection of the nervous system, and the effects of treatment with arsenicals. In 1896 he described the condition now known as Fordyce's disease.

fore \'fō(ə)r, 'fȯ(ə)r\ *adj* : situated in front of something else

fore·arm \'fōr-ˌärm, 'fȯr-\ *n* : the part of the arm between the elbow and the wrist; *also* : the corresponding part in other vertebrates

fore·brain \-ˌbrān\ *n* : the anterior of the three primary divisions of the developing vertebrate brain or the corresponding part of the adult brain that includes esp. the cerebral hemispheres, the thalamus, and the hypothalamus and that esp. in higher vertebrates is the main control center for sensory and associative information processing, visceral functions, and voluntary motor functions — called also *prosencephalon;* see DIENCEPHALON, TELENCEPHALON

forebrain bundle — see MEDIAL FOREBRAIN BUNDLE

fore·con·scious \-ˌkän-chəs\ *n* : PRECONSCIOUS

fore·fin·ger \-ˌfiŋ-gər\ *n* : INDEX FINGER

fore·foot \-ˌfu̇t\ *n* **1** : one of the anterior feet esp. of a quadruped **2** : the front part of the human foot

fore·gut \-ˌgət\ *n* **1** : the anterior part of the alimentary canal of a vertebrate embryo that develops into the pharynx, esophagus, stomach, and extreme anterior part of the intestine **2** : the anterior part of the definitive alimentary canal of an invertebrate animal

fore·head \'fȯr-əd, 'fär-; 'fȯ(ə)r-ˌhed, 'fȯ(ə)r-\ *n* : the part of the face above the eyes — called also *brow, frons*

for·eign \'fȯr-ən, 'fär-\ *adj* **1** : occurring in an abnormal situation in the living body and often introduced from outside ⟨a ~ body lodged in the esophagus⟩ **2** : not recognized by the immune system as part of the self ⟨~ proteins⟩

fore·leg \'fō(ə)r-ˌleg, 'fȯ(ə)r-, -ˌlāg\ *n* : a front leg

fore·limb \-ˌlim\ *n* : a limb (as an arm, fin, wing, or leg) that is situated anteriorly

fore·milk \-ˌmilk\ *n* **1** : first-drawn milk **2** : COLOSTRUM

fo·ren·sic \fə-'ren(t)-sik, -'ren-zik\ *adj* : relating to or dealing with the application of scientific knowledge to legal problems ⟨a ~ pathologist⟩ ⟨~ experts⟩

forensic medicine *n* : a science that deals with the relation and application of medical facts to legal problems — called also *legal medicine*

forensic odontology *n* : a branch of forensic medicine that deals with teeth and marks left by teeth (as in identifying criminal suspects or the remains of a dead person)

forensic psychiatry *n* : the application of psychiatry in courts of law (as for the determination of criminal responsibility or liability to commitment for insanity) — **forensic psychiatrist** *n*

fore·paw \-ˌpȯ\ *n* : the paw of a foreleg

fore·play \-ˌplā\ *n* : erotic stimulation preceding sexual intercourse

fore·plea·sure \-ˌplezh-ər, -ˌplāzh-\ *n* : pleasurable excitement (as that induced by stimulation of erogenous zones) that tends to lead to or release a more intense emotional reaction (as in orgasm) — compare ENDPLEASURE

fore·skin \-ˌskin\ *n* : a retractable fold of skin that covers the glans of the penis — called also *prepuce*

fore·stom·ach \-ˌstəm-ək, -ik\ *n* : the cardiac part of the stomach

fore·wa·ters \-ˌwȯt-ərz, -ˌwät-ərz\ *n pl* : AMNIOTIC FLUID

forge \'fō(ə)rj, 'fȯ(ə)rj\ *vi* **forged; forg·ing** *of a horse* : to make a clicking noise by overreaching so that a hind shoe hits a fore shoe

fork \'fō(ə)rk\ *n* **1** : a forked part, tool, or piece of equipment — see TUNING FORK **2** : the lower part of the human body where the legs diverge from the trunk usu. including the legs

¹form \'fȯ(ə)rm\ *n* **1 a** : the shape and structure of something

as distinguished from its material **b** : a body (as of a person) esp. in its external appearance or as distinguished from the face **2** : a distinguishable group of organisms — used esp. to avoid taxonomic implications

²form *vt* : to give a particular shape to : shape or mold into a certain state or after a particular model ~ *vi* : to become formed or shaped ⟨a clot ~ed over the cut⟩

form·al·de·hyde \fȯr-'mal-də-ˌhīd, fər-\ *n* : a colorless pungent irritating gas CH_2O used chiefly as a disinfectant and preservative and in chemical synthesis

for·ma·lin \'fȯr-mə-lən, -ˌlēn\ *n* : a clear aqueous solution of formaldehyde containing a small amount of methanol

for·mal·in·ized *or Brit* **for·mal·in·ised** \-ˌīzd\ *adj* : FORMOLIZED

for·mate \'fȯ(ə)r-ˌmāt\ *n* : a salt or ester of formic acid

for·ma·tion \fȯr-'mā-shən\ *n* **1** : an act of giving form or shape to something or of taking form : DEVELOPMENT **2** : the manner in which a thing is formed : STRUCTURE

for·ma·tive \'fȯr-mət-iv\ *adj* : capable of alteration by growth and development; *also* : producing new cells and tissues

form·a·zan \'fȯr-mə-ˌzan\ *n* : a hypothetical hydrazone CH_4N_4 related to formic acid and known only in the form of intensely colored derivatives of which some are obtained from colorless compounds by the reducing action of living tissues and serve as indicators of viability by color production; *also* : any of these derivatives

formed element *n* : one of the red blood cells, white blood cells, or blood platelets as contrasted with the fluid portion of the blood

forme fruste \ˌfȯrm-'früest, -'früst\ *n, pl* **formes frustes** \-'früest, -'früst(s)\ : an atypical and usu. incomplete manifestation of a disease

form genus *n* : an artificial taxonomic category established for organisms of which the true relationships are obscure due to incomplete knowledge of structure (as in some fossils) or of development or life history (as in the imperfect fungi and various animal parasites)

for·mic \'fȯr-mik\ *adj* : derived from formic acid

formic acid *n* : a colorless pungent fuming vesicant liquid acid CH_2O_2 found esp. in ants and in many plants and used chiefly in dyeing and finishing textiles

for·mi·ca·tion \ˌfȯr-mə-'kā-shən\ *n* : an abnormal sensation resembling that made by insects creeping in or on the skin

for·mol·ized *or Brit* **for·mol·ised** \'fȯr-(ˌ)mȯ-ˌlīzd, -(ˌ)mō-\ *adj* : treated with a dilute formaldehyde solution esp. for purposes of attenuation ⟨~ influenza vaccine⟩

for·mu·la \'fȯr-myə-lə\ *n, pl* **-las** *or* **-lae** \-ˌlē, -ˌlī\ **1 a** : a recipe or prescription giving method and proportions of ingredients for the preparation of some material (as a medicine) **b** : a milk mixture or substitute for feeding an infant typically consisting of prescribed proportions and forms of cow's milk, water, and sugar; *also* : a batch of this made up at one time to meet an infant's future requirements (as during a 24-hour period) **2** : a symbolic expression showing the composition or constitution of a chemical substance and consisting of symbols for the elements present and subscripts to indicate the relative or total number of atoms present in a molecule ⟨the ~ for ethyl alcohol is C_2H_5OH⟩ — see EMPIRICAL FORMULA, MOLECULAR FORMULA, STRUCTURAL FORMULA

for·mu·lary \'fȯr-myə-ˌler-ē\ *n, pl* **-lar·ies** : a book containing a list of medicinal substances and formulas — see NATIONAL FORMULARY

for·myl \'fȯr-ˌmil\ *n* : the radical HCO– of formic acid that is also characteristic of aldehydes

for·ni·cate \'fȯr-nə-ˌkāt\ *vb* **-cat·ed; -cat·ing** *vi* : to commit fornication ~ *vt* : to commit fornication with — **for·ni·ca·tor** \-ˌkāt-ər\ *n*

\ə\ **abut** \ʼ\ **kitten** \ər\ **further** \a\ **ash** \ā\ **ace** \ä\ **cot, cart**
\au̇\ **out** \ch\ **chin** \e\ **bet** \ē\ **easy** \g\ **go** \i\ **hit** \ī\ **ice** \j\ **job**
\ŋ\ **sing** \ō\ **go** \ȯ\ **law** \ȯi\ **boy** \th\ **thin** \th̲\ **the** \ü\ **loot**
\u̇\ **foot** \y\ **yet** \zh\ **vision** *See also* Pronunciation Symbols page

for·ni·ca·tion \ˌfȯr-nə-'kā-shən\ *n* : consensual sexual intercourse between two persons not married to each other

for·ni·ca·trix \-'kā-triks\ *n, pl* **-tri·ces** \-ˌkə-'trī-ˌsēz\ : a woman who engages in fornication

fornicis — see CRURA FORNICIS

for·nix \'fȯr-niks\ *n, pl* **for·ni·ces** \-nə-ˌsēz\ : an anatomical arch or fold: as **a** : the vault of the cranium **b** : the part of the conjunctiva overlying the cornea **c** : a body of nerve fibers lying beneath the corpus callosum with which they are continuous posteriorly and serving to integrate the hippocampus with other parts of the brain **d** : the vaulted upper part of the vagina surrounding the uterine cervix **e** : the fundus of the stomach **f** : the vault of the pharynx

Fos·a·max \'fä-sə-ˌmaks\ *trademark* — used for a preparation of alendronate

fos·car·net \fäs-'kär-nət\ *n* : a hydrated sodium salt Na₃CO₅P·6H₂O that is an antiviral analog of pyrophosphate and is administered intravenously to individuals infected with HIV to treat retinitis caused by a cytomegalovirus — called also *foscarnet sodium*

fos·sa \'fäs-ə\ *n, pl* **fos·sae** \-ˌē, -ˌī\ : an anatomical pit, groove, or depression 〈the temporal ∼ of the skull〉 〈the ∼ in the liver for the gallbladder〉 — **fos·sate** \-ˌāt\ *adj*

fossa na·vic·u·lar·is \-nə-ˌvik-yə-'lar-əs\ *n* : a depression between the posterior margin of the vaginal opening and the fourchette

fossa oval·is \-ō-'va-ləs, -'vā-, -'vä-\ *n* **1** : a depression in the septum between the right and left atria that marks the position of the foramen ovale in the fetus **2** : SAPHENOUS OPENING

Fos·sar·ia \fäs-'ar-ē-ə, -'er-, fȯs-\ *n* : a widely distributed genus of small freshwater pulmonate snails of the family Lymnaeidae including important intermediate hosts of liver flukes — compare GALBA, LYMNAEA

fos·su·la \'fäs-(y)ə-lə *also* 'fȯs-\ *n, pl* **-lae** \-lē *also* -ˌlī\ : a small or shallow fossa

fou·droy·ant \fü-'drȯi-ənt, fü-drwȧ-yäⁿ\ *adj* : FULMINANT

¹foun·der \'faȯn-dər\ *vb* **foun·dered; foun·der·ing** \-d(ə-)riŋ\ *vi* : to become disabled; *esp* : to go lame ∼ *vt* : to disable (an animal) esp. by inducing laminitis through excessive feeding

²foun·der *n* : LAMINITIS

found·ling \'faȯn-(d)liŋ\ *n* : an infant found after its unknown parents have abandoned it

four·chette *or* **four·chet** \fu̇(ə)r-'shet\ *n* : a small fold of membrane connecting the labia minora in the posterior part of the vulva

fourth cranial nerve \'fō(ə)rth-, 'fȯ(ə)rth-\ *n* : TROCHLEAR NERVE

fourth ventricle *n* : a somewhat rhomboidal ventricle of the posterior part of the brain that connects at the front with the third ventricle through the aqueduct of Sylvius and at the back with the central canal of the spinal cord

fo·vea \'fō-vē-ə\ *n, pl* **fo·ve·ae** \-vē-ˌē, -vē-ˌī\ **1** : a small fossa **2** : a small rodless area of the retina that affords acute vision — **fo·ve·al** \-vē-əl\ *adj* — **fo·ve·ate** \-vē-ˌāt, -ət\ *adj*

fovea cen·tra·lis \-sen-'tral-əs, -'träl-, -'trāl-\ *n* : FOVEA 2

fo·ve·a·tion \ˌfō-vē-'ā-shən\ *n* **1** : the state of being pitted **2** : one of the pits in a pitted surface 〈the pits or ∼s so characteristic of the pockmark —K. F. Maxcy〉

fo·ve·o·la \fō-'vē-ə-lə\ *n, pl* **-lae** \-ˌlē\ *or* **-las** : a small pit; *specif* : one of the pits in the embryonic gastric mucosa from which the gastric glands develop — **fo·ve·o·lar** \-lər\ *adj*

fo·ve·o·late \'fō-vē-ə-lət, 'fō-vē-ə-ˌlāt\ *adj* : having small pits : FOVEATE

fowl cholera \'faȯl-\ *n* : an acute contagious septicemic disease of birds that is marked by fever, weakness, diarrhea, and petechial hemorrhages in the mucous membranes, is caused by a bacterium of the genus *Pasteurella* (*P. multocida* syn. *P. avicida*), and is highly destructive to all types of domestic poultry and most wild birds — called also *chicken cholera*

Fow·ler's solution \'faȯ-lərz-\ *n* : an alkaline aqueous solution of potassium arsenite formerly used in medicine (as in treating some diseases of the blood or skin)

Fowler, Thomas (1736–1801), British physician. Fowler in 1786 published a collection of medical reports on the effectiveness of arsenic in the treatment of agues, fevers, and headaches. One of the remedies discussed was the potassium arsenite solution now known as Fowler's solution.

fowl mite *n* : CHICKEN MITE — see NORTHERN FOWL MITE

fowl paralysis *n* : NEUROLYMPHOMATOSIS

fowl pest *n* **1** : AVIAN INFLUENZA **2** : NEWCASTLE DISEASE

fowl plague *n* : AVIAN INFLUENZA

fowl pox *n* : either of two forms of a disease occurring worldwide esp. in chickens and turkeys that is caused by a poxvirus (species *Fowlpox virus* of the genus *Avipoxvirus*) transmitted by contact or by insect vectors: **a** : a cutaneous form marked by proliferating lesions esp. on skin lacking feathers that progress to pustules, warty growths, and scabs — called also *sorehead* **b** : a more serious diphtheritic form occurring as cheesy lesions of the mucous membranes of the mouth, throat, and eyes that sometimes coalesce into a false membrane

fowl tick *n* : any of several ticks of the genus *Argas* (as *A. persicus*) that attack fowl in the warmer parts of the world causing anemia and transmitting various diseases (as spirochetosis) — called also *chicken tick*

fowl typhoid *n* : an infectious disease of poultry characterized by diarrhea, anemia, and prostration and caused by a bacterium of the genus *Salmonella* (*S. gallinarum*)

fox·glove \'fäks-ˌgləv\ *n* : any plant of the genus *Digitalis*; *esp* : a common European biennial or perennial (*D. purpurea*) cultivated for its showy racemes of dotted white or purple tubular flowers and as a source of digitalis

fp *abbr* freezing point

FP *abbr* **1** family physician; family practitioner **2** family practice

FPC *abbr* fish protein concentrate

fpm *abbr* feet per minute

fps *abbr* foot-pound-second

Fr *symbol* francium

FR *abbr* flocculation reaction

frac·tion \'frak-shən\ *n* : one of several portions (as of a distillate) separable by fractionation 〈gamma globulin is a ∼ of blood plasma〉

frac·tion·al \-shən-ᵊl, -shnəl\ *adj* : of, relating to, or involving a process for separating components of a mixture through differences in physical or chemical properties 〈∼ distillation〉

frac·tion·ate \-shə-ˌnāt\ *vt* **-at·ed; -at·ing** : to separate (as a mixture) into different portions (as by distillation or precipitation)

frac·tion·a·tion \ˌfrak-shə-'nā-shən\ *n* : the action or process of fractionating 〈∼ of blood plasma by the precipitation of blood proteins〉; *also* : the state of being fractionated

¹frac·ture \'frak-chər, -shər\ *n* **1** : the act or process of breaking or the state of being broken; *specif* : the breaking of hard tissue (as bone) — see POTT'S FRACTURE **2** : the rupture (as by tearing) of soft tissue 〈kidney ∼〉

²fracture *vt* **frac·tured; frac·tur·ing** \-chə-riŋ, -shriŋ\ **1** : to cause a fracture in 〈∼ a rib〉 **2** : to cause a rupture or tear in 〈a blow that *fractured* a kidney〉

fragile X syndrome \-'eks-\ *n* : an X-linked inherited disorder that is caused by repeats of a trinucleotide sequence on the X chromosome which are abnormal in number and degree of methylation, that is characterized by moderate to severe mental retardation, by large ears, chin, and forehead, and by enlarged testes in males, and that often has limited or no effect in heterozygous females — called also *fragile X*

fra·gil·i·tas os·si·um \frə-'jil-ət-əs-'äs-ē-əm\ *n* : OSTEOGENESIS IMPERFECTA

fra·gil·i·ty \frə-'jil-ət-ē\ *n, pl* **-ties** : the quality or state of being easily broken or destroyed 〈increased red blood cell ∼ —Sue R. Williams〉 — **frag·ile** \'fraj-əl, -ˌīl\ *adj*

fragility test *n* : a test of the relative fragility of red blood cells made by exposing them to hypotonic solutions and determining the point at which they rupture

fra·gil·o·cyte \frə-'jil-ə-ˌsīt\ *n* : an exceptionally fragile red blood cell (as in congenital hemolytic jaundice)

fra·gil·o·cy·to·sis \frə-ˌjil-ō-(ˌ)sī-'tō-səs\ *n, pl* **-to·ses** \-ˌsēz\ : an abnormal state characterized by the presence of fragilocytes in the blood

frag·ment \'frag-mənt\ *n* : a part broken off or detached

fragmentography — see MASS FRAGMENTOGRAPHY

fraise \'frāz\ *n* : a surgical burr shaped like a cone or hemisphere

fram·be·sia \fram-'bē-zh(ē-)ə\ *or chiefly Brit* **fram·boe·sia** \-zē-ə\ *n* : YAWS

frame \'frām\ *n* **1** : the physical makeup of an animal and esp. a human body : PHYSIQUE, FIGURE **2 a** : a part of a pair of glasses that holds one of the lenses **b frames** *pl* : that part of a pair of glasses other than the lenses

frame·shift \-ˌshift\ *adj* : relating to, being, or causing a mutation in which a number of nucleotides not divisible by three is inserted or deleted so that some triplet codons are read incorrectly during genetic translation ⟨~ mutations⟩ ⟨~ mutagens⟩ — **frameshift** *n*

fran·ci·um \'fran(t)-sē-əm\ *n* : a radioactive element of the alkali-metal group discovered as a disintegration product of actinium and obtained artificially by the bombardment of thorium with protons — symbol *Fr*; see ELEMENT table

fran·gu·la \'fraŋ-gyə-lə\ *n* : the bark of the alder buckthorn used in medicine esp. formerly for its laxative properties

fran·gu·lin \-lən\ *n* : an orange glycoside $C_{21}H_{20}O_9$ obtained esp. from the bark of the alder buckthorn and yielding emodin and rhamnose on hydrolysis

frank \'fraŋk\ *adj* : clinically evident ⟨~ pus⟩ ⟨~ gout⟩

Frank·fort hor·i·zon·tal plane \'fraŋk-fərt-ˌhȯr-ə-'zänt-ᵊl-, -ˌhär-\ *n* : a plane used in craniometry that is determined the highest point on the upper margin of the opening of each external auditory canal and the low point on the lower margin of the left orbit and that is used to orient a human skull or head usu. so that the plane is horizontal — called also *eye-ear plane, Frankfort horizontal, Frankfort plane*

frank·in·cense \'fraŋ-kən-ˌsen(t)s\ *n* : a fragrant gum resin from trees (genus *Boswellia* of the family Burseraceae) of Somalia and southern coastal Arabia that is an important incense resin and has been used in religious rites, perfumery, and embalming — called also *olibanum*

Frank–Star·ling law \'fräŋk-\ *n* : STARLING'S LAW OF THE HEART

Frank, Otto (1865–1944), German physiologist. Frank served as a professor at several German universities, his longest tenure being at Munich. He pioneered in the development of exact physiological recording techniques. In 1904 he published the first study of direct monitoring of heart sounds. He devised a great number of recording instruments. He published the fruits of his research in a handbook of physiological methodology. Areas of his research included the origin of the arterial pulse, a determination of the volume of blood in the heart, and the functioning of the aorta. Frank also made original contributions to the physiology of the ear.

Starling, Ernest Henry (1866–1927), British physiologist. Starling was one of the outstanding physiologists of his time. He served for many years as professor of physiology at University College in London. His foremost contributions to physiology include an understanding of the maintenance of fluid balance in body tissues, the regulatory role of endocrine secretions, and mechanical controls on heart function. Much of his work was in collaboration with the physiologist William Bayliss (1860–1924). In 1902 they isolated a substance that is released into the blood from the epithelial cells of the duodenum, which in turn stimulates secretion into the intestine of pancreatic digestive juice. Two years later Starling coined the term *hormone* as the name for such substances. In 1918 he formulated a law concerning the heart, stating that (other conditions being equal) the greater the filling of the heart during diastole, the greater the following systole. Thus the heart is able to maintain a constant beat despite considerable variations in blood flow.

This law of the heart led to the concept upon which the law of muscle contraction is based.

Frank–Starling law of the heart *n* : STARLING'S LAW OF THE HEART

fra·ter·nal \frə-'tərn-ᵊl\ *adj* : derived from two ova : DIZYGOTIC ⟨~ twins⟩

Fraun·ho·fer lines \'fraùn-ˌhōf-ər-\ *n pl* : the dark lines in the spectrum of sunlight

Fraunhofer, Joseph von (1787–1826), German optician and physicist. Fraunhofer was a master theoretical optician as well as an expert maker of glass lenses and precision optical instruments. He effected the improvement of the homogeneity of optical glass and increased the size of the blanks free of imperfections, thus making possible the construction of large-diameter lenses. He sought to determine precisely the dispersion and index of refraction for different kinds of optical glass so that the construction of lenses could be based on optical theory and calculation. In 1814 he observed the effect of the refracting medium on light and found that the solar spectrum is crossed with many fine lines. He mapped over 570 lines that he observed between the red and violet ends of the spectrum. With these lines, now known as the Fraunhofer lines, as guides, he determined with unprecedented precision the optical constants of various kinds of glass.

FRCP *abbr* Fellow of the Royal College of Physicians

FRCS *abbr* Fellow of the Royal College of Surgeons

¹freck·le \'frek-əl\ *n* : any of the small brownish spots in the skin that are due to augmented melanin production and that increase in number and intensity on exposure to sunlight — called also *ephelis;* compare LENTIGO — **freck·led** \-əld\ *adj*

²freckle *vt* **freck·led; freck·ling** \'frek-(ə-)liŋ\ : to become marked with freckles

free \'frē\ *adj* **fre·er; fre·est 1 a** : relieved from or lacking something and esp. something unpleasant or burdensome ⟨~ from pain⟩ **b** : not bound or confined by force ⟨upon opening the skull a considerable amount of ~ blood is noted —H. G. Armstrong⟩ **2 a** (1) : not united with, attached to, combined with, or mixed with something else ⟨a ~ surface of a bodily part⟩ (2) : having the bare axon exposed in tissue ⟨a ~ nerve ending⟩ **b** : not chemically combined ⟨~ calcium⟩ **c** : not permanently attached but able to move about ⟨a ~ electron in a metal⟩ **3** : having all living connections severed before removal to another site ⟨a ~ graft⟩ ⟨research . . . in ~ flap transfers —B. R. Alford⟩

free–as·so·ci·ate \ˌfrē-ə-'sō-s(h)ē-ˌāt\ *vt* **free–as·so·ci·at·ed; free–as·so·ci·at·ing** : to engage in free association ⟨asked to ~ about his dream —Maya Pines⟩

free association *n* **1 a** : the expression (as by speaking or writing) of the content of consciousness without censorship as an aid in gaining access to unconscious processes esp. in psychoanalysis **b** : the reporting of the first thought that comes to mind in response to a given stimulus (as a word) **2** : an idea or image elicited by free association **3** : a method using free association

¹free–base \'frē-ˌbās\ *vb* **-based; -bas·ing** *vi* : to prepare or use freebase cocaine ~ *vt* : to prepare or use (cocaine) as freebase — **free·bas·er** \-ˌər\ *n*

²freebase *n* : purified solid cocaine (as crack) in a form that is obtained by treating the powdered hydrochloride of cocaine with an alkaloid base (as sodium bicarbonate) and that can be smoked or heated to produce vapors for inhalation; *specif* : cocaine derived from its hydrochloride by treatment with ammonia or a similar alkaloid solution followed by extraction with a solvent (as ether)

free fall \-ˌfȯl\ *n* : the condition of unrestrained motion in a gravitational field; *also* : such motion

free–float·ing \'frē-'flōt-iŋ\ *adj* : felt as an emotion without apparent cause ⟨~ anxiety⟩

\ə\ **abut** \ᵊ\ **kitten** \ər\ **further** \a\ **ash** \ā\ **ace** \ä\ **cot, cart**
\aù\ **out** \ch\ **chin** \e\ **bet** \ē\ **easy** \g\ **go** \i\ **hit** \ī\ **ice** \j\ **job**
\ŋ\ **sing** \ō\ **go** \ȯ\ **law** \ȯi\ **boy** \th\ **thin** \th\ **the** \ü\ **loot**
\ù\ **foot** \y\ **yet** \zh\ **vision** *See also* Pronunciation Symbols page

free induction decay *n* : a time-based electrical signal that is detected in a nuclear magnetic resonance spectrometer, that is produced by induction from the motion of the magnetic moments of nuclei, that decays with time, that can be converted to a more conventional frequency-based signal using analysis by Fourier transforms, and that with a suitable display can be used to extract more information from a test sample or subject than is possible in conventional nuclear magnetic resonance spectroscopy — abbr. *FID*

free–liv·ing \'frē-'liv-iŋ\ *adj* 1 : not fixed to the substrate but capable of motility ⟨a ∼ protozoan⟩ 2 : being metabolically independent : neither parasitic nor symbiotic

free·mar·tin \'frē-ˌmärt-ᵊn\ *n* : a sexually imperfect usu. sterile female calf born as a twin with a male

free radical *n* : an esp. reactive atom or group of atoms that has one or more unpaired electrons; *esp* : one that is produced in the body by natural biological processes or introduced from outside (as in tobacco smoke, toxins, or pollutants) and that can damage cells, proteins, and DNA by altering their chemical structure

free–running *adj* : not involving or subjected to entrainment or resetting periodically by an environmental factor (as photoperiod) ⟨a ∼ circadian rhythm⟩

free·stand·ing \'frē-'stand-iŋ\ *adj* : being independent; *esp* : not part of or affiliated with another organization ⟨a ∼ surgical center⟩ ⟨a ∼ emergency clinic⟩

free–swim·ming \-ˌswim-iŋ\ *adj* : able to swim about : not attached ⟨a ∼ larva of a trematode⟩

freeze \'frēz\ *vb* **froze** \'frōz\; **fro·zen** \'frōz-ᵊn\; **freez·ing** *vi* 1 : to become hardened into a solid (as ice) by loss of heat 2 **a** : to become chilled with cold ⟨almost *froze* to death⟩ **b** : to anesthetize a part esp. by cold ∼ *vt* 1 : to cause to harden into a solid (as ice) by loss of heat 2 : to make extremely cold : CHILL 3 **a** : to act on usu. destructively by frost **b** : to anesthetize by cold

freeze–dry \'frēz-'drī\ *vt* **freeze–dried**; **freeze–dry·ing** : to dry and preserve (as food, vaccines, or tissue) in a frozen state under high vacuum — **freeze–dried** *adj*

freeze–etch \'frēz-ˌech\ *adj* : of, relating to, or used in freeze= etching

freeze–etched *adj* : having been subjected to or prepared by freeze-etching

freeze–etch·ing \'frē-'zech-iŋ\ *n* : preparation of a specimen (as of tissue) for electron microscopic examination by freezing, fracturing along natural structural lines, and preparing a replica (as by simultaneous vapor deposition of carbon and platinum)

freeze fracture *also* **freeze–fracturing** *n* : FREEZE-ETCHING — **freeze–fracture** *vt*

freezing point *n* : the temperature at which a liquid solidifies; *specif* : the temperature at which the liquid and solid states of the substance are in equilibrium at atmospheric pressure : MELTING POINT ⟨the *freezing point* of water is 0° Celsius or 32° Fahrenheit⟩

Frei test \'frī-\ *n* : a serological test for the identification of lymphogranuloma venereum — called also *Frei skin test*
   Frei, Wilhelm Siegmund (1885–1943), German dermatologist. Frei did research in allergic diseases of the skin and experimental syphilis. He described lymphogranuloma venereum and introduced a specific cutaneous diagnostic test for it in 1925.

frem·i·tus \'frem-ət-əs\ *n* : a sensation felt by a hand placed on a part of the body (as the chest) that vibrates during speech

fre·nal \'frēn-ᵊl\ *adj* : of or relating to a frenum

French \'french\ *n, pl* **French** : a unit of measure equal to one-third millimeter used in measuring the outside diameter of a tubular instrument (as a catheter or sound) inserted into a bodily cavity ⟨the catheter shaft size is three ∼ —*Medical Industry Today*⟩ — abbr. *F*

fren·ec·to·my \frə-'nek-tə-mē\ *n, pl* **-mies** : excision of a frenulum

fren·u·lum \'fren-yə-ləm\ *n, pl* **-la** \-lə\ : a connecting fold of membrane serving to support or restrain a part (as the tongue)

fre·num \'frē-nəm\ *n, pl* **frenums** *or* **fre·na** \-nə\ : FRENULUM

fren·zy \'fren-zē\ *n, pl* **frenzies** 1 **a** : a temporary madness **b** : a violent mental or emotional agitation 2 : intense usu. wild and often disorderly compulsive or agitated activity — **fren·zied** \-zēd\ *adj*

freq *abbr* frequency

fre·quen·cy \'frē-kwən-sē\ *n, pl* **-cies** 1 : the number of individuals in a single class when objects are classified according to variations in a set of one or more specified attributes 2 : the number of repetitions of a periodic process in a unit of time

fresh·en \'fresh-ən\ *vt* **fresh·ened; fresh·en·ing** \'fresh-(ə-)niŋ\ *of a milk animal* : to begin lactating

Freud·ian \'froid-ē-ən\ *adj* : of, relating to, or according with the psychoanalytic theories or practices of Freud — **Freudian** *n* — **Freud·ian·ism** \-ə-ˌniz-əm\ *n*
   Freud \'froid\, **Sigmund (1856–1939),** Austrian neurologist and psychiatrist. Freud was the founder of psychoanalysis. He began his study of hysteria with Josef Breuer, whose method of treatment was hypnosis. From 1892 to 1895 Freud developed treatment by the technique of free association of ideas. He came to believe that a complex of repressed and forgotten impressions underlies all abnormal mental states such as hysteria, and that a cure could be affected by a revelation of these impressions. His work in this area convinced him of the fact of infantile sexuality. He also developed a theory that dreams are an unconscious representation of repressed desires, especially sexual desires. In 1900 he published his greatest work, *The Interpretation of Dreams.*

Freudian slip *n* : a slip of the tongue that is motivated by and reveals some unconscious aspect of the mind

Freund's adjuvant \'froin(d)z-, 'froin(t)s-\ *n* : any of several oil and water emulsions that contain antigens and are used to stimulate antibody production in experimental animals
   Freund \'froind\, **Jules Thomas (1890–1960),** American immunologist. Freund was a pioneer in immunological research who developed basic laboratory methods that are now standard. He is known above all for his work on adjuvants that enhance the effectiveness of vaccines. In a 1944 article he discussed such adjuvants as paraffin oil, lanolin= like substances, and killed tubercle bacilli. Other areas of his research were the mechanisms of allergy, antibody formation, toxin-antitoxin reaction, tuberculosis, poliomyelitis, and malaria.

fri·a·ble \'frī-ə-bəl\ *adj* : easily crumbled or pulverized ⟨∼ carcinomatous tissue⟩; *also* : marked by erosion and bleeding ⟨a ∼ cervix with bleeding on contact —Pippa Oakeshott *et al*⟩ — **fri·a·bil·i·ty** \ˌfrī-ə-'bil-ət-ē\ *n, pl* **-ties**

fri·ar's bal·sam \ˌfrī(ə)rz-\ *n* : an alcoholic solution containing essentially benzoin, storax, balsam of Tolu, and aloes used chiefly as a local application (as for small fissures) and after addition to hot water as an inhalant (as in laryngitis) — called also *compound benzoin tincture*

Fried·län·der's bacillus \'frēt-ˌlen-dərz-, 'frēd-\ *or* **Friedländ·er bacillus** *n* : PNEUMOBACILLUS
   Friedländer, Carl (1847–1887), German pathologist. Friedländer was an innovator in bacteriology. He is known chiefly for his work on the organisms associated with pneumonia. He demonstrated that cocci are invariably present in the disease. In 1882 he isolated the organism now known as Friedländer's bacillus, which he believed to be the causative agent in all cases of labor pneumonia. A year later he described a diplococcus associated with pneumonia. Friedländer is also remembered for his original description of thromboangiitis obliterans in 1876.

Fried·man test \'frēd-mən-\ *also* **Friedman's test** *n* : a modification of the Aschheim-Zondek test for pregnancy using rabbits as test animals

Friedman, Maurice Harold (1903–1991), American physiologist. Friedman developed his test for pregnancy with Maxwell Edward Lapham (*b* 1899) and introduced it in 1931.

Fried·reich's ataxia \'frēd-rīks-, 'frēt-rīks-\ *n* : a recessive hereditary degenerative disease affecting the spinal column, cerebellum, and medulla, marked by muscular incoordination and twitching, and usu. becoming manifest in the adult

Friedreich \'frēt-rīk\, **Nikolaus (1825–1882),** German neurologist. Friedreich undertook research on muscle atrophy, muscle hypertrophy, and heart disease. He is known for two original descriptions: the condition now known as Friedreich's ataxia in 1863 and paramyoclonus multiplex in 1881.

Friend virus \'frend-\ *n* : a strain of murine leukemia virus that causes erythroleukemia in mice — called also *Friend leukemia virus*

Friend, Charlotte (1921–1987), American microbiologist. Friend served as professor and director of the center for experimental cell biology at Mt. Sinai Medical School in New York. She did research in immunology, virology, and the relationship between viruses and cancer.

frig·id \'frij-əd\ *adj* **1** : abnormally averse to sexual intercourse — used esp. of women **2** *of a female* : unable to achieve orgasm during sexual intercourse

fri·gid·i·ty \frij-'id-ət-ē\ *n, pl* **-ties** : marked or abnormal sexual indifference esp. in a woman

frig·o·rif·ic \ˌfrig-ə-'rif-ik\ *adj* : causing cold ⟨∼ mixtures⟩

fringe \'frinj\ *n, often attrib* : one of various light or dark bands produced by the interference or diffraction of light

fringed tapeworm \'frinjd-\ *n* : a tapeworm of the genus *Thysanosoma* (*T. actinioides*) found in the intestine and bile ducts of ruminants esp. in the western U.S.

frog \'frȯg, 'fräg\ *n* **1** : any of various smooth-skinned web-footed largely aquatic tailless agile leaping amphibians (as of the suborder Diplasiocoela) **2** : the triangular elastic horny pad in the middle of the sole of the foot of a horse **3** : a condition in the throat that produces hoarseness ⟨had a ∼ in his throat⟩

Fröh·lich's syndrome *or* **Froeh·lich's syndrome** \'frā-liks-, 'frœ-liks-\ *also* **Fröhlich syndrome** *n* : ADIPOSOGENITAL DYSTROPHY

Fröhlich \'frœ-lik\, **Alfred (1871–1953),** Austrian pharmacologist and neurologist. Fröhlich investigated a wide range of topics bearing on pharmacology and neurology including the influence of various therapeutic agents on the central nervous system, the pathways for visceral pain, the contraction of striated muscle fibers, and the effect of pituitrin upon the autonomic nervous system. He published his account of the condition now known as Fröhlich's syndrome in 1901.

frondosum — see CHORION FRONDOSUM

frons \'fränz\ *n, pl* **fron·tes** \'frän-ˌtēz\ : FOREHEAD

front·ad \'frən-ˌtad\ *adv* : toward the front ⟨outside the eye the infraorbital line runs —Nils Holmgren⟩

fron·tal \'frənt-ᵊl\ *adj* **1** : of, relating to, or adjacent to the forehead or the frontal bone **2** : of, relating to, or situated at the front or anteriorly **3** : parallel to the main axis of the body and at right angles to the sagittal plane ⟨a ∼ plane⟩ — **fron·tal·ly** \-ᵊl-ē\ *adv*

frontal artery *n* : SUPRATROCHLEAR ARTERY

frontal bone *n* : a bone that forms the forehead and roofs over most of the orbits and nasal cavity and that at birth consists of two halves separated by a suture; *also* : either of the two halves esp. in a vertebrate in which they do not unite to form a single bone

frontal crest *n* : a median ridge on the internal surface of the vertical part of the human frontal bone

frontal eminence *n* : the prominence of the human frontal bone above each superciliary ridge

frontal gyrus *n* : any of the convolutions of the outer surface of the frontal lobe of the brain — called also *frontal convolution*

fron·ta·lis \ˌfrən-'tā-ləs\ *n* : the muscle of the forehead that forms part of the occipitofrontalis — called also *frontalis muscle*

frontal leukotomy *n* : PREFRONTAL LOBOTOMY

frontal lobe *n* : the anterior division of each cerebral hemisphere having its lower part in the anterior fossa of the skull and bordered behind by the central sulcus

frontal lobotomy *n* : PREFRONTAL LOBOTOMY

frontal nerve *n* : a branch of the ophthalmic nerve supplying the forehead, scalp, and adjoining parts

frontal process *n* **1** : a long plate that is part of the maxillary bone and contributes to the formation of the lateral part of the nose and of the nasal cavity — called also *nasal process* **2** : a process of the zygomatic bone articulating superiorly with the frontal bone, forming part of the orbit anteriorly, and articulating with the sphenoid bone posteriorly

frontal sinus *n* : either of two air spaces lined with mucous membrane each of which lies within the frontal bone above one of the orbits

frontal vein *n* : a vein of the middle of the forehead that unites with the supraorbital vein to form the angular vein near the inner angle of the orbit

frontes *pl of* FRONS

fron·to·oc·cip·i·tal \ˌfrən-tō-äk-'sip-ət-ᵊl, ˌfrän-\ *adj* : of or relating to the forehead and occiput

fron·to·pa·ri·etal \-pə-'rī-ət-ᵊl\ *adj* : of, relating to, or involving both frontal and parietal bones of the skull

frontoparietal suture *n* : CORONAL SUTURE

fron·to·tem·po·ral \-'tem-p(ə-)rəl\ *adj* : of or relating to the frontal and the temporal bones

¹frost·bite \'frȯs(t)-ˌbīt\ *vt* **-bit** \-ˌbit\; **-bit·ten** \-ˌbit-ᵊn\; **-bit·ing** \-ˌbīt-iŋ\ : to affect or injure by frost or frostbite

²frostbite *n* : the superficial or deep freezing of the tissues of some part of the body (as the feet or hands); *also* : the damage to tissues caused by freezing

frost·nip \'frȯs(t)-ˌnip\ *n* : the reversible freezing of superficial skin layers that is usu. marked by numbness and whiteness of the skin

¹froth \'frȯth\ *n, pl* **froths** \'frȯths, 'frȯthz\ : a foamy slaver sometimes accompanying disease or exhaustion

²froth \'frȯth, 'frȯth\ *vt* : to foam at the mouth

frot·tage \frȯ-'täzh\ *n* : FROTTEURISM

frot·teur \frȯ-'tər\ *n* : one who practices frotteurism

frot·teur·ism \-ˌiz-əm\ *n* : the paraphiliac practice of achieving sexual stimulation or orgasm by touching and rubbing against a person without the person's consent and usu. in a public place — called also *frottage*

froze *past of* FREEZE

frozen *past part of* FREEZE

frozen shoulder *n* : a shoulder affected by severe pain, stiffness, and restricted motion — called also *adhesive capsulitis*

FRSC *abbr* Fellow of the Royal Society of Canada

fruc·to·kin·ase \ˌfrək-tō-'kīn-ˌās, -'kin-, -ˌāz, ˌfrük-\ *n* : a kinase that catalyzes the transfer of phosphate groups to fructose

fruc·to·san \'frək-tə-ˌsan, 'frük-\ *n* : a polysaccharide (as inulin) yielding primarily fructose on hydrolysis — called also *levulosan*

fruc·tose \'frək-ˌtōs, 'frük-, 'frúk-, -ˌtōz\ *n* **1** : an optically active sugar $C_6H_{12}O_6$ that differs from glucose in having a ketonic rather than an aldehydic carbonyl group **2** : the very sweet soluble levorotatory D-form of fructose that occurs esp. in fruit juices and honey — called also *levulose*

fructose–1,6–di·phos·phate \-ˌdī-'fäs-ˌfāt\ *n* : a diphosphate ester of fructose $C_6H_{14}O_{12}P_2$ reversibly formed from fructose-6-phosphate as an intermediate in carbohydrate metabolism

---

\ə\ **abut** \ᵊ\ **kitten** \ər\ **further** \a\ **ash** \ā\ **ace** \ä\ **cot, cart** \au̇\ **out** \ch\ **chin** \e\ **bet** \ē\ **easy** \g\ **go** \i\ **hit** \ī\ **ice** \j\ **job** \ŋ\ **sing** \ō\ **go** \ȯ\ **law** \ȯi\ **boy** \th\ **thin** \t͟h\ **the** \ü\ **loot** \u̇\ **foot** \y\ **yet** \zh\ **vision** *See also* Pronunciation Symbols page

E
F

fructose–6–phos·phate \-'fäs-ˌfāt\ n : a phosphate of fructose C₆H₁₃O₉P that is formed as an intermediate in carbohydrate metabolism and can be reversibly converted to glucose-6-phosphate

fruc·to·side \'frək-tə-ˌsīd, 'frük-\ n : a glycoside that yields fructosidic fructose on hydrolysis — **fruc·to·sid·ic** \ˌfrək-tə-'sid-ik, ˌfrük-\ adj

fruc·tos·uria \ˌfrək-tə-'s(y)ùr-ē-ə\ n : the presence of fructose in the urine

fru·giv·o·rous \frü-'jiv-ə-rəs\ adj : feeding on fruit

fruit \'früt\ n, often attrib 1 : the usu. edible reproductive body of a seed plant; esp : one having a sweet pulp associated with the seed ⟨the ∼ of the tree⟩ 2 : a product of fertilization in a plant with its modified envelopes or appendages; specif : the ripened ovary of a seed plant and its contents

fruit·ar·i·an \frü-'ter-ē-ən\ n : one who lives chiefly on fruit

fruit fly n : any of various small dipteran flies (as a drosophila) whose larvae feed on fruit or decaying vegetable matter

fruit·ing body \'früt-iŋ-\ n : a plant organ specialized for producing spores; esp : SPOROPHORE

fruit sugar n : FRUCTOSE 2

fru·se·mide \'frü-sə-ˌmīd\ n, chiefly Brit : FUROSEMIDE

frus·trate \'frəs-ˌtrāt\ vt **frus·trat·ed; frus·trat·ing** : to induce feelings of frustration in

frus·trat·ed adj : filled with a sense of frustration : feeling deep insecurity, discouragement, or dissatisfaction ⟨learned not to resort to aggressiveness when ∼ —Ashley Montagu⟩

frus·tra·tion \(ˌ)frəs-'trā-shən\ n 1 : a deep chronic sense or state of insecurity and dissatisfaction arising from unresolved problems or unfulfilled needs 2 : something that frustrates

FSH abbr follicle-stimulating hormone

ft abbr feet; foot

F₂ \'ef-'tü\ n : F₂ GENERATION; also : F₂ HYBRID

F₂ generation n : the generation produced by interbreeding individuals of an F₁ generation and consisting of individuals that exhibit the result of recombination and segregation of genes controlling traits for which stocks of the P₁ generation differ — called also second filial generation

F₂ hybrid n : an individual of an F₂ generation — called also second generation hybrid

fuch·sin or **fuch·sine** \'fyük-sən, -ˌsēn\ n : a dye that is produced by oxidation of a mixture of aniline and toluidines, that yields a brilliant bluish red, and that is used in carbolfuchsin paint, in Schiff's reagent, and as a biological stain

Fuchs \'füks\, **Leonhard (1501–1566),** German botanist and physician. In 1542 Fuchs published De Historia Stirpium, a manual of herbal plants that stands as a landmark in botany. The work is historically important for its orderly presentation, accurate drawings and precise plant descriptions, and its glossary of botanical terms. Fuchs was especially interested in the medicinal properties of plants, and his book listed the reputed powers of each. The genus Fuchsia was named in his honor by Linnaeus in 1753. Fuchsia also denotes the vivid reddish purple color of the flowers of many plants belonging to the genus.

fuch·si·no·phil·ic \f(y)ük-ˌsin-ə-'fil-ik\ or **fuch·sin·o·phil** \-'sin-ə-ˌfil\ also **fuch·sin·o·phile** \-ˌfīl\ adj : having or involving an affinity for the acid dye fuchsin ⟨∼ cytoplasmic granules⟩ ⟨the ∼ mitochondrial reaction⟩

fu·co·san \'fyü-kə-ˌsan\ n : a polysaccharide occurring in algae of the genus Fucus and in some other brown algae and yielding fucose on hydrolysis

fu·cose \'fyü-ˌkōs, -ˌkōz\ n : an aldose sugar that occurs in bound form in the dextrorotatory D-form in various glycosides and in the levorotatory L-form in some brown algae and in mammalian polysaccharides typical of some blood groups

fu·co·si·dase \ˌfyü-'kō-sə-ˌdās, -ˌdāz\ n : an enzyme existing in stereoisomeric alpha and beta forms that catalyzes the metabolism of fucose and some of its derivatives — see FUCOSIDOSIS

fu·co·si·do·sis \-ˌkō-sə-'dō-səs\ n, pl **-do·ses** \-ˌsēz\ : a disorder of metabolism inherited as a recessive trait and charac-

terized by progressive neurological degeneration, deficiency of the alpha stereoisomer of fucosidase, and accumulation of fucose-containing carbohydrates

fu·cus \'fyü-kəs\ n **1** cap : a genus (family Fucaceae) of cartilaginous brown algae used in the kelp industry **2** : any brown alga of the genus Fucus; broadly : any of various brown algae

fu·gac·i·ty \fyü-'gas-ət-ē\ n, pl **-ties** : the vapor pressure of a vapor assumed to be an ideal gas obtained by correcting the determined vapor pressure and useful as a measure of the escaping tendency of a substance from a heterogeneous system

fugax — see AMAUROSIS FUGAX, PROCTALGIA FUGAX

fu·gi·tive \'fyü-jət-iv\ adj : tending to be inconstant or transient ⟨∼ aches and pains —Berton Roueche⟩

fu·gu \'f(y)ü-(ˌ)gü\ n : any of various very poisonous puffers that contain tetrodotoxin and that are used as food in Japan after the toxin-containing organs are removed

fugue \'fyüg\ n : a disturbed state of consciousness in which the one affected seems to perform acts in full awareness but upon recovery cannot recollect them

ful·gu·ra·tion \ˌfùl-g(y)ə-'rā-shən, ˌfùl-jə-, ˌfəl-\ n : ELECTRODESICCATION — **ful·gu·rate** \'fùl-g(y)ə-ˌrāt, -jə-, 'fəl-\ vt **-rat·ed; -rat·ing**

full–blown adj : fully developed : being in its most extreme or serious form : possessing or exhibiting the characteristic symptoms ⟨a ∼ cold⟩ ⟨∼ hypertension⟩ ⟨a collection of symptoms that isn't quite ∼ AIDS —J. Silberner⟩

full–mouthed \'fùl-'maùthd, 'fəl-, -'maùtht\ adj : having a full complement of teeth — used esp. of sheep and cattle ⟨∼ ewes⟩

ful·mi·nant \'fùl-mə-nənt, 'fəl-\ adj : coming on suddenly with great severity ⟨∼ hepatitis with total hepatocyte necrosis —C. L. Humberston et al⟩

ful·mi·nat·ing \-ˌnāt-iŋ\ adj : FULMINANT ⟨∼ infection⟩ — **ful·mi·na·tion** \ˌfùl-mə-'nā-shən, ˌfəl-\ n

fu·ma·gil·lin \ˌfyü-mə-'jil-ən\ n : a crystalline orally effective antibiotic ester of an unsaturated acid produced by a soil fungus of the genus Aspergillus (A. fumigatus) and used in the treatment of amebiasis

fu·ma·rase \'fyü-mə-ˌrās, -ˌrāz\ n : an enzyme that catalyzes the interconversion (as in the Krebs cycle) of fumaric acid and malic acid or their salts

fu·ma·rate \-ˌrāt\ n : a salt or ester of fumaric acid

fu·mar·ic acid \fyù-ˌmar-ik-\ n : a crystalline acid C₄H₄O₄ formed from succinic acid as an intermediate in the Krebs cycle

fu·mig·a·cin \fyü-'mig-ə-sən\ n : a crystalline antibiotic acid C₃₂H₄₄O₈ obtained from a soil fungus of the genus Aspergillus (A. fumigatus) — called also helvolic acid

fu·mi·gant \'fyü-mi-gənt\ n : a substance used in fumigating

fu·mi·gate \'fyü-mə-ˌgāt\ vt **-gat·ed; -gat·ing** : to apply smoke, vapor, or gas to esp. for the purpose of disinfecting or of destroying pests — **fu·mi·ga·tion** \ˌfyü-mə-'gā-shən\ n — **fu·mi·ga·tor** \'fyü-mə-ˌgāt-ər\ n

¹**func·tion** \'fəŋ(k)-shən\ n : any of a group of related actions contributing to a larger action; esp : the normal and specific contribution of a bodily part to the economy of a living organism — see VITAL FUNCTION — **func·tion·less** \-ləs\ adj

²**function** vi **func·tioned; func·tion·ing** \-sh(ə-)niŋ\ : to have a function ⟨shivering ∼s to maintain the heat of the body⟩

func·tion·al \'fəŋ(k)-shnəl, -shən-ᵊl\ adj **1 a** : of, connected with, or being a function — compare STRUCTURAL 1 **b** : affecting physiological or psychological functions but not organic structure ⟨∼ heart disease⟩ ⟨a ∼ psychosis⟩ — compare ORGANIC 1b **2** : performing or able to perform a regular function — **func·tion·al·ly** \-ē\ adv

functional bleeding n : discharge of blood from the uterus that is not due to any organic lesion

functional food n : NUTRACEUTICAL

functional group n : a characteristic reactive unit of a chemical compound

functional magnetic resonance imaging n : magnetic resonance imaging used to demonstrate correlations between physical changes (as in blood flow) in the brain and mental functioning (as in performing cognitive tasks) — abbr. *fMRI*; called also *functional MRI*

fun·dal \'fən-d⁰l\ *adj* : FUNDIC

fun·da·ment \'fən-də-mənt\ *n* **1** : BUTTOCKS **2** : ANUS

fun·da·men·tal \ˌfən-də-'ment-⁰l\ *n* : the principal musical tone produced by vibration (as of a string or column of air) on which a series of higher overtones is based

fun·dec·to·my \ˌfən-'dek-tə-mē\ *n, pl* **-mies** : excision of a fundus (as of the uterus)

fun·dic \'fən-dik\ *adj* : of or relating to a fundus

fundic gland *n* : one of the tubular glands of the fundus of the stomach secreting pepsin and mucus — compare CHIEF CELL 1

fun·do·pli·ca·tion \ˌfən-dō-plī-'kā-shən\ *n* : a surgical procedure in which the upper portion of the stomach is wrapped around the lower end of the esophagus and sutured in place as a treatment for the reflux of stomach contents into the esophagus — see NISSEN FUNDOPLICATION

fun·dus \'fən-dəs\ *n, pl* **fun·di** \-ˌdī, -ˌdē\ : the bottom of or part opposite the aperture of the internal surface of a hollow organ: as **a** : the greater curvature of the stomach **b** : the lower back part of the bladder **c** : the large upper end of the uterus **d** : the part of the eye opposite the pupil

fun·du·scop·ic *also* **fun·do·scop·ic** \ˌfən-də-'skäp-ik\ *adj* : of, done by, or obtained by ophthalmoscopic examination of the fundus of the eye — **fun·dus·co·py** \ˌfən-'dəs-kə-pē\ *also* **fun·dos·co·py** \-'däs-\ *n, pl* **-pies**

fun·gal \'fən-gəl\ *adj* **1** : of, relating to, or having the characteristics of fungi **2** : caused by a fungus ⟨∼ infections⟩

fun·gate \'fən-ˌgāt\ *vt* **-gat·ed; -gat·ing** : to assume a fungal form or grow rapidly like a fungus ⟨a bulky *fungating* lesion —R. F. Thoeni⟩ — **fun·ga·tion** \ˌfən-'gā-shən\ *n*

fun·ge·mia *or chiefly Brit* **fun·gae·mia** \fən-'jē-mē-ə, fən-'gē-mē-ə\ *n* : the presence of fungi (as yeasts) in the blood

fungi *pl of* FUNGUS

Fun·gi \'fən-ˌjī *also* 'fən-gī\ *n pl* : a kingdom of living things comprising the fungi

fun·gi·cid·al \ˌfən-jə-'sīd-⁰l, ˌfən-gə-\ *adj* : destroying fungi; *broadly* : inhibiting the growth of fungi — **fun·gi·cid·al·ly** \-⁰l-ē\ *adv*

fun·gi·cide \'fən-jə-ˌsīd, 'fən-gə-\ *n* : an agent that destroys fungi or inhibits their growth

fun·gi·ci·din \ˌfən-jə-'sīd-⁰n, ˌfən-gə-\ *n* : NYSTATIN

fun·gi·form \'fən-jə-ˌfȯrm, 'fən-gə-\ *adj* : shaped like a mushroom

fungiform papilla *n* : any of numerous papillae on the upper surface of the tongue that are flat-topped and noticeably red from the richly vascular stroma and usu. contain taste buds

Fungi Im·per·fec·ti \-ˌim-pər-'fek-ˌtī\ *n pl, in former classifications* : a major group of fungi comprising the imperfect fungi — compare DEUTEROMYCETES

fun·gi·sta·sis \ˌfən-jə-'stā-səs *also* ˌfən-gə-, -'sta-; *chiefly Brit* ˌfən-ˌjis-tə-səs\ *n, pl* **-sta·ses** \-ˌsēz\ : inhibition of the growth and reproduction of fungi without destroying them

fun·gi·stat \'fən-jə-ˌstat *also* 'fən-gə-\ *n* : a fungistatic agent

fun·gi·stat·ic \ˌfən-jə-'stat-ik *also* ˌfən-gə-\ *adj* : capable of inhibiting the growth and reproduction of fungi without destroying them ⟨a ∼ agent⟩ — **fun·gi·stat·i·cal·ly** \-i-k(ə-)lē\ *adv*

fun·gi·tox·ic \-'täk-sik\ *adj* : toxic to fungi — **fun·gi·tox·ic·i·ty** \-ˌtäk-'sis-ət-ē\ *n, pl* **-ties**

Fun·gi·zone \'fən-jə-ˌzōn\ *trademark* — used for a preparation of amphotericin B

fun·goid \'fən-ˌgȯid\ *adj* : resembling, characteristic of, caused by, or being a fungus ⟨a ∼ ulcer⟩ ⟨a ∼ growth⟩

fungoides — see MYCOSIS FUNGOIDES

fun·gous \'fən-gəs\ *adj* : FUNGAL

fun·gus \'fən-gəs\ *n, pl* **fun·gi** \'fən-ˌjī *also* 'fən-ˌgī\ *also* **fun·gus·es** \'fən-gə-səz\ *often attrib* **1** : any of the kingdom Fungi of saprophytic and parasitic spore-producing eukaryotic typically filamentous organisms formerly classified as plants

that lack chlorophyll and include molds, rusts, mildews, smuts, mushrooms, and yeasts **2** : infection with a fungus

fu·nic \'fyü-nik\ *adj* : of, relating to, or originating in the umbilical cord

fu·ni·cle \'fyü-nə-kəl\ *n* : FUNICULUS

fu·nic·u·lar \fyù-'nik-yə-lər, fə-\ *adj* : of, relating tō, or being a funiculus

fu·nic·u·li·tis \fyù-ˌnik-yə-'līt-əs, fə-\ *n* : inflammation of the spermatic cord

fu·nic·u·lus \fyù-'nik-yə-ləs, fə-\ *n, pl* **-li** \-ˌlī, -ˌlē\ : any of various bodily structures more or less like a cord in form: as **a** : one of the longitudinal subdivisions of white matter in each lateral half of the spinal cord — see ANTERIOR FUNICULUS, LATERAL FUNICULUS, POSTERIOR FUNICULUS; compare COLUMN a **b** : SPERMATIC CORD

fu·nis \'fyü-nəs\ *n* : UMBILICAL CORD

fun·nel \'fən-⁰l\ *n* : a utensil that is usu. a hollow cone with a tube extending from the smaller end and that is designed to catch and direct a downward flow — see BÜCHNER FUNNEL

funnel chest *n* : a depression of the anterior wall of the chest produced by a sinking in of the sternum — called also *funnel breast, pectus excavatum*

fun·ny bone \'fən-ē-\ *n* : the place at the back of the elbow where the ulnar nerve rests against a prominence of the humerus — called also *crazy bone*

FUO *abbr* fever of undetermined origin

fur \'fər\ *n, often attrib* **1** : the hairy coat of a mammal esp. when fine, soft, and thick **2** : a coat of epithelial debris on the tongue

fu·ran \'fyú(ə)r-ˌan, fyù-'ran\ *also* **fu·rane** \'fyú(ə)r-ˌān, fyù-'rān\ *n* : a flammable liquid C_4H_4O obtained from oils of pines or made synthetically and used esp. in organic synthesis; *also* : a derivative of furan

fu·ra·nose \'fyúr-ə-ˌnōs, -ˌnōz\ *n* : a sugar having an oxygen-containing ring of five atoms

fu·ra·zol·i·done \ˌfyúr-ə-'zäl-ə-ˌdōn\ *n* : an antimicrobial drug $C_8H_7N_3O_5$ used against bacteria and some protozoans esp. in infections of the gastrointestinal tract

fur·co·cer·cous \ˌfər-kō-'sər-kəs\ *adj, of a cercaria* : having the tail forked

fur·cu·la \'fər-kyə-lə\ *n, pl* **-lae** \-ˌlē, -ˌlī\ : an elevation on the embryonic floor of the pharynx from which the epiglottis develops

fur·fur \'fər-fər\ *n* **1** : an exfoliation of a surface esp. of the epidermis : DANDRUFF, SCURF **2** **fur·fu·res** \-f(y)ər-ˌēz\ *pl* : flaky particles (as of scurf)

fur·fu·ra·ceous \ˌfər-f(y)ə-'rā-shəs\ *adj* : consisting of or covered with flaky particles ⟨∼ eczema⟩

fur·fu·ral \'fər-f(y)ə-ˌral\ *n* : a liquid aldehyde $C_5H_4O_2$ of penetrating odor that is usu. made from plant materials and used esp. in making furan or phenolic resins and as a solvent

fur·fur·al·de·hyde \ˌfər-f(y)ə-'ral-də-ˌhīd\ *n* : FURFURAL

fur·fu·ran \'fər-f(y)ə-ˌran\ *n* : FURAN

fu·ri·ous rabies \'fyúr-ē-əs-\ *n* : rabies characterized by spasm of the muscles of throat and diaphragm, choking, salivation, extreme excitement, and evidence of fear often manifested by indiscriminate snapping at objects — compare PARALYTIC RABIES

fu·ro·se·mide \fyù-'rō-sə-ˌmīd\ *n* : a powerful diuretic $C_{12}H_{11}CIN_2O_5S$ used esp. to treat edema — called also *frusemide, fursemide;* see LASIX

furred \'fərd\ *adj* : having a coating consisting chiefly of mucus and dead epithelial cells ⟨a ∼ tongue⟩

fur·row \'fər-(ˌ)ō, -ə(-w)\ *n* **1** : a marked narrow depression or groove **2** : a deep wrinkle

fur·se·mide \'fər-sə-ˌmīd\ *n* : FUROSEMIDE

fu·run·cle \'fyú(ə)r-ˌən-kəl\ *n* : BOIL — **fu·run·cu·lar** \fyú-'rən-kyə-lər\ *adj* — **fu·run·cu·lous** \-ləs\ *adj*

\ə\ **abut** \⁰\ **kitten** \ər\ **further** \a\ **ash** \ā\ **ace** \ä\ **cot, cart**
\aú\ **out** \ch\ **chin** \e\ **bet** \ē\ **easy** \g\ **go** \i\ **hit** \ī\ **ice** \j\ **job**
\ŋ\ **sing** \ō\ **go** \ȯ\ **law** \ȯi\ **boy** \th\ **thin** \th̲\ **the** \ü\ **loot**
\ú\ **foot** \y\ **yet** \zh\ **vision** *See also* Pronunciation Symbols page

E
F

fu·run·cu·loid \fyü-'rəŋ-kyə-ˌlȯid\ *adj* : resembling a furuncle

fu·run·cu·lo·sis \fyü-ˌrəŋ-kyə-'lō-səs\ *n, pl* **-lo·ses** \-ˌsēz\ **1** : the condition of having or tending to develop multiple furuncles **2** : a highly infectious disease of various salmon and trout (genera *Salmo* and *Oncorhynchus*) and their relatives that is caused by a bacterium (*Aeromonas salmonicida* of the family Vibrionaceae)

fu·run·cu·lus \fyü-'rəŋ-kyə-ləs\ *n, pl* **-cu·li** \-ˌlī\ : FURUNCLE

fu·sar·i·um \fyü-'zer-ē-əm\ *n* **1** *cap* : a genus of ascomycetous fungi (family Tuberculariaceae) including important plant pathogens, agents (as *F. solani* and *F. oxysporum*) of infectious conditions in humans and domestic animals, and mycotoxin-producing forms (as *F. moniliforme* and *F. proliferatum*) that contaminate agricultural products (as grain) **2** *pl* **-ia** \-ē-ə\ : any fungus of the genus *Fusarium*

fuse \'fyüz\ *vb* **fused; fus·ing** *vt* : to cause to undergo fusion ⟨~ a joint⟩ ~ *vi* : to undergo fusion

fused \'fyüzd\ *adj* : having atoms in common — used of ring systems in chemical compounds (as an oxazine dye)

fu·sel oil \'fyü-zəl-\ *n* : an acrid oily liquid occurring in insufficiently distilled alcoholic liquors, consisting chiefly of amyl alcohol, and used esp. as a source of alcohols and as a solvent

fu·si·form \'fyü-zə-ˌfȯrm\ *adj* : tapering toward each end ⟨~ bacteria⟩ ⟨a ~ aneurysm⟩

Fu·si·for·mis \ˌfyü-zə-'fȯrm-əs\ *n, in some classifications* : a genus of parasitic anaerobic or microaerophilic nonmotile bacteria of the family Bacteroidaceae now usu. included in the genus *Fusobacterium*

fu·sion \'fyü-zhən\ *n, often attrib* **1 a** : the act or process of liquefying or rendering plastic by heat **b** : the liquid or plastic state induced by heat **2** : a union by or as if by melting together: as **a** : a merging of diverse elements into a unified whole; *specif* : the blending of retinal images in binocular vision **b** : a combination of ingredients achieved by heating and mixing together **c** (1) : a blend of sensations, perceptions, ideas, or attitudes such that the component elements can seldom be identified by introspective analysis (2) : the perception of light from a source that is intermittent above a critical frequency as if the source were continuous — called also *flicker fusion;* compare FLICKER **d** : the surgical immobilization of a joint — see SPINAL FUSION **3** : the union of atomic nuclei to form heavier nuclei resulting in the release of enormous quantities of energy when certain light elements unite — called also *nuclear fusion* — **fu·sion·al** \-ᵊl\ *adj*

fu·so·bac·te·ri·um \ˌfyü-zō-bak-'tir-ē-əm\ *n* **1** *cap* : a genus of gram-negative anaerobic strictly parasitic rod-shaped bacteria of the family Bacteroidaceae that include some pathogens occurring esp. in purulent or gangrenous infections **2** *pl* **-ria** \-ē-ə\ : any bacterium of the genus *Fusobacterium*

fu·so·cel·lu·lar \-'sel-yə-lər\ *adj* : composed of fusiform cells

fu·so·spi·ro·chet·al *or chiefly Brit* **fu·so·spi·ro·chaet·al** \-ˌspī-rə-'kēt-ᵊl\ *adj* : of, relating to, or caused by fusobacteria and spirochetes

fu·so·spi·ro·chet·o·sis *or chiefly Brit* **fu·so·spi·ro·chaet·o·sis** \-ˌkēt-'ō-səs\ *n, pl* **-o·ses** \-ˌsēz\ : ACUTE NECROTIZING ULCERATIVE GINGIVITIS

G

g \'jē\ *n, pl* **g's** *or* **gs** \'jēz\ : a unit of force equal to the force exerted by gravity on a body at rest and used to indicate the force to which a body is subjected when accelerated

g *abbr* **1** gauge **2** gender **3** gingival **4** glucose **5** grain **6** gram **7** gravity; acceleration of gravity

G *abbr* guanine

Ga *symbol* gallium

GABA *abbr* gamma-aminobutyric acid

gab·a·pen·tin \'gab-ə-ˌpen-tin\ *n* : an anticonvulsant drug $C_9H_{17}NO_2$ structurally related to gamma-aminobutyric acid that is administered orally as adjunctive therapy in the treatment of partial seizures — see NEURONTIN

G–ac·tin \'jē-ˌak-tən\ *n* : a globular monomeric form of actin produced in solutions of low ionic concentration — compare F-ACTIN

gad·fly \'gad-ˌflī\ *n, pl* **-flies** : any of various flies (as a horsefly, botfly, or warble fly) that bite or annoy livestock

Gad·i·dae \'gad-ə-ˌdē\ *n pl* : a large family of bony fishes (order Anacanthini) including many important food fishes (as the cod, haddock, and pollacks) and several whose livers yield an oil rich in vitamins A and D

gad·o·lin·i·um \ˌgad-ᵊl-'in-ē-əm\ *n* : a magnetic metallic element of the rare-earth group — symbol *Gd;* see ELEMENT table

Ga·dus \'gā-dəs\ *n* : the type genus of the family Gadidae consisting of the typical codfishes

gage *var of* GAUGE

gag reflex \'gag-\ *n* : reflex contraction of the muscles of the throat caused esp. by stimulation (as by touch) of the pharynx

gain \'gān\ *vi* : to improve in health ⟨the patient ~ed daily⟩

gait \'gāt\ *n* **1** : a manner of walking or moving on foot **2** : a sequence of foot movements (as a walk, trot, pace, or canter) by which a horse or a dog moves forward

gal *abbr* **1** galactose **2** gallon

ga·lac·ta·gogue *or* **ga·lac·to·gogue** \gə-'lak-tə-ˌgäg\ *n* : an agent that promotes the secretion of milk — called also *lactagogue*

ga·lac·tan \gə-'lak-tən, -ˌtan\ *n* : any of several polysaccharides of plant or animal origin (as agar) that yield galactose on hydrolysis

ga·lac·tin \gə-'lak-tən, -(ˌ)tin\ *n* : PROLACTIN

ga·lac·ti·tol \gə-'lak-tə-ˌtȯl\ *n* : a white faintly sweet alcohol $C_6H_{14}O_6$ that occurs in various plants esp. of the snapdragon family (Scrophulariaceae), is formed from galactose by reduction in some living tissues, and accumulates in urine and various tissues (as the lens of the eye) in individuals deficient in certain enzymes (as galactokinase) — called also *dulcitol*

ga·lac·to·cele \-tə-ˌsēl\ *n* : a cystic tumor containing milk or a milky fluid; *esp* : such a tumor of a mammary gland

ga·lac·to·ki·nase \gə-ˌlak-tō-'kīn-ˌās, -'kin-, -ˌāz\ *n* : a kinase that catalyzes the transfer of phosphate groups to galactose

ga·lac·to·lip·id \-'lip-əd\ *n* : a glycolipid that yields galactose on hydrolysis

ga·lac·to·phore \gə-'lak-tə-ˌfō(ə)r, -ˌfȯ(ə)r\ *n* : a duct carrying milk

gal·ac·toph·o·rous \ˌgal-ˌak-'täf-ə-rəs\ *adj* : conveying milk ⟨a ~ duct⟩

ga·lac·to·poi·e·sis \gə-ˌlak-tə-pȯi-'ē-səs\ *n, pl* **-e·ses** \-ˌsēz\ : formation and secretion of milk

¹**ga·lac·to·poi·et·ic** \-pȯi-'et-ik\ *adj* : inducing galactopoiesis ⟨a ~ dose of thyroxine⟩

²**galactopoietic** *n* : a galactopoietic agent

ga·lac·tor·rhea *or chiefly Brit* **ga·lac·tor·rhoea** \gə-ˌlak-tə-'rē-ə\ *n* : a spontaneous flow of milk from the nipple

ga·lac·tos·amine \gə-ˌlak-'tō-sə-ˌmēn, -zə-\ *n* : an amino derivative $C_6H_{13}O_5N$ of galactose that occurs in cartilage

ga·lac·tose \gə-'lak-ˌtōs, -ˌtōz\ *n* : an optically active sugar $C_6H_{12}O_6$ that is less soluble and less sweet than glucose and is known in dextrorotatory, levorotatory, and racemic forms

ga·lac·tos·emia *or chiefly Brit* **ga·lac·tos·aemia** \gə-ˌlak-tə-'sē-mē-ə\ *n* : a metabolic disorder inherited as an autosomal recessive trait in which galactose accumulates in the blood due to deficiency of an enzyme catalyzing its conversion to glucose — **ga·lac·tos·emic** or chiefly Brit **ga·lac·tos·aemic** \-mik\ adj

ga·lac·to·si·dase \gə-ˌlak-'tō-sə-ˌdās, -zə-ˌdāz\ n : an enzyme (as lactase) that hydrolyzes a galactoside

ga·lac·to·side \gə-'lak-tə-ˌsīd\ n : a glycoside that yields galactose on hydrolysis

gal·ac·to·sis \ˌga-ˌlak-'tō-səs\ n, pl **-to·ses** \-ˌsēz\ : a secretion of milk

ga·lac·tos·uria \gə-ˌlak-(ˌ)tō-'s(h)ùr-ē-ə, -'syùr-\ n : an excretion of urine containing galactose

ga·lact·uron·ic acid \gə-ˌlak-t(y)ù-ˌrän-ik-\ n : a crystalline aldehyde acid $C_6H_{10}O_7$ that occurs esp. in polymerized form in pectin

gal·an·gal \gə-'laŋ-gəl\ n **1** : either of two eastern Asian perennial herbs (Alpinia galanga and A. officinarum) of the ginger family with dark green sword-shaped leaves and pungent aromatic rhizomes **2** : the fresh, dried, or ground rhizome of a galangal used in cookery as a spice and sometimes medicinally — called also galangal root

gal·a·nin \'ga-lə-nin\ n : a neurotransmitter that plays a role in regulating various physiological functions (as contraction of gastrointestinal muscle and inhibition of insulin) and is thought to be associated with the urge to eat fatty foods

Gal·ba \'gal-bə, 'gòl-\ n : a widely distributed genus of freshwater snails of the family Lymnaeidae that include important Old World hosts of a liver fluke of the genus Fasciola (F. hepatica) and that are sometimes considered indistinguishable from the genus Lymnaea — compare FOSSARIA

gal·ba·num \'gal-bə-nəm, 'gòl-\ n : a yellowish to green or brown aromatic bitter gum resin derived from several Asian plants (genus Ferula and esp. F. galbaniflua) of the family Umbelliferae and that resembles asafetida and has been used for similar medicinal purposes

ga·lea \'gāl-ē-ə, 'gal-\ n : GALEA APONEUROTICA

galea apo·neu·ro·ti·ca \-ˌap-ō-n(y)ù-'rät-ik-ə\ n : the aponeurosis underlying the scalp and linking the frontalis and occipitalis muscles — called also epicranial aponeurosis

ga·len·ic \gə-'len-ik\ also **ga·len·i·cal** \-i-kəl\ adj **1** cap : of or relating to Galen or his medical principles or method **2** usu galenical : constituting a galenical ⟨galenical preparations⟩

Ga·len \'gā-lən\ (ca 129–ca 199), Greek physician. Galen is universally acclaimed as one of the greatest physicians of ancient times. He was the leading medical authority of the Christian world until the 16th century. He is especially notable because he derived his data from experiments and is now regarded as the father of experimental physiology. Although his observations were generally accurate, because he was allowed to dissect only animals, his statements about humans based on these dissections inevitably contained inaccuracies which were accepted for centuries afterwards. He was the author of 83 treatises; his writings summarized the anatomical knowledge of the time. His work includes descriptions of about 300 muscles and the principal parts of the brain. He also described the treatment of fractures, dislocations, methods of amputation, and the resection of bones. In his practice he used sutures and ligatures, astringents, and cautery. Finally, Galen believed in the curative powers of plants; he used over 500 plant derivatives in his medicinal preparations.

ga·len·i·cal \gə-'len-i-kəl\ n : a standard medicinal preparation (as an extract or tincture) containing usu. one or more active constituents of a plant and made by a process that leaves the inert and other undesirable constituents of the plant undissolved

Ga·len·ism \'gā-lə-ˌniz-əm\ n : the Galenic system of medical practice

Ga·len·ist \'gā-lə-nist\ n : a follower or disciple of the ancient physician Galen

Galen's vein \'gā-lənz-\ n **1** : either of a pair of cerebral veins in the roof of the third ventricle that drain the interior of the brain **2** : GREAT CEREBRAL VEIN

¹gall \'gòl\ n : BILE; esp : bile obtained from an animal and used in the arts or medicine

²gall n : a skin sore caused by chronic irritation

³gall vt : to rub and wear away by friction : CHAFE ⟨the loose saddle ~ed the horse's back⟩

⁴gall n : a swelling of plant tissue usu. due to fungi or insect parasites and sometimes forming an important source of tannin

gall·la \'gal-ə, 'gòl-\ n : any of certain nutgalls from oaks that are used in pharmacy for their astringent properties

gal·la·mine tri·eth·io·dide \'gal-ə-ˌmēn-ˌtrī-ˌeth-'ī-ə-ˌdīd\ n : a substituted ammonium salt $C_{30}H_{60}I_3N_3O_3$ that is used to produce muscle relaxation esp. during anesthesia — called also gallamine

gal·late \'gal-ˌāt, 'gòl-\ n : a salt or ester of gallic acid — see PROPYL GALLATE

gall·blad·der \'gòl-ˌblad-ər\ n : a membranous muscular sac in which bile from the liver is stored — called also cholecyst

gal·lein \'gal-ē-ən, 'gal-ˌēn\ n : a metallic-green crystalline phthalein dye $C_{20}H_{12}O_7$ used esp. in dyeing textiles violet and as an indicator

galli — see CRISTA GALLI

gal·lic acid \ˌgal-ik-, ˌgò-lik-\ n : a white crystalline acid $C_7H_6O_5$ found widely in plants or combined in tannins and used esp. in dyes and writing ink and as a photographic developer

gallicus — see MORBUS GALLICUS

gal·li·pot \'gal-ə-ˌpät\ n : a small usu. ceramic vessel with a small mouth; esp : one used by apothecaries to hold medicines

gal·li·um \'gal-ē-əm\ n : a rare bluish white metallic element that is hard and brittle at low temperatures but melts just above room temperature and expands on freezing and that is used in the form of its hydrated nitrate salt $Ga(NO_3)_3·9H_2O$ to treat hypercalcemia caused by certain cancers — symbol Ga; see ELEMENT table

gall·nut \'gòl-ˌnət\ n : a gall resembling a nut

gal·lon \'gal-ən\ n **1** : a U.S. unit of liquid capacity equal to four quarts or 231 cubic inches or 3.785 liters **2** : a British unit of liquid and dry capacity equal to four quarts or 277.42 cubic inches or 4.544 liters — called also imperial gallon

¹gal·lop \'gal-əp\ vi : to progress or ride at a gallop ~ vt : to cause to gallop

²gallop n **1** : a bounding gait of a quadruped; specif : a fast natural 3-beat gait of the horse **2** : GALLOP RHYTHM

galloping adj, of a disease : progressing rapidly toward a fatal conclusion ⟨~ consumption⟩

gallop rhythm n : an abnormal heart rhythm marked by the occurrence of three distinct sounds in each heartbeat like the sound of a galloping horse — called also gallop

gal·lo·tan·nic acid \ˌgal-ō-ˌtan-ik-, ˌgòl-\ n : TANNIC ACID 1

gal·lo·tan·nin \-'tan-ən\ n : TANNIC ACID 1

gall·sick \'gòl-ˌsik\ adj **1** : affected with anaplasmosis ⟨a herd of ~ cattle⟩ **2** : producing or having the conditions to produce anaplasmosis ⟨~ pastureland⟩

gall sickness n : ANAPLASMOSIS

gall·stone \'gòl-ˌstōn\ n : a calculus (as of cholesterol) formed in the gallbladder or biliary passages — called also biliary calculus, cholelith

galv abbr galvanic; galvanism; galvanized

gal·van·ic \gal-'van-ik\ adj : of, relating to, involving, or producing a direct current of electricity ⟨~ stimulation of flaccid muscles⟩ — compare FARADIC — **gal·van·i·cal·ly** \-i-k(ə-)lē\ adv

Gal·va·ni \gäl-'vä-nē\, **Luigi** (1737–1798), Italian physician and physicist. Galvani is known for his pioneering experiments in the electrical stimulation of frog nerves and muscles. His experiments motivated the discovery of a source of a constant current of electricity by Alessandro Volta.

galvanic skin response *n* : a change in the electrical resistance of the skin that is a physiochemical response to emotional arousal which increases sympathetic nervous system activity — abbr. *GSR*

gal·va·nism \'gal-və-ˌniz-əm\ *n* **1** : a direct current of electricity esp. when produced by chemical action (as in a storage battery) **2** : the therapeutic use of direct electric current (as to relieve pain)

gal·va·ni·za·tion *or Brit* **gal·va·ni·sa·tion** \ˌgal-və-nə-'zā-shən\ *n* : the act or process of galvanizing; *specif* : the application of an electric current to the human body for medical purposes

gal·va·nize *or Brit* **gal·va·nise** \'gal-və-ˌnīz\ *vt* **-nized** *or Brit* **-nised; -niz·ing** *or Brit* **-nis·ing** : to subject to the action of an electric current esp. for the purpose of stimulating physiologically ⟨∼ a muscle⟩

gal·va·no·cau·tery \gal-ˌvan-ə-'kȯt-ə-rē, ˌgal-və-nə-\ *n, pl* **-ter·ies** : ELECTROCAUTERY 2

gal·va·no·far·ad·iza·tion \-ˌfar-əd-ə-'zā-shən\ *n* : therapeutic use of a galvanic and a faradic current simultaneously

gal·va·nom·e·ter \ˌgal-və-'näm-ət-ər\ *n* : an instrument for detecting or measuring a small electric current by movements of a magnetic needle or of a coil in a magnetic field — **gal·va·no·met·ric** \-nō-'me-trik\ *adj*

gal·va·no·scope \gal-'van-ə-ˌskōp, 'gal-və-nə-\ *n* : an instrument for detecting the presence and direction of an electric current by the deflection of a magnetic needle

gal·va·no·tax·is \ˌgal-ˌvan-ə-'tak-səs, ˌgal-və-nə-, -nō-\ *n, pl* **-tax·es** \-ˌsēz\ : a taxis in which a direct electric current is the orienting stimulus

gal·va·no·ther·a·py \-'ther-ə-pē\ *n, pl* **-pies** : the treatment of disease (as arthritis) by galvanism

gal·va·not·ro·pism \ˌgal-və-'nä-trə-ˌpiz-əm\ *n* : a tropism in which electricity is the stimulus — **gal·va·no·tro·pic** \gal-ˌvan-ə-'trō-pik, ˌgal-və-nə-\ *adj*

gal·ziek·te \'gäl-ˌzēk-tə, -ˌsēk-\ *n* : ANAPLASMOSIS

gam·bier *also* **gam·bir** \'gam-ˌbi(ə)r\ *n* : a yellowish catechu that is obtained from a southeast Asian woody vine (*Uncaria gambir*) of the madder family and that is used for chewing with the betel nut and for tanning and dyeing

gam·boge \gam-'bōj, -'büzh\ *n* : an orange to brown gum resin from southeast Asian trees (genus *Garcinia* of the family Guttiferae) that is used as a yellow pigment and cathartic — called also *cambogia*

gam·etan·gi·um \ˌgam-ə-'tan-jē-əm\ *n, pl* **-gia** \-jē-ə\ : a cell or organ in which gametes are developed

ga·mete \'gam-ˌēt *also* gə-'mēt\ *n* : a mature male or female germ cell usu. possessing a haploid chromosome set and capable of initiating formation of a new diploid individual by fusion with a gamete of the opposite sex — called also *sex cell* — **ga·met·ic** \gə-'met-ik, -'mēt-\ *adj* — **ga·met·i·cal·ly** \-i-k(ə-)lē\ *adv*

gamete in·tra·fal·lo·pi·an transfer \-ˌin-trə-fə-'lō-pē-ən-\ *n* : a method of assisting reproduction in cases of infertility in which eggs are obtained from an ovary, mixed with sperm, and inserted into a fallopian tube by a laparoscope — abbr. *GIFT;* called also *gamete intrafallopian tube transfer;* compare ZYGOTE INTRAFALLOPIAN TRANSFER

ga·me·to·cide \gə-'mēt-ə-ˌsīd\ *n* : an agent that destroys the gametocytes of a malaria parasite

ga·me·to·cyte \gə-'mēt-ə-ˌsīt\ *n* : a cell (as of a protozoan causing malaria) that divides to produce gametes

ga·me·to·gen·e·sis \ˌgam-ə-tə-'jen-ə-səs, gə-ˌmēt-ə-\ *n, pl* **-e·ses** \-ˌsēz\ : the production of gametes — **gam·etog·e·nous** \ˌgam-ə-'täj-ə-nəs\ *adj*

gam·etog·e·ny \ˌgam-ə-'täj-ə-nē\ *n, pl* **-nies** : GAMETOGENESIS

gam·etog·o·ny \-'täg-ə-nē\ *n, pl* **-nies** : gamogenesis esp. of protozoans

gam·e·toid \'gam-ə-ˌtoid\ *n* : a multinucleate gamete

ga·me·to·phyte \gə-'mēt-ə-ˌfīt\ *n* : the individual or generation of a plant exhibiting alternation of generations that bears sex organs — compare SPOROPHYTE — **ga·me·to·phyt·ic** \-ˌmēt-ə-'fit-ik\ *adj*

gam·ic \'gam-ik\ *adj* : requiring fertilization : SEXUAL ⟨a ∼ egg⟩ ⟨∼ reproduction⟩

¹gam·ma \'gam-ə\ *n* **1** : the third letter of the Greek alphabet — symbol Γ or γ **2** : a unit of magnetic flux density equal to one nanotesla **3** : GAMMA RAY — usu. used as the attributive form of *gamma ray* ⟨∼ counter⟩ **4** : MICROGRAM 1

²gamma *or* γ- *adj* **1** : of or relating to one of three or more closely related chemical substances ⟨the *gamma* chain of hemoglobin⟩ ⟨γ-yohimbine⟩ — used somewhat arbitrarily to specify ordinal relationship or a particular physical form and esp. one that is allotropic, isomeric, or stereoisomeric (as in *gamma* benzene hexachloride) **2** : third in position in the structure of an organic molecule from a particular group or atom; *also* : occurring at or having a structure characterized by such a position ⟨γ-hydroxy acids⟩ **3** *of streptococci* : producing no hemolysis on blood agar plates

gam·ma–ami·no·bu·tyr·ic acid *also* γ–ami·no·bu·tyr·ic **acid** \ˌgam-ə-ə-ˌmē-(ˌ)nō-byü-ˌtir-ik-, ˌgam-ə-ˌam-ə-(ˌ)nō-\ *n* : an amino acid $C_4H_9NO_2$ that is a neurotransmitter that induces inhibition of postsynaptic neurons — abbr. *GABA*

gamma benzene hexa·chlo·ride \-ˌhek-sə-'klō(ə)r-ˌīd, -'klȯ(ə)r-\ *n* : the gamma isomer of benzene hexachloride that comprises the insecticide lindane and is used in medicine esp. as a scabicide and pediculicide in a one-percent cream, lotion, or shampoo — called also *gamma BHC*

gamma camera *n* : a camera that detects the gamma-ray photons produced by radionuclide decay and is used esp. in medical diagnostic scanning to create a visible record of a radioactive substance injected into the body

gam·ma·cism \'gam-ə-ˌsiz-əm\ *n* : difficulty in pronouncing velar consonants (as \g\ and \k\)

gamma globulin *n* **1 a** : a protein fraction of blood rich in antibodies **b** : a sterile solution of gamma globulin from pooled human blood administered esp. for passive immunity against measles, German measles, hepatitis A, or poliomyelitis **2** : any of numerous globulins of blood plasma or serum that have less electrophoretic mobility at alkaline pH than serum albumins, alpha globulins, or beta globulins and that include most antibodies

gamma hydroxybutyrate *n* : GHB

gamma interferon *n* : an interferon produced by T cells that regulates the immune response (as by the activation of macrophages and natural killer cells) and is used in a form obtained from recombinant DNA in the control of infections associated with chronic granulomatous disease and sometimes in the treatment of other conditions (as basal-cell carcinoma, bowenoid papulosis, leukemia, or rheumatoid arthritis) — called also *interferon gamma;* compare ALPHA INTERFERON, BETA INTERFERON

Gamma Knife *trademark* — used for a medical device that emits a highly focused beam of gamma radiation used in noninvasive surgery

gamma radiation *n* : radiation that is composed of gamma rays and is used in cancer radiotherapy

gamma ray *n* : a photon emitted spontaneously by a radioactive substance; *also* : a high-energy photon — usu. used in pl.

gam·mop·a·thy \gam-'äp-ə-thē\ *n, pl* **-thies** : a disorder characterized by a disturbance in the body's synthesis of antibodies ⟨multiple myeloma is a type of monoclonal ∼⟩

gamo·gen·e·sis \ˌgam-ə-'jen-ə-səs\ *n, pl* **-e·ses** \-ˌsēz\ : sexual reproduction — **gamo·ge·net·ic** \-jə-'net-ik\ *adj* — **gamo·ge·net·i·cal·ly** \-i-k(ə-)lē\ *adv*

gam·one \'gam-ˌōn\ *n* : any of various substances believed to be liberated by eggs or sperms and to affect germ cells of the opposite sex

gam·ont \'gam-ˌänt\ *n* : a protozoan gametocyte

gan·ci·clo·vir \gan-'sī-klə-(ˌ)vir\ *n* : an antiviral drug $C_9H_{13}N_5O_4$ related to acyclovir and used esp. in the treatment of cytomegalovirus retinitis in immunocompromised patients — called also *DHPG*

ganglia *pl of* GANGLION

gan·gli·al \'gaŋ-glē-əl\ *adj* : of, relating to, or resembling a ganglion

gan·gli·at·ed cord \'gaŋ-glē-ˌāt-əd-\ *n* : either of the two main trunks of the sympathetic nervous system of which one lies on each side of the spinal column

gan·gli·form \-glə-ˌfôrm\ *adj* : having the form of a ganglion

gan·gli·o·blast \'gaŋ-glē-ō-ˌblast\ *n* : an embryonic cell that produces gangliocytes

gan·gli·o·cyte \-ˌsīt\ *n* : GANGLION CELL

gan·gli·o·ma \ˌgaŋ-glē-'ō-mə\ *n, pl* **-mas** *also* **-ma·ta** \-mət-ə\ : a tumor of a ganglion

gan·gli·on \'gaŋ-glē-ən\ *n, pl* **-glia** \-glē-ə\ *also* **-gli·ons** **1** : a small cystic tumor (as on the back of the wrist) containing viscid fluid and connected either with a joint membrane or tendon sheath **2 a** : a mass of nerve tissue containing cell bodies of neurons that is located outside the central nervous system and forms an enlargement upon a nerve or upon two or more nerves at their point of junction or separation **b** : a mass of gray matter within the brain or spinal cord : NUCLEUS **2** — see BASAL GANGLION

gan·gli·on·at·ed \-ə-ˌnāt-əd\ *adj* : furnished with ganglia

ganglion cell *n* : a nerve cell having its body outside the central nervous system

gan·gli·on·ec·to·my \ˌgaŋ-glē-ə-'nek-tə-mē\ *n, pl* **-mies** : surgical removal of a nerve ganglion

gan·glio·neu·ro·ma \-(ˌ)ō-n(y)ù-'rō-mə\ *n, pl* **-mas** *also* **-ma·ta** \-mət-ə\ : a neuroma derived from ganglion cells

gan·gli·on·ic \ˌgaŋ-glē-'än-ik\ *adj* : of, relating to, or affecting ganglia or ganglion cells

ganglionic blocking agent *n* : a drug used to produce blockade at a ganglion

gan·gli·on·it·is \ˌgaŋ-glē-ə-'nīt-əs\ *n* : inflammation of a ganglion

gan·gli·o·side \'gaŋ-glē-ə-ˌsīd\ *n* : any of a group of glycolipids that are found esp. in the plasma membrane of cells of the gray matter and have sialic acid, hexoses, and hexosamines in the carbohydrate part and ceramide as the lipid

gan·gli·o·si·do·sis \ˌgaŋ-glē-ō-sī-'dō-səs\ *n, pl* **-do·ses** \-ˌsēz\ : any of several inherited metabolic diseases (as Tay-Sachs disease) characterized by an enzyme deficiency which causes accumulation of gangliosides in the tissues

gan·go·sa \gaŋ-'gō-sə\ *n* : a destructive ulcerative condition believed to be a manifestation of yaws that usu. originates about the soft palate and spreads into the hard palate, nasal structures, and outward to the face, eroding intervening bone, cartilage, and soft tissues — compare GOUNDOU

¹gan·grene \'gaŋ-ˌgrēn, gaŋ-', 'gan-ˌ, gan-'\ *n* : local death of soft tissues due to loss of blood supply

²gangrene *vb* **gan·grened; gan·gren·ing** *vt* : to make gangrenous ∼ *vi* : to become gangrenous

gangrenosum — see PYODERMA GANGRENOSUM

gan·gre·nous \'gaŋ-grə-nəs\ *adj* : affected by, characterized by, or resembling gangrene ⟨a ∼ foot⟩ ⟨∼ septicemia⟩

gangrenous stomatitis *n* : CANCRUM ORIS

gan·ja \'gän-jə, 'gan-\ *n* : a potent preparation of marijuana used esp. for smoking; *broadly* : MARIJUANA

Gan·ser syndrome \'gän-zər-\ *or* **Gan·ser's syndrome** \-zər(z)-\ *n* : a pattern of psychopathological behavior characterized by the giving of approximate answers (as 2 × 2 = about 5) and found in prisoners and in others who consciously or unconsciously seek to give misleading information regarding their mental state

Ganser, Sigbert Joseph Maria (1853–1931), German psychiatrist. In 1898 Ganser described the syndrome that now bears his name.

gap \'gap\ *n* : a break in continuity esp. of structure : HIATUS

gapes \'gāps\ *n pl but sing in constr* : a disease of birds and esp. young birds in which gapeworms invade and irritate the trachea

gape·worm \'gāp-ˌwərm\ *n* : a nematode worm of the genus *Syngamus* (*S. trachea*) that causes gapes of birds

gap junction *n* : an area of contact between adjacent cells characterized by modification of the plasma membranes for intercellular communication or transfer of low molecular= weight substances — **gap–junc·tion·al** \'gap-ˌjəŋk-shən-əl, -shnəl\ *adj*

garden he·lio·trope \-'hē-lē-ə-ˌtrōp, *Brit usu* -'hel-yə-\ *n* : a tall Old World valerian (*Valeriana officinalis*) widely cultivated for its fragrant tiny flowers and for its rhizome and roots which yield the drug valerian

Gard·ner·el·la \ˌgärd-nə-'rel-ə\ *n* : a genus of bacteria of uncertain taxonomic affinities that includes one (*G. vaginalis* syn. *Haemophilus vaginalis*) often present in the flora of the healthy vagina and present in greatly increased numbers in bacterial vaginosis

Gard·ner \'gärd-nər\, Herman L. (*fl* 1955–80), American physician.

Gard·ner's syndrome \'gärd-nərz-\ *n* : a familial polyposis that is characterized by numerous adenomatous polyps in the colon which typically become malignant if left untreated, by osteomas (as of the skull or mandible), and by skin tumors, that is inherited as an autosomal dominant trait, and that is sometimes considered a variant form of familial adenomatous polyposis

gar·get \'gär-gət\ *n* : mastitis of domestic animals; *esp* : chronic bovine mastitis with gross changes in the form and texture of the udder — **gar·gety** \-gət-ē\ *adj*

¹gar·gle \'gär-gəl\ *vb* **gar·gled; gar·gling** \-g(ə-)liŋ\ *vt* **1** : to hold (a liquid) in the mouth or throat and agitate with air from the lungs **2** : to cleanse or disinfect (the oral cavity) by gargling ∼ *vi* : to use a gargle

²gargle *n* : a liquid used in gargling

gar·goyl·ism \'gär-ˌgóil-ˌiz-əm\ *n* : MUCOPOLYSACCHARIDOSIS; *esp* : HURLER'S SYNDROME

gar·lic \'gär-lik\ *n* : a European bulbous herb of the genus *Allium* (*A. sativum*) widely cultivated for its pungent compound bulbs much used in cookery; *also* : one of the bulbs

Gärt·ner's bacillus \'gert-nərz-\ *n* : a motile bacterium of the genus *Salmonella* (*S. enteritidis*) that causes enteritis and is widely distributed in the intestinal tracts of mammals including humans

Gärtner, August Anton Hieronymus (1848–1934), German hygienist and bacteriologist. In 1888 Gärtner described a widely distributed bacterium that is the cause of epidemic diarrheal disease in rodents and gastroenteritis in humans. Although Gärtner originally placed the species in the genus *Bacillus,* it is now classified in the genus *Salmonella* (*S. enteritidis*) and is known by the vernacular name of Gärtner's bacillus.

Gart·ner's duct \'gart-nərz-, 'gert-\ *n* : the remains in the female mammal of a part of the Wolffian duct of the embryo — called also *duct of Gartner*

Gart·ner \'gert-nər\, Hermann Treschow (1785–1827), Danish surgeon and anatomist. Gartner discovered the duct that now bears his name in a sow and in 1822 wrote a detailed description. The structure was apparently first discovered by Marcello Malpighi about 1681.

¹gas \'gas\ *n, pl* **gas·es** *also* **gas·ses** **1** : a fluid (as air) that has neither independent shape nor volume but tends to expand indefinitely **2** : a gaseous product of digestion; *also* : discomfort from this **3** : a gas or gaseous mixture used to produce anesthesia **4** : a substance that can be used to produce a poisonous, asphyxiating, or irritant atmosphere

²gas *vt* **gassed; gas·sing** **1** : to treat chemically with gas **2** : to poison or otherwise affect adversely with gas

GAS *abbr* general adaptation syndrome

gas bacillus *n* : any of several bacteria that form gas in wounds infected with them (esp. *Clostridium perfringens* syn. *C. welchii*)

gas chromatograph *n* : an instrument used to separate a sample into components in gas chromatography

gas chromatography *n* : chromatography in which the sample mixture is vaporized and injected into a stream of carrier gas (as nitrogen or helium) moving through a column containing a stationary phase composed of a liquid or a particu-

G
H

\ə\ abut \ᵊ\ kitten \ər\ further \a\ ash \ā\ ace \ä\ cot, cart \au̇\ out \ch\ chin \e\ bet \ē\ easy \g\ go \i\ hit \ī\ ice \j\ job \ŋ\ sing \ō\ go \ȯ\ law \ȯi\ boy \th\ thin \th̲\ the \ü\ loot \u̇\ foot \y\ yet \zh\ vision *See also* Pronunciation Symbols page

late solid and is separated into its component compounds according to the affinity of the compounds for the stationary phase — abbr. *GC*; compare COLUMN CHROMATOGRAPHY, GAS-LIQUID CHROMATOGRAPHY, THIN-LAYER CHROMATOGRAPHY — **gas chromatographic** *adj*

gas·e·ous \'gas-ē-əs, 'gash-əs\ *adj* : having the form of or being gas; *also* : of or relating to gases

gas gangrene *n* : progressive gangrene marked by impregnation of the dead and dying tissue with gas and caused by one or more toxin-producing bacteria of the genus *Clostridium* that enter the body through wounds and proliferate in necrotic tissue

¹**gash** \'gash\ *vt* : to make a gash in ∼ *vi* : to make a gash : CUT

²**gash** *n* : a deep long cut esp. in flesh

gas·kin \'gas-kən\ *n* : a part of the hind leg of a quadruped between the stifle and the hock

gas–liq·uid chromatography \'gas-'lik-wəd-\ *n* : gas chromatography in which the stationary phase is a liquid — abbr. *GLC* — **gas–liquid chromatographic** *adj*

gas mask *n* : a mask connected to a chemical air filter and used to protect the face and lungs from toxic gases; *broadly* : RESPIRATOR 1

gas·om·e·ter \ga-'säm-ət-ər\ *n* : a laboratory apparatus for holding and measuring gases

gas·o·met·ric \,gas-ə-'me-trik\ *adj* : of or relating to the measurement of gases (as in chemical analysis) — **gas·o·met·ri·cal·ly** \-tri-k(ə-)lē\ *adv* — **gas·om·e·try** \ga-'säm-ə-trē\ *n, pl* **-tries**

gas·se·ri·an ganglion \ga-'sir-ē-ən-\ *n, often cap 1st G* : TRIGEMINAL GANGLION

  Gas·ser \'gä-sər\, **Johann Laurentius (1723–1765),** Austrian anatomist. Gasser was a professor of anatomy at the University of Vienna. In 1765 one of his students, Anton Balthasar Raymund Hirsch (*b* 1743), described in a graduation thesis the gasserian ganglion, naming it in honor of his professor.

gas·ter·oph·i·lo·sis \,gas-tə-,räf-ə-'lō-səs\ *n, pl* **-lo·ses** \-,sēz\ : infestation with horse botflies

Gas·ter·oph·i·lus \-'räf-ə-ləs\ *n* : a genus of botflies including several (esp. *G. intestinalis* in the U.S.) that infest horses and rarely humans

gas·tral \'gas-trəl\ *adj* : of or relating to the stomach or digestive tract

gas·tral·gia \ga-'stral-jə\ *n* : pain in the stomach or epigastrium esp. of a neuralgic type — **gas·tral·gic** \-jik\ *adj*

gas·trec·to·my \ga-'strek-tə-mē\ *n, pl* **-mies** : surgical removal of all or part of the stomach

gas·tric \'gas-trik\ *adj* : of or relating to the stomach

gastrica — see ACHYLIA GASTRICA

gastric artery *n* **1** : a branch of the celiac artery that passes to the cardiac end of the stomach and along the lesser curvature — called also *left gastric artery;* see RIGHT GASTRIC ARTERY **2** : any of several branches of the splenic artery distributed to the greater curvature of the stomach

gastric bypass *n* : a surgical bypass operation performed to restrict food intake and reduce absorption of calories and nutrients in the treatment of severe obesity that typically involves reducing the size of the stomach and reconnecting the smaller stomach to bypass the first portion of the small intestine; *esp* : ROUX-EN-Y GASTRIC BYPASS

gastric gland *n* : any of various glands in the walls of the stomach that secrete gastric juice

gastric juice *n* : a thin watery acid digestive fluid secreted by the glands in the mucous membrane of the stomach and containing 0.2 to 0.4 percent free hydrochloric acid and several enzymes (as pepsin)

gastric pit *n* : any of the numerous depressions in the mucous membrane lining the stomach into which the gastric glands discharge their secretions

gastric ulcer *n* : a peptic ulcer situated in the stomach

gas·trin \'gas-trən\ *n* : any of various polypeptide hormones that are secreted by the gastric mucosa and induce secretion of gastric juice

gas·tri·no·ma \,gas-trə-'nō-mə\ *n, pl* **-mas** *also* **-ma·ta** \-mət-ə\ : a tumor that often involves blood vessels, usu. occurs in the pancreas or the wall of the duodenum, and produces excessive amounts of gastrin which stimulates gastric-acid secretion and consequent formation of ulcers esp. in the duodenum and the jejunum — see ZOLLINGER-ELLISON SYNDROME

gas·tri·tis \ga-'strīt-əs\ *n* : inflammation esp. of the mucous membrane of the stomach

gas·tro·anas·to·mo·sis \,ga-(,)strō-ə-,nas-tə-'mō-səs\ *n, pl* **-mo·ses** \-,sēz\ : the formation by surgical means of a communication between the pyloric and cardiac ends of the stomach when the normal channel is obstructed or contracted

gas·troc·ne·mi·us \,gas-(,)träk-'nē-mē-əs, -trək-\ *n, pl* **-mii** \-mē-,ī\ : the largest and most superficial muscle of the calf of the leg that arises by two heads from the condyles of the femur and has its tendon of insertion incorporated as part of the Achilles tendon — called also *gastrocnemius muscle* — **gas·troc·ne·mi·al** \-mē-əl\ *adj*

gas·tro·coel *also* **gas·tro·coele** \'gas-trə-,sēl\ *n* : ARCHENTERON

gas·tro·co·lic \,gas-trō-'käl-ik, -'kō-lik\ *adj* : of, relating to, or uniting the stomach and colon ⟨a ∼ fistula⟩

gastrocolic omentum *n* : GREATER OMENTUM

gastrocolic reflex *n* : the occurrence of peristalsis following the entrance of food into the empty stomach

Gas·tro·dis·coi·des \,gas-trō-dis-'kói-(,)dēz\ *n* : a genus of amphistome trematode worms including a common intestinal parasite (*G. hominis*) of humans and swine in southeastern Asia

gas·tro·du·o·de·nal \-,d(y)ü-ə-'dēn-ºl, -d(y)ù-'äd-ºn-əl\ *adj* : of, relating to, or involving both the stomach and the duodenum

gastroduodenal artery *n* : an artery that arises from the hepatic artery and divides to form the right gastroepiploic artery and a branch supplying the duodenum and pancreas

gas·tro·du·o·de·ni·tis \-,d(y)ü-ə-(,)dē-'nīt-əs, -d(y)ù-,äd-ºn-'īt-əs\ *n* : inflammation of the stomach and duodenum

gas·tro·du·o·de·nos·to·my \-,d(y)ü-ə-(,)dē-'näs-tə-mē, -d(y)ù-,äd-ºn-'äs-tə-mē\ *n, pl* **-mies** : surgical formation of a passage between the stomach and the duodenum

gas·tro·en·ter·ic \-en-'ter-ik, -in-\ *adj* : GASTROINTESTINAL

gas·tro·en·ter·i·tis \-,ent-ə-'rīt-əs\ *n, pl* **-en·ter·it·i·des** \-'rit-ə-,dēz\ : inflammation of the lining membrane of the stomach and the intestines

gas·tro·en·ter·ol·o·gist \-,en-tə-'räl-ə-jist\ *n* : a specialist in gastroenterology

gas·tro·en·ter·ol·o·gy \-,ent-ə-'räl-ə-jē\ *n, pl* **-gies** : a branch of medicine concerned with the structure, functions, diseases, and pathology of the stomach and intestines — **gas·tro·en·ter·o·log·i·cal** \-rə-'läj-i-kəl\ *or* **gas·tro·en·ter·o·log·ic** \-'läj-ik\ *adj*

gas·tro·en·ter·op·a·thy \-,ent-ə-'räp-ə-thē\ *n, pl* **-thies** : a disease of the stomach and intestines

gas·tro·en·ter·os·to·my \-'räs-tə-mē\ *n, pl* **-mies** : the surgical formation of a passage between the stomach and small intestine

gas·tro·ep·i·plo·ic artery \-,ep-ə-'plō-ik-\ *n* : either of two arteries forming an anastomosis along the greater curvature of the stomach: **a** : one that is larger, arises as one of the two terminal branches of the gastroduodenal artery, and passes from right to left giving off branches to the stomach and greater omentum — called also *right gastroepiploic artery* **b** : one that is smaller, arises as a branch of the splenic artery, and passes from left to right giving off branches to the stomach and to the greater omentum — called also *left gastroepiploic artery*

gas·tro·esoph·a·ge·al *or chiefly Brit* **gas·tro–oe·soph·a·ge·al** \'gas-trō-i-,säf-ə-'jē-əl\ *adj* : of, relating to, or involving stomach and esophagus

gastroesophageal reflux *n* : backward flow of the gastric contents into the esophagus due to improper functioning of a sphincter at the lower end of the esophagus and resulting esp. in heartburn — see HEARTBURN

gas·tro·esoph·a·geal reflux disease *n* : a highly variable chronic condition that is characterized by periodic episodes of gastroesophageal reflux usu. accompanied by heartburn and that may result in histopathologic changes in the esophagus — abbr. *GERD*

gas·tro·gen·ic \ˌgas-trə-'jen-ik\ *or* **gas·trog·e·nous** \ga-'sträj-ə-nəs\ *adj* : of gastric origin ⟨∼ anemia⟩

gas·tro·in·tes·ti·nal \ˌgas-trō-in-'tes-tən-ᵊl, -'tes(t)-nəl\ *adj* : of, relating to, or affecting both stomach and intestine ⟨∼ distress⟩

gastrointestinal series *n* : fluoroscopic and radiographic examination of all or part of the gastrointestinal tract and the esophagus during or following the ingestion or injection of a solution of barium sulfate; *esp* : UPPER GI SERIES

gastrointestinal tract *n* : the stomach and intestine as a functional unit

gas·tro·je·ju·nal \-ji-'jün-ᵊl\ *adj* : of, relating to, or involving both stomach and jejunum ⟨∼ lesions⟩

gas·tro·je·ju·nos·to·my \-ji-(ˌ)jü-'näs-tə-mē\ *n, pl* **-mies** : the surgical formation of a passage between the stomach and jejunum : GASTROENTEROSTOMY

gas·tro·lith \'ga-strə-ˌlith\ *n* : a gastric calculus

gas·trol·o·gist \ga-'sträl-ə-jəst\ *n* : a specialist in gastrology

gas·trol·o·gy \-ə-jē\ *n, pl* **-gies** : the art or science of caring for the stomach either medically or gastronomically

gas·trol·y·sis \-ə-səs\ *n, pl* **-y·ses** \-ˌsēz\ : the surgical operation of freeing the stomach from adhesions

gas·tro·ma·la·cia \ˌgas-trō-mə-'lā-s(h)ē-ə\ *n* : abnormal softening of the stomach walls

gastro–oesophageal *chiefly Brit var of* GASTROESOPHAGEAL

gas·tro·pa·re·sis \ˌgas-trō-pə-'rē-səs\ *n, pl* **gas·tro·pa·re·ses** \-ˌsēz\ : partial paralysis of the stomach ⟨diabetic ∼ is characterized by a triad of postprandial symptoms: nausea, vomiting, and abdominal distension —G. F. Cahill *et al*⟩

gas·tro·pa·thy \ga-'sträp-ə-thē\ *n, pl* **-thies** : a disease of the stomach

gas·tro·pexy \'gas-trə-ˌpek-sē\ *n, pl* **-pex·ies** : a surgical operation in which the stomach is sutured to the abdominal wall

Gas·troph·i·lus \ga-'sträf-ə-ləs\ *n, syn of* GASTEROPHILUS

gas·tro·phren·ic \ˌgas-trə-'fren-ik\ *adj* : of, relating to, or connecting the stomach and diaphragm

gas·tro·pli·ca·tion \ˌgas-trō-plə-'kā-shən\ *n* : a surgical operation for reducing chronic stomach dilatation by plication

Gas·tro·poda \ga-'sträp-ə-də\ *n pl* : a large class of mollusks (as snails) with a univalve shell or none and usu. with a distinct head bearing sensory organs — **gas·tro·pod** \'gas-trə-ˌpäd\ *n or adj*

gas·trop·to·sis \ˌgas-ˌträp-'tō-səs\ *n, pl* **-to·ses** \-ˌsēz\ : abnormal sagging of the stomach into the lower abdomen

gas·tros·chi·sis \ga-'sträs-kə-səs\ *n, pl* **-chi·ses** \-ˌsēz\ : congenital fissure of the ventral abdominal wall

gas·tro·scope \'gas-trə-ˌskōp\ *n* : an endoscope for inspecting the interior of the stomach — **gas·tro·scop·ic** \ˌgas-trə-'skäp-ik\ *adj* — **gas·tros·co·pist** \ga-'sträs-kə-pəst\ *n* — **gas·tros·co·py** \-pē\ *n, pl* **-pies**

gas·tro·splen·ic ligament \ˌgas-trō-ˌsplen-ik-\ *n* : a mesenteric fold passing from the greater curvature of the stomach to the spleen

gas·tros·to·my \ga-'sträs-tə-mē\ *n, pl* **-mies** **1** : the surgical formation of an opening through the abdominal wall into the stomach **2** : the opening made by gastrostomy

gas·trot·o·my \ga-'strät-ə-mē\ *n, pl* **-mies** : surgical incision into the stomach

Gas·trot·ri·cha \ga-'strä-trə-kə\ *n pl* : a small class or other taxon of minute freshwater multicellular animals that superficially resemble infusorians, have cilia on the ventral side, and are related to the rotifers with which they are included in the phylum Aschelminthes — **gas·tro·trich** \'gas-trə-ˌtrik\ *n*

gas·tru·la \'gas-trə-lə\ *n, pl* **-las** *or* **-lae** \-ˌlē, -ˌlī\ : an early metazoan embryo in which the ectoderm, mesoderm, and endoderm are established either by invagination of the blas-

tula (as in fish and amphibians) to form a multilayered cellular cup with a blastopore opening into the archenteron or (as in reptiles, birds, and mammals) by differentiation of the upper layer of the blastodisc into the ectoderm and the lower layer into the endoderm and by the inward migration of cells through the primitive streak to form the mesoderm — compare MORULA — **gas·tru·lar** \-lər\ *adj*

gas·tru·la·tion \ˌgas-trə-'lā-shən\ *n* : the process of becoming or of forming a gastrula — **gas·tru·late** \'gas-trə-ˌlāt\ *vi* **-lat·ed; -lat·ing**

Gatch bed \'gach-\ *n* : HOSPITAL BED

   Gatch, Willis Dew (1878–1954), American surgeon. Gatch did research in experimental and clinical surgery, shock occurring during or after a surgical operation, burns, and diseases of the biliary passages. He introduced his hospital bed in 1909.

¹**gate** \'gāt\ *n* : a molecule or part of a molecule (as an amino acid sequence in a protein) that acts (as by a change in conformation) in response to a stimulus to permit or block passage through a cell membrane

²**gate** *vt* **gat·ed; gat·ing** : to control passage through a cell membrane by way of (a specific channel) by supplying a specific stimulus ⟨a transmembrane ion channel *gated* by the neurotransmitter acetylcholine⟩ — see LIGAND-GATED, VOLTAGE-GATED

gate·keep·er \-ˌkē-pər\ *n* : a health-care professional (as a primary care physician) who regulates access esp. to hospitals and specialists ⟨managed care plans rely on a designated physician ∼ to orchestrate and control the health care of its enrollees —E. A. Halm *et al*⟩

gath·er \'gath-ər, 'geth-\ *vi* **gath·ered; gath·er·ing** \-(ə-)riŋ\ : to swell and fill with pus ⟨the boil is ∼*ing*⟩

gath·er·ing *n* : a suppurating swelling : ABSCESS

gat·ing *n* : an action, process, or mechanism by which the passage of something is controlled

Gau·cher's disease \ˌgō-'shāz-\ *n* : a rare hereditary disorder of lipid metabolism that is caused by an enzyme deficiency of glucocerebrosidase, that is characterized by enormous enlargement of the spleen, pigmentation of the skin, and bone lesions, and that is marked by the presence of large amounts of glucocerebroside in the cells of the reticuloendothelial system — compare NIEMANN-PICK DISEASE, TAY=SACHS DISEASE

   Gau·cher \gō-shā\, **Philippe Charles Ernest (1854–1918),** French physician. Gaucher specialized in skin diseases and syphilology. He described the disease now known as Gaucher's disease in 1882.

¹**gauge** *also* **gage** \'gāj\ *n* **1 a** : measurement according to some standard or system **b** : the dimensions or extent of something **2** : an instrument for or a means of measuring or testing **3** : the diameter of a slender object (as a hypodermic needle)

²**gauge** *also* **gage** *vt* **gauged** *also* **gaged; gaug·ing** *also* **gag·ing** **1 a** : to measure exactly **b** : to determine the capacity or contents of **2 a** : to check for conformity to specifications or limits **b** : to measure off or set out

gaul·the·ria \gȯl-'thir-ē-ə\ *n* **1** *cap* : a genus of evergreen shrubs of the heath family (Ericaceae) that produce small often aromatic fruits resembling berries and include the wintergreen (*G. procumbens*) which is a source of methyl salicylate **2** : a plant of the genus *Gaultheria*

   Gaultier \gō-tyā\, **Jean François (1708–1756),** Canadian physician and botanist. Gaultier made botanical studies of the Quebec region with the Swedish botanist Peter Kalm (1716–1779). Kalm was an associate of Linnaeus, who named the genus *Gaultheria* in honor of Gaultier in 1753.

gaultheria oil *n* : OIL OF WINTERGREEN

gaul·the·rin \'gȯl-thə-rən, gȯl-'thir-ən\ *n* : a glycoside

G
H

\ə\ **abut** \ᵊ\ **kitten** \ər\ **further** \a\ **ash** \ā\ **ace** \ä\ **cot, cart**
\au̇\ **out** \ch\ **chin** \e\ **bet** \ē\ **easy** \g\ **go** \i\ **hit** \ī\ **ice** \j\ **job**
\ŋ\ **sing** \ō\ **go** \ȯ\ **law** \ȯi\ **boy** \th\ **thin** \t̲h̲\ **the** \ü\ **loot**
\u̇\ **foot** \y\ **yet** \zh\ **vision** *See also* Pronunciation Symbols page

$C_{19}H_{26}O_{12}$ of methyl salicylate found esp. in sweet birch and various shrubs of the genus *Gaultheria*

gauss \\'gaus\ *n, pl* **gauss** *also* **gauss·es** : the cgs unit of magnetic flux density that is equal to 1×10^{-4} tesla

  Gauss, Carl Friedrich (1777–1855), German mathematician and astronomer. Gauss is generally regarded as one of the greatest mathematicians of all times. His work on the theory of numbers, published in 1801, is one of the most brilliant achievements in the history of mathematics. Gauss was also a pioneer in applying mathematics to gravitation, electricity, and magnetism. The gauss was named in his honor in 1882.

gauze \\'goz\ *n* : a loosely woven cotton surgical dressing

ga·vage \gə-'väzh, gä-\ *n* : introduction of material into the stomach by a tube

gave *past of* GIVE

gaze \\'gāz\ *vi* **gazed; gaz·ing** : to fix the eyes in a steady and intent look — **gaze** *n*

GB \(')jē-'bē\ *n* : SARIN

GB *abbr* gallbladder

GC *abbr* **1** gas chromatograph; gas chromatography **2** gonococcus

G–CSF *abbr* granulocyte colony-stimulating factor

Gd *symbol* gadolinium

Ge *symbol* germanium

GE *abbr* **1** gastroenterology **2** gradient echo

geel·dik·kop \gēl-'dik-ˌäp\ *n* : a serious photodynamic disease of southern African sheep due to sensitization to light following the ingestion of some plants and characterized by intense jaundice and a severe facial edema

Gei·ger count·er \\'gī-gər-ˌkaun-tər\ *n* : an instrument for detecting the presence and intensity of radiations (as cosmic rays or particles from a radioactive substance) by means of the ionizing effect on an enclosed gas which results in a pulse that is amplified and fed to a device giving a visible or audible indication

  Geiger, Hans (Johannes) Wilhelm (1882–1945), and **Müller** \\'mue-lər\, **Walther** (*fl* 1928), German physicists. Geiger did significant research on atomic theory, radioactivity, and cosmic rays. He developed a number of techniques and instruments for the detection and counting of individual charged particles. With the British physicist Ernest Rutherford (1871–1937), he developed in 1908 the first radiation counter, an instrument that counted alpha particles. With the help of Müller he introduced an improved version of the Geiger counter in 1928. The Geiger=Müller counter marked the introduction of modern electrical devices into radiation research.

Geiger–Mül·ler counter \-'myül-ər-, -'mil-, -'məl-\ *n* : GEIGER COUNTER

Geiger–Müller tube *n* : a gas-filled counting tube with a cylindrical cathode and axial wire electrode for detecting the presence of cosmic rays or radioactive substances by means of the ionizing particles that penetrate its envelope and set up momentary current pulsations in the gas

Geiger tube *n* : GEIGER-MÜLLER TUBE

¹gel \\'jel\ *n* : a colloid in a more solid form than a sol

²gel *vi* **gelled; gel·ling** : to change into or take on the form of a gel — **gel·able** \\'jel-ə-bəl\ *adj*

gel·ate \\'jel-ˌāt\ *vi* **gel·at·ed; gel·at·ing** : GEL

gel·a·tin *also* **gel·a·tine** \\'jel-ət-ən\ *n* **1** : glutinous material obtained from animal tissues by boiling; *esp* : a colloidal protein used as a food, in photography, and in medicine **2 a** : any of various substances (as agar) resembling gelatin **b** : an edible jelly made with gelatin

ge·la·ti·ni·za·tion *or Brit* **ge·la·ti·ni·sa·tion** \jə-ˌlat-ᵊn-ə-'zā-shən, ˌjel-ət-ᵊn-\ *n* : the process of converting into a gelatinous form or into a jelly — **ge·la·ti·nize** *or Brit* **ge·la·ti·nise** \jə-'lat-ᵊn-ˌīz, 'jel-ət-ᵊn-\ *vb* **-nized** *or Brit* **-nised; -niz·ing** *or Brit* **-nis·ing**

gelatinosa — see SUBSTANTIA GELATINOSA

ge·lat·i·nous \jə-'lat-nəs, -ᵊn-əs\ *adj* **1** : resembling gelatin or jelly : VISCOUS **2** : of, relating to, or containing gelatin

gel·ation \je-'lā-shən\ *n* : the formation of a gel from a sol

gel·cap \\'jel-ˌkap\ *n* : a capsule-shaped tablet coated with gelatin for easy swallowing

gel chromatography *n* : GEL FILTRATION

geld \\'geld\ *vt* : CASTRATE 1; *also* : SPAY

geld·ing \\'gel-diŋ\ *n* : a castrated animal; *specif* : a castrated male horse

gel electrophoresis *n* : electrophoresis in which molecules (as proteins and nucleic acids) migrate through a gel and esp. a polyacrylamide gel and separate into bands according to size

gel filtration *n* : chromatography in which the material to be fractionated separates primarily according to molecular size as it moves through a column of a gel and is washed with a solvent so that the fractions appear successively at the end of the column — called also *gel chromatography, molecular sieve chromatography*

gel·ose \\'jel-ōs *also* -ōz\ *n* : a polysaccharide obtained from agar and like gelatin in its ability to form a jelly; *broadly* : a polysaccharide (as agar) occurring in red algae and capable of forming a jelly

gel·se·mine \\'jel-sə-ˌmēn, -mən\ *n* : a crystalline alkaloid $C_{20}H_{22}N_2O_2$ from gelsemium

gel·se·mi·um \jel-'sē-mē-əm\ *n* **1** *cap* : a small genus of woody vines (family Loganiaceae) of Asia and the southern U.S. that include the yellow jessamine (*G. sempervirens*) **2** *pl* **-miums** *or* **-mia** \-mē-ə\ : the root of the yellow jessamine formerly used in medicine

ge·mel·lus \jə-'me-ləs\ *n, pl* **ge·mel·li** \-ˌlī\ *also* **ge·mel·lus·es** : either of two small muscles of the hip that insert into the tendon of the obturator internus: **a** : a superior one originating chiefly from the outer surface of the ischial spine — called also *gemellus superior* **b** : an inferior one originating chiefly from the ischial tuberosity — called also *gemellus inferior*

gem·fi·bro·zil \jem-'fī-brə-(ˌ)zil, -'fib-rə-\ *n* : a drug $C_{15}H_{22}O_3$ that regulates blood serum lipids and is used esp. to lower the levels of triglycerides and increase the levels of HDLs in the treatment of hyperlipidemia — see LOPID

gem·i·nate \\'jem-ə-nət, -ˌnāt\ *adj* : arranged in pairs

gem·i·na·tion \ˌjem-ə-'nā-shən\ *n* : a doubling, duplication, or repetition; *esp* : a formation of two teeth from a single tooth germ

gem·ma \\'jem-ə\ *n, pl* **gem·mae** \-ˌē\ : BUD; *broadly* : an asexual reproductive body that becomes detached from a parent plant

gem·ma·tion \je-'mā-shən\ *n* : asexual reproduction (as in some protozoans) in which a new organism originates as a localized area of growth on or within the parent and subsequently differentiates into a new individual

gem·mule \\'jem-(ˌ)yü(ə)l\ *n* **1** : a theoretical particle in the theory of pangenesis that is shed by a somatic cell and contains all the information necessary to reproduce that cell type (as in an offspring) **2** : a minute thorny process of a nerve-cell dendrite

gen *abbr* **1** general **2** genus

ge·na \\'jē-nə, 'ge-nə\ *n, pl* **ge·nae** \\'jē-ˌnē, 'ge-ˌnī\ : the cheek or lateral part of the head — **ge·nal** \-nəl\ *adj*

gen·der \\'jen-dər\ *n* **1** : SEX 1 **2** : the behavioral, cultural, or psychological traits typically associated with one sex

gender identity *n* : the totality of physical and behavioral traits that are designated by a culture as masculine or feminine

gene \\'jēn\ *n* : a specific sequence of nucleotides in DNA or RNA that is located usu. on a chromosome and that is the functional unit of inheritance controlling the transmission and expression of one or more traits by specifying the structure of a particular polypeptide and esp. a protein or controlling the function of other genetic material — called also *determinant, determiner, factor*

gene complex *n* : a group of genes of an individual or of a potentially interbreeding group that constitute an interacting functional unit ⟨the breakup of adaptive *gene complexes*⟩

gene conversion *n* : a genetic process that is sometimes associated with meiotic recombination in heterozygotes if heteroduplex DNA is formed, that involves the selective enzymatic excision of a mismatched DNA sequence from one heteroduplex strand and replacement with a nucleotide sequence complementary to the other strand so that the two DNA strands are genetically identical, and that results in aberrant gametic ratios (as 3:1 or 1:3 instead of 2:2)

gene flow *n* : the passage and establishment of genes typical of one breeding population into the gene pool of another

gene frequency *n* : the ratio of the number of a specified allele in a population to the total of all alleles at its genetic locus

gene mutation *n* : mutation due to fundamental intramolecular reorganization of a gene — see POINT MUTATION

gene pool *n* : the collection of genes in an interbreeding population that includes each gene at a certain frequency in relation to its alleles : the genetic information of a population of interbreeding organisms ⟨the human *gene pool*⟩

genera *pl of* GENUS

gen·er·al \ˈjen-(ə-)rəl\ *adj* 1 : not confined by specialization or careful limitation ⟨a ∼ surgeon⟩ 2 : belonging to the common nature of a group of like individuals ⟨the ∼ characteristics of a species⟩ 3 : involving or affecting practically the entire organism : not local ⟨∼ nervousness⟩

general adaptation syndrome *n* : the sequence of physiological reactions to prolonged stress that in the classification of Hans Selye includes alarm, resistance, and exhaustion

general anesthesia *n* : anesthesia affecting the entire body and accompanied by loss of consciousness

general anesthetic *n* : an anesthetic used to produce general anesthesia

general hospital *n* 1 : a hospital in which patients with many different types of ailments are given care 2 : a military hospital usu. located in a communications zone that gives treatment to all kinds of cases

gen·er·al·ist \ˈjen-(ə-)rə-ləst\ *n* : an individual whose skills or interests extend to several different medical fields; *esp* : GENERAL PRACTITIONER

generalista — see OSTEITIS FIBROSA CYSTICA GENERALISTA

gen·er·al·iza·tion *or Brit* **gen·er·al·isa·tion** \ˌjen-(ə-)rə-lə-ˈzā-shən\ *n* 1 : the action or process of generalizing 2 : the act or process whereby a learned response is made to a stimulus similar to but not identical with the conditioned stimulus

gen·er·al·ize *or Brit* **gen·er·al·ise** \ˈjen-(ə-)rə-ˌlīz\ *vi* **-ized** *or Brit* **-ised; -iz·ing** *or Brit* **-is·ing** : to spread or extend throughout the body ⟨*generalized* paralysis⟩

gen·er·al·ized *or Brit* **gen·er·al·ised** *adj* : made general; *esp* : not highly differentiated biologically nor strictly adapted to a particular environment ⟨a primitive ∼ mammal⟩

generalized anxiety disorder *n* : an anxiety disorder marked by chronic excessive anxiety and worry that is difficult to control, causes distress or impairment in daily functioning, and is accompanied by three or more associated symptoms (as restlessness, irritability, poor concentration, and sleep disturbances)

generalized seizure *n* : a seizure (as an absence seizure or tonic-clonic seizure) that originates in both cerebral hemispheres — compare PARTIAL SEIZURE

generalized Shwartzman reaction *n* : SHWARTZMAN REACTION a

general paresis *n* : insanity caused by syphilitic alteration of the brain that leads to dementia and paralysis — called also *dementia paralytica, general paralysis of the insane*

general practitioner *n* : a physician or veterinarian whose practice is not limited to a specialty

gen·er·ate \ˈjen-ə-ˌrāt\ *vb* **-at·ed; -at·ing** *vt* : to bring into existence; *esp* : PROCREATE ⟨∼ innumerable offspring⟩ ∼ *vi* : to produce offspring : PROPAGATE

gen·er·a·tion \ˌjen-ə-ˈrā-shən\ *n* **1 a** : a body of living beings constituting a single step in the line of descent from an ancestor **b** : a group of individuals born and living contemporaneously **2** : the average span of time between the birth of parents and that of their offspring **3** : the action or process of producing offspring : PROCREATION — **gen·er·a·tion·al** \-shnəl, -shən-ᵊl\ *adj*

gen·er·a·tive \ˈjen-(ə-)rət-iv, -ə-ˌrāt-\ *adj* : having the power or function of propagating or reproducing ⟨∼ organs⟩

generative cell *n* : a sexual reproductive cell : GAMETE

gen·er·a·tiv·i·ty \ˌjen-(ə-)rə-ˈtiv-ət-ē\ *n, pl* **-ties** : a concern for people besides self and family that usu. develops during middle age; *esp* : a need to nurture and guide younger people and contribute to the next generation — used in the psychology of Erik Erikson

gen·er·a·tor potential \ˈjen-ə-ˌrāt-ər-\ *n* : stationary depolarization of a receptor that occurs in response to a stimulus and is graded according to its intensity and that results in an action potential when the appropriate threshold is reached — called also *receptor potential*

¹**ge·ner·ic** \jə-ˈner-ik\ *adj* 1 : not protected by trademark registration : NONPROPRIETARY ⟨nylon and aspirin are ∼ names⟩ — used esp. in trademark law 2 : relating to or having the rank of a biological genus — **ge·ner·i·cal·ly** \-i-k(ə-)lē\ *adv*

²**generic** *n* : a generic drug — usu. used in pl.

gen·e·sis \ˈjen-ə-səs\ *n, pl* **-e·ses** \-ˌsēz\ : the origin or coming into being of something : the process or mode of origin

gene–splic·ing \ˈjēn-ˈsplī-siŋ\ *n* : the process of preparing recombinant DNA

gene therapy *n* : the insertion of usu. genetically altered genes into cells esp. to replace defective genes in the treatment of genetic disorders or to provide a specialized disease-fighting function (as the destruction of tumor cells) — **gene therapist** *n*

ge·net·ic \jə-ˈnet-ik\ *also* **ge·net·i·cal** \-i-kəl\ *adj* 1 : of, relating to, or involving genetics 2 : of, relating to, caused by, or controlled by genes ⟨a ∼ disease⟩ ⟨∼ material⟩ — compare ACQUIRED 1 — **ge·net·i·cal·ly** \-i-k(ə-)lē\ *adv*

genetic code *n* : the biochemical basis of heredity consisting of codons in DNA and RNA that determine the specific amino acid sequence in proteins and that appear to be uniform for all known forms of life — **genetic coding** *n*

genetic counseling *n* : guidance provided by a medical professional typically to individuals with an increased risk of having offspring with a specific genetic disorder and that includes providing information and advice concerning the probability of producing offspring with the disorder, prenatal diagnostic tests, and available treatments

genetic drift *n* : random changes in gene frequency esp. in small populations when leading to preservation or extinction of particular genes

genetic engineering \-ˌen-jə-ˈnir-iŋ\ *n* : the group of applied techniques of genetics and biotechnology used to cut up and join together genetic material and esp. DNA from one or more species of organism and to introduce the result into an organism in order to change one or more of its characteristics — **genetically engineered** *adj* — **genetic engineer** *n*

genetic fingerprint *n* : DNA FINGERPRINT

genetic fingerprinting *n* : DNA FINGERPRINTING

genetic imprinting *n* : GENOMIC IMPRINTING

ge·net·i·cist \jə-ˈnet-ə-səst\ *n* : a specialist or expert in genetics

genetic load *n* : the decrease in fitness of the average individual in a population due to the presence of deleterious genes or genotypes in the gene pool

genetic map *n* : MAP

genetic marker *n* : a readily recognizable genetic trait, gene, DNA segment, or gene product used for identification purposes esp. when closely linked to a trait or to genetic material that is difficult to identify — called also *marker*

ge·net·ics \jə-ˈnet-iks\ *n pl but sing in constr* **1 a** : a branch of biology that deals with the heredity and variation of organ-

\ə\ **abut** \ᵊ\ **kitten** \ər\ **further** \a\ **ash** \ā\ **ace** \ä\ **cot, cart** \au̇\ **out** \ch\ **chin** \e\ **bet** \ē\ **easy** \g\ **go** \i\ **hit** \ī\ **ice** \j\ **job** \ŋ\ **sing** \ō\ **go** \ȯ\ **law** \ȯi\ **boy** \th\ **thin** \t͟h\ **the** \ü\ **loot** \u̇\ **foot** \y\ **yet** \zh\ **vision** *See also* Pronunciation Symbols page

isms   **b** : a treatise or textbook on genetics   **2** : the genetic makeup and phenomena of an organism, type, group, or condition

ge·ne·to·troph·ic \jə-ˌnet-ə-ˈträf-ik, -ˈtrōf-\ *adj* : relating to or involving genetic predisposing and nutritional precipitating factors — used esp. of certain deficiency diseases

ge·ni·al \ji-ˈnī(-ə)l\ *adj* : of or relating to the chin

genial tubercle *n* : MENTAL TUBERCLE

gen·ic \ˈjēn-ik, ˈjen-\ *adj* : GENETIC 2 — **gen·i·cal·ly** \-i-k(ə-)lē\ *adv*

ge·nic·u·lar artery \jə-ˈnik-yə-lər-\ *n* : any of several branches of the femoral and popliteal arteries that supply the region of the knee — called also *genicular*

ge·nic·u·late \-lət, -ˌlāt\ *adj*   **1** : bent abruptly at an angle like a bent knee   **2** : relating to, comprising, or belonging to a geniculate body or geniculate ganglion ⟨∼ neurons⟩

geniculate body *n* : either of two prominences of the diencephalon that comprise the metathalamus: **a** : LATERAL GENICULATE BODY   **b** : MEDIAL GENICULATE BODY

geniculate ganglion *n* : a small reddish ganglion consisting of sensory and sympathetic nerve cells located at the sharp backward bend of the facial nerve

ge·nic·u·lo·cal·ca·rine \jə-ˌnik-yə-lō-ˈkal-kə-ˌrīn\ *adj* : of or relating to the lateral geniculate body and the calcarine sulcus; *esp* : relating to or comprising the optic radiation from the lateral geniculate body and the pulvinar to the occipital lobe ⟨∼ tracts⟩

ge·nic·u·lum \jə-ˈnik-yə-ləm\ *n, pl* **-la** \-lə\ : a small knee-shaped anatomical structure or abrupt bend

genii *pl of* GENIUS

gen·in \ˈjen-ən, jə-ˈnēn\ *n* : any of various aglycones that occur esp. in some plants and toad venoms

ge·nio·glos·sal \ˌjē-nē-ō-ˈgläs-əl, jə-ˌnī-ə-, -ˈglòs-\ *adj* : of or relating to the chin and tongue

ge·nio·glos·sus \-ˈgläs-əs, -ˈglòs-\ *n, pl* **-glos·si** \-ˌī\ : a fan-shaped muscle that arises from the superior mental spine, inserts on the hyoid bone and into the tongue, and serves to advance and retract and also to depress the tongue

ge·nio·hyo·glos·sus \-ˌhī-ō-ˈgläs-əs, -ˈglòs-\ *n, pl* **-glos·si** \-ˌī\ : GENIOGLOSSUS

ge·nio·hy·oid \-ˈhī-ˌòid\ *adj* : of or relating to the chin and hyoid bone

ge·nio·hy·oid·eus \-ˌhī-ˈòid-ē-əs\ *n, pl* **-oid·ei** \-ē-ˌī\ : GENIO-HYOID MUSCLE

geniohyoid muscle *n* : a slender muscle that arises from the inferior mental spine on the inner side of the symphysis of the lower jaw, is inserted on the hyoid bone, and acts to raise the hyoid bone and draw it forward and to retract and depress the lower jaw — called also *geniohyoid*

ge·nio·plas·ty \ˈjē-nē-ō-ˌplas-tē, jə-ˈnī-ə-\ *n, pl* **-ties** : plastic surgery of the chin

ge·nis·tein \jə-ˈnis-tē-ən, -ˈnis-ˌtēn\ *n* : an isoflavone $C_{15}H_{10}O_5$ found esp. in soybeans and shown in laboratory experiments to have antitumor activity

gen·i·tal \ˈjen-ə-tᵊl\ *adj*   **1** : GENERATIVE   **2** : of, relating to, or being a sexual organ   **3 a** : of, relating to, or characterized by the stage of psychosexual development in psychoanalytic theory following the latency period and during which oral and anal impulses are subordinated to adaptive interpersonal mechanisms   **b** : of, relating to, or characterized by a personality in the genital stage of psychosexual development esp. as typified by normal sexual desires and by concern for the happiness and pleasures of others — compare ANAL 2, ORAL 3 — **gen·i·tal·ly** \-ē\ *adv*

genital cord *n* : a mesenchymal shelf in the female mammalian fetus enclosing the developing uterus and the posterior part of the Wolffian ducts and giving rise to the broad ligaments of the uterus

genital herpes *n* : herpes simplex of the type affecting the genitals — called also *herpes genitalis*

genital herpes simplex *n* : GENITAL HERPES

gen·i·ta·lia \ˌjen-ə-ˈtāl-yə\ *n pl* : the organs of the reproductive system; *esp* : the external genital organs — **gen·i·ta·lic** \-ˈtal-ik, -ˈtāl-\ *adj*

genitalis — see HERPES GENITALIS

gen·i·tal·i·ty \-ˈtal-ə-tē\ *n, pl* **-ties** : possession of full genital sensitivity and capacity to develop orgasmic potency in relation to a sexual partner of the opposite sex

genital ridge *n* : a ridge of embryonic mesoblast developing from the mesonephros and giving rise to the gonad on either side of the body

gen·i·tals \ˈjen-ə-tᵊlz\ *n pl* : GENITALIA

genital tubercle *n* : a conical protuberance on the belly wall of an embryo between the attachment of the umbilical cord and the tail that develops into the penis in the male and the clitoris in the female

genital wart *n* : a wart on the skin or adjoining mucous membrane usu. near the anus and genital organs — called also *condyloma, condyloma acuminatum, venereal wart*

gen·i·to·cru·ral nerve \ˌjən-ə-(ˌ)tō-ˈkrù(ə)r-əl-\ *n* : GENITO-FEMORAL NERVE

gen·i·to·fem·o·ral nerve \-ˈfem-(ə-)rəl-\ *n* : a nerve that arises from the first and second lumbar nerves and is distributed by way of branches to the skin of the scrotum or the labia majora and to the upper anterior aspect of the thigh

gen·i·to·uri·nary \-ˈyùr-ə-ˌner-ē\ *adj* : of, relating to, affecting, or being the organs of reproduction and urination : UROGENITAL

genitourinary system *n* : GENITOURINARY TRACT

genitourinary tract *n* : the system of organs comprising those concerned with the production and excretion of urine and those concerned with reproduction — called also *genitourinary system, urogenital system, urogenital tract*

ge·nius \ˈjē-nyəs, -nē-əs\ *n, pl* **ge·nius·es** *or* **ge·nii** \-nē-ˌī\   **1** : extraordinary intellectual power esp. as manifested in creative activity   **2** : a person endowed with transcendent mental superiority; *specif* : a person with a very high IQ

geno·cide \ˈjen-ə-ˌsīd\ *n* : the deliberate and systematic destruction of a racial, political, or cultural group — compare HOMICIDE — **geno·cid·al** \ˌjen-ə-ˈsīd-ᵊl\ *adj*

ge·no·der·ma·to·sis \ˌjē-nō-ˌdər-mə-ˈtō-səs\ *n, pl* **-to·ses** \-ˌsēz\ : a congenital disease of the skin esp. when genetically determined

ge·no·gram \ˈjē-nə-ˌgram, ˈjen-ə-\ *n* : a diagram outlining the history of the behavior patterns (as of divorce, abortion, or suicide) of a family's members over several generations in order to recognize and understand past influences on current behavior patterns; *also* : a similar diagram detailing the medical history of the members of a family as a means of assessing a family member's risk of developing disease

ge·nome \ˈjē-ˌnōm\ *also* **ge·nom** \-ˌnäm\ *n* : one haploid set of chromosomes with the genes they contain

ge·nom·ic \ji-ˈnō-mik, -ˈnäm-ik\ *adj* : of or relating to a genome or genomics ⟨the ∼ constitution of an organism⟩ ⟨use of ∼ technology to develop new and improved drugs⟩

genomic imprinting *n* : genetic alteration of a gene or its expression that is inferred to take place from the observation that certain genes are expressed differently depending on whether they are inherited from the paternal or maternal parent — called also *genetic imprinting, imprinting*

ge·no·mics \jē-ˈnō-miks, jə-\ *n pl but sing in constr* : a branch of biotechnology concerned with applying the techniques of genetics and molecular biology to the genetic mapping and DNA sequencing of sets of genes or the complete genomes of selected organisms using high-speed methods, with organizing the results in databases, and with applications of the data (as in medicine or biology) — compare PROTEOMICS

ge·no·tox·ic \ˌjē-nə-ˈtäk-sik\ *adj* : damaging to genetic material ⟨environmental exposure to ∼ agents —P. A. Gaspar *et al*⟩ — **ge·no·tox·ic·i·ty** \-ˌtäk-ˈsis-ət-ē\ *n, pl* **-ties**

¹ge·no·type \ˈjē-nə-ˌtīp, ˈjen-ə-\ *n*   **1** : TYPE SPECIES   **2** : all or part of the genetic constitution of an individual or group — compare PHENOTYPE — **ge·no·typ·ic** \ˌjē-nə-ˈtip-ik, ˌjen-ə-\ *also* **ge·no·typ·i·cal** \-i-kəl\ *adj* — **ge·no·typ·i·cal·ly** \-i-k(ə-)lē\ *adv*

²genotype *vt* **-typed; -typ·ing** : to determine the genotype of ⟨50 families were *genotyped* for 20 genetic markers⟩

gen·ta·mi·cin \ˌjent-ə-'mīs-ᵊn\ *n* : a broad-spectrum aminoglycoside antibiotic mixture that is derived from two actinomycetes of the genus *Micromonospora* (*M. purpurea* and *M. echinospora*) and is extensively used in the form of the sulfate in treating infections esp. of the urinary tract

gen·tian \'jen-chən\ *n* **1** : any of two genera (*Gentiana* and *Dasystephana*) of herbs belonging to a family (Gentianaceae, the gentian family) and having opposite smooth leaves and showy usu. blue flowers **2** : the rhizome and roots of a yellow-flowered gentian (*Gentiana lutea*) of southern Europe that is used as a tonic and stomachic — called also *gentian root*

gentian violet *n, often cap G&V* : any of several dyes (as crystal violet) or dye mixtures that consist of one or more methyl derivatives of pararosaniline; *esp* : a dark green or greenish mixture used medicinally that contains not less than 96 percent of the derivative of pararosaniline containing six methyl groups in each molecule and is used esp. as a bactericide, fungicide, and anthelmintic

gen·ti·o·bi·ose \ˌjen-chē-ō-'bī-ˌōs also -ˌōz\ *n* : a crystalline dextrorotatory disaccharide $C_{12}H_{22}O_{11}$ that is composed of two units of glucose

gen·ti·o·pic·rin \-'pik-rən\ *n* : a bitter crystalline glucoside $C_{16}H_{20}O_9$ obtained from gentians and esp. from gentian root

gen·tis·ic acid \jen-'tis-ik-, -ˌtiz-\ *n* : a crystalline acid $C_7H_6O_4$ used medicinally as an analgesic and diaphoretic

ge·nu \'jē-ˌnü, 'jen-(y)ü\ *n, pl* **gen·ua** \'jen-yə-wə\ : an abrupt flexure; *esp* : the bend in the anterior part of the corpus callosum — see GENU VALGUM, GENU VARUM

ge·nus \'jē-nəs, 'jen-əs\ *n, pl* **gen·era** \'jen-ə-rə\ : a class, kind, or group marked by common characteristics or by one common characteristic; *specif* : a category of biological classification ranking between the family and the species, comprising structurally or phylogenetically related species or an isolated species exhibiting unusual differentiation, and designated by a Latin or latinized capitalized singular noun

genu val·gum \-'val-gəm\ *n* : KNOCK-KNEE — compare VALGUS

genu va·rum \-'vär-əm\ *n* : BOWLEG — compare VARUS

geo·med·i·cine \ˌjē-ō-'med-ə-sən, *Brit usu* -'med-sən\ *n* : a branch of medicine that deals with geographic factors in disease — **geo·med·i·cal** \-'med-i-kəl\ *adj*

geo·pa·thol·o·gy \-pa-'thäl-ə-jē\ *n, pl* **-gies** : a science that deals with the relation of geographic factors to peculiarities of specific diseases ⟨∼ of hypertension⟩

ge·o·pha·gia \-'fā-j(ē-)ə\ *n* : GEOPHAGY

ge·oph·a·gism \jē-'äf-ə-ˌjiz-əm\ *n* : GEOPHAGY

ge·oph·a·gy \-ə-jē\ *n, pl* **-gies** : the practice of eating earthy substances (as clay) that in humans is performed esp. to augment a scanty or mineral-deficient diet or as part of a cultural tradition — called also *earth eating;* compare PICA

geo·tac·tic \ˌjē-ō-'tak-tik\ *adj* : of or relating to geotaxis

geo·tax·is \-'tak-səs\ *n, pl* **-tax·es** \-ˌsēz\ : a taxis in which the force of gravity is the directive factor

ge·ot·ri·cho·sis \jē-ˌä-trə-'kō-səs\ *n* : infection of the bronchi or lungs and sometimes the mouth and intestines by a fungus of the genus *Geotrichum* (*G. candidum*)

Ge·ot·ri·chum \jē-'ä-trik-əm\ *n* : a genus of Fungi Imperfecti of the family Moniliaceae comprising fungi that usu. produce arthrospores and including one (*G. candidum*) that causes human geotrichosis

geo·tro·pic \ˌjē-ə-'trō-pik, -'träp-ik\ *adj* : of or relating to geotropism — **geo·tro·pi·cal·ly** \-'trō-pi-k(ə-)lē, -'träp-i-\ *adv*

ge·ot·ro·pism \jē-'ä-trə-ˌpiz-əm\ *n* : a tropism in which gravity is the orienting factor

ge·ra·ni·ol \jə-'rän-ē-ˌȯl, -ˌōl\ *n* : a fragrant liquid unsaturated alcohol $C_{10}H_{18}O$ that occurs both free and combined in many essential oils (as citronella oil) and is used chiefly in perfumes and in soap

ge·rat·ic \jə-'rat-ik\ *adj* : of or relating to old age : GERONTIC

ger·a·tol·o·gy \ˌjer-ə-'täl-ə-jē\ *n, pl* **-gies** : a scientific study of aging and its phenomena

ger·bil *also* **ger·bille** \'jər-bəl\ *n* : any of numerous Old World burrowing desert rodents (*Gerbillus* and related genera) with long hind legs adapted for leaping

GERD *abbr* gastroesophageal reflux disease

¹ge·ri·at·ric \ˌjer-ē-'a-trik, jir-\ *n* **1** **ge·ri·at·rics** *pl but sing in constr* : a branch of medicine that deals with the problems and diseases of old age and aging people — compare GERONTOLOGY **2** : an aged person

²geriatric *adj* **1** : of or relating to geriatrics or its practice ⟨the ∼ department in a hospital⟩ ⟨a ∼ ward⟩ **2** : of, relating to, affecting, or being aged individuals ⟨the ∼ population⟩ ⟨∼ depression⟩ ⟨treated ∼ animals⟩

ger·i·a·tri·cian \ˌjer-ē-ə-'trish-ən, jir-\ *n* : a specialist in geriatrics

ge·ri·a·trist \ˌjer-ē-'a-trəst, jir-; jə-'rī-ə-\ *n* : GERIATRICIAN

ger·i·o·psy·cho·sis \ˌjer-ē-ō-sī-'kō-səs, jir-\ *n, pl* **-cho·ses** \-ˌsēz\ : SENILE DEMENTIA

germ \'jərm\ *n* **1** : a small mass of living substance capable of developing into an organism or one of its parts **2** : MICROORGANISM; *esp* : a microorganism causing disease

Ger·man cockroach \ˌjər-mən-\ *n* : a small active winged cockroach of the genus *Blattella* (*B. germanica*) that is prob. of African origin and is a common household pest in the U.S. — called also *Croton bug*

ger·ma·nin \jər-'mā-nən\ *n* : SURAMIN

ger·ma·ni·um \(ˌ)jər-'mā-nē-əm\ *n* : a grayish white hard brittle metalloid element that resembles silicon and is used as a semiconductor — symbol Ge; see ELEMENT table

German measles *n pl but sing or pl in constr* : an acute contagious disease that is milder than typical measles but is damaging to the fetus when occurring early in pregnancy and that is caused by a togavirus (species *Rubella virus* of the genus *Rubivirus*) — called also *rubella*

germ cell *n* : an egg or sperm cell or one of their antecedent cells

germ center *n* : GERMINAL CENTER

germ-free \'jərm-ˌfrē\ *adj* : free of microorganisms : AXENIC

ger·mi·cid·al \ˌjər-mə-'sīd-ᵊl\ *adj* : of or relating to a germicide; *also* : destroying germs

ger·mi·cide \'jər-mə-ˌsīd\ *n* : an agent that destroys germs

ger·mi·nal \'jərm-nəl, -ən-ᵊl\ *adj* : of, relating to, or having the characteristics of a germ cell or early embryo — **ger·mi·nal·ly** \-ē\ *adv*

germinal cell *n* : an embryonic cell of the early vertebrate nervous system that is the source of neuroblasts and glial cells

germinal center *n* : the lightly staining central proliferative area of a lymphoid follicle

germinal disk *n* **1** : BLASTODISC **2** : the part of the blastoderm that forms the embryo proper of an amniote vertebrate

germinal epithelium *n* : the epithelial covering of the genital ridges and of the gonads derived from them

germinal vesicle *n* : the enlarged nucleus of the egg before completion of meiosis

ger·mi·nate \'jər-mə-ˌnāt\ *vb* **-nat·ed; -nat·ing** *vt* : to cause to sprout or develop ∼ *vi* : to begin to grow : SPROUT — **ger·mi·na·tion** \ˌjər-mə-'nā-shən\ *n*

ger·mi·na·tive \-ˌnāt-iv, -nət-\ *adj* : having the power to germinate ⟨∼ and virulent spores⟩

germinative layer *n* : the innermost layer of the epidermis from which new tissue is constantly formed

germinativum — see STRATUM GERMINATIVUM

ger·mi·no·ma \ˌjər-mə-'nō-mə\ *n, pl* **-mas** : a malignant tumor (as of the ovary, testis, mediastinum, or pineal gland) that originates from undifferentiated embryonic germ cells — see DYSGERMINOMA, SEMINOMA

germ layer *n* : any of the three primary layers of cells differentiated in most embryos during and immediately following gastrulation

germ line *n* : the cellular lineage esp. of a sexually reproducing animal from which eggs and sperm are derived and in which a cell undergoing mutation can be passed to the next generation ⟨the difference between gene therapy of somatic cells and modification of the *germ line* —David Baltimore⟩

germ plasm *n* **1** : germ cells and their precursors serving as the bearers of heredity and being fundamentally independent of other cells **2** : the hereditary material of the germ cells : GENES

germ·proof \'jərm-'prüf\ *adj* : impervious to the penetration or action of germs

germ theory *n* : a theory in medicine: infections, contagious diseases, and various other conditions (as suppurative lesions) result from the action of microorganisms

germ tube *n* : the slender tubular outgrowth first produced by most spores in germination

germ war·fare \-'wȯr-,fe(ə)r\ *n* : the use of harmful microorganisms (as bacteria) as weapons in war

germy \'jər-mē\ *adj* **germ·i·er; -est** : full of germs ⟨~ hands⟩

ger·o·der·ma \,jer-ō-'dər-mə\ *n* : premature aging of the skin (as in Simmonds' disease)

ge·ron·tik \jə-'rän-tik\ *also* **ge·ron·tal** \-təl\ *adj* : of or relating to decadence or old age

ger·on·tol·o·gist \,jer-ən-'täl-ə-jəst\ *n* : a specialist in gerontology

ger·on·tol·o·gy \-ə-jē\ *n, pl* **-gies** : the comprehensive study of aging and the problems of the aged — compare GERIATRIC 1 — **ge·ron·to·log·i·cal** \jə-,ränt-ᵊl-'äj-i-kəl\ *also* **ge·ron·to·log·ic** \-ik\ *adj*

ge·ron·to·phil·ia \jə-,rän-tō-'fil-ē-ə\ *n* : sex attraction toward old persons

ge·ron·to·pho·bia \-'fō-bē-ə\ *n* : morbid fear or dislike of old persons

ge·ron·to·ther·a·py \-'ther-ə-pē\ *n, pl* **-pies** : treatment to improve the health of older persons

Gerst·mann's syndrome \'gerst-mənz-\ *n* : cerebral dysfunction characterized esp. by finger agnosia, disorientation with respect to right and left, agraphia, and acalculia and caused by a lesion in the dominant cerebral hemisphere involving the angular gyrus and adjoining occipital gyri

Gerst·mann \'gerst-män; 'gərst-mən\, **Josef (1887–1969),** Austrian neurologist and psychiatrist. Gerstmann was in charge of a hospital for nervous and mental diseases during World War I, and after the war he occupied a similar position in Vienna where he also served as a university lecturer in neurology and psychiatry. He was the author of more than a hundred papers on neuropsychiatry, including a 1924 article that gave the first description of the brain disorder now called Gerstmann's syndrome.

Gerst·mann–Sträuss·ler–Schein·ker syndrome \'gerst-mən-'s(h)tròis-lər-'shīŋ-kər-\ *n* : a rare spongiform encephalopathy that is related to Creutzfeldt-Jakob disease, is marked by ataxia, dementia, and by accumulation of amyloid plaques in the brain, and that is inherited as an autosomal dominant trait but has been transmitted experimentally to animals — called also *Gerstmann-Sträussler-Scheinker disease, Gerstmann-Sträussler syndrome*

Sträussler, E., and **Scheinker, I.** Austrian physicians. Sträussler and Scheinker were coauthors of an article published in 1936 by Gerstmann that offered the first description of the form of encephalopathy that now bears the names of all three.

ge·stalt \gə-'s(h)tält, -'s(h)tȯlt\ *n, pl* **ge·stalt·en** \-ᵊn\ *or* **ge·stalts** : a structure, arrangement, or pattern of physical, biological, or psychological phenomena so integrated as to constitute a functional unit with properties not derivable by summation of its parts

ge·stalt·ist \gə-'s(h)täl-təst, -'s(h)tȯl-\ *n, often cap* : a specialist in Gestalt psychology

Gestalt psychology *n* : the study of perception and behavior from the standpoint of an individual's response to gestalten with stress on the uniformity of psychological and physiological events and rejection of analysis into discrete events of stimulus, percept, and response — **Gestalt psychologist** *n*

Gestalt therapy *n* : psychotherapy that focuses on gaining self-awareness of emotions, perceptions, and behaviors in the immediate present and on using this awareness to better recognize and satisfy current needs

ges·tate \'jes-,tāt\ *vb* **ges·tat·ed; ges·tat·ing** *vt* : to carry in the uterus during pregnancy ~ *vi* : to be in the process of gestation

ges·ta·tion \je-'stā-shən\ *n* **1** : the carrying of young in the uterus from conception to delivery : PREGNANCY **2** : GESTATION PERIOD — **ges·ta·tion·al** \-shnəl, -shən-ᵊl\ *adj*

gestation period *n* : the length of time during which gestation takes place — called also *gestation*

ges·to·sis \je-'stō-səs\ *n, pl* **-to·ses** \-,sēz\ : any disorder of pregnancy; *esp* : TOXEMIA OF PREGNANCY

get \('ł)get\ *vt* **got** \('ł)gät\; **got** *or* **got·ten** \'gät-ᵊn\; **get·ting** : to catch or become affected by (a disease or bodily condition) ⟨*got* measles from his brother⟩ ⟨*got* her period⟩

GFR *abbr* glomerular filtration rate

GG *abbr* gamma globulin

GH *abbr* growth hormone

ghat·ti gum \'gat-ē-\ *n* : a gum obtained from an East Indian tree (*Anogeissus latifolia* of the family Combretaceae) and related trees and used as a substitute for gum arabic — called also *Indian gum*

GHB \,jē-(,)āch-'bē\ *n* : a fatty acid $C_4H_8O_3$ that is a metabolite of gamma-aminobutyric acid, that is a depressant of the central nervous system, and that is used illicitly to produce sedative and euphoric effects or to stimulate release of growth hormone to increase muscle mass — called also *gamma hydroxybutyrate*

ghost \'gōst\ *n* : a structure (as a cell or tissue) that does not stain normally because of degenerative changes; *specif* : a red blood cell that has lost its hemoglobin

ghost surgery *n* : the practice of performing surgery on another physician's patient by arrangement with the physician but unknown to the patient

ghrel·in \'grel-ən\ *n* : a 28-amino-acid peptide hormone that is secreted primarily by stomach cells with lesser amounts secreted by other cells (as of the hypothalamus), that is a growth hormone secretagogue, and that has been implicated in the stimulation of fat storage and food intake

GHRH *abbr* growth hormone-releasing hormone

GI \('ł)jē-'ī\ *abbr* **1** gastrointestinal **2** glycemic index

gi·ant cell \'jī-ənt-\ *n* : an unusually large cell; *esp* : a large multinucleate often phagocytic cell (as those characteristic of tubercular lesions, various sarcomas, or the megakaryocytes of the red marrow)

giant cell arteritis *n* : arterial inflammation that often involves the temporal arteries and may lead to blindness when the ophthalmic artery and its branches are affected, is characterized by the formation of giant cells, and may be accompanied by fever, malaise, fatigue, anorexia, weight loss, and arthralgia — called also *temporal arteritis*

giant–cell tumor *n* : an osteolytic tumor affecting the metaphyses and epiphyses of long bones, composed of a stroma of spindle cells containing dispersed multinucleate giant cells, and usu. being benign but sometimes malignant — called also *osteoclastoma*

gi·ant·ism \'jī-ənt-,iz-əm\ *n* : GIGANTISM

giant kidney worm *n* : a blood-red nematode worm of the genus *Dioctophyma* (*D. renale*) that sometimes exceeds a yard in length and invades mammalian kidneys esp. of the dog and occas. of humans

giant urticaria *n* : ANGIOEDEMA

giant water bug *n* : any of a family (Belostomatidae and esp. genus *Lethocerus*) of very large predatory bug capable of inflicting a painful bite

giar·dia \jē-'är-dē-ə, 'jär-\ *n* **1** *cap* : a genus of flagellate protozoans inhabiting the intestines of various mammals and including one (*G. lamblia* syn. *G. intestinalis*) that is associated with diarrhea in humans **2** : any flagellate of the genus *Giardia*

Giard \zhē-är\, **Alfred Mathieu (1846–1908),** French biologist. Giard was an all-around naturalist. He was a student of morphology, phylogeny, and ethology and a supporter of both Darwinism and Lamarckism. He investigated a wide range of topics in biology, including regeneration, sexuality, metamorphosis, experimental parthenogenesis, hybridization, autotomy, and mimicry. The genus *Giardia* was named in his honor in 1882 by Johann Kunstler.

giar·di·a·sis \(ˌ)jē-ˌär-'dī-ə-səs, ˌjē-ər-, jär-\ *n, pl* **-a·ses** \-ˌsēz\ : infestation with or disease caused by a flagellate protozoan of the genus *Giardia* (esp. *G. lamblia*) that is often characterized by diarrhea — called also *lambliasis*

gib·bos·i·ty \jib-'äs-ət-ē, gib-\ *n, pl* **-ties** **1** : PROTUBERANCE, SWELLING; *specif* : KYPHOSIS **2** : the quality or state of being gibbous; *specif* : the condition of being humpbacked

gib·bous \'jib-əs, 'gib-\ *adj* **1** : marked by swelling or convexity esp. on one side : PROTUBERANT **2** : having a hump : HUMPBACKED

gib·bus \'jib-əs, 'gib-\ *n* : HUMP; *specif* : the hump of the deformed spine in Pott's disease

gid \'gid\ *n* : a disease esp. of sheep that is caused by the presence in the brain of the coenurus of a tapeworm of the genus *Multiceps* (*M. multiceps*) of the dog and related carnivores and is characterized by cerebral disturbances, dilated pupils, dizziness and circling movements, emaciation, and usu. death — called also *sturdy, turn-sick*

gid·dy \'gid-ē\ *adj* **gid·di·er; -est** **1** : DIZZY **2** : affected with gid \<~ sheep\> — **gid·di·ness** \-nəs\ *n*

Gi·em·sa \gē-'em-zə\ *n* : GIEMSA STAIN — **Giemsa** *adj*
  Giemsa, Gustav (1867–1948), German chemist and pharmacist. For more than thirty years Giemsa did research at an institute for tropical and maritime diseases. He developed staining methods for malarial parasites in 1902 and for spirochetes in 1905 and a method of fixing living tissue utilizing mercuric chloride and alcohol in 1909.

Gi·em·sa stain *also* **Giemsa's stain** \-zə(z)-\ *n* : a stain consisting of a mixture of eosin and methylene azure and used chiefly in differential staining of blood films

GIFT *abbr* gamete intrafallopian transfer; gamete intrafallopian tube transfer

gi·gan·tism \jī-'gan-ˌtiz-əm, jə-; 'jī-gən-\ *n* : development to abnormally large size from excessive growth of the long bones accompanied by muscular weakness and sexual impotence and usu. caused by hyperpituitarism before normal ossification is complete — called also *macrosomia;* compare ACROMEGALY

gi·gan·to·blast \jī-'gant-ə-ˌblast\ *n* : a large nucleated red blood cell

Gi·la monster \'hē-lə-\ *n* : a large orange and black venomous lizard of the genus *Heloderma* (*H. suspectum*) of the southwestern U.S.

gil·bert \'gil-bərt\ *n* : the cgs unit of magnetomotive force equivalent to 5/(2π) or about 0.794 ampere-turn
  Gilbert, William (1544–1603), British physician and physicist. Gilbert was the foremost scientist in Elizabethan England and was physician to the Queen. He was a notable early supporter of the Copernican view of the universe. In 1600 he published a major work on magnetism. Gilbert is regarded as the father of electrical studies.

Gil·bert's disease \zhēl-'berz-\ *n* : a metabolic disorder prob. inherited as an autosomal dominant with variable penetrance and characterized by elevated levels of mostly unconjugated serum bilirubin caused esp. by defective uptake of bilirubin by the liver
  Gil·bert \zhēl-ber\, **Augustin–Nicholas (1858–1927),** French physician. Gilbert is remembered for being one of the foremost clinicians of his time. He was professor of therapeutics at the Faculty of Medicine in Paris, and from 1910 he served as professor of clinical medicine at the Hôtel-Dieu. He carried out work in the chemical activity of the stomach and in the pathology of the liver. With a colleague he identified a form of alcoholic cirrhosis. He is also remembered for his description of hereditary cholemia and his contributions to knowledge of lithiasis in the biliary re-

gion. Among his published articles was one, in 1900, in which he described a type of hereditary jaundice now known as Gilbert's disease.

Gil·christ's disease \'gil-ˌkrists-\ *n* : NORTH AMERICAN BLASTOMYCOSIS
  Gilchrist, Thomas Caspar (1862–1927), American dermatologist. A clinical professor of dermatology, Gilchrist wrote a classic description of generalized blastomycosis in 1896. His other areas of study included the etiology of acne vulgaris, vaccine therapy as applied to cutaneous disease, a form of sarcoma affecting the skin, atrophy of the fatty layer of skin, and hyaline degeneration of cutaneous blood vessels and sweat glands.

¹**gill** \'jil\ *n* : either of two units of capacity: **a** : a British unit equal to ¼ imperial pint or 8.669 cubic inches **b** : a U.S. liquid unit equal to ¼ U.S. liquid pint or 7.218 cubic inches

²**gill** \'gil\ *n* **1** : an organ (as of a fish) for obtaining oxygen from water **2** : one of the radiating plates forming the undersurface of the cap of a mushroom — **gilled** \'gild\ *adj*

gill arch *n* : one of the bony or cartilaginous arches or curved bars extending dorsoventrally and placed one behind the other on each side of the pharynx and supporting the gills of fishes and amphibians; *also* : BRANCHIAL ARCH

gill cleft *n* : GILL SLIT

gill disease *n* : a destructive disease of trout and other fishes (as in hatcheries) marked by swollen eroded gills and usu. anemia and severe general debility and considered due to an unidentified bacterium or to a dietary deficiency

Gilles de la Tourette syndrome *also* **Gilles de la Tourette's syndrome** \ˌzhēl-də-lä-tür-'et(s)-\ *n* : TOURETTE'S SYNDROME

gill slit *n* : one of the openings or clefts between the gill arches in vertebrates that breathe by gills through which water taken in at the mouth passes to the exterior and bathes the gills; *also* : BRANCHIAL CLEFT

gilt \'gilt\ *n* : a young female swine

Gim·ber·nat's ligament \ˌhim-bər-'näts-, ˌgim-\ *n* : the portion of the aponeurosis of the external oblique muscle that is reflected from the inguinal ligament along the iliopectineal line
  Gim·ber·nat y Ar·bós \kim-ber-'nät-ē-är-'bōs\, **Antonio de (1734–1816),** Spanish surgeon and anatomist. Gimbernat was a pioneer in ophthalmology, vascular surgery, and urology. He demonstrated the ligament that now bears his name in 1768, although he did not publish a description of it until 1779.

gin·ger \'jin-jər\ *n* **1 a** : a thickened pungent aromatic rhizome that is used as a spice and sometimes in medicine **b** : the spice usu. prepared by drying and grinding ginger **2** : any of a genus (*Zingiber* of the family Zingiberaceae, the ginger family) of herbs with pungent aromatic rhizomes; *esp* : a widely cultivated tropical herb (*Z. officinale*) that supplies most of the ginger of commerce

gin·ger·root \'jin-jər-ˌ(r)üt, -ˌ(r)ùt\ *n* : GINGER 1a

gin·gi·va \'jin-jə-və, jin-'jī-\ *n, pl* **-vae** \-ˌvē\ : ¹GUM — **gin·gi·val** \'jin-jə-vəl\ *adj*

gingival crevice *n* : a narrow space between the free margin of the gingival epithelium and the adjacent enamel of a tooth — called also *gingival trough*

gingival papilla *n* : INTERDENTAL PAPILLA

gingival trough \-'trόf\ *n* : GINGIVAL CREVICE

gin·gi·vec·to·my \ˌjin-jə-'vek-tə-mē\ *n, pl* **-mies** : the excision of a portion of the gingiva

gin·gi·vi·tis \ˌjin-jə-'vīt-əs\ *n* : inflammation of the gums

gin·gi·vo·plas·ty \'jin-jə-və-ˌplas-tē\ *n, pl* **-ties** : a surgical procedure that involves reshaping the gums for aesthetic or functional purposes

gin·gi·vo·sto·ma·ti·tis \ˌjin-jə-vō-ˌstō-mə-'tīt-əs\ *n, pl* **-tit·i-**

\ə\ **abut** \ʲ\ **kitten** \ər\ **further** \a\ **ash** \ā\ **ace** \ä\ **cot, cart**
\aù\ **out** \ch\ **chin** \e\ **bet** \ē\ **easy** \g\ **go** \i\ **hit** \ī\ **ice** \j\ **job**
\ŋ\ **sing** \ō\ **go** \ò\ **law** \òi\ **boy** \th\ **thin** \t̲h̲\ **the** \ü\ **loot**
\ù\ **foot** \y\ **yet** \zh\ **vision** *See also* Pronunciation Symbols page

des \-'tit-ə-ˌdēz\ *or* -ti·tis·es : inflammation of the gums and of the mouth

gin·gly·mo·ar·thro·dia \ˌjiŋ-glə-(ˌ)mō-är-'thrō-dē-ə, ˌgiŋ-\ *n* : a composite anatomical joint of which one element has an axial or hinge motion and the other a simple gliding motion — gin·gly·mo·ar·thro·di·al \-dē-əl\ *adj*

gin·gly·moid \'jiŋ-glə-ˌmȯid, 'giŋ-\ *adj* : of, relating to, or resembling a ginglymus

gin·gly·mus \-glə-məs\ *n, pl* gin·gly·mi \-ˌmī, -ˌmē\ : a joint (as between the humerus and ulna) allowing motion in one plane only

gink·go bi·lo·ba \'giŋ-(ˌ)kō-ˌbī-'lō-bə, *also* 'giŋk-(ˌ)gō-\ *n* : an extract of the leaves of the ginkgo (*Ginkgo biloba*) that is used as a dietary supplement and is held to enhance mental functioning by increasing blood circulation to the brain — called also *ginkgo*

gin·seng \'jin-ˌseŋ, -ˌsaŋ, -(ˌ)siŋ\ *n* 1 : the aromatic root of a ginseng that is highly valued as a medicine in China though of value chiefly as a demulcent 2 a : a Chinese perennial herb (*Panax schinseng* of the family Araliaceae, the ginseng family) having 5-foliolate leaves, scarlet berries, and an aromatic root valued esp. locally as a medicine b : any of several plants (esp. genus *Panax*) related to or used as substitutes for the Chinese ginseng; *esp* : a No. American woodland herb (*P. quinquefolius*)

gir·dle \'gərd-³l\ *n* : either of two more or less complete bony rings at the anterior and posterior ends of the vertebrate trunk supporting the arms and legs respectively: a : PECTORAL GIRDLE b : PELVIC GIRDLE

girth \'gərth\ *n* : a measure around a body

GI series \ˌjē-'ī-\ *n* : GASTROINTESTINAL SERIES

gi·tal·in \'jit-ə-lən, jə-'tā-lən, jə-'tal-ən\ *n* 1 : a crystalline glycoside $C_{35}H_{56}O_{12}$ obtained from digitalis 2 : an amorphous water-soluble mixture of glycosides of digitalis used similarly to digitalis

gi·tog·e·nin \jə-'täj-ə-nən, jit-ə-'jen-ən\ *n* : a crystalline steroid sapogenin $C_{27}H_{44}O_4$ obtained esp. by hydrolysis of gitonin

gi·to·nin \jə-'tō-nən, 'jit-ə-nən\ *n* : a crystalline steroid saponin $C_{51}H_{82}O_{23}$ occurring with digitonin

gi·tox·i·gen·in \jə-ˌtäk-sə-'jen-ən, (ˌ)ji-ˌtäk-'sij-ə-nən\ *n* : a crystalline steroid lactone $C_{23}H_{34}O_5$ obtained by hydrolysis of gitoxin

gi·tox·in \jə-'täk-sən\ *n* : a poisonous crystalline steroid glycoside $C_{41}H_{64}O_{14}$ that is obtained from digitalis and from lanatoside B by hydrolysis

git·ter cell \'git-ər-\ *n* : an enlarged phagocytic cell of microglial origin having the cytoplasm distended with lipid granules and being characteristic of some organic brain lesions

give \'giv\ *vt* gave \'gāv\; giv·en \'giv-ən\; giv·ing 1 : to administer as a medicine 2 : to cause a person to catch by contagion, infection, or exposure — give birth : to have a baby ⟨*gave birth* last Thursday⟩ — give birth to : to produce as offspring ⟨*gave birth to* a daughter⟩

giz·zard \'giz-ərd\ *n* : the muscular enlargement of the alimentary canal of birds that has usu. thick muscular walls and a tough horny lining for churning and grinding the food

GL *abbr* greatest length

gla·bel·la \glə-'bel-ə\ *n, pl* -bel·lae \-'bel-(ˌ)ē, -ˌī\ : the smooth prominence between the eyebrows — called also *mesophryon* — gla·bel·lar \-'bel-ər\ *adj*

gla·brous \'glā-brəs\ *adj* : having or being a smooth even surface; *specif* : having or being an epidermal covering that is totally or relatively devoid of hairs or down ⟨~ skin⟩

gla·cial acetic acid \'glā-shəl-\ *n* : acetic acid containing usu. less than 1 percent of water, obtained as a pungent caustic hygroscopic liquid that is a good solvent (as for oils and resins), and used formerly as a caustic to remove warts but now only in veterinary medicine for this purpose

glad·i·o·lus \ˌglad-ē-'ō-ləs\ *n, pl* -li \-(ˌ)lē, -ˌlī\ : the large middle portion of the sternum lying between the upper manubrium and the lower xiphoid process — called also *mesosternum*

glairy \'gla(ə)r-ē, 'gle(ə)r-\ *adj* glair·i·er; -est : having a slimy viscid consistency suggestive of an egg white ⟨cough productive of ~ mucoid sputum —*Jour. Amer. Med. Assoc.*⟩

gland \'gland\ *n* 1 : a cell, group of cells, or organ of endothelial origin that selectively removes materials from the blood, concentrates or alters them, and secretes them for further use in the body or for elimination from the body 2 : any of various animal structures (as a lymph node) suggestive of glands though not secretory in function — gland·less \'glan-dləs\ *adj*

glan·dered \'glan-dərd\ *adj* : affected with glanders

glan·der·ous \-d(ə-)rəs\ *adj* 1 : GLANDERED 2 : produced by or resembling the effects of glanders ⟨a ~ condition⟩

glan·ders \-dərz\ *n pl but sing or pl in constr* : a contagious and destructive disease esp. of horses caused by a bacterium of the genus *Pseudomonas* (*P. mallei*) and characterized by caseating nodular lesions esp. of the respiratory mucosae and lungs that tend to break down and form ulcers

glandes *pl of* GLANS

gland of Bartholin *n* : BARTHOLIN'S GLAND

gland of Bow·man \-'bō-mən\ *n* : any of the tubular and often branched glands occurring beneath the olfactory epithelium of the nose — called also *Bowman's gland, olfactory gland*

W. Bowman — see BOWMAN'S CAPSULE

gland of Brunner *n* : BRUNNER'S GLAND

gland of Cowper *n* : COWPER'S GLAND

gland of external secretion *n* : EXOCRINE GLAND

gland of internal secretion *n* : ENDOCRINE GLAND

gland of Lieberkühn *n* : CRYPT OF LIEBERKÜHN

gland of Lit·tré \-lē-'trā\ *n* : any of the urethral glands of the male — called also *Littré's gland*

Lit·tré \lē-trā\, Alexis (1658–1726), French surgeon and anatomist. Littré described the glands of Littré in 1700. He was the first (in 1710) to propose the operation of colostomy for the relief of intestinal obstruction. In 1719 he published the first description of herniation of a diverticulum, which in this case was Meckel's diverticulum.

gland of Moll \-'mōl, -'mȯl, -'mäl\ *n* : any of the small glands near the free margin of each eyelid regarded as modified sweat glands — called also *Moll's gland*

Moll \'mȯl\, Jacob Antonius (1832–1914), Dutch ophthalmologist. In about 1865 Moll wrote the first satisfactory description of the glands that now bear his name.

gland of Ty·son \-'tīs-ᵊn\ *n* : any of the small glands at the base of the glans penis that secrete smegma — called also *preputial gland*

Tyson, Edward (1650–1708), British anatomist. A pioneer in comparative anatomy, Tyson laid down a set of principles and methodology that influenced the field of comparative anatomy for many years after his death. He produced classic anatomical descriptions of such diverse animals as the dolphin, rattlesnake, opossum, shark embryo, and the tapeworm. In 1694 William Cowper published an anatomical work in which he included a description of the glands of the external male genitalia that had been discovered by Tyson and now bear his name.

glan·du·la \'glan-jə-lə\ *n, pl* -lae \-ˌlē, -ˌlī\ : GLAND 1; *esp* : a small gland

glan·du·lar \'glan-jə-lər\ *adj* 1 : of, relating to, or involving glands, gland cells, or their products 2 : having the characteristics or function of a gland ⟨~ tissue⟩

glandular epithelium *n* : the epithelium that forms the secreting surface of a gland

glandular fever *n* : INFECTIOUS MONONUCLEOSIS

glan·du·lous \'glan-jə-ləs\ *adj* : GLANDULAR

glans \'glanz\ *n, pl* glan·des \'glan-ˌdēz\ 1 : a conical vascular body forming the extremity of the penis 2 : a conical vascular body that forms the extremity of the clitoris and is similar to the glans penis

glans cli·tor·i·dis \-klə-'tȯr-ə-(ˌ)dis\ *n* : GLANS 2

glans penis *n* : GLANS 1

Gla·se·ri·an fissure \glə-'zir-ē-ən-\ *n* : PETROTYMPANIC FISSURE

Gla·ser \\'glä-zər\\, **Johann Heinrich (1629–1675),** Swiss anatomist and surgeon. Glaser was a professor of anatomy who notably reformed clinical instruction. One of the first physicians to make hospital rounds, he introduced bedside instruction to his students. He held public dissections that were followed by demonstrations of surgical operations. He also conducted autopsies with his students. As an anatomist Glaser is noteworthy for his studies of the brain, the nervous system, and the bones of the head. A posthumous work, published in 1680, treats the anatomy and physiology of the central nervous system and contains his description of the petrotympanic fissure, which is sometimes called the Glaserian fissure.

Glas·gow Coma Scale \\'glas-(ˌ)kō-, -(ˌ)gō-; 'glaz-(ˌ)gō-\\ *n* : a scale that is used to assess the severity of a brain injury, that consists of values from 3 to 15 obtained by summing the ratings assigned to three variables depending on whether and how the patient responds to certain standard stimuli by opening the eyes, giving a verbal response, and giving a motor response, and that for a low score (as 3 to 5) indicates a poor chance of recovery and for a high score (as 8 to 15) indicates a good chance of recovery

glass \\'glas\\ *n, often attrib* **1 a** : an amorphous inorganic usu. transparent or translucent substance consisting of a mixture of silicates or sometimes borates or phosphates formed by fusion of silica or of oxides of boron or phosphorus with a flux and a stabilizer into a mass that cools to a rigid condition without crystallization **b** : a substance resembling glass esp. in hardness and transparency ⟨organic ∼*es* made from plastics⟩ **2 a** : an optical instrument or device that has one or more lenses and is designed to aid in the viewing of objects not readily seen **b glasses** *pl* : a device used to correct defects of vision or to protect the eyes that consists typically of a pair of glass or plastic lenses and the frame by which they are held in place — called also *eyeglasses*

Glas·ser's disease \\'glas-ərz, 'gles-\\ *n* : swine influenza marked by arthritis

Glässer \\'gles-ər\\, **Karl (*fl* 1906),** German veterinarian. Glässer first described an arthritic form of influenza in pigs in 1906. At the time it was a common disease in Europe. It has since become known as Glasser's disease.

glass eye *n* **1** : an artificial eye made of glass **2** : an eye having a pale, whitish, or colorless iris — **glass–eyed** \\-'īd\\ *adj*

Glau·ber's salt \\ˌglau̇-bər(z)-\\ *also* **Glau·ber salt** \\-bər-\\ *n* : a colorless crystalline sodium sulfate $Na_2SO_4 \cdot 10H_2O$ used esp. in dyeing, as a cathartic, and in solar energy systems — sometimes used in pl.

Glauber, Johann Rudolf (1604–1670), German physician and chemist. Glauber was both an alchemist and a serious chemist. As an alchemist he was a follower of Paracelsus and dealt extensively in secret chemicals and medicinals. As a chemist he made several important contributions. In 1648 he first prepared hydrochloric acid from common salt and sulfuric acid. Substituting potassium nitrate for common salt, he observed the formation of nitric acid. Of the various salts he prepared, the most important is the one now known as Glauber's salt, which he first made in 1656. His observations on dyeing are also noteworthy.

glau·co·ma \\glau̇-'kō-mə, glȯ-\\ *n* : a disease of the eye marked by increased pressure within the eyeball that can result in damage to the optic disk and gradual loss of vision

glau·co·ma·tous \\-'kōm-ət-əs, -'käm-\\ *adj* : of, relating to, or affected with glaucoma

GLC *abbr* gas-liquid chromatography

gleet \\'glēt\\ *n* : a chronic inflammation (as gonorrhea) of a bodily orifice usu. accompanied by an abnormal discharge; *also* : the discharge itself — **gleety** \\-ē\\ *adj* **gleet·i·er; gleet·i·est**

gle·no·hu·mer·al \\ˌglen-(ˌ)ō-'hyüm-(ə-)rəl, ˌglēn-\\ *adj* : of, relating to, or connecting the glenoid cavity and the humerus

glen·oid \\'glen-ˌȯid, 'glēn-\\ *adj* **1** : having the form of a smooth shallow depression — used chiefly of skeletal articulatory sockets **2** : of or relating to the glenoid cavity or glenoid fossa

glenoid cavity *n* : the shallow cavity of the upper part of the scapula by which the humerus articulates with the pectoral girdle

glenoid fossa *n* : the depression in each lateral wall of the skull with which the mandible articulates — called also *mandibular fossa*

glenoid labrum *or* **glen·oid·al labrum** \\gli-'nȯid-ᵊl-\\ *n* : a fibrocartilaginous ligament forming the margin of the glenoid cavity of the shoulder joint that serves to broaden and deepen the cavity and gives attachment to the long head of the biceps brachii — called also *labrum*

glia \\'glē-ə, 'glī-ə\\ *n, pl* **glia** : supporting tissue that is intermingled with the essential elements of nervous tissue esp. in the brain, spinal cord, and ganglia, is of ectodermal origin, and is composed of a network of fine fibrils and of flattened stellate cells with numerous radiating fibrillar processes — see MICROGLIA

gli·a·din \\'glī-əd-ən\\ *n* : PROLAMIN; *esp* : one obtained by alcoholic extraction of gluten from wheat and rye

gli·al \\'glē-əl, 'glī-əl\\ *adj* : of, relating to, or comprising glia ⟨∼ cells⟩

gli·ben·cla·mide \\glī-'ben-klə-ˌmīd, -'ben-\\ *n* : GLYBURIDE

glid·ant \\'glīd-ᵊnt\\ *n* : a substance (as colloidal silica) that enhances the flow of a granular mixture by reducing interparticle friction and that is used in the pharmaceutical production of tablets and capsules

glid·ing joint \\'glī-diŋ-\\ *n* : a diarthrosis in which the articular surfaces glide upon each other without axial motion — called also *arthrodia, plane joint*

glio·blas·to·ma \\ˌglī-(ˌ)ō-bla-'stō-mə\\ *n, pl* **-mas** *also* **-ma·ta** \\-mət-ə\\ : a malignant rapidly growing astrocytoma of the central nervous system and usu. of a cerebral hemisphere — called also *spongioblastoma*

glioblastoma mul·ti·for·me \\-ˌməlt-ə-'fȯrm-ē\\ *n* : GLIOBLASTOMA

Glio·cla·di·um \\ˌglī-ō-'klā-dē-əm\\ *n* : a genus of molds resembling those of the genus *Penicillium* but with the conidia of a spore head becoming surrounded by a slimy deposit that binds them into a rounded mass — see GLIOTOXIN, VIRIDIN

gli·o·ma \\glī-'ō-mə, glē-\\ *n, pl* **-mas** *also* **-ma·ta** \\-mət-ə\\ : a tumor arising from glial cells — **gli·o·ma·tous** \\-mə-təs\\ *adj*

gli·o·ma·to·sis \\glī-ˌō-mə-'tō-səs\\ *n, pl* **-to·ses** \\-ˌsēz\\ : a glioma with diffuse proliferation of glial cells or with multiple foci

gli·o·sis \\glī-'ō-səs\\ *n, pl* **gli·o·ses** \\-ˌsēz\\ : excessive development of glia esp. interstitially — **gli·ot·ic** \\-'ät-ik\\ *adj*

glio·tox·in \\ˌglī-ō-'täk-sən\\ *n* : an antibiotic $C_{13}H_{14}N_2O_4S_2$ that is toxic to higher animals as well as to animal and plant pathogens and that is produced by various fungi (as of the genera *Gliocladium, Aspergillus,* and *Penicillium*)

glip·i·zide \\'glip-ə-ˌzīd\\ *n* : a sulfonylurea $C_{21}H_{27}N_5O_4S$ that lowers blood glucose levels and is used in the control of hyperglycemia associated with type 2 diabetes — see GLUCOTROL

Glis·son's capsule \\'glis-ᵊnz-\\ *n* : an investment of loose connective tissue entering the liver with the portal vessels and sheathing the larger vessels in their course through the organ — called also *capsule of Glisson*

Glisson, Francis (1597–1677), British physician and anatomist. One of the founders of the Royal Society, Glisson was a distinguished anatomist, physiologist, and clinician. His treatise of 1650 on rickets was the fullest account up to that time. In 1654 he clearly described for the first time the capsule that now bears his name and the blood supply of the liver. Glisson is also known for introducing the idea of irritability as a specific property of living tissue.

Gln *abbr* glutamine

\\ə\\ **abut** \\ᵊ\\ **kitten** \\ər\\ **further** \\a\\ **ash** \\ā\\ **ace** \\ä\\ **cot, cart**
\\au̇\\ **out** \\ch\\ **chin** \\e\\ **bet** \\ē\\ **easy** \\g\\ **go** \\i\\ **hit** \\ī\\ **ice** \\j\\ **job**
\\ŋ\\ **sing** \\ō\\ **go** \\ȯ\\ **law** \\ȯi\\ **boy** \\th\\ **thin** \\t̶h̶\\ **the** \\ü\\ **loot**
\\u̇\\ **foot** \\y\\ **yet** \\zh\\ **vision** *See also* Pronunciation Symbols page

glob·al \'glō-bəl\ *adj* **1** : having the shape of a globe **2 a** : of, relating to, or involving the entire world ⟨∼ health conditions⟩ **b** : of, relating to, or involving the globe of the eye ⟨∼ anesthesia in cataract surgery⟩ **3 a** : being comprehensive, all-inclusive, or complete ⟨∼ obstetric care⟩ ⟨transient ∼ amnesia⟩ ⟨akinesia was ∼, although rigidity and dystonia were strikingly unilateral in distribution —Oliver Sacks⟩ **b** : of, relating to, or constituting an organic whole : ORGANISMIC ⟨the newer psychiatry seeks to understand in a ∼ way the dynamic structure of the patient's personality —*Psychological Abstracts*⟩ — **glob·al·ly** \-bə-lē\ *adv*
globe \'glōb\ *n* : EYEBALL
globe·fish \'glōb-ˌfish\ *n* : PUFFER
Glo·bid·i·um \glō-'bid-ē-əm\ *n* : a genus of microscopic parasites of the intestinal mucosa of herbivorous mammals that are commonly regarded as protozoans related to the Sarcosporidia, that form membranous cysts enclosing fusiform spores, and that sometimes produce severe symptoms of gastrointestinal disorder
glo·bin \'glō-bən\ *n* : a colorless protein obtained by removal of heme from a conjugated protein and esp. hemoglobin
glo·boid \'glō-ˌbȯid\ *adj* : SPHEROIDAL
glo·bose \'glō-ˌbōs\ *adj* : GLOBULAR 1
glo·bo·side \'glō-bə-ˌsīd\ *n* : a complex glycolipid that occurs in the red blood cells, serum, liver, and spleen of humans and accumulates in tissues in one of the variants of Tay= Sachs disease
glob·u·lar \'gläb-yə-lər\ *adj* **1 a** : having the shape of a globe or globule **b** : composed of compactly folded polypeptide chains arranged in a spherical form ⟨∼ proteins⟩ **2** : having or consisting of globules — **glob·u·lar·ly** \-lē\ *adv*
glob·ule \'gläb-(ˌ)yü(ə)l\ *n* : a small globular body or mass (as a drop of water or a bead of sweat) ⟨∼s of fat⟩; *specif* : a small spherical pill of compressed sugar usu. saturated with an alcoholic tincture and used in homeopathy
glob·u·lin \'gläb-yə-lən\ *n* : any of a class of simple proteins (as myosin) that are insoluble in pure water but are soluble in dilute salt solutions and that occur widely in plant and animal tissues — see ALPHA GLOBULIN, BETA GLOBULIN, GAMMA GLOBULIN
glob·u·lin·uria \ˌgläb-yə-lən-'(y)ùr-ē-ə\ *n* : the presence of globulin in the urine
glo·bus hys·ter·i·cus \'glō-bəs-his-'ter-i-kəs\ *n* : a choking sensation (as of a lump in the throat) commonly experienced in hysteria
globus pal·li·dus \-'pal-ə-dəs\ *n* : the median portion of the lentiform nucleus — called also *pallidum*
glo·mal \'glō-məl\ *adj* : of or relating to a glomus
glom·an·gi·o·ma \ˌglōm-ˌan-jē-'ō-ma\ *n, pl* **-mas** *also* **-ma·ta** \-mət-ə\ : GLOMUS TUMOR
glome \'glōm\ *n* : a prominent rounded part of the frog of a horse's hoof on each side of the cleft
glo·mec·to·my \glō-'mek-tə-mē\ *n, pl* **-mies** : excision of a glomus (as the carotid body)
glomera *pl of* GLOMUS
glo·mer·u·lar \glə-'mer-(y)ə-lər, glō-\ *adj* : of, relating to, or produced by a glomerulus ⟨∼ nephritis⟩ ⟨∼ capillaries⟩
glomerular capsule *n* : BOWMAN'S CAPSULE
glo·mer·u·li·tis \-ˌmer-(y)ə-'līt-əs\ *n* : inflammation of the glomeruli of the kidney
glo·mer·u·lo·ne·phri·tis \-ˌmer-(y)ə-lō-ni-'frīt-əs\ *n, pl* **-phrit·i·des** \-'frīt-ə-ˌdēz\ : nephritis marked by inflammation of the capillaries of the renal glomeruli
glo·mer·u·lop·a·thy \-(y)ə-'läp-ə-thē\ *n, pl* **-thies** : a disease (as glomerulonephritis) affecting the renal glomeruli
glo·mer·u·lo·sa \-(y)ə-'lō-sə; -zə\ *n, pl* **-sae** \-sē, -sī, -zē, -zī\ : ZONA GLOMERULOSA — **glo·mer·u·lo·sal** \-'lō-səl, -zəl\ *adj*
glo·mer·u·lo·scle·ro·sis \-(y)ə-ˌlō-sklə-'rō-səs\ *n, pl* **-ro·ses** \-ˌsēz\ : nephrosclerosis involving the renal glomeruli
glo·mer·u·lus \glə-'mer-(y)ə-ləs, glō-\ *n, pl* **-li** \-ˌlī, -ˌlē\ : a small convoluted or intertwined mass (as of organisms, nerve fibers, or capillaries): as **a** : a tuft of capillaries that is covered by epithelium, is situated at the point of origin of each vertebrate nephron, and normally passes a protein-free

filtrate from the blood to the surrounding Bowman's capsule — see RENAL CORPUSCLE **b** : the convoluted secretory part of a sweat gland **c** : a dense entanglement of nerve fibers situated in the olfactory bulb and containing the primary synapses of the olfactory pathway
glo·mus \'glō-məs\ *n, pl* **glom·era** \'gläm-ə-rə\ *also* **glo·mi** \'glō-ˌmī, -ˌmē\ : a small arteriovenous anastomosis together with its supporting structures: as **a** : a vascular tuft that suggests a renal glomerulus and that develops from the embryonic aorta in relation to the pronephros **b** : CAROTID BODY **c** : a tuft of the choroid plexus protruding into each lateral ventricle of the brain
glomus ca·rot·i·cum \-kə-'rät-i-kəm\ *n* : CAROTID BODY
glomus coc·cy·ge·um \-käk-'sij-ē-əm\ *n* : a small mass of vascular tissue situated near the tip of the coccyx — called also *coccygeal body, coccygeal gland, Luschka's gland*
glomus jug·u·la·re \-ˌjəg-yə-'lar-ē\ *n* : a mass of chemoreceptors in the adventitia of the dilation in the internal jugular vein where it arises from the transverse sinus in the jugular foramen
glomus tumor *n* : a painful benign tumor that develops by hypertrophy of a glomus — called also *glomangioma*
glos·sal \'gläs-əl, 'glȯs-\ *adj* : of or relating to the tongue ⟨∼ inflammation⟩
glos·si·na \-'sī-nə, -'sē-\ *n* **1** *cap* : an African genus of dipteran flies that have a long slender sharp proboscis and joint antennae bearing feathery appendages and that comprise the tsetse flies **2** : any fly of the genus *Glossina* : TSETSE FLY
glos·si·tis \-'sīt-əs\ *n* : inflammation of the tongue
gloss·odyn·ia \ˌgläs-ō-'din-ē-ə, ˌglȯs-\ *n* : pain localized in the tongue
glos·so·kin·es·thet·ic *or chiefly Brit* **glos·so·kin·aes·thet·ic** \ˌglä-sō-ˌkin-əs-'thet-ik, ˌglȯ-\ *adj* : of or relating to sensations of tongue movement ⟨∼ centers⟩
glos·so·la·lia \ˌgläs-ə-'lā-lē-ə, ˌglȯs-\ *n* : profuse and often emotionally charged speech that mimics coherent speech but is usu. unintelligible to the listener and that is uttered in some states of religious ecstasy and in some schizophrenic states
glos·so·pal·a·tine arch \ˌgläs-ō-'pal-ə-ˌtīn-, ˌglȯs-\ *n* : PALATOGLOSSAL ARCH
glossopalatine nerve *n* : NERVUS INTERMEDIUS
glos·so·pal·a·ti·nus \-ˌpal-ə-'tī-nəs\ *n, pl* **-ni** \-ˌnī, -ˌnē\ : PALATOGLOSSUS
glos·sop·a·thy \glä-'säp-ə-thē\ *n, pl* **-thies** : a disease of the tongue
glos·so·pha·ryn·geal \ˌgläs-ō-fə-'rin-j(ē-)əl, ˌglȯs-, -ˌfar-ən-'jē-əl\ *adj* **1** : of or relating to both tongue and pharynx **2** : of, relating to, or affecting the glossopharyngeal nerve ⟨∼ lesions⟩
glossopharyngeal nerve *n* : a mixed nerve that is either of the ninth pair of cranial nerves, that has sensory fibers arising from the superior and petrosal ganglia and motor fibers arising with those of the vagus nerve from the lateral wall of the medulla, and that supplies chiefly the pharynx, posterior tongue, and parotid gland with motor and sensory fibers including gustatory and autonomic secretory and vasodilator fibers — called also *glossopharyngeal, ninth cranial nerve*
glot·tal \'glät-ᵊl\ *also* **glot·tic** \-ik\ *adj* : of, relating to, or produced in or by the glottis ⟨∼ constriction⟩
glottidis — see RIMA GLOTTIDIS
glot·tis \'glät-əs\ *n, pl* **glot·tis·es** *or* **glot·ti·des** \-ə-ˌdēz\ : the space between one of the true vocal cords and the arytenoid cartilage on one side of the larynx and those of the other side; *also* : the structures that surround this space — compare EPIGLOTTIS
Glu *abbr* glutamic acid; glutamyl
glu·ca·gon \'glü-kə-ˌgän\ *n* : a protein hormone that is produced esp. by the pancreatic islets of Langerhans and that promotes an increase in the sugar content of the blood by increasing the rate of breakdown of glycogen in the liver — called also *hyperglycemic factor, hyperglycemic-glycogenolytic factor*

glu·can \'glü-ˌkan, -kən\ *n* : a polysaccharide (as glycogen or cellulose) that is a polymer of glucose

glu·ca·nase \'glü-kə-ˌnās, -ˌnāz\ *n* : any of various enzymes that digest glucans

glu·cide \'glü-ˌsīd\ *n* : any of a class of carbohydrates comprising both the glycoses and the glycosides

glu·co·ascor·bic acid \ˌglü-kō-ə-ˌskór-bik-\ *n* : an ascorbic acid analog $C_7H_{10}O_7$

glu·co·ce·re·bro·si·dase \-ˌser-ə-'brō-sə-ˌdās, -ˌdāz\ *n* : an enzyme of mammalian tissue that catalyzes the hydrolysis of the glucose part of a glucocerebroside and is deficient in patients affected with Gaucher's disease

glu·co·ce·re·bro·side \-'ser-ə-brō-ˌsīd, -sə-'rē-\ *n* : a lipid composed of a ceramide and glucose that accumulates in the tissues of patients affected with Gaucher's disease

glu·co·cor·ti·coid \-'kórt-i-ˌkóid\ *n* : any of a group of corticosteroids (as cortisol or dexamethasone) that are involved esp. in carbohydrate, protein, and fat metabolism, that tend to increase liver glycogen and blood sugar by increasing gluconeogenesis, that are anti-inflammatory and immunosuppressive, and that are used widely in medicine (as in the alleviation of the symptoms of rheumatoid arthritis) — compare MINERALOCORTICOID

glu·co·gen·e·sis \-'jen-ə-səs\ *n, pl* **-e·ses** \-ˌsēz\ : formation of glucose within the animal body from any product of glycolysis — compare GLUCONEOGENESIS

glu·co·gen·ic \-'jen-ik\ *adj* : tending to produce a pyruvate residue in metabolism which undergoes conversion to a carbohydrate (as glucose) and is eventually stored as a complex carbohydrate (as glycogen) ⟨~ amino acids⟩

glu·co·ki·nase \-'kī-ˌnās, -ˌnāz\ *n* : a hexokinase found esp. in the liver that catalyzes the phosphorylation of glucose in metabolic processes

glu·co·lip·id \-'lip-əd\ *n* : a glycolipid that yields glucose on hydrolysis

glu·co·nate \'glü-kə-ˌnāt\ *n* : a salt or ester of gluconic acid — see CALCIUM GLUCONATE, FERROUS GLUCONATE

glu·co·neo·gen·e·sis \ˌglü-kə-ˌnē-ə-'jen-ə-səs\ *n, pl* **-e·ses** \-ˌsēz\ : formation of glucose within the animal body from precursors other than carbohydrates esp. by the liver and kidney using amino acids from proteins, glycerol from fats, or lactate produced by muscle during anaerobic glycolysis — called also *glyconeogenesis* — **glu·co·neo·gen·ic** \-'jen-ik\ *adj*

glu·con·ic acid \(ˌ)glü-ˌkän-ik-\ *n* : a crystalline acid $C_6H_{12}O_7$ obtained by oxidation of glucose and used chiefly in cleaning metals and as the source of its salts some of which are used medicinally — see GLUCONATE

Glu·co·phage \'glü-kō-ˌfāj\ *trademark* — used for a preparation of the hydrochloride of metformin

glu·co·pro·tein \ˌglü-kō-'prō-ˌtēn, -'prōt-ē-ən\ *n* : GLYCOPROTEIN

glu·co·py·ra·nose \-'pī-rə-ˌnōs, -ˌnōz\ *n* : one of the derivatives of glucose characterized by a pyranose ring

glu·cos·amine \glü-'kō-sə-ˌmēn, -zə-\ *n* : an amino derivative $C_6H_{13}NO_5$ of glucose that occurs esp. as a constituent of polysaccharides (as chitin) in animal supporting structures and some plant cell walls

glu·co·san \'glü-kə-ˌsan\ *n* **1** : any of several intramolecular anhydrides $C_6H_{10}O_5$ of glucose **2** : a hexosan (as dextran or starch) that yields essentially only glucose on hydrolysis

glu·cose \'glü-ˌkōs, -ˌkōz\ *n* : an optically active sugar $C_6H_{12}O_6$ that has an aldehydic carbonyl group; *esp* : the sweet colorless soluble dextrorotatory form that occurs widely in nature and is the usual form in which carbohydrate is assimilated by animals

glucose–1–phosphate *n* : an ester $C_6H_{13}O_9P$ that reacts in the presence of a phosphorylase with aldoses and ketoses to yield disaccharides or with itself in liver and muscle to yield glycogen and phosphoric acid — called also *Cori ester*

glucose phosphate *n* : a phosphate ester of glucose: as **a** : GLUCOSE-1-PHOSPHATE **b** : GLUCOSE-6-PHOSPHATE

glu·cose·phos·phate isomerase \ˌglü-ˌkōs-'fäs-ˌfāt-\ *n* : PHOSPHOHEXOISOMERASE

glucose–6–phosphate *n* : an ester $C_6H_{13}O_9P$ that is formed from glucose and ATP in the presence of a glucokinase and that is an essential early stage in glucose metabolism

glucose–6–phosphate dehydrogenase *n* : an enzyme found esp. in red blood cells that dehydrogenates glucose-6-phosphate in a glucose degradation pathway alternative to the Krebs cycle

glucose–6–phosphate dehydrogenase deficiency *n* : a hereditary metabolic disorder affecting red blood cells that is controlled by a variable gene on the X chromosome, that is characterized by a deficiency of glucose-6-phosphate dehydrogenase conferring marked susceptibility to hemolytic anemia which may be chronic, episodic, or induced by certain foods (as broad beans) or drugs (as primaquine), and that occurs esp. in individuals of Mediterranean or African descent

glucose tolerance test *n* : a test of the body's ability to metabolize glucose that involves the administration of a measured dose of glucose to the fasting stomach and the determination of glucose levels in the blood and urine at measured intervals thereafter and that is used esp. to detect diabetes mellitus

glu·co·si·dase \glü-'kō-sə-ˌdās, -zə-ˌdāz\ *n* : an enzyme (as maltase) that hydrolyzes a glucoside

glu·co·side \'glü-kə-ˌsīd\ *n* : GLYCOSIDE; *esp* : a glycoside that yields glucose on hydrolysis — **glu·co·sid·ic** \ˌglü-kə-'sid-ik\ *adj* — **glu·co·sid·i·cal·ly** \-i-k(ə-)lē\ *adv*

glu·co·sin·o·late \ˌglü-kō-'sin-ə-ˌlāt\ *n* : any of various bitter sulfur-containing glycosides found esp. in cruciferous plants (as broccoli, cabbage, and mustard) that when hydrolyzed form bioactive compounds (as isothiocyanates) including some which are anticarcinogenic

glu·cos·uria \ˌglü-kō-'shúr-ē-ə, -kəs-'yúr-\ *n* : GLYCOSURIA

glu·co·syl \'glü-kə-ˌsil\ *n* : a glycosyl radical $C_6H_{11}O_5$ derived from glucose

glu·co·syl·trans·fer·ase \-'tran(t)s-(ˌ)fər-ˌās, -ˌāz\ *n* : an enzyme that catalyzes the transfer of a glucosyl group; *esp* : one implicated in the formation of dental plaque that catalyzes the formation of glucans — called also *transglucosylase*

Glu·co·trol \'glü-kə-ˌtról\ *trademark* — used for a preparation of glipizide

Glu·co·vance \'glü-kō-ˌvans\ *trademark* — used for a preparation of glyburide and the hydrochloride of metformin

gluc·uro·nate \glü-'kyúr-ə-ˌnāt\ *n* : a salt or ester of glucuronic acid

gluc·uron·ic acid \ˌglü-kyə-ˌrän-ik-\ *n* : a compound $C_6H_{10}O_7$ that occurs esp. as a constituent of glycosaminoglycans (as hyaluronic acid) and combined as a glucuronide

gluc·uron·i·dase \-'rän-ə-ˌdās, -ˌdāz\ *n* : an enzyme that hydrolyzes a glucuronide; *esp* : one that occurs widely (as in the liver and spleen) and hydrolyzes the beta form of a glucuronide

gluc·uro·nide \glü-'kyúr-ə-ˌnīd\ *n* : any of various derivatives of glucuronic acid that are formed esp. as combinations with often toxic aromatic hydroxyl compounds (as phenols) and are excreted in the urine

glue–snif·fing \'glü-ˌsnif-iŋ\ *n* : the deliberate inhalation of volatile organic solvents from plastic glues that may result in symptoms ranging from mild euphoria to disorientation and coma

glu·side \'glü-ˌsīd\ *n* : SACCHARIN

glu·ta·mate \'glüt-ə-ˌmāt\ *n* : a salt or ester of glutamic acid; *specif* : a salt or ester of levorotatory glutamic acid that functions as an excitatory neurotransmitter — see MONOSODIUM GLUTAMATE

glutamate dehydrogenase *n* : an enzyme present esp. in liver mitochondria and cytosol that catalyzes the oxidation of glutamate to ammonia and α-ketoglutaric acid

glu·tam·ic acid \(ˌ)glü-ˌtam-ik-\ *n* : a crystalline amino acid

G
H

\ə\ **abut** \ᵊ\ **kitten** \ər\ **further** \a\ **ash** \ā\ **ace** \ä\ **cot, cart**
\aú\ **out** \ch\ **chin** \e\ **bet** \ē\ **easy** \g\ **go** \i\ **hit** \ī\ **ice** \j\ **job**
\ŋ\ **sing** \ō\ **go** \ó\ **law** \ói\ **boy** \th\ **thin** \th\ **the** \ü\ **loot**
\ú\ **foot** \y\ **yet** \zh\ **vision** *See also* Pronunciation Symbols page

$C_5H_9NO_4$ that is widely distributed in plant and animal proteins and that acts throughout the central nervous system esp. in the form of a salt or ester as a neurotransmitter which excites postsynaptic neurons — abbr. *Glu*

glutamic–ox·a·lo·ace·tic transaminase \-ˌäk-sə-lō-ə-ˌsēt-ik-\ *also* **glutamic–ox·al·ace·tic transaminase** \-ˌäk-sə-lə-ˌsēt-ik-\ *n* : ASPARTATE AMINOTRANSFERASE

glutamic pyruvic transaminase *n* : ALANINE AMINOTRANSFERASE

glu·ta·min·ase \ˈglüt-ə-mə-ˌnās, glü-ˈtam-ə-, -ˌnāz\ *n* : an enzyme that hydrolyzes glutamine to glutamic acid and ammonia

glu·ta·mine \ˈglüt-ə-ˌmēn\ *n* : a crystalline amino acid $C_5H_{10}N_2O_3$ that is found both free and in proteins in plants and animals and that yields glutamic acid and ammonia on hydrolysis — abbr. *Gln*

glu·tamyl \ˈglüt-ə-ˌmil, glü-ˈtam-əl\ *n* : the amino acid radical or residue $-OCCH_2CH_2CH(NH_2)CO-$ of glutamic acid — abbr. *Glu*

glu·tar·al·de·hyde \ˌglüt-ə-ˈral-də-ˌhīd\ *n* : a compound $C_5H_8O_2$ that contains two aldehyde groups and is used as a disinfectant and in fixing biological tissues

glu·tar·ic acid \glü-ˌtar-ik-\ *n* : a crystalline acid $C_5H_8O_4$ used esp. in organic synthesis

glu·ta·ryl \ˈglüt-ə-ˌril, glü-ˈtar-əl\ *n* : the bivalent radical $-OC(CH_2)_3CO-$ of glutaric acid

glu·ta·thi·one \ˌglüt-ə-ˈthī-ˌōn\ *n* : a peptide $C_{10}H_{17}N_3O_6S$ that contains one amino acid residue each of glutamic acid, cysteine, and glycine, that occurs widely in plant and animal tissues, and that plays an important role in biological oxidation-reduction processes and as a coenzyme

glute \ˈglüt\ *n* : GLUTEUS; *esp* : GLUTEUS MAXIMUS — usu. used in pl.

glu·te·al \ˈglüt-ē-əl, glü-ˈtē-\ *adj* : of or relating to the buttocks or the gluteus muscles ⟨the ~ region extends to the anterior superior iliac spine —S. W. Jacob & C. A. Francone⟩

gluteal artery *n* : either of two branches of the internal iliac artery that supply the gluteal region: **a** : the largest branch of the internal iliac artery that sends branches esp. to the gluteal muscles — called also *superior gluteal artery* **b** : a branch that is distributed esp. to the buttocks and the backs of the thighs — called also *inferior gluteal artery*

gluteal nerve *n* : either of two nerves arising from the sacral plexus and supplying the gluteal muscles and adjacent parts: **a** : one arising from the posterior part of the fourth and fifth lumbar nerves and from the first sacral nerve and distributed to the gluteus muscles and to the tensor fasciae latae — called also *superior gluteal nerve* **b** : one arising from the posterior part of the fifth lumbar nerve and from the first and second sacral nerves and distributed to the gluteus maximus — called also *inferior gluteal nerve*

gluteal tuberosity *n* : the lateral ridge of the linea aspera of the femur that gives attachment to the gluteus maximus

glu·telin \ˈglüt-ᵊl-ən, glü-ˈtel-\ *n* : any of a group of simple proteins (as glutenin) that occur esp. in the seeds of cereals and that are insoluble in neutral solvents and soluble in dilute acids or alkalies

glu·ten \ˈglüt-ᵊn\ *n* : a gluey protein substance esp. of wheat flour that causes dough to be sticky — **glu·ten·ous** \ˈglüt-nəs, -ᵊn-əs\ *adj*

glu·te·nin \-ᵊn-ən\ *n* : a glutelin found esp. in wheat and obtained by extracting gluten with dilute alkali

gluten–sensitive enteropathy *n* : CELIAC DISEASE

glutes *pl of* GLUTE

glu·teth·i·mide \glü-ˈteth-ə-ˌmīd, -məd\ *n* : a sedative-hypnotic drug $C_{13}H_{15}NO_2$ that is a derivative of piperidine and has pharmacological properties similar to the barbiturates

glu·te·us \ˈglüt-ē-əs, glü-ˈtē-\ *n, pl* **glu·tei** \ˈglüt-ē-ˌī, -ē-ˌē; glü-ˈtē-ˌī\ : any of three large muscles of the buttocks: **a** : GLUTEUS MAXIMUS **b** : GLUTEUS MEDIUS **c** : GLUTEUS MINIMUS

gluteus max·i·mus \-ˈmak-sə-məs\ *n, pl* **glutei max·i·mi** \-sə-ˌmī\ : the outermost of the three muscles in each but-

tock that arises from the sacrum, coccyx, back part of the ilium and adjacent structures, that is inserted into the fascia lata of the thigh and the gluteal tuberosity of the femur, and that acts to extend and laterally rotate the thigh

gluteus me·di·us \-ˈmē-dē-us\ *n, pl* **glutei me·dii** \-dē-ˌī\ : the middle of the three muscles in each buttock that arises from the outer surface of the ilium, that is inserted into the greater trochanter of the femur, and that acts to abduct and medially rotate the thigh

gluteus min·i·mus \-ˈmin-ə-məs\ *n, pl* **glutei min·i·mi** \-ˌmī\ : the innermost of the three muscles in each buttock that arises from the outer surface of the ilium, that is inserted into the greater trochanter of the femur, and that acts similarly to the gluteus medius

glu·ti·nous \ˈglüt-nəs, -ᵊn-əs\ *adj* : having the quality of glue esp. in physical properties

Gly *abbr* glycine; glycyl

gly·bur·ide \ˈglī-byə-ˌrīd\ *n* : a sulfonylurea $C_{23}H_{28}ClN_3O_5S$ used similarly to glipizide — called also *glibenclamide;* see DIAβETA, GLUCOVANCE, MICRONASE

gly·can \ˈglī-ˌkan\ *n* : POLYSACCHARIDE

gly·ce·mia *or chiefly Brit* **gly·cae·mia** \glī-ˈsē-mē-ə\ *n* : the presence of glucose in the blood — **gly·ce·mic** *or chiefly Brit* **gly·cae·mic** \-ˈsē-mik\ *adj*

glycemic index *n* : a measure of the rate at which an ingested food causes the level of glucose in the blood to rise ⟨the insulin response caused by carbohydrate depends on the *glycemic index* . . . of the food —Trevor Smith⟩; *also* : a ranking of foods according to their glycemic index — abbr. *GI*

glyc·er·al·de·hyde \ˌglis-ə-ˈral-də-ˌhīd\ *n* : a sweet crystalline compound $C_3H_6O_3$ that is formed as an intermediate in carbohydrate metabolism by the breakdown of sugars and that yields glycerol on reduction

gly·cer·ic acid \glis-er-ik-\ *n* : a syrupy acid $C_3H_6O_4$ obtainable by oxidation of glycerol or glyceraldehyde

glyc·er·ide \ˈglis-ə-ˌrīd\ *n* : an ester of glycerol esp. with fatty acids — **glyc·er·id·ic** \ˌglis-ə-ˈrid-ik\ *adj*

glyc·er·in *or* **glyc·er·ine** \ˈglis-(ə)rən\ *n* : GLYCEROL

glyc·er·in·ate \ˈglis-(ə)rə-ˌnāt\ *vt* **-at·ed; -at·ing** : to treat with or preserve in glycerin — **glyc·er·in·ation** \ˌglis-(ə)rə-ˈnā-shən\ *n*

glycerinated gelatin *n* : a jellylike preparation that is made from glycerin, gelatin, and water and that is used as a base for suppositories and ointments

glyc·er·ite \ˈglis-ə-ˌrīt\ *n* : a medicinal preparation made by mixing or dissolving a substance in glycerin

glyc·er·o·gel·a·tin \ˌglis-ə-(ˌ)rō-ˈjel-ət-ən\ *n* : any of several medicated dermatologic preparations made from glycerin and glycerinated gelatin

glyc·er·ol \ˈglis-ə-ˌrȯl, -ˌrōl\ *n* : a sweet syrupy hygroscopic trihydroxy alcohol $C_3H_8O_3$ usu. obtained by the saponification of fats and used esp. as a solvent and plasticizer, as a moistening agent, emollient, and lubricant, and as an emulsifying agent — called also *glycerin*

glyc·er·o·phos·phate \ˌglis-ə-(ˌ)rō-ˈfäs-ˌfāt\ *n* : a salt or ester of either of the glycerophosphoric acids

glyc·er·o·phos·phor·ic acid \-ˌfäs-ˈfȯr-ik-, -ˈfär-; -ˈfäs-f(ə)rik-\ *n* : either of two isomeric dibasic acids $C_3H_9O_6P$ occurring naturally in combined form as lecithin and cephalin and used in medicine in the form of salts

glyc·er·ose \ˈglis-ə-ˌrōs *also* -ˌrōz\ *n* : GLYCERALDEHYDE

glyc·er·yl \ˈglis-(ə)rəl\ *n* : a radical derived from glycerol by removal of hydroxide; *esp* : a trivalent radical CH_2CHCH_2

glyceryl guai·a·col·ate \-ˈg(w)ī-ə-ˌkȯl-ˌāt, -kəl-\ *n* : GUAIFENESIN

gly·cine \ˈglī-ˌsēn, ˈglīs-ᵊn\ *n* : a sweet crystalline nonessential amino acid $C_2H_5NO_2$ that is a neurotransmitter which induces inhibition of postsynaptic neurons, is obtained by hydrolysis of proteins or is prepared synthetically, and is used in the form of its salt as an antacid or in aqueous solution as an irrigating fluid in transurethral surgery — abbr. *Gly;* called also *aminoacetic acid, glycocoll*

gly·cin·uria \ˌglīs-ᵊn-ˈ(y)ùr-ē-ə\ *n* : a kidney disorder characterized by the presence of excessive amounts of glycine in the urine

gly·co·al·ka·loid \ˌglī-kō-ˈal-kə-ˌlȯid\ *n* : a bitter compound (as solanine) occurring in various plants and consisting of a glycoside of an alkaloid

gly·co·bi·ar·sol \ˌglī-kō-(ˌ)bī-ˈär-ˌsȯl, -ˌsōl\ *n* : an antiprotozoal drug $C_8H_9AsBiNO_6$ used esp. in the treatment of intestinal amebiasis

gly·co·ca·lyx \ˌglī-kō-ˈkā-liks *also* -ˈka-\ *n* : a polysaccharide or glycoprotein covering on a cell surface

gly·co·chol·ate \ˌglī-kō-ˈkä-ˌlāt, -ˈkō-; glī-ˈkäk-ə-ˌlāt\ *n* : a salt or ester of glycocholic acid

gly·co·chol·ic acid \ˌglī-kō-ˈkä-lik-, -ˈkō-lik-\ *n* : a crystalline acid $C_{26}H_{43}NO_6$ that occurs in bile esp. of humans and herbivorous animals and that yields glycine and cholic acid on hydrolysis

gly·co·coll \ˈglī-kō-ˌkäl\ *n* : GLYCINE

gly·co·con·ju·gate \ˌglī-kō-ˈkän-ji-gət, -jə-ˌgāt\ *n* : any of a group of compounds (as the glycolipids and glycoproteins) consisting of sugars linked to proteins or lipids

gly·co·gen \ˈglī-kə-jən\ *n* : a white amorphous tasteless polysaccharide $(C_6H_{10}O_5)x$ that constitutes the principal form in which glucose is stored in animal tissues, occurs esp. in the liver and in muscle and also in fungi and yeasts, and resembles starch in molecular structure and in the formation of only glucose on complete hydrolysis — called also *animal starch*

gly·cog·e·nase \glī-ˈkä-jə-ˌnās, -ˌnāz\ *n* : an enzyme that catalyzes the hydrolysis of glycogen

gly·co·gen·e·sis \ˌglī-kə-ˈjen-ə-səs\ *n, pl* **-e·ses** \-ˌsēz\ : the formation and storage of glycogen — compare GLYCOGENOLYSIS — **gly·co·ge·net·ic** \-jə-ˈnet-ik\ *adj*

gly·co·gen·ic \-ˈjen-ik\ *adj* : of, relating to, or involving glycogen or glycogenesis ⟨the ∼ function of the liver⟩

gly·co·gen·ol·y·sis \ˌglī-kə-jə-ˈnäl-ə-səs\ *n, pl* **-y·ses** \-ˌsēz\ : the breakdown of glycogen esp. to glucose in the animal body — compare GLYCOGENESIS — **gly·co·gen·o·lyt·ic** \-jən-ᵊl-ˈit-ik, -ˌjen-\ *adj*

gly·co·ge·no·sis \-ˈnō-səs\ *n, pl* **-no·ses** \-ˌsēz\ : GLYCOGEN STORAGE DISEASE

glycogen storage disease *n* : any of several metabolic disorders (as McArdle's disease or Pompe's disease) that are characterized esp. by abnormal deposits of glycogen in tissue, are caused by enzyme deficiencies in glycogen metabolism, and are usu. inherited as an autosomal recessive trait

gly·col \ˈglī-ˌkȯl, -ˌkōl\ *n* : ETHYLENE GLYCOL; *broadly* : a related alcohol containing two hydroxyl groups

gly·col·al·de·hyde \ˌglī-(ˌ)kȯl-ˈal-də-ˌhīd, -(ˌ)kōl-\ *n* : a compound that exists in solution as the diose $C_2H_4O_2$ but that exists in the anhydrous state only as the crystalline dimer $C_4H_8O_4$

gly·co·late *also* **gly·col·late** \ˈglī-kə-ˌlāt\ *n* : a salt or ester of glycolic acid

gly·col·ic *also* **gly·col·lic** \(ˌ)glī-ˈkäl-ik\ *adj* : containing, involving, or performed using glycolic acid ⟨a ∼ peel⟩

glycolic acid *also* **glycollic acid** *n* : an alpha hydroxy acid $C_2H_4O_3$ that is oxidized to glyoxylic acid in photosynthesis, is used as an agent to produce chemical peels in cutaneous rejuvenation treatments, and is the major toxic metabolite in ethylene glycol poisoning — called also *hydroxyacetic acid*

gly·co·lip·id \ˌglī-kō-ˈlip-əd\ *n* : a lipid (as a ganglioside or a cerebroside) that contains a carbohydrate radical

gly·col·y·sis \glī-ˈkäl-ə-səs\ *n, pl* **-y·ses** \-ˌsēz\ : the enzymatic breakdown of a carbohydrate (as glucose or glycogen) by way of phosphate derivatives with the production of pyruvic or lactic acid and energy stored in high-energy phosphate bonds of ATP — called also *Embden-Meyerhof pathway* — **gly·co·lyt·ic** \ˌglī-kə-ˈlit-ik\ *adj* — **gly·co·lyt·i·cal·ly** \-i-k(ə-)lē\ *adv*

gly·co·neo·gen·e·sis \ˌglī-kə-ˌnē-ə-ˈjen-ə-səs\ *n, pl* **-e·ses** \-ˌsēz\ : GLUCONEOGENESIS

gly·co·pep·tide \ˌglī-kō-ˈpep-ˌtīd\ *n* : GLYCOPROTEIN

gly·co·pro·tein \-ˈprō-ˌtēn, -ˈprōt-ē-ən\ *n* : a conjugated protein in which the nonprotein group is a carbohydrate — called also *glucoprotein;* compare MUCOPROTEIN

gly·co·pyr·ro·late \-ˈpī-rə-ˌlāt\ *n* : a synthetic anticholinergic drug $C_{19}H_{28}BrNO_3$ used in the treatment of gastrointestinal disorders (as peptic ulcer) esp. when associated with hyperacidity, hypermotility, or spasm — see ROBINUL

gly·cos·ami·no·gly·can \ˌglī-kō-sə-ˌmē-nō-ˈglī-ˌkan, -kō-ˌsam-ə-nō-\ *n* : any of various polysaccharides derived from an amino hexose that are constituents of mucoproteins, glycoproteins, and blood-group substances — called also *mucopolysaccharide*

gly·co·si·dase \ˈglī-ˈkō-sə-ˌdās, -zə-ˌdāz\ *n* : an enzyme that catalyzes the hydrolysis of a bond joining a sugar of a glycoside to an alcohol or another sugar unit

gly·co·side \ˈglī-kə-ˌsīd\ *n* : any of numerous sugar derivatives that contain a nonsugar group attached through an oxygen or nitrogen bond and that on hydrolysis yield a sugar (as glucose) — **gly·co·sid·ic** \ˌglī-kə-ˈsid-ik\ *adj* — **gly·co·sid·i·cal·ly** \-i-k(ə-)lē\ *adv*

gly·co·sphin·go·lip·id \ˌglī-kō-ˌsfiŋ-gō-ˈlip-əd\ *n* : any of various lipids (as a cerebroside or a ganglioside) which are derivatives of ceramides, do not contain the phosphorus or the extra nitrogenous base of the sphingomyelins, and do contain a carbohydrate (as glucose), and some of which accumulate in disorders of lipid metabolism (as Tay-Sachs disease)

gly·cos·uria \ˌglī-kō-ˈshur-ē-ə, -kəs-ˈyur-\ *n* : the presence in the urine of abnormal amounts of sugar — called also *glucosuria;* compare GLYCURESIS — **gly·cos·uric** \-ˈshu̇(ə)r-ik, -ˈyu̇(ə)r-\ *adj*

gly·co·syl \ˈglī-kə-ˌsil\ *n* : a monovalent radical derived from a cyclic form of glucose by removal of the hemiacetal hydroxyl group

gly·co·syl·a·tion \ˌglī-ˌkō-sə-ˈlā-shən\ *n* : the process of adding glycosyl groups to a protein to form a glycoprotein — **gly·co·syl·ate** \ˈglī-ˈkō-sə-ˌlāt\ *vt* **-at·ed; -at·ing**

gly·co·syl·trans·fer·ase \-ˈtran(t)s-(ˌ)fər-ˌās, -āz\ *n* : any of a group of enzymes that catalyze the transfer of glycosyl groups in biochemical reactions

gly·co·trop·ic \ˌglī-kō-ˈträp-ik, -ˈtrōp-\ *adj* : antagonizing the action of insulin esp. with regard to the production of hypoglycemia ⟨a ∼ anterior-pituitary fraction⟩

glycu·re·sis \ˌglik-yu̇-ˈrē-səs, ˌglīk-\ *n, pl* **-re·ses** \-ˌsēz\ : physiological excretion of large amounts of sugar in the urine following excessive carbohydrate intake — compare GLYCOSURIA

gly·cyl \ˈglī-səl\ *n* : the amino acid radical or residue H_2NCH_2CO- of glycine — abbr. *Gly*

glyc·yr·rhi·za \ˌglis-ə-ˈrī-zə\ *n* **1** *cap* : a genus of widely distributed perennial herbs of the family Leguminosae that have leathery often prickly pods and that include the licorice (*G. glabra*) **2** : the dried root of licorice that is a source of extracts used esp. to mask unpleasant flavors (as in drugs) or to give a pleasant taste (as to confections) — called also *licorice, licorice root*

glyc·yr·rhi·zic acid \-ˈrī-zik-\ *n* : GLYCYRRHIZIN

glyc·yr·rhi·zin \-ˈrīz-ᵊn\ *n* : a crystalline glycosidic acid $C_{42}H_{62}O_{16}$ constituting the sweet constituent of glycyrrhiza

gly·ox·al \glī-ˈäk-ˌsal\ *n* : a reactive yellow low-melting aldehyde CHOCHO made by catalytic oxidation of ethylene glycol

gly·ox·a·lase \-sə-ˌlās, -ˌlāz\ *n* : an enzyme that accelerates reversibly the conversion in the presence of glutathione of methylglyoxal to lactic acid

gly·ox·a·line \-sə-ˌlēn, -lən\ *n* : IMIDAZOLE

gly·ox·y·late \ˌglī-ˈäk-sə-ˌlāt\ *n* : a salt or ester of glyoxylic acid

gly·ox·yl·ic acid \ˌglī-(ˌ)äk-ˈsil-ik-\ *n* : a syrupy or crystalline aldehyde acid $C_2H_2O_3$ or $C_2H_4O_4$ that is an important inter-

G
H

\ə\ abut \ᵊ\ kitten \ər\ further \a\ ash \ā\ ace \ä\ cot, cart \au̇\ out \ch\ chin \e\ bet \ē\ easy \g\ go \i\ hit \ī\ ice \j\ job \ŋ\ sing \ō\ go \ȯ\ law \ȯi\ boy \th\ thin \th̲\ the \ü\ loot \u̇\ foot \y\ yet \zh\ vision   *See also* Pronunciation Symbols page

mediate compound in plant and animal metabolism and occurs esp. in unripe fruit

gm *abbr* gram

GM and S *abbr* General Medicine and Surgery

GM–CSF *abbr* granulocyte-macrophage colony-stimulating factor

GN *abbr* graduate nurse

gnat \'nat\ *n* : any of various small usu. biting dipteran flies (as a midge or blackfly)

gnath·ic \'nath-ik\ *or* **gna·thal** \'nā-thəl, 'nath-əl\ *adj* : of or relating to the jaw

gnathic index *n* : the anthropometric ratio of the distance from the nasion to the basion to that from the basion to the alveolar point multiplied by 100 — called also *alveolar index*

gna·thi·on \'nā-thē-ˌän, 'na-\ *n* : the midpoint of the lower border of the human mandible — compare LINGUALE

Gna·thob·del·li·da \ˌnā-ˌthäb-'del-ə-də\ *n pl* : an order or other taxon of leeches comprising those lacking a proboscis and having 2-toothed or 3-toothed chitinous jaws (as the medicinal leech and the land leeches) — **gna·thob·del·lid** \-'del-əd\ *adj*

Gna·thos·to·ma \na-'thäs-tə-mə\ *n* : a genus (the type of the family Gnathostomatidae) of spiruroid nematodes comprising parasites living in tumors of the stomach wall of various Old World carnivorous mammals and occas. invading the subcutaneous tissues of humans

gna·thos·to·mi·a·sis \nə-ˌthäs-tə-'mī-ə-səs\ *n, pl* **-a·ses** \-ˌsēz\ : infestation with or disease caused by nematode worms of the genus *Gnathostoma* commonly acquired by eating raw fish

gno·to·bi·ol·o·gy \ˌnō-tə-bī-'äl-ə-jē\ *n, pl* **-gies** : GNOTOBIOTICS

gno·to·bi·ot·ic \ˌnō-tə-(ˌ)bī-'ät-ik, -bē-\ *adj* : of, relating to, living in, or being a controlled environment containing one or a few kinds of organisms : AXENIC ⟨∼ mice⟩ — **gno·to·bi·ote** \-'bī-ˌōt\ *n* — **gno·to·bi·ot·i·cal·ly** \-(ˌ)bī-'ät-ik(-ə)-lē *also* -bē-\ *adv*

gno·to·bi·ot·ics \-'ät-iks\ *n pl but sing in constr* : the raising and study of animals under gnotobiotic conditions

GnRH *abbr* gonadotropin-releasing hormone

goal–di·rec·ted \'gōl-də-ˌrek-təd\ *adj* : aimed toward a goal or toward completion of a task ⟨∼ behavior⟩

Goa powder \ˌgō-ə-\ *n* : a bitter powder found in the wood of a Brazilian leguminous tree (*Andira araroba*) and valued as the chief source of the drug chrysarobin — called also *araroba*

gob·let cell \'gäb-lət-\ *n* : a mucus-secreting epithelial cell (as of columnar epithelium) that is distended with secretion or its precursors at the free end

gog·gles \'gäg-əlz\ *n pl* : protective glasses set in a flexible frame (as of rubber or plastic) that fits snugly against the face

goi·ter *or chiefly Brit* **goi·tre** \'gȯit-ər\ *n* : an enlargement of the thyroid gland that is commonly visible as a swelling of the anterior part of the neck, that often results from insufficient intake of iodine and then is usu. accompanied by hypothyroidism, and that in other cases is associated with hyperthyroidism usu. together with toxic symptoms and exophthalmos — called also *struma* — **goi·trous** \'gȯi-trəs\ *also* **goi·ter·ous** \'gȯit-ə-rəs\ *adj*

goi·tro·gen \'gȯi-trə-jən\ *n* : a substance (as thiourea or thiouracil) that induces goiter formation

goi·tro·gen·e·sis \ˌgȯi-trə-'jen-ə-səs\ *n, pl* **-e·ses** \-ˌsēz\ : the action or process of inducing goiter formation

goi·tro·gen·ic \ˌgȯi-trə-'jen-ik\ *also* **goi·ter·o·gen·ic** \ˌgȯit-ə-rō-'jen-\ *adj* : producing or tending to produce goiter ⟨a ∼ agent⟩ — **goi·tro·ge·nic·i·ty** \ˌgȯi-trə-jə-'nis-ət-ē\ *n, pl* **-ties**

gold \'gōld\ *n, often attrib* : a malleable ductile yellow metallic element that occurs chiefly free or in a few minerals and is used esp. in coins, jewelry, and dentures and in the form of its salts (as gold sodium thiomalate) esp. in the treatment of rheumatoid arthritis — symbol *Au*; see ELEMENT table

gold·en hour \'gōl-dən-'aȯ(-ə)r\ *n* : the hour immediately following traumatic injury in which medical treatment to prevent irreversible internal damage and optimize the chance of survival is most effective

gold·en·seal \'gōl-dən-ˌsēl\ *n* **1** : a perennial American herb of the genus *Hydrastis* (*H. canadensis*) with a thick knotted yellow rootstock and large rounded leaves **2** : HYDRASTIS 2

gold sodium thio·ma·late \-ˌthī-ō-'mal-ˌāt, -'mā-ˌlāt\ *n* : a mixture of two gold salts $C_4H_3AuNa_2O_4S$ and $C_4H_4AuNaO_4S$ injected intramuscularly esp. in the treatment of rheumatoid arthritis — called also *gold thiomalate;* see MYOCHRYSINE

gold sodium thiosulfate *n* : a soluble gold compound $Na_3Au(S_2O_3)_2·2H_2O$ administered by intravenous injection in the treatment of rheumatoid arthritis and lupus erythematosus — called also *sodium aurothiosulfate*

gold thio·glu·cose \-ˌthī-ō-'glü-ˌkōs\ *n* : an organic compound of gold $C_6H_{11}AuO_5S$ injected intramuscularly in the treatment of active rheumatoid arthritis and nondisseminated lupus erythematosus — called also *aurothioglucose*

Gol·gi \'gȯl-(ˌ)jē\ *adj* : of or relating to the Golgi apparatus, Golgi bodies, or the Golgi method of staining nerve tissue ⟨∼ vesicles⟩

Golgi, Camillo (1843 *or* 1844–1926), Italian histologist and pathologist. Among Golgi's many valuable contributions to the histology of the nervous system was his discovery in 1873 of the silver nitrate method of staining nerve tissue, which enabled him in 1880 to demonstrate the existence of the type of nerve cell now known as the Golgi cell. The discovery of Golgi cells led Santiago Ramón y Cajal (1852–1934) to establish in 1892 that the nerve cell is the basic structural unit of the nervous system. The latter discovery was basic to the development of modern neurology. In 1880 Golgi also found and described the Golgi tendon organ. Three years later he discovered in nerve cells an irregular network of fibrils, vesicles, and granules; this cell organelle is now known to be found generally in plant and animal cells and is called the Golgi apparatus or complex. In 1906 Ramón y Cajal and Golgi were awarded the Nobel Prize for Physiology or Medicine.

Golgi apparatus *n* : a cytoplasmic organelle that consists of a stack of smooth membranous saccules and associated vesicles and that is active in the modification and transport of proteins — called also *Golgi complex*

Golgi body *n* : GOLGI APPARATUS; *also* : DICTYOSOME

Golgi cell *n* : a neuron with short dendrites and with either a long axon or an axon that breaks into processes soon after leaving the cell body

Golgi complex *n* : GOLGI APPARATUS

Golgi method *n* : a method of preparing nerve tissue for study using potassium dichromate and silver nitrate that is effective because a few of the neurons are stained completely and stand out from the rest which are not stained at all

Golgi tendon organ *n* : a spindle-shaped sensory end organ within a tendon that provides information about muscle tension — called also *neurotendinous spindle*

go·mer \'gō-mər\ *n, med slang, usu disparaging* : a chronic problem patient who does not respond to treatment

gom·pho·sis \gäm-'fō-səs\ *n* : an immovable articulation in which a hard part is received into a bone cavity (as the teeth into the jaws)

go·nad \'gō-ˌnad\ *n* : a gamete-producing reproductive gland (as an ovary or testis) — **go·nad·al** \gō-'nad-ᵊl\ *adj*

go·nad·ec·to·my \ˌgō-nə-'dek-tə-mē\ *n, pl* **-mies** : surgical removal of an ovary or testis — **go·nad·ec·to·mized** \-ˌmīzd\ *adj*

go·nad·o·troph \gō-'nad-ə-ˌtrōf\ *n* : a cell of the adenohypophysis that secretes a gonadotropic hormone (as luteinizing hormone)

go·nad·o·trop·ic \gō-ˌnad-ə-'träp-ik\ *also* **go·nad·o·tro·phic** \-'trō-fik, -'träf-ik\ *adj* : acting on or stimulating the gonads

go·nad·o·tro·pin \-'trō-pən\ *also* **go·nad·o·tro·phin** \-fən\ *n* : a gonadotropic hormone (as follicle-stimulating hormone) — see HUMAN CHORIONIC GONADOTROPIN

gonadotropin–re·leas·ing hormone \-ri-'lēs-iŋ-\ *n* : a decapeptide hormone produced by the hypothalamus that stimulates the adenohypophysis to release gonadotropins (as luteinizing hormone and follicle-stimulating hormone) — abbr. *GnRH;* called also *luteinizing hormone-releasing factor, luteinizing hormone-releasing hormone*

gone \'gòn *also* \'gän\ *adj* : PREGNANT ⟨she's six months ∼⟩

G₁ phase \ˌjē-'wən-\ *n* : the period in the cell cycle from the end of cell division to the beginning of DNA replication — compare G₂ PHASE, M PHASE, S PHASE

go·ni·al \'gō-nē-əl\ *adj* : of, relating to, or being primitive germ cells

gonial angle *n* : the angle formed by the junction of the posterior and lower borders of the human lower jaw — called also *angle of the jaw, angle of the mandible*

go·ni·om·e·ter \ˌgō-nē-'äm-ət-ər\ *n* : an instrument for measuring angles (as of a joint or the skull) — **go·nio·met·ric** \-nē-ə-'me-trik\ *adj* — **go·ni·om·e·try** \-'äm-ə-trē\ *n, pl* **-tries**

go·ni·on \'gō-nē-ˌän\ *n, pl* **go·nia** \-nē-ə\ : the point on each lower human jaw closest to the vertex of the gonial angle

go·nio·punc·ture \'gō-nē-ə-ˌpəŋ(k)-chər\ *n* : a surgical operation for congenital glaucoma that involves making a puncture into the sclera with a knife at the site of discharge of aqueous fluid at the periphery of the anterior chamber of the eye

go·nio·scope \-ˌskōp\ *n* : an instrument consisting of a contact lens to be fitted over the cornea and an optical system with which the interior of the eye can be viewed — **go·nio·scop·ic** \ˌgō-nē-ə-'skäp-ik\ *adj* — **go·ni·os·co·py** \ˌgō-nē-'äs-kə-pē\ *n, pl* **-pies**

go·ni·ot·o·my \ˌgō-nē-'ät-ə-mē\ *n, pl* **-mies** : surgical relief of glaucoma used in some congenital types and achieved by opening the canal of Schlemm

go·ni·tis \gō-'nīt-əs\ *n* : inflammation of the knee

gon·o·coc·ce·mia *or chiefly Brit* **gon·o·coc·cae·mia** \ˌgä-nə-ˌkäk-'sē-mē-ə\ *n* : the presence of gonococci in the blood — **gon·o·coc·ce·mic** *or chiefly Brit* **gon·o·coc·cae·mic** \-'sē-mik\ *adj*

gon·o·coc·cus \ˌgän-ə-'käk-əs\ *n, pl* **-coc·ci** \-'käk-ˌ(s)ī, -'käk-(ˌ)(s)ē\ : a pus-producing bacterium of the genus *Neisseria* (*N. gonorrhoeae*) that causes gonorrhea — **gon·o·coc·cal** \-'käk-əl\ *or* **gon·o·coc·cic** \-'käk-(s)ik\ *adj*

gon·o·cyte \'gän-ə-ˌsīt\ *n* : a cell that produces gametes; *esp* : GAMETOCYTE

gon·o·duct \-ˌdəkt\ *n* : the duct of a gonad

gon·o·gen·e·sis \ˌgän-ə-'jen-ə-səs\ *n, pl* **-e·ses** \-ˌsēz\ : maturation of germ cells that includes oogenesis and spermatogenesis

gon·or·rhea *or chiefly Brit* **gon·or·rhoea** \ˌgän-ə-'rē-ə\ *n* : a contagious inflammation of the genital mucous membrane caused by the gonococcus — called also *clap* — **gon·or·rhe·al** *or chiefly Brit* **gon·or·rhoe·al** \-'rē-əl\ *adj*

gon·o·tyl \'gän-ə-ˌtil\ *n* : a sucker surrounding the genital opening of some trematode worms

go·ny·au·lax \ˌgō-nē-'ò-ˌlaks\ *n* **1** *cap* : a large genus of phosphorescent marine dinoflagellates that when unusually abundant cause red tide **2** : any dinoflagellate of the genus *Gonyaulax*

Gooch crucible \'güch-\ *n* : a small crucible with a perforated bottom in which precipitates can be collected, dried, and weighed — called also *Gooch filter*

 Gooch, Frank Austin (1852–1929), American chemist. Gooch published a number of papers on procedures in inorganic chemical analysis. In 1878 he introduced the Gooch crucible. He also developed a distillation method for estimating boric acid and a method for the quantitative separation of lithium from other alkali metals.

good cholesterol \'gùd-\ *n* : HDL

Good·pas·ture's syndrome \'gùd-ˌpas-chərz-\ *also* **Good·pas·ture syndrome** \-chər-\ *n* : an autoimmune disorder of unknown cause that is characterized by the presence of circulating antibodies in the blood which attack the basement membrane of the kidney's glomeruli and the lung's alveoli and that is marked initially by coughing, fatigue, difficulty in breathing, and hemoptysis progressing to glomerulonephritis and pulmonary hemorrhages

 Goodpasture, Ernest William (1886–1960), American pathologist. Goodpasture served for many years on the faculty of Vanderbilt University Medical School and as director of the research laboratory there. Known for his viral research, he was the first to study the progression of the herpes simplex virus along neural pathways to the central nervous system. In 1931 he demonstrated that fowl pox virus could be cultivated on the chorioallantoic membrane of the chick embryo and later showed that human viruses could be grown in the same way. He developed methods that made possible the commercial, mass production of vaccines against viral diseases such as smallpox, yellow fever, and influenza. Goodpasture described the syndrome that bears his name in 1919.

goose bumps \'güs-ˌbəmps\ *n pl* : a roughness of the skin produced by erection of its papillae esp. from cold, fear, or a sudden feeling of excitement — called also *goose pimples*

goose·flesh \-ˌflesh\ *n* : GOOSE BUMPS

Gor·di·a·cea \ˌgòr-dē-'ā-sh(ē-)ə\ *n pl, syn of* NEMATOMORPHA

 Gordius \'gòr-dē-əs\, Greek mythological character. Gordius was the king of ancient Phrygia. In his capital city he contrived an intricate knot that lashed a pole to the yoke of his chariot. According to the prophecy of an oracle, the person who could undo the knot would someday be the conqueror of Asia. Alexander the Great marched through the site, and, according to popular legend, he readily solved the problem simply by cutting the knot. Worms of the class Gordiacea are so-called because of the intricate twists and coils they form.

gor·di·a·cean \-'ā-sh(ē-)ən\ *n* : HORSEHAIR WORM

gor·get \'gòr-jət\ *n* : a grooved instrument used esp. formerly to guide the direction of surgical incision in lithotomy

gork \'gòrk\ *n, med slang, usu disparaging* : a terminal patient whose brain is nonfunctional and the rest of whose body can be kept functioning only by the extensive use of mechanical devices and nutrient solutions — **gorked** \'gòrkt\ *adj, med slang, usu disparaging*

gos·sy·pol \'gäs-ə-ˌpól, -ˌpōl\ *n* : a phenolic pigment $C_{30}H_{30}O_8$ in cottonseed that is toxic to some animals

got *past and past part of* GET

gotten *past part of* GET

gouge \'gaùj\ *n* : a chisel with a concavo-convex cross section for removing portions of bone in surgery

goun·dou \'gün-(ˌ)dü\ *n* : a tumorous swelling of the nose involving the nasal bones, occurring in certain tropical areas, and often considered a late lesion of yaws — compare GANGOSA

gout \'gaùt\ *n* : a metabolic disease marked by a painful inflammation of the joints, deposits of urates in and around the joints, and usu. an excessive amount of uric acid in the blood

gouty \'gaùt-ē\ *adj* **1** : diseased with gout ⟨a ∼ person⟩ **2** : of, characteristic of, or caused by gout ⟨a ∼ paroxysm⟩ ⟨∼ concretions⟩ **3** : causing or tending to induce gout ⟨purine-rich ∼ foods⟩ **4** : used or for use during an attack of gout ⟨∼ shoes⟩ — **gout·i·ness** \-nəs\ *n*

gouty arthritis *n* : arthritis associated with gout and caused by the deposition of urate crystals in the articular cartilage of joints

Gow·ers's tract \'gaù-ərz(-)z)-\ *n* : SPINOCEREBELLAR TRACT b

 Gowers, Sir William Richard (1845–1915), British neurologist. Gowers was one of the founders of modern neurology. Early in his career he became interested in the anatomical pathology and diseases of the spinal cord. In 1880 he

G
H

\ə\ **abut** \ᵊ\ **kitten** \ər\ **further** \a\ **ash** \ā\ **ace** \ä\ **cot, cart** \aù\ **out** \ch\ **chin** \e\ **bet** \ē\ **easy** \g\ **go** \i\ **hit** \ī\ **ice** \j\ **job** \ŋ\ **sing** \ō\ **go** \ò\ **law** \òi\ **boy** \th\ **thin** \th̲\ **the** \ü\ **loot** \ù\ **foot** \y\ **yet** \zh\ **vision** *See also* Pronunciation Symbols page

published a work on diseases of the spinal cord in which he described the tract that now bears his name.

gp *abbr* group

GP *abbr* **1** general paresis **2** general practitioner

G₁ phase, G₂ phase — see entries alphabetized as G ONE PHASE, G TWO PHASE

gp120 \ˌjē-(ˌ)pē-ˌwən-ˈtwen-tē\ *n* : a glycoprotein that protrudes from the outer surface of the HIV virion, that has a molecular weight of 120, and that must bind to a CD4 receptor on a T cell bearing such receptors before infection of the cell can occur

G protein \ˈjē-\ *n* : any of a class of cell membrane proteins that are coupled to cell surface receptors and upon stimulation of the receptor by an extracellular molecule (as a hormone or neurotransmitter) bind to GTP to form an active complex which mediates an intracellular event (as activation of adenylate cyclase)

gr *abbr* **1** grain **2** gram **3** gravity

graaf·ian follicle \ˈgräf-ē-ən-, ˈgraf-\ *n, often cap G* : a mature follicle in a mammalian ovary that contains a liquid-filled cavity and that ruptures during ovulation to release an egg — called also *vesicular ovarian follicle*

de Graaf \də-ˈgräf\, **Reinier (1641–1673),** Dutch physician and anatomist. De Graaf is regarded as one of the creators of experimental physiology. In 1672 he produced a treatise on the female reproductive organs that is considered one of the seminal works of biology. De Graaf demonstrated ovulation anatomically, pathologically, and experimentally. The treatise contains the description of the structures now known in English as the graafian follicles. The Swiss anatomist Albrecht von Haller (1708–1777) named them after de Graaf. In 1827 the German embryologist Karl Ernst von Baer (1792–1876) discovered that although the graafian follicles contain the eggs from which organisms develop, they are not the eggs themselves.

grac·ile \ˈgras-əl, -ˌīl\ *adj* : being slender or slight

gracile fasciculus *n, pl* **gracile fasciculi** : FASCICULUS GRACILIS

grac·i·lis \ˈgras-ə-ləs\ *n* : the most superficial muscle of the inside of the thigh that arises from the lower part of the pubic symphysis and the anterior half of the pubic arch and that has its tendon inserted into the inner surface of the shaft of the tibia below the tuberosity, and that acts to adduct the thigh and to flex the leg at the knee and to assist in rotating it medially

grade \ˈgrād\ *n* : a degree of severity of a disease or abnormal condition ⟨a ∼ III carcinoma⟩

gra·di·ent \ˈgrād-ē-ənt\ *n* **1** : change in the value of a quantity (as temperature, pressure, or concentration) with change in a given variable and esp. per unit on a linear scale **2** : a graded difference in physiological activity along an axis (as of the body or an embryonic field) **3** : change in response with distance from the stimulus

gradient echo *n* : a signal that is detected in a nuclear magnetic resonance spectrometer that is analogous to a spin echo but is produced by varying the external magnetic field following application of a single radio-frequency pulse rather than by application of a series of radio-frequency pulses and that can be used to extract more information from a test sample or subject than is possible in conventional nuclear magnetic resonance spectroscopy — usu. used attributively ⟨*gradient-echo* magnetic resonance imaging of the brain⟩

gradient–re·called echo \-ri-ˈkȯld-\ *n* : GRADIENT ECHO

¹grad·u·ate \ˈgraj-(ə-)wət, -ə-ˌwāt\ *n* : a graduated cup, cylinder, or flask for measuring

²grad·u·ate \ˈgraj-ə-ˌwāt\ *vt* **-at·ed; -at·ing** : to mark with degrees of measurement

graduate nurse *n* : a person who has completed the regular course of study and practical hospital training in nursing school — abbr. *GN;* called also *trained nurse*

Graf·en·berg spot \ˈgraf-ən-bərg-, ˈgräf-, ˈgref-\ *n* : G-SPOT

Gräf·en·berg \ˈgref-ən-ˌberk\, **Ernst (1881–1957),** American (German-born) gynecologist. Gräfenberg is credited with the introduction, in 1929, of one of the first intrauter-

ine contraceptive devices. Consisting of a flexible ring of silver wire, it became known as the Gräfenberg ring. He first described a sensitive area of the anterior wall of the vagina in 1944. This area, now called the Grafenberg spot or G-spot, was further described in an article on the role of the urethra in female orgasm in the *International Journal of Sexology* in 1950.

¹graft \ˈgraft\ *vt* : to implant (living tissue) surgically ⟨∼*ed* a new piece of artery into the ruptured portion of the old artery⟩ ∼ *vi* : to perform grafting

²graft *n* **1** : the act of grafting **2** : something grafted; *specif* : living tissue used in grafting

graft–ver·sus–host \-ˌvər-səs-ˈhōst\ *adj* : of, relating to, or caused by graft-versus-host disease ⟨a ∼ response⟩

graft–versus–host disease *n* : a bodily condition that results when T cells from a usu. allogeneic tissue or organ transplant and esp. a bone marrow transplant react immunologically against the recipient's antigens attacking cells and tissues, that affects esp. the skin, gastrointestinal tract, and liver with symptoms including skin rash, fever, diarrhea, liver dysfunction, abdominal pain, and anorexia, and that may be fatal — abbr. *GVHD;* called also *graft-versus-host reaction*

Gra·ham's law \ˈgrā-əmz-, ˈgra(-ə)mz-\ *n* : a statement in chemistry: under constant pressure and temperature two gases diffuse into each other at rates inversely proportional to the square roots of their respective molecular weights or densities

Graham, Thomas (1805–1869), British chemist. Graham ranks as one of the founders of physical chemistry and is regarded in particular as the father of the chemistry of colloids. After studying the molecular diffusion of gases, he wrote his first important paper on the subject in 1829. He explicitly stated Graham's law in another paper in 1833. After examining the diffusion of liquids, he divided particles into two types: colloids and crystalloids. He devised dialysis and proved that the process of liquid diffusion causes partial decomposition of certain compounds.

grain \ˈgrān\ *n* **1 a** : a seed or fruit of a cereal grass **b** : the seeds or fruits of various food plants including the cereal grasses and in commercial and statutory usage other plants (as the soybean) **c** : plants producing grain **2** : a small hard particle or crystal (as of sand or salt) **3** : a unit of avoirdupois, Troy, and apothecaries' weight equal to 0.0648 gram or 0.002286 avoirdupois ounce or 0.002083 Troy ounce — abbr. *gr*

grain alcohol *n* : ETHANOL

grain itch *n* : an itching rash caused by the bite of a mite of the genus *Pyemotes* (*P. ventricosus*) that occurs chiefly on grain, straw, or straw products — compare GROCER'S ITCH

grain mite *n* : any of several mites that frequent esp. stored grain; *esp* : one of the genus *Acarus* (*A. siro*) that causes vanillism and sometimes causes unpleasant odors in imperfectly dry flour or grain

gram *or chiefly Brit* **gramme** \ˈgram\ *n* **1** : a metric unit of mass equal to ¹/₁₀₀₀ kilogram and nearly equal to the mass of one cubic centimeter of water at its maximum density — abbr. *g* **2** : the weight of a gram under standard gravity

gram–atom *n* : GRAM-ATOMIC WEIGHT

gram–atom·ic weight *also Brit* **gramme–atom·ic weight** \-ə-ˈtäm-ik-\ *n* : the mass of one mole of a chemical element equal in grams to the element's atomic weight

gram calorie *n* : CALORIE 1a

gram equivalent *n* : the quantity of a chemical element, group, or compound that has a mass in grams equal to the equivalent weight

gram·i·ci·din \ˌgram-ə-ˈsīd-ᵊn\ *n* : an antibacterial mixture produced by a soil bacterium of the genus *Bacillus* (*B. brevis*) and used topically against gram-positive bacteria in local infections esp. of the eye

gram·i·niv·o·rous \ˌgram-ə-ˈniv-(ə-)rəs\ *adj* : feeding on grass

gramme *chiefly Brit var of* GRAM

gram molecular weight *also Brit* **gramme–molecular**

weight *n* : the mass of one mole of a chemical compound equal in grams to the compound's molecular weight

gram molecule *n* : GRAM MOLECULAR WEIGHT

gram–neg·a·tive \'gram-'neg-ət-iv\ *adj* : not holding the purple dye when stained by Gram's stain — used chiefly of bacteria

gram–pos·i·tive \'gram-'päz-ət-iv, -'päz-tiv\ *adj* : holding the purple dye when stained by Gram's stain — used chiefly of bacteria

Gram's solution \'gramz-\ *n* : a watery solution of iodine and the iodide of potassium used in staining bacteria by Gram's stain

Gram \'gräm\, **Hans Christian Joachim (1853–1938)**, Danish physician. Gram introduced his method for the differential staining of bacteria in 1884. He also devised, in 1922, a method for determining the percentage of fibrin in blood and plasma. Further, he made investigations into the physiology of anemia during pregnancy and the hematoblasts in cases of pernicious anemia.

Gram's stain *or* **Gram stain** \'gram-\ **1** : a method for the differential staining of bacteria that involves fixing the bacterial cells to a slide and staining usu. with the basic dye crystal violet, treating with an iodine solution to fix the dye, washing with acetone or alcohol to decolorize the dye, and counterstaining usu. with a red safranine dye which shows up only if the crystal violet has been decolorized, that results in gram-positive bacteria retaining the purple dye and gram=negative organisms having it decolorized so that the red counterstain shows up, and that is believed to depended on differences in the structure and composition of the bacterial cell walls which facilitate or prevent the decolorization of the crystal violet dye by the alcohol or acetone — called also *Gram's method* **2** : the chemicals used in Gram's stain

gram–vari·able \'gram-'ver-ē-ə-bəl, -'var-\ *adj* : staining irregularly or inconsistently by Gram's stain

grana *pl of* GRANUM

gra·na·tum \grə-'nāt-əm, -'nät-\ *n* : the bark of the stem and of the root of the pomegranate that has sometimes been used to expel tapeworms

gran·di·ose \'gran-dē-ˌōs, ˌgran-dē-'\ *adj* : characterized by affectation of grandeur or splendor or by absurd exaggeration ⟨a paranoid patient with ∼ delusions⟩ — **gran·di·ose·ly** *adv* — **gran·di·os·i·ty** \ˌgran-dē-'äs-ət-ē\ *n, pl* **-ties**

grand mal \'grän(d)-ˌmäl, 'gräⁿ-ˌmäl, -ˌmal; 'gran(d)-ˌmal\ *n* : severe epilepsy characterized by tonic-clonic seizures; *also* : a tonic-clonic seizure

grand multipara \ˌgrand-\ *n* : a woman who has given birth seven or more times

grand rounds *n pl* : rounds involving the formal presentation by an expert of a clinical issue sometimes in the presence of selected patients

gran·u·lar \'gran-yə-lər\ *adj* **1** : consisting of or appearing to consist of granules : having a grainy texture **2** : having or marked by granulations ⟨∼ tissue⟩ — **gran·u·lar·i·ty** \ˌgran-yə-'lar-ət-ē\ *n, pl* **-ties**

granular conjunctivitis *n* : TRACHOMA

granular layer *n* : the deeper layer of the cortex of the cerebellum containing numerous small closely packed cells

granular leukocyte *n* : any of the white blood cells that have granules in their cytoplasm having specific affinity for certain biological stains and that include the eosinophils, basophils, and neutrophils — compare NONGRANULAR LEUKOCYTE

gran·u·late \'gran-yə-ˌlāt\ *vb* **-lat·ed; -lat·ing** *vt* : to form or crystallize (as sugar) into grains or granules ∼ *vi* : to form granulations ⟨as soon as the ulcer is *granulating* and free from slough —R. H. Nyquist⟩

gran·u·la·tion \ˌgran-yə-'lā-shən\ *n* **1** : the act or process of granulating : the condition of being granulated **2 a** : one of the small elevations of a granulated surface: (1) : a minute mass of tissue projecting from the surface of an organ (as on the eyelids in trachoma) (2) : one of the minute red granules made up of loops of newly formed capillaries that form on a raw surface (as of a wound) and that with fibroblasts

are the active agents in the process of healing — see GRANULATION TISSUE **b** : the act or process of forming such elevations or granules

granulation tissue *n* : tissue made up of granulations that temporarily replaces lost tissue in a wound

gran·ule \'gran-(ˌ)yü(ə)l\ *n* **1 a** : a little grain or small particle; *esp* : one of a number of particles forming a larger unit **b** : a small sugar-coated pill **2** : a clump of actinomycetes in a lesion

granule cell *n* : one of the small neurons of the cortex of the cerebellum and cerebrum

gran·u·lo·blast \'gran-yə-lō-ˌblast\ *n* : a cellular precursor of a granulocyte : MYELOBLAST, MYELOCYTE — **gran·u·lo·blas·tic** \-ˌblast-ik\ *adj*

gran·u·lo·blas·to·sis \ˌgran-yə-lō-ˌblas-'tō-səs\ *n, pl* **-to·ses** \-ˌsēz\ : a disorder of avian leukosis characterized by the presence of excessive numbers of immature blood granulocytes in affected birds

gran·u·lo·cyte \'gran-yə-lō-ˌsīt\ *n* : a polymorphonuclear white blood cell (as a basophil, eosinophil, or neutrophil) with granule-containing cytoplasm — compare AGRANULOCYTE — **gran·u·lo·cyt·ic** \ˌgran-yə-lō-'sit-ik\ *adj*

granulocyte colony–stimulating factor *n* : a colony=stimulating factor produced by macrophages, endothelial cells, and fibroblasts that acts to promote the maturation of precursor cells into granulocytes (as neutrophils) — abbr. *G-CSF;* see FILGRASTIM

granulocyte–macrophage colony–stimulating factor *n* : a colony-stimulating factor produced by T cells, macrophages, endothelial cells, and fibroblasts that promotes the differentiation of bone marrow stem cells, stimulates the maturation of precursor cells into granulocytes and macrophages, and activates mature macrophages — abbr. *GM-CSF;* see SARGRAMOSTIM

granulocytic leukemia *n* : MYELOGENOUS LEUKEMIA

gran·u·lo·cy·to·pe·nia \ˌgran-yə-lō-ˌsīt-ə-'pē-nē-ə\ *n* : deficiency of blood granulocytes; *esp* : AGRANULOCYTOSIS — **gran·u·lo·cy·to·pe·nic** \-'pē-nik\ *adj*

gran·u·lo·cy·to·poi·e·sis \-ˌsīt-ə-ˌpȯi-'ē-səs\ *n, pl* **-e·ses** \-ˌsēz\ : GRANULOPOIESIS

gran·u·lo·cy·to·sis \ˌgran-yə-lō-ˌsī-'tō-səs\ *n, pl* **-to·ses** \-ˌsēz\ : an increase in the number of blood granulocytes — compare LYMPHOCYTOSIS, MONOCYTOSIS

gran·u·lo·ma \ˌgran-yə-'lō-mə\ *n, pl* **-mas** *also* **-ma·ta** \-mət-ə\ : a mass or nodule of chronically inflamed tissue with granulations that is usu. associated with an infective process

granuloma an·nu·la·re \-ˌan-yü-'lar-ē, -'ler-\ *n* : a benign chronic rash of unknown cause characterized by one or more flat spreading ringlike spots with lighter centers esp. on the feet, legs, hands, or fingers

granuloma in·gui·na·le \-ˌiŋ-gwə-'nal-ē, -'näl-, -'nāl-\ *n* : a sexually transmitted disease characterized by ulceration and formation of granulations on the genitalia and in the groin area and caused by a bacterium of the genus *Calymmatobacterium* (*C. granulomatis* syn. *Donovania granulomatis*) which is usu. recovered from lesions as Donovan bodies

granuloma py·o·gen·i·cum \-ˌpī-ō-'jen-i-kəm\ *n* : a granuloma that develops usu. at the site of an injury as a response to nonspecific infection

gran·u·lo·ma·to·sis \ˌgran-yə-ˌlō-mə-'tō-səs\ *n, pl* **-to·ses** \-ˌsēz\ : a chronic condition marked by the formation of numerous granulomas

gran·u·lo·ma·tous \-'lō-mə-təs\ *adj* : of, relating to, or characterized by granuloma ⟨chronic ∼ inflammation⟩ — see CHRONIC GRANULOMATOUS DISEASE

granuloma ve·ne·re·um \-və-'nir-ē-əm\ *n* : GRANULOMA INGUINALE

gran·u·lo·pe·nia \ˌgran-yə-lō-'pē-nē-ə\ *n* : GRANULOCYTOPENIA

G
H

\ə\ **abut** \ᵊ\ **kitten** \ər\ **further** \a\ **ash** \ā\ **ace** \ä\ **cot, cart** \au̇\ **out** \ch\ **chin** \e\ **bet** \ē\ **easy** \g\ **go** \i\ **hit** \ī\ **ice** \j\ **job** \ŋ\ **sing** \ō\ **go** \ȯ\ **law** \ȯi\ **boy** \th\ **thin** \t̲h̲\ **the** \ü\ **loot** \u̇\ **foot** \y\ **yet** \zh\ **vision** *See also* Pronunciation Symbols page

gran·u·lo·poi·e·sis \-ˌ(ˌ)lō-ˌpȯi-'ē-səs\ *n, pl* **-e·ses** \-ˌsēz\ : the formation of blood granulocytes typically in the bone marrow — called also *granulocytopoiesis* — **gran·u·lo·poi·et·ic** \-ˌpȯi-'et-ik\ *adj*

gran·u·lo·sa cell \ˌgran-yə-'lō-sə-, -'lō-zə-\ *n* : one of the estrogen-secreting cells of the epithelial lining of a graafian follicle or its follicular precursor

granulosa lutein cell *n* : any of the relatively large pale-staining lutein cells of the corpus luteum that are derived from granulosa cells, have long microvilli projecting from the cell surface, and secrete primarily progesterone — compare THECA LUTEIN CELL

granulosum — see STRATUM GRANULOSUM

gra·num \'grā-nəm, 'grä-nəm\ *n, pl* **gra·na** \-nə\ : one of the lamellar stacks of chlorophyll-containing material in plant chloroplasts

grapes \'grāps\ *n pl* **1** : a cluster of raw red nodules of granulation tissue in the hollow of the fetlock of horses that is characteristic of advanced or chronic grease heel **2** *pl but usu sing in constr* : tuberculous disease of the pleura in cattle — called also *grape disease*

grape sugar \'grāp-\ *n* : DEXTROSE

¹graph \'graf\ *n* : a diagram (as a series of one or more points, lines, line segments, curves, or areas) that represents the variation of a variable in comparison with that of one or more other variables — **graph·ic** \'graf-ik\ *adj*

²graph *vt* **1** : to represent by a graph **2** : to plot on a graph

graph·ite \'graf-ˌīt\ *n* : carbon of a soft black lustrous form that conducts electricity and is used in lead pencils and electrolytic anodes, as a lubricant, and as a moderator in nuclear reactors — called also *plumbago* — **gra·phit·ic** \gra-'fit-ik\ *adj*

gra·phol·o·gy \gra-'fäl-ə-jē\ *n, pl* **-gies** : the study of handwriting esp. for the purpose of character analysis — **graph·o·log·i·cal** \ˌgraf-ə-'läj-i-kəl\ *adj* — **gra·phol·o·gist** \gra-'fäl-ə-jəst\ *n*

grapho·ma·nia \ˌgraf-ō-'mā-nē-ə, -nyə\ *n* : a compulsive urge to write — **grapho·ma·ni·ac** \-nē-ˌak\ *n*

grapho·mo·tor \ˌgraf-ə-'mōt-ər\ *adj* : relating to or affecting movements made in writing

graph·or·rhea *or chiefly Brit* **graph·or·rhoea** \ˌgraf-ə-'rē-ə\ *n* : a symptom of motor excitement exhibited as continual and incoherent writing

grapho·spasm \'graf-ə-ˌspaz-əm\ *n* : WRITER'S CRAMP

GRAS *abbr* generally recognized as safe

grass \'gras\ *n* : MARIJUANA

grass sickness \'gras-ˌ\ *n* : a frequently fatal disease of grazing horses of unknown cause that affects gastrointestinal functioning by causing difficulty in swallowing, interruption of peristalsis, and fecal impaction — called also *grass disease*

grass staggers *n pl but sing in constr* : GRASS TETANY

grass tetany *n* : a disease of cattle and esp. milk cows marked by tetanic staggering, convulsions, coma, and frequently death and caused by reduction of blood calcium and magnesium when overeating on lush pasture — called also *hypomagnesia*; compare MILK FEVER 2, STAGGERS 1

grat·ing \'grāt-iŋ\ *n* : a system of close equidistant and parallel lines or bars ruled on a polished surface to produce spectra by diffraction — called also *diffraction grating*

grating acuity *n* : the aspect of visual acuity involving the ability to distinguish the elements of a fine grating composed of alternating dark and light stripes or squares — compare HYPERACUITY, STEREOACUITY, VERNIER ACUITY

grat·tage \gra-'täzh, grə-\ *n* : the removal of granulations (as in trachoma) by scraping or by friction

grav *abbr* gravida

grave \'grāv\ *adj* : very serious : dangerous to life — used of an illness or its prospects ⟨a ∼ prognosis⟩

grav·el \'grav-əl\ *n* **1** : a deposit of small calculous concretions in the kidneys and urinary bladder — compare MICROLITH **2** : the condition that results from the presence of deposits of gravel

grav·el–blind \'grav-əl-ˌblīnd\ *adj* : having very weak vision

Graves' disease \'grāvz(-əz)-\ *n* : a common form of hyper-thyroidism characterized by goiter and often a slight protrusion of the eyeballs — called also *Basedow's disease, exophthalmic goiter*

Graves, Robert James (1796–1853), British physician. Graves was one of the founders of the Irish school of medicine. He is remembered especially for his reforms in clinical teaching, such as giving advanced medical students actual clinical experience. His description in 1835 of the form of hyperthyroidism that now bears his name was not the first, but it is generally considered to be the first accurate account.

grav·id \'grav-əd\ *adj* : PREGNANT

grav·i·da \'grav-əd-ə\ *n, pl* **-das** *also* **-dae** \-ə-ˌdē\ : a pregnant woman — often used in combination with a number or figure to indicate the number of pregnancies a woman has had ⟨a ∼ four⟩; compare PARA — **gra·vid·ic** \gra-'vid-ik\ *adj*

gravidarum — see HYPEREMESIS GRAVIDARUM

gra·vid·i·ty \gra-'vid-ət-ē\ *n, pl* **-ties** **1** : PREGNANCY ⟨several successive *gravidities* could be observed —*Veterinary Bull.*⟩ **2** : the number of times a female has been pregnant ⟨∼ and parity were highly correlated⟩ ⟨a nulliparous patient of ∼ 4⟩ — compare PARITY 2

gra·vi·me·ter \gra-'vim-ət-ər, 'grav-ə-ˌmēt-ər\ *n* : a device similar to a hydrometer for determining specific gravity

gravi·met·ric \ˌgrav-ə-'me-trik\ *adj* : of or relating to measurement by weight ⟨a ∼ assay of a drug⟩ — **gravi·met·ri·cal·ly** \-tri-k(ə-)lē\ *adv*

gra·vim·e·try \gra-'vim-ə-trē\ *n, pl* **-tries** : the measurement of weight or density

gravior — see ICHTHYOSIS HYSTRIX GRAVIOR

gra·vis \'grav-vəs, 'grä-, 'grā-\ *adj* : tending to be more virulent than average — used esp. of strains of diphtheria bacilli; see ICTERUS GRAVIS, ICTERUS GRAVIS NEONATORUM, MYASTHENIA GRAVIS; compare INTERMEDIUS, MITIS

grav·i·tate \'grav-ə-ˌtāt\ *vi* **-tat·ed; -tat·ing** : to move under the influence of gravitation

grav·i·ta·tion \ˌgrav-ə-'tā-shən\ *n* : a force manifested by acceleration toward each other of two free material particles or bodies or of radiant-energy quanta as if they were particles (as in the bending of rays of starlight passing close to the sun) : an attraction between two bodies that is proportional to the product of their masses, inversely proportional to the square of the distance between them, and independent of their chemical nature or physical state and of intervening matter — **grav·i·ta·tion·al** \-shnəl, -shən-ᵊl\ *adj* — **grav·i·ta·tion·al·ly** \-ē\ *adv*

gravitational field *n* : the space around an object having mass in which the object's gravitational influence can be detected

grav·i·ty \'grav-ət-ē\ *n, pl* **-ties** **1** : WEIGHT 1 — used chiefly in the phrase *center of gravity* **2 a** : the gravitational attraction of the mass of the earth, the moon, or a planet for bodies at or near its surface; *broadly* : GRAVITATION **b** : ACCELERATION OF GRAVITY **c** : SPECIFIC GRAVITY — **gravity** *adj*

gravity drip *n* : the administration of a fluid into the body using an apparatus in which gravity provides the force moving the fluid

¹gray *or chiefly Brit* **grey** \'grā\ *n* : any of a series of neutral colors ranging between black and white — **gray** *or chiefly Brit* **grey** *adj*

²gray \'grā\ *n* : the mks unit of absorbed dose of ionizing radiation equal to an energy of one joule per kilogram of irradiated material — abbr. *Gy*

Gray, Louis Harold (1905–1965), British radiobiologist. In 1933 Gray established a physics laboratory to measure radiation in the treatment of cancer at Mount Vernon Hospital, Middlesex, England. Earlier he and Sir W. H. Bragg had formulated a theory for deducing the energy absorbed by a material exposed to gamma rays from the ionization within a small gas-filled cavity in the material. At Mount Vernon he was to apply his theory to X-rays and later, in modified form, to neutrons. Gray expressed the neutron dose values in energy units, anticipating the International Commission on Radiological Units, which in 1953 adopted the rad as the unit for measuring all types of ionizing radiation. In 1975 the Commission adopted the gray as the physical unit of dose.

gray column *n* : any of the longitudinal columns of gray matter in each lateral half of the spinal cord — called also *gray horn;* compare COLUMN a

gray commissure *n* : a transverse band of gray matter in the spinal cord appearing in sections as the transverse bar of the H-shaped mass of gray matter

gray horn *n* : GRAY COLUMN

gray matter *n* : neural tissue esp. of the brain and spinal cord that contains cell bodies as well as nerve fibers, has a brownish gray color, and forms most of the cortex and nuclei of the brain, the columns of the spinal cord, and the bodies of ganglia — called also *gray substance*

gray·out *or chiefly Brit* **grey·out** \'grā-ˌaůt\ *n* : a transient dimming or haziness of vision resulting from temporary impairment of cerebral circulation — compare BLACKOUT, REDOUT

gray out \ˌgrā-'aůt\ *vi* : to experience a grayout — compare BLACK OUT, RED OUT

gray ramus *n* : RAMUS COMMUNICANS b

gray ramus communicans *n* : RAMUS COMMUNICANS b

gray substance *n* : GRAY MATTER

gray syndrome *n* : a potentially fatal toxic reaction to chloramphenicol esp. in premature infants that is characterized by abdominal distension, cyanosis, vasomotor collapse, and irregular respiration

GRE *abbr* gradient echo; gradient-recalled echo

grease heel \'grēs-, 'grēz-\ *n* : a chronic inflammation of the skin of the fetlocks and pasterns of horses marked by an excess of oily secretion, ulcerations, and in severe cases general swelling of the legs, nodular excrescences, and a foul-smelling discharge and usu. affecting horses with thick coarse legs kept or worked under unsanitary conditions — called also *greasy heel;* see GRAPES 1

great ape \'grāt-'āp\ *n* : any of the recent anthropoid apes that belong to the family Pongidae and include the gorilla, orangutan, and chimpanzees

great cardiac vein *n* : CARDIAC VEIN a

great cerebral vein *n* : a broad unpaired vein formed by the junction of Galen's veins and uniting with the inferior sagittal sinus to form the straight sinus

great·er cornu \'grāt-ər-\ *n* : THYROHYAL

greater curvature *n* : the boundary of the stomach that forms a long usu. convex curve on the left from the opening for the esophagus to the opening into the duodenum — compare LESSER CURVATURE

greater multangular *n* : TRAPEZIUM — called also *greater multangular bone*

greater occipital nerve *n* : OCCIPITAL NERVE a

greater omentum *n* : a part of the peritoneum attached to the greater curvature of the stomach and to the colon and hanging down over the small intestine — called also *caul, gastrocolic omentum;* compare LESSER OMENTUM

greater palatine artery *n* : PALATINE ARTERY 1b

greater palatine foramen *n* : a foramen in each posterior side of the palate giving passage to the greater palatine artery and to a palatine nerve

greater petrosal nerve *n* : a mixed nerve that contains mostly sensory and some parasympathetic fibers, arises in the geniculate ganglion, joins with the deep petrosal nerve at the entrance of the pterygoid canal to form the Vidian nerve, and as part of this nerve sends sensory fibers to the soft palate with some to the eustachian tube and sends parasympathetic fibers forming the motor root of the pterygopalatine ganglion — called also *greater superficial petrosal nerve*

greater sciatic foramen *n* : SCIATIC FORAMEN a

greater sciatic notch *n* : SCIATIC NOTCH a

greater splanchnic nerve *n* : SPLANCHNIC NERVE a

greater superficial petrosal nerve *n* : GREATER PETROSAL NERVE

greater trochanter *also* **great trochanter** *n* : TROCHANTER a

greater tubercle *n* : a prominence on the upper lateral part of the end of the humerus that serves as the insertion for the supraspinatus, infraspinatus, and teres minor — compare LESSER TUBERCLE

greater vestibular gland *n* : BARTHOLIN'S GLAND

greater wing *also* **great wing** *n* : a broad curved winglike expanse on each side of the sphenoid bone — called also *alisphenoid;* compare LESSER WING

great ragweed *n* : RAGWEED b

great saphenous vein *n* : SAPHENOUS VEIN a

great toe *n* : BIG TOE

great trochanter *var of* GREATER TROCHANTER

great white shark *n* : a large shark (*Carcharodon carcharias* of the family Lamnidae) that is bluish when young but becomes whitish with age and has been known to attack humans — called also *white shark*

¹green \'grēn\ *adj* **1** : of the color green **2** *of a wound* : being recently incurred and unhealed **3** : marked by a pale, sickly, or nauseated appearance **4** *of hemolytic streptococci* : tending to produce green pigment when cultured on blood media

²green *n* **1** : a color whose hue is somewhat less yellow than that of growing fresh grass or of the emerald or is that of the part of the spectrum lying between blue and yellow **2** : a pigment or dye that colors green — see JANUS GREEN

green–blind \-ˌblīnd\ *adj* : exhibiting or affected with deuteranopia — **green blind·ness** \-ˌblīn(d)-nəs\ *n*

green·bot·tle fly \'grēn-ˌbät-ᵊl-\ *n* : any of several brilliant coppery green-bodied flies of the family Calliphoridae and esp. one of the genus *Lucilia* (*L. sericata*) — called also *greenbottle*

green hellebore *n* **1** : AMERICAN HELLEBORE **2** : a hellebore of the genus *Helleborus* (*H. viridis*) with palmately divided leaves and solitary nodding flowers whose rhizome and root is a source of various alkaloids

green monkey *n* : a long-tailed African monkey of the genus *Cercopithecus* (*C. aethiops*) that has greenish-appearing hair and is often used in medical research — called also *vervet monkey*

green monkey disease *n* : MARBURG FEVER

green·sick \'grēn-ˌsik\ *adj* : affected with chlorosis

green·sick·ness *n* : CHLOROSIS

green soap *n* : a soft soap made from vegetable oils and used esp. in the treatment of skin diseases

green·stick fracture \'grēn-ˌstik-\ *n* : a bone fracture in a young individual in which the bone is partly broken and partly bent

Greg·a·rin·i·da \ˌgreg-ə-'rin-ə-də\ *n pl* : a large order of parasitic vermiform sporozoan protozoans that usu. occur in insects and other invertebrates — **greg·a·rine** \'greg-ə-ˌrīn, -ˌrēn, -rən\ *n or adj*

Greg·o·ry's powder \'greg-ə-rēz-\ *n* : a laxative powder containing rhubarb, magnesia, and ginger

Gregory, James (1753–1821), British physician. In 1780 Gregory published a volume that contains many of his remedies including the powder that bears his name. He made few original investigations but spent much of his time in public controversy. In general he advocated preventive medicine, stressing especially healthful living and moderation in all things.

grew *past of* GROW

grey, greyout *chiefly Brit var of* GRAY, GRAYOUT

grief \'grēf\ *n* : deep and poignant distress caused by or as if by bereavement; *also* : a cause of such suffering

grieve \'grēv\ *vb* **grieved; griev·ing** *vt* : to feel or show grief over ⟨*grieving* the death of her son⟩ ~ *vi* : to feel grief

grind \'grīnd\ *vt* **ground** \'graůnd\; **grind·ing** **1** : to reduce

---

\ə\ abut \ᵊ\ kitten \ər\ further \a\ ash \ā\ ace \ä\ cot, cart \aů\ out \ch\ chin \e\ bet \ē\ easy \g\ go \i\ hit \ī\ ice \j\ job \ŋ\ sing \ō\ go \ò\ law \òi\ boy \th\ thin \th\ the \ü\ loot \ů\ foot \y\ yet \zh\ vision *See also* Pronunciation Symbols page

to powder or small fragments by friction (as with the teeth) **2** : to press together and move with a rotating or back-and=forth motion — see BRUXISM

grin·de·lia \grin-'dēl-yə, -'dē-lē-ə\ *n* **1 a** *cap* : a large genus of coarse gummy or resinous composite herbs chiefly of western No. America and So. America **b** : a plant of the genus *Grindelia* **2** : the dried leaves or flowering tops of various plants of the genus *Grindelia* (as *G. camporum, G. robusta,* and *G. squarrosa*) sometimes used in teas as a remedy esp. for bronchitis and asthma or applied as a poultice to treat skin eruptions and wounds

Grin·del \'grin-del\, **David Hieronymous** (1776–1836), German botanist. The genus *Grindelia* was named in his honor in 1807 by the German botanist Karl Ludwig Willdenow (1765–1812).

¹gripe \'grīp\ *vb* **griped; grip·ing** *vt* : to cause pinching and spasmodic pain in the bowels of ∼ *vi* : to experience gripes

²gripe *n* : a pinching spasmodic intestinal pain — usu. used in pl.

gripp·al \'grip-əl\ *adj* : of, relating to, or associated with grippe ⟨∼ pneumonia⟩

grippe \'grip\ *n* : an acute febrile contagious virus disease; *esp* : INFLUENZA 1a — **grippy** \'grip-ē\ *adj*

gris·eo·ful·vin \ˌgriz-ē-ō-'fúl-vən, ˌgris-, -'fəl-\ *n* : a fungistatic antibiotic $C_{17}H_{17}ClO_6$ used systemically in treating superficial infections by fungi esp. of the genera *Epidermophyton, Microsporum,* and *Trichophyton*

griseum — see INDUSIUM GRISEUM

gris·tle \'gris-əl\ *n* : CARTILAGE

gro·cer's itch \'grō-sərz-\ *n* : an itching dermatitis that results from prolonged contact with some mites esp. of the family Acaridae, their products, or materials (as feeds) infested with them — called also *baker's itch;* compare GRAIN ITCH

groin \'gróin\ *n* : the fold or depression marking the juncture of the lower abdomen and the inner part of the thigh; *also* : the region of this line

groin pull *n* : a usu. sports-related injury characterized by intense pain in the region of the groin usu. due to abnormal straining or stretching of an adductor muscle of the thigh and esp. the adductor longus

groove \'grüv\ *n* : a long narrow depression occurring naturally on the surface of an organism or an anatomical part

gross \'grōs\ *adj* **1 a** : glaringly or flagrantly obvious **b** : visible without the aid of a microscope : MACROSCOPIC ⟨∼ lesions⟩ — compare OCCULT **2** : growing or spreading with excessive or abnormal luxuriance **3** : of, relating to, or dealing with general aspects or broad distinctions ⟨important to understand the ∼ behavior of the sexually responding animal —A. C. Kinsey⟩ — **gross·ly** *adv*

gross anatomy *n* : a branch of anatomy that deals with the macroscopic structure of tissues and organs — compare HISTOLOGY 1 — **gross anatomist** *n*

gross hematuria *n* : hematuria that produces a visible redness of the urine

ground *past and past part of* GRIND

ground itch \'graúnd-\ *n* : an itching inflammation of the skin marking the point of entrance into the body of larval hookworms

ground substance *n* : a more or less homogeneous matrix that forms the background in which the specific differentiated elements of a system are suspended: **a** : the intercellular substance of tissues **b** : CYTOSOL

group \'grüp\ *n, often attrib* **1** : a number of individuals assembled together or having some unifying relationship **2 a** : an assemblage of related organisms — often used to avoid taxonomic connotations when the kind or degree of relationship is not clearly defined **b** (1) : an assemblage of atoms forming part of a molecule; *esp* : FUNCTIONAL GROUP (2) : an assemblage of elements forming one of the vertical columns of the periodic table

Group A \-'ā\ *n* : the Lancefield group of beta-hemolytic streptococci that comprises all strains of a species of the genus *Streptococcus* (*S. pyogenes*) and that includes the caus-

ative agents of pharyngitis, scarlet fever, septicemia, some skin infections (as pyoderma and erysipelas), rheumatic fever, and glomerulonephritis — usu. used attributively ⟨*Group A* streptococcal infections⟩; compare GROUP B

Group B \-'bē\ *n* : the Lancefield group of usu. beta-hemolytic streptococci that comprises all strains of a species of the genus *Streptococcus* (*S. agalactiae*) and that includes the causative agents of certain infections (as septicemia, pneumonia, and meningitis) esp. of newborn infants — usu. used attributively ⟨affected with *Group B* strep⟩; compare GROUP A

group dynamics *n pl but sing or pl in constr* : the interacting forces within a small human group; *also* : the sociological study of these forces

group home \-ˌhōm\ *n* : a residence for persons (as developmentally disabled individuals or foster children) requiring care, assistance, or supervision

group practice *n* : medicine practiced by a group of associated physicians or dentists (as specialists in different fields) working as partners or as partners and employees

group psychotherapy *n* : GROUP THERAPY

group therapy *n* : therapy in the presence of a therapist in which several patients discuss and share their personal problems — **group therapist** *n*

grow \'grō\ *vb* **grew** \'grü\; **grown** \'grōn\; **grow·ing** *vi* **1 a** : to spring up and develop to maturity **b** : to be able to grow in some place or situation **c** : to assume some relation through or as if through a process of natural growth ⟨the cut edges of the wound *grew* together⟩ **2** : to increase in size by addition of material by assimilation into the living organism or by accretion in a nonbiological process (as crystallization) ∼ *vt* : to cause to grow ⟨*grew* bacteria in culture⟩

grow·ing pains \'grō-iŋ-ˌpānz\ *n pl* : pains occurring in the legs of growing children having no demonstrable relation to growth

growth \'grōth\ *n* **1 a** (1) : a stage in the process of growing (2) : full growth **b** : the process of growing **2 a** : something that grows or has grown **b** : an abnormal proliferation of tissue (as a tumor)

growth cone *n* : the specialized motile tip of an axon of a growing or regenerating nerve cell

growth curve *n* : a curve on a graph representing the growth of a part, organism, or population as a function of time

growth factor *n* : a substance (as a vitamin B_{12} or an interleukin) that promotes growth and esp. cellular growth

growth hormone *n* : a vertebrate polypeptide hormone that is secreted by the anterior lobe of the pituitary gland and regulates growth; *also* : a recombinant version of this hormone — called also *somatotropic hormone, somatotropin;* see HUMAN GROWTH HORMONE

growth hormone–releasing hormone *n* : a neuropeptide released by the hypothalamus that stimulates the release of growth hormone — abbr. *GHRH;* called also *growth hormone-releasing factor*

growth plate *n* : the region in a long bone between the epiphysis and diaphysis where growth in length occurs — called also *physis*

grub \'grəb\ *n* : a soft thick wormlike larva of an insect

¹grunt·ing \'grən-tiŋ\ *n* : abnormal respiration in a horse marked by a laryngeal sound emitted when it is struck or moved suddenly — compare ROARING

²grunting *adj* : sounding like a grunt : resembling a grunt ⟨the breathing is shallow and ∼ —Morris Fishbein⟩

gry·po·sis \grə-'pō-səs, grī-\ *n, pl* **-po·ses** \-ˌsēz\ : abnormal curvature esp. of the fingernail

g's *or* **gs** *pl of* G

GSH *abbr* glutathione (reduced form)

G6PD *abbr* glucose-6-phosphate dehydrogenase

G–spot \'jē-ˌspät\ *n* : a mass of tissue that is held by some physiologists and specialists in human sexual behavior to exist in the anterior vaginal wall and to be highly erogenous but whose existence and function are doubted by others because of insufficient objective evidence — called also *Grafenberg spot*

GSR *abbr* galvanic skin response

GSSG *abbr* glutathione (oxidized form)

G suit \-'süt\ *n* : a suit designed to counteract the physiological effects of acceleration on an aviator or astronaut — called also *anti-G suit*

GSW *abbr* gunshot wound

GTH *abbr* gonadotropic hormone

GTP \ˌjē-ˌtē-'pē\ *n* : an energy-rich nucleotide analogous to ATP that is composed of guanine linked to ribose and three phosphate groups and is necessary for peptide bond formation during protein synthesis — called also *guanosine triphosphate*

G₂ phase \ˌjē-'tü-\ *n* : the period in the cell cycle from the completion of DNA replication to the beginning of cell division — compare G₁ PHASE, M PHASE, S PHASE

GU *abbr* genitourinary

guai·ac \'g(w)ī-ˌak\ *n* : GUAIACUM 3

guai·a·col \'g(w)ī-ə-ˌkȯl, -ˌkōl\ *n* : a fragrant liquid or solid compound $C_7H_8O_2$ obtained by distilling guaiacum or from wood-tar creosote or made synthetically and used chiefly as an expectorant and as a local anesthetic

guaiacolate — see GLYCERYL GUAIACOLATE

guaiac test *n* : a test for blood in urine or feces using a reagent containing guaiacum that yields a blue color when blood is present — see HEMOCCULT

guai·a·cum \'g(w)ī-ə-kəm\ *n* **1** *cap* : a genus (family Zygophyllaceae) of tropical American trees and shrubs having pinnate leaves, usu. blue flowers, and capsular fruit **2** : any tree or shrub of the genus *Guaiacum* **3** : a resin with a faint balsamic odor obtained as tears or masses from the trunk of either of two trees of the genus *Guaiacum* (*G. officinale* or *G. sanctum*) used formerly in medicine as a remedy for gout or rheumatism and now in various tests (as for peroxidases or bloodstains) because of the formation of a blue color on oxidation — see GUAIAC TEST

guai·fen·e·sin \g(w)ī-'fen-ə-sən\ *n* : the glyceryl ether of guaiacol $C_{10}H_{14}O_4$ that is used esp. as an expectorant — called also *glyceryl guaiacolate*

gua·nase \'gwä-ˌnās, -ˌnāz\ *n* : an enzyme present in most animal tissues that hydrolyzes guanine to xanthine and ammonia

gua·neth·i·dine \gwä-'neth-ə-ˌdēn\ *n* : a drug used esp. in the form of its sulfate $C_{10}H_{22}N_4 \cdot H_2SO_4$ to treat severe high blood pressure

gua·ni·dine \'gwän-ə-ˌdēn\ *n* : a base CH_5N_3 that is derived from guanine, is found esp. in young tissues, and is used in organic synthesis and that in the form of its hydrochloride $CH_5N_3 \cdot HCl$ is used as a drug to enhance acetylcholine activity

gua·nine \'gwän-ˌēn\ *n* : a purine base $C_5H_5N_5O$ that codes genetic information in the polynucleotide chain of DNA or RNA — compare ADENINE, CYTOSINE, THYMINE, URACIL

gua·no·sine \'gwän-ə-ˌsēn\ *n* : a nucleoside $C_{10}H_{13}N_5O_5$ composed of guanine and ribose

guanosine 3′,5′-monophosphate *n* : CYCLIC GMP

guanosine triphosphate *n* : GTP

gua·nyl·ate cyclase \'gwän-ᵊl-ˌāt-\ *n* : an enzyme that catalyzes the formation of cyclic GMP from GTP

gua·nyl·ic acid \gwä-'nil-ik-\ *n* : a mononucleotide $C_{10}H_{14}N_5O_8P$ composed of guanine, a phosphate group, and a pentose

gua·ra·na \ˌgwär-ə-'nä\ *n* : a dried paste made from the seeds of a Brazilian climbing shrub (*Paullinia cupana*) containing tannin and caffeine and used in making an astringent drink

guard·ing \'gär-diŋ\ *n* : involuntary reaction to protect an area of pain (as by spasm of muscle on palpation of the abdomen over a painful lesion)

Guar·nie·ri body \gwär-'nyer-ē-\ *also* **Guar·nie·ri's body** \-'nyer-ēz-\ *n* : a minute inclusion body characteristic of smallpox and cowpox

Guarnieri, Giuseppe (1856–1918), Italian pathologist. In 1893 Guarnieri reported his discovery of certain inclusion bodies found in the specific lesions of smallpox and cowpox. Those bodies, now known as Guarnieri bodies, were

thought by him to be the causative organism of these diseases.

gu·ber·nac·u·lum \ˌgü-bər-'nak-yə-ləm\ *n, pl* **-la** \-lə\ : a part or structure that serves as a guide; *esp* : a fibrous cord that connects the fetal testis with the bottom of the scrotum and by failing to elongate in proportion to the rest of the fetus causes the descent of the testis

guide \'gīd\ *n* : a grooved director for a surgical probe or knife

guided imagery *n* : any of various techniques (as a series of verbal suggestions) used to guide another person or oneself in imagining sensations and esp. in visualizing an image in the mind to bring about a desired physical response (as a reduction in stress, anxiety, or pain)

Guil·lain–Bar·ré syndrome \ˌgē-ˌlan-bä-'rā-, -ˌgē-yaⁿ-\ *n* : a polyneuritis of unknown cause characterized esp. by muscle weakness and paralysis — called also *Landry's paralysis*

Guillain \gē-yaⁿ\, Georges Charles (1876–1961), and **Barré \bä-rā\, Jean Alexander (1880–1967),** French neurologists. Guillain published several significant neurological studies concerning the brain and the spinal column. An authority on the spinal column in particular, he made studies of the cerebrospinal fluid and the marrow of the spinal cord. Guillain and Barré published their description of the Guillain-Barré syndrome in 1916.

guil·lo·tine \'gil-ə-ˌtēn, 'gē-ə-ˌtēn\ *n* : a surgical instrument that consists of a ring and handle with a knife blade which slides down the handle and across the ring and that is used for cutting out a protruding structure (as a tonsil) capable of being placed in the ring

Guil·lo·tin \gē-yȯ-taⁿ\, Joseph–Ignace (1738–1814), French surgeon. Guillotin was a member of the National Assembly during the time of the French Revolution. In 1789 he proposed the passage of a law requiring that all death sentences be carried out by decapitation, a practice up to that time reserved for the nobility. At the time decapitation was perceived to be a humane method of execution, and its uniform application was intended as a statement of egalitarian ideals. Various decapitation devices had been in use for centuries, but an improvement was commissioned, and subsequently introduced in 1792. Gradually the device became known as the guillotine as it became associated with the man who had advocated it as a humane instrument of capital punishment. The surgical instrument known as the guillotine is so called because it features a similar sliding-blade action.

guillotine amputation *n* : an emergency surgical amputation (as of a leg) in which the skin is incised around the part being amputated and is allowed to retract, successive layers of muscle are then divided around the part, and finally the bone is divided

guilt \'gilt\ *n* : feelings of culpability esp. for imagined offenses or from a sense of inadequacy : morbid self-reproach often manifest in marked preoccupation with the moral correctness of one's behavior ⟨aggressive responses originating in inner ∼ and uncertainty⟩

guin·ea pig \'gin-ē-\ *n* : a small stout-bodied short-eared nearly tailless domesticated rodent of the genus *Cavia* (*C. cobaya*) often kept as a pet and widely used in biological research — called also *cavy*

guinea worm *n* : a slender tropical nematode worm of the genus *Dracunculus* (*D. medinensis*) that is a human parasite with no known animal reservoir, has an adult female that may attain a length of several feet, and is characterized by a life cycle which includes larval development in copepods of the genus *Cyclops*, ingestions by humans in contaminated drinking water, passage from the intestine to connective tissues of the thorax and abdomen for maturation and mating, and migration of gravid females to subcutaneous tissues and

---

\ə\ **abut** \ᵊ\ **kitten** \ər\ **further** \a\ **ash** \ā\ **ace** \ä\ **cot, cart**
\au̇\ **out** \ch\ **chin** \e\ **bet** \ē\ **easy** \g\ **go** \i\ **hit** \ī\ **ice** \j\ **job**
\ŋ\ **sing** \ō\ **go** \ȯ\ **law** \ȯi\ **boy** \th\ **thin** \t̲h̲\ **the** \ü\ **loot**
\u̇\ **foot** \y\ **yet** \zh\ **vision** *See also* Pronunciation Symbols page

then out through the skin — called also *Medina worm;* see DRACUNCULIASIS

guinea worm disease *n* : DRACUNCULIASIS

Gulf War syndrome \'gəlf-ˌwȯ(ə)r-\ *n* : a syndrome of uncertain cause including fatigue, joint pain, memory loss, skin rash, and headache that has been reported in veterans of the war fought in the Persian Gulf in 1991

gul·let \'gəl-ət\ *n* **1** : ESOPHAGUS; *broadly* : THROAT **2** : an invagination of the protoplasm in various protozoans (as a paramecium) that sometimes functions in the intake of food

gu·lose \'g(y)ü-ˌlōs *also* -ˌlōz\ *n* : a sugar $C_6H_{12}O_6$ stereoisomeric with glucose and obtainable by synthesis from xylose

¹gum \'gəm\ *n* : the tissue that surrounds the necks of teeth and covers the alveolar parts of the jaws; *broadly* : the alveolar portion of a jaw with its enveloping soft tissues

²gum *vt* **gummed; gum·ming** : to chew with the gums

³gum *n* **1** : any of numerous colloidal polysaccharide substances of plant origin that are gelatinous when moist but harden on drying and are salts of complex organic acids — compare MUCILAGE **2** : any of various plant exudates (as a mucilage, oleoresin, or gum resin)

gum acacia *n* : GUM ARABIC

gum ammoniac *n* : AMMONIAC

gum ar·a·bic \-'ar-ə-bik\ *n* : a water-soluble gum obtained from several leguminous plants of the genus *Acacia* (esp. *A. senegal* and *A. arabica*) and used esp. in pharmacy to suspend insoluble substances in water, to prepare emulsions, and to make pills and lozenges — called also *acacia, gum acacia*

gum·boil \'gəm-ˌbȯil\ *n* : an abscess in the gum

gum karaya *n* : KARAYA GUM

gum·line \'gəm-ˌlīn\ *n* : the line separating the gum from the exposed part of the tooth

gum·ma \'gəm-ə\ *n, pl* **gummas** *also* **gum·ma·ta** \'gəm-ət-ə\ : a tumor of gummy or rubbery consistency that is characteristic of the tertiary stage of syphilis — **gum·ma·tous** \-ət-əs\ *adj*

gum·my \'gəm-ē\ *adj* **gum·mi·er; -est** **1** : consisting of or containing gum **2** : being viscous or sticky

gum resin *n* : a product consisting essentially of a mixture of gum and resin usu. obtained by making an incision in a plant and allowing the juice which exudes to solidify

gum tragacanth *n* : TRAGACANTH

gun·cot·ton \'gən-ˌkät-ᵊn\ *n* : any of various cellulose nitrates; *esp* : an explosive consisting of a higher-nitrated product (as one containing at least 13.2 percent nitrogen)

gur·ney \'gər-nē\ *n, pl* **gurneys** : a wheeled cot or stretcher

gus·ta·tion \ˌgəs-'tā-shən\ *n* : the act or sensation of tasting

gus·ta·to·ry \'gəs-tə-ˌtōr-ē, -ˌtȯr-\ *adj* : relating to, affecting, associated with, or being the sense of taste ⟨~ nerves⟩ ⟨~ stimulation⟩ — **gus·ta·to·ri·ly** \ˌgəs-tə-'tōr-ə-lē, -'tȯr-\ *adv*

gustatory cell *n* : TASTE CELL

¹gut \'gət\ *n* **1 a** : ALIMENTARY CANAL; *also* : part of the alimentary canal and esp. the intestine or stomach ⟨the mix of bacteria making up the flora of the ~ —W. E. Leary⟩ **b** : ABDOMEN 1a, BELLY — usu. used in pl.; not often in formal use ⟨his huge ~ hung far below his belt —L. M. Uris⟩ **2** : CATGUT

²gut *vt* **gut·ted; gut·ting** : to take out the bowels of : EVISCERATE

Guth·rie test \'gəth-rē-\ *n* : a test for phenylketonuria in which the plasma phenylalanine of an affected individual reverses the inhibition of a strain of bacteria of the genus *Bacillus* (*B. subtilis*) needing it for growth

Guthrie, Robert (1916–1995), American microbiologist. Guthrie did research in the following fields: the genetics of two bacilli (*Escherichia coli* and *Bacillus subtilis*), cancer chemotherapy, cytology of bacterial endospores, human genetics and the biochemical nature of individuality, and the nutrition of bacteria and invertebrates. He developed the test for phenylketonuria in the early 1960s.

gut·ta–per·cha \ˌgət-ə-'pər-chə\ *n* : a tough plastic substance from the latex of several Malaysian trees (genera *Payena* and *Palaquium*) of the sapodilla family (Sapotaceae) that resem-

bles rubber but contains more resin and is used in dentistry in temporary fillings

gut·tate \'gə-ˌtāt\ *adj* : having small usu. colored spots or drops ⟨~ skin lesions⟩

gut·ter \'gət-ər\ *n* : a depressed furrow between body parts (as on the surface between a pair of adjacent ribs or in the dorsal wall of the body cavity on either side of the spinal column)

gut·tie \'gət-ˌtī\ *n* : colic in young cattle due to strangulation of a loop of intestine

gut·tur·al \'gət-ə-rəl, 'gə-trəl\ *adj* : of or relating to the throat

Gut·zeit test \'güt-ˌsīt-\ *n* : a test for arsenic used esp. in toxicology that is based on the formation of arsine (as in the Marsh test) and the production by the arsine of a brown stain on filter paper moistened with mercuric chloride solution

Gutzeit, Ernst Wilhelm Heinrich (1845–1888), German chemist.

GVH *abbr* graft-versus-host

GVHD *abbr* graft-versus-host disease

Gy *abbr* gray

gym·nas·tics \jim-'nast-iks\ *n pl but sing in constr* : physical exercises designed to develop strength and coordination — **gym·nas·tic** \-'nast-ik\ *adj*

Gym·no·din·i·um \ˌjim-nə-'din-ē-əm\ *n* : a large genus (the type of the family Gymnodiniidae) of marine and freshwater naked dinoflagellates that includes forms which are colorless or tinted yellowish to reddish brown, blue, or green by chromatophores and a few forms which cause red tide

gym·no·sperm \'jim-nə-ˌspərm\ *n* : any of a class or subdivision (Gymnospermae) of woody vascular seed plants (as conifers or cycads) that produce naked seeds not enclosed in an ovary and that in some instances have motile spermatozoids — compare ANGIOSPERM — **gym·no·sper·mous** \ˌjim-nə-'spər-məs\ *adj*

gyn *abbr* gynecologic; gynecologist; gynecology

gyn·an·dro·blas·to·ma \(ˌ)gīn-ˌan-drə-bla-'stō-mə, (ˌ)jin-\ *n, pl* **-mas** *also* **-ma·ta** \-mət-ə\ : a rare tumor of the ovary with both masculinizing and feminizing effects — compare ARRHENOBLASTOMA

¹gy·nan·droid \(')gīn-'an-ˌdrȯid, (')jin-\ *adj* : exhibiting gynandry

²gynandroid *n* : a gynandroid person

gyn·an·dro·morph \(')gīn-'an-drə-ˌmȯrf, (')jin-\ *n* : an abnormal individual exhibiting characters of both sexes in various parts of the body : a sexual mosaic — **gyn·an·dro·mor·phic** \(ˌ)gīn-ˌan-drə-'mȯr-fik, (ˌ)jin-\ *adj* — **gyn·an·dro·mor·phism** \-ˌfiz-əm\ *n* — **gyn·an·dro·mor·phy** \(')gīn-'an-drə-ˌmȯr-fē, (')jin-\ *n, pl* **-phies**

gyn·an·dry \-'an-drē\ *n, pl* **-dries** : HERMAPHRODITISM, INTERSEXUALITY; *specif* : the condition of the pseudohermaphroditic female in which the external genitalia simulate those of the male

gy·ne·cic *or chiefly Brit* **gy·nae·cic** \jī-'nē-sik, ji-'nes-ik\ *adj* : of, relating to, affecting, or treating women or the female sex ⟨~ disorders⟩ ⟨~ practice⟩

gy·ne·co·gen·ic *or chiefly Brit* **gy·nae·co·gen·ic** \ˌgīn-ə-kō-'jen-ik, ˌjin-\ *adj* : tending to induce female characteristics ⟨a ~ hormone⟩

gy·ne·cog·ra·phy *or chiefly Brit* **gy·nae·cog·ra·phy** \ˌgīn-ə-'käg-rə-fē, ˌjin-\ *n, pl* **-phies** : radiographic visualization of the female reproductive tract

gy·ne·coid *or chiefly Brit* **gy·nae·coid** \'gīn-i-ˌkȯid, 'jin-\ *adj* **1** *of the pelvis* : having the rounded form typical of the human female — compare ANDROID, ANTHROPOID, PLATYPELLOID **2** : relating to or characterized by the distribution of body fat chiefly in the region of the hips and thighs ⟨~ obesity⟩ — compare ANDROID

gy·ne·col·o·gist *or chiefly Brit* **gy·nae·col·o·gist** \ˌgīn-ə-'käl-ə-jəst, ˌjin-\ *n* : a specialist in gynecology

gy·ne·col·o·gy *or chiefly Brit* **gy·nae·col·o·gy** \ˌgīn-ə-'käl-ə-jē, ˌjin-\ *n, pl* **-gies** : a branch of medicine that deals with the diseases and routine physical care of the reproductive system of women — **gy·ne·co·log·ic** \ˌgīn-i-kə-'läj-ik, ˌjin-\ *or*

gy·ne·co·log·i·cal \-i-kəl\ *or chiefly Brit* **gy·nae·co·log·ic** *or* **gy·nae·co·log·i·cal** *adj*

gy·ne·co·mas·tia *or chiefly Brit* **gy·nae·co·mas·tia** \ˌgī-nə-kō-ˈmas-tē-ə, ˌjin-ə-\ *n* : excessive development of the breast in the male

gy·no·gam·one \ˌgī-nō-ˈgam-ˌōn, ˌjin-ə-\ *n* : a gamone that occurs in an egg

gy·no·gen·e·sis \-ˈjen-ə-səs\ *n, pl* **-e·ses** \-ˌsēz\ : development in which the embryo contains only maternal chromosomes due to activation of an egg by a sperm that degenerates without fusing with the egg nucleus — compare ANDROGENESIS — **gy·no·ge·net·ic** \-jə-ˈnet-ik\ *adj*

gy·noid \ˈgī-ˌnȯid, ˈjin-ˌȯid\ *adj* : GYNECOID 2

gyp·py tummy \ˈjip-ē-\ *n* : diarrhea contracted esp. by travelers

gyp·sum \ˈjip-səm\ *n* : a widely distributed mineral CaSO₄·2H₂O consisting of hydrous calcium sulfate that is used esp. as a soil amendment and in making plaster of paris

gy·rase \ˈjī-ˌrās, -ˌrāz\ *n* : a bacterial enzyme that catalyzes the breaking and rejoining of bonds linking adjacent nucleotides in circular DNA to generate supercoiled DNA helices

gy·rate \ˈjī-ˌrāt\ *adj* : winding or coiled around : CONVOLUTED

gyrate atrophy *n* : progressive degeneration of the choroid and pigment epithelium of the retina that is inherited as an autosomal recessive trait and is characterized esp. by myopia, constriction of the visual field, night blindness, and cataracts

gy·ra·tion \jī-ˈrā-shən\ *n* : the pattern of convolutions of the brain

gy·rec·to·my \jī-ˈrek-tə-mē\ *n, pl* **-mies** : surgical excision of a cerebral gyrus

Gy·ro·mi·tra \ˌjī-rō-ˈmī-trə, ˌjir-ə-\ *n* : a genus of ascomycetous fungi (family Helvellaceae) that include the false morels and typically contain toxins causing illness or death

gy·rose \ˈjī-ˌrōs\ *adj* : marked with wavy lines : UNDULATE

gy·rus \ˈjī-rəs\ *n, pl* **gy·ri** \-ˌrī\ : a convoluted ridge between anatomical grooves; *esp* : CONVOLUTION

H

h *abbr* **1** height **2** [Latin *hora*] hour — used in writing prescriptions; see QH

H *abbr* heroin

H *symbol* hydrogen

ha·ben·u·la \hə-ˈben-yə-lə\ *n, pl* **-lae** \-lē\ **1** : TRIGONUM HABENULAE **2** : either of two nuclei of which one lies on each side of the pineal gland under the corresponding trigonum habenulae, is composed of two groups of nerve cells, is connected to its contralateral counterpart by the habenular commissure, and forms a correlation center for olfactory stimuli — called also *habenular nucleus* — **ha·ben·u·lar** \-lər\ *adj*

habenular commissure *n* : a band of nerve fibers situated in front of the pineal gland that connects the habenular nucleus on one side with that on the other

hab·it \ˈhab-ət\ *n* **1** : bodily appearance or makeup esp. as indicative of one's capacities and condition ⟨a man of fleshy ∼⟩ **2** : a settled tendency or usual manner of behavior **3 a** : a behavior pattern acquired by frequent repetition or physiological exposure that shows itself in regularity or increased facility of performance ⟨the daily bowel ∼⟩ **b** : an acquired mode of behavior that has become nearly or completely involuntary ⟨locked the door through force of ∼⟩ **c** : ADDICTION ⟨was forced to steal to support his drug ∼⟩ **4** : characteristic mode of growth or occurrence

hab·i·tat \ˈhab-ə-ˌtat\ *n* **1** : the place or environment where a plant or animal naturally occurs ⟨the human pubic region is the natural ∼ of the crab louse⟩ **2** : a housing for a controlled physical environment in which people can live surrounded by inhospitable conditions (as under the sea)

hab·it-form·ing \ˈhab-ət-ˌfȯr-miŋ\ *adj* : inducing the formation of an addiction ⟨a ∼ prescription painkiller⟩

habit spasm *n* : TIC

ha·bit·u·al \hə-ˈbich-(ə-)wəl, ha-, -ˈbich-əl\ *adj* **1** : having the nature of a habit : being in accordance with habit ⟨∼ smoking⟩ **2** : doing, practicing, or acting in some manner by force of habit ⟨∼ liars⟩ — **ha·bit·u·al·ly** \-ē\ *adv*

habitual abortion *n* : spontaneous abortion occurring in three or more successive pregnancies

ha·bit·u·ate \hə-ˈbich-ə-ˌwāt, ha-\ *vb* **-at·ed; -at·ing** *vt* **1** : to cause habituation in ∼ *vi* **1** : to cause habituation ⟨marijuana may be *habituating*⟩ **2** : to undergo habituation ⟨∼ to a stimulus⟩

ha·bit·u·a·tion \-ˌbich-ə-ˈwā-shən\ *n* **1** : the act or process of making habitual or accustomed **2 a** : tolerance to the effects of a drug acquired through continued use **b** : psychological dependence on a drug after a period of use — compare ADDICTION **3** : a form of nonassociative learning characterized by a decrease in responsiveness upon repeated exposure to a stimulus — compare SENSITIZATION 3

hab·i·tus \ˈhab-ət-əs\ *n, pl* **habitus** \-əs, -ə-ˌtüs\ : HABIT; *specif* : body build and constitution esp. as related to predisposition to disease ⟨an ulcer ∼⟩

Hab·ro·ne·ma \ˌhab-rō-ˈnē-mə\ *n* : a genus of parasitic nematode worms of the family Spiruridae that develop in flies of the genera *Musca* and *Stomoxys* and live as adults in the stomach of the horse or the proventriculus of various birds — see HABRONEMIASIS, SUMMER SORES

hab·ro·ne·mi·a·sis \ˌhab-rə-nē-ˈmī-ə-səs\ *n, pl* **-a·ses** \-ˌsēz\ : infestation with or disease caused by roundworms of the genus *Habronema* and characterized in the horse by gastric tumors and inflammation or by summer sores

hab·ro·ne·mo·sis \-ˈmō-səs\ *n, pl* **-mo·ses** \-ˌsēz\ : HABRONEMIASIS

ha·bu \ˈhä-bü\ *n* : a dangerously venomous pit viper of the genus *Trimeresurus* (*T. flavoviridis*) common in the Ryukyu islands

¹hack \ˈhak\ *vi* : to cough in a short dry manner

²hack *n* : a short dry cough

Each boldface word in the list below is a chiefly British variant of the word to its right in small capitals.

haem	HEME	haemangioma	HEMANGIOMA
haemacytometer	HEMACYTOMETER	haemangiomatosis	HEMANGIOMATOSIS
haemadsorbing	HEMADSORBING	haemangiopericytoma	HEMANGIOPERICYTOMA
haemadsorption	HEMADSORPTION	haemangiosarcoma	HEMANGIOSARCOMA
haemadynamometer	HEMADYNAMOMETER	haemarthrosis	HEMARTHROSIS
haemagglutinate	HEMAGGLUTINATE	haematein	HEMATEIN
haemagglutination	HEMAGGLUTINATION	haematemesis	HEMATEMESIS
haemagglutinin	HEMAGGLUTININ	haematic	HEMATIC
haemal	HEMAL	haematidrosis	HEMATIDROSIS
haemangiectasis	HEMANGIECTASIS	haematin	HEMATIN
haemangioblastoma	HEMANGIOBLASTOMA	haematinic	HEMATINIC
		haematoblast	HEMATOBLAST
haemangioendothelioma	HEMANGIOENDOTHELIOMA	haematocele	HEMATOCELE
		haematochezia	HEMATOCHEZIA
		haematochyluria	HEMATOCHYLURIA
		haematocolpos	HEMATOCOLPOS

\ə\ abut \ˈ\ kitten \ər\ further \a\ ash \ā\ ace \ä\ cot, cart
\au̇\ out \ch\ chin \e\ bet \ē\ easy \g\ go \i\ hit \ī\ ice \j\ job
\ŋ\ sing \ō\ go \ȯ\ law \ȯi\ boy \th\ thin \th̷\ the \ü\ loot
\u̇\ foot \y\ yet \zh\ vision *See also* Pronunciation Symbols page

haematocrit	HEMATOCRIT	haemodynamic	HEMODYNAMIC
haematocyst	HEMATOCYST	haemodynami-	HEMODYNAMI-
haematogenic	HEMATOGENIC	cally	CALLY
haematoge-	HEMATOGE-	haemodynam-	HEMODYNAM-
nous	NOUS	ics	ICS
haematoge-	HEMATOGE-	haemoendo-	HEMOENDO-
nously	NOUSLY	thelial	THELIAL
haematogone	HEMATOGONE	haemofilter	HEMOFILTER
haematoid	HEMATOID	haemofiltra-	HEMOFILTRA-
haematoidin	HEMATOIDIN	tion	TION
haematologic	HEMATOLOGIC	haemoflagel-	HEMOFLAGEL-
haematologi-	HEMATOLOGI-	late	LATE
cal	CAL	haemofuscin	HEMOFUSCIN
haematologi-	HEMATOLOGI-	haemoglobin	HEMOGLOBIN
cally	CALLY	haemoglobin-	HEMOGLOBIN-
haematologist	HEMATOLOGIST	aemia	EMIA
haematology	HEMATOLOGY	haemoglobinic	HEMOGLOBINIC
haematoma	HEMATOMA	haemoglobin-	HEMOGLOBIN-
haematometra	HEMATOMETRA	ometer	OMETER
haematomye-	HEMATOMYE-	haemoglobin-	HEMOGLOBIN-
lia	LIA	ometry	OMETRY
haematopa-	HEMATOPA-	haemoglobin-	HEMOGLOBIN-
thologist	THOLOGIST	opathy	OPATHY
haematopa-	HEMATOPA-	haemoglobi-	HEMOGLOBI-
thology	THOLOGY	nous	NOUS
haematoperi-	HEMATOPERI-	haemoglobin-	HEMOGLOBIN-
cardium	CARDIUM	uria	URIA
haematopha-	HEMATOPHA-	haemoglobin-	HEMOGLOBIN-
gous	GOUS	uric	URIC
haematophyte	HEMATOPHYTE	haemogram	HEMOGRAM
haematopoie-	HEMATOPOIE-	haemohistio-	HEMOHISTIO-
sis	SIS	blast	BLAST
haematopoiet-	HEMATOPOIET-	haemokonia	HEMOCONIA
ic	IC	haemolymph	HEMOLYMPH
haematopor-	HEMATOPOR-	haemolysate	HEMOLYSATE
phyrin	PHYRIN	haemolyse	HEMOLYZE
haematopor-	HEMATOPOR-	haemolysin	HEMOLYSIN
phyrinuria	PHYRINURIA	haemolysis	HEMOLYSIS
haematorrha-	HEMATORRHA-	haemolytic	HEMOLYTIC
chis	CHIS	haemometer	HEMOMETER
haematosal-	HEMATOSAL-	haemometric	HEMOMETRIC
pinx	PINX	haemoparasite	HEMOPARASITE
haematoscope	HEMATOSCOPE	haemoparasit-	HEMOPARASIT-
haematoxylin	HEMATOXYLIN	ic	IC
haematozoal	HEMATOZOAL	haemopathy	HEMOPATHY
haematozoan	HEMATOZOAN	haemoperfu-	HEMOPERFU-
haematuria	HEMATURIA	sion	SION
haemerythrin	HEMERYTHRIN	haemopericar-	HEMOPERICAR-
haemic	HEMIC	dium	DIUM
haemin	HEMIN	haemoperito-	HEMOPERITO-
haemoaggluti-	HEMAGGLUTI-	neum	NEUM
nin	NIN	haemopexin	HEMOPEXIN
haemobilia	HEMOBILIA	haemophagia	HEMOPHAGIA
haemoblast	HEMOBLAST	haemophagous	HEMOPHAGOUS
haemoblasto-	HEMOBLASTO-	haemophile	HEMOPHILE
sis	SIS	haemophilia	HEMOPHILIA
haemoccult	HEMOCCULT	haemophiliac	HEMOPHILIAC
haemochorial	HEMOCHORIAL	haemophilic	HEMOPHILIC
haemochroma-	HEMOCHROMA-	haemopneu-	HEMOPNEUMO-
tosis	TOSIS	mothorax	THORAX
haemochroma-	HEMOCHROMA-	haemopoiesis	HEMOPOIESIS
totic	TOTIC	haemopoietic	HEMOPOIETIC
haemochromo-	HEMOCHROMO-	haemoprotein	HEMOPROTEIN
gen	GEN	haemoptoic	HEMOPTOIC
haemoclastic	HEMOCLASTIC	haemoptysis	HEMOPTYSIS
crisis	CRISIS	haemorheologic	HEMORHEO-
haemocoagula-	HEMOCOAGU-		LOGIC
tion	LATION	haemorheologi-	HEMORHEO-
haemocoele	HEMOCOEL	cal	LOGICAL
haemocoelic	HEMOCOELIC	haemorheology	HEMORHEOLO-
haemoconcen-	HEMOCONCEN-		GY
tration	TRATION	haemorrhage	HEMORRHAGE
haemoconia	HEMOCONIA	haemorrhagic	HEMORRHAGIC
haemoconiosis	HEMOCONIOSIS	haemorrhagin	HEMORRHAGIN
haemoculture	HEMOCULTURE	haemorrhoid	HEMORRHOID
haemocuprein	HEMOCUPREIN	haemorrhoidal	HEMORRHOID-
haemocyanin	HEMOCYANIN		AL
haemocyte	HEMOCYTE	haemorrhoid-	HEMORRHOID-
haemocyto-	HEMOCYTO-	ectomy	ECTOMY
blast	BLAST	haemosalpinx	HEMOSALPINX
haemocyto-	HEMOCYTO-	haemosiderin	HEMOSIDERIN
blastic	BLASTIC	haemosiderosis	HEMOSIDEROSIS
haemocyto-	HEMOCYTO-	haemosiderotic	HEMOSIDEROT-
blastosis	BLASTOSIS		IC
haemocyto-	HEMOCYTO-	haemostasis	HEMOSTASIS
genesis	GENESIS	haemostat	HEMOSTAT
haemocytoly-	HEMOCYTOLY-	haemostatic	HEMOSTATIC
sis	SIS	haemotherapy	HEMOTHERAPY
haemocytome-	HEMOCYTOME-	haemothorax	HEMOTHORAX
ter	TER	haemotoxic	HEMOTOXIC
haemodialyser	HEMODIALYZER	haemotoxin	HEMOTOXIN
haemodialysis	HEMODIALYSIS	haemotrophe	HEMOTROPHE
haemodilute	HEMODILUTE	haemozoin	HEMOZOIN
haemodilution	HEMODILUTION		

Hae·ma·dip·sa \ˌhē-mə-ˈdip-sə, ˌhem-ə-\ *n* : a genus of small tropical land leeches of the order Gnathobdellida that are troublesome to humans and animals esp. because their bites result in prolonged bleeding

Hae·ma·moe·ba \-ˈmē-bə\ *n, syn of* PLASMODIUM

Hae·ma·phy·sa·lis \-ˈfi-sə-ləs\ *n* : a cosmopolitan genus of small eyeless ixodid ticks including some that are disease carriers — see KYASANUR FOREST DISEASE

haematobium — see SCHISTOSOMIASIS HAEMATOBIUM

Hae·ma·to·pi·nus \-tə-ˈpī-nəs\ *n* : a genus of sucking lice including the hog louse (*H. suis*), short-nosed cattle louse (*H. eurysternus*), and various other serious pests of domestic animals

hae·ma·tox·y·lon \-ˈtäk-sə-ˌlän\ *n* **1** *cap* : a genus of tropical American bushy and usu. thorny leguminous trees with clusters of small yellow flowers that include the logwood (*H. campechianum*) **2** : the wood or dye of logwood

hae·mo·bar·ton·el·la \ˌhē-mō-ˌbär-tə-ˈnel-ə, ˌhem-ō-\ *n* **1** *cap* : a genus of bacteria of the family Anaplasmataceae that are blood parasites in various mammals **2** *pl* **-lae** \-lē, -lī\ : a bacterium of the genus *Haemobartonella*

hae·mo·bar·ton·el·lo·sis *also* **he·mo·bar·ton·el·lo·sis** \-tə-nə-ˈlō-səs\ *n, pl* **-lo·ses** \-ˌsēz\ : an infection or disease caused by bacteria of the genus *Haemobartonella*

Hae·mo·greg·a·ri·na \ˌhē-mō-ˌgreg-ə-ˈrī-nə, ˌhem-ō-, -ˌrē-nə\ *n* : a genus (the type of the family Haemogregarinidae) of sporozoan parasites of the order Coccidia that at different stages of their life cycle parasitize the circulatory system of vertebrates and the digestive tract of invertebrates — **hae·mo·greg·a·rine** *or* **he·mo·greg·a·rine** \-ˈgreg-ə-ˌrīn, -ˌrēn, -rin\ *adj or n*

hae·mon·cho·sis \ˌhē-ˌmäŋ-ˈkō-səs\ *n, pl* **-cho·ses** \-ˌsēz\ : infestation with or disease that is caused by nematode worms of the genus *Haemonchus* and esp. by the barber's pole worm and that is typically characterized by anemia, digestive disturbances, and emaciation resulting from the blood-sucking habits of the worms

Hae·mon·chus \hē-ˈmäŋ-kəs\ *n* : a widely distributed genus of nematode worms (family Trichostrongylidae) including the barber's pole worm (*H. contortus*) — see HAEMONCHOSIS

hae·moph·i·lus \hē-ˈmäf-ə-ləs\ *n* **1** *cap* : a genus of nonmotile gram-negative facultatively anaerobic rod bacteria of the family Pasteurellaceae that include several important pathogens (as *H. influenzae* associated with human respiratory infections, conjunctivitis, and meningitis and *H. ducreyi* of chancroid) **2** *pl* **-li** \-lē\ : any bacterium of the genus *Haemophilus* — see GARDNERELLA, HIB, CONJUGATE VACCINE

Hae·mo·pro·te·i·dae \ˌhē-mō-(ˌ)prō-ˈtē-ə-ˌdē, ˌhem-ə-\ *n pl* : a family of protozoans of the order Haemosporidia that are related to the malaria parasites but have the schizogonic phases typically in the visceral endothelium of various birds and that include the two genera *Haemoproteus* and *Leucocytozoon*

Hae·mo·pro·te·us \-ˈprō-tē-əs\ *n* : a genus of protozoan parasites of the family Haemoproteidae occurring in the blood of some birds (as pigeons)

Hae·mo·spo·rid·ia \-spə-ˈrid-ē-ə\ *n pl* : an order of minute telosporidian protozoans that are parasitic at some stage of the life cycle in the blood cells of vertebrates and that include the malaria parasites of the family Plasmodiidae, numerous bird parasites of the family Haemoproteidae, and the piroplasms and related pathogens of cattle belonging to the family Babesiidae — **hae·mo·spo·rid·i·an** \-ē-ən\ *adj or n*

haf·ni·um \ˈhaf-nē-əm\ *n* : a metallic element that resembles zirconium chemically, occurs in zirconium minerals, and readily absorbs neutrons — symbol *Hf*; see ELEMENT table

Hag·e·man factor \ˈhag-ə-mən-, ˈhäg-mən-\ *n* : FACTOR XII
    Hageman (*fl* 1963), hospital patient. Hageman was the first patient in whom a deficiency of factor XII was observed, in 1963.

Hai·ding·er's brush·es \ˈhī-diŋ-ərz-ˈbrəsh-əz\ *n pl* : a faint blue and yellow dumbbell-shaped image that is produced in the human eye by the selective absorption of polarized light by the yellow macular pigment of the fovea and can be used to detect polarized light without special equipment

Haidinger, Wilhelm Karl von (1795–1871), Austrian mineralogist. Haidinger is known for his pioneering studies in crystallography, in particular the absorption of light in crystals. In 1848 he designed an instrument with which he made observations of pleochroic minerals, with both transmitted and reflected light. His observations on the connection between absorption and the direction of polarization of transmitted and reflected light led him to develop the theory that a greater absorption (of the whole spectrum of visible light) corresponds to a higher index of refraction. He also discovered the phenomenon which enables the detection of polarized light without instruments.

hair \'ha(ə)r, 'he(ə)r\ *n, often attrib* **1** : a slender threadlike outgrowth of the epidermis of an animal; *esp* : one of the usu. pigmented filaments that form the characteristic coat of a mammal **2** : the hairy covering of an animal or a body part; *esp* : the coating of hairs on a human head — **hair·like** \-,līk\ *adj*

hair ball *n* : a compact mass of hair formed in the stomach esp. of a shedding animal (as a cat) that cleanses its coat by licking — called also *trichobezoar*

hair bulb *n* : the bulbous expansion at the base of a hair from which the hair shaft develops

hair cell *n* : a cell with hairlike processes; *esp* : one of the sensory cells in the auditory epithelium of the organ of Corti

haired \'ha(ə)rd, 'he(ə)rd\ *adj* : having hair esp. of a specified kind — usu. used in combination ⟨red-*haired*⟩

hair follicle *n* : the tubular epithelial sheath that surrounds the lower part of the hair shaft and encloses at the bottom a vascular papilla supplying the growing basal part of the hair with nourishment

hair·less \'ha(ə)r-ləs, 'he(ə)r-\ *adj* : lacking hair — **hair·less·ness** *n*

hair·line \-'līn\ *n* : the outline of scalp hair esp. on the forehead — **hairline** *adj*

hairline fracture *n* : a fracture that appears as a narrow crack along the surface of a bone

hair·pin \'ha(ə)r-,pin, 'he(ə)r-\ *n* : a region in single-stranded RNA or DNA that is double-stranded due to pairing between purine and pyrimidine bases in adjacent sequences of the RNA or DNA that are complementary and inverted — called also *hairpin loop*

hair pull·er \-'pùl-ər\ *n* : an individual affected with trichotillomania

hair·pull·ing \-,pùl-iŋ\ *n* : the often pathological habit of pulling out one's hair one or a few hairs at a time — compare TRICHOTILLOMANIA

hair root *n* : ROOT 2b

hair shaft *n* : the part of a hair projecting beyond the skin

hair·worm \'ha(ə)r-,wərm, 'he(ə)r-\ *n* **1** : any nematode worm of the genus *Capillaria* **2** : HORSEHAIR WORM

hairy \'ha(ə)r-ē, 'he(ə)r-\ *adj* **hair·i·er; -est** **1** : covered with hair or hairlike material **2** : made of or resembling hair — **hair·i·ness** \'har-ē-nəs, 'her-\ *n*

hairy cell leukemia *n* : a chronic leukemia that is usu. of B cell origin and is characterized by malignant cells with a ciliated appearance that replace bone marrow and infiltrate the spleen causing splenomegaly

hairy leukoplakia *n* : a condition that affects the mouth and esp. the edges of the tongue, is characterized by poorly demarcated white raised lesions with a corrugated appearance, is caused by infection with the Epstein-Barr virus, and is associated with HIV infection and AIDS — called also *oral hairy leukoplakia*

hal·a·zone \'hal-ə-,zōn\ *n* : a white crystalline powdery acid $C_7H_5Cl_2NO_4S$ used as a disinfectant for drinking water

Hal·cion \'hal-sē-,än, -ən\ *trademark* — used for a preparation of triazolam

Hal·dol \'hal-,dòl, -,dōl\ *trademark* — used for a preparation of haloperidol

half–blood \'haf-'bləd, 'hàf-\ *or* **half–blood·ed** \-bləd-əd\ *adj* : having half blood or being a half blood

half blood *n* **1** : the relation between persons having only one parent in common **2** : a person so related to another

half–bred \-,bred\ *adj* : having one purebred parent — **half–bred** *n*

half–life \-,līf\ *n* : the time required for half of something to undergo a process: as **a** : the time required for half of the atoms of a radioactive substance to become disintegrated **b** : the time required for half the amount of a substance (as a drug or radioactive tracer) in or introduced into a living system or ecosystem to be eliminated or disintegrated by natural processes ⟨the serum ~ is about 2 days —*Jour. Amer. Med. Assoc.*⟩

half–moon \-,mün\ *n* : LUNULA a

half–val·ue layer \-'val-(,)yü-, -'val-yə-\ *n* : the thickness of an absorbing substance necessary to reduce by one half the initial intensity of the radiation passing through it

half·way house \'haf-'wā-, 'hàf-\ *n* : a center for individuals after institutionalization (as for mental disorder or drug addiction) that is designed to facilitate their readjustment to private life

hal·i·but–liv·er oil \'hal-ə-bət-,liv-ər-, 'häl-\ *n* : a yellowish to brownish fatty oil from the liver of the halibut used chiefly as a source of vitamin A

ha·lide \'hal-,īd, 'hā-,līd\ *n* : a binary compound of a halogen with a more electropositive element or radical

hal·i·ste·re·sis \,hal-ə-stə-'rē-səs, hə-,lis-tə-\ *n, pl* **-re·ses** \-,sēz\ : loss of salts esp. of lime from bone (as in osteomalacia) — **hal·i·ste·ret·ic** \-'ret-ik\ *adj*

hal·i·to·sis \,hal-ə-'tō-səs\ *n, pl* **-to·ses** \-,sēz\ : a condition of having fetid breath

hal·lu·ci·nate \hə-'lüs-°n-,āt\ *vb* **-nat·ed; -nat·ing** *vt* **1** : to affect with visions or imaginary perceptions ⟨the patient is not *hallucinated*⟩ **2** : to perceive or experience as a hallucination ⟨may ~ monsters or attackers —M. J. Horowitz⟩ ~ *vi* : to have hallucinations

hal·lu·ci·na·tion \hə-,lüs-°n-'ā-shən\ *n* **1** : a perception of something (as a visual image or a sound) with no external cause usu. arising from a disorder of the nervous system (as in delirium tremens or in functional psychosis without known neurological disease) or in response to drugs (as LSD) — compare DELUSION 2, ILLUSION 2a **2** : the object of a hallucinatory perception

hal·lu·ci·na·tor \hə-'lüs-°n-,āt-ər\ *n* : a person who has hallucinations

hal·lu·ci·na·to·ry \hə-'lüs-°n-ə-,tōr-ē, -'lüs-nə-, -,tòr-\ *adj* **1** : tending to produce hallucinations ⟨~ drugs⟩ **2** : resembling, involving, or being a hallucination ⟨~ dreams⟩ ⟨a ~ figure⟩ — **hal·lu·ci·na·to·ri·ly** \-,tōr-ə-lē, -,tòr-\ *adv*

hal·lu·ci·no·gen \hə-'lüs-°n-ə-jən\ *n* : a substance and esp. a drug that induces hallucinations

¹**hal·lu·ci·no·gen·ic** \hə-,lüs-°n-ə-'jen-ik\ *adj* : causing hallucinations — **hal·lu·ci·no·gen·i·cal·ly** \-i-k(ə-)lē\ *adv*

²**hallucinogenic** *n* : HALLUCINOGEN

hal·lu·ci·no·sis \hə-,lüs-°n-'ō-səs\ *n, pl* **-no·ses** \-,sēz\ : a pathological mental state characterized by hallucinations

hallucis — see ABDUCTOR HALLUCIS, ADDUCTOR HALLUCIS, EXTENSOR HALLUCIS BREVIS, EXTENSOR HALLUCIS LONGUS, FLEXOR HALLUCIS BREVIS, FLEXOR HALLUCIS LONGUS

hal·lux \'hal-əks\ *n, pl* **hal·lu·ces** \'hal-(y)ə-,sēz\ : the innermost digit (as the big toe in humans) of a hind or lower limb

hallux rig·id·us \-'rij-ə-dəs\ *n* : restricted mobility of the big toe due to stiffness of the metatarsophalangeal joint esp. when due to arthritic changes in the joint

hallux val·gus \-'val-gəs\ *n* : an abnormal deviation of the big toe away from the midline of the body or toward the other toes of the foot that is associated esp. with the wearing of ill-fitting shoes — compare BUNION

ha·lo \'hā-(,)lō\ *n, pl* **halos** *or* **haloes** **1** : a circle of light appearing to surround a luminous body; *esp* : one seen as the result of the presence of glaucoma **2** : a differentiated zone surrounding a central object ⟨the ~ around a boil⟩ **3** : the

G
H

\ə\ **abut** \ʼ\ **kitten** \ər\ **further** \a\ **ash** \ā\ **ace** \ä\ **cot, cart**
\aú\ **out** \ch\ **chin** \e\ **bet** \ē\ **easy** \g\ **go** \i\ **hit** \ī\ **ice** \j\ **job**
\ŋ\ **sing** \ō\ **go** \ò\ **law** \òi\ **boy** \th\ **thin** \th\ **the** \ü\ **loot**
\ù\ **foot** \y\ **yet** \zh\ **vision** *See also* Pronunciation Symbols page

aura of glory, veneration, or sentiment surrounding an idealized person or thing   **4** : an orthopedic device used to immobilize the head and neck (as to treat fracture of neck vertebrae) that consists of a metal band placed around the head and fastened to the skull usu. with metal pins and that is attached by extensions to an inflexible vest — called also *halo brace*

halo effect *n* : generalization from the perception of one outstanding personality trait to an overly favorable evaluation of the whole personality

hal·o·fan·trine \ˌhal-ə-ˈfan-ˌtrēn, -ˌtrīn, -trən\ *n* : an antimalarial drug used in the form of its hydrochloride $C_{26}H_{30}Cl_2F_3NO·HCl$ esp. against chloroquine-resistant falciparum malaria

halo·gen \ˈhal-ə-jən\ *n* : any of the five elements fluorine, chlorine, bromine, iodine, and astatine that form part of group VII A of the periodic table and exist in the free state normally as diatomic molecules — **ha·log·e·nous** \ha-ˈläj-ə-nəs\ *adj*

ha·lo·ge·nate \ˈhal-ə-jə-ˌnāt, ha-ˈläj-ə-\ *vt* **-nat·ed; -nat·ing** : to treat or cause to combine with a halogen — **ha·lo·ge·na·tion** \ˌhal-ə-jə-ˈnā-shən, ha-ˌläj-ə-\ *n*

hal·o·ge·ton \ˌhal-ə-ˈjē-ˌtän\ *n* : a coarse annual herb (*Halogeton glomeratus*) of the goosefoot family (Chenopodiaceae) that in western American ranges is dangerous to sheep and cattle because of its high oxalate content

ha·lom·e·ter \ha-ˈläm-ət-ər\ *n* : an instrument for measuring the average diameter of red blood cells by means of the halos produced around them by diffraction

halo·per·i·dol \ˌhal-ō-ˈper-ə-ˌdȯl, -ˌdōl\ *n* : a butyrophenone antipsychotic drug $C_{21}H_{23}ClFNO_2$ used esp. to treat schizophrenia and to control the involuntary tics and vocalizations of Tourette's syndrome — see HALDOL

halo·phile \ˈhal-ə-ˌfīl\ *n* : an organism that flourishes in a salty environment — **halo·phil·ic** \ˌhal-ə-ˈfil-ik\ *adj*

halo·thane \ˈhal-ə-ˌthān\ *n* : a nonexplosive inhalational anesthetic $C_2HBrClF_3$

Hal·sted radical mastectomy \ˈhal-ˌsted-\ *n* : RADICAL MASTECTOMY — called also *Halsted radical*

Halsted, William Stewart (1852–1922), American surgeon. Halsted served for many years as professor of surgery and surgeon-in-chief at Johns Hopkins Medical School and Hospital. Renowned as a surgeon and clinical teacher, he is credited with pioneering work in physiology and pathology and with innovative surgical techniques. He introduced the wearing of rubber gloves for surgical operations, the use of cocaine for local anesthesia, and a host of surgical techniques and procedures for treating cancers, hernias, goiters, and aneurysms. He made significant physiological and clinical studies of cancer, the thyroid and parathyroid glands, and many other subjects. His procedure for radical mastectomy was first described in a lengthy article on the treatment of wounds that was published in the 1890–91 issue of *Johns Hopkins Hospital Reports.* An expanded description appeared in the 1894–95 issue.

hal·zoun \ˌhal-ˈzün, ˈhal-zün\ *n* : infestation of the larynx and pharynx esp. by tongue worms of the genus *Linguatula* (esp. *L. serrata*) consumed in raw liver

ham \ˈham\ *n* **1** : the part of the leg behind the knee : the hollow of the knee : POPLITEAL SPACE   **2** : a buttock with its associated thigh or with the posterior part of a thigh — usu. used in pl.   **3** : a hock or the hinder part of a hock

hama·dry·ad \ˌham-ə-ˈdrī-əd, -ˌad\ *n* : KING COBRA

ham·a·me·lis \ˌham-ə-ˈmē-ləs\ *n* **1** *cap* : a genus of shrubs or small trees (family Hamamelidaceae) having pinnately veined leaves and clustered flowers with elongated ribbon-shaped petals and including the witch hazels   **2** : the dried leaves of a witch hazel (*Hamamelis virginiana*) of the eastern U.S. used esp. formerly as a tonic and sedative

ha·mar·tia \ˌhäm-ˌär-ˈtē-ə *also* hə-ˈmär-sh(ē-)ə\ *n* : HAMARTOMA

ham·ar·to·ma \ˌham-ˌar-ˈtō-mə\ *n, pl* **-mas** *also* **-ma·ta** \-mət-ə\ : a mass resembling a tumor that represents anomalous development of tissue natural to a part or organ rather

than a true tumor — **ham·ar·toma·tous** \-ˈtäm-ət-əs, -ˈtōm-\ *adj*

¹ha·mate \ˈhā-ˌmāt *also* ˈham-ət\ *adj* : shaped like a hook

²hamate *n* : a bone on the little-finger side of the second row of the carpus in mammals — called also *unciform, unciform bone*

ha·ma·tum \hə-ˈmāt-əm, hā-\ *n, pl* **-ta** \-ə\ *or* **-tums** : HAMATE

ham·mer \ˈham-ər\ *n* : MALLEUS

ham·mer·toe \ˈham-ər-ˌtō\ *n* : a deformed claw-shaped toe and esp. the second that results from permanent angular flexion between one or both phalangeal joints — called also *claw toe*

ham·ster \ˈham(p)-stər\ *n* : any of numerous Old World rodents (*Cricetus* or a related genus) having very large cheek pouches and including several used as laboratory animals

¹ham·string \ˈham-ˌstriŋ\ *n* **1 a** : either of two groups of tendons bounding the upper part of the popliteal space at the back of the knee and forming the tendons of insertion of some muscles of the back of the thigh   **b** : HAMSTRING MUSCLE   **2** : a large tendon above and behind the hock of a quadruped corresponding to the human Achilles tendon

²hamstring *vt* **-strung** \-ˌstrəŋ\; **-string·ing** \-ˌstriŋ-iŋ\ : to cripple by cutting the leg tendons ⟨folklore has it that wolf packs try to ∼ their prey —John Madson⟩

hamstring muscle *n* : any of three muscles at the back of the thigh that function to flex and rotate the leg and extend the thigh: **a** : SEMIMEMBRANOSUS   **b** : SEMITENDINOSUS   **c** : BICEPS b

ham·u·lar \ˈham-yə-lər\ *adj* : HAMATE

ham·u·lus \ˈham-yə-ləs\ *n, pl* **-u·li** \-ˌlī, -ˌlē\ : a hook or hooked process

hand \ˈhand\ *n, often attrib* **1 a** (1) : the terminal part of the vertebrate forelimb when modified (as in humans) as a grasping organ   (2) : the forelimb segment (as the terminal section of a bird's wing) of a vertebrate higher than the fishes that corresponds to the hand irrespective of its form or functional specialization   **b** : a part serving the function of or resembling a hand; *esp* : the hind foot of an ape   **c** : something resembling a hand; *esp* : an indicator or pointer on a dial   **2** : a unit of measure equal to 4 inches or 10.2 centimeters used esp. for the height of horses

hand·ed \ˈhan-dəd\ *adj* **1** : having a hand or hands esp. of a specified kind or number — usu. used in combination ⟨a large-*handed* man⟩   **2** : using a specified hand or number of hands — used in combination ⟨right-*handed*⟩

hand·ed·ness \-nəs\ *n* **1** : a tendency to use one hand rather than the other   **2** : the property of an object (as a molecule) of not being identical with its mirror image   **3** : the property of having either a clockwise or counterclockwise motion (as the corkscrew movement of some microorganisms or their flagella or cilia)

hand, foot and mouth disease *n* : a usu. mild contagious disease esp. of young children that is caused by an enterovirus (species *Human enterovirus A*, esp. serotype Human coxsackievirus A16) and is characterized by vesicular lesions in the mouth, on the hands and feet, and sometimes in the diaper-covered area — compare FOOT-AND-MOUTH DISEASE

hand·i·cap \ˈhan-di-ˌkap\ *n* **1** : a disadvantage that makes achievement unusually difficult   **2** *sometimes offensive* : a physical disability

hand·i·capped \-ˌkapt\ *adj, sometimes offensive* : having a physical or mental disability; *also* : of or reserved for individuals with a physical disability ⟨∼ parking spaces⟩

hand·less \ˈhan-(d)ləs\ *adj* : having no hands

hand·piece \ˈhand-ˌpēs\ *n* : the part of a mechanized device designed to be held or manipulated by hand; *esp* : the handheld part of an electrically powered dental apparatus that holds the revolving instruments (as a bur)

Hand–Schül·ler–Chris·tian disease \ˌhand-ˌshü-lər-ˈkris(h)-chən-\ *n* : an inflammatory histiocytosis associated with disturbances in cholesterol metabolism that occurs chiefly in young children and is marked by cystic defects of the skull and by exophthalmos and diabetes insipidus — called also *Schüller-Christian disease*

Hand, Alfred (1868–1949), American physician. Hand published an early description of the disease in 1893. His description referred to it as a condition characterized by polyuria and tuberculosis. The condition was earlier observed, however, by the British pathologist Thomas Smith (1833–1909) in 1865 and 1876.

Schül·ler \\'shʊl-ər\, **Artur (1874–1958),** Austrian neurologist. Schüller offered his description of the disease in 1915. His description was based on two additional cases and noted the defects in the membranous bones.

Christian, Henry Asbury (1876–1951), American physician. Christian gave a more complete description in 1919 which included all the major characteristics.

hang·nail \\'haŋ-ˌnāl\ *n* : a bit of skin hanging loose at the side or root of a fingernail

hang·over \-ˌō-vər\ *n* : disagreeable physical effects (as headache or nausea) following heavy consumption of alcohol or the use of drugs

hang–up \-ˌəp\ *n* : a source of mental or emotional difficulty

han·sen·osis \ˌhan(t)-sə-'nō-səs\ *n, pl* **-oses** \-ˌsēz\ : LEPROSY

Han·sen \\'hän-sən\, **Gerhard Henrik Armauer (1841–1912),** Norwegian physician. Hansen devoted his professional life to the study of leprosy. He investigated its epidemiology, etiology, prevention, and institutional management. In 1873 he discovered the bacillus (now known as Hansen's bacillus) that causes leprosy.

Han·sen's bacillus \\'han(t)-sənz-\ *n* : a bacterium of the genus *Mycobacterium* (*M. leprae*) that causes leprosy

Hansen's disease *n* : LEPROSY

Han·ta·an virus \\'han-tə-ən-, 'hən-, 'hän-\ *n* : a bunyavirus of the genus *Hantavirus* (species *Hantaan virus*) that causes hemorrhagic fever with renal syndrome and esp. Korean hemorrhagic fever

han·ta·vi·rus \\'han-tə-ˌvī-rəs, 'hən-, 'hän-\ *n* **1** *cap* : a genus of single-stranded RNA viruses of the family *Bunyaviridae* that infect specific rodents as their natural hosts and that include some forms causing hantavirus pulmonary syndrome and hemorrhagic fever with renal syndrome in humans following exposure to the virus in airborne particles of rodent urine, feces, or saliva or directly by the bite of a rodent **2** : any virus (as the Hantaan virus) of the genus *Hantavirus*

hantavirus pulmonary syndrome *n* : an acute respiratory disease caused by various hantaviruses and characterized initially esp. by fever, muscle pain, headache, cough, vomiting, and chills which rapidly progress to pulmonary edema and hypoxia often resulting in death from shock or cardiac complications — compare HEMORRHAGIC FEVER WITH RENAL SYNDROME

H antigen \\'āch-\ *n* : any of various antigens associated with the flagella of motile bacteria and used in serological identification of various bacteria — called also *flagellar antigen;* compare O ANTIGEN

hap·a·lo·nych·ia \ˌhap-ə-lō-'nik-ē-ə\ *n* : abnormal softness of the fingernails or toenails

haph·al·ge·sia \ˌhaf-ᵊl-'jē-zhə, -z(h)ē-ə\ *n* : pain upon physical contact with something which does not usu. induce the sensation of pain

haph·e·pho·bia \ˌhaf-ə-'fō-bē-ə\ *n* : a morbid fear of being touched

hap·lo·dont \\'hap-lə-ˌdänt\ *adj* : having or constituting molar teeth with simple crowns without tubercles — **hap·lo·don·ty** \-ē\ *n, pl* **-ties**

hap·loid \\'hap-ˌlȯid\ *adj* : having the gametic number of chromosomes or half the number characteristic of somatic cells : MONOPLOID — **haploid** *n* — **hap·loi·dy** \-ˌlȯid-ē\ *n, pl* **-dies**

hap·lont \\'hap-ˌlänt\ *n* : an organism with somatic cells having the haploid chromosome number and only the zygote diploid — compare DIPLONT — **hap·lon·tic** \ha-'plänt-ik\ *adj*

hap·lo·scope \\'hap-lə-ˌskōp\ *n* : a simple stereoscope that is

used in the study of depth perception — **hap·lo·scop·ic** \ˌhap-lə-'skäp-ik\ *adj*

hap·lo·type \-ˌtīp\ *n* : a group of alleles of different genes (as of the major histocompatibility complex) on a single chromosome that are closely enough linked to be inherited usu. as a unit

hap·ten \\'hap-ˌten\ *n* : a small separable part of an antigen that reacts specif. with an antibody but is incapable of stimulating antibody production except in combination with an associated protein molecule — **hap·ten·ic** \hap-'ten-ik\ *adj* — **hap·ten·at·ed** \\'hap-tə-ˌnāt-əd\ *adj*

hap·tic \\'hap-tik\ *or* **hap·ti·cal** \-ti-kəl\ *adj* **1** : relating to or based on the sense of touch ⟨the ~ mode of perception —Colin Gordon⟩ **2** : characterized by a predilection for the sense of touch ⟨a ~ person⟩

hap·tics \-tiks\ *n pl but sing in constr* : a science concerned with the sense of touch

hap·to·glo·bin \\'hap-tə-ˌglō-bən\ *n* : any of several forms of an alpha globulin found in blood serum that can combine with free hemoglobin in the plasma and thereby prevent the loss of iron into the urine

hap·to·phore \-ˌfō(ə)r, -ˌfȯ(ə)r\ *adj* : having an ability to enter into combination with specific receptors of a cell ⟨a ~ group of a toxin⟩

har·bor \\'här-bər\ *vt* : to contain or be the home, habitat, or host of ⟨those who ~ the gene for the illness —William Booth⟩ ⟨green monkey (*Cercopithecus aethiops*) may have ~ed the ancestor of the AIDS virus —R. C. Gallo⟩

hard \\'härd\ *adj* **1** : not easily penetrated : not easily yielding to pressure **2 a** *of liquor* : strongly alcoholic; *specif* : having an alcoholic content of more than 22.5 percent **b** : characterized by the presence of salts (as of calcium or magnesium) that prevent lathering with soap ⟨~ water⟩ **3** : of or relating to radiation of relatively high penetrating power ⟨~ X-rays⟩ **4 a** : physically fit ⟨in good ~ condition⟩ **b** : resistant to stress (as disease) **5** : being at once addictive and gravely detrimental to health ⟨such ~ drugs as heroin⟩ **6** : resistant to biodegradation ⟨~ detergents⟩ ⟨~ pesticides like DDT⟩ — **hard·ness** *n*

hard·en·ing \\'härd-niŋ, -ᵊn-iŋ\ *n* : SCLEROSIS 1 ⟨~ of the arteries⟩

har·de·ri·an gland \(')här-'dir-ē-ən-\ *n, often cap H* : an accessory lacrimal gland on the inner side of the orbit in reptiles and birds but usu. degenerate in mammals

Har·der \\'här-dər\, **Johann Jacob (1656–1711),** Swiss anatomist. Harder was at various times professor of physics, anatomy, botany, and medicine at the University of Basle. He was one of the first to write on physiology and toxicology. In 1693 he described an accessory lacrimal gland of the orbit that is present in some animals. The gland is now known as the harderian gland.

Har·der's gland \\'här-dərz-\ *n* : HARDERIAN GLAND

hard of hear·ing \ˌhärd-ə(v)-'hi(ə)r-iŋ\ *adj* : of or relating to a defective but functional sense of hearing

hard pad *n* : a serious and frequently fatal virus disease of dogs now considered to be a form of distemper — called also *hard pad disease*

hard palate *n* : the bony anterior part of the palate forming the roof of the mouth

hard·ware disease \\'här-ˌdwa(ə)r-, -ˌdwe(ə)r-\ *n* : traumatic damage to the viscera of cattle due to ingestion of a foreign body (as a nail or barbed wire)

Har·dy–Wein·berg law \ˌhärd-ē-'wīn-ˌbərg-\ *n* : a fundamental principle of population genetics that is approximately true for small populations and holds with increasing exactness for larger and larger populations: population gene frequencies and population genotype frequencies remain constant from generation to generation if mating is random

---

\ə\ **abut** \ᵊ\ **kitten** \ər\ **further** \a\ **ash** \ā\ **ace** \ä\ **cot, cart**
\au̇\ **out** \ch\ **chin** \e\ **bet** \ē\ **easy** \g\ **go** \i\ **hit** \ī\ **ice** \j\ **job**
\ŋ\ **sing** \ō\ **go** \ȯ\ **law** \ȯi\ **boy** \th\ **thin** \t̲h̲\ **the** \ü\ **loot**
\u̇\ **foot** \y\ **yet** \zh\ **vision** *See also* Pronunciation Symbols page

and if mutation, selection, immigration, and emigration do not occur — called also *Hardy-Weinberg principle*

Hardy, Godfrey Harold (1877–1947), British mathematician. In his time Hardy was probably the leading pure mathematician in Great Britain. In 1908 he published a paper formulating the law of population genetics that the frequencies of both the different kinds of genes and of the different kinds of genotypes which they produce tend to remain constant over generations in large populations under general conditions.

Wein·berg \\'vīn-berk\, **Wilhelm (1862–1937),** German physician and geneticist. Weinberg made important contributions in medicine and human genetics to the study of multiple births, population genetics, and medical statistics. He ranks as one of the founders of population genetics. Independently of Hardy and at about the same time, he discovered the law of population genetics that is now called the Hardy-Weinberg law after both of them. In his studies of population genetics, Weinberg took into account both genetic and environmental factors. He was the first geneticist to partition the total variance of phenotypes into genetic and environmental portions.

hare·lip \\'ha(ə)r-'lip, 'he(ə)r-\ *n, sometimes offensive* : CLEFT LIP — **hare·lipped** \\-'lipt\ *adj*

Har·ley Street \\'här-lē-strēt\ *adj* : relating to, being, or characteristic of the prestigious physicians and surgeons whose offices are located on Harley Street in London ⟨*Harley Street* consultants⟩

har·ma·la \\'här-mə-lə\ *also* **har·mal** \\'här-məl\ *n* : an Old World herb (*Peganum harmala*) with strong-scented seeds that yield several alkaloids and are used as a vermifuge and stimulant

har·ma·line \\'här-mə-lēn\ *n* : a hallucinogenic alkaloid $C_{13}H_{14}N_2O$ found in several plants (*Peganum harmala* of the family Zygophyllaceae and *Banisteriopsis* spp. of the family Malpighiaceae) and used in medicine as a stimulant of the central nervous system

har·ma·lol \\-lȯl, -lōl\ *n* : a brown crystalline phenolic alkaloid $C_{12}H_{12}N_2O$ found in harmala seeds

har·mine \\'här-mēn\ *n* : a hallucinogenic alkaloid $C_{13}H_{12}N_2O$ whose distribution in plants and use in medicine is similar to harmaline

har·poon \\här-'pün\ *n* : a medical instrument with a barbed head used for removing bits of living tissue for examination

Hart·mann's solution \\'härt-mənz-\ *n* : LACTATED RINGER'S SOLUTION

Hartmann, Alexis Frank (1898–1964), American pediatrician. Hartmann spent virtually all of his professional career as professor of pediatrics at Washington University's School of Medicine and as physician-in-chief at St. Louis Children's Hospital. His principal contributions were in the fields of pediatric biochemistry and carbohydrate metabolism. He published papers on neonatal hypoglycemia, hyperinsulinism, juvenile diabetes, galactosemia, and other topics. He is credited with pioneering studies on the use of sodium lactate for the treatment of metabolic acidosis. In 1932 he published two reports describing the use of lactated Ringer's solution for the treatment of acidosis in children.

Hart·nup disease \\'härt-nəp-\ *n* : an inherited metabolic disease that is caused by abnormalities of the renal tubules and is characterized esp. by aminoaciduria involving only monocarboxylic monoamines, a dry red scaly rash, and episodic muscular incoordination due to the effects of the disease on the cerebellum

Hartnup (fl 1950s), British family. Hartnup disease was first described in 1956 in an article published under the names of D. N. Baron, C. E. Dent, H. Harris, E. W. Hart, and J. B. Jepson; all were physicians at London hospitals. The clinical studies of Hartnup disease began in 1951 when a 12-year-old male member of the Hartnup family was admitted to a London hospital under the care of E. W. Hart. At first it was thought that he was suffering from severe pellagra associated with a neurological disorder. Detailed investigation and experimental treatment of his case over sev-

eral years gradually led his physicians to the realization that they were dealing with a distinct and previously undescribed syndrome. Studies of the other members of the family revealed that Hartnup disease is an inherited metabolic disease. The disease affected four out of eight offspring of a marriage between first cousins.

harts·horn \\'härts-hȯ(ə)rn\ *n* : a preparation of ammonia used as smelling salts — see SPIRIT OF HARTSHORN

Har·vei·an \\'här-vē-ən\ *adj* : of, relating to, or commemorating William Harvey ⟨~ physiology⟩

Har·vey \\'här-vē\, **William (1578–1657),** British physician and physiologist. Considered one of the greatest physiologists of all time, Harvey wrote a treatise on the circulation of blood that is perhaps the foremost treatise in the history of physiology. First presented in lecture form in 1616, it was published in 1628. In this treatise, based upon the detailed observations of the anatomy and physiology of eighty species of animals and the dissection of cadavers, Harvey expounded his argument for the circulation of blood and the function of the heart as a pump. In 1651 he published a treatise on embryology in which he formulated the basic principles of epigenesis. One of the foremost physicians in England, he was physician to James I and Charles I.

hash \\'hash\ *n* : HASHISH

Ha·shi·mo·to's thyroiditis *also* **Hashimoto thyroiditis** \\hä-shē-'mō-(‚)tō(z)-\ *n* : a chronic autoimmune thyroiditis that is characterized by thyroid enlargement, thyroid fibrosis, lymphatic infiltration of thyroid tissue, and the production of antibodies which attack the thyroid and that occurs much more often in women than men and increases in frequency of occurrence with age — called also *Hashimoto's disease, Hashimoto's struma, struma lymphomatosa*

Ha·shi·mo·to \\hä-shē-mō-tō\, **Hakaru (1881–1934),** Japanese surgeon. Hashimoto published his description of chronic thyroiditis in 1912.

hash·ish \\'hash-‚ēsh, ha-'shēsh\ *n* : the concentrated resin from the flowering tops of the female hemp plant of the genus *Cannabis* (*C. sativa*) that is smoked, chewed, or drunk for its intoxicating effect — called also *charas;* compare BHANG 2, MARIJUANA

Has·sall's corpuscle \\'has-əlz-\ *n* : one of the small bodies of the medulla of the thymus having granular cells at the center surrounded by concentric layers of modified epithelial cells — called also *thymic corpuscle*

Hassall, Arthur Hill (1817–1894), British physician and chemist. In 1846 Hassall published *The Microscopic Anatomy of the Human Body in Health and Disease* in which he described the bodies that now bear his name.

has·si·um \\'ha-sē-əm\ *n* : a short-lived radioactive element produced artificially — symbol *Hs*; see ELEMENT table

hatch·et \\'hach-ət\ *n* : a dental excavator

hatha yo·ga \\'hət-ə-'yō-gə, 'hät-\ *n* : a form of yoga emphasizing a system of physical postures for balancing, stretching, and strengthening the body

haus·to·ri·um \\hȯ-'stȯr-ē-əm, -'stȯr-\ *n, pl* **-ria** \\-ē-ə\ : a food-absorbing outgrowth of a plant organ (as a hypha or stem) — **haus·to·ri·al** \\-ē-əl\ *adj*

haus·tral \\'hȯ-strəl\ *adj* : of, relating to, or exhibiting haustra ⟨~ contractions⟩

haus·tra·tion \\hȯ-'strā-shən\ *n* **1** : the property or state of having haustra **2** : HAUSTRUM

haus·trum \\'hȯ-strəm\ *n, pl* **haus·tra** \\-strə\ : one of the pouches or sacculations into which the large intestine is divided

ha·ver·sian canal \\hə-‚vər-zhən-\ *n, often cap H* : any of the small canals through which the blood vessels ramify in bone

Ha·vers \\'hā-vərz, 'hav-ərz\, **Clopton (1655?–1702),** British osteologist. In 1691 Havers published the first detailed description of the microscopic structure of the bone lamellae and canals and made important observations on the physiology of bone growth and repair. Although Antoni van Leeuwenhoek had observed the haversian canals in 1686, and Malpighi had mentioned the bone lamellae in

1675, Havers' work is remembered particularly because of its full and systematic treatment.

haversian system *n, often cap H* : a haversian canal with the concentrically arranged laminae of bone that surround it — called also *osteon*

Hav·rix \'hav-riks\ *trademark* — used for a vaccine against hepatitis A containing inactivated virus

haw \'hо̇\ *n* : NICTITATING MEMBRANE; *esp* : an inflamed nictitating membrane of a domesticated mammal

¹**hawk** \'hо̇k\ *vt* : to raise by trying to clear the throat ⟨∼ up phlegm⟩ ∼ *vi* : to make a harsh coughing sound in clearing the throat

²**hawk** *n* : an audible effort to force up phlegm from the throat

hay fever \'hā-,fē-vər\ *n* : an acute allergic reaction to pollen that is usu. seasonal and is marked by sneezing, nasal discharge and congestion, and itching and watering of the eyes — called also *pollinosis*

haz·mat \'haz-,mat\ *n, often attrib* : a material (as radioactive, flammable, explosive, or poisonous material) that would be a danger to life or to the environment if released without necessary precautions being taken ⟨toxic waste hauled away by workers in ∼ suits —Tom Spousta⟩ ⟨∼ storage⟩

Hb *abbr* hemoglobin

H band \'āch-\ *n* : a relatively pale band in the middle of the A band of striated muscle

HBsAg *abbr* hepatitis B surface antigen

HBV *abbr* hepatitis B virus

HCA *abbr* heterocyclic amine

HCFA *abbr* Health Care Financing Administration

HCG *abbr* human chorionic gonadotropin

HCM *abbr* hypertrophic cardiomyopathy

HCT *abbr* hematocrit

HCTZ *abbr* hydrochlorothiazide

HCV *abbr* hepatitis C virus

HD *abbr* **1** Hansen's disease **2** hearing distance

HDL \'āch-'dē-'el\ *n* : a lipoprotein of blood plasma that is composed of a high proportion of protein with little triglyceride and cholesterol and that is associated with decreased probability of developing atherosclerosis — called also *alpha-lipoprotein, good cholesterol, high-density lipoprotein*; compare LDL, VLDL

He *symbol* helium

head \'hed\ *n* **1** : the division of the human body that contains the brain, the eyes, the ears, the nose, and the mouth; *also* : the corresponding anterior division of the body of various animals including all vertebrates, most arthropods, and many mollusks and worms **2** : HEADACHE **3** : a projection or extremity esp. of an anatomical part: as **a** : the rounded proximal end of a long bone (as the humerus) **b** : the end of a muscle nearest the origin **c** : the anterior end of an invertebrate : SCOLEX **4** : the part of a boil, pimple, or abscess at which it is likely to break **5** : the end of a lipid molecule that consists of a polar group and is regarded as being opposite to the tail — **head** *adj*

head·ache \'hed-,āk\ *n* : pain in the head — called also *cephalalgia* — **head·achy** \-,ā-kē\ *adj*

head cold *n* : a common cold centered in the nasal passages and adjacent mucous tissues

head louse *n* : a sucking louse of the genus *Pediculus* (*P. humanus capitis*) that lives on the human scalp

head nurse *n* : CHARGE NURSE; *esp* : one with overall responsibility for the supervision of the administrative and clinical aspects of nursing care

head process *n* : an axial strand of cells that extends forward from the anterior end of the primitive streak in the early vertebrate embryo and is the precursor of the notochord

head·shrink·er \-,shriŋ-kər\ *n* : SHRINK

heal \'hē(ə)l\ *vt* **1** : to make sound or whole esp. in bodily condition **2** : to cure of disease or disorder ⟨∼ injured tissues⟩ ∼ *vi* **1** : to return to a sound state ⟨the wound ∼s⟩ **2** : to effect a cure — **heal·er** \'hē-lər\ *n*

¹**heal·ing** \'hē-liŋ\ *n* **1** : the act or process of curing or of restoring to health **2** : the process of getting well

²**healing** *adj* : tending to heal or cure : CURATIVE ⟨a ∼ art⟩

health \'helth\ *n, often attrib* **1** : the condition of an organism or one of its parts in which it performs its vital functions normally or properly : the state of being sound in body or mind ⟨dental ∼⟩ ⟨mental ∼⟩; *esp* : freedom from physical disease and pain ⟨nursed him back to ∼⟩ — compare DISEASE **2** : the condition of an organism with respect to the performance of its vital functions esp. as evaluated subjectively or nonprofessionally ⟨how is your ∼ today⟩

health care *n* : the maintaining and restoration of health by the treatment and prevention of disease esp. by trained and licensed professionals (as in medicine, dentistry, clinical psychology, and public health) — **health–care** *adj*

health de·part·ment \-də-,pärt-mənt\ *n* : a division of a local or larger government responsible for the oversight and care of matters relating to public health

health·ful \'helth-fəl\ *adj* : beneficial to health of body or mind — **health·ful·ly** \-fə-lē\ *adv* — **health·ful·ness** *n*

health insurance *n* : insurance against loss through illness of the insured; *esp* : insurance providing compensation for medical expenses

Health Insurance Por·ta·bil·i·ty and Accountability Act \-,pȯrt-ə-'bil-ət-ē-ənd-ə-,kau̇nt-ə-'bil-ət-ē-\ *n* : a federal law enacted in 1996 that protects continuity of health coverage when a person changes or loses a job, that limits health plan exclusions for preexisting medical conditions, that requires that patient medical information be kept private and secure, that standardizes electronic transactions involving health information, and that permits tax deduction of health insurance premiums by the self-employed — abbr. *HIPAA*

health main·te·nance or·ga·ni·za·tion \-'mānt-nən(t)s-,ȯrg-(ə-)nə-'zā-shən, -'mānt-ⁿn-ən(t)s-\ *n* : HMO

health of·fi·cer \-,af-ə-sər, -,ȯf-\ *n* : an officer charged with the enforcement of health and sanitation laws

health spa \-,spä, -,spȯ\ *n* : a commercial establishment (as a resort) providing facilities devoted to health and fitness

health vis·i·tor \-,viz-ət-ər, -,viz-tər\ *n, Brit* : a trained person who is usu. a qualified nurse and is employed by a local British authority to visit people (as nursing mothers) in their homes and advise them on health matters

healthy \'hel-thē\ *adj* **health·i·er; -est 1** : enjoying health and vigor of body, mind, or spirit **2** : revealing a state of health ⟨a ∼ complexion⟩ **3** : conducive to health — **health·i·ly** \-thə-lē\ *adv* — **health·i·ness** \-thē-nəs\ *n*

hear \'hi(ə)r\ *vb* **heard** \'hərd\; **hear·ing** \'hi(ə)r-iŋ\ *vt* : to perceive or apprehend by the ear ∼ *vi* : to have the capacity of apprehending sound

hear·ing *n* : the act or power of apprehending sound; *specif* : one of the special senses of vertebrates that is concerned with the perception of sound, is mediated through the organ of Corti in the ear in mammals, is normally sensitive in humans to sound vibrations between 16 and 27,000 hertz but most receptive to those between 2000 and 5000 hertz, is conducted centrally by the cochlear branch of the auditory nerve, and is coordinated esp. in the medial geniculate body

hearing aid \-,ād\ *n* : an electronic device usu. worn by a person for amplifying sound before it reaches the receptor organs

hearing dog *n* : a dog trained to alert its deaf or hearing-impaired owner to sounds (as of a doorbell, alarm, or telephone) — called also *hearing ear dog*

heart \'härt\ *n* **1** : a hollow muscular organ of vertebrate animals that by its rhythmic contraction acts as a force pump maintaining the circulation of the blood and that in the human adult is about five inches (13 centimeters) long and three and one half inches (9 centimeters) broad, is of conical form, is placed obliquely in the chest with the broad end upward and to the right and the apex opposite the interval between the cartilages of the fifth and sixth ribs on the left side, is enclosed in a serous pericardium, and consists as in other

\ə\ **abut** \ᵊ\ **kitten** \ər\ **further** \a\ **ash** \ā\ **ace** \ä\ **cot, cart**
\au̇\ **out** \ch\ **chin** \e\ **bet** \ē\ **easy** \g\ **go** \i\ **hit** \ī\ **ice** \j\ **job**
\ŋ\ **sing** \ō\ **go** \ȯ\ **law** \ȯi\ **boy** \th\ **thin** \t̲h̲\ **the** \ü\ **loot**
\u̇\ **foot** \y\ **yet** \zh\ **vision** *See also* Pronunciation Symbols page

G
H

mammals and in birds of four chambers divided into an upper pair of rather thin-walled atria which receive blood from the veins and a lower pair of thick-walled ventricles into which the blood is forced and which in turn pump it into the arteries **2** : a structure in an invertebrate animal functionally analogous to the vertebrate heart

heart attack *n* : an acute episode of heart disease marked by the death or damage of heart muscle due to insufficient blood supply to the heart muscle usu. as a result of a coronary thrombosis or a coronary occlusion and that is characterized esp. by chest pain — called also *myocardial infarction;* compare ANGINA PECTORIS, CORONARY INSUFFICIENCY, HEART FAILURE 1

heart·beat \'härt-ˌbēt\ *n* : one complete pulsation of the heart

heart block *n* : incoordination of the heartbeat in which the atria and ventricles beat independently due to defective transmission through the bundle of His and which is marked by decreased cardiac output often with cerebral ischemia

heart·burn \-ˌbərn\ *n* : a burning discomfort behind the lower part of the sternum usu. related to spasm of the lower end of the esophagus or of the upper part of the stomach often in association with gastroesophageal reflux — called also *cardialgia, pyrosis;* compare WATER BRASH

heart disease *n* : an abnormal organic condition of the heart or of the heart and circulation

heart failure *n* **1** : a condition in which the heart is unable to pump blood at an adequate rate or in adequate volume — compare ANGINA PECTORIS, CONGESTIVE HEART FAILURE, CORONARY FAILURE, HEART ATTACK **2** : cessation of heartbeat : DEATH

heart–healthy \'härt-ˌhel-thē\ *adj* : conducive to a healthy heart and circulatory system ⟨~ exercise⟩ ⟨a ~ diet⟩

heart–lung ma·chine \ˌhärt-'ləŋ-mə-ˌshēn\ *n* : a mechanical pump that maintains circulation during heart surgery by shunting blood away from the heart, oxygenating it, and returning it to the body

heart murmur *n* : MURMUR

heart rate *n* : a measure of cardiac activity usu. expressed as number of beats per minute — see MAXIMUM HEART RATE

heart valve *n* : any of the valves that control blood flow to and from the heart and that include the atrioventricular valves, the aortic valve, and the pulmonary valve — called also *cardiac valve*

heart·wa·ter \'härt-ˌwȯt-ər, -ˌwät-\ *n* : a serious febrile disease of sheep, goats, and cattle in southern Africa that is caused by a bacterium of the genus *Cowdria* (*C. ruminantium*) transmitted by a bont tick (*Amblyomma hebraeum*) — called also *heartwater disease, heartwater fever*

heart·worm \-ˌwərm\ *n* **1** : a filarial worm of the genus *Dirofilaria* (*D. immitis*) that is esp. common in warm regions, lives as an adult in the right heart esp. of dogs, and discharges active larvae into the circulating blood whence they may be picked up by mosquitoes and transmitted to other hosts and that may infect humans causing local pulmonary infarction but does not achieve sexual maturity in the human organism **2** : infestation with or disease esp. of dogs caused by the heartworm, resulting typically in gasping, coughing, and nervous disorder, and when severe commonly leading to death

¹**heat** \'hēt\ *vi* : to become warm or hot ~ *vt* : to make warm or hot

²**heat** *n* **1 a** : the state of a body or of matter that is perceived as opposed to cold and is characterized by elevation of temperature : a condition of being hot; *esp* : a marked or notable degree of this state : high temperature **b** (1) : a feverish state of the body : pathological excessive bodily temperature (as from inflammation) ⟨knew the throbbing ~ of an abscess⟩ ⟨the ~ of the fever⟩ (2) : a warm flushed condition of the body (as after exercise) : a sensation produced by or like that produced by contact with or approach to heated matter **c** (1) : added energy that causes substances to rise in temperature, fuse, evaporate, expand, or undergo any of various other related changes, that flows to a body by con-

tact with or radiation from bodies at higher temperatures, and that can be produced in a body (as by compression) (2) : the energy associated with the random motions of the molecules, atoms, or smaller structural units of which matter is composed **2** : sexual excitement esp. in a female mammal; *specif* : ESTRUS

heat capacity *n* : the quantity of heat required to raise the temperature of a body one degree — called also *thermal capacity*

heat cramps *n pl* : a condition that is marked by sudden development of cramps in skeletal muscles and that results from prolonged work in high temperatures accompanied by profuse perspiration with loss of sodium chloride from the body

heat ex·chang·er \-iks-ˌchānj-ər\ *n* : a device (as in an apparatus for extracorporeal blood circulation) for transferring heat from one fluid to another without allowing them to mix

heat exhaustion *n* : a condition marked by weakness, nausea, dizziness, and profuse sweating that results from physical exertion in a hot environment — called also *heat prostration;* compare HEATSTROKE

heat of combustion *n* : the heat of reaction resulting from the complete burning of a substance and expressed variously (as in calories per gram or per mole) — see BOMB CALORIMETER

heat prostration *n* : HEAT EXHAUSTION

heat rash *n* : PRICKLY HEAT

heat shock protein *n* : any of a group of proteins that were orig. isolated from certain bacteria exposed to heat, that occur esp. in cells subjected to heat stress, that keep the proteins in the cell from unraveling, and that are either identical with or comprise a class of molecular chaperones

heat·stroke \'hēt-ˌstrōk\ *n* : a condition marked esp. by cessation of sweating, extremely high body temperature, and collapse that results from prolonged exposure to high temperature — compare HEAT EXHAUSTION

heave \'hēv\ *vb* **heaved; heav·ing** *vt* : VOMIT ⟨got carsick and *heaved* his lunch⟩ ~ *vi* : to undergo retching or vomiting

heaves \'hēvz\ *n pl but sing or pl in constr* **1** : chronic emphysema of the horse affecting the alveolae of the lungs and resulting in difficult expiration, heaving of the flanks, and a persistent cough — called also *broken wind* **2** : a spell of retching or vomiting

heavy chain \'hev-ē-'chān\ *n* : either of the two larger of the four polypeptide chains comprising antibodies — compare LIGHT CHAIN

heavy hydrogen *n* : DEUTERIUM

heavy water *n* **1** : the compound D₂O composed of deuterium and oxygen — called also *deuterium oxide* **2** : water having a higher-than-usual proportion of deuterium among its hydrogen atoms

he·be·phre·nia \ˌhē-bə-'frē-nē-ə, -'fren-ē-\ *n* : a disorganized form of schizophrenia characterized esp. by incoherence, delusions which if present lack an underlying theme, and affect that is flat, inappropriate, or silly

¹**he·be·phre·nic** \-'fren-ik *also* -'frēn-ik\ *adj* : of, relating to, or affected with hebephrenia

²**hebephrenic** *n* : a person who is affected with hebephrenia

Heb·er·den's node \'heb-ər-dənz-\ *n* : a bony enlargement of the terminal joint of a finger commonly associated with osteoarthritis — compare BOUCHARD'S NODE

  Heberden, William (1710–1801), British physician. Heberden was an outstanding physician and the author of several medical descriptions that are considered classics. In 1767 he accurately differentiated for the first time chicken pox from smallpox. The following year he presented a classic description of nyctalopia and a description of angina pectoris. In 1802 a collection of 102 of his papers was published. The work contained his description of the hard arthritic nodules now known as Heberden's nodes.

heb·e·tude \'heb-ə-ˌt(y)üd\ *n* : the absence of mental alertness and affect (as in schizophrenia)

hec·tic \'hek-tik\ *adj* **1** : of, relating to, or being a fluctuating but persistent fever (as in tuberculosis) **2** : having a hectic fever ⟨a ~ patient⟩

hec·to·gram *or chiefly Brit* **hec·to·gramme** \'hek-tə-ˌgram\ *n* : a metric unit of mass and weight equal to 100 grams

hec·to·li·ter *or chiefly Brit* **hec·to·li·tre** \'hek-tə-ˌlēt-ər\ *n* : a metric unit of capacity equal to 100 liters

hec·to·me·ter *or chiefly Brit* **hec·to·me·tre** \'hek-tə-ˌmēt-ər, hek-'täm-ət-ər\ *n* : a metric unit of length equal to 100 meters

hede·o·ma oil \ˌhed-ē-'ō-mə-, ˌhēd-\ *n* : PENNYROYAL OIL

he·don·ic \hi-'dän-ik\ *adj* **1** : of, relating to, or characterized by pleasure **2** : of, relating to, or characteristic of hedonism or hedonists — **he·don·i·cal·ly** \-i-k(ə-)lē\ *adv*

he·do·nism \'hēd-ᵊn-ˌiz-əm\ *n* : the doctrine that pleasure or happiness is the sole or chief good in life — **he·do·nist** \-ᵊn-əst\ *n* — **he·do·nis·tic** \ˌhēd-ᵊn-'is-tik\ *adj* — **he·do·nis·ti·cal·ly** \-ti-k(ə-)lē\ *adv*

heel \'hē(ə)l\ *n* **1 a** : the back of the human foot below the ankle and behind the arch **b** : the back of the hind limb of other vertebrates homologous with the human heel **2** : an anatomical structure suggestive of the human heel: as **a** : the hind part of a hoof **b** : either of the projections of a coffin bone **c** : the part of the palm of the hand nearest the wrist

heel bone *n* : CALCANEUS

heel fly *n* : CATTLE GRUB; *esp* : one in the adult stage

Heer·fordt's syndrome \'här-ˌforts-\ *n* : UVEOPAROTID FEVER

Heerfordt, Christian Frederik (1871–1953), Danish ophthalmologist. Heerfordt published his description of uveoparotid fever in 1909.

height \'hīt, 'hītth\ *n* : the distance from the bottom to the top of something standing upright; *esp* : the distance from the lowest to the highest point of an animal body esp. of a human being in a natural standing position or from the lowest point to an arbitrarily chosen upper point ⟨a man six feet in ~⟩ ⟨a dog two feet in ~ at the shoulder⟩

Heim·lich maneuver \ˌhīm-lik-\ *n* : the manual application of sudden upward pressure on the upper abdomen of a choking victim to force a foreign object from the trachea

Heimlich, Henry Jay (*b* 1920), American surgeon. Heimlich wrote a number of medical works for the layman, on such topics as surgery of the stomach, duodenum, and diaphragm and on postoperative care for thoracic surgery. He devised an operation for the replacement of the esophagus and developed the Heimlich maneuver, publishing a monograph on it in 1976.

Heinz body \'hīnts-\ *n* : a cellular inclusion in a red blood cell that consists of damaged aggregated hemoglobin and is associated with some forms of hemolytic anemia

Heinz, Robert (1865–1924), German physician. Heinz did research in dermatology and metallic colloids. In 1890 he described inclusions seen in red blood cells in some cases of hemolytic anemia. These characteristic inclusions are now known as Heinz bodies.

hela cell \'hē-lə-\ *n, often cap H & 1st L* : a cell of a continuously cultured strain isolated from a human uterine cervical carcinoma in 1951 and used in biomedical research esp. to culture viruses

Lacks \'laks\, Henrietta (*fl* 1951), American hospital patient. Lacks was a patient with cancer of the cervix. In 1951 Dr. George O. Gey of Johns Hopkins University Medical School isolated cells from her cervical tumor. The hela (an acronym formed from the first two letters of her names, often given as the pseudonym Helen Lane or rarely as Helen Larson) cells still flourish in research laboratories all over the world.

he·li·an·thate \ˌhē-lē-'an-ˌthāt\ *n* : a salt of helianthin

he·li·an·thin \-'an-thən\ *n* : METHYL ORANGE; *also* : a red compound $C_{14}H_{15}N_3O_3S$ of quinone structure obtained by acidifying methyl orange

he·li·cal \'hel-i-kəl, 'hē-li-\ *adj* : of, relating to, or having the form of a helix ⟨the ~ configuration of DNA⟩; *broadly* : SPIRAL 1a — **he·li·cal·ly** \-k(ə-)lē\ *adv*

he·li·case \'hel-ə-ˌkās, 'hē-lə-\ *n* : any of various enzymes that catalyze the unwinding and separation of double-stranded DNA or RNA during its replication

helices *pl of* HELIX

hel·i·cine artery \'hel-ə-ˌsēn-, 'hē-lə-ˌsīn-\ *n* : any of various convoluted and dilated arterial vessels that empty directly into the cavernous spaces of erectile tissue and function in its erection

helicis — see CAUDA HELICIS

he·lic·i·ty \hē-'lis-ət-ē\ *n, pl* -**ties** **1** : the quality or state of being helical ⟨the degree of ~ in a protein⟩ **2** : the amount or degree of helical curve ⟨a prediction of ~ from the amino acid sequence⟩

hel·i·co·bac·ter \'hel-i-kō-ˌbak-tər\ *n* **1** *cap* : a genus of bacteria formerly placed in the genus *Campylobacter* and including one (*H. pylori*) associated with gastritis and implicated as a causative agent of gastric and duodenal ulcers **2** : any bacterium of the genus *Helicobacter*

he·li·coid \'hel-ə-ˌkoid, 'hē-lə-\ *or* **he·li·coi·dal** \ˌhel-ə-'koid-ᵊl, ˌhē-lə-\ *adj* **1** : forming or arranged in a spiral **2** : having the form of a flat coil or flattened spiral

hel·i·co·trema \ˌhel-ə-kō-'trē-mə\ *n* : the minute opening by which the scala tympani and scala vestibuli communicate at the top of the cochlea of the ear

he·lio·phobe \'hē-lē-ə-ˌfōb\ *n* : one who is abnormally sensitive to the effect of sunlight

he·li·o·sis \ˌhē-lē-'ō-səs\ *n, pl* -**o·ses** \-ˌsēz\ : SUNSTROKE

he·lio·tax·is \ˌhē-lē-ō-'tak-səs\ *n, pl* -**tax·es** \-ˌsēz\ : a taxis in which sunlight is the directive factor

he·lio·ther·a·py \-'ther-ə-pē\ *n, pl* -**pies** : the use of sunlight or of an artificial source of ultraviolet, visible, or infrared radiation for therapeutic purposes

he·li·ot·ro·pism \ˌhē-lē-'ä-trə-ˌpiz-əm\ *n* : phototropism in which sunlight is the orienting stimulus — **he·lio·tro·pic** \-lē-ə-'trōp-ik, -'träp-\ *adj*

he·li·um \'hē-lē-əm\ *n* : a light colorless nonflammable gaseous element found esp. in natural gases and used chiefly for inflating airships and balloons, for filling incandescent lamps, and for cryogenic research — symbol *He*; see ELEMENT table

he·lix \'hē-liks\ *n, pl* **he·li·ces** \'hel-ə-ˌsēz, 'hē-lə-\ *also* **he·lix·es** \'hē-lik-səz\ **1** : the incurved rim of the external ear **2** : a curve traced on a cylinder by the rotation of a point crossing its right sections at a constant oblique angle; *broadly* : SPIRAL 2 — see ALPHA-HELIX, DOUBLE HELIX

hel·le·bore \'hel-ə-ˌbō(ə)r, -ˌbo(ə)r\ *n* **1 a** : any herb of the genus *Helleborus* **b** : the dried roots and rhizome of any medicinal herb of the genus *Helleborus* (as black hellebore *H. niger* or green hellebore *H. viridis*) or a powder or extract of this used by the ancient Greeks and Romans in treating mental and other disorders **2 a** : any of several poisonous herbs of the genus *Veratrum* **b** : the dried rhizome and roots of either of two hellebores of the genus *Veratrum* (the false hellebore *V. viride* of America and *V. album* of Europe) or a powder or extract of this containing alkaloids (as protoveratrine) used as a cardiac and respiratory depressant and also as an insecticide — called also *veratrum, white hellebore*

Hel·leb·o·rus \he-'leb-ə-rəs\ *n* : a genus of Eurasian perennial herbs belonging to the buttercup family having deeply divided leaves and showy flowers — compare HELLEBORE

HELLP syndrome \'help-\ *n* [*h*emolysis *e*levated *l*iver enzymes, and *l*ow *p*latelet count] : a serious disorder of pregnancy of unknown etiology that usu. occurs between the 23rd and 39th weeks, that is characterized by a great reduction in the number of platelets per cubic millimeter, by hemolysis, by abnormal liver function tests, and sometimes by hypertension, and that in the most severe cases requires delivery of the fetus before term

hel·minth \'hel-ˌmin(t)th\ *n, pl* **helminths** : a parasitic worm

G
H

\ə\ **abut** \ᵊ\ **kitten** \ər\ **further** \a\ **ash** \ā\ **ace** \ä\ **cot, cart**
\aù\ **out** \ch\ **chin** \e\ **bet** \ē\ **easy** \g\ **go** \i\ **hit** \ī\ **ice** \j\ **job**
\ŋ\ **sing** \ō\ **go** \ò\ **law** \òi\ **boy** \th\ **thin** \th\ **the** \ü\ **loot**
\ù\ **foot** \y\ **yet** \zh\ **vision** *See also* Pronunciation Symbols page

(as a tapeworm, liver fluke, ascarid, or leech); *esp* : one that parasitizes the intestine of a vertebrate — **hel·min·thic** \hel-'min(t)-thik\ *adj*

hel·min·thi·a·sis \ˌhel-mən-'thī-ə-səs\ *n, pl* **-a·ses** \-ˌsēz\ : infestation with or disease caused by parasitic worms

hel·min·thol·o·gist \ˌhel-mən-'thäl-ə-jəst\ *n* : a specialist in helminthology

hel·min·thol·o·gy \-'thäl-ə-jē\ *n, pl* **-gies** : a branch of zoology concerned with helminths; *esp* : the study of parasitic worms

Helo·der·ma \ˌhē-lō-'dər-mə, ˌhel-ō-\ *n* : the type genus of the lizard family (Helodermatidae) including the Gila monsters

helper–inducer T cell *n* : T4 CELL

help·er T cell \ˌhel-pər-'tē-\ *n* : a T cell that participates in an immune response by recognizing a foreign antigen and secreting lymphokines to activate T cell and B cell proliferation, that usu. carries CD4 molecular markers on its cell surface, and that is reduced to 20 percent or less of normal numbers in AIDS — called also *helper cell, helper lymphocyte, helper T lymphocyte;* compare CYTOTOXIC T CELL, SUPPRESSOR T CELL

hel·vol·ic acid \hel-'väl-ik-\ *n* : FUMIGACIN

he·ma·cy·tom·e·ter *or chiefly Brit* **hae·ma·cy·tom·e·ter** \ˌhē-mə-sī-'täm-ət-ər\ *n* : an instrument for counting blood cells — called also *erythrocytometer, hemocytometer*

hem·ad·sorp·tion *or chiefly Brit* **haem·ad·sorp·tion** \ˌhē-(ˌ)mad-'sórp-shən, -'zórp-\ *n* : adherence of red blood cells to the surface of something (as a virus or cell) — **hem·ad·sorb·ing** *or chiefly Brit* **haem·ad·sorb·ing** \-'sòr-biŋ, -'zòr-\ *adj*

he·ma·dy·na·mom·e·ter *or chiefly Brit* **hae·ma·dy·na·mom·e·ter** \-ˌdī-nə-'mäm-ət-ər\ *n* : a device for measuring blood pressure

hem·ag·glu·ti·na·tion *or chiefly Brit* **haem·ag·glu·ti·na·tion** \ˌhē-mə-ˌglüt-ᵊn-'ā-shən\ *n* : agglutination of red blood cells — **hem·ag·glu·ti·nate** *or chiefly Brit* **haem·ag·glu·ti·nate** \-'glüt-ᵊn-ˌāt\ *vt* **-nat·ed; -nat·ing**

hem·ag·glu·ti·nin \ˌhē-mə-'glüt-ᵊn-ən\ *also* **he·mo·ag·glu·ti·nin** \ˌhē-mō-ə-\ *or chiefly Brit* **haem·ag·glu·ti·nin** *also* **hae·mo·ag·glu·ti·nin** *n* : an agglutinin (as an antibody or viral capsid protein) that causes hemagglutination — compare LEUKOAGGLUTININ

he·mal *or chiefly Brit* **hae·mal** \'hē-məl\ *adj* **1** : of or relating to the blood or blood vessels **2** : relating to or situated on the side of the spinal cord where the heart and chief blood vessels are placed — compare NEURAL 2

hemal arch *n* : a bony or cartilaginous arch extending ventrally from the spinal column; *esp* : the arch formed by a vertebra and an associated pair of ribs

hemal node *n* : HEMOLYMPH NODE

he·man·gi·ec·ta·sis *or chiefly Brit* **hae·man·gi·ec·ta·sis** \ˌhē-ˌman-jē-'ek-tə-səs\ *n, pl* **-ta·ses** \-ˌsēz\ : dilatation of blood vessels

hem·an·gio·blas·to·ma \ˌhē-ˌman-jē-ō-(ˌ)blas-'tō-mə\ *or chiefly Brit* **haem·an·gio·blas·to·ma** *n, pl* **-mas** *also* **-ma·ta** \-mət-ə\ : a hemangioma esp. of the cerebellum that tends to be associated with von Hippel-Lindau disease

he·man·gio·en·do·the·li·o·ma *or chiefly Brit* **hae·man·gio·en·do·the·li·o·ma** \-jē-ō-ˌen-dō-ˌthē-lē-'ō-mə\ *n, pl* **-mas** *also* **-ma·ta** \-mət-ə\ : an often malignant tumor originating by proliferation of capillary endothelium

hem·an·gi·o·ma *or chiefly Brit* **haem·an·gi·o·ma** \ˌhē-ˌman-jē-'ō-mə\ *n, pl* **-mas** *also* **-ma·ta** \-mət-ə\ : a usu. benign tumor made up of blood vessels that typically occurs as a purplish or reddish slightly elevated area of skin

hem·an·gi·o·ma·to·sis *or chiefly Brit* **haem·an·gi·o·ma·to·sis** \-jē-ˌō-mə-'tō-səs\ *n, pl* **-to·ses** \-ˌsēz\ : a condition in which hemangiomas are present in several parts of the body

hem·an·gio·peri·cy·to·ma *or chiefly Brit* **haem·an·gio·peri·cy·to·ma** \-jē-ō-ˌper-ə-ˌsī-'tō-mə\ *n, pl* **-mas** *also* **-ma·ta** \-mət-ə\ : a vascular tumor composed of spindle cells that are held to be derived from pericytes — called also *peritheli·oma*

he·man·gio·sar·co·ma *or chiefly Brit* **hae·man·gio·sar·co·**

ma \-jē-ō-sär-'kō-mə\ *n, pl* **-mas** *also* **-ma·ta** \-mət-ə\ : a malignant hemangioma

he·mar·thro·sis *or chiefly Brit* **hae·mar·thro·sis** \ˌhē-mär-'thrō-səs, ˌhem-är-\ *n, pl* **-thro·ses** \-ˌsēz\ : hemorrhage into a joint

he·ma·tein *or chiefly Brit* **hae·ma·tein** \ˌhē-mə-'tē-ən, 'hē-məˌtēn\ *n* : a reddish brown crystalline compound $C_{16}H_{12}O_6$ constituting the essential dye in logwood extracts

he·ma·tem·e·sis *or chiefly Brit* **hae·ma·tem·e·sis** \ˌhē-mə-'tem-ə-səs *also* ˌhē-mə-tə-'mē-səs\ *n, pl* **-e·ses** \-ˌsēz\ : the vomiting of blood

¹he·mat·ic *or chiefly Brit* **hae·mat·ic** \hi-'mat-ik\ *adj* : of, relating to, or containing blood

²hematic *or chiefly Brit* **haematic** *n* : a drug (as a hematinic or an anticoagulant) having an effect on the blood

he·ma·ti·dro·sis *or chiefly Brit* **hae·ma·ti·dro·sis** \ˌhē-mət-ə-'drō-səs *also* ˌhem-ət-\ *n* : the excretion through the skin of blood or blood pigments

he·ma·tin *or chiefly Brit* **hae·ma·tin** \'hē-mət-ən\ *n* **1** : a brownish black or bluish black derivative $C_{34}H_{33}N_4O_5Fe$ of oxidized heme containing iron with a valence of three; *also* : any of several similar compounds **2** : HEME

he·ma·tin·ic *or chiefly Brit* **hae·ma·tin·ic** \ˌhē-mə-'tin-ik\ *n* : an agent that tends to stimulate blood cell formation or to increase the hemoglobin in the blood — **hematinic** *or chiefly Brit* **hae·ma·tin·ic** *adj*

he·ma·to·blast *or chiefly Brit* **hae·ma·to·blast** \'hē-mət-ə-ˌblast, hi-'mat-ə-\ *n* **1** : PLATELET **2** : an immature blood cell

he·ma·to·cele *or chiefly Brit* **hae·ma·to·cele** \'hē-mət-ə-ˌsēl, hi-'mat-ə-\ *n* : a blood-filled cavity of the body; *also* : the effusion of blood into a body cavity (as the scrotum)

he·ma·to·che·zia *or chiefly Brit* **hae·ma·to·che·zia** \ˌhē-mə-tə-'kē-zē-ə *also* ˌhem-ə-; hi-ˌmat-ə-\ *n* : the passage of blood in the feces — compare MELENA

he·ma·to·chy·lu·ria *or chiefly Brit* **hae·ma·to·chy·lu·ria** \ˌhē-mə-tə-ˌkī-'lù-rē-ə *also* ˌhem-ə-; hi-ˌmat-ə-\ *n* : the simultaneous presence of blood and chyle in the urine

he·ma·to·col·pos *or chiefly Brit* **hae·ma·to·col·pos** \ˌhē-mə-tō-'käl-pəs *also* ˌhem-ə-, -'käl-ˌpäs; hi-ˌmat-ə-\ *n* : an accumulation of blood within the vagina

he·mat·o·crit *or chiefly Brit* **hae·mat·o·crit** \hi-'mat-ə-krət, -ˌkrit\ *n* **1** : an instrument for determining usu. by centrifugation the relative amounts of plasma and corpuscles in blood **2** : the percent of the volume of whole blood that is composed of red blood cells as determined by separation of red blood cells from the plasma usu. by centrifugation ⟨a ~ ranging from 42% to 52% in males and 35% to 47% in females is typically considered normal⟩ — called also *packed cell volume*

he·mat·o·cyst *or chiefly Brit* **hae·mat·o·cyst** \hi-'mat-ə-ˌsist\ *n* : a cyst containing blood

he·ma·to·gen·ic *or chiefly Brit* **hae·ma·to·gen·ic** \ˌhē-mət-ə-'jen-ik\ *adj* : HEMATOGENOUS 2 ⟨~ hepatitis⟩

he·ma·tog·e·nous *or chiefly Brit* **hae·ma·tog·e·nous** \ˌhē-mə-'täj-ə-nəs\ *adj* **1** : concerned with the production of blood or of one or more of its constituents ⟨~ functions of the liver⟩ **2** : taking place or spread by way of the blood ⟨a ~ route of infection⟩ ⟨~ tuberculosis⟩ — **he·ma·tog·e·nous·ly** *or chiefly Brit* **hae·ma·tog·e·nous·ly** *adv*

hem·a·to·gone *or chiefly Brit* **haem·a·to·gone** \'hē-mət-ə-ˌgōn, hi-'mat-ə-ˌgōn\ *n* : HEMOCYTOBLAST

he·ma·toid *or chiefly Brit* **hae·ma·toid** \'hē-mə-ˌtóid *also* 'hem-ə-\ *adj* : resembling blood

he·ma·toi·din *or chiefly Brit* **hae·ma·toi·din** \ˌhē-mə-'tóid-ᵊn *also* ˌhem-ə-\ *n* : BILIRUBIN

he·ma·to·log·ic \ˌhē-mət-ə-ᵊl-'äj-ik\ *also* **he·ma·to·log·i·cal** \-i-kəl\ *or chiefly Brit* **hae·ma·to·log·ic** *also* **hae·ma·to·log·i·cal** *adj* : of or relating to blood or to hematology — **he·ma·to·log·i·cal·ly** *or chiefly Brit* **hae·ma·to·log·i·cal·ly** \-i-k(ə-)lē\ *adv*

he·ma·tol·o·gy *or chiefly Brit* **hae·ma·tol·o·gy** \ˌhē-mə-'täl-ə-jē\ *n, pl* **-gies** : a medical science that deals with the blood and blood-forming organs — **he·ma·tol·o·gist** or chiefly Brit **hae·ma·tol·o·gist** \-jəst\ n

he·ma·to·ma or chiefly Brit **hae·ma·to·ma** \-'tō-mə\ n, pl **-mas** also **-ma·ta** \-mət-ə\ : a mass of usu. clotted blood that forms in a tissue, organ, or body space as a result of a broken blood vessel

he·ma·to·me·tra or chiefly Brit **hae·ma·to·me·tra** \ˌhē-mət-ə-'mē-trə also ˌhem-ət-\ n : an accumulation of blood or menstrual fluid in the uterus

he·ma·to·my·e·lia or chiefly Brit **hae·ma·to·my·e·lia** \hi-ˌmat-ə-ˌmī-'ē-lē-ə, ˌhē-mət-ō-\ n : a hemorrhage into the spinal cord

he·ma·to·pa·thol·o·gy or chiefly Brit **hae·ma·to·pa·thol·o·gy** \hi-ˌmat-ə-pə-'thäl-ə-jē, ˌhē-mət-ō-\ n, pl **-gies** : the medical science concerned with diseases of the blood and related tissues — **he·ma·to·pa·thol·o·gist** or chiefly Brit **hae·ma·to·pa·thol·o·gist** \-ə-jəst\ n

he·ma·to·peri·car·di·um or chiefly Brit **hae·ma·to·peri·car·di·um** \hi-ˌmat-ə-ˌper-ə-'kärd-ē-əm, ˌhē-mət-ō-\ n, pl **-dia** \-ē-ə\ : HEMOPERICARDIUM

he·ma·toph·a·gous or chiefly Brit **hae·ma·toph·a·gous** \ˌhē-mə-'täf-ə-gəs\ adj : feeding on blood ⟨∼ insects⟩

he·ma·to·phyte or chiefly Brit **hae·ma·to·phyte** \'hē-mət-ə-ˌfīt, hi-'mat-ə-\ n : a plant parasite (as a bacterium) of the blood

he·ma·to·poi·e·sis or chiefly Brit **hae·ma·to·poi·e·sis** \hi-ˌmat-ə-pòi-'ē-səs, ˌhē-mət-ō-\ n, pl **-e·ses** \-ˌsēz\ : the formation of blood or of blood cells in the living body — called also hemopoiesis

he·ma·to·poi·et·ic or chiefly Brit **hae·ma·to·poi·et·ic** \-'et-ik\ adj : of, relating to, or involved in the formation of blood cells ⟨∼ stem cells⟩

hematopoietic growth factor n : any of a group of glycoproteins that promote the proliferation and maturation of blood cells; esp : COLONY-STIMULATING FACTOR

he·ma·to·por·phy·rin or chiefly Brit **hae·ma·to·por·phy·rin** \ˌhē-mət-ə-'pòr-fə-rən also ˌhem-ət-\ n : any of several isomeric porphyrins $C_{34}H_{38}O_6N_4$ that are hydrated derivatives of protoporphyrins; esp : the deep red crystalline pigment obtained by treating hematin or heme with acid

he·ma·to·por·phy·rin·u·ria or chiefly Brit **hae·ma·to·por·phy·rin·uria** \-ˌpòr-fə-rən-'(y)ùr-ē-ə\ n : PORPHYRINURIA

he·ma·tor·rha·chis or chiefly Brit **hae·ma·tor·rha·chis** \ˌhē-mə-'tòr-ə-kəs\ n : hemorrhage into the vertebral canal

he·ma·to·sal·pinx or chiefly Brit **hae·ma·to·sal·pinx** \ˌhē-mət-ə-'sal-(ˌ)piŋ(k)s also ˌhem-ət-, hi-ˌmat-ə-\ n, pl **-sal·pin·ges** \-sal-'pin-(ˌ)jēz\ : accumulation of blood in a fallopian tube — called also hemosalpinx

he·ma·to·scope or chiefly Brit **hae·ma·to·scope** \'hē-mət-ə-ˌskōp, hi-'mat-ə-\ n : an instrument for the spectroscopic examination of blood

he·ma·tox·y·lin or chiefly Brit **hae·ma·tox·y·lin** \ˌhē-mə-'täk-sə-lən\ n : a crystalline phenolic compound $C_{16}H_{14}O_6$ found in logwood and used chiefly as a biological stain because of its ready oxidation to hematein

he·ma·to·zo·al or chiefly Brit **hae·ma·to·zo·al** \ˌhē-mət-ə-'zō-əl also ˌhem-ət-, hi-ˌmat-ə-\ adj : of, relating to, or caused by animal parasites of the blood ⟨∼ diseases⟩

he·ma·to·zo·an or chiefly Brit **hae·ma·to·zo·an** \-'zō-ən\ n : a blood-dwelling animal parasite

he·ma·tu·ria or chiefly Brit **hae·ma·tu·ria** \ˌhē-mə-'t(y)ùr-ē-ə\ n : the presence of blood or blood cells in the urine

heme or chiefly Brit **haem** \'hēm\ n : the deep red iron-containing prosthetic group $C_{34}H_{32}N_4O_4Fe$ of hemoglobin and myoglobin that is a ferrous derivative of protoporphyrin and readily oxidizes to hematin or hemin — called also protoheme

hem·er·a·lo·pia \ˌhem-ə-rə-'lō-pē-ə\ n **1** : a defect of vision characterized by reduced visual capacity in bright lights **2** : NIGHT BLINDNESS — not considered good medical usage in this sense

he·me·ryth·rin or chiefly Brit **hae·me·ryth·rin** \ˌhē-mə-'rith-rən\ n : an iron-containing respiratory pigment in the blood of various invertebrates

hemi·ac·e·tal \ˌhem-ē-'as-ə-ˌtal\ n : any of a class of compounds characterized by the group C(OH)(OR) where R is an alkyl group and usu. formed as intermediates in the preparation of acetals from aldehydes or ketones

hemi·al·ge·sia \-al-'jē-zhə, -z(h)ē-ə\ n : diminished sensitivity to pain that affects only one lateral side of the body

hemi·an·al·ge·sia \-ˌan-ᵊl-'jē-zhə, -z(h)ē-ə\ n : loss of sensibility to pain on either lateral side of the body

hemi·an·es·the·sia or chiefly Brit **hemi·an·aes·the·sia** \-ˌan-əs-'thē-zhə\ n : loss of sensation in either lateral half of the body

hemi·an·o·pia \-ə-'nōp-ē-ə\ or **hemi·an·op·sia** \-ə-'näp-sē-ə\ n : blindness in one half of the visual field of one or both eyes — called also hemiopia — **hemi·an·op·tic** \-ə-'näp-tik\ adj

hemi·at·ro·phy \-'a-trə-fē\ n, pl **-phies** : atrophy that affects one half of an organ or part or one side of the whole body ⟨facial ∼⟩ — compare HEMIHYPERTROPHY

hemi·a·zy·gos vein \-(ˈ)ā-'zī-gəs-, -'az-ə-gəs-\ n : a vein that receives blood from the lower half of the left thoracic wall and the left abdominal wall, ascends along the left side of the spinal column, and empties into the azygos vein near the middle of the thorax

hemi·bal·lis·mus \ˌhem-i-ba-'liz-məs\ also **hemi·bal·lism** \-'bal-iz-əm\ n : violent uncontrollable movements of one lateral half of the body usu. due to a lesion in the subthalamic nucleus of the contralateral side of the body

hemi·block \'hem-i-ˌbläk\ n : inhibition or failure of conduction of the muscular excitatory impulse in either of the two divisions of the left branch of the bundle of His

he·mic or chiefly Brit **hae·mic** \'hē-mik\ adj : of, relating to, or produced by the blood or the circulation of the blood ⟨the ∼ system⟩ ⟨a ∼ murmur⟩

hemi·cel·lu·lose \ˌhem-i-'sel-yə-ˌlōs, -ˌlōz\ n : any of various plant polysaccharides less complex than cellulose and easily hydrolyzable to simple sugars and other products — **hemi·cel·lu·los·ic** \-ik\ adj

hemi·ce·re·brum \-sə-'rē-brəm, -'ser-ə-\ n, pl **-brums** or **-bra** \-brə\ : a lateral half of the cerebrum : CEREBRAL HEMISPHERE

hemi·cho·lin·ium \-kō-'lin-ē-əm\ n : any of several blockers of the parasympathetic nervous system that interfere with the synthesis of acetylcholine

hemi·cho·rea \ˌhem-i-kə-'rē-ə\ n : chorea affecting only one lateral half of the body

hemi·col·ec·to·my \-kə-'lek-tə-mē, -kō-\ n, pl **-mies** : surgical excision of part of the colon

hemi·cra·nia \-'krā-nē-ə\ n : pain in one side of the head — compare AMPHICRANIA — **hemi·cra·ni·al** \-nē-əl\ adj

hemi·cra·ni·o·sis \-ˌkrā-nē-'ō-səs\ n : cranial hyperostosis affecting only one lateral half of the head

hemi·de·cor·ti·ca·tion \-(ˌ)dē-ˌkòrt-ə-'kā-shən\ n : removal of the cortex from one lateral half of the cerebrum

hemi·des·mo·some \-'dez-mə-ˌsōm\ n : a specialization of the plasma membrane of an epithelial cell that is similar to half a desmosome and serves to connect the basal surface of the cell to the basement membrane

hemi·di·a·phragm \-'dī-ə-ˌfram\ n : one of the two lateral halves of the diaphragm separating the chest and abdominal cavities

hemi·fa·cial \-'fā-shəl\ adj : involving or affecting one lateral half of the face ⟨∼ spasm⟩

hemi·field \'hem-i-ˌfēld\ n : one of two halves of a sensory field (as of vision) ⟨the parts of each visual ∼ that can be seen with both eyes —R. W. Guillery⟩

hemi·gas·trec·to·my \ˌhem-i-ˌga-'strek-tə-mē\ n, pl **-mies** : surgical removal of one half of the stomach

hemi·glos·sec·to·my \-glä-'sek-tə-mē, -ˌglò-\ n, pl **-mies** : surgical excision of one lateral half of the tongue

---

\ə\ abut \ᵊ\ kitten \ər\ further \a\ ash \ā\ ace \ä\ cot, cart
\aù\ out \ch\ chin \e\ bet \ē\ easy \g\ go \i\ hit \ī\ ice \j\ job
\ŋ\ sing \ō\ go \ò\ law \òi\ boy \th\ thin \th\ the \ü\ loot
\ù\ foot \y\ yet \zh\ vision   See also Pronunciation Symbols page

hemi·hy·per·tro·phy \-hī-'pər-trə-fē\ *n, pl* **-phies** : hypertrophy of one half of an organ or part or of one side of the whole body ⟨facial ∼⟩ — compare HEMIATROPHY

hemi·lam·i·nec·to·my \-ˌlam-ə-'nek-tə-mē\ *n, pl* **-mies** : laminectomy involving the removal of vertebral laminae on only one side

hemi·lat·er·al \-'lat-ə-rəl, -'la-trəl\ *adj* : of or affecting one lateral half of the body

hemi·man·dib·u·lec·to·my \-man-ˌdib-yù-'lek-tə-mē\ *n, pl* **-mies** : surgical removal of one lateral half of the mandible

hemi·me·lia \-'mē-lē-ə\ *n* : a congenital abnormality (as total or partial absence) affecting only the distal half of a limb

hemi·me·lus \-'mē-ləs\ *n* : an individual affected with hemimelia

hemi·me·tab·o·lous \-mə-'tab-ə-ləs\ *adj* : characterized by incomplete metamorphosis ⟨∼ insects⟩ — compare HOLOMETABOLOUS

he·min *or chiefly Brit* **hae·min** \'hē-mən\ *n* : a red-brown to blue-black crystalline salt $C_{34}H_{32}N_4O_4FeCl$ that inhibits the biosynthesis of porphyrin and is used to ameliorate the symptoms of some forms of porphyria — called also *protohemin*

hemi·ne·phrec·to·my \ˌhem-i-ni-'frek-tə-mē\ *n, pl* **-mies** : surgical removal of part of a kidney

hemi·o·pia \ˌhem-ē-'ō-pē-ə\ *or* **hemi·op·sia** \-'äp-sē-ə\ *n* : HEMIANOPIA — **hemi·op·ic** \-'äp-ik, -'ō-pik\ *adj*

hemi·pa·re·sis \ˌhem-i-pə-'rē-səs, -'par-ə-\ *n, pl* **-re·ses** \-ˌsēz\ : muscular weakness or partial paralysis restricted to one side of the body ⟨discharged with a residual partial right ∼ —P. W. Wright⟩ — **hemi·pa·ret·ic** \-pə-'ret-ik\ *adj*

hemi·pel·vec·to·my \-pel-'vek-tə-mē\ *n, pl* **-mies** : amputation of one leg together with removal of the half of the pelvis on the same side of the body

hemi·ple·gia \ˌhem-i-'plē-j(ē-)ə\ *n* : total or partial paralysis of one side of the body that results from disease of or injury to the motor centers of the brain

¹hemi·ple·gic \-'plē-jik\ *adj* : relating to or marked by hemiplegia

²hemiplegic *n* : a hemiplegic individual

He·mip·tera \hi-'mip-tə-rə\ *n pl* : a large order of insects (as the true bugs) that have mouthparts adapted to piercing and sucking and usu. two pairs of wings, undergo an incomplete metamorphosis, and include many important pests — **he·mip·ter·an** \-tə-rən\ *n* — **he·mip·ter·ous** \-tə-rəs\ *adj*

hemi·ret·i·na \ˌhem-i-'ret-ᵊn-ə, -'ret-nə\ *n, pl* **-i·nas** *or* **-i·nae** \-ᵊn-ˌē, -ˌī\ : one half of the retina of one eye — **hemi·ret·i·nal** \-'ret-ᵊn-əl, -'ret-nəl\ *adj*

hemi·sect \'hem-i-ˌsekt\ *vt* : to divide along the mesial plane ⟨the brains were . . . ∼ed by a midline sagittal cut —J. N. Riley & D. W. Walker⟩ — **hemi·sec·tion** \-ˌsek-shən\ *n*

hemi·spasm \-ˌspaz-əm\ *n* : spasm that affects only one lateral side of the body ⟨peripheral facial ∼⟩

hemi·sphere \-ˌsfi(ə)r\ *n* : half of a spherical structure or organ: as **a** : CEREBRAL HEMISPHERE **b** : either of the two lobes of the cerebellum of which one projects laterally and posteriorly from each side of the vermis

hemi·spher·ec·to·my \ˌhem-i-sfi-'rek-tə-mē\ *n, pl* **-mies** : surgical removal of a cerebral hemisphere (as to control severe epileptic seizures)

hemi·spher·ic \-'sfi(ə)r-ik, -'sfer-\ *adj* : of, relating to, or affecting a hemisphere (as a cerebral hemisphere) ⟨∼ lesions⟩ ⟨∼ localization of function⟩

hemi·ter·pene \-'tər-ˌpēn\ *n* : a compound C_5H_8 whose formula represents half that of a terpene; *esp* : ISOPRENE

hemi·tho·rax \-'thō(ə)r-ˌaks, -'thò(ə)r-\ *n, pl* **-tho·rax·es** *or* **-tho·ra·ces** \-'thòr-ə-ˌsēz, -'thór-\ : a lateral half of the thorax

hemi·thy·roid·ec·to·my \-ˌthī-ˌróid-'ek-tə-mē\ *n, pl* **-mies** : surgical removal of one lobe of the thyroid gland

hemi·zy·gote \-'zī-ˌgōt\ *n* : one that is hemizygous

hemi·zy·gous \-'zī-gəs\ *adj* : having or characterized by one or more genes (as in a genetic deficiency or in an X chromosome paired with a Y chromosome) that have no allelic counterparts — **hemi·zy·gos·i·ty** \-zī-'gäs-ə-tē\ *n, pl* **-ties**

hem·lock \'hem-ˌläk\ *n* **1 a** : any of several poisonous herbs (as a poison hemlock or a water hemlock) of the carrot family (Umbelliferae) having finely cut leaves and small white flowers **b** : CONIUM 2 **2** : a drug or lethal drink prepared from the poison hemlock — compare CONIINE

hemoagglutinin *var of* HEMAGGLUTININ

hemobartonellosis *var of* HAEMOBARTONELLOSIS

he·mo·bil·ia *or chiefly Brit* **hae·mo·bil·ia** \ˌhē-mə-'bil-ē-ə\ *n* : bleeding into the bile ducts and gallbladder

he·mo·blast *or chiefly Brit* **hae·mo·blast** \'hē-mə-ˌblast\ *n* : HEMATOBLAST

he·mo·blas·to·sis *or chiefly Brit* **hae·mo·blas·to·sis** \ˌhē-mə-ˌblas-'tō-səs\ *n, pl* **-to·ses** \-ˌsēz\ : abnormal proliferation of the blood-forming tissues

he·moc·cult *or chiefly Brit* **hae·moc·cult** \'hē-mə-ˌkəlt\ *adj* : relating to or being a modified guaiac test in which filter paper impregnated with guaiacum turns blue if occult blood is present ⟨∼ slide testing⟩

he·mo·cho·ri·al *or chiefly Brit* **hae·ma·cho·ri·al** \ˌhē-mə-'kōr-ē-əl, -'kòr-\ *adj, of a placenta* : having the fetal epithelium bathed in maternal blood ⟨humans are ∼⟩

he·mo·chro·ma·to·sis *or chiefly Brit* **hae·mo·chro·ma·to·sis** \ˌhē-mə-ˌkrō-mə-'tō-səs\ *n, pl* **-to·ses** \-ˌsēz\ : a hereditary disorder of metabolism that involves the deposition of iron‑containing pigments in the tissues, is characterized esp. by joint or abdominal pain, weakness, and fatigue, may lead to bronzing of the skin, arthritis, diabetes, cirrhosis, or heart disease if untreated, and typically affects men more often than women — compare HEMOSIDEROSIS — **he·mo·chro·ma·tot·ic** *or chiefly Brit* **hae·mo·chro·ma·tot·ic** \-'tät-ik\ *adj*

he·mo·chro·mo·gen *or chiefly Brit* **hae·mo·chro·mo·gen** \ˌhē-mō-'krō-mə-ˌjen, -jən\ *n* : a colored compound formed from or related to hemoglobin; *esp* : a bright red combination of a nitrogen base (as globin or pyridine) with heme — compare HEMOPROTEIN

he·mo·clas·tic crisis *or chiefly Brit* **hae·mo·clas·tic crisis** \ˌhē-mə-ˌklas-tik-\ *n* : an acute transitory alteration of the blood that sometimes accompanies anaphylactic shock and is marked by intense leukopenia with relative lymphocytosis, alteration in blood coagulability, and fall in blood pressure

he·mo·co·ag·u·la·tion *or chiefly Brit* **hae·mo·co·ag·u·la·tion** \ˌhē-mō-kō-ˌag-yə-'lā-shən\ *n* : coagulation of blood

he·mo·coel *also* **he·mo·coele** *or chiefly Brit* **hae·mo·coele** \'hē-mə-ˌsēl\ *n* : a body cavity (as in arthropods or some mollusks) that normally contains blood and functions as part of the circulatory system — **he·mo·coel·ic** *or chiefly Brit* **hae·mo·coel·ic** \ˌhē-mə-'sē-lik\ *adj*

he·mo·con·cen·tra·tion *or chiefly Brit* **hae·mo·con·cen·tra·tion** \ˌhē-mō-ˌkän(t)-sən-'trā-shən\ *n* : increased concentration of cells and solids in the blood usu. resulting from loss of fluid to the tissues — compare HEMODILUTION 1

he·mo·co·nia *also* **he·mo·ko·nia** *or chiefly Brit* **hae·mo·co·nia** *also* **hae·mo·ko·nia** \ˌhē-mə-'kō-nē-ə\ *n* : small refractive colorless particles in the blood that are prob. granules from the cells in the blood or minute globules of fat — called also *blood dust*

he·mo·co·ni·o·sis *or chiefly Brit* **hae·mo·co·ni·o·sis** \-ˌkō-nē-'ō-səs\ *n, pl* **-o·ses** \-ˌsēz\ : a condition in which there is an abnormally high content of hemoconia in the blood

he·mo·cul·ture *or chiefly Brit* **hae·mo·cul·ture** \'hē-mə-ˌkəl-chər\ *n* : a culture made from blood to detect the presence of pathogenic microorganisms

he·mo·cu·pre·in *or chiefly Brit* **hae·mo·cu·pre·in** \ˌhē-mō-'k(y)ü-prē-ən\ *n* : a blue copper-containing protein obtained from red blood cells

he·mo·cy·a·nin *or chiefly Brit* **hae·mo·cy·a·nin** \ˌhē-mō-'sī-ə-nən\ *n* : a colorless copper-containing respiratory pigment in solution in the blood plasma of various arthropods and mollusks

he·mo·cyte *or chiefly Brit* **hae·mo·cyte** \'hē-mə-ˌsīt\ *n* : a blood cell esp. of an invertebrate animal (as an insect)

he·mo·cy·to·blast *or chiefly Brit* **hae·mo·cy·to·blast** \ˌhē-mə-'sīt-ə-ˌblast\ *n* : a stem cell for blood-cellular elements; *esp* : one considered competent to produce all types of blood cell — called also *lymphoidocyte* — **he·mo·cy·to·blas·tic** *or chiefly Brit* **hae·mo·cy·to·blas·tic** \-ˌsīt-ə-'blast-ik\ *adj*

he·mo·cy·to·blas·to·sis *or chiefly Brit* **hae·mo·cy·to·blas·to·sis** \-ˌsīt-ə-ˌblas-'tō-səs\ *n, pl* **-to·ses** \-ˌsēz\ : lymphocytomatosis of chickens

he·mo·cy·to·gen·e·sis *or chiefly Brit* **hae·mo·cy·to·gen·e·sis** \ˌhē-mō-ˌsīt-ə-'jen-ə-səs\ *n, pl* **-e·ses** \-ˌsēz\ : the part of hematopoiesis concerned with the formation of blood cells

he·mo·cy·tol·y·sis *or chiefly Brit* **hae·mo·cy·tol·y·sis** \-sī-'täl-ə-səs\ *n, pl* **-y·ses** \-ˌsēz\ : a breaking down or dissolution of red blood cells esp. by the action of hypotonic solutions

he·mo·cy·tom·e·ter *or chiefly Brit* **hae·mo·cy·tom·e·ter** \-sī-'täm-ət-ər\ *n* : HEMACYTOMETER

he·mo·di·al·y·sis *or chiefly Brit* **hae·mo·di·al·y·sis** \ˌhē-mō-dī-'al-ə-səs\ *n, pl* **-y·ses** \-ˌsēz\ : DIALYSIS 2a

he·mo·di·a·lyz·er *or chiefly Brit* **hae·mo·di·a·lys·er** \-'dī-ə-ˌlī-zər\ *n* : ARTIFICIAL KIDNEY

he·mo·di·lu·tion *or chiefly Brit* **hae·mo·di·lu·tion** \-dī-'lü-shən, -də-\ *n* **1** : decreased concentration (as after hemorrhage) of cells and solids in the blood resulting from gain of fluid — compare HEMOCONCENTRATION **2** : a medical procedure for producing hemodilution; *esp* : one performed esp. to reduce the number of red blood cells lost during surgery that involves the preoperative withdrawal of one or more units of whole blood, immediate replacement with an equal volume of intravenous fluid (as saline solution), and postoperative reinfusion of withdrawn blood ⟨∼ can be a safe and cost-effective alternative to preoperative autologous donation —P. V. Holland *et al*⟩ — **he·mo·di·lute** *or chiefly Brit* **hae·mo·di·lute** \-'lüt\ *vb* **-lut·ed; -lut·ing**

he·mo·dy·nam·ic *or chiefly Brit* **hae·mo·dy·nam·ic** \-dī-'nam-ik, -də-\ *adj* **1** : of, relating to, or involving hemodynamics **2** : relating to or functioning in the mechanics of blood circulation — **he·mo·dy·nam·i·cal·ly** *or chiefly Brit* **hae·mo·dy·nam·i·cal·ly** \-i-k(ə-)lē\ *adv*

he·mo·dy·nam·ics *or chiefly Brit* **hae·mo·dy·nam·ics** \-iks\ *n pl but sing or pl in constr* **1** : a branch of physiology that deals with the circulation of the blood **2 a** : the forces or mechanisms involved in circulation (as of a particular body part) ⟨renal ∼⟩ **b** : hemodynamic effect (as of a drug)

he·mo·en·do·the·li·al *or chiefly Brit* **hae·mo·en·do·the·li·al** \-ˌen-də-'thē-lē-əl\ *adj, of a placenta* : having the fetal villi reduced to bare capillary loops that are bathed in maternal blood ⟨higher rodents are ∼⟩

he·mo·fil·ter *or chiefly Brit* **hae·mo·fil·ter** \'hē-mō-ˌfil-tər\ *n* : a filter used for hemofiltration

he·mo·fil·tra·tion *or chiefly Brit* **hae·mo·fil·tra·tion** \ˌhē-mō-fil-'trā-shən\ *n* : the process of removing blood from the living body (as of a kidney patient), purifying it by passing it through a system of extracorporeal filters, and returning it to the body

he·mo·fla·gel·late *or chiefly Brit* **hae·mo·fla·gel·late** \-'flaj-ə-lət, -flō-'jel-ət\ *n* : a flagellate (as a trypanosome) that is a blood parasite

he·mo·fus·cin *or chiefly Brit* **hae·mo·fus·cin** \-'fəs-ᵊn\ *n* : a yellowish brown pigment found in small amounts in some normal tissues and increased amounts in some pathological states (as hemochromatosis)

he·mo·glo·bin *or chiefly Brit* **hae·mo·glo·bin** \'hē-mə-ˌglō-bən\ *n* **1** : an iron-containing respiratory pigment of vertebrate red blood cells that functions primarily in the transport of oxygen from the lungs to the tissues of the body, that consists of four polypeptide chains of which two are of the type designated alpha and two are of one of the types designated beta, gamma, or delta and each of which is linked to a heme molecule, that combines loosely and reversibly with oxygen in the lungs or gills to form oxyhemoglobin and with carbon dioxide in the tissues to form carbhemoglobin, that in humans is present normally in blood to the extent of 14 to 16 grams in 100 milliliters expressed sometimes on a scale of 0 to 100 with an average normal value (as 15 grams) taken as 100, and that is determined in blood either colorimetrically or by quantitative estimation of the iron present — see FETAL HEMOGLOBIN, HEMOGLOBIN A; compare CARBOXYHE-

MOGLOBIN, METHEMOGLOBIN **2** : any of numerous iron-containing respiratory pigments of various organisms (as invertebrates and yeasts) — **he·mo·glo·bin·ic** *or chiefly Brit* **hae·mo·glo·bin·ic** \ˌhē-mə-glō-'bin-ik\ *adj* — **he·mo·glo·bi·nous** *or chiefly Brit* **hae·mo·glo·bi·nous** \-'glō-bə-nəs\ *adj*

hemoglobin A *n* : the hemoglobin in the red blood cells of the normal human adult that consists of two alpha chains and two beta chains

hemoglobin C *n* : an abnormal hemoglobin that differs from hemoglobin A in having a lysine residue substituted for the glutamic-acid residue at position 6 in two of the four polypeptide chains making up the hemoglobin molecule

hemoglobin C disease *n* : an inherited hemolytic anemia that occurs esp. in individuals of African descent and is characterized esp. by splenomegaly and the presence of target cells and hemoglobin C in the blood

he·mo·glo·bin·emia *or chiefly Brit* **hae·mo·glo·bin·ae·mia** \-ˌglō-bə-'nē-mē-ə\ *n* : the presence of free hemoglobin in the blood plasma resulting from the solution of hemoglobin out of the red blood cells or from their disintegration

hemoglobin F *n* : FETAL HEMOGLOBIN

he·mo·glo·bin·om·e·ter *or chiefly Brit* **hae·mo·glo·bin·om·e·ter** \-ˌglō-bə-'näm-ət-ər\ *n* : an instrument for the colorimetric determination of hemoglobin in blood — **he·mo·glo·bin·om·e·try** *or chiefly Brit* **hae·mo·glo·bin·om·e·try** \-'näm-ə-trē\ *n, pl* **-tries**

he·mo·glo·bin·op·a·thy *or chiefly Brit* **hae·mo·glo·bin·op·a·thy** \ˌhē-mə-ˌglō-bə-'näp-ə-thē\ *n, pl* **-thies** : a blood disorder (as sickle-cell anemia) caused by a genetically determined change in the molecular structure of hemoglobin

hemoglobin S *n* : an abnormal hemoglobin occurring in the red blood cells in sickle-cell anemia and sickle-cell trait and differing from hemoglobin A in having a valine residue substituted for the glutamic-acid residue in position 6 of two of the four polypeptide chains making up the hemoglobin molecule

he·mo·glo·bin·uria *or chiefly Brit* **hae·mo·glo·bin·uria** \ˌhē-mə-ˌglō-bə-'n(y)ùr-ē-ə\ *n* : the presence of free hemoglobin in the urine — **he·mo·glo·bin·uric** *or chiefly Brit* **hae·mo·glo·bin·uric** \-'n(y)ù(ə)r-ik\ *adj*

he·mo·gram *or chiefly Brit* **hae·mo·gram** \'hē-mə-ˌgram\ *n* : a systematic report of the findings from a blood examination

hemogregarine *var of* HAEMOGREGARINE

he·mo·his·tio·blast *or chiefly Brit* **hae·mo·his·tio·blast** \ˌhē-mō-'hist-ē-ə-ˌblast\ *n* : a hemocytoblast that is a derivative of the reticuloendothelial system

hemokonia *var of* HEMOCONIA

he·mo·lymph *or chiefly Brit* **hae·mo·lymph** \'hē-mə-ˌlim(p)f\ *n* : the circulatory fluid of various invertebrate animals that is functionally comparable to the blood and lymph of vertebrates

hemolymph node *n* : any of several small chiefly retroperitoneal nodes of tissue resembling lymph nodes but having the lymph spaces replaced in whole or in part by blood sinuses — called also *hemal node*

he·mol·y·sate *or* **he·mol·y·zate** *or chiefly Brit* **hae·mol·y·sate** \hi-'mäl-ə-ˌzāt, -ˌsāt\ *n* : a product of hemolysis

he·mo·ly·sin *or chiefly Brit* **hae·mo·ly·sin** \ˌhē-mə-'līs-ᵊn, hi-'mäl-ə-sən\ *n* : a substance that causes the dissolution of red blood cells — called also *hemotoxin;* compare HEMORRHAGIN

he·mo·ly·sis *or chiefly Brit* **hae·mo·ly·sis** \hi-'mäl-ə-səs, ˌhē-mə-'lī-səs\ *n, pl* **-ly·ses** \-ˌsēz\ : lysis of red blood cells with liberation of hemoglobin — see ALPHA HEMOLYSIS, BETA HEMOLYSIS — **he·mo·lyt·ic** *or chiefly Brit* **hae·mo·lyt·ic** \ˌhē-mə-'lit-ik\ *adj*

\ə\ **abut** \ᵊ\ **kitten** \ər\ **further** \a\ **ash** \ā\ **ace** \ä\ **cot, cart**
\aù\ **out** \ch\ **chin** \e\ **bet** \ē\ **easy** \g\ **go** \i\ **hit** \ī\ **ice** \j\ **job**
\ŋ\ **sing** \ō\ **go** \ò\ **law** \òi\ **boy** \th\ **thin** \th\ **the** \ü\ **loot**
\ù\ **foot** \y\ **yet** \zh\ **vision** *See also* Pronunciation Symbols page

hemolytic anemia *n* : anemia caused by excessive destruction (as in chemical poisoning, infection, or sickle-cell anemia) of red blood cells

hemolytic disease of the newborn *n* : ERYTHROBLASTOSIS FETALIS

hemolytic jaundice *n* : a condition characterized by excessive destruction of red blood cells accompanied by jaundice

hemolytic uremic syndrome *n* : any of a group of rare disorders that are characterized by microangiopathic hemolytic anemia, thrombocytopenia, and varying degrees of kidney failure, that are precipitated by a variety of etiologic factors (as infection with toxin-producing bacteria of the genera *Escherichia* or *Shigella*), and that include forms affecting primarily young children or adult females — abbr. *HUS*; see THROMBOTIC THROMBOCYTOPENIC PURPURA

he·mo·lyze *or chiefly Brit* **hae·mo·lyse** \'hē-mə-ˌlīz\ *vb* **-lyzed** *or chiefly Brit* **-lysed; -lyz·ing** *or chiefly Brit* **-lys·ing** *vt* : to cause hemolysis of ~ *vi* : to undergo hemolysis

he·mom·e·ter *or chiefly Brit* **hae·mom·e·ter** \hē-'mäm-ət-ər\ *n* : an instrument for measuring some quality of blood (as hemoglobin content) — **he·mo·met·ric** *or chiefly Brit* **hae·mo·met·ric** \ˌhē-mə-'me-trik\ *adj*

he·mo·par·a·site *or chiefly Brit* **hae·mo·par·a·site** \ˌhē-mō-'par-ə-ˌsīt\ *n* : an animal parasite (as a hemoflagellate or a filarial worm) living in the blood of a vertebrate — **he·mo·par·a·sit·ic** *or chiefly Brit* **hae·mo·par·a·sit·ic** \-ˌpar-ə-'sit-ik\ *adj*

he·mop·a·thy *or chiefly Brit* **hae·mop·a·thy** \hē-'mäp-ə-thē\ *n, pl* **-thies** : a pathological state (as anemia or agranulocytosis) of the blood or blood-forming tissues

he·mo·per·fu·sion *or chiefly Brit* **hae·mo·per·fu·sion** \ˌhē-mō-pər-'fyü-zhən\ *n* : blood cleansing by adsorption on an extracorporeal medium (as activated charcoal) of impurities of larger molecular size than are removed by dialysis

he·mo·peri·car·di·um *or chiefly Brit* **hae·mo·peri·car·di·um** \-ˌper-ə-'kärd-ē-əm\ *n, pl* **-dia** \-ē-ə\ : blood in the pericardial cavity — called also *hematopericardium*

he·mo·peri·to·ne·um *or chiefly Brit* **hae·mo·peri·to·ne·um** \-ˌper-ət-ᵊn-'ē-əm\ *n* : blood in the peritoneal cavity

he·mo·pex·in *or chiefly Brit* **hae·mo·pex·in** \-'pek-sən\ *n* : a glycoprotein that binds heme preventing its excretion in urine and that is part of the beta-globulin fraction of human serum

he·mo·pha·gia *or chiefly Brit* **hae·mo·pha·gia** \-'fā-j(ē-)ə\ *n* **1** : an ingestion of blood **2** : phagocytosis of red blood cells

he·moph·a·gous *or chiefly Brit* **hae·moph·a·gous** \hē-'mäf-ə-gəs\ *adj* : feeding on blood ⟨~ insects⟩

¹**he·mo·phile** *or chiefly Brit* **hae·mo·phile** \'hē-mə-ˌfīl\ *adj* **1** : HEMOPHILIAC **2** : HEMOPHILIC 2

²**hemophile** *or chiefly Brit* **haemophile** *n* **1** : HEMOPHILIAC **2** : a hemophilic organism (as a bacterium)

he·mo·phil·ia *or chiefly Brit* **hae·mo·phil·ia** \ˌhē-mə-'fil-ē-ə\ *n* : a sex-linked hereditary blood defect that occurs almost exclusively in males and is characterized by delayed clotting of the blood and consequent difficulty in controlling hemorrhage even after minor injuries — compare CHRISTMAS DISEASE, HEMORRHAGIC DIATHESIS

hemophilia A *n* : hemophilia caused by the absence of factor VIII from the blood

hemophilia B *n* : CHRISTMAS DISEASE

¹**he·mo·phil·i·ac** *or chiefly Brit* **hae·mo·phil·i·ac** \-'fil-ē-ˌak\ *adj* : of, resembling, or affected with hemophilia

²**hemophiliac** *or chiefly Brit* **haemophiliac** *n* : one affected with hemophilia — called also *bleeder*

¹**he·mo·phil·ic** *or chiefly Brit* **hae·mo·phil·ic** \-'fil-ik\ *adj* **1** : HEMOPHILIAC ⟨a ~ patient⟩ **2** : tending to thrive in blood ⟨~ bacteria⟩

²**hemophilic** *or chiefly Brit* **haemophilic** *n* : HEMOPHILIAC

he·moph·i·lus \hē-'mäf-ə-ləs\ *n* : HAEMOPHILUS 2

He·moph·i·lus \hē-'mäf-ə-ləs\ *n, syn of* HAEMOPHILUS

he·mo·pneu·mo·tho·rax *or chiefly Brit* **hae·mo·pneu·mo·tho·rax** \ˌhē-mə-ˌn(y)ü-mə-'thō(ə)r-ˌaks, -'thȯ(ə)r-\ *n, pl* **-rax·es** *or* **-ra·ces** \-'thōr-ə-ˌsēz, -'thȯr-\ : the accumulation of blood and air in the pleural cavity

he·mo·poi·e·sis *or chiefly Brit* **hae·mo·poi·e·sis** \ˌhē-mə-pȯi-'ē-səs\ *n, pl* **-e·ses** \-ˌsēz\ : HEMATOPOIESIS — **he·mo·poi·et·ic** *or chiefly Brit* **hae·mo·poi·et·ic** \-'et-ik\ *adj*

he·mo·pro·tein *or chiefly Brit* **hae·mo·pro·tein** \-'prō-ˌtēn, -'prōt-ē-ən\ *n* : a conjugated protein (as hemoglobin or cytochrome) whose prosthetic group is a porphyrin combined with iron

He·mo·pro·te·us \ˌhē-mə-'prō-tē-əs\ *n, syn of* HAEMOPROTEUS

he·mop·to·ic *or chiefly Brit* **hae·mop·to·ic** \hi-'mäp-tə-wik\ *adj* : of or produced by hemoptysis

he·mop·ty·sis *or chiefly Brit* **hae·mop·ty·sis** \hi-'mäp-tə-səs\ *n, pl* **-ty·ses** \-ˌsēz\ : expectoration of blood from some part of the respiratory tract

he·mo·rhe·ol·o·gy *or chiefly Brit* **hae·mo·rhe·ol·o·gy** \-rē-'äl-ə-jē\ *n, pl* **-gies** : the science of the physical properties of blood flow in the circulatory system — **he·mo·rheo·log·i·cal** \-ˌrē-ə-'läj-i-kəl\ *also* **he·mo·rheo·log·ic** \-'läj-ik\ *or chiefly Brit* **hae·mo·rheo·log·i·cal** *also* **hae·mo·rheo·log·ic** *adj*

¹**hem·or·rhage** *or chiefly Brit* **haem·or·rhage** \'hem-(ə-)rij\ *n* : a copious discharge of blood from the blood vessels — **hem·or·rhag·ic** *or chiefly Brit* **haem·or·rhag·ic** \ˌhem-ə-'raj-ik\ *adj*

²**hemorrhage** *or chiefly Brit* **haemorrhage** *vi* **-rhaged; -rhag·ing** : to undergo heavy or uncontrollable bleeding

hemorrhagica — see PURPURA HEMORRHAGICA

hemorrhagic dengue *n* : DENGUE HEMORRHAGIC FEVER

hemorrhagic diathesis *n* : an abnormal tendency to spontaneous often severe bleeding — compare HEMOPHILIA, THROMBOCYTOPENIC PURPURA

hemorrhagic fever *n* : any of a diverse group of virus diseases (as Korean hemorrhagic fever, Lassa fever, and Ebola) that are usu. transmitted to humans by arthropods or rodents and are characterized by a sudden onset, fever, aching, bleeding in the internal organs (as of the gastrointestinal tract), petechiae, and shock

hemorrhagic fever with renal syndrome *n* : any of several clinically similar diseases that are caused by hantaviruses (as the Hantaan virus) and are characterized by fever, renal insufficiency, thrombocytopenia, and hemorrhage but not usu. by pulmonary complications — compare HANTAVIRUS PULMONARY SYNDROME

hemorrhagic septicemia *n* : any of several pasteurelloses of domestic animals (as swine plague, shipping fever of cattle and lambs, and fowl cholera) that are caused by a bacterium of the genus *Pasteurella* (*P. multocida*) and are typically marked by internal hemorrhages, fever, mucopurulent discharges, and often pneumonia and diarrhea

hemorrhagic shock *n* : shock resulting from reduction of the volume of blood in the body due to hemorrhage

hemorrhagic stroke *n* : stroke caused by the rupture of a blood vessel with bleeding into the tissue of the brain

hemorrhagicum — see CORPUS HEMORRHAGICUM

hem·or·rhag·in *or chiefly Brit* **haem·or·rhag·in** \ˌhem-ə-'raj-ən\ *n* : a toxic substance occurring usu. as a component of various snake venoms and capable of destroying the blood cells and the walls of small blood vessels — compare HEMOLYSIN

hem·or·rhoid *or chiefly Brit* **haem·or·rhoid** \'hem-(ə-)ˌrȯid\ *n* : a mass of dilated veins in swollen tissue at the margin of the anus or nearby within the rectum — usu. used in pl.; called also *piles*

¹**hem·or·rhoid·al** *or chiefly Brit* **haem·or·rhoid·al** \ˌhem-ə-'rȯid-ᵊl\ *adj* **1** : of, relating to, or involving hemorrhoids **2** : RECTAL

²**hemorrhoidal** *or chiefly Brit* **haemorrhoidal** *n* : a hemorrhoidal part (as an artery or vein)

hemorrhoidal artery *n* : RECTAL ARTERY

hemorrhoidal vein *n* : RECTAL VEIN

hem·or·rhoid·ec·to·my *or chiefly Brit* **haem·or·rhoid·ec·to·my** \ˌhem-ə-ˌrȯi-'dek-tə-mē\ *n, pl* **-mies** : surgical removal of a hemorrhoid

he·mo·sal·pinx *or chiefly Brit* **hae·mo·sal·pinx** \ˌhē-mō-ˈsal-(ˌ)piŋ(k)s\ *n, pl* **-sal·pin·ges** \-sal-ˈpin-(ˌ)jēz\ : HEMATOSALPINX

he·mo·sid·er·in *or chiefly Brit* **hae·mo·sid·er·in** \ˌhē-mō-ˈsid-ə-rən\ *n* : a yellowish brown granular pigment formed by breakdown of hemoglobin, found in phagocytes and in tissues esp. in disturbances of iron metabolism (as in hemochromatosis, hemosiderosis, or some anemias), and composed essentially of colloidal ferric oxide — compare FERRITIN

he·mo·sid·er·o·sis *or chiefly Brit* **hae·mo·sid·er·o·sis** \-ˌsid-ə-ˈrō-səs\ *n, pl* **-o·ses** \-ˌsēz\ : excessive deposition of hemosiderin in bodily tissues as a result of the breakdown of red blood cells — compare HEMOCHROMATOSIS — **he·mo·sid·er·ot·ic** *or chiefly Brit* **hae·mo·sid·er·ot·ic** \-ˈrät-ik\ *adj*

He·mo·spo·rid·ia \-spə-ˈrid-ē-ə\ *n pl, syn of* HAEMOSPORIDIA

he·mo·sta·sis *or chiefly Brit* **hae·mo·sta·sis** \ˌhē-mə-ˈstā-səs\ *n, pl* **-sta·ses** \-ˌsēz\ **1** : stoppage or sluggishness of blood flow **2** : the arrest of bleeding (as by a hemostatic agent)

he·mo·stat *or chiefly Brit* **hae·mo·stat** \ˈhē-mə-ˌstat\ *n* **1** : HEMOSTATIC **2** : an instrument and esp. forceps for compressing a bleeding vessel

¹he·mo·stat·ic *or chiefly Brit* **hae·mo·stat·ic** \ˌhē-mə-ˈstat-ik\ *n* : an agent that checks bleeding; *esp* : one that shortens the clotting time of blood

²hemostatic *or chiefly Brit* **haemostatic** *adj* **1** : of or caused by hemostasis **2** : serving to check bleeding ⟨a ∼ agent⟩

he·mo·ther·a·py *or chiefly Brit* **hae·mo·ther·a·py** \-ˈther-ə-pē\ *n, pl* **-pies** : treatment involving the administration of fresh blood, a blood fraction, or a blood preparation

he·mo·tho·rax *or chiefly Brit* **hae·mo·tho·rax** \ˌhē-mə-ˈthō(ə)r-ˌaks, -ˈthō(ə)r-\ *n, pl* **-tho·rax·es** *or* **-tho·ra·ces** \-ˈthōr-ə-ˌsēz, -ˈthòr-\ : blood in the pleural cavity

he·mo·tox·ic *or chiefly Brit* **hae·mo·tox·ic** \-ˈtäk-sik\ *adj* : destructive to red blood corpuscles ⟨∼ venoms of pit vipers⟩

he·mo·tox·in *or chiefly Brit* **hae·mo·tox·in** \-ˈtäk-sən\ *n* : HEMOLYSIN

he·mot·ro·phe *or chiefly Brit* **hae·mot·ro·phe** \hi-ˈmä-trə-fē\ *n* : the nutrients supplied to the embryo in placental mammals by the maternal bloodstream after formation of the placenta — compare EMBRYOTROPHE, HISTOTROPHE

he·mo·zo·in *or chiefly Brit* **hae·mo·zo·in** \ˌhē-mə-ˈzō-ən\ *n* : an iron-containing pigment which accumulates as cytoplasmic granules in malaria parasites and is a breakdown product of hemoglobin

hemp \ˈhemp\ *n* **1** : a tall widely cultivated Asian herb of the genus *Cannabis* (*C. sativa*) with strong woody fiber used esp. for cordage **2** : the fiber of hemp **3** : a psychoactive drug (as marijuana or hashish) from hemp

hen·bane \ˈhen-ˌbān\ *n* : a poisonous fetid Old World herb of the genus *Hyoscyamus* (*H. niger*) that has sticky hairy dentate leaves and yellowish brown flowers, contains the alkaloids hyoscyamine and scopolamine, and is the source of hyoscyamus — called also *black henbane, insane root*

Hen·der·son–Has·sel·balch equation \ˈhen-dər-sən-ˈhas-əl-ˌbälk-\ *n* : an equation that equates the pH of a buffered solution (as the blood) to the sum of the cologarithm (p) of the dissociation constant (K) of the acid in the buffer and the logarithm of the ratio of the concentration ([ ]) of the salt to that of the acid and that is written

$$pH = pK + \log\frac{[salt]}{[acid]}$$

Henderson, Lawrence Joseph (1878–1942), American biochemist. Henderson is remembered for his discovery of the chemical means by which acid-base equilibria are maintained in nature. In his investigations of body fluids, he discovered that the formation of carbonic acid from carbon dioxide and water in the presence of the salt of the acid (bicarbonates) is the only system in nature that maintains acid-base equilibrium. Henderson developed a chemical equation used to describe these systems, known as physio

logical buffers. This equation is of fundamental importance to biochemistry.

Hasselbalch, Karl Albert (1874–1962), Danish biochemist. In 1916 Hasselbalch converted the equation developed by Lawrence Henderson into logarithmic form. Although the Henderson-Hasselbalch equation is only approximately true, it still remains the most useful mathematical model for treating problems dealing with buffer solutions.

Hen·le's layer \ˈhen-lēz-\ *n* : a single layer of cuboidal epithelium forming the outer boundary of the inner stratum of a hair follicle — compare HUXLEY'S LAYER

Hen·le \ˈhen-lə**, Friedrich Gustav Jacob (1809–1885),** German anatomist and histologist. One of medicine's great anatomists, Henle influenced the development of microscopic anatomy. In 1841 he published the first systematic treatise on histology. He also published the first descriptions of the structure and distribution of human epithelial tissue and of the minute structure of the eye and brain. In the field of pathology he published (1841–53) a two-volume handbook that described diseased organs in relation to their normal physiological functions. This work ushered in the age of modern pathology. The loop of Henle was described in 1862 and the sheath of Henle in 1871.

Henle's loop *n* : LOOP OF HENLE

hen·na \ˈhen-ə\ *n* **1** : an Old World tropical shrub or small tree (*Lawsonia inermis*) of the loosestrife family (Lythraceae) with clusters of fragrant white flowers **2** : a reddish brown dye obtained from the leaves of the henna plant and used esp. on hair and in temporary tattoos

Henoch–Schönlein *adj* : SCHÖNLEIN-HENOCH ⟨∼ purpura⟩

He·noch's purpura \ˈhe-nóks-\ *n* : Schönlein-Henoch purpura that is characterized esp. by gastrointestinal bleeding and pain — compare SCHÖNLEIN'S DISEASE

E. H. Henoch — see SCHÖNLEIN-HENOCH

hen·ry \ˈhen-rē\ *n, pl* **henrys** *or* **henries** : the practical mks unit of inductance equal to the self-inductance of a circuit or the mutual inductance of two circuits in which the variation of one ampere per second results in an induced electromotive force of one volt

Henry, Joseph (1797–1878), American physicist. Henry was a schoolteacher in Albany, New York, and later a professor of mathematics and natural philosophy at Princeton. He conducted a series of investigations into electric phenomena, particularly those related to magnetism. His first major achievement was building a powerful electromagnet, for which he developed insulated wire in order to make a closely wound coil of several layers. He is also credited with constructing primitive versions of the telegraph and the electric motor. In 1846 he became the first secretary and director of the Smithsonian Institution in Washington, D.C. In recognition of his work, his name was given to the henry, the unit of electrical inductance, by international agreement in 1893.

HEPA \ˈhep-ə\ *adj* [*h*igh *e*fficiency *p*articulate *a*ir] : being, using, or containing a filter usu. designed to remove 99.97% of airborne particles measuring 0.3 microns or greater in diameter passing through it ⟨∼ filters⟩ ⟨∼ vacuum cleaners⟩

he·par \ˈhē-ˌpär\ *n* : LIVER

hep·a·ran sulfate \ˈhep-ə-ˌran-\ *n* : a sulfated glycosaminoglycan that accumulates in bodily tissues in abnormal amounts in some mucopolysaccharidoses — called also *heparitin sulfate*

hep·a·rin \ˈhep-ə-rən\ *n* : a glycosaminoglycan sulfuric acid ester that occurs esp. in the liver and lungs, that prolongs the clotting time of blood by preventing the formation of fibrin,

\ə\ **abut** \ᵊ\ kitten \ər\ **further** \a\ **ash** \ā\ **ace** \ä\ **cot, cart**
\au̇\ **out** \ch\ **chin** \e\ **bet** \ē\ **easy** \g\ **go** \i\ **hit** \ī\ **ice** \j\ **job**
\ŋ\ **sing** \ō\ **go** \ȯ\ **law** \ȯi\ **boy** \th\ **thin** \t͟h\ **the** \ü\ **loot**
\u̇\ **foot** \y\ **yet** \zh\ **vision** *See also* Pronunciation Symbols page

G
H

and that is administered parenterally in the form of its sodium salt in vascular surgery and in the treatment of postoperative thrombosis and embolism — see LIQUAEMIN; compare ANTIPROTHROMBIN, ANTITHROMBIN

hep·a·ri·nase \-rə-ˌnās, -ˌnāz\ *n* : an enzyme that breaks down heparin

hep·a·rin·ize *or Brit* **hep·a·rin·ise** \ˈhep-ə-rə-ˌnīz\ *vt* **-ized** *or Brit* **-ised; -iz·ing** *or Brit* **-is·ing** : to treat with heparin ⟨*heparinized* blood⟩ ⟨a *heparinized* laboratory animal⟩ — **hep·a·rin·iza·tion** *or Brit* **hep·a·rin·isa·tion** \-rə-nə-ˈzā-shən\ *n*

hep·a·rin·oid \-ˌnȯid\ *n* : any of various sulfated polysaccharides that have anticoagulant activity resembling that of heparin — **heparinoid** *adj*

hep·a·ri·tin sulfate \ˈhep-ə-ˌrīt-ᵊn-\ *n* : HEPARAN SULFATE

hep·a·tec·to·my \ˌhep-ə-ˈtek-tə-mē\ *n, pl* **-mies** : excision of the liver or of part of the liver — **hep·a·tec·to·mized** *also Brit* **hep·a·tec·to·mised** \-tə-ˌmīzd\ *adj*

he·pat·ic \hi-ˈpat-ik\ *adj* : of, relating to, affecting, or associated with the liver ⟨∼ injury⟩ ⟨∼ insufficiency⟩

hepatic artery *n* : the branch of the celiac artery that supplies the liver with arterial blood

hepatic cell *n* : HEPATOCYTE

hepatic coma *n* : a coma induced by severe liver disease

hepatic duct *n* : a duct conveying the bile away from the liver and in many vertebrates including humans uniting with the cystic duct to form the common bile duct

hepatic flexure *n* : the right-angle bend in the colon on the right side of the body near the liver that marks the junction of the ascending colon and the transverse colon — called also *right colic flexure*

he·pat·i·cos·to·my \hi-ˌpat-i-ˈkäs-tə-mē\ *n, pl* **-mies** : an operation to provide an artificial opening into the hepatic duct

he·pat·i·cot·o·my \-ˈkät-ə-mē\ *n, pl* **-mies** : surgical incision of the hepatic duct

hepatic portal system *n* : a group of veins that carry blood from the capillaries of the stomach, intestine, spleen, and pancreas to the sinusoids of the liver

hepatic portal vein *n* : a portal vein carrying blood from the digestive organs and spleen to the liver where the nutrients carried by the blood are altered by hepatocytes before passing into the systemic circulation

hepaticus — see FETOR HEPATICUS

hepatic vein *n* : any of the veins that carry the blood received from the hepatic artery and from the hepatic portal vein away from the liver and that in humans are usu. three in number and open into the inferior vena cava

hepatis — see PORTA HEPATIS

hep·a·ti·tis \ˌhep-ə-ˈtīt-əs\ *n, pl* **-tit·i·des** \-ˈtit-ə-ˌdēz\ *also* **-ti·tis·es** \-ˈtīt-ə-səz\ **1** : inflammation of the liver **2** : a disease or condition (as hepatitis A or hepatitis B) marked by inflammation of the liver — **hep·a·tit·ic** \-ˈtit-ik\ *adj*

hepatitis A \-ˈā\ *n* : an acute usu. benign hepatitis caused by a single-stranded RNA virus of the family *Picornaviridae* (species *Hepatitis A virus* of the genus *Hepatovirus*) that does not persist in the blood serum and is transmitted esp. in food and water contaminated with infected fecal matter — called also *infectious hepatitis;* see HAVRIX

hepatitis B \-ˈbē\ *n* : a sometimes fatal hepatitis caused by a double-stranded DNA virus (species *Hepatitis B virus* of the genus *Orthohepadnavirus,* family *Hepadnaviridae*) that tends to persist in the blood serum and is transmitted esp. by contact with infected blood (as by transfusion or by sharing contaminated needles in illicit intravenous drug use) or by contact with other infected bodily fluids (as semen) — called also *serum hepatitis*

hepatitis B surface antigen *n* : an antigen that is usu. a surface particle from the hepatitis B virus and that is found in the sera esp. of patients with hepatitis B — abbr. *HBsAg;* called also *Australia antigen*

hepatitis C \-ˈsē\ *n* : hepatitis caused by a single-stranded RNA virus of the family *Flaviviridae* (species *Hepatitis C virus* of the genus *Hepacivirus*) that tends to persist in the blood serum and is usu. transmitted by infected blood (as by injection of an illicit drug, blood transfusion, or exposure to

blood or blood products) and that accounts for most cases of non-A, non-B hepatitis

hepatitis D \-ˈdē\ *n* : hepatitis that is similar to hepatitis B and is caused by coinfection with the hepatitis B virus and hepatitis D virus — called also *delta hepatitis*

hepatitis delta *n* : HEPATITIS D

hepatitis delta virus *n* : HEPATITIS D VIRUS

hepatitis D virus *n* : a subviral particle lacking the protein coat and the surface antigens of the hepatitis B virus that is unable to invade cells except in the presence of the hepatitis B virus and together with this virus causes hepatitis D — called also *delta agent, delta virus*

hepatitis E \-ˈē\ *n* : a hepatitis that is rare in the U.S. but is common in some third-world countries, is usu. contracted from sewage-contaminated water, and is caused by a highly variable single-stranded RNA virus (species *Hepatitis E virus*) of uncertain taxonomic affinities but related to members of the family *Caliciviridae*

hep·a·ti·za·tion \ˌhep-ət-ə-ˈzā-shən\ *n* : conversion of tissue (as of the lungs in pneumonia) into a substance which resembles liver tissue and may become solidified — **hep·a·tized** \ˈhep-ə-ˌtīzd\ *adj*

he·pa·to·bil·i·ary \ˌhep-ət-ō-ˈbil-ē-ˌer-ē, hi-ˌpat-ə-\ *adj* : of, relating to, situated in or near, produced in, or affecting the liver and bile, bile ducts, and gallbladder ⟨∼ disease⟩ ⟨the ∼ system⟩

he·pa·to·blas·to·ma \-blas-ˈtō-mə\ *n, pl* **-mas** *also* **-ma·ta** \-mət-ə\ : a malignant tumor of the liver esp. of infants and young children that is composed of cells resembling embryonic liver cells

he·pa·to·car·cin·o·gen \-kär-ˈsin-ə-jən, -ˈkärs-ᵊn-ə-ˌjen\ *n* : a substance or agent causing cancer of the liver

he·pa·to·car·cin·o·gen·e·sis \-ˌkärs-ᵊn-ō-ˈjen-ə-səs\ *n, pl* **-e·ses** \-ˌsēz\ : the production of cancer of the liver

he·pa·to·car·cin·o·gen·ic \-ˈjen-ik\ *adj* : producing or tending to produce cancer of the liver

he·pa·to·car·ci·no·ge·nic·i·ty \-jə-ˈnis-ət-ē\ *n, pl* **-ties** : the power or tendency to produce cancer of the liver

he·pa·to·car·ci·no·ma \-ˌkärs-ᵊn-ˈō-mə\ *n, pl* **-mas** *also* **-ma·ta** \-mət-ə\ : carcinoma of the liver

he·pa·to·cel·lu·lar \ˌhep-ət-ō-ˈsel-yə-lər, hi-ˌpat-ə-ˈsel-\ *adj* : of or involving hepatocytes ⟨∼ carcinomas⟩ ⟨∼ necrosis⟩

he·pa·to·cyte \hi-ˈpat-ə-ˌsīt, ˈhep-ət-ə-\ *n* : any of the polygonal epithelial parenchymatous cells of the liver that secrete bile — called also *hepatic cell, liver cell*

he·pa·to·gen·ic \ˌhep-ət-ō-ˈjen-ik, hi-ˌpat-ə-\ *or* **hep·a·tog·e·nous** \ˌhep-ə-ˈtäj-ə-nəs\ *adj* : produced or originating in the liver ⟨∼ hypoglycemia⟩ ⟨∼ metabolites⟩

hep·a·tog·ra·phy \ˌhep-ə-ˈtäg-rə-fē\ *n, pl* **-phies** : radiography of the liver

he·pa·to·len·tic·u·lar degeneration \hi-ˌpat-ə-len-ˌtik-yə-lər-, ˌhep-ət-ō-\ *n* : WILSON'S DISEASE

he·pa·to·li·en·og·ra·phy \hi-ˌpat-ə-ˌlī-ən-ˈäg-rə-fē, ˌhep-ət-ō-\ *n, pl* **-phies** : radiographic visualization of the liver and spleen after injection of a radiopaque medium

hep·a·tol·o·gy \ˌhep-ə-ˈtäl-ə-jē\ *n, pl* **-gies** : a branch of medicine concerned with the liver — **hep·a·tol·o·gist** \-ə-jəst\ *n*

hep·a·to·ma \ˌhep-ə-ˈtō-mə\ *n, pl* **-mas** *also* **-ma·ta** \-mət-ə\ : a usu. malignant tumor of the liver — **hep·a·to·ma·tous** \-mət-əs\ *adj*

he·pa·to·meg·a·ly \ˌhep-ət-ō-ˈmeg-ə-lē, hi-ˌpat-ə-ˈmeg-\ *n, pl* **-lies** : enlargement of the liver — **he·pa·to·meg·a·lic** \-ˈmeg-ə-lik\ *adj*

he·pa·to·pan·cre·at·ic \hi-ˌpat-ə-ˌpan-krē-ˈat-ik, ˌhep-ət-ō-, -ˌpan-\ *adj* : of or relating to the liver and the pancreas

hep·a·top·a·thy \ˌhep-ə-ˈtäp-ə-thē\ *n, pl* **-thies** : an abnormal or diseased state of the liver

he·pa·to·por·tal \ˌhep-ət-ō-ˈpȯrt-ᵊl, hi-ˌpat-ə-\ *adj* : of or relating to the hepatic portal system

he·pa·to·re·nal \-ˈrē-nəl\ *adj* : of, relating to, or affecting the liver and the kidneys ⟨fatal ∼ dysfunction⟩

hepatorenal syndrome *n* : functional kidney failure associated with cirrhosis of the liver and characterized typically by jaundice, ascites, hypoalbuminemia, hypoprothrombinemia, and encephalopathy

hep·a·tor·rha·phy \ˌhep-ə-ˈtȯr-ə-fē\ *n, pl* **-phies** : suture of a wound or injury to the liver

hep·a·to·sis \ˌhep-ə-ˈtō-səs\ *n, pl* **-to·ses** \-ˌsēz\ : any noninflammatory functional disorder of the liver

he·pa·to·splen·ic \ˌhep-ət-ō-ˈsplen-ik, hi-ˌpat-ə-\ *adj* : of or affecting the liver and spleen ⟨∼ schistosomiasis⟩

he·pa·to·spleno·meg·a·ly \-splen-ō-ˈmeg-ə-lē\ *n, pl* **-lies** : coincident enlargement of the liver and spleen

hep·a·tot·o·my \ˌhep-ə-ˈtät-ə-mē\ *n, pl* **-mies** : surgical incision of the liver

he·pa·to·tox·ic \ˌhep-ət-ō-ˈtäk-sik, hi-ˌpat-ə-ˈtäk-\ *adj* : relating to or causing injury to the liver ⟨∼ drugs⟩

he·pa·to·tox·ic·i·ty \-täk-ˈsis-ət-ē\ *n, pl* **-ties** **1** : a state of toxic damage to the liver **2** : a tendency or capacity to cause hepatotoxicity

he·pa·to·tox·in \-ˈtäk-sən\ *n* : a substance toxic to the liver

hep·ta·chlor \ˈhep-tə-ˌklō(ə)r, -ˌklȯ(ə)r\ *n* : a persistent cyclodiene chlorinated hydrocarbon pesticide $C_{10}H_5Cl_7$ that causes liver disease in animals and is a suspected human carcinogen

hep·ta·no·ic acid \ˌhep-tə-ˌnō-ik-\ *n* : an oily fatty acid $C_7H_{14}O_2$ used chiefly in making esters — called also *enanthic acid*

hep·tose \ˈhep-ˌtōs, -ˌtōz\ *n* : any of various monosaccharides $C_7H_{14}O_7$ containing seven carbon atoms in a molecule

herb \ˈ(h)ərb\ *n, often attrib* **1** : a seed plant that does not develop persistent woody tissue but dies down at the end of a growing season **2** : a plant or plant part valued for its medicinal, savory, or aromatic qualities

¹herb·al \ˈ(h)ər-bəl\ *n* **1** : a book about plants esp. with reference to their medical properties **2** : HERBAL REMEDY

²herbal *adj* : of, relating to, or made of herbs

herb·al·ism \ˈ(h)ər-bə-ˌliz-əm\ *n* : HERBAL MEDICINE 1

herb·al·ist \-ləst\ *n* **1** : one who collects or grows herbs **2** : one who practices herbal medicine

herbal medicine *n* **1** : the art or practice of using herbs and herbal remedies to maintain health and to prevent, alleviate, or cure disease — called also *herbalism* **2** : HERBAL REMEDY

herbal remedy *n* : a plant or plant part or an extract or mixture of these used to prevent, alleviate, or cure disease — called also *herbal, herbal medicine*

herb doctor *n* : HERBALIST 2

her·bi·cide \ˈ(h)ər-bə-ˌsīd\ *n* : an agent used to destroy or inhibit plant growth — **her·bi·cid·al** \ˌ(h)ər-bə-ˈsīd-ᵊl\ *adj* — **her·bi·cid·al·ly** \-ᵊl-ē\ *adv*

her·bi·vore \ˈ(h)ər-bə-ˌvō(ə)r, -ˌvȯ(ə)r\ *n* : a plant-eating animal; *esp* : UNGULATE

her·biv·o·rous \ˌ(h)ər-ˈbiv-ə-rəs\ *adj* **1** : feeding on plants ⟨∼ mammals⟩ **2** : having a stout body and a long small intestine : ENDOMORPHIC — **her·biv·o·rous·ly** *adv*

her·biv·o·ry \-ˈbiv-ə-rē\ *n, pl* **-ries** : the state or condition of feeding on plants

Her·cep·tin \hər-ˈsep-tən\ *trademark* — used for a preparation of trastuzumab

herd immunity \ˈhərd-\ *n* : a reduction in the probability of infection that is held to apply to susceptible members of a population in which a significant proportion of the individuals are immune because the chance of coming in contact with an infected individual is less

he·red·i·tar·i·an \hə-ˌred-ə-ˈter-ē-ən\ *n* : an advocate of the theory that individual differences in human beings can be accounted for primarily on the basis of genetics — **hereditarian** *adj* — **he·red·i·tar·i·an·ism** \-ē-ə-ˌniz-əm\ *n*

he·red·i·tary \hə-ˈred-ə-ˌter-ē\ *adj* **1** : genetically transmitted or transmittable from parent to offspring — compare ACQUIRED 2, CONGENITAL 2, FAMILIAL **2** : of or relating to inheritance or heredity — **he·red·i·tar·i·ly** \-ˌred-ə-ˈter-ə-lē\ *adv*

hereditary hemorrhagic telangiectasia *n* : a hereditary abnormality that is characterized by multiple telangiectasias and by bleeding into the tissues and mucous membranes be-

cause of abnormal fragility of the capillaries — called also *Rendu-Osler-Weber disease*

hereditary spherocytosis *n* : a disorder of red blood cells that is inherited as a dominant trait and is characterized by anemia, small thick fragile spherocytes which are extremely susceptible to hemolysis, enlargement of the spleen, reticulocytosis, and mild jaundice

he·red·i·ty \hə-ˈred-ət-ē\ *n, pl* **-ties** **1** : the sum of the qualities and potentialities genetically derived from one's ancestors **2** : the transmission of traits from ancestor to descendant through the molecular mechanism lying primarily in the DNA or RNA of the genes — compare MEIOSIS

her·e·do·fa·mil·ial \ˌher-ə-dō-fə-ˈmil-yəl\ *adj* : tending to occur in more than one member of a family and suspected of having a genetic basis ⟨a ∼ disease⟩

Her·ing–Breu·er reflex \ˈher-iŋ-ˈbrȯi-ər-\ *n* : any of several reflexes that control inflation and deflation of the lungs; *esp* : reflex inhibition of inspiration triggered by pulmonary muscle spindles upon expansion of the lungs and mediated by the vagus nerve

Hering, Karl Ewald Konstantin (1834–1918), German physiologist and psychologist. Hering is known for his great influence on contemporary sense physiology and the evolution of modern psychology, especially Gestalt psychology. His early research was on binocular vision. From 1861 to 1864 he published a five-part study on visual space perception. In 1868 with Josef Breuer he discovered the reflex reaction that originates in the lungs and is mediated by the fibers of the vagus nerve and that is now known as the Hering-Breuer reflex. In a series of papers published between 1872 and 1875 he presented his theory of color vision. From that time onward, he devoted most of his career to studying color phenomena.

Breuer, Josef (1842–1925), Austrian physician and physiologist. A major forerunner of psychoanalysis, Breuer is famous for relieving the patient "Anna O." of her hysteria by inducing her to recall, while under hypnosis, traumatic experiences of her early life. He reached the critical insight that neurotic symptoms derive from unconscious processes and that the symptoms can disappear when the processes are made conscious. Sigmund Freud was an early colleague of Breuer, and in 1895 the two men wrote a book on hysteria in which Breuer's method of psychotherapy was described. In 1868 with Karl Hering he described the Hering-Breuer reflex.

Hering theory *n* : a theory of color vision: the sensation of color depends on three processes of which each has two mutually exclusive modes of reaction that are yellow or blue, red or green, and white or black

her·i·ta·bil·i·ty \ˌher-ət-ə-ˈbil-ət-ē\ *n, pl* **-ties** **1** : the quality or state of being heritable **2** : the proportion of observed variation in a particular trait (as intelligence) that can be attributed to inherited genetic factors in contrast to environmental ones

her·i·ta·ble \ˈher-ət-ə-bəl\ *adj* : HEREDITARY ⟨one of several ∼ childhood cancers —W. K. Cavenee *et al*⟩

her·maph·ro·dism \(ˌ)hər-ˈmaf-rə-ˌdiz-əm\ *n* : HERMAPHRODITISM

Her·maph·ro·di·tus \(ˌ)hər-ˌmaf-rə-ˈdīt-əs\, Greek mythological character. Hermaphroditus was the son of Hermes and Aphrodite and renowned for his beauty. A fountain nymph became enamored of him and asked the gods to unite her with him in one body. The result was a creature who was half man and half woman.

her·maph·ro·dite \(ˌ)hər-ˈmaf-rə-ˌdīt\ *n* **1** : an abnormal individual esp. among the higher vertebrates having both male and female reproductive organs — called also *androgyne* **2** : a plant or animal (as a hydra) that normally has both male and female reproductive organs — **hermaphrodite** *adj*

G
H

\ə\ **abut** \ᵊ\ **kitten** \ər\ **further** \a\ **ash** \ā\ **ace** \ä\ **cot, cart** \au̇\ **out** \ch\ **chin** \e\ **bet** \ē\ **easy** \g\ **go** \i\ **hit** \ī\ **ice** \j\ **job** \ŋ\ **sing** \ō\ **go** \ȯ\ **law** \ȯi\ **boy** \th\ **thin** \t̲h̲\ **the** \ü\ **loot** \u̇\ **foot** \y\ **yet** \zh\ **vision** *See also* Pronunciation Symbols page

her·maph·ro·dit·ism \(ͺ)hər-'maf-rə-ͺdīt-ͺiz-əm\ *n* : the condition of being a hermaphrodite — called also *hermaphrodism* — **her·maph·ro·dit·ic** \(ͺ)hər-ͺmaf-rə-'dit-ik\ *adj*

her·met·ic \(ͺ)hər-'met-ik\ *adj* : being airtight or impervious to air — **her·met·i·cal·ly** \-i-k(ə-)lē\ *adv*

Her·mes   Tris·me·gis·tus \'hər-ͺmēz-ͺtris-mə-'jis-təs\, Greek mythological character. Hermes Trismegistus was identified by the Greeks with the Egyptian god Thoth. To him was ascribed authorship of various works on astrology, magic, alchemy, and medicine. It was also believed that he had invented a magic seal to keep vessels airtight, and from his name the adjective *hermetic* meaning airtight was derived.

her·nia \'hər-nē-ə\ *n, pl* **-ni·as** *or* **-ni·ae** \-nē-ͺē, -nē-ͺī\ : a protrusion of an organ or part through connective tissue or through a wall of the cavity in which it is normally enclosed — called also *rupture;* see ABDOMINAL HERNIA, HIATAL HERNIA, STRANGULATED HERNIA — **her·ni·al** \-nē-əl\ *adj*

hernial sac *n* : a protruding pouch of peritoneum that contains a herniated organ or tissue

her·ni·ate \'hər-nē-ͺāt\ *vi* **-at·ed; -at·ing** : to protrude through an abnormal body opening : RUPTURE 〈*herniated* intravertebral disks〉

her·ni·a·tion \ͺhər-nē-'ā-shən\ *n* **1** : the act or process of herniating **2** : HERNIA

her·nio·plas·ty \'hər-nē-ə-ͺplast-ē\ *n, pl* **-ties** : HERNIORRHAPHY

her·ni·or·rha·phy \ͺhər-nē-'ȯr-ə-fē\ *n, pl* **-phies** : an operation for hernia that involves opening the hernial sac, returning the contents to their normal place, obliterating the hernial sac, and closing the opening with strong sutures

her·ni·ot·o·my \-'ät-ə-mē\ *n, pl* **-mies** : the operation of cutting through a band of tissue that constricts a strangulated hernia

he·ro·ic \hi-'rō-ik *also* her-'ō- *or* hē-'rō-\ *adj* **1** : of a kind that is likely to be undertaken only to save life 〈~ surgery〉 〈~ treatment〉 **2** : having a pronounced effect — used chiefly of medicaments or dosage 〈~ doses〉 〈a ~ drug〉

her·o·in \'her-ə-wən\ *n* : a strongly physiologically addictive narcotic $C_{21}H_{23}NO_5$ that is made by acetylation of but is more potent than morphine and that is prohibited for medical use in the U.S. but is used illicitly for its euphoric effects — called also *acetomorphine, diacetylmorphine, diamorphine*

her·o·in·ism \-wə-ͺniz-əm\ *n* : addiction to heroin

her·pan·gi·na \ͺhər-ͺpan-'jī-nə, ͺhər-'pan-jə-nə\ *n* : a contagious disease of children characterized by fever, headache, and a vesicular eruption in the throat and caused by any of numerous coxsackieviruses and echoviruses

her·pes \'hər-(ͺ)pēz\ *n* : any of several inflammatory diseases of the skin caused by herpesviruses and characterized by clusters of vesicles; *esp* : HERPES SIMPLEX

her·pes gen·i·tal·is \ͺhər-(ͺ)pēz-ͺjen-ə-'tal-əs\ *n* : GENITAL HERPES

herpes keratitis *n* : keratitis caused by any of the herpesviruses that produce herpes simplex or shingles

herpes la·bi·al·is \-ͺlā-bē-'al-əs\ *n* : herpes simplex affecting the lips and nose

herpes pro·gen·i·tal·is \-ͺprō-ͺjen-ə-'tal-əs\ *n* : GENITAL HERPES

herpes sim·plex \-'sim-ͺpleks\ *n* : either of two viral diseases caused by herpesviruses of the genus *Simplexvirus* that are marked esp. by watery blisters on the skin or mucous membranes of the lips, mouth, face, or genital region — see HSV-1, HSV-2

Her·pes·vi·ri·dae \-'vir-ə-ͺdē\ *n pl* : a family of double-stranded DNA viruses that consist of a spherical virion having the DNA packaged in a liquid crystalline array in a central core surrounded by an icosahedral capsid, an amorphous layer of proteins, and an envelope consisting of a lipid bilayer closely associated with the amorphous protein layer and that include the cytomegalovirus and Epstein-Barr virus and the causative agents of chicken pox, equine coital exanthema, herpes simplex, infectious bovine rhinotracheitis, infectious laryngotracheitis, malignant catarrhal fever, Mar-

ek's disease, pseudorabies, rhinopneumonitis, roseola infantum, and shingles — see SIMPLEXVIRUS, VARICELLOVIRUS

her·pes·vi·rus \-'vī-rəs\ *n* : any of a family *Herpesviridae* of double-stranded DNA viruses

herpes zos·ter \-'zäs-tər\ *n* : SHINGLES

her·pet·ic \(ͺ)hər-'pet-ik\ *adj* : of, relating to, or resembling herpes 〈~ pain〉 〈~ lesions〉

her·pet·i·form \-'pet-ə-ͺfȯrm\ *adj* : resembling herpes

herpetiformis — see DERMATITIS HERPETIFORMIS

her·pe·tom·o·nas \ͺhər-pə-'täm-ə-nəs, -ͺnas\ *n* **1** *cap* : a genus of flagellates of the family Trypanosomatidae morphologically similar to the genus *Trypanosoma* but exclusively parasites of the gut of insects **2** : any flagellate of the genus *Herpetomonas*; *also* : any member of the family Trypanosomatidae that appears to have two flagella due to precocious duplication of the locomotor apparatus

her·pe·to·pho·bia \ͺhər-pət-ə-'fō-bē-ə\ *n* : a morbid fear of reptiles

Hert·wig's sheath \'hərt-wigz-, 'hert-vik̲s-\ *n* : SHEATH OF HERTWIG

hertz \'hərts, 'herts\ *n* : a unit of frequency equal to one cycle per second — abbr. *Hz*

Herx·heim·er reaction \'hərks-ͺhī-mər-\ *n* : JARISCH-HERXHEIMER REACTION

Heschl's gyrus \'hesh-əlz-\ *n* : a convolution of the temporal lobe that is the cortical center for hearing and runs obliquely outward and forward from the posterior part of the lateral sulcus

    Heschl, Richard Ladislaus (1824–1881), Austrian anatomist. A professor of pathological anatomy, Heschl in 1855 published a textbook on the subject. The text includes his description of the convolution of the temporal lobe that now is known as Heschl's gyrus.

hes·per·i·din \he-'sper-əd-ən\ *n* : a crystalline glycoside $C_{28}H_{34}O_{15}$ found in most citrus fruits and esp. in orange peel

Hes·sel·bach's triangle \'hes-əl-ͺbäks-\ *n* : TRIANGLE OF HESSELBACH

het·a·cil·lin \ͺhet-ə-'sil-ən\ *n* : a semisynthetic oral penicillin $C_{19}H_{23}N_3O_4S$ that is converted to ampicillin in the body and has medical uses similar to those of ampicillin

het·er·a·kid \ͺhet-ə-'rā-kəd\ *n* : any nematode worm of the family (Heterakidae) to which the genus *Heterakis* belongs — **heterakid** *adj*

Het·er·a·kis \-'rā-kəs\ *n* : a genus (the type of the family Heterakidae) of nematode worms including one (*H. gallinae*) that infests esp. chickens and turkeys and serves as an intermediate host and transmitter of the protozoan causing blackhead

het·ero \'het-ə-ͺrō\ *n, pl* **-er·os** : HETEROSEXUAL

het·ero·ag·glu·ti·nin \ͺhet-ə-rō-ə-'glüt-ⁿn-ən\ *n* : a hemagglutinin found in serum and reacting with heterologous red blood cells

het·ero·an·ti·body \-'ant-i-ͺbäd-ē\ *n, pl* **-dies** : an antibody specific for a heterologous antigen

het·ero·an·ti·gen \-'ant-i-jən, -ͺjen\ *n* : an antibody that is produced by an individual of one species and is capable of stimulating an immune response in an individual of another species

het·ero·at·om \'het-ə-rō-ͺat-əm\ *n* : an atom other than carbon in the ring of a heterocyclic compound

het·ero·aux·in \ͺhet-ə-rō-'ȯk-sən\ *n* : INDOLEACETIC ACID

heterocaryon, heterocaryosis, heterocaryotic *var of* HETEROKARYON, HETEROKARYOSIS, HETEROKARYOTIC

het·ero·cel·lu·lar \ͺhet-ə-rō-'sel-yə-lər\ *adj* : composed of more than one kind of cell

het·ero·chro·mat·ic \-krə-'mat-ik\ *adj* **1** : made up of various wavelengths or frequencies 〈white light is ~〉 **2** : of or relating to heterochromatin 〈~ regions of chromosomes〉

het·ero·chro·ma·tin \-'krō-mət-ən\ *n* : densely staining chromatin that appears as nodules in or along chromosomes and contains relatively few genes

het·ero·chro·ma·ti·za·tion \ͺhet-ər-ō-ͺkrō-mə-tə-'zā-shən\ *also* **het·ero·chro·ma·tin·iza·tion** \-mə-tin-i-'zā-\ *also Brit* **het·ero·chro·ma·ti·sa·tion** *also* **het·ero·chro·ma·tin·isa-**

tion *n* : the transformation of or the extent of the transformation of genetically active euchromatin to inactive heterochromatin — **het·ero·chro·ma·tized** *also Brit* **het·ero·chro·ma·tised** \-'krō-mə-ˌtīzd\ *adj*

het·ero·chro·mia \-'krō-mē-ə\ *n* : a difference in coloration in two anatomical structures or two parts of the same structure which are normally alike in color ⟨∼ of the iris⟩

heterochromia ir·i·dis \-'ir-i-dəs\ *n* : a difference in color between the irises of the two eyes or between parts of one iris

het·ero·chro·mo·some \-'krō-mə-ˌsōm, -ˌzōm\ *n* : SEX CHROMOSOME

het·er·och·ro·nism \ˌhet-ə-'räk-rə-ˌniz-əm\ *n* : HETEROCHRONY

het·er·och·ro·ny \-'räk-rə-nē\ *n, pl* **-nies** 1 : deviation from the typical embryological sequence of formation of organs and parts as a factor in evolution 2 : irregularity in time relationships; *specif* : the existence of differences in chronaxies among functionally related tissue elements — **het·er·och·ro·nous** \-'räk-rə-nəs\ *adj*

het·ero·crine \'het-ə-rə-ˌkrin, -ˌkrīn, -ˌkrēn\ *adj* : having both an endocrine and an exocrine secretion

het·ero·cy·cle \'het-ər-ō-ˌsī-kəl\ *n* : a heterocyclic ring system or a heterocyclic compound

¹**het·ero·cy·clic** \ˌhet-ə-rō-'sī-klik, -'sik-lik\ *adj* : relating to, characterized by, or being a ring composed of atoms of more than one kind ⟨∼ chemical compounds⟩

²**heterocyclic** *n* : HETEROCYCLE

heterocyclic amine *n* : an amine containing one or more closed rings of carbon and nitrogen; *esp* : any of various carcinogenic amines that are formed when creatine or creatinine reacts with free amino acids and sugar in meat cooked at high temperature — abbr. *HCA*

het·ero·di·mer \-'dī-mər\ *n* : a protein composed of two polypeptide chains differing in composition in the order, number, or kind of their amino acid residues — **het·ero·di·mer·ic** \-dī-'mer-ik\ *adj*

¹**het·er·odont** \'het-ə-rə-ˌdänt\ *adj* : having the teeth differentiated into incisors, canines, and molars ⟨∼ mammals⟩ — compare HOMODONT

²**heterodont** *n* : any animal (as a human) with heterodont dentition

het·ero·du·plex \ˌhet-ə-rō-'d(y)ü-ˌpleks\ *n* : a nucleic-acid molecule (as DNA) composed of two chains with each derived from a different parent molecule — **heteroduplex** *adj*

het·er·oe·cious \ˌhet-ə-'rē-shəs\ *adj* : passing through the different stages in the life cycle on alternate and often unrelated hosts ⟨∼ insects⟩ — **het·er·oe·cism** \-'rē-ˌsiz-əm\ *n*

het·ero·er·o·tism \ˌhet-ər-ō-'er-ə-ˌtiz-əm\ *n* : ALLOEROTISM — **het·ero·erot·ic** \-i-'rät-ik\ *adj*

het·ero·fer·men·ta·tive \-(ˌ)fər-'ment-ət-iv\ *adj* : producing a fermentation resulting in a number of end products — used esp. of lactic-acid bacteria that ferment carbohydrates and produce volatile acids and carbon dioxide as well as lactic acid — **het·ero·fer·ment·er** \-(ˌ)fər-'ment-ər\ *n*

het·ero·ga·mete \ˌhet-ə-rō-gə-'mēt, -'gam-ˌēt\ *n* : either of a pair of gametes that differ in form, size, or behavior and occur typically as large nonmotile female gametes and small motile sperms

het·ero·ga·met·ic \-gə-'met-ik, -'mēt-\ *adj* : forming two kinds of gametes of which one determines offspring of one sex and the other determines offspring of the opposite sex ⟨the human male is ∼⟩ — **het·ero·gam·e·ty** \-'gam-ət-ē\ *n, pl* **-ties**

het·er·og·a·mous \ˌhet-ə-'räg-ə-məs\ *adj* : having or characterized by fusion of unlike gametes — compare ANISOGAMOUS, ISOGAMOUS

het·er·og·a·my \-mē\ *n, pl* **-mies** 1 : sexual reproduction involving fusion of unlike gametes often differing in size, structure, and physiology 2 : the condition of reproducing by heterogamy

het·ero·ge·ne·ity \ˌhet-ə-rō-jə-'nē-ət-ē, ˌhe-trō-\ *n, pl* **-ties** : the quality or state of being heterogeneous

het·ero·ge·neous \ˌhet-ə-rə-'jē-nē-əs, ˌhe-trə-, -nyəs\ *adj* : not

uniform in structure or composition ⟨tumors which have a ∼ composition by reason of structure and presence of necrosis —*Yr. Bk. of Endocrinology*⟩ — **het·ero·ge·neous·ly** *adv*

het·ero·gen·e·sis \ˌhet-ə-rō-'jen-ə-səs\ *n, pl* **-e·ses** \-ˌsēz\ 1 : ABIOGENESIS 2 : ALTERNATION OF GENERATIONS

het·ero·ge·net·ic \-jə-'net-ik\ *adj* 1 : of, relating to, or characterized by heterogenesis 2 : HETEROPHILE

het·ero·gen·ic \ˌhet-ər-ə-'jen-ic\ *adj* 1 : containing more than one allele of a gene — used of a cell or of population 2 : derived from or involving individuals of a different species ⟨∼ antigens⟩ ⟨∼ transplantation⟩

het·ero·ge·note \ˌhet-ər-ō-'jē-ˌnōt\ *n* : a partially diploid bacterium in which the added genetic material differs from that orig. present and is usu. transferred by transduction — **het·ero·ge·not·ic** \-jə-'nät-ik\ *adj*

het·er·og·e·nous \ˌhet-ə-'räj-ə-nəs\ *adj* 1 : originating in an outside source; *esp* : derived from another species ⟨∼ bone grafts⟩ 2 : HETEROGENEOUS

het·ero·gon·ic \ˌhet-ə-rə-'gän-ik\ *adj* 1 : of, relating to, or marked by allometry 2 a : being or characterized by a course of development in which a generation of parasites is succeeded by a free-living generation ⟨a ∼ life cycle of a nematode worm⟩ — compare HOMOGONIC b : relating to or being the free-living generation of a heterogonic life cycle

het·er·og·o·ny \ˌhet-ə-'räg-ə-nē\ *n, pl* **-nies** 1 : ALTERNATION OF GENERATIONS; *esp* : alternation of a dioecious generation with a parthenogenetic one 2 : ALLOMETRY

het·ero·graft \'het-ə-rō-ˌgräft\ *n* : XENOGRAFT

het·ero·kary·on *also* **het·ero·cary·on** \ˌhet-ə-rō-'kar-ē-ˌän, -ən\ *n* : a cell in the mycelium of a fungus that contains two or more genetically unlike nuclei — compare HOMOKARYON

het·ero·kary·o·sis *also* **het·ero·cary·o·sis** \-ˌkar-ē-'ō-səs\ *n* : the condition of having cells that are heterokaryons

het·ero·kary·ot·ic *also* **het·ero·cary·ot·ic** \-ē-'ät-ik\ *adj* : of, relating to, or consisting of heterokaryons

het·ero·lat·er·al \-'lat-ə-rəl, -'la-trəl\ *adj* : CONTRALATERAL

het·er·ol·o·gous \ˌhet-ə-'räl-ə-gəs\ *adj* 1 : derived from a different species ⟨∼ DNAs⟩ ⟨∼ transplants⟩ — compare AUTOLOGOUS, HOMOLOGOUS 2a 2 : characterized by cross-reactivity ⟨a ∼ vaccine protects against pathogenic antigens that cross-react with antibodies induced by antigens in the vaccine⟩ — **het·er·ol·o·gous·ly** *adv*

het·er·ol·o·gy \-'räl-ə-jē\ *n, pl* **-gies** : a lack of correspondence of apparently similar bodily parts due to differences in fundamental makeup or origin ⟨∼ in nucleic-acid base pairs in phenotypically similar yeasts⟩

het·ero·ly·sin \ˌhet-ə-rō-'līs-ᵊn\ *n* : a hemolysin that is formed in one organism in response to the introduction of the blood of an organism of a different species and has a specific hemolytic action on the blood cells of the introduced kind

het·ero·ly·sis \ˌhet-ə-'räl-ə-səs, -ə-rə-'lī-səs\ *n, pl* **-ly·ses** \-ˌsēz\ 1 : destruction by an outside agent; *specif* : solution (as of a cell) by lysins or enzymes from another source 2 : decomposition of a compound into two oppositely charged particles or ions — compare HOMOLYSIS — **het·ero·lyt·ic** \-lit-ik\ *adj*

het·ero·mer·ic \ˌhet-ə-rə-'mer-ik\ *adj* : consisting of more than one kind of structural subunit ⟨∼ proteins⟩

het·ero·mor·phic \-'mȯr-fik\ *also* **het·ero·mor·phous** \-fəs\ *adj* 1 : deviating from the usual form 2 : unlike in form or size — used specif. of synaptic chromosomes ⟨the X and Y chromosomes constitute a ∼ pair⟩ ⟨∼ bivalents⟩; compare HOMOMORPHIC 2 — **het·ero·mor·phism** \-ˌfiz-əm\ *n*

het·ero·mor·pho·sis \-'mȯr-fə-səs *also* -mȯr-'fō-\ *n, pl* **-pho·ses** \-ˌsēz\ 1 : the production in an organism of an abnormal or misplaced part esp. in place of one that has been lost (as

\ə\ abut \ᵊ\ kitten \ər\ further \a\ ash \ā\ ace \ä\ cot, cart \aú\ out \ch\ chin \e\ bet \ē\ easy \g\ go \i\ hit \ī\ ice \j\ job \ŋ\ sing \ō\ go \ȯ\ law \ȯi\ boy \th\ thin \th\ the \ü\ loot \ú\ foot \y\ yet \zh\ vision *See also* Pronunciation Symbols page

the regeneration of a tail in place of a head) **2 a** : the production of a malformed or malposed tissue or organ **b** : the formation of tissue of a different type from that from which it is derived

het·er·on·o·mous \ˌhet-ə-ˈrän-ə-məs\ *adj* : specialized along different lines of growth or under different controlling forces ⟨in most segmented animals ... the segmentation is ∼ —Libbie H. Hyman⟩ — **het·er·on·o·mous·ly** *adv*

het·ero·phago·some \ˌhet-ə-rō-ˈfag-ə-ˌsōm\ *n* : a cell vacuole formed in the cytoplasm by phagocytosis or pinocytosis

het·er·oph·a·gy \ˌhet-ə-ˈräf-ə-jē\ *n, pl* **-gies** : digestion in a fused vacuole and lysosome of material taken into a cell by phagocytosis or pinocytosis — **het·ero·pha·gic** \-rō-ˈfā-jik\ *adj*

het·ero·phe·my \ˈhet-ə-rə-ˌfē-mē\ *n, pl* **-mies** : unconscious use of words other than those intended

¹het·ero·phile \ˈhet-ə-rə-ˌfīl\ *or* **het·er·o·phil** \-ˌfil\ *also* **het·er·o·phil·ic** \ˌhet-ə-rə-ˈfil-ik\ *adj* : relating to or being any of a group of antigens in organisms of different species that induce the formation of antibodies which will cross-react with the other antigens of the group; *also* : being or relating to any of the antibodies produced and capable of cross-reacting in this way ⟨the detection of ∼ antibodies is the diagnostic method of choice for infectious mononucleosis⟩

²heterophile *or* **heterophil** *n* : NEUTROPHIL — used esp. in veterinary medicine

het·ero·pho·ria \ˌhet-ə-rō-ˈfōr-ē-ə, -ˈfȯr-ē-ə\ *n* : latent strabismus in which one eye tends to deviate either medially or laterally — compare EXOPHORIA — **het·ero·phor·ic** \-ˈfȯr-ik, -ˈfär-ik\ *adj*

Het·ero·phy·es \-ˈfī-(ˌ)ēz\ *n* : a genus (the type of the family Heterophyidae) of small digenetic trematode worms infesting the small intestine esp. of dogs, cats, and humans in Egypt and much of tropical Asia

het·ero·phy·id \-ˈfī-id\ *n* : any trematode worm of the genus *Heterophyes* or of the family (Heterophyidae) to which it belongs — **heterophyid** *adj*

het·ero·pla·sia \-ˈplā-zh(ē-)ə\ *n* : a formation of abnormal tissue or of normal tissue in an abnormal locality

het·ero·plasm \ˈhet-ə-rō-ˌplaz-əm\ *n* : tissue formed or growing where it does not normally occur

het·ero·plas·tic \ˌhet-ə-rə-ˈplas-tik\ *adj* **1** : of or relating to heteroplasia ⟨∼ development⟩ ⟨∼ erythropoietic tissue⟩ **2** : HETEROLOGOUS — **het·er·o·plas·ti·cal·ly** \-ti-k(ə-)lē\ *adv*

het·ero·plas·ty \ˈhet-ə-rə-ˌplas-tē\ *n, pl* **-ties** : XENOGRAFT

het·ero·ploid \ˈhet-ə-rə-ˌplȯid\ *adj* : having a chromosome number that is not a simple multiple of the haploid chromosome number — **heteroploid** *n* — **het·ero·ploi·dy** \-ˌplȯid-ē\ *n, pl* **-dies**

het·ero·poly·mer \ˌhet-ə-rō-ˈpäl-ə-mər\ *n* : COPOLYMER — **het·ero·poly·mer·ic** \-ˌpäl-ə-ˈmer-ik\ *adj*

het·ero·poly·sac·cha·ride \-ˌpäl-i-ˈsak-ə-ˌrīd\ *n* : a polysaccharide consisting of more than one type of monosaccharide

Het·er·op·tera \ˌhet-ə-ˈräp-tə-rə\ *n pl* : a suborder of Hemiptera or sometimes a separate order comprising the true bugs — compare HOMOPTERA — **het·er·op·ter·ous** \-tə-rəs\ *adj*

het·ero·pyk·no·sis *also* **het·ero·pyc·no·sis** \ˌhet-ə-rō-pik-ˈnō-səs\ *n* : the quality or state of some chromosomes or of parts of some chromosomes in a nucleus of taking up more stain and being more tightly coiled or of taking up less stain and being less tightly coiled than is usual — compare ISOPYKNOSIS — **het·ero·pyk·not·ic** *also* **het·ero·pyc·not·ic** \-ˈnät-ik\ *adj*

het·ero·scope \ˈhet-ə-rə-ˌskōp\ *n* : an apparatus for measuring the range of vision in strabismus — **het·er·os·co·py** \ˌhet-ə-ˈräs-kə-pē\ *n, pl* **-pies**

het·ero·sex \ˈhet-ə-rō-ˌseks\ *n* : HETEROSEXUALITY

¹het·er·o·sex·u·al \ˌhet-ə-rō-ˈseksh-(ə-)wəl, -ˈsek-shəl\ *adj* **1 a** : of, relating to, or characterized by a tendency to direct sexual desire toward individuals of the opposite sex — compare HOMOSEXUAL 1 **b** : of, relating to, or involving sexual intercourse between a male and a female ⟨sexual relationships between individuals of opposite sexes are ∼ —A. C. Kin-

sey⟩ — compare HOMOSEXUAL 2 **2** : of or relating to different sexes — **het·ero·sex·u·al·ly** \-ˈseksh-(ə-)wə-lē, -ˈsek-shə-lē\ *adv*

²heterosexual *n* : a heterosexual individual

het·ero·sex·u·al·i·ty \-sek-shə-ˈwal-ət-ē\ *n, pl* **-ties** : the quality or state of being heterosexual

het·er·o·sis \ˌhet-ə-ˈrō-səs\ *n, pl* **-o·ses** \-ˌsēz\ : a marked vigor or capacity for growth that is often shown by crossbred animals or plants — called also *hybrid vigor* — **het·er·ot·ic** \-ˈrät-ik\ *adj*

het·ero·spo·rous \ˌhet-ə-ˈräs-pə-rəs, ˌhet-ə-rō-ˈspōr-əs\ *adj* : producing microspores and megaspores ⟨∼ plants⟩

het·ero·sug·ges·tion \ˌhet-ə-rō-sə(g)-ˈjes(h)-chən\ *n* : suggestion used by one person to influence another — compare AUTOSUGGESTION

het·ero·tax·ia \-ˈtak-sē-ə\ *or* **het·ero·tax·is** \-ˈtak-səs\ *n, pl* **-tax·ias** *or* **-tax·es** \-ˈtak-ˌsēz\ : abnormal arrangement of bodily parts

het·ero·thal·lic \-ˈthal-ik\ *adj* : having two or more morphologically similar haploid phases or types of which individuals from the same type are mutually sterile but individuals from different types are cross-fertile — **het·ero·thal·lism** \-ˈthal-ˌiz-əm\ *n*

het·ero·therm \ˈhet-ə-rə-ˌthərm\ *n* : POIKILOTHERM — **het·ero·therm·ic** \ˌhet-ə-rə-ˈthərm-ik\ *adj* — **het·ero·thermy** \ˈhet-ə-rə-ˌthərm-ē\ *n, pl* **-mies**

het·ero·top·ic \ˌhet-ə-rə-ˈtäp-ik\ *adj* **1** : occurring in an abnormal place ⟨∼ bone formation⟩ **2** : grafted or transplanted into an abnormal position ⟨∼ liver transplantation⟩ — **het·ero·to·pia** \-ˈtō-pē-ə\ *also* **het·er·ot·opy** \ˌhet-ə-ˈrät-ə-pē\ *n, pl* **-pias** *or* **-pies** — **het·ero·top·i·cal·ly** \-rə-ˈtäp-i-k(ə-)lē\ *adv*

het·ero·trans·plant \ˌhet-ə-rō-ˈtran(t)s-ˌplant\ *n* : XENOGRAFT — **het·ero·trans·plant·abil·i·ty** \-ˌtran(t)s-ˌplant-ə-ˈbil-ət-ē\ *n, pl* **-ties** — **het·ero·trans·plant·able** \-ˈtran(t)s-ˈplant-ə-bəl\ *adj* — **het·ero·trans·plan·ta·tion** \-ˌtran(t)s-ˌplan-ˈtā-shən\ *n* — **het·ero·trans·plant·ed** \-ˈtran(t)s-ˈplant-əd\ *adj*

het·ero·tri·cho·sis \-tri-ˈkō-səs\ *n, pl* **-cho·ses** \-ˌsēz\ : a condition of having hair of variegated color

het·ero·tri·mer \-ˈtrī-mər\ *n* : a heterotrimeric molecule

het·ero·tri·mer·ic \-ˌtrī-ˈmer-ik\ *adj* : being a macromolecule composed of three subunits of which at least one differs from the other two ⟨∼ G proteins⟩

het·ero·troph \ˈhet-ə-rə-ˌtrōf, -ˌträf\ *n* : a heterotrophic individual

het·ero·tro·phic \ˌhet-ə-rə-ˈtrō-fik\ *adj* : requiring complex organic compounds of nitrogen and carbon (as that obtained from plant or animal matter) for metabolic synthesis — **het·ero·tro·phi·cal·ly** \-fi-k(ə-)lē\ *adv* — **het·ero·tro·phism** \-ˈtrō-ˌfiz-əm\ *n* — **het·ero·tro·phy** \ˈhet-ə-ˈrä-trə-fē\ *n, pl* **-phies**

het·ero·tro·pia \-ˈtrō-pē-ə\ *n* : STRABISMUS

het·ero·tro·pic \-ˈtrō-pik\ *adj* : characterized by enzyme activity in which the substrate binds to the enzyme at only one site and a different molecule modifies the reaction by binding to an allosteric site ⟨∼ interactions⟩ — compare HOMOTROPIC

het·ero·typ·ic \ˌhet-ə-rō-ˈtip-ik\ *adj* **1** : of or being the reduction division of meiosis as contrasted with typical mitotic division — compare HOMOTYPIC 2 **2** : different in kind, arrangement, or form ⟨∼ aggregations of cells⟩

het·ero·zy·go·sis \ˌhet-ə-rō-(ˌ)zī-ˈgō-səs\ *n, pl* **-go·ses** \-ˌsēz\ **1** : a union of genetically dissimilar gametes forming a heterozygote **2** : HETEROZYGOSITY

het·ero·zy·gos·i·ty \-ˈgäs-ət-ē\ *n, pl* **-ties** : the state of being heterozygous

het·ero·zy·gote \-ˈzī-ˌgōt\ *n* : a heterozygous individual — **het·ero·zy·got·ic** \-(ˌ)zī-ˈgät-ik\ *adj*

het·ero·zy·gous \-gəs\ *adj* : having the two genes at corresponding loci on homologous chromosomes different for one or more loci — compare HOMOZYGOUS

HETP \ˌāch-ˌē-ˌtē-ˈpē\ *n* : an insecticide $C_{12}H_{30}O_{13}P_4$ that is a cholinesterase inhibitor and is obtained synthetically usu. as a yellow liquid mixture containing TEPP

HEW *abbr* Department of Health, Education, and Welfare

hex A \,heks-'ā\ *n* : HEXOSAMINIDASE A

hex·a·canth embryo \'hek-sə-,kan(t)th-\ *n* : ONCOSPHERE

hexachloride — see BENZENE HEXACHLORIDE, GAMMA BENZENE HEXACHLORIDE

hexa·chlo·ro·cy·clo·hex·ane \,hek-sə-,klōr-ō-,sī-klō-'hek-,sān, -,klȯr-\ *n* : a derivative of cyclohexane containing six atoms of chlorine; *esp* : BENZENE HEXACHLORIDE

hexa·chlo·ro·eth·ane \-,klōr-ə-'weth-,ān, -,klȯr-\ *or* **hexa·chlor·eth·ane** \-,klōr-'eth-,, -,klȯr-\ *n* : a toxic crystalline compound C_2Cl_6 used in the control of liver flukes in veterinary medicine

hexa·chlo·ro·phane \-'klōr-ə-,fān, -'klȯr-\ *n, Brit* : HEXACHLOROPHENE

hexa·chlo·ro·phene \-'klōr-ə-,fēn, -'klȯr-\ *n* : a powdered phenolic bacteria-inhibiting agent $C_{13}Cl_6H_6O_2$

hexa·dac·ty·ly \-'dak-tə-lē\ *n, pl* **-lies** : the condition of having six fingers or toes on a hand or foot

hex·a·dec·a·no·ic acid \-,dek-ə-'nō-ik-\ *n* : PALMITIC ACID

hexa·eth·yl tet·ra·phos·phate \-,eth-əl-,te-trə-'fäs-,fāt\ *n* : HETP

hexa·flu·o·re·ni·um \-,flu̇(-ə)r-'ē-nē-əm\ *n* : a cholinesterase inhibitor used in the form of its bromide $C_{36}H_{12}Br_2N_2$ in surgery to extend the skeletal-muscle relaxing activity of succinylcholine

hex·a·mer \'hek-sə-mər\ *n* **1** : a polymer formed from six molecules of a monomer **2** : a structural subunit that is part of a viral capsid and is itself composed of six subunits of similar shape — **hex·a·mer·ic** \,hek-sə-'mer-ik\ *adj*

hexa·me·tho·ni·um \,hek-sə-mə-'thō-nē-əm\ *n* : either of two compounds $C_{12}H_{30}Br_2N_2$ or $C_{12}H_{30}Cl_2N_2$ used as ganglionic blocking agents in the treatment of hypertension

hexa·meth·y·lene·tet·ra·mine \-'meth-ə-,lēn-'te-trə-,mēn\ *n* : METHENAMINE

hex·amine \'hek-sə-,mēn\ *n* : METHENAMINE

Hex·am·i·ta \hek-'sam-ət-ə\ *n* : a genus (the type of the family Hexamitidae) of binucleate zooflagellates that include free-living forms as well as intestinal parasites of birds (as *H. meleagridis*) and of salmonid fishes (as *H. salmonis*) that are associated with enteritides

hex·am·i·ti·a·sis \hek-,sam-ə-'tī-ə-səs\ *n* : infestation with or disease caused by flagellates of the genus *Hexamita*

hex·ane \'hek-,sān\ *n* : any of several isomeric volatile liquid alkanes C_6H_{14} found in petroleum

hexanitrate — see MANNITOL HEXANITRATE

hex·a·no·ic acid \,hek-sə-,nō-ik-\ *n* : CAPROIC ACID

hexa·ploid \'hek-sə-,plȯid\ *adj* : having or being six times the monoploid chromosome number — **hexaploid** *n* — **hexa·ploi·dy** \-,plȯid-ē\ *n, pl* **-dies**

Hex·ap·o·da \hek-'sap-ə-də\ *n pl, in some classifications* : a class or other division of Arthropoda coextensive with the class Insecta — **hexa·pod** \'hek-sə-,päd\ *n or adj*

hexa·va·lent \,hek-sə-'vā-lənt\ *adj* : having a chemical valence of six

hex B \,heks-'bē\ *n* : HEXOSAMINIDASE B

hex·es·trol \'hek-sə-,strȯl, -,strōl\ *or chiefly Brit* **hex·oes·trol** \'hek-sē-,strȯl, -,strōl\ *n* : a synthetic derivative $C_{18}H_{22}O_2$ of diethylstilbestrol

hex·i·tol \'hek-sə-,tȯl, -,tōl\ *n* : any of the alcohols $C_6H_{14}O_6$ that have six hydroxyl groups in each molecule, are obtainable from the corresponding hexoses, and include some (as mannitol and sorbitol) occurring naturally

hexo·bar·bi·tal \,hek-sə-'bär-bə-,tȯl\ *n* : a barbiturate $C_{12}H_{16}N_2O_3$ used as a sedative and hypnotic and in the form of its soluble sodium salt $C_{12}H_{15}N_2NaO_3$ as an intravenous anesthetic of short duration

hexo·bar·bi·tone \-'bar-bə-,tōn\ *n, chiefly Brit* : HEXOBARBITAL

hexo·cy·cli·um me·thyl·sul·fate *or Brit* **hexo·cy·cli·um me·thyl·sul·phate** \-'sī-klē-əm-,meth-əl-'səl-,fāt\ *n* : a white crystalline anticholinergic agent $C_{21}H_{36}N_2O_5S$ that tends to

suppress gastric secretion and has been used in the treatment of peptic ulcers

hexo·ki·nase \,hek-sə-'kī-,nās, -,nāz\ *n* : any of a group of enzymes that accelerate the phosphorylation of hexoses (as in the formation of glucose-6-phosphate from glucose and ATP) in carbohydrate metabolism

hex·os·a·mine \,hek-'säs-ə,mēn\ *n* : an amine (as glucosamine) derived from a hexose by replacement of hydroxyl by the amino group

hex·os·a·min·i·dase \,hek-säs-ə-'min-ə-,dās, -,dāz\ *n* : either of two hydrolytic enzymes that catalyze the splitting off of a hexose from a ganglioside and are deficient in some metabolic diseases: **a** : HEXOSAMINIDASE A **b** : HEXOSAMINIDASE B

hexosaminidase A *n* : the more thermolabile hexosaminidase that is deficient in both Tay-Sachs disease and Sandhoff's disease — called also *hex A*

hexosaminidase B *n* : the more thermostable hexosaminidase that is deficient in Sandhoff's disease but present in elevated quantities in Tay-Sachs disease — called also *hex B*

hex·o·san \'hek-sə-,san\ *n* : a polysaccharide yielding only hexoses on hydrolysis

hex·ose \'hek-,sōs, -,sōz\ *n* : any monosaccharide (as glucose) containing six carbon atoms in the molecule

hexose diphosphate *n* : an ester $C_6H_{10}O_4(OPO_3H_2)_2$ containing two phosphoric groups

hexose monophosphate *n* : an ester $C_6H_{11}O_5(OPO_3H_2)$ containing one phosphoric group

hexose monophosphate shunt *n* : a metabolic pathway of glucose in which glucose-6-phosphate is oxidized enzymatically twice with NADP as a cofactor to form pentose sugars

hexose phosphate *n* : a phosphoric derivative of a hexose (as glucose phosphate) of which two types have been found in living tissues as intermediates of carbohydrate metabolism: **a** : HEXOSE MONOPHOSPHATE **b** : HEXOSE DIPHOSPHATE

hex·u·ron·ic acid \,heks-yə-,rän-ik-\ *n* : a uronic acid (as glucuronic acid) derived from a hexose (as glucose)

hex·yl \'hek-səl\ *n* : an alkyl radical C_6H_{13} derived from a hexane

hex·yl·res·or·cin·ol \,hek-səl-rə-'zȯrs-ᵊn-,ȯl, -,ōl\ *n* : a crystalline phenol $C_{12}H_{18}O_2$ used as an antiseptic (as in a throat lozenge) and as an anthelmintic against ascarids (esp. *Ascaris lumbricoides*), hookworms, and whipworms (esp. *Trichuris trichiura*)

Hf *symbol* hafnium

hg *abbr* hectogram

Hg *symbol* [New Latin *hydrargyrum*] mercury

Hgb *abbr* hemoglobin

HGE \,āch-(,)jē-'ē\ *n* : human granulocytic ehrlichiosis

HGH *abbr* human growth hormone

HHA *abbr* home health aide

HHS *abbr* Department of Health and Human Services

HHV–6 \,āch-(,)āch-(,)vē-'siks\ *n* : a human herpesvirus (species *Human herpesvirus 6* of the genus *Roseolovirus*) that causes roseola infantum

HI *abbr* hemagglutination inhibition

5–HIAA *abbr* 5-hydroxyindoleacetic acid

hi·a·tal \hī-'āt-ᵊl\ *adj* : of, relating to, or involving a hiatus

hiatal hernia *n* : a hernia in which an anatomical part (as the stomach) protrudes through the esophageal hiatus of the diaphragm — called also *hiatus hernia*

hi·a·tus \hī-'āt-əs\ *n* : a gap or passage through an anatomical part or organ; *esp* : a gap through which another part or organ passes

hiatus hernia *n* : HIATAL HERNIA

hiatus semi·lu·nar·is \-,sem-i-lü-'nar-əs\ *n* : a curved fissure in the nasal passages into which the frontal and maxillary sinuses open

---

G
H

Hib \'hib, ˌā-ˌchī-'bē\ *n, often attrib* : a serotype of a bacterium of the genus *Haemophilus* (*H. influenzae* type B) that causes bacterial meningitis and pneumonia esp. in children ⟨~ disease⟩ ⟨a ~ vaccine⟩ — see CONJUGATE VACCINE

hi·ber·nate \'hī-bər-ˌnāt\ *vi* **-nat·ed; -nat·ing** : to pass the winter in a torpid or resting state; *esp* : to pass the winter in a torpid condition in which the body temperature drops to a little above freezing and metabolic activity is reduced nearly to zero — compare ESTIVATE — **hi·ber·na·tion** \ˌhī-bər-'nā-shən\ *n* — **hi·ber·na·tor** \'hī-bər-ˌnāt-ər\ *n*

hi·ber·no·ma \ˌhī-bər-'nō-mə\ *n, pl* **-mas** *also* **-ma·ta** \-mət-ə\ : a rare benign tumor that contains fat cells and resembles the brown fat of hibernating mammals

¹hic·cup *also* **hic·cough** \'hik-(ˌ)əp\ *n* **1** : a spasmodic inhalation with closure of the glottis accompanied by a peculiar sound **2** : an attack of hiccuping — usu. used in pl. but sing. or pl. in constr. ⟨severe ~s is sometimes seen after operation —*Lancet*⟩ ⟨intractable ~ . . . may be successfully treated —*Jour. Amer. Med. Assoc.*⟩

²hiccup *also* **hiccough** *vi* **hic·cuped** *also* **hic·cupped** *or* **hic·coughed; hic·cup·ing** *also* **hic·cup·ping** *or* **hic·cough·ing** : to make a hiccup; *also* : to be affected with hiccups — **hic·cup·er** *also* **hic·cough·er** *n*

hick·ey \'hik-ē\ *n, pl* **hickeys** **1** : PIMPLE **2** : a temporary red mark produced esp. in lovemaking by biting and sucking the skin

Hick·man catheter \'hik-mən-\ *n* : an indwelling venous catheter with a relatively wide bore

hide·bound \'hīd-ˌbau̇nd\ *adj* **1** : having a dry skin lacking in pliancy and adhering closely to the underlying flesh — used of domestic animals **2** : having scleroderma — used of human beings

hi·drad·e·ni·tis \hi-ˌdrad-ᵊn-'īt-əs, ˌhī-\ *n* : inflammation of a sweat gland

hidradenitis sup·pur·a·ti·va \-ˌsəp-yu̇-rə-'tī-və\ *n* : a chronic suppurative inflammatory disease of the apocrine sweat glands

hi·drad·e·no·ma \hī-ˌdrad-ᵊn-'ō-mə\ *n, pl* **-mas** *also* **-ma·ta** \-mət-ə\ : any benign tumor derived from epithelial cells of sweat glands

hidradenoma pa·pil·li·fer·um \-ˌpap-i-lə-'fer-əm\ *n* : a benign solitary tumor of adult women that occurs in the anogenital region

hi·dro·sis \hid-'rō-səs, hī-'drō-\ *n, pl* **-dro·ses** \-ˌsēz\ : excretion of sweat : PERSPIRATION

hi·drot·ic \hid-'rät-ik, hī-'drät-\ *adj* : causing perspiration : DIAPHORETIC 1, SUDORIFIC

¹high \'hī\ *adj* **1** : having a complex organization : greatly differentiated or developed phylogenetically — usu. used in the comparative degree of advanced types of plants and animals ⟨the ~er algae⟩ ⟨the ~er apes⟩; compare LOW **2 a** : exhibiting elation or euphoric excitement ⟨a ~ patient⟩ **b** : being intoxicated; *also* : excited or stupefied by or as if by a drug (as marijuana or heroin)

²high *n* : an excited, euphoric, or stupefied state; *esp* : one produced by or as if by a drug (as heroin)

high blood pressure *n* : HYPERTENSION

high colonic *n* : an enema injected deeply into the colon

high–density lipoprotein *n* : HDL

high enema *n* : an enema in which the injected material reaches the colon — compare LOW ENEMA

high–energy *adj* : yielding a relatively large amount of energy when undergoing hydrolysis ⟨~ phosphate bonds in ATP⟩

high forceps *n* : a rare procedure for delivery of an infant by the use of forceps before engagement has occurred — compare LOW FORCEPS, MIDFORCEPS

high–grade \'hī-ˌgrād\ *adj* : being near the upper, most serious, or most life-threatening extreme of a specified range ⟨~ gliomas⟩ ⟨~ cervical dysplasia⟩ — compare LOW= GRADE

high–per·for·mance liquid chromatography \-pə(r)-'fȯr-mən(t)s-\ *n* : liquid chromatography in which the degree of separation is increased by forcing a solvent under pressure

through a densely packed adsorbent — abbr. *HPLC;* called also *high-pressure liquid chromatography*

high–power \-'pau̇(-ə)r\ *adj* : of, relating to, being, or made with a lens that magnifies an image a relatively large number of times and esp. about 40 times ⟨another ~ view of the liver —*Jour. Amer. Med. Assoc.*⟩ — compare LOW-POWER

high–pres·sure liquid chromatography \-'presh-ər-\ *n* : HIGH-PERFORMANCE LIQUID CHROMATOGRAPHY

high–strung \-'strəŋ\ *adj* : having an extremely nervous or sensitive temperament

hi·lar \'hī-lər\ *adj* : of, relating to, affecting, or located near a hilum ⟨~ lymph nodes of the lung⟩

hill·ock \'hil-ək\ *n* : any small anatomical prominence or elevation — see AXON HILLOCK

Hill reaction \'hil-\ *n* : the light-dependent transfer of electrons by chloroplasts in photosynthesis that results in the cleavage of water molecules and liberation of oxygen

Hill, Robin (fl 1937), British biochemist. Hill discovered the reaction that now bears his name in 1937 while at Cambridge University.

hi·lum \'hī-ləm\ *n, pl* **hi·la** \-lə\ **1** : a scar on a seed (as a bean) marking the point of attachment of the ovule **2** : a notch in or opening from a bodily part suggesting the hilum of a bean esp. when it is where the blood vessels, nerves, or ducts leave and enter: as **a** : the indented part of a kidney **b** : the depression in the medial surface of a lung that forms the opening through which the bronchus, blood vessels, and nerves pass **c** : a shallow depression in one side of a lymph node through which blood vessels pass and efferent lymphatic vessels emerge

hi·lus \-ləs\ *n, pl* **hi·li** \-ˌlī\ : HILUM 2

hind·brain \'hīn(d)-ˌbrān\ *n* : the posterior division of the three primary divisions of the developing vertebrate brain or the corresponding part of the adult brain that includes the cerebellum, pons, and medulla oblongata and that controls the autonomic functions and equilibrium — called also *rhombencephalon;* see METENCEPHALON, MYELENCEPHALON

hind·foot \-ˌfu̇t\ *n* **1** *usu* **hind foot** : one of the posterior feet of a quadruped **2** : the posterior part of the human foot that contains the calcaneus, talus, navicular, and cuboid bones

hind·gut \-ˌgət\ *n* : the posterior part of the embryonic alimentary canal

hind leg \ˌhīn(d)-'\ *n* : the posterior leg of a quadruped

hind limb *n* : a posterior limb esp. of a quadruped

hinge joint \'hinj-\ *n* : a joint between bones (as at the elbow or knee) that permits motion in only one plane; *esp* : GINGLYMUS

hip \'hip\ *n* **1** : the laterally projecting region of each side of the lower or posterior part of the mammalian trunk formed by the lateral parts of the pelvis and upper part of the femur together with the fleshy parts covering them **2** : HIP JOINT

HIPAA *abbr* Health Insurance Portability and Accountability Act

hip bone \-'bōn, -ˌbōn\ *n* : the large flaring bone that makes a lateral half of the pelvis in mammals and is composed of the ilium, ischium, and pubis which are consolidated into one bone in the adult — called also *innominate bone, os coxae, pelvic bone*

HIPC \ˌāch-(ˌ)ī-(ˌ)pē-'sē\ *n* [*health insurance purchasing cooperative*] : a cooperative formed of small businesses or uninsured individuals for the purpose of purchasing health insurance

hip joint *n* : the ball-and-socket joint comprising the articulation between the femur and the hip bone

hipped \'hipt\ *adj* : having hips esp. of a specified kind — often used in combination ⟨broad-*hipped*⟩

Hip·pe·la·tes \ˌhip-ə-'lāt-(ˌ)ēz\ *n* : a genus of small black American eye gnats of the family Chloropidae including some that are held to be vectors of conjunctivitis or yaws

Hip·po·bos·ca \ˌhip-ō-'bäs-kə\ *n* : the type genus of the family Hippoboscidae

Hip·po·bos·ci·dae \-'bäs-(k)ə-ˌdē\ *n pl* : a family of winged or wingless dipteran flies that comprise the louse flies (as the sheep ked), are bloodsucking parasites on birds and mammals, and do not lay eggs but produce well developed larvae from time to time which almost immediately pupate — **hip·po·bos·cid** \-'bäs-(k)əd\ *adj or n*

hip·po·cam·pal \ˌhip-ə-'kam-pəl\ *adj* : of or relating to the hippocampus ⟨∼ function⟩

hippocampal commissure *n* : a triangular band of nerve fibers joining the two crura of the fornix of the rhinencephalon anteriorly before they fuse to form the body of the fornix — called also *lyra, psalterium*

hippocampal convolution *n* : PARAHIPPOCAMPAL GYRUS

hippocampal fissure *n* : HIPPOCAMPAL SULCUS

hippocampal gyrus *n* : PARAHIPPOCAMPAL GYRUS

hippocampal sulcus *n* : a fissure of the mesial surface of each cerebral hemisphere extending from behind the posterior end of the corpus callosum forward and downward to the recurved part of the parahippocampal gyrus — called also *hippocampal fissure*

hip·po·cam·pus \ˌhip-ə-'kam-pəs\ *n, pl* **-pi** \-ˌpī, -ˌ)pē\ : a curved elongated ridge that is an important part of the limbic system, extends over the floor of the descending horn of each lateral ventricle of the brain, consists of gray matter covered on the ventricular surface with white matter, and is involved in forming, storing, and processing memory — see PES HIPPOCAMPI

Hip·po·crat·ic \ˌhip-ə-'krat-ik\ *adj* : of or relating to Hippocrates or to the school of medicine that took his name

Hip·poc·ra·tes \hip-'äk-rə-ˌtēz\ *(ca 460 BC–ca 370 BC)*, Greek physician. Hippocrates has been traditionally regarded as the founder of medicine. A teacher at an early Greek medical school, he strove to make an art and a science out of medicine and remove it from the realm of magic and superstition. Of the large body of works attributed to him, he probably wrote only a fraction. The corpus of Hippocratic writings covered such topics as diet, exercise, regimen, sleep, and external remedies. Hippocratic medicine divided diseases into acute and chronic, epidemic and endemic, malignant and benign. A basic belief of that school was that the four humors of the body (blood, phlegm, yellow bile, and black bile) were the seats of disease. The Hippocratic oath owes much to the teachings and practice of Hippocrates although he probably did not personally write it.

Hippocratic facies *n* : the face as it appears near death and in some debilitating conditions marked by sunken eyes and temples, pinched nose, and tense hard skin — called also *facies Hippocratica*

Hippocratic finger *n* : a clubbed finger

Hippocratic oath \-'ōth\ *n* : an oath that embodies a code of medical ethics and is usu. taken by those about to begin medical practice

Hip·poc·ra·tism \hip-'äk-rə-ˌtiz-əm\ *n* : the medical doctrine of the Hippocratic school

hip pointer *n* : a deep bruise to the iliac crest or to the attachments of the muscles attached to it that occurs esp. in contact sports (as football)

hip·pu·ran \'hip-yù-ˌran\ *n* : a white crystalline iodine-containing powder $C_9H_7INNaO_3\cdot 2H_2O$ used as a radiopaque agent in urography of the kidney — called also *iodohippurate sodium, sodium iodohippurate*

hip·pu·rate \'hip-yù-ˌrāt\ *n* : a salt or ester of hippuric acid

hip·pu·ric acid \hip-ˌyùr-ik-\ *n* : a white crystalline nitrogenous acid $C_9H_9NO_3$ formed in the liver as a detoxification product of benzoic acid and present in the urine of herbivorous animals and in small quantity in human urine

hip·pus \'hip-əs\ *n* : a spasmodic variation in the size of the pupil of the eye caused by a tremor of the iris

Hirsch·sprung's disease \'hirsh-ˌprúŋz-\ *n* : megacolon that is caused by congenital absence of ganglion cells in the muscular wall of the distal part of the colon with resulting loss of peristaltic function in this part and dilatation of the colon proximal to the aganglionic part — called also *congenital megacolon*

Hirschsprung, Harold (1830–1916), Danish pediatrician.

Hirschsprung published a number of important papers on children's diseases, describing such conditions as pyloric stenosis, intussusception, and rickets. As chief physician at a children's hospital in Copenhagen, he noted certain cases of constipation in infants due to enlargement of the colon. He published his description of congenital megacolon in 1888.

hir·sute \'hər-ˌsüt, 'hi(ə)r-, ˌhər-', hi(ə)r-'\ *adj* : very hairy — **hir·sute·ness** *n*

hir·su·ti·es \hir-'sü-shē-ˌēz, hər-\ *n, pl* **hirsuties** : HIRSUTISM

hir·sut·ism \'hər-sə-ˌtiz-əm, 'hi(ə)r-\ *n* : excessive growth of hair of normal or abnormal distribution : HYPERTRICHOSIS

hi·ru·din \hir-'üd-ən, 'hir-(y)əd-ən\ *n* : an anticoagulant extracted from the buccal glands of a leech

Hir·u·din·ea \ˌhir-(y)ə-'din-ē-ə\ *n pl* : a class of hermaphroditic aquatic, terrestrial, and parasitic annelid worms distinguished by a coelom nearly obliterated by connective tissue and reduced to a series of vascular sinuses, by modification of the hindmost segments into a sucking disk, and by the absence of parapodia and setae

hir·u·di·ni·a·sis \ˌhir-(y)ə-də-'nī-ə-səs, hi-ˌrü-d²n-'ī-\ *n, pl* **-a·ses** \-ˌsēz\ : infestation with leeches

Hir·u·din·i·dae \ˌhir-(y)ə-'din-ə-ˌdē\ *n pl* : a family of aquatic leeches that have 5-ringed segments, 5 pairs of eyes, and usu. 3-toothed jaws and that include the common medicinal leech

Hi·ru·do \hi-'rü-(ˌ)dō\ *n* : a genus of leeches that is the type of the family Hirudinidae and includes the common medicinal leech (*H. medicinalis*)

His *abbr* histidine; histidyl

His bundle \'his-\ *n* : BUNDLE OF HIS

His·ma·nal \'his-mə-ˌnal, 'hiz-, -ˌnòl\ *trademark* — used for a preparation of astemizole

his·ta·mi·nase \his-'tam-ə-ˌnās, 'his-tə-mə-, -ˌnāz\ *n* : a widely occurring flavoprotein enzyme that oxidizes histamine and various diamines — called also *diamine oxidase*

his·ta·mine \'his-tə-ˌmēn, -mən\ *n* : a compound $C_5H_9N_3$ esp. of mammalian tissues that causes dilatation of capillaries, contraction of smooth muscle, and stimulation of gastric acid secretion, that is released during allergic reactions, and that is formed by decarboxylation of histidine — **his·ta·min·ic** \ˌhis-tə-'min-ik\ *adj*

histamine cephalalgia *n* : CLUSTER HEADACHE

histamine cephalgia *or* **histaminic cephalgia** *n* : CLUSTER HEADACHE

his·ta·min·er·gic \ˌhis-tə-mə-'nər-jik\ *adj* : liberating or activated by histamine ⟨∼ receptors⟩

his·ta·mi·no·lyt·ic \ˌhis-tə-ˌmin-ə-'lit-ik, hi-ˌstam-ən-ə-\ *adj* : breaking down or tending to break down histamine ⟨∼ action of blood plasma⟩

his·ti·dase \'his-tə-ˌdās, -ˌdāz\ *n* : an enzyme occurring esp. in the liver of vertebrates that is capable of deaminating histidine to form urocanic acid

his·ti·dine \'his-tə-ˌdēn\ *n* : a crystalline essential amino acid $C_6H_9N_3O_2$ formed by the hydrolysis of most proteins — abbr. *His*

his·ti·di·ne·mia *or Brit* **his·ti·di·nae·mia** \ˌhis-tə-də-'nē-mē-ə\ *n* : a recessive autosomal metabolic defect that results in an excess amount of histidine in the blood and urine due to a deficiency of histidase — **his·ti·di·ne·mic** *or Brit* **his·ti·di·nae·mic** \-mik\ *adj*

his·ti·din·uria \-'n(y)ùr-ē-ə\ *n* : the presence of an excessive amount of histidine in the urine (as in pregnancy)

his·ti·dyl \'his-tə-ˌdil\ *n* : the amino acid radical or residue $C_3H_3N_2CH_2CH(NH_2)CO-$ of histidine — abbr. *His*

his·tio·cyte \'his-tē-ə-ˌsīt\ *n* : MACROPHAGE; *esp* : a nonmotile macrophage of extravascular tissues and esp. connective tissue

---

\ə\ **abut** \ᵊ\ **kitten** \ər\ **further** \a\ **ash** \ā\ **ace** \ä\ **cot, cart**
\aù\ **out** \ch\ **chin** \e\ **bet** \ē\ **easy** \g\ **go** \i\ **hit** \ī\ **ice** \j\ **job**
\ŋ\ **sing** \ō\ **go** \ò\ **law** \òi\ **boy** \th\ **thin** \th\ **the** \ü\ **loot**
\ù\ **foot** \y\ **yet** \zh\ **vision** *See also* Pronunciation Symbols page

G
H

his·tio·cyt·ic \ˌhis-tē-ə-ˈsit-ik\ *adj* : of, relating to, or containing macrophages ⟨∼ lymphoma⟩

his·tio·cy·to·ma \ˌhis-tē-ō-sī-ˈtō-mə\ *n, pl* **-mas** *also* **-ma·ta** \-mət-ə\ : a tumor that consists predominantly of macrophages ⟨a malignant fibrous ∼ of the spleen⟩

his·tio·cy·to·sis \-ˈtō-səs\ *n, pl* **-to·ses** \-ˌsēz\ : abnormal multiplication of macrophages ⟨Langerhans cell ∼⟩; *broadly* : a condition characterized by such multiplication

his·to·chem·i·cal \ˌhis-tō-ˈkem-i-kəl\ *adj* : of or relating to histochemistry — **his·to·chem·i·cal·ly** \-k(ə-)lē\ *adv*

his·to·chem·is·try \-ˈkem-ə-strē\ *n, pl* **-tries** : a science that combines the techniques of biochemistry and histology in the study of the chemical constitution of cells and tissues

his·to·com·pat·i·bil·i·ty \ˈhis-(ˌ)tō-kəm-ˌpat-ə-ˈbil-ət-ē\ *n, pl* **-ties** *often attrib* : a state of mutual tolerance between tissues that allows them to be grafted effectively — see MAJOR HISTOCOMPATIBILITY COMPLEX — **his·to·com·pat·ible** \-kəm-ˈpat-ə-bəl\ *adj*

histocompatibility antigen *n* : any of the polymorphic glycoprotein molecules on the surface membranes of cells that aid in the ability of the immune system to determine self from nonself, that bind to and display antigenic peptide fragments for T cell recognition, and that are determined by the major histocompatibility complex

his·to·dif·fer·en·ti·a·tion \-dif-ə-ˌren-chē-ˈā-shən\ *n* : the differentiation of a tissue from an undifferentiated group of cells

his·to·flu·o·res·cence \-ˌflü(ə)r-ˈes-ᵊn(t)s, -ˌflōr-, -ˌflȯr-\ *n* : fluorescence by a tissue upon radiation after introduction of a fluorescent substance into the body and its uptake by the tissue — **his·to·flu·o·res·cent** \-ˈes-ᵊnt\ *adj*

his·to·gen·e·sis \ˌhis-tə-ˈjen-ə-səs\ *n, pl* **-e·ses** \-ˌsēz\ : the formation and differentiation of tissues — **his·to·ge·net·ic** \-jə-ˈnet-ik\ *adj* — **his·to·ge·net·i·cal·ly** \-i-k(ə-)lē\ *adv*

his·to·gram \ˈhis-tə-ˌgram\ *n* : a representation of a frequency distribution by means of rectangles whose widths represent class intervals and whose heights represent corresponding frequencies

his·toid \ˈhis-ˌtȯid\ *adj* **1** : resembling the normal tissues ⟨∼ tumors⟩ **2** : developed from or consisting of but one tissue

his·to·in·com·pat·i·bil·i·ty \ˈhis-(ˌ)tō-ˌin-kəm-ˌpat-ə-ˈbil-ət-ē\ *n, pl* **-ties** : a state of mutual intolerance between tissues (as of a fetus and its mother or a graft and its host) that normally leads to reaction against or rejection of one by the other — **his·to·in·com·pat·ible** \-kəm-ˌpat-ə-bəl\ *adj*

his·tol·o·gist \his-ˈtäl-ə-jəst\ *n* : a specialist in histology

his·tol·o·gy \his-ˈtäl-ə-jē\ *n, pl* **-gies** **1** : a branch of anatomy that deals with the minute structure of animal and plant tissues as discernible with the microscope — compare GROSS ANATOMY **2** : a treatise on histology **3** : tissue structure or organization — **his·to·log·i·cal** \ˌhis-tə-ˈläj-i-kəl\ *or* **his·to·log·ic** \-ˈläj-ik\ *adj* — **his·to·log·i·cal·ly** \-i-k(ə-)lē\ *adv*

his·tol·y·sis \his-ˈtäl-ə-səs\ *n, pl* **-y·ses** \-ˌsēz\ : the breakdown of bodily tissues — **his·to·lyt·ic** \ˌhis-tə-ˈlit-ik\ *adj*

his·tol·y·zate *or* **his·tol·y·sate** \his-ˈtäl-ə-ˌzāt\ *n* : a product of tissue lysis

His·to·mo·nas \ˌhis-tə-ˈmōn-əs\ *n* : a genus of flagellate protozoans (family Mastigamoebidae) that are parasites in the liver and intestinal mucosa esp. of poultry, and are usu. considered to include a single species (*H. meleagridis*) that causes blackhead — **his·to·mo·nad** \-ˈmō-ˌnad\ *n* — **his·to·mo·nal** \-ˈmōn-ᵊl\ *adj*

his·to·mo·ni·a·sis \ˌhis-tə-mə-ˈnī-ə-səs\ *n, pl* **-a·ses** \-ˌsēz\ : infection with or disease caused by protozoans of the genus *Histomonas* : BLACKHEAD 2

his·to·mor·phol·o·gy \ˌhis-tō-mȯr-ˈfäl-ə-jē\ *n, pl* **-gies** : HISTOLOGY — **his·to·mor·pho·log·ic** \-ˌmȯr-fə-ˈläj-ik\ *or* **his·to·mor·pho·log·i·cal** \-i-kəl\ *adj*

his·to·mor·phom·e·try \-mȯr-ˈfäm-ə-trē\ *n, pl* **-tries** : the quantitative study of the microscopic organization and structure of a tissue (as bone) esp. by computer-assisted analysis of images formed by a microscope — **his·to·mor·pho·met·ric** \-ˌmȯr-fə-ˈme-trik\ *also* **his·to·mor·pho·met·ri·cal** \-ˈtri-kəl\ *adj*

his·tone \ˈhis-ˌtōn\ *n* : any of various simple water-soluble proteins that are rich in the basic amino acids lysine and arginine and are complexed with DNA in the nucleosomes of eukaryotic chromatin

his·to·patho·gen·e·sis \ˌhis-tə-ˌpath-ə-ˈjen-ə-səs\ *n, pl* **-e·ses** \-ˌsēz\ : the origin and development of diseased tissue

his·to·pa·thol·o·gist \ˌhis-tō-pə-ˈthäl-ə-jəst, -pa-\ *n* : a pathologist who specializes in the detection of the effects of disease on body tissues; *esp* : one who identifies tumors by their histological characteristics

his·to·pa·thol·o·gy \ˌhis-tō-pə-ˈthäl-ə-jē, -pa-\ *n, pl* **-gies** **1** : a branch of pathology concerned with the tissue changes characteristic of disease **2** : the tissue changes that affect a part or accompany a disease — **his·to·path·o·log·ic** \-ˌpath-ə-ˈläj-ik\ *or* **his·to·path·o·log·i·cal** \-i-kəl\ *adj* — **his·to·path·o·log·i·cal·ly** \-i-k(ə-)lē\ *adv*

his·to·phys·i·ol·o·gy \-ˌfiz-ē-ˈäl-ə-jē\ *n, pl* **-gies** **1** : a branch of physiology concerned with the function and activities of tissues **2** : tissue organization (as of a bodily part) esp. as it relates to function ⟨the ∼ of the thyroid gland⟩ — **his·to·phys·i·o·log·i·cal** \-ē-ə-ˈläj-i-kəl\ *also* **his·to·phys·i·o·log·ic** \-ˈläj-ik\ *adj*

his·to·plas·ma \ˌhis-tə-ˈplaz-mə\ *n* **1** *cap* : a genus of imperfect fungi that includes one (*H. capsulatum*) causing histoplasmosis and another (*H. farciminosum*) causing epizootic lymphangitis **2** : any fungus of the genus *Histoplasma*

his·to·plas·min \-ˈplaz-mən\ *n* : a sterile filtrate of a culture of a fungus of the genus *Histoplasma* (*H. capsulatum*) used in a cutaneous test for histoplasmosis

his·to·plas·mo·ma \-ˌplaz-ˈmō-mə\ *n, pl* **-mas** *also* **-ma·ta** \-mət-ə\ : a granulomatous swelling caused by a fungus of the genus *Histoplasma* (*H. capsulatum*)

his·to·plas·mo·sis \-ˌplaz-ˈmō-səs\ *n, pl* **-mo·ses** \-ˌsēz\ : a respiratory disease with symptoms like those of influenza that is endemic in the Mississippi and Ohio river valleys of the U.S., is caused by infection with a fungus of the genus *Histoplasma* (*H. capsulatum*), and is marked by benign involvement of lymph nodes of the trachea and bronchi usu. without symptoms or by severe progressive generalized involvement of the lymph nodes and macrophage-rich tissues (as of the liver and spleen) with fever, anemia, leukopenia and often with local lesions (as of the skin, mouth, or throat)

his·to·ra·di·og·ra·phy \ˌhis-tō-ˌrā-dē-ˈäg-rə-fē\ *n, pl* **-phies** : microradiography of plant or animal tissue — **his·to·ra·dio·graph·ic** \-dē-ə-ˈgraf-ik\ *adj*

his·to·ry \ˈhis-t(ə-)rē\ *n, pl* **-ries** : an account of a patient's family and personal background and past and present health

his·to·tech·nol·o·gist \ˌhis-tə-tek-ˈnäl-ə-jəst\ *n* : a technician who specializes in histotechnology

his·to·tech·nol·o·gy \-jē\ *n, pl* **-gies** : technical histology concerned esp. with preparing and processing (as by sectioning, fixing, and staining) histological specimens

his·to·tox·ic \ˈhis-tə-ˌtäk-sik\ *adj* : toxic to tissues ⟨∼ agents⟩

histotoxic anoxia *n* : anoxia caused by poisoning of the tissues (as by alcohol) that impairs their ability to utilize oxygen

histotoxic hypoxia *n* : a deficiency of oxygen reaching the bodily tissues due to impairment of cellular respiration esp. by a toxic agent (as cyanide or alcohol)

his·to·trophe *or* **his·to·troph** \ˈhis-tə-ˌträf, -ˌtrȯf\ *n* : all materials supplied for nutrition of the embryo in viviparous animals from sources other than the maternal bloodstream — compare EMBRYOTROPHE, HEMOTROPHE

his·to·tro·pic \ˌhis-tə-ˈtrō-pik, -ˈträp-ik\ *adj* : exhibiting or characterized by histotropism ⟨∼ parasites⟩

his·tot·ro·pism \his-ˈtät-rə-ˌpiz-əm\ *n* : attraction (as of a parasite) to a particular kind of tissue

his·to·zo·ic \ˌhis-tə-ˈzō-ik\ *adj* : living in the tissues of a host ⟨∼ parasites⟩

HIV \ˌā-ˌchī-ˈvē\ *n* : any of several retroviruses and esp. HIV-1 that infect and destroy helper T cells of the immune system causing the marked reduction in their numbers that is diagnostic of AIDS — called also *AIDS virus, human immunodeficiency virus*

hive \\'hīv\ *n* : the raised edematous red patch of skin or mucous membrane characteristic of hives : an urticarial wheal

hives \\'hīvz\ *n pl but sing or pl in constr* : an allergic disorder marked by raised edematous red patches of skin or mucous membrane and usu. by intense itching and caused by contact with a specific precipitating factor (as a food, drug, or inhalant) either externally or internally — called also *urticaria*

HIV–1 \ˌā-ˌchī-ˌvē-'wən\ *n* : a retrovirus of the genus *Lentivirus* (species *Human immunodeficiency virus 1*) that is the most prevalent HIV — called also *HTLV-III, LAV*

HIV–2 \-'tü\ *n* : a retrovirus of the genus *Lentivirus* (species *Human immunodeficiency virus 2*) that causes AIDS esp. in West Africa, that is closely related in structure to SIV of monkeys and may have crossed over to humans, and that is less virulent and has a longer incubation period than HIV-1

hl *abbr* hectoliter

HLA *also* **HL–A** \ˌā-(ˌ)chel-'ā\ *n* [*h*uman *l*eukocyte *a*ntigen] **1** : the major histocompatibility complex in humans **2** : a genetic locus, gene, or antigen of the major histocompatibility complex in humans — often used attributively ⟨*HLA* antigens⟩ ⟨*HLA* typing⟩; often used with one or more letters to designate a locus or with letters and a number to designate an allele at the locus or the antigen corresponding to the locus and allele ⟨relationship . . . between *HLA*-B27 antigen and ankylosing spondylitis —G. E. Ehrlich⟩

HMD *abbr* hyaline membrane disease

HMO \ˌā-(ˌ)chem-'ō\ *n, pl* **HMOs** : an organization that provides comprehensive health care to voluntarily enrolled individuals and families in a particular geographic area by member physicians with limited referral to outside specialists and that is financed by fixed periodic payments determined in advance — called also *health maintenance organization;* compare PPO

HNPCC *abbr* hereditary nonpolyposis colon cancer; hereditary nonpolyposis colorectal cancer

Ho *symbol* holmium

hoarhound *var of* HOREHOUND

hoarse \\'hō(ə)rs, 'hȯ(ə)rs\ *adj* **hoars·er; hoars·est 1** : rough or harsh in sound ⟨a ~ voice⟩ **2** : having a hoarse voice ⟨was ~ from shouting⟩ — **hoarse·ly** *adv* — **hoarse·ness** *n*

¹hob·ble \\'häb-əl\ *vb* **hob·bled; hob·bling** \-(ə-)liŋ\ *vi* : to move along unsteadily or with difficulty; *esp* : to limp along ~ *vt* **1** : to cause to limp : make lame : CRIPPLE **2** : to fasten together the legs of (as a horse) to prevent straying

²hobble *n* : something used to hobble an animal

hob·nail liver \\'häb-ˌnāl-\ *or* **hob·nailed liver** \\'häb-ˌnāld-\ *n* **1** : the liver as it appears in one form of cirrhosis in which it is shrunken and hard and covered with small projecting nodules **2** : the cirrhosis associated with hobnail liver : LAENNEC'S CIRRHOSIS

hock \\'häk\ *n* : the joint or region of the joint that unites the tarsal bones in the hind limb of a digitigrade quadruped (as the horse) and that corresponds to the human ankle but is elevated and bends backward

hock disease *n* : PEROSIS

Hodg·kin's disease \\'häj-kənz-\ *n* : a neoplastic disease that is characterized by progressive enlargement of lymph nodes, spleen, and liver and by progressive anemia

Hodgkin, Thomas (1798–1866), British physician. Hodgkin made important contributions in pathology, including a treatise on the anatomy of diseased tissue that spurred the study of tissue pathology in Great Britain. He is known for his description of aortic regurgitation in 1829 and of Hodgkin's disease in 1832. The latter disease was named in his honor in 1865 by fellow British physician Sir Samuel Wilks (1824–1911).

Hodgkin's lymphoma *n* : HODGKIN'S DISEASE

Hodgkin's paragranuloma *n* : PARAGRANULOMA 2

Hof·meis·ter series \\'hȯf-ˌmī-stər-\ *n* : an arrangement of salts, anions, or cations in descending order of their effect upon a physical phenomenon (as the swelling of gelatin) — called also *lyotropic series*

Hofmeister, Franz (1850–1922), Austro-German chemist.

Hofmeister is known for his work on proteins, metabolism, and the chemistry of colloids. In 1888 he discovered the relative power of different anions to precipitate lyophilic salts. The Hofmeister series is not only fundamental to theories of lyophilic colloids and systems, but it is also important to physiology.

hog cholera \\'häg-, 'hȯg-\ *n* : a highly infectious often fatal disease of swine caused by a flavivirus of the genus *Pestivirus* (species *Classical swine fever virus*) and characterized by fever, loss of appetite, weakness, erythematous lesions esp. in light-skinned animals, and severe leukopenia — called also *swine fever;* see AFRICAN SWINE FEVER

hog gum *n* : TRAGACANTH

hog louse *n* : a large sucking louse of the genus *Haematopinus* (*H. suis*) that is parasitic on the hog and in some areas is associated with the transmission of swine pox

hol·an·dric \hō-'lan-drik, hä-\ *adj* : transmitted by a gene in the nonhomologous portion of the Y chromosome — compare HOLOGYNIC

hold·fast \\'hōl(d)-ˌfast\ *n* : an organ by which a parasitic animal (as a tapeworm) attaches itself to its host

Hol·ger Niel·sen method \\'hōl-gər-'nēl-sən-\ *n* : BACK PRESSURE-ARM LIFT METHOD

Nielsen, Holger (1866–1955), Danish army officer. Nielsen was a lieutenant colonel in the Danish army. He originated the back pressure-arm lift method of artificial respiration and published a description of it in 1932.

ho·lism \\'hō-ˌliz-əm\ *n* **1** : a theory that the universe and esp. living nature is correctly seen in terms of interacting wholes (as of living organisms) that are more than the mere sum of elementary particles **2** : a holistic study or method of treatment

ho·lis·tic \hō-'lis-tik\ *adj* **1** : of or relating to holism **2** : relating to or concerned with wholes or with complete systems rather than with the analysis of, treatment of, or dissection into parts ⟨~ medicine attempts to treat both the mind and the body⟩ — **ho·lis·ti·cal·ly** \-ti-k(ə-)lē\ *adv*

Hol·land·er test \\'häl-ən-dər-\ *n* : a test for function of the vagus nerve (as after vagotomy for peptic ulcer) in which insulin is administered to induce hypoglycemia and gastric acidity tends to increase if innervation by the vagus nerve remains and decrease if severance is complete

Hollander, Franklin (1899–1966), American physiologist. Hollander as a gastrointestinal physiologist made major contributions to the study of gastric secretions. One of his most important studies centered on vagal innervation of the stomach of dogs. This led to the development of a test using insulin to show whether the human vagus nerve is functioning. The test was introduced in a 1942 paper and is now identified with his name.

hol·low \\'häl-(ˌ)ō, -ə(-w)\ *n* : a depressed part of a surface or a concavity ⟨the ~ at the back of the knee⟩

hollow organ *n* : a visceral organ that is a hollow tube or pouch (as the stomach or intestine) or that includes a cavity (as of the heart or bladder) which subserves a vital function

holly — see SEA HOLLY

Holm·gren yarn test \\'hōm-grən-'yärn-, 'hōlm-\ *n* : a method of testing color vision by the use of colored wool yarns — called also *Holmgren test, Holmgren wool test*

Holm·gren \\'hȯlm-ˌgrän\, **Alarik Frithiof (1831–1897),** Swedish physiologist. Holmgren introduced his test for color blindness in an 1874 article.

hol·mi·um \\'hō(l)-mē-əm\ *n* : a metallic element of the rare-earth group that occurs with yttrium and forms highly magnetic compounds — symbol *Ho;* see ELEMENT table

ho·lo·blas·tic \ˌhō-lə-'blas-tik, ˌhäl-ə-\ *adj* : characterized by cleavage planes that divide the whole egg into distinct and separate though coherent blastomeres ⟨~ eggs⟩ ⟨~ cleav-

---

\ə\ **abut** \ˈə\ **kitten** \ər\ **further** \a\ **ash** \ā\ **ace** \ä\ **cot, cart**
\au̇\ **out** \ch\ **chin** \e\ **bet** \ē\ **easy** \g\ **go** \i\ **hit** \ī\ **ice** \j\ **job**
\ŋ\ **sing** \ō\ **go** \ȯ\ **law** \ȯi\ **boy** \th\ **thin** \th̲\ **the** \ü\ **loot**
\u̇\ **foot** \y\ **yet** \zh\ **vision**   *See also* Pronunciation Symbols page

age⟩ — compare MEROBLASTIC — **ho·lo·blas·ti·cal·ly** \-ti-k(ə-)lē\ adv

ho·lo·crine \'hō-lə-krən, -ˌkrīn, -ˌkrēn, 'häl-ə-\ adj : producing or being a secretion resulting from lysis of secretory cells ⟨∼ glands⟩ ⟨∼ secretions⟩ ⟨∼ activity⟩ — compare APOCRINE, ECCRINE, MEROCRINE

ho·lo·en·dem·ic \ˌhō-lō-en-'dem-ik\ adj : affecting all or characterized by the infection of essentially all the inhabitants of a particular area ⟨∼ diseases⟩

ho·lo·en·zyme \ˌhō-lō-'en-ˌzīm\ n : a catalytically active enzyme consisting of an apoenzyme combined with its cofactor

ho·log·a·mous \hō-'läg-ə-məs\ adj : having gametes of essentially the same size and structural features as vegetative cells — **ho·log·a·my** \-mē\ n, pl **-mies**

ho·lo·gram \'hō-lə-ˌgram, 'häl-ə-\ n : a three-dimensional image reproduced from a pattern of interference produced by a split coherent beam of radiation (as from a laser); also : the pattern of interference itself

ho·log·ra·phy \hō-'läg-rə-fē\ n, pl **-phies** : the art or process of making or using a hologram — **ho·lo·graph** \'hō-lə-ˌgraf, 'häl-ə-\ vt — **ho·lo·gra·pher** \hō-'läg-rə-fər\ n — **ho·lo·graph·ic** \ˌhō-lə-'graf-ik, ˌhäl-ə-\ adj — **ho·lo·graph·i·cal·ly** \-i-k(ə-)lē\ adv

ho·lo·gy·nic \ˌhō-lə-'jin-ik, ˌhäl-, -'gī-nik\ adj : inherited solely in the female line presumably through transmission as a recessive factor in the nonhomologous portion of the X chromosome — compare HOLANDRIC — **ho·log·y·ny** \hō-'läj-ə-nē\ n, pl **-nies**

ho·lo·me·tab·o·lous \ˌhō-lō-mə-'tab-ə-ləs, ˌhäl-ō-\ adj : having complete metamorphosis ⟨∼ insects⟩ — compare HEMIMETABOLOUS — **ho·lo·me·tab·o·lism** \-ˌliz-əm\ n

ho·lo·my·ar·i·an \-mī-'ar-ē-ən, -'er-\ adj, of a nematode worm : having the muscle layer continuous or divided into two longitudinal zones without true muscle cells

ho·lo·phyt·ic \-'fit-ik\ adj : obtaining food after the manner of a green plant : PHOTOAUTOTROPHIC ⟨∼ protozoans⟩ — compare HOLOZOIC

ho·lo·sys·tol·ic \-sis-'täl-ik\ adj : relating to an entire systole ⟨a ∼ murmur⟩

ho·lo·type \'hō-lə-ˌtīp, 'häl-ə-\ n **1** : the single specimen designated by an author as the type of a species or lesser taxon at the time of establishing the group **2** : the type of a species or lesser taxon designated at a date later than that of establishing a group or by another person than the author of the taxon

ho·lo·zo·ic \ˌhō-lə-'zō-ik, ˌhäl-ə-\ adj : characterized by food procurement after the manner of most animals by the ingestion of complex organic matter ⟨∼ nutrition⟩ ⟨∼ herbivores and carnivores⟩ — compare HOLOPHYTIC

Hol·ter monitor \'hōl-tər-\ n : a portable device that makes a continuous record of electrical activity of the heart and that can be worn by an ambulatory patient during the course of daily activities in order to detect fleeting episodes of abnormal heart rhythms — **Holter monitoring** n

Holter, Norman Jefferis (1914–1983), American biophysicist. Holter made his first notable contribution during World War II, when, as senior physicist for the U.S. Navy's Bureau of Ships, he conducted important research on the behavior of ocean waves. After the war he and his staff of oceanographic engineers measured wave action and underwater disturbances caused by the atomic testing at the South Pacific atoll of Bikini. During 1952 he recorded for the Atomic Energy Commission the fallout caused by the atmospheric testing of the hydrogen bomb. His later researches ranged from seismography to vitamin C. In medicine he was notable for his work on electrocardiography and his invention of a portable apparatus for monitoring heart activity. Originally known as an ambulatory electrocardiograph, the device is now associated with his name.

Ho·mans' sign \'hō-mənz-\ n : pain in the calf of the leg upon dorsiflexion of the foot with the leg extended that is diagnostic of thrombosis in the deep veins of the area

Homans, John (1877–1954), American surgeon. Homans

was a pioneer in the study of the pancreas. His investigations helped to pave the way for the discovery of insulin as a treatment for diabetes. He also devised an operation for the excision of ulcers in 1929 and wrote a treatise on circulatory diseases of the extremities in 1939. He described Homans' sign in 1941.

hom·at·ro·pine \hō-'ma-trə-ˌpēn\ n : a poisonous crystalline ester of tropine and mandelic acid used in the form of its hydrobromide $C_{16}H_{21}NO_3·HBr$ for dilating the pupil of the eye and in the form of its methyl bromide $C_{16}H_{21}NO_3·CH_3Br$ in combination with hydrocodone in cough suppressant preparations — see HYCODAN

home care \'hōm-\ n : services (as nursing or personal care) provided to a homebound individual (as one who is convalescing, disabled, or terminally ill) ⟨home care as an alternative to institutionalization⟩ ⟨home care providers⟩

home health aide n : a trained and certified health-care worker who provides assistance to a patient in the home with personal care (as hygiene and exercise) and light household duties (as meal preparation) and who monitors the patient's condition — abbr. HHA

ho·meo·box \'hō-mē-ō-ˌbäks\ n : a short usu. highly conserved DNA sequence in various genes and esp. homeotic genes that encodes a homeodomain

ho·meo·do·main \-dō-ˌmān\ n : a domain in a protein that is encoded for by a homeobox, that consists of about 60 amino acid residues which are usu. similar from one such domain to another, and that recognizes and binds to specific DNA sequences in genes regulated by the homeotic gene

ho·meo·mor·phous or Brit **ho·moeo·mor·phous** \ˌhō-mē-ə-'mȯr-fəs\ adj : being alike in size and shape ⟨∼ hooks on a tapeworm⟩

ho·meo·path or Brit **ho·moeo·path** \'hō-mē-ə-ˌpath\ n : a practitioner or adherent of homeopathy

ho·me·op·a·thy or Brit **ho·moe·op·a·thy** \ˌhō-mē-'äp-ə-thē, ˌhäm-ē-\ n, pl **-thies** : a system of medical practice that treats a disease esp. by the administration of minute doses of a remedy that would in healthy persons produce symptoms similar to those of the disease — compare ALLOPATHY 1 — **ho·meo·path·ic** or Brit **ho·moeo·path·ic** \ˌhō-mē-ə-'path-ik\ adj — **ho·meo·path·i·cal·ly** or Brit **ho·moeo·path·i·cal·ly** \-i-k(ə-)lē\ adv

ho·meo·pla·sia or Brit **ho·moeo·pla·sia** \ˌhō-mē-ō-'plāzh(ē-)ə\ n : a growth of tissue similar to normal tissue ⟨endometrial ∼⟩ — **ho·meo·plas·tic** or Brit **ho·moeo·plas·tic** \-'plast-ik\ adj

ho·me·osis also **ho·moe·osis** \ˌhō-mē-'ō-səs\ n : a homeotic change or process in an organism

ho·meo·sta·sis or Brit **ho·moeo·sta·sis** \ˌhō-mē-ō-'stā-səs\ n : the maintenance of relatively stable internal physiological conditions (as body temperature or the pH of blood) in higher animals under fluctuating environmental conditions; also : the process of maintaining a stable psychological state in the individual under varying psychological pressures or stable social conditions in a group under varying social, environmental, or political factors — **ho·meo·stat·ic** or Brit **ho·moeo·stat·ic** \-'stat-ik\ adj — **ho·meo·stat·i·cal·ly** or Brit **ho·moeo·stat·i·cal·ly** \-i-k(ə-)lē\ adv

ho·meo·therm \'hō-mē-ə-ˌthərm\ or **ho·moio·therm** \hō-'mȯi-ə-\ n : a warm-blooded animal — called also homotherm

ho·meo·ther·mic \ˌhō-mē-ə-'thər-mik\ or **ho·moio·ther·mic** \hō-ˌmȯi-ə-\ or **ho·moio·ther·mal** \-'thər-məl\ adj : WARM-BLOODED

ho·meo·therm·ism or **ho·moio·therm·ism** \-'thər-ˌmiz-əm\ n : HOMEOTHERMY

ho·meo·ther·my \'hō-mē-ə-ˌthər-mē\ or **ho·moio·ther·my** \hō-'mȯi-ə-\ n, pl **-mies** : the condition of being warm-blooded : WARM-BLOODEDNESS — called also homeothermism

ho·me·ot·ic also **ho·moe·ot·ic** \ˌhō-mē-'ät-ik\ adj : relating to, caused by, or being a homeotic gene ⟨a ∼ mutant causing replacement of an antenna by a leg in a fruit fly⟩ — **ho·me·ot·i·cal·ly** \-i-k(ə-)lē\ adv

homeotic gene *n* : a gene that produces a usu. major shift in the developmental fate of an organ or body part esp. to a homologous organ or part normally found elsewhere in the organism

home remedy \'hōm-\ *n* : a simply prepared medication or tonic often of unproven effectiveness administered without prescription or professional supervision — compare FOLK MEDICINE

home·sick \'hōm-ˌsik\ *adj* : longing for home and family while absent from them — **home·sick·ness** *n*

ho·mi·cid·al \ˌhäm-ə-'sīd-ᵊl, ˌhō-mə-\ *adj* : of, relating to, or tending toward homicide — **ho·mi·cid·al·ly** \-ᵊl-ē\ *adv*

ho·mi·cide \'häm-ə-ˌsīd, 'hō-mə-\ *n* **1** : a person who kills another **2** : a killing of one human being by another — compare GENOCIDE

hom·i·nid \'häm-ə-nəd, -ˌnid\ *n* : any bipedal primate mammal of the family Hominidae — **hominid** *adj*

Ho·min·i·dae \hō-'min-ə-ˌdē\ *n pl* : a family of bipedal mammals of the order Primates comprising recent humans together with extinct ancestral and related forms — see HOMO 1

hom·i·nine \'häm-ə-ˌnīn\ *n* : any of a subfamily (Homininae) of the family Hominidae comprising large-brained hominids (as *Homo sapiens* and *H. erectus*) in contrast to the small-brained australopithecines (genus *Australopithecus*) — **hom·i·nine** *adj*

hom·i·niv·o·rous \ˌhäm-ə-'niv-(ə-)rəs\ *adj* : feeding on or devouring human beings ⟨the great white shark is ∼⟩

hom·i·ni·za·tion *or chiefly Brit* **hom·i·ni·sa·tion** \ˌhäm-ə-nə-'zā-shən\ *n* : the evolutionary development of human characteristics that differentiate hominids from their primate ancestors — **hom·i·nized** *or chiefly Brit* **hom·i·nised** \'häm-ə-ˌnīzd\ *adj*

hom·i·noid \'häm-ə-ˌnȯid\ *n* : any member of the superfamily Hominoidea; *also* : an animal that resembles humans — **hominoid** *adj*

Hom·i·noi·dea \ˌhäm-ə-'nȯid-ē-ə\ *n pl* **1** *in some classifications* : a major division of the order Primates segregating *Homo* and related fossil forms from the great apes **2** : a superfamily of the primate suborder Anthropoidea including recent hominids, gibbons, and pongids together with extinct ancestral and related forms (as of the genera *Proconsul* and *Dryopithecus*) as distinguished from the lower Old World monkeys — compare CERCOPITHECIDAE

¹ho·mo \'hō-(ˌ)mō\ *n* **1** *cap* : a genus of primate mammals of the family Hominidae that includes modern humans (*H. sapiens*) and several extinct related species (as *H. erectus*) **2** *pl* **homos** : any primate mammal of the genus *Homo*

²homo *n, pl* **homos** *often disparaging* : HOMOSEXUAL — **homo** *adj*

homocaryon, homocaryotic *var of* HOMOKARYON, HOMOKARYOTIC

ho·mo·chi·ral \ˌhō-mō-'kī-rəl\ *adj* : consisting of only one enantiomer ⟨only about 10% of synthetic chiral drugs are marketed in ∼ . . . form —Stu Borman⟩ — **ho·mo·chi·ral·i·ty** \-kī-'ral-ət-ē\ *n, pl* **-ties**

ho·mo·cy·clic \ˌhō-mə-'sī-klik, ˌhäm-ə-, -'sik-lik\ *adj* : ISOCYCLIC

ho·mo·cys·te·ine \ˌhō-mō-'sis-tə-ˌēn, ˌhäm-ō-\ *n* : an amino acid $C_4H_9NO_2S$ that is produced in animal metabolism by the demethylation of methionine and forms a complex with serine that breaks up to produce cysteine and homoserine and that appears to be associated with an increased risk of cardiovascular disease when occurring at high levels in the blood

ho·mo·cys·tine \-'sis-ˌtēn\ *n* : an amino acid $C_8H_{16}N_2O_4S_2$ formed by oxidation of homocysteine and excreted in the urine in homocystinuria

ho·mo·cys·tin·uria \-ˌsis-tin-'(y)ur-ē-ə\ *n* : a metabolic disorder inherited as a recessive autosomal trait, caused by deficiency of an enzyme important in the metabolism of homocystine with resulting accumulation of homocystine in the body and its excretion in the urine, and characterized typi-

cally by mental retardation, dislocation of the crystalline lenses, skeletal abnormalities, and thromboembolic disease

ho·mo·cys·tin·uric \-'(y)ur-ik\ *n* : a person affected with homocystinuria

ho·mo·cy·to·tro·pic \-ˌsīt-ə-'trō-pik\ *adj* : of, relating to, or being any antibody that attaches to cells of the species in which it originates but not to cells of other species

ho·mo·di·mer \-'dī-mər\ *n* : a protein composed of two polypeptide chains that are identical in the order, number, and kind of their amino acid residues — **ho·mo·di·mer·ic** \-dī-'mer-ik\ *adj*

ho·mo·dont \'hō-mə-ˌdänt, 'häm-ə-\ *adj* : having or being teeth that are all of similar form ⟨the porpoise is a ∼ animal⟩ — compare HETERODONT

ho·moe·ol·o·gous \ˌhō-mē-'äl-ə-gəs, ˌhäm-ē-\ *adj* : of similar genetic constitution — used of chromosomes believed to have been completely homologous in an ancestral form — **ho·moeo·logue** *or* **ho·moeo·log** \'hō-mē-ə-ˌlȯg, 'häm-ē-, -ˌläg\ *n*

Each boldface word in the list below is a British variant of the word to its right in small capitals.

homoeomorphous	HOMEOMORPHOUS	**homoeoplasia**	HOMEOPLASIA
homoeopath	HOMEOPATH	**homoeoplastic**	HOMEOPLASTIC
homoeopathic	HOMEOPATHIC	**homoeostasis**	HOMEOSTASIS
homoeopathically	HOMEOPATHICALLY	**homoeostatic**	HOMEOSTATIC
homoeopathy	HOMEOPATHY	**homoeostatically**	HOMEOSTATICALLY

homoeosis, homoeotic *var of* HOMEOSIS, HOMEOTIC

ho·mo·erot·ic \ˌhō-mō-i-'rät-ik\ *adj* : HOMOSEXUAL — **ho·mo·erot·i·cism** \-i-'rät-ə-ˌsiz-əm\ *also* **ho·mo·erot·ism** \-'er-ə-ˌtiz-əm\ *n*

ho·mo·fer·men·ta·tive \ˌhō-mō-fər-'ment-ət-iv, ˌhäm-ō-\ *adj* : producing a fermentation resulting wholly or principally in a single end product — used esp. of economically important lactic-acid bacteria that ferment carbohydrates to lactic acid — **ho·mo·fer·ment·er** \-'ment-ər\ *n*

ho·mo·ga·met·ic \-gə-'met-ik, -'mēt-\ *adj* : forming gametes that all have the same type of sex chromosome

ho·mog·a·my \hō-'mäg-ə-mē\ *n, pl* **-mies** : reproduction within an isolated group perpetuating qualities by which it is differentiated from the larger group of which it is a part; *broadly* : the mating of like with like — **ho·mog·a·mous** \-məs\ *or* **ho·mo·gam·ic** \ˌhō-mə-'gam-ik, ˌhäm-ə-\ *adj*

ho·mo·ge·nate \hō-'mäj-ə-ˌnāt, hə-\ *n* : a product of homogenizing — compare MACERATE

ho·mo·ge·ne·i·ty \ˌhō-mə-jə-'nē-ət-ē, -'nā-ət-, ˌhäm-ə-\ *n, pl* **-ties** : the quality or state of being homogeneous

ho·mo·ge·neous \-'jē-nē-əs, -nyəs\ *adj* : of uniform structure or composition throughout — **ho·mo·ge·neous·ly** *adv* — **ho·mo·ge·neous·ness** *n*

homo·gen·ic \-'jen-ik\ *adj* : having only one allele of a gene or genes — used of a gamete or of a population

ho·mog·e·ni·za·tion *also Brit* **ho·mog·e·ni·sa·tion** \hō-ˌmäj-ə-nə-'zā-shən, hə-\ *n* **1** : the quality or state of being homogenized **2** : the act or process of homogenizing

ho·mog·e·nize *also Brit* **ho·mog·e·nise** \hō-'mäj-ə-ˌnīz, hə-\ *vb* **-nized** *also Brit* **-nised; -niz·ing** *also Brit* **-nis·ing** *vt* **1** : to make homogeneous **2 a** : to reduce to small particles of uniform size and distribute evenly usu. in a liquid **b** : to reduce the particles of so that they are uniformly small and evenly distributed; *specif* : to break up the fat globules of (milk) into very fine particles esp. by forcing through minute openings ∼ *vi* : to become homogenized

ho·mog·e·niz·er *also Brit* **ho·mog·e·nis·er** \-ˌnī-zər\ *n* : one that homogenizes; *esp* : a machine that forces a substance through fine openings against a hard surface for the purpose of blending or emulsification

\ə\ **abut** \ᵊ\ **kitten** \ər\ **further** \a\ **ash** \ā\ **ace** \ä\ **cot, cart** \au̇\ **out** \ch\ **chin** \e\ **bet** \ē\ **easy** \g\ **go** \i\ **hit** \ī\ **ice** \j\ **job** \ŋ\ **sing** \ō\ **go** \ȯ\ **law** \ȯi\ **boy** \th\ **thin** \t̲h̲\ **the** \ü\ **loot** \u̇\ **foot** \y\ **yet** \zh\ **vision** *See also* Pronunciation Symbols page

ho·mog·e·nous \-nəs\ *adj* **1** : HOMOPLASTIC 2 ⟨the value of preserved ∼ bone grafts as compared with autogenous grafts —*Plastic & Reconstructive Surgery*⟩ **2** : HOMOGENEOUS

ho·mo·gen·tis·ic acid \ˌhō-mō-ˌjen-ˈtiz-ik, ˌhäm-ō-\ *n* : a crystalline acid $C_8H_8O_4$ formed as an intermediate in the metabolism of phenylalanine and tyrosine and found esp. in the urine of those affected with alkaptonuria

ho·mo·gon·ic \ˌhō-mə-ˈgän-ik, ˌhäm-ə-, -ˈgōn-\ *adj* : being or characterized by a course of development in which one generation of parasites immediately succeeds another ⟨a ∼ life cycle of a nematode worm⟩ — compare HETEROGONIC 2a

ho·mo·graft \ˈhō-mə-ˌgraft, ˈhäm-ə-\ *n* : a graft of tissue from a donor of the same species as the recipient — called also *homotransplant;* compare XENOGRAFT — **homograft** *vb*

ho·moi·os·mot·ic \ˌhō-ˌmȯi-äz-ˈmät-ik\ *adj* : having a bodily osmotic regulating mechanism and body fluids that differ in osmotic pressure from the surrounding medium or from seawater ⟨∼ animals include all the land and freshwater vertebrates⟩ — compare POIKILOSMOTIC

homoiotherm, homoiothermal, homoiothermic, homoiothermism, homoiothermy *var of* HOMEOTHERM, HOMEOTHERMAL, HOMEOTHERMIC, HOMEOTHERMISM, HOMEOTHERMY

ho·mo·kary·on *also* **ho·mo·cary·on** \ˌhō-mō-ˈkar-ē-ˌän, ˌhäm-ō-, -ən\ *n* : a homokaryotic cell — compare DIKARYON 2, HETEROKARYON

ho·mo·kary·ot·ic *also* **ho·mo·cary·ot·ic** \-ˌkar-ē-ˈät-ik\ *adj* : of, relating to, being, or consisting of cells in the mycelium of a fungus that contain two or more genetically identical cells

ho·mo·lat·er·al \-ˈlat-ər-əl, -ˈla-trəl\ *adj* : IPSILATERAL

ho·mo·lec·i·thal \-ˈles-ə-thəl\ *adj, of an egg* : ISOLECITHAL

homolog *var of* HOMOLOGUE

ho·mol·o·gize *also Brit* **ho·mol·o·gise** \hō-ˈmäl-ə-ˌjīz, hə-\ *vt* **-gized** *also Brit* **-gised; -giz·ing** *also Brit* **-gis·ing** **1** : to make homologous **2** : to demonstrate the homology of

ho·mol·o·gous \hō-ˈmäl-ə-gəs, hə-\ *adj* **1 a** : having the same relative position, value, or structure: as **(1)** : exhibiting biological homology **(2)** : having the same or allelic genes with genetic loci usu. arranged in the same order ⟨∼ chromosomes⟩ **b** : belonging to or consisting of a chemical series whose members exhibit homology **2 a** : derived from or involving organisms of the same species ⟨∼ tissue grafts⟩ — compare AUTOLOGOUS, HETEROLOGOUS 1 **b** : relating to or being immunity or a serum produced by or containing a specific antibody corresponding to a specific antigen — **ho·mol·o·gous·ly** \-lē\ *adv*

homologous serum hepatitis *n* : HEPATITIS B

homologous serum jaundice *n* : HEPATITIS B

ho·mo·logue *or* **ho·mo·log** \ˈhō-mə-ˌlȯg, ˈhäm-ə-, -ˌläg\ *n* : something (as a chemical compound or a chromosome) that is homologous

ho·mol·o·gy \hō-ˈmäl-ə-jē, hə-\ *n, pl* **-gies** **1 a** : likeness in structure between parts of different organisms due to evolutionary differentiation from the same or a corresponding part of a remote ancestor — compare ANALOGY, HOMOMORPHY **b** : correspondence in structure between different parts of the same individual **2 a** : the relation existing between chemical compounds in a series whose successive members have in composition a regular difference esp. of one carbon and two hydrogen atoms CH_2 **b** : the relation existing among elements in the same group of the periodic table **c** : similarity of nucleotide or amino acid sequence (as in nucleic acids or proteins)

ho·mol·y·sis \hō-ˈmäl-ə-səs\ *n, pl* **-y·ses** \-ˌsēz\ : decomposition of a chemical compound into two uncharged atoms or radicals — compare HETEROLYSIS 2 — **ho·mo·lyt·ic** \ˌhō-mə-ˈlit-ik, ˌhäm-ə-\ *adj*

ho·mo·mor·phic \ˌhō-mə-ˈmȯr-fik, ˌhäm-ə-\ *adj* **1** : of, relating to, or characterized by homomorphy **2** : alike in form or size — used specif. of synaptic chromosomes ⟨∼ bivalents⟩; compare HETEROMORPHIC 2

ho·mo·mor·phy \ˈhō-mə-ˌmȯr-fē, ˈhäm-ə-\ *n, pl* **-phies** : similarity of form with different fundamental structure; *specif* : superficial resemblance between organisms of different groups due to evolutionary convergence — compare HOMOLOGY

ho·mo·nom·ous \hō-ˈmän-ə-məs, hə-\ *adj* : having similar structure and arranged in a series ⟨metameric parts are ∼⟩

hom·on·y·mous \hō-ˈmän-ə-məs\ *adj* **1** : affecting the same part of the visual field of each eye ⟨right ∼ hemianopia⟩ **2** : relating to or being diplopia in which the image that is seen by the right eye is to the right of the image that is seen by the left eye

¹ho·mo·phile \ˈhō-mə-ˌfīl\ *adj* : of, relating to, or concerned with homosexuals or homosexuality ⟨∼ lifestyles⟩; *also* : being homosexual

²homophile *n* : HOMOSEXUAL

ho·mo·pho·bia \ˌhō-mə-ˈfō-bē-ə\ *n* : irrational fear of, aversion to, or discrimination against homosexuality or homosexuals — **ho·mo·phobe** \ˈhō-mə-ˌfōb\ *n* — **ho·mo·pho·bic** \ˌhō-mə-ˈfō-bik\ *adj*

ho·mo·plas·tic \ˌhō-mə-ˈplas-tik, ˌhäm-ə-\ *adj* **1** : of or relating to homoplasy **2** : of, relating to, or derived from another individual of the same species ⟨∼ grafts⟩ — **ho·mo·plas·ti·cal·ly** \-ti-k(ə-)lē\ *adv* — **ho·mo·plasty** \ˈhō-mə-ˌplas-tē, ˈhäm-ə-\ *n, pl* **-ties**

ho·mo·pla·sy \ˈhō-mə-ˌplā-sē, ˈhäm-ə-, -ˌplas-ē; hō-ˈmäp-lə-sē\ *n* : correspondence between parts or organs acquired as the result of parallel evolution or convergence

ho·mo·pol·y·mer \ˌhō-mə-ˈpäl-ə-mər, ˌhäm-ə-\ *n* : a polymer consisting of identical monomer units — **ho·mo·pol·y·mer·ic** \-ˌpäl-ə-ˈmer-ik\ *adj*

ho·mo·poly·nu·cleo·tide \ˌhō-mə-ˌpäl-ē-ˈn(y)ü-klē-ə-ˌtīd, ˌhäm-ə-\ *n* : a polynucleotide (as poly(A)) composed of only one type of nucleotide

ho·mo·poly·pep·tide \-ˈpep-ˌtīd\ *n* : a protein with a polypeptide chain made up of only one kind of amino acid residue

ho·mo·poly·sac·char·ide \-ˈsak-ə-ˌrīd\ *n* : a polysaccharide composed of only one kind of monosaccharide ⟨glycogen is a ∼ of glucose⟩

Ho·mop·tera \hō-ˈmäp-tə-rə\ *n pl* : a large suborder of Hemiptera or sometimes a separate order of insects comprising the cicadas, lantern flies, leafhoppers, spittlebugs, treehoppers, aphids, psyllas, whiteflies, and scale insects which have a small prothorax and sucking mouthparts consisting of a jointed beak and which undergo incomplete metamorphosis — compare HETEROPTERA — **ho·mop·ter·an** \-rən\ *n or adj* — **ho·mop·ter·ous** \-rəs\ *adj*

homos *pl of* HOMO

ho·mo·sal·ate \ˌhō-mō-ˈsal-ˌāt, ˌhäm-ō-\ *n* : a salicylate $C_{16}H_{22}O_3$ that is used in sunscreen lotions to absorb ultraviolet rays

Ho·mo sa·pi·ens \ˌhō-(ˌ)mō-ˈsap-ē-ənz, -ˈsä-pē-, -ˌenz\ *n* : MANKIND, HUMANKIND

ho·mo·ser·ine \ˌhō-mō-ˈser-ˌēn, ˌhäm-ō-, -ˈsēr-\ *n* : an amino acid $C_4H_9NO_3$ that is formed in the conversion of methionine to cysteine — see HOMOCYSTEINE

¹ho·mo·sex·u·al \ˌhō-mə-ˈseksh-(ə-)wəl, -ˈsek-shəl\ *adj* **1** : of, relating to, or characterized by a tendency to direct sexual desire toward individuals of one's own sex — compare HETEROSEXUAL 1a **2** : of, relating to, or involving sexual intercourse between individuals of the same sex — compare HETEROSEXUAL 1b — **ho·mo·sex·u·al·ly** \-ē\ *adv*

²homosexual *n* : a homosexual individual and esp. a male

ho·mo·sex·u·al·i·ty \ˌhō-mə-ˌsek-shə-ˈwal-ət-ē\ *n, pl* **-ties** **1** : the quality or state of being homosexual **2** : erotic activity with another of the same sex

ho·mo·spo·rous \ˌhō-mō-ˈspōr-əs, ˌhäm-ə-, -ˈspȯr-; hō-ˈmäs-pə-rəs\ *adj* : producing asexual spores of one kind only

ho·mo·thal·lic \ˌhō-mō-ˈthal-ik\ *adj* : having only one haploid phase that produces two kinds of gametes capable of fusing to form a zygote — **ho·mo·thal·lism** \-ˈthal-ˌiz-əm\ *n*

ho·mo·therm \ˈhō-mə-ˌthərm, ˈhäm-ə-\ *n* : HOMEOTHERM

ho·mo·ther·mal \ˌhō-mə-ˈthər-məl\ *or* **ho·mo·ther·mic** \-mik\ *or* **ho·mo·ther·mous** \-məs\ *adj* : WARM-BLOODED

ho·mo·top·ic \-ˈtäp-ik\ *adj* : relating to or occurring in the same or corresponding places or parts ⟨∼ tumors⟩

ho·mo·trans·plant \ˌhō-mō-ˈtran(t)-ˌsplant, ˌhäm-ō-\ *n* : HOMOGRAFT — **ho·mo·trans·plant** *vt* — **ho·mo·trans·plant·abil·i·ty** \-ˌtran(t)-ˌsplant-ə-ˈbil-ət-ē\ *n, pl* **-ties** — **ho·mo·trans·plant·able** \-ˈtran(t)-ˈsplant-ə-bəl\ *adj* — **ho·mo·trans·plan·ta·tion** \-ˌtran(t)-ˌsplan-ˈtā-shən\ *n*

ho·mo·tro·pic \ˌhō-mə-ˈtrō-pik, ˌhäm-ə-\ *adj* : characterized by enzyme activity in which the substrate binds to the enzyme at two different sites of which one is the normal reactive site and the other is an allosteric site ⟨∼ enzymes⟩ ⟨∼ interaction⟩ — compare HETEROTROPIC

ho·mo·type \ˈhō-mə-ˌtīp, ˈhäm-ə-\ *n* : a part or organ of the same fundamental structure as another ⟨one arm is the ∼ of the other⟩ ⟨the right arm is the ∼ of the right leg⟩

ho·mo·typ·ic \ˌhō-mə-ˈtip-ik, ˌhäm-ə-\ *or* **ho·mo·typ·i·cal** \-ˈtip-i-kəl\ *adj* **1** : of or relating to a homotype **2** : being the equational or typical mitotic division of meiosis — compare HETEROTYPIC 1

ho·mo·va·nil·lic acid \-və-ˈnil-ik-\ *n* : a dopamine metabolite $C_9H_{10}O_4$ excreted in human urine

ho·mo·zy·go·sis \-zī-ˈgō-səs\ *n, pl* **-go·ses** \-ˌsēz\ : HOMOZYGOSITY

ho·mo·zy·gos·i·ty \-ˈgäs-ət-ē\ *n, pl* **-ties** : the state of being homozygous

ho·mo·zy·gote \-ˈzī-ˌgōt\ *n* : a homozygous individual

ho·mo·zy·gous \-ˈzī-gəs\ *adj* : having the two genes at corresponding loci on homologous chromosomes identical for one or more loci — compare HETEROZYGOUS — **ho·mo·zy·gous·ly** *adv*

ho·mun·cu·lus \hō-ˈmən-kyə-ləs\ *n, pl* **-li** \-ˌlī, -ˌlē\ : a miniature adult that in the theory of preformation was held to inhabit the germ cell and to produce a mature individual merely by an increase in size

Hon·du·ras bark \hän-ˈd(y)ùr-əs-ˈbärk\ *n* : CASCARA AMARGA

H₁ antagonist \ˈāch-ˈwən-\ *n* : any of numerous drugs (as cetirizine or loratadine) that bind competitively with histamine to H₁ receptors on cell membranes and are used variously as sedatives, antiemetics, and anticholinergics — called also *H₁ receptor antagonist*

H₁ blocker *n* : H₁ ANTAGONIST

H₁ receptor *n* : a receptor for histamine on cell membranes that modulates the dilation of blood vessels and the contraction of smooth muscle — see H₁ ANTAGONIST

H₁ receptor antagonist *n* : H₁ ANTAGONIST

hon·ey \ˈhən-ē\ *n, pl* **honeys** **1** : a sweet viscid material elaborated out of the nectar of flowers in the honey sac of various bees **2** : any of various preparations consisting of simple mixtures of medicaments with honey — **honey** *adj*

hon·ey·bee \ˈhən-ē-ˌbē\ *n* : a honey-producing bee (*Apis* and related genera); *esp* : a European bee (*A. mellifera*) introduced worldwide and kept in hives for the honey it produces

hon·ey·comb \-ˌkōm\ *n* : RETICULUM 1

honeycomb ringworm *n* : FAVUS

Hong Kong flu \ˈhäŋ-ˈkäŋ-\ *n* : influenza that is caused by a subtype (H3N2) of the orthomyxovirus causing influenza A and that was responsible for about 34,000 deaths in the U.S. in the influenza pandemic of 1968–1969 — called also *Hong Kong influenza;* compare ASIAN FLU, SPANISH FLU

hoof \ˈhùf, ˈhüf\ *n, pl* **hooves** \ˈhüvz, ˈhùvz\ *also* **hoofs** : a horny covering that protects the ends of the toes of numerous plant-eating 4-footed mammals (as horses or cattle); *also* : a hoofed foot

hoof–and–mouth disease *n* : FOOT-AND-MOUTH DISEASE

hoofed \ˈhùft, ˈhüft, ˈhùvd, ˈhùvd\ *or* **hooved** \ˈhùvd, ˈhùvd\ *adj* : furnished with hooves : UNGULATE

hoof pick *n* : a hooked implement used to remove foreign objects from a hoof

hook \ˈhùk\ *n* **1** : an instrument used in surgery to take hold of tissue ⟨a crypt ∼⟩ ⟨a cordotomy ∼⟩ **2** : an anatomical part that resembles a hook

Hooke's law \ˈhùks-\ *n* : a statement in physics: the stress within an elastic solid up to the elastic limit is proportional to the strain responsible for it

Hooke, Robert (1635–1703), British physicist. Hooke was an outstanding scientist who did research in a great number of diverse areas. In 1660 he discovered the law which now bears his name. This law laid the basis for studies of stress and strain in elastic solids.

hook·let \ˈhùk-lət\ *n* : a small hook ⟨a circle of ∼s on the tapeworm scolex⟩

hook·worm \ˈhùk-ˌwərm\ *n* **1** : any of several parasitic nematode worms of the family Ancylostomatidae that have strong buccal hooks or plates for attaching to the host's intestinal lining and that include serious bloodsucking pests **2** : ANCYLOSTOMIASIS

hookworm disease *n* : ANCYLOSTOMIASIS

hoose *also* **hooze** \ˈhüz\ *n* : verminous bronchitis of cattle, sheep, and goats caused by larval strongylid roundworms irritating the bronchial tubes and producing a dry hacking cough — called also *husk, lungworm disease*

hooved *var of* HOOFED

hop \ˈhäp\ *n* **1** : a twining vine (*Humulus lupulus*) of the mulberry family with 3-lobed or 5-lobed leaves and inconspicuous flowers of which the pistillate ones are in glandular cone-shaped catkins **2 hops** *pl* : the ripe dried pistillate catkins of a hop used esp. to impart a bitter flavor to malt liquors and also in medicine as a tonic

HOP *abbr* high oxygen pressure

hor·de·in \ˈhòr-dē-ən\ *n* : a prolamin found in the seeds of barley

hor·de·o·lum \hòr-ˈdē-ə-ləm\ *n, pl* **-o·la** \-lə\ : STY

hore·hound *also* **hoar·hound** \ˈhō(ə)r-ˌhaùnd, ˈhò(ə)r-\ *n* **1** : a European aromatic mint (*Marrubium vulgare*) that is naturalized in the U.S., has pubescent leaves and small axillary flowers, has a very bitter taste, and is used as a tonic and anthelmintic — called also *white horehound* **2** : an extract or confection made from horehound and used as a remedy for coughs and colds

hor·i·zon·tal \ˌhòr-ə-ˈzänt-ᵊl, ˌhär-\ *adj* **1** : relating to or being a transverse plane or section of the body **2** : relating to or being transmission (as of a disease) by physical contact or proximity in contrast with inheritance — compare VERTICAL — **hor·i·zon·tal·ly** \-ᵊl-ē\ *adv*

horizontal cell *n* : any of the retinal neurons whose axons pass along a course in the plexiform layer following the contour of the retina and whose dendrites synapse with the rods and cones

horizontal fissure *n* : a fissure of the right lung that begins at the oblique fissure and runs horizontally dividing the lung into superior and middle lobes

horizontal plate *n* : a plate of the palatine bone that is situated horizontally, joins the bone of the opposite side, and forms the back part of the hard palate — compare PERPENDICULAR PLATE 2

hor·me·sis \hòr-ˈmē-səs\ *n* : a theoretical phenomenon of dose-response relationships in which something (as a heavy metal or ionizing radiation) that produces harmful biological effects at moderate to high doses may produce beneficial effects at low doses — **hor·met·ic** \-ˈmet-ik\ *adj*

Hor·mo·den·drum \ˌhòr-mə-ˈden-drəm\ *n, syn of* CLADOSPORIUM

hor·mon·al \hòr-ˈmōn-ᵊl\ *adj* : of, relating to, or effected by hormones — **hor·mon·al·ly** \-ᵊl-ē\ *adv*

hor·mone \ˈhòr-ˌmōn\ *n* **1 a** : a product of living cells that circulates in body fluids (as blood) or sap and produces a specific often stimulatory effect on the activity of cells usu. remote from its point of origin — called also *internal secretion;* see PLANT HORMONE **b** : a synthetic substance that

\ə\ abut \ᵊ\ kitten \ər\ further \a\ ash \ā\ ace \ä\ cot, cart
\aù\ out \ch\ chin \e\ bet \ē\ easy \g\ go \i\ hit \ī\ ice \j\ job
\ŋ\ sing \ō\ go \ò\ law \òi\ boy \th\ thin \th\ the \ü\ loot
\ù\ foot \y\ yet \zh\ vision *See also* Pronunciation Symbols page

acts like a hormone **2** : SEX HORMONE — **hor·mone·like** \-ₗlīk\ *adj*

hormone replacement therapy *n* : the administration of estrogen often along with a synthetic progestin esp. to ameliorate the symptoms of menopause and reduce the risk of postmenopausal osteoporosis — abbr. *HRT*

hor·mo·no·gen·e·sis \ˌhȯr-ˌmō-nə-ˈjen-ə-səs\ *n, pl* **-e·ses** \-ˌsēz\ : the formation of hormones — **hor·mo·no·gen·ic** \-ˈjen-ik\ *adj*

hor·mo·nol·o·gy \ˌhȯr-mə-ˈnäl-ə-jē\ *n, pl* **-gies** : a branch of science concerned with the study of hormones

hor·mo·no·poi·et·ic \ˌhȯr-ˌmō-nə-pȯi-ˈet-ik\ *adj* : producing hormones ⟨∼ glands⟩

hor·mo·no·ther·a·py \-ˈther-ə-pē\ *n, pl* **-pies** : the therapeutic use of hormones ⟨treated for cancer of the prostate by ∼ —*Jour. Amer. Med. Assoc.*⟩

horn \ˈhȯ(ə)rn\ *n* **1 a** : one of the usu. paired bony processes that arise from the head of many ungulates and that are found in some extinct mammals and reptiles; *esp* : one of the permanent paired hollow sheaths of keratin usu. present in both sexes of cattle and their relatives that function chiefly for defense and arise from a bony core anchored to the skull **b** : the tough fibrous material consisting chiefly of keratin that covers or forms the horns of cattle and related animals, hooves, or other horny parts (as claws or nails) **2** : CORNU — **horned** \ˈhȯ(ə)rnd\ *adj*

horn cell *n* : a nerve cell lying in one of the gray columns of the spinal cord

horned rattlesnake *n* : SIDEWINDER

horned viper *n* : a common desert-dwelling viper (*Aspis cornutus*) of Egypt and Asia Minor characterized by a horny scale resembling a spike above each eye

Hor·ner's syndrome \ˈhȯr-nərz-\ *n* : a syndrome marked by sinking in of the eyeball, contraction of the pupil, drooping of the upper eyelid, and vasodilation and anhidrosis of the face, and caused by paralysis of the cervical sympathetic nerve fibers on the affected side

  Horner, Johann Friedrich (1831–1886), Swiss ophthalmologist. Horner published his description of Horner's syndrome in 1869. The condition had been described previously at least twice and was produced in animals as early as 1727, but Horner's description was the one that attracted attention.

horn fly *n* : a small black European dipteran fly (*Haematobia irritans* of the family Muscidae) that has been introduced into No. America where it is a bloodsucking pest of cattle — called also *cattle fly*

horn·i·fied \ˈhȯr-nə-ˌfīd\ *adj* : converted or changed into horn or horny tissue ⟨∼ skin⟩

horny \ˈhȯr-nē\ *adj* **horn·i·er; -est** **1 a** : composed of or resembling tough fibrous material consisting chiefly of keratin : KERATINOUS ⟨∼ tissue⟩ ⟨after the ∼ material has been ... cut away —Morris Fishbein⟩ **b** : being hard or callused ⟨*horny*-handed⟩ **2** : having horns

horny layer *n* : STRATUM CORNEUM

ho·rop·ter \hə-ˈräp-tər, hȯ-\ *n* : the locus of points in external space whose images are formed on corresponding places of the two retinas and which are seen single — **hor·op·ter·ic** \ˌhȯ-ˌräp-ˈter-ik\ *adj*

hor·rip·i·la·tion \hȯ-ˌrip-ə-ˈlā-shən, hä-\ *n* : a bristling of the hair of the head or body (as from disease, terror, or chilliness) : GOOSE BUMPS — **hor·rip·i·late** \hȯ-ˈrip-ə-ˌlāt, hä-\ *vt* **-lat·ed; -lat·ing**

hor·ror \ˈhȯr-ər, ˈhär-\ *n* : painful and intense fear, dread, or dismay

horror au·to·tox·i·cus \-ˌȯt-ō-ˈtäk-sə-kəs\ *n* : SELF= TOLERANCE

horse \ˈhȯ(ə)rs\ *n, pl* **hors·es** *also* **horse** : a large solid-hoofed herbivorous mammal of the genus *Equus* (*E. caballus*) domesticated since prehistoric times

horse bot *n* : HORSE BOTFLY; *specif* : a larva of a horse botfly

horse botfly *n* : a cosmopolitan botfly of the genus *Gasterophilus* (*G. intestinalis*) that glues its eggs to the hairs esp. of the forelegs of horses from where they are taken into the

mouth and then hatch into young bots, pass into the stomach, and become attached to the lining

horse·fly \ˈhȯrs-ˌflī\ *n, pl* **-flies** : any of the swift usu. large dipteran flies with bloodsucking females that comprise the family Tabanidae

horse·hair worm \-ˌha(ə)r-, -ˌhe(ə)r-\ *n* : any worm of the class or phylum Nematomorpha — called also *gordiacean, horsehair snake*

horse·rad·ish peroxidase \-ˌrad-ish-, -ˌred-\ *n* : a peroxidase that occurs in the root of the horseradish (*Armoracia lapathifolia* of the mustard family), that produces a distinctive color when exposed to an appropriate solution, and that is used as a label for antibody-antigen complexes, as a cytochemical marker in immunohistochemical staining, and as a tracer to follow the course of individual neurons since it is transported by most neural pathways

horse·shoe kidney \-ˌshü\ *n* : a congenital partial fusion of the kidneys resulting in a horseshoe shape

horse·sick·ness \-ˌsik-nəs\ *n* : AFRICAN HORSE SICKNESS

horse tick *n* : a tick attacking horses; *esp* : TROPICAL HORSE TICK

Hor·ton's syndrome \ˈhȯrt-ᵊnz-\ *n* : CLUSTER HEADACHE

  Horton, Bayard Taylor (1895–1980), American physician. Horton is known for classic descriptions of two clinical entities. In 1932 Horton and two colleagues from the Mayo Clinic described giant cell arteritis as a new disease entity. This disease, however, was actually described for the first time two years earlier by an American physician, Max Schmidt, in a study of intracranial aneurysms. In 1939 Horton described the condition now known as a cluster headache or Horton's syndrome.

hosp *abbr* hospital

hos·pice \ˈhäs-pəs\ *n* : a facility or program designed to provide a caring environment for meeting the physical and emotional needs of the terminally ill

hos·pi·tal \ˈhäs-ˌpit-ᵊl\ *n, often attrib* **1** : a charitable institution for the needy, aged, infirm, or young **2 a** : an institution where the sick or injured are given medical or surgical care — when used in British English following a preposition, the article is usu. omitted ⟨came and saw me in ∼ —Robert Graves⟩ **b** : a place for the care and treatment of sick and injured animals

hospital bed *n* : a bed with a frame in three movable sections equipped with mechanical spring parts that permit raising the head end, foot end, or middle as required — called also *Gatch bed*

hospital fever *n* : typhus or fever formerly prevalent in hospitals in association with hospital gangrene

hospital gangrene *n* : gangrene prevalent in crowded hospitals before the development of modern sanitation

hos·pi·tal·ism \ˈhäs-(ˌ)pit-ᵊl-ˌiz-əm\ *n* **1 a** : the factors and influences that adversely affect the health of hospitalized persons **b** : the effect of such factors on mental or physical health **2** : the deleterious physical and mental effects on infants and children resulting from their living in institutions without the benefit of a home environment and parents

hos·pi·tal·ist \ˈhäs-(ˌ)pit-ᵊl-əst\ *n* : a physician who specializes in seeing and treating other physicians' hospitalized patients in order to minimize the number of hospital visits by the patients' regular physicians

hos·pi·tal·iza·tion *or chiefly Brit* **hos·pi·tal·isa·tion** \ˌhäs-(ˌ)pit-ᵊl-ə-ˈzā-shən\ *n* **1** : the act or process of being hospitalized ⟨pain persisted constantly through a two-day period, finally necessitating ∼ —*Jour. Amer. Med. Assoc.*⟩ **2** : the period of stay in a hospital ⟨drug treatment shortened the length of ∼ —*Today's Health*⟩

hospitalization insurance *n* : insurance that provides benefits to cover or partly cover hospital expenses

hos·pi·tal·ize *or chiefly Brit* **hos·pi·tal·ise** \ˈhäs-(ˌ)pit-ᵊl-ˌīz, häs-ˈpit-ᵊl-ˌīz\ *vt* **-ized** *or chiefly Brit* **-ised; -iz·ing** *or chiefly Brit* **-is·ing** : to place in a hospital as a patient ⟨the child was *hospitalized* at once for diagnosis and treatment —*Jour. Amer. Med. Assoc.*⟩

hospital ship *n* : a ship equipped as a hospital; *esp* : one built

G
H

or specifically assigned to assist the wounded, sick, and shipwrecked in time of war

host \'hōst\ *n* **1** : a living animal or plant on or in which a parasite lives — see DEFINITIVE HOST, INTERMEDIATE HOST **2** : the larger, stronger, or dominant one of a commensal or symbiotic pair **3 a** : an individual into which a tissue or part is transplanted from another **b** : an individual in whom an abnormal growth (as a cancer) is proliferating

host cell *n* : a living cell invaded by or capable of being invaded by an infectious agent (as a bacterium or a virus) ⟨HIV makes Tat only after the virus gets inside a *host cell* —John Travis⟩

hos·tel \'häs-tᵊl\ *n, chiefly Brit* : housing maintained by a public or private organization or institution; *esp* : a rest home or rehabilitation center for the chronically ill, the aged, or the physically disabled

hos·til·i·ty \hä-'stil-ət-ē\ *n, pl* **-ties** : conflict, opposition, or resistance in thought or principle — **hos·tile** \'häs-tᵊl, -,tīl\ *adj*

hot \'hät\ *adj* **hot·ter; hot·test** **1 a** : having a relatively high temperature **b** : capable of giving a sensation of heat or of burning, searing, or scalding **c** : having heat in a degree exceeding normal body heat **2 a** : RADIOACTIVE; *esp* : exhibiting a relatively great amount of radioactivity when subjected to radionuclide scanning **b** : dealing with radioactive material

hot flash *n* : a sudden brief flushing and sensation of heat caused by dilation of skin capillaries usu. associated with menopausal endocrine imbalance — called also *hot flush*

Ho·tis test \'hōt-əs-\ *n* : a test for the presence of the common streptococcus of bovine mastitis in milk which is made by incubating a sample of milk with an aniline dye and in which the appearance of yellow patches indicates the presence of the organism

  Hotis, Ralph P. (1890–1935), American agricultural marketing specialist. Hotis was an employee of the U.S. Department of Agriculture and coordinated the testing of the fitness of milk for consumption. The test method was published in 1936 and posthumously named in his honor.

hot line *n* : a usu. toll-free telephone service available to the public for some specific purpose (as to receive advice or information about a particular subject or to talk confidentially about personal problems to a sympathetic listener) ⟨a poison control *hot line*⟩ ⟨an AIDS *hot line*⟩

hot pack *n* : absorbent material (as a blanket or squares of gauze) wrung out in hot water, wrapped around the body or a portion of the body, and covered with dry material to hold in the moist heat ⟨*hot pack* for an infected arm⟩ — compare COLD PACK

hot spot *n* **1** : a patch of painful moist inflamed skin on a domestic animal and esp. a dog that starts as a response to a skin irritant (as an allergen or an insect or tick bite), that is rapidly worsened by scratching, chewing, or licking the affected area, and that may become seriously infected if not promptly cleaned and medicated **2** : a site in genetic material (as DNA or a chromosome) having a high frequency of mutation or recombination

Hot·ten·tot apron \'hät-ᵊn-,tät-'ä-prən\ *n* : an excessive development of the labia minora occurring in Hottentot women

hot–water bottle \,hät-'wȯt-ər-,, -'wät-\ *n* : a stoppered rubber bag or earthenware bottle filled with hot water to provide warmth

hour·glass stomach \'aú(ə)r-,glas\ *n* : a stomach divided into two communicating cavities by a circular constriction usu. caused by the scar tissue around an ulcer

house·break \'haús-,brāk\ *vt* **-broke** \-,brōk\; **-bro·ken** \-,brō-kən\; **-break·ing** : to make housebroken

house·bro·ken \-,brō-kən\ *adj* : trained to excretory habits acceptable in indoor living — used of a household pet

house call \'haús-,kȯl\ *n* : a visit (as by a doctor) to a home to provide medical care

house doctor *n* : a physician who is in residence at an establishment (as a hotel) or on the premises temporarily (as dur-

ing the performance of a play) in the event of a medical emergency

house–dust mite \'haús-,dəst-\ *n* : either of two widely distributed mites of the genus *Dermatophagoides* (*D. farinae* and *D. pteronyssinus*) that commonly occur in house dust and often induce allergic responses esp. in children

house·fly \-,flī\ *n, pl* **-flies** : a cosmopolitan dipteran fly of the genus *Musca* (*M. domestica*) that is often found about human habitations and may act as a mechanical vector of diseases (as typhoid fever); *also* : any of various flies of similar appearance or habitat

house·maid's knee \'haú-,smādz-\ *n* : a swelling over the knee due to an enlargement of the bursa in the front of the patella

house·man \'haú-smən\ *n, pl* **-men** \-smən\ *chiefly Brit* : INTERN

house mouse *n* : a mouse that frequents houses; *esp* : a common nearly cosmopolitan grayish-brown mouse of the genus *Mus* (*M. musculus*) that lives and breeds about buildings, is an important laboratory animal, and is an important pest as a consumer of human food and as a vector of diseases

house of·fi·cer \-,äf-ə-sər, -,óf-\ *n* : an intern or resident employed by a hospital

house physician *n* : a physician and esp. a resident employed by a hospital

house staff *n* : interns, residents, and fellows of a hospital

house surgeon *n* : a surgeon fully qualified in a specialty and resident in a hospital

Houston's valve \'h(y)ü-stənz-\ *n* : any of the usu. three but sometimes four or two permanent transverse semilunar folds of the rectum — called also *plica transversalis recti*

  Houston, John (1802–1845), British surgeon. Houston described the permanent transverse folds of the rectum in 1830. In that same year he reported his discovery of two muscles that compress the dorsal vein of the penis. He was also the author of papers on edema and fevers.

How·ard test \'haú-ərd-\ *n* : a test of renal function that involves the catheterization of each ureter so that the urinary output of each kidney can be determined and analyzed separately

  Howard, John Eager (1902–1985), American internist and endocrinologist. Howard for most of his career was associated with Johns Hopkins Hospital, where he was director of the division of endocrinology and metabolism for many years. His early researches were concerned with the clinical syndrome associated with pheochromocytoma. The Howard test was a product of his research on kidneys and the composition of urine and was designed to determine the differential functional change in a kidney in which a certain type of lesion results in hypertension.

How·ell–Jol·ly body \'haú-əl-zhó-'lē-, -'jäl-ē-\ *n* : one of the basophilic granules that are prob. nuclear fragments, that sometimes occur in red blood cells, and that indicate by their appearance in circulating blood that red cells are leaving the bone marrow while incompletely mature (as in certain anemias)

  Howell, William Henry (1860–1945), American physiologist. Howell was one of the leading physiologists of his time. His early contributions to physiology concerned the circulatory system, nerve tissue, and the components of blood. His later researches dealt with the coagulation of blood. He described what are now known as Howell-Jolly bodies in an article published in 1890.

  Jol·ly \zhó-lē\, **Justin–Marie–Jules (1870–1953),** French histologist. Jolly did research on the morphology of blood and blood-forming tissues and on mammalian embryology. Independently of Howell, he described the Howell-Jolly bodies in a series of articles published 1905–1907.

How·ship's lacuna \'haú-,ships-\ *n* : a groove or cavity usu.

\ə\ **abut** \ᵊ\ **kitten** \ər\ **further** \a\ **ash** \ā\ **ace** \ä\ **cot, cart**
\aú\ **out** \ch\ **chin** \e\ **bet** \ē\ **easy** \g\ **go** \i\ **hit** \ī\ **ice** \j\ **job**
\ŋ\ **sing** \ō\ **go** \ó\ **law** \ói\ **boy** \th\ **thin** \th\ **the** \ü\ **loot**
\ú\ **foot** \y\ **yet** \zh\ **vision**   *See also* Pronunciation Symbols page

containing osteoclasts that occurs in bone which is undergoing reabsorption

Howship, John (1781–1841), British anatomist. Howship was a surgeon at St. George's and Charing Cross hospitals in London. In 1820 he published a treatise on the natural and pathological anatomy of bones. In this work he described the bone pits or cavities now known as Howship's lacunae.

HPI *abbr* history of present illness

HPLC *abbr* high-performance liquid chromatography

HPV \ˌāch-(ˌ)pē-ˈvē\ *n* : HUMAN PAPILLOMAVIRUS

hr *abbr* [Latin *hora*] hour — used in writing prescriptions; see QH

Hr factor \ˈā-ˈchär-\ *n* : a substance present in Rh-negative blood and apparently reciprocally related to the Rh factor

HRT *abbr* hormone replacement therapy

hs *abbr* [Latin *hora somni*] at bedtime — used esp. in writing prescriptions

Hs *symbol* hassium

HS *abbr* house surgeon

HSA *abbr* human serum albumin

H–sub·stance \ˈāch-ˌsəb-stən(t)s\ *n* : a diffusible substance that is thought to be released in the allergic reaction of skin and in the responses of tissue to inflammation and that is held to be similar to histamine or possibly to be histamine itself

HSV \ˌāch-(ˌ)es-ˈvē\ *n* : either of two herpesviruses that cause herpes simplex — see HSV-1, HSV-2

HSV–1 \-ˌvē-ˈwən\ *n* : a herpesvirus of the genus *Simplexvirus* (species *Human herpesvirus 1*) that causes the type of herpes simplex typically involving the lips, mouth, and face

HSV–2 \-ˈtü\ *n* : a herpesvirus of the genus *Simplexvirus* (species *Human herpesvirus 2*) that causes the type of herpes simplex typically involving the genital region

ht *abbr* height

5–HT \ˈfīv-(ˌ)āch-ˈtē\ *n* : SEROTONIN

HTLV \ˌāch-ˌtē-ˌel-ˈvē\ *n* : any of several retroviruses that formerly included the original strain of the AIDS virus before it was grouped with other strains, renamed HIV-1, and made the type species (*Human immunodeficiency virus 1*) of the genus *Lentivirus* — often used with a number or Roman numeral to indicate the type and order of discovery ⟨HTLV⁼ III⟩; called also *human T-cell leukemia virus, human T-cell lymphotropic virus, human T-lymphotropic virus*

HTLV–I \-ˌvē-ˈwən\ *n* : an HTLV (species *Primate T-lymphotropic virus 1* of the genus *Deltaretrovirus*) that is found in association with adult T-cell leukemia and a progressive paralyzing myelopathy

HTLV–III \-ˈthrē\ *n* : HIV-1

H₂ antagonist \-ˈtü-\ *n* : a drug (as cimetidine, famotidine, nizatidine, or ranitidine) that reduces or inhibits the secretion of gastric acid by binding competitively with histamine to H₂ receptors on cell membranes — called also *H₂ receptor antagonist*

H₂ blocker *n* : H₂ ANTAGONIST

H₂ receptor *n* : a receptor for histamine on cell membranes that modulates the stimulation of heart rate and the secretion of gastric acid — called also *H₂ histamine receptor;* see H₂ ANTAGONIST

H₂ receptor antagonist *n* : H₂ ANTAGONIST

hub \ˈhəb\ *n* : the enlarged base by which a hollow needle may be attached to a device (as a syringe)

Hub·bard tank \ˈhəb-ərd-\ *n* : a large tank in which a patient can easily be assisted in exercises while in the water

Hubbard, Leroy Watkins (1857–1938), American orthopedic surgeon. Hubbard devoted the major portion of his career to the study of infantile paralysis. One of his patients was Franklin D. Roosevelt, who suffered from the disease. Roosevelt encouraged him to found and develop the Warm Springs Foundation in Georgia, where Hubbard served as surgeon-in-chief.

hue \ˈhyü\ *n* : the one of the three psychological dimensions of color perception that permits them to be classified as red, yellow, green, blue, or an intermediate between any contiguous pair of these colors and that is correlated with the wave-length or the combination of wavelengths comprising the stimulus — compare BRIGHTNESS, SATURATION 4a

huff \ˈhəf\ *vt* : to inhale (noxious fumes) through the mouth for the euphoric effect produced by the inhalant; *also* : to inhale the noxious fumes of (a substance) for their euphoric effect ⟨teenagers ∼*ing* correction fluid⟩

Huh·ner test \ˈh(y)ü-nər-\ *n* : a test used in sterility studies that involves postcoital examination of fluid aspirated from the vagina and cervix to determine the presence or survival of sperm in these areas

Huhner, Max (1873–1947), American surgeon. Huhner specialized in the study of the genital and urinary organs and their functions. He published his first major study of sterility and its treatment in 1913. The following year he introduced his test for sterility. He also wrote on the diagnosis and treatment of various other sexual disorders, such as impotence.

hum \ˈhəm\ *n* : a sound like that made by humming; *esp* : VENOUS HUM

¹hu·man \ˈhyü-mən, ˈyü-\ *adj* **1 a** : of, relating to, or characteristic of humans ⟨the ∼ body⟩ ⟨∼ biochemistry⟩ **b** : primarily or usu. harbored by, affecting, or attacking humans ⟨∼ diseases⟩ ⟨∼ parasites⟩ **2** : being or consisting of humans ⟨the ∼ race⟩ **3** : consisting of members of the family Hominidae : HOMINID — **hu·man·ness** \-mən-nəs\ *n*

²human *n* : a bipedal primate mammal of the genus *Homo* (*H. sapiens*) : MAN; *broadly* : any living or extinct member of the family Hominidae — **hu·man·like** \-ˌlīk\ *adj*

human being *n* : HUMAN

human botfly *n* : a large fly of the genus *Dermatobia* (*D. hominis*) that has brown wings and a bluish body, is widely distributed in tropical America, and undergoes its larval development subcutaneously in some mammals including humans

human chorionic gonadotropin *n* : a glycoprotein hormone similar in structure to luteinizing hormone that is secreted by the placenta during early pregnancy to maintain corpus luteum function and stimulate placental progesterone production, is found in the urine and blood serum of pregnant women, is commonly tested for as an indicator of pregnancy, is used medically to induce ovulation and to treat male hypogonadism and cryptorchidism, and is produced in certain cancers — abbr. *HCG*

human ecology *n* **1** : a branch of sociology concerned esp. with the study of the spatial and temporal interrelationships between human beings and their economic, social, and political organization **2** : the ecology of human communities and populations esp. as concerned with preservation of environmental quality (as of air or water) through proper application of conservation and civil engineering practices

human ehrlichiosis *n* : any of several ehrlichioses affecting humans; *esp* : HUMAN GRANULOCYTIC EHRLICHIOSIS

human en·gi·neer·ing \-ˌen-jə-ˈni(ə)r-iŋ\ *n* : ERGONOMICS

human factors *n pl but sing in constr* : ERGONOMICS

human factors engineering *n* : ERGONOMICS

human granulocytic ehrlichiosis *n* : an ehrlichiosis of humans that is marked by fever, myalgia, headache, leukemia, and thrombocytopenia and that is caused by a rickettsial bacterium of the genus *Ehrlichia* which is transmitted by ixodid ticks (as the deer tick and American dog tick) — abbr. *HGE*

human growth hormone *n* : the naturally occurring growth hormone of humans or a recombinant version that is used to treat children with growth hormone deficiencies and has been used esp. by athletes to increase muscle mass — abbr. *HGH*; see SOMATROPIN

human immunodeficiency virus *n* : HIV

hu·man·ize *also Brit* **hu·man·ise** \ˈhyü-mə-ˌnīz, ˈyü-\ *vt* **-ized** *also Brit* **-ised; -iz·ing** *also Brit* **-is·ing** : to render (cow's milk) suitable for consumption by human babies — **hu·man·iza·tion** *also Brit* **hu·man·isa·tion** \ˌhyü-mə-nə-ˈzā-shən, ˌyü-\ *n*

hu·man·kind \ˈhyü-mən-ˌkīnd, ˈyü\ *n* : the human race

human leukocyte antigen *n* : any of various proteins that are encoded by genes of the major histocompatibility complex in humans and are found on the surface of many cell types (as white blood cells); *broadly* : HLA 2

hu·man·oid \ˈhyü-mə-ˌnȯid, ˈyü-\ *adj* : having human form or characteristics ⟨∼ dentition⟩ — **humanoid** *n*

human papillomavirus *n* : a double-stranded DNA virus of the genus *Papillomavirus* (species *Human papillomavirus*) that has numerous genotypes causing various human warts (as the common warts of the extremities, plantar warts, and genital warts) including some associated with the production of cervical cancer — called also *HPV*

human relations *n pl but usu sing in constr* **1** : the social and interpersonal relations between human beings **2** : a course, study, or program designed to develop better interpersonal and intergroup adjustments

human T–cell leukemia virus *n* : HTLV

human T–cell leukemia virus type III *n* : HIV-1

human T–cell lym·pho·tro·pic virus \-ˌlim(p)fə-ˈtrō-pik-\ *n* : HTLV

human T–cell lymphotropic virus type III *n* : HIV-1

human T–lymphotropic virus *n* : HTLV

human T–lymphotropic virus type III *n* : HIV-1

¹hu·mec·tant \hyü-ˈmek-tənt\ *adj* : promoting the retention of moisture ⟨∼ properties⟩ ⟨∼ materials⟩

²humectant *n* : a substance (as glycerol or sorbitol) that promotes retention of moisture

hu·mec·ta·tion \ˌhyü-ˌmek-ˈtā-shən\ *n* : the action or process of moistening

hu·mer·al \ˈhyüm-(ə-)rəl\ *adj* : of, relating to, or situated in the region of the humerus or shoulder

humeral circumflex artery — see ANTERIOR HUMERAL CIRCUMFLEX ARTERY, POSTERIOR HUMERAL CIRCUMFLEX ARTERY

hu·mer·us \ˈhyüm-(ə-)rəs\ *n, pl* **hu·meri** \ˈhyü-mə-ˌrī, -ˌrē\ : the longest bone of the upper arm or forelimb extending from the shoulder to the elbow, articulating above by a rounded head with the glenoid fossa, having below a broad articular surface divided by a ridge into a medial pulley-shaped portion and a lateral rounded eminence that articulate with the ulna and radius respectively, and providing various processes and modified surfaces for the attachment of muscles

hu·mic acid \ˈhyü-mik-, ˈyü-\ *n* : any of various organic acids obtained from humus

hu·mid \ˈhyü-məd, ˈyü-\ *adj* : containing or characterized by perceptible moisture esp. to the point of being oppressive ⟨a hot ∼ climate⟩

hu·mid·i·fi·er \hyü-ˈmid-ə-ˌfī(-ə)r, yü-\ *n* : a device for supplying or maintaining humidity

hu·mid·i·fy \-ˌfī\ *vt* **-fied; -fy·ing** : to make humid — **hu·mid·i·fi·ca·tion** \-ˌmid-ə-fə-ˈkā-shən\ *n*

hu·mid·i·stat \hyü-ˈmid-ə-ˌstat, yü-\ *n* : an instrument for regulating or maintaining the degree of humidity

hu·mid·i·ty \hyü-ˈmid-ət-ē, yü-\ *n, pl* **-ties** : a moderate degree of wetness esp. of the atmosphere — see ABSOLUTE HUMIDITY, RELATIVE HUMIDITY

hu·min \ˈhyü-mən\ *n* : any of various dark-colored insoluble usu. amorphous substances formed in many reactions; *esp* : a pigment formed in the acid hydrolysis of protein containing tryptophan — compare MELANOIDIN

hu·mor *or chiefly Brit* **hu·mour** \ˈhyü-mər, ˈyü-\ *n* **1 a** : a normal functioning bodily semifluid or fluid (as the blood or lymph) **b** : a secretion (as a hormone) that is an excitant of activity **2** *in ancient and medieval physiology* : a fluid or juice of an animal or plant; *specif* : one of the four fluids that were believed to enter into the constitution of the body and to determine by their relative proportions a person's health and temperament — see BLACK BILE, BLOOD 3, PHLEGM 1, YELLOW BILE

hu·mor·al \ˈ(h)yüm-(ə-)rəl\ *adj* **1** : of, relating to, proceeding from, or involving a bodily humor (as a hormone) ⟨∼ control of sugar metabolism⟩ **2** : relating to or being the part of immunity or the immune response that involves antibodies secreted by B cells and circulating in bodily fluids ⟨∼

immunity⟩ ⟨∼ immune response⟩ ⟨∼ system of immunity⟩ — compare CELL-MEDIATED

humour *chiefly Brit var of* HUMOR

hump \ˈhəmp\ *n* : a rounded protuberance; *esp* : HUMPBACK

hump·back \-ˌbak, *for 1 also* -ˈbak\ *n* **1** : a humped or crooked back; *also* : KYPHOSIS **2** : HUNCHBACK 2

hump·backed \-ˈbakt\ *adj* : having a humped back

hump sore *n* : infestation of the skin of Zebu cattle by a filarial worm of the genus *Stephanofilaria* (*S. assamensis*); *also* : the hide-damaging lesions caused by such infestation esp. about the hump and neck

Hu·mu·lin \ˈhyü-myü-lən\ *trademark* — used for a preparation of insulin produced by genetic engineering and structurally identical to insulin made by the human pancreas

hu·mus \ˈhyü-məs, ˈyü-\ *n* : a brown or black complex variable material resulting from partial decomposition of plant or animal matter and forming the organic portion of soil

hunch·back \ˈhənch-ˌbak\ *n* **1** : HUMPBACK 1 **2** : a person with a humpback — **hunch·backed** \-ˈbakt\ *adj*

hun·ger \ˈhəŋ-gər\ *n* **1** : a craving, desire, or urgent need for food **2** : an uneasy sensation occasioned normally by the lack of food and resulting directly from stimulation of the sensory nerves of the stomach by the contraction and churning movement of the empty stomach **3** : a weakened disordered condition brought about by prolonged lack of food ⟨die of ∼⟩

hunger pangs *n pl* : pains in the abdominal region which occur in the early stages of hunger or fasting and are correlated with contractions of the empty stomach or intestines

Hun·ner's ulcer \ˈhən-ərz-\ *n* : a painful ulcer affecting all layers of the bladder wall and usu. associated with inflammation of the wall

Hunner, Guy Leroy (1868–1957), American gynecologist. For virtually all of his career Hunner was associated with Johns Hopkins. He made important studies of sterility. In a 1932 article on the treatment of interstitial cystitis he described the lesion now known as Hunner's ulcer.

Hun·ter's canal \ˈhən-tərz-\ *n* : an aponeurotic canal in the middle third of the thigh through which the femoral artery passes

Hunter, John (1728–1793), British anatomist and surgeon. Hunter ranks as one of the greatest surgeons in medical history. He made very important contributions to the practice of surgery which based it on sound biological principles and transformed it into a scientific profession. He also devised an operation for a popliteal aneurysm. An account of the operation, published in 1786 by Sir Everard Home (1756–1832), included a description of Hunter's canal.

Hunter's syndrome *or* **Hunter syndrome** \ˈhən-tər(z)-\ *n* : a mucopolysaccharidosis that is similar to Hurler's syndrome but is inherited as a sex-linked recessive trait and has milder symptoms

Hunter, Charles (1873–1955), Canadian physician. Hunter published his original report on Hunter's syndrome in 1917, basing his findings on case histories of two boys.

Hun·ting·ton's chorea \ˌhənt-iŋ-tənz-\ *n* : HUNTINGTON'S DISEASE

Huntington, George (1850–1916), American neurologist. Huntington was a family doctor who published only one medical document, his description of chronic hereditary chorea. His description of 1872, although not the first, is noted for its detailed recounting of the symptoms, especially the regression that eventually results in dementia. The earliest known description of this type of chorea is by Charles O. Waters (1816–1892), published in 1842 in a work by the American physiologist Robley Dunglison (1798–1869).

Huntington's disease *also* **Huntington disease** *n* : a progressive chorea that is inherited as an autosomal dominant

---

\ə\ abut \ˀ\ kitten \ər\ further \a\ ash \ā\ ace \ä\ cot, cart
\au̇\ out \ch\ chin \e\ bet \ē\ easy \g\ go \i\ hit \ī\ ice \j\ job
\ŋ\ sing \ō\ go \ȯ\ law \ȯi\ boy \th\ thin \t̲h̲\ the \ü\ loot
\u̇\ foot \y\ yet \zh\ vision *See also* Pronunciation Symbols page

trait, that usu. begins in middle age, that is characterized by choreiform movements and mental deterioration leading to dementia, and that is accompanied by atrophy of the caudate nucleus and the loss of certain brain cells with a decrease in the level of several neurotransmitters — called also *Huntington's*

Hur·ler's syndrome \'hər-lərz-, 'hur-\ *or* **Hur·ler syndrome** \'hər-lər-, 'hur-\ *n* : a mucopolysaccharidosis that is inherited as an autosomal recessive trait and is characterized by deformities of the skeleton and features, hepatosplenomegaly, restricted joint flexibility, clouding of the cornea, mental retardation, and deafness — called also *Hurler's disease*

Hur·ler \'hur-lər\, **Gertrud (1889–1965)**, German pediatrician. Hurler published a detailed description of one of the mucopolysaccharidoses in 1919. This hereditary disorder is now also known as Hurler's syndrome, in her honor.

HUS *abbr* hemolytic uremic syndrome

husk \'həsk\ *n* : HOOSE ⟨an outbreak of ∼ was observed in a flock of 200 sheep —*Veterinary Bull.*⟩

hutch·in·so·ni·an teeth \,həch-ən-'sō-nē-ən-\ *n pl, often cap H* : HUTCHINSON'S TEETH

Hutch·in·son's teeth \'həch-ən-sənz-\ *n pl but sing or pl in constr* : peg-shaped teeth having a crescent-shaped notch in the cutting edge and occurring esp. in children with congenital syphilis

Hutchinson, Sir Jonathan (1828–1913), British surgeon and pathologist. Hutchinson was a pioneer in the study of congenital syphilis. He reported his discovery that notched incisor teeth are a sign of congenital syphilis in 1858. He discussed the other elements of Hutchinson's triad in a series of reports published from 1857 to 1860. The triad soon became widely used for the diagnosis of congenital syphilis.

Hutchinson's triad *n* : a triad of symptoms that comprises Hutchinson's teeth, interstitial keratitis, and deafness and occurs in children with congenital syphilis

Hux·ley's layer \'həks-lēz-\ *n* : a layer of the inner stratum of a hair follicle composed of one or two layers of horny flattened epithelial cells with nuclei and situated between Henle's layer and the cuticle next to the hair

Huxley, Thomas Henry (1825–1895), British biologist. Huxley is best remembered as an early proponent and public defender of Darwin's theory of evolution. In 1860 he engaged in a famous debate on the subject with Bishop Samuel Wilberforce at Oxford. One of the most influential scientists of his time, he was particularly influential in the field of scientific education. The author of several seminal textbooks of science, he initiated the first courses in practical training for science teachers. He himself did valuable research in paleontology, taxonomy (especially the classification of birds), and ethnology. He described the layer of the hair follicle now known as Huxley's layer in his first scientific paper, published in 1845.

Huy·ge·ni·an eyepiece \,hī-'gē-nē-ən-, ,hoi-, -'gen-ē-\ *also* **Huy·gens eyepiece** \'hī-gənz-, 'hoi-\ *n* : a compound eyepiece used esp. with achromatic objectives that consists of two plano-convex lenses separated by a diaphragm with the convex sides facing the objective

Huy·gens *or* **Huy·ghens** \'hœi-kəns\, **Christiaan (1629–1695)**, Dutch physicist, astronomer, and mathematician. Huygens was one of the foremost scientists of the 17th century. In 1655 he developed a method of grinding lenses that minimized light aberration. The new lenses that he made enabled him to discover another one of Saturn's satellites and the true shape of the planet's rings. He investigated other astronomical phenomena and experimented further with telescopes. He made lenses of large focal length and invented an achromatic eyepiece. He made the first pendulum-regulated clock in 1657 and investigated the principles of gravity. Above all, Huygens is known for his discoveries concerning light. In 1678 he wrote a treatise in which he discussed the wave nature of light and presented the theory that every point of an advancing wave front generates new

waves. His theory also explained the refraction of light. He also discovered the polarization of light.

HVL *abbr* half-value layer

¹hy·a·line \'hī-ə-lən, -,līn\ *adj* : transparent or nearly transparent and usu. homogeneous

²hyaline *n* **1** *or* **hy·a·lin** \-ə-lən\ : a nitrogenous substance closely related to chitin that forms the main constituent of the walls of hydatid cysts and yields a sugar on decomposition **2** : any of several translucent substances similar to hyaline that collect around cells, are capable of being stained by eosin, and yield a carbohydrate as a cleavage product

hyaline cartilage *n* : translucent bluish white cartilage consisting of cells embedded in an apparently homogeneous matrix, present in joints and respiratory passages, and forming most of the fetal skeleton

hyaline cast *n* : a renal cast of mucoprotein characterized by homogeneity of structure

hyaline degeneration *n* : tissue degeneration chiefly of connective tissues in which structural elements of affected cells are replaced by homogeneous translucent material that stains intensely with acid stains

hyaline membrane disease *n* : RESPIRATORY DISTRESS SYNDROME

hy·a·lin·iza·tion *also Brit* **hy·a·lin·isa·tion** \,hī-ə-lən-ə-'zā-shən\ *n* : the process of becoming hyaline or of undergoing hyaline degeneration; *also* : the resulting state — **hy·a·lin·ized** *also Brit* **hy·a·lin·ised** \'hī-ə-lə-,nīzd\ *adj*

hy·a·li·no·sis \,hī-ə-lə-'nō-səs\ *n, pl* **-no·ses** \-,sēz\ **1** : HYALINE DEGENERATION **2** : a condition characterized by hyaline degeneration

hy·a·li·tis \,hī-ə-'līt-əs\ *n* **1** : inflammation of the vitreous body of the eye **2** : inflammation of the hyaloid membrane of the vitreous body

hy·al·o·gen \hī-'al-ə-jən, -,jen\ *n* : any of several insoluble substances that are related to mucoproteins, are found in many animal structures (as hydatid cysts), and yield hyalines on hydrolysis

hy·a·loid \'hī-ə-,loid\ *adj* : being glassy or transparent ⟨a ∼ appearance⟩

hyaloid membrane *n* : a very delicate membrane enclosing the vitreous body of the eye

hy·al·o·mere \hī-'al-ə-,mi(ə)r\ *n* : the pale portion of a blood platelet that is not refractile — compare CHROMOMERE

Hy·a·lom·ma \,hī-ə-'läm-ə\ *n* : a genus of Old World ticks that attack wild and domestic mammals and sometimes humans, produce severe lesions by their bites, and often serve as vectors of viral and protozoal diseases (as east coast fever)

hy·a·lo·mu·coid \,hī-ə-(,)lō-'myü-,koid\ *n* : a mucoprotein in the vitreous body

hy·a·lo·plasm \hī-'al-ə-,plaz-əm, 'hī-ə-lō-\ *n* : CYTOSOL — **hy·a·lo·plas·mic** \hī-,al-ə-'plaz-mik, ,hī-ə-lō-\ *adj*

hy·al·uro·nate \,hī-ə-'lur-ə-,nāt\ *n* : a salt or ester of hyaluronic acid

hy·al·uron·ic acid \,hīl-yù-,rän-ik-, ,hī-əl-yù-\ *n* : a viscous glycosaminoglycan that occurs esp. in the vitreous body, the umbilical cord, and synovial fluid and as a cementing substance in the subcutaneous tissue

hy·al·uron·i·dase \-'rän-ə-,dās, -,dāz\ *n* : a mucolytic enzyme that splits and lowers the viscosity of hyaluronic acid facilitating the spreading of fluid through tissues either advantageously (as in the absorption of drugs) or disadvantageously (as in the dissemination of infection), that occurs in many normal tissues, in malignant growths, in invasive bacteria, and in certain venoms, and that is used esp. to aid in the dispersion of fluids (as local anesthetics) injected subcutaneously for therapeutic purposes — called also *spreading factor*

H–Y antigen \'āch-'wī-\ *n* : a male histocompatibility antigen determined by genes on the Y chromosome

hy·brid \'hī-brəd\ *n* **1** : an offspring of two animals or plants of different races, breeds, varieties, species, or genera **2** : something heterogeneous in origin or composition ⟨artificial ∼s of DNA and RNA⟩ ⟨somatic cell ∼s of mouse and human cells⟩ — **hybrid** *adj* — **hy·brid·ism** \-brə-₁diz-əm\ *n* — **hy·brid·i·ty** \hī-'brid-ət-ē\ *n, pl* **-ties**

hy·brid·ize *also Brit* **hy·brid·ise** \'hī-brə-₁dīz\ *vb* **-ized** *also Brit* **-ised; -iz·ing** *also Brit* **-is·ing** *vt* : to cause to interbreed or combine so as to produce hybrids ⟨~ two species⟩ ⟨fuse and ~ somatic cells of two different species⟩ ⟨~ two DNAs⟩ ~ *vi* : to produce hybrids — **hy·brid·iza·tion** *also Brit* **hy·brid·isa·tion** \₁hī-brəd-ə-'zā-shən\ *n* — **hy·brid·iz·er** *also Brit* **hy·brid·is·er** *n*

hy·brid·oma \₁hī-brə-'dō-mə\ *n* : a hybrid cell produced by the fusion of an antibody-producing lymphocyte with a tumor cell and used to culture continuously a specific monoclonal antibody

hybrid vig·or \-'vig-ər\ *n* : HETEROSIS

hy·can·thone \hī-'kan-₁thōn\ *n* : a lucanthone analog $C_{20}H_{24}N_2O_2S$ used to treat schistosomiasis

Hy·co·dan \'hī-kə-₁dan\ *trademark* — used for a preparation of the bitartrate of hydrocodone and the methyl bromide of homatropine

hy·dan·to·in \hī-'dan-tə-wən\ *n* **1** : a crystalline weakly acidic imidazole derivative $C_3H_4N_2O_2$ with a sweetish taste that is found in beet juice and used in organic synthesis **2** : a derivative of hydantoin (as phenytoin)

hy·dan·to·in·ate \-wə-₁nāt\ *n* : a salt of hydantoin or of one of its derivatives

hy·da·tid \'hīd-ə-təd, -₁tid\ *n* **1** : the larval cyst of a tapeworm of the genus *Echinococcus* that usu. occurs as a fluid-filled sac containing daughter cysts in which scolices develop but that occas. forms a proliferating spongy mass which actively metastasizes in the host's tissues — called also *hydatid cyst;* see ECHINOCOCCUS 1 **2 a** : an abnormal cyst or cystic structure; *esp* : HYDATIDIFORM MOLE **b** : HYDATID DISEASE

hydatid disease *n* : a form of echinococcosis caused by the development of hydatids of a tapeworm of the genus *Echinococcus* (*E. granulosus*) in the tissues esp. of the liver or lungs of humans and some domestic animals (as sheep and dogs)

hy·da·tid·i·form \₁hī-də-'tid-ə-₁fȯrm\ *adj* : resembling a hydatid or cyst

hydatidiform mole *n* : a mass in the uterus that consists of enlarged edematous degenerated chorionic villi growing in clusters resembling grapes, that typically develops following fertilization of an enucleate egg, and that may or may not contain fetal tissue

hy·da·tid·o·cele \-'tid-ə-₁sēl\ *n* : a tumorous condition of the scrotum caused by local infestation with echinococcus larvae

hydatid of Mor·ga·gni \-mȯr-'gän-yē\ *n* **1** : a small stalked or pedunculated body found between the testicle and the head of the epididymis in the male or attached to the fimbriae of the fallopian tube or the broad ligament in the female and considered to be a remnant of the duct of the pronephros or of the upper end of the Müllerian duct **2** : a small stalkless or sessile body found in the same situation as the hydatid of Morgagni in the male only and considered to be a remnant of the Müllerian duct

G. B. Morgagni — see CRYPT OF MORGAGNI

hy·da·tid·o·sis \₁hī-də-₁ti-'dō-səs\ *n, pl* **-o·ses** \-₁sēz\ : ECHINOCOCCOSIS; *specif* : HYDATID DISEASE

Hyd·er·gine \'hī-dər-₁jēn\ *trademark* — used for a preparation of ergoloid mesylates

hyd·no·car·pic acid \₁hid-nə-'kär-pik-\ *n* : a low-melting unsaturated acid $C_{16}H_{28}O_2$ occurring as the glyceride in chaulmoogra oil and hydnocarpus oil

hyd·no·car·pus \-'kär-pəs\ *n* **1** *cap* : a genus of tropical trees (family Flacourtiaceae) of southeastern Asia having alternate leaves, small flowers, and capsular fruits of which several are sources of chaulmoogra oil and hydnocarpus oil **2** : any tree of the genus *Hydnocarpus*

hydnocarpus oil *n* : a fatty oil obtained from seeds of trees of the genus *Hydnocarpus* (esp. *H. wightiana*) used esp. formerly in the treatment of leprosy

hy·dra \'hī-drə\ *n* : any of numerous small tubular freshwa-

ter hydrozoan polyps (*Hydra* and related genera) having at one end a mouth surrounded by tentacles

hydraemia *chiefly Brit var of* HYDREMIA

hy·dra·gogue *also* **hy·dra·gog** \'hī-drə-₁gäg\ *n* : a cathartic that causes copious watery discharges from the bowels

hy·dral·azine \hī-'dral-ə-₁zēn\ *n* : an antihypertensive drug that is used in the form of its hydrochloride $C_8H_8N_4 \cdot HCl$ and produces peripheral arteriolar dilation by relaxing vascular smooth muscle

hy·dram·ni·os \hī-'dram-nē-₁äs\ *also* **hy·dram·ni·on** \-₁än\ *n* : excessive accumulation of the amniotic fluid — called also *polyhydramnios* — **hy·dram·ni·ot·ic** \hī-₁dram-nē-'ät-ik\ *adj*

hy·dran·en·ceph·a·ly \₁hī-₁dran-en-'sef-ə-lē\ *n, pl* **-lies** : a congenital defect of the brain in which fluid-filled cavities take the place of the cerebral hemispheres

hy·dran·gea \hī-'drān-jə\ *n* **1** *cap* : a large genus of widely distributed shrubs and one woody vine (family Saxifragaceae) with opposite leaves and showy clusters of usu. sterile white, pink, or bluish flowers **2** : any plant of the genus *Hydrangea* **3** : the dried rhizome and roots of the wild plant of the genus *Hydrangea* (*H. arborescens*) formerly used in pharmacy as a diuretic

hy·drar·gyr·ia \₁hī-(₁)drär-'jir-ē-ə\ *n* : MERCURIALISM

hy·drar·gy·rism \hī-'drär-jə-₁riz-əm\ *n* : MERCURIALISM

hy·drar·gy·rum \-rəm\ *n* : MERCURY

hy·drar·thro·sis \₁hī-(₁)drär-'thrō-səs\ *n, pl* **-thro·ses** \-₁sēz\ : a watery effusion into a joint cavity

hy·drase \'hī-₁drās, -₁drāz\ *n* : an enzyme that promotes the addition or removal of water to or from its substrate

hy·dras·tine \hī-'dras-₁tēn, -tən\ *n* : a bitter crystalline alkaloid $C_{21}H_{21}NO_6$ derived from isoquinoline that is an active constituent of hydrastis

hy·dras·ti·nine \hī-'dras-tə-₁nēn, -nən\ *n* : a crystalline base $C_{11}H_{13}NO_3$ formed by the oxidation of hydrastine and formerly used in controlling uterine hemorrhage

hy·dras·tis \hī-'dras-təs\ *n* **1** *cap* : a genus of herbs (family Ranunculaceae) having palmately lobed leaves and small greenish flowers and including the goldenseal (*H. canadensis*) **2** : the dried rhizome and roots of the goldenseal formerly used in pharmacy as a bitter tonic, hemostatic, and antiseptic — called also *goldenseal*

hy·dra·tase \'hī-drə-₁tās, 'hī-drā-, -₁tāz\ *n* : any of several lyases that catalyze the hydration or dehydration of a carbon-oxygen bond

¹hy·drate \'hī-₁drāt\ *n* : a compound (as Glauber's salt) formed by the union of water with some other substance

²hydrate *vb* **hy·drat·ed; hy·drat·ing** *vt* : to cause to take up or combine with water or the elements of water ~ *vi* : to become a hydrate

hy·dra·tion \hī-'drā-shən\ *n* **1** : the act or process of combining or treating with water: as **a** : the introduction of additional fluid into the body ⟨~ sometimes helps to reduce the concentration of toxic substances in the tissues⟩ **b** : a chemical reaction in which water takes part with the formation of only one product ⟨~ of ethylene to ethyl alcohol⟩; *esp* : a reaction in which water takes part in the form of intact molecules **2** : the quality or state of being hydrated; *esp* : the condition of having adequate fluid in the body tissues

hy·drau·lics \hī-'drȯ-liks\ *n pl but sing in constr* : a branch of science that deals with practical applications (as the transmission of energy or the effects of flow) of liquid (as water) in motion — **hy·drau·lic** \-lik\ *adj*

hy·dra·zide \'hī-drə-₁zīd\ *n* : any of a class of compounds resulting from the replacement of hydrogen by an acid group in hydrazine or in one of its derivatives

hy·dra·zine \'hī-drə-₁zēn\ *n* : a colorless fuming corrosive strongly reducing liquid base N_2H_4 used in the production of various materials (as pharmaceuticals and plastics); *also* : an organic base derived from this compound

G
H

\ə\ **abut** \ʰ\ **kitten** \ər\ **further** \a\ **ash** \ā\ **ace** \ä\ **cot, cart** \au̇\ **out** \ch\ **chin** \e\ **bet** \ē\ **easy** \g\ **go** \i\ **hit** \ī\ **ice** \j\ **job** \ŋ\ **sing** \ō\ **go** \ȯ\ **law** \ȯi\ **boy** \th\ **thin** \t̲h̲\ **the** \ü\ **loot** \u̇\ **foot** \y\ **yet** \zh\ **vision** *See also* Pronunciation Symbols page

hy·dra·zi·nol·y·sis \ˌhī-drə-zi-ˈnäl-ə-səs\ *n, pl* **-y·ses** \-ˌsēz\ : the breaking of peptide bonds of a protein by hydrazine with the release of amino acids

hy·dra·zone \ˈhī-drə-ˌzōn\ *n* : any of a class of compounds containing the group >C=NNHR formed by the action of hydrazine or a substituted hydrazine (as phenylhydrazine) on a compound containing a carbonyl group (as an aldehyde or ketone)

hy·dre·mia *or chiefly Brit* **hy·drae·mia** \hī-ˈdrē-mē-ə\ *n* : an abnormally watery state of the blood — **hy·dre·mic** *or chiefly Brit* **hy·drae·mic** \-mik\ *adj*

hy·dren·ceph·a·lo·cele \ˌhī-(ˌ)dren-ˈsef-ə-lō-ˌsēl\ *n* : a hernia through a fissure in the skull in which the hernial sac contains both brain substance and watery fluid

hy·dren·ceph·a·lus \-ˈsef-ə-ləs\ *n, pl* **-li** \-ˌlī\ : HYDROCEPHALUS

hy·dren·ceph·a·ly \-ˈsef-ə-lē\ *n, pl* **-lies** : HYDROCEPHALUS

hy·dride \ˈhī-ˌdrīd\ *n* : a compound of hydrogen with a more electropositive element or group

hy·dri·od·ic acid \ˌhī-drē-ˌäd-ik-\ *n* : an aqueous solution of hydrogen iodide that is a strong acid resembling hydrochloric acid chemically and that is also a strong reducing agent

hy·dro \ˈhī-(ˌ)drō\ *n, pl* **hydros** *Brit* : a hydropathic facility : SPA; *also* : a hotel catering to people using such a facility

hy·droa \hī-ˈdrō-ə\ *n* : an itching usu. vesicular eruption of the skin; *esp* : one induced by exposure to light

hy·dro·al·co·hol·ic \ˌhī-drō-ˌal-kə-ˈhól-ik, -ˈhäl-\ *adj* : of or relating to water and alcohol ⟨∼ solutions⟩

hy·dro·bro·mic acid \ˌhī-drə-ˌbrō-mik-\ *n* : an aqueous solution of hydrogen bromide HBr that is a strong acid resembling hydrochloric acid chemically, that is a weak reducing agent, and that is used esp. for making bromides

hy·dro·bro·mide \-ˈbrō-ˌmīd\ *n* : a salt of hydrogen bromide with an organic base

hy·dro·car·bon \-ˈkär-bən\ *n* : an organic compound (as acetylene, benzene, or butane) containing only carbon and hydrogen and often occurring in petroleum, natural gas, coal, and bitumens

hy·dro·cele \ˈhī-drə-ˌsēl\ *n* : an accumulation of serous fluid in a sacculated cavity (as the scrotum)

hy·dro·ce·lec·to·my \ˌhī-drə-sē-ˈlek-tə-mē\ *n, pl* **-mies** : surgical removal of a hydrocele

¹**hy·dro·ce·phal·ic** \ˌhī-drō-sə-ˈfal-ik, *Brit also* -kə-ˈfal-\ *adj* : relating to, characterized by, or affected with hydrocephalus

²**hydrocephalic** *n* : one affected with hydrocephalus

hy·dro·ceph·a·loid \-ˈsef-ə-ˌlóid, *Brit also* -ˈkef-\ *adj* : resembling hydrocephalus

hy·dro·ceph·a·lus \-ˈsef-ə-ləs, *Brit also* -ˈkef-\ *n, pl* **-li** \-ˌlī\ : an abnormal increase in the amount of cerebrospinal fluid within the cranial cavity that is accompanied by expansion of the cerebral ventricles, enlargement of the skull and esp. the forehead, and atrophy of the brain

hy·dro·ceph·a·ly \ˌhī-drō-ˈsef-ə-lē\ *n, pl* **-lies** : HYDROCEPHALUS

hy·dro·chlo·ric acid \ˌhī-drə-ˌklōr-ik-, -ˌklór-\ *n* : an aqueous solution of hydrogen chloride HCl that is a strong corrosive irritating acid, is normally present in dilute form in gastric juice, and is widely used in industry and in the laboratory — called also *muriatic acid*

hy·dro·chlo·ride \-ˈklō(ə)r-ˌīd, -ˈkló(ə)r-\ *n* : a salt of hydrochloric acid with an organic base used esp. as a vehicle for the administration of a drug

hy·dro·chlo·ro·thi·a·zide \-ˌklōr-ə-ˈthī-ə-ˌzīd, -ˌklór-\ *n* : a diuretic and antihypertensive drug $C_7H_8ClN_3O_4S_2$ — abbr. *HCTZ*; see DYAZIDE, HYDRODIURIL, HYZAAR, ORETIC

hy·dro·cho·le·re·sis \-ˌkō-lər-ˈē-səs, -ˌkä-\ *n, pl* **-re·ses** \-ˌsēz\ : increased production of watery liver bile without necessarily increased secretion of bile solids — compare CHOLERESIS

¹**hy·dro·cho·le·ret·ic** \-ˈet-ik\ *adj* : of, relating to, or characterized by hydrocholeresis

²**hydrocholeretic** *n* : an agent that produces hydrocholeresis

hy·dro·co·done \ˌhī-drō-ˈkō-ˌdōn\ *n* : a habit-forming compound derived from codeine and administered in the form of

its bitartrate $C_{18}H_{21}NO_3 \cdot C_4H_6O_6$ usu. in combination with other drugs (as acetaminophen) as an analgesic or cough sedative — called also *dihydrocodeinone;* see HYCODAN, VICODIN

hy·dro·col·loid \-ˈkäl-ˌóid\ *n* : any of several substances that yield gels with water (as alginic acid salts, agar, carrageenan, and related polysaccharide gums) and that are used esp. as protective colloids and as impression materials in dentistry — **hy·dro·col·loi·dal** \-kə-ˈlóid-ᵊl, -kä-\ *adj*

hy·dro·col·pos \-ˈkäl-ˌpäs\ *n* : an accumulation of watery fluid in the vagina — compare HYDROMETROCOLPOS

hy·dro·cor·ti·sone \-ˈkórt-ə-ˌsōn, -ˌzōn\ *n* : CORTISOL; *esp* : cortisol used pharmaceutically

hy·dro·co·tar·nine \-kō-ˈtär-ˌnēn, -nən\ *n* : a crystalline alkaloid $C_{12}H_{15}NO_3$ obtained from opium and also formed by the reduction of cotarnine

hy·dro·cy·an·ic acid \ˌhī-drō-sī-ˌan-ik-\ *n* : an aqueous solution of hydrogen cyanide HCN that is an extremely poisonous weak acid used esp. in fumigating — called also *prussic acid*

Hy·dro·di·ur·il \-ˈdī-yə-ˌril\ *trademark* — used for a preparation of hydrochlorothiazide

hy·dro·dy·nam·ic \-dī-ˈnam-ik\ *also* **hy·dro·dy·nam·i·cal** \-i-kəl\ *adj* : of, relating to, or involving principles of hydrodynamics

hy·dro·dy·nam·ics \-iks\ *n pl but sing in constr* : a branch of physics that deals with the motion of fluids and the forces acting on solid bodies immersed in fluids and in motion relative to them — compare HYDROSTATICS

hy·dro·flu·me·thi·a·zide \-ˌflü-mə-ˈthī-ə-ˌzīd\ *n* : a diuretic and antihypertensive drug $C_8H_8F_3N_3O_4S_2$ — see SALURON

hy·dro·flu·or·ic acid \-ˌflùr-ik-, -ˌflór-, -ˌflór-\ *n* : an aqueous solution of hydrogen fluoride HF that is a weak poisonous acid, that resembles hydrochloric acid chemically but attacks silica and silicates, and that is used esp. in finishing and etching glass

hy·dro·gel \ˈhī-drə-ˌjel\ *n* : a gel in which the liquid is water ⟨a silicone ∼ used to make soft contact lenses⟩

hy·dro·gen \ˈhī-drə-jən\ *n* : a nonmetallic element that is the simplest and lightest of the elements and that is normally a colorless odorless highly flammable diatomic gas — symbol *H*; see DEUTERIUM, TRITIUM; ELEMENT table — **hy·drog·e·nous** \hī-ˈdräj-ə-nəs\ *adj*

hydrogen arsenide *n* : ARSINE

hy·drog·e·nase \hī-ˈdräj-ə-ˌnās, -ˌnāz\ *n* : an enzyme of various microorganisms that promotes the formation and utilization of gaseous hydrogen

hy·dro·ge·nate \hī-ˈdräj-ə-ˌnāt, ˈhī-drə-jə-\ *vt* **-nat·ed; -nat·ing** : to combine or treat with or expose to hydrogen; *esp* : to add hydrogen to the molecule of (an unsaturated organic compound) — **hy·dro·ge·na·tion** \hī-ˌdräj-ə-ˈnā-shən, ˌhī-drə-jə-\ *n*

hydrogen bond *n* : an electrostatic attraction between a hydrogen atom in one polar molecule (as of water) and a small electronegative atom (as of oxygen, nitrogen, or fluorine) in usu. another molecule of the same or a different polar substance — **hydrogen bonding** *n*

hydrogen bromide *n* : a colorless irritating gas HBr that fumes in moist air and that yields hydrobromic acid when dissolved in water

hydrogen chloride *n* : a colorless pungent poisonous gas HCl that fumes in moist air and yields hydrochloric acid when dissolved in water

hydrogen cyanide *n* **1** : a poisonous usu. gaseous compound HCN that has the odor of bitter almonds **2** : HYDROCYANIC ACID

hydrogen fluoride *n* : a colorless corrosive fuming usu. gaseous compound HF that yields hydrofluoric acid when dissolved in water

hydrogen iodide *n* : an acrid colorless gas HI that fumes in moist air and yields hydriodic acid when dissolved in water

hydrogen ion *n* **1** : the cation H⁺ of acids consisting of a hydrogen atom whose electron has been transferred to the anion of the acid **2** : HYDRONIUM

hydrogen peroxide *n* : an unstable compound H_2O_2 used esp. as an oxidizing and bleaching agent and as an antiseptic

hydrogen sulfide *n* : a flammable poisonous gas H_2S that has an odor suggestive of rotten eggs and is found esp. in many mineral waters and in putrefying matter

¹hy·droid \'hī-ˌdròid\ *adj* : of or relating to a hydrozoan; *esp* : resembling a typical hydra

²hydroid *n* : HYDROZOAN; *esp* : a hydrozoan polyp as distinguished from a medusa

hy·dro·ki·net·ic \ˌhī-drō-kə-'net-ik, *Brit also* -(ˌ)kī-\ *adj* : of or relating to the motions of fluids or the forces which produce or affect such motions — compare HYDROSTATIC

hy·dro·ki·net·ics \-kə-'net-iks, *Brit also* -(ˌ)kī-\ *n pl but usu sing in constr* : a branch of kinetics that deals with liquids

hy·dro·lase \'hī-drə-ˌlās, -ˌlāz\ *n* : a hydrolytic enzyme (as an esterase)

hy·drol·o·gy \hī-'dräl-ə-jē\ *n, pl* **-gies** : the body of medical knowledge and practice concerned with the therapeutic use of bathing and water

hy·dro·ly·sate \hī-'dräl-ə-ˌsāt, ˌhī-drə-'lī-\ *or* **hy·dro·ly·zate** \-ˌzāt\ *n* : a product of hydrolysis

hy·dro·ly·sis \hī-'dräl-ə-səs, ˌhī-drə-'lī-\ *n* : a chemical process of decomposition involving the splitting of a bond and the addition of the hydrogen cation and the hydroxide anion of water — **hy·dro·lyt·ic** \ˌhī-drə-'lit-ik\ *adj* — **hy·dro·lyt·i·cal·ly** \-i-k(ə-)lē\ *adv*

hy·dro·lyze *or chiefly Brit* **hy·dro·lyse** \'hī-drə-ˌlīz\ *vb* **-lyzed** *or chiefly Brit* **-lysed; -lyz·ing** *or chiefly Brit* **-lys·ing** *vt* : to subject to hydrolysis ~ *vi* : to undergo hydrolysis — **hy·dro·lyz·able** *or chiefly Brit* **hy·dro·lys·able** \-ˌlī-zə-bəl\ *adj*

hy·dro·mel \'hī-drə-ˌmel\ *n* : a laxative containing honey and water

hy·dro·men·in·gi·tis \ˌhī-drō-ˌmen-ən-'jīt-əs\ *n, pl* **-git·i·des** \-'jit-ə-ˌdēz\ : meningitis with serous effusion

hy·drom·e·ter \hī-'dräm-ət-ər\ *n* : an instrument for determining the specific gravity of a liquid (as an alcohol or saline solution) and hence its strength — **hy·drom·e·try** \-ə-trē\ *n, pl* **-tries**

hy·dro·me·tra \ˌhī-drō-'mē-trə\ *n* : an accumulation of watery fluid in the uterus

hy·dro·me·tro·col·pos \-ˌmē-trō-'käl-ˌpäs\ *n* : an accumulation of watery fluid in the uterus and vagina — compare HYDROCOLPOS

hy·dro·micro·ceph·a·ly \-ˌmī-krō-'sef-ə-lē, *Brit also* -'kef-\ *n, pl* **-lies** : microcephaly with an increase in cerebrospinal fluid

hy·dro·mor·phone \-'mòr-ˌfōn\ *n* : a ketone $C_{17}H_{19}NO_3$ derived from morphine that is about five times as active biologically as morphine and is administered in the form of its hydrochloride $C_{17}H_{19}NO_3 \cdot HCl$ as an analgesic — called also *dihydromorphinone*

hy·dro·ne·phro·sis \-ni-'frō-səs\ *n, pl* **-phro·ses** \-ˌsēz\ : cystic distension of the kidney caused by the accumulation of urine in the renal pelvis as a result of obstruction to outflow and accompanied by atrophy of the kidney structure and cyst formation

hy·dro·ne·phrot·ic \-ni-'frät-ik\ *adj* : affected with hydronephrosis ⟨~ kidneys⟩

hy·dro·ni·um \hī-'drō-nē-əm\ *n* : a hydrated hydrogen ion H_3O^+

hy·dro·os·mot·ic \ˌhī-drō-äz-'mät-ik, -äs-\ *adj* : of, relating to, or promoting the passage of water through semipermeable membranes ⟨the ~ effect of antidiuretic hormone⟩

hy·drop·a·thy \hī-'dräp-ə-thē\ *n, pl* **-thies** : a method of treating disease by copious and frequent use of water both externally and internally — compare HYDROTHERAPY — **hy·dro·path·ic** \ˌhī-drə-'path-ik\ *adj* — **hy·dro·path·i·cal·ly** \-i-k(ə-)lē\ *adv*

hy·dro·pe·nia \ˌhī-drə-'pē-nē-ə\ *n* : a condition in which the body is deficient in water — **hy·dro·pe·nic** \-'pē-nik\ *adj*

hy·dro·peri·car·di·um \ˌhī-drō-ˌper-ə-'kär-dē-əm\ *n, pl* **-dia** \-dē-ə\ : an excess of watery fluid in the pericardial cavity

hy·dro·peri·to·ne·um \-ˌper-ət-ᵊn-'ē-əm\ *n, pl* **-nea** \-'ē-ə\ *or* **-ne·ums** : ASCITES

hy·dro·per·ox·ide \-pə-'räk-ˌsīd\ *n* : a compound containing the monovalent group –OOH

¹hy·dro·phile \'hī-drə-ˌfīl\ *also* **hy·dro·phil** \-ˌfil\ *adj* : HYDROPHILIC

²hydrophile *n* : a hydrophilic substance

hy·dro·phil·ia \ˌhī-drə-'fil-ē-ə\ *n* : the property of being hydrophilic ⟨the ~ of certain colloids⟩

¹hy·dro·phil·ic \-'fil-ik\ *adj* : of, relating to, or having a strong affinity for water ⟨~ colloids swell in water and are relatively stable⟩ ⟨soft contact lenses are made of ~ plastic, which absorbs water⟩ — compare LIPOPHILIC, LYOPHILIC, OLEOPHILIC — **hy·dro·phi·lic·i·ty** \-fi-'lis-ət-ē\ *n, pl* **-ties**

²hydrophilic *n* : HYDROPHILE

hydrophilic ointment *n* : an ointment base easily removable with water

hy·dro·phobe \'hī-drə-ˌfōb\ *n* : a hydrophobic substance — **hydrophobe** *adj*

hy·dro·pho·bia \ˌhī-drə-'fō-bē-ə\ *n* **1** : a morbid dread of water **2** : RABIES

hy·dro·pho·bic \-'fō-bik\ *adj* **1** : of, relating to, or suffering from hydrophobia **2** : resistant to or avoiding wetting ⟨a ~ lens⟩ **3** : of, relating to, or having a lack of affinity for water ⟨~ colloids are relatively unstable⟩ — compare LYOPHOBIC, OLEOPHOBIC — **hy·dro·pho·bi·cal·ly** \-bi-k(ə-)lē\ *adv* — **hy·dro·pho·bic·i·ty** \-ˌfō-'bis-ət-ē\ *n, pl* **-ties**

hy·droph·thal·mos \ˌhī-ˌdräf-'thal-mäs\ *n* : general enlargement of the eyeball due to a watery effusion within it

hy·drop·ic \hī-'dräp-ik\ *adj* **1** : exhibiting hydrops; *esp* : EDEMATOUS **2** : characterized by swelling and taking up of fluid — used of a type of cellular degeneration

hy·dro·pneu·mo·tho·rax \ˌhī-drə-ˌn(y)ü-mə-'thō(ə)r-ˌaks, -'thó(ə)r-\ *n, pl* **-tho·rax·es** *or* **-tho·ra·ces** \-'thōr-ə-ˌsēz, -'thòr-\ : the presence of gas and serous fluid in the pleural cavity — called also *pneumohydrothorax*

hy·drops \'hī-ˌdräps\ *n, pl* **hy·drop·ses** \-ˌsēz\ **1** : EDEMA **2** : distension of a hollow organ with fluid ⟨~ of the gallbladder⟩ **3** : HYDROPS FETALIS

hydrops fe·tal·is *or Brit* **hydrops foe·tal·is** \-fē-'tal-əs\ *n* : serious and extensive edema of the fetus (as in erythroblastosis fetalis)

hy·dro·qui·nine \ˌhī-drō-'kwī-ˌnīn *also* -'kwin-ˌīn, *esp Brit* -kwin-'ēn, -'kwin-ˌēn\ *n* : a bitter crystalline antipyretic alkaloid $C_{20}H_{26}N_2O_2$ found with quinine in cinchona bark and usu. present in commercial quinine

hy·dro·qui·none \-kwin-'ōn, -'kwin-ˌōn\ *n* : a bleaching agent $C_6H_6O_2$ used topically to remove pigmentation from hyperpigmented areas of skin (as a lentigo or freckle)

hy·dro·rrhea *or chiefly Brit* **hy·dro·rrhoea** \-'rē-ə\ *n* : a profuse watery discharge (as from the nose)

hydros *pl of* HYDRO

hy·dro·sal·pinx \-'sal-(ˌ)piŋ(k)s\ *n, pl* **-sal·pin·ges** \-sal-'pin-(ˌ)jēz\ : abnormal distension of one or both fallopian tubes with fluid usu. due to inflammation

hy·dro·sol \'hī-drə-ˌsäl, -ˌsòl\ *n* : a sol in which the liquid is water — **hy·dro·sol·ic** \ˌhī-drə-'säl-ik\ *adj*

hy·dro·sol·u·ble \ˌhī-drə-'säl-yə-bəl\ *adj* : soluble in water ⟨the ~ tetracyclines⟩

hy·dro·stat·ic \-'stat-ik\ *adj* : of or relating to fluids at rest or to the pressures they exert or transmit — compare HYDROKINETIC — **hy·dro·stat·i·cal·ly** \-i-k(ə-)lē\ *adv*

hydrostatic bed *n* : WATER BED

hy·dro·stat·ics \-iks\ *n pl but sing in constr* : a branch of physics that deals with the characteristics of fluids at rest and esp. with the pressure in a fluid or exerted by a fluid on an immersed body — compare HYDRODYNAMICS

hy·dro·tax·is \ˌhī-drə-'tak-səs\ *n, pl* **-tax·es** \-ˌsēz\ : a taxis in which moisture is the directive factor — **hy·dro·tac·tic** \-'tak-tik\ *adj*

\ə\ abut \ᵊ\ kitten \ər\ further \a\ ash \ā\ ace \ä\ cot, cart
\au̇\ out \ch\ chin \e\ bet \ē\ easy \g\ go \i\ hit \ī\ ice \j\ job
\ŋ\ sing \ō\ go \ȯ\ law \ȯi\ boy \th\ thin \t͟h\ the \ü\ loot
\u̇\ foot \y\ yet \zh\ vision   *See also* Pronunciation Symbols page

G
H

hy·dro·ther·a·peu·tic \-,ther-ə-'pyüt-ik\ *adj* : of, relating to, or involving the methods of hydrotherapy

hy·dro·ther·a·peu·tics \-iks\ *n pl but usu sing in constr* : HYDROTHERAPY

hy·dro·ther·a·pist \-'ther-ə-pəst\ *n* : a specialist in hydrotherapy

hy·dro·ther·a·py \-'ther-ə-pē\ *n, pl* **-pies** : the therapeutic use of water (as in a whirlpool bath) — compare HYDROPATHY

hy·dro·ther·mal \,hī-drə-'thər-məl\ *adj* : of or relating to hot water — **hy·dro·ther·mal·ly** \-mə-lē\ *adv*

hy·dro·tho·rax \-'thō(ə)r-,aks, -'thȯ(ə)r-\ *n, pl* **-tho·rax·es** *or* **-tho·ra·ces** \-'thōr-ə-,sēz, -'thȯr-\ : an excess of serous fluid in the pleural cavity; *esp* : an effusion resulting from failing circulation (as in heart disease or from lung infection)

hy·dro·tro·pic \-'trō-pik, -'träp-ik\ *adj* **1** : exhibiting or characterized by hydrotropism **2** : relating to or causing hydrotropy ⟨the ∼ action of bile salts⟩ — **hy·dro·tro·pi·cal·ly** \-'trō-pi-k(ə-)lē, -'träp-i-\ *adv*

hy·dro·tro·pism \hī-'drä-trə-,piz-əm; ,hī-drə-'trō-,piz-əm, -'trä-\ *n* : a tropism in which water or water vapor is the orienting factor

hy·drot·ro·py \hī-'drä-trə-pē\ *n, pl* **-pies** : solubilization of a sparingly soluble substance in water brought about by an added agent

hy·dro·ure·ter \,hī-drō-'yur-ət-ər\ *n* : abnormal distension of the ureter with urine

hy·drous \'hī-drəs\ *adj* : containing water usu. in chemical association (as in hydrates)

hydrous wool fat *n* : LANOLIN

hy·drox·ide \hī-'dräk-,sīd\ *n* **1** : the monovalent anion OH⁻ consisting of one atom of hydrogen and one of oxygen — called also *hydroxide ion* **2** : an ionic compound of hydroxide with an element or group

hy·droxo·co·bal·amin \hī-'dräk-(,)sō-kō-'bal-ə-mən\ *n* : a member $C_{62}H_{89}CoN_{13}O_{15}P$ of the vitamin B_{12} group used in treating and preventing vitamin B_{12} deficiency

hy·droxy \hī-'dräk-sē\ *adj* : being or containing hydroxyl; *esp* : containing hydroxyl in place of hydrogen — often used in combination ⟨*hydroxy*butyric acid⟩

hy·droxy·ace·tic acid \hī-,dräk-sē-ə-,sēt-ik-\ *n* : GLYCOLIC ACID

hy·droxy·am·phet·amine \-am-'fet-ə-,mēn, -mən\ *n* : a sympathomimetic drug administered in the form of its hydrobromide $C_9H_{13}NO·HBr$ and used esp. as a decongestant and mydriatic

hydroxyanisole — see BUTYLATED HYDROXYANISOLE

hy·droxy·ap·a·tite \hī-,dräk-sē-'ap-ə-,tīt\ *or* **hy·drox·yl·ap·a·tite** \-sə-'lap-ə-,tīt\ *n* : a complex phosphate of calcium $Ca_5(PO_4)_3OH$ that occurs as a mineral and is the chief structural element of vertebrate bone

hy·droxy·ben·zene \hī-,dräk-sē-'ben-,zēn\ *n* : PHENOL 1

hy·droxy·ben·zo·ic acid \-ben-,zō-ik-\ *n* : any of three crystalline derivatives $C_7H_6O_3$ of benzoic acid that contain one hydroxyl group per molecule: as **a** : the colorless para-substituted acid used in making several of its esters that are effective preservatives — called also *parahydroxybenzoic acid* **b** : SALICYLIC ACID

hy·droxy·bu·ty·rate \-'byüt-ə-,rāt\ *n* : a salt or ester of hydroxybutyric acid

hy·droxy·bu·tyr·ic acid \-byü-'tir-ik-\ *or* β**-hy·droxy·bu·tyr·ic acid** \'bät-ə-, *chiefly Brit* 'bēt-ə-\ *n* : a derivative $C_4H_8O_3$ of butyric acid that is excreted in urine in increased quantities in diabetes — called also *oxybutyric acid*

hy·droxy·chlor·o·quine \-'klōr-ə-,kwēn, -kwin\ *n* : a drug derived from quinoline that is administered orally in the form of its sulfate $C_{18}H_{26}ClN_3O·H_2SO_4$ to treat malaria, rheumatoid arthritis, and lupus erythematosus — see PLAQUENIL

25–hy·droxy·cho·le·cal·cif·er·ol \'twent-ē-'fīv-hī-,dräk-sē-,kō-lə-(,)kal-'sif-ə-,rȯl, -,rōl\ *n* : a sterol $C_{27}H_{44}O_2$ that is a metabolite of cholecalciferol formed in the liver, is the circulating form of vitamin D, and has some activity in maintaining calcium homeostasis and preventing rickets

17–hy·droxy·cor·ti·co·ste·roid \,sev-ən-'tēn-hī-,dräk-sē-,kȯrt-i-kō-'sti(ə)r-,ȯid *also* -'ste(ə)r-\ *n* : any of several adrenocorticosteroids (as cortisol) with an –OH group and an $HOCH_2CO^-$ group attached to carbon 17 of the fused ring structure of the steroid

hy·droxy·cor·ti·co·ste·rone \-,kȯrt-i-kō-'käs-tə-,rōn, -i-kō-stə-'; ,kȯrt-i-kō-'sti(ə)r-,ōn, -'ste(ə)r-\ *n* : a hydroxy derivative of corticosterone; *esp* : CORTISOL

hy·droxy·di·one sodium succinate \-'dī-,ōn-\ *n* : a steroid $C_{25}H_{35}NaO_6$ given intravenously as a general anesthetic

6–hy·droxy·do·pa·mine \'siks-hī-,dräk-sē-'dō-pə-,mēn\ *n* : an isomer of norepinephrine that is taken up by catecholaminergic nerve fibers, causes the degeneration of their terminals, and has been used experimentally to study the behavioral and physiological effects of destroying selected groups of neurons in the central nervous systems of experimental animals

5–hy·droxy·in·dole·ace·tic acid \'fīv-hī-,dräk-sē-,in-(,)dōl-ə-,sēt-ik-\ *n* : a metabolite $C_{10}H_9NO_3$ of serotonin that is present in cerebrospinal fluid and in urine — abbr. *5-HIAA*

hy·drox·yl \hī-'dräk-səl\ *n* **1** : the chemical group or ion OH that consists of one atom of hydrogen and one of oxygen and is neutral or positively charged **2** : HYDROXIDE 1 — **hy·drox·yl·ic** \,hī-,dräk-'sil-ik\ *adj*

hy·drox·yl·amine \hī-,dräk-sə-lə-'mēn, ,hī-,dräk-'sil-ə-,mēn\ *n* : a colorless odorless nitrogenous base NH_3O that resembles ammonia in its reactions but is less basic and that is used esp. as a reducing agent

hydroxylapatite *var of* HYDROXYAPATITE

hy·drox·y·lase \hī-'dräk-sə-,lās, -,lāz\ *n* : any of a group of enzymes that catalyze oxidation reactions in which one of the two atoms of molecular oxygen is incorporated into the substrate and the other is used to oxidize NADH or NADPH

hy·drox·y·la·tion \hī-,dräk-sə-'lā-shən\ *n* : the introduction of hydroxyl into an ion or radical usu. by the replacement of hydrogen — **hy·drox·y·late** \-'dräk-sə-,lāt\ *vt* **-lat·ed; -lating**

hydroxyl ion *n* : HYDROXIDE 1

hy·droxy·ly·sine \,hī-,dräk-sē-'lī-,sēn\ *n* : an amino acid $C_6H_{14}N_2O_3$ that is found esp. in collagen

hy·droxy·pro·ges·ter·one \,hī-,dräk-sē-prō-'jes-tə-,rōn\ *or* **17α–hydroxyprogesterone** \,sev-ən-'ten-'al-fə-\ *n* : a synthetic derivative of progesterone used esp. in the form of its caproate $C_{27}H_{40}O_4$ in progestational therapy (as for amenorrhea and abnormal uterine bleeding)

hy·droxy·pro·line \-'prō-,lēn\ *n* : an amino acid $C_5H_9NO_3$ that occurs naturally as a constituent of collagen

8–hy·droxy·quin·o·line \'āt-hī-,dräk-sē-'kwin-°l-,ēn\ *n* : a derivative of quinoline that is used esp. in the form of its sulfate $(C_9H_7NO)_2·H_2SO_4$ as a disinfectant, topical antiseptic, antiperspirant, and deodorant — called also *oxine, oxyquinoline*

hy·droxy·ste·roid \-'sti(ə)r-,ȯid *also* -'ste(ə)r-\ *n* : any of several ketosteroids (as androsterone and dehydroepiandrosterone) found esp. in human urine

hydroxytoluene — see BUTYLATED HYDROXYTOLUENE

5–hy·droxy·tryp·ta·mine \'fīv-hī-,dräk-sē-'trip-tə-,mēn\ *n* : SEROTONIN

hy·droxy·urea \-yu̇-'rē-ə\ *n* : an antineoplastic drug $CH_4N_2O_2$ used esp. to treat melanoma, chronic myelogenous leukemia, and malignant tumors (as of the ovary or neck)

hy·droxy·zine \hī-'dräk-sə-,zēn\ *n* : a compound that is administered usu. in the form of its dihydrochloride $C_{21}H_{27}ClN_2O·2HCl$ or pamoate $C_{21}H_{27}ClN_2O_2·C_{23}H_{16}O_6$ and is used as an antihistamine and tranquilizer — see VISTARIL

Hy·dro·zoa \,hī-drə-'zō-ə\ *n pl* : a class of coelenterates that includes various simple and compound polyps and jellyfishes having no stomodeum or gastric tentacles

hy·dro·zo·an \-'zō-ən\ *n* : any of the class Hydrozoa of coelenterates — **hydrozoan** *adj*

hy·giene \'hī-,jēn *also* hī-'\ *n* **1** : a science of the establishment and maintenance of health — see INDUSTRIAL HY-

GIENE, MENTAL HYGIENE **2** : conditions or practices (as of cleanliness) conducive to health

hy·gien·ic \hī-jē-'en-ik, hī-'jen-, hī-'jēn-\ *adj* : of, relating to, or conducive to health or hygiene — **hy·gien·i·cal·ly** \-i-k(ə-)lē\ *adv*

hy·gien·ics \-iks\ *n pl but sing in constr* : HYGIENE 1

hy·gien·ist \hī-'jēn-əst, -'jen-; 'hī-ˌjēn-\ *n* : a specialist in hygiene; *esp* : one skilled in a specified branch of hygiene ⟨mental ∼⟩ — see DENTAL HYGIENIST

hy·gric \'hī-grik\ *adj* : of, relating to, or containing moisture

hy·grine \'hī-ˌgrēn, -grən\ *n* : a colorless liquid ketonic alkaloid $C_8H_{15}NO$ derived from pyrrolidine and obtained from coca leaves

hy·gro·ma \hī-'grō-mə\ *n, pl* **-mas** *also* **-ma·ta** \-mət-ə\ : a cystic tumor of lymphatic origin

hy·grom·e·ter \hī-'gräm-ət-ər\ *n* : any of several instruments for measuring the humidity of the atmosphere

hy·grom·e·try \-ə-trē\ *n, pl* **-tries** : a branch of physics that deals with the measurement of humidity esp. of the atmosphere — **hy·gro·met·ric** \ˌhī-grə-'me-trik\ *adj*

hy·gro·my·cin B \ˌhī-grə-'mīs-ᵊn-ˌbē\ *n* : an antibiotic $C_{20}H_{37}N_3O_{13}$ obtained from a bacterium of the genus *Streptomyces* (*S. hygroscopicus*) and used as an anthelmintic in swine and chickens

hy·gro·scope \'hī-grə-ˌskōp\ *n* : an instrument that shows changes in humidity (as of the atmosphere)

hy·gro·scop·ic \ˌhī-grə-'skäp-ik\ *adj* : readily taking up and retaining moisture ⟨glycerol is ∼⟩ — **hy·gro·scop·ic·i·ty** \-(ˌ)skäp-'is-ət-ē\ *n, pl* **-ties**

Hy·gro·ton \'hī-grə-ˌtän\ *n* : a preparation of chlorthalidone — formerly a U.S. registered trademark

hy·men \'hī-mən\ *n* : a fold of mucous membrane partly or wholly closing the orifice of the vagina — **hy·men·al** \-mən-ᵊl\ *adj*

hy·men·ec·to·my \ˌhī-mə-'nek-tə-mē\ *n, pl* **-mies** : surgical removal of the hymen

hy·me·no·le·pi·a·sis \ˌhī-mə-(ˌ)nō-lə-'pī-ə-səs\ *n, pl* **-a·ses** \-ˌsēz\ : infestation of the intestines by tapeworms of the genus *Hymenolepis*

hy·me·no·lep·i·did \ˌhī-mə-nō-'lep-ə-ˌdid\ *adj* : of or relating to the genus *Hymenolepis* or the family (Hymenolepididae) to which it belongs

Hy·me·nol·e·pis \ˌhī-mə-'näl-ə-pəs\ *n* : a genus (the type of the family Hymenolepididae) of small taenioid tapeworms including numerous comparatively innocuous parasites of birds and mammals that usu. require insect intermediate hosts but are able in some cases (as in *H. nana* of humans) to complete the life cycle in a single host by means of an oncosphere which hatches in the intestine, invades a villus, and there develops into a cysticercoid which ultimately escapes and develops into an adult tapeworm in the lumen of the intestine

Hy·me·nop·tera \ˌhī-mə-'näp-tə-rə\ *n pl* : an order of highly specialized insects with complete metamorphosis that include the bees, wasps, ants, ichneumon flies, sawflies, gall wasps, and related forms, that often associate in large colonies with complex social organization, and that have usu. four membranous wings and the abdomen generally borne on a slender pedicel

hy·me·nop·ter·an \-t-rən\ *n* : any insect of the order Hymenoptera — **hymenopteran** *adj* — **hy·me·nop·ter·ous** \-tə-rəs\ *adj*

hy·me·nop·ter·ism \-'näp-tə-ˌriz-əm\ *n* : poisoning resulting from the bite or sting of a hymenopteran insect (as a bee or wasp)

hy·me·nop·ter·on \-tə-ˌrän, -rən\ *n, pl* **-tera** \-rə\ *also* **-terons** : HYMENOPTERAN

hy·men·ot·o·my \ˌhī-mə-'nät-ə-mē\ *n, pl* **-mies** : surgical incision of the hymen

hyo·epi·glot·tic \ˌhī-ō-ˌep-ə-'glät-ik\ *adj* : connecting the hyoid bone and epiglottis ⟨the ∼ ligament⟩

hyo·epi·glot·tid·ean \-ˌglä-'tid-ē-ən\ *adj* : HYOEPIGLOTTIC

hyo·glos·sal \-'gläs-ᵊl\ *adj* **1** : of, relating to, or connecting the tongue and hyoid bone **2** : of or relating to the hyoglossus

hyo·glos·sus \-'gläs-əs, -'glós-\ *n, pl* **-si** \-ˌsī\ : a flat muscle on each side of the tongue connecting it with the body and the thyrohyal of the hyoid bone — called also *hyoglossus muscle*

hy·oid \'hī-ˌóid\ *adj* **1** : of or relating to the hyoid bone **2** : of, relating to, or being the second postoral branchial arch from which the hyoid bone of the higher vertebrates is in part formed

hyoid bone *n* : a U-shaped bone or complex of bones that is situated between the base of the tongue and the larynx and that supports the tongue, the larynx, and their muscles — called also *hyoid, lingual bone*

¹hyo·man·dib·u·lar \ˌhī-ō-man-'dib-yə-lər\ *adj* : of or derived from the hyoid arch and mandible; *specif* : being or relating to the dorsal segment of the hyoid arch

²hyomandibular *n* : a bone or cartilage derived from the dorsal hyoid arch that is part of the articulating mechanism of the lower jaw in fishes and forms the columella or stapes of the ear of higher vertebrates

hyo·scine \'hī-ə-ˌsēn\ *n* : SCOPOLAMINE; *esp* : the levorotatory form of scopolamine

hyo·scy·a·mine \ˌhī-ə-'sī-ə-mēn\ *n* : a poisonous crystalline alkaloid $C_{17}H_{23}NO_3$ of which atropine is a racemic mixture; *esp* : its levorotatory form found esp. in the plants belladonna and henbane and used similarly to atropine

hyo·scy·a·mus \-məs\ *n* **1** *cap* : a genus of poisonous Eurasian herbs of the family Solanaceae that have a capsular fruit and include the henbane (*H. niger*) **2** : the dried leaves of the henbane containing the alkaloids hyoscyamine and scopolamine and used as an antispasmodic and sedative

Hyo·stron·gy·lus \-'strän-jə-ləs\ *n* : a genus of nematode worms of the family Trichostrongylidae that includes a common small stomach worm (*H. rubidus*) of swine

hyo·thy·roid \-'thī-ˌróid\ *adj* : THYROHYOID

¹hyp·acu·sic \ˌhip-ə-'k(y)ü-sik, ˌhīp-\ *also* **hyp·acou·sic** \-'kü-\ *adj* : affected with hypoacusis

²hypacusic *also* **hypacousic** *n* : one affected with hypoacusis

hyp·acu·sis \-'k(y)ü-səs\ *n* : HYPOACUSIS

hypaesthesia, hypaesthetic *Brit var of* HYPESTHESIA, HYPESTHETIC

hyp·al·ge·sia \ˌhip-ᵊl-'jē-zhə, ˌhī-pal-, -z(h)ē-ə\ *n* : diminished sensitivity to pain — **hyp·al·ge·sic** \-'jē-sik\ *adj*

hyp·al·gia \hip-'al-j(ē-)ə, hīp-\ *n* : HYPALGESIA

Hy·paque \'hī-ˌpāk\ *trademark* — used for a diatrizoate preparation for use in radiographic diagnosis

hyp·ar·te·ri·al \ˌhip-är-'tir-ē-əl, ˌhīp-\ *adj* : situated below an artery; *specif* : of or being the branches of the bronchi given off below the pulmonary artery

hyp·ax·i·al \(')hip-'ak-sē-əl, (')hīp-\ *adj* : situated beneath the axis of the spinal column

hyp·ax·on·ic \ˌhip-ak-'sän-ik, -'sōn-\ *adj* : HYPAXIAL

hy·pen·gyo·pho·bia \ˌhī-ˌpen-jē-ə-'fō-bē-ə\ *n* : abnormal fear of responsibility

hy·per·acid·i·ty \ˌhī-pə-rə-'sid-ət-ē\ *n, pl* **-ties** : the condition of containing more than the normal amount of acid — **hy·per·ac·id** \ˌhī-pə-'ras-əd\ *adj*

¹hy·per·ac·tive \ˌhī-pə-'rak-tiv\ *adj* : affected with or exhibiting hyperactivity; *broadly* : more active than is usual or desirable

²hyperactive *n* : an individual who is hyperactive

hy·per·ac·tiv·i·ty \ˌhī-pə-ˌrak-'tiv-ət-ē\ *n, pl* **-ties** : a state or condition of being excessively or pathologically active; *esp* : ATTENTION DEFICIT DISORDER

hy·per·acu·ity \ˌhī-pə-rə-'kyü-ət-ē\ *n, pl* **-ities** : greater than normal acuteness esp. of a sense; *specif* : visual acuity that is better than twenty-twenty — compare GRATING ACUITY, STEREOACUITY, VERNIER ACUITY

\ə\ **abut** \ᵊ\ **kitten** \ər\ **further** \a\ **ash** \ā\ **ace** \ä\ **cot, cart** \au̇\ **out** \ch\ **chin** \e\ **bet** \ē\ **easy** \g\ **go** \i\ **hit** \ī\ **ice** \j\ **job** \ŋ\ **sing** \ō\ **go** \ȯ\ **law** \ȯi\ **boy** \th\ **thin** \t̲h̲\ **the** \ü\ **loot** \u̇\ **foot** \y\ **yet** \zh\ **vision** *See also* Pronunciation Symbols page

hy·per·acu·sis \ˌhī-pə-rə-'k(y)ü-səs\ *n* : abnormally acute hearing

hy·per·acute \ˌhī-pə-rə-'kyüt\ *adj* : extremely or excessively acute ⟨∼ hearing⟩

hy·per·adren·a·lin·emia *or chiefly Brit* **hy·per·adren·a·lin·ae·mia** \ˌhī-pə-rə-ˌdren-əl-ə-'nē-mē-ə\ *n* : the presence of an excess of adrenal hormones (as epinephrine) in the blood

hy·per·ad·re·no·cor·ti·cism \'hī-pə-rə-ˌdrē-nō-'kört-ə-ˌsiz-əm\ *n* **1** : the presence of an excess of adrenocortical products in the body **2** : the syndrome resulting from hyperadrenocorticism that is often a complication of medication with adrenal hormones, fractions, or stimulants

hyperaemia, hyperaesthesia, hyperaesthetic *chiefly Brit var of* HYPEREMIA, HYPERESTHESIA, HYPERESTHETIC

hy·per·ag·gres·sive \ˌhī-pə-rə-'gres-əv\ *adj* : extremely or excessively aggressive ⟨∼ patients⟩

hy·per·al·do·ste·ron·emia *or chiefly Brit* **hy·per·al·do·ste·ron·ae·mia** \ˌhī-pə-ral-ˌdäs-tə-ˌrō-'nē-mē-ə, -ˌral-dō-stə-ˌrō-\ *n* : the presence of an excess of aldosterone in the blood

hy·per·al·do·ste·ron·ism \ˌhī-pə-ˌral-'däs-tə-ˌrō-ˌniz-əm, -ˌral-dō-stə-'rō-\ *n* : ALDOSTERONISM

hy·per·al·ge·sia \ˌhī-pə-ral-'jē-zhə, -z(h)ē-ə\ *n* : increased sensitivity to pain or enhanced intensity of pain sensation — **hy·per·al·ge·sic** \-'jē-zik, -sik\ *adj*

hy·per·al·i·men·ta·tion \ˌhī-pə-ˌral-ə-mən-'tā-shən\ *n* : the administration of nutrients by intravenous feeding esp. to patients who cannot ingest food through the alimentary tract

hy·per·ami·no·ac·id·uria \ˌhī-pə-rə-ˌmē-nō-ˌas-ə-'d(y)ùr-ē-ə\ *n* : the presence of an excess of amino acids in the urine

hy·per·am·mo·ne·mia \ˌhī-pə-rə-ˌmō-nē-mē-ə\ *also* **hy·per·am·mon·i·emia** \ˌhī-pə-rə-ˌmō-nē-'yē-mē-ə\ *or chiefly Brit* **hy·per·am·mo·nae·mia** *also* **hy·per·am·mon·i·ae·mia** *n* : the presence of an excess of ammonia in the blood — **hy·per·am·mo·ne·mic** *or chiefly Brit* **hy·per·am·mo·nae·mic** \ˌhī-pe-ˌram-ə-'nē-mik\ *adj*

hy·per·am·y·las·emia *or chiefly Brit* **hy·per·am·y·las·ae·mia** \ˌhī-pə-ˌram-ə-ˌlā-'sē-mē-ə\ *n* : the presence of an excess of amylase in the blood serum

hy·per·arous·al \ˌhī-pə-rə-'raù-zəl\ *n* : excessive arousal ⟨a schizophrenic patient in a state of ∼⟩

hy·per·azo·te·mia *or chiefly Brit* **hy·per·azo·tae·mia** \ˌhī-pə-ˌrā-zō-'tē-mē-ə, -ˌra-zō-\ *n* : the presence of abnormal amounts of nitrogenous substances in the blood

hy·per·bar·ic \ˌhī-pər-'bar-ik\ *adj* **1** : having a specific gravity greater than that of cerebrospinal fluid — used of solutions for spinal anesthesia; compare HYPOBARIC **2** : of, relating to, or utilizing greater than normal pressure esp. of oxygen ⟨a ∼ chamber⟩ ⟨∼ medicine⟩ — **hy·per·bar·i·cal·ly** \-i-k(ə-)lē\ *adv*

hy·per·be·ta·li·po·pro·tein·emia \-ˌbāt-ə-ˌlī-pō-ˌprō-ˌtēn-'ē-mē-ə, -ˌlip-ō-, -ˌprō-tē-ən-\ *or chiefly Brit* **hy·per·be·ta·li·po·pro·tein·ae·mia** \-ˌbē-tə-ˌlip-ō-\ *n* : the presence of excess LDLs in the blood

hy·per·bil·i·ru·bin·emia *or chiefly Brit* **hy·per·bil·i·ru·bin·ae·mia** \-ˌbil-ē-ˌrü-bin-'ē-mē-ə\ *n* : the presence of an excess of bilirubin in the blood — called also *bilirubinemia*

hy·per·brachy·ce·phal·ic \-ˌbrak-ē-sə-'fal-ik\ *adj* : having a very round or broad head with a cephalic index of over 85 — **hy·per·brachy·ce·pha·ly** \-'sef-ə-lē\ *n, pl* **-lies**

hy·per·cal·ce·mia *or chiefly Brit* **hy·per·cal·cae·mia** \ˌhī-pər-ˌkal-'sē-mē-ə\ *n* : the presence of an excess of calcium in the blood — **hy·per·cal·ce·mic** *or chiefly Brit* **hy·per·cal·cae·mic** \-'sē-mik\ *adj*

hy·per·cal·ci·uria \-ˌkal-sē-'yùr-ē-ə\ *also* **hy·per·cal·cin·uria** \-ˌkal-sə-'nùr-ē-ə\ *n* : the presence of an excess amount of calcium in the urine

hy·per·cap·nia \-'kap-nē-ə\ *n* : the presence of an excess of carbon dioxide in the blood — **hy·per·cap·nic** \-nik\ *adj*

hy·per·car·bia \-'kär-bē-ə\ *n* : HYPERCAPNIA

hy·per·ca·thex·is \-kə-'thek-səs, -ka-\ *n, pl* **-thex·es** \-ˌsēz\ : excessive concentration of desire upon a particular object

hy·per·cel·lu·lar \-'sel-yə-lər\ *adj* : of, relating to, or characterized by hypercellularity ⟨∼ bone marrow⟩

hy·per·cel·lu·lar·i·ty \-ˌsel-yə-'lar-ət-ē\ *n, pl* **-ties** : the presence of an abnormal excess of cells (as in bone marrow)

hy·per·ce·men·to·sis \-ˌsē-men-'tō-səs\ *n, pl* **-to·ses** \-ˌsēz\ : excessive formation of cementum at the root of a tooth

hy·per·chlor·emia *or chiefly Brit* **hy·per·chlor·ae·mia** \-ˌklōr-'ē-mē-ə, -ˌklör-\ *n* : the presence of excess chloride ions in the blood — **hy·per·chlor·emic** *or chiefly Brit* **hy·per·chlor·ae·mic** \-'ē-mik\ *adj*

hy·per·chlor·hy·dria \-ˌklōr-'hī-drē-ə, -ˌklör-\ *n* : the presence of a greater than typical proportion of hydrochloric acid in gastric juice that occurs in many normal individuals but is esp. characteristic of various pathological states (as ulceration) — compare ACHLORHYDRIA, HYPOCHLORHYDRIA

hy·per·cho·les·ter·ol·emia \ˌhī-pər-kə-ˌles-tə-rə-'lē-mē-ə\ *or* **hy·per·cho·les·ter·emia** \-tə-'rē-mē-ə\ *or chiefly Brit* **hy·per·cho·les·ter·ol·ae·mia** *or* **hy·per·cho·les·ter·ae·mia** *n* : the presence of excess cholesterol in the blood — see FAMILIAL HYPERCHOLESTEROLEMIA — **hy·per·cho·les·ter·ol·emic** \-tə-rə-'lē-mik\ *or* **hy·per·cho·les·ter·emic** \-tə-'rē-mik\ *or chiefly Brit* **hy·per·cho·les·ter·ol·ae·mic** *or* **hy·per·cho·les·ter·ae·mic** *adj*

hy·per·chro·ma·sia \-krō-'mā-zhə, -z(h)ē-ə\ *n* : HYPERCHROMATISM

hy·per·chro·mat·ic \-krō-'mat-ik\ *adj* : of, relating to, or characterized by hyperchromatism ⟨∼ cell nuclei⟩

hy·per·chro·ma·tism \-'krō-mət-ˌiz-əm\ *n* : the development of excess chromatin or of excessive nuclear staining esp. as a part of a pathological process

hy·per·chro·ma·to·sis \-ˌkrō-mə-'tō-səs\ *n, pl* **-to·ses** \-ˌsēz\ **1** : HYPERCHROMIA 2 **2** : HYPERCHROMATISM

hy·per·chro·mia \-'krō-mē-ə\ *n* **1** : excessive pigmentation (as of the skin) **2** : a state of the red blood cells marked by increase in the hemoglobin content

hy·per·chro·mic \-'krō-mik\ *adj* **1** : of, relating to, or characterized by hyperchromia **2** : of, relating to, or characterized by increased absorption esp. of ultraviolet light ⟨∼ effect in DNA molecules subjected to heat⟩ — **hy·per·chro·mic·i·ty** \-krō-'mis-ət-ē\ *n, pl* **-ties**

hy·per·chro·mic anemia \'hī-pər-ˌkrō-mik-\ *n* : an anemia with increase of hemoglobin in individual red blood cells and reduction in the number of red blood cells — see PERNICIOUS ANEMIA; compare HYPOCHROMIC ANEMIA

hy·per·chy·lo·mi·cro·ne·mia *or chiefly Brit* **hy·per·chy·lo·mi·cro·nae·mia** \ˌhī-pər-ˌkī-lō-ˌmī-krō-'nē-mē-ə\ *n* : the presence of excess chylomicrons in the blood

hy·per·co·ag·u·la·bil·i·ty \-kō-ˌag-yə-lə-'bil-ət-ē\ *n, pl* **-ties** : excessive coagulability — **hy·per·co·ag·u·la·ble** \-kō-'ag-yə-lə-bəl\ *adj*

hy·per·cor·ti·cism \-'kört-i-ˌsiz-əm\ *n* : HYPERADRENOCORTICISM

hy·per·cor·ti·sol·ism \-'kört-i-ˌsól-ˌiz-əm, -ˌsól-\ *n* : hyperadrenocorticism produced by excess cortisol in the body

hy·per·cry·al·ge·sia \-ˌkrī-al-'jē-zhə, -z(h)ē-ə\ *n* : excessive pain due to cold

hy·per·cu·pre·mia *or chiefly Brit* **hy·per·cu·prae·mia** \-k(y)ü-'prē-mē-ə\ *n* : the presence of an excess of copper in the blood

hy·per·cy·the·mia *or chiefly Brit* **hy·per·cy·thae·mia** \-sī-'thē-mē-ə\ *n* : the presence of an excess of red blood cells in the blood : POLYCYTHEMIA — **hy·per·cy·the·mic** *or chiefly Brit* **hy·per·cy·thae·mic** \-'thē-mik\ *adj*

hy·per·dip·loid \-'dip-ˌlóid\ *adj* : having slightly more than the diploid number of chromosomes — **hy·per·dip·loi·dy** \-ˌlóid-ē\ *n, pl* **-dies**

hy·per·dy·nam·ic \-dī-'nam-ik\ *adj* : marked by abnormally increased muscular activity esp. when of organic origin ⟨myocardial infarction, with the remaining left ventricular walls being normal to ∼ —R. A. Nishimura *et al*⟩

hy·per·eme·sis \-'em-ə-səs, -i-'mē-\ *n, pl* **-eme·ses** \-ˌsēz\ : excessive vomiting

hyperemesis grav·i·dar·um \-ˌgrav-ə-'dar-əm\ *n* : excessive vomiting during pregnancy

hy·per·emia *or chiefly Brit* **hy·per·ae·mia** \ˌhī-pə-'rē-mē-ə\ *n* : excess of blood in a body part (as from an increased flow of blood due to vasodilation) : CONGESTION — **hy·per·emic** or chiefly Brit **hy·per·ae·mic** \-mik\ adj

hy·per·en·dem·ic \-en-'dem-ik, -in-\ adj **1** : exhibiting a high and continued incidence — used chiefly of human diseases ⟨∼ malaria⟩ **2** : marked by hyperendemic disease — used of geographic areas ⟨a ∼ focus of plague⟩ — **hy·per·en·de·mic·i·ty** \-,en-,dem-'is-ət-ē, -,dē-'mis-\ n, pl **-ties**

hy·per·er·gia \,hī-pər-'ər-j(ē-)ə\ n : HYPERERGY

hy·per·er·gic \-'ər-jik\ adj : characterized by or exhibiting a greater than normal sensitivity to an allergen ⟨an extensive ∼ tissue response⟩ — compare HYPOERGIC, NORMERGIC

hy·per·er·gy \'hī-pə-,rər-jē\ n, pl **-gies** : the quality or state of being hyperergic

hy·per·es·the·sia or chiefly Brit **hy·per·aes·the·sia** \,hī-pə-res-'thē-zh(ē-)ə\ n : unusual or pathological sensitivity of the skin or of a particular sense to stimulation ⟨tactile ∼ of the leg⟩ — **hy·per·es·thet·ic** or chiefly Brit **hy·per·aes·thet·ic** \-'thet-ik\ adj

hy·per·es·trin·ism \-'res-trən-,iz-əm\ or chiefly Brit **hy·per·oes·trin·ism** \-'rē-strən-\ n : a condition marked by the presence of excess estrins in the body and often accompanied by functional bleeding from the uterus

hy·per·es·tro·gen·ism \-'res-trə-jə-,niz-əm\ or chiefly Brit **hy·per·oes·tro·gen·ism** \-'rē-strə-\ n : a condition marked by the presence of excess estrogens in the body

hy·per·eu·ry·pro·so·pic \,hī-pər-,yū-rē-prə-'sō-pik, -'sä-pik\ adj : having a very short broad face with a facial index below 80 — **hy·per·eu·ry·pro·so·py** \-'präs-ə-pē, -prə-'sō-pē\ n, pl **-pies**

hy·per·ex·cit·abil·i·ty \,hī-pə-rik-,sīt-ə-'bil-ət-ē\ n, pl **-ties** : the state or condition of being unusually or excessively excitable ⟨a period of ∼ of all or most of the reflexes —S. W. Jacob⟩

hy·per·ex·cit·ed \-rik-'sīt-əd\ adj : characterized by unusual or excessive excitement ⟨an acute ∼ state⟩ — **hy·per·ex·cite·ment** \-rik-'sīt-mənt\ n

hy·per·ex·tend \,hī-pə-rik-'stend\ vt : to extend so that the angle between bones of a joint is greater than normal ⟨a ∼ed elbow⟩; also : to extend (as a body part) beyond the normal range of motion — **hy·per·ex·ten·sion** \-'sten-chən\ n

hy·per·ex·ten·si·ble \-rik-'sten(t)-sə-bəl\ adj : having the capacity to be hyperextended or stretched to a greater than normal degree ⟨∼ joints⟩ ⟨∼ skin⟩ — **hy·per·ex·ten·si·bil·i·ty** \-'sten(t)-sə-'bil-ət-ē\ n, pl **-ties**

hy·per·fer·re·mia or chiefly Brit **hy·per·fer·rae·mia** \,hī-pər-fə-'rē-mē-ə\ n : the presence of an excess of iron in the blood — **hy·per·fer·re·mic** or chiefly Brit **hy·per·fer·rae·mic** \-'rē-mik\ adj

hy·per·fer·ri·ce·mia or chiefly Brit **hy·per·fer·ri·cae·mia** \-,fer-i-'sē-mē-ə\ n : HYPERFERREMIA — **hy·per·fer·ri·ce·mic** or chiefly Brit **hy·per·fer·ri·cae·mic** \-'sē-mik\ adj

hy·per·fil·tra·tion \-fil-'trā-shən\ n : a usu. abnormal increase in the filtration rate of the renal glomeruli

hy·per·flex \'hī-pər-,fleks\ vt : to flex so that the angle between the bones of a joint is smaller than normal — **hy·per·flex·ion** \-,flek-shən\ n

hy·per·func·tion \-,fəŋ(k)-shən\ n : excessive or abnormal activity ⟨cardiac ∼⟩ — **hy·per·func·tion·al** \-,fəŋ(k)-shnəl, -shən-ºl\ adj — **hy·per·func·tion·ing** \-sh(ə-)niŋ\ n

hy·per·gam·ma·glob·u·lin·emia or chiefly Brit **hy·per·gam·ma·glob·u·lin·ae·mia** \,hī-pər-,gam-ə-,gläb-yə-lə-'nē-mē-ə\ n : the presence of an excess of gamma globulins in the blood — **hy·per·gam·ma·glob·u·lin·emic** or chiefly Brit **hy·per·gam·ma·glob·u·lin·ae·mic** \-'nē-mik\ adj

hy·per·gas·trin·emia or chiefly Brit **hy·per·gas·trin·ae·mia** \-,gas-trə-'nē-mē-ə\ n : the presence of an excess of gastrin in the blood — **hy·per·gas·trin·emic** or chiefly Brit **hy·per·gas·trin·ae·mic** \-'nē-mik\ adj

hy·per·glob·u·lin·emia or chiefly Brit **hy·per·glob·u·lin·ae·mia** \-,gläb-yə-lə-'nē-mē-ə\ n : the presence of excess globulins in the blood — **hy·per·glob·u·lin·emic** or chiefly Brit **hy·per·glob·u·lin·ae·mic** \-'nē-mik\ adj

hy·per·glu·ca·gon·emia or chiefly Brit **hy·per·glu·ca·gon·**

ae·mia \-,glü-kə-gän-'ē-mē-ə\ n : the presence of excess glucagon in the blood

hy·per·gly·ce·mia or chiefly Brit **hy·per·gly·cae·mia** \,hī-pər-glī-'sē-mē-ə\ n : an excess of sugar in the blood — **hy·per·gly·ce·mic** or chiefly Brit **hy·per·gly·cae·mic** \-mik\ adj

hyperglycemic factor n : GLUCAGON

hy·per·gly·ce·mic–gly·co·gen·o·lyt·ic factor \-,glī-kə-jən-ºl-'it-ik-, -,jen-\ n : GLUCAGON

hy·per·gly·ci·ne·mia or chiefly Brit **hy·per·gly·ci·nae·mia** \,hī-pər-,glī-sə-'nē-mē-ə\ n : a hereditary disorder characterized by the presence of excess glycine in the blood

hy·per·go·nad·ism \,hī-pər-'gō-,nad-,iz-əm\ n : excessive hormonal secretion by the gonads

hy·per·hep·a·rin·emia or chiefly Brit **hy·per·hep·a·rin·ae·mia** \-,hep-ə-rə-'nē-mē-ə\ n : the presence (as from ionizing radiation) of excess heparin in the blood usu. resulting in hemorrhage — **hy·per·hep·a·rin·emic** or chiefly Brit **hy·per·hep·a·rin·ae·mic** \-'nē-mik\ adj

hy·per·hi·dro·sis \-hī-'drō-səs, -hī-'drō-\ also **hy·peri·dro·sis** \-id-'rō-, -ī-'drō-\ n, pl **-dro·ses** \-,sēz\ : generalized or localized excessive sweating — compare HYPOHIDROSIS

hy·per·hor·mon·al \-hór-'mōn-ºl\ adj : of, caused by, or associated with excessive secretion of hormones ⟨∼ female obesity⟩

hy·per·hy·dra·tion \-hī-'drā-shən\ n : an excess of water in the body

hy·per·i·cin \hī-'per-ə-sən\ n : a violet crystalline pigment $C_{30}H_{16}O_8$ from Saint-John's-wort that has a red fluorescence and causes hypericism

hy·per·i·cism \-,siz-əm\ n : a severe dermatitis of domestic herbivorous animals due to photosensitivity resulting from eating Saint-John's-wort — compare FAGOPYRISM

hy·per·im·mune \,hī-pə-rim-'yün\ adj : exhibiting an unusual degree of immunization ⟨∼ swine⟩: **a** of a serum : containing exceptional quantities of antibody **b** of an antibody : having the characteristics of a blocking antibody

hy·per·im·mu·ni·za·tion or Brit **hy·per·im·mu·ni·sa·tion** \-,rim-yə-nə-'zā-shən also -yü-nə-\ n : the process of hyper-immunizing an individual; also : the resulting state

hy·per·im·mu·nize or Brit **hy·per·im·mu·nise** \,hī-pə-'rim-yə-,nīz\ vt **-nized** or Brit **-nised; -niz·ing** or Brit **-nis·ing** : to induce a high level of immunity or of circulating antibodies in (as by a long course of injections of antigen, repeated increasing doses of antigen, or the use of adjuvants along with the antigen) ⟨hyperimmunized the rabbits to various antigens⟩

hy·per·in·fec·tion \,hī-pə-rin-'fek-shən\ n : repeated reinfection with larvae produced by parasitic worms already in the body due to the ability of various parasites to complete the life cycle within a single host — compare AUTOINFECTION

hy·per·in·fla·tion \,hī-pə-rin-'flā-shən\ n : excessive inflation (as of the lungs)

hy·per·ino·se·mia or chiefly Brit **hy·per·ino·sae·mia** \,hī-pə-,rin-ō-'sē-mē-ə\ n : HYPERINOSIS

hy·per·ino·sis \,hī-pə-rin-'ō-səs\ n, pl **-ino·ses** \-,sēz\ : excessive formation of fibrin

hy·per·in·su·lin·emia or chiefly Brit **hy·per·in·su·lin·ae·mia** \,hī-pə-,rin(t)-s(ə-)lə-'nē-mē-ə\ n : the presence of excess insulin in the blood — **hy·per·in·su·lin·emic** or chiefly Brit **hy·per·in·su·lin·ae·mic** \-mik\ adj

hy·per·in·su·lin·ism \,hī-pə-'rin(t)-s(ə-)lə-,niz-əm\ n : the presence of excess insulin in the body resulting in hypoglycemia

hy·per·in·vo·lu·tion \,hī-pə-,rin-və-'lü-shən\ n : unusually rapid return to normal or less than normal size of an organ (as the penis or the uterus) following enlargement

hy·per·ir·ri·ta·bil·i·ty \,hī-pə-,rir-ət-ə-'bil-ət-ē\ n, pl **-ties** : abnormally great or uninhibited response to stimuli — **hy·per·ir·ri·ta·ble** \-'rir-ət-ə-bəl\ adj

---

\ə\ abut \ᵊ\ kitten \ər\ further \a\ ash \ā\ ace \ä\ cot, cart
\aú\ out \ch\ chin \e\ bet \ē\ easy \g\ go \i\ hit \ī\ ice \j\ job
\ŋ\ sing \ō\ go \ó\ law \ói\ boy \th\ thin \th\ the \ü\ loot
\ú\ foot \y\ yet \zh\ vision See also Pronunciation Symbols page

hy·per·ka·le·mia *or chiefly Brit* **hy·per·ka·lae·mia** \ˌhī-pər-kā-ˈlē-mē-ə\ *n* : the presence of an abnormally high concentration of potassium in the blood — called also *hyperpotassemia* — **hy·per·ka·le·mic** *or chiefly Brit* **hy·per·ka·lae·mic** \-ˈlē-mik\ *adj*

hy·per·ke·ra·ti·ni·za·tion \-ˌker-ət-ə-nə-ˈzā-shən, -kə-ˌrat-ᵊn-ə-\ *n* : HYPERKERATOSIS

hy·per·ke·ra·to·sis \-ˌker-ə-ˈtō-səs\ *n, pl* **-to·ses** \-ˈtō-ˌsēz\ 1 : hypertrophy of the stratum corneum layer of the skin 2 a : any of various conditions marked by hyperkeratosis b : a disease of cattle that is marked by thickening and wrinkling of the hide, by formation of papillary outgrowths on the buccal mucous membranes, and often by a watery discharge from eyes and nose, diarrhea, loss of weight, and abortion of pregnant animals and that is caused esp. by ingestion of the chlorinated naphthalene of various lubricating oils, by arsenic poisoning, or by inherited congenital ichthyosis — called also *X-disease, XX disease* — **hy·per·ker·a·tot·ic** \-ˈtät-ik\ *adj*

hy·per·ke·to·ne·mia *or chiefly Brit* **hy·per·ke·to·nae·mia** \-ˌkē-tə-ˈnē-mē-ə\ *n* : KETONEMIA 1

hy·per·ki·ne·mia *or chiefly Brit* **hy·per·ki·nae·mia** \-ki-ˈnē-mē-ə\ *n* : abnormally large cardiac output

hy·per·ki·ne·sia \-kə-ˈnē-zh(ē-)ə, -kī-\ *n* : HYPERKINESIS

hy·per·ki·ne·sis \-ˈnē-səs\ *n* 1 : abnormally increased and sometimes uncontrollable activity or muscular movements : HYPERACTIVITY — compare HYPOKINESIA 2 : a condition esp. of childhood characterized by hyperactivity

hy·per·ki·net·ic \-ˈnet-ik\ *adj* : of, relating to, or affected with hyperkinesis or hyperactivity ⟨the ∼ child⟩

hy·per·lep·tene \-ˈlep-ˌtēn\ *adj* : having a very high narrow forehead with an upper facial index of 60 or over — **hy·per·lep·te·ny** \-tə-nē\ *n, pl* **-nies**

hy·per·lep·to·pro·so·pic \-ˌlep-tō-prə-ˈsō-pik, -ˈsä-\ *adj* : having a very long narrow face with a facial index of 93 and over as measured on the living head and of 95 and over on the skull — **hy·per·lep·to·pro·so·py** \-ˈpräs-ə-pē, -prə-ˈsō-pē\ *n, pl* **-pies**

hy·per·lex·ia \-ˈlek-sē-ə\ *n* : precocious reading ability accompanied by difficulties in acquiring language and social skills — **hy·per·lex·ic** \-sik\ *adj*

hy·per·li·pe·mia \ˌhī-pər-lī-ˈpē-mē-ə\ *or chiefly Brit* **hy·per·lip·ae·mia** \-lip-ˈē-\ *n* : HYPERLIPIDEMIA — **hy·per·li·pe·mic** *or chiefly Brit* **hy·per·lip·ae·mic** \-mik\ *adj*

hy·per·lip·id·emia *or chiefly Brit* **hy·per·lip·id·ae·mia** \-ˌlip-ə-ˈdē-mē-ə\ *n* : the presence of excess fat or lipids in the blood — **hy·per·lip·id·emic** *or chiefly Brit* **hy·per·lip·id·ae·mic** \-mik\ *adj*

hy·per·li·po·pro·tein·emia *or chiefly Brit* **hy·per·li·po·pro·tein·ae·mia** \-ˌlī-pə-ˌprō-tē-ˈnē-mē-ə, -ˌlip-ə-, -ˌprō-tē-ə-ˈnē-\ *n* : the presence of excess lipoprotein in the blood

hy·per·lu·cent \-ˈlüs-ᵊnt\ *adj* : being excessively radiolucent ⟨a ∼ lung⟩ — **hy·per·lu·cen·cy** \-ˈlüs-ᵊn-sē\ *n, pl* **-cies**

hy·per·mag·ne·se·mia *or chiefly Brit* **hy·per·mag·ne·sae·mia** \-ˌmag-ni-ˈsē-mē-ə\ *n* : the presence of excess magnesium in the blood serum

hy·per·ma·ture cataract \ˌhī-pər-mə-ˈt(y)u̇(ə)r-\ *n* : a cataract that has become soft and liquified or dry and shrunken from aging

hy·per·men·or·rhea *or chiefly Brit* **hy·per·men·or·rhoea** \-ˌmen-ə-ˈrē-ə\ *n* : abnormally profuse or prolonged menstrual flow — compare MENORRHAGIA

hy·per·me·tab·o·lism \-mə-ˈtab-ə-ˌliz-əm\ *n* : metabolism at an increased or excessive rate — **hy·per·meta·bol·ic** \-ˌmet-ə-ˈbäl-ik\ *adj*

hy·per·me·tria \-ˈmē-trē-ə\ *n* : a condition of cerebellar dysfunction in which voluntary muscular movements tend to result in the movement of bodily parts (as the arm and hand) beyond the intended goal — compare HYPOMETRIA

hy·per·me·tro·pia \-mə-ˈtrō-pē-ə\ *n* : HYPEROPIA — **hy·per·me·tro·pic** \-ˈtrō-pik, -ˈträp-ik\ *adj*

hy·perm·ne·sia \ˌhī-(ˌ)pərm-ˈnē-zh(ē-)ə\ *n* : abnormally vivid or complete memory or recall of the past (as at times of extreme danger) — **hy·perm·ne·sic** \-ˈnē-zik, -sik\ *adj*

hy·per·mo·bil·i·ty \ˌhī-pər-mō-ˈbil-ət-ē\ *n, pl* **-ties** : an increase in the range of movement of which a bodily part and esp. a joint is capable ⟨∼ of the left temporomandibular joint due to the looseness of the capsular ligaments —W. B. Farrar⟩ — **hy·per·mo·bile** \-ˈmō-bəl, -ˌbīl, -ˌbēl\ *adj*

hy·per·morph \ˈhī-pər-ˌmȯrf\ *n* : a mutant gene having a similar but greater effect than the corresponding wild-type gene — **hy·per·mor·phic** \ˌhī-pər-ˈmȯr-fik\ *adj*

hy·per·mo·til·i·ty \ˌhī-pər-mō-ˈtil-ət-ē\ *n, pl* **-ties** : abnormal or excessive movement; *specif* : excessive motility of all or part of the gastrointestinal tract — compare HYPERPERISTALSIS, HYPOMOTILITY — **hy·per·mo·tile** \-ˈmōt-ᵊl, -ˈmō-ˌtīl\ *adj*

hy·per·myo·to·nia \-ˌmī-ə-ˈtō-nē-ə\ *n* : muscular hypertonicity

hy·per·na·tre·mia *or chiefly Brit* **hy·per·na·trae·mia** \-nā-ˈtrē-mē-ə\ *n* : the presence of an abnormally high concentration of sodium in the blood — **hy·per·na·tre·mic** *or chiefly Brit* **hy·per·na·trae·mic** \-mik\ *adj*

hy·per·neph·roid \-ˈnef-ˌrȯid\ *adj* : resembling the adrenal cortex in histological structure ⟨∼ tumors of the ovary⟩

hy·per·ne·phro·ma \-ni-ˈfrō-mə\ *n, pl* **-mas** *also* **-ma·ta** \-mət-ə\ : a tumor of the kidney resembling the adrenal cortex in its histological structure

hy·per·nu·tri·tion \-n(y)u̇-ˈtrish-ən\ *n* : SUPERALIMENTATION

hyperoestrinism, hyperoestrogenism *chiefly Brit var of* HYPERESTRINISM, HYPERESTROGENISM

hy·per·on·to·morph \-ˈän-tə-ˌmȯrf\ *n* : an ectomorphic body type; *also* : an individual of this type — compare MESO-ONTOMORPH

hy·per·ope \ˈhī-pə-ˌrōp\ *n* : one affected with hyperopia

hy·per·opia \ˌhī-pə-ˈrō-pē-ə\ *n* : a condition in which visual images come to a focus behind the retina of the eye and vision is better for distant than for near objects — called also *farsightedness, hypermetropia* — **hy·per·opic** \-ˈrō-pik, -ˈräp-ik\ *adj*

hy·per·orex·ia \ˌhī-pə-rȯ-ˈrek-sē-ə, -ˈrek-shə\ *n* : BULIMIA

hy·per·or·thog·na·thous \ˌhī-pə-ˌrȯr-ˈthäg-nə-thəs\ *adj* : having a very flat facial profile with a facial angle of 93 degrees or above

hy·per·os·mia \ˌhī-pə-ˈräz-mē-ə\ *n* : extreme acuteness of the sense of smell

hy·per·os·mo·lal·i·ty \ˌhī-pə-ˌräz-mō-ˈlal-ət-ē\ *n, pl* **-ties** : the condition esp. of a bodily fluid of having abnormally high osmolality

hy·per·os·mo·lar·i·ty \-ˈlar-ət-ē\ *n, pl* **-ties** : the condition esp. of a bodily fluid of having abnormally high osmolarity ⟨∼ occurs in dehydration, uremia, and hyperglycemia with or without ketoacidosis —R. W. P. Cutler⟩ — **hy·per·os·mo·lar** \ˌhī-pə-ˌräz-ˈmō-lər\ *adj*

hy·per·os·mot·ic \ˌhī-pə-ˌräz-ˈmät-ik\ *adj* : HYPERTONIC 2 ⟨if a laxative is needed, a ∼ preparation . . . is better than a bowel stimulant —S. E. Goldfinger⟩

hy·per·os·to·sis \ˌhī-pə-ˌräs-ˈtō-səs\ *n, pl* **-to·ses** \-ˈtō-ˌsēz\ : excessive growth or thickening of bone tissue — **hy·per·os·tot·ic** \-ˈtät-ik\ *adj*

hy·per·ox·al·uria \ˌhī-pə-ˌräk-sə-ˈlu̇r-ē-ə\ *n* : the presence of excess oxalic acid or oxalates in the urine — called also *oxaluria*

hy·per·ox·ia \ˌhī-pə-ˈräk-sē-ə\ *n* : a bodily condition characterized by a greater oxygen content of the tissues and organs than normally exists at sea level

hy·per·par·a·site \ˌhī-pər-ˈpar-ə-ˌsīt\ *n* : a parasite that is parasitic upon another parasite — **hy·per·par·a·sit·ic** \-ˌpar-ə-ˈsit-ik\ *adj* — **hy·per·par·a·sit·ism** \-ˈpar-ə-ˌsīt-ˌiz-əm, -sə-ˌtiz-\ *n*

hy·per·para·thy·roid·ism \-ˌpar-ə-ˈthī-ˌrȯid-ˌiz-əm\ *n* : the presence of excess parathyroid hormone in the body resulting in disturbance of calcium metabolism with increase in serum calcium and decrease in inorganic phosphorus, loss of calcium from bone, and renal damage with frequent kidney= stone formation

hy·per·path·ia \-'path-ē-ə\ *n* **1** : disagreeable or painful sensation in response to a normally innocuous stimulus (as touch) **2** : a condition in which the sensations of hyperpathia occur — **hy·per·path·ic** \-'path-ik\ *adj*

hy·per·peri·stal·sis \-ˌper-ə-'stól-səs, -'stäl-, -'stal-\ *n, pl* **-stal·ses** \-ˌsēz\ : excessive or excessively vigorous peristalsis — compare HYPERMOTILITY

hy·per·pha·gia \-'fā-j(ē-)ə\ *n* : abnormally increased appetite for food frequently associated with injury to the hypothalamus — compare POLYPHAGIA — **hy·per·phag·ic** \-'faj-ik\ *adj*

hy·per·pha·lan·gism \-fə-'lan-ˌjiz-əm, -fā-\ *n* : the presence of supernumerary phalanges in fingers or toes

hy·per·phe·nyl·al·a·nin·emia *or chiefly Brit* **hy·per·phe·nyl·al·a·nin·ae·mia** \-ˌfen-ᵊl-ˌal-ə-nə-'nē-mē-ə, -ˌfēn-\ *n* : the presence of excess phenylalanine in the blood (as in phenylketonuria) — **hy·per·phe·nyl·al·a·nin·emic** *or chiefly Brit* **hy·per·phe·nyl·al·a·nin·ae·mic** \-'nē-mik\ *adj*

hy·per·pho·ria \-'fōr-ē-ə, -'fór-\ *n* : latent strabismus in which the visual axis of one eye deviates upward in relation to the other

hy·per·phos·pha·te·mia *or chiefly Brit* **hy·per·phos·pha·tae·mia** \-ˌfäs-fə-'tē-mē-ə\ *n* : the presence of excess phosphate in the blood

hy·per·phos·pha·tu·ria \-ˌfäs-fə-'t(y)ùr-ē-ə\ *n* : the presence of excess phosphate in the urine

hy·per·pi·e·sia \-ˌpī-ē-zh(ē-)ə\ *n* : HYPERTENSION; *esp* : ESSENTIAL HYPERTENSION

hy·per·pi·e·sis \-ˌpī-'ē-səs\ *n, pl* **-e·ses** \-ˌsēz\ : HYPERTENSION; *esp* : ESSENTIAL HYPERTENSION

¹hy·per·pi·et·ic \-ˌpī-'et-ik\ *adj* : marked by hypertension

²hyperpietic *n* : one affected with hypertension

hy·per·pig·men·ta·tion \-ˌpig-mən-'tā-shən, -ˌmen-\ *n* : excess pigmentation in a bodily part or tissue (as the skin) ⟨∼ of deep inflammatory acne lesions —Elizabeth A. Abel *et al*⟩ — **hy·per·pig·ment·ed** \-'pig-mənt-əd, -ˌment-\ *adj*

hy·per·pi·tu·ita·rism \-pə-'t(y)ü-ət-ə-ˌriz-əm, -'t(y)ü-ə-ˌtriz-\ *n* : excessive production of growth hormones by the pituitary gland

hy·per·pi·tu·itary \-pə-'t(y)ü-ə-ˌter-ē\ *adj* : affected with hyperpituitarism

hy·per·pla·sia \ˌhī-pər-'plā-zh(ē-)ə\ *n* : an abnormal or unusual increase in the elements composing a part (as cells composing a tissue) — see BENIGN PROSTATIC HYPERPLASIA — **hy·per·plas·tic** \-'plas-tik\ *adj* — **hy·per·plas·ti·cal·ly** \-ti-k(ə-)lē\ *adv*

hy·per·platy·cne·mic \-ˌplat-i(k)-'nē-mik\ *adj, of a tibia* : much flattened laterally with a platycnemic index of less than 55

hy·per·platy·mer·ic \-ˌplat-i-'mer-ik\ *adj, of a femur* : much flattened laterally with a platymeric index of less than 75

hy·per·ploid \'hī-pər-ˌplóid\ *adj* : having a chromosome number slightly greater than an exact multiple of the monoploid or haploid number — **hyperploid** *n*

hy·per·ploi·dy \-ˌplóid-ē\ *n, pl* **-dies** : the quality or state of being hyperploid

hy·per·pnea *or chiefly Brit* **hy·per·pnoea** \ˌhī-pər-'nē-ə, -ˌpərp-'nē-\ *n* : abnormally rapid or deep breathing — **hy·per·pne·ic** *or chiefly Brit* **hy·per·pnoe·ic** \-'nē-ik\ *adj*

hy·per·po·lar·ize *also Brit* **hy·per·po·lar·ise** \ˌhī-pər-'pō-lə-ˌrīz\ *vb* **-ized** *or chiefly Brit* **-ised; -iz·ing** *or chiefly Brit* **-is·ing** *vt* : to produce an increase in potential difference across (a biological membrane) ⟨a *hyperpolarized* nerve cell⟩ ∼ *vi* : to undergo or produce an increase in potential difference across something — **hy·per·po·lar·iza·tion** *also Brit* **hy·per·po·lar·isa·tion** \-ˌpō-lə-rə-'zā-shən\ *n*

hy·per·po·ne·sis \-pō-'nē-səs\ *n, pl* **-ne·ses** \-ˌsēz\ : a condition marked by excessive activity of motor neurons within the nervous system — **hy·per·po·net·ic** \-'net-ik\ *adj*

hy·per·po·tas·se·mia *or chiefly Brit* **hy·per·po·tas·sae·mia** \-pə-ˌtas-'ē-mē-ə\ *n* : HYPERKALEMIA — **hy·per·po·tas·se·mic** *or chiefly Brit* **hy·per·po·tas·sae·mic** \-'ē-mik\ *adj*

hy·per·pro·duc·tion \-prə-'dək-shən, -prō-\ *n* : excessive production ⟨∼ of lymph . . . might be induced by protein compounds —*Jour. Amer. Med. Assoc.*⟩

hy·per·pro·lac·tin·emia *or chiefly Brit* **hy·per·pro·lac·tin·ae·mia** \-ˌprō-'lak-tə-'nē-mē-ə\ *n* : the presence of an abnormally high concentration of prolactin in the blood — **hy·per·pro·lac·tin·emic** *or chiefly Brit* **hy·per·pro·lac·tin·ae·mic** \-'nē-mik\ *adj*

hy·per·pro·lin·emia *or chiefly Brit* **hy·per·pro·lin·ae·mia** \-ˌprō-lə-'nē-mē-ə\ *n* : a hereditary metabolic disorder characterized by an abnormally high concentration of proline in the blood and often associated with mental retardation

hy·per·pro·tein·emia *or chiefly Brit* **hy·per·pro·tein·ae·mia** \-ˌprōt-ᵊn-'ē-mē-ə, -ˌprō-ˌtēn-, -ˌprōt-ē-ən-\ *n* : abnormal increase in the serum protein of the blood

hy·per·pro·throm·bin·emia *or chiefly Brit* **hy·per·pro·throm·bin·ae·mia** \-prō-ˌthräm-bə-'nē-mē-ə\ *n* : an excess of prothrombin in the blood

hy·per·py·ret·ic \-pī-'ret-ik\ *adj* : of or relating to hyperpyrexia

hy·per·py·rex·ia \-pī-'rek-sē-ə\ *n* : exceptionally high fever (as in a particular disease)

hy·per·py·rex·ic \-'rek-sik\ *adj* : HYPERPYRETIC

hy·per·re·ac·tive \-rē-'ak-tiv\ *adj* : having or showing abnormally high sensitivity to stimuli ⟨cystic fibrosis involves ∼ airways —*Jour. Amer. Med. Assoc.*⟩ ⟨a ∼ patient⟩ — **hy·per·re·ac·tiv·i·ty** \-(ˌ)rē-ˌak-'tiv-ət-ē\ *n, pl* **-ties**

hy·per·re·ac·tor \-rē-'ak-tər\ *n* : one who is hyperreactive (as to a particular drug)

hy·per·re·flex·ia \-rē-'flek-sē-ə\ *n* : overactivity of physiological reflexes

hy·per·re·nin·emia *or chiefly Brit* **hy·per·re·nin·ae·mia** \-ˌrē-nən-'ē-mē-ə *also* -ˌren-ən-\ *n* : the presence of an abnormally high concentration of renin in the blood

hy·per·res·o·nance \-'rez-ᵊn-ən(t)s, -'rez-nən(t)s\ *n* : an exaggerated chest resonance heard in various abnormal pulmonary conditions — **hy·per·res·o·nant** \-'rez-ᵊn-ənt, -'rez-nənt\ *adj*

hy·per·re·spon·sive \-ri-'spän(t)-siv\ *adj* : characterized by an abnormal degree of responsiveness (as to a physical or emotional stimulus) — **hy·per·re·spon·sive·ness** \-nəs\ *n* — **hy·per·re·spon·siv·i·ty** \-ri-ˌspän(t)-'siv-ət-ē\ *n, pl* **-ties**

hy·per·ru·gos·i·ty \-rü-'gäs-ət-ē\ *n, pl* **-ties** : abnormally large or numerous wrinkles or folds

hy·per·sal·i·va·tion \-ˌsal-ə-'vā-shən\ *n* : excessive salivation

hy·per·se·cre·tion \-si-'krē-shən\ *n* : excessive production of a bodily secretion (as gastric acid, mucus, or growth hormone) — **hy·per·se·crete** \-si-'krēt\ *vb* **-cret·ed; -cret·ing** — **hy·per·se·cre·to·ry** \-'sē-krə-ˌtór-ē, *esp Brit* -si-'krēt-(ə-)rē\ *adj*

hy·per·sen·si·tive \ˌhī-pər-'sen(t)-sət-iv, -'sen(t)-stiv\ *adj* **1** : excessively or abnormally sensitive **2** : abnormally susceptible physiologically to a specific agent (as a drug or antigen) — **hy·per·sen·si·tive·ness** *n* — **hy·per·sen·si·tiv·i·ty** \-ˌsen(t)-sə-'tiv-ət-ē\ *n, pl* **-ties**

hy·per·sen·si·ti·za·tion *also Brit* **hy·per·sen·si·ti·sa·tion** \-ˌsen(t)-sət-ə-'zā-shən, -ˌsen(t)-stə-'zā-\ *n* : an act or process of hypersensitizing

hy·per·sen·si·tize *also Brit* **hy·per·sen·si·tise** \-'sen(t)-sə-ˌtīz\ *vt* **-tized** *also Brit* **-tised; -tiz·ing** *also Brit* **-tis·ing** : to make hypersensitive

hy·per·sex·u·al \-'seksh-(ə-)wəl, -'sek-shəl\ *adj* : exhibiting unusual or excessive concern with or indulgence in sexual activity — **hy·per·sex·u·al·i·ty** \-ˌsek-shə-'wal-ət-ē\ *n, pl* **-ties**

hy·per·sid·er·emia *or chiefly Brit* **hy·per·sid·er·ae·mia** \-ˌsid-ə-'rē-mē-ə\ *n* : the presence of an abnormally high concentration of iron in the blood — **hy·per·sid·er·e·mic** *or chiefly Brit* **hy·per·sid·er·ae·mic** \-mik\ *adj*

hy·per·som·nia \-'säm-nē-ə\ *n* **1** : sleep of excessive depth

---

\ə\ **abut** \ᵊ\ **kitten** \ər\ **further** \a\ **ash** \ā\ **ace** \ä\ **cot, cart**
\aù\ **out** \ch\ **chin** \e\ **bet** \ē\ **easy** \g\ **go** \i\ **hit** \ī\ **ice** \j\ **job**
\ŋ\ **sing** \ō\ **go** \ó\ **law** \ói\ **boy** \th\ **thin** \t̲h̲\ **the** \ü\ **loot**
\ù\ **foot** \y\ **yet** \zh\ **vision** *See also* Pronunciation Symbols page

or duration 2 : the condition of sleeping for excessive periods at intervals with intervening periods of normal duration of sleeping and waking — compare NARCOLEPSY

hy·per·sple·nism \-'splē-ˌniz-əm, -'splen-ˌiz-\ *n* : a condition marked by excessive destruction of one or more kinds of blood cells in the spleen — **hy·per·splen·ic** \-'splen-ik\ *adj*

hy·per·sthen·ic \ˌhī-pərs-'then-ik\ *adj* : of, relating to, or characterized by excessive muscle tone

hy·per·sus·cep·ti·bil·i·ty \ˌhī-pər-sə-ˌsep-tə-'bil-ət-ē\ *n, pl* **-ties** : the quality or state of being hypersensitive

hy·per·sus·cep·ti·ble \-sə-'sep-tə-bəl\ *adj* : HYPERSENSITIVE

hy·per·tel·or·ism \-'tel-ər-ˌiz-əm\ *n* : excessive width between two bodily parts or organs (as the eyes)

hy·per·tense \'hī-pər-ˌten)s\ *adj* : excessively tense ⟨a ∼ emotional state⟩

hy·per·ten·sin·ase \-'ten(t)-sə-ˌnās, -ˌnāz\ *n* : ANGIOTENSIN-ASE

hy·per·ten·sin·o·gen \-ˌten-'sin-ə-jən, -ˌjen\ *n* : ANGIOTEN-SINOGEN

hy·per·ten·sion \'hī-pər-ˌten-chən\ *n* **1** : abnormally high arterial blood pressure that is usu. indicated by an adult systolic blood pressure of 140 mm Hg or greater or a diastolic blood pressure of 90 mm Hg or greater, is chiefly of unknown cause but may be attributable to a preexisting condition (as a renal or endocrine disorder), that typically results in a thickening and inelasticity of arterial walls and hypertrophy of the left heart ventricle, and that is a risk factor for various pathological conditions or events (as heart attack, heart failure, stroke, end-stage renal disease, or retinal hemorrhage) — see ESSENTIAL HYPERTENSION, SECONDARY HYPERTENSION, WHITE COAT HYPERTENSION **2** : a systemic condition resulting from hypertension that is either symptomless or is accompanied esp. by dizziness, palpitations, fainting, or headache

¹hy·per·ten·sive \ˌhī-pər-'ten(t)-siv\ *adj* : marked by or due to hypertension ⟨∼ emergencies⟩ ⟨∼ renal disease⟩; *also* : affected with hypertension ⟨a ∼ patient⟩

²hypertensive *n* : one affected with hypertension

hy·per·ten·sor \-'ten(t)-sər, -'ten-ˌsȯ(ə)r\ *n* : a drug that lowers blood pressure

hy·per·the·co·sis \-thē-'kō-səs\ *n* : hyperplasia and luteinization of the theca interna of the graafian follicle

hy·per·the·lia \-'thē-lē-ə\ *n* : the presence of supernumerary nipples

hy·per·ther·mia \ˌhī-pər-'thər-mē-ə\ *n* : exceptionally high fever esp. when induced artificially for therapeutic purposes — **hy·per·ther·mic** \-mik\ *adj*

hy·per·thy·mia \-'thī-mē-ə\ *n* : excessive emotional sensitivity

hy·per·thy·re·o·sis \-ˌthī-rē-'ō-səs\ *also* **hy·per·thy·ro·sis** \-'rō-səs\ *n, pl* **-o·ses** *also* **-ro·ses** \-ˌsēz\ : HYPERTHYROIDISM

¹hy·per·thy·roid \-'thī-ˌrȯid\ *adj* : of, relating to, or affected with hyperthyroidism ⟨a ∼ state⟩ ⟨a ∼ patient⟩

²hyperthyroid *n* : a person affected with hyperthyroidism

hy·per·thy·roid·ism \-ˌrȯid-ˌiz-əm, -rəd-\ *n* : excessive functional activity of the thyroid gland; *also* : the resulting condition marked esp. by increased metabolic rate, enlargement of the thyroid gland, rapid heart rate, and high blood pressure — called also *thyrotoxicosis;* see GRAVES' DISEASE

hy·per·to·nia \ˌhī-pər-'tō-nē-ə\ *n* : HYPERTONICITY

hy·per·ton·ic \-'tän-ik\ *adj* **1** : exhibiting excessive tone or tension ⟨a ∼ baby⟩ ⟨a ∼ bladder⟩ **2** : having a higher osmotic pressure than a surrounding medium or a fluid under comparison ⟨animals that produce urine which is ∼ to their blood⟩ — compare HYPOTONIC 2, ISOTONIC 1

hy·per·to·nic·i·ty \-tə-'nis-ət-ē\ *n, pl* **-ties** : the quality or state of being hypertonic

hy·per·to·nus \-'tō-nəs\ *n* : HYPERTONICITY

hy·per·to·ny \'hī-pər-ˌtō-nē, hī-'pər-tə-nē\ *n, pl* **-nies** : HYPERTONICITY

hy·per·tri·cho·sis \ˌhī-pər-tri-'kō-səs\ *n, pl* **-cho·ses** \-ˌsēz\ : excessive growth of hair

hy·per·tri·glyc·er·i·de·mia *or chiefly Brit* **hy·per·tri·glyc·er·i·dae·mia** \-ˌtrī-ˌglis-ə-ˌrī-'dē-mē-ə\ *n* : the presence of an

excess of triglycerides in the blood — **hy·per·tri·glyc·er·i·de·mic** *or chiefly Brit* **hy·per·tri·glyc·er·i·dae·mic** \-'dē-mik\ *adj*

hy·per·tro·phic \-'trō-fik\ *adj* : of, relating to, or affected with hypertrophy ⟨normal and ∼ hearts⟩ ⟨a ∼ prostate⟩

hypertrophic arthritis *n* : OSTEOARTHRITIS

hypertrophic cardiomyopathy *n* : cardiomyopathy that is characterized by ventricular hypertrophy esp. of the left ventricle which affects the interventricular septum more than the free ventricular wall, that may cause mitral insufficiency or obstructed left ventricle outflow, and that is marked by chest pain, syncope, and palpitations — abbr. *HCM*

¹hy·per·tro·phy \hī-'pər-trə-fē\ *n, pl* **-phies** : excessive development of an organ or part; *specif* : increase in bulk (as by thickening of muscle fibers) without multiplication of parts ⟨ventricular ∼⟩

²hypertrophy *vi* **-phied; -phy·ing** : to undergo hypertrophy

hy·per·tro·pia \ˌhī-pər-'trō-pē-ə\ *n* : elevation of the line of vision of one eye above that of the other : upward strabismus

hy·per·uri·ce·mia *or chiefly Brit* **hy·per·uri·cae·mia** \ˌhī-pər-ˌyu̇r-ə-'sē-mē-ə\ *n* : excess uric acid in the blood (as in gout) — called also *uricacidemia, uricemia* — **hy·per·uri·ce·mic** *or chiefly Brit* **hy·per·uri·cae·mic** \-'sē-mik\ *adj*

hy·per·uri·cos·uria \-ˌyu̇r-i-kō-'shu̇r-ē-ə, -kəs-'yu̇r-\ *n* : the excretion of excessive amounts of uric acid in the urine

hy·per·vari·able \-'ver-ē-ə-bəl, -'var-\ *adj* : relating to or being any of the relatively short polypeptide chain segments in the variable region of an antibody light chain or heavy chain that are extremely variable in the sequence of their amino acid residues and that determine the conformation and specificity of the site which recognizes and combines with an antigen; *also* : relating to, containing, or being a highly variable nucleotide sequence

hy·per·ven·ti·late \-'vent-ᵊl-ˌāt\ *vb* **-lat·ed; -lat·ing** *vi* : to breathe rapidly and deeply : undergo hyperventilation ⟨some swimmers ∼⟩ ∼ *vt* : to subject to hyperventilation ⟨he *hyperventilated* his lungs by deep breathing⟩

hy·per·ven·ti·la·tion \-ˌvent-ᵊl-'ā-shən\ *n* : excessive ventilation; *specif* : excessive rate and depth of respiration leading to abnormal loss of carbon dioxide from the blood — called also *overventilation*

hy·per·vig·i·lance \-'vij-ə-lən(t)s\ *n* : the condition of maintaining an abnormal awareness of environmental stimuli ⟨a person suffering from PTSD may have . . . ∼, heightened startle responses and flashbacks —Ellen L. Bassuk *et al*⟩ — **hy·per·vig·i·lant** \-lənt\ *adj*

hy·per·vis·cos·i·ty \-vis-'käs-ət-ē\ *n, pl* **-ties** : excessive viscosity (as of the blood)

hy·per·vi·ta·min·osis \-ˌvīt-ə-mə-'nō-səs\ *n, pl* **-oses** \-'nō-ˌsēz\ : an abnormal state resulting from excessive intake of one or more vitamins — **hy·per·vi·ta·min·ot·ic** \-'nät-ik\ *adj*

hy·per·vol·emia *or chiefly Brit* **hy·per·vol·ae·mia** \-väl-'ē-mē-ə\ *n* : an excessive volume of blood in the body — **hy·per·vol·emic** *or chiefly Brit* **hy·per·vol·ae·mic** \-'ē-mik\ *adj*

hyp·es·the·sia \ˌhī-pes-'thē-zh(ē-)ə, ˌhip-es-\ *or* **hy·po·es·the·sia** \ˌhī-pō-es-\ *or Brit* **hyp·aes·the·sia** *or* **hy·po·aes·the·sia** *n* : impaired or decreased tactile sensibility — **hyp·es·thet·ic** *or* **hy·po·es·thet·ic** \-'thet-ik\ *or Brit* **hyp·aes·thet·ic** *or* **hy·po·aes·thet·ic** *adj*

hy·pha \'hī-fə\ *n, pl* **hy·phae** \-(ˌ)fē\ : one of the threads that make up the mycelium of a fungus, increase by apical growth, and are coenocytic or transversely septate — **hy·phal** \-fəl\ *adj*

hy·phe·ma *or chiefly Brit* **hy·phae·ma** \hī-'fē-mə\ *n* : a hemorrhage in the anterior chamber of the eye

hy·phyl·line \'hī-fə-ˌlēn\ *n* : DYPHYLLINE

hyp·na·go·gic *also* **hyp·no·go·gic** \ˌhip-nə-'gäj-ik, -'gō-jik\ *adj* : of, relating to, or occurring in the period of drowsiness immediately preceding sleep ⟨∼ hallucinations⟩ — compare HYPNOPOMPIC — **hyp·na·go·gi·cal·ly** \-ji-k(ə-)lē\ *adv*

hyp·no·anal·y·sis \ˌhip-nō-ə-'nal-ə-səs\ *n, pl* **-y·ses** \-ˌsēz\

: the treatment of mental disease by hypnosis and psychoanalytic methods — **hyp·no·an·a·lyt·ic** \-ˌan-ᵊl-ˈit-ik\ adj

hyp·no·an·es·the·sia or chiefly Brit **hyp·no·an·aes·the·sia** \-ˌan-əs-ˈthē-zhə\ n : anesthesia produced by hypnosis

hyp·no·gen·ic \-ˈjen-ik\ adj : producing or concerned with the production of sleep or a hypnotic state ⟨a ∼ site in the brain⟩

hyp·noid \ˈhip-ˌnȯid\ or **hyp·noi·dal** \hip-ˈnȯid-ᵊl\ adj : of or relating to sleep or hypnosis ⟨a ∼ state⟩ ⟨hypnoidal psychotherapy —Margaret Steger⟩

hyp·nol·o·gy \hip-ˈnäl-ə-jē\ n : the scientific study of sleep and hypnotic phenomena

hyp·none \ˈhip-ˌnōn\ n : ACETOPHENONE

hyp·no·pe·dia or chiefly Brit **hyp·no·pae·dia** \ˌhip-nə-ˈpē-dē-ə\ n : instruction of a sleeping person esp. by means of recorded lessons — called also sleep-learning, sleep-teaching — **hyp·no·pe·dic** or chiefly Brit **hyp·no·pae·dic** \-ˈpē-dik\ adj

hyp·no·pom·pic \-ˈpäm-pik\ adj : associated with the semiconsciousness preceding waking ⟨∼ illusions⟩ — compare HYPNAGOGIC

hyp·no·sis \hip-ˈnō-səs\ n, pl **-no·ses** \-ˌsēz\ 1 : a trancelike state of altered consciousness that resembles sleep but is induced by a person whose suggestions are readily accepted by the subject 2 : any of various conditions that resemble sleep 3 : HYPNOTISM 1

hyp·no·ther·a·pist \ˌhip-nō-ˈther-ə-pəst\ n : a specialist in hypnotherapy

hyp·no·ther·a·py \-ˈther-ə-pē\ n, pl **-pies** 1 : treatment by hypnotism 2 : psychotherapy that facilitates suggestion, reeducation, or analysis by means of hypnosis — **hyp·no·ther·a·peu·tic** \-ˌther-ə-ˈpyüt-ik\ adj

¹**hyp·not·ic** \hip-ˈnät-ik\ adj 1 : tending to produce sleep : SOPORIFIC 2 : of or relating to hypnosis or hypnotism — **hyp·not·i·cal·ly** \-i-k(ə-)lē\ adv

²**hypnotic** n 1 : a sleep-inducing agent : SOPORIFIC 2 : one that is or can be hypnotized

hyp·no·tism \ˈhip-nə-ˌtiz-əm\ n 1 : the study or act of inducing hypnosis — compare MESMERISM 2 : HYPNOSIS 1

hyp·no·tist \-təst\ n : an expert in hypnotism : a person who induces hypnosis

hyp·no·tize also Brit **hyp·no·tise** \-ˌtīz\ vt **-tized** also Brit **-tised; -tiz·ing** also Brit **-tis·ing** 1 : to induce hypnosis in 2 : to influence by or as if by suggestion ⟨a voice that ∼s its hearers⟩ — **hyp·no·tiz·abil·i·ty** also Brit **hyp·no·tis·abil·i·ty** \ˌhip-nə-ˌtī-zə-ˈbil-ət-ē\ n, pl **-ties** — **hyp·no·tiz·able** also Brit **hyp·no·tis·able** \ˈhip-nə-ˌtī-zə-bəl\ adj

hyp·no·tox·in \ˌhip-nō-ˈtäk-sən\ n : a neurotoxin found in the tentacles of the Portuguese man-of-war that depresses activity of the central nervous system

¹**hy·po** \ˈhī-(ˌ)pō\ n, pl **hypos** : HYPOCHONDRIA

²**hypo** n, pl **hypos** : SODIUM THIOSULFATE

³**hypo** n, pl **hypos** 1 : HYPODERMIC SYRINGE 2 : HYPODERMIC INJECTION

hy·po·acid·i·ty \ˌhī-pō-ə-ˈsid-ət-ē, -a-ˈsid-\ n, pl **-ties** : abnormally low acidity ⟨gastric ∼⟩

hy·po·acou·sia \-ə-ˈkü-zhə, -zē-ə\ n : HYPOACUSIS

hy·po·ac·tive \-ˈak-tiv\ adj : less than normally active ⟨∼ children⟩ ⟨∼ bowel sounds⟩ — **hy·po·ac·tiv·i·ty** \-ak-ˈtiv-ət-ē\ n, pl **-ties**

hy·po·acu·sis \-ə-ˈk(y)ü-səs\ n : partial loss of hearing — called also hypacusis

hy·po·adren·al·ism \-ə-ˈdren-ᵊl-ˌiz-əm\ n : abnormally decreased activity of the adrenal glands; specif : HYPOADRENOCORTICISM

hy·po·adre·nia \-ə-ˈdrē-nē-ə\ n : HYPOADRENALISM

hy·po·ad·re·no·cor·ti·cism \-ə-ˌdrē-nō-ˈkȯrt-ə-ˌsiz-əm\ n : abnormally decreased activity of the adrenal cortex (as in Addison's disease)

hypoaesthesia, hypoaesthetic Brit var of HYPESTHESIA, HYPESTHETIC

hy·po·ageu·sia \-ə-ˈgü-sē-ə also -ˈjü-, -zē-ə\ n : HYPOGEUSIA

hy·po·al·bu·min·emia or chiefly Brit **hy·po·al·bu·min·ae·mia** \-al-ˌbyü-mə-ˈnē-mē-ə\ n : hypoproteinemia marked by reduction in serum albumins — **hy·po·al·bu·min·emic** or chiefly Brit **hy·po·al·bu·min·ae·mic** \-ˈnē-mik\ adj

hy·po·al·ge·sia \-al-ˈjē-zhə, -z(h)ē-ə\ n : decreased sensitivity to pain

hy·po·al·ler·gen·ic \-ˌal-ər-ˈjen-ik\ adj : having little likelihood of causing an allergic response ⟨∼ food⟩ ⟨∼ makeup⟩

hy·po·ami·no·ac·id·emia or chiefly Brit **hy·po·ami·no·ac·id·ae·mia** \-ə-ˌmē-nō-ˌas-ə-ˈdē-mē-ə\ n : the presence of abnormally low concentrations of amino acids in the blood

hy·po·bar·ic \-ˈbar-ik\ adj : having a specific gravity less than that of cerebrospinal fluid — used of solutions for spinal anesthesia; compare HYPERBARIC 1

hy·po·bar·ism \-ˈbar-iz-əm\ n : a condition which occurs when the ambient pressure is lower than the pressure of gases within the body and which may be marked by the distension of bodily cavities and the release of gas bubbles within bodily tissues

hy·po·blast \ˈhī-pə-ˌblast\ n : the endoderm of an embryo — called also endoblast, entoblast — **hy·po·blas·tic** \ˌhī-pə-ˈblas-tik\ adj

hy·po·bu·lia \-ˈbyü-lē-ə\ n : lowered ability to make decisions or to act — **hy·po·bu·lic** \-lik\ adj

hy·po·cal·ce·mia or chiefly Brit **hy·po·cal·cae·mia** \ˌhī-pō-ˌkal-ˈsē-mē-ə\ n : a deficiency of calcium in the blood — **hy·po·cal·ce·mic** or chiefly Brit **hy·po·cal·cae·mic** \-mik\ adj

hy·po·cal·ci·fi·ca·tion \-ˌkal-sə-fə-ˈkā-shən\ n : decreased or deficient calcification (as of tooth enamel)

hy·po·ca·lor·ic \-kə-ˈlȯr-ik, -ˈlōr-, -ˈlär-; -ˈkal-ə-rik\ adj : characterized by a low number of dietary calories ⟨∼ diets, usually 1,000–1,200 kcal/day —Julie L. Sharpless⟩

hy·po·cap·nia \-ˈkap-nē-ə\ n : a deficiency of carbon dioxide in the blood — **hy·po·cap·nic** \-nik\ adj

hy·po·cat·ala·se·mic or chiefly Brit **hy·po·cat·ala·sae·mic** \-ˌkat-ᵊl-ˌā-ˈsē-mik\ adj : of, relating to, or characterized by a deficiency of catalase in the blood

hy·po·cel·lu·lar \-ˈsel-yə-lər\ adj : containing less than the normal number of cells ⟨∼ bone marrow in chronic lead poisoning⟩ — **hy·po·cel·lu·lar·i·ty** \-ˌsel-yə-ˈlar-ət-ē\ n, pl **-ties**

hy·po·chlor·emia or chiefly Brit **hy·po·chlor·ae·mia** \ˌhī-pō-klȯr-ˈē-mē-ə, -klōr-\ n : abnormal decrease of chlorides in the blood

hy·po·chlor·emic or chiefly Brit **hy·po·chlor·ae·mic** \-klȯr-ˈē-mik, -klōr-\ adj : of, relating to, or characterized by hypochloremia ⟨∼ alkalosis⟩

hy·po·chlor·hy·dria \-klȯr-ˈhī-drē-ə, -klōr-\ n : deficiency of hydrochloric acid in the gastric juice — compare ACHLORHYDRIA, HYPERCHLORHYDRIA — **hy·po·chlor·hy·dric** \-ˈhī-drik\ adj

hy·po·chlo·rite \ˌhī-pə-ˈklō(ə)r-ˌīt, -ˈklȯ(ə)r-\ n : a salt or ester of hypochlorous acid

hy·po·chlo·rous acid \-ˌklōr-əs-, -ˌklȯr-\ n : an unstable strongly oxidizing but weak acid HClO obtained in solution along with hydrochloric acid by reaction of chlorine with water and used esp. in the form of salts as an oxidizing agent, bleaching agent, disinfectant, and chlorinating agent

hy·po·cho·les·ter·ol·emia \ˌhī-pō-kə-ˌles-tə-rə-ˈlē-mē-ə\ or **hy·po·cho·les·ter·emia** \-tə-ˈrē-mē-ə\ or chiefly Brit **hy·po·cho·les·ter·ol·ae·mia** or **hy·po·cho·les·ter·ae·mia** n : an abnormal deficiency of cholesterol in the blood — **hy·po·cho·les·ter·ol·emic** \-ˈlē-mik\ or **hy·po·cho·les·ter·emic** \-ˈrē-mik\ or chiefly Brit **hy·po·cho·les·ter·ol·ae·mic** or **hy·po·cho·les·ter·ae·mic** adj

hy·po·chon·dria \ˌhī-pə-ˈkän-drē-ə\ n : extreme depression of mind or spirits often centered on imaginary physical ailments; specif : HYPOCHONDRIASIS

¹**hy·po·chon·dri·ac** \-drē-ˌak\ adj 1 : HYPOCHONDRIACAL 2 a : situated below the costal cartilages b : of, relating to,

G
H

or being the two abdominal regions lying on either side of the epigastric region and above the lumbar regions

²**hypochondriac** *n* : an individual affected with hypochondria or hypochondriasis ⟨a person can be said to be a ∼ when his or her preoccupation with health or disease is so intense that it disrupts normal living habits —*People*⟩

hy·po·chon·dri·a·cal \-kən-ʹdrī-ə-kəl, -ˌkän-\ *adj* : affected with or produced by hypochondria — **hy·po·chon·dri·a·cal·ly** \-k(ə-)lē\ *adv*

hy·po·chon·dri·a·sis \-ʹdrī-ə-səs\ *n, pl* **-a·ses** \-ˌsēz\ : morbid concern about one's health esp. when accompanied by delusions of physical disease

hy·po·chon·dri·um \-ʹkän-drē-əm\ *n, pl* **-dria** \-drē-ə\ : either hypochondriac region of the body

hy·po·chord·al \-ʹkȯrd-ʲl\ *adj* : ventral to the spinal cord

hy·po·chro·ma·sia \ˌhī-pō-krō-ʹmā-zh(ē-)ə\ *n* : HYPOCHROMIA 2

hy·po·chro·mat·ic \-krō-ʹmat-ik\ *adj* : HYPOCHROMIC

hy·po·chro·mia \ˌhī-pə-ʹkrō-mē-ə\ *n* 1 : deficiency of color or pigmentation 2 : deficiency of hemoglobin in the red blood cells (as in nutritional anemia)

hy·po·chro·mic \-ʹkrō-mik\ *adj* : exhibiting hypochromia ⟨∼ blood cells⟩

hy·po·chro·mic anemia \ˌhī-pə-ˌkrō-mik-\ *n* : an anemia marked by deficient hemoglobin and usu. microcytic red blood cells and associated with lack of available iron — compare HYPERCHROMIC ANEMIA

hy·po·co·ag·u·la·bil·i·ty \ˌhī-pō-kō-ˌag-yə-lə-ʹbil-ət-ē\ *n, pl* **-ties** : decreased or deficient coagulability of blood — **hy·po·co·ag·u·la·ble** \-kōʹag-yə-lə-bəl\ *adj*

hy·po·com·ple·men·te·mia *or chiefly Brit* **hy·po·com·ple·men·tae·mia** \-ˌkäm-plə-(ˌ)men-ʹtē-mē-ə\ *n* : an abnormal deficiency of complement in the blood — **hy·po·com·ple·men·te·mic** *or chiefly Brit* **hy·po·com·ple·men·tae·mic** \-ʹtē-mik\ *adj*

hy·po·con·dy·lar \-ʹkän-də-lər\ *adj* : located under or below a condyle

hy·po·cone \ʹhī-pō-ˌkōn\ *n* : the principal rear inner cusp of a mammalian upper molar

hy·po·con·id \ˌhī-pō-ʹkän-əd\ *n* : the principal rear outer cusp of a mammalian lower molar

hy·po·con·u·lid \-ʹkän-yə-ˌlid\ *n* : the distal cusp located between the hypoconid and the entoconid of a mammalian lower molar

hy·po·cor·ti·cism \-ʹkȯrt-i-ˌsiz-əm\ *n* : HYPOADRENOCORTICISM

hy·po·cu·pre·mia *or chiefly Brit* **hy·po·cu·prae·mia** \-k(y)ü-ʹprē-mē-ə\ *n* : an abnormal deficiency of copper in the blood — **hy·po·cu·pre·mic** *or chiefly Brit* **hy·po·cu·prae·mic** \-ʹprē-mik\ *adj*

hy·po·cu·pro·sis \-k(y)ü-ʹprō-səs\ *n, pl* **-pro·ses** \-ˌsēz\ : HYPOCUPREMIA

hy·po·cy·the·mia *or chiefly Brit* **hy·po·cy·thae·mia** \-sī-ʹthē-mē-ə\ *n* : an abnormal deficiency of red blood cells in the blood

hy·po·der·ma \ˌhī-pə-ʹdər-mə\ *n* 1 *cap* : a cosmopolitan genus (the type of the family Hypodermatidae) of dipteran flies that have larvae parasitic in the tissues of vertebrates and include the heel flies and the common cattle grub (*H. lineatum*) 2 : any insect or maggot of the genus *Hypoderma*

hy·po·der·mal \-ʹdər-məl\ *adj* 1 : of or relating to a hypodermis 2 : lying beneath an outer skin or epidermis ⟨∼ infections of cattle⟩

hy·po·der·mat·ic \-dər-ʹmat-ik\ *adj* : HYPODERMIC — **hy·po·der·mat·i·cal·ly** \-i-k(ə-)lē\ *adv*

hy·po·der·ma·to·sis \-ˌdər-mə-ʹtō-səs\ *n* : infestation with maggots of flies of the genus *Hypoderma*

hy·po·der·ma·sis \-dər-ʹmī-ə-səs\ *n, pl* **-a·ses** \-ˌsēz\ : HYPODERMATOSIS

¹**hy·po·der·mic** \-ʹdər-mik\ *adj* 1 : of or relating to the parts beneath the skin 2 : adapted for use in or administered by injection beneath the skin — **hy·po·der·mi·cal·ly** \-mi-k(ə-)lē\ *adv*

²**hypodermic** *n* 1 : HYPODERMIC INJECTION 2 : HYPODERMIC SYRINGE

hypodermic injection *n* : an injection made into the subcutaneous tissues

hypodermic needle *n* 1 : NEEDLE 2 2 : a hypodermic syringe complete with needle

hypodermic syringe *n* : a small syringe used with a hollow needle for injection of material into or beneath the skin

hypodermic tablet *n* : a water-soluble tablet that contains a specified amount of medication and is intended for hypodermic administration

hy·po·der·mis \ˌhī-pə-ʹdər-məs\ *n* 1 : the cellular layer that underlies and secretes the chitinous cuticle (as of an arthropod) 2 : SUPERFICIAL FASCIA

hy·po·der·moc·ly·sis \-dər-ʹmäk-lə-səs\ *n, pl* **-ly·ses** \-ˌsēz\ : subcutaneous injection of fluids (as saline or glucose solution)

hy·po·der·mo·sis \-dər-ʹmō-səs\ *n, pl* **-mo·ses** \-ˌsēz\ : infestation with warbles

hy·po·dip·loid \ˌhī-pō-ʹdip-ˌlȯid\ *adj* : having slightly fewer than the diploid number of chromosomes — **hy·po·dip·loi·dy** \-ˌlȯid-ē\ *n, pl* **-dies**

hy·po·don·tia \-ʹdän-ch(ē-)ə\ *n* : an esp. congenital condition marked by a less than normal number of teeth : partial anodontia — **hy·po·don·tic** \-ʹdän-tik\ *adj*

hy·po·dy·nam·ic \-dī-ʹnam-ik\ *adj* : marked by or exhibiting a decrease in strength or power ⟨the failing or ∼ heart⟩

hy·po·er·gic \-ʹər-jik\ *adj* : characterized by or exhibiting less than the normal sensitivity to an allergen — compare HYPERERGIC, NORMERGIC

hy·po·er·gy \ʹhī-pō-ˌər-jē\ *n, pl* **-er·gies** : the condition of having less than normal sensitivity to an allergen

hypoesthesia, hypoesthetic *var of* HYPESTHESIA, HYPESTHETIC

hy·po·es·tro·ge·ne·mia \ˌhī-pō-ˌes-trə-jə-ʹnē-mē-ə\ *or chiefly Brit* **hy·po·oes·tro·ge·nae·mia** \-ˌēs-trə-\ *n* : a deficiency of one or more estrogens (as estrone or estradiol) in the blood

hy·po·es·tro·gen·ism \-ʹes-trə-jə-ˌniz-əm\ *or chiefly Brit* **hy·po·oes·tro·gen·ism** \-ʹēs-trə-\ *n* : a deficiency of estrogen in the body ⟨long-term administration of a gonadotropin-releasing hormone agonist induces ∼ and amenorrhea —B. D. Cowan *et al*⟩ — **hy·po·es·tro·gen·ic** \-ˌes-trə-ʹjen-ik\ *or chiefly Brit* **hy·po·oes·tro·gen·ic** \-ˌēs-trə-\ *adj*

hy·po·fer·re·mia *or chiefly Brit* **hy·po·fer·rae·mia** \ˌhī-pō-fə-ʹrē-mē-ə\ *n* : an abnormal deficiency of iron in the blood — **hy·po·fer·re·mic** *or chiefly Brit* **hy·po·fer·rae·mic** \-ʹrē-mik\ *adj*

hy·po·fi·brin·o·gen·emia *or chiefly Brit* **hy·po·fi·brin·o·gen·ae·mia** \-fī-ˌbrin-ə-jə-ʹnē-mē-ə\ *n* : an abnormal deficiency of fibrinogen in the blood — **hy·po·fi·brin·o·gen·emic** *or chiefly Brit* **hy·po·fi·brin·o·gen·ae·mic** \-ʹnē-mik\ *adj*

hy·po·func·tion \ʹhī-pō-ˌfəŋ(k)-shən\ *n* : decreased or insufficient function esp. of an endocrine gland ⟨endocrine ∼ resulting from hypophysial or hypothalamic sarcoidosis —A. T. Cariski⟩

hy·po·ga·lac·tia \ˌhī-pō-gə-ʹlak-tē-ə\ *n* : decreased or deficient secretion of milk

hy·po·gam·ma·glob·u·lin·emia *or chiefly Brit* **hy·po·gam·ma·glob·u·lin·ae·mia** \-ˌgam-ə-ˌgläb-yə-lə-ʹnē-mē-ə\ *n* : a deficiency of gamma globulins and esp. antibodies in the blood; *also* : a state of immunological deficiency characterized by this — **hy·po·gam·ma·glob·u·lin·emic** *or chiefly Brit* **hy·po·gam·ma·glob·u·lin·ae·mic** \-ʹnē-mik\ *adj*

hy·po·gas·tric \ˌhī-pə-ʹgas-trik\ *adj* 1 : of or relating to the lower median abdominal region ⟨∼ arteriograms⟩ 2 : relating to or situated along or near the internal iliac arteries or the internal iliac veins ⟨∼ lymph nodes⟩

hypogastric artery *n* : ILIAC ARTERY 3

hypogastric nerve *n* : a nerve or several parallel nerve bundles situated dorsal and medial to the common and the internal iliac arteries, crossing the branches of the internal iliac artery, and entering the inferior part of the hypogastric plexus

hypogastric plexus *n* : the sympathetic nerve plexus that supplies the pelvic viscera, lies in front of the promontory of the sacrum, and extends down into two lateral portions

hypogastric vein *n* : ILIAC VEIN c

hy·po·gas·tri·um \ˌhī-pə-ˈgas-trē-əm\ *n, pl* **-tria** \-trē-ə\ : the hypogastric region of the abdomen

hy·po·gen·e·sis \-ˈjen-ə-səs\ *n, pl* **-e·ses** \-ˌsēz\ **1** : direct development without alternation of generations **2** : underdevelopment esp. of an organ or function — **hy·po·ge·net·ic** \-jə-ˈnet-ik\ *adj*

hy·po·gen·i·tal·ism \-ˈjen-ə-tə-ˌliz-əm\ *n* : subnormal development of genital organs : genital infantilism

hy·po·geu·sia \-ˈgü-sē-ə *also* -ˈjü-, -zē-ə\ *n* : decreased sensitivity to taste ⟨idiopathic ∼⟩ — called also *hypoageusia*

hy·po·glos·sal \ˌhī-pə-ˈgläs-əl\ *adj* : of or relating to the hypoglossal nerves

hypoglossal nerve *n* : either of the 12th and final pair of cranial nerves which are motor nerves arising from the medulla oblongata and supplying muscles of the tongue and hyoid apparatus in higher vertebrates — called also *hypoglossal, twelfth cranial nerve*

hypoglossal nucleus *n* : a nucleus in the floor of the fourth ventricle of the brain that is the origin of the hypoglossal nerve

hy·po·glos·sus \-ˈglä-səs\ *n, pl* **-glos·si** \-ˌsī, -(ˌ)sē\ : HYPOGLOSSAL NERVE — see ANSA HYPOGLOSSI

hy·po·glot·tis \-ˈglät-əs\ *n, pl* **-tis·es** *or* **-ti·des** \-ə-(ˌ)dēz\ : the underpart of the tongue

hy·po·glu·ce·mia *or chiefly Brit* **hy·po·glu·cae·mia** \ˌhī-pō-glü-ˈsē-mē-ə\ *n* : HYPOGLYCEMIA

hy·po·gly·ce·mia *or chiefly Brit* **hy·po·gly·cae·mia** \ˌhī-pō-glī-ˈsē-mē-ə\ *n* : abnormal decrease of sugar in the blood

¹**hy·po·gly·ce·mic** *or chiefly Brit* **hy·po·gly·cae·mic** \-ˈsē-mik\ *adj* **1** : of, relating to, caused by, or affected with hypoglycemia ⟨a ∼ reaction⟩ ⟨∼ patients⟩ **2** : producing a decrease in the level of sugar in the blood ⟨∼ drugs⟩

²**hypoglycemic** *or chiefly Brit* **hypoglycaemic** *n* **1** : one affected with hypoglycemia **2** : an agent that lowers the level of sugar in the blood

hy·po·gly·cin \-ˈglīs-ᵊn\ *n* : either of two substances from a tropical tree (*Blighia sapida* of the family Sapindaceae) of West Africa that induce hypoglycemia by inhibiting gluconeogenesis in the liver

hy·po·go·nad·al \-gō-ˈnad-ᵊl\ *adj* **1** : relating to or affected with hypogonadism **2** : marked by or exhibiting deficient development of secondary sex characteristics

hy·po·go·nad·ism \-ˈgō-ˌnad-ˌiz-əm\ *n* **1** : functional incompetence of the gonads esp. in the male with subnormal or impaired production of hormones and germ cells **2** : an abnormal condition (as Klinefelter's syndrome) involving gonadal incompetence

hy·po·go·nad·o·trop·ic \-gō-ˌnad-ə-ˈträp-ik\ *or* **hy·po·go·nad·o·tro·phic** \-ˈtrō-fik, -ˈträf-ik\ *adj* : characterized by a deficiency of gonadotropins

hy·po·hi·dro·sis \-hid-ˈrō-səs, -hī-ˈdrō-\ *n, pl* **-dro·ses** \-ˌsēz\ : abnormally diminished sweating — compare HYPERHIDROSIS

hy·po·his·ti·di·ne·mia *or chiefly Brit* **hy·po·his·ti·di·nae·mia** \-ˌhis-tə-də-ˈnē-mē-ə\ *n* : a low concentration of histidine in the blood that is characteristic of rheumatoid arthritis — **hy·po·his·ti·di·ne·mic** *or chiefly Brit* **hy·po·his·ti·di·nae·mic** \-ˈnē-mik\ *adj*

hy·po·hy·dra·tion \-hī-ˈdrā-shən\ *n* : dehydration of the human or animal body

hy·po·in·su·lin·emia *or chiefly Brit* **hy·po·in·su·lin·ae·mia** \-ˌin(t)-s(ə-)lə-ˈnē-mē-ə\ *n* : an abnormally low concentration of insulin in the blood — **hy·po·in·su·lin·emic** *or chiefly Brit* **hy·po·in·su·lin·ae·mic** \-ˈnē-mik\ *adj*

hy·po·in·su·lin·ism \-ˈin(t)-s(ə-)lə-ˌniz-əm\ *n* : deficient secretion of insulin by the pancreas

hy·po·ka·le·mia *or chiefly Brit* **hy·po·ka·lae·mia** \-kā-ˈlē-mē-ə\ *n* : a deficiency of potassium in the blood — called also *hypopotassemia* — **hy·po·ka·le·mic** *or chiefly Brit* **hy·po·ka·lae·mic** \-ˈlē-mik\ *adj*

hy·po·ki·ne·sia \-kə-ˈnē-zh(ē-)ə, -kī-\ *n* : abnormally decreased muscular movement (as in spaceflight) — compare HYPERKINESIS 1

hy·po·ki·ne·sis \-ˈnē-səs\ *n, pl* **-ne·ses** \-ˌsēz\ : HYPOKINESIA

hy·po·ki·net·ic \-ˈnet-ik\ *adj* : characterized by, associated with, or caused by decreased motor activity ⟨∼ obese patients⟩ ⟨∼ hypoxia⟩

hy·po·lem·mal \-ˈlem-əl\ *adj* : located beneath a sheath ⟨∼ nerve terminals⟩

hy·po·ley·dig·ism \-ˈlī-dig-ˌiz-əm\ *n* : decreased or insufficient function of the Leydig cells

hy·po·li·pe·mia \-lī-ˈpē-mē-ə\ *or chiefly Brit* **hy·po·lip·ae·mia** \-lip-ˈē-\ *n* : an abnormally low concentration of fats in the blood

¹**hy·po·li·pe·mic** *or chiefly Brit* **hy·po·lip·ae·mic** \-mik\ *adj* : of or relating to hypolipemia

²**hypolipemic** *or chiefly Brit* **hypolipaemic** *n* : an agent that lowers the concentration of fats in the blood

hy·po·lip·id·emia *or chiefly Brit* **hy·po·lip·id·ae·mia** \-ˌlip-ə-ˈdē-mē-ə\ *n* : a deficiency of lipids in the blood

hy·po·lip·id·emic *or chiefly Brit* **hy·po·lip·id·ae·mic** \-ˈdē-mik\ *adj* : producing or resulting from a decrease in the level of lipids in the blood ⟨a ∼ drug⟩ ⟨∼ effects⟩

hy·po·mag·ne·se·mia *or chiefly Brit* **hy·po·mag·ne·sae·mia** \ˌhī-pə-ˌmag-nə-ˈsē-mē-ə\ *n* : a deficiency of magnesium in the blood esp. of cattle — **hy·po·mag·ne·se·mic** *or chiefly Brit* **hy·po·mag·ne·sae·mic** \-mik\ *adj*

hy·po·mag·ne·sia \-mag-ˈnē-shə, -ˈnē-zhə\ *n* : GRASS TETANY

hy·po·ma·nia \ˌhī-pə-ˈmā-nē-ə, -nyə\ *n* : a mild mania esp. when part of bipolar disorder

hy·po·ma·ni·ac \-ˈmä-nē-ˌak\ *n* : HYPOMANIC

¹**hy·po·man·ic** \-ˈman-ik\ *adj* : of, relating to, or affected with hypomania ⟨depressive periods and ∼ periods may be separated by periods of normal mood —*Diagnostic & Statistical Manual of Mental Disorders*⟩

²**hypomanic** *n* : one affected with hypomania

hy·po·mas·tia \-ˈmas-tē-ə\ *n* : abnormal smallness of the mammary glands

hy·po·men·or·rhea *or chiefly Brit* **hy·po·men·or·rhoea** \-ˌmen-ə-ˈrē-ə\ *n* : decreased menstrual flow

hy·po·mere \ˈhī-pə-ˌmi(ə)r\ *n* : one of the segments from which the walls of the pleuroperitoneal cavity develop

hy·po·me·tab·o·lism \ˌhī-pō-mə-ˈtab-ə-ˌliz-əm\ *n* : a condition (as in myxedema or hypothyroidism) marked by an abnormally low metabolic rate — **hy·po·meta·bol·ic** \-ˌmet-ə-ˈbäl-ik\ *adj*

hy·po·me·tria \-ˈmē-trē-ə\ *n* : a condition of cerebellar dysfunction in which voluntary muscular movements tend to result in the movement of bodily parts (as the arm and hand) short of the intended goal — compare HYPERMETRIA

hy·po·min·er·al·ized *or Brit* **hy·po·min·er·al·ised** \-ˈmin-(ə-)rə-ˌlīzd\ *adj* : relating to or characterized by a deficiency of minerals ⟨∼ defects in tooth enamel⟩

hy·pom·ne·sia \ˌhī-(ˌ)päm-ˈnē-zh(ē-)ə\ *n* : impaired memory

hy·po·mo·bile \ˌhī-pō-ˈmō-bəl, -ˌbīl, -ˌbēl\ *adj* : capable of a smaller range or frequency of movement than normal ⟨a ∼ gut⟩

hy·po·morph \ˈhī-pə-ˌmȯrf\ *n* : a mutant gene having a similar but weaker effect than the corresponding wild-type gene — **hy·po·mor·phic** \ˌhī-pə-ˈmȯr-fik\ *adj*

hy·po·mo·til·i·ty \ˌhī-pō-mō-ˈtil-ət-ē\ *n, pl* **-ties** : abnormal deficiency of movement; *specif* : decreased motility of all or part of the gastrointestinal tract ⟨esophageal ∼⟩ — compare HYPERMOTILITY

hy·po·na·tre·mia *or chiefly Brit* **hy·po·na·trae·mia** \-nā-ˈtrē-mē-ə\ *n* : deficiency of sodium in the blood — **hy·po·na·tre·mic** *or chiefly Brit* **hy·po·na·trae·mic** \-mik\ *adj*

hy·po·nu·tri·tion \-n(y)ü-ˈtrish-ən\ *n* : UNDERNUTRITION

G
H

\ə\ abut \ᵊ\ kitten \ər\ further \a\ ash \ā\ ace \ä\ cot, cart
\au̇\ out \ch\ chin \e\ bet \ē\ easy \g\ go \i\ hit \ī\ ice \j\ job
\ŋ\ sing \ō\ go \ȯ\ law \ȯi\ boy \th\ thin \t̷h\ the \ü\ loot
\u̇\ foot \y\ yet \zh\ vision *See also* Pronunciation Symbols page

hy·po·nych·i·um \-'nik-ē-əm\ *n* **1** : the thickened layer of epidermis beneath the free end of a nail **2** : MATRIX 1b — **hy·po·nych·i·al** \-ē-əl\ *adj*

hypo–oestrogenaemia, hypo–oestrogenic, hypo–oestrogenism *chiefly Brit var of* HYPOESTROGENEMIA, HYPOESTROGENIC, HYPOESTROGENISM

hy·po–on·to·morph \-'än-tə-ˌmȯrf\ *n* : ENDOMORPH

hypoosmolality *var of* HYPOSMOLALITY

hy·po·os·mot·ic \-ˌäz-'mät-ik\ *or* **hy·pos·mot·ic** \ˌhī-ˌpäz-\ *adj* : HYPOTONIC 2

hy·po·ovar·i·an·ism \ˌhī-pō-ō-'var-ē-ə-ˌniz-əm\ *n* : a condition marked by a deficiency of ovarian function : female hypogonadism

hy·po·para·thy·roid \-ˌpar-ə-'thī-ˌrȯid\ *adj* : of or affected by hypoparathyroidism ⟨~ patients⟩

hy·po·para·thy·roid·ism \-ˌpar-ə-'thī-ˌrȯid-ˌiz-əm\ *n* : deficiency of parathyroid hormone in the body; *also* : the resultant abnormal state marked by low serum calcium and a tendency to chronic tetany

hy·po·per·fu·sion \ˌhī-pō-pər-'fyü-zhən\ *n* : decreased blood flow through an organ ⟨cerebral ~⟩

hy·po·pha·lan·gism \-fə-'lan-ˌjiz-əm, -fā-'\ *n* : congenital absence of one or more phalanges

α–hypophamine *var of* ALPHA-HYPOPHAMINE

β–hypophamine *var of* BETA-HYPOPHAMINE

hy·po·pha·ryn·geal \-fə-'rin-j(ē-)əl, -ˌfar-ən-'jē-əl\ *adj* : of, relating to, or affecting the hypopharynx ⟨~ carcinoma⟩

hy·po·phar·ynx \-'far-iŋ(k)s\ *n, pl* **-pha·ryn·ges** \-fə-'rin-(ˌ)jēz\ *also* **-phar·ynx·es** : the laryngeal part of the pharynx extending from the hyoid bone to the lower margin of the cricoid cartilage

hy·po·pho·nia \ˌhī-pə-'fō-nē-ə\ *n* : an abnormally weak voice

hy·po·phos·pha·ta·sia \ˌhī-pō-ˌfäs-fə-'tā-zh(ē-)ə\ *n* : a congenital metabolic disorder characterized by a deficiency of alkaline phosphatase and usu. resulting in demineralization of bone

hy·po·phos·phate \-'fäs-ˌfāt\ *n* : a salt or ester of hypophosphoric acid

hy·po·phos·pha·te·mia *or chiefly Brit* **hy·po·phos·pha·tae·mia** \-ˌfäs-fə-'tē-mē-ə\ *n* : deficiency of phosphates in the blood that is due to inadequate intake, excessive excretion, or defective absorption and that results in various abnormalities (as defects of bone) — **hy·po·phos·pha·te·mic** *or chiefly Brit* **hy·po·phos·pha·tae·mic** \-'tē-mik\ *adj*

hy·po·phos·phite \-'fäs-ˌfīt\ *n* : a salt of hypophosphorous acid; *esp* : one (as the sodium salt) used as a source of assimilable phosphorus

hy·po·phos·phor·ic acid \-fäs-ˌfȯr-ik-, -ˌfär-, -fäs-f(ə-)rik-\ *n* : an unstable acid $H_4P_2O_6$ with four replaceable hydrogen atoms that is usu. obtained in the form of its salts

hy·po·phos·pho·rous acid \-ˌfäs-f(ə-)rəs-, -fäs-ˌfȯr-əs-, -ˌfȯr-\ *n* : a low-melting deliquescent crystalline strong monobasic acid H_3PO_2 usu. obtained by acidifying one of its salts and used as a reducing agent

hy·po·phren·ic \ˌhī-pə-'fren-ik\ *adj* : affected with mental retardation

hy·po·phy·se·al *also* **hy·po·phy·si·al** \(ˌ)hī-ˌpäf-ə-'sē-əl, ˌhī-pə-fə-, -'zē-; ˌhī-pə-'fiz-ē-əl\ *adj* : of or relating to the hypophysis

hypophyseal fossa *n* : the depression in the sphenoid bone that contains the hypophysis

hy·poph·y·sec·to·mize *or chiefly Brit* **hy·poph·y·sec·to·mise** \(ˌ)hī-ˌpäf-ə-'sek-tə-ˌmīz\ *vt* **-mized** *or chiefly Brit* **-mised; -miz·ing** *or chiefly Brit* **-mis·ing** : to remove the pituitary gland from

hy·poph·y·sec·to·my \-mē\ *n, pl* **-mies** : surgical removal of the pituitary gland

hy·po·phys·io·tro·pic \ˌhī-pō-ˌfiz-ē-ō-'trō-pik, -'träp-ik\ *or* **hy·po·phys·io·tro·phic** \-'trō-fik\ *also* **hy·po·phys·eo·tro·pic** *or* **hy·po·phys·eo·tro·phic** *adj* : acting on or stimulating the hypophysis ⟨~ hormones⟩

hy·poph·y·sis \hī-'päf-ə-səs\ *n, pl* **-y·ses** \-ˌsēz\ : PITUITARY GLAND

hypophysis ce·re·bri \-sə-'rē-ˌbrī, -'ser-ə-\ *n* : PITUITARY GLAND

hypopi *pl of* HYPOPUS

hy·po·pi·al \hī-'pō-pē-əl\ *adj* : of, relating to, or consisting of a hypopus ⟨the ~ stage of a mite⟩

hy·po·pig·men·ta·tion \ˌhī-pō-ˌpig-mən-'tā-shən, -ˌmen-\ *n* : diminished pigmentation in a bodily part or tissue (as the skin) — **hy·po·pig·ment·ed** \-'pig-mənt-əd, -ˌment-\ *adj*

hy·po·pi·tu·ita·rism \ˌhī-pō-pə-'t(y)ü-ət-ə-ˌriz-əm, -'t(y)ü-ə-ˌtriz-\ *n* : deficient production of growth hormones by the pituitary gland — **hy·po·pi·tu·itary** \-'t(y)ü-ə-ˌter-ē\ *adj*

hy·po·pla·sia \-'plā-zh(ē-)ə\ *n* : a condition of arrested development in which an organ or part remains below the normal size or in an immature state — **hy·po·plas·tic** \-'plas-tik\ *adj*

hypoplastic anemia *n* : APLASTIC ANEMIA

hypoplastic left heart syndrome *n* : a congenital malformation of the heart in which the left side is underdeveloped resulting in insufficient blood flow

hy·po·ploid \'hī-pō-ˌplȯid\ *adj* : having a chromosome number slightly less than an exact multiple of the monoploid or haploid number — **hypoploid** *n* — **hy·po·ploi·dy** \-ˌplȯid-ē\ *n, pl* **-dies**

hy·po·pnea *or chiefly Brit* **hy·po·pnoea** \ˌhī-pō-'nē-ə\ *n* : abnormally slow or esp. shallow respiration

hy·po·po·tas·se·mia *or chiefly Brit* **hy·po·po·tas·sae·mia** \-pə-ˌtas-'ē-mē-ə\ *n* : HYPOKALEMIA — **hy·po·po·tas·se·mic** *or chiefly Brit* **hy·po·po·tas·sae·mic** \-'ē-mik\ *adj*

hy·po·pro·lac·tin·emia *or chiefly Brit* **hy·po·pro·lac·tin·ae·mia** \-prō-ˌlak-tə-'nē-mē-ə\ *n* : a condition characterized by a deficiency of prolactin in the blood that occurs esp. in panhypopituitarism (as in Sheehan's syndrome)

hy·po·pro·sex·ia \-prə-'sek-sē-ə\ *n* : defective fixing of attention on a stimulus-object

hy·po·pro·tein·emia *or chiefly Brit* **hy·po·pro·tein·ae·mia** \-ˌprōt-ᵊn-'ē-mē-ə, -ˌprō-ˌtēn-, -ˌprōt-ē-ən-\ *n* : abnormal deficiency of protein in the blood — **hy·po·pro·tein·e·mic** *or chiefly Brit* **hy·po·pro·tein·ae·mic** \-'ē-mik\ *adj*

hy·po·pro·throm·bin·emia *or chiefly Brit* **hy·po·pro·throm·bin·ae·mia** \-prō-ˌthräm-bə-'nē-mē-ə\ *n* : deficiency of prothrombin in the blood usu. due to vitamin K deficiency or liver disease (esp. obstructive jaundice) and resulting in delayed clotting of blood or spontaneous bleeding (as from the nose or into the skin) — called also *prothrombinopenia* — **hy·po·pro·throm·bin·e·mic** *or chiefly Brit* **hy·po·pro·throm·bin·ae·mic** \-'nē-mik\ *adj*

hy·po·psel·a·phe·sia \ˌhī-pō-ˌsel-ə-'fē-zē-ə, ˌhī-päp-, -'fē-zhə\ *n* : diminished sense of touch

hyp·o·pus \'hip-ə-pəs\ *n, pl* **hyp·o·pi** \-ˌpī\ : a migratory larva of some mites that is passively distributed by an animal to which it has attached itself and on which it does not feed

hy·po·py·on \hī-'pō-pē-ˌän\ *n* : an accumulation of white blood cells in the anterior chamber of the eye

hy·po·re·ac·tive \ˌhī-pō-rē-'ak-tiv\ *adj* : having or showing abnormally low sensitivity to stimuli ⟨her patellar and Achilles reflexes were ~ —Andres Alcaraz *et al*⟩ ⟨a ~ patient⟩ — **hy·po·re·ac·tiv·i·ty** \-(ˌ)rē-ˌak-'tiv-ət-ē\ *n, pl* **-ties**

hy·po·re·ac·tor \-rē-'ak-tər\ *n* : one who is hyporeactive (as to a particular drug)

hy·po·re·flex·ia \-rē-'flek-sē-ə\ *n* : underactivity of bodily reflexes

hy·po·re·spon·sive \-ri-'spän(t)-siv\ *adj* : characterized by a diminished degree of responsiveness (as to a physical or emotional stimulus) — **hy·po·re·spon·sive·ness** *n*

hy·po·ri·bo·fla·vin·o·sis \-ˌrī-bə-ˌflā-və-'nō-səs\ *n, pl* **-o·ses** \-ˌsēz\ : ARIBOFLAVINOSIS

hypos *pl of* HYPO

hy·po·sal·i·va·tion \-ˌsal-ə-'vā-shən\ *n* : diminished salivation

hy·po·scler·al \ˌhī-pə-'skler-əl\ *adj* : located beneath the sclera of the eye

hy·po·se·cre·tion \ˌhī-pō-si-'krē-shən\ *n* : production of a bodily secretion at an abnormally slow rate or in abnormally small quantities

hy·po·sen·si·tive \-'sen(t)-sət-iv, -'sen(t)-stiv\ *adj* : exhibiting or marked by deficient response to stimulation — **hy·po·sen·si·tiv·i·ty** \-ˌsen(t)-sə-ˈtiv-ət-ē\ *n, pl* **-ties**

hy·po·sen·si·ti·za·tion *or chiefly Brit* **hy·po·sen·si·ti·sa·tion** \-ˌsen(t)-sət-ə-ˈzā-shən, -ˌsen(t)-stə-ˈzā-\ *n* : the state or process of being reduced in sensitivity esp. to an allergen : DESENSITIZATION — **hy·po·sen·si·tize** *or chiefly Brit* **hy·po·sen·si·tise** \-ˈsen(t)-sə-ˌtīz\ *vt* **-tized** *or chiefly Brit* **-tised; -tizing** *or chiefly Brit* **-tis·ing**

hy·pos·mia \hī-ˈpäz-mē-ə, hip-ˈäz-\ *n* : impairment of the sense of smell

hy·pos·mo·lal·i·ty \ˌhī-ˌpäz-mō-ˈlal-ət-ē\ *or* **hy·po·os·mo·lal·i·ty** \ˌhī-pō-ˌäz-\ *n, pl* **-ties** : the condition esp. of a bodily fluid of having abnormally low osmolality

hy·pos·mo·lar·i·ty \ˌhī-ˌpäz-mō-ˈlar-ət-ē\ *n, pl* **-ties** : the condition esp. of a bodily fluid of having abnormally low osmolarity — **hy·pos·mo·lar** \ˌhī-ˌpäz-ˈmō-lər\ *adj*

hyposmotic *var of* HYPOOSMOTIC

hy·po·spa·dia \ˌhī-pə-ˈspäd-ē-ə\ *n* : HYPOSPADIAS

hy·po·spa·di·ac \-ˈspäd-ē-ˌak\ *adj* : characteristic of or affected with hypospadias ⟨a ∼ urethral opening⟩

hy·po·spa·di·as \ˌhī-pə-ˈspäd-ē-əs\ *n* : an abnormality of the penis in which the urethra opens on the underside

hy·po·spa·dy \ˈhī-pə-ˌspäd-ē\ *n, pl* **-dies** : HYPOSPADIAS

hy·pos·ta·sis \hī-ˈpäs-tə-səs\ *n, pl* **-ta·ses** \-ˌsēz\ **1** : the settling of blood in relatively lower parts of an organ or the body due to impaired or absent circulation ⟨the face was discolored by postmortem ∼⟩ **2** : failure of a gene to produce its usual effect when coupled with another gene that is epistatic toward it

hy·po·stat·ic \ˌhī-pə-ˈstat-ik\ *adj* **1 a** *of a gene* : exhibiting hypostasis in the presence of a corresponding epistatic gene **b** *of a hereditary character* : suppressed by epistasis : appearing recessive to another character due to mediation by a hypostatic gene **2** : depending on or due to hypostasis

hypostatic pneumonia *n* : pneumonia that usu. results from the collection of fluid in the dorsal region of the lungs and occurs esp. in those (as the bedridden or elderly) confined to a supine position for extended periods

hy·po·sthe·nia \ˌhī-pəs-ˈthē-nē-ə\ *n* : lack of strength : bodily weakness — **hy·po·sthen·ic** \ˌhī-pəs-ˈthen-ik\ *adj*

hy·pos·the·nu·ria \ˌhī-ˌpäs-thə-ˈn(y)ùr-ē-ə\ *n* : the secretion of urine of low specific gravity due to inability of the kidney to concentrate the urine normally — **hy·pos·the·nu·ric** \-ˈn(y)ùr-ik\ *adj*

hy·po·stome \ˈhī-pə-ˌstōm\ *n* : a rodlike organ that arises at the base of the beak in various mites and ticks

hy·po·styp·sis \ˌhī-pə-ˈstip-səs\ *n* : mild or moderate astringency

hy·po·styp·tic \-ˈstip-tik\ *adj* : mildly or moderately styptic

hyposulfite — see SODIUM HYPOSULFITE

hy·po·ten·sion \ˈhī-pō-ˌten-chən\ *n* **1** : abnormally low pressure of the blood — called also *low blood pressure* **2** : abnormally low pressure of the intraocular fluid

¹hy·po·ten·sive \ˌhī-pō-ˈten(t)-siv\ *adj* **1** : characterized by or due to hypotension ⟨∼ shock⟩ **2** : causing low blood pressure or a lowering of blood pressure ⟨∼ drugs⟩

²hypotensive *n* : one affected with hypotension

hy·po·tet·ra·ploid \-ˈte-trə-ˌplòid\ *adj* : having several chromosomes less than the tetraploid number of the basic genome — **hy·po·tet·ra·ploi·dy** \-ˌplòid-ē\ *n, pl* **-dies**

hy·po·tha·lam·ic \ˌhī-pō-thə-ˈlam-ik\ *adj* : of or relating to the hypothalamus — **hy·po·tha·lam·i·cal·ly** \-i-k(ə-)lē\ *adv*

hy·po·tha·lam·i·co—hy·po·phy·se·al *also* **hy·po·tha·lam·i·co—hy·po·phy·si·al** \ˌhī-pō-thə-ˈlam-i-ˌko-(ˌ)hī-ˌpäf-ə-ˈsē-əl, -ˌhī-pə-fə-, -ˈzē-əl, -ˌhī-pə-ˈfiz-ē-əl\ *adj* : HYPOTHALAMO═HYPOPHYSEAL

hypothalamic releasing factor *n* : any hormone that is secreted by the hypothalamus and stimulates the pituitary gland directly to secrete a hormone — called also *hypothalamic releasing hormone, releasing factor*

hy·po·thal·a·mo—hy·po·phy·se·al *also* **hy·po·thal·a·mo—hy·po·phy·si·al** \ˌhī-pō-ˌthal-ə-mō-(ˌ)hī-ˌpäf-ə-ˈsē-əl, -ˌhī-pə-fə-, -ˈzē-əl; -ˌhī-pə-ˈfiz-ē-əl\ *adj* : of or connecting

the hypothalamus and the pituitary gland ⟨∼ functions⟩ ⟨∼ systems⟩

hy·po·thal·a·mo—neu·ro·hy·po·phy·se·al *or* **hy·po·thal·a·mo—neu·ro·hy·po·phy·si·al** \-ˌn(y)ùr-ō-(ˌ)hī-ˌpäf-ə-ˈsē-əl, -ˌhī-pə-fe-, -ˈzē-əl, -ˌhī-pə-ˈfiz-ē-\ *adj* : of, relating to, or connecting the hypothalamus and the neurohypophysis

hy·po·thal·a·mo—pi·tu·itary \-pə-ˈt(y)ü-ə-ˌter-ē\ *adj* : HYPOTHALAMO-HYPOPHYSEAL

hy·po·thal·a·mot·o·my \ˌhī-pō-ˌthal-ə-ˈmät-ə-mē\ *n, pl* **-mies** : psychosurgery in which lesions are made in the hypothalamus by a knife, ultrasonic energy, radiation, or electricity

hy·po·thal·a·mus \-ˈthal-ə-məs\ *n, pl* **-mi** \-ˌmī\ : a basal part of the diencephalon that lies beneath the thalamus on each side, forms the floor of the third ventricle, and includes vital autonomic regulatory centers (as for the control of food intake)

hy·po·the·nar eminence \ˌhī-pō-ˈthē-ˌnär-, -nər-; hī-ˈpäth-ə-ˌnär-, -nər-\ *n* : the prominent part of the palm of the hand above the base of the little finger

hypothenar muscle *n* : any of four muscles located in the area of the hypothenar eminence: **a** : ABDUCTOR DIGITI MINIMI **b** : FLEXOR DIGITI MINIMI BREVIS **c** : PALMARIS BREVIS **d** : OPPONENS DIGITI MINIMI

hy·po·ther·mia \-ˈthər-mē-ə\ *n* : subnormal temperature of the body ⟨∼, defined as temperature under 36.6°C —*Emergency Medicine*⟩ — **hy·po·ther·mic** \-mik\ *adj*

hy·po·ther·my \ˈhī-pə-ˌthər-mē\ *n, pl* **-mies** : HYPOTHERMIA

hy·poth·e·sis \hī-ˈpäth-ə-səs\ *n, pl* **-e·ses** \-ˌsēz\ : a proposition tentatively assumed in order to draw out its logical or empirical consequences and test its consistency with facts that are known or may be determined ⟨it appears, then, to be a condition of the most genuinely scientific ∼ that it be ... of such a nature as to be either proved or disproved by comparison with observed facts —J. S. Mill⟩

hy·po·thet·i·co—de·duc·tive \ˌhī-pə-ˈthet-i-ˌkō-di-ˈdək-tiv\ *adj* : of or relating to scientific method in which hypotheses suggested by the facts of observation are proposed and consequences deduced from them so as to test the hypotheses and evaluate the consequences

hy·po·thy·mia \ˌhī-pō-ˈthī-mē-ə\ *n* : an abnormal decrease in the intensity with which emotions are experienced : flatness of affect

hy·po·thy·reo·sis \ˌhī-pō-ˌthī-rē-ˈō-səs\ *n* : HYPOTHYROIDISM

hy·po·thy·roid \ˌhī-pō-ˈthī-ˌròid\ *adj* : of, relating to, or affected with hypothyroidism

hy·po·thy·roid·ism \-ˌiz-əm\ *n* : deficient activity of the thyroid gland; *also* : a resultant bodily condition characterized by lowered metabolic rate and general loss of vigor

hy·po·thy·ro·sis \-ˌthī-ˈrō-səs\ *n* : HYPOTHYROIDISM

hy·po·thy·rox·in·emia *or chiefly Brit* **hy·po·thy·rox·in·ae·mia** \ˌhī-pō-thī-ˈräk-sə-ˈnē-mē-ə\ *n* : the presence of an abnormally low concentration of thyroxine in the blood — **hy·po·thy·rox·in·emic** *or chiefly Brit* **hy·po·thy·rox·in·ae·mic** \-ˈnē-mik\ *adj*

hy·po·to·nia \ˌhī-pə-ˈtō-nē-ə, -pō-\ *n* **1** : abnormally low pressure of the intraocular fluid **2** : the state of having hypotonic muscle tone

hy·po·ton·ic \ˌhī-pə-ˈtän-ik, -pō-\ *adj* **1** : having deficient tone or tension ⟨∼ children⟩ **2** : having a lower osmotic pressure than a surrounding medium or a fluid under comparison ⟨a ∼ solution⟩ — compare HYPERTONIC 2, ISOTONIC 1 — **hy·po·ton·i·cal·ly** \-i-k(ə-)lē\ *adv*

hy·po·to·nic·i·ty \-tə-ˈnis-ət-ē\ *n, pl* **-ties** **1** : the state or condition of having hypotonic osmotic pressure **2** : HYPOTONIA 2

hy·po·to·nus \ˌhī-pə-ˈtō-nəs, -pō-\ *n* : HYPOTONIA

hy·pot·ony \hī-ˈpät-ə-nē\ *n, pl* **-onies** : HYPOTONIA

───────────────

\ə\ **abut** \ᵊ\ **kitten** \ər\ **further** \a\ **ash** \ā\ **ace** \ä\ **cot, cart** \aù\ **out** \ch\ **chin** \e\ **bet** \ē\ **easy** \g\ **go** \i\ **hit** \ī\ **ice** \j\ **job** \ŋ\ **sing** \ō\ **go** \ò\ **law** \òi\ **boy** \th\ **thin** \t͟h\ **the** \ü\ **loot** \ù\ **foot** \y\ **yet** \zh\ **vision** *See also* Pronunciation Symbols page

hy·po·trich·ia \ˌhī-pō-ˈtrik-ē-ə\ *n* : HYPOTRICHOSIS

hy·po·tri·cho·sis \-tri-ˈkō-səs\ *n, pl* **-cho·ses** \-ˌsēz\ : congenital deficiency of hair — **hy·po·tri·chot·ic** \-ˈkät-ik\ *adj*

hy·pot·ro·phy \hī-ˈpä-trə-fē\ *n, pl* **-phies** : subnormal growth

hy·po·tro·pia \ˌhī-pō-ˈtrō-pē-ə\ *n* : strabismus in which the line of vision of one eye turns downward

hy·po·tym·pan·ic \ˌhī-pō-tim-ˈpan-ik\ *adj* **1** : located below the middle ear **2** : of or relating to the hypotympanum

hy·po·tym·pa·num \-ˈtim-pə-nəm\ *n, pl* **-na** \-nə\ *also* **-nums** : the lower part of the middle ear — compare EPITYMPANUM

hy·po·uri·ce·mia *or chiefly Brit* **hy·po·uri·cae·mia** \ˌhī-pō-ˌyùr-ə-ˈsē-mē-ə\ *n* : deficient uric acid in the blood — **hy·po·uri·ce·mic** *or chiefly Brit* **hy·po·uri·cae·mic** \-ˈsē-mik\ *adj*

hy·po·uri·cos·uria \-ˌyùr-i-kō-ˈshùr-ē-ə, -kəs-ˈyùr-\ *n* : the excretion of deficient amounts of uric acid in the urine

hy·po·ven·ti·la·tion \-ˌvent-ᵊl-ˈā-shən\ *n* : deficient ventilation of the lungs that results in reduction in the oxygen content or increase in the carbon dioxide content of the blood or both — **hy·po·ven·ti·lat·ed** \-ˈvent-ᵊl-ˌāt-əd\ *adj*

hy·po·vi·ta·min·osis \-ˌvīt-ə-mə-ˈnō-səs\ *n* : AVITAMINOSIS — **hy·po·vi·ta·min·ot·ic** \-ˈnät-ik\ *adj*

hy·po·vo·le·mia *or chiefly Brit* **hy·po·vo·lae·mia** \-väl-ˈē-mē-ə\ *n* : decrease in the volume of the circulating blood — **hy·po·vo·le·mic** *or chiefly Brit* **hy·po·vo·lae·mic** \-ˈē-mik\ *adj*

hy·po·xan·thine \ˌhī-pō-ˈzan-ˌthēn\ *n* : a purine base $C_5H_4N_4O$ found in plant and animal tissues that yields xanthine on oxidation and is an intermediate in uric acid synthesis

hy·po·xan·thine–gua·nine phos·pho·ri·bo·syl·trans·fer·ase \-ˈgwän-ˌēn-ˌfäs-fō-ˌrī-bō-sil-ˈtran(t)s-(ˌ)fər-ˌās, -ˌāz\ *n* : an enzyme that conserves hypoxanthine in the body by limiting its conversion to uric acid and that is lacking in Lesch-Nyhan syndrome — called also *hypoxanthine phosphoribosyltransferase*

hyp·ox·emia *or chiefly Brit* **hyp·ox·ae·mia** \ˌhip-ˌäk-ˈsē-mē-ə, ˌhī-ˌpäk-\ *n* : deficient oxygenation of the blood — **hyp·ox·emic** *or chiefly Brit* **hyp·ox·ae·mic** \-mik\ *adj*

hyp·ox·ia \hip-ˈäk-sē-ə, hī-ˈpäk-\ *n* : a deficiency of oxygen reaching the tissues of the body — **hyp·ox·ic** \-sik\ *adj*

hyps·ar·rhyth·mia *or* **hyps·arhyth·mia** \ˌhips-ā-ˈrith-mē-ə\ *n* : an abnormal encephalogram that is characterized by slow waves of high voltage and a disorganized arrangement of spikes, occurs esp. in infants, and is indicative of a condition that leads to severe mental retardation if left untreated — **hyps·ar·rhyth·mic** *or* **hyps·arhyth·mic** \-mik\ *adj*

hyp·si·brachy·ce·phal·ic \ˌhip-sə-ˌbrak-i-sə-ˈfal-ik\ *adj* : having a high broad head — **hyp·si·brachy·ceph·a·ly** \-ˈsef-ə-lē\ *n, pl* **-lies**

hyp·si·ce·phal·ic \-sə-ˈfal-ik\ *adj* : having a high forehead with a length-height index of 62.6 or higher — compare HYPSICRANIC — **hyp·si·ceph·a·ly** \-ˈsef-ə-lē\ *n, pl* **-lies**

hyp·si·conch \ˈhip-sə-ˌkäŋk, -ˌkänch\ *or* **hyp·si·con·chic** \-ik\ *adj* : having high orbits with an orbital index of 85 or over — **hyp·si·con·chy** \-ē\ *n, pl* **-chies**

hyp·si·cra·nic \ˌhip-sə-ˈkrā-nik\ *or* **hyp·si·cra·ni·al** \-ˈkrā-nē-əl\ *adj* : having a high skull with a length-height index of 75 or over — compare HYPSICEPHALIC — **hyp·si·cra·ny** \ˈhip-sə-ˌkrā-nē\ *n, pl* **-nies**

hyp·si·steno·ce·phal·ic \ˌhip-sə-ˌsten-ə-sə-ˈfal-ik\ *adj* : having an extremely high narrow head — **hyp·si·steno·ceph·a·ly** \-ˈsef-ə-lē\ *n, pl* **-lies**

hyp·so·chrome \ˈhip-sə-ˌkrōm\ *n* : an atom or group that causes a hypsochromic change when introduced into a compound

hyp·so·chro·mic \ˌhip-sə-ˈkrō-mik\ *adj* : of, relating to, causing, or characterized by a visible lightening of color or a shift to spectral colors of shorter wavelength ⟨~ chemical groups⟩ ⟨caused a ~ shift in color⟩

hyp·so·dont \ˈhip-sə-ˌdänt\ *adj* **1** *of teeth* : having high or deep crowns and short roots (as the molar teeth of a horse) — compare BRACHYDONT **2** : having or characterized by hypsodont teeth — **hyp·so·don·ty** \-ē\ *n, pl* **-ties**

hys·sop \ˈhis-əp\ *n* : a European mint (*Hyssopus officinalis*)

having highly aromatic and pungent leaves that have been used to make a tea and as a stimulant and to relieve respiratory symptoms

hys·ter·ec·to·my \ˌhis-tə-ˈrek-tə-mē\ *n, pl* **-mies** : surgical removal of the uterus — see OVARIOHYSTERECTOMY, PANHYSTERECTOMY, RADICAL HYSTERECTOMY, SUPRACERVICAL HYSTERECTOMY — **hys·ter·ec·to·mized** *also Brit* **hys·ter·ec·to·mised** \-tə-ˌmīzd\ *adj*

hys·ter·e·sis \ˌhis-tə-ˈrē-səs\ *n, pl* **-e·ses** \-ˌsēz\ **1** : the lagging of a physical effect on a body behind its cause (as behind changed forces and conditions) ⟨all manometers must be tested for ~ as well as for sensitivity and natural frequency —H. D. Green⟩ **2 a** : the influence of the previous history or treatment of a body on its subsequent response to a given force or changed condition ⟨a study has been made of the phenomenon of rennet ~, in which the time of coagulation of heated milk is progressively greater with increase in the time interval between heating and addition of rennet —J. S. Fruton⟩ **b** : the changed response of a body that results from this influence

hys·te·ria \his-ˈter-ē-ə, -ˈtir-\ *n* **1 a** : a psychoneurosis marked by emotional excitability and disturbances of the psychic, sensory, vasomotor, and visceral functions without an organic basis **b** : a similar condition in domestic animals **2** : behavior exhibiting overwhelming or unmanageable fear or emotional excess

hys·te·ri·a·gen·ic \his-ˌter-ē-ə-ˈjen-ik, -ˌtir-\ *adj* : HYSTEROGENIC ⟨~ animal rations⟩

hys·ter·ic \his-ˈter-ik\ *n* : an individual subject to or affected with hysteria

hys·ter·i·cal \-ˈter-i-kəl\ *also* **hys·ter·ic** \-ˈter-ik\ *adj* : of, relating to, or marked by hysteria ⟨during ~ conditions various functions of the human body are disordered —Morris Fishbein⟩ — **hys·ter·i·cal·ly** \-i-k(ə-)lē\ *adv*

hysterical personality *n* : a personality characterized by superficiality, egocentricity, vanity, dependence, and manipulativeness, by dramatic, reactive, and intensely expressed emotional behavior, and often by disturbed interpersonal relationships

hys·ter·ics \-ˈter-iks\ *n pl but sing or pl in constr* : a fit of uncontrollable laughter or crying : HYSTERIA

hystericus — see GLOBUS HYSTERICUS

hys·ter·i·form \his-ˈter-i-ˌfòrm\ *adj* : resembling hysteria ⟨~ symptoms⟩

hys·tero·col·pec·to·my \ˌhis-tə-(ˌ)rō-käl-ˈpek-tə-mē\ *n, pl* **-mies** : surgical removal of the uterus and vagina

hys·tero–ep·i·lep·sy \-ˈep-ə-ˌlep-sē\ *n, pl* **-sies** : a hysteria characterized by motor convulsions resembling those of epilepsy — **hys·tero–ep·i·lep·tic** \-ˌep-i-ˈlep-tik\ *adj*

hys·ter·o·gen·ic \ˌhis-tə-rō-ˈjen-ik\ *adj* : inducing hysteria

hys·ter·o·gram \ˈhis-tə-rō-ˌgram\ *n* : a radiograph of the uterus

hys·ter·o·graph \-ˌgraf\ *n* : HYSTEROGRAM

hys·ter·og·ra·phy \ˌhis-tə-ˈräg-rə-fē\ *n, pl* **-phies** : examination of the uterus by radiography after the injection of an opaque medium — **hys·ter·o·graph·ic** \ˌhis-tə-rə-ˈgraf-ik\ *adj*

hys·ter·oid \ˈhis-tə-ˌròid\ *adj* : resembling or tending toward hysteria

hys·tero·oo·pho·rec·to·my \ˌhis-tə-(ˌ)rō-ˌō-ə-fə-ˈrek-tə-mē\ *n, pl* **-mies** : surgical removal of the uterus and ovaries

hys·ter·o·pexy \ˈhis-tə-rō-ˌpek-sē\ *n, pl* **-pex·ies** : surgical fixation of a displaced uterus

hys·ter·o·plas·ty \-ˌplas-tē\ *n, pl* **-ties** : plastic surgery of the uterus

hys·ter·or·rha·phy \ˌhis-tə-ˈrór-ə-fē\ *n, pl* **-phies** **1** : a suturing of an incised or ruptured uterus **2** : HYSTEROPEXY

hys·ter·or·rhex·is \ˌhis-tə-rō-ˈrek-səs\ *n, pl* **-rhex·es** \-ˌsēz\ : rupture of the uterus

hys·ter·o·sal·pin·go·gram \-ˌsal-ˈpiŋ-gə-ˌgram\ *n* : a radiograph made by hysterosalpingography

hys·ter·o·sal·pin·gog·ra·phy \-ˌsal-ˌpiŋ-ˈgäg-rə-fē\ *n, pl* **-phies** : examination of the uterus and fallopian tubes by radiography after injection of an opaque medium — called also *uterosalpingography*

hys·ter·o·sal·pin·gos·to·my \-'gäs-tə-mē\ *n, pl* **-mies** : surgical establishment of an anastomosis between the uterus and an occluded fallopian tube

hys·ter·o·scope \'his-tə-rō-ˌskōp\ *n* : an endoscope used for the visual examination of the cervix and interior of the uterus — **hys·ter·o·scop·ic** \ˌhis-tə-rō-'skäp-ik\ *adj* — **hys·ter·os·co·py** \ˌhis-tə-'räs-kə-pē\ *n, pl* **-pies**

hys·ter·o·sto·mat·o·my \ˌhis-tə-rō-ˌstō-'mat-ə-mē\ *n, pl* **-mies** : surgical incision of the uterine cervix

hys·ter·ot·o·my \ˌhis-tə-'rät-ə-mē\ *n, pl* **-mies** : surgical incision of the uterus; *esp* : CESAREAN SECTION

hystrix — see ICHTHYOSIS HYSTRIX GRAVIOR

Hy·trin \'hī-trin\ *trademark* — used for a preparation of terazosin

Hy·zaar \'hī-ˌzär\ *trademark* — used for a preparation of hydrochlorothiazide and the potassium salt of losartan

Hz *abbr* hertz

H zone \'āch-ˌzōn\ *n* : a narrow and less dense zone of myosin filaments bisecting the A band in striated muscle — compare M LINE

I

i *abbr* **1** incisor **2** optically inactive

I *symbol* iodine

IAA *abbr* indoleacetic acid

iat·ric \(ˌ)ī-'a-trik *also* (ˌ)ē-\ *adj* **1** : of or relating to a physician or medical treatment : MEDICAL ⟨outstanding ∼ ability⟩ **2** : being medicinal, healing, or curative ⟨∼ qualities⟩

iat·ro·chem·ist \(ˌ)ī-ə-trō-'kem-əst *also* (ˌ)ē-\ *n* : a person believing in or practicing iatrochemistry

iat·ro·chem·is·try \-'kem-ə-strē\ *n, pl* **-tries** : chemistry combined with medicine — used of a school of medicine of the period about 1525–1660 dominated by the teachings of Paracelsus and stressing the use of chemicals in the treatment of disease; compare IATROPHYSICS — **iat·ro·chem·i·cal** \-'kem-i-kəl\ *adj*

iat·ro·gen·e·sis \-'jen-ə-səs\ *n, pl* **-e·ses** \-ˌsēz\ : inadvertent and preventable induction of disease or complications by the medical treatment or procedures of a physician or surgeon

iat·ro·gen·ic \(ˌ)ī-a-trə-'jen-ik *also* (ˌ)ē-\ *adj* : induced inadvertently by a physician or surgeon or by medical treatment or diagnostic procedures ⟨an ∼ rash⟩ — **iat·ro·gen·i·cal·ly** \-'jen-i-k(ə-)lē\ *adv* — **iat·ro·ge·nic·i·ty** \-jə-'nis-ət-ē\ *n, pl* **-ties**

iat·ro·math·e·mat·ics \-ˌmath-ə-'mat-iks, -math-'mat-\ *n pl but usu sing in constr* : IATROPHYSICS

iat·ro·phys·i·cist \-'fiz-ə-səst\ *n* : a person who specializes in iatrophysics

iat·ro·phys·ics \-'fiz-iks\ *n pl but usu sing in constr* : physics combined with medicine — used of a school of medicine of the 17th century that explained disease and the activities of the body in terms of physics rather than of chemistry; compare IATROCHEMISTRY — **iat·ro·phys·i·cal** \-'fiz-i-kəl\ *adj*

ib *or* **ibid** *abbr* [Latin *ibidem*] in the same place

I band \'ī-\ *n* : a pale band across a striated muscle fiber that consists of actin, is much less birefringent to polarized light than the A bands, is situated between two A bands, and is bisected by a narrow dark-staining Z line — called also *isotropic band*

ibo·ga·ine \i-'bō-gə-ˌēn\ *n* : a crystalline alkaloid hallucinogen $C_{20}H_{26}N_2O$ obtained from the roots, bark, and leaves of a plant (*Tabernanthe iboga*) of the dogbane family (Apocynaceae) that is found in equatorial Africa

ibo·te·nic acid \ˌī-bō-ˌtē-nik-\ *n* : a neurotoxic compound $C_5H_6N_2O_4$ that is structurally similar to kainic acid and is found esp. in fly agaric

IBS *abbr* irritable bowel syndrome

ibu·pro·fen \ˌī-byü-'prō-fən\ *n* : a nonsteroidal antiinflammatory drug $C_{13}H_{18}O_2$ used in over-the-counter preparations to relieve pain and fever and in prescription strength esp. to relieve the symptoms of rheumatoid arthritis and degenerative arthritis — see ADVIL, MOTRIN

ICD *abbr* International Classification of Diseases — usu. used with a number indicating the revision ⟨*ICD*-9⟩

ice \'īs\ *n* **1** : frozen water **2** : methamphetamine in the form of crystals of its hydrochloride salt $C_{10}H_{15}N\cdot HCl$ when used illicitly for smoking — called also *crystal, crystal meth*

ice bag *n* : a waterproof bag to hold ice for local application of cold to the body

Ice·land moss \ˌī-slən(d)-'mòs, ˌī-ˌslan(d)-\ *n* : a lichen of the genus *Cetraria* (*C. islandica*) of mountainous and arctic regions sometimes used in medicine or as food

ice pack *n* : crushed ice placed in a container (as an ice bag) or folded in a towel and applied to the body

ich *also* **ick** \'ik\ *n, pl* **ichs** *also* **icks** : a severe dermatitis of freshwater fish caused by a protozoan of the genus *Ichthyophthirius* (*I. multifiliis*) and esp. destructive in aquariums and hatcheries — called also *ichthyophthiriasis, ichthyophthirius*

ichor \'ī-ˌkò(ə)r\ *n* : a thin watery or blood-tinged discharge (as from an ulcer) — compare SANIES — **ichor·ous** \-kə-rəs\ *adj*

ichs *pl of* ICH

ich·tham·mol \'ik-thə-ˌmòl, -ˌmōl\ *n* : a brownish black viscous tarry liquid prepared from a distillate of bituminous schists by sulfonation followed by neutralization with ammonia and used as an antiseptic and emollient — see ICHTHYOL

ich·thy·ism \'ik-thē-ˌiz-əm\ *or* **ich·thy·is·mus** \ˌik-thē-'iz-məs\ *n, pl* **-isms** *or* **-mus·es** : ICHTHYOTOXISM

ich·thyo·acan·tho·tox·ism \ˌik-thē-ō-ə-ˌkan(t)-thə-'täk-ˌsiz-əm\ *n* : poisoning resulting from a wound inflicted by a venomous fish — compare ICHTHYOHEMOTOXISM, ICHTHYOSARCOTOXISM, ICHTHYOTOXISM

ich·thyo·col·la \ˌik-thē-ə-'käl-ə\ *or* **ich·thyo·col** *or* **ich·thyo·coll** \'ik-thē-ə-ˌkäl\ *n* : ISINGLASS 1

ich·thyo·he·mo·tox·ism *or chiefly Brit* **ich·thyo·hae·mo·tox·ism** \ˌik-thē-ō-ˌhē-mə-'täk-ˌsiz-əm\ *n* : poisoning caused by the ingestion of fish whose blood contains a toxic substance — compare ICHTHYOACANTHOTOXISM, ICHTHYOSARCOTOXISM, ICHTHYOTOXISM

ich·thy·oid \'ik-thē-ˌòid\ *adj* : resembling or characteristic of a fish ⟨an ∼ odor⟩

Ich·thy·ol \'ik-thē-ˌòl, -ˌōl\ *trademark* — used for a preparation of ichthammol

ich·thy·oph·a·gous \ˌik-thē-'äf-ə-gəs\ *adj* : eating or subsisting on fish

ich·thy·oph·thi·ri·a·sis \ˌik-thē-ˌäf-thə-'rī-ə-səs\ *n, pl* **-a·ses** \-ˌsēz\ : ICH

ich·thy·oph·thir·i·us \ˌik-thē-äf-'thir-ē-əs\ *n* **1** *cap* : a genus of oval ciliates (order Holotricha) that are included in a single species (*I. multifiliis*) and are parasitic in the skin of various freshwater fishes where they encyst and multiply causing a severe and sometimes fatal inflammation **2** : ICH

ich·thyo·sar·co·tox·in \ˌik-thē-ō-ˌsär-kə-'täk-sən\ *n* : a toxic substance found in the flesh of fish

ich·thyo·sar·co·tox·ism \-'täk-ˌsiz-əm\ *n* : poisoning caused

---

\ə\ abut \ᵊ\ kitten \ər\ further \a\ ash \ā\ ace \ä\ cot, cart \aù\ out \ch\ chin \e\ bet \ē\ easy \g\ go \i\ hit \ī\ ice \j\ job \ŋ\ sing \ō\ go \ò\ law \òi\ boy \th\ thin \t͟h\ the \ü\ loot \ù\ foot \y\ yet \zh\ vision *See also* Pronunciation Symbols page

by the ingestion of fish whose flesh contains a toxic substance — compare ICHTHYOACANTHOTOXISM, ICHTHYOHEMO- TOXISM, ICHTHYOTOXISM

ich·thy·o·si·form \ˌik-thē-ˈō-sə-ˌfȯrm\ *adj* : resembling ich- thyosis or that of ichthyosis ⟨∼ erythroderma⟩

ich·thy·o·sis \ˌik-thē-ˈō-səs\ *n, pl* **-o·ses** \-ˌsēz\ : any of sever- al congenital diseases of hereditary origin characterized by rough, thick, and scaly skin — called also *fishskin disease*

ichthyosis hys·trix gra·vi·or \-ˈhis-triks-ˈgrav-ē-ˌȯr, -ˈgräv-\ *n* : a rare hereditary abnormality characterized by the for- mation of brown, verrucose, and often linear lesions of the skin

ichthyosis sim·plex \-ˈsim-ˌpleks\ *n* : ICHTHYOSIS VULGARIS

ichthyosis vul·gar·is \-ˌvəl-ˈgar-əs\ *n* : the common heredi- tary form of ichthyosis

ich·thy·ot·ic \ˌik-thē-ˈät-ik\ *adj* : of, relating to, or exhibiting ichthyosis ⟨∼ skin⟩

ich·thyo·tox·in \ˌik-thē-ə-ˈtäk-sən\ *n* : a toxic substance in the blood serum of the eel; *broadly* : any toxic substance de- rived from fish

ich·thyo·tox·ism \-ˈtäk-ˌsiz-əm\ *n* : poisoning from fish — called also *ichthyism;* compare ICHTHYOACANTHOTOXISM, ICHTHYOHEMOTOXISM, ICHTHYOSARCOTOXISM

ick *var of* ICH

ICN *abbr* International Council of Nurses

ICP *abbr* intracranial pressure

ICSH *abbr* interstitial-cell stimulating hormone

ICSI *abbr* intracytoplasmic sperm injection

ICSS *abbr* intracranial self-stimulation

ICT *abbr* **1** inflammation of connective tissue **2** insulin coma therapy

ic·tal \ˈik-təl\ *adj* : of, relating to, or caused by ictus ⟨∼ symptomatology⟩ ⟨∼ speech automatisms⟩

ic·ter·ic \ik-ˈter-ik\ *adj* : of, relating to, or affected with jaun- dice

icteric index *n* : ICTERUS INDEX

ic·tero·ane·mia *or chiefly Brit* **ic·tero·anae·mia** \ˌik-tə-(ˌ)rō- ə-ˈnē-mē-ə\ *n* : a disease characterized by jaundice, anemia, and marked destruction of red blood cells and occurring esp. in swine

ic·ter·o·gen·ic \ˌik-tə-rō-ˈjen-ik, ik-ˌter-ə-\ *adj* : causing or tending to cause jaundice ⟨an ∼ agent in the blood⟩

ic·ter·oid \ˈik-tə-ˌrȯid\ *adj* : resembling jaundice : of a yellow tint like that produced by jaundice

ic·ter·us \ˈik-tə-rəs\ *n* : JAUNDICE

icterus gra·vis \-ˈgrav-əs, -ˈgräv-\ *n* **1** : severe jaundice due esp. to acute yellow atrophy **2** : ICTERUS GRAVIS NEONA- TORUM

icterus gravis neo·na·tor·um \-ˌnē-ō-nā-ˈtȯr-əm\ *n* : severe jaundice in a newborn child due esp. to erythroblastosis fe- talis

icterus index *n* : a figure representing the amount of biliru- bin in the blood as determined by comparing the color of a sample of test serum with a set of color standards ⟨an *icterus index* of 15 or above indicates active jaundice⟩ — called also *icteric index*

icterus neo·na·tor·um \-ˌnē-ō-nā-ˈtȯr-əm\ *n* : jaundice in a newborn infant

ic·tus \ˈik-təs\ *n* **1** : a beat or pulsation esp. of the heart **2** : a sudden attack or seizure esp. of stroke

ICU *abbr* intensive care unit

¹id \ˈid\ *n* : the one of the three divisions of the psyche in psy- choanalytic theory that is completely unconscious and is the source of psychic energy derived from instinctual needs and drives — compare EGO, SUPEREGO

²id *n* : a skin rash that is an allergic reaction to an agent caus- ing an infection ⟨a syphilitic ∼⟩ ⟨tinea pedis and the vesicu- lar ∼s arising from it —*Jour. Amer. Med. Assoc.*⟩ — com- pare BACTERID

id *abbr* [Latin *idem*] the same

ID *abbr* **1** identification **2** inside diameter; internal diame- ter **3** intradermal

IDA *abbr* iron-deficiency anemia

IDDM *abbr* insulin-dependent diabetes mellitus

idea \ī-ˈdē-ə, ˈīd-(ˌ)ē-ə\ *n* **1** : an entity (as a thought, concept, sensation, or image) actually or potentially present to con- sciousness **2** : a formulated thought or opinion

¹ide·al \ī-ˈdē-(ə)l, ˈī-ˌ\ *adj* **1** : existing as an archetypal idea **2 a** : existing as a mental image or in fancy or imagination only **b** : relating to or constituting mental images, ideas, or con- ceptions

²ideal *n* : a standard of perfection, beauty, or excellence ⟨self= criticism and the formation of ∼s are . . . the essential man- ifestations of the superego —G. S. Blum⟩

ide·al·ize *or chiefly Brit* **ide·al·ise** \ī-ˈdē-(ə-)ˌlīz\ *vt* **-ized** *or chiefly Brit* **-ised; -iz·ing** *or chiefly Brit* **-is·ing** : to give ideal form or value to : attribute ideal characteristics of excel- lence to ⟨constantly shifting moods and a tendency to ∼ or devalue other people —*Harvard Mental Health Letter*⟩ — **ide·al·iza·tion** *or chiefly Brit* **ide·al·isa·tion** \ī-ˌdē-(ə-)lə-ˈzā- shən\ *n*

idealogical, idealogy *var of* IDEOLOGICAL, IDEOLOGY

idea of reference *n* : a delusion that the remarks one over- hears and people one encounters seem to be concerned with and usu. hostile to oneself — called also *delusion of reference*

ide·a·tion \ˌīd-ē-ˈā-shən\ *n* : the capacity for or the act of forming or entertaining ideas ⟨suicidal ∼⟩

ide·a·tion·al \-shnəl, -shən-ᵊl\ *adj* : of, relating to, or pro- duced by ideation; *broadly* : consisting of or referring to ideas or thoughts of objects not immediately present to the senses — **ide·a·tion·al·ly** \-ē\ *adv*

idée fixe \(ˌ)ē-ˌdā-ˈfēks\ *n, pl* **idées fixes** \-ˈfēks(-əz)\ : a usu. delusional idea that dominates the whole mental life during a prolonged period (as in certain mental disorders) — called also *fixed idea*

iden·ti·cal \ī-ˈdent-i-kəl, ə-\ *adj* : MONOZYGOTIC ⟨∼ twins⟩

identical points *n pl* : points on the retinas of the two eyes that occupy corresponding positions in respect to the retinal centers

iden·ti·fi·ca·tion \ī-ˌdent-ə-fə-ˈkā-shən, ə-\ *n* **1** : an act of identifying : the state of being identified **2 a** : psychological orientation of the self in regard to something (as a person or group) with a resulting feeling of close emotional association **b** : a largely unconscious process whereby an individual models thoughts, feelings, and actions after those attributed to an object that has been incorporated as a mental image

iden·ti·fy \ī-ˈdent-ə-ˌfī, ə-\ *vb* **-fied; -fy·ing** *vt* : to determine the taxonomic position of (a biological specimen) ∼ *vi* : to undergo or experience psychological identification ⟨∼ with the hero of a novel⟩

iden·ti·ty \ī-ˈden(t)-ət-ē, ə-ˈ\ *n, pl* **-ties** **1** : the distinguishing character or personality of an individual **2** : the relation es- tablished by psychological identification

identity crisis *n* : personal psychosocial conflict esp. in ado- lescence that involves confusion about one's social role and often a sense of loss of continuity to one's personality

ide·ol·o·gy \ˌīd-ē-ˈäl-ə-jē, ˌid-\ *also* **ide·al·o·gy** \-ˈäl-ə-jē, -ˈal-\ *n, pl* **-gies** **1** : a systematic body of concepts esp. about hu- man life or culture **2** : a manner or the content of thinking characteristic of an individual, group, or culture — **ideo- log·i·cal** *also* **idea·log·i·cal** \ˌīd-ē-ə-ˈläj-i-kəl\ *adj* — **ideo- log·i·cal·ly** \-i-k(ə-)lē\ *adv*

ideo·mo·tor \ˌīd-ē-ə-ˈmōt-ər, ˌid-\ *adj* **1** : not reflex but mo- tivated by an idea ⟨∼ muscular activity⟩ **2** : of, relating to, or concerned with ideomotor activity ⟨∼ theory⟩

ideo·pho·bia \-ˈfō-bē-ə\ *n* : fear or distrust of ideas or of rea- son

ID₅₀ *symbol* — used for the dose of an infectious organism required to produce infection in 50 percent of the experi- mental subjects

id·io·chro·mo·some \-ˈkrō-mə-ˌsōm, -ˌzōm\ *n* : SEX CHRO- MOSOME

id·i·o·cy \ˈid-ē-ə-sē\ *n, pl* **-cies** *usu offensive* : extreme mental retardation

id·io·gen·e·sis \ˌid-ē-ə-ˈjen-ə-səs\ *n, pl* **-e·ses** \-ˌsēz\ : sponta- neous origin (as of disease) — **idio·ge·net·ic** \-jə-ˈnet-ik\ *adj*

id·io·glos·sia \-ˈglä-sē-ə, -ˈglȯ-\ *n* : a condition in which words are so poorly articulated that speech is either unintelligible or appears to be a made-up language

id·io·gram \\'id-ē-ə-ˌgram\\ *n* : a diagrammatic representation of a chromosome complement or karyotype

id·io·graph·ic \\ˌid-ē-ə-'graf-ik\\ *adj* : relating to or dealing with the concrete, individual, or unique — compare NOMO-THETIC

id·io·ki·net·ic \\ˌid-ē-ə-kə-'net-ik, -kī-\\ *adj, of movement* : induced by activity of the corticospinal tracts of the brain

id·io·mus·cu·lar \\-'məs-kyə-lər\\ *adj* : relating to muscular tissue exclusively; *esp* : originating in muscle ⟨~ contraction⟩

id·io·path·ic \\ˌid-ē-ə-'path-ik\\ *adj* : arising spontaneously or from an obscure or unknown cause : PRIMARY ⟨~ epilepsy⟩ ⟨~ thrombocytopenic purpura⟩ — **id·io·path·i·cal·ly** \\-'path-i-k(ə-)lē\\ *adv*

idiopathic hypertension *n* : ESSENTIAL HYPERTENSION

id·i·op·a·thy \\ˌid-ē-'äp-ə-thē\\ *n, pl* **-thies** : an idiopathic anomaly or disease

id·io·plasm \\'id-ē-ə-ˌplaz-əm\\ *n* : the part of the protoplasm that functions specif. in hereditary transmission : GERM PLASM 2

id·io·ret·i·nal \\ˌid-ē-ə-'ret-ᵊn-əl, -'ret-nəl\\ *adj* : peculiar to the retina; *specif* : originating subjectively in the retina ⟨~ light⟩

id·io·some \\'id-ē-ə-ˌsōm\\ *n* : any of several specialized cellular organelles: as **a** : ACROSOME **b** : an area of modified cytoplasm surrounding a centrosome

id·io·syn·cra·sy \\ˌid-ē-ə-'sin-krə-sē\\ *n, pl* **-sies** **1** : a peculiarity of physical or mental constitution or temperament **2** : individual hypersensitiveness (as to a drug or food) ⟨anemia accompanying the use of a sulfa drug is usually considered to be due to ~⟩

id·io·syn·crat·ic \\ˌid-ē-ō-(ˌ)sin-'krat-ik\\ *adj* : of, relating to, marked by, or resulting from idiosyncrasy ⟨an ~ response to a drug⟩ ⟨an ~ disease⟩

id·i·ot \\'id-ē-ət\\ *n, usu offensive* : a person affected with extreme mental retardation — **idiot** *adj, usu offensive*

idiot sa·vant \\'ē-ˌdyō-sä-'väⁿ; 'id-ē-ət-sə-'vänt, -'vant\\ *n, pl* **idiots savants** \\-ˌdyō-sä-'väⁿ(z); -əts-sə-'vänt(s), -'vant(s)\\ *or* **idiot savants** : a person affected with a mental disability (as autism or mental retardation) who exhibits exceptional skill or brilliance in some limited field (as mathematics or music) — called also *savant*

id·io·type \\'id-ē-ə-ˌtīp\\ *n* : the molecular structure and conformation in the variable region of an immunoglobulin that confers its antigenic specificity — compare ALLOTYPE, ISO-TYPE — **id·io·typ·ic** \\ˌid-ē-ə-'tip-ik\\ *adj*

id·io·ven·tric·u·lar \\ˌid-ē-ə-ven-'trik-yə-lər, -vən-\\ *adj* : of, relating to, associated with, or arising in the ventricles of the heart independently of the atria ⟨apparent accelerated ~ rhythm occurred in one patient —T. J. Sullivan⟩

id·i·o·zome \\'id-ē-ə-ˌzōm\\ *n* : IDIOSOME

id·i·tol \\'id-ə-ˌtól, -ˌtōl\\ *n* : a sweet crystalline alcohol $C_{12}H_{28}O_{12}$ obtained by a reduction of idose or sorbose

idose \\'īd-ˌōs, 'id- *also* -ˌōz\\ *n* : a sugar $C_6H_{12}O_6$ epimeric with gulose and obtainable along with gulose by synthesis from xylose

idox·uri·dine \\ˌī-ˌdäks-'yúr-ə-ˌdēn\\ *n* : a white crystalline drug $C_9H_{11}IN_2O_5$ that is an analog of pyrimidine and is used to treat keratitis caused by the herpesviruses producing herpes simplex — abbr. *IDU;* called also *iododeoxyuridine, IUDR*

IDU *abbr* idoxuridine

IF *abbr* interferon

IFN *abbr* interferon

ifos·fa·mide \\ˌī-'fäs-fə-ˌmīd\\ *n* : a synthetic cyclophosphamide analog $C_7H_{15}Cl_2H_7O_2P$ that is pharmacologically inert until activated by liver enzymes after being administered by injection for the treatment esp. of testicular cancer

Ig *abbr* immunoglobulin

IgA \\ˌī-ˌjē-'ā\\ *n* **1** : a class of immunoglobulins that include antibodies found in external bodily secretions (as saliva, tears, and sweat) **2** : an immunoglobulin of the class IgA

IgD \\ˌī-ˌjē-'dē\\ *n* **1** : a minor class of immunoglobulins including antibodies that are of unknown function except as receptors for antigen **2** : an immunoglobulin of the class IgD

IgE \\ˌī-ˌjē-'ē\\ *n* **1** : a class of immunoglobulins including antibodies that function esp. in allergic reactions **2** : an immunoglobulin of the class IgE

IGF *abbr* insulin-like growth factor

IGF–1 *abbr* insulin-like growth factor 1

IgG \\ˌī-ˌjē-'jē\\ *n* **1** : a class of immunoglobulins that include the most common antibodies circulating in the blood, that facilitate the phagocytic destruction of microorganisms foreign to the body, that bind to and activate complement, and that are the only immunoglobulins to cross over the placenta from mother to fetus **2** : an immunoglobulin of the class IgG

IgM \\ˌī-ˌjē-'em\\ *n* **1** : a class of immunoglobulins of high molecular weight that include the primary antibodies released into the blood early in the immune response to be replaced later by IgGs of lower molecular weight and that are highly efficient in binding complement **2** : an immunoglobulin of the class IgM

ig·na·tia \\ig-'nā-sh(ē-)ə\\ *n* : the dried ripe seeds of the Saint≈Ignatius's-bean used like nux vomica

Ig·na·tius bean \\ig-'nā-sh(ē-)əs-\\ *n* : SAINT-IGNATIUS'S-BEAN

ig·ni·punc·ture \\'ig-nə-ˌpəŋ(k)-chər\\ *n* : puncture of the body with hot needles for therapeutic purposes

IH *abbr* infectious hepatitis

IL *abbr* interleukin — often used with an identifying number ⟨*IL-2*⟩ ⟨*IL-6*⟩

Ile *abbr* isoleucine; isoleucyl

ilea *pl of* ILEUM

il·e·al \\'il-ē-əl\\ *also* **il·e·ac** \\-ˌak\\ *adj* : of, relating to, or affecting the ileum ⟨~ ulcers⟩ ⟨upper ~ obstruction⟩

il·e·itis \\ˌil-ē-'īt-əs\\ *n, pl* **-it·i·des** \\-'īt-ə-ˌdēz\\ : inflammation of the ileum — see REGIONAL ILEITIS

il·eo·anal \\ˌil-ē-ō-'ān-ᵊl\\ *adj* : of, relating to, or connecting the ileum and anus ⟨an ~ anastomosis⟩

il·eo·ce·cal \\ˌil-ē-ō-'sē-kəl\\ *adj* : of, relating to, or connecting the ileum and cecum ⟨the ~ region⟩ ⟨the ~ orifice⟩

ileocecal valve *n* : the valve formed by two folds of mucous membrane at the opening of the ileum into the large intestine — called also *Bauhin's valve, ileocolic valve, valvula coli*

il·eo·co·lic \\-'kō-lik, -'käl-ik\\ *adj* : relating to, situated near, or involving the ileum and the colon ⟨~ intussusception⟩

ileocolic artery *n* : a branch of the superior mesenteric artery that supplies the terminal part of the ileum and the beginning of the colon

ileocolic valve *n* : ILEOCECAL VALVE

il·eo·co·li·tis \\ˌil-ē-ō-kō-'līt-əs, -kə-'līt-\\ *n* : inflammation of the ileum and colon

il·eo·co·los·to·my \\-kə-'läs-tə-mē\\ *n, pl* **-mies** : a surgical operation producing an artificial opening connecting the ileum and the colon

il·eo·cyto·plas·ty \\-'sīt-ə-ˌplast-ē\\ *n, pl* **-ties** : plastic surgery that involves anastomosing a segment of the ileum to the bladder esp. in order to increase bladder capacity and preserve the function of the kidneys and ureters

il·eo·il·e·al \\-'il-ē-əl\\ *adj* : relating to or involving two different parts of the ileum ⟨an ~ anastomosis⟩ ⟨transient ~ intussusceptions⟩

il·eo·proc·tos·to·my \\-ˌpräk-'täs-tə-mē\\ *n, pl* **-mies** : a surgical operation producing a permanent artificial opening connecting the ileum and rectum

il·eo·sig·moid·os·to·my \\-ˌsig-ˌmóid-'äs-tə-mē\\ *n, pl* **-mies** : a surgical operation producing a permanent artificial opening connecting the ileum and the sigmoid colon

il·e·os·to·my \\ˌil-ē-'äs-tə-mē\\ *n, pl* **-mies** **1** : surgical formation of an artificial anus by connecting the ileum to an open-

\\ə\\ abut \\ᵊ\\ kitten \\ər\\ further \\a\\ ash \\ā\\ ace \\ä\\ cot, cart
\\aú\\ out \\ch\\ chin \\e\\ bet \\ē\\ easy \\g\\ go \\i\\ hit \\ī\\ ice \\j\\ job
\\ŋ\\ sing \\ō\\ go \\ó\\ law \\ói\\ boy \\th\\ thin \\t̲h̲\\ the \\ü\\ loot
\\ú\\ foot \\y\\ yet \\zh\\ vision *See also* Pronunciation Symbols page

ing in the abdominal wall   2 : the artificial opening made by ileostomy

ileostomy bag *n* : a container designed to receive feces discharged through an ileostomy

il·eo·trans·verse \ˌil-ē-ō-tran(t)s-ˈvərs\ *adj* : relating to or involving the ileum and the transverse colon ⟨an ∼ colostomy⟩

Iletin \ˈī-lət-ən\ *trademark* — used for a preparation of insulin

il·e·um \ˈil-ē-əm\ *n, pl* **il·ea** \-ē-ə\ : the last division of the small intestine that constitutes the part between the jejunum and large intestine and in humans forms the last three fifths of the part of the small intestine beyond the end of the duodenum and that is smaller and thinner-walled than the jejunum with fewer circular folds but more numerous Peyer's patches

il·e·us \ˈil-ē-əs\ *n* : obstruction of the bowel; *specif* : a condition that is commonly marked by a painful distended abdomen, vomiting of dark or fecal matter, toxemia, and dehydration and that results when the intestinal contents back up because peristalsis fails although the lumen is not occluded — compare VOLVULUS

ilia *pl of* ILIUM

il·i·ac \ˈil-ē-ˌak\ *also* **il·i·al** \ˈil-ē-əl\ *adj*   **1** : of, relating to, or located near the ilium ⟨the ∼ bone⟩   **2** : of or relating to either of the lowest lateral abdominal regions

iliac artery *n*   **1** : either of the large arteries supplying blood to the lower trunk and hind limbs and arising by bifurcation of the aorta which in humans occurs at the level of the fourth lumbar vertebra to form one vessel for each side of the body — called also *common iliac artery*   **2** : the outer branch of the common iliac artery on either side of the body that passes beneath the inguinal ligament to become the femoral artery — called also *external iliac artery*   **3** : the inner branch of the common iliac artery on either side of the body that soon breaks into several branches and supplies blood chiefly to the pelvic and gluteal areas — called also *hypogastric artery, internal iliac artery*

iliac crest *n* : the thick curved upper border of the ilium

iliac fascia *n* : an aponeurotic layer lining the back part of the abdominal cavity and covering the inner surface of the psoas and iliacus muscles

iliac fossa *n* : the inner concavity of the ilium

iliac node *n* : any of the lymph nodes grouped around the iliac arteries and the iliac veins — see EXTERNAL ILIAC NODE, INTERNAL ILIAC NODE

iliac spine *n* : any of four projections on the ilium: **a** : ANTERIOR INFERIOR ILIAC SPINE **b** : ANTERIOR SUPERIOR ILIAC SPINE **c** : POSTERIOR INFERIOR ILIAC SPINE **d** : POSTERIOR SUPERIOR ILIAC SPINE

ili·a·cus \i-ˈlī-ə-kəs\ *n, pl* **ili·a·ci** \-ə-ˌsī\ : a muscle of the iliac region of the abdomen that flexes the thigh or bends the pelvis and lumbar region forward, has its origin from the iliac fossa, iliac crest, the base of the sacrum, and adjoining parts, and is inserted into the outer side of the tendon of the psoas major, the capsule of the hip joint, and the lesser trochanter of the femur

iliac vein *n* : any of several veins on each side of the body corresponding to and accompanying the iliac arteries: **a** : either of two veins of which one is formed on each side of the body by the union of the external and internal iliac veins and which unite to form the inferior vena cava — called also *common iliac vein*   **b** : a vein that drains the leg and lower part of the anterior abdominal wall, is an upward continuation of the femoral vein, and unites with the internal iliac vein — called also *external iliac vein*   **c** : a vein that drains the pelvis and gluteal and perineal regions, accompanies the internal iliac artery, and unites with the external iliac vein to form the common iliac vein — called also *hypogastric vein, internal iliac vein*

ilial *var of* ILIAC

il·io·coc·cy·geus \ˌil-ē-ō-käk-ˈsij-(ē-)əs\ *n* : a muscle of the pelvis that is a subdivision of the levator ani, has its origin at the pubic symphysis and the tendon which arches over the

obturator internus, inserts on the coccyx and perineal body, and helps support the pelvic viscera — compare PUBOCOCCYGEUS

il·io·cos·ta·lis \-käs-ˈtā-ləs\ *n* : the lateral division of the sacrospinalis muscle that helps to keep the trunk erect and consists of three parts: **a** : ILIOCOSTALIS CERVICIS **b** : ILIOCOSTALIS LUMBORUM **c** : ILIOCOSTALIS THORACIS

iliocostalis cer·vi·cis \-ˈsər-və-səs\ *n* : a muscle that extends from the ribs to the cervical transverse processes and acts to draw the neck to the same side and to elevate the ribs

iliocostalis dor·si \-ˈdor-ˌsī\ *n* : ILIOCOSTALIS THORACIS

iliocostalis lum·bor·um \-ˌləm-ˈbor-əm\ *n* : a muscle that extends from the ilium to the lower ribs and acts to draw the trunk to the same side or to depress the ribs

iliocostalis tho·ra·cis \-thə-ˈrā-səs\ *n* : a muscle that extends from the lower to the upper ribs and acts to draw the trunk to the same side and to approximate the ribs

il·io·fem·o·ral \ˌil-ē-ō-ˈfem-(ə-)rəl\ *adj*   **1** : of or relating to the ilium and the femur   **2** : relating to or involving an iliac vein and a femoral vein ⟨an ∼ bypass graft⟩

iliofemoral ligament *n* : a ligament that extends from the anterior inferior iliac spine to the intertrochanteric line of the femur and divides below into two branches of which one is fixed to the distal part and the other to the proximal part of the intertrochanteric line — called also *Y ligament*

il·io·hy·po·gas·tric nerve \ˌil-ē-ō-ˌhī-pə-ˈgas-trik-\ *n* : a branch of the first lumbar nerve that divides into branches distributed to the skin of the lateral part of the buttocks, the skin of the pubic region, and the muscles of the anterolateral abdominal wall

il·io·in·gui·nal \-ˈiŋ-gwən-ᵊl\ *adj* : of, relating to, or affecting the iliac and inguinal abdominal regions

ilioinguinal nerve *n* : a branch of the first lumbar nerve that is distributed to the muscles of the anterolateral wall of the abdomen, to the skin of the proximal and medial part of the thigh, and to the base of the penis and the scrotum in the male or the mons veneris and labia majora in the female

il·io·lum·bar artery \ˌil-ē-ō-ˈləm-bər-, -ˌbär-\ *n* : a branch of the internal iliac artery that supplies muscles in the lumbar region and the iliac fossa

iliolumbar ligament *n* : a ligament connecting the transverse process of the last lumbar vertebra with the iliac crest

il·io·pec·tin·e·al eminence \ˌil-ē-ō-pek-ˈtin-ē-əl-\ *n* : a ridge on the hip bone marking the junction of the ilium and the pubis

iliopectineal line *n* : a line or ridge on the inner surface of the hip bone marking the border between the true and false pelvis

il·io·pso·as \ˌil-ē-ō-ˈsō-əs, ˌil-ē-ˈäp-sə-wəs\ *n* : a muscle consisting of the iliacus and psoas major muscles

iliopsoas tendon *n* : the tendon that is common to the iliacus and psoas major

il·io·tib·i·al \ˌil-ē-ō-ˈtib-ē-əl\ *adj* : of or relating to the ilium and the tibia ⟨∼ fasciotomy⟩

iliotibial band *n* : a fibrous thickening of the fascia lata that extends from the iliac crest down the lateral part of the thigh to the lateral condyle of the tibia and that provides stability to the knee and assists with flexion and extension of the knee — called also *iliotibial tract*

iliotibial band fric·tion syndrome \-ˈfrik-shən-\ *n* : a sports injury that is marked by diffuse pain in the lateral part of the knee, that occurs esp. in athletes engaged in long distance running, and that is believed to result from inflammation of the iliotibial band due to overuse as it slides across the lateral condyle of the femur as the knee is flexed and extended repeatedly — called also *iliotibial band syndrome*

il·i·um \ˈil-ē-əm\ *n, pl* **il·ia** \-ē-ə\ : the dorsal, upper, and largest one of the three bones composing either lateral half of the pelvis that in humans is broad and expanded above and narrower below where it joins with the ischium and pubis to form part of the acetabulum

¹ill \ˈil\ *adj* **worse** \ˈwərs\ *also* **ill·er** \ˈil-ər\; **worst** \ˈwərst\ **1** : affected with some ailment : not in good health ⟨incurably ∼ with cancer —*Time*⟩ ⟨mentally ∼⟩   **2** : affected with nausea often to the point of vomiting ⟨thought she would be ∼ after the ride on the roller coaster⟩

²**ill** *n* : AILMENT, SICKNESS ⟨chicken pox and other ∼s of childhood⟩

ill–health \ˌil-ˈhelth\ *n* : a condition of inferior health in which some disease or impairment of function is present but is usu. not as serious in terms of curtailing activity as an illness ⟨elderly parents who are in ∼ and need their financial and personal help —E. C. Gottschalk, Jr.⟩

Il·lic·i·um \i-ˈlis(h)-ē-əm\ *n* : a small genus of evergreen trees of the magnolia family (Magnoliaceae) that have aromatic persistent leaves and yellow or purplish flowers and include one (*I. verum*) whose fruit is the source of star anise oil

ill·ness \ˈil-nəs\ *n* : an unhealthy condition of body or mind : SICKNESS

il·lu·mi·nance \il-ˈü-mə-nən(t)s\ *n* : ILLUMINATION 2

il·lu·mi·nant \-nənt\ *n* : an illuminating device or substance (as for a microscope)

il·lu·mi·na·tion \il-ˌü-mə-ˈnā-shən\ *n* **1** : the action of supplying or brightening with light or the resulting state **2** : the luminous flux per unit area on an intercepting surface at any given point — called also *illuminance* — **il·lu·mi·nate** \il-ˈü-mə-ˌnāt\ *vt* **-nat·ed; -nat·ing**

il·lu·mi·na·tor \il-ˈü-mə-ˌnā-tər\ *n* : one that illuminates; *esp* : a device that gives physical light or that is used to direct light to a specific area or that is used to concentrate or reflect light

il·lu·sion \il-ˈü-zhən\ *n* **1** : a misleading image presented as a visual stimulus **2 a** : perception of something objectively existing in such a way as to cause misinterpretation of its actual nature; *esp* : OPTICAL ILLUSION — compare DELUSION 2 **b** : HALLUCINATION 1 **c** : a pattern capable of reversible perspective — **il·lu·sion·al** \-ˈüzh-nəl, -ən-əl\ *adj*

il·lu·so·ry \il-ˈüs-(ə-)rē, -ˈüz-\ *adj* : based on or producing illusion : being deceptive ⟨the search for the ultimate cure-all for a hangover has proved —M. L. Herndon⟩

Il·o·sone \ˈil-ə-ˌsōn\ *trademark* — used for a preparation of the estolate of erythromycin

Il·o·ty·cin \ˌil-ə-ˈtīs-ᵊn\ *n* : a preparation of erythromycin — formerly a U.S. registered trademark

IM *abbr* **1** internal medicine **2** intramuscular; intramuscularly

¹**im·age** \ˈim-ij\ *n* **1 a** : the optical counterpart of an object produced by an optical device (as a lens or mirror) or an electronic device — see REAL IMAGE, VIRTUAL IMAGE **b** : a likeness of an object produced on a photographic material **2** : a mental picture or impression of something ⟨had a negative body ∼ of herself⟩: as **a** (1) : a mental conception held in common by members of a group and symbolic of a basic attitude and orientation ⟨the compassionate small-town family doctor, an ∼ that the AMA deeply admires —*Current Biog.*⟩ (2) : an idealized conception of a person and esp. a parent that is formed by an infant or child, is retained in the unconscious, and influences behavior in later life ⟨the overwhelming influence of the mother ∼ —John Messenger⟩ — called also *imago* **b** : the memory of a perception in psychology that is modified by subsequent experience; *also* : the representation of the source of a stimulus on a receptor mechanism

²**image** *vb* **im·aged; im·ag·ing** *vt* **1** : to call up a mental picture of : IMAGINE **2** : to create a representation of; *also* : to form an image of ⟨the liver was *imaged*⟩ ⟨the animals were anesthetized and *imaged* with a gamma camera —R. T. Proffitt *et al*⟩ ∼ *vi* : to form an image

image in·ten·si·fi·er \-in-ˈten(t)-sə-ˌfī(-ə)r\ *n* : a device used esp. for diagnosis in radiology that provides a more intense image for a given amount of radiation than can be obtained by the usual fluorometric methods — **image in·ten·si·fi·ca·tion** \-in-ˌten(t)s-ə-(ə)fə-ˈkā-shən\ *n*

im·ag·less \ˈim-ij-ləs\ *adj* : characterized by absence of mental images ⟨an ∼ thought⟩

im·ag·ery \ˈim-ij-(ə-)rē\ *n, pl* **-eries** : mental images ⟨eidetic ∼⟩; *esp* : the products of imagination ⟨psychotic ∼⟩

image space *n* : a space that is associated with an optical system and consists of points of which each is an image of a corresponding point in the space in which the objects being imaged reside

¹**imag·i·nal** \im-ˈaj-ən-ᵊl\ *adj* : of, relating to, or involving imagination, images, or imagery

²**ima·gi·nal** \im-ˈā-gən-ᵊl, -ˈäg-ən-\ *adj* : of or relating to the insect imago

imag·i·nary \im-ˈaj-ə-ˌner-ē\ *adj* : existing only in imagination : lacking factual reality ⟨∼ fears⟩ ⟨an ∼ illness⟩

imag·i·na·tion \im-ˌaj-ə-ˈnā-shən\ *n* : an act or process of forming a conscious idea or mental image of something never before wholly perceived in reality by the one forming the images (as through a synthesis of remembered elements of previous sensory experiences or ideas as modified by unconscious defense mechanisms); *also* : the ability or gift of forming such conscious ideas or mental images esp. for the purposes of artistic or intellectual creation

imag·ine \im-ˈaj-ən\ *vb* **imag·ined; imag·in·ing** \-ˈaj-(ə-)niŋ\ *vt* : to form a mental image of (something not present) ∼ *vi* : to use the imagination

imaging *n* : the action or process of producing an image esp. of a part of the body by radiographic techniques ⟨advances in clinical diagnostic ∼⟩ ⟨cardiac ∼⟩ — see MAGNETIC RESONANCE IMAGING

ima·go \im-ˈā-(ˌ)gō, -ˈäg-(ˌ)ō\ *n, pl* **imagoes** *or* **ima·gi·nes** \-ˈā-gə-ˌnēz, -ˈäg-ə-\ **1** : an insect in its final, adult, sexually mature, and typically winged state **2** : IMAGE 2a(2)

im·bal·ance \(ˈ)im-ˈbal-ən(t)s\ *n* : lack of balance : the state of being out of equilibrium or out of proportion: as **a** : loss of parallel relation between the optical axes of the eyes caused by faulty action of the extrinsic muscles and often resulting in diplopia **b** : absence of biological equilibrium ⟨a vitamin ∼⟩ ⟨if the ductus arteriosus fails to close, a circulatory ∼ results —E. B. Steen & Ashley Montagu⟩ **c** : a disproportion between the number of males and females in a population — **im·bal·anced** \-ən(t)st\ *adj*

im·be·cile \ˈim-bə-səl, -ˌsil\ *n, usu offensive* : a person affected with moderate mental retardation — **imbecile** *or* **im·be·cil·ic** \ˌim-bə-ˈsil-ik\ *adj, usu offensive* — **im·be·cil·i·ty** \ˌim-bə-ˈsil-ət-ē\ *n, pl* **-ties** *usu offensive*

imbed *var of* EMBED

im·bi·bi·tion \ˌim-bə-ˈbish-ən\ *n* : the action or process of assimilating, taking into solution, or taking in liquid; *esp* : the taking up of fluid by a colloidal system resulting in swelling — **im·bibe** \im-ˈbīb\ *vb* **im·bibed; im·bib·ing**

im·bri·ca·tion \ˌim-brə-ˈkā-shən\ *n* : an overlapping esp. of successive layers of tissue in the surgical closure of a wound — **im·bri·cate** \ˈim-brə-ˌkāt\ *vt* **-cat·ed; -cat·ing**

im·id·az·ole \ˌim-ə-ˈdaz-ˌōl\ *n* **1** : a white crystalline heterocyclic base $C_3H_4N_2$ that is an antimetabolite related to histidine **2** : any of a large class of derivatives of imidazole including histidine and histamine

im·id·az·o·line \ˌim-ə-ˈdaz-ə-ˌlēn\ *n* : any of three dihydro derivatives $C_3H_6N_2$ of imidazole with adrenergic blocking activity; *also* : a derivative of these

im·id·az·o·lyl \-ə-ˌlil\ *n* : any of four monovalent radicals $C_3H_3N_2$ derived from imidazole by removal of one hydrogen atom

im·ide \ˈim-ˌīd\ *n* : a compound containing the NH group that is derived from ammonia by replacement of two hydrogen atoms by a metal or an equivalent of acid radicals — compare AMIDE — **im·id·ic** \im-ˈid-ik\ *adj*

im·i·do \ˈim-ə-ˌdō\ *adj* : relating to or containing the NH group or its substituted form NR united to one or two groups of acid character

im·ine \ˈim-ˌēn\ *n* : a compound containing the NH group or its substituted form NR that is derived from ammonia by replacement of two hydrogen atoms by a hydrocarbon group or other nonacid organic group

---

\ə\ **abut** \ᵊ\ kitten \ər\ **further** \a\ **ash** \ā\ **ace** \ä\ **cot, cart**
\au̇\ **out** \ch\ **chin** \e\ bet \ē\ **easy** \g\ go \i\ **hit** \ī\ **ice** \j\ **job**
\ŋ\ **sing** \ō\ **go** \ȯ\ **law** \ȯi\ **boy** \th\ **thin** \t͟h\ **the** \ü\ **loot**
\u̇\ **foot** \y\ **yet** \zh\ **vision** *See also* Pronunciation Symbols page

I
J

im·i·no \'im-ə-ˌnō\ *adj* : relating to or containing the NH group or its substituted form NR united to a group other than an acid group

imino acid *n* : an acid that contains an imino group

im·i·no·di·ace·tic acid \ˌim-ə-ˌnō-ˌdī-ə-ˌsēt-ik-\ *n* : an imino acid $C_4H_7NO_4$ that is the source of several derivatives used to visualize the hepatobiliary tract after labeling with a radioisotope of technetium

im·i·no·gly·cin·uria \-ˌglī-sə-'nur-ē-ə\ *n* : an abnormal inherited condition of the kidney associated esp. with hyperprolinemia and characterized by the presence of proline, hydroxyproline, and glycine in the urine

im·i·pen·em \ˌim-ə-'pen-əm\ *n* : a semisynthetic beta-lactam $C_{12}H_{17}N_3O_4S \cdot H_2O$ that is derived from an antibiotic produced by a bacterium of the genus *Streptomyces* (*S. cattleya*) and is effective against gram-negative and gram-positive bacteria

imip·ra·mine \im-'ip-rə-ˌmēn\ *n* : a tricyclic antidepressant drug administered esp. in the form of its hydrochloride $C_{19}H_{24}N_2 \cdot HCl$ or pamoate $(C_{19}H_{24}N_2)_2 \cdot C_{23}H_{16}O_6$ — see TOFRANIL

Im·i·trex \'im-ə-ˌtreks\ *trademark* — used for a preparation of the succinate of sumatriptan

im·ma·ture \ˌim-ə-'t(y)ù(ə)r *also* -'chù(ə)r\ *adj* : lacking complete growth, differentiation, or development ⟨~ blood cells⟩ ⟨emotionally ~⟩ — **im·ma·ture·ly** *adv* — **im·ma·tu·ri·ty** \-'t(y)ùr-ət-ē *also* -'chùr-\ *n, pl* -ties

im·me·di·ate \im-'ēd-ē-ət, *Brit often* -'ē-jit\ *adj* **1 a** : acting or being without the intervention of another object, cause, or agency : being direct ⟨the ~ cause of death⟩ **b** : present to the mind independently of other states or factors ⟨~ awareness⟩ **2** : made or done at once — **im·me·di·ate·ly** *adv*

immediate auscultation *n* : auscultation performed without a stethoscope by laying the ear directly against the patient's body — compare MEDIATE AUSCULTATION

immediate denture *n* : a denture put in place immediately after the extraction of teeth

immediate hypersensitivity *n, pl* -ties : hypersensitivity in which exposure to an antigen produces an immediate or almost immediate reaction

im·med·i·ca·ble \(')im-'(m)ed-i-kə-bəl\ *adj* : INCURABLE ⟨wounds ~ —John Milton⟩

im·mer·sion foot \i-'mər-zhən-, -shən\ *n* : a painful condition of the feet marked by inflammation and stabbing pain and followed by discoloration, swelling, ulcers, and numbness due to prolonged exposure to moist cold usu. without actual freezing

immersion lens *n* : OIL-IMMERSION LENS

immersion objective *n* : OIL-IMMERSION LENS

immersion oil *n* : oil that is used with an oil-immersion lens

im·mis·ci·ble \(')im-'(m)is-ə-bəl\ *adj* : incapable of mixing or attaining homogeneity — used esp. of liquids ⟨~ solvents⟩ — **im·mis·ci·bil·i·ty** \(ˌ)im-ˌ(m)is-ə-'bil-ət-ē\ *n, pl* -ties

im·mo·bile \(')im-'(m)ō-bəl, -ˌbēl, -ˌbīl\ *adj* **1** : incapable of being moved **2** : not moving ⟨keep the patient ~⟩ — **im·mo·bil·i·ty** \ˌim-(ˌ)ō-'bil-ət-ē\ *n, pl* -ties

im·mo·bi·li·za·tion *also Brit* **im·mo·bi·li·sa·tion** \im-ˌō-bə-lə-'zā-shən\ *n* : the act of immobilizing or state of being immobilized: as **a** : quiet rest in bed for a prolonged period used in the treatment of disease (as tuberculosis) **b** : fixation (as by a plaster cast) of a body part usu. to promote healing in normal structural relation

im·mo·bi·lize *also Brit* **im·mo·bi·lise** \im-'ō-bə-ˌlīz\ *vt* -ized *also Brit* -ised; -iz·ing *also Brit* -is·ing : to make immobile; *esp* : to fix (as a body part) so as to reduce or eliminate motion usu. by means of a cast or splint, by strapping, or by strict bed rest ⟨*immobilizing* a fractured bone by a cast and continuous traction⟩ ⟨~ an injury⟩ ⟨~ all patients with a suspected neck or spine injury⟩

¹im·mune \im-'yün\ *adj* **1** : not susceptible or responsive; *esp* : having a high degree of resistance to a disease ⟨~ to diphtheria⟩ **2 a** : having or producing antibodies or lymphocytes capable of reacting with a specific antigen ⟨an ~ se-

rum⟩ **b** : produced by, involved in, or concerned with immunity or an immune response ⟨~ agglutinins⟩

²immune *n* : an immune individual

immune complex *n* : any of various molecular complexes formed in the blood by combination of an antigen and an antibody that tend to accumulate in bodily tissue and are associated with various pathological conditions (as glomerulonephritis, vasculitis, and systemic lupus erythematosus)

immune globulin *n* : globulin from the blood of a person or animal immune to a particular disease — called also *immune serum globulin*

immune response *n* : a bodily response to an antigen that occurs when lymphocytes identify the antigenic molecule as foreign and induce the formation of antibodies and lymphocytes capable of reacting with it and rendering it harmless — called also *immune reaction*

immune serum *n* : ANTISERUM

immune system *n* : the bodily system that protects the body from foreign substances, cells, and tissues by producing the immune response and that includes esp. the thymus, spleen, lymph nodes, special deposits of lymphoid tissue (as in the gastrointestinal tract and bone marrow), lymphocytes including the B cells and T cells, and antibodies

immune therapy *n* : IMMUNOTHERAPY

im·mu·ni·ty \im-'yü-nət-ē\ *n, pl* -ties : the quality or state of being immune; *esp* : a condition of being able to resist a particular disease esp. through preventing development of a pathogenic microorganism or by counteracting the effects of its products — see ACQUIRED IMMUNITY, ACTIVE IMMUNITY, NATURAL IMMUNITY, PASSIVE IMMUNITY

im·mu·ni·za·tion *also Brit* **im·mu·ni·sa·tion** \ˌim-yə-nə-'zā-shən\ *n* : the creation of immunity usu. against a particular disease; *esp* : treatment (as by vaccination) of an organism for the purpose of making it immune to a particular pathogen ⟨~ against polio⟩

im·mu·nize *also Brit* **im·mu·nise** \'im-yə-ˌnīz\ *vt* -nized *also Brit* -nised; -niz·ing *also Brit* -nis·ing : to make immune

im·mu·no·ab·sor·bent *or* **im·mu·no·ab·sor·bant** \ˌim-yə-nō-əb-'sòr-bənt, im-ˌyü-nō-, -əb-'zòr-bənt\ *n* : IMMUNOSORBENT

im·mu·no·ab·sorp·tion \-əb-'sòrp-shən, -'zòrp-\ *n* : IMMUNOADSORPTION — **im·mu·no·ab·sorb** \-əb-'sò(ə)rb, -'zò(ə)rb\ *vt*

im·mu·no·ad·ju·vant \-'aj-ə-vənt\ *n* : a nonspecific substance acting to enhance the immune response to an antigen with which it is administered

im·mu·no·ad·sor·bent \-ad-'sòr-bənt, -'zòr-\ *n* : IMMUNOSORBENT — **immunoadsorbent** *adj*

im·mu·no·ad·sorp·tion \-ad-'sòrp-shən, -'zòrp-\ *n* : the process of using an immunosorbent to purify a substance

im·mu·no·as·say \ˌim-yə-nō-'as-ˌā, im-ˌyü-nō-, -a-'sā\ *n* : a technique or test (as the enzyme-linked immunosorbent assay) used to detect the presence or quantity of a substance (as a protein) based on its capacity to act as an antigen or antibody — **immunoassay** *vt* — **im·mu·no·as·say·able** \-a-'sā-ə-bəl\ *adj*

im·mu·no·bi·ol·o·gist \-bī-'äl-ə-jəst\ *n* : a specialist in immunobiology

im·mu·no·bi·ol·o·gy \-bī-'äl-ə-jē\ *n, pl* -gies : a branch of biology concerned with the physiological reactions characteristic of the immune state — **im·mu·no·bi·o·log·i·cal** \-ˌbī-ə-'läj-i-kəl\ *or* **im·mu·no·bi·o·log·ic** \-'läj-ik\ *adj*

im·mu·no·blast \i-'myü-nə-ˌblast, 'im-yə-nə-\ *n* : a cell formed by transformation of a T cell after antigenic stimulation and giving rise to a population of T cells with specificity against the stimulating antigen

im·mu·no·blas·tic lymphadenopathy \ˌim-yə-nō-ˌblas-tik-, im-ˌyü-nō-\ *n* : a disease characterized by fever, weight loss, sweating spells, rash, itching, proliferation of small blood vessels and of immunoblasts, generalized lymphadenopathy, and enlargement of the liver and spleen

im·mu·no·blot \i-'myü-nə-ˌblät, 'im-yə-nə-, 'im-yə-nō-\ *n* : a blot (as a Western blot) in which a radioactively labeled antibody is used as the molecular probe — **im·mu·no·blot·ting** *n*

¹**im·mu·no·chem·i·cal** \-'kem-i-kəl\ *adj* : of, relating to, or utilizing immunochemistry ⟨∼ studies of blood groups⟩ — **im·mu·no·chem·i·cal·ly** \-i-k(ə-)lē\ *adv*

²**immunochemical** *n* : an immunochemical agent (as an antiserum)

im·mu·no·chem·ist \-'kem-əst\ *n* : a specialist in immunochemistry

im·mu·no·chem·is·try \-'kem-ə-strē\ *n, pl* **-tries** : a branch of chemistry that deals with the chemical aspects of immunology

im·mu·no·che·mo·ther·a·py \-ˌkē-mō-'ther-ə-pē\ *n, pl* **-pies** : the combined use of immunotherapy and chemotherapy in the treatment or control of disease

im·mu·no·com·pe·tence \-'käm-pət-ən(t)s\ *n* : the capacity for a normal immune response ⟨altered the ∼ of the lymphocytes⟩ — **im·mu·no·com·pe·tent** \-ənt\ *adj*

im·mu·no·com·pro·mised \-'käm-prə-ˌmīzd\ *adj* : having the immune system impaired or weakened (as by drugs or illness) ⟨∼ patients⟩

im·mu·no·con·glu·ti·nin \-kən-'glüt-ᵊn-in\ *n* : an autoantibody formed by an organism against its own complement

im·mu·no·con·ju·gate \-'kän-ji-gət, -jə-ˌgāt\ *n* : a complex of an antibody and a toxic agent (as a drug) used to kill or destroy a targeted antigen (as a cancer cell)

im·mu·no·cyte \i-'myü-nə-ˌsīt, 'im-yə-nə-\ *n* : a cell (as a lymphocyte) that has an immunologic function

im·mu·no·cy·to·chem·is·try \ˌim-yə-nə-ˌsīt-ō-'kem-ə-strē, im-ˌyü-nō-\ *n, pl* **-tries** : the application of biochemistry to cellular immunology — **im·mu·no·cy·to·chem·i·cal** \-'kem-i-kəl\ *adj*

im·mu·no·de·fi·cien·cy \-di-'fish-ən-sē\ *n, pl* **-cies** : inability to produce a normal complement of antibodies or immunologically sensitized T cells esp. in response to specific antigens — see AIDS — **im·mu·no·de·fi·cient** \-ənt\ *adj*

im·mu·no·de·pres·sion \-di-'presh-ən\ *n* : IMMUNOSUPPRESSION — **im·mu·no·de·pres·sant** \-di-'pres-ᵊnt\ *n* — **im·mu·no·de·pres·sive** \-di-'pres-iv\ *adj*

im·mu·no·di·ag·no·sis \-ˌdī-ig-'nō-səs, -ˌdī-əg-\ *n, pl* **-no·ses** \-ˌsēz\ : diagnosis (as of cancer) by immunodiagnostic methods

im·mu·no·di·ag·nos·tic \-'näs-tik\ *adj* : of, relating to, or being analytical methods using antibodies as reagents ⟨an ∼ test for cancer⟩

im·mu·no·dif·fu·sion \-dif-'yü-zhən\ *n* : any of several techniques for obtaining a precipitate between an antibody and its specific antigen by suspending one in a gel and letting the other migrate through it from a well or by letting both antibody and antigen migrate through the gel from separate wells to form an area of precipitation

im·mu·no·elec·tro·pho·re·sis \ˌim-yə-nō-ə-ˌlek-trə-fə-'rē-səs, im-ˌyü-nō-\ *n, pl* **-re·ses** \-ˌsēz\ : electrophoretic separation of proteins followed by identification by the formation of precipitates through specific immunologic reactions — **im·mu·no·elec·tro·pho·ret·ic** \-'ret-ik\ *adj* — **im·mu·no·elec·tro·pho·ret·i·cal·ly** \-i-k(ə-)lē\ *adv*

im·mu·no·fer·ri·tin \-'fer-ət-ən\ *n* : an antibody labeled with ferritin

im·mu·no·flu·o·res·cence \-(ˌ)flù(-ə)r-'es-ᵊn(t)s, -flōr-, -flòr-\ *n* : the labeling of antibodies or antigens with fluorescent dyes esp. for the purpose of demonstrating the presence of a particular antigen or antibody in a tissue preparation or smear — **im·mu·no·flu·o·res·cent** \-ᵊnt\ *adj*

im·mu·no·gen \i-'myü-nə-jən, 'im-yə-nə-, -ˌjen\ *n* : an antigen that provokes an immune response (as antibody production)

im·mu·no·gen·e·sis \ˌim-yə-nō-'jen-ə-səs, im-ˌyü-nō-\ *n, pl* **-e·ses** \-ˌsēz\ : immunity production

im·mu·no·ge·net·i·cist \-jə-'net-ə-səst\ *n* : a specialist in immunogenetics

im·mu·no·ge·net·ics \-jə-'net-iks\ *n pl but sing in constr* : a branch of immunology concerned with the interrelations of heredity, disease, and the immune system esp. with regard to

the way in which the genetic information required to produce the diversity of antibodies required by the immune system is stored in the genome, transmitted from one generation to the next, and expressed in the organism — **im·mu·no·ge·net·ic** \-ik\ *adj* — **im·mu·no·ge·net·i·cal·ly** \-i-k(ə-)lē\ *adv*

im·mu·no·gen·ic \ˌim-yə-nō-'jen-ik, im-ˌyü-nō-\ *adj* : relating to or producing an immune response ⟨∼ substances⟩ — **im·mu·no·gen·i·cal·ly** \-i-k(ə-)lē\ *adv*

im·mu·no·ge·nic·i·ty \-jə-'nis-ət-ē\ *n, pl* **-ties** : the quality or state of being immunogenic

im·mu·no·glob·u·lin \-'gläb-yə-lən\ *n* : ANTIBODY — abbr. *Ig*

immunoglobulin A *n* : IGA

immunoglobulin D *n* : IGD

immunoglobulin E *n* : IGE

immunoglobulin G *n* : IGG

immunoglobulin M *n* : IGM

im·mu·no·glob·u·lin·op·a·thy \-ˌgläb-yə-lə-'näp-ə-thē\ *n, pl* **-thies** : GAMMOPATHY

im·mu·no·he·ma·tol·o·gist *or chiefly Brit* **im·mu·no·hae·ma·tol·o·gist** \-ˌhē-mə-'täl-ə-jəst\ *n* : a specialist in immunohematology

im·mu·no·he·ma·tol·o·gy *or chiefly Brit* **im·mu·no·hae·ma·tol·o·gy** \-ˌhē-mə-'täl-ə-jē\ *n, pl* **-gies** : a branch of immunology that deals with the immunologic properties of blood — **im·mu·no·he·ma·to·log·i·cal** \-ˌhē-mət-ᵊl-'äj-ik\ *or* **im·mu·no·he·ma·to·log·ic** \-i-kəl\ *or chiefly Brit* **im·mu·no·hae·ma·to·log·ic** *or* **im·mu·no·hae·ma·to·log·i·cal** *adj*

im·mu·no·he·mo·ly·sis *or chiefly Brit* **im·mu·no·hae·mo·ly·sis** \-hi-'mäl-ə-səs, -ˌhē-mə-'lī-səs\ *n, pl* **-ly·ses** \-ˌsēz\ : hemolysis caused by an abnormal immune response to an antigen

im·mu·no·he·mo·lyt·ic anemia *or chiefly Brit* **im·mu·no·hae·mo·lyt·ic anaemia** \-ˌhē-mə-'lit-ik-\ *n* : hemolytic anemia resulting from immunohemolysis

im·mu·no·his·to·chem·i·cal \-ˌhis-tō-'kem-i-kəl\ *adj* : of or relating to the application of histochemical and immunologic methods to chemical analysis of living cells and tissues — **im·mu·no·his·to·chem·i·cal·ly** \-i-k(ə-)lē\ *adv* — **im·mu·no·his·to·chem·is·try** \-'kem-ə-strē\ *n, pl* **-tries**

im·mu·no·his·tol·o·gy \-his-'täl-ə-jē\ *n, pl* **-gies** : a branch of immunology that deals with the application of immunologic methods to histology — **im·mu·no·his·to·log·i·cal** \-ˌhis-tə-'läj-i-kəl\ *also* **im·mu·no·his·to·log·ic** \-'läj-ik\ *adj* — **im·mu·no·his·to·log·i·cal·ly** \-i-k(ə-)lē\ *adv*

im·mu·no·in·com·pe·tence \-in-'käm-pət-ən(t)s\ *n* : inability of the immune system to function properly — **im·mu·no·in·com·pe·tent** \-pət-ənt\ *adj*

im·mu·no·log·i·cal memory \ˌim-yən-ᵊl-'äj-i-kəl-\ *also* **im·mu·no·log·ic memory** \-'äj-ik-\ *n* : the capacity of the body's immune system to remember an encounter with an antigen due to the activation of B cells or T cells having specificity for the antigen and to react more swiftly to the antigen by means of these activated cells in a later encounter

immunological surveillance *n* : IMMUNOSURVEILLANCE

im·mu·nol·o·gist \ˌim-yə-'näl-ə-jəst\ *n* : a specialist in immunology

im·mu·nol·o·gy \ˌim-yə-'näl-ə-jē\ *n, pl* **-gies** : a science that deals with the immune system and the cell-mediated and humoral aspects of immunity and immune responses — **im·mu·no·log·ic** \-yən-ᵊl-'äj-ik\ *or* **im·mu·no·log·i·cal** \-'äj-i-kəl\ *adj* — **im·mu·no·log·i·cal·ly** \-i-k(ə-)lē\ *adv*

im·mu·no·mod·u·lat·ing \ˌim-yə-nō-'mäj-ə-ˌlāt-iŋ, im-ˌyü-nō-\ *adj* : of, relating to, or being an immunomodulator or its effects or activity ⟨∼ effects⟩ ⟨an ∼ agent⟩ ⟨∼ properties⟩ — **im·mu·no·mod·u·late** \-ˌlāt\ *vt* **-lat·ed; -lat·ing**

im·mu·no·mod·u·la·tion \-ˌmäj-ə-'lā-shən\ *n* : modification of the immune response or the functioning of the immune system by the action of an immunomodulator

---

\ə\ **abut** \ᵊ\ **kitten** \ər\ **further** \a\ **ash** \ā\ **ace** \ä\ **cot, cart** \aú\ **out** \ch\ **chin** \e\ **bet** \ē\ **easy** \g\ **go** \i\ **hit** \ī\ **ice** \j\ **job** \ŋ\ **sing** \ō\ **go** \ò\ **law** \òi\ **boy** \th\ **thin** \th̲\ **the** \ü\ **loot** \ù\ **foot** \y\ **yet** \zh\ **vision** *See also* Pronunciation Symbols page

I
J

im·mu·no·mod·u·la·tor \-'mäj-ə-ˌlāt-ər\ *n* : a chemical agent (as methotrexate or azathioprine) that modifies the immune response or the functioning of the immune system (as by the stimulation of antibody formation or the inhibition of white blood cell activity) — **im·mu·no·mod·u·la·to·ry** *adj*

im·mu·no·par·a·si·tol·o·gist \-ˌpar-ə-sə-'täl-ə-jəst, -ˌsīt-'äl-\ *n* : a specialist in immunoparasitology

im·mu·no·par·a·si·tol·o·gy \-ˌpar-ə-sə-'täl-ə-jē, -ˌsīt-'äl-\ *n, pl* **-gies** : a branch of immunology that deals with animal parasites and their hosts

im·mu·no·patho·gen·e·sis \-ˌpath-ə-'jen-ə-səs\ *n, pl* **-e·ses** \-ˌsēz\ : the development of disease as affected by the immune system — **im·mu·no·path·o·gen·ic** \-'jen-ik\ *adj*

im·mu·no·pa·thol·o·gist \-pə-'thäl-ə-jəst, -pa-\ *n* : a specialist in immunopathology

im·mu·no·pa·thol·o·gy \-pə-'thäl-ə-jē, -pa-\ *n, pl* **-gies** **1** : a branch of medicine that deals with immune responses associated with disease **2** : the pathology of an organism, organ system, or disease with respect to the immune system, immunity, and immune responses — **im·mu·no·path·o·log·ic** \-ˌpath-ə-'läj-ik\ *or* **im·mu·no·path·o·log·i·cal** \-i-kəl\ *adj*

im·mu·no·phar·ma·col·o·gist \-ˌfär-mə-'käl-ə-jəst\ *n* : a pharmacologist who specializes in immunopharmacology

im·mu·no·phar·ma·col·o·gy \-ə-jē\ *n, pl* **-gies** **1** : a branch of pharmacology concerned with the application of immunological techniques and theory to the study of the effects of drugs esp. on the immune system **2** : the immunological effects and significance of a particular drug (as morphine)

im·mu·no·phe·no·type \-'fē-nə-ˌtīp\ *n* : the immunochemical and immunohistological characteristics of a cell or group of cells ⟨the atypical cells . . . have the ~ of activated T cells —T. H. Davis *et al*⟩ — **im·mu·no·phe·no·typ·ic** \-ˌfē-nə-'tip-ik\ *also* **im·mu·no·phe·no·typ·i·cal** \-i-kəl\ *adj* — **im·mu·no·phe·no·typ·i·cal·ly** \-i-k(ə)lē\ *adv*

im·mu·no·phe·no·typ·ing \-'fē-nə-ˌtī-piŋ\ *n* : the process of determining the immunophenotype of a cell or group of cells

im·mu·no·phil·in \-'fil-ən\ *n* : any of a group of proteins that exhibit high specificity in binding to immunosuppressive agents (as cyclosporine)

im·mu·no·po·tent \-'pōt-ᵊnt\ *adj* : stimulating the formation of antibodies esp. in large numbers

im·mu·no·po·ten·ti·a·tion \-pə-ˌten-chē-'ā-shən\ *n* : enhancement of immune responses — **im·mu·no·po·ten·ti·at·ing** \-pə-'ten-chē-ˌāt-iŋ\ *adj* — **im·mu·no·po·ten·ti·a·tor** \-ˌāt-ər\ *n*

im·mu·no·pre·cip·i·ta·tion \-pri-ˌsip-ə-'tā-shən\ *n* : precipitation of a complex of an antibody and its specific antigen — **im·mu·no·pre·cip·i·ta·ble** \-'sip-ət-ə-bəl\ *adj* — **im·mu·no·pre·cip·i·tate** \-'sip-ət-ət, -ə-ˌtāt\ *n* — **im·mu·no·pre·cip·i·tate** \-ə-ˌtāt\ *vt* **-tat·ed; -tat·ing**

im·mu·no·pro·lif·er·a·tive \-prə-'lif-ə-ˌrāt-iv, -prə-'lif-(ə-)rət-iv\ *adj* : of, relating to, or characterized by the production of abnormally increased numbers of antibody-producing cells ⟨~ disorders⟩

im·mu·no·pro·phy·lax·is \-ˌprō-fə-'lak-səs *also* -ˌpräf-ə-\ *n, pl* **-lax·es** \-ˌsēz\ : the prevention of disease by the production of active or passive immunity — **im·mu·no·pro·phy·lac·tic** \-'lak-tik\ *adj*

im·mu·no·ra·dio·met·ric assay \-ˌrād-ē-ō-'me-trik-\ *n* : immunoassay of a substance by combining it with a radiolabeled antibody

im·mu·no·re·ac·tion \-rē-'ak-shən\ *n* : an immunologic reaction between an antigen and an antibody or a T cell sensitized for cell-mediated immunity

im·mu·no·re·ac·tive \-rē-'ak-tiv\ *adj* : reacting to particular antigens or haptens ⟨serum ~ insulin⟩ ⟨~ lymphocytes⟩ — **im·mu·no·re·ac·tiv·i·ty** \-(ˌ)rē-ˌak-'tiv-ət-ē\ *n, pl* **-ties**

im·mu·no·reg·u·la·to·ry \-'reg-yə-lə-ˌtōr-ē, -ˌtȯr-\ *adj* : of or relating to the regulation of the immune system ⟨~ T cells⟩ — **im·mu·no·reg·u·la·tion** \-ˌreg-yə-'lā-shən, -ˌreg-ə-'lā-\ *n*

im·mu·no·se·lec·tion \-sə-'lek-shən\ *n* : selection of cell lines on the basis of their resistance to attack by antibodies and T cells sensitized for cell-mediated immunity ⟨~ of cell variants⟩

¹**im·mu·no·sor·bent** \-'sȯr-bənt, -'zȯr-\ *n* : an immunosorbent preparation

²**immunosorbent** *adj* : relating to or using a substrate consisting of a specific antibody or antigen chemically combined with an insoluble substance (as cellulose) to selectively remove the corresponding specific antigen or antibody from solution

im·mu·no·stain·ing \-ˌstā-niŋ\ *n* : the staining of a specific substance by using an antibody against it which is complexed with a staining medium (as horseradish peroxidase) — **im·mu·no·stain** \-ˌstān\ *vt*

im·mu·no·stim·u·lant \-'stim-yə-lənt\ *n* : an agent that stimulates an immune response — **immunostimulant** *adj*

im·mu·no·stim·u·la·tion \-ˌstim-yə-'lā-shən\ *n* : stimulation of an immune response — **im·mu·no·stim·u·lat·ing** \-'stim-yə-ˌlāt-iŋ\ *adj*

im·mu·no·stim·u·la·to·ry \-'stim-yə-lə-ˌtōr-ē, -ˌtȯr-\ *adj* : of, relating to, or having the capacity to stimulate an immune response ⟨the potent ~ cytokine interleukin-2⟩ ⟨~ effects⟩

im·mu·no·sup·press \-sə-'pres\ *vt* : to suppress the natural immune responses of ⟨a chronically ~ed patient⟩

¹**im·mu·no·sup·pres·sant** \-sə-'pres-ᵊnt\ *n* : a chemical agent (as a drug) that suppresses the immune response

²**immunosuppressant** *adj* : IMMUNOSUPPRESSIVE ⟨~ effects⟩

im·mu·no·sup·pres·sion \-sə-'presh-ən\ *n* : suppression (as by drugs) of natural immune responses

¹**im·mu·no·sup·pres·sive** \ˌim-yə-nō-sə-'pres-iv, im-ˌyü-nō-\ *adj* : causing or characterized by immunosuppression ⟨~ drugs⟩

²**immunosuppressive** *n* : IMMUNOSUPPRESSANT

im·mu·no·sup·pres·sor \-sə-'pres-ər\ *n* : IMMUNOSUPPRESSANT

im·mu·no·sur·veil·lance \-sər-'vā-lən(t)s *also* -'vāl-yən(t)s *or* -'vā-ən(t)s\ *n* : a monitoring process of the immune system which detects and destroys neoplastic cells and which tends to break down in immunosuppressed individuals — called also *immunological surveillance*

im·mu·no·sym·pa·thec·to·my \-ˌsim-pə-'thek-tə-mē\ *n, pl* **-mies** : the destruction of neurons of the sympathetic nervous system in newborn laboratory animals (as mice or rats) by the injection of antiserum to nerve growth factor — **im·mu·no·sym·pa·thec·to·mized** *or chiefly Brit* **im·mu·no·sym·pa·thec·to·mised** \-ˌmīzd\ *adj*

im·mu·no·ther·a·pist \-'ther-ə-pəst\ *n* : a specialist in immunotherapy

im·mu·no·ther·a·py \-'ther-ə-pē\ *n, pl* **-pies** : treatment of or prophylaxis against disease by attempting to produce active or passive immunity — called also *immune therapy* — **im·mu·no·ther·a·peu·tic** \-ˌther-ə-'pyüt-ik\ *adj*

im·mu·no·tox·ic·i·ty \-ˌtäk-'sis-ət-ē\ *n, pl* **-ties** : toxicity to the immune system — **im·mu·no·tox·ic** \-'täk-sik\ *adj*

im·mu·no·tox·i·col·o·gy \-ˌtäk-si-'käl-ə-jē\ *n, pl* **-gies** : the study of the effects of toxic substances on the immune system — **im·mu·no·tox·i·co·log·i·cal** \-kə-'läj-i-kəl\ *adj* — **im·mu·no·tox·i·col·o·gist** \-'käl-ə-jəst\ *n*

im·mu·no·tox·in \'im-yə-nō-ˌtäk-sən, im-'yü-nō-\ *n* : a toxin that is linked to a monoclonal antibody and that is delivered to only those cells (as cancer cells) bearing the antigen targeted by the monoclonal antibody to which it is linked

Imo·di·um \i-'mō-dē-əm\ *trademark* — used for a preparation of the hydrochloride of loperamide

IMP \ˌī-ˌem-'pē\ *n* : INOSINIC ACID

im·pact·ed \im-'pak-təd\ *adj* **1 a** : blocked by material (as feces) that is firmly packed or wedged in position ⟨an ~ colon⟩ **b** : wedged or lodged in a bodily passage ⟨an ~ mass of feces⟩ ⟨an ~ fetus in the birth canal⟩ **2** : characterized by broken ends of bone driven together ⟨an ~ fracture⟩ **3** *of a tooth* : wedged between the jawbone and another tooth ⟨an ~ wisdom tooth⟩

im·pac·tion \im-'pak-shən\ *n* : the act of becoming or the state of being impacted; *specif* : lodgment or an instance of lodgment of something (as a tooth or feces) in a body passage or cavity

impaction fracture *n* : a fracture that is impacted

im·pair \im-'pa(ə)r, -'pe(ə)r\ *vt* : to damage or make worse by or as if by diminishing in some material respect ⟨his health was ∼ed by overwork⟩ — **im·pair·ment** \-'pa(ə)r-mənt\ *n*

impaired *adj* : being in a less than perfect or whole condition: as **a** : disabled or functionally defective — often used in combination ⟨hearing-*impaired*⟩ **b** : intoxicated by alcohol or narcotics ⟨driving while ∼⟩

impaired glucose tolerance *n* : a condition in which an individual has higher than normal levels of glucose in the blood upon fasting or following a carbohydrate-rich meal or ingestion of a glucose test solution but not high enough to be diagnostic of diabetes mellitus

im·pal·pa·ble \(')im-'pal-pə-bəl\ *adj* **1** : incapable of being felt by touch ⟨the pulse was ∼ at the wrist⟩ ⟨preoperative localization of ∼ breast lesions —Jane Barrett⟩ **2** : so finely divided that no grains or grit can be felt ⟨an ∼ powder⟩

im·par \'im-ˌpär\ *adj* : being an unpaired or azygous anatomical part — see TUBERCULUM IMPAR

im·ped·ance \im-'pēd-ᵊn(t)s\ *n* **1** : the apparent opposition in an electrical circuit to the flow of an alternating current that is analogous to the actual electrical resistance to a direct current and that is the ratio of effective electromotive force to the effective current **2** : the ratio of the pressure to the volume displacement at a given surface in a sound-transmitting medium **3** : opposition to blood flow in the circulatory system

im·ped·i·ment \im-'ped-ə-mənt\ *n* : something that impedes ⟨children with deafness or hearing ∼s⟩; *esp* : an impairment (as a stutter or a lisp) that interferes with the proper articulation of speech

im·per·a·tive \im-'per-ət-iv\ *adj* : eliciting a motor response ⟨an ∼ stimulus⟩

im·per·cep·tion \ˌim-pər-'sep-shən\ *n* : selective unawareness of something (as a bodily condition or behavior of others)

imperfecta — see AMELOGENESIS IMPERFECTA, DENTINOGENESIS IMPERFECTA, OSTEOGENESIS IMPERFECTA, OSTEOGENESIS IMPERFECTA CONGENITA, OSTEOGENESIS IMPERFECTA TARDA

im·per·fect fungus \(')im-ˌpər-fikt-\ *n* : any of a large and heterogeneous group of fungi that lack a sexual stage or have an imperfectly known life cycle, that include many which are undoubtedly ascomycetes or more rarely basidiomycetes for which the perfect stage exists but has not been identified, and that are variously considered to comprise the division Deuteromycota, the subdivision Deuteromycotina, or the class Deuteromycetes — called also *deuteromycete*

Imperfecti — see FUNGI IMPERFECTI

im·per·fo·rate \(')im-'pər-f(ə-)rət, -fə-ˌrāt\ *adj* : having no opening or aperture; *specif* : lacking the usual or normal opening ⟨an ∼ hymen⟩ ⟨an ∼ anus⟩

im·pe·ri·al gallon \im-'pir-ē-əl-\ *n* : GALLON 2

im·per·me·able \(')im-'pər-mē-ə-bəl\ *adj* : not permitting passage (as of a fluid) through its substance ⟨the plasma membrane of a red blood cell is relatively ∼ to sodium and calcium ions⟩ — **im·per·me·abil·i·ty** \(ˌ)im-ˌpər-mē-ə-'bil-ət-ē\ *n, pl* -**ties**

im·per·vi·ous \(')im-'pər-vē-əs\ *adj* : not allowing entrance or passage ⟨medication packaged in a container ∼ to air and light⟩ — **im·per·vi·ous·ness** *n*

im·pe·tig·i·nized \ˌim-pə-'tij-ə-ˌnīzd\ *adj* : affected with impetigo on top of an underlying dermatologic condition ⟨∼ eczema⟩ — **im·pe·tig·i·ni·za·tion** \-ˌtij-ə-nə-'zā-shən\ *n*

im·pe·tig·i·nous \ˌim-pə-'tij-ə-nəs\ *adj* : of, relating to, or resembling impetigo ⟨∼ lesions⟩ — **im·pe·tig·i·nous·ly** *adv*

im·pe·ti·go \ˌim-pə-'tē-(ˌ)gō, -'tī-\ *n* : an acute contagious staphylococcal or streptococcal skin disease characterized by vesicles, pustules, and yellowish crusts

impetigo con·ta·gi·o·sa \-kən-ˌtā-jē-'ō-sə\ *n* : IMPETIGO

Im·plac·en·ta·lia \(')im-ˌplas-ᵊn-'tā-lē-ə\ *n pl, in former classifications* : the monotremes and marsupials regarded as a

systematic unit characterized by the absence or rudimentary development of a placenta

¹im·plant \im-'plant\ *vt* **1** : to set permanently in the consciousness or habit patterns **2 a** : to insert or fix in a living site (as for growth, slow release, or formation of an organic union) ⟨subcutaneously ∼ed hormone pellets⟩ **b** : to insert an implant in ⟨100 patients have been ∼ed with nylon ribbons without complications —U. K. Henschke⟩ ∼ *vi* : to undergo implantation : become implanted ⟨failure of embryos to ∼⟩

²im·plant \'im-ˌplant\ *n* : something (as a graft, a small container of radioactive material for treatment of cancer, or a pellet containing hormones to be gradually absorbed) that is implanted esp. in tissue

im·plant·able \im-'plant-ə-bəl\ *adj* : capable of being implanted in the living body ⟨an ∼ pacemaker for the heart⟩

im·plan·ta·tion \ˌim-ˌplan-'tā-shən\ *n* : the act or process of implanting or the state of being implanted: as **a** : the placement of a natural or artificial tooth in an artificially prepared socket in the jawbone **b** *in placental mammals* : the process of attachment of the embryo to the maternal uterine wall — called also *nidation* **c** : medical treatment by the insertion of an implant

im·plant·ee \ˌim-ˌplan-'tē\ *n* : the recipient of an implant

im·plan·tol·o·gist \ˌim-ˌplan-'täl-ə-jəst\ *n* : a dentist who specializes in implantology

im·plan·tol·o·gy \-'täl-ə-jē\ *n, pl* -**gies** : a branch of dentistry dealing with dental implantation

im·plo·sion therapy \im-'plō-zhən-\ *n* : IMPLOSIVE THERAPY

im·plo·sive therapy \im-'plō-siv-\ *n* : exposure therapy in which visualization is utilized by the patient

im·port·ed fire ant \im-ˌpórt-əd-'fī(ə)r-ˌant\ *n* : either of two mound-building So. American fire ants of the genus *Solenopsis* (*S. invicta* and *S. richteri*) that have been introduced into the southeastern U.S., are agricultural pests, and can inflict stings requiring medical attention

im·po·tence \'im-pət-ən(t)s\ *n* **1** : the quality or state of not being potent ⟨drug-resistant bacteria are a virulent indicator of the growing ∼ of antibiotics⟩ **2** : an abnormal physical or psychological state of a male characterized by inability to copulate because of failure to have or maintain an erection — called also *erectile dysfunction*

im·po·ten·cy \-ən-sē\ *n, pl* -**cies** : IMPOTENCE

im·po·tent \'im-pət-ənt\ *adj* **1** : not potent ⟨an ∼ vaccine⟩ **2** : unable to engage in sexual intercourse because of inability to have and maintain an erection; *broadly* : STERILE — usu. used of males

im·preg·nate \im-'preg-ˌnāt, 'im-ˌ\ *vt* -**nat·ed; -nat·ing 1 a** : to make pregnant **b** : to introduce sperm into : FERTILIZE **2** : to cause to be filled, imbued, permeated, or saturated ⟨gauze *impregnated* with white petrolatum⟩ — **im·preg·na·tion** \(ˌ)im-ˌpreg-'nā-shən\ *n*

im·preg·na·tor \im-'preg-ˌnāt-ər\ *n* : one that impregnates; *specif* : an instrument used for artificial insemination

im·pres·sion \im-'presh-ən\ *n* **1** : an imprint in plastic material of the surfaces of the teeth and adjacent portions of the jaw from which a likeness may be produced in dentistry **2** : an esp. marked influence or effect on the senses or the mind

im·print \im-'print, 'im-ˌ\ *vt* **1** : to fix indelibly or permanently (as on the memory) **2** : to subject to or induce by imprinting ⟨an ∼ed preference⟩ ⟨a gene ∼ed to be inactive when inherited from the mother⟩ ∼ *vi* : to undergo imprinting — **im·print·er** \-ər\ *n*

im·print·ing \'im-ˌprint-iŋ, im-'\ *n* **1** : a rapid learning process that takes place early in the life of a social animal (as a greylag goose) and establishes a behavior pattern (as recog-

I

J

\ə\ **abut** \ᵊ\ **kitten** \ər\ **further** \a\ **ash** \ā\ **ace** \ä\ **cot, cart**
\au̇\ **out** \ch\ **chin** \e\ **bet** \ē\ **easy** \g\ **go** \i\ **hit** \ī\ **ice** \j\ **job**
\ŋ\ **sing** \ō\ **go** \ȯ\ **law** \ȯi\ **boy** \th\ **thin** \t̲h̲\ **the** \ü\ **loot**
\u̇\ **foot** \y\ **yet** \zh\ **vision** *See also* Pronunciation Symbols page

nition of and attraction to its own kind or a substitute) **2** : GENOMIC IMPRINTING

im·pu·ber·al \(')im-'pyü-bər-əl\ *adj* : not having reached puberty

im·pu·bic \(')im-'pyü-bik\ *adj* : IMPUBERAL

im·pulse \'im-ˌpəls\ *n* **1** : a wave of excitation transmitted through tissues and esp. nerve fibers and muscles that results in physiological activity or inhibition **2 a** : a sudden spontaneous inclination or incitement to some usu. unpremeditated action ⟨some uncontrollable ∼ . . . may have driven the defendant to the commission of the murderous act —B. N. Cardozo⟩ **b** : a propensity or natural tendency usu. other than rational ⟨the fundamental ∼ of self-expression —Havelock Ellis⟩

im·pul·sion \im-'pəl-shən\ *n* **1** : IMPULSE 1 **2** : COMPULSION

im·pul·sive \im-'pəl-siv\ *adj* **1** : having the power of or actually driving or impelling **2** : actuated by or prone to act on impulse ⟨∼ behavior⟩ **3** : acting momentarily ⟨brief ∼ auditory stimuli⟩ — **im·pul·sive·ly** *adv* — **im·pul·sive·ness** *n* — **im·pul·siv·i·ty** \-ˌpəl-'siv-ət-ē\ *n, pl* **-ties**

im·pure \(')im-'pyü(ə)r\ *adj* : not pure: as **a** : containing something unclean ⟨∼ water⟩ **b** : mixed or impregnated with an extraneous and usu. unwanted substance : ADULTERATED ⟨an ∼ chemical⟩

im·pu·ri·ty \(')im-'pyür-ət-ē\ *n, pl* **-ties** : something that is impure or makes something else impure

Im·u·ran \'im-yə-ˌran\ *trademark* — used for a preparation of azathioprine

in *abbr* inch

In *symbol* indium

in·ac·ti·vate \(')in-'ak-tə-ˌvāt\ *vt* **-vat·ed; -vat·ing** : to make inactive: as **a** : to destroy certain biological activities of ⟨∼ the complement of normal serum by heat⟩ **b** : to cause (as an infective agent) to lose disease-producing capacity ⟨∼ bacteria⟩ — **in·ac·ti·va·tion** \(ˌ)in-ˌak-tə-'vā-shən\ *n* — **in·ac·ti·va·tor** \-ˌvāt-ər\ *n*

in·ac·tive \(')in-'ak-tiv\ *adj* : not active: as **a** : marked by deliberate or enforced absence of activity or effort ⟨forced by illness to lead an ∼ life⟩ **b** *of a disease* : not progressing or fulminating : QUIESCENT **c** (1) : chemically inert ⟨∼ charcoal⟩ (2) : not exhibiting optical activity in polarized light **d** : biologically inert esp. because of the loss of some quality (as infectivity or antigenicity) — **in·ac·tiv·i·ty** \(ˌ)in-ˌak-'tiv-ət-ē\ *n, pl* **-ties**

in·ad·e·qua·cy \(')in-'ad-i-kwə-sē\ *n, pl* **-cies** : the quality or state of being inadequate

¹**in·ad·e·quate** \-i-kwət\ *adj* **1** : not adequate : DEFICIENT ⟨an ∼ dose⟩ ⟨∼ perfusion⟩ ⟨∼ diets⟩ **2** : lacking the capacity for psychological maturity or adequate social adjustment ⟨an ∼ personality⟩ — **in·ad·e·quate·ly** *adv*

²**inadequate** *n* : one who is inadequate esp. in terms of social adjustment

in·ag·glu·ti·na·ble \(')in-ə-'glüt-ᵊn-ə-bəl\ *adj* : not subject to agglutination : not agglutinable — **in·ag·glu·ti·na·bil·i·ty** \(')in-ə-ˌglüt-ᵊn-ə-'bil-ət-ē\ *n, pl* **-ties**

in·an·i·mate \(')in-'an-ə-mət\ *adj* : not animate: **a** : not endowed with life or spirit **b** : lacking consciousness or power of motion

in·a·ni·tion \ˌin-ə-'nish-ən\ *n* : the exhausted condition that results from lack of food and water

in·ap·par·ent \(')in-ə-'par-ənt, -'per-ənt\ *adj* : not apparent; *specif* : not apparent clinically ⟨∼ infections⟩

in·ap·pe·tence \(')in-'ap-ət-ən(t)s\ *n* : loss or lack of appetite ⟨complained of ∼ and slight nausea —*Jour. Amer. Med. Assoc.*⟩

in·ap·pro·pri·ate \ˌin-ə-'prō-prē-ət\ *adj* : ABNORMAL ⟨∼ urinary sodium excretion —K. G. Barry & J. P. Malloy⟩

in ar·ti·cu·lo mor·tis \ˌin-ˌär-'tik-yə-ˌlō-'mȯrt-əs\ *adv or adj* : at the point of death ⟨a patient *in articulo mortis*⟩

in·at·tend \ˌin-ə-'tend\ *vt* : to fail to pay attention to ⟨selectively ∼*ed* the embarrassing aspects of the situation⟩ — **in·at·ten·tion** \-'ten-chən\ *n* — **in·at·ten·tive** \-'tent-iv\ *adj* — **in·at·ten·tive·ness** *n*

in·born \'in-'bȯ(ə)rn\ *adj* : HEREDITARY, INHERITED ⟨∼ errors of metabolism⟩

in·bred \'in-'bred\ *adj* : subjected to or produced by inbreeding

in·breed \'in-'brēd\ *vb* **in·bred** \-'bred\; **in·breed·ing** *vt* : to subject to inbreeding ∼ *vi* : to engage in inbreeding

in·breed·ing \'in-ˌbrēd-iŋ\ *n* : the interbreeding of closely related individuals esp. to preserve and fix desirable characters of and to eliminate unfavorable characters from a stock — compare LINEBREEDING, OUTBREEDING

inbreeding coefficient *n* : COEFFICIENT OF INBREEDING

In·ca bone \'iŋ-kə-\ *n* : the interparietal bone when developed as a separate bone in the skull (as frequently found in Peruvian mummies)

in·ca·pac·i·tant \ˌin-kə-'pas-ə-tənt\ *n* : a chemical or biological agent (as tear gas) used to temporarily incapacitate people or animals (as in war or a riot)

in·car·cer·at·ed \in-'kär-sə-ˌrāt-əd\ *adj, of a hernia* : constricted but not strangulated

in·car·cer·a·tion \in-ˌkär-sə-'rā-shən\ *n* **1** : a confining or state of being confined **2** : abnormal retention or confinement of a body part; *specif* : a constriction of the neck of a hernial sac so that the hernial contents become irreducible

incarnatus — see UNGUIS INCARNATUS

incerta — see ZONA INCERTA

in·cer·tae se·dis \in-'sər-tē-'sē-dəs\ *adv* : in an uncertain position : without assurance of relationship — used of taxa ⟨the enigmatic fossil arthropods were placed *incertae sedis* among the Myriopoda⟩

in·cest \'in-ˌsest\ *n* : sexual intercourse between persons so closely related that they are forbidden by law to marry; *also* : the statutory crime of engaging in such sexual intercourse

in·ces·tu·ous \in-'ses(h)-chə-wəs\ *adj* **1** : constituting or involving incest **2** : of, relating to, or guilty of incest ⟨infantile ∼ wishes of the Oedipus complex⟩

inch \'inch\ *n* : a unit of length equal to 1/36 yard or 2.54 centimeters

in·ci·dence \'in(t)-səd-ən(t)s, -sə-ˌden(t)s\ *n* **1 a** : ANGLE OF INCIDENCE **b** : the arrival of something (as a ray of light) at a surface **2 a** : an act or the fact or manner of occurring or affecting ⟨diseases of domestic ∼ —*Science*⟩ **b** : rate of occurrence or influence; *esp* : the rate of occurrence of new cases of a particular disease in a population being studied — compare PREVALENCE

in·ci·dent \'in(t)-səd-ənt, -sə-ˌdent\ *adj* : falling or striking on something ⟨∼ light rays⟩ ⟨∼ radiation⟩

in·cin·er·ate \in-'sin-ə-ˌrāt\ *vt* **-at·ed; -at·ing** : to cause to burn to ashes

in·cin·er·a·tion \-ˌsin-ə-'rā-shən\ *n* : the act of incinerating or state of being incinerated; *esp* : an analytical procedure of heating an organic substance with free access to air until only its ash remains

in·cip·i·ence \in-'sip-ē-ən(t)s\ *n* : INCIPIENCY

in·cip·i·en·cy \-ən-sē\ *n, pl* **-cies** : the state or fact of being incipient : the beginning of something

in·cip·i·ent \-ənt\ *adj* : beginning to come into being or to become apparent ⟨the ∼ stage of a fever⟩ — **in·cip·i·ent·ly** *adv*

in·ci·sal \in-'sī-zəl\ *adj* : relating to, being, or involving the cutting edge or surface of a tooth (as an incisor)

in·cise \in-'sīz, -'sīs\ *vt* **in·cised; in·cis·ing** : to cut into : make an incision in ⟨*incised* the swollen tissue⟩

incised *adj, of a cut or wound* : made with or as if with a sharp knife or scalpel : clean and well-defined

in·ci·si·form \in-'sīz-ə-ˌfȯrm, -'sīs-\ *adj* : having the form of or resembling a typical incisor tooth ⟨an ∼ canine⟩

in·ci·sion \in-'sizh-ən\ *n* **1** : a cut or wound of body tissue made esp. in surgery **2** : an act of incising something ⟨the surgeon's ∼ of the tissues⟩

in·ci·sion·al \-ən-əl\ *adj* : of, relating to, or resulting from an incision ⟨an ∼ hernia⟩

in·ci·sive \in-'sī-siv\ *adj* : INCISAL; *also* : of, relating to, or situated near the incisors

incisive bone *n* : PREMAXILLA

incisive canal *n* : a narrow branched passage that extends from the floor of the nasal cavity to the incisive fossa and transmits the nasopalatine nerve and a branch of the greater palatine artery

incisive foramen *n* : any of the openings of the incisive canal into the incisive fossa

incisive fossa *n* : a depression on the front of the maxillary bone above the incisor teeth

incisive papilla *n* : a small fold of mucous membrane situated at the anterior end of the raphe of the hard palate near the openings of the incisive canals

in·ci·sor \in-ˈsī-zər\ *n* : a front tooth adapted for cutting; *esp* : any of the eight cutting human teeth that are located between the canines with four in the lower and four in the upper jaw

in·ci·su·ra \ˌin-ˌsī-ˈzhür-ə, ˌin(t)-sə-\ *n, pl* **in·ci·su·rae** \-ē\ **1** : a notch, cleft, or fissure of a body part or organ **2** : a downward notch in the curve recording aortic blood pressure that occurs between systole and diastole and is caused by backflow of blood for a short time before the aortic valve closes — **in·ci·su·ral** \-əl\ *adj*

incisura an·gu·lar·is \-ˌaŋ-gyə-ˈlar-əs\ *n* : a notch or bend in the lesser curvature of the stomach near its pyloric end

in·ci·sure \in-ˈsī-zhər\ *n* : INCISURA 1

in·cit·ant \in-ˈsīt-ᵊnt\ *n* : an inciting agent; *esp* : a factor (as an infective agent) that is the essential causative agent of a particular disease

in·cite \in-ˈsīt\ *vt* **in·cit·ed; in·cit·ing** : to bring into being : induce to exist or occur ⟨organisms that readily *incited* antibody formation⟩

in·cli·na·tion \ˌin-klə-ˈnā-shən, ˌiŋ-\ *n* : a deviation from the true vertical or horizontal; *esp* : the deviation of the long axis of a tooth or of the slope of a cusp from the vertical

in·clu·sion \in-ˈklü-zhən\ *n* : something that is included; *esp* : a passive usu. temporary product of cell activity (as a starch grain) within the cytoplasm or nucleus

inclusion blennorrhea *n* : INCLUSION CONJUNCTIVITIS

inclusion body *n* : an inclusion, abnormal structure, or foreign cell within a cell; *specif* : an intracellular body that is characteristic of some virus diseases and that is the site of virus multiplication

inclusion conjunctivitis *n* : an infectious disease esp. of newborn infants characterized by acute conjunctivitis and the presence of large inclusion bodies and caused by a chlamydia (*C. trachomatis*)

inclusion disease *n* : CYTOMEGALIC INCLUSION DISEASE

in·co·ag·u·la·ble \ˌin-kō-ˈag-yə-lə-bəl\ *adj* : incapable of coagulating — **in·co·ag·u·la·bil·i·ty** \ˌin-kō-ˌag-yə-lə-ˈbil-ət-ē\ *n, pl* **-ties**

in·co·erc·ible \ˌin-kō-ˈər-sə-bəl\ *adj* : incapable of being controlled, checked, or confined ⟨∼ vomiting⟩

in·co·her·ence \ˌin-kō-ˈhir-ən(t)s, -ˈher-\ *n* : the quality or state of being incoherent

in·co·her·ent \-ənt\ *adj* : lacking clarity or intelligibility usu. by reason of some emotional stress ⟨∼ speech⟩ — **in·co·her·ent·ly** *adv*

in·com·pat·i·bil·i·ty \ˌin-kəm-ˌpat-ə-ˈbil-ət-ē\ *n, pl* **-ties** : the quality or state of being incompatible ⟨chemical ∼⟩

in·com·pat·i·ble \ˌin-kəm-ˈpat-ə-bəl\ *adj* **1** : unsuitable for use together because of chemical interaction or antagonistic physiological effects ⟨∼ drugs⟩ **2** *of blood or serum* : unsuitable for use in a particular transfusion because of the presence of agglutinins that act against the recipient's red blood cells

in·com·pen·sat·ed \ˌin-ˈkäm-pən-ˌsāt-əd\ *adj* : lacking physiological compensation

in·com·pen·sa·tion \ˌin-ˌkäm-pən-ˈsā-shən\ *n* : lack of physiological compensation ⟨cardiac ∼⟩ — **in·com·pen·sa·to·ry** \ˌin-kəm-ˈpen(t)-sə-ˌtōr-ē, -ˌtör-ē\ *adj*

in·com·pe·tence \(ˈ)in-ˈkäm-pət-ən(t)s\ *n* **1** : lack of legal qualification **2** : inability of an organ or part to perform its function adequately ⟨∼ of an aortic valve⟩

in·com·pe·ten·cy \-ən-sē\ *n, pl* **-cies** : INCOMPETENCE

in·com·pe·tent \(ˈ)in-ˈkäm-pət-ənt\ *adj* **1** : not legally qualified; *esp* : incapable due to a mental or physical condition **2** : unable to function properly ⟨∼ heart valves⟩ — **in·com·pe·tent·ly** *adv*

in·com·plete \ˌin-kəm-ˈplēt\ *adj* **1** *of insect metamorphosis* : having no pupal stage between the immature stages and the adult with the young insect usu. resembling the adult — compare COMPLETE 1 **2** *of a bone fracture* : not broken entirely across — compare COMPLETE 2 **3** : characterized by incomplete dominance ⟨an ∼ dominant⟩

incomplete antibody *n* : BLOCKING ANTIBODY

incomplete dominance *n* : the property of being expressed or inherited as a semidominant gene or trait

in·con·stant \ˈin-ˈkän(t)-stənt\ *adj* : not always present ⟨an ∼ muscle⟩

in·con·ti·nence \(ˈ)in-ˈkänt-ᵊn-ən(t)s\ *n* **1** : inability or failure to restrain sexual appetite **2** : inability of the body to control the evacuative functions ⟨fecal ∼⟩ — see STRESS INCONTINENCE, URGE INCONTINENCE

in·con·ti·nent \(ˈ)in-ˈkänt-ᵊn-ənt\ *adj* : not continent; *esp* : unable to retain a bodily discharge (as urine) voluntarily

in·co·or·di·nat·ed \ˌin-kō-ˈȯrd-ᵊn-ˌāt-əd\ *also* **in·co·or·di·nate** \ˌin-kō-ˈȯrd-nət, -ᵊn-ət, -ᵊn-ˌāt\ *adj* : not characterized by coordination ⟨∼ movements⟩

in·co·or·di·na·tion \-ˌȯrd-ᵊn-ˈā-shən\ *n* : lack of coordination esp. of muscular movements resulting from loss of voluntary control

in·cor·po·rate \in-ˈkȯr-pə-ˌrāt\ *vt* **-rat·ed; -rat·ing** : to subject to incorporation ⟨*incorporated* his psychiatrist in a system of delusions⟩ — **in·cor·po·ra·tive** \-ˈkȯr-pə-ˌrāt-iv, -p(ə-)rət-\ *adj*

in·cor·po·ra·tion \in-ˌkȯr-pə-ˈrā-shən\ *n* **1** : the process of taking in and uniting with something esp. by chemical reaction ⟨the ∼ of a radioisotope by living cells⟩ **2** : the psychological process of identifying with or introjecting something ⟨the ∼ of the external world in the superego —G. S. Blum⟩

in·cre·ment \ˈin-krə-mənt, ˈin-\ *n* **1 a** : something gained or added ⟨the most common form of leukocytosis is that in which the ∼ is in the neutrophilic leukocytes —W. A. D. Anderson⟩ **b** : one of a series of regular consecutive additions (as of growth or spread of disease) **2** : the amount or degree by which something changes; *esp* : the amount of positive or negative change in the value of one or more of a set of variables — **in·cre·men·tal** \ˌin-krə-ˈment-ᵊl, ˌin-\ *adj* — **in·cre·men·tal·ly** \-ᵊl-ē\ *adv*

incremental lines *n pl* : lines seen in a tooth in section showing the periodic depositions of dentin, enamel, and cementum occurring during the tooth's growth

incremental lines of Ret·zi·us \-ˈret-sē-əs\ *n pl* : incremental lines in the enamel of a tooth

Retzius, Magnus Gustaf (1842–1919), Swedish anatomist and anthropologist. Retzius produced important studies on the histology of the nervous system, and in 1896 he published a two-volume monograph on the gross anatomy of the human brain. The latter was probably the most important work on the brain's gross anatomy published during the 19th century. In 1873 he described the microscopic concentric lines seen in sections of tooth enamel.

in·cre·tion \in-ˈkrē-shən\ *n* **1** : internal secretion : secretion into the blood or tissues rather than into a cavity or outlet of the body **2** : a product of internal secretion : AUTACOID, HORMONE — **in·cre·tion·ary** \-shə-ˌner-ē\ *adj*

in·cre·to·ry \in-ˈkrēt-ə-rē\ *adj* : ENDOCRINE ⟨∼ organs⟩

¹**in·cross** \ˈin-ˌkrȯs\ *n* **1** : an individual produced by crossing inbred lines of the same breed or strain **2** : a mating between individuals from inbred lines of the same breed or strain

²**incross** *vt* : to interbreed (inbred lines of a breed or strain)

incrust *var of* ENCRUST

\ə\ abut \ᵊ\ kitten \ər\ further \a\ ash \ā\ ace \ä\ cot, cart
\au̇\ out \ch\ chin \e\ bet \ē\ easy \g\ go \i\ hit \ī\ ice \j\ job
\ŋ\ sing \ō\ go \ȯ\ law \ȯi\ boy \th\ thin \th̲\ the \ü\ loot
\u̇\ foot \y\ yet \zh\ vision　*See also* Pronunciation Symbols page

in·crus·ta·tion \ˌin-ˌkrəs-ˈtā-shən\ *or* **en·crus·ta·tion** \ˌen-\ *n* **1** : the act of encrusting : the state of being encrusted **2** : a crust or hard coating

in·cu·bate \ˈiŋ-kyə-ˌbāt, ˈin-\ *vb* **-bat·ed; -bat·ing** *vt* **1** : to maintain (as eggs, embryos of animals, or bacteria) under prescribed and usu. controlled conditions favorable for hatching or development esp. in an incubator **2** : to maintain (a chemically active system) under controlled conditions for the development of a reaction ~ *vi* : to undergo incubation ⟨the cultures *incubated* for five days⟩

in·cu·ba·tion \ˌiŋ-kyə-ˈbā-shən, ˌin-\ *n* **1** : the act or process of incubating **2** : INCUBATION PERIOD — **in·cu·ba·tion·al** \-shnəl, -shən-ᵊl\ *adj*

incubation period *n* : the period between the infection of an individual by a pathogen and the manifestation of the disease it causes

in·cu·ba·tor \ˈiŋ-kyə-ˌbāt-ər, ˈin-\ *n* : one that incubates; *esp* : an apparatus with a chamber used to provide controlled environmental conditions esp. for the cultivation of microorganisms or the care and protection of premature or sick babies

in·cu·bus \ˈiŋ-kyə-bəs, ˈin-\ *n, pl* **-bi** \-ˌbī, -ˌbē\ *also* **-bus·es 1** : an evil spirit at one time thought to lie on persons in their sleep; *esp* : one thought to have sexual intercourse with sleeping women — compare SUCCUBUS **2** : NIGHTMARE

in·cu·do·mal·le·al \ˈiŋ-kyə-dō-ˈmal-ē-əl\ *adj* : relating to or connecting the incus and the malleus ⟨the ~ joint⟩

in·cu·do·mal·le·o·lar \-ma-ˈlē-ə-lər\ *adj* : INCUDOMALLEAL

in·cu·do·sta·pe·di·al \-stā-ˈpēd-ē-əl, -stə-\ *adj* : relating to or connecting the incus and the stapedius ⟨the ~ joint⟩

in·cur·able \(ˈ)in-ˈkyùr-ə-bəl\ *adj* : impossible to cure ⟨an ~ disease⟩ — **in·cur·ably** \-blē\ *adv*

in·cus \ˈiŋ-kəs\ *n, pl* **in·cu·des** \iŋ-ˈkyüd-(ˌ)ēz, ˈiŋ-kyə-ˌdēz\ : the middle bone of the chain of three ossicles in the middle ear of a mammal resembling a premolar tooth with the body having a facet which articulates with the malleus and with the longer of the two widely separated crura having a process which articulates with the stapes — called also *ambos, anvil*

IND \ˌī-ˌen-ˈdē\ *abbr* investigational new drug

in·da·lone \ˈin-də-ˌlōn\ *n, often cap* : a preparation of butopyronoxyl — formerly a U.S. registered trademark

ind·amine \ˈin-də-ˌmēn\ *n* : any of a series of organic bases of which the simplest has the formula $C_{12}H_{11}N_3$ and which form salts that are unstable blue and green dyes

in·dane·di·one \ˌin-dān-ˈdī-ˌōn\ *or* **in·dan·di·one** \ˌin-dan-\ *n* : any of a group of synthetic anticoagulants that resemble the coumarins in structure and activity

in·de·cent as·sault \(ˈ)in-ˈdēs-ᵊnt-ə-ˈsȯlt\ *n* : an offensive sexual act or series of acts exclusive of rape committed against another person without consent

indecent exposure *n* : intentional exposure of part of one's body (as the genitalia) in a place where such exposure is likely to be an offense against the generally accepted standards of decency in a community

in·dem·ni·ty \in-ˈdem-nət-ē\ *adj* : FEE-FOR-SERVICE ⟨an ~ plan⟩ ⟨~ insurance⟩

in·de·pen·dent as·sort·ment \ˌin-də-ˈpen-dənt-ə-ˈsȯ(ə)rt-mənt\ *n* : formation of random combinations of chromosomes in meiosis and of genes on different pairs of homologous chromosomes by the passage according to the laws of probability of one of each diploid pair of homologous chromosomes into each gamete independently of each other pair

independent practice association *n* : an organization providing health care by doctors who maintain their own offices and continue to see their own patients but agree to treat enrolled members of the organization for a negotiated lump sum payment or a fixed payment per member or per service provided — abbr. *IPA*

In·der·al \ˈin-də-ˌral\ *trademark* — used for a preparation of the hydrochloride of propranolol

in·de·ter·mi·nate \ˌin-di-ˈtərm-(ə-)nət\ *adj* : relating to, being, or undergoing indeterminate cleavage ⟨an ~ egg⟩

indeterminate cleavage *n* : cleavage in which all the early divisions produce blastomeres with the potencies of the entire zygote — compare DETERMINATE CLEAVAGE

in·dex \ˈin-ˌdeks\ *n, pl* **in·dex·es** *or* **in·di·ces** \-də-ˌsēz\ **1** : INDEX FINGER **2** : a list (as of bibliographical information or citations to a body of literature) arranged usu. in alphabetical order of some specified datum (as author, subject, or keyword) ⟨*Index* Medicus of the U.S. National Library of Medicine⟩ **3 a** : a ratio or other number derived from a series of observations and used as an indicator or measure (as of a condition, property, or phenomenon) ⟨physiochemical ~*es* of the urine, the blood, and the gastric juice —*Jour. Amer. Med. Assoc.*⟩ **b** : the ratio of one dimension of a thing (as an anatomical structure) to another dimension — see CEPHALIC INDEX, CRANIAL INDEX

index case *n* **1** : an instance of a disease or a genetically determined condition that is discovered first and leads to the discovery of others in a family or population **2** : INDEX PATIENT ⟨we first examined the *index case* when he was aged 59 years —Stephanie B. Matthews & Anthony Campbell⟩

index finger *n* : the finger next to the thumb — called also *forefinger*

index of refraction *n* : the ratio of the speed of radiation (as light) in one medium (as a vacuum) to that in another medium — called also *refractive index*

index patient *n* : a patient whose disease or condition provides an index case — called also *index case-patient*

In·di·an co·bra \ˈin-dē-ən-ˈkō-brə\ *n* : a very venomous cobra of the genus *Naja* (*N. naja*) that is found esp. about settled areas and dwellings in southern and eastern Asia and eastward to the Philippines, that is yellowish to dark brown usu. with spectacle-shaped black and white markings on the expansible hood, and that sometimes reaches a length of 6 feet (1.8 meters)

Indian gum *n* **1** : GHATTI GUM **2** : KARAYA GUM

Indian hemp *n* **1** : a No. American dogbane (*Apocynum cannabinum*) with milky juice, tough fibrous bark, and an emetic and cathartic root **2** : HEMP 1

Indian physic *n* : either of two American herbs (*Gillenia trifoliata* and *G. stipulata*) of the rose family with emetic roots

Indian snake root *n* : an Indian plant of the genus *Rauwolfia* (*R. serpentina*) that is a source of reserpine

Indian squill *n* : URGINEA 2a

Indian tick typhus *n* : a disease of India that is caused by a tick-borne member of the genus *Rickettsia* (*R. conorii*) and is prob. identical with or closely related to boutonneuse fever

Indian tobacco *n* **1** : an American wild lobelia (*Lobelia inflata*) with small blue flowers that is the source of the drug lobelia **2** : LOBELIA 2

in·dia rubber \ˈin-dē-ə-\ *n* : RUBBER 1

indica — see CANNABIS INDICA

in·di·can \ˈin-də-ˌkan\ *n* **1** : an indigo-forming substance $C_8H_7NO_4S$ found as a salt in urine and other animal fluids; *also* : its potassium salt $C_8H_6KNO_4S$ **2** : a glucoside $C_{14}H_{17}NO_6$ occurring esp. in the indigo plant and being a source of natural indigo

in·di·can·uria \ˌin-də-ˌkan-ˈ(y)ùr-ē-ə\ *n* : the presence of an abnormally high concentration of indican in the urine

in·di·cate \ˈin-də-ˌkāt\ *vt* **-cat·ed; -cat·ing 1** : to be a fairly certain symptom of : show the presence or existence of ⟨the high fever ~*s* a serious condition⟩ **2** : to call for esp. as treatment for a particular condition ⟨radical surgery is often *indicated* in advanced cancer⟩

in·di·ca·tion \ˌin-də-ˈkā-shən\ *n* **1 a** : a symptom or particular circumstance that indicates the advisability or necessity of a specific medical treatment or procedure ⟨postpartum hemorrhage is the chief ~ for the use of ergot preparations and derivatives —C. H. Thienes⟩ **b** : something that is indicated as advisable or necessary ⟨in case of collapse the immediate ~ is artificial respiration —*Jour. Amer. Med. Assoc.*⟩ **2** : the degree indicated in a specific instance or at a specific time on a graduated physical instrument (as a thermometer)

in·di·ca·tor \ˈin-də-ˌkāt-ər\ *n* : a substance (as a dye) used to show visually usu. by its capacity for color change the condition of a solution with respect to the presence of free acid or alkali or some other substance (as in detecting the end point of a titration) ⟨litmus and phenolphthalein are acid-base ∼s⟩

indices *pl of* INDEX

indicis — see EXTENSOR INDICIS, EXTENSOR INDICIS PROPRIUS

indicus — see COCCULUS INDICUS

in·dif·fer·ence \in-'dif-ərn(t)s, -'dif-(ə-)rən(t)s\ *n* : the quality, state, or fact of being indifferent ⟨a schizophrenic reaction accompanied by apathy and ∼⟩

indifference point *n* **1** : the point in a series of judged magnitudes where there is no constant error of either overestimation or underestimation **2** : a midway point between two opposite sensations (as heat and cold or pleasure and pain) at which neither is felt

in·dif·fer·ent \in-'dif-ərnt, -'dif-(ə-)rent\ *adj* **1** : having or exhibiting a lack of affect, concern, or care **2 a** : not differentiated ⟨∼ tissues of the human body⟩ **b** : capable of development in more than one direction; *esp* : not yet embryologically determined — **in·dif·fer·ent·ly** *adv*

in·dig·e·nous \in-'dij-ə-nəs\ *adj* **1** : having originated in and being produced, growing, or living naturally in a particular region or environment ⟨a disease ∼ to the tropics⟩ ⟨colonization by small numbers of ∼ enteric bacteria —C. M. Kunin *et al*⟩ **2** : being inborn or innate ⟨a type of behavior that is ∼ to human beings⟩ — **in·dig·e·nous·ly** *adv*

in·di·gest·ible \in-(,)dī-'jes-tə-bəl, -də-\ *adj* : not digestible : not easily digested ⟨a diet with much ∼ fiber⟩ — **in·di·gest·ibil·i·ty** \-,jes-tə-'bil-ət-ē\ *n, pl* **-ties**

in·di·ges·tion \-jes(h)-chən\ *n* **1** : inability to digest or difficulty in digesting food : incomplete or imperfect digestion of food **2** : a case or attack of indigestion marked esp. by a burning sensation or discomfort in the upper abdomen

in·di·go \'in-di-,gō\ *n, pl* **-gos** *or* **-goes** **1 a** : a blue dye obtained from indigo plants (as *Indigofera tinctoria* of Africa and India, *I. anil* of So. America, and *I. auriculata* of Arabia and Egypt) **b** : the principal coloring matter $C_{16}H_{10}N_2O_2$ of natural indigo usu. synthesized as a blue powder with a coppery luster — called also *indigotin* **2** : INDIGO PLANT

indigo carmine *n* : a soluble blue dye $C_{16}H_8N_2Na_2O_8S_2$ that is a sodium salt, is used chiefly as a biological stain and food color, and since it is rapidly excreted by the kidneys is used as a dye to mark ureteral structures (as in cystoscopy and catheterization)

indigo plant *n* : a plant that yields indigo; *esp* : any of a genus (*Indigofera*) of leguminous herbs

in·di·go·tin \in-'dig-ət-ən, ,in-di-'gōt-ᵊn\ *n* : INDIGO 1b

in·din·a·vir \(,)in-'din-ə-,vir\ *n* : an antiviral protease inhibitor that is used in the form of its sulfate $C_{36}H_{47}N_5O_4 \cdot H_2SO_4$ in combination therapy with antiretroviral drugs (as AZT and lamivudine) to treat HIV infection — see CRIXIVAN

in·di·rect \in-də-'rekt, -dī-\ *adj* **1** : not direct: as **a** : not resulting directly from an action or cause (as a disease) ⟨∼ effects of malaria⟩ **b** : involving intermediate or intervening parts or pathways ⟨stimulation of one eye elicits narrowing of the pupil of the other eye by an ∼ reaction⟩ ⟨∼ attachment of a muscle through tendons⟩ **2** : involving or being immunofluorescence in which antibodies of two kinds are used of which the first combine with a specific protein and the second contain a fluorescent label and combine with the antibodies of the first type — **indirectly** *adv*

indirect cell division *n* : MITOSIS

in·di·ru·bin \in-də-'rü-bən, 'in-də-,\ *n* : a dark red crystalline pigment $C_{16}H_{10}N_2O_2$ isomeric with indigo (sense 1b) found in natural indigo and sometimes in urine

in·dis·posed \in-dis-'pōzd\ *adj* : being usu. temporarily in poor physical health : slightly ill — **in·dis·po·si·tion** \(,)in-,dis-pə-'zish-ən\ *n*

in·di·um \'in-dē-əm\ *n* : a malleable fusible silvery metallic element that is chiefly trivalent, occurs esp. in sphalerite ores, and is used as a plating for bearings, in alloys having a low melting point, and in making transistors — abbr. *In*; see ELEMENT table

in·di·vid·u·al·ize \in-də-'vij-(ə-)wə-,līz, -'vij-ə-,līz\ *or Brit* **in·di·vid·u·al·ise** *vt* **-ized** *or Brit* **-ised; -iz·ing** *or Brit* **-is·ing** : to adapt to the needs or special circumstances of an individual ⟨∼ dosage for the most beneficial effect⟩ — **in·di·vid·u·al·iza·tion** *or Brit* **in·di·vid·u·al·isa·tion** \-,vij-(ə-)wə-lə-'zā-shən, -,vij-ə-lə-\ *n*

in·di·vid·u·al psychology \in-də-'vij-(ə-)wəl-, -'vij-əl-\ *n* : a modification of psychoanalysis developed by the Austrian psychologist Alfred Adler emphasizing feelings of inferiority and a desire for power as the primary motivating forces in human behavior

in·di·vid·u·a·tion \-,vij-ə-'wā-shən\ *n* **1** : the process in the analytic psychology of C. G. Jung by which the self is formed by integrating elements of the conscious and unconscious mind **2** : regional differentiation along a primary embryonic axis — **in·di·vid·u·ate** \-'vij-ə-,wāt\ *vt* **-at·ed; -at·ing**

In·do·cin \'in-də-sən\ *trademark* — used for a preparation of indomethacin

in·do·cy·a·nine green \,in-dō-'sī-ə-,nēn-'grēn, -'sī-ə-nən-\ *n* : a green dye $C_{43}H_{47}N_2NaO_6S_2$ used esp. in testing liver blood flow and cardiac output

in·dole \'in-,dōl\ *n* : a crystalline compound C_8H_7N that is found along with skatole in the intestines and feces as a decomposition product of proteins containing tryptophan and that can be made synthetically; *also* : a derivative of indole

in·dole·ace·tic acid \'in-,dōl-ə-,sēt-ik-\ *n* : a crystalline compound $C_{10}H_9NO_2$ that is formed from tryptophan in plants and animals, is present in small amounts in normal urine, and acts as a growth hormone in plants — called also *heteroauxin*

in·dole·amine \in-'dōl-ə-'mēn, -'am-,ēn\ *n* : any of various indole derivatives (as serotonin or tryptamine) that contain an amine group

in·do·lent \'in-də-lənt\ *adj* **1** : causing little or no pain ⟨an ∼ tumor⟩ **2 a** : growing or progressing slowly ⟨leprosy is an ∼ infectious disease⟩ **b** : slow to heal ⟨an ∼ ulcer⟩ — **in·do·lence** \-lənt(t)s\ *n*

in·dol·uria \,in-,dōl-'(y)ur-ē-ə\ *n* : the presence of indole in the urine

in·do·lyl \'in-də-,lil\ *n* : any of seven isomeric monovalent radicals C_8H_6N derived from indole by removal of one hydrogen atom

in·do·meth·a·cin \,in-dō-'meth-ə-sən\ *n* : an NSAID $C_{19}H_{16}ClNO_4$ with analgesic and antipyretic properties used esp. to treat painful inflammatory conditions (as rheumatoid arthritis and osteoarthritis) — see INDOCIN

in·do·phe·nol \,in-dō-'fē-,nōl, ,in-(,)dō-fi-'\ *n* : any of various blue or green dyes

In·do·pla·nor·bis \,in-dō-plə-'nór-bəs\ *n* : an Asian genus of freshwater snails of the family Planorbidae of veterinary importance as intermediate hosts of trematode worms (as a bovine blood fluke)

in·dox·yl \in-'däk-səl\ *n* : a crystalline compound C_8H_7NO that has a strong fecal odor and is found in plants and animals or synthesized as a step in indigo manufacture

in·dox·yl·uria \in-,däk-səl-'(y)ur-ē-ə\ *n* : the presence of excess indoxyl and esp. of its sulfate in the urine

in·duce \in-'d(y)üs\ *vt* **in·duced; in·duc·ing** **1** : to cause or bring about ⟨anesthesia *induced* by drugs⟩: as **a** (1) : to cause the embryological formation of ⟨the optic cup ∼s lens tissue in the adjacent ectoderm⟩ (2) : to cause to form through embryonic induction ⟨∼ ectoderm to form a neural tube⟩ **b** : to cause or initiate by artificial means ⟨*induced* abortion⟩ ⟨*induced* labor⟩ **2** : to produce anesthesia in ⟨the patient was *induced* by a mixture of thiopental and curare⟩

in·duc·er \-'d(y)ü-sər\ *n* : one that induces; *specif* : a substance that is capable of activating the transcription of a gene by combining with and inactivating a genetic repressor

\ə\ **abut** \ᵊ\ **kitten** \ər\ **further** \a\ **ash** \ā\ **ace** \ä\ **cot, cart**
\aú\ **out** \ch\ **chin** \e\ **bet** \ē\ **easy** \g\ **go** \i\ **hit** \ī\ **ice** \j\ **job**
\ŋ\ **sing** \ō\ **go** \ó\ **law** \ói\ **boy** \th\ **thin** \th\ **the** \ü\ **loot**
\ú\ **foot** \y\ **yet** \zh\ **vision** *See also* Pronunciation Symbols page

in·duc·ible \in-'d(y)ü-sə-bəl\ *adj* : capable of being formed, activated, or expressed in response to a stimulus esp. of a molecular kind: as **a** : formed by a cell in response to the presence of its substrate ⟨∼ enzymes⟩ — compare CONSTITUTIVE 1a **b** : activated or undergoing expression only in the presence of a particular molecule ⟨an ∼ promoter that turns on its genes only in the presence of lactose⟩ — **in·duc·ibil·i·ty** \in-ˌd(y)ü-sə-'bil-ət-ē\ *n, pl* **-ties**

in·duc·tance \in-'dək-tən(t)s\ *n* **1 a** : a property of an electric circuit by which an electromotive force is induced in it by a variation of current either in the circuit itself or in a neighboring circuit **b** : the measure of this property that is equal to the ratio of the induced electromotive force to the rate of change of the inducing current **2** : a circuit or a device possessing inductance

in·duc·tion \in-'dək-shən\ *n* **1** : the act of causing or bringing on or about ⟨∼ of labor⟩; *specif* : the establishment of the initial state of anesthesia often with an agent other than that used subsequently to maintain the anesthetic state **2** : the process by which an electrical conductor becomes electrified when near a charged body, by which a magnetizable body becomes magnetized when in a magnetic field or in the magnetic flux set up by a magnetomotive force, or by which an electromotive force is produced in a circuit by varying the magnetic field linked with the circuit **3 a** : arousal of a part or area (as of the retina) by stimulation of an adjacent part or area **b** : the process by which the fate of embryonic cells is determined (as by the action of adjacent cells) and morphogenetic differentiation brought about — **in·duct** \in-'dəkt\ *vt*

induction chemotherapy *n* : chemotherapy usu. with high doses of anticancer drugs (as cisplatin or methotrexate) in the initial treatment esp. of advanced cancers in order to make subsequent treatment (as surgery or radiotherapy) more effective

in·duc·tive \in-'dək-tiv\ *adj* **1** : of or relating to inductance or electrical induction **2** : involving the action of an embryological inductor : tending to produce induction ⟨the ∼ effect of chordamesoderm⟩ ⟨∼ reactions in the embryo⟩ — **in·duc·tive·ly** *adv*

in·duc·tor \in-'dək-tər\ *n* : one that inducts; *esp* : ORGANIZER 2 ⟨chordamesoderm acts on embryonic ectoderm as an ∼ of neural tissue⟩

in·duc·to·ri·um \ˌin-ˌdək-'tōr-ē-əm\ *n* : a battery-operated apparatus containing induction coils used for producing a continuous pulsing electric current or a single pulse of current (as for physiological or pharmacological experiments)

in·duc·to·ther·my \in-'dək-tə-ˌthər-mē\ *n, pl* **-mies** : fever therapy by means of an electromagnetic induction field with the body or a part of it acting as a resistance

in·du·line *also* **in·du·lin** \'in-d(y)ə-ˌlēn, -lən\ *n* : any of numerous blue or violet dyes related to the safranines

in·du·rat·ed \'in-d(y)ə-ˌrāt-əd\ *adj* : having become firm or hard esp. by increase of fibrous elements ⟨∼ tissue⟩ ⟨an ulcer with an ∼ border⟩

in·du·ra·tion \ˌin-d(y)ə-'rā-shən\ *n* **1** : an increase in the fibrous elements in tissue commonly associated with inflammation and marked by loss of elasticity and pliability : SCLEROSIS **2** : a hardened mass or formation

in·du·ra·tive \'in-d(y)ə-ˌrāt-iv, in-'d(y)ùr-ət-iv\ *adj* : of, relating to, or producing induration

in·du·si·um \in-'d(y)ü-z(h)ē-əm\ *n, pl* **-sia** \-z(h)ē-ə\ : a membrane serving as a covering; *esp* : INDUSIUM GRISEUM

indusium gris·e·um \-'griz-ē-əm\ *n* : a thin layer of gray matter over the dorsal surface of the corpus callosum

in·dus·tri·al disease \in-ˌdəs-trē-əl-\ *n* : OCCUPATIONAL DISEASE

industrial hygiene *n* : a science concerned with the protection and improvement of the health and well-being of workers in their vocational environment — **industrial hygienist** *n*

industrial psychologist *n* : a psychologist who specializes in workplace problems and issues (as employee satisfaction

and motivation, employee selection, and working conditions)

in·dwell·ing \'in-ˌdwel-iŋ\ *adj* : left within a bodily organ or passage to maintain drainage, prevent obstruction, or provide a route for administration of food or drugs — used of an implanted tube (as a catheter)

ine·bri·ant \in-'ē-brē-ənt\ *n* : INTOXICANT — **inebriant** *adj*

¹**ine·bri·ate** \in-'ē-brē-ˌāt\ *vt* **-at·ed; -at·ing** : to make drunk : INTOXICATE — **ine·bri·a·tion** \-ˌē-brē-'ā-shən\ *n*

²**ine·bri·ate** \in-'ē-brē-ət, -ˌāt\ *adj* **1** : affected by alcohol : DRUNK **2** : addicted to excessive drinking

³**ine·bri·ate** \-ət\ *n* : one who is drunk; *esp* : DRUNKARD

in·e·bri·ety \ˌin-i-'brī-ət-ē\ *n, pl* **-eties** : the state of being inebriated; *esp* : habitual drunkenness

in·elas·tic \ˌin-i-'las-tik\ *adj* : not elastic — **in·elas·tic·i·ty** \-i-ˌlas-'tis-ət-ē, -ˌē-ˌlas-, -'tis-tē\ *n, pl* **-ties**

In·er·mi·cap·si·fer \in-ˌər-mə-'kap-sə-fər\ *n* : a genus of tapeworms of the family Anoplocephalidae that are parasitic in African and Central American rodents and occas. in humans

in·ert \in-'ərt\ *adj* **1** : lacking the power to move **2** : deficient in active properties; *esp* : lacking a usual or anticipated chemical or biological action ⟨an ∼ drug⟩ — **in·ert·ness** *n*

inert gas *n* : NOBLE GAS

in·er·tia \in-'ər-shə, -shē-ə\ *n* **1 a** : a property of matter by which it remains at rest or in uniform motion in the same straight line unless acted upon by some external force **b** : an analogous property of other physical quantities (as electricity) **2** : lack of activity or movement — used esp. of the uterus in labor when its contractions are weak or irregular

in·ex·cit·able \ˌin-ik-'sīt-ə-bəl\ *adj* **1** : not readily excited or aroused **2** *of a nerve* : not subject to excitation : not responsive to stimulation — **in·ex·cit·abil·i·ty** \-ˌsīt-ə-'bil-ət-ē\ *n, pl* **-ties**

in ex·tre·mis \ˌin-ik-'strē-məs, -'strā-\ *adv* : at the point of death

in·fan·cy \'in-fən-sē\ *n, pl* **-cies** **1** : early childhood **2** : the legal status of an infant

in·fant \'in-fənt\ *n* **1 a** : a child in the first year of life : BABY **b** : a child several years of age **2** : a person who is not of full age : MINOR — **infant** *adj*

in·fan·ti·cide \in-'fant-ə-ˌsīd\ *n* **1** : the killing of an infant **2** : one who kills an infant — **in·fan·ti·ci·dal** \-ˌfant-ə-'sīd-ᵊl\ *adj*

in·fan·tile \'in-fən-ˌtīl, -tᵊl, -ˌtēl, -(ˌ)til\ *adj* **1** : of, relating to, or occurring in infants or infancy ⟨∼ eczema⟩ **2** : suitable to or characteristic of an infant; *esp* : very immature

infantile amaurotic idiocy *n* **1** : TAY-SACHS DISEASE **2** : SANDHOFF'S DISEASE

infantile amnesia *n* : inability to remember the feelings and experiences of early childhood

infantile autism *n* : a severe autism that first occurs before 30 months of age — called also *Kanner's syndrome*

infantile myxedema *n* : CRETINISM

infantile paralysis *n* : POLIOMYELITIS

infantile scurvy *n* : acute scurvy during infancy caused by malnutrition — called also *Barlow's disease*

infantile sexuality *n* : needs and strivings in infancy and early childhood that exist according to psychoanalytic theory for libidinal gratification : pregenital eroticism

in·fan·til·ism \'in-fən-ˌtīl-ˌiz-əm, -tə-ˌliz-; in-'fant-tᵊl-ˌiz-\ *n* : retention of childish physical, mental, or emotional qualities in adult life; *esp* : failure to attain sexual maturity

infant mortality *n* : the rate of deaths occurring in the first year of life

infantum — see CHOLERA INFANTUM, ROSEOLA INFANTUM

in·farct \'in-ˌfärkt, in-'\ *n* : an area of necrosis in a tissue or organ resulting from obstruction of the local circulation by a thrombus or embolus

in·farct·ed \in-'färk-təd\ *adj* : affected with infarction ⟨∼ kidney⟩

in·farc·tion \in-'färk-shən\ *n* **1** : the process of forming an infarct ⟨severe stress sometime between the 5th and 20th days after ∼ —*Jour. Amer. Med. Assoc.*⟩ **2** : INFARCT ⟨developed a full-blown ∼ —W. A. Nolen⟩

in·fect \in-ˈfekt\ *vt* **1** : to contaminate with a disease-producing substance or agent (as bacteria) **2 a** : to communicate a pathogen or a disease to **b** *of a pathogenic organism* : to invade (an individual or organ) usu. by penetration — compare INFEST

in·fec·tant \in-ˈfek-tənt\ *n* : an agent of infection (as a bacterium or virus)

in·fec·tion \in-ˈfek-shən\ *n* **1** : an infective agent or material contaminated with an infective agent **2 a** : the state produced by the establishment of an infective agent in or on a suitable host **b** : a disease resulting from infection : INFECTIOUS DISEASE **3** : an act or process of infecting ⟨syphilis ∼ is chiefly venereal⟩; *also* : the establishment of a pathogen in its host after invasion

infection immunity *n* : PREMUNITION

infection stone *n* : a kidney stone composed of struvite

in·fec·ti·os·i·ty \in-ˌfek-shē-ˈäs-ət-ē\ *n, pl* **-ties** : degree of infectiousness

infectiosum — see ERYTHEMA INFECTIOSUM

in·fec·tious \in-ˈfek-shəs\ *adj* **1** : capable of causing infection ⟨a carrier remains ∼ without exhibiting signs of disease⟩ ⟨viruses and other ∼ agents⟩ **2** : communicable by invasion of the body of a susceptible organism ⟨all contagious diseases are also ∼, but it does not follow that all ∼ diseases are contagious —W. A. Hagan⟩ — compare CONTAGIOUS 1 — **in·fec·tious·ly** *adv* — **in·fec·tious·ness** *n*

infectious abortion *n* : CONTAGIOUS ABORTION

infectious anemia *n* **1** : EQUINE INFECTIOUS ANEMIA **2** : FELINE INFECTIOUS ANEMIA

infectious bovine rhinotracheitis *n* : a disease of cattle caused by a herpesvirus of the genus *Varicellovirus* (species *Bovine herpesvirus 1*) and characterized by inflammation and ulceration of the nasal cavities and trachea

infectious bulbar paralysis *n* : PSEUDORABIES

infectious coryza *n* : an acute infectious respiratory disease of chickens that is caused by a bacterium of the genus *Haemophilus* (*H. paragallinarum* syn. *H. gallinarum*) and is characterized by catarrhal inflammation of the mucous membranes of the nasal passages and sinuses frequently with conjunctivitis and subcutaneous edema of the face and wattles and sometimes with pneumonia

infectious disease *n* : a disease caused by the entrance into the body of organisms (as bacteria, protozoans, fungi, or viruses) which grow and multiply there — see COMMUNICABLE DISEASE, CONTAGIOUS DISEASE

infectious enterohepatitis *n* : BLACKHEAD 2

infectious hepatitis *n* : HEPATITIS A

infectious jaundice *n* **1** : HEPATITIS A **2** : WEIL'S DISEASE

infectious laryngotracheitis *n* : a severe highly contagious and often fatal disease of chickens and pheasants that affects chiefly adult birds, is caused by a herpesvirus (species *Gallid herpesvirus 1* of the subfamily *Alphaherpesvirinae*) related to the two viruses causing Marek's disease, and is characterized by inflammation of the trachea and larynx often marked by local necrosis and hemorrhage and by the formation of purulent or cheesy exudate interfering with breathing

infectious mononucleosis *n* : an acute infectious disease associated with Epstein-Barr virus and characterized by fever, swelling of lymph nodes, and lymphocytosis — called also *glandular fever, kissing disease, mono*

in·fec·tive \in-ˈfek-tiv\ *adj* : producing or capable of producing infection : INFECTIOUS

in·fec·tiv·i·ty \ˌin-ˌfek-ˈtiv-ət-ē\ *n, pl* **-ties** : the quality of being infective : the ability to produce infection; *specif* : a tendency to spread rapidly from host to host — compare VIRULENCE b

in·fec·tor \in-ˈfek-tər\ *n* : one that infects

in·fe·cun·di·ty \ˌin-fe-ˈkən-dət-ē\ *n, pl* **-ties** : the condition of not being fecund : STERILITY — **in·fe·cund** \(ˈ)in-ˈfek-ənd, -ˈfēk-\ *adj*

in·fe·ri·or \in-ˈfir-ē-ər\ *adj* **1** : situated below and closer to the feet than another and esp. another similar part of an up-right body esp. of a human being — compare SUPERIOR 1 **2** : situated in a more posterior or ventral position in the body of a quadruped — compare SUPERIOR 2

inferior alveolar artery *n* : a branch of the maxillary artery that is distributed to the mucous membrane of the mouth and through the mandibular canal to the teeth of the lower jaw — called also *inferior dental artery, mandibular artery*

inferior alveolar canal *n* : MANDIBULAR CANAL

inferior alveolar nerve *n* : a branch of the mandibular nerve that passes through the mandibular canal to the mental foramen giving off various branches along the way to the teeth of the lower jaw and finally to the skin of the chin and the skin and mucous membrane of the lower lip — called also *inferior alveolar, inferior dental nerve*

inferior alveolar vein *n* : a tributary of the pterygoid plexus that accompanies the inferior alveolar artery and drains the lower jaw and lower teeth

inferior articular process *n* : ARTICULAR PROCESS b

inferior cardiac nerve *n* : CARDIAC NERVE a

inferior cerebellar peduncle *n* : CEREBELLAR PEDUNCLE c

inferior cervical ganglion *n* : CERVICAL GANGLION c

inferior colliculus *n* : either member of the posterior and lower pair of corpora quadrigemina that are situated next to the pons and together constitute one of the lower centers for hearing — compare SUPERIOR COLLICULUS

inferior concha *n* : NASAL CONCHA a

inferior constrictor *n* : a muscle of the pharynx that is the thickest of its three constrictors, arises from the surface and side of the cricoid and thyroid cartilages, inserts into the median line at the back of the pharynx, and acts to constrict part of the pharynx in swallowing — called also *constrictor pharyngis inferior, inferior pharyngeal constrictor muscle;* compare MIDDLE CONSTRICTOR, SUPERIOR CONSTRICTOR

inferior dental artery *n* : INFERIOR ALVEOLAR ARTERY

inferior dental nerve *n* : INFERIOR ALVEOLAR NERVE

inferior epigastric artery *n* : EPIGASTRIC ARTERY b

inferior extensor retinaculum *n* : EXTENSOR RETINACULUM 1a

inferior ganglion *n* **1** : the lower and larger of the two sensory ganglia of the glossopharyngeal nerve — called also *petrosal ganglion, petrous ganglion;* compare SUPERIOR GANGLION 1 **2** : the lower of the two ganglia of the vagus nerve that forms a swelling just beyond the exit of the nerve from the jugular foramen — called also *inferior vagal ganglion, nodose ganglion;* compare SUPERIOR GANGLION 2

inferior gluteal artery *n* : GLUTEAL ARTERY b

inferior gluteal nerve *n* : GLUTEAL NERVE b

inferior hemorrhoidal artery *n* : RECTAL ARTERY a

inferior hemorrhoidal vein *n* : RECTAL VEIN a

inferior horn *n* : the cornu in the lateral ventricle of each cerebral hemisphere that curves downward into the temporal lobe — compare ANTERIOR HORN 2, POSTERIOR HORN 2

in·fe·ri·or·i·ty \(ˌ)in-ˌfir-ē-ˈȯr-ət-ē, -ˈär-\ *n, pl* **-ties** : a condition or state of being or having a sense of being inferior or inadequate esp. with respect to one's apparent equals or to the world at large

inferiority complex *n* : an acute sense of personal inferiority resulting either in timidity or through overcompensation in exaggerated aggressiveness

inferior laryngeal artery *n* : LARYNGEAL ARTERY a

inferior laryngeal nerve *n* **1** : LARYNGEAL NERVE b — called also *inferior laryngeal* **2** : any of the terminal branches of the inferior laryngeal nerve

inferior longitudinal fasciculus *n* : a band of association fibers in each cerebral hemisphere that interconnects the occipital and temporal lobes and that passes near the lateral walls of the posterior and inferior horns of the lateral ventricle

---

\ə\ abut \ᵊ\ kitten \ər\ further \a\ ash \ā\ ace \ä\ cot, cart \au̇\ out \ch\ chin \e\ bet \ē\ easy \g\ go \i\ hit \ī\ ice \j\ job \ŋ\ sing \ō\ go \ȯ\ law \ȯi\ boy \th\ thin \t͟h\ the \ü\ loot \u̇\ foot \y\ yet \zh\ vision   *See also* Pronunciation Symbols page

in·fe·ri·or·ly *adv* : in a lower position ⟨a focal opacity remained in the vitreous ∼ —H. L. Cantrill *et al*⟩

inferior maxillary bone *n* : JAW 1b

inferior maxillary nerve *n* : MANDIBULAR NERVE

inferior meatus *n* : a space extending along the lateral wall of the nasal cavity between the inferior nasal concha and the floor of the nasal cavity — compare MIDDLE MEATUS, SUPERIOR MEATUS

inferior mesenteric artery *n* : MESENTERIC ARTERY a

inferior mesenteric ganglion *n* : MESENTERIC GANGLION a

inferior mesenteric plexus *n* : MESENTERIC PLEXUS a

inferior mesenteric vein *n* : MESENTERIC VEIN a

inferior mirage *n* : a mirage consisting of an image of a distant object appearing below the real object and usu. somewhat separated from it

in·fe·ri·or·most \-ˌmōst\ *adj* : closest to the feet — used in human anatomy ⟨the ∼ extent of the abdominal cavity —L. L. Langley *et al*⟩

inferior nasal concha *n* : NASAL CONCHA a

inferior nuchal line *n* : NUCHAL LINE c

inferior oblique *n* : OBLIQUE b(2)

inferior olive *n* : a large gray nucleus that forms the interior of the olive on each side of the medulla oblongata and has connections with the thalamus, cerebellum, and spinal cord — called also *inferior olivary nucleus;* see ACCESSORY OLIVARY NUCLEUS; compare SUPERIOR OLIVE

inferior ophthalmic vein *n* : OPHTHALMIC VEIN b

inferior orbital fissure *n* : ORBITAL FISSURE b

inferior pancreaticoduodenal artery *n* : PANCREATICODUODENAL ARTERY a

inferior pectoral nerve *n* : PECTORAL NERVE b

inferior peroneal retinaculum *n* : PERONEAL RETINACULUM b

inferior petrosal sinus *n* : PETROSAL SINUS b

inferior pharyngeal constrictor muscle *n* : INFERIOR CONSTRICTOR

inferior phrenic artery *n* : PHRENIC ARTERY b

inferior phrenic vein *n* : PHRENIC VEIN b

inferior radioulnar joint *n* : DISTAL RADIOULNAR JOINT

inferior ramus *n* : RAMUS b(2), c

inferior rectal artery *n* : RECTAL ARTERY a

inferior rectal vein *n* : RECTAL VEIN a

inferior rectus *n* : RECTUS 2d

inferior sagittal sinus *n* : SAGITTAL SINUS b

inferior temporal gyrus *n* : TEMPORAL GYRUS c

inferior thyroarytenoid ligament *n* : VOCAL LIGAMENT

inferior thyroid artery *n* : THYROID ARTERY b

inferior thyroid vein *n* : THYROID VEIN c

inferior turbinate *n* : NASAL CONCHA a

inferior turbinate bone *also* **inferior tur·bi·nat·ed bone** \-ˈtər-bə-ˌnāt-əd-\ *n* : NASAL CONCHA a

inferior ulnar collateral artery *n* : a small artery that arises from the brachial artery just above the elbow and divides to form or gives off branches that anastomose with other arteries in the region of the elbow — compare SUPERIOR ULNAR COLLATERAL ARTERY

inferior vagal ganglion *n* : INFERIOR GANGLION 2

inferior vena cava *n* : a vein that is the largest vein in the human body, is formed by the union of the two common iliac veins at the level of the fifth lumbar vertebra, and returns blood to the right atrium of the heart from bodily parts below the diaphragm

inferior vermis *n* : VERMIS 1b

inferior vesical *n* : VESICAL ARTERY b

inferior vesical artery *n* : VESICAL ARTERY b

inferior vestibular nucleus *n* : the one of the four vestibular nuclei on each side of the medulla oblongata that is situated between the medial vestibular nucleus and the inferior cerebellar peduncle and that sends fibers down both sides of the spinal cord to synapse with motor neurons of the ventral roots

inferior vocal cords *n pl* : TRUE VOCAL CORDS

in·fe·ro·me·di·al \ˌin-fə-rō-ˈmēd-ē-əl\ *adj* : situated below and in the middle ⟨the ∼ aspect of the orbit⟩

in·fe·ro·tem·po·ral \-ˈtem-p(ə-)rəl\ *adj* **1** : being the inferior or part of the temporal lobe of the cerebral cortex; *also* : situated or occurring in, on, or under this part ⟨the ∼ gyrus⟩ ⟨∼ cortical neurons⟩ ⟨∼ lesions⟩ **2** : of, relating to, or being the lower lateral quadrant of the eye or visual field ⟨extraction of the lens by the ∼ route⟩

in·fer·tile \(ˈ)in-ˈfərt-ᵊl\ *adj* : not fertile; *esp* : incapable of or unsuccessful in achieving pregnancy over a considerable period of time (as a year) in spite of determined attempts by heterosexual intercourse without contraception ⟨∼ couples⟩ ⟨an ∼ male with a low sperm count⟩ ⟨an ∼ female with blocked fallopian tubes⟩ — compare STERILE 1 — **in·fer·til·i·ty** \ˌin-(ˌ)fər-ˈtil-ət-ē\ *n, pl* **-ties**

in·fest \in-ˈfest\ *vt* : to live in or on as a parasite ⟨the flea that ∼s cats⟩ ⟨horses ∼ed with worms⟩ — compare INFECT

in·fes·tant \in-ˈfes-tənt\ *n* : one that infests; *esp* : a visible parasite

in·fes·ta·tion \ˌin-ˌfes-ˈtā-shən\ *n* **1** : the act of infesting something **2** : something that infests **3** : the state of being infested esp. with metazoan ectoparasites

in·fib·u·la·tion \(ˌ)in-ˌfib-yə-ˈlā-shən\ *n* : an act or practice of fastening by ring, clasp, or stitches the labia majora in girls and the foreskin in boys in order to prevent sexual intercourse — **in·fib·u·late** \-ˈfib-yə-ˌlāt\ *vt* **-lat·ed; -lat·ing**

¹in·fil·trate \in-ˈfil-ˌtrāt, ˈin-(ˌ)\ *vb* **-trat·ed; -trat·ing** *vt* **1** : to cause (as a liquid) to permeate something by penetrating its pores or interstices ⟨∼ tissue with a local anesthetic⟩ **2** : to pass into or through (a substance) by filtering or permeating ∼ *vi* : to enter, permeate, or pass through a substance or area

²infiltrate *n* : something that passes or is caused to pass into or through something by permeating or filtering; *esp* : a substance that passes into the bodily tissues and forms an abnormal accumulation ⟨a lung ∼⟩

in·fil·tra·tion \ˌin-(ˌ)fil-ˈtrā-shən\ *n* **1 a** : the act or process of infiltrating **b** : something that infiltrates ⟨anesthetic drug ∼⟩ **2** : an abnormal bodily condition produced or characterized by infiltration

infiltration anesthesia *n* : anesthesia of an operative site accomplished by local injection of anesthetics

in·fil·tra·tive \ˈin-(ˌ)fil-ˌtrāt-iv, in-ˈfil-trət-\ *adj* : relating to or characterized by infiltration ⟨∼ lung disease⟩

in·firm \in-ˈfərm\ *adj* : of poor or deteriorated vitality; *esp* : feeble from age

in·fir·mar·i·an \ˌin-fər-ˈmar-ē-ən\ *n* : a person having charge of an infirmary

in·fir·ma·ry \in-ˈfərm-(ə-)rē\ *n, pl* **-ries** : a place esp. in a school or college for the care and treatment of the sick

in·fir·mi·ty \in-ˈfər-mət-ē\ *n, pl* **-ties** : the quality or state of being infirm; *esp* : an unsound, unhealthy, or debilitated state

in·flame \in-ˈflām\ *vb* **in·flamed; in·flam·ing** *vt* : to cause inflammation in (bodily tissue) ⟨∼ the sinuses⟩ ∼ *vi* : to become affected with inflammation

in·flam·ma·tion \ˌin-flə-ˈmā-shən\ *n* : a local response to cellular injury that is marked by capillary dilatation, leukocytic infiltration, redness, heat, pain, swelling, and often loss of function and that serves as a mechanism initiating the elimination of noxious agents and of damaged tissue

in·flam·ma·to·ry \in-ˈflam-ə-ˌtōr-ē, -ˌtȯr-\ *adj* : accompanied by or tending to cause inflammation ⟨∼ diseases⟩

inflammatory bowel disease *n* : either of two inflammatory diseases of the bowel: **a** : CROHN'S DISEASE **b** : ULCERATIVE COLITIS

in·flat·able \in-ˈflāt-ə-bəl\ *adj* : capable of being inflated ⟨an ∼ prosthesis⟩

in·flate \in-ˈflāt\ *vb* **in·flat·ed; in·flat·ing** *vt* : to swell or distend with air or gas ⟨∼ the lungs⟩ ∼ *vi* : to become inflated — **in·fla·tion** \in-ˈflā-shən\ *n*

in·flec·tion *or chiefly Brit* **in·flex·ion** \in-ˈflek-shən\ *n* : the act or result of curving or bending

in·flu·en·za \ˌin-(ˌ)flü-ˈen-zə\ *n* **1 a** : any of several acute highly contagious respiratory diseases caused by strains of three major orthomyxoviruses now considered to comprise

three species assigned to three separate genera: (1) : INFLU-
ENZA A (2) : INFLUENZA B (3) : INFLUENZA C **b** : any human respiratory infection of undetermined cause — not
used technically **2** : any of numerous febrile usu. virus diseases of domestic animals (as shipping fever of horses)
marked by respiratory symptoms, inflammation of mucous
membranes, and often systemic involvement — **in·flu·en·
zal** \-zəl\ *adj*

influenza A \-'ā\ *n* : a common moderate to severe respiratory disease that affects humans and some other vertebrates
(as swine and birds) sometimes in pandemics following mutation in the causative virus, that in humans is characterized
by sudden onset, fever, prostration, severe aches and pains,
and progressive inflammation of the respiratory mucous
membranes, that is held to have aquatic birds as its natural
and historic host, and that has numerous variants caused by
subtypes (as H1N1, H2N2, or H3N2) of an orthomyxovirus
(species *Influenza A virus* of the genus *Influenzavirus A*) distinguished esp. by mutations of a hemagglutinin (as H1, H2,
or H3) affecting the ability of the virus to infect cells and of a
neuraminidase (as N1 or N2) involved in release of the replicated virus from cells — see AVIAN INFLUENZA, SWINE IN-
FLUENZA; ASIAN FLU, HONG KONG FLU, SPANISH FLU

influenza B \-'bē\ *n* : influenza that is usu. milder than influenza A, that may occur in epidemics but not pandemics, and
that is caused by an orthomyxovirus (species *Influenza B virus* of the genus *Influenzavirus B*) infecting only humans and
esp. children and having relative genetic stability with a single major serotype

influenza C \-'sē\ *n* : influenza that is restricted to humans,
that usu. occurs as a subclinical infection, that occurs in neither epidemics or pandemics, and that is caused by an orthomyxovirus (species *Influenza C virus* of the genus *Influenzavirus C*)

influenza vaccine *n* : a vaccine against influenza; *specif* : a
mixture of strains of formaldehyde-inactivated influenza virus from chick embryo culture

influenza virus *n* : any of the orthomyxoviruses that belong
to three genera (*Influenzavirus A, Influenzavirus B,* and *Influenzavirus C*) and that cause influenza A, influenza B, and influenza C in vertebrates

influenza virus vaccine *n* : INFLUENZA VACCINE

in·fold \in-'fōld\ *vt* : to cover or surround with folds or a covering ⟨~ the hernial sac with sutures⟩ ~ *vi* \'in-,\ : to fold
inward or toward one another ⟨the neural crests ~ and
fuse⟩

in·for·mat·ics \,in-fər-'ma-tiks\ *n pl but sing in constr* : the
collection, classification, storage, retrieval, and dissemination of recorded knowledge — see BIOINFORMATICS

in·formed consent \in-,fȯrmd-\ *n* : consent to surgery by a
patient or to participation in a medical experiment by a subject after achieving an understanding of what is involved

in·for·mo·some \in-'fȯr-mə-,sōm\ *n* : a cellular particle that
is a complex of messenger RNA and protein and is thought
to be the form in which messenger RNA is transported from
the nucleus to the site of protein synthesis in the cytoplasm

in·fra·car·di·ac \,in-frə-'kärd-ē-,ak\ *adj* : situated below the
heart

in·fra·class \'in-frə-,klas\ *n* : a subdivision of a subclass that
is closely equivalent to a superorder

in·fra·cla·vic·u·lar \,in-frə-kla-'vik-yə-lər\ *adj* : situated or
occurring below the clavicle ⟨the radiograph showed an
opacity in the left ~ area of the chest⟩

in·fra·clu·sion \,in-frə-'klü-zhən\ *n* : INFRAOCCLUSION

in·fra·den·ta·le \,in-frə-den-'tā-lē\ *n* : the highest point of
the gum between the two central incisors of the lower jaw

in·fra·di·an \in-'frā-dē-ən\ *adj* : being, characterized by, or
occurring in periods or cycles (as of biological activity) of
less than 24 hours ⟨~ rhythms of growth⟩ — compare CIR-
CADIAN, ULTRADIAN

in·fra·dia·phrag·mat·ic \,in-frə-,dī-ə-frə(g)-'mat-ik, -,frag-\
adj : situated, occurring, or performed below the diaphragm
⟨~ vagotomy⟩ ⟨an ~ abscess⟩

in·fra·gle·noid tubercle \,in-frə-,glē-,nȯid-, -,gle-\ *n* : a tu-

bercle on the scapula for the attachment of the long head of
the triceps muscle

in·fra·glot·tic \,in-frə-'glät-ik\ *adj* : situated below the glottis
⟨~ cancer⟩

¹in·fra·hu·man \,in-frə-'hyü-mən, -'yü-\ *adj* : less or lower
than human; *esp* : ANTHROPOID 1 ⟨~ primate populations⟩

²infrahuman *n* : an animal and esp. a primate that is not human

in·fra·hy·oid \,in-frə-'hī-,ȯid\ *adj* : situated below the hyoid
bone ⟨the fascia of the ~ region⟩

infrahyoid muscle *n* : any of four muscles on each side that
are situated next to the larynx below the hyoid bone and
comprise the sternohyoid, sternothyroid, thyrohyoid, and
omohyoid muscles

in·fra·mam·ma·ry \,in-frə-'mam-ə-rē\ *adj* : situated or occurring below the mammary gland ⟨~ pain⟩

in·fra·man·dib·u·lar \-man-'dib-yə-lər\ *adj* : situated below
the mandible ⟨~ muscles⟩

in·fra·nu·cle·ar \-'n(y)ü-klē-ər\ *adj* : situated below a nucleus of a nerve ⟨an ~ lesion⟩

in·fra·oc·clu·sion \,in-frə-ä-'klü-zhən\ *n* : occlusion in
which one or more teeth fail to project as far as the normal
occlusal plane

in·fra·or·bit·al \,in-frə-'ȯr-bət-ᵊl\ *adj* : situated beneath the
orbit ⟨the ~ prominence of the cheekbones⟩

infraorbital artery *n* : a branch or continuation of the maxillary artery that runs along the infraorbital groove with the
infraorbital nerve and passes through the infraorbital foramen to give off branches which supply the face just below
the eye

infraorbital fissure *n* : ORBITAL FISSURE b

infraorbital foramen *n* : an opening in the maxillary bone
just below the lower rim of the orbit that gives passage to the
infraorbital artery, nerve, and vein

infraorbital groove *n* : a groove in the middle of the posteri-
or part of the bony floor of the orbit that gives passage to the
infraorbital artery, vein, and nerve

infraorbital nerve *n* : a branch of the maxillary nerve that
divides into branches distributed to the skin of the upper
part of the cheek, the upper lip, and the lower eyelid

infraorbital vein *n* : a vein that drains the inferior structures
of the orbit and the adjacent area of the face and that empties into the pterygoid plexus

in·fra·pa·tel·lar \,in-frə-pə-'tel-ər\ *adj* : situated below the
patella or its ligament ⟨the ~ bursa of the knee⟩

¹in·fra·red \,in-frə-'red\ *adj* **1** : lying outside the visible spectrum at its red end — used of radiation having a wavelength
between about 700 nanometers and 1 millimeter **2** : relating to, producing, or employing infrared radiation ⟨~ thera-
py⟩

²infrared *n* : infrared radiation

in·fra·re·nal \,in-frə-'rēn-ᵊl\ *adj* : situated or occurring below the kidneys

in·fra·son·ic \-'sän-ik\ *adj* **1** : having or relating to a frequency below the audibility range of the human ear **2** : utilizing or produced by infrasonic waves or vibrations

in·fra·sound \'in-frə-,saůnd\ *n* : a wave phenomenon of the
same physical nature as sound but with frequencies below
the range of human hearing — compare ULTRASOUND 1

in·fra·spe·cif·ic \,in-frə-spi-'sif-ik\ *adj* : included within a
species ⟨~ categories⟩

in·fra·spi·na·tus \,in-frə-spī-'nāt-əs\ *n, pl* **-na·ti** \-'nā-,tī\ : a
muscle that occupies the chief part of the infraspinous fossa
of the scapula, is inserted into the greater tubercle of the humerus, and rotates the arm laterally

in·fra·spi·nous \,in-frə-'spī-nəs\ *adj* : lying below a spine; *esp*
: lying below the spine of the scapula

infraspinous fossa *n* : the part of the dorsal surface of the
scapula below the spine of the scapula

in·fra·tem·po·ral \ˌin-frə-'tem-p(ə-)rəl\ *adj* : situated below the temporal fossa

infratemporal crest *n* : a transverse ridge on the outer surface of the greater wing of the sphenoid bone that divides it into a superior portion that contributes to the formation of the temporal fossa and an inferior portion that contributes to the formation of the infratemporal fossa

infratemporal fossa *n* : a fossa that is bounded above by the plane of the zygomatic arch, laterally by the ramus of the mandible, and medially by the pterygoid plate, and that contains the masseter and pterygoid muscles and the mandibular nerve

in·fra·ten·to·ri·al \ˌin-frə-ten-'tōr-ē-əl\ *adj* : occurring or made below the tentorium cerebelli 〈an ∼ tumor〉

in·fra·um·bil·i·cal \-ˌəm-'bil-i-kəl *also* -ˌəm-bə-'lī-kəl\ *adj* : situated below the navel

in·fra·ver·sion \ˌin-frə-'vər-zhən\ *n* : INFRAOCCLUSION

infundibula *pl of* INFUNDIBULUM

in·fun·dib·u·lar \ˌin-(ˌ)fən-'dib-yə-lər\ *adj* 1 : INFUNDIBULIFORM 2 : of, relating to, affecting, situated near, or having an infundibulum 〈∼ stenosis〉

infundibular process *n* : NEURAL LOBE

infundibular recess *n* : a funnel-shaped downward prolongation of the floor of the third ventricle of the brain behind the optic chiasma into the infundibulum of the pineal gland

in·fun·dib·u·li·form \-lə-ˌfȯrm\ *adj* : having the form of a funnel or cone

in·fun·dib·u·lo·pel·vic ligament \ˌin-fən-ˌdib-yə-lō-'pel-vik-\ *n* : SUSPENSORY LIGAMENT OF THE OVARY

in·fun·dib·u·lum \ˌin-(ˌ)fən-'dib-yə-ləm\ *n, pl* **-la** \-lə\ : any of various conical or dilated organs or parts: **a** : the hollow conical process of gray matter that is borne on the tuber cinereum and constitutes the stalk of the neurohypophysis by which the pituitary gland is continuous with the brain — called also *neural stalk* **b** : any of the small spaces having walls beset with air sacs in which the bronchial tubes terminate in the lungs **c** : CONUS ARTERIOSUS **d** : the passage by which the anterior ethmoidal air cells and the frontal sinuses communicate with the nose **e** : the abdominal opening of a fallopian tube

in·fuse \in-'fyüz\ *vb* **in·fused; in·fus·ing** *vt* 1 : to steep in liquid (as water) without boiling so as to extract the soluble constituents or principles 2 : to administer or inject by infusion esp. intravenously 〈∼ the blood with glucose〉 〈∼ a solution of lactate〉 ∼ *vi* : to administer a solution by infusion

in·fu·sion \in-'fyü-zhən\ *n* 1 **a** : the introducing of a solution (as of glucose or salt) esp. into a vein; *also* : the solution so used **b** (1) : the steeping or soaking usu. in water of a substance (as a plant drug) in order to extract its soluble constituents or principles — compare DECOCTION 1 (2) : the liquid extract obtained by this process 2 : a watery suspension of decaying organic material 〈culturing soil amebas in lettuce ∼〉

infusion pump *n* : a device that releases a measured amount of a substance in a specific period of time

in·fu·so·ria \ˌin-fyü-'zōr-ē-ə, -'sȯr-\ *n pl, often cap* : organisms that are infusorians — not used technically

in·fu·so·ri·an \-ē-ən\ *n* : any of a heterogeneous group of minute organisms found esp. in water with decomposing organic matter; *esp* : a ciliated protozoan — **infusorian** *adj*

in·gest \in-'jest\ *vt* : to take in for or as if for digestion

in·ges·ta \in-'jes-tə\ *n pl* : material taken into the body by way of the digestive tract

in·ges·tant \-tənt\ *n* : something taken into the body by ingestion; *esp* : an allergen so taken

in·gest·ible \in-'jes-tə-bəl\ *adj* : capable of being ingested 〈∼ capsules〉

in·ges·tion \in-'jes(h)-chən\ *n* : the taking of material (as food) into the digestive system

in·gest·ive \in-'jes-tiv\ *adj* : of or relating to ingestion 〈∼ behavior〉

in·glu·vi·es \in-'glü-vē-ˌēz\ *n, pl* **ingluvies** : CROP

in·glu·vi·itis \in-ˌglü-vē-'īt-əs\ *or* **in·glu·vi·tis** \ˌin-glü-'vīt-əs\ *n* : catarrhal inflammation of the crop in fowls

in·gra·ves·cence \ˌin-grə-'ves-°n(t)s\ *n* : the state of becoming progressively more severe 〈persistence and ∼ of behavior disorders, in spite of improved circumstances —Norman Cameron〉

in·gre·di·ent \in-'grēd-ē-ənt\ *n* : something that enters into a compound or is a component part of any combination or mixture 〈formula which will have just about the same ∼s as mother's milk —Morris Fishbein〉 — **ingredient** *adj*

in·grow·ing \'in-ˌgrō-iŋ\ *adj* : growing or tending inward : INGROWN 〈∼ hairs〉

in·grown \'in-ˌgrōn\ *adj* : grown in; *specif* : having the normally free tip or edge embedded in the flesh 〈an ∼ toenail〉

in·growth \'in-ˌgrōth\ *n* 1 : a growing inward (as to fill a void) 〈∼ of cells〉 2 : something that grows in or into a space 〈lymphoid ∼s〉

in·guen \'iŋ-gwən, -ˌgwen\ *n, pl* **in·gui·na** \-gwə-nə\ : GROIN

in·gui·nal \'iŋ-gwən-°l\ *adj* 1 : of, relating to, or situated in the region of the groin 2 : ILIAC 2 〈the ∼ abdominal region〉 — **in·gui·nal·ly** *adv*

inguinal canal *n* : a passage about one and one half inches (4 centimeters) long that lies parallel to and a half inch above the inguinal ligament: as **a** : a passage in the male through which the testis descends into the scrotum and in which the spermatic cord lies — called also *spermatic canal* **b** : a passage in the female accommodating the round ligament

inguinale — see GRANULOMA INGUINALE, LYMPHOGRANULOMA INGUINALE

inguinal gland *n* : INGUINAL NODE

inguinal hernia *n* : a hernia in which part of the intestine protrudes into the inguinal canal

inguinal ligament *n* : the thickened lower border of the aponeurosis of the external oblique muscle of the abdomen that extends from the anterior superior iliac spine to the pubic tubercle, is continuous with the fascia lata near the thigh, and forms the external pillar of the superficial inguinal ring and a part of the anterior boundary of the femoral ring — called also *Poupart's ligament*

inguinal node *n* : any of the superficial lymphatic nodes of the groin made up of two more or less distinct groups of which one is disposed along the inguinal ligament and the other about the saphenous opening — called also *inguinal gland*

inguinal ring *n* : either of two openings in the fasciae of the abdominal muscles on each side of the body that are the inlet and outlet of the inguinal canal, give passage to the spermatic cord in the male and the round ligament in the female, and are a frequent site of hernia formation : ABDOMINAL RING: **a** : DEEP INGUINAL RING **b** : SUPERFICIAL INGUINAL RING

INH *abbr* isoniazid

¹**in·hal·ant** *also* **in·hal·ent** \in-'hā-lənt\ *n* 1 : something (as an allergen or an anesthetic vapor) that is inhaled 2 : any of various often toxic volatile substances (as spray paint, glue, or paint thinner) whose fumes are sometimes inhaled for their euphoric effect

²**inhalant** *also* **inhalent** *adj* : used for inhaling or constituting an inhalant 〈∼ anesthetics〉

in·ha·la·tion \ˌin-(h)ə-'lā-shən, ˌin-°l-'ā-\ *n* 1 : the act or an instance of inhaling; *specif* : the action of drawing air into the lungs by means of a complex of essentially reflex actions that involve changes in the diaphragm and in muscles of the abdomen and thorax which cause enlargement of the chest cavity and lungs resulting in production of relatively negative pressure within the lungs so that air flows in until the pressure is restored to equality with that of the atmosphere 2 : material (as medication) to be taken in by inhaling — **in·ha·la·tion·al** \-shnəl, -shən-°l\ *adj*

inhalation therapist *n* : a specialist in inhalation therapy

inhalation therapy *n* : the therapeutic use of inhaled gases and esp. oxygen (as in the treatment of respiratory disease)

in·ha·la·tor \'in-(h)ə-ˌlāt-ər, 'in-°l-ˌāt-\ *n* : a device providing a mixture of oxygen and carbon dioxide for breathing that is used esp. in conjunction with artificial respiration — compare INHALER

in·hale \in-ˈhā(ə)l\ *vb* **in·haled; in·hal·ing** *vt* : to draw in by breathing ∼ *vi* : to breathe in

inhalent *var of* INHALANT

in·hal·er \in-ˈhā-lər\ *n* : a device by means of which usu. medicinal material is inhaled — compare INHALATOR

in·her·ent \in-ˈhir-ənt, in-ˈher-\ *adj* : involved in the constitution or essential character of something : belonging by nature ⟨the skin's ∼ elasticity —Kathleen C. Engles⟩ — **in·her·ent·ly** *adv*

in·her·it \in-ˈher-ət\ *vt* : to receive from a parent or ancestor by genetic transmission

in·her·it·able \in-ˈher-ə-bəl\ *adj* : capable of being transmitted from parent to offspring genetically — **in·her·it·abil·i·ty** \-ˌher-ət-ə-ˈbil-ət-ē\ *n, pl* **-ties**

in·her·i·tance \in-ˈher-ət-ən(t)s\ *n* **1** : the reception of genetic qualities by transmission from parent to offspring **2** : all of the genetic characters or qualities transmitted from parent to offspring — compare GENOTYPE 2, PHENOTYPE

in·hib·in \in-ˈhib-ən\ *n* : a glycoprotein hormone that is secreted by the pituitary gland and in the male by the Sertoli cells and in the female by the granulosa cells and that inhibits the secretion of follicle-stimulating hormone

in·hib·it \in-ˈhib-ət\ *vt* **1 a** : to restrain from free or spontaneous activity esp. through the operation of inner psychological or external social constraints ⟨an ∼*ed* person⟩ **b** : to check or restrain the force or vitality of ⟨∼ aggressive tendencies⟩ **2 a** : to reduce or suppress the activity of ⟨a presynaptic neuron can not only excite a postsynaptic neuron but can also ∼ it —H. W. Kendler⟩ **b** : to retard or prevent the formation of **c** : to retard, interfere with, or prevent (a process or reaction) ⟨∼ ovulation⟩

in·hib·it·able \-ə-bəl\ *adj* : capable of being inhibited

in·hi·bi·tion \ˌin-(h)ə-ˈbish-ən\ *n* : the act or an instance of inhibiting or the state of being inhibited: as **a** (1) : a stopping or checking of a bodily action : a restraining of the function of an organ or an agent (as a digestive fluid or enzyme) ⟨∼ of the heartbeat by stimulation of the vagus nerve⟩ ⟨∼ of plantar reflexes⟩ (2) : interference with or retardation or prevention of a process or activity ⟨∼ of bacterial growth⟩ **b** (1) : a desirable restraint or check upon the free or spontaneous instincts or impulses of an individual guided or directed by the social and cultural forces of the environment ⟨the self-control so developed is called ∼ —C. W. Russell⟩ (2) : a neurotic restraint upon a normal or beneficial impulse or activity caused by psychological inner conflicts or by sociocultural forces of the environment ⟨other outspoken neurotic manifestations are general ∼*s* such as inability to think, to concentrate —Muriel Ivimey⟩ ⟨∼*s*, phobias, compulsions, and other neurotic patterns —*Psychological Abstracts*⟩

in·hib·i·tor \in-ˈhib-ət-ər\ *n* : one that inhibits: as **a** : an agent that slows or interferes with a chemical reaction **b** : a substance that reduces the activity of another substance (as an enzyme) **c** : a gene that checks the normal effect of another nonallelic gene when both are present

in·hib·i·to·ry \in-ˈhib-ə-ˌtōr-ē, -ˌtor-\ *adj* : of, relating to, or producing inhibition : tending or serving to inhibit

inhibitory postsynaptic potential *n* : increased negativity of the membrane potential of a neuron on the postsynaptic side of a nerve synapse that is caused by a neurotransmitter (as gamma-aminobutyric acid) which renders the membrane selectively permeable to potassium and chloride ions on the inside but not to sodium ions on the outside and that tends to inhibit the neuron since an added increase in potential in the positive direction is needed for excitation — abbr. IPSP

in·ho·mo·ge·ne·ity \ˌin-ˌhō-mə-jə-ˈnē-ət-ē, -ˈnā-; *esp Brit* -ˌhäm-ə-\ *n, pl* **-ities** : lack of homogeneity — **in·ho·mo·ge·neous** \ˌin-ˌhō-mə-ˈjē-nē-əs\ *adj*

in·i·ac \ˈin-ē-ˌak\ *adj* : relating to the inion

in·i·en·ceph·a·lus \ˌin-ē-in-ˈsef-ə-ləs\ *n* : a teratological fetus with a fissure in the occiput through which the brain protrudes — **in·i·en·ce·phal·ic** \ˌin-ē-ˌen-sə-ˈfal-ik\ *adj*

in·i·en·ceph·a·ly \-ˈsef-ə-lē\ *n, pl* **-lies** : the condition of being an iniencephalus

in·i·on \ˈin-ē-ˌän, -ən\ *n* : OCCIPITAL PROTUBERANCE a

ini·ti·a·tion codon \in-ˌish-ē-ˈā-shən-\ *n* : a codon that stimulates the binding of a transfer RNA which starts protein synthesis — called also *initiator codon;* compare TERMINATOR

ini·ti·a·tor \in-ˈish-ē-ˌāt-ər\ *n* : one that initiates: as **a** : a substance that initiates a chemical reaction **b** : a substance that produces an irreversible change in bodily tissue causing it to respond to other substances which promote the growth of tumors

inj *abbr* injection

in·ject \in-ˈjekt\ *vt* **1** : to force a fluid into (a vessel, cavity, or tissue) for preserving, hardening, or coloring structures **2** : to introduce (as by injection or gravity flow) a fluid into (a living body) esp. for the purpose of restoring fluid balance, treating nutritional deficiencies or disease, or relieving pain; *also* : to treat (an individual) with injections

¹**in·ject·able** \-ˈjek-tə-bəl\ *adj* : capable of being injected ⟨∼ medications⟩

²**injectable** *n* : an injectable substance (as a drug)

in·jec·tant \-ˈjek-tənt\ *n* : an allergen that is injected

injected *adj* : CONGESTED ⟨the tonsils were hypertrophied and ∼ —*Jour. Amer. Med. Assoc.*⟩

in·jec·tion \in-ˈjek-shən\ *n* **1 a** : the act or an instance of injecting a drug or other substance into the body **b** : a solution (as of a drug) intended for injection (as by catheter or hypodermic syringe) either under or through the skin or into the tissues, a vein, or a body cavity **c** : an act or process of injecting vessels or tissues; *also* : a specimen prepared by injection **2** : the state of being injected : CONGESTION — see CIRCUMCORNEAL INJECTION

in·jec·tor \in-ˈjek-tər\ *n* : a device for injecting or making an injection

in·jure \ˈin-jər\ *vt* **in·jured; in·jur·ing** \ˈinj-(ə-)riŋ\ **1** : to inflict bodily hurt on **2** : to impair the soundness of ⟨∼ your health⟩

in·ju·ri·ous \in-ˈjùr-ē-əs\ *adj* : inflicting or tending to inflict injury ⟨∼ to health⟩ — **in·ju·ri·ous·ly** *adv*

in·ju·ry \ˈinj-(ə-)rē\ *n, pl* **-ries** : hurt, damage, or loss sustained

injury potential *n* : the difference in electrical potential between the injured and uninjured parts of a nerve or muscle — called also *demarcation potential*

ink·blot \ˈiŋk-ˌblät\ *n* : any of several plates showing blots of ink for use in psychological testing

inkblot test *n* : any of several psychological tests (as a Rorschach test) based on the interpretation of irregular figures (as blots of ink)

in·lay \ˈin-ˌlā\ *n* **1** : a tooth filling shaped to fit a cavity and then cemented into place **2** : a piece of tissue (as bone) laid into the site of missing tissue to cover a defect

in·let \ˈin-ˌlet, -lət\ *n* : the upper opening of a bodily cavity; *esp* : that of the cavity of the true pelvis bounded by the pelvic brim

in·mate \ˈin-ˌmāt\ *n* : one of a group occupying a single place of residence; *esp* : a person confined (as in a psychiatric hospital) esp. for a long time

in·nards \ˈin-ərdz\ *n pl* : the internal organs of a human being or animal; *esp* : VISCERA

in·nate \in-ˈāt, ˈin-ˌ\ *adj* : existing in, belonging to, or determined by factors present in an individual from birth : NATIVE, INBORN ⟨∼ behavior⟩ — **in·nate·ly** *adv* — **in·nate·ness** *n*

in·ner cell mass \ˌin-ər-\ *n* : the portion of the blastocyst of a mammalian embryo that is destined to become the embryo proper

in·ner–di·rect·ed \ˌin-ər-də-ˈrek-təd, -(ˌ)dī-\ *adj* : directed in

\ə\ abut \ᵊ\ kitten \ər\ further \a\ ash \ā\ ace \ä\ cot, cart \aù\ out \ch\ chin \e\ bet \ē\ easy \g\ go \i\ hit \ī\ ice \j\ job \ŋ\ sing \ō\ go \ò\ law \òi\ boy \th\ thin \t̲h̲\ the \ü\ loot \ù\ foot \y\ yet \zh\ vision   See also Pronunciation Symbols page

thought and action by one's own scale of values as opposed to external norms — compare OTHER-DIRECTED — **in·ner–di·rec·tion** \-'rek-shən\ *n*

inner ear *n* : the essential part of the vertebrate organ of hearing and equilibrium that typically is located in the temporal bone, is innervated by the auditory nerve, and includes the vestibule, the semicircular canals, and the cochlea — called also *internal ear*

in·ner·vate \in-'ər-ˌvāt, 'in-(ˌ)ər-\ *vt* **-vat·ed; -vat·ing** 1 : to supply with nerves 2 : to arouse or stimulate (a nerve or an organ) to activity

in·ner·va·tion \ˌin-(ˌ)ər-'vā-shən, in-ˌər-\ *n* 1 : the process of innervating or the state of being innervated; *esp* : the nervous excitation necessary for the maintenance of the life and functions of the various organs 2 : the distribution of nerves to or in a part — **in·ner·va·tion·al** \-shnəl, -shən-ᵊl\ *adj*

in·no·cent \'in-ə-sənt\ *adj* : lacking capacity to injure : BENIGN ⟨an ∼ tumor⟩ ⟨∼ heart murmurs⟩

in·noc·u·ous \in-'äk-yə-wəs\ *adj* : producing no injury : not harmful — **in·noc·u·ous·ly** *adv*

innominata — see SUBSTANTIA INNOMINATA

in·nom·i·nate artery \in-'äm-ə-nət-\ *n* : BRACHIOCEPHALIC ARTERY

innominate bone *n* : HIP BONE

innominate vein *n* : BRACHIOCEPHALIC VEIN

in·nox·ious \'i(n)-'näk-shəs\ *adj* : INNOCUOUS ⟨an ∼ substance⟩

in·oc·u·la·ble \in-'äk-yə-lə-bəl\ *adj* : susceptible to inoculation : not immune; *also* : transmissible by inoculation ⟨an ∼ disease⟩ — **in·oc·u·la·bil·i·ty** \in-ˌäk-yə-lə-'bil-ət-ē\ *n, pl* **-ties**

in·oc·u·lant \in-'äk-yə-lənt\ *n* : INOCULUM

in·oc·u·late \in-'äk-yə-ˌlāt\ *vb* **-lat·ed; -lat·ing** *vt* 1 : to communicate a disease to (an organism) by inserting its causative agent into the body ⟨12 mice *inoculated* with anthrax⟩ 2 a : to introduce microorganisms or viruses onto or into (an organism, substrate, or culture medium) ⟨*inoculated* a rat with bacteria⟩ b : to introduce (as a microorganism or antiserum) into an organism or onto a culture medium ⟨∼ a pure culture of bacteria into a healthy host⟩ 3 : to introduce immunologically active material (as an antibody or antigen) into esp. in order to treat or prevent a disease ⟨∼ children against diphtheria⟩ ∼ *vi* : to introduce microorganisms, vaccines, or sera by inoculation

in·oc·u·la·tion \in-ˌäk-yə-'lā-shən\ *n* 1 : the act or process or an instance of inoculating: as a : the introduction of a microorganism into a medium suitable for its growth b (1) : the introduction of a pathogen or antigen into a living organism to stimulate the production of antibodies (2) : the introduction of a vaccine or serum into a living organism to confer immunity ⟨travelers in the tropics should have typhoid ∼s⟩ 2 : INOCULUM

in·oc·u·la·tor \in-'äk-yə-ˌlāt-ər\ *n* : one that inoculates

in·oc·u·lum \in-'äk-yə-ləm\ *n, pl* **-la** \-lə\ : material used for inoculation

ino·gen \'in-ə-ˌjen\ *n* : a hypothetical substance formerly supposed to be continually decomposed and reproduced in the muscles and to serve as an oxygen reserve

in·op·er·a·ble \(')in-'äp-(ə-)rə-bəl\ *adj* : not treatable or remediable by or suitable for surgery ⟨an advanced and ∼ cancer⟩ ⟨a developing cataract still ∼⟩ — **in·op·er·a·bil·i·ty** \(ˌ)in-ˌäp-(ə-)rə-'bil-ət-ē\ *n, pl* **-ties**

in·or·gan·ic \ˌin-ˌór-'gan-ik\ *adj* 1 a : being or composed of matter other than plant or animal ⟨an ∼ heart⟩ b : forming or belonging to the inanimate world 2 : of, relating to, or dealt with by a branch of chemistry concerned with substances not usu. classified as organic — **in·or·gan·i·cal·ly** \-i-k(ə-)lē\ *adv*

in·or·gas·mic \ˌin-ór-'gaz-mik\ *adj* : not experiencing or having experienced orgasm ⟨sex therapy for ∼ women⟩

in·os·cu·la·tion \(ˌ)in-ˌäs-kyə-'lā-shən\ *n* : ANASTOMOSIS 1a

ino·se·mia *or chiefly Brit* **ino·sae·mia** \ˌin-ō-'sē-mē-ə\ *n* : the presence of inositol in the blood

ino·sin·ate \in-'ō-sin-ˌāt\ *n* : a salt or ester of inosinic acid

ino·sine \'in-ə-ˌsēn, 'ī-nə-\ *n* : a crystalline nucleoside $C_{10}H_{12}N_4O_5$ formed by partial hydrolysis of inosinic acid or by deamination of adenosine and yielding hypoxanthine and ribose on hydrolysis

ino·sin·ic acid \ˌin-ə-ˌsin-ik-, ˌī-nə-\ *n* : a nucleotide $C_{10}H_{13}N_4O_8P$ that is found in muscle and is formed by deamination of AMP and that yields hypoxanthine, ribose, and phosphoric acid on hydrolysis — called also *IMP*

ino·si·tol \in-'ō-sə-ˌtól, ī-'nō-, -ˌtōl\ *n* : any of several crystalline stereoisomeric cyclic alcohols $C_6H_{12}O_6$; *esp* : MYOINOSITOL

ino·tro·pic \ˌē-nə-'trō-pik, ˌī-nə-, -'träp-ik\ *adj* : relating to or influencing the force of muscular contractions ⟨digitalis is a positive ∼ agent⟩

ino·tro·pism \ˌē-nə-'trō-ˌpiz-əm, ˌī-nə-; i-'nä-trə-ˌpiz-əm\ *n* : modification of muscular contractility

in ovo \in-'ō-(ˌ)vō\ *adv* : in the egg : in embryo

in·pa·tient \'in-ˌpā-shənt\ *n* : a hospital patient who receives lodging and food as well as treatment — compare OUTPATIENT

in·quest \'in-ˌkwest\ *n* : a judicial or official inquiry esp. before a jury to determine the cause of a violent or unexpected death ⟨a coroner's ∼⟩

in·qui·line \'in-kwə-ˌlīn, 'in-, -lən\ *n* : an animal (as the house mouse) that lives habitually in the nest or abode (as a human dwelling) of some other species — **in·qui·lin·ism** \-lə-ˌniz-əm\ *n*

in·sal·i·va·tion \in-ˌsal-ə-'vā-shən\ *n* : the mixing of food with saliva by mastication — **in·sal·i·vate** \in-'sal-ə-ˌvāt\ *vt* **-vat·ed; -vat·ing**

in·sa·lu·bri·ous \ˌin(t)-sə-'lü-brē-əs\ *adj* : not conducive to health : not wholesome ⟨an ∼ climate⟩

in·sane \(')in-'sān\ *adj* 1 : mentally disordered : exhibiting insanity 2 : used by, typical of, or intended for insane persons ⟨an ∼ asylum⟩ — **in·sane·ly** *adv*

insane root *n* 1 : a root believed in medieval times to cause madness in those eating it and usu. identified with either henbane or hemlock 2 : HENBANE

in·san·i·tary \(')in-'san-ə-ˌter-ē\ *adj* : unclean enough to endanger health

in·san·i·ty \in-'san-ət-ē\ *n, pl* **-ties** 1 : a severely disordered state of the mind usu. occurring as a specific disorder (as paranoid schizophrenia) 2 : unsoundness of mind or lack of the ability to understand that prevents one from having the mental capacity required by law to enter into a particular relationship, status, or transaction or that releases one from criminal or civil responsibility

in·scrip·tion \in-'skrip-shən\ *n* : the part of a medical prescription that contains the names and quantities of the drugs to be compounded

in·sect \'in-ˌsekt\ *n* : any arthropod of the class Insecta — **insect** *adj*

In·sec·ta \in-'sek-tə\ *n pl* : a class of Arthropoda comprising segmented animals that as adults have a well-defined head bearing a single pair of antennae, three pairs of mouthparts, and usu. a pair of compound eyes, a 3-segmented thorax each segment of which bears a pair of legs ventrally with the second and third often bearing also a pair of wings, and an abdomen usu. of 7 to 10 visible segments without true jointed legs but often with the last segments modified or fitted with specialized extensions (as claspers, stingers, or ovipositors), that breathe air usu. through a ramifying system of tracheae which open externally through spiracles or gills, that exhibit a variety of life cycles often involving complex metamorphosis, and that include the greater part of all living and extinct animals — **in·sec·tan** \-tən\ *adj*

in·sec·ti·cide \in-'sek-tə-ˌsīd\ *n* : an agent that destroys insects — **in·sec·ti·cid·al** \(ˌ)in-ˌsek-tə-'sīd-ᵊl\ *adj*

in·sec·ti·fuge \-tə-ˌfyüj\ *n* : an insect repellent

In·sec·tiv·o·ra \ˌin-ˌsek-'tiv-ə-rə\ *n pl* : an order of mammals comprising the moles, shrews, hedgehogs, and certain related forms that are mostly small, insectivorous, terrestrial or fossorial, and nocturnal

in·sec·ti·vore \in-'sek-tə-ˌvō(ə)r, -ˌvȯ(ə)r\ *n* **1** : any mammal of the order Insectivora **2** : an insectivorous plant or animal

in·sec·tiv·o·rous \ˌin-ˌsek-'tiv-(ə-)rəs\ *adj* : depending on insects as food

in·se·cure \ˌin(t)-si-'kyu̇(ə)r\ *adj* : characterized by or causing emotional insecurity ⟨an ∼ childhood⟩

in·se·cu·ri·ty \-'kyu̇r-ət-ē\ *n, pl* **-ties** : a feeling of apprehensiveness and uncertainty : lack of assurance or stability

in·sem·i·nate \in-'sem-ə-ˌnāt\ *vt* **-nat·ed; -nat·ing** : to introduce semen into the genital tract of (a female) — **in·sem·i·na·tion** \-ˌsem-ə-'nā-shən\ *n*

in·sem·i·na·tor \-ˌnāt-ər\ *n* : one that inseminates cattle artificially

in·sen·sate \(')in-'sen-ˌsāt, -sət\ *adj* : devoid of sensation or feeling ⟨ulcers developed in the ∼ foot⟩

in·sen·si·ble \-'sen(t)-sə-bəl\ *adj* **1** : incapable or bereft of feeling or sensation: as **a** : UNCONSCIOUS ⟨knocked ∼ by a sudden blow⟩ **b** : lacking sensory perception or ability to react ⟨∼ to pain⟩ **c** : lacking emotional response : APATHETIC **2** : not perceived by the senses ⟨∼ perspiration⟩ — **in·sen·si·bil·i·ty** \(ˌ)in-ˌsen(t)-sə-'bil-ət-ē\ *n, pl* **-ties**

in·sert \in-'sərt\ *vi, of a muscle* : to be in attachment to the part to be moved

inserted *adj* : attached by natural growth (as a muscle or tendon)

in·ser·tion \in-'sər-shən\ *n* **1** : the part of a muscle by which it is attached to the part to be moved — compare ORIGIN 2 **2** : the mode or place of attachment of an organ or part **3 a** : a section of genetic material inserted into an existing gene sequence **b** : the mutational process producing a genetic insertion — **in·ser·tion·al** \-shnəl, -shən-ᵊl\ *adj*

in·sid·i·ous \in-'sid-ē-əs\ *adj* : developing so gradually as to be well established before becoming apparent ⟨an ∼ disease⟩ — **in·sid·i·ous·ly** *adv*

in·sight \'in-ˌsīt\ *n* **1** : understanding or awareness of one's mental or emotional condition; *esp* : recognition that one is mentally ill **2** : immediate and clear understanding (as seeing the solution to a problem or the means to reaching a goal) that takes place without recourse to overt trial-and-error behavior

in·sight·ful \'in-ˌsīt-fəl, in-'\ *adj* : exhibiting or characterized by insight ⟨∼ behavior⟩ — **in·sight·ful·ly** *adv*

insipidus — see CENTRAL DIABETES INSIPIDUS, DIABETES INSIPIDUS, NEPHROGENIC DIABETES INSIPIDUS

in si·tu \(')in-'sī-(ˌ)t(y)ü, -'sē-, -ˌsi- *also* -'si- -(ˌ)chü\ *adv or adj* : in the natural or original position or place ⟨an *in situ* cancer confined to the breast duct⟩ — see CARCINOMA IN SITU

in·so·la·tion \ˌin(t)-(ˌ)sō-'lā-shən, in-ˌsō-\ *n* **1** : exposure to the rays of the sun **2** : SUNSTROKE

in·sol·u·ble \(')in-'säl-yə-bəl\ *adj* : incapable of being dissolved in a liquid; *also* : soluble only with difficulty or to a slight degree

in·som·nia \in-'säm-nē-ə\ *n* : prolonged and usu. abnormal inability to obtain adequate sleep — called also *agrypnia*

¹**in·som·ni·ac** \-nē-ˌak\ *n* : one affected with insomnia

²**insomniac** *adj* : affected with insomnia ⟨an ∼ patient⟩

in·spec·tion \in-'spek-shən\ *n* : visual observation of the body in the course of a medical examination — compare PALPATION 2 — **in·spect** \in-'spekt\ *vb*

in·spi·ra·tion \ˌin(t)-spə-'rā-shən, -(ˌ)spir-'ā-\ *n* : the drawing of air into the lungs

in·spi·ra·tor \'in(t)s-pə-ˌrāt-ər, -(ˌ)pir-ˌāt-\ *n* : a device (as an injector or respirator) by which something (as gas or vapor) is drawn in

in·spi·ra·to·ry \in-'spī-rə-ˌtōr-ē, 'in(t)-sp(ə-)rə-, -ˌtȯr-\ *adj* : of, relating to, used for, or associated with inspiration ⟨∼ muscles⟩ ⟨the ∼ whoop of whooping cough⟩

inspiratory capacity *n* : the total amount of air that can be drawn into the lungs after normal expiration

inspiratory reserve volume *n* : the maximal amount of additional air that can be drawn into the lungs by determined effort after normal inspiration — compare EXPIRATORY RESERVE VOLUME

in·spire \in-'spī(ə)r\ *vb* **in·spired; in·spir·ing** *vt* : to draw in

by breathing : breathe in : INHALE ⟨the volume of air *inspired*⟩ ∼ *vi* : to draw in breath : inhale air into the lungs

in·spi·rom·e·ter \ˌin(t)-spə-'räm-ət-ər\ *n* : an apparatus for measuring air inspired in breathing

in·spis·sat·ed \in-'spis-ˌāt-əd, 'in(t)-spə-ˌsāt-\ *adj* : thick or thickened in consistency ⟨blocked with ∼ bile⟩ ⟨the ∼ juices of an aloe⟩ — **in·spis·sa·tion** \ˌin(t)-spə-'sā-shən, (ˌ)in-ˌspis-'ā-\ *n*

in·spis·sa·tor \in-'spis-ˌāt-ər, 'in(t)-spə-ˌsāt-ər\ *n* : an apparatus for thickening fluids (as blood)

in·sta·bil·i·ty \ˌin(t)-stə-'bil-ət-ē\ *n, pl* **-ties** : the quality or state of being unstable; *esp* : lack of emotional or mental stability

in·star \'in-ˌstär\ *n* : a stage in the life of an arthropod (as an insect) between two successive molts; *also* : an individual in a specified instar

in·step \'in-ˌstep\ *n* : the arched middle portion of the human foot in front of the ankle joint; *esp* : its upper surface

in·still \in-'stil\ *vt* **in·stilled; in·still·ing** : to cause to enter esp. drop by drop ⟨∼ medication into the infected eye⟩

in·stil·la·tion \ˌin(t)-stə-'lā-shən, -(ˌ)stil-'ā-\ *n* **1** : an act of instilling : introduction by instilling ⟨repeated ∼ of penicillin⟩ **2** : something that is instilled or designed for instillation ⟨silver ∼ for use in the eyes of the newborn⟩

in·stinct \'in-ˌstiŋ(k)t\ *n* **1** : a largely inheritable and unalterable tendency of an organism to make a complex and specific response to environmental stimuli without involving reason **2** : behavior that is mediated by reactions below the conscious level

in·stinc·tive \in-'stiŋ(k)-tiv\ *adj* **1** : of, relating to, or being instinct **2** : derived from or prompted by instinct ⟨an ∼ fear⟩ — **in·stinc·tive·ly** *adv*

in·stinc·tiv·ist \-tiv-əst\ *n* : a person who views human behavior and social adaptation as the resultant of the interplay of various instinctive drives (as for survival) with environmental factors (as group relations) — **instinctivist** *or* **in·stinc·tiv·ist·ic** \in-ˌstiŋ(k)-tiv-'ist-ik\ *adj*

in·stinc·tu·al \in-'stiŋ(k)-chə(-wə)l, -'stiŋ(k)sh-wəl\ *adj* : of, relating to, or based on instincts ⟨∼ behavior⟩ ⟨the ∼ society of social insects⟩

in·sti·tu·tion·al·ize *or chiefly Brit* **in·sti·tu·tion·al·ise** \ˌin(t)-stə-'t(y)ü-shnəl-ˌīz, -shən-ᵊl-\ *vt* **-ized** *or chiefly Brit* **-ised; -iz·ing** *or chiefly Brit* **-is·ing** **1** : to place in or commit to an institution (as a nursing home or hospital) offering specialized care (as for mental illness, substance abuse, or terminal illness) **2** : to accustom (a person) so firmly to the care and supervised routine of an institution as to make incapable of managing a life outside — **in·sti·tu·tion·al·iza·tion** *or chiefly Brit* **in·sti·tu·tion·al·isa·tion** \-ˌt(y)ü-shnəl-ə-'zā-shən, -ˌt(y)ü-shən-ᵊl-\ *n*

in·stru·ment \'in(t)-strə-mənt\ *n* : any implement, tool, or utensil (as for surgery)

in·stru·men·tal \ˌin(t)-strə-'ment-ᵊl\ *adj* : OPERANT ⟨∼ learning⟩ ⟨∼ conditioning⟩

in·stru·men·tar·i·um \ˌin(t)-strə-mən-'tar-ē-əm, -ˌmen-\ *n, pl* **-tar·ia** \-ē-ə\ : the equipment needed for a particular surgical, medical, or dental procedure; *also* : the professional instruments of a surgeon, physician, or dentist

in·stru·men·ta·tion \ˌin(t)-strə-mən-'tā-shən, -ˌmen-\ *n* : a use of or operation with instruments; *esp* : the use of one or more instruments in treating a patient (as in the passing of a cystoscope)

in·suf·fi·cien·cy \ˌin(t)-sə-'fish-ən-sē\ *n, pl* **-cies** : the quality or state of not being sufficient: as **a** : lack of adequate supply of something ⟨an ∼ of vitamins⟩ **b** : lack of physical power or capacity; *esp* : inability of an organ or bodily part to function normally ⟨renal ∼⟩ ⟨pulmonary ∼⟩ — compare AORTIC REGURGITATION — **in·suf·fi·cient** \-ənt\ *adj*

in·suf·fla·tion \ˌin(t)-sə-'flā-shən, in-ˌsəf-'lā-\ *n* : the act of

\ə\ abut \ᵊ\ kitten \ər\ further \a\ ash \ā\ ace \ä\ cot, cart
\au̇\ out \ch\ chin \e\ bet \ē\ easy \g\ go \i\ hit \ī\ ice \j\ job
\ŋ\ sing \ō\ go \ȯ\ law \ȯi\ boy \th\ thin \t͟h\ the \ü\ loot
\u̇\ foot \y\ yet \zh\ vision *See also* Pronunciation Symbols page

blowing something (as a gas, powder, or vapor) into a body cavity ⟨∼ of gas into a fallopian tube to determine its patency⟩ — **in·suf·flate** \'in(t)-sə-ˌflāt, in-'səf-ˌlāt\ vt

in·suf·fla·tor \'in(t)-sə-ˌflāt-ər, in-'səf-ˌlāt-ər\ n : a device used in medical insufflation (as of a drug)

in·su·la \'in(t)s-(y)ə-lə, 'in-shə-lə\ n, pl **in·su·lae** \-ˌlē, -ˌlī\ : the lobe in the center of the cerebral hemisphere that is situated deeply between the lips of the sylvian fissure — called also *central lobe, island of Reil*

in·su·lar \-lər\ adj : of or relating to an island of cells or tissue (as the islets of Langerhans or the insula)

in·su·la·tion \ˌin(t)-sə-'lā-shən\ n **1** : the action of separating a conductor from conducting bodies by means of nonconductors so as to prevent transfer of electricity, heat, or sound; *also* : the state resulting from such action **2** : material used to provide insulation — **in·su·late** \'in(t)-sə-ˌlāt\ vt **-lat·ed; -lat·ing**

in·su·la·tor \'in(t)-sə-ˌlāt-ər\ n : a material that is used to provide insulation; *also* : a device made of such material

in·su·lin \'in(t)-s(ə-)lən\ n : a protein hormone that is synthesized in the pancreas from proinsulin and secreted by the beta cells of the islets of Langerhans, that is essential for the metabolism of carbohydrates, lipids, and proteins, that regulates blood sugar levels by facilitating the uptake of glucose into tissues, by promoting its conversion into glycogen, fatty acids, and triglycerides, and by reducing the release of glucose from the liver, and that when produced in insufficient quantities results in diabetes mellitus — see ILETIN

in·su·lin·ase \-ˌās, -ˌāz\ n : an enzyme found esp. in liver that inactivates insulin

insulin coma therapy n : INSULIN SHOCK THERAPY

insulin–dependent diabetes n : TYPE 1 DIABETES

insulin–dependent diabetes mellitus n : TYPE 1 DIABETES — abbr. *IDDM*

in·su·lin·emia or chiefly Brit **in·su·lin·ae·mia** \ˌin(t)-s(ə-)lə-'nē-mē-ə\ n : the presence of an abnormally high concentration of insulin in the blood

in·su·lin–like growth factor \ˌin(t)-s(ə-)lən-ˌlīk-\ n : either of two polypeptides structurally similar to insulin that are secreted either during fetal development or during childhood and that mediate growth hormone activity; *esp* : INSULIN= LIKE GROWTH FACTOR 1

insulin–like growth factor 1 \-'wən\ n : the juvenile form of insulin-like growth factor that produced chiefly by the liver in response to growth hormone with production declining after puberty — abbr. *IGF-1*

in·su·li·no·gen·ic \ˌin(t)-s(ə-)lin-ə-'jen-ik\ adj : of, relating to, or stimulating the production of insulin

in·su·lin·oid \'in(t)-s(ə-)lə-ˌnȯid\ n : any hypoglycemic substance having properties like those of insulin

in·su·lin·o·ma \ˌin(t)-s(ə-)lə-'nō-mə\ n, pl **-mas** also **-ma·ta** \-mət-ə\ : a usu. benign insulin-secreting tumor of the islets of Langerhans

in·su·li·no·tro·pic \ˌin(t)-s(ə-)lin-ə-'trō-pik, -'trä-\ adj : stimulating or affecting the production and activity of insulin ⟨an ∼ hormone⟩

insulin resistance n : reduced sensitivity to insulin by the body's insulin-dependent processes (as glucose uptake, lipolysis, and inhibition of glucose production by the liver) that results in lowered activity of these processes or an increase in insulin production or both and that is typical of type 2 diabetes but often occurs in the absence of diabetes

insulin resistance syndrome n : METABOLIC SYNDROME

insulin shock n : severe hypoglycemia that is associated with the presence of excessive insulin in the system and that if left untreated may result in convulsions and progressive development of coma

insulin shock therapy n : the treatment of mental disorder (as schizophrenia) by insulin in doses sufficient to produce deep coma — called also *insulin coma therapy;* compare IN-SULIN SHOCK

insulin zinc suspension n : a suspension of insulin for injection in a buffered solution containing zinc chloride in which forms of insulin which are relatively slowly and rapidly ab-

sorbed are in the approximate ratio of 3:7 — called also *Lente insulin*

in·su·li·tis \ˌin(t)-sə-'līt-əs\ n : invasion of the pancreatic islets of Langerhans by lymphocytes that produces an inflammatory or autoimmune response and results in destruction of the beta cells of the pancreas

in·su·lo·ma \ˌin(t)-sə-'lō-mə\ n, pl **-mas** also **-ma·ta** \-mət-ə\ : INSULINOMA

in·sult \'in-ˌsəlt\ n **1** : injury to the body or one of its parts ⟨repeated acute vascular ∼s⟩ ⟨any ∼ to the constitution of a patient suffering from active tuberculosis —*Jour. Amer. Med. Assoc.*⟩ **2** : something that causes or has a potential for causing insult to the body ⟨damage resulting from malnutritional ∼s⟩ — **insult** vb

in·sus·cep·ti·ble \ˌin(t)-sə-'sep-tə-bəl\ adj : not susceptible ⟨∼ to disease⟩ — **in·sus·cep·ti·bil·i·ty** \-ˌsep-tə-'bil-ət-ē\ n, pl **-ties**

in·tact \in-'takt\ adj **1** : physically and functionally complete ⟨the sense of touch was ∼⟩ ⟨∼ cell membranes⟩ : as **a** : physically virginal ⟨when ∼ adult females were brought into heat —*Anatomical Record*⟩ **b** : not castrated — used chiefly of a domestic animal ⟨the medication may cause severe problems for ∼ female cats⟩ **2** : mentally unimpaired — **in·tact·ness** n

in·take \'in-ˌtāk\ n **1** : the act or process of taking in ⟨∼ and exhalation of gases⟩ **2** : the amount taken in ⟨reduce fluid ∼ to four cups daily —D. R. Zimmerman⟩

In·tal \'in-ˌtal\ trademark — used for a preparation of cromolyn sodium

in·te·grate \'int-ə-ˌgrāt\ vt **-grat·ed; -grat·ing** : to form or blend into a unified whole : cause to undergo integration ⟨an *integrated* personality⟩ — **in·te·gra·tor** \-ˌgrāt-ər\ n

in·te·gra·tion \ˌint-ə-'grā-shən\ n : the combining and coordinating of separate parts or elements into a unified whole: as **a** : coordination of mental processes into a normal effective personality or with the individual's environment ⟨failure of association and failure of ∼ take place among neurotic individuals —R. M. Dorcus & G. W. Shaffer⟩ **b** : the process by which the different parts of an organism are made a functional and structural whole esp. through the activity of the nervous system and of hormones

in·te·gra·tive \'int-ə-ˌgrāt-iv\ adj : tending to integrate ⟨the ∼ action of the nervous system⟩

integrative medicine n : medicine that integrates the therapies of alternative medicine with those practiced by mainstream medical practitioners

in·te·grin \'int-ə-grən\ n : any of various glycoproteins that are found on cell surfaces (as of white blood cells or platelets), that are composed of two dissimilar polypeptide chains, that are receptors for various proteins which typically bind to the tripeptide ligand consisting of arginine, glycine, and aspartic acid, that promote adhesion of cells (as T cells) to other cells (as endothelial cells) or to extracellular material (as fibronectin or laminin), and that mediate various biological processes (as phagocytosis, wound healing, and embryogenesis)

in·teg·ri·ty \in-'teg-rət-ē\ n, pl **-ties** : an unimpaired condition ⟨personality function depends greatly upon the ∼ of brain function —*Diagnostic & Statistical Manual*⟩

in·teg·u·ment \in-'teg-yə-mənt\ n : an enveloping layer (as a skin, membrane, or husk) of an organism or one of its parts — **in·teg·u·men·ta·ry** \-ˌment-ə-rē, -'men-trē\ adj

in·tel·lect \'int-ᵊl-ˌekt\ n **1** : the power of knowing as distinguished from the power to feel and to will : the capacity for knowledge **2** : the capacity for rational or intelligent thought — **in·tel·lec·tu·al** \ˌint-ᵊl-'ek-ch(ə-w)əl, -'eksh-wəl\ adj — **in·tel·lec·tu·al·ly** adv

in·tel·lec·tion \ˌint-ᵊl-'ek-shən\ n **1** : exercise of the intellect **2** : a specific act of the intellect : IDEA

in·tel·lec·tu·al·ize or chiefly Brit **in·tel·lec·tu·al·ise** \ˌint-ᵊl-'ek-chə(-wə-)ˌlīz, -'eksh-wə-\ vt **-ized** or chiefly Brit **-ised; -iz·ing** or chiefly Brit **-is·ing** **1** : to give rational form or content to **2** : to avoid conscious recognition of the emotional basis of (an act or feeling) by substituting a superficially plausible explanation ⟨conflicts that are *intellectualized* —L. E. Hinsie⟩ — **in·tel·lec·tu·al·iza·tion** *or chiefly Brit* **in·tel·lec·tu·al·isa·tion** \-,ek-chə(-wə)-lə-'zā-shən\ *n*

in·tel·li·gence \in-'tel-ə-jən(t)s\ *n* **1 a** : the ability to learn or understand or to deal with new or trying situations **b** : the ability to apply knowledge to manipulate one's environment or to think abstractly as measured by objective criteria (as tests) **2** : mental acuteness — **in·tel·li·gent** \in-'tel-ə-jənt\ *adj* — **in·tel·li·gent·ly** *adv*

intelligence quotient *n* : IQ

intelligence test *n* : a test designed to determine the relative mental capacity of a person to learn — compare ACHIEVEMENT TEST, APTITUDE TEST

in·tem·per·ance \(')in-'tem-p(ə-)rən(t)s\ *n* : lack of moderation; *esp* : habitual or excessive drinking of intoxicants — **in·tem·per·ate** \-p(ə-)rət\ *adj*

in·tense \in-'ten(t)s\ *adj* **1 a** : existing in an extreme degree ⟨∼ anxiety⟩ **b** : extremely marked or pronounced ⟨a neurodermatitis with ∼ itching and burning of the skin —H. G. Armstrong⟩ **c** : very large or considerable ⟨∼ radiation⟩ **2 a** : feeling deeply esp. by nature or temperament **b** : deeply felt ⟨∼ emotions⟩ — **in·tense·ly** *adv*

in·ten·si·fy \in-'ten(t)-sə-,fī\ *vb* **-fied; -fy·ing** *vt* **1** : to make intense or more intensive **2 a** : to increase the density and contrast of (a photographic image) by special treatment **b** : to make more acute ⟨use of illicit drugs *intensified* the patient's condition⟩ ∼ *vi* : to become intense or more intensive ⟨grow stronger or more acute ⟨the sore throat, headache, and fever *intensified* as the disease progressed⟩ — **in·ten·si·fi·ca·tion** \-,ten(t)s-(ə)fə-'kā-shən\ *n*

intensifying screen *n* : a fluorescent screen placed next to an X-ray photographic film in order to intensify the image initially produced on the film by the action of X-rays

in·ten·si·ty \in-'ten(t)-sət-ē\ *n, pl* **-ties** **1** : the quality or state of being intense; *esp* : extreme degree of strength, force, energy, or feeling **2** : the magnitude of a quantity (as force or energy) per unit (as of surface, charge, mass, or time) **3** : SATURATION 4a

in·ten·sive \in-'ten(t)-siv\ *adj* : of, relating to, or marked by intensity; *esp* : involving the use of large doses or substances having great therapeutic activity — compare AGGRESSIVE 3 — **in·ten·sive·ly** *adv*

intensive care *adj* : having special medical facilities, services, and monitoring devices to meet the needs of gravely ill patients ⟨an *intensive care* unit⟩ — compare ACUTE CARE, CHRONIC CARE — **intensive care** *n*

in·ten·siv·ist \in-'ten(t)-sə-vəst\ *n* : a physician who specializes in the care and treatment of patients in intensive care

in·ten·tion \in-'ten-chən\ *n* **1** : a determination to act in a certain way **2** : a process or manner of healing of incised wounds — see FIRST INTENTION, SECOND INTENTION

intention tremor *n* : a slow tremor of the extremities that increases on attempted voluntary movement and is observed in certain diseases (as multiple sclerosis) of the nervous system

in·ter·ac·i·nar \,int-ə-'ras-ə-nər\ *or* **in·ter·ac·i·nous** \-ə-nəs\ *adj* : situated between or among the acini of a gland

in·ter·ac·tion \,int-ə-'rak-shən\ *n* : mutual or reciprocal action or influence ⟨∼ of the heart and lungs⟩ — **in·ter·ac·tion·al** \-shnəl, -shən-ᵊl\ *adj*

in·ter·al·ve·o·lar \,int-ə-ral-'vē-ə-lər\ *adj* : situated between alveoli esp. of the lungs

in·ter·atri·al \,int-ə-'rā-trē-əl\ *adj* : situated between the atria of the heart

interatrial septum *n* : the wall separating the right and left atria of the heart — called also *atrial septum*

in·ter·aural \,int-ə-'ròr-əl\ *adj* **1** : situated between or connecting the ears ⟨the ∼ plane⟩ **2** : of or relating to sound reception and perception by each ear considered separately ⟨responses of auditory neurons to ∼ time, phase, and intensity differences —E. I. Knudsen *et al*⟩

in·ter·au·ric·u·lar \,int-ə-,rò-'rik-yə-lər\ *adj* : INTERATRIAL

in·ter·body \'int-ər-,bäd-ē\ *adj* : performed between the bodies of two contiguous vertebrae ⟨a lateral resection and ∼ fusion was done —S. J. Larson *et al*⟩

in·ter·brain \'int-ər-,brān\ *n* : DIENCEPHALON

in·ter·breed \,int-ər-'brēd\ *vb* **-bred** \-'bred\; **-breed·ing** *vi* : to breed together: as **a** : CROSSBREED **b** : to breed within a closed population ∼ *vt* : to cause to breed together

in·ter·ca·lat·ed disk \in-'tər-kə-,lāt-əd-\ *n* : any of the specialized regions of the sarcolemma and underlying cytoplasm of cardiac muscle cells that comprise the longitudinal and end-to-end junctions between adjacent cells and that function to connect them mechanically and electrically

intercalated duct *n* : a duct from a tubule or acinus of the pancreas that drains into an intralobular duct

in·ter·cap·il·lary \,int-ər-'kap-ə-,ler-ē, *Brit usu* -kə-'pil-ə-rē\ *adj* : situated between capillaries ⟨∼ thrombi⟩

in·ter·car·pal \,int-ər-'kär-pəl\ *adj* : situated between, occurring between, or connecting carpal bones ⟨an ∼ dislocation⟩ ⟨an ∼ joint⟩ ⟨∼ ligaments⟩

in·ter·cav·ern·ous \,int-ər-'kav-ər-nəs\ *adj* : situated between and connecting the cavernous sinuses behind and in front of the pituitary gland ⟨an ∼ sinus⟩

in·ter·cel·lu·lar \,int-ər-'sel-yə-lər\ *adj* : occurring between cells ⟨∼ spaces⟩ — **in·ter·cel·lu·lar·ly** *adv*

in·ter·ce·re·bral \-sə-'rē-brəl, -'ser-ə-\ *adj* : situated or administered between the cerebral hemispheres ⟨∼ injections⟩

in·ter·cla·vic·u·lar \-kla-'vik-yə-lər, -klə-\ *adj* : situated between the clavicles

in·ter·con·dy·lar \-'kän-də-lər\ *adj* : situated between two condyles ⟨the ∼ eminence of the tibia⟩ ⟨the ∼ fossa or notch separates the condyles of the femur⟩

in·ter·con·dy·loid \-'kän-də-,lòid\ *adj* : INTERCONDYLAR

in·ter·cor·o·nary \-'kòr-ə-,ner-ē, -'kär-\ *adj* : occurring or effected between coronary arteries ⟨∼ arteriolar anastomoses⟩

¹in·ter·cos·tal \,int-ər-'käs-tᵊl\ *adj* : situated or extending between the ribs ⟨∼ vessels⟩ ⟨∼ spaces⟩

²intercostal *n* : an intercostal part or structure (as a muscle or nerve)

intercostal artery *n* : any of the arteries supplying or lying in the intercostal spaces: **a** : any of the arteries branching in front directly from the internal thoracic artery to supply the first five or six intercostal spaces or from its branch comprising the musculophrenic artery to supply the lower intercostal spaces — called also *anterior intercostal artery* **b** : any of the arteries that branch from the costocervical trunk of the subclavian artery to supply the first or first two intercostal spaces or of the nine or 10 arteries that branch from the aorta to supply the lower intercostal spaces — called also *posterior intercostal artery*

intercostal muscle *n* : any of the short muscles that extend between the ribs filling in most of the intervals between them and serving to move the ribs in respiration: **a** : any of 11 muscles on each side between the vertebrae and the junction of the ribs and their cartilages of which each arises from the caudal margin of one rib and is inserted into the cranial margin of the rib below — called also *external intercostal muscle* **b** : any of 11 muscles on each side between the sternum and the line on a rib marking an insertion of the iliocostalis of which each arises from the inner surface of a rib and its corresponding costal cartilage and is inserted into the cranial margin of the rib below — called also *internal intercostal muscle*

intercostal nerve *n* : any of 11 nerves on each side of which each is an anterior division of a thoracic nerve lying between a pair of adjacent ribs

intercostal vein *n* : any of the veins of the intercostal spaces — see SUPERIOR INTERCOSTAL VEIN

in·ter·cos·to·bra·chi·al nerve \,int-ər-,käs-tō-,brā-kē-əl-\ *n*

\ə\ abut \ᵊ\ kitten \ər\ further \a\ ash \ā\ ace \ä\ cot, cart \aù\ out \ch\ chin \e\ bet \ē\ easy \g\ go \i\ hit \ī\ ice \j\ job \ŋ\ sing \ō\ go \ò\ law \òi\ boy \th\ thin \t̲h̲\ the \ü\ loot \ù\ foot \y\ yet \zh\ vision *See also* Pronunciation Symbols page

: a branch of the second intercostal nerve that crosses the axilla and supplies the skin of the inner and back part of the upper half of the arm

in·ter·course \'int-ər-ˌkō(ə)rs, -ˌkȯ(ə)rs\ *n* **1** : connection or dealings between persons or groups **2** : physical sexual contact between individuals that involves the genitalia of at least one person ⟨anal ∼⟩ ⟨oral ∼⟩; *esp* : SEXUAL INTERCOURSE 1 ⟨heterosexual ∼⟩

in·ter·cris·tal \ˌint-ər-'kris-tᵊl\ *adj* : measured between two crests (as of bone) ⟨∼ dimensions of the pelvis⟩

in·ter·crit·i·cal \-'krit-i-kəl\ *adj* : being in the period between attacks ⟨∼ gout⟩

¹in·ter·cross \ˌint-ər-'krȯs\ *vb* : CROSS

²in·ter·cross \'int-ər-ˌkrȯs\ *n* : an instance or a product of crossbreeding

in·ter·cru·ral \ˌint-ər-'kru̇(ə)r-əl\ *adj* : situated or taking place between two crura and esp. in the region of the groin ⟨∼ intercourse⟩

in·ter·cur·rent \ˌint-ər-'kər-ənt, -'kə-rənt\ *adj* : occurring during and modifying the course of another disease ⟨an ∼ infection⟩

in·ter·cus·pal \ˌint-ər-'kəs-pəl\ *adj* : of or relating to intercuspation

in·ter·cus·pa·tion \-ˌkəs-'pā-shən\ *or* **in·ter·cus·pi·da·tion** \-ˌkəs-pə-'dā-shən\ *n* : the meshing together of cusps of opposing teeth in occlusion

in·ter·den·tal \ˌint-ər-'dent-ᵊl\ *adj* : situated or intended for use between the teeth ⟨floss the ∼ spaces⟩ — **in·ter·den·tal·ly** \-ᵊl-ē\ *adv*

interdental papilla *n* : the triangular wedge of gingiva between two adjacent teeth — called also *gingival papilla*

in·ter·dict \'int-ər-ˌdikt\ *n, civil law* : one who has been determined to be incompetent to care for his or her own person or affairs (as by reason of mental incapacity)

in·ter·dic·tion \ˌint-ər-'dik-shən\ *n, civil law* : removal of the right to care for one's own person or affairs (as because of mental incapacity)

in·ter·dig·i·tal \ˌint-ər-'dij-ət-əl\ *adj* : occurring between digits ⟨∼ neuroma⟩

in·ter·dig·i·tate \-'dij-ə-ˌtāt\ *vi* **-tat·ed; -tat·ing** **1** : to become interlocked like the fingers of folded hands ⟨thick myosin filaments ∼ with the thin actin filaments —J. M. Squire⟩ **2** : to undergo intercuspation ⟨these teeth do not ∼ completely —J. A. Glassman⟩ — **in·ter·dig·i·ta·tion** \-ˌdij-ə-'tā-shən\ *n*

in·ter·face \'int-ər-ˌfās\ *n* : a surface forming a common boundary of two bodies, spaces, or phases ⟨∼s between various tissues such as skin, fatty tissue, and muscle —H. P. Schwan⟩ — **interface** *vt* **-faced; -fac·ing** — **in·ter·fa·cial** \ˌint-ər-'fā-shəl\ *adj*

interfacial tension *n* : surface tension at the interface between two liquids

in·ter·fas·cic·u·lar \ˌint-ər-fə-'sik-yə-lər, -fa-\ *adj* : situated between fascicles

in·ter·fem·o·ral \-'fem-(ə-)rəl\ *adj* : situated or performed between the thighs ⟨∼ sexual intercourse⟩

in·ter·fere \ˌint-ə(r)-'fi(ə)r\ *vi* **-fered; -fer·ing** **1** : to strike one foot against the opposite foot or ankle in walking or running — used esp. of horses **2** : to act reciprocally so as to augment, diminish, or otherwise affect one another — used of waves **3** : to be inconsistent with and disturb the performance of previously learned behavior

in·ter·fer·ence \-'fir-ən(t)s\ *n* **1** : the act or process of interfering **2** : the mutual effect on meeting of two wave trains (as of light or sound) that constitutes alternating areas of increased and decreased amplitude (as light and dark lines or louder and softer sound) **3** : partial or complete inhibition or sometimes facilitation of other genetic crossovers in the vicinity of a chromosomal locus where a preceding crossover has occurred **4** : the disturbing effect of new learning on the performance of previously learned behavior with which it is inconsistent — compare NEGATIVE TRANSFER **5** : prevention of typical growth and development of a virus in

a suitable host by the presence of another virus in the same host individual — see INTERFERENCE PHENOMENON

interference phenomenon *n* : the resistance of a particular cell or tissue to infection by a virus that is conferred as a result of prior infection by an unrelated virus

in·ter·fer·om·e·ter \ˌint-ə(r)-fə-'räm-ət-ər, -ˌfir-'äm-\ *n* : an instrument that utilizes the interference of waves (as of light) for precise determination esp. of wavelength, spectral fine structure, indices of refraction, and very small linear displacements — **in·ter·fer·o·met·ric** \-ˌfir-ə-'me-trik\ *adj* — **in·ter·fer·o·met·ri·cal·ly** \-tri-k(ə-)lē\ *adv* — **in·ter·fer·om·e·try** \-fə-'räm-ə-trē, -ˌfir-'äm-\ *n, pl* **-tries**

in·ter·fer·on \ˌint-ə(r)-'fi(ə)r-ˌän\ *n* : any of a group of heat-stable soluble basic antiviral glycoproteins of low molecular weight that are produced usu. by cells exposed to the action of a virus, sometimes to the action of another intracellular parasite (as a bacterium), or experimentally to the action of some chemicals, and that include some used medically as antiviral or antineoplastic agents — see ALPHA INTERFERON, BETA INTERFERON, GAMMA INTERFERON

interferon al·fa \-'al-fə\ *n* : alpha interferon produced by recombinant DNA technology

interferon alpha *n* : ALPHA INTERFERON

interferon gamma *n* : GAMMA INTERFERON

in·ter·fer·tile \ˌint-ər-'fərt-ᵊl\ *adj* : capable of interbreeding — **in·ter·fer·til·i·ty** \-(ˌ)fər-'til-ət-ē\ *n, pl* **-ties**

in·ter·fi·bril·lar \ˌint-ər-'fib-rə-lər, -'fī-brə-lər\ *or* **in·ter·fibril·lary** \-'fib-rə-ˌler-ē, -'fī-brə-ˌler-ē\ *adj* : situated between fibrils

in·ter·fol·lic·u·lar \-fə-'lik-yə-lər, -fä-\ *adj* : situated between follicles ⟨∼ connective tissue⟩

in·ter·fron·tal \-'frənt-ᵊl\ *adj* : lying between the frontal bones ⟨the ∼ cranial suture⟩

in·ter·gan·gli·on·ic \-ˌgaŋ-glē-'än-ik\ *adj* : situated between ganglia

in·ter·ge·nic \-'jē-nik\ *adj* : occurring between genes : involving more than one gene ⟨∼ suppression⟩ ⟨∼ change⟩

in·ter·glob·u·lar \-'gläb-yə-lər\ *adj* : resulting from or situated in an area of faulty dentin formation ⟨∼ dentin⟩ ⟨∼ spaces⟩

in·ter·glu·te·al \-'glüt-ē-əl, -glü-'tē-əl\ *adj* : situated between the buttocks

in·ter·hemi·spher·ic \'int-ər-ˌhem-ə-'sfi(ə)r-ik, -'sfer-\ *also* **in·ter·hemi·spher·al** \-əl\ *adj* : extending or occurring between hemispheres (as of the cerebrum)

in·ter·ic·tal \ˌint-ər-'ik-təl\ *adj* : occurring between seizures (as of epilepsy)

interieur — see MILIEU INTERIEUR

in·ter·in·di·vid·u·al \-ˌin-də-'vij-(ə-)wəl, -'vij-əl\ *adj* : involving or taking place between individuals ⟨∼ conflicts⟩

¹in·te·ri·or \in-'tir-ē-ər\ *adj* : lying, occurring, or functioning within limiting boundaries

²interior *n* : the internal or inner part or cavity of a thing

in·ter·ki·ne·sis \ˌint-ər-kə-'nē-səs, -kī-\ *n, pl* **-ne·ses** \-ˌsēz\ : the period between two mitoses of a nucleus (as between the first and second meiotic divisions) — **in·ter·ki·net·ic** \-kə-'net-ik, -kī-\ *adj*

in·ter·leu·kin \ˌin-tər-'lü-kən\ *n* : any of various compounds of low molecular weight that are produced by lymphocytes, macrophages, and monocytes and that function esp. in regulation of the immune system and esp. cell-mediated immunity

interleukin–1 \-'wən\ *n* : an interleukin produced esp. by monocytes and macrophages that regulates cell-mediated and humoral immune responses by activating lymphocytes and mediates other biological processes (as the onset of fever) usu. associated with infection and inflammation — abbr. *IL-1*

interleukin–6 \-'siks\ *n* : an interleukin that is produced by various cells (as macrophages, fibroblasts, T cells, and tumor cells) and that acts as a pyrogen, induces maturation of B cells and growth of myeloma cells, activates and induces proliferation of T cells, and stimulates synthesis of plasma proteins (as fibrinogen) — abbr. *IL-6*

interleukin–3 \-'thrē\ *n* : an interleukin that is a colony‑stimulating factor produced esp. by T cells stimulated by mitogen or antigen and that promotes the proliferation and differentiation of various stem cells (as hematopoietic stem cells)

interleukin–2 \-'tü\ *n* : an interleukin produced by antigen‑stimulated helper T cells in the presence of interleukin-1 that induces proliferation of immune cells (as T cells and B cells) and has been used experimentally esp. in treating certain cancers — abbr. *IL-2*

in·ter·lo·bar \ˌint-ər-'lō-bər, -ˌbär\ *adj* : situated between the lobes of an organ or structure

interlobar artery *n* : any of various secondary branches of the renal arteries that pass between the Malpighian pyramids and branch to form the arcuate arteries

interlobar vein *n* : any of the veins of the kidney that are formed by convergence of arcuate veins, pass between the Malpighian pyramids, and empty into the renal veins or their branches

in·ter·lob·u·lar \ˌint-ər-'läb-yə-lər\ *adj* : lying between, connecting, or transporting the secretions of lobules ⟨∼ connective tissue⟩ ⟨∼ ducts of the pancreas⟩

interlobular artery *n* : any of the branches of an arcuate artery that pass radially in the cortex of the kidney toward the surface

interlobular vein *n* : any of the veins in the cortex of the kidney that empty into the arcuate veins

in·ter·mam·ma·ry \ˌint-ər-'mam-ə-rē\ *adj* : situated or performed between the breasts ⟨∼ intercourse⟩

in·ter·mar·gin·al \-'märj-ən-ᵊl, -'märj-nəl\ *adj* : situated or occurring between two margins ⟨∼ adhesions⟩

in·ter·mar·riage \ˌint-ər-'mar-ij\ *n* **1** : marriage between members of different groups **2** : marriage within a specific group : ENDOGAMY

¹in·ter·max·il·lary \ˌint-ər-'mak-sə-ˌler-ē, *chiefly Brit* -mak-'sil-ə-rē\ *adj* **1** : lying between maxillae; *esp* : joining the two maxillary bones ⟨∼ sutures⟩ **2** : of or relating to the premaxillae

²intermaxillary *n, pl* **-lar·ies** : PREMAXILLA

intermedia — see MASSA INTERMEDIA, PARS INTERMEDIA

in·ter·me·di·ary \ˌint-ər-'mēd-ē-ˌer-ē\ *n, pl* **-ar·ies 1** : MEDIATOR **2** : an intermediate form, product, or stage — **intermediary** *adj*

intermediary metabolism *n* : the intracellular process by which nutritive material is converted into cellular components — called also *intermediate metabolism*

¹in·ter·me·di·ate \ˌint-ər-'mēd-ē-ət\ *adj* : being or occurring at the middle place, stage, or degree or between extremes ⟨the remaining subjects progressed to some ∼ stage of disease —R. R. Redfield *et al*⟩

²intermediate *n* : one that is intermediate; *esp* : a chemical compound synthesized from simpler compounds and usu. intended to be used in later syntheses of more complex products ⟨pharmaceutical ∼s⟩

intermediate cell mass *n* : NEPHROTOME

intermediate cuneiform *n* : CUNEIFORM BONE 1b

intermediate cuneiform bone *n* : CUNEIFORM BONE 1b

intermediate filament *n* : any of a class of usu. insoluble cellular protein fibers (as a neurofilament or an epithelial‑cell cytoplasmic filament of keratin) composed of various fibrous polypeptides that serve esp. to provide structural stability and strength to the cytoskeleton and are intermediate in diameter between microfilaments and microtubules

intermediate host *n* **1** : a host which is normally used by a parasite in the course of its life cycle and in which it may multiply asexually but not sexually — compare DEFINITIVE HOST **2 a** : RESERVOIR 2 **b** : VECTOR 2

intermediate metabolism *n* : INTERMEDIARY METABOLISM

intermediate temporal artery *n* : TEMPORAL ARTERY 3b

in·ter·me·din \ˌint-ər-'mēd-ᵊn\ *n* : MELANOCYTE-STIMULATING HORMONE

in·ter·me·dio·lat·er·al \ˌint-ər-ˌmē-dē-ō-'lat-ə-rəl, -'la-trəl\ *adj* : of, relating to, or being the lateral column of gray matter in the spinal cord ⟨∼ cell columns⟩

intermedium — see STRATUM INTERMEDIUM

in·ter·me·di·us \ˌint-ər-'mē-dē-əs\ *adj* : tending to be moderately virulent — used esp. of strains of diphtheria bacilli; compare GRAVIS, MITIS

intermedius — see NERVUS INTERMEDIUS, VASTUS INTERMEDIUS

in·ter·mem·bra·nous \-'mem-brə-nəs\ *adj* : situated or occurring between membranes

in·ter·men·in·ge·al \-ˌmen-ən-'jē-əl\ *adj* : situated or occurring between the meninges ⟨∼ hemorrhage⟩

in·ter·men·stru·al \-'men(t)-strə(-wə)l\ *adj* : occurring between menstrual periods ⟨∼ pain⟩

in·ter·mis·sion \ˌint-ər-'mish-ən\ *n* : the space of time between two paroxysms of a disease — compare ARREST, CURE 1, REMISSION

¹in·ter·mi·tot·ic \ˌint-ər-mī-'tät-ik\ *n* : a cell capable of undergoing mitosis — compare POSTMITOTIC

²intermitotic *adj* : of, relating to, or being in the period between mitoses

in·ter·mit·tent \ˌint-ər-'mit-ᵊnt\ *adj* : coming and going at intervals : not continuous ⟨∼ fever⟩ — **in·ter·mit·tence** \-ᵊn(t)s\ *n*

intermittent claudication *n* : cramping pain and weakness in the legs and esp. the calves on walking that disappears after rest and is usu. associated with inadequate blood supply to the muscles (as in Buerger's disease or arteriosclerosis)

intermittent ex·plo·sive disorder \-ik-'splō-siv-, -ziv-\ *n* : a personality disorder characterized by repeated episodes of violent aggressive behavior in an otherwise normal individual that is out of proportion to the events provoking it

intermittent positive pressure breathing *n* : enforced periodic inflation of the lungs by the intermittent application of an increase of pressure to a reservoir of air (as in a bag) supplying the lungs — abbr. *IPPB*

intermittent pulse *n* : a pulse that occas. skips a cardiac beat

in·ter·mo·lec·u·lar \ˌint-ər-mə-'lek-yə-lər\ *adj* : existing or acting between molecules — **in·ter·mo·lec·u·lar·ly** *adv*

in·ter·mus·cu·lar \-'məs-kyə-lər\ *adj* : lying between and separating muscles ⟨∼ fat⟩

¹in·tern *also* **in·terne** \'in-ˌtərn\ *n* : a physician gaining supervised practical experience in a hospital after graduating from medical school — called also *houseman*

²in·tern \'in-ˌtərn\ *vi* : to act as an intern

interna — see OTITIS INTERNA, THECA INTERNA

in·ter·nal \in-'tərn-ᵊl\ *adj* **1** : existing or situated within the limits or surface of something: as **a** : situated near the inside of the body ⟨an ∼ layer of abdominal muscle⟩ **b** : situated on the side toward the midsagittal plane of the body ⟨the ∼ surface of the lung⟩ **2** : present or arising within an organism or one of its parts ⟨an ∼ stimulus⟩ **3** : applied or intended for application through the stomach by being swallowed ⟨an ∼ remedy⟩ — **in·ter·nal·ly** \in-'tərn-ᵊl-ē\ *adv*

internal acoustic meatus *n* : INTERNAL AUDITORY CANAL

internal anal sphincter *n* : ANAL SPHINCTER b

internal auditory artery *n* : a long slender artery that arises from the basilar artery or one of its branches, accompanies the auditory nerve through the internal auditory canal, and is distributed to the inner ear — called also *internal auditory, labyrinthine artery*

internal auditory canal *n* : a short auditory canal in the petrous portion of the temporal bone through which pass the facial and auditory nerves and the nervus intermedius — called also *internal acoustic meatus, internal auditory meatus*

internal capsule *n* : CAPSULE 1b(1)

internal carotid artery *n* : the inner branch of the carotid artery that supplies the brain, eyes, and other internal structures of the head — called also *internal carotid*

internal ear *n* : INNER EAR

internal iliac artery *n* : ILIAC ARTERY 3

\ə\ **abut** \ᵊ\ **kitten** \ər\ **further** \a\ **ash** \ā\ **ace** \ä\ **cot, cart** \au̇\ **out** \ch\ **chin** \e\ **bet** \ē\ **easy** \g\ **go** \i\ **hit** \ī\ **ice** \j\ **job** \ŋ\ **sing** \ō\ **go** \ȯ\ **law** \ȯi\ **boy** \th\ **thin** \t̠h̠\ **the** \ü\ **loot** \u̇\ **foot** \y\ **yet** \zh\ **vision** *See also* Pronunciation Symbols page

internal iliac node *n* : any of the lymph nodes grouped around the internal iliac artery and the internal iliac vein — compare EXTERNAL ILIAC NODE

internal iliac vein *n* : ILIAC VEIN c

internal inguinal ring *n* : DEEP INGUINAL RING

internal intercostal muscle *n* : INTERCOSTAL MUSCLE b — called also *internal intercostal*

in·ter·nal·ize *or chiefly Brit* **in·ter·nal·ise** \in-ˈtərn-ᵊl-ˌīz\ *vt* **-ized** *or chiefly Brit* **-ised; -iz·ing** *or chiefly Brit* **-is·ing** : to give a subjective character to; *specif* : to incorporate (as values or patterns of culture) within the self as conscious or subconscious guiding principles through learning or socialization — **in·ter·nal·iza·tion** *or chiefly Brit* **in·ter·nal·isa·tion** \-ˌtərn-ᵊl-ə-ˈzā-shən\ *n*

internal jugular vein *n* : JUGULAR VEIN a — called also *internal jugular*

internal malleolus *n* : MALLEOLUS b

internal mammary artery *n* : INTERNAL THORACIC ARTERY

internal mammary vein *n* : INTERNAL THORACIC VEIN

internal maxillary artery *n* : MAXILLARY ARTERY

internal medicine *n* : a branch of medicine that deals with the diagnosis and treatment of nonsurgical diseases — abbr. *IM*

internal oblique *n* : OBLIQUE a(2)

internal occipital crest *n* : OCCIPITAL CREST b

internal occipital protuberance *n* : OCCIPITAL PROTUBERANCE b

internal os *n* : the opening of the cervix into the body of the uterus

internal phase *n* : DISPERSED PHASE

internal pterygoid muscle *n* : PTERYGOID MUSCLE b

internal pudendal artery *n* : a branch of the internal iliac artery that is distributed or gives off branches distributed esp. to the external genitalia and the perineum — compare EXTERNAL PUDENDAL ARTERY

internal pudendal vein *n* : any of several veins that receive blood from the external genitalia and the perineum, accompany the internal pudendal artery, and unite to form a single vein that empties into the internal iliac vein

internal respiration *n* : the exchange of gases (as oxygen and carbon dioxide) between the cells of the body and the blood by way of the fluid bathing the cells — compare EXTERNAL RESPIRATION

internal secretion *n* : HORMONE 1a

internal semilunar fibrocartilage *n* : MENISCUS 2a(2)

internal spermatic artery *n* : TESTICULAR ARTERY

internal thoracic artery *n* : a branch of the subclavian artery of each side that runs down along the anterior wall of the thorax and rests against the costal cartilages — called also *internal mammary artery;* compare THORACIC ARTERY

internal thoracic vein *n* : a vein of the trunk on each side of the body that accompanies the corresponding internal thoracic artery and empties into the brachiocephalic vein — called also *internal mammary vein*

in·ter·na·sal \ˌint-ər-ˈnā-zəl\ *adj* : situated between or marking the junction of the nasal bones ⟨the ~ suture⟩

In·ter·na·tion·al System of Units \ˌint-ər-ˈnash-nəl-, -ᵊn°l-\ *n* : an internationally accepted system of units based on the metric system and having the meter, kilogram, second, ampere, kelvin, mole, and candela as base units, the radian and steradian as supplementary units, and deriving all other units from these — abbr. *SI;* called also *International System*

international unit *n* : the amount of specific physiological activity of a standardized preparation (as of a vitamin) that is agreed upon as an international standard esp. for comparison with other biologicals containing the substance in impure form or with a related biologically active substance; *also* : the amount of the biologically active substance in the standard amount of the preparation producing this activity

interne, interneship *var of* INTERN, INTERNSHIP

in·ter·neu·ron \ˌint-ər-ˈn(y)ü-ˌrän, -ˈn(y)u̇(ə)r-ˌän\ *or Brit* **in·ter·neu·rone** \-ˈnyu̇r-ōn\ *n* : a neuron that conveys impulses from one neuron to another — called also *association neuron, associative neuron, internuncial, internuncial neuron;* compare MOTOR NEURON, SENSORY NEURON — **in·ter·neu·ro·nal** \-ˈn(y)u̇r-ən-ᵊl, -nyu̇-ˈrōn-\ *adj*

in·ter·nist \ˈin-ˌtər-nəst\ *n* : a specialist in internal medicine esp. as distinguished from a surgeon

in·ter·no·dal \ˌint-ər-ˈnōd-ᵊl\ *adj* : lying or extending between two nodes ⟨a Schwann cell covers one ~ segment between two nodes of Ranvier⟩ — **in·ter·node** \ˈint-ər-ˌnōd\ *n*

in·tern·ship *also* **in·terne·ship** \ˈin-ˌtərn-ˌship\ *n* **1** : the state or position of being an intern **2 a** : a period of service as an intern **b** : the phase of medical training covered during such service

in·ter·nu·cle·ar \ˌint-ər-ˈn(y)ü-klē-ər\ *adj* : situated or occurring between atomic or biological nuclei

¹**in·ter·nun·ci·al** \ˌint-ər-ˈnən(t)-sē-əl, -ˈnu̇n(t)-\ *adj* : of, relating to, or being interneurons ⟨~ fibers⟩ — **in·ter·nun·ci·al·ly** \-ə-lē\ *adv*

²**internuncial** *n* : INTERNEURON

internuncial neuron *n* : INTERNEURON

internus — see OBLIQUUS INTERNUS, OBLIQUUS INTERNUS ABDOMINIS, OBTURATOR INTERNUS, SPHINCTER ANI INTERNUS, VASTUS INTERNUS

in·ter·ob·serv·er \ˌint-ər-əb-ˈzər-vər\ *adj* : occurring between individuals performing the same and esp. a visual task ⟨~ variability in the interpretation of coronary angiograms —Frank Vieras *et al*⟩

in·ter·oc·clu·sal \-ə-ˈklü-səl, -ä-ˈklü-, -zəl\ *adj* : situated or occurring between the occlusal surfaces of opposing teeth ⟨~ clearance⟩

in·tero·cep·tive \ˌint-ə-rō-ˈsep-tiv\ *adj* : of, relating to, or being stimuli arising within the body and esp. in the viscera

in·tero·cep·tor \-tər\ *n* : a sensory receptor excited by interoceptive stimuli — compare EXTEROCEPTOR

in·ter·o·fec·tive \ˌint-ə-rō-ˈfek-tiv\ *adj* : of, relating to, dependent on, or constituting the autonomic nervous system — compare EXTEROFECTIVE

in·ter·or·bit·al \ˌint-ə-ˈror-bət-ᵊl\ *adj* : situated or extending between the orbits of the eyes ⟨~ area⟩ ⟨~ distance⟩

interorbital breadth *n* : the distance between the dacrya

interossei *pl of* INTEROSSEUS

in·ter·os·se·ous \ˌin-tər-ˈäs-ē-əs\ *adj* : situated between bones ⟨an ~ space⟩

interosseous artery — see COMMON INTEROSSEOUS ARTERY

interosseous membrane *n* : either of two thin strong sheets of fibrous tissue: **a** : one extending between and connecting the shafts of the radius and ulna **b** : one extending between and connecting the shafts of the tibia and fibula

interosseous muscle *n* : INTEROSSEUS

in·ter·os·se·us \ˌin-tər-ˈäs-ē-əs\ *n, pl* **-sei** \-ē-ˌī\ : any of various small muscles arising from the metacarpals and metatarsals and inserted into the bases of the first phalanges: **a** : DORSAL INTEROSSEUS **b** : PALMAR INTEROSSEUS **c** : PLANTAR INTEROSSEUS

interosseus dorsalis *n, pl* **interossei dorsales** : DORSAL INTEROSSEUS

interosseus palmaris *n, pl* **interossei palmares** : PALMAR INTEROSSEUS

interosseus plantaris *n, pl* **interossei plantares** : PLANTAR INTEROSSEUS

in·ter·pal·pe·bral \ˌint-ər-pal-ˈpē-brəl\ *adj* : lying between the eyelids

in·ter·pan·dem·ic \-pan-ˈdem-ik\ *adj* : occurring between pandemics of a disease ⟨an ~ outbreak of influenza⟩

in·ter·pa·ri·etal \ˌint-ər-pə-ˈrī-ət-ᵊl\ *adj* : lying between parietal elements; *esp* : lying between the parietal bones

interparietal bone *n* : a median triangular bone lying at the junction of the parietal and occipital bones and rarely present in humans but conspicuous in various lower mammals — called also *interparietal;* see INCA BONE

in·ter·par·ox·ys·mal \-ˌpar-ək-ˈsiz-məl *also* -pə-ˌräk-\ *adj* : occurring between paroxysms

in·ter·pe·dun·cu·lar \ˌint-ər-pi-ˈdəŋ-kyə-lər\ *adj* : lying between the peduncles of the brain

interpeduncular nucleus *n* : a mass of nerve cells lying between the cerebral peduncles in the midsagittal plane just dorsal to the pons — called also *interpeduncular ganglion*

in·ter·pel·vi·ab·dom·i·nal amputation \ˌint-ər-ˌpel-vē-ab-ˈdäm-(ə-)nəl-\ *n* : amputation of the entire leg including the hip bone

in·ter·per·son·al \-ˈpərs-nəl, -ᵊn-əl\ *adj* : being, relating to, or involving relations between persons — **in·ter·per·son·al·ly** \-ē\ *adv*

interpersonal therapy *n* : psychotherapy that focuses on a patient's interpersonal relationships and that is used esp. to treat depression — abbr. *IPT;* called also *interpersonal psychotherapy*

in·ter·pha·lan·ge·al \ˌint-ər-ˌfā-lən-ˈjē-əl, -ˌfal-ən-ˈjē-əl; -fə-ˈlan-jē-əl, -fā-ˈlan-\ *adj* : situated or occurring between phalanges ⟨an ∼ joint⟩; *also* : of or relating to an interphalangeal joint ⟨∼ flexion⟩ ⟨∼ arthroplasty⟩

in·ter·phase \ˈint-ər-ˌfāz\ *n* : the interval between the end of one mitotic or meiotic division and the beginning of another — called also *resting stage* — **in·ter·pha·sic** \-ik\ *adj*

in·ter·po·lat·ed \in-ˈtər-pə-ˌlāt-əd\ *adj* : occurring between normal heartbeats without disturbing the succeeding beat or the basic rhythm of the heart ⟨an ∼ premature ventricular contraction⟩

in·ter·po·si·tion operation \ˌint-ər-pə-ˈzish-ən-\ *n* : the surgical repositioning of the uterus beneath the bladder for relief of cystocele and uterine prolapse

in·ter·pre·ta·tion \in-ˌtər-prə-ˈtā-shən, -pə-\ *n* : the act or result of giving an explanation of something ⟨∼ of the symptoms of disease⟩; *esp* : an explanation in understandable terms to a patient in psychotherapy of the deeper meaning according to psychological theory of the material related and the behavior exhibited by the patient during treatment — **in·ter·pret** \in-ˈtər-prət, -pət\ *vt* — **in·ter·pre·tive** \-prət-iv, -pət-\ *or* **in·ter·pre·ta·tive** \-prə-ˌtāt-iv, -prət-ət-iv\ *adj*

in·ter·pris·mat·ic \-priz-ˈmat-ik\ *adj* : situated or occurring between prisms esp. of enamel ⟨an ∼ substance⟩

in·ter·prox·i·mal \ˌint-ər-ˈpräk-sə-məl\ *adj* : situated, occurring, or used in the areas between adjoining teeth ⟨∼ space⟩ — **in·ter·prox·i·mal·ly** \-ē\ *adv*

in·ter·pu·pil·lary \ˌint-ər-ˈpyü-pə-ˌler-ē\ *adj* : extending between the pupils of the eyes; *also* : extending between the centers of a pair of spectacle lenses ⟨∼ distance⟩

in·ter·ra·dic·u·lar \-rə-ˈdik-yə-lər, -ra-ˈdik-\ *adj* : situated between the roots of a tooth ⟨the ∼ septum⟩ ⟨∼ areas⟩

in·ter·rupt·ed suture \ˌint-ə-ˈrəp-təd-\ *n* : a suture in which each stitch is separately tied

interruptus — see COITUS INTERRUPTUS

in·ter·scap·u·lar \ˌint-ər-ˈskap-yə-lər\ *adj* : of, relating to, situated in, or occurring in the region between the scapulae ⟨∼ pain⟩

in·ter·seg·men·tal \-seg-ˈment-ᵊl\ *adj* : lying or occurring between segments

in·ter·sen·so·ry \ˌint-ər-ˈsen(t)s-(ə-)rē\ *adj* : involving two or more sensory systems ⟨∼ factors in memory loss⟩

in·ter·sep·tal \-ˈsep-tᵊl\ *adj* : situated between septa

in·ter·sex \ˈint-ər-ˌseks\ *n* : an intersexual individual

in·ter·sex·u·al \ˌint-ər-ˈseksh-(ə-)wəl, -ˈsek-shəl\ *adj* **1** : existing between sexes ⟨∼ hostility⟩ **2** : intermediate in sexual characters between a typical male and a typical female — **in·ter·sex·u·al·i·ty** \-ˌsek-shə-ˈwal-ət-ē\ *n, pl* **-ties** — **in·ter·sex·u·al·ly** \-ˈseksh-(ə-)wə-lē, -(ə-)lē\ *adv*

in·ter·space \ˈint-ər-ˌspās\ *n* : the space between two related body parts whether void or filled by another kind of structure ⟨the skin of the ∼ between the fifth and sixth ribs⟩

in·ter·spe·cif·ic \ˌint-ər-spi-ˈsif-ik\ *also* **in·ter·spe·cies** \-ˈspē-(ˌ)shēz, -(ˌ)sēz\ *adj* : existing or arising between species ⟨an ∼ hybrid⟩ — **in·ter·spe·cif·i·cal·ly** \-i-k(ə-)lē\ *adv*

in·ter·spi·na·lis \ˌint-ər-ˌspī-ˈnal-əs, -ˈnā-ləs\ *n, pl* **-na·les** \-ˌlēz\ : any of various short muscles that have their origin on the superior surface of the spinous process of one verte-bra and their insertion on the inferior surface of the contiguous vertebra above

in·ter·spi·nal ligament \ˌint-ər-ˌspīn-ᵊl-\ *n* : any of the thin membranous ligaments that connect the spinous processes of contiguous vertebrae — called also *interspinous ligament*

in·ter·ster·ile \-ˈster-əl, *chiefly Brit* -ˌīl\ *adj* : incapable of producing offspring by interbreeding — **in·ter·ste·ril·i·ty** \-stə-ˈril-ət-ē\ *n, pl* **-ties**

in·ter·stice \in-ˈtər-stəs\ *n, pl* **-stic·es** \-stə-ˌsēz, -stə-səz\ : a space between closely spaced things (as teeth)

in·ter·stim·u·lus \ˌint-ər-ˈstim-yə-ləs\ *adj* : of, relating to, or being the interval between the presentation of two discrete stimuli

interstitia *pl of* INTERSTITIUM

in·ter·sti·tial \ˌint-ər-ˈstish-əl\ *adj* **1** : situated within but not restricted to or characteristic of a particular organ or tissue — used esp. of fibrous tissue **2** : affecting the interstitial tissues of an organ or part ⟨∼ hepatitis⟩ **3** : occurring in the part of a fallopian tube in the wall of the uterus ⟨∼ pregnancy⟩ — **in·ter·sti·tial·ly** \-ə-lē\ *adv*

interstitial cell *n* : a cell situated between the germ cells of the gonads; *esp* : LEYDIG CELL

interstitial cell of Leydig *n* : LEYDIG CELL

interstitial–cell stimulating hormone *n* : LUTEINIZING HORMONE

interstitial cystitis *n* : a chronic idiopathic cystitis characterized by painful inflammation of the subepithelial connective tissue and often accompanied by Hunner's ulcer

interstitial gland *n* : any of the groups of Leydig cells of the testis

interstitial keratitis *n* : a chronic progressive keratitis of the corneal stroma often resulting in blindness and frequently associated with congenital syphilis

interstitial pneumonia *n* : any of several chronic lung diseases of unknown etiology that affect interstitial tissues of the lung without filling of the alveolae and that may follow damage to the alveolar walls or involve interstitial histological changes

in·ter·sti·tium \ˌint-ər-ˈstish-ē-əm\ *n, pl* **-tia** \-ē-ə\ : interstitial tissue

in·ter·sub·ject \ˈint-ər-ˌsəb-jekt\ *adj* : occurring between subjects in an experiment ⟨∼ variability⟩

in·ter·tar·sal \-ˈtär-səl\ *adj* : situated, occurring, or performed between tarsal bones ⟨a ∼ joint⟩ ⟨∼ arthrotomy⟩

in·ter·tho·ra·co·scap·u·lar amputation \ˌint-ər-ˌthōr-ə-kō-ˌskap-yə-lər-, -ˌthȯr-\ *n* : surgical amputation of the arm with disarticulation of the humerus and removal of the scapula and outer part of the clavicle

in·ter·trans·ver·sa·les \ˌint-ər-ˌtran(t)s-vər-ˈsā-ˌlēz\ *n pl* : INTERTRANSVERSARII

in·ter·trans·ver·sar·ii \-ˌtran(t)s-vər-ˈser-ē-ˌī\ *n pl* : a series of small muscles connecting the transverse processes of contiguous vertebrae and most highly developed in the neck

in·ter·trial \ˌint-ər-ˌtrī(-ə)l\ *adj* : of, relating to, or being an interval between trials of an experiment

in·ter·trig·i·nous \ˌint-ər-ˌtrij-ə-nəs\ *adj* : exhibiting or affected with intertrigo ⟨a candidal ∼ eruption⟩

in·ter·tri·go \-ˈtrī-(ˌ)gō\ *n* : inflammation produced by chafing of adjacent areas of skin

in·ter·tro·chan·ter·ic \ˌint-ər-ˌtrō-kən-ˈter-ik, -ˌkan-\ *adj* : situated, performed, or occurring between trochanters ⟨∼ fractures⟩ ⟨∼ osteotomy⟩

intertrochanteric line *n* : a line on the anterior surface of the femur that runs obliquely from the greater trochanter to the lesser trochanter

in·ter·tu·ber·cu·lar \ˌint-ər-t(y)ù-ˈbər-kyə-lər\ *adj* : situated between tubercles

intertubercular groove *n* : BICIPITAL GROOVE

intertubercular line *n* : an imaginary line passing through

I

J

the iliac crests of the hip bones that separates the umbilical and lumbar regions of the abdomen from the hypogastric and iliac regions

in·ter·tu·bu·lar \ˌint-ər-ˈt(y)ü-byə-lər\ *adj* : lying between tubules ⟨∼ Leydig cells⟩

in·ter·val \ˈint-ər-vəl\ *n* : a space of time between events or states ⟨∼s between pregnancies⟩

in·ter·vas·cu·lar \ˌint-ər-ˈvas-kyə-lər\ *adj* : lying between or surrounded by blood vessels

in·ter·ven·ing variable \ˌint-ər-ˌvē-niŋ-\ *n* : a variable (as memory) whose effect occurs between the treatment in a psychological experiment (as the presentation of a stimulus) and the outcome (as a response), is difficult to anticipate or is unanticipated, and may confuse the results

in·ter·ven·tion \ˌint-ər-ˈven-chən\ *n* : the act or fact or a method of interfering with the outcome or course esp. of a condition or process (as to prevent harm or improve functioning) ⟨relieving a variety of serious arrhythmias by surgical ∼ —G. M. Lawrie *et al*⟩ ⟨develop ∼s to prevent substance abuse —A. Kline *et al*⟩ — **in·ter·vene** \-ˈvēn\ *vi* **-vened; -ven·ing** — **in·ter·ven·tion·al** \-ˈvench-(ə-)nəl\ *adj* — **in·ter·ven·tion·ist** \-ˈven-chə-nist\ *n*

in·ter·ven·tric·u·lar \ˌint-ər-ven-ˈtrik-yə-lər, -vən-\ *adj* : situated between ventricles ⟨an ∼ septal defect⟩

interventricular foramen *n* : the opening from each lateral ventricle into the third ventricle of the brain — called also *foramen of Monro*

interventricular groove *n* : INTERVENTRICULAR SULCUS

interventricular septum *n* : the curved slanting wall that separates the right and left ventricles of the heart and is composed of a muscular lower part and a thinner more membranous upper part

interventricular sulcus *n* : either of the anterior and posterior grooves on the surface of the heart that lie over the interventricular septum and join at the apex — called also *interventricular groove*

in·ter·ver·te·bral \ˌint-ər-ˈvərt-ə-brəl, -(ˌ)vər-ˈtē-\ *adj* : situated between vertebrae — **in·ter·ver·te·bral·ly** \-brə-lē\ *adv*

intervertebral disk *n* : any of the tough elastic disks that are interposed between the centra of adjoining vertebrae and that consist of an outer annulus fibrosus enclosing an inner nucleus pulposus

intervertebral foramen *n* : any of the openings that give passage to the spinal nerves from the vertebral canal and are formed by the juxtaposition of superior and inferior notches in the pedicles of contiguous vertebrae

in·ter·vil·lous \ˌint-ər-ˈvil-əs\ *adj* : situated or occurring between villi ⟨∼ thrombosis⟩

in·tes·ti·nal \in-ˈtes-tən-ᵊl, -ˈtes(t)-nəl, -ˈtes-ᵊn-əl, *Brit often* ˌin-(ˌ)tes-ˈtīn-ᵊl\ *adj* **1 a** : affecting or occurring in the intestine ⟨∼ digestion⟩ ⟨∼ catarrh⟩ **b** : living in the intestine ⟨the ∼ flora⟩ ⟨an ∼ worm⟩ **2** : of, relating to, or being the intestine ⟨the ∼ canal⟩ — **in·tes·ti·nal·ly** \-ē\ *adv*

intestinal artery *n* : any of 12 to 15 arteries that arise from the superior mesenteric artery and divide repeatedly into interconnected branches which encircle and supply the jejunum and ileum

intestinal flu *n* : an acute usu. transitory attack of gastroenteritis that is marked by nausea, vomiting, diarrhea, and abdominal cramping and is typically caused by a virus (as the Norwalk virus) or a bacterium (as E. coli) — not usu. used technically

intestinal gland *n* : CRYPT OF LIEBERKÜHN

intestinal juice *n* : a fluid that is secreted in small quantity in the small intestine, is highly variable in constitution, and contains esp. various enzymes (as erepsin, lipase, lactase, enterokinase, and amylase) and mucus — called also *succus entericus*

intestinal lipodystrophy *n* : WHIPPLE'S DISEASE

in·tes·tine \in-ˈtes-tən\ *n* : the tubular portion of the alimentary canal that lies posterior to the stomach from which it is separated by the pyloric sphincter and consists of a slender but long anterior part made up of the duodenum, jejunum, and ileum which function in digestion and assimilation of nutrients and a broader shorter posterior part made up of the cecum, colon, and rectum which serve chiefly to extract moisture from the by-products of digestion and evaporate them into feces — often used in pl. ⟨the movement of digested food through your ∼s —*Mayo Clinic Health Letter*⟩; see LARGE INTESTINE, SMALL INTESTINE

in·ti·ma \ˈint-ə-mə\ *n, pl* **-mae** \-ˌmē, -ˌmī\ *or* **-mas** : the innermost coat of an organ (as a blood vessel) consisting usu. of an endothelial layer backed by connective tissue and elastic tissue — called also *tunica intima* — **in·ti·mal** \-məl\ *adj*

in·to·cos·trin \ˌint-ə-ˈkäs-trən\ *n* : a standardized preparation of purified curare formerly used in medicine (as for the relaxation of skeletal muscles)

in·toed \ˈin-ˈtōd\ *adj* : having the toes turned inward — **in·toe·ing** \-ˌtō-iŋ\ *n*

in·tol·er·ance \(ˈ)in-ˈtäl-(ə)-rən(t)s\ *n* **1** : lack of an ability to endure ⟨an ∼ to light⟩ **2** : exceptional sensitivity (as to a food or drug); *specif* : inability to properly metabolize or absorb a substance ⟨glucose ∼⟩

in·tol·er·ant \(ˈ)in-ˈtäl-(ə)-rənt\ *adj* : exhibiting physiological intolerance ⟨people who are lactose ∼⟩

in·tor·sion *or* **in·tor·tion** \in-ˈtȯr-shən\ *n* : inward rotation (as of a body part) about an axis or a fixed point; *esp* : rotation of the eye around its anteroposterior axis so that the upper part moves toward the nose — compare EXTORSION — **in·tor·sion·al** \-ˈtȯr-sh(ə-)nəl\ *adj* — **in·tort·ed** \-ˈtȯrt-əd\ *adj*

in·tox·i·cant \in-ˈtäk-si-kənt\ *n* : something that intoxicates; *esp* : an alcoholic drink — called also *inebriant* — **intoxicant** *adj*

in·tox·i·cate \-sə-ˌkāt\ *vt* **-cat·ed; -cat·ing** **1** : POISON **2** : to excite or stupefy by alcohol or a drug esp. to the point where physical and mental control is markedly diminished

in·tox·i·cat·ed \-sə-ˌkāt-əd\ *adj* : affected by an intoxicant and esp. by alcohol

in·tox·i·ca·tion \in-ˌtäk-sə-ˈkā-shən\ *n* **1** : an abnormal state that is essentially a poisoning ⟨hypokalemia potentiates digoxin ∼ —W. H. Abelmann *et al*⟩ ⟨no evidence of cocaine ∼ —Margaret M. McCarron *et al*⟩ ⟨acute carbon monoxide ∼⟩ **2** : the condition of being drunk : INEBRIATION

In·tox·im·e·ter \ˌin-ˌtäk-ˈsim-ət-ər\ *trademark* — used for a device used to measure the degree of an individual's intoxication by means of chemical tests of the breath

in·tra–ab·dom·i·nal \ˌin-trə-ab-ˈdäm-ən-ᵊl, ˌin-(ˌ)trä-, -əb-, -ˈdäm-nᵊl\ *adj* : situated within, occurring within, or administered by entering the abdomen ⟨∼ pressure⟩ ⟨an ∼ injection⟩ — **in·tra–ab·dom·i·nal·ly** \-ē\ *adv*

in·tra–al·ve·o·lar \ˌin-trə-al-ˈvē-ə-lər, ˌin-(ˌ)trä-\ *adj* : situated or occurring within an alveolus

in·tra–am·ni·ot·ic \-ˌam-nē-ˈät-ik\ *adj* : situated within, occurring within, or administered by entering the amnion — **in·tra–am·ni·ot·i·cal·ly** \-i-k(ə-)lē\ *adv*

in·tra–aor·tic \-ā-ˈȯrt-ik\ *adj* **1** : situated or occurring within the aorta **2** : of, relating to, or used in intra-aortic balloon counterpulsation ⟨an ∼ balloon pump⟩

intra–aortic balloon counterpulsation *n* : counterpulsation in which cardiocirculatory assistance is provided by a balloon inserted in the thoracic aorta which is inflated during diastole and deflated just before systole

in·tra–ar·te·ri·al \-är-ˈtir-ē-əl\ *adj* : situated or occurring within, administered into, or involving entry by way of an artery ⟨∼ chemotherapy⟩ ⟨an ∼ catheter⟩ — **in·tra–ar·te·ri·al·ly** \-ē-ə-lē\ *adv*

in·tra–ar·tic·u·lar \-är-ˈtik-yə-lər\ *adj* : situated within, occurring within, or administered by entering a joint — **in·tra–ar·tic·u·lar·ly** *adv*

in·tra–atom·ic \-ə-ˈtäm-ik\ *adj* : existing within an atom ⟨∼ energy⟩

in·tra–atri·al \-ˈā-trē-əl\ *adj* : situated or occurring within an atrium esp. of the heart ⟨an ∼ block⟩

in·tra–ax·o·nal \-ˈak-sən-ᵊl; -ak-ˈsän-, -ˈsōn-\ *adj* : situated or occurring within an axon ⟨∼ transport⟩ — **in·tra–ax·o·nal·ly** \-ē\ *adv*

in·tra·bron·chi·al \-'bräŋ-kē-əl\ *adj* : situated or occurring within the bronchial tubes 〈~ foreign bodies〉

in·tra·buc·cal \-'bək-əl\ *adj* : situated or occurring within the mouth or cheeks

in·tra·can·a·lic·u·lar \-ˌkan-ᵊl-'ik-yə-lər\ *adj* : situated or occurring within a canaliculus 〈~ biliary stasis〉

in·tra·cap·il·lary \-'kap-ə-ˌler-ē, *Brit usu* -kə-'pil-ə-rē\ *adj* : situated or occurring within a capillary of the circulatory system

in·tra·cap·su·lar \-'kap-sə-lər\ *adj* **1** : situated or occurring within a capsule **2** *of a cataract operation* : involving removal of the entire lens and its capsule — compare EXTRACAPSULAR 2

in·tra·car·di·ac \-'kärd-ē-ˌak *also* **in·tra·car·di·al** \-ē-əl\ *adj* : situated within, occurring within, introduced into, or involving entry into the heart 〈~ surgery〉 〈an ~ catheter〉 — **in·tra·car·di·al·ly** \-ē-ə-lē\ *adv*

in·tra·ca·rot·id \-kə-'rät-əd\ *adj* : situated within, occurring within, or administered by entering a carotid artery

in·tra·car·ti·lag·i·nous \-ˌkärt-ᵊl-'aj-ə-nəs\ *adj* : ENDOCHONDRAL 〈~ ossification in bone development〉

in·tra·cav·i·tary \-'kav-ə-ˌter-ē\ *adj* : situated or occurring within a body cavity; *esp* : of, relating to, or being treatment (as of cancer) characterized by the insertion of esp. radioactive substances in a cavity 〈treatment of cervical cancer by ~ irradiation〉 — **in·tra·cav·i·tar·i·ly** \-ˌkav-ə-'ter-ə-lē\ *adv*

in·tra·cav·i·ty \-'kav-ət-ē\ *adj* : INTRACAVITARY

in·tra·cel·lu·lar \-'sel-yə-lər\ *adj* : existing, occurring, or functioning within a cell 〈~ enzymes〉 〈~ localization of RNA synthesis〉 〈~ parasites〉 — **in·tra·cel·lu·lar·ly** *adv*

in·tra·cer·e·bel·lar \-ˌser-ə-'bel-ər\ *adj* : situated or occurring within the cerebellum

in·tra·ce·re·bral \-sə-'rē-brəl, -'ser-ə-\ *adj* : situated within, occurring within, or administered by entering the cerebrum 〈~ bleeding〉 — **in·tra·ce·re·bral·ly** \-brə-lē\ *adv*

in·tra·chro·mo·som·al \-ˌkrō-mə-'sō-məl, -'zō-məl\ *adj* : situated or occurring within a chromosome 〈~ effects on crossing-over〉

in·tra·cis·ter·nal \ˌin-trə-sis-'tər-nəl\ *adj* : situated within, occurring within, or administered by entering a cisterna 〈~ granules〉 〈an ~ injection〉 — **in·tra·cis·ter·nal·ly** *adv*

in·tra·cor·ne·al \-'kȯr-nē-əl\ *adj* : occurring within, situated within, or implanted in the cornea 〈~ hemorrhage〉 〈an ~ lens〉

in·tra·co·ro·nal \-'kȯr-ən-ᵊl, -'kär-; -kə-'rōn-\ *adj* : situated or made within the crown of a tooth 〈an ~ attachment〉 — **in·tra·co·ro·nal·ly** *adv*

in·tra·cor·o·nary \-'kȯr-ə-ˌner-ē, -'kär-\ *adj* : situated within, occurring within, or administered by entering the heart

in·tra·cor·po·re·al \-kȯr-'pōr-ē-əl, -'pȯr-\ *adj* : situated or occurring within the body 〈an ~ mechanical heart〉

in·tra·cor·pus·cu·lar \-kȯr-'pəs-kyə-lər\ *adj* : situated or occurring within a corpuscle and esp. a blood corpuscle

in·tra·cor·ti·cal \-'kȯrt-i-kəl\ *adj* : situated or occurring within a cortex and esp. the cerebral cortex 〈~ injection〉 〈~ noradrenergic fibers〉

in·tra·cra·ni·al \-'krā-nē-əl\ *adj* : situated or occurring within the cranium 〈~ pressure〉; *also* : affecting or involving intracranial structures — **in·tra·cra·ni·al·ly** \-nē-ə-lē\ *adv*

in·trac·ta·ble \(')in-'trak-tə-bəl\ *adj* **1** : not easily managed or controlled (as by antibiotics or psychotherapy) 〈an ~ child〉 〈activity against many ~ *Proteus* and *Pseudomonas* species of bacteria —*Annual Report Pfizer*〉 **2** : not easily relieved or cured 〈~ pain〉 〈~ bleeding in duodenal ulcer —*Jour. Amer. Med. Assoc.*〉 — **in·trac·ta·bil·i·ty** \(ˌ)in-ˌtrak-tə-'bil-ət-ē\ *n, pl* **-ties**

in·tra·cu·ta·ne·ous \ˌin-trə-kyù-'tā-nē-əs, -(ˌ)trā-\ *adj* : INTRADERMAL 〈~ lesions〉 — **in·tra·cu·ta·ne·ous·ly** *adv*

intracutaneous test *n* : INTRADERMAL TEST

in·tra·cy·to·plas·mic \-ˌsīt-ə-'plaz-mik\ *adj* : lying or occurring in the cytoplasm 〈~ membranes〉 〈~ inclusions〉

intracytoplasmic sperm injection *n* : injection by a microneedle of a single sperm into an egg that has been surgically removed from an ovary followed by transfer of the egg to an incubator where fertilization takes place and then by implantation of the fertilized egg into a female's uterus — abbr. ICSI

in·tra·der·mal \ˌin-trə-'dər-məl, -(ˌ)trä-\ *adj* : situated, occurring, or done within or between the layers of the skin; *also* : administered by entering the skin 〈~ injections〉 — **in·tra·der·mal·ly** \-mə-lē\ *adv*

intradermal test *n* : a test for immunity or hypersensitivity made by injecting a minute amount of diluted antigen into the skin — called also *intracutaneous test;* compare PATCH TEST, PRICK TEST, SCRATCH TEST

in·tra·der·mo·re·ac·tion \ˌin-trə-ˌdər-mō-rē-'ak-shən\ *n* : an intradermal reaction

in·tra·di·a·lyt·ic \-ˌdī-ə-'lit-ik\ *adj* : occurring or carried out during hemodialysis 〈~ hypotension〉

in·tra·duc·tal \ˌin-trə-'dəkt-ᵊl\ *adj* : situated within, occurring within, or introduced into a duct 〈~ carcinoma〉

in·tra·du·o·de·nal \-ˌd(y)ü-ə-'dēn-ᵊl, -d(y)ù-'äd-ᵊn-əl\ *adj* : situated in or introduced into the duodenum 〈~ infusions of fat〉 — **in·tra·du·o·de·nal·ly** *adv*

in·tra·du·ral \-'d(y)ùr-əl\ *adj* : situated, occurring, or performed within or between the membranes of the dura mater — **in·tra·dur·al·ly** *adv*

in·tra·em·bry·on·ic \-ˌem-brē-'än-ik\ *adj* : situated or occurring within the embryo

in·tra·epi·der·mal \-ˌep-ə-'dər-məl\ *adj* : located or occurring within the epidermis

in·tra·ep·i·the·li·al \-ˌep-ə-'thē-lē-əl\ *adj* : occurring in or situated among the cells of the epithelium

in·tra·eryth·ro·cyt·ic \-i-ˌrith-rə-'sit-ik\ *adj* : situated or occurring within the red blood cells

in·tra·esoph·a·ge·al *or Brit* **in·tra·oe·soph·a·ge·al** \-i-ˌsäf-ə-'jē-əl\ *adj* : occurring within the esophagus 〈~ pressure〉

intrafallopian — see GAMETE INTRAFALLOPIAN TRANSFER, ZYGOTE INTRAFALLOPIAN TRANSFER

in·tra·fa·mil·ial \-fə-'mil-yəl\ *adj* : occurring within a family 〈~ conflict〉 〈~ spread of cholera〉

in·tra·fis·sur·al \-'fish-ə-rəl\ *adj* : situated within a fissure (as of the brain)

in·tra·fol·lic·u·lar \-fə-'lik-yə-lər, -fä-\ *adj* : situated within a follicle

in·tra·fu·sal \-'fyü-zəl\ *adj* : situated within a muscle spindle 〈~ muscle fibers〉 — compare EXTRAFUSAL

in·tra·gas·tric \-'gas-trik\ *adj* : situated or occurring within the stomach 〈~ intubation〉 — **in·tra·gas·tri·cal·ly** \-i-k(ə-)lē\ *adv*

in·tra·gen·ic \-'jen-ik\ *adj* : being or occurring within a gene 〈~ recombination〉 〈~ mutation〉

in·tra·glan·du·lar \-'glan-jə-lər\ *adj* : situated or performed within a gland

in·tra·glu·te·al \-'glüt-ē-əl, -glü-'tē-əl\ *adj* : situated within or introduced into the gluteal muscle 〈~ injection〉

in·tra·group \-'grüp\ *also* **in·tra·group·al** \-'grü-pəl\ *adj* : being or occurring within a single group 〈increased ~ hostility —J. B. Carroll〉

in·tra·he·pat·ic \-hi-'pat-ik\ *adj* : situated or occurring within or originating in the liver 〈~ cholestasis〉 — **in·tra·he·pat·i·cal·ly** \-i-k(ə-)lē\ *adv*

in·tra·hos·pi·tal \-'häs-ˌpit-ᵊl\ *adj* : occurring within a hospital 〈an ~ epidemic〉

in·tra·in·di·vid·u·al \-ˌin-də-'vij-(ə-)wəl, -'vij-əl\ *adj* : being or occurring within the individual 〈~ changes in performance on cognitive tasks —L. J. Harris〉

in·tra·jug·u·lar \-'jəg-yə-lər *also* -'jüg- *or* -'jəg-(ə-)lər\ *adj* : situated within or introduced into the jugular foramen, process, or vein — **in·tra·jug·u·lar·ly** *adv*

in·tra·la·mel·lar \-lə-'mel-ər\ *adj* : situated within a lamella

in·tra·lam·i·nar \-'lam-ə-nər\ *adj* : situated within a lamina 〈the ~ system of nuclei of the thalamus〉

\ə\ abut \ᵊ\ kitten \ər\ further \a\ ash \ā\ ace \ä\ cot, cart \aù\ out \ch\ chin \e\ bet \ē\ easy \g\ go \i\ hit \ī\ ice \j\ job \ŋ\ sing \ō\ go \ȯ\ law \ȯi\ boy \th\ thin \th\ the \ü\ loot \ù\ foot \y\ yet \zh\ vision *See also* Pronunciation Symbols page

in·tra·len·tic·u·lar \-len-ˈtik-yə-lər\ *adj* : located within the lens of the eye ⟨removal of an ∼ foreign body⟩

in·tra·le·sion·al \-ˈlē-zhən-ᵊl\ *adj* : introduced into or performed within a lesion ⟨∼ injection⟩ — **in·tra·le·sion·al·ly** *adv*

in·tra·leu·ko·cyt·ic *or chiefly Brit* **in·tra·leu·co·cyt·ic** \-ˌlü-kə-ˈsit-ik\ *n* : situated or occurring within a leukocyte ⟨∼ urate inclusions⟩

in·tra·lig·a·men·tous \-ˌlig-ə-ˈment-əs\ *adj* : occurring within or introduced into a ligament and esp. the broad ligament of the uterus

in·tra·lo·bar \-ˈlō-bər, -ˌbär\ *adj* : situated within a lobe

in·tra·lob·u·lar \-ˈläb-yə-lər\ *adj* : situated or occurring within a lobule (as of the liver or pancreas)

intralobular vein *n* : CENTRAL VEIN

in·tra·lu·mi·nal \-ˈlü-mən-ᵊl\ *adj* : situated within, occurring within, or introduced into the lumen ⟨∼ inflammation of the esophagus⟩

in·tra·lym·phat·ic \-lim-ˈfat-ik\ *adj* : situated within or introduced into a lymphatic vessel ⟨an ∼ dose of strophanthin⟩ — **in·tra·lym·phat·i·cal·ly** \-i-k(ə-)lē\ *adv*

in·tra·mam·ma·ry \-ˈmam-ə-rē\ *adj* : situated or introduced within the mammary tissue ⟨an ∼ injection⟩

in·tra·med·ul·lary \-ˈmed-ᵊl-ˌer-ē, -ˈmej-ə-ˌler-ē; -mə-ˈdəl-ə-rē\ *adj* : situated or occurring within a medulla ⟨an ∼ tumor of the spinal cord⟩; *esp* : involving use of the marrow space of a bone for support ⟨∼ pinning of a fracture of the thigh⟩

in·tra·mem·brane \-ˈmem-ˌbrān\ *adj* : INTRAMEMBRANOUS 2

in·tra·mem·bra·nous \-ˈmem-brə-nəs\ *adj* **1** : relating to, formed by, or being ossification of a membrane ⟨∼ bone development⟩ — compare ENDOCHONDRAL, PERICHONDRAL **2** : situated within a membrane ⟨∼ proteins⟩

in·tra·mi·to·chon·dri·al \-ˌmīt-ə-ˈkän-drē-əl\ *adj* : situated or occurring within mitochondria ⟨∼ inclusions⟩

in·tra·mo·lec·u·lar \-mə-ˈlek-yə-lər\ *adj* **1** : existing or acting within the molecule ⟨∼ helical regions in RNA⟩ **2** : formed by reaction between different parts of the same molecule — **in·tra·mo·lec·u·lar·ly** *adv*

in·tra·mu·co·sal \-myü-ˈkō-zəl\ *adj* : situated within, occurring within, or administered by entering a mucous membrane ⟨∼ gastric carcinoma⟩

in·tra·mu·ral \-ˈmyur-əl\ *adj* : situated or occurring within the substance of the walls of an organ ⟨∼ infarction⟩ ⟨failure of or delay in ∼ myocardial conduction —*Amer. Jour. of Cardiology*⟩ — **in·tra·mu·ral·ly** \-ə-lē\ *adv*

in·tra·mus·cu·lar \-ˈməs-kyə-lər\ *adj* : situated within, occurring within, or administered by entering a muscle ⟨∼ fat⟩ ⟨an ∼ injection⟩ — **in·tra·mus·cu·lar·ly** *adv*

in·tra·myo·car·di·al \-ˌmī-ə-ˈkärd-ē-əl\ *adj* : situated within, occurring within, or administered by entering the myocardium ⟨an ∼ injection⟩

in·tra·na·sal \-ˈnā-zəl\ *adj* : lying within or administered by way of the nasal structures — **in·tra·na·sal·ly** \-ˈnāz(-ə)-lē\ *adv*

in·tra·na·tal \-ˈnāt-ᵊl\ *adj* : occurring chiefly with reference to the child during the act of birth ⟨an ∼ accident⟩ — compare INTRAPARTUM; NEONATAL, PERINATAL, POSTNATAL, PRENATAL

in·tra·neu·ral \-ˈn(y)ur-əl\ *adj* : situated within, occurring within, or administered by entering a nerve or nervous tissue — **in·tra·neu·ral·ly** *adv*

in·tra·neu·ro·nal \-ˈn(y)ur-ən-ᵊl, -n(y)u-ˈrōn-ᵊl\ *adj* : situated or occurring within a neuron ⟨excess ∼ sodium⟩ ⟨∼ deamination⟩ — **in·tra·neu·ron·al·ly** \-ə-lē\ *adv*

in·tra·nu·cle·ar \-ˈn(y)ü-klē-ər\ *adj* : situated or occurring within a nucleus ⟨cytomegalic cells with prominent ∼ inclusions —L. J. Dorfman⟩ ⟨∼ DNA synthesis⟩

in·tra·nu·cle·o·lar \-n(y)ü-ˈklē-ə-lər\ *adj* : situated or occurring within a nucleolus ⟨∼ structures⟩

in·tra·oc·u·lar \ˌin-trə-ˈäk-yə-lər, -(ˌ)trä-\ *adj* : implanted in, occurring within, or administered by entering the eyeball ⟨∼ injections⟩ ⟨∼ lens implantation⟩ — **in·tra·oc·u·lar·ly** *adv*

intraocular pressure *n* : the pressure within the eyeball that gives it a round firm shape and is caused by the aqueous humor and vitreous body — called also *intraocular tension*

intraoesophageal *Brit var of* INTRAESOPHAGEAL

in·tra·op·er·a·tive \ˌin-trə-ˈäp-(ə-)rət-iv, -(ˌ)trä-, -ˈäp-ə-ˌrāt-\ *adj* : occurring, carried out, or encountered in the course of surgery ⟨∼ irradiation⟩ ⟨∼ infarction⟩ — **in·tra·op·er·a·tive·ly** *adv*

in·tra·oral \-ˈōr-əl, -ˈȯr-, -ˈär-\ *adj* : situated, occurring, or performed within the mouth ⟨∼ ulcerations⟩

in·tra·os·se·ous \-ˈäs-ē-əs\ *adj* : situated within, occurring within, or administered by entering a bone ⟨∼ vasculature⟩ ⟨∼ anesthesia⟩

in·tra·ovar·i·an \-ō-ˈvar-ē-ən, -ō-ˈver-\ *adj* : situated or occurring within the ovary

in·tra·ovu·lar \-ˈäv-yə-lər, -ˈōv-\ *adj* : situated or occurring within the ovum

in·tra·pan·cre·at·ic \-ˌpaŋ-krē-ˈat-ik, -ˌpan-\ *adj* : situated or occurring within the pancreas

in·tra·pa·ren·chy·mal \-pə-ˈreŋ-kə-məl, -ˌpar-ən-ˈkī-\ *adj* : situated or occurring within the parenchyma of an organ

in·tra·par·tum \-ˈpärt-əm\ *adj* : occurring chiefly with reference to a mother during the act of birth ⟨∼ complications⟩ — compare INTRANATAL

in·tra·pel·vic \-ˈpel-vik\ *adj* : situated or performed within the pelvis

in·tra·peri·car·di·ac \-ˌper-ə-ˈkärd-ē-ˌak\ *adj* : INTRAPERICARDIAL

in·tra·peri·car·di·al \-ē-əl\ *adj* : situated within or administered by entering the pericardium ⟨∼ injections⟩ ⟨∼ hemorrhage⟩

in·tra·per·i·to·ne·al \ˌin-trə-ˌper-ət-ᵊn-ˈē-əl\ *adj* : situated within or administered by entering the peritoneum — **in·tra·per·i·to·ne·al·ly** \-ˈē-ə-lē\ *adv*

in·tra·per·son·al \-ˈpərs-nəl, -ᵊn-əl\ *adj* : occurring within the individual mind or self ⟨∼ concerns of the aged⟩

in·tra·pleu·ral \-ˈplur-əl\ *adj* : situated within, occurring within, or administered by entering the pleura or pleural cavity ⟨∼ inoculation⟩ — **in·tra·pleu·ral·ly** \-ə-lē\ *adv*

intrapleural pneumonolysis *n* : PNEUMONOLYSIS b

in·tra·pop·u·la·tion \ˈin-trə-ˌpäp-yə-ˈlā-shən, -(ˌ)trä-\ *adj* : occurring within or taking place between members of a population ⟨∼ allografts⟩ ⟨∼ variation⟩

in·tra·pros·tat·ic \-prä-ˈstat-ik\ *adj* : situated within, occurring within, or administered by entering the prostate gland

in·tra·psy·chic \ˌin-trə-ˈsī-kik, -(ˌ)trä-\ *adj* : being or occurring within the psyche, mind, or personality ⟨∼ conflicts⟩ ⟨∼ trauma⟩ — **in·tra·psy·chi·cal·ly** \-ki-k(ə-)lē\ *adv*

in·tra·pul·mo·nary \-ˈpul-mə-ˌner-ē, -ˈpəl-\ *also* **in·tra·pul·mon·ic** \-pul-ˈmän-ik, -pəl-\ *adj* : situated within, occurring within, or administered by entering the lungs ⟨an ∼ foreign body⟩ ⟨∼ pressure⟩ ⟨an ∼ injection⟩ — **in·tra·pul·mo·nar·i·ly** \-ˌpul-mə-ˈner-ə-ˌlē\ *adv*

in·tra·rec·tal \-ˈrek-tᵊl\ *adj* : situated within, occurring within, or administered by entering the rectum

in·tra·re·nal \-ˈrēn-ᵊl\ *adj* : situated within, occurring within, or administered by entering the kidney ⟨an ∼ obstruction⟩ — **in·tra·re·nal·ly** \-ə-lē\ *adv*

in·tra·ret·i·nal \-ˈret-ᵊn-əl, -ˈret-nəl\ *adj* : situated or occurring within the retina

in·tra·ru·mi·nal \-ˈrü-mən-ᵊl\ *adj* : situated within, occurring within, or administered by entering the rumen

in·tra·scler·al \-ˈskler-əl\ *adj* : situated or occurring within the sclera

in·tra·scro·tal \-ˈskrōt-ᵊl\ *adj* : situated or occurring within the scrotum

in·tra·spe·cies \-ˈspē-(ˌ)shēz, -(ˌ)sēz\ *adj* : INTRASPECIFIC

in·tra·spe·cif·ic \-spi-ˈsif-ik\ *adj* : occurring within a species or involving members of one species ⟨∼ variation⟩ ⟨∼ competition⟩ — **in·tra·spe·cif·i·cal·ly** \-i-k(ə-)lē\ *adv*

in·tra·spi·nal \-ˈspīn-ᵊl\ *adj* : situated within, occurring within, or introduced into the spinal and esp. the vertebral canal ⟨∼ nerve terminals⟩ — **in·tra·spi·nal·ly** \-ē\ *adv*

in·tra·splen·ic \-'splen-ik\ *adj* : situated within or introduced into the spleen — **in·tra·splen·i·cal·ly** \-i-k(ə-)lē\ *adv*

in·tra·sy·no·vi·al \-sə-'nō-vē-əl, -sī-\ *adj* : situated or introduced within a synovial cavity or membrane

in·tra·tes·tic·u·lar \-tes-'tik-yə-lər\ *adj* : situated within, performed within, or administered into a testis — **in·tra·tes·tic·u·lar·ly** *adv*

in·tra·the·cal \-'thē-kəl\ *adj* : introduced into or occurring in the space under the arachnoid membrane of the brain or spinal cord ⟨∼ chemotherapy and cranial irradiation —*Jour. Amer. Med. Assoc.*⟩ — **in·tra·the·cal·ly** \-kə-lē\ *adv*

in·tra·tho·rac·ic \-thə-'ras-ik\ *adj* : situated, occurring, or performed within the thorax ⟨∼ pressure⟩ — **in·tra·tho·rac·i·cal·ly** *adv*

in·tra·thy·roi·dal \-thī-'roid-ᵊl\ *adj* : situated or occurring within the thyroid ⟨∼ iodine stores⟩

in·tra·tra·che·al \-'trā-kē-əl\ *adj* : occurring within or introduced into the trachea — **in·tra·tra·che·al·ly** \-ē\ *adv*

in·tra·tu·bu·lar \-'t(y)ü-byə-lər\ *adj* : situated or occurring within a tubule ⟨∼ androgen binding protein —R. V. Short⟩

in·tra·tym·pan·ic \-tim-'pan-ik\ *adj* : situated or occurring within the middle ear

in·tra·ure·thral \-yù-'rē-thrəl\ *adj* : situated within, introduced into, or done in the urethra ⟨alprostadil is also available as an ∼ pellet —Abraham Morgentaler⟩

in·tra·uter·ine \-'yüt-ə-rən, -ˌrīn\ *adj* : of, situated in, used in, or occurring within the uterus ⟨the ∼ environment⟩ ⟨∼ instillation of saline⟩; *also* : involving or occurring during the part of development that takes place in the uterus ⟨∼ infection⟩ ⟨∼ mortality⟩

intrauterine contraceptive device *n* : INTRAUTERINE DEVICE

intrauterine device *n* : a device (as a spiral of plastic or a ring of stainless steel) inserted and left in the uterus to prevent effective conception — called also *IUCD, IUD*

in·tra·vag·i·nal \-'vaj-ən-ᵊl\ *adj* : situated within, occurring within, or introduced into the vagina — **in·tra·vag·i·nal·ly** \-ē\ *adv*

in·trav·a·sa·tion \(ˌ)in-ˌtrav-ə-'sā-shən\ *n* : the entrance of foreign matter into a vessel of the body and esp. a blood vessel

in·tra·vas·cu·lar \ˌin-trə-'vas-kyə-lər, -(ˌ)trä-\ *adj* : situated in, occurring in, or administered by entry into a blood vessel ⟨∼ thrombosis⟩ ⟨an ∼ injection⟩ ⟨∼ radionuclide therapy⟩ — **in·tra·vas·cu·lar·ly** *adv*

in·tra·ve·nous \ˌin-trə-'vē-nəs\ *adj* 1 : situated within, performed within, occurring within, or administered by entering a vein ⟨an ∼ feeding⟩ ⟨∼ inflammation⟩ 2 : used in intravenous procedures ⟨∼ needles⟩ ⟨an ∼ solution⟩ — **in·tra·ve·nous·ly** *adv*

intravenous pyelogram *n* : a pyelogram in which radiographic visualization is obtained after intravenous administration of a radiopaque medium which collects in and is excreted by the kidneys

in·tra·ven·tric·u·lar \ˌin-trə-ven-'trik-yə-lər, -(ˌ)trä-\ *adj* : situated within, occurring within, or administered into a ventricle — **in·tra·ven·tric·u·lar·ly** *adv*

in·tra·ver·te·bral \-(ˌ)vər-'tē-brəl, -'vərt-ə-brəl\ *adj* : situated within a vertebra — **in·tra·ver·te·bral·ly** *adv*

in·tra·ves·i·cal \-'ves-i-kəl\ *adj* : situated or occurring within the bladder ⟨∼ pressure⟩ ⟨∼ infection⟩

in·tra·vi·tal \-'vīt-ᵊl\ *adj* 1 : performed upon or found in a living subject 2 : having or utilizing the property of staining cells without killing them — compare SUPRAVITAL — **in·tra·vi·tal·ly** \-ᵊl-ē\ *adv*

in·tra·vi·tam \-'vī-ˌtam, -'wē-ˌtäm\ *adj* : INTRAVITAL

intra vitam *adv* : during life : while the subject is still alive ⟨the condition was diagnosed *intra vitam*⟩

in·tra·vit·re·al \-'vi-trē-əl\ *adj* : INTRAVITREOUS ⟨∼ injection⟩

in·tra·vit·re·ous \-əs\ *adj* : situated within, occurring within, or introduced into the vitreous body ⟨∼ hemorrhage⟩

in·trin·sic \in-'trin-zik, -'trin(t)-sik\ *adj* 1 : originating or due to causes or factors within a body, organ, or part ⟨∼ asthma⟩ 2 : originating and included wholly within an organ or part — used esp. of certain muscles ⟨the cricothyroid is an ∼ muscle of the larynx⟩; compare EXTRINSIC 2

intrinsic factor *n* : a substance produced by the normal gastrointestinal mucosa that facilitates absorption of vitamin B_{12}

in·tro·duc·tion \ˌin-trə-'dək-shən\ *n* : an action of putting in or inserting ⟨∼ of contrast material through the catheter —*Scientific Amer. Medicine*⟩ — **in·tro·duce** \-'d(y)üs\ *vt* **-duced; -duc·ing**

in·troi·tal \in-'trō-ət-ᵊl\ *adj* : of or relating to an introitus ⟨the ∼ opening of the vagina⟩

in·troi·tus \in-'trō-ət-əs\ *n, pl* **introitus** : the orifice of a body cavity; *esp* : the vaginal opening

in·tro·ject \ˌin-trə-'jekt\ *vt* 1 : to incorporate (attitudes or ideas) into one's personality unconsciously 2 : to turn toward oneself (the love felt for another) or against oneself (the hostility felt toward another) — **in·tro·jec·tion** \-'jek-shən\ *n* — **in·tro·jec·tive** \-'jek-tiv\ *adj*

in·tro·mis·sion \ˌin-trə-'mish-ən\ *n* : the insertion or period of insertion of the penis in the vagina in copulation

in·tro·mit·tent \-'mit-ᵊnt\ *adj* : adapted for or functioning in intromission — used esp. of the copulatory organ of an animal

in·tron \'in-ˌträn\ *n* : a polynucleotide sequence in a nucleic acid that does not code information for protein synthesis and is removed before translation of messenger RNA — compare EXON — **in·tron·ic** \in-'trän-ik\ *adj*

In·tro·pin \'in-trə-ˌpin\ *trademark* — used for a preparation of the hydrochloride of dopamine

in·tro·pu·ni·tive \ˌin-trə-'pyü-nət-iv, ˌin-ˌtrō-\ *adj* : tending to blame or to inflict punishment on the self ⟨the direction of hostility was less ∼ than in the neurotic group —David MacSweeney & Denis Parr⟩ — compare EXTRAPUNITIVE

in·tro·spect \ˌin-trə-'spekt\ *vt* : to examine (one's own mind or its contents) reflectively ∼ *vi* : to engage in an examination of one's thought process and sensory experience — **in·tro·spec·tive** \-'spek-tiv\ *adj* — **in·tro·spec·tive·ly** *adv*

in·tro·spec·tion \-'spek-shən\ *n* : an examination of one's own thoughts and feelings — **in·tro·spec·tion·al** \-shnəl, -shən-ᵊl\ *adj*

in·tro·spec·tion·ism \-shə-ˌniz-əm\ *n* : a doctrine that psychology must be based essentially on data derived from introspection — compare BEHAVIORISM

¹in·tro·spec·tion·ist \-shə-nəst\ *n* 1 : a person esp. given to introspection 2 : an adherent of introspectionism

²introspectionist *or* **in·tro·spec·tion·is·tic** \-ˌspek-shə-'nist-ik\ *adj* : of or relating to introspectionism

in·tro·ver·sion \ˌin-trə-'vər-zhən, -shən\ *n* 1 : the act of directing one's attention toward or getting gratification from one's own interests, thoughts, and feelings 2 : the state or tendency toward being wholly or predominantly concerned with and interested in one's own mental life — compare EXTROVERSION — **in·tro·ver·sive** \-'vər-siv, -ziv\ *adj* — **in·tro·ver·sive·ly** *adv*

¹in·tro·vert \'in-trə-ˌvərt\ *vt* : to turn inward or in upon itself: as **a** : to concentrate or direct upon oneself **b** : to produce psychological introversion in

²introvert *n* : one whose personality is characterized by introversion; *broadly* : a reserved or shy person — compare EXTROVERT

in·tro·vert·ed \'in-trə-ˌvərt-əd\ *also* **in·tro·vert** \'in-trə-ˌvərt\ *adj* : marked by or suggesting introversion ⟨an uncommunicative and ∼ person⟩; *broadly* : being a reserved or shy person — compare EXTROVERTED

in·tu·bate \'in-(ˌ)t(y)ü-ˌbāt, -tə-\ *vt* **-bat·ed; -bat·ing** : to per-

\ə\ abut \ᵊ\ kitten \ər\ further \a\ ash \ā\ ace \ä\ cot, cart \aù\ out \ch\ chin \e\ bet \ē\ easy \g\ go \i\ hit \ī\ ice \j\ job \ŋ\ sing \ō\ go \ò\ law \òi\ boy \th\ thin \ṯh\ the \ü\ loot \ù\ foot \y\ yet \zh\ vision *See also* Pronunciation Symbols page

form intubation on ⟨the trachea is *intubated* with a cuffed endotracheal tube —A. M. Siegler⟩

in·tu·ba·tion \ˌin-(ˌ)t(y)ü-ˈbā-shən, -tə-\ *n* : the introduction of a tube into a hollow organ (as the trachea or intestine) to keep it open or restore its patency if obstructed — compare EXTUBATION

in·tu·ition \ˌin-t(y)ù-ˈish-ən\ *n* 1 : immediate apprehension or cognition without reasoning or inferring 2 : knowledge or conviction gained by intuition 3 : the power or faculty of gaining direct knowledge or cognition without evident rational thought and inference — **in·tu·it** \in-ˈt(y)ü-ət\ *vt* — **in·tu·ition·al** \ˌin-t(y)ù-ˈish-nəl, -ən-ᵊl\ *adj* — **in·tu·itive** \inˈt(y)ü-ət-iv\ *adj* — **in·tu·itive·ly** *adv*

in·tu·mes·cence \-ˈmes-ᵊn(t)s\ *n* 1 a : the action or process of becoming enlarged or swollen b : the state of being swollen 2 : something (as a tumor) that is swollen or enlarged — **in·tu·mesce** \-ˈmes\ *vi* **-mesced; -mesc·ing**

in·tu·mes·cent \-ᵊnt\ *adj* : marked by intumescence

in·tus·sus·cept \ˌint-ə-sə-ˈsept\ *vt* : to cause to turn inward esp. upon itself or to be received in some other thing or part; *esp* : to cause (an intestine) to undergo intussusception ⟨the bowel became ∼ed⟩ ∼ *vi* : to undergo intussusception ⟨some 3 ft. of the ileum had ∼ed through the ileocecal valve into the cecum —*Veterinary Record*⟩

in·tus·sus·cep·tion \-ˈsep-shən\ *n* 1 : INVAGINATION; *esp* : the slipping of a length of intestine into an adjacent portion usu. producing obstruction 2 : the deposition of new particles of formative material among those already embodied in a tissue or structure (as in the growth of living organisms) — compare ACCRETION, APPOSITION 1 — **in·tus·sus·cep·tive** \-ˈsep-tiv\ *adj*

in·tus·sus·cep·tum \-ˈsep-təm\ *n, pl* **-ta** \-tə\ : the portion of the intestine that passes into another portion in intussusception

in·tus·sus·cip·i·ens \-ˈsip-ē-ˌenz\ *n, pl* **-cip·i·en·tes** \-ˌsip-ē-ˈen-(ˌ)tēz\ : the portion of the intestine that receives the intussusceptum in intussusception

in·u·la \ˈin-yə-lə\ *n* 1 : the dried roots and rhizome of elecampane used as an aromatic stimulant and esp. formerly as a remedy in pulmonary diseases — called also *elecampane, elecampane root* 2 *cap* : a genus of Old World perennial herbaceous or rarely shrubby plants (family Compositae) having large yellow radiate heads and including the elecampane (*I. helenium*) 3 : any plant or root of the genus *Inula*

in·u·lase \ˈin-yə-ˌlās, -ˌlāz\ *also* **in·u·lin·ase** \-yə-lə-ˌnās, -ˌnāz\ *n* : an enzyme obtained esp. from molds (as *Aspergillus niger*) and capable of converting inulin to levulose but without action on starch

in·u·lin \ˈin-yə-lən\ *n* : a white mildly sweet plant polysaccharide that resists digestion in the stomach and small intestine, is extracted commercially esp. from the roots and rhizomes of composite plants (as chicory), and is used as a source of levulose, as a diagnostic agent in a test for kidney function, and as a food additive to improve the flavor and texture of low-fat and low-sugar processed foods

in·unc·tion \in-ˈəŋ(k)-shən\ *n* 1 : an act of applying an oil or ointment; *specif* : the rubbing of an ointment into the skin for therapeutic purposes 2 : OINTMENT, UNGUENT

in·unc·tum \-təm\ *n* : OINTMENT

in utero \in-ˈyüt-ə-ˌrō\ *adv or adj* : in the uterus : before birth ⟨a disease acquired *in utero*⟩ ⟨an *in utero* diagnosis⟩

in vac·uo \in-ˈvak-yə-ˌwō\ *adv* : in a vacuum ⟨serum dried *in vacuo*⟩

in·vade \in-ˈvād\ *vt* **in·vad·ed; in·vad·ing** 1 : to enter and spread within either normally (as in development) or abnormally (as in infection) often with harmful effects ⟨protect the body from *invading* viruses⟩ ⟨branches of a nerve ∼ the skin area⟩ 2 : to affect injuriously and progressively ⟨gangrene ∼s healthy tissue⟩ — **in·vad·er** \-ˈvād-ər\ *n*

in·vag·i·nate \in-ˈvaj-ə-ˌnāt\ *vb* **-nat·ed; -nat·ing** *vt* 1 : to cover or enclose (as within the body) 2 : to fold in so that an outer becomes an inner surface ⟨∼ the sac into the lumen —E. A. Graham⟩ ∼ *vi* : to undergo invagination ⟨a

condition in which a portion of the intestine ∼s into the adjacent segment —*New England Jour. of Medicine*⟩

in·vag·i·na·tion \-ˌvaj-ə-ˈnā-shən\ *n* 1 : an act or process of invaginating: as a : the formation of a gastrula by an infolding of part of the wall of the blastula b : intestinal intussusception 2 : an invaginated part

¹in·va·lid \ˈin-və-ləd, *Brit usu* -ˌlēd\ *adj* 1 : suffering from disease or disability : SICKLY 2 : of, relating to, or suited to one that is sick ⟨an ∼ chair⟩

²invalid *n* : one who is sickly or disabled

³in·va·lid \ˈin-və-ləd, -ˌlid, *Brit usu* -ˌlēd *or* ˌin-və-ˈlēd\ *vt* 1 : to remove from active duty by reason of sickness or disability ⟨was ∼ed out of the army⟩ 2 : to make sickly or disabled ⟨a patient ∼ed by valvular disease⟩

in·va·lid·ism \ˈin-və-ləd-ˌiz-əm\ *n* : a chronic condition of being an invalid

in·val·id·i·ty \ˌin-və-ˈlid-ət-ē, -va-\ *n, pl* **-ties** 1 : incapacity to work because of prolonged illness or disability 2 : INVALIDISM

in·va·sion \in-ˈvā-zhən\ *n* : the act of invading: as a : the penetration of the body of a host by a microorganism b : the spread and multiplication of a pathogenic microorganism or of malignant cells in the body of a host

in·va·sive \-siv, -ziv\ *adj* 1 : tending to spread; *esp* : tending to invade healthy tissue ⟨∼ cancer cells⟩ 2 : involving entry into the living body (as by incision or by insertion of an instrument) ⟨∼ diagnostic techniques⟩ — **in·va·sive·ness** *n*

in·ven·to·ry \ˈin-vən-ˌtōr-ē, -ˌtȯr-\ *n, pl* **-ries** 1 : a questionnaire designed to provide an index of individual interests or personality traits 2 : a list of traits, preferences, attitudes, interests, or abilities that is used in evaluating personal characteristics or skills

in·ver·sion \in-ˈvər-zhən, -shən\ *n* 1 : a reversal of position, order, form, or relationship: as a : a dislocation of a bodily structure in which it is turned partially or wholly inside out ⟨∼ of the uterus⟩ b : the condition (as of the foot) of being turned or rotated inward — compare EVERSION 2 c : RETROFLEXION d : a breaking off of a chromosome section and its subsequent reattachment in inverted position; *also* : a chromosomal section that has undergone this process 2 a : the conversion of dextrorotatory sucrose into a levorotatory mixture of glucose and fructose b : a change from one stereochemical figuration at a chiral center in a usu. organic molecule to the opposite configuration that is brought about by a reaction in which a substitution of one group is made for a different group 3 : HOMOSEXUALITY

inversus — see SITUS INVERSUS

¹in·vert \in-ˈvərt\ *vt* 1 a : to reverse in position, order, or relationship ⟨adjacent sequences of DNA and RNA that are complementary and ∼ed⟩ b : to subject to inversion 2 a : to turn inside out or upside down b : to turn inward ⟨when a foot is ∼ed its forepart tends to approach the midline of the body —*Jour. Amer. Med. Assoc.*⟩ ∼ *vi* : to undergo inversion ⟨a normal nipple that ∼s later in life can be an ominous sign —P. G. Donohue⟩

²in·vert \ˈin-ˌvərt\ *n* : one characterized by inversion; *esp* : HOMOSEXUAL

in·vert·ase \in-ˈvərt-ˌās, ˈin-vərt-, -ˌāz\ *n* : an enzyme found in many microorganisms and plants and in animal intestines that catalyzes the hydrolysis of sucrose — called also *invertin, saccharase, sucrase*

In·ver·te·bra·ta \(ˌ)in-ˌvərt-ə-ˈbrät-ə, -ˈbrāt-ə\ *n pl, in some esp former classifications* : a primary division of the animal kingdom including all except the Vertebrata

¹in·ver·te·brate \(ˈ)in-ˈvərt-ə-brət, -ˌbrāt\ *n* : an animal having no backbone or internal skeleton

²invertebrate *adj* : lacking a spinal column; *also* : of or relating to invertebrate animals

inverted *adj* 1 : turned upside down or inside out ⟨∼ lumen of the intestine⟩ 2 : HOMOSEXUAL

in·vert·in \in-ˈvərt-ᵊn\ *n* : INVERTASE

in·ver·tor \in-ˈvərt-ər\ *n* : a muscle that turns a part (as the foot) inward

invert sugar *n* : a mixture of D-glucose and D-fructose that is sweeter than sucrose, that occurs naturally in fruits and honey, that is usu. made commercially from a solution of cane sugar by hydrolysis (as with acid), and that is used chiefly as a difficultly crystallizable syrup in foods and in medicine

in·vest \in-'vest\ vt **1** : to envelop or cover completely ⟨the pleura ∼s the lung⟩ **2** : to endow with a quality or characteristic ⟨the paranoid personality who ∼s the external world with his . . . ideas and feelings —*Structure & Meaning of Psychoanalysis*⟩

in·ves·ti·ga·tion·al new drug \in-ˌves-ti-'gā-shə-nəl-\ n : a drug that has not been approved for general use by the Food and Drug Administration but is under investigation in clinical trials regarding its safety and efficacy first by clinical investigators and then by practicing physicians using subjects who have given informed consent to participate — abbr. *IND*; called also *investigational drug*

in·vest·ment \in-'ves(t)-mənt\ n **1** : an external covering of a cell, part, or organism **2** : a layer of heat-resistant material in which a dental appliance (as a bridge or inlay) is cast or in which it is embedded before soldering

in·vet·er·ate \in-'vet-ə-rət, -'ve-trət\ adj **1** : marked by long duration or frequent recurrence ⟨∼ bursitis⟩ **2** : confirmed in a habit : HABITUAL 2 ⟨an ∼ smoker⟩

in·vi·a·ble \(')in-'vī-ə-bəl\ adj : incapable of surviving esp. because of a deleterious genetic constitution — **in·vi·a·bil·i·ty** \(ˌ)in-ˌvī-ə-'bil-ət-ē\ n, pl **-ties**

in vi·tro \in-'vē-(ˌ)trō, -'vi-\ adv or adj : outside the living body and in an artificial environment ⟨growth of cells *in vitro*⟩ ⟨*in vitro* studies⟩

in vitro fertilization n : fertilization of an egg in a laboratory dish or test tube; specif : mixture usu. in a laboratory dish of sperm with eggs which have been surgically removed from an ovary that is followed by implantation of one or more of the resulting fertilized eggs into a female's uterus — abbr. *IVF*

in vi·vo \in-'vē-(ˌ)vō\ adv or adj **1** : in the living body of a plant or animal ⟨*in vivo* synthesis of DNA⟩ ⟨microorganisms are not ordinarily destroyed *in vivo* by bacteriostatic drugs —*Jour. Amer. Med. Assoc.*⟩ **2** : in a real-life situation ⟨observing a patient's behavior *in vivo*⟩

in·vo·lu·crum \ˌin-və-'lü-krəm\ n, pl **-cra** \-krə\ : a formation of new bone about a sequestrum (as in osteomyelitis)

in·vol·un·tary \(')in-'väl-ən-ˌter-ē\ adj : not subject to control of the will : REFLEX ⟨∼ contractions⟩

involuntary muscle n : muscle governing reflex functions and not under direct voluntary control; esp : SMOOTH MUSCLE

in·vo·lute \ˌin-və-'lüt\ vi **-lut·ed; -lut·ing** **1** : to return to a former condition ⟨after pregnancy the uterus ∼s⟩ **2** : to become cleared up ⟨the disease ∼s without desquammation —*Annals of N.Y. Academy of Sciences*⟩

in·vo·lu·tion \ˌin-və-'lü-shən\ n **1 a** : an inward curvature or penetration **b** : the formation of a gastrula by ingrowth of cells formed at the dorsal lip **2** : a shrinking or return to a former size ⟨∼ of the uterus after pregnancy⟩ **3** : the regressive alterations of a body or its parts characteristic of the aging process; specif : decline marked by a decrease of bodily vigor and in women by menopause

¹in·vo·lu·tion·al \ˌin-və-'lüsh-nəl, -ən-°l\ adj **1** : of or relating to involutional melancholia ⟨∼ depression⟩ **2** : of or relating to the climacterium and its associated bodily and psychic changes ⟨the ∼ time of life⟩

²involutional n : one who is affected with involutional melancholia

involutional melancholia n : agitated depression occurring at about the time of menopause or andropause that was formerly considered a distinct disorder but is now subsumed under major depressive disorder — called also *involutional psychosis*

in·vo·lu·tion·ary \ˌin-və-'lü-shə-ˌner-ē\ adj : INVOLUTIONAL 2

involution form n : an irregular or atypical bacterium formed under unfavorable conditions (as in old cultures)

in·volve \in-'välv, -'vòlv also -'väv or -'vòv\ vt **in·volved; in-**

volv·ing : to affect with a disease or condition : include in an area of damage, trauma, or insult ⟨all the bones of the skull were *involved* in the proliferative process⟩ ⟨herpes *involved* the trigeminal nerve⟩ ⟨severely *involved* patients were isolated⟩ ⟨lacerations *involved* the muscles⟩

in·volve·ment \in-'välv-mənt, -'vòlv-\ n : inclusion in an area affected by disease, trauma, or insult ⟨syphilitic ∼ of the brain⟩ ⟨the extent of ∼ of the lung —Morris Fishbein⟩

Io symbol ionium

Iod·amoe·ba \(ˌ)ī-ˌöd-ə-'mē-bə\ n : a genus of amebas commensal in the intestine of mammals including humans and distinguished by uninucleate cysts containing a large glycogen vacuole that stains characteristically with iodine

¹io·date \'ī-ə-ˌdāt, -ə-dət\ n : a salt of iodic acid

²io·date \'ī-ə-ˌdāt\ vt **io·dat·ed; io·dat·ing** : to impregnate or treat with iodine

iod·ic \ī-'äd-ik\ adj : of, relating to, or containing iodine; esp : containing iodine with a valence of five

iodic acid \ī-ˌäd-ik-\ n : a crystalline oxidizing solid HIO_3 formed by oxidation of iodine

io·dide \'ī-ə-ˌdīd\ n : a salt of hydriodic acid; also : the monovalent anion I^- of such a salt

iodimetric, iodimetrically, iodimetry var of IODOMETRIC, IODOMETRICALLY, IODOMETRY

io·din·ate \'ī-ə-də-ˌnāt\ vt **-at·ed; -at·ing** : to treat or cause to combine with iodine or a compound of iodine — **io·din·ation** \ˌī-ə-də-'nā-shən\ n

io·din·at·ed casein \'ī-ə-də-ˌnāt-əd-\ n : an iodine-containing preparation that is made from casein, resembles the thyroid hormone in physiological activity, and is used in animal feeds (as to increase milk production of cows) — called also *iodocasein*

io·dine \'ī-ə-ˌdīn, -əd-ⁿn, -ə-ˌdēn\ n, often attrib **1** : a nonmetallic halogen element obtained usu. as heavy shining blackish gray crystals and used esp. in medicine (as in antisepsis and in the treatment of goiter and cretinism) and in photography and chemical analysis — symbol *I*; see ELEMENT table **2** : a tincture of iodine used esp. as a topical antiseptic

iodine–131 \-ˌwən-ˌthərt-ē-'wən\ n : a heavy radioactive isotope of iodine that has the mass number 131 and a half-life of eight days, emits beta particles and gamma rays, and is used esp. in the form of its sodium salt in the diagnosis of thyroid disease and the treatment of goiter

iodine–125 \-ˌwən-ˌtwen(t)-ē-'fīv\ n : a light radioactive isotope of iodine that has a mass number of 125 and a half-life of 60 days, gives off soft gamma rays, and is used as a tracer in thyroid studies and as therapy in hyperthyroidism

iodine pent·ox·ide \-ˌpent-'äk-ˌsīd\ n : a white crystalline solid I_2O_5 used to oxidize carbon monoxide quantitatively to carbon dioxide

io·din·o·phil \ˌī-ə-'din-ə-ˌfil\ adj : taking up or coloring readily with iodine

io·dip·amide \ˌī-ə-'dip-ə-ˌmīd\ n : a radiopaque substance used in the form of its disodium salt $C_{20}H_{12}I_6N_2Na_2O_6$ or its meglumine salt $C_{34}H_{48}I_6N_4O_{16}$ esp. in cholecystography

io·dism \'ī-ə-ˌdiz-əm\ n : an abnormal local and systemic condition resulting from overdosage with, prolonged use of, or sensitivity to iodine or iodine compounds and marked by ptyalism, coryza, frontal headache, emaciation, and skin eruptions

io·dize or Brit **io·dise** \'ī-ə-ˌdīz\ vt **io·dized** or Brit **io·dised; io·diz·ing** or Brit **io·dis·ing** : to treat with iodine or an iodide ⟨*iodized* salt⟩

iodized oil n : a viscous oily liquid that has an odor like garlic, is made by treating a fatty vegetable oil with iodine or hydriodic acid, and is used as a contrast medium in X-ray photography

io·do \ī-'ō-(ˌ)dō, 'ī-ə-ˌdō\ adj : containing iodine

\ə\ abut \ᵊ\ kitten \ər\ further \a\ ash \ā\ ace \ä\ cot, cart \aú\ out \ch\ chin \e\ bet \ē\ easy \g\ go \i\ hit \ī\ ice \j\ job \ŋ\ sing \ō\ go \ò\ law \òi\ boy \th\ thin \th̲\ the \ü\ loot \ú\ foot \y\ yet \zh\ vision   See also Pronunciation Symbols page

I

J

io·do·ac·e·tate \ī-ˌōd-ō-ˈas-ə-ˌtāt, ī-ˌäd-\ *n* : a salt or ester of iodoacetic acid

io·do·ace·tic acid \-ə-ˌsēt-ik-\ *n* : a crystalline acid $C_2H_3IO_2$ used in biochemical research esp. because of its inhibiting effect on many enzymes (as in glycolysis in muscle extracts)

io·do·al·phi·on·ic acid \-ˌal-fē-ˈän-ik-\ *n* : a radiopaque liquid $C_{15}H_{12}I_2O_3$ used esp. for cholecystography

io·do·ca·sein \ī-ˌōd-ə-kā-ˈsēn, ī-ˌäd-, -ˈkā-sē-ən\ *n* : IODINATED CASEIN

io·do·chlor·hy·droxy·quin \ī-ˌōd-ə-ˌklōr-hī-ˈdräk-sē-ˌkwin, ī-ˌäd-ə-, -ˌklōr-\ *n* : an antimicrobial and mildly irritant drug C_9H_5ClINO formerly used esp. as an antidiarrheal but now used mainly as an antiseptic

io·do·de·oxy·uri·dine \ī-ˌōd-ə-ˌdē-ˌäk-sē-ˈyur-ə-ˌdēn\ *or* **5–io·do·de·oxy·uri·dine** \ˌfīv-\ *n* : IDOXURIDINE

io·do·form \ī-ˈōd-ə-ˌfȯrm, -ˈäd-\ *n* : a yellow crystalline volatile compound CHI_3 with a penetrating persistent odor that is used as an antiseptic dressing

io·do·gor·go·ic acid \ī-ˌōd-ə-ˌgȯr-ˌgō-ik-, ī-ˌäd-\ *n* : DIIODOTYROSINE

io·do·hip·pur·ate sodium \-ˈhip-yə-ˌrāt, -hi-ˈpyur-ˌāt-\ *n* : HIPPURAN

io·do·meth·a·mate \-ˈmeth-ə-ˌmāt\ *n* : a radiopaque substance used in the form of its sodium salt $C_8H_3I_2NNaO_5$ in urography

io·dom·e·try \ˌī-ə-ˈdäm-ə-trē\ *also* **io·dim·e·try** \-ˈdim-\ *n, pl* **-tries 1** : the volumetric determination of iodine usu. by titration with a standard solution of sodium thiosulfate using starch as indicator **2** : a method of quantitative analysis involving the use of a standard solution of iodine or the liberation of iodine from an iodide — **io·do·met·ric** *also* **io·di·met·ric** \-ˈme-trik\ *adj* — **io·do·met·ri·cal·ly** *also* **io·di·met·ri·cal·ly** \-tri-k(ə-)lē\ *adv*

io·do·phile \ī-ˈōd-ə-ˌfīl, -ˈäd-\ *n* : one (as a cell) that is iodophilic

io·do·phil·ic \ī-ˌōd-ə-ˈfil-ik, ī-ˌäd-\ *also* **iodophile** *adj* : staining in a characteristic manner with iodine

io·do·phor \ī-ˈōd-ə-ˌfō(ə)r, ī-ˈäd-\ *n* : a complex of iodine and a surface-active agent that releases iodine gradually and serves as a disinfectant

io·do·phtha·lein \ī-ˌōd-ə-ˈthal-ē-ən, ī-ˈäd-, -ˈthal-ˌēn, -ˈthāl-\ *n* : a derivative of phenolphthalein or its soluble blue-violet crystalline disodium salt $C_{20}H_8L_4Na_2O_4$ used to render the gallbladder opaque to X-rays and formerly to treat typhoid carriers — called also *tetraiodophenolphthalein*

io·do·pro·tein \-ˈprō-ˌtēn, -ˈprōt-ē-ən\ *n* : an iodine-containing protein — compare THYROPROTEIN

io·dop·sin \ˌī-ə-ˈdäp-sən\ *n* : a photosensitive violet pigment in the retinal cones that is similar to rhodopsin but more labile, is formed from vitamin A, and is important in photopic vision

io·do·pyr·a·cet \ī-ˌōd-ə-ˈpir-ə-ˌset, ī-ˌäd-\ *n* : a salt $C_8H_{19}I_2N_2O_3$ used as a radiopaque medium esp. in urography — called also *diodone*

io·do·quin·ol \ī-ˌōd-ə-ˈkwin-ˌȯl, -ˌä-, -ˌōl\ *n* : a drug $C_9H_5I_2NO$ used esp. in the treatment of amebic dysentery — called also *diiodohydroxyquin, diiodohydroxyquinoline*

IOM *abbr* Institute of Medicine

ion \ˈī-ən, ˈī-ˌän\ *n* **1** : an atom or group of atoms that carries a positive or negative electric charge as a result of having lost or gained one or more electrons — see ANION, CATION **2** : a charged subatomic particle (as a free electron)

ion channel *n* : a cell membrane channel that is selectively permeable to certain ions (as of calcium or sodium)

ion ex·change \-iks-ˈchānj\ *n* : a reversible interchange of one kind of ion present on an insoluble solid with another of like charge present in a solution surrounding the solid with the reaction being used esp. for softening or demineralizing water, purifying chemicals, or separating substances

ion–exchange chromatography *n* : chromatography in which the separation and deposition of components in the liquid phase is achieved by differences in their rate of migration through a column, layer, or impregnated paper containing an ion-exchange material and by the exchange of ions in

solution for those of like charge in the ion-exchange material

ion ex·chang·er \-iks-ˈchān-jər\ *n* **1** : a solid agent (as a synthetic resin) used in ion exchange **2** : an apparatus or piece of equipment used for ion exchange

ion exchange resin *n* : an insoluble material of high molecular weight that contains either acidic groups for exchanging cations or basic groups for exchanging anions and is used in ion-exchange processes and in medicine (as for reducing the sodium content of the body or the acidity of the stomach)

ion·ic \ī-ˈän-ik\ *adj* **1** : of, relating to, existing as, or characterized by ions ⟨~ gases⟩ ⟨the ~ charge⟩ **2** : based on or functioning by means of ions ⟨~ conduction⟩ — **ion·i·cal·ly** \-i-k(ə-)lē\ *adv*

io·ni·um \ī-ˈō-nē-əm\ *n* : a natural radioactive isotope of thorium having a mass number of 230

ionization chamber *n* : a partially evacuated tube provided with electrodes so that its conductivity due to the ionization of the residual gas reveals the presence of ionizing radiation

ionization constant *n* : a constant that depends upon the equilibrium between the ions and the molecules that are not ionized in a solution or liquid — symbol *K;* called also *dissociation constant*

ion·ize *or chiefly Brit* **ion·ise** \ˈī-ə-ˌnīz\ *vb* **ion·ized** *or chiefly Brit* **ion·ised; ion·iz·ing** *or chiefly Brit* **ion·is·ing** *vt* : to convert wholly or partly into ions ~ *vi* : to become ionized — **ion·iz·able** *or chiefly Brit* **ion·is·able** \-ˌnī-zə-bəl\ *adj* — **ion·iza·tion** *or chiefly Brit* **ion·isa·tion** \ˌī-ə-nə-ˈzā-shən\ *n*

ion·o·gen·ic \ˌī-ˌän-ə-ˈjen-ik\ *adj* : capable of ionizing ⟨~ phosphate groups of RNA⟩

ion·og·ra·phy \ˌī-ə-ˈnäg-rə-fē\ *n, pl* **-phies** : electrochromatography involving the migration of ions (as on wet filter paper) — **ion·o·graph·ic** \ˌī-ə-nə-ˈgraf-ik\ *adj*

io·none \ˈī-ə-ˌnōn\ *n* : either of two oily liquid isomeric ketones $C_{13}H_{20}O$ that have a strong odor of violets, are found esp. in the essential oil of an Australian shrub (*Boronia megastigma*) but are usu. obtained from citral, and are used esp. in perfumes

ion·o·phore \ī-ˈän-ə-ˌfō(ə)r, -ˈfȯ(ə)r\ *n* : a compound that facilitates transmission of an ion (as of calcium) across a lipid barrier (as in a plasma membrane) by combining with the ion or by increasing the permeability of the barrier to it — **io·noph·or·ous** \ˌī-ə-ˈnäf-ə-rəs\ *adj*

ion·to·pho·re·sis \(ˌ)ī-ˌänt-ə-fə-ˈrē-səs\ *n, pl* **-re·ses** \-ˌsēz\ : the introduction of an ionized substance (as a drug) through intact skin by the application of a direct electric current — **ion·to·pho·rese** \-ˈrēs\ *vt* **-resed; -res·ing** — **ion·to·pho·ret·ic** \-ˈret-ik\ *adj* — **ion·to·pho·ret·i·cal·ly** \-i-k(ə-)lē\ *adv*

io·pa·no·ic acid \ˌī-ə-pə-ˈnō-ik-\ *n* : a white crystalline powder $C_{11}H_{12}I_3NO_2$ administered orally as a radiopaque medium in cholecystography

io·phen·dyl·ate \ˌī-ə-ˈfen-də-ˌlāt\ *n* : a colorless to pale yellow liquid $C_{19}H_{29}IO_2$ administered by injection as a radiopaque medium esp. in myelography

io·phen·ox·ic acid \ˌī-ə-ˌfen-ˌäk-sik-\ *n* : a compound $C_{11}H_{11}I_3O_3$ administered as a radiopaque medium in cholecystography

io·ta·cism \ī-ˈōt-ə-ˌsiz-əm\ *n* **1** : a speech defect marked by use of the sound \ē\ in place of other vowel sounds **2** : a speech defect marked by inability to correctly pronounce the sound \ē\

io·thal·a·mate \ˌī-ə-ˈthal-ə-ˌmāt\ *n* : any of several salts of iothalamic acid that are administered by injection as radiopaque media

io·tha·lam·ic acid \ˌī-ə-thə-ˌlam-ik-\ *n* : a white odorless powder $C_{11}H_9I_3N_2O_4$ used as a radiopaque medium

IP *abbr* intraperitoneal; intraperitoneally

IPA *abbr* independent practice association

ip·e·cac \ˈip-i-ˌkak\ *also* **ipe·ca·cu·a·nha** \ˌip-i-ˌkak-ü-ˈan-ə\ *n* **1** : the dried rhizome and roots of either of two tropical American plants (*Cephaelis acuminata* and *C. ipecacuanha*) of the madder family used esp. as a source of emetine and cephaeline; *also* : either of these plants **2** : an emetic and expectorant preparation of ipecac; *esp* : IPECAC SYRUP

ipecac spurge *n* : a spurge of the genus *Euphorbia* (*E. ipecacuanhae*) of the eastern U.S. with a root that is emetic and purgative

ipecac syrup *n* : an emetic and expectorant liquid preparation that is widely used to induce vomiting in accidental poisoning, that contains the alkaloids emetine and cephaeline, and that is prepared by extracting the ether-soluble alkaloids from powdered ipecac and mixing them with glycerol and a syrup — called also *syrup of ipecac*

ipo·date \\'ī-pə-ˌdāt\ *n* : a compound that is administered in the form of its sodium salt $C_{12}H_{12}I_3N_2NaO_2$ or its calcium salt $C_{24}H_{24}CaI_6N_4O_4$ for use as a radiopaque medium in cholecystography and cholangiography

ip·o·moea \ˌip-ə-'mē-ə\ *n* **1** *cap* : a genus of herbaceous vines (family Convolvulaceae) that comprise forms (as the morning glories and the sweet potato, *I. batatas*) having showy bell- or funnel-shaped flowers and that include some which are sources of cathartic resins or psychoactive alkaloids (as lysergic acid amide) **2** *also* **ip·o·mea** : a plant or flower of the genus *Ipomoea* **3** *usu* **ipomea** : the dried root of a scammony (*Ipomoea orizabensis*)

IPPB *abbr* intermittent positive pressure breathing

ip·ra·tro·pi·um bromide \ˌip-rə-ˌtrō-pē-əm-\ *n* : an anticholinergic bronchodilator $C_{20}H_{30}BrNO_3 \cdot H_2O$ used esp. in the treatment of chronic obstructive pulmonary disease — see COMBIVENT

ipri·fla·vone \ˌī-pri-'flā-ˌvōn\ *n* : a semisynthetic isoflavone $C_{18}H_{16}O_3$ used to prevent postmenopausal bone loss

iprin·dole \i-'prin-ˌdōl\ *n* : an antidepressant drug $C_{19}H_{28}N_2$

ipro·ni·a·zid \ˌī-prə-'nī-ə-zəd\ *n* : a derivative $C_9H_{13}N_3O$ of isoniazid that is a monoamine oxidase inhibitor used as an antidepressant and formerly used in treating tuberculosis

ipro·ver·a·tril \ˌī-prə-'ver-ə-tril\ *n* : VERAPAMIL

ip·sa·tion \ip-'sā-shən\ *n* : MASTURBATION

ip·si·lat·er·al \ˌip-si-'lat-ə-rəl, -'la-trəl\ *adj* : situated or appearing on or affecting the same side of the body — compare CONTRALATERAL — **ip·si·lat·er·al·ly** \-ē\ *adv*

IPSP *abbr* inhibitory postsynaptic potential

IPT *abbr* interpersonal psychotherapy; interpersonal therapy

IQ \ˌī-'kyü\ *n* [*intelligence quotient*] : a number used to express the apparent relative intelligence of a person: as **a** : the ratio of the mental age (as reported on a standardized test) to the chronological age multiplied by 100 **b** : a score determined by one's performance on a standardized intelligence test relative to the average performance of others of the same age

Ir *symbol* iridium

IR *abbr* infrared

iri·dal \'ir-əd-ᵊl, 'īr-\ *adj* : of, relating to, or affecting the iris of the eye : IRIDIC ⟨an ∼ tumor⟩

iri·dec·to·my \ˌir-ə-'dek-tə-mē, ˌīr-\ *n, pl* **-mies** : the surgical removal of part of the iris of the eye

irid·en·clei·sis \ˌir-ə-den-'klī-səs, ˌīr-\ *n, pl* **-clei·ses** \-ˌsēz\ : a surgical procedure esp. for relief of glaucoma in which a small portion of the iris is implanted in a corneal incision to facilitate drainage of aqueous humor

iri·de·re·mia \ˌir-ə-də-'rē-mē-ə\ *n* : a congenital abnormality marked by partial or complete absence of the iris

irides *pl of* IRIS

ir·i·des·cent \ˌir-ə-'des-ᵊnt\ *adj* : having or exhibiting a display of colors producing rainbow effects — **ir·i·des·cence** \-ᵊn(t)s\ *n*

iri·di·ag·no·sis \ˌir-ə-ˌdī-ig-'nō-səs, ˌīr-\ *n, pl* **-no·ses** \-ˌsēz\ : diagnosis of disease by examination of the iris

irid·i·al \ī-'rid-ē-əl, i-\ *adj* : IRIDIC

irid·ic \ī-'rid-ik *also* i-\ *adj* : of or relating to the iris of the eye ⟨the pigmented ∼ epithelium⟩

iridica — see PARS IRIDICA RETINAE

iri·din \'ir-əd-ən, 'īr-\ *n* **1** : a crystalline glucoside $C_{24}H_{26}O_{13}$ occurring esp. in orrisroot **2** : an oleoresin prepared from the common blue flag for use as a purgative and liver stimulant

iridis — see HETEROCHROMIA IRIDIS, RUBEOSIS IRIDIS

irid·i·um \ir-'id-ē-əm\ *n* : a silver-white hard brittle very heavy metallic element of the platinum group used esp. in hardening platinum for alloys (as for surgical instruments) — symbol *Ir*; see ELEMENT table

iri·di·za·tion \ˌir-ə-də-'zā-shən, ˌīr-\ *n* : a semblance of a halo around a light observed by persons affected with glaucoma

iri·do·cap·su·lot·o·my \ˌir-ə-dō-ˌkap-sə-'lät-ə-mē, ˌīr-\ *n, pl* **-mies** : surgical incision through the iris and the capsular membrane surrounding the lens of the eye

iri·do·cho·roid·itis \ˌir-ə-dō-ˌkōr-ȯi-'dīt-əs, ˌīr-, -ˌkȯr-\ *n* : inflammation of the iris and the choroid

iri·do·cy·cli·tis \-ˌsī-'klīt-əs, -si-\ *n* : inflammation of the iris and the ciliary body

iri·do·cy·clo·cho·roid·itis \-ˌsī-klō-ˌkōr-ȯi-'dīt-əs, -ˌsik-lō-, -ˌkȯr-\ *n* : simultaneous inflammation of the iris, the ciliary body, and the choroid of the eye

iri·do·di·ag·no·sis \-ˌdī-ig-'nō-səs\ *n, pl* **-no·ses** \-ˌsēz\ : IRIDIAGNOSIS

iri·do·di·al·y·sis \-dī-'al-ə-səs\ *n, pl* **-y·ses** \-ˌsēz\ : separation of the iris from its attachments to the ciliary body

iri·do·do·ne·sis \-də-'nē-səs\ *n, pl* **-ne·ses** \-ˌsēz\ : tremulousness of the iris caused by dislocation or removal of the lens : HIPPUS

ir·i·dol·o·gist \ˌī-rə-'däl-ə-jəst\ *n* : a practitioner of iridology

ir·i·dol·o·gy \ˌī-rə-'däl-ə-jē\ *n, pl* **-gies** : the study of the iris of the eye for indications of bodily health and disease

iri·do·ple·gia \ˌir-ə-dō-'plē-j(ē-)ə, ˌīr-\ *n* : paralysis of the sphincter of the iris

iri·dos·chi·sis \ˌir-ə-'däs-kə-səs, ˌīr-\ *n, pl* **-chi·ses** \-ˌsēz\ *or* **-chi·sis·es** : separation of the stroma of the iris into two layers with disintegration of the anterior layer into fibrils

iri·do·scle·rot·o·my \ˌir-ə-dō-sklə-'rät-ə-mē, ˌīr-\ *n, pl* **-mies** : incision of the sclera and the iris

iri·dot·a·sis \ˌir-ə-'dät-ə-səs, ˌīr-\ *n, pl* **-a·ses** \-ˌsēz\ : stretching of the iris in the treatment of glaucoma

iri·dot·o·my \ˌir-ə-'dät-ə-mē, ˌīr-\ *n, pl* **-mies** : incision of the iris

iri·do·vi·rus \ˌir-ə-dō-'vī-rəs, ˌīr-\ *n* : any of a family (Iridoviridae) of double-stranded DNA viruses that contain an outer icosahedral capsid and that infect insects, frogs, and fish — see AFRICAN SWINE FEVER

iris \'ī-rəs\ *n, pl* **iris·es** *or* **iri·des** \'ī-rə-ˌdēz, 'ir-ə-\ **1** : the opaque muscular contractile diaphragm that is suspended in the aqueous humor in front of the lens of the eye, is perforated by the pupil and is continuous peripherally with the ciliary body, has a deeply pigmented posterior surface which excludes the entrance of light except through the pupil and a colored anterior surface which determines the color of the eyes **2** : IRIS DIAPHRAGM

iris bom·bé \-ˌbäm-'bā\ *n* : a condition in which the iris is bowed forward by an accumulation of fluid between the iris and the lens

iris diaphragm *n* : an adjustable diaphragm of thin opaque plates that can be turned by a ring so as to change the diameter of a central opening usu. to regulate the aperture of a lens (as in a microscope)

Irish moss \ˌī(ə)r-ish-'mȯs\ *n* **1** : the dried and bleached plants of a red alga (esp. *Chondrus crispus*) that are used as an agent for thickening or emulsifying or as a demulcent (as in cookery or pharmacy) — called also *chondrus* **2** : a red alga (esp. *Chondrus crispus*) that is a source of Irish moss — called also *carrageen*

Irish moss extractive *n* : CARRAGEENAN

iris scissors *n pl* : a small pair of scissors constructed for use in operations (as iridectomy) on the eyeball

iri·tis \ī-'rīt-əs\ *n* : inflammation of the iris of the eye

iron \'ī(-ə)rn\ *n* **1** : a heavy malleable ductile magnetic silver-white metallic element that readily rusts in moist air, occurs

I

J

native in meteorites and combined in most igneous rocks, is the most used of metals, and is vital to biological processes (as in transport of oxygen in the body) — symbol *Fe*; see ELEMENT table   **2** : iron chemically combined ⟨~ in the blood⟩ — **iron** *adj*

iron–deficiency anemia *n* : anemia that is caused by a deficiency of iron and characterized by hypochromic microcytic red blood cells

iron–59 \-ˌfif-tē-ˈnīn\ *n* : a heavy radioisotope of iron that has a mass number of 59 and a half-life of 45.1 days, emits beta particles and gamma rays, and is used as a tracer in the study of iron metabolism

iron lung *n* : a device for artificial respiration in which rhythmic alternations in the air pressure in a chamber surrounding a patient's chest force air into and out of the lungs esp. when the nerves governing the chest muscles fail to function because of poliomyelitis — called also *Drinker respirator*

iron oxide *n* : any of several oxides of iron; *esp* : FERRIC OXIDE

iron sulfate *n* : a sulfate of iron; *esp* : FERROUS SULFATE

ir·ra·di·ance \ir-ˈād-ē-ən(t)s\ *n* : the density of radiation incident on a given surface usu. expressed in watts per square centimeter or square meter

ir·ra·di·ate \ir-ˈād-ē-ˌāt\ *vt* **-at·ed; -at·ing** : to affect or treat by radiant energy (as heat); *specif* : to treat by exposure to radiation (as ultraviolet light or gamma rays)

ir·ra·di·a·tion \ir-ˌād-ē-ˈā-shən\ *n* **1 a** : the radiation of a physiologically active agent from a point of origin within the body; *esp* : the spread of a nervous impulse beyond the usual conduction path **b** : apparent enlargement of a light or bright object or surface when displayed against a dark background **2 a** : exposure to radiation (as ultraviolet light, X-rays, or alpha particles) **b** : application of radiation (as X-rays or gamma rays) esp. for therapeutic purposes **3** : IRRADIANCE

ir·ra·di·a·tor \ir-ˈād-ē-ˌāt-ər\ *n* : one that irradiates; *esp* : an apparatus for applying radiations (as X-rays)

ir·ra·tio·nal \(ˈ)ir-ˈ(r)ash-nəl, -ən-ᵊl\ *adj* : not rational: as **a** : lacking usual or normal mental clarity or coherence ⟨was ~ for several days after the accident⟩ **b** : not governed by or according to reason ⟨~ fears⟩ — **ir·ra·tio·nal·i·ty** \(ˌ)ir-ˌ(r)ash-ə-ˈnal-ət-ē\ *n, pl* **-ties** — **ir·ra·tio·nal·ly** \(ˈ)ir-ˈ(r)ash-nə-lē, -ən-ᵊl-ē\ *adv*

ir·re·duc·ible \ˌir-i-ˈd(y)ü-sə-bəl\ *adj* : impossible to bring into a desired or normal state ⟨an ~ hernia⟩ — **ir·re·duc·ibil·i·ty** \-ˌd(y)ü-sə-ˈbil-ət-ē\ *n, pl* **-ties**

ir·reg·u·lar \(ˈ)ir-ˈ(r)eg-yə-lər\ *adj* **1** : lacking perfect symmetry of form : not straight, smooth, even, or regular ⟨~ teeth⟩ **2 a** : lacking continuity or regularity of occurrence, activity, or function ⟨~ breathing⟩ **b** *of a physiological function* : failing to occur at regular or normal intervals ⟨~ menstruation⟩ ⟨have your bowels been ~⟩ **c** *of an individual* : failing to defecate at regular or normal intervals ⟨was constipated and very ~⟩ — **ir·reg·u·lar·ly** *adv*

ir·reg·u·lar·i·ty \(ˌ)ir-ˌ(r)eg-yə-ˈlar-ət-ē\ *n, pl* **-ties** **1** : the quality or state of being irregular ⟨hormonal ~⟩ **2** : occasional constipation ⟨more fiber in one's diet may help relieve ~⟩

ir·re·me·di·a·ble \ˌir-i-ˈmēd-ē-ə-bəl\ *adj* : impossible to remedy or cure

ir·re·spi·ra·ble \i(r)-ˈres-p(ə-)rə-bəl, -ri-ˈspī-rə-\ *adj* : unfit for breathing ⟨an ~ vapor⟩

ir·re·spon·si·ble \ˌir-i-ˈspän(t)-sə-bəl\ *adj* : not responsible : mentally inadequate to bear responsibility — **ir·re·spon·si·bil·i·ty** \-ˌspän(t)-sə-ˈbil-ət-ē\ *n, pl* **-ties**

ir·re·vers·ible \ˌir-i-ˈvər-sə-bəl\ *adj* : incapable of being reversed : not reversible ⟨an ~ medical procedure⟩: as **a** : impossible to make run or take place backward ⟨~ chemical syntheses⟩ **b** *of a colloid* : incapable of undergoing transformation from sol to gel or vice versa **c** *of a pathological process* : of such severity that recovery is impossible ⟨~ brain damage⟩ — **ir·re·vers·ibil·i·ty** \-ˌvər-sə-ˈbil-ət-ē\ *n, pl* **-ties** — **ir·re·vers·ibly** \-ˈvər-sə-blē\ *adv*

ir·ri·gate \ˈir-ə-ˌgāt\ *vt* **-gat·ed; -gat·ing** : to flush (a body

part) with a stream of liquid ⟨~ the wound with saline to remove debris⟩ ⟨the eye was *irrigated* for 10 minutes following chemical exposure⟩ — **ir·ri·ga·tion** \ˌir-ə-ˈgā-shən\ *n*

ir·ri·ga·tor \ˈir-ə-ˌgāt-ər\ *n* : an apparatus used for irrigation ⟨a dental ~⟩

ir·ri·ta·bil·i·ty \ˌir-ət-ə-ˈbil-ət-ē\ *n, pl* **-ties** **1** : the property of protoplasm and of living organisms that permits them to react to stimuli **2 a** : quick excitability to annoyance, impatience, or anger **b** : abnormal or excessive excitability of an organ or part of the body (as the stomach or bladder)

ir·ri·ta·ble \ˈir-ət-ə-bəl\ *adj* : characterized by irritability: as **a** : easily exasperated or excited **b** : responsive to stimuli

irritable bowel syndrome *n* : a chronic functional disorder of the colon that is of unknown etiology but is often considered to be of psychophysiological origin and that is characterized by diarrhea or constipation or diarrhea alternating with constipation, abdominal pain or discomfort, abdominal bloating, and passage of mucus in the stool — abbr. *IBS;* called also *irritable colon, irritable colon syndrome, mucous colitis, spastic colon*

irritable heart *n* : NEUROCIRCULATORY ASTHENIA

¹ir·ri·tant \ˈir-ə-tənt\ *adj* : causing irritation; *specif* : tending to produce inflammation

²irritant *n* : something that irritates or excites; *specif* : an agent by which irritation is produced ⟨a chemical ~⟩

ir·ri·tate \ˈir-ə-ˌtāt\ *vb* **-tat·ed; -tat·ing** *vt* **1** : to provoke impatience, anger, or displeasure in **2** : to cause (an organ or tissue) to be irritable : produce irritation in ⟨harsh soaps may ~ the skin⟩ **3** : to produce excitation in (as a nerve) : cause (as a muscle) to contract ~ *vi* : to induce irritation

ir·ri·ta·tion \ˌir-ə-ˈtā-shən\ *n* **1 a** : the act of irritating **b** : something that irritates **c** : the state of being irritated **2** : a condition of irritability, soreness, roughness, or inflammation of a bodily part

ir·ri·ta·tive \ˈir-ə-ˌtāt-iv\ *adj* **1** : serving to excite : IRRITATING ⟨an ~ agent⟩ **2** : accompanied with or produced by irritation ⟨~ coughing⟩

ir·ru·ma·tion \ˌir-ü-ˈmā-shən\ *n* : FELLATIO — **ir·ru·mate** \ˈir-ü-ˌmāt\ *vt* **-mat·ed; -mat·ing** — **ir·ru·ma·tor** \-ˌmāt-ər\ *n*

isa·tin \ˈī-sət-ən\ *n* : an orange red crystalline compound $C_8H_5NO_2$ obtained esp. by oxidation of indigo or by various syntheses and used as a reagent

is·aux·e·sis \ˌīs-ȯg-ˈzē-səs, -ȯk-ˈsē-\ *n, pl* **-e·ses** \-ˌsēz\ : ISOGONY — **is·aux·et·ic** \-ˈzet-ik, -ˈset-\ *adj*

isch·emia *or chiefly Brit* **isch·ae·mia** \is-ˈkē-mē-ə\ *n* : deficient supply of blood to a body part (as the heart or brain) that is due to obstruction of the inflow of arterial blood (as by the narrowing of arteries by spasm or disease) — **isch·emic** *or chiefly Brit* **isch·ae·mic** \-mik\ *adj* — **isch·emi·cal·ly** *or chiefly Brit* **isch·ae·mi·cal·ly** \-mi-k(ə-)lē\ *adv*

ischemic contracture *n* : shortening and degeneration of a muscle resulting from deficient blood supply

ischemic stroke *n* : stroke caused by thrombosis or embolism

ischia *pl of* ISCHIUM

is·chi·al \ˈis-kē-əl\ *adj* : of, relating to, or situated near the ischium

is·chi·al·gia \ˌis-kē-ˈal-j(ē-)ə\ *n* : pain in the hip

ischial spine *n* : a thin pointed triangular eminence that projects from the dorsal border of the ischium and gives attachment to the gemellus superior on its external surface and to the coccygeus, levator ani, and pelvic fascia on its internal surface

ischial tuberosity *n* : a bony swelling on the posterior part of the superior ramus of the ischium that gives attachment to various muscles and bears the weight of the body in sitting

is·chi·at·ic \ˌis-kē-ˈat-ik\ *adj* : ISCHIAL

is·chi·ec·to·my \ˌis-kē-ˈek-tə-mē\ *n, pl* **-mies** : surgical removal of a segment of the hip bone including the ischium

is·chio·cap·su·lar \ˌis-kē-ō-ˈkap-sə-lər\ *adj* : ISCHIOFEMORAL

is·chio·cav·er·no·sus \-ˌkav-ər-ˈnō-səs\ *n, pl* **-no·si** \-ˌsī\ : a muscle on each side that arises from the ischium near the crus of the penis or clitoris and is inserted on the crus near the pubic symphysis

is·chio·coc·cy·geus \-käk-'sij-ē-əs\ *n, pl* **-cy·gei** \-ē-ˌī\ : COC-CYGEUS

is·chio·fem·o·ral \-'fem-(ə-)rəl\ *adj* : of, relating to, or being an accessory ligament of the hip joint passing from the ischium below the acetabulum to blend with the joint capsule

is·chi·op·a·gus \ˌis-kē-'äp-ə-gəs\ *n* : congenitally united twins that are fused at the hip

is·chio·pu·bic \ˌis-kē-ō-'pyü-bik\ *adj* : of or relating to the ischium and the pubis

ischiopubic ramus *n* : the flattened inferior projection of the hip bone below the obturator foramen consisting of the united inferior rami of the pubis and ischium

is·chio·rec·tal \ˌis-kē-ō-'rek-t⁀l\ *adj* : of, relating to, or adjacent to both ischium and rectum ⟨a pelvic ~ abscess⟩

is·chi·um \'is-kē-əm\ *n, pl* **is·chia** \-ə\ : the dorsal and posterior of the three principal bones composing either half of the pelvis consisting in humans of a thick portion, a large rough eminence on which the body rests when sitting, and a forwardly directed ramus which joins that of the pubis

isch·uria \isk-'yùr-ē-ə\ *n* : stoppage or reduction in the flow of urine either from blockage of a passage with resulting retention in the bladder or from disease of the kidneys

is·ethi·o·nate \ˌīs-i-'thī-ə-ˌnāt\ *n* : a salt or ester of isethionic acid

is·ethi·on·ic acid \ˌīs-ˌē-thē-'än-ik-\ *n* : a crystalline sulfonic acid $C_2H_6O_4S$ used esp. in making surface-active agents

Ishi·ha·ra \ˌish-ē-'här-ə\ *adj* : of, relating to, or used in an Ishihara test ⟨~ plates⟩ ⟨the ~ method⟩

Ishi·ha·ra \ē-shē-hä-rä\, **Shinobu (1879–1963),** Japanese ophthalmologist. Ishihara introduced his test for color blindness in 1917. The test calls for the discernment of figures or patterned lines formed from colored dots placed in a field of dots of another color. Ishihara also published studies of Daltonism and trachoma.

Ishihara test *n* : a widely used test for color blindness that consists of a set of plates covered with colored dots which the test subject views in order to find a number composed of dots of one color which a person with various defects of color vision will confuse with surrounding dots of color

isin·glass \'īz-⁀n-ˌglas, 'ī-ziŋ-\ *n* **1** : a semitransparent whitish very pure gelatin prepared from the air bladders of fishes (as sturgeons) and used esp. as a clarifying agent and in jellies and glue — called also *ichthyocolla* **2** : MICA

is·land \'ī-lənd\ *n* : an isolated anatomical structure, tissue, or group of cells

islandicus — see LICHEN ISLANDICUS

island of Lang·er·hans \-'län-ər-ˌhänz, -ˌhän(t)s\ *n* : ISLET OF LANGERHANS

island of Reil \-'rī(ə)l\ *n* : INSULA

Reil, Johann Christian (1759–1813), German anatomist. Reil was a leading medical educator and clinician. He described the island of Reil in 1796.

is·let \'ī-lət\ *n* : a small isolated mass of one type of tissue within a different type; *specif* : ISLET OF LANGERHANS

islet cell *n* : one of the endocrine cells making up an islet of Langerhans

islet of Lang·er·hans \-'län-ər-ˌhänz, -ˌhän(t)s\ *n* : any of the groups of small slightly granular endocrine cells that form anastomosing trabeculae among the tubules and alveoli of the pancreas and secrete insulin and glucagon — called also *islet*

Lang·er·hans \'län-ər-ˌhäns\, **Paul (1847–1888),** German pathologist. Langerhans is notable for his studies of human and animal histology. He was among the first investigators to successfully explore this new area of research using staining techniques and other innovative methods. Most important was his work on the pancreas. He described the cell islands of the pancreas in a paper published in 1869. This paper presented the first careful and detailed description of the histology of the pancreas. The islets of Langerhans were first given that name in 1893 by the French histologist G. E.

Laguesse. Langerhans also studied the anatomy of the skin and its innervation.

iso·ag·glu·ti·na·tion \'ī-(ˌ)sō-ə-ˌglüt-⁀n-'ā-shən\ *n* : agglutination of an agglutinogen of one individual by the serum of another of the same species

iso·ag·glu·ti·nin \ˌī-(ˌ)sō-ə-'glüt-⁀n-ən\ *n* : an antibody produced by one individual that causes agglutination of cells (as red blood cells) of other individuals of the same species

iso·ag·glu·tin·o·gen \'ī-(ˌ)sō-ˌag-lü-'tin-ə-jən\ *n* : an antigenic substance capable of provoking formation of or reacting with an isoagglutinin

iso·al·lele \ˌī-(ˌ)sō-ə-'lē(ə)l\ *n* : either of a pair of alleles each of which produces such a similar result that a special test (as combination with another allelic mutant) is needed to distinguish them

iso·al·lox·a·zine \ˌī-(ˌ)sō-ə-'läk-sə-ˌzēn\ *n* : a yellow solid $C_{10}H_6N_4O_2$ that is the precursor of various flavins (as riboflavin)

iso·am·yl alcohol \ˌī-sō-ˌam-əl-\ *n* : a primary amyl alcohol that has a disagreeable odor and pungent taste and is obtained from fusel oil

isoamyl nitrite *n* : AMYL NITRITE

iso·an·dros·ter·one \ˌī-(ˌ)sō-an-'dräs-tə-ˌrōn\ *n* : EPIAN-DROSTERONE

iso·an·ti·body \ˌī-(ˌ)sō-'ant-i-ˌbäd-ē\ *n, pl* **-bod·ies** : ALLOAN-TIBODY

iso·an·ti·gen \-'ant-i-jən\ *n* : ALLOANTIGEN — **iso·an·ti·gen·ic** \ˌī-(ˌ)sō-ˌant-i-'jen-ik\ *adj* — **iso·an·ti·ge·nic·i·ty** \-ˌant-i-jə-'nis-ət-ē\ *n, pl* **-ties**

iso·bar \'ī-sə-ˌbär\ *n* : one of two or more atoms or elements having the same atomic weights or mass numbers but different atomic numbers

iso·bar·ic \ˌī-sə-'bär-ik, -'bar-\ *adj* **1** : of or relating to an isobar **2** : having the same specific gravity as cerebrospinal fluid ⟨~ anesthesia for spinal injection⟩

iso·bor·ne·ol \ˌī-sō-'bȯr-nē-ˌȯl, -ˌōl\ *n* : a volatile crystalline alcohol $C_{10}H_{17}OH$ that is stereoisomeric with borneol and yields camphor on oxidation

iso·bor·nyl thio·cyano·ace·tate \ˌī-sō-'bȯr-nil-ˌthī-ō-ˌsī-ə-nō-'as-ət-ˌāt, -sī-'an-ō-\ *n* : a yellow oily liquid $C_{13}H_{19}N_2OS$ used as a pediculicide

iso·bu·tyl \ˌī-sō-'byüt-⁀l\ *n* : the monovalent alkyl group $(CH_3)_2CHCH_2$

isobutyl alcohol *n* : a branched-chain primary butyl alcohol $C_4H_{11}O$ synthetically made usu. from carbon monoxide and hydrogen

isobutyl nitrite *n* : BUTYL NITRITE

iso·bu·tyr·ic acid \ˌī-sō-byü-'tir-ik-\ *n* : a colorless liquid acid $C_4H_8O_2$ used chiefly in making esters for use as flavoring materials

iso·ca·lo·ric \-kə-'lȯr-ik, -'lōr-, -'lär-; -'kal-ə-rik\ *adj* : having similar caloric values ⟨~ diets⟩ — **iso·ca·lo·ri·cal·ly** \-ri-k(ə-)lē\ *adv*

iso·car·box·az·id \ˌī-sō-ˌkär-'bäk-sə-zəd\ *n* : a hydrazide monoamine oxidase inhibitor $C_{12}H_{13}N_3O_2$ used as an antidepressant — see MARPLAN

iso·chor·ic \ˌī-sə-'kȯr-ik\ *adj* : of, maintained under, or performed under constant volume ⟨~ conditions⟩

iso·chro·mat·ic \ˌī-sō-krō-'mat-ik\ *adj* : of or corresponding to constant color ⟨perception of depth in ~ stereograms containing random dots of color⟩ ⟨a purely ~ stimulus⟩

iso·chro·mo·some \-'krō-mə-ˌsōm, -ˌzōm\ *n* : a chromosome produced by transverse splitting of the centromere so that both arms are from the same side of the centromere, are of equal length, and possess identical genes

iso·chro·nism \ī-'säk-rə-ˌniz-əm, ī-sə-'krō-\ *n* : the state of having the same chronaxie ⟨~ between a muscle and its nerve⟩ — **iso·chron·ic** \ˌī-sə-'krän-ik\ *adj*

\ə\ abut \⁀\ kitten \ər\ further \a\ ash \ā\ ace \ä\ cot, cart
\aù\ out \ch\ chin \e\ bet \ē\ easy \g\ go \i\ hit \ī\ ice \j\ job
\ŋ\ sing \ō\ go \ȯ\ law \ȯi\ boy \th\ thin \t̲h̲\ the \ü\ loot
\ù\ foot \y\ yet \zh\ vision *See also* Pronunciation Symbols page

I

J

iso·cit·rate \ˌī-sō-'si-ˌtrāt\ n : any salt or ester of isocitric acid; also : ISOCITRIC ACID

isocitrate de·hy·dro·ge·nase \-ˌdē-(ˌ)hī-'dräj-e-ˌnās, -(')dē-'hī-drə-jə-, -ˌnāz\ n : either of two enzymes which catalyze the oxidation of isocitric acid to alpha-ketoglutaric acid (as in the Krebs cycle) and of which one uses NAD as an electron acceptor and the other NADP — called also *isocitric dehydrogenase*

iso·cit·ric acid \ˌī-sə-ˌsi-trik-\ n : a crystalline isomer of citric acid that occurs esp. as an intermediate stage in the Krebs cycle

isocitric dehydrogenase n : ISOCITRATE DEHYDROGENASE

iso·cor·tex \ˌī-sō-'kȯr-ˌteks\ n : NEOPALLIUM

iso·cy·a·nide \-'sī-ə-ˌnīd\ n : any of a class of compounds that are isomeric with the normal cyanides, that have the structure RNC, and that are in general colorless volatile poisonous liquids of strong offensive odor — called also *carbylamine, isonitrile*

iso·cy·clic \-'sī-klik, -'sik-lik\ adj : having or being a ring composed of atoms of only one element; esp : CARBOCYCLIC

iso·dose \'ī-sə-ˌdōs\ adj : of or relating to points or zones in a medium that receive equal doses of radiation ⟨an ∼ chart⟩ ⟨∼ curves obtained in different parallel planes —*Physical Rev.*⟩

iso·dy·nam·ic \ˌī-sō-dī-'nam-ik\ adj : ISOCALORIC ⟨the lactose and sugar . . . were replaced by an ∼ quantity of pure butterfat —*Jour. Amer. Med. Assoc.*⟩

iso·elec·tric \ˌī-sō-i-'lek-trik\ adj 1 : having or representing the same or connecting points with the same electrical potential ⟨an ∼ electroencephalogram⟩ ⟨∼ maps of the body surface⟩ 2 : being the pH at which the electrolyte will not migrate in an electrical field ⟨proteins migrating through a gel to a location with pH of their ∼ point⟩

isoelectric focusing n : an electrophoretic technique for separating proteins by causing them to migrate under the influence of an electric field through a medium (as a gel) having a pH gradient to locations with pH values corresponding to their isoelectric points

iso·elec·tro·fo·cus·ing \ˌī-sō-i-ˌlek-trō-'fō-kəs-iŋ\ n : ISOELECTRIC FOCUSING

iso·en·zyme \-'en-ˌzīm\ n : any of two or more chemically distinct but functionally similar enzymes — called also *isozyme* — **iso·en·zy·mat·ic** \ˌī-sō-ˌen-zə-'mat-ik, -zī-\ adj — **iso·en·zy·mic** \-en-'zī-mik\ adj

iso·eth·a·rine \-'eth-ə-ˌrēn\ n : a beta-adrenergic bronchodilator administered by oral inhalation esp. in the form of its hydrochloride $C_{13}H_{21}NO_3 \cdot HCl$ to treat asthma and bronchospasm

iso·fla·vone \-'flā-ˌvōn\ n : a bioactive ketone $C_{15}H_{10}O_2$ noted for its numerous derivatives that are found in plants (as the soybean) and have antioxidant and estrogenic activity; *also* : any of these derivatives (as daidzein or genistein)

iso·fluro·phate \-'flùr-ə-ˌfāt\ n : a volatile irritating liquid ester $C_6H_{14}FO_3P$ that acts as a nerve gas by inhibiting cholinesterases and as a miotic and is used chiefly in treating glaucoma — called also *DFP, diisopropyl fluorophosphate*

iso·form \'ī-sə-ˌfȯrm\ n : any of two or more functionally similar proteins that have a similar but not identical amino acid sequence and are either encoded by different genes or by RNA transcripts from the same gene which have had different exons removed

iso·ga·mete \ˌī-sō-gə-'mēt, -'gam-ˌēt\ n : a gamete indistinguishable in form, size, or behavior from another gamete with which it can unite to form a zygote — **iso·ga·met·ic** \-gə-'met-ik\ adj

isog·a·mous \ī-'säg-ə-məs\ adj : having or involving isogametes — compare ANISOGAMOUS, HETEROGAMOUS — **isog·a·my** \-mē\ n, pl **-mies**

iso·ge·ne·ic \ˌī-sō-jə-'nē-ik, -'nā-\ adj : SYNGENEIC ⟨an ∼ graft⟩

iso·gen·ic \-'jen-ik\ adj : characterized by essentially identical genes ⟨identical twins are ∼⟩

isog·o·ny \ī-'säg-ə-nē\ n, pl **-nies** : relative growth in such a way that the rate of growth of each part is the same as that of the whole — called also *isauxesis*

iso·graft \'ī-sə-ˌgraft\ n : a homograft between genetically identical or nearly identical individuals — **isograft** vt

iso·hem·ag·glu·ti·na·tion or chiefly Brit **iso·haem·ag·glu·ti·na·tion** \ˌī-sō-ˌhē-me-ˌglüt-ᵊn-'ā-shən\ n : isoagglutination of red blood cells

iso·hem·ag·glu·ti·nin or chiefly Brit **iso·haem·ag·glu·ti·nin** \-ˌhē-mə-'glüt-ᵊn-ən\ n : a hemagglutinin causing isoagglutination

iso·hem·ag·glu·tin·o·gen or chiefly Brit **iso·haem·ag·glu·tin·o·gen** \-ˌhē-mə-glü-'tin-ə-jən\ n : an antigen inducing the production of or reacting with specific isohemagglutinins

iso·he·mo·ly·sin or chiefly Brit **iso·hae·mo·ly·sin** \ˌī-sō-ˌhē-mə-'līs-ᵊn\ n : a hemolysin that causes isohemolysis

iso·he·mol·y·sis or chiefly Brit **iso·hae·mol·y·sis** \ˌī-sō-hi-'mäl-ə-səs\ n, pl **-y·ses** \-ˌsēz\ : lysis of the red blood cells of one individual by antibodies in the serum of another of the same species

iso·hy·dric \ˌī-sō-'hī-drik\ adj : having the same or constant pH ⟨∼ solutions⟩ ⟨cells cultured under ∼ conditions⟩

isohydric shift \-'shift\ n : the set of chemical reactions in a red blood cell by which oxygen is released to the tissues and carbon dioxide is taken up while the blood remains at constant pH

iso·im·mune \ˌī-sō-im-'yün\ adj : of, relating to, or characterized by isoimmunization ⟨∼ sera⟩

iso·im·mu·ni·za·tion or chiefly Brit **iso·im·mu·ni·sa·tion** \ˌī-sō-ˌim-yə-nə-'zā-shən\ n : production by an individual of antibodies against constituents of the tissues of another individual of the same species (as when transfused with blood from one belonging to a different blood group)

iso·ion·ic point \ˌī-sō-ī-'än-ik-\ n : the hydrogen-ion concentration expressed usu. as the pH value at which the ionization of an amphoteric substance as an acid equals the ionization as a base and becomes identical with the isoelectric point in the absence of foreign inorganic ions

iso·lant \'ī-sə-lənt\ n : ISOLATE 1, 2

¹iso·late \'ī-sə-ˌlāt\ vt **-lat·ed; -lat·ing** : to set apart from others: as **a** : to separate (one with a contagious disease) from others not similarly infected **b** : to separate (as a chemical compound) from all other substances : obtain pure or in a free state

²iso·late \'ī-sə-lət, -ˌlāt\ n 1 : an individual (as a spore or single organism), a viable part of an organism (as a cell), or a strain that has been isolated (as from diseased tissue, contaminated water, or the air); *also* : a pure culture produced from such an isolate 2 : a relatively homogeneous population separated from related populations by geographic, biologic, or social factors or by human intervention 3 : a socially withdrawn individual

iso·la·tion \ˌī-sə-'lā-shən\ n 1 : the action of isolating or condition of being isolated ⟨∼ of a virus⟩ ⟨put the patient in ∼⟩ 2 : a segregation of a group of organisms from related forms in such a manner as to prevent crossing 3 : a psychological defense mechanism consisting of the separating of ideas or emotions connected with them

iso·lec·i·thal \ˌī-sō-'les-i-thəl\ adj, of an egg : having the yolk small in amount and nearly uniformly distributed — compare CENTROLECITHAL, TELOLECITHAL

Iso·lette \ˌī-sə-'let\ trademark — used for an incubator for premature infants that provides controlled temperature and humidity and an oxygen supply

iso·leu·cine \ˌī-sō-'lü-ˌsēn\ n : a crystalline essential amino acid $C_6H_{13}NO_2$ isomeric with leucine — abbr. *Ile*

iso·leu·cyl \-'lü-ˌsil\ n : the amino acid radical or residue $CH_3CH_2CH(CH_3)CH(NH_2)CO-$ of isoleucine — abbr. *Ile*

isol·o·gous \ī-'säl-ə-gəs\ adj 1 : relating to or being any of two or more compounds of related structure that differ in some way other than the number of methylene groups they contain 2 : SYNGENEIC

iso·logue or **iso·log** \'ī-sə-ˌlȯg, -ˌläg\ n : any of two or more isologous compounds

iso·ly·ser·gic acid \ˌī-sō-lə-ˌsər-jik-, -(ˌ)lī-\ n : an acid

$C_{16}H_{16}N_2O_2$ that is isomeric with lysergic acid and is the parent compound of several ergotic alkaloids

iso·mal·tose \-'mȯl-ˌtōs, -ˌtōz\ *n* : a syrupy disaccharide $C_{12}H_{22}O_{11}$ isomeric with maltose

iso·mer \'ī-sə-mər\ *n* **1** : any of two or more compounds, radicals, or ions that contain the same number of atoms of the same elements but differ in structural arrangement and properties **2** : a nuclide isomeric with one or more others

isom·er·ase \ī-'säm-ə-ˌrās, -ˌrāz\ *n* : an enzyme that catalyzes the conversion of its substrate to an isomeric form

iso·mer·ic \ˌī-sə-'mer-ik\ *adj* : of, relating to, or exhibiting isomerism — **iso·mer·i·cal·ly** \-i-k(ə-)lē\ *adv*

isom·er·ide \ī-'säm-ə-ˌrīd\ *n* : ISOMER

isom·er·ism \ī-'säm-ə-ˌriz-əm\ *n* **1** : the relation of two or more chemical species that are isomers **2** : the relation of two or more nuclides with the same mass numbers and atomic numbers but different energy states and rates of radioactive decay

isom·er·ize *also Brit* **isom·er·ise** \ī-'säm-ə-ˌrīz\ *vb* **-ized** *also Brit* **-ised; -iz·ing** *also Brit* **-is·ing** *vi* : to become changed into an isomeric form ~ *vt* : to cause to isomerize — **isom·er·i·za·tion** *also Brit* **isom·er·i·sa·tion** \-ˌsäm-ə-rə-'zā-shən\ *n*

iso·me·thep·tene \ˌī-sō-me-'thep-ˌtēn\ *n* : a vasoconstrictive and antispasmodic drug administered esp. in the form of its mucate $C_{24}H_{48}N_2O_8$

iso·met·ric \ˌī-sə-'me-trik\ *adj* **1** : of, relating to, or characterized by equality of measure; *esp* : relating to or being a crystallographic system characterized by three equal axes at right angles **2** : of, relating to, involving, or being muscular contraction (as in isometrics) against resistance, without significant change of length of muscle fibers, and with marked increase in muscle tone — compare ISOTONIC 2 **3** : ISOVOLUMETRIC — **iso·met·ri·cal·ly** \-tri-k(ə-)lē\ *adv*

iso·met·rics \ˌī-sə-'me-triks\ *n pl but sing or pl in constr* : isometric exercise or an isometric system of exercises

iso·morph \'ī-sə-ˌmȯrf\ *n* : something identical with or similar to something else in form or structure; *esp* : one of two or more substances related by isomorphism — **iso·mor·phous** \ˌī-sə-'mȯr-fəs\ *adj*

iso·mor·phic \ˌī-sə-'mȯr-fik\ *adj* : being of identical or similar form or shape or structure

iso·mor·phism \ˌī-sə-'mȯr-ˌfiz-əm\ *n* **1** : similarity in organisms of different ancestry resulting from evolutionary convergence **2** : similarity of crystalline form between chemical compounds **3** : a correspondence that is held to exist between a mental process (as perception) and physiological processes

iso·ni·a·zid \ˌī-sə-'nī-ə-zəd\ *n* : a crystalline compound $C_6H_7N_3O$ used in treating tuberculosis — called also *isonicotinic acid hydrazide*

iso·nic·o·tin·ic acid \ˌī-sō-ˌnik-ə-ˌtin-ik-, -ˌtēn-\ *n* : a crystalline acid $C_6H_6NO_2$ used chiefly in making isoniazid

isonicotinic acid hydrazide *n* : ISONIAZID

iso·nip·e·caine \ˌī-sō-'nip-ə-ˌkān\ *n* : MEPERIDINE

iso·ni·trile \-'nī-trəl, -ˌtrēl\ *n* : ISOCYANIDE

iso·os·mot·ic \ˌī-sō-äz-'mät-ik\ *adj* : ISOTONIC 1

Iso·paque \ˌī-sō-'pāk\ *trademark* — used for a preparation of metrizoate sodium

isop·a·thy \ī-'säp-ə-thē\ *n, pl* **-thies** : medical treatment based on the hypothesis that it is beneficial to administer the causative agent or its products or an extract from a healthy animal of the part or organ affected

iso·peri·stal·tic \ˌī-sō-ˌper-ə-'stȯl-tik, -'stäl-, -'stal-\ *adj* : performed or arranged so that the grafted or anastomosed parts exhibit peristalsis in the same direction ⟨~ gastroenterostomy⟩ — **iso·peri·stal·ti·cal·ly** \-ti-k(ə-)lē\ *adv*

iso·phane \'ī-sō-ˌfān\ *adj* : of, relating to, or being a ratio of protamine to insulin equal to that in a solution made by mixing equal parts of a solution of the two in which all the protamine precipitates and a solution of the two in which all the insulin precipitates

isophane insulin *n* : an isophane mixture of protamine and insulin — called also *isophane*

iso·pre·cip·i·tin \ˌī-sō-pri-'sip-ət-ən\ *n* : a precipitin formed by an individual of one species that is specific for antigens of allogeneic individuals

iso·preg·nen·one \-'preg-nen-ˌōn\ *n* : DYDROGESTERONE

iso·pren·a·line \ˌī-sə-'pren-ᵊl-ən\ *n* : ISOPROTERENOL

iso·prene \'ī-sə-ˌprēn\ *n* : a flammable liquid unsaturated hydrocarbon C_5H_8 used esp. in synthetic rubber

iso·pren·oid \ˌī-sə-'prē-ˌnȯid\ *adj* : relating to, containing, or being a branched-chain group characteristic of isoprene — **isoprenoid** *n*

iso·pro·pa·mide iodide \ˌī-sō-ˌprō-pə-ˌmēd-\ *n* : an anticholinergic $C_{23}H_{33}IN_2O$ used esp. for its antispasmodic and antisecretory effect on the gastrointestinal tract — called also *isopropamide*

iso·pro·pa·nol \-'prō-pə-ˌnȯl, -ˌnōl\ *n* : ISOPROPYL ALCOHOL

iso·pro·pyl \ˌī-sə-'prō-pəl\ *n* : the alkyl group isomeric with normal propyl

isopropyl alcohol *n* : a volatile flammable alcohol C_3H_8O used esp. as a solvent and rubbing alcohol — called also *isopropanol*

iso·pro·pyl·ar·te·re·nol \-ˌärt-ə-'rē-ˌnȯl, -ˌnōl\ *n* : ISOPROTERENOL

isopropyl my·ris·tate \-mə-'ris-ˌtāt\ *n* : an ester $C_{17}H_{34}O_2$ of isopropyl alcohol and myristic acid that is used as an emollient to promote absorption through the skin

iso·pro·ter·e·nol \ˌī-sə-prō-'ter-ə-ˌnȯl, -nəl\ *n* : a sympathomimetic agent used in the form of its hydrochloride $C_{11}H_{17}NO_3 \cdot HCl$ or sulfate $(C_{11}H_{17}NO_3)_2 \cdot H_2SO_4$ esp. as a bronchodilator in the treatment of asthma, bronchitis, and emphysema — called also *isoprenaline, isopropylarterenol*; see ISUPREL

isop·ter \ī-'säp-tər\ *n* : a contour line in a representation of the visual field around the points representing the macula lutea that passes through the points of equal visual acuity

iso·pyc·nic \ˌī-sō-'pik-nik\ *adj* **1** : of, relating to, or marked by equal or constant density **2** : being or produced by a technique (as centrifugation) in which the components of a mixture are separated on the basis of differences in density

iso·pyk·no·sis *also* **iso·pyc·no·sis** \ˌī-sō-pik-'nō-səs\ *n* : the quality or state of some chromosomes or of parts of some chromosomes in a nucleus of staining uniformly and being coiled to the same degree — compare HETEROPYKNOSIS — **iso·pyk·not·ic** *also* **iso·pyc·not·ic** \-'nät-ik\ *adj*

iso·quin·o·line \ˌī-sō-'kwin-ᵊl-ˌēn\ *n* : a low-melting nitrogenous base C_9H_7N that is associated with its isomer quinoline in coal tar and that is the parent structure in many alkaloids (as narcotine and papaverine)

Isor·dil \'ī-sȯr-ˌdil\ *trademark* — used for a preparation of isosorbide dinitrate

iso·sex·u·al \ˌī-sə-'seksh-(ə-)wəl, -'sek-shəl\ *adj* : of, relating to, or being bodily processes or development of an individual consistent with the sex of the individual ⟨~ precocious puberty⟩

is·os·mot·ic \ˌī-ˌsäz-'mät-ik, -ˌsäs-\ *adj* : ISOTONIC 1 — **is·os·mot·i·cal·ly** \-'mät-i-k(ə-)lē\ *adv*

iso·sor·bide \ˌī-sō-'sȯr-ˌbīd\ *n* **1** : a diuretic $C_6H_{10}O_4$ **2** : ISOSORBIDE DINITRATE

iso·sor·bide di·ni·trate \-dī-'nī-ˌtrāt\ *n* : a coronary vasodilator $C_6H_8N_2O_8$ used esp. in the treatment of angina pectoris — see ISORDIL

Isos·po·ra \ī-'säs-pə-rə\ *n* : a genus of coccidian protozoans closely related to the genus *Eimeria* and including the only coccidian (*I. hominis*) known to be parasitic in humans

iso·stere \'ī-sə-ˌsti(ə)r\ *also* **iso·ster** \'ī-sə-ˌster\ *n* : one of two or more substances (as carbon monoxide and molecular nitrogen) that exhibit similarity of some properties as a result of having the same number of total or valence electrons in the same arrangement and that consist of different atoms and not necessarily the same number of atoms — **iso·ster·ic**

\ə\ **abut** \ᵊ\ **kitten** \ər\ **further** \a\ **ash** \ā\ **ace** \ä\ **cot, cart** \aů\ **out** \ch\ **chin** \e\ **bet** \ē\ **easy** \g\ **go** \i\ **hit** \ī\ **ice** \j\ **job** \ŋ\ **sing** \ō\ **go** \ȯ\ **law** \ȯi\ **boy** \th\ **thin** \t͟h\ **the** \ü\ **loot** \ů\ **foot** \y\ **yet** \zh\ **vision** *See also* Pronunciation Symbols page

\ˌī-sə-'sti(ə)r-ik, -'ster-\ *adj* — **isos·ter·ism** \ī-'säs-tə-ˌriz-əm\ *n*

isos·the·nu·ria \ī-ˌsäs-thə-'n(y)ùr-ē-ə\ *n* : a condition in which the kidneys produce urine with the specific gravity of protein-free blood plasma

iso·tac·tic \ˌī-sə-'tak-tik\ *adj* : having or relating to a stereochemical regularity of structure in the repeating units of a polymer

iso·therm \'ī-sə-ˌthərm\ *n* : a line on a chart representing changes of volume or pressure under conditions of constant temperature

iso·ther·mal \ˌī-sə-'thər-məl\ *adj* **1** : of, relating to, or marked by equality of temperature **2** : of, relating to, or marked by changes of volume or pressure under conditions of constant temperature — **iso·ther·mal·ly** \-mə-lē\ *adv*

iso·thio·cy·a·nate \ˌī-sō-ˌthī-ō-'sī-ə-ˌnāt\ *n* : a compound containing the monovalent group –NCS : a salt or ester of isothiocyanic acid

iso·thio·cy·an·ic acid \-ˌsī-ˌan-ik-\ *n* : thiocyanic acid regarded as having the formula HNCS and usu. prepared in the form of esters

iso·thio·pen·dyl \ˌī-sō-ˌthī-ō-'pen-ˌdil\ *n* : an antihistaminic drug $C_{16}H_{19}N_3S$

iso·tone \'ī-sə-ˌtōn\ *n* : one of two or more nuclides having the same number of neutrons

iso·ton·ic \ˌī-sə-'tän-ik\ *adj* **1** : of, relating to, or exhibiting equal osmotic pressure ⟨∼ solutions⟩ — compare HYPERTONIC 2, HYPOTONIC 2 **2** : of, relating to, or being muscular contraction in the absence of significant resistance, with marked shortening of muscle fibers, and without great increase in muscle tone — compare ISOMETRIC 2 — **iso·ton·i·cal·ly** \-i-k(ə-)lē\ *adv* — **iso·to·nic·i·ty** \-tō-'nis-ət-ē\ *n, pl* -ties

iso·tope \'ī-sə-ˌtōp\ *n* **1** : any of two or more species of atoms of a chemical element with the same atomic number and position in the periodic table and nearly identical chemical behavior but with differing atomic mass or mass number and different physical properties **2** : NUCLIDE — **iso·to·pic** \ˌī-sə-'täp-ik, -'tō-pik\ *adj* — **iso·to·pi·cal·ly** \-'täp-i-k(ə-)lē, -'tō-pi-\ *adv* — **iso·to·py** \'ī-sə-ˌtō-pē, ī-'sät-ə-pē\ *n, pl* -pies

iso·trans·plant \ˌī-sō-'tran(t)s-ˌplant\ *n* : a graft between syngeneic individuals — **iso·trans·plan·ta·tion** \-ˌtran(t)s-ˌplan-'tā-shən\ *n* — **iso·trans·plant·ed** \-'plant-əd\ *adj*

iso·tret·i·noin \ˌī-sō-'tret-ə-ˌnóin\ *n* : a cis isomer of retinoic acid that is a synthetic derivative of vitamin A, that inhibits sebaceous gland function and keratinization, and that is administered in the treatment of severe inflammatory acne but is contraindicated in pregnancy because of its implication as a cause of birth defects — see ACCUTANE

iso·tro·pic \ˌī-sə-'trō-pik, -'träp-ik\ *adj* **1** : exhibiting properties (as velocity of light transmission) with the same values when measured along axes in all directions ⟨an ∼ crystal⟩ **2** : lacking predetermined axes ⟨an ∼ egg⟩ — **isot·ro·py** \ī-'sä-trə-pē\ *n, pl* -pies

isotropic band *n* : I BAND

iso·type \'ī-sə-ˌtīp\ *n* : any of the categories of antibodies determined by their physicochemical properties (as molecular weight) and antigenic characteristics that occur in all individuals of a species — compare ALLOTYPE, IDIOTYPE — **iso·typ·ic** \ˌī-sə-'tip-ik\ *adj*

iso·val·er·ate \ˌī-sō-'val-ə-ˌrāt\ *n* : a salt or ester of isovaleric acid

iso·va·ler·ic acid \ˌī-sō-və-ˌlir-ik-, -ˌler-\ *n* : a liquid acid $C_5H_{10}O_2$ that has a disagreeable odor, that occurs esp. in valerian root in the free state and in some essential oils and marine-animal oils in the form of esters, and that is used chiefly in making esters for use in flavoring materials

isovaleric ac·i·de·mia \-ˌas-ə-'dē-mē-ə\ *n* : a metabolic disorder characterized by the presence of an abnormally high concentration of isovaleric acid in the blood causing acidosis, coma, and an unpleasant body odor

iso·vol·ume \'ī-sə-ˌväl-yəm, -ˌ(ˌ)yüm\ *adj* : ISOVOLUMETRIC

iso·vol·u·met·ric \ˌī-sə-ˌväl-yù-'me-trik\ *adj* : of, relating to, or characterized by unchanging volume; *esp* : relating to or being an early phase of ventricular systole in which the cardiac muscle exerts increasing pressure on the contents of the ventricle without significant change in the muscle fiber length and the ventricular volume remains constant

iso·vo·lu·mic \-və-'lü-mik\ *adj* : ISOVOLUMETRIC

is·ox·a·zole \(ˌ)īs-'äk-sə-ˌzōl\ *n* **1** : a liquid heterocyclic compound C_3H_3NO isomeric with oxazole and having a penetrating odor like that of pyridine **2** : a derivative of isoxazole

is·ox·az·o·lyl \(ˌ)īs-ˌäk-'saz-ə-ˌlil\ *adj* : relating to or being any of a group of semisynthetic penicillins (as oxacillin and cloxacillin) that are resistant to beta-lactamase, stable in acids, and active against gram-positive bacteria

is·ox·su·prine \ī-'säk-sə-ˌprēn\ *n* : a sympathomimetic drug $C_{18}H_{23}NO_3$ used chiefly as a vasodilator

iso·zyme \'ī-sə-ˌzīm\ *n* : ISOENZYME — **iso·zy·mic** \ˌī-sə-'zī-mik\ *adj*

is·pa·ghul \'is-pə-ˌgül, -ˌgəl\ *n* : an Old World plantain of the genus *Plantago* (*P. ovata*) with mucilaginous seeds that are used as a demulcent and a purgative

is·sue \'ish-(ˌ)ü, *chiefly Brit* 'is-(ˌ)yü\ *n* **1** : PROGENY **2 a** : a discharge (as of blood) from the body that is caused by disease or other physical disorder or that is produced artificially ⟨a woman having an ∼ of blood twelve years, which had spent all her living upon physicians —Lk 8:43 (AV)⟩ **b** : an incision made to produce such a discharge

issue pea *n* : a small globular object (as a dried garden pea or a wooden bead) formerly placed in an abscess or ulcer so as to induce or increase a suppurative discharge

isth·mic \'is-mik\ *adj* : of, relating to, or taking place in an isthmus ⟨∼ ectopic pregnancy⟩ ⟨∼ obstruction⟩

isthmica — see SALPINGITIS ISTHMICA NODOSA

isth·mus \'is-məs\ *n* : a contracted anatomical part or passage connecting two larger structures or cavities: as **a** : an embryonic constriction separating the midbrain from the hindbrain **b** : the lower portion of the uterine corpus

isthmus of the fauces *n* : FAUCES

Isu·prel \'ī-sù-ˌprel\ *trademark* — used for a preparation of the hydrochloride of isoproterenol

it·a·con·ate \ˌit-ə-'kän-ˌāt\ *n* : a salt or ester of itaconic acid

it·a·con·ic acid \ˌit-ə-ˌkän-ik-\ *n* : a crystalline dicarboxylic acid $C_5H_6O_4$ obtained usu. by fermentation of sugars with molds of the genus *Aspergillus*

itai–itai \ē-'tī-i-ˌtī\ *n* : an extremely painful condition caused by poisoning following the ingestion of cadmium and characterized by bone decalcification — called also *itai-itai disease*

itch \'ich\ *n* **1** : an uneasy irritating sensation in the upper surface of the skin usu. held to result from mild stimulation of pain receptors **2** : a skin disorder accompanied by an itch; *esp* : a contagious eruption caused by an itch mite of the genus *Sarcoptes* (*S. scabiei*) that burrows in the skin and causes intense itching — **itch** *vb* — **itch·i·ness** \'ich-ē-nəs\ *n* — **itchy** \-ē\ *adj*

¹itch·ing *adj* : having, producing, or marked by an uneasy sensation in the skin ⟨an ∼ skin eruption⟩

²itching *n* : ITCH 1

itch mite *n* : any of several minute parasitic mites that burrow into the skin of humans and animals and cause itch; *esp* : a mite of any of several varieties of a species of the genus *Sarcoptes* (*S. scabiei*) that causes the itch, is about ¹⁄₆₀ inch (0.4 millimeter) long, and has a round-ovate body and 3-jointed legs and mandibles resembling minute needles

iter \'īt-ər, 'it-\ *n* : an anatomical passage; *specif* : AQUEDUCT OF SYLVIUS

itis \'īt-əs\ *n* : a disease characterized by inflammation ⟨arthritis, tendinitis and all those other ∼es —*Sports Illustrated*⟩

ITP *abbr* idiopathic thrombocytopenic purpura

it·ra·con·a·zole \ˌit-rə-'kän-ə-ˌzōl, -ˌzól\ *n* : a triazole antifungal agent $C_{35}H_{38}Cl_2N_8O_4$ used orally esp. to treat blastomycosis and histoplasmosis — see SPORANOX

IU *abbr* **1** immunizing unit **2** international unit

IUCD \ˌī-ˌyü-ˌsē-ˈdē\ *n* : INTRAUTERINE DEVICE
IUD \ˌī-ˌü-ˈdē\ *n* : INTRAUTERINE DEVICE
IUDR \ˌī-ˌyü-ˌdē-ˈär\ *n* : IDOXURIDINE
IV \ˈī-ˈvē\ *n, pl* **IVs** : an apparatus used to administer a fluid (as of medication, blood, or nutrients) intravenously; *also* : a fluid administered by IV
IV *abbr* **1** intravenous; intravenously **2** intraventricular
iver·mec·tin \ˌī-vər-ˈmek-tən\ *n* : a drug mixture of two structurally similar semisynthetic macrocyclic lactones that is used in veterinary medicine as an anthelmintic, acaricide, and insecticide and in human medicine to treat onchocerciasis
IVF *abbr* in vitro fertilization
ivo·ry \ˈīv-(ə-)rē\ *n, pl* **-ries** : the hard creamy-white modified dentin that composes the tusks of a tusked mammal and esp. the elephant — **ivory** *adj*

IVP *abbr* intravenous pyelogram
Ix·o·des \ik-ˈsō-(ˌ)dēz\ *n* : a widespread genus of ixodid ticks (as the deer tick) many of which are bloodsucking parasites of humans and animals, and sometimes cause paralysis or other severe reactions
ix·od·i·cide \ik-ˈsäd-i-ˌsīd, -ˈsōd-\ *n* : an agent that destroys ticks
ixo·did \ik-ˈsäd-id, -ˈsōd-\ *adj* : of or relating to the family Ixodidae ⟨∼ ticks⟩ — **ixodid** *n*
Ix·od·i·dae \ik-ˈsäd-ə-ˌdē\ *n pl* : a family of ticks (as the deer tick, American dog tick, and lone star tick) that have a hard outer shell and feed on two or three hosts during the life cycle
Ix·o·doi·dea \ˌik-sə-ˈdȯi-dē-ə\ *n pl* : a superfamily of the order Acari comprising the ticks — compare ARGASIDAE, IXODIDAE — **ix·o·doid** \ˈik-sə-ˌdȯid\ *adj*

J

J *symbol* mechanical equivalent of heat
jaag·siek·te *also* **jag·siek·te** *or* **jaag·ziek·te** *or* **jag·ziek·te** \ˈyäg-ˌsēk-tə, -ˌzēk-\ *n* : a chronic contagious pneumonitis of sheep and sometimes goats that is caused by a retrovirus (species *Ovine pulmonary adenocarcinoma virus* of the genus *Betaretrovirus*) and that is characterized by proliferation of the pulmonary alveolar epithelium and occlusion of the alveoli and terminal bronchioles — called also *ovine pulmonary adenocarcinoma, ovine pulmonary adenomatosis, pulmonary adenomatosis*
jab·o·ran·di \ˌzhab-ə-ˌran-ˈdē, -ˈran-dē\ *n* : the dried leaves of two So. American shrubs of the genus *Pilocarpus* (*P. jaborandi* and *P. microphyllus*) of the rue family that are a source of pilocarpine
jack bean \ˈjak-ˌbēn\ *n* **1** : an annual tropical American plant of the genus *Canavalia*; *esp* : a plant (*C. ensiformis*) having long pods with white seeds and grown esp. for forage **2** : the seed of the jack bean that is a source of canavalin and urease
jack·et \ˈjak-ət\ *n* **1** : a rigid covering that envelops the upper body and provides support, correction, or restraint **2** : JACKET CROWN
jacket crown *n* : an artificial crown that is placed over the remains of a natural tooth
jack·so·ni·an \jak-ˈsō-nē-ən\ *adj, often cap* : of, relating to, associated with, or resembling Jacksonian epilepsy
Jack·son \ˈjak-sən\, **John Hughlings (1835–1911),** British neurologist. Jackson was a pioneer in the study of epilepsy, speech defects, and nervous system disorders that arise from injury to the brain and spinal cord. In 1864 he confirmed Broca's discovery concerning the location of the speech center in the brain. In 1863 Jackson discovered epileptic convulsions, now known as Jacksonian epilepsy, that progress through the body in a series of spasms. In 1875 he was able to trace the convulsions to lesions of the motor region of the cerebral cortex.
Jacksonian epilepsy *n* : epilepsy that is characterized by progressive spreading of the abnormal movements or sensations from a focus affecting a muscle group on one side of the body to adjacent muscles or by becoming generalized and that corresponds to the spread of epileptic activity in the motor cortex
Ja·cob·son's cartilage \ˈjā-kəb-sənz-\ *n* : VOMERONASAL CARTILAGE
Jacobson, Ludwig Levin (1783–1843), Danish anatomist. Jacobson was a specialist in comparative anatomy. He discovered the vomeronasal organ and the vomeronasal cartilage in 1809. He published an article on the anatomy of the ear in 1818 that contained his descriptions of the scala tympani, the tympanic nerve, and the tympanic plexus.

Jacobson's nerve *n* : TYMPANIC NERVE
Jacobson's organ *n* : VOMERONASAL ORGAN
jac·ti·ta·tion \ˌjak-tə-ˈtā-shən\ *n* : a tossing to and fro or jerking and twitching of the body or its parts : excessive restlessness esp. in certain psychiatric disorders — **jac·ti·tate** \ˈjak-tə-ˌtāt\ *vt* **-tat·ed; -tat·ing**
Jaf·fé reaction \yä-ˈfā-, zhä-\ *also* **Jaf·fé's reaction** \-ˈfāz-\ *n* : a reaction between creatinine and picric acid in alkaline solution that results in the formation of a red compound and is used to measure the amount of creatinine (as in creatinuria)
Jaf·fé \yä-ˈfā\, **Max (1841–1911),** German biochemist. Jaffé was a professor of pharmacology who was known for his studies in physiological chemistry. His achievements included discovery of urobilin in the urine (1868), discovery of urobilin in the intestines (1871), isolation of indican in the urine (1877), and his reaction for the determination of creatinine (1886).
jagsiekte *or* **jagziekte** *var of* JAAGSIEKTE
jail fever \ˈjāl-\ *n* : TYPHUS a
jake leg \ˈjā-ˌkleg, -ˌklāg\ *n* : a paralysis caused by drinking improperly distilled or contaminated liquor
Ja·kob–Creutz·feldt disease \ˌyä-(ˌ)kȯb-ˈkrȯits-ˌfelt-\ *n* : CREUTZFELDT-JAKOB DISEASE
jal·ap \ˈjal-əp, ˈjäl-\ *n* **1 a** : the dried tuberous root of a Mexican plant of the genus *Ipomoea* (*I. purga*); *also* : a powdered purgative drug prepared from this root that contains resinous glycosides **b** : the root or derived drug of plants related to the one supplying jalap — see TAMPICO JALAP **2** : a plant yielding jalap
jala·pin \ˈjal-ə-pən, ˈjäl-\ *n* : a cathartic glucosidic constituent of the resins of scammony and jalap (*Exogonium purga*)
JAMA *abbr* Journal of the American Medical Association
Ja·mai·ca gin·ger \jə-ˌmā-kə-ˈjin-jər\ *n* : the powdered root of ginger used esp. formerly as an intestinal stimulant and carminative
ja·mais vu \ˌzhà-ˌme-ˈvœ, ˌjä-ˌmä-ˈvü\ *n* : a disorder of memory characterized by the illusion that the familiar is being encountered for the first time — compare PARAMNESIA b
James·ian \ˈjām-zē-ən\ *adj* : of, relating to, or resembling William James or his philosophical or psychological teachings
James \ˈjāmz\, **William (1842–1910),** American psychologist and philosopher. James is generally regarded as one of the great authorities in psychology. He founded in 1876 the first laboratory for psychological research in the U.S. and

---

\ə\ abut \ᵊ\ kitten \ər\ further \a\ ash \ā\ ace \ä\ cot, cart
\aú\ out \ch\ chin \e\ bet \ē\ easy \g\ go \i\ hit \ī\ ice \j\ job
\ŋ\ sing \ō\ go \ȯ\ law \ȯi\ boy \th\ thin \t͟h\ the \ü\ loot
\ú\ foot \y\ yet \zh\ vision *See also* Pronunciation Symbols page

studied the relationship between psychology and physiology. In 1890 he published *Principles of Psychology*, a seminal study that firmly placed psychology upon a physiological foundation and helped to establish it as an independent science. About this same time he independently developed what is now known as the James-Lange theory.

James–Lange theory \\'jāmz-'läŋ-ə-\\ *n* : a theory in psychology: the affective component of emotion follows rather than precedes the attendant physiological changes
  Lange, Carl Georg (1834–1900), Danish physician and psychologist. Lange produced several noteworthy studies in medicine and psychology. In 1885 he published a major psychophysiological work on vasomotor disturbances and conditioned reflexes during periods of emotional stress. In this study he introduced his version of the James-Lange theory. Lange developed the theory independent of James and at almost the same time.

James·town weed \\'jāmz-ˌtaùn-\\ *n* : JIMSONWEED
jani·ceps \\'jan-ə-ˌseps, 'jān-\\ *n* : a teratological double fetus joined at the thorax and skull and having two equal faces looking in opposite directions
Ja·nus green \\'jā-nəs-'grēn\\ *n* : a basic azine dye used esp. as a biological stain (as for mitochondria)
Jap·a·nese B encephalitis \\ˌjap-ə-ˌnēz-'bē-\\ *n* : an encephalitis that occurs epidemically in Japan and other Asian countries in the summer, is caused by a single-stranded RNA virus of the genus *Flavivirus* (species *Japanese encephalitis virus*) transmitted by mosquitoes (esp. *Culex tritaeniorhyncus*), and usu. produces a subclinical infection but may cause acute meningoencephalomyelitis
Japanese encephalitis *n* : JAPANESE B ENCEPHALITIS
Japanese glanders *n* : EPIZOOTIC LYMPHANGITIS
japonica — see SCHISTOSOMIASIS JAPONICA
ja·ra·ra·ca \\ˌzhä-rä-'rä-kə\\ *n* : a poisonous snake (*Bothrops jararaca*) of So. America
jar·gon \\'jär-gən, -ˌgän\\ *n* **1** : the technical terminology or characteristic idiom of a special activity, group, profession, or field of study ⟨medical ∼⟩ **2** : unintelligible, meaningless, or incoherent speech (as that associated with Wernicke's aphasia or some forms of schizophrenia)
Ja·risch–Herx·hei·mer reaction \\'yä-rish-'herks-ˌhī-mər-\\ *n* : an increase in the symptoms of a spirochetal disease (as syphilis, Lyme disease, or relapsing fever) occurring in some persons when treatment with spirocheticidal drugs is started — called also *Herxheimer reaction*
  Jarisch, Adolf (1850–1902), Austrian dermatologist. Jarisch published his description of the Jarisch-Herxheimer reaction in 1895, seven years before Herxheimer published his own description.
  Herxheimer, Karl (1861–1944), German dermatologist. Herxheimer published his description of the Jarisch-Herxheimer reaction in 1902. In that same year he also described acrodermatitis chronica atrophicans.
Jar·vik-7 \\'jär-vik-'sev-ən\\ *n* : an air-driven artificial heart that remains tethered to an external console after implantation and that was formerly implanted in human patients in a clinical study — called also *Jarvik heart*
  Jarvik, Robert Koffler (*b* 1946), American physician and inventor. The son of a surgeon, Jarvik developed an early interest in surgical instruments, designing while still in his teens a surgical stapler to close wounds. By the time he received his MD degree, he had studied mechanical drawing and earned a master's degree in occupational biomechanics. In 1976 he began working in the artificial organs division at the University of Utah's medical center. He proceeded to design a series of mechanical hearts. First tested on animals, one of these hearts kept a calf alive for 268 days. In December 1982 the model designated as *Jarvik-7* was for the first time implanted in a human being, a terminally ill cardiac patient, who went on to live for another 112 days with the plastic and aluminum device.
Jat·ro·pha \\'ja-trə-fə\\ *n* : a widely distributed mainly tropical American genus of herbs, shrubs, and trees (family Euphor-

biaceae) which usu. have lobed leaves and inconspicuous flowers and of which a number including the physic nut (*J. curcas*) yield oils of medicinal value
jaun·dice \\'jon-dəs, 'jän-\\ *n* **1** : a yellowish pigmentation of the skin, tissues, and certain body fluids caused by the deposition of bile pigments that follows interference with normal production and discharge of bile (as in certain liver diseases) or excessive breakdown of red blood cells (as after internal hemorrhage or in various hemolytic states) — called also *icterus* **2** : any disease or abnormal condition (as hepatitis A or leptospirosis) that is characterized by jaundice — called also *icterus*
jaun·diced \\-dəst\\ *adj* : affected with jaundice ⟨a deeply ∼ patient⟩
Ja·velle water \\zha-'vel-, zhə-\\ *n* : an aqueous solution of sodium hypochlorite used as a disinfectant or a bleaching agent
jaw \\'jo\\ *n* **1** : either of two complex cartilaginous or bony structures in most vertebrates that border the mouth, support the soft parts enclosing it, and usu. bear teeth on their oral margin: **a** : an upper structure more or less firmly fused with the skull — called also *upper jaw, maxilla* **b** : a lower structure that consists of a single bone or of completely fused bones and that is hinged, movable, and articulated by a pair of condyles with the temporal bone of either side — called also *inferior maxillary bone, lower jaw, mandible* **2** : the parts constituting the walls of the mouth and serving to open and close it — usu. used in pl. **3** : any of various organs of invertebrates that perform the function of the vertebrate jaws
jaw·bone \\'jo-'bōn, -ˌbōn\\ *n* : JAW 1; *esp* : MANDIBLE
jawed \\'jod\\ *adj* : having jaws ⟨∼ fishes⟩ — usu. used in combination ⟨square-*jawed*⟩
jaw·less \\'jo-ləs\\ *adj* : having no jaw
Jaws of Life \\'joz-əv-'līf\\ *trademark* — used for a hydraulic tool that is used esp. to free victims trapped inside wrecked motor vehicles
JCAH *abbr* Joint Commission on Accreditation of Hospitals
JCAHO *abbr* Joint Commission on Accreditation of Healthcare Organizations
J chain \\'jā-ˌchān\\ *n* : a relatively short polypeptide chain with a molecular weight of about 35,000 daltons and a high number of cysteine residues that is found in antibodies of the IgM and IgA classes
jejuna *pl of* JEJUNUM
je·ju·nal \\ji-'jün-ᵊl\\ *adj* : of or relating to the jejunum
je·ju·ni·tis \\ˌjej-ü-'nīt-əs\\ *n* : inflammation of the jejunum
je·ju·no·gas·tric \\ji-ˌjü-nə-'gas-trik, ˌjej-ü-nə-\\ *adj* : GASTROJEJUNAL
je·ju·no·il·e·al \\ji-ˌjün-ō-'il-ē-əl, ˌjej-ü-nō-\\ *adj* : of, relating to, or connecting the jejunum and the ileum ⟨the ∼ region⟩
jejunoileal bypass *n* : a surgical bypass operation performed esp. to reduce absorption in the small intestine that involves joining the first part of the jejunum with the more distal segment of the ileum
je·ju·no·il·e·it·is \\ji-ˌjü-nō-ˌil-ē-'īt-əs, ˌjej-ü-nō-\\ *n* : inflammation of the jejunum and the ileum
je·ju·no·il·e·os·to·my \\ji-ˌjü-nō-ˌil-ē-'äs-tə-mē, ˌjej-ü-nō-\\ *n*, *pl* **-mies** : the formation of an anastomosis between the jejunum and the ileum
je·ju·nos·to·my \\ji-ˌjü-'näs-tə-mē, ˌjej-ü-\\ *n*, *pl* **-mies 1** : the surgical formation of an opening through the abdominal wall into the jejunum **2** : the opening made by jejunostomy
je·ju·num \\ji-'jü-nəm\\ *n*, *pl* **je·ju·na** \\-nə\\ : the section of the small intestine that comprises the first two fifths beyond the duodenum and that is larger, thicker-walled, and more vascular and has more circular folds and fewer Peyer's patches than the ileum
jel·ly \\'jel-ē\\ *n*, *pl* **jellies 1** : a soft somewhat elastic food product made usu. with gelatin or pectin; *esp* : a fruit product made by boiling sugar and the juice of fruit **2** : a substance resembling jelly in consistency: as **a** : a transparent

elastic gel   **b** : a semisolid medicated or cosmetic preparation often having a gum base and usu. intended for local application ⟨ephedrine ∼⟩   **c** : a jellylike preparation used in electrocardiography to obtain better conduction of electricity ⟨electrode ∼⟩

jel·ly·fish \ˈjel-ē-ˌfish\ *n* : a free-swimming marine coelenterate that is the sexually reproducing form of a hydrozoan or scyphozoan and has a nearly transparent saucer-shaped body and extensible marginal tentacles studded with stinging cells

Jen·ne·ri·an \ji-ˈnir-ē-ən\ *adj* : of or relating to Edward Jenner : by the method of Jenner ⟨∼ vaccination⟩

Jen·ner \ˈjen-ər\, **Edward (1749–1823)**, British physician. Jenner made one of the great achievements in medicine: he discovered vaccination. He started by investigating the truth of the folk wisdom that people who have contracted cowpox are immune to smallpox. In 1796 he performed his first successful vaccination. A healthy person was inoculated with cowpox and thereby contracted the disease. He was then inoculated with smallpox, but he proved to be immune to the disease. Jenner published his results in 1798. He devoted his life to vaccination. His vaccination was the first use of an attenuated virus for immunization. He coined the term *virus*; he described the natural history of the cowpox virus; and he published the first description of anaphylaxis. For these reasons he is considered the father of both immunology and virology.

Jen·ner's stain \ˈjen-ərz-\ *n* : MAY-GRÜNWALD STAIN

je·quir·i·ty bean \jə-ˈkwir-ət-ē-\ *n*   **1** : the poisonous scarlet and black seed of the rosary pea often used for beads   **2** : ROSARY PEA 1

jerk \ˈjərk\ *n* : an involuntary spasmodic muscular movement due to reflex action; *esp* : one induced by an external stimulus — see KNEE JERK

jessamine — see YELLOW JESSAMINE

Je·su·its' bark \ˈjezh-(ə-)wəts-ˈbärk, ˈjez-\ *n* : CINCHONA 3

jet fa·tigue \ˈjet-fə-ˌtēg\ *n* : JET LAG

jet in·jec·tor \ˈjet-in-ˌjek-tər\ *n* : a device used to inject subcutaneously a fine stream of fluid under high pressure without puncturing the skin — **jet in·jec·tion** \-ˌjek-shən\ *n*

jet lag \ˈjet-ˌlag\ *n* : a condition that is characterized by various psychological and physiological effects (as fatigue and irritability), occurs following long flight through several time zones, and prob. results from disruption of circadian rhythms in the human body — called also *jet fatigue* — **jet–lagged** *adj*

jig·ger \ˈjig-ər\ *n* : CHIGGER

jim·jams \ˈjim-ˌjamz\ *n pl*   **1** : DELIRIUM TREMENS   **2** : JITTERS

jim·son·weed *also* **jimp·son·weed** \ˈjim(p)-sən-ˌwēd\ *n* : a poisonous tall annual weed of the genus *Datura* (*D. stramonium*) that has rank-smelling foliage, large white or violet trumpet-shaped flowers, and prickly round fruits and that is a source of stramonium — called also *Jamestown weed*

jit·ters \ˈjit-ərz\ *n pl* : a state of extreme nervousness or nervous shaking — **jit·ter** \ˈjit-ər\ *vi* — **jit·teri·ness** \ˈjit-ə-rē-nəs\ *n* — **jit·tery** *adj*

JND *abbr* just noticeable difference

job \ˈjäb\ *n* : plastic surgery for cosmetic purposes ⟨an eye ∼⟩

Jo·cas·ta complex \jō-ˈkas-tə-\ *n* : libidinal fixation of a mother for her son

Jocasta, Greek mythological character. In mythology Jocasta was the wife of Laius, the king of Thebes. After Laius was slain, she married Oedipus, who had assumed the throne. Eventually she learned that Oedipus was her long-lost son and the murderer of her husband. An unwitting partner in incest, she committed suicide.

jock itch \ˈjäk-\ *n* : ringworm of the crotch : TINEA CRURIS — called also *jockey itch*

jock·strap \ˈjäk-ˌstrap\ *n* : ATHLETIC SUPPORTER

jog·ger's nipple \ˈjäg-ərz-, ˈjȯg-\ *n* : pain and often dermatitis due to chafing of the nipples by clothing worn while jogging — called also *jogger's nipples*

Joh·ne's bacillus \ˈyō-ˌnēz-, -nəz-\ *n* : a bacillus of the genus *Mycobacterium* (*M. paratuberculosis*) that causes Johne's disease

Joh·ne \ˈyō-nə\, **Heinrich Albert (1839–1910)**, German bacteriologist. Johne developed a method for staining bacterial capsules in 1894. He discovered Johne's bacillus in 1895.

Johne's disease *n* : a chronic often fatal enteritis esp. of cattle that is caused by Johne's bacillus and is characterized by persistent diarrhea and gradual emaciation — called also *paratuberculosis*

joh·nin \ˈyō-nən\ *n* : a sterile solution of the growth products of Johne's bacillus made in the same manner as tuberculin and used to identify Johne's disease by skin tests, conjunctival reactions, or intravenous injection

john·ny *also* **john·nie** \ˈjän-ē\ *n, pl* **johnnies** : a short-sleeved collarless gown with an opening in the back for wear by persons (as hospital patients) undergoing medical examination or treatment

joint \ˈjȯint\ *n* : the point of contact between elements of an animal skeleton whether movable or rigidly fixed together with the surrounding and supporting parts (as membranes, tendons, or ligaments) ⟨the capsule of the shoulder ∼⟩ — **out of joint** *of a bone* : having the head slipped from its socket

joint capsule *n* : a ligamentous sac that surrounds the articular cavity of a freely movable joint, is attached to the bones, completely encloses the joint, and is composed of an outer fibrous membrane and an inner synovial membrane — called also *articular capsule, capsular ligament*

joint·ed \ˈjȯint-əd\ *adj* : having joints

joint evil \-ˈē-vəl, *Brit often* ˈē-(ˌ)vil\ *n* : NAVEL ILL

joint fluid *n* : SYNOVIAL FLUID

joint ill *n* : NAVEL ILL

joint mouse \-ˌmaȯs\ *n* : a loose fragment (as of cartilage) within a synovial space

joint oil *n* : SYNOVIAL FLUID

joule \ˈjü(ə)l\ *n* : a unit of work or energy equal to the work done by a force of one newton acting through a distance of one meter

Joule, James Prescott (1818–1889), British physicist. Joule is famous for his experiments on heat. In a series of investigations he demonstrated that heat is a form of energy (regardless of the substance that is heated) and later determined quantitatively the amount of mechanical and electrical energy expended in the generation of heat energy. In 1843 he published his value for the amount of work required to produce a unit of heat, now known as the mechanical equivalent of heat. He established the principle that various forms of energy—mechanical, electrical, and heat—are basically the same and are interchangeable. This principle forms the basis of conservation of energy. The joule unit of work or energy was named in his honor in 1882.

Joule's equivalent *n* : MECHANICAL EQUIVALENT OF HEAT

juga *pl of* JUGUM

¹ju·gal \ˈjü-gəl\ *adj* : MALAR

²jugal *n* : ZYGOMATIC BONE — called also *jugal bone*

ju·glone \ˈjü-ˌglōn\ *n* : a reddish yellow crystalline compound $C_{10}H_6O_3$ that is obtained esp. from green shucks of walnuts and has fungicidal and antibiotic properties

¹jug·u·lar \ˈjəg-yə-lər *also* ˈjüg- *or* -(ə-)lər\ *adj*   **1** : of or relating to the throat or neck   **2** : of or relating to the jugular vein ⟨∼ pulsations⟩

²jugular *n* : JUGULAR VEIN

jugulare — see GLOMUS JUGULARE

jugular foramen *n* : a large irregular opening from the posterior cranial fossa that is bounded anteriorly by the petrous part of the temporal bone and posteriorly by the jugular

\ə\ abut \ᵊ\ kitten \ər\ further \a\ ash \ā\ ace \ä\ cot, cart \aȯ\ out \ch\ chin \e\ bet \ē\ easy \g\ go \i\ hit \ī\ ice \j\ job \ŋ\ sing \ō\ go \ȯ\ law \ȯi\ boy \th\ thin \th\ the \ü\ loot \u̇\ foot \y\ yet \zh\ vision   See also Pronunciation Symbols page

notch of the occipital bone and that transmits the inferior petrosal sinus, the glossopharyngeal, vagus, and accessory nerves, and the internal jugular vein

jugular fossa *n* : a depression on the basilar surface of the petrous portion of the temporal bone that contains a dilation of the internal jugular vein

jugular ganglion *n* : SUPERIOR GANGLION

jugular notch \-ˈnäch\ *n* **1** : SUPRASTERNAL NOTCH **2 a** : a notch in the inferior border of the occipital bone behind the jugular process that forms the posterior part of the jugular foramen **b** : a notch in the petrous portion of the temporal bone that corresponds to the jugular notch of the occipital bone and with it makes up the jugular foramen

jugular process *n* : a quadrilateral or triangular process of the occipital bone on each side that articulates with the temporal bone and is situated lateral to the condyle of the occipital bone on each side articulating with the atlas

jugular trunk *n* : either of two major lymph vessels that drain the head and neck: **a** : one on the right that empties into the right lymphatic duct or into the right subclavian vein where it joins the right internal jugular vein **b** : one on the left that empties into the thoracic trunk

jugular vein *n* : any of several veins of each side of the neck: as **a** : a vein that collects the blood from the interior of the cranium, the superficial part of the face, and the neck, runs down the neck on the outside of the internal and common carotid arteries, and unites with the subclavian vein to form the brachiocephalic vein — called also *internal jugular vein* **b** : a smaller and more superficial vein that collects most of the blood from the exterior of the cranium and deep parts of the face and opens into the subclavian vein — called also *external jugular vein* **c** : a vein that commences near the hyoid bone and joins the terminal part of the external jugular vein or the subclavian vein — called also *anterior jugular vein*

jug·u·lo·di·gas·tric \ˌjəg-yə-lō-ˌdī-ˈgas-trik\ *adj* : relating to or being lymph nodes in the region of the internal jugular vein and the digastric muscles of the jaw

jug·u·lo·omo·hy·oid \-ō-mō-ˈhī-ˌȯid\ *adj* : relating to or being a lymph node located on the internal jugular vein above the omohyoid muscle

ju·gum \ˈjü-gəm\ *n, pl* **ju·ga** \-gə\ *or* **jugums** : an anatomical ridge or groove connecting two structures

juice \ˈjüs\ *n* **1** : the extractable fluid contents of cells or tissues **2 a** : a natural bodily fluid (as blood, lymph, or a secretion) — see GASTRIC JUICE, INTESTINAL JUICE, PANCREATIC JUICE **b** : the liquid or moisture contained in something

ju·jube \ˈjü-ˌjüb, *esp for 2* ˈjü-jü-ˌbē\ *n* **1 a** : an edible drupaceous fruit of any of several trees (genus *Ziziphus*) of the buckthorn family; *esp* : one of an Asian tree (*Z. jujuba*) **b** : a tree producing this fruit **2** : a fruit-flavored gumdrop or lozenge; *esp* : one that is made from the jujube fruit and has been used as a remedy for various throat conditions

jump·er \ˈjəm-pər\ *n* : one affected with latah or by the condition exhibited by the jumping Frenchmen of Maine

jump·ing French·men of Maine \ˌjəmp-iŋ-ˌfrench-mən-əv-ˈmān\ *n pl* : individuals who exhibit a nervous condition characterized by involuntary jumping movements upon being startled, sometimes echolalia, suggestibility and impairment of the will, and inability to concentrate and who are usu. of French descent and from lumbering regions of Maine

jumping gene *n* : TRANSPOSABLE ELEMENT; *esp* : TRANSPOSON

junc·tion \ˈjəŋ(k)-shən\ *n* : a place or point of meeting ⟨the structure of the synaptic ∼ as revealed by electron microscopy⟩ — see NEUROMUSCULAR JUNCTION — **junc·tion·al** \-shnəl, -shən-ᵊl\ *adj*

junctional epidermolysis bullosa *n* : any of several forms of epidermolysis bullosa that are marked esp. by usu. severe blister formation between the epidermis and basement membrane often accompanied by involvement of the mucous membranes (as of the mouth or esophagus) and that are inherited as an autosomal recessive trait

junctional nevus *n* : a nevus that develops at the junction of the dermis and epidermis and is potentially cancerous — called also *junction nevus*

junctional rhythm *n* : a cardiac rhythm resulting from impulses coming from a locus of tissue in the area of the atrioventricular node

junctional tachycardia *n* : tachycardia associated with the generation of impulses in a locus in the region of the atrioventricular node

junction nevus *n* : JUNCTIONAL NEVUS

¹Jung·ian \ˈyu̇ŋ-ē-ən\ *n* : an adherent of the psychological doctrines of C. G. Jung

> **Jung** \ˈyu̇ŋ\, **Carl Gustav (1875–1961),** Swiss psychologist and psychiatrist. Jung founded the variation in psychoanalysis known as analytic psychology. For a time he was associated with Sigmund Freud, but gradually he modified Freud's methods, putting less emphasis on sex. Eventually he broke with Freud over the question of the nature of libido and trauma. He introduced and developed the idea that there are two fundamental types of human beings, the introvert and the extrovert. Later he differentiated four functions of the mind: thinking, feeling, sensation, and intuition. In any given person one or more of these functions will predominate.

²Jungian *adj* : of, relating to, or characteristic of C. G. Jung or his psychological doctrines which stress the opposition of introversion and extroversion and the concept of mythology and cultural and racial inheritance in the psychology of individuals

jun·gle fever \ˈjəŋ-gəl-\ *n* : a severe form of malaria or yellow fever — compare JUNGLE YELLOW FEVER

jungle rot \ˈjəŋ-gəl-ˌrät\ *n* : any of various esp. pyogenic skin infections contracted in tropical environments

jungle yellow fever *n* : yellow fever endemic in or near forest or jungle areas in Africa and So. America and transmitted by mosquitoes other than members of the genus *Aedes* and esp. by those of the genus *Haemagogus*

Ju·nin virus \hü-ˈnēn-\ *n* : a single-stranded RNA virus of the genus *Arenavirus* (species *Junin virus*) that is the causative agent of a hemorrhagic fever endemic to agricultural regions of Argentina and that is transmitted to humans chiefly by rodents (esp. genus *Calomys*)

ju·ni·per \ˈjü-nə-pər\ *n* : an evergreen shrub or tree (genus *Juniperus*) of the cypress family (Cupressaceae); *esp* : one having a prostrate or shrubby habit (as *Juniperus communis*)

juniper–berry oil \-ˌber-ē-\ *n* : JUNIPER OIL

juniper oil *n* : an acrid essential oil obtained from the fruit of the common juniper (*Juniperus communis*) and formerly used as a diuretic, stimulant, carminative, and antiseptic

juniper tar *n* : a dark tarry liquid used topically in treating skin diseases and obtained by distillation from the wood of a Eurasian juniper (*Juniperus oxycedrus*) — called also *cade oil, juniper tar oil*

junk DNA \ˈjəŋk-\ *n* : a region of DNA (as spacer DNA) that usu. consists of a repeating DNA sequence, does not code for protein, and has no known function

jury mast \ˈju̇(ə)r-ē-ˌmast\ *n* : a device for supporting the head in cases of deterioration of the cervical spine (as in Pott's disease) that consists of a rod one end of which is secured to the back of the body and the other extended above the head to form a hook from which a sling is suspended

just no·tice·able dif·fer·ence \ˌjəst-ˌnōt-ə-sə-bəl-ˈdif-(ə-)rən(t)s\ *n* : the minimum amount of change in a physical stimulus required for a subject to detect reliably a difference in the level of stimulation

jus·to ma·jor \ˈjəs-tō-ˈmā-jər\ *adj, of pelvic dimensions* : greater than normal

justo mi·nor \-ˈmī-nər\ *adj, of pelvic dimensions* : smaller than normal

jute \ˈjüt\ *n* : the glossy fiber of either of two East Indian plants (*Corchorus olitorius* and *C. capsularis*) of the linden family (Tiliaceae) formerly used in absorbent dressings

¹ju·ve·nile \ˈjü-və-ˌnīl, -vən-ᵊl\ *adj* **1** : physiologically immature or undeveloped ⟨∼ fish⟩ **2** : of, relating to, characteristic of, or affecting children or young people ⟨∼ arthritis⟩ **3** : reflecting psychological or intellectual immaturity ⟨∼ behavior⟩

²**juvenile** *n* **1** : a young person; *esp* : one below the legally established age (as of 18) of adulthood **2** : a young individual resembling an adult of its kind except in size and reproductive activity

juvenile amaurotic idiocy *n* : BATTEN DISEASE

juvenile delinquency *n* **1** : conduct by a juvenile characterized by antisocial behavior that is beyond parental control and therefore subject to legal action **2** : a violation of the law committed by a juvenile and not punishable by death or life imprisonment

juvenile delinquent *n* : a person whose behavior has been labeled juvenile delinquency; *esp* : a person whose transgressions of the law have been adjudged to constitute juvenile delinquency because the violator is below the legally established age of adulthood

juvenile diabetes *n* : TYPE 1 DIABETES

juvenile myoclonic epilepsy *n* : epilepsy that typically begins during adolescence or late childhood and is marked by myoclonic seizures which occur shortly after awakening and are often followed by tonic-clonic seizures or sometimes by absence seizures

juvenile–onset diabetes *n* : TYPE 1 DIABETES

jux·ta–ar·tic·u·lar \ˌjək-stə-är-'tik-yə-lər\ *adj* : situated near a joint ⟨∼ inflammatory tissue⟩

jux·ta·cor·ti·cal \-'kȯrt-i-kəl\ *adj* : situated or occurring near the cortex of an organ or tissue

jux·ta·glo·mer·u·lar \-glə-'mer-(y)ə-lər, -glō-\ *adj* : situated near a kidney glomerulus

juxtaglomerular apparatus *n* : a functional unit near a kidney glomerulus that controls renin release and is composed of juxtaglomerular cells and a macula densa

juxtaglomerular cell *n* : any of a group of cells that are situated in the wall of each afferent arteriole of a kidney glomerulus near its point of entry adjacent to a macula densa and that produce and secrete renin

jux·ta·med·ul·lary \ˌjək-stə-'med-ᵊl-ˌer-ē, -'mej-ə-ˌler-ē, -mə-'dəl-ə-rē\ *adj* : situated or occurring near the edge of the medulla of the kidney ⟨∼ nephrons⟩ ⟨∼ circulation⟩

jux·ta·po·si·tion \ˌjək-stə-pə-'zish-ən\ *n* : the act or an instance of placing two or more things side by side; *also* : the state of being so placed — **jux·ta·pose** \'jək-stə-ˌpōz\ *vt* **-posed; -pos·ing**

jux·ta·py·lor·ic \-pī-'lȯr-ik\ *adj* : situated near the pylorus ⟨a ∼ gastric ulcer⟩

jux·ta·res·ti·form body \-'res-tə-ˌfȯrm-\ *n* : a part of the inferior cerebellar peduncle containing nerve fibers that reciprocally connect the cerebellum and the vestibular nuclei of the medulla oblongata

K

K *symbol* **1** dissociation constant; ionization constant **2** [New Latin *kalium*] potassium **3** kelvin

ka *abbr* [German *kathode*] cathode

Kahn test \'kän-\ *n* : a serum-precipitation reaction for the diagnosis of syphilis — called also *Kahn, Kahn reaction*
  Kahn, Reuben Leon (1887–1979), American immunologist. Kahn's research on blood reactions led him to attempt an improvement of the Wassermann test for syphilis. He achieved success in 1923, publishing a description of his test (which yields quicker, more accurate results) in the same year. Later Kahn discovered that by adjusting the temperature, salt concentration, and serum dilution used in his test, the reaction could also indicate the presence of the agents of tuberculosis, malaria, or leprosy in the blood sample. He called this universal serologic reaction and published an explanation of it in 1951.

kai·nate \'kī-ˌnāt, 'kā-\ *n* : KAINIC ACID

kai·nic acid \ˌkī-nik-, ˌkā-\ *n* : an excitatory neurotoxin $C_{10}H_{15}NO_4$ that is a glutamate analog orig. isolated from a dried red alga (*Digenia simplex*), that binds selectively to a subset of glutamate receptors which serve as ligand-gated ion channels on neurons, and that is used as an anthelmintic and experimentally to induce seizures and neurodegeneration in laboratory animals

kak·ke \'kak-ē\ *n* : BERIBERI

kak·or·rhaph·io·pho·bia \ˌkak-ə-ˌraf-ē-ə-'fō-bē-ə\ *n* : abnormal fear of failure

kala–azar \ˌkäl-ə-ə-ˌzär, ˌkal-\ *n* : a severe parasitic disease chiefly of Asia marked by fever, progressive anemia, leukopenia, and enlargement of the spleen and liver and caused by a flagellate of the genus *Leishmania* (*L. donovani*) that is transmitted by the bite of sand flies and proliferates in reticuloendothelial cells — called also *dumdum fever;* see LEISHMAN-DONOVAN BODY

ka·li·um \'kā-lē-əm\ *n* : POTASSIUM

ka·li·ure·sis \ˌkā-lē-yù-'rē-səs, ˌkal-ē-\ *also* **kal·ure·sis** \ˌkāl-(y)ù-'rē-, ˌkal-\ *n, pl* **-ure·ses** \-ˌsēz\ : excretion of potassium in the urine esp. in excessive amounts — **ka·li·uret·ic** \-'ret-ik\ *adj*

kal·li·din \'kal-əd-ən\ *n* : either of two vasodilator kinins formed from blood plasma globulin by the action of kallikrein: **a** : BRADYKININ **b** : one that has the same amino acid sequence as bradykinin with a terminal lysine added

kal·li·kre·in \ˌkal-ə-'krē-ən, kə-'lik-rē-ən\ *n* : a hypotensive protease that liberates kinins from blood plasma proteins and is used therapeutically for vasodilation

Kall·mann syndrome \'kȯl-mən-\ *or* **Kall·mann's syndrome** \-mən(z)-\ *n* : a hereditary condition marked by hypogonadism caused by a deficiency of gonadotropins and anosmia caused by failure of the olfactory lobes to develop
  Kallmann, Franz Josef (1897–1965), American geneticist and psychiatrist. Kallmann held positions as a professor of psychiatry at Columbia University and as chief psychiatrist at a state psychiatric institute in New York. He was best known for demonstrating how hereditary factors could play a major role in the development of psychoses. In 1952 he produced an important study that investigated the role of heredity in determining homosexuality.

kaluresis *var of* KALIURESIS

ka·ma·la \'käm-ə-lə\ *n* **1** : an East Indian tree (*Mallotus philippinensis*) of the spurge family **2** : an orange red cathartic powder from kamala capsules used for dyeing silk and wool or as a vermifuge chiefly in veterinary practice

kana·my·cin \ˌkan-ə-'mīs-ᵊn\ *n* : a broad-spectrum antibiotic from a Japanese soil bacterium of the genus *Streptomyces* (*S. kanamyceticus*)

Kan·ner's syndrome \'kan-ərz-\ *n* : INFANTILE AUTISM
  Kanner, Leo (1894–1981), American psychiatrist. For most of his career Kanner was associated with Johns Hopkins University as a professor of psychiatry and as a child psychiatrist. The author of many books, he published a textbook on child psychiatry in 1957 and a history of the study and care of the mentally retarded in 1964.

Kan·trex \'kan-ˌtreks\ *trademark* — used for a preparation of kanamycin

---

\ə\ abut \ᵊ\ kitten \ər\ further \a\ ash \ā\ ace \ä\ cot, cart \aù\ out \ch\ chin \e\ bet \ē\ easy \g\ go \i\ hit \ī\ ice \j\ job \ŋ\ sing \ō\ go \ȯ\ law \ȯi\ boy \th\ thin \t̲h̲\ the \ü\ loot \ù\ foot \y\ yet \zh\ vision   *See also* Pronunciation Symbols page

K
L

ka·olin \\'kā-ə-lən\\ *n* : a fine usu. white clay that is used in ceramics and refractories, as a filler or extender, and in medicine esp. as an adsorbent in the treatment of diarrhea (as in food poisoning or dysentery)

Kao·pec·tate \\,kā-ō-'pek-,tāt\\ *trademark* — used for a preparation of kaolin used as an antidiarrheal

Ka·po·si's sarcoma \\'kap-ə-zēz-, kə-'pō-, -sēz-\\ *n* : a neoplastic disease affecting esp. the skin and mucous membranes, characterized esp. by the formation of pink to reddish-brown or bluish tumorous plaques, macules, papules, or nodules esp. on the lower extremities, and formerly limited primarily to elderly men in whom it followed a benign course but now being a major and sometimes fatal disease associated with immunodeficient individuals with AIDS — abbr. *KS*

  Ka·po·si \\'kȯ-pō-shē\\, **Moritz (1837–1902),** Hungarian dermatologist. Kaposi taught and practiced at a leading clinic of dermatology in Vienna. He was the author of a number of original descriptions of skin diseases including the condition now known as Kaposi's sarcoma.

kap·pa \\'kap-ə\\ *n* : a cytoplasmic factor in certain paramecia that mediates production of paramecin and thereby makes the medium in which such microorganisms are grown toxic to members of strains not possessing the factor — see PARAMECIN

kap·pa chain *or* κ **chain** \\'kap-ə-\\ *n* : a polypeptide chain of one of the two types of light chain that are found in antibodies and can be distinguished antigenically and by the sequence of amino acids in the chain — compare LAMBDA CHAIN

ka·ra·ya \\kə-'rī-ə\\ *n* : KARAYA GUM

karaya gum *n* : any of several laxative vegetable gums that are similar to tragacanth and are often used as substitutes for it, that are obtained from tropical Asian trees (genera *Sterculia* of the family Sterculiaceae and *Cochlospermum* of the family Bixaceae), and that include esp. one derived from an Indian tree (*S. urens*) — called also *gum karaya, karaya, sterculia gum*

ka·rez·za \\kä-'ret-sə\\ *n* : COITUS RESERVATUS

Kar·ta·ge·ner's syndrome \\kär-'tä-gə-nərz-, ,kär-tə-'gā-nərz-\\ *n* : an abnormal condition inherited as an autosomal recessive trait and characterized by situs inversus, abnormalities in the protein structure of cilia, and chronic bronchiectasis and sinusitis

  Kar·ta·ge·ner \\'kär-tä-,gā-nər\\, **Manes (1897–1975),** Swiss physician. Kartagener published his description of Kartagener's syndrome in 1933. He also published various papers on pulmonary and blood-circulation diseases.

Kar·win·skia \\kär-'winz-kē-ə\\ *n* : a genus of shrubs or small trees (family Rhamnaceae) that are chiefly native to Mexico and the southwestern U.S., have flowers with small hooded short-clawed petals and fleshy drupes, and include one (*K. humboldtiana*) with a fruit that has been known to poison birds (as domestic chickens)

  Kar·win·sky Von Kar·win \\kär-'vin-skē-fȯn-'kär-vin\\, **Wilhelm (d 1855),** German traveler. The genus *Karwinskia* was named in Karwinsky's honor in 1832.

kar·yo·clas·tic \\,kar-ē-ō-'klas-tik\\ *or* **kar·yo·cla·sic** \\-'klā-sik\\ *adj* **1** : KARYORRHECTIC **2** : causing the interruption of mitosis

kar·yo·cyte \\'kar-ē-ō-,sīt\\ *n* : NORMOBLAST

kar·y·og·a·my \\,kar-ē-'äg-ə-mē\\ *n, pl* **-mies** : the fusion of cell nuclei (as in fertilization) — **kar·yo·gam·ic** \\,kar-ē-ō-'gam-ik\\ *adj*

kar·yo·gram \\'kar-ē-ō-,gram\\ *n* : KARYOTYPE; *esp* : a diagrammatic representation of the chromosome complement of an organism

kar·yo·ki·ne·sis \\,kar-ē-ō-kə-'nē-səs, -kī-\\ *n, pl* **-ne·ses** \\-,sēz\\ **1** : the nuclear phenomena characteristic of mitosis **2** : the whole process of mitosis — compare CYTOKINESIS — **kar·yo·ki·net·ic** \\-'net-ik\\ *adj*

kar·y·ol·o·gy \\,kar-ē-'äl-ə-jē\\ *n, pl* **-gies** **1** : the minute cytological characteristics of the cell nucleus esp. with regard to the chromosomes of a single cell or of the cells of an organism or group of organisms **2** : a branch of cytology concerned with the karyology of cell nuclei — **kar·y·o·log·i·cal** \\-ē-ə-'läj-i-kəl\\ *also* **kar·y·o·log·ic** \\-ik\\ *adj* — **kar·y·o·log·i·cal·ly** \\-i-k(ə-)lē\\ *adv*

kar·y·o·lymph \\'kar-ē-ō-,lim(p)f\\ *n* : NUCLEAR SAP

kar·y·ol·y·sis \\,kar-ē-'äl-ə-səs\\ *n, pl* **-y·ses** \\-,sēz\\ : dissolution of the cell nucleus with loss of its affinity for basic stains sometimes occurring normally but usu. in necrosis — compare KARYORRHEXIS — **kar·y·o·lyt·ic** \\,kar-ē-ō-'lit-ik\\ *adj*

kar·yo·met·ric \\,kar-ē-ō-'met-rik\\ *adj* : relating to or involving quantitative measurements of cell nuclei ⟨∼ studies of tissue culture cells⟩ — **kar·y·om·e·try** \\-'äm-ə-trē\\ *n, pl* **-tries**

kar·y·on \\'kar-ē-,än\\ *n* : the nucleus of a cell

kar·yo·plasm \\'kar-ē-ō-,plaz-əm\\ *n* : NUCLEOPLASM

kar·yo·pyk·no·sis \\,kar-ē-(,)ō-pik-'nō-səs\\ *n* : shrinkage of the cell nuclei of epithelial cells (as of the vagina) with breakup of the chromatin into unstructured granules — **kar·yo·pyk·not·ic** \\-'nät-ik\\ *adj*

karyopyknotic index *n* : an index that is calculated as the percentage of epithelial cells with karyopyknotic nuclei exfoliated from the vagina and is used in the hormonal evaluation of a patient

kar·y·or·rhec·tic \\,kar-ē-ȯr-'ek-tik\\ *adj* : of or relating to karyorrhexis

kar·y·or·rhex·is \\,kar-ē-ȯr-'ek-səs\\ *n, pl* **-rhex·es** \\-,sēz\\ : a degenerative cellular process involving fragmentation of the nucleus and the breakup of the chromatin into unstructured granules — compare KARYOLYSIS

kar·yo·some \\'kar-ē-ə-,sōm\\ *n* : a mass of chromatin in a cell nucleus that resembles a nucleolus

kar·yo·the·ca \\,kar-ē-ō-'thē-kə\\ *n* : NUCLEAR MEMBRANE

kar·yo·tin \\'kar-ē-ə-,tin, -ət-ən\\ *n* : the reticular usu. stainable material of the cell nucleus

¹kar·yo·type \\'kar-ē-ə-,tīp\\ *n* : the chromosomal characteristics of a cell; *also* : the chromosomes themselves or a representation of them — **kar·yo·typ·ic** \\,kar-ē-ə-'tip-ik\\ *adj* — **kar·yo·typ·i·cal·ly** \\-i-k(ə-)lē\\ *adv*

²karyotype *vt* **-typed; -typ·ing** : to determine or analyze the karyotype of ⟨*karyotyped* a newborn infant with a suspected genetic anomaly⟩

kar·yo·typ·ing \\-,tīp-iŋ\\ *n* : the action or process of studying karyotypes or of making representations of them

ka·su·ga·my·cin \\kä-,sü-gə-'mīs-ᵊn\\ *n* : an aminoglycoside antibiotic produced by a bacterium of the genus *Streptomyces* (*S. kasugaensis*)

kat *var of* KHAT

katabolic, katabolism *var of* CATABOLIC, CATABOLISM

kata·ther·mom·e·ter \\,kat-ə-thə(r)-'mäm-ət-ər\\ *n* : a large-bulbed alcohol thermometer used to measure the cooling effect of particular atmospheric conditions (as on the human body) by increasing its temperature to well above the ambient temperature and then determining the time required for the indicated temperature to fall from one predetermined value to another

Ka·ta·ya·ma \\,kät-ə-'yä-mə\\ *n, in former classifications* : a genus of Asian freshwater snails including important intermediate hosts of a human trematode worm of the genus *Schistosoma* (*S. japonicum*) and now considered part of the genus *Oncomelania*

Katayama syndrome *n* : SCHISTOSOMIASIS JAPONICA; *specif* : an acute form usu. occurring several weeks after initial infection with the causative schistosome (*Schistosoma japonicum*) — called also *Katayama disease, Katayama fever*

ka·tha·rom·e·ter \\,ka-thə-'räm-ət-ər\\ *n* : an apparatus for determining the composition of a gas mixture by measuring thermal conductivity that has been used to determine the basal metabolic rate by measuring the rate of production of carbon dioxide based on the composition of expired air

katharsis *var of* CATHARSIS

kath·i·so·pho·bia \\,kath-i-sō-'fō-bē-ə\\ *n* : fear of sitting down

kat·zen·jam·mer \\'kat-sən-,jam-ər\\ *n* **1** : HANGOVER **2** : emotional distress or depression

ka·va \'käv-ə\ *n* **1** : an Australasian shrubby pepper (*Piper methysticum*) from whose crushed root an intoxicating beverage is made; *also* : the beverage **2** : a preparation consisting of the ground dried rhizome and roots of the kava plant that is used as a dietary supplement chiefly to relieve stress, anxiety, and sleeplessness and in folk medicine esp. as a diuretic and urogenital antiseptic and that has been linked to cases of severe liver injury

kava kava \'käv-ə-'käv-ə\ *n* : KAVA

Ka·wa·sa·ki disease \ˌkä-wə-'sä-kē-\ *also* **Ka·wa·sa·ki's disease** \-kēz-\ *n* : an acute febrile disease of unknown cause affecting esp. infants and children that is characterized by a reddish macular rash esp. on the trunk, conjunctivitis, inflammation of mucous membranes (as of the tongue), erythema of the palms and soles followed by desquamation, edema of the hands and feet, and swollen lymph nodes in the neck — called also *mucocutaneous lymph node disease, mucocutaneous lymph node syndrome*

Ka·wa·sa·ki \kä-wä-sä-kē\, **Tomisaku (***fl* 1961), Japanese pediatrician. Kawasaki first discovered mucocutaneous lymph node syndrome in Japanese children in 1961. In 1967 he published his findings based upon 50 case studies, all of which involved Japanese children five years old and younger. Since that original report, however, Kawasaki disease has been observed in other countries and in patients who are considerably older.

Kawasaki syndrome *also* **Ka·wa·sa·ki's syndrome** *n* : KAWASAKI DISEASE

Kay·ser–Flei·scher ring \'kī-zər-'flī-shər-ˌriŋ\ *n* : a brown or greenish brown ring of copper deposits around the cornea that is characteristic of Wilson's disease

Kayser, Bernhard (1869–1954), and **Fleischer, Bruno Otto (1874–1965)**, German ophthalmologists. Kayser described the corneal ring that is a diagnostic symptom of Wilson's disease in 1902. Fleischer published his own description.

kb *abbr* kilobase
kc *abbr* kilocycle
kcal *abbr* kilocalorie; kilogram calorie
kc/s *abbr* kilocycles per second
kD *abbr* kilodalton
K–Dur \'kā-ˌdúr\ *trademark* — used for a sustained-release preparation of potassium chloride for oral administration
ked \'ked\ *n* : SHEEP KED
keel \'kēl\ *n* : acute septicemic salmonellosis or paratyphoid of ducklings marked by sudden collapse and death of apparently healthy birds — called also *keel disease*
Kee·ley cure \'kē-lē-\ *n* : a method of treatment for alcoholism that was formerly used

Keeley, Leslie E. (1832–1900), American physician. Keeley is remembered for implementing a kind of institutional care as a treatment method for chronic alcoholism and drug addiction. Around 1879 he developed his treatment which consisted chiefly of injecting institutionalized patients with a chloride of gold and allowing them unlimited access to liquor. Keeley claimed a very high rate of success with only a few relapses. The medical establishment dismissed him as a charlatan.

kef \'kef, 'kēf, 'kāf\ *n* **1** : a state of dreamy tranquillity **2** : a smoking material (as marijuana) that produces kef
Ke·gel exercises \'kā-gəl-, 'kē-\ *n pl* : repetitive contractions by a woman of the muscles that are used to stop the urinary flow in urination in order to increase the tone of the pubococcygeal muscle esp. to control incontinence or to enhance sexual responsiveness during intercourse

Kegel, Arnold Henry (*b* 1894), American gynecologist.
Kell \'kel\ *adj* : of, relating to, or being a group of allelic red⸗ blood-cell antigens of which some are important causes of transfusion reactions and some forms of erythroblastosis fetalis ⟨~ blood group system⟩ ⟨~ blood typing⟩

Kell, medical patient. Kell was a female patient in whose blood antibodies to an antigen of the Kell blood group were first found. The discovery of the group was first reported in 1946.

Kel·ler \'kel-ər\ *adj* : relating to or being an operation to correct hallux valgus by excision of the proximal part of the proximal phalanx of the big toe with resulting shortening of the toe ⟨~ procedure⟩ ⟨~ arthroplasty⟩

Keller, William Lorden (1874–1959), American surgeon. Keller was an army surgeon who developed a number of new surgical procedures. He devised operations for hallux valgus (1904), varicose veins (1905), chronic empyema (1922), recurrent dislocation of the shoulder (1925), and stricture of the rectum and anus (1933) caused by contracture of the muscles around their circumference.

kellin *var of* KHELLIN
ke·loid *also* **che·loid** \'kē-ˌlóid\ *n* : a thick scar resulting from excessive growth of fibrous tissue and occurring esp. after burns or radiation injury — **keloid** *adj*
ke·loi·dal \kē-'lóid-ᵊl\ *adj* : resembling or being a keloid ⟨a ~ scar is contracted fibrous tissue —*Jour. Amer. Med. Assoc.*⟩
kelp \'kelp\ *n* **1** : any of various large brown seaweeds (orders Laminariales and Fucales) and esp. laminarias of which some are used for food esp. in China and Japan and as sources of alginates, iodine, and medicinal substances **2** : the ashes of seaweed used esp. as a source of iodine
kel·vin \'kel-vən\ *n* : the base unit of temperature in the International System of Units that is equal to 1/273.16 of the Kelvin scale temperature of the triple point of water and also to the Celsius degree

Thom·son \'täm(p)-sən\, **Sir William (1st Baron Kelvin of Largs) (1824–1907)**, British physicist. One of the most influential scientists of the 19th century, Thomson made important contributions in almost every branch of the physical sciences. He was a prolific inventor. He created the first physics laboratory in Great Britain and was the first to teach physics in a lab. He developed the Kelvin scale in 1848. From 1848 on he did thermodynamic research, often in collaboration with James P. Joule. Between 1851–54 Thomson helped to formulate the first two laws of thermodynamics. During the next few years he laid the theoretical foundations for submarine telegraphic transmission. He was the leading scientist involved in the laying of the transatlantic cable. He also made discoveries in electromagnetism and investigated wave motion and vortex motion.

Kelvin *adj* : relating to, conforming to, or being the Kelvin scale
Kelvin scale *n* : a temperature scale that has the kelvin as its unit of measurement and according to which absolute zero (−273.15°C) is 0 K and water freezes at 273.15 K and boils at 373.15 K
Ken·a·cort \'ken-ə-ˌkórt\ *n* : a preparation of triamcinolone — formerly a U.S. registered trademark
Ken·ne·dy's disease \'ken-əd-ēz-\ *also* **Ken·ne·dy disease** \-əd-ē-\ *n* : a progressive muscular and neurological disorder that is characterized esp. by muscular weakness and atrophy and by neural degeneration, that is inherited as an X-linked recessive trait, and that chiefly affects adult males — called also *spinal and bulbar muscular atrophy*

Kennedy, William Robert (*b* 1927), American neurologist. Kennedy enjoyed a long association with the University of Minnesota's medical center in Minneapolis, rising to rank of professor of neurology. His major area of research was neuromuscular disorders. The neuromuscular disorder that bears his name was described in an article published in 1980 that he coauthored with M. Alter and J. H. Sung.

ken·nel cough \'ken-ᵊl-\ *n* : tracheobronchitis of dogs or cats
Ken·ny method \'ken-ē-\ *n* : a method of treating poliomyelitis consisting basically of application of hot fomentations and rehabilitation of muscular activity by passive movement and then guided active coordination — called also *Kenny treatment*

\ə\ **abut** \ᵊ\ **kitten** \ər\ **further** \a\ **ash** \ā\ **ace** \ä\ **cot, cart**
\aú\ **out** \ch\ **chin** \e\ **bet** \ē\ **easy** \g\ **go** \i\ **hit** \ī\ **ice** \j\ **job**
\ŋ\ **sing** \ō\ **go** \ó\ **law** \ói\ **boy** \th\ **thin** \t͟h\ **the** \ü\ **loot**
\ú\ **foot** \y\ **yet** \zh\ **vision** *See also* Pronunciation Symbols page

K
L

Kenny, Elizabeth (1880–1952), Australian nurse. Sister Kenny first developed an interest in the treatment of paralysis while she was a military nurse during World War I. In 1933 she opened a clinic for the treatment of paralytic patients, most of whom suffered from poliomyelitis. She introduced the Kenny method for the treatment of poliomyelitis in 1937. Thereafter she worked for the general adoption of her method.

keno·tox·in \'ken-ə-ˌtäk-sən\ *n* : a toxin formerly supposed to be produced in the body during activity which causes fatigue

Ke·nya typhus \'ken-yə-, 'kēn-\ *n* : a tick-borne rickettsial disease that occurs esp. in Kenya and is apparently identical with boutonneuse fever — called also *Kenya fever, Kenya tick typhus*

keph·a·lin *var of* CEPHALIN

Ke·pone \'kē-ˌpōn\ *n* : a neurotoxic organochlorine pesticide $C_{10}Cl_{10}O$ — formerly a U.S. registered trademark

ker·a·sin \'ker-ə-sən\ *n* : a cerebroside $C_{48}H_{93}NO_8$ that occurs esp. in Gaucher's disease and that yields lignoceric acid on hydrolysis

ker·a·tan sulfate \'ker-ə-ˌtan-\ *n* : any of several sulfated glycosaminoglycans that have been found esp. in the cornea, cartilage, and bone — called also *keratosulfate*

ker·a·tec·to·my \ˌker-ə-'tek-tə-mē\ *n, pl* **-mies** : surgical excision of part of the cornea — see PHOTOREFRACTIVE KERATECTOMY

ke·rat·ic precipitates \kə-'rat-ik-\ *n pl* : accumulations on the posterior surface of the cornea esp. of macrophages and epithelial cells that occur in chronic inflammatory conditions — called also *keratitis punctata*

ker·a·tin \'ker-ət-ən\ *n* : any of various sulfur-containing fibrous proteins that form the chemical basis of horny epidermal tissues (as hair and nails) and are typically not digested by enzymes of the gastrointestinal tract — see PSEUDOKERATIN

ker·a·tin·ase \'ker-ət-ə-ˌnās, -ˌnāz\ *n* : a proteolytic enzyme that digests keratin, is present in keratin-consuming organisms (as clothes moth larvae), and is used in depilatories

ke·ra·ti·ni·za·tion *or Brit* **ke·ra·ti·ni·sa·tion** \ˌker-ət-ə-nə-'zā-shən, kə-ˌrat-ᵊn-ə-\ *n* : conversion into keratin or keratinous tissue

ke·ra·ti·nize *or Brit* **ke·ra·ti·nise** \'ker-ət-ə-ˌnīz, kə-'rat-ᵊn-ˌīz\ *vb* **-nized** *or Brit* **-nised; -niz·ing** *or Brit* **-nis·ing** *vt* : to make keratinous ⟨tissues *keratinized* by friction⟩ ~ *vi* : to become keratinous or converted into keratin ⟨a *keratinizing* scar⟩

ke·ra·ti·no·cyte \kə-'rat-ᵊn-ə-ˌsīt, ˌker-ə-'tin-\ *n* : an epidermal cell that produces keratin

ke·ra·ti·no·lyt·ic \ˌker-ət-ə-nə-'lit-ik, kə-ˌrat-ᵊn-ə-\ *adj* : causing the lysis of keratin ⟨~ enzymes⟩ — **ke·ra·ti·nol·y·sis** \ˌker-ət-ə-'näl-ə-səs\ *n, pl* **-y·ses** \-ˌsēz\

ke·ra·ti·no·phil·ic \ˌker-ət-ə-nə-'fil-ik, kə-ˌrat-ᵊn-ə-\ *adj* : exhibiting affinity for keratin (as in hair, skin, feathers, or horns) — used chiefly of fungi capable of growing on such materials

ke·ra·ti·nous \kə-'rat-ᵊn-əs, ˌker-ə-'tī-nəs\ *adj* : composed of or containing keratin : HORNY

ker·a·ti·tis \ˌker-ə-'tīt-əs\ *n, pl* **-tit·i·des** \-'tit-ə-ˌdēz\ : inflammation of the cornea of the eye characterized by burning or smarting, blurring of vision, and sensitivity to light and caused by infectious or noninfectious agents — called also *corneitis;* compare KERATOCONJUNCTIVITIS

keratitis punc·ta·ta \-ˌpəŋk-'tät-ə, -'tāt-\ *n* : KERATIC PRECIPITATES

ker·a·to·ac·an·tho·ma \ˌker-ət-ō-ˌak-ˌan-'thō-mə\ *n, pl* **-mas** *also* **-ma·ta** \-mət-ə\ : a rapidly growing skin tumor that occurs esp. in elderly individuals, resembles a carcinoma of squamous epithelial cells but does not spread, and tends to heal spontaneously with some scarring if left untreated

ker·a·to·cele \'ker-ət-ō-ˌsēl\ *n* : hernia of Descemet's membrane through perforations in the cornea

ker·a·to·con·junc·ti·vi·tis \'ker-ə-(ˌ)tō-kən-ˌjən(k)-tə-'vīt-əs\ *n* : combined inflammation of the cornea and conjunctiva; *esp* : EPIDEMIC KERATOCONJUNCTIVITIS — compare KERATITIS

keratoconjunctivitis sic·ca \-'sik-ə\ *n* : DRY EYE

ker·a·to·co·nus \ˌker-ət-ō-'kō-nəs\ *n* : cone-shaped protrusion of the cornea

ker·a·to·der·ma \-'dər-mə\ *n* : a horny condition of the skin

keratoderma blen·nor·rhag·i·cum \-ˌblen-ór-'aj-i-kəm\ *n* : KERATOSIS BLENNORRHAGICA

ker·a·to·der·mia \ˌker-ət-ō-'dər-mē-ə\ *n* : KERATODERMA

ker·a·to·gen·ic \ˌker-ət-ō-'jen-ik\ *adj* : capable of inducing proliferation of epidermal tissues

ker·a·tog·e·nous \ˌker-ə-'täj-ə-nəs\ *adj* : producing horn or horny tissue

ker·a·to·hy·a·lin \-'hī-ə-lən\ *also* **ker·a·to·hy·a·line** \-lən, -ˌlēn\ *n* : a colorless translucent protein that occurs esp. in granules of the stratum granulosum of the epidermis and stains deeply with hematoxylin

ker·a·tol·y·sis \ˌker-ə-'täl-ə-səs\ *n, pl* **-y·ses** \-ˌsēz\ **1** : the process of breaking down or dissolving keratin **2** : a skin disease marked by peeling of the horny layer of the epidermis

¹ker·a·to·lyt·ic \ˌker-ət-ō-'lit-ik\ *adj* : relating to or causing keratolysis

²keratolytic *n* : a keratolytic agent (as salicylic acid)

ker·a·to·ma \ˌker-ə-'tō-mə\ *n, pl* **-mas** *also* **-ma·ta** \-mət-ə\ : a hard thickened area of skin produced by hypertrophy of the horny layers

ker·a·to·ma·la·cia \ˌker-ət-ō-mə-'lā-s(h)ē-ə\ *n* : a softening and ulceration of the cornea of the eye resulting from severe systemic deficiency of vitamin A — compare XEROPHTHALMIA

ker·a·tome \'ker-ə-ˌtōm\ *n* : a surgical instrument used for making an incision in the cornea in cataract operations

ker·a·tom·e·ter \ˌker-ə-'täm-ət-ər\ *n* : an instrument for measuring the curvature of the cornea

ker·a·tom·e·try \ˌker-ə-'täm-ə-trē\ *n, pl* **-tries** : measurement of the form and curvature of the cornea — **ker·a·to·me·tric** \ˌker-ət-ə-'me-trik\ *adj*

ker·at·o·mil·eu·sis \ˌker-ət-ō-mil-'(y)ü-səs\ *n* : keratoplasty in which a piece of the cornea is removed, frozen, shaped to correct refractive error, and reinserted

ker·a·top·a·thy \ˌker-ə-'täp-ə-thē\ *n, pl* **-thies** : any noninflammatory disease of the eye — see BAND KERATOPATHY

ker·a·to·pha·kia \ˌker-ət-ō-'fā-kē-ə\ *n* : keratoplasty in which corneal tissue from a donor is frozen, shaped, and inserted into the cornea of a recipient

ker·a·to·plas·tic \ˌker-ət-ō-'plas-tik\ *adj* : promoting keratinization and thickening of keratin layers ⟨the ~ action of salicylic acid in low concentrations⟩

ker·a·to·plas·ty \'ker-ət-ō-ˌplas-tē\ *n, pl* **-ties** : plastic surgery on the cornea; *esp* : corneal grafting

ker·a·to·pros·the·sis \ˌker-ət-ō-präs-'thē-səs, -'präs-thə-\ *n, pl* **-the·ses** \-ˌsēz\ : a plastic replacement for an opacified inner part of a cornea

ker·a·to·scope \'ker-ət-ō-ˌskōp\ *n* : an instrument for examining the cornea esp. to detect irregularities of its anterior surface — **ker·a·tos·co·py** \ˌker-ə-'täs-kə-pē\ *n, pl* **-pies**

ker·a·to·sis \ˌker-ə-'tō-səs\ *n, pl* **-to·ses** \-ˌsēz\ **1** : a disease of the skin marked by overgrowth of horny tissue **2** : an area of the skin affected with keratosis — **ker·a·tot·ic** \-'tät-ik\ *adj*

keratosis blen·nor·rhag·i·ca \-ˌblen-ór-'aj-i-kə\ *n* : a disease that is characterized by a scaly rash esp. on the palms and soles and is associated esp. with Reiter's syndrome — called also *keratoderma blennorrhagicum*

keratosis fol·li·cu·lar·is \-ˌfäl-ə-kyə-'ler-əs\ *n* : DARIER'S DISEASE

keratosis pi·la·ris \-pi-'ler-əs\ *n* : a condition marked by the formation of hard conical elevations in the openings of the sebaceous glands esp. of the thighs and arms that resemble permanent goose bumps

ker·a·to·sul·fate *or chiefly Brit* **ker·a·to·sul·phate** \ˌker-ət-ō-'səl-ˌfāt\ *n* : KERATAN SULFATE

ker·a·tot·o·mist \ˌker-ə-'tät-ə-məst\ *n* : a surgeon who performs keratotomies

ker·a·tot·o·my \-ə-mē\ *n, pl* **-mies** : incision of the cornea — see RADIAL KERATOTOMY

ke·rau·no·pho·bia \ke-ˌrȯ-nə-'fō-bē-ə\ *n* : abnormal fear of lightning or thunder

ke·ri·on \'kir-ē-ˌän\ *n* : inflammatory ringworm of the hair follicles of the beard and scalp usu. accompanied by secondary bacterial infection and marked by spongy swelling and the exudation of sticky pus from the hair follicles

ker·ma \'kər-mə\ *n* : the ratio of the sum of the initial kinetic energies of all charged particles liberated by uncharged ionizing particles (as neutrons) in an element of volume of irradiated matter to the mass of matter in the element of volume

ker·mes mineral \'kər-(ˌ)mēz-\ *n* : a soft brown-red powder consisting essentially of oxides and sulfides of antimony and formerly used as an alterative, diaphoretic, and emetic

ker·nic·ter·us \kər-'nik-tə-rəs\ *n* : a condition marked by the deposit of bile pigments in the nuclei of the brain and spinal cord and by degeneration of nerve cells that occurs usu. in infants as a part of the syndrome of erythroblastosis fetalis — **ker·nic·ter·ic** \-rik\ *adj*

Ker·nig sign \'ker-nig-\ *or* **Kernig's sign** \'ker-nigz-\ *n* : an indication usu. present in meningitis that consists of pain and resistance on attempting to extend the leg at the knee with the thigh flexed at the hip

Kernig, Vladimir Mikhailovich (1840–1917), Russian physician. Kernig first described his sign for cerebrospinal meningitis in 1882. In 1907 he published a full description.

ker·o·sene *also* **ker·o·sine** \'ker-ə-ˌsēn, ˌker-ə-', 'kar-, ˌkar-\ *n* : a flammable hydrocarbon oil usu. obtained by distillation of petroleum and used for a fuel and as a solvent and thinner (as in insecticide emulsions)

ke·ta·mine \'kēt-ə-ˌmēn\ *n* : a general anesthetic that is administered intravenously and intramuscularly in the form of its hydrochloride $C_{13}H_{16}ClNO·HCl$

ke·tene \'kē-ˌtēn\ *n* : a colorless poisonous gas C_2H_2O of penetrating odor used esp. as an acetylating agent; *also* : any of various derivatives of this compound

ke·thox·al \kē-'thäk-səl\ *n* : an antiviral agent $C_6H_{12}O_4$

ket·im·ine \'kēt-im-ˌēn\ *n* : a Schiff base of the general formula $R_2C = NH$ or $R_2C = NR'$ formed by condensation of a ketone with ammonia or a primary amine

ke·to \'kēt-(ˌ)ō\ *adj* : of or relating to a ketone; *also* : containing a ketone group

keto acid *n* : a compound that is both a ketone and an acid

ke·to·ac·i·do·sis \ˌkēt-ō-ˌas-ə-'dō-səs\ *n, pl* **-do·ses** \-ˌsēz\ : acidosis accompanied by ketosis ⟨diabetic ∼⟩

ke·to·ac·i·dot·ic \-'dät-ik\ *adj* : affected with ketoacidosis ⟨a ∼ diabetic⟩

ke·to·bem·i·done \ˌkēt-ō-'bem-ə-ˌdōn\ *n* : a highly addictive narcotic ketone $C_{15}H_{21}NO_2$ related chemically to meperidine

ke·to·co·na·zole \kē-tō-'kō-nə-ˌzōl\ *n* : a synthetic broad-spectrum antifungal agent $C_{26}H_{28}Cl_2N_4O_4$ used to treat chronic internal and cutaneous disorders — see NIZORAL

ke·to·gen·e·sis \ˌkēt-ō-'jen-ə-səs\ *n, pl* **-e·ses** \-ˌsēz\ : the production of ketone bodies (as in diabetes mellitus) — **ke·to·gen·ic** \-'jen-ik\ *adj*

ketogenic diet *n* : a diet supplying a large amount of fat and minimal amounts of carbohydrate and protein and used esp. formerly in epilepsy to produce a ketosis and alter the degree of bodily alkalinity

ke·to·glu·ta·rate \ˌkēt-ō-glü-'tä-ˌrāt, -'glüt-ə-ˌrāt\ *n* : a salt or ester of ketoglutaric acid

α–ketoglutarate, α–ketoglutaric acid *var of* ALPHA-KETOGLUTARATE, ALPHA-KETOGLUTARIC ACID

ke·to·glu·tar·ic acid \-glü-ˌtar-ik-\ *n* : either of two crystalline keto derivatives $C_5H_6O_5$ of glutaric acid; *esp* : ALPHA-KETOGLUTARIC ACID

ke·to·hep·tose \ˌkēt-ō-'hep-ˌtōs, -ˌtōz\ *n* : a heptose of a ketonic nature

ke·to·hex·ose \-'hek-ˌsōs, -ˌsōz\ *n* : a hexose (as fructose or sorbose) of a ketonic nature

ke·tol \'kē-ˌtȯl, -ˌtōl\ *n* : a compound that is both a ketone and an alcohol — **ke·tol·ic** \kē-'tȯl-ik\ *adj*

ke·tol·y·sis \kē-'täl-ə-səs\ *n, pl* **-y·ses** \-ˌsēz\ : the decomposition of ketones — **ke·to·lyt·ic** \ˌkēt-ō-'lit-ik\ *adj*

ke·tone \'kē-ˌtōn\ *n* : an organic compound (as acetone) with a carbonyl group attached to two carbon atoms

ketone body *n* : any of the three compounds acetoacetic acid, acetone, and the beta derivative of hydroxybutyric acid which are normal intermediates in lipid metabolism and accumulate in the blood and urine in abnormal amounts in conditions of impaired metabolism (as diabetes mellitus) — called also *acetone body*

ke·to·ne·mia *or chiefly Brit* **ke·to·nae·mia** \ˌkēt-ə-'nē-mē-ə\ *n* **1** : a condition marked by an abnormal increase of ketone bodies in the circulating blood — called also *hyperketonemia* **2** : KETOSIS 2 — **ke·to·ne·mic** *or chiefly Brit* **ke·to·nae·mic** \-'nē-mik\ *adj*

ke·ton·ic \kē-'tän-ik, -'tōn-\ *adj* : of, relating to, or being ketones or ketone bodies

ke·to·nize *or Brit* **ke·to·nise** \'kē-tō-ˌnīz\ *vb* **-nized** *or Brit* **-nised; -niz·ing** *or Brit* **-nis·ing** *vt* : to convert into a ketone ∼ *vi* : to become converted into a ketone — **ke·to·ni·za·tion** *or Brit* **ke·to·ni·sa·tion** \ˌkēt-ə-nə-'zā-shən\ *n*

ke·ton·uria \ˌkēt-ə-'n(y)ur-ē-ə\ *n* : the presence of excess ketone bodies in the urine in conditions (as diabetes mellitus and starvation acidosis) involving reduced or disturbed carbohydrate metabolism — called also *acetonuria*

ke·to·pen·tose \ˌkēt-ō-'pen-ˌtōs, -ˌtōz\ *n* : a five-carbon sugar containing the keto group CO

ke·to·pro·fen \ˌkēt-ō-'prō-fən\ *n* : an analgesic nonsteroidal anti-inflammatory drug $C_{16}H_{14}O_3$ that is used to treat dysmenorrhea and the symptoms of rheumatoid arthritis and osteoarthritis

ke·tose \'kē-ˌtōs, -ˌtōz\ *n* : a sugar (as fructose) containing one ketone group per molecule

ke·to·sis \kē-'tō-səs\ *n, pl* **-to·ses** \-ˌsēz\ **1** : an abnormal increase of ketone bodies in the body in conditions of reduced or disturbed carbohydrate metabolism (as in uncontrolled diabetes mellitus) — compare ACIDOSIS, ALKALOSIS **2** : a nutritional disease of cattle and sometimes sheep, goats, or swine that is marked by reduction of blood sugar and the presence of ketone bodies in the blood, tissues, milk, and urine and is associated with digestive and nervous disturbances — **ke·tot·ic** \-'tät-ik\ *adj*

ke·to·ste·roid \ˌkēt-ō-'sti(ə)r-ˌȯid *also* -'ste(ə)r-\ *n* : a steroid (as cortisone or estrone) containing a ketone group; *esp* : 17-KETOSTEROID

17–ketosteroid \'sev-ən-ˌtēn-\ *n* : any of the ketosteroids (as androsterone, dehydroepiandrosterone, and estrone) that have the keto group attached to carbon atom 17 of the steroid ring structure, are present in normal human urine, and may be an indication of a tumor of the adrenal cortex or ovary when present in excess

Ke·ty method \'kēt-ē-\ *n* : a method of determining coronary blood flow by measurement of nitrous oxide levels in the blood of a patient breathing nitrous oxide

Kety, Seymour Solomon (1915–2000), American physiologist. Kety's areas of research included brain circulation and metabolism, the dynamics of the exchange of substances between capillaries and tissues, and the biochemistry of mental states. His most important research concerned the measurement of blood flow and metabolism in the human brain by the use of low concentrations of nitrous oxide and the analysis of its concentration in arterial and cerebral venous blood during the short time in which it is equilibrating with the brain.

kg *abbr* kilogram

kgm *abbr* kilogram-meter

khat *also* **kat** *or* **qat** *or* **quat** \'kät\ *n* : a shrub (*Catha edulis*)

K
L

\ə\ abut \ᵊ\ kitten \ər\ further \a\ ash \ā\ ace \ä\ cot, cart
\aū\ out \ch\ chin \e\ bet \ē\ easy \g\ go \i\ hit \ī\ ice \j\ job
\ŋ\ sing \ō\ go \ȯ\ law \ȯi\ boy \th\ thin \th̲\ the \ü\ loot
\ū̇\ foot \y\ yet \zh\ vision *See also* Pronunciation Symbols page

cultivated in the Middle East and Africa for its leaves and buds that are the source of a habituating stimulant when chewed or used as a tea

khel·lin *also* **kel·lin** \'kel-ən\ *n* : a crystalline compound $C_{14}H_{12}O_5$ obtained from the fruit of a Middle Eastern plant (*Ammi visnaga*) of the family Umbelliferae and used as an antispasmodic in asthma and a coronary vasodilator in angina pectoris

kibe \'kīb\ *n* : an ulcerated chilblain esp. on the heel

kid·ney \'kid-nē\ *n, pl* **kidneys 1** : one of a pair of vertebrate organs situated in the body cavity near the spinal column that excrete waste products of metabolism, in humans are bean-shaped organs about 4½ inches (11½ centimeters) long lying behind the peritoneum in a mass of fatty tissue, and consist chiefly of nephrons by which urine is secreted, collected, and discharged into the pelvis of the kidney whence it is conveyed by the ureter to the bladder — compare MESO-NEPHROS, METANEPHROS, PRONEPHROS **2** : any of various excretory organs of invertebrate animals

kidney basin *n* : a shallow kidney-shaped basin used esp. for the collection of bodily discharges

kidney stone *n* : a calculus in the kidney — called also *renal calculus*

kidney worm *n* : any of several nematode worms parasitic in the kidneys: as **a** : GIANT KIDNEY WORM **b** : a common and destructive black-and-white worm of the genus *Stephanurus* (*S. dentatus*) that is related to the gapeworm but attains a length of two inches (five centimeters) and is parasitic in the kidneys, lungs, and other viscera of the hog in warm regions — called also *lardworm*

Kien·böck's disease \'kēn-ˌbeks-\ *n* : osteochondrosis affecting the lunate bone — called also *lunatomalacia*

Kien·böck \'kēn-ˌbœk\, **Robert (1871–1953),** Austrian radiologist. Kienböck pioneered in radiology. From 1910–11 he published descriptions of dislocation of the hand and a slowly progressive chronic osteitis involving the lunate bone. The latter is now known as Kienböck's disease.

killed \'kild\ *adj* : being or containing a virus that has been inactivated (as by chemicals) so that it is no longer infectious ⟨~ vaccines⟩

kil·ler bee \'kil-ər-ˌbē\ *n* : AFRICANIZED BEE

killer cell *n* : a lymphocyte (as a cytotoxic T cell or a natural killer cell) with cytotoxic activity

killer T cell *n* : CYTOTOXIC T CELL

killer T lymphocyte *n* : CYTOTOXIC T CELL

ki·lo·base \'kil-ə-ˌbās\ *n* : a unit of measure of the length of a nucleic-acid chain (as of DNA or RNA) that equals one thousand base pairs

ki·lo·cal·o·rie \-ˌkal-(ə-)rē\ *n* : CALORIE 1b

kilo·cy·cle \'kil-ə-ˌsī-kəl\ *n* : 1000 cycles; *esp* : KILOHERTZ

ki·lo·dal·ton \-ˌdȯlt-ᵊn\ *n* : a unit of molecular mass equal to 1000 daltons — abbr. *kD*

ki·lo·gram *or chiefly Brit* **ki·lo·gramme** \'kil-ə-ˌgram, 'kē-lə-\ *n* **1** : the base unit of mass in the International System of Units that is equal to the mass of a prototype agreed upon by international convention and that is nearly equal to the mass of 1000 cubic centimeters of water at the temperature of its maximum density **2** : a unit of force equal to the weight of a kilogram mass under a gravitational attraction equal to that of the earth

kilogram calorie *n* : CALORIE 1b

kilogram–meter *or chiefly Brit* **kilogramme–metre** *n* : the mks gravitational unit of work and energy equal to the work done by a kilogram force acting through a distance of one meter in the direction of the force : about 7.235 foot-pounds

ki·lo·hertz \'kil-ə-ˌhərts, 'kē-lə-, -ˌhe(ə)rts\ *n* : 1000 hertz

ki·lo·joule \'kil-ə-ˌjü(ə)l\ *n* : 1000 joules; *also* : a unit equivalent to 0.239 nutritional calories

kilo·li·ter *or chiefly Brit* **kilo·li·tre** \'kil-ə-ˌlēt-ər\ *n* : 1000 liters

ki·lo·me·ter *or chiefly Brit* **kilo·me·tre** \'kil-ə-ˌmēt-ər, kə-ˈläm-ət-ər\ *n* : 1000 meters

ki·lo·rad \'kil-ə-ˌrad\ *n* : 1000 rads

ki·lo·volt \-ˌvōlt\ *n* : a unit of potential difference equal to 1000 volts

kilo·watt \'kil-ə-ˌwät\ *n* : 1000 watts

kilowatt–hour *n* : a unit of work or energy equal to that expended by one kilowatt in one hour

kinaesthesia, kinaesthesis, kinaesthetic, kinaesthetically *chiefly Brit var of* KINESTHESIA, KINESTHESIS, KINESTHETIC, KINESTHETICALLY

ki·nase \'kī-ˌnās, -ˌnāz\ *n* : any of various enzymes that catalyze the transfer of phosphate groups from a high-energy phosphate-containing molecule (as ATP or ADP) to a substrate — called also *phosphokinase*

kin·dle \'kin-dᵊl\ *vi* **kin·dled; kin·dling** : to bring forth young — used chiefly of a rabbit

kind·ling \'kin-dliŋ\ *n* : the electrophysiological changes that occur in the brain as a result of repeated intermittent exposure to a subthreshold electrical or chemical stimulus (as one causing seizures) so that there develops a usu. permanent decrease in the threshold of excitability

kin·dred \'kin-drəd\ *n* : a group of related individuals : a genealogical group ⟨incidence of cancer among members of a ~⟩

ki·ne·mat·ics \ˌkin-ə-ˈmat-iks, ˌkī-nə-\ *also* **ci·ne·mat·ics** \ˌsin-ə-\ *n pl but sing in constr* **1** : a branch of physics that deals with aspects of motion apart from considerations of mass and force **2** : the properties and phenomena of an object or system in motion of interest to kinematics ⟨the ~ of the human ankle joint⟩ — **ki·ne·mat·ic** \-ik\ *or* **ki·ne·mat·i·cal** \-i-kəl\ *adj* — **ki·ne·mat·i·cal·ly** \-i-k(ə-)lē\ *adv*

kinematic viscosity *n* : the ratio of the coefficient of viscosity to the density of a fluid

kineplastic, kineplasty *var of* CINEPLASTIC, CINEPLASTY

kin·e·sim·e·ter \ˌkin-ə-ˈsim-ət-ər, ˌkīn-\ *n* : an instrument for measuring bodily movements

ki·ne·sin \ki-ˈnē-sən\ *n* : an ATPase similar to dynein that functions as a motor protein in the intracellular transport esp. of cell organelles and molecules (as mitochondria and proteins) along microtubules

ki·ne·si·ol·o·gist \kə-ˌnē-sē-ˈäl-ə-jəst, kī-, -zē-\ *n* : an individual skilled in or applying kinesiology

ki·ne·si·ol·o·gy \kə-ˌnē-sē-ˈäl-ə-jē, kī-, -zē-\ *n, pl* **-gies** : the study of the principles of mechanics and anatomy in relation to human movement — **ki·ne·si·o·log·ic** \-ō-ˈläj-ik\ *or* **ki·ne·si·o·log·i·cal** \-i-kəl\ *adj*

ki·ne·sis \kə-ˈnē-səs, kī-\ *n, pl* **ki·ne·ses** \-ˌsēz\ : a movement that lacks directional orientation and depends upon the intensity of stimulation

ki·ne·si·ther·a·py \kə-ˌnē-sē-ˈther-ə-pē, kī-\ *n, pl* **-pies** : the therapeutic and corrective application of passive and active movements (as by massage) and of exercise

ki·ne·so·pho·bia \kə-ˌnē-sō-ˈfō-bē-ə, kī-\ *n* : a pathological fear of motion

kin·es·the·sia \ˌkin-əs-ˈthē-zh(ē-)ə, ˌkī-nəs-\ *or* **kin·es·the·sis** \-ˈthē-səs\ *or chiefly Brit* **kin·aes·the·sia** *or* **kin·aes·the·sis** *n, pl* **-the·sias** *or* **-the·ses** \-ˌsēz\ : a sense mediated by end organs located in muscles, tendons, and joints and stimulated by bodily movements and tensions; *also* : sensory experience derived from this sense — see MUSCLE SENSE — **kin·es·thet·ic** *or chiefly Brit* **kin·aes·thet·ic** \-ˈthet-ik\ *adj* — **kin·es·thet·i·cal·ly** *or chiefly Brit* **kin·aes·thet·i·cal·ly** \-i-k(ə-)lē\ *adv*

ki·net·ic \kə-ˈnet-ik, kī-\ *adj* : of or relating to the motion of material bodies and the forces and energy associated therewith — **ki·net·i·cal·ly** *adv*

kinetic energy *n* : energy associated with motion

ki·net·i·cist \kə-ˈnet-ə-səst, kī-\ *n* : a specialist in kinetics

ki·net·ics \kə-ˈnet-iks, kī-\ *n pl but sing or pl in constr* **1 a** : a branch of science that deals with the effects of forces upon the motions of material bodies or with changes in a physical or chemical system **b** : the rate of change in such a system **2** : the mechanism by which a physical or chemical change is effected

ki·neto·car·dio·gram \kə-ˌnet-ō-ˈkärd-ē-ə-ˌgram, kī-\ *n* : a graphic recording of the vibration of the precordium — **ki-**

neto·car·dio·graph·ic \-ˌkärd-ē-ə-ˈgraf-ik\ adj — ki·neto·car·di·og·ra·phy \-ˌkärd-ē-ˈäg-rə-fē\ n, pl -phies

ki·neto·chore \kə-ˈnet-ə-ˌkō(ə)r, kī-, -ˌkó(ə)r\ n 1 : CENTROMERE 2 : a specialized structure on the centromere to which the microtubular spindle fibers attach during mitosis and meiosis

ki·neto·nu·cle·us \kə-ˌnet-ō-ˈn(y)ü-klē-əs, kī-\ n : KINETOPLAST

ki·neto·plast \kə-ˈnet-ə-ˌplast, kī-\ n : an extranuclear DNA-containing organelle of kinetoplastid protozoans that is usu. found in an elongated mitochondrion located adjacent to the basal body — ki·neto·plas·tic \-ˌnet-ə-ˈplas-tik\ adj

ki·neto·plas·tid \kə-ˌnet-ə-ˈplas-tid, kī-\ n : any protozoan of the order Kinetoplastida — called also protomonad — ki·netoplastid adj

Ki·neto·plas·ti·da \-ˈplas-təd-ə\ n pl : an order of flagellate protozoans of the subphylum Mastigophora that have a kinetoplast and typically one or two flagella — compare BODO, LEISHMANIA, TRYPANOSOMA

kin·e·to·sis \ˌkin-ə-ˈtō-səs, ˌkīn-\ n, pl -to·ses \-ˌsēz\ : MOTION SICKNESS

ki·neto·some \kə-ˈnet-ə-ˌsōm, kī-\ n : BASAL BODY — ki·neto·som·al \-ˌnet-ə-ˈsō-məl\ adj

king co·bra \ˈkiŋ-ˈkō-brə\ n : a large and very venomous cobra of the genus Ophiophagus (O. hannah syn. Naja hannah) of southeastern Asia and the Philippines that may attain a length of 18 feet (5.5 meters) — called also hamadryad

king·dom \ˈkiŋ-dəm\ n 1 : any of the three primary divisions into which natural objects are grouped — see ANIMAL KINGDOM, MINERAL KINGDOM, PLANT KINGDOM 2 : a major category (as Protista) in biological taxonomy that ranks above the phylum and below the domain

king's evil \ˈkiŋz-ˈē-vəl, -vil\ n, often cap K&E : SCROFULA

ki·nin \ˈkī-nən\ n 1 : any of various polypeptide hormones that are formed locally in the tissues and cause dilation of blood vessels and contraction of smooth muscle 2 : CYTOKININ

ki·ni·nase \ˈkī-nə-ˌnās, -ˌnāz\ n : an enzyme in blood that destroys a kinin

ki·nin·o·gen \kī-ˈnin-ə-jən\ n : an inactive precursor of a kinin — ki·nin·o·gen·ic \(ˌ)kī-ˌnin-ə-ˈjen-ik\ adj

¹kink \ˈkiŋk\ n 1 : a short tight twist or curl caused by a doubling or winding of something upon itself 2 : a cramp in some part of the body

²kink vi : to form a kink ~ vt : to make a kink in ⟨blood vessels have been ~ed and shut off —Benjamin Spock⟩

ki·no \ˈkē-(ˌ)nō\ n 1 : any of several dark red to black tannin-containing dried juices or extracts obtained from various tropical trees; esp : the dried juice obtained usu. from the trunk of an Indian and Sri Lankan tree (Pterocarpus marsupium) as brown or black fragments and used as an astringent in diarrhea 2 : a tree that produces kino (esp. Pterocarpus marsupium)

ki·no·cil·i·um \ˌkī-nō-ˈsil-ē-əm\ n, pl -cil·ia \-ē-ə\ : a motile cilium; esp : one that occurs alone at the end of a sensory hair cell of the inner ear among numerous nonmotile stereocilia

kino gum n : KINO 1

ki·no·plasm \ˈkī-nə-ˌplaz-əm, ˈkin-ə-\ also ki·no·plas·ma \-ˈplaz-mə\ n : an active protoplasmic component held to form filaments and mobile structures (as cilia or spindle fibers) — ki·no·plas·mic \-ˈplaz-mik\ adj

Ki·no·rhyn·cha \ˌkī-nō-ˈriŋ-kə, ˌkin-ō-\ n pl : a class of Aschelminthes or a separate phylum comprising minute marine worms of uncertain systematic position having certain resemblances to arthropods and annelids but prob. more closely related to the nematodes

kin selection \ˈkin-\ n : a theory of natural selection which states that a usu. altruistic behavior or attribute that lowers the fitness of a particular individual is selected for if it increases the probability of survival and reproduction of related kin who possess some or all of the same genes as the altruistic individual

Kirsch·ner wire \ˈkərsh-nər-ˌwir\ n : metal wire inserted through bone and used to achieve internal traction or immobilization of bone fractures

Kirsch·ner \ˈkirsh-nər\, Martin (1879–1942), German surgeon. Kirschner was responsible for developing a number of innovative surgical operations. He developed an operation for hernia (1910), an operation on the patella (1911), and the first successful surgical treatment of pulmonary embolism (1924). In 1909 he introduced the use of wires for skeletal traction in the treatment of fracture.

kiss·ing bug \ˈkis-iŋ-ˌbəg\ n : CONENOSE

kissing disease n : INFECTIOUS MONONUCLEOSIS

kiss of life n, chiefly Brit : artificial respiration by the mouth-to-mouth method

KJ abbr knee jerk

Kjel·dahl \ˈkel-ˌdäl\ adj : of, relating to, or being a method for determining the amount of nitrogen (as in an organic substance) by digesting a sample with boiling concentrated sulfuric acid and other reagents, adding an excess of alkali, distilling, collecting the ammonia expelled, and determining the ammonia by titration ⟨~ analysis⟩ ⟨~ apparatus⟩ — kjel·dahl·iza·tion \ˌkel-ˌdäl-ə-ˈzā-shən\ n — kjel·dahl·ize \ˈkel-ˌdäl-ˌīz\ vt -ized; -iz·ing

Kjeldahl, Johann Gustav Christoffer (1849–1900), Danish chemist. Kjeldahl was the director of research at the chemical laboratory of the Carlsberg brewery. He introduced his method for the estimation of nitrogen in organic substances in 1883. In 1888 he constructed the Kjeldahl flask as an aid for simplifying the Kjeldahl method. The method is very important for agriculture, medicine, and drug manufacturing, and it is still used essentially as Kjeldahl developed it.

Kjeldahl flask n : a round-bottomed usu. long-necked glass flask for use in digesting the sample in the Kjeldahl method of nitrogen analysis

kl abbr kiloliter

kleb·si·el·la \ˌkleb-zē-ˈel-ə\ n 1 cap : a genus of nonmotile gram-negative rod-shaped and frequently encapsulated bacteria of the family Enterobacteriaceae that include causative agents of respiratory and urinary infections — see PNEUMOBACILLUS 2 : any bacterium of the genus Klebsiella

Klebs \ˈkläps\, (Theodor Albrecht) Edwin (1834–1913), German bacteriologist. Klebs is notable for his work on the bacterial theory of infection. During the Franco-Prussian War he made one of the first comprehensive studies of the pathology and bacteriology of gunshot wounds. He investigated tuberculosis throughout his career, and in 1873 he successfully produced tuberculosis in cattle. He also did research on the bacteriology of malaria and anthrax. In 1883 he made his most important discovery: the causative organism of diphtheria, now known as the Klebs-Löffler bacillus.

Klebs–Löff·ler bacillus \ˈkläps-ˈlef-lər-, ˈklebz-\ n : a bacterium of the genus Corynebacterium (C. diphtheriae) that causes human diphtheria

Löff·ler \ˈlœf-lər\, Friedrich August Johannes (1852–1915), German bacteriologist. Löffler contributed greatly to the advancement of bacteriology. In 1882 he discovered the bacterium of the genus Pseudomonas (P. mallei) that causes glanders. He discovered the cause of swine erysipelas and swine plague in 1885. With Paul Frosch (1860–1928) he determined in 1897 that foot-and-mouth disease is caused by a virus. This marked the first time that the cause of an animal disease was attributed to a virus. They developed a serum against the disease in 1899. The diphtheria bacillus discovered by Klebs in 1883 was isolated in the following year by Löffler, who also published the first full description of the microorganism which is now known as the Klebs-Löffler bacillus.

klee·blatt·schä·del \ˈklä-ˌblät-ˌshäd-ᵊl\ n : CLOVERLEAF SKULL

K
L

Klein·ian \'klī-nē-ən\ *adj* : of, relating to, or according with the psychoanalytic theories or practices of Melanie Klein — **Kleinian** *n*

Klein \'klīn\, **Melanie (1882–1960),** Austrian psychoanalyst. Klein made major contributions to psychoanalysis, and her work had great influence on the developing science of child psychology and psychiatry. She did pioneering research on the psychoanalysis of young children.

klep·to·lag·nia \ˌklep-tə-'lag-nē-ə\ *n* : sexual arousal and gratification produced by committing an act of theft

klep·to·ma·nia \ˌklep-tə-'mā-nē-ə, -nyə\ *n* : a persistent neurotic impulse to steal esp. without economic motive

klep·to·ma·ni·ac \-nē-ˌak\ *n* : an individual exhibiting kleptomania

klieg eyes *or* **kleig eyes** \'klēg-\ *n pl* : a condition marked by conjunctivitis and watering of the eyes resulting from excessive exposure to intense light

Kline·fel·ter's syndrome \'klīn-ˌfel-tərz-\ *also* **Kline·fel·ter syndrome** \-tər-\ *n* : an abnormal condition in a male characterized by two X chromosomes and one Y chromosome, infertility, smallness of the testes, sparse facial and body hair, and gynecomastia

Klinefelter, Harry Fitch (*b* 1912), American physician. Klinefelter specialized in endocrinology and rheumatology. Klinefelter's syndrome was described in 1942.

Kline reaction \'klīn-\ *n* : KLINE TEST

Kline test *n* : a rapid precipitation test for the diagnosis of syphilis

Kline, Benjamin Schoenbrun (*b* 1886), American pathologist. Kline specialized in experimental pathology and also studied spirochetal gangrene and lobar pneumonia. He developed the Kline test in 1926.

kli·no·ki·ne·sis \ˌklī-nō-kə-'nē-səs, -kī-\ *n* : movement that is induced by stimulation and that involves essentially random alteration of direction — **kli·no·ki·net·ic** \-'net-ik\ *adj*

Klip·pel–Feil syndrome \kli-'pel-'fīl-\ *n* : congenital fusion of the cervical vertebrae resulting in a short and relatively immobile neck

Klippel, Maurice (1858–1942), and **Feil, André** (*b* 1884), French neurologists. Klippel and Feil described the Klippel–Feil syndrome in 1912.

Klor–Con \'klȯr-ˌkän\ *trademark* — used for a preparation of potassium chloride or potassium bicarbonate

Klump·ke's paralysis \'klümp-kēz-\ *n* : atrophic paralysis of the forearm and the hand due to injury to the eighth cervical and first thoracic nerves

Dé·jé·rine–Klump·ke \dā-zhā-rēn-klüm-kē\, **Augusta (1859–1927),** French neurologist. Déjérine-Klumpke was a specialist in the pathology of the nervous system. With her husband, neurologist Joseph Jules Déjérine (1849–1917), she did research on the anatomy of the nerve centers. After his death she founded a neurological laboratory at the University of Paris. She published descriptions of Klumpke's paralysis in 1885 and of lead palsy in 1889.

Klü·ver–Bu·cy syndrome \'klü-vər-'b(y)ü-sē-, 'klev-ər-, 'klüē-vər-\ *n* : a group of symptoms that are caused by bilateral removal of the temporal lobes, that include excessive reactivity to visual stimuli, hypersexuality, diminished emotional responses, and memory deficits, and that have been induced experimentally in monkeys and have occurred in human patients who have severe injuries to the temporal lobes or who have undergone temporal lobe lobectomy

Klüver, Heinrich (1897–1979), American neurologist and psychologist. For many years Klüver served as professor of psychology of the University of Chicago. As an editor, he was associated with several journals of psychology. In addition to having numerous articles to his credit, he was the author of book-length monographs including *Mescal* (1928) and *Mescal and Mechanisms of Hallucinations* (1966). In 1937 he and P. C. Bucy first described the syndrome that bears their names in an article on the effects of bilateral temporal lobectomy in rhesus monkeys. Klüver is also credited with developing a technique for staining nervous

system tissue and the discovery of free porphyrins in the central nervous system.

Bucy, Paul Clancy (1904–1992), American neurologist. Bucy held successive positions as professor of neurology and neurosurgery at the medical schools of the University of Chicago, University of Illinois, and Northwestern University. His last position was clinical professor of neurology and neurosurgery at the Bowmen-Gray Medical School in Winston-Salem, North Carolina. Topics he researched included spinal cord injury, the structure and function of the cerebral cortex, and intracranial tumors.

km *abbr* kilometer

knee \'nē\ *n* **1 a** : a joint in the middle part of the human leg that is the articulation between the femur, tibia, and patella — called also *knee joint* **b** : the part of the leg that includes this joint **2 a** : the joint in the hind leg of a 4-footed vertebrate that corresponds to the human knee **b** : the carpal joint of the foreleg of a 4-footed vertebrate — **kneed** \'nēd\ *adj*

knee·cap \'nē-ˌkap\ *n* : PATELLA

knee jerk *n* : an involuntary forward jerk or kick produced by a light blow or sudden strain upon the patellar ligament of the knee that causes a reflex contraction of the quadriceps muscle — called also *patellar reflex*

knee joint *n* : KNEE 1a

knee·pan \'nē-ˌpan\ *n* : PATELLA

knee–sprung \'nē-ˌsprəŋ\ *adj, of a horse* : having the knees bent when they should normally be straight; *esp* : having the knees protruding too far forward

Kne·mi·do·kop·tes \ˌnē-mə-dō-'käp-(ˌ)tēz\ *n* : a genus of itch mites of the family Sarcoptidae that attack birds and that include one (*K. gallinae*) causing a mangy condition and another (*K. mutans*) causing scaly leg of fowl

knife \'nīf\ *n, pl* **knives** \'nīvz\ **1** : any of various instruments used in surgery primarily to sever tissues: as **a** : a cutting instrument consisting of a sharp blade attached to a handle **b** : an instrument that cuts by means of an electric current **2** : SURGERY **3** — usu. used in the phrase *under the knife* ⟨went under the ~ yesterday⟩ ⟨was afraid of the ~⟩

knit \'nit\ *vb* **knit** *or* **knit·ted; knit·ting** *vt* : to cause to grow together ⟨time and rest will ~ a fractured bone⟩ ~ *vi* : to grow together ⟨fractures in old bones ~ slowly⟩

knob \'näb\ *n* : a rounded protuberance or lump — **knob·by** \'näb-ē\ *adj*

knock \'näk\ *n* **1** : a sharp blow ⟨a ~ to the head⟩ **2** : a sharp pounding noise

knock–knee \'näk-'nē, -ˌnē\ *n* : a condition in which the legs curve inward at the knees — called also *genu valgum* — **knock–kneed** \-'nēd\ *adj*

knock·out \'näk-ˌaút\ *adj* : having all or part of a gene eliminated or inactivated by genetic engineering ⟨~ mice predisposed to diabetes mellitus serve as animal models in the study of human diabetes⟩

knockout drops *n pl* : drops of a solution of a drug (as chloral hydrate) put into a drink and designed to produce unconsciousness or stupefaction

knot \'nät\ *n* **1** : an interlacing of the parts of one or more flexible bodies (as threads or sutures) in a lump to prevent their spontaneous separation — see SURGEON'S KNOT **2** : a usu. firm or hard lump, swelling, or protuberance in or on a part of the body or a bone or process ⟨a ~ in a gland⟩ ⟨a bone with two or three ~s⟩ — compare SURFER'S KNOT — **knot** *vb* **knot·ted; knot·ting**

knuck·le \'nək-əl\ *n* **1 a** : the rounded prominence formed by the ends of the two adjacent bones at a joint — used esp. of those at the joints of the fingers **b** : the joint of a knuckle **2** : a sharply flexed loop of intestines incarcerated in a hernia

Koch·er's forceps \'kō-kərz-\ *n* : a strong forceps for controlling bleeding in surgery having serrated blades with interlocking teeth at the tips

Koch·er \'kȯk-ər\, **Emil Theodor (1841–1917),** Swiss surgeon. Kocher spent virtually all of his career at the university surgical clinic at Bern. He made important contributions to the understanding of the physiology and pathology of the thyroid and the treatment of goiter occurring with and without hyperthyroidism. In 1876 he performed the first excision of the thyroid gland for the treatment of goiter; he published a description of his surgical procedure in 1878. Later, in 1883, he reported his discovery of a characteristic cretinoid pattern in patients after total excision of the thyroid gland. In 1878 he performed a successful drainage of a gallbladder, utilizing the forceps that have since become associated with his name. He also published in 1892 a textbook of operative surgery that remained a standard reference for many years. He was awarded the Nobel Prize for Physiology or Medicine in 1909.

Koch's bacillus \\'kōks-, 'käch-əz-\\ *or* **Koch bacillus** \\'kōk-, 'käch-\\ *n* : a bacillus of the genus *Mycobacterium* (*M. tuberculosis*) that causes human tuberculosis

Koch \\'kók\\, **(Heinrich Hermann) Robert (1843–1910)**, German bacteriologist. Koch is usually hailed as the founder of modern bacteriology. He is responsible for devising or adapting many of the basic principles and techniques (particularly staining methods) of bacteriology. He is most famous for isolating and obtaining in 1876 a pure culture of the bacterium (*Bacillus anthracis*) that causes anthrax, for discovering the cholera vibrio (*Vibrio cholerae*) in 1883, and for identifying and isolating the tubercle bacillus (*Mycobacterium tuberculosis*) in 1882. Koch published an epochal work on the etiology of traumatic infectious disease in 1878, and was the first (in 1887) to demonstrate that a specific microorganism is the cause of a specific disease. In 1890 he introduced tuberculin for the diagnosis of tuberculosis. Koch's postulates were first described in 1882 and then elaborated upon in 1884. The Koch-Weeks bacillus was discovered by Koch in 1883, and he described the Koch phenomenon in 1891. Koch was awarded the Nobel Prize for Physiology or Medicine in 1905.

Koch's phenomenon *also* **Koch phenomenon** *n* : the response of a tuberculous animal to reinfection with tubercle bacilli marked by necrotic lesions that develop rapidly and heal quickly and caused by hypersensitivity to products of the tubercle bacillus

Koch's postulates *n pl* : a statement of the steps required to establish a microorganism as the cause of a disease: (1) it must be found in all cases of the disease; (2) it must be isolated from the host and grown in pure culture; (3) it must reproduce the original disease when introduced into a susceptible host; (4) it must be found present in the experimental host so infected — called also *Koch's laws*

Koch–Weeks bacillus \\-'wēks-\\ *n* : a bacterium of the genus *Haemophilus* (*H. aegyptius*) associated with an infectious form of human conjunctivitis — compare PFEIFFER'S BACILLUS

Weeks, John Elmer (1853–1949), American ophthalmologist. Weeks founded a clinical laboratory for ophthalmology which came to be known for its outstanding work in bacteriological and pathological studies. His personal accomplishments included the development of a method for using X-rays to locate foreign bodies in the eye, an operation for the surgical reconstruction of the orbit, methods for the surgical treatment of trachoma and glaucoma, and the invention of a new instrument for the extraction of cataracts. In 1886, independently of Robert Koch, he isolated the bacterium, now known as the Koch-Weeks bacillus, which causes an infectious form of conjunctivitis. He confirmed the identification by successfully inoculating one of his own eyes.

Koch–Weeks conjunctivitis *n* : conjunctivitis caused by the Koch-Weeks bacillus

Kohs blocks \\'kōs-ˌbläks\\ *n pl* : a set of small variously colored blocks that are used to form test patterns in psychodiagnostic examination

Kohs, Samuel Calmin (1890–1984), American psychologist. Kohs spent his career in clinical and educational psychology. He introduced his block test in 1918.

koi·lo·cyte \\'kói-lə-ˌsīt\\ *n* : a vaculoated pyknotic epithelial cell that has either a clear cytoplasm or a perinuclear halo

and that tends to be associated with certain human papillomavirus infections (as genital warts)

koi·lo·cy·to·sis \\ˌkói-lə-sī-'tō-səs\\ *n* : the presence of koilocytes usu. in the anogenital region or the uterine cervix

koil·onych·ia \\ˌkói̇l-ō-'nik-ē-ə\\ *n* : abnormal thinness and concavity of fingernails occurring esp. in hypochromic anemias — called also *spoon nails*

koilo·ster·nia \\-'stər-nē-ə\\ *n* : FUNNEL CHEST

ko·jic acid \\'kō-jik-\\ *n* : a crystalline water-soluble toxic antibiotic $C_6H_6O_4$ produced by fermentation esp. by fungi of the genus *Aspergillus* and having some antibacterial properties

ko·la nut *also* **co·la nut** \\'kō-lə-\\ *n* : the bitter caffeine-containing chestnut-sized seed of a kola tree used esp. as a masticatory and in beverages

kola tree *or* **cola tree** *n* : an African tree (genus *Cola*, esp. *C. nitida* and *C. acuminata* of the family Sterculiaceae) cultivated in various tropical areas for its kola nuts

Kol·mer reaction \\'kōl-mər-\\ *n* : a complement fixation test for the diagnosis of syphilis — called also *Kolmer, Kolmer test*

Kolmer, John Albert (1886–1962), American physician. Kolmer investigated the fields of bacteriology, immunology, chemotherapy, and syphilology. He developed the Kolmer test in 1922 as a modification of the Wassermann test.

kom·bu·cha \\ˌkäm-'bü-shə, -chə\\ *n* : a gelatinous mass of symbiotic bacteria (as *Acetobacter xylinum*) and yeasts (as of the genera *Brettanomyces* and *Saccharomyces*) grown to produce a fermented beverage held to confer health benefits; *also* : the beverage prepared by fermenting kombucha with black tea and sugar

kombucha mushroom *n* : KOMBUCHA

ko·nim·e·ter \\kō-'nim-ət-ər\\ *n* : a device for estimating the dust content of air (as in a mine or a cement mill)

ko·nio·cor·tex \\ˌkō-nē-ō-'kór-ˌteks\\ *n* : granular-appearing cerebral cortex esp. characteristic of sensory areas

Kop·lik's spots \\'käp-liks-\\ *or* **Kop·lik spots** \\-lik-\\ *n pl* : small bluish white dots surrounded by a reddish zone that appear on the mucous membrane of the cheeks and lips before the appearance of the skin eruption in a case of measles

Koplik, Henry (1858–1927), American pediatrician. Koplik was a specialist in the diseases of infancy and childhood. He discovered the bacterium (*Bordetella pertussis*) that causes whooping cough, and he established the first milk distribution center for poor infants in the U.S. He was the first to note Koplik's spots and published his description of them in 1896.

Korean hemorrhagic fever *n* : a hemorrhagic fever that is endemic to Asia and esp. Korea, Manchuria, and Siberia, is caused by the Hantaan virus, and is characterized by acute renal failure in addition to the usual symptoms of the hemorrhagic fevers — called also *epidemic hemorrhagic fever*

Korff's fiber \\'kórfs-\\ *n* : any of the thick argyrophilic fibers in the developing tooth that arise from the dental papilla, pass between the cells of the odontoblast layer, and form the matrix of the dentin — called also *von Korff fiber*

Korff, Karl von, 20th-century German anatomist and histologist.

Ko·rot·koff sounds *also* **Ko·rot·kow sounds** *or* **Ko·rot·kov sounds** \\kò-'ròt-kòf-ˌsaundz\\ *n pl* : arterial sounds heard through a stethoscope applied to the brachial artery distal to the cuff of a sphygmomanometer that change with varying cuff pressure and that are used to determine systolic and diastolic blood pressure

Korotkoff, Nikolai Sergeievich (1874–1920), Russian physician. Korotkoff introduced the auscultation method of determining blood pressure in 1905.

Kor·sa·koff \\'kór-sə-ˌkóf\\ *adj* : relating to or affected with Korsakoff's psychosis ⟨studies of ~ patients⟩

Korsakoff *or* **Korsakov Sergei Sergeievich (1853–1900),**

\\ə\\ abut \\ᵊ\\ kitten \\ər\\ further \\a\\ ash \\ā\\ ace \\ä\\ cot, cart \\au̇\\ out \\ch\\ chin \\e\\ bet \\ē\\ easy \\g\\ go \\i\\ hit \\ī\\ ice \\j\\ job \\ŋ\\ sing \\ō\\ go \\ò\\ law \\òi\\ boy \\th\\ thin \\th̲\\ the \\ü\\ loot \\u̇\\ foot \\y\\ yet \\zh\\ vision *See also* Pronunciation Symbols page

Russian psychiatrist. Korsakoff was one of the founders of the Russian school of psychiatry. After service at a clinic for nervous diseases, he published his classic description of the syndrome now known as Korsakoff's psychosis or Korsakoff's syndrome.

Kor·sa·koff's psychosis \-ˌkȯfs-\ *n* : an abnormal mental condition that is usu. a sequel of chronic alcoholism, is often associated with polyneuritis, and is characterized by an impaired ability to acquire new information and by an irregular memory loss for which the patient often attempts to compensate through confabulation

Korsakoff's syndrome *or* **Korsakoff syndrome** *n* : KORSAKOFF'S PSYCHOSIS

kos·so \ˈkä-(ˌ)sō\ *or* **kous·so** \ˈkü-\ *or* **ko·so** \ˈkō-\ *n* : BRAYERA

Kr *symbol* krypton

Krab·be's disease \ˈkrab-ēz-\ *n* : a rapidly progressive demyelinating familial leukoencephalopathy with onset in infancy characterized by irritability followed by tonic convulsions, quadriplegia, blindness, deafness, dementia, and death

Krabbe \ˈkräb-ə\, **Knud H. (1885–1961),** Danish neurologist. Krabbe wrote many studies on the morphogenesis of the brain in various classes of animals. He also demonstrated that cerebrovascular malformation is the cause of many meningeal hemorrhages. He described Krabbe's disease in articles in 1913 and 1916.

krad \ˈkā-ˌrad\ *n, pl* **krad** *also* **krads** : KILORAD

Krae·pe·lin·i·an \ˌkrep-ə-ˈlin-ē-ən *also* ˌkrap-\ *adj* : of or relating to Emil Kraepelin or to his system of classifying mental disorders

Krae·pe·lin \ˈkrep-ə-ˌlēn\, **Emil (1856–1926),** German psychiatrist. Kraepelin was one of the foremost psychiatrists of his time. In 1883 he published an influential psychiatry textbook that introduced his classification of mental disorders. His system was later modified, but basically it remains in use today. In 1899 he made an important differentiation between manic-depressive psychosis (now usu. called bipolar disorder) and schizophrenia. He also made noteworthy pioneering efforts to apply the methods of experimental psychology to clinical study.

krait \ˈkrīt\ *n* : any of several brightly banded extremely venomous nocturnal elapid snakes of the genus *Bungarus* that occur in Pakistan, India, southeastern Asia, and adjacent islands

kra·me·ria \krə-ˈmir-ē-ə\ *n* **1** *cap* : a genus of shrubs that are usu. placed with the legumes (family Leguminosae) or sometimes in their own family (Krameriaceae) and include two (*K. triandra* and *K. argentea*) with astringent roots formerly used in pharmacy **2** : the dried roots of either of two plants of the genus *Krameria* (*K. triandra* and *K. argentea*) — called also *rhatany*

Kra·mer \ˈkrä-mər\, **Johann Georg Heinrich (d 1742),** Austrian botanist. Kramer was also a military surgeon and had the advanced idea that scurvy can be cured by the inclusion of lemons and limes in the diet. The genus *Krameria* was named in his honor by Linnaeus in 1758.

krau·ro·sis \krȯ-ˈrō-səs\, *n, pl* **-ro·ses** \-ˌsēz\ : atrophy and shriveling of the skin or mucous membrane esp. of the vulva where it is often a precancerous lesion — **krau·rot·ic** \-ˈrät-ik\ *adj*

kraurosis vul·vae \-ˈvəl-vē\ *n* : kraurosis of the vulva

Krau·se's corpuscle \ˈkraȯ-zəz-\ *n* : any of various rounded sensory end organs occurring in mucous membranes (as of the conjunctiva or genitals) — called also *corpuscle of Krause*

Krause, Wilhelm Johann Friedrich (1833–1910), German anatomist. A professor of anatomy at several German universities, Krause published a handbook of human anatomy and a treatise on end organs of motor nerves. Krause's corpuscle was described for the first time in 1860.

Krause's end–bulb *n* : KRAUSE'S CORPUSCLE

Krause's membrane *n* : one of the isotropic cross bands in a striated muscle fiber that consists of disks of sarcoplasm linking the individual fibrils — called also *membrane of Krause*

kre·bi·o·zen \krə-ˈbī-ə-zən\ *n* : a drug used in the treatment of cancer esp. in the 1950s that was of unproved effectiveness, is not now used in the U.S., and was of undisclosed formulation but was reported to contain creatine

Krebs cycle \ˈkrebz-\ *n* : a sequence of reactions in the living organism in which oxidation of acetic acid or acetyl equivalent provides energy for storage in phosphate bonds (as in ATP) — called also *citric acid cycle, tricarboxylic acid cycle*

Krebs, Sir Hans Adolf (1900–1981), German-British biochemist. Krebs made major contributions to the understanding of metabolic processes. In 1932 he discovered with the German biochemist Kurt Henseleit a series of chemical reactions occurring in mammalian tissue by which ammonia is converted to urea. In 1937 he discovered an essential series of intermediate reactions in the oxidation of foodstuffs: the citric acid cycle. Now known as the Krebs cycle, these reactions have proved to be of vital importance in our understanding of metabolic processes in the cell. In 1953 he was awarded the Nobel Prize for Physiology or Medicine for his researches in metabolic processes.

Kro·may·er lamp \ˈkrō-mī-ər-ˌlamp\ *n* : a small water-cooled mercury-vapor lamp used in ultraviolet therapy

Kromayer, Ernst L. F. (1862–1933), German dermatologist. Kromayer introduced his mercury-vapor lamp around 1911.

Kru·ken·berg tumor \ˈkrü-kən-ˌbərg-\ *n* : a metastatic ovarian tumor of mucin-producing epithelial cells usu. derived from a primary gastrointestinal tumor

Kru·ken·berg \-ˌberk\, **Friedrich Ernst (1871–1946),** German pathologist. Krukenberg published his original description of the Krukenberg tumor in 1896.

kryp·ton \ˈkrip-ˌtän\ *n* : a colorless relatively inert gaseous element found in air at about one part per million — symbol *Kr*; see ELEMENT table

KS *abbr* Kaposi's sarcoma

KUB *abbr* kidney, ureter, and bladder

Kufs' disease \ˈkȯfs-\ *n* : a hereditary lipid metabolism defect with onset usu. in adolescence and characterized by progressive convulsions, paralysis, ataxia, and dementia

Kufs, H. (1871–1955), German neurologist.

Ku·gel·berg–Wel·an·der disease \ˈkü-gəl-ˌbərg-ˈvel-ən-dər-\ *n* : muscular weakness and atrophy that is caused by degeneration of motor neurons in the ventral horn of the spinal cord, is usu. inherited as an autosomal recessive trait, and that becomes symptomatic during childhood or adolescence typically progressing slowly during adulthood — compare WERDNIG-HOFFMANN DISEASE

Kugelberg, Eric Klas Henrik (1913–1983), and **Welander, Lisa (1909–2001),** Swedish neurologists. Kugelberg and Welander described the form of muscular atrophy that bears their names in 1956. The disease had been described earlier, in 1942, by another Swedish neurologist, Karl Gunnar Vilhelm Wohlfart (1910–1961).

Küm·mell's disease \ˈk(y)ü-məlz-, ˈkim-əlz-\ *n* : a syndrome following compression fracture of a vertebra that involves spinal pain, intercostal neuralgia, and motor disturbances of the legs

Küm·mell \ˈkᴜ-məl\, **Hermann (1852–1937),** German surgeon. Kümmell discovered in 1891 a syndrome that results from traumatic spondylitis and published a description of Kümmell's disease in 1892.

Kupf·fer cell \ˈkᴜp-fər-\ *also* **Kupf·fer's cell** \-fərz-\ *n* : a fixed macrophage of the walls of the liver sinusoids that is stellate with a large oval nucleus and the cytoplasm commonly packed with fragments resulting from phagocytic action

Kupffer, Karl Wilhelm von (1829–1902), German anatomist. Kupffer described the large stellate cells in the lining of the sinusoids of the liver first in 1876 and again in 1899. His observations led to a better understanding of the reticuloendothelial system.

ku·ru \ˈkᴜ(ə)r-(ˌ)ü\ *n* : a rare progressive fatal spongiform encephalopathy that is caused by a prion, resembles Creutzfeldt-Jakob disease, and has occurred among tribespeople in eastern New Guinea who engaged in a form of ritual cannibalism — called also *laughing death, laughing sickness*

Kuss·maul breathing \\'kùs-ˌmaùl-\ *or* **Kuss·maul's breath·ing** \-ˌmaùlz-\ *n* : abnormally slow deep respiration characteristic of air hunger and occurring esp. in acidotic states — called also *Kussmaul respiration*

Kussmaul, Adolf (1822–1902), German physician. Kussmaul made notable contributions to clinical medicine. In 1873 he introduced the concept of paradoxical pulse in a clinical description of obstructive pericarditis. The following year he described the labored breathing in diabetic coma that is now known as Kussmaul breathing.

Kveim test \\'kvām-\ *n* : an intradermal test for sarcoidosis in which an antigen prepared from the lymph nodes or spleen of human sarcoidosis patients is injected intracutaneously and which is positive when an infiltrated area, papule, nodule, or superficial necrosis appears around the site of injection or a skin biopsy yields typical tubercles and giant cell formations upon histological examination

Kveim, Morten Ansgar (1892–1966), Norwegian physician. Kveim introduced his test for sarcoidosis in 1941.

kwa·shi·or·kor \ˌkwäsh-ē-'ȯr-kȯr, -ȯ(r)-'kȯr\ *n* : severe malnutrition chiefly affecting young children esp. of impoverished regions that is characterized by failure to grow and develop, changes in the pigmentation of the skin and hair, edema, fatty degeneration of the liver, anemia, and apathy and is caused by a diet excessively high in carbohydrate and extremely low in protein — compare PELLAGRA

Kwell \\'kwel\ *trademark* — used for a preparation of lindane

Kya·sa·nur For·est disease \ˌkya-sə-'nùr-'fȯr-əst-\ *n* : a disease caused by a single-stranded RNA virus of the genus *Flavivirus* (species *Kyasanur Forest disease virus*) that is characterized by fever, headache, diarrhea, and intestinal bleeding and is transmitted by immature ticks of the genus *Haemaphysalis*

ky·mo·gram \\'kī-mə-ˌgram\ *n* : a record made by a kymograph

ky·mo·graph \-ˌgraf\ *n* : a device which graphically records motion or pressure; *esp* : a recording device including an electric motor or clockwork that drives a usu. slowly revolving drum which carries a roll of plain or smoked paper and also having an arrangement for tracing on the paper by means of a stylus a graphic record of motion or pressure (as of the organs of speech, blood pressure, or respiration) often in relation to particular intervals of time — **ky·mo·graph·ic** \ˌkī-mə-'graf-ik\ *adj* — **ky·mog·ra·phy** \kī-'mäg-rə-fē\ *n, pl* **-phies**

kyn·uren·ic acid \ˌkīn-yù-ˌren-ik-, ˌkin-\ *n* : a crystalline acid $C_{10}H_7NO_3$ that is formed from kynurenine as one of the normal products of tryptophan metabolism and that is excreted in the urine in certain metabolic disorders

kyn·uren·ine \ˌkīn-yù-'ren-ˌēn, ˌkin-, -'yù-rən-\ *n* : an amino acid $C_{10}H_{12}N_4O_3$ occurring in the urine of various animals as one of the normal products of tryptophan metabolism

ky·pho·plas·ty \\'kī-fō-ˌplas-tē\ *n, pl* **-ties** : a medical procedure that is similar to vertebroplasty in the use of acrylic cement to stabilize and reduce pain associated with a vertebral compression fracture but that additionally restores vertebral height and lessens spinal deformity by injecting the cement into a cavity created in the fractured bone by the insertion and inflation of a special balloon

ky·pho·sco·li·o·sis \ˌkī-fō-ˌskō-lē-'ō-səs\ *n, pl* **-o·ses** \-ˌsēz\ : backward and lateral curvature of the spine

ky·pho·sco·li·ot·ic \-'ät-ik\ *adj* : of, relating to, or marked by kyphoscoliosis ⟨~ paraplegias⟩

ky·pho·sis \kī-'fō-səs\ *n, pl* **-pho·ses** \-ˌsēz\ : exaggerated outward curvature of the thoracic region of the spinal column resulting in a rounded upper back — compare LORDOSIS, SCOLIOSIS — **ky·phot·ic** \-'fät-ik\ *adj*

L

L *abbr* **1** left **2** levorotatory **3** light **4** liquid **5** liter **6** lumbar — used esp. with a number from 1 to 5 to indicate a vertebra or segment of the spinal cord in the lumbar region

L *symbol* lithium

l- *prefix* **1** \ˌlē-(ˌ)vō, ˌel, 'el\ : levorotatory — usu. printed in italic ⟨*l*-tartaric acid⟩ **2** \ˌel, 'el\ : having a similar configuration at a selected carbon atom to the configuration of levorotatory glyceraldehyde — usu. printed as a small capital ⟨L-fructose⟩ ⟨L-tryptophan⟩

La *symbol* lanthanum

lab \\'lab\ *n* : LABORATORY

La·bar·raque's solution \ˌla-bə-'raks-\ *n* : JAVELLE WATER

La·bar·raque \lä-bä-räk\, **Antoine–Germain (1777–1850),** French chemist and pharmacist. Labarraque was a pharmacist who served in the French army. He did much to improve the sanitary conditions in hospitals and army barracks and is remembered for his outstanding services during a cholera epidemic in 1832. In 1825 he introduced a solution of chlorinated soda for use as a disinfectant; it is sometimes known as Labarraque's solution.

¹la·bel \\'lā-bəl\ *n* : a usu. radioactive isotope used in labeling

²label *vt* **la·beled** *or* **la·belled; la·bel·ing** *or* **la·bel·ling** \\'lā-b(ə-)liŋ\ **1** : to distinguish (an element or atom) by using an isotope distinctive in some manner (as in mass or radioactivity) for tracing through chemical reactions or biological processes **2** : to distinguish (as a compound or cell) by introducing a traceable constituent (as a dye or labeled atom)

la·bet·a·lol \lə-'bet-ə-ˌlȯl, -ˌlōl\ *n* : a beta-adrenergic blocking agent used in the form of its hydrochloride $C_{19}H_{24}O_3 \cdot HCl$ to treat hypertension

labia *pl of* LABIUM

la·bi·al \\'lā-bē-əl\ *adj* **1** : of, relating to, or situated near the lips or labia **2** : uttered with the participation of one or both lips ⟨the ~ sounds \f\, \p\, and \ü\⟩ — **la·bi·al·ly** \-ē\ *adv*

labial artery *n* : either of two branches of the facial artery of which one is distributed to the upper and one to the lower lip

labial gland *n* : one of the small tubular mucous and serous glands lying beneath the mucous membrane of the lips

labialis — see HERPES LABIALIS

la·bi·al·ism \\'lā-bē-ə-ˌliz-əm\ *n* : a speech defect characterized by the substitution of one labial sound for another or of a labial for another type of sound

la·bia ma·jo·ra \ˌlā-bē-ə-mə-'jōr-ə, -'jȯr-ə\ *n pl* : the outer fatty folds of the vulva bounding the vestibule

labia mi·no·ra \-mə-'nōr-ə, -'nȯr-ə\ *n pl* : the inner highly vascular largely connective-tissue folds of the vulva bounding the vestibule — called also *nymphae*

labii — see LEVATOR LABII SUPERIORIS, LEVATOR LABII SUPERIORIS ALAEQUE NASI, QUADRATUS LABII SUPERIORIS

la·bile \\'lā-ˌbīl, -bəl\ *adj* : readily or frequently changing: as **a** : readily or continually undergoing chemical, physical, or biological change or breakdown ⟨a ~ antigen⟩ **b** : characterized by wide fluctuations (as in blood pressure or glucose tolerance) ⟨~ hypertension⟩ ⟨~ diabetes⟩ **c** : emotionally unstable — **la·bil·i·ty** \lā-'bil-ət-ē\ *n, pl* **-ties**

labile factor *n* : FACTOR V

la·bi·lize *or chiefly Brit* **la·bi·lise** \\'lā-bə-ˌlīz\ *vt* **-lized** *or chief-*

\ə\ abut \ᵊ\ kitten \ər\ further \a\ ash \ā\ ace \ä\ cot, cart \aù\ out \ch\ chin \e\ bet \ē\ easy \g\ go \i\ hit \ī\ ice \j\ job \ŋ\ sing \ō\ go \ȯ\ law \ȯi\ boy \th\ thin \t̲h̲\ the \ü\ loot \ù\ foot \y\ yet \zh\ vision   *See also* Pronunciation Symbols page

ly Brit -lised; -liz·ing or chiefly Brit -lis·ing : to render labile (as in chemical structure) — la·bi·li·za·tion or chiefly Brit la·bi·li·sa·tion \ˌlā-bə-lə-ˈzā-shən\ n

la·bio–buc·cal \ˌlā-bē-ō-ˈbək-əl\ adj : of, relating to, or lying against the inner surface of the lips and cheeks; also : administered to labio-buccal tissue ⟨a ~ injection⟩

la·bio·cli·na·tion \ˌlā-bē-ō-kli-ˈnā-shən\ n : outward inclination of a front tooth toward the lips

la·bio·den·tal \ˌlā-bē-ō-ˈdent-ᵊl\ adj : uttered with the participation of the lip and teeth ⟨the ~ sounds \f\ and \v\⟩

la·bio·gin·gi·val \-ˈjin-jə-vəl\ adj : of or relating to the lips and gums

la·bio·glos·so·pha·ryn·geal \-ˌgläs-ō-ˌfar-ən-ˈjē-əl, -ˌglòs-, -fə-ˈrin-j(ē-)əl\ adj : of, relating to, or affecting the lips, tongue, and pharynx

la·bio·lin·gual \-ˈliŋ-g(yə-)wəl\ adj 1 : of or relating to the lips and the tongue 2 : of or relating to the labial and lingual aspects of a tooth ⟨~ measurement of an incisor⟩ — la·bio·lin·gual·ly \-ē\ adv

la·bio·scro·tal \-ˈskrōt-ᵊl\ adj : relating to or being a swelling or ridge on each side of the embryonic rudiment of the penis or clitoris which develops into one of the scrotal sacs in the male and one of the labia majora in the female

la·bi·um \ˈlā-bē-əm\ n, pl la·bia \-ə\ 1 : any of the folds at the margin of the vulva — compare LABIA MAJORA, LABIA MINORA 2 : a lower mouthpart of an insect that is formed by the second pair of maxillae united in the midline

¹la·bor or Brit la·bour \ˈlā-bər\ n : the physical activities involved in parturition consisting essentially of a prolonged series of involuntary contractions of the uterine musculature together with both reflex and voluntary contractions of the abdominal wall ⟨drugs that induce ~⟩ ⟨went into ~ after a fall⟩; also : the period of time during which such labor takes place

²labor or Brit labour vi : to be in the labor of giving birth

lab·o·ra·to·ri·an \ˌlab-(ə-)rə-ˈtōr-ē-ən, -ˈtòr-\ n : a laboratory worker

lab·o·ra·to·ry \ˈlab-(ə-)rə-ˌtōr-ē, -ˌtòr-, Brit usu lə-ˈbär-ə-t(ə-)rē\ n, pl -ries often attrib : a place equipped for experimental study in a science or for testing and analysis

la·bored \ˈlā-bərd\ adj : produced or performed with difficulty or strain ⟨~ breathing⟩

labor room n : a hospital room where a woman in labor stays before being taken to the delivery room

la·brum \ˈlā-brəm\ n 1 : an upper or anterior mouthpart of an arthropod consisting of a single median piece in front of or above the mandibles 2 : a fibrous ring of cartilage attached to the rim of a joint; esp : GLENOID LABRUM

lab·y·rinth \ˈlab-ə-ˌrin(t)th, -rən(t)th\ n : a tortuous anatomical structure; esp : the inner ear or its bony or membranous part — see BONY LABYRINTH, MEMBRANOUS LABYRINTH

lab·y·rin·thec·to·my \ˌlab-ə-ˌrin-ˈthek-tə-mē\ n, pl -mies : surgical removal of the labyrinth of the ear — lab·y·rin·thec·to·mized \-tə-ˌmīzd\ adj

lab·y·rin·thine \-ˈrin(t)-thən; -ˈrin-ˌthīn, -ˌthēn\ adj : of, relating to, affecting, or originating in the inner ear ⟨human ~ lesions⟩

labyrinthine artery n : INTERNAL AUDITORY ARTERY

labyrinthine sense n : a complex sense concerned with the perception of bodily position and motion, mediated by end organs in the vestibular system and the semicircular canals, and stimulated by alterations in the pull of gravity and by head movements

lab·y·rin·thi·tis \ˌlab-ə-rin-ˈthīt-əs\ n : inflammation of the labyrinth of the inner ear — called also otitis interna

lab·y·rin·thot·o·my \ˌlab-ə-rin-ˈthät-ə-mē\ n, pl -mies : surgical incision into the labyrinth of the inner ear

lac·er·ate \ˈlas-ə-ˌrāt\ vt -at·ed; -at·ing : to tear or rend roughly : wound jaggedly ⟨a lacerated spleen⟩

lac·er·a·tion \ˌlas-ə-ˈrā-shən\ n 1 : the act of lacerating 2 : a torn and ragged wound

la·cer·tus fi·bro·sus \lə-ˈsərt-əs-fī-ˈbrō-səs\ n : BICIPITAL APONEUROSIS

lacerum — see FORAMEN LACERUM

Lach·e·sis \ˈlak-ə-səs\ n : a genus of American pit vipers comprising the bushmaster and related snakes that are sometimes included in the genus Trimeresurus

Each boldface word in the list below is a variant of the word to its right in small capitals.

lachrymal	LACRIMAL	lachrymator	LACRIMATOR
lachrymate	LACRIMATE	lachrymatory	LACRIMATORY
lachrymation	LACRIMATION		

lac operon \ˈlak-\ n : the operon which controls lactose metabolism and has been isolated from E. coli

¹lac·ri·mal also lach·ry·mal \ˈlak-rə-məl\ adj 1 : of, relating to, associated with, located near, or constituting the glands that produce tears 2 : of or relating to tears ⟨~ effusions⟩

²lacrimal n : a lacrimal anatomical part (as a lacrimal bone)

lacrimal apparatus n : the bodily parts which function in the production of tears including the lacrimal glands, lacrimal ducts, lacrimal sacs, nasolacrimal ducts, and lacrimal puncta

lacrimal artery n : a large branch of the ophthalmic artery that arises near the optic foramen, passes along the superior border of the lateral rectus, and supplies the lacrimal gland

lacrimal bone n : a small thin bone making up part of the front inner wall of each orbit and providing a groove for the passage of the lacrimal ducts

lacrimal canal n : LACRIMAL DUCT 1

lacrimal canaliculus n : LACRIMAL DUCT 1

lacrimal caruncle n : a small reddish follicular elevation at the medial angle of the eye

lacrimal duct n 1 : a short canal leading from a minute orifice on a small elevation at the medial angle of each eyelid to the lacrimal sac — called also lacrimal canal, lacrimal canaliculus 2 : any of several small ducts that carry tears from the lacrimal gland to the fornix of the conjunctiva

lac·ri·ma·le \ˌlak-rə-ˈmā-(ˌ)lē, -ˈma-\ n : the point where the posterior edge of the lacrimal bone intersects the suture between the frontal bone and the lacrimal bone

lacrimal gland n : an acinous gland that is about the size and shape of an almond, secretes tears, and is situated laterally and superiorly to the bulb of the eye in a shallow depression on the inner surface of the frontal bone — called also tear gland

lacrimalis — see PLICA LACRIMALIS

lacrimal nerve n : a small branch of the ophthalmic nerve that enters the lacrimal gland with the lacrimal artery and supplies the lacrimal gland and the adjacent conjunctiva and the skin of the upper eyelid

lacrimal punc·tum \-ˈpəŋk-təm\ n : the opening of either the upper or the lower lacrimal duct at the inner canthus of the eye

lacrimal sac \-ˈsak\ n : the dilated oval upper end of the nasolacrimal duct that is situated in a groove formed by the lacrimal bone and the frontal process of the maxilla, is closed at its upper end, and receives the lacrimal ducts

lac·ri·ma·tion also lach·ry·ma·tion \ˌlak-rə-ˈmā-shən\ n : the secretion of tears; specif : abnormal or excessive secretion of tears due to local or systemic disease — lac·ri·mate also lach·ry·mate vi -mat·ed; -mat·ing

lac·ri·ma·tor also lach·ry·ma·tor \ˈlak-rə-ˌmāt-ər\ n : a tear-producing substance (as tear gas)

lac·ri·ma·to·ry also lach·ry·ma·to·ry \ˈlak-ri-mə-ˌtōr-ē, -ˌtòr-\ adj : of, relating to, or prompting tears ⟨~ fumes⟩

La Crosse encephalitis \lə-ˈkròs-\ n : an encephalitis typically affecting children that is caused by the La Crosse virus transmitted esp. by a mosquito of the genus Aedes (A. triseriatus)

La Crosse virus n : a virus that causes La Crosse encephalitis and that belongs to a strain of a single-stranded RNA virus of the genus Bunyavirus (species California encephalitis virus)

lact·aci·de·mia or chiefly Brit lact·aci·dae·mia \ˌlakt-ˌas-ə-ˈdē-mē-ə\ n : the presence of excess lactic acid in the blood — called also lacticemia

lac·ta·gogue \ˈlak-tə-ˌgäg\ n : GALACTAGOGUE

lact·al·bu·min \ˌlak-ˌtal-ˈbyü-mən\ *n* : an albumin that is found in milk and is similar to serum albumin; *esp* : a protein fraction from whey that includes lactoglobulin and is used in foods and in preparing protein hydrolysates

lac·tam \ˈlak-ˌtam\ *n* : any of a class of amides of amino carboxylic acids that are formed by the loss of a molecule of water from the amino and carboxyl groups, that are characterized by the carbonyl-imido group –CONH– in a ring, and that include many antibiotics — compare LACTIM, LACTONE

β–lactam, β–lactamase *var of* BETA-LACTAM, BETA= LACTAMASE

lac·tase \ˈlak-ˌtās, -ˌtāz\ *n* : an enzyme that hydrolyzes esp. lactose to glucose and galactose and occurs esp. in the intestines of young mammals and in yeasts

¹lac·tate \ˈlak-ˌtāt\ *n* : a salt or ester of lactic acid

²lactate *vi* **lac·tat·ed; lac·tat·ing** : to secrete milk

lactated *adj* : containing or combined with milk or a milk product ⟨∼ baby food⟩ ⟨a ∼ solution⟩

lactate dehydrogenase *n* : any of a group of isoenzymes that catalyze the conversion of pyruvic acid to lactic acid, are found esp. in the liver, kidneys, striated muscle, and the myocardium, and tend to accumulate in the body when these organs or tissues are diseased or injured — called also *lactic dehydrogenase*

lactated Ringer's solution *n* : a sterile aqueous solution that is similar to Ringer's solution but contains sodium lactate in addition to calcium chloride, sodium chloride, and potassium chloride — called also *Hartmann's solution, lactated Ringer's, Ringer's lactate, Ringer's lactate solution*

   S. Ringer — see RINGER'S FLUID

lac·ta·tion \lak-ˈtā-shən\ *n* **1** : the secretion and yielding of milk by the mammary gland **2** : one complete period of lactation extending from about the time of parturition to weaning — **lac·ta·tion·al** \-shən-ᵊl\ *adj* — **lac·ta·tion·al·ly** \-ē\ *adv*

lactation tetany *n* : MILK FEVER 1

¹lac·te·al \ˈlak-tē-əl\ *adj* **1** : relating to, consisting of, producing, or resembling milk ⟨∼ fluid⟩ **2 a** : conveying or containing a milky fluid (as chyle) ⟨a ∼ channel⟩ **b** : of or relating to the lacteals ⟨impaired ∼ function⟩

²lacteal *n* : any of the lymphatic vessels arising from the villi of the small intestine and conveying chyle to the thoracic duct

lac·te·nin \ˈlak-tə-nən\ *n* : a nitrogenous substance present in milk that inhibits bacterial growth

lac·tic \ˈlak-tik\ *adj* **1 a** : of or relating to milk **b** : obtained from sour milk or whey **2** : involving the production of lactic acid ⟨∼ fermentation⟩

lactic acid *n* : a hygroscopic organic acid $C_3H_6O_3$ that is known in three optically isomeric forms: **a** *or* L**–lactic acid** \ˈel-\ : the dextrorotatory form present normally in blood and muscle tissue as a product of the anaerobic metabolism of glucose and glycogen **b** *or* D**–lactic acid** \ˈdē-\ : the levorotatory form obtained by biological fermentation of sucrose **c** *or* DL**–lactic acid** \ˈdē-ˈel-\ : the racemic form present in food products and made usu. by bacterial fermentation (as of whey or raw sugar) but also synthetically, and used chiefly in foods and beverages, in medicine, in tanning and dyeing, and in making esters for use as solvents and plasticizers

lactic acidosis *n* : a condition characterized by the accumulation of lactic acid in bodily tissues

lactic dehydrogenase *n* : LACTATE DEHYDROGENASE

lac·ti·ce·mia *or chiefly Brit* **lac·ti·cae·mia** \ˌlak-tə-ˈsē-mē-ə\ *n* : LACTACIDEMIA

lac·tif·er·ous \lak-ˈtif-(ə-)rəs\ *adj* : secreting or conveying milk

lactiferous duct *n* : any of the milk-carrying ducts of the mammary gland that open on the nipple

lactiferous sinus *n* : an expansion in a lactiferous duct at the base of the nipple in which milk accumulates

lac·tim \ˈlak-ˌtim\ *n* : any of a class of hydroxy imides tautomeric with lactams and characterized by the enolic group –C(OH)=N–

Lac·to·bac·il·la·ce·ae \ˌlak-tō-ˌbas-ə-ˈlā-sē-ˌē\ *n pl* : a large family of rod-shaped or spherical gram-negative bacteria that are usu. nonmotile and require little or no oxygen, that do not form spores, that require carbohydrates for growth and ferment them chiefly to lactic acid, and that include the lactic acid bacteria — see LACTOBACILLUS

lac·to·ba·cil·lus \ˌlak-tō-bə-ˈsil-əs\ *n* **1** *cap* : a genus of gram-positive nonmotile lactic-acid-forming bacteria of the family Lactobacillaceae including various commercially important lactic acid bacteria **2** *pl* **-li** \-ˌī *also* -ˌē\ : any bacterium of the genus *Lactobacillus*

Lactobacillus ca·sei factor \-ˈkā-sē-ˌī-\ *n* : FOLIC ACID

lac·to·chrome \ˈlak-tə-ˌkrōm\ *n* : RIBOFLAVIN

lac·to·fer·rin \ˌlak-tō-ˈfer-ən\ *n* : a red iron-binding protein synthesized by neutrophils and glandular epithelial cells, found in many human secretions (as tears and milk), and retarding bacterial and fungal growth

lac·to·fla·vin \ˌlak-tō-ˈflā-vən\ *n* : RIBOFLAVIN

lac·to·gen \ˈlak-tə-jən, -ˌjen\ *n* : any hormone (as prolactin) that stimulates the production of milk — see PLACENTAL LACTOGEN

lac·to·gen·e·sis \ˌlak-tō-ˈjen-ə-səs\ *n, pl* **-e·ses** \-ˌsēz\ : initiation of lactation

lac·to·gen·ic \ˌlak-tō-ˈjen-ik\ *adj* : stimulating lactation — **lac·to·gen·i·cal·ly** \-i-k(ə-)lē\ *adv*

lactogenic hormone *n* : LACTOGEN; *esp* : PROLACTIN

lac·to·glob·u·lin \-ˈgläb-yə-lən\ *n* : a crystalline protein fraction that is obtained from the whey of milk

lac·tom·e·ter \lak-ˈtäm-ət-ər\ *n* : a hydrometer for determining the specific gravity of milk — **lac·to·met·ric** \ˌlak-tə-ˈme-trik\ *adj*

lac·tone \ˈlak-ˌtōn\ *n* : any of various cyclic esters formed from hydroxy acids — compare LACTAM, SULTONE — **lac·ton·ic** \lak-ˈtän-ik\ *adj*

lac·to·nize *or chiefly Brit* **lac·to·nise** \ˈlak-tə-ˌnīz\ *vb* **-nized** *or chiefly Brit* **-nised; -niz·ing** *or chiefly Brit* **-nis·ing** *vt* : to convert into a lactone ∼ *vi* : to become converted into a lactone — **lac·to·ni·za·tion** *or chiefly Brit* **lac·to·ni·sa·tion** \ˌlak-tə-nə-ˈzā-shən\ *n*

lac·to–ovo \ˈlak-tō-ˈō-vō\ *adj* : of, relating to, or following the diet of lacto-ovo vegetarians ⟨a ∼ regimen⟩

lacto–ovo vegetarian *n* : a vegetarian whose diet includes milk, eggs, vegetables, fruits, grains, and nuts — called also *ovo-lacto vegetarian;* compare LACTO-VEGETARIAN — **lacto–ovo–vegetarian** *adj*

lac·to·per·ox·i·dase \ˌlak-tō-pə-ˈräk-sə-ˌdās, -ˌdāz\ *n* : a peroxidase that is found in milk and saliva and is used to catalyze the iodination of tyrosine-containing proteins (as thyroglobulin)

lac·to·phos·phate \ˌlak-tō-ˈfäs-ˌfāt\ *n* : a mixture of a lactate and a phosphate

lac·to·pro·tein \-ˈprō-ˌtēn, -ˈprōt-ē-ən\ *n* : any of the proteins in milk (as lactalbumin or lactoglobulin)

lac·tose \ˈlak-ˌtōs, -ˌtōz\ *n* : a disaccharide sugar $C_{12}H_{22}O_{11}$ that is present in milk, yields glucose and galactose upon hydrolysis, yields esp. lactic acid upon fermentation, and is used chiefly in foods, medicines, and culture media (as for the manufacture of penicillin) — called also *milk sugar*

lac·tos·uria \ˌlak-tō-ˈs(h)ùr-ē-ə, -tōs-ˈyùr-\ *n* : the presence of lactose in the urine

lac·to–veg·e·tar·i·an \ˌlak-tō-ˌvej-ə-ˈter-ē-ən\ *n* : a vegetarian whose diet includes milk, vegetables, fruits, grains, and nuts — compare LACTO-OVO VEGETARIAN — **lacto–vegetarian** *adj*

lac·tu·ca·ri·um \ˌlak-tə-ˈkar-ē-əm, -ˈker-\ *n* : the dried milky juice of a wild lettuce (*Lactuca virosa*) of central and southern Europe that resembles opium in physical properties and was formerly used as a sedative

lac·tu·lose \ˈlak-t(y)ù-ˌlōs, -ˌlōz\ *n* : a cathartic disaccharide

\ə\ **abut** \ᵊ\ **kitten** \ər\ **further** \a\ **ash** \ā\ **ace** \ä\ **cot, cart** \aù\ **out** \ch\ **chin** \e\ **bet** \ē\ **easy** \g\ **go** \i\ **hit** \ī\ **ice** \j\ **job** \ŋ\ **sing** \ō\ **go** \ò\ **law** \òi\ **boy** \th\ **thin** \t̲h̲\ **the** \ü\ **loot** \ù\ **foot** \y\ **yet** \zh\ **vision**   *See also* Pronunciation Symbols page

K
L

$C_{12}H_{22}O_{11}$ used to treat chronic constipation and disturbances of function in the central nervous system accompanying severe liver disease

la·cu·na \lə-'k(y)ü-nə\ *n, pl* **la·cu·nae** \-'kyü-(ˌ)nē, -'kü-ˌnī\ : a small cavity, pit, or discontinuity in an anatomical structure: as **a** : one of the follicles in the mucous membrane of the urethra **b** : one of the minute cavities in bone or cartilage occupied by the osteocytes — **la·cu·nar** \-'k(y)ü-nər\ *adj*

Lae·laps \'lē-ˌlaps\ *n* : a large genus (family Laelaptidae) of mites that are parasitic on murid rodents and include some vectors of disease

Laen·nec's cirrhosis *or* **Laën·nec's cirrhosis** \'lā-neks-\ *n* : hepatic cirrhosis in which increased connective tissue spreads out from the portal spaces compressing and distorting the lobules, causing impairment of liver function, and ultimately producing the typical hobnail liver — called also *portal cirrhosis*

    Laen·nec \lä-en-ek\, **René–Théophile–Hyacinthe (1781–1826),** French physician. Laennec is usually regarded as one of the great clinicians of all time and as the father of chest medicine. A foremost authority on tuberculosis, he established that all phthisis is tuberculous. He described pneumothorax and distinguished pneumonia from the various kinds of bronchitis and from pleurisy. He is also credited with inventing the stethoscope; his primitive device was a wooden cylinder about a foot long. For three years he studied patients' chest sounds and correlated them with the diseases found on autopsy. In 1819 he published his findings in a work on auscultation with the aid of a stethoscope. It was in that work he described Laennec's cirrhosis.

la·e·trile \'lā-ə-(ˌ)tril, -trəl\ *n, often cap* : a drug that is derived esp. from pits of the apricot (*Prunus armeniaca* of the rose family), that contains amygdalin, and that has been used in the treatment of cancer although of unproved effectiveness

Each boldface word in the list below is a British variant of the word to its right in small capitals.

laevo	LEVO	laevorotatory	LEVOROTATORY
laevocardia	LEVOCARDIA	laevothyroxine	LEVOTHYROX-
laevocardio-	LEVOCARDIO-		INE
gram	GRAM	laevulinate	LEVULINATE
laevo–	LEVO=	laevulinic acid	LEVULINIC
dihydroxy-	DIHYDROXY-		ACID
phenylala-	PHENYLALA-	laevulosaemia	LEVULOSEMIA
nine	NINE	laevulosan	LEVULOSAN
laevodopa	LEVODOPA	laevulose	LEVULOSE
laevorotation	LEVOROTATION	laevulosuria	LEVULOSURIA

La·fora body \lä-'fōr-ə-\ *n* : any of the cytoplasmic inclusion bodies found in neurons of parts of the central nervous system in Lafora disease and consisting of a complex of glycoprotein and glycosaminoglycan

    Lafora, Gonzalo Rodriguez (1886–1971), Spanish neurologist. Early in his career Lafora served as a histopathologist at a government mental hospital in Washington. Later in Madrid he lectured in neuropathology and directed a laboratory for brain physiology. He published experimental studies on the function of the corpus callosum and produced a full-length work on neurosyphilis.

Lafora disease *or* **Lafora's disease** \-əz-\ *n* : an inherited form of myoclonic epilepsy that typically begins during adolescence or late childhood and is characterized by progressive neurological deterioration and the presence of Lafora bodies in parts of the central nervous system

¹**lag** \'lag\ *vb* **lagged; lag·ging** *vi* : to move, function, or develop with comparative slowness ⟨the child *lagged* in perceptual development⟩ ⟨symptoms may ∼ behind the radiographic changes —Carol J. Johns & Theresa M. Michele⟩ ∼ *vt* : to lag behind ⟨current that ∼*s* the voltage⟩

²**lag** *n* **1** : the act or the condition of lagging **2** : comparative slowness or retardation (as in growth or development) **3 a** : a space of time esp. between related events or phenomena — see LAG PHASE **b** : the time between the application of a stimulus and the occurrence of the response it causes

la·ge·na *or Brit* **la·gae·na** \lə-'jē-nə\ *n, pl* **-nae** \-nē\ **1** : the

upper extremity of the scala media that is attached to the cupula at the upper part of the helicotrema **2** : an organ of vertebrates below the mammals that corresponds to the cochlea

Lag·o·chi·las·ca·ris \ˌlag-ō-kī-'las-kə-rəs\ *n* : a genus of nematode worms including one (*L. minor*) that is normally parasitic in the intestine of wild felines but sometimes occurs as a subcutaneous parasite of humans in Trinidad and Suriname

lag·oph·thal·mos *or* **lag·oph·thal·mus** \ˌlag-ˌäf-'thal-məs\ *n* : pathological incomplete closure of the eyelids : inability to close the eyelids fully

lag phase \'lag-ˌfāz\ *n* : the period of time between the introduction of a microorganism into a culture medium and the time it begins to increase exponentially — called also *lag period;* compare LOG PHASE

la grippe \lä-'grip\ *n* : INFLUENZA

¹**Laing·ian** \'laŋ-ē-ən\ *adj* : of, relating to, or characteristic of R. D. Laing or his psychological doctrines

    Laing \'laŋ\, **Ronald David (1927–1989),** British psychiatrist. Laing began psychoanalytic research at London's Tavistock Institute of Human Relations in 1960. From his clinical experiences there and previously at other psychiatric clinics he developed radical and controversial theories of psychosis and psychoanalysis. His theories centered on the belief that mental illnesses (such as schizophrenia) are an individual's natural and often therapeutic response to the stress and constraints imposed by family and society.

²**Laingian** *n* : an adherent of the psychological doctrines of R. D. Laing

LAK \'lak; ˌel-(ˌ)ā-'kā\ *n* : LYMPHOKINE-ACTIVATED KILLER CELL

LAK cell *n* : LYMPHOKINE-ACTIVATED KILLER CELL

lake \'lāk\ *vb* **laked; lak·ing** *vt* : to cause (blood) to undergo a physiological change in which the hemoglobin becomes dissolved in the plasma ∼ *vi, of blood* : to undergo the process by which hemoglobin becomes dissolved in the plasma

laky \'lā-kē\ *adj* **lak·i·er; -est** *of blood* : having undergone the process by which hemoglobin becomes dissolved in the plasma

lal·la·tion \la-'lā-shən\ *n* **1** : infantile speech whether in infants or in older speakers (as from mental retardation) **2** : a defective articulation of the letter *l*, the substitution of \l\ for another sound, or the substitution of another sound for \l\ — compare LAMBDACISM 2

la·lop·a·thy \la-'läp-ə-thē\ *n, pl* **-thies** : a disorder of speech

La·marck·ian \lə-'märk-ē-ən\ *adj* : of or relating to Lamarckism

    La·marck \lä-'märk\, **Jean–Baptiste–Pierre–Antoine de Monet de (1744–1829),** French botanist and biologist. Lamarck produced voluminous botanical writings and also made substantial contributions to comparative anatomy and the study of invertebrates. In 1801 he introduced his classification of invertebrates, a classification that remains largely accepted. From 1815 to 1822 he published his major work, a multivolume natural history of invertebrates. He is credited with being the first to distinguish invertebrates as a taxonomic group from vertebrates. In 1809 he published a work summarizing his views on zoological philosophy. Here he presented two major "laws": (1) organs are improved with repeated use and weakened by disuse (2) new characteristics are acquired through interaction with the environment and are passed on to progeny. Although his general idea of evolutionary change was later controverted by Darwin, Lamarck is important because his thesis denied the old notion of the immutability of species, thereby preparing the way for later explanations of the transformation and evolution of plants and animals.

La·marck·ian·ism \-kē-ə-ˌniz-əm\ *n* : LAMARCKISM

La·marck·ism \lə-'mär-ˌkiz-əm\ *n* : a theory of organic evolution asserting that environmental changes cause structural changes in animals and plants that are transmitted to offspring

La·maze \lə-'mäz\ *adj* : relating to or being a method of childbirth that involves psychological and physical preparation by the mother in order to suppress pain and facilitate delivery without drugs

La·maze \lȧ-ˈmȧz\, **Fernand (1890–1957),** French obstetrician. Lamaze was the director of an obstetric clinic in France. In 1951 he attended a gynecologic conference where he learned for the first time a method of psychophysical conditioning aimed at the suppression of pain during a normal childbirth. After further study of psychophysical conditioning in the Soviet Union, he added a rapid accelerated breathing technique to the Soviet childbirth program and began implementing his modified method of natural childbirth in France.

lamb·da \ˈlam-də\ *n* **1** : the point of junction of the sagittal and lambdoid sutures of the skull **2** : PHAGE LAMBDA

lambda chain *or* λ **chain** *n* : a polypeptide chain of one of the two types of light chain that are found in antibodies and can be distinguished antigenically and by the sequence of amino acids in the chain — compare KAPPA CHAIN

lamb·da·cism \ˈlam-də-ˌsiz-əm\ *n* **1** : excessive use of the letter *l* or the sound \l\ (as in alliteration) **2** : a defective articulation of \l\, the substitution of other sounds for it, or the substitution of \l\ for another sound — compare LALLATION 2, PARALAMBDACISM

lambda phage *n* : PHAGE LAMBDA

lamb·doid \ˈlam-ˌdȯid\ *or* **lamb·doi·dal** \ˌlam-ˈdȯid-ᵊl\ *adj* : having the Λ or λ shape of the Greek letter lambda; *esp* : of, relating to, or being the lambda-shaped suture that connects the occipital and parietal bones

lam·bert \ˈlam-bərt\ *n* : the centimeter-gram-second unit of brightness equal to the brightness of a perfectly diffusing surface that radiates or reflects one lumen per square centimeter

Lam·bert \ˈläm-ˌbert\, **Johann Heinrich (1728–1777),** German mathematician, physicist, and philosopher. Largely self-educated, Lambert investigated geometry and astronomy, doing so by means of instruments which he himself designed and built. He also made significant contributions to the knowledge of heat and light. In 1760 he demonstrated for the first time how to measure quantitatively the intensity of light. The cgs unit of measurement for light intensity, the lambert, is named in his honor.

Lam·bert–Ea·ton syndrome \ˈlam-bərt-ˈēt-ᵊn-\ *n* : an autoimmune disorder that is caused by impaired presynaptic release of acetylcholine at nerve synapses, that resembles myasthenia, that is characterized by weakness usu. affecting the limbs but not the ocular and bulbar muscles, and that is often associated with carcinoma of the lung — called also *Eaton-Lambert syndrome, Lambert-Eaton myasthenic syndrome*

Lambert, Edward Howard (b 1915), and **Eaton, Lealdes McKendree (1905–1958),** American physicians. Lambert and Eaton spent the bulk of their careers at the Mayo Clinic in Rochester, Minnesota. At the Mayo Medical School Lambert served for many years as professor of physiology and in later years also as professor of neurology. Eaton rose to the position of professor of neurology and head of the Clinic's neurologic section. Lambert's areas of research included neurophysiology, electromyography, and various human neuromuscular disorders. Eaton's own research topics included myasthenia gravis and polymyositis. Lambert and Eaton were the principal authors of a 1956 article describing the syndrome which now bears their names.

lamb·ing paralysis \ˈlam-iŋ-\ *n* : PREGNANCY DISEASE

Lam·blia \ˈlam-blē-ə\ *n, syn of* GIARDIA

Lambl \ˈläm-bᵊl\, **Wilhelm Dusan (1824–1895),** Austrian physician. Lambl was the first to describe the causative agent (*Giardia lamblia*) of giardiasis in humans. The description was included in a collection of medical reports published in 1860 by the hospital where he was in residence.

lam·bli·a·sis \lam-ˈblī-ə-səs\ *n, pl* **-a·ses** \-ˌsēz\ : GIARDIASIS

lame \ˈlām\ *adj* **lam·er; lam·est** : having a body part and esp. a limb so disabled as to impair freedom of movement : physically disabled — **lame·ly** *adv* — **lame·ness** *n*

la·mel·la \lə-ˈmel-ə\ *n, pl* **la·mel·lae** \-ˈmel-ˌlē, -ˌlī\ *also* **lamellas** **1** : an organ, process, or part resembling a plate: as **a** : one of the bony concentric layers surrounding the haversian canals in bone **b** (1) : one of the incremental layers of cementum laid down in a tooth (2) : a thin sheetlike organic structure in the enamel of a tooth extending inward from a surface crack **2** : a small medicated disk prepared from gelatin and glycerin for use esp. in the eyes ⟨*lamellae* of atropine⟩

la·mel·lar \lə-ˈmel-ər\ *adj* **1** : composed of or arranged in lamellae ⟨~ bone⟩ **2** : LAMELLIFORM

lamellar ichthyosis *n* : a rare inherited form of ichthyosis characterized by large coarse scales

la·mel·late \ˈlam-ə-lət, lə-ˈme-lət, -ˌlāt\ *adj* **1** : composed of or furnished with lamellae **2** : LAMELLIFORM — **la·mel·late·ly** *adv* — **lam·el·la·tion** \ˌlam-ə-ˈlā-shən\ *n*

lam·el·lat·ed \ˈlam-ə-ˌlāt-əd\ *adj* : LAMELLATE ⟨~ bone⟩

la·mel·li·form \lə-ˈmel-i-ˌfȯrm\ *adj* : having the form of a thin plate

la·mel·li·po·di·um \lə-ˌmel-i-ˈpō-dē-əm\ *n, pl* **-po·dia** \-dē-ə\ : any of the motile sheetlike cytoplasmic extensions characteristic of some migrating cells (as macrophages)

lame sickness *n* : LAMSIEKTE

lam·i·na \ˈlam-ə-nə\ *n, pl* **-nae** \-ˌnē, -ˌnī\ *or* **-nas** : a thin plate or layer esp. of an anatomical part: as **a** : the part of the neural arch of a vertebra extending from the pedicle to the median line **b** : one of the narrow thin parallel plates of soft vascular sensitive tissue that cover the pododerm of a horse's hoof and fit between corresponding horny laminae on the inside of the wall of the hoof

lamina cri·bro·sa \-kri-ˈbrō-sə\ *n, pl* **laminae cri·bro·sae** \-ˌsē, -ˌsī\ : any of several anatomical structures having the form of a perforated plate: as **a** : CRIBRIFORM PLATE 1 **b** : the part of the sclera of the eye penetrated by the fibers of the optic nerve **c** : a perforated plate that closes the internal auditory canal

lamina du·ra \-ˈd(y)ùr-ə\ *n* : the thin hard layer of bone that lines the socket of a tooth and that appears as a dark line in radiography — called also *cribriform plate*

laminagram, laminagraph, laminagraphic, laminagraphy *var of* LAMINOGRAM, LAMINOGRAPH, LAMINOGRAPHIC, LAMINOGRAPHY

lam·i·nal \ˈlam-ən-ᵊl\ *adj* : LAMINAR

lamina pro·pria \-ˈprō-prē-ə\ *n, pl* **laminae pro·pri·ae** \-prē-ˌē, -ˌī\ : a highly vascular layer of connective tissue under the basement membrane lining a layer of epithelium

lam·i·nar \ˈlam-ə-nər\ *adj* : arranged in, consisting of, or resembling laminae

lam·i·nar·ia \ˌlam-ə-ˈner-ē-ə, -ˈnar-\ *n* : any of a genus (*Laminaria*) of large chiefly perennial kelps of which some have been used to dilate the cervix in performing an abortion

lam·i·nar·in \ˌlam-ə-ˈner-ən, -ˈnar-\ *n* : a polysaccharide that is found in various brown algae and yields only glucose on hydrolysis

lam·i·nar·in·ase \-ˌās, -ˌāz\ *n* : a glycoside hydrolase that hydrolyzes laminarin and lichenin

lamina spi·ral·is \-spə-ˈral-əs, -ˈrāl-\ *n* : SPIRAL LAMINA

lam·i·nat·ed \ˈlam-ə-ˌnāt-əd\ *adj* : composed or arranged in layers or laminae ⟨~ membranes⟩

lamina ter·mi·nal·is \-ˌtər-mi-ˈnal-əs, -ˈnāl-\ *n* : a thin layer of gray matter in the telencephalon that extends backward from the corpus callosum above the optic chiasma and forms the median portion of the rostral wall of the third ventricle of the cerebrum

lam·i·na·tion \ˌlam-ə-ˈnā-shən\ *n* : a laminated structure or arrangement

lam·i·nec·to·my \ˌlam-ə-ˈnek-tə-mē\ *n, pl* **-mies** : surgical removal of the posterior arch of a vertebra

lam·i·nin \ˈlam-ə-nən\ *n* : a glycoprotein that is a component

K
L

of connective tissue basement membrane and that promotes cell adhesion

lam·i·ni·tis \‚lam-ə-ˈnīt-əs\ *n* : inflammation of a lamina esp. in the hoof of a horse, cow, or goat that is typically caused by excessive ingestion of a dietary substance (as carbohydrate) — called also *founder*

lam·i·no·gram *or* **lam·i·na·gram** \ˈlam-ə-nə-‚gram\ *n* : a radiograph of a layer of the body made by means of a laminograph; *broadly* : TOMOGRAM

lam·i·no·graph *or* **lam·i·na·graph** \-‚graf\ *n* : an X-ray machine that makes radiography of body tissue possible at any desired depth; *broadly* : TOMOGRAPH — **lam·i·no·graph·ic** *or* **lam·i·na·graph·ic** \‚lam-ə-nə-ˈgraf-ik\ *adj* — **lam·i·nog·ra·phy** \‚lam-ə-ˈnäg-rə-fē\ *or* **lam·i·nag·ra·phy** \‚lam-ə-ˈnag-rə-fē\ *n, pl* **-phies**

lam·i·not·o·my \‚lam-ə-ˈnät-ə-mē\ *n, pl* **-mies** : surgical division of a vertebral lamina

la·miv·u·dine \lə-ˈmiv-yü-‚dēn\ *n* : an antiviral drug $C_8H_{11}N_3O_3S$ that is a synthetic nucleoside analog acting against HIV by inhibiting reverse transcriptase — see EPIVIR

lamp \ˈlamp\ *n* : any of various devices for producing light or heat — see KROMAYER LAMP, SLIT LAMP

lam·pas \ˈlam-pəs\ *n* : a congestion of the mucous membrane of the hard palate just posterior to the incisor teeth of the horse due to irritation and bruising from harsh coarse feeds

lamp·brush \ˈlamp-‚brəsh\ *adj* : of, relating to, or characterized by lampbrush chromosomes ⟨∼ loops⟩

lamp·brush chromosome \‚lamp-‚brəsh-\ *n* : a greatly enlarged diplotene chromosome that has apparently filamentous granular loops extending from the chromomeres and is characteristic of some animal oocytes

lam·siek·te \ˈlam-‚sēk-tə, ˈläm-\ *or* **lam·ziek·te** \-‚zēk-\ *n* : botulism of phosphorus-deficient cattle esp. in southern Africa due to ingestion of bones and carrion containing clostridial toxins — called also *lame sickness*

lanae — see ADEPS LANAE

la·nat·o·side \lə-ˈnat-ə-‚sīd\ *n* : any of three poisonous crystalline cardiac steroid glycosides occurring in the leaves of a foxglove (*Digitalis lanata*): **a** : the glycoside $C_{49}H_{76}O_{19}$ yielding digitoxin, glucose, and acetic acid on hydrolysis — called also *digilanid A, lanatoside A* **b** : the glycoside $C_{49}H_{76}O_{20}$ yielding gitoxin, glucose, and acetic acid on hydrolysis — called also *digilanid B, lanatoside B* **c** : the bitter glycoside $C_{49}H_{76}O_{20}$ yielding digoxin, glucose, and acetic acid on hydrolysis and used similarly to digitalis — called also *digilanid C, lanatoside C*

¹lance \ˈlan(t)s\ *n* : LANCET

²lance *vt* **lanced; lanc·ing** : to open with or as if with a lancet : make an incision in or into ⟨∼ a boil⟩ ⟨∼ a vein⟩

Lance·field group \ˈlan(t)s-‚fēld-\ *also* **Lance·field's group** \-‚fēldz-\ *n* : any of the serologically distinguishable groups into which most streptococci can be divided and which are based on the polysaccharide antigens present in the streptococcal cell walls — see GROUP A, GROUP B

Lancefield, Rebecca Craighill (1895–1981), American bacteriologist. Lancefield specialized in immunochemical studies of streptococci. In 1928 she published a study of the chemical composition and antigenicity of hemolytic streptococci. In 1933 she introduced a new method of classifying streptococci into groups according to the ability of antigens in their cell walls to induce the formation of antibodies which caused precipitation of the streptococci from solution. These groups are now known as the Lancefield groups.

lance·let \ˈlan(t)-slət\ *n* : any vertebrate animal of the subphylum Cephalochordata — called also *amphioxus*

lan·ce·o·late \ˈlan(t)-sē-ə-‚lāt\ *adj* : shaped like the head of a lance or spear

lan·cet \ˈlan(t)-sət\ *n* : a sharp-pointed and commonly two-edged surgical instrument used to make small incisions (as in a vein or a boil) — called also *lance*

lancet fluke *n* : a small liver fluke of the genus *Dicrocoelium*

(*D. dendriticum* syn. *D. lanceolatum*) widely distributed in sheep and cattle and rarely infecting humans

lan·ci·nat·ing \ˈlan(t)-sə-‚nāt-iŋ\ *adj* : characterized by piercing or stabbing sensations ⟨∼ pain⟩

land leech \ˈland-‚lēch\ *n* : any of various bloodsucking leeches chiefly of moist tropical regions that live on land and are often troublesome to humans and other animals; *esp* : a leech of the gnathobdellid genus *Haemadipsa*

land·mark \-‚märk\ *n* **1** : an anatomical structure used as a point of orientation in locating other structures (as in surgical procedures) **2** : a point on the body or skeleton from which anthropological measurements are taken

Lan·dolt ring \ˈlän-dōlt-‚riŋ\ *n* : one of a series of incomplete rings or circles used in some eye charts to determine visual discrimination or acuity

Landolt, Edmond (1846–1926), French ophthalmologist. Landolt and Louis de Wecker (1832–1906) published from 1880 to 1889 a multivolume treatise on ophthalmology that was once considered a definitive work on the subject. Landolt spent his career applying optics in the study of physiology. In addition to devising the Landolt ring, he described the histological formation on the outer nuclear layer of the retina.

Lan·dry's paralysis \ˈlan-drēz-\ *n* : GUILLAIN-BARRÉ SYNDROME

Lan·dry \län-ˈdrē\, **Jean–Baptiste–Octave (1826–1865),** French physician. Landry published a treatise on diseases of the nervous system in 1855. Four years later he produced a treatise on paralyses and described Landry's paralysis.

Lang·er·hans cell \ˈläŋ-ər-‚hän(t)s-\ *n* : a dendritic cell of the interstitial spaces of the mammalian epidermis that functions as an antigen-presenting cell which binds antigen entering through the skin and transports it to the lymph nodes

P. Langerhans — see ISLET OF LANGERHANS

Lang·hans cell \ˈläŋ-‚hän(t)s-\ *n* : any of the cells of cuboidal epithelium that make up the cytotrophoblast

Langhans, Theodor (1839–1915), German pathologist and anatomist. Langhans described the cytotrophoblast and the cells that form it in 1870. He is also remembered for his descriptions of the giant cells found in tuberculosis tubercles (1867) and of the giant cells found in the lesions of Hodgkin's disease (1872).

Langhans giant cell *n* : any of the large cells found in the lesions of some granulomatous conditions (as leprosy and tuberculosis) and containing a number of peripheral nuclei arranged in a circle or in the shape of a horseshoe

Langhans' layer *n* : CYTOTROPHOBLAST

lan·o·lin \ˈlan-ᵊl-ən\ *n* : a yellowish sticky unctuous mass of refined wool grease that can be absorbed by the skin, contains from 25 to 30 percent incorporated water, and is used chiefly in ointments and cosmetics — called also *adeps lanae, hydrous wool fat*

la·nos·ter·ol \lə-ˈnäs-tə-‚ròl, -‚rōl\ *n* : a crystalline sterol $C_{30}H_{50}O$ that occurs in wool grease and yeast

Lan·ox·in \lə-ˈnäk-sən\ *trademark* — used for a preparation of digoxin

Lan·sing virus \ˈlan-siŋ-\ *n* : a strain of a serotype of the poliovirus that is pathogenic for monkeys and rodents and has been extensively used in studying poliomyelitis — called also *Lansing strain*

lan·so·praz·ole \lan-ˈsō-prə-‚zōl\ *n* : a benzimidazole derivative $C_{16}H_{14}F_3N_3O_2S$ that inhibits gastric acid secretion and is used similarly to omeprazole — see PREVACID

lan·tha·nide \ˈlan(t)-thə-‚nīd\ *n* : any in a series of elements of increasing atomic numbers beginning with lanthanum (57) or cerium (58) and ending with lutetium (71)

lan·tha·non \-‚nän\ *n* : LANTHANIDE

lan·tha·num \-nəm\ *n* : a white soft malleable metallic element that occurs in rare-earth minerals — symbol *La*; see ELEMENT table

lan·tho·pine \ˈlan(t)-thə-‚pēn, -pən\ *n* : a crystalline alkaloid $C_{23}H_{25}NO_4$ found in opium

la·nu·gi·nous \lə-ˈn(y)ü-jə-nəs\ *adj* : covered with down or fine soft hair

la·nu·go \lə-'n(y)ü-(ˌ)gō\ *n* : a dense cottony or downy growth of hair; *specif* : the soft downy hair that covers the fetus of some mammals

lap *abbr* laparotomy

la·pac·tic \lə-'pak-tik\ *adj* : CATHARTIC, LAXATIVE

lap·a·ro·scope \'lap(-ə)-rə-ˌskōp\ *n* : a usu. rigid endoscope that is inserted through an incision in the abdominal wall and is used to examine visually the interior of the peritoneal cavity — called also *peritoneoscope*

lap·a·ros·co·pist \ˌlap-ə-'räs-kə-pəst\ *n* : a physician or surgeon who performs laparoscopies

lap·a·ros·co·py \ˌlap-ə-'räs-kə-pē\ *n, pl* **-pies** **1** : visual examination of the inside of the abdomen by means of a laparoscope — called also *peritoneoscopy* **2** : an operation (as tubal ligation or gallbladder removal) involving laparoscopy — **lap·a·ro·scop·ic** \-rə-'skäp-ik\ *adj* — **lap·a·ro·scop·i·cal·ly** \-i-k(ə)lē\ *adv*

lap·a·rot·om·ize *or Brit* **lap·a·rot·om·ise** \ˌlap-ə-'rät-ə-ˌmīz\ *vt* **-ized** *or Brit* **-ised; -iz·ing** *or Brit* **-is·ing** : to perform a laparotomy on

lap·a·rot·o·my \ˌlap-ə-'rät-ə-mē\ *n, pl* **-mies** : surgical section of the abdominal wall

lap·in·ized *or Brit* **lap·in·ised** \'lap-ə-ˌnīzd\ *adj* : attenuated by passage through rabbits ⟨a ∼ virus⟩

La·place's law \lä-'plä-səz-\ *n* : LAW OF LAPLACE

lap·pa \'lap-ə\ *n* : the root of a burdock (*Actium lappa*) formerly used as a diuretic and alterative

larch agaric \'lärch-\ *n* : AGARIC 1

lard \'lärd\ *n* : ADEPS

lard·worm \-ˌwərm\ *n* : KIDNEY WORM b

Lar·gac·til \lär-'gak-til\ *n* : a preparation of the hydrochloride of chlorpromazine — formerly a U.S. registered trademark

large bowel \'lärj-\ *n* : LARGE INTESTINE

large calorie *n* : CALORIE 1b

large–cell carcinoma *n* : a non-small cell lung cancer usu. arising in the bronchi and composed of large undifferentiated cells — called also *large-cell lung carcinoma*

large intestine *n* : the more terminal division of the vertebrate intestine that is wider and shorter than the small intestine, typically divided into cecum, colon, and rectum, and concerned esp. with the resorption of water and the formation of feces

large–mouthed bowel worm \'lärj-ˌmauṫht-, -ˌmauṫhd-\ *n* : BOWEL WORM

lark·spur \'lärk-ˌspər\ *n* **1** : DELPHINIUM 2 **2** : the dried ripe seeds of a European plant of the genus *Delphinium* (*D. ajacis*) from which an acetic tincture is sometimes prepared for use against ectoparasites (as lice)

Lar·o·tid \'lar-ə-ˌtid\ *n* : a preparation of amoxicillin — formerly a U.S. registered trademark

Lar·sen's syndrome \'lär-sənz-\ *n* : a syndrome characterized by cleft palate, flattened facies, multiple congenital joint dislocations, and deformities of the foot

    Larsen, Loren Joseph (*b* 1914), American orthopedic surgeon. While he was on the staff of a university hospital in San Francisco in 1944 and 1945, Larsen treated a child patient suffering from severely deformed clubfeet, dislocated knees, hips, and elbows, and accompanying facial abnormalities. Observing these common characteristics in five other cases, he summarized and reported his findings on this previously unrecognized clinical entity in an article published in 1950. Later reports confirmed and supplemented the original findings, and Larsen's name subsequently became attached to the syndrome.

lar·va \'lär-və\ *n, pl* **lar·vae** \-(ˌ)vē, -ˌvī\ *also* **larvas** **1** : the immature, wingless, and often wormlike feeding form that hatches from the egg of many insects, alters chiefly in size while passing through several molts, and is finally transformed into a pupa or chrysalis from which the adult emerges **2** : the early form of an animal (as a frog) that at birth or hatching is fundamentally unlike its parent and must metamorphose before assuming the adult characters — **lar·val** \-vəl\ *adj*

larvacide *var of* LARVICIDE

larval mi·grans \-'mī-ˌgranz\ *n* : CREEPING ERUPTION

larva migrans *n, pl* **larvae mi·gran·tes** \-ˌmī-'gran-ˌtēz\ : CREEPING ERUPTION

lar·vi·cide *also* **lar·va·cide** \'lär-və-ˌsīd\ *n* : an agent for killing larvae — **lar·vi·cid·al** \ˌlär-və-'sīd-ᵊl\ *adj* — **lar·vi·cid·al·ly** \-ē\ *adv* — **lar·vi·cid·ing** \'lär-və-ˌsīd-iŋ\ *n*

lar·vip·a·rous \lär-'vip-ə-rəs\ *adj* : bearing and bringing forth young that are larvae — used esp. of specialized dipteran flies and some mollusks; compare OVIPAROUS, OVOVIVIPAROUS, VIVIPAROUS

lar·vi·phag·ic \ˌlär-və-'faj-ik\ *adj* : LARVIVOROUS

lar·vi·pos·it \'lär-və-ˌpäz-ət\ *vi* : to bear and deposit living larvae instead of eggs — compare OVIPOSIT — **lar·vi·po·si·tion** \ˌlär-və-pə-'zi-shən\ *n*

lar·viv·o·rous \lär-'viv-ə-rəs\ *adj* : feeding upon larvae esp. of insects ⟨∼ fishes used in the control of mosquito populations⟩

¹la·ryn·geal \lə-'rin-j(ē-)əl, ˌlar-ən-'jē-əl\ *adj* : of, relating to, affecting, or used on the larynx — **la·ryn·geal·ly** \-ē\ *adv*

²laryngeal *n* : an anatomical part (as a nerve or artery) that supplies or is associated with the larynx

laryngeal artery *n* : either of two arteries supplying blood to the larynx: **a** : a branch of the inferior thyroid artery that supplies the muscles and mucous membranes of the dorsal part of the larynx — called also *inferior laryngeal artery* **b** : a branch of the superior thyroid artery or sometimes of the external carotid artery that supplies the muscles, mucous membranes, and glands of the larynx and anastomoses with the branch from the opposite side — called also *superior laryngeal artery*

laryngeal nerve *n* : either of two branches of the vagus nerve supplying the larynx: **a** : one that arises from the ganglion of the vagus situated below the jugular foramen in front of the transverse processes of the first two cervical vertebrae and that passes down the neck to supply the cricothyroid muscle — called also *superior laryngeal nerve* **b** : one that arises below the larynx, loops under the subclavian artery on the right side and under the arch of the aorta on the left, and returns upward to the larynx to supply all the muscles of the thyroid except the cricothyroid — called also *inferior laryngeal nerve, recurrent laryngeal nerve, recurrent nerve;* see INFERIOR LARYNGEAL NERVE 2

laryngeal saccule *n* : a membranous sac in the larynx located between the false vocal cords and the inner surface of the thyroid cartilage and containing mucus-secreting glands whose secretion lubricates the vocal cords — called also *laryngeal pouch, laryngeal sac*

lar·yn·gect \'lar-ən-ˌjekt\ *n* : LARYNGECTOMEE

lar·yn·gec·to·mee \ˌlar-ən-jek-tə-'mē\ *n* : a person who has undergone laryngectomy

lar·yn·gec·to·my \-'jek-tə-mē\ *n, pl* **-mies** : surgical removal of all or part of the larynx — **lar·yn·gec·to·mized** \-tə-ˌmīzd\ *adj*

larynges *pl of* LARYNX

lar·yn·gis·mus stri·du·lus \ˌlar-ən-'jiz-məs-'strij-ə-ləs\ *n, pl* **lar·yn·gis·mi stri·du·li** \-ˌmī-'strij-ə-ˌlī\ : a sudden spasm of the larynx that occurs in children esp. in rickets and is marked by difficult breathing with prolonged noisy inspiration — compare LARYNGOSPASM

¹lar·yn·git·ic \ˌlar-ən-'jit-ik\ *adj* **1** : of, relating to, or characteristic of laryngitis **2** : affected with laryngitis

²laryngitic *n* : an individual affected with laryngitis

lar·yn·gi·tis \ˌlar-ən-'jīt-əs\ *n, pl* **-git·i·des** \-'jit-ə-ˌdēz\ : inflammation of the larynx

la·ryn·go·cele \lə-'riŋ-gə-ˌsēl\ *n* : an air-containing evagination of laryngeal mucous membrane having its opening communicating with the ventricle of the larynx

la·ryn·go·fis·sure \lə-ˌriŋ-gō-'fish-ər\ *n* : surgical opening of

---

K
L

\ə\ **abut** \ᵊ\ **kitten** \ər\ **further** \a\ **ash** \ā\ **ace** \ä\ **cot, cart**
\aů\ **out** \ch\ **chin** \e\ **bet** \ē\ **easy** \g\ **go** \i\ **hit** \ī\ **ice** \j\ **job**
\ŋ\ **sing** \ō\ **go** \ȯ\ **law** \ȯi\ **boy** \th\ **thin** \tẖ\ **the** \ü\ **loot**
\ů\ **foot** \y\ **yet** \zh\ **vision** *See also* Pronunciation Symbols page

the larynx by an incision through the thyroid cartilage esp. for the removal of a tumor

lar·yn·gog·ra·phy \ˌlar-ən-ˈgäg-rə-fē\ *n, pl* **-phies** : X-ray depiction of the larynx after use of a radiopaque material

laryngol *abbr* laryngological

la·ryn·go·log·i·cal \lə-ˌriŋ-gə-ˈläj-i-kəl\ *also* **la·ryn·go·log·ic** \-ˈläj-ik\ *adj* : of or relating to laryngology or the larynx

lar·yn·gol·o·gist \ˌlar-ən-ˈgäl-ə-jəst\ *n* : a physician specializing in laryngology

lar·yn·gol·o·gy \ˌlar-ən-ˈgäl-ə-jē\ *n, pl* **-gies** : a branch of medicine dealing with diseases of the larynx and nasopharynx

la·ryn·go·pha·ryn·geal \lə-ˌriŋ-gō-ˌfar-ən-ˈjē-əl, -fə-ˈrin-j(ē-)əl\ *adj* : of or common to both the larynx and the pharynx ⟨∼ cancer⟩

la·ryn·go·phar·yn·gi·tis \-ˌfar-ən-ˈjīt-əs\ *n, pl* **-git·i·des** \-ˈjit-ə-ˌdēz\ : inflammation of both the larynx and the pharynx

la·ryn·go·phar·ynx \-ˈfar-iŋ(k)s\ *n* : the lower part of the pharynx lying behind or adjacent to the larynx — compare NASOPHARYNX

la·ryn·go·plas·ty \lə-ˈriŋ-gə-ˌplas-tē\ *n, pl* **-ties** : plastic surgery to repair laryngeal defects

la·ryn·go·scope \lə-ˈriŋ-gə-ˌskōp *also* -ˈrin-jə-\ *n* : an endoscope for visually examining the interior of the larynx — **la·ryn·go·scop·ic** \-ˌriŋ-gə-ˈskäp-ik, -ˌrin-jə-\ *or* **la·ryn·go·scop·i·cal** \-i-kəl\ *adj* — **la·ryn·go·scop·i·cal·ly** \-i-k(ə-)lē\ *adv*

lar·yn·gos·co·py \ˌlar-ən-ˈgäs-kə-pē\ *n, pl* **-pies** : examination of the interior of the larynx (as with a laryngoscope)

la·ryn·go·spasm \lə-ˈriŋ-gə-ˌspaz-əm\ *n* : spasmodic closure of the larynx — compare LARYNGISMUS STRIDULUS

lar·yn·got·o·my \ˌlar-ən-ˈgät-ə-mē\ *n, pl* **-mies** : surgical incision of the larynx

la·ryn·go·tra·che·al \lə-ˌriŋ-gō-ˈtrā-kē-əl\ *adj* : of or common to the larynx and trachea ⟨∼ stenosis⟩

la·ryn·go·tra·che·itis \-ˌtrā-kē-ˈīt-əs\ *n* : inflammation of both larynx and trachea — see INFECTIOUS LARYNGOTRACHEITIS

la·ryn·go·tra·cheo·bron·chi·tis \-ˌtrā-kē-ō-brän-ˈkīt-əs, -brän-\ *n, pl* **-chit·i·des** \-ˈkit-ə-ˌdēz\ : inflammation of the larynx, trachea, and bronchi; *specif* : an acute severe infection of these parts marked by swelling of the tissues and excessive secretion of mucus leading to more or less complete obstruction of the respiratory passages

lar·ynx \ˈlar-iŋ(k)s\ *n, pl* **la·ryn·ges** \lə-ˈrin-(ˌ)jēz\ *or* **lar·ynx·es** : the modified upper part of the respiratory passage of air-breathing vertebrates that is bounded above by the glottis, is continuous below with the trachea, has a complex cartilaginous or bony skeleton capable of limited motion through the action of associated muscles, and in humans, most other mammals, and a few lower forms has a set of elastic vocal cords that play a major role in sound production and speech — called also *voice box*

la·sal·o·cid \lə-ˈsal-ə-ˌsid\ *n* : an antibiotic $C_{34}H_{54}O_8$ used as a veterinary coccidiostat

¹la·ser \ˈlā-zər\ *n* : a device that utilizes the natural oscillations of atoms or molecules between energy levels for generating coherent electromagnetic radiation usu. in the ultraviolet, visible, or infrared regions of the spectrum

²laser *vt* : to subject to the action of a laser : treat with a laser ⟨cutting a corneal flap to remove tissue and then ∼*ing* the area under it —Jenny Manzer⟩

la·ser–as·sist·ed in–situ keratomileusis \ˈlā-zər-ə-ˈsis-təd-\ *n* : LASIK

lash \ˈlash\ *n* : EYELASH

LA·SIK \ˈlā-sik\ *n* : a surgical operation to reshape the cornea for correction of nearsightedness, farsightedness, or astigmatism that involves the use of a microkeratome to separate the surface layer of the cornea creating a hinged flap providing access to the inner cornea where varying degrees of tissue are removed by an excimer laser followed by replacement of the corneal flap — called also *laser-assisted insitu keratomileusis*

La·six \ˈlā-siks, -ziks\ *trademark* — used for a preparation of furosemide

L–as·par·a·gi·nase \ˈel-as-ˈpar-ə-jə-ˌnās, -ˌnāz\ *n* : an enzyme that breaks down the physiologically commoner form of asparagine, is obtained esp. from bacteria, and is used esp. to treat leukemia

Las·sa fever \ˌlas-ə-\ *n* : a disease esp. of Africa that is caused by the Lassa virus and is characterized by a high fever, headaches, mouth ulcers, muscle aches, small hemorrhages under the skin, heart and kidney failure, and a high mortality rate

Lassa virus *n* : a single-stranded RNA virus of the genus *Arenavirus* (species *Lassa virus*) that causes Lassa fever

las·si·tude \ˈlas-ə-ˌt(y)üd\ *n* : a condition of weariness, debility, or fatigue ⟨a disease typically accompanied by chronic ∼⟩

lat \ˈlat\ *n* : LATISSIMUS DORSI — usu. used in pl.

lata — see FASCIA LATA

latae — see FASCIA LATA, TENSOR FASCIAE LATAE

la·tah \ˈlät-ə\ *n* : a neurotic condition marked by automatic obedience, echolalia, and echopraxia observed esp. among the Malayan people

la·tan·o·prost \lə-ˈtan-ə-ˌpräst\ *n* : a prostaglandin analog $C_{26}H_{40}O_5$ used topically to reduce elevated intraocular pressure — see XALATAN

la·ten·cy \ˈlāt-ᵊn-sē\ *n, pl* **-cies** **1** : the quality or state of being latent; *esp* : the state or period of living or developing in a host without producing symptoms — used of an infective agent or disease ⟨the infamous ∼ of the virus causing herpes simplex⟩ **2** : LATENCY PERIOD 1 **3** : the interval between stimulation and response — called also *latent period*

latency period *n* **1** : a stage of psychosexual development that follows the phallic stage and precedes the genital stage, extends from about the age of five or six to the beginning of puberty, and during which sexual urges often appear to lie dormant — called also *latency* **2** : LATENT PERIOD

la·tent \ˈlāt-ᵊnt\ *adj* : existing in hidden or dormant form: as **a** : present or capable of living or developing in a host without producing visible symptoms of disease ⟨a ∼ virus⟩ ⟨a ∼ infection⟩ **b** : not consciously expressed ⟨∼ anxiety⟩ **c** : relating to or being the latent content of a dream or thought — **la·tent·ly** *adv*

latent content *n* : the underlying meaning of a dream or thought that is exposed in psychoanalysis by interpretation of its symbols or by free association — compare MANIFEST CONTENT

latent heat *n* : heat given off or absorbed in a process (as fusion or vaporization) other than a change of temperature

la·ten·ti·a·tion \lā-ˌten-chē-ˈā-shən\ *n* : pharmacological modification of an active drug (as to delay or prolong its action) that produces a compound which reverts to the original active compound when subjected to biological processes after administration

latent learning *n* : learning that is not demonstrated by behavior at the time it is held to take place but that is inferred to exist based on a greater than expected number of favorable or desired responses at a later time when reinforcement is given

latent period *n* **1** : the period between exposure to a disease-causing agent or process and the appearance of symptoms ⟨the *latent period* between exposure to a tumorigenic dose of radioactivity and the appearance of tumors⟩ **2** : LATENCY 3 ⟨smooth muscle has a longer *latent period* than striated muscle⟩

late–on·set diabetes \ˌlāt-ˌän-(ˌ)set-, -ˌón-\ *n* : TYPE 2 DIABETES

lat·er·ad \ˈlat-ə-ˌrad\ *adv* : toward the side

lat·er·al \ˈlat-ə-rəl, ˈla-trəl\ *adj* : of or relating to the side; *esp, of a body part* : lying at or extending toward the right or left side : lying away from the median axis of the body ⟨the lungs are ∼ to the heart⟩ ⟨the ∼ branch of the axillary artery⟩

lateral arcuate ligament *n* : a fascial band that is formed by part of the quadratus lumborum muscle, extends from the tip of the transverse process of the first lumbar vertebra to the twelfth rib, and provides attachment for part of the diaphragm — compare MEDIAL ARCUATE LIGAMENT, MEDIAN ARCUATE LIGAMENT

lateral brachial cutaneous nerve *n* : a continuation of the posterior branch of the axillary nerve that supplies the skin of the lateral aspect of the upper arm over the distal part of the deltoid muscle and the adjacent head of the triceps brachii

lateral check ligament *n* : CHECK LIGAMENT 2a

lateral collateral ligament *n* **1** : a ligament that connects the lateral epicondyle of the femur with the lateral side of the head of the fibula and that helps to stabilize the knee by preventing lateral dislocation — called also *fibular collateral ligament, LCL;* compare MEDIAL COLLATERAL LIGAMENT **2** : RADIAL COLLATERAL LIGAMENT

lateral column *n* **1** : a lateral extension of the gray matter in each lateral half of the spinal cord present in the thoracic and upper lumbar regions — called also *lateral horn;* compare DORSAL HORN, VENTRAL HORN **2** : LATERAL FUNICULUS

lateral condyle *n* : a condyle on the outer side of the lower extremity of the femur; *also* : a corresponding eminence on the upper part of the tibia that articulates with the lateral condyle of the femur — compare MEDIAL CONDYLE

lateral cord *n* : a cord of nerve tissue that is formed by union of the superior and middle trunks of the brachial plexus and that forms one of the two roots of the median nerve — compare MEDIAL CORD, POSTERIOR CORD

lateral corticospinal tract *n* : a band of nerve fibers that descends in the posterolateral part of each side of the spinal cord and consists mostly of fibers arising in the motor cortex of the contralateral side of the brain and crossing over in the decussation of pyramids with some fibers arising in the motor cortex of the same side — called also *crossed pyramidal tract*

lateral crest *n* : SACRAL CREST b

lateral cricoarytenoid *n* : CRICOARYTENOID 1

lateral cuneiform *n* : CUNEIFORM BONE 1c

lateral cuneiform bone *n* : CUNEIFORM BONE 1c

lateral decubitus *n* : a position in which a patient lies on his or her side and which is used esp. in radiography and in making a lumbar puncture

lateral epicondyle *n* : EPICONDYLE a

lateral epicondylitis *n* : TENNIS ELBOW

lateral femoral circumflex artery *n* : an artery that branches from the deep femoral artery or from the femoral artery itself and that supplies the muscles of the lateral part of the thigh and hip joint — compare MEDIAL FEMORAL CIRCUMFLEX ARTERY

lateral femoral circumflex vein *n* : a vein that accompanies the lateral femoral circumflex artery and empties into the femoral vein or sometimes into one of its tributaries and that corresponds to the deep femoral artery — compare MEDIAL FEMORAL CIRCUMFLEX VEIN

lateral femoral cutaneous nerve *n* : a nerve that arises from the lumbar plexus by the association of branches from the dorsal parts of the ventral divisions of the second and third lumbar nerves and that supplies the anterior and lateral aspects of the thigh down to the knee — compare POSTERIOR FEMORAL CUTANEOUS NERVE

lateral fissure *n* : SYLVIAN FISSURE

lateral funiculus *n* : a longitudinal division on each side of the spinal cord comprising white matter between the dorsal and ventral roots — compare ANTERIOR FUNICULUS, POSTERIOR FUNICULUS

lateral gastrocnemius bursa *n* : a bursa of the knee joint that is situated between the lateral head of the gastrocnemius muscle and the joint capsule

lateral geniculate body *n* : a part of the metathalamus that consists of an oval elevation situated on the posterolateral surface of the thalamus, is the terminus of most fibers of the optic tract, and receives nerve impulses from the retinas

which are relayed to the visual area by way of the geniculocalcarine tracts — compare MEDIAL GENICULATE BODY

lateral geniculate nucleus *n* : a nucleus of the lateral geniculate body

lateral horn *n* : LATERAL COLUMN 1

lateral humeral epicondylitis *n* : TENNIS ELBOW

lateral inhibition *n* : a visual process in which the firing of a retinal cell inhibits the firing of surrounding retinal cells and which is held to enhance the perception of areas of contrast

lateralis — see RECTUS LATERALIS, VASTUS LATERALIS

lat·er·al·i·ty \ˌlat-ə-ˈral-ət-ē\ *n, pl* **-ties** : preference in use of homologous parts on one lateral half of the body over those on the other : dominance in function of one of a pair of lateral homologous parts ⟨studies of the ∼ of individuals in the performance of different tasks —K. C. Garrison⟩

lat·er·al·iza·tion *also Brit* **lat·er·al·isa·tion** \ˌlat-ə-rə-lə-ˈzā-shən, ˌla-trə-lə-\ *n* : localization of function or activity (as of verbal processes in the brain) on one side of the body in preference to the other — **lat·er·al·ize** *also Brit* **lat·er·al·ise** \ˈlat-ə-rə-ˌlīz, ˈla-trə-ˌlīz\ *vt* **-ized** *also Brit* **-ised; -iz·ing** *also Brit* **-is·ing**

lateral lemniscus *n* : a band of nerve fibers that arises in the cochlear nuclei and terminates in the inferior colliculus and the lateral geniculate body of the opposite side of the brain

lateral ligament *n* : any of various ligaments (as the lateral collateral ligament of the knee) that are in a lateral position or that prevent lateral dislocation of a joint

lateral malleolus *n* : MALLEOLUS a

lateral meniscus *n* : MENISCUS 2a(1)

lateral nucleus *n* : any of a group of nuclei of the thalamus situated in the dorsolateral region extending from its anterior to posterior ends

lateral pectoral nerve *n* : PECTORAL NERVE a

lateral plantar artery *n* : PLANTAR ARTERY a

lateral plantar nerve *n* : PLANTAR NERVE a

lateral plantar vein *n* : PLANTAR VEIN a

lateral plate *n* : an unsegmented sheet of mesoderm on each side of the vertebrate embryo from which the coelom and its linings develop

lateral popliteal nerve *n* : COMMON PERONEAL NERVE

lateral pterygoid muscle *n* : PTERYGOID MUSCLE a

lateral pterygoid nerve *n* : PTERYGOID NERVE a

lateral pterygoid plate *n* : PTERYGOID PLATE a

lateral rectus *n* : RECTUS 2b

lateral reticular nucleus *n* : a nucleus of the reticular formation that is situated in the ventrolateral part of the medulla oblongata, receives fibers esp. from the dorsal horn of the spinal cord, and sends axons to the cerebellum on the same side of the body

lateral sacral artery *n* : either of two arteries on each side which arise from the posterior division of the internal iliac artery and of which one passes superiorly and the other inferiorly supplying muscles and skin in the area

lateral sacral crest *n* : SACRAL CREST b

lateral sacral vein *n* : any of several veins that accompany the corresponding lateral sacral arteries and empty into the internal iliac veins

lateral semilunar cartilage *n* : MENISCUS 2a(1)

lateral sinus *n* : TRANSVERSE SINUS

lateral spinothalamic tract *n* : SPINOTHALAMIC TRACT b

lateral sulcus *n* : SYLVIAN FISSURE

lateral thoracic artery *n* : THORACIC ARTERY b

lateral umbilical ligament *n* : MEDIAL UMBILICAL LIGAMENT

lateral ventricle *n* : an internal cavity in each cerebral hemisphere that consists of a central body and three cornua including an anterior one curving forward and outward, a posterior one curving backward, and an inferior one curving

\ə\ **abut** \ᵊ\ **kitten** \ər\ **further** \a\ **ash** \ā\ **ace** \ä\ **cot, cart** \au̇\ **out** \ch\ **chin** \e\ **bet** \ē\ **easy** \g\ **go** \i\ **hit** \ī\ **ice** \j\ **job** \ŋ\ **sing** \ō\ **go** \ȯ\ **law** \ȯi\ **boy** \th\ **thin** \th̶\ **the** \ü\ **loot** \u̇\ **foot** \y\ **yet** \zh\ **vision** *See also* Pronunciation Symbols page

downward — see ANTERIOR HORN 2, INFERIOR HORN, POS-
TERIOR HORN 2

lateral vestibular nucleus *n* : the one of the four vestibular nuclei on each side of the medulla oblongata that is situated on the inner side of the inferior cerebellar peduncle beneath the floor of the fourth ventricle and that sends fibers down the same side of the spinal cord through the vestibulospinal tract — called also *Deiters' nucleus*

lat·er·al·ward \-wərd\ *adv* : in a lateral direction

la·tex \'lā-ˌteks\ *n, pl* **la·ti·ces** \'lāt-ə-ˌsēz, 'lat-\ *or* **la·tex·es** : a milky usu. white fluid that is usu. made up of various gum resins, fats, or waxes and often a complex mixture of other substances frequently including poisonous compounds, is produced by cells of various seed plants (as of the milkweed, spurge, and poppy families), and is the source of rubber, gutta-percha, chicle, and balata

latex agglutination test *n* : a test for a specific antibody and esp. rheumatoid factor in which the corresponding antigen is adsorbed on spherical polystyrene latex particles which undergo agglutination upon addition of the specific antibody — called also *latex fixation test, latex test*

lath·y·rism \'lath-ə-ˌriz-əm\ *n* : a diseased condition of humans, domestic animals, and esp. horses that results from poisoning by an amino acid found in some legumes of the genus *Lathyrus* (esp. *L. sativus*) and is characterized esp. by spastic paralysis of the hind or lower limbs

lath·y·rit·ic \ˌlath-ə-'rit-ik\ *adj* : of, relating to, affected with, or characteristic of lathyrism ⟨~ rats⟩ ⟨~ cartilage⟩

lath·y·ro·gen \'lath-ə-rə-jən, -ˌjen\ *n* : any of a group of nucleophilic compounds (as β-aminopropionitrile) that tend to cause lathyrism and inhibit the formation of links between chains of collagen

lath·y·ro·gen·ic \ˌlath-ə-rə-'jen-ik\ *adj* : having the capacity to cause lathyrism ⟨a ~ diet⟩ ⟨~ agents⟩

latices *pl of* LATEX

la·tis·si·mus dor·si \lə-'tis-ə-məs-'dȯr-ˌsī\ *n, pl* **la·tis·si·mi dorsi** \-ˌmī-\ : a broad flat superficial muscle of the lower part of the back that originates mostly in a broad aponeurosis attached to the spinous processes of the vertebrae of the lower back, the supraspinal ligament, and the crest of the ilium, that is inserted into the bicipital groove of the humerus, and that extends, adducts, and rotates the arm medially and draws the shoulder downward and backward

la·trine fly \lə-'trēn-\ *n* : a fly of the genus *Fannia* (*F. scalaris*) that breeds in excrement and occas. causes myiasis in humans

lat·ro·dec·tism \ˌla-trə-'dek-ˌtiz-əm\ *n* : poisoning due to the bite of a spider of the genus *Latrodectus*

Lat·ro·dec·tus \-'dek-təs\ *n* : a genus of nearly cosmopolitan spiders of the family Theridiidae that includes most of the well-known venomous spiders (as the black widow, *L. mactans*), that are of medium size and dark or black in color and often marked with red, and that have a large globular usu. glossy abdomen and long and wiry legs

lats *pl of* LAT

LATS *abbr* long-acting thyroid stimulator

lat·tice \'lat-əs\ *n* : a regular geometrical arrangement of points or objects over an area or in space: as **a** : the geometrical arrangement of atoms in a crystal — called also *space lattice* **b** : a geometrical arrangement of fissionable material in a nuclear reactor

latum — see CONDYLOMA LATUM

laud·able pus \'lȯd-ə-bəl-\ *n* : pus discharged freely (as from a wound) and formerly supposed to facilitate the elimination of unhealthy humors from the injured body

lau·dan·i·dine \lȯ-'dan-ə-ˌdēn, -dən\ *n* : a crystalline levorotatory alkaloid $C_{20}H_{25}NO_4$ obtained from opium or by resolution of laudanine into its optically active forms

lau·da·nine \'lȯd-³n-ˌēn\ *n* : a poisonous crystalline optically inactive alkaloid $C_{20}H_{25}NO_4$ obtained from opium

lau·dan·o·sine \lȯ-'dan-ə-ˌsēn, -sən\ *n* : a poisonous crystalline alkaloid $C_{21}H_{27}NO_4$ that is obtained from opium and produces tetanic convulsions

lau·da·num \'lȯd-nəm, -³n-əm\ *n* **1** : any of various formerly used preparations of opium **2** : a tincture of opium

laugh·ing death \'laf-iŋ-\ *n* : KURU

laughing gas *n* : NITROUS OXIDE

laughing sickness *n* : KURU

lau·rate \'lȯr-ˌāt\ *n* : a salt or ester of lauric acid

Lau·rence–Moon–Biedl syndrome \'lȯr-ən(t)s-'mün-'bēd-³l-, 'lär-\ *n* : an inherited disorder affecting esp. males and characterized by obesity, mental retardation, the presence of extra fingers or toes, subnormal development of the genital organs, and sometimes by retinitis pigmentosa

Laurence, John Zachariah (1830–1874), British physician, and **Moon, Robert Charles (1844–1914),** American ophthalmologist. Laurence and Moon were the coauthors of the first description of the Laurence-Moon-Biedl syndrome. Their 1866 description was based on four cases of retinitis pigmentosa occurring in the same family.

Biedl, Artur (1869–1933), German physician. Biedl published a description of the syndrome in 1922 that elaborated upon the earlier description by Laurence and Moon. Biedl is best known for his classic work (1910) on endocrine secretion in which he established that the adrenal cortex is essential for life.

Lau·rer's canal \'laü-rərz-\ *n* : a muscular duct in some trematode worms that arises from the oviduct between the ovary and the omphalomesenteric duct and passes to the dorsal surface

Laurer, Johann Friedrich (1798–1873), German pharmacologist. Laurer described Laurer's canal in an article published in 1830.

lau·ric acid \ˌlȯr-ik-, ˌlär-\ *n* : a crystalline fatty acid $C_{12}H_{24}O_2$ found esp. in coconut oil and used in making soaps, esters, and lauryl alcohol — called also *dodecanoic acid*

lau·ryl \'lȯr-əl, 'lär-\ *n* : the monovalent group $C_{12}H_{25}$– derived from lauryl alcohol — see SODIUM LAURYL SULFATE

lauryl alcohol \ˌlȯr-əl-, ˌlär-\ *n* : a compound $C_{12}H_{26}O$; *also* : a liquid mixture of this and other alcohols used esp. in making detergents (as sodium lauryl sulfate)

LAV \'el-ˌā-'vē\ *n* : HIV-1

¹la·vage \lə-'väzh, *Brit usu* 'lav-ij\ *n* : the act or action of washing; *esp* : the therapeutic washing out of an organ or part ⟨gastric ~⟩

²lavage *vt* **la·vaged; la·vag·ing** **1** : to wash or wash out therapeutically ⟨*lavaged* the bladder with water⟩ ⟨the incisions were *lavaged* with sterile saline⟩ **2** : to perform lavage on ⟨she was intubated, *lavaged,* and received activated charcoal —R. Rasmussen & P. E. McKinney⟩

la·va·tion \lā-'vā-shən\ *n* : the act or an instance of washing or cleansing — **la·va·tion·al** \-shnəl, -shən-³l\ *adj*

lav·en·der oil \'lav-ən-dər-\ *n* : a colorless to yellowish aromatic essential oil obtained from the flowers of various lavenders (esp. *Lavandula officinalis* of the Mediterranean region) and used chiefly as a perfume and also in medicine as a stimulant

Lav·er·a·nia \ˌlav-ə-'rā-nyə\ *n, in some classifications* : a genus of malaria parasites of the family Plasmodiidae that is now usu. included in the genus *Plasmodium*

La·ve·ran \lȧv-rän\, **Charles–Louis–Alphonse (1845–1922),** French physician and parasitologist. Laveran began his career as an army surgeon and for a time taught military medicine. In 1880, while stationed in Algeria, he discovered the plasmodium parasite (*Plasmodium falciparum*) that causes falciparum malaria in humans. Some parasitologists classify the organism in a separate genus, *Laverania,* named in his honor. (Later, Sir Ronald Ross discovered that the malarial vector is the mosquito.) The author of over 600 scientific books and papers, Laveran went on to develop research in tropical medicine and did productive studies of trypanosomiasis, leishmaniasis, and other protozoal diseases and disease agents. From 1897, while at the Pasteur Institute in Paris, he did research on parasitic blood diseases in humans and animals. In 1907 he was awarded the Nobel Prize for Physiology or Medicine, and with the prize money he established the Laboratory of Tropical Diseases at the Institute.

law \\'lȯ\ *n* : a statement of order or relation holding for certain phenomena that so far as is known is invariable under the given conditions

lawn \\'lȯn, 'län\ *n* : a relatively even layer of bacteria covering the surface of a culture medium

law of conservation of energy *n* : CONSERVATION OF ENERGY

law of conservation of matter *n* : CONSERVATION OF MASS

law of constant proportions *n* : LAW OF DEFINITE PROPORTIONS

law of def·i·nite pro·por·tions \\-'def-(ə-)nət-prə-'pȯr-shənz\ *n* : a statement in chemistry: every definite compound always contains the same elements in the same proportions by weight

law of dominance *n* : MENDEL'S LAW 3

law of effect *n* : a statement in psychology: in trial-and-error learning satisfying or successful behavior is repeated whereas unsatisfying or unsuccessful behavior is not

law of gravitation *n* : a statement in physics: any particle in the universe attracts any other particle with a force that is proportional to the product of the masses of the two particles and inversely proportional to the square of the distance between them

law of independent assortment *n* : MENDEL'S LAW 2

law of La·place \\-lä-'pläs\ *n* : a law in physics that in medicine is applied in the physiology of blood flow: under equilibrium conditions the pressure tangent to the circumference of a vessel storing or transmitting fluid equals the product of the pressure across the wall and the radius of the vessel for a sphere and half this for a tube — called also *Laplace's law*

La·place \lá-plás\, **Pierre–Simon (1749–1827),** French astronomer and mathematician. Laplace has often been called the Newton of France. He successfully applied the Newtonian theory of gravitation to the solar system by accounting for all of the observed deviations of the planets from their theoretical orbits. By 1786 he was able to prove that the eccentricities and inclinations of planetary orbits to each other will always remain small, constant, and self-correcting. He also investigated tides, specific heats, capillary action, electricity, and the equilibrium of a rotating fluid mass. By demonstrating that the attractive force of a mass upon a particle (regardless of direction) could be obtained directly by differentiating a single function, he established the mathematical basis for the scientific study of heat, magnetism, and electricity.

law of mass action *n* : a statement in chemistry: the rate of a chemical reaction is directly proportional to the molecular concentrations of the reacting substances

law of multiple proportions *n* : a statement in chemistry: when two elements combine in more than one proportion to form two or more compounds the weights of one element that combine with a given weight of the other element are in the ratios of small whole numbers

law of partial pressures *n* : a statement in physics and chemistry: the component of the total pressure contributed by each ingredient in a mixture of gases or vapors is equal to the pressure that it would exert if alone in the same enclosure — called also *Dalton's law*

law of refraction *n* : a law in physics: in the refraction of radiation at the interface between two isotropic media the incident ray and the corresponding refracted ray are coplanar with the refracting surface at the point of incidence and the ratio of the sine of the angle of incidence to the sine of the angle of refraction is equal to the index of refraction

law of segregation *n* : MENDEL'S LAW 1

law of the minimum *n* : a law in physiology: when a process is conditioned by several factors its rate is limited by the factor present in the minimum

law of thermodynamics *n* **1** : CONSERVATION OF ENERGY — called also *first law of thermodynamics* **2** : a law in physics: mechanical work can be derived from the heat in a body

only when the body is able to communicate with another at a lower temperature and its actual spontaneous processes result in an increase of total entropy — called also *second law of thermodynamics* **3** : a law in physics: at the absolute zero of temperature the entropy of any pure crystalline substance is zero and its derivative with respect to temperature is zero — called also *third law of thermodynamics*

law·ren·ci·um \lȯ-'ren(t)-sē-əm\ *n* : a short-lived radioactive element that is produced artificially from californium — symbol *Lr*; see ELEMENT table

Law·rence \\'lȯr-ən(t)s, 'lär-\, **Ernest Orlando (1901–1958),** American physicist. Lawrence was associated with the University of California, Berkeley, for virtually all of his research career. He was responsible for the establishment of the Radiation Laboratory at Berkeley and was appointed its director in 1936. He first conceived of the cyclotron, a subatomic particle accelerator, in 1929, and in 1939 he was awarded the Nobel Prize for Physics for its invention. Using the cyclotron Lawrence produced radioactive phosphorus and other isotopes for medical use, including iodine for the first therapeutic treatment of hyperthyroidism. In 1961 element 103 was named lawrencium in his honor.

lax \\'laks\ *adj* **1** *of the bowels* : LOOSE 3 **2** : having loose bowels

lax·a·tion \lak-'sā-shən\ *n* : a bowel movement ⟨the danger of absorption of toxic amounts of mercury if ∼ does not occur after taking calomel —*U.S. Dispensatory,* 27th ed.⟩

¹**lax·a·tive** \\'lak-sət-iv\ *adj* **1** : having a tendency to loosen or relax; *specif* : relieving constipation **2** : LAX 2 — **lax·a·tive·ly** *adv*

²**laxative** *n* : a usu. mild laxative drug

lax·i·ty \\'lak-sət-ē\ *n, pl* **-ties** : the quality or state of being loose ⟨a certain ∼ of the bowels⟩ ⟨ligamentous ∼⟩

lay·er \\'lā-ər, 'le(-ə)r\ *n* **1** : one thickness, course, or fold laid or lying over or under another **2** : STRATUM 1 ⟨the outer ∼s of the skin⟩ — **layer** *vb*

layer of Lang·hans \\-'läŋ-ˌhän(t)s\ *n* : CYTOTROPHOBLAST

T. Langhans — see LANGHANS CELL

la·zar \\'laz-ər, 'lā-zər\ *n* : LEPER

Laz·a·rus \\'laz-(ə-)rəs\, Biblical character. Lazarus was a diseased beggar in a parable told by Jesus in the Gospel according to St. Luke. Apparently he was invented only for the purposes of the parable and has no historical basis. During the Middle Ages, however, he acquired the identity of an actual person, becoming in the process St. Lazarus, the patron saint of beggars and lepers.

laz·a·ret·to \ˌlaz-ə-'ret-(ˌ)ō\ *or* **laz·a·ret** \-'ret, -'ret\ *n, pl* **-rettos** *or* **-rets 1** *usu lazaretto* : an institution (as a hospital) for those with contagious diseases **2** : a building or a ship used for detention in quarantine

lazar house *n* : LAZARETTO 1; *esp* : a hospital for lepers

la·zy eye \\'lā-zē-\ *n* : AMBLYOPIA; *also* : an eye affected with amblyopia

lazy–eye blindness *n* : AMBLYOPIA

lb *abbr* pound

LC *abbr* liquid chromatography

L cell \\'el-ˌsel\ *n* : a fibroblast cell of a strain isolated from mice and used esp. in virus research

L chain *n* : LIGHT CHAIN

LCL \ˌel-(ˌ)sē-'el\ *n* : LATERAL COLLATERAL LIGAMENT

LCMV *abbr* lymphocytic choriomeningitis virus

LD *abbr* **1** learning disability; learning disabled **2** lethal dose

LD50 *or* **LD₅₀** \\'el-ˌdē-'fif-tē\ *n* : the amount of a toxic agent (as a poison, virus, or radiation) that is sufficient to kill 50 percent of a population of animals usu. within a certain time — called also *median lethal dose*

LDH *abbr* lactate dehydrogenase; lactic dehydrogenase

LDL \\'el-ˌdē-'el\ *n* : a lipoprotein of blood plasma that is

K
L

\ə\ **abut** \ˈ\ **kitten** \ər\ **further** \a\ **ash** \ā\ **ace** \ä\ **cot, cart**
\aů\ **out** \ch\ **chin** \e\ **bet** \ē\ **easy** \g\ **go** \i\ **hit** \ī\ **ice** \j\ **job**
\ŋ\ **sing** \ō\ **go** \ȯ\ **law** \ȯi\ **boy** \th\ **thin** \th̲\ **the** \ü\ **loot**
\ů\ **foot** \y\ **yet** \zh\ **vision** *See also* Pronunciation Symbols page

composed of a moderate proportion of protein with little tri-glyceride and a high proportion of cholesterol and that is associated with increased probability of developing atherosclerosis — called also *bad cholesterol, beta-lipoprotein, low-density lipoprotein;* compare HDL, VLDL

L–do·pa \ 'el-'dō-pə\ *n* : the levorotatory form of dopa that is obtained esp. from broad beans or prepared synthetically, is converted to dopamine in the brain, and is used in treating Parkinson's disease — called also *levodopa*

LE *abbr* lupus erythematosus

leach \'lēch\ *vt* **1** : to subject to the action of percolating liquid (as water) in order to separate the soluble components **2** : to dissolve out by the action of a percolating liquid ~ *vi* : to pass out or through by percolation — **leach·abil·i·ty** \,lē-chə-'bil-ət-ē\ *n, pl* **-ties** — **leach·able** \'lē-chə-bəl\ *adj*

leach·ate \'lē-,chāt\ *n* : a solution or product obtained by leaching ⟨toxic ~s from improperly managed landfills⟩

¹lead \'lēd\ *n* : a flexible or solid insulated conductor connected to or leading out from an electrical device (as an electroencephalograph)

²lead \'led\ *n, often attrib* **1** : a heavy soft malleable ductile plastic but inelastic bluish white metallic element found mostly in combination and used esp. in pipes, cable sheaths, batteries, solder, and shields against radioactivity — symbol *Pb*; see ELEMENT table **2** : WHITE LEAD **3** : TETRAETHYL LEAD

lead acetate \'led-\ *n* : a poisonous soluble lead salt $PbC_4H_6O_4·3H_2O$ used in medicine esp. formerly as an astringent — called also *sugar of lead*

lead arsenate *n* : an arsenate of lead; *esp* : either of the two salts $PbHAsO_4$ and $Pb_3(AsO_4)_2$ formerly used as insecticides

lead carbonate *n* : a carbonate of lead; *esp* : a poisonous basic salt $Pb_3(OH)_2(CO_3)_2$ that was formerly used as a white pigment in paints, that was a common cause of painter's colic, and that may cause lead poisoning esp. in children who come in contact with or ingest paint from older surfaces which contain it

lead chromate *n* : a chromate of lead; *esp* : CHROME YELLOW

lead dioxide *n* : a poisonous compound PbO_2 used esp. as an oxidizing agent and as an electrode in batteries

lead·ed \'led-əd\ *adj* : affected with lead poisoning ⟨~ miners⟩

lead monoxide \'led-\ *n* : a yellow to brownish red poisonous compound PbO used in rubber manufacture and glassmaking — see LITHARGE, MASSICOT

lead palsy *n* : localized paralysis caused by lead poisoning esp. of the extensor muscles of the forearm resulting in wrist-drop

lead poisoning *n* : chronic intoxication that is produced by the absorption of lead into the system and is characterized esp. by fatigue, abdominal pain, nausea, diarrhea, loss of appetite, anemia, a dark line along the gums, and muscular paralysis or weakness of limbs — called also *plumbism, saturnism*

lead tetraethyl *n* : TETRAETHYL LEAD

leaf \'lēf\ *n* : a thin layer or sheet of tissue ⟨the anterior ~ of the coronary ligament⟩

leaf·let \'lē-flət\ *n* : a leaflike organ, structure, or part ⟨lipid molecules in a bimolecular ~⟩; *esp* : any of the flaps of the biscuspid valve or the tricuspid valve

leaky \'lē-kē\ *adj* : relating to or being a mutant gene that changes the structure of the protein and esp. an enzyme that it determines so that some but not all of its biological activity is lost; *also* : being such a protein with subnormal activity

learn \'lərn\ *vb* **learned** \'lərnd, 'lərnt\ *also* **learnt** \'lərnt\; **learn·ing** *vt* : to acquire (a change in behavior) by learning ~ *vi* : to acquire a behavioral tendency by learning — **learn·er** *n*

learn·ing *n* : the process of acquiring a modification in a behavioral tendency by experience (as exposure to conditioning) in contrast to modifications occurring because of development or a temporary physiological condition (as fatigue)

of the organism; *also* : the modified behavioral tendency itself

learning disability *n* : any of various disorders (as dyslexia or dysgraphia) that interfere with an individual's ability to learn resulting in impaired functioning in verbal language, reasoning, or academic skills (as reading, writing, and mathematics) and are thought to be caused by difficulties in processing and integrating information — **learning disabled** *adj*

least *superlative of* LITTLE

least splanchnic nerve \'lēst-\ *n* : SPLANCHNIC NERVE c

Le·boy·er \lə-bȯi-'ā\ *adj* : of or relating to a method of childbirth designed to reduce trauma for the newborn esp. by avoiding the use of forceps and bright lights in the delivery room and by giving the newborn a warm bath ⟨the ~ technique⟩

Le·boy·er \lə-bwȧ-yā\, **Frédéric** (*b* 1918), French obstetrician. After an early association with the University of Paris clinic, Leboyer devoted himself exclusively to a private practice in obstetrics. A visit to India in 1958 led him to begin questioning Western methods of childbirth. Dissatisfied with modern hospital delivery room methods, he advocated a series of procedures that included dimmed lighting, soft sounds, gentle massaging of the infant, a delayed severing of the umbilical cord, and a warm-water bath. Leboyer first presented his philosophy and methods in book form in 1974. The Leboyer method was received with a wide-ranging mixture of acclaim and criticism. It triggered a number of studies of the mental and emotional development of children delivered by the Leboyer method.

LE cell \'el-'ē-,sel\ *n* : a polymorphonuclear leukocyte that is found esp. in patients with lupus erythematosus, has a characteristic histologic appearance, and has phagocytosed another cell's damaged nucleus that has combined with a specific antibody — called also *lupus erythematosus cell*

Le Cha·te·lier's principle \lə-,shät-əl-'yāz-\ *n* : a statement in physics and chemistry: if the equilibrium of a system is disturbed by a change in one or more of the determining factors (as temperature, pressure, or concentration) the system tends to adjust itself to a new equilibrium by counteracting as far as possible the effect of the change — called also *Le Chatelier's law*

Le Cha·te·lier \lə-shät-əl-yā\, **Henry–Louis (1850–1936)**, French chemist. A professor of chemistry, Le Chatelier was a noted authority on metallurgy, cements, glasses, fuels, and explosives. He first formulated what is now known as Le Chatelier's principle in 1884. His principle made possible the predicting of the effect a change of conditions will have on chemical reaction, and it proved to be invaluable to the chemical industry for the development of the most efficient chemical processes.

lec·i·thal \'les-ə-thəl\ *adj* : having a yolk — often used in combination ⟨iso*lecithal*⟩ ⟨telo*lecithal*⟩

lec·i·thin \'les-ə-thən\ *n* : any of several waxy hygroscopic phospholipids in which phosphatidic acid has formed an ester with choline and which are widely distributed in animals and plants, form colloidal solutions in water, and have emulsifying, wetting, and antioxidant properties; *also* : a mixture of or a substance rich in lecithins — called also *phosphatidylcholine*

lec·i·thin·ase \-thə-,nās, -,nāz\ *n* : PHOSPHOLIPASE

lec·i·tho·pro·tein \'les-ə-thō-'prō-,tēn, -'prōt-ē-ən\ *n* : any of a class of compounds of lecithin or other phosphatide with protein

lec·tin \'lek-tən\ *n* : any of a group of proteins esp. of plants that are not antibodies and do not originate in an immune system but bind specifically to carbohydrate-containing receptors on cell surfaces (as of red blood cells)

¹leech \'lēch\ *n* : any of numerous carnivorous or bloodsucking annelid worms that comprise the class Hirudinea, that typically have a flattened segmented lance-shaped body with well-marked external annulations, a sucker at each end, a mouth within the anterior sucker, and a large stomach with pouches of large capacity at the sides, that are hermaphroditic usu. with direct development, and that occur chiefly in freshwater although a few are marine and some tropical forms are terrestrial — see MEDICINAL LEECH

²**leech** *vt* **1** : to treat as a physician : CURE, HEAL **2** : to bleed by the use of leeches

leech·craft \'lēch-ˌkraft\ *n* : the art of healing : medical knowledge and skill

leech·dom \'lēch-dəm\ *n* : a medical formula or remedy : MEDICINE ⟨∼s without number are listed for every conceivable condition from cancer to demoniacal possession —Harvey Graham⟩

LE factor \ˈel-ˈē-\ *n* : an antibody found in the serum esp. of patients with systemic lupus erythematosus

Le·Fort I \lə-ˈfȯrt-ˈwən\ *n* : an operation for reconstruction of the midface in which the teeth-bearing part of the maxilla is separated from its bony attachments and repositioned

Le Fort \lə-fȯr\, **Léon–Clémont (1829–1893)**, French surgeon. Le Fort served as professor of surgery in Paris and surgeon to the Hôtel Dieu. He published monographs on the resection of the knee, military surgery, and maternity care and a manual of operative medicine.

LeFort III \-ˈthrē\ *n* : an operation for reconstruction of the midface in which the maxilla, nasal bones, and both zygomatic bones are separated from their bony attachments and repositioned

LeFort II \-ˈtü\ *n* : an operation for reconstruction of the midface in which the maxilla and adjacent nasal bones are separated from their bony attachments and repositioned

left \'left\ *adj* : of, relating to, or being the side of the body in which the heart is mostly located; *also* : located nearer to this side than to the right

left atrioventricular valve *n* : MITRAL VALVE

left brain *n* : the left cerebral hemisphere of the human brain esp. when viewed in terms of its predominant thought processes (as analytic and logical thinking) — **left–brained** \'left-ˈbrānd\ *adj*

left colic artery *n* : COLIC ARTERY c

left colic flexure *n* : SPLENIC FLEXURE

left–eyed \'left-ˈīd\ *adj* : using the left eye in preference (as in using a monocular microscope)

left–foot·ed \-ˈfu̇t-əd\ *adj* : stronger or more adept with the left foot (as in kicking a ball)

left gastric artery *n* : GASTRIC ARTERY 1

left gastroepiploic artery *n* : GASTROEPIPLOIC ARTERY b

left–hand \'left-ˈhand, ˈlef-ˈtand\ *adj* **1** : situated on the left **2** : LEFT-HANDED

left hand *n* **1** : the hand on a person's left side **2** : the left side

left–hand·ed \'left-ˈhan-dəd, ˈlef-ˈtan-\ *adj* **1** : using the left hand habitually or more easily than the right **2** : relating to, designed for, or done with the left hand **3** : having a direction contrary to that of movement of the hands of a watch viewed from in front **4** : LEVOROTATORY — **left–handed** *adv*

left–hand·ed·ness \-nəs\ *n* : the quality or state of being left-handed

left heart *n* : the left atrium and ventricle : the half of the heart that receives oxygenated blood from the pulmonary circulation and passes it to the aorta

left lymphatic duct *n* : THORACIC DUCT

left pulmonary artery *n* : PULMONARY ARTERY c

left subcostal vein *n* : SUBCOSTAL VEIN b

leg \'leg, 'lāg\ *n* : a limb of an animal used esp. for supporting the body and for walking: as **a** : either of the two lower human limbs that extend from the top of the thigh to the foot and esp. the part between the knee and the ankle **b** : any of the rather generalized segmental appendages of an arthropod used in walking and crawling

le·gal age \'lē-gəl-\ *n* : the age at which a person enters into full adult legal rights and responsibilities (as of making contracts or wills)

legal blindness *n* : blindness as recognized by law which in most states of the U.S. means that the better eye using the best possible methods of correction has visual acuity of 20/200 or worse or that the visual field is restricted to 20 degrees or less — **le·gal·ly blind** *adj*

legal medicine *n* : FORENSIC MEDICINE

Legg–Cal·vé–Per·thes disease \'leg-ˌkal-ˈvā-ˈpər-ˌtēz-\ *n* : osteochondritis affecting the bony knob at the upper end of the femur — called also *Legg-Perthes disease, Perthes disease*

Legg, Arthur Thornton (1874–1939), American orthopedic surgeon. Legg published the first description of Legg=Calvé-Perthes disease in February 1910. He is also remembered for introducing an operation for correcting weakness of the abductor muscles of the thigh in cases of infantile paralysis.

Cal·vé \kál-vā\, **Jacques (1875–1954)**, French surgeon. Calvé published independently a description of Legg-Calvé=Perthes disease in July 1910.

Per·thes \'per-(ˌ)tes\, **Georg Clemens (1869–1927)**, German surgeon. Perthes published his description of Legg=Calvé-Perthes disease in October 1910. A pioneer in radiotherapy, he studied the biological effects of X-ray treatment in surgery. He used deep X-ray therapy for the first time in 1903.

leg·ged \'leg-əd, 'lāg-, *Brit usu* 'legd\ *adj* : having a leg or legs esp. of a specified kind or number — often used in combination ⟨a four-*legged* animal⟩

Legg–Perthes disease *n* : LEGG-CALVÉ-PERTHES DISEASE

leg·he·mo·glo·bin *or chiefly Brit* **leg·hae·mo·glo·bin** \'leg-ˈhē-mə-ˌglō-bən\ *n* : a plant hemoglobin found in the root nodules of legumes and reported to function as an oxygen-carrying pigment in symbiotic nitrogen fixation

le·gion·el·la \ˌlē-jə-ˈnel-ə\ *n* **1** *cap* : a genus of gram-negative rod-shaped bacteria (family Legionellaceae) that includes the causative agent (*L. pneumophila*) of Legionnaires' disease **2** *pl* **-lae** \-ˌē\ *also* **-las** : a bacterium of the genus *Legionella*

le·gion·el·lo·sis \ˌlē-jə-ˌnel-ˈō-səs\ *n* : LEGIONNAIRES' DISEASE

Le·gion·naires' bacillus \ˌlē-jə-ˈna(ə)rz-, -ˈne(ə)rz-\ *n* : a bacterium of the genus *Legionella* (*L. pneumophila*) that causes Legionnaires' disease

Legionnaires' disease *also* **Legionnaire's disease** *n* : pneumonia that is caused by a bacterium of the genus *Legionella* (*L. pneumophila*), that is characterized by symptoms resembling influenza (as malaise, headache, and muscular aches) followed by high fever, cough, diarrhea, lobar pneumonia, and mental confusion, and that may be fatal esp. in elderly and immunocompromised individuals — see PONTIAC FEVER

le·gume \'leg-ˌyüm, li-ˈgyüm\ *n* **1** : the fruit or seed of leguminous plants (as peas or beans) used for food **2** : any plant of the family Leguminosae

le·gu·min \li-ˈgyü-mən\ *n* : a globulin found as a characteristic constituent of the seeds of leguminous plants

Le·gu·mi·no·sae \li-ˌgyü-mə-ˈnō-(ˌ)sē\ *n pl* : a large family of dicotyledonous herbs, shrubs, and trees having fruits that are legumes or loments, bearing nodules on the roots that contain nitrogen-fixing bacteria, and including important food and forage plants (as peas, beans, or clovers) — **le·gu·mi·nous** \li-ˈgyü-mə-nəs, le-\ *adj*

leio·myo·blas·to·ma \ˌlī-ō-ˌmī-ō-blas-ˈtō-mə\ *n, pl* **-mas** *also* **-ma·ta** \-mət-ə\ : LEIOMYOMA; *esp* : one resembling epithelium

leio·my·o·ma \ˌlī-ō-mī-ˈō-mə\ *n, pl* **-mas** *also* **-ma·ta** \-mət-ə\ : a benign tumor (as a fibroid) consisting of smooth muscle fibers — **leio·my·o·ma·tous** \-mət-əs\ *adj*

leio·myo·sar·co·ma \ˌlī-ō-ˌmī-ō-sär-ˈkō-mə\ *n, pl* **-mas** *also* **-ma·ta** \-mət-ə\ : a sarcoma composed in part of smooth muscle cells

---

\ə\ abut \ˈə\ kitten \ər\ further \a\ ash \ā\ ace \ä\ cot, cart
\au̇\ out \ch\ chin \e\ bet \ē\ easy \g\ go \i\ hit \ī\ ice \j\ job
\ŋ\ sing \ō\ go \ȯ\ law \ȯi\ boy \th\ thin \th\ the \ü\ loot
\u̇\ foot \y\ yet \zh\ vision *See also* Pronunciation Symbols page

K
L

lei·ot·ri·chous \lī-'ä-trə-kəs\ *adj* : having straight smooth hair

Leish·man body \'lēsh-mən-\ *n* : LEISHMAN-DONOVAN BODY

Leish·man–Don·o·van body \-'dän-ə-vən-\ *n* : a protozoan of the genus *Leishmania* (esp. *L. donovani*) in its nonmotile stage that is found esp. in cells of the skin, spleen, and liver of individuals affected with leishmaniasis and esp. kala-azar — compare DONOVAN BODY

Leishman, Sir William Boog (1865–1926), British bacteriologist. Leishman is famous for his work on kala-azar and antityphoid inoculation. His researches into tropical diseases began when he was with the British Army Medical Service in India. In 1900 he detected the parasite that causes kala-azar. His discovery was confirmed three years later by Charles Donovan. In that year, 1903, Sir Ronald Ross introduced the term *leishmania*. Leishman continued to work on kala-azar and other tropical diseases and by 1913 had perfected the protective vaccine against typhoid fever. During World War I he concentrated on the diseases resulting from trench warfare. He also spent much time researching the parasite of tick fever.

Donovan, Charles (1863–1951), British surgeon. A surgeon in the Indian Medical Service, Donovan made significant contributions to tropical medicine as a result of his service in India. He is known mainly for his discovery of the causative organism of kala-azar. It was first discovered in 1900 by Sir William Leishman, who tentatively identified it as a trypanosome in 1903. In the same year Donovan independently discovered the same organism. In 1905 he discovered the Donovan body, the causative agent of granuloma inguinale.

leish·man·ia \lēsh-'man-ē-ə, -'mān-\ *n* **1** *cap* : a genus of kinetoplastid flagellate protozoans of the family Trypanosomatidae that are parasitic in the tissues of vertebrates, are transmitted by sand flies (genera *Phlebotomus* and *Lutzomyia*), occur parasitically as a minute ovoid or spherical nonflagellated body with a definite kinetoplast and usu. an intracellular axoneme, and include one (*L. donovani*) causing kala-azar and another (*L. tropica*) causing oriental sore **2** : any protozoan of the genus *Leishmania; broadly* : any protozoan of the family Trypanosomatidae having the typical intracellular form of a leishmania — **leish·man·ial** \-ē-əl\ *adj*

leish·man·i·a·sis \ˌlēsh-mə-'nī-ə-səs\ *n, pl* **-a·ses** \-ˌsēz\ : infection with or disease (as kala-azar or oriental sore) caused by leishmanias

leish·man·i·form \ˌlēsh-'man-ə-ˌfȯrm\ *adj* : resembling a leishmania

leish·man·i·o·sis \ˌlēsh-mən-ē-'ō-səs\ *n, pl* **-o·ses** \-ˌsēz\ : LEISHMANIASIS

Lem·nian earth \'lem-nē-ən-'ərth\ *n* : a gray to yellow or red clay obtained from the Greek island of Lemnos and formerly used in medicine as an adsorbent and protective

lem·nis·cus \lem-'nis-kəs\ *n, pl* **-nis·ci** \-'nis-ˌ(k)ī, -'nis-ˌkē\ : a band of fibers and esp. nerve fibers — called also *fillet;* see LATERAL LEMNISCUS, MEDIAL LEMNISCUS — **lem·nis·cal** \-kəl\ *adj*

lem·on \'lem-ən\ *n* : an acid fruit that contains citric acid and vitamin C, is botanically a many-seeded pale yellow oblong berry, and is produced by a small thorny tree of the genus *Citrus* (*C. limon*); *also* : this tree — **lemon** *adj*

lemon balm *n* : a bushy perennial Old World mint of the genus *Melissa* (*M. officinalis*) often cultivated for its fragrant lemon-flavored leaves and tops that have been used to make a diaphoretic tea

lemon oil *n* : a fragrant yellow essential oil obtained from the peel of lemons usu. by expression and used chiefly as a flavoring agent (as in medicinal preparations) and in perfumes

length·en·ing reaction \'leŋ(k)th-(ə-)niŋ-, 'len(t)th-\ *n* : reflex relaxation of a muscle when it is subjected to excessive and vigorous stretching

length–height index \'leŋ(k)th-'hīt-, 'len(t)th-\ *n* : the ratio of the height of the skull esp. as measured between basion and bregma to its length

¹len·i·tive \'len-ət-iv\ *adj* : alleviating pain or harshness

²lenitive *n* : a lenitive medicine or application

Len·nox–Gas·taut syndrome \'len-əks-gas-'tō-\ *n* : an epileptic syndrome esp. of young children that is marked by tonic, atonic, and myoclonic seizures and by atypical absence seizures, that is associated with mental retardation, that is prob. caused by various forms of brain damage (as from cerebral hemorrhage, encephalitis, or developmental or metabolic disorder), and that is characterized between seizures by an EEG having a slow spike and wave pattern

Lennox, William Gordon (1884–1960), American neurologist. Lennox served for many years on the neurology faculty at Harvard University Medical School. Concurrently he was on the staff of Boston's Children's Hospital, serving as chief of the Seizure Division from 1947. In 1939 he organized the National Epilepsy League, a lay organization devoted to combating societal discrimination against epileptics. He devoted his career to researching epilepsy and migraine, focusing on such topics as blood chemistry, cerebral circulation, the electrical activity of the brain, and metabolism. With Frederic A. Gibbs he demonstrated the value of electroencephalography in the diagnosis and treatment of epilepsy. He is also credited with establishing the effectiveness of trimethadione in the treatment of absence seizures in children. He published numerous books and articles on epilepsy, including *Epilepsy and Related Disorders* (1960), in which he described Lennox-Gastaut syndrome.

Gas·taut \gȧs-tō\, **Henri Jean–Pascal (1915–1995),** French neurologist. Gastaut served on the medical faculty of Marseilles University, eventually becoming its dean. He also acted as chief neurobiologist for public hospitals in Marseilles. From the early 1960s he was director of the Regional Center for Epileptic Children and director of the neurobiological research unit at the National Institutes of Health. His research centered on electroencephalography and epilepsy. The author of many books, monographs, and articles, he published the first description of what is now known as Lennox-Gastaut syndrome in 1957 in an article coauthored with M. Vigoroux, C. Trevisan, and H. Regis.

lens *also* **lense** \'lenz\ *n* **1** : a curved piece of glass or plastic used singly or combined in eyeglasses or an optical instrument (as a microscope) for forming an image by focusing rays of light **2** : a device for directing or focusing radiation other than light (as sound waves, radio microwaves, or electrons) **3** : a highly transparent biconvex lens-shaped or nearly spherical body in the eye that focuses light rays entering the eye typically onto the retina, lies immediately behind the pupil, is made up of slender curved rod-shaped ectodermal cells in concentric lamellae surrounded by a tenuous mesoblastic capsule, and alters its focal length by becoming more or less spherical in response to the action of the ciliary muscle on a peripheral suspensory ligament — **lensed** *adj* — **lens·less** *adj*

lens·om·e·ter \len-'zäm-ət-ər\ *n* : an instrument used to determine the optical properties (as the focal length and axis) of ophthalmic lenses

lens placode *n* : an ectodermal placode from which the lens of the embryonic eye develops

Len·te insulin \'len-tā-\ *n* : INSULIN ZINC SUSPENSION

len·ti·co·nus \ˌlen-tə-'kō-nəs\ *n* : a rare abnormal and usu. congenital condition of the lens of the eye in which the surface is conical esp. on the posterior side

len·tic·u·lar \len-'tik-yə-lər\ *adj* **1** : having the shape of a double-convex lens **2** : of or relating to a lens esp. of the eye **3** : relating to or being the lentiform nucleus of the brain

lenticular ganglion *n* : CILIARY GANGLION

lenticular nucleus *n* : LENTIFORM NUCLEUS

lenticular process *n* : the tip of the long process of the incus which articulates with the stapes

len·tic·u·lo·stri·ate artery \(ˌ)len-ˌtik-yə-lō-'strī-ˌāt-\ *n* : a branch of the middle cerebral artery supplying the corpus striatum

len·ti·form \\'len-ti-ˌfȯrm\ *adj* : LENTICULAR

lentiform nucleus *n* : the one of the four basal ganglia in each cerebral hemisphere that comprises the larger and external nucleus of the corpus striatum including the outer reddish putamen and two inner pale yellow globular masses constituting the globus pallidus — called also *lenticular nucleus*

len·tig·i·no·sis \(ˌ)len-ˌtij-ə-'nō-səs\ *n* : a condition marked by the presence of numerous lentigines

len·ti·go \len-'tī-(ˌ)gō, -'tē-\ *n, pl* **len·tig·i·nes** \len-'tij-ə-ˌnēz\ **1** : a small melanotic spot in the skin in which the formation of pigment is unrelated to exposure to sunlight and which is potentially malignant; *esp* : NEVUS — compare FRECKLE **2** : FRECKLE

lentigo ma·lig·na \-mə-'lig-nə\ *n* : a precancerous lesion on the skin esp. in areas exposed to the sun (as the face) that is flat, mottled, and brownish with an irregular outline and grows slowly over a period of years

lentigo se·nil·is \-sə-'nil-əs\ *n* : AGE SPOTS

len·ti·vi·rus \'len-tə-ˌvī-rəs\ *n* **1** *cap* : a genus of single-stranded RNA viruses of the family *Retroviridae* that include SIV and the causative agents of AIDS, equine infectious anemia, and ovine progressive pneumonia **2** : any of the genus *Lentivirus* of the family *Retroviridae* — **len·ti·vi·ral** \-rəl\ *adj*

le·o·nine \'lē-ə-ˌnīn\ *adj* : of or relating to leprotic leontiasis

le·on·ti·a·sis \ˌlē-ən-'tī-ə-səs\ *n, pl* **-a·ses** \-ˌsēz\ : leprosy affecting the flesh of the face and giving it an appearance suggestive of a lion

leontiasis os·sea \-'äs-ē-ə\ *n* : an overgrowth of the bones of the head producing enlargement and distortion of the face

lep·er \'lep-ər\ *n* : an individual affected with leprosy

LE phenomenon \'el-'ē-\ *n* : the process which a white blood cell undergoes in becoming an LE cell

lep·i·dop·tera \ˌlep-ə-'däp-tə-rə\ *n pl* **1** *cap* : a large order of insects comprising the butterflies, moths, and skippers that as adults have four broad or lanceolate wings usu. covered with overlapping and often brightly colored scales and that as larvae are caterpillars **2** : insects of the order Lepidoptera — **lep·i·dop·ter·an** \-rən\ *n or adj* — **lep·i·dop·ter·ous** \-tə-rəs\ *adj*

lep·o·thrix \'lep-ə-ˌthriks\ *n, pl* **lepothrixes** *also* **le·pot·ri·ches** \lə-'pä-trə-ˌkēz\ : TRICHOMYCOSIS

lep·ra \'lep-rə\ *n* : LEPROSY

lepra reaction *n* : one of the acute episodes of chills and fever, malaise, and skin eruption occurring in the chronic course of leprosy

lep·re·chaun·ism \'lep-rə-ˌkän-ˌiz-əm, -ˌkȯn-\ *n* : a rare inherited disorder characterized by mental and physical retardation, by endocrine disorders, by hirsutism, and esp. by a facies marked by large wide-set eyes and large low-set ears

lep·rid \'lep-rəd\ *n* : a skin lesion characteristic of neural leprosy

lep·ro·lin \'lep-rə-ˌlin\ *n* : LEPROMIN

lep·rol·o·gist \le-'präl-ə-jəst\ *n* : a specialist in leprology

lep·rol·o·gy \-jē\ *n, pl* **-gies** : the study of leprosy and its treatment

lep·ro·ma \le-'prō-mə\ *n, pl* **-mas** *also* **-ma·ta** \-mət-ə\ : a nodular lesion of leprosy

le·pro·ma·tous \lə-'präm-ət-əs, -'prō-mət-\ *adj* : of, relating to, characterized by, or affected with lepromas or lepromatous leprosy \⟨~ patients⟩ ⟨the ~ type of leprosy⟩

lepromatous leprosy *n* : the one of the two major forms of leprosy that is characterized by the formation of lepromas, the presence of numerous Hansen's bacilli in the lesions, and a negative skin reaction to lepromin and that remains infectious to others until treated — compare TUBERCULOID LEPROSY

lep·ro·min \le-'prō-mən\ *n* : an extract of human leprous tissue used in a skin test for leprosy infection — called also *leprolin*

lep·ro·pho·bia \ˌlep-rə-'fō-bē-ə\ *n* : a pathological fear of leprosy that may be expressed as a delusion that one is actually suffering from leprosy

lep·ro·sar·i·um \ˌlep-rə-'ser-ē-əm\ *n, pl* **-i·ums** *or* **-ia** \-ē-ə\ : a hospital for leprosy patients

lep·ro·ser·ie *also* **lep·ro·sery** \'lep-rə-ˌser-ē\ *n, pl* **-ser·ies** : LEPROSARIUM

lep·ro·stat·ic \ˌlep-rə-'stat-ik\ *n* : an agent that inhibits the growth of Hansen's bacillus

lep·ro·sy \'lep-rə-sē\ *n, pl* **-sies** : a chronic disease caused by infection with an acid-fast bacillus of the genus *Mycobacterium* (*M. leprae*) and characterized by the formation of nodules on the surface of the body and esp. on the face or by the appearance of tuberculoid macules on the skin that enlarge and spread and are accompanied by loss of sensation followed sooner or later in both types if not treated by involvement of nerves with eventual paralysis, wasting of muscle, and production of deformities and mutilations — called also *hansenosis, Hansen's disease, lepra;* see LEPROMATOUS LEPROSY, TUBERCULOID LEPROSY

lep·rot·ic \le-'prät-ik\ *adj* : of, caused by, or infected with leprosy ⟨~ lesions⟩

lep·rous \'lep-rəs\ *adj* **1** : infected with leprosy **2** : of, relating to, or associated with leprosy or a leper ⟨~ neuritis⟩

lep·tan·dra \lep-'tan-drə\ *n, often cap* : CULVER'S ROOT 2

lep·ta·zol \'lep-tə-ˌzȯl, -ˌzōl\ *n, chiefly Brit* : PENTYLENETETRAZOL

lep·tene \'lep-ˌtēn\ *adj* : having a high, a narrow, or a high narrow forehead with an upper facial index of 55.0 to 59.9 as measured on the skull and of 53.0 to 56.9 on the living head

lepti *pl of* LEPTUS

lep·tin \'lep-tən\ *n* : a peptide hormone that is produced by fat cells and plays a role in body weight regulation by acting on the hypothalamus to suppress appetite and burn fat stored in adipose tissue

lep·to \'lep-ˌtō\ *n* : LEPTOSPIROSIS

lep·to·ce·pha·lia \ˌlep-tō-se-'fā-lē-ə, *Brit also* -ke-'fā-\ *n* : LEPTOCEPHALY

lep·to·ceph·a·ly \ˌlep-tō-'sef-ə-lē, *Brit also* -'kef-\ *n, pl* **-lies** : abnormal narrowness and tallness of the skull

lep·to·men·in·ge·al \ˌlep-tō-ˌmen-ən-'jē-əl\ *adj* : of or involving the leptomeninges ⟨~ infection⟩

lep·to·me·nin·ges \-mə-'nin-(ˌ)jēz\ *n pl* : the pia mater and the arachnoid considered together as investing the brain and spinal cord — called also *leptomeninx, pia-arachnoid*

lep·to·men·in·gi·tis \-ˌmen-ən-'jīt-əs\ *n, pl* **-git·i·des** \-'jit-ə-ˌdēz\ : inflammation of the pia mater and the arachnoid membrane

lep·to·me·ninx \-'mē-ˌniŋ(k)s, -'men-iŋ(k)s\ *n* : LEPTOMENINGES

¹lep·tom·o·nad \lep-'täm-ə-ˌnad\ *adj* : of or relating to the genus *Leptomonas*

²leptomonad *n* : LEPTOMONAS 2

lep·tom·o·nas \lep-'täm-ə-nəs\ *n* **1** *cap* : a genus of flagellate protozoans of the family Trypanosomatidae that are parasites esp. of the digestive tract of insects and that occur as elongated flagellates with a single anterior flagellum and no undulating membrane **2** *pl* **leptomonas a** : any flagellate protozoan of the genus *Leptomonas* **b** : PROMASTIGOTE

lep·to·ne·ma \ˌlep-tə-'nē-mə\ *n* : a chromatin thread or chromosome at the leptotene stage at meiotic prophase

lep·to·phos \'lep-tō-ˌfäs\ *n* : an organophosphorus pesticide $C_{12}H_{10}BrCl_2O_2PS$ that has been associated with the occurrence of neurological damage in individuals exposed to it esp. in the early and mid 1970s

lep·to·pro·so·pic \ˌlep-tō-prə-'sō-pik, -'säp-ik\ *adj* : having a long, a narrow, or a long narrow face with a facial index of 88.0 to 92.9 as measured on the living head and of 90.0 to 94.9 on the skull

lep·tor·rhine \'lep-tə-ˌrīn\ *adj* : having a long narrow nose with a nasal index of less than 47 on the skull or of less than 70 on the living head

---

\ə\ abut \ᵊ\ kitten \ər\ further \a\ ash \ā\ ace \ä\ cot, cart
\au̇\ out \ch\ chin \e\ bet \ē\ easy \g\ go \i\ hit \ī\ ice \j\ job
\ŋ\ sing \ō\ go \ȯ\ law \ȯi\ boy \th\ thin \t̲h̲\ the \ü\ loot
\u̇\ foot \y\ yet \zh\ vision *See also* Pronunciation Symbols page

lep·to·scope \'lep-tə-ˌskōp\ n : an optical instrument used to determine the thickness of plasma membranes

¹**lep·to·some** \-ˌsōm\ *or* **lep·to·som·ic** \ˌlep-tə-'sō-mik\ *also* **lep·to·so·mat·ic** \ˌlep-tə-sō-'mat-ik\ *adj* : ASTHENIC 2, ECTO-MORPHIC

²**leptosome** n : an ectomorphic individual

lep·to·spi·ra \ˌlep-tō-'spī-rə\ n **1** *cap* : a genus of extremely slender aerobic spirochetes (family Leptospiraceae) that are free-living or parasitic in mammals and include a number of important pathogens (as *L. icterohaemorrhagiae* of Weil's disease or *L. canicola* of canicola fever) **2** *pl* **-ra** *or* **-ras** *or* **-rae** \-rē\ : LEPTOSPIRE

lep·to·spi·ral \-'spī-rəl\ *adj* : of, relating to, caused by, or involving leptospires ⟨∼ infection⟩ ⟨∼ disease⟩

leptospiral jaundice n : WEIL'S DISEASE

lep·to·spire \'lep-tə-ˌspī(ə)r\ n : any spirochete of the genus *Leptospira* — called also *leptospira*

lep·to·spi·ri·cid·al \ˌlep-tə-ˌspī-rə-'sīd-ᵊl\ *adj* : destructive to leptospires

lep·to·spi·ro·sis \ˌlep-tə-spī-'rō-səs\ n, pl **-ro·ses** \-ˌsēz\ : any of several diseases of humans and domestic animals (as cattle and dogs) that are caused by infection with spirochetes of the genus *Leptospira* — called also *lepto;* see STUTTGART DISEASE, WEIL'S DISEASE

lep·to·spir·uria \ˌlep-tə-spīr-'(y)ùr-ē-ə\ n : a condition marked by the presence of leptospires in the urine

lep·to·staph·y·line \-'staf-ə-ˌlīn, -lən\ *adj* : having a palate which is narrow and high with a palatal index of less than 80 on the skull

¹**lep·to·tene** \'lep-tə-ˌtēn\ n : a stage of meiotic prophase immediately preceding synapsis in which the chromosomes appear as fine discrete threads

²**leptotene** *also* **lep·to·te·nic** \ˌlep-tə-'tē-nik\ *adj* : relating to or being the leptotene of meiotic prophase

lep·to·thrix \'lep-tə-ˌthriks\ n **1** *cap* : a genus of sheathed filamentous bacteria of uncertain taxonomic affiliation that often have the sheath encrusted with oxides of iron or manganese — see LEPTOTRICHIA **2** *pl* **lep·to·trich·ia** \ˌlep-tə-'trik-ē-ə\ *also* **lep·tot·ri·ches** \lep-'tä-trə-ˌkēz\ : any bacterium of the genus *Leptothrix*

Lep·to·trich·ia \ˌlep-tə-'trik-ē-ə\ n : a genus of long filamentous gram-negative anaerobic rod bacteria of the family Bacteroidaceae that are sometimes placed in the genus *Leptothrix*

lep·tus \'lep-təs\ n, pl **leptuses** *also* **lep·ti** \-ˌtī\ *often cap* : any of several 6-legged larval mites — often used as if the name of a genus

Le·riche's syndrome \lə-'rēsh-əz-\ n : occlusion of the descending continuation of the aorta in the abdomen typically resulting in impotence, the absence of a pulse in the femoral arteries, and weakness and numbness in the lower back, buttocks, hips, thighs, and calves

Le·riche \lə-rēsh\, **René (1879–1955),** French surgeon. Leriche was a pioneer in neurological and vascular surgery. He is celebrated for devising several new operations. He introduced such surgical procedures as surgical removal of the sheath of an artery containing sympathetic nerve fibers for the relief of paresthesia and vasomotor disturbances in 1916, excision of an artery for arterial thrombosis in 1937, and obliteration of the abdominal aorta in 1940.

¹**les·bi·an** \'lez-bē-ən\ *adj* : of or relating to homosexuality between females

²**lesbian** n : a female homosexual

les·bi·an·ism \'lez-bē-ə-ˌniz-əm\ n : female homosexuality

Lesch–Ny·han syndrome \'lesh-'nī-ən-\ n : a rare and usu. fatal genetic disorder of male children that is inherited as an X-linked recessive trait and is characterized by hyperuricemia, mental retardation, spasticity, compulsive biting of the lips and fingers, and a deficiency of hypoxanthine-guanine phosphoribosyltransferase — called also *Lesch-Nyhan disease*

Lesch, Michael (b 1939), and **Nyhan, William Leo (b 1926),** American pediatricians. Nyhan held the position of professor of pediatrics at several medical schools, including

Johns Hopkins. He had a major interest in the disorders of amino acid metabolism and routinely analyzed blood and urine for amino acids. The urine of a pair of patients, two brothers, was found to contain urate crystals. In addition, the brothers were suffering from an obvious but unknown neurological disorder. Nyhan, aided by Lesch, a student research assistant, began investigating urate metabolism and the characteristics of the previously unrecognized genetic disorder exhibited by their two cases. Lesch published a description of the Lesch-Nyhan syndrome in 1964. This report laid the groundwork for the discovery in 1967 of the absence of hypoxanthine-guanine phosphoribosyltransferase in children affected with the syndrome.

¹**le·sion** \'lē-zhən\ n : an abnormal change in structure of an organ or part due to injury or disease; *esp* : one that is circumscribed and well defined — **le·sioned** \-zhənd\ *adj*

²**lesion** vt : to produce lesions in (as an animal's brain)

less, lesser *comparative of* LITTLE

less·er cornu \'les-ər-\ n : CERATOHYAL

lesser curvature n : the boundary of the stomach that in humans forms a relatively short concave curve on the right from the opening for the esophagus to the opening into the duodenum — compare GREATER CURVATURE

lesser housefly n, *chiefly Brit* : LITTLE HOUSEFLY

lesser multangular n : TRAPEZOID — called also *lesser multangular bone*

lesser occipital nerve n : OCCIPITAL NERVE b

lesser omentum n : a part of the peritoneum attached to the liver and to the lesser curvature of the stomach and supporting the hepatic vessels — compare GREATER OMENTUM

lesser petrosal nerve n : the continuation of the tympanic nerve beyond the inferior ganglion of the glossopharyngeal nerve that passes into the cranial cavity through the petrosal bone and out again to terminate in the otic ganglion which it supplies with preganglionic parasympathetic fibers

lesser sciatic foramen n : SCIATIC FORAMEN b

lesser sciatic notch n : SCIATIC NOTCH b

lesser splanchnic nerve n : SPLANCHNIC NERVE b

lesser stomach worm n : a small threadlike nematode worm of the genus *Ostertagia* (*O. ostertagi*) often present in immense numbers in the pyloric part of a sheep's stomach

lesser trochanter n : TROCHANTER b

lesser tubercle n : a prominence on the upper anterior part of the end of the humerus that serves as the insertion for the subscapularis — compare GREATER TUBERCLE

lesser wing n : an anterior triangular process on each side of the sphenoid bone in front of and much smaller than the corresponding greater wing — compare ORBITOSPHENOID

let·down \'let-ˌdaùn\ n : a physiological response of a lactating mammal to suckling and allied stimuli whereby increased intramammary pressure forces previously secreted milk from the acini and finer tubules into the main collecting ducts from where it can be drawn through the nipple

let down \-'daùn\ vt : to release (formed milk) within the mammary gland or udder

¹**le·thal** \'lē-thəl\ *adj* : of, relating to, or causing death ⟨a ∼ injury⟩; *also* : capable of causing death ⟨∼ chemicals⟩ ⟨a ∼ dose⟩ — **le·thal·i·ty** \lē-'thal-ət-ē\ n, pl **-ties** — **le·thal·ly** *adv*

²**lethal** n **1** : an abnormality of genetic origin causing the death of the organism possessing it usu. before maturity **2** : LETHAL GENE

lethal gene n : a gene that in some (as homozygous) conditions may prevent development or cause the death of an organism or its germ cells — called also *lethal factor, lethal mutant, lethal mutation*

lethargica — see ENCEPHALITIS LETHARGICA

le·thar·gic encephalitis \lə-'thär-jik-, le-\ n : ENCEPHALITIS LETHARGICA

leth·ar·gy \'leth-ər-jē\ n, pl **-gies** **1** : abnormal drowsiness **2** : the quality or state of being lazy, sluggish, or indifferent — **lethargic** *adj*

Let·ter·er–Si·we disease \'let-ər-ər-'sē-və-\ n : an acute disease of children characterized by fever, hemorrhages, and other evidences of a disturbance in the reticuloendothelial system and by severe bone lesions esp. of the skull

Letterer, Erich (1895–1982), German physician. Letterer first described Letterer-Siwe disease in 1924. The author of several textbooks on pathology, he described the disease from the viewpoint of a pathologist.

Siwe, Sture August (1897–1966), Swedish pediatrician. Siwe presented another, independent description of Letterer-Siwe disease in 1933, this time from the clinical point of view.

Leu *abbr* leucine; leucyl

leucemia *or chiefly Brit* **leucaemia** *var of* LEUKEMIA

leu·cine \'lü-₁sēn\ *n* : a white crystalline essential amino acid $C_6H_{13}NO_2$ obtained by the hydrolysis of most dietary proteins — abbr. *Leu*

leucine aminopeptidase *n* : an aminopeptidase that cleaves terminal amino acid residues and esp. leucine from protein chains, is found in all bodily tissues, and is increased in the serum in some conditions or diseases (as pancreatic carcinoma)

leu·cine–en·keph·a·lin \'lü-₁sēn-en-'kef-ə-lən\ *n* : a pentapeptide having a terminal leucine residue that is one of the two enkephalins occurring naturally in the brain — called also *Leu-enkephalin*

leu·ci·no·sis \₁lü-sə-'nō-səs\ *n, pl* **-no·ses** \-₁sēz\ *or* **-no·sis·es** : a condition characterized by an abnormally high concentration of leucine in bodily tissues and the presence of leucine in the urine

leu·cin·uria \₁lü-sə-'n(y)ùr-ē-ə\ *n* : the presence of leucine in the urine

Each boldface word in the list below is a chiefly British variant of the word to its right in small capitals.

leucoagglu-tinin	LEUKOAGGLU-TININ	leuconychia	LEUKONYCHIA
leucoblast	LEUKOBLAST	leucopenia	LEUKOPENIA
leucoblastosis	LEUKOBLASTO-SIS	leucopenic	LEUKOPENIC
		leucoplakia	LEUKOPLAKIA
leucocidin	LEUKOCIDIN	leucoplakic	LEUKOPLAKIC
leucocyte	LEUKOCYTE	leucopoiesis	LEUKOPOIESIS
leucocythae-mia	LEUKOCYTHE-MIA	leucopoietic	LEUKOPOIETIC
		leucorrhoea	LEUKORRHEA
leucocytic	LEUKOCYTIC	leucorrhoeal	LEUKORRHEAL
leucocytogene-sis	LEUKOCYTO-GENESIS	leucosarcoma	LEUKOSARCO-MA
leucocytoid	LEUKOCYTOID	leucosarcoma-tosis	LEUKOSARCO-MATOSIS
leucocytosis	LEUKOCYTOSIS	leucosis	LEUKOSIS
leucocytotic	LEUKOCYTOTIC	leucotactic	LEUKOTACTIC
leucoderma	LEUKODERMA	leucotactically	LEUKOTACTI-CALLY
leucodystrophy	LEUKODYS-TROPHY	leucotaxine	LEUKOTAXINE
leucoencephal-alitis	LEUKOENCEPH-ALITIS	leucotaxis	LEUKOTAXIS
		leucotic	LEUKOTIC
leucoencepha-lopathy	LEUKOENCEPH-ALOPATHY	leucotome	LEUKOTOME
		leucotomy	LEUKOTOMY
leucokeratosis	LEUKOKERA-TOSIS	leucotoxin	LEUKOTOXIN
		leucotrichia	LEUKOTRICHIA
leucoma	LEUKOMA	leucovirus	LEUKOVIRUS
leucomaine	LEUKOMAINE		

leu·co·cy·to·zo·on \₁lü-kō-₁sīt-ə-'zō-₁än, -ən\ *n* **1** *cap* : a genus of sporozoans parasitic in birds — see HAEMOPROTEI-DAE **2** *pl* **-zoa** \-'zō-ə\ : any sporozoan of the genus *Leucocytozoon*

leu·co·cy·to·zoo·no·sis \-₁zō-ə-'nō-səs\ *n, pl* **-no·ses** \-₁sēz\ : a disease caused by infection of birds (as turkeys, chickens, ducks, and geese) by sporozoans of the genus *Leucocytozoon* transmitted by arthropods (as blackflies)

leu·co·nos·toc \₁lü-kə-'näs-₁täk\ *n* **1** *cap* : a genus of gram-positive nonmotile coccal bacteria that do not form spores, usu. occur in pairs and chains, and are facultative anaerobes and that include several pests in sugar refineries that produce slime in sugar solutions **2** : any bacterium of the genus *Leuconostoc*

leu·cov·o·rin \lü-'käv-ə-rən\ *n* : a metabolically active form of folic acid that has been used in cancer therapy to protect normal cells against methotrexate — called also *citrovorum factor, folinic acid*

leu·cyl \'lü-səl, -₁sil\ *n* : the amino acid radical or residue $(CH_3)_2CHCH_2CH(NH_2)CO-$ of leucine — abbr. *Leu*

Leu–en·keph·a·lin \₁lü-en-'kef-ə-lən\ *n* : LEUCINE-ENKEPH-ALIN

Each boldface word in the list below is a chiefly British variant of the word to its right in small capitals.

leukaemia	LEUKEMIA	leukaemogenic	LEUKEMOGEN-IC
leukaemic	LEUKEMIC		
leukaemid	LEUKEMID	leukaemoge-nicity	LEUKEMOGE-NICITY
leukaemogen	LEUKEMOGEN		
leukaemogene-sis	LEUKEMOGEN-ESIS	leukaemoid	LEUKEMOID

leuk·ane·mia *or chiefly Brit* **leuk·anae·mia** \₁lük-ə-'nē-mē-ə\ *n* : a blood disease with characteristics of leukemia combined with pernicious anemia

leu·ka·phe·re·sis \₁lü-kə-fə-'rē-səs\ *n, pl* **-phe·re·ses** \-₁sēz\ : a procedure by which the white blood cells are removed from a donor's blood which is then transfused back into the donor — called also *leukopheresis*

leu·ke·mia \lü-'kē-mē-ə\ *also* **leu·ce·mia** \lü-'kē- *also* lü-'sē-\ *or chiefly Brit* **leu·kae·mia** *also* **leu·cae·mia** *n* : an acute or chronic disease of unknown cause in humans and other warm-blooded animals that involves the blood-forming organs, is characterized by an abnormal increase in the number of white blood cells in the tissues of the body with or without a corresponding increase of those in the circulating blood, and is classified according to the type of white blood cell most prominently involved — see ACUTE LYMPHOBLASTIC LEUKEMIA, ACUTE MYELOGENOUS LEUKEMIA, CHRONIC LYMPHOCYTIC LEUKEMIA, CHRONIC MYELOGENOUS LEUKEMIA, FELINE LEUKEMIA, LYMPHOBLASTIC LEUKEMIA, LYMPHOCYTIC LEUKEMIA, MONOCYTIC LEUKEMIA, MYELOGENOUS LEUKEMIA, PROMYELOCYTIC LEUKEMIA

¹leu·ke·mic *or chiefly Brit* **leu·kae·mic** \lü-'kē-mik\ *adj* **1** : of, relating to, or affected by leukemia ⟨∼ mice⟩ **2** : characterized by an increase in white blood cells ⟨∼ blood⟩

²leukemic *or chiefly Brit* **leukaemic** *n* : an individual affected with leukemia

leu·ke·mid *or chiefly Brit* **leu·kae·mid** \lü-'kē-məd\ *n* : a skin lesion of leukemia

leu·ke·mo·gen *or chiefly Brit* **leu·kae·mo·gen** \lü-'kē-mə-jən, -₁jen\ *n* : a substance tending to induce the development of leukemia

leu·ke·mo·gen·e·sis *or chiefly Brit* **leu·kae·mo·gen·e·sis** \lü-₁kē-mə-'jen-ə-səs\ *n, pl* **-e·ses** \-₁sēz\ : induction or production of leukemia — **leu·ke·mo·gen·ic** *or chiefly Brit* **leu·kae·mo·gen·ic** \-'jen-ik\ *adj* — **leu·ke·mo·ge·nic·i·ty** *or chiefly Brit* **leu·kae·mo·ge·nic·i·ty** \-jə-'nis-ət-ē\ *n, pl* **-ties**

leu·ke·moid *or chiefly Brit* **leu·kae·moid** \lü-'kē-mòid\ *adj* : resembling leukemia but not involving the same changes in the blood-forming organs ⟨a ∼ reaction in malaria⟩

leu·ker·gy \'lü-(₁)kər-jē\ *n, pl* **-gies** : the clumping of white blood cells that accompanies some inflammations and infections

leu·kin \'lü-kən\ *n* : a heat-stable extract of polymorphonuclear leukocytes that is active against some bacteria (esp. *Bacillus anthracis*)

leu·ko·ag·glu·ti·nin *or chiefly Brit* **leu·co·ag·glu·ti·nin** \₁lü-kō-ə-'glüt-ᵊn-ən\ *n* : an antibody that agglutinates leukocytes — compare HEMAGGLUTININ

leu·ko·blast *or chiefly Brit* **leu·co·blast** \'lü-kə₁blast\ *n* : a developing leukocyte : a cellular precursor of a leukocyte — compare LYMPHOBLAST, MYELOBLAST

leu·ko·blas·to·sis *or chiefly Brit* **leu·co·blas·to·sis** \₁lü-kō-blas-'tō-səs\ *n, pl* **-to·ses** \-₁sēz\ : LEUKOSIS

leu·ko·ci·din *or chiefly Brit* **leu·co·ci·din** \₁lü-kə-'sīd-ᵊn\ *n* : a heat-stable substance (as that produced by some bacteria) capable of killing or destroying leukocytes

leu·ko·cyte *or chiefly Brit* **leu·co·cyte** \'lü-kə-₁sīt\ *n* **1**

\ə\ **abut** \ᵊ\ **kitten** \ər\ **further** \a\ **ash** \ā\ **ace** \ä\ **cot, cart**
\aú\ **out** \ch\ **chin** \e\ **bet** \ē\ **easy** \g\ **go** \i\ **hit** \ī\ **ice** \j\ **job**
\ŋ\ **sing** \ō\ **go** \ò\ **law** \òi\ **boy** \th\ **thin** \t͟h\ **the** \ü\ **loot**
\ù\ **foot** \y\ **yet** \zh\ **vision** *See also* Pronunciation Symbols page

K
L

: WHITE BLOOD CELL   **2** : a cell (as a macrophage) of the tissues comparable to or derived from a leukocyte

leu·ko·cy·the·mia *or chiefly Brit* **leu·co·cy·thae·mia** \ˌlü-kə-ˌsī-ˈthē-mē-ə\ *n* : LEUKEMIA; *esp* : GRANULOBLASTOSIS

leu·ko·cyt·ic *or chiefly Brit* **leu·co·cyt·ic** \ˌlü-kə-ˈsit-ik\ *adj*   **1** : of, relating to, or involving leukocytes   **2** : characterized by an excess of leukocytes

leu·ko·cy·to·gen·e·sis *or chiefly Brit* **leu·co·cy·to·gen·e·sis** \ˌlü-kə-ˌsīt-ə-ˈjen-ə-səs\ *n, pl* **-e·ses** \-ˌsēz\ : LEUKOPOIESIS

leu·ko·cy·toid *or chiefly Brit* **leu·co·cy·toid** \ˌlü-kə-ˈsīt-ˌȯid\ *adj* : resembling a leukocyte

leu·ko·cy·to·sis *or chiefly Brit* **leu·co·cy·to·sis** \ˌlü-kə-sī-ˈtō-səs, -kə-sə-\ *n, pl* **-to·ses** \-ˌsēz\ : an increase in the number of white blood cells in the circulating blood that occurs normally (as after meals) or abnormally (as in some infections) — **leu·ko·cy·tot·ic** *or chiefly Brit* **leu·co·cy·tot·ic** \-ˈtät-ik\ *adj*

leu·ko·der·ma *or chiefly Brit* **leu·co·der·ma** \ˌlü-kə-ˈdər-mə\ *n* : a skin abnormality that is characterized by a usu. congenital lack of pigment in spots or bands and produces a patchy whiteness — compare VITILIGO

leu·ko·dys·tro·phy *or chiefly Brit* **leu·co·dys·tro·phy** \ˌlü-kō-ˈdis-trə-fē\ *n, pl* **-phies** : any of several inherited diseases (as adrenoleukodystrophy) characterized by progressive degeneration of myelin in the brain, spinal cord, and peripheral nerves

leu·ko·en·ceph·a·li·tis *or chiefly Brit* **leu·co·en·ceph·a·li·tis** \ˌlü-kō-in-ˌsef-ə-ˈlīt-əs\ *n, pl* **-lit·i·des** \-ˈlit-ə-ˌdēz\ : inflammation of the white matter of the brain

leu·ko·en·ceph·a·lop·a·thy *or chiefly Brit* **leu·co·en·ceph·a·lop·a·thy** \-in-ˌsef-ə-ˈläp-ə-thē\ *n, pl* **-thies** : any of various diseases affecting the brain's white matter; *esp* : PROGRESSIVE MULTIFOCAL LEUKOENCEPHALOPATHY

leu·ko·ker·a·to·sis *or chiefly Brit* **leu·co·ker·a·to·sis** \-ˌker-ə-ˈtō-səs\ *n, pl* **-to·ses** \-ˌsēz\ : severely keratinized or ulcerated leukoplakia

leu·ko·ma *or chiefly Brit* **leu·co·ma** \lü-ˈkō-mə\ *n* : a dense white opacity in the cornea of the eye

leu·ko·maine *or chiefly Brit* **leu·co·maine** \ˈlü-kə-ˌmān\ *n* : a basic substance normally produced in the living animal body as a decomposition product of protein matter — compare PTOMAINE

leu·kon \ˈlü-ˌkän\ *n* : the white blood cells and their precursors

leuk·onych·ia *or chiefly Brit* **leuc·onych·ia** \ˌlü-kō-ˈnik-ē-ə\ *n* : a white spotting, streaking, or discoloration of the fingernails caused by injury or ill health

leu·ko·pe·nia *or chiefly Brit* **leu·co·pe·nia** \ˌlü-kō-ˈpē-nē-ə\ *n* : a condition in which the number of white blood cells circulating in the blood is abnormally low and which is most commonly due to a decreased production of new cells in conjunction with various infectious diseases, as a reaction to various drugs or other chemicals, or in response to irradiation — **leu·ko·pe·nic** *or chiefly Brit* **leu·co·pe·nic** \-ˈpē-nik\ *adj*

leu·ko·phe·re·sis \-fə-ˈrē-səs\ *n, pl* **-re·ses** \-ˌsēz\ : LEUKAPHERESIS

leu·ko·pla·kia *or chiefly Brit* **leu·co·pla·kia** \ˌlü-kō-ˈplā-kē-ə\ *n* : a condition commonly considered precancerous in which thickened white patches of epithelium occur on the mucous membranes esp. of the mouth, vulva, and renal pelvis; *also* : a lesion or lesioned area of leukoplakia — **leu·ko·pla·kic** *or chiefly Brit* **leu·co·pla·kic** \-ˈplā-kik\ *adj*

leu·ko·poi·e·sis *or chiefly Brit* **leu·co·poi·e·sis** \-pȯi-ˈē-səs\ *n, pl* **-e·ses** \-ˌsēz\ : the formation of white blood cells — called also *leukocytogenesis* — **leu·ko·poi·et·ic** *or chiefly Brit* **leu·co·poi·et·ic** \-ˈet-ik\ *adj*

leu·kor·rhea *or chiefly Brit* **leu·cor·rhoea** \ˌlü-kə-ˈrē-ə\ *n* : a white, yellowish, or greenish white viscid discharge from the vagina resulting from inflammation or congestion of the uterine or vaginal mucous membrane — **leu·kor·rhe·al** *or chiefly Brit* **leu·cor·rhoe·al** \-ˈrē-əl\ *adj*

leu·ko·sar·co·ma *or chiefly Brit* **leu·co·sar·co·ma** \ˌlü-kō-sär-ˈkō-mə\ *n, pl* **-mas** *also* **-ma·ta** \-mət-ə\ : lymphosarcoma

accompanied by leukemia — **leu·ko·sar·co·ma·to·sis** *or chiefly Brit* **leu·co·sar·co·ma·to·sis** \-sär-ˌkō-mə-ˈtō-səs\ *n, pl* **-to·ses** \-ˌsēz\

leu·ko·sis *or chiefly Brit* **leu·co·sis** \lü-ˈkō-səs\ *n, pl* **-ko·ses** *or chiefly Brit* **-co·ses** \-ˌsēz\ : LEUKEMIA; *esp* : any of various leukemic diseases of poultry — **leu·kot·ic** *or chiefly Brit* **leu·cot·ic** \-ˈkät-ik\ *adj*

leu·ko·tac·tic *or chiefly Brit* **leu·co·tac·tic** \ˌlü-kō-ˈtak-tik\ *adj* : tending to attract leukocytes ⟨psoriatic scale contains ~ substances —G. S. Lazarus *et al*⟩ — **leu·ko·tac·ti·cal·ly** *or chiefly Brit* **leu·co·tac·ti·cal·ly** \-ti-k(ə-)lē\ *adv*

leu·ko·tax·ine *or chiefly Brit* **leu·co·tax·ine** \ˌlü-kə-ˈtak-ˌsēn, -sən\ *n* : a crystalline polypeptide that is obtained from the fluid at sites of inflammation in the body and that increases the permeability of capillaries and migration of leukocytes

leu·ko·tax·is *or chiefly Brit* **leu·co·tax·is** \ˌlü-kə-ˈtak-səs\ *n, pl* **-tax·es** \-ˌsēz\ : the quality or state of being leukotactic : the ability to attract leukocytes

leu·ko·tome *or chiefly Brit* **leu·co·tome** \ˈlü-kə-ˌtōm\ *n* : a cannula through which a wire is inserted and used to cut the white matter in the brain in lobotomy

leu·kot·o·my *or chiefly Brit* **leu·cot·o·my** \lü-ˈkät-ə-mē\ *n, pl* **-mies** : LOBOTOMY

leu·ko·tox·in *or chiefly Brit* **leu·co·tox·in** \ˌlü-kō-ˈtäk-sən\ *n* : a substance specif. destructive to leukocytes

leu·ko·trich·ia *or chiefly Brit* **leu·co·trich·ia** \ˌlü-kə-ˈtrik-ē-ə\ *n* : whiteness of the hair

leu·ko·tri·ene \ˌlü-kə-ˈtrī-ˌēn\ *n* : any of a group of eicosanoids that are generated in basophils, mast cells, macrophages, and human lung tissue by lipoxygenase-catalyzed oxygenation esp. of arachidonic acid and that participate in allergic responses (as bronchoconstriction in asthma) — see SLOW-REACTING SUBSTANCE OF ANAPHYLAXIS

leu·ko·vi·rus *or chiefly Brit* **leu·co·vi·rus** \ˈlü-kō-ˌvī-rəs\ *n* : any of various retroviruses (as the Rous sarcoma virus) that cause tumors in animals

leu·pep·tin \lü-ˈpep-tən\ *n* : any of a group of tripeptides that inhibit proteases

leu·pro·lide \lü-ˈprō-ˌlīd\ *n* : a synthetic analog of gonadotropin-releasing hormone used in the form of its acetate $C_{59}H_{84}N_{16}O_{12} \cdot C_2H_4O_2$ to treat cancer of the prostate gland — see LUPRON

leu·ro·cris·tine \ˌlur-ō-ˈkris-ˌtēn\ *n* : VINCRISTINE

Lev·a·di·ti stain *or* **Lev·a·di·ti's stain** \ˌlev-ə-ˈdē-ˌtē(z)-\ *n* : a silver nitrate stain used to demonstrate in section the spirochete of the genus *Treponema* (*T. pallidum*) that causes syphilis

> **Lev·a·di·ti** \le-vá-dē-tē\, **Constantin (1874–1935),** French bacteriologist. Levaditi spent most of his career in research at the Pasteur Institute in Paris, where he was in charge of the laboratory for many years. In 1906 he introduced the silver nitrate staining method and used it to study the causative spirochete (*Treponema pallidum*) of syphilis in the livers of newborns affected with the disease.

lev·al·lor·phan \ˌlev-ə-ˈlȯr-ˌfan, -fən\ *n* : a drug $C_{19}H_{25}NO$ related to morphine that is used to counteract morphine poisoning

lev·am·fet·amine \ˌlev-am-ˈfet-ə-ˌmēn\ *n* : the levorotatory form of amphetamine formerly used as an anorectic agent — compare LEVMETAMFETAMINE

le·vam·i·sole \lə-ˈvam-ə-ˌsōl\ *n* : an anthelmintic drug administered in the form of its hydrochloride $C_{11}H_{12}N_2S \cdot HCl$ that also possesses immunostimulant properties and is used esp. in the treatment of colon cancer

lev·an \ˈlev-ˌan\ *n* : any of a group of levorotatory polysaccharides $(C_6H_{10}O_5)_n$ composed of levulose units of the furanose type and formed esp. from sucrose solutions by the action of various bacteria (as *Bacillus subtilis* or *B. mesentericus*) — compare DEXTRAN

Le·vant storax \lə-ˈvant-\ *n* : STORAX 1

Levant wormseed *n*   **1** : the buds of a European plant of the genus *Artemisia* (*A. cina*) used as an anthelmintic — compare SANTONICA   **2** : the plant bearing Levant wormseed

Le·va·quin \\'lev-ə-kwən\\ *trademark* — used for a preparation of levofloxacin

lev·ar·ter·e·nol \\,lev-är-'tir-ə-,nól, -'ter-, -,nōl\\ *n* : levorotatory norepinephrine

le·va·tor \\li-'vāt-ər\\ *n, pl* **lev·a·to·res** \\,lev-ə-'tōr-(,)ēz\\ *or* **le·va·tors** \\li-'vāt-ərz\\ : a muscle that serves to raise a body part — compare DEPRESSOR a

levator an·gu·li oris \\-'aŋ-gyə-,lī-'ór-əs\\ *n* : a facial muscle that arises from the maxilla, inclines downward to be inserted into the corner of the mouth, and draws the lips up and back — called also *caninus*

levator ani \\-'ā-,nī\\ *n* : a broad thin muscle that is attached in a sheet to each side of the inner surface of the pelvis and descends to form the floor of the pelvic cavity where it supports the viscera and surrounds structures which pass through it and inserts into the sides of the apex of the coccyx, the margins of the anus, the side of the rectum, and the central tendinous point of the perineum — see ILIOCOCCYGEUS, PUBOCOCCYGEUS

levatores cos·tar·um \\-,käs-'tär-əm, -'tär-\\ *n pl* : a series of 12 muscles on each side that arise from the transverse processes of the seventh cervical and upper 11 thoracic vertebrae, that pass obliquely downward and laterally to insert into the outer surface of the rib immediately below or in the case of the lowest four muscles of the series divide into two fasciculi of which one inserts as described and the other inserts into the second rib below, and that raise the ribs increasing the volume of the thoracic cavity and extend, bend, and rotate the spinal column

levator la·bii su·pe·ri·or·is \\-'lā-bē-,ī-sù-,pir-ē-'ór-əs\\ *n* : a facial muscle arising from the lower margin of the orbit and inserting into the muscular substance of the upper lip which it elevates — called also *quadratus labii superioris*

levator labii superioris alae·que na·si \\-ā-'lē-kwē-'nā-,zī\\ *n* : a muscle that arises from the nasal process of the maxilla, that passes downward and laterally, that divides into a part inserting into the alar cartilage and one inserting into the upper lip, and that dilates the nostril and raises the upper lip

levator pal·pe·brae su·pe·ri·or·is \\-,pal-'pē-,brē-sù-,pir-ē-'ór-əs\\ *n* : a thin flat extrinsic muscle of the eye arising from the lesser wing of the sphenoid bone, passing forward and downward over the superior rectus, and inserting into the tarsal plate of the skin of the upper eyelid which it raises

levator pros·ta·tae \\-'präs-tə-,tē\\ *n* : a part of the pubococcygeus comprising the more medial and ventral fasciculi that insert into the tissue in front of the anus and serve to support and elevate the prostate gland

levator scap·u·lae \\-'skap-yə-,lē\\ *n* : a back muscle that arises in the transverse processes of the first four cervical vertebrae and descends to insert into the vertebral border of the scapula which it elevates

levator ve·li pal·a·ti·ni \\-'vē-,lī-,pal-ə-'tī-,nī\\ *n* : a muscle arising from the temporal bone and the cartilage of the eustachian tube and descending to insert into the midline of the soft palate which it elevates esp. to close the nasopharynx while swallowing is taking place to prevent regurgitation of liquid or solid matter through the nose

Le·Veen shunt \\lə-'vēn-'shənt\\ *n* : a plastic tube that passes from the jugular vein to the peritoneal cavity where a valve permits absorption of ascitic fluid which is carried back to venous circulation by way of the superior vena cava

LeVeen, Harry Henry (1914–1996), American surgeon. LeVeen served as professor of surgery at the State University of New York and later at the Medical University of South Carolina. His major areas of research included vascular surgery, liver physiology, and portal circulation. Experimental testing of the LeVeen shunt was first done using animals in 1972. Use of the LeVeen shunt on human beings began in 1976.

lev·el \\'lev-əl\\ *n* **1** : a characteristic and fairly uniform concentration of a constituent of the blood or other body fluid ⟨a normal blood-sugar ∼⟩ **2 a** : a degree of ability or aptitude or measure of performance **b** : a grade of mental and

emotional development or maturity ⟨evidence as to ∼s of personality development (e.g., anal, oral) —G. P. Murdock⟩

lev·i·gate \\'lev-ə-,gāt\\ *vt* **-gat·ed; -gat·ing** : to grind to a fine smooth powder while in moist condition ⟨by first *levigating* the zinc oxide with a small amount of glycerin a smooth paste is obtained —*Art of Compounding*⟩ — **lev·i·ga·tion** \\,lev-ə-'gā-shən\\ *n*

Le·vin tube \\lə-'vēn-, lə-'vin-\\ *n* : a tube designed to be passed into the stomach or duodenum through the nose

Levin, Abraham Louis (1880–1940), American physician. The author of numerous articles on gastroenterology, Levin introduced his nasal gastroduodenal tube in 1921. He was also the first to call attention to the function of the liver in reducing blood sugar.

Le·vi·tra \\lə-'vē-trə\\ *trademark* — used for a preparation of the hydrated hydrochloride of vardenafil

lev·met·am·fet·amine \\,lev-met-,am-'fet-ə-,mēn\\ *n* : the levorotatory form of methamphetamine used as a nasal decongestant — compare LEVAMFETAMINE

le·vo *or Brit* **lae·vo** \\'lē-(,)vō\\ *adj* : LEVOROTATORY

le·vo·car·dia *or Brit* **lae·vo·car·dia** \\,lē-və-'kärd-ē-ə\\ *n* : normal position of the heart when associated with situs inversus of other abdominal viscera and usu. with structural defects of the heart itself

le·vo·car·dio·gram *or Brit* **lae·vo·car·dio·gram** \\-'kärd-ē-ə-,gram\\ *n* : the part of an electrocardiogram recording activity of the left side of the heart — compare DEXTROCARDIOGRAM

le·vo·di·hy·droxy·phe·nyl·al·a·nine *or Brit* **lae·vo–di·hy·droxy·phe·nyl·al·a·nine** \\,lē-vō-,dī-hī-,dräk-sē-,fen-ᵊl-'al-ə-,nēn, -,fēn-\\ *n* : L-DOPA

le·vo·do·pa \\'lev-ə-,dō-pə, ,lē-və-'dō-pə\\ *or Brit* **lae·vo·do·pa** \\,lē-və-\\ *n* : L-DOPA

Le·vo–Dro·mo·ran \\,lē-vō-'drō-mə-,ran\\ *trademark* — used for a preparation of levorphanol

le·vo·flox·a·cin \\,lē-və-'fläk-sə-sən\\ *n* : a broad-spectrum antibacterial agent that is the levorotatory isomer of ofloxacin — see LEVAQUIN

le·vo·nor·ges·trel \\,lē-və-nór-'jes-trəl\\ *n* : the levorotatory form of norgestrel used in birth control pills and contraceptive implants — see NORPLANT

Levo·phed \\'lev-ə-,fed\\ *trademark* — used for a preparation of norepinephrine

Le·vo·prome \\'lē-və-,prōm\\ *trademark* — used for a preparation of methotrimeprazine

le·vo·pro·poxy·phene \\,lē-və-prō-'päk-si-,fēn\\ *n* : a drug used esp. in the form of its napsylate $C_{22}H_{29}NO_2 \cdot C_{10}H_8SO_3$ as an antitussive

le·vo·ro·ta·tion *or Brit* **lae·vo·ro·ta·tion** \\,lē-və-rō-'tā-shən\\ *n* : left-handed or counterclockwise rotation — used of the plane of polarization of light

le·vo·ro·ta·to·ry \\-'rōt-ə-,tōr-ē, -,tòr-\\ *or* **le·vo·ro·ta·ry** \\-'rōt-ə-rē\\ *or Brit* **lae·vo·ro·ta·to·ry** *or* **lae·vo·ro·ta·ry** *adj* : turning toward the left or counterclockwise; *esp* : rotating the plane of polarization of light to the left — compare DEXTROROTATORY

lev·or·pha·nol \\lev-'ór-fə-,nól\\ *n* : an addictive drug used esp. in the form of its hydrated tartrate $C_{17}H_{23}NO \cdot C_4H_6O_6 \cdot 2H_2O$ as a potent analgesic with properties similar to morphine — see LEVO-DROMORAN

Le·vo·throid \\'lē-və-,thròid\\ *trademark* — used for a preparation of the sodium salt of levothyroxine

le·vo·thy·rox·ine *or Brit* **lae·vo·thy·rox·ine** \\,lē-vō-thī-'räk-,sēn, -sən\\ *n* : the levorotatory isomer of thyroxine that is administered in the form of its sodium salt $C_{15}H_{10}I_4NNaO_4$ in the treatment of hypothyroidism — see LEVOTHROID, LEVOXYL, SYNTHROID

Le·vox·yl \\lə-'väk-səl\\ *trademark* — used for a preparation of the sodium salt of levothyroxine

---

\\ə\ **abut** \\ᵊ\ **kitten** \\ər\ **further** \\a\ **ash** \\ā\ **ace** \\ä\ **cot, cart**
\\aù\ **out** \\ch\ **chin** \\e\ **bet** \\ē\ **easy** \\g\ **go** \\i\ **hit** \\ī\ **ice** \\j\ **job**
\\ŋ\ **sing** \\ō\ **go** \\ò\ **law** \\òi\ **boy** \\th\ **thin** \\t͟h\ **the** \\ü\ **loot**
\\ù\ **foot** \\y\ **yet** \\zh\ **vision** *See also* Pronunciation Symbols page

K
L

lev·u·li·nate \'lev-yə-lə-ˌnāt\ *or Brit* **lae·vu·li·nate** \'lēv-\ *n* : a salt of levulinic acid

lev·u·lin·ic acid \ˌlev-yə-ˌlin-ik-\ *or Brit* **lae·vu·lin·ic acid** \ˌlēv-\ *n* : a crystalline keto acid $C_5H_8O_3$ obtained by action of dilute acids on hexoses (as levulose) and on substances (as starch or sucrose) that yield hexoses on hydrolysis

lev·u·lo·san \'lev-yə-lō-ˌsan\ *or Brit* **lae·vu·lo·san** \'lēv-\ *n* : FRUCTOSAN

lev·u·lose \'lev-yə-ˌlōs, -ˌlōz\ *or Brit* **lae·vu·lose** \'lēv-\ *n* : FRUCTOSE 2

lev·u·los·emia \ˌlev-yə-lō-'sē-mē-ə\ *or Brit* **lae·vu·los·ae·mia** \ˌlēv-\ *n* : the presence of fructose in the blood

lev·u·los·uria \ˌlev-yə-lōs-'(y)ùr-ē-ə\ *or Brit* **lae·vu·los·uria** \ˌlēv-yə-lōs-'yùr-\ *n* : the presence of fructose in the urine

Lew·is \'lü-əs\ *adj* : of or relating to the Lewis blood groups ⟨∼ antigens⟩

Lewis, H. D. G., British hospital patient. The Lewis antigen was first recognized in the blood of Mrs. Lewis in 1946.

Lewis blood group *n* : any of a system of blood groups controlled by a pair of dominant-recessive alleles and characterized by antigens which are released into body fluids, are adsorbed onto the surface of red blood cells, and tend to interreact with the antigens produced by secretors although they are genetically independent of them

lew·is·ite \'lü-ə-ˌsīt\ *n* : a colorless or brown vesicant liquid $C_2H_2AsCl_3$ developed as a poison gas for war use

Lewis, Winford Lee (1878–1943), American chemist. As an officer in the U.S. Army Chemical Warfare Service during World War I, Lewis developed the poisonous gas lewisite in 1918. Later in life he did research for the Institute of American Meat Packers.

Lewy body \'lü-ē-, 'lā-vē-\ *n* : an eosinophilic inclusion body found in the cytoplasm of neurons of the cortex and brain stem in Parkinson's disease and some forms of dementia

Lew·ey \'lü-ē\, **Frederic Henry** (*orig.* **Friedrich Heinrich Lewy**) **(1885–1950),** American neurologist. Born in Berlin, Germany, Lewey oversaw German army field hospitals in France, Russia, and Turkey during World War I. He served as professor of clinical neurology at the University of Berlin's medical school from 1923 to 1933, researching occupational diseases of the nervous system and becoming director of the neurological institute in 1930. After emigrating to the U.S. in 1934, he became professor of neurophysiology at the University of Pennsylvania's medical school. From 1940 he was also professor of neuropathology in its graduate school. While there he did research on avitaminotic diseases of the nervous system. In 1913, before a convention of the German Society of Neurologists, he described in detail the eosinophilic inclusion bodies that he had discovered in the brains of patients with Parkinson's disease. By 1919 his name had become associated with these bodies.

Ley·den jar \'līd-ᵊn-\ *n* : the earliest form of electrical capacitor consisting essentially of a glass jar coated part way up both inside and outside with metal foil and having the inner coating connected to a conducting rod passed through the insulating stopper

Ley·dig cell \'lī-dig-\ *also* **Ley·dig's cell** \-dig(z)-\ *n* : a cell of interstitial tissue of the testis that is usu. considered the chief source of testicular androgens and esp. testosterone — called also *cell of Leydig, interstitial cell of Leydig*

Ley·dig \'lī-diḵ\, **Franz von (1821–1908),** German anatomist. Leydig's interests included comparative anatomy, histology, and physiology. In 1850 he discovered and described the interstitial cell in a detailed account of the male sex organs. In 1857 he published a major text on the histology of humans and animals that is historically important as a major account of histology's development up to that time. The Wolffian duct was discovered and described by him in 1892.

Ley·dig's duct \'lī-digz-\ *n* : WOLFFIAN DUCT

LFA–1 \ˌel-(ˌ)ef-(ˌ)ā-'wən\ *n* [*l*ymphocyte *f*unction-associated *a*ntigen-1] : an integrin that is a heterodimeric protein on the surface of leukocytes and that functions in the adhesion of lymphocytes to other cells

LFD *abbr* least fatal dose

L–form \'el-ˌfȯrm\ *n* : a variant form of some bacteria that usu. lacks a cell wall — called also *L-phase*

LGL syndrome \ˌel-(ˌ)jē-ˌel-\ *n* : a preexcitation syndrome characterized by atrial tachycardia together with a short P-R interval and a QRS complex of normal duration — called also *Lown-Ganong-Levine syndrome*

Lown \'laùn\, **Bernard** (*b* 1921), American cardiologist. Lown enjoyed a long association with Harvard University's School of Public Health, rising to the rank of professor of cardiology and becoming director of the School's cardiovascular research laboratory. His research centered on sudden cardiac death and the identification of potential victims and on the role of neural and psychological factors leading to life-threatening disturbances of heart rhythm. He was cofounder and copresident of International Physicians for the Prevention of Nuclear War, which was awarded the Nobel Peace Prize in 1985.

Gan·ong \'gan-ˌȯn\, **William Francis** (*b* 1924), American physiologist. Ganong spent the bulk of his career at the Medical School at the University of California, San Francisco, rising to the position of professor of physiology. He specialized in neuroendocrinology, investigating the interrelation between endocrine and brain function.

Le·vine \lə-'vīn, -'vēn\, **Samuel Albert (1891–1966),** American cardiologist. Levine served for many years as a cardiologist at Boston's Peter Bent Brigham Hospital, which in 1965 established the Samuel Albert Levine Cardiac Center in his honor. Concurrently, he served on the faculty of Harvard Medical School, which also honored him by establishing the Samuel A. Levine Professorship of Medicine in 1954. Levine's works included *Coronary Thrombosis* (1929) and (with Bernard Lown) *Current Concepts in Digitalis Therapy* (1954). With Lown and William Ganong he coauthored the 1952 article describing the syndrome that now bears their names.

LH *abbr* luteinizing hormone

LHRH *abbr* luteinizing hormone-releasing hormone

Li *symbol* lithium

li·bid·i·nal \lə-'bid-ᵊn-əl, -'bid-nᵊl\ *adj* : of or relating to the libido — **li·bid·i·nal·ly** \-ē\ *adv*

li·bid·i·nize *or chiefly Brit* **li·bid·i·nise** \-ə-ˌnīz\ *vt* **-nized** *or chiefly Brit* **-nised; -niz·ing** *or chiefly Brit* **-nis·ing** : to feel toward or treat as if a source or avenue of sexual gratification : invest with libido — **li·bid·i·ni·za·tion** *or chiefly Brit* **li·bid·i·ni·sa·tion** \lə-ˌbid-ə-nə-'zā-shən\ *n*

li·bid·i·nous \-ᵊn-əs, -'bid-nəs\ *adj* **1** : having or marked by lustful desires **2** : LIBIDINAL ⟨∼ ties between individuals⟩

li·bi·do \lə-'bēd-(ˌ)ō *also* 'lib-ə-ˌdō *or* lə-'bī-(ˌ)dō\ *n, pl* **-dos** **1** : instinctual psychic energy that in psychoanalytic theory is derived from primitive biological urges (as for sexual pleasure or self-preservation) and that is expressed in conscious activity **2** : sexual drive

libitum — see AD LIBITUM

Lib·man–Sacks endocarditis \'lib-mən-'saks-\ *n* : a noninfectious form of verrucous endocarditis associated with systemic lupus erythematosus — called also *Libman-Sacks disease, Libman-Sacks syndrome*

Libman, Emanuel (1872–1946), and **Sacks, Benjamin (1896–1939),** American physicians. Libman spent almost all of his medical career at New York's Mount Sinai Hospital, which during his tenure became a center for cardiology. He began studying infant diarrheas, and while visiting the laboratory of the noted bacteriologist Theodor Escherich in 1898, he discovered a causative bacterium. He continued research in this area, studying streptococci, pneumococci, meningococci, typhoid, paracolitis, and pyocyaneus infections. Also interested in blood cultures, he did the first extensive clinical studies on blood transfusions. In 1923–24 Libman and Sacks recognized a form of endocarditis now known as Libman-Sacks endocarditis.

li·brary \'lī-ˌbrer-ē\ *n, pl* **-brar·ies** : a collection of cloned DNA fragments that are maintained in a suitable cellular environment and that represent the genetic material of a par-

ticular organism or tissue ⟨inserting segments from a ∼ of human DNA into yeast cells —*Science News*⟩
Lib·ri·um \'lib-rē-əm\ *trademark* — used for a preparation of the hydrochloride of chlordiazepoxide
lice *pl of* LOUSE
li·cense *or chiefly Brit* **li·cence** \'līs-ᵊn(t)s\ *n* : a permission granted by competent authority to engage in a business or occupation or in an activity otherwise unlawful ⟨a ∼ to practice medicine⟩ — **license** *or chiefly Brit* **licence** *vt* **li·censed** *or chiefly Brit* **li·cenced; li·cens·ing** *or chiefly Brit* **li·cenc·ing**
licensed practical nurse *n* : a person who has undergone training and obtained a license (as from a state) to provide routine care for the sick — called also *LPN*
licensed vo·ca·tion·al nurse \-vō-,kā-shən-ᵊl-\ *n* : a licensed practical nurse authorized by license to practice in the states of California or Texas — called also *LVN*
li·cen·sure \'līs-ᵊn-shər, -,shùr\ *n* **1** : the state or condition of having a license granted by official or legal authority to perform medical acts and procedures not permitted by persons without such a license ⟨applicant must have RN ∼⟩; *also* : the granting of such licenses ⟨a state board of medical ∼⟩ **2** : approval of a drug or medical procedure by official or legal authority for use in the practice of medicine ⟨the ∼ was based on the results of randomized clinical trials of the vaccine's protective efficacy —E. D. Shapiro *et al*⟩
li·cen·ti·ate \lī-'sen-chē-ət\ *n* : a person who has a license to practice a profession
li·chen \'lī-kən\ *n* **1** : any of several skin diseases characterized by the eruption of flat papules; *esp* : LICHEN PLANUS **2** : any of numerous complex plantlike organisms made up of an alga and a fungus growing in symbiotic association on a solid surface (as a rock)
li·chen·i·fi·ca·tion \lī-,ken-ə-fə-'kā-shən, ,lī-kən-\ *n* : the process by which skin becomes hardened and leathery or lichenoid usu. as a result of chronic irritation; *also* : a patch of skin so modified
li·chen·i·fied \lī-'ken-ə-,fīd, 'lī-kən-\ *adj* : showing or characterized by lichenification ⟨∼ eczema⟩
li·chen·in \'lī-kə-nən\ *n* : a gelatinous polysaccharide $(C_6H_{10}O_5)_n$ composed of glucose units and found esp. in several species of moss and lichen and in cereal grains and bulbs
lichen is·lan·di·cus \-ī-'sland-i-kəs\ *n* : ICELAND MOSS
li·chen·oid \'lī-kə-,nòid\ *adj* : resembling lichen ⟨a ∼ eruption⟩ ⟨∼ dermatitis⟩
lichenoides — see PITYRIASIS LICHENOIDES ET VARIOLIFORMIS ACUTA
lichen pi·lar·is \-pi-'lar-əs\ *n* : KERATOSIS PILARIS
lichen pla·nus \-'plā-nəs\ *n* : a skin disease characterized by an eruption of wide flat papules covered by a horny glazed film, marked by intense itching, and often accompanied by lesions on the oral mucosa
lichen scle·ro·sus et atro·phi·cus \-sklə-'rō-səs-et-,ā-'trō-fi-kəs\ *n* : a chronic skin disease that is characterized by the eruption of flat white hardened papules with central hair follicles often having black keratotic plugs
lichen sim·plex chron·i·cus \-'sim-,pleks-'krän-i-kəs\ *n* : dermatitis marked by one or more clearly defined patches produced by chronic rubbing of the skin
lichen spi·nu·lo·sus \-,spin-yə-'lō-səs, -,spīn-\ *n* : a skin disease characterized by the eruption of follicular papules from which keratotic spines protrude
lichen trop·i·cus \-'träp-i-kəs\ *n* : PRICKLY HEAT
lic·o·rice *or chiefly Brit* **li·quo·rice** \'lik(-ə)-rish, -rəs\ *n* **1** : a European leguminous plant of the genus *Glycyrrhiza* (*G. glabra*) with pinnate leaves and spikes of blue flowers **2 a** : GLYCYRRHIZA **2 b** : an extract of glycyrrhiza commonly prepared in the form of a gummy or rubbery paste
licorice powder *n* : a laxative composed of powdered senna and licorice, sulfur, fennel oil, and sugar
licorice root *n* : GLYCYRRHIZA 2
lid \'lid\ *n* : EYELID
li·do·caine \'līd-ə-,kān\ *n* : a crystalline compound $C_{14}H_{22}N_2O$ used as a local anesthetic often in the form of its

hydrochloride $C_{14}H_{22}N_2O·HCl$ — called also *lignocaine;* see XYLOCAINE
li·do·fla·zine \,līd-ə-'flā-,zēn\ *n* : a drug $C_{30}H_{35}F_2N_3O$ used as a coronary vasodilator
Lie·ber·kühn's gland \'lē-bər-,künz-\ *n* : CRYPT OF LIEBERKÜHN
Lie·ber·mann–Bur·chard reaction \'lē-bər-mən-'bùr-,kärt-\ *n* : a test for unsaturated steroids (as cholesterol) and triterpenes based on the formation of a series of colors (as pink to blue to green) with acetic anhydride in the presence of concentrated sulfuric acid — called also *Liebermann= Burchard test*
   Lie·ber·mann \'lē-bər-,män\, **Carl Theodore (1842–1914),** German chemist. Liebermann is most famous for his work with fellow chemist Carl Graebe (1841–1927). Their work on artificial dyes gave considerable impetus to the development of the modern dye industry. Liebermann was the author of more than 350 scientific papers. He investigated quercetin and naphthalene compounds and prepared halogen and phenol derivatives. H. Burchard may have been one of his many student research assistants.
lie detector \'lī-di-,tek-tər\ *n* : a polygraph for detecting physiological evidence (as change in heart rate) of the tension that accompanies lying
li·en \'lī-ən, 'lī-,en\ *n* : SPLEEN — **li·en·al** \-ᵊl\ *adj*
lienal vein *n* : SPLENIC VEIN
li·en·cu·lus \lī-'en-kyə-ləs\ *n, pl* **-cu·li** \-,lī\ : a small accessory or supplementary spleen
li·eno·re·nal ligament \,lī-ə-nō-'rēn-ᵊl-\ *n* : a mesenteric fold passing from the spleen to the left kidney and affording support to the splenic artery and vein — called also *phrenicolienal ligament*
li·en·ter·ic \,lī-ən-'ter-ik\ *adj* : containing or characterized by the passage of undigested or partially digested food — used of feces or diarrhea
li·en·tery \'lī-ən-,ter-ē, lī-'en-tə-rē\ *n, pl* **-ter·ies** : lienteric diarrhea
Lie·se·gang rings \'lē-zə-,gäŋ-\ *n pl* : a series of usu. concentric bands of a precipitate that are separated by clear spaces and that are often formed in gels by periodic or rhythmic precipitation — called also *Liesegang phenomenon*
   Liesegang, Raphael Eduard (1869–1947), German chemist. Liesegang was an outstanding colloid chemist. Investigating the chemical reactions occurring in gels, he discovered the periodic precipitation reactions in gels that are now known as Liesegang rings.
life \'līf\ *n, pl* **lives** \'līvz\ **1 a** : the quality that distinguishes a vital and functional plant or animal from a dead body **b** : a state of living characterized by capacity for metabolism, growth, reaction to stimuli, and reproduction **2 a** : the sequence of physical and mental experiences that make up the existence of an individual **b** : a specific part or aspect of the process of living ⟨sex ∼⟩ ⟨adult ∼⟩ — **life·less** \'līf-ləs\ *adj*
life cycle *n* **1** : the series of stages in form and functional activity through which an organism passes between successive recurrences of a specified primary stage **2** : LIFE HISTORY 1a
life expectancy *n* : an expected number of years of life based on statistical probability
life history *n* **1 a** : a history of the changes through which an organism passes in its development from the primary stage to its natural death **b** : one series of the changes in a life history **2** : the history of an individual's development in his or her social environment
life instinct *n* : EROS
¹life·sav·ing \'līf-,sā-viŋ\ *adj* : designed for or used in saving lives ⟨∼ drugs⟩
²lifesaving *n* : the skill or practice of saving or protecting the lives esp. of drowning persons

---

\ə\ **abut** \ᵊ\ **kitten** \ər\ **further** \a\ **ash** \ā\ **ace** \ä\ **cot, cart**
\aù\ **out** \ch\ **chin** \e\ **bet** \ē\ **easy** \g\ **go** \i\ **hit** \ī\ **ice** \j\ **job**
\ŋ\ **sing** \ō\ **go** \ò\ **law** \òi\ **boy** \th\ **thin** \th\ **the** \ü\ **loot**
\ù\ **foot** \y\ **yet** \zh\ **vision** *See also* Pronunciation Symbols page

K
L

life science n : a branch of science (as biology, medicine, or anthropology) that deals with living organisms and life processes — usu. used in pl.

life scientist n : a person who specializes in or is expert in one or more of the life sciences

life space n : the physical and psychological environment of an individual or group

life span \ˈlīf-ˌspan\ n **1** : the duration of existence of an individual **2** : the average length of life of a kind of organism or of a material object esp. in a particular environment or under specified circumstances

life–support adj : providing support necessary to sustain life; esp : of, relating to, or being a life-support system ⟨∼ equipment⟩

life support n : equipment, material, and treatment needed to keep a seriously ill or injured patient alive ⟨research shows that if basic *life support* is used on serious trauma victims within four minutes and advanced *life support* within eight, nearly 50% of them survive —Nancy Gibbs *et al*⟩ ⟨was on full *life support* for three weeks —Richard Hoffer⟩

life–support system n : a system that provides all or some of the items (as oxygen, food, water, and disposition of carbon dioxide and body wastes) necessary for maintaining life or health: as **a** : one used to maintain the health of a person or animal in outer space, underwater, or in a mine **b** : one used to maintain the life of an injured or ill person unable to maintain certain physiological processes without artificial support

Li–Frau·me·ni syndrome \ˈlē-fraù-ˈmē-nē-\ n : a rare familial syndrome that is characterized esp. by a high risk of developing early breast cancer and sarcomas of soft tissue

  Li, Frederick P. (b 1940), American epidemiologist. Li held the concurrent positions of professor of clinical cancer epidemiology at the Harvard School of Public Health and epidemiologist at the National Cancer Institute. His research centered on the identification of persons at high risk of cancer and the genetic and environmental causes of cancer susceptibility.
  Fraumeni, Joseph F., Jr. (b 1933), American epidemiologist. Fraumeni enjoyed a long association with the National Cancer Institute, eventually becoming director of the institute's Epidemiology and Biostatistics Program. At the same time he served as attending physician at the Clinical Center of the National Institutes of Health. His research focused on the epidemiology of cancer and the environmental and genetic determinants of the disease.

lift \ˈlift\ n **1** : FACE-LIFT **2** : BREAST LIFT — **lift** vt

lig·a·ment \ˈlig-ə-mənt\ n **1** : a tough band of tissue that serves to connect the articular extremities of bones or to support or retain an organ in place and is usu. composed of coarse bundles of dense white fibrous tissue parallel or closely interlaced, pliant, and flexible, but not extensible **2** : any of various folds or bands of pleura, peritoneum, or mesentery connecting parts or organs

ligamenta, ligamenta flava, ligamenta nuchae pl of LIGAMENTUM, LIGAMENTUM FLAVUM, LIGAMENTUM NUCHAE

ligament of Coo·per \-ˈkü-pər\ n : COOPER'S LIGAMENT

ligament of the ovary n : a rounded cord of fibrous and muscular tissue extending from each superior angle of the uterus to the inner extremity of the ovary of the same side — called also *ovarian ligament;* see SUSPENSORY LIGAMENT OF THE OVARY

ligament of Treitz \-ˈtrīts\ n : a band of smooth muscle extending from the junction of the duodenum and jejunum to the left crus of the diaphragm and functioning as a suspensory ligament

  Treitz, Wenzel (1819–1872), Austrian physician. Treitz was a professor of anatomy and pathology at Krakow and later at Prague. In 1857 he rendered a classic description of the suspensory ligament of the duodenum which is now known as the ligament of Treitz.

ligament of Zinn \-ˈzin, -ˈtsin\ n : the common tendon of the inferior rectus and the internal rectus muscles of the eye — called also *tendon of Zinn*

  Zinn \ˈtsin\, Johann Gottfried (1727–1759), German anatomist and botanist. Zinn was a professor of medicine and director of the botanical gardens at Göttingen. In 1755 he published a monograph on the anatomy of the human eye. It included the first accurate descriptions of the ligament of Zinn and the zonule of Zinn.

lig·a·men·to·pexy \ˌlig-ə-ˈmen-tə-ˌpek-sē\ n, pl **-pex·ies** : a fixation or suspension of the uterus by shortening or suturing the round ligaments

lig·a·men·tous \ˌlig-ə-ˈment-əs\ adj **1** : of or relating to a ligament ⟨∼ laxity⟩ **2** : forming or formed of a ligament ⟨∼ connections⟩ — **lig·a·men·tous·ly** adv

lig·a·men·tum \ˌlig-ə-ˈment-əm\ n, pl **-ta** \-ə\ : LIGAMENT

ligamentum ar·te·rio·sum \-är-ˌtir-ē-ˈō-səm\ n : a cord of tissue that connects the pulmonary trunk and the aorta and that is the vestige of the ductus arteriosus

ligamentum fla·vum \-ˈflā-vəm\ n, pl **ligamenta fla·va** \-və\ : any of a series of ligaments of yellow elastic tissue connecting the laminae of adjacent vertebrae from the axis to the sacrum

ligamentum nu·chae \-ˈn(y)ü-kē\ n, pl **ligamenta nuchae** : a medium ligament of the back of the neck that is rudimentary in humans but highly developed and composed of yellow elastic tissue in many quadrupeds where it assists in supporting the head

ligamentum te·res \-ˈtē-ˌrēz\ n : ROUND LIGAMENT; esp : ROUND LIGAMENT 1

ligamentum ve·no·sum \-vē-ˈnō-səm\ n : a cord of tissue connected to the liver that is the vestige of the ductus venosus

li·gand \ˈlig-ənd, ˈlīg-\ n : a group, ion, or molecule coordinated to a central atom or molecule in a complex — **li·gand·ed** \-əd\ adj

ligand–gated adj : permitting or blocking passage through a cell membrane in response to a chemical stimulus ⟨a ∼ ion channel triggered by ATP —J. M. Besson⟩

li·gase \ˈlī-ˌgās, -ˌgāz\ n : SYNTHETASE

li·gate \ˈlī-ˌgāt, līˈ-\ vt **li·gat·ed; li·gat·ing** **1** : to tie with a ligature **2** : to join together (as DNA or protein chains) by a chemical process ⟨the DNA fragments were enzymatically *ligated*⟩

li·ga·tion \līˈ-ˈgā-shən\ n **1 a** : the surgical process of tying up an anatomical channel (as a blood vessel) **b** : the process of joining together chemical chains (as of DNA or protein) **2** : something that binds : LIGATURE

¹lig·a·ture \ˈlig-ə-ˌchù(ə)r, -chər, -ˌt(y)ù(ə)r\ n **1** : something that is used to bind; specif : a filament (as a thread) used in surgery (as for tying blood vessels) **2** : the action or result of binding or tying ⟨the ∼ of an artery⟩

²ligature vt **-tured; -tur·ing** : to tie up or bind ⟨*ligaturing* the blood vessels —*Veterinary Record*⟩

¹light \ˈlīt\ n **1 a** : the sensation aroused by stimulation of the visual receptors **b** : an electromagnetic radiation in the wavelength range including infrared, visible, ultraviolet, and X-rays and traveling in a vacuum with a speed of about 186,281 miles (300,000 kilometers) per second; specif : the part of this range that is visible to the human eye **2** : a source of light

²light or **lite** adj : made with a lower calorie content or with less of some ingredient (as salt, fat, or alcohol) than usual ⟨∼ salad dressing⟩

light adaptation n : the adjustments including narrowing of the pupillary opening and decrease in rhodopsin by which the retina of the eye is made efficient as a visual receptor under conditions of strong illumination — compare DARK ADAPTATION — **light–adapt·ed** \ˈlīt-ə-ˌdap-təd\ adj

light chain n : either of the two smaller of the four polypeptide chains that are subunits of antibodies — called also *L chain;* compare HEAVY CHAIN

light·en·ing \ˈlīt-ᵊn-iŋ, ˈlīt-niŋ\ n : a sense of decreased weight and abdominal tension felt by a pregnant woman on descent of the fetus into the pelvic cavity prior to labor

light flux n : LUMINOUS FLUX

light guide *n* : an optical fiber used esp. for telecommunication with light waves

light–head·ed·ness \'līt-'hed-əd-nəs\ *n* : the condition of being dizzy or on the verge of fainting ⟨dizziness or ∼, particularly when one arises to a standing position, is a predictable consequence of any medication tending to lower blood pressure —*Harvard Med. School Health Letter*⟩ — **light–head·ed** *adj*

light microscope *n* : an ordinary microscope that uses light as distinguished from an electron microscope — **light microscopy** *n, pl* **-pies**

light·ning pains \'līt-niŋ-\ *n pl* : intense shooting or lancinating pains occurring in tabes dorsalis

light sensitization *n* : PHOTOSENSITIZATION 2

light therapy *n* : PHOTOTHERAPY; *esp* : the use of strong light (as of 10,000 lux intensity) for the treatment of depression and gloom (as in seasonal affective disorder) — called also **light treatment**

lig·nan \'lig-,nan\ *n* : any of a class of propyl phenolic dimers including many found in plants and noted for having antioxidant and estrogenic activity

lig·nin \'lig-nən\ *n* : an amorphous polymeric substance related to cellulose that together with cellulose forms the woody cell walls of plants and the cementing material between them

lig·no·caine \'lig-nə-,kān\ *n, Brit* : LIDOCAINE

lig·no·cel·lu·lose \,lig-nō-'sel-yə-,lōs, -,lōz\ *n* : any of several closely related substances constituting the essential part of woody cell walls and consisting of cellulose intimately associated with lignin — **lig·no·cel·lu·los·ic** \-,sel-yə-'lō-sik, -zik\ *adj*

lig·no·cer·ic acid \,lig-nō-,ser-ik-, -,sir-\ *n* : a crystalline fatty acid $C_{24}H_{48}O_2$ that is found esp. in wood tar (as from beechwood) and in the form of esters in many fats, fatty oils, and waxes and is derived from kerasin

lig·num \'lig-nəm\ *n, pl* **lignums** *also* **lig·na** \-nə\ : woody tissue

lig·num vi·tae \,lig-nəm-'vīt-ē\ *n, pl* **lignum vitaes 1** : any of several tropical American trees of the genus *Guaiacum* with very hard heavy wood; *esp* : either of two (*G. officinale* or *G. sanctum*) that are sources of guaiacum resin **2** : the wood of a lignum vitae

lig·u·la \'lig-yə-lə\ *n* **1** *cap* : a genus of tapeworms of the family Diphyllobothriidae that lack external evidence of segmentation, that as adults are usu. extremely short-lived internal parasites of fish-eating birds but include one (*L. intestinalis*) found rarely in humans, and that develop almost to maturity in the body cavity of freshwater fishes **2** : a larval tapeworm developing reproductive organs and living in the body cavity of a fish

lily of the val·ley \'lil-ē-əv-thə-'val-ē\ *n, pl* **lil·ies of the valley 1** : an erect low-growing perennial herb of the genus *Convallaria* (*C. majalis*) that has two large oblong lanceolate leaves and a raceme of fragrant nodding bell-shaped white flowers and is the source of convallaria, convallamarin, convallarin, and convallatoxin **2** : the dried rhizome and roots of the lily of the valley used as a cardiac tonic

limb \'lim\ *n* **1** : one of the projecting paired appendages (as an arm, wing, fin, or parapodium) of an animal body made up of diverse tissues (as epithelium, muscle, and bone) derived from two or more germ layers and concerned esp. with movement and grasping but sometimes modified into sensory or sexual organs; *esp* : a human leg or arm **2** : a branch or arm of something (as an anatomical part) ⟨the descending ∼ of Henle's loop⟩

lim·bal \'lim-bəl\ *adj* : of or relating to the limbus ⟨a ∼ incision⟩

limb bud *n* : a proliferation of embryonic tissue shaped like a mound from which a limb develops

lim·ber·neck \'lim-bər-,nek\ *n* : a botulism of birds (esp. poultry) characterized by paralysis of the neck muscles and pharynx that interferes with swallowing and with raising or controlling the head

lim·bic \'lim-bik\ *adj* : of, relating to, or being the limbic system of the brain

limbic lobe *n* : the marginal medial portion of the cortex of a cerebral hemisphere

limbic system *n* : a group of subcortical structures (as the hypothalamus, the hippocampus, and the amygdala) of the brain that are concerned esp. with emotion and motivation

lim·bus \'lim-bəs\ *n* : a border distinguished by color or structure; *esp* : the marginal region of the cornea of the eye by which it is continuous with the sclera

¹lime \'līm\ *n* : a caustic powdery white highly infusible solid that consists of calcium oxide often together with magnesia — called also *quicklime;* see LIMEWATER — **lime** *adj*

²lime *n* : the small globose yellowish green fruit of a spiny tropical tree of the genus *Citrus* (*C. aurantifolia*) that has a usu. acid juicy pulp used as a flavoring agent and as a source of vitamin C; *also* : a tree that bears limes

lime liniment *n* : CARRON OIL

li·men \'lī-mən\ *n* : THRESHOLD ⟨appetites and needs . . . smouldering below the ∼ of awareness —R. M. Lindner⟩

lime·wa·ter \'līm-,wȯt-ər, -,wät-\ *n* : an alkaline water solution of calcium hydroxide used topically as an astringent or protective in various dermatologic lotions

lim·i·nal \'lim-ən-°l\ *adj* **1** : of or relating to a sensory threshold ⟨∼ research⟩ **2** : situated at a sensory threshold : barely perceptible ⟨observation of ∼ hues is beset with difficulties —Elsie Murray⟩

lim·o·nene \'lim-ə-,nēn\ *n* : a liquid terpene hydrocarbon $C_{10}H_{16}$ that has an odor like a lemon, exists in dextrorotatory, levorotatory, and racemic forms, and occurs in many essential oils — compare DIPENTENE

¹limp \'limp\ *vi* **1** : to walk lamely; *esp* : to walk favoring one leg **2** : to go unsteadily

²limp *n* : a limping movement or gait

lin·a·mar·in \,lin-ə-'mar-ən\ *n* : a bitter crystalline toxic cyanogenetic glucoside $C_{10}H_{17}NO_6$ occurring esp. in flax and the lima bean — called also *phaseolunatin*

Lin·co·cin \liŋ-'kō-sən\ *trademark* — used for a preparation of the hydrated hydrochloride of lincomycin

lin·co·my·cin \,liŋ-kə-'mīs-°n\ *n* : an antibiotic effective esp. against gram-positive bacteria that is obtained from an actinomycete of the genus *Streptomyces* (*S. lincolnensis*) and is used in the form of its hydrated hydrochloride $C_{18}H_{34}N_2O_6S \cdot HCl \cdot H_2O$

linc·tus \'liŋk-təs\ *n, pl* **linc·tus·es** : a syrupy or sticky preparation containing medicaments exerting a local action on the mucous membrane of the throat

lin·dane \'lin-,dān\ *n* : an insecticide consisting of not less than 99 percent gamma benzene hexachloride that is used esp. in agriculture and is biodegraded very slowly

Lin·dau's disease \'lin-,daůz-\ *n* : VON HIPPEL–LINDAU DISEASE

line \'līn\ *n* **1** : something (as a ridge, seam, mark, or streak) that is distinct, elongated, and narrow — see LINEA **2** : a strain produced and maintained esp. by selective breeding or biological culture **3** : a narrow short synthetic tube (as of plastic) that is inserted approximately one inch into a vein (as of the arm) to provide temporary intravenous access for the administration of fluid, medication, or nutrients

lin·ea \'lin-ē-ə\ *n, pl* **lin·e·ae** \-ē-,ē\ : a line or linear body structure

linea al·ba \-'al-bə\ *n, pl* **lineae al·bae** \-bē\ : a median vertical tendinous line on the mammalian abdomen formed of fibers from the aponeuroses of the two rectus abdominis muscles and extending from the xiphoid process to the pubic symphysis — see ADMINICULUM LINEAE ALBAE

linea as·pe·ra \-'as-pə-rə\ *n, pl* **lineae as·pe·rae** \-rē\ : a longitudinal ridge on the posterior surface of the middle third of the femur

---

\ə\ **abut** \ə\ **kitten** \ər\ **further** \a\ **ash** \ā\ **ace** \ä\ **cot, cart**
\aů\ **out** \ch\ **chin** \e\ **bet** \ē\ **easy** \g\ **go** \i\ **hit** \ī\ **ice** \j\ **job**
\ŋ\ **sing** \ō\ **go** \ȯ\ **law** \ȯi\ **boy** \th\ **thin** \t͟h\ **the** \ü\ **loot**
\ů\ **foot** \y\ **yet** \zh\ **vision** *See also* Pronunciation Symbols page

K
L

lineae al·bi·can·tes \-,al-bə-'kan-,tēz\ *n pl* : whitish marks in the skin esp. of the abdomen and breasts that often follow pregnancy

lin·e·age \'lin-ē-ij *also* 'lin-ij\ *n* **1** : descent in a line from a common progenitor **2** : a group of individuals descended from a common ancestor ⟨replication in T cell ∼*s*⟩

lin·ear \'lin-ē-ər\ *adj* : of, relating to, or resembling a line — **lin·ear·i·ty** \,lin-ē-'ar-ət-ē\ *n, pl* **-ties** — **lin·ear·ly** \'lin-ē-ər-lē\ *adv*

linear accelerator *n* : an accelerator in which particles are propelled in a straight line and receive successive increments of energy through the application of alternating potentials to a series of electrodes and gaps

linea semi·lu·nar·is \-,sem-i-lü-'ner-əs, -'nar-\ *n, pl* **lineae semi·lu·nar·es** \-'ner-,ēz, -'nar-\ : a curved line on the ventral abdominal wall parallel to the midline and halfway between it and the side of the body that marks the lateral border of the rectus abdominis muscle — called also *semilunar line*

line·bred \'līn-'bred\ *adj* : subjected to or produced by linebreeding

line·breed \-'brēd\ *vb* **-bred** \-'bred\; **-breed·ing** *vi* : to practice linebreeding ∼ *vt* : to interbreed (animals) by linebreeding; *also* : to produce by linebreeding

line·breed·ing \-iŋ\ *n* : the interbreeding of individuals within in a particular line of descent usu. to perpetuate desirable characters — compare INBREEDING, OUTBREEDING

line of sight *n* **1** : a line from an observer's eye to a distant point **2** : LINE OF VISION

line of vision *n* : a straight line joining the fovea of the eye with the fixation point — called also *visual axis*

lin·gua \'liŋ-gwə\ *n, pl* **lin·guae** \-,gwē, -,gwī\ : a tongue or an organ resembling a tongue in structure or function

lin·gual \'liŋ-g(yə-)wəl\ *adj* **1** : of, relating to, or resembling the tongue **2** : lying near or next to the tongue ⟨a ∼ blood vessel⟩; *esp* : relating to or being the surface of a tooth next to the tongue

lingual artery *n* : an artery arising from the external carotid artery between the superior thyroid and facial arteries and supplying the tongue — see DEEP LINGUAL ARTERY

lingual bone *n* : HYOID BONE

lin·gua·le \liŋ-'gwä-lē, -'gwā-\ *n* : the midpoint of the upper border of the human mandible — compare GNATHION

lingual gland *n* : any of the mucous, serous, or mixed glands that empty their secretions onto the surface of the tongue

lin·gual·ly \'liŋ-gwə-lē\ *adv* : toward the tongue ⟨a tooth displaced ∼⟩

lingual nerve *n* : a branch of the mandibular division of the trigeminal nerve supplying the anterior two thirds of the tongue and responding to stimuli of pressure, touch, and temperature

lingual tonsil *n* : a variable mass or group of small nodules of lymphoid tissue lying at the base of the tongue just anterior to the epiglottis

Lin·guat·u·la \liŋ-'gwa-chə-lə\ *n* : a genus of tongue worms that includes a cosmopolitan parasite (*L. serrata*) of the nasal and respiratory passages of various canines, sheep and goats, the horse, and occas. humans

lin·guat·u·lid \liŋ-'gwa-chə-ləd, -,lid\ *n* : any tongue worm of the genus *Linguatula*; *broadly* : TONGUE WORM

lin·guat·u·lo·sis \liŋ-,gwa-chə-'lō-səs\ *n, pl* **-lo·ses** \-,sēz\ : infestation with or disease caused by tongue worms

lin·gui·form \'liŋ-gwə-,fòrm\ *adj* : having the form of a tongue : tongue-shaped

lin·gu·la \'liŋ-gyə-lə\ *n, pl* **lin·gu·lae** \-,lē\ : a tongue-shaped process or part: as **a** : a ridge of bone in the angle between the body and the greater wing of the sphenoid **b** : an elongated prominence of the superior vermis of the cerebellum **c** : a dependent projection of the upper lobe of the left lung — **lin·gu·lar** \-lər\ *adj*

lin·guo·ver·sion \,liŋ-gwə-'vər-zhən\ *n* : displacement of a tooth to the lingual side of its proper occlusal position

lin·i·ment \'lin-ə-mənt\ *n* : a liquid or semifluid preparation that is applied to the skin as an anodyne or a counterirritant — called also *embrocation*

¹li·nin \'lī-nən\ *n* : a bitter white crystallizable substance with purgative qualities obtained from the purging flax

²linin *n* : the feebly staining portion of the reticulum of the nucleus of a resting cell in which chromatin granules appear to be embedded

li·ni·tis plas·ti·ca \lə-'nīt-əs-'plas-ti-kə\ *n* : carcinoma of the stomach characterized by thickening and diffuse infiltration of the wall rather than localization of the tumor in a discrete lump

link·age \'liŋ-kij\ *n* **1** : the manner in which atoms or radicals are connected by chemical bonds in a molecule **2** : the relationship between genes on the same chromosome that causes them to be inherited together — compare MENDEL'S LAW 2

linkage group *n* : a set of genes at different loci on the same chromosome that except for crossing-over tend to act as a single pair of genes in meiosis instead of undergoing independent assortment

linked \'liŋ(k)t\ *adj* : marked by linkage and esp. genetic linkage ⟨∼ genes⟩

Lin·nae·an *or* **Lin·ne·an** \lə-'nē-ən, -'nā-; 'lin-ē-ən\ *adj* : of, relating to, or following the systematic methods of the Swedish botanist Linné who established the system of binomial nomenclature

Lin·né \li-'nā\, **Carl von** (*Latin* **Carolus Lin·nae·us** \li-'nā-əs, -'nē-\) **(1707–1778)**, Swedish botanist. Linnaeus is credited with being the first to establish principles for classifying organisms into genera and species and to formulate a uniform system of nomenclature. He was the first to adhere rigorously to the use of two names, one for genus and one for species, for naming plants and animals. A student of botany and medicine, he successfully practiced in both fields before ultimately deciding on botany, his true calling. In 1735 he published the first of his nomenclatorial systems, *Systema Naturae*. The system was based mainly on flower parts, and although artificial, it had the great merit of enabling the botanist to rapidly place a plant in a named category. In 1753 he published *Species Plantarum*, in which the specific names of flowering plants and ferns are fully set forth. A born classifier, he not only systematized the plant and animal kingdoms, but he even drew up a classification of minerals and wrote a treatise on the kinds of diseases then known.

Li·nog·na·thus \li-'näg-nə-thəs\ *n* : a cosmopolitan genus of sucking lice including parasites of several domestic mammals

li·no·le·ate \lə-'nō-lē-,āt\ *n* : a salt or ester of linoleic acid

lin·ole·ic acid \,lin-ə-,lē-ik-, -,lā-\ *n* : a liquid unsaturated fatty acid $C_{18}H_{32}O_2$ found esp. in semidrying oils (as peanut oil) and essential for the nutrition of some animals — called also *linolic acid*

lin·ole·nate \,lin-ə-'lē-,nāt, -'lā-,nāt\ *n* : a salt or ester of linolenic acid

lin·ole·nic acid \-,lē-nik-, -,lā-\ *n* : a liquid unsaturated fatty acid $C_{18}H_{30}O_2$ found esp. in drying oils (as linseed oil) and essential for the nutrition of some animals

li·no·lic acid \li-'nō-lik-\ *n* : LINOLEIC ACID

lin·seed \'lin-,sēd\ *n* : FLAXSEED

linseed oil *n* : a yellowish drying oil obtained from flaxseed and used in liniments, pastes, and green soap and in veterinary medicine as a laxative

lint \'lint\ *n* **1** : a soft fleecy material used for poultices and dressings for wounds and made from linen usu. by scraping **2** *Brit* : sterile cotton cloth used for dressings

li·o·thy·ro·nine \,lī-ō-'thī-rə-,nēn\ *n* : TRIIODOTHYRONINE

lip \'lip\ *n* **1** : either of the two fleshy folds which surround the opening of the mouth in humans and many other vertebrates and in humans are organs of speech essential to certain articulations; *also* : the pinkish or reddish margin of a human lip composed of nonglandular mucous membrane and usu. exposed when the mouth takes on its natural set **2** : an edge of a wound **3** : either of a pair of fleshy folds surrounding an orifice **4** : an anatomical part or structure (as a labium) resembling a lip — **lip-like** \'lip-ˌlik\ *adj*

li·pase \'lip-ˌās, 'līp-, -ˌāz\ *n* : any enzyme (as one secreted by the pancreas) that catalyzes the breakdown of fats and lipoproteins usu. into fatty acids and glycerol

li·pec·to·my \li-'pek-tə-mē, lī-\ *n, pl* **-mies** : the excision of subcutaneous fatty tissue esp. as a cosmetic surgical procedure

li·pe·mia *or chiefly Brit* **li·pae·mia** \li-'pē-mē-ə\ *n* : the presence of an excess of fats or lipids in the blood; *specif* : HYPERCHOLESTEROLEMIA — **li·pe·mic** *or chiefly Brit* **li·pae·mic** \-mik\ *adj*

lip·id \'lip-əd\ *also* **lip·ide** \-ˌīd\ *n* : any of various substances that are soluble in nonpolar organic solvents (as chloroform and ether), that with proteins and carbohydrates constitute the principal structural components of living cells, and that include fats, waxes, phospholipids, cerebrosides, and related and derived compounds

li·pid·ic \li-'pid-ik\ *adj* : of or relating to lipids ⟨∼ inclusions⟩

lip·id·o·lyt·ic \ˌlip-id-ə-'lit-ik\ *adj* : causing the chemical breakdown of lipids ⟨∼ enzymes⟩

lip·i·do·sis \ˌlip-ə-'dō-səs\ *n, pl* **-do·ses** \-ˌsēz\ : a disorder of fat metabolism esp. involving the deposition of fat in an organ (as the liver or spleen) — called also *lipoidosis;* compare LIPODYSTROPHY

lip·in \'lip-ən\ *n* : LIPID; *esp* : a complex lipid (as a phosphatide or a cerebroside)

Lip·io·dol \li-'pī-ə-ˌdȯl\ *trademark* — used for a preparation of iodized poppy-seed oil for use as a radiopaque diagnostic aid

Lip·i·tor \'lip-ə-tȯr\ *trademark* — used for a preparation of the calcium salt of atorvastatin

li·po·ate \li-'pō-ˌāt, lī-\ *n* : a salt or ester of lipoic acid

li·po·at·ro·phy \ˌlip-ō-'a-trə-fē\ *n, pl* **-phies** : an allergic reaction to insulin medication that is manifested as a loss of subcutaneous fat — **li·po·atro·phic** \-(ˈ)ā-'trō-fik\ *adj*

li·po·blast \'lip-ə-ˌblast, 'līp-\ *n* : a connective-tissue cell destined to become a fat cell

li·po·ca·ic \ˌlip-ə-'kā-ik, ˌlīp-\ *n* : a lipotropic preparation from the pancreas

li·po·chon·dri·on \ˌlip-ō-'kän-drē-ən, ˌlīp-\ *n, pl* **-dria** \-drē-ə\ : DICTYOSOME

li·po·chon·dro·dys·tro·phy \-ˌkän-drə-'dis-trə-fē\ *n, pl* **-phies** : MUCOPOLYSACCHARIDOSIS; *esp* : HURLER'S SYNDROME

li·po·chrome \'lip-ə-ˌkrōm, 'līp-\ *n* : any of the naturally occurring pigments soluble in fats or in solvents for fats; *esp* : CAROTENOID

li·po·cyte \-ˌsīt\ *n* : FAT CELL

li·po·dys·tro·phy \ˌlip-ō-'dis-trə-fē, ˌlīp-\ *n, pl* **-phies** : a disorder of fat metabolism esp. involving loss of fat from or deposition of fat in tissue — compare LIPIDOSIS

lipodystrophy syndrome *n* : a group of side effects of antiretroviral therapy for HIV infection that include high triglyceride levels in the blood, diabetes, and redistribution of fat in the body resulting in changes in bodily conformation and that are believed to result esp. from treatment with protease inhibitors

li·po·fi·bro·ma \ˌlip-ō-fī-'brō-mə, ˌlīp-\ *n, pl* **-mas** *also* **-ma·ta** \-mət-ə\ : a lipoma containing fibrous tissue

li·po·fus·cin \ˌlip-ə-'fəs-ᵊn, ˌlīp-ō-, -'fyü-sᵊn\ *n* : a brownish lipochrome found esp. in tissue (as of the heart) of the aged

li·po·fus·cin·o·sis \-ˌfəs-ə-'nō-səs, -ˌfyüs-\ *n* : a storage disease (as Batten disease) marked by abnormal accumulation of lipofuscins

li·po·gen·e·sis \-'jen-ə-səs\ *n, pl* **-e·ses** \-ˌsēz\ **1** : formation of fat in the living body esp. when excessive or abnormal **2** : the formation of fatty acids from acetyl coenzyme A in the living body — **li·po·ge·net·ic** \-jə-'net-ik\ *adj*

li·po·gen·ic \ˌlip-ə-'jen-ik, ˌlīp-\ *also* **li·pog·e·nous** \li-'päj-ə-nəs\ *adj* : producing or tending to produce fat ⟨a ∼ diet⟩

li·po·ic acid \li-ˌpō-ik-, lī-\ *n* : any of several microbial growth factors; *esp* : a crystalline compound $C_8H_{14}O_2S_2$ that

is essential for the oxidation of alpha-keto acids (as pyruvic acid) in metabolism — called also *protogen*

¹li·poid \'lip-ˌȯid, 'līp-\ *or* **li·poi·dal** \li-'pȯid-ᵊl\ *adj* : resembling fat

²lipoid *n* : LIPID

lipoidica — see NECROBIOSIS LIPOIDICA, NECROBIOSIS LIPOIDICA DIABETICORUM

li·poid·o·sis \ˌlip-ˌȯid-'ō-səs, ˌlīp-\ *n, pl* **-o·ses** \-ˌsēz\ : LIPIDOSIS

li·pol·y·sis \li-'päl-ə-səs, lī-\ *n, pl* **-y·ses** \-ˌsēz\ : the hydrolysis of fat — **li·po·lyt·ic** \ˌlip-ə-'lit-ik, ˌlīp-\ *adj*

li·po·ma \li-'pō-mə, lī-\ *n, pl* **-mas** *also* **-ma·ta** \-mət-ə\ : a tumor of fatty tissue — **li·po·ma·tous** \-mət-əs\ *adj*

li·po·ma·to·sis \ˌlip-ō-mə-'tō-səs, ˌlīp-\ *n, pl* **-to·ses** \-ˌsēz\ : any of several abnormal conditions marked by local or generalized deposits of fat or replacement of other tissue by fat; *specif* : the presence of multiple lipomas

li·po·mi·cron \ˌlip-ō-'mī-ˌkrän, ˌlīp-\ *n* : any fat particle (as a chylomicron) in the blood

li·po·phage \'lip-ə-ˌfāj, 'līp-\ *n* : a cell (as a phagocyte) that takes up fat

li·po·pha·gic \ˌlip-ə-'fā-jik, ˌlīp-\ *adj* : of, relating to, or characterized by the destruction of adipose tissue with cellular uptake of the breakdown products (as by lipophages) ⟨∼ disease of the knee joint —*Jour. Amer. Med. Assoc.*⟩

li·po·phan·er·o·sis \ˌlip-ō-ˌfan-ə-'rō-səs, ˌlīp-\ *n, pl* **-o·ses** \-ˌsēz\ : fatty degeneration of cells involving the formation of visible lipid droplets

li·po·phil·ic \ˌlip-ə-'fil-ik, ˌlīp-\ *adj* : having an affinity for lipids (as fats) ⟨a ∼ metabolite⟩ — compare HYDROPHILIC, LYOPHILIC, OLEOPHILIC — **li·po·phi·lic·i·ty** \-fi-'lis-ət-ē\ *n, pl* **-ties**

li·po·poly·sac·cha·ride \ˌlip-ō-ˌpäl-i-'sak-ə-ˌrīd, ˌlī-pō-\ *n* : a large molecule consisting of lipids and sugars joined by chemical bonds — abbr. *LPS*

li·po·pro·tein \-'prō-ˌtēn, -'prōt-ē-ən\ *n* : any of a large class of conjugated proteins composed of a complex of protein and lipid — see HDL, LDL, VLDL

li·po·sar·co·ma \-sär-'kō-mə\ *n, pl* **-mas** *also* **-ma·ta** \-mət-ə\ : a sarcoma arising from immature fat cells of the bone marrow

li·po·sis \li-'pō-səs, lī-\ *n, pl* **li·po·ses** \-ˌsēz\ : OBESITY

li·po·sol·u·ble \ˌlip-ō-'säl-yə-bəl, ˌlīp-\ *adj* : FAT-SOLUBLE ⟨∼ vitamins⟩ — **li·po·sol·u·bil·i·ty** \-ˌsäl-yə-'bil-ət-ē\ *n, pl* **-ties**

li·po·some \'lip-ə-ˌsōm, 'lī-pə-\ *n* **1** : one of the fatty droplets in the cytoplasm of a cell **2** : an artificial vesicle that is composed of one or more concentric phospholipid bilayers and is used esp. to deliver microscopic substances (as DNA or drugs) to body cells — **li·po·so·mal** \ˌlip-ə-'sō-məl, ˌlī-pə-\ *adj*

li·po·suc·tion \-ˌsək-shən\ *n* : surgical removal of local fat deposits (as in the thighs) esp. for cosmetic purposes by applying suction through a small tube inserted into the body — called also *suction lipectomy* — **liposuction** *vt*

li·po·suc·tion·ist \ˌlip-ə-'sək-shən-ist, ˌlī-pə-\ *n* : a surgeon who performs liposuction

li·po·thy·mia \ˌlī-pə-'thī-mē-ə, ˌlip-ə-\ *n* : a condition or feeling of faintness — **li·po·thy·mic** \-mik\ *adj*

li·po·tro·pic \ˌlip-ō-'trō-pik, ˌlīp-, -'träp-ik\ *also* **li·po·tro·phic** \-'trō-fik\ *adj* : promoting the physiological utilization of fat ⟨∼ dietary factors⟩ — **li·po·tro·pism** \-'trō-ˌpiz-əm\ *n*

li·po·tro·pin \ˌlip-ō-'trō-pən, ˌlīp-\ *n* : either of two protein hormones of the adenohypophysis of the pituitary gland that function in the mobilization of fat reserves; *esp* : BETA-LIPOTROPIN

li·po·vac·cine \ˌlip-ō-vak-'sēn, ˌlī-pō-, -'vak-ˌsēn\ *n* : a vaccine whose fluid medium is an oil

li·pox·i·dase \li-'päk-sə-ˌdās, -ˌdāz\ *n* : LIPOXYGENASE

\ə\ **abut** \ᵊ\ **kitten** \ər\ **further** \a\ **ash** \ā\ **ace** \ä\ **cot, cart**
\au̇\ **out** \ch\ **chin** \e\ **bet** \ē\ **easy** \g\ **go** \i\ **hit** \ī\ **ice** \j\ **job**
\ŋ\ **sing** \ō\ **go** \ȯ\ **law** \ȯi\ **boy** \th\ **thin** \t̲h̲\ **the** \ü\ **loot**
\u̇\ **foot** \y\ **yet** \zh\ **vision** See also Pronunciation Symbols page

K
L

li·pox·y·gen·ase \li-ˈpäk-sə-jə-ˌnās, lī-, -ˌnāz\ *n* : a crystallizable enzyme that catalyzes the oxidation primarily of unsaturated fatty acids or unsaturated fats by oxygen and secondarily of carotenoids to colorless substances and that occurs esp. in soybeans and cereals

Lippes loop \ˈlip-ēz-\ *n* : an S-shaped plastic intrauterine device

Lippes, Jack (*b* 1924), American obstetrician and gynecologist. A specialist in reproduction physiology, Lippes did research in such areas as the physiology of human oviductal fluid, immunology of the genital tract, and intrauterine contraception. He invented the Lippes loop and first introduced it around 1962.

lip–read \ˈlip-ˌrēd\ *vb* **-read** \-ˌred\; **-read·ing** \-ˌrēd-iŋ\ *vt* : to understand by lipreading ∼ *vi* : to use lipreading
lip–read·er \-ˌrēd-ər\ *n* : a person who lip-reads
lip·read·ing \-ˌrēd-iŋ\ *n* : the interpreting of spoken words by watching the speaker's lip and facial movements without hearing the voice
li·pu·ria \li-ˈp(y)ùr-ē-ə\ *n* : the presence of fat in urine
liq *abbr* **1** liquid **2** liquor
Li·quae·min \ˈlik-wə-ˌmin\ *n* : a preparation of heparin — formerly a U.S. registered trademark
liq·ue·fa·cient \ˌlik-wə-ˈfā-shənt\ *n* : something that serves to liquefy or to promote liquefaction
liq·ue·fac·tion \ˌlik-wə-ˈfak-shən\ *n* **1** : the process of making or becoming liquid **2** : the state of being liquid
li·queur \li-ˈkər, -ˈk(y)ú(ə)r\ *n* : a usu. sweetened alcoholic beverage variously flavored (as with fruit or aromatics)
¹liq·uid \ˈlik-wəd\ *adj* **1** : flowing freely like water **2** : having the properties of a liquid : being neither solid nor gaseous
²liquid *n* : a fluid (as water) that has no independent shape but has a definite volume and does not expand indefinitely and that is only slightly compressible
liq·uid·am·bar \ˌlik-wə-ˈdam-bər\ *n* **1 a** *cap* : a genus of trees of the witch hazel family (Hamamelidaceae) with a spiny globose fruit that is a cluster of many woody capsules **b** : any tree of the genus *Liquidambar* **2** : STORAX 2
liquid chromatography *n* : chromatography in which the mobile phase is a liquid — abbr. *LC*
liquid crystal *n* : an organic liquid whose physical properties resemble those of a crystal in the formation of loosely ordered molecular arrays similar to a regular crystalline lattice and the anisotropic refraction of light
liquid measure *n* : a unit or series of units for measuring liquid capacity
liquid paraffin *n* : MINERAL OIL 2
liquid petrolatum *n* : MINERAL OIL 2
liquid protein diet *n* : a reducing diet consisting of high= protein liquids
liquid storax *n* : STORAX 1
Li·qui·prin \ˈlik-wə-ˌprin\ *n* : a preparation of acetaminophen — formerly a U.S. registered trademark
li·quor \ˈlik-ər\ *n* : a liquid substance: as **a** : a usu. distilled rather than fermented alcoholic beverage **b** : a solution of a medicinal substance usu. in water — compare TINCTURE **c** : BATH 2b(1)
li·quor am·nii \ˈlī-ˌkwòr-ˈam-nē-ˌī, ˈli-\ *n* : AMNIOTIC FLUID
li·quor fol·li·cu·li \ˈlī-ˌkwòr-fä-ˈlik-yə-ˌlī, ˈli-\ *n* : the fluid surrounding the ovum in the ovarian follicle
liquorice *chiefly Brit var of* LICORICE
li·sin·o·pril \li-ˈsin-ə-ˌpril, lī-\ *n* : an antihypertensive drug $C_{21}H_{31}N_3O_5·2H_2O$ that is an ACE inhibitor — see PRINIVIL, ZESTRIL
¹lisp \ˈlisp\ *vi* **1** : to pronounce the sibilants \s\ and \z\ imperfectly esp. by giving them the sounds \th\ and \th͟\ **2** : to speak with a lisp ∼ *vt* : to utter with a lisp
²lisp *n* : a speech defect or affectation characterized by lisping
lisp·er \ˈlisp-ər\ *n* : one who lisps
Lis·sau·er's tract \ˈlis-aù-ərz-\ *n* : DORSOLATERAL TRACT
Lissauer, Heinrich (1861–1891), German neurologist. Lissauer published a description of the dorsolateral tract in the spinal cord in 1885. He died before he could publish his observations on an atypical general paresis marked by apha-

sia, convulsions, and monoplegia. His description was published posthumously in 1901.
lis·sen·ceph·a·ly \ˌlis-en-ˈsef-ə-lē\ *n, pl* **-lies** : the condition of having a smooth cerebrum without convolutions — **lis·sen·ce·phal·ic** \-sə-ˈfal-ik\ *adj*
Lis·ter bag *also* **Lys·ter bag** \ˈlis-tər-ˌbag\ *n* : a canvas water bag used esp. for supplying military troops with chemically purified drinking water

Lyster, William John Le Hunte (1869–1947), American army surgeon. Lyster had a career as a surgeon in the U.S. Army medical corps. Interested in the field of public health, he began experiments in water purification with the use of sodium hypochlorite. In 1917 he introduced a rubber-lined heavy canvas bag with a tight-fitting cover. A dose of chlorine solution added to the water effected purification within 30 minutes. The Lister bag quickly became a standard piece of army equipment and was used extensively in both world wars.

lis·ter·el·la \ˌlis-tə-ˈrel-ə\ *n* : LISTERIA 2

Lis·ter \ˈlis-tər\, **Joseph** (1827–1912), British surgeon and medical scientist. One of the greatest surgeons in medical history, Lister successfully introduced antisepsis into the operating room and as a result revolutionized modern surgery. Building on Louis Pasteur's studies of bacteria, he studied sepsis and suppuration and the use of chemicals to prevent surgical infection. In 1865 he began using carbolic acid as an antiseptic. In 1877, in an operation involving a compound fracture, he conclusively demonstrated that his practice of antisepsis greatly reduced the rate of mortality due to surgery. Although his work was highly controversial originally, by the time of his death the principle of antisepsis was universally accepted.

Listerella *n, syn of* LISTERIA
lis·te·ria \lis-ˈtir-ē-ə\ *n* **1** *cap* : a genus of small gram-positive flagellated rod-shaped bacteria that do not form spores, are aerobic or facultatively anaerobic, and have a tendency to grow in chains and that include one (*L. monocytogenes*) causing listeriosis **2** : any bacterium of the genus *Listeria* — called also *listerella* — **lis·te·ri·al** \lis-ˈtir-ē-əl\ *adj* — **lis·te·ric** \-ik\ *adj*
lis·te·ri·o·sis \(ˌ)lis-ˌtir-ē-ˈō-səs\ *also* **lis·ter·el·lo·sis** \ˌlis-tə-rə-ˈlō-səs\ *n, pl* **-ri·o·ses** *also* **-lo·ses** \-ˌsēz\ : a serious disease of animals and humans that is caused by a bacterium of the genus *Listeria* (*L. monocytogenes*), that in animals causes severe encephalitis accompanied by disordered movements and is often fatal, that is contracted by humans esp. from contaminated food (as processed meats or unpasteurized milk or cheese), that in otherwise healthy people typically takes the form of a mild flulike illness or has no noticeable symptoms, that in neonates, the elderly, and the immunocompromised often causes serious sometimes fatal illness with symptoms including meningitis and sepsis, and that in pregnant women usu. causes only mild illness in the mother but often results in miscarriage, stillbirth, or premature birth — see CIRCLING DISEASE
lis·ter·ism \ˈlis-tə-ˌriz-əm\ *n, often cap* : the practice of antiseptic surgery
lite *var of* ²LIGHT
li·ter *or chiefly Brit* **li·tre** \ˈlēt-ər\ *n* : a metric unit of capacity equal to the volume of one kilogram of water at 4°C (39°F) and at standard atmospheric pressure of 760 millimeters of mercury
li·tharge \ˈlith-ˌärj, lith-ˈ\ *n* : lead monoxide obtained in flake or powdered form; *broadly* : LEAD MONOXIDE — compare MASSICOT
li·the·mia *or chiefly Brit* **li·thae·mia** \lith-ˈē-mē-ə\ *n* : a condition in which excess uric acid is present in the blood — **li·the·mic** *or chiefly Brit* **li·thae·mic** \-mik\ *adj*
lith·ia \ˈlith-ē-ə\ *n* : a white crystalline oxide of lithium Li_2O
li·thi·a·sis \lith-ˈī-ə-səs\ *n, pl* **-a·ses** \-ˌsēz\ : the formation of stony concretions in the body (as in the urinary tract or gallbladder) — often used in combination ⟨chole*lithiasis*⟩
lith·i·um \ˈlith-ē-əm\ *n* **1** : a soft silver-white element of the alkali metal group that is the lightest metal known and that

is used in chemical synthesis and in storage batteries — symbol *Li*; see ELEMENT table   **2** : a lithium salt and esp. lithium carbonate used in psychiatric medicine

lithium carbonate *n* : a crystalline salt Li_2CO_3 used in the glass and ceramic industries and in medicine in the treatment of mania and hypomania in bipolar disorder

lith·o·cho·lic acid \ˌlith-ə-ˌkō-lik-\ *n* : a crystalline bile acid $C_{24}H_{40}O_3$ found esp. in humans and the ox

lith·o·gen·ic \ˌlith-ə-ˈjen-ik\ *adj* : of, promoting, or undergoing the formation of calculi ⟨a ∼ diet⟩ — **lith·o·gen·e·sis** \-ˈjen-ə-səs\ *n, pl* **-e·ses** \-ˌsēz\

lith·o·kel·y·pho·pe·di·on \ˌlith-ō-ˌkel-i-fə-ˈpē-dē-ˌän\ *n* : a fetus and its surrounding membranes which have both been calcified in the body of the mother

lith·ol·a·paxy \lith-ˈäl-ə-ˌpak-sē, ˈlith-ə-lə-\ *n, pl* **-pax·ies** : LITHOTRIPSY

lith·o·pe·di·on \ˌlith-ə-ˈpē-dē-ˌän\ *n* : a fetus calcified in the body of the mother

Lith·o·sper·mum \ˌlith-ə-ˈspər-məm\ *n* : a genus of herbs of the borage family (Boraginaceae) having polished white stony nutlets and including one (*L. ruderale*) used by some American Indians to make a tea held to prevent conception

lith·o·tome \ˈlith-ə-ˌtōm\ *n* : a knife used for lithotomy

li·thot·o·mist \lith-ˈät-ə-məst\ *n* : a specialist in lithotomy

li·thot·o·my \lith-ˈät-ə-mē\ *n, pl* **-mies** : surgical incision of the urinary bladder for removal of a calculus

lith·o·trip·sy \ˈlith-ə-ˌtrip-sē\ *n, pl* **-sies** : the breaking of a calculus (as by shock waves or crushing with a surgical instrument) in the urinary system into pieces small enough to be voided or washed out — called also *litholapaxy, lithotrity*

lith·o·trip·ter *also* **lith·o·trip·tor** \ˈlith-ə-ˌtrip-tər\ *n* : a device for performing lithotripsy; *esp* : a noninvasive device that pulverizes calculi by focusing shock waves on a patient immersed in a water bath

lith·o·trite \ˈlith-ə-ˌtrīt\ *n* : LITHOTRIPTER

li·thot·ri·ty \lith-ˈät-rə-tē\ *n, pl* **-ties** : LITHOTRIPSY

li·thu·ria \lith-ˈ(y)ùr-ē-ə\ *n* : an excess of uric acid or of its salts in the urine

lit·mus \ˈlit-məs\ *n* : a coloring matter from lichens that turns red in acid solutions and blue in alkaline solutions and is used as an acid-base indicator

litmus paper *n* : paper colored with litmus and used as an acid-base indicator

li·tre \ˈlēt-ər\ *chiefly Brit var of* LITER

¹lit·ter \ˈlit-ər\ *n* **1** : a device (as a stretcher) for carrying a sick or injured person   **2** : the offspring at one birth of a multiparous animal

²litter *vt* : to give birth to a litter of (young) ∼ *vi* : to give birth to a litter

lit·tle \ˈlit-ᵊl\ *adj* **lit·tler** \ˈlit-ᵊl-ər, ˈlit-lər\ *or* **less** \ˈles\ *or* **lesser** \ˈles-ər\; **lit·tlest** \ˈlit-ᵊl-əst, ˈlit-ləst\ *or* **least** \ˈlēst\ : not big: as   **a** : small in size or extent ⟨has ∼ feet⟩   **b** *of a plant or animal* : small in comparison with related forms — used in vernacular names

little finger *n* : the fourth and smallest finger of the hand counting the index finger as the first

little housefly *n* : a fly of the genus *Fannia* (*F. canicularis*) that is smaller than the housefly (*Musca domestica*) — called also *lesser housefly*

Little League elbow \-ˈlēg-\ *n* : inflammation of the medial epicondyle and adjacent tissues of the elbow esp. in preteen and teenage baseball players who make too strenuous use of the muscles of the forearm — called also *Little Lea·guer's elbow* \-ˈlē-gərz-\; compare TENNIS ELBOW

Lit·tle's disease \ˈlit-ᵊlz-\ *n* : a form of spastic cerebral palsy marked by spastic diplegia in which the legs are typically more severely affected than the arms; *broadly* : CEREBRAL PALSY

Little, William John (1810–1894), British physician. Little was the first eminent British orthopedic surgeon. In 1861 he presented the first complete description of congenital cerebral spastic paralysis, which came to be called Little's disease and is now known to be a form of spastic cerebral palsy. He also established that there is a relationship between a

mother's abnormal parturition and the occurrence of nervous disorders in the child.

little stroke *n* : a usu. transient blockage of one or more arteries in the cerebrum causing temporary numbness or impaired function of a part, slowed mentation, speech defects, dizziness, and nausea

little toe *n* : the outermost and smallest digit of the foot

lit·to·ral cell \ˈlit-ə-rəl-, -ˌral-\ *n* : one of the reticuloendothelial cells lining the sinuses of the various reticular organs of the body

Lit·tré's gland \lē-ˈtrāz-\ *n* : GLAND OF LITTRÉ

lit·tri·tis \li-ˈtrīt-əs\ *n* : inflammation of the glands of Littré

¹live \ˈliv\ *vi* **lived; liv·ing**   **1** : to be alive : have the life of an animal or plant   **2** : to continue alive ⟨*lived* for 50 years⟩   **3** : to maintain oneself ⟨∼s on a vegetarian diet⟩   **4** : to conduct or pass one's life ⟨a parasite *living* in the body of a host⟩

²live \ˈlīv\ *adj* : having life : LIVING

live birth \ˈlīv-\ *n* : birth in such a state that processes of life are manifested after the emergence of the whole body : birth of a live fetus — compare STILLBIRTH

live–born \ˈlīv-ˈbó(ə)rn\ *adj* : born alive — compare STILLBORN

li·ve·do \li-ˈvē-dō\ *n* : a bluish usu. patchy discoloration of the skin

livedo ra·ce·mo·sa \-ˌras-ə-ˈmō-sə, -ˌrās-\ *n* : LIVEDO RETICULARIS

livedo re·tic·u·lar·is \-ri-ˌtik-yə-ˈler-əs, -ˈlar-\ *n* : a condition of the peripheral blood vessels characterized by reddish blue mottling of the skin esp. of the extremities usu. upon exposure to cold

liv·er \ˈliv-ər\ *n* **1 a** : a large very vascular glandular organ of vertebrates that secretes bile and causes important changes in many of the substances contained in the blood which passes through it (as by converting sugars into glycogen which it stores up until required and by forming urea), that in humans is the largest gland in the body, weighs from 40 to 60 ounces (1100 to 1700 grams), is a dark red color, and occupies the upper right portion of the abdominal cavity immediately below the diaphragm, that is divided by fissures into five lobes, and that receives blood both from the hepatic artery and the portal vein and returns it to the systemic circulation by the hepatic veins   **b** : any of various large compound glands associated with the digestive tract of invertebrate animals and prob. concerned with the secretion of digestive enzymes   **2** : the liver of an animal (as a calf or pig) eaten as food or used as a source of pharmaceutical products (as liver extract)   **3** : disease or disorder of the liver : BILIOUSNESS

liver cell *n* : HEPATOCYTE

liver extract *n* : an extract of the water-soluble constituents of fresh mammalian liver used in treatment of anemia

liver fluke *n* : any of various trematode worms that invade the mammalian liver; *esp* : one of the genus *Fasciola* (*F. hepatica*) that is a major parasite of the liver, bile ducts, and gallbladder of cattle and sheep, causes fascioliasis in humans, and uses snails of the genus *Lymnaea* as an intermediate host — see CHINESE LIVER FLUKE

liv·er·ish \ˈliv-(ə-)rish\ *adj* : suffering from liver disorder : BILIOUS — **liv·er·ish·ness** *n*

liver of sulfur *n* : SULFURATED POTASH

liver rot *n* : a disease that is caused by liver flukes esp. in sheep and cattle and is marked by sluggishness, anemia, and wasting and by great local damage to the liver — see DISTOMATOSIS; compare BLACK DISEASE

liver spots *n pl* : AGE SPOTS

liv·ery \ˈliv-ə-rē\ *adj* : suggesting liver disorder : LIVERISH

lives *pl of* LIFE

liv·e·tin \ˈliv-ət-ən\ *n* : a protein obtained from egg yolk

K
L

\ə\ **abut** \ᵊ\ **kitten** \ər\ **further** \a\ **ash** \ā\ **ace** \ä\ **cot, cart** \aù\ **out** \ch\ **chin** \e\ **bet** \ē\ **easy** \g\ **go** \i\ **hit** \ī\ **ice** \j\ **job** \ŋ\ **sing** \ō\ **go** \ó\ **law** \ói\ **boy** \th\ **thin** \th̲\ **the** \ü\ **loot** \ù\ **foot** \y\ **yet** \zh\ **vision**   *See also* Pronunciation Symbols page

liv·id \'liv-əd\ *adj* : discolored by bruising : BLACK-AND=BLUE

li·vid·i·ty \liv-'id-ət-ē\ *n, pl* **-ties** : the condition of being livid ⟨postmortem ∼⟩

living will *n* : a document in which the signer requests to be allowed to die rather than be kept alive by artificial means in the event of becoming disabled beyond a reasonable expectation of recovery — see ADVANCE DIRECTIVE

li·vor mor·tis \'lī-ˌvȯr-'mȯrt-əs, -vər-\ *n* : hypostasis of the blood following death that causes a purplish red discoloration of the skin

lix·iv·i·ate \lik-'siv-ē-ˌāt\ *vt* **-at·ed; -at·ing** : to extract a soluble constituent from (a solid mixture) by washing or percolation — **lix·iv·i·a·tion** \(ˌ)lik-ˌsiv-ē-'ā-shən\ *n*

lix·iv·i·um \lik-'siv-ē-əm\ *n, pl* **-ia** \-ē-ə\ *or* **-iums** : a solution (as lye) obtained by lixiviation

LLQ *abbr* left lower quadrant (abdomen)

LMP *abbr* last menstrual period

Loa \'lō-ə\ *n* : a genus of African filarial worms of the family Dipetalonematidae that infect the subcutaneous tissues and blood of humans, include the eye worm (*L. loa*) causing Calabar swellings, are transmitted by the bite of flies of the genus *Chrysops,* and are associated with some allergic manifestations (as hives)

¹load \'lōd\ *n* **1 a** : a mass or weight put on something **b** : the amount of stress put on something ⟨this normal instinctive fear which adds its ∼ to the nervous system —H. G. Armstrong⟩ **c** : an amount of something (as food or water) added to the body or available for use in some physiological process ⟨the cell's response to an increased metabolic ∼ —*Emergency Medicine*⟩ **2** : the number or quantity (as of patients) to be accommodated or treated ⟨the patient ∼ of physicians in private practice —*Jour. Amer. Med. Assoc.*⟩ **3** : the amount of a deleterious microorganism, parasite, growth, or substance present in a human or animal body ⟨measure viral ∼ in the blood⟩ ⟨the worm ∼ in rats⟩ — called also *burden* **4** : GENETIC LOAD

²load *vt* **1** : to put a load in or on ⟨rabbits were ∼ed with . . . pyruvate by intravenous injections —*Experiment Station Record*⟩ **2** : to weight (as a test or experimental situation) with factors influencing validity or outcome **3** : to change by adding an adulterant or drug ⟨patent medicines were ∼ed with narcotics —D. W. Maurer & V. H. Vogel⟩

load·ing *n* **1 a** : the amount or degree to which something is or can be loaded **b** : administration of a factor or substance to the body or a bodily system in sufficient quantity to test capacity to deal with it **2** : the relative contribution of each component factor in a psychological test or in an experimental, clinical, or social situation

loading dose *n* : a large initial dose of a substance or series of such doses given to rapidly achieve a therapeutic concentration in the body

lo·a·i·a·sis \ˌlō-ə-'ī-ə-səs\ *or* **lo·i·a·sis** \ˌlō-'ī-\ *n, pl* **-a·ses** \-ˌsēz\ : infestation with or disease caused by an eye worm of the genus *Loa* (*L. loa*) that migrates through the subcutaneous tissue and across the cornea of the eye — compare CALABAR SWELLING

loa loa \'lō-ə-'lō-ə\ *n* : LOAIASIS

lo·bar \'lō-bər, -ˌbär\ *adj* : of or relating to a lobe

lobar pneumonia *n* : acute pneumonia involving one or more lobes of the lung characterized by sudden onset, chill, fever, difficulty in breathing, cough, and blood-stained sputum, marked by consolidation, and normally followed by resolution and return to normal of the lung tissue

lo·bate \'lō-ˌbāt\ *also* **lo·bat·ed** \-ˌbāt-əd\ *adj* **1** : having lobes **2** : resembling a lobe — **lo·ba·tion** \lō-'bā-shən\ *n*

lobe \'lōb\ *n* : a curved or rounded projection or division: as **a** : a more or less rounded projection of a body organ or part ⟨the ∼ of the ear⟩ **b** : a division of a body organ (as the brain, lungs, or liver) marked off by a fissure on the surface

lo·bec·to·my \lō-'bek-tə-mē\ *n, pl* **-mies** : surgical removal of a lobe of an organ (as a lung) or gland (as the thyroid); *specif* : excision of a lobe of the lung — compare LOBOTOMY

lobed \'lōbd\ *adj* : having lobes ⟨cells with ∼ nuclei⟩

lobe·less \'lōb-ləs\ *adj* : lacking lobes ⟨∼ ears⟩

lo·be·lia \lō-'bēl-yə, -'bē-lē-ə\ *n* **1** *cap* : any of a genus (*Lobelia* of the family Lobeliaceae, the lobelia family) of widely distributed herbaceous plants (as Indian tobacco) **2** : the leaves and tops of Indian tobacco used esp. formerly as an expectorant and antispasmodic

L'Obel *or* **Lo·bel** \lō-'bel\, **Mathias de (1538–1616),** Flemish botanist. L'Obel ranks among the great botanists who preceded Linnaeus. In 1570 he published a work describing more than 1200 plants. He classified plants according to leaf structure, and he apparently tried to incorporate into his classification concepts of genus and family. The genus *Lobelia* was named in his honor in 1702 by the French botanist Charles Plumier (1646–1704).

lo·be·line \'lō-bə-ˌlēn\ *n* : a crystalline alkaloid $C_{22}H_{27}NO_2$ that is obtained from Indian tobacco (*Lobelia inflata*) and is used chiefly as a respiratory stimulant and as a smoking deterrent

lobi *pl of* LOBUS

lo·bo·pod \'lō-bə-ˌpäd\ *n* : LOBOPODIUM

lo·bo·po·di·um \ˌlō-bə-'pō-dē-əm\ *n, pl* **-dia** \-dē-ə\ *or* **-diums** : a broad thick pseudopodium with a core of endoplasm

lo·bot·o·mize *or chiefly Brit* **lo·bot·o·mise** \lō-'bät-ə-ˌmīz\ *vt* **-mized** *or chiefly Brit* **-mised; -miz·ing** *or chiefly Brit* **-mising** : to sever the frontal lobes of the brain of

lo·bot·o·my \lō-'bät-ə-mē\ *n, pl* **-mies** : surgical severance of nerve fibers connecting the frontal lobes to the thalamus performed esp. formerly for the relief of some mental disorders — called also *leukotomy;* compare LOBECTOMY

lob·ster claw \'läb-stər-ˌklȯ\ *n* : an incompletely dominant genetic anomaly in humans marked by variable reduction of the skeleton of the extremities and cleaving of the hands and feet into two segments resembling lobster claws

lob·u·lar \'läb-yə-lər\ *adj* : of, relating to, affecting, or resembling a lobule ⟨∼ fatty degeneration of the liver —Leopold Bellak⟩ — **lob·u·lar·ly** *adv*

lobular pneumonia *n* : BRONCHOPNEUMONIA

lob·u·lat·ed \'läb-yə-ˌlāt-əd\ *adj* : made up of, provided with, or divided into lobules ⟨a ∼ tumor⟩

lob·u·la·tion \ˌläb-yə-'lā-shən\ *n* **1 a** : the quality or state of being lobulated **b** : the formation of or division into lobules **2** : LOBULE

lob·ule \'läb-(ˌ)yü(ə)l\ *n* **1** : a small lobe ⟨the ∼ of the ear⟩ **2** : a subdivision of a lobe; *specif* : one of the small masses of tissue of which various organs (as the liver) are made up

lob·u·lus \'läb-yə-ləs\ *n, pl* **lob·u·li** \-ˌlī\ **1** : LOBE **2** : LOBULE

lo·bus \'lō-bəs\ *n, pl* **lo·bi** \-ˌbī\ : LOBE

¹lo·cal \'lō-kəl\ *adj* : involving or affecting only a restricted part of the organism ⟨∼ inflammation⟩ — compare SYSTEMIC a — **lo·cal·ly** \-kə-lē\ *adv*

²local *n* : LOCAL ANESTHETIC; *also* : LOCAL ANESTHESIA

local anesthesia *n* : loss of sensation in a limited and usu. superficial area esp. from the effect of a local anesthetic

local anesthetic *n* : an anesthetic for use on a limited and usu. superficial area of the body

lo·cal·iza·tion *also Brit* **lo·cal·isa·tion** \ˌlō-kə-lə-'zā-shən\ *n* **1** : restriction (as of a lesion) to a limited area of the body **2** : restriction of functional centers (as of sight, smell, or speech) to a particular section of the brain

lo·cal·ize *also Brit* **lo·cal·ise** \'lō-kə-ˌlīz\ *vb* **-ized** *also Brit* **-ised; -iz·ing** *also Brit* **-is·ing** *vt* : to make local; *esp* : to fix in or confine to a definite place or part ⟨hot applications helped to ∼ the infection⟩ ∼ *vi* : to accumulate in or be restricted to a specific or limited area ⟨this parasite ∼s and grows in the muscle —Morris Fishbein⟩

lo·chia \'lō-kē-ə, 'lä-\ *n, pl* **lochia** : a discharge from the uterus and vagina following delivery — **lo·chi·al** \-əl\ *adj*

loci *pl of* LOCUS

loci cerulei, loci coerulei *pl of* LOCUS CERULEUS, LOCUS COERULEUS

locked \'läkt\ *adj, of the knee joint* : having a restricted mobility and incapable of complete extension

locked–in \\ˈläk-ˈtin\ *adj* : affected with or characterized by the locked-in syndrome ⟨a ~ patient⟩

locked–in syndrome *n* : the condition of an awake and sentient patient who because of motor paralysis throughout the body is unable to communicate except possibly by coded eye movements

Locke's solution *also* **Locke solution** \ˈläk(s)-\ *n* : a solution isotonic with blood plasma that contains the chlorides of sodium, potassium, and calcium and sodium bicarbonate and dextrose and is used similarly to physiological saline
  Locke, Frank Spiller (1871–1949), British physiologist. Locke introduced his solution in 1894.

lock·jaw \ˈläk-ˌjȯ\ *n* : an early symptom of tetanus characterized by spasm of the jaw muscles and inability to open the jaws; *also* : TETANUS 1a

¹**lo·co** \ˈlō-(ˌ)kō\ *n, pl* **locos** *or* **locoes** 1 : LOCOWEED 2 : LOCOISM

²**loco** *vt* : to poison with locoweed

lo·co·ism \ˈlō-kō-ˌiz-əm\ *n* 1 : a disease of horses, cattle, and sheep caused by chronic poisoning with locoweeds and characterized by motor and sensory nerve damage resulting in peculiarities of gait, impairment of vision, lassitude or extreme excitement, emaciation, and ultimately paralysis and death if not controlled 2 : any of several intoxications of domestic animals (as selenosis) that are sometimes mistaken for locoweed poisoning

lo·co·mo·tion \ˌlō-kə-ˈmō-shən\ *n* : an act or the power of moving from place to place : progressive movement (as of an animal body)

lo·co·mo·tive \ˌlō-kə-ˈmōt-iv\ *adj* : LOCOMOTOR 1 ⟨~ organs include flagella, cilia, pseudopodia, and limbs⟩

lo·co·mo·tor \ˌlō-kə-ˈmōt-ər\ *adj* 1 : of, relating to, or functioning in locomotion 2 : affecting or involving the locomotor organs

locomotor ataxia *n* : TABES DORSALIS

lo·co·mo·to·ry \ˌlō-kə-ˈmōt-ə-rē\ *adj* 1 : LOCOMOTOR ⟨parasites without ~ organs⟩ 2 : capable of moving independently from place to place ⟨small ~ animals⟩

lo·co·re·gion·al \-ˈrēj-ən-ᵊl, -nəl\ *adj* : restricted to a localized region of the body ⟨~ anesthesia⟩ ⟨chemotherapy for breast cancer by ~ irradiation⟩

lo·co·weed \ˈlō-(ˌ)kō-ˌwēd\ *n* : any of several leguminous plants (genera *Astragalus* and *Oxytropis*) of western No. America that cause locoism in livestock

loc·u·lar \ˈläk-yə-lər\ *adj* : having or composed of loculi — often used in combination ⟨multi*locular*⟩

loc·u·lat·ed \ˈläk-yə-ˌlāt-əd\ *adj* : having, forming, or divided into loculi ⟨a ~ pocket of pleural fluid —*Jour. Amer. Med. Assoc.*⟩

loc·u·la·tion \ˌläk-yə-ˈlā-shən\ *n* 1 : the condition of being or the process of becoming loculated ⟨a gradual ~ of bony tissue⟩ 2 : a group of loculi usu. isolated from surrounding structures (as by a fibrous tissue septum) ⟨the development of ~s in empyema⟩

loc·u·lus \ˈläk-yə-ləs\ *n, pl* **-li** \-ˌlī *also* -ˌlē\ : a small chamber or cavity esp. in a plant or animal body ⟨the medullary cavity was opened up . . . it was curetted out and the various *loculi* joined —*Lancet*⟩

lo·cum \ˈlō-kəm\ *n, chiefly Brit* : LOCUM TENENS

lo·cum–te·nen·cy \ˌlō-kəm-ˈtē-nən-sē, -ˈten-ən-\ *n, pl* **-cies** : the position or duties of a locum tenens

lo·cum te·nens \ˌlō-kəm-ˈtē-ˌnenz, -nenz\ *n, pl* **locum te·nen·tes** \-ti-ˈnen-ˌtēz\ : a medical practitioner who temporarily takes the place of another

lo·cus \ˈlō-kəs\ *n, pl* **lo·ci** \ˈlō-ˌsī, -ˌkī *also* -ˌkē\ 1 : a place or site of an event, activity, or thing ⟨the integrity of the tissues determines the extent and ~ of the damage —Sylvia E. Hines⟩ 2 : the position in a chromosome of a particular gene or allele

lo·cus coe·ru·le·us *also* **lo·cus ce·ru·le·us** \ˌlō-kə(s)-si-ˈrü-lē-əs\ *n, pl* **loci coe·ru·lei** *also* **loci ce·ru·lei** \-lē-ˌī\ : a blue area of the brain stem with many norepinephrine-containing neurons

lod score \ˈläd-ˌskō(ə)r, ˈlȯd-, -ˌskȯ(ə)r\ *n* [*logarithmic odds*

score] : a statistic that is used to detect genetic linkage and that is equal to the logarithm to base 10 of the ratio of the probability that the data in a linkage experiment would be obtained if the genetic loci under investigation were linked to the probability that the data would be obtained if the loci were not linked

Loef·fler's syndrome \ˈlef-lərz-\ *n* : a mild pneumonitis marked by transitory pulmonary infiltration and eosinophilia and usu. considered to be basically an allergic reaction — called also *Loeffler's pneumonia*
  Löf·fler \ˈlœf-lər\, **Wilhelm (1887–1972)**, Swiss physician. Löffler first described Loeffler's syndrome in 1932.

log·a·rith·mic phase \ˌläg-ə-ˈrith-mik-, ˌlȯg-\ *n* : LOG PHASE

log·o·pe·dia *or chiefly Brit* **log·o·pae·dia** \ˌlȯg-ə-ˈpē-dē-ə, ˌläg-\ *n* : LOGOPEDICS

log·o·pe·dics *or chiefly Brit* **log·o·pae·dics** \-ˈpē-diks\ *n pl but sing or pl in constr* : the scientific study and treatment of speech defects — **log·o·pe·dic** *or chiefly Brit* **log·o·pae·dic** \-dik\ *adj*

log·o·pe·dist *or chiefly Brit* **log·o·pae·dist** \-ˈpē-dəst\ *n* : a specialist in logopedics

log·or·rhea *or chiefly Brit* **log·or·rhoea** \ˌlȯg-ə-ˈrē-ə, ˌläg-\ *n* : pathologically excessive and often incoherent talkativeness or wordiness that is characteristic esp. of the manic phase of bipolar disorder — **log·or·rhe·ic** *or chiefly Brit* **log·or·rhoe·ic** \-ˈrē-ik\ *adj*

log·o·ther·a·py \ˌlȯg-ə-ˈther-ə-pē, ˌläg-\ *n, pl* **-pies** : a highly directive existential psychotherapy that emphasizes the importance of meaning in the patient's life esp. as gained through spiritual values

log phase \ˈlȯg-, ˈläg-\ *n* : the period of growth of a population of cells (as of a microorganism) in a culture medium during which numbers increase exponentially and which is represented by a part of the growth curve that is a straight line segment if the logarithm of numbers is plotted against time — called also *logarithmic phase*; compare LAG PHASE

log·wood \ˈlȯg-ˌwud, ˈläg-\ *n* 1 a : a Central American and West Indian leguminous tree (*Haematoxylon campechianum*) b : the very hard brown or brownish red heartwood of logwood 2 : a dye extracted from the heartwood of logwood — see HEMATOXYLIN

loiasis *var of* LOAIASIS

loin \ˈlȯin\ *n* 1 : the part of the body of a human or a quadruped that is situated on each side of the spinal column between the hip bone and the false ribs 2 **loins** *pl* a : the upper and lower abdominal regions and the region about the hips b (1) : the pubic region (2) : the generative organs — not usu. used technically in senses 2a, b

loin disease *n* : aphosphorosis of cattle often complicated by botulism

Lo·mo·til \ˈlō-mə-ˌtil, lō-ˈmōt-ᵊl\ *trademark* — used for a preparation of the hydrochloride of diphenoxylate and the sulfate of atropine

lo·mus·tine \lō-ˈməs-ˌtēn\ *n* : an antineoplastic drug $C_9H_{16}ClN_3O_2$ used esp. in the treatment of brain tumors and Hodgkin's disease

lone star tick \ˈlōn-ˌstär-\ *n* : an ixodid tick of the genus *Amblyomma* (*A. americanum*) of the southern, central, and eastern U.S. that attacks mammals and birds, is a vector of several diseases (as Rocky Mountain spotted fever and ehrlichiosis), and in which the adult female has a single white spot on the back

long–act·ing thyroid stimulator \ˈlȯŋ-ˌakt-iŋ-\ *n* : a protein that often occurs in the plasma of patients with Graves' disease and that is an IgG immunoglobulin — abbr. *LATS*

long bone *n* : any of the elongated bones supporting a vertebrate limb and consisting of an essentially cylindrical shaft that contains bone marrow and ends in enlarged heads for articulation with other bones

K
L

\ə\ **abut** \ᵊ\ **kitten** \ər\ **further** \a\ **ash** \ā\ **ace** \ä\ **cot, cart**
\au̇\ **out** \ch\ **chin** \e\ **bet** \ē\ **easy** \g\ **go** \i\ **hit** \ī\ **ice** \j\ **job**
\ŋ\ **sing** \ō\ **go** \ȯ\ **law** \ȯi\ **boy** \th\ **thin** \th̲\ **the** \ü\ **loot**
\u̇\ **foot** \y\ **yet** \zh\ **vision** *See also* Pronunciation Symbols page

long–chain *adj* : having a relatively long chain of atoms and esp. carbon atoms in the molecule ⟨∼ hydrocarbons⟩

long ciliary nerve *n* : any of two or three nerves that are given off by the nasociliary nerve as it crosses the optic nerve, pass through the posterior part of the sclera, and run forward between the sclera and the choroid to be distributed to the iris and cornea — compare SHORT CILIARY NERVE

lon·gev·i·ty \län-ˈjev-ət-ē, lȯn-\ *n, pl* **-ties** **1** : a long duration of individual life ⟨attributed his ∼ to daily exercise and a healthy diet⟩ **2** : length of life ⟨studies in ∼⟩

long head *n* : the longest of the three heads of the triceps muscle that arises from the infraglenoid tubercle of the scapula

longi *pl of* LONGUS

lon·gis·si·mus \län-ˈjis-i-məs\ *n, pl* **lon·gis·si·mi** \-ˌmī\ : the intermediate division of the sacrospinalis muscle that consists of the longissimus capitis, longissimus cervicis, and longissimus thoracis; *also* : any of these three muscles

longissimus cap·i·tis \-ˈkap-ət-əs\ *n* : a long slender muscle between the longissimus cervicis and the semispinalis capitis that arises by tendons from the upper thoracic and lower cervical vertebrae, is inserted into the posterior margin of the mastoid process, and extends the head and bends and rotates it to one side — called also *trachelomastoid muscle*

longissimus cer·vi·cis \-ˈsər-və-səs\ *n* : a slender muscle medial to the longissimus thoracis that arises by long thin tendons from the transverse processes of the upper four or five thoracic vertebrae, is inserted by similar tendons into the transverse processes of the second to sixth cervical vertebrae, and extends the spinal column and bends it to one side

longissimus dor·si \-ˈdȯr-sī\ *n* : LONGISSIMUS THORACIS

longissimus tho·ra·cis \-thə-ˈrā-səs\ *n* : a muscle that arises as the middle and largest division of the sacrospinalis muscle, that is attached by some of its fibers to the lumbar vertebrae, that is inserted into all the thoracic vertebrae and the lower 9 or 10 ribs, and that depresses the ribs and with the longissimus cervicis extends the spinal column and bends it to one side — called also *longissimus dorsi*

lon·gi·tu·di·nal \ˌlän-jə-ˈt(y)üd-ᵊn-əl, -nəl, *Brit also* ˌlän-gə-ˈtyüd-\ *adj* **1** : of, relating to, or occurring in the lengthwise dimension ⟨a ∼ bone fracture⟩ **2** : extending along or relating to the anteroposterior axis of a body or part ⟨a trypanosome which reproduces by ∼ fission⟩ **3** : involving the repeated observation or examination of a set of subjects over time with respect to one or more study variables (as general health, the state of a disease, or mortality) ⟨a ∼ study of heart transplant recipients over a five-year period⟩ — **lon·gi·tu·di·nal·ly** \-ē\ *adv*

longitudinal fissure *n* : the deep groove that divides the cerebrum into right and left hemispheres

lon·gi·tu·di·na·lis linguae \ˌlän-jə-ˌt(y)üd-ə-ˈnā-ləs-\ *n* : either of two bands of muscle comprising the intrinsic musculature of the tongue of which one is situated near the dorsal surface and one near the inferior surface of the tongue — called also *longitudinalis*

long–nosed cattle louse \ˈlȯn-ˈnōzd-\ *n* : a widely distributed sucking louse of the genus *Linognathus* (*L. vituli*) that feeds on cattle

long posterior ciliary artery *n* : either of usu. two arteries of which one arises from the ophthalmic artery on each side of the optic nerve, passes forward along the optic nerve accompanying the short posterior ciliary arteries, pierces the sclera passing forward on the same side of the eyeball between the sclera and the choroid to the ciliary muscle, and at the junction of the ciliary process and the iris divides into upper and lower branches which anastomose with the branches of the contralateral artery to form a ring of arteries around the iris — compare SHORT POSTERIOR CILIARY ARTERY

long QT syndrome *n* : any of several inherited cardiac arrhythmias that are characterized by abnormal duration and shape of the QT interval and that place the subject at risk for torsades de pointes — abbr. *LQTS*

long saphenous vein *n* : SAPHENOUS VEIN a

long·sight·ed \-ˈsīt-əd\ *adj* : FARSIGHTED — **long·sight·ed·ness** *n*

long terminal repeat *n* : an identical sequence of several hundred base pairs at each end of the DNA synthesized by the reverse transcriptase of a retrovirus that controls integration of the viral DNA into the host DNA and expression of the genes of the virus — called also *LTR;* compare TANDEM REPEAT

long–term memory *n* : memory that involves the storage and recall of information over a long period of time (as days, weeks, or years)

long–term nonprogressor *n* : an HIV-infected individual who remains symptom-free over the long term and does not progress to develop AIDS — called also *nonprogressor*

long–term potentiation *n* : a long-lasting strengthening of the response of a postsynaptic nerve cell to stimulation across the synapse that occurs with repeated stimulation and is thought to be related to learning and long-term memory — abbr. *LTP*

lon·gus \ˈlȯn-gəs\ *n, pl* **lon·gi** \-gī\ : a long structure (as a muscle) in the body — see ABDUCTOR POLLICIS LONGUS, ADDUCTOR LONGUS, EXTENSOR CARPI RADIALIS LONGUS, EXTENSOR DIGITORUM LONGUS, EXTENSOR HALLUCIS LONGUS, EXTENSOR POLLICIS LONGUS, FLEXOR DIGITORUM LONGUS, FLEXOR HALLUCIS LONGUS, FLEXOR POLLICIS LONGUS, PALMARIS LONGUS, PERONEUS LONGUS

longus cap·i·tis \-ˈkap-ət-əs\ *n* : a muscle of either side of the front and upper portion of the neck that arises from the third to sixth cervical vertebrae, is inserted into the basilar portion of the occipital bone, and bends the neck forward

Lon·i·ten \ˈlän-ət-ᵊn\ *trademark* — used for a preparation of minoxidil

loop \ˈlüp\ *n* **1** : a curving or doubling of a line so as to form a closed or partly open curve within itself through which another line can be passed **2 a** : something (as an anatomical part) shaped like a loop — see LOOP OF HENLE; LIPPES LOOP **b** : a surgical electrode in the form of a loop **3** : a fingerprint in which some of the papillary ridges make a single backward turn without any twist **4** : a wire usu. of platinum bent at one end into a small loop (usu. four millimeters in inside diameter) and used in transferring microorganisms

loop diuretic *n* : a diuretic that inhibits reabsorption in the ascending limb of the loop of Henle causing greatly increased excretion of sodium chloride in the urine and to a lesser extent of potassium

loop·ful \ˈlüp-ˌfu̇l\ *n* : the amount held in a loop; *esp* : the amount taken up in a standard four millimeter loop used by bacteriologists ⟨place a ∼ of . . . culture on a clean slide —*Methods for Medical Laboratory Technicians*⟩

loop of Hen·le \-ˈhen-lē\ *n* : the U-shaped part of a vertebrate nephron that lies between and is continuous with the proximal and distal convoluted tubules, that leaves the cortex of the kidney descending into the medullary tissue and then bending back and reentering the cortex, and that functions in water resorption — called also *Henle's loop*

F. G. J. Henle — see HENLE'S LAYER

loose \ˈlüs\ *adj* **loos·er; loos·est** **1 a** : not rigidly fastened or securely attached **b** (1) : having worked partly free from attachments ⟨a ∼ tooth⟩ (2) : having relative freedom of movement **c** : produced freely and accompanied by raising of mucus ⟨a ∼ cough⟩ **2 a** : not dense, close, or compact in structure or arrangement ⟨∼ connective tissue⟩ **b** : not solid : WATERY ⟨∼ stools⟩ **3** : OVERACTIVE; *specif* : marked by frequent voiding esp. of watery stools ⟨∼ bowels⟩ **4** : not tightly drawn or stretched ⟨∼ skin⟩ — **loose·ly** *adv* — **loose·ness** *n*

lo·per·a·mide \lō-ˈper-ə-ˌmīd\ *n* : a synthetic antidiarrheal agent that slows intestinal peristalsis and is administered in the form of its hydrochloride $C_{29}H_{33}ClN_2O_2 \cdot HCl$ to control acute nonspecific diarrhea or chronic diarrhea associated with inflammatory bowel disease or to reduce fecal volume discharged from ileostomies — see IMODIUM

¹loph·o·dont \ˈläf-ə-ˌdänt\ *adj* : having or constituting molar teeth with transverse ridges on the grinding surface — compare BUNODONT

²**lophodont** *n* : an animal (as an ungulate) having lophodont teeth

Lo·phoph·o·ra \lə-'fäf-ə-rə\ *n* : a genus of spineless cacti including the peyote (*L. williamsii*) which yields lophophorine

lo·phoph·o·rine \lə-'fäf-ə-ˌrēn, -rin\ *n* : an oily psychoactive alkaloid $C_{13}H_{17}NO_3$ derived from peyote

lo·phot·ri·chous \lə-'fä-trə-kəs\ *or* **lo·phot·ri·chate** \-kət\ *adj* : having a tuft of flagella at one end

Lo·pid \'lō-pid\ *trademark* — used for a preparation of gemfibrozil

Lo·pres·sor \lō-'pres-ər, -ˌór\ *trademark* — used for a preparation of the tartrate of metoprolol

lo·rat·a·dine \lə-'rat-ə-ˌdēn, -ˌdin\ *n* : a long-acting H₁ antagonist $C_{22}H_{23}ClN_2O_2$ used esp. to relieve the symptoms of seasonal allergic rhinitis — see CLARITIN

lor·az·e·pam \lòr-'az-ə-ˌpam\ *n* : an anxiolytic benzodiazepine $C_{15}H_{10}Cl_2N_2O_2$ — see ATIVAN

lor·do·sis \lòr-'dō-səs\ *n* : exaggerated forward curvature of the lumbar and cervical regions of the spinal column — compare KYPHOSIS, SCOLIOSIS — **lor·dot·ic** \-'dät-ik\ *adj*

lo·ri·ca \lə-'rī-kə\ *n, pl* **lo·ri·cae** \lə-'rī-ˌkē, -ˌsē\ : a hard protective case or shell (as of a rotifer)

lo·sar·tan \lō-'sär-ˌtan\ *n* : an antihypertensive drug that is administered in the form of its potassium salt $C_{22}H_{22}ClKN_6O$ and blocks the effects of angiotensin II — see COZAAR, HYZAAR

lose \'lüz\ *vt* **lost** \'lóst\; **los·ing** **1** : to become deprived of or lacking in ⟨~ consciousness⟩ ⟨*lost* her sense of smell⟩; *also* : to part with in an unforeseen or accidental manner ⟨~ a leg in an auto crash⟩ **2 a** : to suffer deprivation through the death or removal of or final separation from (a person) ⟨*lost* a son in the war⟩ **b** : to fail to keep (a patient) from dying ⟨have *lost* many fewer pneumonia cases since penicillin came into use⟩ **3** : to fail to keep, sustain, or maintain ⟨~ one's balance⟩ **4** : to free oneself from : get rid of ⟨dieting to ~ weight⟩

loss·less \'lós-ləs\ *adj* : occurring or functioning without loss ⟨~ electrical transmission in a nerve fiber⟩

Lo·ten·sin \lō-'ten-sən\ *trademark* — used for a preparation of the hydrochloride of benazepril

lo·tion \'lō-shən\ *n* **1** : a liquid usu. aqueous medicinal preparation containing one or more insoluble substances and applied externally for skin disorders **2** : a liquid cosmetic preparation usu. containing a cleansing, softening, or astringent agent and applied to the skin ⟨hand ~⟩ ⟨aftershave ~⟩

Lo·trel \'lō-ˌtrel\ *trademark* — used for a preparation of the besylate of amlodipine and the hydrochloride of benazepril

Lo·tri·min \'lō-trə-min\ *trademark* — used for a preparation of clotrimazole

Lou Geh·rig's disease \ˌlü-ˌge(ə)r-igz-, -ˌga(ə)r-\ *n* : AMYOTROPHIC LATERAL SCLEROSIS

Gehrig, Lou (1903–1941), American baseball player. Gehrig began playing for the New York Yankees in 1925. He soon became a fine first baseman and an outstanding hitter. He compiled a lifetime major-league average of .340. He was the American League home-run champion in 1931, 1934, and 1936 and was named the American League's most valuable player in 1927, 1931, 1934, and 1936. Nicknamed the "Iron Horse," he played a total of 2130 consecutive games in 14 seasons. His career ended in 1939 when he learned that he was suffering from a rare form of paralysis—amyotrophic lateral sclerosis. In the years following his death the disease became popularly known as Lou Gehrig's disease.

loupe \'lüp\ *n* : a magnifying lens worn esp. by surgeons performing microsurgery; *also* : two such lenses mounted on a single frame ⟨examine the cornea with a binocular ~⟩

loup·ing ill \'laù-piŋ-, 'lō-\ *n* : a variable tick-borne disease of sheep and other domestic animals that affects primarily the central nervous system and is caused by a flavivirus (genus *Flavivirus*)

louse \'laùs\ *n, pl* **lice** \'līs\ : any of the small wingless usu. flattened insects that are parasitic on warm-blooded animals and constitute the orders Anoplura and Mallophaga

louse–borne typhus \-ˌbórn-\ *n* : TYPHUS a

louse fly *n* : any dipteran insect of the family Hippoboscidae

lou·si·cide \'laù-sə-ˌsīd\ *n* : a louse-killing insecticide : PEDICULICIDE — **lou·si·cid·al** \ˌlaù-sə-'sīd-ᵊl\ *adj*

lous·i·ness \'laù-zē-nəs\ *n* : PEDICULOSIS

lousy \'laù-zē\ *adj* **lous·i·er; -est** : infested with lice

lov·age \'ləv-ij\ *n* : any of several aromatic perennial herbs of the carrot family; *esp* : a European herb (*Levisticum officinale*) sometimes cultivated for its rhizomes which are used as a carminative in domestic remedies, for its stalks and foliage which are used as a potherb, a substitute for celery, for a tea, for its seeds which are used for flavoring and in confectionery, and for its flowering tops which yield an oil used in flavoring and perfumery

lov·a·stat·in \'lō-və-ˌstat-ᵊn, 'ləv-ə-\ *n* : a drug $C_{24}H_{36}O_5$ that decreases the level of cholesterol in the bloodstream by inhibiting the liver enzyme that controls cholesterol synthesis and is used in the treatment of hypercholesterolemia — see MEVACOR

love han·dles \'ləv-ˌhan-dᵊlz\ *n pl* : fatty bulges along the sides at the waist

love object *n* : a person on whom affection is centered or on whom one is dependent for affection or needed help

low \'lō\ *adj* **low·er** \'lō-(ə)r\; **low·est** \'lō-əst\ : having a relatively less complex organization : not greatly differentiated or developed phylogenetically — usu. used in the comparative degree of less advanced types of plants and animals ⟨the ~*er* vertebrates⟩; compare HIGH 1

low–back \-'bak\ *adj* : of, relating to, suffering, or being pain in the lowest portion of the back ⟨a ~ patient⟩ ⟨~ pain⟩

low blood pressure *n* : HYPOTENSION 1

low–den·si·ty lipoprotein \'lō-'den(t)-sət-ē-\ *n* : LDL

low enema *n* : an enema in which the injected material goes no higher than the rectum — compare HIGH ENEMA

lower *n* : the lower member of a pair; *esp* : a lower denture

lower jaw *n* : JAW 1b

lower respiratory *adj* : of, relating to, or affecting the lower respiratory tract ⟨*lower respiratory* infections⟩

lower respiratory tract *n* : the part of the respiratory system including the larynx, trachea, bronchi, and lungs — compare UPPER RESPIRATORY TRACT

low·est splanchnic nerve \'lō-əst-\ *n* : SPLANCHNIC NERVE c

Lowe syndrome *or* **Lowe's syndrome** \'lō(z)-\ *n* : OCULOCEREBRORENAL SYNDROME

low forceps *n* : a procedure for delivery of an infant by the use of forceps when the head is visible at the outlet of the birth canal — called also *outlet forceps;* compare HIGH FORCEPS, MIDFORCEPS

low–grade \'lō-'grād\ *adj* : being near that extreme of a specified range which is lowest, least intense, or least competent ⟨a ~ fever⟩ ⟨a ~ infection⟩ — compare HIGH-GRADE

low–melt·ing \'lō-'melt-iŋ\ *adj* : melting at a relatively low temperature

Lown–Gan·ong–Le·vine syndrome \'laùn-'gan-ˌóŋ-lə-'vīn-, -'vēn-\ *n* : LGL SYNDROME

low–power *adj* : of, relating to, or being a lens that magnifies an image a relatively small number of times and esp. 10 times ⟨find the diameter of the ~ field of the microscope⟩ — compare HIGH-POWER

low–salt diet *n* : LOW-SODIUM DIET

low–sodium diet *n* : a diet restricted to foods naturally low in sodium content and prepared without added salt that is used esp. in the management of hypertension, heart failure, and kidney or liver dysfunction

low vision *n* : impaired vision in which there is a significant

K
L

\ə\ abut \ᵊ\ kitten \ər\ further \a\ ash \ā\ ace \ä\ cot, cart
\aù\ out \ch\ chin \e\ bet \ē\ easy \g\ go \i\ hit \ī\ ice \j\ job
\ŋ\ sing \ō\ go \ó\ law \ói\ boy \th\ thin \t͟h\ the \ü\ loot
\ù\ foot \y\ yet \zh\ vision   *See also* Pronunciation Symbols page

reduction in visual function that cannot be corrected by conventional glasses but which may be improved with special aids or devices

loxa bark \\'läk-sə-, 'lō-hə-\\ *n* : PALE BARK

Lox·os·ce·les \\läk-'säs-ə-,lēz\\ *n* : a genus of spiders (family Loxoscelidae) native to So. America that includes the brown recluse spider (*L. reclusa*)

lox·os·ce·lism \\läk-'säs-ə-,liz-əm\\ *n* : a painful condition resulting from the bite of a spider of the genus *Loxosceles* and esp. the brown recluse spider (*L. reclusa*) that is characterized by local necrosis of tissue and sometimes systemic symptoms of poisoning

loz·enge \\'läz-ənj\\ *n* : a small usu. sweetened solid piece of medicated material of any of various shapes that is designed to be held in the mouth for slow dissolution and often contains a demulcent ⟨sore throat ~*s*⟩ — called also *pastille, troche*

L–PAM \\'el-,pam\\ *n* : MELPHALAN

L–phase \\'el-,fāz\\ *n* : L-FORM

LPN \\'el-'pē-'en\\ *n* : LICENSED PRACTICAL NURSE

LPS *abbr* lipopolysaccharide

LQTS *abbr* long QT syndrome

Lr *symbol* lawrencium

LRCP *abbr* Licentiate of the Royal College of Physicians

LRCS *abbr* Licentiate of the Royal College of Surgeons

LRF *abbr* luteinizing hormone-releasing factor

LSD \\,el-,es-'dē\\ *n* : a semisynthetic illicit organic compound $C_{20}H_{25}N_3O$ which is derived from ergot and the use of which may involve hazardous complications including distorted perceptions of reality, mood shifts, and impulsive behavior — called also *acid, lysergic acid diethylamide, lysergide*

LSD–25 \\-,twent-ē-'fīv\\ *n* : LSD

LTH *abbr* luteotropic hormone

LTP *abbr* long-term potentiation

LTR \\,el-(,)tē-'är\\ *n* : LONG TERMINAL REPEAT

L–tryp·to·phan \\'el-'trip-tə-,fan\\ *n* : the levorotatory form of tryptophan that is a precursor of serotonin and was formerly used in some health food preparations in the belief that it promoted sleep and relieved depression — see EOSINO-PHILIA-MYALGIA SYNDROME

Lu *symbol* lutetium

lubb–dupp *also* **lub–dup** *or* **lub–dub** \\,ləb-'dəp, -'dəb\\ *n* : the characteristic sounds of a normal heartbeat as heard in auscultation

¹lu·bri·cant \\'lü-bri-kənt\\ *adj* : serving to lubricate a surface or part

²lubricant *n* : a substance that serves to lubricate a surface or part ⟨normally, the intestinal passage requires no artificial ~ —E. B. Steen & Ashley Montagu⟩

lu·bri·cate \\'lü-bri-,kāt\\ *vt* **-cat·ed; -cat·ing** : to make smooth, slippery, or oily in motion, action, or appearance ⟨~ the eye⟩ ⟨~ the skin⟩ — **lu·bri·ca·tion** \\,lü-brə-'kā-shən\\ *n*

lu·can·thone \\lü-'kan-,thōn\\ *n* : an antischistosomal drug administered in the form of its hydrochloride $C_{20}H_{24}N_2OS \cdot HCl$ — called also *miracil D*

lu·cent \\'lüs-⁰nt\\ *adj* **1** : glowing with light **2** : marked by clarity or translucence ⟨a ~ membrane⟩ — see RADIOLUCENT

lu·cid \\'lü-səd\\ *adj* : having, showing, or characterized by an ability to think clearly and rationally — **lu·cid·i·ty** *n, pl* **-ties**

lucida — see CAMERA LUCIDA

lucid interval *n* : a temporary period of rationality between periods of insanity or delirium

lucidum — see STRATUM LUCIDUM, TAPETUM LUCIDUM

lu·cif·er·ase \\lü-'sif-ə-,rās, -,rāz\\ *n* : an enzyme that catalyzes the oxidation of luciferin

lu·cif·er·in \\-(ə-)rən\\ *n* : any of various organic substances in luminescent organisms that furnish practically heatless light in undergoing oxidation promoted by luciferase

Lu·cil·ia \\lü-'sil-ē-ə\\ *n* : a genus of blowflies whose larvae are sometimes the cause of intestinal myiasis and infest open wounds

lüc·ken·schä·del \\'lュe-kən-,shä-d⁰l\\ *n* : a condition characterized by incomplete ossification of the bones of the skull

lude \\'lüd\\ *n* : a pill of methaqualone — usu. used in pl.

Lud·wig's angina \\'lüd-(,)vigz-\\ *n* : an acute streptococcal or sometimes staphylococcal infection of the deep tissues of the floor of the mouth and adjoining parts of the neck and lower jaw that is marked by severe rapid swelling which may close the respiratory passage and that is accompanied by chills and fever

Lud·wig \\'lüt-vik\\, **Wilhelm Friedrich von (1790–1865)**, German surgeon. Ludwig began his career as a military physician. He saw considerable action in Russia during the Napoleonic campaign of 1812. After the war he became a professor of surgery and obstetrics at Tübingen, Germany. He also served as physician to German royal families. He published his description of Ludwig's angina in 1836.

Lu·er syringe \\'lü-ər-\\ *n* : a glass syringe with a glass piston that has the apposing surfaces ground and that is used esp. for hypodermic injection

Luer (*d* 1883), German instrument maker. Luer is known to have worked in Paris.

lu·es \\'lü-(,)ēz\\ *n, pl* **lues** : SYPHILIS

¹lu·et·ic \\lü-'et-ik\\ *adj* : SYPHILITIC — **lu·et·i·cal·ly** \\-i-k(ə-)lē\\ *adv*

²luetic *n* : an individual affected with syphilis

lu·e·tin \\'lü-ət-ən\\ *n* : a sterile emulsion of a killed culture of a spirochete of the genus *Treponema* (*T. pallidum*) used in a skin test for syphilis

Lu·gol's solution \\lü-'gólz-\\ *n* : any of several deep brown solutions of iodine and potassium iodide in water or alcohol that are used in medicine (as for the internal administration of iodine) and as microscopic stains — called also *Lugol's iodine, Lugol's iodine solution*

Lu·gol \\lǖ-gól\\, **Jean Guillaume Auguste (1786–1851)**, French physician. Lugol did research on skin diseases, scrofula, and the therapeutic use of iodine. He introduced Lugol's solution for the treatment of tubercular conditions, particularly scrofula, in 1829.

lum·ba·go \\,ləm-'bā-(,)gō\\ *n* : acute or chronic pain (as that caused by muscle strain) in the lower back

lum·bar \\'ləm-bər, -,bär\\ *adj* **1** : of, relating to, or constituting the loins or the vertebrae between the thoracic vertebrae and sacrum ⟨the ~ region⟩ **2** : of, relating to, or being the abdominal region lying on either side of the umbilical region and above the corresponding iliac region

lumbar artery *n* : any artery of the usu. four or occas. five pairs that arise at the level of the lumbar vertebrae from the back of the aorta or in the case of the fifth pair from an artery arising from the aorta and that supply the muscles of the loins, the skin of the sides of the abdomen, and the spinal cord

lumbar ganglion *n* : any of the small ganglia of the lumbar part of the sympathetic nervous system

lum·bar·i·za·tion \\,ləm-bə-rə-'zā-shən\\ *n* : a condition marked by fusion of the first sacral and last lumbar vertebrae

lumbar nerve *n* : any nerve of the five pairs of spinal nerves of the lumbar region of which one on each side passes out below each lumbar vertebra and the upper four unite by connecting branches into a lumbar plexus

lumbar plexus *n* : a plexus embedded in the psoas major and formed by the anterior or ventral divisions of the four upper lumbar nerves of which the first is usu. supplemented by a communication from the twelfth thoracic nerve

lumbar puncture *n* : puncture of the subarachnoid space in the lumbar region of the spinal cord to withdraw cerebrospinal fluid or inject anesthetic drugs — called also *spinal tap*

lumbar vein *n* : any vein of the four pairs collecting blood from the muscles and integument of the loins, the walls of the abdomen, and adjacent parts and emptying into the dorsal part of the inferior vena cava — see ASCENDING LUMBAR VEIN

lumbar vertebra *n* : any of the vertebrae situated between the thoracic vertebrae above and the sacrum below that in humans are five in number

lum·bo·dor·sal fascia \\,ləm-bō-'dȯr-səl-\ *n* : a large fascial band on each side of the back extending from the iliac crest and the sacrum to the ribs and the intermuscular septa of the muscles of the neck, adhering medially to the spinous processes of the vertebrae, and continuing laterally with the aponeuroses of certain of the abdominal muscles

lumborum — see ILIOCOSTALIS LUMBORUM, QUADRATUS LUMBORUM

lum·bo·sa·cral \\,ləm-bō-'sak-rəl, -'sā-krəl\ *adj* : of, relating to, or being the lumbar and sacral regions or parts ⟨the ∼ spinal cord⟩

lumbosacral joint *n* : the joint between the fifth lumbar vertebra and the sacrum

lumbosacral plexus *n* : a network of nerves comprising the lumbar plexus and the sacral plexus

lumbosacral trunk *n* : a nerve trunk that is formed by the fifth lumbar nerve and a smaller branch of the fourth lumbar nerve and that connects the lumbar plexus to the sacral plexus

lum·bri·cal \\'ləm-bri-kəl\ *adj* : being one of or constituting the lumbricales ⟨the outer ∼ muscles⟩

lum·bri·ca·lis \\,ləm-brə-'kā-ləs\ *n, pl* **-les** \-,lēz\ **1** : any of the four small muscles of the palm of the hand that arise from tendons of the flexor digitorum profundus, are inserted at the base of the digit to which the tendon passes, and flex the proximal phalanx and extend the two distal phalanges of each finger **2** : any of four small muscles of the foot homologous to the lumbricales of the hand that arise from tendons of the flexor digitorum longus and are inserted into the first phalanges of the four small toes of which they flex the proximal phalanges and extend the two distal phalanges

Lum·bri·ci·dae \ləm-'bris-ə-,dē\ *n pl* : a family of segmented worms containing most of the earthworms of Eurasia and No. America — **lum·bri·cid** \'ləm-brə-,sid\ *adj or n*

Lum·bri·cus \'ləm-brə-kəs\ *n* : a genus of earthworms that is the type of the family Lumbricidae

lu·men \'lü-mən\ *n, pl* **lu·mi·na** \-mə-nə\ *or* **lumens** **1** : the cavity of a tubular organ ⟨the ∼ of a blood vessel⟩ **2** : the bore of a tube (as of a hollow needle or catheter) **3** : a unit of luminous flux equal to the light emitted in a steradian by a uniform point source of one candle intensity

lu·mi·chrome \'lü-mə-,krōm\ *n* : a blue fluorescent crystalline compound $C_{12}H_{10}N_4O_2$ that is formed from riboflavin by ultraviolet irradiation in neutral or acid solution

lu·mi·fla·vin \\,lü-mə-'flā-vən\ *n* : a yellow-green fluorescent crystalline compound $C_{13}H_{12}N_4O_2$ that is formed from riboflavin by ultraviolet irradiation in alkaline solution

lu·mi·nal *also* **lu·me·nal** \'lü-mən-ᵊl\ *adj* : of or relating to a lumen ⟨∼ scarring⟩

Lu·mi·nal \'lü-mə-,nal, -,nȯl\ *trademark* — used for a preparation of the sodium salt of phenobarbital

lu·mi·nance \'lü-mə-nən(t)s\ *n* **1** : the quality or state of being luminous **2** : the luminous intensity of a surface in a given direction per unit of projected area

lu·mi·nes·cence \\,lü-mə-'nes-ᵊn(t)s\ *n* : the low-temperature emission of light produced esp. by physiological processes (as in the firefly), by chemical action, by friction, or by electrical action; *also* : light produced by luminescence — **lu·mi·nesce** \-'nes\ *vi* **-nesced; -nesc·ing** — **lu·mi·nes·cent** \-ᵊnt\ *adj*

lu·mi·nif·er·ous \\,lü-mə-'nif-(ə-)rəs\ *adj* : transmitting, producing, or yielding light

lu·mi·nol \'lü-mə-,nȯl, -,nōl\ *n* : an almost white to yellow crystalline compound $C_8H_7N_3O_2$ that gives a brilliant bluish luminescence when it is treated in alkaline solution with an oxidizing agent (as hydrogen peroxide) and that is used in chemical analysis

lu·mi·nom·e·ter \\,lü-mə-'näm-ət-ər\ *n* : a sensitive photometer used for measuring very low light levels (as those produced in a luminescent process)

lu·mi·nos·i·ty \\,lü-mə-'näs-ət-ē\ *n, pl* **-ties** **1** : the quality or state of being luminous **2 a** : the relative quantity of light

b : the comparative degree to which light of a given wavelength induces the sensation of brightness when perceived

lu·mi·nous \'lü-mə-nəs\ *adj* **1** : emitting or reflecting usu. steady, suffused, or glowing light **2** : of or relating to light or to luminous flux

luminous flux *n* : radiant flux in the visible-wavelength range usu. expressed in lumens instead of watts — called also *light flux*

luminous intensity *n* : the intensity of a light source as measured by the luminous flux per unit solid angle and usu. expressed in candles

lu·mi·rho·dop·sin \\,lü-mi-rō-'däp-sən\ *n* : an intermediate compound that is formed in the bleaching of rhodopsin by light and that rapidly converts to metarhodopsin

lu·mis·ter·ol \lü-'mis-tə-,rȯl, -,rōl\ *n* : a crystalline compound stereoisomeric with ergosterol from which it is formed by ultraviolet irradiation as an intermediate product in the production of tachysterol and vitamin D_2

lump \'ləmp\ *n* **1** : a piece or mass of indefinite size and shape **2** : an abnormal mass or swelling ⟨presenting as a neck ∼⟩

lump·ec·to·my \\,ləm-'pek-tə-mē\ *n, pl* **-mies** : excision of a breast tumor with a limited amount of associated tissue — called also *tylectomy;* compare QUADRANTECTOMY

lumpy jaw \\,ləm-pē-\ *also* **lump jaw** *n* : ACTINOMYCOSIS; *esp* : actinomycosis of the head in cattle

lumpy skin disease *n* : a highly infectious disease of African cattle that is caused by a poxvirus (genus *Capripoxvirus*), is marked by mild fever, loss of weight, and the development of inflammatory nodules in the skin and mucous membranes tending to become necrotic and ulcerous, and that may be transmitted by insects

lu·na·cy \'lü-nə-sē\ *n, pl* **-cies** : INSANITY; *also* : intermittent insanity once believed to be related to phases of the moon

lu·nar \'lü-nər *also* -,när\ *adj* : LUNATE

lunar caustic *n* : silver nitrate esp. when fused and molded into sticks or small cones for use as a caustic

¹lu·nate \'lü-,nāt\ *adj* : shaped like a crescent

²lunate *n* : LUNATE BONE

lunate bone *n* : a crescent-shaped bone that is the middle bone in the proximal row of the carpus between the scaphoid bone and the triquetral bone and that has a deep concavity on the distal surface articulating with the capitate — called also *lunate, semilunar bone*

lunate sulcus *n* : a sulcus of the cerebrum on the lateral part of the occipital lobe that marks the front boundary of the visual area

¹lu·na·tic \'lü-nə-,tik\ *adj* : INSANE

²lunatic *n* : an insane individual

lu·na·to·ma·la·cia \\,lü-nə-tō-mə-'lā-sh(ē-)ə\ *n* : KIENBÖCK'S DISEASE

lunatus — see SULCUS LUNATUS

lung \'ləŋ\ *n* **1 a** : one of the usu. two compound saccular organs that constitute the basic respiratory organ of air-breathing vertebrates, that normally occupy the entire lateral parts of the thorax and consist essentially of an inverted tree of intricately branched bronchioles communicating with thin-walled terminal alveoli swathed in a network of delicate capillaries where the actual gaseous exchange of respiration takes place, and that in humans are somewhat flattened with a broad base resting against the diaphragm and have the right lung divided into three lobes and the left into two lobes **b** : any of various respiratory organs of invertebrates **2** : a mechanical device for regularly introducing fresh air into and withdrawing stale air from the lungs : RESPIRATOR — see IRON LUNG — **lunged** *adj*

lung·er \'ləŋ-ər\ *n* : one affected with a chronic disease of the lungs; *esp* : one who is tubercular

lung fever *n* : PNEUMONIA

\ə\ abut \ᵊ\ kitten \ər\ further \a\ ash \ā\ ace \ä\ cot, cart \au̇\ out \ch\ chin \e\ bet \ē\ easy \g\ go \i\ hit \ī\ ice \j\ job \ŋ\ sing \ō\ go \ȯ\ law \ȯi\ boy \th\ thin \t͟h\ the \ü\ loot \u̇\ foot \y\ yet \zh\ vision *See also* Pronunciation Symbols page

K
L

lung fluke *n* : a fluke invading the lungs; *esp* : either of two Old World forms of the genus *Paragonimus* (*P. westermanii* and *P. kellicotti*) that produce lesions in humans which are comparable to those of tuberculosis and that are acquired by eating inadequately cooked freshwater crustaceans which act as intermediate hosts

lung plague *n* : contagious pleuropneumonia of cattle — called also *lung sickness*

lung·worm \-ˌwərm\ *n* : any of various nematodes esp. of the family Metastrongylidae that infest the lungs and air passages of mammals: as   **a** : a nematode of the genus *Dictyocaulus*   **b** : a lungworm of the genus *Metastrongylus* (*M. apri* syn. *M. elongatus*) that infests swine and causes bronchitis

lungworm disease *n* : HOOSE

lung·wort \-ˌwərt, -ˌwô(ə)rt\ *n*   **1** : any of several plants formerly used in the treatment of respiratory disorders; *esp* : a European herb (*Pulmonaria officinalis*) of the borage family (Boraginaceae) with rough hairy leaves and bluish flowers   **2** : a widely distributed lichen (*Lobaria pulmonaria*) formerly used in the treatment of bronchitis and now to some extent in perfumes and in tanning extracts

lu·nu·la \ˈlü-nyə-lə\ *n, pl* **-lae** \-ˌlē also -ˌlī\ : a crescent-shaped body part: as   **a** : the whitish mark at the base of a fingernail — called also *half-moon*   **b** : the crescentic unattached border of a semilunar valve

lu·nule \ˈlü-(ˌ)nyü(ə)l\ *n* : LUNULA

lu·pa·nine \ˈlü-pə-ˌnēn, -ˌnīn\ *n* : a bitter crystalline poisonous alkaloid $C_{15}H_{24}N_2O$ found in various lupines

lu·pine *also* **lu·pin** \ˈlü-pən\ *n* : any of a genus (*Lupinus*) of leguminous herbs some of which cause lupinosis and others are cultivated for green manure, fodder, or their edible seeds; *also* : an edible lupine seed

lu·pin·ine \ˈlü-pə-ˌnēn, -pi-, -nən\ *n* : a crystalline weakly poisonous alkaloid $C_{10}H_{19}NO$ found esp. in lupines

lu·pi·no·sis \ˌlü-pə-ˈnō-səs\ *n, pl* **-no·ses** \-ˌsēz\ : acute liver atrophy of domestic animals (as sheep) due to poisoning by ingestion of various lupines

lu·poid \ˈlü-ˌpȯid\ *adj* : resembling lupus

lupoid hepatitis *n* : chronic active hepatitis associated with lupus erythematosus

Lu·pron \ˈlü-ˌprän\ *trademark* — used for a preparation of the acetate of leuprolide

lu·pu·lin \ˈlü-pyə-lən\ *n* : a fine yellow resinous substance of the female catkin of the hop (*Humulus lupulus* of the mulberry family) from which humulon and lupulon are obtained

lu·pu·lon \ˈlü-pyə-ˌlän\ *also* **lu·pu·lone** \-ˌlōn\ *n* : a bitter crystalline antibiotic $C_{26}H_{38}O_4$ that is obtained from lupulin and is effective against fungi and various bacteria

lu·pus \ˈlü-pəs\ *n* : any of several diseases (as lupus vulgaris or systemic lupus erythematosus) characterized by skin lesions

lupus band test *n* : a test to determine the presence of antibodies and complement deposits at the junction of the dermal and epidermal skin layers of patients with systemic lupus erythematosus

lupus er·y·the·ma·to·sus \-ˌer-ə-ˌthē-mə-ˈtō-səs\ *n* : a disorder characterized by skin inflammation; *esp* : SYSTEMIC LUPUS ERYTHEMATOSUS

lupus erythematosus cell *n* : LE CELL

lupus ne·phri·tis \-ni-ˈfrīt-əs\ *n* : glomerulonephritis associated with systemic lupus erythematosus that is typically characterized by proteinuria and hematuria and that often leads to renal failure

lupus per·nio \-ˈpər-nē-ō\ *n* : SARCOIDOSIS

lupus vul·gar·is \-ˌvəl-ˈgar-əs, -ˈger-\ *n* : a tuberculous disease of the skin marked by formation of soft brownish nodules with ulceration and scarring

LUQ *abbr* left upper quadrant (abdomen)

Lur·ide \ˈlur-ˌīd\ *trademark* — used for a preparation of sodium fluoride

Lusch·ka's gland \ˈlush-kəz-\ *n* : GLOMUS COCCYGEUM
  Luschka, Hubert von (1820–1875), German anatomist. Luschka was a professor of anatomy at Tübingen. From

1863 to 1869 he published a three-volume textbook of human anatomy, the second volume of which contains his description of Luschka's gland.

lute \ˈlüt\ *n* : a substance (as cement or clay) for packing a joint (as in laboratory apparatus) or coating a porous surface to produce imperviousness to gas or liquid — **lute** *vt* **lut·ed; lut·ing**

lutea — see MACULA LUTEA

lu·te·al \ˈlüt-ē-əl\ *adj* : of, relating to, characterized by, or involving the corpus luteum or its formation ⟨the ~ phase of the menstrual cycle⟩ ⟨~ activity⟩

lutecium *var of* LUTETIUM

lu·tein \ˈlüt-ē-ən, ˈlü-ˌtēn\ *n* : an orange xanthophyll $C_{40}H_{56}O_2$ occurring in plants usu. with carotenes and chlorophylls and in animal fat, egg yolk, and the corpus luteum

lutein cell *n* : any of the plump cells of the corpus luteum that contain lipid droplets and are derived from granulosa cells and the cells of the theca interna — see GRANULOSA LUTEIN CELL, THECA LUTEIN CELL

lu·tein·iza·tion *or chiefly Brit* **lu·tein·isa·tion** \ˌlüt-ē-ən-ə-ˈzā-shən, ˌlü-ˌtēn-\ *n* : the process of forming corpora lutea — **lu·tein·ize** *also Brit* **lu·tein·ise** \ˈlüt-ē-ə-ˌnīz, ˈlü-ˌtē-ˌnīz\ *vb* **-ized** *also Brit* **-ised; -iz·ing** *also Brit* **-is·ing**

luteinizing hormone *n* : a glycoprotein hormone that is secreted by the adenohypophysis and that in the female stimulates ovulation and the development of the corpora lutea and together with follicle-stimulating hormone the secretion of estrogen from developing ovarian follicles and in the male the development of interstitial tissue in the testis and the secretion of testosterone — abbr. *LH*; called also *interstitial-cell stimulating hormone, lutropin*

luteinizing hormone–releasing factor *n* : GONADOTROPIN-RELEASING HORMONE

luteinizing hormone–releasing hormone *n* : GONADOTROPIN-RELEASING HORMONE

lu·te·o·lin \ˈlüt-ē-ə-lin, -lən\ *n* : a yellow crystalline pigment $C_{15}H_{10}O_6$ occurring usu. as a glycoside in many plants

lu·teo·ly·sin \ˌlü-tē-ō-ˈlīs-ᵊn\ *n* : a substance that is the postulated causative agent of luteolysis and may be a prostaglandin

lu·te·ol·y·sis \ˌlü-tē-ˈäl-ə-səs\ *n, pl* **-y·ses** \-ˌsēz\ : regression of the corpus luteum

lu·teo·lyt·ic \ˌlüt-ē-ə-ˈlit-ik\ *adj* : of, relating to, or producing luteolysis ⟨~ effects⟩ ⟨a ~ agent⟩

lu·te·o·ma \ˌlüt-ē-ˈō-mə\ *n, pl* **-mas** *also* **-ma·ta** \-mət-ə\ : an ovarian tumor derived from a corpus luteum — **lu·te·o·ma·tous** \-mət-əs\ *adj*

lu·teo·tro·pic \ˌlüt-ē-ə-ˈtrō-pik, -ˈträp-ik\ *or* **lu·teo·tro·phic** \-ˈtrō-fik, -ˈträf-ik\ *adj* : acting on the corpora lutea

luteotropic hormone *or* **luteotrophic hormone** *n* : PROLACTIN

lu·teo·tro·pin \ˌlüt-ē-ə-ˈtrō-pən\ *or* **lu·teo·tro·phin** \-fən\ *n* : PROLACTIN

lu·te·tium *also* **lu·te·cium** \lü-ˈtē-sh(ē-)əm\ *n* : a metallic element of the rare-earth group — symbol *Lu*; see ELEMENT table

luteum — see CORPUS LUTEUM

lu·tro·pin \lü-ˈtrō-pən\ *n* : LUTEINIZING HORMONE

lu·tu·trin \ˈlü-tə-ˌtrin\ *n* : a substance obtained from the corpus luteum of sows' ovaries and used as a uterine relaxant

Lu·vox \ˈlü-ˌväks\ *trademark* — used for a preparation of the maleate of fluvoxamine

lux \ˈləks\ *n, pl* **lux** *or* **lux·es** : a unit of illumination equal to the direct illumination on a surface that is everywhere one meter from a uniform point source of one candle intensity or equal to one lumen per square meter — called also *meter-candle*

lux·ate \ˈlək-ˌsāt\ *vt* **lux·at·ed; lux·at·ing** : to throw out of place or out of joint : DISLOCATE ⟨the . . . fractured and *luxated* teeth were removed —*Dental Abstracts*⟩ ⟨a *luxated* patella⟩

lux·a·tion \ˌlək-ˈsā-shən\ *n* : dislocation of an anatomical part

LV *abbr* left ventricle

LVN \\'el-'vē-'en\\ *n* : LICENSED VOCATIONAL NURSE

ly·ase \\'lī-ˌās, -ˌāz\\ *n* : an enzyme (as a decarboxylase) that forms double bonds by removing groups from a substrate other than by hydrolysis or that adds groups to double bonds

ly·can·thrope \\'lī-kən-ˌthrōp, lī-'kan-\\ *n* : an individual affected with lycanthropy

ly·can·thro·py \\lī-'kan(t)-thrə-pē\\ *n, pl* **-pies** : a delusion that one has become or has assumed the characteristics of a wolf

ly·co·pene \\'lī-kə-ˌpēn\\ *n* : a red pigment C₄₀H₅₆ isomeric with carotene that occurs in many ripe fruits (as the tomato)

ly·co·pen·emia *or chiefly Brit* **ly·co·pen·ae·mia** \\lī-kə-pē-'nē-mē-ə\\ *n* : an excess of lycopene in the blood

Ly·co·per·da·les \\lī-kō-pər-'dā-(ˌ)lēz\\ *n pl* : a small order of basidiomycetes comprising fungi (as the puffballs) having a fleshy often globose fruiting body filled at maturity with a mass of dustlike spores

Ly·co·per·don \\lī-kō-'pər-ˌdän\\ *n* : a genus of fungi of a family (Lycoperdaceae) of the order Lycoperdales whose fruiting body tapers toward a base consisting of spongy mycelium and whose spores have been used in folk medicine to treat nosebleeds

ly·co·pin \\'lī-kə-ˌpin\\ *n* : LYCOPENE

ly·co·po·dine \\lī-kə-'pō-ˌdēn\\ *n* : an alkaloid C₁₆H₂₅NO obtained from several members of the genus *Lycopodium*

ly·co·po·di·um \\lī-kə-'pōd-ē-əm\\ *n* **1 a** *cap* : a large genus of erect or creeping club mosses with reduced or scalelike evergreen leaves **b** : any club moss of the genus *Lycopodium* **2** : a fine yellowish flammable powder composed of lycopodium spores and used as a dusting powder for the skin and for the surface of hand-rolled pills

lycopodium powder *n* : LYCOPODIUM 2

Ly·co·pus \\'lī-kə-pəs\\ *n* : a small genus of mints that are not aromatic and include the bugleweeds

ly·co·rine \\'lī-kə-ˌrīn, li-'kōr-ən\\ *n* : a poisonous crystalline alkaloid C₁₆H₁₇NO₄ found in the bulbs of the common daffodil and several other plants of the amaryllis family (Amaryllidaceae)

lye \\'lī\\ *n* **1** : a strong alkaline liquor rich in potassium carbonate leached from wood ashes and used esp. in making soap and washing; *broadly* : a strong alkaline solution (as of sodium hydroxide or potassium hydroxide) **2** : a solid caustic (as sodium hydroxide)

Ly·ell's syndrome \\'lī-əlz-\\ *n* : TOXIC EPIDERMAL NECROLYSIS

  Lyell, Alan (*fl* 1950–1972), British dermatologist. Lyell's best known paper described toxic epidermal necrolysis, a disease to which his name has subsequently been attached. He also wrote the chapter on skin diseases for a 1971 medical textbook.

ly·ing–in \\ˌlī-iŋ-'in\\ *n, pl* **lyings–in** *or* **lying–ins** : the state attending and consequent to childbirth : CONFINEMENT

Lyme arthritis \\'līm-\\ *n* : arthritis as a symptom of or caused by Lyme disease; *also* : LYME DISEASE

Lyme disease *n* : an acute inflammatory disease that is usu. characterized initially by the skin lesion erythema migrans and by fatigue, fever, and chills and if left untreated may later manifest itself in cardiac and neurological disorders, joint pain, and arthritis and that is caused by a spirochete of the genus *Borrelia* (*B. burgdorferi*) transmitted by the bite of a tick esp. of the genus *Ixodes* (*I. scapularis* syn. *I. dammini* in the eastern and midwestern U.S., *I. pacificus* esp. in some parts of the Pacific coastal states of the U.S., and *I. ricinus* in Europe) — called also *Lyme, Lyme borreliosis*

Lym·naea \\lim-'nē-ə, 'lim-nē-ə\\ *n* : a genus of snails formerly almost coextensive with the family Lymnaeidae but now comprising comparatively few species of dextrally coiled freshwater snails that include some medically important intermediate hosts of flukes — compare FOSSARIA, GALBA

Lym·nae·idae \\lim-'nē-ə-ˌdē\\ *n pl* : a family of thin-shelled air-breathing freshwater snails (suborder Basommatophora) that have an elongate ovoidal shell with a large opening and a simple lip and that include numerous species important as intermediate hosts of trematode worms — see FOSSARIA, GALBA, LYMNAEA — **lym·nae·id** \\-'nē-id\\ *adj or n*

lymph \\'lim(p)f\\ *n* : a usu. clear coagulable fluid that passes from intercellular spaces of body tissue into the lymphatic vessels, is discharged into the blood by way of the thoracic duct and right lymphatic duct, and resembles blood plasma in containing white blood cells and esp. lymphocytes but normally few red blood cells and no platelets — see CHYLE; compare CEREBROSPINAL FLUID

lymph·ad·e·nec·to·my \\ˌlim-ˌfad-ⁿn-'ek-tə-mē\\ *n, pl* **-mies** : surgical removal of a lymph node

lymph·ad·e·ni·tis \\ˌlim-ˌfad-ⁿn-'īt-əs\\ *n* : inflammation of lymph nodes — **lymph·ad·e·nit·ic** \\-'it-ik\\ *adj*

lym·phad·e·noid \\(ˌ)lim-'fad-ⁿn-ˌóid\\ *adj* : resembling or having the properties of a lymph node

lymph·ad·e·no·ma \\ˌlim-ˌfad-ⁿn-'ō-mə\\ *n, pl* **-mas** *also* **-ma·ta** \\-mət-ə\\ **1** : LYMPHOMA **2** : HODGKIN'S DISEASE

lymph·ad·e·nop·a·thy \\ˌlim-ˌfad-ⁿn-'äp-ə-thē\\ *n, pl* **-thies** : abnormal enlargement of the lymph nodes — **lymph·ad·e·no·path·ic** \\ˌlim-ˌfad-ⁿn-ō-'path-ik\\ *adj*

lymphadenopathy–associated virus *n* : HIV-1

lymph·ad·e·no·sis \\ˌlim-ˌfad-ⁿn-'ō-səs\\ *n, pl* **-no·ses** \\-ˌsēz\\ : any of certain abnormalities or diseases affecting the lymphatic system: as **a** : leukosis involving lymphatic tissues **b** : LYMPHOCYTIC LEUKEMIA

lymph·a·gogue \\'lim-fə-ˌgäg\\ *n* : an agent that promotes lymph production or lymph flow

lymph·an·gi·ec·ta·sia \\ˌlim-ˌfan-jē-ek-'tā-zh(ē-)ə\\ *or* **lymph·an·gi·ec·ta·sis** \\-'ek-tə-səs\\ *n, pl* **-ta·sias** *or* **-ta·ses** \\-ˌsēz\\ : dilatation of the lymphatic vessels — **lymph·an·gi·ec·tat·ic** \\-ek-'tat-ik\\ *adj*

lymph·an·gio·ad·e·nog·ra·phy \\ˌlim-ˌfan-jē-ō-ˌad-ⁿn-'äg-rə-fē\\ *n, pl* **-phies** : LYMPHANGIOGRAPHY

lymph·an·gio·en·do·the·li·o·ma \\ˌlim-ˌfan-jē-ō-ˌen-dō-ˌthē-lē-'ō-mə\\ *n, pl* **-mas** *also* **-ma·ta** \\-mət-ə\\ : a tumor composed of lymphoid and endothelial tissue

lymph·an·gio·gram \\(ˌ)lim-'fan-jē-ə-ˌgram\\ *n* : an X-ray picture made by lymphangiography

lymph·an·gi·og·ra·phy \\ˌlim-ˌfan-jē-'äg-rə-fē\\ *n, pl* **-phies** : X-ray depiction of lymphatic vessels and lymph nodes after use of a radiopaque material — called also *lymphography* — **lymph·an·gio·graph·ic** \\ˌlim-ˌfan-jē-ə-'graf-ik\\ *adj*

lymph·an·gi·o·ma \\ˌlim-ˌfan-jē-'ō-mə\\ *n, pl* **-mas** *also* **-ma·ta** \\-mət-ə\\ : a tumor formed of dilated lymphatic vessels — **lymph·an·gi·o·ma·tous** \\-mət-əs\\ *adj*

lymph·an·gio·sar·co·ma \\ˌlim-ˌfan-jē-ō-(ˌ)sär-'kō-mə\\ *n, pl* **-mas** *also* **-ma·ta** \\-mət-ə\\ : a sarcoma arising from the endothelial cells of lymphatic vessels

lymph·an·gi·ot·o·my \\ˌlim-ˌfan-jē-'ät-ə-mē\\ *n, pl* **-mies** : incision of a lymphatic vessel

lym·phan·gi·tis \\ˌlim-ˌfan-'jīt-əs\\ *n, pl* **-git·i·des** \\-'jit-ə-ˌdēz\\ : inflammation of the lymphatic vessels

lymphangitis ep·i·zo·ot·i·ca \\-ˌep-ə-zō-'ät-i-kə\\ *n* : EPIZOOTIC LYMPHANGITIS

¹lym·phat·ic \\lim-'fat-ik\\ *adj* **1 a** : of, relating to, or produced by lymph, lymphoid tissue, or lymphocytes ⟨~ nodules⟩ ⟨~ infiltration⟩ **b** : conveying lymph ⟨a ~ channel⟩ **2** : lacking physical or mental energy — **lym·phat·i·cal·ly** \\-i-k(ə-)lē\\ *adv*

²lymphatic *n* : a vessel that contains or conveys lymph, that originates as an interfibrillar or intercellular cleft or space in a tissue or organ, and that if small has no distinct walls or walls composed only of endothelial cells and if large resembles a vein in structure — called also *lymphatic vessel, lymph vessel;* see THORACIC DUCT

lymphatic capillary *n* : any of the smallest lymphatic vessels that are blind at one end and collect lymph in organs and tissues — called also *lymph capillary*

lymphatic duct *n* : any of the lymphatic vessels that are part

K,
L

\\ə\\ **abut** \\ᵊ\\ **kitten** \\ər\\ **further** \\a\\ **ash** \\ā\\ **ace** \\ä\\ **cot, cart**
\\au\\ **out** \\ch\\ **chin** \\e\\ **bet** \\ē\\ **easy** \\g\\ **go** \\i\\ **hit** \\ī\\ **ice** \\j\\ **job**
\\ŋ\\ **sing** \\ō\\ **go** \\ó\\ **law** \\ói\\ **boy** \\th\\ **thin** \\th\\ **the** \\ü\\ **loot**
\\ú\\ **foot** \\y\\ **yet** \\zh\\ **vision** *See also* Pronunciation Symbols page

of the system collecting lymph from the lymphatic capillaries and pouring it into the subclavian veins by way of the right lymphatic duct and the thoracic duct — called also *lymph duct*

lymphatic leukemia *n* : LYMPHOCYTIC LEUKEMIA

lym·phat·i·co·ve·nous \lim-ˌfat-i-kō-ˈvē-nəs\ *adj* : of, relating to, or connecting the veins and lymphatic vessels ⟨∼ anastomoses⟩

lymphatic system *n* : the part of the circulatory system that is concerned esp. with scavenging fluids and proteins that have escaped from cells and tissues and returning them to the blood, with the phagocytic removal of cellular debris and foreign material, and with immune responses, that overlaps and parallels the system of blood vessels in function and shares some constituents with it, and that consists esp. of the thymus, spleen, tonsils, lymph, lymph nodes, lymphatic vessels, lymphocytes, and bone marrow where stem cells differentiate into precursors of B cells and T cells — called also *lymphoid system, lymph system*

lymphaticus — see STATUS LYMPHATICUS

lymphatic vessel *n* : LYMPHATIC

lym·pha·tism \ˈlim(p)-fə-ˌtiz-əm\ *n* : STATUS LYMPHATICUS

lym·phat·o·gogue \lim-ˈfat-ə-ˌgäg\ *n* : LYMPHAGOGUE

lymph capillary *n* : LYMPHATIC CAPILLARY

lymph duct *n* : LYMPHATIC DUCT

lymph·ede·ma *or chiefly Brit* **lymph·oe·de·ma** \ˌlim(p)-fi-ˈdē-mə\ *n* : edema due to faulty lymphatic drainage — **lymph·edem·a·tous** *or chiefly Brit* **lymph·oe·dem·a·tous** \ˌlim(p)-fi-ˈdem-ət-əs\ *adj*

lymph follicle *n* : LYMPH NODE; *esp* : LYMPH NODULE

lymph gland *n* : LYMPH NODE

lymph heart *n* : a contractile muscular expansion of a lymphatic vessel in some lower vertebrates that serves to drive the lymph toward the veins

lymph node *n* : any of the rounded masses of lymphoid tissue that are surrounded by a capsule of connective tissue, are distributed along the lymphatic vessels, and contain numerous lymphocytes which filter the flow of lymph passing through the node — called also *lymph gland*

lymph nodule *n* : a small simple lymph node

lym·pho·blast \ˈlim(p)-fə-ˌblast\ *n* : a lymphocyte that has enlarged following stimulation by an antigen, has the capacity to recognize the stimulating antigen, and is undergoing proliferation and differentiation either to an effector state in which it functions to eliminate the antigen or to a memory state in which it functions to recognize the future reappearance of the antigen — called also *lymphocytoblast;* compare LEUKOBLAST — **lym·pho·blas·tic** \ˌlim(p)-fə-ˈblas-tik\ *adj*

lymphoblastic leukemia *n* : lymphocytic leukemia characterized by an abnormal increase in the number of lymphoblasts; *specif* : ACUTE LYMPHOBLASTIC LEUKEMIA

¹lym·pho·blas·toid \ˌlim(p)-fə-ˈblas-ˌtȯid\ *adj* : resembling a lymphoblast ⟨human ∼ cell lines from tissue infected with Epstein-Barr virus⟩

²lymphoblastoid *n* : a lymphoblastoid cell

lym·pho·blas·to·ma \ˌlim(p)-fə-blas-ˈtō-mə\ *n, pl* **-mas** *also* **-ma·ta** \-mət-ə\ : any of several diseases of lymph nodes marked by the formation of tumorous masses composed of mature or immature lymphocytes

lym·pho·blas·to·sis \-ˌblas-ˈtō-səs\ *n, pl* **-to·ses** \-ˌsēz\ : the presence of lymphoblasts in the peripheral blood (as in acute lymphocytic leukemia or infectious mononucleosis)

lym·pho·cele \ˈlim(p)-fə-ˌsēl\ *n* : a cyst containing lymph

lym·pho·cyte \ˈlim(p)-fə-ˌsīt\ *n* : any of the colorless weakly motile cells that originate from stem cells and differentiate in lymphoid tissue (as of the thymus or bone marrow), that are the typical cellular elements of lymph, that include the cellular mediators of immunity, and that constitute 20 to 30 percent of the white blood cells of normal human blood — see B CELL, T CELL — **lym·pho·cyt·ic** \ˌlim(p)-fə-ˈsit-ik\ *adj*

lymphocyte function–associated antigen–1 *n* : LFA-1

lymphocyte transformation *n* : a transformation caused in lymphocytes by a mitosis-inducing agent (as phytohemagglutinin) or by a second exposure to an antigen and charac-

terized by an increase in size and in the amount of cytoplasm, by visibility of nucleoli in the nucleus, and after about 72 hours by a marked resemblance to blast cells

lymphocytic choriomeningitis *n* : an acute disease caused by an arenavirus (genus *Arenavirus*) and characterized by fever, nausea and vomiting, headache, stiff neck, and slow pulse, marked by the presence of numerous lymphocytes in the cerebrospinal fluid, and transmitted esp. by rodents

lymphocytic leukemia *n* : leukemia of either of two types marked by an abnormal increase in the number of white blood cells (as lymphocytes) which accumulate in bone marrow, lymphoid tissue (as of the lymph nodes and spleen), and circulating blood — called also *lymphatic leukemia, lymphoid leukemia;* see ACUTE LYMPHOBLASTIC LEUKEMIA, CHRONIC LYMPHOCYTIC LEUKEMIA

lym·pho·cy·to·blast \ˌlim(p)-fō-ˈsīt-ə-ˌblast\ *n* : LYMPHOBLAST

lym·pho·cy·to·gen·e·sis \-ˌsīt-ə-ˈjen-ə-səs\ *n, pl* **-e·ses** \-ˌsēz\ : LYMPHOPOIESIS

lym·pho·cy·toid \ˌlim(p)-fō-ˈsīt-ˌȯid\ *adj* : resembling a lymphocyte ⟨∼ cell lines⟩

lym·pho·cy·to·lyt·ic \ˌlim(p)-fō-ˌsīt-ə-ˈlit-ik\ *adj* : causing the dissolution or disintegration of lymphocytes

lym·pho·cy·to·ma \ˌlim(p)-fō-sī-ˈtō-mə\ *n, pl* **-mas** *also* **-ma·ta** \-mət-ə\ **1** : a tumor in which lymphocytes are the dominant cellular elements **2** : LYMPHOID LEUKOSIS

lym·pho·cy·to·ma·to·sis \-ˌsī-ˌtō-mə-ˈtō-səs\ *n, pl* **-to·ses** \-ˌsēz\ : an abnormal condition characterized by the formation of lymphocytomas; *specif* : LYMPHOID LEUKOSIS

lym·pho·cy·to·pe·nia \ˌlim(p)-fō-ˌsīt-ə-ˈpē-nē-ə\ *n* : a decrease in the normal number of lymphocytes in the circulating blood — **lym·pho·cy·to·pe·nic** \-ˈpē-nik\ *adj*

lym·pho·cy·to·poi·e·sis \-ˌpȯi-ˈē-səs\ *n, pl* **-e·ses** \-ˌsēz\ : formation of lymphocytes usu. in the lymph nodes — **lym·pho·cy·to·poi·et·ic** \-ˌpȯi-ˈet-ik\ *adj*

lym·pho·cy·to·sis \ˌlim(p)-fə-ˌsī-ˈtō-səs, -fə-sə-\ *n, pl* **-to·ses** \-ˌsēz\ : an increase in the number of lymphocytes in the blood usu. associated with chronic infections or inflammations — compare GRANULOCYTOSIS, MONOCYTOSIS — **lym·pho·cy·tot·ic** \-ˈtät-ik\ *adj*

lym·pho·cy·to·tox·ic \ˌlim(p)-fə-ˌsīt-ə-ˈtäk-sik\ *adj* **1** : being or relating to toxic effects on lymphocytes ⟨∼ assays⟩ **2** : being toxic to lymphocytes ⟨a ∼ antibody⟩ — **lym·pho·cy·to·tox·ic·i·ty** \-ˌtäk-ˈsis-ət-ē\ *n, pl* **-ties**

lymphoedema, lymphoedematous *chiefly Brit var of* LYMPHEDEMA, LYMPHEDEMATOUS

lym·pho·ep·i·the·li·al \ˌlim(p)-fō-ˌep-ə-ˈthē-lē-əl\ *adj* : consisting of lymphocytes and epithelial cells ⟨∼ tissues⟩

lym·pho·gen·e·sis \ˌlim(p)-fə-ˈjen-ə-səs\ *n, pl* **-e·ses** \-ˌsēz\ : the production of lymph

lym·phog·e·nous \lim-ˈfäj-ə-nəs\ *also* **lym·pho·gen·ic** \ˌlim(p)-fə-ˈjen-ik\ *adj* **1** : producing lymph or lymphocytes **2** : arising, resulting from, or spread by way of lymphocytes or lymphatic vessels ⟨∼ leukemia⟩ ⟨∼ metastases⟩

lym·pho·gram \ˈlim(p)-fə-ˌgram\ *n* : LYMPHANGIOGRAM

lym·pho·gran·u·lo·ma \ˈlim(p)-fō-ˌgran-yə-ˈlō-mə\ *n, pl* **-mas** *also* **-ma·ta** \-mət-ə\ **1** : a nodular swelling of a lymph node **2** : LYMPHOGRANULOMA VENEREUM

lymphogranuloma in·gui·na·le \-ˌiŋ-gwə-ˈnäl-ē, -ˈnal-, -ˈnāl-\ *n* : LYMPHOGRANULOMA VENEREUM

lym·pho·gran·u·lo·ma·to·sis \-ˌlō-mə-ˈtō-səs\ *n, pl* **-to·ses** \-ˌsēz\ : the development of benign or malignant lymphogranulomas in various parts of the body; *also* : a condition characterized by lymphogranulomas

lym·pho·gran·u·lo·ma·tous \ˌlim(p)-fō-ˌgran-yə-ˈlō-mət-əs\ *adj* : of, relating to, or characterized by lymphogranulomas

lymphogranuloma ve·ne·re·um \-və-ˈnir-ē-əm\ *n* : a contagious venereal disease that is caused by various strains of a bacterium of the genus *Chlamydia* (*C. trachomatis*) and is marked by painful swelling and inflammation of the lymph nodes esp. in the region of the groin — called also *lymphogranuloma inguinale, lymphopathia venereum*

lym·phog·ra·phy \lim-ˈfäg-rə-fē\ *n, pl* **-phies** : LYMPHANGIOGRAPHY — **lym·pho·graph·ic** \ˌlim-fə-ˈgraf-ik\ *adj*

lym·pho·he·ma·to·poi·et·ic *or chiefly Brit* **lym·pho·hae·ma·to·poi·et·ic** \lim(p)-fō-hi-ˌmat-ə-pȯi-ˈet-ik, -ˌhē-mət-ō-\ *adj* : of, relating to, or involved in the production of lymphocytes and cells of blood, bone marrow, spleen, lymph nodes, and thymus

lym·phoid \ˈlim-ˌfȯid\ *adj* **1** : of, relating to, or being tissue (as the lymph nodes or thymus) containing lymphocytes **2** : of, relating to, or resembling lymph

lymphoid cell *n* : any of the cells responsible for the production of immunity mediated by cells or antibodies and including lymphocytes, lymphoblasts, and plasma cells

lymphoid leukemia *n* : LYMPHOCYTIC LEUKEMIA

lymphoid leukosis *n* : a neoplastic disease of chickens that is caused by a retrovirus and is characterized by the formation of nodular or diffuse lymphoid tumors composed mostly of B cells and occurring esp. in the bursa of Fabricius, liver, and spleen and sometimes in the kidneys and gonads

lym·phoid·o·cyte \lim-ˈfȯid-ə-ˌsīt\ *n* : HEMOCYTOBLAST

lymphoid system *n* : LYMPHATIC SYSTEM

lym·pho·kine \ˈlim(p)-fə-ˌkīn\ *n* : any of various substances (as an interleukin) of low molecular weight that are not antibodies, are secreted by T cells in response to stimulation by antigens, and have a role (as the activation of macrophages or the enhancement or inhibition of antibody production) in cell-mediated immunity

lym·pho·kine–ac·ti·vat·ed killer cell \-ˌak-tə-ˌvāt-əd-\ *n* : a lymphocyte (as a natural killer cell) that has been turned into a tumor-killing cell by being cultured with interleukin-2 — called also *LAK*

lym·phol·y·sis \lim-ˈfäl-ə-səs\ *n, pl* **-y·ses** \-ˌsēz\ : the destruction of lymph cells — **lym·pho·lyt·ic** \ˌlim(p)-fə-ˈlit-ik\ *adj*

lym·pho·ma \lim-ˈfō-mə\ *n, pl* **-mas** *also* **-ma·ta** \-mət-ə\ : a usu. malignant tumor of lymphoid tissue — **lym·pho·ma·tous** \-mət-əs\ *adj*

lym·pho·ma·gen·e·sis \lim-ˌfō-mə-ˈjen-ə-səs\ *n, pl* **-e·ses** \-ˌsēz\ : the growth and development of a lymphoma — **lym·pho·ma·gen·ic** \-ˈjen-ik\ *adj*

lym·pho·ma·toid \lim-ˈfō-mə-ˌtȯid\ *adj* : characterized by or resembling lymphomas ⟨a ∼ tumor⟩

lymphomatosa — see STRUMA LYMPHOMATOSA

lym·pho·ma·to·sis \(ˌ)lim-ˌfō-mə-ˈtō-səs\ *n, pl* **-to·ses** \-ˌsēz\ : the presence of multiple lymphomas in the body; *specif* : LYMPHOID LEUKOSIS

lym·pho·ma·tot·ic \-ˈtät-ik\ *adj* : of or relating to lymphomatosis

lym·pho·path·ia ve·ne·re·um \ˌlim(p)-fə-ˈpath-ē-ə-və-ˈnir-ē-əm\ *n* : LYMPHOGRANULOMA VENEREUM

lym·pho·pe·nia \ˌlim(p)-fə-ˈpē-nē-ə\ *n* : reduction in the number of lymphocytes circulating in the blood of humans or animals — **lym·pho·pe·nic** \-ˈpē-nik\ *adj*

lym·pho·plas·mo·cyt·ic *or* **lym·pho·plas·ma·cyt·ic** \-ˌplaz-mə-ˈsit-ik\ *adj* : of, relating to, or consisting of lymphocytes and plasma cells ⟨diffuse ∼ infiltration of the small intestine —*Science*⟩

lym·pho·poi·e·sis \ˌlim(p)-fə-pȯi-ˈē-səs\ *n, pl* **-e·ses** \-ˌsēz\ : the formation of lymphocytes or lymphatic tissue — **lym·pho·poi·et·ic** \-pȯi-ˈet·ik\ *adj*

lym·pho·pro·lif·er·a·tive \ˌlim(p)-fō-prə-ˈlif-ə-ˌrāt-iv, -ˈlif-ə-rət-iv\ *adj* : of or relating to the proliferation of lymphoid tissue ⟨Marek's disease is a ∼ disorder⟩ ⟨∼ syndrome⟩ — **lym·pho·pro·lif·er·a·tion** \-prə-ˌlif-ə-ˈrā-shən\ *n*

lym·pho·re·tic·u·lar \ˌlim(p)-fō-ri-ˈtik-yə-lər\ *adj* : RETICULOENDOTHELIAL ⟨∼ malignancies⟩

lymphoreticular system *n* : RETICULOENDOTHELIAL SYSTEM

lym·pho·re·tic·u·lo·sis \ˌlim(p)-fō-ri-ˌtik-yə-ˈlō-səs\ *n, pl* **-lo·ses** \-ˌsēz\ : hyperplasia of reticuloendothelial tissue and esp. of the lymph nodes

lym·phor·rhage \ˈlim(p)-fə-rij\ *n* : a deposit of lymphocytes in muscle

lym·pho·sar·co·ma \ˌlim(p)-fō-sär-ˈkō-mə\ *n, pl* **-mas** *also* **-ma·ta** \-mət-ə\ : a malignant lymphoma that tends to metastasize freely

lym·pho·sar·co·ma·tous \-mət-əs\ *adj* : being, affected with, or characterized by lymphosarcomas ⟨∼ masses⟩

lym·pho·scin·tig·ra·phy \ˌlim(p)-fō-sin-ˈtig-rə-fē\ *n, pl* **-phies** : scintigraphy of the lymphatic system

lym·pho·tox·in \ˌlim(p)-fō-ˈtäk-sən\ *n* : a lymphokine that lyses various cells and esp. tumor cells — **lym·pho·tox·ic** \-ˈtäk-sik\ *adj*

lym·pho·tro·pic \-ˈtrō-pik, -ˈträp-ik\ *adj* : having an affinity for lymphocytes ⟨human ∼ retroviruses⟩ ⟨Epstein-Barr virus ... is a ∼ herpesvirus —Michael Steinitz *et al*⟩ — see HUMAN T-CELL LYMPHOTROPIC VIRUS, HUMAN T-LYMPHOTROPIC VIRUS

lymph system *n* : LYMPHATIC SYSTEM

lymph·uria \ˌlim(p)f-ˈ(y)ùr-ē-ə\ *n* : the presence of lymph in the urine

lymph vessel *n* : LYMPHATIC

lyn·es·tre·nol \lin-ˈes-trə-ˌnȯl, -ˌnōl\ *n* : a progestational steroid $C_{20}H_{28}O$ used esp. in birth control pills

lyo·chrome \ˈlī-ə-ˌkrōm\ *n* : FLAVIN

Ly·on hypothesis \ˈlī-ən-\ *n* : a hypothesis explaining why the phenotypic effect of the X chromosome is the same in the mammalian female which has two X chromosomes as it is in the male which has only one X chromosome: one of each two somatic X chromosomes in mammalian females is selected at random and inactivated early in embryonic development

Lyon, Mary Frances (b 1925), British geneticist. Lyon first proposed in 1962 a hypothesis to explain the variegated gene expression seen in female mice that were heterozygous for sex-linked genes. She proposed that in a given somatic cell of a female mouse only the genes on one of the two X chromosomes were active. The genes on one of the X chromosomes might be active in one part of a tissue, while in another part the genes on the other might function. The determination as to which X chromosome was to be active in a particular cell line was believed to occur early in embryonic development.

lyo·phile \ˈlī-ə-ˌfil\ *also* **lyo·phil** \-ˌfil\ *adj* **1** : LYOPHILIC **2 a** : of or relating to freeze-drying **b** *or* **lyo·philed** \-ˌfīld\ : obtained by freeze-drying

lyo·phil·ic \ˌlī-ə-ˈfil-ik\ *adj* : marked by strong affinity between a dispersed phase and the liquid in which it is dispersed ⟨a ∼ colloid⟩ — compare LYOPHOBIC, HYDROPHILIC, LIPOPHILIC, OLEOPHILIC

ly·oph·i·lize *or Brit* **ly·oph·i·lise** \lī-ˈäf-ə-ˌlīz\ *vt* **-lized** *or Brit* **-lised; -liz·ing** *or Brit* **-lis·ing** : FREEZE-DRY — **ly·oph·i·li·za·tion** *or Brit* **ly·oph·i·li·sa·tion** \-ˌäf-ə-lə-ˈzā-shən\ *n*

ly·oph·i·liz·er *or Brit* **ly·oph·i·lis·er** \lī-ˈäf-ə-ˌlīz-ər\ *n* : a device used to carry out the process of freeze-drying

lyo·pho·bic \ˌlī-ə-ˈfō-bik\ *adj* : marked by lack of strong affinity between a dispersed phase and the liquid in which it is dispersed — compare LYOPHILIC, HYDROPHOBIC 3, OLEOPHOBIC

lyo·sorp·tion \ˌlī-ō-ˈsȯrp-shən\ *n* : the adsorption of a solvent on the surface of a solute or of a dispersing medium of a colloid on the surface of the dispersed material

lyo·tro·pic \ˌlī-ə-ˈtrō-pik, -ˈträp-ik\ *adj* : of, relating to, or being a liquid crystal that is prepared by mixing two substances of which one (as water) is polar in nature and that may assume a series of states from that of a solid to a true solution depending on the proportions of the two substances in the mixture — **ly·ot·ro·py** \lī-ˈä-trə-pē\ *n, pl* **-pies**

lyotropic series *n* : HOFMEISTER SERIES

ly·pres·sin \lī-ˈpres-ᵊn\ *n* : a vasopressin in which the eighth amino acid residue in its polypeptide chain is a lysine residue (as in pigs) rather than an arginine residue (as in most mammals including humans) and which is used esp. as a nasal spray in the control of diabetes mellitus — called also *lysine vasopressin;* compare ARGININE VASOPRESSIN

\ə\ **abut** \ᵊ\ **kitten** \ər\ **further** \a\ **ash** \ā\ **ace** \ä\ **cot, cart** \aù\ **out** \ch\ **chin** \e\ **bet** \ē\ **easy** \g\ **go** \i\ **hit** \ī\ **ice** \j\ **job** \ŋ\ **sing** \ō\ **go** \ȯ\ **law** \ȯi\ **boy** \th\ **thin** \t͟h\ **the** \ü\ **loot** \ù\ **foot** \y\ **yet** \zh\ **vision** *See also* Pronunciation Symbols page

K
L

ly·ra \\'lī-rə\\ *n* : HIPPOCAMPAL COMMISSURE

Lys *abbr* lysine; lysyl

ly·sate \\'lī-ˌsāt\\ *n* : a product of lysis

lyse \\'līs, 'līz\\ *vb* **lysed; lys·ing** *vt* : to cause to undergo lysis : produce lysis in ⟨cells were *lysed*⟩ ∼ *vi* : to undergo lysis

Ly·sen·ko·ism \\lə-'sen-kō-ˌiz-əm\\ *n* : a biological doctrine asserting the fundamental influence of somatic and environmental factors on heredity in contradiction of orthodox genetics — called also *Michurinism*

  Ly·sen·ko \\lə-'sen-kō\\, **Trofim Denisovich (1898–1976),** Soviet biologist and agronomist. Lysenko was the virtual dictator of biology in the Soviet Union from the 1930s through the early 1960s. He was Director of the Institute of Genetics of the Academy of Sciences of the U.S.S.R. from 1940 to 1965. His biological theories came to be officially adopted and mandated throughout the Soviet Union despite their virtually total rejection elsewhere. He attacked Mendelian genetics and advocated a revised form of Lamarckism, the doctrine of the inheritance of acquired characteristics. He denied the existence of genes and plant hormones and asserted that all parts of an organism have a role in heredity. He held that the application of his genetic theories would result in the development of new types of crops and increased agricultural production. In the face of overwhelming scientific challenges and the ultimate loss of political support, he was stripped of all authority in 1965 and his doctrines were repudiated.

ly·ser·gic acid \\lə-ˌsər-jik-, (ˌ)lī-\\ *n* : a crystalline acid $C_{16}H_{16}N_2O_2$ that is an ergotic alkaloid; *also* : LSD

lysergic acid amide *n* : an ergotic alkaloid $C_{16}H_{17}N_3O$ with psychotomimetic properties less potent than those of LSD

lysergic acid di·eth·yl·am·ide \\-ˌdī-ˌeth-ə-'lam-ˌīd\\ *n* : LSD

ly·ser·gide \\lə-'sər-ˌjīd, lī-\\ *n* : LSD

ly·sim·e·ter \\lī-'sim-ət-ər\\ *n* : a device for measuring the solubility of a substance — **ly·si·met·ric** \\ˌlī-sə-'me-trik\\ *adj* — **ly·sim·e·try** \\lī-'sim-ə-trē\\ *n, pl* **-tries**

ly·sin \\'līs-ᵊn\\ *n* : a substance (as an antibody) capable of causing lysis

ly·sine \\'lī-ˌsēn\\ *n* : a crystalline essential amino acid $C_6H_{14}N_2O_2$ obtained from the hydrolysis of various proteins — abbr. *Lys*

lysine vasopressin *n* : LYPRESSIN

ly·sis \\'lī-səs\\ *n, pl* **ly·ses** \\-ˌsēz\\ **1** : the gradual decline of a disease process (as fever) — compare CRISIS 1 **2** : a process of disintegration or dissolution (as of cells)

ly·so·ceph·a·lin \\ˌlī-sō-'sef-ə-lin\\ *n* : a phosphatidylethanolamine from which a fatty acid group has been removed (as by action of cobra venom) and that is used as a hemolytic agent

ly·so·gen \\'lī-sə-jən\\ *n* : a lysogenic bacterium or bacterial strain

ly·so·gen·e·sis \\ˌlī-sə-'jen-ə-səs\\ *n, pl* **-eses** \\-ˌsēz\\ **1** : the production of lysins or of the phenomenon of lysis **2** : LYSOGENY

ly·so·gen·ic \\ˌlī-sə-'jen-ik\\ *adj* **1** : harboring a prophage as hereditary material ⟨∼ bacteria⟩ **2** : TEMPERATE 2 ⟨∼ viruses⟩ — **ly·so·ge·nic·i·ty** \\-jə-'nis-ət-ē\\ *n, pl* **-ties**

ly·sog·e·nize *also Brit* **ly·sog·e·nise** \\lī-'säj-ə-ˌnīz\\ *vt* **-nized** *also Brit* **-nised; -niz·ing** *also Brit* **-nis·ing** : to render lysogenic — **ly·sog·e·ni·za·tion** *also Brit* **ly·sog·e·ni·sa·tion** \\-ˌsäj-ə-nə-'zā-shən\\ *n*

ly·sog·e·ny \\lī-'säj-ə-nē\\ *n, pl* **-nies** : the state of being lysogenic

Ly·sol \\'lī-ˌsȯl, -ˌsōl\\ *trademark* — used for a disinfectant consisting of a brown emulsified solution containing cresols

ly·so·lec·i·thin \\ˌlī-sə-'les-ə-thən\\ *n* : LYSOPHOSPHATIDYL-CHOLINE

ly·so·phos·pha·tide \\ˌlī-sō-'fäs-fə-ˌtīd\\ *n* : a phosphatide from which one fatty acid residue has been removed (as by the action of cobra venom)

ly·so·phos·pha·ti·dyl·cho·line \\-ˌfäs-fə-ˌtīd-ᵊl-'kō-ˌlēn, -(ˌ)fäs-ˌfat-əd-ᵊl-\\ *n* : a hemolytic substance produced by the removal of a fatty acid group (as by the action of cobra venom) from a lecithin — called also *lysolecithin*

ly·so·some \\'lī-sə-ˌsōm\\ *n* : a saclike cellular organelle that contains various hydrolytic enzymes — **ly·so·som·al** \\ˌlī-sə-'sō-məl\\ *adj* — **ly·so·som·al·ly** \\-mə-lē\\ *adv*

ly·so·staph·in \\ˌlī-sə-'staf-ən\\ *n* : an antimicrobial enzyme that is obtained from a strain of staphylococcus and is effective against other staphylococci

ly·so·zyme \\'lī-sə-ˌzīm\\ *n* : a basic bacteriolytic protein that hydrolyzes peptidoglycan and is present in egg white and in saliva and tears — called also *muramidase*

lys·sa \\'lis-ə\\ *n* : RABIES — **lys·sic** \\-ik\\ *adj*

Lyster bag *var of* LISTER BAG

ly·syl \\'lī-səl\\ *n* : the amino acid radical or residue $H_2N(CH_2)_4CH(NH_2)CO–$ of lysine — abbr. *Lys*

lyt·ic \\'lit-ik\\ *adj* : of or relating to lysis or a lysin; *also* : productive of or effecting lysis (as of cells) ⟨∼ viruses⟩ ⟨∼ action on cells⟩ — **lyt·i·cal·ly** \\-i-k(ə-)lē\\ *adv*

Lyt·ta \\'lit-ə\\ *n* : a widespread genus of blister beetles (family Meloidae) containing the Spanish fly (*L. vesicatoria*)

lyx·o·fla·vin \\ˌlik-sə-'flā-vən\\ *n* : a yellow crystalline compound $C_{17}H_{20}N_4O_6$ isolated from heart muscle and stereoisomeric with riboflavin but derived from lyxose

lyx·ose \\'lik-ˌsōs, -ˌsōz\\ *n* : a crystalline aldose sugar $C_5H_{10}O_5$ that is the epimer of xylose

M

m *abbr* **1** Mach **2** male **3** married **4** masculine **5** mass **6** meter **7** [Latin *mille*] thousand **8** million **9** minim **10** minute **11** molal **12** molality **13** molar **14** molarity **15** mole **16** mucoid **17** muscle

m- *abbr* meta-

M \\'em\\ *n, pl* **M's** *or* **Ms** : an antigen of human blood that shares a common genetic locus with the N antigen

M *abbr* **1** [Latin *misce*] mix — used in writing prescriptions **2** mitosis — see M PHASE

mA *abbr* milliampere

MA *abbr* mental age

mac *abbr* macerate

MAC *abbr* **1** maximum allowable concentration **2** Mycobacterium avium complex

Ma·ca·ca \\mə-'käk-ə\\ *n* : a genus of Old World monkeys including the rhesus monkey (*M. mulatta*) and other macaques

ma·caque \\mə-'kak, -'käk\\ *n* : any of numerous short-tailed Old World monkeys of the genus *Macaca* and related genera chiefly of southern Asia; *esp* : RHESUS MONKEY

McArdle's disease, McBurney's point — see entries alphabetized as MC-

Mac·Con·key's agar *or* **Mac·Con·key agar** \\mə-'kän-kē(z)-\\ *n* : an agar culture medium containing bile salts and lactose that is used esp. to isolate coliform bacteria

  MacConkey, Alfred Theodore (1861–1931), British bacteriologist. MacConkey introduced the use of an agar culture medium for the isolation of coliform bacteria in 1900. He is also known for introducing a method for staining the capsules of pneumococcus and pneumobacillus.

Mace \\'mās\\ *trademark* — used for a temporarily disabling liquid that when sprayed in the face of a person causes tears, dizziness, immobilization, and sometimes nausea

¹mac·er·ate \\'mas-ə-ˌrāt\\ *vb* **-at·ed; -at·ing** *vt* : to soften (as tissue) by steeping or soaking so as to separate into constituent elements ~ *vi* : to undergo maceration ⟨allow the drug to ~ in hot water for one hour⟩

²**mac·er·ate** \'mas-ə-rət\ *n* : a product of macerating : something prepared by maceration ⟨examining the chromosomes in a liver ~⟩ — compare HOMOGENATE

macerated *adj, of a dead fetus* : having undergone reddening, loss of skin, and distortion of the features during retention in the uterus ⟨two years later a 10 inch ~ fetus . . . was delivered —*Jour. Amer. Med. Assoc.*⟩

mac·er·a·tion \ˌmas-ə-'rā-shən\ *n* **1** : an act or the process of macerating something; *esp* : the extraction of a drug by allowing it to stand in contact with a solvent **2** : the condition of being macerated ⟨the fetus was recovered in an advanced state of ~⟩

mac·er·a·tive \'mas-ə-ˌrāt-iv\ *adj* : characterized or accompanied by maceration ⟨~ degeneration of tissue⟩

Mach \'mäk\ *n* : a usu. high speed expressed by a Mach number ⟨an airplane flying at ~ 2⟩

Mach \'mäk\, **Ernst (1838–1916)**, Austrian physicist and philosopher. Mach established the basic principles of scientific positivism. In the 1870s he made classic studies on the perception of bodily rotation. Mach was also a pioneer in the study of supersonic projectiles and jets. In 1887 he described in a paper on projectiles in flight the angle between the axis of the projectile and the envelope of the waves produced. This angle forms the basis for the Mach number.

Ma·cha·do–Jo·seph disease \mə-ˌshä-dō-ˌjō-səf-, -ˌchä-, -dü-, -zəf-\ *n* : ataxia of any of several phenotypically variant forms that are inherited as autosomal dominant traits, have an onset early in adult life, tend to occur in families of Portuguese and esp. Azorean ancestry, and are characterized by progressive degeneration of the central nervous system

Ma·cha·do \mä-'shä-dü\ and **Jo·seph** \zhü-'zef\ **(***fl* **1970s)**, Azorean-Portuguese families. A hereditary form of ataxia was found in the Machado family of Massachusetts and described by K. K. Nakano *et al* in an article published in 1972. In that same year a variant form of the disease was found in the Joseph family of California and described in a separate article published by B. I. Woods and H. H. Schaumburg. The disease has been traced to Joseph Antone, a Portuguese seaman who emigrated from the Azores to California in 1845.

Mach number \'mäk-\ *n* : a number representing the ratio of the speed of a body to the speed of sound in a surrounding medium (as air) ⟨a *Mach number* of 2 indicates a speed that is twice that of sound⟩

Ma·chu·po virus \mä-'chü-pō-\ *n* : a single-stranded RNA virus of the genus *Arenavirus* (species *Machupo virus*) that causes a hemorrhagic fever endemic to Bolivia where its natural reservoir is a murid rodent (*Calomys callosus*)

mack·er·el shark \'mak-(ə-)rəl-\ *n* : any of a family (Lamnidae) of large aggressive pelagic sharks that include the great white shark

Mac·leod's syndrome \mə-'klaůdz-\ *n* : abnormally increased translucence of one lung usu. accompanied by reduction in ventilation and in perfusion with blood

Macleod, William Mathieson (1911–1977), British physician. Macleod was a specialist in pulmonology and thoracic medicine. He described the condition now known as Macleod's syndrome in an article published in 1954.

mac·ra·can·tho·rhyn·chi·a·sis \ˌmak-rə-ˌkan(t)-thə-riŋ-'kī-ə-səs\ *n, pl* **-a·ses** \-ˌsēz\ : infestation with or disease caused by an acanthocephalan worm of the genus *Macracanthorhynchus*

Mac·ra·can·tho·rhyn·chus \-'riŋ-kəs\ *n* : a genus of intestinal worms of the phylum or class Acanthocephala that include the common acanthocephalan (*M. hirudinaceus*) of swine

mac·ro \'mak-(ˌ)rō\ *adj* **1** : large, thick, or excessively developed ⟨~ layer of the cerebral cortex⟩ **2 a** : of or involving large quantities : intended for use with large quantities ⟨a ~ procedure in analysis⟩ ⟨carrying out a test on a ~ scale⟩ **b** : GROSS 1b ⟨the ~ appearance of a specimen⟩

mac·ro·ad·e·no·ma \ˌmak-rō-ˌad-ᵊn-'ō-mə\ *n, pl* **-mas** *also*

-ma·ta \-mət-ə\ : an adenoma of the pituitary gland that is greater than ten millimeters in diameter

mac·ro·ag·gre·gate \-'ag-ri-gət\ *n* : a relatively large particle (as of soil or a protein) — **mac·ro·ag·gre·gat·ed** \-ˌgāt-əd\ *adj*

mac·ro·al·bu·min·uria \-al-ˌbyü-mə-'n(y)ůr-ē-ə\ *n* : albuminuria characterized by a relatively high rate of urinary excretion of albumin typically greater than 300 milligrams per 24-hour period — compare MICROALBUMINURIA

mac·ro·anal·y·sis \-ə-'nal-ə-səs\ *n, pl* **-y·ses** \-ˌsēz\ : chemical analysis not on a small or minute scale : qualitative or quantitative analysis dealing with quantities usu. of the order of grams — compare MICROANALYSIS

mac·ro·an·gi·op·a·thy \-ˌan-jē-'äp-ə-thē\ *n, pl* **-thies** : an angiopathy affecting blood vessels of large and medium size

Mac·rob·del·la \ˌmak-ˌräb-'del-ə\ *n* : a genus of large active aquatic bloodsucking leeches including one (*M. decora*) that has been used medicinally in No. America

mac·ro·bi·ot·ic \ˌmak-rō-bī-'ät-ik, -bē-\ *adj* : of, relating to, or being a diet that consists of whole cereals and grains supplemented esp. with beans and vegetables and that in its esp. former more restrictive forms has been linked to nutritional deficiencies

macrobiotics *n pl but sing in constr* : a macrobiotic dietary system

mac·ro·blast \'mak-rə-ˌblast\ *n* **1** : MEGALOBLAST **2** : an erythroblast destined to produce macrocytes

mac·ro·ceph·a·lous \ˌmak-rō-'sef-ə-ləs\ *or* **mac·ro·ce·phal·ic** \-sə-'fal-ik\ *adj* : having or being an exceptionally large head or cranium

mac·ro·ceph·a·lus \-'sef-ə-ləs\ *n, pl* **-li** \-ˌlī\ : a macrocephalous person or skull

mac·ro·ceph·a·ly \-'sef-ə-lē\ *n, pl* **-lies** : the quality or state of being macrocephalous

mac·ro·chem·is·try \-'kem-ə-strē\ *n, pl* **-tries** : chemistry studied or applied without the use of the microscope or of microanalysis

mac·ro·co·nid·i·um \-kə-'nid-ē-əm\ *n, pl* **-ia** \-ē-ə\ : a large usu. multinucleate conidium of a fungus — compare MICROCONIDIUM

mac·ro·cra·ni·al \-'krā-nē-əl\ *adj* : having a large or long skull

mac·ro·cy·cle \'mak-rō-ˌsī-kəl\ *n* : a macrocyclic chemical ring

mac·ro·cy·clic \ˌmak-rō-'sik-lik, -'sī-klik\ *adj* : containing or being a chemical ring that consists usu. of 15 or more atoms ⟨a ~ antibiotic⟩ — **macrocyclic** *n*

mac·ro·cyst \'mak-rō-ˌsist\ *n* : a large cyst ⟨an approximately 5-cm ~ in the head of the pancreas was present —R. J. Churchill *et al*⟩ — compare MICROCYST

mac·ro·cyte \'mak-rə-ˌsīt\ *n* : an exceptionally large red blood cell occurring chiefly in anemias (as pernicious anemia) — called also *megalocyte*

mac·ro·cyt·ic \ˌmak-rə-'sit-ik\ *adj* : of or relating to macrocytes; *specif, of an anemia* : characterized by macrocytes in the blood ⟨pernicious anemia is a ~ anemia⟩

mac·ro·cy·to·sis \ˌmak-rə-sī-'tō-səs, -rə-sə-\ *n, pl* **-to·ses** \-ˌsēz\ : the occurrence of macrocytes in the blood

mac·ro·dont \'mak-rə-ˌdänt\ *adj* : having large teeth usu. with a dental index of over 44

mac·ro·fau·na \'mak-rō-ˌfȯn-ə, -ˌfän-\ *n* : animals large enough to be seen by the naked eye ⟨aquatic ~⟩ — compare MICROFAUNA — **mac·ro·fau·nal** \-ᵊl\ *adj*

mac·ro·flo·ra \-ˌflȯr-ə, -ˌflȯr-ə\ *n* : plants large enough to be seen by the naked eye ⟨the ~ of a sewage filtration bed⟩ — compare MICROFLORA — **mac·ro·flo·ral** \-əl\ *adj*

mac·ro·ga·mete \ˌmak-rō-gə-'mēt, -'gam-ˌēt\ *n* : the larger and usu. female gamete of a heterogamous organism — compare MICROGAMETE

\ə\ **abut** \ᵊ\ **kitten** \ər\ **further** \a\ **ash** \ā\ **ace** \ä\ **cot, cart** \aů\ **out** \ch\ **chin** \e\ **bet** \ē\ **easy** \g\ **go** \i\ **hit** \ī\ **ice** \j\ **job** \ŋ\ **sing** \ō\ **go** \ȯ\ **law** \ȯi\ **boy** \th\ **thin** \t͟h\ **the** \ü\ **loot** \ů\ **foot** \y\ **yet** \zh\ **vision** *See also* Pronunciation Symbols page

M
N

mac·ro·ga·me·to·cyte \-gə-'mēt-ə-ˌsīt\ *n* : a gametocyte producing macrogametes

mac·ro·gen·i·to·so·mia \ˌmak-rō-ˌjen-i-tə-'sō-mē-ə\ *n* : premature excessive development of the external genitalia

macrogenitosomia pre·cox *or* **macrogenitosomia prae·cox** \-'prē-ˌkäks\ *n* : MACROGENITOSOMIA

mac·ro·glia \ma-'kräg-lē-ə, ˌmak-rō-'glī-ə\ *n* : glia made up of astrocytes — **mac·ro·gli·al** \-əl\ *adj*

mac·ro·glob·u·lin \ˌmak-rō-'gläb-yə-lən\ *n* : a highly polymerized globulin (as IgM) of high molecular weight

mac·ro·glob·u·lin·emia *or chiefly Brit* **mac·ro·glob·u·lin·ae·mia** \-ˌgläb-yə-lə-'nē-mē-ə\ *n* : a disorder characterized by increased blood serum viscosity and the presence of macroglobulins in the serum — **mac·ro·glob·u·lin·emic** *or chiefly Brit* **mac·ro·glob·u·lin·ae·mic** \-mik\ *adj*

mac·ro·glos·sia \ˌmak-rō-'gläs-ē-ə, -'glós-\ *n* : pathological and commonly congenital enlargement of the tongue

mac·ro·lec·i·thal \-'les-i-thəl\ *adj* : MEGALECITHAL

mac·ro·lide \'mak-rə-ˌlīd\ *n* : any of several antibiotics (as erythromycin) containing a macrocyclic lactone ring that are produced by actinomycetes of the genus *Streptomyces* and inhibit bacterial protein synthesis

mac·ro·ma·nia \ˌmak-rō-'mā-nē-ə, -nyə\ *n* : a delusion that things (as parts of one's body) are larger than they really are — **mac·ro·ma·ni·a·cal** \-mə-'nī-ə-kəl\ *adj*

mac·ro·mas·tia \ˌmak-rō-'mas-tē-ə\ *n* : excessive development of the mammary glands

mac·ro·mere \'mak-rō-ˌmi(ə)r\ *n* : any of the large blastomeres that occur in the hemisphere of a telolecithal egg containing the vegetal pole and that are formed by unequal segmentation — compare MICROMERE

mac·ro·meth·od \-ˌmeth-əd\ *n* : a method (as of analysis) not involving the use of very small quantities of material — compare MICROMETHOD

mac·ro·mol·e·cule \ˌmak-rō-'mäl-i-ˌkyü(ə)l\ *n* : a very large molecule (as of a protein, nucleic acid, or rubber) built up from smaller chemical structures — compare MICROMOLECULE — **mac·ro·mo·lec·u·lar** \-mə-'lek-yə-lər\ *adj*

mac·ro·mu·tant \ˌmak-rō-'myüt-ənt\ *n* : an organism that has undergone macromutation

mac·ro·mu·ta·tion \-myü-'tā-shən\ *n* : complex mutation involving concurrent alteration of numerous characters

mac·ro·nod·u·lar \-'näj-ə-lər\ *adj* : characterized by large nodules ⟨~ cirrhosis⟩

mac·ro·nor·mo·blast \-'nòr-mə-ˌblast\ *n* : PRONORMOBLAST — **mac·ro·nor·mo·blas·tic** \-ˌnòr-mə-'blas-tik\ *adj*

mac·ro·nu·cle·us \ˌmak-rō-'n(y)ü-klē-əs\ *n, pl* **-clei** \-ˌī\ *also* **-cle·us·es** : a relatively large densely staining nucleus of most ciliate protozoans that is derived from micronuclei and controls various nonreproductive functions — compare MICRONUCLEUS — **mac·ro·nu·cle·ar** \ˌmak-rō-'n(y)ü-klē-ər\ *adj*

mac·ro·nu·tri·ent \-'n(y)ü-trē-ənt\ *n* : a chemical element or substance (as protein, carbohydrate, or fat) required in relatively large quantities in nutrition

mac·ro·or·chid·ism \-'òr-kə-ˌdiz-əm\ *n* : the condition (as in fragile X syndrome) of having large testicles

macro–osmatic *var of* MACROSMATIC

mac·ro·phage \'mak-rə-ˌfāj, -ˌfäzh\ *n* : a phagocytic tissue cell of the immune system that may be fixed or freely motile, is derived from a monocyte, functions in the destruction of foreign antigens (as bacteria and viruses), and serves as an antigen-presenting cell — see HISTIOCYTE, MONONUCLEAR PHAGOCYTE SYSTEM — **mac·ro·phag·ic** \ˌmak-rə-'faj-ik\ *adj*

macrophage colony–stimulating factor *n* : a colony=stimulating factor produced by macrophages, endothelial cells, and fibroblasts that stimulates production and maturation of macrophages — abbr. *M-CSF*

macrophagic system *n* : RETICULOENDOTHELIAL SYSTEM

mac·ro·pol·y·cyte \ˌmak-rō-'päl-i-ˌsīt\ *n* : an exceptionally large neutrophil with a much-lobulated nucleus that appears in the blood in pernicious anemia

mac·rop·sia \ma-'kräp-sē-ə\ *also* **mac·rop·sy** \'ma-ˌkräp-sē\ *n, pl* **-sias** *also* **-sies** : a condition of the eye in which objects appear to be unnaturally large — compare MICROPSIA

mac·rop·tic \ma-'kräp-tik\ *adj* : affected with macropsia

mac·ro·scop·ic \ˌmak-rə-'skäp-ik\ *adj* : large enough to be observed by the naked eye — compare MICROSCOPIC 2, SUBMICROSCOPIC, ULTRAMICROSCOPIC 1 — **mac·ro·scop·i·cal·ly** \-i-k(ə-)lē\ *adv*

mac·ro·sec·tion \'mak-rō-ˌsek-shən\ *n* : a tissue section prepared and mounted for inspection of the macroscopic structure of tissues and organs rather than microscopic examination ⟨~s of emphysematous lung⟩

mac·ros·mat·ic \ˌmak-ˌräz-'mat-ik\ *also* **mac·ro·os·mat·ic** \ˌmak-rō-ˌäz-\ *adj* : having the sense or organs of smell highly developed ⟨dogs are ~ animals⟩

mac·ro·so·mia \ˌmak-rə-'sō-mē-ə\ *n* : GIGANTISM — **mac·ro·so·mic** \-'sō-mik\ *adj*

mac·ro·splanch·nic \-'splaŋk-nik\ *adj* : ENDOMORPHIC

mac·ro·spore \'mak-rō-ˌspōr\ *n* : the larger of two forms of spores produced by certain protozoans (as radiolarians) — called also *megaspore;* compare MICROSPORE 2

mac·ro·sto·mia \ˌmak-rə-'stō-mē-ə\ *n* **1** : the condition of having an abnormally large mouth **2** : an abnormally large mouth

mac·ro·struc·ture \'mak-rō-ˌstrək-chər\ *n* : the structure (as of a body part) revealed by visual examination with little or no magnification — **mac·ro·struc·tur·al** \ˌmak-rō-'strək-chə-rəl, -'strək-shə-rəl\ *adj*

mac·ro·tia \mak-'rō-sh(ē-)ə\ *n* : excessive largeness of the ears

mac·ro·tome \'mak-rə-ˌtōm\ *n* : an apparatus for making large sections of anatomical specimens

mac·u·la \'mak-yə-lə\ *n, pl* **-lae** \-ˌlē, -ˌlī\ *also* **-las** **1** : any spot or blotch; *esp* : MACULE 2 **2** : an anatomical structure having the form of a spot differentiated from surrounding tissues: as **a** : MACULA ACUSTICA **b** : MACULA LUTEA

macula acu·sti·ca \-ə-'küs-ti-kə\ *n, pl* **maculae acu·sti·cae** \-ti-ˌsē\ : either of two small areas of sensory hair cells in the ear that are covered with gelatinous material on which are located crystals or concretions of calcium carbonate and that are associated with the perception of equilibrium: **a** : one located in the saccule — called also *macula sacculi* **b** : one located in the utricle — called also *macula utriculi*

macula den·sa \-'den-sə\ *n* : a group of modified epithelial cells in the distal convoluted tubule of the kidney that lie adjacent to the afferent arteriole just before it enters the glomerulus and control renin release by relaying information about the sodium concentration in the fluid passing through the convoluted tubule to the renin-producing juxtaglomerular cells of the afferent arteriole

macula lu·tea \-'lüt-ē-ə\ *n, pl* **maculae lu·te·ae** \-ē-ˌē, -ē-ˌī\ : a small yellowish area lying slightly lateral to the center of the retina that constitutes the region of maximum visual acuity and is made up almost wholly of retinal cones — called also *yellow spot*

mac·u·lar \'mak-yə-lər\ *adj* **1** : of, relating to, or characterized by a spot or spots ⟨a ~ skin rash⟩ **2** : of, relating to, affecting, or mediated by the macula lutea ⟨~ vision⟩ ⟨the ~ area of the retina⟩

macular degeneration *n* : progressive deterioration of the macula lutea resulting in a gradual loss of the central part of the field of vision; *esp* : AGE-RELATED MACULAR DEGENERATION

macula sac·cu·li \-'sak-yə-ˌlī\ *n* : MACULA ACUSTICA a

mac·u·late \'mak-yə-lət\ *adj* : marked with spots

mac·u·la·tion \ˌmak-yə-'lā-shən\ *n* **1** : a blemish in the form of a discrete spot ⟨acne scars and ~s⟩ **2** : the arrangement of spots and markings on an animal or plant

macula utri·cu·li \-yü-'trik-yə-ˌlī\ *n* : MACULA ACUSTICA b

mac·ule \'mak-(ˌ)yü(ə)l\ *n* **1** : MACULA 2 **2** : a patch of skin that is altered in color but usu. not elevated and that is a characteristic feature of various diseases (as smallpox)

mac·u·lo·pap·u·lar \ˌmak-yə-(ˌ)lō-'pap-yə-lər\ *adj* : combining the characteristics of macules and papules ⟨a ~ rash⟩

mac·u·lo·pap·ule \-ˈpap-(ˌ)yü(ə)l\ *n* : a maculopapular elevation of the skin

mac·u·lop·a·thy \ˌmak-yə-ˈläp-ə-thē\ *n*, *pl* **-thies** : any pathological condition of the macula lutea of the eye

mad \ˈmad\ *adj* **mad·der; mad·dest** **1** : arising from, indicative of, or marked by mental disorder **2** : affected with rabies : RABID

Mad·a·gas·car periwinkle \ˌmad-ə-ˈgas-kər-, -ˌkär-\ *n* : ROSY PERIWINKLE

mad·a·ro·sis \ˌmad-ə-ˈrō-səs\ *n*, *pl* **-ro·ses** \-ˌsēz\ : loss of the eyelashes or of the hair of the eyebrows — **mad·a·rot·ic** \-ˈrät-ik\ *adj*

mad cow disease \-ˈkaü-\ *n* : BOVINE SPONGIFORM ENCEPHALOPATHY

mad·der \ˈmad-ər\ *n* **1** : a Eurasian herb (*Rubia tinctorum* of the family Rubiaceae, the madder family) with whorled leaves, clusters of small yellowish flowers, and red to black berries; *broadly* : any of several related herbs (genus *Rubia*) **2** : the root of the Eurasian madder formerly used in dyeing; *also* : an alizarin dye prepared from it

mad–doctor \ˈmad-ˌ\ *n* : PSYCHIATRIST

Mad·dox rod \ˈmad-əks-ˌräd\ *n* : a transparent cylindrical glass rod or one of a series of such rods placed one above another for use in testing the eyes for heterophoria

   Maddox, Ernest Edmund (1860–1933), British ophthalmologist. Maddox did research on refraction, ocular muscles, and the relation between accommodation and convergence. In 1898 he devised an instrument, consisting of parallel cylindrical glass rods (now called Maddox rods), for testing and measuring the degree of heterophoria.

mad itch *n* : PSEUDORABIES

mad·man \ˈmad-ˌman, -mən\ *n* : a man who is or acts as if insane

mad·ness \ˈmad-nəs\ *n* **1** : INSANITY **2** : any of several ailments of animals marked by frenzied behavior; *specif* : RABIES

mad·stone \ˈmad-ˌstōn\ *n* : a stony concretion (as a hair ball taken from the stomach of a deer) supposed formerly in folklore and by some physicians to counteract the poisonous effects of the bite of an animal (as one affected with rabies)

Ma·du·ra foot \ˈmad-(y)ə-rə-, mə-ˈd(y)ür-ə-\ *n* : maduromycosis of the foot

mad·u·ro·my·co·sis \ˈmad-(y)ə-rō-mī-ˈkō-səs\ *n*, *pl* **-co·ses** \-ˌsēz\ : a destructive chronic disease usu. restricted to the feet, marked by swelling and deformity resulting from the formation of granulomatous nodules drained by sinuses connecting with the exterior, and caused by various actinomycetes (as of the genus *Nocardia*) and fungi (as of the genus *Madurella*) — called also *mycetoma;* see MADURA FOOT; compare NOCARDIOSIS — **mad·u·ro·my·cot·ic** \-ˈkät-ik\ *adj*

mad·wom·an \ˈmad-ˌwùm-ən\ *n* : a woman who is or acts as if insane

mae·di \ˈmī-(ˌ)thē\ *n* : ovine progressive pneumonia esp. as manifested by respiratory symptoms — compare VISNA

maf·e·nide \ˈmaf-ə-ˌnīd\ *n* : a sulfonamide applied topically in the form of its acetate $C_7H_{10}N_2O_2S \cdot C_2H_4O_2$ as an antibacterial ointment esp. in the treatment of burns — see SULFAMYLON

ma·ga·i·nin \mə-ˈgā-ə-nən, -ˈgā-nən\ *n* : any of a group of peptide antibiotics isolated from the skin of frogs esp. of the genus *Xenopus*

ma·gen·stras·se \ˈmä-gən-ˌs(h)trä-sə\ *n* : a groove in the stomach along the lesser curvature that is the route food and liquids tend to take in moving toward the pylorus and that is a frequent site of peptic ulcer formation

ma·gen·ta \mə-ˈjent-ə\ *n* : FUCHSIN

mag·got \ˈmag-ət\ *n* : a soft-bodied legless grub that is the larva of a dipteran fly (as the housefly) and develops usu. in decaying organic matter or as a parasite in plants or animals

maggot therapy *n* : treatment of infected wounds and draining sinuses (as in osteomyelitis) formerly applied by means of maggots that excrete allantoin

mag·ic bul·let \ˈmaj-ik-ˈbùl-ət\ *n* : a substance or therapy capable of destroying pathogenic agents (as bacteria or cancer cells) or providing a remedy for a disease or condition without deleterious side effects

magic mushroom *n* : any fungus containing hallucinogenic alkaloids (as psilocybin)

ma·gis·tral \ˈmaj-ə-strəl, mə-ˈjis-trəl\ *adj* : concocted or prescribed by a physician to meet the needs of a particular case — compare OFFICINAL

mag·ma \ˈmag-mə\ *n* **1** : a crude mixture of mineral or organic matter in the state of a thin paste **2** : a suspension of a large amount of precipitated material (as in milk of magnesia) in a small volume of a watery vehicle

magna — see CISTERNA MAGNA, THERAPIA STERILISANS MAGNA

Mag·na·my·cin \ˌmag-nə-ˈmīs-ᵊn\ *n* : a preparation of carbomycin — formerly a U.S. registered trademark

mag·ne·sia \mag-ˈnē-shə, -ˈnē-zhə\ *n* : MAGNESIUM OXIDE

magnesia magma *n* : MILK OF MAGNESIA

mag·ne·sium \mag-ˈnē-zē-əm, -zhəm\ *n* : a silver-white light malleable ductile metallic element that occurs abundantly in nature (as in bones and seeds and in the form of chlorophyll in the green parts of plants) and is used in metallurgical and chemical processes, in photography, in signaling, and in the manufacture of pyrotechnics because of the intense white light it produces on burning, and in construction esp. in the form of light alloys — symbol *Mg*; see ELEMENT table

magnesium carbonate *n* : a carbonate of magnesium; *esp* : the very white crystalline normal salt $MgCO_3$ that occurs naturally, is prepared artificially by precipitation, and is used chiefly in paint and printing ink, as a filler, as an addition to table salt to prevent caking, and in medicine as an antacid and laxative

magnesium chloride *n* : a bitter crystalline salt $MgCl_2$ used esp. to replenish body electrolytes

magnesium citrate *n* : a crystalline salt used in the form of a lemony acidulous effervescent solution as a saline laxative

magnesium hydroxide *n* : a slightly alkaline crystalline compound $Mg(OH)_2$ that is obtained by hydration of magnesia or by precipitation (as from seawater by lime in the production of magnesium chloride) as a white nearly insoluble powder and is used chiefly in medicine as an antacid and laxative — see MILK OF MAGNESIA

magnesium oxide *n* : a white highly infusible compound MgO used esp. in refractories, cements, insulation, and fertilizers, in rubber manufacture, and in medicine as an antacid and mild laxative

magnesium silicate *n* : a silicate that is approximately $Mg_2Si_3O_8 \cdot nH_2O$, is obtained by precipitation as a white powder, and is used chiefly in medicine as a gastric antacid adsorbent and coating (as in the treatment of ulcers)

magnesium sulfate *n* : a white anhydrous salt $MgSO_4$ that occurs naturally in hydrated form as Epsom salts and that in the hydrated form $MgSO_4 \cdot 7H_2O$ is administered orally to relieve constipation or by injection to treat magnesium deficiency, to control convulsions associated with eclampsia, and to treat symptoms (as hypertension and convulsions) associated with nephritis in children

mag·net \ˈmag-nət\ *n* : a body having the property of attracting iron and producing a magnetic field external to itself; *specif* : a mass of iron, steel, or alloy that has this property artificially imparted

¹mag·net·ic \mag-ˈnet-ik\ *adj* **1** : of or relating to a magnet or to magnetism **2** : of, relating to, or characterized by the earth's magnetism **3** : magnetized or capable of being magnetized **4** : actuated by magnetic attraction — **mag·net·i·cal·ly** \-i-k(ə-)lē\ *adv*

²magnetic *n* : a magnetic substance

magnetic field *n* : the portion of space near a magnetic body or a current-carrying body in which the magnetic forces due

M
N

\ə\ **abut** \ᵊ\ **kitten** \ər\ **further** \a\ **ash** \ā\ **ace** \ä\ **cot, cart** \aú\ **out** \ch\ **chin** \e\ **bet** \ē\ **easy** \g\ **go** \i\ **hit** \ī\ **ice** \j\ **job** \ŋ\ **sing** \ō\ **go** \ò\ **law** \òi\ **boy** \th\ **thin** \t̲h̲\ **the** \ü\ **loot** \ù\ **foot** \y\ **yet** \zh\ **vision** *See also* Pronunciation Symbols page

to the body or current can be detected ⟨the *magnetic field* of the heart⟩

magnetic mo·ment \-'mō-mənt\ *n* : a vector quantity that is a measure of the torque exerted on a magnetic system (as a bar magnet or dipole) when placed in a magnetic field and that for a magnet is the product of the distance between its poles and the strength of either pole

magnetic resonance *n* : the absorption of energy exhibited by particles (as atomic nuclei or electrons) in a static magnetic field when the particles are exposed to electromagnetic radiation of certain frequencies — abbr. *MR*; see NUCLEAR MAGNETIC RESONANCE

magnetic resonance angiography *n* : magnetic resonance imaging used to visualize noninvasively the heart, blood vessels, or blood flow in the circulatory system — abbr. *MRA;* called also *MR angiography*

magnetic resonance imaging *n* : a noninvasive diagnostic technique that produces computerized images of internal body tissues and is based on nuclear magnetic resonance of atoms within the body induced by the application of radio waves — called also *MRI*

magnetic resonance spectroscopy *n* : a noninvasive technique that is similar to magnetic resonance imaging but uses a stronger field and is used to monitor body chemistry (as in metabolism or blood flow) rather than anatomical structures — abbr. *MRS*

mag·ne·tism \'mag-nə-ˌtiz-əm\ *n* : a class of physical phenomena that include the attraction for iron observed in lodestone and a magnet, are inseparably associated with moving electricity, are exhibited by both magnets and electric currents, and are characterized by fields of force

mag·ne·ti·za·tion *also Brit* **mag·ne·ti·sa·tion** \ˌmag-nət-ə-'zā-shən\ *n* : an instance of magnetizing or the state of being magnetized; *also* : the degree to which a body is magnetized

mag·ne·tize *also Brit* **mag·ne·tise** \'mag-nə-ˌtīz\ *vt* **-tized** *also Brit* **-tised; -tiz·ing** *also Brit* **-tis·ing** : to induce magnetic properties in — **mag·ne·tiz·able** *also Brit* **mag·ne·tis·able** \-ˌtī-zə-bəl\ *adj*

mag·ne·to·car·dio·gram \mag-ˌnēt-ō-'kärd-ē-ə-ˌgram, -ˌnet-\ *n* : a recording of a magnetocardiograph

mag·ne·to·car·dio·graph \-'kärd-ē-ə-ˌgraf\ *n* : an instrument for recording the changes in the magnetic field around the heart that is used to supplement information given by an electrocardiograph — **mag·ne·to·car·dio·graph·ic** \-ˌkärd-ē-ə-'graf-ik\ *adj* — **mag·ne·to·car·di·og·ra·phy** \-ˌkärd-ē-'äg-rə-fē\ *n, pl* **-phies**

mag·ne·to·en·ceph·a·lo·gram \mag-ˌnēt-ō-in-'sef-ə-lə-ˌgram, -ˌnet-\ *n* : a record made by magnetoencephalography

mag·ne·to·en·ceph·a·log·ra·phy \-in-ˌsef-ə-'läg-rə-fē\ *n, pl* **-phies** : a noninvasive technique that detects and records the magnetic field associated with electrical activity in the brain

mag·ne·tom·e·ter \ˌmag-nə-'täm-ət-ər\ *n* : an instrument used to detect the presence of a metallic object or to measure the intensity of a magnetic field — **mag·ne·to·met·ric** \ˌmag-ˌnēt-ə-'me-trik, -ˌnet-\ *adj* — **mag·ne·tom·e·try** \ˌmag-nə-'täm-ə-trē\ *n, pl* **-tries**

mag·ne·ton \'mag-nə-ˌtän\ *n* : a unit of measurement of the magnetic moment of a particle (as an atom or atomic nucleus) that is equal to 0.927×10^{-20} ergs per oersted for atoms and 0.505×10^{-23} ergs per oersted for atomic nuclei

mag·ne·to·tac·tic \ˌmag-ˌnēt-ō-'tak-tik\ *adj* : exhibiting movement in response to a magnetic field ⟨~ bacteria⟩

mag·ne·to·tax·is \-'tak-səs\ *n, pl* **-tax·es** \-ˌsēz\ : a taxis in which a magnetic field is the directive factor

mag·ne·tron \'mag-nə-ˌträn\ *n* : a diode vacuum tube in which the flow of electrons is controlled by an externally applied magnetic field to generate power at microwave frequencies

mag·ni·fi·ca·tion \ˌmag-nə-fə-'kā-shən\ *n* **1** : the act of magnifying **2 a** : the state of being magnified **b** : the apparent enlargement of an object by an optical instrument that is the ratio of the dimensions of an image formed by the

instrument to the corresponding dimensions of the object — called also *power*

mag·ni·fy \'mag-nə-ˌfī\ *vb* **-fied; -fy·ing** *vt* : to enlarge in appearance ~ *vi* : to have the power of causing objects to appear larger than they are

mag·ni·tude \'mag-nə-ˌt(y)üd\ *n* : relative size or extent

mag·no·cel·lu·lar \ˌmag-nō-'sel-yə-lər\ *adj* : being or containing neurons with large cell bodies ⟨motion and depth perception processed by the ~ visual pathway⟩ — compare PARVOCELLULAR

mag·no·lia \mag-'nōl-yə\ *n* **1** *cap* : a genus (family Magnoliaceae, the magnolia family) of No. American and Asian shrubs and trees including some whose bark has been used esp. as a bitter tonic and diaphoretic in folk medicine **2 a** : any shrub or tree of the genus *Magnolia* **b** : the dried bark of a magnolia

magnum — see FORAMEN MAGNUM

magnus — see ADDUCTOR MAGNUS, SERRATUS MAGNUS

ma·ho·nia \mə-'hō-nē-ə\ *n* **1** *cap* : a genus of No. American and Asian shrubs (family Berberidaceae) that have unarmed branches and pinnate leaves and are sometimes included in the genus *Berberis* **2** : any shrub of the genus *Mahonia*

ma huang \'mä-'hwäng\ *n* : any of several Chinese plants of the genus *Ephedra* (esp. *E. sinica*) yielding ephedrine; *also* : a preparation of the young canes or rhizome and roots of ma huang used in herbal medicine for its ephedrine content

maid·en·hair \'mād-ᵊn-ˌha(ə)r, -ˌhe(ə)r\ *n* : any of the genus *Adiantum* of ferns including two No. American forms (*A. pedatum* and the Venushair, *A. capillus-veneris*) that have been used in the preparation of expectorants and demulcents — called also *maidenhair fern*

maid·en·head \'mād-ᵊn-ˌhed\ *n* : HYMEN

Mail·lard reaction \mə-'lärd-, -'yär-\ *n* : a nonenzymatic reaction between sugars and proteins that occurs upon heating and that produces browning of some foods (as meat and bread)

Mail·lard \må-yår\, **Louis Camille (1878–1936),** French biochemist. Maillard first observed the reaction that now bears his name in 1912.

maim \'mām\ *vt* **1** : to commit the felony of mayhem upon **2** : to wound seriously : MUTILATE, DISABLE

main·line \'mān-'līn\ *vb* **-lined; -lin·ing** *vt, slang* : to take by or as if by injecting into a principal vein ~ *vi, slang* : to mainline a narcotic drug (as heroin)

main line *n, slang* : a principal vein of the circulatory system

main·stream \ˌmān-ˌstrēm\ *adj* : relating to or being tobacco smoke that is drawn (as from a cigarette) directly into the mouth of the smoker and is usu. inhaled into the lungs — compare SIDESTREAM

main·te·nance \'mānt-nən(t)s, -ᵊn-ən(t)s\ *adj* : designed or adequate to maintain a patient in a stable condition : serving to maintain a gradual process of healing or to prevent a relapse ⟨a ~ dose⟩ ⟨~ chemotherapy⟩

maize oil \'māz-\ *n* : CORN OIL

ma·joon \mə-'jün\ *n* : an East Indian narcotic confection that is made of hemp leaves, henbane, datura seeds, poppy seeds, honey, and ghee and that produces effects like those of hashish and opium

ma·jor \'mā-jər\ *adj* : involving grave risk : SERIOUS ⟨a ~ illness⟩ ⟨a ~ surgical procedure⟩ — compare MINOR

majora — see LABIA MAJORA

major basic protein *n* : a toxic cationic protein that is the principal protein found in the granules of eosinophils and that is capable of damaging tissue (as of the eye) if released into extracellular spaces — abbr. *MBP*

major depression *n* : an episode of depression characteristic of major depressive disorder; *also* : MAJOR DEPRESSIVE DISORDER

¹major depressive *adj* : of, relating to, or affected with major depressive disorder ⟨a *major depressive* episode⟩ ⟨*major depressive* patients⟩

²major depressive *n* : an individual affected with or subject to episodes of major depressive disorder

major depressive disorder *n* : a mood disorder having a clinical course involving one or more episodes of serious psychological depression that last two or more weeks each, do not have intervening episodes of mania or hypomania, and are characterized by a loss of interest or pleasure in almost all activities and by some or all of disturbances of appetite, sleep, or psychomotor functioning, a decrease in energy, difficulties in thinking or making decisions, loss of self-esteem or feelings of guilt, and suicidal thoughts or attempts — compare BIPOLAR DISORDER

major histocompatibility complex *n* : a group of genes in mammals that function esp. in determining the histocompatibility antigens found on cell surfaces and that in humans comprise the alleles occurring at four loci on the short arm of chromosome 6 — abbr. *MHC*

major labia *n pl* : LABIA MAJORA

major–medical *adj* : of, relating to, or being a form of insurance designed to pay all or part of the medical bills of major illnesses usu. after deduction of a fixed initial sum

major surgery *n* : surgery involving a risk to the life of the patient; *specif* : an operation upon an organ within the cranium, chest, abdomen, or pelvic cavity — compare MINOR SURGERY

mal \'mäl, 'mal\ *n* : DISEASE, SICKNESS

mal·ab·sorp·tion \ˌmal-əb-'sorp-shən, -'zorp-\ *n* : faulty absorption of nutrient materials from the alimentary canal — called also *malassimilation* — **mal·ab·sorp·tive** \-tiv\ *adj*

malabsorption syndrome *n* : a syndrome resulting from malabsorption that is typically characterized by weakness, diarrhea, muscle cramps, edema, and loss of weight

malachite green *n* : a triphenylmethane basic dye used as a biological stain and as an antiseptic

ma·la·cia \mə-'lā-sh(ē-)ə\ *n* : abnormal softening of a tissue — often used in combination ⟨osteo*malacia*⟩ — **ma·la·cic** \-sik\ *adj*

mal·a·co·pla·kia *also* **mal·a·ko·pla·kia** \ˌmal-ə-kō-'plā-kē-ə\ *n* : inflammation of the mucous membrane of a hollow organ (as the urinary bladder) characterized by the formation of soft granulomatous lesions

mal·a·cot·ic \ˌmal-ə-'kät-ik\ *adj, of a tooth* : exhibiting malacia : being soft

mal·ad·ap·ta·tion \ˌmal-ˌad-ˌap-'tā-shən\ *n* : poor or inadequate adaptation ⟨psychological ∼⟩ — **mal·adap·tive** \ˌmal-ə-'dap-tiv\ *adj* — **mal·adap·tive·ly** *adv*

mal·a·die de Ro·ger \ˌmal-ə-'dē-də-rō-'zhā\ *n* : a small usu. asymptomatic defect in the septum between the ventricles

Ro·ger \rò-zhā\, **Henri–Louis (1809–1891),** French physician. Roger made his principal contribution in pediatrics and was the first to give systematic clinical instruction in this field. His early research centered on auscultation, a subject on which he wrote a monograph. In 1879 he described an abnormal congenital opening between the ventricles of the heart; this congenital defect is now known as the maladie de Roger. He was not the first to describe this defect, but he was the first to make clinicopathologic observations based on a number of cases.

mal·ad·just·ment \ˌmal-ə-'jəs(t)-mənt\ *n* : poor, faulty, or inadequate adjustment; *esp* : failure to reach a satisfactory adjustment between one's desires and the conditions of one's life ⟨emotional ∼s⟩ ⟨symptoms of ∼ . . . in early childhood —*Psychological Abstracts*⟩ — **mal·ad·just·ed** \-əd\ *adj* — **mal·ad·jus·tive** \-iv\ *adj*

mal·ad·min·is·tra·tion \ˌmal-əd-ˌmin-ə-'strā-shən\ *n* : incorrect administration (as of a drug)

mal·a·dy \'mal-əd-ē\ *n, pl* **-dies** : DISEASE, SICKNESS ⟨a fatal ∼⟩

mal·aise \mə-'lāz, ma-, -'lez\ *n* : an indefinite feeling of debility or lack of health often indicative of or accompanying the onset of an illness ⟨fever, ∼, and other flulike symptoms —Larry Thompson⟩

malakoplakia *var of* MALACOPLAKIA

mal·align·ment \ˌmal-ə-'līn-mənt\ *n* : incorrect or imperfect alignment (as of teeth) — **mal·aligned** \-'līnd\ *adj*

ma·lar \'mā-lər, -ˌlär\ *adj* : of or relating to the cheek, the side of the head, or the zygomatic bone

malar bone *n* : ZYGOMATIC BONE — called also *malar*

ma·lar·ia \mə-'ler-ē-ə\ *n* **1** : an acute or chronic disease caused by the presence of sporozoan parasites of the genus *Plasmodium* in the red blood cells, transmitted from an infected to an uninfected individual by the bite of anopheline mosquitoes, and characterized by periodic attacks of chills and fever that coincide with mass destruction of blood cells and the release of toxic substances by the parasite at the end of each reproductive cycle ⟨∼ remains the greatest single cause of debilitation and death throughout the world —*Jour. Amer. Med. Assoc.*⟩ — see FALCIPARUM MALARIA, VIVAX MALARIA **2** : any of various diseases of birds and mammals that are more or less similar to malaria of human beings and are caused by blood protozoans

ma·lar·i·ae malaria \mə-'ler-ē-(ˌ)ē-\ *n* : malaria caused by a malaria parasite (*Plasmodium malariae*) and marked by recurrence of paroxysms at 72-hour intervals — called also *quartan malaria*

¹ma·lar·i·al \mə-'ler-ē-əl\ *adj* : of, relating to, or infected by malaria ⟨a ∼ region⟩

²malarial *n* : an individual who is infected with malaria

malarial cachexia *n* : a generalized state of debility that is marked by anemia, jaundice, splenomegaly, and emaciation and results from long-continued chronic malarial infection

malarial fever *n* : MALARIA 1

malarial mosquito *or* **malaria mosquito** *n* : a mosquito of the genus *Anopheles* (esp. *A. quadrimaculatus*) that transmits the malaria parasite

malaria parasite *n* : a protozoan of the sporozoan genus *Plasmodium* that is transmitted to humans or to certain other mammals or birds by the bite of a mosquito in which its sexual reproduction takes place, that multiplies asexually in the vertebrate host by schizogony in the red blood cells or in certain tissue cells, and that causes destruction of red blood cells and the febrile disease malaria or produces gametocytes by sporogony which if taken up by a suitable mosquito initiate a new sexual cycle — see MEROZOITE, OOKINETE, PHANEROZOITE, SCHIZONT, SPOROZOITE

ma·lar·i·ol·o·gist \mə-ˌler-ē-'äl-ə-jəst\ *n* : a specialist in the study, treatment, or prevention of malaria

ma·lar·i·ol·o·gy \-'äl-ə-jē\ *n, pl* **-gies** : the scientific study of malaria — **ma·lar·i·o·log·i·cal** \mə-ˌler-ē-ə-'läj-i-kəl\ *adj*

ma·lar·i·om·e·try \-'äm-ə-trē\ *n, pl* **-tries** : the determination of the endemic level of malarial infection in an area or a population — **ma·lar·i·o·met·ric** \mə-ˌler-ē-ə-'me-trik\ *adj*

ma·lar·io·ther·a·py \mə-ˌler-ē-ō-'ther-ə-pē\ *n, pl* **-pies** : the treatment of disease by raising the body temperature through infecting the patient with malaria

ma·lar·i·ous \mə-'ler-ē-əs\ *adj* : characterized by the presence of or infected with malaria ⟨∼ regions⟩ ⟨a ∼ patient⟩

Mal·as·se·zia \ˌmal-ə-'sā-zē-ə\ *n* : a genus of lipophilic typically nonpathogenic yeastlike imperfect fungi including one (*M. furfur* syn. *Pityrosporum oribiculare*) that causes tinea versicolor and another (*M. ovalis* syn. *Pityrosporum ovale*) that is associated with seborrheic dermatitis

mal·as·sim·i·la·tion \ˌmal-ə-ˌsim-ə-'lā-shən\ *n* : MALABSORPTION

ma·late \'mal-ˌāt, 'mā-ˌlāt\ *n* : a salt or ester of malic acid

malate dehydrogenase *n* : an enzyme that catalyzes reversibly the oxidation of malate in the presence of NAD — called also *malic enzyme*

mal·a·thi·on \ˌmal-ə-'thī-ən, -ˌän\ *n* : a thiophosphate insecticide $C_{10}H_{19}O_6PS_2$ with a lower mammalian toxicity than parathion

mal de ca·de·ras \ˌmal-də-kə-'der-əs\ *n* : an infectious disease of horses in So. America caused by a protozoan parasite of the genus *Trypanosoma* (*T. equinum*) in the blood and characterized by rapid emaciation, anemia, blood-colored urine, paresis, and edema — called also *derrengadera*

M
N

\ə\ abut \ᵊ\ kitten \ər\ further \a\ ash \ā\ ace \ä\ cot, cart
\aù\ out \ch\ chin \e\ bet \ē\ easy \g\ go \i\ hit \ī\ ice \j\ job
\ŋ\ sing \ō\ go \ò\ law \òi\ boy \th\ thin \t̲h̲\ the \ü\ loot
\ù\ foot \y\ yet \zh\ vision *See also* Pronunciation Symbols page

mal del pin·to \-del-'pin-tō\ *n* : PINTA

mal de mer \ˌmal-də-'me(ə)r\ *n* : SEASICKNESS

mal·des·cent \ˌmal-di-'sent\ *n* : an improper or incomplete descent of a testis into the scrotum — **mal·des·cend·ed** \-'send-əd\ *adj*

mal·de·vel·op·ment \ˌmal-di-'vel-əp-mənt\ *n* : abnormal growth or development : DYSPLASIA

mal·di·ges·tion \-di-'jes(h)-chən, -dī-\ *n* : imperfect or impaired digestion

¹**male** \'mā(ə)l\ *n* : an individual that produces small usu. motile gametes (as sperm or spermatozoa) which fertilize the eggs of a female

²**male** *adj* **1** : of, relating to, or being the sex that produces gametes which fertilize the eggs of female **2** : designed for fitting into a corresponding hollow part

ma·le·ate \'mā-lē-ˌāt, -lē-ət\ *n* : a salt or ester of maleic acid

male bond·ing \-'bänd-iŋ\ *n* : bonding between males through shared activities excluding females

male climacteric *n* : ANDROPAUSE

male fern *n* : a fern (*Dryopteris filix-mas*) of Europe and No. America producing an oleoresin that is used in expelling tapeworms — see ASPIDIUM

ma·le·ic acid \mə-ˌlē-ik-, -ˌlā-\ *n* : a crystalline dicarboxylic acid $C_4H_4O_4$ that is isomeric with fumaric acid and is used esp. in organic synthesis

male menopause *n* : ANDROPAUSE

male–pattern baldness *n* : androgenetic alopecia in the male characterized by loss of hair on the crown and temples

male pronucleus *n* : the nucleus that remains in a male gamete after the meiotic reduction division and that contains only one half of the number of chromosomes characteristic of its species — compare FEMALE PRONUCLEUS

mal·for·ma·tion \ˌmal-fȯr-'mā-shən, -fər-\ *n* : irregular, anomalous, abnormal, or faulty formation or structure ⟨congenital ~s⟩

mal·formed \(')mal-'fȯ(ə)rmd\ *adj* : characterized by malformation : badly or imperfectly formed ⟨a ~ limb⟩

mal·func·tion \(')mal-'fəŋ(k)-shən\ *vi* : to function imperfectly or badly : fail to operate in the normal or usual manner ⟨~ing kidneys⟩ — **malfunction** *n*

ma·lic \'mal-ik, 'mā-lik\ *adj* : involved in and esp. catalyzing a reaction in which malic acid participates ⟨~ dehydrogenase⟩

malic acid *n* : any of three optical isomers of a crystalline dicarboxylic acid $C_4H_6O_5$; *esp* : the one found in various plant juices and formed as an intermediate in the Krebs cycle

malic enzyme *n* : MALATE DEHYDROGENASE

maligna — see LENTIGO MALIGNA

ma·lig·nan·cy \mə-'lig-nən-sē\ *n, pl* **-cies** **1** : the quality or state of being malignant **2 a** : exhibition (as by a tumor) of malignant qualities : VIRULENCE **b** : a malignant tumor

ma·lig·nant \mə-'lig-nənt\ *adj* **1** : tending to produce death or deterioration ⟨~ malaria⟩; *esp* : tending to infiltrate, metastasize, and terminate fatally ⟨~ tumors⟩ — compare BENIGN 1 **2** : of unfavorable prognosis : not responding favorably to treatment ⟨psychotic reactions with a ~ trend⟩

malignant catarrhal fever *n* : an acute infectious often fatal disease of cattle, some other bovines, and deer that is caused by any of several herpesviruses (genus *Rhadinovirus*) and is characterized by fever, depression, enlarged lymph nodes, discharge from the eyes and nose, and lesions affecting most organ systems — called also *catarrhal fever, malignant catarrh*

malignant edema *n* : an acute often fatal toxemia of wild and domestic animals that follows wound infection by an anaerobic toxin-producing bacterium of the genus *Clostridium* (*C. septicum*) and is characterized by anorexia, intoxication, fever, and soft fluid-filled swellings — compare BLACK DISEASE, BLACKLEG; BRAXY 1

malignant hypertension *n* : essential hypertension characterized by acute onset, severe symptoms, rapidly progressive course, and poor prognosis

malignant hyperthermia *n* : a rare inherited condition characterized by a rapid, extreme, and often fatal rise in body temperature following the administration of general anesthesia

malignant jaundice *n* : ACUTE YELLOW ATROPHY

malignant malaria *n* : FALCIPARUM MALARIA

malignant malnutrition *n* : KWASHIORKOR

malignant melanoma *n* : MELANOMA 2

malignant neutropenia *n* : AGRANULOCYTOSIS

malignant pustule *n* : localized anthrax of the skin taking the form of a pimple surrounded by a zone of edema and hyperemia and tending to become necrotic and ulcerated

malignant tertian malaria *n* : FALCIPARUM MALARIA

malignant transformation *n* : the transformation that a cell undergoes to become a rapidly dividing tumor-producing cell; *also* : the transformation of a mass of cells or a tissue into a rapidly growing tumor ⟨*malignant transformation* of certain warts⟩

ma·lig·ni·za·tion \mə-ˌlig-nə-'zā-shən\ *n* : a process or instance of becoming malignant ⟨~ of a tumor⟩

ma·lin·ger \mə-'liŋ-gər\ *vi* **-gered; -ger·ing** \-g(ə-)riŋ\ : to pretend or exaggerate incapacity or illness so as to avoid duty or work

ma·lin·ger·er \-ər\ *n* : an individual who malingers

mallei *pl of* MALLEUS

mal·le·in \'mal-ē-ən\ *n* : a product containing toxic principles of the bacillus of glanders and used to test for the presence of infection with that organism

mal·le·in·i·za·tion \ˌmal-ē-ə-nə-'zā-shən\ *n* : injection with mallein as a test for glanders

mal·leo·in·cu·dal \ˌmal-ē-ō-in-'kyüd-ᵊl, -'iŋ-kyə-dəl\ *adj* : of or relating to the malleus and incus

mal·le·o·lar \mə-'lē-ə-lər\ *adj* : of or relating to a malleolus esp. of the ankle

mal·le·o·lus \mə-'lē-ə-ləs\ *n, pl* **-li** \-ˌlī\ : an expanded projection or process at the distal extremity of each bone of the leg: **a** : the expanded lower extremity of the fibula situated on the lateral side of the leg at the ankle — called also *external malleolus, lateral malleolus* **b** : a strong pyramid-shaped process of the tibia that projects distally on the medial side of its lower extremity at the ankle — called also *internal malleolus, medial malleolus*

mal·let finger \'mal-ət-\ *n* : involuntary flexion of the distal phalanx of a finger caused by avulsion of the extensor tendon

mal·le·us \'mal-ē-əs\ *n, pl* **mal·lei** \-ē-ˌī, -ē-ˌē\ : the outermost of the chain of three ossicles in the middle ear of a mammal consisting of a head, neck, short process, long process, and handle with the short process and handle being fastened to the tympanic membrane and the head articulating with the head of the incus — called also *hammer*

Mal·loph·a·ga \mə-'läf-ə-gə\ *n pl* : an order of wingless insects comprising the biting lice — **mal·loph·a·gan** \-gən\ *adj or n*

Mal·lo·ry's triple stain \'mal-(ə-)rēz-\ *n* : a stain containing acid fuchsin, aniline blue, and orange G that is used esp. for the study of connective tissue — called also *Mallory's stain*

  Mallory, Frank Burr (1862–1941), American pathologist. Mallory spent almost all of his career on the staff of Harvard Medical School and in the pathology department of Boston City Hospital. A pioneer in histopathology and pathologic techniques, he developed many differential tissue stains that came into wide use. He introduced his stain for connective tissue in 1900.

mal·nour·ished \(')mal-'nər-isht, -'nə-risht\ *adj* : UNDERNOURISHED

mal·nour·ish·ment \-'nər-ish-mənt, -'nə-rish-\ *n* : MALNUTRITION

mal·nu·tri·tion \ˌmal-n(y)ü-'trish-ən\ *n* : faulty nutrition due to inadequate or unbalanced intake of nutrients or their impaired assimilation or utilization — **mal·nu·tri·tion·al** \-ᵊl\ *adj*

mal·oc·clu·ded \ˌmal-ə-'klüd-əd\ *adj* : characterized by malocclusion ⟨~ teeth⟩

mal·oc·clu·sion \ˌmal-ə-'klü-zhən\ *n* : improper occlusion; *esp* : abnormality in the coming together of teeth

mal·o·nate \\'mal-ə-ˌnāt\\ *n* : a salt or ester of malonic acid

ma·lo·nic acid \\mə-'lōn-ik-, -'län-\\ *n* : a crystalline dicarboxylic acid CH₂(COOH)₂ used esp. in the form of its diethyl ester in organic synthesis (as of barbiturates and vitamins of the B complex)

mal·o·nyl \\'mal-ə-ˌnil\\ *n* : the divalent radical –OCCH₂CO– of malonic acid

malonyl CoA \\-ˌkō-'ā\\ *n* : a compound C₂₆H₃₈N₇O₁₉P₃S that is formed by carboxylation of acetyl coenzyme A and is an intermediate in fatty acid synthesis

mal·o·nyl·urea \\-'(y)ùr-ē-ə\\ *n* : BARBITURIC ACID

Mal·pi·ghi·an \\mal-'pig-ē-ən, -'pē-gē-\\ *adj* : of, relating to, or discovered by Marcello Malpighi

Malpighi \\mäl-'pē-gē\\, **Marcello (1628–1694),** Italian anatomist. Malpighi is widely regarded as the founder of histology and one of the great microscopists. One of the first scientists to use the microscope to study tissues, he studied the fine anatomy of the human lung, brain, spinal cord, and secretory glands. In 1661 he made the major discovery of the capillary anastomoses between the arteries and the veins. This important link completed William Harvey's theory of the circulation of the blood. He described the deep layers of the epidermis in 1665. The following year he produced a classic treatise on the structure of the liver, cerebral cortex, kidney, and spleen. Several of the structural units of these organs now bear his name.

Malpighian body *n* : RENAL CORPUSCLE; *also* : MALPIGHIAN CORPUSCLE 2

Malpighian corpuscle *n* **1** : RENAL CORPUSCLE **2** : any of the small masses of adenoid tissue formed around the branches of the splenic artery in the spleen

Malpighian layer *n* : the deepest part of the epidermis that consists of the stratum basale and stratum spinosum and is the site of mitotic activity

Malpighian pyramid *n* : RENAL PYRAMID

mal·posed \\ˌmal-'pōzd\\ *adj* : characterized by malposition ⟨∼ teeth⟩

mal·po·si·tion \\ˌmal-pə-'zish-ən\\ *n* : wrong or faulty position ⟨fetal ∼s⟩ — **mal·po·si·tion·ing** \\-'zish-(ə-)niŋ\\ *n*

¹**mal·prac·tice** \\(ˈ)mal-'prak-təs\\ *n* : a dereliction of professional duty or a failure to exercise an accepted degree of professional skill or learning by a physician rendering professional services which results in injury, loss, or damage

²**malpractice** *vi* **-ticed; -tic·ing** : to engage in or commit malpractice

mal·pre·sen·ta·tion \\ˌmal-ˌprē-zen-'tā-shən, -ˌprez-ᵊn-\\ *n* : abnormal presentation of the fetus at birth

mal·ro·ta·tion \\ˌmal-rō-'tā-shən\\ *n* : improper rotation of a bodily part and esp. of the intestines ⟨ascites associated with ∼ of the intestines —*Biol. Abstracts*⟩ — **mal·ro·ta·ted** \\-'rō-ˌtāt-əd\\ *adj*

malt \\'mòlt\\ *n* : grain softened by steeping in water, allowed to germinate, and used esp. in brewing and distilling

Mal·ta fever \\ˌmòl-tə-\\ *n* : BRUCELLOSIS a

malt·ase \\'mòl-ˌtās, -ˌtāz\\ *n* : an enzyme that catalyzes the hydrolysis of maltose to glucose

Mal·thu·sian \\mal-'th(y)ü-zhən, mòl-\\ *adj* : of or relating to Malthus or to his theory that population tends to increase at a faster rate than its means of subsistence and that unless it is checked by moral restraint or by disease, famine, war, or other disaster widespread poverty and degradation inevitably result — **Malthusian** *n*

Mal·thus \\'mòl-thəs\\, **Thomas Robert (1766–1834),** British economist and demographer. Malthus presented his theory of population in *An Essay on the Principle of Population,* which was first published in 1798 but later expanded and documented. An economic pessimist, he viewed poverty as unfortunate as well as inevitable. His thinking later had a profound influence upon Charles Darwin.

Mal·thu·sian·ism \\-ˌiz-əm\\ *n* : the doctrines of Malthus esp. with respect to the difference between the rates of increase of a population and its food supply and to the long-term effects of this difference on the population

malt·ose \\'mòl-ˌtōs, -ˌtōz\\ *n* : a crystalline dextrorotatory fer-

mentable disaccharide sugar C₁₂H₂₂O₁₁ formed esp. from starch by amylase (as in saliva and malt), as an intermediate reducing product in metabolism, and in brewing and distilling and used chiefly in foods and in biological culture media

mal·union \\ˌmal-'yün-yən\\ *n* : incomplete or faulty union (as of the fragments of a fractured bone)

mal·unit·ed \\-yù-'nīt-əd\\ *adj* : united in a position of abnormality or deformity — used of the fragments of a broken bone

mam·ba \\'mäm-bə, 'mam-\\ *n* : any of several venomous elapid snakes (genus *Dendroaspis*) of sub-Saharan Africa that are related to the cobras but lack a dilatable hood; *esp* : a southern African snake (*D. angusticeps*) that has a light or olive⹀green phase and a black phase, that attains in the latter phase a length of 12 feet (3.66 meters), and that is noted for the quickness with which it inflicts its often fatal bite

mam·e·lon \\'mam-ə-lən\\ *n* : one of the three rounded protuberances on the cutting ridge of a recently erupted incisor tooth

mamillary, mamillated, mamillation, mamilliform, mamillothalamic tract *var of* MAMMILLARY, MAMMILLATED, MAMMILATION, MAMMILLIFORM, MAMMILLOTHALAMIC TRACT

mam·ma \\'mam-ə\\ *n, pl* **mam·mae** \\'mam-ˌē, -ˌī\\ : a mammary gland and its accessory parts

mam·mal \\'mam-əl\\ *n* : any of the higher vertebrate animals comprising the class Mammalia — **mam·ma·li·an** \\mə-'mā-lē-ən, ma-\\ *adj or n*

Mam·ma·lia \\mə-'mā-lē-ə\\ *n pl* : the highest class of the subphylum Vertebrata comprising humans and all other animals that nourish their young with milk secreted by mammary glands, that have the skin usu. more or less covered with hair, a mandible articulating directly with the squamosal, a chain of small ear bones, a brain with four optic lobes, a muscular diaphragm separating the heart and lungs from the abdominal cavity, only a left arch of the aorta, warm blood containing red blood cells without nuclei except in the fetus, and embryos developing both an amnion and an allantois, and that except in the monotremes reproduce viviparously

mam·mal·o·gist \\mə-'mal-ə-jəst, -'mäl-\\ *n* : a person who specializes in mammalogy

mam·mal·o·gy \\mə-'mal-ə-jē, ma-'mal-, -'mäl-\\ *n, pl* **-gies** : a branch of zoology dealing with mammals

mam·ma·plas·ty *or* **mam·mo·plas·ty** \\'mam-ə-ˌplast-ē\\ *n, pl* **-ties** : plastic surgery of the breast

¹**mam·ma·ry** \\'mam-ə-rē\\ *adj* : of, relating to, lying near, or affecting the mammae

²**mammary** *n, pl* **-maries** : MAMMARY GLAND

mammary artery — see INTERNAL THORACIC ARTERY

mammary gland *n* : any of the large compound sebaceous glands that in female mammals are modified to secrete milk, are situated ventrally in pairs, and usu. terminate in a nipple

mammary ridge *n* : either of a pair of longitudinal ectodermal thickenings in the mammalian embryo that extend from the base of the anterior to the posterior limb buds and are the source of the mammary glands — called also *milk line*

mam·mate \\'mam-ˌāt\\ *adj* : MAMMIFEROUS

mam·mec·to·my \\ma-'mek-tə-mē\\ *n, pl* **-mies** : MASTECTOMY

mam·mif·er·ous \\mə-'mif-(ə-)rəs, ma-\\ *adj* : having mammary glands : MAMMALIAN

mam·mi·form \\'mam-ə-ˌfòrm\\ *adj* : having the form of a breast or nipple : MAMMILLARY

mam·mil·la·ry *or* **mam·il·la·ry** \\'mam-ə-ˌler-ē, ma-'mil-ə-rē\\ *adj* **1** : of, relating to, or resembling the breasts **2** : studded with breast-shaped protuberances

mammillary body *n* : either of two small rounded eminences on the underside of the brain behind the tuber cinereum

M
N

\\ə\\ **abut** \\ᵊ\\ **kitten** \\ər\\ **further** \\a\\ **ash** \\ā\\ **ace** \\ä\\ **cot, cart**
\\aù\\ **out** \\ch\\ **chin** \\e\\ **bet** \\ē\\ **easy** \\g\\ **go** \\i\\ **hit** \\ī\\ **ice** \\j\\ **job**
\\ŋ\\ **sing** \\ō\\ **go** \\ò\\ **law** \\òi\\ **boy** \\th\\ **thin** \\th̲\\ **the** \\ü\\ **loot**
\\ù\\ **foot** \\y\\ **yet** \\zh\\ **vision** *See also* Pronunciation Symbols page

forming the terminals of the anterior pillars of the fornix — called also *corpus albicans*

mam·mil·lat·ed *or* **mam·il·lat·ed** \\'mam-ə-ˌlāt-əd\\ *adj* **1** : having nipples or small protuberances **2** : having the form of a bluntly rounded protuberance

mam·mil·la·tion *or* **mam·il·la·tion** \\-'lā-shən\\ *n* **1** : a mammillated or mammilliform protuberance **2** : the condition of having nipples or protuberances resembling nipples

mam·mil·li·form *or* **ma·mil·li·form** \\mə-'mil-ə-ˌfòrm, ma-\\ *adj* : nipple-shaped

mam·mil·lo·tha·lam·ic tract *or* **ma·mil·lo·tha·lam·ic tract** \\mə-ˌmil-ō-thə-'lam-ik-\\ *n* : a bundle of nerve fibers that runs from the mammillary body to the anterior nucleus of the thalamus — called also *mammillothalamic fasciculus*

mam·mi·tis \\ma-'mīt-əs\\ *n, pl* **mam·mit·i·des** \\-'mit-ə-ˌdēz\\ : MASTITIS

mam·mo·gen \\'mam-ə-jən, -ˌjen\\ *n* : any mammogenic hormone; *esp* : PROLACTIN

mam·mo·gen·ic \\ˌmam-ə-'jen-ik\\ *adj* : stimulating or inducing mammary development — **mam·mo·gen·i·cal·ly** \\-i-k(ə-)lē\\ *adv*

mam·mo·gram \\'mam-ə-ˌgram\\ *n* **1** : a photograph of the breasts made by X-rays **2** : the procedure for producing a mammogram

mam·mo·graph \\-ˌgraf\\ *n* : MAMMOGRAM 1

mam·mog·raph·er \\ma-'mäg-rə-fər, mə-\\ *n* : a physician or radiological technologist who prepares and interprets mammograms

mam·mog·ra·phy \\-fē\\ *n, pl* **-phies** : X-ray examination of the breasts (as for early detection of cancer) — **mam·mo·graph·ic** \\ˌmam-ə-'graf-ik\\ *adj*

mammoplasty *var of* MAMMAPLASTY

mam·mo·tro·pic \\ˌmam-ə-'trō-pik, -'träp-ik\\ *or* **mam·mo·tro·phic** \\-'trō-fik, -'träf-ik\\ *n* : stimulating growth of the mammary glands or lactation

mam·mo·tro·pin \\-'trōp-ᵊn\\ *also* **mam·mo·tro·phin** \\-'trō-fən\\ *n* : PROLACTIN

man \\'man\\ *n, pl* **men** \\'men\\ : a bipedal primate mammal of the genus *Homo* (*H. sapiens*) that is anatomically related to the great apes (family Pongidae) but is distinguished by greater development of the brain with resulting capacity for articulate speech and abstract reasoning, by marked erectness of body carriage with corresponding alteration of muscular balance and loss of prehensile powers of the foot, and by shortening of the arm with accompanying increase in thumb size and ability to place the thumb next to each of the fingers, that is usu. considered to occur in a variable number of freely interbreeding races, and that is the sole living representative of the family Hominidae; *broadly* : any living or extinct member of the family Hominidae

man·a·can \\'man-ə-kən\\ *n* : MANACA ROOT

man·a·ca root \\'man-ə-kə-,rüt\\ *n* : the dried root of a shrub (*Brunfelsia hopeana*) of Brazil and the West Indies that has been used to treat rheumatism and syphilis — called also *manaca, vegetable mercury*

man·age \\'man-ij\\ *vt* **man·aged; man·ag·ing** : to conduct the management of ⟨poorly *managed* diabetes⟩

man·aged care \\ˌman-ijd-\\ *n* : a system of providing health care (as by an HMO or a PPO) that is designed to control costs through managed programs in which the physician accepts constraints on the amount charged for medical care and the patient is limited in the choice of a physician

managed care organization *n* : a company (as an HMO or PPO) offering health-care plans with cost controls using managed care — called also *MCO*

man·age·ment \\'man-ij-mənt\\ *n* : the whole system of care and treatment of a disease or a sick individual ⟨the ∼ of contagious diseases⟩

man·ci·nism \\'man-sə-ˌniz-əm\\ *n* : the condition of being left-handed

Man·del·amine \\man-'del-ə-mēn\\ *trademark* — used for a preparation of the mandelate of methenamine

man·del·ate \\'man-də-ˌlāt\\ *n* : a salt or ester of mandelic acid

man·del·ic acid \\man-ˌdel-ik-\\ *n* : an optically active crystal-line hydroxy acid $C_8H_8O_3$ that is obtainable in the levorotatory D-form from amygdalin by hydrolysis but is usu. made in the racemic form by reaction of benzaldehyde with hydrocyanic acid and then hydrochloric acid and that is used chiefly in the form of its salts as a bacteriostatic agent for genitourinary tract infections

man·de·lo·ni·trile \\ˌman-də-lō-'nī-trəl, -ˌtrīl\\ *n* : a yellow oily liquid C_8H_7NO that can be prepared by hydrolysis of amygdalin and yields a small amount of hydrogen cyanide when mixed with alcohol and water

man·di·ble \\'man-də-bəl\\ *n* **1 a** : JAW 1; *esp* : JAW 1b **b** : the lower jaw with its investing soft parts **2** : any of various invertebrate mouthparts serving to hold or bite food materials; *esp* : either member of the anterior pair of mouth appendages of an arthropod often forming strong biting jaws

man·dib·u·la \\man-'dib-yə-lə\\ *n, pl* **-lae** \\-ˌlē\\ : MANDIBLE

¹man·dib·u·lar \\-yə-lər\\ *adj* : of, relating to, or located near a mandible

²mandibular *n* : MANDIBULAR NERVE

mandibular angle *n* : an angle formed by the junction at the gonion of the posterior border of the ramus and the inferior border of the body of the mandible

mandibular arch *n* : the first branchial arch of the vertebrate embryo from which in humans are developed the lower lip, the mandible, the masticatory muscles, and the anterior part of the tongue

mandibular artery *n* : INFERIOR ALVEOLAR ARTERY

mandibular canal *n* : a bony canal within the mandible that gives passage to blood vessels and nerves supplying the lower teeth — called also *inferior alveolar canal*

mandibular foramen *n* : the opening on the medial surface of the ramus of the mandible that leads into the mandibular canal and transmits blood vessels and nerves supplying the lower teeth

mandibular fossa *n* : GLENOID FOSSA

mandibular gland *n* : SUBMANDIBULAR GLAND

mandibular nerve *n* : the one of the three major branches or divisions of the trigeminal nerve that supplies sensory fibers to the lower jaw, the floor of the mouth, the anterior two-thirds of the tongue, and the lower teeth and supplies motor fibers to the muscles of mastication — called also *inferior maxillary nerve, mandibular;* compare MAXILLARY NERVE, OPHTHALMIC NERVE

mandibular notch *n* : a curved depression on the upper border of the lower jaw between the coronoid process and the condyloid process — called also *sigmoid notch*

man·di·bu·lo·fa·cial dysostosis \\man-ˌdib-yə-lō-ˌfā-shəl-\\ *n* : a dysostosis of the face and lower jaw inherited as an autosomal dominant trait and characterized by bilateral malformations, deformities of the outer and middle ear, and a usu. smaller lower jaw — called also *Treacher Collins syndrome*

man·drag·o·ra \\man-'drag-ə-rə\\ *n* **1** : MANDRAKE 1 **2** *cap* : a small genus of Eurasian herbs of the family Solanaceae with basal leaves, bell-shaped flowers, and fleshy berries and that includes the mandrake

man·drake \\'man-ˌdrāk\\ *n* **1 a** : a Mediterranean solanaceous herb of the genus *Mandragora* (*M. officinarum*) that has greenish yellow or purple flowers, globose yellow fruits formerly supposed to have aphrodisiac properties, and a large usu. forked root resembling a human in form and formerly credited with magical properties **b** (1) : the root of this plant that contains hyoscyamine and was formerly used esp. to promote conception, as a cathartic, or as a narcotic and soporific (2) : a solution of mandrake root (as in wine) formerly used as a narcotic **2 a** : MAYAPPLE **b** : PODO-PHYLLUM 2

man·drel *also* **man·dril** \\'man-drəl\\ *n* : the shaft and bearings on which a tool (as a dental grinding disk) is mounted

man·drin \\'man-drən\\ *n* : a stylet for a catheter

man–eat·er \\'man-ˌēt-ər\\ *n* : one that has or is thought to have an appetite for human flesh: as **a** : MACKEREL SHARK; *esp* : GREAT WHITE SHARK **b** : a large feline (as a lion or tiger) that has acquired the habit of feeding on human flesh — **man–eat·ing** \\-ˌēt-iŋ\\ *adj*

man–eater shark *n* : MACKEREL SHARK; *esp* : GREAT WHITE SHARK

man–eating shark *n* : MAN-EATER SHARK

ma·neu·ver *or chiefly Brit* **ma·noeu·vre** \mə-'n(y)ü-vər\ *n* **1** : a movement, procedure, or method performed to achieve a desired result and esp. to restore a normal physiological state or to promote normal function ⟨the simplest ~ to actuate the normal eustachian tube is to swallow —H. G. Armstrong⟩ — see HEIMLICH MANEUVER, VALSALVA MANEUVER **2** : a manipulation to accomplish a change of position; *specif* : rotational or other movement applied to a fetus within the uterus to alter its position and facilitate delivery — see SCANZONI MANEUVER

man·ga·nese \'maŋ-gə-ˌnēz, -ˌnēs\ *n* : a grayish white usu. hard and brittle metallic element that resembles iron but is not magnetic — symbol *Mn*; see ELEMENT table

man·gan·ic \man-'gan-ik, maŋ-\ *adj* : of, relating to, or derived from manganese; *esp* : containing this element with a valence of three or six

man·ga·nous \-nəs\ *adj* : of, relating to, or derived from manganese; *esp* : containing this element with a valence of two

mange \'mānj\ *n* : any of various more or less severe, persistent, and contagious skin diseases that are marked esp. by eczematous inflammation and loss of hair and that affect domestic animals or sometimes humans; *esp* : a skin disease caused by a minute parasitic mite of *Sarcoptes, Psoroptes, Chorioptes,* or related genera that burrows in or lives on the skin or by one of the genus *Demodex* that lives in the hair follicles or sebaceous glands — see CHORIOPTIC MANGE, DEMODECTIC MANGE, SARCOPTIC MANGE, SCABIES

mange mite *n* : any of the small parasitic mites that infest the skin of animals and cause mange

man·go fly \'maŋ-gō-\ *n* : any of various horseflies of the genus *Chrysops* that are vectors of filarial worms

man·gy \'mān-jē\ *adj* **man·gi·er; -est** **1** : infected with mange ⟨a ~ dog⟩ **2** : relating to, characteristic of, or resulting from mange ⟨a ~ appearance⟩ ⟨a ~ itch⟩

ma·nia \'mā-nē-ə, -nyə\ *n* : excitement of psychotic proportions manifested by mental and physical hyperactivity, disorganization of behavior, and elevation of mood; *specif* : the manic phase of bipolar disorder

ma·ni·ac \'mā-nē-ˌak\ *n* : an individual affected with or exhibiting insanity

ma·ni·a·cal \mə-'nī-ə-kəl\ *also* **ma·ni·ac** \'mā-nē-ak\ *adj* : affected with or exhibiting insanity : MAD, INSANE ⟨a ~ killer⟩ — **ma·ni·a·cal·ly** \mə-'nī-ə-k(ə-)lē\ *adv*

¹man·ic \'man-ik\ *adj* : affected with, relating to, or resembling mania — **man·i·cal·ly** \-i-k(ə-)lē\ *adv*

²manic *n* : an individual affected with mania

manic depression *n* : BIPOLAR DISORDER

¹man·ic–de·pres·sive \ˌman-ik-di-'pres-iv\ *adj* : characterized by or affected with either mania or depression or alternating mania and depression (as in bipolar disorder)

²manic–depressive *n* : a manic-depressive individual

manic–depressive illness *n* : BIPOLAR DISORDER

manic–depressive psychosis *n* : BIPOLAR DISORDER

manic–depressive reaction *n* : BIPOLAR DISORDER

man·i·fes·ta·tion \ˌman-ə-fə-'stā-shən, -ˌfes-\ *n* : a perceptible, outward, or visible expression (as of a disease or abnormal condition) ⟨the ~s of shock⟩

man·i·fest con·tent \'man-ə-ˌfest-'kän-ˌtent\ *n* : the content of a dream as it is recalled by the dreamer in psychoanalysis — compare LATENT CONTENT

man·i·kin \'man-i-kən\ *n* : a model of the human body commonly in detachable pieces for exhibiting the parts and organs, their position, and relations

ma·nip·u·late \mə-'nip-yə-ˌlāt\ *vt* **-lat·ed; -lat·ing** **1** : to treat or operate with the hands or by mechanical means esp. in a skillful manner ⟨~ the fragments of a broken bone into correct position⟩ **2 a** : to manage or utilize skillfully **b** : to control or play upon by artful, unfair, or insidious means esp. to one's own advantage — **ma·nip·u·la·tive** \-'nip-yə-ˌlāt-iv, -lət-\ *adj* — **ma·nip·u·la·tive·ness** *n*

ma·nip·u·la·tion \mə-ˌnip-yə-'lā-shən\ *n* **1** : the act, process, or an instance of manipulating esp. a body part by manual examination and treatment; *esp* : adjustment of faulty structural relationships by manual means (as in the reduction of fractures or dislocations or the breaking down of adhesions) **2** : the condition of being manipulated ⟨vulnerability to psychological ~ —M. W. Straight⟩

man·kind \'man-'kīnd, -ˌkīnd\ *n sing but sing or pl in constr* : the human race : the totality of human beings

man·na \'man-ə\ *n* **1** : the sweetish dried exudate of a European ash (esp. *Fraxinus ornus*) that contains mannitol and has been used as a laxative and demulcent **2** : a product that is similar to manna and is excreted by a scale insect (*Trabutina mannipara*) feeding on the tamarisk

man·nan \'man-ˌan, -ən\ *n* : any of several polysaccharides that are polymers of mannose and occur esp. in plant cell walls and in some microorganisms (as yeast)

manna sugar *n* : MANNITOL

man·ner·ism \'man-ə-ˌriz-əm\ *n* : a characteristic and often unconscious mode or peculiarity of action, bearing, or treatment; *esp* : any pointless and compulsive activity performed repeatedly

man·nite \'man-ˌīt\ *n* : MANNITOL

man·ni·tol \'man-ə-ˌtól, -ˌtōl\ *n* : a slightly sweet crystalline alcohol $C_6H_{14}O_6$ found in many plants and used esp. as a diuretic and in testing kidney function

mannitol hexa·ni·trate \-ˌhek-sə-'nī-ˌtrāt\ *n* : an explosive crystalline ester $C_6H_8(NO_3)_6$ made by nitration of mannitol and used mixed with a carbohydrate (as lactose) in the treatment of angina pectoris and vascular hypertension

man·no·hep·tu·lose \ˌman-ō-'hep-t(y)ù-ˌlōs, -ˌlōz\ *n* : a ketose that occurs esp. in the urine of individuals who have eaten avocados

man·no·nic acid \mə-ˌnän-ik-, -ˌnōn-\ *n* : a syrupy acid $C_6H_{12}O_7$ formed by oxidizing mannose

man·nose \'man-ˌōs, -ˌōz\ *n* : an aldose $C_6H_{12}O_6$ whose dextrorotatory enantiomer occurs esp. as a structural unit of mannans from which it can be recovered by hydrolysis

man·nos·i·do·sis \mə-ˌnō-sə-'dō-səs\ *n, pl* **-do·ses** \-ˌsēz\ : a rare inherited metabolic disease characterized by deficiency of an enzyme catalyzing the metabolism of mannose with resulting accumulation of mannose in the body and marked esp. by facial and skeletal deformities and by mental retardation

man·nu·ron·ic acid \ˌman-yə-ˌrän-ik-\ *n* : an acid $C_6H_{10}O_7$ related to mannose and obtained by hydrolysis of alginic acid

manoeuvre *chiefly Brit var of* MANEUVER

ma·nom·e·ter \mə-'näm-ət-ər\ *n* **1** : an instrument (as a pressure gauge) for measuring the pressure of gases and vapors **2** : SPHYGMOMANOMETER — **mano·met·ric** \ˌman-ə-'me-trik\ *adj* — **mano·met·ri·cal·ly** \-tri-k(ə-)lē\ *adv* — **ma·nom·e·try** \mə-'näm-ə-trē\ *n, pl* **-tries**

man·op·to·scope \man-'äp-tə-ˌskōp\ *n* : a device for determining the dominance in function of one eye over the other

man·rem \'man-'rem\ *n* : a unit of measurement of absorbed radiation that is equal to one rem absorbed by one individual

man·slaugh·ter \'man-ˌslòt-ər\ *n* : the slaying of a human being; *specif* : the unlawful killing of a human being without express or implied malice

Man·son·el·la \ˌman(t)-sə-'nel-ə\ *n* : a genus of filarial worms of the superfamily Filarioidea including one (*M. ozzardi*) that is common and apparently nonpathogenic in human visceral fat and mesenteries in So. and Central America

Man·son \'man-sən\, **Sir Patrick (1844–1922)**, British parasitologist. Manson is remembered as the father of tropical medicine. In 1877 he was the first to prove the connection between insects and tropical disease: he demonstrated that culex mosquitoes are carriers of filaria larvae. He found filaria in individuals affected with elephantiasis. In 1894 he first put forth his mosquito-malaria hypothesis. His research helped Sir Ronald Ross to elucidate the transmission of malaria by mosquitoes. The schistosome (*Schistosoma mansoni*) that causes schistosomiasis mansoni is but one of many pathogenic parasites that he discovered and whose life cycle he worked out.

mansoni — see SCHISTOSOMIASIS MANSONI

Man·so·nia \man-'sō-nē-ə\ *n* : a widespread genus of mosquitoes that carry filarial worms and whose larvae and pupae obtain oxygen directly from plants underwater

Man·son's disease \'man(t)-sənz-\ *n* : SCHISTOSOMIASIS MANSONI

man·tle \'man-tᵊl\ *n* **1** : something that covers, enfolds, or envelops **2** : CEREBRAL CORTEX

Man·toux test \ˌman-ˌtü-, ˌmän-\ *n* : an intradermal test for hypersensitivity to tuberculin that indicates past or present infection with tubercle bacilli — see TUBERCULIN TEST

Man·toux \mäⁿ-tü\, **Charles (1877–1947),** French physician. Mantoux introduced his test for tuberculosis in 1908. He is also remembered for reviving the use of pneumothorax induced intentionally by artificial means for the treatment of pulmonary tuberculosis and for advocating radiological examination of the lungs.

man·u·al \'man-yə-(-wə)l\ *adj* **1 a** : of, relating to, or involving the hands ⟨∼ dexterity⟩ **b** : done or performed by hand and not by machine ⟨∼ removal of nits and lice —Jerome Potts⟩ **2** : using signs and the manual alphabet in teaching the deaf — compare ORAL 2

manual alphabet *n* : an alphabet esp. for the deaf in which letters are represented by finger positions and that is used in finger spelling

man·u·al·ist \'man-yə-wə-ləst\ *n* : a person who uses or advocates the use of the manual method in teaching the deaf

manual method *n* : a method of teaching the deaf that mainly employs signs and the manual alphabet

ma·nu·bri·al \mə-'n(y)ü-brē-əl\ *adj* : of, relating to, or shaped like a manubrium ⟨a mediastinal ∼ mass developed three months later —P. L. Gerfo *et al*⟩

ma·nu·bri·um \mə-'n(y)ü-brē-əm\ *n, pl* **-bria** \-brē-ə\ *also* **-bri·ums** : an anatomical process or part shaped like a handle: as **a** : the uppermost segment of the sternum of humans and many other mammals that is a somewhat triangular flattened bone with anterolateral borders which articulate with the clavicles **b** : the process of the malleus of the ear

manubrium ster·ni \-'stər-ˌnī\ *n* : MANUBRIUM a

ma·nus \'mā-nəs, 'mä-\ *n, pl* **ma·nus** \-nəs, -ˌnüs\ : the part of the vertebrate forelimb from the carpus to the distal end

man·u·stu·pra·tion \ˌman-yù-stü-'prā-shən\ *n* : MASTURBATION

many·plies \'men-ē-ˌplīz\ *n pl but usu sing in constr* : OMASUM

MAO *abbr* monoamine oxidase

MAOI *abbr* monoamine oxidase inhibitor

MAO inhibitor \'em-ˌā-'ō-\ *n* : MONOAMINE OXIDASE INHIBITOR

¹map \'map\ *n* : the arrangement of genes on a chromosome — called also *genetic map*

²map *vb* **mapped; map·ping** *vt* : to locate (a gene) on a chromosome ⟨mutants which have been genetically *mapped*⟩ ∼ *vi, of a gene* : to be located ⟨a repressor ∼*s* near the corresponding structural gene⟩

ma·ple syr·up urine disease \'mā-pəl-'sər-əp-, -'sir-əp-\ *n* : a hereditary aminoaciduria caused by a deficiency of decarboxylase leading to high concentrations of valine, leucine, isoleucine, and alloisoleucine in the blood, urine, and cerebrospinal fluid and characterized by an odor of maple syrup to the urine, vomiting, hypertonicity, severe mental retardation, seizures, and eventually death unless the condition is treated with dietary measures

ma·pro·ti·line \mə-'prō-tə-ˌlēn\ *n* : an antidepressant drug used in the form of its hydrochloride $C_{20}H_{23}N\cdot HCl$ to relieve

major depression (as in bipolar disorder) and anxiety associated with depression

map unit *n* : a unit representing a recombination frequency of one percent between genes and used as a measure of distance between genes in the construction of genetic maps

ma·ran·ta \mə-'ran-tə\ *n* **1 a** *cap* : a genus (family Marantaceae) of tropical American herbs with tuberous starchy roots **b** : any plant of the genus *Maranta* : ARROWROOT 1a **2** : the edible starch obtained from the roots of a plant of the genus *Maranta* (*M. arundinacea*) : ARROWROOT 2

ma·ran·tic \mə-'ran-tik\ *adj* : of, relating to, or marked by marasmus : MARASMIC ⟨∼ infants⟩ ⟨∼ disease⟩

ma·ras·ma \mə-'raz-mə\ *n* : MARASMUS

ma·ras·mic \-mik\ *adj* : of, relating to, or marked by marasmus : MARANTIC ⟨∼ infants exhibiting kwashiorkor⟩

ma·ras·mus \mə-'raz-məs\ *n* : severe malnutrition affecting infants and children esp. of impoverished regions that is characterized by poor growth, loss of subcutaneous fat, muscle atrophy, apathy, and pronounced weight loss and is usu. caused by a diet deficient in calories and proteins but sometimes by disease (as dysentery or giardiasis)

mar·ble bone \'mär-bəl-\ *n* : OSTEOPETROSIS b

marble bone disease *n* : OSTEOPETROSIS a, b

marble bones *n pl but sing in constr* : OSTEOPETROSIS a

mar·ble·iza·tion \ˌmär-bə-lə-'zā-shən\ *n* : the process of becoming or the condition of being veined or marked like marble ⟨examination revealed ∼ of both lower extremities —*Jour. Amer. Med. Assoc.*⟩ — called also *marmoration*

Mar·burg fever \'mär-bərg-\ *n* : an often fatal hemorrhagic fever that is caused by the Marburg virus, is an acute febrile illness often progressing to severe hemorrhaging, is spread esp. by contact with the body fluids (as blood or saliva) of infected individuals, and was orig. reported in humans infected by green monkeys — called also *green monkey disease, Marburg hemorrhagic fever, Marburg disease*

Marburg virus *n* : an African single-stranded RNA virus of the family *Filoviridae* (species *Marburg virus*) that causes Marburg fever

marc \'märk\ *n* : an insoluble residue remaining after extraction of a solution (as a drug) with a solvent

march \'märch\ *n* : the progression of epileptic activity through the motor centers of the cerebral cortex that is manifested in localized convulsions in first one and then an adjacent part of the body ⟨the Jacksonian ∼ of convulsions⟩

Mar·ek's disease \'mar-iks-, 'mer-\ *n* : a highly contagious virus disease of poultry that is characterized esp. by proliferation of lymphoid cells and is caused by either of two herpesviruses (*Gallid herpesvirus 2* and *Gallid herpesvirus 3*)

Mar·ek \'mò-rek\, **Jozsef (1867–1952),** Hungarian veterinarian. Marek first described the cancerous disease known as Marek's disease in 1907.

Ma·rey's law \mə-'rāz-\ *n* : a statement in physiology: heart rate is related inversely to arterial blood pressure

Ma·rey \má-rā\, **Étienne–Jules (1830–1904),** French physiologist. Marey contributed greatly to the development of experimental physiology. In 1860 he invented the sphygmograph, an instrument for recording the features of the pulse and variation in blood pressure on a graph. In 1861 he formulated Marey's law. He was the first to realize the relationship between blood pressure and heart rate.

Mar·e·zine \'mar-ə-ˌzēn\ *n* : a preparation of the hydrochloride of cyclizine — formerly a U.S. registered trademark

mar·fa·noid \'mär-fə-ˌnòid\ *adj* : exhibiting the typical characteristics of Marfan syndrome ⟨the ∼ habitus⟩

Mar·fan syndrome \'mär-ˌfan\ *or* **Mar·fan's syndrome** \-ˌfanz\ *n* : a disorder of connective tissue that is inherited as a simple dominant trait, is caused by a defect in the gene controlling the production of fibrillin, and is characterized by abnormal elongation of the long bones and often by ocular and circulatory defects

Mar·fan \mär-fäⁿ\, **Antonin Bernard Jean (1858–1942),** French pediatrician. Marfan concerned himself with the prevention, diagnosis, and treatment of children's diseases. In 1892 he described spastic paralysis in children with hereditary syphilis. In 1896 he described a syndrome marked by arachnodactyly, ectopia of the crystalline lens, and abnormal flexibility of the joints. The syndrome now bears his name.

mar·gar·ic acid \mär-ˌgar-ik-\ *n* **1** : a crystalline synthetic fatty acid $C_{17}H_{34}O_2$ intermediate between palmitic acid and stearic acid **2** : a mixture of palmitic acid and stearic acid obtained from various natural fats, oils, and waxes

mar·ga·rine \ˈmärj-(ə-)rən, -ə-ˌrēn\ *n* : a food product made usu. from vegetable oils churned with ripened skim milk to a smooth emulsion, often fortified with vitamins A and D, and used as a substitute for butter

Mar·gar·o·pus \mär-ˈgar-ə-pəs\ *n* : a genus of ixodid ticks that in some classifications includes an American cattle tick (*M. annulatus* syn. *Boophilus annulatus*) causing Texas fever

mar·gin \ˈmär-jən\ *n* **1** : the outside limit or edge of something (as a bodily part or a wound) **2** : the part of consciousness at a particular moment that is felt only vaguely and dimly

mar·gin·al \ˈmärj-nəl, -ən-ᵊl\ *adj* **1** : of, relating to, or situated at a margin or border **2** : located at the fringe of consciousness ⟨~ sensations⟩

mar·gin·at·ed \ˈmärj-jə-ˌnāt-əd\ *adj* : having a margin distinct in appearance or structure ⟨a sharply ~ lesion⟩

mar·gin·ation \ˌmärj-jə-ˈnā-shən\ *n* **1** : the act or process of forming a margin; *specif* : the adhesion of white blood cells to the walls of damaged blood vessels **2** : the action of finishing a dental restoration or a filling for a cavity ⟨~ of an amalgam with a bur⟩

Ma·rie–Strüm·pell disease *also* **Ma·rie–Strüm·pell's disease** \mä-ˈrē-ˈstrüm-pəl(z)-\ *n* : ANKYLOSING SPONDYLITIS

Ma·rie \má-rē\, **Pierre (1853–1940)**, French neurologist. Marie began his career in neurology under the tutelage of the celebrated neurologist Jean-Martin Charcot at the Salpêtrière clinic. Known for his astute clinical judgments, he was responsible for a number of classic descriptions. From 1886 to 1891 he produced the first description and study of acromegaly. His study of this disorder of the pituitary gland constituted a fundamental contribution to the developing science of endocrinology. In 1906 he published three papers on aphasia that generated controversy because his views on language disorders challenged the widely accepted views of Paul Broca. Marie published his description of ankylosing spondylitis in 1898.

Strüm·pell \ˈshtrüm-pəl\, **Ernst Adolf Gustav Gottfried von (1853–1925)**, German neurologist. Strümpell was at various times professor of medicine at Leipzig, Breslau, and Vienna. He is credited with classic descriptions of polioencephalomyelitis in children (1885) and pseudosclerosis of the brain (1898). In 1883–1884 he published a two-volume text on the pathology and treatment of internal diseases. The second volume included his original description of ankylosing spondylitis. The disease was described independently by Pierre Marie in 1898; it is now sometimes called Marie-Strümpell disease.

mar·i·jua·na *also* **mar·i·hua·na** \ˌmar-ə-ˈwän-ə *also* -ˈhwän-\ *n* **1** : HEMP 1 **2** : the dried leaves and flowering tops of the pistillate hemp plant that yield THC and are sometimes smoked in cigarettes for their intoxicating effect — compare BHANG, CANNABIS, HASHISH

Mar·i·nol \ˈmar-ə-ˌnȯl\ *trademark* — used for a preparation of dronabinol

mar·jo·ram \ˈmärj-(ə-)rəm\ *n* : any of various usu. fragrant and aromatic mints (genera *Origanum* and *Majorana*) often used in cookery; *esp* : SWEET MARJORAM

mark \ˈmärk\ *n* **1** : a narrow deep hollow on the surface of the crown of a horse's incisor tooth that gradually becomes obliterated by the wearing away of the crown and therefore is indicative of the animal's age and usu. disappears from the lower central incisors about the sixth year while traces may remain in the upper until the eleventh **2** : an impression or trace made or occurring on something — see BIRTHMARK, STRAWBERRY MARK **3** : a cut (as an ear notch) made on livestock for identification — **marked** *adj*

mark·er \ˈmär-kər\ *n* : something that serves to identify, predict, or characterize ⟨a surface ~ on a cell that acts as an antigen⟩: as **a** : BIOMARKER **b** : GENETIC MARKER — called also *marker gene*

mar·mo·rat·ed \ˈmär-mȯr-ˌāt-əd\ *adj* : veined or streaked like marble

mar·mo·ra·tion \ˌmär-mȯr-ˈā-shən\ *n* : MARBLEIZATION

mar·mot \ˈmär-mət\ *n* : any of various stout-bodied short-legged burrowing rodents (genus *Marmota*) with coarse fur, a short bushy tail, and very small ears that are important reservoirs of sylvatic plague

Mar·o·teaux–La·my syndrome \mär-ō-ˈtō-lä-ˈmē-\ *n* : a mucopolysaccharidosis that is inherited as an autosomal recessive trait and that is similar to Hurler's syndrome except that intellectual development is not retarded

Mar·o·teaux \má-rō-tō\, **Pierre (b 1926)**, French physician. Maroteaux served as director of genetics research at a medical research institute in Paris. His major field of interest was constitutional diseases of the bones.

La·my \lá-mē\, **Maurice Emile Joseph (1895–1975)**, French physician. After a tenure as executive officer of a children's hospital in Paris, Lamy served from 1950 to 1967 as a professor at an institute for genetics research in Paris. He published works on scarlet fever immunity, twins, hereditary illnesses, and a handbook of medical genetics.

Mar·plan \ˈmär-ˌplan\ *trademark* — used for a preparation of isocarboxazid

mar·row \ˈmar-(ˌ)ō, -ə-(w)\ *n* **1** : BONE MARROW **2** : the substance of the spinal cord

Mar·seilles fever \mär-ˈsā-\ *n* : BOUTONNEUSE FEVER

marsh gas \ˈmärsh-\ *n* : METHANE

marsh·mal·low \ˈmärsh-ˌmel-ō, -ˌmel-ə(w), -ˌmal-\ *n* : a European perennial herb of the genus *Althaea* (*A. officinalis*) naturalized in the eastern U.S. whose pink flowers, velvety leaves, and mucilaginous root are used in herbal medicine and whose root was formerly used in confectionary — see ALTHAEA 2

marshmallow root *n* : ALTHAEA 2

Marsh test \ˈmärsh-\ *n* : a sensitive test for arsenic in which a solution to be tested is treated with hydrogen so that if arsenic is present gaseous arsine is formed and then decomposed to a black deposit of arsenic (as when the gas is passed through a heated glass tube)

Marsh, James Ernest (1794–1846), British chemist. Marsh spent considerable time studying poisons and their effects. He introduced his test for arsenic in 1836.

Mar·su·pi·a·lia \mär-ˌsü-pē-ˈā-lē-ə\ *n pl* : an order or other taxon of mammals comprising kangaroos, wombats, bandicoots, opossums, and related animals that with few exceptions develop no placenta and usu. have a pouch on the abdomen of the female containing the teats and serving to carry the young — **mar·su·pi·al** \mär-ˈsü-pē-əl\ *adj or n*

mar·su·pi·al·iza·tion *or chiefly Brit* **mar·su·pi·al·isa·tion** \mär-ˌsü-pē-ə-li-ˈzā-shən\ *n* : the operation of marsupializing

mar·su·pi·al·ize *or chiefly Brit* **mar·su·pi·al·ise** \mär-ˈsü-pē-ə-ˌlīz\ *vt* **-ized** *or chiefly Brit* **-ised; -iz·ing** *or chiefly Brit* **-is·ing** : to open (as the bladder or a cyst) and sew by the edges to the abdominal wound to permit further treatment (as of an enclosed tumor) or to discharge pathological matter (as from a hydatid cyst)

mar·su·pi·um \mär-ˈsü-pē-əm\ *n, pl* **-pia** \-pē-ə\ : an abdominal pouch formed by a fold of the skin and enclosing the mammary glands of most marsupials

Mar·ti·not·ti cell *or* **Mar·ti·not·ti's cell** \ˌmär-ti-ˈnät-ē(z)-\ *n* : a multipolar fusiform nerve cell in the deepest layer of the cerebral cortex with axons ascending into the layer of pyramidal cells

Mar·ti·not·ti \ˌmär-tē-ˈnȯt-tē\, **Giovanni (1857–1928)**, Italian pathologist. Martinotti held the position of professor of

M
N

anatomy and pathology successively at Modena, Siena, and Bologna. In 1889 he described certain cells in the cerebral cortex with ascending axons; they are now known as Martinotti cells.

Mar·ti·us yellow \\'mär-sh(ē-)əs-\ *n* : a yellow dye $C_{10}H_6N_2O_5$ that is used chiefly as a biological stain
Martius, Carl Alexander von (1838–1920), German chemist. Martius was involved in the synthetic organic dye industry, having been one of the founders of an aniline dye factory in Berlin in 1867.

masc *abbr* masculine

mas·cu·line \\'mas-kyə-lən\ *adj* **1** : MALE 1 **2** : having the qualities distinctive of or appropriate to a male **3** : having a mannish bearing or quality

masculine pro·test \-'prō-,test\ *n* : a tendency attributed esp. to the human female in the psychology of Alfred Adler to escape from the female role by assuming a masculine role and by dominating others; *broadly* : any tendency to compensate for feelings of inferiority or inadequacy by exaggerated overt aggressive behavior

mas·cu·lin·i·ty \,mas-kyə-'lin-ət-ē\ *n, pl* **-ties** : the quality, state, or degree of being masculine ⟨measurement of ~ or femininity —*Psychological Abstracts*⟩

mas·cu·lin·ize *also Brit* **mas·cu·lin·ise** \\'mas-kyə-lə-,nīz\ *vt* **-ized** *also Brit* **-ised; -iz·ing** *also Brit* **-is·ing** : to give a preponderantly masculine character to; *esp* : to cause (a female) to take on male characteristics — **mas·cu·lin·iza·tion** *also Brit* **mas·cu·lin·isa·tion** \,mas-kyə-lə-nə-'zā-shən\ *n*

mas·cu·lin·ovo·blas·to·ma \,mas-kyə-lə-,nō-vō-blas-'tō-mə\ *n, pl* **-mas** *also* **-ma·ta** \-mət-ə\ : a tumor of the ovary that tends to cause masculinization

ma·ser \\'mā-zər\ *n* : a device that utilizes the natural oscillations of atoms or molecules between energy levels for generating electromagnetic radiation in the microwave region of the spectrum

MASH *abbr* mobile army surgical hospital

¹mask \\'mask\ *n* **1** : a protective covering for the face **2 a** : any of various devices that cover the mouth and nose and are used to prevent inhalation of dangerous substances, to facilitate delivery of a gas (as oxygen or a general anesthetic), or to prevent the dispersal of exhaled infective material — see GAS MASK, OXYGEN MASK **3** : a cosmetic preparation for the skin of the face that produces a tightening effect as it dries

²mask *vt* **1** : to prevent (an atom or group of atoms) from showing its ordinary reactions ⟨to ~ hydroxyl in a sugar by converting it into methoxyl⟩ **2** : to modify or reduce the effect or activity of (as a process or a reaction) **3** : to make indistinct or imperceptible ⟨flavorings used in pharmacy to ~ the taste of medications⟩ **4** : to raise the audibility threshold of (a sound) by the simultaneous presentation of another sound

masked *adj* : failing to present or produce the usual symptoms : not obvious : LATENT ⟨~ depression⟩ ⟨a ~ virus⟩

mas·och·ism \\'mas-ə-,kiz-əm, 'maz-\ *n* : a sexual perversion characterized by pleasure in being subjected to pain or humiliation esp. by a love object — compare ALGOLAGNIA, SADISM — **mas·och·is·tic** \,mas-ə-'kis-tik, ,maz-\ *adj* — **mas·och·is·ti·cal·ly** \,mas-ə-'kis-ti-k(ə-)lē, ,maz-\ *adv*
Sa·cher–Ma·soch \'zäk-ər-'mäz-ȯk\, **Leopold von (1836–1895)**, Austrian novelist. Sacher-Masoch is most famous for his erotic novels. In these novels the characters dwell at length on sexual pleasure derived from pain. The subject matter reflects Sacher-Masoch's personal life. He had two wives and several mistresses with whom he acted out the sexual fantasies described in his fictional works. By 1893 *masochism* was an established medical term.

mas·och·ist \-kəst\ *n* : an individual who is given to masochism

mass \\'mas\ *n* **1** : the property of a body that is a measure of its inertia, that is commonly taken as a measure of the amount of material it contains, that causes it to have weight in a gravitational field, and that along with length and time constitutes one of the fundamental quantities on which all

physical measurements are based **2** : a homogeneous pasty mixture compounded for making pills, lozenges, and plasters ⟨blue ~⟩

¹mas·sage \mə-'säzh, -'säj\ *n* : manipulation of tissues (as by rubbing, stroking, kneading, or tapping) with the hand or an instrument esp. for therapeutic purposes

²massage *vt* **mas·saged; mas·sag·ing** : to treat by means of massage

mas·sa in·ter·me·dia \'mas-ə-,in-tər-'mē-dē-ə\ *n* : an apparently functionless mass of gray matter in the midline of the third ventricle that is found in many but not all human brains and is formed when the surfaces of the thalami protruding inward from opposite sides of the third ventricle make contact and fuse

mas·sa·sau·ga \,mas-ə-'sȯg-ə\ *n* : a medium-sized rattlesnake of the genus *Sistrurus* (*S. catenatus*) that has nine large scales on the head, grows to a length of about 18 to 39 inches (46 to 100 centimeters), and is distributed from southern Ontario across the central U.S. to northeastern New Mexico and southeastern Arizona

mas·se·ter \mə-'sēt-ər, ma-\ *n* : a large muscle that raises the lower jaw and assists in mastication, arises from the zygomatic arch and the zygomatic process of the temporal bone, and is inserted into the mandibular ramus and gonial angle — **mas·se·ter·ic** \,mas-ə-'ter-ik\ *adj*

mas·seur \ma-'sər, mə-\ *n* : a man who practices massage and physiotherapy

mas·seuse \-'sə(r)z, -'süz\ *n* : a woman who practices massage and physiotherapy

mass frag·men·tog·ra·phy \-,frag-mən-'täg-rə-fē\ *n, pl* **-phies** : the combination of gas chromatography and mass spectrometry used to isolate and quantify ionic fragments characteristic of particular compounds by examining a selection of ions having specific mass-to-charge ratios rather than examining a range of such ratios

mas·si·cot \\'mas-ə-,kät, -,kō(t)\ *n* : lead monoxide obtained as a yellow powder at temperatures below the melting point of the oxide — compare LITHARGE

mas·sive \\'mas-iv\ *adj* **1** : large in comparison to what is typical — used esp. of medical dosage or of an infective agent ⟨a ~ dose of penicillin⟩ **2** : being extensive and severe — used of a pathologic condition ⟨a ~ hemorrhage⟩ ⟨a ~ collapse of a lung⟩

mass number *n* : an integer that approximates the mass of an isotope and that designates the number of nucleons in the nucleus ⟨the symbol for carbon of *mass number* 14 is ^{14}C or C^{14}⟩ — compare ATOMIC MASS

mas·so·ther·a·pist \,mas-ō-'ther-ə-pəst\ *n* : a person who practices massotherapy

mas·so·ther·a·py \-pē\ *n, pl* **-pies** : the practice of therapeutic massage

mass spectrograph *n* : an instrument used to separate and often to determine the masses of isotopes

mass spectrometer *n* : a mass spectroscope that detects ions by means of electronic amplification

mass spectrometrist *n* : MASS SPECTROSCOPIST

mass spectrometry *n* : an instrumental method for identifying the chemical constitution of a substance by means of the separation of gaseous ions according to their differing mass and charge — called also *mass spectroscopy* — **mass spectrometric** *adj* — **mass spectrometrically** *adv*

mass spectroscope *n* : an instrument that separates a stream of charged particles or gaseous ions according to their mass and charge

mass spectroscopist *n* : a person who analyzes elements and compounds using a mass spectrometer or a mass spectrograph

mass spectroscopy *n* : MASS SPECTROMETRY — **mass spectroscopic** *adj* — **mass spectroscopically** *adv*

mass spectrum *n* : the spectrum of a stream of gaseous ions separated according to their mass and charge

MAST *abbr* military antishock trousers

Mas·tad·e·no·vi·rus \ma-'stad-ə-nō-,vī-rəs\ *n* : a genus of double-stranded DNA viruses of the family *Adenoviridae*

that infect only mammals and include the causative agents of epidemic keratoconjunctivitis and pharyngoconjunctival fever

mas·tal·gia \mas-'tal-jə\ *n* : MASTODYNIA

mast cell \'mast-\ *n* : a granulocyte that occurs esp. in connective tissue and has basophilic granules containing substances (as histamine and heparin) which mediate allergic reactions

mas·tec·to·mee \ma-ˌstek-tə-'mē\ *n* : an individual who has had a mastectomy

mas·tec·to·my \ma-'stek-tə-mē\ *n, pl* **-mies** : surgical removal of all or part of the breast and sometimes associated lymph nodes and muscles — see MODIFIED RADICAL MASTECTOMY, PARTIAL MASTECTOMY, RADICAL MASTECTOMY, SIMPLE MASTECTOMY

mas·ter gland \'mas-tər-\ *n* : PITUITARY GLAND

mas·tic \'mas-tik\ *n* : an aromatic resinous exudation obtained usu. in the form of yellowish to greenish lustrous transparent brittle tears from incisions in a small southern European tree (*Pistacia lentiscus*) of the sumac family and used chiefly in varnishes (as for lining dental cavities)

mas·ti·cate \'mas-tə-ˌkāt\ *vb* **-cat·ed; -cat·ing** *vt* **1** : to grind, crush, and chew (food) with or as if with the teeth in preparation for swallowing **2** : to soften or reduce to pulp by crushing or kneading ~ *vi* : to make the motions involved in masticating food — **mas·ti·ca·tion** \ˌmas-tə-'kā-shən\ *n*

¹**mas·ti·ca·to·ry** \'mas-ti-kə-ˌtōr-ē, -ˌtȯr-\ *adj* **1** : used for or adapted to chewing ⟨the ~ muscles⟩ **2** : of, relating to, or involving the organs of mastication ⟨~ paralysis⟩

²**masticatory** *n, pl* **-ries** : a substance chewed to increase saliva

Mas·ti·goph·o·ra \ˌmas-tə-'gäf-ə-rə\ *n pl* : a subphylum of protozoans comprising forms typically having one or more flagella and reproducing asexually usu. by binary fission — **mas·ti·goph·o·ran** \-rən\ *adj or n*

mas·tit·ic \ma-'stit-ik\ *adj* : of, relating to, or associated with mastitis ⟨~ milk⟩

mas·ti·tis \ma-'stīt-əs\ *n, pl* **-tit·i·des** \-'tit-ə-ˌdēz\ : inflammation of the mammary gland or udder usu. caused by infection — called also *mammitis;* see BLUE BAG, BOVINE MASTITIS, GARGET, SUMMER MASTITIS

mas·to·cyte \'mas-tə-ˌsīt\ *n* : MAST CELL

mas·to·cy·to·gen·e·sis \ˌmas-tə-ˌsīt-ə-'jen-ə-səs\ *n, pl* **-e·ses** \-ˌsēz\ : the formation of mast cells — **mas·to·cy·to·ge·net·ic** \-jə-'net-ik\ *adj*

mas·to·cy·to·ma \ˌmas-tə-ˌsī-'tō-mə\ *n, pl* **-mas** *also* **-ma·ta** \-mət-ə\ : a tumorous mass produced by proliferation of mast cells

mas·to·cy·to·sis \-'tō-səs\ *n, pl* **-to·ses** \-ˌsēz\ : excessive proliferation of mast cells in the tissues

mas·to·dyn·ia \ˌmas-tə-'dī-nē-ə\ *n* : pain in the breast — called also *mastalgia*

mas·tog·ra·phy \ma-'stäg-rə-fē\ *n, pl* **-phies** : MAMMOGRAPHY

¹**mas·toid** \'mas-ˌtȯid\ *adj* : of, relating to, or being the mastoid process; *also* : occurring in the region of the mastoid process

²**mastoid** *n* : a mastoid bone or process

mastoid air cell *n* : MASTOID CELL

mas·toi·dal \ma-'stȯid-ᵊl\ *adj* : MASTOID

mas·toi·da·le \ˌmas-ˌtȯid-'ā-lē\ *n* : the lowest point of the mastoid process

mastoid antrum *n* : TYMPANIC ANTRUM

mastoid cell *n* : one of the small cavities in the mastoid process that develop after birth and are filled with air — called also *mastoid air cell*

mas·toid·ec·to·my \ˌmas-ˌtȯid-'ek-tə-mē\ *n, pl* **-mies** : surgical removal of the mastoid cells or of the mastoid process of the temporal bone

mas·toid·itis \ˌmas-ˌtȯid-'īt-əs\ *n, pl* **-it·i·des** \-'it-ə-ˌdēz\ : inflammation of the mastoid and esp. of the mastoid cells

mas·toid·ot·o·my \ˌmas-ˌtȯid-'ät-ə-mē\ *n, pl* **-mies** : incision of the mastoid

mastoid process *n* : the process of the temporal bone be-

hind the ear that is well developed and of somewhat conical form in adults but inconspicuous in children

mas·to·mys \'mas-tə-ˌmis\ *n* **1** *cap, in some classifications* : a genus of rodents comprising the multimammate mice **2** *pl* **mastomys** : MULTIMAMMATE MOUSE

mas·top·a·thy \ma-'stäp-ə-thē\ *n, pl* **-thies** : a disorder of the breast; *esp* : a painful disorder of the breast

mas·to·pexy \'mas-tō-ˌpek-sē, 'mas-tə-\ *n, pl* **-pex·ies** : BREAST LIFT

mas·tot·o·my \ma-'stät-ə-mē\ *n, pl* **-mies** : incision of the breast

mas·tur·bate \'mas-tər-ˌbāt\ *vb* **-bat·ed; -bat·ing** *vi* : to practice masturbation ~ *vt* : to practice masturbation on — **mas·tur·ba·tor** \-ˌbāt-ər\ *n*

mas·tur·bat·ic \ˌmas-tər-'bat-ik\ *adj* : involving masturbation

mas·tur·ba·tion \ˌmas-tər-'bā-shən\ *n* : erotic stimulation esp. of one's own genital organs commonly resulting in orgasm and achieved by manual or other bodily contact exclusive of sexual intercourse, by instrumental manipulation, occas. by sexual fantasies, or by various combinations of these agencies

mas·tur·ba·to·ry \'mas-tər-bə-ˌtōr-ē, -ˌtȯr-\ *adj* : of, relating to, or associated with masturbation ⟨~ fantasies⟩

¹**mat** *or* **matt** *or* **matte** \'mat\ *adj* **1** : lacking or deprived of luster or gloss : having a usu. smooth even surface free from shine or highlights **2** : having a coarse rough rugose or granular surface ⟨bacteria that form ~ colonies on agar⟩

²**mat** *n* : a mat colony of bacteria

mate *vb* **mated; mat·ing** *vt* : to pair or join for breeding ~ *vi* : COPULATE

ma·té *or* **ma·te** \'mä-ˌtā\ *n* **1** : an aromatic beverage used chiefly in So. America and esp. in Paraguay that has stimulant properties like those of coffee **2** : a So. American holly (*Ilex paraguayensis*) whose leaves and shoots are used in making maté; *also* : these leaves and shoots

mater — see DURA MATER, PIA MATER

ma·te·ria al·ba \mə-ˌtir-ē-ə-'al-bə\ *n pl* : a soft whitish deposit of epithelial cells, white blood cells, and microorganisms esp. at the gumline

ma·te·ria med·i·ca \mə-ˌtir-ē-ə-'med-i-kə\ *n* **1** : substances used in the composition of medical remedies : DRUGS, MEDICINE **2 a** : a branch of medical science that deals with the sources, nature, properties, and preparation of drugs **b** : a treatise on materia medica

ma·ter·nal \mə-'tərn-ᵊl\ *adj* **1** : of, relating to, belonging to, or characteristic of a mother ⟨~ instinct⟩ **2 a** : related through a mother ⟨his ~ aunt⟩ **b** : inherited or derived from the female parent ⟨~ genes⟩ — **ma·ter·nal·ly** \-ᵊl-ē\ *adv*

maternal inheritance *n* : matroclinous inheritance; *specif* : inheritance of characters transmitted through extranuclear elements (as mitochondrial DNA) in the cytoplasm of the egg

maternal rubella *n* : German measles in a pregnant woman that may cause developmental anomalies in the fetus when occurring during the first trimester

¹**ma·ter·ni·ty** \mə-'tər-nət-ē\ *n, pl* **-ties** : a hospital facility designed for the care of women before and during childbirth and for the care of newborn babies

²**maternity** *adj* **1** : being or providing care during and immediately before and after childbirth ⟨~ care⟩ ⟨a ~ unit⟩ **2** : designed for wear during pregnancy ⟨~ clothes⟩ **3** : effective for the period close to and including childbirth ⟨~ leave⟩

ma·ter·no·fe·tal *or chiefly Brit* **ma·ter·no·foe·tal** \me-ˌtər-nō-'fēt-ᵊl\ *adj* : involving a fetus and its mother ⟨the human ~ interface⟩

\ə\ **abut** \ᵊ\ **kitten** \ər\ **further** \a\ **ash** \ā\ **ace** \ä\ **cot, cart**
\aȯ\ **out** \ch\ **chin** \e\ **bet** \ē\ **easy** \g\ **go** \i\ **hit** \ī\ **ice** \j\ **job**
\ŋ\ **sing** \ō\ **go** \ȯ\ **law** \ȯi\ **boy** \th\ **thin** \t̲h̲\ **the** \ü\ **loot**
\ u̇\ **foot** \y\ **yet** \zh\ **vision** *See also* Pronunciation Symbols page

M

N

ma·ti·co \mə-'tē-(ˌ)kō\ *n* **1** : a shrubby tropical wild American pepper (*Piper angustifolium*) with slender elongated aromatic leaves that are rich in volatile oil, gums, and tannins **2** : the leaves of the matico used esp. formerly in medicine chiefly as a stimulant and hemostatic

mat·ing \'māt-iŋ\ *n* **1** : the act of pairing or matching esp. sexually **2** : the period during which a seasonally breeding animal is capable of mating

mating group *n* : a sexually reproducing group in which mating within the group is favored at the expense of mating outside the group — called also *mating isolate*

mating type *n* : a strain or clone or other isolate made up of organisms (as certain fungi or protozoans) incapable of sexual reproduction with one another but capable of such reproduction with members of other strains of the same organism and often capable of behaving as male in respect to one strain and as female in respect to another — see MINUS, PLUS

ma·tri·cal \'mā-tri-kəl\ *adj* : of or relating to a matrix

mat·ri·car·ia \ˌma-trə-'kar-ē-ə\ *n* **1** *cap* : a genus of chiefly Old World aromatic herbs (family Compositae) that have heads with white ray flowers and yellow disk flowers and include one (*M. recutita*) that is a source of chamomile **2** *pl* **matricaria** *or* **matricarias** : any plant of the genus *Matricaria*

ma·tri·cide \'ma-trə-ˌsīd, 'mā-\ *n* **1** : murder of a mother by her son or daughter **2** : one that murders his or her mother

mat·ri·cli·nous \ˌma-trə-'klī-nəs\ *adj* : MATROCLINOUS

ma·tri·lin·eal \ˌma-trə-'lin-ē-əl, ˌmā-\ *adj* : relating to, based on, or tracing descent through the maternal line ⟨a ~ society⟩

ma·trix \'mā-triks\ *n, pl* **ma·tri·ces** \'mā-trə-ˌsēz *also* 'ma-\ *or* **matrixes** **1 a** : the extracellular substance in which tissue cells (as of connective tissue) are embedded ⟨mineralization of bone ~⟩ **b** : the thickened epithelium at the base of a fingernail or toenail from which new nail substance develops — called also *nail bed, nail matrix* **2** : something (as a surrounding or pervading substance or element) within which something else originates or takes form or develops **3** : a mass by which something is enclosed or in which something is embedded ⟨membrane-bound organelles suspended in the cytoplasmic ~⟩ ⟨chromatin fibers attach to the nuclear ~⟩ **4 a** : a strip or band placed so as to serve as a retaining outer wall of a tooth in filling a cavity **b** : a metal or porcelain pattern in which an inlay is cast or fused **5** : the substrate on or within which a fungus grows

mat·ro·cli·nal \ˌma-trə-'klī-nᵊl\ *adj* : MATROCLINOUS

mat·ro·clin·ic \ˌma-trə-'klin-ik\ *adj* : MATROCLINOUS

mat·ro·cli·nous \ˌma-trə-'klī-nəs\ *adj* : derived or inherited from the mother or maternal line — see MATERNAL INHERITANCE; compare PATROCLINOUS

mat·ro·cli·ny \'ma-trə-ˌklī-nē\ *n, pl* **-nies** : the quality or state of being matroclinous

ma·tron \'mā-trən\ *n, Brit* : a woman superintendent of a medical institution (as a hospital)

matt *or* **matte** *var of* ¹MAT

mat·ter \'mat-ər\ *n* **1** : material (as feces or urine) discharged or for discharge from the living body ⟨an obstruction interfering with passage of ~ from the intestine⟩ **2** : material discharged by suppuration : PUS

mat·tery \'mat-ə-rē\ *adj* : producing or containing pus or material resembling pus ⟨eyes all ~⟩

mat·toid \'mat-ȯid\ *n* : a borderline psychopath

mat·tress suture \'ma-trəs-\ *n* : a surgical stitch in which the suture is passed back and forth through both edges of a wound so that the needle is reinserted each time on the side of exit and passes through to the side of insertion — called also *mattress stitch*

mat·u·rate \'mach-ə-ˌrāt\ *vb* **-rat·ed; -rat·ing** : MATURE

mat·u·ra·tion \ˌmach-ə-'rā-shən\ *n* **1 a** : the process of becoming mature **b** : the emergence of personal and behavioral characteristics through growth processes **c** : the final stages of differentiation of cells, tissues, or organs **d** : the achievement of intellectual or emotional maturity **2 a** : the

entire process by which diploid gamete-producing cells are transformed into haploid gametes that includes both meiosis and physiological and structural changes fitting the gamete for its future role **b** : SPERMIOGENESIS 2 — **ma·tur·a·tive** \mə-'t(y)ùr-ət-iv\ *adj*

mat·u·ra·tion·al \-əl\ *adj* : of, relating to, or involved in maturation ⟨~ changes⟩ — **mat·u·ra·tion·al·ly** *adv*

maturation division *n* : a meiotic division

maturation factor *n* : VITAMIN B₁₂

maturation promoting factor *n* : a protein complex that in its active form causes eukaryotic cells to undergo mitosis — abbr. *MPF*

¹**ma·ture** \mə-'t(y)ù(ə)r *also* -'chù(ə)r\ *adj* **ma·tur·er; -est** **1** : having completed natural growth and development ⟨a ~ ovary⟩ **2** : having undergone maturation ⟨~ germ cells⟩

²**mature** *vb* **ma·tured; ma·tur·ing** *vt* : to bring to maturity or completion ~ *vi* : to become fully developed or ripe — **ma·tur·er** *n*

ma·tu·ri·ty \mə-'t(y)ùr-ət-ē *also* -'chùr-\ *n, pl* **-ties** : the quality or state of being mature; *esp* : full development

maturity–onset diabetes *n* : TYPE 2 DIABETES

maturity–onset diabetes of the young *n* : type 2 diabetes of a relatively mild form that is inherited as an autosomal dominant trait and occurs in late adolescence or early adulthood — abbr. *MODY*

Mau·me·né test \ˌmō-mə-'nā-\ *n* : a test for determining the degree of unsaturation of a fatty oil by observing the rise in temperature produced when concentrated sulfuric acid is added to the oil

Mau·me·né \mō-mə-nā\, **Edmé Jules (1818–1891)**, French chemist. A professor of chemistry, Maumené wrote several general textbooks on chemistry, a number of full-length works on fermentation, wine, and winemaking, and many essays on hydrates and manganese. In 1850 he developed a test to detect the presence of sugar in various liquids.

Mau·rer's dots \'maùr-ərz-\ *n pl* : coarse granulations present in red blood cells invaded by the falciparum malaria parasite — compare SCHÜFFNER'S DOTS

Maurer, Georg (*b* 1909), German physician.

maw·worm \'mȯ-ˌwərm\ *n* : a parasitic worm of the stomach or intestine; *esp* : a parasitic nematode

max *abbr* maximum

Max·ib·o·lin \mak-'sib-ə-lin, ˌmak-si-'bō-lən\ *trademark* — used for a preparation of ethylestrenol

max·il·la \mak-'sil-ə\ *n, pl* **max·il·lae** \-'sil-(ˌ)ē, -ˌī\ *or* **maxillas** **1** : JAW 1a **2 a** : an upper jaw esp. of humans or other mammals in which the bony elements are closely fused **b** : either of two membrane bone elements of the upper jaw that lie lateral to the premaxillae and that in higher vertebrates including humans bear most of the teeth **3** : one of the first or second pair of mouthparts posterior to the mandibles in insects, myriopods, crustaceans and closely related arthropods

¹**max·il·lary** \'mak-sə-ˌler-ē, *chiefly Brit* mak-'sil-ə-rē\ *adj* : of, relating to, being, or associated with a maxilla ⟨~ teeth⟩ ⟨~ sinusitis⟩

²**maxillary** *n, pl* **-lar·ies** **1** : MAXILLA 2b **2** : a maxillary part (as a nerve or blood vessel)

maxillary air sinus *n* : MAXILLARY SINUS

maxillary artery *n* : an artery supplying the deep structures of the face (as the nasal cavities, palate, tonsils, and pharynx) and sending a branch to the meninges of the brain — called also *internal maxillary artery;* compare FACIAL ARTERY

maxillary bone *n* : MAXILLA 2b

maxillary nerve *n* : the one of the three major branches or divisions of the trigeminal nerve that supplies sensory fibers to the skin areas of the middle part of the face, the upper jaw and its teeth, and the mucous membranes of the palate, nasal cavities, and nasopharynx — called also *maxillary division, superior maxillary nerve;* compare MANDIBULAR NERVE, OPHTHALMIC NERVE

maxillary process *n* : a triangular embryonic process that grows out from the dorsal end of the mandibular arch on each side and forms the lateral part of the upper lip, the cheek, and the upper jaw except the premaxilla

maxillary sinus *n* : an air cavity in the body of the maxilla that communicates with the middle meatus of the nose — called also *antrum of Highmore*

maxillary vein *n* : a short venous trunk of the face that is formed by the union of veins from the pterygoid plexus and that joins with the superficial temporal vein to form a vein which contributes to the formation of the external jugular vein

max·il·lec·to·my \ˌmak-sə-ˈlek-tə-mē\ *n, pl* **-mies** : surgical removal of the maxilla

max·il·lo·al·ve·o·lar index \mak-ˌsil-(ˌ)ō-al-ˈvē-ə-lər-, ˌmak-sə-(ˌ)lō-\ *n* : the ratio multiplied by 100 of the distance between the most lateral points on the external border of opposite sides of the alveolar arch to its length

max·il·lo·fa·cial \-ˈfā-shəl\ *adj* : of, relating to, treating, or affecting the maxilla and the face ⟨∼ surgery⟩

¹**max·il·lo·tur·bi·nal** \-ˈtər-bə-nəl\ *adj* : of or relating to the maxilla and the inferior nasal concha

²**maxilloturbinal** *n* : NASAL CONCHA a

max·i·mal \ˈmak-s(ə-)məl\ *adj* **1** : most complete or effective ⟨∼ dental protection⟩ ⟨∼ vasodilation⟩ **2** : being an upper limit ⟨the ∼ levels achieved with subcutaneous injections —W. S. Hoffman⟩ — **max·i·mal·ly** \-ē\ *adv*

maximal oxygen consumption *or* **maximum oxygen consumption** *n* : VO₂ MAX

maximal oxygen uptake *or* **maximum oxygen uptake** *n* : VO₂ MAX

max·i·mum \ˈmak-s(ə-)məm\ *n, pl* **max·i·ma** \-sə-mə\ *or* **maximums 1 a** : the greatest quantity or value attainable or attained **b** : the period of highest, greatest, or utmost development **2** : an upper limit allowed (as by a legal authority) or allowable (as by the circumstances of a particular case) — **maximum** *adj*

maximum dose *n* : the largest dose of a medicine or drug consistent with safety

maximum heart rate *n* : the age-related number of beats per minute of the heart when working at its maximum that is usu. estimated as 220 minus one's age ⟨reached 90 percent of his *maximum heart rate* when tested on a treadmill⟩

maximum per·mis·si·ble concentration \-pər-ˈmis-ə-bəl-\ *n* : the maximum concentration of radioactive material in body tissue that is regarded as acceptable and not producing significant deleterious effects on the human organism — abbr. *MPC*

maximum permissible dose *n* : the amount of ionizing radiation a person may be exposed to supposedly without being harmed

maximus — see GLUTEUS MAXIMUS

max VO₂ *n* : VO₂ MAX

max·well \ˈmak-swel\ *n* : the cgs electromagnetic unit of magnetic flux equal to the flux per square centimeter of normal cross section in a region where the magnetic induction is one gauss : 10⁻⁸ weber

  Maxwell, James Clerk (1831–1879), British physicist. Maxwell is ranked as the foremost physical scientist of the 19th century. His greatest achievement was the synthesis of the contributions of Faraday, Gauss, and Ampère into a single coherent electromagnetic theory. Of his several academic appointments the most important was the post of professor of experimental physics at Cambridge. He made contributions of fundamental importance to many branches of physics. The maxwell, a unit of magnetic flux, was named in his honor.

Max·zide \ˈmak(s)-ˌzīd\ *trademark* — used for a preparation of triamterene and hydrochlorothiazide

may·ap·ple \ˈmā-ˌap-ᵊl\ *n, often cap* **1** : a No. American herb of the genus *Podophyllum* (*P. peltatum*) having a poisonous rootstock and rootlets that are a source of the drug podophyllum **2** : the yellow egg-shaped edible but often tasteless fruit of the mayapple

Ma·ya·ro virus \mä-ˈyä-rō-\ *n* : a So. American togavirus of the genus *Alphavirus* (species *Mayaro virus*) that is the causative agent of a febrile disease

May–Grün·wald stain \ˈmā-ˈgrün-wöld-\ *n* : a stain for blood consisting of a saturated solution of eosin in methylene blue added to methyl alcohol — called also *Jenner's stain*

  May \ˈmī\, **Richard (1863–1936),** and **Grünwald** \ˈgrün-ˌvält\, **Ludwig (b 1863),** German physicians. May and Grünwald introduced their staining solution in an article published in 1902.

may·hem \ˈmā-ˌhem, ˈmā-əm\ *n* : willful and permanent crippling, mutilation, or disfiguring of any part of another's body; *also* : the crime of engaging in mayhem ⟨physicians, accused . . . of sterilizing her through trickery, were ordered held for trial on charges of conspiracy to commit ∼ —*Associated Press*⟩

may·tan·sine \ˈmā-ˌtan-ˌsēn\ *n* : an antineoplastic agent C₃₄H₄₆ClN₃O₁₀ isolated from several members of a genus (*Maytenus* of the family Celastraceae) of tropical American shrubs and trees

maze \ˈmāz\ *n* : a path complicated by at least one blind alley and used in learning experiments and in intelligence tests

ma·zin·dol \ˈmā-zin-ˌdōl\ *n* : an adrenergic drug C₁₆H₁₃ClN₂O used as an appetite suppressant

ma·zo·pla·sia \ˌmā-zə-ˈplā-zh(ē-)ə\ *n* : a degenerative condition of breast tissue

Maz·zi·ni test \mə-ˈzē-nē-\ *n* : a flocculation test for the diagnosis of syphilis

  Mazzini, Louis Yolando (1894–1973), American serologist. Mazzini began his career in medical research as a serologist in the department of bacteriology and pathology at Indiana University. Later he served for a number of years as chief of serology and bacteriology at the Indiana board of health. In 1947 he founded his own serodiagnostic laboratory that specialized in blood tests for syphilis. At the same time he was also on the faculty of the medical school at Indiana University. Starting in 1933 he began developing his own flocculation test for syphilis after experimenting with the Wassermann and other tests. The test that he developed possessed greater specificity and sensitivity than the others, especially in early and latent syphilis and neurosyphilis.

MB *abbr* [New Latin *medicinae baccalaureus*] bachelor of medicine

M band \ˈem-ˌband\ *n* : M LINE

mbar *abbr* millibar

MBC *abbr* minimal bactericidal concentration; minimum bactericidal concentration

MBD *abbr* minimal brain dysfunction

MBP *abbr* **1** major basic protein **2** myelin basic protein

mc *abbr* **1** megacycle **2** millicurie

MC *abbr* **1** medical corps **2** [New Latin *magister chirurgiae*] master of surgery

Mc·Ar·dle's disease \mək-ˈärd-ᵊlz-\ *n* : glycogen storage disease that is inherited as an autosomal recessive trait, is marked esp. by muscle weakness and myoglobinuria, and is caused by deficiency of a phosphorylase normally present in skeletal muscle — called also *McArdle's syndrome*

  McArdle, Brian (1911–2002), British physician. McArdle served on the staff of the department of chemical pathology at a London hospital. He was the author of articles on diseases of the muscle. In 1951 he published a paper on myopathy due to a defect in muscle glycogen breakdown. His report was based on the study of a 30-year-old male who had had the disease since childhood.

MCAT *abbr* Medical College Admissions Test

Mc·Bur·ney's point \mək-ˈbər-nēz-\ *n* : a point on the abdominal wall that lies between the navel and the right anterior superior iliac spine and that is the point where most pain is elicited by pressure in acute appendicitis

M
N

\ə\ **abut** \ᵊ\ **kitten** \ər\ **further** \a\ **ash** \ā\ **ace** \ä\ **cot, cart**
\aù\ **out** \ch\ **chin** \e\ **bet** \ē\ **easy** \g\ **go** \i\ **hit** \ī\ **ice** \j\ **job**
\ŋ\ **sing** \ō\ **go** \ò\ **law** \òi\ **boy** \th\ **thin** \t̲h̲\ **the** \ü\ **loot**
\ù\ **foot** \y\ **yet** \zh\ **vision** *See also* Pronunciation Symbols page

McBurney, Charles (1845–1913), American surgeon. A pioneer in the diagnosis and treatment of appendicitis, McBurney first described the pressure point used in the diagnosis of appendicitis in 1889. It was subsequently named in his honor.

mcg *abbr* microgram

MCh *abbr* [New Latin *magister chirurgiae*] master of surgery

MCH *abbr* **1** maternal and child health **2** mean corpuscular hemoglobin (concentration)

MCHC *abbr* mean corpuscular hemoglobin concentration

mCi *abbr* millicurie

MCL \ˌem-(ˌ)sē-ˈel\ *n* : MEDIAL COLLATERAL LIGAMENT

MCO \ˌem-(ˌ)sē-ˈō\ *n* : MANAGED CARE ORGANIZATION

M–CSF *abbr* macrophage colony-stimulating factor

MCV *abbr* mean corpuscular volume

Md *symbol* mendelevium

MD \ˌem-ˈdē\ *abbr or n* **1** [Latin *medicinae doctor*] : an earned academic degree conferring the rank and title of doctor of medicine **2** : a person who has a doctor of medicine

MD *abbr* **1** medical department **2** muscular dystrophy

MDA \ˌem-(ˌ)dē-ˈā\ *n* : a synthetic amphetamine derivative $C_{10}H_{13}NO_2$ used illicitly for its mood-enhancing and hallucinogenic properties — called also *methylenedioxyamphetamine*

MDI *abbr* metered-dose inhaler

MDMA \ˌem-(ˌ)dē-(ˌ)em-ˈā\ *n* : ECSTASY 2

MDR *abbr* minimum daily requirement

MDS *abbr* master of dental surgery

Me *abbr* methyl

ME *abbr* **1** medical examiner **2** myalgic encephalomyelitis

mea·dow mushroom \ˈmed-ˌō-\ *n* : a common edible agaric of the genus *Agaricus* (*A. campestris*) that occurs naturally in moist organically rich soil and is often cultivated

meal \ˈmē(ə)l\ *n* : the portion of food taken at one time to satisfy appetite

mean corpuscular hemoglobin concentration \ˈmēn-\ *n* : the number of grams of hemoglobin per unit volume and usu. 100 milliliters of packed red blood cells that is found by multiplying the number of grams of hemoglobin per unit volume of the original blood sample of whole blood by 100 and dividing by the hematocrit — abbr. *MCHC*

mean corpuscular volume *n* : the volume of the average red blood cell in a given blood sample that is found by multiplying the hematocrit by 100 and dividing by the estimated number of red blood cells — abbr. *MCV*

mean so·lar sec·ond \-ˌsō-lər-ˈsek-ənd, -ənt\ *n* : an mks unit of time equal to 1/86,400 of a mean solar day

mea·sle \ˈmē-zəl\ *n* : CYSTICERCUS; *specif* : one found in the muscles of a domesticated mammal

mea·sles \ˈmē-zəlz\ *n pl but sing or pl in constr* **1 a** : an acute contagious disease that is caused by a paramyxovirus of the genus *Morbillivirus* (species *Measles virus*), that commences with catarrhal symptoms, conjunctivitis, cough, and Koplik's spots on the oral mucous membrane, and that is marked by the appearance on the third or fourth day of an eruption of distinct red circular spots which coalesce in a crescentic form, are slightly raised, and after the fourth day of the eruption gradually decline — called also *rubeola* **b** : any of various eruptive diseases (as German measles) **2** : infestation with or disease caused by larval tapeworms in the muscles and tissues; *specif* : infestation of cattle and swine with cysticerci of tapeworms that as adults parasitize humans — compare MEASLE

mea·sly \ˈmēz-(ə-)lē\ *adj* **mea·sli·er; -est** **1** : infected with measles **2 a** : containing larval tapeworms **b** : infected with trichinae

mea·sur·able \ˈmezh-(ə-)rə-bəl, ˈmāzh-\ *adj* : capable of being measured ⟨such ∼ factors as the amount of nitrogen in air⟩; *specif* : large or small enough to be measured ⟨found in ∼ amounts⟩ ⟨∼ radiation⟩ — **mea·sur·ably** *adv*

¹**mea·sure** \ˈmezh-ər, ˈmāzh-\ *n* **1** : an instrument or utensil for measuring **2** : a standard or unit of measurement; *also* : a system of such measures ⟨metric ∼⟩

²**measure** *vb* **mea·sured; mea·sur·ing** \ˈmezh-(ə-)riŋ, ˈmāzh-\

vt **1** : to allot or apportion in measured amounts **2** : to ascertain the measurements of **3** : to serve as a measure of ⟨a thermometer ∼s temperature⟩ ∼ *vi* : to have a specified measurement

mea·sure·ment \ˈmezh-ər-mənt, ˈmāzh-\ *n* **1** : the act or process of measuring **2** : a figure, extent, or amount obtained by measuring **3** : MEASURE 2

me·a·tal \mē-ˈāt-ᵊl\ *adj* : of, relating to, or forming a meatus

me·ato·plas·ty \mē-ˈat-ə-ˌplast-ē\ *n, pl* **-ties** : plastic surgery of a meatus ⟨urethral ∼⟩

me·a·tot·o·my \ˌmē-ə-ˈtät-ə-mē\ *n, pl* **-mies** : incision of the urethral meatus esp. to enlarge it

me·atus \mē-ˈāt-əs\ *n, pl* **me·atus·es** \-ə-səz\ *or* **me·atus** \-ˈāt-əs, -ˈā-ˌtüs\ : a natural body passage : CANAL, DUCT

me·ban·a·zine \me-ˈban-ə-ˌzēn\ *n* : a monoamine oxidase inhibitor $C_8H_{12}N_2$ used as an antidepressant

Meb·a·ral \ˈmeb-ə-ˌral\ *trademark* — used for a preparation of mephobarbital

me·ben·da·zole \me-ˈbend-ə-ˌzōl\ *n* : a broad-spectrum anthelmintic agent $C_{16}H_{13}N_3O_3$

me·bu·ta·mate \me-ˈbyüt-ə-ˌmāt\ *n* : a central nervous system depressant $C_{10}H_{20}N_2O_4$ used to treat mild hypertension

mec·a·myl·a·mine \ˌmek-ə-ˈmil-ə-ˌmēn\ *n* : a drug administered orally in the form of its hydrochloride $C_{11}H_{21}N \cdot HCl$ as a ganglionic blocking agent to effect a rapid lowering of severely elevated blood pressure

Mec·ca balsam \ˈmek-ə-\ *n* : BALM OF GILEAD 2

me·chan·i·cal \mi-ˈkan-i-kəl\ *adj* **1** : relating to the quantitative relations of force and matter ⟨∼ pressure exerted by the bubbles in the tissues —H. G. Armstrong⟩ **2** : caused by, resulting from, or relating to physical as opposed to biological or chemical processes or change ⟨∼ injury⟩ ⟨∼ asphyxiation⟩ — **me·chan·i·cal·ly** \-i-k(ə-)lē\ *adv*

mechanical equivalent of heat *n* : the value of a unit quantity of heat in terms of mechanical work units with its most probable value in cgs measure being 4.1855×10^7 ergs per calorie — symbol *J;* called also *Joule's equivalent*

mechanical heart *n* : a mechanism designed to maintain the flow of blood to the tissues of the body esp. during a surgical operation on the heart

mechanical stage *n* : a stage on a compound microscope equipped with a mechanical device for moving a slide lengthwise and crosswise or for registering the slide's position by vernier for future exact repositioning

mechanical ventilation *n* : artificial ventilation of the lungs (as by positive end-expiratory pressure) using means external to the body ⟨the patient was sufficiently obtunded to require intubation and *mechanical ventilation* —Susan M. Pond *et al*⟩

me·chan·ics \mi-ˈkan-iks\ *n pl but sing or pl in constr* : a branch of physical science that deals with energy and forces and their effect on material bodies

mech·a·nism \ˈmek-ə-ˌniz-əm\ *n* **1** : a piece of machinery **2 a** : a bodily process or function ⟨the ∼ of healing⟩ **b** : the combination of mental processes by which a result is obtained ⟨psychological ∼s⟩ **3** : the fundamental physical or chemical processes involved in or responsible for an action, reaction, or other natural phenomenon — **mech·a·nis·tic** \ˌmek-ə-ˈnis-tik\ *adj*

mechanism of defense *n* : DEFENSE MECHANISM 1

mech·a·no·chem·is·try \ˌmek-ə-nō-ˈkem-ə-strē\ *n, pl* **-tries** : chemistry that deals with the conversion of chemical energy into mechanical work (as in the contraction of a muscle) — **mech·a·no·chem·i·cal** \-ˈkem-i-kəl\ *adj*

mech·a·no·re·cep·tor \-ri-ˈsep-tər\ *n* : a neural end organ (as a tactile receptor) that responds to a mechanical stimulus (as a change in pressure) — **mech·a·no·re·cep·tion** \-ˈsep-shən\ *n* — **mech·a·no·re·cep·tive** \-ˈsep-tiv\ *adj*

mech·a·no·sen·so·ry \-ˈsen(t)-sə-rē\ *adj* : of, relating to, or functioning in the sensing of mechanical stimuli ⟨∼ cells⟩ ⟨∼ neurons⟩

mech·a·no·ther·a·pist \-ˈther-ə-pəst\ *n* : a person who practices mechanotherapy

mech·a·no·ther·a·py \-'ther-ə-pē\ *n, pl* **-pies** : the treatment of disease by manual, physical, or mechanical means

mech·lor·eth·amine \ˌmek-ˌlōr-'eth-ə-ˌmēn, -ˌlòr-\ *n* : a nitrogen mustard administered by injection in the form of its hydrochloride $C_5H_{11}Cl_2N·HCl$ in the palliative treatment of neoplastic diseases (as Hodgkin's disease and leukemia)

mech·o·lyl \'mek-ə-ˌlil\ *n, often cap* : a preparation of the chloride of methacholine

Me·cis·to·cir·rus \mə-ˌsis-tō-'sir-əs\ *n* : a genus of nematode worms of the family Trichostrongylidae including a common parasite (*M. digitatus*) of the abomasum of domesticated ruminants and the stomach of swine in both of which it may cause serious loss of blood and digestive disturbances esp. in young animals

Meck·el–Gru·ber syndrome \'mek-əl-'grü-bər-\ *n* : a syndrome inherited as an autosomal recessive trait and typically characterized by occipital encephalocele, microcephaly, cleft palate, polydactyly, and polycystic kidneys — called also *Meckel's syndrome*

Meckel, Johann Friedrich, the Younger (1781–1833), German anatomist. One of the greatest anatomists of his time, Meckel, grandson of J. F. Meckel the Elder, made major contributions to comparative and pathological anatomy. Another major area of research for him was embryology. He presented the first detailed analysis of congenital malformations. From 1817 to 1826 he published the first systematic work on human abnormalities in general. A description of Meckel's cartilage was part of an 1805 treatise on comparative and human anatomy. Meckel's diverticulum was described in an 1809 article devoted to the subject. **Gruber, Georg Benno Otto (1884–1977),** German pathologist. A professor of medicine at Innsbruck and then at Göttingen, Gruber specialized in the study of deformities. Also known as a historian of medicine, he published works on the history of pathological anatomy and teratology. He also published studies on the concept of illness and on such specific diseases as polyarteritis nodosa.

Meck·el's cartilage \'mek-əlz-\ *n* : the cartilaginous bar of the embryonic mandibular arch of which the distal end ossifies to form the malleus and most of the rest disappears in development, with the part adjacent to the malleus being replaced by fibrous membrane comprising the sphenomandibular ligament and the connective tissue covering most of the remaining part ossifying to form much of the mandible

J. F. Meckel the Younger — see MECKEL-GRUBER SYNDROME

Meckel's cave *n* : a space beneath the dura mater containing the trigeminal ganglion — called also *Meckel's cavity*

Meckel, Johann Friedrich, the Elder (1724–1774), German anatomist. Meckel was an anatomist known for his considerable powers of observation and skill in preparing anatomical specimens. In 1748 he published a treatise in which he described the trigeminal nerve. This treatise also contained his description of the cavity containing the trigeminal ganglion, the space now known as Meckel's cave. A preliminary description of the ganglion now known as the pterygopalatine ganglion was included in this treatise, but a fuller treatment was presented the following year.

Meckel's diverticulum *n* : the proximal part of the omphalomesenteric duct when persistent as a blind fibrous tube connected with the lower ileum

J. F. Meckel the Younger — see MECKEL-GRUBER SYNDROME

Meckel's ganglion *n* : PTERYGOPALATINE GANGLION

J. F. Meckel the Elder — see MECKEL'S CAVE

mec·li·zine *or Brit* **mec·lo·zine** \'mek-lə-ˌzēn\ *n* : a drug used usu. in the form of its hydrated hydrochloride $C_{25}H_{27}ClN_2·2HCl·H_2O$ to treat nausea and vertigo — see ANTIVERT

mec·lo·fen·a·mate sodium \ˌmek-lō-'fen-ə-ˌmāt\ *n* : a mild analgesic and anti-inflammatory drug $C_{14}H_{10}Cl_2NNaO_2·H_2O$ used orally to treat rheumatoid arthritis and osteoarthritis — called also *meclofenamate*

mec·lo·fe·nam·ic acid \ˌmek-lō-fə-ˌnam-ik-\ *n* : an acid $C_{14}H_{11}Cl_2NO_2$ used as an anti-inflammatory agent

me·com·e·ter \mi-'käm-ət-ər\ *n* : an instrument for measuring a newborn child

meconate — see MORPHINE MECONATE

me·con·ic acid \mi-ˌkän-ik-\ *n* : a crystalline acid $C_7H_4O_7$ obtained from opium

mec·o·nin \'mek-ə-hən\ *also* **mec·o·nine** \-ˌnēn\ *n* : a crystalline lactone $C_{10}H_{10}O_4$ found in opium

me·co·ni·um \mi-'kō-nē-əm\ *n* : a dark greenish mass of desquamated cells, mucus, and bile that accumulates in the bowel of a fetus and is typically discharged shortly after birth

meconium ileus *n* : congenital intestinal obstruction by thickened viscous meconium that is often associated with cystic fibrosis of newborn infants

¹**med** \'med\ *adj* : MEDICAL ⟨∼ school⟩ ⟨∼ students⟩

²**med** *n* : MEDICATION 2 — usu. used in pl. ⟨giving out bedtime ∼s —Susanna Kaysen⟩

me·daz·e·pam \me-'daz-ə-ˌpam\ *n* : a drug used in the form of its hydrochloride $C_{16}H_{15}ClN_2·HCl$ esp. formerly as a tranquilizer

¹**med·e·vac** *also* **med·i·vac** \'med-ə-ˌvak\ *n* **1** : emergency evacuation of the sick or wounded (as from a combat area) **2** : a helicopter used for medevac

²**medevac** *vt* **-vacked; -vack·ing** : to transport in a medevac helicopter

¹**media** *pl of* MEDIUM

²**me·dia** \'mēd-ē-ə\ *n, pl* **me·di·ae** \-ē-ˌē\ : the middle coat of the wall of a blood or lymph vessel consisting chiefly of circular muscle fibers — called also *tunica media*

media — see AERO-OTITIS MEDIA, COLICA MEDIA, OTITIS MEDIA, SCALA MEDIA, SEROUS OTITIS MEDIA

me·di·ad \'mēd-ē-ˌad\ *adv* : toward the median line or plane of a body or part

me·di·al \'mēd-ē-əl\ *adj* **1** : lying or extending in the middle; *esp, of a body part* : lying or extending toward the median axis of the body ⟨the ∼ surface of the tibia⟩ **2** : of or relating to the media of a blood vessel ⟨necrosis and lipid deposition with ∼ involvement⟩ — **me·di·al·ly** \-ə-lē\ *adv*

medial accessory olivary nucleus *n* : ACCESSORY OLIVARY NUCLEUS b

medial angle of the eye *n* : the angle formed by the eyelids near the nose

medial arcuate ligament *n* : an arched band of fascia that covers the upper part of the psoas major muscle, extends from the body of the first or second lumbar vertebra to the transverse process of the first and sometimes also the second lumbar vertebra, and provides attachment for part of the lumbar portion of the diaphragm — compare LATERAL ARCUATE LIGAMENT

medial check ligament *n* : CHECK LIGAMENT 2b

medial collateral ligament *n* **1** : a ligament that connects the medial epicondyle of the femur with the medial condyle and medial surface of the tibia and that helps to stabilize the knee by preventing lateral dislocation — called also *MCL, tibial collateral ligament;* compare LATERAL COLLATERAL LIGAMENT **2** : ULNAR COLLATERAL LIGAMENT

medial condyle *n* : a condyle on the inner side of the lower extremity of the femur; *also* : a corresponding eminence on the upper part of the tibia that articulates with the medial condyle of the femur — compare LATERAL CONDYLE

medial cord *n* : a cord of nerve tissue that is continuous with the anterior division of the inferior trunk of the brachial plexus and that is one of the two roots forming the median nerve — compare LATERAL CORD, POSTERIOR CORD

medial cuneiform *n* : CUNEIFORM BONE 1a

medial cuneiform bone *n* : CUNEIFORM BONE 1a

medial epicondyle *n* : EPICONDYLE b

M

N

\ə\ abut \ᵊ\ kitten \ər\ further \a\ ash \ā\ ace \ä\ cot, cart
\aú\ out \ch\ chin \e\ bet \ē\ easy \g\ go \i\ hit \ī\ ice \j\ job
\ŋ\ sing \ō\ go \ò\ law \òi\ boy \th\ thin \t̲h̲\ the \ü\ loot
\ú\ foot \y\ yet \zh\ vision *See also* Pronunciation Symbols page

medial femoral circumflex artery *n* : an artery that branches from the deep femoral artery or from the femoral artery itself and that supplies the muscles of the medial part of the thigh and hip joint — compare LATERAL FEMORAL CIRCUMFLEX ARTERY

medial femoral circumflex vein *n* : a vein accompanying the medial femoral circumflex artery and emptying into the femoral vein or sometimes into one of its tributaries and corresponding to the deep femoral artery — compare LATERAL FEMORAL CIRCUMFLEX VEIN

medial forebrain bundle *n* : a prominent tract of nerve fibers that connects the subcallosal area of the cerebral cortex with the lateral areas of the hypothalamus and that has fibers passing to the tuber cinereum, the brain stem, and the mammillary bodies

medial geniculate body *n* : a part of the metathalamus consisting of a small oval tubercle situated between the pulvinar, colliculi, and cerebral peduncle that receives nerve impulses from the inferior colliculus and relays them to the auditory area — compare LATERAL GENICULATE BODY

medialis — see RECTUS MEDIALIS, VASTUS MEDIALIS

medial lemniscus *n* : a band of nerve fibers that transmits proprioceptive impulses from the spinal cord to the thalamus

medial longitudinal fasciculus *n* : any of four longitudinal bundles of white matter of which there are two on each side that extend from the midbrain to the upper parts of the spinal cord where they are located close to the midline ventral to the gray commissure and that are composed of fibers esp. from the vestibular nuclei

medial malleolus *n* : MALLEOLUS b

medial meniscus *n* : MENISCUS 2a(2)

medial pectoral nerve *n* : PECTORAL NERVE b

medial plantar artery *n* : PLANTAR ARTERY b

medial plantar nerve *n* : PLANTAR NERVE b

medial plantar vein *n* : PLANTAR VEIN b

medial popliteal nerve *n* : TIBIAL NERVE

medial pterygoid muscle *n* : PTERYGOID MUSCLE b

medial pterygoid nerve *n* : PTERYGOID NERVE b

medial pterygoid plate *n* : PTERYGOID PLATE b

medial rectus *n* : RECTUS 2c

medial semilunar cartilage *n* : MENISCUS 2a(2)

medial umbilical ligament *n* : a fibrous cord sheathed in peritoneum and extending from the pelvis to the navel that is a remnant of part of the umbilical artery in the fetus — called also *lateral umbilical ligament*

medial vestibular nucleus *n* : the one of the four vestibular nuclei on each side of the medulla oblongata that sends ascending fibers to the oculomotor and trochlear nuclei in the cerebrum on the opposite side of the brain and sends descending fibers down both sides of the spinal cord to synapse with motor neurons of the ventral horns

me·di·al·ward \ˈmēd-ē-əl-wərd\ *adj* : occurring or situated in a medial direction — **medialward** *adv*

¹**me·di·an** \ˈmēd-ē-ən\ *n* **1** : a medial part (as a vein or nerve) **2 a** : a value in an ordered set of values below and above which there is an equal number of values or which is the arithmetic mean of the two middle values if there is no one middle number **b** : a vertical line that divides the histogram of a frequency distribution into two parts of equal area

²**median** *adj* : situated in the middle; *specif* : lying in a plane dividing a bilateral animal into right and left halves

median antebrachial vein *n* : a vein that is usu. present in the forearm, that drains the plexus of veins in the palm of the hand, and that runs up the little-finger side of the forearm to join the median cubital vein or may divide into two branches to join the cephalic and basilic veins or may be missing as a recognizably distinct vessel

median arcuate ligament *n* : a tendinous arch that lies in front of the aorta and that connects the attachments of the lumbar portion of the diaphragm to the lumbar vertebrae on each side — compare LATERAL ARCUATE LIGAMENT

median cubital vein *n* : a continuation of the cephalic vein of the forearm that passes obliquely toward the inner side of

the arm in the bend of the elbow to join with the ulnar veins in forming the basilic vein and is often selected for venipuncture

median eminence *n* : a raised area in the floor of the third ventricle of the brain produced by the infundibulum of the hypothalamus

median lethal dose *n* : LD50

median nerve *n* : a nerve that arises by two roots from the brachial plexus and passes down the middle of the front of the arm

median nuchal line *n* : OCCIPITAL CREST a

median plane *n* : MIDSAGITTAL PLANE

median sacral crest *n* : SACRAL CREST a

median sacral vein *n* : an unpaired vein that accompanies the middle sacral artery and usu. empties into the left common iliac vein

median umbilical ligament *n* : a fibrous cord extending from the urinary bladder to the navel that is the remnant of the fetal urachus

mediastina *pl of* MEDIASTINUM

me·di·as·ti·nal \ˌmēd-ē-ə-ˈstī-nəl\ *adj* : of, relating to, or affecting the mediastinum ⟨∼ fibrosis⟩

me·di·as·ti·ni·tis \ˌmēd-ē-ˌas-tə-ˈnīt-əs\ *n, pl* **-nit·i·des** \-ˈnit-ə-ˌdēz\ : inflammation of the tissues of the mediastinum

me·di·as·ti·no·peri·car·di·tis \ˌmē-dē-ˌas-tə-(ˌ)nō-ˌper-ə-ˌkär-ˈdīt-əs\ *n, pl* **-dit·i·des** \-ˈdit-ə-ˌdēz\ : inflammation of the mediastinum and the pericardium

me·di·as·ti·no·scope \ˌmē-dē-as-ˈtin-ə-ˌskōp\ *n* : an endoscope used in mediastinoscopy

me·di·as·ti·nos·co·py \ˌmē-dē-ˌas-tə-ˈnäs-kə-pē\ *n, pl* **-pies** : examination of the mediastinum through an incision above the sternum

me·di·as·ti·not·o·my \-ˈnät-ə-mē\ *n, pl* **-mies** : surgical incision into the mediastinum

me·di·as·ti·num \ˌmēd-ē-ə-ˈstī-nəm\ *n, pl* **-na** \-nə\ **1** : the space in the chest between the pleural sacs of the chest that contains all the viscera of the chest except the lungs and pleurae; *also* : this space with its contents **2** : MEDIASTINUM TESTIS

mediastinum testis *n* : a mass of connective tissue at the back of the testis that is continuous externally with the tunica albuginea and internally with the interlobular septa and encloses the rete testis

¹**me·di·ate** \ˈmēd-ē-ət\ *adj* **1** : occupying a middle position **2** : acting through an intervening agency : exhibiting indirect causation, connection, or relation

²**me·di·ate** \ˈmēd-ē-ˌāt\ *vt* **-at·ed; -at·ing** : to transmit or carry (as a physical process or effect) as an intermediate mechanism or agency

mediate auscultation *n* : auscultation performed with the aid of a stethescope — compare IMMEDIATE AUSCULTATION

me·di·a·tion \ˌmēd-ē-ˈā-shən\ *n* : the act or process of mediating something (as a physical process) — **me·di·a·tion·al** \-shnəl, -shən-ᵊl\ *adj*

me·di·a·tor \ˈmēd-ē-ˌāt-ər\ *n* : one that mediates; *esp* : a mediating agent (as an enzyme or hormone) in a chemical or biological process ⟨substance P, a neuropeptide ∼ of analgesic stimuli in peripheral sensory nerves —D. R. Robinson⟩

me·di·a·to·ry \ˈmēd-ē-ə-ˌtōr-ē, -ˌtȯr-\ *adj* : of or relating to mediation

med·ic \ˈmed-ik\ *n* : a person engaged in medical work; *esp* : CORPSMAN

medica — see MATERIA MEDICA

med·i·ca·ble \ˈmed-i-kə-bəl\ *adj* : CURABLE, REMEDIABLE

Med·ic·aid \ˈmed-i-ˌkād\ *n* : a program of medical aid designed for those unable to afford regular medical service and financed jointly by the state and federal governments

¹**med·i·cal** \ˈmed-i-kəl\ *adj* **1** : of, relating to, or concerned with physicians or the practice of medicine often as distinguished from surgery **2** : requiring or devoted to medical treatment ⟨a ∼ emergency⟩ — **med·i·cal·ly** \-k(ə-)lē\ *adv*

²**medical** *n* : a medical examination

med·i·cal·ese \ˌmed-i-kə-ˈlēz\ *n* : the specialized terminology of the medical profession

medical examiner *n* **1** : a usu. appointed public officer with duties similar to those of a coroner but who is required to have specific medical training (as in pathology) and is qualified to conduct medical examinations and autopsies **2** : a physician employed to make medical examinations (as of applicants for military service or of claimants of workers' compensation) **3** : a physician appointed to examine and license candidates for the practice of medicine in a political jurisdiction (as a state)

med·i·cal·ize *or Brit* **med·i·cal·ise** \'med-ə-kə-ˌlīz\ *vt* **-ized** *or Brit* **-ised; -iz·ing** *or Brit* **-is·ing** : to view or treat as a medical concern, problem, or disorder ⟨those who seek to dispose of social problems by *medicalizing* them —Liam Hudson⟩ ⟨the Western model of *medicalized* birth . . . in order to reduce potential risk —Judith Fitzpatrick⟩ — **med·i·cal·iza·tion** *or Brit* **med·i·cal·isa·tion** \ˌmed-ə-kə-lə-'zā-shən\ *n*

medical jurisprudence *n* : FORENSIC MEDICINE

medical mall \-'mȯl\ *n* : a facility offering comprehensive ambulatory medical services (as primary and secondary care, diagnostic procedures, outpatient surgery, and rehabilitation) ⟨*medical malls* offering most services found in a hospital except the overnight beds —Joel Engelhardt⟩

medical psychology *n* : theories of personality and behavior not necessarily derived from academic psychology that provide a basis for psychotherapy in psychiatry and in general medicine — called also *medicopsychology*

medical record *n* : a record of a patient's medical information (as medical history, care or treatments received, test results, diagnoses, and medications taken)

medical transcriptionist *n* : a typist who transcribes dictated medical reports

me·di·ca·ment \mi-'dik-ə-mənt, 'med-i-kə-\ *n* : a substance used in therapy

medicamentosa — see RHINITIS MEDICAMENTOSA

med·i·ca·men·tous \mi-ˌdik-ə-'ment-əs, ˌmed-i-kə-\ *adj* : of, relating to, or caused by a medicament (as a drug) ⟨~ dermatitis⟩

med·i·cant \'med-i-kənt\ *n* : a medicinal substance

Medi·care \'med-i-ˌke(ə)r, -ˌka(ə)r\ *n* : a government program of medical care esp. for the elderly

med·i·cas·ter \'med-i-ˌkas-tər\ *n* : a medical charlatan : QUACK

med·i·cate \'med-ə-ˌkāt\ *vt* **-cat·ed; -cat·ing** **1** : to treat medicinally **2** : to impregnate with a medicinal substance ⟨*medicated* soap⟩

med·i·ca·tion \ˌmed-ə-'kā-shən\ *n* **1** : the act or process of medicating **2** : a medicinal substance : MEDICAMENT

¹**me·dic·i·nal** \mə-'dis-nəl, -ᵊn-əl\ *adj* : of, relating to, or being medicine : tending or used to cure disease or relieve pain — **me·dic·i·nal·ly** \-ē\ *adv*

²**medicinal** *n* : a medicinal substance : MEDICINE

medicinal leech *n* : a large European freshwater leech of the genus *Hirudo* (*H. medicinalis*) that is a source of hirudin, is now sometimes used to drain blood (as from a hematoma), and was formerly used to bleed patients thought to have excess blood

med·i·cine \'med-ə-sən, *Brit usu* 'med-sən\ *n* **1** : a substance or preparation used in treating disease **2 a** : the science and art dealing with the maintenance of health and the prevention, alleviation, or cure of disease **b** : the branch of medicine concerned with the nonsurgical treatment of disease

medicine cabinet *n* : MEDICINE CHEST

medicine chest *n* : a cupboard used esp. for storing medicines or first-aid supplies

medicine dropper *n* : DROPPER

medicine glass *n* : a small glass vessel graduated (as in ounces, drams, or milliliters) for measuring medicine

me·dic·i·ner \mə-'dis-ᵊn-ər, 'med-(ə-)sən-ər\ *n* : PHYSICIAN

med·i·co \'med-i-ˌkō\ *n, pl* **-cos** : a medical practitioner : PHYSICIAN; *also* : a medical student

med·i·co·le·gal \ˌmed-i-kō-'lē-gəl\ *adj* : of or relating to both medicine and law

med·i·co·psy·chol·o·gy \-sī-'käl-ə-ˌjē\ *n, pl* **-gies** : MEDICAL PSYCHOLOGY

med·i·gap \'med-ə-ˌgap\ *n, often attrib* : supplemental health insurance that covers costs (as of medical care or a hospital stay) not covered by Medicare ⟨~ coverage⟩ ⟨~ plans⟩

Me·di·na worm \mə-'dē-nə-\ *n* : GUINEA WORM

me·dio·car·pal \ˌmēd-ē-ō-'kär-pəl\ *adj* : located between the two rows of the bones of the carpus ⟨the ~ joint⟩

me·dio·lat·er·al \-'lat-ə-rəl, -'la-trəl\ *adj* : relating to, extending along, or being a direction or axis from side to side or from median to lateral — **me·dio·lat·er·al·ly** \-ē\ *adv*

me·dio·ne·cro·sis \-ni-'krō-səs\ *n, pl* **-cro·ses** \-ˌsēz\ : necrosis of the media of a blood vessel ⟨cystic ~ of the aorta⟩

Med·i·ter·ra·nean anemia \ˌmed-ə-tə-'rā-nē-ən-, -nyən-\ *n* : THALASSEMIA

Mediterranean fever *n* : any of several febrile conditions often endemic in parts of the Mediterranean region; *specif* : BRUCELLOSIS a

me·di·um \'mēd-ē-əm\ *n, pl* **mediums** *or* **me·dia** \-ē-ə\ **1** : a means of effecting or conveying something: as **a** : a substance regarded as the means of transmission of a force or effect **b** : a surrounding or enveloping substance **2** *pl media* **a** : a nutrient system for the artificial cultivation of cells or organisms and esp. bacteria **b** : a fluid or solid in which organic structures are placed (as for preservation or mounting)

medius — see CONSTRICTOR PHARYNGIS MEDIUS, GLUTEUS MEDIUS, PEDUNCULUS CEREBELLARIS MEDIUS, SCALENUS MEDIUS

medivac *var of* MEDEVAC

MED·LARS \'med-ˌlärz\ *service mark* — used for a computer system for the search and retrieval of biomedical abstracts and bibliographical information from various databases (as the MEDLINE database)

MED·LINE \'med-ˌlīn\ *service mark* — used for an online computer database of abstracts and references from biomedical journals that is searched by the MEDLARS system

med·ro·ges·tone \ˌmed-rō-'jes-ˌtōn\ *n* : a synthetic progestogen $C_{23}H_{32}O_2$ that has been used in the treatment of fibroid uterine tumors

Med·rol \'med-ˌrȯl\ *trademark* — used for a preparation of methylprednisolone

me·droxy·pro·ges·ter·one acetate \me-ˌdräk-sē-prō-'jes-tə-ˌrōn-\ *n* : a synthetic steroid progestational hormone $C_{24}H_{34}O_4$ that is used esp. in the treatment of amenorrhea and abnormal uterine bleeding, in conjunction with conjugated estrogens to relieve the symptoms of menopause and to prevent osteoporosis, and as an injectable contraceptive — called also *medroxyprogesterone;* see DEPO-PROVERA

meds *pl of* MED

me·dul·la \mə-'dəl-ə, -'dùl-\ *n, pl* **-las** *or* **-lae** \-(ˌ)ē, -ˌī\ **1** *pl* **medullae** **a** : BONE MARROW **b** : MEDULLA OBLONGATA **2 a** : the inner or deep part of an organ or structure ⟨the adrenal ~⟩ **b** : MYELIN SHEATH

medulla ob·lon·ga·ta \-ˌäb-ˌlȯŋ-'gät-ə\ *n, pl* **medulla oblongatas** *or* **medullae ob·lon·ga·tae** \-'gät-ē, -ˌgä-ˌtī\ : the somewhat pyramidal last part of the vertebrate brain developed from the posterior portion of the hindbrain and continuous posteriorly with the spinal cord, enclosing the fourth ventricle, and containing nuclei associated with most of the cranial nerves, major fiber tracts and decussations that link spinal with higher centers, and various centers mediating the control of involuntary vital functions (as respiration)

medullaris — see CONUS MEDULLARIS

med·ul·lary \'med-ᵊl-ˌer-ē, 'mej-ə-ˌler-ē; mə-'dəl-ə-rē\ *adj* **1 a** : of or relating to the medulla of any body part or organ **b** : containing, consisting of, or resembling bone marrow **c** : of or relating to the medulla oblongata or the spinal cord **d** : of, relating to, or formed of the dorsally located embryonic ectoderm destined to sink below the surface and be-

M
N

come neural tissue **2** : resembling bone marrow in consistency — used of cancers

medullary canal *n* : the marrow cavity of a bone

medullary cavity *n* : MEDULLARY CANAL

medullary cystic disease *n* : a progressive familial kidney disease that is characterized by renal medullary cysts and that manifests itself in anemia and uremia

medullary fold *n* : NEURAL FOLD

medullary groove *n* : NEURAL GROOVE

medullary nailing *n* : the fixing of a fractured long bone by inserting a steel nail into the marrow cavity of the bone

medullary plate *n* : the longitudinal dorsal zone of epiblast in the early vertebrate embryo that constitutes the primordium of the neural tissue

medullary sarcoma *n* : a sarcoma of extremely soft vascular consistency

medullary sheath *n* : MYELIN SHEATH

medullary velum *n* : a thin white plate of nervous tissue forming part of the roof of the fourth ventricle

medulla spi·na·lis \-ˌspī-'nā-ləs\ *n* : SPINAL CORD

med·ul·lat·ed \'med-ᵊl-ˌāt-əd, 'mej-ə-ˌlāt-\ *adj* **1** : MYELINATED **2** : having a medulla — used of fibers other than nerve fibers

med·ul·la·tion \ˌmed-ᵊl-'ā-shən, ˌmej-ə-'lā-\ *n* : the formation of a medullary sheath or medulla

med·ul·lec·to·my \ˌmed-ᵊl-'ek-tə-mē, ˌmej-ə-lek-\ *n, pl* **-mies** : surgical excision of a medulla (as of the adrenal glands)

me·dul·lin \me-'dəl-ən, 'med-ᵊl-in, 'mej-ə-lin\ *n* : a renal prostaglandin effective in reducing blood pressure

me·dul·lo·blast \mə-'dəl-ə-ˌblast, 'mej-ə-lə-\ *n* : a primitive undifferentiated nerve cell of the neural tube that is capable of developing into either a neuroblast or a spongioblast and that is found in medulloblastomas

me·dul·lo·blas·to·ma \mə-ˌdəl-ō-ˌblas-'tō-mə\ *n, pl* **-to·mas** *also* **-to·ma·ta** \-'tō-mət-ə\ : a malignant tumor of the central nervous system arising in the cerebellum esp. in children — **me·dul·lo·blas·to·ma·tous** \-'tō-mət-əs\ *adj*

mef·e·nam·ic acid \ˌmef-ə-ˌnam-ik-\ *n* : a drug $C_{15}H_{15}NO_2$ used as an anti-inflammatory and analgesic agent

mef·lo·quine \'mef-lə-ˌkwēn\ *n* : an antimalarial drug similar to quinine that is administered in the form of its hydrochloride $C_{17}H_{16}F_6N_2O \cdot HCl$ esp. for the prevention and treatment of falciparum malaria

meg *abbr* megacycle

mega·ce·phal·ic \ˌmeg-ə-sə-'fal-ik\ *adj* : large-headed; *specif* : having a cranial capacity in excess of the mean — **mega·ceph·a·ly** \-'sef-ə-lē\ *n, pl* **-lies**

mega·cin \'meg-ə-sin\ *n* : an antibacterial protein produced by some strains of a bacterium of the genus *Bacillus* (*B. megaterium*)

mega·co·lon \'meg-ə-ˌkō-lən\ *n* : extreme dilation of the colon that may be congenital or acquired — see HIRSCHSPRUNG'S DISEASE

mega·cu·rie \'meg-ə-ˌkyu̇r-ē, -kyu̇-'rē\ *n* : one million curies

mega·cy·cle \-ˌsī-kəl\ *n* : MEGAHERTZ

mega·dont \-ˌdänt\ *adj* : MACRODONT — **mega·don·ty** \-ˌdänt-ē\ *n, pl* **-ties**

mega·dose \-ˌdōs\ *n* : a large dose (as of a vitamin)

mega·dos·ing \-ˌdō-siŋ\ *n* : the administration of megadoses for therapy or prophylaxis

mega·du·o·de·num \ˌmeg-ə-ˌd(y)ü-ə-'dē-nəm; -d(y)u̇-'äd-ᵊn-əm\ *n, pl* **-de·na** \-'dē-nə; -ᵊn-ə\ *or* **-de·nums** : a congenital or acquired dilation and elongation of the duodenum with hypertrophy of all layers that presents as a feeling of gastric fullness, epigastric pain, belching, heartburn, and nausea with vomiting sometimes of food eaten 24 hours before

mega·esoph·a·gus *or chiefly Brit* **mega·oe·soph·a·gus** \-i-'säf-ə-gəs\ *n, pl* **-gi** \-ˌgī, -ˌjī\ : dilation and hypertrophy of the lower portion of the esophagus ⟨~ secondary to advanced achalasia —Suil Kim *et al*⟩

mega·hertz \'meg-ə-ˌhərts\ *n* : one million hertz — abbr. *MHz*

mega·kary·o·blast \ˌmeg-ə-'kar-ē-ō-ˌblast\ *n* : a large cell with large reticulate nucleus that gives rise to megakaryocytes

mega·kary·o·cyte \ˌmeg-ə-'kar-ē-ō-ˌsīt\ *n* : a large cell that has a lobulated nucleus, is found esp. in the bone marrow, and is the source of blood platelets — **mega·kary·o·cyt·ic** \-ō-ˌsit-ik\ *adj*

mega·lec·i·thal \-'les-ə-thəl\ *adj, of an egg* : containing very large amounts of yolk

meg·a·lo·blast \'meg-ə-lō-ˌblast\ *n* : a large erythroblast that appears in the blood esp. in pernicious anemia — **meg·a·lo·blas·tic** \ˌmeg-ə-lō-'blas-tik\ *adj*

megaloblastic anemia *n* : an anemia (as pernicious anemia) characterized by the presence of megaloblasts in the circulating blood

meg·a·lo·ceph·a·ly \ˌmeg-ə-lō-'sef-ə-lē\ *n, pl* **-lies** : largeness and esp. abnormal largeness of the head

meg·a·lo·cor·nea \-'kȯr-nē-ə\ *n* : abnormal largeness of the corneas

meg·a·lo·cyte \'meg-ə-lə-ˌsīt\ *n* : MACROCYTE — **meg·a·lo·cyt·ic** \ˌmeg-ə-lə-'sit-ik\ *adj*

meg·a·lo·ma·nia \ˌmeg-ə-lō-'mā-nē-ə, -nyə\ *n* : a delusional mental disorder that is marked by feelings of personal omnipotence and grandeur

meg·a·lo·ma·ni·ac \-'mā-nē-ˌak\ *n* : one affected with or exhibiting megalomania

meg·a·lo·ma·ni·a·cal \-mə-'nī-ə-kəl\ *or* **megalomaniac** *also* **meg·a·lo·man·ic** \-'man-ik\ *adj* : belonging to, exhibiting, or affected with megalomania ⟨ruled by a ~ tyrant⟩ — **meg·a·lo·ma·ni·a·cal·ly** \-ə-k(ə-)lē\ *adv*

mega·mol·e·cule \'meg-ə-ˌmäl-ə-ˌkyül\ *n* : an extremely large molecule

megaoesophagus *chiefly Brit var of* MEGAESOPHAGUS

mega·rad \'meg-ə-ˌrad\ *n* : one million rads — abbr. *Mrad*

mega·spore \'meg-ə-ˌspō(ə)r, -ˌspȯ(ə)r\ *n* **1** : a spore in heterosporous plants that gives rise to female gametophytes and is generally larger than a microspore **2** : MACROSPORE — **mega·spor·ic** \ˌmeg-ə-'spȯr-ik, -'spȯr-\ *adj*

mega·unit \-ˌyü-nət\ *n* : one million units

mega·vi·ta·min \-ˌvīt-ə-mən, *Brit usu* -ˌvit-\ *adj* : relating to or consisting of very large doses of vitamins and esp. doses many times greater than the Recommended Daily Allowances ⟨~ therapy⟩

mega·vi·ta·mins \-mənz\ *n pl* : a large quantity of vitamins

mega·volt \-ˌvōlt, -ˌvȯlt\ *n* : one million volts

mega·volt·age \-ˌvōl-tij\ *n, often attrib* : voltage greater than one megavolt ⟨the use of ~ radiotherapy in carcinoma of the lung —J. J. Stein⟩

mega·watt \'meg-ə-ˌwät\ *n* : one million watts — abbr. *MW*

me·ges·trol acetate \me-'jes-ˌtrȯl-\ *n* : a synthetic progestational hormone $C_{24}H_{32}O_4$ used in palliative treatment of advanced carcinoma of the breast and in endometriosis

meg·lu·mine \'meg-lù-ˌmēn, meg-'lü-\ *n* : a crystalline base $C_7H_{17}NO_5$ used to prepare salts used in radiopaque and therapeutic substances — see IODIPAMIDE

meg·ohm \'meg-ˌōm\ *n* : one million ohms

me·grim \'mē-grəm\ *n* **1 a** : MIGRAINE **b** : VERTIGO **2** : any of numerous diseases of animals marked by disturbance of equilibrium and abnormal gait and behavior — usu. used in pl.

Meh·lis' gland \'mā-lis-\ *n* : one of the large unicellular glands surrounding the ootype of a flatworm and possibly playing a part in eggshell formation; *also* : the group of such glands in a worm

Mehlis, Karl Friedrich Eduard (1796–1832), German physician. Mehlis was a practicing mine physician. His lasting contributions were in helminthology.

mei·bo·mian gland \mī-'bō-mē-ən-\ *n, often cap M* : one of the long sebaceous glands of the eyelids that discharge a fatty secretion which lubricates the eyelids — called also *tarsal gland;* see CHALAZION

Mei·bom \'mī-ˌbōm\, **Heinrich (1638–1700),** German physician. A professor of medicine at Helmstadt, Germany, Meibom accurately described the sebaceous glands of the eyelids in 1666. Although they are now identified with Meibom, the glands had been figured by the Italian anatomist Giulio Casserio (1561–1616) in 1609, and their existence has been known since the time of Galen.

mei·bo·mi·a·ni·tis \mī-₁bō-mē-ə-ˈnīt-əs\ *n* : inflammation of the meibomian glands

meio·cyte \ˈmī-ə-₁sīt\ *n* : a cell undergoing meiosis

mei·o·sis \mī-ˈō-səs\ *n, pl* **mei·o·ses** \-₁sēz\ : the cellular process that results in the number of chromosomes in gamete-producing cells being reduced to one half and that involves a reduction division in which one of each pair of homologous chromosomes passes to each daughter cell and a mitotic division — compare MITOSIS 1 — **mei·ot·ic** \mī-ˈät-ik\ *adj* — **mei·ot·i·cal·ly** \-i-k(ə-)lē\ *adv*

meio·stoma·tous \₁mī-ə-ˈstäm-ət-əs, -ˈstōm-\ *adj, of a larval nematode* : having the oral structures reduced or simplified as compared with related forms

meio·stome \ˈmī-ə-₁stōm\ *n* : a meiostomatous nematode

Meiss·ner's corpuscle \ˈmīs-nərz-\ *n* : any of the small elliptical tactile end organs in hairless skin containing numerous transversely placed tactile cells and fine flattened nerve terminations — called also *corpuscle of Meissner*

Meissner, Georg (1829–1905), German anatomist and physiologist. Meissner conducted in 1851 intensive comparative microscopic investigations on the fibers and cells of the common trunk of the vestibular and cochlear nerves. In 1852 he studied the tactile corpuscles of the skin which now bear his name. He published other papers dealing with the problems of microscopy, particularly those relating to the skin. In 1857 he published a description of the nerve plexus in the submucosa of the intestinal wall.

Meissner's plexus *n* : a plexus of ganglionated nerve fibers lying between the muscular and mucous coats of the intestine — compare MYENTERIC PLEXUS

meit·ner·i·um \mīt-ˈnir-ē-əm, -ˈner-\ *n* : a short-lived radioactive element that is artificially produced — symbol *Mt*; see ELEMENT table

Meit·ner \ˈmīt-nər, Lise (1878–1968),** German physicist. One of the first women to pursue a career in physics, Meitner received a PhD in the subject from the University of Vienna before being hired by Max Planck as an assistant at the Institute for Theoretical Physics at the University of Berlin. Beginning in 1918, she was head of the physics department at Berlin's Kaiser-Wilhelm Institut. With German physical chemist Otto Hahn, Meitner discovered an isotope of protactinium, the parent element of actinium, in 1918. With Hahn and Otto von Baeyer, she studied beta emissions from thorium, radium, and uranium, while conducting her own studies on the range of radioactive particles. Forced in 1938 to flee Berlin for Stockholm, she assumed a post at the Nobel Institute. With physicist O. R. Frisch, she became the first to realize that recent experiments by Hahn and others in which uranium had been bombarded with neutrons had resulted in the splitting of the uranium nucleus into two nuclei of smaller masses accompanied by the release of a massive amount of energy. In a 1939 paper they introduced the term *fission* for this nuclear process. After 1947 Meitner did her research at Sweden's Royal Institute for Technology and a laboratory at the Royal Academy for Engineering Sciences. In 1997 the International Union of Pure and Applied Chemistry formally approved *meitnerium* as the name for element 109.

Mek·er burn·er \ˈmek-ər-₁bər-nər\ *n* : a laboratory gas burner that differs from a typical Bunsen burner in having a constriction in the tube and a grid at the top of the burner causing the flame of burning gas to consist of a number of short blue inner cones and a large single outer cone and to be hotter generally than the flame of a Bunsen burner

Méker \ˈmā-kā(r)\, **Georges (*fl* 1897–1914),** French chemist. Méker introduced the Meker burner in an article published in 1909.

¹mel \ˈmel\ *n* : HONEY

²mel *n* : a subjective unit of tone pitch equal to ¹/₁₀₀₀ of the pitch of a tone having a frequency of 1000 hertz — used esp. in audiology

melaena *chiefly Brit var of* MELENA

mel·a·leu·ca \₁mel-ə-ˈl(y)ü-kə\ *n* **1** *cap* : a genus of Australian and southeast Asian trees and shrubs of the myrtle family (Myrtaceae) that includes the cajeput (*M. leucadendron*) **2** : any tree or shrub of the genus *Melaleuca*

mel·a·mine \ˈmel-ə-₁mēn\ *n* **1** : a white crystalline organic base $C_3H_6N_6$ with a high melting point that is used esp. in making resins by reaction with aldehydes **2** : a resin made from melamine or a plastic made from such a resin

melanaemia *chiefly Brit var of* MELANEMIA

mel·an·cho·lia \₁mel-ən-ˈkō-lē-ə\ *n* : a mental condition and esp. a manic-depressive condition characterized by extreme depression, bodily complaints, and often hallucinations and delusions

mel·an·cho·li·ac \-lē-₁ak\ *n* : one affected with melancholia

¹mel·an·chol·ic \₁mel-ən-ˈkäl-ik\ *adj* **1** : of, relating to, or subject to melancholy : DEPRESSED **2** : of or relating to melancholia

²melancholic *n* **1** : a melancholy person **2** : MELANCHOLIAC

mel·an·cho·lious \-ˈkō-lē-əs, -kōl-yəs\ *adj* : MELANCHOLIC

mel·an·choly \ˈmel-ən-₁käl-ē\ *n, pl* **-chol·ies** **1 a** : an abnormal state attributed to an excess of black bile and characterized by irascibility or depression **b** : BLACK BILE **c** : MELANCHOLIA **2** : depression or dejection of spirits — **melancholy** *adj*

mel·ane·mia *or chiefly Brit* **mel·anae·mia** \₁mel-ə-ˈnē-mē-ə\ *n* : an abnormal condition in which the blood contains melanin

Me·la·nia \me-ˈlā-nē-ə\ *n, syn of* THIARA

¹me·lan·ic \mə-ˈlan-ik\ *adj* **1** : MELANOTIC **2** : affected with or characterized by melanism

²melanic *n* : a melanic individual

mel·a·nif·er·ous \₁mel-ə-ˈnif-ə-rəs\ *adj, of a body structure* : containing black pigment

mel·a·nin \ˈmel-ə-nən\ *n* : any of various black, dark brown, reddish brown, or yellow pigments of animal or plant structures (as skin, hair, the choroid, or a raw potato when exposed to air); *esp* : any of numerous animal pigments that are essentially polymeric derivatives of indole formed by enzymatic modification of tyrosine

mel·a·nism \ˈmel-ə-₁niz-əm\ *n* **1** : an increased amount of black or nearly black pigmentation (as of skin, feathers, or hair) of an individual or kind of organism **2** : intense human pigmentation in skin, eyes, and hair — **mel·a·nis·tic** \₁mel-ə-ˈnis-tik\ *adj*

mel·a·nize *or chiefly Brit* **mel·a·nise** \ˈmel-ə-₁nīz\ *vt* **-nized** *or chiefly Brit* **-nised; -niz·ing** *or chiefly Brit* **-nis·ing** : to convert into or infiltrate with melanin ⟨*melanized* cell granules⟩ — **mel·a·ni·za·tion** *or chiefly Brit* **mel·a·ni·sa·tion** \₁mel-ə-nə-ˈzā-shən\ *n*

me·la·no \mə-ˈlä-nō, ˈmel-ə-₁nō\ *n* : a melanistic individual — compare ALBINO

me·la·no·blast \mə-ˈlan-ə-₁blast, ˈmel-ə-nō-\ *n* : a cell that is a precursor of a melanocyte or melanophore — compare MELANOCYTE — **me·la·no·blas·tic** \mə-₁lan-ə-ˈblas-tik, ₁mel-ə-nō-\ *adj*

me·la·no·blas·to·ma \mə-₁lan-ə-blas-ˈtō-mə, ₁mel-ə-nō-\ *n, pl* **-mas** *also* **-ma·ta** \-mət-ə\ : a malignant tumor derived from melanoblasts

mel·a·no·car·ci·no·ma \-₁kärs-°n-ˈō-mə\ *n, pl* **-mas** *also* **-ma·ta** \-mət-ə\ : MELANOMA 2

me·la·no·cyte \mə-ˈlan-ə-₁sīt, ˈmel-ə-nō-\ *n* : an epidermal cell that produces melanin — compare MELANOBLAST

melanocyte–stimulating hormone *n* : either of two vertebrate hormones of the pituitary gland that darken the skin by stimulating melanin dispersion in pigment-containing cells — abbr. *MSH*; called also *intermedin, melanophore-stimulating hormone, melanotropin*

M
N

\ə\ **abut** \ᵊ\ **kitten** \ər\ **further** \a\ **ash** \ā\ **ace** \ä\ **cot, cart**
\aú\ **out** \ch\ **chin** \e\ **bet** \ē\ **easy** \g\ **go** \i\ **hit** \ī\ **ice** \j\ **job**
\ŋ\ **sing** \ō\ **go** \ó\ **law** \ói\ **boy** \th\ **thin** \th̲\ **the** \ü\ **loot**
\ú\ **foot** \y\ **yet** \zh\ **vision** *See also* Pronunciation Symbols page

me·la·no·cyt·ic \mə-ˌlan-ə-ˈsit-ik, ˌmel-ə-nō-\ *adj* : similar to or characterized by the presence of melanocytes ⟨∼ cells⟩ ⟨∼ hyperplasia⟩

me·la·no·cy·to·ma \-sī-ˈtō-mə\ *n, pl* **-mas** *also* **-ma·ta** \-mət-ə\ : a benign tumor composed of melanocytes

me·la·no·derm \mə-ˈlan-ə-ˌdərm, ˈmel-ə-nō-\ *n* : an individual with a dark skin; *specif* : a black-skinned or brown-skinned person

mel·a·no·der·ma \ˌmel-ə-nō-ˈdər-mə, mə-ˌlan-\ *n* : abnormally intense pigmentation of the skin — **mel·a·no·der·mic** \-ˈdər-mik\ *adj*

me·la·no·ep·i·the·li·o·ma \-ˌep-ə-ˌthē-lē-ˈō-mə\ *n, pl* **-mas** *also* **-ma·ta** \-mət-ə\ : MELANOMA 2

me·la·no·gen \mə-ˈlan-ə-jən, ˈmel-ə-nō-\ *n* : a precursor of melanin

me·la·no·gen·e·sis \mə-ˌlan-ə-ˈjen-ə-səs, ˌmel-ə-nō-\ *n, pl* **-e·ses** \-ˌsēz\ : the formation of melanin

me·la·no·ge·net·ic \-jə-ˈnet-ik\ *adj* : of or relating to melanogenesis

me·la·no·gen·ic \-ˈjen-ik\ *adj* **1** : of, relating to, or characteristic of melanogenesis **2** : producing melanin

¹**mel·a·noid** \ˈmel-ə-ˌnȯid\ *adj* **1** : characterized or darkened by melanins ⟨a ∼ lesion⟩ **2** : relating to or occurring in melanosis ⟨∼ symptoms⟩

²**melanoid** *n* **1** : a melanistic individual **2** : a pigment (as one contributing esp. to the yellow color of the skin) that is a disintegration product of a melanin

mel·a·noi·din \ˌmel-ə-ˈnȯid-ᵊn\ *n* : any of various colored substances formed from proteins or amino acids (as in the presence of glucose) — compare HUMIN

mel·a·no·ma \ˌmel-ə-ˈnō-mə\ *n, pl* **-mas** *also* **-ma·ta** \-mət-ə\ **1** : a benign or malignant skin tumor containing dark pigment **2** : a tumor of high malignancy that starts in melanocytes of normal skin or moles and metastasizes rapidly and widely — called also *malignant melanoma, melanocarcinoma, melanoepithelioma, melanosarcoma*

mel·a·no·ma·to·sis \-ˌnō-mə-ˈtō-səs\ *n, pl* **-to·ses** \-ˌsēz\ : the condition of having multiple melanomas in the body

me·la·no·phage \mə-ˈlan-ə-ˌfāj, ˈmel-ə-nə-\ *n* : a melanin-containing cell which obtains the pigment by phagocytosis

me·la·no·phore \mə-ˈlan-ə-ˌfō(ə)r, ˈmel-ə-nə-, -ˌfȯ(ə)r\ *n* : a chromatophore esp. of fishes, amphibians, and reptiles that contains melanin : a black or brown pigment cell — **me·la·no·phor·ic** \-ˌlan-ə-ˈfȯr-ik, -ˈfȯr-\ *adj*

melanophore–stimulating hormone *n* : MELANOCYTE-STIMULATING HORMONE

me·la·no·pla·kia \mə-ˌlan-ə-ˈplā-kē-ə, ˌmel-ə-nō-\ *n* : the occurrence of pigmented patches on the oral mucous membrane

me·la·no·sar·co·ma \-sär-ˈkō-mə\ *n, pl* **-mas** *also* **-ma·ta** \-mət-ə\ : MELANOMA 2

mel·a·no·sis \ˌmel-ə-ˈnō-səs\ *n, pl* **-no·ses** \-ˈnō-ˌsēz\ : a condition characterized by abnormal deposition of melanins or sometimes other pigments in the tissues of the body

melanosis co·li \-ˈkō-ˌlī\ *n* : dark brownish black pigmentation of the mucous membrane of the colon due to the deposition of pigment in macrophages

me·la·no·som·al \mə-ˌlan-ə-ˈsō-məl, ˌmel-ə-nō-\ *adj* : of or relating to a melanosome or its activity

me·la·no·some \mə-ˈlan-ə-ˌsōm, ˈmel-ə-nō-\ *n* : a melanin-producing granule in a melanocyte

mel·a·not·ic \ˌmel-ə-ˈnät-ik\ *adj* : having or characterized by black pigmentation ⟨a ∼ sarcoma⟩

me·la·no·tro·pic \mə-ˌlan-ə-ˈtrō-pik, ˌmel-ə-nō-, -ˈträp-ik\ *also* **me·la·no·tro·phic** \-ˈtrō-fik\ *adj* : promoting the formation and deposit of melanin ⟨∼ activity⟩ ⟨∼ agents⟩

me·la·no·tro·pin \-ˈtrō-pən\ *n* : MELANOCYTE-STIMULATING HORMONE

mel·an·uria \ˌmel-ə-ˈn(y)ùr-ē-ə\ *n* : the presence of melanins in the urine — **mel·an·uric** \-ik\ *adj*

me·lar·so·prol \me-ˈlar-sə-ˌprȯl\ *n* : a drug $C_{12}H_{15}AsN_6OS_2$ used in the treatment of trypanosomiasis esp. in advanced stages

me·las·ma \mə-ˈlaz-mə\ *n* : a dark pigmentation of the skin (as in Addison's disease) — **me·las·mic** \-mik\ *adj*

mel·a·to·nin \ˌmel-ə-ˈtō-nən\ *n* : a vertebrate hormone $C_{13}H_{16}N_2O_2$ that is derived from serotonin, is secreted by the pineal gland esp. in response to darkness, and has been linked to the regulation of circadian rhythms

me·le·na *or chiefly Brit* **me·lae·na** \mə-ˈlē-nə\ *n* : the passage of dark tarry stools containing decomposing blood that is usu. an indication of bleeding in the upper part of the alimentary canal and esp. the esophagus, stomach, and duodenum — compare HEMATOCHEZIA — **me·le·nic** \mə-ˈlē-nik\ *adj*

mel·en·ges·trol acetate \ˌmel-ən-ˈjes-ˌtrȯl-, -ˌtrōl-\ *n* : a progestational and antineoplastic agent $C_{25}H_{32}O_4$ that has been used as a growth-stimulating feed additive for beef cattle

me·lez·i·tose \mə-ˈlez-ə-ˌtōs *also* -ˌtōz\ *n* : a nonreducing trisaccharide sugar $C_{18}H_{32}O_{16}\cdot2H_2O$ that is less sweet than sucrose, that is obtained esp. from exudations of various trees (as the larch or Douglas fir) or from honey made from such exudations, and that on partial hydrolysis yields glucose and turanose

mel·i·bi·ose \ˌmel-ə-ˈbī-ˌōs *also* -ˌōz\ *n* : a disaccharide sugar $C_{12}H_{22}O_{11}$ formed by partial hydrolysis of raffinose

mel·i·oi·do·sis \ˌmel-ē-ˌȯi-ˈdō-səs\ *n, pl* **-do·ses** \-ˌsēz\ : a highly fatal bacterial disease closely related to glanders that occurs primarily in rodents of southeastern Asia but is readily transmitted to other mammals including humans by the rat flea or under certain conditions by dissemination in air of the causative bacterium of the genus *Pseudomonas* (*P. pseudomallei*)

me·lis·sa \mə-ˈlis-ə\ *n* **1** *cap* : a genus of Old World mints having clusters of small white or yellowish flowers and including the lemon balm (*M. officinalis*) **2** : the leaves and tops of the lemon balm that are a source of citral and have been used as a diaphoretic in the form of a tea

me·lis·sic acid \mə-ˌlis-ik-\ *n* : a crystalline fatty acid $C_{30}H_{60}O_2$ found free or in the form of its ester with myricyl alcohol in beeswax and other waxes and also obtained by oxidation of myricyl alcohol

me·lis·syl alcohol \mə-ˈlis-ᵊl-\ *n* : MYRICYL ALCOHOL

mel·i·ten·sis \ˌmel-ə-ˈten(t)-səs\ *adj* : of, derived from, or caused by a bacterium of the genus *Brucella* (*B. melitensis*) ⟨∼ proteins⟩ ⟨∼ fever⟩

mel·i·tose \ˈmel-ə-ˌtōs *also* -ˌtōz\ *n* : RAFFINOSE

me·lit·tin \mə-ˈlit-ᵊn\ *n* : a toxic protein in bee venom that causes localized pain and inflammation but also has a moderate antibacterial and antifungal effect

mel·i·tu·ria *or* **mel·li·tu·ria** \ˌmel-ə-ˈt(y)ùr-ē-ə\ *n* : the presence of any sugar in the urine

Mel·la·ril \ˈmel-ə-ˌril\ *trademark* — used for a preparation of thioridazine

mellitus — see DIABETES MELLITUS, INSULIN-DEPENDENT DIABETES MELLITUS, NON-INSULIN-DEPENDENT DIABETES MELLITUS

melo·ma·nia \ˌmel-ō-ˈmā-nē-ə\ *n* : an inordinate liking for music or melody : excessive or abnormal attraction to music

melo·ma·ni·ac \ˌmel-ō-ˈmā-nē-ˌak\ *n* **1** : an individual exhibiting melomania **2** : an individual (as a person or dog) that is inordinately and abnormally affected by musical or other tones in certain ranges of sound

mel·on–seed body \ˈmel-ən-ˌsēd-\ *n* : a white or brownish oval mass of fibrous synovial tissue that sometimes occurs loose in numbers in the cavity of inflamed joints

Me·loph·a·gus \mə-ˈläf-ə-gəs\ *n* : a genus of wingless hippoboscid flies that includes the sheep ked (*M. ovinus*)

mel·o·plas·ty \ˈmel-ə-ˌplast-ē\ *n, pl* **-ties** : the restoration of a cheek by plastic surgery

melo·rhe·os·to·sis \ˌmel-ə-ˌrē-äs-ˈtō-səs\ *n, pl* **-to·ses** \-ˌsēz\ *or* **-to·sis·es** : an extremely rare form of osteosclerosis of unknown etiology characterized by asymmetrical or local enlargement and sclerotic changes in the long bones of one extremity

Mel·ox·ine \mə-ˈläk-ˌsēn\ *trademark* — used for a preparation of methoxsalen

mel·pha·lan \\'mel-fə-ˌlan\\ *n* : an antineoplastic drug $C_{13}H_{18}Cl_2N_2O_2$ that is a derivative of nitrogen mustard and is used esp. in the treatment of multiple myeloma — called also *L-PAM, phenylalanine mustard, sarcolysin*

melt·ing point \\'mel-tiŋ-ˌ\\ *n* : the temperature at which a solid melts

mem·ber \\'mem-bər\\ *n* : a body part or organ ⟨the thyroid gland may be the offending ∼ —H. A. Overstreet⟩: as **a** : LIMB **b** : PENIS

membra *pl of* MEMBRUM

mem·bra·na \\mem-'brā-nə, -'brä-\\ *n, pl* **mem·bra·nae** \\-ˌnē, -ˌnī\\ : MEMBRANE

mem·bra·na·ceous \\ˌmem-brə-'nā-shəs\\ *adj* : MEMBRANOUS

mem·bra·nal \\'mem-brə-nəl\\ *adj* : relating to or characteristic of cellular membranes

membrana nic·ti·tans \\-'nik-tə-ˌtanz\\ *n* : NICTITATING MEMBRANE

mem·brane \\'mem-ˌbrān\\ *n* **1** : a thin soft pliable sheet or layer esp. of animal or plant origin **2** : a limiting protoplasmic surface or interface — see NUCLEAR MEMBRANE, PLASMA MEMBRANE — **mem·braned** \\'mem-ˌbrānd\\ *adj*

membrane bone *n* : a bone that ossifies directly in connective tissue without previous existence as cartilage — compare CARTILAGE BONE

membrane filter *n* : a filter esp. of cellulose acetate that has pores of any of various maximum diameters so as to prevent the passage of microorganisms (as viruses or bacteria) of greater than a particular size

mem·bra·nel·lar \\ˌmem-brə-'nel-ər\\ *adj* : of, relating to, or constituting a membranelle

mem·bra·nelle \\'mem-brə-ˌnel\\ *also* **mem·bra·nel·la** \\ˌmem-brə-'nel-ə\\ *n, pl* **-nelles** *also* **-nel·lae** \\-'nel-ē\\ : a flattened vibrating organ like a membrane composed of a row of fused cilia in various ciliates

membrane of Descemet *n* : DESCEMET'S MEMBRANE

membrane of Krause *n* : KRAUSE'S MEMBRANE

membrane potential *n* : the potential difference between the interior of a cell and the interstitial fluid beyond the membrane — see INHIBITORY POSTSYNAPTIC POTENTIAL

mem·bra·noid \\'mem-brə-ˌnȯid\\ *adj* : resembling a membrane

mem·bra·nol·o·gist \\ˌmem-brə-'näl-ə-jəst\\ *n* : a specialist in membranology

mem·bra·nol·o·gy \\-'näl-ə-jē\\ *n, pl* **-gies** : the study of the membranes of cells and cell structures

mem·bra·no·pro·lif·er·a·tive glomerulonephritis \\mem-ˌbrā-nō-prə-'lif-ər-ət-iv-\\ *n* : a slowly progressive chronic glomerulonephritis characterized by proliferation of mesangial cells and irregular thickening of glomerular capillary walls and narrowing of the capillary lumina

mem·bra·nous \\'mem-brə-nəs\\ *adj* **1** : of, relating to, or resembling membranes ⟨a ∼ lining⟩ **2** : characterized or accompanied by the formation of a usu. abnormal membrane or membranous layer ⟨∼ croup⟩ — **mem·bra·nous·ly** *adv*

membranous glomerulonephritis *n* : a form of glomerulonephritis characterized by thickening of glomerular capillary basement membranes and nephrotic syndrome

membranous labyrinth *n* : the sensory structures of the inner ear including the receptors of the labyrinthine sense and the cochlea — see BONY LABYRINTH

membranous semicircular canal *n* : SEMICIRCULAR DUCT

membranous urethra *n* : the part of the male urethra that is situated between the layers of the urogenital diaphragm and that connects the parts of the urethra passing through the prostate gland and the penis

mem·brum \\'mem-brəm\\ *n, pl* **-bra** \\-brə\\ : MEMBER; *esp* : PENIS

mem·o·ry \\'mem-(ə-)rē\\ *n, pl* **-ries** **1 a** : the power or process of reproducing or recalling what has been learned and retained esp. through associative mechanisms **b** : the store of things learned and retained from an organism's activity or experience as indicated by modification of structure or behavior or by recall and recognition **2** : a capacity for showing effects as the result of past treatment or for returning to

a former condition — used esp. of a material (as metal or plastic)

memory cell *n* : a long-lived lymphocyte that carries the antibody or receptor for a specific antigen after a first exposure to the antigen and that remains in a less than mature state until stimulated by a second exposure to the antigen at which time it mounts a more effective immune response than a cell which has not been exposed previously

memory span *n* : the greatest amount (as the longest series of letters or digits) that can be perfectly reproduced by a subject after a single presentation by the experimenter

memory trace *n* : ENGRAM

men *pl of* MAN

men·ac·me \\men-'ak-mē\\ *n* : the portion of a woman's life during which menstruation occurs

men·a·di·one \\ˌmen-ə-'dī-ˌōn, -dī-'\\ *n* : a yellow crystalline compound $C_{11}H_8O_2$ with the biological activity of natural vitamin K — called also *vitamin K_3*

me·naph·thone \\mə-'naf-ˌthōn\\ *n, Brit* : MENADIONE

men·a·quin·one \\ˌmen-ə-'kwin-ˌōn\\ *n* : VITAMIN K 1b; *also* : a synthetic derivative of vitamin K_2

men·ar·che \\'men-ˌär-kē\\ *n* : the beginning of the menstrual function; *esp* : the first menstrual period of an individual — **men·ar·che·al** \\ˌmen-'är-kē-əl\\ *or* **men·ar·chal** \\men-'är-kəl\\ *also* **men·ar·chi·al** \\men-'är-kē-əl\\ *adj*

¹**mend** \\'mend\\ *vt* : to restore to health : CURE ⟨time will ∼ the broken bone⟩ ∼ *vi* : to improve in health; *also* : HEAL

²**mend** *n* : an act of mending or repair — **on the mend** : getting better or improving esp. in health

Men·de·le·ev's law *or* **Men·de·lé·ef's law** *also* **Men·de·ley·ev's law** \\ˌmen-də-'lā-efs-\\ *n* : PERIODIC LAW

Mendeleyev, Dmitry Ivanovich (1834–1907), Russian chemist. Mendeleyev made a fundamental contribution to chemistry by proving that all chemical elements are related members of a single ordered system. He was a professor of chemistry at St. Petersburg, and in his later years he served as director of his government's bureau of weights and measures. In 1869 he devised his original version of a periodic table in which all known elements are arranged according to their atomic weights. In his improved table of 1871 he left gaps for elements not yet discovered but which had predictable properties. He also formulated a periodic law stating that the chemical properties of the elements are periodic functions of their atomic weights. His periodic table became the framework for a great part of chemical theory and proved to be highly useful in the interpretation of the processes of radioactive decay. The table also served to unify much of modern physics. The radioactive element mendelevium was named in his honor when it was first produced by scientists in 1955.

men·de·le·vi·um \\ˌmen-də-'lē-vē-əm, -'lā-\\ *n* : a radioactive element that is artificially produced — symbol *Md*; see ELEMENT table

Men·de·lian \\men-'dē-lē-ən, -'dēl-yən\\ *adj* : of, relating to, or according with Mendel's laws or Mendelism — **Mendelian** *n* — **Men·de·lian·ist** \\-əst\\ *n*

Men·del \\'mend-ᵊl\\, **Gregor Johann (1822–1884),** Austrian botanist and geneticist. Mendel was the discoverer of several basic laws of genetics now known as Mendel's laws. A monk at an Augustinian monastery, in 1856 he began experimenting with plants in his garden. His experiments in crossing several varieties of peas led to his discovery of the basic principles of genetics. In 1866 he published the results of his work in a landmark article. He theorized that the occurrence of the visible alternative characters in plants, in their constant varieties and their offspring, is due to the presence of paired elementary units of heredity. Mendel realized that these units—genes—obey simple statistical laws.

\\ə\\ **abut** \\ᵊ\\ **kitten** \\ər\\ **further** \\a\\ **ash** \\ā\\ **ace** \\ä\\ **cot, cart**
\\aȯ\\ **out** \\ch\\ **chin** \\e\\ **bet** \\ē\\ **easy** \\g\\ **go** \\i\\ **hit** \\ī\\ **ice** \\j\\ **job**
\\ŋ\\ **sing** \\ō\\ **go** \\ȯ\\ **law** \\ȯi\\ **boy** \\th\\ **thin** \\th\\ **the** \\ü\\ **loot**
\\ȯ\\ **foot** \\y\\ **yet** \\zh\\ **vision** *See also* Pronunciation Symbols page

He is credited with laying the mathematical foundation of the science of genetics.

Mendelian factor *n* : GENE

Mendelian inheritance *n* : inheritance of characters specif. transmitted by genes in accord with Mendel's law — called also *particulate inheritance;* compare BLENDING INHERITANCE, QUANTITATIVE INHERITANCE

Men·de·lian·ism \ˌmen-ˈdē-lē-ə-ˌniz-əm\ *n* : MENDELISM

Men·del·ism \ˈmen-dᵊl-ˌiz-əm\ *n* : the principles or the operations of Mendel's laws; *also* : MENDELIAN INHERITANCE — **Men·del·ist** \-dᵊl-əst\ *adj or n*

men·del·ize \ˈmen-də-ˌlīz\ *vi* **-ized; -iz·ing** *often cap* : to be inherited in conformity with Mendel's laws ⟨*mendelizing* genes⟩

Men·del's law \ˌmen-dᵊlz-\ *n* **1** : a principle in genetics: hereditary units occur in pairs that separate during gamete formation so that every gamete receives but one member of a pair — called also *law of segregation* **2** : a principle in genetics limited and modified by the subsequent discovery of the phenomenon of linkage: the different pairs of hereditary units are distributed to the gametes independently of each other, the gametes combine at random, and the various combinations of hereditary pairs occur in the zygotes according to the laws of chance — called also *law of independent assortment* **3** : a principle in genetics proved subsequently to be subject to many limitations: because one of each pair of hereditary units dominates the other in expression, characters are inherited as alternatives on an all-or-nothing basis — called also *law of dominance*

men·go·vi·rus \ˈmen-gō-ˌvī-rəs\ *n* : a picornavirus (species *Encephalomyocarditis virus* of the genus *Cardiovirus*) that causes encephalomyocarditis

Mé·nière's disease \mən-ˈye(ə)rz-, ˈmen-yərz-\ *n* : a disorder of the membranous labyrinth of the inner ear that is marked by recurrent attacks of dizziness, tinnitus, and hearing loss — called also *Ménière's syndrome*

Mé·nière \mā-nyer\, **Prosper (1799–1862),** French physician. Ménière specialized in otolaryngology. He published a treatise on diseases of the ear in 1853. In 1861 he published the first detailed description of the form of vertigo now known as Ménière's disease. While others had made peripheral studies of the disorder, he was the first to identify the semicircular canals of the ear as the site of the lesion. A truly complete description of the disease was published in 1874 by the famed neurologist Jean Martin Charcot (1825–1893). Not until 1928 was an operation for the disease developed by Walter Dandy (1886–1946).

men·in·ge·al \ˌmen-ən-ˈjē-əl\ *adj* : of, relating to, or affecting the meninges ⟨~ hemorrhage⟩ ⟨~ infection⟩

meningeal artery *n* : any of several arteries supplying the meninges of the brain and neighboring structures; *esp* : MIDDLE MENINGEAL ARTERY

meningeal vein *n* : any of several veins draining the meninges of the brain and neighboring structures

meninges *pl of* MENINX

me·nin·gi·o·ma \mə-ˌnin-jē-ˈō-mə\ *n, pl* **-mas** *also* **-ma·ta** \-ˈō-mət-ə\ : a slow-growing encapsulated tumor arising from the meninges and often causing damage by pressing upon the brain and adjacent parts

men·in·gism \ˈmen-ən-ˌjiz-əm, mə-ˈnin-\ *n* : MENINGISMUS

men·in·gis·mus \ˌmen-ən-ˈjiz-məs\ *n, pl* **-gis·mi** \-ˌmī\ : a state of meningeal irritation with symptoms suggesting meningitis that often occurs at the onset of acute febrile diseases esp. in children

men·in·git·ic \-ˈjit-ik\ *adj* : of, relating to, or like that of meningitis

men·in·gi·tis \ˌmen-ən-ˈjīt-əs\ *n, pl* **-git·i·des** \-ˈjit-ə-ˌdēz\ **1** : inflammation of the meninges and esp. of the pia mater and the arachnoid **2** : a disease that may be either a mild illness caused by any of numerous viruses (as various coxsackieviruses) or a more severe usu. life-threatening illness caused by a bacterium (esp. the meningococcus or the serotype designated B of *Hemophilus influenzae*), that may be associated with fever, headache, vomiting, malaise, and stiff neck, and

that if untreated in bacterial forms may progress to confusion, stupor, convulsions, coma, and death

me·nin·go·cele *also* **me·nin·go·coele** \me-ˈniŋ-gə-ˌsēl, mə-ˈnin-jə-\ *n* : a protrusion of meninges through a defect in the skull or spinal column (as in spina bifida) forming a cyst filled with cerebrospinal fluid

me·nin·go·coc·ce·mia *or Brit* **me·nin·go·coc·cae·mia** \mə-ˌniŋ-gō-käk-ˈsē-mē-ə, -ˌnin-jə-\ *n* : an abnormal condition characterized by the presence of meningococci in the blood

me·nin·go·coc·cus \mə-ˌniŋ-gə-ˈkäk-əs, -ˌnin-jə-\ *n, pl* **-coc·ci** \-ˈkäk-ˌ(s)ī, -ˌ(s)ē\ : a bacterium of the genus *Neisseria* (*N. meningitidis*) that causes cerebrospinal meningitis — **me·nin·go·coc·cal** \-ˈkäk-əl\ *also* **me·nin·go·coc·cic** \-ˈkäk-(s)ik\ *adj*

me·nin·go·en·ceph·a·lit·ic \mə-ˌniŋ-(ˌ)gō-ən-ˌsef-ə-ˈlit-ik, -ˌnin-(ˌ)jō-\ *adj* : relating to or characteristic of meningoencephalitis ⟨~ lesions⟩

me·nin·go·en·ceph·a·li·tis \-ən-ˌsef-ə-ˈlīt-əs\ *n, pl* **-lit·i·des** \-ˈlit-ə-ˌdēz\ : inflammation of the brain and meninges — called also *encephalomeningitis*

me·nin·go·en·ceph·a·lo·cele \-in-ˈsef-ə-lō-ˌsēl\ *n* : a protrusion of meninges and brain through a defect in the skull

me·nin·go·en·ceph·a·lo·my·eli·tis \-in-ˌsef-ə-lō-ˌmī-ə-ˈlīt-əs\ *n, pl* **-elit·i·des** \-ə-ˈlit-ə-ˌdēz\ : inflammation of the meninges, brain, and spinal cord

me·nin·go·my·eli·tis \-ˌmī-ə-ˈlīt-əs\ *n, pl* **-elit·i·des** \-ə-ˈlit-ə-ˌdēz\ : inflammation of the spinal cord and its enveloping membranes

me·nin·go·my·elo·cele \-ˈmī-ə-lō-ˌsēl\ *n* : a protrusion of meninges and spinal cord through a defect in the spinal column

me·nin·go·pneu·mo·nit·is \-ˌn(y)ü-mə-ˈnīt-əs\ *n, pl* **-ni·ti·des** \-ˈnit-ə-ˌdēz\ : inflammation of both the lungs and the meninges

me·nin·go·vas·cu·lar \-ˈvas-kyə-lər\ *adj* : of, relating to, or affecting the meninges and the cerebral blood vessels ⟨~ neurosyphilis⟩

me·ninx \ˈmē-niŋ(k)s, ˈmen-iŋ(k)s\ *n, pl* **me·nin·ges** \mə-ˈnin-(ˌ)jēz\ : any of the three membranes that envelop the brain and spinal cord and include the arachnoid, dura mater, and pia mater

me·nis·cal \mə-ˈnis-kəl\ *adj* : of or relating to a meniscus ⟨a ~ tear⟩ ⟨~ lesions⟩

men·is·cec·to·my \ˌmen-i-ˈsek-tə-mē\ *n, pl* **-mies** : surgical excision of a meniscus of the knee or temporomandibular joint

me·nis·co·cyte \mə-ˈnis-kə-ˌsīt\ *n* : SICKLE CELL 1

me·nis·co·cy·to·sis \mə-ˌnis-kō-ˌsī-ˈtō-səs\ *n, pl* **-to·ses** \-ˌsēz\ : SICKLE-CELL ANEMIA

me·nis·cus \mə-ˈnis-kəs\ *n, pl* **me·nis·ci** \-ˈnis-ˌ(k)ī, -ˌkē\ *also* **me·nis·cus·es** **1** : a crescent or crescent-shaped body **2** : a fibrous cartilage within a joint: **a** : either of two crescent-shaped lamellae of fibrocartilage that border and partly cover the articulating surfaces of the tibia and femur at the knee : SEMILUNAR CARTILAGE: (1) : one mostly between the lateral condyles of the tibia and femur — called also *external semilunar fibrocartilage, lateral meniscus, lateral semilunar cartilage* (2) : one mostly between the medial condyles of the tibia and femur — called also *internal semilunar fibrocartilage, medial meniscus, medial semilunar cartilage* **b** : a thin oval ligament of the temporomandibular joint that is situated between the condyle of the mandible and the mandibular fossa and separates the joint into two cavities **3** : a concavo-convex lens **4** : the curved upper surface of a liquid column that is concave when the containing walls are wetted by the liquid and convex when not

Men·kes' disease \ˈmeŋ-kəz-, -kə-səz-\ *n* : a disorder of copper metabolism that is inherited as a recessive X-linked trait and is characterized by a deficiency of copper in the liver and of copper-containing proteins (as ceruloplasmin) which results in mental retardation, brittle kinky hair, and a fatal outcome early in life — called also *Menkes' syndrome*

Men·kes \ˈmeŋ-kəs\, **John Hans (b 1928),** American (Austrian-born) pediatric neurologist. For most of his career Menkes was affiliated with the medical school of the University of California–Los Angeles, where over the course of more than two decades starting in 1966, he held a number of professorships in pediatrics, neurology, and psychiatry. In 1997 he was named director of pediatric neurology at Los Angeles' Cedars-Sinai Medical Center. His writings included the fifth edition of *Textbook of Child Neurology* (1995) and numerous articles in pediatric and neurological journals. Notable was his description in 1954 of a progressive familial infantile cerebral dysfunction that is marked by urine with the distinctive odor of maple syrup. Equally notable was his description in 1962 of a hereditary disorder of copper metabolism that has kinky hair as a distinctive feature. This disorder of copper metabolism is commonly known as Menkes' disease or Menkes' syndrome. Menkes was also the author of several plays, screenplays, and novels.

meno·met·ror·rha·gia \ˌmen-ō-ˌmē-trə-ˈrā-j(ē-)ə, -ˈrä-, -zhə\ *n* : a combination of menorrhagia and metrorrhagia

meno·pause \ˈmen-ə-ˌpȯz, ˈmēn-\ *n* **1 a** (1) : the natural cessation of menstruation occurring usu. between the ages of 45 and 55 with a mean in Western cultures of approximately 51 (2) : the physiological period in the life of a woman in which such cessation and the accompanying regression of ovarian function occurs — called also *climacteric;* compare PERI-MENOPAUSE **b** : cessation of menstruation from other than natural causes (as from surgical removal of the ovaries) **2** : ANDROPAUSE — **meno·paus·al** \ˌmen-ə-ˈpȯ-zəl, ˌmēn-\ *adj*

Men·o·pon \ˈmen-ə-ˌpän\ *n* : a genus of biting lice that includes the shaft louse (*M. gallinae*) of poultry

men·or·rha·gia \ˌmen-ə-ˈrā-j(ē-)ə, -ˈrä-zhə; -ˈräj-ə, -ˈräzh-\ *n* : abnormally profuse menstrual flow — compare HYPER-MENORRHEA, METRORRHAGIA — **men·or·rhag·ic** \-ˈraj-ik\ *adj*

men·or·rhea *or Brit* **men·or·rhoea** \ˌmen-ə-ˈrē-ə\ *n* : normal menstrual flow

men·ses \ˈmen-ˌsēz\ *n pl but sing or pl in constr* : the menstrual flow

menstrua *pl of* MENSTRUUM

men·stru·al \ˈmen(t)-strə-(wə)l\ *adj* : of or relating to menstruation — **men·stru·al·ly** *adv*

menstrual cycle *n* : the whole cycle of physiological changes from the beginning of one menstrual period to the beginning of the next

menstrual extraction *n* : a procedure for early termination of pregnancy by withdrawing the uterine lining and a fertilized egg if present by means of suction — called also *menstrual regulation*

men·stru·ate \ˈmen(t)-strə-ˌwāt, ˈmen-ˌstrāt\ *vi* **-at·ed; -at·ing** : to undergo menstruation

men·stru·a·tion \ˌmen(t)-strə-ˈwā-shən, men-ˈstrā-\ *n* : a discharging of blood, secretions, and tissue debris from the uterus that recurs in nonpregnant human and other primate females of breeding age at approximately monthly intervals and that is considered to represent a readjustment of the uterus to the nonpregnant state following proliferative changes accompanying the preceding ovulation; *also* : PERIOD 1b

men·stru·ous \ˈmen(t)-strə-(wə)s\ *adj* : of, relating to, or undergoing menstruation

men·stru·um \ˈmen(t)-strə-(wə)m\ *n, pl* **-stru·ums** *or* **-strua** \-str(ə-w)ə\ : a substance that dissolves a solid or holds it in suspension : SOLVENT

men·su·ra·tion \ˌmen(t)-sə-ˈrā-shən; ˌmen-chə-\ *n* : the act of measuring

menta *pl of* MENTUM

¹men·tal \ˈment-ᵊl\ *adj* **1 a** : of or relating to the mind; *specif* : of or relating to the total emotional and intellectual response of an individual to external reality **b** : of or relating to intellectual as contrasted with emotional activity **2 a** : of, relating to, or affected by a psychiatric disorder ⟨a ~ patient⟩ **b** : intended for the care or treatment of persons affected by psychiatric disorders ⟨~ hospitals⟩ — **men·tal·ly** \-ᵊl-ē\ *adv*

²mental *adj* : of or relating to the chin : GENIAL

mental age *n* : a measure used in psychological testing that expresses an individual's mental attainment in terms of the number of years it takes an average child to reach the same level

mental alienation *n* : mental disorder or derangement : INSANITY

mental artery *n* : a branch of the inferior alveolar artery on each side that emerges from the mental foramen and supplies blood to the chin — called also *mental branch*

mental capacity *n* **1** : sufficient understanding and memory to comprehend in a general way the situation in which one finds oneself and the nature, purpose, and consequence of any act or transaction into which one proposes to enter **2** : the degree of understanding and memory the law requires to uphold the validity of or to charge one with responsibility for a particular act or transaction ⟨*mental capacity* to commit crime requires that the accused know right from wrong⟩

mental competence *n* : MENTAL CAPACITY

mental deficiency *n* : MENTAL RETARDATION

mental disorder *n* : a mental or bodily condition marked primarily by sufficient disorganization of personality, mind, and emotions to seriously impair the normal psychological functioning of the individual — called also *mental illness*

mentales *pl of* MENTALIS

mental foramen *n* : a foramen for the passage of blood vessels and a nerve on the outside of the lower jaw on each side near the chin

mental health *n* : the condition of being sound mentally and emotionally that is characterized by the absence of mental disorder (as neurosis or psychosis) and by adequate adjustment esp. as reflected in feeling comfortable about oneself, positive feelings about others, and ability to meet the demands of life; *also* : the field of mental health : MENTAL HYGIENE

mental hygiene *n* : the science of maintaining mental health and preventing the development of mental disorder (as psychosis or neurosis)

mental illness *n* : MENTAL DISORDER

mental incapacity *n* **1** : an absence of mental capacity **2** : an inability through mental disorder or mental retardation of any sort to carry on the everyday affairs of life or to care for one's person or property with reasonable discretion

mental incompetence *n* : MENTAL INCAPACITY

men·ta·lis \men-ˈtā-ləs\ *n, pl* **men·ta·les** \-ˌlēz\ : a muscle that originates in the incisive fossa of the mandible, inserts in the skin of the chin, and raises the chin and pushes up the lower lip

men·tal·ist \ˈment-ᵊl-əst\ *n* : an adherent or advocate of a mentalistic school of psychology or psychiatry

men·tal·is·tic \ˌment-ᵊl-ˈis-tik\ *adj* : of or relating to any school of psychology or psychiatry that in contrast to behaviorism values subjective data (as those gained by introspection) in the study and explanation of behavior — **men·tal·ism** \ˈment-ᵊl-ˌiz-əm\ *n*

men·tal·i·ty \men-ˈtal-ət-ē\ *n, pl* **-ties** **1** : mental power or capacity **2** : mode or way of thought

mental nerve *n* : a branch of the inferior alveolar nerve that emerges from the bone of the mandible near the mental protuberance and divides into branches which are distributed to the skin of the chin and to the skin and mucous membranes of the lower lip

mental protuberance *n* : the bony protuberance at the front of the lower jaw forming the chin

mental retardation *n* : subaverage intellectual ability equivalent to or less than an IQ of 70 that is accompanied by significant deficits in abilities (as in communication or self-care) necessary for independent daily living, is present from birth or infancy, and is manifested esp. by delayed or abnor-

M
N

\ə\ **abut** \ᵊ\ **kitten** \ər\ **further** \a\ **ash** \ā\ **ace** \ä\ **cot, cart**
\aú\ **out** \ch\ **chin** \e\ **bet** \ē\ **easy** \g\ **go** \i\ **hit** \ī\ **ice** \j\ **job**
\ŋ\ **sing** \ō\ **go** \ȯ\ **law** \ȯi\ **boy** \th\ **thin** \th̲\ **the** \ü\ **loot**
\ú\ **foot** \y\ **yet** \zh\ **vision** *See also* Pronunciation Symbols page

mal development, by learning difficulties, and by problems in social adjustment — **mentally retarded** *adj*

mental spine *n* : either of two small elevations on the inner surface of each side of the symphysis of the lower jaw of which the superior one on each side provides attachment for the genioglossus and the inferior for the geniohyoid muscle

mental test *n* : any of various standardized procedures applied to an individual in order to ascertain ability or evaluate behavior in comparison with other individuals or with the average of any class of individuals

mental tubercle *n* : a prominence on each side of the mental protuberance of the mandible — called also *genial tubercle*

men·ta·tion \men-'tā-shən\ *n* : mental activity ⟨unconscious ∼⟩

Men·tha \'men-thə\ *n* : a widely distributed genus of aromatic herbs of the mint family (Labiatae) which have white or pink flowers and some of which (as the spearmint and peppermint) are used in flavoring and cookery

men·thol \'men-ˌthȯl, -ˌthōl\ *n* : a crystalline alcohol $C_{10}H_{20}O$ that occurs esp. in mint oils, has the odor and cooling properties of peppermint, and is used in flavoring and in medicine (as locally to relieve pain, itching, and nasal congestion)

men·tho·lat·ed \'men(t)-thə-ˌlāt-əd\ *adj* : containing or impregnated with menthol ⟨a ∼ salve⟩

men·thyl \'men-thəl, -ˌthil\ *n* : the monovalent radical $C_{10}H_{19}$ derived from menthol by removal of the hydroxyl group

menti — see SYMPHYSIS MENTI

men·ti·cide \'ment-ə-ˌsīd\ *n* : a systematic and intentional undermining of a person's conscious mind : BRAINWASHING

mentis — see COMPOS MENTIS, NON COMPOS MENTIS

men·to·la·bi·al \ˌmen-tō-'lā-bē-əl\ *adj* : of, relating to, or lying between the chin and lower lip ⟨the ∼ sulcus⟩

men·ton \'men-ˌtän\ *n* **1** : the lowest point in the median plane of the chin **2** : GNATHION

men·tum \'ment-əm\ *n, pl* **men·ta** \-ə\ : CHIN

mep·a·crine \'mep-ə-ˌkrēn, -krən\ *n, chiefly Brit* : QUINACRINE

mep·a·zine \'mep-ə-ˌzēn\ *n* : a phenothiazine $C_{19}H_{22}N_2S$ formerly used as a tranquilizer

me·pen·zo·late bromide \mə-'pen-zə-ˌlāt-\ *n* : an anticholinergic drug $C_{21}H_{26}BrNO_3$

me·per·i·dine \mə-'per-ə-ˌdēn\ *n* : a synthetic narcotic drug used in the form of its hydrochloride $C_{15}H_{21}NO_2 \cdot HCl$ as an analgesic, sedative, and antispasmodic — called also *isonipecaine, pethidine*

me·phen·e·sin \mə-'fen-ə-sən\ *n* : a crystalline compound $C_{10}H_{14}O_3$ used chiefly in the treatment of neuromuscular conditions — called also *myanesin*

meph·en·ox·a·lone \ˌmef-ə-'näk-sə-ˌlōn\ *n* : a tranquilizing drug $C_{11}H_{13}NO_4$

me·phen·ter·mine \mə-'fen-tər-ˌmēn\ *n* : an adrenergic drug administered often in the form of its sulfate $C_{11}H_{17}N \cdot H_2SO_4$ as a vasopressor and nasal decongestant

me·phen·y·to·in \mə-'fen-i-ˌtō-ən\ *n* : an anticonvulsant drug $C_{12}H_{14}N_2O_2$ — see MESANTOIN

me·phit·ic \mə-'fit-ik\ *adj* : having a foul odor

mepho·bar·bi·tal \ˌmef-ō-'bär-bə-ˌtäl\ *n* : a crystalline barbiturate $C_{13}H_{14}N_2O_3$ used as a sedative and in the treatment of epilepsy

Meph·y·ton \'mef-ə-ˌtän\ *trademark* — used for a preparation of vitamin K_1

me·piv·a·caine \me-'piv-ə-ˌkān\ *n* : a drug used esp. in the form of its hydrochloride $C_{15}H_{22}N_2O \cdot HCl$ as a local anesthetic

mep·ro·bam·ate \ˌmep-rō-'bam-ˌāt *also* mə-'prō-bə-ˌmāt\ *n* : a bitter carbamate $C_9H_{18}N_2O_4$ used as a tranquilizer — see EQUANIL, MEPROSPAN, MILTOWN

Mep·ro·span \'mep-rō-ˌspan\ *n* : a preparation of meprobamate — formerly a U.S. registered trademark

me·pyr·a·mine \me-'pir-ə-ˌmēn\ *n, chiefly Brit* : PYRILAMINE

mEq *abbr* milliequivalent

mer \'mər, 'mer\ *n* : the repeating structural unit of a polymer — often prefixed with a number indicating the number of units in the polymer ⟨synthesized two 20-*mers*⟩

me·ral·gia \mə-'ral-j(ē-)ə\ *n* : pain esp. of a neuralgic kind in the thigh

meralgia par·es·thet·i·ca *or Brit* **meralgia par·aes·thet·i·ca** \-ˌpar-əs-'thet-i-kə\ *n* : an abnormal condition characterized by pain and paresthesia in the outer surface of the thigh

mer·al·lu·ride \mə-'ral-yə-ˌrīd, -ˌrid\ *n* : a chemical combination of a mercurial compound $C_9H_{16}HgN_2O_6$ and theophylline formerly used as a diuretic

mer·bro·min \ˌmər-'brō-mən\ *n* : a green crystalline mercurial compound $C_{20}H_8Br_2HgNa_2O_6$ used as a topical antiseptic and germicide in the form of its red solution — see MERCUROCHROME

mer·cap·tal \(ˌ)mər-'kap-ˌtal\ *n* : any of a class of compounds formed by the reaction of thiols with aldehydes or ketones

mer·cap·tan \(ˌ)mər-'kap-ˌtan\ *n* : THIOL 1

mer·cap·tide \-ˌtīd\ *n* : a metallic derivative of a thiol

mer·cap·to \-ˌtō\ *adj* : being or containing the group SH

mer·cap·to·ace·tic acid \ˌmər-ˌkap-tō-ə-ˌsēt-ik-\ *n* : THIOGLYCOLIC ACID

mer·cap·to·eth·a·nol \ˌmər-ˌkap-tō-'eth-ə-ˌnȯl\ *n* : a reducing agent C_2H_6OS used to break disulfide bonds in proteins (as for the destruction of their physiological activity)

mer·cap·tol \(ˌ)mər-'kap-ˌtȯl, -ˌtōl\ *n* : a mercaptal formed from a ketone and analogous to a ketal

mer·cap·tom·er·in \(ˌ)mər-ˌkap-'täm-ə-rən\ *n* : a mercurial compound $C_{16}H_{25}HgNNa_2O_6S$ formerly used as a diuretic

mer·cap·to·pu·rine \(ˌ)mər-ˌkap-tə-'pyu̇(ə)r-ˌēn\ *n* : an antimetabolite $C_5H_4N_4S$ that interferes esp. with the metabolism of purine bases and the biosynthesis of nucleic acids and that is sometimes useful in the treatment of acute leukemia

mer·cap·tu·ric acid \ˌmər-ˌkap-'t(y)u̇r-ik-\ *n* : an acid $C_5H_8O_3S$–R formed from cysteine and an aromatic compound in the body and usu. excreted in the urine (as in the form of a glucuronide)

Mer·cier's bar \mer-sē-'āz-'bär\ *n* : TORUS URETERICUS

Mer·cier \mer-syā\, **Louis–Auguste (1811–1882),** French urologist. Mercier specialized in urogenital surgery and was known for his research in the anatomy of the bladder and urethra. In 1854 he described the transverse ridge that extends between the openings of the ureters on the inner surface of the bladder and forms the posterior boundary of the trigone; it is now sometimes called Mercier's bar.

mer·co·cre·sols \ˌmər-kō-'krē-ˌsȯlz, -ˌsōlz\ *n pl but sing in constr* : a mixture consisting of equal parts of organic mercury and cresol derivatives that is used as a topical antiseptic

mer·cu·mat·i·lin \ˌmər-kyu̇-'mat-ᵊl-ən, ˌmər-ˌkyü-mə-'til-ən\ *n* : a chemical combination of a mercury-containing acid $C_{14}H_{14}HgO_6$ and theophylline formerly used as a diuretic

¹mer·cu·ri·al \(ˌ)mər-'kyu̇r-ē-əl\ *adj* : of, relating to, containing, or caused by mercury ⟨∼ salves⟩

²mercurial *n* : a pharmaceutical or chemical containing mercury ⟨the diuretic action of ∼s⟩

mer·cu·ri·a·lis \(ˌ)mər-ˌkyü-rē-'ā-ləs, -'a-lis\ *n* : an herb (*Mercurialis annua*) of the spurge family formerly dried for use as a purgative, diuretic, and antisyphilitic

mer·cu·ri·al·ism \(ˌ)mər-'kyu̇r-ē-ə-ˌliz-əm\ *n* : chronic poisoning with mercury (as from industrial contacts with the metal or its fumes) — called also *hydrargyria, hydrargyrism*

mer·cu·ric \(ˌ)mər-'kyu̇(ə)r-ik\ *adj* : of, relating to, or containing mercury; *esp* : containing mercury with a valence of two

mercuric chloride *n* : a heavy crystalline poisonous compound $HgCl_2$ used as a disinfectant and fungicide and in photography — called also *bichloride, bichloride of mercury, corrosive sublimate, mercury bichloride*

mercuric cyanide *n* : the mercury cyanide $Hg(CN)_2$ which has been used as an antiseptic

mercuric iodide *n* : a red crystalline poisonous salt HgI_2 which becomes yellow when heated above 126°C (259°F) and has been used as a topical antiseptic

mercuric oxide *n* : either of two forms of a slightly water‐soluble crystalline poisonous compound HgO: **a** : a yellow finely divided powder obtained usu. by precipitation from solutions of mercuric chloride and sodium hydroxide and used in antiseptic ointments   **b** : a bright red coarse powder obtained by precipitation from hot solutions or by heating a nitrate of mercury and used similarly to the yellow form

Mer·cu·ro·chrome \(ˌ)mər-ˈkyúr-ə-ˌkrōm\ *trademark* — used for a preparation of merbromin

mer·cu·ro·phyl·line \ˌmər-kyə-rō-ˈfil-ˌēn, -ən\ *n* : a chemical combination of a mercurial compound $C_{14}H_{24}HgNNaO_5$ and theophylline formerly used as a diuretic

mer·cu·rous \(ˌ)mər-ˈkyúr-əs, ˈmər-kyə-rəs\ *adj* : of, relating to, or containing mercury; *esp* : containing mercury with a valence of one

mercurous chloride *n* : CALOMEL

mercurous iodide *n* : a yellow amorphous powder Hg_2I_2 formerly used to treat syphilis

mer·cu·ry \ˈmər-kyə-rē, -k(ə-)rē\ *n, pl* **-ries**   **1** : a heavy silver-white poisonous metallic element that is liquid at ordinary temperatures and used esp. in scientific instruments — symbol *Hg;* called also *quicksilver;* see ELEMENT table   **2** : a pharmaceutical preparation containing mercury or a compound of it

   Mercury, Roman mythological character. In Roman mythology Mercury became identified with the Greek god Hermes. This god was known especially as the fleet-footed messenger of the gods. He was also the god of science and the arts and the patron of travelers and athletes. He is typically represented in art as a young man wearing a winged helmet and winged sandals and bearing a caduceus. The metal mercury was named after him most probably because he symbolizes mobility.

mercury bichloride *n* : MERCURIC CHLORIDE

mercury chloride *n* : a chloride of mercury: as   **a** : CALOMEL   **b** : MERCURIC CHLORIDE

mer·cu·ry–va·por lamp \-ˌvā-pər-\ *n* : an electric lamp in which the discharge takes place through mercury vapor and which has been used therapeutically as a source of ultraviolet radiation

mer·cy kill·ing \ˈmər-sē-ˌkil-iŋ\ *n* : EUTHANASIA

me·rid·i·an \mə-ˈrid-ē-ən\ *n*   **1** : an imaginary circle or closed curve on the surface of a sphere or globe-shaped body (as the eyeball) that lies in a plane passing through the poles   **2** : any of the pathways along which the body's vital energy flows according to the theory of acupuncture — **meridian** *adj*

me·rid·i·o·nal \mə-ˈrid-ē-ən-ᵊl\ *adj* : of, relating to, or situated on or along a meridian ⟨∼ differences in the acuity of vision⟩ ⟨∼ and circular fibers of the ciliary muscle⟩

me·ris·tic \mə-ˈrist-ik\ *adj*   **1** : of, relating to, or divided into segments (as metameres) ⟨∼ organization of body structures⟩   **2** : characterized by or involving modification in number or in geometrical relation of body parts ⟨∼ variation⟩ — **me·ris·ti·cal·ly** \-i-k(ə-)lē\ *adv*

Mer·kel cell *also* **Merkel's cell** \ˈmər-kəl(z)-\ *n* : a cell that occurs in the basal part of the epidermis, is characterized by dense granules in its cytoplasm, is closely associated with the unmyelinated tip of a nerve fiber, and prob. functions in tactile sensory perception

   Mer·kel \ˈmer-kəl\, **Friedrich Siegmund (1845–1919),** German anatomist. A professor of anatomy, Merkel produced a multivolume work on human anatomy. He also introduced the use of xylene and celloidin into histological techniques and was the first to use in anatomical illustration the now-standard color scheme: red for the arteries, blue for the veins, and yellow for the nerves. In 1880 he described the composite nervous and epithelial structures that are known as Merkel's disks or corpuscles. The epithelial cells associated with these structures are now commonly called Merkel cells.

Merkel's disk *n* : the disklike expansion of the end of a nerve fiber together with a closely associated Merkel cell that has a presumed tactile function — called also *Merkel's corpuscle*

mero·blas·tic \ˌmer-ə-ˈblas-tik\ *adj* : characterized by or being incomplete cleavage as a result of the presence of an im-

peding mass of yolk material (as in the eggs of birds) — compare HOLOBLASTIC — **mero·blas·ti·cal·ly** \-ti-k(ə-)lē\ *adv*

mero·crine \ˈmer-ə-krən, -ˌkrīn, -ˌkrēn\ *adj* : producing a secretion that is discharged without major damage to the secreting cells ⟨∼ glands⟩; *also* : of or produced by a merocrine gland ⟨a ∼ secretion⟩ — compare APOCRINE, ECCRINE, HOLOCRINE

mero·gen·e·sis \ˌmer-ə-ˈjen-ə-səs\ *n, pl* **-e·ses** \-ˌsēz\ : the production of segmental parts

mer·o·gon \ˈmer-ə-ˌgän\ *also* **mer·o·gone** \-ˌgōn\ *n* : a product of merogony

me·rog·o·ny \mə-ˈräg-ə-nē\ *n, pl* **-nies** : development of an embryo by a process that is genetically equivalent to male parthenogenesis and that involves segmentation and differentiation of an egg or egg fragment deprived of its own nucleus but having a functional male nucleus introduced — **mer·o·gon·ic** \ˌmer-ə-ˈgän-ik\ *adj*

mero·my·o·sin \ˌmer-ə-ˈmī-ə-sən\ *n* : either of two structural subunits of myosin that are obtained esp. by tryptic digestion

me·rot·o·my \mə-ˈrät-ə-mē\ *n, pl* **-mies** : division (as of a cell) into parts

mero·zo·ite \ˌmer-ə-ˈzō-ˌīt\ *n* : a small ameboid sporozoan trophozoite (as of a malaria parasite) produced by schizogony that is capable of initiating a new sexual or asexual cycle of development

mero·zy·gote \-ˈzī-ˌgōt\ *n* : an incomplete bacterial zygote having only a fragment of the genome from one of the two parent cells

mer·sal·yl \(ˌ)mər-ˈsal-il\ *n* : an organic mercurial $C_{13}H_{16}HgNNaO_6$ administered by injection in combination with theophylline as a diuretic

Mer·thi·o·late \(ˌ)mər-ˈthī-ə-ˌlāt, -lət\ *n* : a preparation of thimerosal — formerly a U.S. registered trademark

me·sad \ˈmē-ˌzad, -ˌsad\ *also* **me·si·ad** \-zē-ˌad, -sē-\ *adv* : toward or on the side toward the mesial plane

mesal *var of* MESIAL

mes·an·gi·al \ˌmes-ˈan-jē-əl, ˌmēs-\ *adj* : of or relating to the mesangium ⟨∼ thickening⟩ ⟨∼ cells⟩

mes·an·gi·um \ˌmes-ˈan-jē-əm, ˌmēs-\ *n, pl* **-gia** \-jē-ə\ : a thin membrane that gives support to the capillaries surrounding the tubule of a nephron

Mes·an·to·in \mes-ˈan-tō-in\ *trademark* — used for a preparation of mephenytoin

mes·aor·ti·tis \ˌmes-ˌā-ȯr-ˈtīt-əs, ˌmēs-\ *n, pl* **-tit·i·des** \-ˈtit-ə-ˌdēz\ : inflammation of the middle layer of the aorta

mes·ar·ter·i·tis \-ˌärt-ə-ˈrīt-əs\ *n, pl* **-it·i·des** \-ˈrit-ə-ˌdēz\ : inflammation of the middle layer of an artery

me·sat·i·ce·phal·ic \me-ˌsat-ə-si-ˈfal-ik\ *adj* : MESOCEPHALIC

me·sat·i·ceph·a·ly \-ˈsef-ə-lē\ *n, pl* **-lies** : MESOCEPHALY

me·sat·i·pel·lic \-ˈpel-ik\ *adj* : having a pelvis of moderate size with a pelvic index of 90.0 to 94.9

mes·ax·on \mez-ˈak-ˌsän, mēz-, mēs-, mes-\ *n* : the double-layered membrane of a neurilemma that envelops a nerve axon

mes·cal \me-ˈskal, mə-\ *n*   **1** : PEYOTE 2   **2 a** : a usu. colorless Mexican liquor distilled esp. from the central leaves of any of various fleshy-leaved agaves   **b** : a plant from which mescal is produced

mescal button *n* : PEYOTE BUTTON

mes·ca·line \ˈmes-kə-lən, -ˌlēn\ *n* : a hallucinatory crystalline alkaloid $C_{11}H_{17}NO_3$ that is the chief active principle in peyote buttons

mes·cal·ism \ˈmes-kə-ˌliz-əm, mes-ˈkal-ˌiz-əm\ *n* : intoxication produced by the use of peyote buttons

mes·ec·to·derm \ˌmez-ˈek-tə-ˌdərm, ˌmēz-, ˌmēs-, ˌmes-\ *n* : the part of the mesenchyme derived from ectoderm esp. of the neural crest that gives rise to pigment cells, the meninges,

M
N

\ə\ **abut**   \ᵊ\ **kitten**   \ər\ **further**   \a\ **ash**   \ā\ **ace**   \ä\ **cot, cart**
\au̇\ **out**   \ch\ **chin**   \e\ **bet**   \ē\ **easy**   \g\ **go**   \i\ **hit**   \ī\ **ice**   \j\ **job**
\ŋ\ **sing**   \ō\ **go**   \ȯ\ **law**   \ȯi\ **boy**   \th\ **thin**   \t̲h̲\ **the**   \ü\ **loot**
\u̇\ **foot**   \y\ **yet**   \zh\ **vision**   *See also* Pronunciation Symbols page

and most of the branchial cartilages — **mes·ec·to·der·mal** \-ˌek-tə-'dər-məl\ *or* **mes·ec·to·der·mic** \-'dər-mik\ *adj*

mesencephali — see TECTUM MESENCEPHALI

mes·en·ce·phal·ic \-ˌen(t)-sə-'fal-ik\ *adj* : of or relating to the midbrain ⟨the ~ nucleus of the trigeminal nerve⟩

mes·en·ceph·a·lon \ˌmez-ˌen-'sef-ə-ˌlän, ˌmez-ᵊn-, ˌmēz-, ˌmes-, -lən\ *n* : MIDBRAIN

me·sen·chy·ma \mə-'zeŋ-kə-mə\ *n* : MESENCHYME

mes·en·chy·mal \mə-'zeŋ-kə-məl, -'sen-; ˌmez-ᵊn-'kī-məl, ˌmēz-, ˌmēs-, ˌmes-\ *adj* : of, resembling, or being mesenchyme ⟨~ cells⟩ ⟨~ epithelium⟩

mes·en·chy·ma·tous \ˌmez-ᵊn-'kim-ət-əs, ˌmēz-, ˌmēs-, ˌmes-, -'kī-mət-\ *adj* : MESENCHYMAL

mes·en·chyme \'mez-ᵊn-ˌkīm, 'mēz-, 'mēs-, 'mes-\ *n* : loosely organized undifferentiated mesodermal cells that give rise to such structures as connective tissues, blood, lymphatics, bone, and cartilage — see MESECTODERM

mes·en·chy·mo·ma \ˌmez-ᵊn-ˌkī-'mō-mə, ˌmēz-\ *n, pl* **-mas** *also* **-ma·ta** \-mət-ə\ : a benign or malignant tumor consisting of a mixture of at least two types of embryonic connective tissue

mes·en·do·derm \ˌmez-'en-dō-ˌdərm\ *or* **mes·en·to·derm** \-'en-tō-\ *n* : ENDOMESODERM

mesentera *pl of* MESENTERON

¹**mes·en·ter·ic** \ˌmez-ᵊn-'ter-ik, mes-\ *adj* : of, relating to, or located in or near a mesentery

²**mesenteric** *n* : a mesenteric part; *esp* : MESENTERIC ARTERY

mesenteric artery *n* : either of two arteries arising from the aorta and passing between the two layers of the mesentery to the intestine: **a** : one that arises just above the bifurcation of the abdominal aorta into the common iliac arteries and supplies the left half of the transverse colon, the descending colon, the sigmoid colon, and most of the rectum — called also *inferior mesenteric artery*   **b** : a large artery that arises from the aorta just below the celiac artery at the level of the first lumbar vertebra and supplies the greater part of the small intestine, the cecum, the ascending colon, and the right half of the transverse colon — called also *superior mesenteric artery*

mesenteric ganglion *n* : either of two ganglionic masses of the sympathetic nervous system associated with the corresponding mesenteric plexus: **a** : a variable amount of massed ganglionic tissue of the inferior mesenteric plexus near the origin of the inferior mesenteric artery — called also *inferior mesenteric ganglion*   **b** : a usu. discrete ganglionic mass of the superior mesenteric plexus near the origin of the superior mesenteric artery — called also *superior mesenteric ganglion*

mesenteric node *n* : any of the lymphatic glands of the mesentery — called also *mesenteric gland, mesenteric lymph node*

mesenteric plexus *n* : either of two plexuses of the sympathetic nervous system lying mostly in the mesentery in close proximity to and distributed to the same structures as the corresponding mesenteric arteries: **a** : one associated with the inferior mesenteric artery — called also *inferior mesenteric plexus*   **b** : a subdivision of the celiac plexus that is associated with the superior mesenteric artery — called also *superior mesenteric plexus*

mesenteric vein *n* : either of two veins draining the intestine, passing between the two layers of the mesentery, and associated with the corresponding mesenteric arteries: **a** : one that is a continuation of the superior rectal vein, that returns blood from the rectum, the sigmoid colon, and the descending colon, that accompanies the inferior mesenteric artery, and that usu. empties into the splenic vein — called also *inferior mesenteric vein*   **b** : one that drains blood from the small intestine, the cecum, the ascending colon, the transverse colon, that accompanies the superior mesenteric artery, and that joins with the splenic vein to form the portal vein — called also *superior mesenteric vein*

mes·en·teri·o·lum \ˌmez-ᵊn-ˌter-ē-'ō-ləm, ˌmes-ᵊn-tə-'rī-ə-ləm\ *n, pl* **-o·la** \-lə\ : MESOAPPENDIX

mes·en·ter·i·tis \ˌmez-ᵊn-tə-'rīt-əs, ˌmes-\ *n* : inflammation of the mesentery

mes·en·ter·on \(')mez-'ent-ə-ˌrän, (')mēz-, (')mēs-, (')mes-, -rən\ *n, pl* **-tera** \-ə-rə\ : the part of the alimentary canal that is developed from the archenteron and is lined with hypoblast

mes·en·tery \'mez-ᵊn-ˌter-ē, 'mes-\ *n, pl* **-ter·ies** **1** : one or more vertebrate membranes that consist of a double fold of the peritoneum and invest the intestines and their appendages and connect them with the dorsal wall of the abdominal cavity; *specif* : such membranes connected with the jejunum and ileum in humans   **2** : a fold of membrane comparable to a mesentery and supporting a viscus (as the heart) that is not a part of the digestive tract

mesentoderm *var of* MESENDODERM

mesh \'mesh\ *n* : a flexible netting of fine wire used in surgery esp. in the repair of large hernias and other body defects

mesh·work \'mesh-ˌwərk\ *n* : NETWORK ⟨a vascular ~⟩

mesiad *var of* MESAD

me·si·al \'mē-zē-əl, -sē-\ *also* **me·sal** \-zəl, -səl\ *adj* **1** : being or located in the middle or a median part ⟨the ~ aspect of the metacarpal head⟩   **2** : situated in or near or directed toward the median plane of the body ⟨the heart is ~ to the lungs⟩ — compare DISTAL 1b   **3** : of, relating to, or being the surface of a tooth that is next to the tooth in front of it or that is closest to the middle of the front of the jaw — compare DISTAL 1c, PROXIMAL 1b — **me·si·al·ly** \-ē\ *adv*

me·sio·buc·cal \ˌmē-zē-ō-'bək-ᵊl, -sē-\ *adj* : of or relating to the mesial and buccal surfaces of a tooth — **me·sio·buc·cal·ly** \-ē\ *adv*

me·sio·clu·sion *also* **me·si·oc·clu·sion** \ˌmē-zē-ə-'klü-zhən, -sē-\ *n* : malocclusion characterized by mesial displacement of one or more of the lower teeth

me·sio·dis·tal \ˌmē-zē-ō-'dis-tᵊl\ *adj* : of or relating to the mesial and distal surfaces of a tooth; *esp* : relating to, lying along, containing, or being a diameter joining the mesial and distal surfaces ⟨~ length⟩ — **me·sio·dis·tal·ly** \-ē\ *adv*

me·sio·lin·gual \-'liŋ-g(yə-)wəl\ *adj* : of or relating to the mesial and lingual surfaces of a tooth — **me·sio·lin·gual·ly** \-ē\ *adv*

me·sit·y·lene \mə-'sit-ᵊl-ˌēn\ *n* : an oily hydrocarbon C_9H_{12} that is found in coal tar and petroleum or made synthetically and is a powerful solvent

mes·mer·ism \'mez-mə-ˌriz-əm *also* 'mes-\ *n* : hypnotic induction by the practices of F. A. Mesmer that was believed to involve animal magnetism; *broadly* : HYPNOTISM

Mes·mer \'mes-mər\, **Franz** *or* **Friedrich Anton (1734–1815)**, German physician. Mesmer started a career in orthodox medicine but soon began to explore new theories of medicine. He began experimenting with the use of magnets as curative agents and gradually developed a theory of animal magnetism. He believed in the presence of invisible fluids in the body and that disease resulted from an interruption in the free flow of these fluids. The flow of the fluid could be corrected through magnetic force. Eventually he came to believe that his own body possessed special magnetic forces. In 1778 he began practicing mesmerism in Paris and created a popular sensation. In 1784 his followers started to apply his techniques to hypnosis. Mesmer was regarded as a fraud by contemporary medical authorities.

mes·mer·ist \-rəst\ *n* : a practitioner of mesmerism

mes·mer·ize *or Brit* **mes·mer·ise** \-mə-ˌrīz\ *vt* **-ized** *or Brit* **-ised; -iz·ing** *or Brit* **-is·ing** : to subject to mesmerism; *also* : HYPNOTIZE — **mes·mer·iza·tion** *or Brit* **mes·mer·isa·tion** \ˌmez-mə-ri-'zā-shən\ *n*

me·so \'me-(ˌ)zō, 'mē-, -(ˌ)sō\ *adj, of a molecule or compound* : optically inactive because internally compensated

me·so·ap·pen·di·ce·al \ˌmez-ō-ˌə-ˌpen-də-'sē-əl, ˌmēz-, ˌmēs-, ˌmes-\ *adj* : of or relating to the mesoappendix

me·so·ap·pen·dix \-ə-'pen-diks\ *n, pl* **-dix·es** *or* **-di·ces** \-də-ˌsēz\ : the mesentery of the vermiform appendix

me·so·bili·ru·bin \-'bil-ē-ˌrü-bin\ *n* : a red crystalline pigment $C_{33}H_{40}N_4O_6$ obtained by reduction of bilirubin

me·so·blast \\'mez-ə-ˌblast, 'mēz-, 'mēs-, 'mes-\\ *n* : the embryonic cells that give rise to mesoderm; *broadly* : MESODERM

me·so·blas·te·ma \\ˌmez-ə-blas-'tē-mə, ˌmēz-, ˌmēs-, ˌmes-\\ *n* : MESOBLAST — **me·so·blas·te·mic** \\-blas-'tē-mik\\ *adj*

me·so·blas·tic \\-'blas-tik\\ *adj* : relating to, derived from, or made up of mesoblast

me·so·car·dia \\-'kärd-ē-ə\\ *n* : abnormal location of the heart in the central part of the thorax

me·so·car·di·um \\-'kärd-ē-əm\\ *n* **1** : the transitory mesentery of the embryonic heart **2** : either of two tubular prolongations of the epicardium that enclose the aorta and pulmonary trunk and the venae cavae and pulmonary veins

me·so·ce·cum *or chiefly Brit* **me·so·cae·cum** \\-'sē-kəm\\ *n, pl* **-ce·ca** *or chiefly Brit* **-cae·ca** \\-kə\\ : the fold of peritoneum attached to the cecum

me·so·ceph·al \\-'sef-əl\\ *n* : an individual with a mesocephalic skull

me·so·ce·phal·ic \\-sə-'fal-ik\\ *adj* : having a head of medium proportion with a cephalic index of 76.0 to 80.9

me·so·ceph·a·ly \\-'sef-ə-lē\\ *n, pl* **-a·lies** : the quality or state of being mesocephalic — called also *mesaticephaly*

Me·so·ces·toi·des \\-ˌses-'tȯi-(ˌ)dēz\\ *n* : a genus (the type of the family Mesocestoididae) of atypical unarmed cyclophyllidean tapeworms having the adults parasitic in mammals and birds and a slender threadlike contractile larva free in cavities or encysted in tissues of mammals, birds, and sometimes reptiles — **me·so·ces·toid·id** \\-'tȯi-dəd\\

me·so·chon·dri·um \\-'kän-drē-əm\\ *n, pl* **-dria** \\-drē-ə\\ : the matrix of cartilage

me·so·cne·mic \\-ə-'nē-mik, -ək-'nē-mik\\ *adj, of a shinbone* : rounded with a platycnemic index of 63.0 to 69.9

me·so·coele *also* **me·so·coel** \\'mez-ə-ˌsēl, 'mēz-, 'mēs-, 'mes-\\ *n* : the embryonic cavity of the midbrain

me·so·co·lon \\ˌmez-ə-'kō-lən, ˌmēz-, ˌmēs-, ˌmes-\\ *n* : a mesentery joining the colon to the dorsal abdominal wall

meso·conch \\'mez-ə-ˌkäŋk, 'mēz-, 'mēs-, 'mes-\\ *also* **me·so·chon·chic** \\-'käŋk-ik\\ *adj* : having the orbits moderately rounded with an orbital index of 76.0 to 84.9 — **me·so·con·chy** \\-ˌkäŋ-kē\\ *n, pl* **-chies**

me·so·cra·nic \\-'krā-nik, ˌmēz-, ˌmēs-, ˌmes-\\ *also* **me·so·cra·ni·al** \\-'krā-nē-əl\\ *adj* : having a skull of medium proportions with a cranial index of 75.0 to 79.9 — **me·so·cra·ny** \\'mez-ə-ˌkrā-nē\\ *n, pl* **-nies**

me·so·derm \\'mez-ə-ˌdərm, 'mēz-, 'mēs-, 'mes-\\ *n* : the middle of the three primary germ layers of an embryo that is the source esp. of bone, muscle, connective tissue, and dermis; *broadly* : tissue derived from this germ layer — **me·so·der·mal** \\ˌmez-ə-'dor-məl, ˌmēz-, ˌmēs-, ˌmes-\\ *also* **me·so·der·mic** \\-'dər-mik\\ *adj* — **me·so·der·mal·ly** \\-ē\\ *adv*

me·so·dont \\-ˌdänt\\ *adj* : having medium-sized teeth — **me·so·don·ty** \\-ˌdän-tē\\ *n, pl* **-ties**

me·so·duo·de·num \\ˌmez-ə-ˌd(y)ü-ə-'dē-nəm, ˌmēz-, ˌmēs-, ˌmes-, -d(y)ù-'äd-ᵊn-əm\\ *n, pl* **-de·na** \\-'dē-nə, -ᵊn-ə\\ *or* **-de·nums** : the mesentery of the duodenum usu. not persisting in adult life in humans and other mammals in which the developing intestine undergoes a counterclockwise rotation

me·so·e·soph·a·gus *or chiefly Brit* **me·so·oe·soph·a·gus** \\-i-'säf-ə-gəs\\ *n* : the transitory mesentery of the embryonic esophagus that is later modified into the mediastinum

me·so·gas·ter \\'mez-ə-ˌgas-ter, 'mēz-, 'mēs-, 'mes-\\ *n* : MESOGASTRIUM

me·so·gas·tric \\ˌmez-ə-'gas-trik, ˌmēz-, ˌmēs-, ˌmes-\\ *adj* : of or relating to the mesogastrium

me·so·gas·tri·um \\-'gas-trē-əm\\ *n, pl* **-tria** \\-trē-ə\\ **1** : a ventral mesentery of the embryonic stomach that persists as the falciform ligament and the lesser omentum — called also *ventral mesogastrium* **2** : a dorsal mesentery of the embryonic stomach that gives rise to ligaments between the stomach and spleen and the spleen and kidney — called also *dorsal mesogastrium*

me·so·gna·thion \\-'nā-thē-ˌän, -'nath-ē-ən\\ *n* : the lateral part of the premaxilla bearing the lateral incisor tooth on each side

me·sog·na·thous \\mə-'zäg-nə-thəs, mē-'säg-\\ *also* **me·sog-**

nath·ic \\ˌmez-äg-'nath-ik, ˌmēs-\\ *adj* : having the jaws of medium size and slightly projecting with a gnathic index of 98.0 to 102.9 — **me·sog·na·thy** \\mə-'zäg-nə-thē\\ *n, pl* **-thies**

me·so·ino·si·tol \\ˌmez-ō-in-'ō-sə-ˌtȯl, mē-zō-, -ī-'nō-sə-ˌtȯl\\ *n* : MYOINOSITOL

me·so·lec·i·thal \\ˌmez-ō-'les-ə-thəl, ˌmēz-\\ *adj* : CENTROLECITHAL

me·so·lim·bic \\-'lim-bik\\ *adj* : of, relating to, or being the more central portion of the limbic system of the brain that arises mainly in the ventral tegmental area, consists esp. of dopaminergic neurons, and innervates the amygdala, nucleus accumbens, and olfactory tubercle ⟨the brain's ∼ system is involved with the control of memory and emotion —*Chem. & Engineering News*⟩

me·so·mere \\'mez-ə-ˌmi(ə)r, 'mēz-, 'mēs-, 'mes-\\ *n* : a blastomere of medium size; *also* : an intermediate part of the mesoderm

me·som·er·ism \\mə-'säm-ə-ˌriz-əm, -'zäm-\\ *n* : RESONANCE 3 — **me·so·mer·ic** \\ˌmez-ə-'mer-ik, ˌmēz-\\ *adj*

me·so·me·tri·al \\ˌmez-ə-'mē-trē-əl, ˌmēz-, ˌmēs-, ˌmes-\\ *or* **me·so·me·tric** \\-'me-trik\\ *adj* : of or relating to the mesometrium — **me·so·me·tri·al·ly** \\-ē\\ *adv*

me·so·me·tri·um \\-'mē-trē-əm\\ *n, pl* **-tria** \\-trē-ə\\ : a mesentery supporting the oviduct or uterus

me·so·morph \\'mez-ə-ˌmȯrf, 'mēz-, 'mēs-, 'mes-\\ *n* : a mesomorphic body or person

me·so·mor·phic \\ˌmez-ə-'mȯr-fik, ˌmēz-, ˌmēs-, ˌmes-\\ *adj* **1** *also* **me·so·mor·phous** \\-fəs\\ : relating to, existing in, or being an intermediate state (as of a semicrystalline condition characteristic of liquid crystals) — compare NEMATIC, SMECTIC **2 a** : of or relating to the component in W. H. Sheldon's classification of body types that measures esp. the degree of muscularity and bone development **b** : having a husky muscular body build — compare ECTOMORPHIC 2, ENDOMORPHIC 2

me·so·mor·phism \\-'mȯr-ˌfiz-əm\\ *n* : the quality or state of being mesomorphic

me·so·mor·phy \\'mez-ə-ˌmȯr-fē, 'mēz-\\ *n, pl* **-phies** : a mesomorphic body build or type

me·son \\'mez-ˌän, 'mēz-, 'mēs-, 'mes-\\ *n* : any of a group of unstable elementary particles that are subject to nuclear forces and have masses much greater than that of the electron — **me·son·ic** \\me-'zän-ik, mē-, -'sän-\\ *adj*

me·so·neph·ric \\ˌmez-ə-'nef-rik, ˌmēz-, ˌmēs-, ˌmes-\\ *adj* : of or relating to the mesonephros

mesonephric duct *n* : WOLFFIAN DUCT

me·so·ne·phro·ma \\-ni-'frō-mə\\ *n, pl* **-mas** *also* **-ma·ta** \\-mət-ə\\ : a benign or malignant tumor esp. of the female genital tract held to be derived from the mesonephros

me·so·neph·ros \\ˌmez-ə-'nef-rəs, ˌmēz-, ˌmēs-, ˌmes-, -ˌräs\\ *n, pl* **-neph·roi** \\-ˌrȯi\\ : either member of the second and midmost of the three paired vertebrate renal organs that functions in adult fishes and amphibians but functions only in the embryo of reptiles, birds, and mammals in which it is replaced by a metanephros in the adult — called also *Wolffian body;* compare PRONEPHROS

meso–oesophagus *chiefly Brit var of* MESOESOPHAGUS

me·so·on·to·morph \\-'änt-ə-ˌmȯrf\\ *n* : a body type characterized by a thickset robust powerful build; *also* : an individual of this type — compare HYPERONTOMORPH

me·so·phile \\'mez-ə-ˌfīl, 'mēz-, 'mēs, 'mes-\\ *also* **me·so·phil** \\-ˌfil\\ *n* : an organism growing at a moderate temperature (as bacteria that grow best at about the temperature of the human body) — compare PSYCHROPHILE, THERMOPHILE

me·so·phil·ic \\ˌmez-ə-'fil-ik, ˌmēz-, ˌmēs-, ˌmes-\\ *adj* : growing or thriving best in an intermediate environment (as in one of moderate temperature) ⟨∼ bacteria⟩

me·soph·ry·on \\mə-'zäf-rē-ˌän, -ən\\ *n, pl* **me·soph·rya** \\-rē-ə\\ : GLABELLA

\\ə\\ abut \\ᵊ\\ kitten \\ər\\ further \\a\\ ash \\ā\\ ace \\ä\\ cot, cart
\\aù\\ out \\ch\\ chin \\e\\ bet \\ē\\ easy \\g\\ go \\i\\ hit \\ī\\ ice \\j\\ job
\\ŋ\\ sing \\ō\\ go \\ȯ\\ law \\ȯi\\ boy \\th\\ thin \\th\\ the \\ü\\ loot
\\ù\\ foot \\y\\ yet \\zh\\ vision *See also* Pronunciation Symbols page

M
N

me·so·pic \me-'zäp-ik, mē-'sōp-\ *adj* **1** : having a face on which the root of the nose and central line of the face project moderately **2** : of or relating to vision under conditions of intermediate levels of illumination ⟨∼ vision tests made in a cloudy moonlight illumination —*Science News Letter*⟩

me·so·por·phy·rin \mez-ō-'pȯr-fə-rən, ‚mēz-, ‚mēs-, ‚mes-\ *n* : any one of the isomeric porphyrins $C_{34}H_{38}N_4O_4$ produced from protoporphyrin by reducing the vinyl groups to ethyl groups

me·su·pro·so·pic \-prə-'sōp-ik, -'säp-\ *adj* : having a face of average width with a facial index of 84.0 to 87.9 as measured on the living head or 85.0 to 89.9 on the skull — **me·so·pros·o·py** \-'präs-ə-pē, -prə-'säp-ē\ *n, pl* **-pies**

me·sor·chi·um \mə-'zȯr-kē-əm\ *n, pl* **-chia** \-kē-ə\ : the fold of peritoneum that attaches the testis to the dorsal wall in the fetus

me·so·rec·tum \‚mez-ə-'rek-təm, ‚mēz-, ‚mēs-, ‚mes-\ *n, pl* **-tums** *or* **-ta** \-tə\ : the mesentery that supports the rectum

mes·orid·a·zine \-‚ȯr-'id-ə-‚zēn\ *n* : a phenothiazine tranquilizer $C_{21}H_{26}N_2OS_2$ used in the treatment of schizophrenia, organic brain disorders, alcoholism, and psychoneuroses

¹me·sor·rhine \'mez-ə-‚rīn, 'mēz-\ *also* **me·sor·rhin·ic** \‚mez-ə-'rin-ik, ‚mēz-\ *adj* : having a nose of moderate size with a nasal index of 47.0 to 50.9 on the skull or of 70.0 to 84.9 on the living head — **me·sor·rhi·ny** \'mez-ə-‚rī-nē, 'mēz-\ *n, pl* **-nies**

²mesorrhine *n* : a mesorrhine individual

me·so·sal·pinx \‚mez-ō-'sal-(‚)piŋ(k)s, ‚mēz-, ‚mēs-, ‚mes-\ *n, pl* **-sal·pin·ges** \-sal-'pin-(‚)jēz\ : a fold of the broad ligament investing and supporting the fallopian tube

me·so·sig·moid \-'sig-‚mȯid\ *n* : the mesentery of the sigmoid part of the descending colon

me·so·some \'mez-ə-‚sōm, 'mēz-, 'mēs-, 'mes-\ *n* : an organelle of bacteria that appears in electron micrographs as an invagination of the plasma membrane and is a site of localization of respiratory enzymes

me·so·staph·y·line \-'staf-ə-‚līn\ *adj* : having a palate of moderate size with a palatal index of 80.0 to 84.9

me·so·ster·num \‚mez-ə-'stər-nəm, ‚mēz-, ‚mēs-, ‚mes-\ *n, pl* **-ster·na** \-nə\ : GLADIOLUS

me·so·tar·sal \-'tar-səl\ *adj* : of or relating to the median plane of the tarsus

me·so·ten·don \-'ten-dən\ *n* : a fold of synovial membrane connecting a tendon to its synovial sheath

me·so·the·li·o·ma \‚mez-ə-‚thē-lē-'ō-mə, ‚mēz-, ‚mēs-, ‚mes-\ *n, pl* **-mas** *also* **-ma·ta** \-mət-ə\ : a tumor derived from mesothelial tissue (as that lining the peritoneum or pleura)

me·so·the·li·um \-'thē-lē-əm\ *n, pl* **-lia** \-lē-ə\ : epithelium derived from mesoderm that lines the body cavity of a vertebrate embryo and gives rise to epithelia (as of the peritoneum, pericardium, and pleurae), striated muscle, heart muscle, and several minor structures — **me·so·the·li·al** \-lē-əl\ *adj*

mes·ovar·i·um \‚mez-ō-'var-ē-əm, ‚mēz-, ‚mēs-, ‚mes-\ *n, pl* **-ovar·ia** \-ē-ə\ : the mesentery uniting the ovary with the body wall

mes·ox·a·lyl·urea \-‚äk-sə-lil-'(y)ur-ē-ə\ *n* : ALLOXAN

Me·so·zoa \‚mez-ō-'zō-ə, ‚mēz-, ‚mēs-, ‚mes-\ *n pl* : a phylum or other taxonomic group comprising the mesozoans

me·so·zo·an \-'zō-ən\ *n* : any of the animals that comprise the taxon Mesozoa, that includes small wormlike parasitic forms with an outer layer of somatic cells and an inner mass of reproductive cells, and that are often regarded as intermediate in organization between the protozoans and the metazoans although they may be degenerate descendents of more highly organized forms — **mesozoan** *adj*

mes·sen·ger \'mes-ᵊn-jər\ *n* **1** : a substance (as a hormone) that mediates a biological effect — see FIRST MESSENGER, SECOND MESSENGER **2** : MESSENGER RNA

messenger RNA *n* : an RNA produced by transcription that carries the code for a particular protein from the nuclear DNA to a ribosome in the cytoplasm and acts as a template for the formation of that protein — called also *mRNA;* compare TRANSFER RNA

mes·ter·o·lone \mes-'ter-ə-‚lōn\ *n* : an androgen $C_{20}H_{32}O_2$ used in the treatment of male infertility

Mes·ti·non \'mes-tə-‚nän\ *trademark* — used for a preparation of pyridostigmine

mes·tra·nol \'mes-trə-‚nȯl, -‚nōl\ *n* : a synthetic estrogen $C_{21}H_{26}O_2$ used in birth control pills — see ENOVID, ORTHO-NOVUM

me·su·ran·ic \‚mes-(y)ur-'an-ik, ‚mesh-ər-\ *adj* : having a maxillo-alveolar index of between 110.0 and 114.9 — **me·su·rany** \'mes-yər-‚an-ē\ *n, pl* **-ran·ies**

mes·y·late \'mes-i-‚lāt\ *n* : any of the esters of an acid CH_4SO_3 including some in which it is combined with a drug — called also *methanesulfonate;* see ERGOLOID MESYLATES

met \'met, ‚em-(‚)ē-'tē\ *n, often all cap* : a unit of measure of the rate at which the body expends energy that is based on the energy expenditure while sitting at rest and is equal to 3.5 milliliters of oxygen per kilogram of body weight per minute — called also *metabolic equivalent*

Met *abbr* methionine; methionyl

meta \'met-ə\ *adj* : relating to, characterized by, or being two positions in the benzene ring that are separated by one carbon atom

meta- *or* **met-** *prefix* **1** : isomeric with or otherwise closely related to ⟨*met*aldehyde⟩ **2** : involving substitution at or characterized by two positions in the benzene ring that are separated by one carbon atom — abbr. *m-* ⟨*meta*-xylene or *m*-xylene⟩; compare ORTH- 2, PARA- 2

meta–anal·y·sis \‚met-ə-ə-'nal-ə-səs\ *n* : quantitative statistical analysis that is applied to separate but similar experiments of different and usu. independent researchers and that involves pooling the data and using the pooled data to test the effectiveness of the results ⟨the report . . . on low cholesterol presented a comprehensive ∼ of 32 randomized studies involving 42,000 individuals —*Scientific Amer. Medicine Bull.*⟩

me·tab·a·sis \mə-'tab-ə-səs\ *n, pl* **-a·ses** \-ə-‚sēz\ : a medical change (as of disease, symptoms, or treatment)

meta·bi·o·sis \‚met-ə-bī-'ō-səs\ *n, pl* **-o·ses** \-'ō-sēz\ : a mode of life in which one organism so depends on another that it cannot flourish unless the latter precedes and influences the environment favorably — **meta·bi·ot·ic** \-'ät-ik\ *adj* — **meta·bi·ot·i·cal·ly** \-i-k(ə-)lē\ *adv*

meta·bi·sul·fite *or chiefly Brit* **meta·bi·sul·phite** \-‚bī-'səl-‚fīt\ *n* : a salt containing the bivalent anion $S_2O_5^{2-}$ obtained by heating a bisulfite — see SODIUM METABISULFITE

met·a·bol·ic \‚met-ə-'bäl-ik\ *adj* **1** : of, relating to, or based on metabolism **2** : VEGETATIVE 1a(2) — used esp. of a cell nucleus that is not dividing — **met·a·bol·i·cal·ly** \-i-k(ə-)lē\ *adv*

metabolic acidosis *n* : acidosis resulting from excess acid due to abnormal metabolism, excessive acid intake, or renal retention or from excessive loss of bicarbonate (as in diarrhea)

metabolic alkalosis *n* : alkalosis resulting from excessive alkali intake or excessive acid loss (as from vomiting)

metabolic equivalent *n* : MET

metabolic pathway *n* : PATHWAY 2

metabolic pool *n* : the pool of absorbable substances that are or can be involved in metabolism

metabolic rate *n* : metabolism per unit time esp. as estimated by food consumption, energy released as heat, or oxygen used in metabolic processes — see BASAL METABOLIC RATE

metabolic syndrome *n* : a syndrome marked by the presence of usu. three or more of a group of factors (as high blood pressure, abdominal obesity, high triglyceride levels, low HDL levels, and high fasting levels of blood sugar) that are linked to an increased risk of cardiovascular disease and type 2 diabetes — called also *insulin resistance syndrome, syndrome X*

metabolic water *n* : water produced by living cells as a by-product of oxidative metabolism

me·tab·o·lim·e·ter \me-ˌtab-ə-ˈlim-ət-ər, ˌmet-ə-bə-\ *n* : an instrument for measuring basal metabolism

me·tab·o·lism \mə-ˈtab-ə-ˌliz-əm\ *n* **1 a** : the sum of the processes in the buildup and destruction of protoplasm; *specif* : the chemical changes in living cells by which energy is provided for vital processes and activities and new material is assimilated ⟨methods of determining body and tissue ∼ —*Bull. of the Univ. of Ky.*⟩ — see ANABOLISM, CATABOLISM **b** : the sum of the processes by which a particular substance is handled (as by assimilation and incorporation or by detoxification and excretion) in the living body ⟨the ∼ of iodine in the thyroid⟩ **2** : METAMORPHOSIS 2 — usu. used in combination ⟨holo*metabolism*⟩

me·tab·o·lite \-ˌlīt\ *n* **1** : a product of metabolism: **a** : a metabolic waste usu. more or less toxic to the organism producing it : EXCRETION **b** : a product of one metabolic process that is essential to another such process in the same organism **c** : a metabolic waste of one organism that is markedly toxic to another : ANTIBIOTIC **2** : a substance essential to the metabolism of a particular organism or to a particular metabolic process

me·tab·o·liz·able *also Brit* **me·tab·o·lis·able** \mə-ˈtab-ə-ˌlī-zə-bəl\ *adj* **1** : capable of being utilized in metabolism ⟨∼ nutrients⟩ **2** : producible or produced by metabolic processes ⟨∼ energy⟩ — **me·tab·o·liz·abil·i·ty** *also Brit* **me·tab·o·lis·abil·i·ty** \mə-ˌtab-ə-ˌlī-zə-ˈbil-ət-ē\ *n, pl* -ties

me·tab·o·lize *also Brit* **me·tab·o·lise** \-ˌlīz\ *vb* -lized *also Brit* -lised; -liz·ing *also Brit* -lis·ing *vt* : to subject to metabolism ∼ *vi* : to perform metabolism — **me·tab·o·liz·er** *also Brit* **me·tab·o·lis·er** \-ˌlī-zər\ *n*

me·tab·o·tro·pic \mə-ˌtab-ə-ˈtrō-pik, -ˈträp-ik\ *adj* : relating to or being a receptor for glutamate that when complexed with G protein triggers increased production of certain intracellular messengers ⟨∼ glutamate receptors⟩

¹meta·car·pal \ˌmet-ə-ˈkär-pəl\ *adj* : of, relating to, or being the metacarpus or a metacarpal

²metacarpal *n* : any bone of the metacarpus of the human hand or the front foot in quadrupeds

meta·car·po·pha·lan·ge·al \ˌmet-ə-ˌkär-pō-ˌfā-lən-ˈjē-əl, -ˌfa-, -fə-ˈlan-jē-\ *adj* : of, relating to, or involving both the metacarpus and the phalanges ⟨a ∼ joint⟩

meta·car·pus \ˌmet-ə-ˈkär-pəs\ *n* : the part of the human hand or the front foot in quadrupeds between the carpus and the phalanges that contains five more or less elongated bones when all the digits are present (as in humans) but is modified in many animals by the loss or reduction of some bones or the fusing of adjacent bones

meta·cen·tric \ˌmet-ə-ˈsen-trik\ *adj* : having the centromere medially situated so that the two chromosomal arms are of roughly equal length — compare ACROCENTRIC, TELOCENTRIC — **metacentric** *n*

meta·cer·car·ia \ˌmet-ə-(ˌ)sər-ˈkar-ē-ə, -ˈker-\ *n, pl* -i·ae \-ē-ˌē\ : a tailless encysted late larva of a digenetic trematode that is usu. the form which is infective for the definitive host — **meta·cer·car·i·al** \-ē-əl\ *adj*

meta·ces·tode \-ˈses-ˌtōd\ *n* : a stage of a tapeworm occurring in an intermediate host : a larval tapeworm

meta·chro·ma·sia \ˌmet-ə-krō-ˈmā-zh(ē-)ə\ *n* **1** : the property of various tissues of staining in a different color (as when treatment with a blue aniline dye makes a cellular element red) **2** : the property of various biologic stains that permits a single dye to stain different tissue elements in different colors

meta·chro·ma·sy *or* **meta·chro·ma·cy** \-ˈkrō-mə-sē\ *n, pl* -sies *or* -cies : METACHROMASIA

meta·chro·mat·ic \-krō-ˈmat-ik\ *adj* **1** : staining or characterized by staining in a different color or shade from what is typical ⟨∼ granules⟩ **2** : having the capacity to stain different elements of a cell or tissue in different colors or shades ⟨∼ stains⟩ — **meta·chro·mat·i·cal·ly** \-i-k(ə-)lē\ *adv*

metachromatic leukodystrophy *n* : a hereditary neurological disorder of lipid metabolism characterized by the accumulation of cerebroside sulfates, loss of myelin in the central

nervous system, and progressive deterioration of mental and motor activity

meta·chro·ma·tin \ˌmet-ə-ˈkrō-mət-ən\ *n* : VOLUTIN — **meta·chro·ma·tin·ic** \-ˌkrō-mə-ˈtin-ik\ *adj*

meta·chro·ma·tism \-ˈkrō-mə-ˌtiz-əm\ *n* : METACHROMASIA

me·tach·ro·nous \mə-ˈtak-rə-nəs\ *adj* **1** : not functioning or occurring synchronously ⟨the ∼ beating of cilia⟩ **2** : occurring or starting at different times ⟨∼ cancers of the large bowel —*Jour. Amer. Med. Assoc.*⟩

meta·chro·sis \ˌmet-ə-ˈkrō-səs\ *n, pl* -chro·ses \-ˌsēz\ : the power of some animals (as many fishes and reptiles) to change color voluntarily by the expansion of special pigment cells

meta·cone \ˈmet-ə-ˌkōn\ *n* : the distobuccal cusp of an upper molar

meta·co·nid \ˌmet-ə-ˈkō-nəd\ *n* : the cusp of a lower molar corresponding to a metacone

meta·con·trast \ˌmet-ə-ˈkän-ˌtrast\ *n* : a reduction in the perceived brightness of a visual stimulus when followed immediately by an adjacent visual stimulus

meta·co·nule \-ˈkōn-(ˌ)yül\ *n* : the posterior intermediate cusp of a mammalian upper molar between the hypocone and the metacone

meta·cor·tan·dra·cin \-kȯr-ˈtan-drə-sən\ *n* : PREDNISONE

meta·cor·tan·dra·lone \-kȯr-ˈtan-drə-ˌlōn\ *n* : PREDNISOLONE

meta·cre·sol \-ˈkrē-ˌsȯl, -ˌsōl\ *n* : the meta isomer of cresol that has antiseptic properties

meta·cryp·to·zo·ite \-ˌkrip-tō-ˈzō-ˌīt\ *n* : a member of a second or subsequent generation of tissue-dwelling forms of a malaria parasite derived from the sporozoite without intervening generations of blood parasites — compare CRYPTOZOITE

meta·cy·clic \-ˈsī-klik *also* -ˈsik-lik\ *adj, of a trypanosome* : broad and stocky, produced in an intermediate host, and infective for the definitive host

meta·gen·e·sis \-ˈjen-ə-səs\ *n, pl* -e·ses \-ˌsēz\ : ALTERNATION OF GENERATIONS; *esp* : regular alternation of a sexual and an asexual generation — **meta·ge·net·ic** \-jə-ˈnet-ik\ *adj*

Meta·gon·i·mus \-ˈgän-ə-məs\ *n* : a genus of small intestinal flukes (family Heterophyidae) that includes one (*M. yokogawai*) common in humans, dogs, and cats in parts of eastern Asia as a result of the eating of raw fish containing the larva

Meta·hy·drin \-ˈhī-drin\ *trademark* — used for a preparation of trichlormethiazide

meta·ken·trin \-ˈken-trin\ *n* : LUTEINIZING HORMONE

met·al \ˈmet-ᵊl\ *n* : any of various opaque, fusible, ductile, and typically lustrous substances that are good conductors of electricity and heat, form cations by loss of electrons, and yield basic oxides and hydroxides; *esp* : one that is a chemical element as distinguished from an alloy

met·al·de·hyde \ˌmet-ᵊl-də-ˌhīd\ *n* : a crystalline compound $(C_2H_4O)_n$ that is a cyclic oligomer of acetaldehyde used as a solid fuel for portable stoves and as a lure and poison for snails

me·tal·lic \mə-ˈtal-ik\ *adj* **1** : of, relating to, or being a metal **2** : made of or containing a metal **3** : having properties of a metal

me·tal·lo·en·zyme \mə-ˌtal-ō-ˈen-ˌzīm\ *n* : an enzyme consisting of a protein linked with a specific metal

me·tal·lo·fla·vo·pro·tein \-ˌflā-vō-ˈprō-ˌtēn, -ˈprōt-ē-ən\ *n* : a flavoprotein that contains a metal

¹met·al·loid \ˈmet-ᵊl-ˌȯid\ *n* : an element (as boron, silicon, or arsenic) intermediate in properties between the typical metals and nonmetals

²metalloid *also* **met·al·loi·dal** \ˌmet-ᵊl-ˈȯid-ᵊl\ *adj* **1** : resembling a metal **2** : of, relating to, or being a metalloid

---

\ə\ abut \ᵊ\ kitten \ər\ further \a\ ash \ā\ ace \ä\ cot, cart
\au̇\ out \ch\ chin \e\ bet \ē\ easy \g\ go \i\ hit \ī\ ice \j\ job
\ŋ\ sing \ō\ go \ȯ\ law \ȯi\ boy \th\ thin \th\ the \ü\ loot
\u̇\ foot \y\ yet \zh\ vision *See also* Pronunciation Symbols page

me·tal·lo·por·phy·rin \mə-ˌtal-ō-ˈpȯr-fə-rən\ *n* : a compound (as heme) formed from a porphyrin and a metal ion

me·tal·lo·pro·tein \-ˈprō-ˌtēn, -ˈprōt-ē-ən\ *n* : a conjugated protein in which the prosthetic group is a metal

me·tal·lo·thio·ne·in \-ˌthī-ə-ˈnē-ən\ *n* : any of various metal-binding proteins involved in the metabolism of copper and zinc in body tissue (as of the liver) and in the binding of toxic metals (as cadmium)

meta·mer \ˈmet-ə-ˌmər\ *n* **1** : a chemical compound that is metameric with one or more others **2** : either of two colors of different spectral composition that appear identical to the eye of a single observer under some lighting conditions but different under others or that under constant lighting conditions appear identical to some observers and different to others

meta·mere \ˈmet-ə-ˌmi(ə)r\ *n* : any of a linear series of primitively similar segments into which the body of a higher invertebrate or vertebrate is divisible and which are usu. clearly distinguishable in the embryo, identifiable in somewhat modified form in various invertebrates (as annelid worms), and detectable in the adult higher vertebrate only in specialized segmentally arranged structures (as cranial and spinal nerves or vertebrae) : SOMITE

meta·mer·ic \ˌmet-ə-ˈmer-ik\ *adj* **1** : relating to or exhibiting chemical metamerism : ISOMERIC **2 a** : of, relating to, or exhibiting bodily metamerism ⟨a ∼ animal⟩ **b** : of, relating to, or occurring in a metamere ⟨∼ arrangement of blood vessels⟩ **3** : of, relating to, or being color metamers ⟨a ∼ pair⟩ — **meta·mer·i·cal·ly** \-i-k(ə-)lē\ *adv*

me·tam·er·ism \mə-ˈtam-ə-ˌriz-əm\ *n* **1** : isomerism esp. of chemical compounds of the same type **2** : the condition of having or the stage of evolutionary development characterized by a body made up of metamers that is usu. held to be an essential prelude to the differentiation of the more highly organized animals (as arthropods and vertebrates) through the disproportionate development and elaboration of some segments together with the coalescence, reduction, or loss of others **3** : the phenomenon exhibited by pairs of color metamers ⟨the problem of ∼ in matching artificial with natural teeth⟩

meta·mor·phic \ˌmet-ə-ˈmȯr-fik\ *adj* : of or relating to metamorphosis

meta·mor·phose \-ˌfōz, -ˌfōs\ *vi* **-phosed; -phos·ing** : to undergo metamorphosis

meta·mor·pho·sis \ˌmet-ə-ˈmȯr-fə-səs\ *n, pl* **-pho·ses** \-ˌsēz\ **1** : change of physical form, structure, or substance **2** : a marked and more or less abrupt developmental change in the form or structure of an animal (as a butterfly or a frog) occurring subsequent to birth or hatching

Met·a·mu·cil \ˌmet-ə-ˈmyü-sᵊl\ *trademark* — used for a laxative preparation of a hydrophilic mucilloid from the husk of psyllium seed

meta·my·elo·cyte \ˌmet-ə-ˈmī-ə-lə-ˌsīt\ *n* : any of the most immature granulocytes present in normal blood that are distinguished by typical cytoplasmic granulation in combination with a simple kidney-shaped nucleus

meta·neph·ric \ˌmet-ə-ˈnef-rik\ *adj* : of or relating to the metanephros

meta·neph·rine \-ˈnef-ˌrēn\ *n* : a catabolite of epinephrine that is found in the urine and some tissues

meta·neph·ro·gen·ic \-ˌnef-rə-ˈjen-ik\ *adj* : giving rise to the metanephroi ⟨∼ blastema⟩

meta·neph·ros \-ˈnef-rəs, -ˌräs\ *n, pl* **-neph·roi** \-ˌrȯi\ : either member of the final and most caudal pair of the three successive pairs of vertebrate renal organs that functions as a permanent adult kidney in reptiles, birds, and mammals but is not present at all in lower forms — compare MESONEPHROS, PRONEPHROS

meta·phase \ˈmet-ə-ˌfāz\ *n* : the stage of mitosis and meiosis in which the chromosomes become arranged in the equatorial plane of the spindle

metaphase plate *n* : a plane cell section in the equatorial plane of the metaphase spindle having the chromosomes oriented upon it

meta·phos·pho·ric acid \ˌmet-ə-ˌfäs-ˌfȯr-ik-, -ˌfär-; -ˌfäs-f(ə-)rik-\ *n* : a glassy solid acid HPO_3 or $(HPO_3)_n$ formed by heating orthophosphoric acid but usu. obtained in the form of salts

me·taph·y·se·al *also* **me·taph·y·si·al** \mə-ˌtaf-ə-ˈsē-əl, -ˈzē- *also* ˌmet-ə-ˈfiz-ē-əl\ *adj* : of or relating to a metaphysis ⟨∼ decalcification⟩

me·taph·y·sis \mə-ˈtaf-ə-səs\ *n, pl* **-y·ses** \-ˌsēz\ : the transitional zone at which the diaphysis and epiphysis of a bone come together

meta·pla·sia \ˌmet-ə-ˈplā-zh(ē-)ə\ *n* **1** : transformation of one tissue into another ⟨∼ of cartilage into bone⟩ **2** : abnormal replacement of cells of one type by cells of another

meta·plas·tic \-ˈplas-tik\ *adj* : relating to or produced by metaplasia

meta·pro·tein \ˌmet-ə-ˈprō-ˌtēn, -ˈprōt-ē-ən\ *n* : any of various products derived from proteins through the action of acids or alkalies by which the solubility and sometimes the composition of the proteins is changed

meta·pro·ter·e·nol \-prō-ˈter-ə-ˈnȯl, -ˌnōl\ *n* : a beta-adrenergic bronchodilator that is administered in the form of its sulfate $(C_{11}H_{17}NO_3)_2 \cdot H_2SO_4$ in the treatment of bronchial asthma and reversible bronchospasm associated with bronchitis and emphysema — see ALUPENT

meta·psy·chol·o·gy \ˌmet-ə-sī-ˈkäl-ə-jē\ *n, pl* **-gies** : speculative psychology concerned with postulating the mind's structure (as the ego and id) and processes (as cathexis) which usu. cannot be demonstrated objectively — **meta·psy·cho·log·i·cal** \-ˌsī-kə-ˈläj-i-kəl\ *adj*

meta·ram·i·nol \ˌmet-ə-ˈram-ə-ˌnȯl, -ˌnōl\ *n* : a sympathomimetic drug used in the form of its bitartrate $C_9H_{13}NO_2 \cdot C_4H_6O_6$ esp. as a vasoconstrictor to raise or maintain blood pressure

meta·rho·dop·sin \-rō-ˈdäp-sən\ *n* : either of two intermediate compounds formed in the bleaching of rhodopsin by light

met·ar·te·ri·ole \-ˌär-ˈtir-ē-ˌōl\ *n* : any of the delicate blood vessels that branch from the smallest arterioles and connect with the capillary bed — called also *precapillary*

meta·sta·ble \ˌmet-ə-ˈstā-bəl\ *adj* : having or characterized by only a slight margin of stability ⟨a ∼ compound⟩ — **meta·sta·bil·i·ty** \-stə-ˈbil-ət-ē\ *n, pl* **-ties**

me·tas·ta·sis \mə-ˈtas-tə-səs\ *n, pl* **-ta·ses** \-ˌsēz\ **1 a** : change of position, state, or form **b** : the spread of a disease-producing agency (as cancer cells or bacteria) from the initial or primary site of disease to another part of the body ⟨*metastases* of breast cancer to bone —*Medical Physics*⟩; *also* : the process by which such spreading occurs **2** : a secondary malignant tumor resulting from metastasis

me·tas·ta·size *also Brit* **me·tas·ta·sise** \mə-ˈtas-tə-ˌsīz\ *vi* **-sized** *also Brit* **-sised; -siz·ing** *also Brit* **-sis·ing** : to spread by metastasis ⟨the lesion already had *metastasized* beyond the larynx before a diagnosis of carcinoma was made —*Amer. Practitioner*⟩ — **me·tas·ta·si·za·tion** *also Brit* **me·tas·ta·si·sa·tion** \mə-ˌtas-tə-sə-ˈzā-shən\ *n*

met·a·stat·ic \ˌmet-ə-ˈstat-ik\ *adj* **1** : of, relating to, or caused by metastasis ⟨cutaneous ∼ disease as the first sign of lung cancer⟩ **2** : tending to metastasize ⟨determine what makes some cancer cells more ∼ than others —J. L. Marx⟩ — **met·a·stat·i·cal·ly** \-i-k(ə-)lē\ *adv*

Meta·stron·gyl·i·dae \ˌmet-ə-strän-ˈjil-ə-ˌdē\ *n pl* : a large family of parasitic strongyloid nematode worms including the genera *Dictyocaulus, Metastrongylus,* and *Protostrongylus* — **meta·stron·gyle** \-ˈsträn-ˌjīl, -jəl\ *n* — **meta·stron·gy·lid** \-ˈsträn-jə-lid\ *adj or n*

Meta·stron·gy·lus \-ˈsträn-jə-ləs\ *n* : a genus that is the type of the family Metastrongylidae and includes slender threadlike nematode worms parasitizing as adults the lungs and sometimes other organs of mammals and as larvae various earthworms

¹meta·tar·sal \ˌmet-ə-ˈtär-səl\ *adj* : of, relating to, or being the part of the human foot or of the hind foot in quadrupeds between the tarsus and the phalanges that in humans comprises five elongated bones which form the front of the instep and ball of the foot

²**metatarsal** *n* : a metatarsal bone

meta·tar·sal·gia \-ˌtär-ˈsal-j(ē-)ə\ *n* : a cramping burning pain below and between the metatarsal bones where they join the toe bones — see MORTON'S TOE

meta·tar·sec·to·my \-ˌtär-ˈsek-tə-mē\ *n, pl* **-mies** : surgical removal of the metatarsus or a metatarsal bone

meta·tar·so·pha·lan·ge·al joint \-ˌtär-sō-ˌfā-lən-ˈjē-əl-, -ˌfal-ən-, -fə-ˈlan-jē-\ *n* : any of the joints between the metatarsals and the phalanges

meta·tar·sus \ˌmet-ə-ˈtär-səs\ *n* : the part of the human foot or of the hind foot in quadrupeds that is between the tarsus and phalanges, contains when all the digits are present (as in humans) five more or less elongated bones but is modified in many animals with loss or reduction of some bones or fusing of others, and in humans forms the instep

meta·thal·a·mus \-ˈthal-ə-məs\ *n, pl* **-mi** \-ˌmī\ : the part of the diencephalon on each side that comprises the lateral and medial geniculate bodies

me·tath·e·sis \mə-ˈtath-ə-səs\ *n, pl* **-e·ses** \-ˌsēz\ : DOUBLE DECOMPOSITION

meta·troph \ˈmet-ə-ˌträf, -ˌtròf\ *n* : a metatrophic organism

meta·tro·phic \ˌmet-ə-ˈtròf-ik, -ˈträf-\ *adj* : requiring complex organic sources of carbon and nitrogen for metabolic synthesis : HETEROTROPHIC

meta·tro·pic dwarfism \ˌmet-ə-ˌtrō-pik-\ *n* : a congenital skeletal dysplasia characterized by short limbs and spinal deformity

met·ax·a·lone \mə-ˈtak-sə-ˌlōn\ *n* : a drug $C_{12}H_{15}NO_3$ used as a skeletal muscle relaxant

meta·zoa \ˌmet-ə-ˈzō-ə\ *n pl* **1** *cap* : a major taxonomic group comprising the metazoans — compare PROTOZOA **2** : animals that are metazoans

meta·zo·an \-ˈzō-ən\ *n* : any of the animals that comprise the taxon Metazoa, that have the body when adult composed of numerous cells differentiated into tissues and organs and usu. a digestive cavity lined with specialized cells, and that usu. include the coelenterates and all higher animals but sometimes also include the sponges and mesozoans — **meta·zoan** *adj*

met·en·ceph·a·lon \ˌmet-ˌen-ˈsef-ə-ˌlän, -lən\ *n* : the anterior segment of the developing vertebrate hindbrain or the corresponding part of the adult brain composed of the cerebellum and pons — **met·en·ce·phal·ic** \-ˌen(t)-sə-ˈfal-ik\ *adj*

Met–en·keph·a·lin \ˌmet-en-ˈkef-ə-lin\ *n* : METHIONINE-EN-KEPHALIN

me·te·or·ism \ˈmēt-ē-ə-ˌriz-əm\ *n* : gaseous distension of the stomach or intestine : TYMPANITES

¹**me·ter** *or chiefly Brit* **me·tre** \ˈmēt-ər\ *n* : the base unit of length in the International System of Units that is equal to the distance traveled in a vacuum by light in 1/299,792,458 second or to about 39.37 inches

²**meter** *n* : an instrument for measuring and sometimes recording the time or amount of something

meter angle *n* : the angle between the lines of vision and the median plane when the eyes are focused on a point at a distance of one meter in that plane

meter–candle *or chiefly Brit* **metre–candle** *n* : LUX

me·tered–dose inhaler \ˌmē-tər(d)-ˌdōs-\ *n* : a pocket-size handheld inhaler that delivers a standardized dose of medication for bronchodilation — abbr. MDI

meter–kilogram–second *or chiefly Brit* **metre–kilogram–second** *also* **metre–kilogramme–second** *adj* : MKS

met·es·trous \(ˈ)met-ˈes-trəs\ *or chiefly Brit* **met·oes·trous** \(ˈ)met-ˈē-strəs\ *adj* : of or relating to metestrus

met·es·trus \(ˈ)met-ˈes-trəs\ *or chiefly Brit* **met·oes·trus** \-ˈē-strəs\ *n* : the period of regression that follows estrus

met·for·min \met-ˈfòr-mən\ *n* : an antidiabetic drug used in the form of its hydrochloride $C_4H_{11}N_5$·HCl esp. to treat type 2 diabetes in patients unresponsive to or intolerant of approved sulfonylurea drugs — see GLUCOPHAGE, GLUCOVANCE

¹**meth** \ˈmeth\ *n, Brit* : METHS

²**meth** *n* : METHAMPHETAMINE

metha·cho·line \ˌmeth-ə-ˈkō-ˌlēn\ *n* : a parasympathomimetic drug administered in the form of its crystalline chloride $C_8H_{18}ClNO_2$ esp. to diagnose hypersensitivity of the bronchial air passages (as in asthma) — see MECHOLYL, PROVOCHOLINE

meth·ac·ry·late \(ˈ)meth-ˈak-rə-ˌlāt\ *n* **1** : a salt or ester of methacrylic acid **2** : an acrylic resin or plastic made from a derivative of methacrylic acid; *esp* : METHYL METHACRYLATE

methacrylate resin *n* : METHACRYLATE 2

meth·acryl·ic acid \ˌmeth-ə-ˌkril-ik-\ *n* : an acid $C_4H_6O_2$ used esp. in making acrylic resins or plastics

metha·cy·cline \ˌmeth-ə-ˈsī-ˌklēn\ *n* : a semisynthetic tetracycline $C_{22}H_{22}N_2O_8$ with longer duration of action than most other tetracyclines and used in the treatment of gonorrhea esp. in penicillin-sensitive subjects

meth·a·done \ˈmeth-ə-ˌdōn\ *also* **meth·a·don** \-ˌdän\ *n* : a synthetic addictive narcotic drug used esp. in the form of its hydrochloride $C_{21}H_{27}NO$·HCl for the relief of pain and as a substitute narcotic in the treatment of heroin addiction — called also *amidone*

methaemalbumin, methaemoglobin, methaemoglobinaemia, methaemoglobinuria *chiefly Brit var of* METHEMALBUMIN, METHEMOGLOBIN, METHEMOGLOBINEMIA, METHEMOGLOBINURIA

meth·am·phet·amine \ˌmeth-am-ˈfet-ə-ˌmēn, ˌmeth-əm-, -mən\ *n* : an amine $C_{10}H_{15}N$ that is used medically in the form of its crystalline hydrochloride $C_{10}H_{15}N$·HCl esp. to treat attention deficit disorder and obesity and that is often abused illicitly as a stimulant — called also *meth, methedrine, methylamphetamine, speed*

meth·an·dro·sten·o·lone \ˌmeth-ˌan-drō-ˈsten-ə-ˌlōn\ *n* : an anabolic steroid $C_{20}H_{28}O_2$

meth·ane \ˈmeth-ˌān, *Brit usu* ˈmē-ˌthān\ *n* : a colorless odorless flammable gaseous saturated hydrocarbon CH_4 that is lighter than air and forms explosive mixtures with air or oxygen, that is a product of decomposition of organic matter in marshes and mines or of the carbonization of coal, and that is used as a fuel and raw material in chemical synthesis — called also *marsh gas*

methane series *n* : a homologous series of saturated open-chain hydrocarbons C_nH_{2n+2} of which methane is the first and lowest member — compare ALKANE

meth·ane·sul·fo·nate \ˌmeth-ˌān-ˈsəl-fə-ˌnāt\ *or chiefly Brit* **me·thane·sul·pho·nate** \ˌmē-ˌthān-\ *n* : MESYLATE

me·than·o·gen \mə-ˈthan-ə-ˌjen\ *n* : any of various anaerobic microorganisms that produce methane from carbon dioxide and hydrogen, are classified as bacteria (as of the family Methanobacteriaceae) or as archaea, and include some found in the rumina of herbivores (as domestic cattle) that utilize cellulose

me·than·o·gen·e·sis \mə-ˌthan-ə-ˈjen-ə-səs\ *n, pl* **-e·ses** \-ˌsēz\ : the production of methane esp. through the action of methanogens

me·than·o·gen·ic \-ˈjen-ik\ *adj* : of or relating to the methanogens or methanogenesis

meth·a·nol \ˈmeth-ə-ˌnòl, -ˌnōl\ *n* : a light volatile pungent flammable poisonous liquid alcohol CH_3OH formed in the destructive distillation of wood or made synthetically and used esp. as a solvent, antifreeze, or denaturant for ethyl alcohol and in the synthesis of other chemicals — called also *carbinol, methyl alcohol, wood alcohol*

meth·a·no·lic \ˌmeth-ə-ˈnō-lik, -ˈnäl-ik\ *adj* : containing methanol usu. as solvent ⟨∼ solutions⟩

meth·a·nol·y·sis \-ˈnäl-ə-səs\ *n, pl* **-y·ses** \-ˌsēz\ : alcoholysis with methanol

meth·an·the·line \meth-ˈan(t)-thə-ˌlēn, -lən\ *n* : an anticho-

M
N

\ə\ abut \ᵊ\ kitten \ər\ **further** \a\ ash \ā\ ace \ä\ cot, cart \aú\ **out** \ch\ **chin** \e\ bet \ē\ **easy** \g\ go \i\ **hit** \ī\ **ice** \j\ **job** \ŋ\ sing \ō\ go \ò\ law \òi\ boy \th\ thin \t͟h\ the \ü\ **loot** \ù\ **foot** \y\ **yet** \zh\ **vision** *See also* Pronunciation Symbols page

linergic drug usu. administered in the form of its crystalline bromide $C_{21}H_{26}BrNO_3$ in the treatment of peptic ulcers

meth·a·phen·i·lene \ˌmeth-ə-'fen-ᵊl-ˌēn\ *n* : a chemical compound $C_{15}H_{20}N_2S$ formerly used as an antihistamine

meth·a·pyr·i·lene \-'pir-ə-ˌlēn\ *n* : an antihistamine drug $C_{14}H_{19}N_3S$ formerly used as a mild sedative in proprietary sleep-inducing drugs

meth·aqua·lone \me-'thak-wə-ˌlōn\ *n* : a sedative and hypnotic nonbarbiturate drug $C_{16}H_{14}N_2O$ that is habit-forming — see QUAALUDE

meth·ar·bi·tal \me-'thär-bə-ˌtol, -ˌtal\ *n* : an anticonvulsant barbiturate $C_9H_{14}N_2O_3$

meth·a·zol·amide \ˌmeth-ə-'zol-ə-ˌmīd\ *n* : a sulfonamide $C_5H_8N_4O_3S_2$ that inhibits the production of carbonic anhydrase, reduces intraocular pressure, and is used in the treatment of glaucoma — see NEPTAZANE

meth·dil·a·zine \meth-'dil-ə-ˌzēn, -'dīl-ə-ˌzīn\ *n* : a phenothiazine antihistamine used in the form of its hydrochloride $C_{18}H_{20}N_2S·HCl$ as an antipruritic

meth·e·drine \'meth-ə-drən, -drēn\ *n* : METHAMPHETAMINE

met·hem·al·bu·min *or chiefly Brit* **met·haem·al·bu·min** \ˌmet-ˌhēm-al-'byü-mən\ *n* : an albumin complex with hematin found in plasma during diseases (as blackwater fever) that are associated with extensive hemolysis

met·he·mo·glo·bin *or chiefly Brit* **met·hae·mo·glo·bin** \(')met-'hē-mə-ˌglō-bən\ *n* : a soluble brown crystalline basic blood pigment that is found in normal blood in much smaller amounts than hemoglobin, that is formed from blood, hemoglobin, or oxyhemoglobin by oxidation, and that differs from hemoglobin in containing ferric iron and in being unable to combine reversibly with molecular oxygen — called also *ferrihemoglobin*

met·he·mo·glo·bi·ne·mia *or chiefly Brit* **met·hae·mo·glo·bi·nae·mia** \ˌmet-ˌhē-mə-ˌglō-bə-'nē-mē-ə\ *n* : the presence of methemoglobin in the blood due to conversion of part of the hemoglobin to this inactive form

met·he·mo·glo·bin·uria *or chiefly Brit* **met·hae·mo·glo·bin·uria** \-bə-'n(y)ùr-ē-ə\ *n* : the presence of methemoglobin in the urine

me·the·na·mine \mə-'thē-nə-ˌmēn, -mən\ *n* : a crystalline compound used in the form of its mandelate $C_6H_{12}N_4·C_8H_8O_3$ or hippurate $C_6H_{12}N_4·C_9H_9NO_3$ as a urinary antiseptic esp. to treat bacteriuria associated with cystitis and pyelitis — called also *hexamethylenetetramine, hexamine;* see MANDELAMINE

meth·ene \'me-ˌthēn\ *n* **1** : METHYLENE **2** : a complex unsaturated derivative of methane of the general formula R—CH=R′

me·the·no·lone \mə-'thē-nə-lōn, me-'then-ə-\ *n* : a hormone $C_{20}H_{30}O_2$ that is an anabolic steroid

Meth·er·gine \'meth-ər-jən\ *trademark* — used for a preparation of the maleate of methylergonovine

meth·i·cil·lin \ˌmeth-ə-'sil-ən\ *n* : a semisynthetic penicillin $C_{17}H_{19}N_2O_6NaS$ that is esp. effective against beta-lactamase producing staphylococci

me·thi·ma·zole \me-'thī-mə-ˌzōl, mə-\ *n* : a drug $C_4H_6N_2S$ used to inhibit activity of the thyroid gland

meth·io·dal sodium \mə-'thī-ə-ˌdal-\ *n* : a crystalline salt CH_2ISO_3Na used as a radiopaque contrast medium in intravenous urography

me·thi·o·nine \mə-'thī-ə-ˌnēn\ *n* : a crystalline sulfur-containing essential amino acid $C_5H_{11}NO_2S$ that occurs in the L-form as a constituent of many proteins (as casein and egg albumin), that is important esp. as a source of sulfur for the biosynthesis of cysteine and as a source of methyl groups for transmethylation reactions (as in the biosynthesis of choline, creatine, and adrenaline), and that is used as a dietary supplement for human beings and their domestic mammals and poultry and in the treatment of fatty infiltration of the liver — abbr. *Met*

methionine–en·keph·a·lin \-en-'kef-ə-lin\ *n* : a pentapeptide having a terminal methionine residue that is one of the two enkephalins occurring naturally in the brain — called also *Met-enkephalin*

me·thi·o·nyl \mə-'thī-ə-ˌnil\ *n* : the amino acid radical or residue $CH_3S(CH_2)_2CH(NH_2)CO–$ of methionine — abbr. *Met*

meth·is·a·zone \me-'this-ə-ˌzōn\ *n* : an antiviral drug $C_{10}H_{10}N_4OS$ that has been used in the preventive treatment of smallpox

me·thix·ene \me-'thik-ˌsēn\ *n* : an anticholinergic drug $C_{20}H_{23}NS$ used as an antispasmodic in the treatment of functional bowel hypermotility and spasm

meth·o·car·ba·mol \ˌmeth-ə-'kär-bə-ˌmol\ *n* : a skeletal muscle relaxant drug $C_{11}H_{15}NO_5$

meth·od \'meth-əd\ *n* : a procedure or process for attaining an object: as **a** : a systematic procedure, technique, or mode of inquiry employed by or proper to a particular discipline — see SCIENTIFIC METHOD **b** : a way, technique, or process of or for doing something

meth·o·hex·i·tal \ˌmeth-ə-'hek-sə-ˌtol, -ˌtal\ *n* : a barbiturate with a short period of action usu. used in the form of its sodium salt $C_{14}H_{17}N_2NaO_3$ as an intravenous general anesthetic

meth·o·hex·i·tone \-ˌtōn\ *n, Brit* : METHOHEXITAL

me·tho·ni·um \mə-'thō-nē-əm\ *n* : any of several bivalent doubled substituted ammonium ions (as decamethonium or hexamethonium) in which the two quaternary nitrogen atoms are separated by a polymethylene chain ⟨∼ salts used in the treatment of hypertension⟩

meth·o·prene \'meth-ə-ˌprēn\ *n* : an insecticide $C_{19}H_{34}O_3$ that arrests growth at the larval stage of development

meth·o·trex·ate \ˌmeth-ə-'trek-ˌsāt\ *n* : a toxic drug $C_{20}H_{22}N_8O_5$ that is an analog of folic acid and is used to treat certain cancers, severe psoriasis, and rheumatoid arthritis — called also *amethopterin*

meth·o·tri·mep·ra·zine \ˌmeth-ō-ˌtrī-'mep-rə-ˌzēn\ *n* : a nonnarcotic analgesic and tranquilizer $C_{19}H_{24}N_2OS$ — see LEVOPROME

me·thox·amine \me-'thäk-sə-ˌmēn, -mən\ *n* : a sympathomimetic amine used in the form of its hydrochloride $C_{11}H_{17}NO_3·HCl$ esp. to raise or maintain blood pressure (as during surgery) by its vasoconstrictor effects — see VASOXYL

me·thox·sa·len \me-'thäk-sə-lən\ *n* : a drug $C_{12}H_8O_4$ used to increase the production of melanin in the skin upon exposure to ultraviolet light and in the treatment of vitiligo — called also *8-methoxypsoralen, xanthotoxin;* see MELOXINE

me·thoxy \me-'thäk-sē\ *adj* : relating to or containing methoxyl

me·thoxy·chlor \me-'thäk-si-ˌklō(ə)r, -ˌklò(ə)r\ *n* : a chlorinated hydrocarbon insecticide $C_{16}H_{15}Cl_3O_2$

me·thoxy·flu·rane \me-ˌthäk-sē-'flù(ə)r-ˌān\ *n* : a potent nonexplosive inhalational general anesthetic $C_3H_4Cl_2F_2O$

meth·ox·yl \me-'thäk-səl\ *n* : a monovalent radical $CH_3O–$ composed of methyl united with oxygen

8–meth·oxy·psor·a·len \'āt-ˌmeth-ˌäk-sē-'sòr-ə-lən\ *n* : METHOXSALEN

meths \'meths\ *n pl but sing in constr* : methylated spirits esp. as an illicit beverage

meth·sco·pol·amine \ˌmeth-skō-'päl-ə-ˌmēn, -mən\ *n* : an anticholinergic quaternary ammonium derivative of scopolamine that is usu. used in the form of its bromide $C_{18}H_{24}BrNO_4$ for its inhibitory effect on gastric secretion and gastrointestinal motility esp. in the treatment of peptic ulcer and gastric disorders — see PAMINE

meth·sux·i·mide \-'sək-si-ˌmīd\ *n* : an anticonvulsant drug $C_{12}H_{13}NO_2$ used esp. in the control of absence seizures

meth·y·clo·thi·azide \-ē-ˌklō-'thī-ə-ˌzīd\ *n* : a thiazide drug $C_9H_{11}Cl_2N_3O_4S_2$ used as a diuretic and antihypertensive agent

meth·yl \'meth-əl, *Brit also* 'mē-ˌthīl\ *n* : an alkyl group CH_3 that is derived from methane by removal of one hydrogen atom — **me·thyl·ic** \mə-'thil-ik\ *adj*

meth·yl·al \'meth-ə-ˌlal\ *n* : a volatile flammable liquid $C_3H_8O_2$ of pleasant ethereal odor used as a hypnotic and anesthetic and in organic synthesis

methyl alcohol *n* : METHANOL

me·thyl·amine \ˌmeth-ə-lə-'mēn, -'lam-ən; mə-'thil-ə-ˌmēn\

n : a flammable explosive gas CH_5N with a strong ammoniacal odor used esp. in organic synthesis (as of insecticides)

me·thyl·am·phet·amine \ˌmeth-əl-ˌam-ˈfet-ə-ˌmēn\ *n* : METHAMPHETAMINE

meth·yl·ase \ˈmeth-ə-ˌlās, -ˌlāz\ *n* : an enzyme (as DNA methyltransferase) that catalyzes methylation (as of RNA or DNA)

methylated spirit *n* : ethyl alcohol denatured with methanol — often used in pl. with sing. constr.

meth·yl·ation \ˌmeth-ə-ˈlā-shən\ *n* : introduction of the methyl group into a chemical compound; *esp* : DNA METHYLATION — **meth·yl·ate** \ˈmeth-ə-ˌlāt\ *vt* **-at·ed; -at·ing**

meth·yl·ben·zene \ˌmeth-əl-ˈben-ˌzēn\ *n* : TOLUENE

meth·yl·ben·ze·tho·ni·um chloride \ˌmeth-əl-ˌben-zə-ˌthō-nē-əm-\ *n* : a quaternary ammonium salt $C_{28}H_{44}ClNO_2$ used as a bactericide and antiseptic esp. in the treatment of diaper rash — called also *methylbenzethonium*

methyl bromide *n* : a poisonous gaseous compound CH_3Br used chiefly as a fumigant against rodents, worms, and insects

meth·yl·cel·lu·lose \ˌmeth-əl-ˈsel-yə-ˌlōs, -ˌlōz\ *n* : any of various gummy products of cellulose methylation that swell in water and are used esp. as emulsifiers, adhesives, thickeners, and bulk laxatives

methyl chloride *n* : a sweet-smelling gaseous compound CH_3Cl made usu. by the action of hydrochloric acid on methanol and used chiefly as a refrigerant and methylating agent — called also *chloromethane*

methyl chloroform *n* : TRICHLOROETHANE a

meth·yl·cho·lan·threne \-kə-ˈlan-ˌthrēn\ *n* : a potent carcinogenic hydrocarbon $C_{21}H_{16}$ obtained from certain bile acids and cholesterol as well as synthetically — compare CHOLANTHRENE

methyl cyanide *n* : ACETONITRILE

meth·yl·cyt·o·sine \ˌmeth-əl-ˈsīt-ə-ˌsēn\ *n* : a methylated pyrimidine base $C_5H_7N_3O$ found in the nucleic acids (as some DNAs and transfer RNAs) of some organisms

N–**meth·yl**–D–**as·par·tate** \ˈen-ˌmeth-əl-ˌdē-ə-ˈspär-ˌtāt\ *n* : NMDA

meth·yl·di·hy·dro·mor·phi·none \-ˌdī-ˌhī-drə-ˈmȯr-fə-ˌnōn\ *n* : METOPON

meth·yl·do·pa \ˌmeth-əl-ˈdō-pə\ *n* : an antihypertensive drug $C_{10}H_{13}NO_4$

meth·y·lene \ˈmeth-ə-ˌlēn, -lən\ *n* : a bivalent hydrocarbon radical CH_2 derived from methane by removal of two hydrogen atoms

methylene azure *n* : a dye obtained by oxidation of methylene blue and used in biological stains (as Giemsa)

methylene blue *n* : a basic thiazine dye $C_{16}H_{18}ClN_3S·3H_2O$ used in the treatment of methemoglobinemia, as an antidote in cyanide poisoning, as a biological stain, and as an oxidation-reduction indicator

methylene chloride *n* : a nonflammable liquid CH_2Cl_2 formerly used as an inhalation anesthetic but now used esp. as a solvent, paint remover, and aerosol propellant — called also *dichloromethane*

meth·y·lene·di·oxy·am·phet·amine \ˌmeth-ə-ˌlēn-(ˌ)dī-ˌäk-sē-am-ˈfet-ə-ˌmēn, -mən\ *also* **3,4–methylenedioxyamphetamine** \ˌthrē-ˌfō(ə)r-\ *n* : MDA

meth·y·lene·di·oxy·meth·am·phet·amine *also* **3,4–methylenedioxymethamphetamine** \-ˌmeth-am-ˈfet-ə-ˌmēn, -ˌmeth-əm-, -mən\ *n* : ECSTASY 2

meth·yl·er·go·no·vine \ˌmeth-əl-ˌər-gə-ˈnō-ˌvēn\ *n* : an oxytocic drug usu. used in the form of its maleate $C_{20}H_{25}N_3O_2·C_4H_4O_4$ for the same applications and with the same effects as ergonovine — see METHERGINE

meth·yl·glu·ca·mine \-ˈglü-kə-ˌmēn\ *n* : MEGLUMINE

meth·yl·gly·ox·al \-glī-ˈäk-sal\ *n* : a yellow pungent volatile oil $C_3H_4O_2$ that polymerizes readily and is formed as an intermediate in the metabolism or fermentation of carbohydrates and lactic acid — called also *pyruvaldehyde*

methyl green *n* : a basic triphenylmethane dye made by adding methyl chloride to crystal violet and used chiefly as a biological stain

meth·yl·hex·ane·amine \ˌmeth-əl-ˌhek-sān-ˈam-ēn\ *n* : an amine base $C_7H_{17}N$ used as a local vasoconstrictor of nasal mucosa in the treatment of nasal congestion

meth·yl·iso·cy·a·nate \-ˌī-sō-ˈsī-ə-ˌnāt\ *n* : an extremely toxic chemical CH_3NCO that is used esp. in the manufacture of pesticides and was the cause of numerous deaths and injuries in a leak at a chemical plant in Bhopal, India, in 1984 — abbr. *MIC*

meth·yl·ma·lon·ic acid \ˌmeth-əl-mə-ˌlän-ik-\ *n* : a structural isomer of succinic acid present in minute amounts in healthy human urine but excreted in large quantities in the urine of individuals with a vitamin B_{12} deficiency

methylmalonic aciduria *n* : a metabolic defect which is controlled by an autosomal recessive gene and in which methylmalonic acid is not converted to succinic acid with chronic metabolic acidosis resulting

methyl mercaptan *n* : a pungent gas CH_4S produced in the intestine by the decomposition of certain proteins and responsible for the characteristic odor of fetor hepaticus

meth·yl·mer·cury \ˌmeth-əl-ˈmər-kyə-rē, *Brit also* ˌmē-ˌthīl-\ *n, pl* **-cu·ries** : any of various toxic compounds of mercury containing the complex CH_3Hg- that often occur as pollutants formed as industrial by-products or pesticide residues, tend to accumulate in living organisms (as fish) esp. in higher levels of a food chain, are rapidly and easily absorbed through the human intestinal wall, and cause neurological dysfunction in humans — see MINAMATA DISEASE

methyl methacrylate *n* : a volatile flammable liquid ester $C_5H_8O_2$ that polymerizes readily and is used esp. as a monomer for acrylic resin

meth·yl·mor·phine \ˌmeth-əl-ˈmȯr-ˌfēn\ *n* : CODEINE

methyl orange *n* : a basic azo dye $C_{14}H_{14}N_3NaO_3S$ that is used chiefly as an acid-base indicator and whose dilute solution is yellow when neutral and pink when acid

meth·yl·para·ben \ˌmeth-əl-ˈpar-ə-ˌben\ *n* : a crystalline compound $C_8H_8O_3$ used as an antifungal preservative (as in pharmaceutical ointments and cosmetic creams and lotions)

meth·yl·para·fy·nol \-ˌpar-ə-ˈfī-ˌnȯl\ *n* : a sedative and hypnotic drug $C_6H_{10}O$

methyl parathion *n* : a potent synthetic organophosphate insecticide $C_8H_{10}NO_5PS$ that is more toxic than parathion

meth·yl·phe·ni·date \ˌmeth-əl-ˈfen-ə-ˌdāt, -ˈfē-nə-\ *n* : a mild stimulant of the central nervous system that is administered orally in the form of its hydrochloride $C_{14}H_{19}NO_2·HCl$ to treat narcolepsy and hyperactivity disorders (as attention deficit disorder) in children — see CONCERTA, RITALIN

meth·yl·pred·nis·o·lone \-pred-ˈnis-ə-ˌlōn\ *n* : a glucocorticoid $C_{22}H_{30}O_5$ that is a derivative of prednisolone and is used as an anti-inflammatory agent; *also* : any of several of its salts (as an acetate) used similarly — see MEDROL

methyl red *n* : a basic azo dye $C_{15}H_{15}N_3O_2$ used similarly to methyl orange as an acid-base indicator

meth·yl·ros·an·i·line chloride \ˌmeth-əl-rō-ˈzan-°l-ən-\ *n* : CRYSTAL VIOLET

methyl salicylate *n* : a liquid ester $C_8H_8O_3$ that is obtained from the leaves of a wintergreen (*Gaultheria procumbens*) or the bark of a birch (*Betula lenta*), but is usu. made synthetically, and that is used as a flavoring and as a counterirritant — see BIRCH OIL, OIL OF WINTERGREEN

methylsulfate — see HEXOCYCLIUM METHYLSULFATE, PENTAPIPERIDE METHYLSULFATE

meth·yl·tes·tos·ter·one \-te-ˈstäs-tə-ˌrōn\ *n* : a synthetic androgen $C_{20}H_{30}O_2$ administered orally esp. in the treatment of male testosterone deficiency

meth·yl·thio·ura·cil \-ˌthī-ō-ˈyur-ə-ˌsil\ *n* : a crystalline compound $C_5H_6N_2OS$ used in the suppression of hyperactivity of the thyroid

meth·yl·trans·fer·ase \-ˈtran(t)s-fər-ˌās, -ˌāz\ *n* : any of several transferases that promote transfer of a methyl group

---

\ə\ abut \ᵊ\ kitten \ər\ **fur**ther \a\ **a**sh \ā\ **a**ce \ä\ cot, cart
\aü\ **ou**t \ch\ **ch**in \e\ b**e**t \ē\ **ea**sy \g\ **g**o \i\ h**i**t \ī\ **i**ce \j\ **j**ob
\ŋ\ si**ng** \ō\ **g**o \ȯ\ l**aw** \ȯi\ b**oy** \th\ **th**in \t̲h̲\ **th**e \ü\ l**oo**t
\ u̇\ f**oo**t \y\ **y**et \zh\ vi**s**ion *See also* Pronunciation Symbols page

M
N

from one compound to another — see DNA METHYLTRANS‑FERASE

α‑meth·yl·ty·ro·sine \ˌal-fə-ˌmeth-əl-'tī-rə-ˌsēn\ n : a compound $C_{10}H_{13}NO_3$ that inhibits the synthesis of catecholamines but not of serotonin

methyl violet n : any of several basic dyes (as crystal violet or gentian violet) that are methyl derivatives of pararosaniline

meth·yl·xan·thine \ˌmeth-əl-'zan-ˌthēn\ n : a methylated xanthine derivative (as caffeine, theobromine, or theophylline)

meth·y·pry·lon \ˌmeth-ə-'prī-ˌlän\ or Brit **meth·y·pry·lone** \-ˌlōn\ n : a sedative and hypnotic drug $C_{10}H_{17}NO_2$

meth·y·ser·gide \ˌmeth-ə-'sər-ˌjīd\ n : a serotonin antagonist used in the form of its maleate $C_{21}H_{27}N_3O_2 \cdot C_4H_4O_4$ esp. in the treatment and prevention of migraine headaches

me·ti·amide \mə-'tī-ə-ˌmīd\ n : an antihistamine drug $C_9H_{16}N_4S_2$ that has been used experimentally in the treatment of peptic ulcers

met·myo·glo·bin \'met-ˌmī-ə-ˌglō-bən\ n : a reddish brown crystalline pigment that is formed by oxidation of myoglobin

met·o·clo·pra·mide \ˌmet-ə-'klō-prə-ˌmīd\ n : an antiemetic drug administered in the form of its hydrated hydrochloride $C_{14}H_{22}ClN_3O_2 \cdot HCl \cdot H_2O$

met·o·cur·ine iodide \-'kyùr-ˌēn-\ n : a crystalline iodine‑containing powder $C_{40}H_{48}I_2N_2O_6$ that is derived from the dextrorotatory form of tubocurarine and is a potent skeletal muscle relaxant — called also *metocurine*

metoestrus *chiefly Brit var of* METESTRUS

me·to·la·zone \me-'tō-lə-ˌzōn\ n : a diuretic and antihypertensive drug $C_{16}H_{16}ClN_3O_3S$

me·top·ic \mə-'täp-ik\ adj : of or relating to the forehead : FRONTAL; esp : of, relating to, or being a suture uniting the frontal bones in the fetus and sometimes persistent after birth

met·o·pim·a·zine \ˌmet-ə-'pim-ə-ˌzēn\ n : an antiemetic drug $C_{22}H_{27}N_3O_3S_2$

me·to·pi·on \mə-'tō-pē-ən\ n : a point situated midway between the frontal eminences of the skull

Met·o·pir·one \ˌmet-ə-'pir-ˌōn\ trademark — used for a preparation of metyrapone

met·o·pism \'met-ə-ˌpiz-əm\ n : the condition of having a persistent metopic suture

Me·to·pi·um \mə-'tō-pē-əm\ n : a genus of trees and shrubs of the cashew family (Anacardiaceae) that includes the poisonwood (*M. toxiferum*) of southern Florida and the West Indies

met·o·pon \'met-ə-ˌpän\ n : a narcotic drug that is derived from morphine and is used in the form of its hydrochloride $C_{18}H_{21}NO_3 \cdot HCl$ to relieve pain — called also *methyldihydromorphinone*

met·o·pro·lol \me-'tō-prə-ˌlōl, -ˌlōl\ n : a beta-blocker used in the form of its tartrate $(C_{15}H_{25}NO_3)_2 \cdot C_4H_6O_6$ or succinate $(C_{15}H_{25}NO_3)_2 \cdot C_4H_6O_4$ to treat hypertension, angina pectoris, and congestive heart failure — see LOPRESSOR, TOPROL

me·tra \'mē-trə\ n, pl **me·trae** \-trē\ : UTERUS

me·tra·term \'mē-trə-ˌtərm\ n : the distal muscular portion of the uterus of a flatworm

Met·ra·zol \'me-trə-ˌzól, -ˌzōl\ n : a preparation of pentylenetetrazol — formerly a U.S. registered trademark

metre *chiefly Brit var of* METER

metre–candle *chiefly Brit var of* METER-CANDLE

metre–kilogram–second also **metre–kilogramme–second** var of METER-KILOGRAM-SECOND

me·treu·ryn·ter \ˌmē-trür-'int-ər\ n : COLPEURYNTER

me·tri·al \'mē-trē-əl\ adj : of or relating to the uterus — often used in combination ⟨endo*metrial*⟩

met·ric \'me-trik\ adj : of, relating to, or using the metric system ⟨a ∼ study⟩ — **met·ri·cal·ly** \-tri-k(ə-)lē\ adv

met·ri·cal \-tri-kəl\ adj : of, relating to, or subject to measurement ⟨∼ genetic traits⟩

metric system n : a decimal system of weights and measures based on the meter and on the kilogram — compare CGS, MKS

met·rio·cra·nic \ˌme-trē-ə-'krā-nik\ adj : having a skull of moderate height in proportion to its width with a breadth‑height index of 92.0 to 97.9 — **met·rio·cra·ny** \'me-trē-ə-ˌkrā-nē\ n, pl **-nies**

me·tri·tis \mə-'trīt-əs\ n : inflammation of the uterus

me·triz·a·mide \me-'triz-a-ˌmīd\ n : a radiopaque medium $C_{18}H_{22}I_3N_3O_8$

met·ri·zo·ate sodium \ˌme-tri-ˌzō-āt-\ n : a radiopaque medium $C_{12}H_{10}I_3N_2NaO_4$ — see ISOPAQUE

me·trol·o·gy \me-'träl-ə-jē\ n, pl **-gies** 1 : the science of weights and measures or of measurement 2 : a system of weights and measures — **met·ro·log·i·cal** \ˌme-trə-'läj-i-kəl\ adj — **met·ro·log·i·cal·ly** \-k(ə-)lē\ adv — **me·trol·o·gist** \me-'träl-ə-jəst\ n

met·ro·ni·da·zole \ˌme-trə-'nīd-ə-ˌzōl\ n : an antiprotozoal and antibacterial drug $C_6H_9N_3O_3$ used esp. to treat vaginal trichomoniasis, amebiasis, and infections by anaerobic bacteria — see FLAGYL

met·ro·nom·ic \ˌme-trə-'näm-ik\ adj : of, relating to, or being a drug or regimen of drugs administered in low doses at regular intervals over a prolonged period of time ⟨∼ cyclophosphamide⟩ ⟨∼ chemotherapy⟩

me·tror·rha·gia \ˌme-trə-'rā-j(ē-)ə, -'rā-zhə; -'rāj-ə, -'räzh-\ n : irregular uterine bleeding esp. between menstrual periods — compare MENORRHAGIA — **me·tror·rhag·ic** \-'raj-ik\ adj

me·tu·re·depa \mə-ˌtür-ə-'dep-ə, ˌmet-yə-rə-\ n : an antineoplastic drug $C_{11}H_{22}N_3O_3P$

me·tyr·a·pone \mə-'tir-ə-ˌpōn also -'tīr-\ n : a metabolic hormone $C_{14}H_{14}N_2O$ that inhibits biosynthesis of cortisol and corticosterone and is used to test for normal functioning of the pituitary gland — see METOPIRONE

Met·zen·baum scissors \'met-sən-ˌbòm-, -ˌbaùm-\ n : surgical scissors having curved blades with blunt ends

    Metzenbaum, Myron Firth (1876–1944), American surgeon. Metzenbaum specialized in oral surgery and reconstructive surgery of the head and neck. His many papers included descriptions of his methods for the reconstruction of the nose and larynx. His original surgical methods included one for resetting the dislocated nasal cartilage in young children. He also developed a method for administering ether as an anesthetic, and he was a pioneer in the inducement of twilight sleep in patients undergoing general surgery. Metzenbaum is also remembered for his original research on radium.

Mev·a·cor \'mev-ə-ˌkòr\ trademark — used for a preparation of lovastatin

me·val·o·nate \mə-'val-ə-ˌnāt\ n : a salt of mevalonic acid

mev·a·lon·ic acid \ˌmev-ə-ˌlän-ik-\ n : a branched dihydroxy acid $C_6H_{12}O_4$ that is a precursor of squalene in the biosynthetic pathway forming sterols (as cholesterol)

Mex·i·can bedbug \ˌmek-si-kən-\ n : CONENOSE

Mexican fever n : TEXAS FEVER

Mexican spotted fever n : ROCKY MOUNTAIN SPOTTED FEVER

Mexican tea n : a rank-scented tropical American pigweed of the genus *Chenopodium* (*C. ambrosioides*) that is the source of chenopodium oil

Mexican typhus n : MURINE TYPHUS

me·ze·re·on \mə-'zir-ē-ən\ n : a small European shrub of the genus *Daphne* (*D. mezereum* of the family Thymelaeaceae, the mezereon family) with fragrant lilac purple flowers and poisonous emetic leaves, fruit, and bark

me·ze·re·um \-ē-əm\ n 1 : MEZEREON 2 : the dried bark of various European shrubs of the genus *Daphne* and esp. mezereon used externally as a vesicant and irritant

mg abbr milligram

Mg symbol magnesium

mgm abbr milligram

MHC abbr major histocompatibility complex

mho \'mō\ n, pl **mhos** : a unit of conductance equal to the reciprocal of the ohm : SIEMENS

MHPG \ˌem-(ˌ)āch-(ˌ)pē-'jē\ n : a metabolite of norepinephrine that is reported for some patients to fall to lower levels during periods of depression

MHz *abbr* megahertz

MI *abbr* **1** mitral incompetence; mitral insufficiency **2** myocardial infarction

Mi·a·neh fever \ˌmē-ə-ˈnä-\ *n* : a form of relapsing fever endemic to the Middle East

mi·an·ser·in \mī-ˈan-sər-in\ *n* : a drug administered in the form of its hydrochloride $C_{18}H_{20}N_2 \cdot HCl$ esp. as an antidepressant

mi·as·ma \mī-ˈaz-mə, mē-\ *n, pl* **-mas** *also* **-ma·ta** \-mət-ə\ : a vaporous exhalation (as of a marshy region or of putrescent matter) formerly believed to cause disease (as malaria) — **mi·as·mal** \-məl\ *adj* — **mi·as·mat·ic** \ˌmī-əz-ˈmat-ik\ *adj* — **mi·as·mic** \mī-ˈaz-mik, mē-\ *adj*

MIC *abbr* **1** methylisocyanate **2** minimal inhibitory concentration; minimum inhibitory concentration

mi·ca \ˈmī-kə\ *n* : any of various colored or transparent mineral silicates crystallizing in monoclinic forms that readily separate into very thin leaves — **mi·ca·ceous** \mī-ˈkā-shəs\ *adj*

Mi·ca·tin \ˈmī-kə-ˌtin\ *trademark* — used for a preparation of the nitrate of miconazole

mice *pl of* MOUSE

mi·cel·la \mī-ˈsel-ə\ *n, pl* **-cel·lae** \-ˈsel-ē\ : MICELLE

mi·cel·lar \mī-ˈsel-ər\ *adj* : of, relating to, or characterized by micelles

mi·celle \mī-ˈsel\ *n* : a unit of structure built up from polymeric molecules or ions: as **a** : an ordered region in a fiber (as of cellulose or rayon) **b** : a molecular aggregate that constitutes a colloidal particle

Mi·chae·lis constant \mī-ˈkā-ləs-, mə-\ *n* : a constant that is a measure of the kinetics of an enzyme reaction and that is equivalent to the concentration of substrate at which the reaction takes place at one half its maximum rate

> **Michaelis, Leonor (1875–1949),** German-American biochemist. Michaelis made major contributions to both biochemistry and medicine. In 1913 he derived the Michaelis constant, a measure of the affinity of an enzyme for the substance on which it acts.

Mi·chae·lis–Men·ten kinetics \-ˈmen-tən-\ *n pl but sing or pl in constr* : the behavior of an enzyme-catalyzed reaction with a single substrate esp. as exhibited by plotting the velocity of the reaction against the concentration of the substrate which yields a hyperbolic curve approaching a horizontal asymptote rather than yielding a straight line as in nonenzymatic reactions and which has an equation of the form

$$v = \frac{V}{K_m + s}$$

where v is the velocity of the reaction, V is the asymptotic value of the velocity, K_m is the Michaelis constant, and s is the concentration of the substrate

Mi·chel clip \mē-ˈshel-\ *n* : a small clip used to close surgical incisions

> **Mi·chel** \mē-shel\, **Gaston (1874–1937),** French surgeon. Michel taught surgery in Nancy, France. In 1911 he published an important study on pancreatitis. His other contributions included studies of lesions of the spinal column.

Mi·chu·rin·ism \mə-ˈchùr-ə-ˌniz-əm\ *n* : LYSENKOISM

> **Mi·chu·rin** \mi-ˈchür-in\, **Ivan Vladimirovich (1855–1935),** Russian horticulturist and geneticist. In his time Michurin was highly regarded by the Soviet government for his work in the crossbreeding of plants. He developed better strains and new varieties of fruits, vegetables, and grains. His theories of hybridization required acceptance of the inheritance of acquired characteristics and were widely promulgated in Soviet science.

Mickey Finn \ˌmik-ē-ˈfin\ *n* : a drink of liquor doctored with a purgative or a drug

mi·con·a·zole \mī-ˈkän-ə-ˌzōl\ *n* : an antifungal agent administered esp. in the form of its nitrate $C_{18}H_{14}Cl_4N_2O \cdot HNO_3$ — see MICATIN

mi·cren·ceph·a·ly \ˌmī-ˌkren-ˈsef-ə-lē\ *n, pl* **-lies** : the condition of having an abnormally small brain

mi·cro \ˈmī-(ˌ)krō\ *adj* **1** : very small; *esp* : MICROSCOPIC **2** involving minute quantities or variations

mi·cro·ab·scess \-ˌab-ses\ *n* : a very small abscess ⟨lesion is characterized by . . . multiple ~es in a fresh or an organizing thrombus —V. A. McKusick *et al*⟩

mi·cro·ad·e·no·ma \-ˌad-ᵊn-ˈō-mə\ *n, pl* **-mas** *also* **-ma·ta** \-mət-ə\ : a very small adenoma

mi·cro·aero·phile \-ˈar-ə-ˌfīl, -ˈer-\ *n* : an organism requiring very little free oxygen

mi·cro·aero·phil·ic \-ˌar-ə-ˈfil-ik, -ˌer-\ *adj* : requiring very little free oxygen ⟨~ bacteria⟩ — **mi·cro·aero·phil·i·cal·ly** \-i-k(ə-)lē\ *adv*

mi·cro·ag·gre·gate \-ˈag-ri-gət\ *n* : an aggregate of microscopic particles (as of fibrin) formed esp. in stored blood

mi·cro·al·bu·min·uria \-al-ˌbyü-mə-ˈn(y)ùr-ē-ə\ *n* : albuminuria characterized by a relatively low rate of urinary excretion of albumin typically between 30 and 300 milligrams per 24-hour period — compare MACROALBUMINURIA

mi·cro·am·me·ter \-ˈam-ˌēt-ər\ *n* : an instrument for measuring electric current in microamperes

mi·cro·am·pere \ˈmī-krō-ˌam-ˌpi(ə)r\ *n* : a unit of current equal to one millionth of an ampere

mi·cro·anal·y·sis \ˌmī-krō-ə-ˈnal-ə-səs\ *n, pl* **-y·ses** \-ˌsēz\ : chemical analysis on a small or minute scale that usu. requires special, very sensitive, or small-scale apparatus — compare MACROANALYSIS — **mi·cro·an·a·lyt·i·cal** \-ˌan-ᵊl-ˈit-i-kəl\ *also* **mi·cro·an·a·lyt·ic** \-ˈit-ik\ *adj*

mi·cro·an·a·lyz·er *or chiefly Brit* **mi·cro·an·a·lys·er** \-ˈan-ᵊl-ˌī-zər\ *n* : an electronic instrument used for determining the chemical composition of a very small sample or a very small part of a large sample

mi·cro·anat·o·mist \-ə-ˈnat-ə-məst\ *n* : HISTOLOGIST

mi·cro·anat·o·my \-ə-ˈnat-ə-mē\ *n, pl* **-mies** : HISTOLOGY 1, 3 — **mi·cro·ana·tom·i·cal** \-ˌan-ə-ˈtäm-i-kəl\ *adj*

mi·cro·an·eu·rysm *also* **mi·cro·an·eu·rism** \-ˈan-yə-ˌriz-əm\ *n* : a saccular enlargement of the venous end of a retinal capillary associated esp. with diabetic retinopathy — **mi·cro·an·eu·rys·mal** \-ˌan-yə-ˈriz-məl\ *adj*

mi·cro·an·gi·og·ra·phy \-ˌan-jē-ˈäg-rə-fē\ *n, pl* **-phies** : minutely detailed angiography — **mi·cro·an·gio·graph·ic** \-ˌan-jē-ə-ˈgraf-ik\ *adj*

mi·cro·an·gi·op·a·thy \-ˈäp-ə-thē\ *n, pl* **-thies** : a disease of very fine blood vessels ⟨thrombotic ~⟩ — **mi·cro·an·gio·path·ic** \-ˌan-jē-ə-ˈpath-ik\ *adj*

mi·cro·ar·ray \-ə-ˈrā\ *n* : a supporting material (as a glass or plastic slide) onto which numerous molecules or molecular fragments usu. of DNA or protein are attached in a regular pattern for use in biochemical or genetic analysis; *esp* : DNA MICROARRAY

mi·cro·ar·te·ri·og·ra·phy \- är-ˌtir-ē-ˈäg-rə-fē\ *n, pl* **-phies** : minutely detailed arteriography

mi·cro·bac·te·ri·um \-bak-ˈtir-ē-əm\ *n* **1** *cap* : a genus of minute nonmotile gram-positive thermotolerant bacteria closely related to or included in the family Corynebacteriaceae that are common in dairy products and the mammalian intestinal tract **2** *pl* **-ria** \-ē-ə\ : any of numerous minute heat-resistant bacteria; *specif* : any bacterium of the genus *Microbacterium*

mi·cro·bal·ance \ˈmī-krō-ˌbal-ən(t)s\ *n* : a balance designed to measure very small weights with great precision

mi·crobe \ˈmī-ˌkrōb\ *n* : MICROORGANISM, GERM — used esp. of pathogenic bacteria

mi·cro·beam \ˈmī-krō-ˌbēm\ *n* : a beam of radiation of small cross section ⟨a laser ~⟩

mi·cro·bi·al \mī-ˈkrō-bē-əl\ *adj* : of, relating to, caused by, or being microbes ⟨~ infection⟩ ⟨~ agents⟩ — **mi·cro·bi·al·ly** \-ē\ *adv*

\ə\ abut \ᵊ\ kitten \ər\ further \a\ ash \ā\ ace \ä\ cot, cart
\aù\ out \ch\ chin \e\ bet \ē\ easy \g\ go \i\ hit \ī\ ice \j\ job
\ŋ\ sing \ō\ go \ò\ law \òi\ boy \th\ thin \t̲h̲\ the \ü\ loot
\ù\ foot \y\ yet \zh\ vision *See also* Pronunciation Symbols page

M
N

mi·cro·bic \mī-'krō-bik\ *also* **mi·cro·bi·an** \-bē-ən\ *adj* : MI-CROBIAL

mi·cro·bi·ci·dal \mī-,krō-bə-'sīd-ᵊl\ *adj* : destructive to microbes

mi·cro·bi·cide \mī-'krō-bə-,sīd\ *n* : an agent that destroys microbes

mi·cro·bio·as·say \,mī-krō-,bī-ō-'as-,ā, -a-'sā\ *n* : bioassay in which the test organism is a microorganism

mi·cro·bi·ol·o·gist \,mī-krō-bī-'äl-ə-jəst\ *n* : a specialist in microbiology

mi·cro·bi·ol·o·gy \,mī-krō-bī-'äl-ə-jē\ *n, pl* **-gies** : a branch of biology dealing esp. with microscopic forms of life (as bacteria, protozoans, viruses, and fungi) — **mi·cro·bi·o·log·i·cal** \'mī-krō-,bī-ə-'läj-i-kəl\ *also* **mi·cro·bi·o·log·ic** \-'läj-ik\ *adj* — **mi·cro·bi·o·log·i·cal·ly** \-i-k(ə-)lē\ *adv*

mi·cro·bi·o·ta \-bī-'ōt-ə\ *n* : the microscopic flora and fauna of a region

mi·cro·bi·ot·ic \-bī-'ät-ik\ *adj* : of, relating to, or constituting a microbiota

mi·cro·bism \'mī-,krō-,biz-əm\ *n* : the state of being infested with microbes

mi·cro·blast \'mī-krō-,blast\ *n* : a small erythroblast destined to produce an atypically small red blood cell

mi·cro·body \'mī-krō-,bäd-ē\ *n, pl* **-bod·ies** : PEROXISOME

mi·cro·bu·rette *or* **mi·cro·bu·ret** \,mī-krō-byù-'ret\ *n* : a burette (as one with a capacity of 10 milliliters or less) for use esp. in microanalysis

mi·cro·burn·er \'mī-krō-,bər-nər\ *n* : a burner giving a very small flame for use esp. in microanalysis

mi·cro·cal·ci·fi·ca·tion \-,kal-sə-fə-'kā-shən\ *n* : a tiny abnormal deposit of calcium salts esp. in the breast that in the human female is often an indicator of breast cancer

mi·cro·cal·o·rim·e·ter \,mī-krō-,kal-ə-'rim-ət-ər\ *n* : an instrument for measuring very small quantities of heat — **mi·cro·ca·lo·ri·met·ric** \-,kal-ə-rə-'me-trik; -kə-,lór-ə-, -,lōr-, -,lär-\ *adj* — **mi·cro·cal·o·rim·e·try** \-,kal-ə-'rim-ə-trē\ *n, pl* **-tries**

mi·cro·cap·sule \'mī-krō-,kap-səl, -(,)sül\ *n* : a tiny capsule containing material (as a medicine) that is released when the capsule is broken, melted, or dissolved

¹**mi·cro·ce·phal·ic** \,mī-krō-sə-'fal-ik\ *adj* : having a small head; *specif* : having an abnormally small head

²**microcephalic** *n* : an individual with an abnormally small head

mi·cro·ceph·a·lus \-'sef-ə-ləs\ *n, pl* **-li** \-,lī\ : MICROCEPHALY

mi·cro·ceph·a·ly \-'sef-ə-lē\ *n, pl* **-lies** : a condition of abnormal smallness of the head usu. associated with mental retardation

mi·cro·chem·i·cal \-'kem-i-kəl\ *adj* : of, relating to, or using the methods of microchemistry — **mi·cro·chem·i·cal·ly** \-i-k(ə-)lē\ *adv*

mi·cro·chem·ist \-'kem-əst\ *n* : a specialist in microchemistry

mi·cro·chem·is·try \-'kem-ə-strē\ *n, pl* **-tries** : chemistry dealing with the manipulation of very small quantities of matter for purposes of preparation, characterization, or analysis

mi·cro·chro·mo·some \-'krō-mə-,sōm, -,zōm\ *n* : any of the smaller chromosomes of a species that exhibits chromosomal polymorphism in size

mi·cro·cin·e·ma·tog·ra·phy \-,sin-ə-mə-'täg-rə-fē\ *n, pl* **-phies** : photomicrography in which the product is a motion picture — called also *cinephotomicrography* — **mi·cro·cine·mat·o·graph·ic** \-,mat-ə-'graf-ik\ *adj*

mi·cro·cir·cu·la·tion \'mī-krō-,sər-kyə-'lā-shən\ *n* : blood circulation in the microvascular system; *also* : the microvascular system itself — **mi·cro·cir·cu·la·to·ry** \,mī-krō-'sər-kyə-lə-,tōr-ē, -,tòr-\ *adj*

Mi·cro·coc·ca·ce·ae \-kə-'kā-sē-ē, -kä-'kā-\ *n pl* : a family of heterotrophic spherical or elliptical gram-positive usu. nonmotile bacteria that usu. lack endospores, divide in two or three planes forming pairs, tetrads, or masses of cells, are aerobic or facultatively anaerobic, and produce yellow, orange, or red pigment and that include pathogenic toxin-

producing forms (as *Staphylococcus aureus*) as well as numerous harmless commensals and saprophytes

mi·cro·coc·cal \,mī-krō-'käk-əl\ *adj* : relating to or characteristic of micrococci ⟨~ enzymes⟩

mi·cro·coc·cin \-'käk-sən\ *n* : an antibiotic obtained from a bacterium of the genus *Micrococcus* isolated from sewage

mi·cro·coc·cus \,mī-krō-'käk-əs\ *n* **1** *cap* : a large genus (the type genus of the family Micrococcaceae) of nonmotile gram-positive spherical bacteria that occur in tetrads or irregular clusters and include nonpathogenic forms found on human and animal skin **2** *pl* **-coc·ci** \-'käk-,(s)ī\ : a small spherical bacterium; *esp* : any bacterium of the genus *Micrococcus*

mi·cro·col·o·ny \'mī-krō-,käl-ə-nē\ *n, pl* **-nies** : a microscopic colony of cells; *specif* : a minute colony of bacteria growing under suboptimal conditions — **mi·cro·co·lo·nial** \,mī-krō-kə-'lō-nē-əl, -nyəl\ *adj*

mi·cro·co·nid·i·um \-kə-'nid-ē-əm\ *n, pl* **-nid·ia** \-ē-ə\ : a conidium of the smaller of two types produced by the same species and often differing in shape (as in members of the genus *Fusarium*) — compare MACROCONIDIUM — **mi·cro·co·nid·i·al** \-ē-əl\ *adj*

mi·cro·cor·nea \-'kòr-nē-ə\ *n* : abnormal smallness of the cornea

mi·cro·cou·lomb \-'kü-,läm\ *n* : a unit of electrical charge equal to one millionth of a coulomb

mi·cro·crys·tal \'mī-krō-,kris-tᵊl\ *n* : a crystal visible only under the microscope

mi·cro·crys·tal·line \,mī-krō-'kris-tə-lən *also* -,līn *or* -,lēn\ *adj* : of, relating to, or consisting of microcrystals — **mi·cro·crys·tal·lin·i·ty** \-,kris-tə-'lin-ət-ē\ *n, pl* **-ties**

mi·cro·cul·ture \'mī-krō-,kəl-chər\ *n* : a microscopic culture of cells or organisms ⟨a ~ of lymphocytes⟩ — **mi·cro·cul·tur·al** \,mī-krō-'kəlch-(ə-)rəl\ *adj*

mi·cro·cu·rie \'mī-krō-,kyü(ə)r-ē, ,mī-krō-kyù-'rē\ *n* : a unit of quantity or of radioactivity equal to one millionth of a curie

mi·cro·cyst \'mī-krə-,sist\ *n* : a very small cyst — compare MACROCYST — **mi·cro·cys·tic** \,mī-krə-'sis-tik\ *adj*

mi·cro·cyte \'mī-krə-,sīt\ *n* : an abnormally small red blood cell present esp. in some anemias

mi·cro·cy·the·mia *or chiefly Brit* **mi·cro·cy·thae·mia** \,mī-krō-sī-'thē-mē-ə\ *n* : the presence of abnormally small red blood cells in the blood — **mi·cro·cy·the·mic** *or chiefly Brit* **mi·cro·cy·thae·mic** \-'thē-mik\ *adj*

mi·cro·cyt·ic \-'sit-ik\ *adj* : of, relating to, being, or characterized by the presence of microcytes

microcytic anemia *n* : an anemia characterized by the presence of microcytes in the blood

mi·cro·cy·to·sis \-sī-'tō-səs\ *n, pl* **-to·ses** \-,sēz\ : decrease in the size of red blood cells

mi·cro·cy·to·tox·ic·i·ty test \-,sīt-ō-,täk-'sis-ət-ē-\ *n* : a procedure using microscopic quantities of materials (as complement and lymphocytes in cell-mediated immunity) to determine cytotoxicity (as to cancer cells or cells of transplanted tissue) — called also *microcytotoxicity assay*

mi·cro·de·ter·mi·na·tion \-di-,tər-mə-'nā-shən\ *n* : a quantitative chemical analysis in which the amount of a substance presumed to be present in a sample in very small quantities is ascertained — called also *microestimation*

mi·cro·dis·sec·tion \,mī-krō-dis-'ek-shən, -dī-'sek-\ *n* : dissection under the microscope; *specif* : dissection of cells and tissues by means of fine needles that are precisely manipulated by levers — **mi·cro·dis·sect·ed** \-təd\ *adj*

mi·cro·dis·tri·bu·tion \-,dis-trə-'byü-shən\ *n* : the precise distribution of one or more kinds of organisms in a microenvironment or in part of an ecosystem ⟨~ of soil mites⟩

mi·cro·dont \'mī-krə-,dänt\ *adj* : having small teeth — **mi·cro·dont·ism** \-,iz-əm\ *n*

mi·cro·dose \'mī-krō-,dōs\ *n* : an extremely small dose

mi·cro·do·sim·e·try \,mī-krō-dō-'sim-ə-trē\ *n, pl* **-tries** : dosimetry involving microdoses of radiation or minute amounts of radioactive materials

mi·cro·drop \'mī-krō-ˌdräp\ *n* : a very small drop or minute droplet (as 0.1 to 0.01 of a drop)

mi·cro·drop·let \-lət\ *n* : MICRODROP

mi·cro·elec·trode \ˌmī-krō-i-'lek-ˌtrōd\ *n* : a minute electrode; *esp* : one that is inserted in a living biological cell or tissue in studying its electrical characteristics

mi·cro·elec·tro·pho·re·sis \-ˌlek-trə-fə-'rē-səs\ *n, pl* **-re·ses** \-ˌsēz\ : electrophoresis in which the movement of single particles is observed in a microscope; *also* : electrophoresis in which micromethods are used — **mi·cro·elec·tro·pho·ret·ic** \-'ret-ik\ *adj* — **mi·cro·elec·tro·pho·ret·i·cal·ly** \-i-k(ə-)lē\ *adv*

mi·cro·el·e·ment \ˌmī-krō-'el-ə-mənt\ *n* : TRACE ELEMENT

mi·cro·em·bo·lism \-'em-bə-ˌliz-əm\ *n* : a small embolus (as one consisting of an aggregation of platelets) that blocks an arteriole or the terminal part of an artery

mi·cro·em·bo·lus \-'em-bə-ləs\ *n, pl* **-li** \-ˌlī\ : an extremely small embolus

mi·cro·en·cap·su·late \-in-'kap-sə-ˌlāt\ *vt* **-lat·ed; -lat·ing** : to enclose in a microcapsule ⟨*microencapsulated* aspirin⟩ — **mi·cro·en·cap·su·la·tion** \-in-ˌkap-sə-'lā-shən\ *n*

mi·cro·en·vi·ron·ment \-in-'vī-rən-mənt, -'vī(-ə)rn-\ *n* : a small or relatively small usu. distinctly specialized and effectively isolated habitat or environment (as of a nerve cell) — see MICROHABITAT — **mi·cro·en·vi·ron·men·tal** \-ˌvī-rən-'ment-ᵊl\ *adj*

mi·cro·es·ti·ma·tion \-es-tə-'mā-shən\ *n* : MICRODETERMI-NATION ⟨∼ of fatty acids in blood⟩

mi·cro·evo·lu·tion \'mī-krō-ˌev-ə-'lü-shən *also* -ˌē-və-\ *n* : comparatively minor evolutionary change involving the accumulation of variations in populations usu. below the species level — **mi·cro·evo·lu·tion·ary** \-shə-ˌner-ē\ *adj*

mi·cro·far·ad \'mī-krō-ˌfa(ə)r-ˌad, -ˌfar-əd\ *n* : a unit of capacitance equal to one millionth of a farad

mi·cro·fau·na \ˌmī-krō-'fôn-ə, -'fän-\ *n* : minute animals; *esp* : those invisible to the naked eye ⟨the soil ∼⟩ — compare MACROFAUNA — **mi·cro·fau·nal** \-'fôn-ᵊl, -'fän-\ *adj*

mi·cro·fi·bril \-'fīb-rəl, -'fib-\ *n* : an extremely fine fibril — **mi·cro·fi·bril·lar** \-rə-lər\ *adj*

mi·cro·fil·a·ment \ˌmī-krō-'fil-ə-mənt\ *n* : any of the minute actin-containing protein filaments that are widely distributed in the cytoplasm of eukaryotic cells, help maintain their structural framework, and play a role in the movement of cell components — **mi·cro·fil·a·men·tous** \-ˌfil-ə-'ment-əs\ *adj*

mi·cro·fil·a·re·mia *or chiefly Brit* **mi·cro·fil·a·rae·mia** \-ˌfil-ə-'rē-mē-ə\ *n* : the presence of microfilariae in the blood of one affected with some forms of filariasis

mi·cro·fi·lar·ia \ˌmī-krō-fi-'lar-ē-ə, -'ler-\ *n, pl* **-i·ae** \-ē-ˌē\ : a minute larval filaria — **mi·cro·fi·lar·i·al** \-ē-əl\ *adj*

mi·cro·flo·ra \ˌmī-krə-'flōr-ə, -'flór-\ *n* **1** : a small or strictly localized flora (as of a microenvironment) ⟨intestinal ∼⟩ **2** : microscopic flora — compare MACROFLORA — **mi·cro·flo·ral** \-əl\ *adj*

mi·cro·flu·o·rom·e·try \-ˌflu(ə)r-'äm-ə-trē\ *n, pl* **-tries** : the detection and measurement of the fluorescence produced by minute quantities of materials (as in cells) — **mi·cro·flu·o·rom·e·ter** \-'äm-ət-ər\ *n* — **mi·cro·flu·o·ro·met·ric** \-ə-'me-trik\ *adj*

mi·cro·ga·mete \-'gam-ˌēt, -gə-'mēt\ *n* : the smaller and usu. male gamete of an organism producing two types of gametes — compare MACROGAMETE

mi·cro·ga·me·to·cyte \-gə-'mēt-ə-ˌsīt\ *n* : a gametocyte producing microgametes

mi·cro·ge·nia \-'jē-nē-ə\ *n* : abnormal smallness of the chin

mi·crog·lia \mī-'kräg-lē-ə\ *n* : glia consisting of small cells with few processes that are scattered throughout the central nervous system, have a phagocytic function as part of the reticuloendothelial system, and are now usu. considered to be of mesodermal origin — **mi·crog·li·al** \-lē-əl\ *adj*

β₂-mi·cro·glob·u·lin \ˌbāt-ə-ˌtü-ˌmī-krō-'gläb-yə-lən, *chiefly Brit* ˌbē-tə-\ *n* : a beta globulin of low molecular weight that is present at a low level in plasma, is normally excreted in the urine, is homologous in structure to part of an antibody,

comprises the light chain in certain histocompatibility antigens, and occurs at elevated levels in blood serum or urine in some pathological conditions (as tubulointerstitial disease)

mi·cro·glos·sia \ˌmī-krō-'gläs-ē-ə, -'glós-\ *n* : abnormal smallness of the tongue

mi·cro·gna·thia \ˌmī-krō-'nā-thē-ə, -'nath-ē-ə, ˌmī-ˌkräg-\ *n* : abnormal smallness of one or both jaws

mi·cro·gram \'mī-krə-ˌgram\ *n* **1** : one millionth of a gram **2** : MICROGRAPH 1

mi·cro·graph \-ˌgraf\ *n* **1** : a graphic reproduction (as a photograph) of the image of an object formed by a microscope **2** : an instrument for measuring minute movements by magnifying and recording photographically the corresponding vibrations of a diaphragm moving in unison with the original object — **micrograph** *vt*

mi·crog·ra·phy \mī-'kräg-rə-fē\ *n, pl* **-phies 1** : examination or study with the microscope **2** : the art or process of producing micrographs

mi·cro·gy·ria \ˌmī-krō-'jī-rē-ə\ *n* : abnormal smallness of the brain's convolutions — **mi·cro·gy·ric** \-'jī-rik\ *adj*

mi·cro·hab·i·tat \ˌmī-krō-'hab-ə-ˌtat\ *n* : the microenvironment in which an organism lives ⟨the kidneys, heart, and sinuses are the usual ∼s of the sporocysts of the schistosome⟩

mi·cro·he·mat·o·crit *or chiefly Brit* **mi·cro·hae·mat·o·crit** \-hi-'mat-ə-ˌkrit\ *n* **1** : a procedure for determining the ratio of the volume of packed red blood cells to the volume of whole blood by centrifuging a minute quantity of blood in a capillary tube coated with heparin **2** : a hematocrit value obtained by microhematocrit ⟨a ∼ of 37 percent⟩

mi·cro·het·er·o·ge·ne·ity \-ˌhet-ə-rō-jə-'nē-ət-ē\ *n, pl* **-ities** : variation in the chemical structure of a substance (as the amino acid sequence of a protein) that does not produce a major change in its properties

mi·crohm \'mī-ˌkrōm\ *n* : one millionth of an ohm

mi·cro·in·cin·er·a·tion \ˌmī-krō-in-ˌsin-ə-'rā-shən\ *n* : a technique employing high temperatures (as 600–650°C) for driving off the organic constituents of cells or tissue fragments leaving the inorganic matter for chemical identification

mi·cro·in·farct \-in-'färkt\ *n* : a very small infarct

mi·cro·in·jec·tion \ˌmī-krō-in-'jek-shən\ *n* : injection under the microscope; *specif* : injection esp. by a micropipette into a tissue or a single cell — **mi·cro·in·ject** \-in-'jekt\ *vt*

mi·cro·in·va·sive \-in-'vā-siv\ *adj* : of, relating to, or characterized by very slight invasion into adjacent tissues by malignant cells of a carcinoma in situ ⟨no ∼ lesions were found in the sample⟩ — **mi·cro·in·va·sion** \-'vā-zhən\ *n*

mi·cro·ion·to·pho·re·sis \-ˌ(ˌ)ī-änt-ə-fə-'rē-səs\ *n, pl* **-re·ses** \-ˌsēz\ : a process for observing or recording the effect of an ionized substance on nerve cells that involves inserting a double micropipette into the brain close to a nerve cell, injecting an ionized fluid through one barrel of the pipette, and using a concentrated saline solution in the other tube as an electrical conductor to pick up and transmit back to an oscilloscope any change in neural activity — **mi·cro·ion·to·pho·ret·ic** \-'ret-ik\ *adj* — **mi·cro·ion·to·pho·ret·i·cal·ly** \-i-k(ə-)lē\ *adv*

mi·cro·ker·a·tome \-'ker-ə-ˌtōm\ *n* : a small keratome used for fine surgical procedures on the cornea

mi·cro·lec·i·thal \ˌmī-krō-'les-ə-thəl\ *adj* : having little yolk ⟨a ∼ egg⟩

mi·cro·li·ter *or chiefly Brit* **mi·cro·li·tre** \ˌmī-krō-'lēt-ər\ *n* : a unit of capacity equal to one millionth of a liter

mi·cro·lith \'mī-krō-ˌlith\ *n* : a microscopic calculus or concretion ⟨rupture of ∼s into blood vessels —*Modern Medicine*⟩ — compare GRAVEL 1

mi·cro·li·thi·a·sis \ˌmī-krō-lith-'ī-ə-səs\ *n, pl* **-a·ses** \-ˌsēz\ : the formation or presence of microliths or gravel

mi·crol·o·gy \mī-'kräl-ə-jē\ *n, pl* **-gies** : a science dealing

M
N

with the handling and preparation of microscopic objects for study

mi·cro·ma·nip·u·la·tion \ˌmī-krō-mə-ˌnip-yə-'lā-shən\ *n* : the technique or practice of manipulating cells or tissues (as by microdissection or microinjection) — **mi·cro·ma·nip·u·late** \-'nip-yə-ˌlāt\ *vt* **-lat·ed; -lat·ing**

mi·cro·ma·nip·u·la·tor \-'nip-yə-ˌlāt-ər\ *n* : an instrument for micromanipulation

mi·cro·ma·nom·e·ter \-mə-'näm-ət-ər\ *n* : a manometer designed to measure minute differences of pressure

mi·cro·mas·tia \-'mast-ē-ə\ *n* : postpubertal immaturity and abnormal smallness of the breasts

mi·cro·me·lia \-'mē-lē-ə\ *n* : a condition characterized by abnormally small and imperfectly developed extremities — **mi·cro·me·lic** \-'mē-lik\ *adj*

mi·cro·mer·al \-'mir-əl\ *or* **mi·cro·mer·ic** \-'mir-ik\ *adj* : of or relating to a micromere

mi·cro·mere \'mī-krō-ˌmi(ə)r\ *n* : one of the smaller blastomeres resulting from the unequal segmentation of an egg — compare MACROMERE

mi·cro·me·tas·ta·sis \ˌmī-krō-mə-'tas-tə-səs\ *n, pl* **-ta·ses** \-ˌsēz\ : the spread of cancer cells from a primary site and the formation of microscopic tumors at secondary sites; *also* : one of those microscopic tumors — **mi·cro·met·a·stat·ic** \-ˌmet-ə-'stat-ik\ *adj*

¹**mi·crom·e·ter** \mī-'kräm-ət-ər\ *n* : an instrument used with a telescope or microscope for measuring minute distances

²**mi·cro·me·ter** *or chiefly Brit* **mi·cro·me·tre** \'mī-krō-ˌmēt-ər\ *n* : MICRON

mi·cro·meth·od \'mī-krō-ˌmeth-əd\ *n* : a method (as of microanalysis) that requires only very small quantities of material or that involves the use of the microscope — compare MACROMETHOD

mi·cro·met·ric \ˌmī-krō-'me-trik\ *adj* : relating to or made by a micrometer

mi·crom·e·try \mī-'kräm-ə-trē\ *n, pl* **-tries** : measurement with a micrometer

mi·cro·mi·cro·cu·rie \'mī-krō-'mī-krō-ˌkyu̇(ə)r-ē\ *n* : one millionth of a microcurie

mi·cro·mi·cro·far·ad \-ˌfar-əd\ *n* : PICOFARAD

mi·cro·mi·cro·gram \-ˌgram\ *n* : PICOGRAM

mi·cro·mole \'mī-krə-ˌmōl\ *n* : one millionth of a mole — **mi·cro·mo·lar** \ˌmī-krə-'mō-lər\ *adj*

mi·cro·mol·e·cule \ˌmī-krō-'mäl-ə-ˌkyül\ *n* : a molecule (as of an amino acid or a fatty acid) of relatively low molecular weight — compare MACROMOLECULE — **mi·cro·mo·lec·u·lar** \-mə-'lek-yə-lər\ *adj*

mi·cro·mono·spo·ra \-ˌmän-ə-'spȯr-ə\ *n* **1** *cap* : a genus of actinomycetes that have well developed, branching, septate mycelia bearing single spores that are sessile or on short or long sporophores and that include several antibiotic-producing forms (as *M. purpurea,* the source of gentamicin) **2** *pl* **-rae** \-rē\ : any bacterium of the genus *Micromonospora*

mi·cro·mor·phol·o·gy \ˌmī-krə-mȯr-'fäl-ə-jē\ *n, pl* **-gies** : minute morphological detail esp. as determined by electron microscopy; *also* : the study of such detail — **mi·cro·mor·pho·log·ic** \-ˌmȯr-fə-'läj-ik\ *or* **mi·cro·mor·pho·log·i·cal** \-i-kəl\ *adj* — **mi·cro·mor·pho·log·i·cal·ly** \-i-k(ə)lē\ *adv*

mi·cron \'mī-ˌkrän\ *n* : a unit of length equal to one millionth of a meter — called also *micrometer, mu*

Mi·cro·nase \'mī-krō-ˌnās, -ˌnāz\ *trademark* — used for a preparation of glyburide

mi·cro·nee·dle \'mī-krō-ˌnēd-ᵊl\ *n* **1** : a needle for micromanipulation **2 microneedles** *pl* : long thin microscopic particles of material ⟨inhaled asbestos ∼s —Jack De Ment⟩

mi·cron·ize *also Brit* **mi·cron·ise** \'mī-krə-ˌnīz\ *vt* **-ized** *also Brit* **-ised; -iz·ing** *also Brit* **-is·ing** : to pulverize extremely fine; *esp* : to pulverize into particles a few microns in diameter ⟨*micronized* graphite⟩ ⟨*micronized* penicillin⟩ — **mi·cron·iza·tion** *also Brit* **mi·cron·isa·tion** \ˌmī-krə-nə-'zā-shən\ *n*

mi·cro·nod·u·lar \ˌmī-krō-'näj-ə-lər\ *adj* : characterized by the presence of extremely small nodules ⟨∼ . . . opacities

whose greatest diameter is between 1.5 and 3 mm —E. P. Pendergrass *et al*⟩

mi·cro·nu·cle·ar \-'n(y)ü-klē-ər\ *adj* : of or relating to a micronucleus

mi·cro·nu·cle·us \ˌmī-krō-'n(y)ü-klē-əs\ *n* : a minute nucleus; *specif* : one regarded as primarily concerned with reproductive and genetic functions in most ciliated protozoans — compare MACRONUCLEUS

mi·cro·nu·tri·ent \-'n(y)ü-trē-ənt\ *n* **1** : TRACE ELEMENT **2** : an organic compound (as a vitamin) essential in minute amounts to the growth and health of an animal

mi·cro·nych·ia \ˌmī-krə-'nik-ē-ə\ *n* : the presence of one or more abnormally small fingernails or toenails

mi·cro·or·gan·ic \ˌmī-krō-ȯr-'gan-ik\ *adj* : MICROORGANISMAL ⟨new ∼ antibiotics⟩

mi·cro·or·gan·ism \-'ȯr-gə-ˌniz-əm\ *n* : an organism of microscopic or ultramicroscopic size

mi·cro·or·gan·is·mal \-ˌȯr-gə-'niz-məl\ *adj* : of, relating to, or characteristic of microorganisms ⟨a ∼ agent⟩

mi·cro·par·a·site \ˌmī-krō-'par-ə-ˌsīt\ *n* : a parasitic microorganism — **mi·cro·par·a·sit·ic** \-ˌpar-ə-'sit-ik\ *adj*

mi·cro·pe·nis \-'pē-nəs\ *n, pl* **-pe·nes** \-(ˌ)nēz\ *or* **-pe·nis·es** : MICROPHALLUS

mi·cro·per·fu·sion \-pər-'fyü-zhən\ *n* : an act or instance of forcing a fluid through a small organ or tissue by way of a tubule or blood vessel — **mi·cro·per·fused** \-'fyüzd\ *adj*

mi·cro·phage \'mī-krə-ˌfāj\ *also* -ˌfäzh\ *n* : a small phagocyte

mi·croph·a·gous \mī-'kräf-ə-gəs\ *adj* : feeding on minute particles (as bacteria) ⟨∼ ciliates⟩ ⟨∼ habit⟩ — **mi·croph·a·gy** \-ə-jē\ *n, pl* **-gies**

mi·cro·pha·kia \ˌmī-krō-'fā-kē-ə\ *n* : abnormal smallness of the lens of the eye

mi·cro·phal·lus \-'fal-əs\ *n* : smallness of the penis esp. to an abnormal degree — called also *micropenis*

mi·cro·phone \'mī-krə-ˌfōn\ *n* : an instrument whereby sound waves are caused to generate or modulate an electric current usu. for the purpose of transmitting or recording sound (as speech or music)

¹**mi·cro·phon·ic** \ˌmī-krə-'fän-ik\ *adj* **1** : of or relating to a microphone : serving to intensify sounds **2** : of or relating to the cochlear microphonic

²**microphonic** *n* : COCHLEAR MICROPHONIC

mi·cro·pho·to·graph \-'fōt-ə-ˌgraf\ *n* **1** : a small photograph that is normally magnified for viewing **2** : PHOTOMICROGRAPH — **microphotograph** *vt* — **mi·cro·pho·tog·ra·pher** \-fə-'täg-rə-fər\ *n* — **mi·cro·pho·to·graph·ic** \-ˌfōt-ə-'graf-ik\ *adj* — **mi·cro·pho·tog·ra·phy** \-fə-'täg-rə-fē\ *n, pl* **-phies**

mi·cro·pho·tom·e·ter \-fō-'täm-ət-ər\ *n* : an instrument for measuring the amount of light transmitted or reflected by small areas or for measuring the relative densities of spectral lines on a photographic film or plate — **mi·cro·pho·to·met·ric** \-ˌfōt-ə-'me-trik\ *adj* — **mi·cro·pho·to·met·ri·cal·ly** \-tri-k(ə)lē\ *adv* — **mi·cro·pho·tom·e·try** \-fō-'täm-ə-trē\ *n, pl* **-tries**

mi·croph·thal·mia \ˌmī-ˌkräf-'thal-mē-ə\ *n* : abnormal smallness of the eye usu. occurring as a congenital anomaly

mi·croph·thal·mic \-'thal-mik\ *adj* : exhibiting microphthalmia : having small eyes

mi·croph·thal·mos \-'thal-məs, -ˌmäs\ *or* **mi·croph·thal·mus** \-məs\ *n, pl* **-moi** \-ˌmȯi\ *or* **-mi** \-ˌmī\ : MICROPHTHALMIA

mi·cro·phys·i·ol·o·gist \ˌmī-krō-ˌfiz-ē-'äl-ə-jəst\ *n* : a specialist in microphysiology

mi·cro·phys·i·ol·o·gy \-ˌfiz-ē-'äl-ə-jē\ *n, pl* **-gies** : physiology of minute quantities or on a microscopic scale — **mi·cro·phys·i·o·log·i·cal** \-ˌfiz-ē-ə-'läj-i-kəl\ *adj*

mi·cro·phyte \'mī-krə-ˌfīt\ *n* : a microscopic plant (as a bacterium, fungus, or alga) — **mi·cro·phyt·ic** \ˌmī-krə-'fit-ik\ *adj*

mi·cro·pi·no·cy·to·sis \ˌmī-krō-ˌpī-nō-ˌsī-'tō-səs\ *n, pl* **-to·ses** \-'tō-ˌsēz\ : the incorporation of macromolecules or other chemical substances into cells by membrane invagination and the pinching off of relatively minute vesicles

mi·cro·pi·no·cy·tot·ic \-'tät-ik\ *adj* : of or relating to micropinocytosis

¹mi·cro·pi·pette *or* **mi·cro·pi·pet** \-pī-'pet\ *n* **1** : a pipette for the measurement of minute volumes **2** : a small and extremely fine-pointed pipette used in making microinjections

²micropipette *vt* **-pet·ted; -pet·ting** : to measure or inject by means of a micropipette

mi·cro·pop·u·la·tion \'mī-krō-ˌpäp-yə-'lā-shən\ *n* **1** : a population of microorganisms **2** : a population of organisms within a small area

mi·cro·po·rous \-ˌpōr-əs, -ˌpȯr-\ *adj* : characterized by very small pores or channels with diameters in the micron or nanometer range ⟨a cell monolayer grown on a ∼ substrate⟩

mi·cro·probe \-ˌprōb\ *n* : a device for microanalysis that operates by exciting radiation in a minute area or volume of material so that the composition may be determined from the emission spectrum

mi·cro·pro·jec·tor \ˌmī-krō-prə-'jek-tər\ *n* : a projector utilizing a compound microscope for projecting on a screen a greatly enlarged image of a microscopic object — **mi·cro·pro·jec·tion** \-'jek-shən\ *n*

mi·crop·sia \mī-'kräp-sē-ə\ *also* **mi·crop·sy** \'mī-ˌkräp-sē\ *n, pl* **-sias** *also* **-sies** : a pathological condition in which objects appear to be smaller than they are in reality — compare MACROPSIA

mi·crop·tic \mī-'kräp-tik\ *adj* : of, relating to, or affected with micropsia

mi·cro·punc·ture \ˌmī-krō-'pəŋ(k)-chər\ *n* : an extremely small puncture (as of a nephron); *also* : an act of making such a puncture

mi·cro·pyle \'mī-krə-ˌpīl\ *n* : a differentiated area of surface in an egg through which a sperm enters — **mi·cro·py·lar** \ˌmī-krə-'pī-lər\ *adj*

mi·cro·ra·dio·gram \ˌmī-krō-'rā-dē-ə-ˌgram\ *n* : MICRORADIOGRAPH

mi·cro·ra·dio·graph \ˌmī-krō-'rād-ē-ə-ˌgraf\ *n* : an X-ray photograph prepared by microradiography

mi·cro·ra·di·og·ra·phy \-ˌrā-dē-'äg-rə-fē\ *n, pl* **-phies** : radiography in which an X-ray photograph is prepared showing minute internal structure — see HISTORADIOGRAPHY — **mi·cro·ra·dio·graph·ic** \-ˌrā-dē-ə-'graf-ik\ *adj*

mi·cro·res·pi·rom·e·ter \-ˌres-pə-'räm-ət-ər\ *n* : an apparatus for the quantitative study of the respiratory activity of minute amounts of living material (as individual cells or protozoans) — **mi·cro·res·pi·rom·e·try** \-ə-trē\ *n, pl* **-tries**

mi·cro·sat·el·lite \-'sat-ᵊl-ˌīt\ *n* : any of numerous short segments of DNA that are distributed throughout the genome, that consist of repeated sequences of usu. two to five nucleotides, and that are often useful markers in studies of genetic linkage because they tend to vary from one individual to another — compare MINISATELLITE

mi·cro·scis·sors \'mī-krō-ˌsiz-ərz\ *n pl but sing or pl in constr* : extremely small scissors for use in microsurgery

mi·cro·scope \'mī-krə-ˌskōp\ *n* **1** : an optical instrument consisting of a lens or combination of lenses for making enlarged images of minute objects; *esp* : COMPOUND MICROSCOPE — see LIGHT MICROSCOPE, PHASE-CONTRAST MICROSCOPE, POLARIZING MICROSCOPE, REFLECTING MICROSCOPE, ULTRAVIOLET MICROSCOPE **2** : an instrument using radiations other than light or using vibrations for making enlarged images of minute objects ⟨an acoustic ∼⟩ — see ELECTRON MICROSCOPE, SCANNING ELECTRON MICROSCOPE, X-RAY MICROSCOPE

mi·cro·scop·ic \ˌmī-krə-'skäp-ik\ *or* **mi·cro·scop·i·cal** \-i-kəl\ *adj* **1** : of, relating to, or conducted with the microscope or microscopy **2** : so small or fine as to be invisible or indistinguishable without the use of a microscope — compare MACROSCOPIC, SUBMICROSCOPIC, ULTRAMICROSCOPIC 1 — **mi·cro·scop·i·cal·ly** \-i-k(ə-)lē\ *adv*

microscopic anatomy *n* : HISTOLOGY 1, 3

mi·cros·co·pist \mī-'kräs-kə-pəst\ *n* : a specialist in microscopy

mi·cros·co·py \mī-'kräs-kə-pē\ *n, pl* **-pies** : the use of or investigation with the microscope

mi·cro·sec·ond \'mī-krō-ˌsek-ənd, -ənt\ *n* : one millionth of a second

mi·cro·sec·tion \-ˌsek-shən\ *n* : a thin section (as of tissue) prepared for microscopic examination — **microsection** *vt*

mi·cro·slide \-ˌslīd\ *n* : a slip of glass on which a preparation is mounted for microscopic examination

mi·cros·mat·ic \ˌmī-ˌkräz-'mat-ik\ *adj* : having the sense of smell feebly developed

mi·cro·some \'mī-krə-ˌsōm\ *n* **1** : any of various minute cellular structures (as a ribosome) **2** : a particle in a particulate fraction that is obtained by heavy centrifugation of broken cells and consists of various amounts of ribosomes, fragmented endoplasmic reticulum, and mitochondrial cristae — **mi·cro·som·al** \ˌmī-krə-'sō-məl\ *adj*

mi·cro·so·mia \ˌmī-krə-'sō-mē-ə\ *n* : abnormal smallness of the body

mi·cro·spec·tro·graph \-'spek-trə-ˌgraf\ *n* : a microspectroscope equipped (as with a camera) to make a graphic record of the observed spectrum — **mi·cro·spec·tro·graph·ic** \-ˌspek-trə-'graf-ik\ *adj* — **mi·cro·spec·trog·ra·phy** \-ˌspek-'träg-rə-fē\ *n, pl* **-phies**

mi·cro·spec·tro·pho·tom·e·ter \ˌmī-krə-ˌspek-trə-fō-'täm-ət-ər\ *n* : a spectrophotometer adapted to the examination of light transmitted by a very small specimen (as a single organic cell) — **mi·cro·spec·tro·pho·to·met·ric** \-ˌfōt-ə-'me-trik\ *adj* — **mi·cro·spec·tro·pho·tom·e·try** \-fō-'täm-ə-trē\ *n, pl* **-tries**

mi·cro·spec·tro·scope \-'spek-trə-ˌskōp\ *n* : a spectroscope arranged for attachment to a microscope for observation of the spectrum of light from minute portions of an object — **mi·cro·spec·tro·scop·ic** \-ˌspek-trə-'skäp-ik\ *adj* — **mi·cro·spec·tros·co·py** \-ˌspek-'träs-kə-pē\ *n, pl* **-pies**

mi·cro·sphere \-ˌsfir\ *n* : a spherical shell that is usu. made of a biodegradable or resorbable plastic polymer, that has a very small diameter usu. in the micron or nanometer range, and that is often filled with a substance (as a drug or antibody) for release as the shell is degraded

mi·cro·sphe·ro·cy·to·sis \-ˌsfir-ō-ˌsī-'tō-səs, -ˌsfer-\ *n, pl* **-to·ses** \-'tō-ˌsēz\ : spherocytosis esp. when marked by very small spherocytes

mi·cro·splanch·nic \-'splaŋk-nik\ *adj* : ECTOMORPHIC

microspora *pl of* MICROSPORUM

mi·cro·spore \'mī-krə-ˌspō(ə)r, -ˌspȯ(ə)r\ *n* **1** : any of the spores in heterosporous plants that give rise to male gametophytes and are generally smaller than the megaspore **2** : the smaller of two forms of spores produced by various protozoans (as radiolarians) — compare MACROSPORE

Mi·cro·spo·rid·ia \ˌmī-krō-spə-'rid-ē-ə\ *n pl* : an order of spore-forming protozoans (class Microsporea) that are parasites of various invertebrate and vertebrate animals, that typically invade and destroy host cells, and that include some (as of the genera *Enterocytozoon* and *Nosema*) that cause infections in immunocompromised humans — **mi·cro·spo·rid·i·an** \-ē-ən\ *adj or n*

mi·cro·spo·rid·i·o·sis \-spə-ˌrid-ē-'ō-səs\ *n, pl* **-o·ses** \-ˌsēz\ : infection with or disease caused by microsporidian protozoans

mi·cros·po·ron \mī-'kräs-pə-ˌrän\ *n* : MICROSPORUM 2

Microsporon *n, syn of* MICROSPORUM

mi·cro·spo·ro·sis \ˌmī-krə-spə-'rō-səs\ *n, pl* **-ro·ses** \-ˌsēz\ : ringworm caused by fungi of the genus *Microsporum*

mi·cros·po·rum \mī-'kräs-pə-rəm\ *n* **1** *cap* : a genus of fungi of the family Moniliaceae producing both small, nearly oval single-celled spores and large spindle-shaped multicellular spores with a usu. rough outer wall and including several that cause ringworm, tinea capitis, and tinea corporis **2** *pl* **-ra** : any fungus of the genus *Microsporum*

\ə\ abut \ᵊ\ kitten \ər\ further \a\ ash \ā\ ace \ä\ cot, cart
\aù\ out \ch\ chin \e\ bet \ē\ easy \g\ go \i\ hit \ī\ ice \j\ job
\ŋ\ sing \ō\ go \ȯ\ law \ȯi\ boy \th\ thin \th̶\ the \ü\ loot
\ù\ foot \y\ yet \zh\ vision *See also* Pronunciation Symbols page

M
N

mi·cro·sto·mia \‚mī-krō-'stō-mē-ə\ *n* : abnormal smallness of the mouth

mi·cro·struc·ture \'mī-krō-‚strək-chər\ *n* : microscopic structure (as of a cell) — **mi·cro·struc·tur·al** \‚mī-krō-'strək-chə-rəl, -'strək-shrəl\ *adj*

mi·cro·sur·geon \'mī-krō-‚sər-jən\ *n* : a specialist in microsurgery

mi·cro·sur·gery \‚mī-krō-'sərj-(ə-)rē\ *n, pl* **-ger·ies** : minute dissection or manipulation (as by a micromanipulator or laser beam) of living structures (as cells or tissues) for surgical or experimental purposes — **mi·cro·sur·gi·cal** \-'sər-ji-kəl\ *adj* — **mi·cro·sur·gi·cal·ly** \-ji-k(ə-)lē\ *adv*

mi·cro·sy·ringe \-sə-'rinj\ *n* : a hypodermic syringe equipped for the precise measurement and injection of minute quantities of fluid

mi·cro·tech·nique \‚mī-krō-tek-'nēk\ *also* **mi·cro·tech·nic** \'mī-krō-‚tek-nik, ‚mī-krō-tek-'nēk\ *n* : any of various methods of handling and preparing material for microscopic observation and study

mi·cro·throm·bus \-'thräm-bəs\ *n, pl* **-bi** \-‚bī\ : a very small thrombus

mi·cro·tia \mī-'krō-sh(ē-)ə\ *n* : abnormal smallness of the external ear

mi·cro·ti·ter *or Brit* **mi·cro·ti·tre** \'mī-krō-‚tīt-ər\ *n* : a titer determined by microtitration

mi·cro·ti·tra·tion \-tī-'trā-shən\ *n* : microanalytical titration

mi·cro·ti·tra·tor \-'tī-‚trāt-ər\ *n* : an apparatus used for microtitration

¹**mi·cro·tome** \'mī-krə-‚tōm\ *n* : an instrument for cutting sections (as of organic tissues) for microscopic examination ⟨bone-sectioning ∼s⟩

²**microtome** *vt* **-tomed; -tom·ing** : to cut in sections with a microtome

mi·crot·o·my \mī-'krät-ə-mē\ *n, pl* **-mies** : the technique of using the microtome or of preparing with its aid objects for microscopic study

mi·cro·trau·ma \'mī-krō-‚traù-mə, -‚trò-\ *n* : a very slight injury or lesion

mi·cro·tu·bule \‚mī-krō-'t(y)ü-(‚)byü(ə)l\ *n* : any of the minute tubules in eukaryotic cytoplasm that are composed of the protein tubulin and form an important component of the cytoskeleton, mitotic spindle, cilia, and flagella — **mi·cro·tu·bu·lar** \-byə-lər\ *adj*

Mi·cro·tus \mī-'krōt-əs\ *n* : a genus of rodents of the family Cricetidae comprising the voles of the northern hemisphere

mi·cro·unit \'mī-krō-‚yü-nət\ *n* : one millionth of a standard unit and esp. an international unit ⟨∼s of insulin⟩

mi·cro·vas·cu·lar \‚mī-krō-'vas-kyə-lər\ *adj* : of, relating to, or constituting the part of the circulatory system made up of minute vessels (as venules or capillaries) that average less than 0.3 millimeters in diameter — **mi·cro·vas·cu·la·ture** \-lə-‚chú(ə)r, -‚t(y)ù(ə)r\ *n*

mi·cro·ves·i·cle \-'ves-i-kəl\ *n* : a very small vesicle ⟨nerve endings characterized by the presence of ∼s —J. J. Nordmann⟩

mi·cro·ves·sel \-'ves-əl\ *n* : a blood vessel (as a capillary, arteriole, or venule) of the microcirculatory system

mi·cro·vil·lus \-'vil-əs\ *n, pl* **-vil·li** \-‚lī\ : a microscopic projection of a tissue, cell, or cell organelle; *esp* : any of the fingerlike outward projections of some cell surfaces — **mi·cro·vil·lar** \-'vil-ər\ *adj* — **mi·cro·vil·lous** \-'vil-əs\ *adj*

mi·cro·volt \'mī-krə-‚vōlt\ *n* : one millionth of a volt

mi·cro·watt \-‚wät\ *n* : one millionth of a watt

mi·cro·wave \-‚wāv\ *n, often attrib* : a comparatively short electromagnetic wave; *esp* : one between about 1 millimeter and 1 meter in wavelength

microwave sickness *n* : a condition of impaired health reported esp. in the Russian medical literature that is characterized by headaches, anxiety, sleep disturbances, fatigue, and difficulty in concentrating and by changes in the cardiovascular and central nervous systems and that is held to be caused by prolonged exposure to low-intensity microwave radiation

microwave spectroscope *n* : an apparatus for observing and measuring the absorption of different substances for microwaves as a function of wavelength and thus obtaining the microwave spectra of the substances — **microwave spectroscopy** *n*

mi·cro·zoa \‚mī-krə-'zō-ə\ *n pl* : microscopic animals and esp. protozoans; *also* : microscopic animal life — **mi·cro·zo·an** \-'zō-ən\ *adj or n*

mi·crur·gy \'mī-‚krùr-jē\ *n, pl* **-gies** : MICROMANIPULATION; *broadly* : the practice of using minute tools in a magnified field — **mi·crur·gi·cal** \‚mī-'krùr-ji-kəl\ *also* **mi·crur·gic** \-jik\ *adj*

Mi·cru·rus \mī-'krùr-əs\ *n* : a genus of small venomous elapid snakes comprising the American coral snakes

mic·tion \'mik-shən\ *n* : URINATION

mic·tu·rate \'mik-chə-‚rāt, 'mik-tə-\ *vi* **-rat·ed; -rat·ing** : URINATE

mic·tu·ri·tion \‚mik-chə-'rish-ən, ‚mik-tə-\ *n* : URINATION — **mic·tu·ri·tion·al** \-əl\ *adj*

MID *abbr* minimal infective dose

mid-ax·il·lary line \'mid-'ak-sə-‚ler-ē-\ *n* : an imaginary line through the axilla parallel to the long axis of the body and midway between its ventral and dorsal surfaces

mid·azo·lam \mi-'dā-zō-‚lam, 'mi-dā-\ *n* : a benzodiazepine tranquilizer administered in the form of its hydrochloride $C_{18}H_{13}ClFN_3 \cdot HCl$ esp. to produce sedation before an operation

mid·brain \'mid-‚brān\ *n* : the middle division of the three primary divisions of the developing vertebrate brain or the corresponding part of the adult brain that includes a ventral part containing the cerebral peduncles and a dorsal tectum containing the corpora quadrigemina and that surrounds the aqueduct of Sylvius connecting the third and fourth ventricles — called also *mesencephalon*

mid·ca·pac·i·ty \-kə-'pas-ət-ē\ *n, pl* **-ties** : the pulmonary volume when the lungs are in the state of contraction characteristic of the end of a normal quiet exhalation equal to the sum of the volumes occupied by the residual volume, supplemental air, and dead space

mid·car·pal \-'kär-pəl\ *adj* : being between the proximal and distal carpals — used esp. of an anatomical articulation

mid·cla·vic·u·lar line \-kla-'vik-yə-lər-, -klə-\ *n* : an imaginary line parallel to the long axis of the body and passing through the midpoint of the clavicle on the ventral surface of the body

mid·dle age \‚mid-ᵊl-'āj\ *n* : the period of life from about 40 to about 60 years of age — **middle-aged** \‚mid-ᵊl-'ājd\ *adj*

mid·dle–ag·er \-'ā-jər\ *n* : a middle-aged person

middle cardiac nerve *n* : CARDIAC NERVE b

middle cardiac vein *n* : CARDIAC VEIN b

middle cerebellar peduncle *n* : CEREBELLAR PEDUNCLE b

middle cerebral artery *n* : CEREBRAL ARTERY b

middle cervical ganglion *n* : CERVICAL GANGLION b

middle coat *n* : MEDIA

middle colic artery *n* : COLIC ARTERY b

middle concha *n* : NASAL CONCHA b

middle constrictor *n* : a fan-shaped muscle of the pharynx that arises from the ceratohyal and thyrohyal of the hyoid bone and from the stylohyoid ligament, inserts into the median line at the back of the pharynx, and acts to constrict part of the pharynx in swallowing — called also *constrictor pharyngis medius, middle pharyngeal constrictor muscle;* compare INFERIOR CONSTRICTOR, SUPERIOR CONSTRICTOR

middle cranial fossa *n* : CRANIAL FOSSA b

middle ear *n* : the intermediate portion of the ear of higher vertebrates consisting typically of a small air-filled membrane-lined chamber in the temporal bone continuous with the nasopharynx through the eustachian tube, separated from the external ear by the tympanic membrane and from the inner ear by fenestrae, and containing a chain of three ossicles that extends from the tympanic membrane to the oval window and transmits vibrations to the inner ear — called also *tympanic cavity;* see INCUS, MALLEUS, STAPES

middle finger *n* : the midmost of the five digits of the hand

middle fossa *n* : CRANIAL FOSSA b

middle hemorrhoidal artery *n* : RECTAL ARTERY b
middle hemorrhoidal vein *n* : RECTAL VEIN b
middle meatus *n* : a curved anteroposterior passage in each nasal cavity that is situated below the middle nasal concha and extends along the entire superior border of the inferior nasal concha — compare INFERIOR MEATUS, SUPERIOR MEATUS
middle meningeal artery *n* : a branch of the first portion of the maxillary artery that is the largest artery supplying the dura mater, enters the cranium through the foramen spinosum, and divides into anterior and posterior branches in a groove in the greater wing of the sphenoid bone
middle nasal concha *n* : NASAL CONCHA b
middle peduncle *n* : CEREBELLAR PEDUNCLE b
middle pharyngeal constrictor muscle *n* : MIDDLE CONSTRICTOR
middle piece *n* : the portion of a sperm cell that lies between the nucleus and the flagellum
middle rectal artery *n* : RECTAL ARTERY b
middle rectal vein *n* : RECTAL VEIN b
middle sacral artery *n* : a small artery that arises from the back of the abdominal part of the aorta just before it forks into the two common iliac arteries and that descends near the midline in front of the fourth and fifth lumbar vertebrae, the sacrum, and the coccyx to the glumus coccygeum
middle scalene *n* : SCALENUS b
middle temporal artery *n* : TEMPORAL ARTERY 2b
middle temporal gyrus *n* : TEMPORAL GYRUS b
middle temporal vein *n* : TEMPORAL VEIN a(2)
middle thyroid vein *n* : THYROID VEIN b
middle turbinate *n* : NASAL CONCHA b
middle turbinate bone *also* **middle tur·bi·nat·ed bone** \-'tər-bə-ˌnāt-əd-\ *n* : NASAL CONCHA b
mid·dor·sal \(ˈ)mid-'dȯr-səl\ *adj* : of, relating to, or situated in the middle part or median line of the back
mid·epi·gas·tric \-ˌep-i-'gas-trik\ *adj* : of, relating to, or located in the middle of the epigastric region of the abdomen ⟨~ tenderness⟩
mid·face \'mid-ˌfās, ˌmid-'fās\ *n* : the middle of the face including the nose and its associated bony structures — **mid·fa·cial** \ˌmid-'fā-shəl\ *adj*
mid·for·ceps \-'fȯr-səps, -ˌseps\ *n* : a procedure for delivery of an infant by the use of forceps after engagement has occurred but before the head has reached the lower part of the birth canal — compare HIGH FORCEPS, LOW FORCEPS
midge \'mij\ *n* : any of numerous tiny dipteran flies (esp. families Ceratopogonidae, Cecidomyiidae, and Chironomidae) many of which are capable of giving painful bites and some of which are vectors or intermediate hosts of parasites of humans and various other vertebrates — see BITING MIDGE
midg·et \'mij-ət\ *n, sometimes offensive* : a very small person; *specif* : a person of unusually small size who is physically well-proportioned
midg·et·ism \-ˌiz-əm\ *n* : the state of being a midget
mid·gut \'mid-ˌgət\ *n* **1** : the middle part of the alimentary canal of a vertebrate embryo that in humans gives rise to the more distal part of the duodenum and to the jejunum, ileum, cecum and appendix, ascending colon, and much of the transverse colon **2** : the mesodermal intermediate part of the intestine of an invertebrate animal
mid·life \(ˈ)mid-'līf\ *n* : MIDDLE AGE
midlife crisis *n* : a period of emotional turmoil in middle age caused by the realization that one is no longer young and characterized esp. by a strong desire for change
mid·line \'mid-ˌlīn, ˌmid-'līn\ *n* : a median line; *esp* : the median line or median plane of the body or some part of the body
mid·preg·nan·cy \(ˌ)mid-'preg-nən-sē\ *n, pl* **-cies** : the middle period of a term of pregnancy
mid·riff \'mid-ˌrif\ *n* **1** : DIAPHRAGM 1 **2** : the mid-region of the human torso
mid·sag·it·tal \(ˈ)mid-'saj-ət-ᵊl\ *adj* : median and sagittal
midsagittal plane *n* : the median vertical longitudinal plane

that divides a bilaterally symmetrical animal into right and left halves — called also *median plane*
mid·sec·tion \'mid-ˌsek-shən\ *n* : a section midway between the extremes; *esp* : MIDRIFF 2
mid·stream \ˌmid-'strēm\ *adj* : of, relating to, or being urine passed during the middle of an act of urination and not at the beginning or end ⟨a ~ specimen⟩
mid·tar·sal \-'tär-səl\ *adj* : of, relating to, or being the articulation between the two rows of tarsal bones
midtarsal amputation *n* : amputation of the forepart of the foot through the midtarsal joint
mid·tri·mes·ter \-(ˈ)trī-'mes-tər\ *adj* : of, performed during, or occurring during the fourth through sixth months of human pregnancy ⟨~ spontaneous abortion⟩
mid·ven·tral \-'ven-trəl\ *adj* : of, relating to, or being the middle of the ventral surface — **mid·ven·tral·ly** \-ē\ *adv*
mid·wife \'mid-ˌwīf\ *n* : a person who assists women in childbirth — see NURSE-MIDWIFE
mid·wife·ry \ˌmid-'wif-(ə-)rē, -'wīf-; 'mid-ˌwīf-\ *n, pl* **-ries** : the art or act of assisting at childbirth; *also* : OBSTETRICS — see NURSE-MIDWIFERY
mi·fep·ris·tone \ˌmi-fə-'pris-ˌtōn, mi-'fep-ri-ˌstōn\ *n* : RU-486
mi·graine \'mī-ˌgrān, *Brit often* 'mē-\ *n* **1** : a condition that is marked by recurrent usu. unilateral severe headache often accompanied by nausea and vomiting and followed by sleep, that tends to occur in more than one member of a family, and that is of uncertain origin though attacks appear to be precipitated by dilatation of intracranial blood vessels **2** : an episode or attack of migraine ⟨suffers from ~s⟩ — called also *sick headache* — **mi·grain·ous** \-ˌgrā-nəs\ *adj*
mi·grain·eur \ˌmē-gre-'nər\ *n* : an individual who experiences migraines
mi·grain·oid \'mī-ˌgrā-ˌnȯid, mī-'grā-\ *adj* : resembling migraine
migrans — see ERYTHEMA CHRONICUM MIGRANS, LARVAL MIGRANS, LARVA MIGRANS
migrantes — see LARVA MIGRANS
mi·grate \'mī-ˌgrāt, mī-'\ *vi* **mi·grat·ed; mi·grat·ing** : to move from one place to another: as **a** : to move from one site to another in a host organism esp. as part of a life cycle ⟨filarial worms ~ within the human body⟩ **b** *of an atom or group* : to shift position within a molecule — **mi·gra·to·ry** \'mī-grə-ˌtōr-ē, -ˌtȯr-\ *adj*
mi·gra·tion \mī-'grā-shən\ *n* : the act, process, or an instance of migrating ⟨~ of larval nematodes to the lungs⟩
migration inhibitory factor *n* : a lymphokine which inhibits the migration of macrophages away from the site of interaction between lymphocytes and antigens
mi·ka·my·cin \ˌmī-kə-'mīs-ᵊn\ *n* : an antibiotic complex isolated from a bacterium of the genus *Streptomyces* (*S. mitakaensis*)
Mi·ku·licz cell \'mē-kù-ˌlich-\ *n* : a round or oval macrophage with a small nucleus that is found in the nodules of rhinoscleroma and contains the causative bacterium (*Klebsiella rhinoscleromatis*)
Mikulicz–Ra·dec·ki \-ra-'det-skē\, **Johann von (1850–1905)**, Polish surgeon. Mikulicz served as professor of surgery at universities in Kraków, Königsberg, and Breslau. He is remembered as a pioneer in modern surgery who developed surgical operations for a wide variety of diseases. The published reports of his surgical innovations include descriptions of his operation for complete prolapse of the rectum (1888) and his operation for the treatment of disease of the paranasal sinuses (1887). He also wrote articles discussing radiation therapy, blood transfusions, and treatments for tuberculosis and hyperthyroidism. In a noteworthy article of 1876 he described round or oval macrophages that have small nuclei and are present in the nodules of rhinoscleroma; they are now known as Mikulicz cells.

\ə\ **abut** \ᵊ\ kitten \ər\ **further** \a\ ash \ā\ ace \ä\ cot, cart \aù\ **out** \ch\ chin \e\ bet \ē\ easy \g\ go \i\ hit \ī\ ice \j\ job \ŋ\ sing \ō\ go \ȯ\ law \ȯi\ boy \th\ thin \th\ the \ü\ loot \ù\ foot \y\ yet \zh\ vision *See also* Pronunciation Symbols page

M
N

Mikulicz resection *n* : an operation for removal of part of the intestine and esp. the colon in stages that involves bringing the diseased portion out of the body, closing the wound around the two parts of the loop which have been sutured together, and cutting off the diseased part leaving a double opening which is later joined by crushing the common wall and closed from the exterior

Mi·ku·licz's disease \'mē-kù-,lich-əz-\ *n* : abnormal enlargement of the lacrimal and salivary glands

Mikulicz's syndrome *n* : Mikulicz's disease esp. when occurring as a complication of another disease (as leukemia or sarcoidosis)

mild \'mī(ə)ld\ *adj* **1** : moderate in action or effect ⟨a ∼ drug⟩ **2** : not severe ⟨a ∼ case of the flu⟩

mil·dew \'mil-,d(y)ü\ *n* **1** : a superficial usu. whitish growth produced esp. on organic matter or living plants by fungi (as of the families Erysiphaceae and Peronosporaceae) **2** : a fungus producing mildew

mild mercurous chloride *n* : CALOMEL — called also *mild mercury chloride*

mild silver protein *n* : SILVER PROTEIN a

milia *pl of* MILIUM

mil·i·ar·ia \,mil-ē-'ar-ē-ə, -'er-\ *n* : an inflammatory disorder of the skin characterized by redness, eruption, burning or itching, and the release of sweat in abnormal ways (as by the eruption of vesicles) due to blockage of the ducts of the sweat glands; *esp* : PRICKLY HEAT — **mil·i·ar·i·al** \-əl\ *adj*

miliaria crys·tal·li·na \-,kris-tə-'lē-nə\ *n* : SUDAMINA

mil·i·ary \'mil-ē-,er-ē\ *adj* **1** : resembling or suggesting a small seed or many small seeds ⟨a ∼ aneurysm⟩ ⟨∼ tubercles⟩ **2** : characterized by the formation of numerous small lesions ⟨∼ pneumonia⟩

miliary tuberculosis *n* : acute tuberculosis in which minute tubercles are formed in one or more organs of the body by tubercle bacilli usu. spread by way of the blood

mi·lieu \mēl-'yə(r), -'yü; 'mēl-,yü, mē-lyœ\ *n, pl* **milieus** *or* **mi·lieux** \-'yə(r)(z), -'yüz; -,yü(z), -lyœ(z)\ : ENVIRONMENT

mi·lieu in·te·ri·eur \mēl-,yœ-aⁿ-tä-rē-'œr\ *n* : the bodily fluids regarded as an internal environment in which the cells of the body are nourished and maintained in a state of equilibrium

milieu therapy *n* : psychiatric treatment involving manipulation of the environment of a patient for therapeutic purposes

mil·i·tary an·ti·shock trou·sers \'mil-ə-,ter-ē-,an-ti-'shäk-'traù-zərz, -,an-,tī-\ *n pl* : a garment for the lower half of the body that by applying pressure to this part increases the amount of blood in the upper half of the body — abbr. *MAST*

mil·i·um \'mil-ē-əm\ *n, pl* **mil·ia** \-ē-ə\ : a small pearly firm noninflammatory elevation of the skin (as of the face) due to retention of keratin in an oil gland duct blocked by a thin layer of epithelium — called also *whitehead;* compare BLACKHEAD 1

¹milk \'milk\ *n* **1** : a fluid secreted by the mammary glands of females for the nourishment of their young; *esp* : cow's milk used as a food by humans **2** : LACTATION 2 ⟨cows in ∼⟩

²milk *vt* **1 a** : to draw milk from the breasts or udder of **b** : to draw (milk) from the breast or udder **2** : to induce (a snake) to eject venom ∼ *vi* : to draw or yield milk

milk·er's nodules \'mil-kərz-\ *n pl but sing in constr* : a mild virus infection characterized by reddish blue nodules on the hands, arms, face, or neck acquired by direct contact with the udders of cows infected with a poxvirus (species *Pseudocowpox virus* of the genus *Parapoxvirus*) — called also *paravaccinia, pseudocowpox*

milk fever *n* **1** : a febrile disorder following parturition **2** : a disease of newly lactating cows, sheep, or goats that is caused by excessive drain on the body mineral reserves during the establishment of the milk flow — called also *parturient apoplexy, parturient paresis;* compare GRASS TETANY

milk leg *n* : postpartum thrombophlebitis of a femoral vein — called also *phlegmasia alba dolens*

milk line *n* : MAMMARY RIDGE

Milk·man's syndrome \'milk-mənz-\ *n* : an abnormal condition marked by porosity of bone and tendency to spontaneous often symmetrical fractures

Milkman, Louis Arthur (1895–1951), American radiologist. Milkman published his description of a kind of advanced osteomalacia in 1930. Although this disease had been known to others for some years, his classic description led the profession to associate his name with it.

milk of bismuth *n* : a thick white suspension of bismuth hydroxide and bismuth subcarbonate in water used esp. in the treatment of diarrhea

milk of magnesia *n* : a milk-white suspension of magnesium hydroxide in water used as an antacid and laxative — called also *magnesia magma*

milk sickness *n* : an acute disease characterized by weakness, vomiting, and constipation and caused by eating dairy products or meat from cattle affected with trembles

milk sugar *n* : LACTOSE

milk this·tle \-'this-əl\ *n* : a tall thistle (*Silybum marianum*) that is the source of silymarin, has large clasping white-blotched leaves and large purple flower heads with bristly receptacles, and is native to southern Europe but has been widely introduced elsewhere including the U.S.

milk tooth *n* : a temporary tooth of a young mammal; *esp* : one of the human dentition including four incisors, two canines, and four molars in each jaw which fall out during childhood and are replaced by the permanent teeth — called also *baby tooth, deciduous tooth, primary tooth*

milk·weed \'milk-,wēd\ *n* : any of various plants that secrete latex; *esp* : any plant of the genus *Asclepias* (family Asclepiadaceae, the milkweed family) including several whose dried roots were formerly used medicinally

milky \'mil-kē\ *adj* **milk·i·er; -est** **1** : resembling milk in color or consistency ⟨∼ secretion⟩ **2** : consisting of, containing, or abounding in milk — **milk·i·ness** *n*

Mil·ler–Ab·bott tube \'mil-ər-'ab-ət-\ *n* : a double-lumen balloon-tipped rubber tube used for the purpose of decompression in treating intestinal obstruction

Miller, Thomas Grier (1886–1981), and **Abbott, William Osler (1902–1943),** American physicians. Miller and Abbott introduced their intestinal tube in 1934. Three years later Abbott devised another tube, this one for use in the postoperative care of gastroenterostomy cases.

mill fever \'mil-\ *n* : BYSSINOSIS

mil·li·am·me·ter \,mil-ē-'am-,ēt-ər\ *n* : an instrument for measuring electric currents in milliamperes — compare AMMETER

mil·li·am·pere \,mil-ē-'am-,pi(ə)r\ *n* : one thousandth of an ampere — abbr. *mA*

mil·li·bar \'mil-ə-,bär\ *n* : a unit of atmospheric pressure equal to 1/1000 bar or 1000 dynes per square centimeter — abbr. *mbar*

mil·li·cu·rie \,mil-ə-'kyu̇(ə)r-(,)ē, -kyu̇-'rē\ *n* : one thousandth of a curie — abbr. *mCi*

mil·li·equiv·a·lent \,mil-ē-i-'kwiv(-ə)-lənt\ *n* : one thousandth of an equivalent of a chemical element, radical, or compound — abbr. *mEq*

mil·li·gauss \'mil-ə-,gaùs\ *n* : one thousandth of a gauss

mil·li·gram *or chiefly Brit* **mil·li·gramme** \-,gram\ *n* : one thousandth of a gram — abbr. *mg*

milligram–hour *or chiefly Brit* **milligramme–hour** *n* : a unit in which the therapeutic dosage of radium is expressed and which consists in exposure to the action of one milligram of radium for one hour

mil·li·lam·bert \,mil-ə-'lam-bərt\ *n* : one thousandth of a lambert — abbr. *mL*

mil·li·li·ter *or chiefly Brit* **mil·li·li·tre** \'mil-ə-,lēt-ər\ *n* : one thousandth of a liter — abbr. *ml*

mil·li·me·ter *or chiefly Brit* **mil·li·me·tre** \'mil-ə-,mēt-ər\ *n* : one thousandth of a meter — abbr. *mm*

mil·li·mi·cron \,mil-ə-'mī-,krän\ *n* : NANOMETER

mil·li·mol·ar \-'mō-lər\ *adj* : of, relating to, or containing a millimole — **mil·li·mo·lar·i·ty** \-mə-'lar-ət-ē\ *n, pl* **-ities**

mil·li·mole \\'mil-ə-ˌmōl\ *n* : one thousandth of a mole — abbr. *mmol, mmole*

mil·li·nor·mal \ˌmil-ē-'nȯr-məl\ *adj* : having a concentration that is one thousandth that of a normal solution

mil·li·os·mol *or* **mil·li·os·mole** \ˌmil-ē-'äz-ˌmōl, -'äs-\ *n* : one thousandth of an osmol

mil·li·os·mo·lal·i·ty \-ˌäz-mō-'lal-ət-ē, -ˌäs-\ *n, pl* **-ties** : the concentration of an osmotic solution when measured in milliosmols per 1000 grams of solvent — **mil·li·os·mo·lal** \-äz-'mō-ləl, -äs-\ *adj*

mil·li·os·mo·lar \-äz-'mō-lər, -äs-\ *adj* : relating to or being a solution whose concentration is measured in milliosmols per liter of solution ⟨a 70 ~ solution⟩

mil·li·pede \\'mil-ə-ˌpēd\ *n* : any of a class (Diplopoda) of arthropods having usu. a cylindrical segmented body, two pairs of legs on most segments, and including some forms that secrete toxic substances causing skin irritation but that unlike centipedes possess no poison fangs

mil·li·rad \-ˌrad\ *n* : one thousandth of a rad — abbr. *mrad*

mil·li·rem \\'mil-ə-ˌrem\ *n* : one thousandth of a rem — abbr. *mrem*

mil·li·roent·gen \ˌmil-ə-'rent-gən, -'ränt-, -jən; -'ren-chən, -'rän-\ *n* : one thousandth of a roentgen — abbr. *mR*

mil·li·sec·ond \\'mil-ə-ˌsek-ənd, -ənt\ *n* : one thousandth of a second — abbr. *ms, msec*

mil·li·sie·vert \\'mil-ə-ˌsē-vərt\ *n* : one thousandth of a sievert — abbr. *mSv*

mil·li·unit \\'mil-ə-ˌyü-nət\ *n* : one thousandth of a standard unit and esp. of an international unit

mil·li·volt \-ˌvōlt\ *n* : one thousandth of a volt — abbr. *mV*

mil·li·volt·me·ter \ˌmil-ə-'vōlt-ˌmēt-ər\ *n* : an instrument for measuring potential differences in millivolts

mil·li·watt \\'mil-ə-ˌwät\ *n* : one thousandth of a watt — abbr. *mW*

Mil·lon's reagent \mē-'lōnz-\ *or* **Mil·lon reagent** \mē-'lōn-\ *n* : a solution that is usu. made by dissolving mercury in concentrated nitric acid and diluting with water and that when heated with phenolic compounds gives a red coloration used as a test esp. for tyrosine and proteins containing tyrosine

  Mil·lon \mē-lōⁿ\, **Auguste–Nicolas–Eugène (1812–1867),** French chemist and physician. Millon devoted his career to the military, first as a surgeon and then as a chemist. In 1848 he demonstrated that urea could be quantitatively analyzed, and in 1849 he formulated the solution now known as Millon's reagent.

Mi·lon·tin \mi-'län-tin\ *n* : a preparation of phensuximide — formerly a U.S. registered trademark

mil·ri·none \\'mil-rə-ˌnōn\ *n* : an inotropic vasodilator agent administered in the form of its lactate $C_{12}H_9N_3O\cdot C_3H_6O_3$ esp. in short-term intravenous therapy for congestive heart failure

Mil·roy's disease \\'mil-ˌrȯiz-\ *n* : a hereditary lymphedema esp. of the legs

  Milroy, William Forsyth (1855–1942), American physician. Milroy specialized in internal medicine and was an authority on diseases of the heart and lungs. His most important topic of research was chronic hereditary edema of the legs. From one patient he was able to trace the disease back through six generations of his family, learning that 22 individuals had been affected with the edema. He published his findings in 1892.

milt \\'milt\ *n* : the sperm-containing fluid of a male fish

Mil·town \\'mil-ˌtaun\ *trademark* — used for a preparation of meprobamate

Mil·wau·kee brace \mil-'wȯ-kē-, -'wä-\ *n* : an orthopedic brace that extends from the pelvis to the neck and is used esp. in the treatment of scoliosis

milz·brand \\'milts-ˌbränt\ *n* : ANTHRAX

mi·met·ic \mə-'met-ik, mī-\ *adj* : simulating the action or effect of — usu. used in combination ⟨sympatho*mimetic* drugs⟩ ⟨adrenocortico*mimetic* activity⟩

¹mim·ic \\'mim-ik\ *n* : one that mimics ⟨a ~ of a naturally occurring hormone⟩

²mimic *vt* **mim·icked** \-ikt\; **mim·ick·ing** : to imitate or resem-

ble closely: as **a** : to imitate the symptoms of ⟨an acute inflammatory process located in the ileocecal region ~s acute appendicitis *—Merck Manual*⟩ **b** : to produce an effect and esp. a physiological effect similar to ⟨chemically unrelated to the hormone that it ~s *—Chem. & Engineering News*⟩

mim·ic·ry \\'mim-i-krē\ *n, pl* **-ries** : an instance of mimicking something

min *abbr* **1** minim **2** minimum **3** minute

Min·a·mata disease \ˌmin-ə-'mät-ə-\ *n* : a toxic neuropathy caused by the ingestion of methylmercury compounds (as in contaminated seafood) and characterized by impairment of cerebral functions, constriction of the visual field, and progressive weakening of muscles

mind \\'mīnd\ *n* **1** : the element or complex of elements in an individual that feels, perceives, thinks, wills, and esp. reasons **2** : the conscious mental events and capabilities in an organism **3** : the organized conscious and unconscious adaptive mental activity of an organism

mind–set \\'mīn(d)-ˌset\ *n* : a mental inclination, tendency, or habit

¹min·er·al \\'min-(ə-)rəl\ *n* : a solid homogeneous crystalline chemical element or compound that results from the inorganic processes of nature

²mineral *adj* **1** : of or relating to minerals; *also* : INORGANIC **2** : impregnated with mineral substances

min·er·al·iza·tion *also Brit* **min·er·al·isa·tion** \ˌmin(-ə)-rəl-ə-'zā-shən\ *n* **1** : the action of mineralizing **2** : the state of being mineralized ⟨~ of bone⟩

min·er·al·ize *also Brit* **min·er·al·ise** \\'min-(ə)-rə-ˌlīz\ *vt* **-ized** *also Brit* **-ised; -iz·ing** *also Brit* **-is·ing** : to impregnate or supply with minerals or an inorganic compound

mineral kingdom *n* : a basic group of natural objects that includes inorganic objects — compare ANIMAL KINGDOM, PLANT KINGDOM

min·er·al·o·cor·ti·coid \ˌmin(-ə)-rə-lō-'kȯrt-ə-ˌkȯid\ *n* : a corticosteroid (as aldosterone) that affects chiefly the electrolyte and fluid balance in the body — compare GLUCOCORTICOID

mineral oil *n* **1** : a liquid product of mineral origin that has the viscosity of an oil **2** : a transparent oily liquid obtained usu. by distilling petroleum and used chiefly in medicine for treating constipation and esp. formerly as a demulcent and solvent for nose and throat medication — called also *liquid petrolatum, white mineral oil*

mineral water *n* : water naturally or artificially infused with mineral salts or gases (as carbon dioxide)

mineral wax *n* : a wax of mineral origin: as **a** : OZOKERITE **b** : CERESIN

min·er's anemia \\'mī-nərz-\ *n* : ANCYLOSTOMIASIS

miner's asthma *n* : PNEUMOCONIOSIS

miner's consumption *n* : PNEUMOCONIOSIS

miner's cramps *n pl* : HEAT CRAMPS

miner's elbow *n* : bursitis of the elbow that tends to occur in miners who work in small tunnels and rest their weight on their elbows

miner's phthisis *n* : an occupational respiratory disease (as pneumoconiosis or anthracosilicosis) of miners

mini·lap·a·rot·o·my \ˌmin-ē-ˌlap-ə-'rät-ə-mē\ *n, pl* **-mies** : a ligation of the Fallopian tubes performed through a small incision in the abdominal wall

min·im \\'min-əm\ *n* : either of two units of capacity equal to ¹⁄₆₀ fluid dram: as **a** : a U.S. unit of liquid capacity equivalent to 0.003760 cubic inch or 0.061610 milliliter **b** : a British unit of liquid capacity and dry measure equivalent to 0.003612 cubic inch or 0.059194 milliliter

minima *pl of* MINIMUM

minimae — see VENAE CORDIS MINIMAE

min·i·mal \\'min-ə-məl\ *adj* : relating to or being a minimum : constituting the least possible with respect to size, number,

M
N

\ə\ **abut** \ᵊ\ **kitten** \ər\ **further** \a\ **ash** \ā\ **ace** \ä\ **cot, cart**
\au̇\ **out** \ch\ **chin** \e\ **bet** \ē\ **easy** \g\ **go** \i\ **hit** \ī\ **ice** \j\ **job**
\ŋ\ **sing** \ō\ **go** \ȯ\ **law** \ȯi\ **boy** \th\ **thin** \th̶\ **the** \ü\ **loot**
\u̇\ **foot** \y\ **yet** \zh\ **vision** *See also* Pronunciation Symbols page

degree, or certain stated conditions ⟨tuberosity fractures heal with ∼ . . . treatment —J. S. Keene *et al*⟩ ⟨residents receive a ∼ level of personal care —A. S. Oser⟩ ⟨side effects are ∼⟩

minimal brain damage *n* : ATTENTION DEFICIT DISORDER

minimal brain dysfunction *n* : ATTENTION DEFICIT DISORDER — abbr. *MBD*

minimal infective dose *n* : the smallest quantity of infective material that regularly produces infection — abbr. *MID*

minimal inhibitory concentration *n* : the smallest concentration of an antibiotic that regularly inhibits growth of a bacterium in vitro — abbr. *MIC;* called also *minimum inhibitory concentration*

minimal medium *n* : a medium that contains only inorganic salts, a simple carbon source (as carbon dioxide or glucose), and water

minimi — see ABDUCTOR DIGITI MINIMI, EXTENSOR DIGITI MINIMI, FLEXOR DIGITI MINIMI BREVIS, GLUTEUS MINIMUS, OPPONENS DIGITI MINIMI

¹**min·i·mum** \'min-ə-məm\ *n, pl* **-i·ma** \-ə-mə\ *or* **-i·mums** **1** : the least quantity assignable, admissible, or possible **2** : the lowest degree or amount of variation (as of temperature) reached or recorded

²**minimum** *adj* : of, relating to, or constituting a minimum ⟨meet the ∼ psychiatric needs of the country —E. A. Strecker⟩ ⟨establishing ∼ standards for medical education —*CIBA Symposia*⟩

minimum dose *n* : the smallest dose of a medicine or drug that will produce an effect

minimum inhibitory concentration *n* : MINIMAL INHIBITORY CONCENTRATION

minimum lethal dose *n* : the smallest dose experimentally found to kill any one animal of a test group

minimum sep·a·ra·ble \-'sep-(ə-)rə-bəl\ *n* : the least separation at which two parallel lines are recognized by the eye as separate — compare MINIMUM VISIBLE, VISUAL ACUITY

minimum visible *n* : the least area perceivable as distinct by the eye — compare MINIMUM SEPARABLE, VISUAL ACUITY

minimus — see GLUTEUS MINIMUS

mini·pill \'min-ē-ˌpil\ *n* : a birth control pill that is intended to minimize side effects, contains a very low dose of a progestogen and esp. norethindrone but no estrogen, and is taken daily

Mini·press \-ˌpres\ *trademark* — used for a preparation of prazosin

mini·sat·el·lite \-'sat-ᵊl-ˌīt\ *n* : any of numerous DNA segments located mainly near the ends of chromosomes that consist of repeating sequences of at least five but usu. not more than 100 nucleotides and that are useful in DNA fingerprinting — compare MICROSATELLITE

mini–stroke \-ˌstrōk\ *n* : TRANSIENT ISCHEMIC ATTACK

Min·ne·so·ta Mul·ti·pha·sic Personality Inventory \ˌmin-ə-'sōt-ə-ˌməl-ti-'fā-zik-, -ˌməl-ˌtī-\ *n* : a test of personal and social adjustment based on a complex scaling of the answers to an elaborate true or false test

Mi·no·cin \mi-'nō-sin\ *trademark* — used for a preparation of minocycline

min·o·cy·cline \ˌmin-ō-'sī-klēn\ *n* : a broad-spectrum tetracycline antibiotic administered in the form of its hydrochloride $C_{23}H_{27}N_3O_7 \cdot HCl$

mi·nom·e·ter \mi-'näm-ət-ər, mī-\ *n* : an instrument for the detection and measurement of stray radiations from X-ray generators and radioactive materials

¹**mi·nor** \'mī-nər\ *adj* : not serious or involving risk to life ⟨∼ illness⟩ ⟨a ∼ operation⟩ — compare MAJOR

²**minor** *n* : a person of either sex under the age of legal qualification for adult rights and responsibilities that has traditionally been 21 in the U.S. but is now 18 in many states or sometimes less under certain circumstances (as marriage or pregnancy)

minora — see LABIA MINORA

minor labia *n pl* : LABIA MINORA

minor surgery *n* : surgery involving little risk to the life of the patient; *specif* : an operation on the superficial structures of the body or a manipulative procedure that does not involve a serious risk — compare MAJOR SURGERY

min·ox·i·dil \min-'äk-sə-ˌdil\ *n* : a peripheral vasodilator $C_9H_{15}N_5O$ used orally to treat hypertension and topically in a propylene glycol solution to promote hair regrowth esp. in male-pattern baldness — see LONITEN, ROGAINE

mint \'mint\ *n* : any of a family (Labiatae, the mint family) of aromatic plants with a square stem and a four-lobed ovary which produces four one-seeded nutlets in fruit; *esp* : any of the genus *Mentha*

mi·nus \'mī-nəs\ *adj* : relating to or being one of the two mating types required for successful fertilization in sexual reproduction in some lower plants (as a fungus) — compare PLUS

min·ute \'min-ət\ *n* : a 60th part of an hour of time or of a degree

minute volume *n* : CARDIAC OUTPUT

mio·lec·i·thal \ˌmī-ō-'les-ə-thəl\ *adj* : MICROLECITHAL

mi·o·sis *also* **my·o·sis** \mī-'ō-səs, mē-\ *n, pl* **mi·o·ses** *also* **my·o·ses** \-ˌsēz\ : excessive smallness or contraction of the pupil of the eye

¹**mi·ot·ic** *also* **my·ot·ic** \-'ät-ik\ *n* : an agent that causes miosis

²**miotic** *also* **myotic** *adj* : relating to or characterized by miosis

mi·ra·cid·i·um \ˌmir-ə-'sid-ē-əm, ˌmī-rə-\ *n, pl* **-cid·ia** \-ē-ə\ : the free-swimming ciliated first larva of a digenetic trematode that seeks out and penetrates a suitable snail intermediate host in which it develops into a sporocyst — **mi·ra·cid·i·al** \-ē-əl\ *adj*

mir·a·cil D \'mir-ə-ˌsil-'dē\ *n* : LUCANTHONE

mir·a·cle drug \'mir-ə-kəl-\ *n* : a drug usu. newly discovered that elicits a dramatic response in a patient's condition — called also *wonder drug*

mi·rage \mə-'räzh\ *n* : an optical effect that is sometimes seen at sea, in the desert, or over a hot pavement, that may have the appearance of a pool of water or a mirror in which distant objects are seen inverted, and that is caused by the bending or reflection of rays of light by a layer of heated air of varying density

mire \'mī(ə)r\ *n* : any of the objects on the arm of an ophthalmometer that are used to measure astigmatism by the reflections they produce in the cornea when illuminated

mi·rex \'mī-ˌreks\ *n* : an organochlorine insecticide $C_{10}Cl_{12}$ formerly used esp. against ants that is a suspected carcinogen

mir·ror \'mir-ər\ *n* : a polished or smooth surface (as of glass) that forms images by reflection

mirror image *n* : something that has its parts reversely arranged in comparison with another similar thing or that is reversed with reference to an intervening axis or plane

mirror writing *n* : backward writing resembling in slant and order of letters the reflection of ordinary writing in a mirror

mis·an·drist \'mis-ˌan-drist\ *n* : a person who hates men — compare MISOGYNIST — **misandrist** *adj* — **mis·an·dry** \-drē\ *n, pl* **-dries**

mis·an·thrope \'mis-ᵊn-ˌthrōp\ *n* : a person who hates or distrusts humankind

mis·an·throp·ic \ˌmis-ᵊn-'thräp-ik\ *adj* **1** : of, relating to, or characteristic of a misanthrope **2** : marked by a hatred or contempt for humankind

mis·an·thro·py \mis-'an(t)-thrə-pē\ *n, pl* **-pies** : a hatred or distrust of humankind

mis·car·riage \mis-'kar-ij\ *n* : spontaneous expulsion of a human fetus before it is viable and esp. between the 12th and 28th weeks of gestation — compare ABORTION 1a

mis·car·ry \(')mis-'kar-ē\ *vi* **-ried; -ry·ing** : to suffer miscarriage of a fetus ⟨*miscarried* several times before a viable offspring was born⟩ — compare ABORT

mis·ce·ge·na·tion \(ˌ)mis-ˌej-ə-'nā-shən, ˌmis-i-jə-'nā-\ *n* : a mixture of races; *esp* : marriage or cohabitation between a white person and a member of another race — **mis·ce·ge·na·tion·al** \-shnəl, -shən-ᵊl\ *adj*

mis·ci·ble \'mis-ə-bəl\ *adj* : capable of being mixed; *specif* : capable of mixing in any ratio without separation of two phases ⟨∼ liquids⟩ — **mis·ci·bil·i·ty** \ˌmis-ə-'bil-ət-ē\ *n, pl* **-ties**

mis·di·ag·nose \\(')mis-'dī-ig-ˌnōs, -ˌnōz\ *vt* **-nosed; -nos·ing** : to diagnose incorrectly

mis·di·ag·no·sis \\(ˌ)mis-ˌdī-ig-'nō-səs\ *n, pl* **-no·ses** \-ˌsēz\ : an incorrect diagnosis

miso·gy·nic \ˌmis-ə-'jin-ik, -'gīn-\ *adj* : MISOGYNISTIC

mi·sog·y·nist \mə-'säj-ə-nəst\ *n* : a person who hates women — compare MISANDRIST — **misogynist** *adj* — **mi·sog·y·ny** \mə-'säj-ə-nē\ *n, pl* **-nies**

mi·sog·y·nis·tic \mə-ˌsäj-ə-'nis-tik\ *adj* : having or showing a hatred and distrust of women

miso·ne·ism \ˌmis-ə-'nē-ˌiz-əm\ *n* : a hatred, fear, or intolerance of innovation or change

miso·pe·dia *or Brit* **miso·pae·dia** \ˌmis-ə-'pē-dē-ə\ *n* : a hatred of children

misophobia *var of* MYSOPHOBIA

mi·so·pros·tol \ˌmī-sō-'präs-ˌtōl, -ˌtȯl\ *n* : a synthetic prostaglandin analog $C_{22}H_{38}O_5$ used to prevent stomach ulcers associated with NSAID use and to induce abortion in conjunction with RU-486

mis·per·cep·tion \ˌmis-pər-'sep-shən\ *n* : a false perception

missed abortion \'mist-\ *n* : an intrauterine death of a fetus that is not followed by its immediate expulsion

missed labor *n* : a retention of a fetus in the uterus beyond the normal period of pregnancy

¹**mis·sense** \'mis-ˌsen(t)s\ *adj* : relating to or being a genetic mutation involving alteration of one or more codons so that different amino acids are determined ⟨~ mutations⟩ ⟨a ~ suppressor⟩ — compare ANTISENSE, NONSENSE

²**missense** *n* : missense genetic mutation — compare NON-SENSE

mis·sion·ary position \'mish-ə-ˌner-ē-\ *n* : a coital position in which the female lies on her back with the male on top and with his face opposite hers

mis·tle·toe \'mis-əl-ˌtō, *chiefly Brit* 'miz-\ *n* : any of various parasitic or semiparasitic plants (family Loranthaceae, the mistletoe family) that have thick leathery mostly opposite and sometimes scaly leaves and include some formerly used in preparations with oxytocic, antispasmodic, or heart=stimulating properties: as **a** : a European semiparasitic green shrub (*Viscum album*) having somewhat poisonous leaves, stems, and waxy-white glutinous berries that have been used in folk medicine **b** : any of various American plants (genus *Phoradendron* and esp. *P. serotinum* syn. *P. flavescens*) resembling the true mistletoe of Europe

mite \'mīt\ *n* : any of numerous small to very minute arachnids of the order Acari that have a body without a constriction between the cephalothorax and abdomen, mandibles generally chelate or adapted for piercing, usu. four pairs of short legs in the adult and but three in the young larvae, and often breathing organs in the form of tracheae and that include parasites of insects and vertebrates some of which are important disease vectors, parasites of plants in which they frequently cause gall formation, pests of various stored products, and completely innocuous free-living aquatic and terrestrial forms — see ITCH MITE

mith·ra·my·cin \ˌmith-rə-'mīs-ᵊn\ *n* : PLICAMYCIN

mith·ri·da·tism \ˌmith-rə-'dāt-ˌiz-əm\ *n* : tolerance to a poison acquired by taking gradually increased doses of it

Mith·ra·da·tes VI Eu·pa·tor \ˌmith-rə-'dāt-ēz-'siks-'yü-pə-ˌtȯr\ (*d* 63 BC), king of Pontus. Mithradates the Great ruled from 120–63 BC. A great military leader, a brave warrior, and a cunning politician, he was one of the few serious threats to Roman domination in the ancient world. A revolt of his own soldiers led him to attempt to take his own life. According to legend, he was ever suspicious of treachery, so he had consumed doses of poison in increasingly greater amounts in order to build up a tolerance. When he vainly sought to commit suicide, he found that he had become totally immune to poison. He finally resorted to ordering a follower to stab him to death.

mi·ti·cide \'mīt-ə-ˌsīd\ *n* : an agent used to kill mites — **mi·ti·cid·al** \ˌmīt-ə-'sīd-ᵊl\ *adj*

mit·i·gate \'mit-ə-ˌgāt\ *vt* **-gat·ed; -gat·ing** : to make less severe or painful

mit·i·ga·tion \ˌmit-ə-'gā-shən\ *n* **1** : the act of mitigating or state of being mitigated ⟨the cure, prevention, or ~ of disease —*Encyc. Americana*⟩ **2** : something that mitigates ⟨a large number of drugs and ~s . . . at the clinic —*Jour. Amer. Med. Assoc.*⟩

mi·tis \'mīt-əs\ *adj* : tending to be less virulent than the average — used esp. of strains of diphtheria bacilli; compare GRAVIS, INTERMEDIUS

mitochondrial DNA *n* : an extranuclear double-stranded DNA found exclusively in mitochondria that in most eukaryotes is a circular molecule and is maternally inherited — called also *mtDNA*

mi·to·chon·dri·on \ˌmīt-ə-'kän-drē-ən\ *n, pl* **-dria** \-drē-ə\ : any of various round or long cellular organelles of most eukaryotes that are found outside the nucleus, produce energy for the cell through cellular respiration, and are rich in fats, proteins, and enzymes — called also *chondriosome* — **mi·to·chon·dri·al** \-drē-əl\ *adj* — **mi·to·chon·dri·al·ly** \-ē\ *adv*

mi·to·gen \'mīt-ə-jən\ *n* : a substance that induces mitosis

mi·to·gen·e·sis \ˌmīt-ə-'jen-ə-səs\ *n, pl* **-e·ses** \-ˌsēz\ : the production of cell mitosis

mi·to·ge·net·ic \-jə-'net-ik\ *adj* : MITOGENIC

mi·to·gen·ic \-'jen-ik\ *adj* : of, producing, or stimulating mitosis ⟨~ activity⟩ ⟨~ agents⟩ — **mi·to·ge·nic·i·ty** \-jə-'nis-ət-ē\ *n, pl* **-ties**

mi·to·my·cin \ˌmīt-ə-'mīs-ᵊn\ *n* **1** : a complex of antibiotic substances which is produced by a Japanese bacterium of the genus *Streptomyces* (*S. caespitosus*) **2** : a component $C_{15}H_{18}N_4O_5$ of mitomycin that inhibits DNA synthesis and is used as an antineoplastic in the palliative treatment of some carcinomas — called also *mitomycin C*

mi·to·sis \mī-'tō-səs\ *n, pl* **-to·ses** \-ˌsēz\ **1** : a process that takes place in the nucleus of a dividing cell, involves typically a series of steps consisting of prophase, metaphase, anaphase, and telophase, and results in the formation of two new nuclei each having the same number of chromosomes as the parent nucleus — compare MEIOSIS **2** : cell division in which mitosis occurs — **mi·tot·ic** \-'tät-ik\ *adj* — **mi·tot·i·cal·ly** \-i-k(ə-)lē\ *adv*

mi·to·some \'mīt-ə-ˌsōm\ *n* **1** : a threadlike cytoplasmic inclusion; *esp* : one held to be derived from the preceding mitotic spindle **2** : NEBENKERN

mi·to·spore \-ˌspō(ə)r, -ˌspȯ(ə)r\ *n* : a haploid or diploid spore produced by mitosis

mitotic index *n* : the number of cells per thousand cells actively dividing at a particular time

mi·to·xan·trone \ˌmīt-ō-'zan-ˌtrōn\ *n* : an antineoplastic drug that is used in the form of its dihydrochloride $C_{22}H_{28}N_4O_6·2HCl$ either alone or in combination in the treatment of some leukemias and carcinomas

mi·tral \'mī-trəl\ *adj* **1** : resembling a miter **2** : of, relating to, being, or adjoining a mitral valve or orifice

mitral cell *n* : any of the pyramidal cells of the olfactory bulb about which terminate numerous fibers from the olfactory cells of the nasal mucosa

mitral insufficiency *n* : inability of the mitral valve to close perfectly permitting blood to flow back into the atrium and leading to varying degrees of heart failure — called also *mitral incompetence*

mitral orifice *n* : the left atrioventricular orifice

mitral regurgitation *n* : backward flow of blood into the atrium due to mitral insufficiency

mitral stenosis *n* : a condition usu. the result of disease in which the mitral valve is abnormally narrow

mitral valve *n* : a valve in the heart that guards the opening between the left atrium and the left ventricle, prevents the blood in the ventricle from returning to the atrium, and consists of two triangular flaps attached at their bases to the fibrous ring which surrounds the opening and connected at

M
N

\ə\ **abut** \ᵊ\ **kitten** \ər\ **further** \a\ **ash** \ā\ **ace** \ä\ **cot, cart** \au̇\ **out** \ch\ **chin** \e\ **bet** \ē\ **easy** \g\ **go** \i\ **hit** \ī\ **ice** \j\ **job** \ŋ\ **sing** \ō\ **go** \ȯ\ **law** \ȯi\ **boy** \th\ **thin** \th\ **the** \ü\ **loot** \u̇\ **foot** \y\ **yet** \zh\ **vision** *See also* Pronunciation Symbols page

their margins with the ventricular walls by the chordae tendineae and papillary muscles — called also *bicuspid valve, left atrioventricular valve*

mitral valve prolapse *n* : a valvular heart disorder in which one or both mitral valve flaps close incompletely during systole usu. producing either a click or murmur and sometimes minor mitral regurgitation and which is often a benign symptomless condition but may be marked by varied symptoms (as chest pain, fatigue, dizziness, dyspnea, or palpitations) leading in some cases to endocarditis or ventricular tachycardia — abbr. *MVP;* called also *Barlow's syndrome*

mit·tel·schmerz \'mit-³l-ˌshmertz\ *n* : abdominal pain occurring between the menstrual periods and usu. considered to be associated with ovulation

mixed \'mikst\ *adj* **1** : combining features or exhibiting symptoms of more than one condition or disease ⟨a ~ tumor⟩ **2** : producing more than one kind of secretion ⟨~ salivary glands⟩

mixed connective tissue disease *n* : a syndrome characterized by symptoms of various rheumatic diseases (as systemic lupus erythematosus, scleroderma, and polymyositis) and by high concentrations of antibodies to extractable nuclear antigens

mixed dementia *n* : dementia involving both Alzheimer's disease and vascular dementia

mixed glioma *n* : a glioma consisting of more than one cell type

mixed nerve *n* : a nerve containing both sensory and motor fibers

mixo·sco·pia \ˌmik-sə-'skō-pē-ə\ *or* **mix·os·co·py** \mik-'säs-kə-pē\ *n, pl* **-pias** *or* **-pies** : the obtainment of sexual gratification from observing coitus — **mixo·scop·ic** \ˌmik-sə-'skäp-ik\ *adj*

mixt *abbr* mixture

mix·ture \'miks-chər\ *n* : a product of mixing: as **a** : a portion of matter consisting of two or more components in varying proportions that retain their own properties **b** : an aqueous liquid medicine : POTION; *specif* : a preparation in which insoluble substances are suspended in watery fluids by the addition of a viscid material (as gum, sugar, or glycerol)

Mi·ya·ga·wa·nel·la \ˌmē-ə-ˌgä-wə-'nel-ə\ *n, syn of* CHLAMYDIA

Mi·ya·ga·wa \ˌmē-ə-ˌgä-wə, mē-yä-gä-wä\, **Yoneji (1885–1959),** Japanese bacteriologist. Miyagawa specialized in microscopic research on infectious diseases. His most notable discovery was a sexually transmitted disease, lymphogranuloma venereum, that is distinct from syphilis and is caused by a chlamydia. Miyagawa cultured this microorganism and a closely related one for the first time in 1935. In 1938 the genus *Miyagawanella* was named in his honor to include these two species. Unfortunately, the name was not validly published and the genus was later redescribed with the name *Chlamydia.*

mks \ˌem-(ˌ)kā-'es\ *adj, often cap M&K&S* : of, relating to, or being a system of units based on the meter as the unit of length, the kilogram as the unit of mass, and the mean solar second as the unit of time ⟨the ~ system⟩ ⟨~ units⟩

ml *abbr* milliliter

mL *abbr* millilambert

MLD *abbr* **1** median lethal dose **2** minimum lethal dose

M line \'em-ˌlīn\ *n* : a thin dark line across the center of the H zone of a striated muscle fiber — called also *M band*

MLT *abbr* medical laboratory technician

mm *abbr* millimeter

mm Hg \'mil-ə-ˌmēt-ər-əv-'mər-kyə-rē, -k(ə-)rē\ *n* : a unit of pressure equal to the pressure exerted by a column of mercury 1 millimeter high at 0°C and under the acceleration of gravity and nearly equivalent to 1 torr (about 133.3 pascals)

M–mode *adj* : of, relating to, or being an ultrasonographic technique that is used for studying the movement of internal body structures

mmol *also* **mmole** *abbr* millimole

MMPI *abbr* Minnesota Multiphasic Personality Inventory

MMR *abbr* measles-mumps-rubella (vaccine)

Mn *symbol* manganese

MN *abbr* master of nursing

mne·me \'nē-(ˌ)mē\ *n* : the persistent or recurrent effect of past experience of the individual or of the race — **mne·mic** \-mik\ *adj*

mne·mon \'nē-ˌmän\ *n* : a theoretical fundamental unit of memory

¹mne·mon·ic \ni-'män-ik\ *adj* **1** : assisting or intended to assist memory; *also* : of or relating to mnemonics **2** : of or relating to memory — **mne·mon·i·cal·ly** \-i-k(ə-)lē\ *adv*

²mnemonic *n* : a mnemonic device or code

mne·mon·ics \ni-'män-iks\ *n pl but sing in constr* : a technique of improving the memory

mne·mo·tech·ni·cal \ˌnē-mō-'tek-ni-kəl\ *or* **mne·mo·tech·nic** \-nik\ *adj* : MNEMONIC — **mne·mo·tech·ni·cal·ly** \-ni-k(ə-)lē\ *adv*

mo *abbr* month

Mo *symbol* molybdenum

MO *abbr* medical officer

mo·bile \'mō-bəl, -ˌbīl\ *adj* **1** : capable of moving or being moved about readily ⟨globular proteins that are ~ and rod-shaped proteins that form solid structures⟩ ⟨the tongue . . . is clearly the most ~ articulator —G. A. Miller⟩ **2** : characterized by an extreme degree of fluidity ⟨ether and mercury are ~ liquids⟩ — **mo·bil·i·ty** \mō-'bil-ət-ē\ *n, pl* **-ties**

mo·bi·li·za·tion *also Brit* **mo·bi·li·sa·tion** \ˌmō-bə-lə-'zā-shən\ *n* **1** : the act or process of mobilizing ⟨~ of glycogen⟩ **2** : the state of being mobilized

mo·bi·lize *also Brit* **mo·bi·lise** \'mō-bə-ˌlīz\ *vb* **-lized** *also Brit* **-lised; -liz·ing** *also Brit* **-lis·ing** *vt* **1** : to put into movement or circulation : make mobile; *specif* : to release (something stored in the body) for body use ⟨the body ~s its antibodies⟩ **2** : to assemble (as resources) and make ready for use ⟨the sympathetic nervous system . . . ~s the bodily resources as a means of preparing for fight or flight —H. G. Armstrong⟩ **3** : to separate (an organ or part) from associated structures so as to make more accessible for operative procedures **4** : to develop to a state of acute activity ⟨ego feeling and ego attitude . . . ~ hostile feelings toward others —Abram Kardiner⟩ ~ *vi* : to undergo mobilization : assemble and organize for action — **mo·bi·liz·able** *also Brit* **mo·bi·lis·able** \'mō-bə-ˌlī-zə-bəl\ *adj*

Mö·bius syndrome *or* **Moe·bius syndrome** \'mü-bē-əs-, 'mœ-, 'mər-, 'mē-\ *n* : congenital bilateral paralysis of the facial muscles associated with other neurological disorders

Mö·bius \'mœ̄-bē-ùs\, **Paul Julius (1853–1907),** German neurologist. Möbius is remembered for his series of pathological studies of great men (Goethe, Schopenhauer, Nietzsche, Schumann, and Rousseau). He also wrote several books on nervous diseases and in 1879 published a work on hereditary nervous diseases. His descriptions include Möbius syndrome (1884) and an atrophic type of progressive muscular dystrophy found in children.

moc·ca·sin \'mäk-ə-sən\ *n* **1** : WATER MOCCASIN **2** : a snake (as of the genus *Natrix*) resembling a water moccasin

mo·dal·i·ty \mō-'dal-ət-ē\ *n, pl* **-ties** **1** : one of the main avenues of sensation (as vision) **2 a** : a usu. physical therapeutic agency **b** : an apparatus for applying a modality

¹mod·el \'mäd-³l\ *n* **1 a** : a pattern of something to be made : a cast of a tooth or oral cavity **2** : something (as a similar object or a construct) used to help visualize or explore something else (as the living human body) that cannot be directly observed or experimented on — see ANIMAL MODEL **3** : a system of postulates, data, and inferences presented as a mathematical description of an entity or state of affairs

²model *vt* **mod·eled** *or* **mod·elled; mod·el·ing** *or* **mod·el·ling** \'mäd-liŋ, -³l-iŋ\ : to produce (as by computer) a representation or simulation of

¹mod·er·ate \'mäd-(ə-)rət\ *adj* **1** : avoiding extremes of behavior : observing reasonable limits ⟨a ~ drinker⟩ **2** : not severe in effect or degree ⟨~ alcohol consumption⟩ ⟨the abdomen was mildly distended with ∼ tenderness —Timothy Melester *et al*〉 〈∼ developmental disabilities〉

²**mod·er·ate** \ˈmäd-ə-ˌrāt\ *vt* **-at·ed; -at·ing** : to reduce the speed or energy of (neutrons) — **mod·er·a·tion** \ˌmäd-ə-ˈrā-shən\ *n*

mod·er·a·tor \ˈmäd-ə-ˌrāt-ər\ *n* : a substance (as graphite, deuterium in heavy water, or beryllium) used for slowing down neutrons in a nuclear reactor

mod·i·fi·ca·tion \ˌmäd-ə-fə-ˈkā-shən\ *n* **1** : the act or result of modifying something **2** : a change in an organism that is not inherited and that is caused by the influence of its environment

modified milk *n* : milk altered in composition (as by the addition of lactose) esp. for use in infant feeding

modified radical mastectomy *n* : a mastectomy that is similar to a radical mastectomy but does not include removal of the pectoral muscles — compare SIMPLE MASTECTOMY

mod·i·fi·er \ˈmäd-ə-ˌfī(-ə)r\ *n* **1** : one that modifies **2** : a gene that modifies the effect of another

mod·i·fy \ˈmäd-ə-ˌfī\ *vt* **-fied; -fy·ing** : to make a change in 〈∼ behavior by the use of drugs〉 — **mod·i·fi·abil·i·ty** \ˌmäd-ə-ˌfī-ə-ˈbil-ət-ē\ *n, pl* **-ties** — **mod·i·fi·able** \-ˈfī-ə-bəl\ *adj*

mo·di·o·lar \mə-ˈdī-ə-lər\ *adj* : of or relating to the modiolus of the ear

mo·di·o·lus \mə-ˈdī-ə-ləs\ *n, pl* **-li** \-ˌlī\ : a central bony column in the cochlea of the ear

MODS *abbr* multiple organ dysfunction syndrome

mod·u·late \ˈmäj-ə-ˌlāt\ *vt* **-lat·ed; -lat·ing** : to adjust to or keep in proper measure or proportion 〈∼ an immune response〉 〈∼ cell activity〉 — **mod·u·la·to·ry** \-lə-ˌtōr-ē, -ˌtȯr-\ *adj*

mod·u·la·tion \ˌmäj-ə-ˈlā-shən\ *n* **1** : the act or process of modulating **2** : a reversible change in histological structure due to physiological factors

mod·u·la·tor \ˈmäj-ə-ˌlāt-ər\ *n* **1** : one that modulates **2** : any of the nerve fibers that carry impulses from single retinal cones and are believed to be responsible for the transmission of discrete sensations of color

mod·u·lus \ˈmäj-ə-ləs\ *n, pl* **-li** \-ˌlī, -ˌlē\ : a constant or coefficient that expresses usu. numerically the degree to which a substance or body possesses a property (as elasticity)

MODY *abbr* maturity-onset diabetes of the young

Moebius syndrome *var of* MÖBIUS SYNDROME

mogi·graph·ia \ˌmäj-ə-ˈgraf-ē-ə\ *n* : WRITER'S CRAMP

MOH *abbr* medical officer of health

Mohs' chemosurgery \ˈmōz-, ˈmōs-, ˈmō-zəz-\ *n* : MOHS' TECHNIQUE

Mohs' scale \ˈmōz-, ˈmōs-, ˈmō-səz-\ *n* **1** : a scale of hardness for minerals in which 1 represents the hardness of talc; 2, gypsum; 3, calcite; 4, fluorite; 5, apatite; 6, orthoclase; 7, quartz; 8, topaz; 9, corundum; and 10, diamond **2** : a revised and expanded version of the original Mohs' scale which provides finer distinctions between the harder materials and in which 1 represents the hardness of talc; 2, gypsum; 3, calcite; 4, fluorite; 5, apatite; 6, orthoclase; 7, vitreous pure silica; 8, quartz; 9, topaz; 10, garnet; 11, fused zirconium oxide; 12, fused alumina; 13, silicon carbide; 14, boron carbide; and 15, diamond

Mohs \ˈmōs\, **Friedrich (1773–1839),** German mineralogist. Mohs's chief scientific contribution was establishing systematic mineralogy on a new basis. He was placed in charge of several important mineral collections, of which he later published systematic descriptions. In the early 1820s he developed a new method of mineral classification that focused on the arrangements of minerals in crystal systems based on external symmetry. In 1812 he introduced the Mohs' scale of hardness for minerals. By the 1820s the scale had been widely adopted by other mineralogists.

Mohs' technique *n* : a chemosurgical technique for the removal of skin malignancies in which excision is made to a depth at which the tissue is microscopically free of cancer — called also *Mohs' chemosurgery*

Mohs \ˈmōz\, **Frederic Edward (1910–2002),** American

surgeon. Mohs served for many years as professor of surgery and chief of the chemosurgery clinic at the University of Wisconsin. He discovered and developed the clinical use of chemosurgery for the microscopically controlled excision of cancer of the skin, lip, parotid gland, and other external structures.

moi·ety \ˈmȯi-ət-ē\ *n, pl* **-eties** : one of the portions into which something is divided 〈the hemoglobin molecule contains four heme *moieties* —Lionel Whitby〉

moist \ˈmȯist\ *adj* **1** : slightly or moderately wet **2 a** : marked by a discharge or exudation of liquid 〈∼ eczema〉 **b** : suggestive of the presence of liquid — used of sounds heard in auscultation 〈∼ rales〉

moist gangrene *n* : gangrene that develops in the presence of combined arterial and venous obstruction, is usu. accompanied by an infection, and is characterized by a watery discharge usu. of foul odor

mol *var of* ³MOLE

mol *abbr* molecular; molecule

mol·al \ˈmō-ləl\ *adj* : of, relating to, or containing a mole 〈the ∼ volume of a gas is 22.4 liters at standard conditions〉; *esp* : of, relating to, or containing a mole of solute per 1000 grams of solvent 〈a ∼ solution〉 — **mo·lal·i·ty** \mō-ˈlal-ət-ē\ *n, pl* **-ties**

¹**mo·lar** \ˈmō-lər\ *n* : a tooth with a rounded or flattened surface adapted for grinding; *specif* : one of the mammalian teeth behind the incisors and canines sometimes including the premolars but more exactly restricted to the three posterior pairs in each human jaw on each side which are not preceded by milk teeth

²**molar** *adj* **1 a** : pulverizing by friction 〈∼ teeth〉 **b** : of, relating to, or located near the molar teeth 〈∼ gland〉 **2** : of, relating to, possessing the qualities of, or characterized by a hydatidiform mole 〈∼ pregnancy〉

³**molar** *adj* **1** : of or relating to a mass of matter as distinguished from the properties or motions of molecules or atoms **2** : of or relating to larger units of behavior esp. as relatable to a prior deprivation or motivational pattern of the organism 〈interest in such ∼ problems of personality as the ego functions —R. R. Holt〉 — compare MOLECULAR 2

⁴**molar** *adj* **1** : of or relating to a mole of a substance 〈the ∼ volume of a gas〉 **2** : containing one mole of solute in one liter of solution

mo·lar·i·form \mō-ˈlar-ə-ˌfȯrm\ *adj* : resembling a molar tooth esp. in shape

mo·lar·i·ty \mō-ˈlar-ət-ē\ *n, pl* **-ties** : molar concentration

¹**mold** *or chiefly Brit* **mould** \ˈmōld\ *n* : a cavity in which a fluid or malleable substance is shaped

²**mold** *or chiefly Brit* **mould** *vt* : to give shape to esp. in a mold

³**mold** *or chiefly Brit* **mould** *vi* : to become moldy

⁴**mold** *or chiefly Brit* **mould** *n* **1** : a superficial often woolly growth produced esp. on damp or decaying organic matter or on living organisms **2** : a fungus (as of the order Mucorales) that produces mold

mold·ing *or chiefly Brit* **mould·ing** \ˈmōl-diŋ\ *n* : an act or process of molding; *specif* : the shaping of the fetal head to allow it to pass through the birth canal during parturition

moldy *or chiefly Brit* **mouldy** \ˈmōl-dē\ *adj* **mold·i·er** *or chiefly Brit* **mould·i·er; -est** : covered with a mold-producing fungus 〈∼ bread〉

¹**mole** \ˈmōl\ *n* : a pigmented spot, mark, or small permanent protuberance on the human body; *esp* : NEVUS

²**mole** *n* : an abnormal mass in the uterus: **a** : a blood clot containing a degenerated fetus and its membranes **b** : HYDATIDIFORM MOLE

³**mole** *also* **mol** \ˈmōl\ *n* : the base unit in the International System of Units for the amount of pure substance that contains the same number of elementary entities as there are at-

M
N

\ə\ **abut** \ᵊ\ **kitten** \ər\ **further** \a\ **ash** \ā\ **ace** \ä\ **cot, cart**
\au̇\ **out** \ch\ **chin** \e\ **bet** \ē\ **easy** \g\ **go** \i\ **hit** \ī\ **ice** \j\ **job**
\ŋ\ **sing** \ō\ **go** \ȯ\ **law** \ȯi\ **boy** \th\ **thin** \t͟h\ **the** \ü\ **loot**
\u̇\ **foot** \y\ **yet** \zh\ **vision** *See also* Pronunciation Symbols page

oms in exactly 12 grams of the isotope carbon 12 ⟨a ∼ of photons⟩ ⟨a ∼ of sodium chloride⟩

mo·lec·u·lar \mə-ˈlek-yə-lər\ *adj* **1** : of, relating to, or produced by molecules ⟨∼ oxygen⟩ **2** : relating to or emphasizing individual responses or structures of behavior ⟨proceed by more and more detailed analysis to the ∼ facts of perception —G. A. Miller⟩ — compare ³MOLAR 2 — **mo·lec·u·lar·i·ty** \-ˌlek-yə-ˈlar-ət-ē\ *n, pl* **-ties** — **mo·lec·u·lar·ly** \mə-ˈlek-yə-lər-lē\ *adv*

molecular biologist *n* : a specialist in molecular biology

molecular biology *n* : a branch of biology dealing with the ultimate physicochemical organization of living matter and esp. with the molecular basis of inheritance and protein synthesis

molecular chaperone *n* : CHAPERONE

molecular clock *n* : a measure of evolutionary change over time at the molecular level that is based on the theory that specific DNA sequences or the proteins they encode spontaneously mutate at constant rates and that is used chiefly for estimating how long ago two related organisms diverged from a common ancestor

molecular distillation *n* : distillation that is carried out under a high vacuum in an apparatus so designed as to permit molecules escaping from the warm liquid to reach the cooled surface of the condenser before colliding with other molecules and consequently returning to the liquid and that is used in the purification of substances of low volatility (as in the separation of vitamin A and vitamin E from fish-liver oils)

molecular formula *n* : a chemical formula for a compound existing as discrete molecules that gives the total number of atoms of each element in a molecule ⟨the *molecular formula* for water is H_2O⟩ — see STRUCTURAL FORMULA; compare EMPIRICAL FORMULA

molecular geneticist *n* : a specialist in molecular genetics

molecular genetics *n pl but sing in constr* : a branch of genetics dealing with the structure and activity of genetic material at the molecular level

molecular heat *n* : the heat capacity per mole of any pure substance : the specific heat in calories per degree per gram multiplied by the molecular weight — compare ATOMIC HEAT

molecular layer *n* **1** : the outer layer of the cortex of the cerebellum and cerebrum consisting of a mass of unmyelinated fibers rich in synapses **2** : either of the two plexiform layers of the retina

molecular sieve chromatography \-ˈsiv-\ *n* : GEL FILTRATION

molecular weight *n* : the mass of a molecule that may be calculated as the sum of the atomic weights of its constituent atoms

mol·e·cule \ˈmäl-i-ˌkyü(ə)l\ *n* : the smallest particle of a substance that retains all the properties of the substance and is composed of one or more atoms

mo·li·men \mə-ˈlī-mən\ *n, pl* **mo·lim·i·na** \mə-ˈlim-ə-nə\ : the periodic symptoms (as tension or discomfort) associated with the physiological stress preceding or accompanying menstruation

mol·in·done \mō-ˈlin-ˌdōn\ *n* : an antipsychotic drug used in the form of its hydrochloride $C_{16}H_{24}N_2O_2 \cdot HCl$ esp. in the treatment of schizophrenia

Mo·lisch test \ˈmō-lish-\ *n* : a test for carbohydrate (as sugar) in which a reddish violet color is formed by reaction with alpha-naphthol in the presence of concentrated sulfuric acid — called also *Molisch reaction*

Molisch, Hans (1856–1937), German botanist. Molisch's extensive studies of plants embraced several disciplines: comparative anatomy, morphology, physiology, and microchemistry. He devised his test for carbohydrate in 1886.

Moll's gland \ˈmälz-\ *n* : GLAND OF MOLL

mollusc *var of* MOLLUSK

Mol·lus·ca \mə-ˈləs-kə\ *n pl* : a large phylum of invertebrate animals (as snails, clams, and mussels) that have a soft unseg-

mented body lacking segmented appendages and commonly protected by a calcareous shell

mollusca contagiosa *pl of* MOLLUSCUM CONTAGIOSUM

mol·lus·ci·cide \mə-ˈləs-(k)ə-ˌsīd\ *also* **mol·lus·ca·cide** \-ˈləs-kə-\ *n* : an agent for destroying mollusks (as snails) — **mol·lus·ci·cid·al** \-ˌləs-(k)ə-ˈsīd-ᵊl\ *also* **mol·lus·ca·cid·al** \-ˌləs-kə-\ *adj*

mol·lus·cous \mə-ˈləs-kəs\ *adj* : of, relating to, or having the properties of a molluscum ⟨∼ tubercles⟩

mol·lus·cum \mə-ˈləs-kəm\ *n, pl* **-ca** \-kə\ : any of several skin diseases marked by soft pulpy nodules; *esp* : MOLLUSCUM CONTAGIOSUM

molluscum body *n* : any of the rounded cytoplasmic bodies found in the central opening of the nodules characteristic of molluscum contagiosum — called also *molluscum corpuscle*

molluscum con·ta·gi·o·sum \-kən-ˌtā-jē-ˈō-səm\ *n, pl* **mollusca con·ta·gi·o·sa** \-sə\ : a mild chronic disease of the skin caused by a poxvirus (species *Molluscum contagiosum virus* of the genus *Molluscipoxvirus*) and characterized by the formation of small nodules with a central opening and contents resembling curd

molluscum corpuscle *n* : MOLLUSCUM BODY

molluscum se·ba·ce·um \-sə-ˈbā-s(h)ē-əm\ *n* : KERATOACANTHOMA

mol·lusk *or* **mol·lusc** \ˈmäl-əsk\ *n* : any invertebrate animal of the phylum Mollusca — **mol·lus·can** *also* **mol·lus·kan** \mə-ˈles-kən, mä-\ *adj*

Mo·lo·ney test \mə-ˈlō-nē-\ *n* : a test for determining hypersensitivity to diphtheria toxoid by intradermal injection of a small amount in dilute solution

Moloney, Paul Joseph (1870–1939), Canadian immunologist. Moloney introduced the Moloney test in an article published in 1927.

Moloney virus *n* : a strain of murine leukemia virus that causes lymphocytic leukemia in mice — called also *Moloney leukemia virus, Moloney murine leukemia virus*

Moloney, John Bromley (b 1924), American biologist. Moloney devoted his career to research at the National Cancer Institute. He studied the biological and biochemical properties of tumor viruses and leukemia agents, giving particular attention to the Moloney virus and the Rous sarcoma virus.

¹molt \ˈmōlt\ *or chiefly Brit* **moult** *vi* : to shed hair, feathers, shell, horns, or an outer layer periodically ∼ *vt* : to cast off (an outer covering) periodically; *specif* : to throw off (the old cuticle) — used of arthropods

²molt *or chiefly Brit* **moult** *n* : the act or process of molting; *specif* : ECDYSIS

mo·lyb·date \mə-ˈlib-ˌdāt\ *n* : a salt of molybdenum containing the group MoO_4 or Mo_2O_7

mo·lyb·de·num \-də-nəm\ *n* : a metallic element that resembles chromium and tungsten in many properties, is used esp. in strengthening and hardening steel, and is a trace element in plant and animal metabolism — symbol *Mo*; see ELEMENT table

mo·lyb·dic \mə-ˈlib-dik\ *adj* : of, relating to, or containing molybdenum esp. with one of its higher valences

molybdic acid *n* : an acid H_2MoO_4 used as a reagent in chemical analysis

mo·lyb·dous \-dəs\ *adj* : of, relating to, or containing molybdenum esp. with one of its lower valences

mo·men·tum \mō-ˈment-əm, mə-ˈment-\ *n, pl* **mo·men·ta** \-ˈment-ə\ *or* **momentums** : a property of a moving body that the body has by virtue of its mass and motion and that is equal to the product of the body's mass and velocity; *broadly* : a property of a moving body that determines the length of time required to bring it to rest when under the action of a constant force

mo·met·a·sone fu·ro·ate \mō-ˈmet-ə-ˌsōn-ˈfyùr-ə-ˌwāt\ *n* : a synthetic corticosteroid $C_{27}H_{30}Cl_2O_6$ used topically in a cream or ointment base to treat inflammatory and pruritic dermatoses or intranasally in aqueous suspension to relieve the nasal symptoms of allergic rhinitis — see NASONEX

mom·ism \ˈmäm-ˌiz-əm\ *n* : an excessive popular adoration and oversentimentalizing of mothers that is held to be oedipal in nature

mo·nad \'mō-,nad\ *n* **1** : a flagellated protozoan (as of the genus *Monas*) **2** : a monovalent element or radical **3** : any of the four chromatids that make up a tetrad in meiosis

Mon·a·di·na \,män-ə-'dī-nə\ *n pl, in some esp former classifications* : a group nearly equivalent to Mastigophora

monamine *var of* MONOAMINE

mo·nar·da \mə-'närd-ə\ *n* **1** *cap* : a genus of coarse No. American mints with whorls of showy flowers including one (*M. punctata*) that has been used as a carminative **2** : any plant of the genus *Monarda*

monarticular *var of* MONOARTICULAR

Mo·nas \'mō-,nas, 'män-,as\ *n* : a genus of small single or colonial aquatic flagellates (order Protomonadina) that often have one long primary flagellum and two shorter secondary ones

mon·as·ter \män-'as-tər, mōn-\ *n* **1** : METAPHASE PLATE **2** : a single aster formed in an aberrant type of mitosis

mon·atom·ic \,män-ə-'täm-ik\ *adj* **1** : consisting of one atom; *esp* : having but one atom in the molecule **2** : MONOVALENT 1

mon·au·ral \(')mä-'nȯr-əl\ *adj* : of, relating to, affecting, or designed for use with one ear ⟨∼ hearing aid systems⟩ — **mon·au·ral·ly** \-ə-lē\ *adv*

Möncke·berg's sclerosis \'mủŋk-ə-,bərgz-, 'meŋk-\ *n* : arteriosclerosis characterized by the formation of calcium deposits in the mediae of esp. the peripheral arteries

　Möncke·berg \'mœŋk-ə-,berk\, **Johann Georg (1877–1925),** German pathologist. Mönckeberg in 1903 described for the first time a form of sclerosis affecting the middle coat of the arterial walls especially of the extremities. In 1924 he published a follow-up report.

Mon·day disease \'mən-dē-, -(,)dā-\ *n* : MONDAY MORNING DISEASE

Monday fever *n* : byssinosis esp. in its early stages of development

Monday morning disease *n* : azoturia of horses caused by heavy feeding during a period of inactivity — called also *Monday disease*

monecious *var of* MONOECIOUS

mo·nen·sin \mō-'nen-sən\ *n* : an antibiotic $C_{36}H_{62}O_{11}$ obtained from a bacterium of the genus *Streptomyces* (*S. cinnamonensis*) and used as an antiprotozoal, antibacterial, and antifungal agent and as an additive to cattle feed

mo·ne·ra \mə-'nir-ə\ *n pl* **1** *cap, in some classifications* : a kingdom or other major division of living things comprising the prokaryotes **2** : living things that are prokaryotes

mo·ne·ran \mə-'nir-ən\ *n* : PROKARYOTE — **moneran** *adj*

mon·es·trous \(')mä-'nes-trəs\ *or chiefly Brit* **mon·oes·trous** \(')mä-'nēs-\ *adj* : experiencing estrus once each year or breeding season

Mon·gol \'mäŋ-gəl; 'män-,gōl, 'mäŋ-\ *n* **1** : a person of Mongoloid racial stock **2** *often not cap, usu offensive* : one affected with Down syndrome

¹Mon·go·lian \män-'gōl-yən, mäŋ-, -'gō-lē-ən\ *adj* **1** : MONGOLOID 1 **2** *often not cap, usu offensive* : MONGOLOID 2

²Mongolian *n* **1** : MONGOL 1 **2** *often not cap, usu offensive* : one affected with Down syndrome

Mongolian fold *n* : EPICANTHIC FOLD

Mongolian gerbil *n* : a gerbil (*Meriones unguiculatus*) of Mongolia and northern China that has a high capacity for temperature regulation and is used as an experimental laboratory animal

mon·go·lian·ism \män-'gōl-yə-,niz-əm, mäŋ-, -'gō-lē-ə-\ *n, usu offensive* : DOWN SYNDROME

Mongolian spot *n* : a bluish pigmented area near the base of the spine that is present at birth esp. in Asian, southern European, American Indian, and black infants and that usu. disappears during childhood — called also *blue spot, Mongol spot*

Mon·gol·ic fold \män-'gäl-ik-, mäŋ-\ *n* : EPICANTHIC FOLD

mon·gol·ism \'mäŋ-gə-,liz-əm\ *n, usu offensive* : DOWN SYNDROME

¹Mon·gol·oid \'mäŋ-gə-,lȯid\ *adj* **1** : of, constituting, or characteristic of a major racial stock native to Asia as classified according to physical features (as the presence of an epicanthic fold) that includes peoples of northern and eastern Asia, Malaysians, Eskimos, and often American Indians **2** *often not cap, usu offensive* : of, relating to, or affected with Down syndrome

²Mongoloid *n* **1** : a person of Mongoloid racial stock **2** *often not cap, usu offensive* : one affected with Down syndrome

Mongoloid fold *n* : EPICANTHIC FOLD

mongoloid idiocy *n, usu offensive* : DOWN SYNDROME

Mongol spot *n* : MONGOLIAN SPOT

mo·nie·zia \,män-ē-'ez-ē-ə\ *n* **1** *cap* : a genus of cyclophyllidean tapeworms (family Anoplocephalidae) parasitizing the intestine of various ruminants and having a cysticercoid larva in oribatid mites **2** : any tapeworm of the genus *Moniezia*

　Mo·niez \mȯn-yā\, **Romain–Louis (1852–1936),** French parasitologist. Moniez gained an international reputation in parasitology for his major contributions in the field. In 1880 he published an important study on the anatomy and histology of the larval forms of the cestodes. Particular attention was paid to the genus *Echinococcus,* but the study also examined another genus of tapeworms now included in the genus *Moniezia.*

mo·nil·e·thrix \mə-'nil-ə-,thriks\ *n, pl* **mon·i·let·ri·ches** \,män-ə-'le-trə-,kēz\ : an inherited disease of the hair in which each hair appears as if strung with small beads or nodes

mo·nil·ia \mə-'nil-ē-ə\ *n* **1** *pl* **monilias** *or* **monilia** *also* **mo·nil·i·ae** \-ē-,ē\ : any fungus of the genus *Candida* **2** *pl* **monilias** : CANDIDIASIS

Mo·nil·ia \mə-'nil-ē-ə\ *n, syn of* CANDIDA

Mo·nil·i·a·ce·ae \mə-,nil-ē-'ā-sē-,ē\ *n pl* : a family of imperfect fungi of the order Moniliales having white or brightly colored hyphae and similarly colored spores that are produced directly on the mycelium and not aggregated in fruiting bodies

mo·nil·i·al \mə-'nil-ē-əl\ *adj* : of, relating to, or caused by a fungus of the genus *Candida* ⟨∼ vaginitis⟩

Mo·nil·i·a·les \mə-,nil-ē-'ā-(,)lēz\ *n pl* : an order of imperfect fungi lacking conidiophores or having conidiophores that are superficial and free or gathered in tufts or cushion‑shaped masses but never enclosed in a fruiting body that is a pycnidium or a compact often saucer-shaped mass of threads with the conidiophores lacking tufts

mo·nil·i·a·sis \,mō-nə-'lī-ə-səs, ,män-ə-\ *n, pl* **-a·ses** \-,sēz\ : CANDIDIASIS

mo·nil·i·form \mə-'nil-ə-,fȯrm\ *adj* : jointed or constricted at regular intervals so as to resemble a string of beads

Mo·nil·i·for·mis \mə-,nil-ə-'fȯr-məs\ *n* : a genus of acanthocephalan worms usu. parasitic in rodents but occas. found in dogs, cats, or rarely humans

mo·nil·iid \mə-'nil-ē-əd\ *n* : a secondary commonly generalized dermatitis resulting from hypersensitivity developed in response to a primary focus of infection with a fungus of the genus *Candida*

¹mon·i·tor \'män-ət-ər\ *n* : one that monitors; *esp* : a device for observing or measuring a biologically important condition or function ⟨a heart ∼⟩

²monitor *vt* **mon·i·tored; mon·i·tor·ing** \'män-ət-ə-riŋ, 'män-ə-triŋ\ **1** : to watch, observe, or check closely or continuously ⟨∼ a patient's vital signs⟩ **2** : to test for intensity of radiations esp. if due to radioactivity

mon·key \'məŋ-kē\ *n* : a nonhuman primate mammal with the exception usu. of the lemurs and tarsiers; *esp* : any of the smaller longer-tailed primates as contrasted with the apes

mon·key·pox \'məŋ-kē-,päks\ *n* : a rare virus disease esp. of rain forest areas of central and western Africa that is caused

M
N

\ə\ **abut** \ᵊ\ **kitten** \ər\ **further** \a\ **ash** \ā\ **ace** \ä\ **cot, cart**
\aủ\ **out** \ch\ **chin** \e\ **bet** \ē\ **easy** \g\ **go** \i\ **hit** \ī\ **ice** \j\ **job**
\ŋ\ **sing** \ō\ **go** \ȯ\ **law** \ȯi\ **boy** \th\ **thin** \t̲h̲\ **the** \ü\ **loot**
\ủ\ **foot** \y\ **yet** \zh\ **vision**　*See also* Pronunciation Symbols page

by a poxvirus of the genus *Orthopoxvirus* (species *Monkeypox virus*), that occurs in wild rodents and primates and in captive monkeys, and that when transmitted to humans resembles smallpox but is milder

monks·hood \\'məŋ(k)s-ˌhu̇d\\ *n* : any plant of the genus *Aconitum*; *esp* : a Eurasian herb (*A. napellus*) often cultivated for its showy white or purplish flowers that is extremely poisonous in all its parts — see ACONITE 2

mono \\'män-(ˌ)ō\\ *n* : INFECTIOUS MONONUCLEOSIS

mono·ac·e·tin \\ˌmän-ō-'as-ət-ən\\ *n* : ACETIN a

¹mono·ac·id \\-'as-əd\\ *or* **mono·acid·ic** \\-ə-'sid-ik\\ *adj* 1 : able to react with only one molecule of a monobasic acid to form a salt or ester : characterized by one hydroxyl group — used of bases and sometimes of alcohols 2 : containing only one hydrogen atom replaceable by a basic atom or radical — used esp. of acid salts

²monoacid *n* : an acid having only one acid hydrogen atom

mono·am·ide \\-'am-ˌīd\\ *n* : an amide containing only one amido group

mono·am·ine \\ˌmän-ō-ə-'mēn, -'am-ˌēn\\ *also* **mon·am·ine** \\ˌmän-ə-'mēn, -'am-ˌēn\\ *n* : an amine RNH_2 that has one organic substituent attached to the nitrogen atom; *esp* : one (as serotonin) that is functionally important in neural transmission

monoamine oxidase *n* : an enzyme that deaminates monoamines oxidatively and that functions in the nervous system by breaking down monoamine neurotransmitters

monoamine oxidase inhibitor *n* : any of various antidepressant drugs which increase the concentration of monoamines in the brain by inhibiting the action of monoamine oxidase

mono·am·in·er·gic \\ˌmän-ō-ˌam-ə-'nər-jik\\ *adj* : liberating or involving monoamines (as serotonin or norepinephrine) in neural transmission ⟨~ neurons⟩ ⟨~ mechanisms⟩

mono·ar·tic·u·lar \\ˌmän-ō-är-'tik-yə-lər\\ *or* **mon·ar·tic·u·lar** \\ˌmän-är-\\ *adj* : affecting only one joint of the body ⟨acute ~ arthritis⟩ — compare OLIGOARTICULAR, POLYARTICULAR

mono·bac·tam \\ˌmän-ō-'bak-tam\\ *n* : any of the class of beta-lactam antibiotics (as aztreonam) with a monocyclic ring structure

mono·ba·sic \\ˌmän-ə-'bā-sik\\ *adj, of an acid* : having only one replaceable hydrogen atom

monobasic sodium phosphate *n* : SODIUM PHOSPHATE 1

mono·ben·zone \\-'ben-ˌzōn\\ *n* : a drug $C_{13}H_{12}O_2$ applied topically as a melanin inhibitor in the treatment of hyperpigmentation

mono·blast \\'män-ə-ˌblast\\ *n* : a motile cell of the spleen and bone marrow that gives rise to the monocyte of the circulating blood

mono·bro·mat·ed \\ˌmän-ō-'brō-ˌmāt-əd\\ *adj* : having one bromine atom introduced into each molecule ⟨~ camphor⟩

mono·bro·min·at·ed \\-'brō-mə-ˌnāt-əd\\ *adj* : MONOBROMATED

mono·bro·min·a·tion \\-ˌbrō-mə-'nā-shən\\ *n* : the introduction of one bromine atom into an organic compound

mono·car·box·yl·ic \\-ˌkär-(ˌ)bäk-'sil-ik\\ *adj* : containing one carboxyl group

mono·cel·lu·lar \\-'sel-yə-lər\\ *adj* : having or involving a single kind of cell

mono·cen·tric \\-'sen-trik\\ *adj* : having a single centromere ⟨~ chromosomes⟩ — compare POLYCENTRIC

mono·chlo·ro·ace·tic acid \\-ˌklōr-ō-ə-ˌsēt-ik-\\ *also* **mono·chlor·ace·tic acid** \\-ˌklōr-ə-ˌsēt-ik-\\ *n* : a crystalline acid $C_2H_3ClO_2$ obtained by direct chlorination of acetic acid and used in organic synthesis (as of dyes, coumarin, pharmaceuticals, weed killers, insecticides, and cosmetics) — called also *chloroacetic acid*; compare TRICHLOROACETIC ACID

mono·chord \\'män-ə-ˌkȯ(ə)rd\\ *n* : an instrument that has been used to test hearing acuity and that consists of a single string stretched over a sounding board and a movable bridge set on a graduated scale

mono·cho·ri·on·ic \\ˌmän-ō-ˌkōr-ē-'än-ik\\ *also* **mono·cho·ri-**

al \\-'kōr-ē-əl\\ *adj, of twins* : sharing or developed with a common chorion

mono·chro·ic \\-'krō-ik\\ *adj* : MONOCHROMATIC

mono·chro·ma·cy *also* **mono·chro·ma·sy** \\-'krō-mə-sē\\ *n, pl* **-cies** *also* **-sies** : MONOCHROMATISM

mono·chro·mat \\ˌmän-ə-krō-ˌmat, ˌmän-ə-'\\ *n* 1 : an individual who is completely color-blind 2 : an optical part (as a microscope objective) that is used only in a limited range of wavelengths

mono·chro·mat·ic \\ˌmän-ə-krō-'mat-ik\\ *adj* 1 : having or consisting of one color or hue 2 : consisting of radiation of a single wavelength or of a very small range of wavelengths 3 : of, relating to, or exhibiting monochromatism — **mono·chro·ma·tic·i·ty** \\-ˌkrō-mə-'tis-ət-ē\\ *n, pl* **-ties**

mono·chro·ma·tism \\-'krō-mə-ˌtiz-əm\\ *n* : complete color blindness in which all colors appear as shades of gray — called also *monochromacy*

mono·chro·ma·tor \\ˌmän-ə-'krō-ˌmāt-ər\\ *n* : a device for isolating a narrow portion of a spectrum

mon·o·cle \\'män-i-kəl\\ *n* : an eyeglass for one eye

mono·clin·ic \\ˌmän-ə-'klin-ik\\ *adj, of a crystal* : having one oblique intersection of the axes

¹mono·clo·nal \\ˌmän-ə-'klōn-ᵊl\\ *adj* : produced by, being, or composed of cells derived from a single cell ⟨a ~ tumor⟩; *esp* : relating to or being an antibody derived from a single cell in large quantities for use against a specific antigen (as a cancer cell)

²monoclonal *n* : a monoclonal antibody

monoclonal gammopathy *n* : any of various disorders marked by proliferation of a single clone of antibody-producing lymphoid cells resulting in an abnormal increase of a monoclonal antibody in the blood serum and urine and that include both benign or asymptomatic conditions and neoplastic conditions (as multiple myeloma and Waldenström's macroglobulinemia) — see M PROTEIN 2

mono·con·tam·i·nate \\ˌmän-ō-kən-'tam-ə-ˌnāt\\ *vt* **-nat·ed; -nat·ing** : to infect (a germ-free organism) with one kind of pathogen — **mono·con·tam·i·na·tion** \\-kən-ˌtam-ə-'nā-shən\\ *n*

mono·cro·ta·line \\-'krōt-ᵊl-ˌīn, -ᵊl-ən\\ *n* : a poisonous crystalline alkaloid $C_{16}H_{23}NO_6$ found in a leguminous plant of the genus *Crotalaria* (*C. spectabilis*) and in other plants of the same genus

mono·crot·ic \\-'krät-ik\\ *adj, of the pulse* : having a simple beat and forming a smooth single-crested curve on a sphygmogram — compare DICROTIC 1

mon·oc·u·lar \\mä-'näk-yə-lər, mə-\\ *adj* 1 : of, involving, or affecting a single eye ⟨~ vision⟩ 2 : suitable for use with only one eye ⟨a ~ microscope⟩ — **mon·oc·u·lar·ly** *adv*

mono·cy·clic \\ˌmän-ō-'sī-klik, -'sik-lik\\ *adj* : containing one ring in the molecular structure ⟨a ~ terpene⟩

mono·cyte \\'män-ə-ˌsīt\\ *n* : a large white blood cell with finely granulated chromatin dispersed throughout the nucleus that is formed in the bone marrow, enters the blood, and migrates into the connective tissue where it differentiates into a macrophage — **mono·cyt·ic** \\ˌmän-ə-'sit-ik\\ *adj* — **mono·cyt·oid** \\-'sī-ˌtȯid\\ *adj*

monocytic leukemia *n* : leukemia characterized by the presence of large numbers of monocytes in the circulating blood

mono·cy·to·pe·nia \\ˌmän-ə-ˌsīt-ə-'pē-nē-ə\\ *n* : a deficiency in circulating monocytes

mono·cy·to·sis \\-sī-'tō-səs\\ *n, pl* **-to·ses** \\-ˌsēz\\ : an abnormal increase in the number of monocytes in the circulating blood — compare GRANULOCYTOSIS, LYMPHOCYTOSIS

mono·dis·perse \\ˌmän-ō-dis-'pərs\\ *adj* : characterized by particles of uniform size in a dispersed phase — compare POLYDISPERSE

mo·noe·cious *also* **mo·ne·cious** \\mə-'nē-shəs, (')mä-\\ *adj* : having male and female sex organs in the same individual — **mo·noe·cious·ly** *adv*

mono·en·er·get·ic \\ˌmän-ō-ˌen-ər-'jet-ik\\ *adj* 1 : having equal energy — used of particles or radiation quanta 2 : composed of monoenergetic particles or radiation quanta

mono·es·ter \'män-ō-ˌes-tər\ n : an ester (as of a dibasic acid) that contains only one ester group

monoestrous *chiefly Brit var of* MONESTROUS

mono·eth·a·nol·amine \ˌmän-ō-ˌeth-ə-'näl-ə-ˌmēn, -'nōl-\ n : ETHANOLAMINE

mono·fac·to·ri·al \-fak-'tōr-ē-əl, -'tór-\ adj : MONOGENIC

mono·fil \'män-ə-ˌfil\ n : MONOFILAMENT

mono·fil·a·ment \ˌmän-ə-'fil-ə-mənt\ n : a single untwisted synthetic filament (as of nylon) used to make surgical sutures

mono·fla·gel·late \-'flaj-ə-lət, -flə-'jel-ət\ adj : UNIFLAGEL-LATE

mono·func·tion·al \-'fəŋk-sh(ə-)nəl\ adj : of, relating to, or being a compound with one reactive site in a molecule (as in polymerization) ⟨formaldehyde is a ∼ reagent⟩

mo·nog·a·mist \mə-'näg-ə-məst\ n : a person who practices or upholds monogamy

mo·nog·a·my \-mē\ n, pl **-mies** : the state or custom of being married to one person at a time or of having only one mate at a time — **mo·nog·a·mous** \mə-'näg-ə-məs\ *also* **mono·gam·ic** \ˌmän-ə-'gam-ik\ adj

mono·gas·tric \ˌmän-ə-'gas-trik\ adj : having a stomach with only a single compartment (as in humans)

Mono·ge·nea \ˌmän-ə-ə-'jē-nē-ə\ n pl : a class, subclass, or suborder of parasitic platyhelminthic worms that were formerly usu. classified as trematodes but are currently considered to be more closely related to the tapeworms and that comprise flatworms ordinarily living as ectoparasites on a single usu. fish host throughout the entire life cycle — compare DIGE-NEA

mono·ge·ne·an \-'jē-nē-ən\ n : a monogenetic flatworm — **monogenean** adj

mono·ge·net·ic \-jə-'net-ik\ adj 1 : relating to or involving the origin of diverse individuals or kinds by descent from a single ancestral individual or kind ⟨the entire present human population is ∼⟩ 2 : of, relating to, or being any platyhel-minthic worm of the taxon Monogenea

mono·gen·ic \-'jen-ik, -'jēn-\ adj : of, relating to, or controlled by a single gene and esp. by either of an allelic pair — **mono·gen·i·cal·ly** \-i-k(ə-)lē\ adv

mono·glyc·er·ide \ˌmän-ō-'glis-ə-ˌrīd\ n : any of various esters of glycerol in which only one of the three hydroxyl groups is esterified and which are often used as emulsifiers

mono·go·nad·ic \-gō-'nad-ik\ adj, of a tapeworm : having a single set of reproductive organs in each segment

mo·nog·o·ny \mə-'näg-ə-nē\ n, pl **-nies** : asexual reproduction

mono·graph \'män-ə-ˌgraf\ n 1 : a learned detailed treatise covering a small area of a field of learning ⟨this ∼ covers the development of intravenous anesthesia from 1872 —*Jour. Amer. Med. Assoc.*⟩ 2 : a description (as in the *U.S. Pharmacopeia*) of the name, chemical formula, and uniform method for determining the strength and purity of a drug — **monograph** vt

mono·hy·brid \ˌmän-ō-'hī-brəd\ n : an individual or strain heterozygous for one specified gene — **monohybrid** adj

mono·hy·drate \-'hī-ˌdrāt\ n : a hydrate containing one molecule of water — **mono·hy·drat·ed** \-əd\ adj

mono·hy·dric \-'hī-drik\ adj : MONOHYDROXY

mono·hy·droxy \-(ˌ)hī-'dräk-sē\ adj : containing one hydroxyl group in the molecule

mono·ide·ism \-'īd-ē-ˌiz-əm\ n : a state of prolonged absorption in a single idea (as in mental depression, trance, hypnosis) — compare POLYIDEISM

mono·ide·is·tic \-ˌīd-ē-'ist-ik\ adj : of, relating to, or characterized by monoideism

mono·iodo·ty·ro·sine \-ī-ˌōd-ə-'tī-rə-ˌsēn, -ī-ˌäd-ə-\ n : an iodinated tyrosine $C_9H_{10}INO_3$ that is produced in the thyroid gland by the substitution of one iodine atom in the amino acid for an atom of hydrogen, that undergoes further iodination to produce diiodotyrosine, and that combines with diiodotyrosine to form triiodothyronine

mono·kary·on \-'kar-ē-ˌän, -ən\ n : a mononuclear spore or cell of a fungus that produces a dikaryon in its life cycle

mono·kary·ot·ic \-ˌkar-ē-'ät-ik\ adj : of, relating to, or consisting of monokaryons ⟨∼ mycelia⟩

mono·lay·er \'män-ō-ˌlā-ər, -ˌle(-ə)r\ n : a single continuous layer or film that is one cell or molecule in thickness — **mono·lay·er·ing** \-iŋ\ n

mono·loc·u·lar \ˌmän-ō-'läk-yə-lər\ adj : UNILOCULAR

mono·ma·nia \ˌmän-ə-'mā-nē-ə, -nyə\ n : mental disorder esp. when limited in expression to one idea or area of thought

mono·ma·ni·ac \-nē-ˌak\ n : an individual affected by monomania

mono·ma·ni·a·cal \-mə-'nī-ə-kəl\ *also* **monomaniac** adj : relating to, characterized by, or affected with monomania

mono·me·lic \-'mē-lik\ adj : relating to or affecting only one limb ⟨∼ tumors of the leg⟩

mono·mer \'män-ə-mər\ n : a chemical compound that can undergo polymerization — **mo·no·mer·ic** \ˌmän-ə-'mer-ik, ˌmō-nə-\ adj

mono·mo·lec·u·lar \ˌmän-ō-mə-'lek-yə-lər\ adj 1 : being only one molecule thick ⟨a ∼ film⟩ 2 : relating to or being a process whose rate is directly proportional to the amount or concentration of the material undergoing the process

mono·mor·phic \-'mór-fik\ adj : having but a single form, structural pattern, or genotype ⟨a ∼ species of insect⟩ — **mono·mor·phism** \-ˌfiz-əm\ n

mono·neu·ri·tis \-n(y)ù-'rīt-əs\ n, pl **-rit·i·des** \-'rit-ə-ˌdēz\ or **-ri·tis·es** : neuritis of a single nerve

mononeuritis mul·ti·plex \-'məl-tə-ˌpleks\ n : neuritis that affects several separate nerves — called also *mononeuropa-thy multiplex*

mono·neu·rop·a·thy \-n(y)ù-'räp-ə-thē\ n, pl **-thies** : a nerve disease affecting only a single nerve

mononeuropathy multiplex n : MONONEURITIS MULTI-PLEX

¹**mono·nu·cle·ar** \ˌmän-ō-'n(y)ü-klē-ər\ adj 1 : having only one nucleus ⟨a ∼ cell⟩ 2 : MONOCYCLIC

²**mononuclear** n : a mononuclear cell; *esp* : MONOCYTE

mononuclear leukocyte n : NONGRANULAR LEUKOCYTE — used esp. in the clinical literature

mononuclear phagocyte system n : a system of cells comprising all free and fixed macrophages together with their ancestral cells including monocytes and their precursors in the bone marrow — compare RETICULOENDOTHELIAL SYSTEM

mono·nu·cle·at·ed \-'n(y)ü-klē-ˌāt-əd\ *also* **mono·nu·cle·ate** \-klē-ət, -ˌāt\ adj : MONONUCLEAR 1

mono·nu·cle·o·sis \-ˌn(y)ü-klē-'ō-səs\ n : an abnormal increase of mononuclear white blood cells in the blood; *specif* : INFECTIOUS MONONUCLEOSIS

mono·nu·cle·o·tide \-'n(y)ü-klē-ə-ˌtīd\ n : a nucleotide that is derived from one molecule each of a nitrogenous base, a sugar, and a phosphoric acid

mono·ox·y·gen·ase \-'äk-si-jə-ˌnās, -ˌnāz\ n : any of several oxygenases that bring about the incorporation of one atom of molecular oxygen into a substrate

mono·pha·sic \-'fā-zik\ adj 1 : having a single phase; *specif* : relating to or being a record of a nerve impulse that is negative or positive but not both ⟨a ∼ action potential⟩ — compare DIPHASIC b, POLYPHASIC 1 2 : having a single period of activity followed by a period of rest in each 24-hour period ⟨humans are naturally ∼ beings⟩

mono·pho·bia \-'fō-bē-ə\ n : a morbid dread of being alone

mono·phos·phate \-'fäs-ˌfāt\ n : a phosphate containing a single phosphate group

mono·phy·let·ic \ˌmän-ō-fī-'let-ik\ adj : of or relating to a single stock; *specif* : developed from a single common ancestral form — **mono·phy·ly** \'män-ə-ˌfī-lē\ n, pl **-lies**

monophyletic theory n : a theory in physiology: all the cel-

\ə\ abut \ᵊ\ kitten \ər\ further \a\ ash \ā\ ace \ä\ cot, cart
\aù\ out \ch\ chin \e\ bet \ē\ easy \g\ go \i\ hit \ī\ ice \j\ job
\ŋ\ sing \ō\ go \ó\ law \ói\ boy \th\ thin \t͟h\ the \ü\ loot
\ù\ foot \y\ yet \zh\ vision *See also* Pronunciation Symbols page

M
N

lular elements of the blood derive from a common stem cell — compare POLYPHYLETIC THEORY

mono·phy·odont \-'fī-ə-ˌdänt\ *adj* : having but one set of teeth of which none are replaced at a later stage of growth — compare DIPHYODONT, POLYPHYODONT

mono·ple·gia \-'plē-j(ē-)ə\ *n* : paralysis affecting a single limb, body part, or group of muscles — **mono·ple·gic** \-jik\ *adj*

¹mono·ploid \'män-ə-ˌplȯid\ *n* : a monoploid individual or organism

²monoploid *adj* **1** : HAPLOID **2** : having or being the basic haploid number of chromosomes in a polyploid series of organisms

mono·po·lar \ˌmän-ō-'pō-lər\ *adj* : UNIPOLAR — **mono·po·lar·i·ty** \-pō-'lar-ət-ē\ *n, pl* **-ties**

mono·po·lar·ly \-lē\ *adv* : by means of unipolar leads ⟨EEGs were recorded ∼ —H. L. Meltzer *et al*⟩

¹mon·or·chid \mä-'nȯr-kəd\ *adj* : having only one testis or only one testis descended into the scrotum — compare CRYPTORCHID

²monorchid *n* : a monorchid individual

mon·or·chid·ism \-ˌiz-əm\ *also* **mon·or·chism** \mä-'nȯr-ˌkiz-əm\ *n* : the quality or state of being monorchid — compare CRYPTORCHIDISM

mono·rhi·nic \ˌmän-ō-'rī-nik, -'rin-ik\ *adj* : affecting or applied to only one nostril

mono·sac·cha·ride \ˌmän-ə-'sak-ə-ˌrīd\ *n* : a sugar not decomposable to simpler sugars by hydrolysis — called also *simple sugar*

mono·sac·cha·rose \-'sak-ə-ˌrōs\ *n* : MONOSACCHARIDE

mono·ose \'mä-ˌnōs\ *n* : MONOSACCHARIDE

mono·sex·u·al \ˌmän-ō-'seksh-(ə-)wəl\ *adj* : being or relating to a male or a female rather than a bisexual — **mono·sex·u·al·i·ty** \-ˌsek-shə-'wal-ət-ē\ *n, pl* **-ties**

mono·so·di·um glu·ta·mate \ˌmän-ə-ˌsōd-ē-əm-'glüt-ə-ˌmāt\ *n* : a crystalline salt $C_5H_8NO_4Na$ derived from glutamic acid that is used to enhance the flavor of food and medicinally to reduce ammonia levels in blood and tissues in ammoniacal azotemia (as in hepatic insufficiency) — abbr. *MSG;* called also *sodium glutamate;* see CHINESE RESTAURANT SYNDROME

monosodium urate *n* : a salt of uric acid that precipitates out in cartilage as tophi in gout

mono·some \'män-ə-ˌsōm\ *n* **1** : a chromosome lacking a synaptic mate; *esp* : an unpaired X chromosome **2** : a single ribosome

¹mono·so·mic \ˌmän-ə-'sō-mik\ *adj* : having one less than the diploid number of chromosomes — **mono·so·my** \'män-ə-ˌsō-mē\ *n, pl* **-mies**

²monosomic *n* : a monosomic individual

mono·spe·cif·ic \ˌmän-ō-spə-'sif-ik\ *adj* : specific for a single antigen or receptor site on an antigen — **mono·spec·i·fic·i·ty** \-ˌspes-ə-'fis-ət-ē\ *n, pl* **-ties**

mono·sper·mic \-'spər-mik\ *adj* : involving or resulting from a single sperm cell ⟨∼ fertilization⟩

mono·sper·my \'män-ō-ˌspər-mē\ *n, pl* **-mies** : the entry of a single fertilizing sperm into an egg — compare DISPERMY, POLYSPERMY

mon·os·tot·ic \ˌmän-ˌäs-'tät-ik\ *adj* : relating to or affecting a single bone

mono·stra·tal \ˌmän-ō-'strāt-ᵊl\ *adj* : arranged in a single stratum

mono·sub·sti·tut·ed \-'səb-stə-ˌt(y)üt-əd\ *adj* : having one substituent atom or group in a molecule ⟨∼ acetylenes⟩ — **mono·sub·sti·tu·tion** \-ˌsəb-stə-'t(y)ü-shən\ *n*

mono·symp·tom·at·ic \-ˌsim(p)-tə-'mat-ik\ *adj* : exhibiting or manifested by a single principal symptom ⟨a ∼ phobia⟩

mono·syn·ap·tic \ˌmän-ō-sə-'nap-tik\ *adj* : having or involving a single neural synapse — **mono·syn·ap·ti·cal·ly** \-ti-k(ə-)lē\ *adv*

mono·ter·pene \ˌmän-ə-'tər-ˌpēn\ *n* : any of a class of terpenes $C_{10}H_{16}$ containing two isoprene units per molecule; *also* : a derivative of a monoterpene

mono·ther·a·py \-'ther-ə-pē\ *n, pl* **-pies** : the use of a single drug to treat a particular disorder or disease ⟨propranolol as ∼ for angina pectoris⟩

mo·not·o·cous \mä-'nät-ə-kəs\ *adj* : producing a single egg or young at one time ⟨∼ ovulation⟩ — compare POLYTOCOUS

Mono·trema·ta \ˌmän-ə-'trem-ət-ə, -'trēm-\ *n pl* : an order of egg-laying mammals comprising the platypuses and the echidnas

mono·treme \'män-ə-ˌtrēm\ *n* : any mammal (as a platypus) of the order Monotremata

mo·not·ri·chous \mə-'nä-tri-kəs\ *adj* : having a single flagellum at one pole — used of bacteria

mono·typ·ic \ˌmän-ə-'tip-ik\ *adj* : including a single representative — used esp. of a genus with only one species

mono·un·sat·u·rate \ˌmän-ō-ˌən-'sach-ə-rət\ *n* : a monounsaturated oil or fatty acid

mono·un·sat·u·rat·ed \ˌmän-ō-ˌən-'sach-ə-ˌrāt-əd\ *adj, of an oil, fat, or fatty acid* : containing one double or triple bond per molecule ⟨canola and olive oils are rich in ∼ fatty acids⟩ — compare POLYUNSATURATED

mono·va·lent \ˌmän-ə-'vā-lənt\ *adj* **1** : having a chemical valence of one **2** : containing antibodies specific for or antigens of a single strain of a microorganism ⟨a ∼ vaccine⟩

mon·ovu·lar \(')mä-'näv-yə-lər, -'nōv-\ *adj* : MONOZYGOTIC

mono·xen·ic \ˌmän-ə-'zen-ik\ *adj* : relating to or being a culture in which one organism is grown or contaminated with only one other organism ⟨grown under ∼ conditions⟩

mon·ox·e·nous \mə-'näk-sə-nəs\ *adj, of a parasite* : living on only one kind of host throughout its life cycle

mon·ox·ide \mə-'näk-ˌsīd\ *n* : an oxide containing one atom of oxygen per molecule — see CARBON MONOXIDE

Mon·o·zoa \ˌmän-ə-'zō-ə, ˌmōn-\ *n pl, syn of* CESTODARIA

mono·zo·ic \-'zō-ik\ *adj* : MONOZOOTIC

mono·zo·ot·ic \ˌmän-ō-zə-'wät-ik\ *adj* : consisting of a single differentiated unit — used of cestodarians; compare POLYZOOTIC

mono·zy·gote \-'zī-ˌgōt\ *n* : one of two or more individuals derived from a single egg ⟨an identical twin is a ∼⟩

mono·zy·got·ic \ˌmän-ə-zī-'gät-ik\ *adj* : derived from a single egg ⟨∼ twins⟩ — **mono·zy·gos·i·ty** \-'gäs-ət-ē\ *n, pl* **-ties**

mono·zy·gous \ˌmän-ə-'zī-gəs, (')mä-'näz-ə-gəs\ *adj* : MONOZYGOTIC

mons \'mänz\ *n, pl* **mon·tes** \'män-ˌtēz\ : a body part or area raised above or demarcated from surrounding structures (as the papilla of mucosa through which the ureter enters the bladder)

mons pubis *n, pl* **mon·tes pubis** \ˌmän-ˌtēz-\ : a rounded eminence of fatty tissue upon the pubic symphysis esp. of the human female — see MONS VENERIS

mon·ster \'män(t)-stər\ *n* : an animal or plant of abnormal form or structure; *esp* : a fetus or offspring with a major developmental abnormality

mon·stros·i·ty \män-'sträs-ət-ē\ *n, pl* **-ties** **1 a** : a malformation of a plant or animal **b** : MONSTER **2** : the quality or state of deviating greatly from the natural form or character — **mon·strous** \'män(t)-strəs\ *adj*

mons ve·ne·ris \-'ven-ə-rəs\ *n, pl* **mon·tes veneris** \ˌmän-ˌtēz-\ : the mons pubis of a female

Mon·teg·gia fracture \män-'tej-ə-\ *or* **Mon·teg·gia's fracture** \-'tej-əz-\ *n* : a fracture in the proximal part of the ulna with dislocation of the head of the radius

 Monteggia, Giovanni Battista (1762–1815), Italian surgeon. Monteggia is remembered for his description (circa 1810) of a form of dislocation of the hip in which the head of the femur is displaced toward the anterior superior iliac spine.

mon·te·lu·kast \ˌmänt-ə-'lü-ˌkast\ *n* : a leukotriene antagonist administered in the form of its sodium salt $C_{35}H_{35}ClNNaO_3S$ in tablet form to treat asthma or to relieve the symptoms of seasonal allergic rhinitis — see SINGULAIR

Mon·te·zu·ma's re·venge \ˌmänt-ə-ˌzü-məz-ri-'venj\ *n* : diarrhea contracted in Mexico esp. by tourists

 Montezuma II (1466–1520), Aztec emperor of Mexico. Montezuma was emperor of the Aztecs at the time of the

Spanish conquest. Montezuma tried to appease the Spanish but failed and was captured by them and deposed. During the ensuing Aztec revolt he was either killed by his own people or murdered by the Spanish. For the injustice done to him, he continues to wreak vengeance against the latter‑day hordes of invading tourists.

Mont·gom·ery's gland \(ˌ)mən(t)-ˈgəm-(ə-)rēz-, män(t)-ˈgäm-\ *n* : an apocrine gland in the areola of the mammary gland

Montgomery, William Fetherston (1797–1859), British obstetrician. In 1837 Montgomery published an article describing the sebaceous glands of the areola, which are now known as Montgomery's glands. He also described the enlarged sebaceous glands observed on the surface of the areola during pregnancy. These tubercles had been observed previously by Giovanni Morgagni but have been since identified with Montgomery.

month·lies \ˈmən(t)th-lēz\ *n pl* : a menstrual period

mon·tic·u·lus \män-ˈtik-yə-ləs\ *n* : the median dorsal ridge of the cerebellum formed by the vermis

mood \ˈmüd\ *n* : a conscious state of mind or predominant emotion : affective state : FEELING 3

mood disorder *n* : any of several psychological disorders characterized by abnormalities of emotional state and including esp. major depressive disorder, dysthymia, and bipolar disorder — called also *affective disorder*

moon \ˈmün\ *n* : LUNULA a

moon blindness *n* : a recurrent inflammation of the eye of the horse — called also *periodic ophthalmia*

moon facies *n* : the full rounded facies characteristic of hyperadrenocorticism — called also *moon face*

Moon's molar *or* **Moon molar** *n* : a first molar tooth which has become dome-shaped due to malformation by congenital syphilis; *also* : MULBERRY MOLAR

Moon, Henry (1845–1892), British surgeon. Moon described the irregular first molars found in congenital syphilis in 1876.

MOPP \ˌem-ˌō-ˌpē-ˈpē\ *n* : a drug regimen that includes mechlorethamine, vincristine, procarbazine, and prednisone and is used in the treatment of some forms of cancer (as Hodgkin's disease)

Mor·ax–Ax·en·feld bacillus \ˈmȯr-äks-ˈäk-sən-ˌfeld-\ *n* : a rod-shaped bacterium of the genus *Moraxella* (*M. lacunata*) that causes Morax-Axenfeld conjunctivitis

Mor·ax \ˈmȯr-aks\, **Victor (1866–1935),** French ophthalmologist. Morax published a general summary of ophthalmology and several papers dealing specifically with the conjunctiva and the cornea. In 1896 he isolated a bacterium of the genus *Moraxella* which causes a chronic conjunctivitis. **Ax·en·feld** \ˈäk-sən-ˌfelt\, **Karl Theodor Paul Polykarpos (1867–1930),** German ophthalmologist. Axenfeld presented a classic account of a form of choroiditis due especially to metastasis in 1894. In 1896, independently of Morax, he isolated the bacterium of the genus *Moraxella* and described the chronic conjunctivitis that it causes. This conjunctivitis is now known as the Morax-Axenfeld conjunctivitis.

Morax–Axenfeld conjunctivitis *n* : a chronic conjunctivitis caused by a rod-shaped bacterium of the genus *Moraxella* (*M. lacunata*) and now occurring rarely but formerly more prevalent in persons living under poor hygienic conditions

Mor·ax·el·la \ˌmȯr-ak-ˈsel-ə\ *n* : a genus of short rod-shaped gram-negative bacteria of the family Neisseriaceae that includes the causative agent (*M. lacunata*) of Morax-Axenfeld conjunctivitis

morbi *pl of* MORBUS

mor·bid \ˈmȯr-bəd\ *adj* **1 a** : of, relating to, or characteristic of disease **b** : affected with or induced by disease ⟨a ~ condition⟩ ⟨~ alteration of tissues⟩ **c** : productive of disease ⟨~ substances⟩ **2** : abnormally susceptible to or characterized by gloomy or unwholesome feelings

morbid anatomy *n* : PATHOLOGICAL ANATOMY

mor·bid·i·ty \mȯr-ˈbid-ət-ē\ *n, pl* **-ties 1** : a diseased state or symptom ⟨lumbar puncture, if improperly performed, may be followed by a significant ~ —*Jour. Amer. Med. Assoc.*⟩ **2**

: the incidence of disease : the rate of sickness (as in a specified community or group) ⟨while TB mortality has declined fairly steadily, ~ has been rising —*Time*⟩ — compare MORTALITY 2

mor·bif·ic \mȯr-ˈbif-ik\ *adj* : causing disease : generating a sickly state

mor·bil·li \mȯr-ˈbil-ˌī\ *n pl* : MEASLES 1

mor·bil·li·form \mȯr-ˈbil-ə-ˌfȯrm\ *adj* : resembling the eruption of measles ⟨a ~ pruritic rash⟩

mor·bil·li·vi·rus \-ˌvī-rəs\ *n* **1** *cap* : a genus of single-stranded RNA viruses of the family *Paramyxoviridae* that includes the causative agents of measles, canine distemper, and rinderpest **2** : any of the genus *Morbillivirus* of paramyxoviruses

mor·bus \ˈmȯr-bəs\ *n, pl* **mor·bi** \-ˌbī\ : DISEASE — see CHOLERA MORBUS

morbus cae·ru·le·us *or* **morbus coe·ru·le·us** \-sə-ˈrü-lē-əs\ *n* : congenital heart disease with cyanosis

morbus cor·dis \-ˈkȯrd-əs\ *n* : HEART DISEASE

morbus cox·ae se·nil·is \-ˈkäk-sē-se-ˈnil-əs\ *n* : osteoarthritis of the hip occurring esp. in late middle and old age

morbus gal·li·cus \-ˈgal-i-kəs\ *n* : SYPHILIS

mor·cel·la·tion \ˌmȯr-sə-ˈlā-shən\ *n* **1** : division and removal in small pieces (as of a tumor) **2** : the surgical cutting of the skull into small pieces and leaving them in place to allow more even or symmetrical expansion of the brain and skull during growth

mor·celle·ment \ˌmȯr-sel-ˈmäⁿ\ *n* : MORCELLATION

mor·dant \ˈmȯrd-ᵊnt\ *n* : a chemical that fixes a dye in or on a substance by combining with the dye to form an insoluble compound — **mordant** *vt*

mor·gan \ˈmȯr-gən\ *n* **1** : a unit of inferred distance between genes on a chromosome that is used in constructing genetic maps and is equal to the distance for which the frequency of crossing-over is 100 percent **2** : CENTIMORGAN

Morgan, Thomas Hunt (1866–1945), American geneticist. Morgan spent much of his career as a professor of experimental biology at Columbia University. He became a pioneer in the developing science of genetics. In 1908 and 1909 he began a series of experiments first with mice and rats and then with fruit flies of the genus *Drosophila*. During the next several years he discovered many mutant traits, such as eye colors, body colors, and wing variations, and determined the modes of heredity. He and the members of his experimental laboratory made such advances in genetics as a clear understanding of sex-linkage, final proof of the chromosome theory of heredity, establishment of the linear arrangement of genes in the chromosome, the demonstration of interference in crossing-over, and the discovery of chromosomal inversions. He was awarded the Nobel Prize for Physiology or Medicine in 1933.

morgue \ˈmȯ(ə)rg\ *n* : a place where the bodies of persons found dead are kept until identified and claimed by relatives or are released for burial

mor·i·bund \ˈmȯr-ə-(ˌ)bənd, ˈmär-\ *adj* : being in the state of dying : approaching death ⟨in the ~ patient deepening stupor and coma are the usual preludes to death —Norman Cameron⟩

mo·ric·i·zine \mə-ˈris-ə-ˌzēn\ *n* : an antiarrhythmic drug used in the form of its hydrochloride $C_{22}H_{25}N_3O_4S \cdot HCl$ esp. in the treatment of life-threatening ventricular arrhythmias

morn·ing–af·ter pill \ˌmȯr-niŋ-ˈaf-tər-\ *n* : an oral drug typically containing high doses of estrogen taken up to usu. three days after unprotected sexual intercourse that interferes with pregnancy by inhibiting ovulation or by blocking implantation of a fertilized egg in the human uterus

morn·ing breath \ˈmȯr-niŋ-\ *n* : halitosis upon awakening from sleep that is caused by the buildup of bacteria in the mouth due to decreased saliva production

---

\ə\ **abut** \ᵊ\ **kitten** \ər\ **further** \a\ **ash** \ā\ **ace** \ä\ **cot, cart**
\aů\ **out** \ch\ **chin** \e\ **bet** \ē\ **easy** \g\ **go** \i\ **hit** \ī\ **ice** \j\ **job**
\ŋ\ **sing** \ō\ **go** \ȯ\ **law** \ȯi\ **boy** \th\ **thin** \th\ **the** \ü\ **loot**
\ů\ **foot** \y\ **yet** \zh\ **vision** *See also* Pronunciation Symbols page

morning sickness *n* : nausea and vomiting that occurs typically in the morning esp. during the earlier months of pregnancy

mo·ron \'mō(ə)r-ˌän, 'mȯ(ə)r-\ *n, usu offensive* : a mildly mentally retarded person — **mo·ron·ic** \mə-'rän-ik, mȯ-\ *adj, usu offensive*

Moro reflex \'mȯr-ō-\ *n* : a reflex reaction of infants upon being startled (as by a loud noise or a bright light) that is characterized by extension of the arms and legs away from the body and to the side and then by drawing them together as if in an embrace

  Moro, Ernst (1874–1951), German pediatrician. Moro is remembered for his isolation of a bacterium of the genus *Lactobacillus* (*L. acidophilus*) in 1900 and for his introduction of a percutaneous tuberculin reaction as a diagnostic test in 1908. The characteristic reflex reaction of young infants to a sudden startling stimulus is named in his honor.

Moro test *n* : a diagnostic skin test which was formerly used to detect infection or past infection by the tubercle bacillus, which involves rubbing an ointment containing tuberculin directly on the skin, and in which a positive result is indicated by the appearance of reddish papules after one or two days

morph *abbr* **1** morphological **2** morphology

mor·phal·lax·is \ˌmȯr-fə-'lak-səs\ *n, pl* **-lax·es** \-ˌsēz\ : regeneration of a part or organism from a fragment by reorganization without cell proliferation — compare EPIMORPHOSIS

mor·phea *also Brit* **mor·phoea** \mȯr-'fē-ə\ *n, pl* **mor·phe·ae** *also Brit* **mor·phoe·ae** \-'fē-ē\ : localized scleroderma

mor·phia \'mȯr-fē-ə\ *n* : MORPHINE

mor·phine \'mȯr-ˌfēn\ *n* : a bitter crystalline addictive narcotic base $C_{17}H_{19}NO_3$ that is the principal alkaloid of opium and is used in the form of its hydrated sulfate $(C_{17}H_{19}NO_3)_2 \cdot H_2SO_4 \cdot 5H_2O$ or hydrated hydrochloride $C_{17}H_{19}NO_3 \cdot HCl \cdot 3H_2O$ as an analgesic and sedative

  Mor·pheus \'mȯr-fē-əs, -ˌf(y)üs\, Greek mythological character. Morpheus was one of the sons of Hypnos, the god of sleep. As a dream-god Morpheus made human shapes appear to dreamers. His two brothers were responsible for sending forms of animals and inanimate things.

morphine mec·o·nate \-'mek-ə-ˌnāt\ *n* : the morphine salt of meconic acid that occurs naturally in opium

mor·phin·ism \'mȯr-ˌfē-ˌniz-əm, -fə-\ *n* : a disordered condition of health produced by habitual use of morphine

mor·phin·ist \-nəst\ *n* : an individual addicted to the use of morphine

mor·phin·iza·tion \ˌmȯr-fē-nə-'zā-shən, -fə-\ *n* : the act or process of treating with morphine; *also* : the condition of being under the influence of morphine — **mor·phin·ized** \'mȯr-fē-ˌnīzd, -fə-\ *adj*

mor·phi·no·ma·ni·ac \-nō-'mā-nē-ˌak\ *n* : an individual who has a habitual and uncontrollable craving for morphine — **morphinomaniac** *adj*

mor·phi·no·mi·met·ic \-mə-'met-ik, -mī-\ *adj* : resembling opiates in their affinity for opiate receptors in the brain ⟨the enkephalins are ∼ pentapeptides⟩

mor·pho·dif·fer·en·ti·a·tion \ˌmȯr-fō-ˌdif-ə-ˌren-chē-'ā-shən\ *n* : structure or organ differentiation (as in tooth development)

morphoea *Brit var of* MORPHEA

mor·pho·gen \'mȯr-fə-jən, -ˌjen\ *n* : a diffusible chemical substance that exerts control over morphogenesis esp. by forming a gradient in concentration

mor·pho·gen·e·sis \ˌmȯr-fə-'jen-ə-səs\ *n, pl* **-e·ses** \-ˌsēz\ : the formation and differentiation of tissues and organs — compare ORGANOGENESIS

mor·pho·ge·net·ic \-jə-'net-ik\ *adj* : relating to or concerned with the development of normal organic form ⟨∼ movements of early embryonic cells⟩ — **mor·pho·ge·net·i·cal·ly** \-i-k(ə-)lē\ *adv*

mor·pho·gen·ic \-'jen-ik\ *adj* : MORPHOGENETIC

mor·pho·line \'mȯr-fə-ˌlēn, -lən\ *n* : an oily cyclic secondary amine C_4H_9NO made from ethylene oxide and ammonia and used chiefly as a solvent and emulsifying agent

mor·pho·log·i·cal \ˌmȯr-fə-'läj-i-kəl\ *also* **mor·pho·log·ic** \-'läj-ik\ *adj* : of, relating to, or concerned with form or structure — **mor·pho·log·i·cal·ly** \-i-k(ə-)lē\ *adv*

morphological index *n* : the ratio of the volume of the human trunk to the sum of the lengths of one arm and one leg multiplied by 100

mor·phol·o·gist \mȯr-'fäl-ə-jəst\ *n* : a person specializing in morphology

mor·phol·o·gy \mȯr-'fäl-ə-jē\ *n, pl* **-gies** **1** : a branch of biology that deals with the form and structure of animals and plants esp. with respect to the forms, relations, metamorphoses, and phylogenetic development of organs apart from their functions — see ANATOMY 1; compare PHYSIOLOGY 1 **2** : the form and structure of an organism or any of its parts

mor·pho·met·rics \ˌmȯr-fə-'me-triks\ *n pl* **1** : MORPHOMETRY **2** : morphometric measurements

mor·phom·e·try \mȯr-'fäm-ə-trē\ *n, pl* **-tries** : the quantitative measurement of the form esp. of living systems or their parts — **mor·pho·met·ric** \ˌmȯr-fə-'me-trik\ *adj*

mor·pho·phys·io·log·i·cal \ˌmȯr-fō-ˌfiz-ē-ə-'läj-i-kəl\ *adj* : of, relating to, or concerned with biological interrelationships between form and function — **mor·pho·phys·i·ol·o·gy** \-ē-'äl-ə-jē\ *n, pl* **-gies**

Mor·quio's disease \'mȯr-kē-ˌōz-\ *n* : an autosomal recessive mucopolysaccharidosis characterized by excretion of keratan sulfate in the urine, dwarfism, a short neck, protruding sternum, kyphosis, a flat nose, prominent upper jaw, and a waddling gait

  Morquio, Luis (1867–1935), Uruguayan physician. Morquio held positions as a director of a pediatric clinic and as a professor of medicine at Montevideo. He published his description of Morquio's disease in 1929.

mor·rhu·ate sodium \'mȯr-ə-ˌwāt-\ *n* : a pale-yellow granular salt of morrhuic acid administered in solution intravenously as a sclerosing agent esp. in the treatment of varicose veins

mor·rhu·ic acid \ˌmȯr-ə-wik-\ *n* : a mixture of fatty acids obtained from cod-liver oil

mor·tal \'mȯrt-ᵊl\ *adj* **1** : having caused or being about to cause death : FATAL ⟨a ∼ injury⟩ **2** : of, relating to, or connected with death ⟨∼ agony⟩

mor·tal·i·ty \mȯr-'tal-ət-ē\ *n, pl* **-ties** **1** : the quality or state of being mortal **2 a** : the number of deaths in a given time or place **b** : the proportion of deaths to population : DEATH RATE — called also *mortality rate;* compare FERTILITY 2, MORBIDITY 2

mor·tar \'mȯrt-ər\ *n* : a strong vessel in which material is pounded or rubbed with a pestle

mor·ti·cian \mȯr-'tish-ən\ *n* : UNDERTAKER

mor·ti·fi·ca·tion \ˌmȯrt-ə-fə-'kā-shən\ *n* : local death of tissue in the animal body : NECROSIS, GANGRENE

mor·ti·fied \'mȯrt-ə-ˌfīd\ *adj* : GANGRENOUS

mor·ti·fy \'mȯrt-ə-ˌfī\ *vi* **-fied; -fy·ing** : to become necrotic or gangrenous

mortis — see ALGOR MORTIS, IN ARTICULO MORTIS, RIGOR MORTIS

Mor·ton Mains disease \'mȯrt-ᵊn-'mānz-\ *n* : cobalt deficiency disease of sheep and cattle in New Zealand — compare ²PINE

Mor·ton's neuroma \ˌmȯrt-ᵊnz-\ *n* : a neuroma formed in conjunction with Morton's toe

  Morton, Thomas George (1835–1903), American surgeon. Morton published the first complete description of a form of metatarsalgia involving compression of a branch of the plantar nerve in 1876. Although it had been already observed, the condition has since become identified with him.

Morton's toe *n* : metatarsalgia that is caused by compression of a branch of the plantar nerve between the heads of the metatarsal bones — called also *Morton's disease, Morton's foot*

¹**mor·tu·ary** \'mȯr-chə-ˌwer-ē\ *adj* **1** : of or relating to the burial of the dead **2** : of, relating to, or characteristic of death

²**mortuary** *n, pl* **-ar·ies** : a place in which dead bodies are kept and prepared for burial or cremation

mor·u·la \'mȯr-(y)ə-lə, 'mär-\ *n, pl* **-lae** \-ˌlē, -ˌlī\ : a globular solid mass of blastomeres formed by cleavage of a zygote that typically precedes the blastula — compare GASTRULA — **mor·u·lar** \-lər\ *adj* — **mor·u·la·tion** \ˌmȯr-(y)ə-'lā-shən, ˌmär-\ *n*

mor·u·loid \-ˌlȯid\ *adj* : having a segmented appearance suggesting that of a morula or mulberry ⟨a ~ bacterial colony⟩

¹**mo·sa·ic** \mō-'zā-ik\ *n* : an organism or one of its parts composed of cells of more than one genotype : CHIMERA

²**mosaic** *adj* **1** : exhibiting mosaicism **2** : DETERMINATE — **mo·sa·i·cal·ly** \-'zā-ə-k(ə-)lē\ *adv*

mo·sa·i·cism \mō-'zā-ə-ˌsiz-əm\ *n* : the condition of possessing cells of two or more different genetic constitutions

mOsm *abbr* milliosmol

mos·qui·to \mə-'skēt-(ˌ)ō, -ə-(-w)\ *n, pl* **-toes** *also* **-tos** : any of numerous dipteran flies of the family Culicidae that have a rather narrow abdomen, usu. a long slender rigid proboscis, and narrow wings with a fringe of scales on the margin and usu. on each side of the wing veins, that have in the male broad feathery antennae and mouthparts not fitted for piercing and in the female slender antennae and a set of needlelike organs in the proboscis with which they puncture the skin of animals to suck the blood, that lay their eggs on the surface of stagnant water, that include many species which pass through several generations in the course of a year and hibernate as adults or winter in the egg state, and that include some species which are the only vectors of certain diseases — see AEDES, ANOPHELES, CULEX

mos·qui·to·cide \mə-'skēt-ə-ˌsīd\ *n* : an agent used to destroy mosquitoes

mosquito forceps *n* : a very small surgical forceps — called also *mosquito clamp*

moss \'mȯs\ *n* **1** : any of a class (Musci) of bryophytic plants having a small leafy often tufted stem bearing sex organs at its tip — see SPHAGNUM **2** : any of various plants resembling mosses in appearance or habit of growth — see CLUB MOSS, ICELAND MOSS, IRISH MOSS

Moss·man fever \'mȯs-mən-\ *n* : a form of tsutsugamushi disease occurring in northern Australia

mossy fiber \'mȯ-sē-\ *n* : any of the complexly ramifying nerve fibers that surround some nerve cells of the cerebellar cortex

moth·er \'məth-ər\ *n* : a female parent

mother cell *n* : a cell that gives rise to other cells usu. of a different sort ⟨a sperm *mother cell*⟩

mother yaw *n* : the initial superficial lesion of yaws appearing at the site of infection after an incubation period of several weeks

mo·tif \mō-'tēf\ *n* : a distinctive usu. recurrent molecular sequence (as of amino acids or base pairs) or structural elements (as of secondary protein structures) ⟨a simple protein ~ consisting of two alpha helices⟩

¹**mo·tile** \'mōt-ᵊl, 'mō-ˌtīl\ *adj* : exhibiting or capable of movement ⟨~ cilia⟩

²**motile** *n* : a person whose prevailing mental imagery is motor rather than visual or auditory and takes the form of inner feelings of action — compare AUDILE, TACTILE, VISUALIZER

mo·til·in \mō-'til-ən\ *n* : a polypeptide hormone secreted by the small intestine that increases gastrointestinal motility and stimulates the production of pepsin

mo·til·i·ty \mō-'til-ət-ē\ *n, pl* **-ties** : the quality or state of being motile : CONTRACTILITY ⟨gastrointestinal ~⟩

mo·tion \'mō-shən\ *n* **1** : an act, process, or instance of changing place : MOVEMENT **2 a** : an evacuation of the bowels **b** : the matter evacuated — often used in pl. ⟨blood in the ~s —*Lancet*⟩

motion sickness *n* : sickness induced by motion (as in travel by air, car, or ship) and characterized by nausea — called also *kinetosis*

mo·ti·vate \'mōt-ə-ˌvāt\ *vt* **-vat·ed; -vat·ing** : to provide with a motive or serve as a motive for ⟨~ patients to change unhealthy lifestyles⟩ — **mo·ti·va·tive** \-ˌvāt-iv\ *adj*

mo·ti·va·tion \ˌmōt-ə-'vā-shən\ *n* **1 a** : the act or process of motivating **b** : the condition of being motivated **2** : a motivating force, stimulus, or influence (as a drive or incentive) ⟨lacks the ~ to lose weight⟩ — **mo·ti·va·tion·al** \-shnəl, -shən-ᵊl\ *adj* — **mo·ti·va·tion·al·ly** \-ē\ *adv*

mo·tive \'mōt-iv\ *n* : something (as a need or desire) that causes a person to act

mo·to·neu·ron \ˌmōt-ə-'n(y)ü-ˌrän, -'n(y)u̇(ə)r-ˌän\ *or chiefly Brit* **mo·to·neu·rone** \-ˌrōn, -ˌōn\ *n* : MOTOR NEURON — **mo·to·neu·ro·nal** \-'n(y)u̇r-ən-ᵊl, -n(y)u̇-'rōn-ᵊl\ *adj*

mo·tor \'mōt-ər\ *adj* **1** : causing or imparting motion **2** : of, relating to, or being a motor neuron or a nerve containing motor neurons ⟨~ fibers⟩ ⟨~ cells⟩ **3** : of, relating to, concerned with, or involving muscular movement ⟨~ areas of the brain⟩

motor amusia *n* : AMUSIA 1

motor aphasia *n* : the inability to speak or to organize the muscular movements of speech — called also *aphemia, Broca's aphasia*

motor area *n* : any of various areas of cerebral cortex believed to be associated with the initiation, coordination, and transmission of motor impulses to lower centers; *specif* : a region immediately anterior to the central sulcus having an unusually thick zone of cortical gray matter and communicating with lower centers chiefly through the corticospinal tracts — see PRECENTRAL GYRUS

motor center *n* : a nervous center that controls or modifies (as by inhibiting or reinforcing) a motor impulse

motor cortex *n* : the cortex of a motor area; *also* : the motor areas as a functional whole

motor end plate *n* : the terminal arborization of a motor axon on a muscle fiber

mo·to·ri·al \mō-'tōr-ē-əl\ *adj* : MOTOR

mo·tor·ic \mō-'tȯr-ik, -'tär-\ *adj* : MOTOR 3 ⟨~ and verbal behavior⟩ — **mo·tor·i·cal·ly** \-i-k(ə-)lē\ *adv*

mo·to·ri·um \mō-'tōr-ē-əm\ *n, pl* **-ria** \-ē-ə\ **1** : the part of an organism and esp. the part of its nervous system that is concerned with movement as distinguished from that concerned with sensation **2** : a differentiated cytoplasmic area in certain protozoans that acts as a coordinating center analogous to the brain of higher animals

motor neuron *n* : a neuron that passes from the central nervous system or a ganglion toward or to a muscle and conducts an impulse that causes movement — called also *motoneuron;* compare INTERNEURON, SENSORY NEURON

motor paralysis *n* : paralysis of the voluntary muscles

motor point *n* : a small area on a muscle at which a minimal amount of electrical stimulation will cause the muscle to contract

motor protein *n* : a protein (as dynein, kinesin, or myosin) that moves itself along a filament or polymeric molecule using energy generated by the hydrolysis of ATP

motor root *n* : a nerve root containing only motor fibers; *specif* : VENTRAL ROOT — compare SENSORY ROOT

motor unit *n* : a motor neuron together with the muscle fibers on which it acts

Mo·trin \'mō-trən\ *trademark* — used for a preparation of ibuprofen

mot·tled enamel \ˌmät-ᵊld-\ *n* : spotted tooth enamel typically caused by drinking water containing excessive fluorides during the time the teeth are calcifying

mou·lage \mü-'läzh\ *n* : a mold of a lesion or defect used as a guide in applying medical treatment (as in radiotherapy) or in performing reconstructive surgery esp. on the face

mould, moulding, mouldy *chiefly Brit var of* MOLD, MOLDING, MOLDY

moult *chiefly Brit var of* MOLT

¹**mount** \'mau̇nt\ *vt* : to prepare for examination or display;

M
N

\ə\ **abut** \ᵊ\ **kitten** \ər\ **further** \a\ **ash** \ā\ **ace** \ä\ **cot, cart**
\au̇\ **out** \ch\ **chin** \e\ **bet** \ē\ **easy** \g\ **go** \i\ **hit** \ī\ **ice** \j\ **job**
\ŋ\ **sing** \ō\ **go** \ȯ\ **law** \ȯi\ **boy** \th\ **thin** \t̲h̲\ **the** \ü\ **loot**
\u̇\ **foot** \y\ **yet** \zh\ **vision** *See also* Pronunciation Symbols page

specif : to place (an object) on a slide for microscopic examination ⟨∼ a specimen⟩

²**mount** *n* **1** : a glass slide with its accessories on which objects are placed for examination with a microscope **2** : a specimen mounted on a slide for microscopic examination

moun·tain fever \'maùnt-ᵊn-\ *n* **1** : any of various febrile diseases occurring in mountainous regions **2** : EQUINE INFECTIOUS ANEMIA

mountain sickness *n* : altitude sickness experienced esp. above 10,000 feet (about 3000 meters) and caused by insufficient oxygen in the air

moun·tant \'maùnt-ᵊnt\ *n* : any substance in which a specimen is suspended between a slide and a cover glass for microscopic examination

moun·te·bank \'maùnt-i-ˌbaŋk\ *n* : an itinerant hawker of pills and patent medicines esp. from a platform : QUACK ⟨bought an unction of a ∼ —Shak.⟩

mounting medium *n* : a medium in which a biological specimen is mounted for preservation or display

mouse \'maùs\ *n, pl* **mice** \'mīs\ **1** : any of numerous small rodents with pointed snout, rather small ears, elongated body, and slender hairless or sparsely haired tail, including all the smaller members of the genus *Mus* (as the medically significant house mouse, *M. musculus*) and many members of other rodent genera and families having little more in common than their relatively small size **2** : a dark-colored swelling caused by a blow; *specif* : BLACK EYE

mouse·pox \'maùs-ˌpäks\ *n* : a highly contagious disease of mice that is caused by a poxvirus of the genus *Orthopoxvirus* (species *Ectromelia virus*) — called also *ectromelia*

mouth \'maùth\ *n, pl* **mouths** \'maùthz\ : the natural opening through which food passes into the animal body and which in vertebrates is typically bounded externally by the lips and internally by the pharynx and encloses the tongue, gums, and teeth

mouth breath·er \-ˌbrē-thər\ *n* : one who habitually inhales and exhales through the mouth rather than through the nose

mouth·part \'maùth-ˌpärt\ *n* : a structure or appendage near the mouth esp. of an insect

mouth–to–mouth *adj* : of, relating to, or being a method of artificial respiration in which the rescuer's mouth is placed tightly over the victim's mouth in order to force air into the victim's lungs by blowing forcefully enough every few seconds to inflate them ⟨∼ resuscitation⟩

mouth·wash \'maùth-ˌwòsh, -ˌwäsh\ *n* : a liquid preparation (as an antiseptic solution) for cleansing the mouth and teeth — called also *collutorium*

mov·able kidney \'mü-və-bəl-\ *n* : NEPHROPTOSIS

move \'müv\ *vb* **moved; mov·ing** *vi* **1** : to go or pass from one place to another **2** *of the bowels* : to eject fecal matter : EVACUATE ∼ *vt* **1** : to change the place or position of **2** : to cause (the bowels) to void

move·ment \'müv-mənt\ *n* **1** : the act or process of moving **2 a** : an act of voiding the bowels **b** : matter expelled from the bowels at one passage : STOOL

moxa \'mäk-sə\ *n* **1** : a soft woolly mass prepared from the ground young leaves of a Eurasian artemisia (esp. *Artemisia vulgaris*) that is used in traditional Chinese and Japanese medicine typically in the form of sticks or cones which are ignited and placed on or close to the skin or used to heat acupuncture needles **2** : any of various substances applied and ignited like moxa as a counterirritant

moxa·lac·tam \ˌmäk-sə-'lak-ˌtam\ *n* : a cephalosporin antibiotic administered parenterally in the form of its disodium salt $C_{20}H_{18}N_6Na_2O_9S$

mox·i·bus·tion \ˌmäk-si-'bəs-chən\ *n* : the therapeutic use of moxa

mp *abbr* melting point

MPC *abbr* maximum permissible concentration

MPD *abbr* multiple personality disorder

MPF *abbr* maturation promoting factor

MPH *abbr* master of public health

M phase \'em-ˌfāz\ *n* : the period in the cell cycle during which cell division takes place — called also *D phase;* compare G_1 PHASE, G_2 PHASE, S PHASE

M protein \'em-\ *n* **1** : an antigenic protein of Group A streptococci that is found on the cell wall extending into the surrounding capsule, is variable among the different serotypes, and confers streptococcal virulence by protecting the cell from phagocytotic action — called also *M substance* **2** : a monoclonal antibody that is produced by plasma cells abnormally proliferating from a single clone and that is characteristic of monoclonal gammopathy

MPTP \ˌem-(ˌ)pē-(ˌ)tē-'pē\ *n* [1-*m*ethyl-4-*p*henyl-1,2,3,6=*t*etrahydro*p*yridine] : a neurotoxin $C_{12}H_{15}N$ that destroys dopamine-producing neurons of the substantia nigra and causes symptoms (as tremors and rigidity) similar to those of Parkinson's disease

mR *abbr* milliroentgen

MR *abbr* magnetic resonance

MRA *abbr* magnetic resonance angiography

mrad *abbr* millirad

Mrad *abbr* megarad

MR angiography \ˌem-'är-\ *n* : MAGNETIC RESONANCE ANGIOGRAPHY

mrem *abbr* millirem

MRI \ˌem-(ˌ)är-'ī\ *n* : MAGNETIC RESONANCE IMAGING; *also* : a procedure in which magnetic resonance imaging is used

mRNA \'em-ˌär-'en-'ā\ *n* : MESSENGER RNA

MRS *abbr* magnetic resonance spectroscopy

MRSA \ˌem-ˌär-ˌes-'ā\ *n* [*m*ethicillin-*r*esistant *S*taphylococcus *a*ureus] : any of several bacterial strains of the genus *Staphylococcus* (*S. aureus*) that are resistant to beta-lactam antibiotics (as methicillin and nafcillin) and that are typically benign colonizers of the skin and mucous membranes (as of the nostrils) but may cause severe infections (as by entrance through a surgical wound) esp. in immunocompromised individuals

ms *abbr* millisecond

MS *abbr* **1** mass spectrometry **2** master of science **3** multiple sclerosis

MSc *abbr* master of science

msec *abbr* millisecond

MSG *abbr* monosodium glutamate

MSH *abbr* melanocyte-stimulating hormone

MSN *abbr* master of science in nursing

M substance \'em-ˌ\ *n* : M PROTEIN 1

mSv *abbr* millisievert

MSW *abbr* master of social work

Mt *symbol* meitnerium

MT *abbr* medical technologist

MTD *abbr* maximum tolerated dose

mtDNA \ˌem-(ˌ)tē-ˌdē-(ˌ)en-'ā\ *n* : MITOCHONDRIAL DNA

mu \'myü, 'mü\ *n, pl* **mu** : MICRON

mu·cate \'myü-ˌkāt\ *n* : a salt of mucic acid esp. when formed by combination with a drug that is an organic base and used as a vehicle for administration of the drug

mu·cic acid \ˌmyü-sik-\ *n* : an optically inactive crystalline acid $C_6H_{10}O_8$ obtained from galactose or lactose by oxidation with nitric acid

mu·ci·car·mine \ˌmyü-sə-'kär-mən, -ˌmīn\ *n* : a stain consisting of carmine in solution with aluminum chloride that is used for detecting mucin

mu·cif·er·ous \myü-'sif-(ə-)rəs\ *adj* : producing or filled with mucus ⟨∼ ducts⟩

mu·ci·fi·ca·tion \ˌmyü-sə-fə-'kā-shən\ *n* : the transformation of epithelial cells into mucus-secreting cells ⟨vaginal ∼⟩

mu·ci·fy \'myü-sə-ˌfī\ *vi* **-fied; -fy·ing** : to undergo mucification

mu·ci·gen \-jən, -ˌjen\ *n* : MUCINOGEN

mu·ci·lage \'myü-s(ə-)lij\ *n* **1** : a gelatinous substance of various plants (as legumes or seaweeds) that contains protein and polysaccharides and is similar to plant gums **2** : an aqueous usu. viscid solution (as of a gum) used in pharmacy as an excipient and in medicine as a demulcent

mu·ci·lag·i·nous \ˌmyü-sə-'laj-ə-nəs\ *adj* : relating to, resembling, containing, or secreting mucilage

mu·cil·loid \\'myü-sə-ˌlȯid\\ *n* : a mucilaginous substance

mu·cin \\'myüs-ᵊn\\ *n* : any of a group of mucoproteins that are found in various human and animal secretions and tissues (as in saliva, the lining of the stomach, and the skin) and that are white or yellowish powders when dry and viscid when moist ⟨gastric ∼⟩

mu·cin·o·gen \\myü-'sin-ə-jən, -ˌjen\\ *n* : any of various substances which undergo conversion into mucins — called also *mucigen*

mu·cin·oid \\'myü-sᵊn-ˌȯid\\ *adj* : resembling mucin

mu·ci·no·lyt·ic \\ˌmyü-sᵊn-ō-'lit-ik\\ *adj* : tending to break down or lower the viscosity of mucin-containing body secretions or components ⟨a ∼ enzyme⟩

mu·ci·no·sis \\ˌmyü-sə-'nō-səs\\ *n, pl* **-no·ses** \\-ˌsēz\\ : a condition characterized by the presence of abnormally high concentrations of mucins in the skin

mu·ci·nous \\'myü-sᵊn-əs\\ *adj* : of, relating to, resembling, or containing mucin ⟨∼ fluid⟩ ⟨∼ carcinoma⟩

mu·cip·a·rous \\myü-'sip-ə-rəs\\ *adj* : secreting mucus ⟨∼ cells⟩

mu·co·buc·cal fold \\ˌmyü-kō-'bək-əl-\\ *n* : the fold formed by the oral mucosa where it passes from the mandible or maxilla to the cheek

mu·co·cele \\'myü-kə-ˌsēl\\ *n* : a swelling like a sac that is due to distension of a hollow organ or cavity with mucus ⟨a ∼ of the appendix⟩; *specif* : a dilated lacrimal sac

mu·co·cil·i·ary \\ˌmyü-kō-'sil-ē-ˌer-ē\\ *adj* : of, relating to, or involving cilia of the mucous membranes of the respiratory system ⟨∼ transport in the lung⟩

mu·co·cu·ta·ne·ous \\ˌmyü-kō-kyu̇-'tā-nē-əs\\ *adj* : made up of or involving both typical skin and mucous membrane ⟨the ∼ junction of the mouth⟩ ⟨∼ candidiasis⟩

mucocutaneous lymph node disease *n* : KAWASAKI DISEASE

mucocutaneous lymph node syndrome *n* : KAWASAKI DISEASE

mu·co·epi·der·moid \\ˌmyü-kō-ˌep-ə-'dər-ˌmȯid\\ *adj* : of, relating to, or consisting of both mucous and squamous epithelial cells; *esp* : being a tumor of the salivary glands made up of mucous and epithelial elements ⟨∼ carcinoma⟩

mu·co·floc·cu·lent \\-'fläk-yə-lənt\\ *adj* : consisting of or containing flaky shreds of mucus

mu·co·gin·gi·val \\-'jin-jə-vəl\\ *adj* : of, relating to, or being the junction between the oral mucosa and the gingiva ⟨the ∼ line⟩

¹mu·coid \\'myü-ˌkȯid\\ *adj* **1** : resembling mucus **2** : forming large moist sticky colonies — used of dissociated strains of bacteria

²mucoid *n* : MUCOPROTEIN

mucoid degeneration *n* : tissue degeneration marked by conversion of cell substance into a glutinous substance like mucus

mucoid tissue *n* : MUCOUS TISSUE

mu·coi·tin·sul·fu·ric acid *or chiefly Brit* **mu·coi·tin·sul·phu·ric acid** \\myü-'kō-ət-ᵊn-ˌsəl-ˌfyu̇r-ik, -'kȯit-ᵊn-\\ *n* : an acidic glycosaminoglycan found esp. in the cornea of the eye and in gastric mucosa

mu·co·lip·i·do·sis \\ˌmyü-kō-ˌlip-ə-'dō-səs\\ *n, pl* **-do·ses** \\-ˌsēz\\ : any of several metabolic disorders that are marked by the accumulation of glycosaminoglycans and lipids in tissues and by lysosomal enzymes which are produced in deficient amounts or which fail to be incorporated into lysosomes, that are inherited as autosomal recessive traits, and that have characteristics (as mental retardation) resembling Hurler's syndrome

mu·co·lyt·ic \\ˌmyü-kə-'lit-ik\\ *adj* : hydrolyzing glycosaminoglycans : tending to break down or lower the viscosity of mucin-containing body secretions or components ⟨∼ enzymes⟩

Mu·co·myst \\'myü-kə-ˌmist\\ *trademark* — used for a preparation of acetylcysteine

mu·co·pep·tide \\ˌmyü-kō-'pep-ˌtīd\\ *n* : PEPTIDOGLYCAN

mu·co·peri·os·te·al \\-ˌper-ē-'äs-tē-əl\\ *adj* : of or relating to the mucoperiosteum

mu·co·peri·os·te·um \\-'äs-tē-əm\\ *n* : a periosteum backed with mucous membrane (as that of the palatine surface of the mouth)

mu·co·poly·sac·cha·ride \\ˌmyü-kō-ˌpäl-i-'sak-ə-ˌrīd\\ *n* : GLYCOSAMINOGLYCAN

mu·co·poly·sac·cha·ri·do·sis \\-ˌsak-ə-rī-'dō-səs\\ *n, pl* **-do·ses** \\-ˌsēz\\ : any of a group of genetically determined disorders (as Hunter's syndrome and Hurler's syndrome) of glycosaminoglycan metabolism that are characterized by the accumulation of glycosaminoglycans in the tissues and their excretion in the urine — called also *gargoylism, lipochondrodystrophy*

mu·co·pro·tein \\ˌmyü-kə-'prō-ˌtēn, -'prōt-ē-ən\\ *n* : any of a group of various complex conjugated proteins (as mucins) that contain glycosaminoglycans (as chondroitin sulfate or mucoitinsulfuric acid) combined with amino acid units or polypeptides and that occur in body fluids and tissues — called also *mucoid;* compare GLYCOPROTEIN

mu·co·pu·ru·lent \\-'pyu̇r-(y)ə-lənt\\ *adj* : containing both mucus and pus ⟨∼ discharge⟩

mu·co·pus \\ˌmyü-kō-ˌpəs\\ *n* : mucus mixed with pus

mu·cor \\'myü-ˌkȯ(ə)r\\ *n* **1** *cap* : a genus (the type of the family Mucoraceae) of molds that are distinguished from molds of the genus *Rhizopus* by having round usu. cylindrical or pear-shaped sporangia not clustered and not limited in location to the points where rhizoids develop and that include several (as *M. corymbifer*) causing infections in humans and animals **2** : any mold of the genus *Mucor*

Mu·co·ra·ce·ae \\ˌmyü-kə-'rā-sē-ˌē\\ *n pl* : a large family of chiefly saprophytic molds of the order Mucorales having a well-developed branching mycelium that lacks septa and including many molds (as members of the genera *Rhizopus* and *Mucor*) that are destructive to food products (as bread, fruits, or vegetables) — **mu·co·ra·ceous** \\-'rā-shəs\\ *adj*

Mu·co·ra·les \\-'rā-(ˌ)lēz\\ *n pl* : an order of mostly saprophytic fungi of the subclass Zygomycetes that reproduce asexually by spores borne within sporangia and sexually by homothallic or heterothallic zygospores and that include many common domestic molds

mu·cor·my·co·sis \\ˌmyü-kər-mī-'kō-səs\\ *n, pl* **-co·ses** \\-ˌsēz\\ : mycosis caused by fungi of the genus *Mucor* usu. primarily involving the lungs and invading other tissues by means of metastatic lesions — **mu·cor·my·cot·ic** \\-'kät-ik\\ *adj*

mu·co·sa \\myü-'kō-zə\\ *n, pl* **-sae** \\-(ˌ)zē, -ˌzī\\ *or* **-sas** : MUCOUS MEMBRANE — **mu·co·sal** \\-zəl\\ *adj*

mucosae — see MUSCULARIS MUCOSAE

mucosal disease *n* : BOVINE VIRAL DIARRHEA

mu·co·san·guin·eous \\ˌmyü-kō-san-'gwin-ē-əs, -saŋ-\\ *adj* : containing mucus and blood ⟨∼ feces⟩

mu·co·se·rous \\-'sir-əs\\ *adj* : containing or producing both mucous and serous matter

mu·co·si·tis \\ˌmyü-kə-'sīt-əs\\ *n* : inflammation of a mucous membrane

mu·cos·i·ty \\myü-'käs-ət-ē\\ *n, pl* **-ties** : the quality or state of being mucous

mu·co·stat·ic \\ˌmyü-kə-'stat-ik\\ *adj* **1** : of, relating to, or representing the mucosal tissues of the jaws as they are in a state of rest ⟨a ∼ impression taken without displacing any tissue⟩ **2** : stopping the secretion of mucus

mu·cous \\'myü-kəs\\ *adj* **1** : covered with or as if with mucus ⟨a ∼ surface⟩ **2** : of, relating to, or resembling mucus ⟨a ∼ secretion⟩ **3** : secreting or containing mucus ⟨∼ glands of the intestine⟩

mucous cell *n* : a cell that secretes mucus

mucous colitis *n* : IRRITABLE BOWEL SYNDROME; *esp* : irritable bowel syndrome characterized by the passage of unusually large amounts of mucus

mucous membrane *n* : a membrane rich in mucous glands; *specif* : one that lines body passages and cavities which com-

---

\\ə\\ **abut** \\ᵊ\\ **kitten** \\ər\\ **further** \\a\\ **ash** \\ā\\ **ace** \\ä\\ **cot, cart**
\\au̇\\ **out** \\ch\\ **chin** \\e\\ **bet** \\ē\\ **easy** \\g\\ **go** \\i\\ **hit** \\ī\\ **ice** \\j\\ **job**
\\ŋ\\ **sing** \\ō\\ **go** \\ȯ\\ **law** \\ȯi\\ **boy** \\th\\ **thin** \\th̲\\ **the** \\ü\\ **loot**
\\u̇\\ **foot** \\y\\ **yet** \\zh\\ **vision** *See also* Pronunciation Symbols page

M
N

municate directly or indirectly with the exterior (as the alimentary, respiratory, and genitourinary tracts), that functions in protection, support, nutrient absorption, and secretion of mucus, enzymes, and salts, and that consists of a deep vascular connective-tissue stroma which in many parts of the alimentary canal contains a thin but definite layer of nonstriated muscle and a superficial epithelium which has an underlying basement membrane and varies in kind and thickness but is always soft and smooth and kept lubricated by the secretions of the cells and numerous glands embedded in the membrane — called also *mucosa;* compare SEROUS MEMBRANE

mucous neck cell *n* : a mucous cell in the neck of a gastric gland

mucous patch *n* : a broad flat syphilitic condyloma that is often marked by a yellowish discharge and that occurs on moist skin or mucous membranes

mucous tissue *n* : a gelatinous connective tissue that contains stellate cells with long processes in a soft matrix and that occurs in the umbilical cord and in the embryo and in myxomas

mu·co·vis·ci·do·sis \ˌmyü-kō-ˌvis-ə-ˈdō-səs\ *n, pl* **-do·ses** \-ˌsēz\ : CYSTIC FIBROSIS

mu·cro \ˈmyü-ˌkrō\ *n, pl* **mu·cro·nes** \myü-ˈkrō-(ˌ)nēz\ : an abrupt sharp terminal point or tip or process — **mu·cro·nate** \ˈmyü-krə-ˌnāt\ *adj*

Mu·cu·na \myü-ˈkü-nə\ *n* : a genus of tropical herbs and woody vines of the family Leguminosae with clusters of showy flowers that includes cowhage (*M. pruritum*)

mu·cus \ˈmyü-kəs\ *n* : a viscid slippery secretion that is usu. rich in mucins and is produced by mucous membranes which it moistens and protects

mud bath \ˈməd-\ *n* : an immersion of the body or a part of it in mud (as for the alleviation of rheumatism or gout)

mud fever *n* **1** : a chapped inflamed condition of the skin of the legs and belly of a horse due to irritation from mud or drying resulting from washing off mud spatters and closely related or identical in nature to grease heel **2** : BLUE COMB **3** : a mild leptospirosis that occurs chiefly in European agricultural and other workers in wet soil, is caused by infection with a spirochete of the genus *Leptospira* (*L. grippotyphosa*) present in native field mice, and is marked by fever and headache without accompanying jaundice

muellerian *var of* MÜLLERIAN

Muellerian duct *var of* MÜLLERIAN DUCT

Muel·le·ri·us \myü-ˈlir-ē-əs\ *n* : a genus of lungworms of the family Metastrongylidae that include forms (as *M. capillaris* syn. *M. minutissimus*) infecting the lungs of sheep and goats and having larval stages in various snails and slugs

Mül·ler \ˈmʊel-ər\, **Fritz (Johann Friedrich Theodor) (1822–1897),** German zoologist. Working mostly in So. America, Müller made major contributions to the anatomy of invertebrates including the coelenterates, annelids, and crustaceans, to entomology, and to botany. From 1878 onward Müller published a series of articles reporting the mimicry that exists among similar, unpalatable species of insects. This is now known as Müllerian mimicry.

MUFA \ˈməf-ə, ˈm(y)ü-fə\ *n* : a monounsaturated fatty acid

mul·ber·ry \ˈməl-ˌber-ē, -b(ə-)rē\ *n, pl* **-ries** : any of a genus (*Morus* of the family Moraceae, the mulberry family) of trees with an edible usu. purple fruit that includes one (*M. nigra*) with a fruit whose juice is sometimes used for its medicinal properties; *also* : the fruit

mulberry calculus *n* : a mulberry-shaped urinary calculus of calcium oxalate

mulberry mass *n* : MORULA

mulberry molar *n* : a first molar tooth whose occlusal surface is pitted due to congenital syphilis with nodules replacing the cusps — see MOON'S MOLAR

mule \ˈmyü(ə)l\ *n* : a hybrid between a horse and a donkey; *esp* : the offspring of a male donkey and a mare

mules·ing \ˈmyül-ziŋ\ *n* : the use of Mules operation to reduce the occurrence of blowfly strike — **mulesed** \ˈmyülzd\ *adj*

Mules operation \ˈmyülz-\ *n* : removal of excess loose skin from either side of the crutch of a sheep to reduce the incidence of blowfly strike

Mules, J. H. W. Australian sheep grazier. Mules, a grazier at Woodside, South Australia, first proposed the Mules operation in 1931. Since that time the operation has become a standard procedure especially in Australia and New Zealand.

¹mull \ˈməl\ *vt* : to grind or mix thoroughly (as in a mortar) : PULVERIZE ⟨the alloy, after removal from the amalgamator, was ~ed in the palm of the hand —*Jour. of Amer. Dental Assoc.*⟩

²mull *n* **1** : a soft fine sheer fabric of cotton, silk, or rayon **2** : an ointment of high melting point intended to be spread on muslin or mull and used like a plaster ⟨zinc ~⟩

mull·er \ˈməl-ər\ *n* : a stone or piece of wood, metal, or glass having a usu. flat base and often a handle and held in the hand to pound, grind, or mix a material (as a drug) or to polish a surface : PESTLE

Mül·ler cell *also* **Mül·ler's cell** \ˈmyül-ər(z)-, ˈmil-, ˈməl-\ *n* : FIBER OF MÜLLER

mül·le·ri·an *also* **muel·le·ri·an** \myü-ˈlir-ē-ən, mi-, mə-\ *adj, often cap* **1** : discovered by or named after the German physiologist Johannes Peter Müller **2** : discovered by or named after the German anatomist Heinrich Müller

Mül·ler \ˈmʊel-ər\, **Heinrich (1820–1864),** German anatomist. Müller discovered rhodopsin in 1851. In 1856 with Rudolph A. von Kölliker (1817–1905) he demonstrated that each contraction of a frog's heart produces an electric current. In 1858 he published classic descriptions of three eye muscles: the superior and inferior muscles of the tarsal plate, the muscle that bridges the inferior orbital fissure, and the innermost fibers of the circular portion of the ciliary muscle.

Müller, Johannes Peter (1801–1858), German physiologist and anatomist. Müller is generally acclaimed as one of the greatest biologists of all time. In 1834–40 he published a handbook of physiology that ranks as the first great text on that subject produced in the 19th century. In histology he described the microscopic anatomy of a large series of secreting glands. He was the first to classify the excretory system of the glands as an independent system of tubes; he noted that the blood vessels formed only a capillary network. He described the Müllerian duct in 1825.

Müllerian duct *also* **Muellerian duct** *n* : either of a pair of ducts parallel to the Wolffian ducts in vertebrate animals and giving rise in the female to the oviducts — called also *paramesonephric duct*

J. P. Müller — see MÜLLERIAN

müllerian in·hib·it·ing substance \-in-ˌhib-ət-iŋ-\ *n* : a glycoprotein hormone produced by the Sertoli cells of the male during fetal development that causes regression and atrophy of the Müllerian ducts

J. P. Müller — see MÜLLERIAN

Müllerian tubercle *n* : an elevation on the wall of the embryonic urogenital sinus where the Müllerian ducts enter

J. P. Müller — see MÜLLERIAN

Müller's muscle *n* : the circular muscle fibers comprising the inner set of muscle fibers of the ciliary muscle of the eye

H. Müller — see MÜLLERIAN

¹mult·an·gu·lar \ˌməl-ˈtaŋ-gyə-lər\ *adj* : having many angles ⟨a ~ bone⟩

²multangular *n* : a multangular bone — see TRAPEZIUM, TRAPEZOID

mul·ti·an·gu·lar \ˌməl-tē-ˈaŋ-gyə-lər, ˌməl-ˌtī-\ *adj* : MULTANGULAR

mul·ti·cel·lu·lar \-ˈsel-yə-lər\ *adj* : having or consisting of many cells — **mul·ti·cel·lu·lar·i·ty** \-ˌsel-yə-ˈlar-ət-ē\ *n, pl* **-ties**

mul·ti·cen·ter \ˈməl-tē-ˌsen-tər, ˈməl-ˌtī-\ *adj* : involving more than one medical or research institution ⟨a ~ clinical study⟩

mul·ti·cen·tric \ˌməl-tē-ˈsen-trik, ˌməl-ˌtī-\ *adj* : having multiple centers of origin ⟨a ~ tumor⟩ — **mul·ti·cen·tri·cal·ly**

\-tri-k(ə-)lē\ *adv* — **mul·ti·cen·tric·i·ty** \-sen-'tris-ət-ē\ *n, pl* **-ties**

mul·ti·ceps \'məl-tə-ˌseps\ *n* **1** *cap* : a genus of cyclophyllidean tapeworms of the family Taeniidae that have a coenurus larva parasitic in ruminants, rodents, and rarely humans and that include the parasite of gid (*M. multiceps*) and other worms typically parasitic on carnivores **2** : COENURUS

mul·ti·chain \'məl-tē-ˌchān, -ˌtī-\ *adj* : containing more than one chain ⟨∼ proteins⟩

mul·ti·clo·nal \ˌməl-tē-'klō-nəl, -ˌtī-\ *adj* : POLYCLONAL

mul·ti·cus·pid \-'kəs-pəd\ *adj* : having several cusps ⟨a ∼ tooth⟩

mul·ti·cys·tic \-'sis-tik\ *adj* : POLYCYSTIC

mul·ti·den·tate \-'den-ˌtāt\ *adj* : being, containing, or involving a ligand that can form bonds at more than one point

mul·ti·dose \'məl-ti-ˌdōs\ *adj* : utilizing or containing more than one dose ⟨∼ regimens⟩ ⟨a ∼ vial⟩

mul·ti·drug \-ˌdrəg\ *adj* : utilizing or relating to more than one drug ⟨∼ therapy⟩

multidrug–resistant *adj* : resistant to more than one drug ⟨∼ tuberculosis⟩

mul·ti·en·zyme \ˌməl-tē-'en-ˌzīm, -ˌtī-\ *adj* : composed of or involving two or more enzymes or subunits similar to enzymes that function in a biosynthetic pathway ⟨a ∼ complex⟩

mul·ti·fac·to·ri·al \-fak-'tōr-ē-əl, -'tor-\ *adj* **1** : having characters or a mode of inheritance dependent on a number of genes at different loci **2** *or* **mul·ti·fac·tor** \-'fak-tər\ : having, involving, or produced by a variety of elements or causes ⟨a ∼ study⟩ ⟨a disease with a ∼ etiology⟩ — **mul·ti·fac·to·ri·al·ly** \-ē-ə-lē\ *adv* — **mul·ti·fac·to·ri·al·i·ty** \-ˌtōr-ē-'al-ət-ē, -ˌtor-\ *n, pl* **-ties**

mul·tif·i·dus \ˌməl-'tif-ə-dəs\ *n, pl* **-di** \-ˌdī\ : a muscle of the fifth and deepest layer of the back filling up the groove on each side of the spinous processes of the vertebrae from the sacrum to the skull and consisting of many fasciculi that pass upward and inward to the spinous processes and help to erect and rotate the spine

mul·ti·fo·cal \ˌməl-ti-'fō-kəl\ *adj* **1** : having more than one focal length ⟨∼ lenses⟩ **2** : arising from or occurring in more than one focus or location ⟨∼ seizures⟩

multifocal leukoencephalopathy — see PROGRESSIVE MULTIFOCAL LEUKOENCEPHALOPATHY

mul·ti·form \'məl-ti-ˌform\ *adj* : having or occurring in many forms — **mul·ti·for·mi·ty** \ˌməl-ti-'for-mət-ē\ *n, pl* **-ties**

multiforme — see ERYTHEMA MULTIFORME, GLIOBLASTOMA MULTIFORME

mul·ti·gene \ˌməl-tē-'jēn, -ˌtī-\ *adj* : relating to or determined by a group of genes which were orig. copies of the same gene but evolved by mutation to become different from each other ⟨a ∼ family of proteins with a common evolutionary origin —Vann Bennett *et al*⟩

mul·ti·gen·ic \ˌməl-ti-'jen-ik, -ˌjēn-\ *adj* : MULTIFACTORIAL 1 ⟨∼ chromosomal blocks —*Advances in Genetics*⟩

mul·ti·glan·du·lar \-'glan-jə-lər\ *adj* : POLYGLANDULAR

mul·ti·grav·i·da \-'grav-əd-ə\ *n, pl* **-dae** \-ə-ˌdē\ *also* **-das** : a woman who has been pregnant more than once — compare MULTIPARA

mul·ti·han·di·capped \ˌməl-tē-'han-di-ˌkapt, -ˌtī-\ *adj, sometimes offensive* : affected by more than one mental or physical disability

mul·ti·hos·pi·tal \-'häs-ˌpit-ᵊl\ *adj* : involving or affiliated with more than one hospital ⟨a ∼ group of researchers⟩

mul·ti–in·farct dementia \-'in-ˌfärkt-, -in-'färkt-\ *n* : irreversible dementia that results from a series of small strokes in which cerebral infarction occurs and in which mental deterioration is usu. characterized by stepwise progression

mul·ti·lay·er \'məl-ti-ˌlā-ər, -ˌle(ə)r\ *n* : a layer built up of two or more layers and esp. monolayers

mul·ti·lay·ered \ˌməl-ti-'lā-ərd, -'le(-ə)rd\ *or* **mul·ti·lay·er** \-'lā-ər, -'le(-ə)r\ *adj* : having or involving several distinct layers, strata, or levels ⟨∼ epidermis⟩ ⟨a ∼ personality⟩

mul·ti·lobed \-'lōbd\ *adj* : having two or more lobes

mul·ti·loc·u·lar \ˌməl-ti-'läk-yə-lər\ *adj* : having or divided into many small chambers or vesicles ⟨a ∼ cyst⟩

mul·ti·mam·mate mouse \-'mam-ˌāt-\ *n* : any of several common African rodents of the genus *Rattus* that have 12 rather than the usual five or six mammae on each side, are vectors of disease, and are used in medical research — called also *multimammate rat*

mul·ti·mo·dal \ˌməl-ti-'mōd-ᵊl\ *adj* : relating to, having, or utilizing more than one mode or modality (as of stimulation or treatment) ⟨∼ cancer therapy involving surgery, immunotherapy, and radiation⟩

mul·ti·neu·ro·nal \-'n(y)ùr-ən-ᵊl, -n(y)ù-'rōn-ᵊl\ *adj* : made up of or involving more than one neuron ⟨∼ activity⟩

mul·ti·nod·u·lar \-'näj-ə-lər\ *adj* : having many nodules ⟨∼ goiter⟩

mul·ti·nu·cle·ate \-'n(y)ü-klē-ət\ *or* **mul·ti·nu·cle·at·ed** \-klē-ˌāt-əd\ *adj* : having more than two nuclei

mul·ti·or·gan \-'or-gən\ *adj* : of, involving, or affecting more than one organ ⟨∼ failure⟩

mul·ti·or·gas·mic \-ˌor-'gaz-mik\ *adj* : experiencing one orgasm after another with little or no recovery period between them

mul·ti·p·a·ra \ˌməl-'tip-ə-rə\ *n, pl* **-ras** *or* **-rae** \-ˌrē\ : a woman who has borne more than one child — see GRAND MULTIPARA; compare MULTIGRAVIDA

mul·ti·par·i·ty \ˌməl-ti-'par-ət-ē\ *n, pl* **-ties** **1** : the production of two or more young at a birth **2** : the condition of having borne a number of children

mul·tip·a·rous \ˌməl-'tip-ər-əs\ *adj* **1** : producing many or more than one at a birth **2** : having experienced one or more previous parturitions — compare PRIMIPAROUS

Multiphasic — see MINNESOTA MULTIPHASIC PERSONALITY INVENTORY

mul·ti·ple \'məl-tə-pəl\ *adj* **1** : consisting of, including, or involving more than one ⟨∼ births⟩ **2** : affecting many parts of the body at once

multiple allele *n* : an allele of a genetic locus having more than two allelic forms within a population

multiple allelism *n* : the state of having more than two alternative contrasting characters controlled by multiple alleles at a single genetic locus

multiple factor *n* : POLYGENE

multiple fission *n* : division of a cell into more than two parts — compare BINARY FISSION

multiple myeloma *n* : a disease of bone marrow that is characterized by the presence of numerous myelomas in various bones of the body — called also *myelomatosis*

multiple organ dysfunction syndrome *n* : progressive dysfunction of two or more major organ systems in a critically ill patient that makes it impossible to maintain homeostasis without medical intervention and that is typically a complication of sepsis and is a major factor in predicting mortality — abbr. *MODS*

multiple personality *n* : MULTIPLE PERSONALITY DISORDER

multiple personality disorder *n* : a dissociative disorder that is characterized by the presence of two or more distinct and complex identities or personality states each of which becomes dominant and controls behavior from time to time to the exclusion of the others — abbr. *MPD;* called also *alternating personality, dissociative identity disorder*

multiple sclerosis *n* : a demyelinating disease marked by patches of hardened tissue in the brain or the spinal cord and associated esp. with partial or complete paralysis and jerking muscle tremor

multiplex — see ARTHROGRYPOSIS MULTIPLEX CONGENITA, MONONEURITIS MULTIPLEX, PARAMYOCLONUS MULTIPLEX

mul·ti·plic·i·ty \ˌməl-tə-'plis-ət-ē\ *n, pl* **-ties** **1** : the quality or state of being multiple or various **2** : the ratio of the

M

N

number of infectious particles (as of a bacteriophage) to the number of cells at risk ⟨monolayer cultures . . . were infected at an effective ∼ of approximately 100 —J. J. Holland⟩

mul·ti·po·lar \ˌməl-ti-ˈpō-lər, -ˌtī-\ *adj* **1** : having several poles ⟨∼ mitoses⟩ **2** : having several dendrites ⟨∼ nerve cells⟩ — **mul·ti·po·lar·i·ty** \-ˌpō-ˈlar-ət-ē\ *n, pl* **-ties**

mul·tip·o·tent \ˌməl-ˈtip-ət-ənt\ *adj* : having the potential of becoming any of several mature cell types ⟨∼ stem cells⟩

mul·ti·po·ten·tial \ˌməl-ti-pə-ˈten-chəl, -ˌtī-\ *adj* : MULTIPOTENT

mul·ti·re·sis·tant \ˌməl-tē-ri-ˈzis-tənt, -ˌtī-\ *adj* : biologically resistant to several toxic agents ⟨∼ falciparum malaria⟩ — **mul·ti·re·sis·tance** \-tən(t)s\ *n*

mul·ti·spe·cial·ty \-ˈspesh-əl-tē\ *adj* : providing service in or staffed by members of several medical specialties ⟨∼ health centers⟩

mul·ti·syn·ap·tic \-sə-ˈnap-tik\ *adj* : relating to or consisting of more than one synapse ⟨∼ pathways in the central nervous system⟩

mul·ti·sys·tem \-ˌsis-təm\ *also* **mul·ti·sys·tem·ic** \-sis-ˈtem-ik\ *adj* : relating to, consisting of, or involving more than one bodily system ⟨systemic lupus erythematosus is a ∼ disease⟩

¹**mul·ti·va·lent** \ˌməl-ti-ˈvā-lənt, -ˌtī-\ *adj* **1** : POLYVALENT **2** : represented more than twice in the somatic chromosome number ⟨∼ chromosomes⟩

²**multivalent** *n* : a multivalent group of chromosomes

mul·ti·ve·sic·u·lar \-və-ˈsik-yə-lər, -ve-\ *adj* : having, containing, or composed of many vesicles ⟨a ∼ cyst⟩

multivesicular body *n* : a lysosome that is a membranous sac containing numerous small endocytic vesicles

mul·ti·ves·sel \-ˈves-əl\ *adj* : affecting more than one blood vessel ⟨patients with ∼ coronary artery disease⟩

¹**mul·ti·vi·ta·min** \-ˈvīt-ə-mən, *Brit also* -ˈvit-\ *adj* : containing several vitamins and esp. all known to be essential to health ⟨a ∼ formula⟩

²**multivitamin** *n* : a multivitamin preparation

mum·mi·fi·ca·tion \ˌməm-i-fə-ˈkā-shən\ *n* **1** : the process of mummifying or the state of being mummified **2** : the devitalization of a tooth pulp followed by amputation of the coronal portion leaving the remainder of the devitalized tissue in the tooth canal **3** : DRY GANGRENE

mum·mi·fy \ˈməm-i-ˌfī\ *vb* **-fied; -fy·ing** *vt* **1** : to embalm and dry as or as if a mummy **2 a** : to make into or like a mummy **b** : to cause to dry up and shrivel ∼ *vi* : to dry up and shrivel like a mummy ⟨a *mummified* fetus⟩

mumps \ˈməm(p)s\ *n pl but sing or pl in constr* : an acute contagious virus disease caused by a paramyxovirus of the genus *Rubulavirus* (species *Mumps virus*) and marked by fever and by swelling esp. of the parotid gland — called also *epidemic parotitis*

Mun·chau·sen syndrome \ˈmən-ˌchau̇-zən-\ *or* **Mun·chau·sen's syndrome** \-zənz-\ *n* : a psychological disorder characterized by the feigning of the symptoms of a disease or injury in order to undergo diagnostic tests, hospitalization, or medical or surgical treatment

Münch·hau·sen \ˈmᵫnk-ˌhau̇-zən\, **Karl Friedrich Hieronymous, Freiherr von (1720–1797),** German soldier. As a retired cavalry officer Münchhausen acquired a reputation as a raconteur of preposterous stories about his adventures as a soldier, hunter, and sportsman. From 1781 to 1783 a collection of such tales was published, with authorship generally attributed to the baron. An English version of the tales was published in 1785 under the title *Baron Munchausen's Narrative of His Marvellous Travels and Campaigns in Russia.* Only years later in 1824 was it revealed that the author of the English edition was Rudolph Erich Raspe (1737–1794). Other authors used these stories as source material to exaggerate still further or to compose other tall tales of a similar mode. Gradually Münchhausen's name became associated with the amusingly preposterous story or the lie winningly told.

Munchausen syndrome by proxy *also* **Munchausen's syndrome by proxy** \-bī-ˈpräk-sē\ *n* : a psychological disor-

der in which a parent and typically a mother harms her child (as by poisoning), falsifies the child's medical history, or tampers with the child's medical specimens in order to create a situation that requires or seems to require medical attention

mu·pir·o·cin \myü-ˈpir-ō-sən, -ˈpir-ə-\ *n* : an antibacterial drug $C_{26}H_{44}O_9$ that inhibits bacterial protein synthesis and is used in the topical treatment of impetigo caused by some bacteria of the genera *Streptococcus* and *Staphylococcus* — see BACTROBAN

mu·ral \ˈmyu̇r-əl\ *adj* : attached to and limited to a wall or a cavity ⟨a ∼ thrombus⟩ ⟨∼ abscesses⟩

mu·ram·ic acid \myu̇-ˈram-ik-\ *n* : an amino sugar $C_9H_{17}NO_7$ that is a lactic acid derivative of glucosamine and is found esp. in bacterial cell walls

mu·ram·i·dase \myu̇-ˈram-ə-ˌdās, -ˌdāz\ *n* : LYSOZYME

mu·rar·i·um \myu̇-ˈrar-ē-əm, -ˈrer-\ *n* : a place for rearing mice or rats under controlled conditions

mu·rein \ˈmyu̇r-ē-ən, ˈmyu̇(ə)r-ˌēn\ *n* : PEPTIDOGLYCAN

mu·rex·ide \myu̇-ˈrek-ˌsīd\ *n* : a red crystalline compound $C_8H_8N_6O_6$ having a green luster, forming purple-red solutions with water, formerly used as a dye, and formed in the murexide test for uric acid

murexide test *n* : a reaction giving rise to murexide when uric acid or a related compound is heated with nitric acid and the product is treated with ammonia — called also *murexide reaction*

mu·ri·ate \ˈmyu̇r-ē-ˌāt\ *n* : CHLORIDE 1

mu·ri·at·ic acid \ˌmyu̇r-ē-ˌat-ik-\ *n* : HYDROCHLORIC ACID

mu·rid \ˈmyu̇r-id\ *n* : any rodent of the family Muridae — **murid** *adj*

Mu·ri·dae \ˈmyu̇r-ə-ˌdē\ *n pl* : a very large family of relatively small rodents (superfamily Muroidea) that include various orig. Old World rodents (as the house mouse and the common rats) that are now cosmopolitan in distribution and that in recent classifications often include the cricetid rodents as a subfamily (Cricetinae)

¹**mu·rine** \ˈmyu̇(ə)r-ˌīn\ *adj* **1 a** : of or relating to the genus *Mus* or to its subfamily (Murinae) that includes most of the rats and mice which habitually live in intimate association with humans ⟨∼ rodents⟩ **b** : of, relating to, or produced by the house mouse ⟨a ∼ odor⟩ **2** : affecting or transmitted by rats or mice ⟨∼ rickettsial diseases⟩

²**murine** *n* : a murine animal

murine leukemia virus *n* : a retrovirus (species *Murine leukemia virus* of the genus *Gammaretrovirus*) that includes several strains producing leukemia in mice — see FRIEND VIRUS, MOLONEY VIRUS

murine typhus *n* : a mild febrile disease that is marked by headache and rash, is caused by a bacterium of the genus *Rickettsia* (*R. typhi*), is widespread in nature in rodents, and is transmitted to humans by a flea — called also *endemic typhus*

mur·mur \ˈmər-mər\ *n* : an atypical sound of the heart typically indicating a functional or structural abnormality — called also *heart murmur*

Mur·ray Val·ley encephalitis \ˈmər-ē-ˈval-ē-\ *n* : an encephalitis that is caused by a single-stranded RNA virus of the genus *Flavivirus* (species *Murray Valley encephalitis virus*) closely related to Japanese B encephalitis, that tends to affect children seriously, and that occurred in Australia in epidemics of the 1920s and early 1950s

mur·ri·na \mə-ˈrī-nə\ *n* : a disease of Central American horses and mules attributed to a protozoan blood parasite of the genus *Trypanosoma* (*T. hippicum*), characterized by emaciation, anemia, edema, conjunctivitis, fever, and paralysis of the hind legs, and often considered identical to surra

Mus \ˈməs\ *n* : a genus of rodents that is the type of the family Muridae and includes the house mouse (*M. musculus*) and a few related small forms distinguished by the square-notched tip of the upper incisors as seen in profile

Mus·ca \ˈməs-kə\ *n* : a genus of flies that is the type of the family Muscidae and is now restricted to the common housefly (*M. domestica*) and closely related flies

mus·cae vo·li·tan·tes \'məs-ˌ(k)ē-ˌväl-ə-'tan-ˌtēz\ *n pl* : spots before the eyes due to cells and cell fragments in the vitreous body and lens — compare FLOATER

mus·ca·rine \'məs-kə-ˌrēn\ *n* : a toxic ammonium base [C₉H₂₀NO₂]⁺ that is biochemically related to acetylcholine, is found esp. in fly agaric, acts directly on smooth muscle, and when ingested produces profuse salivation and sweating, abdominal colic with evacuation of bowels and bladder, contracted pupils and blurring of vision, excessive bronchial secretion, bradycardia, and respiratory depression

mus·ca·rin·ic \-kə-ˌrin-ik\ *adj* : relating to, resembling, producing, or mediating the effects (as a slowed heart rate, increased secretion by exocrine glands, and increased activity of smooth muscle) that are produced on organs and tissues by acetylcholine liberated by postganglionic nerve fibers of the parasympathetic nervous system and that are mimicked by muscarine ⟨∼ receptors⟩ ⟨atropine is a ∼ antagonist⟩ — compare NICOTINIC

Mus·ci·dae \'məs-ə-ˌdē\ *n pl* : a family of dipteran flies including the housefly (*Musca domestica*) — **mus·cid** \'məs-əd\ *adj or n*

mus·cle \'məs-əl\ *n, often attrib* **1** : a body tissue consisting of long cells that contract when stimulated and produce motion — see CARDIAC MUSCLE, SMOOTH MUSCLE, STRIATED MUSCLE **2** : an organ that is essentially a mass of muscle tissue attached at either end to a fixed point and that by contracting moves or checks the movement of a body part — see AGONIST 1, ANTAGONIST a, SYNERGIST 2

mus·cle–bound \'məs-əl-ˌbau̇nd\ *adj* : having some of the muscles tense and enlarged and of impaired elasticity sometimes as a result of excessive exercise

muscle fiber *n* : any of the elongated cells characteristic of muscle

muscle plate *n* : MYOTOME 1

muscle sense *n* : the part of kinesthesia mediated by end organs located in muscles

muscle spasm *n* : persistent involuntary hypertonicity of one or more muscles usu. of central origin and commonly associated with pain and excessive irritability

muscle spindle *n* : a sensory end organ in a muscle that is sensitive to stretch in the muscle, consists of small striated muscle fibers richly supplied with nerve fibers, and is enclosed in a connective tissue sheath — called also *stretch receptor*

muscle sugar *n* : INOSITOL

muscle tone *n* : TONUS 2

Mus·coi·dea \məs-'kȯid-ē-ə\ *n pl* : a superfamily of dipteran flies including the houseflies and many related flies (as of the families Muscidae, Gasterophilidae, Calliphoridae, and Tachinidae) that have the head freely movable and the abdomen usu. oval and bristly — **mus·coid** \'məs-ˌkȯid\ *adj*

mus·cu·lar \'məs-kyə-lər\ *adj* **1 a** : of, relating to, or constituting muscle **b** : of, relating to, or performed by the muscles **2** : having well-developed musculature — **mus·cu·lar·ly** \'məs-kyə-lər-lē\ *adv*

muscular coat *n* : an outer layer of smooth muscle surrounding a hollow or tubular organ (as the bladder, esophagus, large intestine, small intestine, stomach, ureter, uterus, and vagina) that often consists of an inner layer of circular fibers serving to narrow the lumen of the organ and an outer layer of longitudinal fibers serving to shorten its length — called also *muscularis externa, tunica muscularis*

muscular dystrophy *n* : any of a group of hereditary diseases characterized by progressive wasting of muscles — called also *progressive muscular dystrophy;* see BECKER MUSCULAR DYSTROPHY, DUCHENNE MUSCULAR DYSTROPHY

mus·cu·la·ris \ˌməs-kyə-'lar-əs\ *n* **1** : the smooth muscular layer of the wall of various more or less contractile organs (as the bladder) **2** : the thin layer of smooth muscle that forms part of a mucous membrane (as in the esophagus)

muscularis ex·ter·na \-eks-'tər-nə\ *n* : MUSCULAR COAT

muscularis mu·co·sae \-myü-'kō-sē\ *also* **muscularis mu·co·sa** \-sə\ *n* : MUSCULARIS 2

mus·cu·lar·i·ty \ˌməs-kyə-'lar-ət-ē\ *n, pl* **-ties** : the quality or state of being muscular

muscular rheumatism *n* : FIBROSITIS

mus·cu·la·ture \'məs-kyə-lə-ˌchu̇(ə)r, -chər, -ˌt(y)u̇(ə)r\ *n* : the muscles of all or a part of the animal body

mus·cu·li pec·ti·na·ti \'məs-kyə-ˌlī-ˌpek-ti-'nā-ˌtī\ *n pl* : small muscular ridges on the inner wall of the auricular appendage of the left and the right atria of the heart

mus·cu·lo·apo·neu·rot·ic \ˌməs-kyə-lō-ˌap-ə-n(y)u̇-'rät-ik\ *adj* : of, relating to, or affecting muscular and aponeurotic tissue

mus·cu·lo·cu·ta·ne·ous \-kyu̇-'tā-nē-əs\ *adj* : of, relating to, supplying, or consisting of both muscle and skin ⟨use of ∼ flaps in breast reconstruction⟩ ⟨∼ circulation⟩

musculocutaneous nerve *n* **1** : a large branch of the brachial plexus supplying various parts of the upper arm (as flexor muscles) and forearm (as the skin) **2** : SUPERFICIAL PERONEAL NERVE

mus·cu·lo·fas·cial \-'fash-(ē-)əl\ *adj* : relating to or consisting of both muscular and fascial tissue ⟨∼ supports of the uterus⟩

mus·cu·lo·fi·brous \-'fī-brəs\ *adj* : relating to or consisting of both muscular and fibrous connective tissue ⟨the ∼ capsule of the spleen⟩

mus·cu·lo·mem·bra·nous \-'mem-brə-nəs\ *adj* : relating to or consisting of both muscle and membrane ⟨the vagina is a ∼ tube —L. L. Langley *et al*⟩

mus·cu·lo·phren·ic artery \-'fren-ik-\ *n* : a branch of the internal thoracic artery that gives off branches to the seventh, eighth, and ninth intercostal spaces as anterior intercostal arteries, to the pericardium, to the diaphragm, and to the abdominal muscles — called also *musculophrenic, musculophrenic branch*

musculorum — see DYSTONIA MUSCULORUM DEFORMANS

mus·cu·lo·skel·e·tal \ˌməs-kyə-lō-'skel-ət-ᵊl\ *adj* : of, relating to, or involving both musculature and skeleton ⟨∼ defects⟩ ⟨the ∼ organization of the arm⟩

mus·cu·lo·spi·ral nerve \-'spī-rəl-\ *n* : RADIAL NERVE

mus·cu·lo·ten·di·nous \-'ten-də-nəs\ *adj* : of, relating to, or affecting muscular and tendinous tissue ⟨the ∼ junction⟩

musculotendinous cuff *n* : ROTATOR CUFF

mus·cu·lo·tro·pic \-'trō-pik, -'träp-ik\ *adj* : having a direct usu. stimulatory effect on muscle ⟨∼ drugs⟩

mus·cu·lus \'məs-kyə-ləs\ *n, pl* **-li** \-ˌlī\ : MUSCLE

mush·room \'məsh-ˌru̇m, -ˌru̇m\ *n* **1** : an enlarged complex fleshy fruiting body of a fungus (as most basidiomycetes) that arises from an underground mycelium and consists typically of a stem bearing a spore-bearing structure; *esp* : one that is edible — compare TOADSTOOL **2** : FUNGUS 1

mu·si·co·gen·ic \ˌmyü-zi-kō-'jen-ik\ *adj* : of, relating to, or being epileptic seizures precipitated by music ⟨those afflicted with ∼ convulsions are not affected by pure tones —R. J. Joynt *et al*⟩

mu·si·co·ther·a·py \-'ther-ə-pē\ *n, pl* **-pies** : MUSIC THERAPY

mu·sic therapy \'myü-zik-\ *n* : the treatment of disease (as mental illness) by means of music — **music therapist** *n*

mus·sel poisoning \'məs-əl-,\ *n* : a toxic reaction following the eating of mussels; *esp* : a severe often fatal intoxication following the consumption of mussels that have fed on red tide flagellates and esp. gonyaulax and stored up a dangerous alkaloid in their tissues

mus·si·ta·tion \ˌməs-ə-'tā-shən\ *n* : movement of the lips as if in speech but without accompanying sound

must \'məst\ *n* : the expressed juice of fruit and esp. grapes before and during fermentation

mus·tard \'məs-tərd\ *n* **1** : a pungent yellow condiment consisting of the pulverized seeds of the black mustard or sometimes the white mustard either dry or made into a paste and serving as a stimulant and diuretic or in large doses as an

---

\ə\ **abut** \ᵊ\ **kitten** \ər\ **further** \a\ **ash** \ā\ **ace** \ä\ **cot, cart**
\au̇\ **out** \ch\ **chin** \e\ **bet** \ē\ **easy** \g\ **go** \i\ **hit** \ī\ **ice** \j\ **job**
\ŋ\ **sing** \ō\ **go** \ȯ\ **law** \ȯi\ **boy** \th\ **thin** \th̲\ **the** \ü\ **loot**
\u̇\ **foot** \y\ **yet** \zh\ **vision** *See also* Pronunciation Symbols page

M
N

emetic and as a counterirritant when applied to the skin as a poultice **2** : any of several herbs (genus *Brassica* of the family Cruciferae, the mustard family) with lobed leaves, yellow flowers, and linear beaked pods — see BLACK MUSTARD 1, WHITE MUSTARD **3 a** : MUSTARD GAS **b** : NITROGEN MUSTARD

mustard gas *n* : an irritant oily liquid $C_4H_8Cl_2S$ used esp. as a chemical weapon that causes blistering, attacks the eyes and lungs, and is a systemic poison — called also *dichlorethyl sulfide, sulfur mustard*

mustard oil *n* **1** : a colorless to pale yellow pungent irritating essential oil that is obtained by distillation from the seeds usu. of black mustard after expression of the fatty oil and maceration with water, that consists largely of allyl isothiocyanate, and that is used esp. in liniments and medicinal plasters — compare SINIGRIN **2 a** : ALLYL ISOTHIOCYANATE **b** : an isothiocyanate ester

mustard plaster *n* : a counterirritant and rubefacient plaster containing powdered mustard — called also *mustard paper*

mu·ta·bil·i·ty \ˌmyüt-ə-ˈbil-ət-ē\ *n, pl* **-ties** **1** : the quality or state of being mutable or capable of mutation **2** : an instance of being mutable

mu·ta·ble \ˈmyüt-ə-bəl\ *adj* **1** : capable of change or of being changed in form, quality, or nature **2** : capable of or liable to mutation

mu·ta·fa·cient \ˌmyüt-ə-ˈfā-shənt\ *adj* : MUTAGENIC

mu·ta·gen \ˈmyüt-ə-jən\ *n* : a substance (as a chemical or various radiations) that tends to increase the frequency or extent of mutation

mu·ta·gen·e·sis \ˌmyüt-ə-ˈjen-ə-səs\ *n, pl* **-e·ses** \-ˌsēz\ : the occurrence or induction of mutation

mu·ta·gen·ic \-ˈjen-ik\ *adj* : inducing or capable of inducing genetic mutation ⟨some chemicals and X-rays are ∼ agents⟩ — **mu·ta·gen·i·cal·ly** \-i-k(ə-)lē\ *adv*

mu·ta·ge·nic·i·ty \-jə-ˈnis-ət-ē\ *n, pl* **-ties** : the capacity to induce mutations

mu·ta·gen·ize \ˈmyüt-ə-jə-ˌnīz\ *vt* **-ized; -iz·ing** : MUTATE ⟨∼ strains of E. coli⟩ ⟨*mutagenized* genes⟩

¹mu·tant \ˈmyüt-ᵊnt\ *adj* : of, relating to, or produced by mutation

²mutant *n* : a mutant individual

mu·ta·ro·tase \ˌmyüt-ə-ˈrō-ˌtās, -ˌtāz\ *n* : an isomerase found esp. in mammalian tissues that catalyzes the interconversion of anomeric forms of some sugars

mu·ta·ro·tate \-ˈrō-ˌtāt\ *vi* **-tat·ed; -tat·ing** : to undergo mutarotation

mu·ta·ro·ta·tion \-rō-ˈtā-shən\ *n* : a change in optical rotation shown by various solutions (as of sugars) on standing as a result of chemical change — called also *birotation*

mu·tase \ˈmyü-ˌtās, -ˌtāz\ *n* : any of various enzymes that catalyze molecular rearrangements and esp. those involving the transfer of phosphate from one hydroxyl group to another in the same molecule

mu·tate \ˈmyü-ˌtāt, myü-ˈ\ *vb* **mu·tat·ed; mu·tat·ing** *vi* : to undergo mutation ∼ *vt* : to cause to undergo mutation — **mu·ta·tive** \ˈmyü-ˌtāt-iv, ˈmyüt-ət-\ *adj*

mu·ta·tion \myü-ˈtā-shən\ *n* **1** : a relatively permanent change in hereditary material involving either a physical change in chromosome relations or a biochemical change in the codons that make up genes; *also* : the process of producing a mutation **2** : an individual, strain, or trait resulting from mutation — **mu·ta·tion·al** \-shnəl, -shən-ᵊl\ *adj* — **mu·ta·tion·al·ly** \-ē\ *adv*

mu·ta·tion·ism \-ˌiz-əm\ *n* : the theory that mutation is a fundamental factor in evolution

mu·ta·tion·ist \-əst\ *n* : a believer in or upholder of mutationism

mu·ta·tor gene \ˈmyü-ˌtāt-ər-\ *n* : a gene that increases the rate of mutation of one or more other genes — called also *mutator*

¹mute \ˈmyüt\ *adj* **mut·er; mut·est** : unable to speak : lacking the power of speech — **mute·ness** *n*

²mute *n* : one who cannot or does not speak

mu·ti·late \ˈmyüt-ᵊl-ˌāt\ *vt* **-lat·ed; -lat·ing** : to cut off or permanently destroy a limb or essential part of ⟨∼ a body⟩; *also* : CASTRATE 1

mu·ti·la·tion \ˌmyüt-ᵊl-ˈā-shən\ *n* **1** : deprivation of a limb or essential part esp. by excision ⟨the ∼ of a body⟩ **2** : an instance of mutilating

mut·ism \ˈmyüt-ˌiz-əm\ *n* : the condition of being mute whether from physical, functional, or psychological cause

mu·tu·al·ism \ˈmyüch-(ə-)wə-ˌliz-əm, ˈmyü-chə-ˌliz-\ *n* : mutually beneficial association between different kinds of organisms — **mu·tu·al·ist** \-ləst\ *n* — **mu·tu·al·is·tic** \ˌmyüch-(ə-)wə-ˈlis-tik, ˌmyü-chə-ˈlis-\ *adj*

¹muz·zle \ˈməz-əl\ *n* **1** : the projecting jaws and nose of an animal : SNOUT **2** : a fastening or covering for the mouth of an animal used to prevent eating or biting

²muzzle *vt* **muz·zled; muz·zling** \-(ə-)liŋ\ : to fit with a muzzle

mV *abbr* millivolt

Mv *symbol* mendelevium

MVP *abbr* mitral valve prolapse

mW *abbr* milliwatt

MW *abbr* megawatt

my·al·gia \mī-ˈal-j(ē-)ə\ *n* : pain in one or more muscles — **my·al·gic** \-jik\ *adj*

myalgic encephalomyelitis *n, chiefly Brit* : CHRONIC FATIGUE SYNDROME — abbr. *ME*

My·am·bu·tol \mī-ˈam-byù-ˌtȯl, -ˌtōl\ *trademark* — used for a preparation of the dihydrochloride of ethambutol

my·an·e·sin \mī-ˈan-ə-sən\ *n* : MEPHENESIN

my·as·the·nia \ˌmī-əs-ˈthē-nē-ə\ *n* : muscular debility; *also* : MYASTHENIA GRAVIS — **my·as·then·ic** \-ˈthen-ik\ *adj*

myasthenia gra·vis \-ˈgrav-əs, -ˈgräv-\ *n* : a disease characterized by progressive weakness and exhaustibility of voluntary muscles without atrophy or sensory disturbance and caused by an autoimmune attack on acetylcholine receptors at neuromuscular junctions

my·a·to·nia \ˌmī-ə-ˈtō-nē-ə\ *n* : lack of muscle tone : muscular flabbiness

my·ce·li·al \mī-ˈsē-lē-əl\ *adj* : of, relating to, or characterized by mycelium

my·ce·li·oid \-lē-ˌȯid\ *adj* : resembling mycelium

my·ce·li·um \mī-ˈsē-lē-əm\ *n, pl* **-lia** \-lē-ə\ : the mass of interwoven filamentous hyphae that forms esp. the vegetative body of a fungus and is often submerged in another body (as of soil or organic matter or the tissues of a host); *also* : a similar mass of filaments formed by some bacteria (as of the genus *Streptomyces*)

my·ce·tism \ˈmī-sə-ˌtiz-əm\ *n* : MYCETISMUS

my·ce·tis·mus \ˌmī-sə-ˈtiz-məs\ *n, pl* **-mi** \-ˌmī\ : mushroom poisoning

my·ce·to·ma \ˌmī-sə-ˈtō-mə\ *n, pl* **-mas** *also* **-ma·ta** \-mət-ə\ **1** : a condition marked by invasion of the deep subcutaneous tissues with fungi or actinomycetes: **a** : MADUROMYCOSIS **b** : NOCARDIOSIS **2** : a tumorous mass occurring in mycetoma — **my·ce·to·ma·tous** \-mət-əs\ *adj*

My·ce·to·zoa \ˌmī-ˌsēt-ə-ˈzō-ə\ *n pl* : an order of rhizopod protozoans that includes the slime molds when they are regarded as animals — **my·ce·to·zo·an** \-ˈzō-ən\ *adj or n*

My·co·bac·te·ri·a·ce·ae \ˌmī-kō-bak-ˌtir-ē-ˈā-sē-ˌē\ *n pl* : a family of rod-shaped bacteria of the order Actinomycetales that are rarely filamentous and only occas. have slight branching

my·co·bac·te·ri·ol·o·gy \-ˌäl-ə-jē\ *n, pl* **-gies** : bacteriology concerned esp. with bacteria of the genus *Mycobacterium*

my·co·bac·te·ri·o·sis \-ˈō-səs\ *n, pl* **-o·ses** \-ˌsēz\ : a disease caused by bacteria of the genus *Mycobacterium*

my·co·bac·te·ri·um \-ˈtir-ē-əm\ *n* **1** *cap* : a genus of nonmotile acid-fast aerobic bacteria of the family Mycobacteriaceae that are usu. slender and difficult to stain and that include the causative agents of tuberculosis (*M. tuberculosis*) and leprosy (*M. leprae*) as well as numerous purely saprophytic forms **2** *pl* **-ria** \-ē-ə\ : any bacterium of the genus *Mycobacterium* or a closely related genus — **my·co·bac·te·ri·al** \-ē-əl\ *adj*

Mycobacterium avi·um complex \-ˈā-vē-əm-, -ˈä-\ *n* : two bacteria of the genus *Mycobacterium* (*M. avium* and *M. intra-*

cellulare) that account for most mycobacterial infections in humans other than tuberculosis, that usu. affect the lungs but may involve the lymph nodes, bones, joints, and skin, and that may cause disseminated disease in immunosuppressed conditions (as AIDS) — abbr. *MAC*

Mycobacterium avium–in·tra·cel·lu·la·re complex \-,in-trə-,sel-yə-'lär-ē-\ *n* : MYCOBACTERIUM AVIUM COMPLEX

my·co·bac·tin \,mī-kə-'bak-tin\ *n* : any of several iron= chelating growth factors derived from mycobacteria and used esp. to culture Johne's bacillus

my·co·cide \'mī-kə-,sīd\ *n* : a fungicide that destroys molds

my·col·ic acid \mī-,käl-ik-\ *n* : any of several hydroxy fatty acids that have very long branched chains and are obtained esp. from the wax of the tubercle bacillus

my·col·o·gy \mī-'käl-ə-jē\ *n, pl* **-gies** **1** : a branch of biology dealing with fungi **2** : fungal life — **my·co·log·i·cal** \,mī-kə-'läj-i-kəl\ *adj* — **my·col·o·gist** \mī-'käl-ə-jəst\ *n*

my·co·my·cin \,mī-kə-'mīs-ᵊn\ *n* : a highly unsaturated antibiotic acid $C_{13}H_{10}O_2$ obtained from an actinomycete of the genus *Nocardia* (*N. acidophilus*)

my·co·phage \'mī-kə-,fāj\ *n* : a virus that attacks fungi

my·co·phe·no·lic acid \,mī-kō-fi-,nō-lik-, -,näl-ik-\ *n* : a crystalline antibiotic $C_{17}H_{20}O_6$ obtained from fungi of the genus *Penicillium*

my·co·plas·ma \,mī-kō-'plaz-mə\ *n* **1** *cap* : the type genus of the family Mycoplasmataceae containing minute pleomorphic gram-negative chiefly nonmotile bacteria that are mostly parasitic usu. in mammals — see PLEUROPNEUMONIA 2 **2** *pl* **-mas** *also* **-ma·ta** \-mət-ə\ : any bacterium of the genus *Mycoplasma* or of the family Mycoplasmataceae — called also *pleuropneumonia-like organism, PPLO* — **my·co·plas·mal** \-məl\ *adj*

My·co·plas·ma·ta·ce·ae \-,plaz-mə-'tā-sē-,ē\ *n pl* : a family (coextensive with the order Mycoplasmatales) of minute pleomorphic gram-negative nonmotile bacteria that have complex life cycles, are mostly parasitic usu. in mammals, and are classified into the genera *Mycoplasma* and *Ureaplasma*

my·co·sis \mī-'kō-səs\ *n, pl* **my·co·ses** \-,sēz\ : infection with or disease caused by a fungus

mycosis fun·goi·des \-fəŋ-'gȯid-,ēz\ *n* : a form of lymphoma characterized by a chronic patchy red scaly irregular and often eczematous dermatitis that progresses over a period of years to form elevated plaques and then tumors

my·co·stat \'mī-kə-,stat\ *n* : an agent that inhibits the growth of molds

my·co·stat·ic \,mī-kə-'stat-ik\ *adj* : of or relating to a mycostat ⟨∼ vapors⟩

My·co·stat·in \-'stat-ᵊn\ *trademark* — used for a preparation of nystatin

my·cos·ter·ol \mī-'käs-tə-,rȯl, -,rōl\ *n* : any of a class of sterols obtained from fungi

my·cot·ic \mī-'kät-ik\ *adj* : of, relating to, or characterized by mycosis ⟨∼ dermatitis⟩

mycotic stomatitis *n* : thrush of cattle and other ruminants

my·co·tox·ic \,mī-kə-'täk-sik\ *adj* : of, relating to, or caused by a mycotoxin ⟨a ∼ disease⟩ — **my·co·tox·ic·i·ty** \-täk-'sis-ət-ē\ *n, pl* **-ties**

my·co·tox·i·col·o·gy \-,täk-sə-'käl-ə-jē\ *n, pl* **-gies** : toxicology of toxins produced by fungi

my·co·tox·i·co·sis \-'kō-səs\ *n, pl* **-co·ses** \-'kō-,sēz\ : poisoning caused by a mycotoxin

my·co·tox·in \-'täk-sən\ *n* : a poisonous substance produced by a fungus and esp. a mold — see AFLATOXIN

My·dri·a·cyl \mə-'drī-ə-,sil\ *trademark* — used for a preparation of tropicamide

my·dri·a·sis \mə-'drī-ə-səs\ *n, pl* **-a·ses** \-,sēz\ : excessive or prolonged dilation of the pupil of the eye

¹myd·ri·at·ic \,mid-rē-'at-ik\ *adj* : causing or involving dilation of the pupil of the eye

²mydriatic *n* : a drug that produces dilation of the pupil of the eye

my·ec·to·my \mī-'ek-tə-mē\ *n, pl* **-mies** : surgical excision of part of a muscle

my·el·en·ceph·a·lon \,mī-ə-len-'sef-ə-,län, -lən\ *n* : the posterior part of the developing vertebrate hindbrain or the corresponding part of the adult brain composed of the medulla oblongata — **my·el·en·ce·phal·ic** \-,len(t)-sə-'fal-ik\ *adj*

my·el·ic \mī-'el-ik\ *adj* : of or relating to the spinal cord

my·e·lin \'mī-ə-lən\ *n* : a soft white somewhat fatty material that forms a thick myelin sheath about the protoplasmic core of a myelinated nerve fiber — **my·e·lin·ic** \,mī-ə-'lin-ik\ *adj*

my·e·lin·at·ed \'mī-ə-lə-,nāt-əd\ *adj* : having a myelin sheath ⟨∼ nerve fibers⟩

my·e·li·na·tion \,mī-ə-lə-'nā-shən\ *n* **1** : the process of acquiring a myelin sheath **2** : the condition of being myelinated

myelin basic protein *n* : a protein that is a constituent of myelin and is often found in higher than normal amounts in the cerebrospinal fluid of individuals affected with some demyelinating disease (as multiple sclerosis) — abbr. *MBP*

my·e·lin·iza·tion *also Brit* **my·e·lin·isa·tion** \,mī-ə-,lin-ə-'zā-shən\ *n* : MYELINATION

my·e·li·noc·la·sis \,mī-ə-lə-'näk-lə-səs\ *n, pl* **-la·ses** \-,sēz\ : the process of destruction of myelin leading to demyelination — **my·e·li·no·clas·tic** \-,lin-ə-'klast-ik\ *adj*

my·e·li·nol·y·sis \-'näl-ə-səs\ *n, pl* **-y·ses** \-,sēz\ : DEMYELINATION — see CENTRAL PONTINE MYELINOLYSIS

my·e·li·no·tox·ic \,mī-ə-,lin-ə-'täk-sik\ *adj* : destructive of myelin ⟨a substance that is ∼ in vitro⟩

myelin sheath *n* : a layer of myelin surrounding some nerve fibers — called also *medullary sheath*

my·e·li·tis \,mī-ə-'līt-əs\ *n, pl* **my·e·lit·i·des** \-'lit-ə-,dēz\ : inflammation of the spinal cord or of the bone marrow — **my·e·lit·ic** \-'lit-ik\ *adj*

my·e·lo·ar·chi·tec·ton·ic \,mī-ə-lō-,är-kə-,tek-'tän-ik\ *adj* : of or relating to myeloarchitectonics

my·e·lo·ar·chi·tec·ton·ics \-iks\ *n pl but sing in constr* : cytological architectonics of the brain, spinal cord, or bone marrow

my·e·lo·blast \'mī-ə-lə-,blast\ *n* : a large mononuclear nongranular bone marrow cell; *esp* : one that is a precursor of a myelocyte — compare LEUKOBLAST — **my·e·lo·blas·tic** \,mī-ə-lə-'blas-tik\ *adj*

my·e·lo·blas·te·mia *or chiefly Brit* **my·e·lo·blas·tae·mia** \,mī-ə-lō-blas-'tē-mē-ə\ *n* : the presence of myeloblasts in the circulating blood (as in myelogenous leukemia)

myeloblastic leukemia *n* : MYELOGENOUS LEUKEMIA

my·e·lo·blas·to·ma \-blas-'tō-mə\ *n, pl* **-mas** *also* **-ma·ta** \-mət-ə\ : a myeloma consisting of myeloblasts

my·e·lo·blas·to·sis \-blas-'tō-səs\ *n, pl* **-to·ses** \-,sēz\ : the presence of an abnormally large number of myeloblasts in the tissues, organs, or circulating blood

my·e·lo·cele \'mī-ə-lə-,sēl\ *n* : spina bifida in which the neural tissue of the spinal cord is exposed

my·e·lo·coele \'mī-ə-lə-,sēl\ *n* : the central canal of the spinal cord

my·e·lo·cyte \'mī-ə-lə-,sīt\ *n* : a bone marrow cell; *esp* : a motile cell with cytoplasmic granules that gives rise to the blood granulocytes and occurs abnormally in the circulating blood (as in myelogenous leukemia) — **my·e·lo·cyt·ic** \,mī-ə-lə-'sit-ik\ *adj*

myelocytic leukemia *n* : MYELOGENOUS LEUKEMIA

my·e·lo·cy·to·ma \,mī-ə-lō-sī-'tō-mə\ *n, pl* **-mas** *also* **-ma·ta** \-mət-ə\ : a tumor esp. of fowl in which the typical cellular element is a myelocyte or a cell of similar differentiation

my·e·lo·cy·to·sis \-sī-'tō-səs\ *n, pl* **-to·ses** \-,sēz\ : the presence of excess numbers of myelocytes esp. in the blood or bone marrow

my·e·lo·dys·pla·sia \-dis-'plā-zh(ē-)ə\ *n* **1** : a developmental anomaly of the spinal cord **2** : MYELODYSPLASTIC SYNDROME — **my·e·lo·dys·plas·tic** \-'plas-tik\ *adj*

\ə\ abut \ᵊ\ kitten \ər\ further \a\ ash \ā\ ace \ä\ cot, cart \au̇\ out \ch\ chin \e\ bet \ē\ easy \g\ go \i\ hit \ī\ ice \j\ job \ŋ\ sing \ō\ go \ȯ\ law \ȯi\ boy \th\ thin \th̶\ the \ü\ loot \u̇\ foot \y\ yet \zh\ vision *See also* Pronunciation Symbols page

M
N

myelodysplastic syndrome *n* : any of a group of bone marrow disorders that are marked esp. by an abnormal reduction in one or more types of circulating blood cells due to defective growth and maturation of blood-forming cells in the bone marrow and that sometimes progress to acute myelogenous leukemia — called also *myelodysplasia*

my·e·lo·fi·bro·sis \ˌmī-ə-lō-fī-ˈbrō-səs\ *n, pl* **-bro·ses** \-ˌsēz\ : an anemic condition in which bone marrow becomes fibrotic and the liver and spleen usu. exhibit a development of blood-cell precursors — **my·e·lo·fi·brot·ic** \-ˈbrät-ik\ *adj*

my·e·log·e·nous \ˌmī-ə-ˈläj-ə-nəs\ *also* **my·e·lo·gen·ic** \ˌmī-ə-lə-ˈjen-ik\ *adj* : of, relating to, originating in, or produced by the bone marrow ⟨∼ sarcoma⟩

myelogenous leukemia *n* : leukemia characterized by proliferation of myeloid tissue (as of the bone marrow and spleen) and an abnormal increase in the number of granulocytes, myelocytes, and myeloblasts in the circulating blood — called also *granulocytic leukemia, myeloblastic leukemia, myelocytic leukemia, myeloid leukemia;* see ACUTE MYELOGENOUS LEUKEMIA, ACUTE NONLYMPHOCYTIC LEUKEMIA, CHRONIC MYELOGENOUS LEUKEMIA

my·e·lo·gram \ˈmī-ə-lə-ˌgram\ *n* **1** : a differential study of the cellular elements present in bone marrow usu. made on material obtained by sternal biopsy **2** : a radiograph of the spinal cord made by myelography

my·e·lo·graph·ic \ˌmī-ə-lə-ˈgraf-ik\ *adj* : of, relating to, or made by means of a myelogram or myelography — **my·e·lo·graph·i·cal·ly** \-i-k(ə-)lē\ *adv*

my·e·log·ra·phy \ˌmī-ə-ˈläg-rə-fē\ *n, pl* **-phies** : radiographic visualization of the spinal cord after injection of a contrast medium into the spinal subarachnoid space

my·e·loid \ˈmī-ə-ˌlȯid\ *adj* **1** : of or relating to the spinal cord **2** : of, relating to, or resembling bone marrow

myeloid leukemia *n* : MYELOGENOUS LEUKEMIA

my·e·lo·li·po·ma \ˌmī-ə-lō-lī-ˈpō-mə, -lip-ˈō-mə\ *n, pl* **-mas** *also* **-ma·ta** \-mət-ə\ : a benign tumor esp. of the adrenal glands that consists of fat and hematopoietic tissue

my·e·lo·ma \ˌmī-ə-ˈlō-mə\ *n, pl* **-mas** *also* **-ma·ta** \-mət-ə\ : a primary tumor of the bone marrow formed of any one of the bone marrow cells (as myelocytes or plasma cells) and usu. involving several different bones at the same time — see MULTIPLE MYELOMA

my·e·lo·ma·to·sis \ˌmī-ə-lō-mə-ˈtō-səs\ *n, pl* **-to·ses** \-ˌsēz\ : MULTIPLE MYELOMA

my·e·lo·ma·tous \ˌmī-ə-ˈlō-mət-əs, -ˈläm-ət-əs\ *adj* : of or relating to a myeloma or to myelomatosis

my·e·lo·me·nin·go·cele \ˌmī-ə-lō-mə-ˈniŋ-gə-ˌsēl, -mə-ˈninjə-\ *n* : spina bifida in which neural tissue of the spinal cord and the investing meninges protrude from the spinal column forming a sac under the skin

my·e·lo·mono·cyte \-ˈmän-ə-ˌsīt\ *n* : a myelomonocytic blood cell

my·e·lo·mono·cyt·ic \-ˌmän-ə-ˈsit-ik\ *adj* : relating to or being a blood cell that has the characteristics of both monocytes and granulocytes

myelomonocytic leukemia *n* : a kind of monocytic leukemia in which the cells resemble granulocytes

my·e·lo·path·ic \-ˈpath-ik\ *adj* : of or relating to a myelopathy : resulting from abnormality of the spinal cord or the bone marrow ⟨∼ anemia⟩

my·e·lop·a·thy \ˌmī-ə-ˈläp-ə-thē\ *n, pl* **-thies** : any disease or disorder of the spinal cord or bone marrow

my·e·lo·per·ox·i·dase \ˌmī-ə-lō-pə-ˈräk-sə-ˌdās, -ˌdāz\ *n* : a green peroxidase of phagocytic cells (as neutrophils and monocytes) that is held to assist in bactericidal activity by catalyzing the oxidation of ionic halogen to free halogen

my·e·lo·phthi·sic anemia \-ˈtiz-ik-, -ˈtī-sik-\ *n* : anemia in which the blood-forming elements of the bone marrow are unable to reproduce normal blood cells and which is commonly caused by specific toxins or by overgrowth of tumor cells

my·e·lo·plax \ˈmī-ə-lə-ˌplaks, mī-ˈel-ə-\ *n* : any of the large multinucleate cells in bone marrow

my·e·lo·poi·e·sis \ˌmī-ə-lō-(ˌ)pȯi-ˈē-səs\ *n, pl* **-poi·e·ses** \-ˈē-

ˌsēz\ **1** : production of bone marrow or bone marrow cells **2** : production of blood cells in bone marrow; *esp* : formation of blood granulocytes

my·e·lo·poi·et·ic \-(ˌ)pȯi-ˈet-ik\ *adj* : of or relating to myelopoiesis

my·e·lo·pro·lif·er·a·tive \ˈmī-ə-lō-prə-ˈlif-ə-ˌrāt-iv, -rət-\ *adj* : of, relating to, or being a disorder (as leukemia) marked by excessive proliferation of bone marrow elements and esp. blood cell precursors

my·e·lo·ra·dic·u·li·tis \-rə-ˌdik-yə-ˈlīt-əs, -ra-\ *n* : inflammation of the spinal cord and the spinal nerve roots

my·e·lo·scle·ro·sis \-sklə-ˈrō-səs\ *n, pl* **-ro·ses** \-ˌsēz\ **1** : sclerosis of the bone marrow **2** : MYELOFIBROSIS

my·e·lo·sis \ˌmī-ə-ˈlō-səs\ *n, pl* **-lo·ses** \-ˌsēz\ **1** : the proliferation of bone marrow tissue to produce the changes in cell distribution typical of myelogenous leukemia **2** : MYELOGENOUS LEUKEMIA

my·e·lo·spon·gi·um \ˌmī-ə-lō-ˈspän-jē-əm, -ˈspən-\ *n, pl* **-gia** \-jē-ə\ : a network in the embryonic central nervous system derived from the spongioblasts and giving rise to the glia

my·e·lo·sup·pres·sion \-sə-ˈpresh-ən\ *n* : suppression of the bone marrow's production of blood cells and platelets

my·e·lo·sup·pres·sive \-sə-ˈpres-iv\ *adj* : causing myelosuppression ⟨∼ chemotherapy⟩ ⟨a ∼ drug⟩

my·e·lot·o·my \ˌmī-ə-ˈlät-ə-mē\ *n, pl* **-mies** : surgical incision of the spinal cord; *esp* : section of crossing nerve fibers at the midline of the spinal cord and esp. of sensory fibers for the relief of intractable pain

my·e·lo·tox·ic \ˌmī-ə-lō-ˈtäk-sik\ *adj* : destructive to bone marrow or any of its elements ⟨a ∼ agent⟩ — **my·e·lo·tox·ic·i·ty** \-ˌtäk-ˈsis-ət-ē\ *n, pl* **-ties**

my·en·ter·ic \ˌmī-ən-ˈter-ik\ *adj* : of or relating to the muscular coat of the intestinal wall

myenteric plexus *n* : a network of nerve fibers and ganglia between the longitudinal and circular muscle layers of the intestine — called also *Auerbach's plexus;* compare MEISSNER'S PLEXUS

myenteric plexus of Auerbach *n* : MYENTERIC PLEXUS

myenteric reflex *n* : a reflex that is responsible for the wave of peristalsis moving along the intestine and that involves contraction of the digestive tube above and relaxation below the place where it is stimulated by an accumulated mass of food

my·en·ter·on \mī-ˈen-tə-ˌrän\ *n* : the muscular coat of the intestine

my·ia·sis \mī-ˈī-ə-səs, mē-\ *n, pl* **my·ia·ses** \-ˌsēz\ : infestation with fly maggots

My·lan·ta \mī-ˈlan-tə\ *trademark* — used for an antacid and antiflatulent preparation of aluminum hydroxide, magnesium hydroxide, and simethicone

Myl·e·ran \ˈmil-ə-ˌran\ *trademark* — used for a preparation of busulfan

My·li·con \ˈmī-lə-ˌkän\ *trademark* — used for a preparation of simethicone

¹my·lo·hy·oid \ˌmī-lō-ˈhī-ˌȯid\ *adj* : of, indicating, or adjoining the mylohyoid muscle

²mylohyoid *n* : MYLOHYOID MUSCLE

my·lo·hy·oi·de·us \-hī-ˈȯid-ē-əs\ *n, pl* **-dei** \-ē-ˌī\ : MYLOHYOID MUSCLE

mylohyoid line *n* : a ridge on the inner side of the bone of the lower jaw extending from the junction of the two halves of the bone in front to the last molar on each side and giving attachment to the mylohyoid muscle and to the superior constrictor of the pharynx — called also *mylohyoid ridge*

mylohyoid muscle *n* : a flat triangular muscle on each side of the mouth that is located above the anterior belly of the digastric muscle, extends from the inner surface of the mandible to the hyoid bone, and with its mate on the opposite side forms the floor of the mouth — called also *mylohyoid, mylohyoideus*

mylohyoid ridge *n* : MYLOHYOID LINE

myo·blast \ˈmī-ō-ˌblast\ *n* : an undifferentiated cell capable of giving rise to muscle cells

myo·blas·to·ma \ˌmī-ə-(ˌ)blas-ˈtō-mə\ *n, pl* **-mas** *also* **-ma·ta**

\-mət-ə\ : a tumor that is composed of cells resembling primitive myoblasts and is associated with striated muscle

myo·car·dia *pl of* MYOCARDIUM

myo·car·di·ac \-'kärd-ē-ˌak\ *adj* : MYOCARDIAL

myo·car·di·al \ˌmī-ə-'kärd-ē-əl\ *adj* : of, relating to, or involving the myocardium — **myo·car·di·al·ly** \-ē-\ *adv*

myocardial infarction *n* : HEART ATTACK

myocardial insufficiency *n* : inability of the myocardium to perform its function : HEART FAILURE

myo·car·dio·graph \ˌmī-ə-'kärd-ē-ə-ˌgraf\ *n* : a recording instrument for making a tracing of the action of the heart muscles — **myo·car·dio·graph·ic** \-ˌkärd-ē-ə-'graf-ik\ *adj*

myo·car·di·op·a·thy \-ˌkärd-ē-'äp-ə-thē\ *n, pl* **-thies** : disease of the myocardium

myo·car·di·tis \ˌmī-ə-(ˌ)kär-'dīt-əs\ *n* : inflammation of the myocardium

myo·car·di·um \ˌmī-ə-'kärd-ē-əm\ *n, pl* **-dia** \-ē-ə\ : the middle muscular layer of the heart wall

myo·car·do·sis \-ˌkär-'dō-səs\ *n, pl* **-do·ses** \-'dō-ˌsēz\ : a noninflammatory disease of the myocardium

Myo·chry·sine \ˌmī-ō-'krī-ˌsēn, -sən\ *trademark* — used for a preparation of gold sodium thiomalate

myo·clo·nia \ˌmī-ə-'klō-nē-ə\ *n* : MYOCLONUS

myo·clon·ic \-'klän-ik\ *adj* : of, relating to, characterized by, or being myoclonus ⟨~ seizures⟩

myoclonic epilepsy *n* : epilepsy marked by myoclonic seizures: as **a** : JUVENILE MYOCLONIC EPILEPSY **b** : LAFORA DISEASE

my·oc·lo·nus \ˌmī-'äk-lə-nəs\ *n* : irregular involuntary contraction of a muscle usu. resulting from functional disorder of controlling motor neurons; *also* : a condition characterized by myoclonus

myoclonus epilepsy *n* : MYOCLONIC EPILEPSY

myo·coele *or* **myo·coel** \'mī-ə-ˌsēl\ *n* : the cavity of a myotome

myo·com·ma \ˌmī-ə-'kä-mə\ *n, pl* **-ma·ta** \-mət-ə\ *also* **-mas** : MYOSEPTUM

myo·cyte \'mī-ə-ˌsīt\ *n* : a contractile cell; *specif* : a muscle cell

myo·dy·nam·ics \ˌmī-ō-dī-'nam-iks\ *n pl but often sing in constr* : the physiology of muscular contraction

myo·ede·ma *or Brit* **myo·oe·de·ma** \ˌmī-ō-i-'dē-mə\ *n, pl* **-mas** *also* **-ma·ta** \-mət-ə\ : the formation of a lump in a muscle when struck a slight blow that occurs in states of exhaustion or in certain diseases

myo·elas·tic \-i-'las-tik\ *adj* : made up of muscular and elastic tissues ⟨~ lung fibers⟩

myo·elec·tric \ˌmī-ō-i-'lek-trik\ *also* **myo·elec·tri·cal** \-tri-kəl\ *adj* : of, relating to, or utilizing electricity generated by muscle — **myo·elec·tri·cal·ly** \-tri-k(ə-)lē\ *adv*

myo·epi·the·li·al \-ˌep-ə-'thē-lē-əl\ *adj* : of, relating to, or being large contractile cells of epithelial origin which are located at the base of the secretory cells of various glands (as the salivary and mammary glands)

myo·epi·the·li·o·ma \-ˌep-ə-ˌthē-lē-'ō-mə\ *n, pl* **-mas** *also* **-ma·ta** \-mət-ə\ : a tumor arising from myoepithelial cells esp. of the sweat glands

myo·epi·the·li·um \-ˌep-ə-'thē-lē-əm\ *n, pl* **-lia** : tissue made up of myoepithelial cells

myo·fas·cial \-'fash-(ē-)əl\ *adj* : of or relating to the fasciae of muscles ⟨~ pain⟩

myo·fi·ber *or* **myo·fi·bre** \'mī-ō-ˌfī-bər\ *n* : MUSCLE FIBER

myo·fi·bril \ˌmī-ō-'fīb-rəl, -'fib-\ *n* : one of the longitudinal parallel contractile elements of a muscle cell that are composed of myosin and actin — **myo·fi·bril·lar** \-rə-lər\ *adj*

myo·fi·bril·la \-fī-'bril-ə, -fi-; -'fī-bri-lə, -'fi-\ *n, pl* **-lae** \-ˌlē\ : MYOFIBRIL

myo·fi·bro·blast \-'fīb-rə-ˌblast, -'fib-\ *n* : a fibroblast that has developed some of the functional and structural characteristics (as the presence of myofilaments) of smooth muscle cells

myo·fi·bro·ma \-fī-'brō-mə\ *n, pl* **-mas** *also* **-ma·ta** \-mət-ə\ : a tumor composed of fibrous and muscular tissue

myo·fil·a·ment \-'fil-ə-mənt\ *n* : one of the individual filaments of actin or myosin that make up a myofibril

myo·func·tion·al \-'fəŋ(k)-shnəl, -shən-ᵊl\ *adj* : of, relating to, or concerned with muscle function esp. in the treatment of orthodontic problems

myo·ge·lo·sis \ˌmī-ō-jə-'lō-səs\ *n, pl* **-lo·ses** \-ˌsēz\ *also* **-lo·sis·es** : an area of abnormal hardening in a muscle

my·o·gen \'mī-ə-jən, -ˌjen\ *n* : a mixture of albumins obtained by extracting muscle with cold water

myo·gen·e·sis \ˌmī-ə-'jen-ə-səs\ *n, pl* **-e·ses** \-ˌsēz\ : the development of muscle tissue

myo·gen·ic \ˌmī-ə-'jen-ik\ *also* **my·og·e·nous** \mī-'äj-ə-nəs\ *adj* **1** : originating in muscle ⟨~ pain⟩ **2** : taking place or functioning in ordered rhythmic fashion because of inherent properties of cardiac muscle rather than by reason of specific neural stimuli ⟨a ~ heartbeat⟩ — compare NEUROGENIC 2b — **myo·ge·nic·i·ty** \-jə-'nis-ət-ē\ *n, pl* **-ties**

myo·glo·bin \ˌmī-ə-'glō-bən, 'mī-ə-ˌ\ *n* : a red iron-containing protein pigment in muscles that is similar to hemoglobin but differs in the globin portion of its molecule, in the smaller size of its molecule (as in the mammalian heart muscle which has only one fourth the molecular weight of the hemoglobin in the blood of the same animal), in its greater tendency to combine with oxygen, and in its absorption of light at longer wavelengths — called also *myohemoglobin*

myo·glo·bin·uria \-ˌglō-bin-'(y)ùr-ē-ə\ *n* : the presence of myoglobin in the urine — called also *myohemoglobinuria*

myo·gram \'mī-ə-ˌgram\ *n* : a graphic representation of the phenomena (as velocity and intensity) of muscular contractions

myo·graph \-ˌgraf\ *n* : an apparatus for producing myograms — **myo·graph·ic** \ˌmī-ə-'graf-ik\ *adj* — **myo·graph·i·cal·ly** \-ik-(ə-)lē\ *adv*

my·og·ra·phy \mī-'äg-rə-fē\ *n, pl* **-phies** : the use of a myograph

myo·he·ma·tin *or chiefly Brit* **myo·hae·ma·tin** \ˌmī-ō-'hē-mət-ən\ *n* : CYTOCHROME

myo·he·mo·glo·bin *or chiefly Brit* **myo·hae·mo·glo·bin** \-'hē-mə-ˌglō-bən\ *n* : MYOGLOBIN

myo·he·mo·glo·bin·uria *or chiefly Brit* **myo·hae·mo·glo·bin·uria** \-ˌhē-mə-ˌglō-bin-'(y)ùr-ē-ə\ *n* : MYOGLOBINURIA

¹my·oid \'mī-ˌòid\ *adj* : resembling muscle

²myoid *n* : an inner structural part of a retinal rod or cone containing numerous cell organelles

myo·ino·si·tol \ˌmī-ō-in-'ō-sə-ˌtòl, -ˌtōl\ *n* : a biologically active inositol that is a component of many phospholipids and occurs widely in plants, animals, and microorganisms — called also *mesoinositol*

myo·in·ti·mal \-'int-ə-məl\ *adj* : of, relating to, or being the smooth muscle cells of the intima of a blood vessel ⟨vasoconstriction and ~ proliferation —D. A. Calhoun *et al*⟩

myo·ki·nase \-'kī-ˌnās, -ˌnāz\ *n* : a crystallizable enzyme that promotes the reversible transfer of phosphate groups in ADP with the formation of ATP and adenylic acid and that occurs in muscle and other tissues

my·ol·o·gy \mī-'äl-ə-jē\ *n, pl* **-gies** : a scientific study of muscles — **my·o·log·ic** \ˌmī-ə-'läj-ik\ *or* **my·o·log·i·cal** \-i-kəl\ *adj*

my·ol·y·sis \mī-'äl-ə-səs\ *n, pl* **-y·ses** \-ˌsēz\ **1** : destruction or disintegration of muscle tissue ⟨~ is typical in sea snake and tiger snake envenomations —A. Barelli *et al*⟩ **2** : a laparoscopic procedure for treating uterine fibroids that involves coagulation (as by electric current) of blood vessels supplying the fibroid with subsequent shrinkage of the fibroid — **myo·lyt·ic** \ˌmī-ə-'lit-ik\ *adj*

my·o·ma \mī-'ō-mə\ *n, pl* **-mas** *also* **-ma·ta** \-mət-ə\ : a tumor consisting of muscle tissue — **my·o·ma·tous** \-mət-əs\ *adj*

\ə\ abut \ᵊ\ kitten \ər\ **further** \a\ ash \ā\ ace \ä\ cot, cart
\aù\ **out** \ch\ **chin** \e\ bet \ē\ **easy** \g\ go \i\ hit \ī\ ice \j\ job
\ŋ\ **sing** \ō\ go \ò\ law \òi\ boy \th\ **thin** \t̲h̲\ **the** \ü\ loot
\ù\ **foot** \y\ yet \zh\ **vision** *See also* Pronunciation Symbols page

myo·mec·to·my \ˌmī-ə-ˈmek-tə-mē\ *n, pl* **-mies** : surgical excision of a myoma or fibroid

myo·me·tri·al \-ˈmē-trē-əl\ *adj* : of, relating to, or affecting the myometrium

myo·me·tri·tis \-mə-ˈtrīt-əs\ *n* : inflammation of the uterine myometrium

myo·me·tri·um \ˌmī-ə-ˈmē-trē-əm\ *n* : the muscular layer of the wall of the uterus

myo·ne·cro·sis \-nə-ˈkrō-səs, -ne-\ *n, pl* **-cro·ses** \-ˌsēz\ : necrosis of muscle

my·o·neme \ˈmī-ə-ˌnēm\ *n* : a contractile fibril in the body of a protozoan

myo·neu·ral \ˌmī-ə-ˈn(y)ùr-əl\ *adj* : of, relating to, or connecting muscles and nerves ⟨~ effects⟩ ⟨competitive ~ blockade⟩

myoneural junction *n* : NEUROMUSCULAR JUNCTION

myo–oedema *Brit var of* MYOEDEMA

myo·path·ic \ˌmī-ə-ˈpath-ik\ *adj* **1** : involving abnormality of the muscles ⟨a ~ syndrome⟩ **2** : of or relating to myopathy ⟨~ dystrophy⟩

my·op·a·thy \mī-ˈäp-ə-thē\ *n, pl* **-thies** : a disorder of muscle tissue or muscles

my·ope \ˈmī-ˌōp\ *n* : a myopic individual — called also *myopic*

myo·peri·car·di·tis \ˌmī-ō-ˌper-ə-ˌkär-ˈdīt-əs\ *n, pl* **-dit·i·des** \-ˈdit-ə-ˌdēz\ : inflammation of both the myocardium and pericardium

my·o·pia \mī-ˈō-pē-ə\ *n* : a condition in which the visual images come to a focus in front of the retina of the eye because of defects in the refractive media of the eye or of abnormal length of the eyeball resulting esp. in defective vision of distant objects — called also *nearsightedness;* compare ASTIGMATISM 2, EMMETROPIA

¹**my·o·pic** \-ˈō-pik, -ˈäp-ik\ *adj* : affected by myopia : of, relating to, or exhibiting myopia — **my·o·pi·cal·ly** \-(ə-)lē\ *adv*

²**myopic** *n* : MYOPE

myo·plasm \ˈmī-ə-ˌplaz-əm\ *n* : the contractile portion of muscle tissue — compare SARCOPLASM — **myo·plas·mic** \ˌmī-ə-ˈplaz-mik\ *adj*

¹**myo·re·lax·ant** \ˌmī-ō-ri-ˈlak-sənt\ *n* : a drug that causes relaxation of muscle

²**myorelaxant** *adj* : relating to or causing relaxation of muscle ⟨~ effects⟩

myo·re·lax·ation \-ˌrē-ˌlak-ˈsā-shən, -ri-ˌlak-, *esp Brit* -ˌrel-ək-\ *n* : relaxation of muscle

myo·sar·co·ma \-sär-ˈkō-mə\ *n, pl* **-mas** *also* **-ma·ta** \-mət-ə\ : a sarcomatous myoma

myo·sep·tum \-ˈsep-təm\ *n, pl* **-sep·ta** \-tə\ : the septum between adjacent myotomes — called also *myocomma*

my·o·sin \ˈmī-ə-sən\ *n* **1** : ACTOMYOSIN **2** : a fibrous globulin of muscle that can split ATP and that reacts with actin to form actomyosin

myosis *var of* MIOSIS

myo·si·tis \ˌmī-ə-ˈsīt-əs\ *n* : muscular discomfort or pain from infection or an unknown cause

myositis os·sif·i·cans \-ä-ˈsif-ə-ˌkanz\ *n* : myositis accompanied by ossification of muscle tissue or bony deposits in the muscles

myo·tat·ic \ˌmī-ə-ˈtat-ik\ *adj* : relating to or involved in a muscular stretch reflex

myotatic reflex *n* : STRETCH REFLEX

myotic *var of* MIOTIC

myo·tome \ˈmī-ə-ˌtōm\ *n* **1** : the portion of an embryonic somite from which skeletal musculature is produced — called also *muscle plate* **2** : an instrument for myotomy — **myo·to·mal** \ˌmī-ə-ˈtō-məl\ *adj*

my·ot·o·my \mī-ˈät-ə-mē\ *n, pl* **-mies** : incision or division of a muscle

myo·to·nia \ˌmī-ə-ˈtō-nē-ə\ *n* : tonic spasm of one or more muscles; *also* : a condition characterized by such spasms — **myo·ton·ic** \-ˈtän-ik\ *adj*

myotonia con·gen·i·ta \-kän-ˈjen-ə-tə\ *n* : an inherited condition that is characterized by delay in the ability to relax muscles after forceful contractions but not by wasting of muscle — called also *Thomsen's disease*

myotonia dys·tro·phi·ca \-dis-ˈträf-i-kə, -ˈtrōf-\ *n* : MYOTONIC DYSTROPHY

myotonic dystrophy *n* : an inherited condition that is characterized by delay in the ability to relax muscles after forceful contraction, wasting of muscles, formation of cataracts, premature baldness, atrophy of the gonads, endocrine and cardiac abnormalities, and often mental retardation and that is inherited as an autosomal dominant trait — abbr. *DM;* called also *Steinert's disease*

myotonic muscular dystrophy *n* : MYOTONIC DYSTROPHY

my·ot·o·nus \mī-ˈät-ə-nəs\ *n* : sustained spasm of a muscle or muscle group

myo·tox·ic \ˌmī-ō-ˈtäk-sik\ *adj* : having or being a toxic effect on muscle ⟨a ~ drug⟩ — **myo·tox·ic·i·ty** \-ˌtäk-ˈsis-ət-ē\ *n, pl* **-ties**

myo·trop·ic \ˌmī-ə-ˈträp-ik *also* -ˈtrōp-\ *adj* : affecting or tending to invade muscles ⟨a ~ infection⟩

myo·tube \ˈmī-ə-ˌt(y)üb\ *n* : a developmental stage of a muscle fiber composed of a syncytium formed by fusion of myoblasts

myr·ia·me·ter \ˈmir-ē-ə-ˌmēt-ər\ *n* : a metric unit of length equal to 10,000 meters

myriapod *var of* MYRIOPOD

Myr·i·ap·o·da \ˌmir-ē-ˈap-ə-də\ *n pl, syn of* MYRIOPODA

myr·i·cyl alcohol \ˈmir-ə-ˌsil-\ *n* : a crystalline alcohol C₃₀H₆₂O occurring in the form of esters (as the palmitate) in beeswax and other waxes — called also *melissyl alcohol*

my·rin·ga \mə-ˈriŋ-gə\ *n* : TYMPANIC MEMBRANE

myr·in·gi·tis \ˌmir-ən-ˈjīt-əs\ *n* : inflammation of the tympanic membrane

my·rin·go·plas·ty \mə-ˈriŋ-gə-ˌplas-tē\ *n, pl* **-ties** : a plastic operation for the repair of perforations in the tympanic membrane

my·rin·go·tome \-ˌtōm\ *n* : an instrument used in myringotomy

myr·in·got·o·my \ˌmir-ən-ˈgät-ə-mē\ *n, pl* **-mies** : incision of the tympanic membrane — called also *tympanotomy*

myr·io·pod *also* **myr·ia·pod** \ˈmir-ē-ə-ˌpäd\ *n* : any arthropod of the group Myriopoda — **myriopod** *also* **myriapod** *adj*

Myr·i·op·o·da \ˌmir-ē-ˈäp-ə-də\ *n pl* : a group of arthropods having the body made up of numerous similar segments nearly all of which bear true jointed legs and including the millipedes and centipedes

my·ris·tate \mi-ˈris-ˌtāt\ *n* : a salt or ester of myristic acid — see ISOPROPYL MYRISTATE

my·ris·ti·ca \mi-ˈris-ti-kə\ *n* **1** *cap* : a large genus of tropical trees (family Myristicaceae) which produce fleshy fruits and which include the nutmeg (*M. fragrans*) **2** : NUTMEG 1

my·ris·tic acid \mi-ˌris-tik-, mī-\ *n* : a crystalline fatty acid C₁₄H₂₈O₂ occurring esp. in the form of glycerides in most fats — called also *tetradecanoic acid*

myristica oil *n* : NUTMEG OIL

my·ris·ti·cin \mi-ˈris-tə-sən\ *n* : a crystalline phenolic ether C₁₁H₁₂O₃ that has a strong odor and occurs in various essential oils (as nutmeg oil)

my·ris·tin \mi-ˈris-tən, mī-\ *n* : a glycerol ester of myristic acid

my·ro·sin \ˈmir-ə-sən, ˈmīr-\ *n* : an enzyme occurring in various plants of the mustard family (Cruciferae) that hydrolyzes the glucoside sinigrin

my·ro·sin·ase \-sə-ˌnās, -ˌnāz\ *n* : MYROSIN

myrrh \ˈmər\ *n* : a yellowish to reddish brown aromatic bitter gum resin that is obtained from various trees (genus *Commiphora*) esp. of East Africa and Arabia (as *C. myrrha* or *C. abyssinica*) and has been used in the manufacture of dentifrices and as a carminative and a stimulating tonic — compare BDELLIUM

my·so·phil·ia \ˌmī-sə-ˈfil-ē-ə\ *n* : abnormal attraction to filth

my·so·pho·bia *or* **mi·so·pho·bia** \-ˈfō-bē-ə\ *n* : abnormal fear of or distaste for uncleanliness or contamination — **my·so·pho·bic** \-ˈfō-bik\ *adj*

my·ta·cism \\'mīt-ə-ˌsiz-əm\\ *n* : excessive or wrong use of the sound of the letter *m*

mytho·ma·nia \\ˌmith-ə-'mā-nē-ə, -nyə\\ *n* : an excessive or abnormal propensity for lying and exaggerating

¹**mytho·ma·ni·ac** \\-'mā-nē-ˌak\\ *n* : an individual affected with or exhibiting mythomania

²**mythomaniac** *adj* : of, relating to, or affected with mythomania

myx·ede·ma *or chiefly Brit* **myx·oe·de·ma** \\ˌmik-sə-'dē-mə\\ *n* : severe hypothyroidism characterized by firm inelastic edema, dry skin and hair, and loss of mental and physical vigor — **myx·ede·ma·tous** *or chiefly Brit* **myx·oe·de·ma·tous** \\-'dem-ət-əs, -'dē-mət-\\ *adj*

myxo·bac·ter \\'mik-sə-ˌbak-tər\\ *n* : MYXOBACTERIUM

Myxo·bac·ter·a·les \\ˌmik-sə-ˌbak-tə-'rā-(ˌ)lēz\\ *n pl* : an order of higher bacteria having long slender nonflagellated vegetative cells that form colonies capable of creeping slowly over a layer of slime secreted by the cells, forming spores usu. in distinct fruiting bodies, and living chiefly as saprophytes on substrates rich in carbohydrates

Myxo·bac·te·ri·a·ce·ae \\-tir-ē-'ā-sē-ˌē\\ *n pl, syn of* MYXO-BACTERALES

myxo·bac·te·ri·um \\-'tir-ē-əm\\ *n, pl* **-ria** \\-ē-ə\\ : any bacterium of the order Myxobacterales — called also *myxobacter, slime bacterium* — **myxo·bac·te·ri·al** \\-ē-əl\\ *adj*

myxo·chon·dro·ma \\ˌmik-sə-ˌkän-'drō-mə\\ *n, pl* **-mas** *also* **-ma·ta** \\-mət-ə\\ : a benign tumor with characteristics of both a chondroma and a myxoma

myxo·coc·cus \\-'käk-əs\\ *n* **1** *cap* : a genus of myxobacteria in which the rod-shaped vegetative cells are transformed into ovoid to spherical spores **2** *pl* **-coc·ci** \\-'käk-ˌ(s)ī\\ : any myxobacterium of the genus *Myxococcus*

myxo·cyte \\'mik-sə-ˌsīt\\ *n* : a stellate cell that is characteristic of mucous tissue

myxoedema, myxoedematous *chiefly Brit var of* MYXEDEMA, MYXEDEMATOUS

myxo·fi·bro·sar·co·ma \\ˌmik-sō-ˌfī-brō-sär-'kō-mə\\ *n, pl* **-mas** *also* **-ma·ta** \\-mət-ə\\ : a fibrosarcoma with myxomatous elements

myx·oid \\'mik-ˌsȯid\\ *adj* : resembling mucus

myx·o·ma \\mik-'sō-mə\\ *n, pl* **-mas** *also* **-ma·ta** \\-mət-ə\\ : a soft tumor made up of gelatinous connective tissue resembling that found in the umbilical cord — **myx·o·ma·tous** \\-mət-əs\\ *adj*

myx·o·ma·to·sis \\mik-ˌsō-mə-'tō-səs\\ *n, pl* **-to·ses** \\-ˌsēz\\ : a condition characterized by the presence of myxomas in the body; *specif* : a severe virus disease of rabbits that is caused by a poxvirus (species *Myxoma virus* of the genus *Leporipoxvirus*), is transmitted by mosquitoes, biting flies, and direct contact, and has been used in the biological control of wild rabbit populations

myxo·my·cete \\ˌmik-sō-'mī-ˌsēt, ˌmik-sō-(ˌ)mī-'\\ *n* : SLIME MOLD

Myxo·my·ce·tes \\-mī-'sēt-ēz\\ *n pl* : a class of organisms of uncertain systematic position that include the slime molds and are sometimes considered to be protozoans but are now usu. regarded as lower fungi or placed in a separate division and that exist vegetatively as complex mobile plasmodia, reproduce by means of spores which in almost all cases are borne in characteristic fruiting bodies, and have complex variable life cycles — **myxo·my·ce·tous** \\-'sēt-əs\\ *adj*

Myxo·phy·ce·ae \\ˌmik-sə-'fī-sē-ˌē\\ *n pl, in former classifications* : a class of algae now designated as the cyanobacteria

myxo·sar·co·ma \\-sär-'kō-mə\\ *n, pl* **-mas** *also* **-ma·ta** \\-mət-ə\\ : a sarcoma with myxomatous elements — **myxo·sar·co·ma·tous** \\-mət-əs\\ *adj*

myxo·spore \\'mik-sō-ˌspō(ə)r, -ˌspȯ(ə)r\\ *n* : a spore in the fruiting body of a slime mold

Myxo·spo·rid·ia \\ˌmik-sə-spə-'rid-ē-ə\\ *n pl* : an order of sporozoans (subclass Cnidosporidia) that are mostly parasitic in fishes and include various serious pathogens — **myxo·spo·rid·i·an** \\-ē-ən\\ *adj or n*

myxo·vi·rus \\'mik-sə-ˌvī-rəs\\ *n* : any of the viruses now classified in the families *Orthomyxoviridae* and *Paramyxoviridae* that were formerly included in a now rejected family (Myxoviridae) — **myxo·vi·ral** \\ˌmik-sə-'vī-rəl\\ *adj*

my·zo·rhyn·chus \\ˌmī-zə-'riŋ-kəs\\ *n, pl* **-chi** \\-ˌkī\\ : an apical sucker on the scolex of various tapeworms that is often stalked

N

n \\'en\\ *n, pl* **n's** *or* **ns** \\'enz\\ **1** : the haploid or gametic number of chromosomes — compare X **2** *cap* : an antigen of human blood that shares a common genetic locus with the M antigen

N *abbr* **1** nasal **2** newton **3** *usu ital* normal (sense 4a) — used of solutions ⟨0.1 *N* hydrochloric acid⟩

N *symbol* **1** nitrogen — usu. italicized when used as a prefix ⟨*N*-allylnormorphine⟩ **2** index of refraction

Na *symbol* sodium

NA *abbr* **1** Nomina Anatomica **2** numerical aperture **3** nurse's aide

na·bo·thi·an cyst \\nə-'bō-thē-ən-\\ *n* : a mucous gland of the uterine cervix esp. when occluded and dilated — called also *nabothian follicle*

    Na·both \\'nä-ˌbȯt\\, **Martin (1675–1721),** German anatomist and physician. Naboth described the mucous glands of the uterine cervix in 1707. At the same time he noted small cysts in these glands caused by blockage of the outflow of the secretion but he thought that they were ova.

na·cre·ous \\'nā-krē-əs, -k(ə-)rəs\\ *adj* : having a pearly appearance ⟨∼ bacterial colonies⟩

NAD \\ˌen-ˌā-'dē\\ *n* : a coenzyme $C_{21}H_{27}N_7O_{14}P_2$ of numerous dehydrogenases that occurs in most cells and plays an important role in all phases of intermediary metabolism as an oxidizing agent or when in the reduced form as a reducing agent for various metabolites — called also *diphosphopyridine nucleotide, DPN, nicotinamide adenine dinucleotide*

NAD *abbr* no appreciable disease

NADH \\ˌen-ˌā-ˌdē-'āch\\ *n* : the reduced form of NAD

na·do·lol \\nā-'dō-ˌlȯl, -ˌlōl\\ *n* : a beta-blocker $C_{17}H_{27}NO_4$ used in the treatment of hypertension and angina pectoris

NADP \\ˌen-ˌā-ˌdē-'pē\\ *n* : a coenzyme $C_{21}H_{28}N_7O_{17}P_3$ of numerous dehydrogenases (as that acting on glucose-6-phosphate) that occurs esp. in red blood cells and plays a role in intermediary metabolism similar to NAD but acting often on different metabolites — called also *nicotinamide adenine dinucleotide phosphate, TPN, triphosphopyridine nucleotide*

NADPH \\ˌen-ˌā-ˌdē-ˌpē-'āch\\ *n* : the reduced form of NADP

Nae·gle·ria \\nā-'glir-ē-ə\\ *n* : a genus of diphasic ameboid protozoans that are characterized by a predominate ameboid stage and a minute flagellate stage with two flagella, that occur esp. in stagnant water and are often coprozoic, and that include one (*N. fowleri*) causing meningoencephalitis in humans

nae·paine \\'nē-ˌpān\\ *n* : a drug $C_{14}H_{22}N_2O_2$ formerly used as a local anesthetic

naevocarcinoma *chiefly Brit var of* NEVOCARCINOMA

naevoid, naevus *chiefly Brit var of* NEVOID, NEVUS

\\ə\\ abut \\ᵊ\\ kitten \\ər\\ further \\a\\ ash \\ā\\ ace \\ä\\ cot, cart \\au̇\\ out \\ch\\ chin \\e\\ bet \\ē\\ easy \\g\\ go \\i\\ hit \\ī\\ ice \\j\\ job \\ŋ\\ sing \\ō\\ go \\ȯ\\ law \\ȯi\\ boy \\th\\ thin \\t͟h\\ the \\ü\\ loot \\u̇\\ foot \\y\\ yet \\zh\\ vision *See also* Pronunciation Symbols page

naf·cil·lin \naf-'sil-ən\ *n* : a semisynthetic penicillin that is resistant to beta-lactamase and is used esp. in the form of its hydrated sodium salt $C_{21}H_{21}N_2NaO_5S \cdot H_2O$ as an antibiotic

naf·ox·i·dine \-'äk-sə-₁dēn\ *n* : an antiestrogen administered in the form of its hydrochloride $C_{29}H_{31}NO_2 \cdot HCl$

na·ga·na *also* **n'ga·na** \nə-'gä-nə\ *n* : a highly fatal disease of domestic animals in tropical Africa caused by a flagellated protozoan of the genus *Trypanosoma* and transmitted by tsetse and other biting flies; *broadly* : trypanosomiasis of domestic animals

Na·ga sore \'näg-ə-\ *n* : TROPICAL ULCER

nail \'nā(ə)l\ *n* **1** : a horny sheath of thickened and condensed epithelial stratum lucidum that grows out from a vascular matrix of dermis and protects the upper surface of the end of each finger and toe of humans and most other primates and that is strictly homologous with the hoof or claw of other mammals from which it differs chiefly in shape and size — called also *nail plate* **2** : a structure (as a claw) that terminates a digit and corresponds to a nail **3** : a rod (as of metal) used to fix the parts of a broken bone in normal relation ⟨a medullary ∼⟩

nail bed *n* : the vascular epidermis upon which most of the fingernail or toenail rests that has a longitudinally ridged surface often visible through the nail; *also* : MATRIX 1b

nail–biting *n* : habitual biting at the fingernails usu. being symptomatic of emotional tensions and frustrations — called also *onychophagia, onychophagy*

nail fold *n* : the fold of the dermis at the margin of a fingernail or toenail

nail·ing \'nā-liŋ\ *n* : the act or process of fixing the parts of a broken bone by means of a nail ⟨intramedullary ∼⟩

nail matrix *n* : MATRIX 1b

nail plate *n* : NAIL 1

Nai·ro·bi sheep disease \nī-'rō-bē-\ *n* : a severe and frequently fatal gastroenteritis of sheep or sometimes goats that occurs in parts of Kenya and is caused by a single-stranded RNA virus of the family *Bunyaviridae* (species *Nairobi sheep virus* of the genus *Nairovirus*) transmitted by the bite of an African tick esp. of the genus *Rhipicephalus* (*R. appendiculatus*) — called also *Nairobi disease*

na·ive *or* **na·ïve** \nä-'ēv\ *adj* **na·iv·er; -est** **1** : not previously subjected to experimentation or a particular experimental situation ⟨∼ laboratory rats⟩ **2** : not having previously used a particular drug (as marijuana) **3** : not having been exposed previously to an antigen ⟨a ∼ immune system⟩ ⟨∼ T cells⟩

Na·ja \'nä-jə\ *n* : a genus of elapid snakes comprising the true cobras

na·ked \'nā-kəd\ *adj* **1** : lacking some natural external covering (as of hair or myelin) — used of the animal body or one of its parts ⟨∼ nerve endings⟩ ⟨viroids are ∼: the RNA strand is not encapsulated in a protein coat —Roger Lewin⟩ **2** : unaided by any optical device or instrument ⟨visible to the ∼ eye⟩

na·ku·ru·i·tis \nə-₁kü-rü-'īt-əs\ *n* : a cobalt deficiency disease of sheep and cattle in eastern Africa

na·led \'nā-₁led\ *n* : a short-lived organophosphate insecticide $C_4H_7Br_2Cl_2O_4P$ of moderate toxicity to warm-blooded animals that is used esp. to control crop pests and mosquitoes

na·li·dix·ic acid \₁nā-lə-₁dik-sik-\ *n* : an antibacterial agent $C_{12}H_{12}N_2O_3$ that is used esp. in the treatment of genitourinary infections — see NEGGRAM

Nal·line \'nal-₁ēn\ *trademark* — used for a preparation of the hydrochloride of nalorphine

na·lor·phine \nal-'ȯr-₁fēn\ *n* : a white crystalline compound that is derived from morphine and is used in the form of its hydrochloride $C_{19}H_{21}NO_3 \cdot HCl$ as a respiratory stimulant to counteract poisoning by morphine and similar narcotic drugs — called also *N-allylnormorphine;* see NALLINE

nal·ox·one \nal-'äk-₁sōn, 'nal-ək-₁sōn\ *n* : a potent synthetic antagonist of narcotic drugs and esp. morphine that is administered in the form of its hydrochloride $C_{19}H_{21}NO_4 \cdot HCl$ — see NARCAN

nal·trex·one \nal-'trek-₁sōn\ *n* : a synthetic opiate antagonist administered in the form of its hydrochloride $C_{20}H_{23}NO_4 \cdot HCl$ esp. to maintain detoxified opiate addicts in a drug-free state

nan·dro·lone \'nan-drə-₁lōn\ *n* : a semisynthetic anabolic steroid $C_{18}H_{26}O_2$ derived from testosterone and used in the form of its esters to control metastatic breast cancer and to treat certain anemias and postmenopausal osteoporosis — called also *19-nortestosterone*

na·nism \'nan-₁iz-əm, 'nān-\ *n* : the condition of being abnormally or exceptionally small in stature : DWARFISM

nano·ce·phal·ic \₁nan-ō-si-'fal-ik\ *adj* : having an abnormally small head

nano·cu·rie \'nan-ə-₁kyu̇(ə)r-ē, -kyu̇-'rē\ *n* : one billionth of a curie — abbr. *nCi*

nano·gram *or chiefly Brit* **nano·gramme** \'nan-ə-₁gram\ *n* : one billionth of a gram — abbr. *ng*

nano·li·ter *or chiefly Brit* **nan·o·li·tre** \'nan-ə-₁lēt-ər\ *n* : one billionth of a liter — abbr. *nl*

nano·me·ter *or chiefly Brit* **nano·me·tre** \'nan-ə-₁mēt-ər\ *n* : one billionth of a meter — abbr. *nm*

nano·mole \-₁mōl\ *n* : one billionth of a mole — abbr. *nmol, nmole* — **nano·mo·lar** \-₁mō-lər\ *adj*

nano·par·ti·cle \-₁pärt-i-kəl\ *n* : a microscopic particle whose size is measured in nanometers ⟨drugs bound to biodegradable polymeric ∼s⟩

nano·scale \-₁skāl\ *adj* : having dimensions measured in nanometers ⟨∼ macromolecular structures⟩

nanosec *abbr* nanosecond

nano·sec·ond \-₁sek-ənd, -ənt\ *n* : one billionth of a second — abbr. *ns, nsec*

na·no·so·mia \₁nan-ə-'sō-mē-ə, ₁nān-\ *n* : DWARFISM

nano·sphere \'nan-ə-₁sfir\ *n* : a spherical particle whose diameter is measured in nanometers ⟨lipid-based ∼s⟩

nano·tes·la \-₁tes-lə\ *n* : a unit of magnetic flux density equal to 10^{-9} tesla — abbr. *nT*

nano·tube \-₁t(y)üb\ *n* : a microscopic tube whose diameter is measured in nanometers

nape \'nāp *also* 'nap\ *n* : the back of the neck

na·phaz·o·line \nə-'faz-ə-₁lēn\ *n* : a base derived from naphthalene and imidazoline and used topically in the form of its hydrochloride $C_{14}H_{14}N_2 \cdot HCl$ esp. to relieve nasal congestion and itching and redness of the eyes

naph·tha \'naf-thə, 'nap-\ *n* : any of various volatile often flammable liquid hydrocarbon mixtures used chiefly as solvents and diluents

naph·tha·lene \-₁lēn\ *n* : a crystalline aromatic hydrocarbon $C_{10}H_8$ usu. obtained by distillation of coal tar and used esp. in organic synthesis and formerly as a topical and intestinal antiseptic — **naph·tha·len·ic** \₁naf-thə-'len-ik, ₁nap-, -'lēn-\ *adj*

naph·tha·lene·sul·fon·ic acid *or chiefly Brit* **naph·tha·lene·sul·phon·ic acid** \-₁səl-₁fän-ik-, -₁fōn-\ *n* : either of two crystalline acids $C_{10}H_8SO_3$ obtained by sulfonation of naphthalene and used in the synthesis of dyes and naphthols

naphthoate — see PAMAQUINE NAPHTHOATE

naph·thol \'naf-₁thȯl, 'nap-, -₁thōl\ *n* : either of two isomeric derivatives $C_{10}H_8O$ of naphthalene found in coal tar or made synthetically: **a** : one used chiefly in synthesizing dyes — called also *alpha-naphthol* **b** : one used chiefly as an intermediate (as for dyes and pharmaceuticals) and esp. formerly in medicine as an antiseptic and parasiticide — called also *beta-naphthol*

naph·thol·sul·fon·ic acid *or chiefly Brit* **naph·thol·sul·phon·ic acid** \-₁səl-₁fän-ik-, -₁fōn-\ *n* : any of several sulfonic acids derived from the naphthols and used as dye intermediates

naph·tho·qui·none *also* **naph·tha·qui·none** \₁naf-thə-kwin-'ōn, ₁nap-, -'kwin-₁ōn\ *n* : any of three isomeric yellow to red crystalline compounds $C_{10}H_6O_2$ derived from naphthalene; *esp* : one that occurs naturally in the form of derivatives (as vitamin K)

naph·thyl \'naf-thəl, 'nap-\ *n* : either of two monovalent hydrocarbon radicals $C_{10}H_7$ derived from naphthalene by removal of a hydrogen atom in the alpha or the beta position

naph·thyl·amine \naf-'thil-ə-ˌmēn, nap-\ *n* : either of two isomeric crystalline bases $C_{10}H_9N$ that are used esp. in synthesizing dyes; *esp* : one (β–**naphthylamine**) with the amino group in the beta position that has been demonstrated to cause bladder cancer in individuals exposed to it while working in the dye industry

α–naphthylthiourea *var of* ALPHA-NAPHTHYLTHIOUREA

nap·kin \'nap-kən\ *n* **1** *chiefly Brit* : DIAPER **2** : SANITARY NAPKIN

nap·ra·path \'nap-rə-ˌpath\ *n* : a practitioner of naprapathy

na·prap·a·thy \nə-'prap-ə-thē\ *n, pl* **-thies** : a system of treatment by manipulation of connective tissue and adjoining structures (as ligaments, joints, and muscles) and by dietary measures that is held to facilitate the recuperative and regenerative processes of the body

Na·pro·syn \nə-'prōs-ᵊn\ *trademark* — used for a preparation of naproxen

na·prox·en \nə-'präk-sᵊn\ *n* : an anti-inflammatory analgesic antipyretic drug $C_{14}H_{14}O_3$ administered esp. to treat arthritis often in the form of its sodium salt $C_{14}H_{13}NaO_3$ — see ALEVE, NAPROSYN

nap·syl·ate \'nap-sə-ˌlāt\ *n* : a salt of naphthalenesulfonic acid esp. with an organic base (as a drug) used as a vehicle for administration of the drug

Naqua \'nak-wə\ *trademark* — used for a preparation of trichlormethiazide

Nar·can \'när-ˌkan\ *trademark* — used for a preparation of naloxone

nar·ce·ine \'när-sē-ˌēn, -ən\ *n* : a bitter crystalline narcotic amphoteric alkaloid $C_{23}H_{27}NO_8$ found in opium and also obtainable from narcotine

nar·cism \'när-ˌsiz-əm\ *n* : NARCISSISM

Nar·cis·sus \när-'sis-əs\, Greek mythological character. Narcissus was a youth of renowned beauty. Transfixed by his own beauty, he contemplated his reflection in a pool of water. The more he looked, the more he liked what he saw. Held captive by his self-love, he never strayed from the pool, but gradually wasted away and died. The gods then transformed him into the flower which is now called narcissus after him.

nar·cis·sism \'när-sə-ˌsiz-əm\ *n* **1** : love of or sexual desire for one's own body **2** : the state or stage of development in psychoanalytic theory in which there is considerable erotic interest in one's own body and ego and which in abnormal forms persists through fixation or reappears through regression

nar·cis·sist \-səst\ *n* : an individual showing symptoms of or suffering from narcissism

nar·cis·sis·tic \ˌnär-sə-'sis-tik\ *adj* : of or relating to narcissism — **nar·cis·sis·ti·cal·ly** \-ti-k(ə-)lē\ *adv*

narcissistic personality disorder *n* : a personality disorder characterized esp. by an exaggerated sense of self-importance, persistent need for admiration, lack of empathy for others, excessive pride in achievements, and snobbish, disdainful, or patronizing attitudes

nar·cis·tic \när-'sis-tik\ *adj* : NARCISSISTIC

nar·co·anal·y·sis \ˌnär-kō-ə-'nal-ə-səs\ *n, pl* **-y·ses** \-ˌsēz\ : psychotherapy that is performed under sedation for the recovery of repressed memories together with the emotion accompanying the experience and that is designed to facilitate an acceptable integration of the experience in the patient's personality

nar·co·an·es·the·sia *or chiefly Brit* **nar·co·an·aes·the·sia** \ˌan-əs-'thē-zhə\ *n* : anesthesia produced by a narcotic drug (as morphine)

nar·co·di·ag·no·sis \-ˌdī-ig-'nō-səs\ *n, pl* **-no·ses** \-ˌsēz\ : the use of sedative or hypnotic drugs for diagnostic purposes (as in psychiatry)

nar·co·hyp·no·sis \-hip-'nō-səs\ *n, pl* **-no·ses** \-ˌsēz\ : a hypnotic state produced by drugs and sometimes used in psychotherapy

nar·co·lep·sy \'när-kə-ˌlep-sē\ *n, pl* **-sies** : a condition characterized by brief attacks of deep sleep often occurring with cataplexy and hypnagogic hallucinations — compare HYPERSOMNIA 2

¹nar·co·lep·tic \ˌnär-kə-'lep-tik\ *adj* : of, relating to, or affected with narcolepsy

²narcoleptic *n* : an individual who is subject to attacks of narcolepsy

nar·co·ma·nia \-'mā-nē-ə\ *n* : an uncontrollable desire for narcotics

nar·cose \'när-ˌkōs\ *adj* : marked by a condition of stupor

nar·co·sis \när-'kō-səs\ *n, pl* **-co·ses** \-ˌsēz\ : a state of stupor, unconsciousness, or arrested activity produced by the influence of narcotics or other chemicals or physical agents — see NITROGEN NARCOSIS

nar·co·sug·ges·tion \ˌnär-kō-sə(g)-'jes(h)-chən\ *n* : the psychoanalytic use of suggestion in subjects who have received sedative or hypnotic drugs

nar·co·syn·the·sis \-'sin(t)-thə-səs\ *n, pl* **-the·ses** \-ˌsēz\ : NARCOANALYSIS

nar·co·ther·a·py \-'ther-ə-pē\ *n, pl* **-pies** : psychotherapy carried out with the aid of sedating or hypnotic drugs

¹nar·cot·ic \när-'kät-ik\ *n* **1** : a drug (as codeine, methadone, or morphine) that in moderate doses dulls the senses, relieves pain, and induces profound sleep but in excessive doses causes stupor, coma, or convulsions **2** : a drug (as marijuana or LSD) subject to restriction similar to that of addictive narcotics whether in fact physiologically addictive and narcotic or not

²narcotic *adj* **1** : having the properties of or yielding a narcotic **2** : of, induced by, or concerned with narcotics **3** : of, involving, or intended for narcotic addicts

nar·cot·i·cism \när-'kät-ə-ˌsiz-əm\ *n* : addiction to habit-forming drugs

nar·co·tine \'när-kə-ˌtēn, -tən\ *n* : a crystalline alkaloid $C_{22}H_{23}NO_7$ that is found in opium and possesses antispasmodic but no narcotic properties

nar·co·tism \'när-kə-ˌtiz-əm\ *n* **1** : NARCOSIS **2** : NARCOTICISM

nar·co·ti·za·tion \ˌnär-kət-ə-'zā-shən\ *n* : the act or process of inducing narcosis

nar·co·tize *also Brit* **nar·co·tise** \'när-kə-ˌtīz\ *vb* **-tized** *also Brit* **-tised; -tiz·ing** *also Brit* **-tis·ing** *vt* **1** : to treat with or subject to a narcotic **2** : to put into a state of narcosis ~ *vi* : to act as a narcotizing agent

nar·co·tol·ine \'när-kə-ˌtōl-ˌēn, -ˌtōl-, -ən\ *n* : a crystalline alkaloid $C_{21}H_{21}NO_7$ found in the seed capsules of the opium poppy

Nar·dil \'när-ˌdil\ *trademark* — used for a preparation of phenelzine

na·res \'na(ə)r-(ˌ)ēz, 'ne(ə)r-\ *n pl* : the pair of openings of the nose

narrow–angle glaucoma *n* : ANGLE-CLOSURE GLAUCOMA

nar·row–spec·trum \'nar-(ˌ)ō-'spek-trəm, 'nar-ə-\ *adj* : effective against only a limited range of organisms ⟨~ antibiotics effective only against gram-negative bacteria⟩ — compare BROAD-SPECTRUM

Na·sa·cort \'nā-zə-ˌkòrt\ *trademark* — used for a preparation of the acetonide of triamcinolone

¹na·sal \'nā-zəl\ *n* : a nasal part (as a bone)

²nasal *adj* : of or relating to the nose ⟨~ inflammation⟩ — **na·sal·ly** \'nāz-(ə-)lē\ *adv*

nasal bone *n* : either of two bones of the skull of vertebrates above the fishes that lie in front of the frontal bones and in humans are oblong in shape forming by their junction the bridge of the nose and partly covering the nasal cavity

nasal breadth *n* **1** *on the skull* : the distance between the two most lateral points on the rim of the nasal opening **2** *on the living body* : the distance between the two most lateral points on the wings of the nostrils

---

\ə\ **abut** \ᵊ\ **kitten** \ər\ **further** \a\ **ash** \ā\ **ace** \ä\ **cot, cart** \aú\ **out** \ch\ **chin** \e\ **bet** \ē\ **easy** \g\ **go** \i\ **hit** \ī\ **ice** \j\ **job** \ŋ\ **sing** \ō\ **go** \ò\ **law** \òi\ **boy** \th\ **thin** \t͟h\ **the** \ü\ **loot** \ú\ **foot** \y\ **yet** \zh\ **vision** *See also* Pronunciation Symbols page

nasal cartilage *n* : any of the cartilages forming the anterior part of the nose

nasal cavity *n* : the vaulted chamber that lies between the floor of the cranium and the roof of the mouth of higher vertebrates extending from the external nares to the pharynx, being enclosed by bone or cartilage and usu. incompletely divided into lateral halves by the septum of the nose, and having its walls lined with mucous membrane that is rich in venous plexuses and ciliated in the lower part which forms the beginning of the respiratory passage and warms and filters the inhaled air and that is modified as sensory epithelium in the upper olfactory part

nasal concha *n* : any of three thin bony plates on the lateral wall of the nasal fossa on each side with or without their covering of mucous membrane: **a** : a separate curved bony plate that is the largest of the three and separates the inferior and middle meatuses of the nose — called also *inferior concha, inferior nasal concha, inferior turbinate, inferior turbinate bone, maxilloturbinal* **b** : the lower of two thin bony processes of the ethmoid bone on the lateral wall of each nasal fossa that separates the superior and middle meatuses of the nose — called also *middle concha, middle nasal concha, middle turbinate, middle turbinate bone, nasoturbinal* **c** : the upper of two thin bony processes of the ethmoid bone on the lateral wall of each nasal fossa that forms the upper boundary of the superior meatus of the nose — called also *superior concha, superior nasal concha, superior turbinate, superior turbinate bone*

nasal duct *n* : NASOLACRIMAL DUCT

nasal fossa *n* : either lateral half of the nasal cavity

nasal height *n* : the height of the nose from the nasion to the point where the nasal septum joins the upper lip

nasal index *n* : the ratio of nasal breadth to nasal height multiplied by 100

na·sa·lis \nā-ˈzā-ləs, -ˈsā-\ *n* : a small muscle on each side of the nose that constricts the nasal aperture by the action of a triangular transverse portion which draws the lateral part of the aperture upward and a quadrangular alar portion which draws it downward

nasal nerve *n* : NASOCILIARY NERVE

nasal notch *n* : the rough surface on the anterior lower border of the frontal bone between the orbits which articulates with the nasal bones and the maxillae

nasal process *n* : FRONTAL PROCESS 1

nasal sac *n* : OLFACTORY PIT

nasal septum *n* : the bony and cartilaginous partition between the nasal passages

nasal spine *n* : any of several median bony processes adjacent to the nasal passages: as **a** : ANTERIOR NASAL SPINE **b** : POSTERIOR NASAL SPINE

na·scent \ˈnas-ᵊnt, ˈnās-\ *adj* **1** : coming or having recently come into existence : beginning to develop ⟨∼ polypeptide chains⟩ **2** : of, relating to, or being an atom or substance at the moment of its formation usu. with the implication of greater reactivity than otherwise ⟨∼ hydrogen⟩

nasi — see ALA NASI, LEVATOR LABII SUPERIORIS ALAEQUE NASI

na·si·on \ˈnā-zē-ˌän\ *n* : the middle point of the nasofrontal suture

Na·smyth's membrane \ˈnā-smiths-\ *n* : the thin cuticular remains of the enamel organ which surrounds the enamel of a tooth during its fetal development and for a brief period after birth

Nasmyth, Alexander (*d* 1848), British anatomist and dentist. Nasmyth served as oral surgeon to Queen Victoria and Prince Albert. In 1839, in an article on the structure and diseases of teeth, he described the cuticle of the dental enamel, now known as Nasmyth's membrane.

na·so·al·ve·o·lar \ˌnā-zō-al-ˈvē-ə-lər\ *adj* : of, relating to, or affecting the nose and one or more alveoli of the maxilla ⟨a ∼ cyst⟩

na·so·bas·i·lar \-ˈbaz-(ə-)lər, -ˈbas- *also* -ˈbāz- *or* -ˈbās-\ *adj* : of or relating to the nasion and the basion

na·so·cil·i·ary \-ˈsil-ē-ˌer-ē\ *adj* : nasal and ciliary

nasociliary nerve *n* : a branch of the ophthalmic nerve distributed in part to the ciliary ganglion and in part to the mucous membrane and skin of the nose — called also *nasal nerve*

na·so·fron·tal \-ˈfrənt-ᵊl\ *adj* : of or relating to the nasal and frontal bones

nasofrontal suture *n* : the cranial suture between the nasal and frontal bones

na·so·gas·tric \-ˈgas-trik\ *adj* : of, relating to, being, or performed by intubation of the stomach by way of the nasal passages ⟨insertion of a ∼ tube⟩ ⟨∼ suction⟩

na·so·la·bi·al \-ˈlā-bē-əl\ *adj* : of, relating to, located between, or affecting the nose and the upper lip ⟨a ∼ cyst⟩

nasolabial fold *n* : the crease that runs from the ala of the nose to the corner of the mouth of the same side

na·so·lac·ri·mal *also* **na·so·lach·ry·mal** \-ˈlak-rə-məl\ *adj* : of or relating to the lacrimal apparatus and nose

nasolacrimal duct *n* : a duct that transmits tears from the lacrimal sac to the inferior meatus of the nose — called also *nasal duct*

na·so·max·il·lary \-ˈmak-sə-ˌler-ē, *chiefly Brit* -mak-ˈsil-ə-rē\ *adj* : of, relating to, or located between the nasal bone and the maxilla ⟨∼ fracture⟩

nasomaxillary suture *n* : the suture uniting the nasal bone and the maxilla

Na·so·nex \ˈnā-zə-ˌneks\ *trademark* — used for a preparation of mometasone furoate used intranasally

na·so·pal·a·tine \-ˈpal-ə-ˌtīn\ *adj* : of, relating to, or connecting the nose and the palate

nasopalatine nerve *n* : a parasympathetic and sensory nerve that arises in the pterygopalatine ganglion, passes through the sphenopalatine foramen, across the roof of the nasal cavity to the nasal septum, and obliquely downward to and through the incisive canal, and innervates esp. the glands and mucosa of the nasal septum and the anterior part of the hard palate

na·so·pha·ryn·geal \ˌnā-zō-fə-ˈrin-j(ē-)əl, -ˌfar-ən-ˈjē-əl\ *adj* : of, relating to, or affecting the nose and pharynx or the nasopharynx ⟨∼ cancer⟩ ⟨∼ secretions⟩

nasopharyngeal tonsil *n* : PHARYNGEAL TONSIL

na·so·phar·yn·gi·tis \-ˌfar-ən-ˈjīt-əs\, *n, pl* **-git·i·des** \-ˈjit-ə-ˌdēz\ : inflammation of the nose and pharynx

na·so·pha·ryn·go·scope \-fə-ˈrin-gə-ˌskōp\ *n* : an endoscope for visually examining the nasal passages and pharynx — **na·so·pha·ryn·go·scop·ic** \-fə-ˌrin-gə-ˈskäp-ik\ *adj* — **na·so·phar·yn·gos·co·py** \-ˌfar-ən-ˈgäs-kə-pē\ *n, pl* **-pies**

na·so·phar·ynx \-ˈfar-in(k)s\ *n, pl* **-pha·ryn·ges** \-fə-ˈrin-(ˌ)jēz\ *also* **-phar·ynx·es** : the upper part of the pharynx continuous with the nasal passages — compare LARYNGOPHARYNX

na·so·scope \ˈnā-zə-ˌskōp\ *n* : RHINOSCOPE

na·so·si·nus·itis \ˌnā-zō-ˌsī-n(y)ə-ˈsīt-əs\ *also* **na·so·sin·u·itis** \-ˌsin-yü-ˈīt-əs\ *n* : inflammation of the nasal sinuses

na·so·spi·na·le \ˌnā-zō-spī-ˈnā-lē\ *n* : the point of intersection of a line uniting the lowest points on the margin of each nasal opening with the midsagittal plane

na·so·tra·che·al \-ˈtrā-kē-əl\ *adj* : of, relating to, being, or performed by means of intubation of the trachea by way of the nasal passage

na·so·tra·cheo·bron·chi·al \-ˌtrā-kē-ō-ˈbrän-kē-əl\ *adj* : of, relating to, being, or performed by means of intubation of a bronchus by way of the nasal passages and trachea ⟨∼ aspiration⟩

na·so·tur·bi·nal \-ˈtər-bə-nəl\ *n* : NASAL CONCHA b

na·tal \ˈnāt-ᵊl\ *adj* : of or relating to birth ⟨lowering the ∼ death rate —*Jour. Amer. Med. Assoc.*⟩

Na·tal aloes \nə-ˈtal-, -ˈtäl-\ *n pl* : a commercial variety of aloes

na·tal·i·ty \nā-ˈtal-ət-ē, nə-\ *n, pl* **-ties** : BIRTHRATE

Natal sore *n* : ORIENTAL SORE

na·tes \ˈnā-ˌtēz\ *n pl* : BUTTOCKS

Na·tion·al For·mu·lary \ˌnash-(ə-)nəl-ˈfòr-myə-ˌler-ē\ *n* : a periodically revised book of officially established and recognized drug names and standards — abbr. *NF*

National Health Service *n* : a government organization in Great Britain that provides at public expense all hospital, medical, dental, and related supportive or ancillary services and appliances and prescription drugs

na·tive \'nāt-iv\ *adj* **1** : belonging to or associated with one by birth **2** : living or growing naturally in a particular region **3 a** : constituting the original substance or source **b** : found in nature esp. in an unadulterated form ⟨conversion of a ∼ protein to a denatured protein⟩ — **na·tive·ly** *adv*

na·tri·um \'nā-trē-əm\ *n* : SODIUM

na·tri·ure·sis \ˌnā-trē-(y)ə-'rē-səs\ *also* **na·tru·re·sis** \-trə-'rē-səs\ *n* : excessive loss of cations and esp. sodium in the urine — **na·tri·uret·ic** \-'ret-ik\ *adj or n*

nat·u·ral \'nach-(ə-)rəl\ *adj* **1** : having, constituting, or relating to a classification based on features existing in nature **2** : of or relating to nature as an object of study and research **3** : relating to or being natural food

natural childbirth *n* : a system of managing childbirth in which the mother receives preparatory education in order to remain conscious during and assist in delivery with minimal or no use of drugs or anesthetics

natural family plan·ning \-'plan-iŋ\ *n* : a method of birth control that involves abstention from sexual intercourse during the period of ovulation which is determined through observation and measurement of bodily signs (as cervical mucus and body temperature) — abbr. *NFP*

natural food *n* : food that has undergone minimal processing and contains no preservatives or artificial additives

natural history *n* : the natural development of something (as an organism or disease) over a period of time ⟨increasing knowledge of the *natural histories* of tumors —H. S. N. Greene⟩

natural immunity *n* : immunity that is possessed by a group (as a race, strain, or species) and occurs in an individual as part of its natural biologic makeup and that is sometimes considered to include that acquired passively in utero or from mother's milk or actively by exposure to infection — compare ACQUIRED IMMUNITY, ACTIVE IMMUNITY, PASSIVE IMMUNITY

natural killer cell *n* : a large granular lymphocyte capable esp. of destroying tumor cells or virally infected cells without prior exposure to the target cell and without having it presented with or marked by a histocompatibility antigen — called also *NK cell*

natural selection *n* : a natural process that results in the survival and reproductive success of individuals or groups best adjusted to their environment and that leads to the perpetuation of genetic qualities best suited to that particular environment

na·tu·ro·path *also* **na·ture·o·path** \'nā-chə-rə-ˌpath, nə-'t(y)ùr-ə-\ *n* : a practitioner of naturopathy

na·tu·rop·a·thy *also* **na·ture·op·a·thy** \ˌnā-chə-'räp-ə-thē\ *n*, *pl* **-thies** : a system of treatment of disease that avoids drugs and surgery and emphasizes the use of natural agents (as air, water, and herbs) and physical means (as tissue manipulation and electrotherapy) — **na·tu·ro·path·ic** *also* **na·ture·o·path·ic** \ˌnā-chə-rə-'path-ik, nə-ˌt(y)ùr-ə-\ *adj*

nau·path·ia \nȯ-'path-ē-ə\ *n* : SEASICKNESS

nau·sea \'nȯ-zē-ə, -sē-ə; 'nȯ-zhə, -shə\ *n* : a stomach distress with distaste for food and an urge to vomit

¹nau·se·ant \'nȯ-z(h)ē-ənt, -s(h)ē-\ *n* : an agent that induces nausea; *esp* : an expectorant that liquefies and increases the secretion of mucus

²nauseant *adj* : inducing nausea : NAUSEATING

nau·se·ate \'nȯ-z(h)ē-ˌāt, -s(h)ē-\ *vb* **-at·ed; -at·ing** *vi* : to become affected with nausea ∼ *vt* : to affect with nausea

nau·seous \'nȯ-shəs, 'nȯ-zē-əs\ *adj* **1** : causing nausea **2** : affected with nausea

Nav·ane \'nav-ˌān\ *trademark* — used for a preparation of thiothixene

na·vel \'nā-vəl\ *n* : a depression in the middle of the abdomen

that marks the point of former attachment of the umbilical cord to the embryo — called also *umbilicus*

navel ill *n* : a serious septicemia of newborn animals caused by pus-producing bacteria entering the body through the umbilical cord or opening and typically marked by joint inflammation or arthritis accompanied by generalized pyemia, rapid debilitation, and commonly death — called also *joint evil, joint ill, pyosepticemia*

navel string *n* : UMBILICAL CORD

¹na·vic·u·lar \nə-'vik-yə-lər\ *n* : a navicular bone: **a** : the one of the seven tarsal bones of the human foot that is situated on the big-toe side between the talus and the cuneiform bones — called also *scaphoid* **b** : SCAPHOID 2 **c** : a small bone enclosed within the hoof of the horse behind the junction of the coffin bone and short pastern bone

²navicular *adj* **1** : resembling or having the shape of a boat ⟨a ∼ bone⟩ **2** : of, relating to, or involving a navicular bone ⟨∼ fractures⟩

navicular disease *n* : inflammation of the navicular bone and forefoot of the horse resulting in a shortened stride and persistent lameness and regarded as due to repeated bruising or strain esp. in individuals exhibiting a hereditary predisposition

navicular fossa *n* : the dilated terminal portion of the urethra in the glans penis

navicularis — see FOSSA NAVICULARIS

Nb *symbol* niobium

NB *abbr* newborn

NBRT *abbr* National Board for Respiratory Therapy

NCA *abbr* neurocirculatory asthenia

nCi *abbr* nanocurie

NCI *abbr* National Cancer Institute

NCQA *abbr* National Committee for Quality Assurance

Nd *symbol* neodymium

ND *abbr* doctor of naturopathy

NDT *abbr* neurodevelopmental treatment

Ne *symbol* neon

near point *n* : the point nearest the eye at which an object is accurately focused on the retina when the maximum degree of accommodation is employed — compare FAR POINT; see RANGE OF ACCOMMODATION

near·sight·ed \'ni(ə)r-'sīt-əd\ *adj* : able to see near things more clearly than distant ones : MYOPIC — **near·sight·ed·ly** *adv*

near·sight·ed·ness *n* : MYOPIA

ne·ar·thro·sis \ˌnē-är-'thrō-səs\ *n, pl* **-thro·ses** \-ˌsēz\ : a false joint : PSEUDARTHROSIS

ne·ben·kern \'nā-bən-ˌkərn, -ˌke(ə)rn\ *n* : a two-stranded helical structure of the proximal tail region of a spermatozoon that is derived from mitochondria

neb·u·la \'neb-yə-lə\ *n, pl* **-las** *or* **-lae** \-ˌlē, -ˌlī\ : a slight cloudy opacity of the cornea

neb·u·li·za·tion *or Brit* **neb·u·li·sa·tion** \ˌneb-yə-lə-'zā-shən\ *n* **1** : reduction of a medicinal solution to a fine spray **2** : treatment (as of respiratory diseases) by means of a fine spray

neb·u·lize *or Brit* **neb·u·lise** \'neb-yə-ˌlīz\ *vt* **-lized** *or Brit* **-lised; -liz·ing** *or Brit* **-lis·ing** : to reduce to a fine spray ⟨a *nebulized* medication⟩

neb·u·liz·er *or Brit* **neb·u·lis·er** \-ˌlī-zər\ *n* : ATOMIZER; *specif* : an atomizer equipped to produce an extremely fine spray for deep penetration of the lungs

Ne·ca·tor \nə-'kāt-ər\ *n* : a genus of common hookworms that have buccal teeth resembling flat plates, that include internal parasites of humans and various other mammals, and that are prob. of African origin though first identified in No. America — compare ANCYLOSTOMA

ne·ca·to·ri·a·sis \nə-ˌkāt-ə-'rī-ə-səs\ *n, pl* **-a·ses** \-ˌsēz\ : infestation by hookworms of the genus *Necator*

\ə\ **abut** \ᵊ\ kitten \ər\ **further** \a\ ash \ā\ ace \ä\ cot, cart \au̇\ out \ch\ chin \e\ bet \ē\ easy \g\ go \i\ hit \ī\ ice \j\ job \ŋ\ sing \ō\ go \ȯ\ law \ȯi\ boy \th\ thin \th\ the \ü\ loot \u̇\ foot \y\ yet \zh\ vision   *See also* Pronunciation Symbols page

neck \'nek\ *n* **1 a** : the usu. narrowed part of an animal that connects the head with the body; *specif* : the cervical region of a vertebrate **b** : the part of a tapeworm immediately behind the scolex from which new proglottids are produced **2** : a relatively narrow part suggestive of a neck: as **a** : a narrow part of a bone ⟨the ∼ of the femur⟩ **b** : CERVIX 2 **c** : the part of a tooth between the crown and the root

nec·ro \'nek-(ˌ)rō\ *n* : NECROTIC ENTERITIS

nec·ro·bac·il·lo·sis \ˌnek-rō-ˌbas-ə-'lō-səs\ *n, pl* **-lo·ses** \-ˌsēz\ : any of several infections or diseases (as bullnose or calf diphtheria) that are either localized (as in foot rot) or disseminated through the body of the infected animal and that are characterized by inflammation and ulcerative or necrotic lesions from which a bacterium of the genus *Fusobacterium* (*F. necrophorum* syn. *Sphaerophorus necrophorus*) has been isolated — see QUITTOR

nec·ro·bi·o·sis \-bī-'ō-səs\ *n, pl* **-o·ses** \-ˌsēz\ : death of a cell or group of cells within a tissue whether normal (as in various epithelial tissues) or part of a pathologic process — compare NECROSIS

necrobiosis li·poid·i·ca \-li-'pȯid-i-kə\ *n* : a disease of the skin that is characterized by the formation of multiple necrobiotic lesions esp. on the legs and that is often associated with diabetes mellitus

necrobiosis lipoidica dia·bet·i·co·rum \-ˌdī-ə-ˌbet-i-'kȯr-əm\ *n* : NECROBIOSIS LIPOIDICA

nec·ro·bi·ot·ic \ˌnek-rə-bī-'ät-ik\ *adj* : of, relating to, or being in a state of necrobiosis

nec·ro·gen·ic \-'jen-ik\ *adj* : causing necrosis ⟨∼ X-ray burns —*Jour. of Amer. Dental Assoc.*⟩

nec·ro·phile \'nek-tə-ˌfīl\ *also* **nec·ro·phil** \-ˌfil\ *n* : one that is affected with necrophilia

nec·ro·phil·ia \ˌnek-rə-'fil-ē-ə\ *n* : obsession with and usu. erotic interest in or stimulation by corpses

¹**nec·ro·phil·i·ac** \-'fil-ē-ˌak\ *adj* : of, relating to, or marked by necrophilia

²**necrophiliac** *n* : NECROPHILE

nec·ro·phil·ic \-'fil-ik\ *adj* : NECROPHILIAC

ne·croph·i·lism \nə-'kräf-ə-ˌliz-əm, ne-\ *n* : NECROPHILIA

ne·croph·i·list \-ləst\ *n* : NECROPHILE

ne·croph·i·lous \-ləs\ *adj* : NECROPHILIAC

ne·croph·i·ly \-lē\ *n, pl* **-lies** : NECROPHILIA

nec·ro·phobe \'nek-rə-ˌfōb\ *n* : one who exhibits necrophobia

nec·ro·pho·bia \ˌnek-rə-'fō-bē-ə\ *n* : an exaggerated fear of death or horror of dead bodies — **nec·ro·pho·bic** \-'fō-bik\ *adj*

¹**nec·rop·sy** \'nek-ˌräp-sē\ *n, pl* **-sies** : AUTOPSY; *esp* : an autopsy performed on an animal

²**necropsy** *vt* **-sied; -sy·ing** : to perform an autopsy esp. on an animal

nec·rose \'nek-ˌrōs, -ˌrōz, ne-'krōz\ *vb* **nec·rosed; nec·ros·ing** *vi* : to undergo necrosis ⟨tissues subjected to prolonged pressure may ∼ to form bedsores⟩ ∼ *vt* : to affect with or cause to undergo necrosis

nec·ro·sin \'nek-rə-sən\ *n* : a toxic substance associated with euglobulin in injured tissue and inflammatory exudates that induces leukopenia and hastens blood coagulation and is regarded by some as a proteolytic enzyme

ne·cro·sis \nə-'krō-səs, ne-\ *n, pl* **ne·cro·ses** \-ˌsēz\ : death of living tissue; *specif* : death of a portion of tissue differentially affected by local injury (as loss of blood supply, corrosion, burning, or the local lesion of a disease) — compare NECROBIOSIS

nec·ro·sper·mia \ˌnek-rə-'spər-mē-ə\ *n* : a condition in which the spermatozoa in seminal fluid are dead or motionless

ne·crot·ic \nə-'krät-ik, ne-\ *adj* : affected with, characterized by, or producing necrosis ⟨a ∼ gallbladder⟩

necrotic enteritis *n* : either of two often fatal infectious diseases marked esp. by intestinal inflammation and necrosis and by diarrhea: **a** : one affecting young swine and caused by a bacterium of the genus *Salmonella* (*S. choleraesuis*) — called also *necro* **b** : one affecting poultry and esp. young

chickens and turkeys and caused by a bacterium of the genus *Clostridium* (*C. perfringens*)

necrotic rhinitis *n* : BULLNOSE

nec·ro·tiz·ing *or chiefly Brit* **nec·ro·tis·ing** \'nek-rə-ˌtī-zin\ *adj* : causing, associated with, or undergoing necrosis ⟨∼ infections⟩ ⟨∼ tissue⟩

necrotizing angiitis *n* : NECROTIZING VASCULITIS

necrotizing fasciitis *n* : a severe soft tissue infection typically by Group A streptococci or by a mixture of aerobic and anaerobic bacteria that is marked by edema and necrosis of subcutaneous tissues with involvement of the fascia and widespread undermining of adjacent tissue, by painful red swollen skin over affected areas, and by polymorphonuclear leukocytosis and that usu. occurs as a complication of surgery, injury, or infection by extension from the initially affected site

necrotizing papillitis *n* : necrosis of the papillae of the kidney — called also *necrotizing renal papillitis*

necrotizing ulcerative gingivitis *n* : ACUTE NECROTIZING ULCERATIVE GINGIVITIS

necrotizing vasculitis *n* : an inflammatory condition of the blood vessels characterized by necrosis of vascular tissue — called also *necrotizing angiitis, systemic necrotizing vasculitis*

ne·crot·o·my \ne-'krät-ə-mē, nə-\ *n, pl* **-mies** **1** : dissection of dead bodies **2** : surgical removal of necrosed bone

nec·ro·tox·in \'nek-rə-ˌtäk-sən\ *n* : a substance produced by some bacteria of the genus *Staphylococcus* which destroys tissue cells

nec·ro·zoo·sper·mia \ˌnek-rə-ˌzō-ə-'spər-mē-ə\ *n* : NECROSPERMIA

nec·tu·rus \nek-'t(y)ùr-əs\ *n* **1** *cap* : a genus of large No. American gilled aquatic salamanders (family Proteidae) which are used as laboratory animals **2** *pl* **-ri** \-ˌrī\ *or* **-rus·es** : a salamander of the genus *Necturus*

ne·do·cro·mil sodium \nə-'däk-rə-mil, ˌned-ə-'krō-\ *n* : an anti-inflammatory disodium salt $C_{19}H_{15}NNa_2O_7$ that is administered either as an aerosol by oral inhalation for the treatment of mild to moderate asthma or as eyedrops for the treatment of itching associated with allergic conjunctivitis — called also *nedocromil*

¹**nee·dle** \'nēd-ᵊl\ *n* **1** : a small slender usu. steel instrument designed to carry sutures when sewing tissues in surgery **2** : a slender hollow instrument for introducing material into or removing material from the body parenterally

²**needle** *vt* **nee·dled; nee·dling** \'nēd-lin, -ᵊl-in\ : to puncture, operate on, or inject with a needle ⟨*needling* a cataract⟩

needle bath *n* : a bath in which water is forcibly projected on the body in fine jets

needle biopsy *n* : any of several methods (as fine needle aspiration or core biopsy) for obtaining a sample of cells or tissue by inserting a hollow needle through the skin and withdrawing the sample from the tissue or organ to be examined

nee·dle·stick \'nēd-ᵊl-ˌstik\ *n* : an accidental puncture of the skin with an unsterilized instrument (as a syringe) — called also *needlestick injury*

ne·en·ceph·a·lon \ˌnē-in-'sef-ə-ˌlän, -lən\ *n* : the part of the brain having the most recent phylogenetic origin; *specif* : the cerebral cortex and parts developed in relation to it — compare PALEENCEPHALON

¹**neg·a·tive** \'neg-ət-iv\ *adj* **1** : marked by denial, prohibition, or refusal ⟨received a ∼ answer⟩ **2** : marked by features (as hostility, withdrawal, or pessimism) that hinder or oppose constructive treatment or development ⟨a ∼ outlook⟩ **3 a** : being, relating to, or charged with electricity of which the electron is the elementary unit **b** : having more electrons than protons ⟨∼ ions⟩ **c (1)** : having lower electrical potential and constituting the part toward which the current flows from the external circuit ⟨the ∼ pole⟩ **(2)** : being the electron-emitting electrode of an electron tube **4 a** : not affirming the presence of a condition, substance, or organism suspected to be present; *also* : having a test result indicating the absence esp. of a condition, substance, or organism ⟨she is HIV ∼⟩ **b** : directed or moving away from a source of stimulation ⟨∼ tropism⟩ **5** : having the light and dark parts

in approximately inverse relation to those of the original photographic subject — **neg·a·tive·ly** adv

²**negative** n **1** : a negative photographic image on transparent material used for printing positive pictures; also : the material that carries such an image **2** : a negative result (as of a test); also : a test yielding such a result

negative afterimage n : a visual afterimage in which light portions of the original sensation are replaced by dark portions and dark portions are replaced by light portions — compare POSITIVE AFTERIMAGE

negative catalysis n : catalysis in which the catalyst has an inhibiting effect on the reaction

negative catalyst n : an agent that retards a chemical reaction

negative eugenics n pl but usu sing in constr : improvement of the genetic makeup of a population by preventing the reproduction of the obviously unfit

negative feedback n : feedback that tends to stabilize a process by reducing its rate or output when its effects are too great

negative lens n : DIVERGING LENS

negative phase n : a phase of lowered resistance that may follow the injection of foreign antigen in active immunization

negative pressure n : pressure that is less than existing atmospheric pressure

negative reinforcement n : psychological reinforcement by removal of an unpleasant stimulus when a desired response occurs

negative staining n : a method of demonstrating the form of small objects (as bacteria) by surrounding them with a stain that they do not take up so that they appear as sharply outlined unstained bright bodies on a colored ground

negative transfer n : the impeding of learning or performance in a situation by the carryover of learned responses from another situation — compare INTERFERENCE 4

neg·a·tiv·ism \'neg-ət-iv-,iz-əm\ n **1** : an attitude of mind marked by skepticism about nearly everything affirmed by others **2** : a tendency to refuse to do, to do the opposite of, or to do something at variance with what is asked

neg·a·tiv·ist·ic \,neg-ət-iv-'is-tik\ adj : of, relating to, or characterized by negativism

neg·a·tiv·i·ty \,neg-ə-'tiv-ə-tē\ n, pl -**ties** : the quality or state of being negative

neg·a·tron \'neg-ə-,trän\ also **neg·a·ton** \-,tän\ n : ELECTRON

Neg·Gram \'neg-,gram\ trademark — used for a preparation of nalidixic acid

Ne·gri body \'nā-grē-\ n : an inclusion body found in the nerve cells in rabies

Negri, Adelchi (1876–1912), Italian physician and pathologist. Negri conducted research in histology, hematology, cytology, protozoology, and hygiene. During histological research undertaken to clarify the etiology of rabies, he discovered in animals suffering from rabies that certain cells of the nervous system contain intracellular bodies with an internal structure so evident and regular as to constitute a characteristic feature. He announced his discovery of the Negri bodies in 1903.

Ne·gro \'nē-(,)grō\ n, pl **Negroes** sometimes offensive : a member of a race of humankind native to Africa and classified according to physical features (as dark skin pigmentation) — **Negro** adj, sometimes offensive

Neis·se·ria \nī-'sir-ē-ə\ n : a genus (the type of the family Neisseriaceae) of parasitic bacteria that grow in pairs and occas. tetrads, thrive best at 98.6°F (37°C) in the animal body or serum media, and include the gonococcus (N. gonorrhoeae) and meningococcus (N. meningitidis)

Neis·ser \'nī-sər\, Albert Ludwig Sigesmund (1855–1916), German dermatologist. Neisser discovered the bacillus that causes gonorrhea in 1879. In 1885 the genus Neisseria, named in his honor, was described, and this microorganism and related bacteria were placed in it.

Neis·ser·i·a·ce·ae \nī-,sir-ē-ē-'ā-sē-,ē\ n pl : a small family of spherical nonmotile gram-negative bacteria of the order Eu-

bacteriales that are obligate parasites of warm-blooded vertebrates

neis·se·ri·an \nī-'sir-ē-ən\ or **neis·se·ri·al** \-ē-əl\ adj : of, relating to, or caused by bacteria of the genus Neisseria ⟨a ∼ culture⟩ ⟨∼ infections⟩

nel·fin·a·vir \nel-'fin-ə-,vir\ n : a protease inhibitor that is administered in the form of its mesylate $C_{32}H_{45}N_3O_4S$·CH_4O_3S in the treatment of HIV infection — see VIRACEPT

ne·ma \'nē-mə, 'nem-ə\ n : NEMATODE

nemacide var of NEMATOCIDE

nem·a·thel·minth \,nem-ə-'thel-,min(t)th\ n : any wormlike animal of the phylum Nemathelminthes

Nem·a·thel·min·thes \-,thel-'min(t)-(,)thēz\ n pl, in some classifications : a phylum including the nematodes and horsehair worms and sometimes the acanthocephalans, rotifers, gastrotrichs, and minute marine organisms of a related class (Kinorhyncha) which are all more or less wormlike animals with a cylindrical unsegmented body covered by an ectoderm without cilia that secretes an external cuticle

ne·mat·ic \ni-'mat-ik\ adj : of, relating to, or being the phase of a liquid crystal characterized by arrangement of the long axes of the molecules in parallel lines but not layers ⟨∼ polypeptide liquid crystals⟩ — compare SMECTIC

nem·a·to·cid·al also **nem·a·ti·cid·al** \,nem-ət-ə-'sīd-ᵊl, ni-,mat-ə-\ adj : capable of destroying nematodes

nem·a·to·cide also **nem·a·ti·cide** \'nem-ət-ə-,sīd, ni-'mat-ə-\ or **nem·a·cide** \'nem-ə-\ n : a substance or preparation used to destroy nematodes

nem·a·to·cyst \'nem-ət-ə-,sist, ni-'mat-ə-\ n : one of the minute stinging organelles of various coelenterates — called also stinging cell

Nem·a·to·da \,nem-ə-'tō-də\ n pl : a phylum related to the Aschelminthes and comprising elongated cylindrical worms without an epithelial coelomic lining, with dorsal and ventral nerve cords, and with lateral excretory ducts that are parasites of humans, animals, or plants or free-living dwellers in soil or water and are known as roundworms, eelworms, or nematodes

¹**nem·a·tode** \'nem-ə-,tōd\ adj : of or relating to the phylum Nematoda

²**nematode** n : any worm of the phylum Nematoda

nem·a·to·di·a·sis \,nem-ə-(,)tō-'dī-ə-səs\ n, pl -**a·ses** \-,sēz\ : infestation with or disease caused by nematode worms

nem·a·to·di·ri·a·sis \,nem-ə-,tō-di-'rī-ə-səs\ n, pl -**a·ses** \-,sēz\ : an infestation of the small intestine esp. of sheep by nematode worms of the genus Nematodirus that is characterized primarily by the scours

Nem·a·to·di·rus \,nem-ə-tə-'dī-rəs\ n : a genus of reddish nematode worms of the family Strongylidae having slender elongated necks and being parasitic in the small intestine of ruminants and sometimes other mammals

Nem·a·toi·dea \,nem-ə-'tȯid-ē-ə\ n pl, syn of NEMATODA

nem·a·tol·o·gist \,nem-ə-'täl-ə-jəst\ n : a specialist in nematology

nem·a·tol·o·gy \,nem-ə-'täl-ə-jē\ n, pl -**gies** : a branch of zoology that deals with nematodes — **nem·a·to·log·i·cal** \,nem-ət-ᵊl-'äj-i-kəl\ adj

Nem·a·to·mor·pha \,nem-ə-tə-'mȯr-fə, nə-,mat-ə-\ n pl : a phylum that is related to the phylum Aschelminthes and comprises the horsehair worms which were formerly often grouped with the nematodes but are distinguished from these by possession of a true body cavity, gonads discontinuous with their ducts, and an atrophied digestive tract in the adult — **nem·a·to·morph** \'nem-ət-ə-,mȯrf, nə-'mat-ə-\ n or adj

Nem·bu·tal \'nem-byə-,tȯl\ trademark — used for the sodium salt of pentobarbital

nem·bu·tal·ized \-,īzd\ adj : anesthetized with pentobarbital ⟨∼ dogs were operated upon⟩

M
N

\ə\ **abut** \ᵊ\ **kitten** \ər\ **further** \a\ **ash** \ā\ **ace** \ä\ **cot, cart**
\aù\ **out** \ch\ **chin** \e\ **bet** \ē\ **easy** \g\ **go** \i\ **hit** \ī\ **ice** \j\ **job**
\ŋ\ **sing** \ō\ **go** \ȯ\ **law** \ȯi\ **boy** \th\ **thin** \t̲h̲\ **the** \ü\ **loot**
\ù\ **foot** \y\ **yet** \zh\ **vision**   See also Pronunciation Symbols page

nem·ic \'nem-ik\ *adj* : of or relating to nematodes

neo·ars·phen·a·mine \ˌnē-ō-ärs-'fen-ə-ˌmēn\ *n* : a yellow powder $C_{13}H_{13}As_2N_2NaO_4S$ similar to arsphenamine in structure and use — called also *neosalvarsan*

neo·blas·tic \ˌnē-ə-'blas-tik\ *adj* : relating to or constituting new growth

neo·cer·e·bel·lar \ˌnē-ō-ˌser-ə-'bel-ər\ *adj* : of or relating to the neocerebellum

neo·cer·e·bel·lum \-'bel-əm\ *n, pl* **-bellums** *or* **-bel·la** \-'bel-ə\ : the phylogenetically youngest part of the cerebellum associated with the cerebral cortex in the integration of voluntary limb movements and comprising most of the cerebellar hemispheres and the superior vermis — compare PALEOCEREBELLUM

neo·cin·cho·phen \ˌnē-ō-'siŋ-kə-ˌfen\ *n* : a white crystalline compound $C_{19}H_{17}NO_2$ used as an analgesic and in the treatment of gout

neo·cor·tex \ˌnē-ō-'kȯr-ˌteks\ *n, pl* **-cor·ti·ces** \-'kȯrt-ə-ˌsēz\ *or* **-cor·tex·es** : the large 6-layered dorsal region of the cerebral cortex that is unique to mammals; *broadly* : the mammalian cerebral cortex

neo·cor·ti·cal \-'kȯrt-i-kəl\ *adj* : of or relating to the neocortex

neo–Dar·win·ian \-där-'win-ē-ən\ *adj* : of or relating to neoDarwinism

C. R. Darwin — see DARWINIAN

neo–Dar·win·ism \-'där-wə-ˌniz-əm\ *n* : a theory of evolution that is a synthesis of Darwin's theory in terms of natural selection and modern population genetics — **neo–Dar·win·ist** \-nəst\ *n*

neo·dym·i·um \ˌnē-ō-'dim-ē-əm\ *n* : a yellow metallic element of the rare-earth group — symbol *Nd*; see ELEMENT table

neo·for·ma·tion \-fȯr-'mā-shən\ *n* : a new growth; *specif* : TUMOR — **neo·for·ma·tive** \-'fȯr-mət-iv\ *adj*

¹neo–Freud·ian \-'frȯid-ē-ən\ *adj, often cap N* : of or relating to a school of psychoanalysis that differs from Freudian orthodoxy in emphasizing the importance of social and cultural factors in the development of an individual's personality

S. Freud — see FREUDIAN

²neo–Freudian *n, often cap N* : a member of or advocate of a neo-Freudian school of psychoanalysis

neo·ge·net·ic \ˌnē-ō-jə-'net-ik\ *or* **neo·gen·ic** \-'jen-ik\ *adj* : of, relating to, or characterized by the process of regeneration or of producing a new formation — **neo·gen·e·sis** \-'jen-ə-səs\ *n, pl* **-e·ses** \-ˌsēz\

neo·hes·per·i·din di·hy·dro·chal·cone \ˌnē-ō-hes-'per-ə-dən-ˌdī-ˌhī-drō-'kal-ˌkōn\ *n* : a sweetening agent $C_{28}H_{36}O_{15}$ that is found in grapefruit, is 1000 to 1500 times sweeter than sucrose, and is used esp. in chewing gum and toothpastes

neo·in·ti·ma \-'int-ə-mə\ *n* : a new or thickened layer of arterial intima formed esp. on a prosthesis or in atherosclerosis by migration and proliferation of cells from the media — **neo·in·ti·mal** \-məl\ *adj*

ne·ol·o·gism \nē-'äl-ə-ˌjiz-əm\ *n* **1** : a new word, usage, or expression **2** : a word coined by a psychotic that is meaningless except to the coiner

neo·morph \'nē-ə-ˌmȯrf\ *n* **1** : a structure that is not derived from a similar structure in an ancestor **2** : a mutant gene having a function distinct from that of any nonmutant gene of the same locus

neo·my·cin \ˌnē-ə-'mīs-ᵊn\ *n* : a broad-spectrum highly toxic mixture of aminoglycoside antibiotics produced by a bacterium of the genus *Streptomyces* (*S. fradiae*); *specif* : a commercial preparation that is composed chiefly of two stereoisomers of neomycin administered in the form of their sulfate $C_{23}H_{46}N_6O_{13}\cdot2\frac{1}{2}H_2SO_4$ and that is used either alone or in combination with one or more other drugs esp. to treat infections (as impetigo or conjunctivitis) topically, to irrigate the bladder, and to produce intestinal antisepsis prior to certain surgeries

ne·on \'nē-ˌän\ *n* : a colorless odorless primarily inert gaseous element found in minute amounts in air and used in electric lamps — symbol *Ne*; see ELEMENT table

neo·na·tal \ˌnē-ō-'nāt-ᵊl\ *adj* : of, relating to, or affecting the newborn and esp. the human infant during the first month after birth ⟨∼ jaundice⟩ ⟨∼ death⟩ — compare PRENATAL, INTRANATAL, POSTNATAL — **neo·na·tal·ly** \-ᵊl-ē\ *adv*

ne·o·nate \'nē-ə-ˌnāt\ *n* : a newborn infant; *esp* : an infant less than a month old

neo·na·tol·o·gist \ˌnē-ə-nāt-'äl-ə-jəst\ *n* : a specialist in neonatology

neo·na·tol·o·gy \ˌnē-ə-nāt-'äl-ə-jē\ *n, pl* **-gies** : a branch of medicine concerned with the care, development, and diseases of newborn infants

neonatorum — see ERYTHROBLASTOSIS NEONATORUM, ICTERUS GRAVIS NEONATORUM, ICTERUS NEONATORUM, OPHTHALMIA NEONATORUM, SCLEREMA NEONATORUM

neo·pal·li·al \ˌnē-ō-'pal-ē-əl\ *adj* : of, relating to, or mediated by the neopallium

neo·pal·li·um \-ē-əm\ *n, pl* **-lia** \-ē-ə\ : the phylogenetically new part of the cerebral cortex that develops from the area between the piriform lobe and the hippocampus, comprises the nonolfactory region of the cortex, and attains its maximum development in humans where it makes up the greater part of the cerebral hemisphere on each side — called also *isocortex;* compare ARCHIPALLIUM

neo·pho·bia \ˌnē-ə-'fō-bē-ə\ *n* : dread of or aversion to novelty — **neo·pho·bic** \-bik\ *adj*

ne·o·pine \'nē-ə-ˌpēn, -pən\ *n* : an opium alkaloid $C_{18}H_{21}NO_3$ isomeric with codeine

neo·pla·sia \ˌnē-ə-'plā-zh(ē-)ə\ *n* **1** : the process of tumor formation **2** : a tumorous condition of the body

neo·plasm \'nē-ə-ˌplaz-əm\ *n* : a new growth of tissue serving no physiological function : TUMOR

neo·plas·tic \ˌnē-ə-'plas-tik\ *adj* : of, relating to, or constituting a neoplasm or neoplasia — **neo·plas·ti·cal·ly** \-ti-k(ə-)lē\ *adv*

neo·sal·var·san \ˌnē-ō-'sal-vər-ˌsan\ *n* : NEOARSPHENAMINE

neo·sti·bo·san \-'stī-bə-ˌsan\ *n* : ETHYLSTIBAMINE

neo·stig·mine \ˌnē-ō-'stig-ˌmēn\ *n* : a cholinergic drug used in the form of its bromide $C_{12}H_{19}BrN_2O_2$ or a methyl sulfate derivative $C_{13}H_{22}N_2O_6S$ esp. in the diagnosis and treatment of myasthenia gravis and in the treatment of urinary bladder or bowel atony — see PROSTIGMIN

neo·stri·a·tum \ˌnē-ō-(ˌ)strī-'āt-əm\ *n, pl* **-tums** *or* **-ta** \-ə\ : the phylogenetically newer part of the corpus striatum consisting of the caudate nucleus and putamen — **neo·stri·a·tal** \-'āt-ᵊl\ *adj*

Neo–Sy·neph·rine \ˌnē-ō-sin-'ef-rən, -ˌrēn\ *trademark* — used for a preparation of the hydrochloride of phenylephrine

neo·thal·a·mus \ˌnē-ō-'thal-ə-məs\ *n, pl* **-mi** \-ˌmī\ : the phylogenetically more recent part of the thalamus including the lateral nuclei and the pulvinar together with the geniculate bodies

neo·vas·cu·lar \ˌnē-ō-'vas-kyə-lər\ *adj* : of, relating to, or being neovascularization — **neo·vas·cu·lar·i·ty** \-ˌvas-kyə-'lar-ət-ē\ *n, pl* **-ties**

neo·vas·cu·lar·i·za·tion *also Brit* **neo·vas·cu·lar·i·sa·tion** \-ˌvas-kyə-lə-rə-'zā-shən\ *n* : vascularization esp. in abnormal quantity (as in some conditions of the retina) or in abnormal tissue (as a tumor)

nep·e·ta·lac·tone \ˌnep-ət-ə-'lak-ˌtōn\ *n* : a compound $C_{10}H_{14}O_2$ that is the chief constituent of the essential oil of catnip

neph·e·lom·e·ter \ˌnef-ə-'läm-ət-ər\ *n* : an instrument for measuring cloudiness: as **a** : a set of barium chloride or barium sulfate standards used for estimating the turbidity of a fluid and thereby the number of bacteria in suspension **b** : an instrument for determining the concentration or particle size of suspensions by means of transmitted or reflected light — **neph·e·lo·met·ric** \ˌnef-ə-lō-'me-trik\ *adj*

neph·e·lom·e·try \-'läm-ə-trē\ *n, pl* **-tries** : the measurement of the intensity of reflected light by means of a nephelometer esp. as applied to studies of turbidity (as in the determination of particle size or of the amount of suspended matter in chemical analysis)

ne·phral·gia \ni-'fral-jə\ *n* : pain in a kidney

ne·phrec·to·mize *also Brit* **ne·phrec·to·mise** \ni-'frek-tə-ˌmīz\ *vb* **-mized** *also Brit* **-mised; -miz·ing** *also Brit* **-mis·ing** *vt* : to perform nephrectomy upon ~ *vi* : to remove a kidney

ne·phrec·to·my \ni-'frek-tə-mē\ *n, pl* **-mies** : the surgical removal of a kidney

neph·ric \'nef-rik\ *adj* : RENAL

ne·phrid·i·um \ni-'frid-ē-əm\ *n, pl* **-ia** \-ē-ə\ : an excretory organ that is characteristic of various coelomate invertebrates (as annelid worms, mollusks, brachiopods, and some arthropods), occurs paired in each body segment or as a single pair serving the whole body, typically consists of a tube opening at one end into the coelom and discharging at the other end on the exterior of the body, is often lengthened and convoluted, and has glandular walls — **ne·phrid·i·al** \-ē-əl\ *adj*

¹ne·phrit·ic \ni-'frit-ik\ *adj* **1** : RENAL **2** : of, relating to, or affected with nephritis

²nephritic *n* : an individual affected with nephritis

ne·phri·tis \ni-'frīt-əs\ *n, pl* **ne·phrit·i·des** \-'frit-ə-ˌdēz\ : acute or chronic inflammation of the kidney affecting the structure (as of the glomerulus or parenchyma) and caused by infection, a degenerative process, or vascular disease — compare NEPHROSCLEROSIS, NEPHROSIS

neph·ri·to·gen·ic \ˌnef-rət-ə-'jen-ik, ni-ˌfrit-ə-\ *adj* : causing nephritis ⟨~ types of streptococci⟩

neph·ro·blas·to·ma \ˌnef-rō-blas-'tō-mə\ *n, pl* **-mas** *also* **-ma·ta** \-mət-ə\ : WILMS' TUMOR

neph·ro·cal·ci·no·sis \-ˌkal-si-'nō-səs\ *n, pl* **-no·ses** \-ˌsēz\ : a condition marked by calcification of the tubules of the kidney

neph·ro·cap·sec·to·my \-ˌkap-'sek-tə-mē\ *n, pl* **-mies** : surgical excision of the capsule of the kidney

neph·ro·coel *or* **neph·ro·coele** \'nef-rə-ˌsēl\ *n* : the cavity of a nephrotome

neph·ro·gen·e·sis \ˌnef-rə-'jen-ə-səs\ *n, pl* **-e·ses** \-ˌsēz\ : development or growth of the kidney

neph·ro·gen·ic \ˌnef-rə-'jen-ik\ *adj* **1** : originating in the kidney : caused by factors originating in the kidney ⟨~ hypertension⟩ **2** : developing into or producing kidney tissue ⟨strands of ~ cells⟩

nephrogenic diabetes insipidus *n* : diabetes insipidus that is caused by partial or complete failure of the kidneys to respond to vasopressin

neph·ro·gram \'nef-rə-ˌgram\ *n* : an X-ray of the kidney

ne·phrog·ra·phy \ni-'fräg-rə-fē\ *n, pl* **-phies** : radiology of the kidney

neph·ro·li·thi·a·sis \ˌnef-rō-li-'thī-ə-səs\ *n, pl* **-a·ses** \-ˌsēz\ : a condition marked by the presence of renal calculi

neph·ro·li·thot·o·my \-li-'thät-ə-mē\ *n, pl* **-mies** : the surgical operation of removing a calculus from the kidney

ne·phrol·o·gist \ni-'fräl-ə-jəst\ *n* : a specialist in nephrology

ne·phrol·o·gy \ni-'fräl-ə-jē\ *n, pl* **-gies** : a medical specialty concerned with the kidneys and esp. with their structure, functions, or diseases

ne·phrol·y·sis \ni-'fräl-ə-səs\ *n, pl* **-y·ses** \-ˌsēz\ : the surgical operation of freeing the kidney from surrounding adhesions

ne·phro·ma \ni-'frō-mə\ *n, pl* **-mas** *also* **-ma·ta** \-mət-ə\ : a malignant tumor of the renal cortex

neph·ro·mere \'nef-rə-ˌmi(ə)r\ *n* : a segment of the mesoblast giving rise to a part of the kidney

neph·ron \'nef-ˌrän\ *n* : a single excretory unit esp. of the vertebrate kidney typically consisting of a Malpighian corpuscle, proximal convoluted tubule, loop of Henle, distal convoluted tubule, collecting tubule, and vascular and supporting tissues and discharging by way of a renal papilla into the renal pelvis

ne·phrop·a·thy \ni-'fräp-ə-thē\ *n, pl* **-thies** : an abnormal state of the kidney; *esp* : one associated with or secondary to some other pathological process — **neph·ro·path·ic** \ˌnef-rə-'path-ik\ *adj*

neph·ro·pexy \'nef-rə-ˌpek-sē\ *n, pl* **-pex·ies** : surgical fixation of a floating kidney

neph·rop·to·sis \ˌnef-ˌräp-'tō-səs\ *n, pl* **-to·ses** \-ˌsēz\ : abnormal mobility of the kidney : floating kidney

ne·phror·rha·phy \nef-'ror-ə-fē\ *n, pl* **-phies** **1** : the fixation of a floating kidney by suturing it to the posterior abdominal wall **2** : the suturing of a kidney wound

neph·ro·scle·ro·sis \ˌnef-rō-sklə-'rō-səs\ *n, pl* **-ro·ses** \-ˌsēz\ : hardening of the kidney; *specif* : a condition that is characterized by sclerosis of the renal arterioles with reduced blood flow and contraction of the kidney, that is associated usu. with hypertension, and that terminates in renal failure and uremia — compare NEPHRITIS — **neph·ro·scle·rot·ic** \-'rät-ik\ *adj*

neph·ro·scope \'nef-rə-ˌskōp\ *n* : an endoscope used for inspecting and passing instruments into the interior of the kidney — **neph·ros·co·py** \ni-'fräs-kə-pē\ *n*

ne·phro·sis \ni-'frō-səs\ *n, pl* **ne·phro·ses** \-ˌsēz\ : a noninflammatory disease of the kidneys chiefly affecting function of the nephrons; *esp* : NEPHROTIC SYNDROME — compare NEPHRITIS

neph·ros·to·gram \ni-'fräs-tə-ˌgram\ *n* : a radiograph of the renal pelvis after injection of a radiopaque substance through an opening formed by nephrostomy

neph·ro·stome \'nef-rə-ˌstōm\ *also* **ne·phros·to·ma** \ni-'fräs-tə-mə\ *n, pl* **-stomes** *also* **-sto·ma·ta** \-mət-ə\ : the ciliated funnel-shaped coelomic opening of a typical nephridium

ne·phros·to·my \ni-'fräs-tə-mē\ *n, pl* **-mies** : the surgical formation of an opening between a renal pelvis and the outside of the body

ne·phrot·ic \ni-'frät-ik\ *adj* : of, relating to, affected by, or associated with nephrosis ⟨~ edema⟩ ⟨a ~ patient⟩

nephrotic syndrome *n* : an abnormal condition that is marked by deficiency of albumin in the blood and its excretion in the urine due to altered permeability of the glomerular basement membranes (as by a toxic chemical agent)

neph·ro·tome \'nef-rə-ˌtōm\ *n* : the modified part of a somite of a vertebrate embryo that develops into a segmental excretory tubule of the primitive kidney — called also *intermediate cell mass*

neph·ro·to·mo·gram \ˌnef-rō-'tō-mə-ˌgram\ *n* : a radiograph made by nephrotomography

neph·ro·to·mog·ra·phy \-tō-'mäg-rə-fē\ *n, pl* **-phies** : tomographic visualization of the kidney usu. combined with intravenous nephrography — **neph·ro·to·mo·graph·ic** \-ˌtō-mə-'graf-ik\ *adj*

ne·phrot·o·my \ni-'frät-ə-mē\ *n, pl* **-mies** : surgical incision of a kidney (as for the extraction of a stone)

neph·ro·tox·ic \ˌnef-rə-'täk-sik\ *adj* : poisonous to the kidney ⟨~ drugs⟩; *also* : resulting from or marked by poisoning of the kidney ⟨~ effects⟩ — **neph·ro·tox·ic·i·ty** \-täk-'sis-ət-ē\ *n, pl* **-ties**

neph·ro·tox·in \-'täk-sən\ *n* : a cytotoxin that is destructive to kidney cells

Nep·ta·zane \'nep-tə-ˌzān\ *trademark* — used for a preparation of methazolamide

nep·tu·ni·um \nep-'t(y)ü-nē-əm\ *n* : a radioactive metallic element that is chemically similar to uranium and is obtained in nuclear reactors as a by-product in the production of plutonium — symbol *Np*; see ELEMENT table

Nep·tune \'nep-ˌt(y)ün\, Roman mythological character. Neptune was originally the god of fresh water. Later he became identified with the Greek god Poseidon, a deity of the sea. In art Neptune is usually represented as a bearded man holding a trident and sometimes a fish. The planet Neptune was named after him and the element neptunium was named after the planet.

Nernst equation \'nernst-\ *n* : an equation used to find the potential difference across a semipermeable membrane through which an ion diffuses between solutions where its concentration differs and that for a temperature of 37°C

\ə\ **abut** \ᵊ\ **kitten** \ər\ **further** \a\ **ash** \ā\ **ace** \ä\ **cot, cart**
\au̇\ **out** \ch\ **chin** \e\ **bet** \ē\ **easy** \g\ **go** \i\ **hit** \ī\ **ice** \j\ **job**
\ŋ\ **sing** \ō\ **go** \ȯ\ **law** \ȯi\ **boy** \th\ **thin** \t͟h\ **the** \ü\ **loot**
\u̇\ **foot** \y\ **yet** \zh\ **vision** *See also* Pronunciation Symbols page

M
N

(98.6°F) gives a result in millivolts equal to plus or minus 61.5 times the logarithm of the ratio of the concentration of the ion on one side of the membrane to its concentration on the other

Nernst, Walther Hermann (1864–1941), German physical chemist. One of the founders of modern physical chemistry, Nernst was a professor of chemistry first at Göttingen and then at Berlin. His research topics included the thermodynamics of chemical equilibrium, the theory of galvanic cells, the mechanism of photochemistry, and the properties of vapors at high temperature and of solids at low temperature. In 1888 he published his derivation of the law of diffusion for electrolytes in the simple case when only two kinds of ions are present. The formulation is now known as the Nernst equation. In 1889 in a more extensive study he developed the fundamental relationship between electromotive force and ionic concentration. Perhaps his most notable contribution was his formulation of the third law of thermodynamics in 1906, for which he was awarded the Nobel Prize for Chemistry in 1920.

ner·o·li oil \'ner-ə-lē-\ *n* : a fragrant pale yellow essential oil obtained from orange flowers and used in perfume and as a flavoring — called also *orange-flower oil*

Ner·o·la \'ner-ə-lə\, **Princess of (Anna Maria de La Tremoille) (***d* **1722)**, Italian princess. Born in France of noble birth, Anna Maria became the wife of an Italian duke. She introduced neroli oil into France around 1670.

nerve \'nərv\ *n* **1** : any of the filamentous bands of nervous tissue that connect parts of the nervous system with the other organs, conduct nervous impulses, and are made up of axons and dendrites together with protective and supportive structures and that for the larger nerves have the fibers gathered into funiculi surrounded by a perineurium and the funiculi enclosed in a common epineurium **2** **nerves** *pl* : a state or condition of nervous agitation or irritability **3** : the sensitive pulp of a tooth

nerve block *n* **1** : an interruption of the passage of impulses through a nerve (as with pressure or narcotization) — called also *nerve blocking* **2** : BLOCK ANESTHESIA

nerve canal *n* : ROOT CANAL 1

nerve cavity *n* : PULP CAVITY

nerve cell *n* : NEURON; *also* : CELL BODY

nerve center *n* : CENTER

nerve cord *n* : the dorsal tubular cord of nervous tissue above the notochord of a chordate that in vertebrates includes or develops an anterior enlargement comprising the brain and a more posterior part comprising the spinal cord with the two together making up the central nervous system

nerve deafness *n* : hearing loss or impairment resulting from injury to or loss of function of the organ of Corti or the auditory nerve — called also *perceptive deafness;* compare CENTRAL DEAFNESS, CONDUCTION DEAFNESS

nerve ending *n* : the structure in which the distal end of the axon of a nerve fiber terminates — called also *nerve end*

nerve fiber *n* : any of the processes (as an axon or a dendrite) of a neuron

nerve gas *n* : an organophosphate chemical weapon that interferes with normal nerve transmission and induces intense bronchial spasm with resulting inhibition of respiration — compare WAR GAS

nerve growth factor *n* : a protein that promotes development of the sensory and sympathetic nervous systems and is required for maintenance of sympathetic neurons — abbr. *NGF*

nerve impulse *n* : the progressive physicochemical change in the membrane of a nerve fiber that follows stimulation and serves to transmit a record of sensation from a receptor or an instruction to act to an effector — called also *nervous impulse*

nerve of Her·ing \-'her-iŋ\ *n* : a nerve that arises from the main trunk of the glossopharyngeal nerve and runs along the internal carotid artery to supply afferent fibers esp. to the baroreceptors of the carotid sinus

Hering, Heinrich Ewald (1866–1948), German physiolo-

gist. Hering was appointed professor of general and experimental pathology at Prague in 1901 and from 1913 was director of an institute of pathological physiology at Cologne. In 1923, while studying a reflex whereby pressure on the carotid artery at the level of the cricoid cartilage results in a slowing of the pulse rate, he identified the origin of the reflex in the nerve endings in the carotid sinus, the region where the common carotid artery forks to form the internal and external carotid arteries. In 1924 he published the first description of the structure and function of the nerve (now called the nerve of Hering) which innervates this region.

nerve of Lan·ci·si \-län-'chē-zē\ *n* : either of a pair of longitudinal elevations near the middle line of the upper surface of the corpus callosum

Lancisi, Giovanni Maria (1654–1720), Italian physician. The foremost Italian physician of his time, Lancisi served as professor of anatomy and medicine and as personal physician to several popes. He described the nerve of Lancisi in 1711.

nerve of Wris·berg \-'riz-ˌbərg, *Ger* -'vris-ˌberk\ *n* **1** : NERVUS INTERMEDIUS **2** : a small nerve of the upper arm arising from the brachial plexus and distributed esp. to the skin of the medial side

H. A. Wrisberg — see CARTILAGE OF WRISBERG

nerve sheath *n* : NEURILEMMA

nerve trunk *n* : a bundle of nerve fibers enclosed in a connective tissue sheath

nervi *pl of* NERVUS

¹ner·vine \'nər-ˌvēn\ *adj* : tending to soothe nervous excitement ⟨a ∼ tonic⟩

²nervine *n* : a tonic that soothes nervous excitement

ner·vi ner·vo·rum \ˌnər-ˌvī-ˌnər-'vōr-əm\ *n pl* : small nerve filaments innervating the sheath of a larger nerve

nerv·ing \'nər-viŋ\ *n* : the removal of part of a nerve trunk in chronic inflammation in order to cure lameness (as of a horse) by destroying sensation in the parts supplied

ner·von \'nər-ˌvän\ *or* **ner·vone** \-ˌvōn\ *n* : a crystalline cerebroside $C_{48}H_{91}NO_8$ found together with a hydroxy derivative in the brain

ner·von·ic acid \nər-ˌvän-ik-\ *n* : a crystalline unsaturated fatty acid $C_{23}H_{45}COOH$ obtained from nervon by hydrolysis

nervosa — see ANOREXIA NERVOSA, BULIMIA NERVOSA, PARS NERVOSA

ner·vous \'nər-vəs\ *adj* **1** : of, relating to, or composed of neurons ⟨the ∼ layer of the eye⟩ **2 a** : of or relating to the nerves; *also* : originating in or affected by the nerves ⟨∼ energy⟩ **b** : easily excited or irritated — **ner·vous·ly** *adv* — **ner·vous·ness** *n*

nervous breakdown *n* : an attack of mental or emotional disorder esp. when of sufficient severity to require hospitalization

nervous impulse *n* : NERVE IMPULSE

nervous system *n* : the bodily system that in vertebrates is made up of the brain and spinal cord, nerves, ganglia, and parts of the receptor organs and that receives and interprets stimuli and transmits impulses to the effector organs — see AUTONOMIC NERVOUS SYSTEM, CENTRAL NERVOUS SYSTEM, PERIPHERAL NERVOUS SYSTEM

ner·vus \'nər-vəs, 'ner-\ *n, pl* **ner·vi** \'nər-ˌvī, 'ner-ˌvē\ : NERVE 1

nervus er·i·gens \-'er-i-ˌjenz\ *n, pl* **nervi er·i·gen·tes** \-ˌer-i-'jen-(ˌ)tēz\ : PELVIC SPLANCHNIC NERVE

nervus in·ter·me·di·us \-ˌint-ər-'mēd-ē-əs\ *n* : the branch of the facial nerve that contains sensory and parasympathetic fibers and that supplies the anterior tongue and parts of the palate and fauces — called also *glossopalatine nerve, nerve of Wrisberg*

nervus ra·di·a·lis \-ˌrā-dē-'ā-ləs\ *n, pl* **nervi ra·di·a·les** \-(ˌ)lēz\ : RADIAL NERVE

nervus ter·mi·na·lis \-ˌtər-mə-'nā-ləs\ *n, pl* **nervi ter·mi·na·les** \-(ˌ)lēz\ : a group of ganglionated nerve fibers that arise in the cerebral hemisphere near where the nerve tract leading from the olfactory bulb joins the temporal lobe and that pass anteriorly along this tract and the olfactory bulb through the cribriform plate to the nasal mucosa — called also *terminal nerve*

Nes·a·caine \'nes-ə-ˌkān\ *trademark* — used for a preparation of chloroprocaine

ness·ler·ize *also Brit* **ness·ler·ise** \'nes-lə-ˌrīz\ *vt* **-ized** *also Brit* **-ised; -iz·ing** *also Brit* **-is·ing** : to treat or test with Nessler's reagent — **ness·ler·iza·tion** *also Brit* **ness·ler·isa·tion** \ˌnes-lə-rə-ˈzā-shən\ *n*

Ness·ler \'nes-lər\, **Julius (1827–1905),** German agricultural chemist. Nessler developed his test reagent for ammonia in 1856. He was also an authority on wine growing.

Ness·ler's reagent \'nes-lərz-\ *n* : an alkaline solution of potassium mercuric iodide used in chemical analysis esp. in a test for ammonia in aqueous solution (as when distilled from water, blood, or urine) with which it forms a yellowish brown color or precipitate — called also *Nessler's solution*

nest \'nest\ *n* : an isolated collection or clump of cells in tissue of a different structure ⟨a ∼ of sarcomatous cells⟩

net \'net\ *n* : NETWORK ⟨in the portal system, blood passes through two capillary ∼s —E. B. Steen & Ashley Montagu⟩

net·tle \'net-ᵊl\ *n* **1** : any plant of the genus *Urtica* (family Urticaceae, the nettle family) **2** : any of various prickly or stinging plants other than one of the genus *Urtica*

nettle rash *n* : an eruption on the skin caused by or resembling the condition produced by stinging with nettles : HIVES

net·work \'net-ˌwərk\ *n* **1** : a fabric or structure of cords or wires that cross at regular intervals and are knotted or secured at the crossings **2** : a system of lines or channels resembling a network ⟨a ∼ of veins⟩

Neu·po·gen \'nü-pə-jən, 'nyü-\ *trademark* — used for a preparation of filgrastim

neu·ral \'n(y)ùr-əl\ *adj* **1** : of, relating to, or affecting a nerve or the nervous system **2** : situated in the region of or on the same side of the body as the brain and spinal cord : DORSAL — compare HEMAL 2 — **neu·ral·ly** \-ə-lē\ *adv*

neural arch *n* : the cartilaginous or bony arch enclosing the spinal cord on the dorsal side of a vertebra — called also *vertebral arch*

neural canal *n* **1** : VERTEBRAL CANAL **2** : the cavity or system of cavities in a vertebrate embryo that form the central canal of the spinal cord and the ventricles of the brain

neural crest *n* : the ridge of one of the folds forming the neural tube that gives rise to the spinal ganglia and various structures of the autonomic nervous system — called also *neural ridge;* compare NEURAL PLATE

neural fold *n* : the lateral longitudinal fold on each side of the neural plate that by folding over and fusing with the opposite fold gives rise to the neural tube

neu·ral·gia \n(y)ù-'ral-jə\ *n* : acute paroxysmal pain radiating along the course of one or more nerves usu. without demonstrable changes in the nerve structure — compare NEURITIS — **neu·ral·gic** \-jik\ *adj*

neu·ral·gi·form \n(y)ù-'ral-jə-ˌfòrm\ *adj* : resembling neuralgia or that of neuralgia ⟨∼ pains⟩

neural groove *n* : the median dorsal longitudinal groove formed in the vertebrate embryo by the neural plate after the appearance of the neural folds — called also *medullary groove*

neural lobe *n* : the expanded distal portion of the neurohypophysis — called also *infundibular process, pars nervosa*

neural plate *n* : a thickened plate of ectoderm along the dorsal midline of the early vertebrate embryo that gives rise to the neural tube and crests

neural process *n* : the lateral half of the neural arch of a vertebra that is equivalent to the pedicle and lamina together

neural ridge *n* : NEURAL CREST

neural spine *n* : the spinous process of the neural arch of a vertebra

neural stalk *n* : INFUNDIBULUM a

neural tube *n* : the hollow longitudinal dorsal tube that is formed by infolding and subsequent fusion of the opposite ectodermal folds in the vertebrate embryo and gives rise to the brain and spinal cord

neural tube defect *n* : any of various congenital defects (as anencephaly and spina bifida) caused by incomplete closure of the neural tube during the early stages of embryonic development

neur·amin·ic acid \ˌn(y)ùr-ə-ˌmin-ik-\ *n* : an amino acid $C_9H_{17}NO_8$ that is essentially a carbohydrate and occurs in the form of acyl derivatives

neur·amin·i·dase \ˌn(y)ùr-ə-ˈmin-ə-ˌdās, -ˌdāz\ *n* : a hydrolytic enzyme that occurs on the surface of the pneumococcus, the orthomyxoviruses, and some paramyxoviruses and that cleaves terminal acetylated neuraminic acids from sugar residues (as in glycoproteins and mucoproteins)

neur·aprax·ia \ˌn(y)ùr-ə-ˈprak-sē-ə, ˌn(y)ùr-(ˌ)ā-\ *n* : an injury to a nerve that interrupts conduction causing temporary paralysis but not degeneration and that is followed by a complete and rapid recovery

neur·as·the·nia \ˌn(y)ùr-əs-ˈthē-nē-ə\ *n* : a condition that is characterized esp. by physical and mental exhaustion usu. with accompanying symptoms (as headaches, insomnia, and irritability), is believed to result from psychological factors (as depression or emotional stress or conflict), and is sometimes considered similar to or identical with chronic fatigue syndrome

neur·as·then·i·ac \-ˈthen-ē-ˌak\ *n* : NEURASTHENIC

¹neur·as·then·ic \-ˈthen-ik\ *adj* : of, relating to, or having neurasthenia

²neurasthenic *n* : an individual affected with neurasthenia

neur·ax·is \n(y)ùr-ˈak-səs\ *n, pl* **neur·ax·es** \-ˌsēz\ : CENTRAL NERVOUS SYSTEM

neur·ax·on \-ˈak-ˌsän\ *also* **neur·ax·one** \-ˌsōn\ *n* **1** : AXON **2** : CENTRAL NERVOUS SYSTEM

neur·ec·to·derm \n(y)ùr-ˈek-tə-ˌdərm\ *n* : ectoderm destined to give rise to neural tissues

neu·rec·to·my \n(y)ù-ˈrek-tə-mē\ *n, pl* **-mies** : the surgical excision of part of a nerve

neur·en·ter·ic \ˌn(y)ùr-en-ˈter-ik\ *adj* : being or relating to a canal that in embryos of many vertebrates and tunicates temporarily connects the neural tube and the primitive intestine

neu·rer·gic \n(y)ùr-ˈər-jik\ *adj* : of or relating to the action of a nerve

neu·ri·lem·ma \ˌn(y)ùr-ə-ˈlem-ə\ *n* : the plasma membrane surrounding a Schwann cell of a myelinated nerve fiber and separating layers of myelin — **neu·ri·lem·mal** \-ˈlem-əl\ *adj*

neu·ri·lem·mo·ma *or* **neu·ri·le·mo·ma** *or* **neu·ro·lem·mo·ma** \-lə-ˈmō-mə\ *n, pl* **-mas** *also* **-ma·ta** \-ˈmət-ə\ : a tumor of the myelinated sheaths of nerve fibers that consist of Schwann cells in a matrix — called also *neurinoma, schwannoma*

neu·ril·i·ty \n(y)ù-ˈril-ət-ē\ *n, pl* **-ties** : the special properties and functions of the nerves

neu·rine \'n(y)ù-ˌrēn\ *also* **neu·rin** \-rən\ *n* : a syrupy poisonous quaternary ammonium hydroxide $CH_2{=}CHN(CH_3)_3OH$ that is found in the brain, in bile, and in putrefying flesh

neu·ri·no·ma \ˌn(y)ùr-ə-ˈnō-mə\ *n, pl* **-mas** *also* **-ma·ta** \-ˈmət-ə\ : NEURILEMMOMA

neu·rite \'n(y)ù-ˌrīt\ *n* : AXON; *also* : DENDRITE

neu·ri·tis \n(y)ù-ˈrīt-əs\ *n, pl* **-rit·i·des** \-ˈrit-ə-ˌdēz\ *or* **-ri·tis·es** : an inflammatory or degenerative lesion of a nerve marked esp. by pain, sensory disturbances, and impaired or lost reflexes — compare NEURALGIA — **neu·rit·ic** \-ˈrit-ik\ *adj*

neu·ro \'n(y)ù-ˌrō\ *adj* : NEUROLOGICAL

neu·ro·ac·tive \ˌn(y)ùr-ō-ˈak-tiv\ *adj* : stimulating neural tissue ⟨injected a ∼ substance into the blood⟩

neu·ro·anat·o·mist \-ə-ˈnat-ə-məst\ *n* : a specialist in neuroanatomy

neu·ro·anat·o·my \-ə-ˈnat-ə-mē\ *n, pl* **-mies** : the anatomy of nervous tissue and the nervous system — **neu·ro·ana·tom·i-**

M
N

\ə\ **abut** \ᵊ\ **kitten** \ər\ **further** \a\ **ash** \ā\ **ace** \ä\ **cot, cart**
\aù\ **out** \ch\ **chin** \e\ **bet** \ē\ **easy** \g\ **go** \i\ **hit** \ī\ **ice** \j\ **job**
\ŋ\ **sing** \ō\ **go** \ò\ **law** \òi\ **boy** \th\ **thin** \th̶\ **the** \ü\ **loot**
\ù\ **foot** \y\ **yet** \zh\ **vision** *See also* Pronunciation Symbols page

cal \-ˌan-ə-'täm-i-kəl\ *also* **neu·ro·ana·tom·ic** \-ik\ *adj* — **neu·ro·ana·tom·i·cal·ly** \-i-k(ə-)lē\ *adv*

neu·ro·ar·throp·a·thy \-är-'thräp-ə-thē\ *n, pl* **-thies** : a joint disease (as Charcot's joint) that is associated with a disorder of the nervous system

neu·ro·be·hav·ior·al *or chiefly Brit* **neu·ro·be·hav·iour·al** \-bi-'hā-vyə-rəl\ *adj* : of or relating to the relationship between the action of the nervous system and behavior ⟨∼ disorders such as aphasia, alexia, and childhood learning disabilities⟩

neu·ro·bi·ol·o·gist \-bī-'äl-ə-jəst\ *n* : a specialist in neurobiology

neu·ro·bi·ol·o·gy \-bī-'äl-ə-jē\ *n, pl* **-gies** : a branch of science that deals with the anatomy, physiology, and pathology of the nervous system — **neu·ro·bi·o·log·i·cal** \-ˌbī-ə-'läj-i-kəl\ *also* **neu·ro·bi·o·log·ic** \-ik\ *adj* — **neu·ro·bi·o·log·i·cal·ly** \-i-k(ə-)lē\ *adv*

neu·ro·bio·tax·is \-ˌbī-ō-'tak-səs\ *n, pl* **-tax·es** \-ˌsēz\ : a hypothetical directed and oriented shift of nerve cells in the course of phylogeny toward a region of maximum stimulation that has been held to explain cephalization and brain evolution — **neu·ro·bio·tac·tic** \-'tak-tik\ *or* **neu·ro·bio·tac·ti·cal** \-ti-kəl\ *adj*

neu·ro·blast \'n(y)ùr-ə-ˌblast\ *n* : a cellular precursor of a nerve cell; *esp* : an undifferentiated embryonic nerve cell — **neu·ro·blas·tic** \ˌn(y)ùr-ə-'blas-tik\ *adj*

neu·ro·blas·to·ma \ˌn(y)ùr-ō-blas-'tō-mə\ *n, pl* **-mas** *also* **-ma·ta** \-mət-ə\ : a malignant tumor formed of embryonic ganglion cells — **neu·ro·blas·to·mal** \-'tō-məl\ *adj*

neu·ro·bor·rel·i·o·sis \-bə-ˌrel-ē-'ō-səs\ *n, pl* **-o·ses** \-ˌsēz\ : a disease of the central nervous system caused by infection with a spirochete of the genus *Borrelia; esp* : a late stage of Lyme disease typically involving the skin, joints, and central nervous system

neu·ro·car·dio·gen·ic syncope \ˌn(y)ùr-ō-ˌkärd-ē-(ˌ)ō-'jen-ik-\ *n* : VASOVAGAL SYNCOPE

neu·ro·cen·trum \-'sen-trəm\ *n, pl* **-trums** *or* **-tra** \-trə\ : either of the two dorsal elements of a vertebra that unite to form a neural arch from which the vertebral spine is developed — **neu·ro·cen·tral** \-'sen-trəl\ *adj*

neu·ro·chem·ist \-'kem-əst\ *n* : a specialist in neurochemistry

neu·ro·chem·is·try \-'kem-ə-strē\ *n, pl* **-tries   1** : the study of the chemical makeup and activities of nervous tissue **2** : chemical processes and phenomena related to the nervous system — **neu·ro·chem·i·cal** \-'kem-i-kəl\ *adj or n* — **neu·ro·chem·i·cal·ly** \-i-k(ə-)lē\ *adv*

neu·ro·cir·cu·la·to·ry \ˌn(y)ùr-ō-'sər-kyə-lə-ˌtōr-ē, -ˌtòr-\ *adj* : of or relating to the nervous and circulatory systems

neurocirculatory asthenia *n* : a condition marked by shortness of breath, fatigue, rapid pulse, and heart palpitation sometimes with extra beats that occurs chiefly with exertion and is not due to physical disease of the heart — called also *cardiac neurosis, effort syndrome, irritable heart, soldier's heart*

neu·ro·coele *also* **neu·ro·coel** \'n(y)ùr-ə-ˌsēl\ *n* : the cavity or system of cavities in the interior of the vertebrate central nervous system comprising the central canal of the spinal cord and the ventricles of the brain

neu·ro·cog·ni·tive \ˌn(y)ùr-ō-'käg-nət-iv\ *adj* : of, relating to, or involving the nervous system and cognitive abilities ⟨∼ deficits in fragile X syndrome⟩

neu·ro·cra·ni·um \ˌn(y)ùr-ō-'krā-nē-əm\ *n, pl* **-ni·ums** *or* **-nia** \-nē-ə\ : the portion of the skull that encloses and protects the brain — **neu·ro·cra·ni·al** \-nē-əl\ *adj*

neu·ro·crine \'n(y)ùr-ə-krən, -ˌkrīn, -ˌkrēn\ *adj* : NEUROENDOCRINE

neu·ro·cu·ta·ne·ous \ˌn(y)ùr-ō-kyù-'tā-nē-əs\ *adj* : of, relating to, or affecting the skin and nerves ⟨a ∼ syndrome⟩

neu·ro·cys·ti·cer·co·sis \ˌsis-tə-(ˌ)sər-'kō-səs\ *n, pl* **-co·ses** \-ˌsēz\ : infection of the central nervous system with cysticerci of the pork tapeworm (*Taenia solium*)

neu·ro·cyte \'n(y)ùr-ə-ˌsīt\ *n* : CELL BODY; *broadly* : NEURON

neu·ro·cy·tol·o·gy \ˌn(y)ùr-ō-sī-'täl-ə-jē\ *n, pl* **-gies** : the cytology of the nervous system — **neu·ro·cy·to·log·i·cal** \-ˌsīt-ə-'läj-i-kəl\ *adj*

neu·ro·cy·tol·y·sin \-sī-'täl-ə-sən\ *n* : a toxic substance in the venom of some snakes (as the cobras and coral snakes) which causes the lysis of nerve cells

neu·ro·cy·to·ma \-sī-'tō-mə\ *n, pl* **-mas** *also* **-ma·ta** \-mət-ə\ : any of various tumors of nerve tissue arising in the central or sympathetic nervous system

neu·ro·de·gen·er·a·tive \-di-'jen-ə-ˌrāt-iv, -di-'jen-(ə-)rət-\ *adj* : relating to or characterized by degeneration of nervous tissue — **neu·ro·de·gen·er·a·tion** \-di-ˌjen-ə-'rā-shən, -ˌdē-\ *n*

n·ro·den·drite \-'den-ˌdrīt\ *n* : DENDRITE

neu·ro·den·dron \-'den-ˌdrän\ *n* : DENDRITE

neu·ro·der·ma·tit·ic \-ˌdər-mə-'tit-ik\ *adj* : of, relating to, or exhibiting neurodermatitis

neu·ro·der·ma·ti·tis \-ˌdər-mə-'tīt-əs\ *n, pl* **-ti·tis·es** *or* **-tit·i·des** \-'tit-ə-ˌdēz\ : a chronic allergic disorder of the skin characterized by patches of an itching lichenoid eruption and occurring esp. in persons of nervous and emotional instability

neu·ro·der·ma·to·sis \-'tō-səs\ *n, pl* **-to·ses** \-ˌsēz\ : dermatosis caused by or related to psychosomatic or neurogenic factors

neu·ro·de·vel·op·ment \-di-'vel-əp-mənt\ *n* : the development of the nervous system — **neu·ro·de·vel·op·men·tal** \-ˌvel-əp-'ment-ᵊl\ *adj*

neu·ro·di·ag·nos·tic \-ˌdī-ig-'näs-tik, -ˌdī-əg-\ *adj* : of or relating to the diagnosis of diseases of the nervous system ⟨∼ imaging in patients with leg pain —Silvia E. Hines⟩

neu·ro·dy·nam·ic \-dī-'nam-ik\ *adj* : of, relating to, or involving communication between different parts of the nervous system — **neu·ro·dy·nam·ics** \-iks\ *n pl but sing or pl in constr*

neu·ro·ec·to·derm \-'ek-tə-ˌdərm\ *n* : embryonic ectoderm that gives rise to nervous tissue — **neu·ro·ec·to·der·mal** \-ˌek-tə-'dərm-əl\ *adj*

neu·ro·ef·fec·tor \-i-'fek-tər, -ˌtò(ə)r\ *adj* : of, relating to, or involving both neural and effector components ⟨∼ junctions⟩

neu·ro·elec·tric \-i-'lek-trik\ *also* **neu·ro·elec·tri·cal** \-tri-kəl\ *adj* : of or relating to the electrical phenomena (as potentials or signals) generated by the nervous system — **neu·ro·elec·tric·i·ty** \-ˌlek-'tris-ət-ē, -ˌtris-tē\ *n, pl* **-ties**

neu·ro·em·bry·ol·o·gist \-ˌem-brē-'äl-ə-jəst\ *n* : a specialist in neuroembryology

neu·ro·em·bry·ol·o·gy \-'äl-ə-jē\ *n, pl* **-gies** : a branch of embryology dealing with the development of the nervous system — **neu·ro·em·bry·o·log·ic** \-ˌem-brē-ə-'läj-ik\ *or* **neu·ro·em·bry·o·log·i·cal** \-i-kəl\ *adj*

neu·ro·en·do·crine \-'en-də-krən, -ˌkrīn, -ˌkrēn\ *adj* **1** : of, relating to, or being a hormonal substance that influences the activity of nerves **2** : of, relating to, or functioning in neurosecretion

neu·ro·en·do·cri·nol·o·gist \-ˌen-də-kri-'näl-ə-jəst, -(ˌ)krī-\ *n* : a specialist in neuroendocrinology

neu·ro·en·do·cri·nol·o·gy \-ˌen-də-kri-'näl-ə-jē, -(ˌ)krī-\ *n, pl* **-gies** : a branch of science dealing with neurosecretion and the physiological interaction between the central nervous system and the endocrine system — **neu·ro·en·do·cri·no·log·i·cal** \-ˌkrin-ᵊl-'äj-i-kəl, -ˌkrīn-, -ˌkrēn-\ *also* **neu·ro·en·do·cri·no·log·ic** \-'äj-ik\ *adj*

neu·ro·ep·i·the·li·al \ˌn(y)ùr-ō-ˌep-ə-'thē-lē-əl\ *adj* **1** : of or relating to neuroepithelium **2** : having qualities of both neural and epithelial cells

neu·ro·ep·i·the·li·o·ma \-ˌthē-lē-'ō-mə\ *n, pl* **-mas** *also* **-ma·ta** \-mət-ə\ : a neurocytoma or glioma esp. of the retina

neu·ro·ep·i·the·li·um \-'thē-lē-əm\ *n, pl* **-lia** \-lē-ə\ **1** : the part of the embryonic ectoderm that gives rise to the nervous system **2** : the modified epithelium of an organ of special sense

neu·ro·fi·bril \ˌn(y)ùr-ō-'fīb-rəl, -'fib-\ *n* : a fine proteinaceous fibril that is found in cytoplasm (as of a neuron or a paramecium) and is capable of conducting excitation —

neu·ro·fi·bril·lary \-rə-ˌler-ē\ *also* **neu·ro·fi·bril·lar** \-rə-lər\ *adj*

neu·ro·fi·bril·la \-fī-ˈbril-ə, -fi-; -ˈfī-bri-lə, -ˈfi-\ *n, pl* **-lae** \-ē, -lē\ : NEUROFIBRIL

neurofibrillary tangle *n* : a pathological accumulation of paired helical filaments composed of abnormally formed tau protein that is found chiefly in the cytoplasm of nerve cells of the brain and esp. the cerebral cortex and hippocampus and that occurs typically in Alzheimer's disease

neu·ro·fi·bro·ma \-fī-ˈbrō-mə\ *n, pl* **-mas** *also* **-ma·ta** \-mət-ə\ : a fibroma composed of nervous and connective tissue and produced by proliferation of Schwann cells

neu·ro·fi·bro·ma·to·sis \-fī-ˌbrō-mə-ˈtō-səs\ *n, pl* **-to·ses** \-ˌsēz\ : a disorder inherited as an autosomal dominant trait and characterized by brown spots on the skin, neurofibromas of peripheral nerves, and deformities of subcutaneous tissues and bone — abbr. *NF;* called also *Recklinghausen's disease, von Recklinghausen's disease*

neu·ro·fi·bro·sar·co·ma \-ˌfī-brō-sär-ˈkō-mə\ *n, pl* **-mas** *also* **-ma·ta** \-mət-ə\ : a malignant neurofibroma

neu·ro·fil·a·ment \-ˈfil-ə-mənt\ *n* : a microscopic filament of protein that is found in the cytoplasm of neurons and that with neurotubules makes up the structure of neurofibrils — **neu·ro·fil·a·men·tous** \-ˌfil-ə-ˈment-əs\ *adj*

neu·ro·gen \ˈn(y)uṙ-ə-jən, -ˌjen\ *n* : a hypothetical specific primary organizer that induces formation of neural structures in an embryo

neu·ro·gen·e·sis \ˌn(y)uṙ-ə-ˈjen-ə-səs\ *n, pl* **-e·ses** \-ˌsēz\ : development of nerves, nervous tissue, or the nervous system — **neu·ro·ge·net·ic** \-jə-ˈnet-ik\ *adj*

neu·ro·ge·net·i·cist \-jə-ˈnet-ə-səst\ *n* : a specialist or expert in neurogenetics

neu·ro·ge·net·ics \-jə-ˈnet-iks\ *n pl but sing in constr* : a branch of genetics dealing with the nervous system and esp. with its development

neu·ro·gen·ic \ˌn(y)uṙ-ə-ˈjen-ik\ *also* **neu·rog·e·nous** \n(y)u̇-ˈräj-ə-nəs\ *adj* **1 a** : originating in nervous tissue ⟨a ∼ tumor⟩ **b** : induced, controlled, or modified by nervous factors ⟨∼ intestinal lesions⟩ ⟨a ∼ suckling reflex⟩; *esp* : disordered because of abnormally altered neural relations ⟨the ∼ kidney⟩ **2 a** : constituting the neural component of a bodily process ⟨∼ factors in disease⟩ **b** : taking place or viewed as taking place in ordered rhythmic fashion under the control of a network of nerve cells scattered in the cardiac muscle ⟨a ∼ heartbeat⟩ — compare MYOGENIC 2 — **neu·ro·gen·i·cal·ly** \-ˈjen-i-k(ə-)lē\ *adv*

neu·ro·glan·du·lar \ˌn(y)uṙ-ō-ˈglan-jə-lər\ *adj* : of, relating to, or composed of nervous and glandular tissue ⟨the pituitary gland is ∼⟩ ⟨∼ responses⟩

neu·ro·glia \n(y)u̇-ˈrō-glē-ə, -ˈräg-lē-ə; ˌn(y)uṙ-ə-ˈglē-ə, -ˈglī-\ *n* : GLIA — **neu·ro·gli·al** \-əl\ *adj*

neu·ro·gram \ˈn(y)uṙ-ə-ˌgram\ *n* **1** : the postulated modified neural structure resulting from activity and serving to retain whatever has been learned : a neural engram **2** : a visualization (as by electrical recording) of the state of a peripheral nerve — **neu·ro·gram·mic** \-ˌgram-ik\ *adj*

neu·rog·ra·phy \n(y)u̇-ˈräg-rə-fē\ *n, pl* **-phies 1** : the postulated formation of neurograms **2** : the postulated system of engrams present in an individual's brain

neu·ro·his·tol·o·gist \ˌn(y)uṙ-ō-his-ˈtäl-ə-jəst\ *n* : a specialist in neurohistology

neu·ro·his·tol·o·gy \-ə-jē\ *n, pl* **-gies** : a branch of histology concerned with the nervous system — **neu·ro·his·to·log·i·cal** \-ˌhis-tə-ˈläj-i-kəl\ *also* **neu·ro·his·to·log·ic** \-ˈläj-ik\ *adj*

neu·ro·hor·mon·al \ˌn(y)uṙ-ō-hȯr-ˈmōn-ᵊl\ *adj* **1** : involving both neural and hormonal mechanisms **2** : of, relating to, or being a neurohormone

neu·ro·hor·mone \-ˈhȯr-ˌmōn\ *n* : a hormone (as acetylcholine or norepinephrine) produced by or acting on nervous tissue

neu·ro·hu·mor *or chiefly Brit* **neu·ro·hu·mour** \ˌn(y)uṙ-ō-ˈhyü-mər, -ˈyü-\ *n* : NEUROHORMONE; *esp* : NEUROTRANSMITTER — **neu·ro·hu·mor·al** *or chiefly Brit* **neu·ro·hu·mour·al** \-mə-rəl\ *adj*

neu·ro·hy·po·phy·se·al *or* **neu·ro·hy·po·phy·si·al** \-(ˌ)hī-ˌpäf-ə-ˈsē-əl, -ˌhī-pə-fə-, -ˈzē-; -ˌhī-pə-ˈfiz-ē-əl\ *adj* : of, relating to, or secreted by the neurohypophysis ⟨∼ hormones⟩

neu·ro·hy·poph·y·sis \-hī-ˈpäf-ə-səs\ *n, pl* **-y·ses** \-ˌsēz\ : the portion of the pituitary gland that is derived from the embryonic brain, is composed of the infundibulum and neural lobe, and is concerned with the secretion of various hormones — called also *posterior pituitary gland;* compare ADENOHYPOPHYSIS

neu·roid \ˈn(y)u̇-ˌrȯid\ *adj* : resembling a nerve or nerve tissue

neu·ro·im·ag·ing \ˌn(y)uṙ-ō-ˈim-ə-jiŋ\ *n* : a clinical specialty concerned with producing images of the brain by noninvasive techniques (as computed tomography, magnetic resonance imaging, and positron-emission tomography); *also* : imaging of the brain by these techniques

neu·ro·im·mu·nol·o·gy \ˌn(y)uṙ-ō-ˌim-yə-ˈnäl-ə-jē\ *n, pl* **-gies** : a branch of immunology that deals esp. with the interrelationships of the nervous system and immune responses and autoimmune disorders (as multiple sclerosis) — **neu·ro·im·mu·no·log·i·cal** \-nə-ˈläj-i-kəl\ *adj*

neu·ro·ker·a·tin \-ˈker-ət-ən\ *n* : a pseudokeratin present in nerve tissue (as in the myelin sheath of a myelinated nerve fiber)

neu·ro·kyme \ˈn(y)uṙ-ə-ˌkīm\ *n* : the kinetic energy of neural activity

neurol *abbr* **1** neurological **2** neurology

neurolemmoma *var of* NEURILEMMOMA

neu·ro·lept·an·al·ge·sia \ˈn(y)uṙ-ə-ˌlep-ˌtan-ᵊl-ˈjē-zhə, -z(h)ē-ə\ *or* **neu·ro·lep·to·an·al·ge·sia** \ˌn(y)uṙ-ə-ˈlep-tō-ˌan-\ *n* : joint administration of a tranquilizing drug and an analgesic esp. for relief of surgical pain — **neu·ro·lept·an·al·ge·sic** \-ˈje-zik, -sik\ *adj*

neu·ro·lep·tic \ˌn(y)uṙ-ə-ˈlep-tik\ *n* : ANTIPSYCHOTIC — **neuroleptic** *adj*

neu·ro·lin·guis·tics \-liŋ-ˈgwis-tiks\ *n pl but sing in constr* : the study of the relationships between the human nervous system and language esp. with respect to the correspondence between disorders of language and the nervous system — **neu·ro·lin·guis·tic** \-tik\ *adj*

neu·ro·log·i·cal \-ˈläj-i-kəl\ *or* **neu·ro·log·ic** \-ik\ *adj* : of or relating to neurology — **neu·ro·log·i·cal·ly** \-i-k(ə-)lē\ *adv*

neu·rol·o·gist \n(y)u̇-ˈräl-ə-jəst\ *n* : a person specializing in neurology; *esp* : a physician skilled in the diagnosis and treatment of disease of the nervous system

neu·rol·o·gy \-jē\ *n* : a branch of medicine concerned esp. with the structure, functions, and diseases of the nervous system

neu·ro·lym·pho·ma·to·sis \ˌn(y)uṙ-ō-(ˌ)lim-ˌfō-mə-ˈtō-səs\ *n* : infiltration by lymphoid cells of the peripheral nerves esp. in the legs and wings of chickens approaching maturity and affected with Marek's disease — called also *fowl paralysis, range paralysis*

neu·rol·y·sis \n(y)u̇-ˈräl-ə-səs\ *n, pl* **-y·ses** \-ˌsēz\ **1 a** : the breaking down of nervous tissue (as from disease or injury) **b** : destruction of nervous tissue (as by the use of chemicals or radio frequencies) to temporarily or permanently block nerve pathways esp. to relieve pain or spasticity ⟨phenolic ∼ of the celiac plexus to treat intractable pancreatic cancer pain⟩ **2** : the surgical operation of freeing a nerve from perineural adhesions

neu·ro·lyt·ic \ˌn(y)uṙ-ə-ˈlit-ik\ *adj* : of, relating to, or causing neurolysis ⟨injection of ∼ agents⟩

neu·ro·ma \n(y)u̇-ˈrō-mə\ *n, pl* **-mas** *also* **-ma·ta** \-mət-ə\ **1** : a tumor or mass growing from a nerve and usu. consisting of nerve fibers **2** : a mass of nerve tissue in an amputation stump resulting from abnormal regrowth of the stumps of severed nerves — called also *amputation neuroma*

\ə\ abut \ᵊ\ kitten \ər\ further \a\ ash \ā\ ace \ä\ cot, cart \au̇\ out \ch\ chin \e\ bet \ē\ easy \g\ go \i\ hit \ī\ ice \j\ job \ŋ\ sing \ō\ go \ȯ\ law \ȯi\ boy \th\ thin \t͟h\ the \ü\ loot \u̇\ foot \y\ yet \zh\ vision　*See also* Pronunciation Symbols page

neu·ro·ma·la·cia \ˌn(y)ùr-ō-mə-ˈlā-sh(ē-)ə\ *n* : pathological softening of nervous tissue

neu·ro·mech·a·nism \-ˈmek-ə-ˌniz-əm\ *n* : a bodily regulatory mechanism that is based in the structure and functioning of the nervous system

neu·ro·mel·a·nin \-ˈmel-ə-nən\ *n* : a melanin pigment found esp. in some dopaminergic neurons of the human substantia nigra

neu·ro·mere \ˈn(y)ùr-ə-ˌmi(ə)r\ *n* : a metameric segment of the vertebrate nervous system ⟨the ∼s of the spinal cord are identified by the exits of the spinal nerves⟩

neu·ro·met·rics \ˌn(y)ùr-ō-ˈme-triks\ *n pl but sing in constr* : the quantitative study of the electrical activity of the brain and nervous system

neu·ro·mi·me·sis \-mə-ˈmē-səs, -mī-\ *n, pl* **-e·ses** \-ˌsēz\ : neurotic simulation of organic disease that occurs in some forms of hysterical neurosis — **neu·ro·mi·met·ic** \-ˈmet-ik\ *adj*

neu·ro·mod·u·la·tor \-ˈmäj-ə-ˌlāt-ər\ *n* : something (as a polypeptide) that potentiates or inhibits the transmission of a nerve impulse but is not the actual means of transmission itself — **neu·ro·mod·u·la·to·ry** \-lə-ˌtōr-ē, -ˌtȯr-\ *adj*

neu·ro·mo·tor \ˌn(y)ùr-ə-ˈmōt-ər\ *adj* : relating to efferent nervous impulses

neuromotor apparatus *n* : a system of noncontractile cytoplasmic fibrils that is often associated with a motorium in various protozoans and may be analogous to the nervous system of higher forms — called also *neuromotor system*

neu·ro·mus·cu·lar \ˌn(y)ùr-ō-ˈməs-kyə-lər\ *adj* : of or relating to nerves and muscles; *esp* : jointly involving nervous and muscular elements ⟨∼ disease⟩

neuromuscular junction *n* : the junction of an efferent nerve fiber and the muscle fiber plasma membrane — called also *myoneural junction*

neuromuscular spindle *n* : MUSCLE SPINDLE

neu·ro·my·al \-ˈmī-əl\ *adj* : NEUROMUSCULAR

neu·ro·my·eli·tis \-ˌmī-ə-ˈlīt-əs\ *n* **1** : inflammation of the medullary substance of the nerves **2** : inflammation of both spinal cord and nerves

neu·ro·my·op·a·thy \-ˌmī-ˈäp-ə-thē\ *n, pl* **-thies** : a disease of nerves and associated muscle tissue

neu·ro·my·o·si·tis \-ˌmī-ō-ˈsīt-əs\ *n* : neuritis associated with inflammation of a muscle

neu·ron \ˈn(y)ü-ˌrän, ˈn(y)ù(ə)r-ˌän\ *also* **neu·rone** \-ˌrōn, -ˌōn\ *n* : one of the cells that constitute nervous tissue, that have the property of transmitting and receiving nervous impulses, and that are composed of somewhat reddish or grayish protoplasm with a large nucleus containing a conspicuous nucleolus, irregular cytoplasmic granules, and cytoplasmic processes which are highly differentiated frequently as multiple dendrites or usu. as solitary axons and which conduct impulses toward and away from the nerve cell body — called also *nerve cell* — **neu·ro·nal** \ˈn(y)ùr-ən-ᵊl, n(y)ù-ˈrōn-ᵊl\ *also* **neu·ron·ic** \n(y)ù-ˈrän-ik\ *adj*

neuron doctrine *n* : a theory in anatomy and physiology: the nervous system is composed of nerve cells each of which is a structural unit in contact with other units but not in continuity, a genetic unit derived from a single embryonic neuroblast, a functional unit or unit of conduction with the nervous pathways being chains of such units, and a trophic unit with the nerve processes degenerating when severed from the cell body and being replaced by outgrowths from the cell body — called also *neuron theory*

neu·ro·neu·ro·nal \ˌn(y)ùr-ō-ˈn(y)ùr-ən-ᵊl, -n(y)ù-ˈrōn-ᵊl\ *adj* : between nerve cells or nerve fibers ⟨∼ synapses⟩

neu·ro·ne·vus *or chiefly Brit* **neu·ro·nae·vus** \-ˈnē-vəs\ *n, pl* **-ne·vi** *or chiefly Brit* **-nae·vi** \-ˌvī\ : an intradermal nevus that is composed of cells resembling or sometimes held to be derived from neural structures in the skin

neu·ron·i·tis \ˌn(y)ùr-ə-ˈnīt-əs\ *n* : inflammation of neurons; *esp* : neuritis involving nerve roots and nerve cells within the spinal cord

neu·ro·nog·ra·phy \ˌn(y)ùr-ə-ˈnäg-rə-fē\ *n, pl* **-phies** : the mapping of neuron connections by electrographically recording neural action in nerve tissue that has been treated with strychnine

neu·ro·no·pha·gia \ˌn(y)ù-ˌrō-nə-ˈfā-j(ē-)ə, ˌn(y)ùr-ˌän-ə-\ *also* **neu·ro·noph·a·gy** \ˌn(y)ùr-ə-ˈnäf-ə-jē\ *n, pl* **-gias** *also* **-gies** : destruction of neurons by phagocytic cells

neu·ro·no·tro·pic \-ˈtrō-pik, -ˈträp-ik\ *adj* : having an affinity for neurons : NEUROTROPIC

Neu·ron·tin \ˈnùr-än-tin\ *trademark* — used for a preparation of gabapentin

neu·ro·oph·thal·mol·o·gy \ˌn(y)ùr-ō-ˌäf-thə(l)-ˈmäl-ə-jē\ *n, pl* **-gies** : the neurological study of the eye — **neu·ro-oph·thal·mo·log·ic** \-mə-ˈläj-ik\ *or* **neu·ro-oph·thal·mo·log·i·cal** \-ˈläj-i-kəl\ *adj*

neu·ro·otol·o·gy \-ō-ˈtäl-ə-jē\ *or* **neu·ro·tol·o·gy** \-ˌtäl-ə-jē\ *n, pl* **-gies** : the neurological study of the ear — **neu·ro·oto·log·ic** \ˌn(y)ùr-ō-ˌōt-ə-ˈläj-ik\ *or* **neu·ro·oto·log·i·cal** \-ˈläj-i-kəl\ *adj*

neu·ro·par·a·lyt·ic \-ˌpar-ə-ˈlit-ik\ *adj* : of, relating to, causing, or characterized by paralysis or loss of sensation due to a lesion in a nerve ⟨∼ disease⟩

neu·ro·path \ˈn(y)ùr-ə-ˌpath\ *n* : an individual subject to nervous disorders or to neuroses

neu·ro·path·ic \ˌn(y)ùr-ə-ˈpath-ik\ *adj* : of, relating to, characterized by, or being a neuropathy ⟨∼ pain⟩ ⟨∼ disorders⟩ — **neu·ro·path·i·cal·ly** \-i-k(ə-)lē\ *adv*

neu·ro·patho·gen·e·sis \-ˌpath-ə-ˈjen-ə-səs\ *n, pl* **-e·ses** \-ˌsēz\ : the pathogenesis of a nervous disease

neu·ro·patho·gen·ic \-ˈjen-ik\ *adj* : causing or capable of causing disease of nervous tissue ⟨∼ viruses⟩ — **neu·ro·patho·ge·nic·i·ty** \-jə-ˈnis-ət-ē\ *n, pl* **-ties**

neu·ro·pa·thol·o·gist \-pə-ˈthäl-ə-jəst\ *n* : a specialist in neuropathology

neu·ro·pa·thol·o·gy \-pə-ˈthäl-ə-jē, -pa-\ *n, pl* **-gies** : pathology of the nervous system — **neu·ro·patho·log·ic** \-ˌpath-ə-ˈläj-ik\ *or* **neu·ro·patho·log·i·cal** \-i-kəl\ *adj* — **neu·ro·patho·log·i·cal·ly** \-k(ə-)lē\ *adv*

neu·rop·a·thy \n(y)ù-ˈräp-ə-thē\ *n, pl* **-thies** : an abnormal and usu. degenerative state of the nervous system or nerves; *also* : a systemic condition (as muscular atrophy) that stems from a neuropathy

neu·ro·pep·tide \ˌn(y)ùr-ə-ˈpep-ˌtīd\ *n* : an endogenous peptide (as an endorphin or an enkephalin) that influences neural activity or functioning

neuropeptide Y \-ˈwī\ *n* : a neurotransmitter composed of 36 amino acid residues that has a vasoconstrictive effect on blood vessels and is held to play a role in regulating eating behavior

neu·ro·phar·ma·ceu·ti·cal \ˈn(y)ùr-ō-ˌfär-mə-ˈsüt-i-kəl\ *n* : a drug used to treat neuropsychiatric, neuropsychological, or nervous-system disorders (as depression, obesity, schizophrenia, or Alzheimer's disease)

neu·ro·phar·ma·col·o·gist \-ˌfär-mə-ˈkäl-ə-jəst\ *n* : a specialist in neuropharmacology

neu·ro·phar·ma·col·o·gy \ˈn(y)ùr-ō-ˌfär-mə-ˈkäl-ə-jē\ *n, pl* **-gies** **1** : a branch of medical science dealing with the action of drugs on and in the nervous system **2** : the properties and reactions of a drug on and in the nervous system ⟨the ∼ of lithium⟩ — **neu·ro·phar·ma·co·log·i·cal** \-kə-ˈläj-i-kəl\ *also* **neu·ro·phar·ma·co·log·ic** \-ik\ *adj*

neu·ro·phil·ic \ˌn(y)ùr-ə-ˈfil-ik\ *adj* : NEUROTROPIC

neu·ro·phy·sin \-ˈfī-sᵊn\ *n* : any of several brain hormones that bind with and carry either oxytocin or vasopressin

neu·ro·phys·i·ol·o·gist \-ˌfiz-ē-ˈäl-ə-jəst\ *n* : a specialist in neurophysiology

neu·ro·phys·i·ol·o·gy \ˌn(y)ùr-ō-ˌfiz-ē-ˈäl-ə-jē\ *n, pl* **-gies** : physiology of the nervous system — **neu·ro·phys·i·o·log·i·cal** \-ē-ə-ˈläj-i-kəl\ *also* **neu·ro·phys·i·o·log·ic** \-ik\ *adj* — **neu·ro·phys·i·o·log·i·cal·ly** \-i-k(ə-)lē\ *adv*

neu·ro·pil \ˈn(y)ùr-ə-ˌpil\ *also* **neu·ro·pile** \-ˌpīl\ *n* : a fibrous network of delicate unmyelinated nerve fibers interrupted by numerous synapses and found in concentrations of nervous tissue esp. in parts of the brain where it is highly developed — **neu·ro·pi·lar** \-ˌpī-lər\ *adj*

neu·ro·pi·lem \ˌn(y)ůr-ə-'pī-ləm\ *or* **neu·ro·pi·le·ma** \-lə-mə\ *n* : NEUROPIL

neu·ro·plasm \'n(y)ůr-ə-ˌplaz-əm\ *n* : the cytosol of a nerve cell as distinguished from the neurofibrils — **neu·ro·plas·mat·ic** \ˌn(y)ůr-ə-ˌplaz-'mat-ik\ *or* **neu·ro·plas·mic** \-'plaz-mik\ *adj*

¹neu·ro·ple·gic \ˌn(y)ůr-ə-'plē-jik\ *adj* : of, relating to, or being a tranquilizing agent which acts by suppressing the transmission of nerve impulses ⟨∼ drugs⟩

²neuroplegic *n* : a neuroplegic drug

neu·ro·po·di·um \-'pōd-ē-əm\ *n, pl* **-dia** \-ē-ə\ : one of the delicate terminal branches of an axon

neu·ro·pore \'n(y)ůr-ə-ˌpō(ə)r, -ˌpò(ə)r\ *n* : either of the openings to the exterior at the anterior and posterior ends of the neural tube of a vertebrate embryo

neu·ro·pro·tec·tant \ˌnyůr-ō-prə-'tek-tənt\ *n* : a neuroprotective drug that protects against or helps repair the damaging effects of a stroke

neu·ro·pro·tec·tive \ˌn(y)ůr-ō-prə-'tek-tiv\ *adj* : serving to protect neurons from injury or degeneration ⟨the ∼ effects of nimodipine⟩ — **neu·ro·pro·tec·tion** \-'tek-shən\ *n*

neu·ro·psy·chi·a·trist \-sə-'kī-ə-trəst, -sī-\ *n* : a specialist in neuropsychiatry

neu·ro·psy·chi·a·try \-sə-'kī-ə-trē, -sī-\ *n, pl* **-tries** : a branch of medicine concerned with both neurology and psychiatry — **neu·ro·psy·chi·at·ric** \-ˌsī-kē-'a-trik\ *adj* — **neu·ro·psy·chi·at·ri·cal·ly** \-tri-k(ə-)lē\ *adv*

neu·ro·psy·chic \ˌn(y)ůr-ə-'sī-kik\ *also* **neu·ro·psy·chi·cal** \-ki-kəl\ *adj* : of or relating to both the mind and the nervous system as affecting mental processes

neu·ro·psy·chol·o·gist \-sī-'käl-ə-jəst\ *n* : a specialist in neuropsychology

neu·ro·psy·chol·o·gy \-sī-'käl-ə-jē\ *n, pl* **-gies** : a science concerned with the integration of psychological observations on behavior and the mind with neurological observations on the brain and nervous system — **neu·ro·psy·cho·log·i·cal** \-ˌsī-kə-'läj-i-kəl\ *adj* — **neu·ro·psy·cho·log·i·cal·ly** \-i-k(ə-)lē\ *adv*

neu·ro·psy·cho·phar·ma·col·o·gy \-ˌsī-kō-ˌfär-mə-'käl-ə-jē\ *n, pl* **-gies** : a branch of medical science combining neuropharmacology and psychopharmacology

neu·ro·ra·di·ol·o·gist \-ˌrād-ē-'äl-ə-jəst\ *n* : a specialist in neuroradiology

neu·ro·ra·di·ol·o·gy \-ˌrād-ē-'äl-ə-jē\ *n, pl* **-gies** : radiology of the nervous system — **neu·ro·ra·dio·log·i·cal** \-ē-ə-'läj-i-kəl\ *also* **neu·ro·ra·dio·log·ic** \-ik\ *adj*

neu·ro·re·lapse \-ri-'laps, -'rē-ˌlaps\ *n* : syphilitic meningitis that sometimes follows apparently successful but inadequate treatment of early syphilis

neu·ro·ret·i·ni·tis \-ˌret-ᵊn-'īt-əs\ *n, pl* **-nit·i·des** \-'nit-ə-ˌdēz\ : inflammation of the optic nerve and the retina

neu·ror·rha·phy \n(y)ů-'rór-ə-fē\ *n, pl* **-phies** : the surgical suturing of a divided nerve

neu·ro·sci·ence \ˌn(y)ůr-ō-'sī-ən(t)s\ *n* : a branch (as neurophysiology) of science that deals with the anatomy, physiology, biochemistry, or molecular biology of nerves and nervous tissue and esp. their relation to behavior and learning — **neu·ro·sci·en·tif·ic** \-ˌsī-ən-'tif-ik\ *adj*

neu·ro·sci·en·tist \-'sī-ənt-əst\ *n* : a specialist or expert in neuroscience

neu·ro·se·cre·tion \-si-'krē-shən\ *n* **1** : the process of producing a secretion by nerve cells **2** : a secretion produced by neurosecretion — **neu·ro·se·cre·to·ry** \-'sē-krə-ˌtór-ē, *esp Brit* -si-'krēt-(ə-)rē\ *adj*

neu·ro·sen·so·ry \-'sen(t)s-(ə-)rē\ *adj* : of or relating to afferent nerves ⟨∼ control of feeding behavior⟩

neu·ro·sis \n(y)ů-'rō-səs\ *n, pl* **-ro·ses** \-ˌsēz\ : a mental and emotional disorder that affects only part of the personality, is accompanied by a less distorted perception of reality than in a psychosis, does not result in disturbance of the use of language, and is accompanied by various physical, physiological, and mental disturbances (as visceral symptoms, anxieties, or phobias)

neu·ro·some \'n(y)ůr-ə-ˌsōm\ *n* **1** : the cell body of a neuron

2 : one of various small particles in the cytoplasm of a neuron

neu·ros·po·ra \n(y)ů-'räs-pə-rə\ *n* **1** *cap* : a genus (family Sphaeriaceae) of ascomycetous fungi which are used extensively in genetic research and have black perithecia and persistent asci and some of which have salmon pink or orange spore masses and are severe pests in bakeries **2** : any ascomycetous fungus of the genus *Neurospora*

neu·ro·stim·u·la·tor \ˌn(y)ůr-ō-'stim-yə-ˌlāt-ər\ *n* : a device that provides electrical stimulation to nerves (as to relieve intractable pain or to suppress tremors)

neu·ro·sur·geon \ˌn(y)ůr-ō-'sər-jən, 'n(y)ůr-ō-ˌsər-jən\ *n* : a surgeon specializing in neurosurgery

neu·ro·sur·gery \-'sərj-(ə-)rē\ *n, pl* **-ger·ies** : surgery of nervous structures (as nerves, the brain, or the spinal cord) — **neu·ro·sur·gi·cal** \-'sər-ji-kəl\ *adj* — **neu·ro·sur·gi·cal·ly** \-ji-k(ə-)lē\ *adv*

neu·ro·syph·i·lis \-'sif-(ə-)ləs\ *n* : syphilis of the central nervous system

¹neu·ro·syph·i·lit·ic \-ˌsif-ə-'lit-ik\ *adj* : of or relating to neurosyphilis

²neurosyphilitic *n* : an individual affected with neurosyphilis

neu·ro·ten·di·nous \-'ten-di-nəs\ *adj* : of or relating to a nerve and tendon; *esp* : being any of various nerve endings in tendons

neurotendinous spindle *n* : GOLGI TENDON ORGAN

neu·ro·ten·sin \-'ten(t)-sən\ *n* : a protein composed of 13 amino acid residues that causes hypertension and vasodilation and is present in the brain

¹neu·rot·ic \n(y)ů-'rät-ik\ *adj* **1 a** : of, relating to, or involving the nerves ⟨a ∼ disorder⟩ **b** : being a neurosis : NERVOUS ⟨a ∼ disease⟩ **2** : affected with, relating to, or characterized by neurosis ⟨a ∼ person⟩ — **neu·rot·i·cal·ly** \-i-k(ə-)lē\ *adv*

²neurotic *n* **1** : one affected with a neurosis **2** : an emotionally unstable individual

neu·rot·i·cism \n(y)ů-'rät-ə-ˌsiz-əm\ *n* : a neurotic character, condition, or trait

neu·ro·to·gen·ic \n(y)ů-ˌrät-ə-'jen-ik\ *adj* : tending to produce neurosis ⟨∼ effects⟩

neurotology *var of* NEURO-OTOLOGY

neu·ro·tome \'n(y)ůr-ə-ˌtōm\ *n* : NEUROMERE

neu·rot·o·my \n(y)ů-'rät-ə-mē\ *n, pl* **-mies** **1** : the dissection or cutting of nerves **2** : the division of a nerve (as to relieve neuralgia)

neu·ro·tox·ic \ˌn(y)ůr-ə-'täk-sik\ *adj* : toxic to the nerves or nervous tissue — **neu·ro·tox·ic·i·ty** \-ˌtäk-'sis-ət-ē\ *n, pl* **-ties**

neu·ro·tox·i·col·o·gist \-ˌtäk-sə-'käl-ə-jəst\ *n* : a specialist in the study of neurotoxins and their effects

neu·ro·tox·i·col·o·gy \-ə-jē\ *n, pl* **-gies** : the study of neurotoxins and their effects — **neu·ro·tox·i·co·log·i·cal** \-kə-'läj-ə-kəl\ *adj*

neu·ro·tox·in \-'täk-sən\ *n* : a poisonous protein complex that acts on the nervous system

neu·ro·trans·mis·sion \-tran(t)s-'mish-ən, -tranz-\ *n* : the transmission of nerve impulses across a synapse

neu·ro·trans·mit·ter \ˌn(y)ůr-ō-tran(t)s-'mit-ər, -tranz-\ *n* : a substance (as norepinephrine or acetylcholine) that transmits nerve impulses across a synapse — see FALSE NEUROTRANSMITTER

neu·ro·trau·ma \-'trò-mə, -'traů-\ *n* : injury to a nerve or to the nervous system

neu·ro·trope \'n(y)ůr-ə-ˌtrōp\ *n* : a neurotropic agent

neu·ro·troph·ic \ˌn(y)ůr-ə-'träf-ik, -'tròf-\ *adj* **1** : relating to or dependent on the influence of nerves on the nutrition of tissue **2** : NEUROTROPIC

neurotrophic factor *n* : any of a group of neuropeptides (as nerve growth factor) that regulate the growth, differentia-

---

\ə\ **abut** \ᵊ\ **kitten** \ər\ **further** \a\ **ash** \ā\ **ace** \ä\ **cot, cart** \aů\ **out** \ch\ **chin** \e\ **bet** \ē\ **easy** \g\ **go** \i\ **hit** \ī\ **ice** \j\ **job** \ŋ\ **sing** \ō\ **go** \ò\ **law** \òi\ **boy** \th\ **thin** \t̲h̲\ **the** \ü\ **loot** \ů\ **foot** \y\ **yet** \zh\ **vision** *See also* Pronunciation Symbols page

tion, and survival of certain neurons in the peripheral and central nervous systems

neu·ro·tro·phin \-'trō-fən\ *n* : NEUROTROPHIC FACTOR

neu·ro·trop·ic \ˌn(y)ur-ə-'träp-ik\ *adj* : having an affinity for or localizing selectively in nerve tissue ⟨∼ stains⟩ ⟨∼ viruses⟩ — compare DERMOTROPIC, PANTROPIC

neu·rot·ro·pism \n(y)ù-'rä-trə-ˌpiz-əm\ *n* : the quality or state of being neurotropic

neu·ro·tu·bule \ˌn(y)ur-ō-'t(y)ü-(ˌ)byü(ə)l\ *n* : one of the tubular elements sometimes considered to be a fundamental part of the nerve-cell axon

neu·ro·vac·cine \-vak-'sēn, -'vak-ˌ\ *n* : a smallpox vaccine virus cultivated in vivo in the brains of rabbits

neu·ro·vac·cin·ia \-vak-'sin-ē-ə\ *n* : the disease or condition produced by infection (as by inoculation) with neurovaccine

neu·ro·vas·cu·lar \-'vas-kyə-lər\ *adj* : of, relating to, or involving both nerves and blood vessels

neu·ro·veg·e·ta·tive \-'vej-ə-ˌtāt-iv\ *adj* : AUTONOMIC 1b ⟨∼ dermatoses⟩

neu·ro·vi·rol·o·gy \-vī-'räl-ə-jē\ *n, pl* **-gies** : virology concerned with viral infections of the nervous system

neu·ro·vir·u·lence \-'vir-(y)ə-lən(t)s\ *n* : the tendency or capacity of a microorganism to cause disease of the nervous system — **neu·ro·vir·u·lent** \-lənt\ *adj*

neu·ro·vis·cer·al \-'vis-ə-rəl\ *adj* : of, relating to, or affecting the viscera and the autonomic nervous system that innervates them ⟨a ∼ storage disorder or sphingolipidosis⟩

neu·ru·la \'n(y)ur-(y)ə-lə\ *n, pl* **-lae** \-ˌlē\ *or* **-las** : an early vertebrate embryo which follows the gastrula and in which nervous tissue begins to differentiate and the basic pattern of the vertebrate begins to emerge — **neu·ru·lar** \-lər\ *adj* — **neu·ru·la·tion** \ˌn(y)ur-(y)ə-'lā-shən\ *n*

¹neu·ter \'n(y)üt-ər\ *n* : a spayed or castrated animal (as a cat)

²neuter *vt* : CASTRATE 1, ALTER ⟨a ∼ed cat⟩

¹neu·tral \'n(y)ü-trəl\ *n* : a neutral color

²neutral *adj* **1** : not decided or pronounced as to characteristics **2 a** : totally lacking in saturation : ACHROMATIC **b** : not decided in color : nearly achromatic : of low saturation **3** : neither acid nor basic : neither acid nor alkaline; *specif* : having a pH value of 7.0 ⟨a ∼ solution contains both hydrogen ions and hydroxide ions at the same concentration 1.00×10^{-7} —Linus Pauling⟩ **4** : not electrically charged

neutral dye *n* : a salt formed by interaction of an acid dye (as eosin) and a basic dye (as methylene blue) — called also *neutral stain*

neutral fat *n* : TRIGLYCERIDE

neu·tral·iza·tion *also Brit* **neu·tral·isa·tion** \ˌn(y)ü-trə-lə-'zā-shən\ *n* **1** : an act or process of neutralizing **2** : the quality or state of being neutralized

neu·tral·ize *also Brit* **neu·tral·ise** \'n(y)ü-trə-ˌlīz\ *vb* **-ized** *also Brit* **-ised; -iz·ing** *also Brit* **-is·ing** *vt* **1** : to make chemically neutral **2 a** : to counteract the activity or effect of : make ineffective **b** : to counteract the refractive power of (a lens) by combining it with one or more other lenses **3** : to make electrically inert by combining equal positive and negative quantities ∼ *vi* : to undergo neutralization — **neu·tral·iz·er** *also Brit* **neu·tral·is·er** *n*

neutral red *n* : a basic phenazine dye used chiefly as a biological stain and acid-base indicator

neutral stain *n* : NEUTRAL DYE

neu·tri·no \n(y)ü-'trē-(ˌ)nō\ *n, pl* **-nos** : an uncharged elementary particle that is believed to be massless or to have a very small mass, that has any of three forms, and that interacts only rarely with other particles

neu·tro·clu·sion \ˌn(y)ü-trə-'klü-zhən\ *n* : the condition in which the anteroposterior occlusal relations of the teeth are normal

neu·tro·cyte \'n(y)ü-trə-ˌsīt\ *n* : NEUTROPHIL

neu·tron \'n(y)ü-ˌträn\ *n* : an uncharged elementary particle that has a mass nearly equal to that of the proton and is present in all known atomic nuclei except the hydrogen nucleus

neu·tro·pe·nia \ˌn(y)ü-trə-'pē-nē-ə\ *n* : leukopenia in which the decrease in white blood cells is chiefly in neutrophils — **neu·tro·pe·nic** \-'pē-nik\ *adj*

¹neu·tro·phil \'n(y)ü-trə-ˌfil\ *or* **neu·tro·phil·ic** \ˌn(y)ü-trə-'fil-ik\ *also* **neu·tro·phile** \ˌn(y)ü-trə-ˌfil\ *adj* : staining to the same degree with acid or basic dyes ⟨∼ granulocytes⟩

²neutrophil *also* **neutrophile** *n* : a granulocyte that is the chief phagocytic white blood cell

neu·tro·phil·ia \ˌn(y)ü-trə-'fil-ē-ə\ *n* : leukocytosis in which the increase in white blood cells is chiefly in neutrophils

ne·vi·ra·pine \nə-'vir-ə-ˌpēn, -'vī-rə-\ *n* : an antiretroviral drug $C_{15}H_{14}N_4O$ that inhibits reverse transcriptase and is administered orally in combination with at least one other antiretroviral in the treatment of infection by HIV-1 and AIDS

ne·vo·car·ci·no·ma *or chiefly Brit* **nae·vo·car·ci·no·ma** \ˌnē-vō-ˌkärs-ᵊn-'ō-mə\ *n, pl* **-mas** *also* **-ma·ta** \-mət-ə\ : a carcinoma developing from a nevus

ne·void *or chiefly Brit* **nae·void** \'nē-ˌvóid\ *adj* : resembling a nevus ⟨a ∼ tumor⟩; *also* : accompanied by nevi or similar superficial lesions ⟨∼ lesions⟩

ne·vus *or chiefly Brit* **nae·vus** \'nē-vəs\ *n, pl* **ne·vi** *or chiefly Brit* **nae·vi** \-ˌvī\ : a congenital or acquired usu. highly pigmented area on the skin that is either flat or raised : MOLE — see BLUE NEVUS, JUNCTIONAL NEVUS, SPIDER NEVUS

nevus flam·me·us \-'flam-ē-əs\ *n* : PORT-WINE STAIN

¹new·born \'n(y)ü-'bó(ə)rn\ *adj* **1** : recently born ⟨a ∼ child⟩ **2** : affecting or relating to the newborn

²new·born \-ˌbó(ə)rn\ *n, pl* **newborn** *or* **newborns** : a newborn individual : NEONATE

New·cas·tle disease \'n(y)ü-ˌkas-əl-, n(y)ü-'\ *n* : a contagious mild to fatal virus disease of birds and esp. the domestic chicken that is caused by a paramyxovirus of the genus *Rubulavirus* (species *Newcastle disease virus*), that is marked by highly variable respiratory, digestive, and nervous clinical signs (as sneezing, coughing, diarrhea, incoordination, tremors, and twitching of the head) and that is esp. destructive to young birds although all ages may be attacked — called also *pseudoplague*

new drug *n* : a drug that has not been declared safe and effective by qualified experts under the conditions prescribed, recommended, or suggested in the label and that may be a new chemical formula or an established drug prescribed for use in a new way

New Lat·in \-'lat-ᵊn\ *n* : Latin as used since the end of the medieval period esp. in scientific description and classification

new·ton \'n(y)üt-ᵊn\ *n* : the unit of force in the metric system equal to the force required to impart an acceleration of one meter per second per second to a mass of one kilogram

Newton, Sir Isaac (1642–1727), British physicist and mathematician. One of the greatest figures in the history of science, Newton made great fundamental discoveries in mathematics and physical science including the method of fluxions (now known as differential calculus); laws concerning the composition of white light and the transmission of light through various media, upon which he built the foundation for the science of optics; and the law of gravitation. The newton unit of force was named in his honor in 1904.

New·to·ni·an \n(y)ü-'tō-nē-ən\ *adj* : of, relating to, or following Sir Isaac Newton, his discoveries, or his doctrines ⟨∼ dynamics⟩

Newton's law of cool·ing \-'kü-liŋ\ *n* : a statement in physics: the rate at which an exposed body changes temperature through radiation is approximately proportional to the difference between its temperature and that of its surroundings

Newton's rings *n pl* : colored rings due to light interference that are seen about the contact of a convex lens with a plane surface or of two lenses differing in curvature

new variant Creutzfeldt–Jakob disease *n* : VARIANT CREUTZFELDT-JAKOB DISEASE — abbr. *nvCJD*

Nex·i·um \'nek-sē-əm\ *trademark* — used for a preparation of the magnesium salt of esomeprazole

nex·us \'nek-səs\ *n, pl* **nex·us·es** \-sə-səz\ *or* **nex·us** \-səs, -ˌsüs\ **1** : a connection or link **2** : a connected group or series

NF *abbr* **1** National Formulary **2** neurofibromatosis

NFP *abbr* natural family planning

ng *abbr* nanogram

NG *abbr* nasogastric

n'gana *var of* NAGANA

NGF *abbr* nerve growth factor

NGU *abbr* nongonococcal urethritis

NHS *abbr* National Health Service

Ni *symbol* nickel

ni·a·cin \'nī-ə-sən\ *n* : a crystalline acid $C_6H_5NO_2$ that is a member of the vitamin B complex occurring usu. in the form of a complex of niacinamide in various animal and plant parts (as blood, liver, yeast, bran, and legumes) and is effective in preventing and treating human pellagra and blacktongue of dogs — called also *nicotinic acid*

ni·a·cin·amide \,nī-ə-'sin-ə-,mīd\ *n* : a bitter crystalline basic amide $C_6H_6N_2O$ that is a member of the vitamin B complex and is formed from and converted to niacin in the living organism, that occurs naturally usu. as a constituent of coenzymes, and that is used similarly to niacin — called also *nicotinamide*

ni·al·amide \nī-'al-ə-,mīd\ *n* : a synthetic antidepressant drug $C_{16}H_{18}N_4O_2$ that is an inhibitor of monoamine oxidase

ni·car·di·pine \nī-'kär-də-,pēn\ *n* : a calcium channel blocker administered orally in the form of its hydrochloride $C_{26}H_{29}N_3O_6 \cdot HCl$ to treat angina pectoris and hypertension

niche \'nich *sometimes* 'nish *or* 'nēsh\ *n* : CRATER ⟨typical ~ formation resulting from an ulcer⟩

¹nick \'nik\ *n* : a break in one strand of two-stranded DNA caused by a missing phosphodiester bond

²nick *vt* : to produce a nick in (DNA) ⟨circular DNA that has been ~ed and closed⟩

nick·el \'nik-əl\ *n* : a silver-white hard malleable ductile metallic element capable of a high polish and resistant to corrosion that is used chiefly in alloys and as a catalyst — symbol *Ni*; see ELEMENT table

nick·ing \'nik-iŋ\ *n* : localized constriction of a retinal vein by the pressure from an artery crossing it seen esp. in arterial hypertension

Ni·co·ti·ana \ni-,kō-shē-'an-ə\ *n* : a genus of American and Asian herbs or shrubs of the family Solanaceae that have viscid foliage, tubular flowers, and a many-seeded capsule and that include the cultivated tobacco (*N. tabacum*)

nic·o·tin·amide \,nik-ə-'tē-nə-,mīd, -'tin-ə-\ *n* : NIACINAMIDE

nicotinamide adenine dinucleotide *n* : NAD

nicotinamide adenine dinucleotide phosphate *n* : NADP

nic·o·tin·ate \,nik-ə-'tē-,nāt\ *n* : a salt or ester of niacin

nic·o·tine \'nik-ə-,tēn\ *n* : a poisonous alkaloid $C_{10}H_{14}N_2$ that is the chief active principle of tobacco and that is used as an insecticide

    Ni·cot \nē-kō\, **Jean (1530?–1600),** French diplomat. While French ambassador to Portugal, Nicot introduced tobacco to France by sending tobacco seeds as a gift to the French court in 1560. Linnaeus named the plant genus *Nicotiana* in his honor in 1753.

nic·o·tin·ic \,nik-ə-'tē-nik, -'tin-ik\ *adj* : relating to, resembling, producing, or mediating the effects that are produced by acetylcholine liberated by nerve fibers at autonomic ganglia and at the neuromuscular junctions of voluntary muscle and that are mimicked by nicotine which increases activity in small doses and inhibits it in larger doses ⟨~ receptors⟩ — compare MUSCARINIC

nicotinic acid *n* : NIACIN

nic·o·tin·ism \'nik-ə-,tē-,niz-əm, ,nik-ə-'tē-,niz-əm\ *n* : the effect of the excessive use of tobacco

nic·o·tin·uric acid \,nik-ə-,tē-,n(y)ùr-ik-\ *n* : a crystalline acid $C_8H_8N_2O_3$ found in the urine of some animals as a product of the metabolism of niacin

nictitans — see MEMBRANA NICTITANS

nic·ti·tate \'nik-tə-,tāt\ *vi* **-tat·ed; -tat·ing** : WINK

nictitating membrane *n* : a thin membrane found in many vertebrate animals at the inner angle or beneath the lower lid of the eye and capable of extending across the eyeball — called also *membrana nictitans, third eyelid*

NICU \,en-,ī-(,)sē-'yü, 'nik-(,)yü\ *abbr* neonatal intensive care unit

ni·dal \'nīd-ᵊl\ *adj* : of or relating to a nidus

ni·da·tion \nī-'dā-shən\ *n* **1** : the development of the epithelial membrane lining the inner surface of the uterus following menstruation **2** : IMPLANTATION b

NIDDK *abbr* National Institute of Diabetes and Digestive and Kidney Diseases

NIDDM *abbr* non-insulin-dependent diabetes mellitus

ni·dus \'nī-dəs\ *n, pl* **ni·di** \,dī\ *or* **ni·dus·es** **1** : a place or substance in tissue where the germs of a disease or other organisms lodge and multiply **2** : a place where something originates or is fostered or develops ⟨hysterical symptoms often grow from an organic ~, congenital or acquired —D. N. Parfitt⟩

Niel·sen method \'nēl-sən-\ *n* : BACK PRESSURE-ARM LIFT METHOD

    H. Nielsen — see HOLGER NIELSEN METHOD

Nie·mann–Pick disease \'nē-,män-'pik-\ *n* : an error in lipid metabolism that is inherited as an autosomal recessive trait, is characterized by accumulation of phospholipid in macrophages of the liver, spleen, lymph glands, and bone marrow, and leads to gastrointestinal disturbances, malnutrition, enlargement of the spleen, liver, and lymph nodes, and abnormalities of the blood-forming organs — compare GAUCHER'S DISEASE, TAY-SACHS DISEASE

    Niemann, Albert (1880–1921), and **Pick, Ludwig (1868–1944),** German physicians. Niemann published the first description of a form of xanthomatosis in 1914. In 1926 Pick described the same condition but in much greater detail. Because of their respective contributions the disease is now known as Niemann-Pick disease.

ni·fed·i·pine \nī-'fed-ə-,pēn\ *n* : a calcium channel blocker $C_{17}H_{18}N_2O_6$ that is a coronary vasodilator used esp. in the treatment of angina pectoris — see ADALAT, PROCARDIA

ni·fur·ox·ime \,nī-fyùr-'äk-,sēm\ *n* : a pale yellow crystalline antifungal agent $C_5H_4N_2O_4$ often used in combination with furazolidone

night blindness *n* : reduced visual capacity in faint light (as at night) — called also *nyctalopia* — **night–blind** \'nīt-,blīnd\ *adj*

night·mare \'nīt-,ma(ə)r, -,me(ə)r\ *n* : a frightening dream accompanied by a sense of oppression or suffocation that usu. awakens the sleeper

night·shade \'nīt-,shād\ *n* **1** : any plant of the genus *Solanum* (family Solanaceae, the nightshade family) which includes some poisonous weeds, various ornamental garden plants, and important crop plants (as the potato and eggplant) **2** : BELLADONNA 1

night sweat *n* : profuse sweating during sleep that is sometimes a symptom of febrile disease

night ter·ror \-'ter-ər\ *n* : a sudden awakening in dazed terror that occurs in children during slow-wave sleep, is often preceded by a sudden shrill cry uttered in sleep, and is not remembered when the child awakes — usu. used in pl.; called also *pavor nocturnus*

night vision *n* : ability to see in dim light (as provided by moon and stars)

ni·gra \'nī-grə\ *n* : SUBSTANTIA NIGRA

ni·gral \-grəl\ *adj* : of, relating to, or being the substantia nigra ⟨~ cell firing⟩

nigricans — see ACANTHOSIS NIGRICANS

ni·gro·stri·a·tal \,nī-grō-strī-'āt-ᵊl\ *adj* : of, relating to, or joining the corpus striatum and the substantia nigra ⟨the ~ dopamine pathway degenerates in Parkinson's disease —S. H. Snyder *et al*⟩

nigrum — see PIGMENTUM NIGRUM

NIH *abbr* National Institutes of Health

ni·hi·lism \'nī-(h)ə-,liz-əm, 'nē-\ *n* **1** : NIHILISTIC DELUSION

\ə\ **abut** \ᵊ\ **kitten** \ər\ **further** \a\ **ash** \ā\ **ace** \ä\ **cot, cart**
\au̇\ **out** \ch\ **chin** \e\ **bet** \ē\ **easy** \g\ **go** \i\ **hit** \ī\ **ice** \j\ **job**
\ŋ\ **sing** \ō\ **go** \ȯ\ **law** \ȯi\ **boy** \th\ **thin** \t̲h̲\ **the** \ü\ **loot**
\u̇\ **foot** \y\ **yet** \zh\ **vision** *See also* Pronunciation Symbols page

M N

2 : skepticism as to the value of a drug or method of treatment — **ni·hi·lis·tic** \ˌnī-(h)ə-ˈlis-tik, ˌnē-\ *adj*

nihilistic delusion *n* : the belief that oneself, a part of one's body, or the real world does not exist or has been destroyed

nik·eth·amide \ni-ˈketh-ə-ˌmīd\ *n* : a bitter viscous liquid or crystalline compound $C_{10}H_{14}N_2O$ used chiefly in aqueous solution as a respiratory stimulant

Nile blue \ˈnīl-\ *n* : a dye used chiefly in the form of its sulfate as a biological stain (as for staining neutral fat red in the presence of dilute sulfuric acid)

NIMH *abbr* National Institute of Mental Health

ni·mo·di·pine \ni-ˈmōd-ə-ˌpēn\ *n* : a calcium channel blocker $C_{21}H_{26}N_2O_7$

Nine Mile fever \ˈnīn-ˈmīl-\ *n* : a rickettsial disease identical with or closely related to Q fever that affects humans and various mammals in parts of the northwestern U.S.

nin·hy·drin \nin-ˈhī-drən\ *n* : a poisonous crystalline oxidizing agent $C_9H_6O_4$ used esp. as an analytical reagent

ninhydrin reaction *n* : a reaction of ninhydrin with amino acids or related amino compounds used for the colorimetric determination of amino acids, peptides, or proteins by measuring the intensity of the blue to violet to red color formed or for the quantitative determination of amino acids by measuring the amount of carbon dioxide produced

ninth cranial nerve \ˈninth-\ *n* : GLOSSOPHARYNGEAL NERVE

ni·o·bi·um \nī-ˈō-bē-əm\ *n* : a lustrous light gray ductile metallic element that resembles tantalum chemically and is used in alloys — symbol *Nb;* called also *columbium;* see ELEMENT table

NIOSH *abbr* National Institute of Occupational Safety and Health

Ni·pah virus \ˈnē-pə-\ *n* : a single-stranded RNA virus of the family *Paramyxoviridae* (species *Nipah virus* of the genus *Henipavirus*) that has caused epidemics of respiratory disease in pigs and an often fatal encephalitis in humans in Malaysia, Singapore, and Bangladesh

nip·per \ˈnip-ər\ *n* **1** : any of various devices (as pincers) for gripping, breaking, or cutting (as nails or cuticle) — usu. used in pl. **2** : an incisor of a horse; *esp* : one of the middle four incisors — compare CORNER TOOTH, DIVIDER

nip·ple \ˈnip-əl\ *n* **1** : the protuberance of a mammary gland upon which in the female the lactiferous ducts open and from which milk is drawn **2 a** : an artificial teat through which a bottle-fed infant nurses **b** : a device with an orifice through which the discharge of a liquid can be regulated

Nip·po·stron·gy·lus \ˌnip-ō-ˈsträn-jə-ləs\ *n* : a genus of strongyloid nematode worms that comprise intestinal parasites of rodents (as *N. muris* of rats) and are much used in biological research

Ni·pride \ˈnī-ˌprīd\ *n* : a preparation of sodium nitroprusside — formerly a U.S. registered trademark

ni·sin \ˈnīs-ᵊn\ *n* : a polypeptide antibiotic that is produced by a bacterium of the genus *Streptococcus* (*S. lactis*) and is used as a food preservative esp. for cheese and canned fruits and vegetables

Nis·sen fundoplication \ˈnis-ᵊn-\ *n* : fundoplication in which the fundus of the stomach is wrapped completely around the lower end of the esophagus

　Nissen, Rudolph (1896–1981), Swiss (German-born) surgeon. From 1920 to 1933 Nissen held a series of surgical positions at the universities of Breslau, Freiburg, Munich, and Berlin. From 1933 to 1939 he served as professor of surgery and head of the department at the University of Istanbul. After extended stays at hospitals in New York City, he emigrated to Basel, Switzerland, to become professor of surgery at the university and chief surgeon at Burgerspital. He authored or coauthored over 30 books on surgery and 475 papers on thoracic and abdominal surgery. He first performed the fundoplication associated with his name in 1951 on a patient with a hole in the esophageal sphincter; in 1956 he proposed the surgical procedure for the treatment of reflux of gastric contents due to improper functioning of the

lower esophageal sphincter. Nissen is also credited with performing the first total pneumonectomy in 1931.

Nissl bodies \ˈnis-əl-\ *n pl* : discrete granular bodies of variable size that occur in the cell body and dendrites but not the axon of neurons, are composed of RNA and polyribosomes, are stained with basic dyes (as methylene blue), and give a striped appearance to the cell — called also *Nissl granules, tigroid substance*

　Nissl, Franz (1860–1919), German neurologist. Nissl discovered a granular basophilic substance that is found in the nerve cell body and the dendrites. He published his research in 1894, and since then the granules have come to be known as Nissl bodies or Nissl granules. Also known for his many contributions to the preparation and microscopic inspection of nervous tissue, he used methylene blue or toluidine blue dyes in order to achieve maximum delineation of cellular structure.

Nissl stain *n* : any of various stains that stain Nissl substance

Nissl substance *n* : the nucleoprotein material of Nissl bodies — called also *chromidial substance*

ni·sus \ˈnī-səs\ *n, pl* **ni·sus** \-səs, -ˌsüs\ : a mental or physical effort to attain an end

nit \ˈnit\ *n* : the egg of a louse or other parasitic insect; *also* : the insect itself when young

ni·ter *or chiefly Brit* **ni·tre** \ˈnīt-ər\ *n* **1** : POTASSIUM NITRATE **2** *archaic* : CHILE SALTPETER

ni·trate \ˈnī-ˌtrāt, -trət\ *n* : a salt or ester of nitric acid

ni·tra·tion \nī-ˈtrā-shən\ *n* : the process of treating or combining with nitric acid or a nitrate; *esp* : conversion of an organic compound into a nitro compound or a nitrate — **nitrate** *vb* **ni·trat·ed; ni·trat·ing**

ni·tric \ˈnī-trik\ *adj* : of, relating to, or containing nitrogen esp. with a higher valence than in corresponding nitrous compounds

nitric acid *n* : a corrosive liquid inorganic acid HNO_3 used esp. as an oxidizing agent, in nitrations, and in making organic compounds

nitric oxide *n* : a poisonous colorless gas NO that occurs as a common air pollutant formed by the oxidation of atmospheric nitrogen and that is also formed by the oxidation of arginine in the mammalian body where it acts as a mediator of intracellular and intercellular communication regulating numerous biological processes (as vasodilation and neurotransmission)

nitric oxide synthase *n* : any of various enzymes that catalyze the oxidation of arginine to form nitric oxide and citruline

ni·trid·a·tion \ˌnī-trə-ˈdā-shən\ *n* : conversion into a nitride

ni·tride \ˈnī-ˌtrīd\ *n* : a binary compound of nitrogen with a more electropositive element

ni·tri·fi·ca·tion \ˌnī-trə-fə-ˈkā-shən\ *n* : the oxidation (as by bacteria) of ammonium salts to nitrites and the further oxidation of nitrites to nitrates

ni·tri·fy·ing \ˈnī-trə-ˌfī-iŋ\ *adj* : active in nitrification ⟨∼ bacteria⟩

ni·trile \ˈnī-trəl, -ˌtrēl\ *n* : an organic cyanide containing the group CN which on hydrolysis yields an acid with elimination of ammonia

ni·trite \ˈnī-ˌtrīt\ *n* : a salt or ester of nitrous acid

ni·tri·toid reaction \ˈnī-trə-ˌtòid-\ *n* : an acute reaction that sometimes occurs to certain drugs (as gold sodium thiomalate) and that resembles poisoning by nitrite esp. in the presence of flushing, tachycardia, and faintness — called also *nitritoid crisis*

¹ni·tro \ˈnī-(ˌ)trō\ *adj* : containing or being the monovalent group NO_2 united through nitrogen

²nitro *n, pl* **nitros** : any of various nitrated products; *specif* : NITROGLYCERIN

ni·tro·ben·zene \ˌnī-trō-ˈben-ˌzēn, -ben-ˈ\ *n* : a poisonous yellow insoluble oil $C_6H_5NO_2$ with an almond odor that is used esp. as a solvent, as a mild oxidizing agent, and in making aniline

ni·tro·cel·lu·lose \-ˈsel-yə-ˌlōs, -ˌlōz\ *n* : CELLULOSE NITRATE

ni·tro·chlo·ro·form \-'klōr-ə-ˌfȯrm, -'klȯr-\ *n* : CHLOROPIC-RIN

Ni·tro–Dur \'nī-trō-ˌdər\ *trademark* — used for a preparation of nitroglycerin

ni·tro·fu·ran \ˌnī-trō-'fyu̇(ə)r-ˌan, -fyu̇-'ran\ *n* : any of several derivatives of furan that contain a nitro group and are used as bacteria-inhibiting agents

ni·tro·fu·ran·to·in \-fyu̇-'ran-tə-wən\ *n* : a nitrofuran derivative $C_8H_6N_4O_5$ that is a broad-spectrum antimicrobial agent used esp. in treating urinary tract infections

ni·tro·fu·ra·zone \-'fyu̇r-ə-ˌzōn\ *n* : a pale yellow crystalline compound $C_6H_6N_4O_4$ used chiefly externally as a bacteriostatic or bactericidal dressing (as for wounds and infections)

ni·tro·gen \'nī-trə-jən\ *n* : a common nonmetallic element that in the free form is normally a colorless odorless tasteless insoluble inert diatomic gas comprising 78 percent of the atmosphere by volume and that in the combined form is a constituent of biologically important compounds (as proteins, nucleic acids, and alkaloids) and hence of all living cells as well as of industrially important substances (as cyanides, fertilizers, dyes, and antibiotics) — symbol *N*; see ELEMENT table

ni·tro·ge·nase \nī-'träj-ə-ˌnās, 'nī-trə-jə-, -ˌnāz\ *n* : an iron- and molybdenum-containing enzyme of various nitrogen-fixing microorganisms (as some bacteria) that catalyzes the reduction of molecular nitrogen to ammonia

nitrogen balance *n* : the difference between nitrogen intake and nitrogen excretion in the animal body such that a greater intake results in a positive balance and an increased excretion causes a negative balance — see NITROGEN EQUILIBRIUM

nitrogen base *or* **nitrogenous base** *n* : a nitrogen-containing molecule with basic properties; *esp* : one that is a purine or pyrimidine

nitrogen cycle *n* : a continuous series of natural processes by which nitrogen passes through successive stations in air, soil, and organisms and which principally involves nitrogen fixation, nitrification, decay, and denitrification

nitrogen dioxide *n* : a poisonous strongly oxidizing reddish brown gas NO_2

nitrogen equilibrium *n* : nitrogen balance when intake and excretion of nitrogen are equal — called also *nitrogenous equilibrium*

nitrogen fixation *n* **1** : the industrial conversion of free nitrogen into combined forms useful esp. as starting materials for fertilizers or explosives **2** : the metabolic assimilation of atmospheric nitrogen by soil microorganisms and esp. rhizobia and its release for plant use by nitrification in the soil on the death of the microorganisms

nitrogen–fixing *adj* : capable of nitrogen fixation ⟨∼ bacteria⟩

nitrogen mustard *n* : any of various toxic blistering compounds analogous to mustard gas but containing nitrogen instead of sulfur; *esp* : MECHLORETHAMINE

nitrogen narcosis *n* : a state of euphoria and confusion similar to that of alcohol intoxication which occurs when nitrogen in normal air enters the bloodstream at increased partial pressure (as in deepwater diving) ⟨divers typically begin to experience the effects of *nitrogen narcosis* at depths of 100 feet⟩ — called also *rapture of the deep*

ni·trog·e·nous \nī-'träj-ə-nəs\ *adj* : of, relating to, or containing nitrogen in combined form (as in nitrates or proteins) ⟨∼ wastes in urine⟩

nitrogenous equilibrium *n* : NITROGEN EQUILIBRIUM

nitrogen tri·chlor·ide \-(ˈ)trī-'klōr(ə)r-ˌīd, -'klō(ə)r-\ *n* : a pungent volatile explosive yellow oil NCl_3 that was formerly used in bleaching and aging flour but was discontinued because of deleterious effects (as epilepsy) produced in laboratory animals fed on bread made from the bleached flour

ni·tro·glyc·er·in *or* **ni·tro·glyc·er·ine** \ˌnī-trə-'glis-(ə-)rən\ *n* : a heavy oily explosive poisonous liquid $C_3H_5N_3O_9$ used chiefly in making dynamites and in medicine as a vasodilator (as in angina pectoris) — called also *trinitrin, trinitroglycerin*; see NITRO-DUR, NITROSTAT

ni·tro·hy·dro·chlo·ric acid \ˌnī-trō-ˌhī-drə-ˌklōr-ik-, -ˌklȯr-\ *n* : AQUA REGIA

ni·tro·mer·sol \-'mər-ˌsȯl, -ˌsōl\ *n* : a brownish-yellow to yellow solid organic mercurial $C_7H_5HgNO_3$ that is a derivative of orthocresol used esp. formerly as an antiseptic and disinfectant

ni·trom·e·ter \nī-'träm-ət-ər\ *n* : an apparatus for collecting and measuring the volume of a gas (as nitrogen) that is liberated from a substance during analysis — called also *azotometer*

ni·tron \'nī-ˌträn\ *n* : a compound $C_{20}H_{16}N_4$ used in the qualitative and quantitative determination of nitric acid with which it forms an insoluble nitrate

ni·tro·prus·side \ˌnī-trō-'prəs-ˌīd\ *n* : a salt containing the anion $[Fe(CN)_5NO]^{2-}$ composed of five cyanogen groups and one nitrosyl group coordinated with iron — see SODIUM NITROPRUSSIDE

ni·tro·sa·mine \nī-'trō-sə-ˌmēn\ *also* **ni·tro·so·amine** \-sō-ə-ˌmēn, -'am-ˌēn\ *n* : any of various neutral compounds which are characterized by the group NNO and of which some are powerful carcinogens

ni·tro·sate \'nī-trə-ˌsāt\ *vt* **-sat·ed; -sat·ing** : to introduce the nitroso group into (a compound) : convert into a nitroso compound

ni·tro·sa·tion \ˌnī-trə-'sā-shən\ *n* : the process of converting into a nitroso compound

ni·tro·so \nī-'trō-(ˌ)sō\ *adj* : containing or being the monovalent group –NO — used esp. of organic compounds

ni·tro·so·di·meth·yl·amine \-ˌdī-ˌmeth-əl-'am-ˌēn, -ə-'mēn\ *n* : DIMETHYLNITROSAMINE

ni·tro·so·gua·ni·dine \-ˌ'gwän-ə-ˌdēn\ *n* : an explosive compound CH_4N_4O often used as a mutagen in biological research

ni·tro·so·urea \-yu̇-'rē-ə\ *n* : any of a group of lipid-soluble drugs that function as alkylating agents, have the ability to enter the central nervous system, and are effective in the treatment of some brain tumors and meningeal leukemias

Ni·tro·stat \'nī-trə-ˌstat\ *trademark* — used for a preparation of nitroglycerin

ni·tro·syl \nī-'trō-ˌsil\ *n* : the nitroso group — used esp. in names of inorganic compounds

nitrosyl chloride *n* : an orange-red corrosive gaseous compound NOCl that has an odor like chlorine and is used chiefly in bleaching flour and in chemical synthesis

ni·trous \'nī-trəs\ *adj* : of, relating to, or containing nitrogen esp. with a lower valence than in corresponding nitric compounds

nitrous acid *n* : an unstable acid HNO_2 known only in solution or in the form of its salts

nitrous oxide *n* : a colorless gas N_2O that when inhaled produces loss of sensibility to pain preceded by exhilaration and sometimes laughter and is used esp. as an anesthetic in dentistry — called also *laughing gas*

ni·tryl \'nī-ˌtril\ *n* : the nitro group — used esp. in names of inorganic compounds ⟨∼ chloride NO_2Cl⟩

ni·zat·i·dine \nī-'zat-ə-ˌdīn, -ˌdēn\ *n* : an H_2 antagonist $C_{12}H_{21}N_5O_2S_2$ that inhibits gastric acid secretion and is used in the treatment of duodenal ulcers — see AXID

Ni·zo·ral \'nī-zə-ˌral\ *trademark* — used for a preparation of ketoconazole

NK cell \ˌen-'kā-\ *n* : NATURAL KILLER CELL

nl *abbr* nanoliter

nm *abbr* nanometer

NMDA \ˌen-(ˌ)em-(ˌ)dē-'ā\ *n* : a synthetic amino acid $C_5H_9NO_4$ that binds selectively to a subset of glutamate receptors on neurons where the binding of glutamate results in the opening of calcium channels — called also *N-methyl-D-aspartate*

nmol *also* **nmole** *abbr* nanomole

M
N

\ə\ **abut** \ᵊ\ **kitten** \ər\ **further** \a\ **ash** \ā\ **ace** \ä\ **cot, cart**
\au̇\ **out** \ch\ **chin** \e\ **bet** \ē\ **easy** \g\ **go** \i\ **hit** \ī\ **ice** \j\ **job**
\ŋ\ **sing** \ō\ **go** \ȯ\ **law** \ȯi\ **boy** \th\ **thin** \th\ **the** \ü\ **loot**
\u̇\ **foot** \y\ **yet** \zh\ **vision** *See also* Pronunciation Symbols page

NMR *abbr* nuclear magnetic resonance

NNK \,en-(,)en-'kā\ *n* : a nitrosamine $C_{10}H_{13}N_3O_2$ in tobacco smoke that is derived from nicotine and is a powerful carcinogen

no *abbr* number

No *symbol* nobelium

no·bel·i·um \nō-'bel-ē-əm\ *n* : a radioactive element produced artificially — symbol *No*; see ELEMENT table

> **No·bel** \nō-'bel\, **Alfred Bernhard (1833–1896)**, Swedish inventor and philanthropist. A manufacturer of explosives, Nobel developed many inventions, his first in 1863 being a detonator for liquid nitroglycerin. Later, after considerable experimentation, he patented dynamite in 1867. His invention transformed the manufacture of explosives. He is most famous for bequeathing his fortune for the establishment of the Nobel Prizes. Nobelium was discovered in 1957.

no·ble gas \'nō-bəl-\ *n* : any of a group of rare gases that include helium, neon, argon, krypton, xenon, and sometimes radon and that exhibit great stability and extremely low reaction rates — called also *inert gas*

no·car·dia \nō-'kärd-ē-ə\ *n* **1** *cap* : a genus of aerobic actinomycetous bacteria that form limited mycelia which tend to break up into rod-shaped cells and occas. form spores by fragmentation but develop neither conidia nor endospores and that include various pathogens as well as some soil⸗ dwelling saprophytes **2** : any bacterium of the genus *Nocardia* — **no·car·di·al** \-əl\ *adj*

> **No·card** \nò-kär\, **Edmond–Isidore–Étienne (1850–1903)**, French veterinarian and biologist. Nocard was an instructor at a veterinary school near Paris and later became its director. As an assistant to Pasteur, he worked on communicable diseases in mammals. In 1885 he described the organism causing pseudotuberculosis in sheep, cattle, and horses. He developed a method for the early diagnosis of glanders in horses, and in 1888 he published a description of bovine glanders. The genus of fungi now known as *Nocardia* was named in his honor because the first species to be described was isolated by Nocard from glanders in cattle.

no·car·di·o·sis \nō-,kärd-ē-'ō-səs\ *n, pl* **-o·ses** \-,sēz\ : actinomycosis caused by actinomycetes of the genus *Nocardia* and characterized by production of spreading granulomatous lesions — compare MADUROMYCOSIS

no·ce·bo \,nō-'sē-(,)bō\ *n* : a harmless substance that when taken by a patient is associated with harmful effects due to negative expectations or the psychological condition of the patient

no·ci·cep·tive \,nō-si-'sep-tiv\ *adj* **1** *of a stimulus* : PAINFUL, INJURIOUS **2** : of, induced by, or responding to a nociceptive stimulus — used esp. of receptors or protective reflexes

no·ci·cep·tor \-'sep-tər\ *n* : a receptor for injurious or painful stimuli : a pain sense organ

no·ci·fen·sor \-'fen(t)-sər\ *adj* : of, relating to, or constituting a system of cutaneous nerve fibers held to mediate diffuse pain sensations

no·ci·per·cep·tion \-pər-'sep-shən\ *n* : perception of injurious stimuli

no code \'nō-\ *n* **1** : an order not to revive or sustain a patient who experiences a life-threatening event (as heart stoppage) ⟨dislikes putting a *no code* on patients —Gail A. Campbell⟩ **2** : a patient assigned a no code ⟨whether a . . . patient should be made a *no code* —Sabrina D. Jarvis⟩

noc·tu·ria \näk-'t(y)ùr-ē-ə\ *n* : urination at night esp. when excessive — called also *nycturia*

noc·tur·nal \näk-'tərn-ᵊl\ *adj* **1** : of, relating to, or occurring at night ⟨~ myoclonus⟩ **2** : characterized by nocturnal activity ⟨a ~ form of filariasis⟩

nocturnal emission *n* : an involuntary discharge of semen during sleep often accompanied by an erotic dream — compare WET DREAM

nocturnus — see PAVOR NOCTURNUS

noc·u·ous \'näk-yə-wəs\ *adj* : likely to cause injury ⟨a ~ stimulus⟩

nod·al \'nōd-ᵊl\ *adj* : being, relating to, or located at or near a node — **nod·al·ly** \'nōd-ᵊl-ē\ *adv*

nodal point *n* : either of two points so located on the axis of a lens or optical system that any incident ray directed through one will produce a parallel emergent ray directed through the other

node \'nōd\ *n* **1 a** : a pathological swelling or enlargement (as of a rheumatic joint) **b** : a body part resembling a knot; *esp* : a discrete mass of one kind of tissue enclosed in tissue of a different kind — see ATRIOVENTRICULAR NODE, LYMPH NODE **2** : a point, line, or surface of a vibrating body that is free or relatively free of vibratory motion

node–negative *adj* : being or having cancer that has not spread to nearby lymph nodes ⟨~ breast cancer⟩

node of Ran·vier \-'rän-vē-,ā\ *n* : a small gap in the myelin sheath of a myelinated nerve fiber

> **Ran·vier** \rä*ⁿ*-vyā\, **Louis–Antoine (1835–1922)**, French histologist. Ranvier was one of the foremost histologists of his time. He is credited with transforming histology from a descriptive into an experimental science. Most of his research focused on detailed nerve and skin structure. He discovered in 1871 the interruptions of the myelin sheaths, which are now known as the nodes of Ranvier. Ranvier also produced a major study on cicatrization. With the French bacteriologist André-Victor Cornil (1837–1908) he produced a manual of histopathology that ranks as one of the landmarks of medicine in the 19th century.

nodosa — see PERIARTERITIS NODOSA, POLYARTERITIS NODOSA, SALPINGITIS ISTHMICA NODOSA

no·dose \'nō-,dōs\ *adj* : having numerous or conspicuous protuberances — **no·dos·i·ty** \nō-'däs-ət-ē\ *n, pl* **-ties**

nodose ganglion *n* : INFERIOR GANGLION 2

nodosum — see ERYTHEMA NODOSUM

nod·u·lar \'näj-ə-lər\ *adj* : of, relating to, characterized by, or occurring in the form of nodules ⟨~ lesions⟩ ⟨~ melanoma⟩ — **nod·u·lar·i·ty** \,näj-ə-'lar-ət-ē\ *n, pl* **-ties**

nodular disease *n* : infestation with or disease caused by nodular worms of the genus *Oesophagostomum* esp. in sheep — called also *nodule worm disease*

nodular worm *n* : any of several nematode worms of the genus *Oesophagostomum* that are parasitic in the large intestine of ruminants and swine where they cause swellings of the intestinal wall resembling abscesses — called also *nodule worm*

nod·u·la·tion \,näj-ə-'lā-shən\ *n* : the formation or presence of nodules ⟨lung X-rays showing evidence of ~⟩

nod·ule \'näj-(,)ü(ə)l\ *n* : a small mass of rounded or irregular shape: as **a** : a small abnormal knobby bodily protuberance (as a tumorous growth or a calcification near an arthritic joint) **b** : the nodulus of the cerebellum

nod·u·lo·cys·tic \,näj-ə-lə-'sis-tik\ *adj* : characterized by the formation of nodules and cystic lesions ⟨~ acne⟩

nod·u·lus \'näj-ə-ləs\ *n, pl* **nod·u·li** \-,lī\ : NODULE; *esp* : a prominence on the inferior surface of the cerebellum forming the anterior end of the vermis

no·et·ic \nō-'et-ik\ *adj* : of, relating to, or based on the intellect

noise pollution \'nóiz-\ *n* : environmental pollution consisting of annoying or harmful noise (as of automobiles or jet airplanes) — called also *sound pollution*

Nol·va·dex \'näl-və-,deks\ *trademark* — used for a preparation of the citrate of tamoxifen

no·ma \'nō-mə\ *n* : a spreading invasive gangrene chiefly of the lining of the cheek and lips that is usu. fatal and occurs most often in persons severely debilitated by disease or profound nutritional deficiency — see CANCRUM ORIS

no·men·cla·ture \'nō-mən-,klā-chər *also* nō-'men-klə-,chù(ə)r, -'men-, -klə-chər, -klə-,t(y)ù(ə)r\ *n* : a system of terms used in a particular science; *esp* : an international system of standardized New Latin names used in biology for kinds and groups of kinds of animals and plants — see BINOMIAL NOMENCLATURE — **no·men·cla·tur·al** \,nō-mən-'klāch-(ə-)rəl\ *adj* — **no·men·cla·tur·al·ly** \-ē\ *adv*

No·mi·na An·a·tom·i·ca \'näm-ə-nə-,an-ə-'täm-i-kə, 'nō-mə-nə-\ *n* : the Latin anatomical nomenclature that was prepared by revising the Basle Nomina Anatomica, adopted in

1955 at the Sixth International Congress of Anatomists, and modified at subsequent Congresses — abbr. *NA*

no·mo·gen·e·sis \ˌnō-mə-'jen-ə-səs\ *n, pl* **-e·ses** \-ˌsēz\ : a theory of evolution that regards evolutionary change as due to inherent orderly processes fundamental to organic nature and independent of environmental influences

no·mo·gram \'näm-ə-ˌgram, 'nō-mə-\ *n* : a graphic representation that consists of several lines marked off to scale and arranged in such a way that by using a straightedge to connect known values on two lines an unknown value can be read at the point of intersection with another line

no·mo·graph \-ˌgraf\ *n* : NOMOGRAM — **no·mo·graph·ic** \ˌnäm-ə-'graf-ik, ˌnō-mə-\ *adj* — **no·mog·ra·phy** \nō-'mäg-rə-fē\ *n, pl* **-phies**

no·mo·thet·ic \ˌnäm-ə-'thet-ik, ˌnō-mə-\ *adj* : relating to, involving, or dealing with abstract, general, or universal statements or laws — compare IDIOGRAPHIC

no·mo·top·ic \-'tō-pik, -'täp-ik\ *adj* : occurring in the normal place

non·ab·sorb·able \ˌnän-əb-'sȯr-bə-bəl, -'zȯr-\ *adj* : not capable of being absorbed ⟨∼ silk sutures⟩ ⟨∼ antibiotics⟩

non·ac·id \(')nän-'as-əd\ *adj* : not acid : being without acid properties ⟨a ∼ chemical group⟩

non·adap·tive \-ə-'dap-tiv, -a-'\ *adj* : not serving to adapt the individual to the environment ⟨∼ traits⟩

non·ad·dict \(')nän-'ad-ikt\ *n* : one who is not addicted to a drug

non·ad·dict·ing \ˌnän-ə-'dikt-iŋ\ *adj* : NONADDICTIVE

non·ad·dic·tive \-ə-'dik-tiv\ *adj* : not causing addiction ⟨∼ painkillers⟩

non·ad·di·tive \(')nän-'ad-ət-iv\ *adj* : of, relating to, or being a genetic effect that is not additive — **non·ad·di·tiv·i·ty** \ˌnän-ˌad-ə-'tiv-ət-ē\ *n, pl* **-ties**

non·al·le·lic \ˌnän-ə-'lē-lik, -'lel-ik\ *adj* : not behaving as alleles toward one another ⟨∼ genes⟩

non·al·ler·gen·ic \-ˌal-ər-'jen-ik\ *adj* : not causing an allergic reaction ⟨∼ proteins⟩

non·al·ler·gic \-ə-'lər-jik\ *adj* : not allergic ⟨∼ individuals⟩; *also* : not caused by an allergic reaction ⟨∼ rhinitis⟩

non·am·bu·la·to·ry \(')nän-'am-byə-lə-ˌtōr-ē, -ˌtȯr-\ *adj* : not able to walk about ⟨∼ patients⟩

non·a·no·ic acid \ˌnän-ə-ˌnō-ik-\ *n* : PELARGONIC ACID

non–A, non–B hepatitis \ˌnän-'ā-ˌnän-'bē-\ *n* : hepatitis clinically and immunologically similar to hepatitis A and hepatitis B but caused by different viruses; *esp* : HEPATITIS C

non·an·ti·bi·ot·ic \-ˌant-i-bī-'ät-ik, -ˌan-ˌtī-; -ˌant-i-bē-\ *adj* : not antibiotic ⟨∼ drugs⟩

non·an·ti·gen·ic \-ˌant-i-'jen-ik\ *adj* : not antigenic ⟨∼ materials⟩

non·aque·ous \-'ā-kwē-əs, -'ak-wē-\ *adj* : not aqueous : made from, with, or by means of a liquid other than water ⟨∼ solutions⟩

non·ar·tic·u·lar \-är-'tik-yə-lər\ *adj* : affecting or involving soft tissues (as muscles and connective tissues) rather than joints ⟨∼ rheumatic disorders⟩

non·as·so·cia·tive \-ə-'sō-s(h)ē-ˌāt-iv, -shət-iv\ *adj* : not associative; *esp* : relating to or being learning (as habituation and sensitization) that is not associative learning

non·ato·pic \-(')ā-'täp-ik, -'tō-pik\ *adj* : not affected with atopy ⟨∼ patients⟩

non·au·di·to·ry \(')nän-'ȯd-ə-ˌtōr-ē, -ˌtȯr-\ *adj* : not relating to or functioning in hearing ⟨the ∼ part of the inner ear⟩

non·bac·te·ri·al \-bak-'tir-ē-əl\ *adj* : not of, relating to, caused by, or being bacteria ⟨∼ pneumonia⟩

non·bar·bi·tu·rate \-bär-'bich-ə-rət, -ˌrāt; -ˌbär-bə-'t(y)ur-ət, -ˌāt\ *adj* : not derived from barbituric acid ⟨∼ sedatives⟩

non·bi·o·log·i·cal \-ˌbī-ə-'läj-i-kəl\ *adj* : not biological ⟨∼ parents⟩ ⟨∼ factors⟩

non·cal·ci·fied \-'kal-sə-ˌfīd\ *adj* : not calcified ⟨a ∼ lesion⟩

non·ca·lo·ric \-kə-'lȯr-ik, -'lōr-; -'lär-; -'kal-ə-rik\ *adj* : not providing calories when consumed as part of a diet ⟨∼ beverages⟩ ⟨a ∼ fat substitute⟩

non·can·cer·ous \-'kan(t)s-(ə-)rəs\ *adj* : not affected with or being cancer ⟨∼ patients⟩ ⟨∼ tumors⟩

non·car·bo·hy·drate \-ˌkär-bō-'hī-ˌdrāt, -bə-, -drət\ *n* : a substance that is not a carbohydrate; *esp* : one (as an aglycone) combined with a carbohydrate (as a sugar)

non·car·cin·o·gen \-kär-'sin-ə-jən, -'kärs-ᵊn-ə-ˌjen\ *n* : a noncarcinogenic substance or agent

non·car·ci·no·gen·ic \-ˌkärs-ᵊn-ō-'jen-ik\ *adj* : not causing cancer

non·car·di·ac \-'kärd-ē-ˌak\ *adj* : not cardiac: as **a** : not affected with heart disease ⟨∼ geriatric patients⟩ **b** : not relating to the heart or heart disease ⟨∼ disorders⟩

non·ca·se·at·ing \-'kā-sē-ˌāt-iŋ\ *adj* : not exhibiting caseation ⟨∼ granulomas⟩

non·cel·lu·lar \(')nän-'sel-yə-lər\ *adj* : not made up of or divided into cells

non·chro·mo·som·al \ˌnän-ˌkrō-mə-'sō-məl\ *adj* **1** : not situated on a chromosome ⟨∼ DNA⟩ **2** : not involving chromosomes ⟨∼ mutations⟩

non·cod·ing \(')nän-'kōd-iŋ\ *adj* : not specifying the genetic code ⟨∼ introns⟩

non·co·ital \-'kō-ət-ᵊl, -kō-'ēt-\ *adj* : not involving heterosexual copulation

non·com·e·do·gen·ic \-ˌkäm-ə-dō-'jen-ik\ *adj* : not tending to clog pores (as by the formation of blackheads) ⟨a ∼ cosmetic⟩

non·com·mu·ni·ca·ble \-kə-'myü-ni-kə-bəl\ *adj* : not capable of being communicated; *specif* : not transmissible by direct contact ⟨a ∼ disease⟩

non·com·pet·i·tive \-kəm-'pet-ət-iv\ *adj* : involving or acting in inhibition of an enzyme by affecting its intrinsic catalytic activity rather than by competition with the substrate for the active site

non·com·pli·ance \-kəm-'plī-ən(t)s\ *n* : failure or refusal to comply (as in the taking of prescribed medication) — **non·com·pli·ant** \-ənt\ *adj*

non com·pos men·tis \ˌnän-ˌkäm-pə-'sment-əs, ˌnōn-\ *adj* : not of sound mind

non·con·duc·tor \ˌnän-kən-'dək-tər\ *n* : a substance that conducts heat, electricity, or sound only in very small degree

non·con·scious \(')nän-'kän-chəs\ *adj* : not conscious ⟨∼ psychic processes —A. A. Brill⟩

non·con·ta·gious \ˌnän-kən-'tā-jəs\ *adj* : not contagious

non·con·trac·tile \-kən-'trak-tᵊl, -ˌtīl\ *adj* : not contractile ⟨∼ fibers⟩

non·con·trib·u·to·ry \-kən-'trib-yə-ˌtōr-ē, -ˌtȯr-\ *adj* : making no contribution to a medical diagnosis ⟨the patient's past history was ∼⟩

non·con·vul·sive \ˌnän-kən-'vəl-siv\ *adj* : not convulsive ⟨∼ seizures⟩

non·cor·o·nary \(')nän-'kȯr-ə-ˌner-ē, -'kär-\ *adj* : not affecting, affected with disease of, or involving the coronary vessels of the heart ⟨∼ patients⟩ ⟨∼ cardiomyopathy⟩

non·cross·over \(')nän-'krȯ-ˌsō-vər\ *adj* : having or being chromosomes that have not participated in genetic crossing-over

non·cy·to·tox·ic \-ˌsīt-ə-'täk-sik\ *adj* : not toxic to cells ⟨∼ drug concentrations⟩

non·de·form·ing \ˌnän-di-'fȯr-miŋ\ *adj* : not causing deformation ⟨∼ arthritis⟩

non·de·pressed \-di-'prest\ *adj* : not depressed ⟨∼ adults⟩

¹non·di·a·bet·ic \-ˌdī-ə-'bet-ik\ *adj* : not affected with diabetes ⟨∼ persons⟩

²nondiabetic *n* : an individual not affected with diabetes

non·di·ag·nos·tic \-ˌdī-ig-'näs-tik, -əg-\ *adj* : not diagnostic ⟨a ∼ lung scan⟩ ⟨a ∼ physical exam⟩

non·di·a·lyz·able *or Brit* **non·di·a·lys·able** \-ˌdī-ə-'lī-zə-bəl\ *adj* : not dialyzable ⟨∼ antigens⟩

non·dif·fus·ible \-dif-'yü-zə-bəl\ *adj* : not diffusible ⟨∼ anions⟩

non·di·rec·tive \ˌnän-də-'rek-tiv, -(ˌ)dī-\ *adj* : of, relating to,

\ə\ **abut** \ᵊ\ **kitten** \ər\ **further** \a\ **ash** \ā\ **ace** \ä\ **cot, cart** \aȯ\ **out** \ch\ **chin** \e\ **bet** \ē\ **easy** \g\ **go** \i\ **hit** \ī\ **ice** \j\ **job** \ŋ\ **sing** \ō\ **go** \ȯ\ **law** \ȯi\ **boy** \th\ **thin** \th\ **the** \ü\ **loot** \u̇\ **foot** \y\ **yet** \zh\ **vision** *See also* Pronunciation Symbols page

M
N

or being psychotherapy, counseling, or interviewing in which the counselor refrains from interpretation or explanation but encourages the client (as by repeating phrases) to talk freely

non·dis·junc·tion \ˌnän-dis-'jəŋ(k)-shən\ *n* : failure of homologous chromosomes or sister chromatids to separate subsequent to metaphase in meiosis or mitosis so that one daughter cell has both and the other neither of the chromosomes — **non·dis·junc·tion·al** \-shnəl, -shən-əl\ *adj*

non·dis·sem·i·nat·ed \'nän-dis-'em-ə-ˌnāt-əd\ *adj* : not disseminated ⟨∼ lupus erythematosus⟩

non·di·vid·ing \ˌnän-də-'vīd-iŋ\ *adj* : not undergoing cell division ⟨∼ cells⟩

non·drowsy \-'draú-zē\ *adj* : not causing or accompanied by drowsiness ⟨∼ antihistamines⟩

non·drug \(')nän-'drəg\ *adj* : not relating to, being, or employing drugs ⟨∼ treatment⟩

non·dry·ing \-'drī-iŋ\ *adj* : not drying; *esp* : being a natural or synthetic oil (as olive oil) characterized by low saturation and consequent inability to solidify readily when exposed in a thin film to the air

non·elas·tic \-i-'las-tik\ *adj* : not elastic ⟨∼ fibrous tissue⟩

non·elec·tro·lyte \ˌnän-ə-'lek-trə-ˌlīt\ *n* : a substance that does not readily ionize when dissolved or melted and is a poor conductor of electricity

non·emer·gen·cy \-i-'mər-jən-sē\ *adj* : not being or requiring emergency care ⟨∼ surgery⟩ ⟨∼ patients⟩

non·en·zy·mat·ic \-ˌen-zə-'mat-ik\ *or* **non·en·zy·mic** \-en-'zī-mik\ *also* **non·en·zyme** \-'en-ˌzīm\ *adj* : not involving the action of enzymes ⟨∼ cleavage of protein⟩ — **non·en·zy·mat·i·cal·ly** \-ˌen-zə-'mat-i-k(ə-)lē\ *adv*

non·ero·sive \-i-'rō-siv, -ziv\ *adj* : not characterized by erosion of tissue ⟨∼ arthritis⟩

non·es·sen·tial \-i-'sen-chəl\ *adj* : being a substance synthesized by the body in sufficient quantity for normal health and growth ⟨a ∼ fatty acid⟩ — compare ESSENTIAL

nonessential amino acid *n* : any of various alpha-amino acids which are required for normal health and growth, which can be synthesized within the body or derived in the body from essential amino acids, and which include alanine, asparagine, aspartic acid, cysteine, glutamic acid, glutamine, glycine, proline, serine, and tyrosine

non·fa·mil·ial \ˌnän-fə-'mil-yəl\ *adj* : not familial ⟨∼ colon cancer⟩

non·fat \'nän-'fat\ *adj* : lacking fat solids : having fat solids removed ⟨∼ milk⟩

non·fa·tal \-'fāt-əl\ *adj* : not fatal ⟨∼ infections⟩

non·fe·brile \-'feb-ˌrīl *also* -'fēb-\ *adj* : not marked or affected by a fever ⟨∼ illnesses⟩ ⟨∼ patients⟩; *also* : not occurring with a fever ⟨∼ seizures⟩

non·fil·a·men·tous \-ˌfil-ə-'ment-əs\ *adj* : not filamentous ⟨∼ bacteria⟩

non·flag·el·lat·ed \-'flaj-ə-ˌlāt-əd\ *adj* : not having flagella

non·func·tion·al \-'fəŋ(k)-shnəl, -shən-əl\ *adj* : not performing or able to perform a regular function ⟨a ∼ muscle⟩

non·ge·net·ic \-jə-'net-ik\ *adj* : not genetic ⟨∼ diseases⟩

non·glan·du·lar \-'glan-jə-lər\ *adj* : not glandular ⟨the ∼ mucosa⟩

non·gono·coc·cal \ˌnän-ˌgän-ə-'käk-əl\ *adj* : not caused by a gonococcus ⟨∼ pelvic inflammatory disease⟩

nongonococcal urethritis *n* : urethritis caused by a microorganism other than a gonococcus; *esp* : urethritis that is sexually transmitted and is caused esp. by a bacterium of the genus *Chlamydia* (*C. trachomatis*) or a mycoplasma of the genus *Ureaplasma* (*U. urealyticum*) — called also *nonspecific urethritis*

non·gran·u·lar \-'gran-yə-lər\ *adj* : not granular; *esp* : characterized by or being cytoplasm which does not contain granules ⟨∼ white blood cells⟩

nongranular leukocyte *n* : any of the white blood cells that usu. lack granules in their cytoplasm having an affinity for specific biological stains and that include the lymphocytes and monocytes — called also *monouclear leukocyte;* compare GRANULAR LEUKOCYTE

non·grav·id \ˌnän-'grav-əd\ *adj* : not pregnant

non·heal·ing \-'hē-liŋ\ *adj* : not healing ⟨∼ ulcers⟩

non·heme *or chiefly Brit* **non·haem** \'nän-'hēm\ *adj* : not containing or being iron that is bound in a porphyrin ring like that of heme ⟨the ferredoxins are ∼ iron proteins⟩

non·he·mo·lyt·ic *or chiefly Brit* **non·hae·mo·lyt·ic** \-ˌhē-mə-'lit-ik\ *adj* : not causing or characterized by hemolysis ⟨a ∼ streptococcus⟩

non·hem·or·rhag·ic *or chiefly Brit* **non·haem·or·rhag·ic** \-ˌhem-ə-'raj-ik\ *adj* : not causing or associated with hemorrhage ⟨∼ shock⟩

non·he·red·i·tary \-hə-'red-ə-ˌter-ē\ *adj* : not hereditary

non·her·i·ta·ble \-'her-ət-ə-bəl\ *adj* : not heritable ⟨∼ diseases⟩

non·his·tone \(')nän-'his-ˌtōn\ *adj* : relating to or being any of the eukaryotic proteins (as DNA polymerase) that form complexes with DNA but are not considered histones

non–Hodg·kin's lymphoma \-'häj-kənz-\ *n* : any of various malignant lymphomas (as Burkitt's lymphoma) that are not classified as Hodgkin's disease and that usu. have malignant cells derived from B cells or T cells

non·ho·mol·o·gous \'nän-hō-'mäl-ə-gəs, -hə-\ *adj* : being of unlike genetic constitution — used of chromosomes of one set containing nonallelic genes

non·hor·mo·nal \-hòr-'mōn-əl\ *adj* : not hormonal

non·hos·pi·tal \-'häs-ˌpit-əl\ *adj* : not relating to, associated with, or occurring within a hospital ⟨∼ clinics⟩

non·hos·pi·tal·ized *or chiefly Brit* **non·hos·pi·tal·ised** \-'häs-ˌpit-əl-ˌīzd\ *adj* : not hospitalized ⟨∼ patients⟩

non·hy·gro·scop·ic \-ˌhī-grə-'skäp-ik\ *adj* : not hygroscopic

non·iden·ti·cal \ˌnän-(ˌ)ī-'dent-i-kəl, ˌnän-ə-'dent-\ *adj* : not identical; *esp* : FRATERNAL

¹non·im·mune \-im-'yün\ *adj* : not immune

²nonimmune *n* : an individual that lacks immunity to a particular disease

non·in·fect·ed \'nän-in-'fek-təd\ *adj* : not having been subjected to infection

non·in·fec·tious \-in-'fek-shəs\ *adj* : not infectious ⟨∼ causes of chronic diarrhea —E. T. Ryan *et al*⟩

non·in·fec·tive \-tiv\ *adj* : not infective ⟨∼ leukemia⟩

non·in·flam·ma·to·ry \-in-'flam-ə-ˌtōr-ē\ *adj* : not inflammatory ⟨∼ lesions⟩

non·in·sti·tu·tion·al·ized *also Brit* **non·in·sti·tu·tion·al·ised** \-ˌin(t)-stə-'t(y)ü-shnəl-ˌīzd, -shən-əl-\ *adj* : not institutionalized; *esp* : not having been placed in a special institution

non–insulin–dependent diabetes *n* : TYPE 2 DIABETES

non–insulin–dependent diabetes mellitus *n* : TYPE 2 DIABETES — abbr. *NIDDM*

non·in·va·sive \ˌnän-in-'vā-siv, -ziv\ *adj* **1** : not tending to spread; *specif* : not tending to infiltrate and destroy healthy tissue ⟨∼ cancer of the bladder⟩ **2** : not being or involving an invasive medical procedure ⟨∼ imaging techniques that do not require the injection of dyes⟩ — **non·in·va·sive·ly** *adv* — **non·in·va·sive·ness** *n*

non·ir·ra·di·at·ed \-ir-'ād-ē-ˌāt-əd\ *adj* : not having been exposed to radiation

non·isch·emic *or chiefly Brit* **non·isch·ae·mic** \-is-'kē-mik\ *adj* : not marked by or resulting from ischemia ⟨∼ tissue⟩

non·ke·ra·ti·nized \-'ker-ət-ə-ˌnīzd, -kə-'rat-ən-ˌīzd\ *adj* : not keratinous ⟨∼ epithelium⟩

non·ke·tot·ic \-kē-'tät-ik\ *adj* : not associated with ketosis ⟨∼ diabetes⟩

non·liv·ing \-'liv-iŋ\ *adj* : not having or characterized by life

non·lym·pho·cyt·ic \-ˌlim(p)-fə-'sit-ik\ *adj* : not lymphocytic — see ACUTE NONLYMPHOCYTIC LEUKEMIA

non·lym·phoid \-'lim-ˌfòid\ *adj* : not derived from or being lymphoid tissue ⟨∼ cells⟩; *also* : not composed of lymphoid cells ⟨a ∼ tumor⟩

non·ma·lig·nant \-mə-'lig-nənt\ *adj* : not malignant ⟨a ∼ tumor⟩

non·med·ul·lat·ed \-'med-əl-ˌāt-əd, -'mej-ə-ˌlāt-\ *adj* : UNMYELINATED ⟨∼ nerve fibers⟩

non·mel·a·no·ma \-ˌmel-ə-'nō-mə\ *n, often attrib* : a tumor that is not a melanoma ⟨~ cells⟩ ⟨~ skin cancer⟩

non·met·al \(')nän-'met-ᵊl\ *n* : a chemical element (as boron, carbon, or nitrogen) that lacks the characteristics of a metal and that is able to form anions, acidic oxides, acids, and stable compounds with hydrogen

non·me·tal·lic \ˌnän-mə-'tal-ik\ *adj* **1** : not metallic **2** : of, relating to, or being a nonmetal

non·met·a·stat·ic \-ˌmet-ə-'stat-ik\ *adj* : not metastatic ⟨~ tumors⟩

non·mi·cro·bi·al \-mī-'krō-bē-əl\ *adj* : not microbial ⟨~ diseases⟩

non·mo·tile \-'mōt-ᵊl, -'mō-ˌtīl\ *adj* : not motile ⟨~ gametes⟩ ⟨~ gram-negative bacterial rods⟩

non·mu·tant \-'myüt-ᵊnt\ *adj* : not mutant

non·my·e·lin·at·ed \-'mī-ə-lə-ˌnāt-əd\ *adj* : UNMYELINATED

non·my·eloid \-'mī-ə-ˌlȯid\ *adj* : not being, involving, or affecting bone marrow ⟨~ malignancies⟩

non·nar·cot·ic \-när-'kät-ik\ *adj* : not narcotic ⟨~ analgesics⟩

non·neo·plas·tic \-ˌnē-ə-'plas-tik\ *adj* : not being or not caused by neoplasms ⟨~ diseases⟩

non·ner·vous \-'nər-vəs\ *adj* : not nervous ⟨~ tissue⟩

non·neu·ro·nal \-'n(y)ùr-ən-ᵊl, -n(y)ù-'rōn-ᵊl\ *adj* : of, relating to, or being cells other than neurons ⟨~ cells⟩

non·nu·cle·at·ed \-'n(y)ü-klē-ˌāt-əd\ *adj* : not nucleated ⟨~ bacterial cells⟩

non·nu·tri·tive \-'n(y)ü-trət-iv\ *adj* : not relating to or providing nutrition ⟨~ sweeteners⟩

non·obese \-ō-'bēs\ *adj* : not obese ⟨~ diabetics⟩

non·ob·struc·tive \-əb-'strək-tiv\ *adj* : not causing or characterized by obstruction (as of a bodily passage) ⟨~ renal calculi⟩

non·oc·clu·sive \-ə-'klü-siv\ *adj* : not causing or characterized by occlusion ⟨~ mesenteric infarction⟩

non·of·fi·cial \-ə-'fish-əl\ *adj* : UNOFFICIAL; *esp* : not described in the current *U.S. Pharmacopeia* and *National Formulary* and never having been described therein — compare OFFICIAL

non·ol·fac·to·ry \-äl-'fak-t(ə-)rē, -ōl-\ *adj* : not olfactory

non·opaque \-ō-'pāk\ *adj* : not opaque; *esp* : allowing the passage of radiation (as X-rays)

non·op·er·a·tive \-'äp-(ə-)rət-iv, -'äp-ə-ˌrāt-\ *adj* : not involving an operation ⟨~ treatment⟩

non·or·gas·mic \ˌnän-ȯr-'gaz-mik\ *adj* : not capable of experiencing orgasm ⟨~ women⟩

no·nox·y·nol-9 \nä-'näk-sə-ˌnōl-'nīn, -ˌnȯl-\ *n* : a spermicide used in contraceptive products that consists of a mixture of compounds having the general formula $C_{15}H_{23}$-$(OCH_2CH_2)_nOH$ with an average of nine ethylene oxide groups per molecule

non·par·a·sit·ic \-ˌpar-ə-'sit-ik\ *adj* : not parasitic; *esp* : not caused by parasites ⟨~ diseases⟩

non·par·ous \ˌnän-'par-əs\ *adj* : NULLIPAROUS

non·pa·ter·ni·ty \ˌnän-pə-'tər-nət-ē\ *n, pl* **-ties** : the condition of not being the father of a particular child

non·patho·gen·ic \ˌnän-ˌpath-ə-'jen-ik\ *adj* : not capable of inducing disease — compare AVIRULENT

non·per·mis·sive \ˌnän-pər-'mis-iv\ *adj* : being or relating to a cell, medium, or environmental condition which does not support the replication of a mutant gene of a virus or bacteriophage ⟨~ host cells⟩ ⟨~ temperatures⟩

non·per·sis·tent \ˌnän-pər-'sis-tənt, -'zis-\ *adj* : not persistent: as **a** : decomposed rapidly by environmental action ⟨~ insecticides⟩ **b** : capable of being transmitted by a vector for only a relatively short time ⟨~ viruses⟩

non·phy·si·cian \-fə-'zish-ən\ *n* : a person who is not a legally qualified physician

non·pig·ment·ed \-'pig-mənt-əd\ *adj* : not pigmented

non·poi·son·ous \-'pȯiz-nəs, -ᵊn-əs\ *adj* : not poisonous

non·po·lar \-'pō-lər\ *adj* : not polar ⟨a ~ molecule⟩ ⟨a ~ group⟩; *esp* : consisting of molecules not having a dipole

non·pol·yp·o·sis \-ˌpäl-i-'pō-səs\ *adj* : characterized by the absence of polyps ⟨hereditary ~ colorectal cancer⟩

non·preg·nant \-'preg-nənt\ *adj* : not pregnant

non·pre·scrip·tion \ˌnän-pri-'skrip-shən\ *adj* : available for purchase without a doctor's prescription ⟨~ drugs⟩

non·pro·duc·tive \-prə-'dək-tiv\ *adj, of a cough* : not effective in raising mucus or exudate from the respiratory tract : DRY 2

non·pro·gres·sor \-prə-'gres-ər\ *n* : LONG-TERM NONPROGRESSOR

non·pro·pri·etary \-prə-'prī-ə-ˌter-ē\ *adj* : not proprietary ⟨a drug's ~ name⟩

non·pro·tein \'nän-'prō-ˌtēn, -'prōt-ē-ən\ *adj* : not being or derived from protein ⟨the ~ part of an enzyme⟩

non·psy·chi·at·ric \-ˌsī-kē-'a-trik\ *adj* : not psychiatric ⟨~ patients⟩ ⟨~ medical personnel —L. S. Holsenbeck⟩

¹**non·psy·chi·a·trist** \-sə-'kī-ə-trəst, -sī-\ *adj* : not specializing in psychiatry ⟨~ physicians⟩

²**nonpsychiatrist** *n* : a physician who does not specialize in psychiatry

non·psy·chot·ic \-sī-'kät-ik\ *adj* : not psychotic ⟨~ emotional disorders⟩

non·ra·dio·ac·tive \-ˌrād-ē-ō-'ak-tiv\ *adj* : not radioactive

non·re·ac·tive \-rē-'ak-tiv\ *adj* : not reactive ⟨dilated ~ pupils⟩; *esp* : not exhibiting a positive reaction in a particular laboratory test ⟨the serum was ~ in the VDRL test⟩

non·re·com·bi·nant \ˌnän-(ˌ)rē-'käm-bə-nənt\ *adj* : not exhibiting the result of genetic recombination ⟨~ progeny⟩

non·re·duc·ing \-ri-'d(y)üs-iŋ\ *adj* : not reducing; *esp* : not readily reducing a mild oxidizing agent (as Fehling solution) ⟨sucrose is a ~ sugar⟩ — compare REDUCING SUGAR

non·re·duc·tion \-ri-'dək-shən\ *n* : the failure of homologous chromosomes to break apart into separate sets in the reduction division of meiosis with the result that some gametes have the diploid number of chromosomes

non–REM sleep \-ˌrem-\ *n* : SLOW-WAVE SLEEP

non·re·nal \-'rēn-ᵊl\ *adj* : not renal; *esp* : not resulting from dysfunction of the kidneys ⟨~ alkalosis⟩

non·re·spond·er \-ri-'spän-dər\ *n* : one (as a person or a cell) that does not respond (as to medical treatment or to an antigen)

non·rheu·ma·toid \-'rü-mə-ˌtȯid\ *adj* : not relating to, affected with, or being rheumatoid arthritis

non·rhyth·mic \-'rith-mik\ *adj* : not rhythmic ⟨~ contractions⟩

¹**non·schizo·phren·ic** \-ˌskit-sə-'fren-ik\ *adj* : not relating to, affected with, or being schizophrenia ⟨~ patients⟩

²**nonschizophrenic** *n* : a nonschizophrenic individual

non·se·cre·tor \-si-'krēt-ər\ *n* : an individual of blood group A, B, or AB who does not secrete the antigens characteristic of these blood groups in bodily fluids (as saliva)

non·se·cre·to·ry \-'sē-krə-ˌtȯr-ē, *esp Brit* -si-'krēt-ə-rē\ *adj* : not secretory ⟨~ cells⟩

non·se·dat·ing \-si-'dāt-iŋ\ *adj* : not producing sedation ⟨prescribed a ~ antihistamine⟩

¹**non·sed·a·tive** \-'sed-ət-iv\ *adj* : NONSEDATING ⟨a ~ anxiolytic drug⟩

²**nonsedative** *n* : a nonsedating drug

non·sed·i·ment·able \ˌnän-sed-ə-'ment-ə-bəl\ *adj* : not capable of being sedimented under specified conditions (as of centrifugation) ⟨~ RNA⟩

non·se·lec·tive \-sə-'lek-tiv\ *adj* : not selective; *esp* : not limited (as to a single body part or organism) in action or effect ⟨~ anti-infective agents⟩

non·self \'nän-'self\ *n* : material that is foreign to the body of an organism — **nonself** *adj*

¹**non·sense** \'nän-ˌsen(t)s, 'nän(t)-sən(t)s\ *n* : genetic information consisting of one or more codons that do not code for any amino acid and usu. cause termination of the molecular chain in protein synthesis — compare ANTISENSE, MISSENSE

\ə\ abut \ᵊ\ kitten \ər\ further \a\ ash \ā\ ace \ä\ cot, cart
\aù\ out \ch\ chin \e\ bet \ē\ easy \g\ go \i\ hit \ī\ ice \j\ job
\ŋ\ sing \ō\ go \ȯ\ law \ȯi\ boy \th\ thin \t̲h̲\ the \ü\ loot
\ù\ foot \y\ yet \zh\ vision   *See also* Pronunciation Symbols page

M
N

²**nonsense** *adj* : consisting of one or more codons that are genetic nonsense ⟨∼ mutations⟩

non·sen·si·tive \-'sen(t)-sət-iv\ *adj* : not sensitive

non·sep·tate \-'sep-ₜtāt\ *adj* : not divided by or having a septum ⟨a ∼ mycelium⟩

non·sex chromosome \'nän-'seks-\ *n* : AUTOSOME

non·sex·u·al \(�')nän-'seksh-(ə-)wəl\ *adj* : not sexual ⟨∼ reproduction⟩

non–small cell lung cancer \ₜnän-ₜsmȯl-\ *n* : any carcinoma (as an adenocarcinoma or squamous cell carcinoma) of the lungs that is not a small-cell lung cancer — called also *non-small cell cancer, non-small cell carcinoma, non-small cell lung carcinoma;* see LARGE-CELL CARCINOMA

non·smok·er \-'smō-kər\ *n* : a person who does not smoke tobacco

non·spe·cif·ic \-spi-'sif-ik\ *adj* : not specific: as **a** : not caused by a specific agent ⟨∼ adenitis⟩ ⟨∼ enteritis⟩ **b** : having a general purpose or effect ⟨∼ therapy⟩ — **non·spe·cif·i·cal·ly** \-'sif-i-k(ə-)lē\ *adv*

nonspecific urethritis *n* : NONGONOCOCCAL URETHRITIS

nonspecific vaginitis *n* : BACTERIAL VAGINOSIS

non·spore–form·ing \-'spȯr-ₜfȯr-miŋ\ *adj* : not producing spores ⟨∼ bacteria⟩

non·ste·roi·dal \ₜnän-stə-'rȯid-ᵊl\ *also* **non·ste·roid** \(ᵋ')nän-'sti(ə)r-ₜȯid *also* -'ste(ə)r-\ *adj* : of, relating to, or being a compound and esp. a drug that is not a steroid ⟨a ∼ antiinflammatory drug⟩ — see NSAID — **nonsteroid** *n*

non·stress test \'nän-'stres-\ *n* : a test of fetal well-being that is performed by ultrasound monitoring of the increase in fetal heartbeat following fetal movement

non·stri·at·ed \'nän-'strī-ₜāt-əd\ *adj* : being without striations

nonstriated muscle *n* : SMOOTH MUSCLE

non·sug·ar \-'shùg-ər\ *n* : a substance that is not a sugar; *esp* : AGLYCONE

non·sup·pu·ra·tive \-'səp-yə-ₜrāt-iv\ *adj* : not characterized by or accompanied by suppuration ⟨∼ inflammation⟩

non·sur·gi·cal \-'sər-ji-kəl\ *adj* : not surgical ⟨∼ hospital care⟩ — **non·sur·gi·cal·ly** \-ji-k(ə-)lē\ *adv*

non·sys·tem·ic \-sis-'tem-ik\ *adj* : not systemic

non·tast·er \-'tā-stər\ *n* : a person unable to taste the chemical phenylthiocarbamide

non·ther·a·peu·tic \-ₜther-ə-'p(y)üt-ik\ *adj* : not relating to or being therapy ⟨∼ procedures⟩

non·throm·bo·cy·to·pe·nic \-ₜthräm-bə-ₜsīt-ə-'pē-nik\ *adj* : not relating to, affected with, or associated with thrombocytopenia ⟨∼ purpura⟩

non·tox·ic \-'täk-sik\ *adj* **1** : not toxic ⟨∼ chemicals⟩ **2** *of goiter* : not associated with hyperthyroidism

non·trau·mat·ic \-trə-'mat-ik, -trō-, -traù-\ *adj* : not causing, caused by, or associated with trauma and esp. traumatic injury ⟨∼ surgery⟩ ⟨sudden ∼ death in conditioned runners —B. F. Waller *et al*⟩

non·trop·i·cal sprue \-'träp-i-kəl-\ *n* : CELIAC DISEASE

non·tu·ber·cu·lous \-t(y)ù-'bər-kyə-ləs\ *adj* : not causing, caused by, or affected with tuberculosis ⟨∼ mycobacteria⟩

non·union \-'yün-yən\ *n* : failure of the fragments of a broken bone to knit together

non·vas·cu·lar \-'vas-kyə-lər\ *adj* : lacking blood vessels or a vascular system ⟨a ∼ layer of the skin⟩

non·vec·tor \-'vek-tər\ *n* : an organism (as an insect) that does not transmit a particular pathogen (as a virus) ⟨∼ anophelines⟩

non·ven·om·ous \-'ven-ə-məs\ *adj* : not venomous

non·vi·a·ble \-'vī-ə-bəl\ *adj* : not capable of living, growing, or developing and functioning successfully ⟨∼ embryos⟩

non·vol·a·tile \-'väl-ət-ᵊl, *esp Brit* -ə-ₜtīl\ *adj* : not volatile

¹**no·o·tro·pic** \ₜnō-ə-'trō-pik, -'träp-ik\ *adj* : of, relating to, or promoting the enhancement of cognition and memory and the facilitation of learning ⟨∼ drugs⟩

²**nootropic** *n* : a nootropic substance and esp. a drug — called also *smart drug*

NOPHN *abbr* National Organization for Public Health Nursing

nor·adren·a·line *also* **nor·adren·a·lin** \ₜnȯr-ə-'dren-ᵊl-ən\ *n* : NOREPINEPHRINE

nor·ad·ren·er·gic \ₜnȯr-ₜad-rə-'nər-jik\ *adj* : liberating, activated by, or involving norepinephrine in the transmission of nerve impulses ⟨a progressive deterioration of central ∼ pathways —C. D. Wise & Larry Stein⟩ ⟨∼ synapses⟩ — compare ADRENERGIC 1, CHOLINERGIC 1

nor·epi·neph·rine \ₜnȯr-ₜep-ə-'nef-rən, -ₜrēn\ *n* : a catecholamine $C_8H_{11}NO_3$ that is the chemical means of transmission across synapses in postganglionic neurons of the sympathetic nervous system and in some parts of the central nervous system, is a vasopressor hormone of the adrenal medulla, and is a precursor of epinephrine in its major biosynthetic pathway — called also *arterenol, noradrenaline;* see LEVOPHED

nor·eth·in·drone \nȯr-'eth-ən-ₜdrōn, ₜnȯr-eth-'in-\ *n* : a synthetic progestational hormone $C_{20}H_{26}O_2$ used in birth control pills often in the form of its acetate $C_{22}H_{28}O_3$ — see ORTHO-NOVUM

nor·ethis·ter·one \ₜnȯr-ə-'this-tə-ₜrōn\ *n, chiefly Brit* : NORETHINDRONE

nor·ethyn·o·drel \ₜnȯr-ə-'thīn-ō-ₜdrel, -'thin-, -'eth-in-\ *n* : a progesterone derivative $C_{20}H_{26}O_2$ used in birth control pills and in the treatment of endometriosis and hypermenorrhea — see ENOVID

nor·flox·a·cin \nȯr-'fläk-sə-ₜsin\ *n* : a fluoroquinolone $C_{16}H_{18}FN_3O_3$ used topically to treat conjunctivitis and orally to treat various bacterial infections (as of the urinary tract)

nor·ges·ti·mate \nȯr-'jes-tə-ₜmāt\ *n* : a progestogen $C_{23}H_{31}NO_3$ that is used in combination with an estrogen (as ethinyl estradiol) in birth control pills — see ORTHO TRI-CYCLEN

nor·ges·trel \nȯr-'jes-trəl\ *n* : a synthetic progestogen $C_{21}H_{28}O_2$ having two optically active forms of which the biologically active levorotatory form is used in birth control pills — see LEVONORGESTREL

nor·leu·cine \(ᵋ')nȯr-'lü-ₜsēn\ *n* : a crystalline amino acid $C_6H_{13}NO_2$ isomeric with leucine

norm \'nȯ(ə)rm\ *n* : an established standard or average: as **a** : a set standard of development or achievement usu. derived from the average or median achievement of a large group **b** : a pattern or trait taken to be typical in the behavior of a social group

¹**nor·mal** \'nȯr-məl\ *adj* **1 a** : according with, constituting, or not deviating from a norm, rule, or principle **b** : conforming to a type, standard, or regular pattern **2** : occurring naturally and not because of disease, inoculation, or any experimental treatment ⟨∼ immunity⟩ **3 a** : of, relating to, or characterized by average intelligence or development **b** : free from mental disorder : SANE **c** : characterized by balanced well-integrated functioning of the organism as a whole **4 a** *of a solution* : having a concentration of one gram equivalent of solute per liter **b** : containing neither basic hydrogen nor acid hydrogen ⟨∼ phosphate of silver⟩ **c** : not associated ⟨∼ molecules⟩ **d** : having a straight-chain structure ⟨∼ pentane⟩ — **nor·mal·ly** \'nȯr-mə-lē\ *adv*

²**normal** *n* : a subject who is normal

nor·mal·cy \'nȯr-məl-sē\ *n, pl* **-cies** : the state or fact of being normal

nor·mal·i·ty \nȯr-'mal-ət-ē\ *n, pl* **-ties** **1** : the quality or state of being normal **2** *of a solution* : concentration expressed in gram equivalents of solute per liter

nor·mal·ize *or Brit* **nor·mal·ise** \'nȯr-mə-ₜlīz\ *vt* **-ized** *or Brit* **-ised; -iz·ing** *or Brit* **-is·ing** : to make conform to or reduce to a norm or standard ⟨∼ blood pressure⟩ — **nor·mal·iza·tion** *or Brit* **nor·mal·isa·tion** \ₜnȯr-mə-lə-'zā-shən\ *n*

normal saline solution *n* : PHYSIOLOGICAL SALINE

normal salt solution *n* : PHYSIOLOGICAL SALINE

nor·mer·gic \(ᵋ')nȯr-'mər-jik\ *adj* : having the degree of sensitivity toward an allergen typical of age group and community — compare HYPERERGIC, HYPOERGIC

nor·mer·gy \'nȯr-mər-jē\ *n, pl* **-gies** : the quality or state of being normergic

nor·meta·neph·rine \ₜnȯr-ₜmet-ə-'nef-rən, -ₜrēn\ *n* : a metabolite of norepinephrine $C_9H_{13}NO_3$ found esp. in the urine

nor·mo·ac·tive \\ˌnȯr-mō-ˈak-tiv\\ *adj* : normally active ⟨∼ children⟩; *also* : indicating normal activity ⟨∼ bowel sounds⟩

nor·mo·blast \\ˈnȯr-mə-ˌblast\\ *n* : an immature red blood cell containing hemoglobin and a pyknotic nucleus and normally present in bone marrow but appearing in the blood in many anemias — compare ERYTHROBLAST — **nor·mo·blas·tic** \\-ˌblas-tik\\ *adj*

nor·mo·cal·ce·mia *or chiefly Brit* **nor·mo·cal·cae·mia** \\ˌnȯr-mō-kal-ˈsē-mē-ə\\ *n* : the presence of a normal concentration of calcium in the blood — **nor·mo·cal·ce·mic** *or chiefly Brit* **nor·mo·cal·cae·mic** \\-mik\\ *adj*

nor·mo·chro·mia \\ˌnȯr-mə-ˈkrō-mē-ə\\ *n* : the color of red blood cells that contain a normal amount of hemoglobin

nor·mo·chro·mic \\-ˈkrō-mik\\ *adj* : characterized by normochromia ⟨∼ blood⟩

normochromic anemia *n* : an anemia marked by reduced numbers of normochromic red blood cells in the circulating blood

nor·mo·cyte \\ˈnȯr-mə-ˌsīt\\ *n* : a red blood cell that is normal in size and in hemoglobin content

nor·mo·cyt·ic \\ˌnȯr-mə-ˈsit-ik\\ *adj* : characterized by red blood cells that are normal in size and usu. also in hemoglobin content ⟨∼ blood⟩

normocytic anemia *n* : an anemia marked by reduced numbers of normal red blood cells in the circulating blood

nor·mo·gly·ce·mia *or chiefly Brit* **nor·mo·gly·cae·mia** \\ˌnȯr-mō-glī-ˈsē-mē-ə\\ *n* : the presence of a normal concentration of glucose in the blood — **nor·mo·gly·ce·mic** *or chiefly Brit* **nor·mo·gly·cae·mic** \\-mik\\ *adj*

nor·mo·ka·le·mic *or chiefly Brit* **nor·mo·ka·lae·mic** \\ˌnȯr-mō-kā-ˈlē-mik\\ *adj* : having or characterized by a normal concentration of potassium in the blood ⟨∼ patients⟩

nor·mo·ten·sion \\ˌnȯr-mō-ˈten-chən\\ *n* : normal blood pressure

¹**nor·mo·ten·sive** \\ˌnȯr-mō-ˈten(t)-siv\\ *adj* : having normal blood pressure ⟨∼ offspring of hypertensive parents⟩

²**normotensive** *n* : an individual with normal blood pressure

nor·mo·ther·mia \\ˌnȯr-mō-ˈthər-mē-ə\\ *n* : normal body temperature — **nor·mo·ther·mic** \\-mik\\ *adj*

nor·mo·ton·ic \\-ˈtän-ik\\ *adj* : relating to or characterized by normal tone or tension ⟨a ∼ muscle⟩

nor·mo·vol·emia *or chiefly Brit* **nor·mo·vol·ae·mia** \\ˌnȯr-mō-ˌväl-ˈē-mē-ə\\ *n* : a normal volume of blood in the body — **nor·mo·vol·emic** *or chiefly Brit* **nor·mo·vol·ae·mic** \\-mik\\ *adj*

Nor·plant \\ˈnō(ə)r-ˌplant\\ *trademark* — used for contraceptive implants of encapsulated levonorgestrel

Nor·pra·min \\ˈnȯr-prə-mən\\ *trademark* — used for a preparation of the hydrochloride of desipramine

Nor·rie disease *also* **Nor·rie's disease** \\ˈnō(ə)r-(ˌ)ē(z)-\\ *n* : a rare congenital X-linked disease that affects males and is characterized esp. by retinal malformation and opacification of the vitreous body leading to blindness, by progressive mental deterioration, and by deafness

Norrie, Gordon (1855–1941), Danish ophthalmologist. Norrie described the congenital disease that bears his name in a 1927 article on the causes of blindness in children.

19–nor·tes·tos·ter·one \\(ˈ)nīn-ˈtēn-ˌnȯr-te-ˈstäs-tə-ˌrōn\\ *n* : NANDROLONE

North American blastomycosis \\ˈnȯrth-\\ *n* : blastomycosis that involves esp. the skin, lymph nodes, and lungs and that is caused by infection with a fungus of the genus *Blastomyces* (*B. dermatitidis*) — called also *Gilchrist's disease*

North·ern blot \\ˈnȯr-thərn\\ *n* : a blot consisting of a sheet of cellulose nitrate or nylon that contains spots of RNA for identification by a suitable molecular probe — compare SOUTHERN BLOT, WESTERN BLOT — **Northern blot·ting** \\-ˈblät-iŋ\\ *n*

northern cattle grub *n* : an immature form or adult of a warble fly of the genus *Hypoderma* (*H. bovis*) — called also *cattle grub;* see BOMB FLY

northern fowl mite *n* : a parasitic mite (*Ornithonyssus sylvi-*

arum, family Macronyssidae) that is a pest of birds and esp. poultry and pigeons in both Europe and No. America

northern rat flea *n* : a common and widely distributed flea of the genus *Nosopsyllus* (*N. fasciatus*) that is parasitic on rats and transmits murine typhus and possibly plague

nor·trip·ty·line \\nȯr-ˈtrip-tə-ˌlēn\\ *n* : a tricyclic antidepressant administered in the form of its hydrochloride $C_{19}H_{21}N·HCl$ — see AVENTYL

nor·va·line \\(ˈ)nȯr-ˈval-ˌēn, -ˈvā-ˌlēn\\ *n* : an amino acid $C_5H_{11}NO_2$ isomeric with valine and usu. made synthetically

Nor·vasc \\ˈnȯr-ˌvask\\ *trademark* — used for a preparation of the besylate of amlodipine

Nor·vir \\ˈnȯr-ˌvir\\ *trademark* — used for a preparation of ritonavir

Nor·walk virus \\ˈnȯ(ə)r-ˌwȯk-\\ *n* : a single-stranded RNA virus of the family *Caliciviridae* (species *Norwalk virus*) that was first discovered in Norwalk, Ohio, and causes an infectious human gastroenteritis — called also *Norwalk agent*

Nor·way rat \\ˈnȯ(ə)r-wā-\\ *n* : BROWN RAT

Nor·wood procedure \\ˈnȯ(ə)r-ˌwu̇d-\\ *n* : a complex surgical procedure esp. for the palliative treatment of hypoplastic left heart syndrome — called also *Norwood operation*

Norwood, William I. (b 1941), American surgeon. In 1979 Norwood developed the first successful treatment for hypoplastic left heart syndrome.

nose \\ˈnōz\\ *n* **1 a** : the part of the face that bears the nostrils and covers the anterior part of the nasal cavity; *broadly* : this part together with the nasal cavity **b** : the anterior part of the head above or projecting beyond the muzzle **2** : the sense of smell : OLFACTION **3** : OLFACTORY ORGAN

nose·bleed \\-ˌblēd\\ *n* : an attack of bleeding from the nose — called also *epistaxis*

nose botfly *n* : a widely distributed botfly of the genus *Gasterophilus* (*G. haemorrhoidalis*) that has a red tip on the abdomen and is parasitic in the larval stage esp. on horses and mules — called also *nose fly*

nose job *n* : RHINOPLASTY

No·se·ma \\nō-ˈsē-mə\\ *n* : a genus (the type of the family Nosematidae) of microsporidian protozoans that includes various parasites esp. of insects and other invertebrates

nose·piece \\ˈnōz-ˌpēs\\ *n* **1** : the end piece of a microscope body to which an objective is attached and which often consists of a revolving holder for two or more objectives **2** : the bridge of a pair of eyeglasses

nos·o·co·mi·al \\ˌnäs-ə-ˈkō-mē-əl\\ *adj* : acquired or occurring in a hospital ⟨∼ infection⟩ — **nos·o·co·mi·al·ly** \\-ē\\ *adv*

noso·ge·og·ra·phy \\ˌnäs-ō-jē-ˈäg-rə-fē\\ *n, pl* **-phies** : the geography of disease : GEOMEDICINE — **noso·geo·graph·ic** \\-ˌjē-ə-ˈgraf-ik\\ *or* **noso·geo·graph·i·cal** \\-i-kəl\\ *adj*

no·sog·ra·phy \\nō-ˈsäg-rə-fē\\ *n, pl* **-phies** : a description or classification of diseases — **noso·graph·ic** \\ˌnäs-ə-ˈgraf-ik\\ *adj*

no·sol·o·gist \\nō-ˈsäl-ə-jəst\\ *n* : a specialist in nosology

no·sol·o·gy \\nō-ˈsäl-ə-jē, -ˈzäl-\\ *n, pl* **-gies** **1** : a classification or list of diseases **2** : a branch of medical science that deals with classification of diseases — **no·so·log·i·cal** \\ˌnō-sə-ˈläj-i-kəl\\ *or* **no·so·log·ic** \\-ik\\ *adj* — **no·so·log·i·cal·ly** \\-i-k(ə-)lē\\ *adv*

noso·pho·bia \\ˌnäs-ə-ˈfō-bē-ə\\ *n* : an abnormal fear of disease

Nos·o·psyl·lus \\ˌnäs-ə-ˈsil-əs\\ *n* : a genus of fleas that includes the northern rat flea (*N. fasciatus*)

nos·tal·gia \\nä-ˈstal-jə, nə-, nō-; nə-ˈstäl-\\ *n* **1** : the state of being homesick **2** : a wistful or excessively sentimental sometimes abnormal yearning for return to or of some past period or irrecoverable condition — **nos·tal·gic** \\-jik\\ *adj* — **nos·tal·gi·cal·ly** \\-ji-k(ə-)lē\\ *adv*

nos·tril \\ˈnäs-trəl\\ *n* **1** : either of the external nares; *broadly* : either of the nares with the adjoining passage on the same

\\ə\\ abut \\ᵊ\\ kitten \\ər\\ further \\a\\ ash \\ā\\ ace \\ä\\ cot, cart
\\au̇\\ out \\ch\\ chin \\e\\ bet \\ē\\ easy \\g\\ go \\i\\ hit \\ī\\ ice \\j\\ job
\\ŋ\\ sing \\ō\\ go \\ȯ\\ law \\ȯi\\ boy \\th\\ thin \\th̲\\ the \\ü\\ loot
\\u̇\\ foot \\y\\ yet \\zh\\ vision *See also* Pronunciation Symbols page

M
N

side of the nasal septum **2** : either fleshy lateral wall of the nose

nos·trum \'näs-trəm\ *n* : a medicine of secret composition recommended by its preparer but usu. without scientific proof of its effectiveness

notch \'näch\ *n* : a V-shaped indentation (as on a bone) — see ACETABULAR NOTCH, SCIATIC NOTCH, VERTEBRAL NOTCH — **notched** \'nächt\ *adj*

no·ti·fi·able \'nōt-ə-ˌfī-ə-bəl, ˌnōt-ə-'\ *adj* : required by law to be reported to official health authorities ⟨a ∼ disease⟩

no·ti·fi·ca·tion \ˌnōt-ə-fə-'kā-shən\ *n* : the act or an instance of notifying; *esp* : the act of reporting the occurrence of a communicable disease or of an individual affected with such a disease

no·ti·fy \'nōt-ə-ˌfī\ *vt* **-fied; -fy·ing 1** *Brit* : to report the occurrence of (a case of communicable disease) or the occurrence of communicable disease in (an individual) ⟨all cases of disease should be *notified* by the treating consultant —*Practitioner*⟩ **2** : to give formal notice to ⟨the Broward County Public Health Unit . . . was *notified* of three children . . . hospitalized with encephalitis attributed to cat scratch disease —*Jour. Amer. Med. Assoc.*⟩

no·to·chord \'nōt-ə-ˌkȯ(ə)rd\ *n* : a longitudinal flexible rod of cells that in the lowest chordates (as a lancelet or a lamprey) and in the embryos of the higher vertebrates forms the supporting axis of the body, that is almost obliterated in the adult of the higher vertebrates as the bodies of the vertebrae develop, and that arises as an outgrowth from the dorsal lip of the blastopore extending forward between epiblast and hypoblast in the middorsal line — **no·to·chord·al** \ˌnōt-ə-'kȯrd-ᵊl\ *adj*

No·to·ed·res \ˌnōt-ō-'ed-ˌrēz\ *n* : a genus of mites of the family Sarcoptidae containing mange mites that attack various mammals including occas. but rarely seriously humans usu. through contact with cats

no·to·ed·ric \-'ed-rik\ *adj* **1** : of or relating to the genus *Notoedres* **2** : caused by mites of the genus *Notoedres*

nour·ish \'nər-ish, 'nə-rish\ *vt* : to furnish or sustain with nutriment : FEED

nour·ish·ing *adj* : giving nourishment : NUTRITIOUS

nour·ish·ment \'nər-ish-mənt, 'nə-rish-\ *n* **1** : FOOD 1, NUTRIMENT **2** : the act of nourishing or the state of being nourished

no·vo·bi·o·cin \ˌnō-və-'bī-ə-sən\ *n* : a highly toxic antibiotic that is a weak dibasic acid $C_{31}H_{36}N_2O_{11}$ and is used in some serious cases of staphylococcal and urinary tract infection

No·vo·cain \'nō-və-ˌkān\ *trademark* — used for a preparation of the hydrochloride of procaine

no·vo·caine \-ˌkān\ *n* : procaine in the form of its hydrochloride; *broadly* : a local anesthetic

noxa \'näk-sə\ *n, pl* **nox·ae** \-ˌsē, -ˌsī\ : something that exerts a harmful effect on the body

nox·ious \'näk-shəs\ *adj* : physically harmful or destructive to living beings ⟨∼ wastes⟩

Np *symbol* neptunium

NP *abbr* **1** neuropsychiatric; neuropsychiatry **2** nurse practitioner

NPN *abbr* nonprotein nitrogen

NPO *abbr* [Latin *nil per os*] nothing by mouth

NPT *abbr* normal pressure and temperature

nr *abbr* near

NR *abbr* no refill

NREM sleep \'en-ˌrem-\ *n* : SLOW-WAVE SLEEP

ns *abbr* nanosecond

n's *or* **ns** *pl of* N

NSAID \'en-ˌsed *also* -ˌsād\ *n* : a nonsteroidal antiinflammatory drug (as ibuprofen)

nsec *abbr* nanosecond

NSU *abbr* nonspecific urethritis

nT *abbr* nanotesla

NTD *abbr* neural tube defect

NTP *abbr* normal temperature and pressure

nu·bile \'n(y)ü-bəl, -ˌbīl\ *adj* : sexually mature; *esp* : of marriageable condition or age — used of young women — **nu·bil·i·ty** \n(y)ü-'bil-ət-ē\ *n, pl* **-ties**

nuchae — see LIGAMENTUM NUCHAE

nu·chal \'n(y)ü-kəl\ *adj* : of, relating to, or lying in the region of the nape

nuchal line *n* : any of several ridges on the outside of the skull: as **a** : one on each side that extends laterally in a curve from the external occipital protuberance to the mastoid process of the temporal bone — called also *superior nuchal line* **b** : OCCIPITAL CREST a **c** : one on each side that extends laterally from the middle of the external occipital crest below and roughly parallel to the superior nuchal line — called also *inferior nuchal line*

nu·cle·ar \'n(y)ü-klē-ər\ *adj* **1** : of, relating to, or constituting a nucleus **2** : of, relating to, or utilizing the atomic nucleus, atomic energy, the atomic bomb, or atomic power

nuclear atom *n* : a conceptual model of the atom developed by Ernest Rutherford in which a small positively charged nucleus is surrounded by planetary electrons

nuclear chemistry *n* : RADIOCHEMISTRY

nuclear family *n* : a family group that consists only of father, mother, and children — see EXTENDED FAMILY

nuclear fission *n* : FISSION 2b

nuclear fusion *n* : FUSION 3

nuclear magnetic resonance *n* **1** : the magnetic resonance of an atomic nucleus **2** : chemical analysis that uses nuclear magnetic resonance esp. to study molecular structure — abbr. *NMR*; see MAGNETIC RESONANCE IMAGING

nuclear medicine *n* : a branch of medicine dealing with the use of radioactive materials in the diagnosis and treatment of disease

nuclear membrane *n* : a double membrane enclosing a cell nucleus and having its outer part continuous with the endoplasmic reticulum — called also *karyotheca*

nuclear reticulum *n* : the diffuse intermeshed granular threads that represent the chromosomes in the resting nucleus — called also *nuclear network*

nuclear sap \-'sap\ *n* : the clear homogeneous ground substance of a cell nucleus — called also *karyolymph*

nu·cle·ase \'n(y)ü-klē-ˌās, -ˌāz\ *n* : any of various enzymes that promote hydrolysis of nucleic acids

nu·cle·ate \'n(y)ü-klē-ˌāt\ *vb* **-at·ed; -at·ing** *vt* **1** : to form into a nucleus **2** : to act as a nucleus for **3** : to supply nuclei to ∼ *vi* **1** : to form a nucleus **2** : to act as a nucleus **3** : to begin to form

nu·cle·at·ed \'n(y)ü-klē-ˌāt-əd\ *or* **nu·cle·ate** \-klē-ət\ *adj* : having a nucleus or nuclei ⟨∼ cells⟩

nu·cle·a·tion \ˌn(y)ü-klē-'ā-shən\ *n* **1** : the formation of nuclei **2** : the action of a nucleus in starting a process (as condensation, crystallization, or precipitation)

nuclei *pl of* NUCLEUS

nu·cle·ic acid \n(y)ü-ˌklē-ik-, -ˌklā-\ *n* : any of various acids (as an RNA or a DNA) composed of nucleotide chains

nu·cle·in \'n(y)ü-klē-ən\ *n* **1** : NUCLEOPROTEIN **2** : NUCLEIC ACID

nu·cleo·cap·sid \ˌn(y)ü-klē-ō-'kap-səd\ *n* : the nucleic acid and surrounding protein coat of a virus

nu·cleo·cy·to·plas·mic \-ˌsīt-ə-'plaz-mik\ *adj* : of or relating to the nucleus and cytoplasm

nu·cleo·his·tone \-'his-ˌtōn\ *n* : a nucleoprotein in which the protein is a histone

¹nu·cle·oid \'n(y)ü-klē-ˌȯid\ *adj* : resembling a nucleus

²nucleoid *n* : the DNA-containing area of a prokaryotic cell (as a bacterium)

nu·cle·o·lar \n(y)ü-'klē-ə-lər *also* ˌn(y)ü-klē-'ō-lər\ *adj* : of, relating to, or constituting a nucleolus ⟨∼ proteins⟩

nucleolar organizer *n* : NUCLEOLUS ORGANIZER

nu·cle·o·lo·ne·ma \(ˌ)n(y)ü-ˌklē-ə-lə-'nē-mə *also* **nu·cle·o·lo·neme** \-'klē-ə-lə-ˌnēm\ *pl* **-nemas** *or* **-ne·ma·ta** \-'nē-mət-ə\ *also* **-nemes** : a filamentous network consisting of small granules in some nucleoli

nu·cle·o·lus \n(y)ü-'klē-ə-ləs\ *n, pl* **-li** \-ˌlī\ : a spherical body of the nucleus of most eukaryotes that becomes enlarged during protein synthesis, is associated with a nucleolus organizer, and contains the DNA templates for ribosomal RNA — called also *plasmosome*

nucleolus organizer *n* : the specific part of a chromosome with which a nucleolus is associated esp. during its reorganization after nuclear division — called also *nucleolar organizer*

nu·cle·on \'n(y)ü-klē-ˌän\ *n* : a nuclear particle: **a** : PROTON **b** : NEUTRON — **nu·cle·on·ic** \ˌn(y)ü-klē-'än-ik\ *adj*

nu·cle·on·ics \ˌn(y)ü-klē-'än-iks\ *n pl but sing or pl in constr* : a branch of physical science that deals with nucleons or with all phenomena of the atomic nucleus

nu·cleo·phile \'n(y)ü-klē-ə-ˌfīl\ *n* : a nucleophilic substance (as an electron-donating reagent)

nu·cleo·phil·ic \ˌn(y)ü-klē-ə-'fil-ik\ *adj* **1** *of an atom, ion, or molecule* : having an affinity for atomic nuclei : being an electron donor **2** : involving a nucleophilic species ⟨a ∼ reaction⟩ — **nu·cleo·phil·i·cal·ly** \-i-k(ə-)lē\ *adv* — **nu·cleo·phi·lic·i·ty** \-klē-ō-fil-'is-ət-ē\ *n, pl* **-ties**

nu·cleo·plasm \'n(y)ü-klē-ə-ˌplaz-əm\ *n* : the protoplasm of a nucleus; *esp* : NUCLEAR SAP — **nu·cleo·plas·mat·ic** \ˌn(y)ü-klē-ō-ˌplaz-'mat-ik\ *or* **nu·cleo·plas·mic** \-klē-ə-'plaz-mik\ *adj*

nu·cleo·prot·amine \ˌn(y)ü-klē-ō-'prōt-ə-ˌmēn\ *n* : a nucleoprotein derived from a protamine

nu·cleo·pro·tein \ˌn(y)ü-klē-ō-'prō-ˌtēn, -'prōt-ē-ən\ *n* : a compound that consists of a protein (as a histone) conjugated with a nucleic acid (as a DNA) and that is the principal constituent of the hereditary material in chromosomes

nu·cle·o·sid·ase \ˌn(y)ü-klē-ə-'sī-ˌdās, -ˌdāz\ *n* **1** : an enzyme that promotes the hydrolysis of a nucleoside **2** : a phosphorylase that promotes reversibly the reaction of a nucleoside with phosphate forming a base and a phosphate of ribose or deoxyribose — called also *nucleoside phosphorylase*

nu·cle·o·side \'n(y)ü-klē-ə-ˌsīd\ *n* : a compound (as guanosine or adenosine) that consists of a purine or pyrimidine base combined with deoxyribose or ribose and is found esp. in DNA or RNA — compare NUCLEOTIDE

nucleoside phosphorylase *n* : NUCLEOSIDASE 2

nu·cleo·some \-ˌsōm\ *n* : any of the repeating globular subunits of chromatin that consist of a complex of DNA and histone and are thought to be present only during interphase — **nu·cleo·so·mal** \ˌn(y)ü-klē-ə-'sō-məl\ *adj*

nu·cleo·tid·ase \ˌn(y)ü-klē-ō-'tīd-ˌās, -ˌāz\ *n* : a phosphatase that promotes hydrolysis of a nucleotide (as into a nucleoside and phosphoric acid)

nu·cle·o·tide \'n(y)ü-klē-ə-ˌtīd\ *n* : any of several compounds that consist of a ribose or deoxyribose sugar joined to a purine or pyrimidine base and to a phosphate group and that are the basic structural units of RNA and DNA — compare NUCLEOSIDE

nu·cleo·ti·dyl·trans·fer·ase \ˌn(y)ü-klē-ə-'tīd-ə-ᵊl-'tran(t)s-(ˌ)fər-ˌās, -ˌāz\ *n* : any of several enzymes that catalyze the transfer of a nucleotide residue from one compound to another

nu·cleo·tox·ic \-'täk-sik\ *adj* : toxic to the nuclei of cells ⟨∼ agents that disrupt mitosis⟩

nu·cle·us \'n(y)ü-klē-əs\ *n, pl* **nu·clei** \-klē-ˌī\ *also* **nu·cle·us·es 1** : a cellular organelle of eukaryotes that is essential to cell functions (as reproduction and protein synthesis), is composed of nuclear sap and a nucleoprotein-rich network from which chromosomes and nucleoli arise, and is enclosed in a definite membrane **2** : a mass of gray matter or group of nerve cells in the central nervous system **3** : a characteristic and stable complex of atoms or groups in a molecule; *esp* : RING 2 ⟨the naphthalene ∼⟩ **4** : the positively charged central portion of an atom that comprises nearly all of the atomic mass and that consists of protons and neutrons except in hydrogen which consists of one proton only

nucleus ac·cum·bens \-ə-'kəm-bənz\ *n* : a nucleus forming the floor of the caudal part of the anterior prolongation of the lateral ventricle of the brain

nucleus am·big·u·us \-am-'big-yə-wəs\ *n* : an elongated nucleus in the medulla oblongata that is a continuation of a group of cells in the ventral horn of the spinal cord and gives rise to the motor fibers of the glossopharyngeal, vagus, and accessory nerves supplying striated muscle of the larynx and pharynx

nucleus basalis *n* : the gray matter of the substantia innominata of the forebrain that consists mostly of cholinergic neurons

nucleus basalis of Mey·nert \-əv-'mī-(ˌ)nert\ *n* : NUCLEUS BASALIS

Meynert, Theodor Hermann (1833–1892), Austrian psychiatrist and neurologist. Meynert was a professor of psychiatry and later of neurology at Vienna. He was an early advocate of the use of minimal restraint in asylums for the mentally ill. He is credited with classic descriptions of several structures of the brain. Collected in book form in 1868, they included the first description of interneurons.

nucleus cu·ne·a·tus \-ˌkyü-nē-'āt-əs\ *n* : the nucleus in the medulla oblongata in which the fibers of the fasciculus cuneatus terminate and synapse with a component of the medial lemniscus — called also *cuneate nucleus*

nucleus dor·sa·lis \-dòr-'sā-ləs\ *n, pl* **nuclei dor·sa·les** \-ˌlēz\ : an elongated longitudinal strand of neurons in the spinal cord with its axons passing into the cerebellar tract — called also *Clarke's column*

nucleus grac·i·lis \-'gras-ə-ləs\ *n* : a nucleus in the posterior part of the medulla oblongata in which the fibers of the fasciculus gracilis terminate

nucleus of origin *n* : a group of cell bodies in the brain from which nerve fibers of a cranial nerve arise or at which they terminate — compare SUPERFICIAL ORIGIN

nucleus pul·po·sus \-ˌpəl-'pō-səs\ *n, pl* **nuclei pul·po·si** \-ˌsī\ : an elastic pulpy mass lying in the center of each intervertebral fibrocartilage and regarded as a remnant of the notochord

nu·clide \'n(y)ü-ˌklīd\ *n* : a species of atom characterized by the constitution of its nucleus and hence by the number of protons, the number of neutrons, and the energy content — **nu·clid·ic** \n(y)ü-'klid-ik\ *adj*

nude mouse \'n(y)üd-\ *n* : a mouse of a hairless strain bred for laboratory use that lacks a thymus and mature T cells and is used esp. in immunological research

Nuel's space \n(y)ü-'elz-\ *n* : a fluid-filled space within the organ of Corti — called also *space of Nuel*

Nu·el \nūē-el\, **Jean–Pierre (1847–1920),** Belgian physician. Nuel served as professor of otology and physiology at several Belgian medical schools. In 1873 he published the results of his observations on the microscopic anatomy of the cochlea. This work contains his description of the space found within the organ of Corti that now bears his name.

null cell \'nəl-\ *n* : a lymphocyte in the blood that does not have on its surface the receptors typical of either mature B cells or T cells

nul·li·grav·i·da \ˌnəl-ə-'grav-əd-ə\ *n, pl* **-dae** \ə-ˌdī, -ˌdē\ *also* **-das** : a woman who has never been pregnant — compare NULLIPARA

nul·lip·a·ra \ˌnə-'lip-ə-rə\ *n, pl* **-ras** *or* **-rae** \-ˌrē\ : a woman who has never borne a child — compare NULLIGRAVIDA

nul·li·par·i·ty \ˌnəl-ə-'par-ət-ē\ *n, pl* **-ties** : the condition of being nulliparous

nul·lip·a·rous \ˌnə-'lip-ə-rəs\ *adj* : of, relating to, or being a female that has not borne offspring

¹nul·li·so·mic \ˌnəl-ə-'sō-mik\ *adj* : having two less than the diploid number of chromosomes due to loss of one chromosome pair

²nullisomic *n* : a nullisomic individual

numb \'nəm\ *adj* : devoid of sensation esp. as a result of cold or anesthesia

numb·ness *n* : reduced sensibility to touch ⟨facial ∼⟩

nu·mer·i·cal aperture \n(y)ü-'mer-i-kəl-\ *n* : a number that

\ə\ abut \ᵊ\ kitten \ər\ further \a\ ash \ā\ ace \ä\ cot, cart \aù\ out \ch\ chin \e\ bet \ē\ easy \g\ go \i\ hit \ī\ ice \j\ job \ŋ\ sing \ō\ go \ò\ law \òi\ boy \th\ thin \th̲\ the \ü\ loot \ù\ foot \y\ yet \zh\ vision *See also* Pronunciation Symbols page

M
N

indicates the resolving power of a microscope objective and is equal to the product of the index of refraction of the medium (as immersion oil) in front of the objective and the sine of half the angle formed by two rays emanating from the object upon which the microscope is focused and entering the objective at either end of a diameter of the objective

num·mu·lar \'nəm-yə-lər\ *adj* **1** : circular or oval in shape ⟨~ lesions⟩ **2** : characterized by circular or oval lesions or drops ⟨~ dermatitis⟩ ⟨~ sputum⟩

nun·na·tion \ˌnə-'nā-shən\ *n* : overly frequent or abnormal use (as in stammering) of the sound of the letter *n*

¹**nurse** \'nərs\ *n* **1** : a woman who suckles an infant not her own : WET NURSE **2** : a person who cares for the sick or infirm; *specif* : a licensed health-care professional who practices independently or is supervised by a physician, surgeon, or dentist and who is skilled in promoting and maintaining health — see LICENSED PRACTICAL NURSE, LICENSED VOCATIONAL NURSE, REGISTERED NURSE

²**nurse** *vb* **nursed; nurs·ing** *vt* **1 a** : to nourish at the breast : SUCKLE **b** : to take nourishment from the breast of : suck milk from **2 a** : to care for and wait on (as an injured or infirm person) **b** : to attempt a cure of (as an ailment) by care and treatment ~ *vi* **1 a** : to feed an offspring from the breast **b** : to feed at the breast : SUCK **2** : to act or serve as a nurse

nurse–anes·the·tist \-ə-'nes-thət-əst, *Brit* -'nēs-\ *n* : a registered nurse who has completed two years of additional training in anesthesia and is qualified to serve as an anesthetist under the supervision of a physician

nurse clinician *n* : NURSE PRACTITIONER

nurse–midwife *n, pl* **nurse–midwives** : a registered nurse with additional training as a midwife who is certified to deliver infants and provide prenatal and postpartum care, newborn care, and some routine care (as gynecological exams) of women

nurse–midwifery *n, pl* **nurse–midwiferies** : the profession or nursing specialty of a nurse-midwife

nurse practitioner *n* : a registered nurse who through advanced training is qualified to assume some of the duties and responsibilities formerly assumed only by a physician — abbr. *NP;* called also *nurse clinician*

nurs·ery \'nərs-(ə-)rē\ *n, pl* **-er·ies** : the department of a hospital where newborn infants are cared for

nurse's aide *n* : a worker who assists trained nurses in a hospital by performing general services (as making beds or giving baths)

nurs·ing *n* **1** : the profession of a nurse ⟨schools of ~⟩ **2** : the duties of a nurse ⟨proper ~ is difficult work⟩

nursing bottle *n* : a bottle with a rubber nipple used in supplying food to infants

nursing home *n* : a privately operated establishment where maintenance and personal or nursing care are provided for persons (as the aged or the chronically ill) who are unable to care for themselves properly — compare REST HOME

nursing sister *n, Brit* : GRADUATE NURSE

nurs·ling \'nər-sliŋ\ *n* : a nursing child

nur·tur·ance \'nər-chə-rən(t)s\ *n* : affectionate care and attention — **nur·tur·ant** \-rənt\ *adj*

nut·gall \'nət-ˌgȯl\ *n* : a gall that resembles a nut; *esp* : a gall produced on an oak (esp. *Quercus infectoria*) and used as a source of tannic acid

nut·meg \'nət-ˌmeg, -ˌmāg\ *n* **1** : an aromatic seed that is used as a spice and is produced by a tree of the genus *Myristica* (*M. fragrans* of the family Myristicaceae, the nutmeg family) native to the Moluccas — called also *myristica* **2** : a tree that produces nutmegs

nutmeg butter *n* : a soft yellowish or orange fat of nutmeg odor obtained from nutmegs and used chiefly in ointments

nutmeg liver *n* : a liver appearing mottled like a nutmeg when cut because of congestion and associated with impaired circulation esp. from heart or lung disease

nutmeg oil *n* : a colorless or pale yellow essential oil of nutmeg odor distilled from nutmegs and used as a flavoring

agent in pharmacology and formerly as a carminative and local stimulant — called also *myristica oil*

nu·tra·ceu·ti·cal *also* **nu·tri·ceu·ti·cal** \ˌn(y)ü-trə-'sü-ti-kəl\ *n* : a foodstuff (as a fortified food or a dietary supplement) that is held to provide health or medical benefits in addition to its basic nutritional value — called also *functional food*

Nu·tra·Sweet \'n(y)ü-trə-ˌswēt\ *trademark* — used for a preparation of aspartame

¹**nu·tri·ent** \'n(y)ü-trē-ənt\ *adj* : furnishing nourishment

²**nutrient** *n* : a nutritive substance or ingredient

nu·tri·lite \'n(y)ü-trə-ˌlīt\ *n* : a substance (as a vitamin or growth factor) required in small quantities for normal metabolism and growth and obtained by an organism in its food

nu·tri·ment \'n(y)ü-trə-mənt\ *n* : something that nourishes or promotes growth, provides energy, repairs body tissues, and maintains life

nu·tri·tion \n(y)ü-'trish-ən\ *n* **1** : the act or process of nourishing or being nourished; *specif* : the sum of the processes by which an animal or plant takes in and utilizes food substances **2** : FOOD 1, NOURISHMENT — **nu·tri·tion·al** \-'trish-nəl, -ən-°l\ *adj* — **nu·tri·tion·al·ly** \-ē\ *adv*

nutritional anemia *n* : anemia (as hypochromic anemia) that results from inadequate intake or assimilation of materials essential for the production of red blood cells and hemoglobin — called also *deficiency anemia*

nu·tri·tion·ist \-'trish-(ə-)nəst\ *n* : a specialist in the study of nutrition

nu·tri·tious \n(y)ü-'trish-əs\ *adj* : providing nourishment

nu·tri·tive \'n(y)ü-trət-iv\ *adj* **1** : of or relating to nutrition **2** : NOURISHING

nu·tri·ture \'n(y)ü-trə-ˌchü(ə)r, -chər\ *n* : bodily condition with respect to nutrition and esp. with respect to a given nutrient (as zinc)

nux vom·i·ca \'nəks-'väm-i-kə\ *n, pl* **nux vomica** **1** : the poisonous seed of an Asian tree of the genus *Strychnos* (*S. nux=vomica*) that contains several alkaloids and esp. strychnine and brucine; *also* : the tree yielding nux vomica **2** : a drug containing nux vomica

nvCJD *abbr* new variant Creutzfeldt-Jakob disease

nyc·ta·lope \'nik-tə-ˌlōp\ *n* : one affected with night blindness

nyc·ta·lo·pia \ˌnik-tə-'lō-pē-ə\ *n* : NIGHT BLINDNESS

nyc·to·pho·bia \ˌnik-tə-'fō-bē-ə\ *n* : abnormal fear of darkness

nyc·tu·ria \nik-'t(y)ùr-ē-ə\ *n* : NOCTURIA

ny·li·drin \'nī-li-drən\ *n* : a synthetic adrenergic drug that acts as a peripheral vasodilator and is usu. administered in the form of its hydrochloride $C_{19}H_{25}NO_2 \cdot HCl$

ny·lon \'nī-ˌlän\ *n* : any of numerous strong tough elastic synthetic polyamide materials that are fashioned into fibers, filaments, bristles, or sheets ⟨~ sutures and prosthetic devices⟩

nymph \'nim(p)f\ *n* **1** : any of various hemimetabolous insects in an immature stage and esp. a late larva (as of a true bug) in which rudiments of the wings and genitalia are present; *broadly* : any insect larva that differs chiefly in size and degree of differentiation from the imago **2** : a mite or tick in the first eight-legged form that immediately follows the last larval molt **3** : a nymphal stage in the life cycle of an insect or acarid — **nymph·al** \'nim(p)-fəl\ *adj*

nym·phae \'nim(p)-(ˌ)fē\ *n pl* : LABIA MINORA

nym·pho \'nim(p)-(ˌ)fō\ *n, pl* **nymphos** : one affected by nymphomania : NYMPHOMANIAC

nym·pho·lep·sy \'nim(p)-fə-ˌlep-sē\ *n, pl* **-sies** : a frenzy of erotic emotion

nym·pho·ma·nia \ˌnim(p)-fə-'mā-nē-ə, -nyə\ *n* : excessive sexual desire by a female — compare SATYRIASIS

¹**nym·pho·ma·ni·ac** \-nē-ˌak\ *n* : one affected with nymphomania

²**nymphomaniac** *or* **nym·pho·ma·ni·a·cal** \-mə-'nī-ə-kəl\ *adj* : of, affected with, or characterized by nymphomania

nys·tag·mic \nis-'tag-mik\ *adj* : of, relating to, characterized by, or being nystagmus

nys·tag·mo·graph \nis-'tag-mə-ˌgraf\ *n* : an instrument used for nystagmography

nys·tag·mog·ra·phy \‚nis-‚tag-'mäg-rə-fē\ *n, pl* **-phies** : the recording of the movements of the eyeballs in nystagmus — **nys·tag·mo·graph·ic** \nis-‚tag-mə-'graf-ik\ *adj*

nys·tag·moid \nis-'tag-‚mȯid\ *adj* : characterized by or being oscillatory eye movements resembling nystagmus ⟨rapid lateral ∼ movements —W. S. Weidorn⟩

nys·tag·mus \nis-'tag-məs\ *n* : involuntary usu. rapid movement of the eyeballs (as from side to side) occurring normally with dizziness during and after bodily rotation or abnormally following head injury or as a symptom of disease

nys·ta·tin \'nis-tət-ən\ *n* : an antibiotic that is derived from a soil actinomycete of the genus *Streptomyces* (*S. noursei*) and is used esp. in the treatment of candidiasis — called also *fungicidin*

O

o- *abbr* orth-; ortho-

O \'ō\ *n* : the one of the four ABO blood groups characterized by the absence of antigens designated by the letters A and B and by the presence of antibodies against these antigens

O *abbr* **1** opening **2** [Latin *octarius*] pint — used in writing prescriptions

O *symbol* oxygen

OA *abbr* osteoarthritis

O antigen *n* : an antigen that occurs in the body of a gram-negative bacterial cell — called also *somatic antigen;* compare H ANTIGEN

oat cell \'ōt-\ *n* : any of the small round or oval cells with a high ratio of nuclear protoplasm to cytoplasm that resemble oat grains and are characteristic of small-cell lung cancer

oat–cell cancer *n* : SMALL-CELL LUNG CANCER

oat–cell carcinoma *n* : SMALL-CELL LUNG CANCER

oath — see HIPPOCRATIC OATH

OB *abbr* **1** obstetric **2** obstetrician **3** obstetrics

obe·li·al \ō-'bē-lē-əl\ *adj* : of or relating to the obelion

obe·li·on \ō-'bē-lē-‚än, -ən\ *n, pl* **obe·lia** \-lē-ə\ : a point on the sagittal suture that lies between two small openings through the superior dorsal aspect of the parietal bones and is used in craniometric determinations

obese \ō-'bēs\ *adj* : having excessive body fat : affected by obesity

obe·si·ty \ō-'bē-sət-ē\ *n, pl* **-ties** : a condition that is characterized by excessive accumulation and storage of fat in the body and that in an adult is typically indicated by a body mass index of 30 or greater

obex \'ō-‚beks\ *n* : a thin triangular lamina of gray matter in the roof of the fourth ventricle of the brain

ob–gyn \‚ō-(‚)bē-'jin, -(‚)jē-(‚)wī-'en\ *n, pl* **ob–gyns** : a physician who specializes in obstetrics and gynecology

OB–GYN *abbr* obstetrics-gynecology

ob·ject \'äb-(‚)jekt, -jikt\ *n* **1** : something material that may be perceived by the senses **2** : something mental or physical toward which thought, feeling, or action is directed

¹ob·jec·tive \əb-'jek-tiv, äb-\ *adj* **1** : of, relating to, or being an object, phenomenon, or condition in the realm of sensible experience independent of individual thought and perceptible by all observers ⟨∼ reality⟩ **2** : perceptible to persons other than the affected individual ⟨an ∼ symptom of disease⟩ — compare SUBJECTIVE 2b — **ob·jec·tive·ly** *adv*

²objective *n* **1** : a lens or system of lenses that forms an image of an object **2** : something toward which effort is directed

objective vertigo *n* : vertigo characterized by a sensation that the external world is revolving — compare SUBJECTIVE VERTIGO

object libido *n* : libido directed toward someone or something other than the self — compare EGO-LIBIDO

ob·li·gate \'äb-li-gət, -lə-‚gāt\ *adj* **1** : restricted to one particularly characteristic mode of life or way of functioning ⟨the infant is an ∼ nose breather —*Jour. Amer. Med. Assoc.*⟩ ⟨an ∼ parasite⟩ **2** : biologically essential for survival ⟨∼ parasitism⟩ — **ob·li·gate·ly** *adv*

oblig·a·to·ry \ə-'blig-ə-‚tōr-ē, ä-, -‚tȯr- *also* 'äb-li-gə-\ *adj* : OBLIGATE 1 — **oblig·a·to·ri·ly** \ə-‚blig-ə-'tōr-ə-lē, ä-, -'tȯr- *also* ‚äb-li-gə-\ *adv*

¹oblique \ō-'blēk, ə-, -'blīk\ *adj* **1** : neither perpendicular nor parallel : being on an incline **2** : situated obliquely and having one end not inserted on bone ⟨∼ muscles⟩ — **oblique·ly** *adv*

²oblique *n* : any of several oblique muscles: as **a** : either of two flat muscles on each side that form the middle and outer layers of the lateral walls of the abdomen, that have aponeuroses extending medially to ensheathe the rectus muscles and fusing in the midventral line in the linea alba, and that act to compress the abdominal contents and to assist in expelling the contents of various visceral organs (as in urination, defecation, parturition, and expiration): (1) : one that forms the outer layer of the lateral abdominal wall — called also *external oblique, obliquus externus, obliquus externus abdominis* (2) : one situated under the external oblique in the lateral and ventral part of the abdominal wall — called also *internal oblique, obliquus internus, obliquus internus abdominis* **b** (1) : a long thin muscle that arises just above the margin of the optic foramen, is inserted on the upper part of the eyeball, and moves the eye downward and laterally — called also *superior oblique, obliquus superior oculi* (2) : a short muscle that arises from the orbital surface of the maxilla, is inserted slightly in front of and below the superior oblique, and moves the eye upward and laterally — called also *inferior oblique, obliquus inferior oculi* **c** (1) : a muscle that arises from the superior surface of the transverse process of the atlas, passes medially upward to insert into the occipital bone, and functions to extend the head and bend it to the side — called also *obliquus capitis superior, obliquus superior* (2) : a muscle that arises from the apex of the spinous process of the axis, inserts into the transverse process of the atlas, and rotates the atlas turning the face in the same direction — called also *obliquus capitis inferior, obliquus inferior*

oblique fissure *n* : either of two fissures of the lungs of which the one on the left side of the body separates the superior lobe of the left lung from the inferior lobe and the one on the right separates the superior and middle lobes of the right lung from the inferior lobe

oblique popliteal ligament *n* : a strong broad flat fibrous ligament that passes obliquely across and strengthens the posterior part of the knee and is derived esp. from the tendon of the semimembranosus muscle — compare ARCUATE POPLITEAL LIGAMENT

oblique vein of Mar·shall \-'mär-shəl\ *n* : OBLIQUE VEIN OF THE LEFT ATRIUM

Marshall, John (1818–1891), British anatomist and surgeon. Marshall enjoyed a long association with the medical faculty of University College, London, where he was at various times a demonstrator of anatomy, a surgeon, professor of surgery, and professor of clinical surgery. In an 1850 paper on veins he described the oblique vein of the left atrium. He is also known for his early operations for excision of varicose veins.

oblique vein of the left atrium *n* : a small vein that passes

O
P

\ə\ abut \ᵊ\ kitten \ər\ further \a\ ash \ā\ ace \ä\ cot, cart
\au̇\ out \ch\ chin \e\ bet \ē\ easy \g\ go \i\ hit \ī\ ice \j\ job
\ŋ\ sing \ō\ go \ȯ\ law \ȯi\ boy \th\ thin \t͟h\ the \ü\ loot
\u̇\ foot \y\ yet \zh\ vision   See also Pronunciation Symbols page

obliquely down the posterior surface of the left atrium, empties into the coronary sinus, and is a remnant of the left duct of Cuvier — called also *oblique vein, oblique vein of left atrium, oblique vein of Marshall*

obliq·ui·ty \ō-ˈblik-wət-ē, ə-\ *n, pl* **-ties** : the quality or state of being oblique : deviation from parallelism or perpendicularity; *also* : the amount of such deviation

ob·li·quus \ō-ˈblī-kwəs\ *n, pl* **ob·li·qui** \-ˌkwī\ : OBLIQUE

obliquus cap·i·tis inferior \-ˈkap-ət-əs-\ *n* : OBLIQUE c(2)

obliquus capitis superior *n* : OBLIQUE c(1)

obliquus ex·ter·nus \-ek-ˈstər-nəs\ *n* : OBLIQUE a(1)

obliquus externus ab·dom·i·nis \-ab-ˈdäm-ə-nəs\ *n* : OBLIQUE a(1)

obliquus inferior *n* : OBLIQUE c(2)

obliquus inferior oculi *n* : OBLIQUE b(2)

obliquus in·ter·nus \-in-ˈtər-nəs\ *n* : OBLIQUE a(2)

obliquus internus ab·dom·i·nis \-ab-ˈdäm-ə-nəs\ *n* : OBLIQUE a(2)

obliquus superior *n* : OBLIQUE c(1)

obliquus superior oculi *n* : OBLIQUE b(1)

obliterans — see ARTERIOSCLEROSIS OBLITERANS, ENDARTERITIS OBLITERANS, THROMBOANGIITIS OBLITERANS

oblit·er·ate \ə-ˈblit-ə-ˌrāt, ō-\ *vt* **-at·ed; -at·ing** : to cause to disappear (as a bodily part or a scar) or collapse (as a duct conveying body fluid) ⟨a blood vessel *obliterated* by inflammation⟩ — **oblit·er·a·tion** \-ˌblit-ə-ˈrā-shən\ *n*

obliterating endarteritis *n* : ENDARTERITIS OBLITERANS

oblit·er·a·tive \ə-ˈblit-ə-ˌrāt-iv, ō-, -ə-rət-\ *adj* : inducing or characterized by obliteration; *esp* : causing or accompanied by closure or collapse of a lumen ⟨~ arterial disease⟩

ob·lon·ga·ta \ˌäb-ˌlȯŋ-ˈgät-ə\ *n, pl* **-tas** *or* **-tae** \-ē\ : MEDULLA OBLONGATA

ob·nub·i·la·tion \äb-ˌn(y)ü-bə-ˈlā-shən\ *n* : mental cloudiness and torpidity ⟨had a headache, slight nuchal rigidity, and ~ —*Jour. Amer. Med. Assoc.*⟩

OBS *abbr* **1** obstetrician **2** obstetrics

ob·ser·va·tion \ˌäb-sər-ˈvā-shən, -zər-\ *n* **1** : the noting of a fact or occurrence (as in nature) often involving the measurement of some magnitude with suitable instruments ⟨temperature ~s⟩; *also* : a record so obtained **2** : close watch or examination (as to monitor or diagnose a condition) ⟨postoperative ~⟩ ⟨psychiatric ~⟩

ob·sess \əb-ˈses, äb-\ *vt* : to preoccupy intensely or abnormally ⟨was ~ed with success⟩ ~ *vi* : to engage in obsessive thinking ⟨solve problems rather than ~ about them —Carol Tavris⟩

ob·ses·sion \äb-ˈsesh-ən, əb-\ *n* : a persistent disturbing preoccupation with an often unreasonable idea or feeling; *also* : something that causes such preoccupation — compare COMPULSION, PHOBIA — **ob·ses·sion·al** \-ˈsesh-nəl, -ən-ᵊl\ *adj*

obsessional neurosis *n* : an obsessive-compulsive disorder in which obsessive thinking predominates with little need to perform compulsive acts

¹ob·ses·sive \äb-ˈses-iv, əb-\ *adj* : of, relating to, causing, or characterized by obsession : deriving from obsession ⟨~ behavior⟩ — **ob·ses·sive·ly** *adv* — **ob·ses·sive·ness** *n*

²obsessive *n* : an obsessive individual

¹obsessive–compulsive *adj* : relating to or characterized by recurring obsessions and compulsions esp. as symptoms of an obsessive-compulsive disorder

²obsessive–compulsive *n* : an individual affected with an obsessive-compulsive disorder

obsessive–compulsive disorder *n* : a psychoneurotic disorder in which the patient is beset with obsessions or compulsions or both and suffers extreme anxiety or depression through failure to think the obsessive thoughts or perform the compelling acts — abbr. *OCD;* called also *obsessive=compulsive neurosis, obsessive-compulsive reaction*

ob·so·lete \ˌäb-sə-ˈlēt, ˈäb-sə-ˌ\ *adj* : no longer active or distinct ⟨~ cases of infection⟩ ⟨~ pulmonary lesions⟩

obstet *abbr* **1** obstetric **2** obstetrics

ob·stet·ric \əb-ˈste-trik, äb-\ *or* **ob·stet·ri·cal** \-tri-kəl\ *adj*

: of, relating to, or associated with childbirth or obstetrics — **ob·stet·ri·cal·ly** \-tri-k(ə-)lē\ *adv*

obstetric forceps *n* : a forceps for grasping the fetal head or other part to facilitate delivery in difficult labor

ob·ste·tri·cian \ˌäb-stə-ˈtrish-ən\ *n* : a physician or veterinarian specializing in obstetrics

ob·stet·rics \əb-ˈste-triks, äb-\ *n pl but sing or pl in constr* : a branch of medical science that deals with birth and with its antecedents and sequelae

ob·stet·rist \-ˈtrəst\ *n* : OBSTETRICIAN

ob·sti·na·cy \ˈäb-stə-nə-sē\ *n, pl* **-cies** : the quality or state of being obstinate ⟨the ~ of tuberculosis⟩

ob·sti·nate \ˈäb-stə-nət\ *adj* **1** : adhering to an opinion, purpose, or course in spite of reason, arguments, or persuasion **2** : not easily subdued, remedied, or removed ⟨~ fever⟩

ob·sti·pa·tion \ˌäb-stə-ˈpā-shən\ *n* : severe and obstinate constipation

ob·struct \əb-ˈstrəkt, äb-\ *vt* : to block or close up by an obstacle ⟨veins ~ed by clots⟩

ob·struc·tion \əb-ˈstrək-shən, äb-\ *n* **1 a** : an act of obstructing **b** : a condition of being clogged or blocked ⟨intestinal ~⟩ **2** : something that obstructs ⟨dislodge an airway ~⟩

ob·struc·tive \-tiv\ *adj* : relating to, characterized by, causing, or resulting from obstruction ⟨~ uropathy⟩

obstructive jaundice *n* : jaundice due to obstruction of the biliary passages (as by gallstones or tumor)

obstructive sleep apnea *n* : sleep apnea that is caused by recurring interruption of breathing during sleep because of obstruction of the upper airway by weak or malformed pharyngeal tissues, that occurs esp. in obese middle-aged and elderly men, and that results in hypoxemia and in chronic lethargy during the day — called also *obstructive sleep apnea syndrome*

ob·stru·ent \ˈäb-strə-wənt\ *adj* : OBSTRUCTIVE

ob·tund \äb-ˈtənd\ *vt* : to reduce the intensity or sensitivity of : make dull ⟨~ed reflexes⟩ ⟨agents that ~ pain⟩

ob·tun·da·tion \ˌäb-(ˌ)tən-ˈdā-shən\ *n* : the state or condition of being obtunded ⟨mental ~⟩

¹ob·tund·ent \äb-ˈtən-dənt\ *adj* : blunting irritation or lessening pain

²obtundent *n* : an agent that blunts pain or dulls sensibility

ob·tu·ra·tion \ˌäb-t(y)ə-ˈrā-shən\ *n* : obstruction of a bodily passage ⟨intestinal ~⟩

ob·tu·ra·tor \ˈäb-t(y)ə-ˌrāt-ər\ *n* **1 a** : either of two muscles arising from the obturator membrane and adjacent bony surfaces: (1) : OBTURATOR EXTERNUS (2) : OBTURATOR INTERNUS **b** : OBTURATOR NERVE **2 a** : a prosthetic device that closes or blocks up an opening (as a fissure in the palate) **b** : a device that blocks the opening of an instrument (as a sigmoidoscope) that is being introduced into the body

obturator artery *n* : an artery that arises from the internal iliac artery or one of its branches, passes out through the obturator canal, and divides into two branches which are distributed to the muscles and fasciae of the hip and thigh

obturator canal *n* : the small patent opening of the obturator foramen through which nerves and vessels pass and which is formed by the obturator groove covered over by part of the obturator membrane

obturator ex·ter·nus \-ek-ˈstər-nəs\ *n* : a flat triangular muscle that arises esp. from the medial side of the obturator foramen made up of the rami of the pubis and ischium and from the medial part of the obturator membrane, that inserts by a tendon into the trochanteric fossa of the femur, and that acts to rotate the thigh laterally

obturator foramen *n* : an opening that is the largest foramen in the human body, is situated between the ischium and pubis of the hip bone, and is closed by the obturator membrane except for the obturator canal

obturator groove *n* : a groove in the inferior surface of the superior ramus of the pubis that is converted to the obturator canal when covered over by part of the obturator membrane

obturator in·ter·nus \-in-ˈtər-nəs\ *n* : a muscle that arises from the margin of the obturator foramen and from the obturator membrane, that inserts into the greater trochanter of the femur by way of tendons passing through the greater sciatic foramen, and that acts to rotate the thigh laterally when it is extended and to abduct it in the flexed position

obturator membrane *n* : a firm fibrous membrane covering most of the obturator foramen except for the obturator canal and serving as origin of the obturator externus and obturator internus

obturator nerve *n* : a branch of the lumbar plexus that arises from the second, third, and fourth lumbar nerves and that supplies the hip and knee joints, the adductor muscles of the thigh, and the skin

obturator vein *n* : a tributary of the internal iliac vein that accompanies the obturator artery

ob·tuse \äb-'t(y)üs, əb-\ *adj* **ob·tus·er; -est** **1** : lacking sharpness or quickness of sensibility or intellect **2** : not pointed or acute ⟨~ pain⟩

occipita *pl of* OCCIPUT

¹**oc·cip·i·tal** \äk-'sip-ət-³l\ *adj* : of, relating to, or located within or near the occiput or the occipital bone

²**occipital** *n* : OCCIPITAL BONE

occipital artery *n* : an artery that arises from the external carotid artery opposite to the origin of the facial artery, that passes posteriorly to the base of the skull where it turns upward and ascends within the superficial fascia of the scalp, and that supplies or gives off branches supplying structures and esp. muscles of the back of the neck and head

occipital bone *n* : a compound bone that forms the posterior part of the skull and surrounds the foramen magnum, bears the condyles for articulation with the atlas, is composed of four united elements, is much curved and roughly trapezoidal in outline, ends in front of the foramen magnum in the basilar process, and bears on its external surface behind the foramen magnum the two curved transverse superior and inferior nuchal lines as well as the median external occipital crest and external occipital protuberance

occipital condyle *n* : an articular surface on the occipital bone on each side of the foramen magnum by which the skull articulates with the atlas

occipital crest *n* : either of the two ridges on the occipital bone connecting the occipital protuberances and foramen magnum: **a** : a median ridge on the outer surface of the occipital bone that with the external occipital protuberance gives attachment to the ligamentum nuchae — called also *external occipital crest, median nuchal line* **b** : a median ridge similarly situated on the inner surface of the occipital bone that bifurcates near the foramen magnum to give attachment to the falx cerebelli — called also *internal occipital crest*

occipital fontanel *n* : a triangular fontanel at the meeting of the sutures between the parietal and occipital bones

occipital foramen *n* : FORAMEN MAGNUM

oc·cip·i·ta·lis \äk-ˌsip-ə-'tā-ləs\ *n* : the posterior belly of the occipitofrontalis that arises from the lateral two-thirds of the superior nuchal lines and from the mastoid part of the temporal bone, inserts into the galea aponeurotica, and acts to move the scalp

occipital lobe *n* : the posterior lobe of each cerebral hemisphere that is separated medially from the parietal lobe by the parieto-occipital sulcus, is indistinctly separated more laterally from the temporal and parietal lobes, bears the visual areas, and has the form of a 3-sided pyramid

occipital nerve *n* : either of two nerves that arise mostly from the second cervical nerve: **a** : the medial branch of the second cervical nerve that innervates the scalp at the top of the head — called also *greater occipital nerve* **b** : one arising from the second cervical nerve or from the loop between the second and third cervical nerves and innervating the scalp esp. in the lateral area of the head behind the ear — called also *lesser occipital nerve*

occipital protuberance *n* : either of two prominences on the occipital bone: **a** : a prominence on the outer surface of the occipital bone midway between the upper border and

the foramen magnum that with the external occipital crest gives attachment to the ligamentum nuchae — called also *external occipital protuberance, inion* **b** : a prominence similarly situated on the inner surface of the occipital bone — called also *internal occipital protuberance*

occipital sinus *n* : a single or paired venous sinus that arises near the margin of the foramen magnum by the union of several small veins, follows the internal occipital crest along the attached margin of the falx cerebelli, and empties into the confluence of sinuses or sometimes into one of the transverse sinuses

oc·cip·i·to·fron·ta·lis \äk-ˌsip-ət-ō-frən-'tā-ləs\ *n* : a fibrous and muscular sheet on each side of the vertex of the skull that extends from the eyebrow to the occiput, that is composed of the frontalis muscle in front and the occipitalis muscle in back with the galea aponeurotica in between, and that acts to draw back the scalp to raise the eyebrow and wrinkle the forehead — called also *epicranius*

oc·cip·i·to·pa·ri·etal \-pə-'rī-ət-³l\ *adj* : of or relating to the occipital and parietal bones of the skull ⟨the ~ regions⟩

oc·cip·i·to·tem·po·ral \-'tem-p(ə-)rəl\ *adj* : of, relating to, or distributed to the occipital and temporal lobes of a cerebral hemisphere ⟨the ~ cortex⟩

oc·ci·put \'äk-sə-(ˌ)pət\ *n, pl* **occiputs** *or* **oc·cip·i·ta** \äk-'sip-ət-ə\ : the back part of the head or skull

oc·clude \ə-'klüd, ä-\ *vb* **oc·clud·ed; oc·clud·ing** *vt* **1** : to close up or block off : OBSTRUCT ⟨a thrombus *occluding* a coronary artery⟩ **2** : to bring (upper and lower teeth) into occlusion **3** : to take in and retain (a substance) in the interior rather than on an external surface : SORB ⟨proteins in precipitating may ~ alcohol⟩ ~ *vi* **1** : to come into contact with cusps of the opposing teeth fitting together ⟨his teeth do not ~ properly⟩ **2** : to become occluded

oc·clu·sal \ə-'klü-səl, ä-, -zəl\ *adj* : of, relating to, or being the grinding or biting surface of a tooth; *also* : of or relating to occlusion of the teeth ⟨~ abnormalities⟩ — **oc·clu·sal·ly** \-ē\ *adv*

occlusal disharmony *n* : a condition in which incorrect positioning of one or more teeth causes an abnormal increase in or change of direction of the force applied to one or more teeth when the upper and lower teeth are occluded

occlusal plane *n* : an imaginary plane formed by the occlusal surfaces of the teeth when the jaw is closed

oc·clu·sion \ə-'klü-zhən\ *n* **1** : the act of occluding or the state of being occluded : a shutting off or obstruction of something ⟨a coronary ~⟩; *esp* : a blocking of the central passage of one reflex by the passage of another **2 a** : the bringing of the opposing surfaces of the teeth of the two jaws into contact; *also* : the relation between the surfaces when in contact **b** : the transient approximation of the edges of a natural opening ⟨~ of the eyelids⟩ **3** : SORPTION; *esp* : sorption of gases

oc·clu·sive \-siv\ *adj* : causing or characterized by occlusion ⟨~ arterial disease⟩

occlusive dressing *n* : a dressing that seals a wound to protect against infection

oc·cult \ə-'kəlt, 'äk-ˌəlt\ *adj* : not manifest or detectable by clinical methods alone ⟨~ carcinoma⟩; *also* : not present in macroscopic amounts ⟨~ blood in a stool specimen⟩ ⟨fecal ~ blood testing⟩ — compare GROSS 1b

occulta — see SPINA BIFIDA OCCULTA

oc·cu·pa·tion·al \ˌäk-yə-'pā-shnəl, -shən-³l\ *adj* : relating to or being an occupational disease ⟨~ deafness⟩ — **oc·cu·pa·tion·al·ly** \-ē\ *adv*

occupational disease *n* : an illness caused by factors arising from one's occupation ⟨dermatitis is often an *occupational disease*⟩ — called also *industrial disease*

occupational medicine *n* : a branch of medicine concerned with the prevention and treatment of occupational diseases

---

\ə\ **abut** \ə\ **kitten** \ər\ **further** \a\ **ash** \ā\ **ace** \ä\ **cot, cart** \au̇\ **out** \ch\ **chin** \e\ **bet** \ē\ **easy** \g\ **go** \i\ **hit** \ī\ **ice** \j\ **job** \ŋ\ **sing** \ō\ **go** \ȯ\ **law** \ȯi\ **boy** \th\ **thin** \t̲h̲\ **the** \ü\ **loot** \u̇\ **foot** \y\ **yet** \zh\ **vision** *See also* Pronunciation Symbols page

O
P

occupational neurosis *n* : a condition that is caused by overuse of a muscle or set of muscles in repetitive performance of an operation (as in milking or dancing) and that is marked by loss of ability to constrain the muscles to perform the particular operation normal

occupational therapist *n* : a person trained in or engaged in the practice of occupational therapy

occupational therapy *n* : therapy based on engagement in meaningful activities of daily life (as self-care skills, education, work, or social interaction) esp. to enable or encourage participation in such activities despite impairments or limitations in physical or mental functioning

OCD *abbr* obsessive-compulsive disorder

ocel·lus \ō-ˈsel-əs\ *n, pl* **ocel·li** \-ˈsel-ˌī, -ˌē\ : a minute simple eye or eyespot of an invertebrate — **ocel·lar** \ō-ˈsel-ər\ *adj*

och·lo·pho·bia \ˌäk-lə-ˈfō-bē-ə\ *n* : morbid fear of crowds

och·ra·tox·in \ˌō-krə-ˈtäk-sən\ *n* : a mycotoxin produced by a fungus of the genus *Aspergillus* (*A. ochraceus*)

ochro·no·sis \ˌō-krə-ˈnō-səs\ *n, pl* **-no·ses** \-ˌsēz\ : a condition often associated with alkaptonuria and marked by pigment deposits in cartilages, ligaments, and tendons — **ochro·not·ic** \-ˈnät-ik\ *adj*

oc·ta·dec·a·di·e·no·ic acid \ˌäk-tə-ˌdek-ə-ˌdī-ə-ˌnō-ik-\ *n* : any of several unsaturated fatty acids $C_{18}H_{32}O_2$ some of which (as linoleic acid) occur in fats and oils

oc·ta·dec·a·no·ic acid \-ˌdek-ə-ˌnō-ik-\ *n* : STEARIC ACID

oc·ta·dec·e·no·ic acid \-ˌdes-ə-ˌnō-ik-\ *n* : any of several unsaturated fatty acids $C_{18}H_{34}O_2$ of which some (as oleic acid and vaccenic acid) occur in fats and oils

oc·ta·meth·yl·py·ro·phos·phor·a·mide \-ˌmeth-əl-ˌpī-rō-ˌfäs-ˈfor-ə-ˌmīd\ *n* : an almost odorless viscous liquid anticholinesterase $C_8H_{24}N_4O_3P_2$ that is marketed as a systemic insecticide and has been used to treat myasthenia gravis — called also *OMPA, schradan*

oc·ta·no·ate \ˌäk-tə-ˈnō-ət, -ˌāt\ *n* : CAPRYLATE

oc·ta·no·ic acid \ˌäk-tə-ˌnō-ik-\ *n* : CAPRYLIC ACID

oc·ta·pep·tide \ˌäk-tə-ˈpep-ˌtīd\ *n* : a protein fragment or molecule (as oxytocin or vasopressin) that consists of eight amino acids linked in a polypeptide chain

octaploid *var of* OCTOPLOID

oc·ta·va·lent \ˌäk-tə-ˈvā-lənt\ *adj* : having a valence of eight

oc·to·ge·nar·i·an \ˌäk-tə-jə-ˈner-ē-ən\ *n* : a person whose age is in the eighties — **octogenarian** *adj*

oc·to·pa·mine \äk-ˈtō-pə-ˌmēn, -mən\ *n* : an adrenergic biogenic amine $C_8H_{11}NO_2$ that is found in some invertebrates and vertebrates and has been used to treat hypotension

¹**oc·to·ploid** *also* **oc·ta·ploid** \ˈäk-tə-ˌploid\ *adj* : having a chromosome number eight times the basic haploid chromosome number — **oc·to·ploi·dy** \-ˌploid-ē\ *n, pl* **-dies**

²**octoploid** *also* **octaploid** *n* : an octoploid individual

oc·tose \ˈäk-ˌtōs\ *n* : any of a class of synthetic monosaccharides $C_8H_{16}O_8$ containing eight carbon atoms in a molecule

oc·tre·o·tide \äk-ˈtrē-ə-ˌtīd\ *n* : a long-acting synthetic analog of somatostatin that is a cyclic octapeptide, is administered esp. by subcutaneous injection in the form of its acetate $C_{49}H_{66}N_{10}O_{10}S_2$, and is used to treat acromegaly and to treat severe diarrhea associated with metastatic carcinoid tumors and vipomas

¹**oc·u·lar** \ˈäk-yə-lər\ *adj* : of or relating to the eye ⟨the ∼ adnexa include the eyelids and the lacrimal glands⟩

²**ocular** *n* : EYEPIECE

oc·u·lar·ist \ˈäk-yə-lə-rəst\ *n* : a person who makes and fits artificial eyes

ocular micrometer *n* : EYEPIECE MICROMETER

oculi — see OBLIQUUS INFERIOR OCULI, OBLIQUUS SUPERIOR OCULI, ORBICULARIS OCULI, RECTUS OCULI

oc·u·list \ˈäk-yə-ləst\ *n* **1** : OPHTHALMOLOGIST **2** : OPTOMETRIST

oc·u·lo·ce·re·bro·re·nal syndrome \ˌäk-yə-(ˌ)lō-sə-ˌrē-brō-ˈrēn-ᵊl-, -ˌser-ə-brō-\ *n* : a rare human developmental disorder that is inherited as an X-linked recessive trait and that is marked by congenital cataracts, glaucoma, and abnormal nystagmus affecting the eyes, by severe mental retardation, generalized hypotonia, and absence of or reduction in certain tendon reflexes due to defects in the central nervous system, and by acidosis and hyperaminoaciduria due to defects in the renal tubules — called also *Lowe syndrome*

oc·u·lo·cu·ta·ne·ous \ˌäk-yə-(ˌ)lō-kyú-ˈtā-nē-əs\ *adj* : relating to or affecting both the eyes and the skin ⟨∼ albinism⟩

oc·u·lo·glan·du·lar \-ˈglan-jə-lər\ *adj* : affecting or producing symptoms in the eye and lymph nodes ⟨∼ fever produced by the herpes simplex virus⟩ — see PARINAUD'S OCULOGLANDULAR SYNDROME

oc·u·lo·gy·ral illusion \ˌäk-yə-lō-ˌjī-rəl-\ *n* : the apparent motion of an object that is fixed in relation to an observer whose semicircular canals have been stimulated by rotational motion — called also *oculogyric illusion*

oc·u·lo·gy·ric \-ˈjī-rik\ *adj* : relating to or involving circular movements of the eyeballs

oculogyric crisis *n* : a spasmodic attack that occurs in some nervous diseases and is marked by fixation of the eyeballs in one position usu. upward — called also *oculogyric spasm*

¹**oc·u·lo·mo·tor** \ˌäk-yə-lə-ˈmōt-ər\ *adj* **1** : moving or tending to move the eyeball **2** : of or relating to the oculomotor nerve

²**oculomotor** *n* : an oculomotor part; *esp* : OCULOMOTOR NERVE

oculomotor nerve *n* : either nerve of the third pair of cranial nerves that are motor nerves with some associated autonomic fibers, arise from the midbrain, supply muscles of the eye except the superior oblique and the lateral rectus with motor fibers, and supply the ciliary body and iris with autonomic fibers by way of the ciliary ganglion — called also *third cranial nerve*

oculomotor nucleus *n* : a nucleus that is situated under the aqueduct of Sylvius rostral to the trochlear nucleus and is the source of the motor fibers of the oculomotor nerve

oc·u·lo·plas·tic \-ˈplas-tik\ *adj* : of, relating to, or being plastic surgery of the eye and associated structures

oc·u·lus \ˈäk-yə-ləs\ *n, pl* **-li** \-yə-ˌlī\ : EYE 1

od *abbr* [Latin *omnes dies*] every day — used in writing prescriptions

¹**OD** \(ˈ)ō-ˈdē\ *n* **1** : an overdose of a narcotic **2** : an individual who has taken an OD

²**OD** *vi* **OD'd** *or* **ODed; OD'·ing; OD's** : to become ill or die of an OD

OD *abbr* **1** doctor of optometry **2** [Latin *oculus dexter*] right eye — used in writing prescriptions

ODD *abbr* oppositional defiant disorder

Od·di's sphincter \ˈäd-ēz-\ *n* : SPHINCTER OF ODDI

odon·tal·gia \(ˌ)ō-ˌdän-ˈtal-j(ē-)ə\ *n* : TOOTHACHE — **odon·tal·gic** \-jik\ *adj*

odon·ti·a·sis \(ˌ)ō-ˌdän-ˈtī-ə-səs\ *n, pl* **-a·ses** \-ˌsēz\ : cutting of the teeth : TEETHING

odon·ti·tis \-ˈtīt-əs\ *n, pl* **odon·tit·i·des** \-ˈtit-ə-ˌdēz\ : inflammation of a tooth

odon·to·blast \ō-ˈdänt-ə-ˌblast\ *n* : one of the elongated radially arranged outer cells of the dental pulp that secrete dentin — **odon·to·blas·tic** \-ˌdänt-ə-ˈblas-tik\ *adj*

odon·to·cele \-ˌsēl\ *n* : a cyst in the alveolus of a tooth

odon·to·clast \-ˌklast\ *n* : one of the large multinucleate cells that are active during the absorption of the roots of the milk teeth

odon·to·gen·e·sis \ō-ˌdänt-ə-ˈjen-ə-səs\ *n, pl* **-e·ses** \-ˌsēz\ : the formation and development of teeth

odon·to·gen·ic \ō-ˌdänt-ə-ˈjen-ik\ *adj* **1** : forming or capable of forming teeth ⟨∼ tissues⟩ **2** : containing or arising from odontogenic tissues ⟨∼ tumors⟩

odon·tog·ra·phy \(ˌ)ō-ˌdän-ˈtäg-rə-fē\ *n, pl* **-phies** : scientific description of the teeth (as of their gross structure); *also* : a treatise on this subject

odon·toid \ō-ˈdän-ˌtoid\ *adj* **1** : having the form of a tooth **2** : of or relating to the dens

odontoid process *n* : DENS

odon·tol·o·gist \(ˌ)ō-ˌdän-ˈtäl-ə-jəst\ *n* : a specialist in odontology

odon·tol·o·gy \(ˌ)ō-ˌdän-ˈtäl-ə-jē\ *n, pl* **-gies** **1** : a science dealing with the teeth, their structure and development, and their diseases **2** : FORENSIC ODONTOLOGY — **odon·to·log·i·cal** \-ˌdänt-ᵊl-ˈäj-i-kəl\ *adj*

odon·to·ma \(ˌ)ō-ˌdän-ˈtō-mə\ *n, pl* **-mas** *also* **-ma·ta** \-ˌmət-ə\ : a tumor originating from a tooth and containing dental tissue (as enamel, dentin, or cementum)

odon·tome \ō-ˈdän-ˌtōm\ *n* : ODONTOMA

odon·tot·o·my \(ˌ)ō-ˌdän-ˈtät-ə-mē\ *n, pl* **-mies** : the operation of cutting into a tooth

odor *or chiefly Brit* **odour** \ˈōd-ər\ *n* **1** : a quality of something that stimulates the olfactory organ : SMELL **2** : a sensation resulting from adequate chemical stimulation of the olfactory organ ⟨a disagreeable ∼⟩ — **odored** *or chiefly Brit* **odoured** *adj* — **odor·less** *or chiefly Brit* **odour·less** *adj*

odor·ant \ˈōd-ə-rənt\ *n* : an odorous substance; *esp* : one added to a toxic odorless substance to warn of its presence

odor·if·er·ous \ˌōd-ə-ˈrif-(ə-)rəs\ *adj* : yielding an odor : ODOROUS

odor·im·e·try \-ˈrim-ə-trē\ *n, pl* **-tries** : the measurement of the intensity of odors

odor·i·phore \ō-ˈdär-ə-ˌfō(ə)r\ *n* : OSMOPHORE

odor·ous \ˈōd-ə-rəs\ *adj* : having an odor: as **a** : having a sweet or pleasant odor **b** : having a bad odor

odour, odoured, odourless *chiefly Brit var of* ODOR, ODORED, ODORLESS

odyno·pha·gia \ō-ˌdin-ə-ˈfā-j(ē-)ə\ *n* : pain produced by swallowing

oedema, oedematous *chiefly Brit var of* EDEMA, EDEMATOUS

oe·di·pal \ˈed-ə-pəl, ˈēd-\ *adj, often cap* : of, relating to, or resulting from the Oedipus complex — **oe·di·pal·ly** \-pə-lē\ *adv, often cap*

Oe·di·pus \ˈed-i-pəs, ˈēd-\, Greek mythological character. In Greek mythology Oedipus was the son of Laius and Jocasta, the king and queen of Thebes. Because at his birth an oracle had predicted that he would someday murder his father and marry his mother, Oedipus was abandoned by his parents, but he survived to maturity. Through a highly improbable series of circumstances, he fulfilled the prophecy: he unknowingly slew his father and later married his widowed mother, thereby succeeding his father to the throne. When the truth was eventually revealed to all, Jocasta committed suicide and Oedipus blinded himself.

¹Oedipus *adj* : OEDIPAL

²Oedipus *n* : OEDIPUS COMPLEX

Oedipus complex *n* **1** : a child's positive libidinal feelings toward the parent of the opposite sex and hostile or jealous feelings toward the parent of the same sex that develop usu. between the ages of three and six and that may be a source of adult personality disorder when unresolved — used esp. of the male child; see ELECTRA COMPLEX **2** : the unresolved oedipal feelings persisting into adult life

oe·no·ther·a·py \ˌē-nə-ˈther-ə-pē\ *n, pl* **-pies** : a use of wine for therapeutic purposes

oer·sted \ˈər-stəd\ *n* : the cgs unit of magnetic field strength equal to the intensity of a magnetic field in a vacuum in which a unit magnetic pole experiences a mechanical force of one dyne in the direction of the field

Oer·sted \ˈœr-steth, -stəd; ˈə(r)-stəd\, **Hans Christian (1777–1851),** Danish physicist. Oersted was a professor of physics at the University of Copenhagen, and in 1820 he reported his discovery that a compass needle—a magnet—moved to a position at right angles to the direction of an electric current. This discovery established that a relationship exists between electricity and magnetism, and it marked the foundation of the science of electromagnetism, to which Ampère and Faraday later made significant contributions. The cgs unit of magnetic field strength was named in Oersted's honor.

Each boldface word in the list below is a chiefly British variant of the word to its right in small capitals.

oesophageal	ESOPHAGEAL
oesophagecto·my	ESOPHAGECTO·MY
oesophagitis	ESOPHAGITIS
oesophagogas·trectomy	ESOPHAGOGAS·TRECTOMY

oesophagogas·tric	ESOPHAGOGAS·TRIC	oesophago·scope	ESOPHAGO·SCOPE
oesophagogas·troscopy	ESOPHAGOGAS·TROSCOPY	oesophago·scopic	ESOPHAGO·SCOPIC
oesophagogas·trostomy	ESOPHAGOGAS·TROSTOMY	oesophagosco·pist	ESOPHAGOSCO·PIST
oesophagojeju·nostomy	ESOPHAGOJEJU·NOSTOMY	oesophagosco·py	ESOPHAGOSCO·PY
oesophagomy·otomy	ESOPHAGOMY·OTOMY	oesophagosto·my	ESOPHAGOSTO·MY
oesophago·plasty	ESOPHAGOPLAS·TY	oesophagoto·my	ESOPHAGOTO·MY
		oesophagus	ESOPHAGUS

oe·soph·a·go·stome *also* **esoph·a·go·stome** \i-ˈsäf-ə-gə-ˌstōm\ *n* : a nematode worm of the genus *Oesophagostomum*

oe·soph·a·go·sto·mi·a·sis *also* **esoph·a·go·sto·mi·a·sis** \i-ˌsäf-ə-(ˌ)gō-stə-ˈmī-ə-səs\ *n, pl* **-a·ses** \-ˌsēz\ : infestation with or disease caused by nematode worms of the genus *Oesophagostomum* : NODULAR DISEASE

Oe·soph·a·gos·to·mum \i-ˌsäf-ə-ˈgäs-tə-məm\ *n* : a genus of nematode worms of the family Strongylidae comprising the nodular worms of ruminants and swine and other worms affecting primates including humans esp. in Africa

Each boldface word in the list below is a chiefly British variant of the word to its right in small capitals.

oestradiol	ESTRADIOL	oestrogenicity	ESTROGENICITY
oestral cycle	ESTRAL CYCLE	oestrone	ESTRONE
oestrin	ESTRIN	oestrous	ESTROUS
oestrinization	ESTRINIZATION	oestrual	ESTRUAL
oestriol	ESTRIOL	oestruate	ESTRUATE
oestrogen	ESTROGEN	oestruation	ESTRUATION
oestrogenic	ESTROGENIC	oestrum	ESTRUM
oestrogeni·cally	ESTROGENI·CALLY	oestrus	ESTRUS

oes·tri·a·sis \e-ˈstrī-ə-səs, ē-\ *n, pl* **-a·ses** \-ˌsēz\ : infestation with or disease caused by botflies of the genus *Oestrus*

Oes·tri·dae \ˈes-tri-ˌdē, ˈēs-\ *n pl* : a family of dipteran flies consisting of the botflies and formerly including also the warble flies — **oes·trid** \-trəd\ *adj or n*

Oes·trus \ˈes-trəs, ˈēs-\ *n* : the type genus of the family *Oestridae* that includes the sheep botfly

of·fi·cial \ə-ˈfish-əl\ *adj* : prescribed or recognized as authorized; *specif* : described by the *U.S. Pharmacopeia* or the *National Formulary* — compare NONOFFICIAL, UNOFFICIAL — **of·fi·cial·ly** \-ˈfish-(ə-)lē\ *adv*

¹of·fi·ci·nal \ə-ˈfis-ᵊn-əl, ȯ-, ä-; ˌȯf-ə-ˈsīn-ᵊl, ˌäf-\ *adj* **1 a** : available without special preparation or compounding ⟨∼ medicine⟩ — compare MAGISTRAL **b** : OFFICIAL **2** *of a plant* : MEDICINAL ⟨∼ herbs⟩ ⟨∼ rhubarb⟩

²officinal *n* : an officinal drug, medicine, or plant

off-la·bel \ˌȯf-ˈlā-bəl\ *adj* : of, relating to, or being an approved drug legally prescribed or a medical device legally used by a physician for a purpose (as the treatment of children or of a certain disease or condition) for which it has not been specifically approved (as by the U.S. Food and Drug Administration) ⟨the ∼ use of oral contraceptives to treat dysmenorrhea⟩

off·spring \ˈȯf-ˌspriŋ\ *n, pl* **offspring** *also* **offsprings** : the progeny of an animal or plant : YOUNG

oflox·a·cin \ō-ˈfläk-sə-sən, ə-\ *n* : a fluoroquinolone $C_{18}H_{20}FN_3O_4$ that is a broad-spectrum antibacterial agent administered orally or intravenously or in topical solution for otic or ophthalmic use — see LEVOFLOXACIN

Ogil·vie's syndrome \ˈō-gəl-vēz-\ *n* : distension of the colon that is similar to that occurring as a consequence of bowel obstruction but in which no physical obstruction exists and that occurs esp. in seriously ill individuals and as a complication of abdominal surgery

Ogilvie, Sir William Heneage (1887–1971), British surgeon. Ogilvie's major professional association was with Guy's Hospital in London. He also served as an examiner in surgery for the universities of Oxford and Cambridge and

O
P

\ə\ abut \ᵊ\ kitten \ər\ further \a\ ash \ā\ ace \ä\ cot, cart
\aú\ out \ch\ chin \e\ bet \ē\ easy \g\ go \i\ hit \ī\ ice \j\ job
\ŋ\ sing \ō\ go \ȯ\ law \ȯi\ boy \th\ thin \t̲h̲\ the \ü\ loot
\ú\ foot \y\ yet \zh\ vision *See also* Pronunciation Symbols page

as editor of the journal *Practitioner*. He wrote a number of surgical treatises, contributed chapters to textbooks on surgery, and published monographs on bone fractures and hernias. His description of Ogilvie's syndrome was the subject of a 1948 article.

ohm \'ōm\ *n* : the practical mks unit of electrical resistance equal to the resistance of a circuit in which a potential difference of one volt produces a current of one ampere — **ohm·ic** \'ō-mik\ *adj*

Ohm, Georg Simon (1789–1854), German physicist. Ohm is best remembered for his discovery of a law of electricity that is now called Ohm's law in his honor. He summarized his discovery in a pamphlet published in 1827. His work exerted great influence on the theory and applications of current electricity. The physical unit measuring electrical resistance was officially designated the *ohm* by the Paris Electrical Congress of 1881.

ohm·me·ter \'ō(m)-ˌmēt-ər\ *n* : an instrument for indicating resistance in ohms directly

Ohm's law \'ōmz-\ *n* : a law in electricity: the strength or intensity of an unvarying electric current is directly proportional to the electromotive force and inversely proportional to the resistance of the circuit

OI *abbr* opportunistic infection

oid·i·o·my·co·sis \ˌō-ˌid-ē-ō-ˌmī-'kō-səs\ *n, pl* **-co·ses** \-ˌsēz\ : infection with or disease caused by fungi of the genus *Oidium*

oid·i·um \ō-'id-ē-əm\ *n* **1** *cap* : a genus of imperfect fungi of the family Moniliaceae including many which are now considered to be conidial stages of various powdery mildews **2** *pl* **oid·ia** \-ē-ə\ : any fungus of the genus *Oidium* **3** *pl* **oidia** : ARTHROCONIDIUM

oil \'ȯi(ə)l\ *n* **1** : any of numerous unctuous combustible substances that are liquid or can be liquefied easily on warming, are soluble in ether but not in water, and leave a greasy stain on paper or cloth — see ESSENTIAL OIL, FATTY OIL, VOLATILE OIL **2** : a substance (as a cosmetic preparation) of oily consistency ⟨bath ∼⟩ — **oil** *adj*

oil gland *n* : a gland (as of the skin) that produces an oily secretion; *specif* : SEBACEOUS GLAND

oil–immersion lens *n* : an objective lens designed to work with a drop of liquid (as oil or water) between the lens and cover glass — called also *immersion lens, immersion objective, oil-immersion objective*

oil of turpentine *n* : TURPENTINE 2a

oil of vitriol *n* : concentrated sulfuric acid

oil of wintergreen *n* : a preparation of methyl salicylate obtained by distilling the leaves of wintergreen (*Gaultheria procumbens*) — called also *gaultheria oil, wintergreen oil*; compare BIRCH OIL

oil·seed rape \'ȯi(ə)l-ˌsēd-\ *n, chiefly Brit* : a rape plant grown for the oil in its seeds; *specif* : CANOLA 1

oil–soluble *adj* : FAT-SOLUBLE

oily \'ȯi-lē\ *adj* **oil·i·er; -est** **1** : of, relating to, or consisting of oil **2** : excessively high in naturally secreted oils ⟨∼ hair⟩ ⟨∼ skin⟩

oint·ment \'ȯint-mənt\ *n* : a salve or unguent for application to the skin; *specif* : a semisolid medicinal preparation usu. having a base of fatty or greasy material

ol *abbr* oleum

OL *abbr* [Latin *oculus laevus*] left eye — used in writing prescriptions

olan·za·pine \ō-'lan-zə-ˌpēn\ *n* : an antipsychotic drug C₁₇H₂₀N₄S administered orally esp. in short-term treatment of schizophrenia and acute manic episodes of bipolar disorder — see ZYPREXA

old–man's beard \ˌōl(d)-ˌmanz-\ *n* : a greenish gray pendulous lichen of the genus *Usnea* (*U. barbata*) that grows on trees and is a source of usnic acid

old tuberculin *n* : tuberculin prepared by boiling, filtering, and concentrating a broth culture of tubercle bacilli and orig. introduced as a proposed curative agent for tuberculosis but now used in skin tests to detect tubercular infection

olea *pl of* OLEUM

ole·ag·i·nous \ˌō-lē-'aj-ə-nəs\ *adj* : resembling or having the properties of oil; *also* : containing or producing oil

ole·an·der \'ō-lē-ˌan-dər, ˌō-lē-'\ *n* : a poisonous evergreen shrub (*Nerium oleander*) of the dogbane family (Apocynaceae) with fragrant white to red flowers that contains oleandrin and was formerly used in medicine

ole·an·do·my·cin \ˌō-lē-ˌan-də-'mīs-ᵊn\ *n* : an antibiotic C₃₅H₆₁NO₁₂ produced by a bacterium of the genus *Streptomyces* (*S. antibioticus*)

ole·an·drin \ˌō-lē-'an-drən\ *n* : a poisonous crystalline glycoside C₃₂H₄₈O₉ found in oleander leaves and resembling digitalis in its action

ole·ate \'ō-lē-ˌāt\ *n* **1** : a salt or ester of oleic acid **2** : a liquid or semisolid preparation of a medicinal dissolved in an excess of oleic acid ⟨mercury ∼⟩ ⟨∼ of quinine⟩

olec·ra·non \ō-'lek-rə-ˌnän\ *n* : the large process of the ulna that projects behind the elbow, forms the bony prominence of the elbow, and receives the insertion of the triceps muscle

olecranon fossa *n* : the fossa at the distal end of the humerus into which the olecranon fits when the arm is in full extension — compare CORONOID FOSSA

ole·fin \'ō-lə-fən\ *n* : ALKENE — **ole·fin·ic** \ˌō-lə-'fin-ik\ *adj*

ole·ic \ō-'lē-ik, -'lā-\ *adj* : of or relating to oleic acid

oleic acid *n* : a monounsaturated fatty acid C₁₈H₃₄O₂ found in natural fats and oils

ole·in \'ō-lē-ən\ *n* : an ester of glycerol and oleic acid — called also *triolein*

ole·o·phil·ic \ˌō-lē-ō-'fil-ik\ *adj* : having or relating to strong affinity for oils : HYDROPHOBIC 3 — compare HYDROPHILIC, LIPOPHILIC, LYOPHILIC

ole·o·pho·bic \-'fō-bik\ *adj* : having or relating to a lack of strong affinity for oils : HYDROPHILIC — compare HYDROPHOBIC 3, LYOPHOBIC

oleo·res·in \ˌō-lē-ō-'rez-ᵊn\ *n* **1** : a natural plant product (as copaiba or turpentine) containing chiefly essential oil and resin **2** : a preparation consisting essentially of oil holding resin in solution — **oleo·res·in·ous** \-'rez-ᵊn-əs, -'rez-nəs\ *adj*

oleo·tho·rax \-'thō(ə)r-ˌaks, -'thȯ(ə)r-\ *n, pl* **-tho·rax·es** or **-tho·ra·ces** \-'thȯr-ə-ˌsēz, -'thȯr-\ : a state in which oil is present in the pleural cavity usu. as a result of injection — compare PNEUMOTHORAX

oleo·vi·ta·min \-'vīt-ə-mən, *Brit usu* -'vit-\ *n* : a preparation containing one or more fat-soluble vitamins or derivatives in oil (as a fish-liver oil or an edible vegetable oil) ⟨∼ A⟩

oles·tra \ō-'les-trə\ *n* : a noncaloric fat substitute consisting of a series of compounds that are sucrose esters of six to eight fatty acids resistant to absorption by the digestive system due to their large size

ole·um \'ō-lē-əm\ *n, pl* **olea** \-lē-ə\ : OIL 1

ol·fac·tion \äl-'fak-shən, ōl-\ *n* **1** : the sense of smell **2** : the act or process of smelling

ol·fac·tom·e·ter \ˌäl-ˌfak-'täm-ət-ər, ˌōl-\ *n* : an instrument for measuring the sensitivity of the sense of smell in regard to intensity, concentration, or quality of an odor

ol·fac·tom·e·try \ˌäl-ˌfak-'täm-ə-trē, ˌōl-\ *n, pl* **-tries** : the testing and measurement of the sensitivity of the sense of smell — **ol·fac·to·met·ric** \-tə-'me-trik\ *adj*

ol·fac·to·ry \äl-'fak-t(ə-)rē, ōl-\ *adj* : of, relating to, or connected with the sense of smell

olfactory area *n* **1** : the sensory area for olfaction lying in the parahippocampal gyrus **2** : the area of nasal mucosa in which the olfactory organ is situated

olfactory bulb *n* : a bulbous anterior projection of the olfactory lobe that is the place of termination of the olfactory nerves

olfactory cell *n* : a sensory cell specialized for the reception of sensory stimuli caused by odors; *specif* : any of the spindle-shaped neurons that are buried in the nasal mucous membrane of vertebrates and that have a round nucleus and two slender processes of which the inner constitutes an olfactory nerve fiber and the short outer one is modified peripherally to form the actual sensory receptor — see OLFACTORY ORGAN

olfactory cortex *n* : a group of cortical areas of the cerebrum that include parts of the perforated substance, lateral olfactory gyrus, amygdala, and piriform lobe and that are prob. concerned with the subjective evaluation of olfactory stimuli

olfactory epithelium *n* : the nasal mucosa containing olfactory cells

olfactory gland *n* : GLAND OF BOWMAN

olfactory gyrus *n* : either a lateral or a medial gyrus on each side of the brain by which the olfactory tract on the corresponding side communicates with the olfactory area

olfactory lobe *n* : a lobe of the brain that rests on the lower surface of a temporal lobe and projects forward from the anterior lower part of each cerebral hemisphere, that is continuous anteriorly with the olfactory nerve, that consists of an olfactory bulb, an olfactory tract, and an olfactory trigone, and that is well developed in most vertebrates but is reduced to a narrow elongated body in humans

olfactory nerve *n* : either of the pair of nerves that are the first cranial nerves, that serve to conduct sensory stimuli from the olfactory organ to the brain, and that arise from the olfactory cells as discrete bundles of unmyelinated fibers passing in small groups (in humans, about 20) through the cribriform plate of the ethmoid bone and terminating in the olfactory bulb — called also *first cranial nerve*

olfactory organ *n* : an organ of chemical sense that receives stimuli interpreted as odors from volatile and soluble substances in low dilution, that lies in the walls of the upper part of the nasal cavity, and that forms a mucous membrane continuous with the rest of the lining of the nasal cavity and made up of tall columnar sustentacular cells containing golden brown pigment interspersed with olfactory cells the outer processes of which project between the sustentacular cells as small vesicles surmounted by delicate sensory filaments and the inner ends of which are continuous with fibers of the olfactory nerves

olfactory pit *n* : a depression on the head of an embryo that becomes converted into a nasal passage — called also *nasal sac*

olfactory placode *n* : a thick plate of cells derived from the neural ectoderm in the head region of the vertebrate embryo and developing into the olfactory region of the nasal cavity

olfactory tract *n* : a tract of nerve fibers in the olfactory lobe on the inferior surface of the frontal lobe of the brain that passes from the olfactory bulb to the olfactory trigone

olfactory trigone *n* : a triangular area of gray matter on each side of the brain forming the junction of an olfactory tract with a cerebral hemisphere near the optic chiasma

olfactory tubercle *n* : a small area of gray matter behind the olfactory trigone that is noted for receiving dopaminergic neurons from the substantia nigra and the reticular formation which have been implicated in schizoaffective disorders.

ol·fac·ty \äl-'fak-tē, ōl-\ *n, pl* **-ties** : an arbitrary unit used in olfactometry for measuring the strength of an odorous stimulus

olib·a·num \ō-'lib-ə-nəm\ *n* : FRANKINCENSE

ol·i·ge·mia *or chiefly Brit* **ol·i·gae·mia** \,äl-ə-'gē-mē-ə, -'jē-\ *n* : a condition in which the total volume of the blood is reduced — **ol·i·ge·mic** *or chiefly Brit* **ol·i·gae·mic** \-mik\ *adj*

oli·go \'äl-i-gō, 'ō-li-\ *n* : OLIGONUCLEOTIDE

oli·go·ar·tic·u·lar \,äl-i-gō-är-'tik-yə-lər, ə-,lig-ə-\ *adj* : affecting a few joints ⟨∼ arthritis⟩ — compare MONOARTICULAR, POLYARTICULAR

oli·go·chro·me·mia *or chiefly Brit* **oli·go·chro·mae·mia** \-krō-'mē-mē-ə\ *n* : deficiency of hemoglobin in the blood

oli·go·clon·al \-'klōn-ºl\ *adj* **1** : cloned or derived from one or a few cells or molecules ⟨∼ T cells⟩ ⟨∼ lymphomas⟩ **2** : of, relating to, or being any small group of proteins that migrate close together during electrophoresis producing closely placed bands on the electrophoretogram ⟨∼ immunoglobulins⟩ — **oli·go·clo·nal·i·ty** \-klō-'nal-ət-ē\ *n, pl* **-ties**

oli·go·cy·the·mia *or chiefly Brit* **oli·go·cy·thae·mia** \-,sī-'thē-mē-ə\ *n* : deficiency in the total number of red blood cells present in the body — compare ANEMIA 1 — **oli·go·cy·the·mic** *or chiefly Brit* **oli·go·cy·thae·mic** \-'thē-mik\ *adj*

oli·go·dac·tyl·ism \-'dak-tə-,liz-əm\ *n* : the presence of fewer than five digits on a hand or foot

oli·go·dac·ty·ly \-'dak-tə-lē\ *n, pl* **-lies** : OLIGODACTYLISM

oli·go·den·dro·cyte \-'den-drə-,sīt\ *n* : a glial cell resembling an astrocyte but smaller with few and slender processes having few branches

oli·go·den·drog·lia \-den-'dräg-lē-ə, -'drōg-\ *n* : glia made up of oligodendrocytes that forms the myelin sheath around axons in the central nervous system — **oli·go·den·drog·li·al** \-lē-əl\ *adj*

oli·go·den·dro·gli·o·ma \-,den-drō-glī-'ō-mə\ *n, pl* **-mas** *also* **-ma·ta** \-mət-ə\ : a tumor of the nervous system composed of oligodendroglia

oli·go·de·oxy·nu·cle·o·tide \-(,)dē-,äk-sē-'n(y)ü-klē-ə-,tīd\ *n* : an oligonucleotide consisting of deoxyribose-containing nucleotides

oli·go·de·oxy·ri·bo·nu·cle·o·tide \-,rī-bō-'n(y)ü-klē-ə-,tīd\ *n* : OLIGODEOXYNUCLEOTIDE

oli·go·dy·nam·ic \-dī-'nam-ik\ *adj* **1** : active in very small quantities ⟨an ∼ germicide⟩ **2 a** : produced by minute quantities ⟨∼ action of silver in disinfecting water⟩ **b** : of or relating to the action of such quantities **3** : of, relating to, or being produced by the specific activity of an oligodynamic substance ⟨∼ effects of metals on bacterial growth⟩

oli·go·fruc·tose \-'frak-,tōs, -'frük-, -'frúk-, -,tōz\ *n* : a short-chain polysaccharide that is produced by partial enzymatic hydrolysis of inulin and is used similarly to inulin in processed foods

oli·go·gene \'äl-i-gō-,jēn, ə-'lig-ə-\ *n* : a gene that exerts a major effect on a character either as one of two Mendelian alternatives or as one of a few genes controlling a qualitative character — **oli·go·gen·ic** \,äl-i-gō-'jen-ik, ə-,lig-ə-, -'jē-nik\ *adj*

oli·go·hy·dram·ni·os \,äl-i-gō-,hī-'dram-nē-,äs, ə-,lig-ə-\ *n* : deficiency of amniotic fluid sometimes resulting in an embryonic defect through adherence between embryo and amnion

oli·go·lec·i·thal \-'les-ə-thəl\ *adj, of an egg* : having little yolk ⟨echinoderm eggs are ∼⟩

oli·go·men·or·rhea *or chiefly Brit* **oli·go·men·or·rhoea** \-,men-ə-'rē-ə\ *n* : abnormally infrequent or scanty menstrual flow

oligo·mer \ə-'lig-ə-mər\ *n* : a polymer or polymer intermediate containing relatively few structural units — **oligo·mer·ic** \-,lig-ə-'mer-ik\ *adj* — **oligo·mer·iza·tion** \-mə-rə-'zā-shən\ *n*

oli·go·my·cin \,äl-i-gō-'mīs-ºn, ,ō-li-\ *n* : any of several antibiotic substances produced by an actinomycete of the genus *Streptomyces* (*S. diastatochromogenes* or a closely related species) and used esp. in biochemical research to inhibit oxidative phosphorylation

oli·go·nu·cle·o·tide \-'n(y)ü-klē-ə-,tīd\ *n* : a relatively short single-stranded nucleic-acid chain (as an oligodeoxynucleotide or oligoribonucleotide) usu. consisting of up to approximately 20 nucleotides

oli·go·pep·tide \,äl-i-gō-'pep-,tīd, ,ō-li-\ *n* : a protein fragment or molecule that usu. consists of less than 25 amino acid residues linked in a polypeptide chain

oli·go·phre·nia \-'frē-nē-ə\ *n* : MENTAL RETARDATION

¹oli·go·phren·ic \-'fren-ik\ *adj* : of, relating to, or exhibiting mental retardation

²oligophrenic *n* : a mentally retarded individual

oli·go·ri·bo·nu·cle·o·tide \-,rī-bō-'n(y)ü-klē-ə-,tīd\ *n* : an oligonucleotide consisting of ribonucleotides

oli·go·sac·cha·ride \,äl-i-gō-'sak-ə-,rīd, ,ō-li-\ *n* : a saccharide (as a disaccharide) that contains a known small number of monosaccharide units

oli·go·si·a·lia \-sī-'ā-lē-ə\ *n* : an abnormal deficiency of saliva

O
P

\ə\ **abut** \ᵊ\ **kitten** \ər\ **further** \a\ **ash** \ā\ **ace** \ä\ **cot, cart**
\aú\ **out** \ch\ **chin** \e\ **bet** \ē\ **easy** \g\ **go** \i\ **hit** \ī\ **ice** \j\ **job**
\ŋ\ **sing** \ō\ **go** \ó\ **law** \ói\ **boy** \th\ **thin** \t͟h\ **the** \ü\ **loot**
\ú\ **foot** \y\ **yet** \zh\ **vision**   *See also* Pronunciation Symbols page

oli·go·sper·mia \-'spər-mē-ə\ *n* : deficiency of sperm in the semen — **oli·go·sper·mic** \-'spər-mik\ *adj*

oli·go·trich·ia \-'trik-ē-ə\ *n* : deficiency in the growth of hair esp. when congenital

ol·i·gu·ria \ˌäl-ə-'g(y)ùr-ē-ə\ *n* : reduced excretion of urine — **ol·i·gur·ic** \-ik\ *adj*

ol·i·vary \'äl-ə-ˌver-ē\ *adj* **1** : shaped like an olive **2** : of, relating to, situated near, or comprising one or more of the olives, inferior olives, or superior olives ⟨the ∼ complex⟩

olivary body *n* : OLIVE 2

olivary nucleus *n* **1** : INFERIOR OLIVE **2** : SUPERIOR OLIVE

ol·ive \'äl-iv, -əv\ *n* **1** : an Old World evergreen tree (*Olea europaea* of the family Oleaceae, the olive family) cultivated for its drupaceous fruit that is an important food and source of oil; *also* : the fruit **2** : an oval eminence on each ventrolateral aspect of the medulla oblongata that contains the inferior olive of the same side — called also *olivary body*

olive oil *n* : a pale yellow to yellowish green nondrying oil obtained from the pulp of olives usu. by expression and used chiefly as a salad oil and in cooking, in toilet soaps, and as an emollient

ol·i·vo·cer·e·bel·lar \ˌäl-i-vō-ˌser-ə-'bel-ər\ *adj* : of or relating to the cerebellum and the olivary nuclei

olivocerebellar tract *n* : a tract of fibers that arises in the olive on one side, crosses to the olive on the other, and enters the cerebellum by way of the inferior cerebellar peduncle

ol·i·vo·pon·to·cer·e·bel·lar atrophy \-ˌpän-tō-ˌser-ə-'bel-ər-\ *n* : an inherited disease esp. of mid to late life that is characterized by ataxia, hypotonia, dysarthria, and degeneration of the cerebellar cortex, middle cerebellar peduncles, and inferior olives — called also *olivopontocerebellar degeneration*

ol·i·vo·spi·nal \-'spīn-ᵊl\ *adj* : of or relating to the olivary nuclei and the spinal cord

olivospinal tract *n* : a tract of fibers on the peripheral aspect of the ventral side of the cervical part of the spinal cord that communicates with the inferior olive

olo·li·u·qui \ˌō-lō-lē-'ü-kē\ *n* : a woody stemmed Mexican vine (*Rivea corymbosa*) of the morning glory family having seeds with hallucinogenic properties

ol·sal·a·zine \ōl-'sal-ə-ˌzēn\ *n* : a disodium salicylate salt $C_{14}H_8N_2Na_2O_6$ that is administered orally and is converted in the body to an aminosalicylic acid having an anti-inflammatory effect used in the treatment of ulcerative colitis — called also *olsalazine sodium*

oma·sal \ō-'mā-səl\ *adj* : of or relating to the omasum

oma·si·tis \ˌō-mə-'sīt-əs\ *n* : inflammation of the omasum

oma·sum \ō-'mā-səm\ *n, pl* **oma·sa** \-sə\ : the third chamber of the ruminant stomach that is situated between the reticulum and the abomasum — called also *manyplies, psalterium;* compare RUMEN

ome·ga *or* ω- \ō-'meg-ə, -'mā-gə, *esp Brit* 'ō-meg-ə\ *adj* : of, relating to, or being a chemical group or position at the end of a molecular chain ⟨∼ oxidation of fatty acids⟩

ome·ga–6 \-'siks\ *adj* : being or composed of polyunsaturated fatty acids in which the first double bond in the hydrocarbon chain occurs between the sixth and seventh carbon atoms from the end of the molecule most distant from the carboxylic acid group and which are found esp. in vegetable oils, nuts, beans, seeds, and grains — **omega–6** *n*

ome·ga–3 \-'thrē\ *adj* : being or composed of polyunsaturated fatty acids in which the first double bond in the hydrocarbon chain occurs between the third and fourth carbon atoms from the end of the molecule most distant from the carboxylic acid group and which are found esp. in fish (as tuna and salmon), fish oils, green leafy vegetables, and some vegetable oils — **omega–3** *n*

omenta *pl of* OMENTUM

omen·tal \ō-'ment-əl\ *adj* : of, relating to, or formed from an omentum

omen·tec·to·my \ˌō-men-'tek-tə-mē\ *n, pl* **-mies** : excision or resection of all or part of an omentum — called also *epiploectomy*

omen·to·pexy \ō-'ment-ə-ˌpek-sē\ *n, pl* **-pex·ies** : the operation of suturing the omentum esp. to another organ

omen·to·plas·ty \-ˌplast-ē\ *n, pl* **-ties** : the use of a piece or flap of tissue from an omentum as a graft

omen·tor·rha·phy \ˌō-men-'tór-ə-fē\ *n, pl* **-phies** : surgical repair of an omentum by suturing

omen·tum \ō-'ment-əm\ *n, pl* **-ta** \-ə\ *or* **-tums** : a fold of peritoneum connecting or supporting abdominal structures (as the stomach and liver) — see GREATER OMENTUM, LESSER OMENTUM

omen·tum·ec·to·my \ō-ˌmen-təm-'ek-tə-mē\ *n, pl* **-mies** : OMENTECTOMY

omep·ra·zole \ō-'mep-rə-ˌzōl, -'mē-prə-, -ˌzòl\ *n* : a benzimidazole derivative $C_{17}H_{19}N_3O_3S$ that inhibits gastric acid secretion and is used in the short-term treatment of duodenal and gastric ulcers as well as the treatment of gastroesophageal reflux, erosive esophagitis, and disorders (as Zollinger-Ellison syndrome) involving gastric acid hypersecretion — see PRILOSEC

om·ni·fo·cal \ˌäm-ni-'fō-kəl\ *adj* : of, relating to, or being a bifocal eyeglass that is so ground as to permit smooth transition from one correction to the other

om·niv·o·rous \äm-'niv-(ə-)rəs\ *adj* : eating both animal and plant matter — **om·niv·o·rous·ly** *adv* — **om·niv·o·rous·ness** *n*

omo·hy·oid \ˌō-mō-'hī-ˌòid\ *adj* : of or relating to the shoulder and the hyoid bone

omohyoid muscle *n* : a muscle that arises from the upper border of the scapula, is inserted in the body of the hyoid bone, and acts to draw the hyoid bone in a caudal direction — called also *omohyoid*

omo·hy·oi·de·us \-hī-'òid-ē-əs\ *n, pl* **-dei** \-ē-ˌī\ : OMOHYOID MUSCLE

OMPA \'ō-ˌem-ˌpē-'ā\ *n* : OCTAMETHYLPYROPHOSPHORAMIDE

om·pha·lec·to·my \ˌäm(p)-fə-'lek-tə-mē\ *n, pl* **-mies** : surgical excision of the navel — called also *umbilectomy*

omphali *pl of* OMPHALOS

om·phal·ic \(')äm-'fal-ik\ *adj* : of or relating to the navel

om·pha·li·tis \ˌäm(p)-fə-'līt-əs\ *n, pl* **-lit·i·des** \-'līt-ə-ˌdēz\ : inflammation of the navel

om·pha·lo·cele \äm-'fal-ə-ˌsēl, 'äm(p)-fə-lə-\ *n* : protrusion of abdominal contents through an opening at the navel occurring esp. as a congenital defect

om·pha·lo·mes·en·ter·ic \ˌäm(p)-fə-lō-ˌmez-ᵊn-'ter-ik, -ˌmes-\ *adj* : of or relating to the navel and mesentery ⟨∼ vessels⟩

omphalomesenteric artery *n* : an artery that arises in a vertebrate embryo from the aorta or one of the aortic trunks of the embryo, is distributed by numerous branches over the yolk sac, and is usu. paired — called also *vitelline artery*

omphalomesenteric duct *n* : the duct by which the yolk sac or umbilical vesicle remains connected with the alimentary tract of the vertebrate embryo — called also *vitelline duct, yolk stalk*

omphalomesenteric vein *n* : any of the veins in a vertebrate embryo that return the blood from the yolk sac to the heart or later to the portal vein and in mammals have their function of bringing nutriment to the embryo superseded early by that of the umbilical vein — called also *vitelline vein*

om·pha·lo·phle·bi·tis \-fli-'bīt-əs\ *n, pl* **-bit·i·des** \-'bit-ə-ˌdēz\ : a condition (as navel ill) characterized by or resulting from inflammation and infection of the umbilical vein

om·pha·lo·pleure \'äm(p)-fə-lō-ˌplù(ə)r\ *n* : an embryonic membrane constituted in part of the yolk sac wall

om·pha·los \'äm(p)-fə-ˌläs, -ləs\ *n, pl* **-pha·li** \-ˌlī, -ˌlē\ : NAVEL

om·pha·lo·site \-fə-lə-ˌsīt\ *n* : the member of a pair of conjoined twins of unequal size that is smaller and parasitic and that receives its blood supply by way of the larger twin — compare AUTOSITE

Omsk hemorrhagic fever \'ämsk-\ *n* : an acute tick-borne disease occurring in central Russia and caused by a single=

stranded RNA virus of the genus *Flavivirus* (species *Omsk hemorrhagic fever virus*)

on \'ȯn, 'än\ *prep* : regularly using or showing the effects of using ⟨is ~ an ACE inhibitor to control hypertension⟩ ⟨was ~ drugs for two years before entering rehab⟩

onan·ism \'ō-nə-ˌniz-əm\ *n* **1** : MASTURBATION **2** : COITUS INTERRUPTUS — **onan·is·tic** \ˌō-nə-'nis-tik\ *adj*
   Onan \'ō-nən\, Biblical character. In the Book of Genesis Onan was commanded by his father to impregnate the widow of his slain brother and to raise the offspring of the union. In order to avoid raising descendants for his late brother, however, Onan engaged in coitus interruptus.

onan·ist \'ō-nə-nəst\ *n* : an individual that practices onanism

On·cho·cer·ca \ˌäŋ-kə-'sər-kə\ *n* : a genus of long slender filarial worms of the family Dipetalonematidae that are parasites of subcutaneous and connective tissues of mammals with their adults enclosed in fibrous nodules and their larvae free in the tissues — **on·cho·cer·cal** \-kəl\ *adj*

on·cho·cer·ci·a·sis \ˌäŋ-kō-ˌsər-'kī-ə-səs\ *n, pl* **-a·ses** \-ˌsēz\ : infestation with or disease caused by filarial worms of the genus *Onchocerca*; *esp* : a human disease that is marked by subcutaneous nodules, dermatitis, and visual impairment and is caused by a worm (*O. volvulus*) which is found in Africa and tropical America and transmitted by the bite of a female blackfly — called also *onchocercosis, river blindness*; see CRAW-CRAW

on·cho·cer·co·ma \-'kō-mə\ *n* : the subcutaneous nodule of onchocerciasis that contains encysted parasites

on·cho·cer·co·sis \-'kō-səs\ *n, pl* **-co·ses** \-ˌsēz\ : ONCHOCERCIASIS

onchosphere *var of* ONCOSPHERE

on·co·cyte *also* **on·ko·cyte** \'äŋ-kō-ˌsīt\ *n* : an acidophilic granular cell esp. of the parotid gland

on·co·cy·to·ma *also* **on·ko·cy·to·ma** \ˌäŋ-kō-sī-'tō-mə\ *n, pl* **-mas** *also* **-ma·ta** \-mət-ə\ : a tumor (as of the parotid gland) consisting chiefly or entirely of oncocytes

on·co·fe·tal *or Brit* **on·co·foe·tal** \-'fēt-ᵊl\ *adj* : of, relating to, or occurring in both tumorous and fetal tissues

on·co·gen \'äŋ-kə-jən, -ˌjen\ *n* : a substance or agent causing oncogenesis

on·co·gene \'äŋ-kō-ˌjēn\ *n* : a gene having the potential to cause a normal cell to become cancerous

on·co·gen·e·sis \ˌäŋ-kō-'jen-ə-səs\ *n, pl* **-e·ses** \-ˌsēz\ : the induction or formation of tumors

on·co·gen·ic \-'jen-ik\ *also* **on·cog·e·nous** \äŋ-'käj-ə-nəs\ *adj* **1** : relating to tumor formation **2** : tending to cause tumors ⟨an ~ virus⟩ ⟨~ tars⟩ — **on·co·gen·i·cal·ly** \-i-k(ə-)lē\ *adv* — **on·co·ge·nic·i·ty** \-jə-'nis-ət-ē\ *n*

on·co·graph \'äŋ-kō-ˌgraf\ *n* : a recording device attached to an oncometer

on·col·o·gist \än-'käl-ə-jəst, äŋ-\ *n* : a specialist in oncology

on·col·o·gy \-jē\ *n, pl* **-gies** : the study of tumors — **on·co·log·i·cal** \ˌäŋ-kə-'läj-i-kəl\ *also* **on·co·log·ic** \-ik\ *adj*

on·col·y·sis \-'käl-ə-səs\ *n, pl* **-y·ses** \-ˌsēz\ : the destruction of tumor cells — **on·co·lyt·ic** \ˌäŋ-kə-'lit-ik\ *adj* — **on·co·lyt·i·cal·ly** \-i-k(ə-)lē\ *adv*

On·co·me·la·nia \ˌäŋ-kō-mi-'lā-nē-ə\ *n* : a genus of amphibious snails (family Bulimidae) of Asian and Pacific island freshwaters that comprises forms which are intermediate hosts of a schistosome (*Schistosoma japonicum*)

on·com·e·ter \äŋ-'käm-ət-ər, än-\ *n* : an instrument for measuring variations in size or volume of the internal organs of the body — **on·co·met·ric** \ˌäŋ-kə-'me-trik\ *adj*

on·co·pro·tein \ˌäŋ-kō-'prō-ˌtēn, ˌän-, -'prōt-ē-ən\ *n* : a protein that is coded for by a viral oncogene which has been integrated into the genome of a eukaryotic cell and that is involved in the regulation or synthesis of proteins linked to tumorigenic cell growth

on·cor·na·vi·rus \ˌäŋ-ˌkȯ(ə)r-nə-'vī-rəs\ *n* : ONCOVIRUS

on·co·sphere *also* **on·cho·sphere** \'äŋ-kō-ˌsfi(ə)r\ *n* : a tapeworm embryo that has six hooks and is the earliest differentiated stage of a cyclophyllidean tapeworm — called also *hexacanth embryo*

on·cot·ic pressure \(')än-'kät-ik-, (')än-\ *n* : the pressure exerted by plasma proteins on the capillary wall

On·co·vin \'äŋ-kō-ˌvin\ *n* : a preparation of vincristine — formerly a U.S. registered trademark

on·co·vi·rus \'äŋ-kō-ˌvī-rəs\ *n* : any of the tumor-forming RNA viruses formerly grouped in a subfamily (Oncovirinae) of the family (Retroviridae) of retroviruses but now assigned to various genera throughout the family

on·dan·se·tron \än-'dän-si-ˌträn, ōn-\ *n* : an antiemetic drug administered orally or parenterally in the form of its hydrated hydrochloride $C_{18}H_{19}N_3O \cdot HCl \cdot 2H_2O$ to prevent nausea and vomiting esp. when a consequence of chemotherapy or surgery — see ZOFRAN

one–egg \'wən-ˌeg\ *adj* : MONOZYGOTIC ⟨~ twins⟩

onei·ric \ō-'nī-rik\ *adj* **1** : of or relating to dreams **2** : of, relating to, or characterized by oneirism

onei·rism \ō-'nī-ˌriz-əm\ *n* : a dreamlike mental state experienced while awake

onio·ma·nia \ˌō-nē-ō-'mā-nē-ə\ *n* : an abnormal impulse for buying things

oni·um \'ō-nē-əm\ *adj* : being or characterized by a usu. complex cation ⟨~ salts⟩

onkocyte, onkocytoma *var of* ONCOCYTE, ONCOCYTOMA

on·lay \'ȯn-ˌlā, 'än-\ *n* **1** : a metal covering attached to a tooth to restore one or more of its surfaces **2** : a graft applied to the surface of a tissue (as bone)

on·o·mato·ma·nia \ˌän-ə-ˌmat-ə-'mā-nē-ə, -ˌmät-\ *n* : an abnormal obsession with words or names; *esp* : a mania for repeating certain words or sounds

on·set \'ȯn-ˌset, 'än-\ *n* : the initial existence or symptoms of a disease ⟨the ~ of scarlet fever⟩

on·to·gen·e·sis \ˌänt-ə-'jen-ə-səs\ *n, pl* **-gen·e·ses** \-ˌsēz\ : ONTOGENY

on·to·ge·net·ic \-jə-'net-ik\ *adj* : of, relating to, or appearing in the course of ontogeny ⟨~ variation⟩ — **on·to·ge·net·i·cal·ly** \-i-k(ə-)lē\ *adv*

on·to·gen·ic \ˌänt-ə-'jen-ik\ *adj* : ONTOGENETIC — **on·to·gen·i·cal·ly** \-i-k(ə-)lē\ *adv*

on·tog·e·ny \än-'täj-ə-nē\ *n, pl* **-nies** : the development or course of development of an individual organism — called also *ontogenesis*; compare PHYLOGENY 2

on·ych·a·tro·phia \ˌän-i-kə-'trō-fē-ə\ *n* : an atrophic or undeveloped condition of the nails

on·ych·aux·is \ˌän-ik-'ȯk-səs\ *n, pl* **-aux·es** \-ˌsēz\ : abnormal thickening of the nails

on·ych·ec·to·my \ˌän-ik-'ek-tə-mē\ *n, pl* **-mies** : surgical excision of a fingernail or toenail

onych·ia \ō-'nik-ē-ə\ *n* : inflammation of the matrix of a nail often leading to suppuration and loss of the nail

on·y·chi·tis \ˌän-i-'kīt-əs\ *n, pl* **-chit·i·des** \-'kit-ə-ˌdēz\ : ONYCHIA

on·y·cho·cryp·to·sis \ˌän-i-kō-ˌkrip-'tō-səs\ *n, pl* **-to·ses** \-ˌsēz\ : ONYXIS

on·y·cho·dys·tro·phy \-'dis-trə-fē\ *n, pl* **-phies** : any deformity of a nail

on·y·cho·gry·po·sis \-ˌgri-'pō-səs\ *n, pl* **-po·ses** \-ˌsēz\ : an abnormal condition of the nails characterized by marked hypertrophy and increased curvature

on·y·cho·het·ero·to·pia \-ˌhet-ə-rō-'tō-pē-ə\ *n* : a condition characterized by abnormal location of the nails

on·y·chol·y·sis \ˌän-ə-'käl-ə-səs\ *n, pl* **-y·ses** \-ˌsēz\ : a loosening of a nail from the nail bed beginning at the free edge and proceeding to the root

on·y·cho·ma \ˌän-ə-'kō-mə\ *n, pl* **-mas** *or* **-ma·ta** \-mət-ə\ : a tumor originating from a nail bed

on·y·cho·ma·de·sis \ˌän-i-kō-mə-'dē-səs\ *n, pl* **-de·ses** \-ˌsēz\ : loosening and shedding of the nails

on·y·cho·my·co·sis \-mī-'kō-səs\ *n, pl* **-co·ses** \-ˌsēz\ : a fungal disease of the nails

on·y·cho·pha·gia \-'fā-j(ē-)ə\ *n* : NAIL-BITING

on·y·choph·a·gy \ˌän-i-'käf-ə-jē\ *n, pl* **-gies** : NAIL-BITING

on·y·chor·rhex·is \ˌän-i-kə-'rek-səs\ *n, pl* **-rhex·es** \-ˌsēz\ : longitudinal ridging and splitting of the nails

on·y·cho·schiz·ia \-'skit-sē-ə, -'skiz-ē-ə\ *n* : a condition of the nails marked by lamination in two or more layers and by scaling away in thin flakes

on·y·cho·sis \ˌän-ə-'kō-səs\ *n, pl* **-cho·ses** \-ˌsēz\ : a disease of the nails

on·y·cho·til·lo·ma·nia \ˌän-i-kə-ˌtil-ə-'mā-nē-ə, -nyə\ *n* : an obsessive-compulsive disorder marked by the picking at or pulling out of one's fingernails or toenails

onyx·is \ō-'nik-səs\ *n* : an ingrown nail

oo·blast \'ō-ə-ˌblast\ *n* : a cellular precursor of an ovum

oo·cy·e·sis \ˌō-ə-sī-'ē-səs\ *n, pl* **-e·ses** \-ˌsēz\ : extrauterine pregnancy in an ovary

oo·cyst \'ō-ə-ˌsist\ *n* : ZYGOTE; *specif* : a sporozoan zygote undergoing sporogenous development

oo·cyte \'ō-ə-ˌsīt\ *n* : an egg before maturation : a female gametocyte — called also *ovocyte*

oog·a·mous \ō-'äg-ə-məs\ *adj* **1** : characterized by fusion of a small actively motile male gamete and a large immobile female gamete **2** : having oogamous reproduction — **oog·a·my** \-mē\ *n, pl* **-mies**

oo·gen·e·sis \ˌō-ə-'jen-ə-səs\ *n, pl* **-e·ses** \-ˌsēz\ : formation and maturation of the egg — called also *ovogenesis* — **oo·ge·net·ic** \-jə-'net-ik\ *adj*

oo·go·ni·um \ˌō-ə-'gō-nē-əm\ *n* : a descendant of a primordial germ cell that gives rise to oocytes — **oo·go·ni·al** \-nē-əl\ *adj*

oo·ki·nete \ˌō-ə-'kī-ˌnēt, -kə-'nēt\ *n* : a motile zygote in various protozoans (as the malaria parasite)

oo·lem·ma \ˌō-ə-'lem-ə\ *n* **1** : ZONA PELLUCIDA **2** : VITELLINE MEMBRANE

oo·pho·rec·to·mize *or chiefly Brit* **oo·pho·rec·to·mise** \ˌō-ə-fə-'rek-tə-ˌmīz\ *vt* **-mized** *or chiefly Brit* **-mised; -miz·ing** *or chiefly Brit* **-mis·ing** : OVARIECTOMIZE

oo·pho·rec·to·my \ˌō-ə-fə-'rek-tə-mē\ *n, pl* **-mies** : the surgical removal of an ovary — called also *ovariectomy*

oo·pho·ri·tis \ˌō-ə-fə-'rīt-əs\ *n* : inflammation of one or both ovaries — called also *ovaritis*

oo·pho·ro·cys·tec·to·my \ˌō-ə-ˌfôr-ə-ˌsis-'tek-tə-mē\ *n, pl* **-mies** : surgical removal of an ovarian cyst

oophorus — see CUMULUS OOPHORUS

oo·plasm \'ō-ə-ˌplaz-əm\ *n* : the cytoplasm of an egg — **oo·plas·mic** \-mik\ *adj*

oo·spore \'ō-ə-ˌspō(ə)r, -ˌspo(ə)r\ *n* : ZYGOTE; *esp* : a spore produced by heterogamous fertilization that yields a sporophyte

oo·tid \'ō-ə-ˌtid\ *n* : an egg cell after meiosis — compare SPERMATID

oo·type \-ˌtīp\ *n* : the part of the oviduct of most flatworms in which the eggs are furnished with a shell

opaca — see AREA OPACA

opac·i·fi·ca·tion \ō-ˌpas-ə-fə-'kā-shən\ *n* : an act or the process of becoming or rendering opaque ⟨∼ of the cornea⟩ ⟨∼ of the bile passages for radiographic examination⟩

opac·i·fy \ō-'pas-ə-ˌfī\ *vb* **-fied; -fy·ing** *vt* : to cause (as the cornea or internal organs) to become opaque or radiopaque ∼ *vi* : to become opaque or radiopaque

opac·i·ty \ō-'pas-ət-ē\ *n, pl* **-ties** **1** : the quality or state of a body that makes it impervious to the rays of light; *broadly* : the relative capacity of matter to obstruct by absorption or reflection the transmission of radiant energy (as X-rays, infrared radiation, or sound) **2** : an opaque spot in a normally transparent structure (as the lens of the eye)

opal·es·cent \ˌō-pə-'les-²nt\ *adj* : reflecting an iridescent light ⟨saliva is a viscous ∼ fluid⟩ — **opal·es·cence** \-²n(t)s\ *n* — **opal·es·cent·ly** \-²nt-lē\ *adv*

opaque \ō-'pāk\ *adj* : exhibiting opacity : not pervious to radiant energy — **opaque·ness** *n*

OPD *abbr* outpatient department

¹open \'ō-pən\ *adj* **1 a** : not covered, enclosed, or scabbed over ⟨an ∼ lesion⟩ ⟨an ∼ running ulcer⟩ **b** : not involving or encouraging a covering (as by bandages or overgrowth of tissue) or enclosure ⟨∼ treatment of burns⟩ **c** : relating to or being a compound fracture **d** : being an operation or surgical procedure in which an incision is made such that the tissues and organs are fully exposed — compare OPEN-HEART **2** : shedding the infective agent to the exterior ⟨∼ tuberculosis⟩ — compare CLOSED 3 **3 a** : unobstructed by congestion or occlusion ⟨∼ sinuses⟩ **b** : not constipated ⟨∼ bowels⟩ **4** : using a minimum of physical restrictions and custodial restraints on the freedom of movement of the patients or inmates ⟨an ∼ psychiatric ward⟩

²open *vb* **opened; open·ing** *vt* **1 a** : to make available for entry or passage by removing (as a cover) or clearing away (as an obstruction) **b** : to free (a body passage) of congestion or occlusion ⟨an inhalator for ∼*ing* congested nasal passages⟩ ⟨∼ clogged arteries⟩ **2** : to make one or more openings in ⟨∼*ed* the boil⟩ ∼ *vi* : to spread out ⟨the wound ∼*ed*⟩

open–an·gle glaucoma \ˌō-pən-'aŋ-gəl-\ *n* : a progressive form of glaucoma in which the drainage channel for the aqueous humor composed of the attachment at the edge of the iris and the junction of the sclera and cornea remains open and in which serious reduction in vision occurs only in the advanced stages of the disease due to tissue changes along the drainage channel — compare ANGLE-CLOSURE GLAUCOMA

open chain *n* : an arrangement of atoms represented in a structural formula by a chain whose ends are not joined so as to form a ring

open–heart *adj* : of, relating to, or performed on a heart temporarily stopped and relieved of circulatory function and surgically opened for repair of defects or damage ⟨∼ surgery⟩

open·ing \'ōp-(ə-)niŋ\ *n* **1** : an act or instance of making or becoming open **2** : something (as an anatomical aperture) that is open or opens

open–label *adj* : being or relating to a clinical trial in which both the researchers and the patients know who receives the drug and who receives a placebo ⟨long-term ∼ studies⟩ — compare DOUBLE-BLIND, SINGLE-BLIND

open read·ing frame \-'rēd-iŋ-\ *n* : a reading frame that does not contain a nucleotide triplet which stops translation before formation of a complete polypeptide — abbr. *ORF*

open reduction *n* : realignment of a fractured bone after incision into the fracture site — compare CLOSED REDUCTION

op·er·a·ble \'äp-(ə-)rə-bəl\ *adj* **1** : fit, possible, or desirable to use **2** : likely to result in a favorable outcome upon surgical treatment — **op·er·a·bil·i·ty** \ˌäp-(ə-)rə-'bil-ət-ē\ *n, pl* **-ties**

¹op·er·ant \'äp-ə-rənt\ *adj* : of, relating to, or being an operant or operant conditioning ⟨∼ behavior⟩ — compare RESPONDENT — **op·er·ant·ly** *adv*

²operant *n* : behavior (as bar pressing by a rat to obtain food) that operates on the environment to produce rewarding and reinforcing effects

operant conditioning *n* : conditioning in which the desired behavior or increasingly closer approximations to it are followed by a rewarding or reinforcing stimulus — compare CLASSICAL CONDITIONING

op·er·ate \'äp-(ə-)ˌrāt\ *vb* **-at·ed; -at·ing** *vi* : to perform surgery ∼ *vt* : to perform surgery on ⟨*operated* the growth⟩

op·er·at·ing \'äp-(ə-)ˌrāt-iŋ\ *adj* : of, relating to, or used for operations ⟨a hospital ∼ room⟩ ⟨∼ scissors⟩

operating the·atre \-ˌthē-ət-ər\ *n, Brit* : a room where operations are performed

op·er·a·tion \ˌäp-ə-'rā-shən\ *n* : a procedure performed on a living body usu. with instruments for the repair of damage or the restoration of health and esp. one that involves incision, excision, or suturing

op·er·a·tive \'äp-(ə-)rət-iv, 'äp-ə-ˌrāt-\ *adj* : of, relating to, involving, or resulting from an operation ⟨∼ treatment⟩ ⟨∼ mortality rates⟩

op·er·a·tor \'äp-(ə-)ˌrāt-ər\ *n* **1** : one (as a dentist or surgeon) who performs surgical operations **2** : a binding site in a DNA chain at which a genetic repressor binds to inhibit the initiation of transcription of messenger RNA by one or more nearby structural genes — called also *operator gene;* compare OPERON

op·er·a·to·ry \\'äp-(ə-)rə-ˌtōr-ē, -ˌtȯr-\\ *n, pl* **-ries** : a working space (as of a dentist or surgeon) : SURGERY

oper·cu·lec·to·my \\ō-ˌpər-kyə-'lek-tə-mē\\ *n, pl* **-mies** : surgical excision of the mucosa over an unerupted tooth

oper·cu·lum \\ō-'pər-kyə-ləm\\ *n, pl* **-la** \\-lə\\ *also* **-lums** : any of several parts of the cerebrum bordering the sylvian fissure and concealing the insula

op·er·on \\'äp-ə-ˌrän\\ *n* : a group of closely linked genes that produces a single messenger RNA molecule in transcription and that consists of structural genes and regulating elements (as an operator and promoter)

ophid·io·pho·bia \\ō-ˌfid-ē-(ˌ)ō-'fō-bē-ə\\ *n* : abnormal fear of snakes

ophid·ism \\'äf-i-ˌdiz-əm, 'ōf-\\ *n* : poisoning by snake venom

Ophi·oph·a·gus \\ˌō-fē-'äf-ə-gəs\\ *n* : a genus of elapid snakes that includes the king cobra (*O. hannah*)

ophry·on \\'äf-rē-ˌän, 'ōf-\\ *n* : a craniometric point in the median line of the forehead and immediately above the orbits

oph·thal·mia \\äf-'thal-mē-ə, äp-\\ *n* : inflammation of the conjunctiva or the eyeball

ophthalmia neo·na·to·rum \\-ˌnē-ə-nə-'tōr-əm\\ *n* : acute inflammation of the eyes of a newborn from infection during passage through the birth canal

¹**oph·thal·mic** \\-mik\\ *adj* **1** : of, relating to, or situated near the eye **2** : supplying or draining the eye or structures in the region of the eye

²**ophthalmic** *n* : OPHTHALMIC NERVE

ophthalmic artery *n* : a branch of the internal carotid artery following the optic nerve through the optic foramen into the orbit and supplying the eye and adjacent structures

ophthalmic division *n* : OPHTHALMIC NERVE

ophthalmic ganglion *n* : CILIARY GANGLION

ophthalmic glass *n* : glass similar to optical glass but annealed in rolled sheets and used primarily for spectacle lens blanks

ophthalmic nerve *n* : the one of the three major branches or divisions of the trigeminal nerve that supply sensory fibers to the lacrimal gland, eyelids, ciliary muscle, nose, forehead, and adjoining parts — called also *ophthalmic, ophthalmic division;* compare MANDIBULAR NERVE, MAXILLARY NERVE

ophthalmic optician *n, Brit* : OPTOMETRIST

ophthalmic vein *n* : either of two veins that pass from the orbit: **a** : one that begins at the inner angle of the orbit and passes through its superior part and through the superior orbital fissure to empty into the cavernous sinus — called also *superior ophthalmic vein* **b** : one that drains a venous network in the floor and medial wall of the orbit and passes posteriorly dividing into two parts of which one passes through the inferior orbital fissure to join the pterygoid plexus of veins and the other passes through the superior orbital fissure and empties into the cavernous sinus — called also *inferior ophthalmic vein*

oph·thal·mi·tis \\ˌäf-ˌthal-'mīt-əs, ˌäp-, -thəl-\\ *n* : OPHTHALMIA

oph·thal·mo·dy·na·mom·e·try \\äf-ˌthal-mō-ˌdī-nə-'mäm-ə-trē, äp-\\ *n, pl* **-tries** : measurement of the arterial blood pressure in the retina

oph·thal·mo·graph \\äf-'thal-mə-ˌgraf, äp-\\ *n* : an instrument that photographs the movements of the eyes during reading

oph·thal·mol·o·gist \\ˌäf-thə(l)-'mäl-ə-jəst, ˌäp-, -ˌthal-\\ *n* : a physician who specializes in ophthalmology — compare OPTICIAN 2, OPTOMETRIST

oph·thal·mol·o·gy \\-'mäl-ə-jē\\ *n, pl* **-gies** : a branch of medical science dealing with the structure, functions, and diseases of the eye — **oph·thal·mo·log·ic** \\-mə-'läj-ik\\ *or* **oph·thal·mo·log·i·cal** \\-i-kəl\\ *adj* — **oph·thal·mo·log·i·cal·ly** \\-i-k(ə-)lē\\ *adv*

oph·thal·mom·e·ter \\-'mäm-ət-ər\\ *n* : an instrument for measuring the eye; *specif* : KERATOMETER

oph·thal·mom·e·try \\-'mäm-ə-trē\\ *n, pl* **-tries** : the measuring of the corneal curvatures of the eye and of their devia-

tions from normal (as in astigmatism) usu. by means of an ophthalmometer

oph·thal·mo·my·ia·sis \\äf-ˌthal-mō-mī-'ī-ə-səs\\ *n, pl* **-ia·ses** \\-ˌsēz\\ : infestation of the eye with fly larvae (as *Oestrus ovis*)

oph·thal·mo·plas·tic \\-'plas-tik\\ *adj* : of or relating to plastic surgery of the eye or its adnexa ⟨an ~ surgeon⟩

oph·thal·mo·ple·gia \\-'plē-j(ē-)ə\\ *n* : paralysis of some or all of the muscles of the eye — **oph·thal·mo·ple·gic** \\-jik\\ *adj*

oph·thal·mo–re·ac·tion \\-rē-'ak-shən\\ *n* : a serological diagnostic reaction in a test formerly used that involved placing a test antigen (as tuberculin) on the mucous membrane of the eye with infection being indicated by a positive response characterized by hyperemia, swelling, and lacrimation

oph·thal·mo·scope \\äf-'thal-mə-ˌskōp\\ *n* : an instrument for viewing the interior of the eye consisting of a concave mirror with a hole in the center through which the observer examines the eye, a source of light that is reflected into the eye by the mirror, and lenses in the mirror which can be rotated into the opening in the mirror to neutralize the refracting power of the eye being examined and thus make the image of the fundus clear — **oph·thal·mo·scop·ic** \\-ˌthal-mə-'skäp-ik\\ *adj* — **oph·thal·mo·scop·i·cal·ly** \\-i-k(ə-)lē\\ *adv*

oph·thal·mos·co·py \\äf-thal-'mäs-kə-pē\\ *n, pl* **-pies** : examination of the eye with an ophthalmoscope

oph·thal·mo·ste·re·sis \\äf-ˌthal-mō-ster-'ē-səs\\ *n* : loss or absence of an eye

oph·thal·mo·trope \\äf-'thal-mə-ˌtrōp\\ *n* : a mechanical eye for demonstrating the movement of the eye muscles

oph·thal·mo·tro·pom·e·ter \\äf-ˌthal-mō-trō-'päm-ət-ər\\ *n* : an instrument for measuring ocular movements

oph·thal·mo·vas·cu·lar \\-'vas-kyə-lər\\ *adj* : of or relating to the blood vessels of the eye

¹**opi·ate** \\'ō-pē-ət, -ˌāt\\ *n* **1** : a drug (as morphine, heroin, and codeine) containing or derived from opium and tending to induce sleep and to alleviate pain; *broadly* : NARCOTIC 1 **2** : OPIOID 1

²**opiate** *adj* **1** : of, relating to, or being opium or an opium derivative **2** : of, relating to, binding, or being an opiate ⟨~ receptors⟩

opin·ion \\ə-'pin-yən\\ *n* : a formal expression of judgment or advice by an expert ⟨wanted a second ~ on the advisability of performing the operation⟩

¹**opi·oid** \\'ō-pē-ˌȯid\\ *adj* **1** : possessing some properties characteristic of opiate narcotics but not derived from opium **2** : of, involving, or induced by an opioid

²**opioid** *n* **1** : any of a group of endogenous neural polypeptides (as an endorphin or enkephalin) that bind esp. to opiate receptors and mimic some of the pharmacological properties of opiates — called also *opioid peptide* **2** : a synthetic drug (as methadone) possessing narcotic properties similar to opiates but not derived from opium; *broadly* : OPIATE 1

op·is·thap·tor \\ˌäp-is-'thap-tər\\ *n* : the posterior and usu. complex adhesive organ of a monogenetic trematode

opis·the·nar \\ə-'pis-thə-ˌnär\\ *n* : the back of the hand

opis·thi·on \\ə-'pis-thē-ˌän\\ *n, pl* **-thia** \\-thē-ə\\ *or* **-thions** : the median point of the posterior border of the foramen magnum

opis·tho·cra·ni·on \\ə-ˌpis-thō-'krā-nē-ˌän\\ *n* : the posteriormost point in the midsagittal plane of the occiput

op·is·thog·na·thism \\ˌäp-əs-'thäg-nə-ˌthiz-əm\\ *n* : the condition of being markedly opisthognathous

op·is·thog·na·thous \\ˌäp-əs-'thäg-nə-thəs\\ *adj* : having retreating jaws

opis·thor·chi·a·sis \\ə-ˌpis-ˌthȯr-'kī-ə-səs\\ *n* : infestation with or disease caused by liver flukes of the genus *Opisthorchis*

Opis·thor·chi·idae \\ə-ˌpis-ˌthȯr-'kī-ə-ˌdē\\ *n pl* : a family of digenetic trematodes including the genera *Clonorchis* and *Opisthorcis* and comprising trematodes that are parasitic as

---

\\ə\\ **abut** \\ᵊ\\ **kitten** \\ər\\ **further** \\a\\ **ash** \\ā\\ **ace** \\ä\\ **cot, cart**
\\aů\\ **out** \\ch\\ **chin** \\e\\ **bet** \\ē\\ **easy** \\g\\ **go** \\i\\ **hit** \\ī\\ **ice** \\j\\ **job**
\\ŋ\\ **sing** \\ō\\ **go** \\ȯ\\ **law** \\ȯi\\ **boy** \\th\\ **thin** \\t̶h̶\\ **the** \\ü\\ **loot**
\\ů\\ **foot** \\y\\ **yet** \\zh\\ **vision** *See also* Pronunciation Symbols page

O
P

adults in the bile ducts of various birds and mammals including humans, that are ingested with fish as encysted metacercaria and freed in the digestive tract to make their way into the liver, and that are distinguished by the absence of a cirrus pouch and the presence of the ovary anterior to the testes

Op·is·thor·chis \ˌäp-əs-ˈthȯr-kəs\ n : the type genus of the family Opisthorchiidae including several trematodes that are casual or incidental parasites of the human liver

opis·tho·ton·ic \ə-ˌpis-thə-ˈtän-ik\ adj : characteristic of or affected with opisthotonos ⟨an ∼ posture⟩

op·is·thot·o·nos \ˌäp-əs-ˈthät-ᵊn-əs\ n : a condition of spasm of the muscles of the back, causing the head and lower limbs to bend backward and the trunk to arch forward

opis·thot·o·nus \-ᵊn-əs\ n : OPISTHOTONOS

opi·um \ˈō-pē-əm\ n : a highly addictive drug that consists of the dried milky juice from the seed capsules of the opium poppy obtained from incisions made in the unripe capsules of the plant, that has a brownish yellow color, a faint smell, and a bitter and acrid taste, that is a stimulant narcotic usu. producing a feeling of well-being, hallucinations, and drowsiness terminating in coma or death if the dose is excessive, that was formerly used in medicine to soothe pain but is now often replaced by derivative alkaloids (as morphine or codeine) or synthetic substitutes, and that is smoked illicitly as an intoxicant with harmful effects

opium poppy n : an annual Eurasian poppy (*Papaver somniferum*) cultivated since antiquity as the source of opium, for its edible oily seeds, or for its showy flowers

op·o·del·doc \ˌäp-ə-ˈdel-ˌdäk\ n : any of various soap liniments; esp : an unofficial camphorated soap liniment of a soft semisolid consistency

opo·ther·a·py \-ˈther-ə-pē\ n, pl **-pies** : ORGANOTHERAPY

op·po·nens \ə-ˈpō-ˌnenz\ n, pl **-nen·tes** \ˌäp-ə-ˈnen-(ˌ)tēz\ or **-nens** : any of several muscles of the hand or foot that tend to draw one of the lateral digits across the palm or sole toward the others

opponens dig·i·ti min·i·mi \-ˈdij-ə-ˌtī-ˈmin-ə-ˌmī\ n : a triangular muscle of the hand that arises from the hamate and adjacent flexor retinaculum, is inserted along the ulnar side of the metacarpal of the little finger, and functions to abduct, flex, and rotate the fifth metacarpal in opposing the little finger and thumb

opponens pol·li·cis \-ˈpäl-ə-səs\ n : a small triangular muscle of the hand that is located below the abductor pollicis brevis, arises from the trapezium and the flexor retinaculum of the hand, is inserted along the radial side of the metacarpal of the thumb, and functions to abduct, flex, and rotate the metacarpal of the thumb in opposing the thumb and fingers

op·po·nent \ə-ˈpō-nənt\ n : a muscle that opposes or counteracts and limits the action of another

op·por·tun·ist \ˌäp-ər-ˈt(y)ü-nəst\ n : an opportunistic microorganism

op·por·tu·nist·ic \-t(y)ü-ˈnis-tik\ adj 1 : of, relating to, or being a microorganism that is usu. harmless but can become pathogenic when the host's resistance to disease is impaired 2 : of, relating to, or being an infection or disease caused by an opportunistic organism ⟨Pneumocystis carinii pneumonia and other ∼ infections that kill AIDS patients —*N.Y. Times*⟩

op·pos·able \ə-ˈpō-zə-bəl\ adj : capable of being placed against one or more of the remaining digits of a hand or foot ⟨an ∼ thumb⟩ — **op·pos·abil·i·ty** \-ˌpō-zə-ˈbil-ət-ē\ n, pl **-ties**

op·pose \ə-ˈpōz\ vt **op·posed; op·pos·ing** : to place the ball of (a first digit) against the corresponding part of a second digit of the same hand or foot ⟨some monkeys ∼ the big toe⟩

op·po·si·tion·al de·fi·ant disorder \ˌäp-ə-ˈzish-nəl-di-ˈfī-ənt-, -ən-ᵊl-\ n : a disruptive behavior pattern of childhood and adolescence characterized by defiant, disobedient, and hostile behavior esp. toward adults in positions of authority — abbr. *ODD*

op·sin \ˈäp-sən\ n : any of various colorless proteins that in combination with retinal or a related prosthetic group form

a visual pigment (as rhodopsin) in a reaction which is reversed by light

op·son·ic \äp-ˈsän-ik\ adj : of, relating to, or involving opsonin ⟨the ∼ action of a serum⟩

opsonic index n : the ratio of the phagocytic index of a tested serum to that of normal serum taken as the unit

op·son·i·fi·ca·tion \(ˌ)äp-ˌsän-ə-fə-ˈkā-shən\ n : the action or the effect of opsonins in making bacteria more readily phagocytosed

op·so·nin \ˈäp-sə-nən\ n : any of various proteins (as complement or antibodies) that bind to foreign particles and microorganisms (as bacteria) making them more susceptible to the action of phagocytes

op·son·iza·tion \ˌäp-sə-nə-ˈzā-shən, -ˌnī-ˈzā-\ n : the process of modifying (as a bacterium) by the action of opsonins — **op·son·ize** \ˈäp-sə-ˌnīz\ vt **-ized; -iz·ing**

op·so·no·cy·to·pha·gic test \ˌäp-sə-ˌnō-ˌsīt-ə-ˌfā-jik-\ n : a test for immunity to or infection by a pathogenic organism (as of brucellosis or whooping cough) based on the assumption that the serum of an immune or infected individual contains specific opsonins capable of facilitating phagocytosis of the organism in question

opt abbr optician

¹**op·tic** \ˈäp-tik\ adj 1 a : of or relating to vision ⟨∼ phenomena⟩ b : dependent chiefly on vision for orientation ⟨humans are basically ∼ animals⟩ 2 a : of or relating to the eye : OCULAR b : affecting the eye or an optic structure

²**optic** n 1 : any of the elements (as lenses, mirrors, or light guides) of an optical instrument or system — usu. used in pl. 2 : an optical instrument

op·ti·cal \ˈäp-ti-kəl\ adj 1 : of or relating to the science of optics 2 a : of or relating to vision : VISUAL b : using the properties of light to aid vision ⟨an ∼ instrument⟩ 3 : of, relating to, or utilizing light ⟨∼ microscopy⟩

optical activity n : ability of a chemical substance to rotate the plane of vibration of polarized light to the right or left

optical antipode n : ENANTIOMER

optical axis n : a straight line perpendicular to the front of the cornea of the eye and extending through the center of the pupil — called also *optic axis*

optical center n : a point on the axis of a lens that is so located that any ray of light passing through it in passing through the lens suffers no net deviation and that may be within, without, or on either surface of the lens

optical density n : ABSORBANCE

optical fiber n : a single fiber-optic strand

optical glass n : flint or crown glass of well-defined characteristics used esp. for making lenses

optical illusion n : visual perception of a real object in such a way as to misinterpret its actual nature

optical isomer n : one of two or more forms of a compound exhibiting optical isomerism

optical isomerism n : stereoisomerism in which the isomers have different effects on polarized light and in which asymmetry of the molecule as a whole or the presence of one or more asymmetrical atoms is responsible for such effects

op·ti·cal·ly \ˈäp-ti-k(ə-)lē\ adv 1 : by means of sight : with or to the eye ⟨as viewed ∼⟩ 2 : with reference to or by means of optics : with reference to optical properties ⟨object deformation was ... measured ∼ —G. N. Duda *et al*⟩

optically active adj : capable of rotating the plane of vibration of polarized light to the right or left : either dextrorotatory or levorotatory — used of compounds, molecules, or atoms

optically inactive adj : INACTIVE c(2)

optical maser n : LASER

optical path n : the path followed by a ray of light through an optical system

optical rotation n : the angle through which the plane of vibration of polarized light that traverses an optically active substance is rotated

optic angle n 1 : the angle formed by the optical axes of the two eyes when directed to the same point 2 : VISUAL ANGLE

optic atrophy *n* : degeneration of the optic nerve

optic axis *n* : OPTICAL AXIS

optic canal *n* : OPTIC FORAMEN

optic chiasma *n* : the X-shaped partial decussation on the undersurface of the hypothalamus through which the optic nerves are continuous with the brain — called also *optic chiasm*

optic cup *n* : the optic vesicle after invaginating to form a 2-layered cup from which the retina and pigmented layer of the eye will develop — called also *eyecup*

optic disk *n* : BLIND SPOT

optic foramen *n* : the passage through the orbit of the eye in the lesser wing of the sphenoid bone that is traversed by the optic nerve and ophthalmic artery — called also *optic canal;* see CHIASMATIC GROOVE

optic groove *n* : CHIASMATIC GROOVE

op·ti·cian \äp-'tish-ən\ *n* **1** : a maker of or dealer in optical items and instruments **2** : a person who reads prescriptions for visual correction, orders lenses, and dispenses eyeglasses and contact lenses — compare OPHTHALMOLOGIST, OPTOMETRIST

op·ti·cian·ry \-rē\ *n, pl* **-ries** : the profession or practice of an optician

op·ti·cist \'äp-tə-səst\ *n* : a specialist in optics

optic lobe *n* : SUPERIOR COLLICULUS

optic nerve *n* : either of the pair of sensory nerves that comprise the second pair of cranial nerves, arise from the ventral part of the diencephalon, form an optic chiasma before passing to the eye and spreading over the anterior surface of the retina, and conduct visual stimuli to the brain — called also *second cranial nerve*

optic neuritis *n* : inflammation of the optic nerve

optic papilla *n* : a slight elevation that is nearly coextensive with the optic disk and is produced by the thick bundles of the fibers of the optic nerve in entering the eyeball

optic radiation *n* : any of several neural radiations concerned with the visual function; *esp* : one made up of fibers from the pulvinar and the lateral geniculate body to the cuneus and other parts of the occipital lobe

op·tics \'äp-tiks\ *n pl but sing or pl in constr* **1** : a science that deals with the genesis and propagation of light, the changes that it undergoes and produces, and other phenomena closely associated with it **2** : optical properties

optic stalk *n* : the constricted part of the optic vesicle by which it remains continuous with the embryonic forebrain

optic tectum *n* : SUPERIOR COLLICULUS

optic thalamus *n* : LATERAL GENICULATE BODY

optic tract *n* : the portion of each optic nerve between the optic chiasma and the diencephalon proper

optic vesicle *n* : an evagination of each lateral wall of the embryonic vertebrate forebrain from which the nervous structures of the eye develop

op·ti·mal \'äp-tə-məl\ *adj* : most desirable or satisfactory : OPTIMUM ⟨~ concentrations of a drug⟩ — **op·ti·mal·i·ty** \äp-tə-'mal-ət-ē\ *n, pl* **-ties** — **op·ti·mal·ly** \-mə-lē\ *adv*

op·ti·mism \'äp-tə-ˌmiz-əm\ *n* : an inclination to put the most favorable construction upon actions and events or to anticipate the best possible outcome — **op·ti·mist** \-məst\ *n* — **op·ti·mis·tic** \ˌäp-tə-'mis-tik\ *adj*

op·ti·mum \'äp-tə-məm\ *n, pl* **-ma** \-mə\ *also* **-mums** **1** : the amount or degree of something that is most favorable to some end; *esp* : the most favorable condition for the growth and reproduction of an organism **2** : greatest degree attained or attainable under implied or specified conditions — **optimum** *adj*

op·to·gram \'äp-tə-ˌgram\ *n* : an image of an external object fixed on the retina by the photochemical action of light on the rhodopsin

op·to·ki·net·ic \ˌäp-tō-kə-'net-ik, -kī-\ *adj* : of, relating to, or involving movements of the eyes ⟨~ nystagmus⟩

op·tom·e·ter \äp-'täm-ət-ər\ *n* : an instrument for measuring the power and range of vision

op·tom·e·trist \äp-'täm-ə-trəst\ *n* : a specialist licensed to practice optometry — compare OPHTHALMOLOGIST, OPTICIAN 2

op·tom·e·try \-trē\ *n, pl* **-tries** : the health-care profession concerned esp. with examining the eye for defects and faults of refraction, with prescribing corrective lenses or eye exercises, with diagnosing diseases of the eye, and with treating such diseases or referring them for treatment — **op·to·met·ric** \ˌäp-tə-'me-trik\ *adj*

op·to·phone \'äp-tə-ˌfōn\ *n* : an instrument that is designed to enable the blind to read and that scans printed type and translates the light variations into sound variations

op·to·type \-ˌtīp\ *n* : figures or letters of different sizes used in testing the acuity of vision — usu. used in pl.

OPV *abbr* oral polio vaccine

OR *abbr* operating room

ora *pl of* ²OS

orad \'ōr-ˌad, 'ȯr-\ *adv* : toward the mouth or oral region

orae serratae *pl of* ORA SERRATA

oral \'ōr-əl, 'ȯr-, 'är-\ *adj* **1 a** : of, relating to, or involving the mouth : BUCCAL ⟨the ~ mucous membrane⟩ **b** : given or taken through or by way of the mouth ⟨an ~ vaccine⟩ ⟨an ~ suspension of a drug⟩ **c** : acting on the mouth ⟨~ diseases⟩ **2** : emphasizing lipreading and the development of vocal expression in teaching the deaf — compare MANUAL 2 **3 a** : of, relating to, or characterized by the first stage of psychosexual development in psychoanalytic theory during which libidinal gratification is derived from intake (as of food), by sucking, and later by biting **b** : of, relating to, or characterized by personality traits of passive dependence and aggressiveness — compare ANAL 2, GENITAL 3, PHALLIC 2 — **oral·i·ty** \ȯ-'ral-ət-ē, ō-\ *n, pl* **-ties** — **oral·ly** *adv*

oral cavity *n* : the cavity of the mouth; *esp* : the part of the mouth behind the gums and teeth that is bounded above by the hard and soft palates and below by the tongue and by the mucous membrane connecting it with the inner part of the mandible

oral contraceptive *n* : BIRTH CONTROL PILL

oral contraceptive pill *n* : BIRTH CONTROL PILL

ora·le \ō-'rä-lē\ *n* : the point where a line drawn tangent to the inner margin of the sockets of the two middle incisors of the upper jaw and projected onto the hard palate intersects the midsagittal plane

oral hairy leukoplakia *n* : HAIRY LEUKOPLAKIA

oral·ism \'ōr-ə-ˌliz-əm, 'ȯr-, 'är-\ *n* : advocacy or use of the oral method of teaching the deaf

oral·ist \-ləst\ *n* : a person who advocates or uses the oral method of teaching the deaf

oral membrane *n* : BUCCOPHARYNGEAL MEMBRANE

oral·o·gy \ō-'ral-ə-jē, ȯ-\ *n, pl* **-gies** : STOMATOLOGY

oral plate *n* : BUCCOPHARYNGEAL MEMBRANE

oral sex *n* : oral stimulation of the genitals : CUNNILINGUS, FELLATIO

oral surgeon *n* : a specialist in oral surgery

oral surgery *n* **1** : a branch of dentistry that deals with the diagnosis and treatment of oral conditions requiring surgical intervention **2** : a branch of surgery that deals with conditions of the jaws and mouth structures requiring surgery

oral suspension *n* : a suspension consisting of undissolved particles of one or more medicinal agents mixed with a liquid vehicle for oral administration ⟨nystatin powder for *oral suspension*⟩

oral tolerance *n* : the capacity of the immune system to recognize substances taken in through the digestive system and to weaken or suppress the immune response to them

oral tol·er·iza·tion \-ˌtä-lə-rə-'zā-shən\ *n* : treatment of an autoimmune disease by feeding to the affected individual the autoantigen inducing the immune response and causing the disease in order to suppress the immune response by invoking oral tolerance

---

\ə\ **abut** \ᵊ\ **kitten** \ər\ **further** \a\ **ash** \ā\ **ace** \ä\ **cot, cart** \au̇\ **out** \ch\ **chin** \e\ **bet** \ē\ **easy** \g\ **go** \i\ **hit** \ī\ **ice** \j\ **job** \ŋ\ **sing** \ō\ **go** \ȯ\ **law** \ȯi\ **boy** \th\ **thin** \th̲\ **the** \ü\ **loot** \u̇\ **foot** \y\ **yet** \zh\ **vision** *See also* Pronunciation Symbols page

O

P

or·ange \'är-inj, 'òr-\ *n*   **1 a** : a globose berry with a yellowish to reddish orange rind and a sweet edible pulp   **b** : any of various rather small evergreen trees (genus *Citrus*) with ovate leaves, hard yellow wood, fragrant white flowers, and fruits that are oranges   **2** *often cap* : AGENT ORANGE

orange–flower oil *n* : NEROLI OIL

Orange G *n* : an acid azo dye used chiefly in dyeing wool and leather and as a biological stain

orange oil *n* : an essential oil from orange peel or orange flowers: as   **a** : a yellow to deep orange oil obtained from the peel of the sweet fruit of the common cultivated orange (*Citrus sinensis*) and used chiefly as a flavor and perfume — called also *sweet orange oil*   **b** : a similar but bitter pale yellow or yellowish brown oil from the peel of the fruit of the sour orange (*Citrus aurantium*) — called also *bitter orange oil*

orange stick *n* : ORANGEWOOD STICK

orange II \-'tü\ *n* : an acid azo dye used chiefly in dyeing wool and leather, in making pigments, and as a biological stain

or·ange·wood stick \'är-inj-,wùd-'stik, 'òr-\ *n* : a thin stick like a pencil usu. of orangewood and with pointed and rounded ends for manicuring — called also *orange stick*

ora ser·ra·ta \,òr-ə-sə-'rät-ə, -'rāt-\ *n, pl* **orae ser·ra·tae** \,òr-ē-sə-'rāt-ē\ : the dentate border of the retina

or·bic·u·lar \òr-'bik-yə-lər\ *adj* : encircling a part or opening

or·bic·u·lar·is \òr-,bik-yə-'ler-əs\ *n, pl* **-lar·es** \-(,)ēz\ : a muscle encircling an orifice

orbicularis oculi *n, pl* **orbiculares oculi** : the muscle encircling the opening of the orbit and functioning to close the eyelids

orbicularis oris \-'òr-əs\ *n, pl* **orbiculares oris** : a muscle made up of several layers of fibers passing in different directions that encircles the mouth and controls most movements of the lips (as compressing, closing, or pursing movements)

orbicular ligament *n* : ANNULAR LIGAMENT b

orbiculus cil·i·ar·is \-,sil-ē-'er-əs\ *n* : a circular tract in the eye that extends from the ora serrata forward to the posterior or part of the ciliary processes — called also *ciliary ring, pars plana*

or·bit \'òr-bət\ *n* : the bony cavity perforated for the passage of nerves and blood vessels that occupies the lateral front of the skull immediately beneath the frontal bone on each side and encloses and protects the eye and its appendages — called also *eye socket, orbital cavity* — **or·bit·al** \-ᵊl\ *adj*

or·bit·al \'òr-bət-ᵊl\ *n* : a subdivision of a nuclear shell containing zero, one, or two electrons

orbital cavity *n* : ORBIT

or·bi·ta·le \,òr-bə-'tā-lē\ *n, pl* **-lia** \-lē-ə\ : the lowest point on the lower edge of the cranial orbit

orbital fissure *n* : either of two openings transmitting nerves and blood vessels to or from the orbit: **a** : one situated superiorly between the greater wing and the lesser wing of the sphenoid bone — called also *superior orbital fissure, supraorbital fissure*   **b** : one situated inferiorly between the greater wing of the sphenoid bone and the maxilla — called also *inferior orbital fissure, infraorbital fissure, sphenomaxillary fissure*

orbital index *n* : the ratio of the greatest height of the orbital cavity to its greatest width multiplied by 100 where the width is measured from the dacryon to the farthest point on the opposite border and the height is measured along a line perpendicular to the width — see HYPSICONCH, MESOCONCH

orbital plate *n*   **1** : the part of the frontal bone forming most of the top of the orbit   **2** : a thin plate of bone forming the lateral wall enclosing the ethmoidal air cells and forming part of the side of the orbit next to the nose

orbital process *n* : a process of the palatine bone that forms part of the floor of the orbit

or·bi·to·fron·tal \,òr-bit-ə-'frənt-ᵊl\ *adj* : located in, supplying, or being the part of the cerebral cortex in the basal region of the frontal lobe near the orbit ⟨the ~ branch of the middle cerebral artery⟩ ⟨~ blood flow⟩ ⟨the ~ cortex⟩

or·bi·to·nom·e·ter \,òr-bit-ə-'näm-ət-ər\ *n* : an instrument

for measuring the resistance of the eye to pressure exerted into the orbit — **or·bi·to·nom·e·try** \-ə-trē\ *n, pl* **-tries**

¹or·bi·to·sphe·noid \,òr-bit-ō-'sfē-,nòid\ *adj* : being or relating to a paired element of the skull between the presphenoid and frontal bone that in humans forms the lesser wing of the sphenoid

²orbitosphenoid *n* : an orbitosphenoid bone or process (as the lesser wing of the human sphenoid bone)

or·bito·stat \'òr-bit-ə-,stat\ *n* : a device used for measuring the axis of the orbit

or·bi·tot·o·my \,òr-bə-'tät-ə-mē\ *n, pl* **-mies** : surgical incision of the orbit

or·bi·vi·rus \'òr-bi-,vī-rəs\ *n*   **1** *cap* : a genus of double-stranded RNA viruses of the family *Reoviridae* that have a genome composed of 10 segments with the core RNA particles having characteristic ring-shaped capsomers and that include the causative agents of African horse sickness and bluetongue   **2** : any of the genus *Orbivirus* of reoviruses

or·ce·in \'òr-sē-ən\ *n* : a purple nitrogenous dye that is the essential coloring matter of cudbear and archil and that is used as a biological stain

or·chi·dec·to·my \,òr-kə-'dek-tə-mē\ *n, pl* **-mies** : ORCHIECTOMY

or·chi·do·pexy \'òr-kə-dō-,pek-sē\ *n, pl* **-pex·ies** : surgical fixation of a testis — called also *orchiopexy*

or·chi·ec·to·my \,òr-kē-'ek-tə-mē\ *also* **or·chec·to·my** \òr-'kek-tə-mē\ *n, pl* **-mies** : surgical excision of a testis or of both testes — called also *orchidectomy*

orchil *var of* ARCHIL

or·chi·o·pexy \'òr-kē-ō-,pek-sē\ *n, pl* **-pex·ies** : ORCHIDOPEXY

or·chit·ic \òr-'kit-ik\ *adj* : of, relating to, causing, or affected with orchitis

or·chi·tis \òr-'kīt-əs\ *n* : inflammation of a testis

or·cin·ol \'òr-sə-,nòl, -,nōl\ *n* : a crystalline dihydroxy phenol $CH_3C_6H_3(OH)_2$ obtained from various lichens that is used as an analytical reagent

¹or·der \'òrd-ər\ *vt* **or·dered; or·der·ing** \'òrd-(ə-)riŋ\ : to give a prescription for : PRESCRIBE ⟨the doctor ~ed bed rest⟩

²order *n* : a category of taxonomic classification ranking above the family and below the class

or·der·ly \-lē\ *n, pl* **-lies** : a hospital attendant who does routine or heavy work (as carrying supplies or moving patients)

orec·tic \òr-'ek-tik\ *adj* : of or relating to orexis ⟨~ energy⟩

Or·e·gon grape \'òr-i-gən-, ,är-, -,gän-\ *n* : an evergreen shrub of the genus *Mahonia* (*M. aquifolium*) having a rhizome and roots from which various alkaloids (as berberine) are obtained

Oret·ic \òr-'et-ik\ *trademark* — used for a preparation of hydrochlorothiazide

orex·is \òr-'ek-səs\ *n* : the feeling and striving aspect of the mind or of an act as contrasted with the intellectual aspect

orf \'ò(r)f\ *n, chiefly Brit* : SORE MOUTH 1

ORF *abbr* open reading frame

org *abbr* organic

or·gan \'òr-gən\ *n* : a differentiated structure (as a heart or kidney) consisting of cells and tissues and performing some specific function in an organism

or·gan·elle \,òr-gə-'nel\ *n* : a specialized cellular part (as a mitochondrion or ribosome) that is analogous to an organ

¹or·gan·ic \òr-'gan-ik\ *adj*   **1 a** : of, relating to, or arising in a bodily organ   **b** : affecting the structure of the organism ⟨~ disease⟩ — compare FUNCTIONAL 1b   **2 a** (1) : of, relating to, or derived from living organisms   (2) : relating to, yielding, dealing in, or involving the use of food produced with the use of feed or fertilizer of plant or animal origin without employment of chemically formulated fertilizers, growth stimulants, antibiotics, or pesticides ⟨~ stores⟩   **b** (1) : of, relating to, or containing carbon compounds   (2) : relating to, being, or dealt with by a branch of chemistry concerned with the carbon compounds of living beings and most other carbon compounds — **or·gan·i·cal·ly** \-i-k(ə-)lē\ *adv* — **or·ga·nic·i·ty** \,òr-gə-'nis-ət-ē\ *n, pl* **-ties**

²organic *n* : an organic substance: as   **a** : a fertilizer of plant or animal origin **b** : a pesticide whose active component is an organic compound or a mixture of organic compounds

organic brain syndrome *n* : any acute or chronic mental dysfunction (as delirium or senile dementia) resulting chiefly from physical changes in brain structure and characterized esp. by impaired cognition — called also *organic brain disorder, organic mental syndrome*

or·gan·i·cism \or-'gan-ə-ˌsiz-əm\ *n* : a theory that disease is always associated with a structural lesion of an organ

or·gan·i·cist \-səst\ *n* : an advocate of organicism — **or·gan·i·cis·tic** \ˌor-ˌgan-ə-'sis-tik\ *adj*

or·gan·ism \'or-gə-ˌniz-əm\ *n* : an individual constituted to carry on the activities of life by means of organs separate in function but mutually dependent : a living being — **or·gan·is·mic** \ˌor-gə-'niz-mik\ *also* **or·gan·is·mal** \-məl\ *adj* — **or·gan·is·mi·cal·ly** \-mi-k(ə-)lē\ *adv*

or·ga·ni·za·tion *also Brit* **or·ga·ni·sa·tion** \ˌorg-(ə-)nə-'zā-shən\ *n* **1 a** : the act or process of organizing or of being organized **b** : the condition of being organized **2** : the formation of fibrous tissue from a clot or exudate by invasion of connective tissue cells and capillaries from adjoining tissues accompanied by phagocytosis of superfluous material and multiplication of connective tissue cells

organization center *n* : a region in a developing embryo that serves as an organizer

or·ga·nize *also Brit* **or·ga·nise** \'or-gə-ˌnīz\ *vb* **-nized** *also Brit* **-nised; -niz·ing** *also Brit* **-nis·ing** *vt* **1 a** : to cause to develop an organic structure **b** : to cause to undergo organization ⟨an *organized* blood clot⟩ **2** : to arrange or form into a coherent unit or functioning whole ∼ *vi* : to undergo organization ⟨an *organizing* pneumonitis⟩

or·ga·niz·er *also Brit* **or·ga·nis·er** \-ˌnī-zər\ *n* **1** : one that organizes **2** : a region of a developing embryo (as the chordamesoderm of the dorsal lip of the vertebrate blastopore) or a substance produced by such a region that is capable of inducing a specific type of development in undifferentiated tissue — called also *inductor*

organ neurosis *n* : any psychosomatic disorder (as a conversion disorder)

or·gan·o·chlo·rine \or-ˌgan-ə-'klō(ə)r-ˌēn, -'klo(ə)r-, -ən\ *adj* : of, relating to, or being a chlorinated hydrocarbon and esp. one used as a pesticide (as aldrin, DDT, or dieldrin) — **organochlorine** *n*

organ of Cor·ti \-'kort-ē\ *n* : a complex epithelial structure in the cochlea that in mammals is the chief part of the ear by which sound is directly perceived and that rests on the internal surface of the basilar membrane and contains two spiral rows of rods of Corti which arch over a spiral tunnel of Corti and support on the inner side a single row of columnar hair cells and on the outer side several rows having their bases surrounded by nerve-cell arborizations — compare ARCH OF CORTI

Corti, Alfonso Giacomo Gaspare (1822–1876), Italian anatomist. Corti is remembered for his pioneering investigations of the mammalian cochlea. Inspired by the color effect of chromic acid solutions, which were used as fixing agents, he introduced carmine staining into microscopic anatomy. This method enabled Corti to distinguish and describe the individual components of the membranous cochlea. A number of these components including the organ of Corti, the tunnel of Corti, and the rods of Corti are now identified with his name. Corti published his research in 1851.

organ of Jacobson *n* : VOMERONASAL ORGAN

L. L. Jacobson — see JACOBSON'S CARTILAGE

organ of Ro·sen·mül·ler \-'rō-zən-ˌmyü-lər\ *n* : EPOOPHORON

Ro·sen·mül·ler \'röz-ᵊn-ˌmʋel-ər\, **Johann Christian (1771–1820),** German anatomist. Rosenmüller served as professor of anatomy and surgery at a German university. He is remembered for classic descriptions of three anatomical features: the palpebral part of the lacrimal gland (1797), the epoophoron (1802), and the lateral recess of the phar-

ynx situated dorsal and cranial to the eustachian tube (1808). In 1808 he published a handbook of anatomy.

or·gan·o·gel \or-'gan-ə-ˌjel\ *n* : a gel formed by the coagulation of an organosol

or·gan·o·gen·e·sis \ˌor-gə-nō-'jen-ə-səs, or-ˌgan-ə-\ *n, pl* **-e·ses** \-ˌsēz\ : the origin and development of bodily organs — compare MORPHOGENESIS — **or·gan·o·ge·net·ic** \-jə-'net-ik\ *adj*

or·ga·nog·e·ny \ˌor-gə-'näj-ə-nē\ *n, pl* **-nies** : ORGANOGENESIS

or·ga·nog·ra·phy \ˌor-gə-'näg-rə-fē\ *n, pl* **-phies** : a descriptive study of the organs of plants or animals

¹or·gan·oid \'or-gə-ˌnoid\ *adj* : resembling an organ in structural appearance or qualities — used esp. of abnormal masses (as tumors)

²organoid *n* **1** : ORGANELLE **2** : any of various minute organized body structures (as a nematocyst)

or·gan·o·lep·tic \ˌor-gə-nō-'lep-tik, or-ˌgan-ə-\ *adj* **1** : being, affecting, or relating to qualities (as taste, color, odor, and feel) of a substance (as a food or drug) that stimulate the sense organs **2** : involving use of the sense organs ⟨∼ evaluation of foods⟩ — **or·gan·o·lep·ti·cal·ly** \-ti-k(ə-)lē\ *adv*

or·gan·ol·o·gy \ˌor-gə-'näl-ə-jē\ *n, pl* **-gies** : the study of the organs of plants and animals

or·ga·no·meg·a·ly \ˌor-gə-nō-'meg-ə-lē\ *n, pl* **-lies** : abnormal enlargement of the viscera — called also *splanchnomegaly, visceromegaly*

or·gan·o·mer·cu·ri·al \or-ˌgan-ō-(ˌ)mər-'kyur-ē-əl\ *n* : an organic compound or a pharmaceutical preparation containing mercury — **organomercurial** *adj*

or·gan·o·mer·cu·ry \-'mər-k(y)ə-ˌrē\ *adj* : of, relating to, or being an organic compound of mercury ⟨∼ compounds⟩

or·gan·o·me·tal·lic \-mə-'tal-ik\ *adj* : of, relating to, or being an organic compound that usu. contains a metal or metalloid bonded directly to carbon — **organometallic** *n*

or·gan·o·phos·phate \or-ˌgan-ə-'fäs-ˌfāt\ *n* : an organophosphorus compound — **organophosphate** *adj*

or·gan·o·phos·pho·rus \-'fäs-f(ə-)rəs\ *also* **or·gan·o·phos·pho·rous** \-fäs-'fōr-əs, -'for-\ *adj* : of, relating to, or being a phosphorus-containing organic pesticide (as malathion) that acts by inhibiting cholinesterase — **organophosphorus** *n*

or·gan·o·sol \or-'gan-ə-ˌsäl, -ˌsol\ *n* : a sol in which an organic liquid forms the dispersion medium

or·gan·o·ther·a·peu·tic \ˌor-gə-nō-ˌther-ə-'pyüt-ik, or-ˌgan-ə-\ *adj* : of, relating to, or used in organotherapy

or·gan·o·ther·a·py \ˌor-gə-nō-'ther-ə-pē, or-ˌgan-ə-\ *n, pl* **-pies** : treatment of disease by the use of animal organs or their extracts — called also *opotherapy*

or·gan·o·tro·phic \-'trō-fik, -'träf-ik\ *adj* : obtaining energy by the oxidation of organic compounds ⟨∼ bacteria⟩

or·gan·o·trop·ic \ˌor-gə-nō-'träp-ik, or-ˌgan-ə-\ *adj* : having an affinity for particular bodily tissues or organs (as the viscera) ⟨∼ drugs⟩ — **or·gan·o·trop·i·cal·ly** \-i-k(ə-)lē\ *adv*

or·gan·o·tro·pism \-'trō-ˌpiz-əm\ *n* : the quality or state of being organotropic

¹or·gasm \'or-ˌgaz-əm\ *n* : the climax of sexual excitement that is usu. accompanied by ejaculation of semen in the male and by vaginal contractions in the female — **or·gas·mic** \or-'gaz-mik\ *also* **or·gas·tic** \-'gas-tik\ *adj*

²orgasm *vi* : to experience an orgasm ⟨able to ∼ during intercourse —Shere Hite⟩

orib·a·tid \o-'rib-ət-əd, ˌor-ə-'bat-əd\ *n* : any of a superfamily (Oribatoidea) of small oval eyeless nonparastic mites having a heavily sclerotized integument with a leathery appearance — **oribatid** *adj*

ori·ent \'ōr-ē-ˌent, 'or-\ *vt* **1** : to set or arrange in any determinate position esp. in relation to the points of the compass **2** : to acquaint with or adjust according to the existing situa-

O

P

\ə\ abut \ᵊ\ kitten \ər\ further \a\ ash \ā\ ace \ä\ cot, cart
\au̇\ out \ch\ chin \e\ bet \ē\ easy \g\ go \i\ hit \ī\ ice \j\ job
\ŋ\ sing \ō\ go \ȯ\ law \oi\ boy \th\ thin \t̲h̲\ the \ü\ loot
\u̇\ foot \y\ yet \zh\ vision *See also* Pronunciation Symbols page

tion or environment **3** : to cause the axes of the molecules of to assume the same direction

ori·en·tal cockroach \ˌōr-ē-'ent-ᵊl-, ˌȯr-\ n : a dark or blackish brown medium-sized cockroach (*Blatta orientalis*) prob. originating in Asia but now nearly cosmopolitan in warm and temperate areas esp. about dwellings — called also *oriental roach*

oriental rat flea n : a flea of the genus *Xenopsylla* (*X. cheopis*) that is widely distributed on rodents and is a vector of plague

oriental sore n : a skin disease caused by a protozoan of the genus *Leishmania* (*L. tropica*) that is marked by persistent granulomatous and ulcerating lesions and occurs widely in Asia and in tropical regions — called also *Natal sore*

ori·en·ta·tion \ˌōr-ē-ən-'tā-shən, ˌȯr-, -ˌen-\ n **1 a** : the act or process of orienting or of being oriented **b** : the state of being oriented **2** : a usu. general or lasting direction of thought, inclination, or interest — see SEXUAL ORIENTATION **3** : change of position by organs, organelles, or organisms in response to external stimulus **4** : awareness of the existing situation with reference to time, place, and identity of persons ⟨psychological ∼⟩ — **ori·en·ta·tion·al** \-shnəl, -shən-ᵊl\ adj — **ori·en·ta·tion·al·ly** \-ē\ adv

oriented adj : having psychological orientation ⟨the patient was alert and ∼⟩

or·i·fice \'ȯr-ə-fəs, 'är-\ n : an opening through which something may pass — **or·i·fi·cial** \ˌȯr-ə-'fish-əl, ˌär-\ adj

orig·a·num oil \ə-'rig-ə-nəm-\ n : an essential oil obtained from various aromatic plants of the mint or vervain families (esp. genus *Origanum* of the mint family) that was formerly used in pharmacology

or·i·gin \'ȯr-ə-jən, 'är-\ n **1** : the point at which something begins or rises or from which it derives **2** : the more fixed, central, or larger attachment of a muscle — compare INSERTION 1

oris — see CANCRUM ORIS, LEVATOR ANGULI ORIS, ORBICULARIS ORIS

or·li·stat \'ȯr-li-stat\ n : a pancreatic lipase inhibitor $C_{29}H_{53}NO_5$ that prevents the digestion of fat and is administered orally in the treatment of obesity — see XENICAL

Or·mond's disease \'ȯr-ˌmändz-\ n : RETROPERITONEAL FIBROSIS

> **Ormond, John Kelso (1886–1978)**, American urologist. Ormond for many years was in charge of the department of urology at a Detroit hospital before engaging in private practice. In 1948 he published a description of ureteral obstruction resulting from fibrosis of retroperitoneal tissue. From 1952 to 1955 Ormond directed the urological department of a medical center in India.

or·ni·thine \'ȯr-nə-ˌthēn\ n : a crystalline amino acid $C_5H_{12}N_2O_2$ that functions esp. in urea production as a carrier by undergoing conversion to citrulline and then arginine in reaction with ammonia and carbon dioxide followed by recovery along with urea by enzymatic hydrolysis of arginine

ornithine   car·ba·moyl·trans·fer·ase \-ˌkär-bə-ˌmȯil-'tran(t)s-(ˌ)fər-ˌās, -ˌāz\ n : ORNITHINE TRANSCARBAMYLASE

ornithine decarboxylase n : an enzyme that catalyzes the decarboxylation of ornithine to form putrescine

ornithine trans·car·ba·moy·lase \-ˌtran(t)s-ˌkär-bə-'mȯi-ˌläs, -ˌtranz-\ n : ORNITHINE TRANSCARBAMYLASE

ornithine transcarbamylase n : an enzyme of hepatic mitochondria that catalyzes the conversion of ornithine to citrulline as part of urea formation and that when deficient in the body results in hyperammonemia, vomiting, coma, seizures, and sometimes death — called also *ornithine carbamoyltransferase, ornithine transcarbamoylase*

Or·ni·thod·o·ros \ˌȯr-nə-'thäd-ə-rəs\ n : a genus of ticks of the family Argasidae containing forms that act as carriers of relapsing fever as well as of Q fever

Or·ni·thon·ys·sus \ˌȯr-nə-'thän-ə-səs, -thə-'nis-əs\ n : a genus of mites (family Macronyssidae) that are parasitic on vertebrates and include the rat mite (*O. bacoti*) and two serious pests (*O. bursa* and *O. sylviarum*) of domestic fowl

or·ni·tho·sis \ˌȯr-nə-'thō-səs\ n, pl **-tho·ses** \-ˌsēz\ : PSITTACOSIS; esp : a form of the disease occurring in or originating in birds (as the turkeys and pigeons) that do not belong to the family (Psittacidae) containing the parrots

or·nith·uric acid \ˌȯr-nə-ˌthyur-ik-\ n : a crystalline acid $C_{19}H_{20}N_2O_4$ secreted in the urine of birds and reptiles

oro·an·tral \ˌōr-ō-'an-trəl, ˌȯr-\ adj : of, relating to, or connecting the mouth and the maxillary sinus ⟨an ∼ fistula⟩

oro·fa·cial \-'fā-shəl\ adj : of or relating to the mouth and face ⟨∼ abnormalities⟩ ⟨∼ musculature⟩

oro·gas·tric \-'gas-trik\ adj : traversing or affecting the alimentary tract from the mouth to the stomach ⟨the use of ∼ versus nasogastric feeding tubes in infants⟩

oro·man·dib·u·lar \-man-'dib-yə-lər\ adj : of or affecting the mouth and mandible ⟨∼ dystonia⟩

oro·na·sal \-'nā-zəl\ adj : of or relating to the mouth and nose; esp : connecting the mouth and the nasal cavity ⟨∼ fistulae⟩

oro·pha·ryn·geal \-ˌfar-ən-'jē-əl, -fə-'rin-j(ē-)əl\ adj **1** : of or relating to the oropharynx **2** : of or relating to the mouth and pharynx

oropharyngeal airway n : a tube used to provide free passage of air between the mouth and pharynx of an unconscious person

oro·phar·ynx \-'far-in(k)s\ n, pl **-pha·ryn·ges** \-fə-'rin-(ˌ)jēz\ also **-phar·ynx·es** : the part of the pharynx that is below the soft palate and above the epiglottis and is continuous with the mouth

oro·so·mu·coid \ˌȯr-ə-sō-'myü-ˌkȯid\ n : a plasma glycoprotein believed to be associated with inflammation

oro·tate \'ȯr-ə-ˌtāt\ n : a salt of orotic acid; also : the anion of such a salt

orot·ic acid \ȯr-ˌät-ik-\ n : a crystalline acid $C_4H_4N_2O_4$ that occurs in milk and is a growth factor for various microorganisms (as *Lactobacillus bulgaricus*) and a precursor of the pyrimidine bases of nucleotides

oro·tra·che·al \ˌȯr-ō-'trā-kē-əl\ adj : relating to or being intubation of the trachea by way of the mouth

Oroya fever \ȯr-'ȯi-ə-\ n : the acute first stage of bartonellosis characterized by high fever and severe anemia

or·phan disease \'ȯr-fən-\ n : a disease which affects a relatively small number of individuals and for which no drug therapy has been developed because the small market would make the research and the drug unprofitable

orphan drug n : a drug that is not developed or marketed because its extremely limited use (as in the treatment of a rare disease) makes it unprofitable

or·phen·a·drine \ȯr-'fen-ə-drən, -ˌdrēn\ n : a drug used in the form of its citrate $C_{18}H_{23}NO\cdot C_6H_8O_7$ or hydrochloride $C_{18}H_{23}NO\cdot HCl$ as a muscle relaxant and antispasmodic

or·ris·root \'ȯr-əs-ˌrüt, 'är-əs-, -ˌrut\ n : the fragrant rootstock of any of three European irises (*Iris pallida, I. florentina,* and *I. germanica*) used in pulverized form in perfumery and pharmacology — called also *orris*

ORS abbr oral rehydration salts; oral rehydration solution

orth- or **ortho-** prefix **1** : hydrated or hydroxylated to the highest degree ⟨*ortho*phosphoric acid⟩ **2** : involving substitution at or characterized by or having the relationship of two neighboring positions in the benzene ring — abbr. *o-* ⟨*ortho*-xylene or *o*-xylene⟩; compare META- 2, PARA- 2

or·the·sis \ȯr-'thē-səs\ n, pl **or·the·ses** \-ˌsēz\ : a device (as a brace) used in orthopedics

or·thet·ics \ȯr-'thet-iks\ n pl but sing in constr : ORTHOTICS

¹**or·tho** \'ȯr-(ˌ)thō\ adj **1** : derived from or being an acid in the highest hydrated or hydroxylated form known **2** : relating to, characterized by, or being two neighboring positions in the benzene ring

²**ortho** adj : ORTHOCHROMATIC

or·tho·bo·ric acid \ˌȯr-thə-ˌbōr-ik-\ n : BORIC ACID

or·tho·caine \'ȯr-thə-ˌkān\ n : a white crystalline powder $C_8H_9NO_3$ used as a local anesthetic

¹**or·tho·ce·phal·ic** \ˌȯr-thō-sə-'fal-ik\ adj : having a head with a length-height index of 74.9 or less on the skull or of 62.9 or

less on the living head — **or·tho·ceph·a·ly** \-thə-'sef-ə-lē\ *n, pl* **-lies**

²orthocephalic *n* : an orthocephalic individual

or·tho·chro·mat·ic \ˌȯr-thə-krō-'mat-ik\ *adj* **1** : of, relating to, or producing tone values of light and shade in a photograph that correspond to the tones in nature **2** : sensitive to all colors except red **3** : staining in the normal way ⟨~ tissue⟩ ⟨an ~ erythroblast⟩

or·tho·cra·nic \-'krā-nik\ *adj* : ORTHOCEPHALIC — **or·tho·cra·ny** \-nē\ *n, pl* **-nies**

or·tho·cre·sol \-'krē-ˌsȯl, -ˌsōl\ *n* : the ortho isomer of cresol

or·tho·di·a·gram \-'dī-ə-ˌgram\ *n* : a tracing showing the outer contours and exact size of an organ (as the heart) made by illuminating the edge of the organ with parallel X-rays through a small movable aperture and marking the outer edge of the shadow cast upon a fluoroscopic screen

or·tho·di·a·graph \-ˌgraf\ *n* : a fluoroscopic device used in making orthodiagrams

or·tho·di·ag·ra·phy \-dī-'ag-rə-fē\ *n, pl* **-phies** : the making of orthodiagrams — **or·tho·di·a·graph·ic** \-ˌdī-ə-'graf-ik\ *adj*

orth·odon·tia \ˌȯr-thə-'dän-ch(ē-)ə\ *n* **1** : ORTHODONTICS **2** : dental appliances (as braces) used in orthodontic treatment

orth·odon·tics \-'dänt-iks\ *n pl but sing in constr* **1** : a branch of dentistry dealing with irregularities of the teeth and their correction (as by means of braces) **2** : the treatment provided by an orthodontist — **orth·odon·tic** \-ik\ *adj* — **orth·odon·ti·cal·ly** \-i-k(ə-)lē\ *adv*

or·tho·don·tist \ˌȯr-thə-'dänt-əst\ *n* : a specialist in orthodontics

or·tho·dox sleep \'ȯr-thə-ˌdäks-\ *n* : SLOW-WAVE SLEEP

or·tho·drom·ic \ˌȯr-thə-'dräm-ik\ *adj* **1** : proceeding or conducting in a normal direction — used esp. of a nerve impulse or fiber ⟨~ neural stimulation⟩ **2** : characterized by orthodromic conduction ⟨in ~ tachycardia, the atrial impulse conducts in an antegrade direction from the atria through the AV node —Norris Lai & Melvyn Rubenfire⟩ — **or·tho·drom·i·cal·ly** \-i-k(ə-)lē\ *adv*

or·tho·gen·e·sis \ˌȯr-thə-'jen-ə-səs\ *n, pl* **-e·ses** \-ˌsēz\ : variation of organisms in successive generations that in some evolutionary theories takes place in some predestined direction and results in progressive evolutionary trends independent of external factors — **or·tho·ge·net·ic** \-jə-'net-ik\ *adj*

or·thog·na·thism \ȯr-'thäg-nə-ˌthiz-əm\ *or* **or·thog·na·thy** \-nə-thē\ *n, pl* **-thisms** *or* **-thies** : the quality or state of not having the lower parts of the face projecting — **or·thog·na·thous** \-nə-thəs\ *adj*

or·thog·nath·ic \ˌȯr-thəg-'nath-ik, -ˌthäg-\ *adj* : correcting deformities of the jaw and the associated malocclusion ⟨~ surgery⟩

or·thog·o·nal \ȯr-'thäg-ən-ᵊl\ *adj* **1 a** : lying or intersecting at right angles **b** : being, using, or made with three ECG leads whose axes are perpendicular to each other and to the frontal, horizontal, and sagittal axes of the body ⟨the three ~ leads were recorded simultaneously on magnetic tape —Massoud Nemati *et al*⟩ **2** : statistically independent ⟨mental ability may be classified into several ~ . . . factors —O. D. Duncan⟩

or·tho·grade \'ȯr-thə-ˌgrād\ *adj* **1** : walking with the body upright or vertical — compare PRONOGRADE **2** : ANTEROGRADE 2

or·tho·kera·tol·o·gist \ˌȯr-thō-ˌker-ə-'täl-ə-jəst\ *n* : a person who performs orthokeratology

or·tho·kera·tol·o·gy \-'täl-ə-jē\ *n, pl* **-gies** : a treatment for defects of vision by altering the shape of the cornea through the application of a series of differently shaped hard contact lenses

or·tho·mo·lec·u·lar \ˌȯr-thə-mə-'lek-yə-lər\ *adj* : relating to, based on, using, or being a theory according to which disease may be cured by providing the optimum amounts of substances (as vitamins) normally present in the body ⟨~ therapy⟩ ⟨~ psychiatry⟩

Or·tho·myxo·vi·ri·dae \ˌȯr-thō-ˌmik-sə-'vir-ə-ˌdē\ *n pl* : a

family of single-stranded RNA viruses that have a spherical or filamentous virion with numerous surface glycoprotein projections, a helical nucleocapsid, and a genome consisting of six to eight segments of RNA and that include the viruses causing influenza A, influenza B, and influenza C and a genus (*Thogotovirus*) of tick-borne viruses that occas. infect humans

or·tho·myxo·vi·rus \ˌȯr-thō-'mik-sə-ˌvī-rəs\ *n* : any of the family *Orthomyxoviridae* of single-stranded RNA viruses that include the causative agents of influenza in vertebrates — see INFLUENZA VIRUS

Or·tho–No·vum \ˌȯr-thō-'nō-vəm\ *trademark* — used for a preparation of norethindrone and either ethinyl estradiol or mestranol

or·tho·pe·dic *or chiefly Brit* **or·tho·pae·dic** \ˌȯr-thə-'pēd-ik\ *adj* **1** : of, relating to, or employed in orthopedics ⟨~ surgery⟩ ⟨~ casts⟩ **2** : marked by or affected with a deformity, disorder, or injury of the skeleton and associated structures — **or·tho·pe·di·cal·ly** *or chiefly Brit* **or·tho·pae·di·cal·ly** \-i-k(ə-)lē\ *adv*

or·tho·pe·dics *or chiefly Brit* **or·tho·pae·dics** \-'pēd-iks\ *n pl but sing or pl in constr* : a branch of medicine concerned with the correction or prevention of deformities, disorders, or injuries of the skeleton and associated structures (as tendons and ligaments)

or·tho·pe·dist *or chiefly Brit* **or·tho·pae·dist** \-'pēd-əst\ *n* : a specialist in orthopedics

or·tho·pho·ria \ˌȯr-thə-'fōr-ē-ə\ *n* : a normal condition of balance of the ocular muscles of the two eyes in which their lines of vision meet at the object toward which they are directed

or·tho·phos·phate \ˌȯr-thə-'fäs-ˌfāt\ *n* : a salt or ester of orthophosphoric acid

or·tho·phos·pho·ric acid \ˌȯr-thə-ˌfäs-'fȯr-ik-, -, 'fär-; -ˌfäs-f(ə-)rik-\ *n* : PHOSPHORIC ACID 1

or·thop·nea *or chiefly Brit* **or·thop·noea** \ȯr-'thäp-nē-ə *also* ˌȯr-ˌthäp-'nē-ə\ *n* : difficulty in breathing that occurs when lying down and is relieved upon changing to an upright position (as in congestive heart failure) — **or·thop·ne·ic** *or chiefly Brit* **or·thop·noe·ic** \-ik\ *adj*

or·tho·pox·vi·rus \'ȯr-thō-päks-ˌvī-rəs, ȯr-thō-'päks-\ *n* **1** *cap* : a genus of poxviruses that are brick-shaped measuring about 200 by 200 by 250 nanometers, that hybridize extensively within the genus and sometimes with the DNA of members of other poxvirus genera, and that include the vaccina virus and the causative agents of cowpox, monkeypox, mousepox, and smallpox **2** : any of the genus *Orthopoxvirus* of poxviruses

or·tho·praxy \'ȯr-thə-ˌprak-sē\ *n, pl* **-prax·ies** : the correction of physical deformities by means of mechanical appliances

or·tho·psy·chi·a·trist \ˌȯr-thə-sə-'kī-ə-trəst, -(ˌ)sī-\ *n* : a specialist in orthopsychiatry

or·tho·psy·chi·a·try \-sə-'kī-ə-trē, -(ˌ)sī-\ *n, pl* **-tries** : prophylactic psychiatry concerned esp. with incipient mental and behavioral disorders in youth — **or·tho·psy·chi·at·ric** \-ˌsī-kē-'a-trik\ *adj*

or·thop·tic \ȯr-'thäp-tik\ *adj* : of or relating to orthoptics

or·thop·tics \-tiks\ *n pl but sing or pl in constr* : the treatment or the art of treating defective visual habits, defects of binocular vision, and muscle imbalance (as strabismus) by reeducation of visual habits, exercise, and visual training

or·thop·tist \-təst\ *n* : a person specializing in orthoptics

or·tho·rhom·bic \ˌȯr-thə-'räm-bik\ *adj* : of, relating to, or constituting a system of crystallization characterized by three unequal axes at right angles to each other

or·tho·scope \'ȯr-thə-ˌskōp\ *n* : an instrument for examining the superficial parts of the eye through a layer of water which neutralizes the corneal refraction

O
P

\ə\ **abut** \ᵊ\ **kitten** \ər\ **further** \a\ **ash** \ā\ **ace** \ä\ **cot, cart** \aú\ **out** \ch\ **chin** \e\ **bet** \ē\ **easy** \g\ **go** \i\ **hit** \ī\ **ice** \j\ **job** \ŋ\ **sing** \ō\ **go** \ȯ\ **law** \ȯi\ **boy** \th\ **thin** \t͟h\ **the** \ü\ **loot** \ú\ **foot** \y\ **yet** \zh\ **vision** *See also* Pronunciation Symbols page

or·tho·scop·ic \ˌȯr-thə-'skäp-ik\ *adj* : giving an image in correct and normal proportions with a minimum of distortion

or·tho·sis \ȯr-'thō-səs\ *n, pl* **or·tho·ses** \-ˌsēz\ : ORTHOTIC

or·tho·stat·ic \ˌȯr-thə-'stat-ik\ *adj* : of, relating to, or caused by erect posture ⟨∼ hypotension⟩

orthostatic albuminuria *n* : albuminuria that occurs only when a person is in an upright position and disappears upon lying down for a short time

or·tho·stat·ism \ˌȯr-thō-'stat-ˌiz-əm\ *n* : an erect standing position of the body

¹or·thot·ic \ȯr-'thät-ik\ *adj* **1** : of or relating to orthotics ⟨∼ research⟩ **2** : designed for the support of weak or ineffective joints or muscles ⟨∼ devices⟩ ⟨∼ shoe inserts⟩

²orthotic *n* : a support or brace for weak or ineffective joints or muscles — called also *orthosis*

or·thot·ics \-iks\ *n pl but sing in constr* : a branch of mechanical and medical science that deals with the support and bracing of weak or ineffective joints or muscles

or·thot·ist \-əst\ *n* : a person specializing in orthotics

or·tho·top·ic \ˌȯr-thə-'täp-ik\ *adj* : of or relating to the grafting of tissue in a natural position ⟨∼ transplant⟩ — **or·tho·top·i·cal·ly** \-i-k(ə-)lē\ *adv*

Or·tho Tri–Cy·clen \ˌȯr-thō-ˌtrī-'sī-klən\ *trademark* — used for a preparation of norgestimate and ethinyl estradiol

or·tho·volt·age \'ȯr-thō-ˌvōl-tij\ *n* : X-ray voltage of about 150 to 500 kilovolts

ory·ze·nin \ō-'rī-zə-nən\ *n* : a glutelin found in the seeds of rice

¹os \'äs\ *n, pl* **os·sa** \'äs-ə\ : BONE — see OS CALCIS, OS COXAE

²os \'ōs\ *n, pl* **ora** \'ōr-ə, 'ȯr-ə\ : ORIFICE — see INTERNAL OS, PER OS

Os *symbol* osmium

OS *abbr* [Latin *oculus sinister*] left eye — used in writing prescriptions

osa·zone \'ō-sə-ˌzōn, 'äs-ə-\ *n* : any of a class of basic compounds that contain two adjacent hydrazone groups

os cal·cis \-'kal-səs\ *n, pl* **ossa calcis** : CALCANEUS

os·cil·late \'äs-ə-ˌlāt\ *vi* **-lat·ed; -lat·ing 1** : to swing backward and forward like a pendulum **2** : to move or travel back and forth between two points — **os·cil·la·to·ry** \'äs-ə-lə-ˌtōr-ē, -ˌtȯr-\ *adj*

os·cil·la·tion \ˌäs-ə-'lā-shən\ *n* **1** : the action or state of oscillating **2** : a flow of electricity changing periodically from a maximum to a minimum; *esp* : a flow periodically changing direction

os·cil·la·tor \'äs-ə-ˌlāt-ər\ *n* : a device or mechanism for producing or controlling oscillations; *esp* : one (as a radiofrequency generator) for producing an alternating current

os·cil·lo·gram \ä-'sil-ə-ˌgram, ə-\ *n* : a record made by an oscillograph or oscilloscope

os·cil·lo·graph \-ˌgraf\ *n* : an instrument for recording alternating current waveforms or other electrical oscillations — **os·cil·lo·graph·ic** \ä-ˌsil-ə-'graf-ik, ˌäs-ə-lə-\ *adj* — **os·cil·lo·graph·i·cal·ly** \-i-k(ə-)lē\ *adv* — **os·cil·log·ra·phy** \ˌäs-ə-'läg-rə-fē\ *n, pl* **-phies**

os·cil·lom·e·ter \ˌäs-ə-'läm-ət-ər\ *n* : an instrument for measuring the changes in pulsations in the arteries esp. of the extremities — **os·cil·lo·met·ric** \ˌäs-ə-lō-'me-trik\ *adj* — **os·cil·lom·e·try** \-'läm-ə-trē\ *n, pl* **-tries**

os·cil·lop·sia \-'läp-sē-ə\ *n* : a visual disturbance in which objects appear to oscillate

os·cil·lo·scope \ä-'sil-ə-ˌskōp, ə-\ *n* : an instrument in which the variations in a fluctuating electrical quantity appear temporarily as a visible waveform on the fluorescent screen of a cathode-ray tube — called also *cathode-ray oscilloscope* — **os·cil·lo·scop·ic** \ä-ˌsil-ə-'skäp-ik, ˌäs-ə-lə-\ *adj* — **os·cil·lo·scop·i·cal·ly** \-i-k(ə-)lē\ *adv*

os cox·ae \-'käk-ˌsē\ *n, pl* **ossa coxae** : HIP BONE

osel·tam·i·vir \ō-ˌsel-'tam-ə-ˌvir\ *n* : an antiviral drug administered orally in the form of its phosphate $C_{16}H_{28}N_2O_4 \cdot H_3PO_4$ in the treatment and prevention of influenza A and B

Os·good–Schlat·ter's disease \'äz-ˌgud-'shlät-ərz-\ *n* : an

osteochondritis of the tuberosity of the tibia that occurs esp. among adolescent males

Osgood, Robert Bayley (1873–1956), American orthopedic surgeon. Osgood was a professor of orthopedic surgery and chief of staff of the orthopedic department at a Boston hospital. He published several texts on orthopedic surgery and was one of the authors of a 1909 monograph on diseases of the bones. In 1903 he described painful lesions of the tibial tuberosity in children and adolescents.

Schlatter, Carl (1864–1934), Swiss surgeon. A professor of surgery at Zurich, Schlatter is best known for performing the first successful total gastrectomy in 1897. He published, also in 1903, an independent description of the same disease described by Osgood. The disease is now known as Osgood=Schlatter's disease.

Os·ler's maneuver *or* **Os·ler maneuver** \'äs-lər(z)-, 'ōs-\ *n* : a sphygmomanometric procedure of disputed usefulness in detecting false cases of hypertension in the elderly that involves inflating the cuff above the systolic blood pressure and that is held to indicate pseudohypertension if the arteries remain palpable presumably due to inelasticity and sclerosis

W. Osler — see RENDU-OSLER-WEᵦER DISEASE

Osm *abbr* osmol

os·mate \'äz-ˌmāt\ *n* : a salt or ester of osmic acid

os·mic acid \ˌäz-mik-\ *n* : OSMIUM TETROXIDE

os·mics \'äz-miks\ *n pl but sing in constr* : a science that deals with the sense of smell : the study of odors

os·mio·phil·ic \ˌäz-mē-ə-'fil-ik\ *adj* : reacting to or staining with osmium tetroxide usu. by the formation of a black deposit ⟨a strongly ∼ biological membrane⟩ — **os·mi·oph·i·ly** \ˌäz-mē-'äf-ə-lē\ *n, pl* **-lies**

os·mi·um \'äz-mē-əm\ *n* : a hard brittle blue-gray or blue-black polyvalent metallic element of the platinum group with a high melting point that is the heaviest metal known and that is used esp. as a catalyst and in hard alloys — symbol *Os*; see ELEMENT table

osmium tetroxide *n* : a crystalline compound OsO_4 that is an oxide of osmium, has a poisonous irritating vapor, and is used chiefly as a catalyst, as an oxidizing and hydroxylating agent (as in the conversion of alkenes to glycols), and as a biological fixative and stain (as for fatty substances in cytology) — called also *osmic acid*

os·mol *or* **os·mole** \'äz-ˌmōl, 'äs-\ *n* : a standard unit of osmotic pressure based on a one molal concentration of an ion in a solution

os·mo·lal·i·ty \ˌäz-mō-'lal-ət-ē, ˌäs-\ *n, pl* **-ties** : the concentration of an osmotic solution esp. when measured in osmols or milliosmols per 1000 grams of solvent — **os·mo·lal** \äz-'mō-ləl, äs-\ *adj*

os·mo·lar·i·ty \ˌäz-mō-'lar-ət-ē, ˌäs-\ *n, pl* **-ties** : the concentration of an osmotic solution esp. when measured in osmols or milliosmols per liter of solution — **os·mo·lar** \äz-'mō-lər, äs-\ *adj*

os·mom·e·ter \äz-'mäm-ət-ər, äs-\ *n* : an apparatus for measuring osmotic pressure — **os·mo·met·ric** \ˌäz-mə-'me-trik, ˌäs-\ *adj*

os·mom·e·try \-ə-trē\ *n, pl* **-tries** : the measurement of osmotic pressure ⟨molecular weight was determined by ∼⟩

os·mo·phil·ic \ˌäz-mə-'fil-ik\ *adj* also **os·mo·phile** \'äz-mə-ˌfīl\ *adj* : living or thriving in a medium of high osmotic pressure ⟨∼ yeasts that ferment maple syrup⟩

os·mo·phore \'äz-mə-ˌfō(ə)r\ *n* : a group (as an aldehyde group) to whose presence in a molecule the odor of a compound is attributed — **os·mo·phor·ic** \ˌäz-mə-'fȯr-ik\ *adj*

os·mo·re·cep·tor \ˌäz-mō-ri-'sep-tər\ *n* : any of a group of cells sensitive to plasma osmolality that are held to exist in the brain and to regulate water balance in the body by controlling thirst and the release of vasopressin

os·mo·reg·u·la·tion \ˌäz-mō-ˌreg-yə-'lā-shən, ˌäs-\ *n* : regulation of osmotic pressure esp. in the body of a living organism

os·mo·reg·u·la·tor \-'reg-yə-ˌlāt-ər\ *n* : a body mechanism concerned with the maintenance of constant osmotic pressure relationships

os·mo·reg·u·la·to·ry \-'reg-yə-lə-ˌtōr-ē, -ˌtȯr-\ *adj* : of, relating to, or concerned with the maintenance of constant osmotic pressure

os·mo·scope \'äz-mə-ˌskōp\ *n* : an instrument for detecting and for measuring odors

os·mo·sis \äz-'mō-səs, äs-\ *n, pl* **os·mo·ses** \-ˌsēz\ : movement of a solvent through a semipermeable membrane (as of a living cell) into a solution of higher solute concentration that tends to equalize the concentrations of solute on the two sides of the membrane

os·mot·ic \-'mät-ik\ *adj* : of, relating to, or having the properties of osmosis — **os·mot·i·cal·ly** \-i-k(ə-)lē\ *adv*

osmotic pressure *n* : the pressure produced by or associated with osmosis and dependent on molar concentration and absolute temperature: as **a** : the maximum pressure that develops in a solution separated from a solvent by a membrane permeable only to the solvent **b** : the pressure that must be applied to a solution to just prevent osmosis

osmotic shock *n* : a rapid change in the osmotic pressure (as by transfer to a medium of different concentration) affecting a living system

os·phre·si·ol·o·gy \äs-ˌfrē-zē-'äl-ə-jē\ *n, pl* **-gies** : the study of odors and the sense of smell

ossa *pl of* ¹**OS**

ossea — see LEONTIASIS OSSEA

os·se·in \'äs-ē-ən\ *n* : the chief organic substance of bone tissue that remains as a residue after removal of the mineral matters from cleaned degreased bone by dilute acid and is used in making gelatin : the collagen of bones

os·se·let \'äs-(ə-)lət\ *n* : an exostosis on the leg of a horse; *esp* : one on the lateral or anterior aspect of the fetlock occurring chiefly in horses subjected to severe strain while young

os·seo·in·te·gra·tion \ˌäs-ē-ō-ˌint-ə-'grā-shən\ *n* : the firm anchoring of a surgical implant (as in dentistry or in bone surgery) by the growth of bone around it without fibrous tissue formation at the interface — **os·seo·in·te·grat·ed** \-'int-ə-ˌgrāt-əd\ *adj*

os·seo·mu·coid \ˌäs-ē-ō-'myü-ˌkȯid\ *n* : a mucoprotein found in bone

os·se·ous \'äs-ē-əs\ *adj* : of, relating to, or composed of bone — **os·se·ous·ly** *adv*

osseous labyrinth *n* : BONY LABYRINTH

os·si·cle \'äs-i-kəl\ *n* : a small bone or bony structure; *esp* : any of three small bones of the middle ear including the malleus, incus, and stapes — **os·sic·u·lar** \ä-'sik-yə-lər\ *adj*

os·si·cu·lec·to·my \ˌäs-i-kyə-'lek-tə-mē\ *n, pl* **-mies** : the surgical removal of an ossicle of the middle ear

os·si·cu·lot·o·my \-'lät-ə-mē\ *n, pl* **-mies** : the surgical division of one or more of the ossicles of the middle ear

os·sic·u·lum \ä-'sik-yə-ləm\ *n, pl* **-la** \-lə\ : OSSICLE

os·sif·ic \ə-'sif-ik\ *adj* : tending to form bone : making bone

ossificans — see MYOSITIS OSSIFICANS

os·si·fi·ca·tion \ˌäs-ə-fə-'kā-shən\ *n* **1 a** : the process of bone formation usu. beginning at particular centers in each prospective bone and involving the activities of special osteoblasts that segregate and deposit inorganic bone substance about themselves — compare CALCIFICATION a **b** : an instance of this process **2 a** : the condition of being altered into a hard bony substance ⟨∼ of soft tissue⟩ **b** : a mass or particle of ossified tissue : a calcareous deposit in the tissues ⟨∼s in the aortic wall⟩ — **os·si·fi·ca·to·ry** \'äs-ə-fə-kə-ˌtōr-ē, -ˌtȯr-; *esp Brit* ˌäs-ə-fə-'kāt-(ə-)rē\ *adj*

os·si·fy \'äs-ə-ˌfī\ *vb* **-fied; -fy·ing** *vi* : to form or be transformed into bone ⟨cartilage ossified postnatally⟩ ∼ *vt* : to change (as cartilage) into bone ⟨osteoblasts ∼ the tissue⟩

ossium — see FRAGILITAS OSSIUM

ost *abbr* osteopathic

os·te·al \'äs-tē-əl\ *adj* : of, relating to, or resembling bone; *also* : affecting or involving bone or the skeleton

os·tec·to·my \äs-'tek-tə-mē\ *n, pl* **-mies** : surgical removal of all or part of a bone

os·te·itis \ˌäs-tē-'īt-əs\ *n, pl* **-it·i·des** \-'it-ə-ˌdēz\ : inflammation of bone — called also *ostitis* — **os·te·it·ic** \-'it-ik\ *adj*

osteitis de·for·mans \-di-'fȯr-ˌmanz\ *n* : PAGET'S DISEASE 2

osteitis fi·bro·sa \-fī-'brō-sə\ *n* : a disease of bone that is characterized by fibrous degeneration of the bone and the formation of cystic cavities and that results in deformities of the affected bones and sometimes in fracture — called also *osteodystrophia fibrosa*

osteitis fibrosa cys·ti·ca \-'sis-tə-kə\ *n* : OSTEITIS FIBROSA

osteitis fibrosa cystica gen·er·al·is·ta \-ˌjen-ə-rə-'list-ə\ *n* : OSTEITIS FIBROSA

os·teo·ar·thri·tis \ˌäs-tē-ō-är-'thrīt-əs\ *n, pl* **-thrit·i·des** \-'thrit-ə-ˌdēz\ : arthritis typically with onset during middle or old age that is characterized by degenerative and sometimes hypertrophic changes in the bone and cartilage of one or more joints and a progressive wearing down of apposing joint surfaces with consequent distortion of joint position and is marked symptomatically esp. by pain, swelling, and stiffness — abbr. *OA;* called also *degenerative arthritis, degenerative joint disease, hypertrophic arthritis;* compare RHEUMATOID ARTHRITIS — **os·teo·ar·thrit·ic** \-'thrit-ik\ *adj*

os·teo·ar·throp·a·thy \-är-'thräp-ə-thē\ *n, pl* **-thies** : a disease of joints or bones; *specif* : a hypertrophic condition that is marked esp. by clubbing of the fingers and toes, painful swollen joints, and periostitis and subperiosteal bone formation chiefly affecting the long bones (as the radius or fibula) and that usu. occurs secondary to another disease (as bronchiectasis, bronchogenic carcinoma, mesothelioma, or cirrhosis) — called also *acropachy*

os·teo·ar·thro·sis \-är-'thrō-sis\ *n* : OSTEOARTHRITIS — **os·teo·ar·throt·ic** \-'thrät-ik\ *adj*

os·teo·ar·throt·o·my \-är-'thrät-ə-mē\ *n, pl* **-mies** : surgical removal of the articulating end of a bone

os·teo·ar·tic·u·lar \-är-'tik-yə-lər\ *adj* : relating to, involving, or affecting bones and joints ⟨∼ diseases⟩ ⟨∼ grafts⟩

os·teo·blast \'äs-tē-ə-ˌblast\ *n* : a bone-forming cell

os·teo·blas·tic \ˌäs-tē-ə-'blas-tik\ *adj* **1** : relating to or involving the formation of bone **2** : composed of or being osteoblasts

os·teo·blas·to·ma \-bla-'stō-mə\ *n, pl* **-mas** *also* **-ma·ta** \-mət-ə\ : a benign tumor of bone

os·teo·cal·cin \-'kal-sən\ *n* : a protein that is found in the extracellular matrix of bone and in the serum of circulating blood, is produced by osteoblasts esp. in the presence of vitamin K but is not a collagen, and when present at excessive levels in serum may be indicative of various disorders (as Paget's disease or postmenopausal osteoporosis) of bone metabolism

os·teo·car·ti·lag·i·nous \-ˌkärt-ᵊl-'aj-ə-nəs\ *adj* : relating to or composed of bone and cartilage ⟨an ∼ nodule⟩

os·teo·chon·dral \-'kän-drəl\ *also* **os·teo·chon·drous** \-drəs\ *adj* : relating to or composed of bone and cartilage

os·teo·chon·dri·tis \-ˌkän-'drīt-əs\ *n* : inflammation of bone and cartilage

osteochondritis dis·se·cans \-'dis-ə-ˌkanz\ *n* : partial or complete detachment of a fragment of bone and cartilage at a joint

os·teo·chon·dro·dys·pla·sia \-ˌkän-drō-ˌdis-'plā-zh(ē-)ə\ *n* : abnormal growth or development of cartilage and bone

os·teo·chon·dro·ma \-ˌkän-'drō-mə\ *n, pl* **-mas** *also* **-ma·ta** \-mət-ə\ : a benign tumor containing both bone and cartilage and usu. occurring near the end of a long bone

os·teo·chon·drop·a·thy \-ˌkän-'dräp-ə-thē\ *n, pl* **-thies** : a disease involving both bone and cartilage

os·teo·chon·dro·sar·co·ma \-ˌkän-drō-sär-'kō-mə\ *n, pl* **-mas** *also* **-ma·ta** \-mət-ə\ : a sarcoma composed of bone and cartilage

os·teo·chon·dro·sis \-ˌkän-'drō-səs\ *n, pl* **-dro·ses** \-ˌsēz\ : a disease esp. of children and young animals in which an ossification center esp. in the epiphyses of long bones undergoes degeneration followed by calcification — **os·teo·chon·drot·ic** \-'drät-ik\ *adj*

\ə\ abut \ᵊ\ kitten \ər\ **further** \a\ **ash** \ā\ **ace** \ä\ **cot, cart**
\au̇\ **out** \ch\ **chin** \e\ **bet** \ē\ **easy** \g\ **go** \i\ **hit** \ī\ **ice** \j\ **job**
\ŋ\ **sing** \ō\ **go** \ȯ\ **law** \ȯi\ **boy** \th\ **thin** \t̲h̲\ **the** \ü\ **loot**
\u̇\ **foot** \y\ **yet** \zh\ **vision** *See also* Pronunciation Symbols page

O

P

osteochondrous *var of* OSTEOCHONDRAL

os·te·oc·la·sis \ˌäs-tē-ə-'äk-lə-səs\ *n, pl* **-la·ses** \-lə-ˌsēz\ : the breaking of a bone as a step in the correction of a deformity

os·teo·clast \'äs-tē-ə-ˌklast\ *n* **1** : any of the large multinucleate cells closely associated with areas of bone resorption (as in a fracture that is healing) — compare CHONDROCLAST **2** : an instrument for performing osteoclasis — **os·teo·clas·tic** \ˌäs-tē-ə-'klas-tik\ *adj*

os·teo·clas·to·ma \ˌäs-tē-ō-klas-'tō-mə\ *n, pl* **-mas** *also* **-ma·ta** \-mət-ə\ : GIANT-CELL TUMOR

os·teo·cra·ni·um \-'krā-nē-əm\ *n, pl* **-niums** *or* **-nia** \-nē-ə\ : the bony cranium; *esp* : the parts of the cranium that arise in membrane bone — compare CHONDROCRANIUM

os·teo·cyte \'äs-tē-ə-ˌsīt\ *n* : a cell that is characteristic of adult bone and is isolated in a lacuna of the bone substance

os·teo·den·tin \ˌäs-tē-ō-'dent-ᵊn\ *n* : a modified dentin approaching true bone in structure

os·teo·dys·tro·phia \-dis-'trō-fē-ə\ *n* : OSTEODYSTROPHY

osteodystrophia de·for·mans \-di-'fȯr-ˌmanz\ *n* : PAGET'S DISEASE 2

osteodystrophia fi·bro·sa \-fī-'brō-sə\ *n* : OSTEITIS FIBROSA

os·teo·dys·tro·phic \-(ˌ)dis-'trō-fik\ *adj* : of, relating to, or marked by osteodystrophy

os·teo·dys·tro·phy \-'dis-trə-fē\ *n, pl* **-phies** : defective ossification of bone usu. associated with disturbed calcium and phosphorus metabolism

os·teo·fi·bro·sis \-fī-'brō-səs\ *n, pl* **-bro·ses** \-ˌsēz\ : fibrosis of bone

os·teo·gen·e·sis \ˌäs-tē-ə-'jen-ə-səs\ *n, pl* **-e·ses** \-ˌsēz\ : development and formation of bone

osteogenesis im·per·fec·ta \-ˌim-pər-'fek-tə\ *n* : a hereditary disease caused by defective or deficient collagen production and marked by extreme brittleness of the long bones and a bluish color of the whites of the eyes — called also *fragilitas ossium, osteopsathyrosis*

osteogenesis imperfecta con·gen·i·ta \-kən-'jen-ət-ə\ *n* : a severe and often fatal form of osteogenesis imperfecta characterized by usu. multiple fractures in utero

osteogenesis imperfecta tar·da \-'tär-də\ *n* : a less severe form of osteogenesis imperfecta which is not apparent at birth

os·teo·gen·ic \ˌäs-tē-ə-'jen-ik\ *also* **os·teo·ge·net·ic** \-jə-'net-ik\ *adj* **1** : of, relating to, or functioning in osteogenesis; *esp* : producing bone ⟨the ~ layer of the periosteum⟩ **2** : originating in bone

osteogenic sarcoma *n* : OSTEOSARCOMA

os·te·og·e·nous \ˌäs-tē-'äj-ə-nəs\ *adj* : OSTEOGENIC 1

¹os·te·oid \'äs-tē-ˌȯid\ *adj* : resembling bone ⟨~ tissue⟩

²osteoid *n* : uncalcified bone matrix

osteoid osteoma *n* : a small benign painful tumor of bony tissue occurring esp. in the extremities of children and young adults

os·teo·lath·y·rism \ˌäs-tē-ō-'lath-ə-ˌriz-əm\ *n* : a form of lathyrism produced experimentally in laboratory animals that is characterized esp. by skeletal deformities and the formation of aortic aneurisms

os·te·ol·o·gist \ˌäs-tē-'äl-ə-jəst\ *n* : a specialist in osteology

os·te·ol·o·gy \ˌäs-tē-'äl-ə-jē\ *n, pl* **-gies** **1** : a branch of anatomy dealing with the bones **2** : the bony structure of an organism — **os·te·o·log·i·cal** \-tē-ə-'läj-i-kəl\ *adj*

os·te·ol·y·sis \ˌäs-tē-'äl-ə-səs\ *n, pl* **-y·ses** \-ˌsēz\ : dissolution of bone esp. when associated with resorption

os·te·o·lyt·ic \ˌäs-tē-ə-'lit-ik\ *adj* : of, relating to, characterized by, or causing osteolysis ⟨~ lesions⟩ ⟨~ metastases⟩

os·te·o·ma \ˌäs-tē-'ō-mə\ *n, pl* **-mas** *also* **-ma·ta** \-mət-ə\ : a benign tumor composed of bone tissue

os·teo·ma·la·cia \ˌäs-tē-ō-mə-'lā-sh(ē-)ə\ *n* : a disease of adults that is characterized by softening of the bones and is analogous to rickets in the young — **os·teo·ma·la·cic** \-'lā-sik\ *adj*

os·te·o·ma·toid \ˌäs-tē-'ō-mə-ˌtȯid\ *adj* : resembling an osteoma

os·te·o·ma·tous \ˌäs-tē-'ō-mət-əs\ *adj* : of, relating to, or being an osteoma

os·te·om·e·try \ˌäs-tē-'äm-ə-trē\ *n, pl* **-tries** : the measurement of bones; *esp* : anthropometric measurement of the human skeleton — **os·teo·met·ric** \ˌäs-tē-ə-'me-trik\ *adj*

os·teo·my·elit·ic \ˌäs-tē-ō-ˌmī-ə-'lit-ik\ *adj* : of, relating to, characterized by, or caused by osteomyelitis ⟨~ lesions⟩

os·teo·my·eli·tis \-ˌmī-ə-'līt-əs\ *n, pl* **-elit·i·des** \-ə-'lit-ə-ˌdēz\ : an infectious usu. painful inflammatory disease of bone that is often of bacterial origin and may result in death of bone tissue

os·te·on \'äs-tē-ˌän\ *also* **os·te·one** \-ˌōn\ *n* : HAVERSIAN SYSTEM — **os·te·on·al** \ˌäs-tē-'än-ᵊl, -'ōn-\ *adj*

os·teo·ne·cro·sis \ˌäs-tē-ō-nə-'krō-səs\ *n, pl* **-cro·ses** \-ˌsēz\ : necrosis of bone; *esp* : AVASCULAR NECROSIS

os·teo·path \'äs-tē-ə-ˌpath\ *n* : a practitioner of osteopathy

os·te·op·a·thist \ˌäs-tē-'äp-ə-thəst\ *n* : OSTEOPATH

os·te·op·a·thy \ˌäs-tē-'äp-ə-thē\ *n, pl* **-thies** **1** : a disease of bone **2** : a system of medical practice based on a theory that diseases are due chiefly to loss of structural integrity which can be restored by manipulation of the parts supplemented by therapeutic measures (as use of medicine or surgery) — **os·teo·path·ic** \ˌäs-tē-ə-'path-ik\ *adj* — **os·teo·path·i·cal·ly** \-i-k(ə-)lē\ *adv*

os·teo·pe·nia \ˌäs-tē-ō-'pē-nē-ə\ *n* : reduction in bone volume to below normal levels esp. due to inadequate replacement of bone lost to normal lysis — **os·teo·pe·nic** \-'nik\ *adj*

os·teo·peri·os·ti·tis \ˌäs-tē-ō-ˌper-ē-ˌäs-'tīt-əs\ *n* : inflammation of a bone and its periosteum

os·teo·pe·tro·sis \-pə-'trō-səs\ *n, pl* **-tro·ses** \-ˌsēz\ : a condition characterized by abnormal thickening and hardening of bone: as **a** : a rare hereditary disease characterized by extreme density and hardness and abnormal fragility of the bones with partial or complete obliteration of the marrow cavities — called also *Albers-Schönberg disease, marble bone disease, marble bones* **b** : avian leukosis of chickens marked by great enlargement and excessive calcification of the long bones esp. of the legs and by more or less complete obliteration of the marrow cavities — called also *marble bone, marble bone disease*

os·teo·pe·trot·ic \-pə-'trät-ik\ *adj* : of, relating to, characterized by, or affected with osteopetrosis

os·teo·pha·gia \-'fā-j(ē-)ə\ *n* : the eating or chewing of bones by herbivorous animals (as cattle) craving phosphorus

os·teo·phyte \'äs-tē-ə-ˌfīt\ *n* : a pathological bony outgrowth — **os·teo·phyt·ic** \ˌäs-tē-ə-'fit-ik\ *adj*

os·teo·plas·tic \ˌäs-tē-ə-'plas-tik\ *adj* : of, relating to, or being osteoplasty

osteoplastic flap *n* : a surgically excised portion of the skull folded back on a hinge of skin to expose the underlying tissues (as in a craniotomy)

os·teo·plas·ty \'äs-tē-ə-ˌplas-tē\ *n, pl* **-ties** : plastic surgery on bone; *esp* : replacement of lost bone tissue or reconstruction of defective bony parts

os·teo·poi·ki·lo·sis \ˌäs-tē-ō-ˌpȯi-kə-'lō-səs\ *n* : an asymptomatic hereditary bone disorder characterized by numerous sclerotic foci giving the bones a mottled or spotted appearance

os·teo·po·ro·sis \ˌäs-tē-ō-pə-'rō-səs\ *n, pl* **-ro·ses** \-ˌsēz\ : a condition that affects esp. older women and is characterized by decrease in bone mass with decreased density and enlargement of bone spaces producing porosity and brittleness — **os·teo·po·rot·ic** \-'rät-ik\ *adj*

os·teo·psath·y·ro·sis \ˌäs-tē-ō-ˌäp-ˌsath-ə-'rō-səs\ *n, pl* **-ro·ses** \-ˌsēz\ : OSTEOGENESIS IMPERFECTA

os·teo·ra·dio·ne·cro·sis \ˌäs-tē-ō-ˌrā-dē-ō-nə-'krō-səs\ *n, pl* **-cro·ses** \-ˌsēz\ : necrosis of bone following irradiation

os·teo·sar·co·ma \-sär-'kō-mə\ *n, pl* **-mas** *also* **-ma·ta** \-mət-ə\ : a sarcoma derived from bone or containing bone tissue — called also *osteogenic sarcoma*

os·teo·scle·ro·sis \-sklə-'rō-səs\ *n, pl* **-ro·ses** \-ˌsēz\ : abnormal hardening of bone or of bone marrow

os·teo·scle·rot·ic \-'rät-ik\ *adj* : of, relating to, characterized by, or affected with osteosclerosis

osteosclerotic anemia *n* : a form of myelophthisic anemia associated with osteosclerotic changes in the bones

os·teo·syn·the·sis \-'sin(t)-thə-səs\ *n, pl* **-the·ses** \-ˌsēz\ : the operation of uniting the ends of a fractured bone by mechanical means (as a wire or metal plate)

os·te·o·tome \'äs-tē-ə-ˌtōm\ *n* : a chisel without a bevel that is used for cutting bone

os·te·ot·o·my \ˌäs-tē-'ät-ə-mē\ *n, pl* **-mies** : a surgical operation in which a bone is divided or a piece of bone is excised (as to correct a deformity)

Os·ter·ta·gia \ˌäs-tər-'tā-j(ē-)ə\ *n* : a genus of slender brown nematode worms of the family Trichostrongylidae that are parasitic in the abomasum of ruminants

os·ti·al \'äs-tē-əl\ *adj* : of or relating to an ostium ⟨∼ defects⟩

os·ti·tis \ˌäs-'tīt-əs\ *n* : OSTEITIS

os·ti·um \'äs-tē-əm\ *n, pl* **os·tia** \-tē-ə\ : a mouthlike opening in a bodily part (as a fallopian tube or a blood vessel) ⟨stenosis of coronary *ostia* —R. L. Cecil & R. F. Loeb⟩

ostium pri·mum \-'prī-məm\ *n* : an opening between the two embryonic atria of the heart that exists temporarily at the bottom of the developing interatrial septum and is eventually closed off by this septum and replaced by the ostium secundum

ostium se·cun·dum \-sə-'kən-dəm\ *n* : an opening in the upper part of the developing embryonic interatrial septum corresponding to the foramen ovale of the fetus

os·to·mate \'äs-tə-ˌmāt\ *n* : an individual who has undergone an ostomy

os·to·my \'äs-tə-mē\ *n, pl* **-mies** : an operation (as a colostomy, ileostomy, or urostomy) to create an artificial passage for bodily elimination

OT *abbr* **1** occupational therapist; occupational therapy **2** old tuberculin

ot·ac·a·ri·a·sis \ˌōt-ˌak-ə-'rī-ə-səs\ *n, pl* **-a·ses** \-ˌsēz\ : infestation of the ear with mites; *also* : an ear disease (as otodectic mange) resulting from this

otal·gia \ō-'tal-j(ē-)ə\ *n* : EARACHE

otal·gic \-jik\ *n* : a remedy for earache

OTC *abbr* over-the-counter

oth·er–di·rect·ed \ˌəth-ər-də-'rek-təd, -dī-\ *adj* : directed in thought and action primarily by external norms rather than by one's own scale of values — compare INNER-DIRECTED — **oth·er–di·rect·ed·ness** *n*

otic \'ōt-ik\ *adj* : of, relating to, or located in the region of the ear : AUDITORY, AURICULAR

otic capsule *n* : a mesenchymal shell around the auditory vesicle that becomes cartilaginous and bony and develops into the petrous portion of the sphenoid bone

otic ganglion *n* : a small parasympathetic ganglion that is associated with the mandibular nerve, is located just below the foramen ovale of the sphenoid bone, receives preganglionic fibers from the glossopharyngeal nerve by way of the lesser petrosal nerve, and sends postganglionic fibers to the parotid gland by way of the auriculotemporal nerve

otic pit *n* : AUDITORY PIT

otic placode *n* : AUDITORY PLACODE

otic vesicle *n* : AUDITORY VESICLE

oti·tis \ō-'tīt-əs\ *n, pl* **otit·i·des** \ō-'tit-ə-ˌdēz\ : inflammation of the ear — **otit·ic** \-'tit-ik\ *adj*

otitis ex·ter·na \-ek-'stər-nə\ *n* : inflammation of the external auditory canal; *specif* : SWIMMER'S EAR

otitis in·ter·na \-in-'tər-nə\ *n* : inflammation of the inner ear; *specif* : LABYRINTHITIS

otitis me·dia \-'mēd-ē-ə\ *n* : acute or chronic inflammation of the middle ear; *esp* : an acute inflammation esp. in infants or young children that is caused by a virus or bacterium, usu. occurs as a complication of an upper respiratory infection, and is marked by earache, fever, hearing loss, and sometimes rupture of the tympanic membrane — see SEROUS OTITIS MEDIA

oto·ac·a·ri·a·sis \ˌōt-ō-ˌak-ə-'rī-ə-səs\ *n, pl* **-a·ses** \-ˌsēz\ : OTACARIASIS

Oto·bi·us \ō-'tō-bē-əs\ *n* : a genus of argasid ticks that includes the spinose ear tick

oto·car·i·a·sis \ˌōt-ō-kə-'rī-ə-səs\ *n, pl* **-a·ses** \-ˌsēz\ : OTACARIASIS

oto·ceph·a·ly \ˌōt-ə-'sef-ə-lē\ *n, pl* **-lies** : congenital malformation of the head characterized in severe cases by cyclopia, absence of a lower jaw, and joining of the ears below the face — **oto·ce·phal·ic** \-si-'fal-ik\ *adj*

oto·co·nia \-'kō-nē-ə\ *n pl* : small crystals of calcium carbonate in the saccule and utricle of the ear that under the influence of acceleration in a straight line cause stimulation of the hair cells by their movement relative to the gelatinous supporting substrate containing the embedded cilia of the hair cells — called also *statoconia*

oto·cyst \'ōt-ə-ˌsist\ *n* **1** : a fluid-containing organ of many invertebrates that contains an otolith **2** : AUDITORY VESICLE

Oto·dec·tes \ˌōt-ō-'dek-ˌtēz\ *n* : a genus of mites with suckers on the legs that includes one (*O. cynotis*) causing otodectic mange — **oto·dec·tic** \-'dek-tik\ *adj*

otodectic mange *n* : ear mange caused by a mite (*O. cynotis*) of the genus *Otodectes*

otog·e·nous \ō-'täj-ə-nəs\ *adj* : originating in the ear

oto·lar·yn·gol·o·gist \ˌōt-ō-ˌlar-ən-'gäl-ə-jəst\ *n* : a specialist in otolaryngology — called also *otorhinolaryngologist*

oto·lar·yn·gol·o·gy \-ə-jē\ *n, pl* **-gies** : a medical specialty concerned esp. with the ear, nose, and throat — called also *otorhinolaryngology* — **oto·lar·yn·go·log·i·cal** \-ˌlar-ən-gə-'läj-i-kəl\ *adj*

oto·lith \'ōt-ᵊl-ˌith\ *n* : a calcareous concretion in the inner ear of a vertebrate or in the otocyst of an invertebrate that is esp. conspicuous in many bony fishes where it forms a hard body and in most of the higher vertebrates where it is represented by a mass of small calcareous otoconia — called also *statolith* — **oto·lith·ic** \ˌōt-ᵊl-'ith-ik\ *adj*

otol·o·gist \ō-'täl-ə-jəst\ *n* : a specialist in otology

otol·o·gy \-jē\ *n, pl* **-gies** : a science that deals with the ear and its diseases — **oto·log·ic** \ˌōt-ə-'läj-ik\ *also* **oto·log·i·cal** \-'läj-i-kəl\ *adj* — **oto·log·i·cal·ly** \-i-k(ə-)lē\ *adv*

oto·my·co·sis \ˌōt-ō-mī-'kō-səs\ *n, pl* **-co·ses** \-ˌsēz\ : disease of the ear produced by the growth of fungi in the external auditory canal — **oto·my·cot·ic** \-'kät-ik\ *adj*

oto·neu·rol·o·gy \-n(y)ů-'räl-ə-jē\ *n, pl* **-gies** : neurological otology — **oto·neu·ro·log·i·cal** \-ˌn(y)ůr-ə-'läj-i-kəl\ *adj*

oto·plas·ty \'ōt-ə-ˌplas-tē\ *n, pl* **-ties** : plastic surgery of the external ear

oto·rhi·no·lar·yn·gol·o·gist \ˌōt-ō-ˌrī-nō-ˌlar-ən-'gäl-ə-jəst\ *n* : OTOLARYNGOLOGIST

oto·rhi·no·lar·yn·gol·o·gy \ˌōt-ō-ˌrī-nō-ˌlar-ən-'gäl-ə-jē\ *n, pl* **-gies** : OTOLARYNGOLOGY — **oto·rhi·no·lar·yn·go·log·i·cal** \-gə-'läj-i-kəl\ *adj*

otor·rha·gia \ˌōt-ə-'rā-j(ē-)ə\ *n* : hemorrhage from the ear

otor·rhea *or chiefly Brit* **otor·rhoea** \ˌōt-ə-'rē-ə\ *n* : a discharge from the external ear

oto·scle·ro·sis \ˌōt-ō-sklə-'rō-səs\ *n, pl* **-ro·ses** \-ˌsēz\ : growth of spongy bone in the inner ear where it gradually obstructs the oval window or round window or both and causes progressively increasing deafness

oto·scle·rot·ic \-sklə-'rät-ik\ *adj* : of, relating to, or affected by otosclerosis

oto·scope \'ōt-ə-ˌskōp\ *n* : an instrument fitted with lighting and magnifying lens systems and used to facilitate visual examination of the auditory canal and eardrum — **oto·scop·ic** \ˌōt-ə-'skäp-ik\ *adj*

otos·co·py \ō-'täs-kə-pē\ *n, pl* **-pies** : visual examination of the auditory canal and the eardrum with an otoscope

ot·os·te·al \ˌōt-'äs-tē-əl\ *adj* : of or relating to the bones of the ear

oto·tox·ic \ˌōt-ə-'täk-sik\ *adj* : producing, involving, or being adverse effects on organs or nerves involved in hearing or

---

\ə\ abut \ᵊ\ kitten \ər\ **further** \a\ ash \ā\ ace \ä\ cot, cart \aů\ out \ch\ **chin** \e\ bet \ē\ **easy** \g\ go \i\ hit \ī\ ice \j\ job \ŋ\ **sing** \ō\ **go** \ȯ\ **law** \ȯi\ **boy** \th\ **thin** \t̲h̲\ **the** \ü\ **loot** \ů\ **foot** \y\ yet \zh\ **vision** *See also* Pronunciation Symbols page

O
P

balance ⟨an ∼ drug⟩ — **oto·tox·ic·i·ty** \-täk-'sis-ət-ē\ *n, pl* **-ties**

OTR *abbr* registered occupational therapist

oua·bain \wä-'bā-ən, 'wä-₁bān\ *n* : a poisonous glycoside $C_{29}H_{44}O_{12}$ obtained from several African shrubs or trees of the dogbane family and used medically like digitalis and in Africa as an arrow poison

ounce \'aủn(t)s\ *n* **1 a** : a unit of troy weight equal to $\frac{1}{12}$ troy pound or 31.103 grams **b** : a unit of avoirdupois weight equal to $\frac{1}{16}$ avoirdupois pound or 28.350 grams **2** : FLUID OUNCE

out·break \'aủt-₁brāk\ *n* **1** : a sudden rise in the incidence of a disease ⟨an ∼ of measles⟩ **2** : a sudden increase in numbers of a harmful organism and esp. an insect within a particular area ⟨an ∼ of locusts⟩

out·bred \'aủt-₁bred\ *adj* : subjected to or produced by outbreeding

out·breed \-'brēd\ *vt* **out·bred** \-'bred\; **out·breed·ing** \-'brēd-iŋ\ **1** : to subject to outbreeding **2** : to increase in numbers faster than the increase in (a resource or a competing population) ⟨humans may ∼ their food supply⟩

out·breed·ing \'aủt-₁brēd-iŋ\ *n* : the interbreeding of individuals or stocks that are relatively unrelated — compare INBREEDING, LINEBREEDING

¹**out·cross** \'aủt-₁krόs\ *n* **1** : a cross between relatively unrelated individuals **2** : the progeny of an outcross

²**outcross** *vt* : to cross with a relatively unrelated individual or strain

out·cross·ing *n* : a mating of individuals of different strains but usu. of the same breed

out·er·course \'aủt-ər-₁kō(ə)rs, -₁kό(ə)rs\ *n* : physical sexual activity between individuals that typically includes stimulation of the genitalia but does not involve penetration of the vagina or anus with the penis ⟨some people do not include oral sex in ∼ because it can cause transmission of sexually transmitted diseases and HIV⟩

out·er ear \'aủt-ər-\ *n* : the outer visible portion of the ear that collects and directs sound waves toward the tympanic membrane by way of a canal which extends inward through the temporal bone

out·growth \'aủt-₁grōth\ *n* **1** : the process of growing out ⟨in vitro, dopamine modifies axonal and dendritic ∼ —Linda C. Mayes⟩ **2** : something that grows directly out of something else ⟨an ∼ of hair⟩ ⟨a bony ∼⟩

out·let \'aủt-₁let, -lət\ *n* **1** : an opening or a place through which something is let out ⟨the pelvic ∼⟩ **2** : a means of release or satisfaction for an emotion or impulse ⟨counseling provides an ∼ for expressing and evaluating their feelings —Vicki Glaser⟩

outlet forceps *n* : LOW FORCEPS

outlet of the pelvis *n* : PELVIC OUTLET

out–of–body \₁aủt-ə(v)-'bäd-ē\ *adj* : relating to or involving a feeling of separation from one's body and of being able to view oneself and others from an external perspective ⟨an ∼ experience⟩

out·pa·tient \'aủt-₁pā-shənt\ *n* : a patient who is not hospitalized overnight but who visits a hospital, clinic, or associated facility for diagnosis or treatment — compare INPATIENT

out·pock·et·ing \'aủt-₁päk-ət-iŋ\ *n* : EVAGINATION 2

out·pouch·ing \-₁paủch-iŋ\ *n* : EVAGINATION 2

out·put \'aủt-₁pủt\ *n* : the amount of energy or matter discharged usu. within a specified time by a bodily system or organ ⟨renal ∼⟩ ⟨urinary ∼⟩ — see CARDIAC OUTPUT

ova *pl of* OVUM

ov·al·bu·min \₁äv-al-'byü-mən, ₁ōv-\ *n* : the principal albumin of white of egg — called also *egg albumin*

ovale — see FORAMEN OVALE

ova·le malaria \ō-'vä-lē-\ *n* : a relatively mild form of malaria caused by a protozoan of the genus *Plasmodium* (*P. ovale*) that is characterized by tertian chills and febrile paroxysms and that usu. ends spontaneously

ovalis — see FENESTRA OVALIS, FOSSA OVALIS

ovalo·cyte \ō-'val-ə-₁sīt, 'ō-və-lō-₁sīt\ *n* : ELLIPTOCYTE — **ovalo·cyt·ic** \-₁sit-ik\ *adj*

ovalo·cy·to·sis \-₁sī-'tō-səs\ *n, pl* **-to·ses** \-₁sēz\ : ELLIPTOCYTOSIS

oval window \'ō-vəl-\ *n* : an oval opening between the middle ear and the vestibule having the base of the stapes or columella attached to its membrane — called also *fenestra ovalis, fenestra vestibuli*

ovar·i·an \ō-'var-ē-ən, -'ver-\ *also* **ovar·i·al** \-ē-əl\ *adj* : of, relating to, affecting, or involving an ovary ⟨∼ functions⟩

ovarian artery *n* : either of two arteries in the female that correspond to the testicular arteries in the male, arise from the aorta below the renal arteries with one on each side, and are distributed to the ovaries with branches supplying the ureters, the fallopian tubes, the labia majora, and the groin

ovarian follicle *n* : FOLLICLE 3

ovarian ligament *n* : LIGAMENT OF THE OVARY

ovarian vein *n* : either of two veins in the female with one on each side that drain a venous plexus in the broad ligament of the same side, correspond to the testicular veins in the male, and empty on the right into the inferior vena cava and on the left into the left renal vein

ovari·ec·to·mize *or chiefly Brit* **ovari·ec·to·mise** \ō-₁var-ē-'ek-tə-₁mīz, -₁ver-\ *vt* **-mized** *or chiefly Brit* **-mised; -miz·ing** *or chiefly Brit* **-mis·ing** : to surgically remove an ovary from

ovari·ec·to·my \ō-₁var-ē-'ek-tə-mē, -₁ver-\ *n, pl* **-mies** : OOPHORECTOMY

ovar·io·hys·ter·ec·to·my \ō-₁var-ē-ō-₁his-tə-'rek-tə-mē\ *n, pl* **-mies** : surgical removal of the ovaries and the uterus

ovar·io·tes·tis \-'tes-təs\ *n, pl* **-tes·tes** \-₁tēz\ : OVOTESTIS

ovar·i·ot·o·my \ō-₁var-ē-'ät-ə-mē, -₁ver-\ *n, pl* **-mies** **1** : surgical incision of an ovary **2** : OOPHORECTOMY

ova·ri·tis \₁ō-və-'rīt-əs\ *n, pl* **-rit·i·des** \-'rit-ə-₁dēz\ : OOPHORITIS

ova·ry \'ōv-(ə-)rē\ *n, pl* **-ries** : one of the typically paired essential female reproductive organs that produce eggs and in vertebrates female sex hormones, that occur in the adult human as oval flattened bodies about one and a half inches (four centimeters) long suspended from the dorsal surface of the broad ligament of either side, that arise from the mesonephros, and that consist of a vascular fibrous stroma enclosing developing egg cells

over·achiev·er \₁ō-və-rə-'chē-vər\ *n* : one who achieves success over and above the standard or expected level esp. at an early age — **over·achieve** *vi* **-achieved; -achiev·ing**

over·ac·tive \₁ō-və-'rak-tiv\ *adj* : excessively or abnormally active ⟨an ∼ mind⟩ ⟨∼ glands⟩ — **over·ac·tiv·i·ty** \-₁rak-'tiv-ət-ē\ *n, pl* **-ties**

over·ag·gres·sive \₁ō-və-rə-'gres-iv\ *adj* : excessively aggressive ⟨an ∼ personality⟩

overate *past of* OVEREAT

over·bite \'ō-vər-₁bīt\ *n* : the projection of the upper anterior teeth over the lower when the jaws are in the position they occupy in occlusion — compare OVERJET

over·breathe \₁ō-vər-'brēth\ *vi* **-breathed; -breath·ing** : HYPERVENTILATE

over·com·pen·sa·tion \-₁käm-pən-'sā-shən, -₁pen-\ *n* : excessive compensation; *specif* : excessive reaction to a feeling of inferiority, guilt, or inadequacy leading to an exaggerated attempt to overcome the feeling — **over·com·pen·sate** \-'käm-pən-₁sāt\ *vb* **-sat·ed; -sat·ing** — **over·com·pen·sa·to·ry** \-kəm-'pen(t)-sə-₁tōr-ē, -₁tόr-\ *adj*

over·cor·rect \-kə-'rekt\ *vt* : to apply a correction to in excess of that required (as for satisfactory performance); *specif* : to correct (a lens) beyond the point of achromatism or so that there is aberration of a kind opposite to that of the uncorrected lens — **over·cor·rec·tion** \-kə-'rek-shən\ *n*

over·de·ter·mined \-di-'tər-mənd\ *adj* : having more than one determining psychological factor : affording an outlet for more than a single wish or need ⟨an ∼ dream symbol⟩ — **over·de·ter·mi·na·tion** \-di-₁tər-mə-'nā-shən\ *n*

over·di·ag·no·sis \-₁dī-ig-'nō-səs, -əg-\ *n, pl* **-no·ses** \-₁sēz\ : the diagnosis of a condition or disease (as Lyme disease) more often than it is actually present — **over·di·ag·nose** \-'dī-ig-₁nōs, -₁nōz, -₁dī-ig-', -əg-\ *vt* **-nosed; -nos·ing**

over·dig·i·tal·iza·tion *or Brit* **over·dig·i·tal·isa·tion** \ˌō-vər-ˌdij-ət-ᵊl-ə-ˈzā-shən\ *n* : excessive use of digitalis; *also* : the bodily state produced by this

over·dis·ten·sion *or* **over·dis·ten·tion** \-dis-ˈten-chən\ *n* : excessive distension ⟨gastric ∼⟩ ⟨∼ of the alveoli⟩ — **over·dis·tend·ed** \-dis-ˈten-dəd\ *adj*

over·dom·i·nance \-ˈdäm(-ə)-nən(t)s\ *n* : the property of having a heterozygote that produces a phenotype more extreme or better adapted than that of the homozygote — **over·dom·i·nant** \-nənt\ *adj*

over·dos·age \-ˈdō-sij\ *n* **1** : the administration or taking of an excessive dose ⟨guard against ∼ of this drug⟩ **2** : the condition of being overdosed ⟨the symptoms of acute ∼ —Henry Borsook⟩

¹**over·dose** \ˈō-vər-ˌdōs\ *n* : too great a dose (as of a therapeutic agent) ⟨an ∼ of exposure to the sun —Morris Fishbein⟩; *also* : a lethal or toxic amount (as of a drug)

²**over·dose** \ˌō-vər-ˈdōs\ *vb* **-dosed; -dos·ing** *vt* : to give an overdose or too many doses to ∼ *vi* : to take or experience an overdose — usu. used *with on*

over·eat \ˌō-və-ˈrēt\ *vi* **over·ate** \-ˈrāt\; **over·eat·en** \-ˈrēt-ᵊn\; **over·eat·ing** : to eat to excess — **over·eat·er** *n*

overeating disease *n* : ENTEROTOXEMIA

over·ex·ert \ˌō-və-rig-ˈzərt\ *vt* : to exert (oneself) too much ∼ *vi* : to exert oneself to excess — **over·ex·er·tion** \-ˈzər-shən\ *n*

over·ex·pose \ˌō-və-rik-ˈspōz\ *vt* **-posed; -pos·ing** : to expose excessively ⟨skin *overexposed* to sunlight⟩ — **over·ex·po·sure** \-ˈspō-zhər\ *n*

over·ex·pres·sion \-rik-ˈspresh-ən\ *n* : excessive expression of a gene by producing too much of its effect or product ⟨we now suspect that many, if not most, cancers arise through the ∼ . . . of key cellular regulatory genes —J. D. Watson *et al*⟩ — **over·ex·press** \-rik-ˈspres\ *vt*

over·ex·tend \ˌō-və-rik-ˈstend\ *vt* : to extend too far ⟨∼ the back⟩ — **over·ex·ten·sion** \-ˈsten-chən\ *n*

over·fa·tigue \ˌō-vər-fə-ˈtēg\ *n* : excessive fatigue esp. when carried beyond the recuperative capacity of the individual

over·feed \ˌō-vər-ˈfēd\ *vb* **-fed** \-ˈfed\; **-feed·ing** *vt* : to feed to excess ∼ *vi* : to eat to excess

over·flow \ˈō-vər-ˌflō\ *n* : an excessive flow or amount

over·grow \ˌō-vər-ˈgrō\ *vi* **-grew** \-ˈgrü\; **-grown** \-ˈgrōn\; **-grow·ing** : to grow or increase beyond the normal or natural size or numbers ⟨when a scar ∼s into a keloid —Morris Fishbein⟩

over·growth \ˈō-vər-ˌgrōth\ *n* **1 a** : excessive growth or increase in numbers ⟨an ∼ of bacteria . . . may achieve pathogenic proportions —*Jour. Amer. Med. Assoc.*⟩ ⟨an ∼ of yeast in the mouth⟩ **b** : HYPERTROPHY, HYPERPLASIA **2** : something (as cells or tissue) grown over something else

over·hang \ˈō-vər-ˌhaŋ\ *n* : a portion of a filling that extends beyond the normal contour of a tooth

over·hy·dra·tion \ˌō-vər-hī-ˈdrā-shən\ *n* : a condition in which the body contains an excessive amount of fluids

over·iden·ti·fi·ca·tion \-ī-ˌdent-ə-fə-ˈkā-shən\ *n* : excessive psychological identification ⟨∼ with his father⟩ — **over·iden·ti·fy** \-ī-ˈdent-ə-ˌfī\ *vi* **-fied; -fy·ing**

over·jet \ˈō-vər-ˌjet\ *n* : displacement of the mandibular teeth sideways when the jaws are held in the position they occupy in occlusion — compare OVERBITE

over·lie \ˌō-vər-ˈlī\ *vt* **-lay** \-ˈlā\; **-lain** \-ˈlān\; **-ly·ing** \-ˈlī-iŋ\ : to cause the death of by lying upon

over·med·i·cate \-ˈmed-i-ˌkāt\ *vb* **-cat·ed; -cat·ing** *vt* : to administer too much medication to : prescribe too much medication for ∼ *vi* : to administer or prescribe too much medication — **over·med·i·ca·tion** \-ˌmed-i-ˈkā-shən\ *n*

over·nu·tri·tion \ˌō-vər-n(y)ü-ˈtrish-ən\ *n* : excessive food intake esp. when viewed as a factor in pathology

over·pop·u·la·tion \ˌō-vər-ˌpäp-yə-ˈlā-shən\ *n* : the condition of having a population so dense as to cause environmental deterioration, an impaired quality of life, or a population crash — **over·pop·u·lat·ed** \-ˈpäp-yə-ˌlāt-əd\ *adj*

over·pre·scribe \-pri-ˈskrīb\ *vb* **-scribed; -scrib·ing** *vi* : to prescribe excessive or unnecessary medication ∼ *vt* : to pre-

scribe (medication) unnecessarily or to excess — **over·pre·scrip·tion** \-pri-ˈskrip-shən\ *n*

over·pro·duce \-prə-ˈd(y)üs, -prō-\ *vt* **-duced; -duc·ing** : to produce to excess ⟨mice genetically altered to ∼ betaᵃ amyloid —Richard Saltus⟩ — **over·pro·duc·tion** \-ˈdək-shən\ *n*

over·pro·na·tion \-prō-ˈnā-shən\ *n* : excessive pronation of the foot in walking or running that predisposes the individual to injuries on the medial side of the lower extremities and that causes heavier wear on shoes on the inner margin — **over·pro·nate** \-ˈprō-ˌnāt\ *vi* **-nat·ed; -nat·ing** — **over·pro·na·tor** \-ˈprō-ˌnāt-ər\ *n*

over·pro·tect \-prə-ˈtekt\ *vt* : to protect unduly ⟨∼ed children⟩ — **over·pro·tec·tive** \-ˈtek-tiv\ *adj*

over·pro·tec·tion \-prə-ˈtek-shən\ *n* : undue or excessive protection or shielding; *specif* : excessive restriction of a child's behavior allegedly in the interest of his or her health and welfare by an anxious, insecure, or domineering parent

over·reach \-ˈrēch\ *vi, of a horse* : to strike the toe of the hind foot against the heel or quarter of the forefoot

over·re·act \ˌō-və(r)-rē-ˈakt\ *vi* : to react excessively or too strongly ⟨the body's immune system ∼s to the endotoxin —Tina Adler⟩ — **over·re·ac·tion** \-ˈak-shən\ *n*

over·se·da·tion \ˌō-vər-si-ˈdā-shən\ *n* : excessive sedation

over·shoot \ˈō-vər-ˌshüt\ *n* : a rapid change in electrical potential and reversal of polarity that occurs during an action potential when a cell or tissue is stimulated

over·shot \ˈō-vər-ˌshät\ *adj* **1** : having the upper jaw extending beyond the lower **2** : projecting beyond the lower jaw

over·stim·u·la·tion \ˌō-vər-ˌstim-yə-ˈlā-shən\ *n* : excessive stimulation ⟨∼ of the pancreas⟩ — **over·stim·u·late** \-ˈstim-yə-ˌlāt\ *vt* **-lat·ed; -lat·ing**

over·strain \-ˈstrān\ *n* : excessive mental or physical strain; *also* : a condition resulting from this — **overstrain** *vb*

overt \ō-ˈvərt, ˈō-ˌvərt *also* ˈō-vərt\ *adj* : open to view : readily perceived ⟨∼ behavior⟩ — **overt·ly** *adv*

over–the–counter *adj* : sold lawfully without prescription ⟨an ∼ painkiller⟩

over·tone \ˈō-vər-ˌtōn\ *n* : one of the higher tones produced simultaneously with the fundamental and that with the fundamental comprise a complex musical tone

over·ven·ti·la·tion \ˌō-vər-ˌvent-ᵊl-ˈā-shən\ *n* : HYPERVENTILATION

over·weight \-ˈwāt\ *adj* : weighing in excess of the normal for one's age, height, and build ⟨∼ adolescents⟩ ⟨∼ adults typically have a body mass index of 25 to 29.9⟩ — **overweight** *n*

over·work \ˌō-vər-ˈwərk\ *vt* : to cause to work too hard, too long, or to exhaustion ∼ *vi* : to work too much or too long — **overwork** *n*

ovi·cid·al \ˌō-və-ˈsīd-ᵊl\ *adj* : capable of killing eggs

ovi·cide \ˈō-və-ˌsīd\ *n* : an agent that kills eggs; *esp* : an insecticide effective against the egg stage

ovi·du·cal \ˌō-və-ˈd(y)ü-kəl\ *adj* : OVIDUCTAL

ovi·duct \ˈō-və-ˌdəkt\ *n* : a tube that allows for the passage of eggs from an ovary

ovi·duc·tal \ˌō-və-ˈdək-tᵊl\ *adj* : of, relating to, or affecting an oviduct ⟨∼ carcinomas⟩ ⟨∼ surgery⟩

ovi·form \ˈō-və-ˌform\ *adj* : shaped like an egg

ovi·gen·e·sis \ˌō-və-ˈjen-ə-səs\ *n, pl* **-e·ses** \-ˌsēz\ : OOGENESIS

ovi·ge·net·ic \-jə-ˈnet-ik\ *adj* : OOGENETIC

ovig·er·ous \ō-ˈvij-(ə-)rəs\ *adj* : bearing or modified for the purpose of bearing eggs

ovine \ˈō-ˌvīn\ *adj* : of, relating to, or resembling sheep ⟨∼ growth hormone⟩

ovine progressive pneumonia *n* : a chronic disease esp. of sheep caused by a retrovirus of the genus *Lentivirus* (species *Visna/maedi virus*) and occurring in a respiratory form that

---

\ə\ **abut** \ᵊ\ **kitten** \ər\ **further** \a\ **ash** \ā\ **ace** \ä\ **cot, cart**
\aú\ **out** \ch\ **chin** \e\ **bet** \ē\ **easy** \g\ **go** \i\ **hit** \ī\ **ice** \j\ **job**
\ŋ\ **sing** \ō\ **go** \ò\ **law** \òi\ **boy** \th\ **thin** \th̲\ **the** \ü\ **loot**
\ú\ **foot** \y\ **yet** \zh\ **vision** *See also* Pronunciation Symbols page

O

P

affects the lungs and udder and produces progressive wasting and in an encephalitic form that affects the central nervous system and joints and leads eventually to paralysis — see MAEDI, VISNA

ovine pulmonary adenocarcinoma *n* : JAAGSIEKTE

ovine pulmonary adenomatosis *n* : JAAGSIEKTE

ovin·ia \ō-'vin-ē-ə\ *n* : SHEEP POX

ovi·par·i·ty \ˌō-və-'par-ət-ē\ *n, pl* **-ties** : the quality or state of being oviparous

ovip·a·rous \ō-'vip-(ə-)rəs\ *adj* : producing eggs that develop and hatch outside the maternal body; *also* : involving the production of such eggs — compare LARVIPAROUS, OVOVIVIPAROUS, VIVIPAROUS — **ovip·a·rous·ness** *n*

ovi·pos·it \'ō-və-ˌpäz-ət, ˌō-və-'\ *vi* : to lay eggs — used esp. of insects; compare LARVIPOSIT

ovi·po·si·tion \ˌō-və-pə-'zish-ən\ *n* : the act or an instance of ovipositing — **ovi·po·si·tion·al** \-'zish-nəl, -ən-ᵊl\ *adj*

ovi·pos·i·tor \'ō-və-ˌpäz-ət-ər, ˌō-və-'\ *n* : a specialized organ (as of an insect) for depositing eggs

ovi·sac \'ō-və-ˌsak\ *n* : GRAAFIAN FOLLICLE

ovo·cyte \'ō-və-ˌsīt\ *n* : OOCYTE

ovo·fla·vin \ˌō-və-'flā-vən\ *n* : RIBOFLAVIN

ovo·gen·e·sis \-'jen-ə-səs\ *n, pl* **-e·ses** \-ˌsēz\ : OOGENESIS

ovo·glob·u·lin \-'gläb-yə-lən\ *n* : a globulin present in egg white

¹ovoid \'ō-ˌvóid\ *adj* : shaped like an egg ⟨an ~ tumor⟩

²ovoid *n* : an ovoid radium applicator placed within the vagina for radiotherapy

ovo–lac·to \'ō-vō-'lak-tō\ *adj* : LACTO-OVO ⟨an ~ entree⟩

ovo–lacto vegetarian *n* : LACTO-OVO VEGETARIAN

ovo·lec·i·thin \ˌō-vō-'les-ə-thən\ *n* : lecithin obtained from egg yolk

ovo·mu·cin \ˌō-və-'myü-sən\ *n* : a mucin present in egg white

ovo·mu·coid \-'myü-ˌkóid\ *n* : a mucoprotein present in egg white

ovo·plasm \'ō-və-ˌplaz-əm\ *n* : the cytoplasm of an unfertilized egg

ovo·tes·tis \ˌō-vō-'tes-təs\ *n, pl* **-tes·tes** \-ˌtēz\ : a hermaphrodite gonad containing both ovarian and testicular tissue

ovo·vi·tel·lin \-vī-'tel-ən\ *n* : VITELLIN

ovo·vi·vi·par·i·ty \-ˌvī-və-'par-ət-ē, -ˌviv-ə-\ *n, pl* **-ties** : the condition of being ovoviviparous

ovo·vi·vip·a·rous \-ˌvī-'vip-(ə-)rəs\ *adj* : producing eggs that develop within the maternal body and hatch within or immediately after extrusion from the parent — compare LARVIPAROUS, OVIPAROUS, VIVIPAROUS

ovu·lar \'äv-yə-lər *also* 'ōv-\ *adj* : of or relating to an ovule or ovum

ovu·la·tion \ˌäv-yə-'lā-shən *also* ˌōv-\ *n* : the discharge of a mature ovum from the ovary — **ovu·late** \'äv-yə-ˌlāt *also* 'ōv-\ *vi* **-lat·ed; -lat·ing**

ovu·la·to·ry \'äv-yə-lə-ˌtōr-ē, -ˌtòr- *also* 'ōv-\ *adj* : of, relating to, or involving ovulation ⟨the ~ cycle⟩

ovule \'äv-(ˌ)yü(ə)l *also* 'ōv-\ *n* **1** : an outgrowth of the ovary of a seed plant that after fertilization develops into a seed **2** : a small egg; *esp* : one in an early stage of growth — **ovu·lar** \-yə-lər\ *adj*

ovum \'ō-vəm\ *n, pl* **ova** \-və\ : a female gamete : MACROGAMETE; *esp* : a mature egg that has undergone reduction, is ready for fertilization, and takes the form of a relatively large inactive gamete providing a comparatively great amount of reserve material and contributing most of the cytoplasm of the zygote

Ow·ren's disease \'ō-renz-\ *n* : PARAHEMOPHILIA

 Owren, Paul A. (1905–1990), Norwegian hematologist. Owren conducted research on diseases of the blood, blood coagulation, thrombosis, coronary artery disease, and anticoagulin therapy. In 1947 he published a monograph on blood coagulation in which he reported on his study of an abnormal bleeding tendency in a woman caused by a deficiency of a newly discovered coagulation-promoting globulin. He called this globulin factor V. The condition caused by a deficiency of factor V is called parahemophilia or Owren's disease.

ox·a·cil·lin \ˌäk-sə-'sil-ən\ *n* : a semisynthetic penicillin administered in the form of its hydrated sodium salt $C_{19}H_{18}N_3NaO_5S \cdot H_2O$ to treat infections caused by penicillin-resistant staphylococci

oxalacetic acid *var of* OXALOACETIC ACID

¹ox·a·late \'äk-sə-ˌlāt\ *n* : a salt or ester of oxalic acid

²oxalate *vt* **-lat·ed; -lat·ing** : to add an oxalate to (blood or plasma) to prevent coagulation

ox·a·le·mia *or Brit* **ox·a·lae·mia** \ˌäk-sə-'lē-mē-ə\ *n* : the presence of an excess of oxalic acid in the blood

ox·al·ic acid \(ˌ)äk-ˌsal-ik-\ *n* : a poisonous strong acid $(COOH)_2$ or $H_2C_2O_4$ that occurs in various plants as oxalates and is used esp. as a bleaching or cleaning agent and as a chemical intermediate

ox·a·lo·ac·e·tate \ˌäk-sə-lō-'as-ə-ˌtāt\ *also* **ox·al·ac·e·tate** \ˌäk-sə-'las-\ *n* : a salt or ester of oxaloacetic acid

ox·a·lo·ace·tic acid \ˌäk-sə-lō-ə-ˌsēt-ik-\ *also* **ox·al·ace·tic acid** \ˌäk-sə-lə-ˌsēt-ik-\ *n* : a crystalline acid $C_4H_4O_5$ that is formed by reversible oxidation of malic acid (as in carbohydrate metabolism via the Krebs cycle) and in reversible transamination reactions (as from aspartic acid)

ox·a·lo·sis \ˌäk-sə-'lō-səs\ *n* : an abnormal condition characterized by hyperoxaluria and the formation of calcium oxalate deposits in tissues throughout the body

ox·a·lo·suc·cin·ic acid \'äk-sə-lō-sək-ˌsin-ik-, ˌäk-'sal-ō-\ *n* : a tricarboxylic acid $C_6H_6O_7$ that is formed as an intermediate in the metabolism of fats and carbohydrates

ox·al·uria \ˌäk-səl-'(y)ùr-ē-ə\ *n* : HYPEROXALURIA

ox·a·lyl \'äk-sə-ˌlil\ *n* : the bivalent group –COCO– of oxalic acid

ox·a·lyl·urea \ˌäk-sə-ˌlil-yù-'rē-ə\ *n* : PARABANIC ACID

ox·an·a·mide \äk-'san-ə-ˌmīd\ *n* : a tranquilizing drug $C_8H_{15}NO_2$

ox·an·dro·lone \äk-'san-drə-ˌlōn\ *n* : an androgenic anabolic steroid $C_{19}H_{30}O_3$ administered orally esp. to promote weight gain (as after extensive surgery or a chronic infection) and to relieve bone pain in osteoporosis

ox·a·pro·zin \ˌäk-sə-'prō-zən\ *n* : an NSAID drug $C_{18}H_{15}NO_3$ administered orally to treat osteoarthritis and rheumatoid arthritis — see DAYPRO

ox·az·e·pam \äk-'saz-ə-ˌpam\ *n* : a benzodiazepine tranquilizer $C_{15}H_{11}ClN_2O_2$

ox·a·zine \'äk-sə-ˌzēn\ *n* : any of several parent compounds C_4H_5NO containing a ring composed of four carbon atoms, one oxygen atom, and one nitrogen atom

oxazine dye *n* : a dye containing at least one fused oxazine ring in which the oxygen atom and the nitrogen atom are in the para or 1,4-positions

ox·a·zol·i·dine \ˌäk-sə-'zō-lə-ˌdēn, -'zä-\ *n* : the heterocyclic compound C_3H_7NO; *also* : an anticonvulsant derivative (as trimethadione) of this compound

ox bile ex·tract \'äks-ˌbīl-ˌek-ˌstrakt\ *n* : BILE SALT 2

ox·gall \-ˌgól\ *n* : BILE SALT 2

ox·i·dant \'äk-səd-ənt\ *n* : OXIDIZING AGENT — **oxidant** *adj*

ox·i·dase \'äk-sə-ˌdās, -ˌdāz\ *n* : any of various enzymes that catalyze oxidations; *esp* : one able to react directly with molecular oxygen

ox·i·da·tion \ˌäk-sə-'dā-shən\ *n* **1** : the act or process of oxidizing **2** : the state or result of being oxidized

oxidation–reduction *n* : a chemical reaction in which one or more electrons are transferred from one atom or molecule to another — called also *oxidoreduction, redox*

oxidation–reduction potential *n* : the standard potential of an atom or ion that undergoes oxidation at the anode or reduction at the cathode in an electrochemical cell as compared to the potential of a standard hydrogen electrode when it is undergoing the same process — called also *redox potential*

ox·i·da·tive \'äk-sə-ˌdāt-iv\ *adj* : of, relating to, or characterized by oxidation — **ox·i·da·tive·ly** *adv*

oxidative phosphorylation *n* : the synthesis of ATP by phosphorylation of ADP for which energy is obtained by electron transport and which takes place in the mitochondria during aerobic respiration

oxidative stress *n* : physiological stress on the body that is caused by the cumulative damage done by free radicals inadequately neutralized by antioxidants and that is held to be associated with aging

ox·ide \'äk-ˌsīd\ *n* : a binary compound of oxygen with a more electropositive element or chemical group

ox·i·dize *also Brit* **ox·i·dise** \'äk-sə-ˌdīz\ *vb* **-dized** *also Brit* **-dised; -diz·ing** *also Brit* **-dis·ing** *vt* **1** : to combine with oxygen **2** : to dehydrogenate esp. by the action of oxygen **3** : to change (a compound) by increasing the proportion of the electronegative part or change (an element or ion) from a lower to a higher positive valence : remove one or more electrons from (an atom, ion, or molecule) ~ *vi* : to become oxidized — **ox·i·diz·able** \-ˌdī-zə-bəl\ *adj*

oxidized cellulose *n* : an acid degradation product of cellulose that is usu. obtained by oxidizing cotton or gauze with nitrogen dioxide, is a useful hemostatic (as in surgery), and is absorbed by body fluids (as when used to pack wounds)

oxidizing agent *n* : a substance that oxidizes something esp. chemically (as by accepting electrons) — called also *oxidant;* compare REDUCING AGENT

ox·i·do·re·duc·tase \'äk-səd-ō-ri-ˈdək-ˌtās, -ˌtāz\ *n* : an enzyme that catalyzes an oxidation-reduction reaction

ox·i·do·re·duc·tion \-'dək-shən\ *n* : OXIDATION-REDUCTION

ox·ime \'äk-ˌsēm\ *n* : any of various compounds obtained chiefly by the action of hydroxylamine on aldehydes and ketones and characterized by the bivalent group C=NOH

ox·im·e·ter \äk-ˈsim-ət-ər\ *n* : an instrument for measuring continuously the degree of oxygen saturation of the circulating blood — **ox·i·met·ric** \ˌäk-sə-ˈme-trik\ *adj*

ox·im·e·try \-ə-trē\ *n, pl* **-tries** : measurement of the blood's oxygen saturation by means of an oximeter

ox·ine \'äk-ˌsēn\ *n* : 8-HYDROXYQUINOLINE

oxo \'äk-(ˌ)sō\ *adj* : containing oxygen

ox·o·ni·um \äk-ˈsō-nē-əm\ *n* : an ion formed from hydronium by replacement of one or more hydrogens with other usu. organic substituents; *also* : HYDRONIUM

oxo·phen·ar·sine \ˌäk-sə-fen-ˈär-ˌsēn, -sən\ *n* : an arsenical formerly used in the form of its hydrochloride C₆H₄AsNO₂·HCl to treat syphilis

oxo·trem·o·rine \ˌäk-sō-ˈtrem-ə-ˌrēn, -rən\ *n* : a synthetic cholinergic agent C₁₂H₁₈N₂O used esp. in pharmacological research (as to induce tremors characteristic of Parkinson's disease)

ox·pren·o·lol \ˌäks-ˈpren-ə-ˌlȯl\ *n* : a beta-adrenergic blocking agent used in the form of its hydrochloride C₁₅H₂₃NO₃·HCl as a coronary vasodilator

ox·tri·phyl·line \ˌäks-tri-ˈfil-ˌēn, -ˈtrif-ə-ˌlēn\ *n* : the choline salt C₁₂H₂₁N₅O₃ of theophylline used chiefly as a bronchodilator

ox warble *n* : the maggot of an ox warble fly

ox warble fly *n* : either of two warble flies of the genus *Hypoderma*: **a** : COMMON CATTLE GRUB **b** : NORTHERN CATTLE GRUB

oxy \'äk-sē\ *adj* : containing oxygen or additional oxygen — often used in combination ⟨*oxy*hemoglobin⟩

oxy·ac·id \'äk-sē-ˌas-əd\ *n* : an acid (as sulfuric acid) that contains oxygen — called also *oxygen acid*

oxy·ben·zone \ˌäk-sē-ˈben-ˌzōn\ *n* : a sunscreen C₁₄H₁₂O₃ that absorbs UVB radiation and some UVA radiation

oxy·bi·o·tin \-ˈbī-ət-ən\ *n* : a compound C₁₀H₁₆N₂O₄ that contains an oxygen atom in place of the sulfur atom in the biotin molecule and that is less active biologically than biotin

oxy·bu·ty·nin \ˌäk-sē-ˈbyüt-ᵊn-ən\ *n* : an antispasmodic and anticholinergic drug C₂₂H₃₁NO₃ administered transdermally as a skin patch or orally in the form of its hydrochloride C₂₂H₃₁NO₃·HCl to relax the smooth muscles of the bladder in the treatment of urge incontinence, frequent urination, and urinary urgency

oxy·bu·tyr·ic acid \-byü-ˈtir-ik\ *n* : HYDROXYBUTYRIC ACID

oxy·cal·o·rim·e·ter \-ˌkal-ə-ˈrim-ət-ər\ *n* : a calorimeter in which the energy content of a substance is determined by the direct measurement of the oxygen consumed

oxy·ceph·a·ly \-ˈsef-ə-lē\ *n, pl* **-lies** : congenital deformity of the skull due to early synostosis of the parietal and occipital bones with compensating growth in the region of the anterior or frontanel resulting in a pointed or pyramidal skull — called also *acrocephaly, turricephaly* — **oxy·ce·phal·ic** \-si-ˈfal-ik\ *adj*

oxy·chlo·ride \-ˈklō(ə)r-ˌīd, -ˈklȯ(ə)r-\ *n* : a compound of oxygen and chlorine with an element or radical : a basic chloride

oxy·chlo·ro·sene \-ˈklōr-ə-ˌsēn, -ˈklȯr-\ *n* : a topical antiseptic C₂₀H₃₄O₃S·HOCl

oxy·chro·ma·tin \-ˈkrō-mət-ən\ *n* : chromatin which stains readily with acid dyes — compare BASICHROMATIN

oxy·co·done \-ˈkō-ˌdōn\ *n* : a narcotic analgesic used esp. in the form of its hydrochloride C₁₈H₂₁NO₄·HCl — see OXYCONTIN

Oxy·Con·tin \-ˈkän-tin\ *trademark* — used for a preparation of the hydrochloride of oxycodone

ox·y·gen \'äk-si-jən\ *n* : a colorless tasteless odorless gaseous element that constitutes 21 percent of the atmosphere and is found in water, in most rocks and minerals, and in numerous organic compounds, that is capable of combining with all elements except the inert gases, that is active in physiological processes, and that is involved esp. in combustion processes — symbol O; see ELEMENT table — **ox·y·gen·ic** \ˌäk-si-ˈjen-ik\ *adj*

oxygen acid *n* : OXYACID

ox·y·gen·ase \'äk-si-jə-ˌnās, -ˌnāz\ *n* : an enzyme that catalyzes the reaction of an organic compound with molecular oxygen

ox·y·gen·ate \'äk-si-jə-ˌnāt, äk-ˈsij-ə-\ *vt* **-at·ed; -at·ing** : to impregnate, combine, or supply with oxygen ⟨*oxygenated* blood⟩ ⟨better to ~ the patient first —*Anesthesia Digest*⟩ — **ox·y·gen·ation** \ˌäk-si-jə-ˈnā-shən, äk-ˌsij-ə-\ *n*

ox·y·gen·ator \'äk-si-jə-ˌnāt-ər, äk-ˈsij-ə-\ *n* : one that oxygenates; *specif* : an apparatus that oxygenates the blood extracorporeally (as during open-heart surgery)

oxygen capacity *n* : the amount of oxygen which a quantity of blood is able to absorb

oxygen debt \-'det\ *n* : a cumulative deficit of oxygen available for oxidative metabolism that develops during periods of intense bodily activity and must be made good when the body returns to rest

oxygen de·mand \-di-ˈmand\ *n* : BIOCHEMICAL OXYGEN DEMAND

oxygen dissociation curve \-ˈkərv\ *n* : a curve determined by plotting on a graph the partial pressure of oxygen in blood as the abscissa and the percentage of hemoglobin combined with oxygen in the form of oxyhemoglobin as the ordinate

ox·y·ge·ni·um \ˌäk-sə-ˈjē-nē-əm\ *n* : OXYGEN

ox·y·gen·ize *also Brit* **ox·y·gen·ise** \'äk-si-jə-ˌnīz, äk-ˈsij-ə-\ *vt* **-ized** *also Brit* **-ised; -iz·ing** *also Brit* **-is·ing** : OXYGENATE

oxygen mask *n* : a device worn over the nose and mouth through which oxygen is supplied from a storage tank

oxygen tent *n* : a canopy which can be placed over a bedridden person and within which a flow of oxygen can be maintained

oxy·he·mo·glo·bin *or chiefly Brit* **oxy·hae·mo·glo·bin** \ˌäk-si-ˈhē-mə-ˌglō-bən\ *n* : hemoglobin loosely combined with oxygen that it releases to the tissues

oxy·he·mo·graph *or chiefly Brit* **oxy·hae·mo·graph** \-ˌgraf\ *n* : OXIMETER

ox·y·mel \'äk-si-ˌmel\ *n* : a mixture of honey and dilute acetic acid used as an expectorant

oxy·me·taz·o·line \ˌäk-si-mə-ˈtaz-ə-ˌlēn\ *n* : a sympathomimetic drug with vasoconstrictive activity that is used in the form of its hydrochloride C₁₆H₂₄N₂O·HCl chiefly as a topical nasal decongestant

O
P

\ə\ **abut** \ᵊ\ **kitten** \ər\ **further** \a\ **ash** \ā\ **ace** \ä\ **cot, cart**
\aů\ **out** \ch\ **chin** \e\ **bet** \ē\ **easy** \g\ **go** \i\ **hit** \ī\ **ice** \j\ **job**
\ŋ\ **sing** \ō\ **go** \ȯ\ **law** \ȯi\ **boy** \th\ **thin** \th̲\ **the** \ü\ **loot**
\ů\ **foot** \y\ **yet** \zh\ **vision** *See also* Pronunciation Symbols page

oxy·mor·phone \-'mȯr-ˌfōn\ *n* : a semisynthetic narcotic analgesic drug used in the form of its hydrochloride $C_{17}H_{19}NO_4 \cdot HCl$ and having uses, activity, and side effects like those of morphine

oxy·myo·glo·bin \ˌäk-si-'mī-ə-ˌglō-bən\ *n* : a pigment formed by the combination of myoglobin with oxygen

oxy·neu·rine \-'n(y)u̇r-ˌēn, -ən\ *n* : BETAINE

ox·yn·tic \äk-'sint-ik\ *adj* : secreting acid — used esp. of the parietal cells of the gastric glands

oxy·phen·bu·ta·zone \ˌäk-sē-ˌfen-'byüt-ə-ˌzōn\ *n* : a phenylbutazone derivative $C_{19}H_{20}N_2O_3$ having anti-inflammatory, analgesic, and antipyretic effects

oxy·phen·cy·cli·mine \-'sī-klə-ˌmēn\ *n* : an anticholinergic drug with actions similar to atropine usu. used in the form of its hydrochloride $C_{20}H_{28}N_2O_3 \cdot HCl$ as an antispasmodic esp. in the treatment of peptic ulcer

oxy·phile \'äk-si-ˌfīl\ *also* **oxy·phil** \-ˌfil\ *n* : ACIDOPHIL

oxy·phil·ic \ˌäk-si-'fil-ik\ *also* **oxyphil** *or* **oxyphile** *adj* : ACIDOPHILIC

oxy·pho·nia \ˌäk-si-'fō-nē-ə\ *n* : shrillness or high pitch of the voice

oxy·quin·o·line \-'kwin-ᵊl-ˌēn\ *n* : 8-HYDROXYQUINOLINE

Oxy·spi·ru·ra \ˌäk-si-spī-'ru̇r-ə\ *n* : a genus of spiruroid nematode worms of the family Thelaziidae comprising the eye worms of birds and esp. domestic poultry

oxy·tet·ra·cy·cline \-ˌte-trə-'sī-ˌklēn\ *n* : a yellow crystalline broad-spectrum antibiotic $C_{22}H_{24}N_2O_9$ produced by a soil actinomycete of the genus *Streptomyces* (*S. rimosus*) — see TERRAMYCIN

oxy·thi·a·mine \-'thī-ə-mən, -ˌmēn\ *also* **oxy·thi·a·min** \-mən\ *n* : a chemical compound $C_{12}H_{16}ClN_3O_2S$ that differs from thiamine in having the amino group in the pyrimidine ring replaced by a hydroxyl group and that is a thiamine antagonist producing symptoms of thiamine deficiency

¹**oxy·to·cic** \ˌäk-si-'tō-sik\ *adj* : hastening parturition; *also* : inducing contraction of uterine smooth muscle

²**oxytocic** *n* : a substance that stimulates contraction of uterine smooth muscle or hastens childbirth

oxy·to·cin \-'tōs-ᵊn\ *n* **1** : an octapeptide hormone $C_{43}H_{66}N_{12}O_{12}S_2$ secreted by the anterior lobe of the pituitary gland that stimulates esp. the contraction of uterine muscle and the secretion of milk — called also *alpha-hypophamine* **2** : a synthetic version of oxytocin used esp. to initiate or increase uterine contractions (as in the induction of labor) — see PITOCIN

oxy·uri·a·sis \ˌäk-si-yu̇-'rī-ə-səs\ *n, pl* **-a·ses** \-ˌsēz\ : infestation with or disease caused by pinworms (as of the genera *Enterobius* and *Oxyuris*)

oxy·uric \-'yu̇r-ik\ *adj* : of, relating to, or caused by pinworms of the genus *Oxyuris* or a related genus

oxy·uri·cide \-'yu̇r-ə-ˌsīd\ *n* : a substance that destroys pinworms

oxy·urid \-'yu̇r-əd\ *n* : any nematode worm of the family Oxyuridae — **oxyurid** *adj*

Oxy·uri·dae \-'yu̇r-ə-ˌdē\ *n pl* : a family of nematode worms that have a distinct posterior enlargement of the pharynx and no preanal suckers in the male and that are chiefly parasites of the vertebrate intestinal tract — see PINWORM

oxy·uris \-'yu̇r-əs\ *n* **1** *cap* : a genus (the type of the family Oxyuridae) of parasitic nematodes with a long slender tail and a well-developed posterior pharyngeal enlargement **2** : any nematode worm of the genus *Oxyuris* or a related genus (as *Enterobius*) : PINWORM

oz *abbr* ounce; ounces

oze·na *or chiefly Brit* **ozae·na** \ō-'zē-nə\ *n* : a chronic disease of the nose accompanied by a fetid discharge and marked by atrophic changes in the nasal structures

ozo·ke·rite \ˌō-zō-'ki(ə)r-ˌīt\ *also* **ozo·ce·rite** \-'si(ə)r-\ *n* : a waxy mineral mixture of hydrocarbons that is colorless or white when pure and often of unpleasant odor and is used esp. in making ceresin

ozon·a·tor \'ō-(ˌ)zō-ˌnāt-ər\ *n* : OZONIZER

ozone \'ō-ˌzōn\ *n* : a triatomic very reactive form of oxygen that is a bluish irritating gas of pungent odor, that is formed naturally in the atmosphere by a photochemical reaction and is a major air pollutant in the lower atmosphere but a beneficial component of the upper atmosphere, and that is used for oxidizing, bleaching, disinfecting, and deodorizing — **ozo·nic** \ō-'zō-nik, -'zän-ik\ *adj*

ozon·ide \'ō-(ˌ)zō-ˌnīd\ *n* : a compound of ozone; *specif* : a compound formed by the addition of ozone to the double or triple bond of an unsaturated organic compound

ozon·iza·tion *also Brit* **ozon·isa·tion** \ˌō-(ˌ)zō-nə-'zā-shən\ *n* **1** : the combining of ozone with organic or inorganic substances **2** : the production of ozone in an ozonizer

ozon·ize *also Brit* **ozon·ise** \'ō-(ˌ)zō-ˌnīz\ *vt* **-ized** *also Brit* **-ised; -iz·ing** *also Brit* **-is·ing** **1** : to convert (oxygen) into ozone **2** : to treat, impregnate, or combine with ozone

ozon·iz·er *also Brit* **ozon·is·er** \-ˌnī-zər\ *n* : a device for producing ozone usu. by the discharge of an electric current through oxygen or air — called also *ozonator*

ozon·ol·y·sis \ˌō-(ˌ)zō-'näl-ə-səs\ *n, pl* **-y·ses** \-ə-ˌsēz\ : the cleavage of an unsaturated organic compound at the position of unsaturation by conversion to the ozonide followed by decomposition (a by hydrolysis)

P

P *abbr* **1** parental **2** part **3** percentile **4** pharmacopoeia **5** pint **6** pole **7** population **8** position **9** positive **10** posterior **11** pressure **12** pulse **13** pupil

P *symbol* phosphorus

p- *abbr* para- ⟨*p*-dichlorobenzene⟩

Pa *symbol* protactinium

PA \ˌpē-'ā\ *n* : PHYSICIAN'S ASSISTANT

PA *abbr* pernicious anemia

PABA \'pab-ə, ˌpē-ˌā-ˌbē-ˌā\ *n* : PARA-AMINOBENZOIC ACID

pab·u·lum \'pab-yə-ləm\ *n* : FOOD; *esp* : a suspension or solution of nutrients in a state suitable for absorption

PAC *abbr* physician's assistant, certified

pac·chi·o·ni·an body \ˌpak-ē-'ō-nē-ən-\ *n* : ARACHNOID GRANULATION

Pac·chi·o·ni \ˌpäk-ē-'ō-nē\, **Antonio (1665–1726),** Italian anatomist. Pacchioni wrote several papers on the structure and function of the dura mater. In 1705 he published his major treatise on the subject, including a description of the arachnoid granulations now sometimes called pacchionian bodies.

pace·mak·er \'pā-ˌsmā-kər\ *n* **1** : a group of cells or a body part (as the sinoatrial node of the heart) that serves to establish and maintain a rhythmic activity **2** : an electrical device for stimulating or steadying the heartbeat or reestablishing the rhythm of an arrested heart — called also *pacer*

pace·mak·ing \'pā-ˌsmā-kiŋ\ *n* : the act or process of serving as a pacemaker

pac·er \'pā-sər\ *n* : PACEMAKER 2 ⟨electronic cardiac ∼s⟩

pa·chom·e·ter \pa-'käm-ət-ər\ *n* : a device for measuring the thickness of an object ⟨corneal ∼ that accurately measures corneal thickness —P. S. Binder *et al*⟩

pachy·ce·pha·lia \ˌpak-ē-sə-'fā-lē-ə\ *or* **pachy·ceph·a·ly** \ˌpak-i-'sef-ə-lē\ *n, pl* **-lias** *or* **-lies** : thickness of the skull or head

pachy·der·ma·tous \ˌpak-i-'dər-mət-əs\ *adj* : abnormally thickened — used esp. of skin

pachy·der·mia \-'dər-mē-ə\ *n* : abnormal thickness of tissue (as of skin or of the laryngeal mucous membrane) — **pachy·der·mi·al** \-'dər-mē-əl\ *adj*

pachy·der·mic \-'dər-mik\ *adj* : PACHYDERMATOUS

pachy·lepto·men·in·gi·tis \,pak-i-,lep-tō-,men-ən-'jīt-əs\ *n, pl* **-git·i·des** \-'jit-ə-,dēz\ : simultaneous inflammation of the pia mater and dura mater

pachy·men·in·gi·tis \-,men-ən-'jīt-əs\ *n, pl* **-git·i·des** \-'jit-ə-,dēz\ : inflammation of the dura mater

pachy·me·ninx \-'mē-niŋ(k)s, -'men-iŋ(k)s\ *n, pl* **-me·nin·ges** \-mə-'nin-(,)jēz\ : DURA MATER

pachy·ne·ma \,pak-i-'nē-mə\ *n* : PACHYTENE

pachy·o·nych·ia \,pak-ē-ō-'nik-ē-ə\ *n* : extreme usu. congenital thickness of the nails

pachy·tene \'pak-i-,tēn\ *n* : the stage of meiotic prophase which immediately follows the zygotene and in which the paired chromosomes are thickened and visibly divided into chromatids — **pachytene** *adj*

pac·i·fi·er \'pas-ə-,fī(-ə)r\ *n* **1** : a usu. nipple-shaped device for babies to suck or bite on **2** : TRANQUILIZER

pac·ing \'pā-siŋ\ *n* : the act or process of regulating or changing the timing or intensity of cardiac contractions (as by an artificial pacemaker)

Pa·cin·i·an corpuscle \pə-,sin-ē-ən-\ *also* **Pa·ci·ni's corpus·cle** \pə-'chē-nēz-\ *n* : a pressure-sensitive mechanoreceptor that is an oval capsule terminating some sensory nerve fibers esp. in the skin (as of the hands and feet) — see CORPUSCLE OF HERBST

Pacini, Filippo (1812–1883), Italian anatomist. Pacini devoted his medical career to microscopic research. In 1831, while dissecting a hand, he observed the corpuscles around the branches of the median nerve to the digits. These corpuscles, now known as Pacinian corpuscles, had been originally described in 1741, but Pacini was the first to describe their distribution in the body, their microscopic structure, and their nerve connections. He also related the function of the corpuscles to the sensation of touch and deep pressure.

¹pack \'pak\ *n* **1** : a container shielded with lead or mercury for holding radium in large quantities esp. for therapeutic application **2 a** : absorbent material saturated with water or other liquid for therapeutic application to the body or a body part — see COLD PACK, HOT PACK; compare ICE PACK **b** : a folded square or compress of gauze or other absorbent material used esp. to maintain a clear field in surgery, to plug cavities, to check bleeding by compression, or to apply medication

²pack *vt* : to cover or surround with a pack ⟨~ed it away from the operative field with gauze packs —R. P. Parsons⟩; *specif* : to envelop (a patient) in a wet or dry sheet or blanket

packed cell volume *n* : HEMATOCRIT 2 — abbr. *PCV*

packed red blood cells *n pl* : a concentrated preparation of red blood cells that is obtained from whole blood by removing the plasma (as by centrifugation) and is used in transfusion

pack·ing \'pak-iŋ\ *n* **1** : the therapeutic application of a pack ⟨hemorrhage . . . could not be controlled by suture or ~ —Jour. Amer. Med. Assoc.⟩ **2** : the material used in packing

pac·li·tax·el \,pak-li-'tak-səl\ *n* : an antineoplastic agent $C_{47}H_{51}NO_{14}$ that was orig. derived from the bark of a yew tree (*Taxus brevifolia* of the family Taxaceae) of the western U.S. and British Columbia but that is now typically derived as a semisynthetic product of the English yew (*T. baccata*) and is used to treat ovarian cancer which has not responded to conventional chemotherapy — see TAXOL

PaCO₂ *abbr* partial pressure of arterial carbon dioxide

PACU *abbr* postanesthesia care unit

pad \'pad\ *n* **1** : a usu. square or rectangular piece of often folded typically absorbent material (as gauze) fixed in place over some part of the body as a dressing or other protective covering **2** : a part of the body or of an appendage that resembles or is suggestive of a cushion : a thick fleshy resilient part: as **a** : the sole of the foot or underside of the toes of an animal (as a dog) that is typically thickened so as to form a cushion **b** : the underside of the extremities of the fingers; *esp* : the ball of the thumb

PAD *abbr* peripheral arterial disease

pad·dle \'pad-ᵊl\ *n* : a flat electrode that is the part of a defibrillator placed on the chest of a patient and through which a shock of electricity is discharged — called also *paddle electrode*

pad·i·mate O \'pad-i-,māt-'ō\ *n* : a sunscreen $C_{17}H_{27}NO_2$ effective against UVB that is an aminobenzoate derivative

Each boldface word in the list below is a chiefly British variant of the word to its right in small capitals.

paederast	PEDERAST	paedodontic	PEDODONTIC
paederastic	PEDERASTIC	paedodontics	PEDODONTICS
paederasty	PEDERASTY	paedodontist	PEDODONTIST
paediatric	PEDIATRIC	paedology	PEDOLOGY
paediatrician	PEDIATRICIAN	paedophile	PEDOPHILE
paediatrics	PEDIATRICS	paedophilia	PEDOPHILIA
paediatrist	PEDIATRIST	paedophiliac	PEDOPHILIAC
paedodontia	PEDODONTIA	paedophilic	PEDOPHILIC

pae·do·gen·e·sis *also* **pe·do·gen·e·sis** \,pēd-ō-'jen-ə-səs\ *n, pl* **-e·ses** \-,sēz\ : reproduction by young or larval animals — **pae·do·ge·net·ic** *also* **pe·do·ge·net·ic** \-jə-'net-ik\ *adj*

pae·do·mor·phic *or* **pe·do·mor·phic** \,pēd-ə-'mor-fik\ *adj* : of, relating to, or involving paedomorphosis or paedomorphism

pae·do·mor·phism *or* **pe·do·mor·phism** \-,fiz-əm\ *n* : retention in the adult of infantile or juvenile characters

pae·do·mor·pho·sis *or* **pe·do·mor·pho·sis** \-'mor-fə-səs\ *n, pl* **-pho·ses** \-,sēz\ : phylogenetic change that involves retention of juvenile characters by the adult

PAF *abbr* platelet-activating factor

pag·et·oid \'paj-ə-,toid\ *adj* : belonging to or typical of Paget's disease ⟨~ symptoms⟩

Pag·et \'paj-ət\, **Sir James (1814–1899),** British surgeon. Along with the German biologist Rudolf Virchow, Paget is considered one of the founders of the science of pathology. In 1834 he discovered in human muscle the parasitic worm that causes trichinosis. A professor of anatomy and surgery, he wrote classic descriptions of breast cancer, of a chronic precancerous eczema of the nipple (1874), and of osteitis deformans (1877). Both of these last two conditions are often called Paget's disease.

Pag·et's disease \,paj-əts-\ *n* **1** : a rare form of breast cancer initially manifested as a scaly red rash on the nipple and areola **2** : a chronic disease of bones characterized by their great enlargement and rarefaction with bowing of the long bones and deformation of the flat bones — called also *osteitis deformans, osteodystrophia deformans*

pa·go·pha·gia \,pā-gə-'fā-j(ē-)ə\ *n* : the compulsive eating of ice that is a common symptom of a lack of iron

PAH \,pē-(,)ā-'āch\ *n* : POLYCYCLIC AROMATIC HYDROCARBON

PAH *abbr* para-aminohippurate; para-aminohippuric acid

pai·dol·o·gy \pī-'däl-ə-jē, pē-, pā-\ *n, pl* **-gies** : PEDOLOGY

¹pain \'pān\ *n* **1 a** : a state of physical, emotional, or mental lack of well-being or physical, emotional, or mental uneasiness that ranges from mild discomfort or dull distress to acute often unbearable agony, may be generalized or localized, and is the consequence of being injured or hurt physically or mentally or of some derangement of or lack of equilibrium in the physical or mental functions (as through disease), and that usu. produces a reaction of wanting to avoid, escape, or destroy the causative factor and its effects ⟨was in constant ~⟩ **b** : a basic bodily sensation that is induced by a noxious stimulus, is received by naked nerve endings, is characterized by physical discomfort (as pricking, throbbing, or aching), and typically leads to evasive action **2 pains** *pl* : the protracted series of involuntary contractions of the uterine musculature that constitute the major factor

\ə\ **abut** \ᵊ\ **kitten** \ər\ **further** \a\ **ash** \ā\ **ace** \ä\ **cot, cart** \aú\ **out** \ch\ **chin** \e\ **bet** \ē\ **easy** \g\ **go** \i\ **hit** \ī\ **ice** \j\ **job** \ŋ\ **sing** \ō\ **go** \ó\ **law** \ói\ **boy** \th\ **thin** \th̲\ **the** \ü\ **loot** \ú\ **foot** \y\ **yet** \zh\ **vision** *See also* Pronunciation Symbols page

O
P

in parturient labor and that are often accompanied by considerable pain ⟨her ∼s had begun⟩

²**pain** *vt* : to make suffer or cause distress to ∼ *vi* : to give or have a sensation of pain

pain·ful \'pān-fəl\ *adj* **pain·ful·ler** \-fə-lər\; **pain·ful·lest** : feeling or giving pain — **pain·ful·ly** \-f(ə-)lē\ *adv*

pain·kill·er \-ˌkil-ər\ *n* : something (as a drug) that relieves pain — **pain·kill·ing** \-iŋ\ *adj*

pain·less \'pān-ləs\ *adj* **1** : not experiencing pain **2** : not causing pain : not accompanied by pain : not painful ⟨∼ surgery⟩ — **pain·less·ly** *adv*

pain spot *n* : one of many small localized areas of the skin that respond to stimulation (as by pricking or burning) by giving a sensation of pain

paint·er's colic \'pānt-ərz-\ *n* : intestinal colic associated with obstinate constipation due to chronic lead poisoning

pair–bond \'pa(ə)r-ˌbänd, 'pe(ə)r-\ *n* : an exclusive union with a single mate at any one time : a monogamous relationship — **pair–bond·ing** *n*

paired–associate learning *n* : the learning of items (as syllables, digits, or words) in pairs so that one member of the pair evokes recall of the other — compare ASSOCIATIVE LEARNING

paired associates *n pl* : a pair of items (as words or digits) used in paired-associate learning — **paired–associate** *adj*

pa·ja·ro·el·lo \ˌpä-hə-rə-'we-(ˌ)lō\ *n* : a venomous tick of the genus *Ornithodoros* (*O. coriaceus*) whose bite causes painful swelling — called also *pajaroello tick*

Each boldface word in the list below is a British or chiefly British variant of the word to its right in small capitals.

palae–encephalon	PALEENCEPHA-LON	**palaeopallial**	PALEOPALLIAL
palaeocerebel-lar	PALEOCEREBEL-LAR	**palaeopallium**	PALEOPALLIUM
palaeocerebel-lum	PALEOCEREBEL-LUM	**palaeopathologist**	PALEOPATHOLO-GIST
palaeocortex	PALEOCORTEX	**palaeopatholo-gy**	PALEOPATHOL-OGY
		palaeostriatum	PALEOSTRIATUM

pal·a·tal \'pal-ət-ᵊl\ *adj* : of, relating to, forming, or affecting the palate ⟨∼ itching⟩ — **pal·a·tal·ly** \-ᵊl-ē\ *adv*

palatal bar *n* : a connector extending across the roof of the mouth to join the parts of a maxillary partial denture

palatal index *n* : the ratio of the length of the hard palate to its breadth multiplied by 100 — called also *palatomaxillary index*

palatal myoclonus *n* : an abnormal condition that is associated with neurological trauma and is characterized by rapid involuntary contraction of the muscles of the soft palate and often of adjacent structures

palatal process *n* : PALATINE PROCESS

pal·ate \'pal-ət\ *n* : the roof of the mouth separating the mouth from the nasal cavity — see HARD PALATE, SOFT PALATE

palate bone *n* : PALATINE BONE

palati — see TENSOR PALATI

¹**pal·a·tine** \'pal-ə-ˌtīn\ *adj* : of, relating to, or lying near the palate

²**palatine** *n* : PALATINE BONE

palatine aponeurosis *n* : a thin fibrous lamella attached to the posterior part of the hard palate that supports the soft palate, includes the tendon of the tensor veli palatini, and supports the other muscles of the palate

palatine arch *n* : PILLAR OF THE FAUCES

palatine artery *n* **1** : either of two arteries of each side of the face: **a** : an inferior artery that arises from the facial artery and divides into two branches of which one supplies the soft palate and the palatine glands and the other supplies esp. the tonsils and the eustachian tube — called also *ascending palatine artery* **b** : a superior artery that arises from the maxillary artery and sends branches to the soft palate, the palatine glands, the mucous membrane of the hard palate, and the gums — called also *greater palatine artery* **2** : any of the branches of the palatine arteries

palatine bone *n* : a bone of extremely irregular form on each

side of the skull that is situated in the posterior part of the nasal cavity between the maxilla and the pterygoid process of the sphenoid bone and that consists of a horizontal plate which joins the bone of the opposite side and forms the back part of the hard palate and a vertical plate which is extended into three processes and helps to form the floor of the orbit, the outer wall of the nasal cavity, and several adjoining parts — called also *palate bone, palatine*

palatine foramen *n* : any of several foramina in the palatine bone giving passage to the palatine vessels and nerves — see GREATER PALATINE FORAMEN

palatine gland *n* : any of numerous small mucous glands in the palate opening into the mouth

palatine nerve *n* : any of several nerves arising from the pterygopalatine ganglion and supplying the roof of the mouth, parts of the nose, and adjoining parts

palatine process *n* : a process of the maxilla that projects medially, articulates posteriorly with the palatine bone, and forms with the corresponding process on the other side the anterior three-fourths of the hard palate — called also *palatal process*

palatine suture *n* : either of two sutures in the hard palate: **a** : a transverse suture lying between the horizontal plates of the palatine bones and the maxillae **b** : a median suture lying between the maxillae in front and continued posteriorly between the palatine bones

palatine tonsil *n* : TONSIL 1a

palatini — see LEVATOR VELI PALATINI, TENSOR VELI PALATINI

pal·a·ti·tis \ˌpal-ə-'tīt-əs\ *n* : inflammation of the palate

pal·a·to·glos·sal arch \ˌpal-ət-ō-ˌgläs-əl-, -ˌglòs-\ *n* : the more anterior of the two ridges of soft tissue at the back of the mouth on each side that curves downward from the uvula to the side of the base of the tongue forming a recess for the palatine tonsil as it diverges from the palatopharyngeal arch and that is composed of part of the palatoglossus with its covering of mucous membrane — called also *anterior pillar of the fauces, glossopalatine arch*

pal·a·to·glos·sus \-'gläs-əs, -'glòs-əs\ *n, pl* **-glos·si** \-(ˌ)ī\ : a thin muscle that arises from the soft palate on each side, contributes to the structure of the palatoglossal arch, and is inserted into the side and dorsum of the tongue — called also *glossopalatinus*

pal·a·to·gram \'pal-ət-ə-ˌgram\ *n* : a record of the movement of the tongue and palate in the articulation of sounds

pal·a·tog·ra·phy \ˌpal-ə-'täg-rə-fē\ *n, pl* **-phies** : the making or use of palatograms — **pal·a·to·graph·ic** \ˌpal-ət-ə-'graf-ik\ *adj*

pal·a·to·max·il·lary \ˌpal-ət-ō-'mak-sə-ˌler-ē, *chiefly Brit* -mak-'sil-ə-rē\ *adj* : of, relating to, or involving the palate and maxilla ⟨∼ defects⟩

palatomaxillary index *n* : PALATAL INDEX

pal·a·to·pha·ryn·geal arch \-ˌfar-ən-'jē-əl-, -fə-'rin-j(ē-)əl-\ *n* : the more posterior of the two ridges of soft tissue at the back of the mouth on each side that curves downward from the uvula to the side of the pharynx forming a recess for the palatine tonsil as it diverges from the palatoglossal arch and that is composed of part of the palatopharyngeus with its covering of mucous membrane — called also *posterior pillar of the fauces, pharyngopalatine arch*

pal·a·to·pha·ryn·ge·us \-ˌfar-ən-'jē-əs; -fə-'rin-j(ē-)əs\ *n* : a longitudinal muscle of the pharynx that arises from the soft palate, contributes to the structure of the palatopharyngeal arch, and is inserted into the thyroid cartilage and the wall of the pharynx — called also *pharyngopalatinus*

pal·a·to·plas·ty \'pal-ət-ə-ˌplas-tē\ *n, pl* **-ties** : plastic surgery for repair of the palate (as in cleft palate)

pal·a·tos·chi·sis \ˌpal-ə-'täs-kə-səs\ *n, pl* **-chi·ses** \-ˌsēz\ *also* **-chi·sis·es** : CLEFT PALATE

pale \'pā(ə)l\ *adj* **pal·er; pal·est** : deficient in color or intensity of color ⟨a ∼ face⟩ — **pale·ness** \-nəs\ *n*

pale bark *n* : cinchona bark from a tree of the genus *Cinchona* (*C. officinalis*) that contains an exceptionally high percentage of quinine — called also *loxa bark*

pa·le·en·ceph·a·lon \ˌpā-lē-in-'sef-ə-ˌlän\ *or Brit* **pal·ae·en·ceph·a·lon** \ˌpal-ē-\ *n, pl* **-la** \-lə\ : the phylogenetically older part of the brain consisting of all parts except the cerebral cortex and closely related structures — compare NEENCEPHALON

pa·leo·cer·e·bel·lar \ˌpā-lē-ō-ˌser-ə-'bel-ər\ *or Brit* **pal·aeo·cer·e·bel·lar** \ˌpal-ē-\ *adj* : of or relating to the paleocerebellum

pa·leo·cer·e·bel·lum \-'bel-əm\ *or Brit* **pal·aeo·cer·e·bel·lum** \ˌpal-ē-\ *n, pl* **-bel·lums** *or* **-bel·la** \-'bel-ə\ : a phylogenetically old part of the cerebellum concerned with maintenance of normal postural relationships and made up chiefly of the anterior lobe of the vermis and of the pyramid — compare NEOCEREBELLUM

pa·leo·cor·tex *or Brit* **pal·aeo·cor·tex** \-'kór-ˌteks\ *n, pl* **-cor·ti·ces** \-'kórt-ə-ˌsēz\ *or* **-cor·tex·es** : the part of the cerebral cortex that is evolutionarily older than the neocortex and that is composed esp. of the olfactory cortex

pa·leo·pal·li·al \ˌpā-lē-ō-'pal-ē-əl\ *or Brit* **pal·aeo·pal·li·al** \ˌpal-ē-ō-\ *adj* : of, relating to, or mediated by the paleopallium

pa·leo·pal·li·um *or Brit* **pal·aeo·pal·li·um** \-'pal-ē-əm\ *n, pl* **-lia** \-ē-ə\ *or* **-li·ums** : a phylogenetically old part of the cerebral cortex that develops along the lateral aspect of the hemispheres and gives rise to the olfactory lobes in higher forms

pa·leo·pa·thol·o·gist \ˌpā-lē-ō-pə-'thäl-ə-jəst\ *or chiefly Brit* **pal·aeo·pa·thol·o·gist** \ˌpal-ē-ō-pa-\ *n* : a specialist in paleopathology

pa·leo·pa·thol·o·gy *or chiefly Brit* **pal·aeo·pa·thol·o·gy** \-jē\ *n, pl* **-gies** : a branch of pathology concerned with diseases of former times as determined esp. from fossil or other remains

pa·leo·stri·a·tum *or Brit* **pal·aeo·stri·a·tum** \-strī-'āt-əm\ *n, pl* **-ta** \-tə\ : the phylogenetically older part of the corpus striatum consisting of the globus pallidus

pali·la·lia \ˌpal-ə-'lā-lē-ə\ *n* : a speech defect marked by abnormal repetition of syllables, words, or phrases

pal·in·drome \'pal-ən-ˌdrōm\ *n* : a palindromic sequence of DNA

pal·in·dro·mic \ˌpal-ən-'drō-mik\ *adj* **1** : RECURRENT ⟨~ rheumatism⟩ **2** : of, relating to, or consisting of a double-stranded sequence of DNA in which the order of the nucleotides is the same on each side but running in opposite directions

pal·in·gen·e·sis \ˌpal-ən-'jen-ə-səs\ *n, pl* **-e·ses** \-ˌsēz\ : the appearance in an individual during its development of characters or structures that have been maintained essentially unchanged throughout the evolutionary history of the group to which it belongs

pal·in·ge·net·ic \-jə-'net-ik\ *adj* **1** : of or relating to palingenesis **2** : of, relating to, or being biological characters (as the gill slits in a human embryo) that are derivations from distant ancestral forms rather than adaptations of recent origin

pal·i·sade worm \ˌpal-ə-'sād-\ *n* : BLOODWORM

pal·la·di·um \pə-'lād-ē-əm\ *n* : a silver-white ductile malleable metallic element of the platinum group that is used esp. in electrical contacts, as a catalyst, and in alloys — symbol *Pd*; see ELEMENT table

pall·es·the·sia *or Brit* **pall·aes·the·sia** \ˌpal-es-'thē-zh(ē-)ə\ *n* : awareness or perception of vibration esp. as transmitted through skin and bones

pallia *pl of* PALLIUM

pal·li·ate \'pal-ē-ˌāt\ *vt* **-at·ed; -at·ing** : to reduce the violence of (a disease) : ease without curing — **pal·li·a·tion** \ˌpal-ē-'ā-shən\ *n*

¹pal·lia·tive \'pal-ē-ˌāt-iv, 'pal-yət-\ *adj* : serving to palliate ⟨~ surgery⟩ — **pal·lia·tive·ly** *adv*

²palliative *n* : something that palliates

pal·li·dal \'pal-əd-ᵊl\ *adj* : of, relating to, or involving the globus pallidus ⟨a severe ~ lesion⟩

pal·li·do·fu·gal \ˌpal-əd-ō-'fyü-gəl, ˌpal-i-'däf-yə-gəl\ *adj, of a nerve fiber or impulse* : passing out of the globus pallidus

pal·li·dot·o·my \ˌpal-i-'dät-ə-mē\ *n, pl* **-mies** : the surgical in-

activation of the globus pallidus or a part of it in the treatment of involuntary movements (as in Parkinson's disease)

pal·li·dum \'pal-əd-əm\ *n* : GLOBUS PALLIDUS

pallidum — see TREPONEMA PALLIDUM IMMOBILIZATION TEST

pallidus — see GLOBUS PALLIDUS

pal·li·um \'pal-ē-əm\ *n, pl* **-lia** \-ē-ə\ *or* **-li·ums** : CEREBRAL CORTEX

pal·lor \'pal-ər\ *n* : deficiency of color esp. of the face : PALENESS ⟨patients in hemorrhagic shock may exhibit extreme ~ —*Scientific Amer. Medicine*⟩

palm \'pä(l)m\ *n* : the somewhat concave part of the human hand between the bases of the fingers and the wrist or the corresponding part of the forefoot of a lower mammal

pal·mar \'pal-mər, 'pä(l)m-ər\ *adj* : of, relating to, or involving the palm of the hand ⟨~ surfaces⟩

palmar aponeurosis *n* : an aponeurosis of the palm of the hand that consists of a superficial longitudinal layer continuous with the tendon of the palmaris longus and of a deeper transverse layer — called also *palmar fascia*

palmar arch *n* : either of two loops of blood vessels in the palm of the hand: **a** : a deeply situated transverse artery that is composed of the terminal part of the radial artery joined to a branch of the ulnar artery and that supplies principally the deep muscles of the hand, thumb, and index finger — called also *deep palmar arch* **b** : a superficial arch that is the continuation of the ulnar artery which anastomoses with a branch derived from the radial artery and that sends branches mostly to the fingers — called also *superficial palmar arch*

palmar fascia *n* : PALMAR APONEUROSIS

palmar interosseus *n* : any of three small muscles of the palmar surface of the hand each of which arises from, extends along, and inserts on the side of the second, fourth, or fifth finger facing the middle finger and which acts to adduct its finger toward the middle finger, flex its metacarpophalangeal joint, and extend its distal two phalanges — called also *interosseus palmaris, palmar interosseous muscle*

pal·mar·is \pal-'mar-əs, -'mer-\ *n, pl* **pal·mar·es** \-ˌēz\ : either of two muscles of the palm of the hand: **a** : PALMARIS BREVIS **b** : PALMARIS LONGUS — see PALMAR INTEROSSEUS

palmaris brev·is \-'brev-əs\ *n* : a short transverse superficial muscle of the ulnar side of the palm of the hand that arises from the flexor retinaculum and palmar aponeurosis, inserts into the skin on the ulnar edge of the palm, and functions to tense and stabilize the palm (as in making a fist or catching a ball)

palmaris lon·gus \-'lón-gəs\ *n* : a superficial muscle of the forearm lying on the medial side of the flexor carpi radialis that arises esp. from the medial epicondyle of the humerus, inserts esp. into the palmar aponeurosis, and acts to flex the hand

pal·mi·tate \'pal-mə-ˌtāt, 'pä(l)m-ə-\ *n* : a salt or ester of palmitic acid

pal·mit·ic acid \(ˌ)pal-ˌmit-ik-, (ˌ)pä(l)-\ *n* : a waxy crystalline saturated fatty acid $C_{16}H_{32}O_2$ occurring free or in the form of esters (as glycerides) in most fats and fatty oils and in several essential oils and waxes — called also *hexadecanoic acid*

pal·mi·tin \'pal-mət-ən, 'pä(l)m-ət-ən\ *n* : the triglyceride $C_{51}H_{98}O_6$ of palmitic acid that occurs as a solid with stearin and olein in animal fats — called also *tripalmitin*

pal·mit·ole·ic acid \ˌpal-mət-ō-ˌlē-ik-, ˌpäm-ət-\ *n* : a crystalline unsaturated fatty acid $C_{16}H_{30}O_2$ occurring in the form of glycerides esp. in marine animal oils (as of cod, seals, and whales) and yielding palmitic acid on hydrogenation

pal·mo·plan·tar \ˌpal-mō-'plant-ər, ˌpä(l)m-ō-\ *adj* : of, relating to, or affecting both the palms of the hands and the soles of the feet ⟨~ psoriasis⟩

\ə\ abut \ᵊ\ kitten \ər\ further \a\ ash \ā\ ace \ä\ cot, cart
\aú\ out \ch\ chin \e\ bet \ē\ easy \g\ go \i\ hit \ī\ ice \j\ job
\ŋ\ sing \ō\ go \ó\ law \ói\ boy \th\ thin \th̶\ the \ü\ loot
\ú\ foot \y\ yet \zh\ vision *See also* Pronunciation Symbols page

O
P

pal·pa·ble \'pal-pə-bəl\ *adj* : capable of being touched or felt; *esp* : capable of being examined by palpation ⟨the tip of the spleen was questionably ∼ —*Jour. Amer. Med. Assoc.*⟩

pal·pate \'pal-ˌpāt\ *vb* **-pat·ed; -pat·ing** *vt* : to examine by touch : explore by palpation ∼ *vi* : to use the technique of palpation

pal·pa·tion \pal-'pā-shən\ *n* **1** : an act of touching or feeling **2** : physical examination in medical diagnosis by pressure of the hand or fingers to the surface of the body esp. to determine the condition (as of size or consistency) of an underlying part or organ ⟨∼ of the liver⟩ ⟨∼ of cervical lymph glands⟩ — compare INSPECTION

pal·pa·to·ry \'pal-pə-ˌtō-rē\ *adj* : of, involving, or used for palpation

pal·pe·bra \'pal-pə-brə, pal-'pē-brə\ *n, pl* **pal·pe·brae** \-brē\ : EYELID

palpebrae — see LEVATOR PALPEBRAE SUPERIORIS

pal·pe·bral \pal-'pē-brəl, *Brit also* 'pal-pə-brəl\ *adj* : of, relating to, or located on or near the eyelids ⟨∼ ptosis⟩

palpebral fissure *n* : the space between the margins of the eyelids — called also *rima palpebrarum*

palpebrarum — see RIMA PALPEBRARUM, XANTHELASMA PALPEBRARUM

pal·pi·tate \'pal-pə-ˌtāt\ *vi* **-tat·ed; -tat·ing** : to beat rapidly and strongly — used esp. of the heart when its pulsation is abnormally rapid

pal·pi·ta·tion \ˌpal-pə-'tā-shən\ *n* : a rapid pulsation; *esp* : an abnormally rapid beating of the heart when excited by violent exertion, strong emotion, or disease

pal·sied \'pol-zēd\ *adj* : affected with palsy

pal·sy \'pol-zē\ *n, pl* **pal·sies 1** : PARALYSIS — used chiefly in combination ⟨oculomotor ∼⟩; see BELL'S PALSY, CEREBRAL PALSY **2** : a condition that is characterized by uncontrollable tremor or quivering of the body or one or more of its parts — not used technically

pa·lu·dal \pə-'lüd-ᵊl, 'pal-yəd-ᵊl\ *adj* : of or relating to marshes or fens

pal·u·dism \'pal-yə-ˌdiz-əm\ *n* : MALARIA

pal·u·drine \'pal-ə-drən\ *n* : PROGUANIL

L–PAM \'el-ˌpam\ *n* : MELPHALAN

2–PAM \ˌtü-ˌpē-ˌā-'em\ *n* : PRALIDOXIME

pam·a·quine \'pam-ə-ˌkwin, -ˌkwēn\ *n* : a toxic antimalarial drug $C_{19}H_{29}N_3O$; *also* : PAMAQUINE NAPHTHOATE

pamaquine naph·tho·ate \-'naf-thə-ˌwāt\ *n* : an insoluble salt $C_{42}H_{45}N_3O_7$ of pamaquine obtained as a yellow to orange-yellow powder

pam·id·ro·nate \ˌpam-i-'drō-ˌnāt, -'id-rō-\ *n* : a disodium bisphosphonate bone-resorption inhibitor $C_3H_9NNa_2O_7P_2$ administered as an intravenous infusion in the treatment of hypercalcemia associated with malignancy — called also *pamidronate disodium*

Pam·ine \'pam-ˌēn\ *trademark* — used for a preparation of the bromide salt of methscopolamine

pam·o·ate \'pam-ə-ˌwāt\ *n* : any of various salts or esters of an acid $C_{23}H_{16}O_6$ that include some used as drugs — see HYDROXYZINE

pam·pin·i·form plexus \pam-'pin-ə-ˌform-\ *n* : a venous plexus that is associated with each testicular vein in the male and each ovarian vein in the female — called also *pampiniform venous plexus*

Pan \'pan\ *n* : a genus of anthropoid apes containing the chimpanzee

PAN *abbr* peroxyacetyl nitrate

pan·a·cea \ˌpan-ə-'sē-ə\ *n* : a remedy for all ills or difficulties — **pan·a·ce·an** \-'sē-ən\ *adj*

Pan·a·dol \'pan-ə-ˌdol\ *trademark* — used for a preparation of acetaminophen

pan·ag·glu·ti·na·ble \ˌpan-ə-'glüt-ᵊn-ə-bəl\ *adj, of a red blood cell* : agglutinable by all human sera in the presence of viruses or bacteria — **pan·ag·glu·ti·na·bil·i·ty** \-ˌglüt-ᵊn-ə-'bil-ət-ē\ *n, pl* **-ties**

pan·ag·glu·ti·na·tion \-ə-ˌglüt-ᵊn-'ā-shən\ *n* : agglutination of panagglutinable red blood cells

pan·a·ri·ti·um \ˌpan-ə-'rish-ē-əm\ *n, pl* **-tia** \-ē-ə\ **1** : WHITLOW **2** : FOOT ROT

pan·ar·ter·i·tis \ˌpan-ˌärt-ə-'rīt-əs\ *n* : inflammation involving all coats of an artery

pan·au·to·nom·ic \-ˌot-ə-'näm-ik\ *adj* : of or relating to the entire autonomic nervous system ⟨∼ dysfunction⟩

pan·car·di·tis \-kär-'dīt-əs\ *n* : general inflammation of the heart

Pan·coast's syndrome \'pan-ˌkōsts-\ *n* : a complex of symptoms associated with Pancoast's tumor which includes Horner's syndrome and neuralgia of the arm resulting from pressure on the brachial plexus

Pancoast, Henry Khunrath (1875–1939), American radiologist. One of the pioneers in radiology, Pancoast exerted a major influence in the development of radiology as a science. In 1902 he became head of the X-ray department at the University of Pennsylvania medical school, and from 1912 he held the post of professor of roentgenology (later called radiology). His major contributions included his collective studies on the healthy chest, the X-ray diagnosis of intracranial disease, and his studies on silicosis and pneumoconiosis. He described Pancoast's tumor in 1932.

Pancoast's tumor *or* **Pancoast tumor** *n* : a malignant tumor formed at the upper extremity of the lung

pan·cre·as \'paŋ-krē-əs, 'pan-\ *n, pl* **-cre·as·es** *also* **-cre·ata** \pan-'krē-ət-ə\ : a large lobulated gland that in humans lies in front of the upper lumbar vertebrae and behind the stomach and is somewhat hammer-shaped and firmly attached anteriorly to the curve of the duodenum with which it communicates through one or more pancreatic ducts and that consists of (1) tubular acini secreting digestive enzymes which pass to the intestine and function in the breakdown of proteins, fats, and carbohydrates; (2) modified acinar cells that form islets of Langerhans between the tubules and secrete the hormones insulin and glucagon; and (3) a firm connective-tissue capsule that extends supportive strands into the organ

pan·cre·atec·to·mized \ˌpaŋ-krē-ə-'tek-tə-ˌmīzd, ˌpan-\ *adj* : having undergone a pancreatectomy

pan·cre·atec·to·my \ˌpaŋ-krē-ə-'tek-tə-mē, ˌpan-\ *n, pl* **-mies** : surgical excision of all or part of the pancreas ⟨a total ∼⟩

pan·cre·at·ic \ˌpaŋ-krē-'at-ik, ˌpan-\ *adj* : of, relating to, or produced in the pancreas ⟨∼ amylase⟩

pancreatic artery *n* : any of the branches of the splenic artery that supply the pancreas

pancreatic cholera *n* : VERNER-MORRISON SYNDROME

pancreatic duct *n* : a duct connecting the pancreas with the intestine: **a** : the chief duct of the pancreas that runs from left to right through the body of the gland, passes out its neck, and empties into the duodenum either through an opening shared with the common bile duct or through one close to it — called also *duct of Wirsung, Wirsung's duct* **b** : ACCESSORY PANCREATIC DUCT

pancreatic fibrosis *n* : CYSTIC FIBROSIS

pancreatic juice *n* : a clear alkaline secretion of pancreatic enzymes (as trypsin and lipase) that flows into the duodenum and acts on food already acted on by the gastric juice and saliva

pan·cre·at·i·co·du·o·de·nal \ˌpaŋ-krē-ˌat-i-(ˌ)kō-ˌd(y)ü-ə-'dē-nəl, ˌpan-, -d(y)ú-'äd-ᵊn-əl\ *adj* : of or relating to the pancreas and the duodenum ⟨∼ resection⟩

pancreaticoduodenal artery *n* : either of two arteries that supply the pancreas and duodenum forming an anastomosis giving off numerous branches to these parts: **a** : one arising from the superior mesenteric artery — called also *inferior pancreaticoduodenal artery* **b** : one arising from the gastroduodenal artery — called also *superior pancreaticoduodenal artery*

pancreaticoduodenal vein *n* : any of several veins that drain the pancreas and duodenum accompanying the inferior and superior pancreaticoduodenal arteries

pan·cre·at·i·co·du·o·de·nec·to·my \-ˌd(y)ü-ə-ˌdē-'nek-tə-mē, -d(y)ú-ˌäd-ə-'nek-tə-mē\ *n, pl* **-mies** : partial or complete excision of the pancreas and the duodenum — called also *pancreatoduodenectomy*

pan·cre·at·i·co·du·o·de·nos·to·my \-'näs-tə-mē\ *n, pl* **-mies** : surgical formation of an artificial opening connecting the pancreas to the duodenum

pan·cre·at·i·co·gas·tros·to·my \-ga-'sträs-tə-mē\ *n, pl* **-mies** : surgical formation of an artificial passage connecting the pancreas to the stomach

pan·cre·at·i·co·je·ju·nos·to·my \-ji-,jü-'näs-tə-mē, -,jej-ü-\ *n, pl* **-mies** : surgical formation of an artificial passage connecting the pancreas to the jejunum

pan·cre·atin \pan-'krē-ət-ən; 'paŋ-krē-, 'pan-\ *n* : a mixture of enzymes from the pancreatic juice; *also* : a preparation containing such a mixture obtained from the pancreas of the domestic swine or ox and used as a digestant

pan·cre·ati·tis \,paŋ-krē-ə-'tīt-əs, ,pan-\ *n, pl* **-atit·i·des** \-'tit-ə-,dēz\ : inflammation of the pancreas

pan·cre·at·o·bil·i·ary \,paŋ-krē-ət-ō-'bil-ē-,er-ē, ,pan-\ *adj* : of, relating to, or affecting the pancreas and the bile ducts and gallbladder ⟨the ∼ system⟩ ⟨∼ diseases⟩ ⟨∼ surgery⟩

pan·cre·at·o·du·o·de·nec·to·my \-,d(y)ü-ə-,dē-'nek-tə-mē, -d(y)ù-,äd-ə-'nek-tə-mē\ *n, pl* **-mies** : PANCREATICODUODE-NECTOMY

pan·creo·zy·min \,pan-krē-ō-'zī-mən\ *n* : CHOLECYSTOKI-NIN

pan·cu·ro·ni·um bromide \,pan-kyə-'rō-nē-əm-\ *n* : a neuromuscular blocking agent $C_{35}H_{60}Br_2N_2O_4$ used as a skeletal muscle relaxant — called also *pancuronium*

pan·cy·to·pe·nia \,pan-,sīt-ə-'pē-nē-ə\ *n* : an abnormal reduction in the number of red blood cells, white blood cells, and blood platelets in the blood; *also* : a disorder (as aplastic anemia) characterized by such a reduction — **pan·cy·to·pe·nic** \-'pē-nik\ *adj*

pan·de·mia \pan-'dē-mē-ə\ *n* : PANDEMIC

¹**pan·dem·ic** \pan-'dem-ik\ *adj* : occurring over a wide geographic area and affecting an exceptionally high proportion of the population ⟨∼ malaria⟩ ⟨∼ influenza⟩

²**pandemic** *n* : a pandemic outbreak of a disease

pan·dic·u·la·tion \pan-,dik-yə-'lā-shən\ *n* : a stretching and stiffening esp. of the trunk and extremities (as when fatigued and drowsy or after waking from sleep)

Pan·dy's test \'pan-dēz-\ *n* : a test to determine the presence of protein in the cerebrospinal fluid in which a drop of cerebrospinal fluid is added to a special reagent and the formation of a cloudy precipitate indicates a positive test

   Pán·dy \'pän-dē\, **Kálmán** (1868–1945), Hungarian neurologist. Pándy introduced his test for protein in cerebrospinal fluid in 1910.

pan·el \'pan-ᵊl\ *n* : a list or group of persons selected for some service: as **a** : a list of physicians from among whom a patient may make a choice in accordance with various British health and insurance plans **b** : the patients cared for by a doctor under such a plan

pan·en·ceph·a·li·tis \,pan-in-,sef-ə-'līt-əs\ *n, pl* **-lit·i·des** \-'lit-ə-,dēz\ : inflammation of the brain affecting both white and gray matter — see SUBACUTE SCLEROSING PANENCEPH-ALITIS

pan·en·do·scope \-'en-də-,skōp\ *n* : a cystoscope fitted with an obliquely forward telescopic system that permits wide-angle viewing of the interior of the urinary bladder — **pan·en·do·scop·ic** \-,en-də-'skäp-ik\ *adj* — **pan·en·dos·co·py** \-en-'däs-kə-pē\ *n, pl* **-pies**

Pa·neth cell \'pä-net-\ *n* : any of the granular epithelial cells with large acidophilic nuclei occurring at the base of the crypts of Lieberkühn in the small intestine and appendix

   Paneth, Josef (1857–1890), Austrian physiologist. A professor of physiology in Vienna, Paneth published a description of the granular cells in the crypts of Lieberkühn in 1888.

pang \'paŋ\ *n* : a brief piercing spasm of pain — see BIRTH PANG, HUNGER PANGS

pan·gen \'pan-,jen\ *also* **pan·gene** \-,jēn\ *n* : a hypothetical heredity-controlling particle of protoplasm

pan·gen·e·sis \(')pan-'jen-ə-səs\ *n, pl* **-e·ses** \-,sēz\ : a

disproven hypothetical mechanism of heredity in which the cells throw off particles that collect in the reproductive products or in buds so that the egg or bud contains particles from all parts of the parent — **pan·ge·net·ic** \,pan-jə-'net-ik\ *adj*

pan·hy·po·pi·tu·ita·rism \(')pan-,hī-pō-pə-'t(y)ü-ət-ə-,riz-əm, -'t(y)ü-ə-,triz-əm\ *n* : generalized secretory deficiency of the anterior lobe of the pituitary gland; *also* : a disorder (as Simmonds' disease) characterized by such deficiency

pan·hy·po·pi·tu·itary \-'t(y)ü-ə-,ter-ē\ *adj* : of, relating to, or resulting from panhypopituitarism ⟨∼ dwarfism⟩

pan·hys·ter·ec·to·my \(')pan-,his-tə-'rek-tə-mē\ *n, pl* **-mies** : surgical excision of the uterus and uterine cervix — called also *total hysterectomy;* compare RADICAL HYSTERECTOMY

¹**pan·ic** \'pan-ik\ *n* **1** : a sudden overpowering fright; *also* : acute extreme anxiety **2** : a sudden unreasoning terror often accompanied by mass flight ⟨widespread ∼ in the streets⟩

²**panic** *vb* **pan·icked** \-ikt\; **pan·ick·ing** *vt* : to affect with panic ∼ *vi* : to be affected with panic

panic attack *n* : an episode of intense fear or apprehension that is of sudden onset and may occur for no apparent reason or as a reaction to an identifiable triggering stimulus (as a stressful event); *specif* : one that is accompanied by usu. four or more bodily or cognitive symptoms (as heart palpitations, dizziness, shortness of breath, or feelings of unreality) and that typically peaks within 10 minutes of onset

panic disorder *n* : an anxiety disorder characterized by recurrent unexpected panic attacks followed by a month or more of worry about their recurrence, implications, or consequences or by a change in behavior related to the panic attacks

pan·leu·ko·pe·nia *or chiefly Brit* **pan·leu·co·pe·nia** \,pan-,lü-kə-'pē-nē-ə\ *n* : an acute usu. fatal epizootic disease esp. of cats that is caused by a single-stranded RNA virus of the genus *Parvovirus* (species *Feline panleukopenia virus*) and is characterized by fever, diarrhea, and dehydration and by extensive destruction of white blood cells — called also *cat distemper, cat fever, cat plague, cat typhoid, feline distemper, feline enteritis, feline panleukopenia*

pan·mic·tic \(')pan-'mik-tik\ *adj* : of, relating to, or exhibiting panmixia ⟨a ∼ population⟩

pan·mix·ia \-'mik-sē-ə\ *also* **pan·mixy** \-'mik-sē\ *n, pl* **-mix·ias** *also* **-mix·ies** : random mating within a breeding population

pan·my·e·lop·a·thy \-,mī-ə-'läp-ə-thē\ *n, pl* **-thies** : an abnormal condition of all the blood-forming elements of the bone marrow

pan·my·e·lo·phthi·sis \-,mī-ə-lō-'t(h)ī-səs, -'t(h)is-əs\ *n, pl* **-phthi·ses** \-'t(h)ī-,sēz, -'t(h)is-,ēz\ : wasting or degeneration of the blood-forming elements of the bone marrow

pan·nic·u·li·tis \pə-,nik-yə-'līt-əs\ *n* **1** : inflammation of the subcutaneous layer of fat **2** : a syndrome characterized by recurring fever and usu. painful inflammatory and necrotic nodules in the subcutaneous tissues esp. of the thighs, abdomen, or buttocks — called also *relapsing febrile nodular nonsuppurative panniculitis, Weber-Christian disease*

pan·nic·u·lus \pə-'nik-yə-ləs\ *n, pl* **-u·li** \-yə-,lī\ : a sheet or layer of tissue; *esp* : PANNICULUS ADIPOSUS

panniculus ad·i·po·sus \-,ad-ə-'pō-səs\ *n* : any superficial fascia bearing deposits of fat

panniculus car·no·sus \-kär-'nō-səs\ *n* : a thin sheet of striated muscle lying within or just beneath the superficial fascia, serving to produce local movement of the skin, and well developed in many lower mammals but in humans represented primarily by the platysma

pan·nier \'pan-yər, 'pan-ē-ər\ *n* : a covered basket holding surgical instruments and medicines for a military ambulance

pan·nus \'pan-əs\ *n, pl* **pan·ni** \'pan-,ī\ **1** : a vascular tissue

O
P

\ə\ abut \ᵊ\ kitten \ər\ further \a\ ash \ā\ ace \ä\ cot, cart \aú\ out \ch\ chin \e\ bet \ē\ easy \g\ go \i\ hit \ī\ ice \j\ job \ŋ\ sing \ō\ go \ò\ law \òi\ boy \th\ thin \t͟h\ the \ü\ loot \ù\ foot \y\ yet \zh\ vision *See also* Pronunciation Symbols page

causing a superficial opacity of the cornea and occurring esp. in trachoma **2** : a sheet of inflammatory granulation tissue that spreads from the synovial membrane and invades the joint in rheumatoid arthritis ultimately leading to fibrous ankylosis

pan·o·pho·bia \ˌpan-ə-ˈfō-bē-ə\ *n* : a condition of vague non-specific anxiety : generalized fear

pan·oph·thal·mi·tis \(ˈ)pan-ˌäf-thəl-ˈmīt-əs, -ˌäp-\ *n* : inflammation involving all the tissues of the eyeball

pan·op·tic \(ˈ)pan-ˈäp-tik\ *adj* : permitting everything to be seen ⟨microscopic study of tissues treated with a ∼ stain⟩

pan·sex·u·al·ism \-ˈseksh-(ə-)wə-ˌliz-əm\ *or* **pan·sex·u·al·i·ty** \-ˌsek-shə-ˈwal-ət-ē\ *n, pl* **-isms** *or* **-ties 1** : the suffusion of all experience and conduct with erotic feeling **2** : the view that all desire and interest are derived from the sex instinct ⟨the reproach of ∼ which has so often been levelled against psychoanalysis —*Psychiatry*⟩

pan·sex·u·al·ist \-ləst\ *n* : an adherent of pansexualism

pan·si·nus·itis \-ˌsī-n(y)ə-ˈsīt-əs\ *n* : inflammation of all the sinuses on one or both sides of the nose

pan·sper·mia \ˌpan-ˈspər-mē-ə\ *n* : a theory propounded in the 19th century in opposition to the theory of spontaneous generation and holding that reproductive bodies of living organisms exist throughout the universe and develop wherever the environment is favorable

Pan·stron·gy·lus \ˌpan-ˈsträn-jə-ləs\ *n* : a genus of triatomid bugs that is sometimes considered a subgenus of the genus *Triatoma* and includes some important vectors (as *P. megistus* or *Triatoma megista*) which transmit the causative trypanosome of Chagas' disease to humans

pan·sys·tol·ic \(ˈ)pan-sis-ˈtäl-ik\ *adj* : persisting throughout systole ⟨a ∼ heart murmur⟩

pant \ˈpant\ *vi* : to breathe quickly, spasmodically, or in a labored manner

pan·ta·pho·bia \ˌpant-ə-ˈfō-bē-ə, ˌpant-ˌā-\ *n* : total absence of fear

pan·te·the·ine \ˌpant-ə-ˈthē-ən, -ˌēn\ *n* : a growth factor $C_{11}H_{22}N_2O_4S$ that is essential for various microorganisms (as *Lactobacillus bulgaricus*) and that is a constituent of coenzyme A

pan·to·caine \ˈpant-ə-ˌkān\ *n* : TETRACAINE

pan·to·graph \ˈpant-ə-ˌgraf\ *n* : an instrument for copying (as from a radiograph) on a predetermined scale consisting of four light rigid bars jointed in parallelogram form

pan·to·ic acid \pan-ˌtō-ik-\ *n* : an unstable dihydroxy acid $C_6H_{12}O_4$ that is a constituent of pantothenic acid and used in its synthesis

pan·to·pho·bia \ˌpant-ə-ˈfō-bē-ə\ *n* : PANOPHOBIA

pan·to·pra·zole \pan-ˈtō-prə-ˌzōl\ *n* : a benzimidazole derivative that inhibits gastric acid secretion and is administered in the form of its sodium salt $C_{16}H_{14}F_2N_3NaO_4S$ to treat erosive esophagitis and disorders (as Zollinger-Ellison syndrome) involving gastric acid hypersecretion — see PROTONIX

pan·to·the·nate \ˌpant-ə-ˈthen-ˌāt, pan-ˈtäth-ə-ˌnāt\ *n* : a salt or ester of pantothenic acid — see CALCIUM PANTOTHENATE

pan·to·then·ic acid \ˌpant-ə-ˌthen-ik-\ *n* : a viscous oily acid $C_9H_{17}NO_5$ that belongs to the vitamin B complex, occurs usu. combined (as in coenzyme A) in all living tissues and esp. liver, is made synthetically, and is essential for the growth of various animals and microorganisms

pan·to·yl \ˈpant-ə-wil\ *n* : the acid group $C_6H_{11}O_3$– of pantoic acid

pan·trop·ic \(ˈ)pan-ˈträp-ik\ *adj* : affecting various tissues without showing special affinity for one of them ⟨a ∼ virus⟩ — compare DERMOTROPIC, NEUROTROPIC

pan·zo·ot·ic \-zə-ˈwät-ik\ *n* : a disease affecting animals of many species esp. over a wide area

PaO₂ *abbr* partial pressure of arterial oxygen

pap \ˈpap\ *n* : a soft food (as for infants)

pa·pa·in \pə-ˈpā-ən, -ˈpī-\ *n* : a crystallizable protease in the juice of the green fruit of the papaya obtained usu. as a brownish powder and used chiefly as a tenderizer for meat and in medicine as a digestant and as a topical agent in the debridement of necrotic tissue

pa·pa·in·ase \pə-ˈpā-ə-ˌnās, pə-ˈpī-ə-, -ˌnāz\ *n* : any of several proteases (as papain, ficin, and bromelain) that are found in plants, are activated by reducing agents (as cysteine or glutathione), and are inactivated by oxidizing agents (as hydrogen peroxide or iodine) toward which other proteases are stable

Pa·pa·ni·co·laou smear \ˌpäp-ə-ˈnē-kə-ˌlaù-, ˌpap-ə-ˈnik-ə-\ *n* : PAP SMEAR

Papanicolaou, George Nicholas (1883–1962), American anatomist and cytologist. Papanicolaou devoted his medical research almost entirely to the physiology of reproduction and exfoliative cytology. In 1917 he began studying the vaginal discharge of the guinea pig, examining specifically the histological and physiological changes that occur during a typical estrous cycle. In 1923 he turned to the cytological examination of the vaginal fluid of women as a way of detecting uterine cancer. In 1943 he published his findings after studying 179 cases of uterine cancer. His monograph *Diagnosis of Uterine Cancer by Vaginal Smear* treated a variety of physiological and pathological states, including abortion, amenorrhea, ectopic pregnancy, endometrial hyperplasia, menopause, the menstrual cycle, prepuberty, and puerperium. The Papanicolaou smear rapidly achieved wide acceptance as a means of cancer diagnosis.

Papanicolaou test *n* : PAP SMEAR

papataci fever, papatasi fever *var of* PAPPATACI FEVER

Pa·pa·ver \pə-ˈpav-ər, -ˈpāv-\ *n* : a genus (the type of the family Papaveraceae) of chiefly bristly hairy herbs that includes the opium poppy (*P. somniferum*)

pa·pav·er·ine \pə-ˈpav-ə-ˌrēn, -(ə-)rən\ *n* : a crystalline alkaloid $C_{20}H_{21}NO_4$ that constitutes about one percent of opium, that is made synthetically from vanillin, and that is used usu. in the form of its hydrochloride $C_{20}H_{21}NO_4 \cdot HCl$ esp. as a vasodilator because of its ability to relax smooth muscle

pa·paw *or* **paw·paw** *n* **1** \pə-ˈpò\ : PAPAYA **2** \ˈpäp-(ˌ)ò, ˈpóp-\ : a No. American tree (*Asimina triloba* of the family Annonaceae) with purple flowers and a yellow edible fruit; *also* : its fruit

pa·pa·ya \pə-ˈpī-ə\ *n* : a tropical American tree of the genus *Carica* (*C. papaya*) with large oblong yellow edible fruit; *also* : its fruit which is the source of papain

pa·pay·o·tin \pə-ˈpī-ət-ən\ *n* : PAPAIN

pa·per·bark \ˈpā-pər-ˌbärk\ *n* : CAJEPUT

paper chromatography *n* : chromatography that uses paper strips or sheets as the adsorbent stationary phase through which a solution flows and is used esp. to separate amino acids — compare COLUMN CHROMATOGRAPHY, THIN-LAYER CHROMATOGRAPHY

pa·pil·la \pə-ˈpil-ə\ *n, pl* **pa·pil·lae** \-ˈpil-(ˌ)ē, -ˌī\ : a small projecting body part similar to a nipple in form: as **a** : a vascular process of connective tissue extending into and nourishing the root of a hair, feather, or developing tooth **b** : any of the vascular protuberances of the dermal layer of the skin extending into the epidermal layer and often containing tactile corpuscles **c** : RENAL PAPILLA **d** : any of the small protuberances on the upper surface of the tongue — see CIRCUMVALLATE PAPILLA, FILIFORM PAPILLA, FUNGIFORM PAPILLA, INTERDENTAL PAPILLA, OPTIC PAPILLA

papilla of Vater *n* : AMPULLA OF VATER

pap·il·lary \ˈpap-ə-ˌler-ē, *esp Brit* pə-ˈpil-ə-rē\ *adj* : of, relating to, or resembling a papilla : PAPILLOSE

papillary carcinoma *n* : a carcinoma characterized by a papillary structure

papillary layer *n* : the superficial layer of the dermis raised into papillae that fit into corresponding depressions on the inner surface of the epidermis

papillary muscle *n* : one of the small muscular columns attached at one end to the chordae tendineae and at the other to the wall of the ventricle and that maintain tension on the chordae tendineae as the ventricle contracts

pap·il·late \ˈpap-ə-ˌlāt, pə-ˈpil-ət\ *adj* : covered with or bearing papillae

pap·il·lec·to·my \ˌpap-ə-ˈlek-tə-mē\ *n, pl* **-mies** : the surgical removal of a papilla

pap·il·le·de·ma *or chiefly Brit* **pap·il·loe·de·ma** \ˌpap-əl-ə-ˈdē-mə\ *n* : swelling and protrusion of the blind spot of the eye caused by edema — called also *choked disk*

pa·pil·li·form \pə-ˈpil-ə-ˌförm\ *adj* : resembling a papilla

pap·il·li·tis \ˌpap-ə-ˈlīt-əs\ *n* : inflammation of a papilla; *esp* : inflammation of the optic disk — see NECROTIZING PAPILLITIS

pap·il·lo·ma \ˌpap-ə-ˈlō-mə\ *n, pl* **-mas** *also* **-ma·ta** \-mət-ə\ : a benign tumor (as a wart or condyloma) resulting from an overgrowth of epithelial tissue on papillae of vascularized connective tissue (as of the skin) — see PAPILLOMAVIRUS

pap·il·lo·ma·to·sis \-ˌlō-mə-ˈtō-səs\ *n, pl* **-to·ses** \-ˌsēz\ : a condition marked by the presence of numerous papillomas

pap·il·lo·ma·tous \-ˈlō-mət-əs\ *adj* **1** : resembling or being a papilloma **2** : marked or characterized by papillomas

pap·il·lo·ma·vi·rus \ˌpap-ə-ˈlō-mə-ˌvī-rəs\ *n* **1** *cap* : the sole genus in a family (*Papillomaviridae*) of double-stranded DNA viruses that contain a single molecule of DNA, have a capsid composed of 72 capsomers, and cause papillomas in mammals **2** : any of the genus *Papillomavirus* of double-stranded DNA viruses

pap·il·lose \ˈpap-ə-ˌlōs\ *adj* : covered with, resembling, or bearing papillae — **pap·il·los·i·ty** \ˌpap-ə-ˈläs-ət-ē\ *n, pl* **-ties**

Pa·po·va·vi·ri·dae \pə-ˌpō-və-ˈvir-ə-ˌdē\ *n pl* : a former family of double-stranded DNA viruses that included the polyomaviruses and the papillomaviruses before they were placed in their own families

pa·po·va·vi·rus \pə-ˈpō-və-ˌvī-rəs\ *n* : any of the papillomaviruses and polyomaviruses

pap·pa·ta·ci fever *also* **pa·pa·ta·ci fever** \ˌpäp-ə-ˈtäch-ē-\ *or* **pa·pa·ta·si fever** \-ˈtä-sē-\ *n* : SANDFLY FEVER

Pap smear \ˈpap-\ *n* : a method or a test based on it for the early detection of cancer esp. of the uterine cervix that involves staining exfoliated cells by a special technique which differentiates diseased tissue — called also *Papanicolaou smear, Papanicolaou test, Pap test*

G. N. Papanicolaou — see PAPANICOLAOU SMEAR

pap·u·la \ˈpap-yə-lə\ *n, pl* **pap·u·lae** \-ˌlē\ **1** : PAPULE **2** : a small papilla

pap·u·lar \ˈpap-yə-lər\ *adj* : consisting of or characterized by papules ⟨a ~ rash⟩ ⟨~ lesions⟩

pap·u·la·tion \ˌpap-yə-ˈlā-shən\ *n* **1** : a stage in some eruptive conditions marked by the formation of papules **2** : the formation of papules

pap·ule \ˈpap-(ˌ)yül\ *n* : a small solid usu. conical elevation of the skin caused by inflammation, accumulated secretion, or hypertrophy of tissue elements

pap·u·lo·ne·crot·ic \ˌpap-yə-lō-nə-ˈkrät-ik\ *adj* : marked by the formation of papules that tend to break down and form open sores ⟨~ tuberculids⟩

pap·u·lo·pus·tu·lar \-ˈpəs-chə-lər, -ˈpəs-t(y)ə-\ *adj* : consisting of both papules and pustules ⟨~ acne⟩

pap·u·lo·sis \ˌpap-yə-ˈlō-səs\ *n* : the condition of having papular lesions

pap·u·lo·ve·sic·u·lar \ˌpap-yə-lō-və-ˈsik-yə-lər\ *adj* : marked by the presence of both papules and vesicles ⟨a ~ rash⟩

pap·y·ra·ceous \ˌpap-ə-ˈrā-shəs\ *adj* : of, relating to, or being the flattened remains of one of twin fetuses which has died in the uterus and been compressed by the growth of the other

par \ˈpär\ *n* : a usual standard of physical condition or health ⟨his insulin production . . . is not up to ~ —P. G. Donohue⟩

¹para \ˈpar-ə\ *n, pl* **par·as** *or* **par·ae** \ˈpar-ˌē\ : a woman delivered of a specified number of children — used in combination with a term or figure to indicate the number ⟨multip*ara*⟩ ⟨a 36-year-old *para* 5⟩; compare GRAVIDA

²para \ˈpar-ə\ *adj* **1** : relating to, characterized by, or being two positions in the benzene ring that are separated by two carbon atoms **2** : of, relating to, or being a diatomic molecule (as of hydrogen) in which the nuclei of the atoms are spinning in opposite directions

para- \ˌpar-ə, ˈpar-ə\ *or* **par-** *prefix* **1** : closely related to ⟨*par*-

aldehyde⟩ **2** : involving substitution at or characterized by two opposite positions in the benzene ring that are separated by two carbon atoms ⟨*para*dichlorobenzene⟩ — abbr. *p-*; compare META- 2, ORTH- 2

para–ami·no·ben·zo·ic acid \ˈpar-ə-ə-ˌmē-nō-ˌben-ˌzō-ik-, ˈpar-ə-ˌam-ə-(ˌ)nō-\ *n* : a colorless para-substituted aminobenzoic acid that is a growth factor of the vitamin B complex and is used as a sunscreen — called also *PABA*

para–ami·no·hip·pu·rate \-ˈhip-yə-ˌrāt\ *n* : a salt of para-aminohippuric acid

para–ami·no·hip·pu·ric acid \-hi-ˌpyùr-ik-\ *n* : a crystalline acid administered intravenously in the form of its sodium salt $C_9H_9N_2NaO_3$ in testing kidney function

para–ami·no·sal·i·cyl·ic acid \-ˌsal-ə-ˌsil-ik-\ *n* : the white crystalline para-substituted isomer of aminosalicylic acid that is made synthetically and is used in the treatment of tuberculosis

para–an·es·the·sia *or chiefly Brit* **para–an·aes·the·sia** \-ˌan-əs-ˈthē-zhə\ *n* : anesthesia of both sides of the lower part of the body

para–aor·tic \-ā-ˈort-ik\ *adj* : close to the aorta ⟨~ lymph nodes⟩

para–api·cal \-ˈā-pi-kəl *or* -ˈap-i-\ *adj* : close to the apex of the heart ⟨~ regions⟩

par·a·ban·ic acid \ˌpar-ə-ˌban-ik-\ *n* : a crystalline nitrogenous cyclic diacid $C_3H_2N_2O_3$ made esp. by oxidation of uric acid — called also *oxalylurea*

para·ba·sal body \-ˌbā-səl-, -zəl-\ *n* : a cytoplasmic body closely associated with the kinetoplast of certain flagellates

para·ben \ˈpar-ə-ben\ *n* : either of two antifungal agents used as preservatives in foods and pharmaceuticals: **a** : METHYLPARABEN **b** : PROPYLPARABEN

para·bi·ont \ˌpar-ə-ˈbī-ˌänt\ *n* : either of the organisms joined in parabiosis

para·bi·o·sis \ˌpar-ə-(ˌ)bī-ˈō-səs, -bē-\ *n, pl* **-o·ses** \-ˌsēz\ : the anatomical and physiological union of two organisms either natural (as in conjoined twins) or artificially produced — **para·bi·ot·ic** \-ˈät-ik\ *adj* — **para·bi·ot·i·cal·ly** \-i-k(ə-)lē\ *adv*

para·blast \ˈpar-ə-ˌblast\ *n* **1** : MESOBLAST; *esp* : the part of the mesoblast giving rise to vascular structures **2** : blastomeres that give rise to extraembryonic membranes — **para·blas·tic** \-ˌblas-tik\ *adj*

para·car·mine \ˌpar-ə-ˈkär-mən, -ˌmīn\ *n* : a carmine microscopy stain containing calcium chloride and often aluminum chloride

para·ca·sein \-kā-ˈsēn, -ˈkā-sē-ən\ *n* : CASEIN b

Par·a·cel·sian \ˌpar-ə-ˈsel-sən\ *adj* : of, relating to, or conforming to the practice or theories of Paracelsus according to whose teachings the activities of the human body are chemical, health depends on the proper chemical composition of the organs and fluids, and the object of chemistry is to prepare medicines

Par·a·cel·sus \ˌpar-ə-ˈsel-səs\ (*orig.* **Philippus Aureolus Theophrastus Bombastus von Hohenheim**) **(1493–1541)**, German alchemist and physician. One of the most remarkable and notorious men of his time, Paracelsus is credited with a major part in applying chemistry to medicine. His introduction of many new chemical remedies—including those containing mercury, sulfur, iron, and copper sulfate—stimulated the development of pharmaceutical chemistry. An argumentative, vitriolic iconoclast, he challenged the medical establishment and questioned the blind adherence to the Galenic and Arabic traditions in medicine. He denounced the widespread belief that the stars and planets control the parts of the human body. He stressed the healing power of nature and raged against the worthless nostrums and treatments of his day. His own notable medical achievements include the best clinical description of

O
P

\ə\ **abut** \ˈə\ **kitten** \ər\ **further** \a\ **ash** \ā\ **ace** \ä\ **cot, cart**
\aù\ **out** \ch\ **chin** \e\ **bet** \ē\ **easy** \g\ **go** \i\ **hit** \ī\ **ice** \j\ **job**
\ŋ\ **sing** \ō\ **go** \ò\ **law** \òi\ **boy** \th\ **thin** \th\ **the** \ü\ **loot**
\ù\ **foot** \y\ **yet** \zh\ **vision** *See also* Pronunciation Symbols page

syphilis up to that time, the discovery that silicosis results from the inhalation of airborne mine dust, and the first realization that goiter is related to the presence of minerals and especially lead in drinking water.

para·cen·te·sis \ˌpar-ə-(ˌ)sen-ˈtē-səs\ *n, pl* **-te·ses** \-ˌsēz\ : a surgical puncture of a bodily cavity (as of the abdomen) with a trocar, aspirator, or other instrument usu. to draw off an abnormal effusion for diagnostic or therapeutic purposes

para·cen·tral \ˌpar-ə-ˈsen-trəl\ *adj* : lying near a center or central part ⟨hemorrhages located near the fovea . . . caused a ∼ scotoma —D. M. McFadden *et al*⟩

para·cen·tric \-ˈsen-trik\ *adj* : being an inversion that occurs in a single arm of one chromosome and does not involve the chromomere — compare PERICENTRIC

para·cer·vi·cal \-ˈsər-vi-kəl\ *adj* : located or administered next to the uterine cervix ⟨∼ injection⟩

par·ac·et·al·de·hyde \ˌpar-ˌas-ə-ˈtal-də-ˌhīd\ *n* : PARALDEHYDE

para·cet·a·mol \ˌpar-ə-ˈsēt-ə-ˌmól\ *n, Brit* : ACETAMINOPHEN

para·chlo·ro·phe·nol \-ˌklōr-ə-ˈfē-ˌnōl, -ˌklór-ə-, -ˈfē-ˌnòl, -fi-ˈnōl\ *n* : a chlorinated phenol C_6H_5ClO used as a germicide

para·chol·era \-ˈkäl-ə-rə\ *n* : a disease clinically resembling Asiatic cholera but caused by a different vibrio

¹**para·chord·al** \-ˈkórd-ᵊl\ *adj* : situated at the side of the notochord

²**parachordal** *n* : either of a pair of cartilaginous rods that develop on each side of the notochord beneath the posterior part of the embryonic brain and participate in formation of the parachordal plate

parachordal plate *n* : a cartilaginous plate that is formed of the fused parachordals and anterior notochord and gives rise to the ethmoid bone and certain other bones of the vertebrate skull — called also *basilar plate*

Para·coc·cid·i·oi·des \ˌpar-ə-(ˌ)käk-ˌsid-ē-ˈóid-ˌēz\ *n* : a genus of imperfect fungi that includes the causative agent (*P. brasiliensis*) of South American blastomycosis

para·coc·cid·i·oi·do·my·co·sis \-(ˌ)käk-ˌsid-ē-ˌóid-ō-(ˌ)mī-ˈkō-sis\ *n, pl* **-co·ses** \-ˌsēz\ : SOUTH AMERICAN BLASTOMYCOSIS

para·col·ic \-ˈkō-lik, -ˈkäl-ik\ *adj* : adjacent to the colon ⟨∼ lymph nodes⟩

paracolic gutter *n* : either of two grooves formed by the peritoneum and lying respectively lateral to the ascending and descending colons

para·co·lon \-ˈkō-lən\ *n* : any of several coliform bacteria that do not ferment lactose, are causative agents of a number of human gastroenteritides, and have sometimes been grouped in a separate genus (*Paracolobactrum*) but are now assigned to other genera (as *Escherichia*)

para·cone \ˈpar-ə-ˌkōn\ *n* : the anterior of the three cusps of a primitive upper molar that in higher forms is the principal anterior and external cusp

para·co·nid \ˌpar-ə-ˈkō-nəd\ *n* : the cusp of a primitive lower molar that corresponds to the paracone of the upper molar and that in higher forms is the anterior and internal cusp

para·cre·sol \-ˈkrē-ˌsól, -ˌsōl\ *n* : the para isomer of cresol

para·crine \ˈpar-ə-krən, -ˌkrīn\ *adj* : of, relating to, promoted by, or being a substance secreted by a cell and acting on adjacent cells ⟨∼ stimulation of tumor growth —M. B. Rettig *et al*⟩ — compare AUTOCRINE

par·acu·sis \ˌpar-ə-ˈk(y)ü-səs\ *n, pl* **-acu·ses** \-ˌsēz\ : a disorder in the sense of hearing — **par·acu·sic** \-sik\ *adj or n*

para·cys·ti·tis \ˌpar-ə-sis-ˈtīt-əs\ *n, pl* **-tit·i·des** \-ˈtit-ə-ˌdēz\ : inflammation of the connective tissue about the bladder

para·den·tal \-ˈdent-ᵊl\ *adj* : adjacent to a tooth ⟨an inflammatory ∼ cyst⟩

para·den·ti·tis \-ˌden-ˈtīt-əs\ *n* : PERIODONTITIS

para·den·ti·um \-ˈdent-ē-əm, -ˈden-ch(ē-)əm\ *n, pl* **-tia** \-ē-ə, -ch(ē-)ə\ : the paradental tissues including the gums, the alveolar process, and the periodontal membrane

para·den·to·sis \-ˌden-ˈtō-səs\ *n, pl* **-to·ses** \-ˈtō-ˌsēz\ : PERIODONTOSIS

para·di·chlo·ro·ben·zene *also* **p–di·chlo·ro·ben·zene** \ˌpar-ə-ˌdī-ˌklōr-ə-ˈben-ˌzēn, -ˌklór-, -ben-ˈ\ *n* : a white crystalline compound $C_6H_4Cl_2$ made by chlorinating benzene and used chiefly as a moth repellent and deodorizer — called also *PDB*

para·did·y·mis \-ˈdid-ə-məs\ *n, pl* **-y·mi·des** \-ə-mə-ˌdēz\ : a group of coiled tubules situated in front of the lower end of the spermatic cord above the enlarged upper extremity of the epididymis and considered to be a remnant of tubes of the mesonephros

par·a·don·to·sis \-ˌdän-ˈtō-səs\ *n, pl* **-to·ses** \-ˈtō-ˌsēz\ : PERIODONTOSIS

par·a·dox \ˈpar-ə-ˌdäks\ *n* : an instance of a paradoxical phenomenon or reaction

par·a·dox·i·cal \ˌpar-ə-ˈdäk-si-kəl\ *also* **par·a·dox·ic** \-sik\ *adj* : not being the normal or usual kind ⟨a ∼ embolism⟩

paradoxical sleep *n* : REM SLEEP

paradoxus — see PULSUS PARADOXUS

para·esoph·a·ge·al *or Brit* **para–oe·soph·a·ge·al** \-i-ˌsäf-ə-ˈjē-əl\ *adj* : adjacent to the esophagus; *esp* : relating to or being a hiatal hernia in which the connection between the esophagus and the stomach remains in its normal location but part or all of the stomach herniates through the hiatus into the thorax

paraesthesia, paraesthetic *chiefly Brit var of* PARESTHESIA, PARESTHETIC

par·af·fin \ˈpar-ə-fən\ *n* **1 a** : a waxy crystalline flammable substance obtained esp. from distillates of wood, coal, petroleum, or shale oil that is a complex mixture of hydrocarbons and is used chiefly in coating and sealing, in candles, in rubber compounding, and in pharmaceuticals and cosmetics **b** : any of various mixtures of similar hydrocarbons including mixtures that are semisolid or oily **2** : ALKANE — **par·af·fin·ic** \ˌpar-ə-ˈfin-ik\ *adj*

paraffin oil *n* : any of various hydrocarbon oils (as mineral oil) obtained from petroleum

par·af·fin·o·ma \ˌpar-ə-fə-ˈnō-mə\ *n, pl* **-mas** *also* **-ma·ta** \-mət-ə\ : a granuloma caused by the introduction (as by injection) of paraffin into the tissues

para·floc·cu·lus \ˌpar-ə-ˈfläk-yə-ləs\ *n, pl* **-li** \-ˌlī\ : a lateral accessory part of the flocculus of the cerebellum

para·fol·lic·u·lar \-fə-ˈlik-yə-lər\ *adj* : located in the vicinity of or surrounding a follicle ⟨∼ cells of the thyroid⟩

para·form \ˈpar-ə-ˌfórm\ *n* : PARAFORMALDEHYDE

para·form·al·de·hyde \ˌpar-ə-fòr-ˈmal-də-ˌhīd, -fər-\ *n* : a white powder $(CH_2O)_x$ that consists of a polymer of formaldehyde and is used esp. as a fungicide

para·fo·vea \-ˈfō-vē-ə\ *n, pl* **-fo·ve·ae** \-ˈfō-vē-ē, -vē-ˌī\ : the area surrounding the fovea and containing both rods and cones

para·fo·ve·al \-ˈfō-vē-əl\ *adj* **1** : surrounding the fovea ⟨∼ regions of the retina⟩ **2** : dependent on parts of the retina external to the fovea ⟨∼ vision⟩ ⟨∼ threshold of reaction⟩

para·fuch·sin \-ˈfyük-sən\ *n* : the chloride of pararosaniline base used as a biological stain

para·gan·gli·o·ma \-ˌgan·glī-ˈō-mə\ *n, pl* **-mas** *also* **-ma·ta** \-mət-ə\ : a ganglioma derived from chromaffin cells — compare PHEOCHROMOCYTOMA

para·gan·gli·on \-ˈgaŋ-glē-ən\ *n, pl* **-glia** \-glē-ə\ : one of numerous collections of chromaffin tissue associated with the collateral and chain ganglia of the sympathetic nerves and similar in structure to the medulla of the adrenal glands — **para·gan·gli·on·ic** \-ˌgaŋ-glē-ˈän-ik\ *adj*

par·ag·glu·ti·na·tion \ˌpar-ə-ˌglüt-ᵊn-ˈā-shən\ *n* : CROSS AGGLUTINATION

par·a·gon·i·mi·a·sis \ˌpar-ə-ˌgän-ə-ˈmī-ə-səs\ *n, pl* **-a·ses** \-ˌsēz\ : infestation with or disease caused by a lung fluke of the genus *Paragonimus* (*P. westermanii*) that invades the lung where it produces chronic bronchitis with cough and reddish or brownish sputum and that occas. also enters other viscera or the brain

Par·a·gon·i·mus \ˌpar-ə-ˈgän-ə-məs\ *n* : a genus of digenetic trematodes of the family Troglotrematidae comprising forms normally parasitic in the lungs of mammals including humans

para·gram·ma·tism \-'gram-ə-ˌtiz-əm\ *n* : PARAPHASIA

para·gran·u·lo·ma \-ˌgran-yə-'lō-mə\ *n, pl* **-mas** *also* **-ma·ta** \-mət-ə\ **1** : a granuloma esp. of the lymph glands that is characterized by inflammation and replacement of the normal cell structure by an infiltrate **2** : a benign form of Hodgkin's disease in which paragranulomas of the lymph glands are a symptom — called also *Hodgkin's paragranuloma*

para·graph·ia \-'graf-ē-ə\ *n* : a condition (as in some mental disorders) in which words or letters other than those intended are written

para·he·mo·phil·ia *or chiefly Brit* **para·hae·mo·phil·ia** \-ˌhē-mə-'fil-ē-ə\ *n* : a congenital deficiency of factor V in the blood that is associated with hemorrhagic diathesis and abnormally slow clotting time — called also *Owren's disease*

para·hip·po·cam·pal gyrus \-ˌhip-ə-'kam-pəl-\ *n* : a convolution on the inferior surface of the cerebral cortex of the temporal lobe that borders the hippocampus and contains elements of both archipallium and neopallium — called also *hippocampal convolution, hippocampal gyrus*

para·hor·mone \-'hor-ˌmōn\ *n* : a substance that functions as a hormone but is of relatively nonspecific nature ⟨the likely role of neurotensin as a ∼ in the gastrointestinal tract —J. P. Vincent⟩

para·hy·droxy·ben·zo·ic acid \-hī-ˌdräk-sē-ben-ˌzō-ik-\ *n* : HYDROXYBENZOIC ACID a

para·in·flu·en·za virus \-ˌin-flü-ˌen-zə-\ *n* : any of several single-stranded RNA viruses (genera *Respirovirus* and *Rubulavirus*) of the family *Paramyxoviridae* that are associated with or responsible for some respiratory infections esp. in children — called also *parainfluenza*

para·ker·a·to·sis \ˌpar-ə-ˌker-ə-'tō-səs\ *n, pl* **-to·ses** \-ˌsēz\ : an abnormality of the horny layer of the skin resulting in a disturbance in the process of keratinization — **para·ker·a·tot·ic** \-'tät-ik\ *adj*

para·ki·net·ic \-kə-'net-ik, -kī-\ *adj* : of, relating to, or affected with a disorder of motor function resulting in abnormal movements

para·la·lia \-'lā-lē-ə\ *n* : a speech disorder marked by distortions of sounds or substitution of letters

para·lamb·da·cism \-'lam-də-ˌsiz-əm\ *n* : inability to pronounce the sound of *l* or difficulty in pronouncing it that usu. results in some other sound (as of *t, r,* or *w*) being substituted — compare LAMBDACISM 2

par·al·de·hyde \pa-'ral-də-ˌhīd, pə-\ *n* : a colorless liquid polymer $C_6H_{12}O_3$ derived from acetaldehyde and used esp. as an anticonvulsant, hypnotic, and sedative — called also *paracetaldehyde*

para·lex·ia \ˌpar-ə-'lek-sē-ə\ *n* : a disturbance in reading ability marked by the transposition of words or syllables and usu. associated with brain injury

par·al·lax \'par-ə-ˌlaks\ *n* : the apparent displacement or the difference in apparent direction of an object as seen from two different points not on a straight line with the object ⟨motion ∼ governs the way objects appear to move when the eyes or head are shifted —Edmund Andrews⟩

par·al·lel·ism \'par-ə-ˌlel-ˌiz-əm, -ləl-\ *n* : a philosophical or psychological doctrine that there is a one-to-one correspondence between events in the mind and events in the brain but that the two sets of events exist without interacting in a causal way — called also *psychophysical parallelism*

par·al·lel·om·e·ter \ˌpar-ə-ˌle-'läm-ət-ər\ *n* : a device to test the parallelism of flat surfaces esp. in aligning attachments and abutments of dental prostheses

para·lo·gia \ˌpar-ə-'lō-j(ē-)ə\ *n* : a reasoning disorder characterized by expression of illogical or delusional thoughts

paralysant, paralysation, paralyse, paralyser *Brit var of* PARALYZANT, PARALYZATION, PARALYZE, PARALYZER

pa·ral·y·sis \pə-'ral-ə-səs\ *n, pl* **-y·ses** \-ˌsēz\ : complete or partial loss of function esp. when involving the power of motion or of sensation in any part of the body — see HEMIPLEGIA, PARAPLEGIA, PARESIS 1

paralysis agi·tans \-'aj-ə-ˌtanz\ *n* : PARKINSON'S DISEASE

¹par·a·lyt·ic \ˌpar-ə-'lit-ik\ *adj* **1** : affected with or character-

ized by paralysis **2** : of, relating to, causing, or resembling paralysis

²paralytic *n* : one affected with paralysis

paralytica — see DEMENTIA PARALYTICA

paralytic dementia *n* : GENERAL PARESIS

paralytic ileus *n* : ileus resulting from failure of peristalsis

paralytic rabies *n* : rabies marked by sluggishness and by early paralysis esp. of the muscles of jaw and throat — called also *dumb rabies;* compare FURIOUS RABIES

paralytic shell·fish poisoning \-'shel-ˌfish-\ *n* : food poisoning that results from consumption of shellfish and esp. 2-shelled mollusks (as clams, mussels, or scallops) contaminated with dinoflagellates causing red tide and that is characterized by paresthesia, nausea, vomiting, abdominal cramping, muscle weakness, and sometimes paralysis which may lead to respiratory failure

¹par·a·ly·zant *or Brit* **par·a·ly·sant** \'par-ə-ˌlīz-ᵊnt, pə-'ral-ə-zənt\ *adj* : causing paralysis

²paralyzant *or Brit* **paralysant** *n* : an agent that causes paralysis

par·a·lyze *or Brit* **par·a·lyse** \'par-ə-ˌlīz\ *vt* **-lyzed** *or Brit* **-lysed; -lyz·ing** *or Brit* **-lys·ing** : to affect with paralysis — **par·a·ly·za·tion** *or Brit* **par·a·ly·sa·tion** \ˌpar-ə-lə-'zā-shən\ *n*

par·a·lyz·er *or Brit* **par·a·lys·er** \-ˌlī-zər\ *n* **1** : one that paralyzes **2** : INHIBITOR a

para·mag·net·ic \ˌpar-ə-mag-'net-ik\ *adj* : being or relating to a magnetizable substance (as aluminum) that has a small but positive susceptibility which varies little with magnetizing force — **para·mag·ne·tism** \-'mag-nə-ˌtiz-əm\ *n*

para·mas·toid \-'mas-ˌtoid\ *adj* : situated beside or adjacent to the mastoid process ⟨a ∼ process⟩

par·a·me·cin \-'mēs-ᵊn\ *n* : a toxic substance that is secreted into the ambient medium by paramecia and that possess the cytoplasmic factor kappa

par·a·me·cium \ˌpar-ə-'mē-sh(ē-)əm, -sē-əm\ *n* **1** *cap* : a genus of ciliate protozoans that have an elongate body rounded at the anterior end and an oblique funnel-shaped buccal groove bearing the mouth at the extremity **2** *pl* **-cia** \-sh(ē-)ə, -sē-ə\ *also* **-ciums** : any ciliate protozoan of the genus *Paramecium*

para·me·di·an \-'mēd-ē-ən\ *adj* : situated adjacent to the midline ⟨a ∼ scar on the abdomen⟩

para·med·ic \ˌpar-ə-'med-ik\ *also* **para·med·i·cal** \-i-kəl\ *n* **1** : a person who works in a health field in an auxiliary capacity to a physician (as by giving injections and taking X-rays) **2** : a specially trained medical technician certified to provide a wide range of emergency medical services (as defibrillation and the intravenous administration of drugs) before or during transport to the hospital — compare EMT

para·med·i·cal \ˌpar-ə-'med-i-kəl\ *also* **para·med·ic** \-ik\ *adj* : concerned with supplementing the work of highly trained medical professionals ⟨∼ aides and technicians⟩

para·me·so·neph·ric duct \-ˌmez-ə-'nef-rik-, -ˌmēz-, -ˌmēs-, -ˌmes-\ *n* : MÜLLERIAN DUCT

para·metha·di·one \-ˌmeth-ə-'dī-ˌōn\ *n* : a liquid compound $C_7H_{11}NO_3$ that is a derivative of trimethadione and is sometimes used in the treatment of absence seizures

para·meth·a·sone \-'meth-ə-ˌzōn\ *n* : a glucocorticoid with few mineralocorticoid side effects that is used for its antiinflammatory and antiallergic actions esp. in the form of its acetate $C_{24}H_{31}FO_6$

para·me·tri·al \-'mē-trē-əl\ *adj* : located near the uterus

para·me·tri·tis \-mə-'trīt-əs\ *n* : inflammation of the parametrium

para·me·tri·um \-'mē-trē-əm\ *n, pl* **-tria** \-trē-ə\ : the connective tissue and fat adjacent to the uterus

par·am·ne·sia \ˌpar-ˌam-'nē-zhə, -əm-\ *n* : a disorder of memory: as **a** : a condition in which the proper meaning of

---

\ə\ **abut** \ᵊ\ **kitten** \ər\ **further** \a\ **ash** \ā\ **ace** \ä\ **cot, cart**
\au̇\ **out** \ch\ **chin** \e\ **bet** \ē\ **easy** \g\ **go** \i\ **hit** \ī\ **ice** \j\ **job**
\ŋ\ **sing** \ō\ **go** \ȯ\ **law** \ȯi\ **boy** \th\ **thin** \t͟h\ **the** \ü\ **loot**
\u̇\ **foot** \y\ **yet** \zh\ **vision** *See also* Pronunciation Symbols page

words cannot be remembered   **b** : the illusion of remembering scenes and events when experienced for the first time — called also *déjà vu;* compare JAMAIS VU

Par·a·moe·cium \ˌpar-ə-ˈmē-sh(ē-)əm, -sē-əm\ *n, syn of* PARAMECIUM

para·mo·lar \-ˈmō-lər\ *adj* : of, relating to, or being a supernumerary tooth esp. on the buccal side of a permanent molar or a cusp or tubercle located esp. on the buccal aspect of a molar and representing such a tooth

para·mor·phine \-ˈmȯr-ˌfēn\ *n* : THEBAINE

par·am·phis·tome \ˌpar-ˌam-ˈfis-ˌtōm, ˌpar-əm-\ *n* : a digenetic trematode of the genus *Paramphistomum* or of the family (Paramphistomidae) to which it belongs

Par·am·phis·to·mum \-ˈfis-tə-məm\ *n* : a genus (the type of the family Paramphistomidae) of conical amphistome digenetic trematodes with a large ventral sucker at the posterior end of the body — see WATSONIUS

para·mu·cin \ˌpar-ə-ˈmyüs-ᵊn\ *n* : a mucoprotein found esp. in ovarian cysts

par·am·y·loid·osis \ˌpar-ˌam-ə-ˌlȯi-ˈdō-səs\ *n, pl* **-oses** \-ˌsēz\ : amyloidosis characterized by the accumulation of an atypical form of amyloid in the tissues

par·am·y·lum \(ˈ)pa(ə)r-ˈam-ə-ləm\ *n* : a reserve carbohydrate of various protozoans and algae that resembles starch

para·my·oc·lo·nus mul·ti·plex \ˌpar-ə-ˌmī-ˈäk-lə-nəs-ˈməlt-ə-ˌpleks\ *n* : a nervous disease characterized by clonic spasms with tremor in corresponding muscles on the two sides

para·myo·to·nia \ˌpar-ə-ˌmī-ə-ˈtō-nē-ə\ *n* : an abnormal state characterized by tonic muscle spasm

Para·vi·ri·dae \ˌpar-ə-ˌmik-sə-ˈvir-ə-ˌdē\ *n pl* : a family of large single-stranded RNA viruses that have a helical nucleocapsid and lipid-containing envelope and that include the parainfluenza viruses, respiratory syncytial virus, and the causative agents of canine distemper, measles, mumps, Newcastle disease, and rinderpest — see MORBILLIVIRUS, RUBULAVIRUS

para·myxo·vi·rus \ˌpar-ə-ˈmik-sə-ˌvī-rəs\ *n* : any of the family *Paramyxoviridae* of single-stranded RNA viruses — compare MYXOVIRUS

para·na·sal \-ˈnā-zəl\ *adj* : adjacent to the nasal cavities; *esp* : of, relating to, or affecting the paranasal sinuses ⟨~ pain⟩

paranasal sinus *n* : any of various sinuses (as the maxillary sinus and frontal sinus) in the bones of the face and head that are lined with mucous membrane derived from and continuous with the lining of the nasal cavity

par·a·nee \ˌpar-ə-ˈnē\ *n* : the object or victim of paranoid thinking : one on whom paranoid delusions are projected

para·neo·plas·tic \ˌpar-ə-ˌnē-ə-ˈplas-tik\ *adj* : caused by or resulting from the presence of cancer in the body but not the physical presence of cancerous tissue in the part or organ affected ⟨~ effects on the central nervous system⟩

para·neph·ric \ˌpar-ə-ˈnef-rik\ *adj* **1** : adjacent to the kidney   **2** : relating to or being an adrenal gland

pa·ran·gi \pə-ˈran-jē\ *n* : YAWS

para·noia \ˌpar-ə-ˈnȯi-ə\ *n* **1** : a psychosis characterized by systematized delusions of persecution or grandeur usu. without hallucinations   **2** : a tendency on the part of an individual or group toward excessive or irrational suspiciousness and distrustfulness of others

¹para·noi·ac \-ˈnȯi-ˌak, -ˈnȯi-ik\ *also* **para·no·ic** \-ˈnō-ik\ *adj* : of, relating to, affected with, or characteristic of paranoia or paranoid schizophrenia

²paranoiac *also* **paranoic** *n* : PARANOID

¹para·noid \ˈpar-ə-ˌnȯid\ *also* **para·noi·dal** \ˌpar-ə-ˈnȯid-ᵊl\ *adj* **1** : characterized by or resembling paranoia or paranoid schizophrenia   **2** : characterized by suspiciousness, persecutory trends, or megalomania

²paranoid *n* : one affected with paranoia or paranoid schizophrenia — called also *paranoiac*

para·noid·ism \-ˌiz-əm\ *n* : the state or condition of being paranoid

paranoid personality disorder *n* : a personality disorder characterized by a pervasive pattern of distrust and suspi-

cion of others resulting in a tendency to attribute the motives of others to malevolence

paranoid schizophrenia *n* : schizophrenia characterized esp. by persecutory or grandiose delusions or hallucinations or by delusional jealousy

paranoid schizophrenic *n* : an individual affected with paranoid schizophrenia

para·nor·mal \ˌpar-ə-ˈnȯr-məl\ *adj* : not understandable in terms of known scientific laws and phenomena ⟨experiments in ~ cognition of drawings —*Psychological Abstracts*⟩ — **para·nor·mal·ly** \-ē\ *adv*

para–oesophageal *chiefly Brit var of* PARAESOPHAGEAL

para·ol·fac·to·ry \ˌpar-ə-äl-ˈfak-t(ə-)rē, -ōl-ˈfak-\ *n* : a small area of the cerebral cortex situated on the medial side of the frontal lobe below the corpus callosum and considered part of the limbic system

para·ox·on \-ˈäk-ˌsän\ *n* : a phosphate ester $C_{10}H_{14}NO_6P$ that is formed from parathion in the body and that is a potent anticholinesterase

para·pa·re·sis \ˌpar-ə-pə-ˈrē-səs, ˌpar-ə-ˈpar-ə-səs\ *n, pl* **-re·ses** \-ˌsēz\ : partial paralysis affecting the lower limbs

para·pa·ret·ic \-pə-ˈret-ik\ *adj* : of, relating to, or affected with paraparesis ⟨~ patients⟩

para·pe·de·sis \-pə-ˈdē-səs\ *n, pl* **-de·ses** \-ˌsēz\ : passage of an excretion or secretion (as bile) through an abnormal channel (as blood vessels instead of the bile ducts)

para·per·tus·sis \-(ˌ)pər-ˈtəs-əs\ *n* : a human respiratory disease closely resembling whooping cough but milder and less often fatal and caused by a different bacterium of the genus *Bordetella* (*B. parapertussis*)

para·pha·ryn·geal space \-ˌfar-ən-ˈjē-əl-, -fə-ˈrin-j(ē-)əl-\ *n* : a space bounded medially by the superior constrictor of the pharynx, laterally by the medial pterygoid muscle, posteriorly by the cervical vertebrae, and below by the muscles arising from the styloid process

par·a·pha·sia \-ˈfā-zh(ē-)ə\ *n* : aphasia in which the patient uses wrong words or uses words or sounds in senseless combinations — called also *paragrammatism* — **par·a·pha·sic** \-ˈfā-zik\ *adj*

para·phen·yl·ene·di·amine \-ˌfen-ᵊl-ˌēn-ˈdī-ə-ˌmēn\ *n* : the para isomer of phenylenediamine that is used esp. in dyeing hair and sometimes causes an allergic reaction

para·phil·ia \-ˈfil-ē-ə\ *n* : a pattern of recurring sexually arousing mental imagery or behavior that involves unusual and esp. socially unacceptable sexual practices (as sadism, masochism, fetishism, or pedophilia)

¹para·phil·iac \-ˈfil-ē-ˌak\ *or* **para·phil·ic** \-ˈfil-ik\ *adj* : of, relating to, or characterized by paraphilia ⟨~ neuroses⟩

²paraphiliac *or* **paraphilic** *n* : an individual who engages in paraphilia

para·phi·mo·sis \-fī-ˈmō-səs, -fi-\ *n, pl* **-mo·ses** \-ˌsēz\ : a condition in which the foreskin is retracted behind the glans penis and cannot be brought back to its original position

para·phra·sia \-ˈfrā-zh(ē-)ə\ *n* : a speech defect characterized by incoherence in arrangement of words

para·phre·nia \-ˈfrē-nē-ə\ *n* **1** : the group of paranoid disorders   **2** : any of the paranoid disorders; *also* : SCHIZOPHRENIA

¹para·phren·ic \-ˈfren-ik\ *adj* : of, relating to, or affected with paraphrenia

²paraphrenic *n* : an individual affected with paraphrenia

pa·raph·y·se·al \pə-ˌraf-ə-ˈsē-əl, -ˈzē-\ *or* **par·a·phys·i·al** \ˌpar-ə-ˈfiz-ē-əl\ *adj* : of or relating to a paraphysis ⟨~ cysts⟩

pa·raph·y·sis \pə-ˈraf-ə-səs\ *n, pl* **-y·ses** \-ˌsēz\ **1** : one of the slender sterile often septate filaments of many cryptogamic plants (as fungi) that are borne among the spore- or gamete-forming organs, are single or branched, and are composed of one or more cells   **2** : a median evagination of the roof of the telencephalon anterior to the epiphysis of certain lower vertebrates that is present only in the embryo of higher vertebrates

para·ple·gia \ˌpar-ə-ˈplē-j(ē-)ə\ *n* : paralysis of the lower half of the body with involvement of both legs usu. due to disease of or injury to the spinal cord

¹**para·ple·gic** \-'plē-jik\ *adj* : of, relating to, or affected with paraplegia

²**paraplegic** *n* : an individual affected with paraplegia

para·prax·is \-'prak-səs\ *n, pl* **-prax·es** \-'prak-ˌsēz\ : a faulty act (as a Freudian slip) of purposeful behavior

para·pro·fes·sion·al \-prə-'fesh-nəl, -ən-ᵊl\ *n* : a trained aide who assists a professional person (as a doctor) — **paraprofessional** *adj*

para·pro·tein \-'prō-ˌtēn, -'prōt-ē-ən\ *n* : any of various abnormal serum globulins with unique physical and electrophoretic characteristics

para·pro·tein·emia *or chiefly Brit* **para·pro·tein·ae·mia** \-ˌprō-tē-'nē-mē-ə, -ˌprōt-ē-ə-'nē-\ *n* : the presence of a paraprotein in the blood

para·pso·ri·a·sis \-sə-'rī-ə-səs\ *n, pl* **-a·ses** \-ˌsēz\ : a rare skin disease characterized by red scaly patches similar to those of psoriasis but causing no sensations of pain or itch

para·psy·cho·log·i·cal \-ˌsī-kə-'läj-i-kəl\ *adj* : of or relating to parapsychology

para·psy·chol·o·gist \-(ˌ)sī-'käl-ə-jəst\ *n* : a specialist in parapsychology

para·psy·chol·o·gy \ˌpar-ə-(ˌ)sī-'käl-ə-jē\ *n, pl* **-gies** : a field of study concerned with the investigation of evidence for paranormal psychological phenomena (as telepathy, clairvoyance, and psychokinesis)

para·quat \'par-ə-ˌkwät\ *n* : an herbicide containing a salt of a cation $[C_{12}H_{14}N_2]^{2+}$ that is used esp. as a weed killer and that is extremely toxic to the liver, kidneys, and lungs if ingested

para·rec·tus \ˌpar-ə-'rek-təs\ *adj* : situated or performed along the side of the rectus muscle ⟨a ∼ incision⟩

para·re·nal \-'rēn-ᵊl\ *adj* : adjacent to the kidney

para·ros·an·i·line \ˌpar-ə-ˌrō-'zan-ᵊl-ən\ *n* : a white crystalline base $C_{19}H_{19}N_3O$ that is the parent compound of many dyes; *also* : its red chloride used esp. as a biological stain

para·sa·cral \-'sak-rəl, -'sā-krəl\ *adj* : adjacent to the sacrum

para·sag·it·tal \-'saj-ət-ᵊl\ *adj* : situated alongside of or adjacent to a sagittal location or a sagittal plane

Par·as·ca·ris \(ᵊ)par-'as-kə-rəs\ *n* : a genus of nematode worms of the family Ascaridae including a large roundworm (*P. equorum*) that is parasitic in horses

para·sex·u·al \ˌpar-ə-'seksh-(ə-)wəl, -'sek-shəl\ *adj* : relating to or being reproduction that results in recombination of genes from different individuals but does not involve meiosis and formation of a zygote by fertilization as in sexual reproduction ⟨the ∼ cycle in some fungi⟩ — **para·sex·u·al·i·ty** \-ˌsek-shə-'wal-ət-ē\ *n, pl* **-ties**

par·a·site \'par-ə-ˌsīt\ *n* : an organism living in, with, or on another organism in parasitism

par·a·sit·emia *or chiefly Brit* **par·a·sit·ae·mia** \ˌpar-ə-ˌsī-'tē-mē-ə\ *n* : a condition in which parasites are present in the blood — used esp. to indicate the presence of parasites without clinical symptoms ⟨an afebrile ∼ of malaria⟩

¹**par·a·sit·ic** \ˌpar-ə-'sit-ik\ *also* **par·a·sit·i·cal** \-i-kəl\ *adj* **1** : relating to or having the habit of a parasite : living on another organism **2** : caused by or resulting from the effects of parasites — **par·a·sit·i·cal·ly** \-i-k(ə-)lē\ *adv*

²**parasitic** *n* : PARASITICIDE

parasitica — see SYCOSIS PARASITICA

par·a·sit·i·ci·dal \-ˌsit-ə-'sīd-ᵊl\ *adj* : destructive to parasites ⟨the ∼ action of a substance⟩

par·a·sit·i·cide \-'sit-ə-ˌsīd\ *n* : a parasiticidal agent

par·a·sit·ism \'par-ə-sə-ˌtiz-əm, -ˌsīt-ˌiz-\ *n* **1** : an intimate association between organisms of two or more kinds; *esp* : one in which a parasite obtains benefits from a host which it usu. injures **2** : PARASITOSIS

par·a·sit·ize *also Brit* **par·a·sit·ise** \-sə-ˌtīz, -ˌsīt-ˌīz\ *vt* **-ized** *also Brit* **-ised**; **-iz·ing** *also Brit* **-is·ing** : to infest or live on or with as a parasite — **par·a·sit·iza·tion** *also Brit* **par·a·sit·isa·tion** \ˌpar-ə-sət-ə-'zā-shən, -ˌsīt-\ *n*

¹**par·a·sit·oid** \'par-ə-sə-ˌtóid, -ˌsīt-ˌóid\ *adj* **1** : resembling a parasite **2** : being a parasitoid

²**parasitoid** *n* : an insect and esp. a wasp that completes its larval development within the body of another insect which it eventually kills and that is free-living as an adult

Par·a·si·toi·dea \ˌpar-ə-sə-'tóid-ē-ə, -sī-\ *n pl* : a superfamily of mites that is characterized by a small simple hypostome and the absence of eyes and comprises numerous families including the economically and medically important Dermanyssidae

par·a·si·tol·o·gist \-'täl-ə-jəst\ *n* : a specialist in parasitology; *esp* : one who deals with the worm parasites of animals

par·a·si·tol·o·gy \ˌpar-ə-sə-'täl-ə-jē, -ˌsīt-'äl-\ *n, pl* **-gies** : a branch of biology dealing with parasites and parasitism esp. among animals — **par·a·si·to·log·i·cal** \-ˌsit-ᵊl-'äj-i-kəl, -ˌsīt-\ *also* **par·a·si·to·log·ic** \-ik\ *adj* — **par·a·si·to·log·i·cal·ly** \-i-k(ə-)lē\ *adv*

par·a·si·to·pho·bia \ˌpar-ə-ˌsīt-ə-'fō-bē-ə\ *n* : a delusion that one is infested with parasites

par·a·sit·o·sis \-sə-'tō-səs, -ˌsīt-'ō-\ *n, pl* **-o·ses** \-ˌsēz\ : infestation with or disease caused by parasites

par·a·si·to·trop·ic \ˌpar-ə-ˌsīt-ə-'träp-ik\ *adj* : having an affinity for parasites ⟨a ∼ drug⟩

para·spe·cif·ic \-spi-'sif-ik\ *adj* : having or being curative actions or properties in addition to the specific one considered medically useful ⟨determine the ∼ actions of an antivenin⟩

para·spi·nal \-'spīn-ᵊl\ *adj* : adjacent to the spinal column ⟨∼ muscles⟩ ⟨∼ tissues⟩

para·ster·nal \-'stər-nəl\ *adj* : adjacent to the sternum — **para·ster·nal·ly** \-ē\ *adv*

¹**para·sym·pa·thet·ic** \ˌpar-ə-ˌsim-pə-'thet-ik\ *adj* : of, relating to, being, or acting on the parasympathetic nervous system ⟨∼ fibers of the vascular wall⟩ ⟨∼ drugs⟩

²**parasympathetic** *n* **1** : a parasympathetic nerve ⟨this sacral group of ∼s supplies fibers to the external genitalia —A. C. Guyton⟩ **2** : PARASYMPATHETIC NERVOUS SYSTEM

parasympathetic nervous system *n* : the part of the autonomic nervous system that contains chiefly cholinergic fibers, that tends to induce secretion, to increase the tone and contractility of smooth muscle, and to slow the heart rate, and that consists of (1) a cranial part made up of preganglionic fibers leaving and passing the midbrain by the oculomotor nerves and the hindbrain by the facial, glossopharyngeal, vagus, and accessory nerves and passing to the ciliary, sphenopalatine, submandibular, and otic ganglia of the head or to ganglionated plexuses of the thorax and abdomen and postganglionic fibers passing from these ganglia to end organs of the head and upper trunk and (2) a sacral part made up of preganglionic fibers emerging and passing in the sacral nerves and passing to ganglionated plexuses of the lower trunk and postganglionic fibers passing from these plexuses chiefly to the viscera of the lower abdomen and the external genital organs — called also *parasympathetic system;* compare SYMPATHETIC NERVOUS SYSTEM

para·sym·pa·thet·i·co·mi·met·ic \-ˌthet-i-(ˌ)kō-mə-'met-ik, -mī-\ *adj* : PARASYMPATHOMIMETIC

parasympathetic system *n* : PARASYMPATHETIC NERVOUS SYSTEM

¹**para·sym·pa·tho·lyt·ic** \ˌpar-ə-ˌsim-pə-thō-'lit-ik\ *adj* : tending to oppose the physiological results of parasympathetic nervous activity or of parasympathomimetic drugs — compare SYMPATHOLYTIC

²**parasympatholytic** *n* : a parasympatholytic substance

¹**para·sym·pa·tho·mi·met·ic** \ˌpar-ə-ˌsim-pə-(ˌ)thō-mī-'met-ik, -mə-\ *adj* : simulating parasympathetic nervous action in physiological effect — compare SYMPATHOMIMETIC

²**parasympathomimetic** *n* : a parasympathomimetic agent (as a drug)

para·syph·i·lis \-'sif-(ə-)ləs\ *n* : any of several diseases (as tabes dorsalis or general paresis) of the central nervous system that develop in the late stages of untreated syphilis and were

\ə\ abut \ᵊ\ kitten \ər\ further \a\ ash \ā\ ace \ä\ cot, cart \aú\ out \ch\ chin \e\ bet \ē\ easy \g\ go \i\ hit \ī\ ice \j\ job \ŋ\ sing \ō\ go \ó\ law \ói\ boy \th\ thin \th̲\ the \ü\ loot \ú\ foot \y\ yet \zh\ vision *See also* Pronunciation Symbols page

formerly believed to be only indirectly related to it — **para·syph·i·lit·ic** \-ˌsif-ə-'lit-ik\ *adj*

para·sys·to·le \-'sis-tə-(ˌ)lē\ *n* : an irregularity in cardiac rhythm caused by an ectopic pacemaker in addition to the normal one

para·tax·ic \ˌpar-ə-'tak-sik\ *adj* : relating to or being thinking in which a cause and effect relationship is attributed to events occurring at about the same time but having no logical relationship — compare PROTOTAXIC

para·tax·is \-'tak-səs\ *n, pl* **-tax·es** \-ˌsēz\ : the parataxic mode of thinking

para·ten·on \ˌpar-ə-'ten-ən, -(ˌ)än\ *n* : the areolar tissue filling the space between a tendon and its sheath

para·thi·on \ˌpar-ə-'thī-ən, -ˌän\ *n* : an extremely toxic thiophosphate insecticide $C_{10}H_{14}NO_5PS$

par·a·thor·mone \ˌpar-ə-'thȯr-ˌmōn\ *n* : PARATHYROID HORMONE

¹para·thy·roid \-'thī-ˌrȯid\ *n* : PARATHYROID GLAND

²parathyroid *adj* **1** : adjacent to a thyroid gland **2** : of, relating to, or produced by the parathyroid glands

para·thy·roid·ec·to·my \-ˌrȯid-'ek-tə-mē\ *n, pl* **-mies** : partial or complete excision of the parathyroid glands — **para·thy·roid·ec·to·mized** \-ˌmīzd\ *adj*

parathyroid gland *n* : any of usu. four small endocrine glands that are adjacent to or embedded in the thyroid gland, are composed of irregularly arranged secretory epithelial cells lying in a stroma rich in capillaries, and produce parathyroid hormone

parathyroid hormone *n* : a hormone of the parathyroid gland that regulates the metabolism of calcium and phosphorus in the body — abbr. *PTH;* called also *parathormone*

para·thy·ro·pri·val \ˌpar-ə-ˌthī-rō-'prī-vəl\ *adj* : of, relating to, or caused by functional deficiency of the parathyroid glands ⟨∼ tetany⟩

para·thy·ro·priv·ic \-'priv-ik\ *adj* : PARATHYROPRIVAL

para·thy·ro·trop·ic \-'träp-ik\ *adj* : acting on or stimulating the parathyroid glands ⟨a ∼ hormone⟩

para·to·nia \ˌpar-ə-'tō-nē-ə\ *n* : a disorder of muscle tone

para·tra·che·al \-'trā-kē-əl\ *adj* : adjacent to the trachea ⟨bilateral hilar and ∼ lymph nodes —T. E. Goffman *et al*⟩

para·tro·phic \ˌpar-ə-'trō-fik, -'träf-ik\ *adj* : deriving nourishment parasitically from other organisms ⟨∼ bacteria⟩

para·tu·ber·cu·lo·sis \-t(y)ù-ˌbər-kyə-'lō-səs\ *n, pl* **-lo·ses** \-ˌsēz\ : JOHNE'S DISEASE — **para·tu·ber·cu·lous** \-t(y)ù-'bər-kyə-ləs\ *adj*

¹para·ty·phoid \ˌpar-ə-'tī-ˌfȯid, -(ˌ)tī-'\ *adj* **1** : resembling typhoid fever **2** : of or relating to paratyphoid or its causative organisms ⟨∼ infection⟩

²paratyphoid *n* : any of numerous salmonelloses (as necrotic enteritis) that resemble typhoid fever and are commonly contracted by eating contaminated food — called also *paratyphoid fever*

para·um·bil·i·cal \-ˌəm-'bil-i-kəl, *Brit usu* -ˌəm-bə-'lī-kəl\ *adj* : adjacent to the navel ⟨∼ pain⟩

para·ure·thral \-yù-'rē-thrəl\ *adj* : adjacent to the urethra

paraurethral gland *n* : any of several small glands that open into the female urethra near its opening and are homologous to glandular tissue in the prostate gland in the male — called also *Skene's gland*

para·vac·cin·ia \-vak-'sin-ē-ə\ *n* : MILKER'S NODULES

para·vag·i·nal \-'vaj-ən-ᵊl\ *adj* : adjacent to the vagina or a vaginal part — **para·vag·i·nal·ly** \-ē\ *adv*

para·ven·tric·u·lar nucleus \-ven-'trik-yə-lər-, -vən-\ *n* : a discrete band of nerve cells in the anterior part of the hypothalamus that produce vasopressin and esp. oxytocin and that innervate the neurohypophysis

para·ver·bal \-'vər-bəl\ *adj* : being nonverbal communication ⟨∼ techniques in the therapy of childhood —*Jour. Amer. Med. Assoc.*⟩

para·ver·te·bral \-(ˌ)vər-'tē-brəl, -'vərt-ə-\ *adj* : situated, occurring, or performed beside or adjacent to the spinal column ⟨∼ ganglia⟩ — **para·ver·te·bral·ly** \-ē\ *adv*

par·ax·i·al \(')par-'ak-sē-əl\ *adj* : relating to or being the space in the immediate neighborhood of the optical axis of a lens or mirror ⟨∼ rays⟩ — **par·ax·i·al·ly** \-ē\ *adv*

par·e·gor·ic \ˌpar-ə-'gȯr-ik, -'gōr-, -'gär-\ *n* : camphorated tincture of opium used esp. to relieve pain

pa·rei·ra bra·va \pə-'rer-ə-'brä-və\ *n* : the root of a So. American vine (*Chondodendron tomentosum* of the family Menispermaceae) that was formerly used as a diuretic, tonic, and aperient — called also *pareira*

pa·ren·chy·ma \pə-'reŋ-kə-mə\ *n* : the essential and distinctive tissue of an organ or an abnormal growth as distinguished from its supportive framework

pa·ren·chy·mal \pə-'reŋ-kə-məl, ˌpar-ən-'kī-məl\ *adj* : PARENCHYMATOUS ⟨hepatocytes are ∼ cells of the liver⟩

par·en·chy·ma·tous \ˌpar-ən-'kīm-ət-əs, -'kim-\ *adj* : of, relating to, made up of, or affecting parenchyma ⟨∼ renal disease⟩

par·ent \'par-ənt, 'per-\ *n* **1** : one that begets or brings forth offspring **2** : the material or source from which something is derived — **parent** *adj* — **pa·ren·tal** \pə-'rent-ᵊl\ *adj*

parental generation *n* : a generation that supplies the parents of a subsequent generation; *esp* : P_1 GENERATION — see FILIAL GENERATION, F_2 GENERATION

¹par·en·ter·al \pə-'rent-ə-rəl\ *adj* : situated or occurring outside the intestine ⟨∼ drug administration by intravenous, intramuscular, or subcutaneous injection⟩; *esp* : introduced otherwise than by way of the intestines ⟨enteric versus ∼ feeding⟩ — **par·en·ter·al·ly** \-rə-lē\ *adv*

²parenteral *n* : an agent (as a drug or solution) intended for parenteral administration

par·ent·ing \'par-ənt-iŋ, 'per-\ *n* : the raising of a child by its parents

pa·re·sis \pə-'rē-səs, 'par-ə-\ *n, pl* **pa·re·ses** \-ˌsēz\ **1** : slight or partial paralysis **2** : GENERAL PARESIS

par·es·the·sia *or chiefly Brit* **par·aes·the·sia** \ˌpar-es-'thē-zh(ē-)ə\ *n* : a sensation of pricking, tingling, or creeping on the skin having no objective cause and usu. associated with injury or irritation of a sensory nerve or nerve root — **par·es·thet·ic** *or chiefly Brit* **par·aes·thet·ic** \-'thet-ik\ *adj*

paresthetica — see MERALGIA PARESTHETICA

¹pa·ret·ic \pə-'ret-ik\ *adj* : of, relating to, or affected with paresis

²paretic *n* : an individual affected with paresis

par·fo·cal \(')pär-'fō-kəl\ *adj* : having corresponding focal points all in the same plane : having sets of objectives or eyepieces so mounted that they may be interchanged without varying the focus of the instrument (as a microscope) with which they are used — **par·fo·cal·i·ty** \-fō-'kal-ət-ē\ *n, pl* **-ties**

par·gy·line \'pär-jə-ˌlēn\ *n* : a monoamine oxidase inhibitor that is used in the form of its hydrochloride $C_{11}H_{13}N \cdot HCl$ esp. as an antihypertensive

par·i·es \'par-ē-ˌēz, 'per-\ *n, pl* **pa·ri·etes** \pə-'rī-ə-ˌtēz\ : the wall of a cavity or hollow organ — usu. used in pl.

¹pa·ri·etal \pə-'rī-ət-ᵊl\ *adj* **1** : of or relating to the walls of a part or cavity — compare VISCERAL **2** : of, relating to, or located in the upper posterior part of the head; *specif* : relating to the parietal bones

²parietal *n* : a parietal part (as a bone)

parietal bone *n* : either of a pair of membrane bones of the roof of the skull between the frontal and occipital bones that are large and quadrilateral in outline, meet in the sagittal suture, and form much of the top and sides of the cranium

parietal cell *n* : any of the large oval cells of the gastric mucous membrane that secrete hydrochloric acid and lie between the chief cells and the basement membrane

parietal emissary vein *n* : a vein that passes from the superior sagittal sinus inside the skull through a foramen in the parietal bone to connect with veins of the scalp

parietalis — see DECIDUA PARIETALIS

parietal lobe *n* : the middle division of each cerebral hemisphere that is situated behind the central sulcus, above the sylvian fissure, and in front of the parieto-occipital sulcus and that contains an area concerned with bodily sensations

parietal pericardium *n* : the tough thickened membranous outer layer of the pericardium that is attached to the central part of the diaphragm and the posterior part of the sternum — compare EPICARDIUM

parietal peritoneum *n* : the part of the peritoneum that lines the abdominal wall — compare VISCERAL PERITONEUM

parietes *pl of* PARIES

pa·ri·e·to·mas·toid \pə-ˌrī-ət-ō-ˈmas-ˌtȯid\ *adj* : of or relating to the parietal bone and the mastoid portion of the temporal bone

pa·ri·e·to·oc·cip·i·tal \-äk-ˈsip-ət-ᵊl\ *adj* : of, relating to, or situated between the parietal and occipital bones or lobes

parieto–occipital sulcus *n* : a fissure near the posterior end of each cerebral hemisphere separating the parietal and occipital lobes — called also *parieto-occipital fissure*

pa·ri·e·to·tem·po·ral \-ˈtem-p(ə-)rəl\ *adj* : of or relating to the parietal and temporal bones or lobes

Par·i·naud's oc·u·lo·glan·du·lar syndrome \ˌpar-i-ˈnōz-ˌäk-yə-lō-ˈglan-jə-lər-\ *n* : conjunctivitis that is often unilateral, is usu. characterized by dense local infiltration by lymphoid tissue with tenderness and swelling of the preauricular lymph nodes, and is usu. associated with a bacterial infection (as in cat scratch disease and tularemia) — called also *Parinaud's conjunctivitis*

  Pa·ri·naud \pȧ-rē-nō\, **Henri (1844–1905),** French ophthalmologist. In 1889 Parinaud described an infectious tuberculous conjunctivitis that can be transmitted from animals to humans. This conjunctivitis is now known as Parinaud's oculoglandular syndrome.

Parinaud's syndrome *n* : paralysis of the upward movements of the two eyes that is associated esp. with a lesion or compression of the superior colliculi of the midbrain

Par·is green \ˌpar-əs-\ *n* : a very poisonous copper-based bright green powder $Cu(C_2H_3O_2)_2 \cdot 3Cu(AsO_2)_2$ that is used as an insecticide and pigment

par·i·ty \ˈpar-ət-ē\ *n, pl* **-ties** **1** : the state or fact of having borne offspring ⟨diagnosis of ∼ or nulliparity⟩ **2** : the number of times a female has given birth counting multiple births as one and usu. including stillbirths ⟨gravidity and ∼ were highly correlated⟩ — compare GRAVIDITY 2

Par·ker's fluid \ˈpär-kərz-\ *n* : a mixture of 100 parts 70 percent alcohol and one part formaldehyde used for hardening and preserving tissues for microscopic study

  Parker, George Howard (1864–1955), American zoologist. Parker was a member of Harvard's faculty in the zoological department for almost all of his long academic career.

¹par·kin·so·nian \ˌpär-kən-ˈsō-nē-ən, -nyən\ *adj* **1** : of or similar to that of parkinsonism **2** : affected with parkinsonism and esp. Parkinson's disease

  Par·kin·son \ˈpär-kən-sən\, **James (1755–1824),** British surgeon. Parkinson published a monograph on paralysis agitans in 1817. His classic description established the disease as a clinical entity, and ever since his name has been closely identified with it.

²parkinsonian *n* : an individual affected with parkinsonism and esp. Parkinson's disease

parkinsonian syndrome *n* : PARKINSON'S DISEASE

par·kin·son·ism \ˈpär-kən-sə-ˌniz-əm\ *n* **1** : PARKINSON'S DISEASE **2** : any of several neurological conditions that resemble Parkinson's disease and that result from a deficiency or blockage of dopamine caused by degenerative disease, drugs, or toxins

Par·kin·son's disease \ˈpär-kən-sənz-\ *also* **Par·kin·son disease** \-sən-\ *n* : a chronic progressive neurological disease chiefly of later life that is linked to decreased dopamine production in the substantia nigra and is marked esp. by tremor of resting muscles, rigidity, slowness of movement, impaired balance, and a shuffling gait — called also *paralysis agitans, parkinsonian syndrome, parkinsonism, Parkinson's, Parkinson's syndrome*

par·odon·tal \ˌpar-ə-ˈdänt-ᵊl\ *adj* : PERIODONTAL 2 — **par·odon·tal·ly** \-ē\ *adv*

par·odon·ti·um \ˌpar-ə-ˈdän-ch(ē-)əm\ *n* : PERIODONTIUM

pa·role \pə-ˈrōl\ *n* : a conditional release given to a psychiatric patient in a hospital before discharge enabling the patient to visit freely various designated areas on the hospital grounds or beyond its limits — **pa·rol·able** *adj* — **parole** *vt* **pa·roled; pa·rol·ing**

pa·rol·ee \pə-ˌrō-ˈlē, -ˈrō-(ˌ); ˌpar-ə-ˈlē\ *n* : an individual released on parole

par·ol·fac·to·ry area \ˌpar-ˌäl-ˈfak-tə-rē-, -ˌōl-\ *n* : SUBCALLOSAL AREA

par·o·mo·my·cin \ˌpar-ə-mō-ˈmīs-ᵊn\ *n* : a broad-spectrum aminoglycoside antibiotic that is obtained from a bacterium of the genus *Streptomyces* (*S. rimosus paromomycinus*) and is usu. used in the form of its sulfate $C_{23}H_{45}N_5O_{14} \cdot H_2SO_4$ to treat intestinal amebiasis

par·o·nych·ia \ˌpar-ə-ˈnik-ē-ə\ *n* : inflammation of the tissues adjacent to the nail of a finger or toe usu. accompanied by infection and pus formation — compare WHITLOW

par·ooph·o·ron \ˌpar-ō-ˈäf-ə-ˌrän\ *n* : a group of rudimentary tubules in the broad ligament between the epoophoron and the uterus that constitutes a remnant of the lower part of the mesonephros in the female corresponding to the paradidymis of the male

par·os·mia \ˌpar-ˈäz-mē-ə\ *n* : a distortion of the sense of smell (as when affected with a cold)

pa·rotic \pə-ˈrät-ik\ *adj* : adjacent to the ear

¹pa·rot·id \pə-ˈrät-əd\ *adj* : of, relating to, being, produced by, or located near the parotid gland ⟨∼ acinar cells⟩

²parotid *n* : PAROTID GLAND

parotid duct *n* : the duct of the parotid gland opening on the inner surface of the cheek opposite the second upper molar tooth — called also *Stensen's duct*

pa·rot·i·dec·to·my \pə-ˌrät-ə-ˈdek-tə-mē\ *n, pl* **-mies** : surgical removal of the parotid gland

parotid gland *n* : a salivary gland that is situated on each side of the face below and in front of the ear, in humans is the largest of the salivary glands, is of pure serous type, and communicates with the mouth by the parotid duct

par·o·tit·ic \ˌpar-ə-ˈtit-ik\ *adj* : of, relating to, or having mumps

par·o·ti·tis \-ˈtīt-əs\ *n* **1** : inflammation and swelling of one or both parotid glands or other salivary glands (as in mumps) **2** : MUMPS

par·ous \ˈpar-əs\ *adj* **1** : having produced offspring **2** : of or characteristic of the parous female ⟨∼ relaxation of the vaginal outlet —W. H. Masters & V. E. Johnson⟩

par·o·var·i·um \ˌpar-ō-ˈvar-ē-əm, -ˈver-\ *n* : EPOOPHORON — **par·o·var·i·an** \-ē-ən\ *adj*

par·ox·e·tine \pə-ˈräk-sə-ˌtēn\ *n* : a drug that enhances serotonin activity and is usu. administered in the form of its hydrochloride $C_{19}H_{20}FNO_3 \cdot HCl$ to treat depression — see PAXIL

par·ox·ysm \ˈpar-ək-ˌsiz-əm *also* pə-ˈräk-\ *n* **1** : a sudden attack or spasm (as of a disease) **2** : a sudden recurrence of symptoms or an intensification of existing symptoms ⟨pain occurred in frequent ∼s —*Therapeutic Notes*⟩

par·ox·ys·mal \ˌpar-ək-ˈsiz-məl *also* pə-ˌräk-\ *adj* : of, relating to, or marked by paroxysms ⟨the hypertension may be either sustained or ∼ —D. A. Calhoun *et al*⟩

paroxysmal dyspnea *n* : CARDIAC ASTHMA

paroxysmal nocturnal hemoglobinuria *n* : a form of hemolytic anemia that is characterized by an abnormally strong response to the action of complement, by acute episodes of hemolysis esp. at night with hemoglobinuria noted upon urination after awakening, venous occlusion, and often leukopenia and thrombocytopenia — abbr. *PNH*

paroxysmal tachycardia *n* : tachycardia that begins and ends abruptly and that is initiated by a premature supraventricular beat originating in the atrium or in the atrioventricular node or bundle of His or by a premature ventricular beat

---

\ə\ abut \ᵊ\ kitten \ər\ further \a\ ash \ā\ ace \ä\ cot, cart
\au̇\ out \ch\ chin \e\ bet \ē\ easy \g\ go \i\ hit \ī\ ice \j\ job
\ŋ\ sing \ō\ go \ȯ\ law \ȯi\ boy \th\ thin \t̲h̲\ the \ü\ loot
\u̇\ foot \y\ yet \zh\ vision *See also* Pronunciation Symbols page

O
P

par·rot fever \\'par-ət-\ *n* : PSITTACOSIS

pars \\'pärs\ *n, pl* **par·tes** \\'pär-(ˌ)tēz\ : an anatomical part

pars com·pac·ta \-käm-'pak-tə\ *n* : the large dorsal part of gray matter of the substantia nigra that is next to the tegmentum

pars dis·ta·lis \-dis-'tä-ləs\ *n* : the anterior part of the adenohypophysis that is the major secretory part of the gland

pars in·ter·me·dia \-int-ər-'mē-dē-ə\ *n* : a thin slip of tissue fused with the neurohypophysis and representing the remains of the posterior wall of Rathke's pouch

pars irid·i·ca ret·i·nae \-i-'rid-i-kə-'ret-³n-ˌē\ *n* : the two deep purple cellular layers of columnar epithelium that cover the posterior surface of the iris of the eye and are continuous with the retina

pars·ley \\'pär-slē\ *n* : a southern European annual or biennial herb (*Petroselinum crispum*) of the carrot family having leaves which are used as a culinary herb or garnish and a root and seeds which have been used medicinally

pars ner·vo·sa \-nər-'vō-sə\ *n* : NEURAL LOBE

pars pla·na \-'plä-nə\ *n* : ORBICULUS CILIARIS

pars re·tic·u·la·ta \-ri-ˌtik-yə-'lät-ə, -'lät-\ *n* : the ventral part of gray matter of the substantia nigra continuous with the globus pallidus

pars tu·ber·a·lis \-ˌt(y)ü-bə-'rä-ləs\ *n* : a thin plate of cells that is an extension of the adenohypophysis on the ventral or anterior aspect of the infundibulum

part \\'pärt\ *n* **1** : one of several or many like units into which something is divided or of which it is composed : a proportional division or ingredient ⟨mix the powder with three ∼s of water⟩ **2** : a portion of an animal body: as **a** : an essential anatomical element : ORGAN, MEMBER ⟨the chief ∼s of the digestive system are the esophagus, stomach, intestine, and associated glands⟩ **b** : an indefinite area or one lacking or not considered in respect to a natural boundary ⟨bathe the affected ∼ with warm water⟩

partes *pl of* PARS

par·then·i·ta \pär-'then-ət-ə\ *n, pl* **-i·tae** \-ə-ˌtē\ : a juvenile trematode worm

par·the·no·gen·e·sis \ˌpär-thə-nō-'jen-ə-səs\ *n, pl* **-e·ses** \-ˌsēz\ : reproduction by development of an unfertilized usu. female gamete that occurs esp. among lower plants and invertebrate animals

par·the·no·ge·net·ic \-jə-'net-ik\ *also* **par·the·no·gen·ic** \-'jen-ik\ *adj* : of, characterized by, or produced by parthenogenesis — **par·the·no·ge·net·i·cal·ly** \-i-k(ə-)lē\ *adv*

par·tial–birth abortion \\'pär-shəl-\ *n* : DILATION AND EXTRACTION

partial denture *n* : a usu. removable artificial replacement of one or more teeth

partial epilepsy *n* : FOCAL EPILEPSY

par·tial·ism \\'pär-shə-ˌliz-əm\ *n* : concentration of libidinal interest on one part of the body (as breasts or buttocks)

partial mastectomy *n* : a mastectomy in which only a tumor and a wedge of surrounding healthy tissue are removed

partial pressure *n* : the pressure exerted by a (specified) component in a mixture of gases

partial seizure *n* : a seizure (as of Jacksonian epilepsy or temporal lobe epilepsy) that originates in a localized part of the cerebral cortex, that involves motor, sensory, autonomic, or psychic symptoms (as twitching of muscles, localized numbness, or auras), and that may or may not progress to a generalized seizure — called also *focal seizure;* compare GENERALIZED SEIZURE

par·ti·cle \\'pärt-i-kəl\ *n* **1** : one of the minute subdivisions of matter (as an atom or molecule); *also* : ELEMENTARY PARTICLE **2** : a minute quantity or fragment

¹par·tic·u·late \pär-'tik-yə-lət\ *adj* **1** : of, relating to, or existing in the form of minute separate particles ⟨dust, smoke, and other ∼ matter⟩ **2** : of or relating to particulate inheritance ⟨the ∼ theory of heredity —Julian Huxley⟩

²particulate *n* : a particulate substance ⟨emission of ∼s by car engines⟩ ⟨cytoplasmic ∼s in the cell⟩

particulate inheritance *n* : MENDELIAN INHERITANCE

par·ti·tion \pär-'tish-ən\ *n* : the distribution of a substance between two immiscible phases in contact at equilibrium and esp. between two liquids — **partition** *vt*

partition chromatography *n* : a process for the separation of mixtures in columns or on filter paper based on partition of a solute between two solvents one of which is immobilized by the substance in the column or by the paper

partition coefficient *n* : the ratio of the amounts of a substance distributed between two immiscible phases (as two liquids or a stationary and a mobile phase in chromatography) at equilibrium — called also *distribution coefficient*

¹par·tu·ri·ent \pär-'t(y)ùr-ē-ənt\ *adj* **1** : bringing forth or about to bring forth young **2** : of or relating to parturition ⟨∼ pangs⟩ **3** : typical of parturition ⟨the ∼ uterus⟩

²parturient *n* : a parturient individual ⟨∼s are at high risk for aspiration —R. M. Meyer⟩

parturient apoplexy *n* : MILK FEVER 2

parturient paresis *n* : MILK FEVER 2

par·tu·ri·tion \ˌpärt-ə-'rish-ən, ˌpär-chə-, ˌpär-tyù-\ *n* : the action or process of giving birth to offspring — **par·tu·ri·tion·al** \-əl\ *adj*

pa·ru·lis \pə-'rü-ləs\ *n, pl* **-li·des** \-lə-ˌdēz\ : an abscess in the gum : GUMBOIL

par·um·bil·i·cal vein \ˌpar-ˌəm-'bil-i-kəl-, *Brit usu* -ˌəm-bə-'lī-\ *n* : any of several small veins that connect the veins of the anterior abdominal wall with the portal vein and the internal and common iliac veins

parv·al·bu·min \ˌpär-val-'byü-mən; -'val-ˌbyü-, -byə-\ *n* : a small calcium-binding protein in vertebrate skeletal muscle

par·vo \\'pär-ˌvō\ *n* : PARVOVIRUS 2

Par·vo·bac·te·ri·a·ce·ae \ˌpär-vō-(ˌ)bak-ˌtir-ē-'ā-sē-ˌē\ *n pl, syn of* BRUCELLACEAE

par·vo·cel·lu·lar *also* **par·vi·cel·lu·lar** \ˌpär-və-'sel-yə-lər\ *adj* : characterized by relatively small cell bodies ⟨the ∼ layers of the lateral geniculate nucleus⟩ — compare MAGNOCELLULAR

Par·vo·vi·ri·dae \ˌpär-vō-'vir-ə-ˌdē\ *n pl* : a family of small single-stranded DNA viruses that have a virion 18 to 26 nanometers in diameter without an encompassing envelope and a capsid composed of 60 copies of a protein and that include the causative agents of panleukopenia, fifth disease, and parvovirus

par·vo·vi·rus \\'pär-vō-ˌvī-rəs\ *n* **1 a** *cap* : a genus of the family *Parvoviridae* that includes the causative agents of panleukopenia in cats and parvovirus in canines **b** : any of the family *Parvoviridae* and esp. of the genus *Parvovirus* of single-stranded DNA viruses **2** : a highly contagious febrile disease of canines and esp. dogs that is caused by a single-stranded DNA virus of the genus *Parvovirus* (species *Canine parvovirus*), is spread esp. by contact with infected feces, and is marked by loss of appetite, lethargy, often bloody diarrhea and vomiting, and sometimes death — called also *parvo*

par·vule \\'pär-(ˌ)vyül\ *n* : a very small pill

PAS \\'pē-ˌā-'es\ *adj* : PERIODIC ACID-SCHIFF

PAS *abbr* para-aminosalicylic acid

PASA *abbr* para-aminosalicylic acid

pas·cal \pas-'kal\ *n* : a unit of pressure in the mks system equivalent to one newton per square meter or to 1.45×10^{-4} pounds per square inch

Pas·cal \pás-kál\, **Blaise (1623–1662)**, French mathematician, physicist, and religious philosopher. A mathematical prodigy as a child, Pascal completed an original treatise on conic sections by the time he was 16. He undertook the study of geometry, hydrodynamics, and hydrostatic and atmospheric pressure. From 1651 to 1654 he composed treatises on the weight and density of air, on Pascal's triangle, and on the equilibrium of liquid solutions. In this last treatise he formulated Pascal's law of pressure. He is also credited with laying the foundations for the theory of probability. Pascal is a major figure in French literature and religious philosophy.

Pas·cal's law \pas-'kalz-\ *n* : a statement in physics: a force applied to an enclosed fluid at equilibrium is transmitted uniformly and with undiminished intensity in all directions throughout the fluid

pasque·flow·er \\'pask-ˌflaủ(-ə)r\\ *n* : any of several perennial herbs of the genus *Anemone* having palmately compound leaves and large usu. white or purple flowers and including several (esp. *A. pulsatilla* syn. *Pulsatilla vulgaris*) used as sources of pulsatilla

pass \\'pas\\ *vt* : to emit or discharge from a bodily part and esp. from the bowels : EVACUATE 2, VOID

¹**pas·sage** \\'pas-ij\\ *n* **1** : the action or process of passing from one place, condition, or stage to another ⟨the ∼ of air from the lungs —*Encyc. Americana*⟩ **2** : an anatomical channel ⟨the nasal ∼*s*⟩ **3** : a movement or an evacuation of the bowels **4 a** : an act or action of passing something or undergoing a passing ⟨∼ of a catheter through the urethra⟩ **b** : incubation of a pathogen (as a virus) in a tissue culture, a developing egg, or a living organism to increase the amount of pathogen or to alter its characteristics ⟨several ∼*s* of the virus through mice⟩

²**passage** *vt* **pas·saged; pas·sag·ing** : to subject to passage ⟨the virus has been *passaged* in series seven times —*Jour. Amer. Med. Assoc.*⟩

pas·sive \\'pas-iv\\ *adj* **1 a** (1) : lethargic or lacking in energy or will (2) : tending not to take an active or dominant part ⟨a ∼ spouse⟩ **b** : induced by an outside agency ⟨∼ exercise of a paralyzed leg⟩ **2 a** : of, relating to, or characterized by a state of chemical inactivity **b** : not involving expenditure of chemical energy ⟨∼ transport across a plasma membrane⟩ — **pas·sive·ly** *adv* — **pas·sive·ness** *n*

¹**passive–aggressive** *adj* : being, marked by, or displaying behavior characterized by expression of negative feelings, resentment, and aggression in an unassertive way (as through procrastination, stubbornness, and unwillingness to communicate) ⟨a ∼ personality⟩ — **passive–aggressively** *adv*

²**passive–aggressive** *n* : a passive-aggressive individual

passive congestion *n* : congestion caused by obstruction to the return flow of venous blood — called also *passive hyperemia*

passive immunity *n* : immunity acquired by transfer of antibodies (as by injection of serum from an individual with active immunity) — compare ACQUIRED IMMUNITY, NATURAL IMMUNITY — **passive immunization** *n*

passive smoke *n* : SECONDHAND SMOKE

passive smoking *n* : the involuntary inhalation of tobacco smoke (as from another's cigarette) esp. by a nonsmoker — **passive smoker** *n*

passive transfer *n* : a local transfer of skin sensitivity from an allergic to a normal individual by injection of the allergic individual's serum that is used esp. for identifying specific allergens when a high degree of sensitivity is suspected — called also *Prausnitz-Küstner reaction*

pas·siv·ism \\'pas-iv-ˌiz-əm\\ *n* : MASOCHISM

pas·siv·i·ty \\pa-'siv-ət-ē\\ *n, pl* **-ties** : the quality or state of being passive or submissive

pass out *vi* : to lose consciousness ⟨three men *passed out* from heat exhaustion —F. J. Bell⟩

paste \\'pāst\\ *n* : a soft plastic mixture or composition; *esp* : an external medicament that has a stiffer consistency than an ointment and is less greasy because of its higher percentage of powdered ingredients

pas·tern \\'pas-tərn\\ *n* **1** : a part of the foot of an equine extending from the fetlock to the top of the hoof **2** : a part of the leg of an animal other than an equine that corresponds to the pastern

pastern bone *n* : either of two bones in the foot of an equine between the cannon bone and the coffin bone

pastern joint *n* : the joint between the two pastern bones

Pas·teur effect \\pas-'tər-\\ *n* : the inhibiting effect of oxygen upon a fermentative process (as one carried on by facultative anaerobic organisms)

Pas·teur \\pás-tœr\\, **Louis (1822–1895),** French chemist and bacteriologist. Pasteur made contributions that rank with the greatest in modern science. His achievements include pioneer work in modern stereochemistry that proved that racemic acid is a mixture of two optically different

forms of tartaric acid; the investigation of problems encountered in the fermentation of wine and beer; and the demonstration that lactic, alcoholic, and other fermentations are caused by minute organisms. He also disproved the theory of spontaneous generation. He saved the French silk industry by discovering the bacilli that were the cause of two diseases of silkworms and developed the means of preventing the spread of these diseases. He discovered bacteria to be the cause of anthrax and developed in 1881 a method of inoculating animals with attenuated cultures of the bacteria causing fowl cholera. Finally, in 1885 he developed a preventive and curative treatment for rabies.

pas·teu·rel·la \\ˌpas-tə-'rel-ə\\ *n* **1** *cap* : a genus of gram-negative facultatively anaerobic nonmotile rod bacteria of the family Pasteurellaceae that stain differentially at the poles of the cell and include several important pathogens esp. of domestic animals — see HEMORRHAGIC SEPTICEMIA, YERSINIA **2** *pl* **-las** *or* **-lae** \\-ˌlī\\ : any bacterium of the genus *Pasteurella*

Pas·teu·rel·la·ce·ae \\ˌpas-tər-ə-'lā-sē-ˌē, -ˌī\\ *n pl* : a family of gram-negative coccoid to rod-shaped pleomorphic bacteria that are nonmotile and mesophilic and do not form spores — see ACTINOBACILLUS, HAEMOPHILUS, PASTEURELLA

pas·teu·rel·lo·sis \\ˌpas-tə-rə-'lō-səs\\ *n, pl* **-lo·ses** \\-ˌsēz\\ : infection with or disease caused by bacteria of the genus *Pasteurella* — see HEMORRHAGIC SEPTICEMIA

pas·teur·iza·tion *also Brit* **pas·teur·isa·tion** \\ˌpas-chə-rə-'zā-shən, ˌpas-tə-\\ *n* **1** : partial sterilization of a substance and esp. a liquid (as milk) at a temperature and for a period of exposure that destroys objectionable organisms without major chemical alteration of the substance **2** : partial sterilization of perishable food products (as fruit or fish) with radiation (as gamma rays)

pas·teur·ize *also Brit* **pas·teur·ise** \\'pas-chə-ˌrīz, 'pas-tə-\\ *vt* **-ized** *also Brit* **-ised; -iz·ing** *also Brit* **-is·ing** : to subject to pasteurization — **pas·teur·iz·er** *also Brit* **pas·teur·is·er** *n*

Pasteur treatment *n* : a method of aborting rabies by stimulating production of antibodies through successive inoculations with attenuated virus of gradually increasing strength

pas·tille \\pas-'tē(ə)l\\ *also* **pas·til** \\'pas-t²l\\ *n* : LOZENGE

past–point \\'past-'pȯint\\ *vi* : to point (as in a past-pointing test) to one side or the other of an object at which one intends to point with a finger or the hand

past–pointing test *n* : a test for defective functioning of the vestibular nerve in which a subject is asked to point at an object with eyes open and then closed first after rotation in a chair to the right and then to the left and which indicates an abnormality if the subject does not past-point in the direction of rotation

PAT *abbr* paroxysmal atrial tachycardia

Pa·tau syndrome \\pä-'taủ-\\ *or* **Patau's syndrome** \\-'taủz-\\ *n* : TRISOMY 13

  Patau, Klaus (fl 1960), American (German-born) geneticist. Associated with the University of Wisconsin at Madison, Patau and his colleagues in 1960 became the first to attribute the syndrome of trisomy to the chromosome numbered 13.

patch \\'pach\\ *n* **1 a** : a piece of material used medically usu. to cover a wound or repair a defect — see PATCH GRAFT **b** : a usu. disk-shaped piece of material that is worn on the skin and contains a substance (as a drug) that is absorbed at a constant rate through the skin and into the bloodstream ⟨a nicotine ∼⟩ — called also *skin patch* **c** : a shield worn over the socket of an injured or missing eye **2** : a circumscribed region of tissue (as on the skin or in a section from an organ) that differs from the normal color or composition ⟨sometimes great white ∼*es* develop on the tongue, the cheeks, and the gums —Morris Fishbein⟩ — **patch** *vt* — **patchy** \\-ē\\ *adj* **patch·i·er; -est**

O

P

patch graft *n* : a graft of living or synthetic material used to repair a defect in a blood vessel

patch test *n* : a test for determining allergic sensitivity that is made by applying to the unbroken skin small pads soaked with the allergen to be tested and that indicates sensitivity when irritation develops at the point of application — compare INTRADERMAL TEST, PRICK TEST, SCRATCH TEST

pa·tel·la \pə-ˈtel-ə\ *n, pl* **-lae** \-ˈtel-(ˌ)ē, -ˌī\ *or* **-las** : a thick flat triangular movable bone that forms the anterior point of the knee, protects the front of the joint, increases the leverage of the quadriceps, and is usu. regarded as a sesamoid bone since it is developed in the tendon of the quadriceps and in structure is similar to other sesamoid bones — called also *kneecap, kneepan* — **pa·tel·lar** \-ər\ *adj*

patellar ligament *n* : the part of the tendon of the quadriceps that extends from the patella to the tibia — called also *patellar tendon*

patellar reflex *n* : KNEE JERK

patellar tendon *n* : PATELLAR LIGAMENT

pat·el·lec·to·my \ˌpat-ə-ˈlek-tə-mē\ *n, pl* **-mies** : surgical excision of the patella

pa·tel·lo·fem·o·ral \pə-ˌtel-ō-ˈfem-(ə-)rəl\ *adj* : of or relating to the patella and femur ⟨a ~ articulation⟩

pa·ten·cy \ˈpat-ᵊn-sē, ˈpāt-\ *n, pl* **-cies** : the quality or state of being open or unobstructed ⟨evaluating arterial ~⟩

pa·tent \ˈpat-ᵊnt, *Brit usu* ˈpāt-\ *n* **1** : protected by a trademark or a trade name so as to establish proprietary rights analogous to those conveyed by a patent : PROPRIETARY ⟨~ drugs⟩ **2** \ˈpāt-\ : affording free passage : being open and unobstructed ⟨the nose ~ with no pathological discharge —*Jour. Amer. Med. Assoc.*⟩

pa·tent ductus arteriosus \ˈpāt-ᵊnt-\ *n* : an abnormal condition in which the ductus arteriosus fails to close after birth

pat·ent medicine \ˈpat-ᵊnt-, *Brit usu* ˈpāt-\ *n* : a packaged nonprescription drug which is protected by a trademark and whose contents are incompletely disclosed; *also* : any drug that is a proprietary

pa·tent period \ˈpāt-ᵊnt-\ *n* : the period of time in the course of a parasitic disease (as malaria) during which the parasitic organisms can be demonstrated in the body

pa·ter·ni·ty test \pə-ˈtər-nət-ē-\ *n* : a test esp. of DNA or genetic traits to determine whether a given man could be the biological father of a given child — **paternity testing** *n*

path \ˈpath, ˈpàth\ *n, pl* **paths** \ˈpaᵺz, ˈpaths, ˈpàᵺz, ˈpàths\ **1** : the way or route traversed by something ⟨the sweat glands are the chief ~s by which water reaches the surface of the skin —Morris Fishbein⟩ **2** : PATHWAY 1

path *abbr* pathological; pathology

path·er·ga·sia \ˌpath-ˌər-ˈgā-zh(ē-)ə\ *n* : psychological maladjustment associated with major abnormalities in structure or function

path·er·gy \ˈpath-ər-jē\ *n, pl* **-gies** : an abnormal response to an allergen including both abnormally mild and abnormally severe reactions

path·e·tism \ˈpath-ə-ˌtiz-əm\ *n* : HYPNOTISM 1

path·ic \ˈpath-ik\ *n* : CATAMITE

Path·i·lon \ˈpath-ə-ˌlän\ *n* : a preparation of tridihexethyl chloride — formerly a U.S. registered trademark

patho·bi·ol·o·gy \ˌpath-ō-bī-ˈäl-ə-jē\ *n, pl* **-gies** : PATHOLOGY 1, 2

patho·gen \ˈpath-ə-jən\ *n* : a specific causative agent (as a bacterium or virus) of disease

patho·gen·e·sis \ˌpath-ə-ˈjen-ə-səs\ *n, pl* **-e·ses** \-ˌsēz\ : the origination and development of a disease — called also *pathogeny*

patho·ge·net·ic \-jə-ˈnet-ik\ *adj* **1** : of or relating to pathogenesis **2** : PATHOGENIC 2

patho·gen·ic \-ˈjen-ik\ *adj* **1** : PATHOGENETIC 1 **2** : causing or capable of causing disease ⟨~ microorganisms⟩ — **patho·gen·i·cal·ly** \-i-k(ə-)lē\ *adv*

patho·ge·nic·i·ty \-jə-ˈnis-ət-ē\ *n, pl* **-ties** : the quality or state of being pathogenic : degree of pathogenic capacity

pa·thog·e·ny \pə-ˈthäj-ə-nē, pa-\ *n, pl* **-nies** : PATHOGENESIS

patho·gnom·ic \ˌpath-ə(g)-ˈnäm-ik\ *adj* : PATHOGNOMONIC

pa·tho·gno·mon·ic \ˌpath-ə(g)-nō-ˈmän-ik\ *adj* : distinctively characteristic of a particular disease or condition ⟨erosions, which are virtually ~ of GERD —Barbara Baker⟩

pathol *abbr* pathological; pathologist; pathology

patho·log·i·cal \ˌpath-ə-ˈläj-i-kəl\ *also* **patho·log·ic** \-ik\ *adj* **1** : of or relating to pathology ⟨a ~ laboratory⟩ **2** : altered or caused by disease ⟨~ tissue⟩ — **patho·log·i·cal·ly** \-i-k(ə-)lē\ *adv*

pathological anatomist *n* : a person who specializes in pathological anatomy

pathological anatomy *n* : a branch of anatomy concerned with structural changes accompanying disease

pathological fracture *n* : a fracture of a bone weakened by disease

pathological liar *n* : an individual who habitually tells lies so exaggerated or bizarre that they are suggestive of mental disorder

pa·thol·o·gist \pə-ˈthäl-ə-jəst, pa-\ *n* : a specialist in pathology; *specif* : a physician who interprets and diagnoses the changes caused by disease in tissues and body fluids

pa·thol·o·gize *or chiefly Brit* **pa·thol·o·gise** \-ˌjīz\ *vt* **-gized** *or chiefly Brit* **-gised; -giz·ing** *or chiefly Brit* **-gis·ing** : to view or characterize as medically or psychologically abnormal ⟨natural hormonal shifts have been *pathologized* —Joyce C. Mills⟩ ⟨*pathologizing* childhood behavior —Ruth Shalit⟩ — **pa·thol·o·gi·za·tion** *or chiefly Brit* **pa·thol·o·gi·sa·tion** \pə-ˌthäl-ə-jə-ˈzā-shən\ *n*

pa·thol·o·gy \-jē\ *n, pl* **-gies** **1** : the study of the essential nature of diseases and esp. of the structural and functional changes produced by them **2** : the anatomic and physiological deviations from the normal that constitute disease or characterize a particular disease **3** : a treatise on or compilation of abnormalities ⟨a new ~ of the eye⟩

patho·mi·me·sis \ˌpath-ō-mə-ˈmē-səs\ *n* : imitation of disease esp. unconsciously in some forms of hysteria

patho·mor·phol·o·gy \ˌpath-ō-mòr-ˈfäl-ə-jē\ *n, pl* **-gies** : morphology of abnormal conditions — **patho·mor·pho·log·i·cal** \-ˌmòr-fə-ˈläj-i-kəl\ *or* **patho·mor·pho·log·ic** \-ik\ *adj*

patho·phys·i·ol·o·gy \-ˌfiz-ē-ˈäl-ə-jē\ *n, pl* **-gies** : the physiology of abnormal states; *specif* : the functional changes that accompany a particular syndrome or disease — **patho·phys·i·o·log·i·cal** \-ē-ə-ˈläj-i-kəl\ *or* **patho·phys·i·o·log·ic** \-ik\ *adj* — **patho·phys·i·ol·o·gist** \-ē-ˈäl-ə-jəst\ *n*

pa·tho·sis \pə-ˈthō-səs, pa-\ *n, pl* **pa·tho·ses** \-ˌsēz\ : a diseased state : an abnormal condition ⟨dental ~⟩

path·way \ˈpath-ˌwā, ˈpàth-\ *n* **1** : a line of communication over interconnecting neurons extending from one organ or center to another; *also* : a network of interconnecting neurons along which a nerve impulse travels **2** : the sequence of usu. enzyme-catalyzed reactions by which one substance is converted into another ⟨metabolic ~s⟩

pa·tient \ˈpā-shənt\ *n* **1** : a sick individual esp. when awaiting or under the care and treatment of a physician or surgeon ⟨the hospital is equipped to handle 500 ~s⟩ **2** : a client for medical service (as of a physician or dentist) ⟨a good practice with a large number of ~s⟩

pat·ri·cide \ˈpa-trə-ˌsīd\ *n* : murder of a father by his son or daughter

pat·ri·lin·eal \ˌpa-trə-ˈlin-ē-əl\ *adj* : relating to, based on, or tracing descent through the paternal line ⟨~ society⟩

pat·ro·cli·nal \ˌpa-trə-ˈklī-nᵊl\ *adj* : PATROCLINOUS

pat·ro·cli·nous \-ˈklī-nəs\ *adj* : derived or inherited from the father or paternal line — compare MATROCLINOUS

pat·ro·cli·ny \ˌpa-trə-ˌklī-nē\ *n, pl* **-nies** : the quality or state of being patroclinous

pat·ro·gen·e·sis \ˌpa-trə-ˈjen-ə-səs\ *n* : ANDROGENESIS

pat·tern \ˈpat-ərn\ *n* **1** : a model for making a mold used to form a casting **2** : a reliable sample of traits, acts, tendencies, or other observable characteristics of a person, group, or institution ⟨~s of behavior⟩ **3** : an established mode of behavior or cluster of mental attitudes, beliefs, and values that are held in common by members of a group

pat·tern·ing *n* : physical therapy esp. for neurological impairment based on a theory holding that repeated manipulation of body parts to simulate normal motor neurological activity (as crawling or walking) promotes neurological development or repair

pat·u·lin \'pach-ə-lən\ n : a very toxic colorless crystalline antibiotic $C_7H_6O_4$ produced by several molds (as *Aspergillus clavatus* and *Penicillium patulum*) — called also *clavacin, claviformin*

pat·u·lous \'pach-ə-ləs\ adj : spread widely apart : wide open or distended ⟨a ∼ eustachian tube⟩ — **pat·u·lous·ness** n

Paul–Bun·nell test \'pȯl-'bən-əl-\ n : a test for heterophile antibodies used in the diagnosis of infectious mononucleosis — called also *Paul-Bunnell reaction*

Paul, John Rodman (1893–1971), and **Bunnell, Walls Willard (1902–1965),** American physicians. Paul served for many years on the medical faculty at Yale University. He undertook major research on several microbial diseases. In a systematic study of familial rheumatic fever, he determined that a streptococcus infection precipitated the disease. He published a book-length study of the epidemiology of rheumatic fever in 1930. With Bunnell he developed in 1932 a laboratory test for infectious mononucleosis based on their discovery of heterophile antibodies in the sera of persons with the disease.

paunch \'pȯnch, 'pänch\ n : RUMEN

pave·ment epithelium \'pāv-mənt-\ n : an epithelium made up of a single layer of flat cells

pa·vil·ion \pə-'vil-yən\ n 1 : PINNA 2 : a detached or semidetached part of a hospital devoted to a special use ⟨a maternity ∼⟩ ⟨a nuclear medicine ∼⟩

Pav·lov·ian \pav-'lō-vē-ən, -'lȯ-; -'lȯ-fē-\ adj : of or relating to Ivan Pavlov or to his work and theories ⟨∼ conditioning⟩

Pav·lov \'päv-lȯf, 'pav-, -ˌlȯv\, **Ivan Petrovich (1849–1936),** Russian physiologist. Pavlov is most famous for developing the concept of the conditioned reflex. In his classic experiment he trained a hungry dog to salivate at the sound of a bell by conditioning the dog to associate the sound of the bell with the sight of food. His earlier research had been concerned with cardiac physiology and the regulation of blood pressure. Carefully dissecting the fine cardiac nerves, he demonstrated that the strength of the heartbeat was controlled by nerves leaving the cardiac plexus. He later turned his attention to the study of the secretory activity of digestion. Having devised with the German physiologist Rudolph Heidenhain an operation to prepare what is now often called a Pavlov pouch, he was able to isolate the stomach from salivary and pancreatic secretions and thereby study the gastrointestinal secretions in a normal animal over its life span. This research led him to formulate the laws of the conditioned reflex. In 1904 he was awarded the Nobel Prize for Physiology or Medicine for his research on the physiology of digestive secretions.

Pavlov pouch n : an isolated portion of the stomach separated by surgical operation from the main part, open to the exterior, and used for study of gastric secretion

pav·or noc·tur·nus \'pav-ˌȯr-näk-'tər-nəs\ n : NIGHT TERROR

pawpaw var of PAPAW

Pax·il \'pak-səl\ trademark — used for a preparation of the hydrochloride of paroxetine

pay–bed \'pā-ˌbed\ n, Brit : hospital accommodations and services for which the patient is charged

Pb symbol lead

PBB \ˌpē-ˌbē-'bē\ n : POLYBROMINATED BIPHENYL

PBI abbr protein-bound iodine

PBL abbr peripheral blood lymphocyte

PBMC abbr peripheral blood mononuclear cell

PC abbr 1 percent; percentage 2 [Latin *post cibos*] after meals — used in writing prescriptions 3 professional corporation 4 purified concentrate

PCB \ˌpē-ˌsē-'bē\ n : POLYCHLORINATED BIPHENYL

pCi abbr picocurie

PCL \ˌpē-(ˌ)sē-'el\ n : POSTERIOR CRUCIATE LIGAMENT

PCOS abbr polycystic ovary syndrome

PCP \ˌpē-ˌsē-'pē\ n 1 : PHENCYCLIDINE 2 : PENTACHLOROPHENOL 3 : a health-care professional and esp. a physician who is authorized (as by an HMO) to provide primary care

PCP abbr Pneumocystis carinii pneumonia

PCR abbr polymerase chain reaction

Pcs abbr preconscious

PCV abbr packed cell volume

PCWP abbr pulmonary capillary wedge pressure

Pd symbol palladium

PD abbr 1 interpupillary distance 2 Parkinson's disease 3 peritoneal dialysis

PDB \ˌpē-ˌdē-'bē\ n : PARADICHLOROBENZENE

PDGF abbr platelet-derived growth factor

PDR abbr *Physicians' Desk Reference*

PE abbr 1 physical examination 2 pulmonary embolism

peach–ker·nel oil \'pēch-ˌkərn-ᵊl-\ n : PERSIC OIL b

peak flow meter \'pēk-ˌflō-\ n : a device that measures the maximum rate of air flow out of the lungs during forced expiration and that is used esp. for monitoring lung capacity of individuals with asthma (as to indicate bronchial narrowing) — called also *peak expiratory flow meter*

pea·nut oil \'pē-nət-\ n : a colorless to yellow nondrying fatty oil that is obtained from peanuts and is used chiefly as a salad oil, in margarine, in soap, and as a vehicle in pharmaceutical preparations and cosmetics — called also *arachis oil*

pearl \'pərl\ n 1 : PERLE 2 : one of the rounded concentric masses of squamous epithelial cells characteristic of certain tumors 3 : a miliary leproma of the iris 4 : a rounded abnormal mass of enamel on a tooth

pearl disease n : tuberculosis of serous membranes (as the pleura or peritoneum) that is characterized by small rounded grayish elevated lesions and occurs chiefly in cattle — called also *pearly disease*

pearly tumor n : CHOLESTEATOMA 1

pec \'pek\ n : PECTORALIS — usu. used in pl.

pec·cant \'pek-ənt\ adj : causing disease ⟨specific virtues . . . of drugs, as opposed to the unspecific adjustment of "∼ humours," were recognized in the 16th and 17th centuries —Joseph Needham⟩

peck·ing order \'pek-iŋ-\ also **peck order** \'pek-ˌ\ n : the basic pattern of social organization within a flock of poultry in which each bird pecks another lower in the scale without fear of retaliation and submits to pecking by one of higher rank — compare CANNIBALISM 3, DOMINANCE a

pec·tase \'pek-ˌtās, -ˌtāz\ n : PECTINESTERASE

pec·ten \'pek-tən\ n, pl **pec·ti·nes** \-tə-ˌnēz\ : a body part that resembles a comb; esp : a folded vascular pigmented membrane projecting into the vitreous body in the eye of a bird or reptile

pec·te·no·sis \ˌpek-tə-'nō-səs\ n, pl **-no·ses** \-'nō-ˌsēz\ or **-no·sis·es** : a condition that affects the middle third of the anal canal and is characterized by the formation of a thick hardened ring of fibrous tissue with resulting stenosis and contracture

pec·tic \'pek-tik\ adj : of, relating to, or derived from pectin

pectic acid n : any of various water-insoluble substances formed by hydrolyzing the methyl ester groups of pectins

pectic substance n : any of a group of complex colloidal carbohydrate derivatives of plant origin that contain a large proportion of units derived from galacturonic acid and include protopectins, pectins, pectinic acids, and pectic acids

pec·tin \'pek-tən\ n 1 : any of various water-soluble substances that bind adjacent cell walls in plant tissues and yield a gel which is the basis of fruit jellies 2 : a commercial product rich in pectins and used chiefly in making jelly and other foods, in pharmaceutical products esp. for the control of diarrhea, and in cosmetics

pec·tin·ase \'pek-tə-ˌnās, -ˌnāz\ n : an enzyme or complex of

O

P

\ə\ **abut** \ᵊ\ **kitten** \ər\ **further** \a\ **ash** \ā\ **ace** \ä\ **cot, cart** \au̇\ **out** \ch\ **chin** \e\ **bet** \ē\ **easy** \g\ **go** \i\ **hit** \ī\ **ice** \j\ **job** \ŋ\ **sing** \ō\ **go** \ȯ\ **law** \ȯi\ **boy** \th\ **thin** \th̲\ **the** \ü\ **loot** \u̇\ **foot** \y\ **yet** \zh\ **vision** *See also* Pronunciation Symbols page

enzymes that catalyzes the hydrolysis of pectic substances; *esp* : the polygalacturonase that is active toward pectic acid

¹**pec·ti·nate** \'pek-tə-ˌnāt\ *adj* : having narrow parallel projections or divisions suggestive of the teeth of a comb

²**pectinate** *n* : a salt or ester of a pectinic acid

pectinati — see MUSCULI PECTINATI

pec·tin·e·al \pek-'tin-ē-əl\ *adj* : of, relating to, or located near the pubic bone

pectineal line *n* **1** : ILIOPECTINEAL LINE **2** : a ridge on the posterior surface of the femur that runs downward from the lesser trochanter and gives attachment to the pectineus

pectines *pl of* PECTEN

pec·tin·es·ter·ase \ˌpek-tə-'nes-tə-ˌrās, -ˌrāz\ *n* : an enzyme that catalyzes the hydrolysis of pectins into pectic acids and methanol — called also *pectase*

pec·tin·e·us \pek-'tin-ē-əs\ *n, pl* **-tin·ei** \-ē-ˌī, -ē-ˌē\ : a flat quadrangular muscle of the upper front and inner aspect of the thigh that arises mostly from the iliopectineal line of the pubis and is inserted along the pectineal line of the femur

pec·tin·ic acid \pek-ˌtin-ik-\ *n* : any of the colloidal polysaccharides of acidic nature that are obtained by partial hydrolysis of protopectins and are intermediate in methyl ester content between pectic acids and the usual pectin

pec·tin·i·form septum \pek-'tin-i-ˌfȯrm-\ *n* : a pectinate band of connective tissue extending between the corpora cavernosa of the penis or the clitoris

pec·ti·no·lyt·ic \ˌpek-ti-nō-'lit-ik\ *adj* : producing hydrolysis of pectins ⟨∼ aerobic bacteria⟩

pec·ti·za·tion \ˌpek-tə-'zā-shən\ *n* : the act or process of changing from a sol to a gel

pec·to·lyt·ic \ˌpek-tə-'lit-ik\ *adj* : producing hydrolysis of pectic substances ⟨∼ enzymes⟩

¹**pec·to·ral** \'pek-t(ə-)rəl\ *n* **1** : a pectoral part or organ; *esp* : PECTORALIS **2** : a medicinal substance for treating diseases of the respiratory tract

²**pectoral** *adj* **1** : of, relating to, or occurring in or on the chest ⟨∼ arch⟩ **2** : relating to or good for diseases of the respiratory tract ⟨a ∼ syrup⟩

pectoral girdle *n* : the bony or cartilaginous arch supporting the forelimbs of a vertebrate that corresponds to the pelvic girdle of the hind limbs but is usu. not attached to the spinal column and that consists in lower forms of a single cartilage on each side which in higher forms becomes ossified, divided into the scapula above and the precoracoid and coracoid below, and complicated by the addition or substitution of one or more membrane bones and which in humans is highly modified with the scapula alone of the original elements well developed, the coracoid being represented only by the coracoid process of the scapula, and the precoracoid being replaced by the clavicle that connects the scapula with the sternum and is the only bony connection of the arm bones with the rest of the skeleton — called also *shoulder girdle*

pec·to·ra·lis \ˌpek-tə-'rā-ləs\ *n, pl* **-ra·les** \-ˌlēz\ : either of the muscles that connect the ventral walls of the chest with the bones of the upper arm and shoulder of which in humans there are two on each side: **a** : a larger one that arises from the clavicle, the sternum, the cartilages of most or all of the ribs, and the aponeurosis of the external oblique muscle and is inserted by a strong flat tendon into the posterior bicipital ridge of the humerus — called also *pectoralis major* **b** : a smaller one that lies beneath the larger, arises from the third, fourth, and fifth ribs, and is inserted by a flat tendon into the coracoid process of the scapula — called also *pectoralis minor*

pectoralis major *n* : PECTORALIS a

pectoralis minor *n* : PECTORALIS b

pectoralis muscle *n* : PECTORALIS

pectoral muscle *n* : PECTORALIS

pectoral nerve *n* : either of two nerves that arise from the brachial plexus on each side or from the nerve trunks forming it and that supply the pectoral muscles: **a** : one lateral to the axillary artery — called also *lateral pectoral nerve, superior pectoral nerve* **b** : one medial to the axillary artery — called also *inferior pectoral nerve, medial pectoral nerve*

pec·to·ril·o·quy \ˌpek-tə-'ril-ə-kwē\ *n, pl* **-quies** : the sound of words heard through the chest wall and usu. indicating a cavity or consolidation of lung tissue — compare BRONCHOPHONY

pectoris — see ANGINA PECTORIS

pec·tose \'pek-ˌtōs, -ˌtōz\ *n* : PROTOPECTIN

pec·tous \'pek-təs\ *adj* **1** : of, relating to, or consisting of protopectin or pectin **2** : resembling a jelly esp. in consistency

pec·tus ex·ca·va·tum \'pek-təs-ˌek-skə-'vāt-əm\ *n* : FUNNEL CHEST

ped·al \'ped-ºl *also* 'pēd-\ *adj* : of or relating to the foot

pedal bone *n* : COFFIN BONE

ped·er·ast \'ped-ə-ˌrast\ *or chiefly Brit* **pae·der·ast** \'pēd-\ *n* : one that practices pederasty

ped·er·as·ty \'ped-ə-ˌras-tē\ *or chiefly Brit* **pae·der·as·ty** \'pēd-\ *n, pl* **-ties** : anal intercourse esp. with a boy as the passive partner — **ped·er·as·tic** \ˌped-ə-'ras-tik\ *or chiefly Brit* **pae·der·as·tic** \ˌpēd-\ *adj*

pedes *pl of* PES

pe·di·at·ric *or chiefly Brit* **pae·di·at·ric** \ˌpēd-ē-ə-'a-trik\ *adj* : of or relating to pediatrics

pe·di·a·tri·cian *or chiefly Brit* **pae·di·a·tri·cian** \ˌpēd-ē-ə-'trish-ən\ *n* : a specialist in pediatrics — called also *pediatrist*

pe·di·at·rics *or chiefly Brit* **pae·di·at·rics** \ˌpēd-ē-'a-triks\ *n pl but sing or pl in constr* : a branch of medicine dealing with the development, care, and diseases of children

pe·di·a·trist *or chiefly Brit* **pae·di·a·trist** \'pēd-ē-ə-trəst\ *n* : PEDIATRICIAN

ped·i·cle \'ped-i-kəl\ *n* : a basal attachment: as **a** : the basal part of each side of the neural arch of a vertebra connecting the laminae with the centrum **b** : the narrow basal part by which various organs (as kidney or spleen) are continuous with other body structures **c** : the narrow base of a tumor **d** : the part of a pedicle flap left attached to the original site

ped·i·cled \-kəld\ *adj* : having a pedicle ⟨a ∼ tumor⟩

pedicle flap *n* : a flap which is left attached to the original site by a narrow base of tissue to provide a blood supply during grafting — called also *pedicle graft*

pe·dic·u·lar \pi-'dik-yə-lər\ *adj* : of, relating to, or infested with lice

pe·dic·u·lat·ed \pi-'dik-yə-ˌlāt-əd\ *adj* : PEDICLED ⟨∼ tumors⟩

pediculi *pl of* PEDICULUS

pe·dic·u·li·cide \pi-'dik-yə-lə-ˌsīd\ *n* : an agent for destroying lice — **pe·dic·u·li·cid·al** \pi-ˌdik-yə-lə-'sīd-ºl\ *adj*

Ped·i·cu·li·dae \ˌped-ə-'kyü-lə-ˌdē\ *n pl* : a family of lice of the order Anoplura that includes the head louse (*Pediculus humanus capitis*), the body louse (*P. humanus corporis*), and the crab louse (*Pthirus pubis*) which are the only lice that attack humans

Pe·dic·u·loi·des \pi-ˌdik-yə-'lȯi-(ˌ)dēz\ *n, syn of* PYEMOTES

pe·dic·u·lo·sis \pi-ˌdik-yə-'lō-səs\ *n, pl* **-lo·ses** \-ˌsēz\ : infestation with lice — called also *lousiness*

pediculosis cap·i·tis \-'kap-ət-əs\ *n* : infestation of the scalp by head lice

pediculosis cor·po·ris \-'kȯr-pə-rəs\ *n* : infestation by body lice

pediculosis pubis *n* : infestation by crab lice

pe·dic·u·lous \pi-'dik-yə-ləs\ *adj* : infested with lice : LOUSY

pe·dic·u·lus \pi-'dik-yə-ləs\ *n* **1** *cap* : the type genus of the family Pediculidae that includes the body louse (*P. humanus corporis*) and head louse (*P. humanus capitis*) infesting humans **2** *pl* **pe·dic·u·li** \-ˌlī\ *or* **pediculus** : any louse of the genus *Pediculus*

ped·i·cure \'ped-i-ˌkyu̇(ə)r\ *n* **1** : a person who provides care for the feet, toes, and nails **2 a** : care of the feet, toes, and nails **b** : a single treatment of the feet, toes, or nails

ped·i·gree \'ped-ə-ˌgrē\ *n* : a record of the ancestry of an individual ⟨the ∼ of a diabetic patient⟩

Ped·i·lan·thus \ˌped-ə-'lan(t)-thəs\ *n* : a genus of tropical American plants (family Euphorbiaceae) that resemble cacti and include the redbird cactus (*P. tithymaloides*)

pedis — see DORSALIS PEDIS, TINEA PEDIS

pe·do·don·tia *or chiefly Brit* **pae·do·don·tia** \ˌpēd-ə-'dän-ch(ē-)ə\ *n* : PEDODONTICS

pe·do·don·tics *or chiefly Brit* **pae·do·don·tics** \ˌpēd-ə-'dänt-iks\ *n pl but sing or pl in constr* : a branch of dentistry that is concerned with the dental care of children — **pe·do·don·tic** *or chiefly Brit* **pae·do·don·tic** *adj*

pe·do·don·tist *or chiefly Brit* **pae·do·don·tist** \ˌpēd-ə-'dänt-əst\ *n* : a specialist in pedodontics

pedogenesis, pedogenetic *var of* PAEDOGENESIS, PAEDOGENETIC

pe·dol·o·gy *or chiefly Brit* **pae·dol·o·gy** \pē-'däl-ə-jē\ *n, pl* **-gies** : the scientific study of the life and development of children

pedomorphic, pedomorphism, pedomorphosis *var of* PAEDOMORPHIC, PAEDOMORPHISM, PAEDOMORPHOSIS

pe·do·phile \'pēd-ə-ˌfīl, 'ped-\ *or chiefly Brit* **pae·do·phile** \'pēd-\ *n* : one affected with pedophilia — called also *pedophiliac*

pe·do·phil·ia \ˌpēd-ə-'fil-ē-ə, ˌped-\ *or chiefly Brit* **pae·do·phil·ia** \ˌpēd-\ *n* : sexual perversion in which children are the preferred sexual object

¹**pe·do·phil·i·ac** \-'fil-ē-ˌak\ *or* **pe·do·phil·ic** \-'fil-ik\ *or chiefly Brit* **pae·do·phil·i·ac** \ˌpēd-ə-'fil-ē-ˌak\ *or* **pae·do·phil·ic** \-'fil-ik\ *adj* : of, relating to, or affected with pedophilia

²**pedophiliac** *or chiefly Brit* **paedophiliac** *n* : PEDOPHILE

pe·do·phil·ic *or chiefly Brit* **pae·do·phil·ic** \-'fil-ik\ *adj* : PEDOPHILIAC

pe·dun·cle \'pē-ˌdən-kəl, pi-'\ *n* **1** : a band of white matter joining different parts of the brain — see CEREBELLAR PEDUNCLE, CEREBRAL PEDUNCLE **2** : a narrow stalk by which a tumor or polyp is attached — **pe·dun·cu·lar** \pi-'dən-kyə-lər\ *adj*

pe·dun·cu·lat·ed \pi-'dən-kyə-ˌlāt-əd\ *also* **pe·dun·cu·late** \-lət\ *adj* : having, growing on, or being attached by a peduncle ⟨a ∼ tumor⟩

pe·dun·cu·lot·o·my \pi-ˌdən-kyə-'lät-ə-mē\ *n, pl* **-mies** : surgical incision of a cerebral peduncle for relief of involuntary movements

pe·dun·cu·lus ce·re·bel·la·ris inferior \pi-'dən-kyə-ləs-ˌser-ə-bel-'er-əs-\ *n* : CEREBELLAR PEDUNCLE c

pedunculus cerebellaris me·di·us \-'mē-dē-əs\ *n* : CEREBELLAR PEDUNCLE b

pedunculus cerebellaris superior *n* : CEREBELLAR PEDUNCLE a

¹**peel** \'pēl\ *vt* **1** : to strip off an outer layer of **2** : to remove (as skin or a blemish) by stripping ∼ *vi* **1** : to come off in sheets or scales ⟨sunburned skin ∼s⟩ **2** : to lose an outer layer (as of skin) ⟨his face is ∼ing⟩

²**peel** *n* : CHEMICAL PEEL

PEEP *abbr* positive end-expiratory pressure

peep·er \'pē-pər\ *n* : VOYEUR

Peep·ing Tom \ˌpē-piŋ-'täm\ *n* : a pruriently prying person : VOYEUR — **Peeping Tom·ism** \-'täm-ˌiz-əm\ *n*

Peeping Tom, British legendary character. According to popular legend, Tom was a prying tailor who was struck blind (or, in some versions, struck dead) as he watched Lady Godiva when she rode naked through the streets of Coventry, England, as a protest against the heavy taxes imposed upon the citizens of Coventry.

peer re·view organization \'pir-ri-'vyü-\ *n* : any of a group of organizations staffed by local practicing physicians that were established by the Tax Equity and Fiscal Responsibility Act of 1982 to evaluate the quality, necessity, cost, and adherence to professional standards of medical care provided to Medicare patients as a prerequisite for payment of the medical services by Medicare — abbr. *PRO*

Peg·a·none \'peg-ə-ˌnōn\ *trademark* — used for a preparation of ethotoin

pel·age \'pel-ij\ *n* : the hairy covering of a mammal

pel·ar·gon·ic acid \ˌpel-är-ˌgän-ik-\ *n* : an oily fatty acid $C_9H_{18}O_2$ found esp. in fusel oil and rancid fats and made synthetically by oxidation of oleic acid

pe·li·o·sis \ˌpel-ē-'ō-səs, ˌpē-lē-\ *n, pl* **-o·ses** \-ˌsēz\ *or* **-o·sis·es** : PURPURA — **pe·li·ot·ic** \-'ät-ik\ *adj*

peliosis hepatitis *n* : an abnormal condition characterized by the occurrence of numerous small blood-filled cystic lesions throughout the liver

Pel·i·zae·us–Merz·bach·er disease \ˌpel-ēt-'sä-əs-'merts-ˌbäk-ər-\ *n* : a familial degenerative disease of the central nervous system that is characterized by slowly progressive demyelination of white matter resulting in mental deterioration and the occurrence of various motor disorders (as ataxia and nystagmus)

Pelizaeus, Friedrich (1850–1917), and **Merzbacher, Ludwig (1875–1942),** German neurologists. In 1885 Pelizaeus described a congenital and familial disease that is due to atrophy of the white matter of the brain and whose characteristics include speech disturbances, loss of coordination, and mental retardation. Merzbacher independently described the same disease in 1908.

pel·la·gra \pə-'lag-rə, -'lāg-, -'läg-\ *n* : a disease marked by dermatitis, gastrointestinal disorders, mental disturbance, and memory loss and associated with a diet deficient in niacin and protein — compare KWASHIORKOR

pel·la·gra·gen·ic \-ˌlag-rə-'jen-ik, -ˌlāg-, -ˌläg-\ *adj* : producing pellagra

pellagra–preventive factor *n* : NIACIN

pel·la·grin \pə-'lag-rən, -'lāg-, -'läg-\ *n* : one that is affected with pellagra

pel·la·groid \-ˌroid\ *adj* : resembling pellagra

pel·la·grous \-rəs\ *adj* : of, relating to, or affected with pellagra ⟨∼ insanity⟩ ⟨∼ symptoms⟩ ⟨∼ patients⟩

pel·let \'pel-ət\ *n* : a usu. small rounded or spherical body; *specif* : a small cylindrical or ovoid compressed mass (as of a hormone) that is implanted subcutaneously for slow absorption into bodily tissues

pel·le·tier·ine \ˌpel-ə-'tir-ˌēn, -ən\ *n* **1** : a liquid alkaloid $C_8H_{15}NO$ found in the bark of the pomegranate **2** : a mixture of alkaloids from the bark of the pomegranate used esp. in the form of its tannate as a vermifuge

Pel·le·tier \pel-ə-tyā\, **Pierre–Joseph (1788–1842),** French chemist. Pelletier was one of the founders of the chemistry of alkaloids. Much of his work was done in collaboration with fellow chemist Joseph-Bienaimé Caventou (1795–1877). The two chemists first isolated chlorophyll in 1817. Pelletier developed an interest in alkaloids, and with Caventou he undertook a search for alkaloids. In 1820 they discovered brucine, cinchonine, colchicine, quinine, strychnine, and veratrine. Their discoveries allowed medicine to move away from the use of crude plant extracts and toward the use of natural and synthetic compounds found or formulated by chemists. In 1877 pelletierine was first isolated and named in Pelletier's honor.

pel·li·cle \'pel-i-kəl\ *n* : a thin skin or film: as **a** : an outer membrane of some protozoans (as euglenoids or paramecia) **b** : a bacterial growth in the form of a sheet on the surface of a liquid medium **c** : a thin layer of salivary glycoproteins coating the surface of the teeth

pel·lic·u·lar \pe-'lik-yə-lər\ *adj* : of, relating to, or having the characteristics of a pellicle

pellucida — see AREA PELLUCIDA, ZONA PELLUCIDA

pellucidum — see SEPTUM PELLUCIDUM

pel·oid \'pel-ˌoid\ *n* : mud prepared and used for therapeutic purposes ⟨natural therapeutic resources, including mineral waters and ∼s —*Jour. Amer. Med. Assoc.*⟩

pel·ta·tin \pel-'tāt-ᵊn\ *n* : either of two lactones that occur as glycosides in the rootstock of the mayapple (*Podophyllum peltatum*) and have some antineoplastic activity: **a** *or* α–**peltatin** \'al-fə-\ : one $C_{21}H_{20}O_8$ containing two hydroxyl groups **b** *or* β–**peltatin** \'bāt-ə-, *chiefly Brit* 'bēt-ə-\ : one $C_{22}H_{22}O_8$ containing only one hydroxyl group with the other replaced by a methoxyl group

pelves *pl of* PELVIS

\ə\ **abut** \ᵊ\ **kitten** \ər\ **further** \a\ **ash** \ā\ **ace** \ä\ **cot, cart** \aů\ **out** \ch\ **chin** \e\ **bet** \ē\ **easy** \g\ **go** \i\ **hit** \ī\ **ice** \j\ **job** \ŋ\ **sing** \ō\ **go** \ȯ\ **law** \ȯi\ **boy** \th\ **thin** \th\ **the** \ü\ **loot** \ů\ **foot** \y\ **yet** \zh\ **vision** *See also* Pronunciation Symbols page

O
P

¹**pel·vic** \'pel-vik\ *adj* : of, relating to, or located in or near the pelvis ⟨∼ organs⟩ ⟨∼ pain⟩

²**pelvic** *n* : a pelvic part

pelvic bone *n* : HIP BONE

pelvic brim *n* : the bony ridge in the cavity of the pelvis that marks the boundary between the false pelvis and the true pelvis

pelvic cavity *n* : the cavity of the pelvis comprising in humans a broad upper and a more contracted lower part — compare FALSE PELVIS, TRUE PELVIS; ABDOMEN 1c

pelvic colon *n* : SIGMOID COLON

pelvic diaphragm *n* : the muscular floor of the pelvis

pelvic fascia *n* : the fascia lining the pelvic cavity

pelvic girdle *n* : a bony or cartilaginous arch that supports the hind limbs of a vertebrate, that corresponds to the pectoral girdle of the forelimbs but is usu. more rigid and firmly attached to the spinal column, and that consists in lower forms of a single cartilage which is replaced in higher forms including humans by paired hip bones articulating solidly with the sacrum dorsally and with one another at the pubic symphysis

pelvic index *n* : the ratio of the transverse diameter to the dorsoventral diameter of the opening formed by the pelvic brim multiplied by 100

pelvic inflammatory disease *n* : infection of the female reproductive tract (as the fallopian tubes and ovaries) that results from microorganisms (as *Neisseria gonorrhea* or *Chlamydia trachomatis*) transmitted esp. during sexual intercourse but also by other means (as during surgery, abortion, or parturition), is marked esp. by lower abdominal pain, an abnormal vaginal discharge, and fever, and is a leading cause of infertility in women — abbr. *PID*

pelvic outlet *n* : the irregular bony opening bounded by the lower border of the pelvis and closed by muscle and other soft tissues through which the terminal parts of the excretory, reproductive, and digestive systems pass to communicate with the surface of the body — called also *outlet of the pelvis*

pelvic plexus *n* : a plexus of the autonomic nervous system that is formed by the hypogastric plexus, by branches from the sacral part of the sympathetic chain, and by the visceral branches of the second, third, and fourth sacral nerves and that is distributed to the viscera of the pelvic region

pelvic splanchnic nerve *n* : any of the groups of parasympathetic fibers that originate with cells in the second, third, and fourth sacral segments of the spinal cord, pass through the inferior portion of the hypogastric plexus, and supply the descending colon, rectum, anus, bladder, prostate gland, and external genitalia — called also *nervus erigens*

pel·vi·graph \'pel-və-ˌgraf\ *n* : a recording pelvimeter

pel·vim·e·ter \pel-'vim-ət-ər\ *n* : an instrument for measuring the dimensions of the pelvis

pel·vim·e·try \pel-'vim-ə-trē\ *n, pl* **-tries** : measurement of the pelvis (as by a pelvimeter or by X-ray examination) — **pel·vi·met·ric** \ˌpel-və-'me-trik\ *adj*

pel·vio·li·thot·o·my \ˌpel-vē-ō-lith-'ät-ə-mē\ *n, pl* **-mies** : PYELOLITHOTOMY

pel·vi·rec·tal abscess \ˌpel-və-'rek-t°l-\ *n* : an abscess occurring between the levator ani muscle and the rectum

pel·vis \'pel-vəs\ *n, pl* **pel·vis·es** \-və-səz\ *or* **pel·ves** \-ˌvēz\ **1** : a basin-shaped structure in the skeleton of many vertebrates that is formed by the pelvic girdle together with the sacrum and often various coccygeal and caudal vertebrae and that in humans is composed of the two hip bones bounding it on each side and in front while the sacrum and coccyx complete it behind **2** : PELVIC CAVITY **3** : RENAL PELVIS

pel·vi·scope \'pel-və-ˌskōp\ *n* : an endoscope for visually examining the interior of the pelvis

pem·o·line \'pem-ə-ˌlēn\ *n* : a synthetic drug $C_9H_8N_2O_2$ that is a mild stimulant of the central nervous system and has been used to treat attention deficit disorder and narcolepsy

¹**pem·phi·goid** \'pem(p)-fə-ˌgȯid\ *adj* : resembling pemphigus

²**pemphigoid** *n* : any of several diseases that resemble pemphigus; *esp* : BULLOUS PEMPHIGOID

pem·phi·gus \'pem(p)-fi-gəs, pem-'fī-gəs\ *n, pl* **-gus·es** *or* **-gi** \-ˌjī\ : any of several autoimmune diseases characterized by the formation of successive eruptions of large blisters on apparently normal skin and mucous membranes often in association with sensations of itching or burning

pemphigus er·y·the·ma·to·sus \-ˌer-i-ˌthē-mə-'tō-səs\ *n* : a relatively benign form of chronic pemphigus that is characterized by the eruption esp. on the face and trunk of lesions resembling those which occur in systemic lupus erythematosus

pemphigus fo·li·a·ce·us \-ˌfō-lē-'ā-s(h)ē-əs\ *n* : a form of chronic pemphigus characterized by numerous flaccid blisters which rupture to produce widespread exfoliation of the skin

pemphigus vul·gar·is \-vəl-'gar-əs\ *n* : a severe and often fatal form of chronic pemphigus

Pen·brit·in \pen-'brit-ᵊn\ *n* : a preparation of ampicillin — formerly a U.S. registered trademark

pen·ci·clo·vir \ˌpen-'sī-klō-ˌvir\ *n* : an antiviral drug $C_{10}H_{15}N_5O_3$ that is applied topically esp. to treat recurrent herpes labialis

pen·cil \'pen(t)-səl\ *n* **1** : a small medicated or cosmetic roll or stick for local applications ⟨a menthol ∼⟩ **2** : an aggregate of rays of radiation (as light) esp. when diverging from or converging to a point

pen·du·lar \'pen-jə-lər, 'pen-d(y)ə-\ *adj* : characterized by or being regular rhythmic movement esp. from side to side

pendular nystagmus *n* : nystagmus marked by rhythmic side-to-side or up-and-down movements of constant speed

pen·du·lous \-ləs\ *adj* : inclined or hanging downward

pe·nec·to·my \pē-'nek-tə-mē\ *n, pl* **-mies** : surgical removal of the penis

penes *pl of* PENIS

pen·e·tram·e·ter \ˌpen-ə-'tram-ət-ər\ *n* : an instrument for measuring the penetrating power of radiation (as X-rays) by comparing transmission through different absorbers — called also *penetrometer*

pen·e·trance \'pen-ə-trən(t)s\ *n* : the proportion of individuals of a particular genotype that express its phenotypic effect in a given environment — compare EXPRESSIVITY

pen·e·trate \'pen-ə-ˌtrāt\ *vb* **-trat·ed; -trat·ing** *vt* **1** : to pass into or through ⟨enzymes that help the sperm ∼ the zona pellucida —Anna Maria Gillis⟩ **2** : to insert the penis into the vagina in copulation ∼ *vi* : to pass, extend, pierce, or diffuse into or through something ⟨*penetrating* percutaneous nephroscopy or ureteroscopy —R. A. Riehle *et al*⟩

pen·e·trat·ing *adj* : having the power of entering, piercing, or pervading ⟨treat hemorrhage from both ∼ injury and blunt trauma —*Jour. Amer. Med. Assoc.*⟩ — **pen·e·trat·ing·ly** \-ˌtrāt-iŋ-lē\ *adv*

pen·e·tra·tion \ˌpen-ə-'trā-shən\ *n* **1** : the depth to which something penetrates **2** : the act or process of penetrating

pen·e·trom·e·ter \ˌpen-ə-'träm-ət-ər\ *n* **1** : an instrument for measuring the firmness or consistency of a substance **2** : PENETRAMETER

pen·flur·i·dol \ˌpen-'flúr-i-ˌdȯl\ *n* : a tranquilizing drug $C_{28}H_{27}ClF_5NO$

pe·ni·al \'pē-nē-əl\ *adj* : PENILE

pen·i·cil·la·mine \ˌpen-ə-'sil-ə-ˌmēn\ *n* : an amino acid $C_5H_{11}NO_2S$ that is obtained from penicillins and is used esp. to treat cystinuria, rheumatoid arthritis, and metal poisoning (as by copper or lead)

pen·i·cil·lary \ˌpen-ə-'sil-ə-rē\ *adj* : of, relating to, or being a penicillus ⟨a ∼ artery⟩

pen·i·cil·late \ˌpen-ə-'sil-ət, -ˌāt\ *adj* : furnished with a tuft of fine filaments

penicilli *pl of* PENICILLUS

penicillia *pl of* PENICILLIUM

pen·i·cil·lic acid \ˌpen-ə-ˌsil-ik-\ *n* : a crystalline antibiotic unsaturated keto acid $C_8H_{10}O_4$ or the tautomeric hydroxy lactone produced by several molds of the genera *Penicillium* and *Aspergillus*

pen·i·cil·lin \ˌpen-ə-'sil-ən\ *n* **1** : a mixture of relatively nontoxic antibiotic acids produced esp. by molds of the genus

Penicillium (as *P. notatum* or *P. chrysogenum*) and having a powerful bacteriostatic effect against various chiefly gram-positive bacteria (as staphylococci, gonococci, pneumococci, hemolytic streptococci, or some meningococci) **2** : any of numerous often hygroscopic and unstable amido acids (as penicillin G, penicillin O, and penicillin V) that have a structure in which a four-membered lactam ring shares a nitrogen and a carbon atom with a thiazolidine ring to which it is fused and that are components of the penicillin mixture or are produced biosynthetically by the use of different strains of molds or different media or are synthesized chemically **3** : a salt or ester of a penicillin acid or a mixture of such salts or esters

pen·i·cil·lin·ase \-'sil-ə-ˌnās, -ˌnāz\ *n* : BETA-LACTAMASE

penicillin F \-'ef\ *n* : a penicillin $C_{14}H_{20}N_2O_4S$ that was the first of the penicillins isolated in Great Britain

penicillin G \-'jē\ *n* : the penicillin $C_{16}H_{18}N_2O_4S$ that constitutes the principal or sole component of most commercial preparations and is used chiefly in the form of its stable salts (as the sodium salt $C_{16}H_{17}N_2NaO_4S$ or potassium salt $C_{16}H_{17}KN_2O_4S$) — called also *benzylpenicillin;* see PENICILLIN G BENZATHINE, PENICILLIN G PROCAINE

penicillin G ben·za·thine \-'ben-zə-ˌthēn, -thən\ *n* : an aqueous suspension of a relatively insoluble salt of penicillin G that provides a low but persistent serum level of penicillin G following intramuscular injection — called also *benzathine penicillin G*

penicillin G procaine *n* : an aqueous suspension of equimolar amounts of penicillin G and procaine that provides a low but persistent serum level of penicillin G following intramuscular injection — called also *procaine penicillin G*

penicillin O \-'ō\ *n* : a penicillin $C_{13}H_{18}N_2O_4S_2$ that is similar to penicillin G in antibiotic activity but that is obtained by growing the penicillia in a culture medium that contains a precursor

penicillin V \-'vē\ *n* : a crystalline nonhygroscopic acid that is used in the form of its potassium salt $C_{16}H_{17}KN_2O_5S$ and has antibacterial action similar to penicillin G and is more resistant to inactivation by gastric acids — called also *phenoxymethyl penicillin*

pen·i·cil·li·o·sis \ˌpen-ə-ˌsil-ē-'ō-səs\ *n, pl* **-o·ses** \-ˌsēz\ : infection with or disease caused by molds of the genus *Penicillium*

pen·i·cil·li·um \ˌpen-ə-'sil-ē-əm\ *n* **1** *cap* : a genus of fungi (as the blue molds) that have been grouped with the imperfect fungi but are now often placed with the ascomycetes and that are found chiefly on moist nonliving organic matter (as decaying fruit), are characterized by the erect branching conidiophores ending in tufts of club-shaped cells from which conidia are formed in chains, and include molds useful in economic fermentation and the production of antibiotics **2** *pl* **-lia** \-ē-ə\ : any mold of the genus *Penicillium*

pen·i·cil·lo·ic acid \ˌpen-ə-sə-ˌlō-ik-\ *n* : any of several acids having the general formula $RCONH(C_6H_{10}NS)(COOH)_2$ which are obtained from the penicillins by hydrolytic opening of the lactam ring (as by the action of a beta-lactamase)

pen·i·cil·lo·yl–poly·ly·sine \ˌpen-ə-'sil-ō-ˌil-ˌpäl-i-'lī-ˌsēn\ *n* : a preparation of a penicillic acid and polylysine which is used in a skin test to determine hypersensitivity to penicillin

pen·i·cil·lus \ˌpen-ə-'sil-əs\ *n, pl* **-li** \-ˌī\ **1** : one of the small straight arteries of the red pulp of the spleen **2** : the branching penicillate conidiophore in fungi of various genera (as *Penicillium*)

pe·nile \'pē-ˌnīl\ *adj* : of, relating to, or affecting the penis ⟨a ~ prosthesis⟩ ⟨~ lesions⟩

pe·nis \'pē-nəs\ *n, pl* **pe·nes** \'pē-(ˌ)nēz\ *or* **pe·nis·es** : the male copulatory organ of a higher vertebrate animal that in mammals including humans usu. functions as the channel by which urine leaves the body and is typically a cylindrical organ that is suspended from the pubic arch, contains a pair of large lateral corpora cavernosa and a smaller ventromedial corpus cavernosum containing the urethra, and has a terminal glans enclosing the ends of the corpora cavernosa,

covered by mucous membrane, and sheathed by a foreskin continuous with the skin covering the body of the organ

penis en·vy \-ˌen-vē\ *n* : the supposed coveting of the penis by a young human female which is held in psychoanalytic theory to lead to feelings of inferiority and defensive or compensatory behavior

pen·nate \'pen-ˌāt\ *adj* : having a structure like that of a feather; *esp* : being a muscle in which fibers extend obliquely from either side of a central tendon

pen·ni·form \'pen-i-ˌfôrm\ *adj* : PENNATE

pen·ny·roy·al \ˌpen-ē-'rôi(-ə)l, 'pen-i-ˌrīl\ *n* : any of several mints; *esp* : an aromatic American mint (*Hedeoma pulegioides*) that yields pennyroyal oil

pennyroyal oil *n* : a yellowish aromatic essential oil obtained from an American pennyroyal (*Hedeoma pulegioides*) and used as an insect repellent and in folk medicine as an emmenagogue, carminative, and stimulant — called also *hedeoma oil*

pen·ny·weight \'pen-ē-ˌwāt\ *n* : a unit of weight equal to 24 grains

pe·nol·o·gist \pi-'näl-ə-jəst\ *n* : a specialist in penology

pe·nol·o·gy \pi-'näl-ə-jē\ *n, pl* **-gies** : a branch of criminology dealing with prison management and the treatment of offenders — **pe·no·log·i·cal** \ˌpē-nə-'läj-i-kəl\ *adj*

pe·no·scro·tal \ˌpē-nō-'skrōt-ᵊl\ *adj* : of or relating to the penis and scrotum ⟨a ~ urethroplasty⟩

penoscrotal raphe *n* : the ridge on the surface of the scrotum that divides it into two lateral halves and is continued forward on the underside of the penis and backward along the midline of the perineum to the anus

Pen·rose drain \'pen-ˌrōz-\ *n* : CIGARETTE DRAIN

Penrose, Charles Bingham (1862–1925), American gynecologist. Penrose founded the Gynecean Hospital of Philadelphia in 1887, and until 1899 he served as the hospital's chief surgeon. During the same period he was professor of gynecology at the University of Pennsylvania Medical School and gynecologist at the university hospital. He wrote a textbook on the diseases of women, and in 1890 he published a paper on abdominal surgery in which he introduced the Penrose drain.

pen·ta·ba·sic \ˌpent-ə-'bā-sik\ *adj* **1** *of an acid* : having five hydrogen atoms capable of replacement by basic atoms or radicals **2** *of a salt* : containing five atoms of a monovalent metal or their equivalent

pen·ta·chlo·ro·phe·nate \ˌpent-ə-ˌklōr-ə-'fē-ˌnāt\ *n* : a salt of pentachlorophenol

pen·ta·chlo·ro·phe·nol \ˌpent-ə-ˌklōr-ə-'fē-ˌnōl, -ˌnôl-, -ˌklôr-, -fi-'\ *n* : a crystalline compound C_6Cl_5OH used esp. as a wood preservative, insecticide, and fungicide — called also *PCP*

pen·ta·dac·tyl \ˌpent-ə-'dak-tᵊl\ *adj* : having five digits on each hand or foot ⟨~ mammals⟩

pen·ta·eryth·ri·tol \ˌpent-ə-i'rith-rə-ˌtôl, -ˌtōl\ *n* : a crystalline alcohol $C_5H_{12}O_4$ that is used chiefly in making synthetic resins, synthetic drying oils, and explosives

pentaerythritol tet·ra·ni·trate \-ˌte-trə-'nī-ˌtrāt, -ˌtrət\ *n* : a crystalline ester $C_5H_8N_4O_{12}$ made by nitrating pentaerythritol and used in the treatment of angina pectoris

pen·ta·gas·trin \ˌpent-ə-'gas-trən\ *n* : a pentapeptide $C_{37}H_{49}N_7O_9S$ that stimulates gastric acid secretion

pen·tal·o·gy \pen-'tal-ə-jē\ *n, pl* **-gies** : a combination of five closely related usu. simultaneous defects or symptoms ⟨a ~ of congenital birth defects⟩

pen·ta·mer \'pent-ə-mər\ *n* : a polymer formed from five molecules of a monomer

pen·ta·me·tho·ni·um \ˌpent-ə-me-'thō-nē-əm\ *n* : an organic ion $[C_{11}H_{28}N_2]^{2+}$ used in the form of its salts (as the bromide and iodide) for its ganglionic blocking activity in the treatment of hypertension

---

\ə\ abut \ᵊ\ kitten \ər\ further \a\ ash \ā\ ace \ä\ cot, cart
\aù\ out \ch\ chin \e\ bet \ē\ easy \g\ go \i\ hit \ī\ ice \j\ job
\ŋ\ sing \ō\ go \ò\ law \òi\ boy \th\ thin \th\ the \ü\ loot
\ù\ foot \y\ yet \zh\ vision   *See also* Pronunciation Symbols page

O

P

pen·ta·meth·y·lene·di·amine \-ˌmeth-ə-ˌlēn-ˈdī-ə-ˌmēn\ *n* : CADAVERINE

pent·am·i·dine \pen-ˈtam-ə-ˌdēn, -dən\ *n* : a diamidine used chiefly in the form of its salt $C_{23}H_{36}N_4O_{10}S_2$ to treat protozoal infections (as leishmaniasis) and to prevent Pneumocystis carinii pneumonia in HIV-infected individuals

pen·tane \ˈpen-ˌtān\ *n* : any of three isomeric alkanes C_5H_{12} occurring in petroleum; *esp* : the volatile flammable liquid straight-chain isomer that has been used to produce anesthesia

pen·ta·no·ic acid \ˌpent-ə-ˌnō-ik-\ *n* : VALERIC ACID a

pen·ta·pep·tide \ˌpent-ə-ˈpep-ˌtīd\ *n* : a polypeptide that contains five amino acid residues

pen·ta·pip·er·ide methylsulfate \ˌpent-tə-ˈpip-ə-ˌrīd-\ *n* : PENTAPIPERIUM METHYLSULFATE

pen·ta·pi·per·i·um meth·yl·sul·fate \ˌpent-ə-pī-ˈper-ē-əm-ˌmeth-əl-ˈsəl-ˌfāt\ *n* : a synthetic quaternary ammonium anticholinergic and antisecretory agent $C_{20}H_{33}NO_6S$ used esp. in the treatment of peptic ulcer

¹pen·ta·ploid \ˈpen-tə-ˌplȯid\ *adj* : having or being a chromosome number that is five times the basic number — **pen·ta·ploi·dy** \ˈpen-tə-ˌplȯid-ē\ *n, pl* **-dies**

²pentaploid *n* : a pentaploid individual

pen·ta·quine \-ˌkwēn\ *also* **pen·ta·quin** \-kwən\ *n* : an antimalarial drug used esp. in the form of its pale yellow crystalline phosphate $C_{18}H_{27}N_3O \cdot H_3PO_4$

Pen·ta·stom·i·da \ˌpent-ə-ˈstäm-əd-ə\ *n pl* : any of a group of parasitic animals that are considered a class of the phylum Arthropoda or a separate phylum, that lack eyes, a circulatory system, and a respiratory system, that live as adults in the respiratory passages or body cavity of reptiles, birds, or mammals and undergo larval development in similar hosts, and that comprise the tongue worms — **pen·tas·to·mid** \pen-ˈtas-tə-məd\ *n*

pen·ta·tom·ic \ˌpent-ə-ˈtäm-ik\ *adj* **1** : consisting of five atoms **2** : having five replaceable atoms or radicals

Pen·ta·tricho·mo·nas \ˌpent-ə-ˌtrik-ə-ˈmō-nəs, -tri-ˈkäm-ə-nəs\ *n* : a genus of flagellates related to *Trichomonas* but possessing five anterior flagella and often regarded as indistinguishable from a subgenus of *Trichomonas*

pen·ta·va·lent \ˌpent-ə-ˈvā-lənt\ *adj* : having a valence of five

pen·taz·o·cine \pen-ˈtaz-ə-ˌsēn\ *n* : a synthetic analgesic drug $C_{19}H_{27}NO$ that is less addictive than morphine — see TALWIN

pen·tene \ˈpen-ˌtēn\ *n* : either of the two normal amylenes obtained from gasoline

pen·to·bar·bi·tal \ˌpent-ə-ˈbär-bə-ˌtȯl\ *n* : a granular barbiturate used esp. in the form of its sodium salt $C_{11}H_{17}N_2NaO_3$ or calcium salt $(C_{11}H_{17}N_2O_3)_2Ca$ as a sedative, hypnotic, and antispasmodic

pen·to·bar·bi·tone \-ˌtōn\ *n, Brit* : PENTOBARBITAL

pen·to·lin·i·um tartrate \ˌpent-ə-ˈlin-ē-əm-\ *n* : a quaternary ammonium ganglionic blocking agent $C_{23}H_{42}N_2O_{12}$ used as an antihypertensive drug

pen·to·san \ˈpent-ə-ˌsan\ *n* : any of various polysaccharides that yield only pentoses on hydrolysis and are widely distributed in plants

pen·tose \ˈpen-ˌtōs, -ˌtōz\ *n* : a monosaccharide $C_5H_{10}O_5$ (as ribose) that contains five carbon atoms in a molecule

pen·to·side \ˈpent-ə-ˌsīd\ *n* : a glycoside that yields a pentose on hydrolysis

pen·tos·uria \ˌpen-tōs-ˈ(y)ùr-ē-ə\ *n* : the excretion of pentoses in the urine; *specif* : a rare hereditary anomaly characterized by regular excretion of pentoses

Pen·to·thal \ˈpen-tə-ˌthȯl\ *trademark* — used for a preparation of thiopental

pent·ox·ide \pent-ˈäk-ˌsīd\ *n* : an oxide containing five atoms of oxygen in the molecule — see IODINE PENTOXIDE

pent·ox·i·fyl·line \ˌpen-ˌtäk-ˈsif-ə-ˌlēn\ *n* : a methylxanthine derivative $C_{13}H_{18}N_4O_3$ that reduces blood viscosity, increases microcirculatory blood flow, and is used to treat intermittent claudication resulting from occlusive arterial disease — see TRENTAL

pen·tyl \ˈpent-ᵊl\ *n* : AMYL

pen·tyl·ene·tet·ra·zol \ˌpent-i-ˌlēn-ˈte-trə-ˌzȯl, -ˌzōl\ *n* : a white crystalline drug $C_6H_{10}N_4$ used as a respiratory and circulatory stimulant and for producing a state of convulsion in treating certain mental disorders — called also *leptazol*; see METRAZOL

pe·num·bra \pə-ˈnəm-brə\ *n, pl* **-brae** \-(ˌ)brē, -ˌbrī\ *or* **-bras** : a blurred area in a radiograph at the edge of an anatomical structure — **pe·num·bral** \-brəl\ *adj*

PEP *abbr* phosphoenolpyruvate

Pep·cid \ˈpep-səd\ *trademark* — used for a preparation of famotidine

pe·po \ˈpē-(ˌ)pō\ *n, pl* **pepos** : the dried ripe seeds of the pumpkin (*Cucurbita pepo*) used as an anthelmintic and taeniafuge — called also *pumpkin seed*

pep·per \ˈpep-ər\ *n* **1 a** : a woody Indian vine of the genus *Piper* (*P. nigrum*) that is widely cultivated in the tropics for its red berries from which black pepper and white pepper are prepared **b** (1) : BLACK PEPPER (2) : WHITE PEPPER **2** : CAPSICUM 2

pep·per·mint \-ˌmint, -mənt\ *n* : a mint of the genus *Mentha* (*M. piperita*) with dark green leaves and spikes of small pink flowers from which an aromatic oil is obtained — **pep·per·minty** \-ˌmint-ē\ *adj*

peppermint oil *n* : an oil that has a strong peppermint odor and produces a cooling sensation in the mouth, is obtained from peppermint, and is used chiefly as a flavoring agent and as a carminative

peppermint spirit *n* : an alcoholic solution of peppermint oil

pep pill \ˈpep-ˌ\ *n* : any of various stimulant drugs (as amphetamine) in pill or tablet form

pep·si·gogue \ˈpep-sə-ˌgäg\ *adj* : inducing the secretion of pepsin

pep·sin \ˈpep-sən\ *n* **1** : a crystallizable protease that in an acid medium digests most proteins to polypeptides (as by dissolving coagulated egg albumin or causing casein to precipitate from skim milk), that is secreted by glands in the mucous membrane of the stomach of higher animals, and that in combination with dilute hydrochloric acid is the chief active principle of gastric juice **2** : a preparation containing pepsin obtained as a powder or scales from the stomach esp. of the hog and used esp. as a digestant

pep·sin·o·gen \pep-ˈsin-ə-jən\ *n* : a granular zymogen of the gastric glands that is readily converted into pepsin in a slightly acid medium

pep·tic \ˈpep-tik\ *adj* **1** : relating to or promoting digestion : DIGESTIVE **2** : of, relating to, producing, or caused by pepsin ⟨∼ digestion⟩

peptic ulcer *n* : an ulcer in the wall of the stomach or duodenum resulting from the digestive action of the gastric juice on the mucous membrane when the latter is rendered susceptible to its action (as from infection with the bacterium *Helicobacter pylori* or the chronic use of NSAIDs)

pep·ti·dase \ˈpep-tə-ˌdās, -ˌdāz\ *n* : an enzyme that hydrolyzes simple peptides or their derivatives — compare PROTEASE

pep·tide \ˈpep-ˌtīd\ *n* : any of various amides that are derived from two or more amino acids by combination of the amino group of one acid with the carboxyl group of another and are usu. obtained by partial hydrolysis of proteins — **pep·tid·ic** \pep-ˈtid-ik\ *adj*

peptide bond *n* : the chemical bond between carbon and nitrogen in a peptide linkage

peptide linkage *n* : the bivalent group CONH that unites the amino acid residues in a peptide

pep·tid·er·gic \ˌpep-tīd-ˈər-jik\ *adj* : being, relating to, releasing, or activated by neurotransmitters that are short peptide chains ⟨∼ neurons⟩ ⟨∼ receptors⟩

pep·ti·do·gly·can \ˌpep-təd-ō-ˈglī-ˌkan\ *n* : a polymer that is composed of polysaccharide and peptide chains and is found esp. in bacterial cell walls — called also *mucopeptide, murein*

pep·ti·dyl transferase \ˈpep-tə-dil-\ *n* : an enzyme that catalyzes the addition of amino acid residues to the growing polypeptide chain in protein synthesis by means of peptide bonds

pep·tize *also Brit* **pep·tise** \'pep-,tīz\ *vt* **pep·tized** *also Brit* **pep·tised; pep·tiz·ing** *also Brit* **pep·tis·ing** : to cause to disperse in a medium; *specif* : to bring into colloidal solution — **pep·ti·za·tion** \,pep-tə-'zā-shən\ *also Brit* **pep·ti·sa·tion** \,pep-,tī-'zā-\ *n* — **pep·tiz·er** *also Brit* **pep·tis·er** \'pep-,tī-zer\ *n*

Pep·to–Bis·mol \,pep-(,)tō-'biz-,môl\ *trademark* — used for a preparation of bismuth subsalicylate

pep·to·coc·cus \,pep-tə-'käk-əs\ *n* **1** *cap* : a genus of anaerobic gram-positive coccal bacteria that do not form spores and are now considered to comprise a single species (*P. niger*) **2** *pl* **-coc·ci** \-'käk-,(s)ī\ : any bacterium of the genus *Peptococcus*

pep·tone \'pep-,tōn\ *n* **1** : any of various protein derivatives that are formed by the partial hydrolysis of proteins (as by enzymes of the gastric and pancreatic juices or by acids or alkalies), that are not coagulated by heat, and that are soluble in water but unlike proteoses are not precipitated from solution by saturation with ammonium sulfate **2** : a complex water-soluble product that contains peptones and other protein derivatives, is obtained by digesting protein (as meat) with an enzyme (as pepsin or trypsin), and is used chiefly in nutrient media in bacteriology

pep·to·ne·mia *or chiefly Brit* **pep·to·nae·mia** \,pep-tō-'nē-mē-ə\ *n* : the presence of peptones in the blood

pep·to·niz·a·tion *also Brit* **pep·to·nis·a·tion** \,pep-tə-nə-'zā-shən\ *n* : the process of peptonizing : PROTEOLYSIS

pep·to·nize *also Brit* **pep·to·nise** \'pep-tə-,nīz\ *vt* **-nized** *also Brit* **-nised; -niz·ing** *also Brit* **-nis·ing** **1** : to convert into peptone; *esp* : to digest or dissolve by a proteolytic enzyme **2** : to combine with peptone

pep·to·noid \'pep-tə-,nòid\ *n* : a substance resembling peptone

per \'pər\ *prep* : by the means or agency of : by way of : through ⟨enter through the mouth lining and ∼ the bloodstream to the stomach —*Sydney (Australia) Bull.*⟩ ⟨blood ∼ rectum⟩ — see PER OS

per *abbr* **1** period; periodic **2** person

per·ace·tic acid \,pər-ə-,sēt-ik-\ *n* : a corrosive toxic strongly oxidizing unstable pungent liquid acid $C_2H_4O_3$ used chiefly in a solution in acetic acid or an inert solvent in bleaching, in organic synthesis, and as a fungicide and disinfectant

per·ac·id \(,)pər-'as-əd\ *n* : an acid (as perchloric acid or permanganic acid) derived from the highest oxidation state of an element

per·acute \,pər-ə-'kyüt\ *adj* : very acute and violent ⟨anthrax occurs in four forms: ∼, acute, subacute and chronic —G. W. Stamm⟩

per·bo·rate \(,)pər-'bō(ə)r-,āt, -'bò(ə)r-\ *n* : a salt that is a compound of a borate with hydrogen peroxide

perc \'pərk\ *n* : PERCHLOROETHYLENE

per·ceive \pər-'sēv\ *vt* **per·ceived; per·ceiv·ing** : to become aware of through the senses — **per·ceiv·able** \-'sē-və-bəl\ *adj* — **per·ceiv·ably** \-blē\ *adv* — **per·ceiv·er** *n*

per·cen·tile \pər-'sen-,tīl\ *n* : a value on a scale of one hundred that indicates the percent of a distribution that is equal to or below it ⟨a ∼ score of 95 is a score equal to or better than 95 percent of the scores⟩

per·cept \'pər-,sept\ *n* : an impression of an object obtained by use of the senses : SENSE-DATUM

per·cep·ti·ble \pər-'sep-tə-bəl\ *adj* : capable of being perceived esp. by the senses ⟨barely ∼ motion⟩ ⟨sound ∼ by the human ear⟩ — **per·cep·ti·bil·i·ty** \-,sep-tə-'bil-ət-ē\ *n, pl* **-ties** — **per·cep·ti·bly** \-blē\ *adv*

per·cep·tion \pər-'sep-shən\ *n* : awareness of the elements of environment through physical sensation ⟨color ∼⟩ ⟨some sensation of ∼ of the extremity after amputation is felt by 98% of patients —*Orthopedics & Traumatic Surgery*⟩ — compare SENSATION 1a

per·cep·tive \pər-'sep-tiv\ *adj* : responsive to sensory stimulus ⟨a ∼ eye⟩ — **per·cep·tive·ly** *adv* — **per·cep·tive·ness** *n* — **per·cep·tiv·i·ty** \(,)pər-,sep-'tiv-ət-ē\ *n, pl* **-ties**

perceptive deafness *n* : NERVE DEAFNESS

per·cep·tu·al \(,)pər-'sep-chə(-wə)l, -'sepsh-wəl\ *adj* : of, relating to, or involving perception esp. in relation to immediate sensory experience ⟨auditory ∼ deficits⟩ — **per·cep·tu·al·ly** \-ē\ *adv*

per·chlo·rate \(')pər-'klō(ə)r-,āt, -'klò(ə)r-, -ət\ *n* : a salt or ester of perchloric acid

per·chlo·ric acid \(,)pər-,klōr-ik-, -,klòr-\ *n* : a fuming corrosive strong acid $HClO_4$ that is the highest oxyacid of chlorine and a powerful oxidizing agent when heated

per·chlo·ride \(')pər-'klō(ə)r-,īd\ *n* : a chloride (as perchloroethylene) containing a relatively high proportion of chlorine

per·chlo·ro·eth·y·lene \,pər-,klōr-ō-'eth-ə-,lēn\ *also* **per·chlor·eth·y·lene** \-,klōr-'eth-\ *n* : a toxic nonflammable carcinogenic liquid C_2Cl_4 often used as a solvent in dry cleaning and for removal of grease from metals — called also *perc, tetrachloroethylene*

Per·co·cet \'pər-kō-,set\ *trademark* — used for a preparation of acetaminophen and the hydrochloride of oxycodone

Per·co·dan \'pər-kə-,dan\ *trademark* — used for a preparation containing aspirin and the hydrochloride of oxycodone

¹per·co·late \'pər-kə-,lāt\ *vb* **-lat·ed; -lat·ing** *vt* **1** : to cause (a solvent) to pass through a permeable substance (as a powdered drug) esp. for extracting a soluble constituent **2** : to be diffused through ∼ *vi* **1** : to ooze or trickle through a permeable substance **2** : to become percolated

²per·co·late \-,lāt, -lət\ *n* : a product of percolation

per·co·la·tion \,pər-kə-'lā-shən\ *n* **1** : the slow passage of a liquid through a filtering medium **2** : a method of extraction or purification by means of filtration **3** : the process of extracting the soluble constituents of a powdered drug by passage of a liquid through it

per·co·la·tor \'pər-kə-,lāt-ər\ *n* : an apparatus for the extraction of a drug with a liquid solvent by downward displacement

per·co·morph liver oil \'pər-kə-,mòrf-\ *n* : a fatty oil that is obtained from the fresh livers of bony fishes of an order (Percomorphi) including perches, basses, mackerels, and numerous related forms and that is administered to infants as a source of vitamins A and D

per·cuss \pər-'kəs\ *vt* : to tap sharply; *esp* : to practice percussion on ⟨∼ all four quadrants of the abdomen before starting palpation —Herrick Peterson⟩ ∼ *vi* : to percuss a body part ⟨∼ing with the ends of our fingers over the lungs —Robert Chawner⟩

per·cus·sion \pər-'kəsh-ən\ *n* **1** : the act or technique of tapping the surface of a body part to learn the condition of the parts beneath by the resulting sound **2** : massage consisting of the striking of a body part with light rapid blows — called also *tapotement*

per·cus·sor \pər-'kəs-ər\ *n* : PLEXOR

per·cu·ta·ne·ous \,pər-kyù-'tā-nē-əs\ *adj* : effected or performed through the skin ⟨∼ removal of renal calculi —G. M. Preminger *et al*⟩ — **per·cu·ta·ne·ous·ly** *adv*

percutaneous transluminal angioplasty *n* : a surgical procedure used to enlarge the lumen of a partly occluded blood vessel (as one with atherosclerotic plaques on the walls) by passing a balloon catheter through the skin, into the vessel, and through the vessel to the site of the lesion where the tip of the catheter is inflated to expand the lumen of the vessel

percutaneous transluminal coronary angioplasty *n* : percutaneous transluminal angioplasty of a coronary artery — called also *PTCA*

Per·di·em \pər-'dē-,em, -əm\ *trademark* — used for a laxative preparation of psyllium seed husks and senna

pe·ren·ni·al \pə-'ren-ē-əl\ *adj* : present at all seasons of the year ⟨∼ rhinitis⟩

perf *abbr* perforated; perforation

per·fec·tion·ism \pər-'fek-shə-,niz-əm\ *n* : a disposition to regard anything short of perfection as unacceptable; *esp* : the setting of unrealistically demanding goals accompanied

O

P

\ə\ abut \ᵊ\ kitten \ər\ further \a\ ash \ā\ ace \ä\ cot, cart \aú\ out \ch\ chin \e\ bet \ē\ easy \g\ go \i\ hit \ī\ ice \j\ job \ŋ\ sing \ō\ go \ò\ law \òi\ boy \th\ thin \th\ the \ü\ loot \ù\ foot \y\ yet \zh\ vision See also Pronunciation Symbols page

by a disposition to regard failure to achieve them as unacceptable and a sign of personal worthlessness

¹**per·fec·tion·ist** \-sh(ə-)nəst\ *n* : an individual who exhibits or adheres to perfectionism

²**perfectionist** *also* **per·fec·tion·is·tic** \pər-ˌfek-shə-'nis-tik\ *adj* : of, relating to, or characterized by perfectionism

per·fect stage \'pər-fikt-\ *n* : a stage in the life cycle of a fungus at which sexual spores are produced

per·fo·rate \'pər-fə-ˌrāt\ *vb* **-rat·ed; -rat·ing** *vt* **1** : to make a hole through ⟨an ulcer ∼*s* the duodenal wall⟩ **2** : to enter or extend through ⟨the nerve ∼*s* the dura mater⟩ ∼ *vi* : to penetrate a surface ⟨the wound in the forearm was *perforating* —*Jour. Amer. Med. Assoc.*⟩

per·fo·rat·ed \-fə-ˌrāt-əd\ *adj* : having a hole or series of holes : characterized by perforation ⟨a ∼ eardrum⟩

perforated substance *n* : any of three small areas on the lower surface of the brain that are perforated by many small openings for blood vessels and that are situated two anteriorly at the commencement of the sylvian fissure and one posteriorly between the mammillary bodies in front and the cerebral peduncles laterally — called also *perforated space, perforate space*

per·fo·ra·tion \ˌpər-fə-'rā-shən\ *n* **1** : the act or process of perforating; *specif* : the penetration of a body part through accident or disease ⟨spontaneous ∼ of the sigmoid colon in the presence of diverticulosis —*Jour. Amer. Med. Assoc.*⟩ **2 a** : a rupture in a body part caused esp. by accident or disease **b** : a natural opening in an organ or body part

per·fo·ra·tor \'pər-fə-ˌrāt-ər\ *n* : one that perforates: as **a** : an instrument used to perforate tissue (as bone) **b** : a nerve or blood vessel forming a connection between a deep system and a superficial one

per·fo·ra·to·ri·um \ˌpər-fə-rə-'tōr-ē-əm, -'tȯr-\ *n, pl* **-ria** \-ē-ə\ : ACROSOME

per·for·mance test \pər-'fȯr-mən(t)s-\ *n* : a test of capacity to achieve a desired result; *esp* : an intelligence test (as by a maze or picture completion) requiring little use of language

per·fus·ate \(ˌ)pər-'fyü-ˌzāt, -zət\ *n* : a fluid (as a solution pumped through the heart) that is perfused

per·fuse \(ˌ)pər-'fyüz\ *vt* **per·fused; per·fus·ing** **1** : SUFFUSE ⟨the skin was *perfused* by blood⟩ **2 a** : to cause to flow or spread : DIFFUSE **b** : to force a fluid through (an organ or tissue) esp. by way of the blood vessels ⟨∼ a liver with salt solution⟩

per·fu·sion \-'fyü-zhən\ *n* : an act or instance of perfusing; *specif* : the pumping of a fluid through an organ or tissue ⟨believes that intermittent injection . . . is better and safer than continuous ∼ —*Yr. Bk. of Urology*⟩

per·fu·sion·ist \pər-'fyüzh-(ə-)nəst\ *n* : a certified medical technician responsible for extracorporeal oxygenation of the blood during open-heart surgery and for the operation and maintenance of equipment (as a heart-lung machine) controlling it

per·go·lide \'pər-gə-ˌlīd\ *n* : an agonist of dopamine receptors that is an ergot derivative and is used in the form of its mesylate $C_{19}H_{26}N_2S \cdot CH_4O_3S$ esp. in the treatment of Parkinson's disease

per·hex·i·line \ˌpər-'hek-sə-ˌlīn\ *n* : a drug $C_{19}H_{35}N$ used as a coronary vasodilator

peri·ad·e·ni·tis \ˌper-ē-ˌad-ᵊn-'īt-əs\ *n* : inflammation of the tissues around a gland

peri·anal \-'ān-ᵊl\ *adj* : of, relating to, occurring in, or being the tissues surrounding the anus ⟨a ∼ abscess⟩

peri·aor·tal \-ā-'ȯrt-ᵊl\ *adj* : PERIAORTIC

peri·aor·tic \-ā-'ȯrt-ik\ *adj* : of, relating to, occurring in, or being the tissues surrounding the aorta

peri·api·cal \-'ā-pi-kəl *also* -'ap-i-kəl\ *adj* : of, relating to, occurring in, affecting, or being the tissues surrounding the apex of the root of a tooth ⟨∼ infection⟩

peri·aq·ue·duc·tal \-'ak-wə-ˌdək-tᵊl\ *adj* : of, relating to, or being the gray matter which surrounds the aqueduct of Sylvius

peri·ar·te·ri·al \-är-'tir-ē-əl\ *adj* : of, relating to, occurring in, or being the tissues surrounding an artery ⟨∼ fibrosis⟩

peri·ar·te·ri·o·lar \-är-ˌtir-ē-'ō-lər\ *adj* : of, relating to, occurring in, or being the tissues surrounding an arteriole

peri·ar·ter·i·tis no·do·sa \ˌper-ē-ˌärt-ə-'rīt-əs-nō-'dō-sə\ *n* : POLYARTERITIS NODOSA

peri·ar·thri·tis \-är-'thrīt-əs\ *n, pl* **-thrit·i·des** \-'thrit-ə-ˌdēz\ : inflammation of the structures (as the muscles, tendons, and bursa of the shoulder) around a joint

peri·ar·tic·u·lar \-är-'tik-yə-lər\ *adj* : of, relating to, occurring in, or being the tissues surrounding a joint ⟨∼ pain⟩

peri·au·ric·u·lar \-ȯ-'rik-yə-lər\ *adj* : of, relating to, occurring in, or being the tissues surrounding the external ear

periaxialis — see ENCEPHALITIS PERIAXIALIS DIFFUSA

peri·blast \'per-ə-ˌblast\ *n* : the nucleated cytoplasmic layer surrounding the blastodisc of an egg undergoing discoidal cleavage

peri·bron·chi·al \ˌper-ə-'brän-kē-əl\ *adj* : of, relating to, occurring in, affecting, or being the tissues surrounding a bronchus ⟨a ∼ growth⟩

peri·bron·chi·o·lar \-ˌbrän-kē-'ō-lər\ *adj* : of, relating to, occurring in, or being the tissues surrounding a bronchiole ⟨∼ edema⟩

peri·bron·chi·o·li·tis \-ˌbrän-kē-ō-'līt-əs\ *n* : inflammation of the tissues surrounding the bronchioles

peri·bron·chi·tis \-ˌbrän-'kīt-əs, -ˌbrän-\ *n, pl* **-chit·i·des** \-'kit-ə-ˌdēz\ : inflammation of the tissues surrounding the bronchi

pericaecal *chiefly Brit var of* PERICECAL

peri·cal·lo·sal \-ka-'lō-səl\ *adj* : of, relating to, occurring in, or being the tissues surrounding the corpus callosum ⟨a ∼ aneurysm⟩

peri·can·a·lic·u·lar \-ˌkan-ᵊl-'ik-yə-lər\ *adj* : of, relating to, occurring in, or being the tissues surrounding a canaliculus

peri·cap·il·lary \-'kap-ə-ˌler-ē, *Brit usu* -kə-'pil-ə-rē\ *adj* : of, relating to, occurring in, or being the tissues surrounding a capillary ⟨∼ infiltration⟩

pericardia *pl of* PERICARDIUM

peri·car·di·al \ˌper-ə-'kärd-ē-əl\ *adj* : of, relating to, or affecting the pericardium; *also* : situated around the heart

pericardial cavity *n* : the fluid-filled space between the two layers of the pericardium

pericardial fluid *n* : the serous fluid that fills the pericardial cavity and protects the heart from friction

pericardial fric·tion rub \-'frik-shən-ˌrəb\ *n* : the auscultatory sound produced by the rubbing together of inflamed pericardial membranes in pericarditis — called also *pericardial rub*

peri·car·di·ec·to·my \ˌper-ə-ˌkärd-ē-'ek-tə-mē\ *n, pl* **-mies** : surgical excision of the pericardium

peri·car·dio·cen·te·sis \ˌper-ə-ˌkärd-ē-ō-(ˌ)sen-'tē-səs\ *n, pl* **-te·ses** \-ˌsēz\ : surgical puncture of the pericardium esp. to aspirate pericardial fluid

peri·car·dio·phren·ic artery \ˌper-ə-ˌkärd-ē-ə-'fren-ik-\ *n* : a branch of the internal thoracic artery that descends through the thorax accompanying the phrenic nerve between the pleura and the pericardium to the diaphragm

peri·car·di·os·to·my \ˌper-ə-ˌkärd-ē-'äs-tə-mē\ *n, pl* **-mies** : surgical formation of an opening into the pericardium

peri·car·di·ot·o·my \-'ät-ə-mē\ *n, pl* **-mies** : surgical incision of the pericardium

peri·car·dit·ic \ˌper-ə-ˌkär-'dit-ik\ *adj* : of or relating to pericarditis

peri·car·di·tis \-ˌkär-'dīt-əs\ *n, pl* **-dit·i·des** \-'dit-ə-ˌdēz\ : inflammation of the pericardium — see ADHESIVE PERICARDITIS

peri·car·di·um \ˌper-ə-'kärd-ē-əm\ *n, pl* **-dia** \-ē-ə\ : the conical sac of serous membrane that encloses the heart and the roots of the great blood vessels of vertebrates and consists of an outer fibrous coat that loosely invests the heart and is prolonged on the outer surface of the great vessels except the inferior vena cava and a double inner serous coat of which one layer is closely adherent to the heart while the other lines the inner surface of the outer coat with the intervening space being filled with pericardial fluid

pericaryon *var of* PERIKARYON

peri·ce·cal *or chiefly Brit* **peri·cae·cal** \ˌper-ə-ˈsē-kəl\ *adj* : situated near or surrounding the cecum

peri·cel·lu·lar \-ˈsel-yə-lər\ *adj* : of, relating to, occurring in, or being the tissues surrounding a cell

peri·ce·ment·al \-si-ˈment-əl\ *adj* **1** : around the cement layer of a tooth **2** : of, relating to, or involving the periodontal membrane

peri·ce·men·ti·tis \-ˌsē-ˌmen-ˈtīt-əs\ *n* : PERIODONTITIS

peri·ce·men·tum \-si-ˈment-əm\ *n* : PERIODONTAL MEMBRANE

peri·cen·tric \-ˈsen-trik\ *adj* : of, relating to, or involving the centromere of a chromosome ⟨∼ inversion⟩ — compare PARACENTRIC

peri·chol·an·gi·tis \-ˌkōl-ˌan-ˈjīt-əs, -ˌkäl-\ *n* : inflammation of the tissues surrounding the bile ducts

peri·chon·dral \ˌper-ə-ˈkän-drəl\ *adj* : relating to, formed by, or being ossification that occurs peripherally beneath the perichondrium of a cartilage — compare ENDOCHONDRAL, INTRAMEMBRANOUS 1

peri·chon·dri·al \-ˈkän-drē-əl\ *adj* : of or relating to the perichondrium

peri·chon·dri·tis \-ˌkän-ˈdrīt-əs\ *n* : inflammation of a perichondrium

peri·chon·dri·um \ˌper-ə-ˈkän-drē-əm\ *n, pl* **-dria** \-drē-ə\ : the membrane of fibrous connective tissue that invests cartilage except at joints

peri·chord \ˈper-ə-ˌkȯrd\ *n* : the sheath of the notochord — **peri·chord·al** \ˌper-ə-ˈkȯrd-əl\ *adj*

Peri–Co·lace \ˌper-ə-ˈkō-ˌlās\ *trademark* — used for a preparation of casanthranol and the sodium salt of docusate

peri·co·li·tis \ˌper-ə-kō-ˈlīt-əs, -kə-\ *n* : inflammation of tissues around the colon

peri·con·cep·tion·al \ˌper-ə-kən-ˈsep-shə-nəl\ *adj* : of, relating to, or done during the period from before conception to early pregnancy ⟨∼ folic acid supplementation⟩

peri·co·ro·nal \ˌper-ə-ˈkȯr-ən-əl, -ˈkär-; -kə-ˈrōn-əl\ *adj* : occurring about or surrounding the crown of a tooth ⟨∼ infection⟩

peri·cor·o·ni·tis \-ˌkȯr-ə-ˈnīt-əs, -ˌkär-\ *n, pl* **-nit·i·des** \-ˈnit-ə-ˌdēz\ : inflammation of the gum about the crown of a partially erupted tooth

peri·cra·ni·um \ˌper-ə-ˈkrā-nē-əm\ *n, pl* **-nia** \-nē-ə\ : the external periosteum of the skull — **peri·cra·ni·al** \-nē-əl\ *adj*

peri·cyst \ˈper-ə-ˌsist\ *n* : the enclosing wall of fibrous tissue laid down by the host about various parasites (as a hydatid)

peri·cys·tic \ˌper-ə-ˈsis-tik\ *adj* : occurring about or surrounding a cyst or bladder ⟨a ∼ membrane⟩

peri·cyte \ˈper-ə-ˌsīt\ *n* : a cell of the connective tissue about capillaries or other small blood vessels

peri·den·tal \ˌper-ə-ˈdent-əl\ *adj* : PERIODONTAL

peri·den·ti·tis \-ˌden-ˈtīt-əs\ *n* : PERIODONTITIS

peri·den·ti·um \-ˈden-tē-əm, -ˈden-chəm\ *n, pl* **-tia** \-tē-ə, -chə\ : PERIODONTIUM

peri·derm \ˈper-ə-ˌdərm\ *n* : the outer layer of the epidermis of the skin esp. of the embryo

peri·du·ral \ˌper-i-ˈd(y)ur-əl\ *adj* : occurring or applied about the dura mater

peridural anesthesia *n* : EPIDURAL ANESTHESIA

peri·en·ter·ic \ˌper-ē-en-ˈter-ik\ *adj* : around the intestine

peri·esoph·a·ge·al *or chiefly Brit* **peri·oe·soph·a·ge·al** \-i-ˌsäf-ə-ˈjē-əl\ *adj* : of, relating to, occurring in, or being the tissues surrounding the esophagus

peri·esoph·a·gi·tis *or chiefly Brit* **peri·oe·soph·a·gi·tis** \-i-ˌsäf-ə-ˈjīt-əs\ *n* : inflammation of the tissues surrounding the esophagus

peri·fo·cal \ˌper-ə-ˈfō-kəl\ *adj* : of, relating to, occurring in, or being the tissues surrounding a focus (as of infection) ⟨∼ proliferation of fibroblasts⟩ — **peri·fo·cal·ly** \-ē\ *adv*

peri·fol·lic·u·lar \ˌper-ə-fə-ˈlik-yə-lər, -fä-\ *adj* : of, relating to, occurring in, or being the tissues surrounding a follicle

peri·fol·lic·u·li·tis \-ˌlik-yə-ˈlīt-əs\ *n* : inflammation of the tissues surrounding the hair follicles

peri·gan·gli·on·ic \-ˌgaŋ-glē-ˈän-ik\ *adj* : surrounding a ganglion

peri·hep·a·ti·tis \-ˌhep-ə-ˈtīt-əs\ *n, pl* **-tit·i·des** \-ˈtit-ə-ˌdēz\ : inflammation of the peritoneal capsule of the liver

peri·kary·on *also* **peri·cary·on** \-ˈkar-ē-ˌän, -ən\ *n, pl* **-karya** *also* **-carya** \-ē-ə\ : CELL BODY — **peri·kary·al** \-ē-əl\ *adj*

peri·ky·ma·ta \-ˈkī-mət-ə\ *n pl* : minute transverse ridges on the surface of the enamel of a tooth which correspond to the incremental lines of Retzius

peri·lab·y·rin·thi·tis \-ˌlab-ə-ˌrin-ˈthīt-əs\ *n* : inflammation of the tissues surrounding the labyrinth of the ear

peri·lymph \ˈper-ə-ˌlim(p)f\ *n* : the fluid between the membranous and bony labyrinths of the ear

peri·lym·phat·ic \ˌper-ə-lim-ˈfat-ik\ *adj* : relating to or containing perilymph ⟨∼ fistulas⟩

peri·men·o·paus·al \ˌper-ē-ˌmen-ə-ˈpȯ-zəl, -ˌmēn-\ *adj* : relating to, being in, or occurring in perimenopause ⟨∼ women⟩ ⟨∼ bleeding⟩

peri·men·o·pause \-ˈmen-ə-ˌpȯz, -ˈmēn-\ *n* : the period around the onset of menopause that is often marked by various physical signs (as hot flashes and menstrual irregularity)

pe·rim·e·ter \pə-ˈrim-ət-ər\ *n* **1 a** : the boundary of a closed plane figure **b** : the length of a perimeter **2** : an instrument for examining the discriminative powers of different parts of the retina often consisting of an adjustable semicircular arm with a fixation point for the eye and variable stations for the visual stimuli

peri·me·tri·um \ˌper-ə-ˈmē-trē-əm\ *n, pl* **-tria** \-trē-ə\ : the peritoneum covering the fundus and ventral and dorsal aspects of the uterus

pe·rim·e·try \pə-ˈrim-ə-trē\ *n, pl* **-tries** : examination of the eye by means of a perimeter — **peri·met·ric** \ˌper-ə-ˈme-trik\ *adj*

peri·my·si·al \ˌper-ə-ˈmiz(h)-ē-əl\ *adj* : of, relating to, or being perimysium

peri·my·si·um \ˌper-ə-ˈmiz(h)-ē-əm\ *n, pl* **-sia** \-ē-ə\ : the connective-tissue sheath that surrounds a muscle and forms sheaths for the bundles of muscle fibers

perinaeum *var of* PERINEUM

peri·na·tal \-ˈnāt-əl\ *adj* : occurring in, concerned with, or being in the period around the time of birth ⟨∼ mortality⟩ ⟨∼ care⟩ — **peri·na·tal·ly** \-əl-(l)ē\ *adv*

peri·na·tol·o·gist \ˌper-ə-nā-ˈtäl-ə-jəst\ *n* : a specialist in perinatology

peri·na·tol·o·gy \-ˌnā-ˈtäl-ə-jē\ *n, pl* **-gies** : a branch of medicine concerned with perinatal care

per·in·do·pril \pə-ˈrin-də-ˌpril\ *n* : an ACE inhibitor administered in the form of its amine salt $C_{19}H_{32}N_2O_5 \cdot C_4H_{11}N$ to treat essential hypertension

perinea *pl of* PERINEUM

per·i·ne·al \ˌper-ə-ˈnē-əl\ *adj* : of or relating to the perineum

perineal artery *n* : a branch of the internal pudendal artery that supplies the skin of the external genitalia and the superficial parts of the perineum

perineal body *n* : a mass of muscle and fascia that separates the lower end of the vagina and the rectum in the female and the urethra and the rectum in the male

perinei — see TRANSVERSUS PERINEI SUPERFICIALIS

per·i·ne·om·e·ter \ˌper-ə-nē-ˈäm-ət-ər\ *n* : an instrument which measures the strength of contractions of the vaginal muscles

per·i·ne·o·plas·ty \ˌper-ə-ˈnē-ō-ˌplas-tē\ *n, pl* **-ties** : plastic surgery of the perineum

per·i·ne·or·rha·phy \ˌper-ə-nē-ˈȯr-ə-fē\ *n, pl* **-phies** : suture of the perineum usu. to repair a laceration occurring during labor

per·i·ne·ot·o·my \ˌper-ə-nē-ˈät-ə-mē\ *n, pl* **-mies** : surgical incision of the perineum

peri·neph·ric \ˌper-ə-ˈnef-rik\ *adj* : PERIRENAL

peri·ne·phrit·ic \-ni-ˈfrit-ik\ *adj* : of, relating to, or affected with perinephritis

\ə\ abut \ˈə\ kitten \ər\ further \a\ ash \ā\ ace \ä\ cot, cart \au̇\ out \ch\ chin \e\ bet \ē\ easy \g\ go \i\ hit \ī\ ice \j\ job \ŋ\ sing \ō\ go \ȯ\ law \ȯi\ boy \th\ thin \th\ the \ü\ loot \u̇\ foot \y\ yet \zh\ vision *See also* Pronunciation Symbols page

O

P

peri·ne·phri·tis \-ni-'frīt-əs\ *n, pl* **-phrit·i·des** \-'frit-ə-ˌdēz\ : inflammation of the tissues surrounding the kidney

peri·neph·ri·um \-'nef-rē-əm\ *n, pl* **-ria** \-rē-ə\ : the capsule of connective and fatty tissue about the kidney

per·i·ne·um *also* **per·i·nae·um** \ˌper-ə-'nē-əm\ *n, pl* **-nea** *also* **-naea** \-'nē-ə\ : an area of tissue that marks externally the approximate boundary of the pelvic outlet and gives passage to the urogenital ducts and rectum; *also* : the area between the anus and the posterior part of the external genitalia esp. in the female

peri·neu·ral \ˌper-ə-'n(y)ur-əl\ *adj* : occurring about or surrounding nervous tissue or a nerve

peri·neu·ri·al \-'n(y)ur-ē-əl\ *adj* **1** : of or relating to the perineurium **2** : PERINEURAL

peri·neu·ri·tis \-n(y)u-'rīt-əs\ *n, pl* **-rit·i·des** \-'rit-ə-ˌdēz\ *or* **-ri·tis·es** : inflammation of the perineurium — **peri·neu·rit·ic** \-'rit-ik\ *adj*

peri·neu·ri·um \ˌper-ə-'n(y)ur-ē-əm\ *n, pl* **-ria** \-ē-ə\ : the sheath of connective tissue that surrounds a bundle of nerve fibers

peri·nu·cle·ar \-'n(y)ü-klē-ər\ *adj* : situated around or surrounding the nucleus of a cell ⟨∼ structures⟩

peri·oc·u·lar \ˌper-ē-'äk-yə-lər\ *adj* : surrounding the eyeball but within the orbit ⟨∼ space⟩

pe·ri·od \'pir-ē-əd\ *n* **1 a** : a portion of time determined by some recurring phenomenon **b** : a single cyclic occurrence of menstruation **2** : a chronological division ⟨the ∼ of incubation of a disease⟩

per·io·date \(ˈ)pər-'ī-ə-ˌdāt, -'ī-əd-ət\ *n* : a salt of a periodic acid

pe·ri·od·ic \ˌpir-ē-'äd-ik\ *adj* : occurring or recurring at regular intervals ⟨∼ epidemics⟩

per·iod·ic acid \ˌpər-(ˌ)ī-ˌäd-ik-\ *n* : any of the strongly oxidizing iodine-containing acids (as H_5IO_6 or HIO_4)

periodic acid–Schiff \-'shif\ *adj* : relating to, being, or involving a reaction testing for polysaccharides and related substances in which tissue sections are treated with periodic acid and then Schiff's reagent with a reddish violet color indicating a positive test caused by the reaction with Schiff's reagent of aldehydes formed by the oxidation of hydroxyl groups on adjacent carbon atoms or of adjacent hydroxyl and amino groups

periodic breathing *n* : abnormal breathing characterized by an irregular respiratory rhythm; *esp* : CHEYNE-STOKES RESPIRATION

pe·ri·od·ic·i·ty \ˌpir-ē-ə-'dis-ət-ē\ *n, pl* **-ties** : the quality, state, or fact of being regularly recurrent or having periods ⟨the ∼ of peptic ulcer is . . . characteristic of the disease —*Jour. Amer. Med. Assoc.*⟩

periodic law *n* : a law in chemistry: the elements when arranged in the order of their atomic numbers show a periodic variation of atomic structure and of most of their properties — called also *Mendeleev's law*

periodic ophthalmia *n* : MOON BLINDNESS

periodic table *n* : an arrangement of chemical elements based on the periodic law

peri·odon·tal \ˌper-ē-ō-'dänt-ᵊl\ *adj* **1** : investing or surrounding a tooth **2** : of or affecting the periodontium ⟨∼ infection⟩ — **peri·odon·tal·ly** \-ᵊl-ē\ *adv*

periodontal disease *n* : any disease (as gingivitis or periodontitis) affecting the periodontium

periodontal ligament *n* : PERIODONTAL MEMBRANE

periodontal membrane *n* : the fibrous connective-tissue layer covering the cementum of a tooth and holding it in place in the jawbone — called also *pericementum, periodontal ligament*

peri·odon·tia \ˌper-ē-ō-'dänt-ch(ē-)ə\ *n* : PERIODONTICS

peri·odon·tics \-'dänt-iks\ *n pl but sing or pl in constr* : a branch of dentistry that deals with diseases of the supporting and investing structures of the teeth including the gums, cementum, periodontal membranes, and alveolar bone — called also *periodontia, periodontology*

peri·odon·tist \-'dänt-əst\ *n* : a specialist in periodontics — called also *periodontologist*

peri·odon·ti·tis \ˌper-ē-(ˌ)ō-ˌdän-'tīt-əs\ *n* : inflammation of the periodontium and esp. the periodontal membrane — called also *pericementitis*

periodontitis complex *n* : a rare form of chronic periodontitis which is characterized by deep and irregular pocketing around the teeth and by resorption of alveolar bone in a vertical direction and which is sometimes regarded as periodontosis complicated by the occurrence of inflammatory lesions

periodontitis sim·plex \-'sim-ˌpleks\ *n* : the common form of chronic periodontitis usu. resulting from local infection and characterized by destruction of the periodontal membrane, formation of pockets around the teeth, and resorption of alveolar bone in a horizontal direction

peri·odon·tium \ˌper-ē-ō-'dän-ch(ē-)əm\ *n, pl* **-tia** \-ch(ē-)ə\ : the supporting structures of the teeth including the cementum, the periodontal membrane, the bone of the alveolar process, and the gums

peri·odon·to·cla·sia \-ō-ˌdänt-ə-'klā-zh(ē-)ə\ *n* : any periodontal disease characterized by destruction of the periodontium

peri·odon·tol·o·gist \ˌper-ē-ō-ˌdän-'täl-ə-jəst\ *n* : PERIODONTIST

peri·odon·tol·o·gy \-ˌdän-'täl-ə-jē\ *n, pl* **-gies** : PERIODONTICS

peri·odon·to·sis \ˌper-ē-ō-ˌdän-'tō-səs\ *n, pl* **-to·ses** \-ˌsēz\ : a severe degenerative disease of the periodontium which in the early stages of its pure form is characterized by a lack of clinical evidence of inflammation — called also *paradentosis, paradontosis*

perioesophageal, perioesophagitis *chiefly Brit var of* PERIESOPHAGEAL, PERIESOPHAGITIS

peri·onych·i·um \ˌper-ē-ō-'nik-ē-əm\ *n, pl* **-ia** \-ē-ə\ : the tissue bordering the root and sides of a fingernail or toenail

peri·on·yx \ˌper-ē-'än-iks\ *n* : the persistent layer of stratum corneum at the base of a fingernail or toenail

peri·op·er·a·tive \-'äp-(ə-)rət-iv, -'äp-ə-ˌrāt-\ *adj* : relating to, occurring in, or being the period around the time of a surgical operation ⟨∼ morbidity⟩

peri·ople \'per-ē-ˌō-pəl\ *n* : the thin waxy outer layer of a hoof

peri·op·tic \ˌper-ē-'äp-tik\ *adj* : of, relating to, occurring in, or being the tissues surrounding the eyeball

peri·oral \-'ōr-əl, -'ȯr-, -'är-\ *adj* : of, relating to, occurring in, or being the tissues around the mouth

peri·or·bit·al \-'ȯr-bət-ᵊl\ *adj* : of, relating to, occurring in, or being the tissues surrounding or lining the orbit of the eye ⟨∼ edema⟩ ⟨discoloration of the ∼ area —Norman Levine⟩

peri·ost \'per-ē-ˌäst\ *n* : PERIOSTEUM

peri·os·te·al \ˌper-ē-'äs-tē-əl\ *adj* **1** : situated around or produced external to bone **2** : of, relating to, or involving the periosteum ⟨a ∼ sarcoma⟩

periosteal elevator *n* : a surgical instrument used to separate the periosteum from bone

peri·os·te·um \-tē-əm\ *n, pl* **-tea** \-tē-ə\ : the membrane of connective tissue that closely invests all bones except at the articular surfaces

peri·os·ti·tis \-ˌäs-'tīt-əs\ *n* : inflammation of the periosteum

peri·ot·ic \ˌper-ē-'ōt-ik\ *adj* : situated around the ear

peri·ovar·i·an \-ō-'var-ē-ən, -'ver-\ *adj* : being adjacent to or surrounding an ovary ⟨∼ adhesions⟩

peri·pan·cre·at·ic \ˌper-ə-ˌpaŋ-krē-'at-ik, -ˌpan-\ *adj* : of, relating to, occurring in, or being the tissue surrounding the pancreas

peri·pap·il·lary \-'pap-ə-ˌler-ē, *esp Brit* -pə-'pil-ə-rē\ *adj* : situated around the optic papilla

¹peri·par·tum \-'pärt-əm\ *adj* : occurring in or being the period preceding or following parturition ⟨∼ cardiomyopathy⟩

²peripartum *adv* : in the peripartum period ⟨infants were infected with the virus ∼⟩

peri·pha·ryn·geal \-ˌfar-ən-'jē-əl, -fə-'rin-j(ē-)əl\ *adj* : surrounding the pharynx

pe·riph·er·ad \pə-'rif-ə-ˌrad\ *adv* : toward the periphery

pe·riph·er·al \pə-'rif-(ə-)rəl\ *adj* **1** : of, relating to, involving, forming, or located near a periphery or surface part (as of the body) **2** : of, relating to, affecting, or being part of the peripheral nervous system ⟨∼ nerves⟩ **3** : of, relating to, or being the outer part of the visual field ⟨good ∼ vision⟩ **4** : of, relating to, or being blood in the systemic circulation ⟨∼ lymphocytes⟩ ⟨∼ resistance⟩ ⟨∼ blood⟩ — **pe·riph·er·al·ly** \-ē\ *adv*

peripheral arterial disease *n* : damage to or dysfunction of the arteries outside the heart resulting in reduced blood flow; *esp* : narrowing or obstruction (as from atherosclerosis) of an artery (as the iliac artery or femoral artery) supplying the legs that is marked chiefly by intermittent claudication and by numbness and tingling in the legs

peripheral nervous system *n* : the part of the nervous system that is outside the central nervous system and comprises the cranial nerves excepting the optic nerve, the spinal nerves, and the autonomic nervous system

peripheral neuritis *n* : inflammation of one or more peripheral nerves

peripheral neuropathy *n* : a disease or degenerative state (as polyneuropathy) of the peripheral nerves in which motor, sensory, or vasomotor nerve fibers may be affected and which is marked by muscle weakness and atrophy, pain, and numbness

peripheral vascular disease *n* : vascular disease (as Raynaud's disease and Buerger's disease) affecting blood vessels outside of the heart and esp. those vessels supplying the extremities; *esp* : PERIPHERAL ARTERIAL DISEASE

peripheral vascular resistance *n* : vascular resistance to the flow of blood in peripheral arterial vessels that is typically a function of the internal vessel diameter, vessel length, and blood viscosity — called also *peripheral resistance*

pe·riph·ery \pə-'rif-(ə-)rē\ *n, pl* **-er·ies 1** : the outward bounds of something as distinguished from its internal regions or center **2** : the regions (as the sense organs, the muscles, or the viscera) in which nerves terminate

peri·phle·bi·tis \ˌper-ə-fli-'bīt-əs\ *n, pl* **-bit·i·des** \-'bit-ə-ˌdēz\ : inflammation of the outer coat of a vein or of tissues around a vein

Peri·pla·ne·ta \ˌper-ə-plə-'nēt-ə\ *n* : a genus of large cockroaches that includes the American cockroach

peri·plas·mic \-'plaz-mik\ *adj* : of, relating to, occurring in, or being the space between the cell wall and the plasma membrane ⟨the ∼ flagella of spirochetes⟩

peri·plast \'per-ə-ˌplast\ *n* : PLASMA MEMBRANE

Pe·rip·lo·ca \pə-'rip-lə-kə\ *n* : a genus of woody vines of the milkweed family (Asclepiadaceae) found in warm regions of the Old World that have dry many-seeded cylindrical fruits and include the silk vine

pe·rip·lo·cin \pə-'rip-lə-ˌsin, ˌper-ə-'plō-sən\ *n* : a glycoside $C_{36}H_{56}O_{13}$ obtainable from the silk vine

pe·rip·lo·cy·ma·rin \pe-ˌrip-lō-'sī-mə-rən\ *n* : a glycoside $C_{30}H_{46}O_8$ obtainable from the silk vine

peri·por·tal \ˌper-ə-'pōrt-ᵊl, -'pȯrt-ᵊl\ *adj* : of, relating to, occurring in, or being the tissues surrounding a portal vein

peri·pro·ce·dur·al \-prə-'sē-jə-rəl\ *adj* : occurring soon before, during, or soon after the performance of a medical procedure ⟨∼ mortality⟩

peri·pros·tat·ic \-prä-'stat-ik\ *adj* : of, relating to, or occurring in the tissues surrounding the prostate

peri·rec·tal \-'rek-tᵊl\ *adj* : of, relating to, occurring in, or being the tissues surrounding the rectum ⟨a ∼ abscess⟩

peri·re·nal \-'rēn-ᵊl\ *adj* : of, relating to, occurring in, or being the tissues surrounding the kidney ⟨a ∼ abscess⟩

peri·sal·pin·gi·tis \-ˌsal-pən-'jīt-əs\ *n* : inflammation of the tissues surrounding a fallopian tube

peri·scop·ic \ˌper-ə-'skäp-ik\ *adj* : giving a distinct image of objects viewed obliquely as well as those in a direct line

peri·si·nu·ous \-'sin-yə-wəs\ *adj* : of, relating to, or occurring in the tissues surrounding a sinus

peri·si·nu·soi·dal \-ˌsī-n(y)ə-'sȯid-ᵊl\ *adj* : of, relating to, or occurring in the tissue surrounding one or more sinusoids ⟨∼ cells⟩ ⟨∼ fibrosis⟩

peri·sple·ni·tis \-spli-'nīt-əs\ *n* : inflammation of the tissues surrounding the spleen

Pe·ris·so·dac·tyla \pə-ˌris-ə-'dak-tə-lə\ *n pl* : an order of nonruminant ungulate mammals (as the horse, the tapir, or the rhinoceros) that usu. have an odd number of toes, molar teeth with transverse ridges on the grinding surface, and posterior premolars resembling true molars — compare ARTIODACTYLA — **pe·ris·so·dac·tyl** \pə-ˌris-ə-ˌdak-tᵊl\ *n or adj*

peri·stal·sis \ˌper-ə-'stȯl-səs, -'stäl-, -'stal-\ *n, pl* **-stal·ses** \-ˌsēz\ : successive waves of involuntary contraction passing along the walls of a hollow muscular structure (as the esophagus or intestine) and forcing the contents onward — compare SEGMENTATION 2

peri·stal·tic \-tik\ *adj* : of, relating to, resulting from, or being peristalsis ⟨∼ contractions⟩

peri·stome \'per-ə-ˌstōm\ *n* : the area surrounding the mouth or cytostome of a protozoan — **peri·sto·mi·al** \ˌper-ə-'stō-mē-əl\ *adj*

peri·ten·di·ni·tis \ˌper-ə-ˌten-də-'nīt-əs\ *n* : inflammation of the tissues around a tendon

peri·ten·on \-'ten-ən\ *n* : the connective-tissue sheath of a tendon

peri·the·ci·um \-'thē-sē-əm\ *n, pl* **-cia** \-sē-ə\ : a spherical, cylindrical, or flask-shaped hollow fruiting body in various ascomycetous fungi that contains the asci, usu. opens by a terminal pore, and sometimes includes the cleistothecium

peri·the·li·al \ˌper-ə-'thē-lē-əl\ *adj* : of, relating to, or made up of perithelium

peri·the·li·o·ma \-ˌthē-lē-'ō-mə\ *n, pl* **-mas** *also* **-ma·ta** \-mət-ə\ : HEMANGIOPERICYTOMA

peri·the·li·um \-'thē-lē-əm\ *n, pl* **-lia** \-lē-ə\ : a layer of connective tissue surrounding a small vessel (as a capillary)

peritonaeum *chiefly Brit var of* PERITONEUM

peritonea *pl of* PERITONEUM

peri·to·ne·al *or chiefly Brit* **peri·to·nae·al** \ˌper-ət-ᵊn-'ē-əl\ *adj* : of, relating to, or affecting the peritoneum — **peri·to·ne·al·ly** *or chiefly Brit* **peri·to·nae·al·ly** \-ə-lē\ *adv*

peritoneal cavity *n* : a space formed when the parietal and visceral layers of the peritoneum spread apart

peritoneal dialysis *n* : DIALYSIS 2b

peri·to·ne·al·ize \-'ē-ə-ˌlīz\ *vt* **-ized; -iz·ing** : to cover (a surgical surface) with peritoneum

peri·to·neo·cen·te·sis \ˌper-ət-ᵊn-ˌē-ō-ˌsen-'tē-səs\ *n, pl* **-te·ses** \-ˌsēz\ : surgical puncture of the peritoneal cavity to obtain fluid

peri·to·neo·scope \ˌper-ət-ᵊn-'ē-ə-ˌskōp\ *n* : LAPAROSCOPE — **peri·to·neo·scop·ic** \-ˌē-ə-'skäp-ik\ *adj*

peri·to·neo·sco·py \ˌper-ət-ᵊn-ˌē-'äs-kə-pē\ *n, pl* **-pies** : LAPAROSCOPY 1

peri·to·neo·ve·nous shunt \ˌper-ət-ᵊn-ˌē-ō-ˌvē-nəs-\ *n* : a shunt between the peritoneum and the jugular vein for relief of peritoneal ascites

peri·to·ne·um *or chiefly Brit* **peri·to·nae·um** \ˌper-ət-ᵊn-'ē-əm\ *n, pl* **-ne·ums** *or chiefly Brit* **-nae·ums** \-'ē-əmz\ *or* **-nea** *or chiefly Brit* **-naea** \-'ē-ə\ : the smooth transparent serous membrane that lines the cavity of the abdomen of a mammal, is folded inward over the abdominal and pelvic viscera, and consists of an outer layer closely adherent to the walls of the abdomen and an inner layer that folds to invest the viscera — see PARIETAL PERITONEUM, VISCERAL PERITONEUM; compare MESENTERY 1

peri·to·ni·tis \ˌper-ət-ᵊn-'īt-əs\ *n* : inflammation of the peritoneum

peri·to·nize \'per-ət-ᵊn-ˌīz\ *vt* **-nized; -niz·ing** : PERITONEALIZE

peri·ton·sil·lar abscess \ˌper-ə-'tän(t)-sə-lər-\ *n* : QUINSY

peri·tra·che·al \-'trā-kē-əl\ *adj* : situated or occurring in the tissues surrounding the trachea ⟨∼ sarcoma⟩

peri·trich \'per-ə-ˌtrik\ *n* : any ciliate of the order Peritricha

\ə\ abut \ᵊ\ kitten \ər\ further \a\ ash \ā\ ace \ä\ cot, cart \aú\ out \ch\ chin \e\ bet \ē\ easy \g\ go \i\ hit \ī\ ice \j\ job \ŋ\ sing \ō\ go \ȯ\ law \ȯi\ boy \th\ thin \t̲h̲\ the \ü\ loot \ú\ foot \y\ yet \zh\ vision *See also* Pronunciation Symbols page

O
P

Pe·rit·ri·cha \pə-ˈri-tri-kə\ *n pl* : an order of the class Ciliata comprising protozoans with an enlarged disklike ciliated anterior end leading to the cytostome via a counterclockwise zone near the mouth and with reduced body ciliation and often being attached to the substrate by a contractile stalk

pe·rit·ri·chate \-kət, -ˌkāt\ *adj* : PERITRICHOUS 1

peri·trich·ic \ˌper-ə-ˈtrik-ik\ *adj* : PERITRICHOUS

Peri·trich·i·da \-ˈtrik-əd-ə\ *n pl, syn of* PERITRICHA

pe·rit·ri·chous \pə-ˈri-tri-kəs\ *adj* **1** : having or being flagella which are uniformly distributed over the body ⟨∼ bacteria⟩ **2** : having a spiral line of modified cilia around the cytostome ⟨∼ protozoans⟩ — **pe·rit·ri·chous·ly** *adv*

peri·tu·bu·lar \ˌper-ə-ˈt(y)ü-byə-lər\ *adj* : being adjacent to or surrounding a tubule ⟨∼ fibroblasts of the renal cortex —Deborah R. Bosman *et al*⟩

peritubular capillary *n* : any of a network of capillaries surrounding the renal tubules

peri·typh·li·tis \ˌper-ə-tif-ˈlīt-əs\ *n* : inflammation of the connective tissue about the cecum and appendix : APPENDICITIS

peri·um·bil·i·cal \ˌper-ē-ˌəm-ˈbil-i-kəl, *Brit usu* -ˌəm-bə-ˈlī-kəl\ *adj* : situated or occurring adjacent to the navel ⟨pain was initially localized to the ∼ region —A. S. Kochar⟩

peri·un·gual \-ˈəŋ-gwəl, -ˈən-gwəl\ *adj* : situated or occurring around a fingernail or toenail

peri·ure·ter·al \-yü-ˈrēt-ə-rəl\ *adj* : of, relating to, occurring in, or being the tissues surrounding a ureter

peri·ure·thral \-yü-ˈrē-thrəl\ *adj* : of, relating to, occurring in, or being the tissues surrounding the urethra ⟨a ∼ abscess⟩

peri·vas·cu·lar \ˌper-ə-ˈvas-kyə-lər\ *adj* : of, relating to, occurring in, or being the tissues surrounding a blood vessel

perivascular foot *n* : an expanded pedicle of an astrocyte that adheres to a blood vessel

peri·vas·cu·li·tis \-ˌvas-kyə-ˈlīt-əs\ *n* : inflammation of a perivascular sheath ⟨∼ in the retina⟩

peri·ve·nous \ˌper-ə-ˈvē-nəs\ *adj* : of, relating to, occurring in, or being the tissues surrounding a vein

peri·ven·tric·u·lar \-ven-ˈtrik-yə-lər\ *adj* : situated or occurring around a ventricle esp. of the brain ⟨∼ white matter⟩

peri·vis·cer·al \ˌper-ə-ˈvis-ə-rəl\ *adj* : situated about, surrounding, or enclosing the viscera ⟨∼ fluid⟩

peri·vis·cer·i·tis \-ˌvis-ə-ˈrīt-əs\ *n* : inflammation of the tissue surrounding a viscus or the viscera

peri·vi·tel·line space \ˌper-ə-vī-ˈtel-ən-, -ˌēn-, -ˌīn-\ *n* : the fluid-filled space between the fertilization membrane and the ovum after the entry of a sperm into the egg

per·i·win·kle \ˈper-i-ˌwiŋ-kəl\ *n* : any of several trailing or woody evergreen plants of the dogbane family (Apocynaceae); *esp* : ROSY PERIWINKLE

perle \ˈpər(-ə)l\ *n* **1** : a soft gelatin capsule for enclosing volatile or unpleasant-tasting liquids intended to be swallowed **2** : a fragile glass vial that contains a liquid (as amyl nitrite) and that is intended to be crushed and the vapor inhaled

per·lèche \per-ˈlesh\ *n* : a superficial inflammatory condition of the angles of the mouth often with fissuring that is caused esp. by infection or avitaminosis

per·lin·gual \(ˈ)pər-ˈliŋ-g(yə-)wəl\ *adj* : being administered by application to the tongue ⟨∼ medication⟩ — **per·lin·gual·ly** \-ē\ *adv*

per·ma·nent \ˈpərm(-ə)-nənt\ *adj* : of, relating to, or being a permanent tooth ⟨∼ dentition⟩

permanent tooth *n* : one of the second set of teeth of a mammal that follow the milk teeth, typically persist into old age, and in humans are 32 in number including 4 incisors, 2 canines, and 10 premolars and molars in each jaw

per·man·ga·nate \(ˌ)pər-ˈmaŋ-gə-ˌnāt\ *n* **1** : a salt containing the anion MnO_4^-; *esp* : POTASSIUM PERMANGANATE **2** : the anion MnO_4^- of a permanganate

per·man·gan·ic acid \ˌpər-(ˌ)man-ˌgan-ik-, -(ˌ)maŋ-\ *n* : an unstable strong acid $HMnO_4$ known chiefly in purple-colored strongly oxidizing aqueous solutions

per·me·abil·i·ty \ˌpər-mē-ə-ˈbil-ət-ē\ *n, pl* **-ties** : the quality or state of being permeable

per·me·able \ˈpər-mē-ə-bəl\ *adj* : capable of being permeat-

ed; *esp* : having pores or openings that permit liquids or gases to pass through ⟨a ∼ membrane⟩

per·me·ant \ˈpər-mē-ənt\ *adj* : capable of permeating a membrane ⟨a ∼ ion⟩ — **permeant** *n*

per·me·ase \-ˌās, -ˌāz\ *n* : a substance that catalyzes the transport of another substance across a plasma membrane

per·me·ate \ˈpər-mē-ˌāt\ *vb* **-at·ed; -at·ing** *vi* : to diffuse through or penetrate something ∼ *vt* : to pass through the pores or interstices of

per·me·ation \ˌpər-mē-ˈā-shən\ *n* **1** : the quality or state of being permeated **2** : the action or process of permeating

per·meth·rin \pər-ˈmeth-rən\ *n* : a synthetic pyrethroid pesticide $C_{21}H_{20}Cl_2O_3$ used esp. against insects, ticks, and mites

per·mis·sive \pər-ˈmis-iv\ *adj* : supporting genetic replication (as of a virus) ⟨∼ temperatures⟩ ⟨∼ monkey cells⟩

per·mono·sul·fu·ric acid \(ˌ)pər-ˌmän-ō-ˌsəl-ˌfyür-ik-\ *n* : an unstable crystalline strong monobasic acid H_2SO_5

per·ni·cious \pər-ˈnish-əs\ *adj* : highly injurious or destructive : tending to a fatal issue : DEADLY ⟨∼ disease⟩

pernicious anemia *n* : a severe hyperchromic anemia marked by a progressive decrease in number and increase in size and hemoglobin content of the red blood cells and by pallor, weakness, and gastrointestinal and nervous disturbances and associated with reduced ability to absorb vitamin B_{12} due to the absence of intrinsic factor — called also *addisonian anemia*

pernicious malaria *n* : FALCIPARUM MALARIA

per·nio \ˈpər-nē-ˌō\ *n, pl* **per·ni·o·nes** \ˌpər-nē-ˈō-(ˌ)nēz\ : CHILBLAIN — see LUPUS PERNIO

per·ni·o·sis \ˌpər-nē-ˈō-səs\ *n, pl* **-o·ses** \-ˌsēz\ : any skin abnormality resulting from exposure to cold

pe·ro·me·lia \ˌpē-rə-ˈmē-lē-ə\ *n* : congenital malformation of the limbs

pe·ro·ne·al \ˌper-ō-ˈnē-əl, pə-ˈrō-nē-\ *adj* **1** : of, relating to, or located near the fibula **2** : relating to or involving a peroneal part

peroneal artery *n* : a deeply seated artery running along the back part of the fibular side of the leg to the heel, arising from the posterior tibial artery, and ending in branches near the ankle

peroneal muscle *n* : PERONEUS

peroneal muscular atrophy *n* : a chronic inherited progressive muscular atrophy that affects the parts of the legs and feet innervated by the peroneal nerves first and later progresses to the hands and arms — called also *Charcot-Marie-Tooth disease, peroneal atrophy*

peroneal nerve *n* : COMMON PERONEAL NERVE — see DEEP PERONEAL NERVE, SUPERFICIAL PERONEAL NERVE

peroneal retinaculum *n* : either of two bands of fascia that support and bind in place the tendons of the peroneus longus and peroneus brevis muscles as they pass along the lateral aspect of the ankle: **a** : one that is situated more superiorly — called also *superior peroneal retinaculum* **b** : one that is situated more inferiorly — called also *inferior peroneal retinaculum*

peroneal vein *n* : any of several veins that drain the muscles in the lateral and posterior parts of the leg, accompany the peroneal artery, and empty into the posterior tibial veins about two-thirds of the way up the leg

per·o·ne·us \ˌper-ə-ˈnē-əs\ *n, pl* **-nei** \-ˈnē-ˌī\ : any of three muscles of the lower leg: **a** : PERONEUS BREVIS **b** : PERONEUS LONGUS **c** : PERONEUS TERTIUS

peroneus brev·is \-ˈbrev-əs\ *n* : a peroneus muscle that arises esp. from the side of the lower part of the fibula, ends in a tendon that inserts on the tuberosity at the base of the fifth metatarsal bone, and assists in everting and pronating the foot

peroneus lon·gus \-ˈloŋ-gəs\ *n* : a peroneus muscle that arises esp. from the head and side of the fibula, ends in a long tendon that inserts on the side of the first metatarsal bone and the cuneiform bone on the medial side, and aids in everting and pronating the foot

peroneus ter·ti·us \-ˈtər-shē-əs\ *n* : a branch of the extensor digitorum longus muscle that arises esp. from the lower portion of the fibula, inserts on the dorsal surface of the base of the fifth metatarsal bone, and flexes the foot dorsally and assists in everting it

per·oral \(ˌ)pər-ˈȯr-əl, pe(ə)r-, -ˈȯr-, -ˈär-\ *adj* : done, occurring, or obtained through or by way of the mouth ⟨~ administration of a drug⟩ ⟨~ infection⟩ — **per·oral·ly** \-ə-lē\ *adv*

per os \ˌpər-ˈōs\ *adv* : by way of the mouth ⟨medication administered *per os*⟩ ⟨infection *per os*⟩

pe·ro·sis \pə-ˈrō-səs\ *n, pl* **pe·ro·ses** \-ˌsēz\ : a disorder of poultry that is characterized by leg deformity and is caused by a deficiency of vitamins (as biotin or choline) or minerals (as manganese) in the diet — called also *hock disease, slipped tendon*

pe·rot·ic \pə-ˈrät-ik\ *adj* : of, relating to, or affected with perosis

per·ox·i·dase \pə-ˈräk-sə-ˌdās, -ˌdāz\ *n* : an enzyme occurring esp. in plants, milk, and white blood cells and consisting of a protein complex with hematin groups that catalyzes the oxidation of various substances by peroxides

per·ox·i·dat·ic \pə-ˌräk-sə-ˈdat-ik\ *adj* : of or relating to peroxidase ⟨~ activity⟩

per·ox·i·da·tion \-ˈdā-shən\ *n* : the process of peroxidizing a chemical compound

per·ox·ide \pə-ˈräk-ˌsīd\ *n* : a compound (as hydrogen peroxide) in which oxygen is visualized as joined to oxygen

per·ox·i·dize \-sə-ˌdīz\ *vt* **-dized; -diz·ing** : to convert (a compound) into a peroxide

per·ox·i·some \pə-ˈräk-sə-ˌsōm\ *n* : a cytoplasmic cell organelle containing enzymes (as catalase) which act esp. in the production and decomposition of hydrogen peroxide — called also *microbody* — **per·ox·i·som·al** \-ˌräk-sə-ˈsō-məl\ *adj*

per·oxy \pə-ˈräk-sē\ *adj* : containing the bivalent group O—O

per·oxy·ace·tic acid \pə-ˌräk-sē-ə-ˌsēt-ik-\ *n* : PERACETIC ACID

per·oxy·ace·tyl nitrate \pə-ˌräk-sē-ə-ˌsēt-ᵊl-, -ˌas-ət-, -ˌas-ə-ˌtēl-\ *n* : a toxic compound $C_2H_3O_5N$ irritating to the eyes and upper respiratory tract that is formed by the action of sunlight on volatile organic compounds and oxides of nitrogen and is found esp. in smog — abbr. *PAN*

per·oxy·di·sul·fu·ric acid \pə-ˌräk-si-ˌdī-ˌsəl-ˌfyu̇r-ik-\ *n* : PERSULFURIC ACID a

per·oxy·mono·sul·fu·ric acid \-ˌmän-ō-ˌsəl-ˌfyu̇r-ik-\ *n* : PERMONOSULFURIC ACID

per·pen·dic·u·lar plate \ˌpər-pən-ˈdik-yə-lər-\ *n* **1** : a flattened bony lamina of the ethmoid bone that is the largest bony part assisting in forming the nasal septum **2** : a long thin vertical bony plate forming part of the palatine bone — compare HORIZONTAL PLATE

per·phen·a·zine \(ˌ)pər-ˈfen-ə-ˌzēn\ *n* : a phenothiazine tranquilizer $C_{21}H_{26}ClN_3OS$ used esp. to control symptoms (as anxiety, agitation, and delusions) of psychotic conditions

per pri·mam \ˌpər-ˈprē-məm, -ˈprī-\ *adv* : by first intention ⟨a wound that heals *per primam* usually leaves little scarring⟩

per·rec·tal \ˌpər-ˈrek-tᵊl\ *adj* : done or occurring through or by way of the rectum ⟨~ examination⟩ — **per·rec·tal·ly** \-ē\ *adv*

per rectum *adv* : by way of the rectum ⟨a solution injected *per rectum*⟩

per·salt \ˈpər-ˌsȯlt\ *n* **1** : a salt containing a relatively large proportion of the acidic element or group **2** : a salt of a peracid

Per·san·tine \pər-ˈsan-ˌtēn\ *trademark* — used for a preparation of dipyridamole

per·se·cu·tion complex \ˌpər-si-ˈkyü-shən-\ *n* : the feeling of being persecuted esp. without basis in reality

per·se·cu·to·ry \ˈpər-sə-kyü-ˌtōr-ē, pər-ˈsek-yə-, -ˌtȯr-ē\ *adj* : of, relating to, or being feelings of persecution : PARANOID

per·sev·er·ate \pər-ˈsev-ə-ˌrāt\ *vi* **-at·ed; -at·ing** : to manifest the phenomenon of perseveration ⟨the *perseverating* tendency in stutterers in sensorimotor tasks —*Quarterly Jour. of Speech*⟩

per·sev·er·a·tion \pər-ˌsev-ə-ˈrā-shən\ *n* : continual involuntary repetition of a mental act usu. exhibited by speech or by some other form of overt behavior

per·sev·er·a·tive \pər-ˈsev-ə-ˌrāt-iv\ *adj* : characterized by perseveration

per·sic oil \ˈpər-sik-\ *n* : either of two substantially identical colorless or straw-colored nondrying fatty oils obtained by expression: **a** : one expressed from apricot kernels — called also *apricot-kernel oil* **b** : one expressed from peach kernels — called also *peach-kernel oil*

per·sim·mon \pər-ˈsim-ən\ *n* **1** : any tree or shrub of the genus *Diospyros*; *esp* : one (*D. virginiana*) of the eastern U.S. whose bark has been used as an astringent **2** : the usu. orange globular berry of a persimmon that is edible when fully ripe but usu. extremely astringent when unripe

per·sis·tence of vision \pər-ˈsis-tən(t)s-, -ˈzis-\ *n* : a visual phenomenon that is responsible for the apparent continuity of rapidly presented discrete images (as in motion pictures or television) consisting essentially of a brief retinal persistence of one image so that it is overlapped by the next and the whole is centrally interpreted as continuous

per·sis·tent \-tənt\ *adj* **1** : existing or continuing for a long time: as **a** : effective in the open for an appreciable time usu. through slow volatilizing ⟨mustard gas is ~⟩ **b** : degraded only slowly by the environment ⟨~ pesticides⟩ **c** : remaining infective for a relatively long time in a vector after an initial period of incubation ⟨~ viruses⟩ **2** : continuing to exist despite interference or treatment ⟨a ~ cough⟩ ⟨has been in a ~ vegetative state for two years⟩

per·sist·er \-tər\ *n* : a persistent microbe ⟨elimination of ~s may constitute the worst stumbling block for eradication programs —R. J. Dubos⟩

per·so·na \pər-ˈsō-nə, -ˌnä\ *n, pl* **personas** : an individual's social facade or front that esp. in the analytic psychology of C. G. Jung reflects the role in life the individual is playing — compare ANIMA 1

per·son·al·i·ty \ˌpərs-ᵊn-ˈal-ət-ē, ˌpər-ˈsnal-\ *n, pl* **-ties** **1** : the complex of characteristics that distinguishes an individual esp. in relationships with others **2 a** : the totality of an individual's behavioral and emotional tendencies **b** : the organization of the individual's distinguishing character traits, attitudes, or habits

personality disorder *n* : a psychopathological condition or group of conditions in which an individual's entire life pattern is considered deviant or nonadaptive although the individual shows neither neurotic symptoms nor psychotic disorganization

personality inventory *n* : any of several tests that attempt to characterize the personality of an individual by objective scoring of replies to a large number of questions concerning the individual's behavior and attitudes — see MINNESOTA MULTIPHASIC PERSONALITY INVENTORY

personality test *n* : any of several tests that consist of standardized tasks designed to determine various aspects of the personality or the emotional status of the individual examined

per·spi·ra·tion \ˌpər-spə-ˈrā-shən\ *n* **1** : the act or process of perspiring **2** : a saline fluid that is secreted by the sweat glands, that consists chiefly of water containing sodium chloride and other salts, nitrogenous substances (as urea), carbon dioxide, and other solutes, and that serves both as a means of excretion and as a regulator of body temperature through the cooling effect of its evaporation

per·spi·ra·to·ry \pər-ˈspī-rə-ˌtōr-ē, ˈpər-sp(ə-)rə-, -ˌtȯr-\ *adj* : of, relating to, secreting, or inducing perspiration

per·spire \pər-ˈspī(ə)r\ *vi* **per·spired; per·spir·ing** : to emit matter through the skin; *specif* : to secrete and emit perspiration

per·sua·sion \pər-ˈswā-zhən\ *n* : a method of treating neuro-

---

\ə\ **abut** \ᵊ\ **kitten** \ər\ **further** \a\ **ash** \ā\ **ace** \ä\ **cot, cart**
\au̇\ **out** \ch\ **chin** \e\ **bet** \ē\ **easy** \g\ **go** \i\ **hit** \ī\ **ice** \j\ **job**
\ŋ\ **sing** \ō\ **go** \ȯ\ **law** \ȯi\ **boy** \th\ **thin** \t̲h̲\ **the** \ü\ **loot**
\u̇\ **foot** \y\ **yet** \zh\ **vision** *See also* Pronunciation Symbols page

O
P

ses consisting essentially in rational conversation and reeducation

per·sul·fate \(')pər-,səl-,fāt\ *n* : a salt of persulfuric acid; *esp* : a salt of the acid $H_2S_2O_8$

per·sul·fu·ric acid \(,)pər-,səl-,fyùr-ik-°l\ *n* : either of two peroxy acids of sulfur: **a** : a crystalline strongly oxidizing acid $H_2S_2O_8$ **b** : PERMONOSULFURIC ACID

per·tech·ne·tate \pər-'tek-nə-,tāt\ *n* : an anion [TcO_4]⁻ of technetium used esp. in the form of its sodium salt as a radiopharmaceutical in medical diagnostic scanning (as of the thyroid or brain)

Per·thes disease \'pər-,tēz-\ *n* : LEGG-CALVÉ-PERTHES DISEASE

Per·to·frane \'pərt-ə-,frān\ *n* : a preparation of the hydrochloride of desipramine — formerly a U.S. registered trademark

per·tus·sal \pər-'təs-əl\ *adj* : of or relating to whooping cough 〈~ vaccines〉

per·tus·sis \pər-'təs-əs\ *n* : WHOOPING COUGH

peruana — see VERRUGA PERUANA

Peru balsam *n* : BALSAM OF PERU

Pe·ru·vi·an balsam \pə-,rü-vē-ən-\ *n* : BALSAM OF PERU

Peruvian bark *n* : CINCHONA 3

per·vap·o·ra·tion \(,)pər-,vap-ə-'rā-shən\ *n* : the concentration of a colloidal solution whose colloid will not pass through a semipermeable membrane by placing the solution in a bag made of the membrane material and blowing warm air against the surface of the bag

per·verse \pər-'vərs\ *adj* : being, relating to, or characterized by perversion 〈~ sexual behavior〉

per·ver·sion \pər-'vər-zhən, -shən\ *n* **1** : the action of perverting or the condition of being perverted **2** : an aberrant sexual practice or interest esp. when habitual

¹per·vert \pər-'vərt\ *vt* : to cause to engage in perversion or to become perverted

²per·vert \'pər-,vərt\ *n* : one that has been perverted; *specif* : one given to some form of sexual perversion

perverted *adj* : marked by abnormality or perversion 〈~ pancreatic function〉 〈relieve concepts or fears of ~ sexual interest —W. H. Masters & V. E. Johnson〉

pes \'pēz\ *n, pl* **pe·des** \'pē-(,)dēz\ : the distal segment of the hind limb of a vertebrate including the tarsus and foot

pes an·se·ri·nus \-,an-sə-'rī-nəs\ *n* : the combined tendinous insertion on the medial aspect of the tuberosity of the tibia of the sartorius, gracilis, and semitendinosus muscles

pes ca·vus \-'kā-vəs\ *n* : a foot deformity characterized by an abnormally high arch

pes hip·po·cam·pi \-,hip-ə-'kam-,pī\ *n* : the enlarged rostral extremity of the hippocampus

pes·sa·ry \'pes-ə-rē\ *n, pl* **-ries** **1** : a vaginal suppository **2** : a device worn in the vagina to support the uterus, remedy a malposition, or prevent conception

pes·si·mism \'pes-ə-,miz-əm *also* 'pez-\ *n* : an inclination to emphasize adverse aspects, conditions, and possibilities or to expect the worst possible outcome — **pes·si·mis·tic** \,pes-ə-'mis-tik *also* ,pez-\ *adj*

pest \'pest\ *n* **1** : an epidemic disease associated with high mortality; *specif* : PLAGUE 2 **2** : something resembling a pest in destructiveness; *esp* : a plant or animal detrimental to humans or human concerns — **pesty** \'pes-tē\ *adj*

pest·house \-,haùs\ *n* : a shelter or hospital for those infected with a pestilential or contagious disease

pes·ti·ci·dal \,pes-tə-'sīd-°l\ *adj* : of, relating to, or being a pesticide

pes·ti·cide \'pes-tə-,sīd\ *n* : an agent used to destroy pests

pes·tif·er·ous \pes-'tif-(ə-)rəs\ *adj* **1** : carrying or propagating infection : PESTILENTIAL 〈a ~ insect〉 **2** : infected with a pestilential disease

pes·ti·lence \'pes-tə-lən(t)s\ *n* : a contagious or infectious epidemic disease that is virulent and devastating; *specif* : BUBONIC PLAGUE

pes·ti·len·tial \,pes-tə-'len-chəl\ *adj* **1** : causing or tending to cause pestilence **2** : of or relating to pestilence

pes·tis \'pest-əs\ *n* : PLAGUE 2

Pes·ti·vi·rus \'pes-tə-,vī-rəs\ *n* : a genus of single-stranded RNA viruses of the family *Flaviviridae* that includes the causative agents of bovine viral diarrhea and hog cholera

pes·tle \'pes-əl *also* 'pes-t°l\ *n* : a usu. club-shaped implement for pounding or grinding substances in a mortar

PET *abbr* positron-emission tomography

PetCO₂ *abbr* partial pressure of end-tidal carbon dioxide

pe·te·chia \pə-'tē-kē-ə\ *n, pl* **-chi·ae** \-kē-,ī\ : a minute reddish or purplish spot containing blood that appears in skin or mucous membrane as a result of localized hemorrhage

pe·te·chi·al \-kē-əl\ *adj* : relating to, marked by, or causing petechiae or petechiation 〈~ hemorrhage〉 〈a ~ rash〉

pe·te·chi·a·tion \pə-,tē-kē-'ā-shən\ *n* : the state of being covered with petechiae 〈spotty ~ of the intestinal mucosa〉

peth·i·dine \'peth-ə-,dēn, -dən\ *n, chiefly Brit* : MEPERIDINE

pe·tit mal \'pet-ē-,mal, -,mäl\ *n* : epilepsy characterized by absence seizures; *also* : ABSENCE SEIZURE

pe·tri dish \'pē-trē-\ *n* : a small shallow dish of thin glass or plastic with a loose cover used esp. for cultures in bacteriology

Pe·tri \'pā-trē\, **Julius Richard (1852–1921)**, German bacteriologist. Petri was an assistant to the eminent bacteriologist Robert Koch. In 1887 Petri introduced a vessel for growing bacteria that consists of two round rimmed plates, one serving as a cover for the other.

pet·ri·fac·tion \,pe-trə-'fak-shən\ *n* **1** : the process of petrifying 〈calcification or ~ of tissue〉 **2** : something petrified **3** : the quality or state of being petrified

pet·ri·fi·ca·tion \,pe-trə-fə-'kā-shən\ *n* : PETRIFACTION

pet·ri·fy \'pe-trə-,fī\ *vb* **-fied; -fy·ing** *vt* : to convert (organic matter) into stone or a stony substance ~ *vi* : to become stone or like stone

pe·tris·sage \,pā-tri-'säzh\ *n* : massage in which the muscles are kneaded

pet·ro·la·tum \,pe-trə-'lāt-əm, -'lät-\ *n* : a neutral unctuous substance that is practically odorless and tasteless and is insoluble in water, that is obtained from petroleum and differs chemically from paraffin wax in containing unsaturated hydrocarbons or naphthenes as well as alkanes, and that is produced in several forms: **a** : a yellowish to light amber semisolid mass used chiefly as a base for ointments and cosmetics, as a protective dressing, and in lubricating greases — called also *petroleum jelly, yellow petrolatum* **b** : a white or faintly yellowish mass obtained by decolorizing yellow petrolatum and used similarly to it — called also *petroleum jelly, white petrolatum, white petroleum jelly*

pe·tro·leum \pə-'trō-lē-əm, -'trōl-yəm\ *n* : an oily flammable bituminous liquid that may vary from almost colorless to black, occurs in many places in the upper strata of the earth, is a complex mixture of hydrocarbons with small amounts of other substances, and is prepared for use as gasoline, naphtha, or other products by various refining processes

petroleum ben·zin \-'ben-(,)zin\ *n* : a flammable petroleum distillate containing primarily pentanes, hexanes, and heptanes, and used chiefly as a solvent esp. in pharmacy

petroleum ether *n* : a volatile flammable petroleum distillate (as petroleum benzin)

petroleum jelly *n* : PETROLATUM a, b

pe·tro–oc·cip·i·tal \,pe-trō-äk-'sip-ət-°l, ,pē-\ *adj* : of or relating to the occipital bone and the petrous portion of the temporal bone

¹pe·tro·sal \pə-'trō-səl\ *adj* : of, relating to, or situated in the region of the petrous portion of the temporal bone or capsule of the inner ear

²petrosal *n* : PETROSAL BONE

petrosal bone *n* : the petrous portion of the human temporal bone; *also* : a bone corresponding to this in a nonhuman vertebrate

petrosal ganglion *n* : INFERIOR GANGLION 1

petrosal nerve *n* : any of several small nerves passing through foramina in the petrous portion of the temporal bone: as **a** : DEEP PETROSAL NERVE **b** : GREATER PETROSAL NERVE **c** : LESSER PETROSAL NERVE

petrosal sinus *n* : either of two venous sinuses on each side of the base of the brain: **a** : a small superior sinus that connects the cavernous and transverse sinuses of the same side — called also *superior petrosal sinus* **b** : a larger inferior sinus that is situated in a sulcus on each side formed by the junction of the petrous portion of the temporal bone and the basilar portion of the occipital bone and that extends from the posterior inferior end of the cavernous sinus through the jugular foramen to join the internal jugular vein of the same side — called also *inferior petrosal sinus*

pe·tro·si·tis \ˌpe-trə-ˈsīt-əs, ˌpē-\ *n* : inflammation of the petrous portion of the temporal bone

pe·tro·tym·pan·ic \ˌpe-trō-tim-ˈpan-ik, ˌpē-\ *adj* : of or relating to the petrous and tympanic portions of the temporal bone

petrotympanic fissure *n* : a narrow transverse slit dividing the glenoid fossa of the temporal bone — called also *Glaserian fissure*

pe·trous \ˈpe-trəs, ˈpē-\ *adj* : of, relating to, or constituting the exceptionally hard and dense portion of the human temporal bone that contains the internal auditory organs and is a pyramidal process wedged in at the base of the skull between the sphenoid and occipital bones with its lower half exposed on the surface of the skull and pierced by the external auditory canal

petrous ganglion *n* : INFERIOR GANGLION 1

pe·trox·o·lin \pə-ˈträk-sə-lən\ *n* : a mixture of liquid petrolatum and ammonia soap medicated and perfumed esp. for use in ointments

PET scan \ˈpet-\ *n* : a sectional view of the body constructed by positron-emission tomography — **PET scanning** *n*

PET scanner *n* : a medical instrument consisting of integrated X-ray and computing equipment and used for positron-emission tomography

Peutz–Je·ghers syndrome \ˈpɔ(r)ts-ˈjā-gərz-, ˈpo͞ets-\ *n* : a familial polyposis inherited as an autosomal dominant trait and characterized by numerous polyps in the stomach, small intestine, and colon and by melanin-containing spots on the skin and mucous membranes esp. of the lips and gums

Peutz \ˈpo͞ets\, **J. L. A. (1886–1957)**, Dutch physician. Peutz published the first detailed description of Peutz-Jeghers syndrome in 1921. Some of the symptoms had been described by British physician Sir Jonathan Hutchinson in 1896.

Jeghers, Harold Joseph (1904–1990), American physician. Jeghers successively served on the medical faculties of Boston University, Georgetown University, New Jersey College of Medicine and Dentistry, and Tufts University. He also held concurrent positions with several hospitals in Boston, Washington, D.C., and Jersey City, New Jersey. His last position was that of director of St. Vincent Hospital in Worcester, Massachusetts. His topics of research included nutrition, especially vitamin A deficiency, renal function, and skin pigmentation. He published his description of Peutz-Jeghers syndrome with V. A. McKusick and K. H. Katz in 1949.

Pey·er's patch \ˈpī-ərz-\ *n* : any of numerous large oval patches of closely aggregated nodules of lymphoid tissue in the walls of the small intestine esp. in the ileum that partially or entirely disappear in advanced life and in typhoid fever become the seat of ulcers which may perforate the intestines — called also *Peyer's gland*

Peyer, Johann Conrad (1653–1712), Swiss physician and anatomist. Peyer was one of a group of physicians in the late 17th century who made important contributions to the methodology of medical research. They sought to explain the symptoms of a disease in terms of the lesion, which was considered the site of the disease. In 1677 Peyer published the first description of the nodules of lymphoid tissue in the small intestine that are now associated with his name.

pey·o·te \pā-ˈōt-ē\ *also* **pey·otl** \-ˈōt-ᵊl\ *n* **1** : a hallucinogenic drug containing mescaline that is derived from peyote buttons and used esp. in the religious ceremonies of some American Indian peoples **2** : a small spineless cactus of the genus *Lophophora* (*L. williamsii*) of the southwestern U.S.

and Mexico having rounded stems covered with jointed tubercules — called also *mescal*

peyote button *n* : one of the dried discoid tops of the peyote cactus — called also *mescal button*

Pey·ro·nie's disease \ˌpā-rə-ˈnēz-, pā-ˈrō-(ˌ)nēz-\ *n* : the formation of fibrous plaques in one or both corpora cavernosa of the penis resulting in distortion or deflection of the erect organ

La Pey·ro·nie \lä-pā-rȯ-nē\, **François Gigot de (1678–1747)**, French surgeon. La Peyronie is credited with establishing Paris as the surgical center of the world in the 18th century. Using his power and influence as surgeon to Louis XV, La Peyronie helped to raise the general standing of surgeons and surgery in France. He devoted his fortune to the advancement of surgery, helped to found the Academy of Surgery, and left a legacy for the awarding of annual prizes in surgery. In 1743 he described a disease of the penis marked by induration and fibrosis of the corpora cavernosa; it is now known as Peyronie's disease.

pf *abbr* picofarad

Pfan·nen·stiel's incision \ˈ(p)fän-ən-ˌs(h)tēlz-, ˈfan-\ *n* : a long horizontal abdominal incision made below the line of the pubic hair and above the mons veneris down to and through the sheath of the rectus abdominus muscles but not the muscles themselves which are separated in the direction of their fibers — called also *bikini incision*

Pfan·nen·stiel \ˈpfän-ən-ˌshtēl\, **Hermann Johann (1862–1909)**, German gynecologist. Pfannenstiel's incision was publicly introduced in an article published in 1900.

Pfeif·fer·el·la \ˌfī-fə-ˈrel-ə\ *n, syn of* ACTINOBACILLUS

Pfeif·fer \ˈpfī-fər\, **Richard Friedrich Johannes (1858–1945)**, German bacteriologist. An assistant of the renowned bacteriologist Robert Koch, Pfeiffer discovered the bacillus of the genus *Haemophilus* (*H. influenzae*) which was once thought to be the causative agent of influenza and is now known as Pfeiffer's bacillus.

Pfeif·fer's bacillus \ˈfī-fərz-\ *n* : a minute bacillus of the genus *Haemophilus* (*H. influenzae*) associated with acute respiratory infections and meningitis — compare KOCH-WEEKS BACILLUS

Pfie·ster·ia \fē-ˈstir-ē-ə, fis-ˈtir-\ *n* : a genus of dinoflagellates including one (*Pfiesteria piscicida*) found in waters esp. along the middle and southern Atlantic coast of the U.S. that produces a toxin which causes skin lesions in fish, that feeds upon the lesions sometimes causing large fish die-offs, and that may cause symptoms (as skin lesions and memory loss) in humans exposed to the toxin

p53 \ˌpē-ˌfif-tē-ˈthrē\ *n* : a tumor suppressor gene that in a defective form tends to be associated with a high risk of certain cancers (as of the colon, lung, and breast)

pg *abbr* picogram

PG *abbr* prostaglandin

PGA *abbr* pteroylglutamic acid

PGR *abbr* psychogalvanic reaction; psychogalvanic reflex; psychogalvanic response

PGY *abbr* postgraduate year

ph *abbr* **1** pharmacopoeia **2** phosphor **3** phot

pH \(ˈ)pē-ˈāch\ *n* : a measure of acidity and alkalinity of a solution that is a number on a scale on which a value of 7 represents neutrality and lower numbers indicate increasing acidity and higher numbers increasing alkalinity and on which each unit of change represents a tenfold change in acidity or alkalinity and that is the negative logarithm of the effective hydrogen-ion concentration or hydrogen-ion activity in gram equivalents per liter of the solution ⟨instead of saying that the concentration of hydrogen ion in pure water is 1.00×10^{-7}, it is customary to say that the ∼ of pure water is 7 —Linus Pauling⟩; *also* : the condition represented by such a number — compare PK

O

P

PHA *abbr* phytohemagglutinin

phaco·emul·si·fi·ca·tion *also* **phako·emul·si·fi·ca·tion** \ˌfak-ō-iˌməl-sə-fə-ˈkā-shən\ *n* : a cataract operation in which the diseased lens is reduced to a liquid by ultrasonic vibrations and drained out of the eye — **phaco·emul·si·fi·er** \-ˈməl-sə-ˌfī(-ə)r\ *n*

phaco·ma·to·sis \ˌfak-ō-mə-ˈtō-səs\ *n, pl* **-to·ses** \-ˌsēz\ : any of a group of hereditary or congenital diseases (as neurofibromatosis) affecting the central nervous system and characterized by the development of hamartomas

phaeochrome, phaeochromoblast, phaeochromocyte, phaeochromocytoma, phaeophorbide, phaeophytin *Brit var of* PHEOCHROME, PHEOCHROMOBLAST, PHEOCHROMOCYTE, PHEOCHROMOCYTOMA, PHEOPHORBIDE, PHEOPHYTIN

phage \ˈfāj *also* ˈfäzh\ *n* : BACTERIOPHAGE

phag·e·de·na *also* **phag·e·dae·na** \ˌfaj-ə-ˈdē-nə\ *n* : rapidly spreading destructive ulceration of soft tissue

phag·e·de·nic *also* **phag·e·dae·nic** \-ˈden-ik, -ˈdē-nik\ *adj* 1 *of a lesion* : being or marked by phagedena 2 : of, relating to, or resembling phagedena ⟨the ~ form of chancroid⟩

phage lambda *n* : a bacteriophage (species *Enterobacteria phage* λ of the family *Siphoviridae*) of double-stranded DNA that consists of an icosahedral head about 60 nanometers in diameter with 72 capsomers and a flexible tail about 150 nanometers long and eight nanometers wide, that can be integrated as a prophage into the genome of some strains of E. coli, and that is used as a vector to clone DNA from various organisms by replacing nonessential DNA in the bacteriophage with the foreign DNA and introducing the combined DNA into E. coli where it is replicated with the bacterium — called also *bacteriophage lambda, lambda, lambda phage*

phage type *n* : a set of strains of a bacterium susceptible to the same bacteriophages

phage typing *n* : determination of the phage type of a bacterium

phago·cyt·able \ˌfag-ə-ˈsīt-ə-bəl\ *adj* : susceptible to phagocytosis

¹phago·cyte \ˈfag-ə-ˌsīt\ *n* : a cell (as a white blood cell) that engulfs and consumes foreign material (as microorganisms) and debris

²phagocyte *vt* **-cyt·ed; -cyt·ing** : PHAGOCYTOSE

phago·cyt·ic \ˌfag-ə-ˈsit-ik\ *adj* : having the ability to engulf by phagocytosis : capable of functioning as phagocytes

phagocytic index *n* : a measure of phagocytic activity determined by counting the number of bacteria ingested per phagocyte during a limited period of incubation of a suspension of bacteria and phagocytes in serum

phago·cy·tize *also Brit* **phago·cy·tise** \ˈfag-ə-sə-ˌtīz, -ˌsīt-ˌīz\ *vt* **-tized** *also Brit* **-tised; -tiz·ing** *also Brit* **-tis·ing** : PHAGOCYTOSE

phago·cy·tos·able \ˈfag-ə-sə-ˌtōz-ə-bəl, -sī-, -ˌtōs-\ *adj* : capable of being phagocytosed ⟨granulocytes are stimulated . . . by ~ particles —L. D. Grouse⟩

phago·cy·tose \-ˌtōs, -ˌtōz\ *vt* **-tosed; -tos·ing** : to consume by phagocytosis

phago·cy·to·sis \ˌfag-ə-sə-ˈtō-səs, -sī-\ *n, pl* **-to·ses** \-ˌsēz\ : the engulfing and usu. the destruction of particulate matter by phagocytes that serves as an important bodily defense mechanism against infection by microorganisms and against occlusion of mucous surfaces or tissues by foreign particles and tissue debris — **phago·cy·tot·ic** \-ˈtät-ik\ *adj*

pha·gol·y·sis \fə-ˈgäl-ə-səs\ *n, pl* **-y·ses** \-ˌsēz\ : destruction of phagocytes

phago·ly·so·some \ˌfag-ə-ˈlī-sə-ˌsōm\ *n* : a digestive vesicle formed within a cell by the fusion of a phagosome containing ingested material and a lysosome containing hydrolytic enzymes — **phago·ly·so·som·al** \-ˌlī-sə-ˈsō-məl\ *adj*

phago·some \ˈfag-ə-ˌsōm\ *n* : a membrane-bound vesicle that encloses particulate matter taken into the cell by phagocytosis

phakoemulsification *var of* PHACOEMULSIFICATION

phal·a·cro·sis \ˌfal-ə-ˈkrō-səs\ *n, pl* **-cro·ses** \-ˌsēz\ : BALDNESS, ALOPECIA

pha·lan·ge·al \ˌfā-lən-ˈjē-əl, ˌfal-ən-; fə-ˈlan-jē-, fā-\ *adj* : of or relating to a phalanx or the phalanges

pha·lan·gec·to·my \ˌfā-lən-ˈjek-tə-mē, ˌfa-\ *n, pl* **-mies** : surgical excision of a phalanx of a finger or toe

phal·an·gette \ˌfal-ən-ˈjet\ *n* : a distal phalanx of a finger or toe

pha·lanx \ˈfā-ˌlaŋ(k)s, *Brit usu* ˈfal-ˌaŋ(k)s\ *n, pl* **pha·lan·ges** \fə-ˈlan-(ˌ)jēz, fā-, ˈfā-, *Brit usu* fal-ˈan-\ : any of the digital bones of the hand or foot distal to the metacarpus or metatarsus of a vertebrate that in humans are three to each finger and toe with the exception of the thumb and big toe which have only two each

phalli *pl of* PHALLUS

phal·lic \ˈfal-ik\ *adj* 1 : of, relating to, or resembling a penis 2 : of, relating to, or characterized by the stage of psychosexual development in psychoanalytic theory following the anal stage and during which a child becomes interested in his or her own sexual organs — compare ANAL 2, GENITAL 3, ORAL 3

phal·li·cism \ˈfal-ə-ˌsiz-əm\ *n* : the worship of the generative principle as symbolized by the phallus

phal·lism \ˈfa-ˌliz-əm\ *n* : PHALLICISM

phal·loid \ˈfa-ˌlȯid\ *adj* : resembling a penis esp. in shape

phal·loi·din \fa-ˈlȯid-ᵊn\ *also* **phal·loi·dine** \fa-ˈlȯid-ᵊn, ˈfal-ȯi-ˌdēn\ *n* : a very toxic crystalline peptide $C_{35}H_{46}N_8O_{10}S \cdot H_2O$ obtained from the death cap mushroom

phal·lo·plas·ty \ˈfal-ō-ˌplas-tē\ *n, pl* **-ties** : plastic surgery of the penis or scrotum

phal·lus \ˈfal-əs\ *n, pl* **phal·li** \ˈfal-ˌī, -ˌē\ *or* **phal·lus·es** 1 : PENIS 2 : the first embryonic rudiment of the vertebrate penis or clitoris

Phan·er·o·gam·ia \ˌfan-ə-rō-ˈgam-ē-ə\ *n pl, in some esp former classifications* : a division of plants comprising all the seed plants — compare CRYPTOGAMIA

phan·er·o·gen·ic \ˌfan-ə-rō-ˈjen-ik\ *adj* : of known origin — compare CRYPTOGENIC

phan·er·o·ma·nia \-ˈmā-nē-ə\ *n* : a persistent or obsessive picking at some superficial body growth (as in habitual nail-biting)

phan·er·o·sis \ˌfan-ə-ˈrō-səs\ *n, pl* **-o·ses** \-ˌsēz\ : the attaining of visibility — used chiefly of intercellular lipids that become visible fatty droplets as the cells degenerate

phan·ero·zo·ite \ˌfan-ə-rō-ˈzō-ˌīt\ *n* : an exoerythrocytic malaria parasite formed late in the course of an infection — **phan·ero·zo·it·ic** \-zō-ˈit-ik\ *adj*

phan·tasm \ˈfan-ˌtaz-əm\ *n* 1 : a figment of the imagination or disordered mind 2 : an apparition of a living or dead person

phantasy *var of* FANTASY

phan·to·geu·sia \ˌfan-tə-ˈgyü-zē-ə, -ˈjü-, -sē-\ *n* : an often metallic or salty taste in the mouth for which no external stimulus can be found

¹phan·tom *also* **fan·tom** \ˈfant-əm\ *n* 1 : a model of the body or one of its parts 2 : a body of material resembling a body or bodily part in mass, composition, and dimensions and used to measure absorption of radiations

²phantom *also* **fantom** *adj* : not caused by an anatomical lesion ⟨~ respiratory disorders⟩

phantom limb *n* : an often painful sensation of the presence of a limb that has been amputated — called also *phantom pain, phantom sensations*

phantom tumor *n* : a swelling (as of the abdomen) suggesting a tumor

Phar. D. *abbr* doctor of pharmacy

pharm *abbr* pharmaceutical; pharmacist; pharmacy

phar·ma \ˈfär-mə\ *n* : a pharmaceutical company

phar·ma·cal \ˈfär-mə-kəl\ *adj* : PHARMACEUTICAL

¹phar·ma·ceu·ti·cal \ˌfär-mə-ˈsüt-i-kəl\ *also* **phar·ma·ceu·tic** \-ˈsüt-ik\ *adj* : of, relating to, or engaged in pharmacy or the manufacture and sale of pharmaceuticals ⟨a ~ company⟩ — **phar·ma·ceu·ti·cal·ly** \-i-k(ə-)lē\ *adv*

²pharmaceutical *also* **pharmaceutic** *n* : a medicinal drug

phar·ma·ceu·tics \-iks\ *n pl but sing in constr* : the science of preparing, using, or dispensing medicines : PHARMACY

phar·ma·cist \\'fär-mə-səst\ *n* : a person licensed to engage in pharmacy

phar·ma·co·dy·nam·ics \ˌfär-mə-kō-dī-'nam-iks, -də-\ *n pl but sing in constr* : a branch of pharmacology dealing with the reactions between drugs and living systems — **phar·ma·co·dy·nam·ic** \-ik\ *adj* — **phar·ma·co·dy·nam·i·cal·ly** \-i-k(ə)lē\ *adv*

phar·ma·co·ge·net·ics \-jə-'net-iks\ *n pl but sing in constr* : the study of the interrelation of hereditary constitution and response to drugs — **phar·ma·co·ge·net·ic** \-ik\ *adj*

phar·ma·co·ge·no·mics \-jē-'nō-miks\ *n pl but sing in constr* : a biotechnological science that combines the techniques of medicine, pharmacology, and genomics and is concerned with developing drug therapies to compensate for genetic differences in patients which cause varied responses to a single therapeutic regimen — **phar·ma·co·ge·no·mic** \-mik\ *adj*

phar·ma·cog·no·sist \ˌfär-mə-'käg-nə-səst\ *n* : a specialist in pharmacognosy

phar·ma·cog·no·sy \ˌfär-mə-'käg-nə-sē\ *n, pl* **-sies** : a branch of pharmacology dealing esp. with the composition, use, and development of medicinal substances of biological origin and esp. medicinal substances obtained from plants — **phar·ma·cog·nos·tic** \-ˌkäg-'näs-tik\ *or* **phar·ma·cog·nos·ti·cal** \-ti-kəl\ *adj*

phar·ma·co·ki·net·ics \-kō-kə-'net-iks, -kō-kī-\ *n pl but sing in constr* **1** : the study of the bodily absorption, distribution, metabolism, and excretion of drugs **2** : the characteristic interactions of a drug and the body in terms of its absorption, distribution, metabolism, and excretion ⟨evaluated the ∼ of a single theophylline dose —*Jour. Amer. Med. Assoc.*⟩ — **phar·ma·co·ki·net·ic** \-ik\ *adj*

phar·ma·col·o·gist \ˌfär-mə-'käl-ə-jəst\ *n* : a specialist in pharmacology

phar·ma·col·o·gy \ˌfär-mə-'käl-ə-jē\ *n, pl* **-gies** **1** : the science of drugs including their origin, composition, pharmacokinetics, therapeutic use, and toxicology **2** : the properties and reactions of drugs esp. with relation to their therapeutic value — **phar·ma·co·log·i·cal** \-kə-'läj-i-kəl\ *also* **phar·ma·co·log·ic** \-ik\ *adj* — **phar·ma·co·log·i·cal·ly** \-i-k(ə)lē\ *adv*

phar·ma·con \'fär-mə-ˌkän\ *n* : a medicinal substance : DRUG

phar·ma·co·poe·ia *or* **phar·ma·co·pe·ia** \ˌfär-mə-kə-'pē-(y)ə\ *n* **1** : a book describing drugs, chemicals, and medicinal preparations; *esp* : one issued by an officially recognized authority and serving as a standard — compare DISPENSATORY 1 **2** : a collection or stock of drugs — **phar·ma·co·poe·ial** *or* **phar·ma·co·pe·ial** \-(y)əl\ *adj*

phar·ma·co·psy·cho·sis \ˌfär-mə-kō-sī-'kō-səs\ *n, pl* **-cho·ses** \-ˌsēz\ : addiction to a drug

phar·ma·co·ther·a·peu·tic \-ˌther-ə-'pyüt-ik\ *also* **phar·ma·co·ther·a·peu·ti·cal** \-i-kəl\ *adj* : of or relating to pharmacotherapeutics or pharmacotherapy

phar·ma·co·ther·a·peu·tics \-'pyüt-iks\ *n pl but sing or pl in constr* : the study of the therapeutic uses and effects of drugs

phar·ma·co·ther·a·py \ˌfär-mə-kō-'ther-ə-pē\ *n, pl* **-pies** : the treatment of disease and esp. mental disorder with drugs

phar·ma·cy \'fär-mə-sē\ *n, pl* **-cies** **1** : the art, practice, or profession of preparing, preserving, compounding, and dispensing medical drugs **2 a** : a place where medicines are compounded or dispensed ⟨a hospital ∼⟩ **b** : DRUGSTORE **3** : PHARMACOPOEIA 2

Pharm. D. *abbr* doctor of pharmacy

pha·ryn·geal \ˌfar-ən-'jē-əl, fə-'rin-j(ē-)əl\ *adj* **1** : relating to or located in the region of the pharynx **2 a** : innervating the pharynx esp. by contributing to the formation of the pharyngeal plexus ⟨the ∼ branch of the vagus nerve⟩ **b** : supplying or draining the pharynx ⟨the ∼ branch of the maxillary artery⟩

pharyngeal aponeurosis *n* : the middle or fibrous coat of the walls of the pharynx

pharyngeal arch *n* : BRANCHIAL ARCH

pharyngeal bursa *n* : a crypt in the pharyngeal tonsil that represents a communication existing during fetal life between the pharynx and the tip of the notochord

pharyngeal cavity *n* : the cavity of the pharynx that consists of a part continuous anteriorly with the nasal cavity by way of the nasopharynx, a part opening into the oral cavity by way of the isthmus of the fauces, and a part continuous posteriorly with the esophagus and opening into the larynx by way of the epiglottis

pharyngeal cleft *n* : BRANCHIAL CLEFT

pharyngeal membrane *n* : BUCCOPHARYNGEAL MEMBRANE

pharyngeal plexus *n* : a plexus formed by branches of the glossopharyngeal, vagus, and sympathetic nerves supplying the muscles and mucous membrane of the pharynx and adjoining parts

pharyngeal pouch *n* : any of a series of evaginations of ectoderm on either side of the pharynx that meet the corresponding external furrows and give rise to the branchial clefts of the vertebrate embryo

pharyngeal slit *n* : BRANCHIAL CLEFT

pharyngeal tonsil *n* : a mass of lymphoid tissue at the back of the pharynx between the eustachian tubes that is usu. best developed in young children, is commonly atrophied in the adult, and is markedly subject to hypertrophy and adenoid formation esp. in children — called also *nasopharyngeal tonsil*

phar·yn·gec·to·my \ˌfar-ən-'jek-tə-mē\ *n, pl* **-mies** : surgical removal of a part of the pharynx

pharynges *pl of* PHARYNX

pharyngis — see CONSTRICTOR PHARYNGIS INFERIOR, CONSTRICTOR PHARYNGIS MEDIUS, CONSTRICTOR PHARYNGIS SUPERIOR

phar·yn·gi·tis \ˌfar-ən-'jīt-əs\ *n, pl* **-git·i·des** \-'jit-ə-ˌdēz\ : inflammation of the pharynx

pha·ryn·go·con·junc·ti·val fever \fə-ˌriŋ-gō-ˌkän-ˌjən(k)-'tī-vəl-, -kən\ *n* : an acute epidemic illness caused by various adenoviruses of the genus *Mastadenovirus* (esp. serotypes of species *Human adenovirus B, Human adenovirus C,* and *Human adenovirus E*) that usu. affects children of school age and that is characterized typically by fever, pharyngitis, and conjunctivitis

pha·ryn·go·epi·glot·tic fold \-ˌep-ə-'glät-ik-\ *n* : either of two folds of mucous membrane extending from the base of the tongue to the epiglottis with one on each side of the midline

pha·ryn·go·esoph·a·ge·al *or Brit* **pha·ryn·go–oe·soph·a·ge·al** \-i-ˌsäf-ə-'jē-əl\ *adj* : of or relating to the pharynx and the esophagus

pharyngoesophageal diverticulum *n* : ZENKER'S DIVERTICULUM

pha·ryn·go·lar·yn·gec·to·my \fə-ˌriŋ-gō-ˌlar-ən-'jek-tə-mē\ *n, pl* **-mies** : surgical excision of the hypopharynx and larynx

pha·ryn·go·pal·a·tine arch \-'pal-ə-ˌtīn-\ *n* : PALATOPHARYNGEAL ARCH

pha·ryn·go·pal·a·ti·nus \-ˌpal-ə-'tī-nəs\ *n, pl* **-ti·ni** \-ˌnī\ : PALATOPHARYNGEUS

pha·ryn·go·plas·ty \fə-'riŋ-gō-ˌplas-tē\ *n, pl* **-ties** : plastic surgery performed on the pharynx

pha·ryn·go·ple·gia \fə-ˌriŋ-gō-'plē-j(ē-)ə\ *n* : paralysis of the muscles of the pharynx

phar·yn·gos·to·my \ˌfar-iŋ-'gäs-tə-mē\ *n, pl* **-mies** : surgical formation of an artificial opening into the pharynx

phar·yn·got·o·my \ˌfar-iŋ-'gät-ə-mē\ *n, pl* **-mies** : surgical incision into the pharynx

pha·ryn·go·ton·sil·li·tis \fə-ˌriŋ-gō-ˌtän(t)-sə-'līt-əs\ *n* : inflammation of the pharynx and the tonsils

pha·ryn·go·tym·pan·ic tube \-tim-'pan-ik-\ *n* : EUSTACHIAN TUBE

O

P

phar·ynx \'far-iŋ(k)s\ *n, pl* **pha·ryn·ges** \fə-'rin-(ˌ)jēz\ *also* **phar·ynx·es** : the part of the digestive and respiratory tracts situated between the cavity of the mouth and the esophagus and in humans being a conical musculomembranous tube about four and a half inches (11.43 centimeters) long that is continuous above with the mouth and nasal passages, communicates through the eustachian tubes with the ears, and extends downward past the opening into the larynx to the lower border of the cricoid cartilage where it is continuous with the esophagus — see LARYNGOPHARYNX, NASOPHARYNX, OROPHARYNX

phase \'fāz\ *n* **1** : a particular appearance or state in a regularly recurring cycle of changes **2** : a distinguishable part in a course, development, or cycle ⟨the early ∼s of a disease⟩ **3** : a point or stage in the period of a periodic motion or process (as a light wave or a vibration) in relation to an arbitrary reference or starting point in the period **4** : a homogeneous, physically distinct, and mechanically separable portion of matter present in a nonhomogeneous physicochemical system; *esp* : one of the fundamental states of matter usu. considered to include the solid, liquid, and gaseous forms **5** : an individual or subgroup distinguishably different in appearance or behavior from the norm of the group to which it belongs; *also* : the distinguishing peculiarity

phase–contrast *adj* : of or employing the phase-contrast microscope ⟨∼ optics⟩

phase–contrast microscope *n* : a microscope that translates differences in phase of the light transmitted through or reflected by the object into differences of intensity in the image — called also *phase-difference microscope, phase microscope*

phase–contrast microscopy *n* : use of or investigation with the phase-contrast microscope — called also *phase microscopy*

phase–difference microscope *n* : PHASE-CONTRAST MICROSCOPE

phase microscope *n* : PHASE-CONTRAST MICROSCOPE

phase microscopy *n* : PHASE-CONTRAST MICROSCOPY

pha·seo·lu·na·tin \ˌfā-sē-ō-'lü-nə-ˌtin\ *n* : LINAMARIN

pha·sic \'fā-zik\ *adj* **1** : of, relating to, or of the nature of a phase : having phases **2** : reacting rapidly and strongly to a stimulus but quickly adapting and having a short period of excitation ⟨∼ receptors⟩ — **pha·si·cal·ly** \-zi-k(ə-)lē\ *adv*

phas·mid \'fas-mid\ *n* : either of the paired lateral postanal organs characteristic of most parasitic nematodes and usu. regarded as chemoreceptors — see PHASMIDIA

Phas·mid·ia \faz-'mid-ē-ə\ *n pl* : a subclass of Nematoda comprising worms having typically papillose sensory organs, phasmids, lateral cervical papillae, and simple lateral sensory depressions at the anterior end which resemble pores — compare APHASMIDIA — **phas·mid·ian** \-ən\ *n*

PhD \ˌpē-ˌāch-'dē\ *abbr or n* **1** : an earned academic degree conferring the rank and title of doctor of philosophy **2** : a person who has a doctor of philosophy

Phe *abbr* phenylalanine; phenylalanyl

phe·na·caine \'fē-nə-ˌkān, 'fen-ə-\ *n* : a crystalline base that has been used as a local anesthetic in the form of its hydrochloride $C_{18}H_{22}N_2O_2 \cdot HCl$

phen·ac·e·tin \fi-'nas-ət-ən\ *n* : a compound $C_{10}H_{13}NO_2$ formerly used to ease pain or fever but now withdrawn from use because of its link to high blood pressure, heart attacks, cancer, and kidney disease — called also *acetophenetidin*

phen·ace·tu·ric acid \ˌfen-ˌas-ə-ˌt(y)ùr-ik-\ *n* : a crystalline amido acid $C_{10}H_{11}NO_3$ found in the urine of the horse and sometimes in that of humans

phen·an·threne \fə-'nan-ˌthrēn\ *n* : a crystalline aromatic hydrocarbon $C_{14}H_{10}$ of coal tar isomeric with anthracene

phen·an·thri·dine \fi-'nan(t)-thrə-ˌdēn\ *n* : a crystalline base $C_{13}H_9N$ isomeric with acridine

phe·nan·thri·din·i·um \fi-ˌnan(t)-thrə-'din-ē-əm\ *n* : the ion $[C_{13}H_9NH]^+$ derived from phenanthridine and occurring in substituted form in quaternary salts used as trypanocides

phe·nate \'fē-ˌnāt, 'fe-\ *n* : PHENOXIDE

phen·azine \'fen-ə-ˌzēn\ *n* : a yellowish crystalline base

$C_{12}H_8N_2$ that is the parent compound of many dyes and a few antibiotics

phe·naz·o·cine \fi-'naz-ə-ˌsēn\ *n* : a drug $C_{22}H_{27}NO$ related to morphine that has greater pain-relieving and slighter narcotic effect

phen·a·zone \'fen-ə-ˌzōn\ *n* : ANTIPYRINE

phen·cy·cli·dine \(')fen-'sik-lə-ˌdēn, -'sī-klə-, -dən\ *n* : a piperidine derivative used chiefly in the form of its hydrochloride $C_{17}H_{25}N \cdot HCl$ esp. as a veterinary anesthetic and sometimes illicitly as a psychedelic drug to induce vivid mental imagery — called also *angel dust, PCP*

phen·di·met·ra·zine \ˌfen-dī-'me-trə-ˌzēn\ *n* : an appetite suppressant that is a sympathetic amine with pharmacological activity similar to the amphetamines and is administered orally usu. in the form of its bitartrate $C_{12}H_{17}NO \cdot C_4H_6O_6$ to assist weight reduction esp. in the treatment of obesity

phen·el·zine \'fen-ᵊl-ˌzēn\ *n* : a monoamine oxidase inhibitor $C_8H_{12}N_2$ that suppresses REM sleep and is used esp. as an antidepressant drug — see NARDIL

Phen·er·gan \fen-'ər-ˌgan\ *trademark* — used for a preparation of the hydrochloride of promethazine

phe·neth·i·cil·lin \fi-ˌneth-ə-'sil-ən\ *n* : a semisynthetic penicillin administered orally in the form of its potassium salt $C_{17}H_{19}KN_2O_5S$ and used esp. in the treatment of less severe infections caused by bacteria that do not produce beta⸗lactamase

phen·eth·yl alcohol \ˌfen-'eth-əl-\ *n* : PHENYLETHYL ALCOHOL

phe·net·i·dine \fə-'net-ə-ˌdēn\ *also* **phe·net·i·din** \-dən\ *n* : any of three liquid basic amino derivatives $C_8H_{11}NO$ of phenetole used esp. in manufacturing dyestuffs and in the preparation of phenacetin

phen·e·tole \'fen-ə-ˌtōl\ *n* : the aromatic liquid ethyl ether $C_8H_{10}O$ of phenol

phen–fen \'fen-ˌfen\ *n* : FEN-PHEN

phen·for·min \fen-'fòr-mən\ *n* : a biguanide $C_{10}H_{15}N_5$ formerly used to treat diabetes but now withdrawn from use because of its link to life-threatening lactic acidosis

phen·in·di·one \ˌfen-in-'dī-ˌōn\ *n* : an anticoagulant drug $C_{15}H_{10}O_2$

phen·ip·ra·zine \(')fen-'ip-rə-ˌzēn\ *n* : a monoamine oxidase inhibitor $C_9H_{14}N_2$

phen·ir·amine \(')fen-'ir-ə-ˌmēn, -mən\ *n* : a drug used in the form of its maleate $C_{16}H_{20}N_2 \cdot C_4H_4O_4$ as an antihistamine

phen·met·ra·zine \(')fen-'me-trə-ˌzēn\ *n* : a sympathomimetic stimulant used in the form of its hydrochloride $C_{11}H_{15}NO \cdot HCl$ as an appetite suppressant — see PRELUDIN

phe·no·barb \'fē-nō-ˌbärb\ *n* : PHENOBARBITAL; *also* : a pill containing phenobarbital

phe·no·bar·bi·tal \ˌfē-nō-'bär-bə-ˌtól, -ˌtȧl\ *n* : a crystalline barbiturate $C_{12}H_{12}N_2O_3$ that is used orally or is administered by injection in the form of its sodium salt $C_{12}H_{11}N_2NaO_3$ as a hypnotic and sedative — see LUMINAL

phe·no·bar·bi·tone \-bə-ˌtōn\ *n, chiefly Brit* : PHENOBARBITAL

phe·no·copy \'fē-nə-ˌkäp-ē\ *n, pl* **-cop·ies** : a phenotypic variation that is caused by unusual environmental conditions and resembles the normal expression of a genotype other than its own

phe·no·ge·net·ics \ˌfē-nə-jə-'net-iks\ *n pl but sing in constr* : the part of genetics that deals with the mechanisms of development and the differentiation of the concrete qualities controlled by the genes

phe·nol \'fē-ˌnōl, -ˌnól, fi-'\ *n* **1** : a corrosive poisonous crystalline acidic compound C_6H_5OH present in coal tar and wood tar that is used in the manufacture of resins and plastics, dyes, and pharmaceuticals (as aspirin) and as a topical anesthetic in dilute solution — called also *carbolic, carbolic acid, hydroxybenzene* **2** : any of various acidic compounds analogous to phenol and regarded as hydroxyl derivatives of aromatic hydrocarbons

phe·no·lase \'fen-ə-ˌlās, -ˌlāz\ *n* : PHENOL OXIDASE

phe·no·late \'fēn-ᵊl-ˌāt\ *n* : PHENOXIDE

phe·no·lat·ed \\'fēn-ᵊl-‚āt-əd\ *adj* : treated, mixed, or impregnated with phenol

phenol coefficient *n* : a number relating the germicidal efficiency of a compound to phenol regarded as having an arbitrarily assigned value of 1 toward specified bacteria (as typhoid bacteria) under specified conditions

¹**phe·no·lic** \fi-'nō-lik, -'näl-ik\ *adj* : of, relating to, or having the characteristics of a phenol; *also* : containing or derived from a phenol

²**phenolic** *n* : PHENOL 2

phenol oxidase *n* : any of various copper-containing enzymes that promote the oxidation of phenols — called also *phenolase*

phe·nol·phtha·lein \‚fēn-ᵊl-'thal-ē-ən, -'thal-‚ēn, -'thāl-\ *n* : a white or yellowish white crystalline compound $C_{20}H_{14}O_4$ that is used in analysis as an indicator because its solution is brilliant red in alkalies and is decolorized by acids and that is used in medicine as a laxative

phenol red *n* : PHENOLSULFONPHTHALEIN

phe·nol·sul·fo·nate *or chiefly Brit* **phe·nol·sul·pho·nate** \‚fēn-ᵊl-'səl-fə-‚nāt\ *n* : a salt of a phenolsulfonic acid

phe·nol·sul·fon·ic acid *or chiefly Brit* **phe·nol·sul·phon·ic acid** \‚səl-'fän-ik, -'fōn-\ *n* : a sulfonic acid derived from phenol; *esp* : a crystalline acid $C_6H_6O_4S$ used chiefly as an intermediate for dyes and pharmaceuticals

phe·nol·sul·fon·phtha·lein *or chiefly Brit* **phe·nol·sul·phon·phtha·lein** \-‚səl-fän-'thal-ē-ən, -'thal-‚ēn, -'thāl-\ *n* : a red crystalline compound $C_{19}H_{14}O_5S$ used chiefly as a test of kidney function and as an acid-base indicator — called also *phenol red*

phenolsulfonphthalein test *n* : a test in which phenolsulfonphthalein is administered by injection and urine samples are subsequently taken at regular intervals to measure the rate at which it is excreted by the kidneys

phe·nol·tet·ra·io·do·phtha·lein \‚fēn-ᵊl-te-trə-‚ī-‚ōd-ə-'thal-ē-ən, -'thal-‚ēn, -'thāl-\ *n* : PHENTETIOTHALEIN

phe·nom·e·nol·o·gy \fi-‚näm-ə-'näl-ə-jē\ *n, pl* **-gies** : the way in which one perceives and interprets events and one's relationship to them in contrast both to one's objective responses to stimuli and to any inferred unconscious motivation for one's behavior; *also* : a psychology based on the theory that phenomenology determines behavior — **phe·nom·e·no·log·i·cal** \fi-‚näm-ən-ᵊl-'äj-i-kəl\ *adj*

phe·nom·e·non \fi-'näm-ə-‚nän, -nən\ *n, pl* **-na** \-nə, -‚nä\ **1** : an observable fact or event **2 a** : an object or aspect known through the senses rather than by thought or intuition **b** : a fact or event of scientific interest susceptible of scientific description and explanation

phe·no·thi·azine \‚fē-nō-'thī-ə-‚zēn\ *n* **1** : a greenish yellow crystalline compound $C_{12}H_9NS$ used as an anthelmintic and insecticide esp. in veterinary practice — called also *thiodiphenylamine* **2** : any of various phenothiazine derivatives (as chlorpromazine) that are used as tranquilizing agents esp. in the treatment of schizophrenia

phe·no·type \'fē-nə-‚tīp\ *n* : the observable properties of an organism that are produced by the interaction of the genotype and the environment — compare GENOTYPE 2 — **phe·no·typ·ic** \‚fē-nə-'tip-ik\ *also* **phe·no·typ·i·cal** \-i-kəl\ *adj* — **phe·no·typ·i·cal·ly** \-i-k(ə-)lē\ *adv*

phen·ox·ide \fi-'näk-‚sīd\ *n* : a salt of a phenol esp. in its capacity as a weak acid — called also *phenate, phenolate*

phe·noxy \fi-'näk-sē\ *adj* : containing the group $C_6H_5O–$

phe·noxy·ace·tic acid \fi-‚näk-sē-ə-‚sēt-ik-\ *n* : an acid $C_8H_8O_3$ used as a fungicide and in plasters and pads to soften callused skin surfaces

phe·noxy·ben·za·mine \-'ben-zə-‚mēn\ *n* : a drug that blocks the activity of alpha-receptors and is used in the form of its hydrochloride $C_{18}H_{22}ClNO·HCl$ esp. in the treatment of hypertension and sweating due to pheochromocytoma

phe·noxy·meth·yl penicillin \-'meth-əl-\ *n* : PENICILLIN V

phen·pro·cou·mon \‚fen-prō-'kü-‚män\ *n* : an anticoagulant drug $C_{18}H_{16}O_3$

phen·sux·i·mide \‚fen-'sək-si-‚mīd\ *n* : an anticonvulsant

drug $C_{11}H_{11}NO_2$ sometimes used in the treatment of absence seizures — see MILONTIN

phen·ter·mine \'fen-tər-‚mēn\ *n* : an anorectic drug administered in the form of its hydrochloride $C_{10}H_{15}N·HCl$ to treat obesity

phen·tet·io·tha·lein \‚fen-‚tet-ī-ō-'thal-ē-ən, -'thāl-\ *n* : a substance or its disodium salt $C_{20}H_8I_4Na_2O_4$ isomeric with iodophthalein used esp. formerly as a radiopaque medium in cholecystography and in tests of liver function — called also *phenoltetraiodophthalein*

phen·tol·amine \fen-'täl-ə-‚mēn, -mən\ *n* : an adrenergic blocking agent that is administered by injection in the form of its mesylate $C_{17}H_{19}N_3O·CH_4O_3S$ esp. in the diagnosis and treatment of hypertension due to pheochromocytoma — see REGITINE

phe·nyl \'fen-ᵊl, 'fēn-, *Brit also* 'fē-‚nīl\ *n* : a monovalent group C_6H_5 that is an aryl group derived from benzene by removal of one hydrogen atom — often used in combination ⟨*phenyl*alanine⟩

phe·nyl·acet·amide \‚fen-ᵊl-ə-'set-ə-‚mīd, ‚fēn-ᵊl-, -'as-ət-ə-‚mīd\ *n* : ACETANILIDE

phe·nyl·ace·tic acid \‚fen-ᵊl-ə-‚sēt-ik-, ‚fēn-\ *n* : a crystalline acid $C_8H_8O_2$ used chiefly in the manufacture of penicillin

phe·nyl·al·a·nine \‚fen-ᵊl-'al-ə-‚nēn, ‚fēn-\ *n* : an essential amino acid $C_9H_{11}NO_2$ that is obtained in its levorotatory L-form by the hydrolysis of proteins (as lactalbumin), that is essential in human nutrition, and that is converted in the normal body to tyrosine — abbr. *Phe*; see PHENYLKETONURIA, PHENYLPYRUVIC ACID

phenylalanine mustard *or* L–**phenylalanine mustard** \'el-\ *n* : MELPHALAN

phe·nyl·al·a·nyl \‚fen-ᵊl-'al-ə-‚nil\ *n* : the amino acid radical or residue $C_6H_5CH_2CH(NH_2)CO–$ of phenylalanine — abbr. *Phe*

phen·yl·bu·ta·zone \‚fen-ᵊl-'byüt-ə-‚zōn\ *n* : a drug $C_{19}H_{20}N_2O_2$ that is used for its analgesic and anti-inflammatory properties esp. in the treatment of arthritis, gout, and bursitis — see BUTAZOLIDIN

phen·yl·ene \'fen-ᵊl-‚ēn\ *n* : any of three bivalent radicals C_6H_4 derived from benzene by removal of two hydrogen atoms from the ortho, meta, or para positions

phe·nyl·ene·di·amine \'fen-ᵊl-‚ēn-'dī-ə-‚mēn, 'fēn-\ *n* : any of three toxic isomeric crystalline compounds $C_6H_8N_2$ that are derivatives of benzene containing two amino groups attached to carbon atoms in the ortho, meta, or para positions — see QUINOXALINE

phen·yl·eph·rine \‚fen-ᵊl-'ef-‚rēn, -rən\ *n* : a sympathomimetic agent with vasoconstrictive properties that is used in the form of its hydrochloride $C_9H_{13}NO_2·HCl$ esp. as a nasal decongestant and mydriatic and to raise blood pressure — see NEO-SYNEPHRINE

phe·nyl·eth·yl alcohol \'fen-ᵊl-'eth-əl-, 'fēn-\ *n* : a fragrant liquid alcohol $C_8H_{10}O$ that is found in rose oil and neroli oil but is usu. made synthetically and that is used in flavorings and perfumes and as an antibacterial agent in ophthalmic solutions with limited effectiveness — called also *phenethyl alcohol*

phe·nyl·eth·yl·amine \‚fen-ᵊl-‚eth-əl-'am-‚ēn, ‚fēn-\ *n* : a neurotransmitter $C_8H_{11}N$ that is an amine resembling amphetamine in structure and pharmacological properties; *also* : any of various derivatives of phenylethylamine

phe·nyl·eth·y·lene \‚fen-ᵊl-'eth-ə-‚lēn, ‚fēn-\ *n* : STYRENE

phe·nyl·hy·dra·zine \‚fen-ᵊl-'hī-drə-‚zēn, ‚fēn-\ *n* : a toxic liquid nitrogen base $C_6H_8N_2$ that reacts with aldehydes and ketones to form compounds useful in the identification of sugars

phe·nyl·hy·dra·zone \-'hī-drə-‚zōn\ *n* : a hydrazone derived from phenylhydrazine

---

\ə\ **abut** \ᵊ\ **kitten** \ər\ **further** \a\ **ash** \ā\ **ace** \ä\ **cot, cart**
\aù\ **out** \ch\ **chin** \e\ **bet** \ē\ **easy** \g\ **go** \i\ **hit** \ī\ **ice** \j\ **job**
\ŋ\ **sing** \ō\ **go** \ò\ **law** \òi\ **boy** \th\ **thin** \th̲\ **the** \ü\ **loot**
\ù\ **foot** \y\ **yet** \zh\ **vision** *See also* Pronunciation Symbols page

O
P

phe·nyl·ic \fə-'nil-ik\ *adj* : relating to, derived from, or containing phenyl

phe·nyl·ke·ton·uria \ˌfen-ᵊl-ˌkēt-ᵊn-'(y)ùr-ē-ə, ˌfēn-\ *n* : a metabolic disorder that is caused by an enzyme deficiency resulting in the accumulation of phenylalanine and its metabolites (as phenylpyruvic acid) in the blood and their excess excretion in the urine, that is inherited as an autosomal recessive trait, and that causes usu. severe mental retardation, seizures, eczema, and abnormal body odor unless phenylalanine is restricted from the diet beginning at birth — *abbr. PKU*; called also *phenylpyruvic amentia, phenylpyruvic oligophrenia*

¹phe·nyl·ke·ton·uric \-'(y)ùr-ik\ *n* : one affected with phenylketonuria

²phenylketonuric *adj* : of, relating to, or affected with phenylketonuria

phen·yl·mer·cu·ric \ˌfen-ᵊl-mər-'kyùr-ik\ *adj* : being a salt containing the positively charged ion $[C_6H_5Hg]^+$

phenylmercuric acetate *n* : a crystalline salt $C_8H_8HgO_2$ made by reaction of benzene with acetate of bivalent mercury in alcoholic solution and used chiefly as a fungicide and herbicide

phenylmercuric nitrate *n* : a crystalline basic salt that is a mixture of $C_6H_5HgNO_3$ and C_6H_5HgOH used chiefly as a fungicide and antiseptic

phen·yl·pro·pa·nol·amine \ˌfen-ᵊl-ˌprō-pə-'nòl-ə-ˌmēn, -'nōl-; -nò-'lam-ˌēn\ *n* : a sympathomimetic agent that has been used in the form of its hydrochloride $C_9H_{13}NO·HCl$ esp. as a nasal decongestant and appetite suppressant but has been largely withdrawn from use because of its link to hemorrhagic stroke — *abbr. PPA*

phe·nyl·py·ru·vate \ˌfen-ᵊl-pī-'rü-ˌvāt, ˌfēn-\ *n* : a salt or ester of phenylpyruvic acid

phe·nyl·py·ru·vic acid \-pī-ˌrü-vik-\ *n* : a crystalline keto acid $C_9H_8O_3$ found in the urine as a metabolic product of phenylalanine esp. in phenylketonuria

phenylpyruvic amentia *n* : PHENYLKETONURIA

phenylpyruvic oligophrenia *n* : PHENYLKETONURIA

phenyl salicylate *n* : a crystalline ester $C_{13}H_{10}O_3$ used chiefly as a stabilizer for cellulosic plastics and vinyl plastics and as an ingredient of suntan preparations because of its ability to absorb ultraviolet light and also as an analgesic and antipyretic — called also *salol*

phen·yl·thio·car·ba·mide \ˌfen-ᵊl-ˌthī-ō-'kär-bə-ˌmīd\ *n* : a crystalline compound $C_7H_8N_2S$ that is extremely bitter or tasteless depending on the presence or absence of a single dominant gene in the taster — called also *phenylthiourea, PTC*

phen·yl·thio·urea \-ˌthī-ō-yù-'rē-ə\ *n* : PHENYLTHIOCARBAMIDE

phe·nyt·o·in \fə-'nit-ə-wən\ *n* : an anticonvulsant used in the treatment of epilepsy often in the form of its sodium salt $C_{15}H_{11}N_2NaO_2$ — called also *diphenylhydantoin;* see DILANTIN

pheo·chrome *or Brit* **phaeo·chrome** \'fē-ə-ˌkrōm\ *adj* : CHROMAFFIN ⟨~ tissue⟩ ⟨~ tumors⟩

pheo·chro·mo·blast *or Brit* **phaeo·chro·mo·blast** \ˌfē-ō-'krō-mə-ˌblast\ *n* : an embryonic cell destined to give rise to chromaffin tissue esp. of the adrenal medulla

pheo·chro·mo·cyte *or Brit* **phaeo·chro·mo·cyte** \ˌfē-ə-'krō-mə-ˌsīt\ *n* : a chromaffin cell

pheo·chro·mo·cy·to·ma *or Brit* **phaeo·chro·mo·cy·to·ma** \ˌfē-ə-'krō-mə-sə-'tō-mə, -sī-\ *n, pl* **-mas** *also* **-ma·ta** \-mət-ə\ : a tumor that is derived from chromaffin cells and is usu. associated with paroxysmal or sustained hypertension

pheo·phor·bide *or Brit* **phaeo·phor·bide** \ˌfē-ə-'fòr-ˌbīd\ *n* : a blue-black crystalline acid obtained from chlorophyll or pheophytin by treatment with hydrochloric acid

pheo·phy·tin *or Brit* **phaeo·phy·tin** \ˌfē-ə-'fīt-ᵊn\ *n* : a bluish black waxy pigment that can be formed from chlorophyll by replacement of the magnesium with two hydrogen atoms by treatment with a weak acid (as oxalic acid)

phe·ren·ta·sin \fə-'ren-tə-sən\ *n* : a pressor amine present in the blood in severe hypertension

phe·re·sis \fə-'rē-səs\ *n, pl* **phe·re·ses** \-ˌsēz\ : APHERESIS

pher·o·mon·al \ˌfer-ə-'mōn-ᵊl\ *adj* : of or relating to a pheromone — **pher·o·mon·al·ly** \-ē\ *adv*

pher·o·mone \'fer-ə-ˌmōn\ *n* : a chemical substance that is produced by an animal and serves esp. as a stimulus to other individuals of the same species for one or more behavioral responses — called also *ectohormone*

PhG *abbr* graduate in pharmacy

phi·al \'fī(-ə)l\ *n* : VIAL

Phi·a·loph·o·ra \ˌfī-ə-'läf-(ə-)rə\ *n* : a form genus (family Dematiaceae) of imperfect fungi of which some forms are important in human mycotic infections (as chromoblastomycosis)

Phil·a·del·phia chromosome \ˌfil-ə-'del-fē-ə-\ *n* : an abnormally short chromosome 22 that is found in the hematopoietic cells of persons affected with chronic myelogenous leukemia and lacks the major part of its long arm which has usu. undergone translocation to chromosome 9

phil·ter *or chiefly Brit* **phil·tre** \'fil-tər\ *n* : a potion, drug, or charm held to have the power to arouse sexual passion

phil·trum \'fil-trəm\ *n, pl* **phil·tra** \-trə\ : the vertical groove on the median line of the upper lip

phi·mo·sis \fī-'mō-səs, fi-\ *n, pl* **phi·mo·ses** \-ˌsēz\ : tightness or constriction of the orifice of the foreskin arising either congenitally or postnatally (as from balanoposthitis) and preventing retraction of the foreskin over the glans

phi phenomenon \'fī-\ *n* : apparent motion resulting from an orderly sequence of stimuli (as lights flashed in rapid succession a short distance apart on a sign) without any actual motion being presented to the eye — compare APPARENT MOTION

phleb·ec·ta·sia \ˌfleb-ek-'tā-zh(ē-)ə\ *n* : dilation of a vein : VARICOSITY 1, VARICOSIS

phle·bit·ic \fli-'bit-ik\ *adj* : of or relating to phlebitis ⟨a severe ~ condition⟩

phle·bi·tis \fli-'bīt-əs\ *n, pl* **phle·bit·i·des** \-'bit-ə-ˌdēz\ : inflammation of a vein

phle·bo·cly·sis \ˌflē-bō-'klī-səs\ *n, pl* **-cly·ses** \-ˌsēz\ : administration of a large volume of fluid intravenously

phle·bo·gram \'flē-bə-ˌgram\ *n* **1** : a tracing made with a sphygmograph that records the pulse in a vein **2** : a radiograph of a vein after injection of a radiopaque medium

phle·bo·graph \-ˌgraf\ *n* : a sphygmograph adapted for recording the venous pulse

phle·bog·ra·phy \fli-'bäg-rə-fē\ *n, pl* **-phies** : the process of making phlebograms — **phle·bo·graph·ic** \ˌflē-bə-'graf-ik\ *adj*

phle·bo·lith \'flē-bə-ˌlith\ *n* : a calculus in a vein usu. resulting from the calcification of an old thrombus

phle·bol·o·gist \fli-'bäl-ə-jəst\ *n* : a specialist in phlebology

phle·bol·o·gy \fli-'bäl-ə-jē\ *n, pl* **-gies** : a branch of medicine concerned with the veins

phle·bo·ma·nom·e·ter \ˌflē-bō-mə-'näm-ət-ər\ *n* : an instrument for measuring venous blood pressure

phle·bor·rha·phy \fli-'bòr-ə-fē\ *n, pl* **-phies** : the suturing of a vein

phle·bo·scle·ro·sis \ˌflē-bō-sklə-'rō-səs\ *n, pl* **-ro·ses** \-ˌsēz\ : sclerosis of the wall of a vein and esp. of its inner coats — called also *venofibrosis*

phle·bo·scle·rot·ic \-sklə-'rät-ik\ *adj* : of, relating to, or affected by phlebosclerosis

phle·bos·ta·sis \fli-'bäs-tə-səs\ *n, pl* **-ta·ses** \-ˌsēz\ : abnormally slow venous blood circulation

phle·bo·throm·bo·sis \ˌflē-bō-thräm-'bō-səs\ *n, pl* **-bo·ses** \-ˌsēz\ : venous thrombosis accompanied by little or no inflammation — compare THROMBOPHLEBITIS

phle·bot·o·mist \fli-'bät-ə-məst\ *n* : one who practices phlebotomy

phle·bot·o·mize *also Brit* **phle·bot·o·mise** \fli-'bät-ə-ˌmīz\ *vb* **-mized** *also Brit* **-mised; -miz·ing** *also Brit* **-mis·ing** *vt* : to draw blood from : BLEED ~ *vi* : to practice phlebotomy

phle·bot·o·mus \fli-'bät-ə-məs\ *n* **1** *cap* : a genus of small bloodsucking sand flies (family Psychodidae) including one (*P. papatasii*) that is the carrier of sandfly fever and others suspected of carrying other human disease 2 *pl* **-mi** \-ˌmī\ *also* **-mus·es** : any sand fly of the genus *Phlebotomus*

phlebotomus fever *n* : SANDFLY FEVER

phle·bot·o·my \fli-ˈbät-ə-mē\ *n, pl* **-mies** : the letting of blood for transfusion, apheresis, diagnostic testing, or experimental procedures and widely used in the past to treat many types of disease but now limited to the treatment of only a few specific conditions (as hemochromatosis and polycythemia vera) — called also *venesection, venotomy*

Phle·bo·vi·rus \ˈflē-bə-ˌvī-rəs\ *n* : a genus of single-stranded RNA viruses of the family *Bunyaviridae* that includes the causative agents of Rift Valley fever and sandfly fever

phlegm \ˈflem\ *n* **1** : the one of the four humors of ancient and medieval physiology that was believed to be cold and moist and to cause sluggishness **2** : viscid mucus secreted in abnormal quantity in the respiratory passages

phleg·ma·sia \fleg-ˈmā-zh(ē-)ə\ *n, pl* **-si·ae** \-zh(ē-)ē\ : INFLAMMATION

phlegmasia al·ba do·lens \-ˈal-bə-ˈdō-ˌlenz\ *n* : MILK LEG

phlegmasia ce·ru·lea dolens \-sə-ˈrü-lē-ə-\ *n* : severe thrombophlebitis with extreme pain, edema, cyanosis, and possible ischemic necrosis

phleg·mat·ic \fleg-ˈmat-ik\ *adj* **1** : resembling, consisting of, or producing the humor phlegm **2** : having or showing a slow and stolid temperament — **phleg·mat·i·cal·ly** \-i-k(ə-)lē\ *adv*

phleg·mon \ˈfleg-ˌmän\ *n* : a purulent inflammation and infiltration of connective tissue ⟨an acute ∼ of the tongue —R. L. Cecil & R. F. Loeb⟩ — compare ABSCESS

phleg·mon·ous \ˈfleg-mə-nəs\ *adj* : of, relating to, or constituting a phlegmon : accompanied by or characterized by phlegmons ⟨∼ pancreatic lesions⟩ — **phleg·mon·ous·ly** *adv*

phlo·gis·tic \flō-ˈjis-tik\ *adj* : of or relating to inflammations and fevers

phlog·o·gen·ic \ˌfläg-ə-ˈjen-ik\ *also* **phlo·gog·e·nous** \flō-ˈgäj-ə-nəs\ *adj* : producing inflammation ⟨a ∼ substance⟩

phlor·e·tin \ˈflȯr-ət-ən, flə-ˈrēt-ᵊn\ *n* : a crystalline phenolic ketone $C_{15}H_{14}O_5$ that is obtained esp. by hydrolysis of phlorizin and is a potent inhibitor of transport systems for sugars and anions

phlo·ri·zin *or* **phlo·rhi·zin** \ˈflȯr-ə-zən, ˈflȯr-; flə-ˈrīz-ᵊn\ *or* **phlo·rid·zin** \ˈflȯr-əd-zən, ˈflȯr-; flə-ˈrid-zən\ *n* : a bitter crystalline glucoside $C_{21}H_{24}O_{10}$ that is extracted from root bark or bark (as of the apple, pear, or cherry), produces glycosuria if injected hypodermically, and is used chiefly in producing experimental diabetes in animals

phlo·ri·zin·ized *also* **phlo·rhi·zin·ized** \ˈflȯr-ə-zə-ˌnīzd, ˈflȯr-; flə-ˈrīz-ə-ˌnīzd\ *or* **phlo·rid·zin·ized** \-əd-zə-ˌnīzd; -ˈrid-zə-ˌnīzd\ *adj* : having been administered phlorizin ⟨a ∼ dog⟩

phlor·o·glu·cin \ˌflȯr-ə-ˈglüs-ᵊn\ *n* : PHLOROGLUCINOL

phlor·o·glu·cin·ol \-ˈglüs-ᵊn-ˌȯl, -ˌōl\ *n* : a sweet crystalline phenol $C_6H_6O_3$ that occurs in combined form in glycosides (as phlorizin), in resins, and in tannins and that is usu. made from trinitrotoluene by a series of steps

phlox·ine \ˈfläk-ˌsēn, -sən\ *n* : either of two acid dyes or their sodium salts that are derivatives of eosin and are used chiefly as biological stains and organic pigments: **a** : one containing two atoms of chlorine in each molecule — called also *phloxine B* **b** : one containing four atoms of chlorine in each molecule

phlyc·ten·u·lar \flik-ˈten-yə-lər\ *adj* : marked by or associated with phlyctenules ⟨∼ conjunctivitis⟩

phlyc·te·nule \flik-ˈten-(ˌ)yü(ə)l, ˈflik-tə-ˌn(y)ü(ə)l\ *n* : a small vesicle or pustule; *esp* : one on the conjunctiva or cornea of the eye

PHN *abbr* public health nurse

pho·bia \ˈfō-bē-ə\ *n* : an exaggerated and often disabling fear usu. inexplicable to the subject and having sometimes a logical but usu. an illogical or symbolic object, class of objects, or situation — compare COMPULSION, OBSESSION

pho·bi·ac \ˈfō-bē-ˌak\ *n* : PHOBIC

¹pho·bic \ˈfō-bik\ *adj* : of, relating to, affected with, marked by, involving, or constituting a phobia ⟨∼ disorders⟩ ⟨a ∼ person⟩ ⟨∼ anxiety⟩ ⟨∼ situations⟩

²phobic *n* : one who exhibits a phobia

phobic reaction *n* : a psychoneurosis in which the principal symptom is a phobia

pho·bo·pho·bia \ˌfō-bə-ˈfō-bē-ə\ *n* : excessive fear of acquiring a phobia

pho·co·me·lia \ˌfō-kə-ˈmē-lē-ə\ *n* : a congenital deformity in which the limbs are extremely shortened so that the feet and hands arise close to the trunk — **pho·co·me·lic** \-ˈmē-lik\ *adj*

pho·com·e·lus \fō-ˈkäm-ə-ləs\ *n, pl* **-li** \-ˌlī\ : an individual exhibiting phocomelia

phon \ˈfän\ *n* : the unit of loudness on a scale beginning at zero for the faintest audible sound and corresponding to the decibel scale of sound intensity with the number of phons of a given sound being equal to the decibels of a pure 1000= hertz tone judged by the average listener to be equal in loudness to the given sound

phon·as·the·nia \ˌfō-nəs-ˈthē-nē-ə\ *n* : weakness or hoarseness of voice

pho·na·tion \fō-ˈnā-shən\ *n* : the production of vocal sounds and esp. speech — **pho·nate** \ˈfō-ˌnāt\ *vi* **pho·nat·ed; pho·nat·ing**

pho·na·to·ry \ˈfō-nə-ˌtōr-ē\ *adj* : of or relating to the production of speech sounds

pho·neme \ˈfō-ˌnēm\ *n* : a member of the set of the smallest units of speech that serve to distinguish one utterance from another in a language or dialect ⟨the \p\ of English *pat* and the \f\ of English *fat* are two different ∼s⟩ — **pho·ne·mic** \fə-ˈnē-mik, fō-\ *adj* — **pho·ne·mi·cal·ly** \-mi-k(ə-)lē\ *adv*

pho·ne·mics \fə-ˈnē-miks, fō-\ *n pl but sing in constr* **1** : a branch of linguistic analysis that consists of the study of phonemes **2** : the structure of a language in terms of phonemes

pho·nen·do·scope \fō-ˈnen-də-ˌskōp\ *n* : a stethoscope equipped with a diaphragm for intensifying auscultatory sounds

pho·net·ic \fə-ˈnet-ik\ *adj* **1 a** : of or relating to spoken language or speech sounds **b** : of or relating to the science of phonetics **2** : representing the sounds and other phenomena of speech — **pho·net·i·cal·ly** \-i-k(ə-)lē\ *adv*

pho·net·ics \fə-ˈnet-iks\ *n pl but sing in constr* **1 a** : the study and systematic classification of the sounds made in spoken utterance **b** : the practical application of this science to language study **2** : the system of speech sounds of a language or group of languages

pho·ni·at·rics \ˌfō-nē-ˈa-triks\ *n pl but sing in constr* : the scientific study and treatment of defects of the voice — **pho·ni·at·ric** \-trik\ *adj*

pho·ni·a·try \fō-ˈnī-ə-trē\ *n, pl* **-tries** : PHONIATRICS

pho·nic \ˈfän-ik, *except 2b also* ˈfō-nik\ *adj* **1** : of, relating to, or producing sound **2 a** : of or relating to the sounds of speech **b** : of or relating to phonics — **pho·ni·cal·ly** \-(ə-)lē\ *adv*

pho·nics \ˈfän-iks, *1 is also* ˈfō-niks\ *n pl but sing in constr* **1** : the science of sound : ACOUSTICS **2** : a method of teaching beginners to read and pronounce words by learning the phonetic value of letters, letter groups, and esp. syllables

pho·nism \ˈfō-niz-əm\ *n* : a synesthetic auditory sensation

pho·no·car·dio·gram \ˌfō-nə-ˈkärd-ē-ə-ˌgram\ *n* : a graphic record of heart sounds made by means of a phonocardiograph

pho·no·car·dio·graph \-ˌgraf\ *n* : an instrument used for producing a graphic record of heart sounds and consisting of microphones, an amplifier, and recording equipment

pho·no·car·di·og·ra·phy \-ˌkärd-ē-ˈäg-rə-fē\ *n, pl* **-phies** : the recording of heart sounds by means of a phonocardiograph — **pho·no·car·dio·graph·ic** \-ˌkärd-ē-ə-ˈgraf-ik\ *adj*

pho·nol·o·gy \fə-ˈnäl-ə-jē, fō-\ *n, pl* **-gies** **1** : the science of

O
P

\ə\ abut \ᵊ\ kitten \ər\ further \a\ ash \ā\ ace \ä\ cot, cart \au̇\ out \ch\ chin \e\ bet \ē\ easy \g\ go \i\ hit \ī\ ice \j\ job \ŋ\ sing \ō\ go \ȯ\ law \ȯi\ boy \th\ thin \th̲\ the \ü\ loot \u̇\ foot \y\ yet \zh\ vision *See also* Pronunciation Symbols page

speech sounds including esp. the history and theory of sound changes in a language or in two or more related languages **2** : the phonetics and phonemics of a language at a particular time — **pho·no·log·i·cal** \ˌfōn-ᵊl-'äj-i-kəl *also* ˌfän-ᵊl-\ *also* **pho·no·log·ic** \-ik\ *adj* — **pho·no·log·i·cal·ly** \-i-k(ə-)lē\ *adv*

pho·nom·e·ter \fə-'näm-ət-ər\ *n* : an instrument for measuring the intensity of sound or the frequency of its vibration

pho·no·pho·bia \ˌfō-nə-'fō-bē-ə\ *n* : pathological fear of sound or of speaking aloud

pho·no·re·cep·tor \ˌfō-nō-ri-'sep-tər\ *n* : a receptor for sound stimuli

phor·bol \'for-ˌbȯl, -ˌbōl\ *n* : an alcohol $C_{20}H_{28}O_6$ that is the parent compound of tumor-promoting esters occurring in croton oil

pho·ria \'fō-rē-ə\ *n* : any of various tendencies of the lines of vision to deviate from the normal when binocular fusion of the retinal images is prevented

Phor·mia \'for-mē-ə\ *n* : a genus of dipteran flies of the family Calliphoridae including one (*P. regina*) causing myiasis in sheep

pho·rom·e·ter \fə-'räm-ət-ər\ *n* : an instrument for detecting and measuring imbalance in the extrinsic muscles of the eyes

pho·rom·e·try \-ə-trē\ *n, pl* **-tries** : examination of the eyes by means of a phorometer

Pho·rop·tor \fə-'räp-tər\ *trademark* — used for an instrument used to determine the corrective eyeglass lenses needed by an individual

phos·gene \'fäz-ˌjēn\ *n* : a colorless gas $COCl_2$ of unpleasant odor that is a severe respiratory irritant and has been used in chemical warfare

phos·pha·gen \'fäs-fə-jən, -ˌjen\ *n* : any of several organic phosphate compounds (as phosphocreatine or phosphoarginine) occurring esp. in muscle and releasing energy on hydrolysis of the phosphate

phos·pha·tase \'fäs-fə-ˌtās, -ˌtāz\ *n* : an enzyme that accelerates the hydrolysis and synthesis of organic esters of phosphoric acid and the transfer of phosphate groups to other compounds: **a** : ALKALINE PHOSPHATASE **b** : ACID PHOSPHATASE

phosphatase test *n* : a test for the efficiency of pasteurization of milk and other dairy products based on a determination of the activity of the phosphatase that is present in raw milk and is inactivated by proper pasteurization

phos·phate \'fäs-ˌfāt\ *n* **1 a** : a salt or ester of a phosphoric acid **b** : the trivalent anion PO_4^{3-} derived from phosphoric acid H_3PO_4 **2** : an organic compound of phosphoric acid in which the acid group is bound to nitrogen or a carboxyl group in a way that permits useful energy to be released (as in metabolism)

phos·pha·te·mia *or chiefly Brit* **phos·pha·tae·mia** \ˌfäs-fə-'tē-mē-ə\ *n* : the occurrence of phosphate in the blood esp. in excessive amounts

phos·phat·ic \fäs-'fat-ik, -'fāt-\ *adj* : of, relating to, or containing phosphoric acid or phosphates

phos·pha·tide \'fäs-fə-ˌtīd\ *n* : PHOSPHOLIPID — **phos·pha·tid·ic** \ˌfäs-fə-'tid-ik\ *adj*

phosphatidic acid *n* : any of several acids $(RCOO)_2C_3H_5OPO_3H_2$ that are formed from phosphatides by partial hydrolysis and that yield on hydrolysis two fatty-acid molecules RCOOH and one molecule each of glycerol and phosphoric acid

phos·pha·ti·dyl \ˌfäs-fə-'tīd-ᵊl, fäs-'fat-əd-ᵊl\ *n* : any of several monovalent groups $(RCOO)_2C_3H_5OPO(OH)$ that are derived from phosphatidic acids

phos·pha·ti·dyl·cho·line \ˌfäs-fə-ˌtīd-ᵊl-'kō-ˌlēn, (ˌ)fäs-ˌfat-əd-ᵊl-\ *n* : LECITHIN

phos·pha·ti·dyl·eth·a·nol·amine \-ˌeth-ə-'näl-ə-ˌmēn, -'nōl-\ *n* : any of a group of phospholipids that occur esp. in blood plasma and in the white matter of the central nervous system — called also *cephalin*

phos·pha·ti·dyl·ser·ine \-'se(ə)r-ˌēn\ *n* : a phospholipid found in mammalian cells

phos·pha·tu·ria \ˌfäs-fə-'t(y)ùr-ē-ə\ *n* : the excessive discharge of phosphates in the urine

phos·phene \'fäs-ˌfēn\ *n* : a luminous impression that occurs when the retina undergoes nonluminous stimulation (as by pressure on the eyeball when the lid is closed)

phos·phide \-ˌfīd\ *n* : a binary compound of phosphorus with a more electropositive element or group

phos·phine \-ˌfēn\ *n* **1** : a colorless poisonous flammable gas PH_3 that is a weaker base than ammonia and that is used esp. to fumigate stored grain **2** : any of various derivatives of phosphine analogous to amines but weaker as bases

phos·phite \-ˌfīt\ *n* : a salt or ester of phosphorous acid

phos·pho·ar·gi·nine \ˌfäs-(ˌ)fō-'är-jə-ˌnēn\ *n* : a compound $C_6H_{15}N_4O_5P$ of arginine and phosphoric acid that functions in various invertebrates (as crustaceans) in a way similar to that of phosphocreatine in vertebrates

phos·pho·cre·atine \ˌfäs-(ˌ)fō-'krē-ə-ˌtēn\ *n* : a compound $C_4H_{10}N_3O_5P$ of creatine and phosphoric acid that is found esp. in vertebrate muscle where it is an energy source for muscle contraction — called also *creatine phosphate*

phos·pho·di·es·ter \-dī-'es-tər\ *n* : an oligonucleotide with an oxygen atom linking consecutive nucleotides — see PHOSPHODIESTER BOND; compare PHOSPHOROTHIOATE

phos·pho·di·es·ter·ase \-dī-'es-tə-ˌrās, -ˌrāz\ *n* : a phosphatase (as from snake venom) that acts on diesters (as some nucleotides) to hydrolyze only one of the two ester groups

phosphodiester bond *n* : a covalent bond in RNA or DNA that holds a polynucleotide chain together by joining a phosphate group at position 5 in the pentose sugar of one nucleotide to the hydroxyl group at position 3 in the pentose sugar of the next nucleotide — called also *phosphodiester linkage*

phos·pho·enol·pyr·uvate \ˌfäs-fō-ə-ˌnōl-pī-'rü-ˌvāt, -ˌnōl-, -ˌpī(ə)r-'yü-\ *n* : a salt or ester of phosphoenolpyruvic acid — called also *phosphopyruvate*

phos·pho·enol·pyr·uvic acid \-pī-'rü-vik-, -ˌpī(ə)r-ˌyü-vik-\ *n* : the phosphate $H_2C=C(OPO_3H_2)COOH$ of the enol form of pyruvic acid that is formed as an intermediate in carbohydrate metabolism (as in the reversible dehydration of phosphoglyceric acid) — called also *phosphopyruvic acid*

phos·pho·fruc·to·ki·nase \ˌfäs-(ˌ)fō-ˌfrək-tō-'kī-ˌnās, -ˌfrük-, -ˌfrùk-, -ˌnāz\ *n* : an enzyme that functions in carbohydrate metabolism and esp. in glycolysis by catalyzing the transfer of a second phosphate group (as from ATP) to fructose

phos·pho·glu·co·mu·tase \-ˌglü-kō-'myü-ˌtās, -ˌtāz\ *n* : an enzyme of both plants and animals that catalyzes the reversible isomerization of glucose-1-phosphate to glucose-6-phosphate

phos·pho·glu·co·nate \-'glü-kə-ˌnāt\ *n* : a compound formed by dehydrogenation of glucose-6-phosphate as the first step in a glucose degradation pathway alternative to the Krebs cycle

phosphogluconate dehydrogenase *n* : an enzyme that catalyzes the oxidative decarboxylation of phosphogluconate with the generation of NADPH

phos·pho·glyc·er·al·de·hyde \-ˌglis-ə-'ral-də-ˌhīd\ *n* : a phosphate of glyceraldehyde $C_3H_5O_3(H_2PO_3)$ that is formed esp. in anaerobic metabolism of carbohydrates by the splitting of a diphosphate of fructose

phos·pho·glyc·er·ate \ˌfäs-fō-'glis-ə-ˌrāt\ *n* : a salt or ester of phosphoglyceric acid

phos·pho·glyc·er·ic acid \-glis-ˌer-ik-\ *n* : either of two isomeric phosphates $HOOCC_2H_3(OH)OPO_3H_2$ of glyceric acid that are formed as intermediates in photosynthesis and in carbohydrate metabolism

phos·pho·hexo·isom·er·ase \-ˌhek-sō-ī-'säm-ə-ˌrās, -ˌrāz\ *n* : an enzyme that catalyzes the reversible isomerization of glucose-6-phosphate to fructose-6-phosphate — called also *glucosephosphate isomerase, phosphohexose isomerase*

phos·pho·hex·ose isomerase \-'hek-ˌsōs-\ *n* : PHOSPHOHEXOISOMERASE

phos·pho·ino·si·tide \-in-'ō-sə-ˌtīd\ *n* : any of a group of inositol-containing derivatives of phosphatidic acid that do not contain nitrogen and are found in the brain

phos·pho·ki·nase \ˌfäs-fō-'kī-ˌnās, -ˌnāz\ *n* : KINASE

phos·pho·li·pase \-'lī-ˌpās, -ˌpāz\ *n* : any of several enzymes that hydrolyze lecithins or phosphatidylethanolamines — called also *lecithinase*

phos·pho·lip·id \-'lip-əd\ *also* **phos·pho·lip·ide** \-ˌīd\ *n* : any of numerous lipids (as lecithins and phosphatidylethanolamines) in which phosphoric acid as well as a fatty acid is esterified to glycerol and which are found in all living cells and in the bilayers of cell membranes — called also *phosphatide, phospholipin*

phos·pho·lip·in \-'lip-ən\ *n* : PHOSPHOLIPID

phos·pho·mo·lyb·dic acid \-mə-ˌlib-dik-\ *n* : any of several acids obtainable from solutions of phosphoric acid and molybdic acid and used chiefly as precipitants (as for alkaloids); *esp* : the yellow crystalline acid $H_3PMo_{12}O_{40}\cdot xH_2O$ containing twelve atoms of molybdenum in a molecule

phos·pho·mono·es·ter·ase \-ˌmän-ō-'es-tə-ˌrās, -ˌrāz\ *n* : a phosphatase that acts on monoesters

phos·pho·nate \'fäs-fə-ˌnāt\ *n* : a salt or ester of a phosphonic acid

phos·pho·ne·cro·sis \ˌfäs-fō-ni-'krō-səs\ *n, pl* **-cro·ses** : PHOSSY JAW

phos·phon·ic acid \ˌfäs-ˌfän-ik-\ *n* : any of a series of dibasic organic acids $RPO(OH)_2$ that are obtainable from some phosphines by oxidation

phos·pho·ni·um \fäs-'fō-nē-əm\ *n* : a monovalent cation PH_4^+ analogous to ammonium and derived from phosphine; *also* : an organic derivative of phosphonium (as $(C_2H_5)_4P^+$)

phos·pho·pro·tein \ˌfäs-fō-'prō-ˌtēn, -'prōt-ē-ən\ *n* : any of various proteins (as casein) that contain combined phosphoric acid

phos·pho·py·ru·vate \ˌfäs-fō-pī-'rü-ˌvāt, -ˌpī(ə)r-'yü-\ *n* : PHOSPHOENOLPYRUVATE

phos·pho·py·ru·vic acid \-pī-ˌrü-vik-, -ˌpī(ə)r-ˌyü-\ *n* : PHOSPHOENOLPYRUVIC ACID

phos·phor \'fäs-fər, -ˌfȯ(ə)r\ *also* **phos·phore** \-ˌfȯ(ə)r, -ˌfȯ(ə)r, -fər\ *n* : a phosphorescent substance; *specif* : a substance that emits light when excited by radiation

phos·pho·resce \ˌfäs-fə-'res\ *vi* **-resced; -resc·ing** : to exhibit phosphorescence

phos·pho·res·cence \-'res-ᵊn(t)s\ *n* **1** : luminescence that is caused by the absorption of radiation at one wavelength followed by delayed reradiation at a different wavelength and that continues for a noticeable time after the incident radiation stops **2** : an enduring luminescence without sensible heat

phos·pho·res·cent \-ᵊnt\ *adj* : exhibiting phosphorescence

phos·pho·ri·bo·syl·py·ro·phos·phate \ˌfäs-phō-ˌrī-bə-ˌsil-ˌpī-rō-'fäs-ˌfāt\ *n* : a substance that is formed enzymatically from ATP and the phosphate of ribose and that plays a fundamental role in nucleotide synthesis

phosphoribosyltransferase — see HYPOXANTHINE=GUANINE PHOSPHORIBOSYLTRANSFERASE

phos·pho·ric \fäs-'fȯr-ik, -'fär-; 'fäs-f(ə-)rik\ *adj* : of, relating to, or containing phosphorus esp. with a valence higher than in phosphorous compounds

phosphoric acid *n* **1** : a syrupy or deliquescent tribasic acid H_3PO_4 used esp. in preparing phosphates (as for fertilizers), in rust-proofing metals, and esp. formerly as a flavoring in soft drinks — called also *orthophosphoric acid* **2** : a compound (as pyrophosphoric acid or metaphosphoric acid) consisting of phosphate groups linked directly to each other by oxygen

phos·pho·rized *also Brit* **phos·pho·rised** \'fäs-fə-ˌrīzd\ *adj* : containing phosphorus ⟨∼ fat⟩

phos·pho·ro·clas·tic \ˌfäs-fə-rō-'klas-tik\ *adj* : of, relating to, or inducing a reaction in which a phosphate is involved in the splitting of a compound (as pyruvic acid)

phos·pho·rol·y·sis \ˌfäs-fə-'räl-ə-səs\ *n, pl* **-y·ses** \-ˌsēz\ : a reversible reaction analogous to hydrolysis in which phosphoric acid functions in a manner similar to that of water with the formation of a phosphate (as glucose-1-phosphate in the breakdown of liver glycogen) — **phos·pho·ro·lyt·ic** \-rō-'lit-ik\ *adj*

phos·pho·ro·thio·ate \ˌfäs-fə-rō-'thī-ō-ˌāt\ *n* : an oligonucleotide in which the oxygen atom normally linking two con-

secutive nucleotides has been replaced with sulfur and which resists degradation by cellular enzymes — compare PHOSPHODIESTER

phos·pho·rous \'fäs-f(ə-)rəs; fäs-'fōr-əs, -'fȯr-\ *adj* : of, relating to, or containing phosphorus esp. with a valence lower than in phosphoric compounds

phosphorous acid *n* : a deliquescent crystalline acid H_3PO_3 used esp. as a reducing agent and in making phosphites

phos·pho·rus \'fäs-f(ə)rəs\ *n, often attrib* : a nonmetallic multivalent element that occurs widely in combined form esp. as inorganic phosphates in minerals, soils, natural waters, bones, and teeth and as organic phosphates in all living cells and that exists in several allotropic forms — symbol *P*; see ELEMENT table

phosphorus pentoxide *n* : a compound known in various polymeric forms $(P_2O_5)_x$ that is obtained usu. by burning phosphorus in an excess of dry air, occurs as a white powder that reacts vigorously and sometimes explosively with water to form phosphoric acids irritating to the skin and mucous membranes, and is used chiefly as a drying agent, as a condensing agent in organic synthesis, and in making phosphoric acids and derivatives

phosphorus 32 \-ˌthərt-ē-'tü\ *n* : a heavy radioactive isotope of phosphorus having a mass number of 32 and a half-life of 14.3 days that is produced in nuclear reactors and used chiefly in tracer studies (as in biology and in chemical analysis) and in medical diagnosis (as in location of tumors) and therapy (as of polycythemia vera) — symbol P^{32} or ^{32}P

phos·pho·ryl \'fäs-fə-ˌril\ *n* : a usu. trivalent group PO consisting of phosphorus and oxygen

phos·phor·y·lase \fäs-'fōr-ə-ˌlās\ *n* : any of a group of enzymes that catalyze phosphorolysis with the formation of organic phosphates (as glucose-1-phosphate in the breakdown and synthesis of glycogen) and that occur in animal and plant tissues

phos·phor·y·late \-ˌlāt\ *vt* **-lat·ed; -lat·ing** : to cause (an organic compound) to take up or combine with phosphoric acid or a phosphorus-containing group

phos·phor·y·la·tion \ˌfäs-ˌfȯr-ə-'lā-shən\ *n* : the process of phosphorylating a chemical compound either by reaction with inorganic phosphate or by transfer of phosphate from another organic phosphate; *esp* : the enzymatic conversion of carbohydrates into their phosphoric esters in metabolic processes (as the conversion of glucose to glucose-6-phosphate by ATP and hexokinase)

phos·phor·y·la·tive \fäs-'fȯr-ə-ˌlāt-əv\ *adj* : of, relating to, or characterized by phosphorylation

phos·phor·yl·cho·line \ˌfäs-fə-ˌril-'kō-ˌlēn\ *n* : a hapten used medicinally in the form of its chloride $C_5H_{15}ClNO_4P$ to treat hepatobiliary dysfunction

phos·pho·trans·fer·ase \ˌfäs-fō-'tran(t)s-(ˌ)fər-ˌas, -ˌāz\ *n* : any of several enzymes that catalyze the transfer of phosphorus-containing groups from one compound to another

phos·pho·tung·state \ˌfäs-fō-'təŋ-ˌstāt\ *n* : a salt of a phosphotungstic acid

phos·pho·tung·stic acid \-ˌtəŋ-stik-\ *n* : any of several acids obtainable from solutions of phosphoric acid and tungstic acid and used chiefly as precipitants (as for alkaloids and for basic dyes for pigments) and in analytical reagents; *esp* : a greenish yellow crystalline acid $H_3PW_{12}O_{40}\cdot xH_2O$ used as a reagent and as a biological stain

phos·sy jaw \'fäs-sē-\ *n* : a jawbone destroyed by chronic phosphorus poisoning — called also *phosphonecrosis*

phos·vi·tin \'fäs-ˌvīt-ᵊn, -vət-ən\ *n* : a phosphoprotein obtained from egg yolk

phot \'fōt\ *n* : the cgs unit of illumination equal to one lumen per square centimeter

pho·tic \'fōt-ik\ *adj* : of, relating to, or involving light esp. in relation to organisms ⟨∼ stimulation⟩ — **pho·ti·cal·ly** \'fōt-i-k(ə-)lē\ *adv*

pho·tism \'fōt-ᵢiz-əm\ *n* : a synesthetic visual sensation

pho·to·ac·ti·va·tion \ᵢfōt-ō-ᵢak-tə-'vā-shən\ *n* : the process of activating a substance by means of radiant energy and esp. light; *also* : PHOTOCATALYSIS — compare PHOTOINACTIVATION 2 — **pho·to·ac·ti·vate** \-'ak-tə-ᵢvāt\ *vt* **-vat·ed; -vat·ing**

pho·to·ac·tive \-'ak-tiv\ *adj* : physically or chemically responsive to radiant energy and esp. to light — **pho·to·ac·tiv·i·ty** \-ak-'tiv-ət-ē\ *n, pl* **-ties**

pho·to·af·fin·i·ty \-ə-'fin-ət-ē\ *adj* : of, relating to, used in, or utilizing photoaffinity labeling ⟨a ∼ probe⟩ ⟨a ∼ ligand⟩

¹**photoaffinity label** *vt* : to label by photoaffinity labeling

²**photoaffinity label** *n* : a label used in photoaffinity labeling

photoaffinity labeling *n* : a technique of attaching a label to the active site of a large molecule and esp. a protein by using a molecule which binds loosely and reversibly to the large molecule's active site and which has an inactive part that can be converted by photolysis to a highly reactive form causing the complex of the large substrate molecule and the loosely attached label to bind more permanently

pho·to·ag·ing \-'āj-iŋ\ *n* : the cumulative detrimental effects (as wrinkles or dark spots) on skin that result from long-term exposure to sunlight and esp. ultraviolet light — **pho·to·aged** \-'ājd\ *adj*

pho·to·al·ler·gic \ᵢfōt-ō-ə-'lər-jik\ *adj* : of, relating to, caused by, or affected with a photoallergy ⟨∼ dermatitis⟩

pho·to·al·ler·gy \-'al-ər-jē\ *n, pl* **-gies** : an allergic sensitivity to light

pho·to·au·to·troph \ᵢfōt-ō-'ot-ə-ᵢtrōf\ *n* : a photoautotrophic organism

pho·to·au·to·tro·phic \-ᵢot-ə-'trō-fik\ *adj* : autotrophic and utilizing energy from light ⟨green plants are ∼⟩ — **pho·to·au·to·tro·phi·cal·ly** \-fi-k(ə-)lē\ *adv*

pho·to·bi·ol·o·gist \ᵢfōt-ō-(ᵢ)bī-'äl-ə-jəst\ *n* : a specialist in photobiology

pho·to·bi·ol·o·gy \ᵢfōt-ō-(ᵢ)bī-'äl-ə-jē\ *n, pl* **-gies** : a branch of biology that deals with the effects of radiant energy (as light) on living things — **pho·to·bi·o·log·i·cal** \-ᵢbī-ə-'läj-i-kəl\ *also* **pho·to·bi·o·log·ic** \-ik\ *adj*

pho·to·bi·ot·ic \-(ᵢ)bī-'ät-ik\ *adj* : requiring light in order to live or thrive

pho·to·ca·tal·y·sis \ᵢfōt-ō-kə-'tal-ə-səs\ *n, pl* **-y·ses** \-ᵢsēz\ : the acceleration of a chemical reaction by radiant energy (as light) acting either directly or by exciting a substance that in turn catalyzes the main reaction — compare PHOTOINACTIVATION 1

pho·to·cat·a·lyst \-'kat-ᵊl-əst\ *n* : a substance that catalyzes the main reaction in photocatalysis

pho·to·cat·a·lyt·ic \-kat-ᵊl-'it-ik\ *adj* : of or relating to photocatalysis

pho·to·cat·a·lyze *or Brit* **pho·to·cat·a·lyse** \-'kat-ᵊl-ᵢīz\ *vt* **-lyzed** *or Brit* **-lysed; -lyz·ing** *or Brit* **-lys·ing** : to subject to photocatalysis

pho·to·cath·ode \-'kath-ᵢōd\ *n* : a cathode (as in a photoelectric cell) that emits electrons when exposed to light or other radiation

pho·to·chem·i·cal \ᵢfōt-ō-'kem-i-kəl\ *adj* **1** : of, relating to, or resulting from the chemical action of radiant energy and esp. light ⟨∼ smog⟩ **2** : of or relating to photochemistry ⟨∼ studies⟩ — **pho·to·chem·i·cal·ly** \-k(ə-)lē\ *adv*

pho·to·chem·ist \-'kem-əst\ *n* : a specialist in photochemistry

pho·to·chem·is·try \-'kem-ə-strē\ *n, pl* **-tries** **1** : a branch of chemistry that deals with the effect of radiant energy in producing chemical changes **2 a** : photochemical properties ⟨the ∼ of gases⟩ **b** : photochemical processes ⟨the ∼ of vision⟩

pho·to·che·mo·ther·a·py \-ᵢkē-mō-'ther-ə-pē\ *n, pl* **-pies** : treatment esp. for psoriasis in which administration of a photosensitizing drug (as psoralen) is followed by exposure to ultraviolet radiation or sunlight

pho·to·chro·mat·ic \-krō-'mat-ik\ *adj* : PHOTOCHROMIC

¹**pho·to·chro·mic** \ᵢfōt-ə-'krō-mik\ *adj* **1** : capable of changing color on exposure to radiant energy (as light) ⟨eyeglasses with ∼ lenses⟩ **2** : of, relating to, or utilizing the change of color shown by a photochromic substance ⟨a ∼ process⟩ — **pho·to·chro·mism** \-ᵢmiz-əm\ *n*

²**photochromic** *n* : a photochromic substance — usu. used in pl.

pho·to·chro·mo·gen \ᵢfōt-ō-'krō-mə-jən\ *n* : a microorganism esp. of the genus *Mycobacterium* (as *M. kansasii*) that has little or no pigment when grown in the dark but becomes highly pigmented when grown in light

pho·to·chro·mo·ge·nic·i·ty \-ᵢkrō-mə-jə-'nis-ət-ē\ *n, pl* **-ties** : the property of some microorganisms of producing pigment only when grown in the light or after exposure to light — **pho·to·chro·mo·gen·ic** \-'jen-ik\ *adj*

pho·to·co·ag·u·la·tion \-kō-ᵢag-yə-'lā-shən\ *n* : a surgical process of coagulating tissue by means of a precisely oriented high-energy light source (as a laser beam)

pho·to·co·ag·u·la·tor \-kō-'ag-yə-ᵢlāt-ər\ *n* : a device (as a laser) used to produce a high-energy beam of light in photocoagulation

pho·to·con·duc·tive \-kən-'dək-tiv\ *adj* : having, involving, or operating by photoconductivity

pho·to·con·duc·tiv·i·ty \-ᵢkän-ᵢdək-'tiv-ət-ē, -kən-\ *n, pl* **-ties** : electrical conductivity that is affected by exposure to electromagnetic radiation (as light)

pho·to·con·vul·sive \ᵢfōt-ō-kən-'vəl-siv\ *adj* : of, relating to, being, or marked by an abnormal electroencephalographic response to a flickering light ⟨a ∼ response during photic stimulation at frequencies above 8 Hz —K. M. Reese⟩

pho·to·dam·age \-'dam-ij\ *n* : damage (as to skin or DNA) caused by exposure to ultraviolet radiation — **pho·to·dam·aged** \-ijd\ *adj*

pho·to·de·com·po·si·tion \-ᵢdē-ᵢkäm-pə-'zish-ən\ *n* : chemical breaking down (as of a pesticide) by means of radiant energy

pho·to·deg·ra·da·tion \-ᵢdeg-rə-'dā-shən\ *n* : degradation by means of radiant energy (as light) — **pho·to·de·grad·able** \-di-'grād-ə-bəl\ *adj*

pho·to·der·ma·ti·tis \ᵢfōt-ō-ᵢdər-mə-'tīt-əs\ *n, pl* **-ti·tis·es** *or* **-tit·i·des** \-'tit-ə-ᵢdēz\ : any dermatitis caused or precipitated by exposure to light

pho·to·der·ma·to·sis \-ᵢdər-mə-'tō-səs\ *n, pl* **-to·ses** \-ᵢsēz\ : any dermatosis produced by exposure to light

pho·to·dy·nam·ic \-dī-'nam-ik\ *adj* : of, relating to, or having the property of intensifying or inducing a toxic reaction to light (as the destruction of cancer cells stained with a light-sensitive dye) in a living system ⟨∼ action⟩ ⟨∼ therapy⟩ — **pho·to·dy·nam·i·cal·ly** \-i-k(ə-)lē\ *adv*

pho·to·elec·tric \ᵢfōt-ō-i-'lek-trik\ *adj* : involving, relating to, or utilizing any of various electrical effects due to the interaction of radiation (as light) with matter — **pho·to·elec·tri·cal·ly** \-tri-k(ə-)lē\ *adv*

pho·to·elec·tric·i·ty \-i-ᵢlek-'tris-ət-ē\ *n, pl* **-ties** **1** : electricity produced by the action of light **2** : a branch of physics that deals with the electrical effects of light

pho·to·elec·tron \ᵢfōt-ō-i-'lek-ᵢträn\ *n* : an electron released in photoemission — **pho·to·elec·tron·ic** \-ᵢlek-'trän-ik\ *adj*

pho·to·emis·sion \-i-'mish-ən\ *n* : the release of electrons from a usu. solid material (as a metal) by means of energy supplied by incidence of radiation and esp. light — **pho·to·emis·sive** \-'mis-iv\ *adj*

pho·to·flu·o·ro·gram \ᵢfōt-ə-'flur-ə-ᵢgram\ *n* : a photograph made by photofluorography

pho·to·flu·o·ro·graph·ic \ᵢfōt-ō-ᵢflur-ə-'graf-ik\ *adj* : of, relating to, or used in photofluorography

pho·to·flu·o·rog·ra·phy \-(ᵢ)flu(-ə)r-'äg-rə-fē\ *n, pl* **-phies** : the photography of the image produced on a fluorescent screen by X-rays

Pho·to·frin \'fōt-ə-frin\ *trademark* — used for a preparation of porfimer sodium

pho·to·gen·ic \ᵢfōt-ə-'jen-ik\ *adj* **1** : produced or precipitated by light ⟨∼ epilepsy⟩ ⟨∼ dermatitis⟩ **2** : producing or generating light : PHOSPHORESCENT ⟨∼ bacteria⟩

pho·to·in·ac·ti·va·tion \ˌfōt-ō-(ˌ)in-ˌak-tə-ˈvā-shən\ *n* 1 : the retardation or prevention of a chemical reaction by radiant energy (as light) — compare PHOTOCATALYSIS 2 : the inactivation of a substance by radiant energy (as light) — compare PHOTOACTIVATION

pho·to·isom·er·iza·tion *also Brit* **pho·to·isom·er·isa·tion** \ˌfōt-ō-ī-ˌsäm-ə-rə-ˈzā-shən\ *n* : the light-initiated process of change from one isomeric form of a compound, radical, or ion to another

pho·to·ker·a·ti·tis \-ˌker-ə-ˈtīt-əs\ *n, pl* **-tit·i·des** \-ˈtit-ə-ˌdēz\ : keratitis of the cornea caused by exposure to ultraviolet radiation

pho·to·ki·ne·sis \-kə-ˈnē-səs, -kī-\ *n, pl* **-ne·ses** \-ˈnē-ˌsēz\ : motion or activity induced by light — **pho·to·ki·net·ic** \-ˈnet-ik\ *adj*

pho·to·ky·mo·graph \ˌfōt-ō-ˈkī-mə-ˌgraf\ *n* : a kymograph in which the record is made photographically — **pho·to·ky·mo·graph·ic** \-ˌkī-mə-ˈgraf-ik\ *adj*

¹**pho·to·la·bel** \-ˈlā-bəl\ *vt* **-la·beled** *or* **-la·belled; -la·bel·ing** *or* **-la·bel·ling** \-ˈlā-b(ə-)liŋ\ : PHOTOAFFINITY LABEL

²**photolabel** *n* : PHOTOAFFINITY LABEL

photolabeling *or* **photolabelling** *n* : PHOTOAFFINITY LABELING

pho·to·lu·mi·nes·cence \ˌfōt-ō-ˌlü-mə-ˈnes-ᵊn(t)s\ *n* : luminescence in which the excitation is produced by visible or invisible light — **pho·to·lu·mi·nes·cent** \-ˈnes-ᵊnt\ *adj*

pho·tol·y·sis \fō-ˈtäl-ə-səs\ *n, pl* **-y·ses** \-ˌsēz\ : chemical decomposition by the action of radiant energy — compare RADIOLYSIS — **pho·to·lyt·ic** \ˌfōt-ᵊl-ˈit-ik\ *adj* — **pho·to·lyt·i·cal·ly** \-i-k(ə-)lē\ *adv*

pho·to·lyze *or chiefly Brit* **pho·to·lyse** \ˈfōt-ᵊl-ˌīz\ *vb* **-lyzed** *or chiefly Brit* **-lysed; -lyz·ing** *or chiefly Brit* **-lys·ing** *vt* : to cause to undergo photolysis ~ *vi* : to undergo photolysis — **pho·to·lyz·able** *or chiefly Brit* **pho·to·lys·able** \-ˌī-zə-bəl\ *adj*

pho·to·mac·ro·graph \ˌfōt-ō-ˈmak-rə-ˌgraf\ *n* 1 : a photograph in which the object is either unmagnified or slightly magnified up to a limit of magnification often of about 10 diameters 2 : a photomicrograph of very low magnification

pho·to·mac·rog·ra·phy \-mə-ˈkräg-rə-fē\ *n, pl* **-phies** : the making of photomacrographs — **pho·to·mac·ro·graph·ic** \-ˌmak-rə-ˈgraf-ik\ *adj*

¹**pho·tom·e·ter** \fō-ˈtäm-ət-ər\ *n* : an instrument for measuring the intensity of light, luminous flux, illumination or brightness by comparison of two unequal lights from different sources usu. by reducing the illumination of one (as by varying the distance of the source or using a polarizing device) until the two lights appear equal with the amount of adjustment serving as the basis of comparison and the equality of illumination being judged by various means

²**photometer** *vt* : to examine with a photometer

pho·to·met·ric \ˌfōt-ə-ˈme-trik\ *adj* : of or relating to photometry or the photometer — **pho·to·met·ri·cal·ly** \-tri-k(ə-)lē\ *adv*

pho·tom·e·try \fō-ˈtäm-ə-trē\ *n, pl* **-tries** : a branch of science that deals with measurement of the intensity of light; *also* : the practice of using a photometer

pho·to·mi·cro·graph \ˌfōt-ə-ˈmī-krə-ˌgraf\ *n* : a photograph of a microscope image — called also *microphotograph* — **pho·to·mi·cro·graph·ic** \-ˌmī-krə-ˈgraf-ik\ *adj* — **pho·to·mi·cro·graph·i·cal·ly** \-i-k(ə-)lē\ *adv*

pho·to·mi·crog·ra·pher \-mī-ˈkräg-rə-fər\ *n* : a person who makes photomicrographs

pho·to·mi·crog·ra·phy \-mī-ˈkräg-rə-fē\ *n, pl* **-phies** : the making of photomicrographs

pho·to·mi·cro·scope \ˌfōt-ō-ˈmī-krə-ˌskōp\ *n* : a combined microscope, camera, and suitable light source

pho·to·mi·cros·co·py \-mī-ˈkräs-kə-pē\ *n, pl* **-pies** : PHOTOMICROGRAPHY

pho·to·mul·ti·pli·er tube \ˌfōt-ō-ˈməl-tə-ˌplī(-ə)r-\ *n* : a vacuum tube that detects light esp. from dim sources through the use of photoemission and successive instances of secondary emission to produce enough electrons to generate a useful current — called also *photomultiplier*

pho·ton \ˈfō-ˌtän\ *n* 1 : a unit of intensity of light at the reti-

na equal to the illumination received per square millimeter of a pupillary area from a surface having a brightness of one candle per square meter — called also *troland* 2 : a quantum of electromagnetic radiation

pho·ton·ic \fō-ˈtän-ik\ *adj* : of or relating to a photon

pho·to·nu·cle·ar \ˌfōt-ō-ˈn(y)ü-klē-ər\ *adj* : relating to or caused by the incidence of radiant energy (as gamma rays) on atomic nuclei

pho·to·ox·i·da·tion \-ˌäk-sə-ˈdā-shən\ *n* : oxidation under the influence of radiant energy (as light) — **pho·to·ox·i·da·tive** \-ˈäk-sə-ˌdāt-iv\ *adj* — **pho·to·ox·i·dize** *also Brit* **pho·to·ox·i·dise** \-ˈäk-sə-ˌdīz\ *vb* **-dized** *also Brit* **-dised; -diz·ing** *also Brit* **-dis·ing**

pho·to·patch test \ˈfōt-ō-ˌpach-\ *n* : a test of the capability of a particular substance to photosensitize a particular human skin in which the substance is applied to the skin under a patch and the area is irradiated with ultraviolet light

pho·to·pe·ri·od \ˌfōt-ō-ˈpir-ē-əd\ *n* : a recurring cycle of light and dark periods of constant length — **pho·to·pe·ri·od·ic** \-ˌpir-ē-ˈäd-ik\ *adj* — **pho·to·pe·ri·od·i·cal·ly** \-i-k(ə-)lē\ *adv*

pho·to·pe·ri·od·ism \-ˈpir-ē-ə-ˌdiz-əm\ *also* **pho·to·pe·ri·od·ic·i·ty** \-ˌpir-ē-ə-ˈdis-ət-ē\ *n, pl* **-isms** *also* **-ties** : the response or the capacity to respond to photoperiod

pho·to·phe·re·sis \-fə-ˈrē-səs\ *n* : a method of treating disease (as certain lymphomas) esp. of T cell origin that involves pretreating blood in the living patient by administering a photoactive drug (as methoxalen), obtaining a fraction rich in white blood cells, exposing the fraction to damaging ultraviolet radiation, and returning it to the body where it stimulates a therapeutic immunological response

pho·to·phil·ic \ˌfōt-ə-ˈfil-ik\ *or* **pho·toph·i·lous** \fō-ˈtäf-ə-ləs\ *also* **pho·to·phile** \ˈfōt-ə-ˌfil\ *adj* : thriving in full light : requiring abundant light

pho·to·pho·bia \ˌfōt-ə-ˈfō-bē-ə\ *n* 1 : intolerance to light; *esp* : painful sensitiveness to strong light 2 : an abnormal fear of light

pho·to·pho·bic \-ˈfō-bik\ *adj* 1 : shunning or avoiding light 2 : of or relating to photophobia

pho·to·phos·phor·y·la·tion \ˈfōt-ō-ˌfäs-ˌfor-ə-ˈlā-shən\ *n* : the synthesis of ATP from ADP and phosphate that occurs in a plant using radiant energy absorbed during photosynthesis

phot·oph·thal·mia \ˌfōt-äf-ˈthal-mē-ə, ˌfōt-ˌäp-\ *n* : inflammation of the eye and esp. of the cornea and conjunctiva caused by exposure to light of short wavelength (as ultraviolet light)

phot·opic \fōt-ˈō-pik, -ˈäp-ik\ *adj* : relating to or being vision in bright light with light-adapted eyes that is mediated by the cones of the retina

pho·to·pig·ment \ˈfōt-ō-ˌpig-mənt\ *n* : a pigment (as chlorophyll or a compound in the retina) that undergoes a physical or chemical change under the action of light

pho·to·po·ly·mer·iza·tion *also Brit* **pho·to·po·ly·mer·isa·tion** \ˌfōt-ō-pə-ˌlim-ə-rə-ˈzā-shən, -ˌpäl-ə-mə-rə-\ *n* : polymerization under the influence of radiant energy (as light) : photochemical polymerization

pho·to·prod·uct \ˈfōt-ō-ˌpräd-(ˌ)əkt\ *n* : a product of a photochemical reaction

pho·to·pro·duc·tion \ˌfōt-ō-prə-ˈdək-shən\ *n* : the production of a substance (as hydrogen) by a photochemical reaction (as in photosynthetic bacteria)

pho·top·sia \fō-ˈtäp-sē-ə\ *n* : the perception of light (as luminous rays or flashes) that is purely subjective and accompanies a pathological condition esp. of the retina or brain

pho·to·re·ac·tion \-rē-ˈak-shən\ *n* : a photochemical reaction

pho·to·re·ac·ti·va·tion \-rē-ˌak-tə-ˈvā-shən\ *n* : repair of DNA (as of a bacterium) esp. by a light-dependent enzymat-

O

P

ic reaction after damage by ultraviolet irradiation — **pho·to·re·ac·ti·vat·ing** \-'ak-tə-ˌvāt-iŋ\ adj

pho·to·re·cep·tion \-ri-'sep-shən\ n : perception of waves in the range of visible light; specif : VISION 1 — **pho·to·re·cep·tive** \-'sep-tiv\ adj

pho·to·re·cep·tor \-'sep-tər\ n : a receptor for light stimuli

pho·to·re·duc·tion \-ri-'dək-shən\ n : chemical reduction under the influence of radiant energy (as light) : photochemical reduction — **pho·to·re·duce** \-ri-'d(y)üs\ vt **-duced; -duc·ing**

pho·to·re·frac·tive keratectomy \-ri-ˌfrak-tiv-\ n : surgical ablation of part of the corneal surface using an excimer laser in order to correct for myopia — abbr. PRK; compare RADIAL KERATOTOMY

pho·to·scan \'fōt-ō-ˌskan\ n : a photographic representation of variation in tissue state (as of the kidney) determined by gamma ray emission from an injected radioactive substance — **photoscan** vb **-scanned; -scan·ning**

pho·to·scan·ner \-ˌskan-ər\ n : an instrument used for making photoscans

pho·to·scope \-ˌskōp\ n : a photofluorographic screen and camera

pho·to·sen·si·tive \ˌfōt-ō-'sen(t)-sət-iv, -'sen(t)-stiv\ adj **1** : sensitive or sensitized to the action of radiant energy ⟨∼ paper⟩ **2** : being or caused by an abnormal reaction to sunlight ⟨∼ rashes⟩ — **pho·to·sen·si·tiv·i·ty** \-ˌsen(t)-sə-'tiv-ət-ē\ n, pl **-ties**

pho·to·sen·si·ti·za·tion also Brit **pho·to·sen·si·ti·sa·tion** \-ˌsen(t)-sət-ə-'zā-shən, -ˌsen(t)-stə-'zā-\ n **1** : the process of photosensitizing **2** : the condition of being photosensitized; esp : the development of an abnormal capacity to react to sunlight typically by edematous swelling and dermatitis

pho·to·sen·si·tize \-'sen(t)-sə-ˌtīz\ also Brit **pho·to·sen·si·tise** vt **-tized** also Brit **-tised; -tiz·ing** also Brit **-tis·ing** : to make sensitive to the influence of radiant energy and esp. light — **pho·to·sen·si·tiz·er** n

pho·to·sta·ble \-'stā-bəl\ adj : resistant to change under the influence of radiant energy and esp. of light — **pho·to·sta·bil·i·ty** \-stə-'bil-ət-ē\ n, pl **-ties**

pho·to·syn·the·sis \ˌfōt-ō-'sin(t)-thə-səs\ n, pl **-the·ses** : synthesis of chemical compounds with the aid of light sometimes including the near infrared or near ultraviolet; esp : the formation of carbohydrates from carbon dioxide and a source of hydrogen (as water) in chlorophyll-containing cells (as of green plants) exposed to light involving a photochemical release of oxygen through the decomposition of water followed by various enzymatic synthetic reactions that usu. do not require the presence of light — **pho·to·syn·the·size** \-ˌsīz\ also Brit **pho·to·syn·the·sise** vi **-sized** also Brit **-sised; -siz·ing** also Brit **-sis·ing** — **pho·to·syn·thet·ic** \-sin-'thet-ik\ adj — **pho·to·syn·thet·i·cal·ly** \-i-k(ə-)lē\ adv

pho·to·tac·tic \ˌfōt-ō-'tak-tik\ adj : of, relating to, or exhibiting phototaxis — **pho·to·tac·ti·cal·ly** \-ti-kə-lē\ adv

pho·to·tax·is \-'tak-səs\ n, pl **-tax·es** \-ˌsēz\ : a taxis in which light is the directive factor

pho·to·ther·a·py \-'ther-ə-pē\ n, pl **-pies** : the application of light for therapeutic purposes

pho·to·tim·er \'fōt-ō-ˌtī-mər\ n : a photoelectric device that automatically controls photographic exposures (as to X-rays or light)

pho·to·tox·ic \ˌfōt-ō-'täk-sik\ adj **1** : rendering the skin susceptible to damage (as sunburn or blisters) upon exposure to light and esp. ultraviolet light ⟨∼ antibiotics⟩ ⟨a ∼ topical agent⟩ **2** : induced by a phototoxic substance ⟨a ∼ response⟩ — **pho·to·tox·ic·i·ty** \-täk-'sis-ət-ē\ n, pl **-ties**

pho·to·trans·duc·tion \-tran(t)s-'dək-shən\ n : the conversion of a light signal received by a nervous receptor to an electrical signal transmitted to the brain

pho·to·troph·ic \ˌfōt-ə-'träf-ik, -'trōf-\ adj : capable of utilizing carbon dioxide in the presence of light as a source of metabolic carbon ⟨∼ bacteria⟩

pho·to·tro·pic \ˌfōt-ə-'trōp-ik, -'träp-\ adj : of, relating to, or capable of phototropism

pho·tot·ro·pism \fō-'tä-trə-ˌpiz-əm, ˌfōt-ō-'trō-ˌpiz-əm\ n : a

tropism in which light is the orienting stimulus — see HELIOTROPISM **2** : the reversible change in color of a substance produced by the formation of an isomeric modification when exposed to radiant energy (as light)

phrag·mo·plast \'frag-mō-ˌplast\ n : the enlarged barrel-shaped spindle that is characteristic of the later stages of plant mitosis and within which the cell plate forms

phren·em·phrax·is \ˌfren-ˌem-'frak-səs\ n, pl **-phrax·es** \-ˌsēz\ : crushing of the phrenic nerve for therapeutic reasons

¹phren·ic \'fren-ik\ adj : of or relating to the diaphragm

²phrenic n : PHRENIC NERVE

phrenic artery n : any of the several arteries supplying the diaphragm: **a** : either of two arising from the thoracic aorta and distributed over the upper surface of the diaphragm — called also superior phrenic artery **b** : either of two that arise from the abdominal aorta either directly as separate arteries or from the celiac artery or a renal artery or from a common trunk originating in the abdominal aorta or the celiac artery and that supply the underside of the diaphragm and the adrenal glands — called also inferior phrenic artery

phren·i·cec·to·my \ˌfren-ə-'sek-tə-mē\ n, pl **-mies** : surgical removal of part of a phrenic nerve to secure collapse of a diseased lung by paralyzing the diaphragm on one side — compare PHRENICOTOMY

phren·i·cla·sia \ˌfren-ə-'klā-zh(ē-)ə\ or **phren·i·cla·sis** \-'klā-səs\ n, pl **-cla·sias** or **-cla·ses** \-ˌsēz\ : PHRENEMPHRAXIS

phrenic nerve n : a general motor and sensory nerve on each side of the body that arises chiefly from the fourth cervical nerve, passes down through the thorax to the diaphragm, and supplies or gives off branches supplying esp. the pericardium, pleura, and diaphragm — called also phrenic

phren·i·co·ex·er·e·sis \ˌfren-i-kō-ig-'zer-ə-səs\ n, pl **-e·ses** \-ˌsēz\ : surgical removal of part of a phrenic nerve

phren·i·co·li·en·al ligament \-'lī-ə-nəl-\ n : LIENORENAL LIGAMENT

phren·i·cot·o·my \ˌfren-i-'kät-ə-mē\ n, pl **-mies** : surgical division of a phrenic nerve to secure collapse of a diseased lung by paralyzing the diaphragm on one side — compare PHRENICECTOMY

phrenic vein n : any of the veins that drain the diaphragm and accompany the phrenic arteries: **a** : one that accompanies the pericardiophrenic artery and usu. empties into the internal thoracic vein — called also superior phrenic vein **b** : any of two or three veins which follow the course of the inferior phrenic arteries and of which the one on the right empties into the inferior vena cava and the one or two on the left empty into the left renal or suprarenal vein or the inferior vena cava — called also inferior phrenic vein

phre·nol·o·gist \fri-'näl-ə-jəst\ n : a specialist in phrenology

phre·nol·o·gy \fri-'näl-ə-jē\ n, pl **-gies** : the study of the conformation of the skull based on the belief that it is indicative of mental faculties and character

phren·o·sin \'fren-ə-sən\ n : a crystalline cerebroside that yields cerebronic acid on hydrolysis

phric·to·path·ic \ˌfrik-tə-'path-ik\ adj : relating to or accompanied by shuddering ⟨∼ sensations⟩

phry·no·der·ma \ˌfrī-nə-'dər-mə\ n : a rough dry skin eruption marked by keratosis and usu. associated with vitamin A deficiency — called also toad skin

PHS abbr Public Health Service

phthal·ate \'thal-ˌāt\ n : a salt or ester of phthalic acid

phtha·lein \'thal-ē-ən, 'thal-ˌēn, 'thāl-\ n : any of various xanthene dyes (as phenolphthalein or fluorescein) that are intensely colored in alkaline solution

phthal·ic acid \ˌthal-ik-\ n : any of three isomeric acids $C_8H_6O_4$ obtained by oxidation of various benzene derivatives

phthalic anhydride n : a crystalline cyclic acid anhydride $C_8H_4O_3$ that is used esp. in making alkyd resins and is a structural part of thalidomide

phthal·yl·sul·fa·thi·a·zole or chiefly Brit **phthal·yl·sul·pha·thi·a·zole** \'thal-ˌil-ˌsəl-fə-'thī-ə-ˌzōl\ n : a sulfonamide $C_{17}H_{13}N_3O_5S_2$ used in the treatment of intestinal infections

phthi·o·col \\'thī-ə-ˌkȯl, -ˌkōl\ *n* : a yellow crystalline quinone $C_{11}H_8O_3$ with vitamin K activity that is isolated from the human tubercle bacillus and also made synthetically

phthi·o·ic acid \thī-ˌō-ik-\ *n* : a branched-chain optically active fatty acid or mixture of such acids isolated from the human tubercle bacillus that causes the formation of tubercular lesions on injection into animals

phthi·ri·a·sis \thə-'rī-ə-səs, thī-\ *n, pl* **-a·ses** \-ˌsēz\ : PEDICULOSIS; *esp* : infestation with crab lice

Phthir·i·us \'thir-ē-əs\ *n, syn of* PTHIRUS

Phthi·rus \'thī-rəs\ *n, syn of* PTHIRUS

¹**phthi·sic** \'tiz-ik, 'tī-sik\ *n* 1 : PHTHISIS 2 : TUBERCULAR

²**phthisic** *or* **phthi·si·cal** \-i-kəl\ *adj* : of, relating to, or affected with or as if with pulmonary tuberculosis

phthisica — *see* SPES PHTHISICA

phthis·io·gen·e·sis \ˌt(h)iz-ē-ə-'jen-ə-səs\ *n, pl* **-e·ses** \-ˌsēz\ : the development of pulmonary tuberculosis

phthis·io·gen·ic \-'jen-ik\ *adj* : of or relating to phthisiogenesis

phthis·i·ol·o·gist \ˌt(h)iz-ē-'äl-ə-jəst\ *n* : a physician who specializes in phthisiology

phthis·i·ol·o·gy \-jē\ *n, pl* **-gies** : the care, treatment, and study of tuberculosis

phthis·io·pho·bia \ˌt(h)iz-ē-ə-'fō-bē-ə\ *n* : pathological fear of tuberculosis

phthis·io·ther·a·py \-'ther-ə-pē\ *n, pl* **-pies** : the treatment of pulmonary tuberculosis

phthi·sis \'t(h)ī-səs, 't(h)is-əs\ *n, pl* **phthi·ses** \'t(h)ī-ˌsēz, 't(h)is-ˌēz\ : a progressively wasting or consumptive condition; *esp* : pulmonary tuberculosis

phthisis bul·bi \-'bəl-ˌbī\ *n* : wasting and shrinkage of the eyeball following destructive diseases of the eye (as panophthalmitis)

phy·co·bi·lin \ˌfī-kō-'bī-lən, -'bil-ən\ *n* : any of a class of pigments that occur in the cells of algae, are active in photosynthesis, and are proteins combined with pyrrole derivatives related to the bile pigments

phy·co·cy·a·nin \ˌfī-kō-'sī-ə-nən\ *n* : any of various bluish green protein pigments in the cells of cyanobacteria

phy·co·er·y·thrin \-'er-i-thrən\ *n* : any of the red protein pigments in the cells of red algae

phy·col·o·gist \fī-'käl-ə-jəst\ *n* : a specialist in phycology

phy·col·o·gy \-jē\ *n, pl* **-gies** : the study or science of algae — **phy·co·log·i·cal** \ˌfī-kə-'läj-i-kəl\ *adj*

phy·co·my·cete \ˌfī-kō-'mī-ˌsēt, -ˌmī-'sēt\ *n* : any fungus of two subdivisions of lower fungi (Mastigomycotina and Zygomycotina of the division Eumycota) that have a body ranging from an undifferentiated mass of protoplasm to a well-developed and much-branched coenocytic mycelium and that reproduce mainly asexually by the formation of conidia or sporangia but include forms reproducing by nearly every transitional method from simple conjugation to sexual reproduction by the union of egg and sperm — **phy·co·my·ce·tous** \-ˌmī-'sēt-əs\ *adj*

Phy·co·my·ce·tes \ˌfī-kō-ˌmī-'sēt-(ˌ)ēz\ *n pl, in some classifications* : a large class of lower fungi comprising the phycomycetes

phy·co·my·co·sis \-ˌmī-'kō-səs\ *n, pl* **-co·ses** \-'kō-ˌsēz\ : any mycosis caused by a phycomycete (as of the genera *Rhizopus* and *Mucor*)

phyla *pl of* PHYLUM

phy·lac·tic \fī-'lak-tik\ *adj* : serving to protect esp. against disease ⟨∼ treatments⟩

phy·let·ic \fī-'let-ik\ *adj* : of or relating to the course of evolutionary or phylogenetic development — **phy·let·i·cal·ly** \-i-k(ə-)lē\ *adv*

Phyl·lo·both·ri·oi·dea \ˌfil-ō-ˌbäth-rē-'ȯid-ē-ə\ *n pl, syn of* TETRAPHYLLIDEA

phyl·lode \'fil-ˌōd\ *adj* : having a cross section that resembles a leaf ⟨∼ tumors of the breast⟩

phyl·lo·er·y·thrin \ˌfil-ō-'er-ə-thrən, -i-'rith-rən\ *n* : a rose-red photosensitizing porphyrin pigment formed as a degradation product of chlorophyll in the digestive tract of herbivorous animals and normally excreted esp. in the bile but

absorbed by the blood in pathological conditions (as geeldikkop)

phyl·lo·qui·none \ˌfil-ō-kwin-'ōn, -'kwin-ˌōn\ *n* : VITAMIN K 1a

phy·lo·gen·e·sis \ˌfī-lō-'jen-ə-səs\ *n, pl* **-e·ses** \-ˌsēz\ : PHYLOGENY 2

phy·lo·ge·net·ic \ˌfī-lō-jə-'net-ik\ *adj* 1 : of or relating to phylogeny 2 : based on natural evolutionary relationships 3 : acquired in the course of phylogenetic development — **phy·lo·ge·net·i·cal·ly** \-i-k(ə-)lē\ *adv*

phy·log·e·ny \fi-'läj-ə-nē\ *n, pl* **-nies** 1 : the evolutionary history of a kind of organism 2 : the evolution of a genetically related group of organisms as distinguished from the development of the individual organism — called also *phylogenesis;* compare ONTOGENY

phy·lum \'fī-ləm\ *n, pl* **phy·la** \-lə\ : a major group of animals or in some classifications plants sharing one or more fundamental characteristics that set them apart from all other animals and plants and forming a primary category of the animal or plant kingdom ⟨the ∼ Arthropoda⟩

phy·ma \'fī-mə\ *n, pl* **phymas** *or* **phy·ma·ta** \-mət-ə\ : an external nodule or swelling : a skin tumor

phy·mo·sis \fī-'mō-səs, fi-\ *n, pl* **phy·mo·ses** \-'mō-ˌsēz\ : PHIMOSIS

phys *abbr* 1 physical 2 physician 3 physiological

phy·sa·lia \fī-'sā-lē-ə\ *n* 1 *cap* : a genus (family Physaliidae) of large oceanic siphonophores including the Portuguese man-of-wars 2 : any siphonophore of the genus *Physalia*

phy·sa·lif·e·rous \ˌfī-sə-'lif-ə-rəs, ˌfis-ə-\ *adj* : having vacuoles ⟨∼ cells⟩

Phy·sa·lop·tera \ˌfī-sə-'läp-tə-rə, ˌfis-ə-\ *n* : a large genus (family Physalopteridae) of spiruroid nematode worms parasitic in the digestive tract of various vertebrates including humans

physes *pl of* PHYSIS

phys·iat·rics \ˌfiz-ē-'a-triks\ *n pl but sing or pl in constr* : PHYSICAL MEDICINE AND REHABILITATION

phys·iat·rist \ˌfiz-ē-'a-trəst\ *n* : a physician who specializes in physical medicine and rehabilitation

phys·iat·ry \ˌfiz-ē-'a-trē, fə-'zī-ə-trē\ *n* : PHYSICAL MEDICINE AND REHABILITATION

¹**phys·ic** \'fiz-ik\ *n* 1 **a** : the art or practice of healing disease **b** : the practice or profession of medicine 2 : a medicinal agent or preparation; *esp* : PURGATIVE

²**physic** *vt* **phys·icked; phys·ick·ing** : to treat with or administer medicine to; *esp* : PURGE

¹**phys·i·cal** \'fiz-i-kəl\ *adj* 1 : having material existence : perceptible esp. through the senses and subject to the laws of nature 2 **a** : of or relating to physics **b** : characterized or produced by the forces and operations of physics 3 : of or relating to the body — **phys·i·cal·ly** \-k(ə-)lē\ *adv*

²**physical** *n* : PHYSICAL EXAMINATION

physical anthropologist *n* : an anthropologist specializing in physical anthropology

physical anthropology *n* : anthropology concerned with the comparative study of human evolution, variation, and classification esp. through measurement and observation — called also *somatology;* compare CULTURAL ANTHROPOLOGY

physical chemist *n* : a specialist in physical chemistry

physical chemistry *n* : a branch of science applying physical methods and theory to the study of chemical systems

physical examination *n* : an examination of the bodily functions and condition of an individual

physical medicine and rehabilitation *n* : a medical specialty concerned with the prevention, diagnosis, treatment, and management of disabling diseases, disorders, and injuries typically of a musculoskeletal, cardiovascular, neuromuscular, or neurological nature by physical means (as by

---

\ə\ abut \ˈ\ kitten \ər\ further \a\ ash \ā\ ace \ä\ cot, cart
\aů\ out \ch\ chin \e\ bet \ē\ easy \g\ go \i\ hit \ī\ ice \j\ job
\ŋ\ sing \ō\ go \ȯ\ law \ȯi\ boy \th\ thin \t͟h\ the \ü\ loot
\ů\ foot \y\ yet \zh\ vision *See also* Pronunciation Symbols page

O
P

the use of electromyography, electrotherapy, therapeutic exercise, or pharmaceutical pain control) — called also *physiatrics, physiatry*

physical science *n* : any of the natural sciences (as physics, chemistry, and astronomy) that deal primarily with nonliving materials — **physical scientist** *n*

physical sign *n* : an indication of bodily condition that can be directly perceived (as by auscultation) by an examining physician

physical therapist *n* : a specialist in physical therapy — called also *physiotherapist*

physical therapy *n* : the treatment of disease by physical and mechanical means (as massage, regulated exercise, water, light, heat, and electricity) — called also *physiotherapy*

phy·si·cian \fə-'zish-ən\ *n* : a skilled health-care professional trained and licensed to practice medicine; *specif* : a doctor of medicine or osteopathy

physician–assisted suicide *n* : suicide by a patient facilitated by means or information (as a drug prescription or indication of the lethal dosage) provided by a physician who is aware of how the patient intends to use such means or information

physician's as·sis·tant \-ə-'sis-tənt\ *or* **physician assistant** *n* : a specially trained person who is certified to provide basic medical services (as the diagnosis and treatment of common ailments) usu. under the supervision of a licensed physician — called also *PA*

phys·i·cist \'fiz-(ə-)səst\ *n* : a specialist in physics

physic nut *n* : the seed of a small tropical American tree of the genus *Jatropha* (*J. curcas*) containing a strongly purgative oil

phys·i·co·chem·i·cal \ˌfiz-i-kō-'kem-i-kəl\ *adj* **1** : being physical and chemical **2** : of or relating to physical chemistry — **phys·i·co·chem·i·cal·ly** \-k(ə-)lē\ *adv*

phys·ics \'fiz-iks\ *n pl but sing or pl in constr* : a science that deals with matter and energy and their interactions in the fields of mechanics, acoustics, optics, heat, electricity, magnetism, radiation, atomic structure, and nuclear phenomena

phys·i·o·chem·i·cal \ˌfiz-ē-ō-'kem-i-kəl\ *adj* : of or relating to physiological chemistry ⟨∼ processes⟩ — **phys·i·o·chem·i·cal·ly** \-k(ə-)lē\ *adv*

phys·i·og·nom·ic \ˌfiz-ē-ə(g)-'näm-ik\ *also* **phys·i·og·nom·i·cal** \-i-kəl\ *adj* : of, relating to, or characteristic of physiognomy or the physiognomy — **phys·i·og·nom·i·cal·ly** \-i-k(ə-)lē\ *adv*

phys·i·og·no·my \ˌfiz-ē-'ä(g)-nə-mē\ *n, pl* **-mies** **1** : the art of discovering temperament and character from outward appearance **2** : the facial features held to show qualities of mind or character by their configuration or expression

phys·i·o·log·i·cal \ˌfiz-ē-ə-'läj-i-kəl\ *or* **phys·i·o·log·ic** \-ik\ *adj* **1** : of or relating to physiology **2** : characteristic of or appropriate to an organism's healthy or normal functioning **3** : differing in, involving, or affecting physiological factors ⟨a ∼ strain of bacteria⟩ — **phys·i·o·log·i·cal·ly** \-i-k(ə-)lē\ *adv*

physiological age *n* : age judged in terms of physiological development

physiological chemistry *n* : a branch of science dealing with the chemical aspects of physiological and biological systems : BIOCHEMISTRY

physiological clock *n* : BIOLOGICAL CLOCK

physiological dead space *n* : the total dead space in the entire respiratory system including the alveoli — compare ANATOMICAL DEAD SPACE

physiological psychology *n* : PSYCHOPHYSIOLOGY

physiological saline *n* : a solution of a salt or salts that is essentially isotonic with tissue fluids or blood; *esp* : an approximately 0.9 percent solution of sodium chloride — called also *normal saline solution, normal salt solution, physiological saline solution, physiological salt solution*

physiological zero *n* : a temperature that is felt by the skin as neither warm nor cold and that under ordinary conditions usu. falls at about 85° to 90°F (29° to 32°C)

physiologic clock *n* : BIOLOGICAL CLOCK

phys·i·ol·o·gist \ˌfiz-ē-'äl-ə-jəst\ *n* : a specialist in physiology

phys·i·ol·o·gy \ˌfiz-ē-'äl-ə-jē\ *n, pl* **-gies** **1** : a branch of biology that deals with the functions and activities of life or of living matter (as organs, tissues, or cells) and of the physical and chemical phenomena involved — compare ANATOMY 1, MORPHOLOGY 1 **2** : the organic processes and phenomena of an organism or any of its parts or of a particular bodily process ⟨the ∼ of the thyroid gland⟩ **3** : a treatise on physiology

phys·io·neu·ro·sis \ˌfiz-ē-ō-n(y)ù-'rō-səs\ *n, pl* **-ro·ses** \-ˌsēz\ : ACTUAL NEUROSIS

phys·io·pa·thol·o·gy \ˌfiz-ē-ō-pə-'thäl-ə-jē, -pa-\ *n, pl* **-gies** : a branch of biology or medicine that combines physiology and pathology esp. in the study of altered bodily function in disease — **phys·io·path·o·log·ic** \-ˌpath-ə-'läj-ik\ *or* **phys·io·path·o·log·i·cal** \-i-kəl\ *adj*

phys·io·psy·chic \ˌfiz-ē-ō-'sī-kik\ *adj* : of, relating to, or involving the physical and the psychic or their interrelations

phys·io·psy·chol·o·gy \ˌfiz-ē-ō-sī-'käl-ə-jē\ *n, pl* **-gies** : PSYCHOPHYSIOLOGY — **phys·io·psy·cho·log·i·cal** \-ˌsī-kə-'läj-i-kəl\ *adj*

phys·io·ther·a·peu·tic \ˌfiz-ē-ō-ˌther-ə-'pyüt-ik\ *adj* : of or relating to physical therapy

phys·io·ther·a·pist \-'ther-ə-pəst\ *n* : PHYSICAL THERAPIST

phys·io·ther·a·py \ˌfiz-ē-ō-'ther-ə-pē\ *n, pl* **-pies** : PHYSICAL THERAPY

phy·sique \fə-'zēk\ *n* : the form or structure of a person's body : bodily makeup ⟨a muscular ∼⟩

phy·sis \'fī-səs\ *n, pl* **phy·ses** \-ˌsēz\ : GROWTH PLATE

Phy·so·ceph·a·lus \ˌfī-sə-'sef-ə-ləs\ *n* : a genus of nematode worms of the family Thelaziidae including a common parasite (*P. sexalatus*) of the stomach and small intestine of swine

Phy·so·stig·ma \ˌfī-sə-'stig-mə\ *n* : a genus of African woody vines of the legume family including one (*P. venenosum*) whose fruit is the Calabar bean

phy·so·stig·mine \ˌfī-sō-'stig-ˌmēn\ *n* : a tasteless crystalline alkaloid with anticholinesterase activity that is obtained from Calabar beans and is used parenterally in the form of its salicylate $C_{15}H_{21}N_3O_2 \cdot C_7H_6O_3$ esp. to reverse the toxic effects of an anticholinergic agent (as atropine) and topically in the form of its sulfate $(C_{15}H_{21}N_3O_2)_2 \cdot H_2SO_3$ as a miotic in the treatment of glaucoma — called also *eserine*

phy·tan·ic acid \fī-ˌtan-ik-\ *n* : a fatty acid derived from phytol that accumulates in the blood and tissues of patients affected with Refsum's disease

phy·tase \'fī-ˌtās, -ˌtāz\ *n* : an esterase present in grains, alfalfa, and molds that accelerates the hydrolysis of phytic acid into inositol and phosphoric acid

phy·tate \'fī-ˌtāt\ *n* : a salt or ester of phytic acid

phy·tic acid \ˌfīt-ik-\ *n* : an acid $C_6H_{18}P_6O_{24}$ that occurs in cereal grains and that when ingested interferes with the intestinal absorption of various minerals (as calcium and magnesium)

phy·to·be·zoar \ˌfīt-ō-'bē-ˌzō(ə)r\ *n* : a concretion formed in the stomach or intestine and composed chiefly of undigested compacted vegetable fiber

¹phy·to·chem·i·cal \-'kem-i-kəl\ *adj* : of, relating to, or being phytochemistry — **phy·to·chem·i·cal·ly** \-i-k(ə-)lē\ *adv*

²phytochemical *n* : a chemical compound (as a carotenoid or phytosterol) occurring naturally in plants; *esp* : PHYTONUTRIENT

phy·to·chem·ist \-'kem-əst\ *n* : a specialist in phytochemistry

phy·to·chem·is·try \-'kem-ə-strē\ *n, pl* **-tries** : the chemistry of plants, plant processes, and plant products

phy·to·es·tro·gen \-'es-trə-jən\ *or chiefly Brit* **phy·to–oes·tro·gen** *n* : a chemical compound (as genistein) that occurs naturally in plants and has estrogenic properties

phy·to·fla·gel·late \ˌfīt-ō-'flaj-ə-lət, -ˌlāt; -flə-'jel-ət\ *n* : any of various organisms (as dinoflagellates) that are considered a subclass (Phytomastigophora syn. Phytomastigina) usu. of algae by botanists and of protozoans by zoologists and that have many characteristics in common with typical algae

phy·to·gen·e·sis \ˌfīt-ə-ˈjen-ə-səs\ *n, pl* **-e·ses** \-ˌsēz\ : the origin and developmental history of plants

phy·to·gen·ic \ˌfīt-ə-ˈjen-ik\ *adj* : of plant origin

phy·to·hem·ag·glu·ti·nin *or chiefly Brit* **phy·to·haem·ag·glu·ti·nin** \ˈfīt-ō-ˌhē-mə-ˈglüt-ᵊn-ən\ *n* : a proteinaceous hemagglutinin of plant origin used esp. to induce mitosis (as in lymphocytes) — abbr. *PHA*

phy·to·hor·mone \ˈfīt-ə-ˈhȯr-ˌmōn\ *n* : PLANT HORMONE

phy·tol \ˈfī-ˌtȯl, -ˌtōl\ *n* : an oily aliphatic primary alcohol $C_{20}H_{39}OH$ obtained by hydrolysis of chlorophyll and used in synthesizing vitamin E and vitamin K_1

Phy·tom·o·nas \fī-ˈtäm-ə-nəs\ *n* : a genus of flagellates of the family Trypanosomatidae that are morphologically similar to members of the genus *Leptomonas* but alternate between a hemipterous insect and usu. a latex plant as hosts

phy·to·na·di·one \ˌfī-tō-nə-ˈdī-ˌōn\ *n* : VITAMIN K 1a

phy·ton·cide \ˈfī-ˌtän-ˌsīd\ *n* : any of various bactericidal substances obtained from plants (as onion and garlic) — **phy·ton·cid·al** \ˌfī-tän-ˈsīd-ᵊl\ *adj*

phy·to·nu·tri·ent \ˌfīt-ō-ˈn(y)ü-trē-ənt\ *n* : a bioactive plant-derived compound (as resveratrol or sulforaphane) associated with positive health effects

phyto-oestrogen *chiefly Brit var of* PHYTOESTROGEN

phy·to·par·a·site \ˌfīt-ō-ˈpar-ə-ˌsīt\ *n* : a parasitic plant

phy·to·patho·gen \ˌfīt-ō-ˈpath-ə-jən\ *n* : an organism parasitic on a plant host — **phy·to·patho·gen·ic** \-ˌpath-ə-ˈjen-ik\ *adj*

phy·to·pa·thol·o·gist \ˌfīt-ō-pə-ˈthäl-ə-jəst\ *n* : PLANT PATHOLOGIST

phy·to·pa·thol·o·gy \-pə-ˈthäl-ə-jē, -pa-\ *n, pl* **-gies** : PLANT PATHOLOGY — **phy·to·path·o·log·i·cal** \-ˌpath-ə-ˈläj-i-kəl\ *adj*

phy·toph·a·gous \fī-ˈtäf-ə-gəs\ *adj* : feeding on plants

phy·to·phar·ma·col·o·gy \ˌfīt-ō-ˌfär-mə-ˈkäl-ə-jē\ *n, pl* **-gies** : the study of the influences of drugs on the physiological processes of plants — **phy·to·phar·ma·co·log·ic** \-ˌfär-mə-kə-ˈläj-ik\ *adj*

phy·to·pho·to·der·ma·ti·tis \ˌfīt-ō-ˌfōt-ō-ˌdər-mə-ˈtīt-əs\ *n, pl* **-ti·tis·es** *or* **-tit·i·des** \-ˈtit-ə-ˌdēz\ : an inflammatory reaction of skin that has been exposed to sunlight and esp. UVA radiation after being made hypersensitive by contact with any of various plants or plant parts and esp. those (as limes and celery) with high levels of psoralens and that is typically characterized by a burning sensation, blisters, and erythema followed by hyperpigmentation

phy·tos·ter·ol \fī-ˈtäs-tə-ˌrȯl, -ˌrōl\ *n* : any of various sterols derived from plants — compare ZOOSTEROL

phy·to·ther·a·py \ˌfīt-ō-ˈther-ə-pē\ *n, pl* **-pies** : the use of vegetable drugs in medicine

phy·to·tox·ic \ˌfīt-ə-ˈtäk-sik\ *adj* **1** : of or relating to a phytotoxin **2** : poisonous to plants 〈∼ compounds〉 — **phy·to·tox·ic·i·ty** \-täk-ˈsis-ət-ē\ *n, pl* **-ties**

phy·to·tox·in \-ˈtäk-sən\ *n* : a toxin (as ricin) produced by a plant

phy·tyl \ˈfīt-ᵊl\ *n* : the monovalent radical $C_{20}H_{39}$ derived from phytol

pia \ˈpī-ə, ˈpē-ə\ *n* : PIA MATER

¹pia–arach·noid \ˌpī-ə-ə-ˈrak-ˌnȯid, ˌpē-\ *also* **pia–arach·noid·al** \-ə-ˌrak-ˈnȯid-ᵊl\ *or* **pi·arach·noid** \ˌpī-ə-ˈrak-, ˌpē-\ *adj* : of, relating to, or being the leptomeninges

²pia–arachnoid *also* **piarachnoid** *n* : LEPTOMENINGES

Pia·get·ian \ˌpē-ə-ˈjet-ē-ən\ *adj* : of, relating to, or dealing with Jean Piaget or his writings, theories, or methods esp. with respect to child development

Pia·get \pē-ä-zhä\, **Jean (1896–1980),** Swiss psychologist. Piaget was professor of psychology at the University of Geneva and from 1955 served as director of that university's International Center for Epistemology. A leading investigator of thought processes in children, he described the development of the individual's cognitive abilities. He suggested that thinking is a refined, flexible, trial-and-error process. He divided the development of thinking in children into four stages. The first stage, the sensorimotor stage, occurs during the first two years and is marked by an empiri-cal, largely nonverbal intelligence. The second stage occurs between two and seven years of age and is the time when the child perceives that objects can be represented by words, which the child begins to use experimentally. The third stage occurs between seven and twelve years of age and is occupied by logical operations, which the child uses to classify objects by their similarities and differences. The fourth stage occurs from the age of twelve through adulthood, when the individual begins experimenting with formal logical operations and with more flexible kinds of thinking.

pi·al \ˈpī-əl, ˈpē-\ *adj* : of or relating to the pia mater 〈a ∼ artery〉

pia ma·ter \-ˈmāt-ər\ *n* : the delicate and highly vascular membrane of connective tissue investing the brain and spinal cord, lying internal to the arachnoid and dura mater, dipping down between the convolutions of the brain, and sending an ingrowth into the anterior fissure of the spinal cord — called also *pia*

pia–ma·tral \-ˈmā-trəl\ *adj* : of or relating to the pia mater : PIAL

pi·an \pē-ˈan, ˈpyän\ *n* : YAWS

pi·a·nist's cramp \pē-ˈan-əsts-, ˈpē-ə-nəsts-\ *n* : painful spasm of the muscles of the forearm caused by excessive piano playing

piarachnoid *var of* PIA-ARACHNOID

pi·blok·to \pi-ˈbläk-(ˌ)tō\ *n* : a condition among the Inuit that is characterized by attacks of disturbed behavior (as screaming and crying) and that occurs chiefly in winter

pi·ca \ˈpī-kə\ *n* : an abnormal craving for and eating of substances (as chalk, ashes, or bones) not normally eaten that occurs in nutritional deficiency states (as aphosphorosis) in humans or animals or in some forms of mental illness — compare GEOPHAGY

pi·chi \ˈpē-chē\ *n* : a Peruvian shrub (*Fabiana imbricata*) of the nightshade family that has herbage yielding a tonic and diuretic

¹Pick's disease \ˈpiks-\ *also* **Pick disease** \ˈpik-\ *n* : a dementia marked by progressive impairment of intellect and judgment and transitory aphasia, caused by progressive atrophic changes of the cerebral cortex, and usu. commencing in late middle age

Pick, Arnold (1851–1924), Czechoslovakian psychiatrist and neurologist. Pick is best known for his description in 1892 of an atrophy of the cerebral cortex, now known as Pick's disease, and for his 1913 description of agrammatism.

²Pick's disease *n* : pericarditis with adherent pericardium resulting in circulatory disturbances with edema and ascites

Pick, Friedel (1867–1926), Czechoslovakian physician. Pick described the form of pericarditis that is now known as Pick's disease in 1896.

Pick·wick·ian syndrome \(ˈ)pik-ˈwik-ē-ən-\ *n* : obesity accompanied by somnolence and lethargy, hypoventilation, hypoxia, and secondary polycythemia

Pick·wick \ˈpik-ˌwik\, **Samuel,** literary character. Pickwick is the title character in the novel *The Posthumous Papers of the Pickwick Club* (1836–37) by Charles Dickens. In the novel one of the characters, Joe, is described as a "fat and red-faced boy in a state of somnolence." The term *Pickwickian syndrome* was first used by C. S. Burwell in an article on the syndrome in 1956. The name was chosen because Dickens's description was the first description of the syndrome found in literature.

pi·clo·ram \ˈpik-lə-ˌram, ˈpīk-\ *n* : a systemic herbicide $C_6H_3Cl_3N_2O_2$ that breaks down very slowly in the soil

pi·co·cu·rie \ˌpē-kō-ˈkyü(ə)r-(ˌ)ē, -kyü-ˈrē\ *n* : one trillionth of a curie — abbr. *pCi*

pi·co·far·ad \ˌpē-kō-ˈfar-ˌad, -əd\ *n* : one trillionth of a farad — abbr. *pf*

O
P

\ə\ **abut** \ᵊ\ **kitten** \ər\ **further** \a\ **ash** \ā\ **ace** \ä\ **cot, cart**
\au̇\ **out** \ch\ **chin** \e\ **bet** \ē\ **easy** \g\ **go** \i\ **hit** \ī\ **ice** \j\ **job**
\ŋ\ **sing** \ō\ **go** \ȯ\ **law** \ȯi\ **boy** \th\ **thin** \th̲\ **the** \ü\ **loot**
\u̇\ **foot** \y\ **yet** \zh\ **vision** *See also* Pronunciation Symbols page

pi·co·gram \'pē-kō-ˌgram, -kə-\ *n* : one trillionth of a gram — abbr. *pg*

pi·co·li·nate \pi-'kä-lə-ˌnāt, 'pik-(-ə)-li-\ *n* : a salt of picolinic acid

pic·o·line \'pik-ə-ˌlēn, 'pīk-\ *n* : any of the three liquid pyridine bases C_6H_7N used chiefly as solvents and in organic synthesis

pic·o·lin·ic acid \ˌpik-ə-ˌlin-ik-\ *n* : a crystalline acid $C_6H_5NO_2$ isomeric with niacin

pi·co·mo·lar \ˌpē-kō-'mō-lər\ *adj* : of, relating to, or of the order of magnitude of a picomole

pi·co·mole \'pē-kō-ˌmōl, -kə-\ *n* : one trillionth of a mole — abbr. *pmol, pmole*

Pi·cor·na·vi·ri·dae \(ˌ)pē-ˌkȯr-nə-'vir-ə-ˌdē\ *n pl* : a family of small single-stranded RNA viruses that have an icosahedral virion with no envelope and that include the causative agents of avian encephalomyelitis, encephalomyocarditis, hepatitis A, poliomyelitis, foot-and-mouth disease, and hand, foot and mouth disease — see COXSACKIEVIRUS, ECHOVIRUS, ENTEROVIRUS, RHINOVIRUS

pi·cor·na·vi·rus \(ˌ)pē-ˌkȯr-nə-'vī-rəs\ *n* : any of the family *Picornaviridae* of single-stranded RNA viruses

pi·co·sec·ond \'pē-kō-ˌsek-ənd, -ənt\ *n* : one trillionth of a second — abbr. *ps*

pic·ram·ic acid \pi-ˌkram-ik-\ *n* : a red crystalline acid $C_6H_5N_3O_5$ obtained by reducing picric acid and used chiefly in making azo dyes

pic·rate \'pik-ˌrāt\ *n* : a salt or ester of picric acid

pic·ric acid \ˌpik-rik-\ *n* : a bitter toxic explosive yellow crystalline strong acid $C_6H_3N_3O_7$ used esp. as a dye or biological stain, as an antiseptic, and as a precipitant for organic bases and polycyclic hydrocarbons — called also *trinitrophenol*

pic·ro·car·mine \ˌpik-rō-'kär-mən, -ˌmīn\ *n* : a stain for tissue sections made by mixing solutions of carmine and picric acid

pic·ro·lon·ic acid \ˌpik-rə-ˌlän-ik-\ *n* : a yellow crystalline acidic compound $C_{10}H_8N_4O_5$ that yields yellow solutions with alkalies and is used as a precipitant for organic bases (as alkaloids)

pic·ro·podo·phyl·lin \ˌpik-rō-ˌpäd-ə-'fil-ən\ *n* : a bitter crystalline compound obtained from podophyllin

pic·ro·rhi·za \ˌpik-rə-'rī-zə\ *n* : the dried rhizome of a Himalayan herb (*Picrorhiza kurrooa*) of the snapdragon family (Scrophulariaceae) that is used in India as a bitter tonic and antiperiodic

pic·ro·tin \'pik-rət-ən\ *n* : a nonpoisonous bitter crystalline compound $C_{15}H_{18}O_7$ obtained from picrotoxin

pic·ro·tox·in \ˌpik-rō-'täk-sən\ *n* : a poisonous bitter crystalline principle $C_{30}H_{34}O_{13}$ found esp. in cocculus that is a compound of picrotoxinin and picrotin and is a stimulant and convulsant drug administered intravenously as an antidote for poisoning by overdoses of barbiturates

pic·ro·tox·in·in \-'täk-sə-nən\ *n* : a poisonous bitter crystalline compound $C_{15}H_{16}O_6$ obtained from picrotoxin

pic·ryl \'pik-rəl\ *n* : the monovalent radical $-C_6H_2(NO_2)_3$ derived from picric acid by removal of the hydroxyl group

PID *abbr* pelvic inflammatory disease

pie·dra \pē-'ä-drə\ *n* : a fungus disease of the hair marked by the formation of small stony nodules along the hair shafts

Pierre Ro·bin syndrome \ˌpyer-rȯ-'baⁿ-\ *n* : a congenital defect of the face characterized by micrognathia, abnormal smallness of the tongue, cleft palate, and absence of the gag reflex and sometimes accompanied by bilateral eye defects, glaucoma, or retinal detachment

> **Ro·bin** \rȯ-baⁿ\, **Pierre (1867–1950),** French pediatrician.

pi·ezo·chem·is·try \pē-ˌā-zō-'kem-ə-strē, pē-ˌāt-sō-, *esp Brit* pī-ˌē-zō-\ *n, pl* **-tries** : a science dealing with the effect of pressure on chemical phenomena

pi·ezo·elec·tric \pē-ˌā-(ˌ)zō-ə-'lek-trik, pē-ˌāt-(ˌ)sō-, *esp Brit* pī-ˌē-(ˌ)zō-\ *adj* : of, relating to, marked by, or functioning by means of piezoelectricity — **pi·ezo·elec·tri·cal·ly** \-tri-k(ə-)lē\ *adv*

pi·ezo·elec·tric·i·ty \-ˌlek-'tris-ət-ē, -'tris-tē\ *n, pl* **-ties** : electricity or electric polarity due to pressure esp. in a crystalline substance (as quartz)

pi·ezom·e·ter \ˌpē-ə-'zäm-ət-ər, pē-ˌāt-'säm-\ *n* : an instrument for measuring pressure or compressibility; *esp* : one for measuring the change of pressure of a material subjected to hydrostatic pressure — **pi·ezo·met·ric** \pē-ˌā-zə-'me-trik, pē-ˌāt-sə-\ *adj* — **pi·ezom·e·try** \ˌpē-ə-'zäm-ə-trē, pē-ˌāt-'säm-\ *n, pl* **-tries**

pi·geon breast \'pij-ən-\ *n* : a rachitic deformity of the chest marked by sharp projection of the sternum — **pi·geon–breast·ed** \'pij-ən-'bres-təd\ *adj*

pigeon chest *n* : PIGEON BREAST

pi·geon–toed \'pij-ən-'tōd\ *adj* : having the forefoot turned inward toward the midline of the body

pig louse \'pig-\ *n* : HOG LOUSE

pig·ment \'pig-mənt\ *n* : a coloring matter in animals and plants esp. in a cell or tissue; *also* : any of various related colorless substances

pig·men·tary \'pig-mən-ˌter-ē\ *adj* : of, relating to, or containing pigment

pigmentary retinopathy *n* : RETINITIS PIGMENTOSA

pig·men·ta·tion \ˌpig-mən-'tā-shən, -ˌmen-\ *n* : coloration with or deposition of pigment; *esp* : an excessive deposition of bodily pigment

pigment cell *n* : a cell containing a deposition of coloring matter

pig·ment·ed \'pig-ˌment-əd\ *adj* : colored by a deposit of pigment ⟨a ~ wart⟩

pig·men·to·phage \pig-'men-tə-ˌfāj\ *n* : a cell that ingests pigment

pigmentosa — see RETINITIS PIGMENTOSA

pigmentosum — see XERODERMA PIGMENTOSUM

pig·men·tum ni·grum \pig-'ment-əm-'nī-grəm\ *n* : the melanin coloring the choroid of the eye

pigmy *var of* PYGMY

Pi·gnet index \pēn-'yā-\ *n* : a measure of the type of body build obtained by subtracting the sum of the weight in kilograms and the chest circumference in centimeters from the height in centimeters

> **Pi·gnet** \pē-nʸā\, **Maurice–Charles–Joseph** (*b* 1871), French physician. Pignet, who had a career as an army doctor, introduced the Pignet index in 1900. He also is credited with introducing a new method for the chemical analysis of water in 1902.

pig·weed \'pig-ˌwēd\ *n* : any of several plants of the genus *Amaranthus* (as *A. retroflexus* and *A. hybridus*) producing pollen that is an important hay fever allergen

pil *abbr* [Latin *pilula*] pill — used in writing prescriptions

pilaris — see KERATOSIS PILARIS, LICHEN PILARIS, PITYRIASIS RUBRA PILARIS

pi·la·ry \'pī-lə-rē\ *adj* : of or relating to the hair or a hair : HAIRY

pi·las·ter \pi-'las-tər\ *n* : an elongated hardened ridge; *esp* : a longitudinal bony ridge on the back of the femur

pi·las·tered \-tərd\ *adj* : having or borne on pilasters

Pi·la·tes \pə-'lä-tēz\ *trademark* — used for an exercise regimen typically performed with the use of specialized apparatus and designed to improve the overall condition of the body

pile \'pī(ə)l\ *n* **1** : a single hemorrhoid **2 piles** *pl* : HEMORRHOIDS; *also* : the condition of one affected with hemorrhoids

pi·le·us \'pī-lē-əs\ *n, pl* **pi·lei** \-lē-ˌī\ : the convex, concave, or flattened spore-bearing structure of some basidiomycetous fungi that is attached to the top of the stem and typically is expanded with gills or pores on the underside — called also *cap*

pili *pl of* PILUS

pili — see ARRECTOR PILI MUSCLE, ERECTOR PILI MUSCLE

pi·li·at·ed \'pil-ē-ˌāt-əd, 'pīl-\ *adj* : covered with pili ⟨~ bacteria⟩

pi·li·gan \'pē-lē-ˌgän\ *n* : a club moss of the genus *Lycopodium* (*L. saururus*) of Brazil and Argentina with cathartic properties

pill \'pil\ *n* **1** : a usu. medicinal or dietary preparation in a small rounded mass to be swallowed whole **2** *often cap* : BIRTH CONTROL PILL — usu. used with *the* ⟨has been on the ∼ for three years⟩

pil·lar \'pil-ər\ *n* : a body part likened to a pillar or column (as the margin of the external inguinal ring); *specif* : PILLAR OF THE FAUCES

pillar of the fauces *n* : either of two curved folds on each side that bound the fauces and enclose the tonsil — called also *arch of the fauces, palatine arch;* see PALATOGLOSSAL ARCH, PALATOPHARYNGEAL ARCH

pillar of the fornix *n* : either of the anterior and posterior diverging extensions of the fornix of the brain — see MAMMILLARY BODY

pil·let \'pil-ət\ *n* : a small pill : PELLET

pillular, pillule *var of* PILULAR, PILULE

pi·lo·car·pi·dine \ˌpī-lə-'kär-pə-ˌdēn\ *n* : a liquid alkaloid $C_{10}H_{14}N_2O_2$ closely related to pilocarpine and occurring with it in the leaves of jaborandi (*Pilocarpus jaborandi*)

pi·lo·car·pine \ˌpī-lə-'kär-ˌpēn\ *n* : a miotic muscarinic alkaloid that is obtained from jaborandi and is used chiefly in the form of its hydrochloride $C_{11}H_{16}N_2O_2 \cdot HCl$ or nitrate $C_{11}H_{16}N_2O_2 \cdot HNO_3$ esp. in the treatment of glaucoma and xerostomia

pi·lo·car·pus \ˌpī-lə-'kär-pəs\ *n* **1** *cap* : a small genus of tropical American shrubs (family Rutaceae) having clusters of small greenish flowers **2** *pl* **-pus·es** : JABORANDI

pi·lo·erec·tion \ˌpī-lō-i-'rek-shən\ *n* : involuntary erection or bristling of hairs due to a sympathetic reflex usu. triggered by cold, shock, or fright or due to a sympathomimetic agent

pi·lo·mo·tor \ˌpī-lə-'mōt-ər\ *adj* : moving or tending to cause movement of the hairs of the skin ⟨∼ nerves⟩ ⟨∼ erection⟩

pilomotor muscle *n* : ARRECTOR PILI MUSCLE

pilomotor nerve *n* : an autonomic nerve supplying an arrector pili muscle

pi·lo·ni·dal \ˌpī-lə-'nīd-ᵊl\ *adj* **1** : containing hair nested in a cyst — used of congenitally anomalous cysts in the sacrococcygeal area that often become infected and discharge through a channel near the anus **2** : of, relating to, involving, or for use on pilonidal cysts, tracts, or sinuses

pi·lose \'pī-ˌlōs\ *adj* : covered with usu. soft hair

pi·lo·se·ba·ceous \ˌpī-lō-si-'bā-shəs\ *adj* : of or relating to hair and the sebaceous glands

pi·los·i·ty \pī-'läs-ət-ē\ *n, pl* **-ties** : the state of being pilose : HAIRINESS

pil·u·lar *or* **pil·lu·lar** \'pil-yə-lər\ *adj* : of, relating to, or resembling a pill

pil·ule *or* **pil·lule** \'pil-(ˌ)yü(ə)l\ *n* : a little pill

pi·lus \'pī-ləs\ *n, pl* **pi·li** \-ˌlī\ : a hair or a structure (as on the surface of a bacterial cell) resembling a hair

pi·mar·i·cin \pi-'mar-ə-sən\ *n* : an antifungal antibiotic $C_{34}H_{49}NO_{14}$ derived from a bacterium of the genus *Streptomyces* and effective esp. against aspergillus, candida, and mucor infections

pi·mel·ic acid \pi-ˌmel-ik-\ *n* : a crystalline dicarboxylic acid $C_7H_{12}O_4$ obtained usu. by oxidation of unsaturated fats or castor oil

Pi·men·ta \pə-'ment-ə\ *n* : a genus of tropical American aromatic trees of the myrtle family (Myrtaceae) having large leaves and small flowers — see ALLSPICE, BAYBERRY 1

pimenta oil *n* : a colorless to yellow or reddish pungent essential oil obtained from allspice and used chiefly in flavoring — called also *allspice oil, pimento oil*

pi·men·to \pə-'ment-(ˌ)ō\ *n, pl* **pimentos** *or* **pimento** : ALLSPICE

pimento oil *n* : PIMENTA OIL

pim·o·zide \'pim-ə-ˌzīd\ *n* : a tranquilizer $C_{28}H_{29}F_2N_3O$

pim·ple \'pim-pəl\ *n* **1** : a small inflamed elevation of the skin : PAPULE; *esp* : PUSTULE **2** : a swelling or protuberance like a pimple — **pim·pled** \-pəld\ *adj* — **pim·ply** \-p(ə-)lē\ *adj*

¹pin \'pin\ *n* **1** : a metal rod driven into or through a fractured bone to immobilize it **2** : a metal rod driven into the root of

a reconstructed tooth to provide support for a crown or into the jaw to provide support for an artificial tooth

²pin *vt* **pinned; pin·ning** : to fasten, join, or secure with a pin

PIN *abbr* prostatic intraepithelial neoplasia

pin·cers \'pin(t)-sərz, *US often* 'pin-chərz\ *n pl* : FORCEPS

pinch \'pinch\ *vt* : to squeeze or compress (a part of the body) usu. in a painful or discomforting way ⟨a ∼ed nerve caused by entrapment⟩

pin·do·lol \'pin-də-ˌlōl, -ˌlōl\ *n* : a beta-blocker $C_{14}H_{20}N_2O_2$ used in the treatment of hypertension

¹pine \'pīn\ *n* : any tree of the genus *Pinus*

²pine *n* : a dietary deficiency disease of sheep or cattle marked by anemia, malnutrition, and general debility; *specif* : such a disease due to cobalt deficiency — compare MORTON MAINS DISEASE

¹pi·ne·al \'pī-nē-əl, pī-'\ *adj* : of, relating to, or being the pineal gland

²pineal *n* : PINEAL GLAND

pi·ne·al·ec·to·mize *also Brit* **pi·ne·a·lec·to·mise** \ˌpī-nē-ə-'lek-tə-ˌmīz\ *vt* **-mized** *also Brit* **-mised; -miz·ing** *also Brit* **-mis·ing** : to perform a pinealectomy on

pi·ne·al·ec·to·my \ˌpī-nē-ə-'lek-tə-mē, pī-ˌnē-, ˌpin-ē-\ *n, pl* **-mies** : surgical removal of the pineal gland

pineal gland *n* : a small body that arises from the roof of the third ventricle and is enclosed by the pia mater and that functions primarily as an endocrine gland that produces melatonin — called also *pineal, pineal body, pineal organ*

pin·e·a·lo·cyte \'pin-ē-ə-lə-ˌsīt\ *n* : the parenchymatous epithelioid cell of the pineal gland that has prominent nucleoli and long processes ending in bulbous expansions

pin·e·a·lo·ma \ˌpin-ē-ə-'lō-mə\ *n, pl* **-mas** *also* **-ma·ta** \-mət-ə\ : a tumor (as a germinoma) of the pineal gland or pineal region

pineal organ *n* : PINEAL GLAND

pine·ap·ple \'pī-ˌnap-əl\ *n* **1** : a tropical monocotyledonous plant (*Ananas comosus* of the family Bromeliaceae, the pineapple family) that has rigid spiny-margined recurved leaves and a short stalk with a dense oblong head of small abortive flowers **2** : the multiple fruit of the pineapple that consists of the succulent fleshy inflorescence and whose juice is the source of the proteolytic enzyme bromelain

pi·nene \'pī-ˌnēn\ *n* : either of two liquid isomeric unsaturated bicyclic terpene hydrocarbons $C_{10}H_{16}$ of which one is a major constituent of wood turpentine

pine–needle oil *n* : a colorless or yellowish bitter essential oil obtained from the needles of various pines (esp. *Pinus mugo*) and used in medicine chiefly as an inhalant in treating bronchitis

pine tar *n* : tar obtained from the wood of pine trees (genus *Pinus* and esp. *P. palustris*) and used in soaps and in the treatment of skin diseases

pin·guec·u·la \pin-'gwek-yə-lə\ *also* **pin·guic·u·la** \-'gwik-\ *n, pl* **-lae** \-ˌlē, -ˌlī\ : a small yellowish elevation situated near the inner or outer margins of the cornea and occurring esp. in people of advanced age

pink disease \'piŋk-\ *n* : ACRODYNIA

pink·eye \'piŋ-ˌkī\ *n* : an acute highly contagious conjunctivitis of humans and various domestic animals

pink·root \'piŋ-ˌkrüt, -ˌkrůt\ *n* : any of several plants of the genus *Spigelia* related to the nux vomica and used as anthelmintics

pink spot *n* : the appearance of pulp through the attenuated hard tissue of the crown of a tooth affected with resorption of dentin

pin·na \'pin-ə\ *n, pl* **pin·nae** \'pin-ē, -ˌī\ *or* **pinnas** : the largely cartilaginous projecting portion of the external ear — **pin·nal** \'pin-ᵊl\ *adj*

pi·no·cy·tosed \ˌpin-ə-'sī-ˌtōzd, ˌpīn-\ *adj* : having undergone pinocytosis ⟨∼ food⟩

\ə\ abut \ᵊ\ kitten \ər\ further \a\ ash \ā\ ace \ä\ cot, cart \aů\ out \ch\ chin \e\ bet \ē\ easy \g\ go \i\ hit \ī\ ice \j\ job \ŋ\ sing \ō\ go \ò\ law \òi\ boy \th\ thin \t̲h̲\ the \ü\ loot \ů\ foot \y\ yet \zh\ vision   *See also* Pronunciation Symbols page

O
P

pi·no·cy·to·sis \ˌpin-ə-sə-ˈtō-səs, ˌpīn-, -ˌsī-\ *n, pl* **-to·ses** \-ˌsēz\ : the uptake of fluid and dissolved substances by a cell by invagination and pinching off of the cell membrane

pi·no·cy·tot·ic \-ˈtät-ik\ *or* **pi·no·cyt·ic** \ˌpin-ə-ˈsīt-ik, ˌpīn-\ *adj* : of, relating to, or being pinocytosis — **pi·no·cy·tot·i·cal·ly** \-i-k(ə-)lē\ *adv*

pins and needles *n pl* : a pricking tingling sensation in a limb growing numb or recovering from numbness

pint \ˈpīnt\ *n* : any of various measures of liquid capacity equal to one-half quart: as **a** : a U.S. measure equal to 16 fluid ounces, 473.176 milliliters, or 28.875 cubic inches **b** : a British measure equal to 20 fluid ounces, 568.26 milliliters, or 34.678 cubic inches

pin·ta \ˈpint-ə, ˈpin-ˌtä\ *n* : a chronic skin disease that is endemic in tropical America, that occurs successively as an initial papule, a generalized eruption, and a patchy loss of pigment, and that is caused by a spirochete of the genus *Treponema* (*T. careteum*) morphologically indistinguishable from the causative agent of syphilis — called also *mal del pinto, pinto*

pin·tid \ˈpint-əd\ *n* : one of many initially reddish, then brown, slate blue, or black patches on the skin characteristic of the second stage of pinta

pin·to \ˈpin-(ˌ)tō\ *n* : PINTA

Pi·nus \ˈpī-nəs\ *n* : a large and economically important genus (the type of the family Pinaceae) of coniferous evergreen trees chiefly of temperate regions of the northern hemisphere that includes a number which yield products (as pine tar) with medicinal applications

pin·worm \ˈpin-ˌwərm\ *n* : any of numerous small nematode worms of the family Oxyuridae that have the tail of the female prolonged into a sharp point and infest the intestines and esp. the cecum of various vertebrates; *esp* : a worm of the genus *Enterobius* (*E. vermicularis*) that is parasitic in humans

pi·o·glit·a·zone \ˌpī-ə-ˈglit-ə-ˌzōn\ *n* : a thiazolidine derivative administered in the form of its hydrochloride $C_{19}H_{20}N_2O_3S \cdot HCl$ to treat type 2 diabetes by decreasing insulin resistance — see ACTOS

Pi·oph·i·la \pī-ˈäf-ə-lə\ *n* : a genus of dipteran flies (family Piophilidae) that include the cheese fly (*P. casei*)

pip \ˈpip\ *n* : the formation of a scale or crust on the tip and dorsal surface of the tongue of a bird often associated with respiratory diseases; *also* : the scale or crust itself

Pi·per \ˈpī-pər, ˈpip-ər\ *n* : a very large genus (the type of the family Piperaceae) of tropical plants that comprise the true peppers, are mostly climbing jointed shrubs with pulpy fruit, and include the betel (*P. betle*), kava (*P. methysticum*), and matico (*P. angustifolium*) and the sources of cubebs (from *P. cubeba*) and black and white pepper (from *P. nigrum*)

pi·per·a·zine \pī-ˈper-ə-ˌzēn\ *n* : a crystalline heterocyclic base $C_4H_{10}N_2$ or $C_4H_{10}N_2 \cdot 6H_2O$ used esp. as an anthelmintic

pi·per·i·dine \pī-ˈper-ə-ˌdēn\ *n* : a liquid heterocyclic base $C_5H_{11}N$ that has a peppery ammoniacal odor and is obtained usu. by hydrolysis of piperine

pip·er·ine \ˈpip-ə-ˌrēn\ *n* : a white crystalline alkaloid $C_{17}H_{19}NO_3$ that is the chief active constituent of pepper

pi·per·o·caine \pī-ˈper-ə-ˌkān\ *n* : a compound derived from piperidine and benzoic acid that has been used in the form of its hydrochloride $C_{16}H_{23}NO_2 \cdot HCl$ as a local anesthetic

pi·per·o·nyl bu·tox·ide \pī-ˈper-ə-ˌnil-byü-ˈtäk-ˌsīd, -ən-ᵊl-\ *n* : an insecticide $C_{19}H_{30}O_5$ that has the capacity to alter the pharmacological action of some drugs; *also* : an oily liquid containing this compound that is used chiefly as a synergist (as for pyrethrum insecticides)

pip·er·ox·an \ˌpip-ə-ˈräk-ˌsan\ *n* : an adrenolytic drug that has been used in the form of its crystalline hydrochloride $C_{14}H_{19}NO_2 \cdot HCl$ to diagnose pheochromocytoma

pi·pette *also* **pi·pet** \pī-ˈpet\ *n* : a small piece of apparatus which typically consists of a narrow tube into which fluid is drawn by suction (as for dispensing or measurement) and retained by closing the upper end — **pipette** *also* **pipet** *vb* **pi·pet·ted; pi·pet·ting**

pip·sis·se·wa \pip-ˈsis-ə-ˌwȯ\ *n* : any of a genus (*Chimaphila*, esp. *C. umbellata*) of evergreen herbs of the wintergreen family (Pyrolaceae) with astringent leaves used as a tonic and diuretic

pir·ac·e·tam \ˌpī(ə)r-ˈas-ə-ˌtam\ *n* : a derivative $C_6H_{10}N_2O_2$ of pyrrolidine that has been used as a nootropic

pir·i·form *or* **pyr·i·form** \ˈpir-ə-ˌfȯrm\ *adj* **1** : having the form of a pear **2** : of or relating to the piriform lobe ⟨the ~ cortex⟩

piriform aperture *n* : the anterior opening of the nasal cavities in the skull

piriform area *n* : PIRIFORM LOBE

piriform fossa *n* : PIRIFORM RECESS

pir·i·for·mis *or* **pyr·i·for·mis** \ˌpir-ə-ˈfȯr-məs\ *n* : a muscle that arises from the front of the sacrum, passes out of the pelvis through the greater sciatic foramen, is inserted into the upper border of the greater trochanter of the femur, and rotates the thigh laterally

piriform lobe *n* : the lateral olfactory gyrus and the parahippocampal gyrus taken together — called also *piriform area*

piriform recess *n* : a small cavity or pocket between the lateral walls of the pharynx on each side and the upper part of the larynx — called also *piriform fossa, piriform sinus*

Pi·ro·goff's amputation *or* **Pi·ro·goff amputation** \ˌpir-ə-ˈgȯf(s)-\ *n* : amputation of the foot through the articulation of the ankle with retention of part of the calcaneus — compare SYME'S AMPUTATION

Pirogoff, Nikolai Ivanovich (1810–1881), Russian surgeon. Pirogoff is regarded as the greatest Russian surgeon and as one of the founders of modern surgery. He headed the department of surgery and the surgical clinic at a hospital in St. Petersburg. He also served as a professor of pathological anatomy and for a time as an army field surgeon. He introduced his procedure for the amputation of the foot in 1854.

piro·plasm \ˈpir-ə-ˌplaz-əm\ *or* **piro·plas·ma** \ˌpir-ə-ˈplaz-mə\ *n, pl* **piro·plasms** *or* **piro·plas·ma·ta** \ˌpir-ə-ˈplaz-mət-ə\ : BABESIA 2 — **piro·plas·mic** \ˌpir-ə-ˈplaz-mik\ *adj*

Piro·plas·ma \ˌpir-ə-ˈplaz-mə\ *n, syn of* BABESIA

¹piro·plas·mid \-ˈplaz-məd\ *adj* : of or relating to the Babesiidae

²piroplasmid *n* : BABESIA 2

piro·plas·mo·sis \ˌpir-ə-ˌplaz-ˈmō-səs\ *n, pl* **-mo·ses** \-ˌsēz\ : infection with or disease that is caused by protozoans of the genus *Babesia* or the family Babesiidae and that includes Texas fever and east coast fever of cattle and babesiosis of sheep

pi·rox·i·cam \pi-ˈräk-sə-ˌkam\ *n* : a nonsteroidal anti-inflammatory drug $C_{15}H_{13}N_3O_4S$ used in the treatment of rheumatic diseases (as osteoarthritis)

Pir·quet test \pir-ˈkā-\ *n* : a tuberculin test made by applying a drop of tuberculin to a scarified spot on the skin — called also *Pirquet reaction*

Pir·quet von Ce·se·na·ti·co \pir-ˈkā-fən-chā-se-ˈnät-i-kō\, **Clemens Peter (1874–1929),** Austrian physician. Pirquet is remembered for his fundamental work on tuberculosis and allergy. In 1907 he introduced a cutaneous reaction test for the diagnosis of tuberculosis that is now known as the Pirquet test.

Pis·ces \ˈpī-ˌsēz *also* ˈpi-\ *n pl, in some classifications* : a class of vertebrates comprising all the fishes and sometimes the cyclostomes and lancelets

pis·cid·ia \pi-ˈsid-ē-ə\ *n* : the bark of a West Indian leguminous tree (*Piscidia erythrina*) that was formerly used as a narcotic and anodyne

¹pi·si·form \ˈpī-sə-ˌfȯrm\ *adj* : resembling a pea in size or shape ⟨~ granules⟩

²pisiform *n* : a bone on the little-finger side of the carpus that articulates with the triquetral bone — called also *pisiform bone*

¹pit \ˈpit\ *n* : a hollow or indentation esp. in a surface of an organism: as **a** : a natural hollow in the surface of the body **b** : one of the indented scars left in the skin by a pustular disease : POCKMARK **c** : a usu. developmental imperfection in the enamel of a tooth that takes the form of a small pointed depression

²pit vb pit·ted; pit·ting vt : to make pits in; esp : to scar or mark with pits ⟨a face pitted by acne⟩ ~ vi : to become marked with pits; esp : to preserve for a time an indentation made by pressure ⟨a swollen area on the gingiva which ~s readily —A. B. Wade⟩

¹pitch \'pich\ n 1 : a black or dark viscous substance obtained as a residue in the distillation of organic materials and esp. tars 2 : resin obtained from various conifers and often used medicinally

²pitch n : the property of a sound and esp. a musical tone that is determined by the frequency of the waves producing it : highness or lowness of sound

pitch·blende \'pich-ˌblend\ n : a brown to black mineral that consists of massive uraninite, has a distinctive luster, contains radium, and is the chief ore-mineral source of uranium

pitch·er's elbow \'pich-ərz-\ n : pain and disability associated with the tearing of tendons from their attachment on the epicondyle of the humerus often with involvement of tissues within and around the elbow

pith \'pith\ vt 1 : to kill (as cattle) by piercing or severing the spinal cord 2 : to destroy the spinal cord or central nervous system of (as a frog) usu. by passing a wire or needle up and down the vertebral canal

pith·e·coid \'pith-ə-ˌkȯid\ adj : of, relating to, or resembling monkeys ⟨assumed a ~ posture⟩

pith·i·a·tism \'pith-ē-ə-ˌtiz-əm\ n : HYSTERIA 1a

Pi·to·cin \pi-'tō-sən\ trademark — used for a preparation of oxytocin

pi·tot tube \ˌpē-ˌtō-\ n, often cap P : a device that consists of a tube having a short right-angled bend which is placed vertically in a moving body of fluid with the mouth of the bent part directed upstream and that is used with a manometer to measure the velocity of fluid flow (as in a blood vessel)
  Pi·tot \pē-tō\, Henri (1695–1771), French hydraulic engineer. Pitot began his career in the chemical laboratory at the Academy of Sciences in Paris. During his two decades at the academy he published a number of papers addressing minor questions in astronomy, geometry, and mechanics, especially hydraulics. In 1735 he published a paper announcing his invention of the Pitot tube.

Pi·tres·sin \pi-'tres-ᵊn\ trademark — used for a preparation of vasopressin

pitting n 1 : the action or process of forming pits (as in acned skin, a tooth, or a dental restoration) 2 : the formation of a depression or indentation in living tissue that is produced by pressure with a finger or blunt instrument and disappears only slowly following release of the pressure in some forms of edema

pitting edema n : edema in which pitting results in a depression in the edematous tissue which disappears only slowly

pi·tu·i·cyte \pə-'t(y)ü-ə-ˌsīt\ n : one of the pigmented more or less fusiform cells of the stalk and posterior lobe of the pituitary gland that are usu. considered to be derived from glial cells

¹pi·tu·i·tary \pə-'t(y)ü-ə-ˌter-ē\ adj 1 : of or relating to the pituitary gland 2 : caused or characterized by secretory disturbances of the pituitary gland ⟨a ~ dwarf⟩

²pituitary n, pl -tar·ies 1 : PITUITARY GLAND 2 : the cleaned, dried, and powdered posterior lobe of the pituitary gland of cattle that is used in the treatment of uterine atony and hemorrhage, shock, and intestinal paresis

pituitary ba·soph·i·lism \-bā-'säf-ə-ˌliz-əm\ n : CUSHING'S DISEASE

pituitary gland n : a small oval reddish gray very vascular endocrine organ that is attached to the infundibulum of the brain and occupies the sella turcica, that is present in all craniate vertebrates, that consists essentially of an epithelial anterior lobe derived from a diverticulum of the oral cavity and joined to a posterior lobe of nervous origin by a pars intermedia, and that has the several parts associated with various hormones which directly or indirectly affect most basic bodily functions and include substances exerting a control-

ling and regulating influence on other endocrine organs, controlling growth and development, or modifying the contraction of smooth muscle, renal function, and reproduction — called also hypophysis, pituitary body; see ADENOHYPOPHYSIS, NEUROHYPOPHYSIS

pituitary myxedema n : myxedema caused by deficient secretion of thyroid-stimulating hormone

pituitary portal system n : a portal system supplying blood to the anterior lobe of the pituitary gland through veins connecting the capillaries of the median eminence of the hypothalamus with those of the anterior lobe

pi·tu·i·trin \pə-'t(y)ü-ə-trən\ n, often cap : an aqueous extract of the fresh pituitary gland of cattle — formerly a U.S. registered trademark

pit viper n : any of various mostly New World highly specialized venomous snakes (as the rattlesnake, copperhead, water moccasin, and fer-de-lance) that belong to a subfamily (Crotalinae) of the family Viperidae, that have a small depression on each side of the head between the eye and the nostril, and that have hollow perforated fangs usu. folded back in the upper part of the mouth but erected in striking

pit·y·ri·a·sis \ˌpit-ə-'rī-ə-səs\ n, pl -a·ses \-ˌsēz\ 1 : any of several skin diseases marked by the formation and desquamation of fine scales 2 : a disease of domestic animals marked by dry epithelial scales or scurf due to alteration of the function of the sebaceous glands and possibly associated with digestive disorders

pityriasis li·che·noi·des et var·i·o·li·for·mis acu·ta \-ˌlī-kə-'nȯi-ˌdēz-et-ˌvar-ē-ˌō-lə-'fȯr-məs-ə-'k(y)üt-ə\ n : a disease of unknown cause that is characterized by the sudden appearance of polymorphous lesions (as papules, purpuric vesicles, crusts, or ulcerations) resembling chicken pox but tending to persist from a month to as long as years, occurs esp. between the ages of 30 and 50, and is more common in men

pityriasis ro·sea \-'rō-zē-ə\ n : an acute benign and self⸗limited skin eruption of unknown cause that consists of dry, scaly, oval, pinkish or fawn-colored papules, usu. lasts six to eight weeks, and affects esp. the trunk, arms, and thighs

pityriasis ru·bra pi·lar·is \-'rü-brə-pi-'lar-əs\ n : a chronic dermatitis characterized by the formation of papular horny plugs in the hair follicles and pinkish macules which tend to spread and become scaly plaques

pityriasis ste·a·toi·des \-ˌstē-ə-'tȯi-ˌdēz\ n : dandruff characterized by greasy adherent scales

pityriasis ver·si·col·or \-'vər-sə-ˌkəl-ər\ n : TINEA VERSICOLOR

Pit·y·ros·po·rum \ˌpit-ə-'räs-pə-rəm; ˌpit-ər-ō-'spōr-əm, -'spȯr-\ n, syn of MALASSEZIA

pi·val·ic acid \pī-ˌval-ik-\ n : a crystalline acid $(CH_3)_3CCOOH$ isomeric with normal valeric acid

piv·ot \'piv-ət\ n : a usu. metallic pin holding an artificial crown to the root of a tooth

pivot crown n : PIVOT TOOTH

pivot joint n : an anatomical articulation that consists of a bony pivot in a ring of bone and ligament (as that of the dens and atlas) and that permits rotatory movement only — called also trochoid

pivot tooth n : an artificial crown attached to the root of a tooth by a usu. metallic pin — called also pivot crown

pK \'pē-'kā\ n : the cologarithm of the dissociation constant K or –log K that serves as a convenient measure of the strength of an acid ⟨K for acetic acid is 0.000018 or 1.8×10^{-5} from which pK is (5 – 0.25) or 4.75⟩ — compare PH

PK \'pē-'kā\ n : PSYCHOKINESIS

PKC abbr protein kinase C

PKU abbr phenylketonuria

pla·ce·bo \plə-'sē-(ˌ)bō\ n, pl -bos 1 : a usu. pharmacologically inert preparation prescribed more for the mental relief

O
P

of the patient than for its actual effect on a disorder **2** : an inert or innocuous substance used esp. in controlled experiments testing the efficacy of another substance (as a drug)

placebo effect *n* : improvement in the condition of a patient that occurs in response to treatment but cannot be considered due to the specific treatment used

pla·cen·ta \plə-'sent-ə\ *n, pl* **-centas** *or* **-cen·tae** \-'sent-(ˌ)ē\ : the vascular organ in mammals except monotremes and marsupials that unites the fetus to the maternal uterus and mediates its metabolic exchanges through a more or less intimate association of uterine mucosal with chorionic and usu. allantoic tissues permitting exchange of material by diffusion between the maternal and fetal vascular systems but without direct contact between maternal and fetal blood and typically involving the interlocking of fingerlike vascular chorionic villi with corresponding modified areas of the uterine mucosa — see ABRUPTIO PLACENTAE

placentae previae *pl of* PLACENTA PREVIA

¹**pla·cen·tal** \-əl\ *adj* **1** : of, relating to, having, involving, or produced by a placenta ⟨∼ lactogen⟩ ⟨∼ defects⟩ **2** : of or relating to placental mammals

²**placental** *n* : PLACENTAL MAMMAL

placental barrier *n* : a semipermeable membrane made up of placental tissues and limiting the kind and amount of material exchanged between mother and fetus ⟨thiazides cross the *placental barrier* and appear in cord blood —*Resident & Staff Physician*⟩

Plac·en·ta·lia \ˌplas-ᵊn-'tā-lē-ə\ *n pl, syn of* EUTHERIA

placentalis — see AREA PLACENTALIS, DECIDUA PLACENTALIS

placental lactogen *n* : a somatomammotropin that is secreted by the syncytiotrophoblast and that inhibits production of maternal insulin during pregnancy

placental mammal *n* : any mammal of the major taxonomic division Eutheria characterized by the attachment of the developing fetus to the maternal uterus by a placenta

placental sign *n* : a slight bloody discharge from the vagina coinciding with implantation of an embryo in the uterus

placental transmission *n* : passage (as of antibodies or hormones) across the placental barrier

placenta pre·via \-'prē-vē-ə\ *n, pl* **placentae pre·vi·ae** \-vē-ˌē\ : an abnormal implantation of the placenta at or near the internal opening of the uterine cervix so that it tends to precede the child at birth usu. causing severe maternal hemorrhage

pla·cen·ta·tion \ˌplas-ᵊn-'tā-shən, plə-ˌsen-\ *n* **1** : the development of the placenta and attachment of the fetus to the uterus during pregnancy **2** : the morphological type of a placenta

plac·en·ti·tis \ˌplas-ᵊn-'tīt-əs\ *n, pl* **-tit·i·des** \-'tit-ə-ˌdēz\ : inflammation of the placenta

plac·en·tog·ra·phy \ˌplas-ᵊn-'täg-rə-fē\ *n, pl* **-phies** : radiographic visualization of the placenta after injection of a radiopaque medium

plac·en·to·ma \ˌplas-ᵊn-'tō-mə\ *n, pl* **-mas** *or* **-ma·ta** \-mət-ə\ : a tumor developed from retained placental remnants

plac·en·tome \'plas-ᵊn-ˌtōm\ *n* : the whole group of fetal and maternal tissues that are involved in placentation

place theory \'plās-\ *n* : a theory in physiology: the perception of pitch results from the ability of sounds of different pitch to stimulate different areas of the organ of Corti — compare TELEPHONE THEORY

Plac·i·dyl \'plas-ə-ˌdil\ *trademark* — used for a preparation of ethchlorvynol

plac·ode \'pla-ˌkōd\ *n* : a platelike thickening of embryonic ectoderm from which a definitive structure develops ⟨ear ∼⟩ — see LENS PLACODE, OLFACTORY PLACODE

placque *var of* PLAQUE

pla·gi·o·ceph·a·ly \ˌplā-jē-ō-'sef-ə-lē\ *n, pl* **-lies** : a malformation of the head marked by an oblique slant to the main axis of the skull and usu. caused by closure of half of the coronal suture

Pla·gi·or·chis \ˌplā-jē-'ȯr-kəs\ *n* : a large genus (the type of the family Plagiorchiidae) of digenetic trematodes including

parasites of the oviducts or intestine of various wild and domesticated birds and of the intestine of mammals

Pla·gi·o·rhyn·chus \ˌplā-jē-ō-'riŋ-kəs\ *n* : a genus of acanthocephalan worms parasitic in the intestine of domestic fowls and other birds

plague \'plāg\ *n* **1** : an epidemic disease causing a high rate of mortality : PESTILENCE ⟨a ∼ of cholera⟩ **2** : a virulent contagious febrile disease that is caused by a bacterium of the genus *Yersinia* (*Y. pestis* syn. *Pasteurella pestis*), that occurs in bubonic, pneumonic, and septicemic forms, and that is usu. transmitted from rats to humans by the bite of infected fleas (as in bubonic plague) or directly from person to person (as in pneumonic plague) — called also *black death*

plague spot *n* **1** : a hemorrhagic spot on the skin **2** : a locality afflicted with a plague or regarded as a source of contamination

plana *pl of* PLANUM

plana — see PARS PLANA

pla·nar·ia \plə-'nar-ē-ə, -'ner-\ *n* **1** *cap* : the type genus of the family Planariidae comprising planarian worms having two eyes **2** : any worm of the genus *Planaria*; *broadly* : PLANARIAN

pla·nar·i·an \-ē-ən\ *n* : any of the family Planariidae or order Tricladida comprising small soft-bodied ciliated mostly aquatic turbellarian worms — **planarian** *adj*

Plan·a·ri·idae \ˌplan-ə-'rī-ə-ˌdē\ *n pl* : a large family of small soft-bodied usu. leaf-shaped flatworms of the order Tricladida that are almost all free-living in fresh water and often have well-developed eyespots — see PLANARIA

plan·chet \'plan-chət\ *n* : a small metal disk or plate on which a sample of radioactive material is placed (as for quantitative determination of its reactivity)

Planck's constant \'plaŋ(k)s-, 'pläŋ(k)s-\ *n* : a constant that gives the unvarying ratio of the energy of a quantum of radiation to its frequency and that has an approximate value of 6.626×10^{-34} joule second — symbol *h*

Planck \'pläŋk\, **Max Karl Ernst Ludwig (1858–1947),** German physicist. Planck is credited with originating the quantum theory in physics. Throughout his career he taught theoretical physics at a succession of German universities. In 1900 he introduced Planck's constant as a part of his accurate formulation of the distribution of the radiation emitted by a blackbody, which is a perfect absorber of radiant energy. His discoveries established the field of quantum physics. Planck is also remembered for his work relating to thermodynamics and mechanics and to electrical and optical problems associated with radiation of heat and with the quantum theory. He was awarded the Nobel Prize for Physics in 1918.

plane \'plān\ *n* **1 a** : a surface that contains at least three points not all in a straight line and is such that a line drawn through any two points in it lies wholly in the surface **b** : an imaginary plane used to identify parts of the body or a part of the skull — see FRANKFORT HORIZONTAL PLANE, MIDSAGITTAL PLANE **2** : a stage in surgical anesthesia ⟨a light ∼ of anesthesia is maintained with cyclopropane —*Jour. Amer. Med. Assoc.*⟩

plane joint *n* : GLIDING JOINT

plane of polarization *n* : a plane in which electromagnetic radiation vibrates when it is polarized so as to vibrate in a single plane

plane wart *n* : FLAT WART

pla·ni·gram \'plā-nə-ˌgram, 'plan-ə-\ *n* : TOMOGRAM

pla·nig·ra·phy \plə-'nig-rə-fē\ *n, pl* **-phies** : TOMOGRAPHY

pla·nim·e·ter \plā-'nim-ət-ər, plə-\ *n* : an instrument for measuring the area of a plane figure by tracing its boundary line

pla·ni·met·ric \ˌplā-nə-'me-trik\ *adj* : of, relating to, or made by means of a planimeter ⟨∼ measurement⟩ — **pla·nim·e·try** \plā-'nim-ə-trē, plə-\ *n, pl* **-tries**

planing — see ROOT PLANING

Planned Par·ent·hood \'pland-'par-ənt-ˌhu̇d\ *service mark* — used for services and materials promoting the accessibility of effective means of voluntary fertility control

pla·no \'plā-(ˌ)nō\ *adj* : having a flat surface ⟨a ∼ lens⟩

pla·no·cel·lu·lar \ˌplā-nō-'sel-yə-lər\ *adj* : composed of relatively flat cells ⟨∼ cancer of the urinary bladder⟩

pla·no—con·cave \ˌplā-nō-(ˌ)kän-'kāv, -'kän-ˌ\ *adj* : flat on one side and concave on the other ⟨a ∼ lens⟩

pla·no—con·vex \-(ˌ)kän-'veks, -'kän-ˌ, -kən-'\ *adj* : flat on one side and convex on the other ⟨a ∼ lens⟩

Pla·nor·bi·dae \plə-'nȯr-bə-ˌdē\ *n pl* : a family of freshwater pulmonate snails having a single pair of tentacles with an eye at the base of each and gills as well as lungs and including numerous forms important as intermediate hosts of pathogenic trematode worms — see PLANORBIS — **pla·nor·bid** \-bəd\ *adj or n*

Pla·nor·bis \plə-'nȯr-bəs\ *n* : a widely distributed genus of snails that is the type genus of the family Planorbidae, comprises snails having secondarily acquired gills and rather flattened spiral shells, and includes several that are intermediate hosts for schistosomes infecting humans

plantae — see QUADRATUS PLANTAE

plan·ta·go \plan-'tā-(ˌ)gō\ *n* **1** *cap* : a large genus (the type of the family Plantaginaceae) of weeds that have narrow or elliptic leaves and very small inconspicuous flowers, comprise the plantains, and include the Old World fleawort (*P. psyllium*) and two other plants (*P. indica* and *P. ovata*) having indigestible and mucilaginous seeds used as a mild cathartic — see PSYLLIUM SEED **2** : PLANTAIN

plantago seed *n* : PSYLLIUM SEED

plan·tain \'plant-ᵊn\ *n* : any plant of the genus *Plantago*

plan·tar \'plant-ər, 'plan-ˌtär\ *adj* : of, relating to, or typical of the sole of the foot ⟨the ∼ aspect of the foot⟩

plantar arch *n* : an arterial arch in the sole of the foot formed by the lateral plantar artery and a branch of the dorsalis pedis

plantar artery *n* : either of the two terminal branches into which the posterior tibial artery divides: **a** : one that is larger and passes laterally and then medially to join with a branch of the dorsalis pedis to form the plantar arch — called also *lateral plantar artery* **b** : one that is smaller and follows a more medial course as it passes distally supplying or giving off branches which supply the plantar part of the foot and the toes — called also *medial plantar artery*

plantar cal·ca·neo·na·vic·u·lar ligament \-(ˌ)kal-ˌkā-nē-ō-nə-'vik-yə-lər-\ *n* : an elastic ligament of the sole of the foot that connects the calcaneus and navicular bone and supports the head of the talus — called also *spring ligament*

plantar cushion *n* : a thick pad of fibrous tissue behind and under the navicular and coffin bones of the horse

plantar fascia *n* : a very strong dense fibrous membrane of the sole of the foot that lies beneath the skin and superficial layer of fat and binds together the deeper structures

plantar fasciitis *n* : inflammation involving the plantar fascia esp. in the area of its attachment to the calcaneus and causing pain under the heel in walking and running

plantar flexion *n* : movement of the foot that flexes the foot or toes downward toward the sole — compare DORSIFLEXION

plantar interosseus *n* : any of three small muscles of the plantar aspect of the foot each of which lies along the plantar side of one of the third, fourth, and fifth toes facing the second toe, arises from the metatarsal bone of the toe along which it lies, inserts into its proximal phalanx, and acts to flex the proximal phalanx and extend the distal phalanges of its toe and to adduct its toe toward the second toe — called also *interosseus plantaris, plantar interosseus muscle*

plan·tar·is \plan-'tar-əs\ *n, pl* **plan·tar·es** \-ˌēz\ : a small muscle of the calf of the leg that arises from the lower end of the femur and the posterior ligament of the knee joint, is inserted with the Achilles tendon by a very long slender tendon into the calcaneus, and weakly flexes the leg at the knee and the foot at the ankle — see PLANTAR INTEROSSEUS, VERRUCA PLANTARIS

plantar nerve *n* : either of two nerves of the foot that are the two terminal branches into which the tibial nerve divides: **a** : a smaller one that supplies most of the deeper muscles of the foot and the skin on the lateral part of the sole and on the fifth toe as well as on the lateral part of the fourth toe — called also *lateral plantar nerve* **b** : a larger one that accompanies the medial plantar artery and supplies a number of muscles of the medial part of the foot, the skin on the medial two-thirds of the sole, and the skin on the first to fourth toes — called also *medial plantar nerve*

plantar reflex *n* : a reflex movement of flexing the foot and toes that after the first year is the normal response to tickling of the sole — compare BABINSKI REFLEX

plantar vein *n* : either of two veins that accompany the plantar arteries: **a** : one accompanying the lateral plantar artery — called also *lateral plantar vein* **b** : one accompanying the medial plantar artery — called also *medial plantar vein*

plantar wart *n* : a wart on the sole of the foot — called also *verruca plantaris*

plan·ter's wart \'plan-tərz-\ *n* : PLANTAR WART

plant hormone \'plant-\ *n* : an organic substance other than a nutrient that in minute amounts modifies a plant physiological process; *esp* : one produced by a plant and active elsewhere than at the site of production — called also *phytohormone*

plan·ti·grade \'plant-ə-ˌgrād\ *adj* : walking on the sole with the heel touching the ground ⟨humans are ∼ animals⟩ — compare DIGITIGRADE — **plantigrade** *n*

plant kingdom *n* : the one of the three basic groups of natural objects that includes all living and extinct plants — compare ANIMAL KINGDOM, MINERAL KINGDOM

plant pathologist *n* : a specialist in plant pathology — called also *phytopathologist*

plant pathology *n* : a branch of botany concerned with the diseases of plants — called also *phytopathology*

pla·num \'plā-nəm\ *n, pl* **pla·na** \-nə\ : a flat surface of bone esp. of the skull

planum tem·po·ra·le \-ˌtem-pə-'rā-lē\ *n* : an area of the cerebral cortex between Heschl's gyrus and the sylvian fissure that is involved in speech and is usu. larger in the cerebral hemisphere on the left side of the brain

planus — see LICHEN PLANUS

plaque *also* **placque** \'plak\ *n* **1 a** : a localized abnormal patch on a body part or surface and esp. on the skin ⟨psoriatic ∼⟩ **b** : a sticky usu. colorless film on teeth that is formed by and harbors bacteria **c** : an atherosclerotic lesion **d** : a histopathologic lesion of brain tissue that is characteristic of Alzheimer's disease and consists of a dense proteinaceous core composed primarily of beta-amyloid that is often surrounded and infiltrated by a cluster of degenerating axons and dendrites — called also *senile plaque* **2** : a visibly distinct and esp. a clear or opaque area in a bacterial culture produced by damage to or destruction of cells by a virus

Plaque·nil \'plak-ə-ˌnil\ *trademark* — used for a preparation of the sulfate of hydroxychloroquine

plasm \'plaz-əm\ *n* : PLASMA — see GERM PLASM

plas·ma \'plaz-mə\ *n* **1 a** : the fluid part esp. of blood, lymph, or milk that is distinguished from suspended material — see BLOOD PLASMA **b** : the juice that can be expressed from muscle **2** : PROTOPLASM **3** : a mixture of starch and gel used as an ointment base

plas·ma·blast \'plaz-mə-ˌblast\ *n* : a precursor of a plasma cell

plasma cell *n* : a lymphocyte that is a mature antibody-secreting B cell

plasma—cell dyscrasia *n* : MONOCLONAL GAMMOPATHY

plas·ma·cyte \'plaz-mə-ˌsīt\ *n* : PLASMA CELL — **plas·ma·cyt·ic** \ˌplaz-mə-'sit-ik\ *adj*

plas·ma·cy·toid \ˌplaz-mə-'sī-ˌtȯid\ *adj* : resembling or derived from a plasma cell

plas·ma·cy·to·ma *also* **plas·mo·cy·to·ma** \ˌplaz-mə-sī-'tō-

\ə\ abut \ᵊ\ kitten \ər\ further \a\ ash \ā\ ace \ä\ cot, cart \au̇\ out \ch\ chin \e\ bet \ē\ easy \g\ go \i\ hit \ī\ ice \j\ job \ŋ\ sing \ō\ go \ȯ\ law \ȯi\ boy \th\ thin \t͟h\ the \ü\ loot \u̇\ foot \y\ yet \zh\ vision *See also* Pronunciation Symbols page

mə\ *n, pl* **-mas** *also* **-ma·ta** \-mət-ə\ : a myeloma composed of plasma cells

plas·ma·cy·to·sis \ˌplaz-mə-sī-ˈtō-səs\ *n, pl* **-to·ses** \-ˌsēz\ : the presence of abnormal numbers of plasma cells in the blood

plas·ma·gel \ˈplaz-mə-ˌjel\ *n* : gelated protoplasm; *esp* : the outer firm zone of a pseudopodium

plas·ma·gene \-ˌjēn\ *n* : an extranuclear determiner of hereditary characteristics with a capacity for replication similar to that of a nuclear gene

plas·mal \ˈplaz-məl\ *n* : a substance consisting of one or more aldehydes that is of the same type as those related to palmitic acid and stearic acid and is obtained in the form of an acetal (as by treatment of a plasmalogen with alkali)

plas·ma·lem·ma \ˌplaz-mə-ˈlem-ə\ *n* : PLASMA MEMBRANE

plas·mal·o·gen \plaz-ˈmal-ə-jən, -ˌjen\ *n* : any of a group of phospholipids in which a fatty acid group is replaced by a fatty aldehyde and which include lecithins, phosphatidylethanolamines, and phosphatidylserines

plasmal reaction *n* : a modified Feulgen reaction designed to detect aldehyde in tissue

plasma membrane *n* : a semipermeable limiting layer of cell protoplasm consisting of a fluid phospholipid bilayer with intercalated proteins — called also *cell membrane, plasmalemma*

plas·ma·pher·e·sis \ˌplaz-mə-ˈfer-ə-səs, -fə-ˈrē-səs\ *n, pl* **-e·ses** \-ˌsēz\ : a process for obtaining blood plasma without depleting the donor or patient of other blood constituents (as red blood cells) by separating out the plasma from the whole blood and returning the rest to the donor's or patient's circulatory system

plas·ma·sol \ˈplaz-mə-ˌsäl, -ˌsòl, -ˌsōl\ *n* : cytoplasm in the form of a sol esp. in a pseudopodium or ameboid cell

plasmasome *var of* PLASMOSOME

plasma thromboplastin an·te·ced·ent \-ˌant-ə-ˈsēd-ᵊnt\ *n* : a clotting factor whose absence is associated with a form of hemophilia — abbr. *PTA;* called also *factor XI*

plasma thromboplastin component *n* : FACTOR IX — abbr. *PTC*

plas·mat·ic \plaz-ˈmat-ik\ *adj* : of, relating to, or occurring in plasma esp. of blood ⟨∼ fibrils⟩

plas·mic \ˈplaz-mik\ *adj* : PROTOPLASMIC; *also* : PLASMATIC

plas·mid \ˈplaz-məd\ *n* : an extrachromosomal ring of DNA that replicates autonomously and is found esp. in bacteria — compare EPISOME

plas·min \-mən\ *n* : a proteolytic enzyme that dissolves the fibrin of blood clots

plas·min·o·gen \plaz-ˈmin-ə-jən\ *n* : the precursor of plasmin that is found in blood plasma and serum — called also *profibrinolysin*

plasminogen activator *n* : any of a group of substances (as urokinase) that convert plasminogen to plasmin — see TISSUE PLASMINOGEN ACTIVATOR

plasmocytoma *var of* PLASMACYTOMA

plasmodia *pl of* PLASMODIUM

plas·mo·di·al \plaz-ˈmōd-ē-əl\ *also* **plas·mod·ic** \-ˈmäd-ik\ *adj* : of, relating to, or resembling a plasmodium

plas·mo·di·a·sis \ˌplaz-mə-ˈdī-ə-səs\ *n, pl* **-a·ses** \-ˌsēz\ : MALARIA

plas·mo·di·cide \plaz-ˈmōd-ə-ˌsīd\ *n* : an agent used to kill malaria parasites — **plas·mo·di·cid·al** \-ˌmōd-ə-ˈsīd-ᵊl\ *adj*

Plas·mo·di·idae \ˌplaz-mə-ˈdī-ə-ˌdē\ *n pl* : a family of sporozoans of the order Haemosporidia that comprises the malaria parasites, is distinguished by alternation between the blood system of vertebrates and the digestive system of mosquitoes, and is usu. held to include only the genus *Plasmodium* — see LAVERANIA

plas·mo·di·o·sis \plaz-ˌmōd-ē-ˈō-səs\ *n, pl* **-o·ses** \-ˌsēz\ : MALARIA

plas·mo·di·tro·pho·blast \plaz-ˌmōd-ē-ˈtrō-fə-ˌblast\ *n* : the syncytium of a chorion

plas·mo·di·um \plaz-ˈmōd-ē-əm\ *n* **1** *pl* **-dia** \-dē-ə\ **a :** a motile multinucleate mass of protoplasm resulting from fusion of uninucleate ameboid cells; *also* : an organism (as a

stage of a slime mold) that consists of such a structure **b** : SYNCYTIUM 1 **2 a** *cap* : the type genus of the family Plasmodiidae of sporozoans that includes all the malaria parasites affecting humans **b** *pl* **-dia** : any individual malaria parasite

Plas·mod·ro·ma \plaz-ˈmäd-rə-mə\ *n pl, in some former classifications* : a subphylum of Protozoa comprising the classes Mastigophora, Sarcodina, and Sporozoa and characterized by absence of cilia and possession of nuclei of one kind only

plas·mog·a·my \plaz-ˈmäg-ə-mē\ *n, pl* **-mies** : fusion of the cytoplasm of two or more cells as distinguished from fusion of nuclei — called also *plastogamy*

plas·mol·y·sis \plaz-ˈmäl-ə-səs\ *n* : shrinking of the cytoplasm away from the wall of a living cell due to water loss by exosmosis

plas·mo·lyt·ic \ˌplaz-mə-ˈlit-ik\ *adj* : of or relating to plasmolysis

plas·mo·lyz·abil·i·ty *or chiefly Brit* **plas·mo·lys·abil·i·ty** \ˌplaz-mə-ˌlī-zə-ˈbil-ət-ē\ *n, pl* **-ties** : the capability of being plasmolyzed

plas·mo·lyz·able *or chiefly Brit* **plas·mo·lys·able** \ˌplaz-mə-ˈlī-zə-bəl\ *adj* : capable of being plasmolyzed

plas·mo·lyze *or chiefly Brit* **plas·mo·lyse** \ˈplaz-mə-ˌlīz\ *vb* **-lyzed** *or chiefly Brit* **-lysed; -lyz·ing** *or chiefly Brit* **-lys·ing** *vt* : to subject to plasmolysis ∼ *vi* : to undergo plasmolysis

plas·mon \ˈplaz-ˌmän\ *also* **plas·mone** \-ˌmōn\ *n* : the cytoplasm of a cell regarded as a system of hereditary extrachromosomal determinants

plas·mop·ty·sis \plaz-ˈmäp-tə-səs\ *n, pl* **-ty·ses** \-ˌsēz\ : the bursting forth of protoplasm from a cell through rupture of the cell wall

plas·mor·rhex·is \ˌplaz-mə-ˈrek-səs\ *n, pl* **-rhex·es** \-ˌsēz\ : ERYTHROCYTORRHEXIS

plas·mo·some *also* **plas·ma·some** \ˈplaz-mə-ˌsōm\ *n* : NUCLEOLUS

plas·mot·o·my \plaz-ˈmät-ə-mē\ *n, pl* **-mies** : division of the plasmodium of a protozoan into two or more multinucleate parts

plas·tein \ˈplas-ˌtēn, -tē-ən\ *n* : any of several substances that resemble proteins and are precipitated by the action of proteolytic enzymes (as pepsin or papain) on the digestion products of protein

plas·ter \ˈplas-tər\ *n* : a medicated or protective dressing that consists of a film (as of cloth or plastic) spread with a usu. medicated substance ⟨adhesive ∼⟩

plaster cast *n* : a rigid dressing of gauze impregnated with plaster of paris

plaster of par·is \-ˈpar-əs\ *n* : a white powdery slightly hydrated calcium sulfate $CaSO_4 \cdot \frac{1}{2}H_2O$ or $2CaSO_4 \cdot H_2O$ that is made by calcining gypsum, forms a quick-setting paste with water, and is used in medicine chiefly in casts and for surgical bandages

¹plas·tic \ˈplas-tik\ *adj* **1** : made or consisting of a plastic **2** : capable of being deformed continuously and permanently in any direction without breaking or tearing **3 a** : capable of growth, repair, or differentiation ⟨a ∼ tissue⟩ **b** : relating to, characterized by, or exhibiting neural plasticity **4** : of, relating to, or involving plastic surgery ⟨∼ repair⟩

²plastic *n* **1** : a plastic substance; *specif* : any of numerous organic synthetic or processed materials that are mostly thermoplastic or thermosetting polymers of high molecular weight and that can be made into objects, films, or filaments **2** : an object made of plastic

plas·tic·i·ty \pla-ˈstis-ət-ē\ *n, pl* **-ties** **1** : the quality or state of being plastic; *esp* : capacity for being molded or altered **2** : the ability to retain a shape attained by pressure deformation **3** : the capacity of organisms with the same genotype to vary in developmental pattern, in phenotype, or in behavior according to varying environmental conditions **4** : the capacity for continuous alteration of the neural pathways and synapses of the living brain and nervous system in response to experience or injury that involves the formation of new pathways and synapses and the elimination or modification of existing ones

plas·ti·cize *or Brit* **plas·ti·cise** \'plas-tə-ˌsīz\ *vt* **-cized** *or Brit* **-cised; -ciz·ing** *or Brit* **-cis·ing** **1** : to make plastic **2** : to treat with a plastic — **plas·ti·ci·za·tion** *or Brit* **plas·ti·ci·sa·tion** \ˌplas-tə-sə-'zā-shən\ *n*

plas·ti·ciz·er *or Brit* **plas·ti·cis·er** \'plas-tə-ˌsī-zər\ *n* : a chemical added esp. to rubbers and resins to impart flexibility, workability, or stretchability

plastic surgeon *n* : a specialist in plastic surgery

plastic surgery *n* : a branch of surgery concerned with the repair, restoration, or improvement of lost, injured, defective, or misshapen parts of the body chiefly by transfer of tissue; *also* : an operation performed for such a purpose

plas·tid \'plas-təd\ *n* : any of various cytoplasmic organelles of photosynthetic cells that serve in many cases as centers of special metabolic activities — **plas·tid·i·al** \pla-'stid-ē-əl\ *adj*

plas·tog·a·my \pla-'stäg-ə-mē\ *n, pl* **-mies** : PLASMOGAMY

plas·to·qui·none \ˌplas-(ˌ)tō-kwin-'ōn, -'kwin-ˌōn\ *n* : any of a group of substances that occur mostly in plant chloroplasts, are related to vitamin K, and play a role in photosynthetic phosphorylation

plas·ty \'plas-tē\ *n, pl* **plas·ties** : a surgical procedure for the repair, restoration, or replacement (as by a prosthesis) of a part of the body ⟨quadriceps ∼⟩ ⟨total knee ∼⟩

¹plate \'plāt\ *n* **1** : a thin relatively flat piece or lamina (as of bone) that is part of the body **2 a** : a flat glass dish used chiefly for culturing microorganisms; *esp* : PETRI DISH **b** : a culture or culture medium contained in such a dish **3** : a supporting or reinforcing element: as **a** : the part of a denture that fits in the mouth; *broadly* : DENTURE **b** : a thin flat narrow piece of metal (as stainless steel) that is used to repair a bone defect or fracture

²plate *vt* **plat·ed; plat·ing** **1** : to inoculate and culture (microorganisms or cells) on a plate; *also* : to distribute (an inoculum) on a plate or plates for cultivation **2** : to repair (as a fractured bone) with metal plates

pla·teau \pla-'tō, 'pla-ˌ\ *n, pl* **plateaus** *or* **pla·teaux** \-'tōz, -ˌtōz\ : a relatively flat elevated area — see TIBIAL PLATEAU

plate·let \'plāt-lət\ *n* : a minute colorless anucleate disklike body of mammalian blood that is derived from fragments of megakaryocyte cytoplasm, that is released from the bone marrow into the blood, and that assists in blood clotting by adhering to other platelets and to damaged epithelium — called also *blood platelet, thrombocyte*

plate·let–ac·ti·vat·ing factor \-ˌak-tə-ˌvāt-iŋ-\ *n* : phospholipid that is produced esp. by mast cells and basophils, causes the aggregation of blood platelets and the release of bloodplatelet substances (as histamine or serotonin), and is a mediator of inflammation (as in asthma) — abbr. *PAF*

platelet co·fac·tor I \-'kō-ˌfak-tər-'wən\ *n* : FACTOR VIII

platelet cofactor II \-'tü\ *n* : FACTOR IX

platelet–derived growth factor *n* : a mitogenic growth factor that is found esp. in platelets, consists of two polypeptide chains linked by bonds containing two sulfur atoms each, stimulates cell proliferation (as in connective tissue, smooth muscle, and glia), and plays a role in wound healing — abbr. *PDGF*

plate·let·phe·re·sis \-fə-'rē-səs, -'fer-ə-səs\ *n, pl* **-re·ses** \-ˌsēz\ : apheresis used to collect blood platelets

plat·ing \'plāt-iŋ\ *n* **1** : the spreading of a sample of cells or microorganisms on a nutrient medium in a petri dish **2** : the immobilization of a fractured bone by securing a metal plate to it

pla·tin·ic \pla-'tin-ik\ *adj* : of, relating to, or containing platinum esp. with a valence of four — compare PLATINOUS

Plat·i·nol \'plat-ə-ˌnȯl, -ˌnōl\ *trademark* — used for a preparation of cisplatin

plat·i·nous \'plat-nəs, -ᵊn-əs\ *adj* : of, relating to, or containing platinum esp. with a valence of two — compare PLATINIC

plat·i·num \'plat-nəm, -ᵊn-əm\ *n* : a heavy precious grayish white noncorroding ductile malleable metallic element that fuses with difficulty and is used esp. in chemical ware and apparatus, as a catalyst, and in dental and jewelry alloys — symbol *Pt*; see ELEMENT table

plat·ode \'pla-ˌtōd\ *n* : FLATWORM, PLATYHELMINTH

platy·ba·sia \ˌplat-i-'bā-sē-ə\ *n* : a developmental deformity of the base of the skull in which the lower occiput is pushed by the upper cervical spine into the cranial fossa

platy·cne·mia \ˌplat-i(k)-'nē-mē-ə\ *n* : the condition of being platycnemic — called also *platycnemy*

platy·cne·mic \-'nē-mik\ *adj, of a shinbone* : laterally flattened with a platycnemic index of 55.0 to 62.9

platycnemic index *n* : the ratio of the anteroposterior diameter of the shinbone to its lateral diameter multiplied by 100

platy·cne·my \'plat-i(k)-ˌnē-mē\ *n, pl* **-mies** : PLATYCNEMIA

platy·hel·minth \ˌplat-i-'hel-ˌmin(t)th\ *n* : any worm of the phylum Platyhelminthes — called also *flatworm*

Platy·hel·min·thes \ˌplat-i-hel-'min(t)-thēz\ *n pl* : a phylum of soft-bodied bilaterally symmetrical usu. much flattened invertebrates comprising the planarians, flukes, tapeworms, and related worms, having the body unsegmented or composed of a series of proglottids formed by strobilation, built up of ectoderm, endoderm, and mesoderm, and without body cavity, the space between the body wall and the various organs being filled with parenchyma, and distinguished by an excretory system made up of tubules that permeate the body and usu. communicate with the exterior and that end internally in flame cells

platy·hel·min·thic \-hel-'min(t)-thik\ *adj* **1** : of or relating to the phylum Platyhelminthes **2** : of or relating to a platyhelminth

platy·hi·er·ic \ˌplat-i-hī-'er-ik\ *adj* : having a relatively wide sacrum with a sacral index of 106.0 or over — compare DOLICHOHIERIC, SUBPLATYHIERIC

platy·mer·ic \ˌplat-i-'mer-ik\ *adj, of a thigh bone* : laterally flattened with a platymeric index of 75.0 to 84.9

platymeric index *n* : the ratio of the anteroposterior diameter of the femur to its lateral diameter multiplied by 100

platy·pel·lic \ˌplat-i-'pel-ik\ *adj* : having a broad pelvis with a pelvic index of 89.9 or less — **platy·pel·ly** \'plat-i-ˌpel-ē\ *n, pl* **-pel·lies**

platy·pel·loid \-'pel-ˌȯid\ *adj, of the pelvis* : broad and flat : approaching a platypellic condition — compare ANDROID, ANTHROPOID, GYNECOID

¹plat·yr·rhine \'plat-i-ˌrīn\ *adj* **1** : of, relating to, or being any of a division (Platyrrhina) of arboreal New World monkeys characterized by a broad nasal septum, usu. 36 teeth, and often a prehensile tail **2** : having a short broad nose

²platyrrhine *n* : a platyrrhine individual

pla·tys·ma \plə-'tiz-mə\ *n, pl* **-ma·ta** \-'mät-ə\ *also* **-mas** : a broad thin layer of muscle that is situated on each side of the neck immediately under the superficial fascia belonging to the group of facial muscles, that is innervated by the facial nerve, and that draws the lower lip and the corner of the mouth to the side and down and when moved forcefully expands the neck and draws its skin upward — **pla·tys·mal** \-məl\ *adj*

Pla·vix \'plā-viks\ *trademark* — used for a preparation of the bisulfate of clopidogrel

play therapy \'plā-ˌ\ *n* : psychotherapy in which a child is encouraged to reveal feelings and conflicts in play rather than by verbalization

pleasure principle \'ple-zhər-ˌ\ *n* : a tendency for individual behavior to be directed toward immediate satisfaction of instinctual drives and immediate relief from pain or discomfort — compare REALITY PRINCIPLE

pled·get \'plej-ət\ *n* : a compress or small flat mass usu. of gauze or absorbent cotton that is laid over a wound or into a cavity to apply medication, exclude air, retain dressings, or absorb the matter discharged

ple·gia \'plē-j(ē-)ə\ *n* : PARALYSIS

pleiomorphic *var of* PLEOMORPHIC

pleio·tro·pic \ˌplī-ə-'trōp-ik, -'träp-\ *adj* : producing more

\ə\ **abut** \ᵊ\ **kitten** \ər\ **further** \a\ **ash** \ā\ **ace** \ä\ **cot, cart**
\au̇\ **out** \ch\ **chin** \e\ **bet** \ē\ **easy** \g\ **go** \i\ **hit** \ī\ **ice** \j\ **job**
\ŋ\ **sing** \ō\ **go** \ȯ\ **law** \ȯi\ **boy** \th\ **thin** \th̲\ **the** \ü\ **loot**
\u̇\ **foot** \y\ **yet** \zh\ **vision** *See also* Pronunciation Symbols page

O
P

than one effect; *esp* : having multiple phenotypic expressions ⟨a ∼ gene⟩

plei·ot·ro·pism \plī-'ä-trə-ˌpiz-əm\ *n* : a condition produced by a pleiotropic gene

plei·ot·ro·py \plī-'ä-trə-pē\ *n, pl* **-pies** : the quality or state of being pleiotropic

ple·och·ro·ism \plē-'äk-rə-ˌwiz-əm\ *n* : the property of a crystal of showing different colors when viewed by light that vibrates parallel to different axes — **pleo·chro·ic** \ˌplē-ə-'krō-ik\ *adj*

pleo·cy·to·sis \ˌplē-ō-ˌsī-'tō-səs\ *n, pl* **-to·ses** \-ˌsēz\ : an abnormal increase in the number of cells (as lymphocytes) in the cerebrospinal fluid

pleo·mor·phic \ˌplē-ə-'mȯr-fik\ *also* **pleio·mor·phic** \ˌplī-ə-\ *adj* : able to assume different forms : POLYMORPHIC ⟨∼ bacteria⟩ ⟨a ∼ sarcoma⟩

pleo·mor·phism \ˌplē-ə-'mȯr-ˌfiz-əm\ *n* : the quality or state of having or assuming various forms : POLYMORPHISM

pleo·mor·phous \ˌplē-ə-'mȯr-fəs\ *adj* : POLYMORPHIC

ple·op·tics \plē-'äp-tiks\ *n pl but sing in constr* : a system of treating amblyopia by retraining visual habits using guided exercises — **ple·op·tic** \-tik\ *adj*

ple·ro·cer·coid \ˌplir-ō-'sər-ˌkȯid\ *n* : the solid elongate infective larva of some tapeworms esp. of the order Pseudophyllidea usu. occurring in the muscles of fishes

pleth·o·ra \'pleth-ə-rə\ *n* : a bodily condition characterized by an excess of blood and marked by turgescence and a reddish complexion — **ple·tho·ric** \plə-'thȯr-ik, ple-, -'thär-; 'pleth-ə-rik\ *adj*

ple·thys·mo·gram \ple-'thiz-mə-ˌgram, plə-\ *n* : a tracing made by a plethysmograph

ple·thys·mo·graph \-ˌgraf\ *n* : an instrument for determining and registering variations in the size of an organ or limb resulting from changes in the amount of blood present or passing through it — **ple·thys·mo·graph·ic** \-ˌthiz-mə-'graf-ik\ *adj* — **ple·thys·mo·graph·i·cal·ly** \-i-k(ə-)lē\ *adv*

pleth·ys·mog·ra·phy \ˌpleth-iz-'mäg-rə-fē\ *n, pl* **-phies** : the use of the plethysmograph : examination by plethysmograph

pleu·ra \'plu̇r-ə\ *n, pl* **pleu·rae** \'plu̇r-ē\ *or* **pleuras** : either of a pair of two-walled sacs of serous membrane each of which lines one lateral half of the thorax, has an inner visceral layer closely adherent to the corresponding lung, is reflected at the root of the lung to form a parietal layer that adheres to the walls of the thorax, the pericardium, the upper surface of the diaphragm, and adjacent parts, and contains a small amount of serous fluid that minimizes the friction of respiratory movements

pleu·ral \'plu̇r-əl\ *adj* : of or relating to the pleura or the sides of the thorax

pleural cavity *n* : the space that is formed when the two layers of the pleura spread apart — called also *pleural space*

pleural effusion *n* **1** : an exudation of fluid from the blood or lymph into a pleural cavity **2** : an exudate in a pleural cavity

pleural space *n* : PLEURAL CAVITY

pleu·rec·to·my \plu̇-'rek-tə-mē\ *n, pl* **-mies** : surgical excision of part of the pleura

pleu·ri·sy \'plu̇r-ə-sē\ *n, pl* **-sies** : inflammation of the pleura that is typically characterized by sudden onset, painful and difficult respiration, and exudation of fluid or fibrinous material into the pleural cavity — called also *pleuritis;* see DRY PLEURISY, WET PLEURISY

pleurisy root *n* **1** : BUTTERFLY WEED **2** : ASCLEPIAS 3

pleu·rit·ic \plu̇-'rit-ik\ *adj* : of, relating to, or affected with pleurisy ⟨∼ chest pain⟩

pleu·ri·tis \plu̇-'rīt-əs\ *n, pl* **pleu·rit·i·des** \-'rit-ə-ˌdēz\ : PLEURISY

pleu·rod·e·sis \plu̇-'räd-ə-səs\ *n* : obliteration of the pleural cavity by inducing adherence of the visceral and parietal pleural layers (as by the use of sclerosing agents or surgical abrasion) esp. to treat pleural effusion, pneumothorax, and chylothorax

pleu·ro·dyn·ia \ˌplu̇r-ə-'din-ē-ə\ *n* **1** : a sharp pain in the

side usu. located in the intercostal muscles and believed to arise from inflammation of fibrous tissue **2** : EPIDEMIC PLEURODYNIA

pleu·ro·loph·o·cer·cous \ˌplu̇r-ə-ˌläf-ə-'sər-kəs\ *adj* : of, relating to, or being a small cercaria that has a long strong tail, a protrusible oral sucker, and pigmented eyespots

pleu·rol·y·sis \plu̇-'räl-ə-səs\ *n, pl* **-y·ses** \-ˌsēz\ : PNEUMONOLYSIS

pleu·ro·peri·car·di·tis \ˌplu̇r-ō-ˌper-ə-ˌkär-'dīt-əs\ *n, pl* **-dit·i·des** \-'dit-ə-ˌdēz\ : inflammation of the pleura and the pericardium

pleu·ro·peri·to·ne·al \-ˌper-ət-ᵊn-'ē-əl\ *adj* : of or relating to the pleura and the peritoneum

pleu·ro·pneu·mo·nia \ˌplu̇r-ō-n(y)u̇-'mō-nyə\ *n* **1** : pleurisy accompanied by pneumonia **2** : a highly contagious pneumonia usu. associated with pleurisy of cattle, goats, and sheep that is caused by a microorganism of the genus *Mycoplasma* (esp. *M. mycoides*) **3** : a contagious often fatal respiratory disease esp. of young pigs that is caused by a bacterium of the genus *Haemophilus* (*H. pleuropneumoniae*) **4** : pleurisy of horses that is often accompanied by pneumonia and is caused by various microorganisms

pleu·ro·pneu·mo·nia–like organism \-ˌlīk-\ *n* : MYCOPLASMA 2

pleu·ro·pul·mo·nary \ˌplu̇r-ō-'pu̇l-mə-ˌner-ē, -'pəl-\ *adj* : of or relating to the pleura and the lungs ⟨∼ infections⟩

pleu·ro·thot·o·nos \ˌplu̇r-ə-'thät-ᵊn-əs\ *n* : a tonic spasm in which the body is curved laterally

plex·ec·to·my \plek-'sek-tə-mē\ *n, pl* **-mies** : surgical removal of a plexus

plexi·form \'plek-sə-ˌfȯrm\ *adj* : of, relating to, or having the form or characteristics of a plexus ⟨∼ networks⟩

plexiform layer *n* : either of two reticular layers of the retina consisting of nerve cell processes and situated between layers of ganglion cells and cell bodies

plex·im·e·ter \plek-'sim-ət-ər\ *n* : a small hard flat plate (as of ivory) placed in contact with the body to receive the blow in percussion

plex·op·a·thy \plek-'säp-ə-thē\ *n, pl* **-thies** : an injured or disordered condition of a plexus and esp. a nerve plexus ⟨severe neuralgia due to brachial ∼ —Mary Ann Moon⟩

plex·or \'plek-sər\ *n* : a small hammer with a rubber head used in medical percussion

plex·us \'plek-səs\ *n, pl* **plex·us·es** : a network of anastomosing or interlacing blood vessels or nerves

pli·ca \'plī-kə\ *n, pl* **pli·cae** \-ˌkē, -ˌsē\ : a fold or folded part; *esp* : a groove or fold of skin

plicae cir·cu·la·res \-ˌsər-kyə-'lar-(ˌ)ēz\ *n pl* : the numerous permanent crescentic folds of mucous membrane found in the small intestine esp. in the lower part of the duodenum and the jejunum — called also *valvulae conniventes*

plica fim·bri·a·ta \-ˌfim-brē-'āt-ə\ *n, pl* **plicae fim·bri·a·tae** \-'āt-ē\ : a fold resembling a fringe on the under surface of the tongue on either side of the frenulum

pli·cal \'plī-kəl\ *adj* : of, relating to, or having plicae

plica lac·ri·ma·lis \-ˌlak-rə-'mā-ləs\ *n* : an imperfect valve at the opening of the nasolacrimal duct into the inferior meatus of the nose — called also *valve of Hasner*

pli·ca·my·cin \ˌplī-kə-'mīs-ᵊn\ *n* : an antineoplastic agent $C_{52}H_{76}O_{24}$ produced by three bacteria of the genus *Streptomyces* (*S. argillaceus, S. tanashiensis,* and *S. plicatus*) and administered intravenously esp. in the treatment of malignant tumors of the testes or in the treatment of hypercalcemia and hypercalciuria associated with advanced neoplastic disease — called also *mithramycin*

plica po·lon·i·ca \-pə-'län-i-kə\ *n, pl* **plicae po·lon·i·cae** \-ˌsē\ : a state of the hair in which it becomes twisted, matted, and crusted, usu. as a result of neglect, filth, and infestation by vermin

plica semi·lu·na·ris \-ˌsem-i-ˌlü-'nar-əs\ *n, pl* **plicae semi·lu·na·res** \-(ˌ)ēz\ : the vertical fold of conjunctiva that occupies the canthus of the eye nearer the nose and is homologous to the nictitating membrane of lower animals

plica sub·lin·gua·lis \-ˌsəb-(ˌ)lin̬-'gwā-ləs\ *n, pl* **plicae sub-**

lin·gua·les \-(ˌ)lēz\ : a transverse fold of mucous membrane that is situated at the base of the tongue on either side of the frenulum, overlies the sublingual gland, and is studded with 10 or 12 openings of the ducts of Rivinus

¹pli·cate \ˈplī-ˌkāt\ vt **pli·cat·ed; pli·cat·ing** : to perform plication on ⟨the vein graft was then *plicated* by means of . . . sutures placed about 2 mm. apart —*Jour. Amer. Med. Assoc.*⟩

²plicate or **pli·cat·ed** \-ˌkāt-əd\ adj : being folded, tucked, or ridged esp. like a fan

pli·ca·tion \plī-ˈkā-shən\ n **1** : the tightening of stretched or weakened bodily tissues or channels by folding the excess in tucks and suturing ⟨∼ of the neck of the bladder⟩ **2** : the folding of one part on and the fastening of it to another (as areas of the bowel freed from adhesions and left without normal serosal covering)

plica trans·ver·sa·lis rec·ti \-ˌtranz-vər-ˌsā-ləs-ˈrek-ˌtī\ n, pl **plicae trans·ver·sa·les recti** \-ˌsā-lēz-\ : HOUSTON'S VALVE

ploi·dy \ˈplȯid-ē\ n, pl **ploi·dies** : degree of repetition of the basic number of chromosomes

plom·bage \ˌpläm-ˈbäzh\ n : sustained compression of the sides of a pulmonary cavity against each other to effect closure by pressure exerted by packing (as of paraffin or plastic spheres)

PLSS abbr portable life-support system

¹plug \ˈpləg\ n : a piece of material (as wood or alloy) used or serving to fill a hole: as **a** : the piece in a cock that can be turned to regulate the flow of liquid or gas **b** : an obstructing mass of material in a bodily vessel or opening (as of the cervix or a skin lesion) **c** : a filling for a hollow tooth

²plug vt **plugged; plug·ging 1** : to stop, make tight, or secure (as an opening) by or as if by insertion of a plug : close an opening in **2** : to fill a cavity in (a tooth)

plugged \ˈpləgd\ adj : blocked, closed, or obstructed by or as if by a plug ⟨a ∼ lymph vessel⟩

plug·ger \ˈpləg-ər\ n : a dental instrument used for packing, condensing, and consolidating filling material in a tooth cavity

plum·ba·gin \ˌpləm-ˈbā-jən\ n : a yellow crystalline phenolic compound $C_{11}H_8O_3$ with antibacterial and medicinal properties that occurs esp. in the roots of shrubs (genus *Plumbago*) of the legume family

plum·ba·go \ˌpləm-ˈbā-(ˌ)gō\ n, pl **-gos** : GRAPHITE

plum·bic \ˈpləm-bik\ adj : of, relating to, or containing lead esp. with a valence of four

plum·bism \ˈpləm-ˌbiz-əm\ n : LEAD POISONING; esp : chronic lead poisoning

Plum·mer–Vin·son syndrome \ˈpləm-ər-ˈvin(t)-sən-\ n : a condition that is marked esp. by the growth of a mucous membrane across the esophageal lumen, by difficulty in swallowing, and by hypochromic anemia and that is usu. considered to be due to an iron deficiency

Plummer, Henry Stanley (1874–1936), American physician. Plummer made his most important contributions in the study of the thyroid gland and thyroid diseases. He developed a new classification of thyroid diseases that led to a general recognition of the value of iodine in the preoperative treatment of Graves' disease. He published a monograph on the thyroid gland in 1926. His work generated a surge of interest in thyroid function. Plummer also made significant improvements in methods for dilating esophageal strictures, for the relief of cardiospasm, and for removing foreign bodies from air passages. In a 1912 paper on diffuse dilation of the esophagus without cardiospasm, he described a syndrome of dysphagia, glossitis, and hypochromic anemia.

Vinson, Porter Paisley (1890–1959), American surgeon. Vinson's primary area of research centered on the diagnosis and treatment of diseases of the esophagus. He published major works on the subject in 1940 and 1947. In 1919 he published his own report on the syndrome that had been discussed by Plummer in 1912. The syndrome is now known as the Plummer-Vinson syndrome in honor of both men.

plu·mose \ˈplü-ˌmōs\ adj : resembling a feather

plump·er \ˈpləm-pər\ n : an object carried in the mouth to fill out the cheeks

plu·ri·glan·du·lar \ˌplu̇r-ə-ˈglan-jə-lər\ adj : of, relating to, affecting, or derived from more than one gland or kind of gland ⟨∼ insufficiency⟩

plu·ri·grav·i·da \-ˈgrav-əd-ə\ n, pl **-dae** \-ə-ˌdē\ also **-das** : MULTIGRAVIDA

plu·ri·loc·u·lar \-ˈläk-yə-lər\ adj : divided into chambers : MULTILOCULAR

plu·rip·a·ra \plü-ˈrip-ə-rə\ n, pl **-ras** or **-rae** \-ə-ˌrē\ : MULTIPARA

plu·ri·po·ten·cy \ˌplu̇r-ə-ˈpōt-ᵊn-sē\ n, pl **-cies** : PLURIPOTENTIALITY

plu·rip·o·tent \plu̇-ˈrip-ət-ənt\ adj **1** : not fixed as to developmental potentialities; esp : capable of differentiating into one of many cell types ⟨∼ stem cells⟩ **2** : capable of affecting more than one organ or tissue

plu·ri·po·ten·tial \ˌplu̇r-ə-pə-ˈten-chəl\ adj : PLURIPOTENT

plu·ri·po·ten·ti·al·i·ty \-pə-ˌten-chē-ˈal-ət-ē\ n, pl **-ties** : the quality or state of being pluripotent

plus \ˈpləs\ adj : relating to or being a particular one of the two mating types that are required for successful fertilization in sexual reproduction in some lower plants (as a fungus) — compare MINUS

plu·to·ma·nia \ˌplüt-ə-ˈmā-nē-ə\ n : excessive or abnormal desire for wealth

plu·to·nism \ˈplüt-ᵊn-ˌiz-əm\ n : radiation sickness resulting from exposure to plutonium

Plu·to \ˈplüt-(ˌ)ō\, Greek mythological character. Pluto, who was also known as Hades, was the god of the dead and ruler of the underworld. The brother of the gods Zeus, Poseidon, Demeter, Hera, and Hestia, he had Persephone as his consort and queen. The ancients perceived him to be a grim, cold god who justly but mercilessly ruled his shadowy subterranean kingdom.

plu·to·ni·um \plü-ˈtō-nē-əm\ n : a radioactive metallic element similar chemically to uranium that is formed as the isotope 239 by decay of neptunium and found in minute quantities in pitchblende, that undergoes slow disintegration with the emission of an alpha particle to form uranium 235, and that is fissionable with slow neutrons to yield atomic energy — symbol *Pu*; see ELEMENT table

pm abbr premolar

Pm symbol promethium

PM abbr **1** [Latin *post meridiem*] after noon **2** postmortem

PMA abbr Pharmaceutical Manufacturers Association

PMA index \ˈpē-ˈem-ˈā-\ n : a measure of the incidence and severity of gingivitis in a given population based on examination and rating of the degree of involvement of the interdental papilla and the marginal and attached portions of the gingiva in each individual

PMDD abbr premenstrual dysphoric disorder

PMN abbr polymorphonuclear neutrophilic leukocyte

pmol or **pmole** abbr picomole

PMS \ˌpē-(ˌ)em-ˈes\ n : PREMENSTRUAL SYNDROME

PN abbr psychoneurotic

pneu·mat·ic \n(y)u̇-ˈmat-ik\ adj : of, relating to, or using gas (as air): as **a** : moved or worked by air pressure **b** : adapted for holding or inflated with compressed air **c** : having air-filled cavities ⟨∼ bone⟩ — **pneu·mat·i·cal·ly** \-i-k(ə-)lē\ adv

pneu·mat·ics \n(y)u̇-ˈmat-iks\ n pl but sing in constr : a branch of mechanics that deals with the mechanical properties of gases

pneu·ma·ti·za·tion also Brit **pneu·ma·ti·sa·tion** \ˌn(y)ü-mət-ə-ˈzā-shən\ n : the presence or development of air-filled cavities in a bone ⟨∼ of the temporal bone⟩

pneu·ma·tized also Brit **pneu·ma·tised** \ˈn(y)ü-mə-ˌtīzd\ adj : having air-filled cavities

---

\ə\ **abut** \ᵊ\ **kitten** \ər\ **further** \a\ **ash** \ā\ **ace** \ä\ **cot, cart** \au̇\ **out** \ch\ **chin** \e\ **bet** \ē\ **easy** \g\ **go** \i\ **hit** \ī\ **ice** \j\ **job** \ŋ\ **sing** \ō\ **go** \ȯ\ **law** \ȯi\ **boy** \th\ **thin** \th\ **the** \ü\ **loot** \u̇\ **foot** \y\ **yet** \zh\ **vision** *See also* Pronunciation Symbols page

O

P

pneu·ma·to·cele \'n(y)ü-mət-ō-ˌsēl, n(y)ù-'mat-ə-\ *n* : a gas-filled cavity or sac occurring esp. in the lung

pneu·ma·to·gram \-ˌgram\ *n* : PNEUMOGRAM

pneu·ma·to·graph \-ˌgraf\ *n* : PNEUMOGRAPH

pneu·ma·tol·o·gy \ˌn(y)ü-mə-'täl-ə-jē\ *n, pl* **-gies** : a science dealing with the medical uses of air and gases

pneu·ma·to·sis \ˌn(y)ü-mə-'tō-səs\ *n, pl* **-to·ses** \-ˌsēz\ : the presence of air or gas in abnormal places in the body

pneu·ma·tu·ria \ˌn(y)ü-mə-'tùr-ē-ə\ *n* : passage of gas in the urine

pneu·mec·to·my \n(y)ù-'mek-tə-mē\ *n, pl* **-mies** : PNEUMONECTOMY

pneu·mo·ba·cil·lus \ˌn(y)ü-mō-bə-'sil-əs\ *n, pl* **-cil·li** \-ˌī *also* -ē\ : a bacterium of the genus *Klebsiella* (*K. pneumoniae*) associated with inflammations (as pneumonia) of the respiratory tract

pneu·mo·ceph·a·lus \-'sef-ə-ləs\ *n, pl* **-li** \-ˌlī\ : the presence of air within the cranial cavity

pneu·mo·coc·cal \ˌn(y)ü-mə-'käk-əl\ *adj* : of, relating to, caused by, or derived from pneumococci ⟨~ pneumonia⟩

pneu·mo·coc·ce·mia *or chiefly Brit* **pneu·mo·coc·cae·mia** \ˌn(y)ü-mə-ˌkäk-'sē-mē-ə\ *n* : the presence of pneumococci in the circulating blood

pneu·mo·coc·cic \-'käk-sik\ *adj* : PNEUMOCOCCAL

pneu·mo·coc·cus \ˌn(y)ü-mə-'käk-əs\ *n, pl* **-coc·ci** \-'käk-ˌ(s)ī\ : a bacterium of the genus *Streptococcus* (*S. pneumoniae*) that causes an acute pneumonia involving one or more lobes of the lung

pneu·mo·co·lon \ˌn(y)ü-mə-'kō-lən\ *n* : the presence of air in the colon

pneu·mo·co·ni·o·sis \ˌn(y)ü-mō-ˌkō-nē-'ō-səs\ *n, pl* **-o·ses** \-ˌsēz\ : a disease of the lungs caused by the habitual inhalation of irritants (as mineral or metallic particles) — called also *miner's asthma, miner's consumption, pneumonoconiosis;* see BLACK LUNG, SILICOSIS

pneu·mo·cys·tic pneumonia \ˌn(y)ü-mə-'sis-tik-\ *n* : PNEUMOCYSTIS CARINII PNEUMONIA

Pneu·mo·cys·tis \ˌn(y)ü-mə-'sis-təs\ *n* **1** : a genus of microorganisms of uncertain affiliation that are usu. considered protozoans or sometimes fungi and that include one (*P. carinii*) causing pneumonia esp. in immunocompromised individuals **2** : PNEUMOCYSTIS CARINII PNEUMONIA

Pneumocystis ca·ri·nii pneumonia \-kə-'rī-nē-ˌē-\ *n* : a pneumonia chiefly affecting immunocompromised individuals that is caused by a microorganism of the genus *Pneumocystis* (*P. carinii*) which shows up in specially stained preparations of fresh infected lung tissue as cysts containing six to eight oval bodies, that attacks esp. the interstitial and alveolar tissues of the lungs, and that is characterized esp. by a nonproductive cough, shortness of breath, and fever — abbr. *PCP;* called also *pneumocystic pneumonia, Pneumocystis carinii pneumonitis*

pneu·mo·cys·tog·ra·phy \ˌn(y)ü-mə-ˌsis-'täg-rə-fē\ *n, pl* **-phies** : radiography of the urinary bladder after it has been injected with air

pneu·mo·cyte \'n(y)ü-mə-ˌsīt\ *n* : any of the specialized cells that occur in the alveoli of the lungs

pneu·mo·en·ceph·a·li·tis \ˌn(y)ü-mō-in-ˌsef-ə-'līt-əs\ *n, pl* **-lit·i·des** \-'lit-ə-ˌdēz\ : NEWCASTLE DISEASE

pneu·mo·en·ceph·a·lo·gram \-in-'sef-ə-lə-ˌgram\ *n* : a radiograph made by pneumoencephalography

pneu·mo·en·ceph·a·lo·graph \-ˌgraf\ *n* : PNEUMOENCEPHALOGRAM

pneu·mo·en·ceph·a·lo·graph·ic \-in-ˌsef-ə-lə-'graf-ik\ *adj* : of, relating to, or by means of pneumoencephalography

pneu·mo·en·ceph·a·log·ra·phy \-in-ˌsef-ə-'läg-rə-fē\ *n, pl* **-phies** : radiography of the brain after the injection of air into the ventricles

pneu·mo·en·ter·i·tis \-ˌent-ə-'rīt-əs\ *n, pl* **-en·ter·it·i·des** \-'rit-ə-ˌdēz\ *or* **-en·ter·i·tis·es** : pneumonia combined with enteritis

pneu·mo·gas·tric nerve \ˌn(y)ü-mə-'gas-trik-\ *n* : VAGUS NERVE

pneu·mo·gram \'n(y)ü-mə-ˌgram\ *n* : a record of respiratory movements obtained by pneumography

pneu·mo·graph \'n(y)ü-mə-ˌgraf\ *n* : an instrument for recording the thoracic movements or volume change during respiration

pneu·mo·graph·ic \ˌn(y)ü-mə-'graf-ik\ *adj* : of, relating to, or by means of pneumography

pneu·mog·ra·phy \n(y)ü-'mäg-rə-fē\ *n, pl* **-phies** **1** : a description of the lungs **2** : radiography after the injection of air into a body cavity **3** : the process of making a pneumogram

pneu·mo·he·mo·tho·rax *or chiefly Brit* **pneu·mo·hae·mo·tho·rax** \ˌn(y)ü-mō-ˌhē-mə-'thō(ə)r-ˌaks, -'thó(ə)r-\ *n, pl* **-tho·rax·es** *or* **-tho·ra·ces** \-'thōr-ə-ˌsēz, -'thór-\ : accumulation of blood and gas in the pleural cavity

pneu·mo·hy·dro·tho·rax \-ˌhī-drō-'thō(ə)r-ˌaks, -'thó(ə)r-\ *n, pl* **-tho·rax·es** *or* **-tho·ra·ces** \-'thōr-ə-ˌsēz\ : HYDROPNEUMOTHORAX

pneu·mo·li·thi·a·sis \-lith-'ī-ə-səs\ *n, pl* **-a·ses** \-ˌsēz\ : the presence or formation of calculi in the lungs

pneu·mol·o·gy \n(y)ü-'mäl-ə-jē\ *n, pl* **-gies** : PULMONOLOGY

pneu·mol·y·sis \-'mäl-ə-səs\ *n, pl* **-y·ses** \-ˌsēz\ : PNEUMONOLYSIS

pneu·mo·me·di·as·ti·num \ˌn(y)ü-mō-ˌmēd-ē-ə-'stī-nəm\ *n, pl* **-ti·na** \-nə\ **1** : an abnormal state characterized by the presence of gas (as air) in the mediastinum **2** : the induction of pneumomediastinum as an aid to radiography

pneu·mo·my·co·sis \-mī-'kō-səs\ *n, pl* **-co·ses** \-ˌsēz\ : a fungus disease of the lungs; *esp* : aspergillosis in poultry

pneu·mo·nec·to·my \ˌn(y)ü-mə-'nek-tə-mē\ *n, pl* **-mies** : surgical excision of an entire lung or of one or more lobes of a lung — called also *pneumectomy, pulmonectomy;* compare SEGMENTAL RESECTION

pneu·mo·nia \n(y)ù-'mō-nyə\ *n* : a disease of the lungs that is characterized esp. by inflammation and consolidation of lung tissue followed by resolution, is accompanied by fever, chills, cough, and difficulty in breathing, and is caused chiefly by infection — see BRONCHOPNEUMONIA, LOBAR PNEUMONIA, PRIMARY ATYPICAL PNEUMONIA

pneumonia al·ba \-'al-bə\ *n* : a fatal congenital disorder that results from prenatal syphilis and is characterized by extremely pale, fibrotic, and nearly airless lungs

pneu·mon·ic \n(y)ù-'män-ik\ *adj* **1** : of, relating to, or affecting the lungs : PULMONARY **2** : of, relating to, or affected with pneumonia

pneumonic plague *n* : plague of an extremely virulent form that is caused by a bacterium of the genus *Pasteurella* (*P. pestis*), involves chiefly the lungs, and usu. is transmitted from person to person by droplet infection — compare BUBONIC PLAGUE

pneu·mo·ni·tis \ˌn(y)ü-mə-'nīt-əs\ *n, pl* **-nit·i·des** \-'nit-ə-ˌdēz\ **1** : a disease characterized by inflammation of the lungs; *esp* : PNEUMONIA **2** : FELINE PNEUMONITIS

pneu·mo·no·cen·te·sis \ˌn(y)ü-mə-(ˌ)nō-sen-'tē-səs\ *n, pl* **-te·ses** \-ˌsēz\ : surgical puncture of a lung for aspiration

pneu·mo·no·co·ni·o·sis \-ˌkō-nē-'ō-səs\ *n, pl* **-o·ses** \-ˌsēz\ : PNEUMOCONIOSIS

pneu·mo·nol·y·sis \ˌn(y)ü-mə-'näl-ə-səs\ *n, pl* **-y·ses** \-ˌsēz\ : either of two surgical procedures to permit collapse of a lung: **a** : separation of the parietal pleura from the fascia of the chest wall — called also *extrapleural pneumonolysis* **b** : separation of the visceral and parietal layers of the pleura — called also *intrapleural pneumonolysis*

pneu·mo·nos·to·my \ˌn(y)ü-mə-'näs-tə-mē\ *n, pl* **-mies** : surgical formation of an artificial opening (as for drainage of an abscess) into a lung

pneu·mo·no·ul·tra·mi·cro·scop·ic·sil·i·co·vol·ca·no·co·ni·o·sis \'n(y)ü-mə-(ˌ)nō-ˌəl-trə-ˌmī-krə-'skäp-ik-ˌsil-i-(ˌ)kō-väl-ˌkā-nō-ˌkō-nē-'ō-səs\ *n, pl* **-o·ses** \-ˌsēz\ : a pneumoconiosis caused by inhalation of very fine silicate or quartz dust

Pneu·mo·nys·sus \ˌn(y)ü-mə-'nis-əs\ *n* : a genus of mites (family Halarachnidae) that live in the air passages of mammals and include one (*P. caninum*) found in dogs and another (*P. simicola*) found in monkeys

pneu·mop·a·thy \n(y)ü-'mäp-ə-thē\ *n, pl* **-thies** : any disease of the lungs

pneu·mo·peri·car·di·um \ˌn(y)ü-mō-ˌper-ə-'kärd-ē-əm\ *n, pl* **-dia** \-ē-ə\ : an abnormal state characterized by the presence of gas (as air) in the pericardium

pneu·mo·peri·to·ne·um \-ˌper-ət-ᵊn-'ē-əm\ *n, pl* **-ne·ums** or **-nea** \-'ē-ə\ **1** : an abnormal state characterized by the presence of gas (as air) in the peritoneal cavity **2** : the induction of pneumoperitoneum as a therapeutic measure or as an aid to radiography

pneu·mo·scle·ro·sis \-sklə-'rō-səs\ *n, pl* **-ro·ses** \-ˌsēz\ : fibrosis of the lungs

pneu·mo·tacho·gram \ˌn(y)ü-mō-'tak-ə-ˌgram\ *n* : a record of the velocity of the respiratory function obtained by use of a pneumotachograph

pneu·mo·tacho·graph \-ˌgraf\ *n* : a device or apparatus for measuring the rate of the respiratory function

pneu·mo·tax·ic center \ˌn(y)ü-mə-'tak-sik-\ *n* : a neural center in the upper part of the pons that provides inhibitory impulses on inspiration and thereby prevents overdistension of the lungs and helps to maintain alternately recurrent inspiration and expiration

pneu·mo·tho·rax \ˌn(y)ü-mə-'thō(ə)r-ˌaks, -'thó(ə)r-\ *n, pl* **-tho·rax·es** or **-tho·ra·ces** \-'thōr-ə-ˌsēz\ : a condition in which air or other gas is present in the pleural cavity and which occurs spontaneously as a result of disease or injury of lung tissue, rupture of air-filled pulmonary cysts, or puncture of the chest wall or is induced as a therapeutic measure to collapse the lung — see TENSION PNEUMOTHORAX; compare OLEOTHORAX

pneu·mo·tro·pic \ˌn(y)ü-mə-'trōp-ik, -'träp-\ *adj* : turning, directed toward, or having an affinity for lung tissues — used esp. of infective agents — **pneu·mot·ro·pism** \n(y)ü-'mä-trə-ˌpiz-əm\ *n*

PNF *abbr* proprioceptive neuromuscular facilitation

PNH *abbr* paroxysmal nocturnal hemoglobinuria

po *abbr* per os — used esp. in writing prescriptions

Po *symbol* polonium

pock \'päk\ *n* : a pustule in an eruptive disease (as smallpox)

pock·et \'päk-ət\ *n* : a small cavity or space; *esp* : an abnormal cavity formed in diseased tissue ⟨a gingival ∼⟩

pocketing *n* : the formation of pathological pockets ⟨periodontal ∼⟩

pock·mark \'päk-ˌmärk\ *n* : a mark, pit, or depressed scar caused by smallpox or acne — **pock·marked** *adj*

POD *abbr* postoperative day

po·dag·ra \pə-'dag-rə\ *n* **1** : GOUT **2** : a painful condition of the big toe caused by gout

po·dal·ic \pō-'dal-ik\ *adj* : of, relating to, or by means of the feet; *specif* : being an obstetric version in which the fetus is turned so that the feet emerge first in delivery

po·di·a·trist \pə-'dī-ə-trəst\ *n* : a specialist in podiatry

po·di·a·try \pə-'dī-ə-trē, pō-\ *n, pl* **-tries** : the medical care and treatment of the human foot — called also *chiropody* — **po·di·at·ric** \ˌpōd-ē-'a-trik\ *adj*

podo·derm \'päd-ə-ˌdərm\ *n* : the dermal or growing part of the covering of the foot of a hoofed animal as distinguished from the epidermal or horny part

podo·der·ma·ti·tis \ˌpäd-ō-ˌdər-mə-'tīt-əs\ *n, pl* **-ti·ti·des** or **-tit·i·des** \-'tit-ə-ˌdēz\ : a condition (as foot rot) characterized by inflammation of the dermal tissue underlying the horny layers of a hoof

podo·phyl·lin \ˌpäd-ə-'fil-ən\ *n* : a resin obtained from podophyllum and used in medicine as a caustic — called also *podophyllum resin*

podo·phyl·lo·tox·in \ˌpäd-ə-ˌfil-ə-'täk-sən\ *n* : a crystalline polycyclic compound $C_{22}H_{22}O_8$ constituting one of the active principles of podophyllum and podophyllin

podo·phyl·lum \-'fil-əm\ *n* **1** *cap* : a small genus of herbs (family Berberidaceae) that have poisonous rootstocks and large fleshy sometimes edible berries **2** *pl* **-phyl·li** \-'fil-ˌī\ or **-phyllums** : the dried rhizome and rootlet of the mayapple (*Podophyllum peltatum*) that is used as a caustic or as a source of the more effective podophyllin

podophyllum resin *n* : PODOPHYLLIN

po·go·ni·on \pə-'gō-nē-ən\ *n* : the most projecting median point on the anterior surface of the chin

poi·ki·lo·cyte \'pói-ki-lə-ˌsīt, (ˌ)pói-'kil-ə-\ *n* : an abnormally formed red blood cell characteristic of various anemias

poi·ki·lo·cy·to·sis \-sī-tō-səs\ *n, pl* **-to·ses** \-ˌsēz\ : a condition characterized by the presence of poikilocytes in the blood

poi·ki·lo·der·ma \ˌpói-kə-lə-'dər-mə\ *n, pl* **-mas** or **-ma·ta** \-mət-ə\ : any of several disorders characterized by patchy discoloration of the skin

poi·kil·os·mot·ic \ˌpói-kil-äz-'mät-ik\ *adj* : having body fluids with an osmotic pressure similar to that of the surrounding medium ⟨most lower marine invertebrates are ∼⟩ — compare HOMOIOSMOTIC

poi·ki·lo·therm \'pói-ki-lə-ˌthərm, (ˌ)pói-'kil-ə-\ *n* : an organism (as a frog) with a variable body temperature that is usu. slightly higher than the temperature of its environment : a cold-blooded organism — called also *heterotherm*

poi·ki·lo·ther·mic \ˌpói-ki-lō-'thər-mik\ *adj* : of, relating to, or being a poikilotherm : COLD-BLOODED

poi·ki·lo·ther·mism \-'thər-ˌmiz-əm\ *n* : the quality or state of being cold-blooded

poi·ki·lo·ther·my \'pói-ki-lə-ˌthər-mē\ *n, pl* **-mies** : POIKILOTHERMISM

¹point \'póint\ *n* **1** : a narrowly localized place or area **2** : the terminal usu. sharp or narrowly rounded part of something **3** : a definite measurable position in a scale — see BOILING POINT, FREEZING POINT

²point *vi, of an abscess* : to become distended with pus prior to breaking

pointer — see HIP POINTER

point mutation *n* : a gene mutation involving the substitution, addition, or deletion of a single nucleotide base

point–of–service *adj* : of, relating to, or being a health-care insurance plan that allows enrollees to seek care from a physician affiliated with the service provider at a fixed co= payment or to choose a nonaffiliated physician and pay a larger share of the cost — abbr. *POS*

poise \'póiz, 'pwäz\ *n* : a cgs unit of viscosity equal to the viscosity of a fluid that would require a shearing force of one dyne to impart to a one square-centimeter area of an arbitrary layer of the fluid a velocity of one centimeter per second relative to another layer separated from the first by a distance of one centimeter

Poi·seuille's law \pwä-'zə(r)z-, -'zwēz-, -'zə-ēz-\ *n* : a statement in physics: the velocity of the steady flow of a fluid through a narrow tube (as a blood vessel or a catheter) varies directly as the pressure and the fourth power of the radius of the tube and inversely as the length of the tube and the coefficient of viscosity

Poi·seuille \pwà-zœy\, **Jean–Léonard–Marie (1797–1869),** French physiologist and physician. Poiseuille is best known for his research on the physiology of the circulation of blood through the arteries. He published his research in an 1828 dissertation in which he demonstrated that blood pressure rises and falls on expiration and inspiration. His interest in blood circulation led him to study the flow rates of other fluids. In 1840 he formulated the law regarding the flow rate for the laminar flow of fluids in circular tubes. In 1847 he published the results of further experiments using ether and mercury. Gotthilf Hagen, a German hydraulic engineer, discovered Poiseuille's law independently in 1839.

¹poi·son \'pói-zᵊn\ *n* **1** : a substance that through its chemical action usu. kills, injures, or impairs an organism **2** : a substance that inhibits the activity of another substance or the course of a reaction or process ⟨a catalyst ∼⟩

²poison *vt* **poi·soned; poi·son·ing** \'pói-zə-niŋ, -ᵊn-iŋ\ **1** : to injure or kill with poison **2** : to treat, taint, or impregnate with poison

O
P

\ə\ abut \ᵊ\ kitten \ər\ further \a\ ash \ā\ ace \ä\ cot, cart
\aú\ out \ch\ chin \e\ bet \ē\ easy \g\ go \i\ hit \ī\ ice \j\ job
\ŋ\ sing \ō\ go \ó\ law \ói\ boy \th\ thin \th\ the \ü\ loot
\ú\ foot \y\ yet \zh\ vision *See also* Pronunciation Symbols page

³poison *adj* **1** : POISONOUS ⟨a ~ plant⟩ **2** : impregnated with poison ⟨a ~ arrow⟩

poison dog·wood \-'dȯg-ˌwu̇d\ *n* : POISON SUMAC

poison gas *n* : a poisonous gas or a liquid or a solid giving off poisonous vapors designed (as in chemical warfare) to kill, injure, or disable by inhalation or contact

poison hemlock *n* **1** : a large branching biennial poisonous herb of the genus *Conium* (*C. maculatum*) with finely divided leaves and white flowers **2** : WATER HEMLOCK

poison ivy \-'ī-vē\ *n* **1 a** : a climbing plant of the genus *Rhus* (*R. radicans* syn. *Toxicodendron radicans*) that is esp. common in the eastern and central U.S., that has leaves in groups of three, greenish flowers, and white berries, and that produces an acutely irritating oil causing a usu. intensely itching skin rash **b** : any of several plants closely related to poison ivy; *esp* : POISON OAK 1b **2** : a skin rash produced by poison ivy

poison oak \-'ōk\ *n* **1** : any of several plants included in the genus *Rhus* or sometimes in the genus *Toxicodendron* that produce an irritating oil like that of poison ivy: **a** : a bushy plant (*R. diversiloba* syn. *T. diversilobum*) of the Pacific coast **b** : a bushy plant (*R. toxicodendron* syn. *T. pubescens*) of the southeastern U.S. **2** : POISON IVY 1a **3** : a skin rash produced by poison oak

poi·son·ous \'pȯiz-nəs, -°n-əs\ *adj* : having the properties or effects of poison : VENOMOUS

poison pars·ley \-'pär-slē\ *n* : POISON HEMLOCK 1

poison su·mac \-'s(h)ü-ˌmak\ *n* : an American swamp shrub of the genus *Rhus* (*R. vernix* syn. *Toxicodendron vernix*) that has smooth pinnate leaves, greenish flowers, and greenish white berries and produces an irritating oil — called also *poison dogwood*

poi·son·wood \'pȯiz-°n-ˌwu̇d\ *n* : a caustic or poisonous tree of the genus *Metopium* (*M. toxiferum*) of Florida and the West Indies that has compound leaves, clusters of greenish flowers, and orange-yellow fruits

poke·weed \'pōk-ˌkwēd\ *n* : a coarse American perennial herb (*Phytolacca americana* of the family Phytolaccaceae, the pokeweed family) which has stalks of white flowers, dark purple juicy berries, and a poisonous root and from which is obtained a mitogen that has been used to stimulate lymphocyte proliferation

po·lar \'pō-lər\ *adj* **1** : of or relating to one or more poles (as of a spherical body) **2** : exhibiting polarity; *esp* : having a dipole or characterized by molecules having dipoles ⟨a ~ solvent⟩ **3** : being at opposite ends of a spectrum of symptoms or manifestations ⟨~ types of leprosy⟩

polar body *n* : a cell that separates from an oocyte during meiosis: **a** : one containing a nucleus produced in the first meiotic division — called also *first polar body* **b** : one containing a nucleus produced in the second meiotic division — called also *second polar body*

po·lar·im·e·ter \ˌpō-lə-'rim-ət-ər\ *n* **1** : an instrument for determining the amount of polarization of light or the proportion of polarized light in a partially polarized ray **2** : a polariscope for measuring the amount of rotation of the plane of polarization esp. by liquids — **po·lari·met·ric** \pō-ˌlar-ə-'me-trik\ *adj* — **po·lar·im·e·try** \ˌpō-lə-'rim-ə-trē\ *n, pl* **-tries**

po·lari·scope \pō-'lar-ə-ˌskōp\ *n* **1** : an instrument for studying the properties of or examining substances in polarized light **2** : POLARIMETER 2

po·lari·scop·ic \pō-ˌlar-ə-'skäp-ik, pə-\ *adj* : of, relating to, or obtained by the use of a polariscope ⟨~ observations⟩ — **po·lari·scop·i·cal·ly** \-i-k(ə-)lē\ *adv*

po·lar·i·ty \pō-'lar-ət-ē, pə-\ *n, pl* **-ties** **1** : the quality or condition inherent in a body that exhibits contrasting properties or powers in contrasting parts or directions **2** : attraction toward a particular object or in a specific direction **3** : the particular state either positive or negative with reference to the two poles or to electrification

po·lar·iz·abil·i·ty *also Brit* **po·lar·is·abil·i·ty** \ˌpō-lə-ˌrī-zə-'bil-ət-ē\ *n, pl* **-ties** : the capacity (as of a molecule) of being polarized — **po·lar·iz·able** *also Brit* **po·lar·is·able** \-'rī-zə-bəl\ *adj*

po·lar·iza·tion *also Brit* **po·lar·isa·tion** \ˌpō-lə-rə-'zā-shən\ *n* : the action of polarizing or state of being or becoming polarized: as **a** (1) : the action or process of affecting radiation and esp. light so that the vibrations of the wave assume a definite form (2) : the state of radiation affected by this process **b** : an increase in the resistance of an electrolytic cell caused by the deposition of gas on one or both electrodes **c** : MAGNETIZATION

po·lar·ize *also Brit* **po·lar·ise** \'pō-lə-ˌrīz\ *vb* **-ized** *also Brit* **-ised; -iz·ing** *also Brit* **-is·ing** *vt* **1** : to cause (as light waves) to vibrate in a definite pattern **2** : to give physical polarity to ~ *vi* : to become polarized

po·lar·iz·er *also Brit* **po·lar·is·er** \-ˌrīz-ər\ *n* : the part of a polariscope receiving and polarizing the light — compare ANALYZER

polarizing microscope *n* : a microscope equipped to produce polarized light for examination of a specimen

po·lar·o·gram \pō-'lar-ə-ˌgram\ *n* : the current-voltage diagram obtained during polarographic treatment of a solution

po·lar·og·ra·phy \ˌpō-lə-'räg-rə-fē\ *n, pl* **-phies** : a method of qualitative or quantitative analysis based on current-voltage curves obtained during electrolysis of a solution with a steadily increasing electromotive force — **po·laro·graph·ic** \pō-ˌlar-ə-'graf-ik\ *adj* — **po·laro·graph·i·cal·ly** \-i-k(ə-)lē\ *adv*

pole \'pōl\ *n* **1 a** : either of the two terminals of an electric cell, battery, generator, or motor **b** : one of two or more regions in a magnetized body at which the magnetic flux density is concentrated **2** : either of two morphologically or physiologically differentiated areas at opposite ends of an axis in an organism, organ, or cell — see ANIMAL POLE, VEGETAL POLE

Po·len·ske val·ue \pō-'len(t)-skə-ˌval-(ˌ)yü\ *n* : a value similar to a Reichert value that indicates the content in butter or other fat of the volatile water-insoluble acids (as capric acid and lauric acid) — called also *Polenske number*

Polenske, Eduard (*fl* 1889–1912), German chemist. Polenske introduced a method for the detection of coconut oil in butter and lard in an article published in 1911. He developed his method after examining 34 fresh and eight old butters.

po·lice·man \pə-'lēs-mən\ *n, pl* **-men** \-mən\ : an instrument (as a flat piece of rubber on a glass rod) for removing solids from a vessel (as a beaker)

pol·i·clin·ic \'päl-ə-ˌklin-ik\ *n* : a dispensary or department of a hospital at which outpatients are treated — compare POLYCLINIC

pol·i·co·sa·nol *also* **poly·co·sa·nol** \ˌpäl-ē-'kō-sə-ˌnȯl\ *n* : a mixture of primary aliphatic alcohols derived chiefly from the waxy coating of sugarcane and used esp. as a dietary supplement to lower cholesterol levels

po·lio \'pō-lē-ˌō\ *n* : POLIOMYELITIS

po·lio·dys·tro·phy \ˌpō-lē-ō-'dis-trə-fē\ *n, pl* **-phies** : atrophy of the gray matter esp. of the cerebrum

po·lio·en·ceph·a·li·tis \ˌpō-lē-(ˌ)ō-in-ˌsef-ə-'līt-əs\ *n, pl* **-lit·i·des** \-'lit-ə-ˌdēz\ : inflammation of the gray matter of the brain

po·lio·en·ceph·a·lo·my·eli·tis \-in-ˌsef-ə-lō-ˌmī-ə-'līt-əs\ *n, pl* **-elit·i·des** \-'lit-ə-ˌdēz\ : inflammation of the gray matter of the brain and the spinal cord

po·lio·my·eli·tis \ˌpō-lē-(ˌ)ō-ˌmī-ə-'līt-əs\ *n, pl* **-elit·i·des** \-'lit-ə-ˌdēz\ : an acute infectious virus disease caused by the poliovirus, characterized by fever, motor paralysis, and atrophy of skeletal muscles often with permanent disability and deformity, and marked by inflammation of nerve cells in the ventral horns of the spinal cord — called also *infantile paralysis, polio* — **po·lio·my·elit·ic** \-'lit-ik\ *adj*

po·li·o·sis \ˌpō-lē-'ō-səs\ *n, pl* **-o·ses** \-ˌsēz\ : loss of color from the hair

polio vaccine *n* : a vaccine intended to confer immunity to poliomyelitis

po·lio·vi·rus \'pō-lē-(ˌ)ō-ˌvī-rəs\ *n* : a picornavirus of the genus *Enterovirus* (species *Poliovirus*) occurring in three distinct serotypes that cause poliomyelitis — see SABIN VACCINE, SALK VACCINE

po·litz·er bag \'pō-lit-sər-, 'pä-\ *n* : a soft rubber bulb used to inflate the middle ear by increasing air pressure in the nasopharynx

Po·litz·er \'pō-lit-sər\, **Adam (1835–1920)**, Austrian otologist. Politzer was the first professor of otology at Vienna and one of the greatest of all otologists. He devoted his career to the anatomy, physiology, and pathology of the organs of hearing. While he was still a medical student, he described the innervation of the intrinsic muscle of the ear and the variations in air pressure on the middle ear. In 1863 he devised the pneumatic device for inflating the middle ear that is now called the politzer bag. Two years later he published an atlas of the tympanic membrane. In 1878–82 he published a textbook on diseases of the ear that was the standard authority for many years. His two-volume history of otolaryngology that was published in 1907–13 was equally significant. His other achievements included improvement of tuning-fork tests; use of the otoscope in the diagnosis of seromucous exudate in the tympanic cavity; the first recognition of otosclerosis as a separate clinical entity; and investigations into the pathological anatomy of cholesteatoma, congenital deafness, and labyrinthitis.

¹poll \'pōl\ *n* : the head or a part of it; *esp* : the region between the ears of some quadrupeds (as a horse)

²poll *vt* : to cut off or cut short the horns of (cattle)

³poll *adj* : having no horns

pol·la·ki·uria \ˌpäl-ə-kē-'yùr-ē-ə\ *n* : abnormally frequent urination

pol·len \'päl-ən\ *n* : a mass of male spores in a seed plant appearing usu. as a fine dust

pol·lex \'päl-ˌeks\ *n, pl* **pol·li·ces** \'päl-ə-ˌsēz\ : the first digit of the forelimb : THUMB

pollicis — see ABDUCTOR POLLICIS BREVIS, ABDUCTOR POLLICIS LONGUS, ADDUCTOR POLLICIS, EXTENSOR POLLICIS BREVIS, EXTENSOR POLLICIS LONGUS, FLEXOR POLLICIS BREVIS, FLEXOR POLLICIS LONGUS, OPPONENS POLLICIS, PRINCEPS POLLICIS

pol·li·ci·za·tion \ˌpäl-ə-sə-'zā-shən\ *n* : the reconstruction or replacement of the thumb esp. from part of the index finger

pol·li·no·sis *or* **pol·le·no·sis** \ˌpäl-ə-'nō-səs\ *n, pl* **-no·ses** \-ˌsēz\ : HAY FEVER

pol·lut·ant \pə-'lüt-ᵊnt\ *n* : something that pollutes

pol·lute \pə-'lüt\ *vt* **pol·lut·ed; pol·lut·ing** **1** : to make physically impure or unclean **2** : to contaminate (an environment) esp. with man-made waste — **pol·lut·er** *n* — **pol·lut·ive** \-'lüt-iv\ *adj*

pol·lu·tion \pə-'lü-shən\ *n* **1** : the action of polluting or the condition of being polluted **2** : POLLUTANT

polonica — see PLICA POLONICA

po·lo·ni·um \pə-'lō-nē-əm\ *n* : a radioactive metallic element that is similar chemically to tellurium and bismuth, occurs esp. in pitchblende and radium-lead residues, and emits an alpha particle to form an isotope of lead — symbol *Po*; see ELEMENT table

pol·toph·a·gy \ˌpäl-'täf-ə-gē\ *n, pl* **-gies** : thorough chewing of food until it becomes like porridge

poly \'päl-ē\ *n, pl* **pol·ys** \-ēz\ : a polymorphonuclear leukocyte

poly(A) \ˌpäl-ē-'ā\ *n* : RNA or a segment of RNA that is composed of a polynucleotide chain consisting entirely of adenine-containing nucleotides and that codes for polylysine when functioning as messenger RNA in protein synthesis — called also *polyadenylate, polyadenylic acid*

¹poly·ac·id \'päl-ē-ˌas-əd\ *n* **1** : an acid (as phosphoric acid) having more than one acid hydrogen atom **2** : an acid of a large group of oxygen-containing acids

²polyacid *adj* : able to react with more than one molecule of a monoacid to form a salt — used esp. of bases

poly·acryl·amide \ˌpäl-ē-ə-'kril-ə-ˌmīd\ *n* : a polyamide polymer ($-CH_2CHCONH_2-$)$_x$ derived from acrylic acid

polyacrylamide gel *n* : hydrated polyacrylamide that is used esp. to provide a medium for the suspension of a substance to be subjected to gel electrophoresis

¹poly·ade·nyl·ate \ˌpäl-ē-ˌad-ᵊn-'il-ˌāt, -ə-'den-ə-ˌlāt\ *n* : POLY(A)

²polyadenylate *vt* **-at·ed; -at·ing** : to add one or more segments of poly(A) to ⟨some mechanism must exist in the cytoplasm for *polyadenylating* messenger RNA —Benjamin Lewin⟩ — **poly·aden·y·la·tion** \-ə-ˌden-ə-'lā-shən\ *n*

poly·ad·e·nyl·ic acid \-ˌil-ik-\ *n* : POLY(A)

poly·al·co·hol \ˌpäl-ē-'al-kə-ˌhòl\ *n* : an alcohol (as ethylene glycol) that contains more than one hydroxyl group

poly·am·ide \ˌpäl-ē-'am-ˌīd, -əd\ *n* : a compound characterized by more than one amide group; *esp* : a polymer containing a long chain of amides

poly·amine \'päl-ē-ə-ˌmēn, ˌpäl-ē-'am-ˌēn\ *n* : a compound characterized by more than one amino group

poly·an·dry \'päl-ē-ˌan-drē\ *n, pl* **-dries** : the state or practice of having more than one husband or male mate at one time — compare POLYGAMY, POLYGYNY — **poly·an·drous** \ˌpäl-ē-'an-drəs\ *adj*

poly·an·ion \ˌpäl-ē-'an-ˌī-ən\ *n* : a molecule or chemical complex having negative charges at several sites — **poly·an·ion·ic** \-ˌan-(ˌ)ī-'än-ik\ *adj*

poly·ar·ter·i·tis \ˌpäl-ē-ˌärt-ə-'rīt-əs\ *n* : POLYARTERITIS NODOSA

polyarteritis no·do·sa \-nō-'dō-sə\ *n* : an acute inflammatory disease that involves all layers of the arterial wall and is characterized by degeneration, necrosis, exudation, and the formation of inflammatory nodules along the outer layer — called also *periarteritis nodosa*

poly·ar·thral·gia \-är-'thral-j(ē-)ə\ *n* : pain in two or more joints

poly·ar·thri·tis \-är-'thrīt-əs\ *n, pl* **-thrit·i·des** \-'thrit-ə-ˌdēz\ : arthritis involving two or more joints

poly·ar·tic·u·lar \-är-'tik-yə-lər\ *adj* : having or affecting many joints ⟨∼ arthritis⟩ — compare MONOARTICULAR, OLIGOARTICULAR

poly·ba·sic \-'bā-sik, -zik\ *adj* : having more than one hydrogen atom replaceable by basic atoms or radicals — used of acids — **poly·ba·sic·i·ty** \-bā-'sis-ət-ē\ *n, pl* **-ties**

poly·blast \'päl-i-ˌblast\ *n* : a floating macrophage — **poly·blas·tic** \ˌpäl-i-'blas-tik\ *adj*

poly·bro·mi·nat·ed biphenyl \ˌpäl-i-'brō-mə-ˌnāt-əd-\ *n* : any of several compounds that are similar to polychlorinated biphenyls in environmental toxicity and in structure except that various hydrogen atoms are replaced by bromine rather than chlorine — called also *PBB*

poly(C) \ˌpäl-ē-'sē\ *n* : POLYCYTIDYLIC ACID

poly·cat·ion \ˌpäl-i-'kat-ˌī-ən\ *n* : a molecule or chemical complex having positive charges at several sites — **poly·cat·ion·ic** \-ˌkat-(ˌ)ī-'än-ik\ *adj*

poly·cen·tric \-'sen-trik\ *adj* : having several centromeres ⟨∼ chromosomes⟩ — compare MONOCENTRIC

poly·chlo·ri·nat·ed biphenyl \ˌpäl-i-'klōr-ə-ˌnāt-əd-, -'klȯr-\ *n* : any of several compounds that are produced by replacing hydrogen atoms in biphenyl with chlorine, have various industrial applications, and are toxic environmental pollutants which tend to accumulate in animal tissues — called also *PCB*

poly·chon·dri·tis \ˌpäl-ē-(ˌ)kän-'drīt-əs\ *n* : inflammation of cartilage at multiple sites in the body — see RELAPSING POLYCHONDRITIS

poly·chro·ma·sia \-krō-'mā-zh(ē-)ə\ *n* : the quality of being polychromatic; *specif* : POLYCHROMATOPHILIA

poly·chro·mat·ic \-krō-'mat-ik\ *adj* **1** : showing a variety or a change of colors **2** *of a cell or tissue* : exhibiting polychromatophilia

¹poly·chro·ma·to·phil \-krō-'mat-ə-ˌfil, -'krō-mət-ə-\ *n* : a

\ə\ **abut** \ᵊ\ **kitten** \ər\ **further** \a\ **ash** \ā\ **ace** \ä\ **cot, cart**
\aù\ **out** \ch\ **chin** \e\ **bet** \ē\ **easy** \g\ **go** \i\ **hit** \ī\ **ice** \j\ **job**
\ŋ\ **sing** \ō\ **go** \ò\ **law** \òi\ **boy** \th\ **thin** \th̲\ **the** \ü\ **loot**
\ù\ **foot** \y\ **yet** \zh\ **vision** *See also* Pronunciation Symbols page

O
P

young or degenerated red blood cell staining with both acid and basic dyes

²**polychromatophil** *adj* : exhibiting polychromatophilia; *esp* : staining with both acid and basic dyes

poly·chro·mato·phil·ia \-krō-ˌmat-ə-ˈfil-ē-ə\ *n* : the quality of being stainable with more than one type of stain and esp. with both acid and basic dyes

poly·chro·mato·phil·ic \-krō-ˌmat-ə-ˈfil-ik\ *adj* : stainable with more than one type of stain and esp. with both acid and basic dyes ⟨∼ erythroblasts⟩

poly·chro·mia \ˌpäl-i-ˈkrō-mē-ə\ *n* : excessive or abnormal pigmentation of the skin

poly·cis·tron·ic \ˌpäl-i-sis-ˈträn-ik\ *adj* : containing the genetic information of a number of cistrons ⟨∼ messenger RNA⟩

poly·clin·ic \ˌpäl-i-ˈklin-ik\ *n* : a clinic or hospital treating diseases of many sorts — compare POLICLINIC

poly·clo·nal \ˈpäl-i-ˌklōn-ᵊl\ *adj* : produced by or being cells derived from two or more cells of different ancestry or genetic constitution ⟨∼ antibody synthesis⟩

polycosanol *var of* POLICOSANOL

poly·cy·clic \ˌpäl-i-ˈsī-klik, -ˈsik-lik\ *adj* : having more than one cyclic component; *esp* : having two or more usu. fused rings in a molecule

polycyclic aromatic hydrocarbon *n* : any of a class of hydrocarbon molecules with multiple carbon rings that include numerous carcinogenic substances and environmental pollutants — called also *PAH, polynuclear aromatic hydrocarbon*

poly·cys·tic \-ˈsis-tik\ *adj* : having or involving more than one cyst ⟨∼ kidneys⟩ ⟨∼ disease⟩

polycystic kidney disease *n* : either of two hereditary diseases characterized by gradually enlarging bilateral cysts of the kidney which lead to reduced renal functioning: **a** : a disease that is inherited as an autosomal dominant trait, is usu. asymptomatic until middle age, and is marked by side or back pain, hematuria, urinary tract infections, and nephrolithiasis **b** : a disease that is inherited as an autosomal recessive trait, usu. affects infants or children, and results in renal failure

polycystic ovary syndrome *n* : a variable disorder that is marked esp. by amenorrhea, hirsutism, obesity, infertility, and ovarian enlargement and is usu. initiated by an elevated level of luteinizing hormone, androgen, or estrogen which results in an abnormal cycle of gonadotropin release by the pituitary gland — abbr. *PCOS;* called also *polycystic ovarian disease, polycystic ovarian syndrome, polycystic ovary disease, Stein-Leventhal syndrome*

poly·cy·the·mia *or chiefly Brit* **poly·cy·thae·mia** \-(ˌ)sī-ˈthē-mē-ə\ *n* : a condition marked by an abnormal increase in the number of circulating red blood cells; *esp* : POLYCYTHEMIA VERA — compare ERYTHROCYTOSIS

polycythemia ve·ra \-ˈvir-ə\ *n* : chronic polycythemia that is a myeloproliferative disorder of unknown cause characterized by an increase in total blood volume and viscosity and typically accompanied by nosebleed, headache, dizziness, weakness, itchy skin, reddish complexion, distension of the circulatory vessels, and enlargement of the spleen — called also *erythremia, erythrocythemia, Vaquez's disease*

poly·cy·the·mic *or chiefly Brit* **poly·cy·thae·mic** \-ˈthē-mik\ *adj* : relating to or involving polycythemia or polycythemia vera

poly·cyt·i·dyl·ic acid \ˌpäl-i-ˌsit-ə-ˈdil-ik-\ *n* : RNA or a segment of RNA that is composed of a polynucleotide chain consisting entirely of cytosine-containing nucleotides and that codes for a polypeptide chain consisting of proline residues when functioning as messenger RNA in protein synthesis — called also *poly(C);* see POLY I:C

¹**poly·dac·tyl** \ˌpäl-i-ˈdak-tᵊl\ *adj* : characterized by polydactyly ⟨∼ strains of guinea pigs —*Genetics*⟩; *also* : being a gene that determines polydactyly

²**polydactyl** *n* : one having more than the normal number of toes or fingers

poly·dac·tyl·ia \-dak-ˈtil-ē-ə\ *n* : POLYDACTYLY

poly·dac·tyl·ism \-ˈdak-tᵊl-ˌiz-əm\ *n* : POLYDACTYLY

poly·dac·ty·lous \-tə-ləs\ *adj* : POLYDACTYL

poly·dac·ty·ly \-ˈdak-tə-lē\ *n, pl* **-lies** : the condition of having more than the normal number of toes or fingers — called also *polydactylia, polydactylism*

poly·dex·trose \ˌpäl-i-ˈdek-ˌstrōs, -ˌstrōz\ *n* : a polymer of dextrose containing small amounts of bound sorbitol and citric acid that is used to mimic the texture and bulk of fat or sugar in low-calorie foods

poly·dip·sia \ˌpäl-i-ˈdip-sē-ə\ *n* : excessive or abnormal thirst — **poly·dip·sic** \-sik\ *adj*

poly·dis·perse \-dis-ˈpərs\ *adj* : of, relating to, characterized by, or characterized as particles of varied sizes in the dispersed phase of a disperse system — compare MONODISPERSE — **poly·dis·per·si·ty** \-ˈpər-sət-ē\ *n, pl* **-ties**

poly·drug \ˈpäl-ē-ˌdrəg\ *adj* : of, relating to, or being the abuse of more than one drug esp. when illicit; *also* : engaging in polydrug abuse or the distribution of illicit drugs for such abuse ⟨∼ users⟩ ⟨a ∼ smuggling cartel⟩

poly·elec·tro·lyte \ˌpäl-ē-ə-ˈlek-trə-ˌlīt\ *n* : a substance of high molecular weight (as a protein) that is an electrolyte

poly·em·bry·o·ny \-ˈem-brē-ə-nē, -(ˌ)em-ˈbrī-\ *n, pl* **-nies** : the production of two or more embryos from one ovule or egg — **poly·em·bry·on·ic** \-ˌem-brē-ˈän-ik\ *adj*

poly·en·do·crine \-ˈen-də-krən, -ˌkrīn, -ˌkrēn\ *adj* : relating to or affecting more than one endocrine gland ⟨a family history of ∼ disorders⟩

poly·ene \ˈpäl-ē-ˌēn\ *n* : an organic compound containing many double bonds; *esp* : one having the double bonds in a long aliphatic hydrocarbon chain — **poly·enic** \ˌpäl-ē-ˈē-nik\ *adj*

poly·es·trous \ˌpäl-ē-ˈes-trəs\ *or Brit* **poly·oes·trous** \-ˈē-strəs\ *adj* : having more than one period of estrus in a year

poly·eth·yl·ene \ˌpäl-ē-ˈeth-ə-ˌlēn\ *n* : a polymer of ethylene; *esp* : any of various lightweight thermoplastics $(CH_2CH_2)_x$ that are resistant to chemicals and moisture and are used esp. in packaging, insulation, surgical implants, prostheses, and tubing

po·lyg·a·la \pə-ˈlig-ə-lə\ *n* **1** *cap* : a genus of herbs and shrubs (family Polygalaceae) of temperate and warm regions having many colored often showy flowers and including some (as the seneca snakeroot) which have been used in medicine **2** : any plant of the genus *Polygala*

poly·ga·lac·tia \ˌpäl-i-gə-ˈlak-tē-ə, -ˈlak-sh(ē-)ə\ *n* : excessive milk secretion

poly·ga·lac·tu·ro·nase \-ˌga-ˌlak-ˈt(y)ùr-ə-ˌnās, -gə-ˈlak-tyər-ə-, -ˌnāz\ *n* : an enzyme that hydrolyzes the glycosidic linkages of polymerized galacturonic acids (as pectic acid) and that occurs esp. in microorganisms — compare PECTINASE

po·lyg·a·mous \pə-ˈlig-ə-məs\ *adj* **1** : relating to or practicing polygamy **2** : having more than one mate at one time

po·lyg·a·my \-mē\ *n, pl* **-mies** : marriage in which a spouse of either sex may have more than one mate at the same time — compare POLYANDRY, POLYGYNY

poly·gene \ˈpäl-i-ˌjēn\ *n* : any of a group of nonallelic genes that collectively control the inheritance of a quantitative character or modify the expression of a qualitative character — called also *multiple factor;* compare QUANTITATIVE INHERITANCE

poly·gen·ic \ˌpäl-i-ˈjēn-ik, -ˈjen-ik\ *adj* : of, relating to, or resulting from polygenes : MULTIFACTORIAL ⟨a ∼ disorder⟩ — **poly·gen·i·cal·ly** \-i-k(ə-)lē\ *adv*

poly·glan·du·lar \-ˈglan-jə-lər\ *adj* : of, relating to, or involving several glands ⟨∼ therapy⟩

poly·glo·bu·lia \ˌpäl-i-glab-ˈyü-lē-ə\ *n* : POLYCYTHEMIA

poly·glob·u·lism \-ˈgläb-yə-ˌliz-əm\ *n* : POLYCYTHEMIA

poly·gram \ˈpäl-i-ˌgram\ *n* : a tracing made by a polygraph

poly·graph \ˈpäl-i-ˌgraf\ *n* : an instrument for simultaneously recording variations of several different pulsations (as of the pulse, blood pressure, and respiration) — see LIE DETECTOR — **poly·graph·ic** \ˌpäl-i-ˈgraf-ik\ *adj* — **poly·graph·i·cal·ly** \-i-k(ə-)lē\ *adv*

po·lyg·ra·pher \ˈpäl-i-ˌgraf-ər, pə-ˈlig-rə-fər\ *n* : a person who operates a polygraph

po·lyg·ra·phist \ˈpäl-i-ˌgraf-əst, pə-ˈlig-rə-fəst\ *n* : POLYGRA-PHER

po·lyg·y·ny \pə-ˈlij-ə-nē\ *n, pl* **-nies** : the state or practice of having more than one wife or female mate at one time — compare POLYANDRY, POLYGAMY — **po·lyg·y·nous** \-nəs\ *adj*

poly·hy·brid \ˌpäl-i-ˈhī-brəd\ *n* : a hybrid whose parents differ in a number of characters : an individual or group heterozygous for more than one pair of genes — **poly·hy·brid·ism** \-ˈhī-brə-ˌdiz-əm\ *n*

poly·hy·dram·ni·os \-hī-ˈdram-nē-ˌäs\ *n* : HYDRAMNIOS

poly·hy·droxy \-hī-ˈdräk-sē\ *adj* : containing more than one hydroxyl group in the molecule

poly I:C \ˌpäl-ē-ˈī-ˈsē\ *n* : a synthetic 2-stranded RNA composed of one strand of polyinosinic acid and one strand of polycytidylic acid that induces interferon formation and has been used experimentally as an anticancer and antiviral agent — called also *poly I·poly C*

poly·ide·ism \ˌpäl-ē-ˈīd-ē-ˌiz-əm\ *n* : a state of absorption in a group of related ideas or memories — compare MONOIDE-ISM

poly·ino·sin·ic acid \ˌpäl-ē-ˌin-ə-ˌsin-ik-, -ˌī-nə-\ *n* : RNA or a segment of RNA that is composed of a polynucleotide chain consisting entirely of inosinic acid residues — see POLY I:C

poly I·poly C \ˌpäl-ē-ˈī-ˌpäl-ē-ˈsē\ *n* : POLY I:C

poly·ke·tide \ˌpäl-ē-ˈkē-ˌtīd\ *n* : any of a large class of diverse compounds that are characterized by more than two carbonyl groups connected by single intervening carbon atoms, that are produced esp. by certain bacteria and fungi, and that include various substances (as erythromycin and lovastatin) having antibiotic, anticancer, cholesterol-lowering, or immunosuppressive effects

poly·ly·sine \ˌpäl-i-ˈlī-ˌsēn\ *n* : a protein whose polypeptide chain consists entirely of lysine residues

poly·mas·tia \-ˈmas-tē-ə\ *n* : the condition of having more than the normal number of breasts

poly·mas·ti·gote \ˌpäl-i-ˈmas-tə-ˌgōt\ *adj* : having many flagella

poly·men·or·rhea *or Brit* **poly·men·or·rhoea** \-ˌmen-ə-ˈrē-ə\ *n* : menstruation at abnormally frequent intervals

poly·mer \ˈpäl-ə-mər\ *n* : a chemical compound or mixture of compounds formed by polymerization and consisting essentially of repeating structural units

po·ly·mer·ase \pə-ˈlim-ər-ˌās; ˈpä-lə-mə-ˌrās, -ˌrāz\ *n* : any of several enzymes that catalyze the formation of DNA or RNA from precursor substances in the presence of preexisting DNA or RNA acting as a template

polymerase chain reaction *n* : an in vitro technique for rapidly synthesizing large quantities of a given DNA segment that involves separating the DNA into its two complementary strands, binding a primer to each single strand at the end of the given DNA segment where synthesis will start, using DNA polymerase to synthesize two-stranded DNA from each single strand, and repeating the process — abbr. *PCR*

poly·mer·ic \ˌpäl-ə-ˈmer-ik\ *adj* **1** : of, relating to, or constituting a polymer **2** : of, relating to, being, or involving nonallelic often identical genes that collectively control one or more hereditary traits — **poly·mer·i·cal·ly** \-i-k(ə-)lē\ *adv* — **po·ly·mer·ism** \pə-ˈlim-ə-ˌriz-əm, ˈpäl-ə-mə-\ *n*

po·ly·mer·iza·tion *also Brit* **po·ly·mer·isa·tion** \pə-ˌlim-ə-rə-ˈzā-shən, ˌpäl-ə-mə-rə-\ *n* **1** : a chemical reaction in which two or more small molecules combine to form larger molecules that contain repeating structural units of the original molecules — compare ASSOCIATION 4 **2** : reduplication of parts in an organism

po·ly·mer·ize *also Brit* **po·ly·mer·ise** \pə-ˈlim-ə-ˌrīz, ˈpäl-ə-mə-\ *vb* **-ized** *also Brit* **-ised; -iz·ing** *also Brit* **-is·ing** *vt* : to subject to polymerization ∼ *vi* : to undergo polymerization

poly·meth·y·lene \ˌpäl-i-ˈmeth-ə-ˌlēn, -lən\ *n* **1** : a hydrocarbon constituted of methylene groups **2** : a bivalent radical –(CH₂)ₙ– consisting of a series of methylene groups

poly·meth·yl methacrylate \ˈpäl-i-ˌmeth-əl-\ *n* : a thermoplastic resin of polymerized methyl methacrylate that is used

esp. in hard contact lenses and in prostheses to replace bone

poly·mi·cro·bi·al \ˌpäl-i-mī-ˈkrō-bē-əl\ *adj* : of, relating to, or caused by several types of microorganisms ⟨∼ infections⟩

poly·mod·al \-ˈmōd-ᵊl\ *adj* : responding to several different forms of sensory stimulation (as heat, touch, and chemicals) ⟨unmyelinated ∼ nociceptors⟩

poly·morph \ˈpäl-i-ˌmȯrf\ *n* **1** : a polymorphic organism; *also* : one of the several forms of such an organism **2** : any of the crystalline forms of a polymorphic substance **3** : a polymorphonuclear leukocyte

poly·mor·phic \ˌpäl-i-ˈmȯr-fik\ *adj* : of, relating to, or having polymorphism ⟨a ∼ species⟩ ⟨a ∼ genetic locus⟩ ⟨∼ proteins⟩ — **poly·mor·phi·cal·ly** \-fi-k(ə-)lē\ *adv*

polymorphic light eruption *n* : POLYMORPHOUS LIGHT ERUPTION

poly·mor·phism \ˌpäl-i-ˈmȯr-ˌfiz-əm\ *n* : the quality or state of existing in or assuming different forms: as **a** (1) : existence of a species in several forms independent of the variations of sex (2) : existence of a gene in several allelic forms (3) : existence of a molecule (as an enzyme) in several forms in a single species **b** : the property of crystallizing in two or more forms with distinct structure

poly·mor·pho·cel·lu·lar \-ˌmȯr-fə-ˈsel-yə-lər\ *adj* : of, relating to, or consisting of several different forms of cells

¹poly·mor·pho·nu·cle·ar \-ˌmȯr-fə-ˈn(y)ü-klē-ər\ *adj, of a leukocyte* : having the nucleus complexly lobed; *specif* : being a mature neutrophil with a characteristic distinctly lobed nucleus

²polymorphonuclear *n* : POLYMORPH 3

poly·mor·phous \-ˈmȯr-fəs\ *adj* : having, assuming, or occurring in various forms : POLYMORPHIC ⟨∼ skin rashes⟩ — **poly·mor·phous·ly** *adv*

polymorphous light eruption *n* : photodermatosis that is marked esp. by red papules or blisters often accompanied by itching or a burning sensation and in which bodily manifestations do not appear for several hours to several days following sun exposure

polymorphous perverse *adj* : relating to or exhibiting infantile sexual tendencies in which the genitals are not yet identified as the sole or principal sexual organs nor coitus as the goal of erotic activity

poly·my·al·gia \ˌpäl-i-mī-ˈal-j(ē-)ə\ *n* : myalgia affecting several muscle groups; *specif* : POLYMYALGIA RHEUMATICA

polymyalgia rheu·mat·i·ca \-rü-ˈmat-i-kə\ *n* : a disorder of the elderly characterized by muscular pain and stiffness in the shoulders and neck and in the pelvic area

poly·myo·si·tis \-ˌmī-ə-ˈsīt-əs\ *n* : inflammation of several muscles at once; *specif* : an inflammatory disease of unknown cause that affects muscles and esp. skeletal muscles, is characterized typically by weakness usu. of the proximal muscles (as of the pectoral or pelvic girdles or of the neck), muscle and joint pain, pathological muscle changes (as fiber degeneration or infiltration by lymphocytes), pneumonia, and cardiac abnormalities (as arrhythmia or myocarditis) — see DERMATOMYOSITIS

poly·myx·in \ˌpäl-i-ˈmik-sən\ *n* : any of several toxic antibiotics obtained from a soil bacterium of the genus *Bacillus* (*B. polymyxa*) and active against gram-negative bacteria

polymyxin B *n* : the least toxic of the polymyxins used in the form of its sulfate chiefly in the treatment of some localized, gastrointestinal, or systemic infections

polymyxin E *n* : COLISTIN

poly·neu·rit·ic \ˌpäl-i-n(y)ù-ˈrit-ik\ *adj* : of, relating to, or marked by polyneuritis ⟨∼ leprosy⟩

poly·neu·ri·tis \ˌpäl-i-n(y)ù-ˈrīt-əs\ *n, pl* **-rit·i·des** \-ˈrit-ə-ˌdēz\ *or* **-ri·tis·es** : neuritis of several peripheral nerves at the same time (as that caused by vitamin B deficiency, a toxic

O
P

substance, or an infectious disease) — see GUILLAIN-BARRÉ SYNDROME

poly·neu·rop·a·thy \-n(y)ù-'räp-ə-thē\ *n, pl* **-thies** : a disease of nerves; *esp* : a noninflammatory degenerative disease of nerves usu. caused by toxins (as of lead)

poly·nu·cle·ar \ˌpäl-i-'n(y)ü-klē-ər\ *adj* : chemically polycyclic esp. with respect to the benzene ring

polynuclear aromatic hydrocarbon *n* : POLYCYCLIC AROMATIC HYDROCARBON

poly·nu·cle·o·sis \-ˌn(y)ü-klē-'ō-səs\ *n, pl* **-o·ses** \-ˌsēz\ : the presence of an excess of polymorphonuclear leukocytes (as in the circulating blood)

poly·nu·cle·o·tide \-'n(y)ü-klē-ə-ˌtīd\ *n* : a polymeric chain of mononucleotides

polyoestrous *chiefly Brit var of* POLYESTROUS

poly·ol \'päl-ē-ˌól, -ˌōl\ *n* : a compound (as sorbitol or pentaerythritol) containing usu. several alcoholic hydroxyl groups

poly·oma·vi·rus \ˌpäl-ē-'ō-mə-\ *n* **1** *cap* : the sole genus in a family (*Polyomaviridae*) of double-stranded DNA viruses that contain a single molecule of DNA, have a capsid composed of 72 capsomers, and induce tumors usu. in specific mammals and that include simian virus 40 and the causative agent of progressive multifocal leukoencephalopathy **2** : any of the genus *Polyomavirus* of double-stranded DNA viruses

poly·opia \ˌpäl-ē-'ō-pē-ə\ *n* : perception of more than one image of a single object esp. with one eye

poly·or·chi·dism \ˌpäl-ē-'ór-kə-ˌdiz-əm\ *also* **poly·or·chism** \-ˌkiz-əm\ *n* : a condition of having more than two testes

poly·os·tot·ic \ˌpäl-ē-äs-'tät-ik\ *adj* : involving or relating to many bones ⟨∼ dysplasia⟩

poly·ovu·lar \ˌpäl-ē-'äv-yə-lər\ *adj* : of, relating to, producing, or containing more than one ovum ⟨∼ follicle⟩

poly·ovu·la·tion \-ˌäv-yə-'lā-shən\ *n* : the production of more than one ovum at a single ovulation — **poly·ovu·la·to·ry** \-'äv-yə-lə-ˌtōr-ē\ *adj*

pol·yp \'päl-əp\ *n* : a projecting mass of swollen and hypertrophied or tumorous membrane (as in the nasal cavity or the intestine) — called also *polypus*

pol·yp·ec·to·my \ˌpäl-i-'pek-tə-mē\ *n, pl* **-mies** : the surgical excision of a polyp ⟨cervical ∼⟩

poly·pep·tide \ˌpäl-i-'pep-ˌtīd\ *n* : a molecular chain of amino acids — **poly·pep·tid·ic** \-(ˌ)pep-'tid-ik\ *adj*

poly·pha·gia \-'fā-j(ē-)ə\ *n* : excessive appetite or eating — compare HYPERPHAGIA

poly·phar·ma·cy \-'fär-mə-sē\ *n, pl* **-cies** : the practice of administering many different medicines esp. concurrently for the treatment of the same disease

poly·pha·sic \-'fā-zik\ *adj* **1** : of, relating to, or having more than one phase ⟨∼ evoked potentials⟩ — compare DIPHASIC b, MONOPHASIC 1 **2** : having several periods of activity interrupted by intervening periods of rest in each 24 hours ⟨an infant is essentially ∼⟩

poly·phe·nol \ˌpäl-i-'fē-ˌnól, -ˌnól, -fi-'\ *n* : a polyhydroxy phenol; *esp* : an antioxidant phytochemical (as chlorogenic acid) that tends to prevent or neutralize the damaging effects of free radicals — **poly·phe·no·lic** \-fi-'nō-lik, -näl-ik\ *adj*

poly·phy·let·ic \ˌpäl-i-(ˌ)fī-'let-ik\ *adj* : of or relating to more than one stock; *specif* : derived from more than one ancestral line — **poly·phy·let·i·cal·ly** \-i-k(ə-)lē\ *adv*

polyphyletic theory *n* : a theory in physiology: the several cellular elements of the blood originate in two or more distinct stem cells — compare MONOPHYLETIC THEORY

poly·phy·le·tism \ˌpäl-i-'fī-lə-ˌtiz-əm\ *n* **1** : POLYPHYLETIC THEORY **2** : derivation from more than one ancestral line

poly·phy·odont \ˌpäl-i-'fī-ə-ˌdänt\ *adj* : having several or many sets of teeth in succession — compare DIPHYODONT, MONOPHYODONT — **poly·phy·odon·ty** \-ē\ *n, pl* **-ties**

polypi *pl of* POLYPUS

poly·plas·tic \-'plas-tik\ *adj* : assuming or able to assume many forms

¹poly·ploid \'päl-i-ˌplóid\ *adj* : having or being a chromosome number that is a multiple greater than two of the monoploid number

²polyploid *n* : a polyploid individual

poly·ploi·dy \-ˌplóid-ē\ *n, pl* **-dies** : the condition of being polyploid

po·lyp·nea *or Brit* **po·lyp·noea** \pä-'lip-nē-ə, pə-\ *n* : rapid or panting respiration — **po·lyp·ne·ic** *or Brit* **po·lyp·noe·ic** \-nē-ik\ *adj*

pol·yp·oid \'päl-ə-ˌpóid\ *adj* **1** : resembling a polyp ⟨a ∼ intestinal growth⟩ **2** : marked by the formation of lesions suggesting polyps ⟨∼ disease⟩

Po·lyp·o·rus \pə-'lip-ə-rəs\ *n* : a genus (the type of the family Polyporaceae) of fungi having fruiting bodies that are sessile or borne on a stipe and including important pathogens of various trees and in some classifications the fungus (*Fomes officinalis* syn. *P. officinalis*) supplying the drug agaric formerly used to treat excessive perspiration

pol·yp·o·sis \ˌpäl-i-'pō-səs\ *n, pl* **-o·ses** \-ˌsēz\ : a condition characterized by the presence of numerous polyps ⟨∼ of the colon⟩ — see FAMILIAL ADENOMATOUS POLYPOSIS

pol·yp·ous \'päl-ə-pəs\ *adj* : relating to, being, or resembling a polyp

poly·pro·tein \ˌpäl-i-'prō-ˌtēn, -'prōt-ē-ən\ *n* : a large protein that is cleaved into separate smaller proteins with different biological functions

poly·ptych·i·al \ˌpäl-i-'tik-ē-əl\ *adj* : arranged in more than one layer ⟨∼ glandular cells⟩

poly·pus \'päl-ə-pəs\ *n, pl* **poly·pi** \-ˌpī, -ˌpē\ *or* **poly·pus·es** : POLYP

poly·ra·dic·u·lo·neu·rop·a·thy \ˌpäl-i-rə-ˌdik-yə-(ˌ)lō-n(y)ù-'räp-ə-thē\ *n, pl* **-thies** : an inflammatory disorder (as Guillain-Barré syndrome) affecting peripheral nerves and the nerve roots of the spinal nerves and marked by demyelination or axon degeneration

poly·ri·bo·nu·cle·o·tide \ˌpäl-i-ˌrī-bō-'n(y)ü-klē-ə-ˌtīd\ *n* : a polynucleotide in which the mononucleotides are ribonucleotides

poly·ri·bo·some \-'rī-bə-ˌsōm\ *n* : a cluster of ribosomes linked together by a molecule of messenger RNA and forming the site of protein synthesis — called also *polysome* — **poly·ri·bo·som·al** \-ˌrī-bə-'sō-məl\ *adj*

poly·ri·bo·syl·ri·bi·tol phosphate \ˌpäl-i-ˌrī-bə-sil-ˌrī-bə-ˌtól, -ˌtōl-\ *n* : a polysaccharide of the capsule of the Hib bacterium that exhibits activity against phagocytes — see CONJUGATE VACCINE

poly·sac·cha·ride \-'sak-ə-ˌrīd\ *n* : a carbohydrate that can be decomposed by hydrolysis into two or more molecules of monosaccharides; *esp* : one (as cellulose, starch, or glycogen) containing many monosaccharide units and marked by complexity — called also *glycan*

poly·se·ro·si·tis \-ˌsir-ə-'sīt-əs\ *n* : inflammation of several serous membranes (as the pleura, pericardium, and peritoneum) at the same time — called also *Concato's disease*

poly·so·ma·ty \ˌpäl-i-'sō-mət-ē\ *n, pl* **-ties** : the replication in somatic cells of the chromosome number through division of chromosomes without subsequent nuclear division — **poly·so·mat·ic** \-sō-'mat-ik\ *adj*

poly·some \'päl-i-ˌsōm\ *n* : POLYRIBOSOME

¹poly·so·mic \ˌpäl-i-'sō-mik\ *adj* : basically polyploid but having one or a few chromosomes present in a greater or smaller number than is characteristic of the rest of the chromosome complement

²polysomic *n* : a polysomic individual

poly·som·no·gram \-'säm-nə-ˌgram\ *n* : a record of physiological variables during sleep obtained by polysomnography

poly·som·no·graph \-ˌgraf\ *n* : a polygraph used for polysomnography

poly·som·nog·ra·pher \-ˌsäm-'näg-rə-fər\ *n* : a technician trained in polysomnography

poly·som·nog·ra·phy \-fē\ *n, pl* **-phies** : the technique or process of using a polygraph to make a continuous record during sleep of multiple physiological variables (as breathing, heart rate, and muscle activity) — **poly·som·no·graph·ic** \-ˌsäm-nə-'graf-ik\ *adj* — **poly·som·no·graph·i·cal·ly** \-i-k(ə-)lē\ *adv*

poly·so·my \\'päl-i-ˌsō-mē\ *n, pl* **-mies** : the condition of being polysomic

poly·sor·bate \ˌpäl-i-'sȯr-ˌbāt\ *n* : any of several emulsifiers used in the preparation of some pharmaceuticals and foods — see TWEEN

poly·sper·mic \-'spər-mik\ *adj* : of, relating to, or characterized by polyspermy ⟨∼ fertilization⟩

poly·sper·my \'päl-i-ˌspər-mē\ *n, pl* **-mies** : the entrance of several spermatozoa into one egg — compare DISPERMY, MONOSPERMY

poly·sty·rene \ˌpäl-i-'stī(ə)r-ˌēn\ *n* : a polymer of styrene; *esp* : a rigid transparent thermoplastic that has good physical and electrical insulating properties and is used esp. in molded products, foams, and sheet materials

poly·sub·stance \-'səb-stən(t)s\ *n, often attrib* : a group of substances used often indiscriminately by a substance abuser ⟨has a ∼ dependence problem⟩

poly·syn·ap·tic \ˌpäl-i-sə-'nap-tik\ *adj* : involving two or more synapses in the central nervous system ⟨∼ reflexes⟩ — **poly·syn·ap·ti·cal·ly** \-ti-k(ə-)lē\ *adv*

poly·tene \'päl-i-ˌtēn\ *adj* : relating to, being, or having chromosomes each of which consists of many strands with the corresponding chromomeres in contact — **poly·te·ny** \-ˌtē-nē\ *n, pl* **-nies**

poly·tet·ra·flu·or·o·eth·yl·ene \ˌpäl-i-ˌte-trə-ˌflü(-ə)r-ō-'eth-ə-ˌlēn\ *n* : a polymer of tetrafluoroethylene (CF_2–CF_2)$_n$ that is a resin with good resistance to chemicals and heat and that is used to fabricate prostheses — abbr. *PTFE*; see TEFLON

poly·the·lia \ˌpäl-i-'thē-lē-ə\ *n* : the condition of having more than the normal number of nipples

poly·thi·a·zide \-'thī-ə-ˌzīd, -zəd\ *n* : an antihypertensive and diuretic drug $C_{11}H_{13}ClF_3N_3O_4S_3$ — see RENESE

po·lyt·o·cous \pə-'lit-ə-kəs\ *adj* : producing many eggs or young at one time — compare MONOTOCOUS

poly·to·mo·gram \ˌpäl-i-'tō-mə-ˌgram\ *n* : a recording made by polytomography

poly·to·mog·ra·phy \-tō-'mäg-rə-fē\ *n, pl* **-phies** : tomography performed along several sectional planes

poly·typ·ic \ˌpäl-i-'tip-ik\ *also* **poly·typ·i·cal** \-'tip-i-kəl\ *adj* : represented by several or many types or subdivisions ⟨a ∼ species of organisms⟩

poly(U) \ˌpäl-ē-'yü\ *n* : POLYURIDYLIC ACID

poly·un·sat·u·rate \ˌpäl-ē-ˌən-'sach-ə-ˌrət\ *n* : a polyunsaturated oil or fatty acid

poly·un·sat·u·rat·ed \ˌpäl-ē-ˌən-'sach-ə-ˌrāt-əd\ *adj, of an oil, fat, or fatty acid* : having in each molecule many chemical bonds in which two or three pairs of electrons are shared by two atoms — compare MONOUNSATURATED

poly·uria \ˌpäl-ē-'yùr-ē-ə\ *n* : excessive secretion of urine

poly·uri·dyl·ic acid \ˌpäl-ē-ˌyùr-ə-ˌdil-ik-\ *n* : RNA or a segment of RNA that is composed of a polynucleotide chain consisting entirely of uracil-containing nucleotides and that codes for a polypeptide chain consisting of phenylalanine residues when functioning as messenger RNA in protein synthesis — called also *poly(U)*

poly·va·lent \ˌpäl-i-'vā-lənt\ *adj* **1 a** : having a chemical valence greater usu. than two **b** : having variable valence **2** : effective against, sensitive toward, or counteracting more than one exciting agent (as a toxin or antigen) ⟨a ∼ vaccine⟩ — **poly·va·lence** \-lən(t)s\ *n*

poly·vi·nyl \-'vīn-ᵊl\ *adj* : of, relating to, or being a polymerized vinyl compound, resin, or plastic

poly·vi·nyl·pyr·rol·i·done \-ˌvīn-ᵊl-pi-'räl-ə-ˌdōn\ *n* : a water-soluble chemically inert solid polymer (–$CH_2CHC_4H_6NO$–)$_n$ used chiefly in medicine as a vehicle for drugs (as iodine) and esp. formerly as a plasma expander — called also *povidone*

poly·zo·ot·ic \ˌpäl-i-zə-'wät-ik\ *adj* : consisting of a linear series of similar segments ⟨∼ tapeworms⟩ — compare MONOZOOTIC

po·made \pō-'mād, -'mäd\ *n* : a perfumed ointment; *esp* : a fragrant unguent for the hair or scalp

po·man·der \'pō-ˌman-dər, pō-'-\ *n* : a mixture of aromatic substances enclosed in a perforated bag or box and used to scent clothes and linens or formerly carried as a guard against infection; *also* : a clove-studded orange or apple used for the same purposes

po·ma·tum \pō-'māt-əm, -'mät-\ *n* : OINTMENT; *esp* : a perfumed unguent for the hair or scalp

pome·gran·ate \'päm-(ə-)ˌgran-ət, 'pəm-ˌgran-\ *n* **1** : a tart thick-skinned several-celled reddish berry that is about the size of an orange **2** : a widely cultivated tropical Old World tree (*Punica granatum* of the family Punicaceae) bearing pomegranates and having bark and roots which were formerly used in dried form as a taeniacide

Pom·pe's disease \ˌpäm-'pāz-\ *also* **Pom·pe disease** \-'pā-\ *n* : an often fatal glycogen storage disease that results from an enzyme deficiency, is characterized by abnormal accumulation of glycogen esp. in the liver, heart, and muscle, and usu. appears during infancy — called also *acid maltase deficiency*

    Pom·pe \'pòm-pə\, **Johann Cassianius** (*fl* 1932), Dutch physician. Pompe published a description of acid maltase deficiency in 1932.

pom·pho·lyx \'päm(p)-fə-ˌliks\ *n* : a skin disease marked by an eruption of vesicles esp. on the palms and soles

Pon·ceau \ˌpän-'sō\ *n* : any of several azo dyes (as Biebrich scarlet) giving red colors and used as biological stains

pon·der·a·ble \'pän-d(ə-)rə-bəl\ *adj* : capable of being weighed

pon·der·al \'pän-də-rəl\ *adj* : of or relating to weight ⟨∼ data⟩

ponderal index *n* : a measure of relative body mass expressed as the ratio of the cube root of body weight to height multiplied by 100

P₁ generation \'pē-'wən-\ *n* : a generation consisting of stocks which are usu. homozygous for one or more traits and from which the parents used in the first cross of a genetic experiment are selected — compare F_1 GENERATION, F_2 GENERATION

Pon·gi·dae \'pän-gi-ˌdē, 'pän-jə-\ *n pl* : a family of anthropoid apes consisting of the gorilla, orangutan, chimpanzee, and bonobo — **pon·gid** \'pän-jəd, 'pän-gəd\ *adj or n*

pons \'pänz\ *n, pl* **pon·tes** \'pän-ˌtēz\ : a broad mass of chiefly transverse nerve fibers in the mammalian brain stem lying ventral to the cerebellum at the anterior end of the medulla oblongata

pons Va·ro·lii \-və-'rō-lē-ˌī, -lē-ˌē\ *n, pl* **pontes Varolii** : PONS

    Va·ro·lio \vä-'rō-lē-ō\, **Costanzo** (1543–1575), Italian anatomist. A surgeon and professor of anatomy at Bologna, Varolio is remembered for his work on the cranial nerves. In 1573 he published a work which described his new method of dissecting the brain: he separated the brain from the skull and began the dissection from the base. This method allowed for better observation of the structures of the brain, especially the cranial nerves. As a result of his improved method of dissection, he was able to observe and describe for the first time the mass of nerve fibers that is now known as the pons Varolii. His method also allowed him to add to the knowledge of the course and terminations of the cranial nerves in the brain.

Pon·ti·ac fever \'pänt-ē-ˌak-\ *n* : an illness caused by a bacterium of the genus *Legionella* (*L. pneumophila*) that is a less severe form of Legionnaires' disease in which pneumonia does not develop

pon·tic \'pänt-ik\ *n* : an artifical tooth on a dental bridge

pon·tile \'pän-ˌtīl, -tᵊl\ *adj* : PONTINE

pon·tine \'pän-ˌtīn\ *adj* : of or relating to the pons ⟨a study of ∼ lesions⟩

pontine flexure *n* : a flexure of the embryonic hindbrain that serves to delimit the developing cerebellum and medulla oblongata

pontine nucleus *n* : any of various large groups of nerve

O
P

\ə\ **abut** \ᵊ\ **kitten** \ər\ **further** \a\ **ash** \ā\ **ace** \ä\ **cot, cart** \aù\ **out** \ch\ **chin** \e\ **bet** \ē\ **easy** \g\ **go** \i\ **hit** \ī\ **ice** \j\ **job** \ŋ\ **sing** \ō\ **go** \ò\ **law** \òi\ **boy** \th\ **thin** \ṯh\ **the** \ü\ **loot** \ù\ **foot** \y\ **yet** \zh\ **vision** *See also* Pronunciation Symbols page

cells in the basal part of the pons that receive fibers from the cerebral cortex and send fibers to the cerebellum by way of the middle cerebellar peduncles

pontis — see BRACHIUM PONTIS

Pon·to·caine \'pänt-ə-ˌkān\ *trademark* — used for a preparation of the hydrochloride of tetracaine

pon·to·cer·e·bel·lar \ˌpän-tō-ˌser-ə-'bel-ər\ *adj* : of or relating to the pons and the cerebellum

¹pool \'pül\ *vi, of blood* : to accumulate or become static (as in the veins of a bodily part) ⟨blood ∼ed in his legs⟩

²pool *n* : a readily available supply: as **a** : the whole quantity of a particular material present in the body and available for function or the satisfying of metabolic demands — see GENE POOL, METABOLIC POOL **b** : a body product (as blood) collected from many donors and stored for later use

pop·li·te·al \ˌpäp-lə-'tē-əl *also* päp-'lit-ē-əl\ *adj* : of or relating to the back part of the leg behind the knee joint

popliteal artery *n* : the continuation of the femoral artery that after passing through the thigh crosses the popliteal space and soon divides into the anterior and posterior tibial arteries

popliteal fossa *n* : POPLITEAL SPACE

popliteal ligament — see ARCUATE POPLITEAL LIGAMENT, OBLIQUE POPLITEAL LIGAMENT

popliteal nerve — see LATERAL POPLITEAL NERVE, MEDIAL POPLITEAL NERVE

popliteal space *n* : a lozenge-shaped space at the back of the knee joint — called also *popliteal fossa*

popliteal vein *n* : a vein formed by the union of the anterior and posterior tibial veins and ascending through the popliteal space to the thigh where it becomes the femoral vein

pop·li·te·us \ˌpäp-lə-'tē-əs *also* päp-'lit-ē-əl\ *n, pl* **-li·tei** \-ˌī\ : a flat muscle that originates from the lateral condyle of the femur, forms part of the floor of the popliteal space, and functions to flex the leg and rotate the femur medially

pop·per \'päp-ər\ *n, slang* : a vial of amyl nitrite or butyl nitrite esp. when used illicitly as an inhalational aphrodisiac

pop·py \'päp-ē\ *n, pl* **poppies** : any herb of the genus *Papaver* (family Papaveraceae, the poppy family); *esp* : OPIUM POPPY

poppy–seed oil *n* : a pale to reddish drying oil obtained from the seeds esp. of the opium poppy — see LIPIODOL

pop·u·la·tion \ˌpäp-yə-'lā-shən\ *n* **1** : the whole number of people or inhabitants in a country or region **2 a** : a body of persons or individuals having a quality or characteristic in common **b** (1) : the organisms inhabiting a particular locality (2) : a group of interbreeding organisms that represents the level of organization at which speciation begins **3** : a group of individual persons, objects, or items from which samples are taken for statistical measurement

population explosion *n* : a pyramiding of numbers of a biological population; *esp* : the recent great increase in human numbers resulting from both increased survival and exponential population growth

population genetics *n pl but sing in constr* : a branch of genetics concerned with gene frequencies and genotype frequencies in populations under equilibrium and nonequilibrium conditions considering esp. randomness of mating, immigration, emigration, mutation, and selection — see HARDY-WEINBERG LAW

por·ad·e·ni·tis \ˌpȯr-ˌad-ᵊn-'īt-əs\ *n* : LYMPHOGRANULOMA VENEREUM

por·ce·lain \'pōr-s(ə-)lən, 'pȯr-\ *n* : a hard, fine-grained, nonporous, and usu. translucent and white ceramic ware that consists essentially of kaolin, quartz, and feldspar and that has many uses in dentistry

por·cine \'pȯr-ˌsīn\ *adj* : of or derived from swine ⟨∼ heterografts⟩

pore \'pō(ə)r, 'pȯ(ə)r\ *n* : a minute opening esp. in an animal or plant; *esp* : one by which matter passes through a membrane

por·en·ce·pha·lia \ˌpȯr-ˌen-sə-'fā-lē-ə\ *n* : PORENCEPHALY

por·en·ceph·a·lic \-in-'sef-ə-lik\ *adj* : relating to or characterized by porencephaly ⟨a ∼ brain⟩

por·en·ceph·a·ly \ˌpȯr-in-'sef-ə-lē\ *n, pl* **-lies** : the presence of cavities in the brain

por·fi·mer sodium \'pȯr-fə-mər-\ *n* : a photosensitizing mixture of porphyrin oligomers that is administered by intravenous injection to induce photosensitivity in tumor cells (as of esophageal carcinoma) before subjecting them to laser light in photodynamic therapy — see PHOTOFRIN

po·ri·on \'pōr-ē-ˌän\ *n, pl* **po·ria** \-ē-ə\ *or* **porions** : the midpoint on the upper margin of the external auditory canal

pork tapeworm \'pȯ(ə)rk-\ *n* : a tapeworm of the genus *Taenia* (*T. solium*) that infests the human intestine as an adult, has a cysticercus larva that typically develops in swine, and is contracted by humans through ingestion of the larva in raw or imperfectly cooked pork

po·ro·ceph·a·li·a·sis \ˌpō-rō-ˌsef-ə-'lī-ə-səs\ *n, pl* **-a·ses** \-ˌsēz\ : infestation with or disease caused by a tongue worm of the family Porocephalidae

Po·ro·ceph·al·i·dae \-si-'fal-ə-ˌdē\ *n pl* : a family of tongue worms (order Porocephalida) having cylindrical bodies and occurring as adults in the lungs of reptiles and as young in various vertebrates including humans

Po·ro·ceph·a·lus \-'sef-ə-ləs\ *n* : the type genus of the family Porocephalidae of tongue worms

po·ro·ker·a·to·sis \-ˌker-ə-'tō-səs\ *n* : any of several uncommon inherited skin disorders characterized by hypertrophy of the stratum corneum

po·ro·sis \pə-'rō-səs\ *n, pl* **po·ro·ses** \-ˌsēz\ *or* **porosises** : a condition (as of a bone) characterized by porosity; *specif* : rarefaction (as of bone) with increased translucency to X-rays

po·ros·i·ty \pə-'räs-ət-ē, pō-, pȯ-\ *n, pl* **-ties** **1 a** : the quality or state of being porous **b** : the ratio of the volume of interstices of a material to the volume of its mass **2** : PORE

¹po·rot·ic \pə-'rät-ik\ *n* : a medicine favoring the formation of callus

²porotic *adj* : exhibiting or marked by porous structure or osteoporosis ⟨∼ bone⟩ ⟨∼ alteration of teeth⟩

po·rous \'pōr-əs, 'pȯr-\ *adj* **1** : possessing or full of pores ⟨∼ bones⟩ **2** : permeable to fluids

por·phin \'pȯr-fən\ *also* **por·phine** \-ˌfēn\ *n* : a deep purple crystalline compound $C_{20}H_{14}N_4$ that is made synthetically from pyrrole and formaldehyde, contains four pyrrole rings joined by =CH– groups so as to give a heterocyclic arrangement, and forms the essential skeletal structure of the porphyrins, heme, and chlorophyll

por·pho·bi·lin·o·gen \ˌpȯr-fō-bī-'lin-ə-jən\ *n* : a dicarboxylic acid $C_{10}H_{14}N_2O_4$ that is derived from pyrrole, that is found in the urine in acute porphyria, and that on condensation of four molecules yields uroporphyrin and other porphyrins

por·phyr·ia \pȯr-'fir-ē-ə\ *n* : any of several usu. hereditary abnormalities of porphyrin metabolism characterized by excretion of excess porphyrins in the urine and by extreme sensitivity to light

porphyria cu·ta·nea tar·da \-kyü-'tā-nē-ə-'tärd-ə\ *n* : a common porphyria that is marked by an excess of uroporphyrin caused by an enzyme deficiency chiefly of the liver and that is characterized esp. by skin lesions produced by exposure to light, scarring, hyperpigmentation, and hypertrichosis

por·phy·rin \'pȯr-fə-rən\ *n* : any of various compounds with a structure that consists essentially of four pyrrole rings joined by four =CH– groups; *esp* : one (as chlorophyll or hemoglobin) containing a central metal atom and usu. having biological activity

por·phy·rin·uria \ˌpȯr-fə-rə-'n(y)ùr-ē-ə\ *n* : the presence of porphyrin in the urine — called also *hematoporphyrinuria*

por·phy·rop·sin \ˌpȯr-fə-'räp-sən\ *n* : a purple pigment in the retinal rods of freshwater fishes that resembles rhodopsin

por·phy·rox·ine \ˌpȯr-fə-'räk-sən\ *n* : a crystalline opium alkaloid $C_{19}H_{23}NO_4$ whose solution in dilute acid turns red on exposure to air

por·ta \'pȯrt-ə\ *n, pl* **por·tae** \-ē\ : an opening in a bodily part where the blood vessels, nerves, or ducts leave and enter : HILUM

por·ta·ca·val \ˌpȯrt-ə-ˈkā-vəl\ *adj* : extending from the portal vein to the vena cava ⟨∼ anastomosis⟩

portacaval shunt *n* : a surgical shunt by which the portal vein is made to empty into the inferior vena cava in order to bypass a damaged liver

porta hep·a·tis \-ˈhep-ə-təs\ *n* : the fissure running transversely on the underside of the liver where most of the vessels enter or leave — called also *transverse fissure*

¹**por·tal** \ˈpȯrt-ᵊl\ *n* : a communicating part or area of an organism: as **a** : PORTAL VEIN **b** : the point at which something enters the body ⟨∼s of infection⟩

²**portal** *adj* **1** : of or relating to the porta hepatis **2** : of, relating to, or being a portal vein or a portal system ⟨∼ blood⟩ ⟨∼ circulation⟩

portal cirrhosis *n* : LAENNEC'S CIRRHOSIS

portal hypertension *n* : hypertension in the hepatic portal system caused by venous obstruction or occlusion that produces splenomegaly and ascites in its later stages

portal system *n* : a system of veins that begins and ends in capillaries — see HEPATIC PORTAL SYSTEM, PITUITARY PORTAL SYSTEM

portal vein *n* : a large vein that is formed by fusion of other veins, that terminates in a capillary network, and that delivers blood to some area of the body other than the heart; *esp* : HEPATIC PORTAL VEIN

por·tio \ˈpȯr-shē-ˌō, ˈpȯrt-ē-ˌō\ *n, pl* **-ti·o·nes** \ˌpȯr-shē-ˈō-ˌnēz\ : a part, segment, or branch (as of an organ or nerve) ⟨the visible ∼ of the cervix⟩

por·tog·ra·phy \pȯr-ˈtäg-rə-fē\ *n, pl* **-phies** : X-ray visualization of the hepatic portal system made radiopaque by intravenous infusion of a suitable medium

por·to·sys·tem·ic \ˌpȯr-tō-sis-ˈtem-ik\ *adj* : connecting the hepatic portal system and the venous part of the systemic circulation ⟨management of hypertension in the hepatic portal system by ∼ shunting⟩ ⟨diagnosis of spontaneous formation of a ∼ shunt in chronic liver disease⟩

Por·tu·guese man–of–war \ˌpȯr-chə-ˌgēz-ˌman-əv-ˈwȯr\ *n, pl* **Portuguese man–of–wars** \-ˈwȯrz\ *also* **Portuguese men–of–war** \-ˌmen-əv-ˈwȯr\ : any siphonophore of the genus *Physalia* including large tropical and subtropical oceanic forms having a crested bladderlike float which bears a colony comprised of three types of zooids on the lower surface with one of the three having stinging tentacles

port–wine stain \ˈpȯrt-ˌwīn-\ *n* : a reddish purple superficial hemangioma of the skin commonly occurring as a birthmark — called also *nevus flammeus, port-wine mark*

POS *abbr* point-of-service

¹**po·si·tion** \pə-ˈzish-ən\ *n* : a particular arrangement or location; *specif* : an arrangement of the parts of the body considered particularly desirable for some medical or surgical procedure ⟨knee-chest ∼⟩ ⟨lithotomy ∼⟩ — **po·si·tion·al** \pə-ˈzish-ᵊn-əl\ *adj*

²**position** *vt* : to put in proper position

¹**pos·i·tive** \ˈpäz-ət-iv, ˈpäz-tiv\ *adj* **1** : directed or moving toward a source of stimulation ⟨a ∼ taxis⟩ **2** : having rendition of light and shade similar in tone to the tones of the original ⟨a ∼ photographic image⟩ **3 a** (1) : being, relating to, or charged with electricity of which the proton is the elementary unit and which predominates in a glass body after being rubbed with silk (2) : having more protons than electrons ⟨a ∼ ion⟩ **b** (1) : having higher electrical potential and constituting the part from which the current flows to the external circuit ⟨the ∼ terminal of a discharging storage battery⟩ (2) : being an electron-collecting electrode of an electron tube **4 a** : marked by or indicating acceptance, approval, or affirmation **b** : affirming the presence of that sought or suspected to be present ⟨a ∼ test for blood⟩ **5** *of a lens* : converging light rays and forming a real inverted image — **pos·i·tive·ly** \-lē, *for emphasis often* ˌpäz-ə-ˈtiv-\ *adv* — **pos·i·tive·ness** \ˈpäz-ət-iv-nəs, ˈpäz-tiv-\ *n*

²**positive** *n* **1** : a positive photograph or a print from a nega-

tive **2** : a positive result (as of a test); *also* : a test yielding such a result

positive afterimage *n* : a visual afterimage that retains the same light, dark, and color relationships as those appearing in the original image — compare NEGATIVE AFTERIMAGE

positive electron *n* : POSITRON

positive end–expiratory pressure *n* : a technique of assisting breathing by increasing the air pressure in the lungs and air passages near the end of expiration so that an increased amount of air remains in the lungs following expiration — abbr. *PEEP*; compare CONTINUOUS POSITIVE AIRWAY PRESSURE

positive pressure *n* : pressure that is greater than atmospheric pressure ⟨mechanical ventilation of the lungs using *positive pressure*⟩

pos·i·tron \ˈpäz-ə-ˌträn\ *n* : a positively charged particle having the same mass and magnitude of charge as the electron and constituting the antiparticle of the electron — called also *positive electron*

positron–emission tomography *n* : tomography in which an in vivo, noninvasive, cross-sectional image of regional metabolism is obtained by a usu. color-coded cathode-ray tube representation of the distribution of gamma radiation given off in the collision of electrons in cells with positrons emitted by radionuclides incorporated into metabolic substances — abbr. *PET*

po·sol·o·gy \pō-ˈsäl-ə-jē, -ˈzäl-\ *n, pl* **-gies** : a branch of medical science concerned with dosage

post·abor·tal \ˌpōst-ə-ˈbȯrt-ᵊl\ *adj* : POSTABORTION

post·abor·tion \-ə-ˈbȯr-shən\ *adj* : occurring after an abortion ⟨∼ uterine infection⟩

post·ab·sorp·tive \-ab-ˈsȯrp-tiv\ *adj* : being in or typical of the period following absorption of nutrients from the alimentary canal ⟨subjects in the ∼ state⟩

post·ad·e·noid·ec·to·my \-ˌad-ᵊn-ˌȯi-ˈdek-tə-mē\ *adj* : relating to, occurring in, or being the period after an adenoidectomy ⟨∼ bleeding⟩

post·ad·o·les·cence \-ˌad-ᵊl-ˈes-ᵊn(t)s\ *n* : the period following adolescence and preceding adulthood

¹**post·ad·o·les·cent** \-ᵊnt\ *adj* : of, relating to, occurring in, or being in postadolescence

²**postadolescent** *n* : a postadolescent individual

post·anal \-ˈān-ᵊl\ *adj* : situated behind the anus

post·an·es·the·sia *or chiefly Brit* **post·an·aes·the·sia** \-ˌan-əs-ˈthē-zhə\ *adj* : POSTANESTHETIC

postanesthesia care unit *n* : RECOVERY ROOM

post·an·es·thet·ic *or chiefly Brit* **post·an·aes·thet·ic** \-ˈthet-ik\ *adj* : occurring in, used in, or being the period following administration of an anesthetic ⟨∼ encephalopathy⟩

post·an·ox·ic \-an-ˈäk-sik\ *adj* : occurring or being after a period of anoxia ⟨∼ respiratory rhythms⟩

post·au·ric·u·lar \-ȯ-ˈrik-yə-lər\ *adj* : located or occurring behind the auricle of the ear ⟨a ∼ incision⟩

post·ax·i·al \-ˈak-sē-əl\ *adj* : of or relating to the ulnar side of the vertebrate forelimb or the fibular side of the hind limb; *also* : of or relating to the side of an animal or side of one of its limbs that is posterior to the axis of its body or limbs

post·bran·chi·al body \-ˈbraŋ-kē-əl-\ *n* : ULTIMOBRANCHIAL BODY

post·ca·nine \-ˈkā-ˌnīn\ *adj* : of, relating to, or being teeth which are posterior to the canines ⟨∼ dentition⟩

post·cap·il·lary \-ˈkap-ə-ˌler-ē, *Brit usu* -kə-ˈpil-ə-rē\ *adj* : of, relating to, affecting, or being a venule of the circulatory system

post·car·di·nal \-ˈkärd-nəl, -ᵊn-əl\ *adj* : of, relating to, or being a vein on either side in the embryo that drains the mesonephros and the portion of the trunk caudal to the heart

post·car·di·ot·o·my \-ˌkärd-ē-ˈät-ə-mē\ *adj* : occurring or being in the period following open-heart surgery

---

\ə\ **abut** \ᵊ\ **kitten** \ər\ **further** \a\ **ash** \ā\ **ace** \ä\ **cot, cart** \au̇\ **out** \ch\ **chin** \e\ **bet** \ē\ **easy** \g\ **go** \i\ **hit** \ī\ **ice** \j\ **job** \ŋ\ **sing** \ō\ **go** \ȯ\ **law** \ȯi\ **boy** \th\ **thin** \t̲h̲\ **the** \ü\ **loot** \u̇\ **foot** \y\ **yet** \zh\ **vision** *See also* Pronunciation Symbols page

post·ca·va \-'kā-və\ *n* : the inferior vena cava of vertebrates higher than fishes — **post·ca·val** \-vəl\ *adj*

post·cen·tral \'pōst-'sen-trəl\ *adj* : located behind a center or central structure; *esp* : located behind the central sulcus of the cerebral cortex

postcentral gyrus *n* : a gyrus of the parietal lobe located just posterior to the central sulcus, lying parallel to the precentral gyrus of the temporal lobe, and comprising the somatosensory cortex

post·cho·le·cys·tec·to·my syndrome \-ˌkō-lə-(ˌ)sis-'tek-tə-mē-\ *n* : persistent pain and associated symptoms (as indigestion and nausea) following a cholecystectomy

post·ci·bal \-'sī-bəl\ *adj* : occurring after a meal ⟨∼ symptoms⟩

post·co·i·tal \-'kō-ət-ᵊl, -kō-'ēt-ᵊl\ *adj* : occurring, existing, or being administered after coitus ⟨a ∼ contraceptive⟩ — **post·co·ital·ly** \-ᵊl-ē\ *adv*

post·cor·o·nary \-'kȯr-ə-ˌner-ē, -'kär-\ *adj* **1** : relating to, occurring in, or being the period following a heart attack ⟨∼ exercise⟩ **2** : having suffered a heart attack ⟨a ∼ patient⟩

post·cra·ni·al \-'krā-nē-əl\ *adj* : of or relating to the part of the body caudal to the head ⟨a ∼ skeleton⟩ — **post·cra·ni·al·ly** \-ē\ *adv*

post·dam \-'dam\ *n* : a posterior extension of a full denture to accomplish a complete seal between denture and tissues

post·em·bry·o·nal \-em-'brī-ən-ᵊl\ *adj* : POSTEMBRYONIC

post·em·bry·on·ic \-ˌem-brē-'än-ik\ *adj* : occurring after the embryonic stage ⟨∼ growth⟩ — **post·em·bry·on·i·cal·ly** \-i-k(ə-)lē\ *adv*

post·en·ceph·a·lit·ic \-in-ˌsef-ə-'lit-ik\ *adj* : occurring after and presumably as a result of encephalitis ⟨∼ parkinsonism⟩

post·en·ceph·a·li·tis \-'līt-əs\ *n, pl* **-lit·i·des** \-'lit-ə-ˌdēz\ : symptoms or residual abnormality remaining after recovery from epidemic encephalitis

post·ep·i·lep·tic \-ˌep-ə-'lep-tik\ *adj* : occurring or being in the period immediately following an epileptic seizure ⟨∼ confusion⟩

pos·te·ri·ad \pä-'stir-ē-ˌad, pō-\ *adv* : toward the posterior part of the body

¹pos·te·ri·or \pō-'stir-ē-ər, pä-\ *adj* : situated behind: as **a** : situated at or toward the hind part of the body : CAUDAL **b** : DORSAL — used of human anatomy in which the upright posture makes dorsal and caudal identical

²pos·te·ri·or \pä-'stir-ē-ər, pō-\ *n* : a posterior thing or part: as **a** : the rear end of a quadruped **b** : BUTTOCKS

posterior auricular artery *n* : a small branch of the external carotid artery that supplies or gives off branches supplying the back of the ear and the adjacent region of the scalp, the middle ear, tympanic membrane, and mastoid cells — called also *posterior auricular*

posterior auricular vein *n* : a vein formed from venous tributaries in the region behind the ear that joins with the posterior facial vein to form the external jugular vein

posterior brachial cutaneous nerve *n* : a branch of the radial nerve that arises on the medial side of the arm in the axilla and supplies the skin on the dorsal surface almost to the olecranon

posterior cerebral artery *n* : CEREBRAL ARTERY c

posterior chamber *n* : a narrow space in the eye behind the peripheral part of the iris and in front of the suspensory ligament of the lens and the ciliary processes — compare ANTERIOR CHAMBER

posterior column *n* : DORSAL HORN

posterior commissure *n* : a bundle of white matter crossing from one side of the brain to the other just rostral to the superior colliculi and above the opening of the aqueduct of Sylvius into the third ventricle

posterior communicating artery *n* : COMMUNICATING ARTERY b

posterior cord *n* : a cord of nerve tissue that is formed from the posterior divisions of the three trunks of the brachial plexus and that divides into the axillary and radial nerves — compare LATERAL CORD, MEDIAL CORD

posterior cranial fossa *n* : CRANIAL FOSSA a

posterior cricoarytenoid *n* : CRICOARYTENOID 2

posterior cruciate ligament *n* : a cruciate ligament of each knee that is attached medially in back between the condyles of the tibia, that passes upward and forward through the middle of the knee crossing the anterior cruciate ligament to attach to the medial aspect of the femur, that functions to prevent hyperflexion of the knee and to keep the tibia from sliding backward in relation to the femur when the knee is flexed, and that is stronger and less subject to sports injury by tearing than the anterior cruciate ligament — called also *PCL*

posterior elastic lamina *n* : DESCEMET'S MEMBRANE

posterior facial vein *n* : a vein that is formed in the upper part of the parotid gland behind the mandible by the union of several tributaries, gives off a communication with the facial vein as it passes through the parotid gland, and joins with the posterior auricular vein to form the external jugular vein

posterior femoral cutaneous nerve *n* : a nerve that arises from the sacral plexus, leaves the pelvis in company with the sciatic nerve through the greater sciatic foramen, and is distributed to the skin of the perineum and of the back of the thigh and leg — compare LATERAL FEMORAL CUTANEOUS NERVE

posterior fossa *n* : CRANIAL FOSSA a

posterior funiculus *n* : a longitudinal division on each side of the spinal cord comprising white matter between the dorsal root and the posterior median sulcus — compare ANTERIOR FUNICULUS, LATERAL FUNICULUS

posterior gray column *n* : DORSAL HORN

posterior horn *n* **1** : DORSAL HORN **2** : the cornu of the lateral ventricle of each cerebral hemisphere that curves backward into the occipital lobe — compare ANTERIOR HORN 2, INFERIOR HORN

posterior humeral circumflex artery *n* : an artery that branches from the axillary artery in the shoulder, curves around the back of the humerus, and is distributed esp. to the deltoid muscle and shoulder joint — compare ANTERIOR HUMERAL CIRCUMFLEX ARTERY

posterior inferior cerebellar artery *n* : an artery that usu. branches from the vertebral artery below its junction with the contralateral vertebral artery to form the basilar artery and that supplies much of the medulla oblongata, the inferior or portion of the cerebellum, and part of the floor of the fourth ventricle

posterior inferior iliac spine *n* : a projection on the posterior margin of the ilium that is situated below the posterior superior iliac spine and is separated from it by a notch — called also *posterior inferior spine*

posterior intercostal artery *n* : INTERCOSTAL ARTERY b

posterior lobe *n* **1** : NEUROHYPOPHYSIS **2** : the part of the cerebellum between the primary fissure and the flocculonodular lobe

pos·te·ri·or·ly \pō-'stir-ē-ər-lē, pä-\ *adv* : in a posterior direction ⟨ossification of the maxilla extends ∼, superiorly, anteriorly and palatally —W. J. Tulley⟩

posterior median septum *n* : a sheet of glial tissue in the midsagittal plane of the spinal cord that extends from the posterior median sulcus toward the gray commissure and that partitions the posterior part of the spinal cord into right and left halves

posterior median sulcus *n* : a shallow groove along the midline of the posterior part of the spinal cord that separates the two posterior funiculi and is the external boundary of the posterior median septum

pos·te·ri·or·most \pō-'stir-ē-ər-ˌmōst, pä-\ *adj* : farthest back in time, order, or position ⟨the ∼ portion of the orbit⟩

posterior naris *n* : CHOANA

posterior nasal spine *n* : the nasal spine that is formed by the union of processes of the two palatine bones and projects between the choanae

posterior pillar of the fauces *n* : PALATOPHARYNGEAL ARCH

posterior pituitary *n* **1** : NEUROHYPOPHYSIS **2** : an extract of the neurohypophysis of domesticated animals for medicinal use — called also *posterior pituitary extract*

posterior pituitary gland *n* : NEUROHYPOPHYSIS

posterior root *n* : DORSAL ROOT

posterior sacrococcygeal muscle *n* : SACROCOCCYGEUS DORSALIS

posterior scalene *n* : SCALENUS C

posterior spinal artery *n* : SPINAL ARTERY b

posterior spinocerebellar tract *n* : SPINOCEREBELLAR TRACT a

posterior superior alveolar artery *n* : a branch of the maxillary artery that supplies the upper molar and bicuspid teeth

posterior superior alveolar vein *n* : any of several tributaries of the pterygoid plexus that drain the upper posterior teeth and gums

posterior superior iliac spine *n* : a projection at the posterior end of the iliac crest — called also *posterior superior spine*

posterior synechia *n* : SYNECHIA b

posterior temporal artery *n* : TEMPORAL ARTERY 3c

posterior tibial artery *n* : TIBIAL ARTERY a

posterior tibial vein *n* : TIBIAL VEIN a

posterior triangle *n* : a triangular region that is a landmark in the neck, has its apex above at the occipital bone, and is bounded in front by the sternocleidomastoid muscle, behind by the anterior margin of the trapezius, and inferiorly by the middle third of the clavicle — compare ANTERIOR TRIANGLE

posterior ulnar recurrent artery *n* : ULNAR RECURRENT ARTERY b

posterior vein of the left ventricle *n* : a vein that ascends on the surface of the left ventricle facing the diaphragm and that usu. empties into the coronary sinus — called also *posterior vein*

posterior vitreous detachment *n* : VITREOUS DETACHMENT

pos·tero·an·te·ri·or \ˌpäs-tə-rō-an-ˈtir-ē-ər\ *adj* : involving or produced in a direction from the back toward the front (as of the body or an organ) ⟨a ∼ radiograph⟩

pos·tero·ex·ter·nal \ˌpäs-tə-rō-ek-ˈstərn-ᵊl\ *adj* : posterior and external in location or direction

pos·tero·in·fe·ri·or \ˌpäs-tə-rō-in-ˈfir-ē-ər\ *adj* : posterior and inferior in position or direction

pos·tero·in·ter·nal \ˌpäs-tə-rō-in-ˈtərn-ᵊl\ *adj* : posterior and internal in position or direction ⟨a ∼ cusp on a molar⟩

pos·tero·lat·er·al \ˌpäs-tə-rō-ˈlat-ə-rəl, -ˈla-trəl\ *adj* : posterior and lateral in position or direction ⟨the ∼ aspect of the leg⟩ — **pos·tero·lat·er·al·ly** \-ē\ *adv*

pos·tero·me·di·al \ˌpäs-tə-rō-ˈmēd-ē-əl\ *adj* : located on or near the dorsal midline of the body or a body part

pos·tero·me·di·an \-ˈmēd-ē-ən\ *adj* : POSTEROMEDIAL

pos·tero·su·pe·ri·or \ˌpäs-tə-rō-sù-ˈpir-ē-ər\ *adj* : posterior and superior in position or direction

post·erup·tive \ˌpōst-i-ˈrəp-tiv\ *adj* : occurring or forming after eruption (as of the teeth)

post·ex·po·sure \-ik-ˈspō-zhər\ *adj* : occurring after exposure (as to a virus) ⟨∼ vaccination⟩ — **postexposure** *adv*

¹post·fer·til·iza·tion \ˌpōst-ˌfərt-ᵊl-ə-ˈzā-shən\ *adj* : occurring in the period following fertilization ⟨the early ∼ stages of embryonic development —N. A. Wivel & LeRoy Walters⟩

²postfertilization *adv* : after fertilization ⟨changes occurring 48 hours ∼⟩

post·fix \(ˈ)pōst-ˈfiks\ *vt* : to treat again with a different fixative ⟨the tissue was ∼ed in 1 percent osmium tetroxide⟩ — **post·fix·a·tion** \ˌpōst-fik-ˈsā-shən\ *n*

post·gan·gli·on·ic \ˌpōst-ˌgaŋ-glē-ˈän-ik\ *adj* : distal to a ganglion; *specif* : of, relating to, or being an axon arising from a cell body within an autonomic ganglion — compare PREGANGLIONIC

post·gas·trec·to·my \-ga-ˈstrek-tə-mē\ *adj* : occurring in,

being in, or characteristic of the period following a gastrectomy

postgastrectomy syndrome *n* : dumping syndrome following a gastrectomy

post·glen·oid \-ˈglen-ˌòid, -ˈglēn-\ *adj* : situated behind the glenoid fossa ⟨∼ tubercle⟩

post·hem·or·rhag·ic \ˌpōst-ˌhem-ə-ˈraj-ik\ *or chiefly Brit* **post·haem·or·rhag·ic** \-ˌhēm-\ *adj* : occurring after and as the result of a hemorrhage ⟨∼ shock⟩ ⟨∼ anemia⟩

post·he·pat·ic \-hi-ˈpat-ik\ *adj* : occurring or located behind the liver

post·hep·a·tit·ic \-ˌhep-ə-ˈtit-ik\ *adj* : occurring after and esp. as a result of hepatitis ⟨∼ cirrhosis⟩

post·her·pet·ic \-hər-ˈpet-ik\ *adj* : occurring after and esp. as a result of herpes ⟨∼ scars⟩

pos·thi·tis \(ˌ)päs-ˈthīt-əs\ *n, pl* **pos·thit·i·des** \-ˈthit-ə-ˌdēz\ : inflammation of the prepuce

post·hu·mous \ˈpäs-chə-məs *also* -t(y)ə-\ *adj* **1** : born after the death of the father **2** : following or occurring after death — **post·hu·mous·ly** *adv*

post·hyp·not·ic \ˌpōst-(h)ip-ˈnät-ik\ *adj* : of, relating to, or characteristic of the period following a hypnotic trance during which the subject will still carry out suggestions made by the operator during the trance state ⟨∼ suggestion⟩

post·ic·tal \-ˈik-tᵊl\ *adj* : occurring after a sudden attack (as of epilepsy) ⟨∼ drowsiness⟩

posticus — see TIBIALIS POSTICUS

post·im·mu·ni·za·tion \-ˌim-yə-nə-ˈzā-shən\ *adj* : occurring or existing after immunization ⟨∼ antibody levels⟩

post·in·farc·tion \-in-ˈfärk-shən\ *adj* **1** : occurring after and esp. as a result of myocardial infarction ⟨∼ ventricular septal defect⟩ **2** : having suffered myocardial infarction

post·in·fec·tion \-in-ˈfek-shən\ *adj* : relating to, occurring in, or being the period following infection — **postinfection** *adv*

post·in·flu·en·zal \-ˌin-flü-ˈen-zəl\ *adj* : occurring after and esp. as a result of influenza ⟨∼ peripheral neuritis⟩

post·ir·ra·di·a·tion \-ir-ˌād-ē-ˈā-shən\ *adj* : occurring after irradiation ⟨∼ sarcoma⟩ — **postirradiation** *adv*

post·isch·emic \-is-ˈkē-mik\ *adj* : occurring after and esp. as a result of ischemia ⟨∼ renal failure⟩

post·junc·tion·al \-ˈjəŋ(k)-shnəl, -shən-ᵊl\ *adj* : of, relating to, occurring on, or located on the muscle fiber side of a neuromuscular junction ⟨∼ muscarinic receptors⟩

post·lin·gual \-ˈliŋ-g(yə-)wəl\ *adj* : occurring after an individual has developed the use of language ⟨∼ deafness⟩ — **post·lin·gual·ly** \-ē\ *adv*

post·mas·tec·to·my \-ma-ˈstek-tə-mē\ *adj* **1** : occurring after and esp. as a result of a mastectomy ⟨∼ swelling of the arm⟩ **2** : having undergone mastectomy

post·ma·ture \-mə-ˈt(y)ù(ə)r *also* -ˈchù(ə)r\ *adj* : remaining in the uterus for longer than the normal period of gestation ⟨a ∼ fetus⟩

post·ma·tu·ri·ty \-mə-ˈt(y)ùr-ət-ē *also* -ˈchùr-\ *n, pl* **-ties** : the quality or state of being postmature

post·mei·ot·ic \-mī-ˈät-ik\ *adj* **1** : occurring after meiosis ⟨∼ stages⟩ **2** : being in a stage after meiosis ⟨∼ germ cells⟩

post·meno·paus·al \-ˌmen-ə-ˈpò-zəl\ *adj* **1** : having undergone menopause ⟨∼ women⟩ **2** : occurring after menopause ⟨∼ osteoporosis⟩ — **post·meno·paus·al·ly** \-ē\ *adv*

post·mi·tot·ic \-mī-ˈtät-ik\ *n* : a mature cell that is no longer capable of undergoing mitosis — compare INTERMITOTIC — **postmitotic** *adj*

post·mor·tal \-ˈmòrt-ᵊl\ *adj* : occurring after death ⟨∼ wounds⟩ ⟨∼ decomposition⟩ — **post·mor·tal·ly** \-ē\ *adv*

¹post·mor·tem \(ˈ)pōst-ˈmòrt-əm\ *adj* : done, occurring, or collected after death ⟨∼ tissue specimens⟩

²postmortem *n* : AUTOPSY

post–mor·tem *adv* : after death ⟨seven cases examined ∼⟩

O
P

\ə\ abut \ᵊ\ kitten \ər\ further \a\ ash \ā\ ace \ä\ cot, cart
\aú\ out \ch\ chin \e\ bet \ē\ easy \g\ go \i\ hit \ī\ ice \j\ job
\ŋ\ sing \ō\ go \ò\ law \òi\ boy \th\ thin \th\ the \ü\ loot
\ù\ foot \y\ yet \zh\ vision *See also* Pronunciation Symbols page

postmortem examination *n* : AUTOPSY
post·na·sal \\(ˈ)pōst-ˈnā-zəl\ *adj* : lying or occurring posterior to the nose ⟨∼ space⟩ ⟨a discharge of ∼ mucus⟩
postnasal drip *n* : flow of mucous secretion from the posterior part of the nasal cavity onto the wall of the pharynx occurring usu. as a chronic accompaniment of an allergic state or a viral infection
post·na·tal \\(ˈ)pōst-ˈnāt-ᵊl\ *adj* : occurring or being after birth; *specif* : of or relating to an infant immediately after birth ⟨∼ care⟩ — compare INTRANATAL, NEONATAL, PRENATAL — **post·na·tal·ly** \-ᵊl-ē\ *adv*
post·ne·crot·ic cirrhosis \ˌpōst-nə-ˈkrät-ik-\ *n* : cirrhosis of the liver following widespread necrosis of liver cells esp. as a result of hepatitis
post·neo·na·tal \-ˌnē-ō-ˈnāt-ᵊl\ *adj* : of, relating to, or affecting the infant and esp. the human infant usu. from the end of the first month to a year after birth ⟨∼ mortality⟩
post·nor·mal \-ˈnȯr-məl\ *adj* : having, characterized by, or resulting from a position (as of the mandible) that is distal to the normal position ⟨∼ malocclusion⟩ — compare PRENORMAL — **post·nor·mal·i·ty** \-nȯr-ˈmal-ət-ē\ *n, pl* **-ties**
post-op \ˈpōst-ˈäp\ *adj* : POSTOPERATIVE ⟨the second ∼ day⟩ — **post-op** *adv*
post·op·er·a·tive \ˈpōst-ˈäp-(ə-)rət-iv\ *adj* **1** : relating to, occurring in, or being the period following a surgical operation ⟨∼ care⟩ **2** : having recently undergone a surgical operation ⟨a ∼ patient⟩ — **post·op·er·a·tive·ly** *adv*
post·oral \ˌpōst-ˈȯr-əl, -ˈȯr-, -ˈär-\ *adj* : situated behind the mouth
post·or·bit·al \-ˈȯr-bət-ᵊl\ *adj* : situated or occurring behind the orbit of the eye
post·ovu·la·to·ry \-ˈäv-yə-lə-ˌtōr-ē, -ˌtȯr-\ *also* -ˈōv-\ *adj* : occurring, being, or used in the period following ovulation ⟨∼ endometrium⟩ ⟨∼ stages⟩
¹**post·par·tum** \\(ˈ)pōst-ˈpärt-əm\ *adj* **1** : occurring in or being the period following parturition ⟨∼ depression⟩ **2** : being in the postpartum period ⟨∼ mothers⟩
²**postpartum** *adv* : after parturition ⟨a blood sample taken 14 days ∼⟩ ⟨an infection occurred three weeks ∼⟩
post·phle·bit·ic \ˌpōst-flə-ˈbit-ik\ *adj* : occurring after and esp. as the result of phlebitis ⟨∼ edema⟩
postphlebitic syndrome *n* : chronic venous insufficiency with associated pathological manifestations (as pain, edema, stasis dermatitis, varicose veins, and ulceration) following thrombophlebitis of the deep veins of the leg
post·pi·tu·i·tary \-pə-ˈt(y)ü-ə-ˌter-ē\ *adj* : arising in or derived from the posterior lobe of the pituitary gland ⟨∼ extracts⟩
post·pneu·mon·ic \-n(y)ü-ˈmän-ik\ *adj* : occurring after and esp. as a result of pneumonia ⟨∼ bronchitis⟩
post·po·lio \-ˈpō-lē-ˌō\ *adj* : recovered from poliomyelitis; *also* : affected with post-polio syndrome ⟨a ∼ patient⟩
post–polio syndrome *n* : a condition that affects former poliomyelitis patients long after recovery from the disease and that is characterized by muscle weakness, joint and muscle pain, and fatigue
post·pran·di·al \-ˈpran-dē-əl\ *adj* : occurring after a meal ⟨∼ hypoglycemia⟩ — **post·pran·di·al·ly** \-ē\ *adv*
post·pu·ber·tal \-ˈpyü-bərt-ᵊl\ *adj* : occurring after puberty
post·pu·bes·cent \-pyü-ˈbes-ᵊnt\ *adj* : occurring or being in the period following puberty : POSTPUBERTAL
post·ra·di·a·tion \-ˌrād-ē-ˈā-shən\ *adj* : occurring after exposure to radiation
postrema — see AREA POSTREMA
post·res·i·den·cy \-ˈrez-əd-ən-sē\ *adj* : occurring or obtained in the period following medical residency ⟨∼ training⟩
post·spi·nal \-ˈspīn-ᵊl\ *adj* : occurring after spinal anesthesia ⟨a ∼ headache⟩
post·sple·nec·to·my \-spli-ˈnek-tə-mē\ *adj* : occurring after and esp. as a result of a splenectomy ⟨∼ sepsis⟩
post·stim·u·lus \-ˈstim-yə-ləs\ *adj* : of, relating to, occurring in, or being the period immediately after administration of a stimulus (as to a neuron)

post·stroke \-ˈstrōk\ *adj* : occurring in or being in the period following a stroke ⟨∼ depression⟩ ⟨a ∼ patient⟩
post·sur·gi·cal \-ˈsər-ji-kəl\ *adj* : POSTOPERATIVE ⟨∼ swelling⟩ ⟨a ∼ patient⟩
post·syn·ap·tic \ˌpōst-sə-ˈnap-tik\ *adj* **1** : occurring after synapsis ⟨a ∼ chromosome⟩ **2** : relating to, occurring in, or being part of a nerve cell by which a wave of excitation is conveyed away from a synapse ⟨∼ dopamine receptors⟩ — **post·syn·ap·ti·cal·ly** \-ti-k(ə-)lē\ *adv*
post·tran·scrip·tion·al \ˌtran(t)s-ˈkrip-shnəl, -shən-ᵊl\ *adj* : occurring, acting, or existing after genetic transcription ⟨∼ control of messenger-RNA production⟩ — **post·tran·scrip·tion·al·ly** \-ē\ *adv*
post·trans·fu·sion \ˌtran(t)s-ˈfyü-zhən\ *adj* **1** : caused by transfused blood ⟨∼ hepatitis⟩ **2** : occurring after blood transfusion ⟨induction of ∼ shock⟩
post·trans·la·tion·al \ˌtran(t)s-ˈlā-shnəl, -shən-ᵊl\ *adj* : occurring or existing after genetic translation ⟨∼ modification of a molecule⟩ — **post·trans·la·tion·al·ly** \-ē\ *adv*
post·trans·plant \-ˈtran(t)s-ˌplant\ *adj* : occurring or being in the period following transplant surgery ⟨∼ care⟩
post·trans·plan·ta·tion \-ˌtran(t)s-ˌplan-ˈtā-shən\ *adj* : POSTTRANSPLANT
post–trau·mat·ic \-trə-ˈmat-ik, -trȯ-, -traü-\ *adj* : occurring after or as a result of trauma ⟨∼ epilepsy⟩
post–traumatic stress disorder *n* : a psychological reaction that occurs after experiencing a highly stressing event (as wartime combat, physical violence, or a natural disaster) outside the range of normal human experience and that is usu. characterized by depression, anxiety, flashbacks, recurrent nightmares, and avoidance of reminders of the event — abbr. *PTSD;* called also *delayed-stress disorder, delayed-stress syndrome, post-traumatic stress syndrome;* compare COMBAT FATIGUE
post·treat·ment \\(ˈ)pōst-ˈtrēt-mənt\ *adj* : relating to, typical of, or occurring in the period following treatment ⟨∼ examinations⟩ — **posttreatment** *adv*
pos·tu·late \ˈpäs-chə-lət, -ˌlāt\ *n* : a hypothesis advanced as an essential presupposition, condition, or premise of a train of reasoning — see KOCH'S POSTULATES
pos·tur·al \ˈpäs-chə-rəl\ *adj* : of, relating to, or involving posture ⟨∼ tension⟩ ⟨∼ exercises⟩ ⟨∼ muscles⟩; *also* : ORTHOSTATIC ⟨∼ hypotension⟩
postural drainage *n* : drainage of the lungs by placing the patient in an inverted position so that fluids are drawn by gravity toward the trachea
pos·ture \ˈpäs-chər\ *n* **1** : the position or bearing of the body whether characteristic or assumed for a special purpose ⟨erect ∼⟩ **2** : a conscious mental or outward behavioral attitude
post·vac·ci·nal \ˌpōst-ˈvak-sən-ᵊl\ *adj* : occurring after and esp. as a result of vaccination ⟨∼ dermatosis⟩
post·vac·ci·na·tion \-ˌvak-sə-ˈnā-shən\ *adj* : POSTVACCINAL
post·wean·ing \-ˈwē-niŋ\ *adj* : relating to, occurring in, or being the period following weaning
¹**pot** \ˈpät\ *n* : a usu. rounded container
²**pot** *n* : MARIJUANA
potabile — see AURUM POTABILE
¹**po·ta·ble** \ˈpōt-ə-bəl\ *adj* : suitable for drinking ⟨∼ water⟩
²**potable** *n* : a liquid that is suitable for drinking; *esp* : an alcoholic beverage
pot·ash \ˈpät-ˌash\ *n* **1 a** : potassium carbonate esp. from wood ashes **b** : POTASSIUM HYDROXIDE **2** : potassium or a potassium compound esp. as used in agriculture or industry
potash alum *n* : ALUM 1a
po·tas·sic \pə-ˈtas-ik\ *adj* : of, relating to, or containing potassium
po·tas·si·um \pə-ˈtas-ē-əm\ *n* : a silver-white soft light low-melting monovalent metallic element of the alkali metal group that occurs abundantly in nature esp. combined in minerals — symbol K; see ELEMENT table
potassium alum *n* : ALUM 1a
potassium aluminum sulfate *n* : ALUM 1a

potassium an·ti·mo·nyl·tar·trate \-'ant-ə-mə-,nil-'tär-,trāt, -,nēl-\ *n* : TARTAR EMETIC

potassium arsenite *n* : a poisonous hygroscopic salt $KH(AsO_2)_2$ formerly used in medicine

potassium bicarbonate *n* : a crystalline salt $KHCO_3$ that gives a weakly alkaline reaction in aqueous solution and is sometimes used as an antacid and urinary alkalizer — see KLOR-CON

potassium bichromate *n* : POTASSIUM DICHROMATE

potassium bromide *n* : a crystalline salt KBr with a saline taste that is used as a sedative and in photography

potassium carbonate *n* : a white salt K_2CO_3 that forms a strongly alkaline solution and was formerly used as a systemic alkalizer and diuretic and that is now used chiefly in making glass and soap

potassium chlorate *n* : a crystalline salt $KClO_3$ with a cooling saline taste that is used esp. in veterinary medicine as a mild astringent (as in the treatment of stomatitis)

potassium chloride *n* : a crystalline salt KCl that occurs as a mineral and in natural waters and is used esp. in the treatment of potassium deficiency and occas. as a diuretic — see KLOR-CON

potassium citrate *n* : a crystalline salt $K_3C_6H_5O_7$ used chiefly as a systemic and urinary alkalizer and in the treatment of hypokalemia

potassium cyanide *n* : a very poisonous crystalline salt KCN

potassium dichromate *n* : a soluble salt $K_2Cr_2O_7$ forming large orange-red crystals that is used as an oxidizing agent and in the Golgi method of staining nerve tissue — called also *potassium bichromate*

potassium hydroxide *n* : a white deliquescent solid KOH that dissolves in water with much heat to form a strongly alkaline liquid and that is used as a powerful caustic and in the making of pharmaceuticals — called also *caustic potash*

potassium iodide *n* : a crystalline salt KI that is very soluble in water and is used in medicine chiefly as an expectorant

potassium mercuric iodide *n* : a poisonous yellow crystalline salt K_2HgI_4 used as a disinfectant and as a chemical reagent

potassium nitrate *n* : a crystalline salt KNO_3 that is a strong oxidizing agent and is used in medicine chiefly as a diuretic — called also *niter, saltpeter*

potassium perchlorate *n* : a crystalline salt $KClO_4$ that is sometimes used as a thyroid inhibitor

potassium permanganate *n* : a dark purple salt $KMnO_4$ used chiefly as an oxidizing agent and disinfectant

potassium phosphate *n* : any of various phosphates of potassium; *esp* : a salt K_2HPO_4 occurring as colorless or white granules or powder and used as a saline cathartic

potassium sodium tartrate *n* : ROCHELLE SALT

potassium sorbate *n* : a potassium salt $C_6H_7KO_2$ of sorbic acid used esp. as a food preservative

potassium sulfate *n* : a white crystalline compound K_2SO_4 which has been used medicinally as a cathartic

potassium thiocyanate *n* : a hygroscopic crystalline salt KSCN that has been used as an antihypertensive agent

pot·bel·lied \'pät-,bel-ēd\ *adj* : having a potbelly

pot·bel·ly \'pät-,bel-ē\ *n, pl* **-lies** : an enlarged, swollen, or protruding abdomen; *also* : a condition characterized by such an abdomen that is symptomatic of disease or malnourishment

po·ten·cy \'pōt-ᵊn-sē\ *n, pl* **-cies** : the quality or state of being potent: as **a** : chemical or medicinal strength or efficacy ⟨a drug's ∼⟩ **b** : the ability to copulate — usu. used of the male **c** : initial inherent capacity for development of a particular kind ⟨cells with a ∼ for eye formation⟩

po·tent \'pōt-ᵊnt\ *adj* **1** : having force or power **2** : chemically or medicinally effective ⟨a ∼ vaccine⟩ **3** : able to copulate — usu. used of the male — **po·tent·ly** *adv*

po·ten·tia \pə-'ten-chē-ə\ *n* : POTENCY b

¹po·ten·tial \pə-'ten-chəl\ *adj* : existing in possibility : capable of development into actuality — **po·ten·tial·ly** \-'tench-(ə-)lē\ *adv*

²potential *n* **1** : something that can develop or become actual **2 a** : any of various functions from which the intensity or the velocity at any point in a field may be readily calculated; *specif* : ELECTRICAL POTENTIAL **b** : POTENTIAL DIFFERENCE

potential cautery *n* : an agent (as a caustic or escharotic) used to destroy tissue by chemical action — compare ACTUAL CAUTERY

potential dif·fer·ence \-'dif-(ə-)rən(t)s\ *n* : the difference in electrical potential between two points that represents the work involved or the energy released in the transfer of a unit quantity of electricity from one point to the other — compare ACTION POTENTIAL, GENERATOR POTENTIAL, MEMBRANE POTENTIAL, RESTING POTENTIAL

potential energy *n* : the energy that a piece of matter has because of its position or because of the arrangement of parts

po·ten·ti·ate \pə-'ten-chē-,āt\ *vt* **-at·ed; -at·ing** : to make effective or active or more effective or more active; *also* : to augment the activity of (as a drug) synergistically — **po·ten·ti·a·tion** \-,ten-chē-'ā-shən\ *n*

po·ten·ti·a·tor \-,āt-ər\ *n* : a chemical agent or drug that potentiates something (as another drug)

po·ten·ti·om·e·ter \pə-,ten-chē-'äm-ət-ər\ *n* : an instrument for measuring electromotive forces — **po·ten·tio·met·ric** \-ch(ē-)ə-'me-trik\ *adj*

po·tion \'pō-shən\ *n* : a mixed drink (as of liquor) or dose (as of medicine)

Po·to·mac horse fever \pə-'tō-mək-, -mik-\ *n* : an often fatal disease of horses that is marked by fever, loss of appetite, diarrhea, and laminitis, that is caused by a bacterium of the genus *Ehrlichia* (*E. risticii*), and that was discovered in the region of the Potomac River in Maryland but is much more widespread — called also *Potomac fever*

Pott's disease \'päts-\ *n* : tuberculosis of the spine with destruction of bone resulting in curvature of the spine and occas. in paralysis of the lower extremities

Pott, Percivall (1714–1788), British surgeon. The leading surgeon in London in his time, Pott did much to improve the lot and reputation of surgeons. He is best known for three important medical contributions. In 1768 he published a seminal work on fractures and dislocations. In 1779 he described a form of spinal disease that accompanies curvature of the spine; it is now known as Pott's disease. In 1760 he described osteomyelitis of the calvarium.

Pott's fracture *n* : a fracture of the lower part of the fibula often accompanied with injury to the tibial articulation so that the foot is dislocated outward

pouch \'pauch\ *n* : an anatomical structure resembling a bag or pocket ⟨a blind gastric ∼ filled with bile and gastric juice —*Jour. Amer. Med. Assoc.*⟩

pouch of Doug·las \-'dəg-ləs\ *n* : a deep peritoneal recess between the uterus and the upper vaginal wall anteriorly and the rectum posteriorly — called also *cul-de-sac, cul-de-sac of Douglas, Douglas's cul-de-sac, Douglas's pouch*

Douglas, James (1675–1742), British anatomist. Douglas was the author of a number of books and papers on human, comparative, and pathological anatomy. In 1707 he published an important book on muscles. In 1730 he published a detailed study of the peritoneum which contained his original description of the pouch of Douglas.

pou·drage \pü-'dräzh\ *n* : a surgical procedure in which an irritating powder is applied between serous membranes (as in the pericardium or the pleural cavity) to promote their adhesion

¹poul·tice \'pōl-təs\ *n* : a soft usu. heated and sometimes medicated mass spread on cloth and applied to sores or other lesions to supply moist warmth, relieve pain, or act as a counterirritant or antiseptic — called also *cataplasm*

²poultice *vt* **-ticed; -tic·ing** : to apply a poultice to

poul·try mite \'pōl-trē-\ *n* : CHICKEN MITE

\ə\ abut \ᵊ\ kitten \ər\ further \a\ ash \ā\ ace \ä\ cot, cart
\au̇\ out \ch\ chin \e\ bet \ē\ easy \g\ go \i\ hit \ī\ ice \j\ job
\ŋ\ sing \ō\ go \ȯ\ law \ȯi\ boy \th\ thin \ṯẖ\ the \ü\ loot
\u̇\ foot \y\ yet \zh\ vision   *See also* Pronunciation Symbols page

O
P

pound \\'paùnd\ *n, pl* **pounds** *also* **pound** : any of various units of mass and weight: as **a** : a unit of troy weight equal to 12 troy ounces or 5760 grains or 0.3732417216 kilogram formerly used in weighing gold, silver, and a few other costly materials — called also *troy pound* **b** : a unit of avoirdupois weight equal to 16 avoirdupois ounces or 7000 grains or 0.45359237 kilogram — called also *avoirdupois pound*

pound·al \\'paùnd-ᵊl\ *n* : a unit of force equal to the force that would give a free mass of one pound an acceleration of one foot per second per second

Pou·part's ligament \pü-'pärz-\ *n* : INGUINAL LIGAMENT
  Pou·part \pü-pàr\, **François (1661–1709),** French surgeon and naturalist. In 1695 Poupart provided a more extensive description of the inguinal ligament, giving it new significance by showing its relationship to hernia. As a naturalist he did research on invertebrates including locusts, slugs, leeches, worms, and mussels.

pov·er·ty \\'päv-ərt-ē\ *n, pl* **-ties** : debility due to malnutrition ⟨evidence of ∼ in calves⟩

po·vi·done \\'pō-və-‚dōn\ *n* : POLYVINYLPYRROLIDONE

povidone–iodine *n* : a solution of polyvinylpyrrolidone and iodine used as an antibacterial agent in topical application (as in preoperative prepping or a surgical scrub) — see BETADINE

pow·der \\'paùd-ər\ *n* : a product in the form of discrete usu. fine particles; *specif* : a medicine or medicated preparation in the form of a powder ⟨antiseptic ∼⟩ ⟨digestive ∼⟩

pow·er \\'paù(-ə)r\ *n* **1** : an inherent property or effect ⟨a drug that enhances the heart's pumping ∼ —Kathleen Fackelmann⟩ **2** : MAGNIFICATION 2b

power test *n* : a psychological test of knowledge or skill in which the time taken to complete the test is not considered : test of ability apart from speed

pox \\'päks\ *n, pl* **pox** *or* **pox·es** **1** : a virus disease (as chicken pox) characterized by pustules or eruptions **2** *archaic* : SMALLPOX **3** : SYPHILIS

Pox·vi·ri·dae \‚päks-'vir-ə-‚dē\ *n pl* : a family of large brick-shaped or ovoid double-stranded DNA viruses that have a fluffy appearance caused by a covering of tubules and threads and that include the vaccinia virus and the causative agents of cowpox, fowl pox, molluscum contagiosum, monkeypox, mousepox, myxomatosis of rabbits, sheep pox, smallpox, sore mouth of sheep, and swine pox

pox·vi·rus \\'päks-‚vī-rəs\ *n* : any of the family *Poxviridae* of brick-shaped or ovoid double-stranded DNA viruses

pp *abbr* parts per

PP *abbr* pellagra preventive

PPA *abbr* phenylpropanolamine

ppb *abbr* parts per billion

PPD *abbr* purified protein derivative

PP factor \\'pē-'pē-\ *n* : NIACIN

PPI *abbr* proton pump inhibitor

PPLO \‚pē-‚pē-‚el-'ō\ *n, pl* **PPLO** : MYCOPLASMA

ppm *abbr* parts per million

PPO \‚pē-(‚)pē-'ō\ *n, pl* **PPOs** : an organization providing health care that gives economic incentives to the individual purchaser of a health-care contract to patronize certain physicians, laboratories, and hospitals which agree to supervision and reduced fees — called also *preferred provider organization;* compare HMO

ppt *abbr* **1** parts per thousand **2** parts per trillion **3** precipitate

Pr *symbol* praseodymium

prac·ti·cal nurse \\'prak-ti-kəl-\ *n* : a nurse who cares for the sick professionally without having the training or experience required of a registered nurse; *esp* : LICENSED PRACTICAL NURSE

¹prac·tice *or* **prac·tise** \\'prak-təs\ *vb* **prac·ticed** *or* **prac·tised**; **prac·tic·ing** *or* **prac·tis·ing** *vt* : to be professionally engaged in ⟨∼ medicine⟩ ∼ *vi* : to pursue a profession actively

²practice *also* **practise** *n* **1** : the continuous exercise of a profession **2** : a professional business; *esp* : one constituting an incorporeal property ⟨the doctor sold his ∼ and retired⟩

prac·ti·tion·er \prak-'tish-(ə-)nər\ *n* : one who practices a profession and esp. medicine

prac·to·lol \\'prak-tə-‚lòl\ *n* : a beta-blocker $C_{14}H_{22}N_2O_3$ used in the control of arrhythmia

Pra·der–Wil·li syndrome \\'prä-dər-'vil-ē-\ *n* : a genetic disorder characterized by short stature, mental retardation, hypotonia, abnormally small hands and feet, hypogonadism, and uncontrolled appetite leading to extreme obesity
  Prader, Andrea (1919–2001), and **Willi, Heinrich (1900–1971),** Swiss pediatricians. Prader was a professor of pediatrics in Zurich. Her articles and chapters in textbooks dealt with such topics as genetics, growth, endocrinology, and metabolism in children and adolescents. Prader and Willi first described the Prader-Willi syndrome in 1956. Cases of the disorder were not diagnosed in the U.S. until the 1960s.

praecox — see DEMENTIA PRAECOX, EJACULATIO PRAECOX, MACROGENITOSOMIA PRAECOX, PUBERTAS PRAECOX

prag·mat·ics \prag-'mat-iks\ *n pl but sing or pl in constr* : a branch of semiotic that deals with the relation between signs or linguistic expressions and their users

pral·i·dox·ime \‚pral-i-'däk-‚sēm\ *n* : a substance $C_7H_9ClN_2O$ that restores the reactivity of cholinesterase and is used to counteract phosphorylation (as by an organophosphate pesticide) — called also *2-PAM;* see PROTOPAM

pram·i·pex·ole \‚pram-i-'pek-‚sōl\ *n* : a dopamine agonist administered in the form of its dihydrochloride $C_{10}H_{17}N_3S$·2HCl to treat the symptoms of Parkinson's disease

pran·di·al \\'pran-dē-əl\ *adj* : of or relating to a meal

pra·seo·dym·i·um \‚prā-zē-ō-'dim-ē-əm, ‚prā-sē-\ *n* : a yellowish white trivalent metallic element of the rare-earth group — symbol *Pr;* see ELEMENT table

pra·tique \pra-'tēk\ *n* : clearance given an incoming ship by the health authority of a port after compliance with quarantine regulations or on presentation of a clean bill of health

Praus·nitz–Küst·ner reaction \\'praùs-nits-'kùest-nər-\ *n* : PASSIVE TRANSFER
  Prausnitz, Carl Willy (1876–1963), German bacteriologist. Prausnitz's career began with a series of positions at various institutes of hygiene and public health throughout Germany. His research centered on cholera, hay fever, general epidemiology, and the standardization of sera. Several of his publications dealt with hay fever toxins and antitoxins. In 1921 he demonstrated the transferability of local hypersensitivity by the intradermal injection of serum of an allergic person into a normal person.
  Küstner, Heinz (1897–1963), German gynecologist. After holding positions at several medical clinics for women in Germany, Küstner went on to become a professor of obstetrics and gynecology and chief physician at a hospital in Leipzig. His areas of research included endocrinology, pregnancy, puerperal fever, and gynecology. In 1930 he published a study of job-related injuries to the reproductive system incurred by working women.

Prav·a·chol \\'prav-ə-‚kól\ *trademark* — used for a preparation of pravastatin

prav·a·stat·in \\'prav-ə-‚stat-ᵊn\ *n* : a drug $C_{23}H_{35}NaO_7$ that inhibits the production of cholesterol in the body and is used to treat hypercholesterolemia — see PRAVACHOL

pra·ze·pam \\'prā-zə-‚pam\ *n* : a benzodiazepine derivative $C_{19}H_{17}ClN_2O$ used as a tranquilizer

praz·i·quan·tel \‚praz-i-'kwän-‚tel\ *n* : an anthelmintic drug $C_{19}H_{24}N_2O_2$ — see BILTRICIDE

pra·zo·sin \\'prā-zə-‚sin\ *n* : an antihypertensive peripheral vasodilator usu. used in the form of its hydrochloride $C_{19}H_{21}N_5O_4$·HCl — see MINIPRESS

pre·ad·mis·sion \‚prē-əd-'mish-ən\ *adj* : occurring in or relating to the period prior to admission (as to a hospital) ⟨a ∼ physical examination⟩

pre·ad·o·les·cence \-‚ad-ᵊl-'es-ᵊn(t)s\ *n* : the period of human development just preceding adolescence; *specif* : the period between the approximate ages of 9 and 12

¹pre·ad·o·les·cent \-‚ad-ᵊl-'es-ᵊnt\ *adj* **1** : of, characteristic of, or occurring during preadolescence ⟨∼ changes⟩ **2** : being in the stage of preadolescence ⟨a ∼ girl⟩

²**preadolescent** *n* : a preadolescent child

pre·adult \-ə-ˈdəlt, -ˈad-ˌəlt\ *adj* : occurring or existing prior to adulthood

pre·ag·o·nal \(ˈ)prē-ˈag-ən-ᵊl\ *adj* : occurring or existing immediately before death

pre·al·bu·min \ˌprē-al-ˈbyü-mən, -ˈal-ˌbyü-\ *n* : TRANSTHYRETIN

pre·anal \-ˈān-ᵊl\ *adj* : situated in front of the anus

¹**pre·an·es·thet·ic** *or Brit* **pre·an·aes·thet·ic** \-ˌan-əs-ˈthet-ik\ *adj* : used or occurring before administration of an anesthetic ⟨∼ medication⟩ ⟨a ∼ agent⟩

²**preanesthetic** *or Brit* **preanaesthetic** *n* : a substance used to induce an initial light state of anesthesia

pre·aor·tic \-ā-ˈȯrt-ik\ *adj* : situated anterior to the aorta ⟨∼ ganglia⟩ ⟨∼ lymph nodes⟩

pre·au·ric·u·lar \-ȯ-ˈrik-yə-lər\ *adj* : situated or occurring anterior to the auricle of the ear ⟨∼ lymph nodes⟩

pre·ax·i·al \ˌprē-ˈak-sē-əl\ *adj* : situated in front of an axis of the body ⟨∼ muscles⟩

pre·bi·o·log·i·cal \-ˌbī-ə-ˈläj-i-kəl\ *also* **pre·bi·o·log·ic** \-ik\ *adj* : PREBIOTIC

pre·bi·ot·ic \-bī-ˈät-ik\ *adj* : of, relating to, or being chemical or environmental precursors of the origin of life ⟨∼ molecules⟩; *also* : existing or occurring before the origin of life ⟨∼ conditions⟩ — **pre·bi·ot·i·cal·ly** \-i-k(ə-)lē\ *adv*

pre·breathe \(ˈ)prē-ˈbrēth\ *vt* **pre-breathed; pre·breath·ing** : to breathe (pure oxygen) to purge the blood of nitrogen content in preparation for an activity (as a space walk) that involves exposure to a significant change in pressure which might otherwise cause decompression sickness — **pre·breath·ing** \-iŋ\ *n*

pre·can·cer \ˌprē-ˈkan(t)-sər\ *n* : a precancerous lesion or condition ⟨one ∼ called actinic keratosis often disappears after a few weeks of . . . treatment —Elizabeth Morgan⟩

pre·can·cer·o·sis \-ˌkan(t)s-ə-ˈrō-səs\ *n, pl* **-o·ses** \-ˌsēz\ : a condition marked by the presence of one or more precancerous lesions

pre·can·cer·ous \-ˈkan(t)s-(ə-)rəs\ *adj* : tending to become cancerous ⟨a ∼ lesion⟩

¹**pre·cap·il·lary** \-ˈkap-ə-ˌler-ē, *Brit usu* -kə-ˈpil-ə-rē\ *adj* : being on the arterial side of and immediately adjacent to a capillary

²**precapillary** *n, pl* **-lar·ies** : METARTERIOLE

precapillary sphincter *n* : a sphincter of smooth muscle tissue located at the arterial end of a capillary and serving to control the flow of blood to the tissues

pre·car·ti·lage \-ˈkärt-ᵊl-ij, -ˈkärt-lij\ *n* : embryonic tissue from which cartilage is formed

pre·ca·val vein \-ˈkā-vəl-\ *n* : SUPERIOR VENA CAVA

pre·cen·tral \-ˈsen-trəl\ *adj* : situated in front of the central sulcus of the brain ⟨the ∼ motor cortex⟩

precentral gyrus *n* : the gyrus containing the motor area immediately anterior to the central sulcus

pre·cep·tee \ˌprē-ˌsep-ˈtē\ *n* : a person who works for and studies under a preceptor ⟨a ∼ in urology⟩

pre·cep·tor \pri-ˈsep-tər, ˈprē-ˌ\ *n* : a practicing physician who gives personal instruction, training, and supervision to a medical student or young physician

pre·cep·tor·ship \pri-ˈsep-tər-ˌship, ˈprē-ˌ\ *n* **1** : the position of a preceptor **2** : the state of being a preceptee : a period of training under a preceptor

pre·chord·al \ˌprē-ˈkȯrd-ᵊl\ *adj* : situated anterior to the notochord

pre·ci·bal \-ˈsī-bəl\ *adj* : occurring before meals

pre·cip·i·ta·ble \pri-ˈsip-ət-ə-bəl\ *adj* : capable of being precipitated — **pre·cip·i·ta·bil·i·ty** \-ˌsip-ət-ə-ˈbil-ət-ē\ *n, pl* **-ties**

pre·cip·i·tant \pri-ˈsip-ət-ənt\ *n* : something that precipitates; *esp* : a chemical agent that causes the formation of a precipitate

¹**pre·cip·i·tate** \pri-ˈsip-ə-ˌtāt\ *vb* **-tat·ed; -tat·ing** *vt* **1** : to bring about esp. abruptly **2 a** : to cause to separate from solution or suspension **b** : to cause (vapor) to condense and fall or deposit ∼ *vi* **1** : to fall or come suddenly into some condition **2** : to separate from solution or suspension

²**pre·cip·i·tate** \pri-ˈsip-ət-ət, -ə-ˌtāt\ *n* : a substance separated from a solution or suspension by chemical or physical change usu. as an insoluble amorphous or crystalline solid

precipitated chalk *n* : precipitated calcium carbonate used esp. as an ingredient of toothpastes and tooth powders for its polishing qualities

precipitated sulfur *n* : sulfur obtained as a pale yellowish or grayish amorphous or microcrystalline powder by precipitation and used chiefly in treating skin diseases

pre·cip·i·ta·tion \pri-ˌsip-ə-ˈtā-shən\ *n* **1 a** : the process of forming a precipitate from a solution **b** : the process of precipitating or removing solid or liquid particles from a smoke or gas by electrical means **2** : PRECIPITATE

pre·cip·i·tin \pri-ˈsip-ət-ən\ *n* : any of various antibodies which form insoluble precipitates with specific antigens and some of which are used in serological testing

pre·cip·i·tin·o·gen \pri-ˌsip-ə-ˈtin-ə-jən\ *n* : an antigen that stimulates the production of a specific precipitin — **pre·cip·i·tin·o·gen·ic** \-ˌtin-ə-ˈjen-ik\ *adj*

precipitin reaction *n* : the specific reaction of a precipitin with its antigen to give an insoluble precipitate

precipitin test *n* : a serological test using a precipitin reaction to detect the presence of a specific antigen; *specif* : a test used in criminology for determining the human or other source of a blood stain

pre·clin·i·cal \(ˈ)prē-ˈklin-i-kəl\ *adj* **1 a** : of, relating to, concerned with, or being the period preceding clinical manifestations ⟨the ∼ stage of diabetes mellitus⟩ **b** : occurring prior to a clinical trial ⟨∼ animal testing to assess a drug's safety⟩ **2** : of, relating to, or being the period in medical or dental education preceding the clinical study of medicine or dentistry ⟨the ∼ years⟩; *specif* : of or relating to the early period of prescribed medical or dental study devoted to the basic sciences (as anatomy, physiology, and pathology) ⟨∼ studies⟩ **3** : of, relating to, or being a science basic to medicine ⟨research in the ∼ sciences⟩

pre·co·cious \pri-ˈkō-shəs\ *adj* **1** : exceptionally early in development or occurrence ⟨∼ puberty⟩ **2** : exhibiting mature qualities at an unusually early age — **pre·co·cious·ly** *adv* — **pre·co·cious·ness** *n*

pre·coc·i·ty \pri-ˈkäs-ət-ē\ *n, pl* **-ties** : exceptionally early or premature development (as of mental powers or sexual characteristics)

pre·cog·ni·tion \ˌprē-(ˌ)käg-ˈnish-ən\ *n* : clairvoyance relating to an event or state not yet experienced — compare PSYCHOKINESIS, TELEKINESIS — **pre·cog·ni·tive** \-ˈkäg-nət-iv\ *adj*

pre·co·i·tal \-ˈkō-ət-ᵊl, -kō-ˈēt-\ *adj* : used or occurring before coitus

pre·co·ma \-ˈkō-mə\ *n* : a stuporous condition preceding coma ⟨diabetic ∼⟩

pre·con·cep·tion \-kən-ˈsep-shən\ *adj* : occurring prior to conception ⟨∼ genetic counseling⟩

¹**pre·con·scious** \-ˈkän-chəs\ *adj* : not present in consciousness but capable of being recalled without encountering any inner resistance or repression — **pre·con·scious·ly** *adv*

²**preconscious** *n* : the preconscious part of the psyche esp. in psychoanalysis — called also *foreconscious*

pre·con·vul·sive \-kən-ˈvəl-siv\ *adj* : relating to or occurring in the period just prior to a convulsion

pre·cor·a·coid \-ˈkȯr-ə-ˌkȯid, -ˈkär-\ *n* : the anterior and ventral bony or cartilaginous element of the pectoral girdle in front of the coracoid proper that occurs in many amphibians and reptiles and that in humans is replaced by the clavicle

pre·cor·dial \-ˈkȯrd-ē-əl, -ˈkȯr-jəl\ *adj* **1** : situated or occurring in front of the heart **2** : of or relating to the precordium

pre·cor·di·um \-ˈkȯr-dē-əm\ *n, pl* **-dia** \-dē-ə\ : the part of the ventral surface of the body overlying the heart and stomach and comprising the epigastrium and the lower median part of the thorax

precox — see MACROGENITOSOMIA PRECOX

pre·cu·ne·us \-'kyü-nē-əs\ *n, pl* **-nei** \-nē-ˌī\ : a somewhat rectangular convolution bounding the mesial aspect of the parietal lobe of the cerebrum and lying immediately in front of the cuneus

pre·cur·sor \pri-'kər-sər, 'prē-ˌ\ *n* **1** : one that precedes and indicates the onset of another ⟨angina may be the ∼ of a second infarction⟩ **2** : a substance, cell, or cellular component from which another substance, cell, or cellular component is formed esp. by natural processes

pre·cur·so·ry \pri-'kər-sə-rē\ *adj* : having the character of a precursor : PREMONITORY ⟨∼ symptoms of a fever⟩

pre·de·liv·ery \ˌprē-di-'liv-(ə-)rē\ *adj* : PRENATAL

pre·den·tal \-'dent-ᵊl\ *adj* : preliminary to or preparing for a course in dentistry

pre·den·tin \-'dent-ᵊn\ *or* **pre·den·tine** \-'den-ˌtēn, -den-'\ *n* : immature uncalcified dentin consisting chiefly of fibrils

pre·di·a·be·tes \-ˌdī-ə-'bēt-ēz, -'bēt-əs\ *n* : an asymptomatic abnormal state that precedes the development of clinically evident diabetes

¹pre·di·a·bet·ic \-'bet-ik\ *n* : a prediabetic individual

²prediabetic *adj* : of, relating to, or affected with prediabetes ⟨∼ patients⟩

pre·dic·tor \pri-'dik-tər\ *n* : a preliminary symptom or indication (as of the development of a disease) ⟨∼s of multiple sclerosis⟩

pre·di·gest \ˌprēd-ī-'jest, ˌprēd-ə-\ *vt* : to subject to predigestion

pre·di·ges·tion \-'jes(h)-chən\ *n* : artificial or natural partial digestion of food esp. for use in cases of illness or impaired digestion

pre·dis·pose \ˌprēd-is-'pōz\ *vb* **-posed; -pos·ing** *vt* : to make susceptible ⟨malnutrition ∼s one to disease⟩ ∼ *vi* : to bring about susceptibility ⟨conditions that ∼ to infection⟩

pre·dis·po·si·tion \ˌprē-ˌdis-pə-'zish-ən\ *n* : a condition of being predisposed ⟨a hereditary ∼ to disease⟩ — **pre·dis·po·si·tion·al** \-ᵊl\ *adj*

pred·nis·o·lone \pred-'nis-ə-ˌlōn\ *n* : a glucocorticoid $C_{21}H_{28}O_5$ that is a dehydrogenated analog of cortisol and is used often in the form of an ester or methyl derivative esp. as an anti-inflammatory drug in the treatment of arthritis

pred·ni·sone \'pred-nə-ˌsōn *also* -ˌzōn\ *n* : a glucocorticoid $C_{21}H_{26}O_5$ that is a dehydrogenated analog of cortisone and is used as an anti-inflammatory agent, as an antineoplastic agent, and as an immunosuppressant

pre·drug \'prē-ˈdrəg\ *adj* : existing or occurring prior to the administration of a drug ⟨∼ baseline values⟩

pre·eclamp·sia \ˌprē-i-'klam(p)-sē-ə\ *n* : a serious condition developing in late pregnancy that is characterized by a sudden rise in blood pressure, excessive weight gain, generalized edema, proteinuria, severe headache, and visual disturbances and that may result in eclampsia if untreated — compare ECLAMPSIA a, TOXEMIA OF PREGNANCY

¹pre·eclamp·tic \-tik\ *adj* : relating to or affected with preeclampsia ⟨a ∼ patient⟩

²preeclamptic *n* : a woman affected with preeclampsia

pree·mie *or* **pre·mie** \'prē-mē\ *n* : a baby born prematurely

pre·erup·tive \ˌprē-i-'rəp-tiv\ *adj* : occurring or existing prior to an eruption ⟨the ∼ stage of a skin disease⟩

pre·eryth·ro·cyt·ic \-i-ˌrith-rə-'sit-ik\ *adj* : of, relating to, or being exoerythrocytic stages of a malaria parasite that occur before the red blood cells are invaded

pre·ex·ci·ta·tion \-ˌek-ˌsī-'tā-shən, -ˌek-sə-\ *n* : premature activation of part or all of the cardiac ventricle by an electrical impulse from the atrium that typically is conducted along an anomalous pathway (as muscle fibers on the heart surface) bypassing the atrioventricular node, that may produce arrhythmias, and that is characteristic of LGL syndrome and Wolff-Parkinson-White syndrome — **pre·ex·cit·ed** \-ik-'sīt-əd\ *adj*

pre·ex·po·sure \-ik-'spō-zhər\ *adj* : of, relating to, occurring

in, or being the period preceding exposure (as to a stimulus or a pathogen) ⟨∼ immunization⟩

pre·ferred pro·vid·er organization \prə-ˌfərd-prə-'vīd-ər-\ *n* : PPO

pre·for·ma·tion \ˌprē-fȯr-'mā-shən\ *n* : a now discredited theory in biology that every germ cell contains the organism of its kind fully formed and complete in all its parts and that development involves merely an increase in size from microscopic proportions to those of the adult — compare EPIGENESIS — **pre·for·ma·tion·ist** \-shə-nəst\ *n or adj*

pre·for·ma·tion·ism \-ˌiz-əm\ *n* : PREFORMATION

pre·fron·tal \ˌprē-'frənt-ᵊl\ *adj* **1** : situated or occurring anterior to a frontal structure ⟨a ∼ bone⟩ **2** : of, relating to, or constituting the prefrontal lobe or prefrontal cortex of the brain

prefrontal cortex *n* : the gray matter of the anterior part of the frontal lobe that is highly developed in humans and plays a role in the regulation of complex cognitive, emotional, and behavioral functioning

prefrontal leukotomy *n* : PREFRONTAL LOBOTOMY

prefrontal lobe *n* : the anterior part of the frontal lobe that is made up chiefly of association areas, mediates various inhibitory controls, and is bounded posteriorly by the ascending frontal convolution

prefrontal lobotomy *n* : lobotomy of the white matter in the frontal lobe of the brain — called also *frontal leukotomy, frontal lobotomy, prefrontal leukotomy*

pre·gan·gli·on·ic \-ˌgan-glē-'än-ik\ *adj* : anterior or proximal to a ganglion; *specif* : being, affecting, involving, or relating to a usu. myelinated efferent nerve fiber arising from a cell body in the central nervous system and terminating in an autonomic ganglion — compare POSTGANGLIONIC

pre·gen·i·tal \-'jen-ə-tᵊl\ *adj* : of, relating to, or characteristic of the oral, anal, and phallic phases of psychosexual development

preg·nan·cy \'preg-nən-sē\ *n, pl* **-cies** **1** : the condition of being pregnant **2** : an instance of being pregnant

pregnancy disease *n* : a form of ketosis affecting pregnant ewes that is marked by listlessness, staggering, and collapse and is esp. frequent in ewes carrying twins or triplets — called also *twin disease, twin-lamb disease*

pregnancy test *n* : a physiological test to determine the existence of pregnancy in an individual

preg·nane \'preg-ˌnān\ *n* : a crystalline steroid $C_{21}H_{36}$ that is related to cholane and is the parent compound of the corticosteroid and progestational hormones

preg·nane·di·ol \-'dī-ˌȯl\ *n* : a biologically inactive crystalline dihydroxy derivative $C_{21}H_{36}O_2$ of pregnane that is formed by reduction of progesterone and is found esp. in the urine of pregnant women in the form of its glucuronide

preg·nant \'preg-nənt\ *adj* : containing a developing embryo, fetus, or unborn offspring within the body : GESTATING, GRAVID

preg·nene \'preg-ˌnēn\ *n* : an unsaturated derivative $C_{21}H_{34}$ of pregnane containing one double bond in a molecule

preg·nen·in·o·lone \ˌpreg-nen-'in-ᵊl-ˌōn\ *n* : ETHISTERONE

preg·nen·o·lone \preg-'nen-ᵊl-ˌōn\ *n* : an unsaturated hydroxy steroid ketone $C_{21}H_{32}O_2$ that is formed by the oxidation of steroids (as cholesterol) and yields progesterone on dehydrogenation

pre·hen·sile \prē-'hen(t)-səl, -'hen-ˌsīl\ *adj* : adapted for seizing or grasping esp. by wrapping around ⟨∼ tail⟩ — **pre·hen·sil·i·ty** \(ˌ)prē-ˌhen-'sil-ət-ē\ *n, pl* **-ties**

pre·hen·sion \prē-'hen-chən\ *n* : the act of taking hold, seizing, or grasping

pre·hos·pi·tal \ˌprē-'häs-(ˌ)pit-ᵊl\ *adj* : occurring before or during transportation (as of a trauma victim) to a hospital ⟨∼ emergency care⟩

pre·hy·per·ten·sion \ˌprē-'hī-pər-ˌten-chən\ *n* : slightly to moderately elevated arterial blood pressure that in adults is usu. indicated by a systolic blood pressure of 120 to 139 mm Hg or a diastolic blood pressure of 80 to 89 mm Hg and that is considered a risk factor for hypertension — **pre·hy·per·ten·sive** \-'hī-pər-ˌten(t)-siv\ *adj*

pre·im·mu·ni·za·tion \-,im-yə-nə-'zā-shən\ *adj* : existing or occurring in the period before immunization ⟨~ serum⟩

pre·im·plan·ta·tion \-,im-,plan-'tā-shən\ *adj* : of, involving, or being an embryo before uterine implantation

pre·in·cu·bate \-'iŋ-kyə-,bāt, -'in-\ *vt* **-bat·ed; -bat·ing** : to incubate (as a cell or a culture) prior to a treatment or process ⟨red cells were *preincubated* with cholinergic ligands —D. P. Richman *et al*⟩

pre·in·cu·ba·tion \-,iŋ-kyə-'bā-shən, -,in-\ *n* : incubation (as of a cell or culture) prior to a treatment or process

pre·in·fec·tion \-in-'fek-shən\ *n* : an infection that is established in the body but not yet clinically manifested

pre·in·jec·tion \-in-'jek-shən\ *adj* : occurring or existing before an injection ⟨~ care⟩

pre·in·va·sive \-in-'vā-siv\ *adj* : not yet having become invasive — used of malignant cells or lesions remaining in their original focus

pre·leu·ke·mia *or chiefly Brit* **pre·leu·kae·mia** \-lü-'kē-mē-ə\ *n* : the stage of leukemia occurring before the disease becomes overt

pre·leu·ke·mic *or chiefly Brit* **pre·leu·kae·mic** \-mik\ *adj* : occurring before the development of overt leukemia ⟨a ~ latent phase⟩

pre·lin·gual \,prē-'liŋ-g(yə-)wəl\ *adj* : occurring before an individual has developed the use of language ⟨~ deafness⟩ — **pre·lin·gual·ly** \-ē\ *adv*

pre·load \-'lōd\ *n* : the stretched condition of the heart muscle at the end of diastole just before contraction

pre·lo·cal·iza·tion *also Brit* **pre·lo·cal·isa·tion** \-,lō-kə-lə-'zā-shən\ *n* : segregation in the egg or by early cleavage divisions of material destined to form particular tissues or organs

Pre·lu·din \pri-'lüd-ᵊn\ *n* : a preparation of the hydrochloride of phenmetrazine — formerly a U.S. registered trademark

pre·ma·lig·nant \,prē-mə-'lig-nənt\ *adj* : PRECANCEROUS

Prem·a·rin \'prem-ə-rən\ *trademark* — used for a preparation of conjugated estrogens

pre·mar·i·tal \,prē-'mar-ət-ᵊl\ *adj* : existing or occurring before marriage

¹**pre·ma·ture** \-mə-'t(y)ü(ə)r, -'chü(ə)r, *chiefly Brit* ,prem-ə-\ *adj* : happening, arriving, existing, or performed before the proper, usual, or intended time; *esp* : born after a gestation period of less than 37 weeks ⟨~ babies⟩ — **pre·ma·ture·ly** *adv*

²**premature** *n* : PREEMIE

premature beat *n* : EXTRASYSTOLE

premature contact *n* : contact between maloccluded teeth occurring prematurely as the jaws close

premature delivery *n* : expulsion of the human fetus after the 28th week of gestation but before the normal time

premature ejaculation *n* : ejaculation of semen that occurs prior to or immediately after penetration of the vagina by the penis — called also *ejaculatio praecox*

premature ejaculator *n* : a man who experiences premature ejaculation

premature labor *n* : the labor preceding premature delivery

pre·ma·tu·ri·ty \,prē-mə-'t(y)ùr-ət-ē, -'chùr-, *chiefly Brit* ,prem-ə-\ *n, pl* **-ties** **1** : the condition of an infant born viable but before its proper time **2** : PREMATURE CONTACT

pre·max·il·la \,prē-mak-'sil-ə\ *n, pl* **-lae** \-ē\ : either member of a pair of bones of the upper jaw of vertebrates situated between and in front of the maxillae that in humans form the median anterior part of the superior maxillary bones but in most other mammals are distinct and bear the incisor teeth and in birds coalesce to form the principal part of the upper mandible — called also *incisive bone*

¹**pre·max·il·lary** \-'mak-sə-,ler-ē, *chiefly Brit* -mak-'sil-ə-rē\ *adj* **1** : situated in front of the maxillary bones **2** : relating to or being the premaxilla

²**premaxillary** *n* : PREMAXILLA

¹**pre·med** \'prē-'med\ *n* : a premedical student or course of study

²**premed** *adj* : PREMEDICAL

pre·med·i·cal \,prē-'med-i-kəl\ *adj* : preceding and preparing for the professional study of medicine ⟨a ~ course at a university⟩ ⟨a ~ student⟩

pre·med·i·cate \-'med-ə-,kāt\ *vt* **-cat·ed; -cat·ing** : to administer premedication to : treat by premedication

pre·med·i·ca·tion \-,med-ə-'kā-shən\ *n* : preliminary medication; *esp* : medication to induce a relaxed state preparatory to the administration of an anesthetic

pre·mei·ot·ic \-mī-'ät-ik\ *adj* : of, occurring in, or typical of a stage prior to meiosis ⟨~ DNA synthesis⟩ ⟨~ tissue⟩

pre·men·ar·chal \-men-'är-kəl\ *or* **pre·men·ar·che·al** \-kē-əl\ *adj* : of, relating to, or being in the period of life of a female before the first menstrual period occurs

pre·men·ar·che \-'men-,är-kē\ *n* : the period in the life of a female preceding the establishment of menstruation

pre·meno·paus·al \-,men-ə-'pó-zəl, -,mēn-\ *adj* : of, relating to, or being in the period preceding menopause ⟨~ women⟩

pre·meno·pause \-'men-ə-,póz, -'mēn-\ *n* : the premenopausal period of a woman's life; *esp* : the period of irregular menstrual cycles preceding menopause

pre·men·stru·al \,prē-'men(t)-strə(-wə)l\ *adj* : of, relating to, occurring in, or being in the period just preceding menstruation ⟨~ women⟩ — **pre·men·stru·al·ly** \-ē\ *adv*

premenstrual dysphoric disorder *n* : severe premenstrual syndrome marked esp. by depression, anxiety, cyclical mood shifts, and lethargy — abbr. *PMDD*

premenstrual syndrome *n* : a varying constellation of symptoms manifested by some women prior to menstruation that may include emotional instability, irritability, insomnia, fatigue, anxiety, depression, headache, edema, and abdominal pain — called also *PMS*

premenstrual tension *n* : tension occurring as a part of the premenstrual syndrome

pre·men·stru·um \-'men(t)-strə-wəm\ *n, pl* **-stru·ums** *or* **-strua** \-strə-wə\ : the period or physiological state that immediately precedes menstruation

premie *var of* PREEMIE

¹**pre·mo·lar** \-'mō-lər\ *adj* : situated in front of or preceding the molar teeth; *esp* : being or relating to those teeth of a mammal in front of the true molars and behind the canines when the latter are present

²**premolar** *n* **1** : a premolar tooth that in humans is one of two in each side of each jaw — called also *bicuspid* **2** : a milk tooth that occupies the position later taken by a premolar tooth of the permanent dentition

pre·mon·i·to·ry \pri-'män-ə-,tōr-ē, -,tòr-\ *adj* : giving warning ⟨a ~ symptom⟩ ⟨~ aura in epilepsy⟩

pre·mor·bid \,prē-'mòr-bəd\ *adj* : occurring or existing before the occurrence of physical disease or emotional illness ⟨a patient's . . . ~ state of mood —Jaye Hefner *et al*⟩ ⟨~ measurements of lung function —R. F. Lemanske⟩

pre·mor·tal \-'mòrt-ᵊl\ *adj* : PREMORTEM

¹**pre·mor·tem** \-'mòrt-əm\ *adj* : existing or taking place immediately before death ⟨~ infections⟩ ⟨~ findings⟩

²**premortem** *adv* : in the premortem period ⟨the patient was diagnosed ~⟩ ⟨medication administered 24 hours ~⟩

pre·mo·tor \-'mōt-ər\ *adj* : of, relating to, or being the area of the cortex of the frontal lobe lying immediately in front of the motor area of the precentral gyrus

Prem·pro \'prem-,prō\ *trademark* — used for a preparation of conjugated estrogens and medroxyprogesterone acetate

pre·mune \(')prē-'myün\ *adj* : characterized by premunition

pre·mu·ni·tion \,prē-myù-'nish-ən\ *n* **1** : resistance to a disease due to the existence of its causative agent in a state of physiological equilibrium in the host **2** : immunity to a particular infection due to previous presence of the causative agent

pre·mu·nize *or chiefly Brit* **pre·mu·nise** \'prē-myə-,nīz\ *vt*

\ə\ abut \ᵊ\ kitten \ər\ further \a\ ash \ā\ ace \ä\ cot, cart
\aú\ out \ch\ chin \e\ bet \ē\ easy \g\ go \i\ hit \ī\ ice \j\ job
\ŋ\ sing \ō\ go \ò\ law \òi\ boy \th\ thin \th\ the \ü\ loot
\ù\ foot \y\ yet \zh\ vision *See also* Pronunciation Symbols page

O
P

-nized *or chiefly Brit* **-nised; -niz·ing** *or chiefly Brit* **-nis·ing** : to induce premunition in

pre·my·cot·ic \ˌprē-mī-'kät-ik\ *adj* : of, relating to, or being the earliest and nonspecific stage of eczematoid eruptions of mycosis fungoides

pre·my·elo·cyte \-'mī-ə-lə-ˌsīt\ *n* : PROMYELOCYTE

pre·na·tal \-'nāt-ᵊl\ *adj* **1** : occurring, existing, performed, or used before birth ⟨~ care⟩ ⟨the ~ period⟩ ⟨~ testing⟩ ⟨~ vitamins⟩ **2** : providing or receiving prenatal medical care ⟨a ~ clinic⟩ ⟨a ~ patient⟩ — compare INTRANATAL, NEONATAL, POSTNATAL — **pre·na·tal·ly** \-ē\ *adv*

pre·neo·plas·tic \-ˌnē-ə-'plas-tik\ *adj* : existing or occurring prior to the formation of a neoplasm ⟨~ cells⟩

pre·nor·mal \-'nór-məl\ *adj* : having, characterized by, or resulting from a position (as of the mandible) that is proximal to the normal position ⟨~ malocclusion⟩ — compare POST-NORMAL — **pre·nor·mal·i·ty** \-nór-'mal-ət-ē\ *n, pl* **-ties**

pre·oc·cip·i·tal \-äk-'sip-ət-ᵊl\ *adj* : situated or occurring anterior to the occiput or an occipital part (as the occipital lobe of the brain) ⟨~ lesions⟩

pre·oe·di·pal \-'ed-ə-pəl, -'ēd-\ *adj* : of, relating to, occurring in, or being the phase in a child's life prior to the occurrence of oedipal conflict

pre·op \'prē-ˌäp\ *adj* : PREOPERATIVE ⟨a ~ blood workup⟩

pre·op·er·a·tive \(ˈ)prē-'äp-(ə-)rət-iv, -'äp-ə-ˌrāt-\ *adj* : occurring, performed, or administered before and usu. close to a surgical operation ⟨~ care⟩ ⟨~ medication⟩ — **pre·op·er·a·tive·ly** *adv*

pre·op·tic \ˌprē-'äp-tik\ *adj* : situated in front of an optic part or region ⟨~ tracts in the brain⟩

preoptic area *n* : a region of the brain that is situated immediately below the anterior commissure, above the optic chiasma, and anterior to the hypothalamus although it is not clearly demarcated from the hypothalamus and that regulates certain autonomic activities often with the hypothalamus — called also *preoptic region*

preoptic nucleus *n* : any of several groups of nerve cells located in the preoptic area esp. in the lateral and the medial portions

preoptic region *n* : PREOPTIC AREA

pre·ovu·la·to·ry \-'äv-yə-lə-ˌtōr-ē, -ˌtór-, -'ōv-\ *adj* : occurring in, being in, existing in, or typical of the period immediately preceding ovulation ⟨~ oocytes⟩

pre·oxy·gen·ation \-ˌäk-si-jə-'nā-shən, -äk-ˌsij-ə-\ *n* : inhalation of large quantities of essentially pure oxygen usu. as a prelude to some activity or medical procedure in which it is desirable to minimize nitrogen and maximize oxygen in the blood and tissues

¹prep \'prep\ *n* : the act or an instance of preparing a patient for a surgical operation ⟨the nurse had three ~s to do⟩

²prep *vt* **prepped; prep·ping** : to prepare for a surgical operation or examination ⟨the patient for an appendectomy⟩

prep·a·ra·tion \ˌprep-ə-'rā-shən\ *n* **1** : the action or process of preparing **2** : something that is prepared; *specif* : a medicinal substance made ready for use ⟨a ~ for colds⟩

pre·pare \pri-'pa(ə)r, -'pe(ə)r\ *vt* **pre·pared; pre·par·ing 1** : to make ready beforehand ⟨~ a patient for surgery⟩ **2** : to put together : COMPOUND ⟨*prepared* a vaccine from live virus⟩ ⟨*prepared* the doctor's prescription⟩

prepared chalk *n* : finely ground native calcium carbonate that is freed of most of its impurities by elutriation and used esp. in dentistry for polishing

pre·par·tum \ˌprē-'pärt-əm\ *adj* : ANTEPARTUM

pre·pa·tel·lar bursa \-pə-'tel-ər-\ *n* : a synovial bursa situated between the patella and the skin

pre·pa·tent period \-'pāt-ᵊnt-\ *n* : the period between infection with a parasite and the demonstration of the parasite in the body esp. as determined by the recovery of an infective form (as oocysts or eggs) from the blood or feces

pre·phe·nic acid \-ˌfē-nik-\ *n* : a quinonoid dicarboxylic acid $C_{10}H_{10}O_6$ formed as an intermediate in the biosynthesis of aromatic amino acids from shikimic acid

pre·pla·cen·tal \-plə-'sent-ᵊl\ *adj* : existing or arising before the formation of a placenta

pre·pon·tine \-'pän-ˌtīn\ *adj* : of, relating to, occurring in, or being the part of the brain that is anterior to the pons

pre·po·ten·cy \-'pōt-ᵊn-sē\ *n, pl* **-cies** : unusual ability of an individual or strain to transmit its characters to offspring because of homozygosity for numerous dominant genes

pre·po·tent \-'pōt-ᵊnt\ *adj* **1** : exhibiting genetic prepotency : DOMINANT **2** : having priority over other response tendencies esp. by virtue of maturational primacy, recentness of emission or evocation, repetition with positive reinforcement, or greater motivational charge ⟨the ~ response is that with the greatest immediately effective habit strength⟩

pre·po·ten·tial \-pə-'ten-chəl\ *n* : a slow depolarization of a plasma membrane that precedes the action potential ⟨fast ~s were seen and appear similar to those recorded in hippocampal pyramidal cells —*Science*⟩ — compare AFTERPOTENTIAL

pre·pran·di·al \ˌprē-'pran-dē-əl\ *adj* : of, relating to, or suitable for the time just before a meal ⟨~ blood glucose⟩

pre·preg·nan·cy \-'preg-nən-sē\ *adj* : existing or occurring prior to pregnancy ⟨~ weight⟩

pre·psy·chot·ic \-sī-'kät-ik\ *adj* : preceding or predisposing to psychosis : possessing recognizable features prognostic of psychosis ⟨~ behavior⟩ ⟨a ~ personality⟩

pre·pu·ber·al \-'pyü-b(ə-)rəl\ *adj* : PREPUBERTAL

pre·pu·ber·tal \-bərt-ᵊl\ *adj* : of, relating to, occurring in, or being in prepuberty ⟨~ children⟩

pre·pu·ber·ty \-bərt-ē\ *n, pl* **-ties** : the period immediately preceding puberty

pre·pu·bes·cence \-pyü-'bes-ᵊn(t)s\ *n* : PREPUBERTY

¹pre·pu·bes·cent \-'ᵊnt\ *adj* : PREPUBERTAL

²prepubescent *n* : a prepubertal child

pre·puce \'prē-ˌpyüs\ *n* : FORESKIN; *also* : a similar fold investing the clitoris

pre·pu·tial *also* **pre·pu·cial** \prē-'pyü-shəl\ *adj* : of, relating to, or being a prepuce ⟨~ adhesions⟩

preputial gland *n* : GLAND OF TYSON

pre·pu·tium cli·tor·i·dis \prē-'pyü-shəm-kli-'tór-əd-əs\ *n* : the prepuce which invests the clitoris

pre·py·lo·ric \ˌprē-pī-'lōr-ik\ *adj* : situated or occurring anterior to the pylorus ⟨~ ulcers⟩

pre·re·nal \-'rēn-ᵊl\ *adj* : occurring in the circulatory system before the kidney is reached ⟨the usual ~ causes for transient renal insufficiency such as hypotonia and hypovolemia were excluded —Rudolf Pfab *et al*⟩

prerenal azotemia *n* : uremia caused by extrarenal factors

prerenal uremia *n* : PRERENAL AZOTEMIA

pre·rep·li·ca·tive \-'rep-li-ˌkāt-iv\ *adj* : relating to or being the G₁ phase of the cell cycle

pre·re·pro·duc·tive \-ˌrē-prə-'dək-tiv\ *adj* : PREPUBERTAL

pre·ret·i·nal \-'ret-ᵊn-əl\ *adj* : situated or occurring anterior to the retina ⟨~ hemorrhages⟩

pre·sa·cral \-'sak-rəl, -'sāk-\ *adj* : done or effected by way of the anterior aspect of the sacrum ⟨~ nerve block⟩

pres·by·acu·sis \ˌprez-bē-ə-'kyü-səs\ *n, pl* **-acu·ses** \-ˌsēz\ : PRESBYCUSIS

pres·by·cu·sis \ˌprez-bi-'kyü-səs, ˌpres-\ *n, pl* **-cu·ses** \-ˌsēz\ : a lessening of hearing acuteness resulting from degenerative changes in the ear that occur esp. in old age

pres·by·ope \'prez-bē-ˌōp, 'pres-bē-\ *n* : one affected with presbyopia

pres·byo·phre·nia \ˌprez-bē-ə-'frē-nē-ə, ˌpres-\ *n* : a form of senile dementia characterized by loss of memory and sense of location, disorientation, and confabulation — **pres·byo·phren·ic** \-'fren-ik\ *adj*

pres·by·opia \ˌprez-bē-'ō-pē-ə, ˌpres-\ *n* : a visual condition which becomes apparent esp. in middle age and in which loss of elasticity of the lens of the eye causes defective accommodation and inability to focus sharply for near vision

pres·by·opic \-'ō-pik, -'äp-ik\ *adj* : affected with presbyopia

pres·byt·ic \ˌprez-'bit-ik\ *adj* : PRESBYOPIC

pre·schizo·phren·ic \ˌprē-ˌskit-sə-'fren-ik\ *n* : one whose behavior and personality traits are prognostic of schizophrenia — **preschizophrenic** *adj*

pre·scribe \pri-'skrīb\ *vb* **pre·scribed; pre·scrib·ing** *vi* : to write or give medical prescriptions ~ *vt* : to designate or order the use of as a remedy ⟨~ a drug⟩

pre·scrib·er \-ər\ *n* : a person who prescribes

pre·scrip·tion \pri-'skrip-shən\ *n* **1** : a written direction for the preparation, compounding, and administration of a medicine **2** : a prescribed remedy **3** : a written formula for the grinding of corrective lenses for eyeglasses **4** : a written direction for the application of physical therapy measures (as directed exercise or electrotherapy) in cases of injury or disability

prescription drug *n* : a drug that can be obtained only by means of a physician's prescription

pre·se·nile \ˌprē-'sē-ˌnīl\ *adj* **1** : of, relating to, occurring in, or being the period immediately preceding the development of senility in an organism or person ⟨the ~ period of life⟩ **2** : prematurely displaying symptoms of senile dementia

presenile dementia *n* : dementia beginning in middle age and progressing rapidly — compare ALZHEIMER'S DISEASE

pre·sen·il·in \prē-'se-nil-ən\ *n* : any of several proteins of cell membranes that are believed to contribute to the development of Alzheimer's disease

pre·se·nil·i·ty \ˌprē-sə-'nil-ət-ē\ *n, pl* **-ties** **1** : premature senility **2** : the period of life immediately preceding senility

pre·sent \pri-'zent\ *vt* : to show or manifest ⟨patients who ~ symptoms of malaria⟩ ~ *vi* **1 a** : to become manifest ⟨Lyme disease often ~s with erythema migrans, fatigue, fever, and chills⟩ **b** : to come forward as a patient ⟨he ~ed with grossly swollen ankles and large varicose veins —T. E. Greene⟩ **2** : to become directed toward the opening of the uterus — used of a fetus or a part of a fetus ⟨babies which ~ by breech —*Yr. Bk. of Obstetrics & Gynecology*⟩

pre·sen·ta·tion \ˌprē-ˌzen-'tā-shən, ˌprez-ᵊn-\ *n* **1** : the position in which the fetus lies in the uterus in labor with respect to the opening of the uterus ⟨face ~⟩ ⟨a breech ~⟩ **2** : appearance in conscious experience either as a sensory product or as a memory image **3** : a presenting symptom or group of symptoms ⟨clinical ~ of arthritis⟩ **4** : a formal oral report of a patient's medical history

pre·sent·ing \pri-'zent-iŋ\ *adj* : of, relating to, or being a symptom, condition, or sign which is patent upon initial examination of a patient or which the patient discloses to the physician ⟨may be the ~ sign of a severe systemic disease —H. H. Roenigk, Jr.⟩

pre·ser·va·tive \pri-'zər-vət-iv\ *n* : something that preserves or has the power of preserving; *specif* : an additive used to protect against decay, discoloration, or spoilage ⟨a food ~⟩

pre·serve \pri-'zərv\ *vt* **pre·served; pre·serv·ing** **1** : to keep alive, intact, or free from decay **2** : to keep or save from decomposition

pre·so·mite \ˌprē-'sō-ˌmīt\ *adj* : occurring in, being in, or being the period of embryonic development prior to the formation of somites ⟨a ~ human embryo⟩

¹pre·sphe·noid \-'sfē-ˌnȯid\ *n* : a presphenoid bone or cartilage usu. united with the basisphenoid in the adult and in humans forming the anterior part of the body of the sphenoid

²presphenoid *also* **pre·sphe·noi·dal** \-sfi-'nȯid-ᵊl\ *adj* : indicating or relating to a median part of the vertebrate skull anterior to the basisphenoid

pres·sor \'pres-ˌȯr, -ər\ *adj* : raising or tending to raise blood pressure ⟨~ substances⟩; *also* : involving or producing an effect of vasoconstriction ⟨~ reflexes⟩ ⟨a ~ action⟩

pres·so·re·cep·tor \ˌpres-ō-ri-'sep-tər\ *n* : BARORECEPTOR

pres·sure \'presh-ər\ *n* **1** : the burden of mental or physical distress esp. from grief, illness, or adversity **2** : the application of force to something by something else in direct contact with it : COMPRESSION **3 a** : the action of a force against some opposing force : a force in the nature of a thrust distributed over a surface **b** : the force or thrust exerted over a surface divided by the area of the surface **4** : ELECTROMOTIVE FORCE **5** : ATMOSPHERIC PRESSURE **6** : a touch sensation aroused by moderate compression of the skin

pressure bandage *n* : a thick pad of gauze or other material placed over a wound and attached firmly so that it will exert pressure

pressure dressing *n* : PRESSURE BANDAGE

pressure point *n* **1** : a region of the body in which the distribution of soft and skeletal parts is such that a static position (as of a part in a cast or of a bedridden person) tends to cause circulatory deficiency and necrosis due to local compression of blood vessels — compare BEDSORE **2** : a discrete point on the body to which pressure is applied (as in acupressure or reflexology) for therapeutic purposes **3** : a point where a blood vessel runs near a bone and can be compressed (as to check bleeding) by the application of pressure against the bone

pressure sore *n* : BEDSORE

pressure spot *n* : one of the spots on the skin peculiarly sensitive to pressure

pressure suit \-ˌsüt\ *n* : an inflatable suit for high-altitude or space flight to protect the body from low pressure

pressure wave *n* : a wave (as a sound wave) in which the propagated disturbance is a variation of pressure in a material medium (as air)

pre·su·bic·u·lum \ˌprē-sə-'bik-yə-ləm\ *n, pl* **-la** \-lə\ : a part of the parahippocampal gyrus lying between the subiculum and the main olfactory region

pre·sump·tive \pri-'zəm(p)-tiv\ *adj* **1** : expected to develop in a particular direction under normal conditions ⟨~ regions of the blastula⟩ **2** : being the embryonic precursor of ⟨~ neural tissue⟩

pre·sur·gi·cal \ˌprē-'sər-ji-kəl\ *adj* : occurring before, performed before, or preliminary to surgery ⟨~ care⟩

pre·symp·to·mat·ic \-ˌsimp-tə-'mat-ik\ *adj* : relating to, being, or occurring before symptoms appear ⟨~ diagnosis of a hereditary disease⟩

pre·syn·ap·tic \-sə-'nap-tik\ *adj* : relating to, occurring in, or being part of a nerve cell by which a wave of excitation is conveyed to a synapse ⟨~ terminals⟩ ⟨~ inhibition⟩ ⟨a ~ membrane⟩ — **pre·syn·ap·ti·cal·ly** \-ti-k(ə-)lē\ *adv*

pre·sys·to·le \-'sis-tə-(ˌ)lē\ *n* : the interval just preceding cardiac systole

pre·sys·tol·ic \-sis-'täl-ik\ *adj* : of, relating to, or occurring just before cardiac systole ⟨a ~ murmur⟩

pre·tec·tal \-'tek-tᵊl\ *adj* : occurring in or being the transitional zone of the brain stem between the midbrain and the diencephalon that is situated rostral to the superior colliculus and is associated esp. with the analysis and distribution of light impulses

pre·term \-'tərm\ *adj* : of, relating to, being, or born by premature birth ⟨~ infants⟩ ⟨a ~ delivery⟩ ⟨~ labor⟩

pre·ter·mi·nal \-'tərm-nəl, -ən-ᵊl\ *adj* **1** : occurring or being in the period prior to death ⟨~ cancer⟩ ⟨a ~ patient⟩ **2** : situated or occurring anterior to an end (as of a nerve)

¹pre·test \'prē-ˌtest\ *n* : a preliminary test; *esp* : a test of the effectiveness or safety of a product (as a drug) prior to its sale

²pre·test \ˌprē-'test\ *vt* : to subject to a pretest ⟨~ed drugs⟩ ~ *vi* : to perform a pretest

pre·tib·i·al \-'tib-ē-əl\ *adj* : lying or occurring anterior to the tibia ⟨a ~ skin rash⟩

pretibial fever *n* : a rare infectious disease that is characterized by an eruption in the pretibial region, headache, backache, malaise, chills, and fever and that is caused by a spirochete of the genus *Leptospira* (*L. interrogans autumnalis*)

pretibial myxedema *n* : myxedema characterized primarily by a mucoid edema in the pretibial area

pre·to·pha·ceous \-tə-'fā-shəs\ *adj* : occurring before the development of tophi ⟨the ~ stage of gout⟩

pre·trans·plan·ta·tion \-ˌtran(t)s-ˌplan-'tā-shən\ *adj* : occurring or being in the period before transplant surgery ⟨~ hospitalization⟩ ⟨a ~ patient⟩

pre·treat \-'trēt\ *vt* : to subject to pretreatment

O
P

\ə\ **abut** \ᵊ\ **kitten** \ər\ **further** \a\ **ash** \ā\ **ace** \ä\ **cot, cart** \aȯ\ **out** \ch\ **chin** \e\ **bet** \ē\ **easy** \g\ **go** \i\ **hit** \ī\ **ice** \j\ **job** \ŋ\ **sing** \ō\ **go** \ȯ\ **law** \ȯi\ **boy** \th\ **thin** \t͟h\ **the** \ü\ **loot** \u̇\ **foot** \y\ **yet** \zh\ **vision** *See also* Pronunciation Symbols page

¹**pre·treat·ment** \-mənt\ n : preliminary or preparatory treatment ⟨unsuccessful . . . in preventing tumor growth by ∼ with vitamin A in mice —E. L. Felix *et al*⟩

²**pretreatment** *adj* : occurring in or typical of the period prior to treatment ⟨a patient's ∼ blood pressure⟩

pre·tu·ber·cu·lous \-t(y)ü-'bər-kyə-ləs\ *or* **pre·tu·ber·cu·lar** \-lər\ *adj* : occurring in, being in, or being the period preceding the development of lesions definitely identifiable as tuberculous ⟨∼ children⟩

Prev·a·cid \'prev-ə-ˌsid\ *trademark* — used for a preparation of lansoprazole

prev·a·lence \'prev(-ə)-lən(t)s\ n : the percentage of a population that is affected with a particular disease at a given time — compare INCIDENCE 2b

pre·ven·ta·tive \pri-'vent-ət-iv\ *adj or n* : PREVENTIVE

¹**pre·ven·tive** \-'vent-iv\ n : something (as a drug) used to prevent disease

²**preventive** *adj* : devoted to or concerned with the prevention of disease ⟨∼ drug therapy⟩ ⟨∼ psychiatry⟩

preventive medicine n : a branch of medical science dealing with methods (as vaccination) of preventing the occurrence of disease

pre·ven·to·ri·um \ˌprē-vən-'tór-ē-əm\ n, pl **-ria** \-ē-ə\ *also* **-riums** : an establishment where persons (as children) liable to develop disease (as tuberculosis) receive preventive care and treatment

pre·ver·te·bral \-'vərt-ə-brəl, -(ˌ)vər-'tē-brəl\ *adj* : situated or occurring anterior to a vertebra or the spinal column ⟨∼ muscles⟩

prevertebral ganglion n : COLLATERAL GANGLION

pre·ves·i·cal space \-'ves-i-kəl-\ n : RETROPUBIC SPACE

previa — see PLACENTA PREVIA

pre·vi·able \-'vī-ə-bəl\ *adj* : not sufficiently developed to survive outside the uterus ⟨a ∼ fetus⟩

pre·vil·lous \-'vil-əs\ *adj* : relating to, being in, or being the stage of embryonic development before the formation of villi ⟨a ∼ human embryo⟩

pri·a·pism \'prī-ə-ˌpiz-əm\ n : an abnormal, more or less persistent, and often painful erection of the penis; *esp* : one caused by disease rather than sexual desire

Pri·a·pus \prī-'ā-pəs\, Greek mythological character. A god of gardens and fertility, Priapus was the son of Aphrodite, who disowned him because he had a grotesque little body with a huge penis. He was a member of the retinue of the god Dionysus and chased after nymphs.

Price–Jones curve \'prīs-'jōnz-\ n : a graph of the frequency distribution of the diameters of red blood cells in a sample that has been smeared, stained, and magnified for direct observation and counting

Price–Jones, Cecil (1863–1943), British hematologist. Price-Jones developed in 1910 a method for the direct measurement of the diameters of red blood cells and for the recording of the results in the form of a graph that expressed their distribution in a stained sample. In 1924 he reported on anisocytosis in cases of pernicious anemia, and he published a study of the diameters of red blood cells in 1933.

prick·le cell \'prik-əl-\ n : a cell of the stratum spinosum of the skin having numerous intercellular bridges which give the separated cells a prickly appearance in microscopic preparations

prickle cell layer n : STRATUM SPINOSUM

prick·ly heat \'prik-lē-\ n : a noncontagious cutaneous eruption of red pimples with intense itching and tingling caused by inflammation around the sweat ducts — called also *heat rash;* see MILIARIA

prickly juniper n : a European juniper (*Juniperus oxycedrus*) whose wood yields juniper tar by distillation — called also *cade*

prick test \'prik-\ n : a test for allergic susceptibility made by placing a drop of the allergy-producing substance on the skin and making breaks in the skin by lightly pricking the surface (as with a pin) — compare INTRADERMAL TEST, PATCH TEST, SCRATCH TEST

pril·o·caine \'pril-ə-ˌkān\ n : a local anesthetic related to lidocaine and used in the form of its hydrochloride $C_{13}H_{20}N_2O \cdot HCl$ as a nerve block for pain esp. in surgery and dentistry

Pril·o·sec \'pril-ə-ˌsek\ *trademark* — used for a preparation of omeprazole

pri·mal scene \'prī-məl-'sēn\ n : the first instance of parental sexual intercourse that a child observes; *broadly* : sexual intercourse observed by a child

primal scream therapy \-'skrēm-\ n : psychotherapy in which the patient recalls and reenacts a particularly disturbing past experience usu. occurring early in life and expresses normally repressed anger or frustration esp. through spontaneous and unrestrained screams, hysteria, or violence — called also *primal scream, primal therapy*

primam — see PER PRIMAM

pri·ma·quine \'prī-mə-ˌkwēn, 'prim-ə-, -kwin\ n : an antimalarial drug used in the form of its diphosphate $C_{15}H_{21}N_3O \cdot 2H_3PO_4$

¹**pri·ma·ry** \'prī-ˌmer-ē, 'prim-(ə-)rē\ *adj* **1 a** (1) : first in order of time or development (2) : relating to or being the deciduous teeth and esp. the 20 deciduous teeth in the human set **b** (1) : arising spontaneously : IDIOPATHIC ⟨∼ insomnia⟩ ⟨the absence of any pelvic abnormality confirmed the diagnosis of ∼ dysmenorrhea⟩ (2) : being an initial tumor or site esp. of cancer ⟨efforts to find the ∼ tumor have failed —Raphael Feinmesser⟩ **c** : providing primary care ⟨a ∼ physician⟩ **2** : not derivable from other colors, odors, or tastes **3** : belonging to the first group or order in successive divisions, combinations, or ramifications ⟨∼ nerves⟩ **4** : of, relating to, or being the amino acid sequence in proteins ⟨∼ protein structure⟩ — compare SECONDARY 3, TERTIARY 2c **5** : resulting from the substitution of one of two or more atoms or groups in a molecule; *esp* : being or characterized by a carbon atom having a bond to only one other carbon atom

²**primary** n, pl **-ries** : PRIMARY COLOR

primary alcohol n : an alcohol that possesses the group $-CH_2OH$ and can be oxidized so as to form a corresponding aldehyde and acid having the same number of carbon atoms

primary aldosteronism n : aldosteronism caused by an adrenal tumor — called also *Conn's syndrome*

primary amenorrhea n : amenorrhea in which menstruation has not yet occurred by age 16

primary amine n : an amine RNH_2 (as methylamine) having one organic substituent attached to the nitrogen atom

primary atypical pneumonia n : any of a group of pneumonias (as Q fever and psittacosis) caused esp. by a virus, mycoplasma, rickettsia, or chlamydia

primary care n : health care provided by a medical professional (as a general practitioner or a pediatrician) with whom a patient has initial contact and by whom the patient may be referred to a specialist for further treatment — often used attributively ⟨*primary care* physicians⟩ ⟨*primary care* practice⟩ ⟨*primary care* medicine⟩; called also *primary health care;* compare SECONDARY CARE, TERTIARY CARE

primary color n : any of a set of colors (as red, yellow, and blue or red, green, and blue) from which all other colors may be derived

primary fissure n : a fissure of the cerebellum that is situated between the culmen and declive and that marks the boundary between the anterior lobe and the posterior lobe

primary health care n : PRIMARY CARE

primary host n : DEFINITIVE HOST

primary hypertension n : ESSENTIAL HYPERTENSION

primary lesion n : the initial lesion of a disease; *specif* : the chancre of syphilis

primary oocyte n : a diploid oocyte that has not yet undergone meiosis

primary spermatocyte n : a diploid spermatocyte that has not yet undergone meiosis

primary syphilis n : the first stage of syphilis that is marked by the development of a chancre and the spread of the causative spirochete in the tissues of the body

primary tooth n : MILK TOOTH

pri·mate \'prī-ˌmāt\ *n* : any mammal of the order Primates
Pri·ma·tes \prī-'mā-ˌtēz\ *n pl* : an order of eutherian mammals including humans, apes, monkeys, lemurs, and living and extinct related forms that are all thought to be derived from generalized arboreal ancestors and that are in general characterized by increasing perfection of binocular vision, specialization of the appendages for grasping, and enlargement and differentiation of the brain
pri·ma·tol·o·gist \ˌprī-mə-'täl-ə-jəst\ *n* : a specialist in primatology
pri·ma·tol·o·gy \-ə-jē\ *n, pl* **-gies** : the study of members of the order Primates esp. other than recent humans (*Homo sapiens*) — **pri·ma·to·log·i·cal** \-mət-ə-'läj-i-kəl\ *adj*
prime mover \'prīm-'mü-vər\ *n* : AGONIST 1
prim·er \'prī-mər\ *n* : a molecule (as a short strand of RNA or DNA) whose presence is required for formation of another molecule (as a longer chain of DNA)
pri·mi·done \'prī-mə-ˌdōn\ *n* : an anticonvulsant phenobarbital derivative $C_{12}H_{14}N_2O_2$ used esp. to control epileptic seizures
pri·mi·grav·id \ˌprī-mə-'grav-əd\ *adj* : pregnant for the first time
pri·mi·grav·i·da \-'grav-əd-ə\ *n, pl* **-dae** \-ə-ˌdē\ *also* **-das** : an individual pregnant for the first time
pri·mip·a·ra \prī-'mip-ə-rə\ *n, pl* **-ras** *or* **-rae** \-ˌrē\ **1** : an individual bearing a first offspring **2** : an individual that has borne only one offspring
pri·mip·a·rous \-ə-rəs\ *adj* : of, relating to, or being a primipara : bearing young for the first time — compare MULTIPAROUS 2
prim·i·tive \'prim-ət-iv\ *adj* **1** : closely approximating an early ancestral type : little evolved **2** : belonging to or characteristic of an early stage of development ⟨~ cells⟩ — **prim·i·tive·ly** *adv*
primitive groove *n* : a depression or groove in the epiblast of the primitive streak that extends forward to the primitive knot
primitive knot *n* : a knob of cells at the anterior end of the primitive streak that is the point of origin of the embryonic head process — see TAIL BUD
primitive pit *n* : a depression immediately behind the primitive knot in which the primitive groove ends
primitive streak *n* : an elongated band of cells that forms along the axis of an embryo early in gastrulation by the movement of lateral cells toward the axis and that develops a groove along its midline through which cells move to the interior of the embryo to form the mesoderm
pri·mor·di·al \prī-'mȯrd-ē-əl\ *adj* : earliest formed in the growth of an individual or organ : PRIMITIVE ⟨the ~ skeleton⟩
pri·mor·di·um \-ē-əm\ *n, pl* **-dia** \-ē-ə\ : the rudiment or commencement of a part or organ : ANLAGE ⟨the gonadal ~⟩
primum — see OSTIUM PRIMUM
prin·ceps pol·li·cis \'prin-ˌseps-'päl-ə-səs\ *n* : a branch of the radial artery that passes along the ulnar side of the first metacarpal and divides into branches running along the palmar side of the thumb
prin·ci·pal axis \'prin(t)-sə-pəl-\ *n* : the line with respect to which a spherical mirror or lens system is symmetrical and which passes through both the center of the surfaces and their centers of curvature
principal plane *n* : either of the two planes perpendicular to the principal axis and passing through one of the two principal points of an optical system
principal point *n* : either of two points on the principal axis of a lens where the object and image have the same size and are not inverted in relation to each other
prin·ci·ple \'prin(t)-sə-pəl\ *n* **1** : a comprehensive and fundamental law, doctrine, or assumption **2** : an ingredient (as a chemical) that exhibits or imparts a characteristic quality ⟨the active ~ of a drug⟩
Prin·i·vil \'prin-ə-ˌvil\ *trademark* — used for a preparation of lisinopril

P–R interval \'pē-'är-\ *n* : the interval between the beginning of the P wave and the beginning of the QRS complex of an electrocardiogram that represents the time between the beginning of the contraction of the atria and the beginning of the contraction of the ventricles
Prinz·met·al's angina \'prinz-ˌmet-ᵊlz\ *n* : angina pectoris of a variant form that is characterized by chest pain during rest and by an elevated ST segment during pain and that is typically caused by an obstructive lesion in the coronary artery
Prinzmetal, Myron (1908–1987), American cardiologist. Prinzmetal served for many years as attending physician at Los Angeles's Cedars of Lebanon Hospital and as professor of clinical medicine at the University of California, Los Angeles. He published monographs on auricular arrhythmias and related cardiac conditions. He published his first description of Prinzmetal's angina in 1955 with R. A. Massumi as coauthor.
pri·on \'prē-ˌän\ *n* : a protein particle that lacks nucleic acid and has been implicated as the cause of various neurodegenerative diseases (as scrapie, Creutzfeldt-Jakob disease, and bovine spongiform encephalopathy)
prism \'priz-əm\ *n* **1** : a polyhedron with two polygonal faces lying in parallel planes and with the other faces parallelograms **2** : a transparent body that is bounded in part by two nonparallel plane faces and is used to refract or disperse a beam of light **3** : a crystal form whose faces are parallel to one axis; *esp* : one whose faces are parallel to the vertical axis
pris·mat·ic \priz-'mat-ik\ *adj* **1** : relating to, resembling, or constituting a prism **2** : formed by a prism **3** : having such symmetry that a general form with faces cutting all axes at unspecified intercepts is a prism ⟨~ crystals⟩
prism diopter *n* : an arbitrary standard of prismatic deflection equal to that of a prism that deflects a beam of light one centimeter on a plane placed at a distance of one meter
pris·on fever \'priz-ᵊn-\ *n* : TYPHUS a
pri·vate \'prī-vət\ *adj* **1** : of, relating to, or receiving hospital service in which the patient has more privileges than a semiprivate or ward patient **2** : of, relating to, or being private practice ⟨a ~ office⟩ ⟨a ~ practitioner⟩
pri·vate–du·ty \-'d(y)üt-ē\ *adj* : caring for a single patient either in the home or in a hospital ⟨a ~ nurse⟩
private practice *n* **1** : practice of a profession (as medicine) independently and not as an employee **2** : the patients depending on and using the services of a physician in private practice
priv·i·leged communication \'priv-ə-lijd-\ *n* : a communication between parties to a confidential relation (as between physician and patient) such that the recipient cannot be legally compelled to disclose it as a witness
PRK *abbr* photorefractive keratectomy
PRL *abbr* prolactin
prn *abbr* [Latin *pro re nata*] as needed; as the circumstances require — used in writing prescriptions
Pro *abbr* proline; prolyl
PRO *abbr* peer review organization
pro·abor·tion \(')prō-ə-'bȯr-shən\ *adj* : favoring the legalization of abortion — **pro·abor·tion·ist** \-sh(ə-)nəst\ *n*
pro·ac·cel·er·in \ˌprō-ak-'sel-ə-rən\ *n* : FACTOR V
pro·ac·tive \(')prō-'ak-tiv\ *adj* : relating to, caused by, or being interference from previous learning and the recall or performance of later learning ⟨~ inhibition of memory⟩
pro·am·ni·on \-'am-nē-ˌän, -ən\ *n, pl* **-ni·ons** *or* **-nia** \-nē-ə\ : an area in the anterior part of the blastoderm of an early amniote embryo that is free of mesoderm — **pro·am·ni·ot·ic** \-ˌam-nē-'ät-ik\ *adj*
pro·at·las \-'at-ləs\ *n* : a rudimentary vertebra that lies between the atlas and the occipital bone and that occurs as a

O
P

regular feature of the structure of reptiles and may occur as an anomaly in humans

pro·bac·te·rio·phage \-bak-'tir-ē-ə-ˌfāj, -ˌfäzh\ *n* : PROPHAGE

pro·band \'prō-ˌband\ *n* : an individual being studied (as in a genetic investigation) : SUBJECT 1 ⟨the ∼ had four negative sibs⟩ — called also *propositus*

pro·bang \'prō-ˌbaŋ\ *n* : a slender flexible rod with a sponge on one end used esp. for removing obstructions from the esophagus

Pro–Ban·thine \(')prō-'ban-ˌthēn\ *n* : a preparation of propantheline bromide — formerly a U.S. registered trademark

pro·bar·bi·tal \-'bär-bə-ˌtal, -ˌtȯl\ *n* : a barbiturate $C_9H_{14}N_2O_3$ with sedative activity of intermediate duration

¹probe \'prōb\ *n* **1** : a surgical instrument that consists typically of a light slender fairly flexible pointed metal instrument like a small rod that is used typically for locating a foreign body (as a bullet embedded in a part of the body), for exploring a wound or suppurative tract by prodding or piercing, or for penetrating and exploring bodily passages and cavities **2** : a device (as an ultrasound generator) or a substance (as radioactively labeled DNA) used to obtain specific information (as detection of a virus or location of specific segments of a nucleic acid) for diagnostic or experimental purposes ⟨the radioactive ∼ revealed the distribution of molecules in the membrane⟩

²probe *vb* **probed; prob·ing** *vt* : to examine with or as if with a probe ⟨∼ a wound⟩ ∼ *vi* : to search by using a probe ⟨∼ for a bullet⟩

pro·ben·e·cid \prō-'ben-ə-səd\ *n* : a drug $C_{13}H_{19}NO_4S$ that acts on renal tubular function and is used to increase the concentration of some drugs (as penicillin) in the blood by inhibiting their excretion and to increase the excretion of urates in gout

pro·bi·ot·ic \prō-bī-'ät-ik, -bē-\ *n* : a preparation (as a dietary supplement) containing live bacteria (as lactobacilli) that is taken orally to restore beneficial bacteria to the body; *also* : a bacterium in such a preparation — **probiotic** *adj*

prob·it \'präb-ət\ *n* : a unit of measurement of statistical probability based on deviations from the mean of a normal distribution

pro·bos·cis \prə-'bäs-əs, -kəs\ *n, pl* **-bos·cis·es** *also* **-bos·ci·des** \-'bäs-ə-ˌdēz\ : any of various elongated or extensible tubular organs or processes esp. of the oral region of an invertebrate: as **a** : a sucking organ of insects (as houseflies or mosquitoes) that is often also adapted for piercing **b** : one of the complex protrusible holdfasts on the scolex of certain tapeworms

pro·bu·col \'prō-byə-ˌkȯl\ *n* : an antioxidant drug $C_{31}H_{48}O_2S_2$ that is used to reduce levels of serum cholesterol

pro·cain·amide \(ˌ)prō-'kān-ə-ˌmīd, -məd; -ˌkān-'am-əd\ *n* : a base of an amide related to procaine that is used in the form of its hydrochloride $C_{13}H_{21}N_3O·HCl$ as a cardiac depressant esp. in the treatment of ventricular arrhythmias — see PRONESTYL

pro·caine \'prō-ˌkān\ *n* : a basic ester $C_{13}H_{20}N_2O_2$ of para-aminobenzoic acid used in the form of its hydrochloride $C_{13}H_{20}N_2O_2·HCl$ as a local anesthetic — see NOVOCAIN, NOVOCAINE

procaine penicillin G *n* : PENICILLIN G PROCAINE

pro·car·ba·zine \prō-'kär-bə-ˌzēn, -zən\ *n* : an antineoplastic drug that occurs as a white to yellowish crystalline powder, is a monoamine oxidase inhibitor, and is used in the form of its hydrochloride $C_{12}H_{19}N_3O·HCl$ esp. in the palliative treatment of Hodgkin's disease

Pro·car·dia \prō-'kärd-ē-ə\ *trademark* — used for a preparation of nifedipine

procaryote, procaryotic *var of* PROKARYOTE, PROKARYOTIC

pro·ce·dur·al \prə-'sēj-(ə-)rəl\ *adj* : relating to or comprising memory or knowledge concerned with how to manipulate symbols, concepts, and rules to accomplish a task or solve a problem — compare DECLARATIVE

pro·ce·dure \prə-'sē-jər\ *n* **1** : a particular way of accomplishing something or of acting **2** : a step in a procedure; *esp* : a series of steps followed in a regular definite order ⟨a surgical ∼⟩ ⟨a therapeutic ∼⟩

pro·cer·coid \(')prō-'sər-ˌkȯid\ *n* : the solid first parasitic larva of some tapeworms that develops usu. in the body cavity of a copepod

pro·ce·rus \prō-'sir-əs\ *n, pl* **-ri** \-ˌrī\ *or* **-rus·es** : a facial muscle that arises from the nasal bone and a cartilage in the side of the nose and that inserts into the skin of the forehead between the eyebrows

pro·cess \'präs-ˌes, 'prōs-, -əs\ *n* **1 a** : a natural progressively continuing operation or development marked by a series of gradual changes that succeed one another in a relatively fixed way and lead toward a particular result or end ⟨the ∼ of growth⟩ ⟨the ∼ of digestion⟩ **b** : a natural continuing activity or function ⟨such life ∼*es* as breathing and the circulation of the blood⟩ **2** : a prominent or projecting part of an organism or organic structure ⟨a bone ∼⟩ ⟨a nerve cell ∼⟩

pro·ces·sus \prō-'ses-əs\ *n, pl* **processus** : PROCESS 2

processus vag·i·na·lis \-ˌvaj-ə-'nā-ləs\ *n* : a pouch of peritoneum that is carried into the scrotum by the descent of the testicle and which in the scrotum forms the tunica vaginalis

pro·chlor·per·azine \ˌprō-ˌklȯr-'per-ə-ˌzēn\ *n* : a tranquilizing and antiemetic drug $C_{20}H_{24}ClN_3S$ — see COMPAZINE

pro–choice \(')prō-'chȯis\ *adj* : favoring the legalization of abortion — **pro–choic·er** \-'chȯi-sər\ *n*

pro·chro·mo·some \-'krō-mə-ˌsōm, -ˌzōm\ *n* : a condensed heterochromatic portion of a chromosome visible in the resting nucleus

pro·ci·den·tia \ˌprō-sə-'den-ch(ē-)ə, ˌprä-\ *n* : PROLAPSE; *esp* : severe prolapse of the uterus in which the cervix projects from the vaginal opening

proc·li·na·tion \ˌpräk-lə-'nā-shən\ *n* : the condition of being inclined forward ⟨∼ of the upper and lower incisors⟩

¹pro·co·ag·u·lant \(')prō-kō-'ag-yə-lənt\ *n* : a procoagulant substance

²procoagulant *adj* : promoting the coagulation of blood ⟨∼ activity⟩

pro·col·la·gen \-'käl-ə-jən\ *n* : a molecular precursor of collagen

pro·con·ver·tin \-kən-'vərt-ᵊn\ *n* : FACTOR VII

pro·cre·ate \'prō-krē-ˌāt\ *vb* **-at·ed; -at·ing** *vt* : to beget or bring forth (offspring) : PROPAGATE ∼ *vi* : to beget or bring forth offspring : REPRODUCE

pro·cre·ation \ˌprō-krē-'ā-shən\ *n* : the act or process of procreating : REPRODUCTION

pro·cre·ative \'prō-krē-ˌāt-iv\ *adj* **1** : capable of procreating : GENERATIVE **2** : of, relating to, or directed toward procreation ⟨the ∼ process⟩ ⟨∼ instincts⟩

proct·al·gia fu·gax \ˌpräk-'tal-j(ē-)ə-'fyü-ˌgaks\ *n* : a condition characterized by the intermittent occurrence of sudden sharp pain in the rectal area

proc·tec·to·my \präk-'tek-tə-mē\ *n, pl* **-mies** : surgical excision of the rectum

proc·ti·tis \präk-'tīt-əs\ *n* : inflammation of the anus and rectum

proc·toc·ly·sis \präk-'täk-lə-səs\ *n, pl* **-ly·ses** \-ˌsēz\ : slow injection of large quantities of a fluid (as a solution of salt) into the rectum in supplementing the liquid intake of the body

proc·to·co·li·tis \ˌpräk-tō-kə-'līt-əs\ *n* : inflammation of the rectum and colon

proc·to·de·um *or* **proc·to·dae·um** \ˌpräk-tə-'dē-əm\ *n, pl* **-dea** *or* **-daea** \-'dē-ə\ *or* **-de·ums** *or* **-dae·ums** : the posterior ectodermal part of the alimentary canal formed in the embryo by invagination of the outer body wall — **proc·to·de·al** *or* **proc·to·dae·al** \-'dē-əl\ *adj*

proc·tol·o·gist \präk-'täl-ə-jəst\ *n* : a specialist in proctology

proc·tol·o·gy \präk-'täl-ə-jē\ *n, pl* **-gies** : a branch of medicine dealing with the structure and diseases of the anus, rectum, and sigmoid colon — **proc·to·log·ic** \ˌpräk-tə-'läj-ik\ *or* **proc·to·log·i·cal** \-i-kəl\ *adj*

proc·to·pexy \'präk-tə-ˌpek-sē\ *n, pl* **-pex·ies** : the suturing of the rectum to an adjacent structure (as the sacrum)

proc·to·plas·ty \'präk-tə-ˌplas-tē\ *n, pl* **-ties** : plastic surgery of the rectum and anus

¹**proc·to·scope** \'präk-tə-ˌskōp\ *n* : an instrument used for dilating and visually inspecting the rectum and lower portion of the sigmoid colon

²**proctoscope** *vt* **-scoped; -scop·ing** : to use a proctoscope on

proc·to·scop·ic \ˌpräk-tə-'skäp-ik\ *adj* : of or relating to a proctoscope or proctoscopy — **proc·to·scop·i·cal·ly** \-i-k(ə-)lē\ *adv*

proc·tos·co·py \präk-'täs-kə-pē\ *n, pl* **-pies** : dilation and visual inspection of the rectum

proc·to·sig·moid·ec·to·my \ˌpräk-tō-ˌsig-mȯid-'ek-tə-mē\ *n, pl* **-mies** : complete or partial surgical excision of the rectum and sigmoid colon

proc·to·sig·moid·itis \-'īt-əs\ *n* : inflammation of the rectum and sigmoid colon

proc·to·sig·moid·o·scope \-sig-'mȯid-ə-ˌskōp\ *n* : SIGMOID-OSCOPE

proc·to·sig·moid·os·co·py \-ˌsig-ˌmȯi-'däs-kə-pē\ *n, pl* **-pies** : SIGMOIDOSCOPY — **proc·to·sig·moid·o·scop·ic** \-ˌmȯid-ə-'skäp-ik\ *adj*

proc·tot·o·my \präk-'tät-ə-mē\ *n, pl* **-mies** : surgical incision into the rectum

pro·cum·bent \(')prō-'kəm-bənt\ *adj* : a slanting forward ⟨∼ maxillary incisors⟩

pro·dig·i·o·sin \prō-ˌdij-ē-'ō-sⁿn\ *n* : a red antibiotic pigment $C_{20}H_{25}N_3O$ that is produced by a bacterium of the genus *Serratia* (*S. marcescens*) and was formerly used against protozoans (as the parasite of amebic dysentery) and against fungi (as the parasite of coccidioidomycosis)

prod·ro·ma \'prä-drə-mə\ *n, pl* **prodromas** *or* **pro·dro·ma·ta** \prō-'drō-mət-ə\ : PRODROME

pro·dro·mal \(')prō-'drō-məl\ *also* **pro·dro·mic** \-mik\ *adj* : PRECURSORY; *esp* : of, relating to, or marked by prodromes ⟨the ∼ stages of a disease⟩

pro·drome \'prō-ˌdrōm\ *n* : a premonitory symptom of disease — called also *prodroma*

pro·drug \'prō-ˌdrəg\ *n* : a pharmacologically inactive substance that is the modified form of a pharmacologically active drug to which it is converted (as by enzymatic action) in the body ⟨∼s that enhance drug absorption⟩ ⟨a ∼ that is rapidly converted to phenytoin in the body —Danielle G. LeStrange⟩

prod·uct \'präd-(ˌ)əkt\ *n* : a substance produced from one or more other substances as a result of chemical change

pro·duc·tive \prə-'dək-tiv, prō-\ *adj* : raising mucus or sputum (as from the bronchi) ⟨a ∼ cough⟩

pro·en·zyme \(')prō-'en-ˌzīm\ *n* : ZYMOGEN

pro·eryth·ro·blast \(')prō-i-'rith-rə-ˌblast\ *n* : a hemocytoblast that gives rise to erythroblasts — **pro·eryth·ro·blas·tic** \-i-ˌrith-rə-'blas-tik\ *adj*

pro·eryth·ro·cyte \-ˌsīt\ *n* : any immature red blood cell

pro·es·tro·gen \(')prō-'es-trə-jən\ *or chiefly Brit* **pro·oes·tro·gen** \-'ēs-\ *n* : a precursor of an estrogen that must undergo metabolism before becoming an active hormone

pro·es·trous \-'es-trəs\ *or chiefly Brit* **pro·oes·trous** \-'ēs-\ *adj* : of or relating to proestrus

pro·es·trus \-'es-trəs\ *or* **pro·es·trum** \-'es-trəm\ *or chiefly Brit* **pro—oes·trus** *or* **pro—oes·trum** \-'ēs-\ *n* : a preparatory period immediately preceding estrus and characterized by growth of graafian follicles, increased estrogenic activity, and alteration of uterine and vaginal mucosa

pro·fer·ment \-'fər-ˌment\ *n* : an inactive precursor of a ferment : ZYMOGEN

pro·fes·sion \prə-'fesh-ən\ *n* **1** : a calling requiring specialized knowledge and often long and intensive academic preparation **2** : the whole body of persons engaged in a calling

¹**pro·fes·sion·al** \prə-'fesh-nəl, -ən-ᵊl\ *adj* **1** : of, relating to, or characteristic of a profession **2** : engaged in one of the learned professions **3** : characterized by or conforming to the technical or ethical standards of a profession — **pro·fes·sion·al·ly** \-ē\ *adv*

²**professional** *n* : a person who is professional; *esp* : a person who engages in a pursuit or activity professionally

professional corporation *n* : a corporation organized by one or more licensed individuals (as a doctor, dentist, or physical therapist) esp. for the purpose of providing professional services and obtaining tax advantages — abbr. *PC*

professional standards review organization *n* : any of a group of organizations that were established to review the quality and costs of medical care and were replaced by peer review organizations in the Tax Equity and Fiscal Responsibility Act of 1982 — abbr. *PSRO*

pro·fi·bri·no·ly·sin \(')prō-ˌfī-brən-ᵊl-'īs-ᵊn\ *n* : PLASMINO-GEN

¹**pro·file** \'prō-ˌfīl\ *n* **1** : a set of data exhibiting the significant features of something and often obtained by multiple tests ⟨the ∼ of CK isoenzymes in skeletal muscle —A. J. Siegel & D. M. Dawson⟩ **2** : a graphic representation of the extent to which an individual or group exhibits traits as determined by tests or ratings ⟨this group did not give a homogeneous personality ∼ —*Diseases of the Nervous System*⟩

²**profile** *vt* **pro·filed; pro·fil·ing** : to represent in profile or by a profile : produce a profile of (as by writing or graphing)

pro·fla·vine \(')prō-'flā-ˌvēn\ *also* **pro·fla·vin** \-vən\ *n* : a yellow crystalline mutagenic acridine dye $C_{13}H_{11}N_3$; *also* : the orange to brownish red hygroscopic crystalline sulfate used as an antiseptic esp. for wounds — see ACRIFLAVINE

pro·flu·o·ri·da·tion·ist \'prō-ˌflùr-ə-'dā-shən-əst, -ˌflȯr-\ *n* : a person who supports the fluoridation of public water supplies for the prevention of dental caries

pro·found·ly \prə-'faùn-dlē, prō-\ *adv* **1** : totally or completely ⟨∼ deaf persons⟩ **2** : to the greatest possible degree ⟨∼ mentally retarded persons⟩

pro·fun·da artery \prə-'fənd-ə-\ *n* **1** : DEEP BRACHIAL ARTERY **2** : DEEP FEMORAL ARTERY

profunda fem·o·ris \-'fem-ə-rəs\ *n* : DEEP FEMORAL ARTERY

profunda femoris artery *n* : DEEP FEMORAL ARTERY

profundus — see FLEXOR DIGITORUM PROFUNDUS

pro·gen·e·sis \-'jen-ə-səs\ *n, pl* **-e·ses** \-ˌsēz\ : precocious sexual reproduction in a trematode worm in which metacercariae or sometimes cercariae may lay eggs capable of repeating the life cycle — **pro·ge·net·ic** \-jə-'net-ik\ *adj*

progenitalis — see HERPES PROGENITALIS

pro·gen·i·tor \prō-'jen-ət-ər, prə-\ *n* **1** : an ancestor of an individual in a direct line of descent along which some or all of the ancestral genes could theoretically have passed **2** : a biologically ancestral form

prog·e·ny \'präj-(ə-)nē\ *n, pl* **-nies** : offspring of animals or plants

pro·ge·ria \prō-'jir-ē-ə\ *n* : a rare genetic disorder of childhood marked by slowed physical growth and characteristic signs (as baldness, wrinkled skin, and atherosclerosis) of rapid aging with death usu. occurring during puberty

progestagen, progestagenic *var of* PROGESTOGEN, PRO-GESTOGENIC

pro·ges·ta·tion·al \ˌprō-ˌjes-'tā-shnəl, -shən-ᵊl\ *adj* : preceding pregnancy or gestation; *esp* : of, relating to, inducing, or constituting the modifications of the female mammalian system associated esp. with ovulation and corpus luteum formation ⟨∼ hormones⟩

pro·ges·ter·one \prō-'jes-tə-ˌrōn\ *n* : a female steroid sex hormone $C_{21}H_{30}O_2$ that is secreted by the corpus luteum to prepare the endometrium for implantation and later by the placenta during pregnancy to prevent rejection of the developing embryo or fetus; *also* : a synthetic steroid resembling progesterone in action

pro·ges·ter·on·ic \prō-ˌjes-tə-'rän-ik\ *adj* : of, relating to, or induced by progesterone

pro·ges·tin \prō-'jest-ən\ *n* : PROGESTOGEN; *esp* : a synthetic progesterone (as levonorgestrel)

\ə\ abut \ᵊ\ kitten \ər\ further \a\ ash \ā\ ace \ä\ cot, cart \aù\ out \ch\ chin \e\ bet \ē\ easy \g\ go \i\ hit \ī\ ice \j\ job \ŋ\ sing \ō\ go \ȯ\ law \ȯi\ boy \th\ thin \th\ the \ü\ loot \ù\ foot \y\ yet \zh\ vision *See also* Pronunciation Symbols page

O
P

pro·ges·to·gen also **pro·ges·ta·gen** \-'jes-tə-jən\ n : a naturally occurring or synthetic progestational steroid

pro·ges·to·gen·ic also **pro·ges·ta·gen·ic** \prō-ˌjes-tə-'jen-ik\ adj : of, relating to, induced by, or being a progestogen ⟨~ changes⟩ ⟨~ steroids⟩

pro·glot·tid \(')prō-'glät-əd\ n : one of the segments of a tapeworm formed by a process of strobilation in the neck region of the worm, containing both male and female reproductive organs, and surviving briefly after breaking away from the strobila

pro·glot·tis \(')prō-'glät-əs\ n, pl **-glot·ti·des** \-'glät-ə-ˌdēz\ : PROGLOTTID

prog·na·thic \präg-'nath-ik, -'nā-thik\ adj : PROGNATHOUS

prog·na·thism \'präg-nə-ˌthiz-əm, präg-'nā-\ n : prognathous condition

prog·na·thous \'präg-nə-thəs\ adj : having the jaws projecting beyond the upper part of the face

prog·no·sis \präg-'nō-səs\ n, pl **-no·ses** \-ˌsēz\ **1** : the act or art of foretelling the course of a disease **2** : the prospect of survival and recovery from a disease as anticipated from the usual course of that disease or indicated by special features of the case ⟨the ~ is poor because of the accompanying cardiovascular disease —P. A. Mead et al⟩

prog·nos·tic \präg-'näs-tik\ adj : of, relating to, or serving as ground for a prognosis ⟨a ~ sign⟩

prog·nos·ti·cate \präg-'näs-tə-ˌkāt\ vt **-cat·ed; -cat·ing** : to make a prognosis about the probable outcome of — **prog·nos·ti·ca·tion** \-ˌnäs-tə-'kā-shən\ n

¹pro·gram or chiefly Brit **pro·gramme** \'prō-ˌgram, -grəm\ n : a sequence of coded instructions (as genes or behavioral responses) that is part of an organism

²program or chiefly Brit **programme** vt **-grammed** or **-gramed; -gram·ming** or **-gram·ing** **1** : to code in an organism's program **2** : to provide with a biological program ⟨cells programmed to synthesize hemoglobin⟩

programmed cell death n : APOPTOSIS

pro·gran·u·lo·cyte \(')prō-'gran-yə-lō-ˌsīt\ n : PROMYELOCYTE

pro·grav·id \-'grav-əd\ adj : PROGESTATIONAL

pro·gres·sive \prə-'gres-iv\ adj : increasing in extent or severity ⟨a ~ disease⟩ — **pro·gres·sive·ly** adv

progressive multifocal leukoencephalopathy n : a progressive and fatal demyelinating disease of the central nervous system that typically occurs in immunosuppressed individuals due to loss of childhood immunity to a double-stranded DNA virus of the genus Polyomavirus (species JC polyomavirus) ubiquitous in human populations and that is characterized by hemianopia, hemiplegia, alterations in mental state, and eventually coma

progressive muscular dystrophy n : MUSCULAR DYSTROPHY

progressive supranuclear palsy n : an uncommon neurological disorder that is of unknown etiology, that typically occurs from late middle age onward, and that is marked by loss of voluntary vertical eye movement, muscular rigidity and dystonia of the neck and trunk, pseudobulbar paralysis, bradykinesia, and dementia — called also supranuclear palsy

pro·guan·il \ˌprō-'gwän-ᵊl\ n : an antimalarial drug derived from biguanide and administered in the form of its hydrochloride $C_{11}H_{16}ClN_5 \cdot HCl$ — called also chloroguanide

pro·hor·mone \(')prō-'hȯr-ˌmōn\ n : a physiologically inactive precursor of a hormone

pro·in·su·lin \(')prō-'in(t)-s(ə-)lən\ n : a single-chain pancreatic polypeptide precursor of insulin that gives rise to the double chain of insulin by loss of the middle part of the molecule

pro·ject \prə-'jekt\ vt : to attribute or assign (something in one's own mind or a personal characteristic) to a person, group, or object ⟨the patient ~ed hostility onto the therapist⟩ ~ vi : to connect by sending nerve fibers or processes ⟨cells of the lateral geniculate body ~ to the back part of the cerebral cortex⟩

pro·jec·tile vomiting \prə-'jek-tᵊl-, -ˌtīl-\ n : vomiting that is sudden, usu. without nausea, and so vigorous that the vomit is forcefully projected to a distance

pro·jec·tion \prə-'jek-shən\ n **1 a** : the process or technique of reproducing a spatial object or a section of such an object upon a plane or curved surface **b** : a diagram or figure formed by projection; esp : VIEW **2 a** : the act of referring a mental image constructed by the brain from bits of data collected by the sense organs to the actual source of stimulation outside the body **b** : the attribution of one's own ideas, feelings, or attitudes to other people or to objects; esp : the externalization of blame, guilt, or responsibility as a defense against anxiety **3** : the functional correspondence and connection of parts of the cerebral cortex with parts of the organism ⟨the ~ of the retina upon the visual area⟩

projection area n : an area of the cerebral cortex having connection through projection fibers with subcortical centers that in turn are linked with peripheral sense or motor organs

projection fiber n : a nerve fiber connecting some part of the cerebral cortex with lower sensory or motor centers — compare ASSOCIATION FIBER

pro·jec·tive \prə-'jek-tiv\ adj : of, relating to, or being a technique, device, or test (as the Rorschach test) designed to analyze the psychodynamic constitution of an individual by presenting unstructured or ambiguous material (as inkblots, pictures, and sentence elements) that will elicit interpretive responses revealing personality structure

pro·kary·ote also **pro·cary·ote** \(')prō-'kar-ē-ˌōt\ n : any of the typically unicellular microorganisms that lack a distinct nucleus and membrane-bound organelles and that are classified as a kingdom (Prokaryotae syn. Monera) or into two domains (Bacteria and Archaea) — compare EUKARYOTE — **pro·kary·ot·ic** also **pro·cary·ot·ic** \-ˌkar-ē-'ät-ik\ adj

pro·ki·net·ic \ˌprō-kə-'net-ik, -kī-\ adj : stimulating motility of the esophageal and gastrointestinal muscles ⟨~ agents to treat gastroparesis⟩ — **prokinetic** n

pro·la·bi·um \prō-'lā-bē-əm\ n, pl **-bia** \-bē-ə\ : the exposed part of a lip; esp : the protuberant central part of the upper lip

pro·lac·tin \prō-'lak-tən\ n : a protein hormone of the adenohypophysis of the pituitary gland that induces and maintains lactation in the postpartum mammalian female — abbr. PRL; called also luteotropic hormone, luteotropin, mammotropin

pro·la·min or **pro·la·mine** \'prō-lə-mən, -ˌmēn\ n : any of various simple proteins that are found esp. in seeds and are insoluble in dehydrated alcohol or water

pro·lan \'prō-ˌlan\ n : either of two gonadotropic hormones: **a** : FOLLICLE-STIMULATING HORMONE **b** : LUTEINIZING HORMONE

¹pro·lapse \prō-'laps, 'prō-ˌ\ n : the falling down or slipping of a body part from its usual position or relations ⟨~ of the uterus⟩ ⟨~ of an intervertebral disk⟩

²pro·lapse \prō-'laps\ vi **pro·lapsed; pro·laps·ing** : to undergo prolapse

prolapsed adj : having undergone prolapse ⟨a ~ bladder⟩

pro·lap·sus \-səs\ n : PROLAPSE

pro·leu·ko·cyte or chiefly Brit **pro·leu·co·cyte** \(')prō-'lü-kə-ˌsīt\ n : LEUKOBLAST

pro·life \(')prō-'līf\ adj : ANTIABORTION

pro·lif·er \-'lī-fər\ n : ANTIABORTIONIST

proliferans — see RETINITIS PROLIFERANS

pro·lif·er·ate \prə-'lif-ə-ˌrāt\ vb **-at·ed; -at·ing** vi : to grow by rapid production of new parts, cells, buds, or offspring ~ vt : to cause to grow by proliferating

pro·lif·er·a·tion \prə-ˌlif-ə-'rā-shən\ n **1 a** : rapid and repeated production of new parts or of offspring (as in a mass of cells by a rapid succession of cell divisions) **b** : a growth so formed **2** : the action, process, or result of increasing by or as if by proliferation

pro·lif·er·a·tive \prə-'lif-ə-ˌrāt-iv\ adj **1** : capable of or engaged in proliferation **2** : of, marked by, or tending to proliferation

proligerus — see DISCUS PROLIGERUS

pro·line \'prō-ˌlēn\ *n* : an amino acid $C_5H_9NO_2$ that can be synthesized by animals from glutamate — abbr. *Pro*

Pro·lix·in \prō-'lik-sən\ *trademark* — used for a preparation of fluphenazine

pro·lo·ther·a·py \ˌprō-lō-'ther-ə-pē\ *n* : an alternative therapy for treating musculoskeletal pain that involves injecting an irritant substance (as dextrose) into a ligament or tendon to promote the growth of new tissue

pro·lyl \'prō-ˌlil\ *n* : the amino acid radical or residue C_4H_8NCO- of proline — abbr. *Pro*

pro·lym·pho·cyte \(ˈ)prō-'lim(p)-fə-ˌsīt\ *n* : a cell in an intermediate stage of development between a lymphoblast and a lymphocyte

pro·mas·ti·gote \-'mas-ti-ˌgōt\ *n* : a protozoan that belongs to the family Trypanosomatidae and esp. to the genus *Leishmania* and that is in a flagellated usu. extracellular stage characterized by a single anterior flagellum and no undulating membrane — **promastigote** *adj*

pro·ma·zine \'prō-mə-ˌzēn\ *n* : a tranquilizer derived from phenothiazine that is administered in the form of its hydrochloride $C_{17}H_{20}N_2S \cdot HCl$ and is used similarly to chlorpromazine — see SPARINE

pro·mega·kary·o·cyte \ˌprō-ˌmeg-ə-'kar-ē-ō-ˌsīt\ *n* : a cell in an intermediate stage of development between a megakaryoblast and a megakaryocyte

pro·meg·a·lo·blast \(ˈ)prō-'meg-ə-lō-ˌblast\ *n* : a cell that produces megaloblasts and is possibly equivalent to a hemocytoblast — called also *erythrogone*

pro·meta·phase \-'met-ə-ˌfāz\ *n* : a stage sometimes distinguished between the prophase and metaphase of mitosis or meiosis and characterized by disappearance of the nuclear membrane and formation of the spindle

pro·meth·a·zine \(ˈ)prō-'meth-ə-ˌzēn\ *n* : a crystalline antihistamine drug derived from phenothiazine and used chiefly in the form of its hydrochloride $C_{17}H_{20}N_2S \cdot HCl$ — see PHENERGAN

pro·meth·es·trol \-meth-'es-ˌtrōl\ *or Brit* **pro·meth·oes·trol** \-'ēs-\ *n* : a synthetic estrogen $C_{20}H_{26}O_2$

pro·me·thi·um \prə-'mē-thē-əm\ *n* : a radioactive metallic element of the rare-earth group obtained as a fission product of uranium or from neutron-irradiated neodymium — symbol *Pm*; see ELEMENT table

prom·i·nence \'präm(-ə)-nən(t)s\ *n* : an elevation or projection on an anatomical structure (as a bone)

prominens — see VERTEBRA PROMINENS

prom·i·nent \'präm-(ə)nənt\ *adj* : standing out or projecting beyond a surface

pro·mis·cu·i·ty \ˌpräm-əs-'kyü-ət-ē, prə-ˌmis-\ *n, pl* **-ties** : promiscuous sexual behavior

pro·mis·cu·ous \prə-'mis-kyə-wəs\ *adj* : not restricted to one sexual partner

pro·mono·cyte \-'män-ə-ˌsīt\ *n* : a cell in an intermediate stage of development between a monoblast and a monocyte

prom·on·to·ry \'präm-ən-ˌtōr-ē, -ˌtòr-\ *n, pl* **-ries** : a bodily prominence: as **a** : the angle of the ventral side of the sacrum where it joins the vertebra **b** : a prominence on the inner wall of the tympanum of the ear

pro·mote \prə-'mōt\ *vt* **pro·mot·ed; pro·mot·ing** : to cause or contribute to the growth, development, or occurrence of ⟨sugary drinks ~ cavities⟩ ⟨a diet that ~s good health⟩

pro·mot·er \-'mōt-ər\ *n* **1** : a substance that in very small amounts is able to increase the activity of a catalyst **2** : a binding site in a DNA chain at which RNA polymerase binds to initiate transcription of messenger RNA by one or more nearby structural genes **3** : a chemical believed to promote carcinogenicity or mutagenicity

pro·my·elo·cyte \(ˈ)prō-'mī-ə-lə-ˌsīt\ *n* : a cell in bone marrow that is in an intermediate stage of development between a myeloblast and a myelocyte and has the characteristic granulations but lacks the specific staining reactions of a mature granulocyte of the blood — called also *premyelocyte, progranulocyte* — **pro·my·elo·cyt·ic** \(ˌ)prō-ˌmī-ə-lə-'sit-ik\ *adj*

promyelocytic leukemia *n* : a leukemia in which the predominant blood cell type is the promyelocyte

pro·nase \'prō-ˌnās, -ˌnāz\ *n* : a proteolytic enzyme from an actinomycete of the genus *Streptomyces* (*S. griseus*)

pro·nate \'prō-ˌnāt\ *vb* **pro·nat·ed; pro·nat·ing** *vt* : to subject (as the hand or forearm) to pronation ~ *vi* : to assume a position of pronation

pro·na·tion \prō-'nā-shən\ *n* : rotation of an anatomical part towards the midline: as **a** : rotation of the hand and forearm so that the palm faces backwards or downwards **b** : rotation of the medial bones in the midtarsal region of the foot inward and downward so that in walking the foot tends to come down on its inner margin

pro·na·tor \'prō-ˌnāt-ər\ *n* : a muscle that produces pronation

pronator qua·dra·tus \-kwä-'drāt-əs\ *n* : a deep muscle of the forearm passing transversely from the ulna to the radius and serving to pronate the forearm

pronator te·res \-'tir-ˌēz\ *n* : a muscle of the forearm arising from the medial epicondyle of the humerus and the coronoid process of the ulna, inserting into the lateral surface of the middle third of the radius, and serving to pronate and flex the forearm

prone \'prōn\ *adj* : having the front or ventral surface downward; *esp* : lying facedown — **prone** *adv*

pro·neph·ric \(ˈ)prō-'nef-rik\ *adj* : of or relating to a pronephros ⟨the ~ duct⟩

pro·neph·ros \(ˈ)prō-'nef-rəs, -ˌräs\ *n, pl* **-neph·roi** \-ˌrói\ : either member of the first and most anterior pair of the three paired vertebrate renal organs that functions in the adults of amphioxus and some lampreys, functions temporarily in larval fishes and amphibians, and is present but nonfunctional in embryos of reptiles, birds, and mammals — compare MESONEPHROS, METANEPHROS

prone pressure method *n* : a method of artificial respiration consisting essentially of alternate pressure and release of pressure on the back of the thorax of the prone patient by means of which water if present is expelled from the lungs and air is allowed to enter — called also *Schafer method*

Pro·nes·tyl \prō-'nes-til\ *trademark* — used for a preparation of the hydrochloride of procainamide

pro·no·grade \'prō-nə-ˌgrād\ *adj* : walking with the body approximately horizontal ⟨most mammals except humans and the higher apes are ~⟩ — compare ORTHOGRADE 1

pro·nor·mo·blast \(ˈ)prō-'nòr-mə-ˌblast\ *n* : a cell recognized in some theories of erythropoiesis that arises from a myeloblast and gives rise to normoblasts and is approximately equivalent to the erythroblast of other theories — called also *macronormoblast, rubriblast*

pron·to·sil \'prän-tə-ˌsil\ *n* : any of three sulfonamide drugs: **a** : a red azo dye $C_{12}H_{13}N_5O_2S$ that was the first sulfa drug tested clinically — called also *prontosil rubrum* **b** : SULFANILAMIDE **c** : AZOSULFAMIDE

prontosil al·bum \-'al-bəm\ *n* : SULFANILAMIDE

prontosil ru·brum \-'rü-brəm\ *n* : PRONTOSIL a

prontosil soluble *n* : AZOSULFAMIDE

pro·nu·clear \(ˈ)prō-'n(y)ü-klē-ər\ *adj* : of, relating to, or resembling a pronucleus

pro·nu·cle·us \(ˈ)prō-'n(y)ü-klē-əs\ *n, pl* **-clei** \-klē-ˌī\ *also* **-cle·us·es** : the haploid nucleus of a male or female gamete (as an egg or sperm) up to the time of fusion with that of another gamete in fertilization — see FEMALE PRONUCLEUS, MALE PRONUCLEUS

pro–oestrogen, pro–oestrous, pro–oestrum, pro–oestrus *chiefly Brit var of* PROESTROGEN, PROESTROUS, PROESTRUM, PROESTRUS

proof spirit \'prüf-\ *n* **1** : an alcoholic liquor or mixture of alcohol and water containing 50 percent ethanol by volume at 60° F (15.6° C) **2** *Brit* : liquor that weighs $^{12}\!/_{13}$ of an equal

\ə\ abut \ᵊ\ kitten \ər\ further \a\ ash \ā\ ace \ä\ cot, cart
\aú\ out \ch\ chin \e\ bet \ē\ easy \g\ go \i\ hit \ī\ ice \j\ job
\ŋ\ sing \ō\ go \ò\ law \òi\ boy \th\ thin \th\ the \ü\ loot
\ú\ foot \y\ yet \zh\ vision   *See also* Pronunciation Symbols page

measure of distilled water or contains 57.10 percent by volume of alcohol

prop·a·gate \\'präp-ə-ˌgāt\\ *vb* **-gat·ed; -gat·ing** *vt* **1** : to cause to continue or increase by sexual or asexual reproduction **2** : to cause to spread or to be transmitted ~ *vi* : to multiply sexually or asexually — **prop·a·ga·ble** \\'präp-ə-gə-bəl\\ *adj* — **prop·a·ga·tive** \\-ˌgāt-iv\\ *adj*

prop·a·ga·tion \\ˌpräp-ə-'gā-shən\\ *n* : the act or action of propagating: as **a** : increase (as of a kind of organism) in numbers ⟨~ of a pure culture of bacteria⟩ **b** : the spreading or transmission of something ⟨~ of a nerve impulse⟩

pro·pam·i·dine \\prō-'pam-ə-ˌdēn, -dən\\ *n* : an antiseptic drug $C_{17}H_{20}N_4O_2$

pro·pane \\'prō-ˌpān\\ *n* : a heavy flammable gaseous alkane C_3H_8 found in crude petroleum and natural gas and used esp. as fuel and in chemical synthesis

pro·pa·no·ic acid \\ˌprō-pə-ˌnō-ik-\\ *n* : PROPIONIC ACID

pro·pa·nol \\'prō-pə-ˌnȯl, -ˌnōl\\ *n* : PROPYL ALCOHOL

pro·pan·o·lol \\prō-'pan-ə-ˌlȯl, -ˌlōl\\ *n* : PROPRANOLOL

pro·pa·none \\'prō-pə-ˌnōn\\ *n* : ACETONE

pro·pan·the·line bromide \\prō-'pan-thə-ˌlēn-\\ *n* : an anticholinergic drug $C_{23}H_{30}BrNO_3$ used esp. in the treatment of peptic ulcer — called also *propantheline;* see PRO-BANTHINE

pro·par·a·caine \\prō-'par-ə-ˌkān\\ *n* : a drug used in the form of its hydrochloride $C_{16}H_{26}N_2O_3$·HCl as a topical anesthetic

Pro·pe·cia \\prō-'pē-sh(ē-)ə, prə-\\ *trademark* — used for a preparation of finasteride

pro·pene \\'prō-ˌpēn\\ *n* : PROPYLENE

pro·pe·nyl \\'prō-pə-ˌnil\\ *n* : a univalent unsaturated group $CH_3CH=CH–$ derived from propylene by removal of one hydrogen atom

pro·per·din \\prō-'pərd-ᵊn\\ *n* : a blood serum protein that participates in the activation of complement in a pathway which does not involve the presence of antibodies

pro·peri·to·ne·al \\(ˈ)prō-ˌper-ət-ᵊn-'ē-əl\\ *adj* : lying between the parietal peritoneum and the ventral musculature of the body cavity ⟨a ~ herniated mass⟩ ⟨~ fat⟩

pro·phage \\'prō-ˌfāj, -ˌfäzh\\ *n* : an intracellular form of a bacteriophage in which it is harmless to the host, is usu. integrated into the hereditary material of the host, and reproduces when the host does

pro·phase \\-ˌfāz\\ *n* **1** : the initial stage of mitosis and of the mitotic division of meiosis characterized by the condensation of chromosomes consisting of two chromatids, disappearance of the nucleolus and nuclear membrane, and formation of the mitotic spindle **2** : the initial stage of the first division of meiosis in which the chromosomes become visible, homologous pairs of chromosomes undergo synapsis and crossing-over, chiasmata appear, chromosomes condense with homologues visible as tetrads, and the nuclear membrane and nucleolus disappear and which is divided into the five consecutive stages leptotene, zygotene, pachytene, diplotene, and diakinesis — **pro·pha·sic** \\(ˈ)prō-'fā-zik\\ *adj*

¹pro·phy·lac·tic \\ˌprō-fə-'lak-tik *also* ˌpräf-ə-\\ *adj* **1** : guarding from or preventing the spread or occurrence of disease or infection ⟨~ therapy⟩ **2** : tending to prevent or ward off : PREVENTIVE — **pro·phy·lac·ti·cal·ly** \\-ti-k(ə-)lē\\ *adv*

²prophylactic *n* : something (as a medicinal preparation) that is prophylactic; *esp* : a device and esp. a condom for preventing venereal infection or conception

pro·phy·lax·is \\-'lak-səs\\ *n, pl* **-lax·es** \\-'lak-ˌsēz\\ : measures designed to preserve health and prevent the spread of disease : protective or preventive treatment ⟨~ against viral diseases⟩ ⟨a paste containing fluorine for dental ~⟩

pro·pio·lac·tone \\ˌprō-pē-ō-'lak-ˌtōn\\ *or* β**–pro·pio·lac·tone** \\ˌbāt-ə-\\ *n* : a liquid disinfectant $C_3H_4O_2$

pro·pi·o·ma·zine \\ˌprō-pē-'ō-mə-ˌzēn\\ *n* : a phenothiazine used esp. in the form of its hydrochloride $C_{20}H_{24}N_2OS$·HCl as a sedative

pro·pi·o·nate \\'prō-pē-ə-ˌnāt\\ *n* : a salt or ester of propionic acid

pro·pi·oni·bac·te·ri·um \\ˌprō-pē-ˌän-ə-bak-'tir-ē-əm\\ *n* **1** *cap* : a genus (the type of the family Propionibacteriaceae)

of gram-positive nonmotile usu. anaerobic bacteria that form propionic acid by fermenting lactic acid, carbohydrates, and polyalcohols and that include forms found esp. on human skin and in dairy products **2** *pl* **-ria** \\-ē-ə\\ : any bacterium of the genus *Propionibacterium*

pro·pi·on·ic acid \\ˌprō-pē-ˌän-ik-\\ *n* : a liquid sharp-odored fatty acid $C_3H_6O_2$ found in milk and distillates of wood, coal, and petroleum — called also *propanoic acid*

pro·pi·o·nyl \\'prō-pē-ə-ˌnil, -ˌnēl\\ *n* : the monovalent radical $C_2H_5CO–$ of propionic acid

pro·pio·phe·none \\ˌprō-pē-ō-'fē-ˌnōn, -'fen-ˌōn\\ *n* : a flowery-smelling compound $C_9H_{10}O$ used in perfumes and in the synthesis of pharmaceuticals (as ephedrine) and organic compounds

pro·plas·tid \\(ˈ)prō-'plas-təd\\ *n* : a minute cytoplasmic body from which a plastid is formed

pro·po·fol \\'prō-pō-ˌfȯl\\ *n* : a sedating and hypnotic agent $C_{12}H_{18}O$ administered in the form of an injectable emulsion to induce and maintain anesthesia or sedation

pro·pos·i·ta \\prō-'päz-ət-ə\\ *n, pl* **-i·tae** \\-ə-ˌtē\\ : a female proband

pro·pos·i·tus \\prō-'päz-ət-əs\\ *n, pl* **-i·ti** \\-ə-ˌtī\\ : PROBAND

pro·poxy·phene \\prō-'päk-sə-ˌfēn\\ *n* : a narcotic analgesic structurally related to methadone but less addicting that is administered in the form of its hydrochloride $C_{22}H_{29}NO_2$·HCl or hydrated napsylate $C_{22}H_{29}NO_2$·$C_{10}H_8SO_3$·H_2O — called also *dextropropoxyphene;* see DARVOCET-N, DARVON

pro·pran·o·lol \\prō-'pran-ə-ˌlȯl, -ˌlōl\\ *n* : a beta-blocker used in the form of its hydrochloride $C_{16}H_{21}NO_2$·HCl esp. in the treatment of hypertension, cardiac arrhythmias, and angina pectoris and in the prevention of migraine headache — called also *propanolol;* see INDERAL

propria — see LAMINA PROPRIA, SUBSTANTIA PROPRIA, TUNICA PROPRIA

¹pro·pri·e·tary \\p(r)ə-'prī-ə-ˌter-ē\\ *n, pl* **-tar·ies** : something that is used, produced, or marketed under exclusive legal right of the inventor or maker; *specif* : a drug (as a patent medicine) that is protected by secrecy, patent, or copyright against free competition as to name, product, composition, or process of manufacture

²proprietary *adj* **1** : used, made, or marketed by one having the exclusive legal right ⟨a ~ drug⟩ **2** : privately owned and managed and run as a profit-making organization ⟨a ~ clinic⟩

pro·prio·cep·tion \\ˌprō-prē-ō-'sep-shən\\ *n* : the reception of stimuli produced within the organism

pro·prio·cep·tive \\-'sep-tiv\\ *adj* : activated by, relating to, or being stimuli arising within the organism ⟨~ feedback⟩

proprioceptive neuromuscular facilitation *n* : a method of stretching muscles to maximize their flexibility that is often performed with a partner or trainer and that involves a series of contractions and relaxations with enforced stretching during the relaxation phase — abbr. *PNF*

pro·prio·cep·tor \\-'sep-tər\\ *n* : a sensory receptor that is located deep in the tissues (as in skeletal or heart muscle, tendons, the gastrointestinal wall, or the carotid sinus) and that functions in proprioception (as in response to changes of physical tension or chemical condition within the body)

pro·prio·spi·nal \\-'spīn-ᵊl\\ *adj* : distinctively or exclusively spinal ⟨a ~ neuron⟩

proprius — see EXTENSOR DIGITI QUINTI PROPRIUS, EXTENSOR INDICIS PROPRIUS

prop·tosed \\'präp-ˌtōst\\ *adj* : affected with proptosis ⟨a ~ eye⟩

pro·pto·sis \\(ˈ)prō-'tō-səs, präp-'tō-\\ *n, pl* **-pto·ses** \\-ˌsēz\\ : forward projection or displacement esp. of the eyeball

pro·pyl \\'prō-pəl\\ *n* : either of two isomeric alkyl groups C_3H_7 derived from propane — often used in combination

propyl alcohol *n* : either of two isomeric liquid alcohols C_3H_7OH: **a** : the normal alcohol $CH_3CH_2CH_2OH$ that is used chiefly as a solvent and in organic synthesis **b** : ISOPROPYL ALCOHOL

pro·pyl·amine \\ˌprō-pəl-ə-'mēn, -'am-ˌēn\\ *n* **1** : either of two flammable isomeric liquid bases $C_3H_7NH_2$ of ammoniacal fishy odor; *esp* : the normal amine $CH_3CH_2CH_2NH_2$ **2** : an amine in which propyl is attached to the nitrogen atom

pro·pyl·ene \'prō-pə-ˌlēn\ *n* : a flammable gaseous hydrocarbon C_3H_6 obtained by cracking petroleum hydrocarbons and used chiefly in organic synthesis — called also *propene*

propylene glycol *n* : a sweet hygroscopic viscous liquid $C_3H_8O_2$ made esp. from propylene and used esp. as an antifreeze and solvent, in brake fluids, and as a food preservative

propyl gallate *n* : a white crystalline antioxidant $C_{10}H_{12}O_5$ that is used as a preservative

pro·pyl·hex·e·drine \ˌprō-pəl-'hek-sə-ˌdrēn\ *n* : a sympathomimetic drug $C_{10}H_{21}N$ used chiefly as a nasal decongestant

pro·pyl·par·a·ben \-'par-ə-ˌben\ *n* : a crystalline ester $C_{10}H_{12}O_3$ used as a preservative in pharmaceutical and cosmetic preparations

pro·pyl·thio·ura·cil \-ˌthī-ō-'yùr-ə-ˌsil\ *n* : a crystalline compound $C_7H_{10}N_2OS$ used as an antithyroid drug in the treatment of goiter

pro·re·nin \prō-'rēn-ən, -'ren-\ *also* **pro·ren·nin** \-'ren-\ *n* : the precursor of the kidney enzyme renin

Pros·car \'präs-ˌkär\ *trademark* — used for a preparation of finasteride

pro·sco·lex \-'skō-ˌleks\ *n* : ONCOSPHERE

pro·se·cre·tin \(')prō-si-'krēt-ᵊn\ *n* : an inactive precursor of secretin

pro·sec·tor \prō-'sek-tər\ *n* : a person who makes dissections for anatomic demonstrations — **pro·sec·to·ri·al** \ˌpro-ˌsek-'tōr-ē-əl, -'tòr-\ *adj*

pros·en·ceph·a·lon \ˌpräs-ˌen-'sef-ə-ˌlän, -lən\ *n* : FOREBRAIN — **pros·en·ce·phal·ic** \-sə-'fal-ik\ *adj*

pros·op·ag·no·sia \ˌpräs-əp-ag-'nō-zhə\ *n* : a form of visual agnosia characterized by an inability to recognize faces

pros·o·pla·sia \ˌpräs-ə-'plā-zh(ē-)ə\ *n* **1** : differentiation of tissue; *esp* : abnormal differentiation **2** : organization of tissue toward a more complex state

pros·o·plas·tic \-'plas-tik\ *adj* : relating to or produced by prosoplasia

Pros·o·sto·ma·ta \ˌpräs-ə-'stō-mət-ə\ *n pl, in some classifications* : an order of Digenea comprising trematode worms with the mouth at or near the anterior end of the body

pro·spec·tive \prə-'spek-tiv\ *adj* : relating to or being a study (as of the incidence of disease) that starts with the present condition of a population of individuals and follows them into the future — compare RETROSPECTIVE — **pro·spec·tive·ly** \-lē\ *adv*

pros·ta·cy·clin \ˌpräs-tə-'sī-klən\ *n* : a prostaglandin that is a metabolite of arachidonic acid, inhibits aggregation of platelets, and dilates blood vessels

pros·ta·glan·din \ˌpräs-tə-'glan-dən\ *n* : any of various oxygenated unsaturated cyclic fatty acids of animals that are formed as cyclooxygenase metabolites esp. from unsaturated fatty acids (as arachidonic acid) composed of a chain of 20 carbon atoms and that perform a variety of hormonelike actions (as in controlling blood pressure or smooth muscle contraction)

prostaglandin E_1 \-'ē-'wən\ *n* : ALPROSTADIL

prostatae — see LEVATOR PROSTATAE

¹pros·tate \'präs-ˌtāt\ *n* : PROSTATE GLAND

²prostate *adj* : of, relating to, or being the prostate gland

pros·ta·tec·to·my \ˌpräs-tə-'tek-tə-mē\ *n, pl* **-mies** : surgical removal or resection of the prostate gland

prostate gland *n* : a firm partly muscular partly glandular body that is situated about the base of the mammalian male urethra and secretes an alkaline viscid fluid which is a major constituent of the ejaculatory fluid — called also *prostate*

prostate–specific antigen *n* : a protease that is secreted by the epithelial cells of the prostate and is used in the diagnosis of prostate cancer since its concentration in the blood serum tends to be proportional to the clinical stage of the disease — abbr. *PSA*

pros·tat·ic \prä-'stat-ik\ *adj* : of, relating to, or affecting the prostate gland ⟨∼ cancer⟩ ⟨∼ fluid⟩

prostatic intraepithelial neoplasia *n* : the formation of neoplastic epithelial cells in the prostate gland that are be-

lieved to be early precursors of adenocarcinoma — abbr. *PIN*

prostatic urethra *n* : the part of the male urethra from the base of the prostate gland where the urethra begins as the outlet of the bladder to the point where it emerges from the apex of the prostate gland

prostatic utricle *n* : a small blind pouch that projects from the wall of the prostatic urethra into the prostate gland

pros·ta·tism \'präs-tə-ˌtiz-əm\ *n* : disease of the prostate gland; *esp* : a disorder resulting from obstruction of the bladder neck by an enlarged prostate gland

pros·ta·ti·tis \ˌpräs-tə-'tīt-əs\ *n* : inflammation of the prostate gland

pros·ta·to·li·thot·o·my \ˌpräs-tə-(ˌ)tō-lith-'ät-ə-mē\ *n, pl* **-mies** : surgical removal of a calculus from the prostate gland

pros·ta·tor·rhea *or chiefly Brit* **pros·ta·tor·rhoea** \ˌpräs-tə-tə-'rē-ə\ *n* : an abnormal discharge of secretion from the prostate gland esp. when more or less continuous

pros·ta·tot·o·my \ˌpräs-tə-'tät-ə-mē\ *n, pl* **-mies** : surgical incision (as for drainage of an abscess) into the prostate gland

pros·ta·to·ve·sic·u·li·tis \ˌpräs-tə-(ˌ)tō-və-ˌsik-yə-'līt-əs\ *n* : inflammation of the prostate gland and the seminal vesicles

pros·the·sis \präs-'thē-səs, 'präs-thə-\ *n, pl* **-the·ses** \-ˌsēz\ : an artificial device to replace or augment a missing or impaired part of the body ⟨a dental ∼⟩ ⟨silicone breast and limb *prostheses*⟩

pros·thet·ic \präs-'thet-ik\ *adj* **1** : of, relating to, or being a prosthesis ⟨a ∼ device⟩ ⟨∼ limbs⟩; *also* : of or relating to prosthetics ⟨∼ research⟩ **2** : of, relating to, or constituting a nonprotein group of a conjugated protein — **pros·thet·i·cal·ly** \-i-k(ə-)lē\ *adv*

prosthetic dentistry *n* : PROSTHODONTICS

pros·thet·ics \-iks\ *n pl but sing or pl in constr* : the surgical and dental specialty concerned with the design, construction, and fitting of prostheses

prosthetic valve endocarditis *n* : endocarditis caused by or involving a surgically implanted prosthetic heart valve — abbr. *PVE*

pros·the·tist \'präs-thət-əst\ *n* : a specialist in prosthetics

pros·thi·on \'präs-thē-ˌän\ *n* : a point on the alveolar arch midway between the median upper incisor teeth — called also *alveolar point*

prosth·odon·tia \ˌpräs-thə-'dän-ch(ē-)ə\ *n* : PROSTHODONTICS

prosth·odon·tics \ˌpräs-thə-'dänt-iks\ *n pl but sing or pl in constr* : the dental specialty concerned with the making of artificial replacements for missing parts of the mouth and jaw — called also *prosthetic dentistry, prosthodontia* — **prosth·odon·tic** \-ik\ *adj*

prosth·odon·tist \-'dänt-əst\ *n* : a specialist in prosthodontics

Pros·tho·gon·i·mus \ˌpräs-thə-'gän-ə-məs\ *n* : a genus of trematode worms (family Plagiorchiidae) parasitic in the oviducts and bursa of Fabricius and rarely in the intestine or esophagus of domestic and other birds

Pro·stig·min \prō-'stig-mən\ *trademark* — used for a preparation of neostigmine

¹pros·trate \'präs-ˌtrāt\ *adj* : completely overcome ⟨was ∼ from the heat⟩

²prostrate *vt* **pros·trat·ed; pros·trat·ing** : to put into a state of extreme bodily exhaustion ⟨*prostrated* by fever⟩

pros·tra·tion \prä-'strā-shən\ *n* : complete physical or mental exhaustion — see HEAT EXHAUSTION

prot·ac·tin·i·um \ˌprōt-ˌak-'tin-ē-əm\ *also* **pro·to·ac·tin·i·um** \ˌprōt-ō-\ *n* : a shiny metallic radioelement of relatively short life — symbol *Pa*; see ELEMENT table

prot·amine \'prōt-ə-ˌmēn\ *n* : any of various strongly basic proteins of relatively low molecular weight that are rich in

---

\ə\ abut \ᵊ\ kitten \ər\ further \a\ ash \ā\ ace \ä\ cot, cart
\aù\ out \ch\ chin \e\ bet \ē\ easy \g\ go \i\ hit \ī\ ice \j\ job
\ŋ\ sing \ō\ go \ò\ law \òi\ boy \th\ thin \th\ the \ü\ loot
\ù\ foot \y\ yet \zh\ vision *See also* Pronunciation Symbols page

arginine and are found associated esp. with DNA in place of histone in the sperm of various animals (as fish)

protamine zinc insulin *n* : a combination of protamine, zinc, and insulin used in suspension in water for subcutaneous injection in place of insulin because of its prolonged effect — abbr. *PZI*

prot·anom·a·lous \ˌprōt-ə-ˈnäm-ə-ləs\ *adj* : characterized by protanomaly ⟨∼ vision⟩

prot·anom·a·ly \-lē\ *n, pl* **-lies** : deficient color vision in which an abnormally large proportion of red is required to match the spectrum — compare DEUTERANOMALY, TRICHROMATISM

pro·ta·nope \ˈprōt-ə-ˌnōp\ *n* : an individual affected with protanopia

prot·an·opia \ˌprōt-ə-ˈnō-pē-ə\ *n* : a dichromatism in which the spectrum is seen in tones of yellow and blue with confusion of red and green and reduced sensitivity to monochromatic lights from the red end of the spectrum

¹pro·te·an \ˈprōt-ē-ən, prō-ˈtē-\ *adj* : displaying great diversity or variety ⟨a disease with ∼ clinical manifestations⟩

²pro·te·an \ˈprōt-ē-ən\ *n* : any of various insoluble primary protein derivatives that result from a slight modification of the protein molecule esp. by the action of water, very dilute acids, or enzymes

pro·te·ase \ˈprōt-ē-ˌās, -ˌāz\ *n* : any of numerous enzymes that hydrolyze proteins and are classified according to the most prominent functional group (as serine or cysteine) at the active site — called also *proteinase;* compare PEPTIDASE

protease inhibitor *n* : a substance that inhibits the action of a protease; *specif* : any of various drugs (as indinavir or saquinavir) that inhibit the action of HIV protease so that cleavage of viral proteins into mature infectious particles is prevented and that are used esp. in combination with other antiretroviral agents in the treatment of HIV infection

¹pro·tec·tive \prə-ˈtek-tiv\ *adj* : serving to protect the body or one of its parts from disease or injury ⟨a ∼ reflex⟩

²protective *n* : an agent (as a medicine or a dressing) that protects the body or one of its parts (as from irritation or injury) ⟨vitamins are ∼s against certain deficiency diseases⟩

protective colloid *n* : a lyophilic colloid (as gelatin, a natural gum, or a cellulose derivative) that when present in small quantities keeps lyophobic colloids from precipitating under the coagulating action of electrolytes

pro·te·ic \prō-ˈtē-ik\ *adj* : PROTEINACEOUS

pro·teid \ˈprōt-ē-əd, ˈprō-ˌtēd\ *n* : PROTEIN 1

pro·tei·i·form \prō-ˈtē-ə-ˌfòrm\ *adj* : PROTEAN

pro·tein \ˈprō-ˌtēn, ˈprōt-ē-ən\ *n, often attrib* **1** : any of numerous naturally occurring extremely complex substances (as an enzyme or antibody) that consist of amino acid residues joined by peptide bonds, contain the elements carbon, hydrogen, nitrogen, oxygen, usu. sulfur, and occas. other elements (as phosphorus or iron), that are essential constituents of all living cells, that are synthesized from raw materials by plants but assimilated as separate amino acids by animals, that are both acidic and basic and usu. colloidal in nature although many have been crystallized, and that are hydrolyzable by acids, alkalies, proteolytic enzymes, and putrefactive bacteria to polypeptides, to simpler peptides, and ultimately to alpha-amino acids **2** : the total nitrogenous material in plant or animal substances — *esp* : CRUDE PROTEIN

pro·tein·aceous \ˌprōt-ᵊn-ˈā-shəs, ˌprō-ˌtēn-, ˌprōt-ē-ən-\ *adj* : of, relating to, resembling, or being protein ⟨∼ materials⟩

pro·tein·ase \ˈprōt-ᵊn-ˌās, ˈprō-ˌtēn-, ˈprōt-ē-ən-, -ˌāz\ *n* : PROTEASE

pro·tein·ate \-ˌāt\ *n* : a compound of a protein ⟨silver ∼⟩

protein–bound iodine *n* : the amount of iodine expressed in micrograms per 100 milliliters of blood serum that is precipitated with serum proteins and that serves as a measure of the activity of the thyroid gland ⟨the *protein-bound iodine* in the normal human being ranges from 4 to 8 micrograms, in hypothyroidism falls below this range, and in hyperthyroidism rises above it⟩

protein hydrolysate *n* : a mixture of amino acids obtained by the hydrolysis of various animal and plant proteins (as

lactalbumin or soybean protein) and used as a source of amino acids, as a seasoning agent, and in nutrition

pro·tein·ic \prō-ˈtē-nik, ˌprōt-ē-ˈin-ik\ *adj* : PROTEINACEOUS

protein kinase *n* : any of a class of allosteric enzymes that possess a catalytic subunit which transfers a phosphate from ATP to one or more amino acid residues (as serine, threonine, or tyrosine) in a protein's side chain resulting in a conformational change affecting protein function, that play a role in regulating intracellular processes, and that include many which are activated by the binding of a second messenger (as cyclic AMP)

protein kinase C \-ˈsē\ *n* : any of a group of isoenzymes of protein kinase that modify the conformation and activity of various intracellular proteins by catalyzing the phosphorylation of specific serine or threonine amino acid residues in the polypeptide chains of the proteins — abbr. *PKC*

pro·tein·oid \ˈprō-ˌtē-ˌnòid, ˈprōt-ē-ə-ˌnòid, ˈprōt-ᵊn-ˌòid\ *n* : any of various polypeptides which can be obtained by suitable polymerization of mixtures of amino acids

pro·tein·o·sis \ˌprō-ˌtē-ˈnō-səs, -tē-ə-\ *n, pl* **-o·ses** \-ˌsēz\ *or* **-o·sis·es** : the accumulation of abnormal amounts of protein in bodily tissues — see PULMONARY ALVEOLAR PROTEINOSIS

protein shock *n* : a severe reaction produced by the injection of protein (as bacterial or animal proteins) and marked by chills, fever, bronchial spasm, acute emphysema, vomiting, and diarrhea

protein silver *n* : SILVER PROTEIN

pro·tein·uria \ˌprōt-ᵊn-ˈ(y)ùr-ē-ə, ˌprō-ˌtēn-, ˌprōt-ē-ən-\ *n* : the presence of excess protein in the urine — **pro·tein·uric** \-ˈ(y)ùr-ik\ *adj*

pro·teo·clas·tic \ˌprōt-ē-ō-ˈklas-tik\ *adj* : PROTEOLYTIC

pro·teo·gly·can \ˌprōt-ē-ə-ˈglī-ˌkan\ *n* : any of a class of glycoproteins of high molecular weight that are found in the extracellular matrix of connective tissue, are made up mostly of carbohydrate consisting of various polysaccharide side chains linked to a protein, and resemble polysaccharides rather than proteins in their properties

pro·teo·lip·id \-ˈlip-əd\ *also* **pro·teo·lip·ide** \-ˈlip-ˌīd\ *n* : any of a class of proteins that contain a considerable percentage of lipid and are soluble in lipids and insoluble in water

pro·te·ol·y·sin \ˌprōt-ē-ˈäl-ə-sən, -ē-ə-ˈlīs-ᵊn\ *n* : a lysin (as an enzyme) producing proteolysis

pro·te·ol·y·sis \ˌprōt-ē-ˈäl-ə-səs\ *n, pl* **-y·ses** \-ˌsēz\ : the hydrolysis of proteins or peptides with formation of simpler and soluble products (as in digestion)

pro·teo·lyt·ic \ˌprōt-ē-ə-ˈlit-ik\ *adj* : of, relating to, or producing proteolysis ⟨∼ enzymes⟩ — **pro·teo·lyt·i·cal·ly** \-i-k(ə-)lē\ *adv*

pro·teo·lyzed *or Brit* **pro·teo·lysed** \ˈprōt-ē-ə-ˌlīzd\ *adj* : having been subjected to proteolysis ⟨∼ liver⟩

pro·te·ome \ˈprōt-ē-ˌōm\ *n* : the complement of proteins expressed in a cell, tissue, or organism by a genome

pro·te·o·mics \ˌprōt-ē-ˈō-miks\ *n pl but sing in constr* : a branch of biotechnology concerned with applying the techniques of molecular biology, biochemistry, and genetics to analyzing the structure, function, and interactions of the proteins produced by the genes of a particular cell, tissue, or organism, with organizing the information in databases, and with applications of the data (as in medicine or biology) — compare GENOMICS — **pro·te·o·mic** \-mik\ *adj*

pro·te·ose \ˈprōt-ē-ˌōs\ *n* : any of various protein derivatives that are formed by the partial hydrolysis of proteins (as by enzymes of the gastric and pancreatic juices), that are not coagulated by heat, and that are soluble in water but are precipitated from solution by saturation with ammonium sulfate — compare PEPTONE 1

protest — see MASCULINE PROTEST

pro·te·us \ˈprōt-ē-əs\ *n* **1** *cap* : a genus of aerobic gramnegative bacteria of the family Enterobacteriaceae that ferment glucose but not lactose and decompose urea, that are usu. motile by means of peritrichous flagella, and that include saprophytes in decaying organic matter and a common causative agent (*P. mirabilis*) of urinary tract infections **2** *pl* **-tei** \-ˌī\ : any bacterium of the genus *Proteus*

Proteus, Greek mythological character. Proteus was an ancient god of the sea and sometimes identified as a son of Poseidon. His job was to herd Poseidon's flocks of seals and other sea creatures. Possessed of the gift of prophecy, he was generally unwilling to share his knowledge and would escape his questioners by assuming a variety of shapes, including fire and water and the forms of wild beasts.

proth·e·sis \'präth-ə-səs\ *n, pl* **-e·ses** \-ˌsēz\ : PROSTHESIS — **pro·thet·ic** \prä-'thet-ik\ *adj*

pro·throm·base \(')prō-'thräm-ˌbās, -ˌbāz\ *n* : PROTHROM-BIN

pro·throm·bin \(')prō-'thräm-bən\ *n* : a plasma protein produced in the liver in the presence of vitamin K and converted into thrombin by the action of various activators (as thromboplastin) in the clotting of blood — **pro·throm·bic** \-bik\ *adj*

pro·throm·bino·pe·nia \ˌprō-ˌthräm-bin-ə-'pē-nē-ə\ *n* : HY-POPROTHROMBINEMIA

prothrombin time *n* : the time required for a particular specimen of prothrombin to induce blood-plasma clotting under standardized conditions in comparison with a time of between 11.5 and 12 seconds for normal human blood

pro·tide \'prō-ˌtīd, -təd\ *n* : any of a class of compounds comprising the proteins and their hydrolysis products (as amino acids, amines, and amides)

pro·ti·re·lin \prō-'tī-rə-lən\ *n* : THYROTROPIN-RELEASING HORMONE

pro·tist \'prōt-əst, 'prō-ˌtist\ *n* : any of a diverse taxonomic group and esp. a kingdom (Protista syn. Protoctista) of eukaryotic organisms that are unicellular and sometimes colonial or less often multicellular and that typically include the protozoans, most algae, and often some fungi (as slime molds) — **pro·tis·tan** \prō-'tis-tən\ *adj or n*

Pro·tis·ta \prō-'tis-tə\ *n pl* : a major taxonomic group and esp. a kingdom comprising the protists

pro·tis·tol·o·gy \ˌprō-tis-'täl-ə-jē\ *n, pl* **-gies** : a branch of biology concerned with protists — **pro·tis·to·log·i·cal** \prə-ˌtis-tə-'läj-i-kəl\ *adj*

pro·ti·um \'prōt-ē-əm, 'prō-shē-\ *n* : the ordinary light hydrogen isotope of atomic mass 1

protoactinium *var of* PROTACTINIUM

pro·to·cate·chu·ic acid \ˌprōt-ō-ˌkat-ə-ˌkyü-ik-, -ˌchü-\ *n* : a crystalline acid $C_7H_6O_4$ produced from various resins and found in combination in many plant products

pro·to·col \'prōt-ə-ˌkȯl, -ˌkōl, -ˌkäl\ *n* **1** : an official account of a proceeding; *esp* : the notes or records relating to a case, an experiment, or an autopsy **2** : a detailed plan of a scientific or medical experiment, treatment, or procedure ⟨cryotherapy was performed in approximately half of the eyes through a randomization ∼ —*Jour. Amer. Med. Assoc.*⟩

pro·to·cone \'prōt-ō-ˌkōn\ *n* : the central of the three cusps of a primitive upper molar that in higher forms is the principal anterior and internal cusp

pro·to·co·nid \ˌprōt-ō-'kō-nəd\ *n* : an anterior and external cusp of a lower molar that corresponds to the protocone

pro·to·di·as·to·le \ˌprōt-ō-dī-'as-tə-(ˌ)lē\ *n* **1** : the period just before aortic valve closure **2** : the period just after aortic valve closure

pro·to·di·a·stol·ic \-ˌdī-ə-'stäl-ik\ *adj* **1** : of or relating to the early phase of diastole **2** : of or relating to protodiastole

pro·to·fil·a·ment \-'fil-ə-mənt\ *n* : one of several filaments composing a subunit of a microtubule

pro·to·gen \'prōt-ə-jən, -ˌjen\ *n* : LIPOIC ACID

pro·to·heme *or chiefly Brit* **pro·to·haem** \'prōt-ō-ˌhēm\ *n* : HEME

pro·to·he·min *or chiefly Brit* **pro·to·hae·min** \-ˌhē-mən\ *n* : HEMIN

pro·tom·er·ite \prō-'täm-ə-ˌrīt\ *n* : the smaller anterior part of the trophozoite of a gregarine

pro·to·mo·nad \ˌprōt-ō-'mō-ˌnad, -'män-əd\ *n* : KINETO-PLASTID — **protomonad** *adj*

Pro·to·mon·a·di·na \-ˌmän-ə-'dī-nə, -dē-\ *n pl, syn of* KI-NETOPLASTIDA

pro·ton \'prō-ˌtän\ *n* : an elementary particle that is identical with the nucleus of the hydrogen atom, that along with neutrons is a constituent of all other atomic nuclei, that carries a positive charge numerically equal to the charge of an electron, and that has a mass of 1.673×10^{-24} gram — **pro·ton·ic** \prō-'tän-ik\ *adj*

Pro·to·nix \'prōt-ə-ˌniks\ *trademark* — used for a preparation of the sodium salt of pantoprazole

proton pump *n* : a molecular mechanism that transports hydrogen ions across cell membranes

proton pump inhibitor *n* : any of a group of drugs (as omeprazole) that inhibit the activity of proton pumps and are used to inhibit gastric acid secretion in the treatment of ulcers and gastroesophageal reflux disease — abbr. *PPI*

pro·to—on·co·gene \ˌprōt-ō-'äŋ-kə-ˌjēn\ *n* : a gene having the potential for change into an active oncogene

Pro·to·pam \'prōt-ə-ˌpam\ *trademark* — used for a preparation of pralidoxime

pro·to·path·ic \ˌprōt-ə-'path-ik\ *adj* : of, relating to, being, or mediating cutaneous sensory reception that is responsive only to rather gross stimuli — compare EPICRITIC

pro·to·pec·tin \-'pek-tᵊn\ *n* : any of a group of water-insoluble pectic substances occurring in plants and yielding pectin or pectinic acids on hydrolysis — called also *pectose*

pro·to·pine \'prōt-ə-ˌpēn\ *n* : a crystalline alkaloid $C_{20}H_{19}NO_5$ found in small quantities in opium and in many plants of the poppy family

pro·to·plasm \'prōt-ə-ˌplaz-əm\ *n* **1** : the organized colloidal complex of organic and inorganic substances (as proteins and water) that constitutes the living nucleus, cytoplasm, plastids, and mitochondria of the cell and is regarded as the only form of matter in which the vital phenomena (as metabolism and reproduction) are manifested **2** : CYTOPLASM

pro·to·plas·mat·ic \ˌprōt-ə-ˌplaz-'mat-ik\ *adj* : PROTOPLAS-MIC

pro·to·plas·mic \-'plaz-mik\ *adj* : of, relating to, consisting of, or resembling protoplasm

pro·to·plast \'prōt-ə-ˌplast\ *n* : the nucleus, cytoplasm, and plasma membrane of a cell as distinguished from inert walls and inclusions

pro·to·por·phyr·ia \ˌprōt-ō-pȯr-'fir-ē-ə\ *n* : the presence of protoporphyrin in the blood — see ERYTHROPOIETIC PRO-TOPORPHYRIA

pro·to·por·phy·rin \ˌprōt-ō-'pȯr-f(ə-)rən\ *n* : a purple porphyrin acid $C_{34}H_{34}N_4O_4$ obtained from hemin or heme by removal of bound iron

Pro·to·stron·gy·lus \-'strän-jə-ləs\ *n* : a genus of lungworms of the family Metastrongylidae including one (*P. rufescens*) parasitic esp. in sheep and goats — **pro·to·stron·gyle** \-'strän-ˌjil, -jəl\ *n* — **pro·to·stron·gy·line** \-jə-ˌlēn, -ˌlīn\ *adj*

pro·to·tax·ic \-'tak-sik\ *adj* : relating to or being thinking that is lacking in self-awareness and in perception of temporal sequence — compare PARATAXIC

Pro·to·the·ca \ˌprōt-ə-'thē-kə\ *n* : a genus of unicellular algae that resemble algae of the genus *Chlorella* but lack chlorophyll and that include two (*P. zopfii* and *P. wickerhamii*) that cause mastitis in cows and sometimes localized infection (as of the skin) in humans

pro·to·the·co·sis \-thē-'kō-səs\ *n, pl* **-co·ses** \-ˌsēz\ : an infection produced by an alga of the genus *Prototheca*

pro·to·troph \'prōt-ə-ˌtrōf, -ˌträf\ *n* : a prototrophic individual

pro·to·tro·phic \ˌprōt-ə-'trō-fik\ *adj* **1** : deriving nutriment from inorganic sources ⟨∼ bacteria⟩ **2** : not requiring specific nutritional substances for normal metabolism and reproduction : not differing from the wild type in nutritional requirements — used esp. of bacteria and fungi ⟨a yeast ∼ for uracil and leucine⟩; compare AUXOTROPHIC — **pro·tot·ro·phy** \prō-'tä-trə-fē\ *n, pl* **-phies**

\ə\ **abut** \ᵊ\ **kitten** \ər\ **further** \a\ **ash** \ā\ **ace** \ä\ **cot, cart**
\aú\ **out** \ch\ **chin** \e\ **bet** \ē\ **easy** \g\ **go** \i\ **hit** \ī\ **ice** \j\ **job**
\ŋ\ **sing** \ō\ **go** \ȯ\ **law** \ȯi\ **boy** \th\ **thin** \t͟h\ **the** \ü\ **loot**
\ú\ **foot** \y\ **yet** \zh\ **vision** *See also* Pronunciation Symbols page

pro·tot·ro·py \prō-'tä-trə-pē\ *n, pl* **-pies** : tautomerism involving the migration of a proton esp. to a location three atoms distant in an organic molecule — compare ANIONOTROPY, CATIONOTROPY — **pro·to·tro·pic** \ˌprōt-ə-'trō-pik\ *adj*

pro·to·ver·a·trine \ˌprōt-ō-'ver-ə-ˌtrēn, -trən\ *n* **1** : either of two toxic crystalline alkaloids obtained from hellebores of the genus *Veratrum* (esp. *V. viride* of No. America and *V. album* of Europe) and used in the treatment of hypertension — called also respectively *protoveratrine A, protoveratrine B* **2** : a mixture of protoveratrine A and B used to treat hypertension

protozoa *pl of* PROTOZOON

Pro·to·zoa \ˌprōt-ə-'zō-ə\ *n pl* : a phylum or subkingdom of chiefly motile unicellular protists (as amebas, trypanosomes, sporozoans, and paramecia) that consist of a protoplasmic body either naked or enclosed in an outer covering, that have holophytic, saprophytic, or holozoic modes of nourishment, that reproduce asexually by nuclear division usu. with a more or less modified mitosis associated with cytoplasmic binary fission or with multiple fission or budding or often sexually by various means, that have the life cycle simple (as in an ameba) or extremely complex (as in many sporozoans), that are represented in almost every kind of habitat, and that include pathogenic parasites of humans and domestic animals — compare METAZOA 1

pro·to·zo·a·ci·dal \ˌprōt-ə-ˌzō-ə-'sīd-ᵊl\ *adj* : destroying protozoans

pro·to·zo·a·cide \-'zō-ə-ˌsīd\ *n* : an agent that destroys protozoans

pro·to·zo·al \ˌprōt-ə-'zō-əl\ *adj* : of or relating to protozoans

¹**pro·to·zo·an** \-'zō-ən\ *n* : any protist of the phylum or subkingdom Protozoa

²**protozoan** *adj* : of or relating to the phylum or subkingdom Protozoa

pro·to·zo·i·a·sis \ˌprōt-ə-zō-'ī-ə-səs\ *n, pl* **-a·ses** \-ˌsēz\ : infection with or disease caused by protozoan parasites

pro·to·zo·ol·o·gist \-zō-'äl-ə-jəst\ *n* : a specialist in protozoology

pro·to·zo·ol·o·gy \-zō-'äl-ə-jē\ *n, pl* **-gies** : a branch of zoology dealing with protozoans — **pro·to·zoo·log·i·cal** \-ˌzō-ə-'läj-i-kəl\ *adj*

pro·to·zo·on \ˌprōt-ə-'zō-ˌän\ *n, pl* **pro·to·zoa** : PROTOZOAN

pro·tract \prō-'trakt\ *vt* : to extend forward or outward ⟨the mandible is ~ed and retracted in chewing⟩ — compare RETRACT

pro·trac·tion \-'trak-shən\ *n* **1** : the act of moving an anatomical part forward **2** : the state of being protracted; *esp* : protrusion of the jaws

pro·trac·tor \-tər\ *n* : a muscle that extends a part — compare RETRACTOR b

pro·trip·ty·line \prō-'trip-tə-ˌlēn\ *n* : a tricyclic antidepressant drug C₁₉H₂₁N — see VIVACTIL

pro·trude \prō-'trüd\ *vb* **pro·trud·ed; pro·trud·ing** *vt* : to cause to project ⟨the mentalis raises and ~s the lower lip —*Gray's Anatomy*⟩ ~ *vi* : to jut out from the surrounding surface

pro·tru·sion \prō-'trü-zhən\ *n* **1** : the quality or state of protruding ⟨the ~ of a jaw⟩ **2** : something (as an anatomical part) that protrudes

pro·tru·sive \-'trü-siv, -ziv\ *adj* **1** : thrusting forward ⟨~ movements of the jaw⟩ **2** : PROMINENT, PROTUBERANT ⟨a ~ jaw⟩

pro·tu·ber·ance \prō-'t(y)ü-b(ə-)rən(t)s\ *n* **1** : something that is protuberant ⟨a bony ~⟩ **2** : the quality or state of being protuberant

protuberans — see DERMATOFIBROSARCOMA PROTUBERANS

pro·tu·ber·ant \-b(ə-)rənt\ *adj* : bulging beyond the surrounding or adjacent surface : PROMINENT ⟨~ eyes⟩

proud flesh *n* : an excessive growth of granulation tissue (as in an ulcer)

Proust's law \'prüsts-\ *n* : LAW OF DEFINITE PROPORTIONS

   Proust \prüst\, **Joseph–Louis (1754–1826),** French chem-

ist. Proust spent the major part of his professional life in Spain where he taught chemistry and undertook laboratory research. He was an outstanding chemical analyst. In his use of quantitative methods he consistently gave the results of his analyses in terms of percentage weight composition and sometimes the weight of oxygen or sulfur in comparison with the constant weight of the metal under analysis. In 1808 he proved that the relative quantities of any given pure chemical compound's constituent elements remain constant, regardless of the source of the compound. He thereby provided important evidence to support John Dalton's law of definite proportions.

Pro·ven·til \prō-'ven-til\ *trademark* — used for a preparation of the sulfate of albuterol

pro·ven·tric·u·li·tis \ˌprō-ven-ˌtrik-yə-'līt-əs\ *n* : inflammation of the proventriculus of a bird usu. due to nutritional deficiencies or to parasitism

pro·ven·tric·u·lus \ˌprō-ven-'trik-yə-ləs\ *n, pl* **-li** \-ˌlī, -ˌlē\ : the glandular or true stomach of a bird that is situated between the crop and gizzard

pro·vi·ral \(')prō-'vī-rəl\ *adj* : of, relating to, or being a provirus ⟨~ DNA⟩

pro·vi·rus \(')prō-'vī-rəs\ *n* : a form of a virus that is integrated into the genetic material of a host cell and by replicating with it can be transmitted from one cell generation to the next without causing lysis

pro·vi·ta·min \(')prō-'vīt-ə-mən\ *n* : a precursor of a vitamin convertible into the vitamin in an organism ⟨ergosterol is a ~ of vitamin D⟩

provitamin A *n* : a provitamin of vitamin A; *esp* : CAROTENE

prov·o·ca·tion \ˌpräv-ə-'kā-shən\ *n* : the act or process of provoking ⟨a nonspecific irritant that brings about ~ of bronchial asthma⟩

pro·voc·a·tive \prə-'väk-ət-iv\ *adj* : serving or tending to provoke, excite, or stimulate ⟨~ test for coronary spasm —*Jour. Amer. Med. Assoc.*⟩

Pro·vo·cho·line \ˌprō-və-'kō-ˌlēn\ *trademark* — used for a preparation of the chloride of methacholine

pro·voke \prə-'vōk\ *vt* **pro·voked; pro·vok·ing** : to induce (a physical reaction) ⟨ipecac ~s vomiting⟩

prox·e·mics \präk-'sē-miks\ *n pl but sing or pl in constr* : the study of the nature, degree, and effect of the spatial separation individuals naturally maintain (as in various social and interpersonal situations) and of how this separation relates to environmental and cultural factors — **prox·e·mic** \-mik\ *adj*

prox·i·mad \'präk-sə-ˌmad\ *adv* : PROXIMALLY ⟨viable small bowel was clamped ~ —*Jour. Amer. Med. Assoc.*⟩

prox·i·mal \'präk-sə-məl\ *adj* **1 a** : situated next to or near the point of attachment or origin or a central point ⟨the ~ was . . . better than the peripheral stump for a graft —*Annual Rev. of Med.*⟩; *esp* : located toward the center of the body ⟨the ~ end of a bone⟩ — compare DISTAL 1a **b** : of, relating to, or being the mesial and distal surfaces of a tooth **2** : sensory rather than physical or social ⟨~ stimuli⟩ — compare DISTAL 2 — **prox·i·mal·ly** \-ē\ *adv*

proximal convoluted tubule *n* : the convoluted portion of the vertebrate nephron that lies between Bowman's capsule and the loop of Henle, is made up of a single layer of cuboidal cells with striated borders, and functions esp. in the resorption of sugar, sodium and chloride ions, and water from the glomerular filtrate — called also *proximal tubule*

proximal radioulnar joint *n* : a pivot joint between the upper end of the radius and the ring formed by the radial notch of the ulna and its annular ligament that permits rotation of the proximal head of the radius — called also *superior radioulnar joint*

proximal tubule *n* : PROXIMAL CONVOLUTED TUBULE

prox·i·mate \'präk-sə-mət\ *adj* **1 a** : very near **b** : next, preceding, or following; *esp* : relating to or being a proximate cause **2** : determined by proximate analysis **3** : PROXIMAL 1b — **prox·i·mate·ly** *adv*

proximate analysis *n* : quantitative analysis of a mixture (as food) to determine the percentage of components

proximate cause *n* : a cause that directly or with no intervening agency produces an effect ⟨whether the negligence was the *proximate cause* of the pneumonia —*Jour. Amer. Med. Assoc.*⟩

prox·i·mo·lin·gual \ˌpräk-sə-mō-ˈliŋ-g(yə-)wəl\ *adj* : of or relating to the proximal and lingual surfaces of a tooth

Pro·zac \ˈprō-ˌzak\ *trademark* — used for a preparation of the hydrochloride of fluoxetine

pro·zone \ˈprō-ˌzōn\ *n* : the portion of the range of concentration of antibody-antigen mixtures in which one of them although present in excess does not produce its characteristic effect (as agglutination or precipitation)

prozone phenomenon *n* : the reduction in characteristic effect exhibited in the prozone of antibody-antigen mixtures — called also *prozone effect*

PrP *abbr* prion protein

pru·lau·ra·sin \prü-ˈlȯr-ə-sən\ *n* : a cyanogenetic glucoside $C_{14}H_{17}NO_6$ found in the leaves of a European evergreen shrub of the genus *Prunus* (*P. laurocerasus*)

pru·nase \ˈprü-ˌnās\ *n* : an enzyme that accelerates the hydrolysis of prunasin, is found in yeast and in bitter almonds, and is one of two enzymes concerned in the hydrolysis of amygdalin

pru·na·sin \ˈprü-nə-sən\ *n* : a crystalline cyanogenetic glucoside $C_{14}H_{17}NO_6$ found in various plants of the genus *Prunus* and obtained by partial hydrolysis of amygdalin by the enzyme prunase

prune \ˈprün\ *n* : a plum dried or capable of drying without fermentation and often used as a food and as a mild laxative

Pru·nus \ˈprü-nəs\ *n* : a genus of trees and shrubs of the rose family (Rosaceae) that are widely distributed in temperate regions, have showy clusters of usu. white or pink flowers, and include many whose fruit (as the plum, cherry, peach, or apricot) is used for food

pru·rig·i·nous \prü-ˈrij-ə-nəs\ *adj* : resembling, caused by, affected with, or being prurigo ⟨∼ dermatosis⟩

pru·ri·go \prü-ˈrī-(ˌ)gō\ *n* : a chronic inflammatory skin disease marked by a general eruption of small itching papules

pru·rit·ic \-ˈrit-ik\ *adj* : of, relating to, or marked by itching

pru·ri·tus \prü-ˈrīt-əs\ *n* : localized or generalized itching due to irritation of sensory nerve endings — ITCH

pruritus ani \-ˈā-ˌnī\ *n* : pruritus of the anal region

pruritus vul·vae \-ˈvəl-vē\ *n* : pruritus of the vulva

Prus·sian blue \ˈprəsh-ən-ˈblü\ *n* **1** : any of numerous blue iron pigments formerly regarded as the ferric salt of ferrocyanide **2** : a dark blue crystalline hydrated compound $Fe_4[Fe(CN)_6]_3 \cdot xH_2O$ that is a ferrocyanide of iron and is used as a test for ferric iron — called also *ferric ferrocyanide*

prus·si·ate \ˈprəs-ē-ˌāt\ *n* **1** : a salt of hydrocyanic acid : CYANIDE **2 a** : FERROCYANIDE 2 **b** : FERRICYANIDE 2

prus·sic acid \ˌprəs-ik-\ *n* : HYDROCYANIC ACID

ps *abbr* picosecond

PSA *abbr* prostate-specific antigen

psal·te·ri·um \sȯl-ˈtir-ē-əm\ *n, pl* **-ria** \-ē-ə\ **1** : OMASUM **2** : HIPPOCAMPAL COMMISSURE

psam·mo·ma \sa-ˈmō-mə\ *n, pl* **-mas** *or* **-ma·ta** \-mət-ə\ : a hard fibrous tumor of the meninges of the brain and spinal cord containing calcareous matter — **psam·mo·ma·tous** \sa-ˈmō-mət-əs, -ˈmä-\ *adj*

pseud·ar·thro·sis \ˌsüd-är-ˈthrō-səs\ *also* **pseu·do·ar·thro·sis** \ˌsüd-ō-\ *n, pl* **-thro·ses** \-ˈthrō-ˌsēz\ : an abnormal union formed by fibrous tissue between parts of a bone that has fractured usu. spontaneously due to congenital weakness — called also *false joint*

pseud·en·ceph·a·ly \ˌsüd-in-ˈsef-ə-lē\ *n, pl* **-lies** : a severe congenital malformation characterized by the presence of a vascular tumorous mass in place of the brain and the partial or complete absence of the upper part of the skull

pseu·do·acon·i·tine \ˌsüd-ō-ə-ˈkän-ə-ˌtēn, -tən\ *n* : a very poisonous crystallizable alkaloid $C_{36}H_{51}NO_{12}$ found in the root of a plant of the genus *Aconitum* (*A. ferox*)

pseu·do·ag·glu·ti·na·tion \-ə-ˌglüt-ᵊn-ˈā-shən\ *n* : the forming of rouleaux by red blood cells

pseu·do·al·lele \ˌsüd-ō-ə-ˈlē(ə)l\ *n* : any of two or more closely linked genes that act usu. as if a single member of an allelic pair but occas. undergo crossing-over and recombination — **pseu·do·al·le·lic** \-ˈlē-lik, -ˈlel-ik\ *adj* — **pseu·do·al·lel·ism** \-ˈlē(ə)l-ˌiz-əm, -ˈlel-ˌiz-\ *n*

pseu·do·an·eu·rysm \-ˈan-yə-ˌriz-əm\ *n* : a vascular abnormality (as an elongation or buckling of the aorta) that resembles an aneurysm in radiography

pseu·do·ap·pen·di·ci·tis \-ə-ˌpen-də-ˈsīt-əs\ *n* : a condition having symptoms like those of appendicitis but not resulting from inflammation of the appendix

pseudoarthrosis *var of* PSEUDARTHROSIS

pseu·do·bul·bar \-ˈbəl-bər\ *adj* : simulating that (as bulbar paralysis) which is caused by lesions of the medulla oblongata ⟨∼ paralysis⟩

pseu·do·cho·lin·es·ter·ase \ˌsüd-ō-ˌkō-lə-ˈnes-tə-ˌrās, -ˌrāz\ *n* : CHOLINESTERASE 2

pseu·do·chrom·es·the·sia *or chiefly Brit* **pseu·do·chrom·aes·the·sia** \-ˌkrō-mes-ˈthē-zh(ē-)ə\ *n* : association of sounds with certain colors; *specif* : the production of a colored visual sensation in response to certain sounds

pseu·do·co·arc·ta·tion \-(ˌ)kō-ˌärk-ˈtā-shən\ *n* : a congenital abnormality of the aorta that resembles aortic coarctation in radiography but does not significantly block the flow of blood

pseu·do·coel *also* **pseu·do·cele** *or* **pseu·do·coele** \ˈsüd-ō-ˌsēl\ *n* : a body cavity (as in various worms) that is not the product of gastrulation and is not lined with a well-defined mesodermal membrane

¹pseu·do·coe·lom·ate \ˌsüd-ō-ˈsē-lə-ˌmāt\ *adj* : having a body cavity that is a pseudocoel

²pseudocoelomate *n* : a pseudocoelomate organism

pseu·do·cow·pox \-ˈkau̇-ˌpäks\ *n* : MILKER'S NODULES

pseu·do·cri·sis \ˈsüd-ō-ˌkrī-səs\ *n, pl* **-cri·ses** \-ˌsēz\ : a false crisis (as in the course of a febrile disease)

pseu·do·cy·e·sis \-sī-ˈē-səs\ *n, pl* **-e·ses** \-ˌsēz\ : a psychosomatic state that occurs without conception and is marked by some of the physical symptoms (as cessation of menses, enlargement of the abdomen, and apparent fetal movements) and changes in hormonal balance of pregnancy

pseu·do·cyst \ˈsüd-ō-ˌsist\ *n* **1** : a cluster of toxoplasmas in an enucleate host cell **2** : CYSTOID

pseu·do·de·men·tia \ˌsüd-ō-di-ˈmen-chə\ *n* : a condition of extreme apathy which outwardly resembles dementia but is not the result of actual mental deterioration

pseu·do·dom·i·nance \-ˈdäm-ə-ˌnən(t)s\ *n* : appearance of a recessive phenotype in a heterozygote containing the recessive gene on one chromosome and a deletion or only part of the dominant gene on the corresponding part of the homologous chromosome

pseu·do·ephed·rine \-i-ˈfed-rən, *Brit also* -ˈef-ə-drən\ *n* : a crystalline alkaloid $C_{10}H_{15}NO$ that is isomeric with ephedrine and is administered chiefly in the form of its hydrochloride $C_{10}H_{15}NO \cdot HCl$ or sulfate $(C_{10}H_{15}NO)_2 \cdot H_2SO_4$ esp. to relieve nasal congestion

pseu·do·far·cy \-ˈfär-sē\ *n, pl* **-cies** : EPIZOOTIC LYMPHANGITIS

pseudo–foot–and–mouth disease *n* : VESICULAR STOMATITIS

pseu·do·gli·o·ma \-glī-ˈō-mə, -glē-\ *n, pl* **-mas** *also* **-ma·ta** \-mət-ə\ : an inflammatory condition of the eye which resembles glioma of the retina and is marked by a circumscribed suppurative inflammation of the vitreous body

pseu·do·glob·u·lin \-ˈgläb-yə-lən\ *n* : a simple protein insoluble in half-saturated ammonium sulfate or sodium sulfate solutions but soluble in pure water — compare EUGLOBULIN

pseu·do·gout \-ˈgau̇t\ *n* : an arthritic condition which resembles gout but is characterized by the deposition of crystalline salts other than urates in and around the joints

---

\ə\ abut \ᵊ\ kitten \ər\ further \a\ ash \ā\ ace \ä\ cot, cart \au̇\ out \ch\ chin \e\ bet \ē\ easy \g\ go \i\ hit \ī\ ice \j\ job \ŋ\ sing \ō\ go \ȯ\ law \ȯi\ boy \th\ thin \t͟h\ the \ü\ loot \u̇\ foot \y\ yet \zh\ vision   *See also* Pronunciation Symbols page

O
P

pseu·do·hal·lu·ci·na·tion \-hə-ˌlüs-ᵊn-ˈā-shən\ *n* : an externalized sensory image vivid enough to be a hallucination but recognized as unreal

pseu·do·he·mo·phil·ia *or chiefly Brit* **pseu·do·hae·mo·phil·ia** \-ˌhē-mə-ˈfil-ē-ə\ *n* : VON WILLEBRAND'S DISEASE

pseu·do·her·maph·ro·dism \-(ˌ)hər-ˈmaf-rə-ˌdiz-əm\ *n* : PSEUDOHERMAPHRODITISM

pseu·do·her·maph·ro·dite \-(ˌ)hər-ˈmaf-rə-ˌdīt\ *n* : an individual exhibiting pseudohermaphroditism — **pseu·do·her·maph·ro·dit·ic** \-(ˌ)hər-ˌmaf-rə-ˈdit-ik\ *adj*

pseu·do·her·maph·ro·dit·ism \-rə-ˌdīt-ˌiz-əm\ *n* : the condition of having the gonads of one sex and the external genitalia and other sex organs so variably developed that the sex of the individual is uncertain — called also *pseudohermaphrodism*

pseu·do·hy·per·ten·sion \ˌsüd-ō-ˌhī-pər-ˈten-chən\ *n* : a condition esp. of some elderly, diabetic, and uremic individuals in which an erroneous high blood pressure reading is given by sphygmomanometry usu. due to loss of flexibility of the arterial walls

pseu·do·hy·per·tro·phic \-ˌhī-pər-ˈtrō-fik\ *adj* : falsely hypertrophic; *specif* : being a form of muscular dystrophy in which the muscles become swollen with deposits of fat and fibrous tissue — **pseu·do·hy·per·tro·phy** \-ˈhī-ˈpər-trə-fē\ *n*, *pl* **-phies**

pseu·do·hy·po·para·thy·roid·ism \-ˌhī-pō-ˌpar-ə-ˈthī-ˌroid-ˌiz-əm\ *n* : a usu. inherited disorder that clinically resembles hypoparathyroidism but results from the body's inability to respond normally to parathyroid hormone rather than from a deficiency of the hormone itself

pseu·do·iso·chro·mat·ic \-ˌī-sə-krō-ˈmat-ik\ *adj* : falsely or apparently isochromatic; *specif* : of, relating to, using, or being a set of colored plates that include some which appear isochromatic to individuals with color-vision abnormality and that are used in the Ishihara test for color blindness

pseu·do·ker·a·tin \-ˈker-ət-ən\ *n* : a protein (as neurokeratin) that occurs esp. in the skin and nerve sheaths and that like keratins is insoluble but is less resistant to enzymatic action than keratins

pseu·do·leu·ke·mia *or chiefly Brit* **pseu·do·leu·kae·mia** \-lü-ˈkē-mē-ə\ *n* : any abnormal state (as Hodgkin's disease) resembling leukemia in its anatomical changes but lacking the changes in the circulating blood characteristic of the latter — **pseu·do·leu·ke·mic** *or chiefly Brit* **pseu·do·leu·kae·mic** \-mik\ *adj*

Pseu·do·lyn·chia \ˌsüd-ō-ˈliŋ-kē-ə\ *n* : a genus of hippoboscid flies

pseu·do·mega·co·lon \-ˈmeg-ə-ˌkō-lən\ *n* : abnormal dilatation of the colon occurring in adults ⟨∼ resulting from chronic constipation⟩

pseu·do·mem·brane \-ˈmem-ˌbrān\ *n* : FALSE MEMBRANE

pseu·do·mem·bra·nous \-ˈmem-brə-nəs\ *adj* : characterized by the presence or formation of a false membrane ⟨∼ colitis⟩

pseu·do·mo·nad \ˌsüd-ə-ˈmō-ˌnad, -nəd\ *n* : any bacterium of the genus *Pseudomonas*

pseu·do·mo·nal \-ˈmō-nəl\ *adj* : of, relating to, or caused by bacteria of the genus *Pseudomonas* ⟨∼ infection⟩

pseu·do·mo·nas \ˌsüd-ə-ˈmō-nəs, sü-ˈdäm-ə-nəs\ *n* **1** *cap* : a genus (the type of the family Pseudomonadaceae) comprising short rod-shaped motile gram-negative bacteria including some saprophytes, a few animal pathogens, and numerous important plant pathogens **2** *pl* **pseu·do·mo·na·des** \ˌsüd-ə-ˈmō-nə-ˌdēz, -ˈmän-ə-\ : PSEUDOMONAD

pseu·do·mu·cin \-ˈmyüs-ᵊn\ *n* : a mucoprotein occurring in ovarian cysts — **pseu·do·mu·cin·ous** \-əs\ *adj*

pseu·do·neu·rot·ic \-n(y)ù-ˈrät-ik\ *adj* : having or characterized by neurotic symptoms which mask an underlying psychosis ⟨∼ schizophrenia⟩

Pseu·do–nitzsch·ia \ˌsüd-ō-ˈnich-ē-ə\ *n* : a genus of dinoflagellates (order Pennales) including several (as *P. australis*) that occur in algal blooms, produce domoic acid, and cause or have the potential for causing amnesic shellfish poisoning

pseu·do·pa·ral·y·sis \ˌsüd-ə-pə-ˈral-ə-səs\ *n*, *pl* **-y·ses** \-ˌsēz\ : apparent lack or loss of muscular power (as that produced by pain) that is not accompanied by true paralysis

pseu·do·par·a·site \-ˈpar-ə-ˌsīt\ *n* : an object or organism that resembles or is mistaken for a parasite — **pseu·do·par·a·sit·ic** \-ˌpar-ə-ˈsit-ik\ *adj*

pseu·do·par·kin·son·ism \-ˈpär-kən-sə-ˌniz-əm\ *n* : a condition (as one induced by a drug) characterized by symptoms like those of parkinsonism

Pseu·do·phyl·lid·ea \ˌsüd-ō-fi-ˈlid-ē-ə\ *n pl* : an order of the class Cestoda comprising tapeworms with two sucking grooves on the unarmed scolex and the vitellaria scattered throughout the parenchyma and including numerous parasites of fish-eating vertebrates (as the medically important fish tapeworm of humans) — see DIPHYLLOBOTHRIIDAE

pseu·do·phyl·lid·ean \-ē-ən\ *n* : any tapeworm of the order Pseudophyllidea

pseu·do·plague \ˈsüd-ō-ˌplāg\ *n* : NEWCASTLE DISEASE

pseu·do·plasm \-ˌplaz-əm\ *n* : an apparent neoplasm that disappears spontaneously

pseu·do·pod \ˈsüd-ə-ˌpäd\ *n* **1** : PSEUDOPODIUM **2 a** : a slender extension from the edge of a wheal at the site of injection of an allergen **b** : one of the slender processes of some tumor cells extending out from the main mass of a tumor

pseu·dop·o·dal \sü-ˈdäp-əd-ᵊl\ *or* **pseu·do·po·di·al** \ˌsüd-ə-ˈpōd-ē-əl\ *adj* : of, relating to, or resembling a pseudopod or pseudopodium

pseu·do·po·di·um \ˌsüd-ə-ˈpōd-ē-əm\ *n*, *pl* **-dia** \-ē-ə\ **1** : a temporary protrusion or retractile process of the cytoplasm of a cell (as a unicellular organism or a white blood cell of a higher organism) that functions esp. as an organ of locomotion or in taking up food **2** : one of the ameboid protrusions of the active plasmodium of a slime mold

pseu·do·pol·yp \ˈsüd-ō-ˌpäl-əp\ *n* : a projecting mass of hypertrophied mucous membrane (as in the stomach or colon) resulting from local inflammation

pseu·do·preg·nan·cy \ˌsüd-ō-ˈpreg-nən-sē\ *n*, *pl* **-cies** : a condition which resembles pregnancy: as **a** : PSEUDOCYESIS **b** : an anestrous state resembling pregnancy that occurs in various mammals usu. after an infertile copulation — **pseu·do·preg·nant** \-nənt\ *adj*

pseu·do–pseu·do·hy·po·para·thy·roid·ism \ˌsüd-ō-ˌsüd-ō-ˌhī-pō-ˌpar-ə-ˈthī-ˌroid-ˌiz-əm\ *n* : a relatively mild form of pseudohypoparathyroidism that is characterized by normal levels of calcium and phosphorus in the blood

pseu·do·ra·bies \-ˈrā-bēz\ *n* : an acute febrile virus disease of domestic animals (as cattle and swine) that is caused by a herpesvirus of the genus *Varicellovirus* (species *Suid herpesvirus 1*) and that is marked by cutaneous irritation and intense itching followed by encephalomyelitis and pharyngeal paralysis and commonly terminating in death within 48 hours — called also *infectious bulbar paralysis, mad itch*

pseu·do·re·ac·tion \-rē-ˈak-shən\ *n* : a reaction following the injection of a toxin (as in the Schick test) which is caused by something (as impurities in the test medium) other than the toxin itself

pseu·do·sar·co·ma·tous \ˌsüd-ō-sär-ˈkō-mət-əs\ *adj* : resembling but not being a true sarcoma ⟨a ∼ polyp⟩

pseu·do·sci·ence \ˌsüd-ō-ˈsī-ən(t)s\ *n* : a system of theories, assumptions, and methods erroneously regarded as scientific — **pseu·do·sci·en·tif·ic** \-ˌsī-ən-ˈtif-ik\ *adj*

pseu·do·sci·en·tist \-ˈsī-ənt-əst\ *n* : a practitioner of a pseudoscience

pseu·do·scle·ro·sis \-sklə-ˈrō-səs\ *n*, *pl* **-ro·ses** \-ˌsēz\ : a condition having symptoms like those of multiple sclerosis; *esp* : WILSON'S DISEASE

pseu·do·sco·lex \-ˈskō-ˌleks\ *n*, *pl* **-sco·li·ces** \-lə-ˌsēz\ : an altered group of anterior segments that in some tapeworms replaces the scolex and serves as a holdfast

pseu·do·strat·i·fied \-ˈstrat-ə-ˌfīd\ *adj* : of, relating to, or being an epithelium consisting of closely packed cells which appear to be arranged in layers but all of which are in fact attached to the basement membrane — **pseu·do·strat·i·fi·ca·tion** \-ˌstrat-ə-fə-ˈkā-shən\ *n*

pseu·do·tro·pine \-ˈtrō-ˌpēn\ *n* : a crystalline alkaloid $C_8H_{15}NO$ stereoisomeric with tropine and formed by hydrolysis of tropacocaine

pseu·do·tu·ber·cle \-ˈt(y)ü-bər-kəl\ *n* : a nodule or granuloma resembling a tubercle of tuberculosis but due to other causes

pseu·do·tu·ber·cu·lo·sis \-t(y)ù-ˌbər-kyə-ˈlō-səs\ *n, pl* **-lo·ses** \-ˌsēz\ **1** : any of several diseases that are marked by the formation of granulomas resembling tubercular nodules and are caused by a bacterium (as *Yersinia pseudotuberculosis*) other than the tubercle bacillus **2** : CASEOUS LYMPHADENITIS

pseu·do·tu·mor *or Brit* **pseu·do·tu·mour** \-ˈt(y)ü-mər\ *n* : an abnormality (as a temporary swelling) that resembles a tumor — **pseu·do·tu·mor·al** *or Brit* **pseu·do·tu·mour·al** \-mə-rəl\ *adj*

pseudotumor cer·e·bri \-ˈser-ə-ˌbrī\ *n* : an abnormal condition that is characterized by increased intracranial pressure, headaches of varying intensity, and papilledema without any demonstrable intracranial lesion and that tends to occur in overweight women from 20 to 50 years of age — called also *benign intracranial hypertension*

pseu·do·uri·dine \-ˈyùr-ə-ˌdēn\ *n* : a nucleoside $C_9H_{12}O_6N_2$ that is a uracil derivative incorporated as a structural component into transfer RNA

pseu·do·xan·tho·ma elas·ti·cum \ˌsüd-ō-zan-ˈthō-mə-i-ˈlas-ti-kəm\ *n* : a chronic degenerative disease of elastic tissues that is marked by the occurrence of small yellowish papules and plaques on areas of abnormally loose skin

¹psi \ˈsī\ *adj* : relating to, concerned with, or being parapsychological psychic events or powers ⟨~ phenomena⟩

²psi *n* : psi events or phenomena

psi·lo·cin \ˈsī-lə-sən\ *n* : a hallucinogenic tertiary amine $C_{12}H_{16}N_2O$ obtained from a basidiomycetous fungus (*Psilocybe mexicana*)

psi·lo·cy·bin \ˌsī-lə-ˈsī-bən\ *n* : a hallucinogenic indole $C_{12}H_{17}N_2O_4P$ obtained from a basidiomycetous fungus (as *Psilocybe mexicana* or *P. cubensis* syn. *Stropharia cubensis*)

psi·lo·sis \sī-ˈlō-səs\ *n, pl* **psi·lo·ses** \-ˌsēz\ **1** : a falling out of hair **2** : SPRUE

psit·ta·co·sis \ˌsit-ə-ˈkō-səs\ *n, pl* **-co·ses** \-ˌsēz\ : an infectious disease of birds caused by a bacterium of the genus *Chlamydia* (*C. psittaci*), marked by diarrhea and wasting, and transmissible to humans in whom it usu. occurs as an atypical pneumonia accompanied by high fever — called also *parrot fever;* compare ORNITHOSIS — **psit·ta·co·tic** \-ˈkät-ik, -ˈkōt-\ *adj*

pso·as \ˈsō-əs\ *n, pl* **pso·ai** \ˈsō-ˌī\ *or* **pso·ae** \-ˌē\ : either of two internal muscles of the loin: **a** : PSOAS MAJOR **b** : PSOAS MINOR

psoas major *n* : the larger of the two psoas muscles that arises from the anterolateral surfaces of the lumbar vertebrae, passes beneath the inguinal ligament to insert with the iliacus into the lesser trochanter of the femur, and serves esp. to flex the thigh

psoas minor *n* : the smaller of the two psoas muscles that arises from the last dorsal and first lumbar vertebrae and inserts into the brim of the pelvis, that functions to flex the trunk and the lumbar spinal column, and that is often absent

psoas muscle *n* : PSOAS

pso·ra \ˈsō-rə\ *n* : PSORIASIS

pso·ra·len \ˈsòr-ə-lən\ *n* : a substance $C_{11}H_6O_3$ found in some plants that photosensitizes mammalian skin and is used in conjunction with ultraviolet light to treat psoriasis; *also* : any of various derivatives of psoralen having similar properties — see PUVA

pso·ri·a·si·form \sə-ˈrī-ə-si-ˌfórm\ *adj* : resembling psoriasis or a psoriatic lesion

pso·ri·a·sis \sə-ˈrī-ə-səs\ *n, pl* **-a·ses** \-ˌsēz\ : a chronic skin disease characterized by circumscribed red patches covered with white scales

psoriasis ar·thro·path·i·ca \-ˌär-thrə-ˈpath-i-kə\ *n* : PSORIATIC ARTHRITIS

¹pso·ri·at·ic \ˌsōr-ē-ˈat-ik, ˌsòr-\ *adj* : of, relating to, affected with, or accompanied by psoriasis ⟨~ lesions⟩

²psoriatic *n* : an individual affected with psoriasis

psoriatic arthritis *n* : a severe form of arthritis accompanied by inflammation, psoriasis of the skin or nails, and a negative test for rheumatoid factor — called also *psoriasis arthropathica*

psoriatic arthropathy *n* : PSORIATIC ARTHRITIS

Pso·rop·tes \sə-ˈräp-(ˌ)tēz\ *n* : a genus (the type of the family Psoroptidae) of mites having piercing mandibles and suckers with jointed pedicels, living on and irritating the skin of various mammals, and resulting in the development of inflammatory skin diseases (as mange)

pso·rop·tic \sə-ˈräp-tik\ *adj* : of, relating to, caused by, or being mites of the genus *Psoroptes* ⟨~ mange⟩

PSRO *abbr* professional standards review organization

PSVT *abbr* paroxysmal supraventricular tachycardia

psych *abbr* psychology

psy·cha·gogy \ˈsī-kə-ˌgōj-ē *also* -ˌgäj-, *esp Brit* -ˌgäg-\ *n, pl* **-gies** : a psychotherapeutic method of influencing behavior by suggesting desirable life goals

psy·chal·gia \sī-ˈkal-j(ē-)ə\ *n* : mental distress

psychanalysis *var of* PSYCHOANALYSIS

psych·as·the·nia \ˌsī-kas-ˈthē-nē-ə\ *n* : a neurotic state characterized esp. by phobias, obsessions, or compulsions that one knows are irrational — **psych·as·then·ic** \-ˈthen-ik\ *adj*

psy·che \ˈsī-(ˌ)kē\ *n* : the specialized cognitive, conative, and affective aspects of a psychosomatic unity : MIND; *specif* : the totality of the id, ego, and superego including both conscious and unconscious components

¹psy·che·del·ic \ˌsī-kə-ˈdel-ik\ *n* : a psychedelic drug (as LSD)

²psychedelic *adj* **1** : of, relating to, or being drugs (as LSD) capable of producing abnormal psychic effects (as hallucinations) and sometimes psychotic states **2** : produced by or associated with the use of psychedelic drugs ⟨a ~ experience⟩ — **psy·che·del·i·cal·ly** \-ˈdel-i-k(ə-)lē\ *adv*

psy·chi·at·ric \ˌsī-kē-ˈa-trik\ *adj* **1** : relating to or employed in psychiatry ⟨~ disorders⟩ ⟨~ drugs⟩ **2** : engaged in the practice of psychiatry : dealing with cases of mental disorder ⟨~ experts⟩ ⟨~ nursing⟩ ⟨a ~ ward⟩ — **psy·chi·at·ri·cal·ly** \-tri-k(ə-)lē\ *adv*

psy·chi·a·trist \sə-ˈkī-ə-trəst, sī-\ *n* : a physician specializing in psychiatry

psy·chi·a·try \-trē\ *n, pl* **-tries** : a branch of medicine that deals with the science and practice of treating mental, emotional, or behavioral disorders esp. as originating in endogenous causes or resulting from faulty interpersonal relationships

¹psy·chic \ˈsī-kik\ *also* **psy·chi·cal** \-ki-kəl\ *adj* **1** : of or relating to the psyche : PSYCHOGENIC **2** : sensitive to nonphysical or supernatural forces and influences — **psy·chi·cal·ly** \-ki-k(ə-)lē\ *adv*

²psychic *n* : a person apparently sensitive to nonphysical forces

psychic energizer *n* : ANTIDEPRESSANT

psy·cho \ˈsī-(ˌ)kō\ *n, pl* **psychos** : a deranged or psychopathic individual — not used technically — **psycho** *adj*

psy·cho·acous·tics \ˌsī-kō-ə-ˈkü-stiks\ *n pl but sing in constr* : a branch of science dealing with the perception of sound, the sensations produced by sounds, and the problems of communication — **psy·cho·acous·tic** \-stik\ *adj*

psy·cho·ac·tive \ˌsī-kō-ˈak-tiv\ *adj* : affecting the mind or behavior ⟨~ drugs⟩ ⟨THC is the principal ~ ingredient in marijuana⟩

psy·cho·anal·y·sis \ˌsī-kō-ə-ˈnal-ə-səs\ *also* **psych·anal·y·sis** \ˌsī-kə-\ *n, pl* **-y·ses** \-ˌsēz\ **1** : a method of analyzing psychic phenomena and treating mental and emotional disorders

O
P

\ə\ abut \ᵊ\ kitten \ər\ further \a\ ash \ā\ ace \ä\ cot, cart
\aù\ out \ch\ chin \e\ bet \ē\ easy \g\ go \i\ hit \ī\ ice \j\ job
\ŋ\ sing \ō\ go \ò\ law \òi\ boy \th\ thin \t̲h̲\ the \ü\ loot
\ù\ foot \y\ yet \zh\ vision   *See also* Pronunciation Symbols page

that is based on the concepts and theories of Sigmund Freud, that emphasizes the importance of free association and dream analysis, and that involves treatment sessions during which the patient is encouraged to talk freely about personal experiences and esp. about early childhood and dreams **2** : a body of empirical findings and a set of theories on human motivation, behavior, and personality development that developed esp. with the aid of psychoanalysis **3** : a school of psychology, psychiatry, and psychotherapy founded by Sigmund Freud and rooted in and applying psychoanalysis

psy·cho·an·a·lyst \-'an-ᵊl-əst\ *n* : a person who practices or adheres to the principles of psychoanalysis; *specif* : a psychotherapist trained at an established psychoanalytic institute

psy·cho·an·a·lyt·ic \-ˌan-ᵊl-'it-ik\ *also* **psy·cho·an·a·lyt·i·cal** \-i-kəl\ *adj* : of, relating to, or employing psychoanalysis or its principles and techniques — **psy·cho·an·a·lyt·i·cal·ly** \-i-k(ə-)lē\ *adv*

psy·cho·an·a·lyze *or Brit* **psy·cho·an·a·lyse** \-'an-ᵊl-ˌīz\ *vt* **-lyzed** *or Brit* **-lysed; -lyz·ing** *or Brit* **-lys·ing** : to treat by means of psychoanalysis

psy·cho·bi·og·ra·phy \-bī-'äg-rə-fē, -bē-\ *n, pl* **-phies** : a biography written from a psychodynamic or psychoanalytic point of view — **psy·cho·bio·graph·i·cal** \-ˌbī-ə-'graf-i-kəl\ *adj*

psy·cho·bi·o·log·i·cal \-ˌbī-ə-'läj-i-kəl\ *also* **psy·cho·bi·o·log·ic** \-ik\ *adj* : of or relating to psychobiology

psy·cho·bi·ol·o·gist \-bī-'äl-ə-jəst\ *n* : a specialist in psychobiology

psy·cho·bi·ol·o·gy \-bī-'äl-ə-jē\ *n, pl* **-gies** : the study of mental functioning and behavior in relation to other biological processes

psy·cho·ca·thar·sis \-kə-'thär-səs\ *n, pl* **-thar·ses** \-ˌsēz\ : CATHARSIS 2

psy·cho·chem·i·cal \-'kem-i-kəl\ *n* : a psychoactive chemical — **psychochemical** *adj*

psy·cho·chem·is·try \-'kem-ə-strē\ *n, pl* **-tries** : the study of the psychological functions and effects of chemicals

psy·cho·cul·tur·al \-'kəlch(-ə)-rəl\ *adj* : of or relating to the interaction of psychological and cultural factors in the individual's personality or in the characteristics of a group ⟨a ~ study of suicide⟩ — **psy·cho·cul·tur·al·ly** \-ē\ *adv*

psy·cho·di·ag·no·sis \-ˌdī-ig-'nō-səs\ *n, pl* **-no·ses** \-ˌsēz\ : diagnosis employing the principles and techniques of psychodiagnostics

psy·cho·di·ag·nos·tic \-'näs-tik\ *adj* : of, relating to, or employing psychodiagnostics

psy·cho·di·ag·nos·tics \-tiks\ *n pl but sing in constr* : a branch of psychology concerned with the use of tests in the evaluation of personality and the determination of factors underlying human behavior

Psy·cho·di·dae \sī-'käd-ə-ˌdē, -'kōd-\ *n pl* : a family of very small dipteran flies (suborder Nematocera) that have hairy wings resembling those of moths and larvae developing in moss and damp plant matter and that include some of medical importance belonging to the genus *Phlebotomus*

psy·cho·dra·ma \ˌsī-kō-'dräm-ə, -'dram-; 'sī-kō-ˌdräm-ə, -ˌdram-\ *n* : an extemporized dramatization designed to afford catharsis and social relearning for one or more of the participants from whose life history the plot is abstracted — **psy·cho·dra·mat·ic** \-ˌkō-drə-'mat-ik\ *adj*

psy·cho·dy·nam·ics \ˌsī-kō-dī-'nam-iks, -də-\ *n pl but sing or pl in constr* **1** : the psychology of mental or emotional forces or processes developing esp. in early childhood and their effects on behavior and mental states **2** : explanation or interpretation (as of behavior or mental states) in terms of mental or emotional forces or processes **3** : motivational forces acting esp. at the unconscious level — **psy·cho·dy·nam·ic** \-ik\ *adj* — **psy·cho·dy·nam·i·cal·ly** \-i-k(ə-)lē\ *adv*

psy·cho·ed·u·ca·tion·al \-ˌej-ə-'kā-shnəl, -shən-ᵊl\ *adj* : of or relating to the psychological aspects of education; *specif* : relating to or used in the education of children with behavioral disorders or learning disabilities ⟨a ~ clinic⟩

psy·cho·gal·van·ic \-gal-'van-ik\ *adj* : of or relating to the psychogalvanic reflex ⟨a ~ record⟩

psychogalvanic reflex *n* : a momentary decrease in the apparent electrical resistance of the skin resulting from activity of the sweat glands in response to mental or emotional stimulation — called also *psychogalvanic reaction, psychogalvanic response*

psy·cho·gal·va·nom·e·ter \-ˌgal-və-'näm-ət-ər\ *n* : a galvanometer used to detect the psychogalvanic reflex — **psy·cho·gal·va·no·met·ric** \-nō-'me-trik\ *adj*

psy·cho·gen·e·sis \ˌsī-kə-'jen-ə-səs\ *n, pl* **-e·ses** \-ˌsēz\ **1** : the origin and development of mental functions, traits, or states **2** : development from mental as distinguished from physical origins ⟨the ~ of an illness⟩

psy·cho·ge·net·ic \-jə-'net-ik\ *adj* **1** : of or relating to psychogenesis **2** : PSYCHOGENIC — **psy·cho·ge·ne·ti·cal·ly** \-i-k(ə-)lē\ *adv*

psy·cho·ge·net·ics \-iks\ *n pl but sing in constr* : the study of psychogenesis

psy·cho·gen·ic \-'jen-ik\ *adj* : originating in the mind or in mental or emotional conflict ⟨~ impotence⟩ — compare SOMATOGENIC — **psy·cho·gen·i·cal·ly** \-i-k(ə-)lē\ *adv*

psy·cho·ge·nic·i·ty \-jə-'nis-ət-ē\ *n, pl* **-ties** : the quality or state of being psychogenic : PSYCHOGENESIS

psy·cho·ge·ri·at·rics \-ˌjer-ē-'a-triks, -ˌjir-\ *n pl but sing in constr* : a branch of psychiatry concerned with behavioral and emotional disorders among the elderly — **psy·cho·ge·ri·at·ric** \-trik\ *adj*

psy·cho·gno·sis \ˌsī-käg-'nō-səs, -ˌkäg-\ *n, pl* **-no·ses** \-'nō-ˌsēz\ : the study of the psyche in relation to character

psy·cho·gram \'sī-kə-ˌgram\ *n* **1** : a description of the mental functioning of an individual; *esp* : the pattern of responses to a projective technique (as the Rorschach test) **2** : PROFILE 2

psy·cho·graph \'sī-kə-ˌgraf\ *n* **1** : PROFILE 2 **2** : a biography written from a psychodynamic point of view; *also* : a character analysis

psy·cho·graph·ic \ˌsī-kə-'graf-ik\ *adj* : of, relating to, or involving the preparation of psychographs

psy·cho·ki·ne·sis \-kə-'nē-səs, -kī-\ *n, pl* **-ne·ses** \-ˌsēz\ : movement of physical objects by the mind without use of physical means — called also *PK;* compare PRECOGNITION, TELEKINESIS — **psy·cho·ki·net·ic** \-'net-ik\ *adj*

psy·cho·ki·net·ics \-kə-'net-iks, -kī-\ *n pl but sing in constr* : a branch of parapsychology that deals with psychokinesis

psychol *abbr* psychologist; psychology

psy·cho·lep·sy \'sī-kō-ˌlep-sē\ *n, pl* **-sies** : an attack of hopelessness and mental inertia esp. following elation and occurring typically in psychasthenic individuals

¹psy·cho·lep·tic \ˌsī-kō-'lep-tik\ *adj* : of, relating to, or being a tranquilizing drug

²psycholeptic *n* : TRANQUILIZER

psy·cho·lin·guist \ˌsī-kō-'liŋ-gwəst\ *n* : a person specializing in psycholinguistics

psy·cho·lin·guis·tic \-liŋ-'gwis-tik\ *adj* **1** : of or relating to psycholinguistics **2** : of or relating to the psychological aspects of language

psy·cho·lin·guis·tics \ˌsī-kō-liŋ-'gwis-tiks\ *n pl but sing in constr* : the study of the mental faculties involved in the perception, production, and acquisition of language

psy·cho·log·i·cal \ˌsī-kə-'läj-i-kəl\ *also* **psy·cho·log·ic** \-ik\ *adj* **1 a** : relating to, characteristic of, directed toward, influencing, arising in, or acting through the mind esp. in its affective or cognitive functions ⟨~ phenomena⟩ ⟨the ~ aspects of a problem⟩ **b** : directed toward the will or toward the mind specif. in its conative function ⟨~ warfare⟩ **2** : relating to, concerned with, deriving from, or used in psychology ⟨~ research⟩ ⟨~ tests⟩ ⟨a ~ clinic⟩ — **psy·cho·log·i·cal·ly** \-ē\ *adv*

psychological medicine *n* : PSYCHIATRY

psychological primary *n* : any of the set of colors which are perceived as belonging to objects, which include red, yellow, green, and blue and sometimes black and white, and in terms of which all other colors belonging to objects can be described

psy·chol·o·gist \sī-'käl-ə-jəst\ *n* : a specialist in one or more branches of psychology; *esp* : a practitioner of clinical psychology, counseling, or guidance

psy·chol·o·gize *also Brit* **psy·chol·o·gise** \-ˌjīz\ *vb* **-gized** *also Brit* **-gised; -giz·ing** *also Brit* **-gis·ing** *vt* : to explain or interpret in psychological terms ~ *vi* : to speculate in psychological terms or upon psychological motivations

psy·chol·o·gy \-jē\ *n, pl* **-gies** **1** : the science of mind and behavior **2 a** : the mental or behavioral characteristics typical of an individual or group or a particular form of behavior ⟨mob ~⟩ ⟨the ~ of arson⟩ **b** : the study of mind and behavior in relation to a particular field of knowledge or activity ⟨color ~⟩ ⟨the ~ of learning⟩ **3** : a treatise on or a school, system, or branch of psychology

psy·cho·met·ric \ˌsī-kə-ˈme-trik\ *adj* : of or relating to psychometrics — **psy·cho·met·ri·cal·ly** \-tri-k(ə-)lē\ *adv*

psy·cho·me·tri·cian \-mə-ˈtrish-ən\ *n* **1** : a person (as a clinical psychologist) who is skilled in the administration and interpretation of objective psychological tests **2** : a psychologist who devises, constructs, and standardizes psychometric tests

psy·cho·met·rics \-ˈme-triks\ *n pl but sing in constr* **1** : a branch of clinical or applied psychology dealing with the use and application of mental measurement **2** : the technique of mental measurements : the use of quantitative devices for assessing psychological trends

psy·chom·e·trist \sī-ˈkäm-ə-trəst\ *n* : PSYCHOMETRICIAN

psy·chom·e·try \sī-ˈkäm-ə-trē\ *n, pl* **-tries** : PSYCHOMETRICS

psy·cho·mi·met·ic \ˌsī-kō-mə-ˈmet-ik, -mī-\ *adj* : producing effects (as hallucinations or paranoid delusions) that resemble or are identical with psychotic symptoms ⟨~ drugs like mescaline⟩

psy·cho·mo·til·i·ty \-mō-ˈtil-ət-ē\ *n, pl* **-ties** : bodily movement proceeding from mental processes and indicating psychological tendencies and traits

psy·cho·mo·tion \-ˈmō-shən\ *n* : PSYCHOMOTILITY

psy·cho·mo·tor \ˌsī-kō-ˈmōt-ər\ *adj* **1** : of or relating to motor action directly proceeding from mental activity **2** : of or relating to temporal lobe epilepsy ⟨~ seizures⟩

psychomotor epilepsy *n* : TEMPORAL LOBE EPILEPSY

psy·cho·neu·ral \-ˈn(y)ùr-əl\ *adj* : of or relating to the interrelationship of the nervous system and consciousness : relating to the mental functions of the central nervous system

psy·cho·neu·ro·im·mu·nol·o·gist \ˌsī-kō-ˌn(y)ùr-ō-ˌim-yə-ˈnäl-ə-jəst\ *n* : a specialist in psychoneuroimmunology

psy·cho·neu·ro·im·mu·nol·o·gy \-ə-jē\ *n, pl* **-gies** : a field of medicine that deals with the influence of emotional states (as stress) and nervous system activity on immune function esp. in relation to their effect on the onset and progression of disease

psy·cho·neu·ro·log·i·cal \-ˌn(y)ùr-ə-ˈläj-i-kəl\ *also* **psy·cho·neu·ro·log·ic** \-ˈläj-ik\ *adj* : of, relating to, or concerned with psychology and neurology esp. in their clinical aspects — **psy·cho·neu·rol·o·gy** \-n(y)ù-ˈräl-ə-jē\ *n, pl* **-gies**

psy·cho·neu·ro·sis \-n(y)ù-ˈrō-səs\ *n, pl* **-ro·ses** \-ˌsēz\ : NEUROSIS; *esp* : a neurosis based on emotional conflict in which an impulse that has been blocked seeks expression in a disguised response or symptom — compare ACTUAL NEUROSIS

¹psy·cho·neu·rot·ic \-ˈrät-ik\ *adj* : of, relating to, being, or affected with a psychoneurosis ⟨a ~ disorder⟩ ⟨a ~ patient⟩

²psychoneurotic *n* : a psychoneurotic individual

psy·cho·nom·ic \ˌsī-kə-ˈnäm-ik\ *adj* : of, relating to, or constituting the laws of mental functioning

psy·cho·path \ˈsī-kə-ˌpath\ *n* : a mentally ill or unstable individual; *esp* : one having an antisocial personality

psy·cho·path·ia \ˌsī-kə-ˈpath-ē-ə\ *n* : PSYCHOPATHY

¹psy·cho·path·ic \ˌsī-kə-ˈpath-ik\ *adj* : of, relating to, or characterized by psychopathy — **psy·cho·path·i·cal·ly** \-i-k(ə-)lē\ *adv*

²psychopathic *n* : PSYCHOPATH

psychopathic personality *n* **1** : ANTISOCIAL PERSONALITY **2** : an individual having an antisocial personality

psy·cho·patho·log·i·cal \ˌsī-kō-ˌpath-ə-ˈläj-i-kəl\ *or* **psy·cho-**

patho·log·ic \-ik\ *adj* : of, relating to, or exhibiting psychopathology — **psy·cho·patho·log·i·cal·ly** \-i-k(ə-)lē\ *adv*

psy·cho·pa·thol·o·gist \-pə-ˈthäl-ə-jəst, -pa-\ *n* : a specialist in psychopathology

psy·cho·pa·thol·o·gy \ˌsī-kō-pə-ˈthäl-ə-jē, -pa-\ *n, pl* **-gies** **1** : the study of psychological and behavioral dysfunction occurring in mental disorder or in social disorganization **2** : disordered psychological and behavioral functioning (as in mental disorder) ⟨the theory that holidays are associated with an increased incidence of ~ —*Science News*⟩

psy·chop·a·thy \sī-ˈkäp-ə-thē\ *n, pl* **-thies** **1** : MENTAL DISORDER **2** : ANTISOCIAL PERSONALITY

psy·cho·phar·ma·ceu·ti·cal \ˌsī-kō-ˌfär-mə-ˈsüt-i-kəl\ *n* : a drug having an effect on the mental state of the user

psy·cho·phar·ma·co·log·ic \-ˌfär-mə-kə-ˈläj-ik\ *or* **psy·cho·phar·ma·co·log·i·cal** \-i-kəl\ *adj* : of, relating to, or used in psychopharmacology ⟨a ~ agent⟩

psy·cho·phar·ma·col·o·gist \-ˌfär-mə-ˈkäl-ə-jəst\ *n* : a specialist in psychopharmacology

psy·cho·phar·ma·col·o·gy \ˌsī-kō-ˌfär-mə-ˈkäl-ə-jē\ *n, pl* **-gies** : the study of the effect of drugs on the mind and behavior

psy·cho·phys·i·cal \ˌsī-kō-ˈfiz-i-kəl\ *adj* : of or relating to psychophysics; *also* : sharing mental and physical qualities — **psy·cho·phys·i·cal·ly** \-k(ə-)lē\ *adv*

psychophysical parallelism *n* : PARALLELISM

psy·cho·phys·i·cist \-ˈfiz-ə-səst\ *n* : a specialist in psychophysics

psy·cho·phys·ics \ˌsī-kō-ˈfiz-iks\ *n pl but sing in constr* : a branch of psychology concerned with the effect of physical processes (as intensity of stimulation) on the mental processes and esp. sensations of an organism

psy·cho·phys·i·o·log·i·cal \ˌsī-kō-ˌfiz-ē-ə-ˈläj-i-kəl\ *also* **psy·cho·phys·i·o·log·ic** \-ik\ *adj* **1** : of or relating to psychophysiology **2** : combining or involving mental and bodily processes — **psy·cho·phys·i·o·log·i·cal·ly** \-i-k(ə-)lē\ *adv*

psy·cho·phys·i·ol·o·gist \-ˌfiz-ē-ˈäl-ə-jəst\ *n* : a specialist in psychophysiology

psy·cho·phys·i·ol·o·gy \-ē-ˈäl-ə-jē\ *n, pl* **-gies** : a branch of psychology that deals with the effects of normal and pathological physiological processes on mental functioning — called also *physiological psychology, physiopsychology*

psy·cho·quack \ˈsī-kō-ˌkwak\ *n* : a quack psychologist, psychiatrist, or psychotherapist — **psy·cho·quack·ery** \ˌsī-kō-ˈkwak-ə-rē\ *n, pl* **-eries**

psy·cho·sen·so·ri·al \ˌsī-kō-sen-ˈsōr-ē-əl\ *adj* : PSYCHOSENSORY

psy·cho·sen·so·ry \-ˈsen(t)s-(ə-)rē\ *adj* : of or relating to sense perception

psy·cho·sex·u·al \ˌsī-kō-ˈseksh-(ə-)wəl, -ˈsek-shəl\ *adj* **1** : of or relating to the mental, emotional, and behavioral aspects of sexual development **2** : of or relating to mental or emotional attitudes concerning sexual activity **3** : of or relating to the psychophysiology of sex — **psy·cho·sex·u·al·ly** \-ē\ *adv*

psy·cho·sex·u·al·i·ty \-ˌsek-shə-ˈwal-ət-ē\ *n, pl* **-ties** : the psychic factors of sex

psy·cho·sis \sī-ˈkō-səs\ *n, pl* **-cho·ses** \-ˌsēz\ : a serious mental disorder (as schizophrenia) characterized by defective or lost contact with reality often with hallucinations or delusions

psy·cho·so·cial \ˌsī-kō-ˈsō-shəl\ *adj* **1** : involving both psychological and social aspects ⟨~ adjustment in marriage⟩ **2** : relating social conditions to mental health ⟨~ medicine⟩ — **psy·cho·so·cial·ly** \-ˈsōsh-(ə-)lē\ *adv*

psy·cho·so·cio·log·i·cal \-ˌsō-sē-ə-ˈläj-i-kəl, -ˌsō-sh(ē-)ə-\ *adj* : dealing with or measuring both psychological and sociological variables : concerned with the psychological characteristics of a people ⟨a ~ survey⟩

\ə\ **abut** \ᵊ\ **kitten** \ər\ **further** \a\ **ash** \ā\ **ace** \ä\ **cot, cart** \aù\ **out** \ch\ **chin** \e\ **bet** \ē\ **easy** \g\ **go** \i\ **hit** \ī\ **ice** \j\ **job** \ŋ\ **sing** \ō\ **go** \ò\ **law** \òi\ **boy** \th\ **thin** \t̷h\ **the** \ü\ **loot** \ù\ **foot** \y\ **yet** \zh\ **vision** *See also* Pronunciation Symbols page

O

P

psy·cho·so·ci·ol·o·gist \-ˌsō-sē-ˈäl-ə-jəst, -ˌsō-shē-\ *n* : a specialist in psychosociology

psy·cho·so·ci·ol·o·gy \-ə-jē\ *n, pl* **-gies** : the study of problems common to psychology and sociology

¹**psy·cho·so·mat·ic** \ˌsī-kə-sə-ˈmat-ik, -kō-, -sō-\ *adj* **1** : of, relating to, concerned with, or involving both mind and body ⟨the ∼ nature of man —Herbert Ratner⟩ **2 a** : of, relating to, involving, or concerned with bodily symptoms caused by mental or emotional disturbance ⟨∼ illness⟩ ⟨∼ medicine⟩ **b** : exhibiting psychosomatic symptoms ⟨a ∼ patient⟩ — **psy·cho·so·mat·i·cal·ly** \-i-k(ə-)lē\ *adv*

²**psychosomatic** *n* : an individual exhibiting psychosomatic symptoms

psy·cho·so·mat·i·cist \-sə-ˈmat-ə-səst\ *n* : a specialist in psychosomatics

psy·cho·so·mat·ics \ˌsī-kə-sə-ˈmat-iks, -kō-, -sō-\ *n pl but sing in constr* : a branch of medical science dealing with interrelationships between the mind or emotions and the body and esp. with the relation of psychic conflict to somatic symptomatology

psy·cho·stim·u·lant \-ˈstim-yə-lənt\ *n or adj* : ANTIDEPRESSANT

psy·cho·sur·geon \ˌsī-kō-ˈsər-jən\ *n* : a surgeon specializing in psychosurgery

psy·cho·sur·gery \-ˈsərj-(ə-)rē\ *n, pl* **-ger·ies** : cerebral surgery employed in treating psychic symptoms — **psy·cho·sur·gi·cal** \-ˈsər-ji-kəl\ *adj*

psy·cho·syn·the·sis \ˌsī-kō-ˈsin(t)-thə-səs\ *n, pl* **-the·ses** \-ˌsēz\ : a form of psychotherapy combining psychoanalytic techniques with meditation and exercise

psy·cho·tech·ni·cal \ˌsī-kō-ˈtek-ni-kəl\ *also* **psy·cho·tech·nic** \-ˈnik\ *adj* : of or relating to or devoted to the practical applications (as industrial or military problems) of psychology

psy·cho·tech·nics \-ˈtek-niks\ *n pl but sing in constr* : PSYCHOTECHNOLOGY 1

psy·cho·tech·nol·o·gist \-tek-ˈnäl-ə-jəst\ *n* : a specialist in psychotechnology

psy·cho·tech·nol·o·gy \-jē\ *n, pl* **-gies** **1** : the application of psychological methods and results to the solution of practical problems esp. in industry **2** : an application of technology for psychological purposes (as personal growth or behavior change) — **psy·cho·tech·no·log·i·cal** \-ˌtek-nə-ˈläj-i-kəl\ *adj*

psy·cho·ther·a·peu·tic \-ˌther-ə-ˈpyüt-ik\ *adj* : of, relating to, or used in psychotherapy ⟨∼ methods⟩ — **psy·cho·ther·a·peu·ti·cal·ly** \-i-k(ə-)lē\ *adv*

psy·cho·ther·a·peu·tics \-iks\ *n pl but sing or pl in constr* : PSYCHOTHERAPY

psy·cho·ther·a·pist \-ˈther-ə-pəst\ *n* : an individual (as a psychiatrist, clinical psychologist, or psychiatric social worker) who is a practitioner of psychotherapy

psy·cho·ther·a·py \ˌsī-kō-ˈther-ə-pē\ *n, pl* **-pies** **1** : treatment of mental or emotional disorder or maladjustment by psychological means esp. involving verbal communication (as in psychoanalysis, nondirective psychotherapy, reeducation, or hypnosis) **2** : any alteration in an individual's interpersonal environment, relationships, or life situation brought about esp. by a qualified therapist and intended to have the effect of alleviating symptoms of mental or emotional disturbance

¹**psy·chot·ic** \sī-ˈkät-ik\ *adj* : of, relating to, marked by, or affected with psychosis — **psy·chot·i·cal·ly** \-i-k(ə-)lē\ *adv*

²**psychotic** *n* : a psychotic individual

psy·cho·to·gen \sī-ˈkät-ə-jən\ *n* : a chemical agent (as a drug) that induces a psychotic state — **psy·cho·to·gen·ic** \(ˌ)sī-ˌkät-ə-ˈjen-ik\ *adj*

¹**psy·cho·to·mi·met·ic** \sī-ˌkät-ō-mə-ˈmet-ik, -mī-\ *adj* : of, relating to, involving, or inducing psychotic alteration of behavior and personality ⟨∼ drugs⟩ — **psy·cho·to·mi·met·i·cal·ly** \-i-k(ə-)lē\ *adv*

²**psychotomimetic** *n* : a psychotomimetic agent (as a drug)

psy·cho·tox·ic \ˌsī-kə-ˈtäk-sik\ *adj* : having or being a detrimental effect on one's mind, personality, or behavior ⟨a ∼ chemical⟩

¹**psy·cho·tro·pic** \ˌsī-kə-ˈtrō-pik\ *adj* : acting on the mind ⟨∼ drugs⟩

²**psychotropic** *n* : a psychotropic substance (as a drug)

psy·chrom·e·ter \sī-ˈkräm-ət-ər\ *n* : a hygrometer consisting essentially of two similar thermometers with the bulb of one being kept wet so that the cooling that results from evaporation makes it register a lower temperature than the dry one and with the difference between the readings constituting a measure of the dryness of the atmosphere — **psy·chro·met·ric** \ˌsī-krə-ˈme-trik\ *adj* — **psy·chrom·e·try** \sī-ˈkräm-ə-trē\ *n, pl* **-tries**

psy·chro·phile \ˈsī-krō-ˌfīl\ *n* : a psychrophilic organism — compare MESOPHILE, THERMOPHILE

psy·chro·phil·ic \ˌsī-krō-ˈfil-ik\ *adj* : thriving at a relatively low temperature ⟨∼ bacteria⟩

psyl·li·um \ˈsil-ē-əm\ *n* **1** : FLEAWORT **2** : PSYLLIUM SEED

psyllium seed *n* : the seed of a fleawort (esp. *Plantago psyllium*) that has the property of swelling and becoming gelatinous when moist and is used as a mild laxative — called also *fleaseed, plantago seed, psyllium;* see METAMUCIL

pt *abbr* **1** patient **2** pint

Pt *symbol* platinum

PT *abbr* **1** physical therapist **2** physical therapy

PTA *abbr* plasma thromboplastin antecedent

PTC \ˌpē-ˌtē-ˈsē\ *n* : PHENYLTHIOCARBAMIDE

PTC *abbr* plasma thromboplastin component

PTCA \ˌpē-ˌtē-ˌsē-ˈā\ *n* : PERCUTANEOUS TRANSLUMINAL CORONARY ANGIOPLASTY

pter·i·dine \ˈter-ə-ˌdēn\ *n* : a yellow crystalline bicyclic base $C_6H_4N_4$ that is a structural constituent esp. of various animal pigments

pter·in \ˈter-ən\ *n* : any of various compounds that contain the bicyclic ring system characteristic of pteridine

pter·i·on \ˈter-ē-ˌän\ *n* : the point on each side of the skull where the parietal and temporal bones meet the greater wing of the sphenoid

pte·ro·ic acid \tə-ˌrō-ik-\ *n* : a crystalline amino acid $C_{14}H_{12}N_6O_3$ formed with glutamic acid by hydrolysis of folic acid

pter·o·yl·glu·tam·ic acid \ˌter-ə-ˌwil-glü-ˌtam-ik-\ *n* : FOLIC ACID — abbr. *PGA*

pte·ryg·i·um \te-ˈrij-ē-əm\ *n, pl* **-iums** *or* **-ia** \-ē-ə\ **1** : a triangular fleshy mass of thickened conjunctiva occurring usu. at the inner side of the eyeball, covering part of the cornea, and causing a disturbance of vision **2** : a forward growth of the cuticle over the nail

¹**pter·y·goid** \ˈter-ə-ˌgóid\ *adj* : of, relating to, being, or lying in the region of the inferior part of the sphenoid bone

²**pterygoid** *n* : a pterygoid part (as a pterygoid muscle or nerve)

pterygoid canal *n* : an anteroposterior canal in the base of each medial pterygoid plate of the sphenoid bone that gives passage to the Vidian artery and the Vidian nerve — called also *Vidian canal*

pter·y·goi·de·us \ˌter-ə-ˈgóid-ē-əs\ *n, pl* **-dei** \-ē-ˌī\ : PTERYGOID MUSCLE

pterygoid fissure *n* : the angular cleft separating the medial and lateral pterygoid plates of each pterygoid process — called also *pterygoid notch*

pterygoid fossa *n* : a V-shaped depression on the posterior part of each pterygoid process that is formed by the divergence posteriorly of its medial and lateral pterygoid plates and that contains the medial pterygoid muscle and the tensor veli palatini

pterygoid hamulus *n* : a hook-shaped process forming the inferior extremity of each medial pterygoid plate of the sphenoid bone and providing a support around which the tendon of the tensor veli palatini moves

pterygoid lamina *n* : PTERYGOID PLATE

pterygoid muscle *n* : either of two muscles extending from the sphenoid bone to the lower jaw: **a** : a muscle that arises from the greater wing of the sphenoid bone and from the outer surface of the lateral pterygoid plate, is inserted into the condyle of the mandible and the articular disk of the temporomandibular joint, and acts as an antagonist of the masseter, temporalis, and medial pterygoid muscles — called also *external pterygoid muscle, lateral pterygoid muscle* **b** : a muscle that arises from the inner surface of the lateral pterygoid plate and from the palatine and maxillary bones, is inserted into the ramus and the gonial angle, cooperates with the masseter and temporalis in elevating the lower jaw, and controls certain lateral and rotary movements of the jaw — called also *internal pterygoid muscle, medial pterygoid muscle*

pterygoid nerve *n* : either of two branches of the mandibular nerve: **a** : one that is distributed to the lateral pterygoid muscle — called also *lateral pterygoid nerve* **b** : one that is distributed to the medial pterygoid muscle, tensor tympani, and tensor veli palatini — called also *medial pterygoid nerve*

pterygoid notch \-'näch\ *n* : PTERYGOID FISSURE

pterygoid plate *n* : either of two vertical plates making up a pterygoid process of the sphenoid bone: **a** : a broad thin plate that forms the lateral part of the pterygoid process and gives attachment to the lateral pterygoid muscle on its lateral surface and to the medial pterygoid muscle on its medial surface — called also *lateral pterygoid plate* **b** : a long narrow plate that forms the medial part of the pterygoid process, terminates in the pterygoid hamulus, and forms with its lateral surface part of the pterygoid fossa and with its medial surface the lateral boundary of a choana — called also *medial pterygoid plate*

pterygoid plexus *n* : a plexus of veins draining the region of the pterygoid muscles and emptying chiefly into the facial vein by way of the deep facial vein and into the maxillary vein

pterygoid process *n* : a process that extends downward from each side of the sphenoid bone near the union of its body and a greater wing, that consists of the medial and lateral pterygoid plates which are fused above anteriorly and separated below by the pterygoid fissure whose edges articulate with a process of the palatine bone, and that contains on its posterior aspect the pterygoid and scaphoid fossae which give attachment to muscles

pter·y·go·man·dib·u·lar \ˌter-ə-(ˌ)gō-man-'dib-yə-lər\ *adj* : of, relating to, or linking the pterygoid process of the sphenoid bone and the mandible

pterygomandibular raphe *n* : a fibrous seam that descends from the pterygoid hamulus of the medial pterygoid plate to the mylohyoid line of the mandible and that separates and gives rise to the superior constrictor of the pharynx and the buccinator

pter·y·go·max·il·lary \ˌter-ə-gō-'mak-sə-ˌler-ē, *chiefly Brit* -mak-'sil-ə-rē\ *adj* : of, relating to, or connecting the pterygoid process of the sphenoid bone and the maxilla

pterygomaxillary fissure *n* : a vertical gap between the lateral pterygoid plate of the pterygoid process and the maxilla that descends at right angles to the medial end of the inferior orbital fissure and gives passage to part of the maxillary artery and vein

pterygomaxillary fossa *n* : PTERYGOPALATINE FOSSA

pter·y·go·pal·a·tine fossa \ˌter-ə-gō-'pal-ə-ˌtīn-\ *n* : a small triangular space beneath the apex of the orbit that is bounded above by the sphenoid bone and the orbital process of the palatine bone, in front by the maxilla, medially by the palatine bone, and behind by the pterygoid process of the sphenoid bone and that contains among other structures the pterygopalatine ganglion — called also *pterygomaxillary fossa, sphenomaxillary fossa*

pterygopalatine ganglion *n* : an autonomic ganglion of the maxillary nerve that is situated in the pterygopalatine fossa and that receives preganglionic parasympathetic fibers from the facial nerve and sends postganglionic fibers to the nasal mucosa, palate, pharynx, and orbit — called also *Meckel's ganglion, sphenopalatine ganglion*

pter·y·go·spi·nous \ˌter-ə-gō-'spī-nəs\ *adj* : situated or extending between the lateral pterygoid plate and the inferiorly directed spine on the posterior part of the greater wing of the sphenoid bone

PTFE *abbr* polytetrafluoroethylene

PTH *abbr* parathyroid hormone

Pthir·us \'thir-əs\ *n* : a genus of lice of the family Pediculidae that contains the crab louse (*P. pubis*)

pto·maine \'tō-ˌmān, tō-'\ *n* : any of various organic bases formed by the action of putrefactive bacteria on nitrogenous matter and including some which are poisonous — compare LEUKOMAINE

ptomaine poisoning *n* : food poisoning caused by bacteria or bacterial products — not used technically

ptosed \'tōzd\ *adj* : PTOTIC ⟨a ~ kidney⟩

pto·sis \'tō-səs\ *n, pl* **pto·ses** \-ˌsēz\ : a sagging or prolapse of an organ or part ⟨renal ~⟩; *esp* : a drooping of the upper eyelid (as from paralysis of the oculomotor nerve)

ptot·ic \'tät-ik\ *adj* : relating to or affected with ptosis ⟨a ~ eyelid⟩

PTSD *abbr* post-traumatic stress disorder

pty·a·lin \'tī-ə-lən\ *n* : an amylase found in the saliva of many animals that converts starch into sugar

pty·a·lism \-ˌliz-əm\ *n* : an excessive flow of saliva

Pu *symbol* plutonium

pub·ar·che \'pyü-ˌbär-kē\ *n* : the beginning of puberty marked by the first growth of pubic hair

pu·ber·al \'pyü-bər-əl\ *adj* : PUBERTAL

pu·ber·tal \'pyü-bərt-ᵊl\ *adj* : of, relating to, or occurring in puberty ⟨~ development⟩

pu·ber·tas prae·cox \'pyü-bər-ˌtas-'prē-ˌkäks\ *n* : abnormally early sexual maturity

pu·ber·ty \'pyü-bərt-ē\ *n, pl* **-ties** **1** : the condition of being or the period of becoming first capable of reproducing sexually marked by maturing of the genital organs, development of secondary sex characteristics, and in humans and the higher primates by the first occurrence of menstruation in the female **2** : the age at which puberty occurs being typically between 13 and 16 years in boys and 11 and 14 in girls and often construed legally as 14 in boys and 12 in girls

pu·ber·u·lic acid \pyü-ˌber-yə-lik-\ *n* : a crystalline cyclic keto acid $C_8H_6O_6$ that is a metabolic product of several molds of the genus *Penicillium* and that exhibits some germicidal activity against gram-positive bacteria

pu·ber·u·lon·ic acid \pyü-ˌber-yə-ˌlän-ik-\ *n* : a crystalline compound $C_9H_4O_7$ that is formed from molds along with puberulic acid and exhibits mild germicidal activity against gram-positive bacteria

¹pu·bes \'pyü-(ˌ)bēz\ *n, pl* **pubes** **1** : the hair that appears on the lower part of the hypogastric region at puberty — called also *pubic hair* **2** : the lower part of the hypogastric region : the pubic region

²pubes *pl of* PUBIS

pu·bes·cence \pyü-'bes-ᵊn(t)s\ *n* : the quality or state of being pubescent : PUBERTY

pu·bes·cent \-ᵊnt\ *adj* **1** : arriving at or having reached puberty **2** : of or relating to puberty

pu·bic \'pyü-bik\ *adj* : of, relating to, or situated in or near the region of the pubes or the pubis

pubic arch *n* : the notch formed by the inferior rami of the two conjoined pubic bones as they diverge from the midline

pubic bone *n* : PUBIS

pubic crest *n* : the border of a pubis between its pubic tubercle and the pubic symphysis

pubic hair *n* : PUBES 1

pubic louse *n* : CRAB LOUSE

pubic symphysis *n* : the rather rigid articulation of the two pubic bones in the midline of the lower anterior part of the abdomen — called also *symphysis pubis*

pubic tubercle *n* : a rounded eminence on the upper margin of each pubis near the pubic symphysis

pu·bi·ot·o·my \ˌpyü-bē-'ät-ə-mē\ *n, pl* **-mies** : surgical division of a pubis lateral to the pubic symphysis esp. to facilitate delivery

---

\ə\ abut \ᵊ\ kitten \ər\ further \a\ ash \ā\ ace \ä\ cot, cart
\aù\ out \ch\ chin \e\ bet \ē\ easy \g\ go \i\ hit \ī\ ice \j\ job
\ŋ\ sing \ō\ go \ò\ law \òi\ boy \th\ thin \th\ the \ü\ loot
\ù\ foot \y\ yet \zh\ vision   *See also* Pronunciation Symbols page

O
P

pu·bis \'pyü-bəs\ *n, pl* **pu·bes** \-(ˌ)bēz\ : the ventral and anterior of the three principal bones composing either half of the pelvis that in humans consists of two rami diverging posteriorly from the region of the pubic symphysis with the superior ramus extending to the acetabulum of which it forms a part and uniting there with the ilium and ischium and the inferior ramus extending below the obturator foramen where it unites with the ischium — called also *pubic bone*

pub·lic health \ˌpəb-lik-\ *n* : the art and science dealing with the protection and improvement of community health by organized community effort and including preventive medicine and sanitary and social science

public health nurse *n* : VISITING NURSE

pu·bo·cap·su·lar ligament \ˌpyü-bō-ˌkap-sə-lər-\ *n* : PUBOFEMORAL LIGAMENT

pu·bo·coc·cy·geal \ˌpyü-bō-käk-ˈsij-(ē-)əl\ *adj* : of or relating to the pubococcygeus

pu·bo·coc·cy·geus \-käk-ˈsij-(ē-)əs\ *n, pl* **-cy·gei** \-ˈsij-ē-ˌī\ : the inferior subdivision of the levator ani that arises from the dorsal surface of the pubis along a line extending from the lower part of the pubic symphysis to the obturator canal, that inserts esp. into the coccyx, that acts to help support the pelvic viscera, to draw the lower end of the rectum toward the pubis, and to constrict the rectum and in the female the vagina, and that contains bands of fibers comprising the puborectalis, the levator prostatae in the male, and the pubovaginalis in the female — compare ILIOCOCCYGEUS

pu·bo·fem·o·ral ligament \ˌpyü-bō-ˈfem-(ə-)rəl-\ *n* : a ligament of the hip joint that extends from the superior ramus of the pubis to the capsule of the hip joint near the neck of the femur and that acts to prevent excessive extension and abduction of the thigh — called also *pubocapsular ligament*

pu·bo·pros·tat·ic ligament \ˌpyü-bō-präs-ˈtat-ik-\ *n* : any of three strands of pelvic fascia in the male that correspond to the pubovesical ligament in the female and that support the prostate gland and indirectly the bladder passing from the capsule of the prostate gland to the pubic symphysis or to the pubis on one side or the other

pu·bo·rec·ta·lis \ˌpyü-bō-rek-ˈtā-ləs\ *n* : a band of muscle fibers that is part of the pubococcygeus, that passes from the pubic symphysis to interdigitate with the contralateral band of fibers forming a sling around the rectum at its junction with the anal canal, and that acts to hold the rectum and anal canal at right angles to each other except during defecation

pu·bo·vag·i·na·lis \ˌpyü-bō-ˌvaj-ə-ˈnā-ləs\ *n* : the most medial and anterior fasciculi of the pubococcygeal part of the levator ani in the female that correspond to the levator prostatae in the male, pass along the sides of the vagina, insert into the coccyx, and act to constrict the vagina

pu·bo·ves·i·cal ligament \ˌpyü-bō-ˈves-i-kəl-\ *n* : any of three strands of pelvic fascia in the female that correspond to the puboprostatic ligament in the male and that support the bladder passing from its neck to the pubic symphysis or to the pubis on one side

pudenda *pl of* PUDENDUM

¹pu·den·dal \pyù-ˈden-dᵊl\ *adj* : of, relating to, occurring in, or lying in the region of the external genital organs

²pudendal *n* : a pudendal anatomical part (as a vessel or the pudendal nerve)

pudendal artery — see EXTERNAL PUDENDAL ARTERY, INTERNAL PUDENDAL ARTERY

pudendal cleft *n* : the opening between the labia majora — called also *rima pudendi*

pudendal nerve *n* : a nerve that arises from the second, third, and fourth sacral nerves and that supplies the external genitalia, the skin of the perineum, and the anal sphincters

pudendal vein — see INTERNAL PUDENDAL VEIN

pudendi — see RIMA PUDENDI

pu·den·dum \pyù-ˈden-dəm\ *n, pl* **-da** \-də\ : the external genital organs of a human being; *esp* : the external genitals of a woman : VULVA — usu. used in pl.

pu·dic \'pyü-dik\ *adj* : PUDENDAL

pu·er·ile \'pyù-(ə)r-əl, -ˌī'l\ *adj* **1** : marked by or suggesting

childishness and immaturity **2** : being respiration that is like that of a child in being louder than normal ⟨∼ breathing⟩

pu·er·per·al \pyü-ˈər-p(ə-)rəl\ *adj* : of, relating to, or occurring during childbirth or the period immediately following ⟨∼ infection⟩ ⟨∼ depression⟩

puerperal fever *n* : an abnormal condition that results from infection (as by streptococci) of the placental site following delivery or abortion and is characterized in mild form by fever of not over 100.4°F (38.0°C) but may progress to a localized endometritis or spread through the uterine wall and develop into peritonitis or pass into the bloodstream and produce sepsis — called also *childbed fever, puerperal sepsis*

puerperal sepsis *n* : PUERPERAL FEVER

pu·er·pe·ri·um \ˌpyü-ər-ˈpir-ē-əm\ *n, pl* **-ria** \-ē-ə\ : the period between childbirth and the return of the uterus to its normal size

PUFA \'pəf-ə, 'p(y)ü-fə\ *n* : a polyunsaturated fatty acid

¹puff \'pəf\ *vi* **1** : to become distended — SWELL — usu. used with *up* **2** : to form a chromosomal puff

²puff *n* **1** : WINDGALL **2** : an enlarged region of a chromosome that is associated with intensely active genes involved in RNA synthesis

puff adder *n* : a large thick-bodied exceedingly venomous widely distributed African viper (*Bitis arietans*) that inflates its body and hisses loudly when disturbed; *also* : a similar smaller snake (*B. inornata*) of southern Africa

puff·ball \'pəf-ˌból\ *n* : any of various globose and often edible fungi (esp. family Lycoperdaceae) that discharge ripe spores in a smokelike cloud when pressed or struck

puff·er \'pəf-ər\ *n* : any of a family (Tetraodontidae) of chiefly tropical marine bony fishes which can distend themselves to a globular form and most of which are highly poisonous — called also *blowfish, globefish, pufferfish*

pugilistica — see DEMENTIA PUGILISTICA

Pu·lex \'pyü-ˌleks\ *n* : a genus of fleas that is the type genus of the family Pulicidae and includes the most common flea (*P. irritans*) that regularly attacks human beings

Pu·lic·i·dae \pyü-ˈlis-ə-ˌdē\ *n pl* : a large and nearly cosmopolitan family of fleas that includes many of the common fleas attacking human beings and domestic animals — see PULEX

¹pull \'pùl\ *vt* **1** : EXTRACT 1 ⟨∼ a tooth⟩ **2** : to strain or stretch abnormally ⟨∼ a tendon⟩ ⟨∼ a muscle⟩

²pull *n* : an injury resulting from abnormal straining or stretching esp. of a muscle — see GROIN PULL

pul·ley \'pùl-ē\ *n* : TROCHLEA

pul·lo·rum disease \pə-ˈlōr-əm-, -ˈlòr-\ *n* : a destructive typically diarrheic salmonellosis esp. of the domestic chicken caused by a bacterium of the genus *Salmonella* (*S. pullorum*) which is transmitted either through the egg or from chick to chick — called also *pullorum*

pul·lu·late \'pəl-yə-ˌlāt\ *vi* **-lat·ed; -lat·ing** **1** : to bud or sprout **2** : to breed or produce freely — **pul·lu·la·tion** \ˌpəl-yə-ˈlā-shən\ *n*

pulmonale, pulmonalia — see COR PULMONALE

pul·mo·nary \'pùl-mə-ˌner-ē, 'pəl-\ *adj* : relating to, functioning like, associated with, or carried on by the lungs

pulmonary adenomatosis *n* : JAAGSIEKTE

pulmonary alveolar proteinosis *n* : a chronic disease of the lungs characterized by the filling of the alveoli with proteinaceous material and by the progressive loss of lung function

pulmonary arch *n* : either the right or the left sixth aortic arch that in the human fetus persists on the right side as the right pulmonary artery and on the left side as the ductus arteriosus and part of the pulmonary trunk

pulmonary artery *n* : an arterial trunk or either of its two main branches that carry oxygen-deficient blood to the lungs: **a** : a large arterial trunk that arises from the conus arteriosus of the right ventricle, ascends in front of the aorta, and branches into the right and left pulmonary arteries — called also *pulmonary trunk* **b** : a branch of the pulmonary trunk that passes under the arch of the aorta to the right lung where it divides into branches — called also *right pulmonary artery* **c** : a branch of the pulmonary trunk that passes to the left in front of the descending part of the aorta, gives off the ductus arteriosus in the fetus which regresses to the ligamentum arteriosum in the adult, and passes to the left lung where it divides into branches — called also *left pulmonary artery*

pulmonary capillary wedge pressure *n* : WEDGE PRESSURE — abbr. *PCWP*

pulmonary circulation *n* : the passage of venous blood from the right atrium of the heart through the right ventricle and pulmonary arteries to the lungs where it is oxygenated and its return via the pulmonary veins to enter the left auricle and participate in the systemic circulation

pulmonary edema *n* : abnormal accumulation of fluid in the lungs

pulmonary embolism *n* : embolism of a pulmonary artery or one of its branches that is produced by foreign matter and most often a blood clot originating in a vein of the leg or pelvis and that is marked by labored breathing, chest pain, fainting, rapid heart rate, cyanosis, shock, and sometimes death — abbr. *PE*

pulmonary ligament *n* : a supporting fold of pleura that extends from the lower part of the lung on its surface opposite the mediastinum to the pericardium

pulmonary plexus *n* : either of two nerve plexuses associated with each lung that lie on the dorsal and ventral aspects of the bronchi of each lung and distribute fibers mainly from the vagus nerve to the lungs

pulmonary stenosis *n* : abnormal narrowing of the orifice between the pulmonary artery and the right ventricle — called also *pulmonic stenosis*

pulmonary trunk *n* : PULMONARY ARTERY a

pulmonary valve *n* : a valve consisting of three semilunar cusps separating the pulmonary trunk from the right ventricle

pulmonary vein *n* : any of usu. four veins comprising two from each lung that return oxygenated blood from the lungs to the superior part of the left atrium, that may include three veins from the right lung if the veins from all three lobes of the right lung remain separate, and that may include a single trunk from the left lung if its major veins unite before emptying into the left atrium

pulmonary wedge pressure *n* : WEDGE PRESSURE

pul·mo·nec·to·my \ˌpu̇l-mə-ˈnek-tə-mē, ˌpəl-\ *n, pl* **-mies** : PNEUMONECTOMY

pul·mon·ic \pu̇l-ˈmän-ik, ˌpəl-\ *adj* : PULMONARY ⟨∼ lesions⟩

pulmonic stenosis *n* : PULMONARY STENOSIS

pul·mo·nol·o·gist \ˌpu̇l-mə-ˈnäl-ə-jəst, ˌpəl-\ *n* : a specialist in pulmonology

pul·mo·nol·o·gy \-jē\ *n, pl* **-gies** : a branch of medicine concerned with the anatomy, physiology, and pathology of the lungs

pul·mo·tor \ˈpu̇l-ˌmōt-ər, ˈpəl-\ *n* : a respiratory apparatus for pumping oxygen or air into and out of the lungs (as of an asphyxiated person)

pulp \ˈpəlp\ *n* : a mass of soft tissue: as **a** : DENTAL PULP **b** : the characteristic somewhat spongy tissue of the spleen **c** : the fleshy portion of the fingertip

pulp·al \ˈpəl-pəl\ *adj* : of or relating to pulp esp. of a tooth ⟨a ∼ abscess⟩ — **pulp·al·ly** \ˈpəl-pə-lē\ *adv*

pulp canal *n* : ROOT CANAL 1

pulp cavity *n* : the central cavity of a tooth containing the dental pulp and being made up of the root canal and the pulp chamber

pulp chamber *n* : the part of the pulp cavity lying in the crown of a tooth

pulp·ec·to·my \ˌpəl-ˈpek-tə-mē\ *n, pl* **-mies** : the removal of the pulp of a tooth

pulp·i·tis \ˌpəl-ˈpīt-əs\ *n, pl* **pulp·it·i·des** \-ˈpit-ə-ˌdēz\ : inflammation of the pulp of a tooth

pulp·less \ˈpəlp-ləs\ *adj* : having no pulp ⟨∼ teeth⟩

pulposi, pulposus — see NUCLEUS PULPOSUS

pulp·ot·o·my \ˌpəl-ˈpät-ə-mē\ *n, pl* **-mies** : removal in a dental procedure of the coronal portion of the pulp of a tooth in such a manner that the pulp of the root remains intact and viable

pulp stone *n* : a lump of calcified tissue within the dental pulp — called also *denticle*

pulpy \ˈpəl-pē\ *adj* **pulp·i·er; pulp·i·est** : resembling or consisting of pulp ⟨a ∼ mass⟩

pulpy kidney *n* : a destructive enterotoxemia of lambs caused by a bacterium of the genus *Clostridium* (*C. perfringens*) and characterized by softening and degeneration of the kidneys and often by accumulation of fluid about the heart — called also *pulpy kidney disease*

pul·sate \ˈpəl-ˌsāt also ˌpəl-ˈ\ *vi* **pul·sat·ed; pul·sat·ing** : to exhibit a pulse or pulsation ⟨a *pulsating* artery⟩

pul·sa·tile \ˈpəl-sət-ᵊl, -sə-ˌtīl\ *adj* : marked by or occurring in pulsations ⟨a ∼ glandular secretion⟩

pul·sa·til·la \ˌpəl-sə-ˈtil-ə\ *n* : a dried medicinal herb from a pasqueflower (esp. *Anemone pulsatilla* syn. *Pulsatilla vulgaris*) formerly used to treat amenorrhea and dysmenorrhea and still used in India to induce abortion

pul·sa·tion \ˌpəl-ˈsā-shən\ *n* **1** : rhythmic throbbing or vibrating (as of an artery); *also* : a single beat or throb **2** : a periodically recurring alternate increase and decrease of a quantity (as pressure, volume, or voltage)

¹pulse \ˈpəls\ *n* **1 a** : a regularly recurrent wave of distension in arteries that results from the progress through an artery of blood injected into the arterial system at each contraction of the ventricles of the heart **b** : the palpable beat resulting from such pulse as detected in a superficial artery (as the radial artery) ⟨a very soft ∼⟩; *also* : the number of such beats in a specified period of time (as one minute) ⟨a resting ∼ of 70⟩ **2** : PULSATION **3 a** : a transient variation of a quantity (as electric current or voltage) whose value is normally constant — often used of current variations produced artificially and repeated either with a regular period or according to some code **b** : an electromagnetic wave or modulation thereof having brief duration **c** : a brief disturbance transmitted through a medium **4** : a dose of a substance esp. when applied over a short period of time ⟨therapy with ∼s of intravenous methylprednisolone⟩

²pulse *vb* **pulsed; puls·ing** *vi* : to exhibit a pulse or pulsation ∼ *vt* **1** : to cause to pulsate **2 a** : to produce or modulate (as electromagnetic waves) in the form of pulses ⟨*pulsed* waves⟩ **b** : to cause (an apparatus) to produce pulses

pulse–chase \-ˌchās\ *adj* : involving the exposure of cells to a substrate bearing a radioactive label for a predetermined time followed by exposure to a high concentration of unlabeled substrate in order to stop uptake of the labeled substrate and follow its metabolic course ⟨a ∼ experiment⟩

pulsed–field gel electrophoresis \ˌpəls(t)-ˌfē(ə)ld-\ *n* : gel electrophoresis that is used esp. to separate large fragments of DNA and that involves changing the direction of the electric current periodically in order to minimize overlap of the spots due to diffusion — called also *pulsed-field electrophoresis*

pulsed light *n* : high intensity white light that is emitted (as by a xenon flashtube) in a series of flashes of brief duration (as 10 to 20 milliseconds in length) ⟨*pulsed light* therapy to treat skin imperfections and rosacea⟩

pulse–la·bel \ˈpəls-ˌlā-bəl\ *vt* **-la·beled** *or* **-la·belled; -la·bel·ing** *or* **-la·bel·ling** : to cause a pulse of a radiolabeled atom or substance to become incorporated into (as a molecule or cell component) ⟨∼ed DNA⟩

pulse·less \-ləs\ *adj* : having no pulse

pulseless disease *n* : TAKAYASU'S ARTERITIS

pulse oximeter *n* : a device that determines the oxygen saturation of the blood of an anesthetized patient using a sensor attached to a finger, yields a computerized readout, and

\ə\ abut \ᵊ\ kitten \ər\ further \a\ ash \ā\ ace \ä\ cot, cart \au̇\ out \ch\ chin \e\ bet \ē\ easy \g\ go \i\ hit \ī\ ice \j\ job \ŋ\ sing \ō\ go \ȯ\ law \ȯi\ boy \th\ thin \t͟h\ the \ü\ loot \u̇\ foot \y\ yet \zh\ vision *See also* Pronunciation Symbols page

sounds an alarm if the blood saturation becomes less than optimal — **pulse oximetry** *n*

pulse pressure *n* : the pressure that is characteristic of the arterial pulse and represents the difference between diastolic and systolic blood pressures of the heart cycle

pulse rate *n* : the rate of the arterial pulse usu. observed at the wrist and stated in beats per minute

pulse wave *n* : the wave of increased pressure started by the ventricular systole radiating from the semilunar valves over the arterial system at a rate varying between 20 and 30 feet (6.1 and 9.1 meters) per second in different arteries

pul·sion diverticulum \'pəl-shən-\ *n* : a diverticulum pushed out from a hollow organ by pressure from within; *specif* : a diverticulum of the esophagus as a result of the pressure from within resulting in herniation of the mucosa — compare ZENKER'S DIVERTICULUM

pul·sus al·ter·nans \'pəl-səs-'òl-tər-ˌnanz\ *n* : alternation of strong and weak beats of the arterial pulse due to alternate strong and weak ventricular contractions

pulsus par·a·dox·us \-ˌpar-ə-'däk-səs\ *n* : a pulse that weakens abnormally during inspiration and is symptomatic of various abnormalities (as pericarditis)

pul·ta·ceous \ˌpəl-'tā-shəs\ *adj* : having a soft consistency : PULPY

pulv *abbr* [Latin *pulvis*] powder — used in writing prescriptions

pul·ver·i·za·tion *also Brit* **pul·ver·i·sa·tion** \ˌpəl-və-rə-'zā-shən\ *n* : the act or process of pulverizing

pul·ver·ize *also Brit* **pul·ver·ise** \'pəl-və-ˌrīz\ *vb* **-ized** *also Brit* **-ised; -iz·ing** *also Brit* **-is·ing** *vt* : to reduce (as by crushing, beating, or grinding) to very small particles ∼ *vi* : to become pulverized

pul·ver·u·lent \ˌpəl-'ver-(y)ə-lənt\ *adj* **1** : consisting of or reducible to fine powder **2** : being or looking dusty

pul·vi·nar \ˌpəl-'vī-nər\ *n* : a rounded prominence on the back of the thalamus

Pul·vule \'pəl-ˌvyül\ *trademark* — used for a gelatin-based medicinal capsule

pum·ice \'pəm-əs\ *n* : a volcanic glass full of cavities and very light in weight used esp. in powder form for smoothing and polishing

¹pump \'pəmp\ *n* **1** : a device that raises, transfers, or compresses fluids or that attenuates gases esp. by suction or pressure or both **2** : HEART **3** : an act or the process of pumping **4** : an energy source (as light) for pumping atoms or molecules **5** : a mechanism by which atoms, ions, or molecules are transported across cell membranes — see PROTON PUMP, SODIUM PUMP

²pump *vi* : to work a pump : raise or move a fluid with a pump ∼ *vt* **1** : to raise (as water) with a pump **2** : to draw fluid from with a pump **3** : to transport (as ions) against a concentration gradient by the expenditure of energy **4 a** : to excite (as atoms or molecules) esp. so as to cause emission of coherent monochromatic electromagnetic radiation (as in a laser) **b** : to energize (as a laser) by pumping

pump·kin \'pəm(p)-kən\ *n* : the usu. round orange fruit of a vine (*Cucurbita pepo*) of the gourd family that is widely cultivated as food and is the source of pepo

pumpkin seed *n* : PEPO

punch–drunk \'pənch-ˌdrəŋk\ *adj* : suffering cerebral injury from many minute brain hemorrhages as a result of repeated head blows received in boxing — **punch–drunk·en·ness** \-ˌdrəŋ-kən-nəs\ *n*

punctata — see KERATITIS PUNCTATA

¹punc·tate \'pəŋ(k)-ˌtāt\ *adj* : characterized by dots or points ⟨∼ skin lesions⟩ — **punc·ta·tion** \ˌpəŋ(k)-'tā-shən\ *n*

²punctate *n* : a punctate structure or area

punc·ti·form \'pəŋ(k)-tə-ˌfòrm\ *adj* **1** : having the form or character of a point **2** : marked by or composed of points or dots : PUNCTATE **3** : of or relating to tangible points or dots used for representing words for reading by the blind

punc·tum \'pəŋ(k)-təm\ *n, pl* **punc·ta** \-tə\ : a small area marked off from a surrounding surface ⟨insect bites . . . may

show the central tiny hemorrhagic ∼ —*Jour. Amer. Med. Assoc.*⟩ — see LACRIMAL PUNCTUM

¹punc·ture \'pəŋ(k)-chər\ *n* **1** : an act of puncturing **2** : a hole, wound, or perforation made by puncturing

²puncture *vb* **punc·tured; punc·tur·ing** \'pəŋ(k)-chə-riŋ, 'pəŋ(k)-shriŋ\ *vt* : to pierce with or as if with a pointed instrument or object ⟨∼ the skin with a needle⟩ ∼ *vi* : to become punctured

pun·gen·cy \'pən-jən-sē\ *n, pl* **-cies** : the quality or state of being pungent

pun·gent \-jənt\ *adj* : causing a sharp or irritating sensation; *esp* : ACRID — **pun·gent·ly** *adv*

PUO *abbr* pyrexia of unknown origin

pu·pa \'pyü-pə\ *n, pl* **pu·pae** \-(ˌ)pē, -ˌpī\ *or* **pupas** : an intermediate usu. quiescent stage of an insect that occurs between the larva and the imago in forms (as a bee, moth, or beetle) which undergo complete metamorphosis and that is characterized by internal changes by which larval structures are replaced by those typical of the imago — **pu·pal** \'pyü-pəl\ *adj*

pu·pil \'pyü-pəl\ *n* : the contractile usu. round aperture in the iris of the eye

pupillae — see SPHINCTER PUPILLAE

pu·pil·lary *also* **pu·pi·lary** \'pyü-pə-ˌler-ē\ *adj* : of or relating to the pupil of the eye

pupillary reflex *n* : the contraction of the pupil in response to light entering the eye

pu·pil·lo·di·la·tor \ˌpyü-pə-lō-dī-'lāt-ər, -'dī-ˌ\ *adj* : having a dilating effect on or involving dilation of the pupil of the eye

pu·pil·log·ra·phy \ˌpyü-pə-'läg-rə-fē\ *n, pl* **-phies** : the measurement of the reactions of the pupil

pu·pil·lom·e·ter \ˌpyü-pə-'läm-ət-ər\ *n* : an instrument for measuring the diameter of the pupil of the eye — **pu·pil·lom·e·try** \-ə-trē\ *n, pl* **-tries**

pu·pil·lo·mo·tor \ˌpyü-pə-lō-'mōt-ər\ *adj* : having a motor influence on or involving alteration of the pupil of the eye ⟨∼ nerve fibers⟩ ⟨a ∼ reflex⟩

pura — see AQUA PURA

pure \'pyü(ə)r\ *adj* **pur·er; pur·est** **1** : unmixed with any other matter ⟨∼ gold⟩ **2** : free from dust, dirt, or taint ⟨∼ food⟩ **3 a** : of unmixed ancestry : PUREBRED **b** : homozygous in and breeding true for one or more characters — **pure·ness** *n*

pure·bred \-'bred\ *adj* : bred from members of a recognized breed, strain, or kind without outbreeding over many generations — **pure·bred** \-ˌbred\ *n*

pure culture *n* **1** : a culture containing a growth of a single kind of organism free from other organisms **2** : a culture containing the descendants of a single organism whether free from all organisms of other kinds or not

pure line *n* : a homogeneous line of descent: as **a** : a group of closely related individuals of identical genetic constitution (as the offspring of a homozygous self-fertilized parent) : a line of descent theoretically realizable from the inbreeding of completely homozygous and comparable parents **b** : the descendants of a single individual esp. by vegetative multiplication : CLONE

pure tone *n* : a musical tone of a single frequency produced by simple harmonic vibrations and without overtones

pur·ga·tion \ˌpər-'gā-shən\ *n* **1** : the act of purging; *specif* : vigorous evacuation of the bowels (as from the action of a cathartic or an infective agent) **2** : administration of or treatment with a purgative

¹pur·ga·tive \'pər-gət-iv\ *adj* : purging or tending to purge : CATHARTIC — **pur·ga·tive·ly** *adv*

²purgative *n* : a purging medicine : CATHARTIC

¹purge \'pərj\ *vb* **purged; purg·ing** *vt* **1** : to cause evacuation from (as the bowels) or of or from the bowels of ⟨drugs that ∼ the bowels⟩ ⟨*purged* the patient with a cathartic⟩ **2** : to free (itself) of suspended matter usu. by sedimentation — used of a liquid ∼ *vi* **1** : to become purged **2** : to have or produce frequent evacuations **3** : to cause purgation

²purge *n* **1** : something that purges; *esp* : PURGATIVE **2** : an act or instance of purging

purging agaric *n* : a common white basidiomycetous fungus (*Fomitopsis officinalis* syn. *Fomes officinalis* of the family Polyporaceae) that is found in the U.S. and Europe on conifers (as larch and pine) and that has been used in medicine as a purgative — called also *white agaric*

purging flax *n* : a European annual herb (*Linum catharticum*) with white or yellowish white flowers followed by seeds that are cathartic and diuretic — see ¹LININ

pu·ri·fied protein derivative \'pyür-ə-₁fīd-\ *n* : a highly purified preparation of tuberculin used in skin tests (as the Mantoux test) to detect tuberculous infection — abbr. *PPD*

pu·rine \'pyü(ə)r-₁ēn\ *n* **1** : a crystalline base $C_5H_4N_4$ that is the parent of compounds of the uric-acid group **2** : a derivative of purine; *esp* : a base (as adenine or guanine) that is a constituent of DNA or RNA

purine base *n* : any of a group of crystalline bases comprising purine and bases derived from it (as adenine, caffeine, guanine, theobromine, or xanthine) some of which are components of nucleosides and nucleotides

pu·ri·ty \'pyür-ət-ē\ *n* : the quality or state of being pure

Pur·kin·je afterimage \(₁)pər-'kin-jē-\ *n* : a second positive afterimage in a succession of visual afterimages resulting from a brief light stimulus and appearing most distinctly in a hue complementary to that of the original sensation

Pur·ky·ně *or* **Purkinje** \'pür-kin-ye, -yā\, **Jan Evangelista (1787–1869),** Bohemian physiologist. Purkyně was a pioneering physiologist who made major contributions to histology, embryology, and pharmacology and whose discoveries considerably increased our understanding of the composition of cells, the functions of the brain and the heart, mammalian reproduction, and the phenomena of human vision. His best known discoveries include the large nerve cells in the cortex of the cerebellum that are known as Purkinje cells (1837) and the fibrous tissue that conducts the pacemaker stimulus along the inside walls of the ventricles to all parts of the heart (1839); the fibers are known as Purkinje fibers and make up Purkinje's network. He wrote his graduation dissertation in 1823 on the subjective phenomena of human vision. One such phenomenon is now known as the Purkinje phenomenon.

Purkinje cell *n* : any of numerous nerve cells that occupy the middle layer of the cerebellar cortex and are characterized by a large globe-shaped body with massive dendrites directed outward and a single slender axon directed inward — called also *Purkinje neuron*

Purkinje effect *n* : PURKINJE PHENOMENON

Purkinje fiber *n* : any of the modified cardiac muscle fibers with few nuclei, granulated central cytoplasm, and sparse peripheral striations that make up Purkinje's network

Purkinje neuron *n* : PURKINJE CELL

Purkinje phenomenon *n* : a shift of the region of apparent maximal spectral luminosity from yellow with the light-adapted eye toward violet with the dark-adapted eye that is presumably associated with predominance of cone vision in bright and rod vision in dim illumination — called also *Purkinje effect, Purkinje shift*

Purkinje's network *n* : a network of intracardiac conducting tissue made up of syncytial Purkinje fibers that lie in the myocardium and constitute the bundle of His and other conducting tracts which spread out from the sinoatrial node — called also *Purkinje's system, Purkinje's tissue*

pu·ro·my·cin \₁pyür-ə-'mīs-ᵊn\ *n* : an antibiotic $C_{22}H_{29}N_7O_5$ that is obtained from an actinomycete of the genus *Streptomyces* (*S. alboniger*) and is used esp. as a potent inhibitor of protein synthesis in microorganisms and mammalian cells

¹pur·ple \'pər-pəl\ *adj* **pur·pler** \-p(ə-)lər\; **pur·plest** \-p(ə-)ləst\ : of the color purple

²purple *n* **1** : any of various colors that fall about midway between red and blue in hue **2** : a pigment or dye that colors purple — see VISUAL PURPLE

purple bacterium *n* : any of various free-living bacteria that contain bacteriochlorophyll marked by purplish or sometimes reddish or brownish pigments

purple cone·flow·er \-'kōn-₁flaü(-ə)r\ *n* : any of three com-

posite herbs (*Echinacea purpurea, E. pallida,* and *E. angustifolia*) which have usu. reddish purple to pale pink ray flowers and whose various parts (as the dried rhizome, stems, or leaves) are used in the preparation of the dietary supplement echinacea

pur·pu·ra \'pər-p(y)ə-rə\ *n* : any of several hemorrhagic states characterized by patches of purplish discoloration resulting from extravasation of blood into the skin and mucous membranes — see THROMBOCYTOPENIC PURPURA

purpura ful·mi·nans \-'fül-mə-₁nanz, -'fəl-\ *n* : purpura of an often severe progressive form esp. of children that is characterized by widespread necrosis of the skin and that is associated with a severe illness, results from an inherited or acquired defect of a certain biochemical pathway, or is of unknown cause

purpura hem·or·rhag·i·ca \-₁hem-ə-'raj-ə-kə\ *n* : THROMBOCYTOPENIC PURPURA

purpura rheu·mat·i·ca \-rü-'mat-i-kə\ *n* : SCHÖNLEIN'S DISEASE

pur·pu·rate \pər-'pyür-₁āt\ *n* : a salt or ester of purpuric acid

pur·pu·ric \₁pər-'pyür-ik\ *adj* : of, relating to, or affected with purpura

purpuric acid *n* : a nitrogenous acid $C_8H_5N_5O_6$ related to barbituric acid that yields alloxan and uramil on hydrolysis and is known esp. in purple-red salts (as murexide) from which it is obtained as an orange-red powder

pur·pu·rin \'pər-pyə-rən\ *n* **1** : an orange or red crystalline compound $C_{14}H_8O_5$ obtained from madder root along with alizarin or by oxidation of alizarin and used in dyeing **2** *also* **pur·pu·rine** \-rən, -₁rēn\ : any of various colored compounds obtained from chlorophyll or related compounds by the action of cold alcoholic alkali and oxygen

purse–string suture \'pərs-₁striŋ-\ *n* : a surgical suture passed as a running stitch in and out along the edge of a circular wound in such a way that when the ends of the suture are drawn tight the wound is closed like a purse

pu·ru·lence \'pyür-(y)ə-lən(t)s\ *n* : the quality or state of being purulent; *also* : PUS

pu·ru·lent \-lənt\ *adj* **1** : containing, consisting of, or being pus ⟨a ~ discharge⟩ ⟨a ~ lesion⟩ **2** : accompanied by suppuration ⟨~ meningitis⟩

pus \'pəs\ *n* : thick opaque usu. yellowish white fluid matter formed by suppuration and composed of exudate containing leukocytes, tissue debris, and microorganisms

pus basin *n* : KIDNEY BASIN

pus cell *n* : a polymorphonuclear leukocyte

pus·sy \'pəs-ē\ *adj* **pus·si·er; -est** : full of or resembling pus

¹pus·tu·lant \'pəs-chə-lənt, 'pəs-t(y)ə-\ *n* : an agent (as a chemical) that induces pustule formation

²pustulant *adj* : producing pustules

pus·tu·lar \-lər\ *adj* **1** : of, relating to, or resembling pustules ⟨~ eruptions⟩ **2** : covered with pustular prominences : PUSTULATED

pus·tu·lat·ed \-₁lāt-əd\ *adj* : covered with pustules

pus·tule \'pəs-(₁)chü(ə)l, -(₁)t(y)ü(ə)l\ *n* **1** : a small circumscribed elevation of the skin containing pus and having an inflamed base **2** : a small often distinctively colored elevation or spot resembling a blister or pimple

pu·ta·men \pyü-'tā-mən\ *n, pl* **pu·tam·i·na** \-'tam-ə-nə\ : an outer reddish layer of gray matter in the lentiform nucleus — **pu·tam·i·nous** \-'tam-ə-nəs\ *adj*

pu·tre·fac·tion \₁pyü-trə-'fak-shən\ *n* **1** : the decomposition of organic matter; *esp* : the typically anaerobic splitting of proteins by bacteria and fungi with the formation of foul-smelling incompletely oxidized products **2** : the state of being putrefied

pu·tre·fac·tive \-tiv\ *adj* **1** : of or relating to putrefaction **2** : causing or tending to promote putrefaction

O
P

\ə\ abut \ᵊ\ kitten \ər\ further \a\ ash \ā\ ace \ä\ cot, cart \aü\ out \ch\ chin \e\ bet \ē\ easy \g\ go \i\ hit \ī\ ice \j\ job \ŋ\ sing \ō\ go \o\̇ law \o\̇i boy \th\ thin \th\ the \ü\ loot \u\̇ foot \y\ yet \zh\ vision *See also* Pronunciation Symbols page

pu·tre·fy \'pyü-trə-ˌfī\ *vb* **-fied; -fy·ing** *vt* : to make putrid ~ *vi* : to undergo putrefaction

pu·tres·cent \pyü-'tres-ᵊnt\ *adj* **1** : undergoing putrefaction : becoming putrid **2** : of or relating to putrefaction

pu·tres·ci·ble \-'tres-ə-bəl\ *adj* : liable to become putrid — **pu·tres·ci·bil·i·ty** \(ˌ)pyü-ˌtres-ə-'bil-ət-ē\ *n, pl* **-ties**

pu·tres·cine \-'tres-ˌēn\ *n* : a crystalline slightly poisonous ptomaine $C_4H_{12}N_2$ that is formed by decarboxylation of ornithine, occurs widely but in small amounts in living things, and is found esp. in putrid flesh

pu·trid \'pyü-trəd\ *adj* **1** : being in a state of putrefaction **2** : of, relating to, or characteristic of putrefaction ⟨a ~ odor⟩

pu·trid·i·ty \pyü-'trid-ət-ē\ *n, pl* **-ties** : the quality or state of being putrid

PUVA \ˌpē-(ˌ)yü-(ˌ)vē-'ā\ *n* [*p*soralen *u*ltraviolet *A*] : photochemotherapy for psoriasis using psoralen and UVA

PVD *abbr* peripheral vascular disease

PVE *abbr* prosthetic valve endocarditis

PVP *abbr* polyvinylpyrrolidone

pvt *abbr* private

PWA \ˌpē-ˌdəb-əl-(ˌ)yü-'ā\ *n* : a person affected with AIDS

P wave \'pē-ˌwāv\ *n* : a deflection in an electrocardiographic tracing that represents atrial activity of the heart — compare QRS COMPLEX, T WAVE

Px *abbr* **1** pneumothorax **2** prognosis

pyaemia *chiefly Brit var of* PYEMIA

py·ar·thro·sis \ˌpī-är-'thrō-səs\ *n, pl* **-thro·ses** \-ˌsēz\ : the formation or presence of pus within a joint

pycnic, pycnodysostosis, pycnosis, pycnotic *var of* PYKNIC, PYKNODYSOSTOSIS, PYKNOSIS, PYKNOTIC

pyc·nom·e·ter *or* **pyk·nom·e·ter** \pik-'näm-ət-ər\ *n* : a standard vessel often provided with a thermometer for measuring and comparing the densities or specific gravities of liquids or solids — **pyc·no·met·ric** *or* **pyk·no·met·ric** \ˌpik-nə-'me-trik\ *adj* — **pyc·nom·e·try** *or* **pyk·nom·e·try** \ˌpik-'näm-ə-trē\ *n, pl* **-tries**

py·el·ec·ta·sis \ˌpī-əl-'ek-tə-səs\ *n, pl* **-ta·ses** \-ˌsēz\ : dilation of the renal pelvis of a kidney

py·eli·tis \ˌpī-ə-'līt-əs\ *n* : inflammation of the lining of the renal pelvis of a kidney

py·elo·gram \'pī-(ə-)lə-ˌgram\ *n* : a radiograph made by pyelography

py·elog·ra·phy \ˌpī-ə-'läg-rə-fē\ *n, pl* **-phies** : radiographic visualization of the renal pelvis of a kidney after injection of a radiopaque substance through the ureter or into a vein — see RETROGRADE PYELOGRAPHY — **py·elo·graph·ic** \ˌpī-(ə-)lə-'graf-ik\ *adj*

py·elo·li·thot·o·my \ˌpī-(ə-)lō-li-'thät-ə-mē\ *n, pl* **-mies** : surgical incision of the renal pelvis of a kidney for removal of a kidney stone — called also *pelviolithotomy*

py·elo·ne·phri·tis \ˌpī-(ə-)lō-ni-'frīt-əs\ *n, pl* **-phrit·i·des** \-'frit-ə-ˌdēz\ : inflammation of both the parenchyma of a kidney and the lining of its renal pelvis esp. due to bacterial infection — **py·elo·ne·phrit·ic** \-'frit-ik\ *adj*

py·elo·plas·ty \'pī-(ə-)lə-ˌplas-tē\ *n, pl* **-ties** : plastic surgery of the renal pelvis of a kidney

py·e·los·to·my \ˌpī-(ə-)'läs-tə-mē\ *n, pl* **-mies** : the operation of forming an artificial opening in the renal pelvis of a kidney in order to provide a drainage route for urine alternative to the ureter

py·e·lot·o·my \ˌpī-(ə-)'lät-ə-mē\ *n, pl* **-mies** : surgical incision into the renal pelvis of a kidney

py·elo·ure·ter·og·ra·phy \-yù-ˌrēt-ə-'räg-rə-fē\ *n, pl* **-phies** : PYELOGRAPHY

py·elo·ve·nous back·flow \-'vē-nəs-'bak-ˌflō\ *n* : drainage of fluid from the renal pelvis of a kidney into the renal venous system under certain conditions (as in retrograde pyelography) in which abnormal amounts of pressure occur in a direction opposite to normal — called also *pyelovenous reflux*

py·emia *or chiefly Brit* **py·ae·mia** \pī-'ē-mē-ə\ *n* : septicemia accompanied by multiple abscesses and secondary toxemic symptoms and caused by pus-forming microorganisms (as

the bacterium *Staphylococcus aureus*) — called also *septicopyemia* — **py·emic** *or chiefly Brit* **py·ae·mic** \-mik\ *adj*

Py·emo·tes \ˌpī-ə-'mōt-ēz\ *n* : a genus of mites that are usu. ectoparasites of insects but that include one (*P. ventricosus*) which causes grain itch in humans when transferred (as in harvesting) to the skin

pyg·ma·lion·ism \pig-'māl-yən-ˌiz-əm\ *n, often cap* : sexual responsiveness directed toward a statue or other representation esp. when of one's own making

Pyg·ma·lion \pig-'māl-yən, -'mā-lē-ən\, Greek mythological character. According to the most common version of the myth, Pygmalion was a king of Cyprus and a sculptor who created a beautiful ivory statue representing his ideal of womanhood. He then fell in love with his own creation. In answer to his prayer the goddess Aphrodite brought the statue to life.

pyg·my *also* **pig·my** \'pig-mē\ *n, pl* **pygmies** *also* **pigmies** **1** *cap* : any of a small people of equatorial Africa ranging under five feet (1.5 meters) in height **2** : a relatively short or small individual : DWARF — **pygmy** *adj*

pygmy chimpanzee *n* : BONOBO

py·gop·a·gus \pī-'gäp-ə-gəs\ *n, pl* **-gi** \-ˌgī, -ˌjī\ : a twin fetus joined in the sacral region

¹pyk·nic *also* **pyc·nic** \'pik-nik\ *adj* : characterized by shortness of stature, broadness of girth, and powerful muscularity : ENDOMORPHIC 2

²pyknic *also* **pycnic** *n* : a person of pyknic build

pyk·no·dys·os·to·sis *or* **pyc·no·dys·os·to·sis** \ˌpik-nō-ˌdis-äs-'tō-səs\ *n, pl* **-to·ses** \-ˌsēz\ : a rare condition inherited as an autosomal recessive trait and characterized esp. by short stature, fragile bones, shortness of the fingers and toes, failure of the anterior fontanel to close properly, and a receding chin

pyk·no·ep·i·lep·sy \-'ep-ə-ˌlep-sē\ *n, pl* **-sies** : PYKNOLEPSY

pyk·no·lep·sy \'pik-nə-ˌlep-sē\ *n, pl* **-sies** : a condition marked by epileptiform attacks resembling those of petit mal epilepsy

pyknometer, pyknometric, pyknometry *var of* PYCNOMETER, PYCNOMETRIC, PYCNOMETRY

pyk·no·sis *also* **pyc·no·sis** \pik-'nō-səs\ *n, pl* **pyk·no·ses** *also* **pyc·no·ses** \-ˌsēz\ : a degenerative condition of a cell nucleus marked by clumping of the chromosomes, hyperchromatism, and shrinking of the nucleus

pyk·not·ic *also* **pyc·not·ic** \-'nät-ik\ *adj* : of, relating to, or exhibiting pyknosis

py·le·phle·bi·tis \ˌpī-lə-fli-'bīt-əs\ *n, pl* **-bit·i·des** \-'bit-ə-ˌdēz\ : inflammation of the renal portal vein usu. secondary to intestinal disease and with suppuration

py·lon \'pī-ˌlän, -lən\ *n* : a simple temporary artificial leg

py·lo·rec·to·my \ˌpī-lə-'rek-tə-mē\ *n, pl* **-mies** : surgical excision of the pyloric end of the stomach

pylori *pl of* PYLORUS

py·lo·ric \pī-'lōr-ik, pə-, -'lȯr-\ *adj* : of or relating to the pylorus; *also* : of, relating to, or situated in or near the posterior part of the stomach

pyloric glands *n pl* : the short coiled tubular glands of the mucous coat of the stomach occurring chiefly near the pyloric end

pyloric sphincter *n* : the circular fold of mucous membrane containing a ring of circularly disposed muscle fibers that closes the vertebrate pylorus — called also *pyloric valve*

pyloric stenosis *n* : narrowing of the pyloric opening (as from congenital malformation or contraction of scar tissue)

pyloric valve *n* : PYLORIC SPHINCTER

py·lo·ro·du·o·de·nal \pī-ˌlȯr-ō-ˌd(y)ü-ə-'dēn-ᵊl, pə-'lȯr-ə-, -d(y)ù-'äd-ᵊn-əl\ *adj* : of or relating to the pylorus and the duodenum ⟨the ~ junction⟩

py·lo·ro·my·ot·o·my \-mī-'ät-ə-mē\ *n, pl* **-mies** : surgical incision of the muscle fibers of the pyloric sphincter for relief of stenosis caused by muscular hypertrophy

py·lo·ro·plas·ty \pī-'lȯr-ə-ˌplas-tē\ *n, pl* **-ties** : plastic surgery on the pylorus (as to enlarge a stricture)

py·lo·ro·spasm \pī-'lȯr-ə-ˌspaz-əm\ *n* : spasm of the pyloric sphincter often marked by pain and vomiting

py·lo·rus \pī-'lōr-əs, pə-'lòr-\ *n, pl* **py·lo·ri** \-'lō(ə)r-ˌī, -(ˌ)ē\ : the opening from the vertebrate stomach into the intestine — see PYLORIC SPHINCTER

pyo·cele \'pī-ō-ˌsēl\ *n* : a pus-filled cavity (as of the scrotum)

pyo·coc·cus \ˌpī-ō-'käk-əs\ *n, pl* **-coc·ci** \-'käk-(s)ī\ : any coccoid bacterium that tends to form pus

pyo·col·pos \ˌpī-ō-'käl-pəs, -ˌpäs\ *n* : an accumulation of pus in the vagina

pyo·cy·a·nase \ˌpī-ō-'sī-ə-ˌnās, -ˌnāz\ *n* : a mixture of antibiotics once regarded as a specific bacteriolytic enzyme that is obtained from a bacterium of the genus *Pseudomonas* (*P. aeruginosa*) and that is a soluble yellowish green alkaline amorphous substance capable of digesting various other bacteria

pyo·cy·a·ne·us *also* **pyo·cy·a·ne·ous** \ˌpī-ō-sī-'ā-nē-əs\ *or* **pyo·cy·an·ic** \-'an-ik\ *adj* : of, relating to, or produced by a specific bacterium of the genus *Pseudomonas* (*P. aeruginosa*)

pyo·cy·a·nin \ˌpī-ō-'sī-ə-nən\ *or* **pyo·cy·a·nine** \-ˌnēn\ *n* : a toxic blue crystalline pigment $C_{13}H_{10}N_2O$ that is formed in the metabolism of a bacterium of the genus *Pseudomonas* (*P. aeruginosa*), gives a bluish tint to pus infected with this organism, is a quinone imine related to phenazine, and has antibiotic activity esp. toward gram-positive bacteria

pyo·der·ma \ˌpī-ə-'dər-mə\ *also* **pyo·der·mia** \-mē-ə\ *n* : a bacterial skin inflammation marked by pus-filled lesions — **pyo·der·mic** \-mik\ *adj*

pyoderma gan·gre·no·sum \-ˌgaŋ-gri-'nō-səm\ *n* : a chronic noninfectious condition that is marked by the formation of purplish nodules and pustules which tend to coalesce and form ulcers and that is associated with various underlying systemic or malignant diseases (as leukemia, ulcerative colitis, rheumatoid arthritis, or metastatic adenocarcinoma of the intestine)

pyo·der·ma·to·sis \-ˌdər-mə-'tō-səs\ *n, pl* **-to·ses** \-ˌsēz\ : PYODERMA

py·o·gen \'pī-ə-jən, -ˌjen\ *n* : a pus-producing microorganism

pyo·gen·ic \ˌpī-ə-'jen-ik\ *adj* : producing pus ⟨∼ bacteria⟩; *also* : marked by pus production ⟨∼ meningitis⟩

pyogenic membrane *n* : the limiting layer of an abscess or other region of suppuration

pyogenicum — see GRANULOMA PYOGENICUM

pyo·me·tra \ˌpī-ə-'mē-trə\ *n* : an accumulation of pus in the uterine cavity

pyo·myo·si·tis \ˌpī-ō-ˌmī-ə-'sīt-əs\ *n* : infiltrative bacterial inflammation of muscles leading to the formation of abscesses

pyo·ne·phro·sis \-ni-'frō-səs\ *n, pl* **-phro·ses** \-ˌsēz\ : a collection of pus in the kidney

pyo·ne·phrot·ic \-ni-'frät-ik\ *adj* : of, relating to, or affected with pyonephrosis

pyo·pneu·mo·tho·rax \-ˌn(y)ü-mə-'thō(ə)r-ˌaks, -'thò(ə)r-\ *n, pl* **-tho·rax·es** *or* **-tho·ra·ces** \-'thō-rə-ˌsēz\ : a collection of pus and air or other gas in the pleural cavity

py·or·rhea *or chiefly Brit* **py·or·rhoea** \ˌpī-ə-'rē-ə\ *n* **1** : a discharge of pus **2** : an inflammatory condition of the periodontium that is an advanced form of periodontal disease associated esp. with a discharge of pus from the alveoli and loosening of the teeth in their sockets — called also *Riggs' disease*

pyorrhea al·ve·o·lar·is \-ˌal-vē-ə-'lar-əs\ *n* : PYORRHEA 2

py·or·rhe·ic *or chiefly Brit* **py·or·rhoe·ic** \-'rē-ik\ *adj* : of, relating to, or affected with pyorrhea

pyo·sal·pinx \-'sal-(ˌ)piŋks\ *n, pl* **-sal·pin·ges** \-sal-'pin-(ˌ)jēz\ : a collection of pus in an oviduct

pyo·sep·ti·ce·mia *or chiefly Brit* **pyo·sep·ti·cae·mia** \-ˌsep-tə-'sē-mē-ə\ *n* : pyemia and septicemia combined; *specif* : NAVEL ILL — **pyo·sep·ti·ce·mic** *or chiefly Brit* **pyo·sep·ti·cae·mic** \-mik\ *adj*

pyo·tho·rax \-'thō(ə)r-ˌaks, -'thò(ə)r-\ *n, pl* **-tho·rax·es** *or* **-tho·ra·ces** \-'thōr-ə-(ˌ)sēz\ : EMPYEMA

pyr·a·mid \'pir-ə-ˌmid\ *n* **1** : a polyhedron having for its base a polygon and for faces triangles with a common vertex **2** : an anatomical structure resembling a pyramid: as **a** : RENAL PYRAMID **b** : either of two large bundles of motor fibers from the cerebral cortex that reach the medulla ob-

longata and are continuous with the corticospinal tracts of the spinal cord **c** : a conical projection making up the central part of the inferior vermis of the cerebellum

py·ram·i·dal \pə-'ram-əd-ᵊl\ *adj* **1** : of, relating to, or having the form of a pyramid **2** : of, relating to, or affecting an anatomical pyramid esp. of the central nervous system ⟨a crossed ∼ lesion⟩ ⟨a ∼ disorder⟩

pyramidal cell *n* : any of numerous large multipolar pyramid-shaped cells in the cerebral cortex of higher vertebrates

pyramidal decussation *n* : DECUSSATION OF PYRAMIDS

py·ram·i·da·lis \pə-ˌram-ə-'dā-ləs\ *n, pl* **-da·les** \-(ˌ)lēz\ *or* **-dalises** : a small triangular muscle of the lower front part of the abdomen that is situated in front of and in the same sheath with the rectus and functions to tense the linea alba

pyramidal lobe *n* : a conical lobe of the thyroid gland that varies in shape and position but is often found on the cranial part of the isthmus joining the right and left lobes of the gland or on the adjacent part of either lobe and that may project upward to the hyoid bone

pyramidal tract *n* : CORTICOSPINAL TRACT

py·ram·i·dot·o·my \pə-ˌram-ə-'dät-ə-mē\ *n, pl* **-mies** : a surgical procedure in which a corticospinal tract is severed (as for relief of parkinsonism)

pyr·a·mis \'pir-ə-məs\ *n, pl* **py·ram·i·des** \pə-'ram-ə-ˌdēz\ : PYRAMID 2 ⟨removal of the cerebellar ∼⟩

py·ran \'pī(ə)r-ˌan\ *n* : either of two cyclic compounds C_5H_6O that contain five carbon atoms and one oxygen atom in the ring

py·ra·nose \'pī-rə-ˌnōs, -ˌnōz\ *n* : a monosaccharide in the form of a cyclic hemiacetal containing a pyran ring

py·ran·tel \pə-'ran-ˌtel\ *n* : an anthelmintic drug administered in the form of its pamoate $C_{11}H_{14}N_2S \cdot C_{23}H_{16}O_6$ or tartrate $C_{11}H_{14}N_2S \cdot C_4H_6O_6$

pyr·a·zin·amide \ˌpir-ə-'zin-ə-ˌmīd, -məd\ *n* : a tuberculostatic drug $C_5H_5N_3O$

pyr·azine \'pir-ə-ˌzēn\ *n* **1** : a crystalline heterocyclic weakly basic compound $C_4H_4N_2$ **2** : any of various derivatives of pyrazine

pyr·azole \'pir-ə-ˌzōl\ *n* **1** : a crystalline heterocyclic weakly basic compound $C_3H_4N_2$ isomeric with imidazole **2** : any of various derivatives of pyrazole

py·raz·o·line \pī-'raz-ə-ˌlēn\ *n* **1** : a dihydro derivative $C_3H_6N_2$ of pyrazole **2** : any of various derivatives of pyrazoline

py·raz·o·lone \-ˌlōn\ *n* **1** : any of three isomeric carbonyl compounds $C_3H_4N_2O$ derived from pyrazoline **2** : any of various derivatives of the pyrazolones some of which (as antipyrine) have been used as analgesics and antipyretics

py·re·thrin \pī-'rē-thrən, -'reth-rən\ *n* : either of two oily liquid esters $C_{21}H_{28}O_3$ and $C_{22}H_{28}O_5$ that have insecticidal properties and are the active components of pyrethrum

py·re·throid \pī-'rē-ˌthròid, -'reth-ˌròid\ *n* : any of various synthetic compounds that are related to the pyrethrins and resemble them in insecticidal properties — **pyrethroid** *adj*

py·re·thrum \pī-'rē-thrəm, -'reth-rəm\ *n* **1** : any of several chrysanthemums with finely divided often aromatic leaves including ornamentals as well as important sources of insecticides **2** : an insecticide consisting of or derived from the dried heads of any of several Old World chrysanthemums (genus *Chrysanthemum* of the family Compositae)

pyr·e·to·ther·a·py \ˌpir-ə-tō-'ther-ə-pē, ˌpī(ə)r-; pī-ˌret-ō-\ *n, pl* **-pies** : FEVER THERAPY

Py·rex \'pī(ə)r-ˌeks\ *trademark* — used for glass and glassware that contains appreciable oxide of boron and is resistant to heat, chemicals, and electricity

py·rex·ia \pī-'rek-sē-ə\ *n* : abnormal elevation of body temperature : FEVER

O
P

\ə\ abut \ᵊ\ kitten \ər\ further \a\ ash \ā\ ace \ä\ cot, cart \aů\ out \ch\ chin \e\ bet \ē\ easy \g\ go \i\ hit \ī\ ice \j\ job \ŋ\ sing \ō\ go \ò\ law \òi\ boy \th\ thin \t̲h̲\ the \ü\ loot \ů\ foot \y\ yet \zh\ vision   *See also* Pronunciation Symbols page

py·rex·i·al \-sē-əl\ *adj* : of, relating to, or characterized by fever ⟨a ~ patient⟩

py·rex·ic \-sik\ *adj* : PYREXIAL

Pyr·i·ben·za·mine \ˌpir-ə-'ben-zə-ˌmēn\ *n* : a preparation of tripelennamine — formerly a U.S. registered trademark

pyr·i·dine \'pir-ə-ˌdēn\ *n* : a toxic water-soluble flammable liquid base C_5H_5N of pungent odor that is the parent of many naturally occurring organic compounds and is used as a solvent and a denaturant for alcohol and in the manufacture of pharmaceuticals (as antiseptics and antihistamines) and waterproofing agents

pyridine nucleotide *n* : a nucleotide characterized by a pyridine derivative as a nitrogen base; *esp* : NAD

pyr·i·do·stig·mine \ˌpir-əd-ō-'stig-ˌmēn\ *n* : a cholinergic drug that is administered in the form of its bromide $C_9H_{13}BrN_2O_2$ esp. in the treatment of myasthenia gravis — see MESTINON

pyr·i·dox·al \ˌpir-ə-'däk-ˌsal\ *n* : a crystalline aldehyde $C_8H_9NO_3$ of the vitamin B_6 group that in the form of its phosphate is active as a coenzyme

pyr·i·dox·amine \ˌpir-ə-'däk-sə-ˌmēn\ *n* : a crystalline amine $C_8H_{12}N_2O_2$ of the vitamin B_6 group that in the form of its phosphate is active as a coenzyme

pyr·i·dox·ic acid *or* **4—pyr·i·dox·ic acid** \ˌpir-ə-ˌdäk-sik-\ *n* : a crystalline acid $C_8H_9NO_4$ isolated from urine and held to be formed by oxidation of pyridoxal as the major end product of vitamin B_6 metabolism

pyr·i·dox·ine \ˌpir-ə-'däk-ˌsēn, -sən\ *n* : a crystalline phenolic alcohol $C_8H_{11}NO_3$ of the vitamin B_6 group found esp. in cereals and convertible in the body into pyridoxal and pyridoxamine

pyridoxine hydrochloride *n* : the hydrochloride salt $C_8H_{11}NO_3 \cdot HCl$ of pyridoxine that is used therapeutically (as in the treatment of pyridoxine deficiency)

pyriform, pyriformis *var of* PIRIFORM, PIRIFORMIS

py·ril·amine \pī-'ril-ə-ˌmēn\ *n* : an oily liquid base $C_{17}H_{23}N_3O$ or its bitter crystalline maleate $C_{21}H_{27}N_3O_5$ used as an antihistamine drug in the treatment of various allergies

py·ri·meth·amine \ˌpī-rə-'meth-ə-ˌmēn\ *n* : a folic acid antagonist $C_{12}H_{13}ClN_4$ that is used in the treatment of toxoplasmosis and the prevention of malaria

py·rim·i·dine \pī-'rim-ə-ˌdēn, pə-\ *n* **1** : a weakly basic organic compound $C_4H_2N_2$ of penetrating odor that is composed of a single six-membered ring having four carbon atoms with nitrogen atoms in positions one and three **2** : a derivative of pyrimidine having its characteristic ring structure; *esp* : a base (as cytosine, thymine, or uracil) that is a constituent of DNA or RNA

py·ri·thi·one zinc \ˌpir-ə-'thī-ˌōn-\ *n* : ZINC PYRITHIONE

py·ro·cat·e·chol \ˌpī-rō-'kat-ə-ˌkȯl, -ˌkōl\ *n* : a crystalline phenol $C_6H_6O_2$ obtained by pyrolysis of various natural substances (as resins and lignins) but usu. made synthetically and used esp. as a photographic developer and in organic synthesis — called also *catechol*

py·ro·gal·lic acid \-ˌgal-ik-\ *n* : PYROGALLOL

py·ro·gal·lol \-'gal-ˌȯl, -ˌōl; -'gȯ-ˌlȯl, -ˌlōl\ *n* : a poisonous bitter crystalline phenol $C_6H_6O_3$ with weak acid properties that is obtained usu. by pyrolysis of gallic acid and that is used esp. as a mild reducing agent (as in photographic developing) and in medicine as a topical antimicrobial (as in the treatment of psoriasis)

py·ro·gen \'pī-rə-jən\ *n* : a fever-producing substance (as various thermostable products of bacterial metabolism)

py·ro·gen·ic \ˌpī-rō-'jen-ik\ *adj* : producing or produced by fever

py·ro·ge·nic·i·ty \-jə-'nis-ət-ē\ *n, pl* **-ties** : the quality or state of being pyrogenic; *esp* : capacity to produce fever

py·rol·y·sis \pī-'räl-ə-səs\ *n, pl* **-y·ses** \-ˌsēz\ : chemical change brought about by the action of heat — **py·ro·lyt·ic** \ˌpī-rə-'lit-ik\ *adj*

py·ro·ma·nia \ˌpī-rō-'mā-nē-ə, -nyə\ *n* : an irresistible impulse to start fires — **py·ro·ma·ni·a·cal** \-mə-'nī-ə-kəl\ *adj*

py·ro·ma·ni·ac \-nē-ˌak\ *n* : an individual affected with pyromania

py·rone \'pī-ˌrōn\ *n* **1** : either of two isomeric carbonyl compounds $C_5H_4O_2$ derived from pyran **2** : a derivative of either of the pyrones

py·ro·nine \'pī-rə-ˌnēn\ *n* : any of several basic xanthene dyes used chiefly as biological stains

py·ro·ni·no·phil·ic \ˌpī-rə-ˌnē-nə-'fil-ik\ *adj* : staining selectively with pyronines ⟨~ cells⟩

py·ro·pho·bia \ˌpī-rə-'fō-bē-ə\ *n* : morbid dread of fire — **py·ro·pho·bic** \-'fō-bik\ *adj*

py·ro·phos·pha·tase \ˌpī-rō-'fäs-fə-ˌtās, -ˌtāz\ *n* : an enzyme that catalyzes the hydrolysis of a pyrophosphate to form orthophosphate

py·ro·phos·phate \-'fäs-ˌfāt\ *n* : a salt or ester of pyrophosphoric acid

py·ro·phos·pho·ric acid \-fäs-ˌfȯr-ik-, -ˌfär-; -ˌfäs-f(ə-)rik-\ *n* : a crystalline acid $H_4P_2O_7$ that is formed when orthophosphoric acid is heated or that is prepared in the form of salts by heating acid salts of orthophosphoric acid

py·ro·sis \pī-'rō-səs\ *n* : HEARTBURN

py·rox·y·lin \pī-'räk-sə-lən, pə-\ *n* : a flammable mixture of cellulose nitrates usu. with less than 12.5 percent nitrogen that is less explosive than guncotton, soluble in a mixture of ether and alcohol or other organic solvents, and used esp. in making plastics and coatings (as lacquers) — see COLLODION

pyr·role \'pi(ə)r-ˌōl\ *n* : a toxic liquid heterocyclic compound C_4H_5N that has a ring consisting of four carbon atoms and one nitrogen atom, polymerizes readily in air, and is the parent compound of many biologically important substances (as bile pigments, porphyrins, and chlorophyll); *broadly* : a derivative of pyrrole — **pyr·ro·lic** \pir-'ō-lik\ *adj*

pyr·rol·idine \pə-'räl-ə-ˌdēn\ *n* : a liquid heterocyclic secondary amine C_4H_9N obtained from pyrrole by reduction and also prepared synthetically

py·ruv·al·de·hyde \ˌpī-ˌrüv-'ald-ə-ˌhīd\ *n* : METHYLGLYOXAL

py·ru·vate \pī-'rü-ˌvāt\ *n* : a salt or ester of pyruvic acid

pyruvate carboxylase *n* : an enzyme that contains biotin as a prosthetic group and in the presence of acetyl coenzyme A catalyzes the fixation of carbon dioxide by pyruvate to form oxalacetate

pyruvate decarboxylase *n* : a lyase that catalyzes the first step in the final stage of alcoholic fermentation involving the decarboxylation of pyruvate to form an aldehyde and carbon dioxide

pyruvate dehydrogenase *n* : an enzyme that catalyzes the first step in the formation of acetyl coenzyme A from pyruvate by dehydrogenation in preparation for participation in the Krebs cycle

pyruvate kinase *n* : an enzyme that functions in glycolysis by catalyzing esp. the transfer of phosphate from phosphoenolpyruvate to ADP forming pyruvate and ATP

py·ru·vic acid \pī-ˌrü-vik-\ *n* : a 3-carbon acid $C_3H_4O_3$ that is an intermediate in carbohydrate metabolism and can be formed either from glucose after phosphorylation or from glycogen by glycolysis

py·uria \pī-'yu̇r-ē-ə\ *n* : the presence of pus in the urine; *also* : a condition (as pyelonephritis) characterized by pus in the urine

PZI *abbr* protamine zinc insulin

Q

qat *var of* KHAT

qd *abbr* [Latin *quaque die*] every day — used in writing prescriptions

Q fever *n* : a disease that is characterized by high fever, chills, muscular pains, headache, and sometimes pneumonia, that is caused by a rickettsial bacterium of the genus *Coxiella* (*C. burnetii*) of which domestic animals serve as reservoirs, and that is transmitted to humans esp. by inhalation of infective airborne bacteria (as in contaminated dust)

qh *or* **qhr** *abbr* [Latin *quaque hora*] every hour — used in writing prescriptions often with a number indicating the hours between doses ⟨*q4h* means every 4 hours⟩

qid *abbr* [Latin *quater in die*] four times a day — used in writing prescriptions

qi·gong \'chē-'gủn\ *n, often cap* : an ancient Chinese healing art involving meditation, controlled breathing, and movement exercises designed to improve physical and mental well-being and prevent disease — called also *chi kung, ch'i kung*

ql *abbr* [Latin *quantum libet*] as much as you please — used in writing prescriptions

qn *abbr* [Latin *quaque nocte*] every night — used in writing prescriptions

qp *abbr* [Latin *quantum placet*] as much as you please — used in writing prescriptions

QRS \'kyü-'är-'es\ *n* : QRS COMPLEX

QRS complex *n* : the series of deflections in an electrocardiogram that represent electrical activity generated by ventricular depolarization prior to contraction of the ventricles — compare P WAVE, T WAVE

qt *abbr* quart

QT interval \'kyü-'tē-\ *n* : the interval from the beginning of the QRS complex to the end of the T wave on an electrocardiogram that represents the time during which contraction of the ventricles occurs

quaa·lude \'kwā-,lüd\ *n* : a tablet or capsule of methaqualone

¹quack \'kwak\ *n* : a pretender to medical skill : an ignorant or dishonest practitioner — **quack·ish** \-ish\ *adj*

²quack *adj* : of, relating to, characteristic of, or being a quack ⟨scores of ∼ remedies for arthritis —Jane E. Brody⟩

quack·ery \'kwak-(ə-)rē\ *n, pl* **quack·eries** : the practices or pretensions of a quack

quack grass *n* : a European grass of the genus *Agropyron* (*A. repens*) that is naturalized throughout No. America and has roots and rhizome with diuretic properties — called also *couch grass, quitch, twitch, witchgrass*

quad \'kwäd\ *n* : QUADRICEPS — usu. used in pl.

quad·rant \'kwäd-rənt\ *n* **1** : an arc of 90° that is one quarter of a circle **2** : any of the four more or less equivalent segments into which an anatomic structure may be divided by vertical and horizontal partitioning through its midpoint ⟨pain in the lower right ∼ of the abdomen⟩

quad·rant·ec·to·my \,kwäd-rən-'tek-tə-mē\ *n, pl* **-mies** : a partial mastectomy involving excision of a tumor along with the involved quadrant of the breast including the skin and underlying fascia — compare LUMPECTOMY

quad·rate lobe \'kwäd-,rāt-\ *n* : a small lobe of the liver on the underside of the right lobe to the left of the fissure for the gallbladder

qua·dra·tus \kwä-'drāt-əs\ *n, pl* **qua·dra·ti** \-,ī\ : any of several skeletal muscles more or less quadrilateral in outline — see PRONATOR QUADRATUS

quadratus fem·o·ris \-'fem-ə-rəs\ *n* : a small flat muscle of the gluteal region that arises from the ischial tuberosity, inserts into the greater trochanter and adjacent region of the femur, and serves to rotate the thigh laterally

quadratus la·bii su·pe·ri·or·is \-'lā-bē-,ī-sù-'pir-ē-'ôr-əs\ *n* : LEVATOR LABII SUPERIORIS

quadratus lum·bor·um \-ləm-'bôr-əm\ *n* : a quadrilateral-shaped muscle of the abdomen that arises from the iliac crest and the iliolumbar ligament, inserts into the lowest rib and the upper four lumbar vertebrae, and functions esp. to flex the trunk laterally

quadratus plan·tae \-'plan-,tē\ *n* : a muscle of the sole of the foot that arises by two heads from the calcaneus, inserts into the lateral side of the tendons of the flexor digitorum longus, and aids in flexing the toes

quad·ri·ceps \'kwäd-rə-,seps\ *n* : a large extensor muscle of the front of the thigh divided above into four parts which include the rectus femoris, vastus lateralis, vastus intermedius, and vastus medialis, and which unite in a single tendon to enclose the patella as a sesamoid bone at the knee and insert as the patellar ligament into the tuberosity of the tibia — called also *quadriceps femoris, quadriceps muscle*

quadriceps fem·o·ris \-'fem-ə-rəs\ *n* : QUADRICEPS

quadriceps muscle *n* : QUADRICEPS

quadrigemina — see CORPORA QUADRIGEMINA

quad·ri·gem·i·nal bodies \,kwäd-rə-'jem-ən-ᵊl-\ *n pl* : CORPORA QUADRIGEMINA

quad·ri·lat·er·al \,kwäd-rə-'lat-ə-rəl, -'la-trəl\ *adj* : having four sides ⟨a ∼ muscle⟩

qua·drip·a·ra \kwä-'drip-ə-rə\ *n* : a woman who has given birth to four children

quad·ri·pa·re·sis \,kwäd-rə-pə-'rē-səs, -'par-ə-\ *n, pl* **-re·ses** \-,sēz\ : TETRAPARESIS

quad·ri·pa·ret·ic \-pə-'ret-ik\ *adj* : TETRAPARETIC

quad·ri·ple·gia \,kwäd-rə-'plē-j(ē-)ə\ *n* : paralysis of all four limbs — called also *tetraplegia*

¹quad·ri·ple·gic \,kwäd-rə-'plē-jik\ *adj* : of, relating to, or affected with quadriplegia ⟨∼ patients⟩

²quadriplegic *n* : one affected with quadriplegia — called also *tetraplegic*

¹quad·ri·va·lent \,kwäd-rə-'vā-lənt, *in sense 2* kwä-'driv-ə-lənt\ *adj* **1** : TETRAVALENT **2** : composed of four homologous chromosomes synapsed in meiotic prophase

²quadrivalent *n* : a quadrivalent chromosomal group

quad·ru·ped \'kwäd-rə-,ped\ *n* : an animal having four feet — **qua·dru·pe·dal** \kwä-'drü-pəd-ᵊl, ,kwäd-rə-'ped-\ *adj*

qua·dru·plet \kwä-'drəp-lət, -'drüp-; 'kwäd-rəp-\ *n* **1** : one of four offspring born at one birth **2** **quadruplets** *pl* : a group of four offspring born at one birth

quads *pl of* QUAD

qual·i·ta·tive \'kwäl-ə-,tāt-iv\ *adj* : of, relating to, or involving quality or kind ⟨∼ changes⟩ — **qual·i·ta·tive·ly** *adv*

qualitative analysis *n* : chemical analysis designed to identify the components of a substance or mixture

qual·i·ty \'kwäl-ət-ē\ *n, pl* **-ties** : a special or distinguishing attribute: as **a** : TIMBRE **b** : the attribute of an elementary sensation that makes it fundamentally unlike any other sensation **c** : the character of an X-ray beam that determines its penetrating power and is dependent upon its wavelength distribution

quality as·sur·ance \-ə-'shùr-ən(t)s\ *n* : a program for the systematic monitoring and evaluation of the various aspects of a project, service, or facility to ensure that standards of quality are being met

quanta *pl of* QUANTUM

quan·tal \'kwänt-ᵊl\ *adj* **1** : of or relating to a quantum or to quanta (as of energy or a neurotransmitter) ⟨∼ release of acetylcholine⟩ **2** : being or relating to a sensitivity response marked by the presence or absence of a definite reaction ⟨an all-or-none response to a stimulus is ∼⟩

\ə\ abut \ᵊ\ kitten \ər\ further \a\ ash \ā\ ace \ä\ cot, cart
\aù\ out \ch\ chin \e\ bet \ē\ easy \g\ go \i\ hit \ī\ ice \j\ job
\ŋ\ sing \ō\ go \ò\ law \òi\ boy \th\ thin \t͟h\ the \ü\ loot
\ù\ foot \y\ yet \zh\ vision *See also* Pronunciation Symbols page

Q
R

quan·ti·ta·tive \ˈkwän(t)-ə-ˌtāt-iv\ *adj* **1** : of, relating to, or expressible in terms of quantity **2** : of, relating to, or involving the measurement of quantity or amount — **quan·ti·ta·tive·ly** *adv*

quantitative analysis *n* : chemical analysis designed to determine the amounts or proportions of the components of a substance

quantitative character *n* : an inherited character that is expressed phenotypically in all degrees of variation between one often indefinite extreme and another : a character determined by polygenes — compare QUANTITATIVE INHERITANCE

quantitative inheritance *n* : genetic inheritance of a character (as human skin color) controlled by polygenes with each allelic pair of genes at a given locus having a specific quantitative effect — compare BLENDING INHERITANCE, MENDELIAN INHERITANCE

quan·tize *also Brit* **quan·tise** \ˈkwänt-ˌtīz\ *vt* **quan·tized** *also Brit* **quan·tised; quan·tiz·ing** *also Brit* **quan·tis·ing** **1** : to subdivide (as energy) into small but measurable increments **2** : to calculate or express in terms of quantum mechanics — **quan·ti·za·tion** *also Brit* **quan·ti·sa·tion** \ˌkwän-tə-ˈzā-shən\ *n* — **quan·tiz·er** *also Brit* **quan·tis·er** \ˈkwän-ˌtī-zər\ *n*

quan·tum \ˈkwänt-əm\ *n, pl* **quan·ta** \ˈkwänt-ə\ **1** : one of the very small increments or parcels into which many forms of energy are subdivided ⟨a molecule of rhodopsin in the human eye can cause a response to a single ∼ of light⟩ **2** : one of the small molecular packets of a neurotransmitter (as acetylcholine) released into the synaptic cleft in the transmission of a nerve impulse across a synapse

quantum mechanics *n pl but sing or pl in constr* : a theory of matter that is based on the concept of the possession of wave properties by elementary particles, that affords a mathematical interpretation of the structure and interactions of matter on the basis of these properties, and that incorporates within it quantum theory and the uncertainty principle — called also *wave mechanics* — **quantum mechanical** *adj* — **quantum mechanically** *adv*

quantum theory *n* : a theory in physics based on the concept of the subdivision of radiant energy into finite quanta and applied to numerous processes involving transference or transformation of energy in an atomic or molecular scale

quar·an·tin·able \ˈkwȯr-ən-ˌtē-nə-bəl, ˈkwär-\ *adj* : subject to or constituting grounds for quarantine ⟨a ∼ disease⟩

¹quar·an·tine \ˈkwȯr-ən-ˌtēn, ˈkwär-\ *n* **1 a** : a term during which a ship arriving in port and suspected of carrying contagious disease is held in isolation from the shore **b** : a regulation placing a ship in quarantine **c** : a place where a ship is detained during quarantine **2 a** : a restraint upon the activities or communication of persons or the transport of goods that is designed to prevent the spread of disease or pests **b** : a place in which those under quarantine are kept

²quarantine *vb* **-tined; -tin·ing** *vt* : to detain in or exclude by quarantine ∼ *vi* : to establish or declare a quarantine

quarantine flag *n* : a yellow flag hoisted by all ships to request pratique on entering a harbor, by a ship to show that it has contagious or infectious disease aboard, or by a ship that has been quarantined — called also *yellow flag, yellow jack*

quart \ˈkwȯ(ə)rt\ *n* **1** : a British unit of liquid or dry capacity equal to ¼ gallon or 69.355 cubic inches or 1.136 liters **2** : a U.S. unit of liquid capacity equal to ¼ gallon or 57.75 cubic inches or 0.946 liters

¹quar·tan \ˈkwȯrt-ᵊn\ *adj* : occurring every fourth day reckoning inclusively; *specif* : recurring at approximately 72-hour intervals ⟨∼ chills and fever⟩ — compare TERTIAN

²quartan *n* : an intermittent fever that recurs at approximately 72-hour intervals; *esp* : MALARIAE MALARIA

quartan malaria *n* : MALARIAE MALARIA

quar·ter \ˈkwȯ(r)t-ər\ *n* **1** : one limb of a quadruped with the adjacent parts **2** : one teat together with the part of a cow's udder that it drains **3** : the side of a horse's hoof between the toe and the heel

quarter evil *n* : BLACKLEG

quarter ill *n* : BLACKLEG

quartz \ˈkwȯ(ə)rts\ *n* : a mineral SiO_2 consisting of a silica that occurs in colorless and transparent or colored hexagonal crystals and also in crystalline masses

quartz glass *n* : vitreous silica prepared from pure quartz and noted for its transparency to ultraviolet radiation

quartz lamp *n* : a mercury-vapor lamp in a tube of quartz glass that transmits most of the ultraviolet radiation

quas·sia \ˈkwäsh-(ē-)ə, ˈkwäs-ē-ə\ *n* **1** *cap* : a genus of shrubs and trees (family Simaroubaceae) with clusters of scarlet flowers — compare SIMAROUBA **2** : a drug derived from the heartwood and bark of various tropical trees (family Simaroubaceae) and used esp. as a bitter tonic and remedy for roundworms in children and as an insecticide

> **Quas·si** \ˈkwäs-ē\, **Graman** (*fl* 1730), Suriname slave. Quassi was a black slave who obtained his freedom and practiced as a medicine man. Around 1730 he discovered the medicinal value of the bark and heartwood of certain trees in the treatment of malignant fevers common in Suriname. According to tradition, a traveling Swede bought the secret of the cures and brought specimens of the plants back to Sweden. Linnaeus examined the plants and named the genus *Quassia*. Later, the name *quassia* was applied to the drug as well.

quas·sin \ˈkwäs-ᵊn\ *n* : the bitter crystalline principle $C_{22}H_{28}O_6$ of quassia

¹quat *var of* KHAT

²quat \ˈkwät\ *n* : QUATERNARY AMMONIUM COMPOUND

¹qua·ter·na·ry \ˈkwät-ə(r)-ˌner-ē, kwə-ˈtər-nə-rē\ *adj* : consisting of, containing, or being an atom bonded to four other atoms

²quaternary *n, pl* **-ries** : QUATERNARY AMMONIUM COMPOUND

quaternary ammonium compound *n* : any of numerous strong bases and their salts derived from ammonium by replacement of the hydrogen atoms with organic radicals and important esp. as surface-active agents, disinfectants, and drugs — called also *quat, quaternary*

qua·ter·ni·za·tion *or chiefly Brit* **qua·ter·ni·sa·tion** \ˌkwät-ər-nə-ˈzā-shən\ *n* : the process of quaternizing

qua·ter·nize *or chiefly Brit* **qua·ter·nise** \ˈkwät-ər-ˌnīz\ *vt* **-nized** *or chiefly Brit* **-nised; -niz·ing** *or chiefly Brit* **-nis·ing** : to convert (as an amine) into a quaternary compound

que·brach·a·mine \ki-ˈbräch-ə-ˌmēn\ *n* : a crystalline alkaloid $C_{19}H_{26}N_2$ obtained from the dried bark of the quebracho

que·brach·ine \ki-ˈbräch-ˌēn, -ən\ *n* : YOHIMBINE

que·brach·i·tol \ki-ˈbräch-ə-ˌtȯl, -ˌtōl\ *n* : a sweet crystalline compound $C_7H_{14}O_6$ occurring esp. in quebracho bark

que·bra·cho \kä-ˈbräch-(ˌ)ō, ki-\ *n* **1** : a tree of the genus *Aspidosperma* (*A. quebracho*) of the dogbane family (Apocynaceae) which occurs in Argentina and Chile and whose dried bark is used as a respiratory sedative in dyspnea and in asthma — called also *white quebracho* **2** : ASPIDOSPERMA 2

quebracho bark *n* : ASPIDOSPERMA 2

Queck·en·stedt test \ˈkvek-ᵊn-shtet-\ *n* : a test for spinal blockage of the subarachnoid space in which manual pressure is applied to the jugular vein to elevate venous pressure, which indicates the absence of a block when there is a simultaneous increase in cerebrospinal fluid pressure, and which indicates the presence of a block when cerebrospinal fluid pressure remains the same or almost the same — called also *Queckenstedt sign*

> **Queckenstedt, Hans Heinrich Georg (1876–1918),** German physician. Queckenstedt devoted most of his energies to the management of the sick at clinics first in Heidelberg and then in Rostock, Germany. He published papers on iron metabolism in pernicious anemia, on periostitis in typhoid fever, and on the dynamics and constituents of cerebrospinal fluid. He introduced the procedure known as the Queckenstedt test in 1916.

quel·lung \ˈkwel-əŋ, ˈkvel-ůŋ\ *n, often cap* : swelling of the capsule of a microorganism after reaction with antibody

quer·ce·tin \ˈkwər-sət-ən\ *n* : a yellow crystalline pigment

$C_{15}H_{10}O_7$ occurring usu. in the form of glycosides in various plants

quer·ci·mer·i·trin \\ˌkwər-sə-ˈmer-ə-trən\ *n* : a yellow crystalline glucoside $C_{21}H_{20}O_{12}$ occurring in cotton flowers and leaves and in sunflowers and yielding quercetin and glucose on hydrolysis

quer·ci·trin \ˈkwər-sə-ˌtrin\ *n* : a bitter pale yellow crystalline glycoside $C_{21}H_{20}O_{11}$ yielding quercetin and rhamnose on hydrolysis

Quer·cus \ˈkwər-kəs\ *n* : a genus of hardwood often evergreen trees or shrubs (family Fagaceae) that comprise the typical oaks and include sources of nutgall

¹**quer·u·lent** *also* **quer·u·lant** \ˈkwer-(y)ə-lənt *also* ˈkwir-\ *adj* : abnormally given to suspicion and accusation

²**querulent** *n* : one who is querulent

Quete·let index \ket(-ə)-ˈlā-\ *or* **Quete·let's index** \-ˈlāz\ *n* : BODY MASS INDEX

Qué·te·let \kā-tə-lā\, **Lambert Adolphe Jacques (1796–1874)**, Belgian astronomer and statistician. Quételet is remembered chiefly for his application of statistics and probability theory to social phenomena. As an astronomer he is credited with founding in 1828 Brussels's Royal Observatory and developing methods for the simultaneous observation of astronomical, meteorological, and geodetic phenomena from various European locations. As a statistician he collected and analyzed statistics on crime, mortality, and other phenomena for the Dutch and Belgian governments. In 1835 he published his treatise *Sur l'homme* in which he first presented his conception of the "average man," using it as the central value about which measurements of various human traits are distributed according to the normal curve. He used stature, weight, complexion and other physical traits as criteria for determining the "average man" in any given race or population. Quételet's "average man" became a catch phrase in 19th-century discussions on social science.

¹**quick** \ˈkwik\ *adj* **1** : not dead : LIVING, ALIVE **2** : PREGNANT

²**quick** *n* **1 quick** *pl* : living beings **2** : a painfully sensitive spot or area of flesh (as that underlying a fingernail)

quick·en \ˈkwik-ən\ *vi* **quick·ened**; **quick·en·ing** \-(ə-)niŋ\ : to reach the stage of gestation at which fetal motion is felt

quickening *n* : the first motion of a fetus in the uterus felt by the mother usu. somewhat before the middle of the period of gestation

quick·lime \ˈkwik-ˌlīm\ *n* : ¹LIME

quick·sil·ver \-ˌsil-vər\ *n* : MERCURY 1

qui·es·cence \kwī-ˈes-ᵊn(t)s, kwē-\ *n* : the quality or state of being quiescent

qui·es·cent \-ᵊnt\ *adj* **1** : being in a state of arrest ⟨∼ tuberculosis⟩ **2** : causing no symptoms ⟨∼ gallstones⟩

quil·la·ic acid \kwi-ˌlā-ik-\ *n* : a poisonous crystalline triterpenoid sapogenin $C_{30}H_{46}O_5$ obtained by hydrolysis of the saponin from soapbark

quil·la·ja \kwi-ˈlā-yə, -jə\ *n* **1** *cap* : a genus of trees of the rose family (Rosaceae) native to Brazil, Peru, and Chile, distinguished by their saponaceous bark, and including the soapbark (*Q. saponaria*) **2** : SOAPBARK 2

qui·na \ˈkē-nə\ *n* : CINCHONA 2, 3

quin·a·crine \ˈkwin-ə-ˌkrēn\ *n* : an antimalarial drug derived from acridine and used esp. in the form of its dihydrochloride $C_{23}H_{30}ClN_3O \cdot 2HCl \cdot 2H_2O$ — called also *mepacrine;* see ATABRINE

quin·al·bar·bi·tone \ˌkwin-al-ˈbär-bi-ˌtōn\ *n, chiefly Brit* : SECOBARBITAL

quin·al·dine \kwin-ˈal-ˌdēn, -dən\ *n* : an oily liquid base $C_{10}H_9N$ that has a slightly pungent odor, is obtained by condensation of acetaldehyde and aniline and occurs in coal tar, and is used chiefly in the manufacture of dyes and pharmaceuticals

quin·a·mine \ˈkwin-ə-ˌmēn, -mən\ *n* : a crystalline alkaloid $C_{19}H_{24}N_2O_2$ in various cinchona barks

quin·a·pril \ˈkwin-ə-ˌpril\ *n* : an ACE inhibitor administered orally in the form of its hydrochloride $C_{25}H_{30}N_2O_5 \cdot HCl$ to treat hypertension — see ACCUPRIL

quin·az·o·line \kwin-ˈaz-ə-ˌlēn, -lən\ *n* : a yellow crystalline bicyclic compound $C_8H_6N_2$ composed of fused benzene and pyrimidine rings; *also* : a derivative of this compound

quince \ˈkwin(t)s\ *n* : the fruit of a central Asian tree of the genus *Cydonia* (*C. oblonga*) that resembles a hard-fleshed yellow apple; *also* : the tree

Quin·cke's disease \ˈkviŋ-kəz-\ *n* : ANGIOEDEMA

Quincke, Heinrich Irenaeus (1842–1922), German physician. Quincke was a professor of internal medicine at Kiel, Germany, who is remembered for making a number of important observations. In 1868 he made observations on the pulse that were helpful in establishing a diagnosis of aortic regurgitation. In 1870 he observed aneurysm of the hepatic artery. His description of angioedema, published in 1882, was not the first description of the disease but the most complete.

Quincke's edema *n* : ANGIOEDEMA

quin·eth·a·zone \ˌkwin-ˈeth-ə-ˌzōn\ *n* : a diuretic $C_{10}H_{12}ClN_3O_3S$ used in the treatment of edema and hypertension

qui·ne·tum \kwi-ˈnēt-əm\ *n* : a mixture of the alkaloids in varying proportions as they occur naturally in red bark that is used to treat malaria

quin·hy·drone \ˌkwin-ˈhī-ˌdrōn\ *n* : a green crystalline compound $C_{12}H_{10}O_4$ used in pH determinations; *also* : any of various similar compounds

quin·ic acid \ˌkwin-ik-, ˌkwīn-\ *n* : a crystalline acid $C_7H_{12}O_6$ obtained from cinchona bark, coffee beans, and other plant products and made synthetically by hydrolysis of chlorogenic acid

quin·i·cine \ˈkwin-ə-ˌsēn, -sən\ *n* : a bitter poisonous reddish yellow amorphous alkaloid $C_{20}H_{24}N_2O_2$ isomeric with quinine and obtained from cinchona bark or by heating a salt of quinine — called also *quinotoxine*

quin·i·dine \ˈkwin-ə-ˌdēn, -dən\ *n* : a crystalline dextrorotatory stereoisomer of quinine found in some species of cinchona and used chiefly in the form of its hydrated sulfate $(C_{20}H_{24}N_2O_2)_2 \cdot H_2SO_4 \cdot 2H_2O$ to treat irregularities of cardiac rhythm and sometimes in place of quinine as an antimalarial

qui·nine \ˈkwī-ˌnīn *also* ˈkwin-ˌīn, *esp Brit* kwin-ˈēn, ˈkwin-ˌēn\ *n* : a bitter crystalline alkaloid $C_{20}H_{24}N_2O_2$ obtained from cinchona bark that is used as a flavoring agent, has antipyretic and analgesic properties, and is administered orally in the form of its salts (as the hydrated sulfate $(C_{20}H_{24}N_2O_2)_2 \cdot H_2SO_4 \cdot 2H_2O$) as an antimalarial

qui·nin·ic acid \kwi-ˌnin-ik-\ *n* : a yellowish crystalline acid $C_{11}H_9NO_3$ obtained by oxidation of quinine or quinidine

quinoid *var of* QUINONOID

quin·o·line \ˈkwin-ᵊl-ˌēn\ *n* **1** : a pungent oily nitrogenous base C_9H_7N that is obtained usu. by distillation of coal tar or by synthesis from aniline and is the parent compound of many alkaloids, drugs, and dyes **2** : a derivative of quinoline

quin·o·lin·ic acid \ˌkwin-ə-ˌlin-ik-\ *n* : an acid $C_7H_5NO_4$ that is a metabolite of tryptophan and is neurotoxic in high concentrations

8–quin·o·lin·ol \ˈkwin-ə-lə-ˌnȯl, -ˌnōl\ *n* : 8-HYDROXYQUINOLINE

quin·o·lone \ˈkwin-ə-ˌlōn\ *n* : any of a class of synthetic antibacterial drugs that are derivatives of hydroxylated quinolines and inhibit the replication of bacterial DNA; *esp* : FLUOROQUINOLONE

qui·none \kwin-ˈōn, ˈkwin-ˌ\ *n* **1** : either of two isomeric cyclic crystalline compounds $C_6H_4O_2$ that are extremely irritating to the skin and mucous membranes **2** : any of various usu. yellow, orange, or red quinonoid compounds including several that are biologically important as coenzymes, hydrogen acceptors, or vitamins

---

Q
R

qui·no·noid \kwi-'nō-ˌnȯid, 'kwin-ə-ˌnȯid\ *or* **quin·oid** \'kwi-ˌnȯid\ *adj* : resembling quinone; *esp* : having a structure characterized by a benzene nucleus containing two instead of three double bonds within the nucleus and two external double bonds attached to the nucleus either at ortho or para positions (as in the two carbonyl groups of quinones)

quino·tox·ine \ˌkwin-ō-'täk-ˌsēn\ *n* : QUINICINE

qui·no·vin \kwi-'nō-vən\ *n* : a bitter crystalline glycoside found esp. in cinchona

qui·no·vose \kwi-'nō-vōs\ *n* : a sugar $C_6H_{12}O_5$ found by hydrolysis of quinovin

qui·nox·a·line \kwi-'näk-sə-ˌlēn, -ˌlīn\ *n* : a weakly basic bicyclic compound $C_8H_6N_2$ made by condensing the ortho form of phenylenediamine with glyoxal and having fused benzene and pyrazine rings; *also* : any of various derivatives of quinoxaline having antibiotic properties

quin·que·va·lent \ˌkwiŋ-kwi-'vā-lənt\ *adj* : PENTAVALENT

quin·sy \'kwin-zē\ *n, pl* **quin·sies** : an abscess in the connective tissue around a tonsil usu. resulting from bacterial infection and often accompanied by fever, pain, and swelling — called also *peritonsillar abscess*

quint \'kwint\ *n* : QUINTUPLET

quinti — see EXTENSOR DIGITI QUINTI PROPRIUS

quin·tu·plet \kwin-'təp-lət, -'t(y)üp-; 'kwint-əp-\ *n* **1** : one of five children or offspring born at one birth **2 quintuplets** *pl* : a group of five such offspring

qui·nu·cli·dine \kwi-'nük-lə-ˌdēn, -dən\ *n* : a crystalline bicyclic base $C_7H_{13}N$ of which quinine and related alkaloids are derivatives

qui·nu·cli·di·nyl ben·zi·late \kwi-'n(y)ü-klə-ˌdēn-ᵊl-'ben-zə-ˌlāt\ *n* : BZ

quitch \'kwich\ *n* : QUACK GRASS — called also *quitch grass*

quit·tor \'kwit-ər\ *n* : a purulent inflammation (as a necrobacillosis) of the feet esp. of horses and donkeys occurring chiefly in a cartilaginous form characterized by a chronic persistent inflammation of the lateral cartilage of the foot leading to suppuration and the formation of one or more fistulous openings above the coronet and causing marked lameness or in a cutaneous form characterized by an inflammation of the soft tissues just above the hoof involving suppuration and sloughing of the skin before healing

¹quo·tid·i·an \kwō-'tid-ē-ən\ *adj* : occurring every day ⟨∼ fever⟩

²quotidian *n* : something (as an intermittent fever) that occurs each day

quo·tient \'kwō-shənt\ *n* : the numerical ratio usu. multiplied by 100 between a test score and a measurement on which that score might be expected largely to depend

qv *abbr* [Latin *quantum vis*] as much as you will — used in writing prescriptions

Q wave \'kyü-ˌ\ *n* : the short initial downward stroke of the QRS complex in an electrocardiogram formed during the beginning of ventricular depolarization

R

r *abbr* roentgen

R *abbr* **1** Reaumur **2** rough — used in bacteriology

R *symbol* chemical group and esp. an organic chemical group ⟨thiols have the general formula *R*SH⟩

Ra *symbol* radium

RA *abbr* rheumatoid arthritis

rab·bit fever \'rab-ət-\ *n* : TULAREMIA

ra·bep·ra·zole \rə-'bep-rə-ˌzōl\ *n* : a benzimidazole derivative that inhibits gastric acid secretion and is administered in the form of its sodium salt $C_{18}H_{20}NaN_3O_3S$ esp. to treat gastroesophageal reflux disease, duodenal ulcers, and disorders (as Zollinger-Ellison syndrome) involving gastric acid hypersecretion — see ACIPHEX

ra·bic \'rā-bik\ *adj* : of or relating to rabies

ra·bid \'rab-əd *also* 'rā-bəd\ *adj* : affected with rabies ⟨a ∼ dog⟩

ra·bies \'rā-bēz\ *n, pl* **rabies** : an acute virus disease of the nervous system of warm-blooded animals that is caused by a rhabdovirus (species *Rabies virus* of the genus *Lyssavirus*) transmitted in infected saliva usu. through the bite of a rabid animal and that is characterized typically by increased salivation, abnormal behavior, and eventual paralysis and death when untreated — called also *hydrophobia*

race \'rās\ *n* **1 a** : an actually or potentially interbreeding group within a species; *also* : a taxonomic category (as a subspecies) representing such a group **b** : BREED **2** : a category of humankind that shares certain distinctive physical traits

rac·e·mase \'ras-ə-ˌmās\ *n* : any of various enzymes that catalyze racemizations and occur esp. in bacteria ⟨alanine ∼⟩

ra·ce·mate \rā-'sē-ˌmāt, rə-; 'ras-ə-\ *n* : a racemic compound or mixture

ra·ce·mic \rā-'sē-mik, rə-\ *adj* : of, relating to, or constituting a compound or mixture that is composed of equal amounts of dextrorotatory and levorotatory forms of the same compound and is optically inactive — compare DL-

ra·ce·mi·za·tion *also Brit* **ra·ce·mi·sa·tion** \rā-ˌsē-mə-'zā-shən, rə-; ˌras-ə-mə-\ *n* : the action or process of changing from an optically active compound into a racemic compound or mixture — **ra·ce·mize** *also Brit* **ra·ce·mise** \rā-'sē-ˌmīz, rə-; 'ras-ə-\ *vb* **-mized** *also Brit* **-mised; -miz·ing** *also Brit* **-mis·ing**

racemosa — see LIVEDO RACEMOSA

ra·ce·mose \'ras-ə-ˌmōs; rā-'sē-, rə-\ *adj* : having or growing in a form like that of a cluster of grapes ⟨∼ glands⟩

rac·e·phed·rine \ˌras-ə-'fed-rən\ *n* : synthetic racemic ephedrine administered in the form of its hydrochloride

ra·chis·chi·sis \rə-'kis-kə-səs\ *n, pl* **-chi·ses** \-kə-ˌsēz\ : a congenital abnormality (as spina bifida) characterized by a cleft of the spinal column

ra·chit·ic \rə-'kit-ik\ *adj* : of, relating to, or affected by rickets ⟨∼ lesions⟩ ⟨a ∼ child⟩

rachitic rosary *n* : BEADING

ra·chi·tis *also* **rha·chi·tis** \rə-'kīt-əs\ *n, pl* **-chit·i·des** \-'kit-ə-ˌdēz\ : RICKETS

rach·i·to·gen·ic \ˌrak-ət-ə-'jen-ik\ *adj* : leading or tending to the development of rickets ⟨a ∼ diet⟩

ra·cial \'rā-shəl\ *adj* : of, relating to, or based on a race

rad \'rad\ *n* : a unit of absorbed dose of ionizing radiation equal to an energy of 100 ergs per gram of irradiated material

rad *abbr* [Latin *radix*] root — used in writing prescriptions

ra·di·a·bil·i·ty \ˌrād-ē-ə-'bil-ət-ē\ *n, pl* **-ties** : the capability of transmitting radiation (as X-rays) ⟨the ∼ is altered by differences in thickness of the bone —K. H. Thoma⟩

¹ra·di·al \'rād-ē-əl\ *adj* **1** : arranged or having parts arranged like rays **2** : of, relating to, or situated near the radius or the thumb side of the hand or forearm ⟨the ∼ aspect of the hand⟩ **3** : developing uniformly around a central axis ⟨∼ cleavage of an egg⟩ — **ra·di·al·ly** \-ē-ə-lē\ *adv*

²radial *n* : a body part (as an artery) lying near or following the course of the radius

radial artery *n* : the smaller of the two branches into which the brachial artery divides just below the bend of the elbow and which passes along the radial side of the forearm to the wrist then winds backward around the outer side of the carpus and enters the palm between the first and second metacarpal bones to form the deep palmar arch

radial collateral ligament *n* : a ligament of the elbow that connects the lateral epicondyle with the lateral side of the annular ligament and helps to stabilize the elbow joint — called also *lateral collateral ligament;* compare ULNAR COLLATERAL LIGAMENT

radialis — see EXTENSOR CARPI RADIALIS BREVIS, EXTENSOR CARPI RADIALIS LONGUS, FLEXOR CARPI RADIALIS, NERVUS RADIALIS

radial keratotomy *n* : a surgical operation on the cornea for the correction of myopia that involves flattening the cornea by making a series of incisions in a radial pattern resembling the spokes of a wheel — abbr. *RK*; compare PHOTOREFRACTIVE KERATECTOMY

radial nerve *n* : a large nerve that arises from the posterior cord of the brachial plexus and passes spirally down the humerus to the front of the lateral epicondyle where it divides into a superficial branch distributed to the skin of the back of the hand and arm and a deep branch to the underlying extensor muscles — called also *musculospiral nerve, nervus radialis*

radial notch *n* : a narrow depression on the lateral side of the coronoid process of the ulna that articulates with the head of the radius and gives attachment to the annular ligament of the radius

radial symmetry *n* : the condition of having similar parts regularly arranged around a central axis — **radially symmetrical** *adj*

radial tuberosity *n* : an oval eminence on the medial side of the radius distal to the neck where the tendon of the biceps brachii muscle inserts

radial vein *n* : any of several deep veins of the forearm that accompany the radial artery and unite at the elbow with the ulnar veins to form the brachial veins

ra·di·an \ˈrād-ē-ən\ *n* : a unit of plane angular measurement that is equal to the angle at the center of a circle subtended by an arc equal in length to the radius

ra·di·ant \ˈrād-ē-ənt\ *adj* **1** : emitted or transmitted by radiation **2** : emitting or relating to radiant heat

radiant energy *n* : energy traveling as electromagnetic waves

radiant flux *n* : the rate of emission or transmission of radiant energy

radiata — see CORONA RADIATA

¹ra·di·ate \ˈrād-ē-ˌāt\ *vb* **-at·ed; -at·ing** *vi* : to issue in or as if in rays : spread from a central point ⟨back pain *radiating* to both upper legs —Tony Miksanek⟩ ∼ *vt* : IRRADIATE

²ra·di·ate \ˈrād-ē-ət, -ē-ˌāt\ *adj* **1** : having rays or radial parts **2** : characterized by radial symmetry : RADIALLY SYMMETRICAL

radiate ligament *n* : a branching ligament uniting the front of the head of a rib with the bodies of the two vertebrae and the intervertebral disk between them — called also *stellate ligament*

ra·di·a·tion \ˌrād-ē-ˈā-shən\ *n* **1** : energy radiated in the form of waves or particles **2 a** : the action or process of radiating ⟨with ∼ of the pain there may be tenderness over the sciatic nerve —J. A. Key⟩ **b** (1) : the process of emitting radiant energy in the form of waves or particles (2) : the combined processes of emission, transmission, and absorption of radiant energy **3** : a tract of nerve fibers within the brain; *esp* : one concerned with the distribution of impulses arising from sensory stimuli to the relevant coordinating centers and nuclei ⟨the optic ∼s⟩

radiation sickness *n* : sickness that results from exposure to radiation and is commonly marked by fatigue, nausea, vomiting, loss of teeth and hair, and in more severe cases by damage to blood-forming tissue with decrease in red and white blood cells and with bleeding

radiation syndrome *n* : RADIATION SICKNESS

radiation therapist *n* : RADIOTHERAPIST

radiation therapy *n* : RADIOTHERAPY

¹rad·i·cal \ˈrad-i-kəl\ *adj* **1** : designed to remove the root of a

disease or all diseased tissue ⟨∼ surgery⟩ **2** : involving complete removal of an organ ⟨∼ prostatectomy⟩ — compare CONSERVATIVE — **rad·i·cal·ly** \-i-k(ə-)lē\ *adv*

²radical *n* : FREE RADICAL; *also* : a group of atoms bonded together that is considered an entity in various kinds of reactions

radical hysterectomy *n* : the surgical removal of the uterus, parametrium, and uterine cervix along with the partial removal of the pelvic lymph nodes that is typically performed to treat cervical or endometrial cancer — see WERTHEIM OPERATION; compare PANHYSTERECTOMY

radical mastectomy *n* : a mastectomy in which the breast tissue, associated skin, nipple, areola, axillary lymph nodes, and pectoral muscles are removed — called also *Halsted radical mastectomy;* compare MODIFIED RADICAL MASTECTOMY, SIMPLE MASTECTOMY

radices *pl of* RADIX

rad·i·cle \ˈrad-i-kəl\ *n* **1** : the rootlike beginning of an anatomical vessel or part ⟨the ∼ of a vein⟩ **2** : RADICAL

ra·dic·u·lar \rə-ˈdik-yə-lər, ra-\ *adj* **1** : of, relating to, or involving a nerve root ⟨∼ pain⟩ **2** : of, relating to, or occurring at the root of a tooth ⟨a ∼ cyst⟩

ra·dic·u·li·tis \rə-ˌdik-yə-ˈlīt-əs\ *n* : inflammation of a nerve root

ra·dic·u·lo·neu·ri·tis \rə-ˌdik-yə-(ˌ)lō-n(y)ù-ˈrīt-əs\ *n* : inflammation of one or more roots of the spinal nerves

ra·dic·u·lop·a·thy \-ˈläp-ə-thē\ *n, pl* **-thies** : any pathological condition of the nerve roots

radii *pl of* RADIUS

ra·dio·ac·tive \ˌrād-ē-ō-ˈak-tiv\ *adj* : of, caused by, or exhibiting radioactivity ⟨∼ isotopes⟩ — **ra·dio·ac·tive·ly** *adv*

ra·dio·ac·tiv·i·ty \-ak-ˈtiv-ət-ē\ *n, pl* **-ties** : the property possessed by some elements (as uranium) or isotopes (as carbon 14) of spontaneously emitting energetic particles (as electrons or alpha particles) by the disintegration of their atomic nuclei

ra·dio·aero·sol \-ˈar-ə-ˌsäl, -ˈer-, -ˌsòl\ *n* : a radioactive aerosol

ra·dio·al·ler·go·sor·bent \-ə-ˌlər-gō-ˈsòr-bənt\ *adj* : relating to, involving, or being a radioallergosorbent test

radioallergosorbent test *n* : a radioimmunoassay for specific antibodies of immunoglobulin class IgE in which an insoluble matrix containing allergenic antigens is reacted with a sample of antibody-containing serum and then reacted again with antihuman antibodies against individual IgE antibodies to make specific determinations — abbr. *RAST*

ra·dio·as·say \-ˈas-ˌā, -a-ˈsā\ *n* : an assay based on examination of the sample in terms of radiation components

ra·dio·au·to·gram \-ˈòt-ə-ˌgram\ *n* : AUTORADIOGRAPH

ra·dio·au·to·graph \ˌrād-ē-ō-ˈòt-ə-ˌgraf\ *n* : AUTORADIOGRAPH — **radioautograph** *vt* — **ra·dio·au·to·graph·ic** \-ˌòt-ə-ˈgraf-ik\ *adj* — **ra·dio·au·tog·ra·phy** \-ō-ò-ˈtäg-rə-fē\ *n, pl* **-phies**

ra·dio·bi·ol·o·gist \ˌrād-ē-ō-bī-ˈäl-ə-jəst\ *n* : a specialist in radiobiology

ra·dio·bi·ol·o·gy \ˌrād-ē-ō-bī-ˈäl-ə-jē\ *n, pl* **-gies** : a branch of biology dealing with the effects of radiation or radioactive materials on biological systems — **ra·dio·bi·o·log·i·cal** \-ˌbī-ə-ˈläj-i-kəl\ *also* **ra·dio·bi·o·log·ic** \-ik\ *adj* — **ra·dio·bi·o·log·i·cal·ly** \-i-k(ə-)lē\ *adv*

ra·dio·car·bon \ˌrād-ē-ō-ˈkär-bən\ *n* : radioactive carbon; *esp* : CARBON 14

¹ra·dio·chem·i·cal \-ˈkem-i-kəl\ *adj* : of, relating to, being, or using radiochemicals or the methods of radiochemistry ⟨∼ analysis⟩ ⟨∼ purity⟩ — **ra·dio·chem·i·cal·ly** \-k(ə-)lē\ *adv*

²radiochemical *n* : a chemical prepared with radioactive elements esp. for medical research or application (as for use as a tracer in renal or heart function studies)

ra·dio·chem·ist \-ˈkem-əst\ *n* : a specialist in radiochemistry

\ə\ **abut** \ˈ\ **kitten** \ər\ **further** \a\ **ash** \ā\ **ace** \ä\ **cot, cart**
\au̇\ **out** \ch\ **chin** \e\ **bet** \ē\ **easy** \g\ **go** \i\ **hit** \ī\ **ice** \j\ **job**
\ŋ\ **sing** \ō\ **go** \ò\ **law** \ói\ **boy** \th\ **thin** \th̲\ **the** \ü\ **loot**
\u̇\ **foot** \y\ **yet** \zh\ **vision** *See also* Pronunciation Symbols page

Q

R

ra·dio·chem·is·try \ˌrād-ē-ō-ˈkem-ə-strē\ *n, pl* **-tries** : a branch of chemistry dealing with radioactive substances and phenomena including tracer studies — called also *nuclear chemistry*

ra·dio·chro·mato·gram \-krō-ˈmat-ə-ˌgram, -krə-\ *n* : a chromatogram revealing one or more radioactive substances

ra·dio·chro·ma·tog·ra·phy \ˈrād-ē-ō-ˌkrō-mə-ˈtäg-rə-fē\ *n, pl* **-phies** : the process of making a quantitative or qualitative determination of a radioisotope-labeled substance by measuring the radioactivity of the appropriate zone or spot in the chromatogram — **ra·dio·chro·ma·to·graph·ic** \-krə-ˌmat-ə-ˈgraf-ik, -ˌkrō-mət-\ *adj*

ra·dio·chro·mi·um \-ˈkrō-mē-əm\ *n* : radioactive chromium; *esp* : an isotope of chromium of mass number 51

ra·dio·co·balt \-ˈkō-ˌbolt\ *n* : radioactive cobalt; *esp* : COBALT 60

ra·dio·col·loid \-ˈkäl-ˌoid\ *n* : a colloidal aggregate consisting of or containing a radioactive element — **ra·dio·col·loi·dal** \-kə-ˈloid-ᵊl, -kä-\ *adj*

ra·dio·con·trast \-ˈkän-ˌtrast\ *adj* : relating to or being a radioactive contrast medium

ra·dio·den·si·ty \-ˈden(t)-sət-ē\ *n, pl* **-ties** : RADIOPACITY

ra·dio·der·ma·ti·tis \-ˌdər-mə-ˈtīt-əs\ *n, pl* **-ti·tis·es** *or* **-tit·i·des** \-ˈtit-ə-ˌdēz\ : dermatitis resulting from overexposure to sources of radiant energy (as X-rays or radium)

ra·dio·di·ag·no·sis \-ˌdī-ig-ˈnō-səs\ *n, pl* **-no·ses** \-ˌsēz\ : diagnosis by means of radiology — compare RADIOTHERAPY

ra·dio·ecol·o·gist \ˌrād-ē-ō-i-ˈkäl-ə-jəst\ *n* : a specialist in radioecology

ra·dio·ecol·o·gy \ˌrād-ē-ō-i-ˈkäl-ə-jē\ *n, pl* **-gies** : the study of the effects of radiation and radioactive substances on ecological communities — **ra·dio·eco·log·i·cal** \-ˌē-kə-ˈläj-i-kəl, -ˌek-ə-\ *adj*

ra·dio·el·e·ment \-ˈel-ə-mənt\ *n* : a radioactive element whether formed naturally or produced artificially — compare RADIOISOTOPE

ra·dio·en·zy·mat·ic \-ˌen-zə-ˈmat-ik\ *adj* : of, relating to, or produced by a radioactive enzyme — **ra·dio·en·zy·mat·i·cal·ly** \-i-k(ə-)lē\ *adv*

ra·dio–fre·quen·cy \ˈrād-ē-ō-ˈfrē-kwən-sē\ *adj* : of, relating to, using, or induced by radio frequencies ⟨a new . . . procedure that uses ~ heat to collapse veins —Tara Parker-Pope⟩

radio frequency *n* : any of the electromagnetic wave frequencies that lie in a range extending from below 3 kilohertz to about 300 gigahertz and that include the frequencies used in radio and television transmission

ra·dio·gen·ic \ˌrād-ē-ō-ˈjen-ik\ *adj* : produced or caused by radioactivity ⟨~ isotopes⟩ ⟨~ cancer⟩

ra·dio·gold \-ˈgōld\ *n* : radioactive gold; *esp* : an isotope of gold of mass number 198

ra·dio·gram \ˈrād-ē-ō-ˌgram\ *n* : RADIOGRAPH

¹**ra·dio·graph** \-ˌgraf\ *n* : an X-ray or gamma-ray photograph

²**radiograph** *vt* : to make a radiograph of

ra·di·og·ra·pher \ˌrād-ē-ˈäg-rə-fər\ *n* : a person who makes radiographs; *specif* : an X-ray technician

ra·dio·graph·ic \ˌrād-ē-ə-ˈgraf-ik\ *adj* : of or relating to radiography; *specif* : of or relating to the process that depends on the differential absorption of rays transmitted through heterogeneous media ⟨a ~ study revealed shin splints in both legs⟩ — **ra·dio·graph·i·cal·ly** \-i-k(ə-)lē\ *adv*

ra·di·og·ra·phy \ˌrā-dē-ˈäg-rə-fē\ *n, pl* **-phies** : the art, act, or process of making radiographs and sonograms

ra·dio·hu·mer·al bursitis \ˌrād-ē-ō-ˌhyüm-(ə-)rəl-\ *n* : TENNIS ELBOW

ra·dio·im·mu·no·as·say \ˌrād-ē-ō-ˌim-yə-nō-ˈas-ˌā, -im-ˌyü-, -ə-ˈsā\ *n* : immunoassay of a substance (as insulin) that has been radiolabeled — abbr. *RIA* — **ra·dio·im·mu·no·as·say·able** \-ə-bəl\ *adj*

ra·dio·im·mu·no·elec·tro·pho·re·sis \-i-ˌlek-trə-fə-ˈrē-səs\ *n, pl* **-re·ses** \-ˌsēz\ : immunoelectrophoresis in which the substances separated in the electrophoretic system are identified by radioactive labels on antigens or antibodies — **ra·dio·im·mu·no·elec·tro·pho·ret·ic** \-ˈret-ik\ *adj*

ra·dio·im·mu·no·log·i·cal \-ˌim-yə-nə-ˈläj-i-kəl\ *also* **ra·dio-**

im·mu·no·log·ic \-ˈläj-ik\ *adj* : of, relating to, or involving a radioimmunoassay ⟨~ detection of a hormone⟩

ra·dio·im·mu·no·pre·cip·i·ta·tion \-ˌim-yə-nō-pri-ˌsip-ə-ˈtā-shən, -im-ˌyü-\ *n* : immunoprecipitation using antibodies or antigens labeled with a radioisotope

ra·dio·io·dide \-ˈī-ə-ˌdīd\ *n* : an iodide containing radioactive iodine

ra·dio·io·din·ate \-ˈī-ə-də-ˌnāt\ *vt* **-at·ed; -at·ing** : to treat or label with radioactive iodine — **ra·dio·io·din·ation** \-ˌī-ə-də-ˈnā-shən\ *n*

ra·dio·io·dine \-ˈī-ə-ˌdīn, -əd-ᵊn, -ə-ˌdēn\ *n* : radioactive iodine; *esp* : IODINE-131

ra·dio·iron \-ˈī(-ə)rn\ *n* : radioactive iron; *esp* : a heavy isotope having the mass number 59 produced in nuclear reactors or cyclotrons and used in biochemical tracer studies

ra·dio·iso·tope \ˌrād-ē-ō-ˈī-sə-ˌtōp\ *n* : a radioactive isotope — compare RADIOELEMENT — **ra·dio·iso·to·pic** \-ˌī-sə-ˈtäp-ik, -ˈtōp-ik\ *adj* — **ra·dio·iso·to·pi·cal·ly** \-i-k(ə-)lē\ *adv*

radio knife *n* : a needlelike surgical instrument using high-frequency oscillations in the form of a tiny electric arc at the point of cutting through or cutting away tissue and at the same time sterilizing the edges of the wound and sealing cut blood vessels — called also *acusector*

ra·dio·la·bel \-ˈlā-bəl\ *vt* **-la·beled** *or* **-la·belled; -la·bel·ing** *or* **-la·bel·ling** : to label with a radioactive atom or substance ⟨~ed monoclonal antibodies⟩ — **radiolabel** *n*

ra·dio·lead \-ˈled\ *n* : lead formed in the disintegration of radium; *esp* : a radioactive isotope of lead

ra·dio·li·gand \-ˈlig-ənd, -ˈlīg-\ *n* : a substance (as an antigen) that has been radiolabeled esp. for analysis by radioimmunoassay

ra·dio·log·i·cal \ˌrād-ē-ə-ˈläj-i-kəl\ *or* **ra·dio·log·ic** \-ik\ *adj* **1** : of or relating to radiology ⟨~ treatment⟩ **2** : of or relating to esp. nuclear radiation ⟨~ physics⟩; *specif* : producing or capable of producing casualties by nuclear radiation ⟨~ hazards⟩ — **ra·dio·log·i·cal·ly** \-i-k(ə-)lē\ *adv*

ra·di·ol·o·gist \ˌrād-ē-ˈäl-ə-jəst\ *n* : a physician specializing in the use of radiant energy for diagnostic and therapeutic purposes

ra·di·ol·o·gy \-jē\ *n, pl* **-gies** **1** : the science of radioactive substances and high-energy radiations **2** : a branch of medicine concerned with the use of radiant energy (as X-rays or ultrasound) in the diagnosis and treatment of disease

ra·dio·lu·cen·cy \ˌrād-ē-ō-ˈlüs-ᵊn-sē\ *n, pl* **-cies** : the quality or state of being radiolucent

ra·dio·lu·cent \-ˈlüs-ᵊnt\ *adj* : partly or wholly permeable to radiation and esp. X-rays — compare RADIOPAQUE

ra·di·ol·y·sis \ˌrād-ē-ˈäl-ə-səs\ *n, pl* **-y·ses** \-ˌsēz\ : chemical decomposition by the action of radiation — compare PHOTOLYSIS

ra·di·om·e·ter \ˌrād-ē-ˈäm-ət-ər\ *n* : an instrument for measuring the intensity of radiant energy; *also* : an instrument for measuring electromagnetic radiation or sound waves

ra·dio·met·ric \ˌrād-ē-ō-ˈme-trik\ *adj* : relating to, using, or measured by a radiometer — **ra·dio·met·ri·cal·ly** \-tri-k(ə-)lē\ *adv*

ra·di·om·e·try \ˌrā-dē-ˈäm-ə-trē\ *n, pl* **-tries** : the use of the radiometer; *also* : the measurement of radiation

ra·dio·mi·met·ic \ˌrād-ē-ō-mə-ˈmet-ik, -mī-\ *adj* : producing effects similar to those of radiation ⟨~ agents⟩

ra·dio·ne·cro·sis \-nə-ˈkrō-səs, -ne-\ *n, pl* **-cro·ses** \-ˌsēz\ : ulceration or destruction of tissue resulting from irradiation — **ra·dio·ne·crot·ic** \-ˈkrät-ik\ *adj*

ra·dio·nu·clide \-ˈn(y)ü-ˌklīd\ *n* : a radioactive nuclide

ra·di·opac·i·ty \ˌrād-ē-ō-ˈpas-ət-ē\ *n, pl* **-ties** : the quality or state of being radiopaque

ra·dio·paque \-ō-ˈpāk\ *adj* : being opaque to radiation and esp. X-rays ⟨~ dyes⟩ — compare RADIOLUCENT

ra·dio·par·ent \ˌrād-ē-ō-ˈpar-ənt, -ˈper-\ *adj* : RADIOTRANSPARENT

¹**ra·dio·phar·ma·ceu·ti·cal** \ˌrād-ē-ō-ˌfär-mə-ˈsüt-i-kəl\ *n* : a radioactive drug used for diagnostic or therapeutic purposes

²**radiopharmaceutical** *adj* : of, relating to, or being a radiopharmaceutical ⟨~ agents⟩

ra·dio·phar·ma·cist \-'fär-mə-səst\ *n* : a person who special-izes in or who prepares and dispenses radiopharmaceuticals

ra·dio·phar·ma·cy \-sē\ *n, pl* **-cies** : a branch of pharmacy concerned with radiopharmaceuticals; *also* : a pharmacy that supplies radiopharmaceuticals

ra·dio·phos·pho·rus \-'fäs-f(ə-)rəs\ *n* : radioactive phospho-rus; *esp* : PHOSPHORUS 32

ra·dio·pro·tec·tive \-prə-'tek-tiv\ *adj* : serving to protect or aiding in protecting against the injurious effect of radiations ⟨~ drugs⟩ — **ra·dio·pro·tec·tion** \-'tek-shən\ *n*

ra·dio·pro·tec·tor \-'tek-tər\ *also* **ra·dio·pro·tec·tor·ant** \-'tek-tə-rənt\ *n* : a radioprotective chemical agent

ra·dio·re·cep·tor assay \-ri-'sep-tər-\ *n* : an assay for a sub-stance and esp. a hormone in which a mixture of the test sample and a known amount of the radiolabeled substance under test is exposed to a measured quantity of receptors for the substance and the amount in the test sample is deter-mined from the proportion of receptors occupied by radiola-beled molecules of the substance under the assumption that labeled and unlabeled molecules bind to the receptor sites at random

ra·dio·re·sis·tance \-ri-'zis-tən(t)s\ *n* : resistance (as of a cell) to the effects of radiant energy — compare RADIOSEN-SITIVITY

ra·dio·re·sis·tant \-tənt\ *adj* : resistant to the effects of radi-ant energy ⟨~ cancer cells⟩ — compare RADIOSENSITIVE

ra·dio·re·spi·ro·met·ric \-,res-pə-rō-'me-trik\ *adj* : of, relat-ing to, or being a study of metabolism by the measurement of carbon dioxide labeled with carbon 14 from the carbohy-drate substrate

ra·di·os·co·py \,rād-ē-'äs-kə-pē\ *n, pl* **-pies** : direct observa-tion of objects opaque to light by means of some other form of radiant energy (as X-rays)

ra·dio·sen·si·tive \,rād-ē-ō-'sen(t)-sət-iv, -'sen(t)-stiv\ *adj* : sensitive to the effects of radiant energy ⟨~ cancer cells⟩ — compare RADIORESISTANT

ra·dio·sen·si·tiv·i·ty \-,sen(t)-sə-'tiv-ət-ē\ *n, pl* **-ties** : the quality or state of being radiosensitive — compare RADIO-RESISTANCE

ra·dio·sen·si·tiz·er *also Brit* **ra·dio·sen·si·tis·er** \-'sen(t)-sə-,tī-zər\ *n* : a substance or condition capable of increasing the radiosensitivity of a cell or tissue — **ra·dio·sen·si·ti·za·tion** *also Brit* **ra·dio·sen·si·ti·sa·tion** \-,sen(t)-sət-ə-'zā-shən\ *n* — **ra·dio·sen·si·tiz·ing** *also Brit* **ra·dio·sen·si·tis·ing** \-'sen(t)-sə-,tī-ziŋ\ *adj*

ra·dio·so·di·um \-'sōd-ē-əm\ *n* : radioactive sodium; *esp* : a heavy isotope having the mass number 24, produced in nu-clear reactors, and used in the form of a salt (as sodium chlo-ride) chiefly in biochemical tracer studies

ra·dio·ster·il·ized *also Brit* **ra·dio·ster·il·ised** \-'ster-ə-,līzd\ *adj* : sterilized by irradiation (as with X-rays or gamma rays) ⟨~ mosquitoes⟩ ⟨~ syringes⟩ — **ra·dio·ster·il·iza·tion** *also Brit* **ra·dio·ster·il·isa·tion** \-,ster-ə-lə-'zā-shən\ *n*

ra·dio·stron·tium \,rād-ē-ō-'strän-ch(ē-)əm, -'stränt-ē-əm\ *n* : radioactive strontium; *esp* : STRONTIUM 90

ra·dio·sur·gery \-'sərj-(ə-)rē\ *n, pl* **-ger·ies** **1** : surgery by means of a radio knife **2** : STEREOTACTIC RADIOSURGERY — **ra·dio·sur·gi·cal** \-'sər-ji-kəl\ *adj*

ra·dio·te·lem·e·try \-tə-'lem-ə-trē\ *n, pl* **-tries** **1** : TELEME-TRY **2** : BIOTELEMETRY — **ra·dio·tele·met·ric** \-,tel-ə-'me-trik\ *adj*

ra·dio·ther·a·peu·tic \,rād-ē-ō-,ther-ə-'pyüt-ik\ *adj* : of or relating to radiotherapy — **ra·dio·ther·a·peu·ti·cal·ly** \-i-k(ə-)lē\ *adv*

ra·dio·ther·a·peut·ics \-'pyüt-iks\ *n pl but sing in constr* : RADIOTHERAPY

ra·dio·ther·a·peut·ist \-'pyüt-əst\ *n* : RADIOTHERAPIST

ra·dio·ther·a·pist \-'ther-ə-pəst\ *n* : a specialist in radiothera-py

ra·dio·ther·a·py \,rād-ē-ō-'ther-ə-pē\ *n, pl* **-pies** : the treat-ment of disease by means of radiation (as X-rays) — called also *radiation therapy, radium therapy;* compare RADIODI-AGNOSIS

ra·dio·ther·my \'rād-ē-ō-,thər-mē\ *n, pl* **-mies** : diathermy by means of a shortwave radio machine

ra·dio·tho·ri·um \-'thōr-ē-əm, -'thór-\ *n* : a radioactive iso-tope of thorium with the mass number 228

ra·dio·thy·roid·ec·to·my \-,thī-rói-'dek-tə-mē\ *n, pl* **-mies** : the destruction of part of the thyroid gland by administer-ing radioactive iodine in order to reduce thyroid function

ra·dio·tox·emia \-,täk-'sē-mē-ə\ *n* : toxemia resulting from exposure to radiation or a radioactive substance

ra·dio·tox·ic·i·ty \-,täk-'sis-ət-ē\ *n, pl* **-ties** : the toxicity of ra-dioactive substances

ra·dio·trac·er \'rād-ē-ō-,trā-sər\ *n* : a radioactive tracer

ra·dio·trans·par·ent \-tran(t)s-'par-ənt, -'per-\ *adj* : permit-ting the passage of radiation and esp. X-rays ⟨~ gallstones⟩

ra·dio·ul·nar \,rād-ē-ō-'əl-nər\ *adj* : of, relating to, or con-necting the radius and ulna ⟨~ synostosis⟩

radioulnar joint *n* : any of three joints connecting the radius and ulna at their proximal and distal ends and along their shafts — see DISTAL RADIOULNAR JOINT, SUPERIOR RADIO-ULNAR JOINT

ra·dio wave \'rād-ē-ō-,wāv\ *n* : an electromagnetic wave having a frequency in the range that extends from about 3000 hertz to about 300 billion hertz and includes the fre-quencies used for radio and television

ra·di·um \'rād-ē-əm\ *n, often attrib* : an intensely radioactive shining white metallic element that resembles barium chem-ically, that occurs in combination in minute quantities in minerals (as pitchblende or carnotite) principally as the iso-tope of mass number 226 formed from uranium 238, having a half-life of 1620 years, and emitting alpha particles and gamma rays to form radon, and that is used chiefly in lumi-nous materials and in the treatment of cancer — symbol *Ra*; see ELEMENT table

radium emanation *n* : RADON

radium needle *n* : a hollow radium-containing device shaped like a needle and used esp. in medical treatment

radium therapy *n* : RADIOTHERAPY

ra·di·us \'rād-ē-əs\ *n, pl* **ra·dii** \-ē-,ī\ *also* **ra·di·us·es** : the bone on the thumb side of the human forearm or on the cor-responding part of the forelimb of vertebrates above fishes that in humans is movably articulated with the ulna at both ends so as to permit partial rotation about that bone, that bears on its inner aspect somewhat distal to the head a prom-inence for the insertion of the biceps tendon, and that has the lower end broadened for articulation with the proximal bones of the carpus so that rotation of the radius involves also that of the hand

ra·dix \'rād-iks\ *n, pl* **ra·di·ces** \'rād-ə-,sēz, 'rad-\ *or* **ra·dix·es** \'rād-ik-səz\ : the base or root of something (as a plant or a cranial or spinal nerve)

ra·don \'rā-dän\ *n* : a heavy radioactive gaseous element of the group of inert gases formed by disintegration of radium and used similarly to radium in medicine — symbol *Rn;* called also *radium emanation;* see ELEMENT table

rad·u·la \'raj-ə-lə\ *n, pl* **-lae** \-,lē, -,lī\ *also* **-las** : a horny band or ribbon in mollusks other than bivalves that bears minute teeth on its dorsal surface and tears up food and draws it into the mouth and that in some members of the gastropod genus *Conus* is used to inflict a poisonous and sometimes fatal bite — **rad·u·lar** \-lər\ *adj*

raf·fi·nase \'raf-ə-,nās, -,nāz\ *n* : an enzyme that catalyzes the hydrolysis of raffinose and occurs in various molds (as *Aspergillus niger*) and yeasts

raf·fi·nose \'raf-ə-,nōs, -,nōz\ *n* : a crystalline sugar $C_{18}H_{32}O_{16}$ obtained commercially from cottonseed meal and present in sugar beets and many plant products — called also *melitose*

rage \'rāj\ *n* : violent and uncontrolled anger

\ə\ abut \ᵊ\ kitten \ər\ further \a\ ash \ā\ ace \ä\ cot, cart
\aù\ out \ch\ chin \e\ bet \ē\ easy \g\ go \i\ hit \ī\ ice \j\ job
\ŋ\ sing \ō\ go \ò\ law \òi\ boy \th\ thin \t̲h̲\ the \ü\ loot
\ù\ foot \y\ yet \zh\ vision *See also* Pronunciation Symbols page

Q
R

rag·pick·er's disease \'rag-ˌpik-ərz-\ *n* : RAGSORTER'S DISEASE

rag·sort·er's disease \-ˌsȯrt-ərz-\ *n* : pulmonary anthrax caused by inhalation of spores of the anthrax bacillus from contaminated hair and esp. wool

rag·weed \'rag-ˌwēd\ *n* : any of various chiefly No. American weedy herbaceous plants comprising the genus *Ambrosia* and producing highly allergenic pollen responsible for much hay fever and asthma: as   **a** : an annual weed (*A. artemisiifolia*) with finely divided foliage that is common on open or cultivated ground in much of No. America   **b** : a coarse annual (*A. trifida*) with some or all of the leaves usu. deeply and palmately 3-cleft or 5-cleft — called also *great ragweed*

Rail·lie·ti·na \ˌrāl-yə-'tī-nə\ *n* : a large genus of armed cyclophyllidean tapeworms (family Davaineidae) of which the adults are parasitic in birds, rodents, or rarely humans and the larvae are parasitic in various insects

  Rail·liet \rī-yā\, **Louis–Joseph Alcide (1852–1930),** French veterinarian. Railliet was a professor of veterinary science, a naturalist, and a noted helmintologist. He is considered by some a founder of parasitology. He was the author of several works on parasitic diseases in animals. The genus *Raillietina* was named in his honor in 1920.

rain·bow \'rān-ˌbō\ *n, slang* : a combination of the sodium derivatives of amobarbital and secobarbital in a blue and red capsule

rainbow pill *n, slang* : any of a combination of pills (as of amphetamines, laxatives, and thyroid hormones) typically of different colors that were formerly taken to curb appetite and promote weight loss

Rain·ey's corpuscle \'rā-nēz-\ *n* : the crescent-shaped spore of a sporozoan of the order Sarcosporidia

  Rainey, George (1801–1884), British anatomist. A lecturer on anatomy by profession, Rainey also was the author of a book on the formation of shell and bone and of papers on histology, both normal and pathological. In an 1857 article on the process of calcification of tissues, he described Rainey's corpuscles.

rale \'ral, 'räl\ *n* : an abnormal sound heard accompanying the normal respiratory sounds on auscultation of the chest — compare RATTLE 2, RHONCHUS

ral·ox·i·fene \ˌral-'äk-sə-ˌfēn\ *n* : a selective estrogen receptor modulator that is administered orally in the form of its hydrochloride $C_{28}H_{27}NO_4S\cdot HCl$ as prophylaxis against osteoporosis after menopause, that binds with estrogen receptors to act as an estrogen agonist promoting bone mineralization and lipid metabolism, and that is believed to spare breast and uterine tissues the cancer-producing effects of estrogen by acting as an estrogen antagonist in those tissues — see EVISTA

ram \'ram\ *n* : a male sheep

ra·mal \'rā-məl\ *adj* : of or relating to a ramus

Ra·man \'rä-mən\ *adj* : of, relating to, using, or caused by the Raman effect

  Raman, Sir Chandrasekhara Venkata (1888–1970), Indian physicist. Raman discovered in 1928 that when light of one frequency was transmitted through a medium, other frequencies were added and that they were characteristic of the material. The use of the Raman effect in determining fine molecular structure was instrumental in the making of laser spectrometers. In 1930 he was awarded the Nobel Prize for Physics.

Raman effect *n* : a change in frequency undergone by a portion of the light that has been scattered in passage through a transparent liquid, solid, or gas whose characteristics determine the amount of change

Raman scattering *n* : the scattering of light (as from a laser) by a pure substance that gives rise to a characteristic Raman spectrum

Raman spectroscopy *n* : a spectroscopic technique in which the Raman spectrum of a substance is analyzed to determine the properties (as the structure) of the substance

Raman spectrum *n* : the characteristic array of frequencies of light that are observed when a fixed single frequency of light is scattered by a pure substance

rami *pl of* RAMUS

ram·i·fi·ca·tion \ˌram-ə-fə-'kā-shən\ *n*   **1** : the act or process of branching; *specif* : the mode of arrangement of branches   **2** : a branch or offshoot from a main stock or channel ⟨the ∼ of an artery⟩; *also* : the resulting branched structure ⟨make visible the whole ∼ of the dendrite⟩

ram·i·fy \'ram-ə-ˌfī\ *vi* -**fied; -fy·ing** : to split up into branches or constituent parts

ra·mip·ril \rä-'mip-rəl, ra-\ *n* : an ACE inhibitor $C_{23}H_{32}N_2O_5$ used esp. to treat hypertension — see ALTACE

rami·sec·tion \ˌram-i-'sek-shən\ *n* : the surgical severance of one or more rami and esp. the rami communicantes (as for the relief of spastic paralysis)

ra·mose \'rā-ˌmōs\ *adj* : consisting of or having branches

Rams·den eyepiece \'ramz-dən-\ *n* : a nearly achromatic optical system that contains two plano-convex lenses with the convex surfaces facing each other and is used esp. in instruments fitted with micrometer wires or a scale

  Ramsden, Jesse (1735–1800), British instrument maker. Ramsden was a pioneer in the early invention and manufacture of precision instruments. He designed improved, highly accurate sextants and theodolites. He introduced the Ramsden eyepiece in 1779.

ram·u·lus \'ram-yə-ləs\ *n, pl* **ram·u·li** \-ˌlī\ : a small branch

ra·mus \'rā-məs\ *n, pl* **ra·mi** \-ˌmī\ : a projecting part, elongated process, or branch: as   **a** : the posterior more or less vertical part of the lower jaw on each side which articulates with the skull   **b** (1) : the upper more cranial branch of the pubis that extends from the pubic symphysis to the body of the pubis at the acetabulum and forms the cranial part of the obturator foramen — called also *superior ramus*   (2) : the thin flat lower branch of the pubis that extends from the pubic symphysis to unite with the ramus of the ischium in forming the inferior rim of the obturator foramen — called also *inferior ramus*   **c** : a branch of the ischium that extends down and forward from the ischial tuberosity to unite with the inferior ramus of the pubis in forming the inferior rim of the obturator foramen — called also *inferior ramus*   **d** : a branch of a nerve — see RAMUS COMMUNICANS

ramus com·mu·ni·cans \-kə-'myü-nə-ˌkanz\ *n, pl* **rami com·mu·ni·can·tes** \-kə-ˌmyü-nə-'kan-ˌtēz\ : any of the bundles of nerve fibers connecting a sympathetic ganglion with a spinal nerve and being divided into two kinds: **a** : one consisting of myelinated preganglionic fibers — called also *white ramus, white ramus communicans*   **b** : one consisting of unmyelinated postganglionic fibers — called also *gray ramus, gray ramus communicans*

ran *past of* RUN

Ra·na \'rä-nə\ *n* : a nearly cosmopolitan genus (family Ranidae) of frogs including some extensively used in animal research and some that are intermediate hosts of tapeworms and schistosomes

ran·cid \'ran(t)-səd\ *adj* : having a rank smell or taste usu. from chemical change or decomposition ⟨∼ butter⟩

ran·cid·i·fi·ca·tion \ran-ˌsid-ə-fə-'kā-shən\ *n* : the chemical change that produces rancidity

ran·cid·i·fy \ran-'sid-ə-ˌfī\ *vb* -**fied; -fy·ing** *vt* : to make rancid ∼ *vi* : to become rancid

ran·cid·i·ty \ran-'sid-ət-ē\ *n, pl* -**ties** : the quality or state of being rancid; *also* : a rancid odor or flavor

ran·dom·ized controlled trial \'ran-də-ˌmīzd-\ *n* : a clinical trial in which the subjects are randomly distributed into groups which are either subjected to the experimental procedure (as use of a drug) or which serve as controls — called also *randomized clinical trial*

rang *past of* RING

¹range \'rānj\ *n, often attrib*   **1** : the region throughout which a kind of organism or ecological community naturally lives or occurs   **2** : the difference between the least and greatest values of an attribute or of the variable of a frequency distribution

²range *vi* **ranged; rang·ing** **1** : to change or differ within limits ⟨symptoms ∼ in severity from mild to severe⟩ **2** *of an organism* : to live or occur in or be native to a region

range of accommodation *n* : the range through which accommodation is able to adjust the optical system of the eye so that an image falls in sharp focus on the retina : the distance between the near point and the far point of the eye

range paralysis *n* : NEUROLYMPHOMATOSIS

ra·nine artery \'rā-ˌnīn-\ *n* : DEEP LINGUAL ARTERY

ra·nit·i·dine \ra-'nit-ə-ˌdēn\ *n* : an antihistamine that is administered in the form of its hydrochloride $C_{13}H_{22}N_4O_3S$·HCl to inhibit gastric acid secretion (as in the treatment of duodenal ulcers or Zollinger-Ellison syndrome) — see ZANTAC

Ran·kine \'raŋ-kən\ *adj* : being, according to, or relating to an absolute-temperature scale on which the unit of measurement equals a Fahrenheit degree and on which the freezing point of water is 491.67° and the boiling point 671.67°

Rankine, William John Macquorn (1820–1872), British physicist and engineer. Rankine was one of the founders of the science of thermodynamics. In 1843 he published a paper on metal fatigue in railway axles that attracted the attention of physicists and railway engineers and brought about new methods of construction. He published in 1858 a *Manual of Applied Mechanics* that became a classic text for designing engineers and architects, and a year later he introduced a manual on the steam engine that was the first attempt at a systematic treatment of steam-engine theory.

ran·u·la \'ran-yə-lə\ *n* : a cyst formed under the tongue by obstruction of a gland duct

Ra·oult's law \rä-'ülz-\ *n* : a law in physical chemistry: the fraction by which the vapor pressure of a liquid is lowered when a small amount of a substance that is nonvolatile, not capable of being dissociated, and usu. not a high polymer is dissolved in it is equal to the ratio of the number of moles of the solute to the total number of moles of all components of the solution

Ra·oult \rä-ü\, **François–Marie (1830–1901),** French chemist. Raoult is known for developing the theory of solutions. He discovered about 1886 that the freezing point of an aqueous solution is lowered in proportion to the amount of nonelectrolyte dissolved. He recognized that the effect of the amount of solute dissolved on the solvent's freezing point was due to a change in the vapor pressure of the solvent brought about by the presence of the solute. This recognition led to the formulation of Raoult's law. The law made possible the determining of molecular weights of dissolved substances.

rap·a·my·cin \ˌrap-ə-'mīs-³n\ *n* : an immunosuppressive agent $C_{51}H_{79}NO_{13}$

¹rape \'rāp\ *n* : a European herb (*Brassica napus*) of the mustard family grown as a forage crop and for its seeds which yield rapeseed oil and are a bird food — see CANOLA 1

²rape *vt* **raped; rap·ing** : to commit rape on

³rape *n* : unlawful sexual activity and usu. sexual intercourse carried out forcibly or under threat of injury against the will usu. of a female or with a person who is beneath a certain age or incapable of valid consent — compare SEXUAL ASSAULT, STATUTORY RAPE

rape oil *n* : RAPESEED OIL

rape·seed \'rāp-ˌsēd\ *n* : the seed of the rape plant (*Brassica napus* of the mustard family) that is the source of rapeseed oil

rapeseed oil *n* : a nondrying or semidrying oil obtained from rapeseed and turnip seed and used chiefly as a lubricant, illuminant, and food — called also *rape oil*

ra·phe *also* **rha·phe** \'rā-fē\ *n* : the seamlike union of the two lateral halves of a part or organ (as of the tongue, perineum, or scrotum) having externally a ridge or furrow and internally usu. a fibrous connective tissue septum

raphe nucleus *n* : any of several groups of nerve cells situated along or near the median plane of the tegmentum of the midbrain

rap·id eye movement \'rap-əd-\ *n* : a rapid conjugate move-

ment of the eyes associated esp. with REM sleep — called also *REM*

rapid eye movement sleep *n* : REM SLEEP

rapid plasma reagin test *n* : a flocculation test for syphilis employing the antigen used in the VDRL slide test with charcoal particles added so that the flocculation can be seen without the aid of a microscope — called also *RPR card test*

rap·ist \'rā-pəst\ *n* : an individual who commits rape

rap·port \ra-'pō(ə)r, rə-\ *n* **1** : relation characterized by harmony, conformity, accord, or affinity **2** : confidence of a subject in the operator (as in hypnotism, psychotherapy, or mental testing) with willingness to cooperate ⟨the first step in treatment is establishment of a firm ∼ —C. A. H. Watts⟩

rap·ture of the deep \'rap-chər-\ *n* : NITROGEN NARCOSIS

rap·tus \'rap-təs\ *n* : a pathological paroxysm of activity giving vent to impulse or tension (as in an act of violence)

rare earth \ˌrer-'ərth\ *n* **1** : any of a group of similar oxides of metals or a mixture of such oxides occurring together in widely distributed but relatively scarce minerals **2** : RARE EARTH ELEMENT

rare earth element *n* : any of a series of metallic elements of which the oxides are classed as rare earths and which include the elements of the lanthanide series and sometimes yttrium and scandium — called also *rare earth metal*

rar·e·fac·tion \ˌrar-ə-'fak-shən, ˌrer-\ *n* **1** : the action or process of rarefying **2** : the quality or state of being rarefied; *esp* : an increase in porosity ⟨areas of ∼ in the bones⟩ **3** : a state or region of minimum pressure in a medium transversed by compressional waves (as sound waves) ⟨the eardrum vibrates according to the compressions and ∼s of the sound wave⟩ — **rar·e·fac·tion·al** \-shnəl, -shən-³l\ *adj*

rar·e·fy *also* **rar·i·fy** \'rar-ə-ˌfī, 'rer-\ *vb* **-e·fied** *also* **-i·fied; -e·fy·ing** *also* **-i·fy·ing** *vt* : to make rare, thin, porous, or less dense : to expand without the addition of matter ∼ *vi* : to become less dense

ras \'ras\ *n, often attrib* [*ras* sarcoma] : any of a family of genes that undergo mutation to oncogenes and esp. to some commonly linked to human cancers (as of the colon, lung, and pancreas) ⟨∼ oncogenes⟩ ⟨∼ proteins⟩

ra·sce·ta \rə-'sēt-ə\ *n pl* : transverse creases of the skin on the palmar surface of the wrist

rash \'rash\ *n* : an eruption on the body typically with little or no elevation above the surface

ras·pa·to·ry \'ras-pə-ˌtōr-ē\ *n, pl* **-ries** : a file or rasp used (as for scraping bone) in surgery

RAST *abbr* radioallergosorbent test

rat \'rat\ *n* : any of the numerous rodents (family Muridae) of *Rattus* and related genera that differ from the murid mice by their usu. considerably larger size and by features of the teeth and other structures and that include forms (as the brown rat, the black rat, and the roof rat) which live in and about human habitations and in ships, have become naturalized by commerce in most parts of the world, and are destructive pests consuming or destroying vast quantities of food and other goods and acting as vectors of various diseases (as bubonic plague)

rat–bite fever *n* : either of two febrile human diseases usu. transmitted by the bite of a rat: **a** : a septicemia marked by irregular relapsing fever, rashes, muscular pain and arthritis, and great weakness and caused by a bacterium of the genus *Streptobacillus* (*S. moniliformis*) **b** : a disease that is marked by sharp elevation of temperature, swelling of lymph glands, eruption, recurrent inflammation of the bite wound, and muscular pains in the part where the bite wound occurred and that is caused by a bacterium of the genus *Spirillum* (*S. minor* syn. *S. minus*) — called also *sodoku*

rate \'rāt\ *n* **1** : a fixed ratio between two things **2** : a quantity, amount, or degree of something measured per unit of

Q
R

something else — see DEATH RATE, HEART RATE, METABOL-IC RATE, PULSE RATE, SEDIMENTATION RATE

rat flea *n* : any of various fleas that occur on rats: as **a** : NORTHERN RAT FLEA **b** : ORIENTAL RAT FLEA

Rath·ke's pouch \'rät-kəz-\ *n* : a pouch of ectoderm that grows out from the upper surface of the embryonic stomodeum and gives rise to the adenohypophysis of the pituitary gland — called also *Rathke's pocket*

   Rathke, Martin Heinrich (1793–1860), German anatomist. Rathke is regarded as one of the founders of modern embryology. In his early researches he discovered embryonic precursors of gills in the embryos of higher animals that lack gills as adults. He is best known for his discovery of branchial clefts and branchial arches in the embryos of birds and land animals. He followed the embryological history of these structures and found that the branchial clefts disappear eventually and that the blood vessels adapt themselves to the lungs. He also described and compared the development of the air sacs in birds and the larynx in birds and mammals. In 1838 he published an important study of the pituitary gland and in the following year discovered a diverticulum arising from the embryonic buccal cavity. This embryonic structure is now known as Rathke's pouch.

rat·i·cide \'rat-ə-ˌsīd\ *n* : a substance (as red squill) for killing rats — **rat·i·cid·al** \ˌrat-ə-'sīd-ᵊl\ *adj*

ra·tio \'rā-(ˌ)shō, -shē-ˌō\ *n, pl* **ra·tios** : the relationship in quantity, amount, or size between two or more things — see SEX RATIO

¹ra·tion \'rash-ən, 'rā-shən\ *n* : a food allowance for one day

²ration *vt* **ra·tioned; ra·tion·ing** \'rash-(ə-)niŋ, 'rāsh-\ : to supply with or put on rations

ra·tio·nal \'rash-nəl, -ən-ᵊl\ *adj* **1 a** : having reason or understanding **b** : relating to, based on, or agreeable to reason ⟨a ∼ explanation⟩ ⟨∼ behavior⟩ **2** : using medical treatments based on reason or general principles — used esp. of an ancient school of physicians; compare EMPIRICAL 1a — **ra·tio·nal·ly** \-ē\ *adv*

rational–emo·tive therapy \-i-'mōt-iv-\ *n* : cognitive therapy based on a theory of Albert Ellis that a patient can be taught to effect emotional well-being by changing negative and irrational thoughts to positive or rational ones

ra·tio·nal·i·ty \ˌrash-ə-'nal-ət-ē\ *n, pl* **-ties** **1** : the quality or state of being rational **2** : the quality or state of being agreeable to reason

ra·tio·nal·iza·tion *also Brit* **ra·tio·nal·isa·tion** \ˌrash-nə-lə-'zā-shən, -ən-ᵊl-ə-\ *n* : the act, process, or result of rationalizing; *esp* : the provision of plausible reasons to explain to oneself or others behavior for which one's real motives are different and unknown or unconscious

ra·tio·nal·ize *also Brit* **ra·tio·nal·ise** \'rash-nə-ˌlīz, -ən-ᵊl-ˌīz\ *vb* **-ized** *also Brit* **-ised; -iz·ing** *also Brit* **-is·ing** *vt* : to bring into accord with reason or cause something to seem reasonable; *esp* : to attribute (one's actions) to rational and creditable motives without analysis of true and esp. unconscious motives ⟨he tried to ∼ his cruel behavior⟩ ∼ *vi* : to provide plausible but untrue reasons for conduct — **ra·tio·nal·iz·er** *also Brit* **ra·tio·nal·is·er** \-ər\ *n*

rational therapy *n* : RATIONAL-EMOTIVE THERAPY

rat louse *n* : a sucking louse (*Polyplax spinulosa*) that is a widely distributed parasite of rats and transmits murine typhus from rat to rat

rat mite *n* : a widely distributed mite of the genus *Ornithonyssus* (*O. bacoti* syn. *Bdellonyssus bacoti*) that usu. feeds on rodents but may cause dermatitis in and transmit typhus to humans

rats·bane \'rats-ˌbān\ *n* : ARSENIC TRIOXIDE

rat·tle \'rat-ᵊl\ *n* **1** : the sound-producing organ on a rattlesnake's tail **2** : a throat noise caused by air passing through mucus; *specif* : DEATH RATTLE — compare RALE, RHONCHUS

rat·tle·box \-ˌbäks\ *n* : CROTALARIA 2; *esp* : one (*Crotalaria spectabilis*) that is highly toxic to farm animals

rat·tle·snake \'rat-ᵊl-ˌsnāk\ *n* : any of the American pit vipers that have a series of horny interlocking joints at the end of the tail which make a sharp rattling sound when vibrated and that comprise the genera *Sistrurus* and *Crotalus* — see DIAMONDBACK RATTLESNAKE, TIGER RATTLESNAKE, TIMBER RATTLESNAKE

Rat·tus \'rat-əs\ *n* : a genus of rodents of the family Muridae that comprise the common rats and are distinguished from members of the closely related genus *Mus* by bevel-edged upper incisors and comparatively large second and third molars

rat unit *n* : a bioassay unit consisting of the amount of a material (as a vitamin) that under standardized conditions is just sufficient to produce a specified response in all or a designated proportion of a group of experimental rats

Rau·dix·in \raù-'diks-ən, rō-\ *trademark* — used for a preparation of reserpine

rau·wol·fia \raù-'wùl-fē-ə, rō-\ *n* **1** : any of a genus (*Rauvolfia* syn. *Rauwolfia*) of tropical trees and shrubs of the dogbane family (Apocynaceae) that yield medicinal alkaloids (as reserpine) **2** : the dried root or an extract from the root of a rauwolfia (esp. *Rauvolfia serpentina* of Asia) used chiefly in the treatment of hypertension

   Rau·wolf \'raù-ˌvòlf\, **Leonhard (1535–1596),** German botanist. Rauwolf is famous for his botanical studies in the Middle East. He began his outstanding collection of dried plants with specimens from southern France, Switzerland, and northern Italy. Then from 1573 to 1576 he traveled extensively in the Middle East to collect more specimens for his herbarium with the intention of exploring the potential of the local plants for their use as drugs. In 1582 he published an account of his travels and descriptions of the plants that he had collected. In 1703 the botanist Charles Plumier named the genus *Rauwolfia* in his honor.

¹ray \'rā\ *n* : any of numerous elasmobranch fishes (order Hypotremata) having the body flattened dorsoventrally, the eyes on the upper surface, and a much-reduced caudal region having typically a slender process often with venomous spines

²ray *n* **1** : one of the lines of light that appear to radiate from a bright object **2** : a beam of radiant energy (as light) of small cross section **3 a** : a stream of material particles traveling in the same line (as in radioactive phenomena) **b** : a single particle of such a stream — **rayed** \'rād\ *adj*

ray·less goldenrod *n* : a shrubby or herbaceous composite plant (*Haplopappus heterophyllus* syn. *Isocoma wrightii*) that occurs esp. on open saline ground from Texas to Arizona and northern Mexico and causes trembles in cattle

Ray·naud's disease \rā-'nōz-\ *n* : a vascular disorder that is marked by recurrent spasm of the capillaries and esp. those of the fingers and toes upon exposure to cold, that is characterized by pallor, cyanosis, and redness in succession usu. accompanied by pain, and that in severe cases progresses to local gangrene — called also *Raynaud's*

   Ray·naud \re-nō\, **Maurice (1834–1881),** French physician. Raynaud described the vascular disorder now known as Raynaud's disease in his thesis for a medical degree in 1862. In 1874 he published a revised version of the dissertation with additional case reports and experimental studies. He was also very much interested in the history of medicine and wrote a scholarly study of the medical profession in the time of Molière.

Raynaud's phenomenon *n* : the symptoms associated with Raynaud's disease — called also *Raynaud's syndrome*

Rb *symbol* rubidium

RBC *abbr* **1** red blood cells **2** red blood count

RBE *abbr* relative biological effectiveness

rBGH *abbr* recombinant bovine growth hormone

RBRVS *abbr* resource-based relative value scale

rBST *abbr* recombinant bovine somatotropin

RCT *abbr* randomized clinical trial; randomized controlled trial

rd *abbr* rutherford

RD *abbr* **1** reaction of degeneration **2** registered dietitian

RDA *abbr* recommended daily allowance; recommended dietary allowance

RDH *abbr* registered dental hygienist

RDS *abbr* respiratory distress syndrome

Re *symbol* rhenium

re·ab·sorb \ˌrē-əb-ˈsȯ(ə)rb, -ˈzȯ(ə)rb\ *vt* : to take up (something previously secreted or emitted) ⟨sugars ∼ed in the kidney⟩; *also* : RESORB

re·ab·sorp·tion \-ˈsȯrp-shən, -ˈzȯrp-\ *n* : the act, process, or condition of absorbing again or of being absorbed again

re·act \rē-ˈakt\ *vi* **1** : to respond to a stimulus **2** : to undergo chemical reaction ∼ *vt* : to cause to react

re·ac·tance \rē-ˈak-tən(t)s\ *n* : the part of the impedance of an alternating-current circuit that is due to capacitance or inductance or both and that is expressed in ohms

re·ac·tant \-ˈtənt\ *n* : a substance that enters into and is altered in the course of a chemical reaction — **reactant** *adj*

re·ac·tion \rē-ˈak-shən\ *n* **1** : the act or process or an instance of reacting **2** : bodily response to or activity aroused by a stimulus: **a** : an action induced by vital resistance to another action; *esp* : the response of tissues to a foreign substance (as an antigen or infective agent) **b** : depression or exhaustion due to excessive exertion or stimulation **c** : abnormally heightened activity succeeding depression or shock **d** : a mental or emotional disorder forming an individual's response to his or her life situation **3** : the force that a body subjected to the action of a force from another body exerts in the opposite direction **4 a** (1) : chemical transformation or change : the interaction of chemical entities (2) : the state resulting from such a reaction **b** : a process involving change in atomic nuclei

reaction formation *n* : a psychological defense mechanism in which one form of behavior substitutes for or conceals a diametrically opposed repressed impulse in order to protect against it

reaction of degeneration *n* : the reaction to electric stimulation that occurs in muscles in which the nerves have undergone degeneration and that consists in severe cases of a sluggish response to galvanic stimulation of the muscle and no response to faradic stimulation of the muscle or to galvanic or faradic stimulation of the nerve — *abbr. RD*

reaction time *n* : the time elapsing between the beginning of the application of a stimulus and the beginning of an organism's reaction to it

re·ac·ti·vate \(ˈ)rē-ˈak-tə-ˌvāt\ *vt* **-vat·ed; -vat·ing** : to activate again : cause to be again active or more active: as **a** : to cause (as a repressed complex) to reappear in consciousness or behavior ⟨persecution feelings *reactivated* by new social failures⟩ **b** : to cause (a quiescent disease) to become active again in an individual ⟨a herpes infection *reactivated* by physical and emotional stresses⟩ **c** : to restore complement to (an inactivated serum) by addition of fresh normal serum

re·ac·ti·va·tion \-ˌak-tə-ˈvā-shən\ *n* : the act or process of reactivating or condition of being reactivated

re·ac·tive \rē-ˈak-tiv\ *adj* **1 a** : of, relating to, or marked by reaction ⟨∼ symptoms⟩ ⟨a ∼ process⟩ **b** : capable of reacting chemically ⟨highly ∼ materials⟩ **2 a** : readily responsive to a stimulus ⟨the skin of the geriatric is less ∼ than that of younger persons —Louis Tuft⟩ **b** : occurring as a result of stress or emotional upset esp. from factors outside the organism ⟨∼ depression⟩

reactive arthritis *n* : acute arthritis that sometimes develops following a bacterial infection (as with the bacteria of the genera *Shigella, Salmonella,* or *Chlamydia*)

re·ac·tiv·i·ty \(ˌ)rē-ˌak-ˈtiv-ət-ē\ *n, pl* **-ties** : the quality or state of being reactive ⟨skin ∼⟩ ⟨emotional ∼⟩

re·ac·to·gen·ic \(ˌ)rē-ˌak-tə-ˈjen-ik\ *adj* : capable of causing a reaction and esp. an immunological reaction ⟨a highly ∼ vaccine⟩ — **re·ac·to·ge·nic·i·ty** \-jə-ˈnis-ə-tē\ *n, pl* **-ties**

re·ac·tor \rē-ˈak-tər\ *n* **1** : one that reacts: as **a** : a chemical reagent **b** : an individual reacting to a stimulus **c** : an individual reacting positively to a foreign substance (as in a test for disease) ⟨∼s to tuberculin⟩ **2 a** : a piece of equipment in which a chemical reaction and esp. an industrial chemical reaction is carried out **b** : a device for the controlled release of nuclear energy (as for producing heat)

read·ing frame \ˈrēd-iŋ-\ *n* : any of the three possible ways of reading a sequence of nucleotides as a series of triplets — see OPEN READING FRAME

re·ad·just \ˌrē-ə-ˈjəst\ *vi* : to become adjusted or undergo adjustment again — **re·ad·just·ment** \-ˈjəs(t)-mənt\ *n*

re·agent \rē-ˈā-jənt\ *n* **1** : a substance used (as in detecting or measuring a component, in preparing a product, or in developing photographs) because of its chemical or biological activity **2** : REACTOR 1b

re·ag·gre·gate \(ˈ)rē-ˈag-ri-ˌgāt\ *vb* **-gat·ed; -gat·ing** *vt* : to cause (as cells) to re-form into an aggregate or a whole ∼ *vi* : to re-form into an aggregate or a whole ⟨the cells *reaggregated* into organized tissue⟩ — **re·ag·gre·gate** \-gət\ *n* — **re·ag·gre·ga·tion** \(ˌ)rē-ˌag-ri-ˈgā-shən\ *n*

re·agin \rē-ˈā-jən, -gən\ *n* **1** : a substance that is in the blood of individuals with syphilis and is responsible for positive serological reactions for syphilis **2** : an antibody (as IgE in humans) that mediates hypersensitive allergic reactions of rapid onset — **re·agin·ic** \ˌrē-ə-ˈjin-ik, -ˈgin-\ *adj*

real focus \ˈrē(ə)l-\ *n* : a point at which rays (as of light) converge or from which they diverge

real image *n* : an optical image formed of real foci

re·al·i·ty principle \rē-ˈal-ət-ē-\ *n* : the tendency to defer immediate instinctual gratification so as to achieve longer-range goals or so as to meet external demands (as from the physical environment or from a group of psychologically significant individuals) — compare PLEASURE PRINCIPLE

reality testing *n* : the psychological process in which acts are explored and their outcomes determined so that the individual will be aware of these consequences when the stimulus to act in a given fashion recurs

ream·er \ˈrē-mər\ *n* : an instrument used in dentistry to enlarge and clean out a root canal

re·am·i·na·tion \(ˌ)rē-ˌam-ə-ˈnā-shən\ *n* : the restoration of an amino group to a compound from which it had previously been removed

re·am·pu·ta·tion \(ˌ)rē-ˌam-pyə-ˈtā-shən\ *n* : the second of two amputations performed upon the same member

re·anas·to·mo·sis \ˌrē-ə-ˌnas-tə-ˈmō-səs\ *n, pl* **-mo·ses** \-ˌsēz\ : the reuniting (as by surgery or healing) of a divided vessel

re·an·i·mate \(ˈ)rē-ˈan-ə-ˌmāt\ *vt* **-mat·ed; -mat·ing** : to restore to life : REVIVE — **re·an·i·ma·tion** \-ˌan-ə-ˈmā-shən\ *n*

re·as·so·ci·ate \ˌrē-ə-ˈsō-s(h)ē-ˌāt\ *vb* **-at·ed; -at·ing** *vt* : to bring (as strands of DNA) into association again ∼ *vi* : to become reassociated ⟨two single strands of DNA will ∼ to form a double strand —Gina B. Kolata⟩

re·as·so·ci·a·tion \ˌrē-ə-ˌsō-s(h)ē-ˈā-shən\ *n* : the act of reassociating or state of being reassociated ⟨DNA ∼⟩

re·at·tach \ˌrē-ə-ˈtach\ *vi* : to become attached anew ∼ *vt* : to attach again ⟨∼ a severed finger⟩ — **re·at·tach·ment** \-mənt\ *n*

Re·au·mur \ˌrā-ō-ˈmyu̇(ə)r\ *adj* : relating or conforming to a thermometric scale on which the boiling point of water is at 80° above the zero of the scale and the freezing point is at zero ⟨the ∼ thermometer⟩ — *abbr. R*

Ré·au·mur \rā-ō-mūͤr\, **René–Antoine Ferchault de (1683–1757),** French physicist and naturalist. Réaumur devised in 1730 a thermometer with a scale marking 0° as the freezing point and 80° as the boiling point of water. Interested in many areas of science, he isolated gastric juice in 1752 and investigated its role in the digestive process.

re·base \(ˈ)rē-ˈbās\ *vt* **re·based; re·bas·ing** : to modify the base of (a denture) after an initial period of wear in order to produce a good fit

re·bleed \ˈrē-ˌblēd\ *vi* **re·bled** \-ˌbled\; **re·bleed·ing 1** : bleed or hemorrhage again ⟨lesions that are likely to ∼ or need surgical intervention —Anne L. Davis *et al*⟩ ⟨repeat

Q

R

\ə\ **abut** \ᵊ\ **kitten** \ər\ **further** \a\ **ash** \ā\ **ace** \ä\ **cot, cart** \au̇\ **out** \ch\ **chin** \e\ **bet** \ē\ **easy** \g\ **go** \i\ **hit** \ī\ **ice** \j\ **job** \ŋ\ **sing** \ō\ **go** \ȯ\ **law** \ȯi\ **boy** \th\ **thin** \th̲\ **the** \ü\ **loot** \u̇\ **foot** \y\ **yet** \zh\ **vision** *See also* Pronunciation Symbols page

embolization may be successful in patients who ∼ —Michelle L. Wong *et al*〉 **2** *of a hemorrhage* : to occur again 〈intracorneal hemorrhages, like hyphemas, can ∼ —K. H. Baratz *et al*〉 — **rebleed** *n*

re·bound \'rē-₁baůnd, ri-'\ *n* : a spontaneous reaction; *esp* : a return to a previous state or condition following removal of a stimulus or cessation of treatment 〈withdrawal of antihypertensive medication may lead to a ∼ hypertensive crisis —*Emergency Medicine*〉

rebound tenderness *n* : a sensation of pain felt when pressure (as to the abdomen) is suddenly removed

re·breathe \(')rē-'brēth\ *vb* **re·breathed; re·breath·ing** *vt* : to breathe (as reconstituted air) again ∼ *vi* : to inhale previously exhaled air or gases

re·cal·ci·fi·ca·tion \₁rē-₁kal-sə-fə-'kā-shən\ *n* : the restoration of calcium or calcium compounds to decalcified tissue (as bone or blood)

recalcification time *n* : a measure of the time taken for clot formation in recalcified blood

re·cal·ci·fied \(')rē-'kal-sə-₁fīd\ *adj* : having undergone recalcification 〈∼ human plasma〉

re·cal·ci·trant \ri-'kal-sə-trənt\ *adj* : not responsive to treatment 〈severe ∼ psoriasis〉 〈∼ warts〉

re·call \ri-'kȯl, 'rē-₁\ *n* : remembrance of what has been previously learned or experienced — **re·call** \ri-'kȯl\ *vt*

recall dose *n* : BOOSTER SHOT

re·can·a·li·za·tion *also Brit* **re·can·a·li·sa·tion** \(₁)rē-₁kan-ᵊl-ə-'zā-shən\ *n* : the process of restoring flow to or reuniting an interrupted channel of a bodily tube (as an artery or the vas deferens) 〈∼ of an acutely occluded vessel —Nanette Hock〉 — **re·can·a·lize** *also Brit* **re·can·a·lise** \-kə-'nal-₁īz, -'kan-ᵊl-₁īz\ *vt* **-lized** *also Brit* **-lised; -liz·ing** *also Brit* **-lis·ing**

re·ca·pit·u·la·tion \₁rē-kə-₁pich-ə-'lā-shən\ *n* : the supposed repetition in the development of the individual of its phylogenetic history — see RECAPITULATION THEORY

recapitulation theory *n* : BIOGENETIC LAW

re·cep·tive \ri-'sep-tiv\ *adj* **1** : open and responsive to ideas, impressions, or suggestions **2 a** *of a sensory end organ* : fit to receive and transmit stimuli **b** : SENSORY 1 — **re·cep·tive·ness** *n* — **re·cep·tiv·i·ty** \₁rē-₁sep-'tiv-ət-ē, ri-\ *n, pl* **-ties**

receptive aphasia *n* : SENSORY APHASIA

re·cep·tor \ri-'sep-tər\ *n* **1** : a cell or group of cells that receives stimuli : SENSE ORGAN **2** : a chemical group or molecule (as a protein) on the cell surface or in the cell interior that has an affinity for a specific chemical group, molecule, or virus **3** : a cellular entity (as a beta-receptor or alpha-receptor) that is a postulated intermediary between a chemical agent (as a neurohormone) acting on nervous tissue and the physiological or pharmacological response

receptor potential *n* : GENERATOR POTENTIAL

re·cer·ti·fi·ca·tion \(₁)rē-₁sərt-ə-fə-'kā-shən\ *n* : the act of having one's certification renewed — **re·cer·ti·fy** \(')rē-'sərt-ə-₁fī\ *vb* **-fied; -fy·ing**

re·cess \'rē-₁ses, ri-'\ *n* : an anatomical depression or cleft : FOSSA

re·ces·sion \ri-'sesh-ən\ *n* : pathological withdrawal of tissue from its normal position 〈advanced gum ∼〉

¹**re·ces·sive** \ri-'ses-iv\ *adj* **1** : producing little or no phenotypic effect when occurring in heterozygous condition with a contrasting allele 〈∼ genes〉 **2** : expressed only when the determining gene is in the homozygous condition 〈∼ traits〉 — **re·ces·sive·ly** *adv* — **re·ces·sive·ness** *n*

²**recessive** *n* **1** : a recessive character or gene **2** : an organism possessing one or more recessive characters

re·ces·sus \ri-'ses-əs\ *n* : RECESS

re·chal·lenge \(')rē-'chal-ənj\ *n* : a physiological or immunological challenge made subsequent to a previous challenge — **rechallenge** *vt* **-lenged; -leng·ing**

re·cid·i·va·tion \ri-₁sid-ə-'vā-shən\ *n* : RECIDIVISM — **re·cid·i·vate** \ri-'sid-ə-₁vāt\ *vi* **-vat·ed; -vat·ing**

re·cid·i·vism \ri-'sid-ə-₁viz-əm\ *n* : a tendency to relapse into a previous condition or mode of behavior 〈high ∼ rates after cessation of smoking —A. E. Kazdin *et al*〉

re·cid·i·vist \-vəst\ *n* : one who relapses into a previous be-

havior or condition; *esp* : a habitual criminal — **recidivist** *adj* — **re·cid·i·vis·tic** \-₁sid-ə-'vis-tik\ *adj*

rec·i·pe \'res-ə-(₁)pē\ *n* : PRESCRIPTION 1

re·cip·i·ent \ri-'sip-ē-ənt\ *n* : an individual who receives biological material (as blood or an organ) from a donor

re·cip·ro·cal \ri-'sip-rə-kəl\ *adj* **1** : inversely related **2** : of, constituting, or resulting from paired crosses in which the kind that supplies the male parent of the first cross supplies the female parent of the second cross and vice versa **3** : shared, felt, or shown by both sides

reciprocal inhibition *n* **1** : RECIPROCAL INNERVATION **2** : behavior modification in which the patient is exposed to anxiety-producing stimuli while in a controlled state of relaxation so that the anxiety response is gradually inhibited

reciprocal innervation *n* : innervation so that the contraction of a muscle or set of muscles (as of a joint) is accompanied by the simultaneous inhibition of an antagonistic muscle or set of muscles

reciprocal translocation *n* : exchange of parts between nonhomologous chromosomes — called also *segmental interchange*

Reck·ling·hau·sen's disease \'rek-liŋ-₁haů-zənz-\ *n* : NEUROFIBROMATOSIS

Recklinghausen, Friedrich Daniel von (1833–1910), German pathologist. A professor of pathology at the universities of Königsberg, Würzburg, and Strasbourg, Recklinghausen is best known for his descriptions of two disorders: neurofibromatosis, sometimes called Recklinghausen's disease, in 1882; and osteitis fibrosa in 1891. He also rendered classic descriptions of the smallest lymph channels in connective tissue (1862) and of calculi found in the pancreas in cases of diabetes (1864).

rec·og·ni·tion \₁rek-əg-'nish-ən\ *n* : the form of memory that consists in knowing or feeling that a present object has been met before

¹**re·com·bi·nant** \(')rē-'käm-bə-nənt\ *adj* **1** : relating to or exhibiting genetic recombination 〈∼ progeny〉 **2 a** : relating to or containing genetically engineered DNA **b** : produced by genetic engineering 〈∼ bovine growth hormone〉

²**recombinant** *n* : an individual exhibiting recombination

recombinant DNA *n* : genetically engineered DNA usu. incorporating DNA from more than one species of organism

re·com·bi·na·tion \₁rē-₁käm-bə-'nā-shən\ *n* : the formation by the processes of crossing-over and independent assortment of new combinations of genes in progeny that did not occur in the parents — **re·com·bi·na·tion·al** \-shnəl, -shən-ᵊl\ *adj*

re·com·bine \₁rē-kəm-'bīn\ *vb* **-bined; -bin·ing** *vi* : to undergo recombination ∼ *vt* : to cause to undergo recombination

rec·om·mend·ed dai·ly al·low·ance \₁rek-ə-₁mend-əd-₁dā-lē-ə-'laů-ən(t)s\ *n, often cap R&D&A* : the amount of a nutrient (as a vitamin or mineral) that is recommended for daily consumption by the National Research Council of the U.S. National Science Foundation — *abbr.* RDA

recommended dietary allowance *n, often cap R&D&A* : RECOMMENDED DAILY ALLOWANCE — *abbr.* RDA

re·com·pres·sion \₁rē-kəm-'presh-ən\ *n* : a renewed heightening of atmospheric pressure esp. as treatment for decompression sickness

re·con·di·tion \₁rē-kən-'dish-ən\ *vt* **1** : to restore to good condition and esp. to good physical and mental condition 〈∼ an athlete after severe knee injuries〉 **2** : to condition anew; *also* : to reinstate (a response) in an organism 〈∼ an emotional response〉 — **re·con·di·tion·ing** *n*

re·con·sti·tute \(')rē-'kän(t)-stə-₁t(y)üt\ *vt* **-tut·ed; -tut·ing** : to constitute again or anew; *esp* : to restore to a former condition by adding liquid 〈*reconstituted* blood plasma〉

re·con·sti·tu·tion \(₁)rē-₁kän(t)-stə-'t(y)ü-shən\ *n* **1** : the action of reconstituting or state of being reconstituted **2** : regeneration of an organic form by reorganization of existent tissue without blastema formation

re·con·struct \₁rē-kən-'strəkt\ *vt* : to subject (an organ or part) to surgery so as to re-form the structure of or to correct a defect

re·con·struc·tion \ˌrē-kən-ˈstrək-shən\ n : repair of an organ or part by reconstructive surgery ⟨breast ∼⟩

re·con·struc·tive \-tiv\ adj : of, relating to, or being reconstructive surgery ⟨∼ measures⟩

reconstructive surgery n : surgery to restore function or normal appearance by remaking defective organs or parts

re·cov·er \ri-ˈkəv-ər\ vi **re·cov·ered; re·cov·er·ing** \-(ə-)riŋ\ : to regain a normal position or condition (as of health) ⟨∼ing from the effects of a cold⟩

re·cov·er·able \ri-ˈkəv-(ə-)rə-bəl\ adj : permitting recovery : not precluding a return to health ⟨a ∼ disease⟩

re·cov·ered \ri-ˈkəv-ərd\ adj : no longer sick ⟨∼ patients⟩

recovered memory n : a forgotten memory of a traumatic event (as sexual abuse) experienced typically during childhood and recalled many years later that is sometimes held to be an invalid or false remembrance generated by outside influence

re·cov·ery \ri-ˈkəv-(ə-)rē\ n, pl **-er·ies** : the act of regaining or returning toward a normal or healthy state

recovery room n : a hospital room which is equipped with apparatus for meeting postoperative emergencies and in which surgical patients are kept during the immediate postoperative period for care and recovery from anesthesia — abbr. *RR*

rec·re·a·tion·al drug \ˌrek-rē-ˈā-sh(ə-)nəl-\ n : a drug (as cocaine, marijuana, or methamphetamine) used without medical justification for its psychoactive effects often in the belief that occasional use of such a substance is not habit-forming or addictive

recreational therapy n : therapy based on engagement in recreational activities (as sports or music) esp. to enhance the functioning, independence, and well-being of individuals affected with a disabling condition — **recreational therapist** n

re·cru·desce \ˌrē-krü-ˈdes\ vi **-desced; -desc·ing** : to break out or become active again ⟨the epidemic *recrudesced* after a period of quiescence⟩

re·cru·des·cence \ˌrē-krü-ˈdes-ᵊn(t)s\ n : increased severity of a disease after a remission; *also* : recurrence of a disease after a brief intermission — compare RELAPSE

re·cru·des·cent \-ˈdes-ᵊnt\ adj : breaking out again : renewing disease after abatement, suppression, or cessation ⟨a ∼ typhus⟩

re·cruit \ri-ˈkrüt\ vt : to restore or increase the health, vigor, or intensity of

re·cruit·ment \ri-ˈkrüt-mənt\ n **1** : the increase in intensity of a reflex when the initiating stimulus is prolonged without alteration of intensity due to the activation of increasing numbers of motor neurons — compare REINFORCEMENT **2** : an abnormally rapid increase in the sensation of loudness with increasing sound intensity that occurs in deafness of neural origin and esp. in neural deafness of the aged in which soft sounds may be completely inaudible while louder sounds are distressingly loud

re·crys·tal·lize also Brit **re·crys·tal·lise** \(ˈ)rē-ˈkris-tə-ˌlīz\ vb **-lized** also Brit **-lised; -liz·ing** also Brit **-lis·ing** : to crystallize again or repeatedly — **re·crys·tal·li·za·tion** also Brit **re·crys·tal·li·sa·tion** \(ˌ)rē-ˌkris-tə-lə-ˈzā-shən\ n

recta pl of RECTUM

recta — see VASA RECTA

rec·tal \ˈrek-tᵊl\ adj : relating to, affecting, or being near the rectum ⟨∼ bleeding⟩ — **rec·tal·ly** \-ē\ adv

rectal artery n : any of three arteries supplying esp. the rectum: **a** : one arising from the internal pudendal artery and supplying the lower part of the rectum and the perineal region — called also *inferior hemorrhoidal artery, inferior rectal artery* **b** : one arising from the internal iliac artery and supplying the middle part of the rectum — called also *middle hemorrhoidal artery, middle rectal artery* **c** : one that is a continuation of the inferior mesenteric artery and that supplies the upper part of the rectum — called also *superior hemorrhoidal artery, superior rectal artery*

rectal plexus n : RECTAL VENOUS PLEXUS

rectal valve n : any of three or four crescentic folds projecting into the cavity of the rectum

rectal vein n : any of three veins that receive blood from the rectal venous plexus: **a** : one draining the lower part of the rectal venous plexus and emptying into the internal pudendal vein — called also *inferior hemorrhoidal vein, inferior rectal vein* **b** : one draining the bladder, prostate, and seminal vesicle by way of the middle part of the rectal venous plexus and emptying into the internal iliac vein — called also *middle hemorrhoidal vein, middle rectal vein* **c** : one draining the upper part of the rectal venous plexus and forming the first part of the inferior mesenteric vein — called also *superior hemorrhoidal vein, superior rectal vein*

rectal venous plexus n : a plexus of veins that surrounds the rectum and empties esp. into the rectal veins — called also *rectal plexus*

recti pl of RECTUS

rec·ti·fi·ca·tion \ˌrek-tə-fə-ˈkā-shən\ n **1** : the conversion of alternating to direct current **2** : a process by which distilled spirits are blended together or substantially changed by the addition usu. of spirits, flavoring, or coloring material

rec·ti·fy \ˈrek-tə-ˌfī\ vt **-fied; -fy·ing** **1** : to purify (as alcohol) esp. by repeated or fractional distillation **2** : to make (an alternating current) unidirectional

rec·to·cele \ˈrek-tə-ˌsēl\ n : herniation of the rectum through a defect in the intervening fascia into the vagina

rec·to·coc·cyg·e·us \ˌrek-tō-käk-ˈsij-ē-əs\ n, pl **-ei** \-ē-ˌī\ : a band of smooth muscle extending from the coccyx to the posterior wall of the rectum and serving to retract and elevate the rectum

rec·to·co·li·tis \ˌrek-tō-kō-ˈlīt-əs\ n : inflammation of the rectum and colon

rec·to·scope \ˈrek-tə-ˌskōp\ n : PROCTOSCOPE

rec·to·sig·moid \ˌrek-tō-ˈsig-ˌmȯid\ n : the distal part of the sigmoid colon and the proximal part of the rectum

rec·to·sig·moid·o·scope \-sig-ˈmȯid-ə-ˌskōp\ n : SIGMOIDOSCOPE — **rec·to·sig·moid·o·scop·ic** \-ˌmȯid-ə-ˈskäp-ik\ adj — **rec·to·sig·moid·os·co·py** \-ˌmȯi-ˈdäs-kə-pē\ n, pl **-pies**

rec·to·ure·thral \ˌrek-tō-yu̇-ˈrē-thrəl\ adj : of, relating to, or joining the rectum and the urethra ⟨closure of a ∼ fistula⟩

rec·to·uter·ine pouch \ˌrek-tō-ˈyüt-ə-ˌrīn-, -rən-\ n : a sac between the rectum and the uterus that is formed by a folding of the peritoneum — compare RECTOVESICAL POUCH

rec·to·vag·i·nal \-ˈvaj-ən-ᵊl\ adj : of, relating to, or connecting the rectum and the vagina ⟨a ∼ fistula⟩ ⟨the ∼ septum⟩

rec·to·ves·i·cal fascia \ˌrek-tō-ˈves-i-kəl-\ n : a membrane derived from the pelvic fascia and investing the rectum, bladder, and adjacent parts

rectovesical pouch n : a sac between the rectum and the urinary bladder in males that is formed by a folding of the peritoneum — compare RECTOUTERINE POUCH

rec·tum \ˈrek-təm\ n, pl **rectums** or **rec·ta** \-tə\ : the terminal part of the intestine from the sigmoid colon to the anus

rec·tus \ˈrek-təs\ n, pl **rec·ti** \-ˌtī\ **1** : any of several straight muscles (as the rectus abdominis or the rectus femoris) **2** : any of four muscles of the eyeball that arise from the border of the optic foramen and run forward to insert into the sclera of the eyeball: **a** : one that is the thinnest and narrowest and inserts into the superior aspect of the sclera — called also *rectus superior, superior rectus* **b** : one that is the longest, arises by two heads, and inserts into the lateral aspect of the sclera — called also *lateral rectus, rectus lateralis* **c** : one that is the broadest and inserts into the medial aspect of the sclera — called also *medial rectus, rectus medialis* **d** : one that inserts into the inferior aspect of the sclera — called also *inferior rectus, rectus inferior*

rectus ab·dom·i·nis \-ab-ˈdäm-ə-nəs\ n : a long flat muscle on either side of the linea alba extending along the whole length of the front of the abdomen, arising from the pubic

---

\ə\ abut \ᵊ\ kitten \ər\ further \a\ ash \ā\ ace \ä\ cot, cart
\au̇\ out \ch\ chin \e\ bet \ē\ easy \g\ go \i\ hit \ī\ ice \j\ job
\ŋ\ sing \ō\ go \ȯ\ law \ȯi\ boy \th\ thin \t͟h\ the \ü\ loot
\u̇\ foot \y\ yet \zh\ vision *See also* Pronunciation Symbols page

Q
R

crest and symphysis, inserted into the cartilages of the fifth, sixth, and seventh ribs, and acting to flex the spinal column, tense the anterior wall of the abdomen, and assist in compressing the contents of the abdomen

rec·tus cap·i·tis posterior major \-ˈkap-ə-təs-\ *n* : a muscle on each side of the back of the neck that arises from the spinous process of the axis, inserts into the lateral aspect of the inferior nuchal line and the adjacent inferior area of the occipital bone, and acts to extend and rotate the head

rectus capitis posterior minor *n* : a muscle on each side of the back of the neck that arises from the posterior arch of the atlas, inserts esp. into the medial aspect of the inferior nuchal line, and acts to extend the head

rectus fem·o·ris \-ˈfem-ə-rəs\ *n* : a division of the quadriceps muscle lying in the anterior middle region of the thigh, arising from the ilium by two heads, inserted into the tuberosity of the tibia by a narrow flattened tendon, and acting to flex the thigh at the hip and with the rest of the quadriceps to extend the leg at the knee

rectus inferior *n* : RECTUS 2d

rectus lat·e·ra·lis \-ˌlat-ə-ˈrā-ləs, -ˈral-əs\ *n* : RECTUS 2b

rectus me·di·a·lis \-ˌmē-dē-ˈā-ləs, -ˈal-əs\ *n* : RECTUS 2c

rectus oc·u·li \-ˈäk-yə-ˌlī\ *n* : RECTUS 2

rectus superior *n* : RECTUS 2a

re·cum·ben·cy \ri-ˈkəm-bən-sē\ *n, pl* **-cies** : the state of leaning, resting, or reclining; *also* : a recumbent position ⟨dyspnea . . . relieved with ∼ —Elizabeth Dean⟩

re·cum·bent \-bənt\ *adj* : lying down ⟨a patient ∼ on a stretcher⟩

re·cu·per·ate \ri-ˈk(y)ü-pə-ˌrāt\ *vb* **-at·ed; -at·ing** *vt* : to get back or recover ⟨*recuperating* health and strength after pneumonia⟩ ∼ *vi* : to recover health or strength ⟨time to ∼ after major surgery⟩

re·cu·per·a·tion \rē-ˌk(y)ü-pə-ˈrā-shən\ *n* : restoration to health or strength

re·cu·per·a·tive \-ˈk(y)ü-pə-ˌrāt-iv\ *adj* **1** : of or relating to recuperation ⟨∼ powers⟩ **2** : aiding in recuperation : RESTORATIVE ⟨strongly ∼ remedies⟩

re·cur \ri-ˈkər\ *vi* **re·curred; re·cur·ring** : to occur again after an interval ⟨a disease likely to ∼⟩

re·cur·rence \ri-ˈkər-ən(t)s, -ˈkə-rən(t)s\ *n* **1** : return of symptoms of a disease after a remission **2** : reappearance of a tumor after previous removal

re·cur·rent \-ˈkər-ənt, -ˈkə-rənt\ *adj* **1** : running or turning back in a direction opposite to a former course — used of various nerves and branches of vessels in the arms and legs **2** : returning or happening time after time ⟨∼ pain⟩ — **re·cur·rent·ly** *adv*

recurrent fever *n* : RELAPSING FEVER

recurrent laryngeal nerve *n* : LARYNGEAL NERVE b — called also *recurrent laryngeal*

recurrent nerve *n* : LARYNGEAL NERVE b

¹**red** \ˈred\ *adj* **red·der; red·dest** : of the color red

²**red** *n* **1** : a color whose hue resembles that of blood or of the ruby or is that of the long-wave extreme of the visible spectrum **2** : a pigment or dye that colors red — see CONGO RED, NEUTRAL RED, VITAL RED

red alga *n* : any of a division (Rhodophyta) of chiefly marine algae that have predominantly red pigmentation

red bark *n* : a reddish bark that contains quinine and is obtained from a cinchona tree (*Cinchona succirubra*) and its hybrids — called also *red cinchona*

red·bird cac·tus \ˈred-ˌbərd-ˈkak-təs\ *n* : a tropical American spurge of the genus *Pedilanthus* (*P. tithymaloides*) that causes severe poisoning if any part of the plant is eaten

red–blind *adj* : affected with protanopia

red blindness *n* : PROTANOPIA

red blood cell *n* : any of the hemoglobin-containing cells that carry oxygen to the tissues and are responsible for the red color of vertebrate blood — called also *erythrocyte, red blood corpuscle, red cell, red corpuscle;* compare WHITE BLOOD CELL

red blood count *n* : a blood count of the red blood cells — abbr. *RBC*

red bone marrow *n* : BONE MARROW b

red bug \-ˌbəg\ *n, Southern & Midland* : CHIGGER 2

red cell *n* : RED BLOOD CELL

red cinchona *n* : RED BARK; *also* : the cinchona (*Cinchona succirubra*) that yields red bark

red corpuscle *n* : RED BLOOD CELL

Red Cross *n* : a red Greek cross on a white ground adopted by the Geneva convention of 1864 as the emblem to identify noncombat installations, vehicles, and personnel ministering to the sick and wounded in war and now used as the emblem of the International Red Cross and its affiliates not only in war but in disaster relief and other humanitarian services

red dev·ils \-ˈdev-əlz\ *n pl, slang* : REDS

red–green color blindness *n* : deficiency of color vision ranging from imperfect perception of red and green to an ability to see only tones of yellow, blue, and gray — called also *red-green blindness*

re·dia \ˈrēd-ē-ə\ *n, pl* **re·di·ae** \-ē-ˌē\ *also* **re·di·as** : a larva produced within the sporocyst of many trematodes that produces another generation of larvae like itself or develops into a cercaria — **re·di·al** \-ē-əl\ *adj*

red·in·te·gra·tion \ri-ˌdint-ə-ˈgrā-shən, re-\ *n* **1** : revival of the whole of a previous mental state when a phase of it recurs **2** : arousal of any response by a part of the complex of stimuli that orig. aroused that response — **red·in·te·gra·tive** \-ˈdint-ə-ˌgrāt-iv\ *adj*

re·dis·solve \ˌrē-diz-ˈälv, -ˈolv\ *vb* **-solved; -solv·ing** *vt* : to cause to dissolve again ∼ *vi* : to dissolve again

red marrow *n* : BONE MARROW b

red nucleus *n* : a nucleus of gray matter in the tegmentum of the midbrain on each side of the middle line that receives fibers from the cerebellum of the opposite side by way of the superior cerebellar peduncle and gives rise to fibers of the rubrospinal tract of the opposite side

red·out \ˈred-ˌaut\ *n* : a condition in which centripetal acceleration (as that created when an aircraft abruptly enters a dive) drives blood to the head and causes reddening of the visual field and headache — compare BLACKOUT, GRAYOUT

red out *vi* : to experience a redout — compare BLACK OUT, GRAY OUT

¹**re·dox** \ˈrē-ˌdäks\ *adj* : of or relating to oxidation-reduction

²**redox** *n* : OXIDATION-REDUCTION

redox potential *n* : OXIDATION-REDUCTION POTENTIAL

red pulp *n* : a parenchymatous tissue of the spleen that consists of loose plates or cords infiltrated with red blood cells — compare WHITE PULP

re·drape \(ˈ)rē-ˈdrāp\ *vt* **re·draped; re·drap·ing** **1** : to pull (skin) tight during plastic surgery **2** : to drape again with surgical drapes

reds *n pl, slang* : red drug capsules containing the sodium salt of secobarbital — called also *red devils*

red squill *n* **1** : a Mediterranean squill of the genus *Urginea* (*U. maritima*) of the form with a reddish brown bulb — compare WHITE SQUILL **2** : a rat poison derived from the bulb of red squill

red tide *n* : seawater discolored by the presence of large numbers of dinoflagellates esp. of the genera *Gonyaulax* and *Gymnodinium* which produce a toxin poisonous esp. to many forms of marine vertebrate life and to humans who consume contaminated shellfish — see PARALYTIC SHELLFISH POISONING; compare SAXITOXIN

re·duce \ri-ˈd(y)üs\ *vb* **re·duced; re·duc·ing** *vt* **1** : to correct (as a fracture or a herniated mass) by bringing displaced or broken parts back into their normal positions **2 a** : to bring to the metallic state by removal of nonmetallic elements ⟨∼ an ore by heat⟩ **b** : DEOXIDIZE **c** : to combine with or subject to the action of hydrogen **d** (1) : to change (an element or ion) from a higher to a lower oxidation state (2) : to add one or more electrons to (an atom or ion or molecule) ∼ *vi* **1** : to become diminished or lessened; *esp* : to lose weight by dieting **2** : to become reduced ⟨ferrous iron ∼s to ferric iron⟩ **3** : to undergo meiosis

re·duc·ible \ri-ˈd(y)üs-ə-bəl\ *adj* : capable of being reduced

⟨a ∼ hernia⟩ — **re·duc·i·bil·i·ty** \ri-ˌd(y)üs-ə-ˈbil-ət-ē\ *n, pl* **-ties**

reducing *adj* : causing or facilitating reduction

reducing agent *n* : a substance that reduces; *esp* : a substance (as hydrogen, sodium, or hydroquinone) that donates electrons or a share in its electrons to another substance — called also *reductant;* compare OXIDIZING AGENT

reducing sugar *n* : a sugar (as glucose, maltose, or lactose) that is capable of reducing a mild oxidizing agent (as Fehling solution) — see BENEDICT'S TEST; compare NONREDUCING

re·duc·tant \ri-ˈdək-tənt\ *n* : REDUCING AGENT

re·duc·tase \-ˌtās, -ˌtāz\ *n* : an enzyme that catalyzes chemical reduction

re·duc·tion \ri-ˈdək-shən\ *n* **1** : the replacement or realignment of a body part in normal position or restoration of a bodily condition to normal **2** : the process of reducing by chemical or electrochemical means **3** : the psychological diminishment of emotion or needs through activity or adjustment **4** : MEIOSIS; *specif* : production of the gametic chromosome number in the first meiotic division

reduction division *n* : the usu. first division of meiosis in which chromosome reduction occurs; *also* : MEIOSIS

re·duc·tion·ism \ri-ˈdək-shə-ˌniz-əm\ *n* **1** : the attempt to explain all biological processes by the same explanations (as by physical laws) that chemists and physicists use to interpret inanimate matter; *also* : the theory that complete reductionism is possible **2** : a procedure or theory that reduces complex data or phenomena to simple terms — **re·duc·tion·ist** \-sh(ə-)nəst\ *or* **re·duc·tion·is·tic** \-ˌdək-shə-ˈnis-tik\ *adj*

re·duc·tive \ri-ˈdək-tiv\ *adj* : of, relating to, causing, or involving reduction

re·dun·dant \ri-ˈdən-dənt\ *adj* : characterized by or containing an excess or superfluous amount ⟨∼ pharyngeal tissue⟩

re·du·pli·cate \ri-ˈd(y)ü-pli-ˌkāt, ˈrē-\ *vi* **-cat·ed; -cat·ing** : to undergo reduplication ⟨chromosomes ∼⟩

re·du·pli·ca·tion \ri-ˌd(y)ü-pli-ˈkā-shən, ˌrē-\ *n* : an act or instance of doubling ⟨∼ of the chromosomes⟩

re·du·vi·id \ri-ˈd(y)ü-vē-əd\ *n* : any bug of the family Reduviidae — **reduviid** *adj*

Red·u·vi·idae \ˌrej-ə-ˈvī-ə-ˌdē\ *n pl* : a very large and widely distributed family of bloodsucking hemipterous insects comprising the assassin bugs, having a short 3-jointed proboscis that is curved back under the head when at rest, and including vectors of Chagas' disease belonging to the genera *Rhodnius* and *Triatoma*

Re·du·vi·us \ri-ˈd(y)ü-vē-əs\ *n* : the type genus of the family Reduviidae that includes an assassin bug (*R. personatus*) capable of inflicting a painful bite

red water *n* : any of several cattle diseases characterized by hematuria; *esp* : any of several babesioses (as Texas fever) in which hemoglobin liberated by the destruction of red blood cells appears in the urine

red worm *n* : BLOODWORM

Reed–Stern·berg cell \ˈrēd-ˈstərn-bərg-\ *n* : a binucleate or multinucleate acidophilic giant cell found in the tissues in Hodgkin's disease — called also *Sternberg cell, Sternberg=Reed cell*

    Reed, Dorothy (1874–1964), American pathologist. Reed published an article on Hodgkin's disease in 1902. In an analysis of the histological picture she described the proliferation of the endothelial and reticular cells and the formation of the giant binucleate or multinucleate cells. Because these cells had been described by Sternberg independently four years earlier, they are now known as Reed-Sternberg cells.
    Stern·berg \ˈshtern-berk\, **Carl (1872–1935),** Austrian pathologist. Sternberg described the giant binucleate or multinucleate cells found in the lymph nodes in Hodgkin's disease in 1898. He was the first to differentiate Hodgkin's disease and aleukemic leukemia. He also wrote classic descriptions of lymphogranulomatosis (1905) and leukosarcoma (1915).

re·ed·u·cate \(ˈ)rē-ˈej-ə-ˌkāt\ *vt* **-cat·ed; -cat·ing** : to subject to reeducation

re·ed·u·ca·tion \-ˌej-ə-ˈkā-shən\ *n* **1** : training in the use of muscles in new functions or of prosthetic devices in old functions in order to replace or restore lost functions ⟨∼ of the bowel of the chronically constipated patient —C. H. Thienes⟩ ⟨neuromuscular ∼⟩ **2** : training to develop new behaviors (as attitudes or habits) to replace others that are considered undesirable

reef·er \ˈrē-fər\ *n* : a marijuana cigarette; *also* : MARIJUANA 2

re·en·try \(ˈ)rē-ˈen-trē\ *n, pl* **-tries** : a cardiac mechanism that is held to explain certain abnormal heart actions (as tachycardia) and that involves the transmission of a wave of depolarization along an alternate pathway when the original pathway is blocked with return of the impulse along the blocked pathway when the alternate pathway is refractory and then transmission along the open pathway resulting in an abnormality

re·ep·i·the·li·al·iza·tion \(ˈ)rē-ˌep-ə-ˌthē-lē-ə-lə-ˈzā-shən\ *n* : restoration of epithelium over a denuded area (as a burn site) by natural growth or plastic surgery

re–ex·plo·ra·tion \-ˌek-splə-ˈrā-shən\ *n* : a second exploration ⟨intestinal obstruction in which ∼ was done because of persistent ileus —L. R. King & W. W. Scott⟩

re·fec·tion \ri-ˈfek-shən\ *n* **1** : satisfaction of hunger and thirst **2 a** : the eating of feces esp. by the animal producing them **b** : spontaneous recovery of vitamin-depleted animals on a high starch diet presumably resulting from consumption of feces enriched with vitamins synthesized by intestinal bacteria

re·fer \ri-ˈfər\ *vt* **re·ferred; re·fer·ring** **1** : to regard as coming from or localized in a certain portion of the body or of space ⟨pain of appendicitis may be *referred* to any region of the abdomen —*Encyc. Americana*⟩ **2** : to send or direct for diagnosis or treatment ⟨∼ a patient to a specialist⟩

re·fer·able *also* **re·fer·rable** \ˈref-(ə-)rə-bəl, ri-ˈfər-ə-\ *adj* : capable of being considered as being related to or caused by something else ⟨symptoms ∼ to the primary tumor —M. A. Beckles *et al*⟩

ref·er·ence \ˈref-(ə-)rən(t)s\ *adj* : of known potency and used as a standard in the biological assay of a sample of the same drug of unknown strength ⟨a dose of ∼ cod-liver oil⟩

reference — see IDEA OF REFERENCE

re·fer·ral \ri-ˈfər-əl\ *n* **1** : the process of directing or redirecting (as a medical case or a patient) to an appropriate specialist or agency for definitive treatment **2** : an individual that is referred

referred pain *n* : a pain subjectively localized in one region though due to irritation in another region

¹re·fill \(ˈ)rē-ˈfil\ *vt* : to fill (a prescription) a second or subsequent time

²re·fill \ˈrē-ˌfil\ *n* **1** : a replacement in a cavity of removed liquid or other material or a substitution (as of gas) for such material ⟨pneumothorax ∼⟩ **2** : a prescription compounded and dispensed for a second or subsequent time without an order from the physician

re·fill·able \(ˈ)rē-ˈfil-ə-bəl\ *adj* : capable of being refilled ⟨a ∼ prescription⟩

re·fine \ri-ˈfin\ *vt* **re·fined; re·fin·ing** : to free (as sugar or oil) from impurities or unwanted material

re·flect \ri-ˈflekt\ *vt* **1** : to bend or fold back : impart a backward curve, bend, or fold to **2** : to push or lay aside (as tissue or an organ) during surgery in order to gain access to the part to be operated on ⟨the pleura were ∼ed and later closed over the stump⟩ ∼ *vi* : to throw back light or sound : return rays, beams, or waves

re·flec·tance \ri-ˈflek-tən(t)s\ *n* : the fraction of the total radiant flux incident upon a surface that is reflected and that varies according to the wavelength distribution of the incident radiation — called also *reflection coefficient, reflection factor*

\ə\ abut \ᵊ\ kitten \ər\ further \a\ ash \ā\ ace \ä\ cot, cart
\aú\ out \ch\ chin \e\ bet \ē\ easy \g\ go \i\ hit \ī\ ice \j\ job
\ŋ\ sing \ō\ go \ò\ law \òi\ boy \th\ thin \ṯh\ the \ü\ loot
\ù\ foot \y\ yet \zh\ vision *See also* Pronunciation Symbols page

Q

R

reflecting microscope *n* : a microscope in which the image is formed by mirrors instead of lenses

re·flec·tion *also Brit* **re·flex·ion** \ri-ˈflek-shən\ *n* **1** : an instance of reflecting; *esp* : the return of light or sound waves from a surface **2** : the production of an image by or as if by a mirror **3 a** : the action of bending or folding back **b** : a reflected part or a fold ⟨the mesentery is a ∼ of the peritoneum⟩ **4** : something produced by reflecting; *esp* : an image given back by a reflecting surface

reflection coefficient *n* : REFLECTANCE

reflection factor *n* : REFLECTANCE

re·flec·tive \ri-ˈflek-tiv\ *adj* **1** : capable of reflecting light, images, or sound waves **2** : of, relating to, or caused by reflection ⟨∼ glare of the snow⟩

re·flec·tor \ri-ˈflek-tər\ *n* : one that reflects; *esp* : a polished surface for reflecting light or other radiation

¹re·flex \ˈrē-ˌfleks\ *n* **1 a** : reflected heat, light, or color **b** : a mirrored image **2 a** : an automatic and often inborn response to a stimulus that involves a nerve impulse passing inward from a receptor to the spinal cord and thence outward to an effector (as a muscle or gland) without reaching the level of consciousness and often without passing to the brain ⟨the knee-jerk ∼⟩ **b** : the process that culminates in a reflex and comprises reception, transmission, and reaction **c** **reflexes** *pl* : the power of acting or responding with adequate speed

²reflex *adj* **1** : bent, turned, or directed back : REFLECTED **2** : of, relating to, or produced by a reflex without intervention of consciousness

reflexa — see DECIDUA REFLEXA

reflex arc *n* : the complete nervous path that is involved in a reflex

re·flex·ion *Brit var of* REFLECTION

re·flex·ive \ri-ˈflek-siv\ *adj* : characterized by habitual and unthinking behavior; *also* : relating to or consisting of a reflex

re·flex·ly *adv* : in a reflex manner : by means of reflexes ⟨∼ induced contractions⟩ ⟨∼ contracting the iris⟩

re·flexo·gen·ic \ri-ˌflek-sə-ˈjen-ik\ *or* **re·flex·og·e·nous** \ˌrē-ˌflek-ˈsäj-ə-nəs\ *adj* **1** : causing or being the point of origin of reflexes ⟨a ∼ zone⟩ **2** : originating reflexly ⟨∼ components of respiration⟩ ⟨a ∼ erection⟩

re·flex·ol·o·gist \ˌrē-ˌflek-ˈsäl-ə-jəst\ *n* **1** : an individual who interprets behavior as consisting of reflexes **2** : a practitioner of manipulative reflexology

re·flex·ol·o·gy \ˌrē-ˌflek-ˈsäl-ə-jē\ *n, pl* **-gies** **1** : the study and interpretation of behavior in terms of simple and complex reflexes **2** : massage of the feet or hands based on the belief that pressure applied to specific points on these extremities benefits other parts of the body

reflex sympathetic dystrophy *n* : a painful disorder that usu. follows a localized injury, that is marked by burning pain, swelling, and motor and sensory disturbances esp. of an extremity, and that is associated with sympathetic nervous system dysfunction — abbr. *RSD*; see SHOULDER-HAND SYNDROME

¹re·flux \ˈrē-ˌfləks\ *n* **1 a** : a flowing back : REGURGITATION ⟨∼ of gastric acid⟩ ⟨mitral valve ∼⟩ **b** : GASTROESOPHAGEAL REFLUX **2** : a process of refluxing or condition of being refluxed ⟨the sample was hydrolyzed . . . under ∼ for 24 hours —T. Y. Ho *et al*⟩

²reflux *adj* : of, relating to, involving, or caused by reflux ⟨∼ esophagitis⟩

³reflux *vt* : to cause to flow back or return; *esp* : to heat (as under a reflux condenser) so that the vapors formed condense to a liquid that flows back to be heated again ∼ *vi* : to flow back ⟨damage to the esophageal mucous membrane when gastric acid *refluxed* into the esophagus⟩

reflux condenser *n* : a condenser usu. placed upright so that the condensed vapors flow back into the distilling flask and continued boiling of easily volatile substances is possible with little loss from evaporation

re·fo·cus \(ˈ)rē-ˈfō-kəs\ *vt* : to focus again ∼ *vi* : to focus something again

re·fract \ri-ˈfrakt\ *vt* **1** : to subject (as a ray of light) to refraction **2** : to determine the refracting power of or abnormality of refraction in (as an eye or a lens)

re·frac·tile \ri-ˈfrak-tᵊl, -ˌtīl\ *adj* : capable of refracting : REFRACTIVE ⟨∼ crystalline material in the retina⟩

re·frac·tion \ri-ˈfrak-shən\ *n* **1** : the deflection from a straight path undergone by a light ray or a wave of energy in passing obliquely from one medium (as air) into another (as water or glass) in which its velocity is different **2 a** : the refractive power of the eye **b** : the act or technique of determining ocular refraction and identifying abnormalities as a basis for the prescription of corrective lenses

re·frac·tion·ist \-shə-nəst\ *n* : a person (as an optometrist) skilled in the practical application of the laws of refraction esp. to the determination of errors of refraction in the eye

re·frac·tive \ri-ˈfrak-tiv\ *adj* **1** : having power to refract ⟨a ∼ lens⟩ **2** : relating to or due to refraction ⟨∼ phenomena⟩ ⟨∼ dispersion of light⟩ — **re·frac·tive·ly** *adv*

refractive index *n* : INDEX OF REFRACTION

re·frac·tiv·i·ty \ˌrē-ˌfrak-ˈtiv-ət-ē, ri-\ *n, pl* **-ties** : the ability of a substance to refract light expressed quantitatively; *specif* : the index of refraction minus one

re·frac·tom·e·ter \ˌrē-ˌfrak-ˈtäm-ət-ər, ri-\ *n* : an instrument for measuring indices of refraction

re·frac·tom·e·try \-ˈtäm-ə-trē\ *n, pl* **-tries** : the art or process of measuring indices of refraction : the use of the refractometer — **re·frac·to·met·ric** \ri-ˌfrak-tə-ˈme-trik\ *adj*

re·frac·to·ri·ness \ri-ˈfrak-t(ə-)rē-nəs\ *n* : the insensitivity to further immediate stimulation that develops in irritable and esp. nervous tissue as a result of intense or prolonged stimulation

re·frac·to·ry \ri-ˈfrak-t(ə-)rē\ *adj* **1** : resistant to treatment or cure ⟨a ∼ fulminant lesion⟩ ⟨had disease that was extremely ∼ to multiple intensive therapies —Michelle L. Bennett *et al*⟩ **2** : unresponsive to stimulus ⟨the ∼ period of a muscle fiber⟩ **3** : resistant or not responding to an infectious agent : IMMUNE ⟨∼ to reinfection⟩

refractory period *n* : the brief period immediately following the response esp. of a muscle or nerve before it recovers the capacity to make a second response — called also *refractory phase*; see ABSOLUTE REFRACTORY PERIOD, RELATIVE REFRACTORY PERIOD

re·frac·ture \(ˈ)rē-ˈfrak-chər\ *vi* **-tured; -tur·ing** : to break along the line of a previous fracture ⟨excessive stress caused the femur to ∼⟩ — **refracture** *n*

re·fran·gi·bil·i·ty \ri-ˌfran-jə-ˈbil-ət-ē\ *n, pl* **-ties** : the property of being able to be refracted

¹re·frig·er·ant \ri-ˈfrij-(ə-)rənt\ *adj* : allaying heat or fever

²refrigerant *n* : a medicine or an application for allaying fever or its symptoms

re·frig·er·a·tion \ri-ˌfrij-ə-ˈrā-shən\ *n* : a deliberate lowering of the temperature of the body or of a part (as a leg) for therapeutic purposes or to facilitate surgery

re·frin·gent \ri-ˈfrin-jənt\ *adj* : REFRACTIVE

Ref·sum's disease \ˈref-səmz-\ *n* : an autosomal recessive lipidosis characterized by faulty metabolism of phytanic acid resulting in its accumulation in the blood, retinitis pigmentosa, ataxia, deafness, and mental retardation

Ref·sum \ˈref-sùm\, **Sigvald Bernhard (1907–1991)**, Norwegian physician. Refsum served as a professor of neurology and as a specialist in neurology and psychiatry at a succession of Norwegian hospitals. In addition to identifying Refsum's disease, he did research on the genetic aspects of neurology.

re·gen·er·ate \ri-ˈjen-ə-ˌrāt\ *vb* **-at·ed; -at·ing** *vi* **1** : to become formed again **2** : to undergo regeneration ⟨the human bladder and liver can ∼ when injured⟩ ∼ *vt* **1** : to generate or produce anew; *esp* : to replace (a body part) by a new growth of tissue **2** : to produce again chemically sometimes in a physically changed form — **re·gen·er·a·ble** \-ˈjen-(ə-)rə-bəl\ *adj*

re·gen·er·a·tion \ri-ˌjen-ə-ˈrā-shən, ˌrē-\ *n* **1** : an act or the process of regenerating : the state of being regenerated **2** : the renewal, regrowth, or restoration of a body or a bodily part, tissue, or substance after injury or as a normal bodily process ⟨continual ~ of epithelial cells⟩ ⟨~ of the uterine lining⟩ — compare REGULATION 2a

re·gen·er·a·tive \ri-'jen-ə-ˌrāt-iv, -'jen-(ə-)rət-\ *adj* 1 : of, relating to, or marked by regeneration 2 : tending to regenerate

regia — see AQUA REGIA

re·gime \rā-'zhēm, ri- *also* ri-'jēm\ *n* : REGIMEN

reg·i·men \'rej-ə-mən *also* 'rezh-ə-\ *n* : a systematic plan (as of diet, therapy, or medication) esp. when designed to improve and maintain the health of a patient

re·gion \'rē-jən\ *n* 1 : any of the major subdivisions into which the body or one of its parts is divisible ⟨the nine ~s of the abdomen⟩ 2 : an indefinite area surrounding a specified body part ⟨a pain in the ~ of the heart⟩

re·gion·al \'rēj-ən-ᵊl, -nəl\ *adj* : of, relating to, or affecting a particular bodily region ⟨anesthesia by means of a ~ block⟩ — **re·gion·al·ly** \-ē\ *adv*

regional anatomy *n* : a branch of anatomy dealing with regions of the body esp. with reference to diagnosis and treatment of disease or injury — called also *topographic anatomy*

regional anesthesia *n* : anesthesia of a region of the body accomplished by a series of encircling injections of an anesthetic — compare BLOCK ANESTHESIA

regional enteritis *n* : CROHN'S DISEASE

regional ileitis *n* : CROHN'S DISEASE

re·gio·se·lec·tive \ˌrē-jē-ō-sə-'lek-tiv\ *adj* : REGIOSPECIFIC — **re·gio·se·lec·tive·ly** *adv*

re·gio·se·lec·tiv·i·ty \-sə-ˌlek-'tiv-ət-ē, -ˌsē-\ *n, pl* **-ties** : the property of a chemical reaction of producing one structural isomer in preference to others that are theoretically possible

re·gio·spe·cif·ic \-spi-'sif-ik\ *adj* : being a chemical reaction in which one structural isomer is produced exclusively when other isomers are also theoretically possible — **re·gio·spe·cif·i·cal·ly** \-i-k(ə-)lē\ *adv*

re·gio·spec·i·fic·i·ty \-ˌspes-ə-'fis-ə-tē\ *n, pl* **-ties** : the state or condition of being regiospecific

reg·is·tered \'rej-ə-stərd\ *adj* : qualified by formal, official, or legal certification or authentication ⟨a ~ pharmacist⟩

registered nurse *n* : a graduate trained nurse who has been licensed by a state authority after passing qualifying examinations for registration — called also *RN*

reg·is·trar \'rej-ə-ˌsträr\ *n* 1 : an admitting officer at a hospital 2 *Brit* : RESIDENT

reg·is·try \'rej-ə-strē\ *n, pl* **-tries** 1 : a place where data, records, or laboratory samples are kept and usu. are made available for research or comparative study ⟨a cancer ~⟩ 2 : an establishment at which nurses available for employment are listed and through which they are hired

Reg·i·tine \'rej-ə-ˌtēn\ *n* : a preparation of the mesylate of phentolamine — formerly a U.S. registered trademark

re·gress \ri-'gres\ *vi* : to undergo or exhibit regression ⟨a ~ing lesion⟩ ~ *vt* : to induce a state of psychological regression in ⟨~ a hypnotized subject⟩

re·gres·sion \ri-'gresh-ən\ *n* : a trend or shift toward a lower, less severe, or less perfect state: as **a** : progressive decline (as in size or severity) of a manifestation of disease ⟨tumor ~ following radiation⟩ **b** (1) : a gradual loss of differentiation and function by a body part esp. as a physiological change accompanying aging ⟨menopausal ~ of the ovaries⟩ (2) : gradual loss (as in old age) of memories and acquired skills **c** : reversion to an earlier mental or behavioral level or to an earlier stage of psychosexual development in response to organismic stress or to suggestion ⟨a protective ~ towards childhood —Havelock Ellis⟩

re·gres·sive \ri-'gres-iv\ *adj* : relating to, resulting from, producing, or characterized by regression ⟨~ behavior⟩ ⟨~ tissue changes⟩

re·grow \(')rē-'grō\ *vi* **re·grew** \-'grü\; **re·grown** \-'grōn\; **re·grow·ing** : to continue growth after interruption or injury

re·growth \-'grōth\ *n* : an act or instance of regrowing ⟨~ of hair⟩ ⟨tumor ~⟩

reg·u·lar \'reg-yə-lər\ *adj* 1 : having or constituting an isometric system ⟨~ crystals⟩ 2 : conforming to what is usual

or normal: as **a** : recurring or functioning at fixed or normal intervals ⟨~ bowel movements⟩ **b** : having menstrual periods or bowel movements at normal intervals — **reg·u·lar·ly** *adv*

reg·u·lar·i·ty \ˌreg-yə-'lar-ət-ē\ *n, pl* **-ties** : the quality or state of being regular ⟨maintain bowel ~⟩

reg·u·late \'reg-yə-ˌlāt\ *vt* **-lat·ed; -lat·ing** 1 : to control or direct according to rule or law ⟨~ the testing of experimental drugs⟩ 2 : to fix or adjust the time, amount, degree, or rate of — **reg·u·la·to·ry** \-lə-ˌtōr-ē, -ˌtòr-\ *adj*

reg·u·la·tion \ˌreg-yə-'lā-shən, ˌreg-ə-'lā-\ *n* 1 : the act of regulating; *also* : the resulting state or condition 2 **a** : the process of redistributing material (as in an embryo) to restore a damaged or lost part independent of new tissue growth — compare REGENERATION 2 **b** : the mechanism by which an early embryo maintains normal development 3 : the control of the kind and rate of cellular processes by controlling the activity of individual genes

reg·u·la·tive \'reg-yə-ˌlāt-iv, -lət-əv\ *adj* 1 : tending to regulate : having regulation as an aim 2 : INDETERMINATE

reg·u·la·tor \'reg-yə-ˌlāt-ər\ *n* 1 : one that regulates 2 : REGULATORY GENE

regulatory gene *or* **regulator gene** *n* : a gene that regulates the expression of one or more structural genes by controlling the production of a protein (as a genetic repressor) which regulates their rate of transcription

re·gur·gi·tant \(')rē-'gər-jə-tənt\ *adj* : characterized by, allowing, or being a backward flow (as of blood) ⟨~ cardiac valves⟩

re·gur·gi·tate \(')rē-'gər-jə-ˌtāt\ *vb* **-tat·ed; -tat·ing** *vi* : to become thrown or poured back ~ *vt* : to throw or pour back or out from or as if from a cavity ⟨~ swallowed food into the mouth⟩

re·gur·gi·ta·tion \(ˌ)rē-ˌgər-jə-'tā-shən\ *n* : an act of regurgitating; *esp* : the backward flow of blood through a defective heart valve — see AORTIC REGURGITATION

re·hab \'rē-ˌhab\ *n, often attrib* : REHABILITATION; *esp* : a program for rehabilitating esp. drug or alcohol abusers

re·ha·bil·i·tant \ˌrē-(h)ə-'bil-ə-tənt\ *n* : an individual undergoing rehabilitation

re·ha·bil·i·tate \ˌrē-(h)ə-'bil-ə-ˌtāt\ *vt* **-tat·ed; -tat·ing** : to restore or bring to a condition of health or useful and constructive activity ⟨~ patients with hip fractures⟩

re·ha·bil·i·ta·tion \ˌrē-(h)ə-ˌbil-ə-'tā-shən\ *n, often attrib* 1 : the action or process of rehabilitating or of being rehabilitated: as **a** : the physical restoration of a sick or disabled person by therapeutic measures and reeducation to participation in the activities of a normal life within the limitations of the person's physical disability ⟨~ after coronary occlusion⟩ **b** : the process of restoring an individual to a useful and constructive place in society esp. through some form of vocational, correctional, or therapeutic retraining 2 : the result of rehabilitating : the state of being rehabilitated ⟨~ of the patient⟩

re·ha·bil·i·ta·tive \-'bil-ə-ˌtāt-iv\ *adj* : of, relating to, or designed to accomplish rehabilitation ⟨~ treatment⟩

re·ha·bil·i·ta·tor \ˌrē-(h)ə-'bil-ə-ˌtāt-ər\ *n* : a person who is engaged in rehabilitating others

re·ha·bil·i·tee \ˌrē-(h)ə-ˌbil-ə-'tē\ *n* : one who is in the process of being rehabilitated

re·hears·al \ri-'hər-səl\ *n* 1 : a method for improving memory by mentally or verbally repeating over and over the information to be remembered 2 : the repeated mental review of a desired action or behavioral response ⟨preoperative ~ of coping imagery to reduce anxiety⟩

Reh·fuss tube \'rā-fəs-\ *n* : a flexible tube that is used esp. for withdrawing gastric juice from the stomach for analysis and that has a syringe at the upper end and an attachment with a slot at the end passing into the stomach

---

\ə\ **abut** \ᵊ\ **kitten** \ər\ **further** \a\ **ash** \ā\ **ace** \ä\ **cot, cart** \aú\ **out** \ch\ **chin** \e\ **bet** \ē\ **easy** \g\ **go** \i\ **hit** \ī\ **ice** \j\ **job** \ŋ\ **sing** \ō\ **go** \ò\ **law** \òi\ **boy** \th\ **thin** \th̷\ **the** \ü\ **loot** \ú\ **foot** \y\ **yet** \zh\ **vision** *See also* Pronunciation Symbols page

Rehfuss, Martin Emil (1887–1964), American physician. Rehfuss specialized in gastroenterology, and especially in the diagnosis and treatment of diseases of the stomach. Indigestion and practical therapeutics were two topics of particular interest. In 1914 he devised a method of removing portions of a standard test meal from the stomach at certain intervals by using a flexible tube.

re·hy·drate \('rē-'hī-‚drāt\ vt **-drat·ed; -drat·ing** : to restore fluid to (something dehydrated); esp : to restore body fluid lost in dehydration to ⟨~ a patient⟩ — **re·hy·dra·tion** \‚rē-‚hī-'drā-shən\ n

Rei·chert–Meissl num·ber \'rī-kərt-'mī-səl-‚nəm-bər\ n : a Reichert value expressed as the milliliters of tenth-normal alkali required to neutralize the acids obtained from five grams of fat by a specified method of saponification and distillation — called also *Reichert-Meissl value*

Rei·chert \'rī-kərt\, **Emil (1838–1894),** German food scientist. In 1879 Reichert introduced a method for determining the proportion of volatile water-soluble fatty acids present in butter, fats, and oils.

Meissl, Emerich (fl 1879–1882), German chemist. Meissl is known to have written an article on the testing of yeast.

Reichert value n : a value that indicates the content in fat (as butter) of water-soluble volatile fatty acids (as butyric acid or caproic acid); esp : REICHERT-MEISSL NUMBER

Rei·ki \'rā-‚kē\ n : a system of hands-on touching based on the belief that such touching by an experienced practitioner produces beneficial effects by strengthening and normalizing certain vital energy fields held to exist within the body

re·im·plan·ta·tion \‚rē-‚im-‚plan-'tā-shən\ n **1** : the restoration of a bodily tissue or part (as a tooth) to the site from which it was removed **2** : the implantation of a fertilized egg in the uterus after it has been removed from the body and fertilized in vitro — **re·im·plant** \-im-'plant\ vt

rei·nec·kate \'rī-nə-‚kāt\ n : a salt of Reinecke acid

Rei·necke \'rī-nə-kə\, **A. (fl 1863–1867),** German chemist.

Rei·nec·ke acid \'rī-nə-kē-\ n : the monobasic acid HCr(NH₃)₂(SCN)₄ of which Reinecke salt is the ammonium salt

Reinecke salt n : a red crystalline powder NH₄[Cr(NH₃)₂(SCN)₄]·H₂O that is used as a reagent and a precipitant (as for primary and secondary amines)

re·in·farc·tion \‚rē-in-'färk-shən\ n : an infarction occurring subsequent to a previous infarction

re·in·fec·tion \‚rē-in-'fek-shən\ n : infection following recovery from or superimposed on a previous infection of the same type ⟨rescreening aimed at detecting ~ following treatment —Diana Mahoney⟩ — **re·in·fect** \-'fekt\ vt

re·in·force \‚rē-ən-'fō(ə)rs, -'fȯ(ə)rs\ vt **-forced; -forc·ing 1** : to strengthen by additional material or support : make stronger ⟨reinforced with vitamins⟩ **2** : to stimulate (as an experimental animal or a student) by reinforcement; also : to encourage (a response) by reinforcement — **re·in·force·able** \-ə-bəl\ adj

re·in·force·ment \‚rē-ən-'fōr-smənt, -'fȯr-\ n : the action of causing a subject (as a student or an experimental animal) to learn to give or to increase the frequency of a desired response that in classical conditioning involves the repeated presentation of an unconditioned stimulus (as the sight of food) paired with a conditioned stimulus (as the sound of a bell) and that in operant conditioning involves the use of a reward following a correct response or a punishment following an incorrect response; also : the reward, punishment, or unconditioned stimulus used in reinforcement — compare RECRUITMENT 1

re·in·forc·er \-'fōr-sər, -'fȯr-\ n : a stimulus (as a reward or removal of an electric shock) that increases the probability of a desired response in operant conditioning by being applied or removed following the desired response

re·in·fuse \‚rē-in-'fyüz\ vt **-fused; -fus·ing** : to return (as blood or lymphocytes) to the body by infusion after having been previously withdrawn — **re·in·fu·sion** \-'fyü-zhən\ n

re·in·jec·tion \‚rē-in-'jek-shən\ n : an injection made subsequent to a previous injection — **re·in·ject** \-'jekt\ vt

re·in·ner·va·tion \‚rē-‚in-(‚)ər-'vā-shən, -in-‚ər-\ n : restoration of function esp. to a denervated muscle by supplying it with nerves by regrowth or by grafting — **re·in·ner·vate** \-in-'ər-‚vāt, -'in-(‚)ər-\ vt **-vat·ed; -vat·ing**

re·in·oc·u·la·tion \‚rē-in-‚äk-yə-'lā-shən\ n : inoculation a second or subsequent time with the same organism as the original inoculation — **re·in·oc·u·late** \-'äk-yə-‚lāt\ vt **-lat·ed; -lat·ing**

Reinsch test \'rīnsh-\ n : a test for the presence esp. of arsenic, antimony, and mercury in which a strip of clean pure copper foil is heated with the test material in acid solution and then if a black or gray stain appears on the foil, it is heated in a test tube to produce a sublimate deposited in the upper part of the tube in a form characteristic of arsenic, antimony, or mercury if any of these are present

Reinsch, Adolf (1862–1916), German physician. Reinsch was a professor and director of chemical research for the city of Altona, which is now part of Hamburg. He was involved with the bacteriological and chemical testing of Altona's water supply.

re·in·te·gra·tion \‚rē-‚int-ə-'grā-shən\ n : repeated or renewed integration (as of the personality and mental activity after mental illness) — **re·in·te·grate** \-'int-ə-‚grāt\ vt **-grat·ed; -grat·ing** — **re·in·te·gra·tive** \-‚grāt-iv\ adj

Reiss·ner's membrane \'rīs-nərz-\ n : VESTIBULAR MEMBRANE

Reissner, Ernst (1824–1878), German anatomist. A professor of anatomy, Reissner described in 1851 the membrane of the scala media that is now also known as Reissner's membrane.

Rei·ter's syndrome \'rīt-ərz-\ n : a disease that is usu. initiated by infection in genetically predisposed individuals and is characterized usu. by recurrence of arthritis, conjunctivitis, and urethritis — called also *Reiter's disease*

Reiter, Hans Conrad Julius (1881–1969), German bacteriologist. Reiter had a career both as a professor of hygiene at several German universities and as a government public health official. While serving with the German forces during World War I, he discovered the causative organism of Weil's disease. During the war he treated his first patient suffering from a disease marked by urethritis, conjunctivitis, and arthritis. This disease is now known as Reiter's syndrome. He published reports of his field hospital discoveries in 1916. He identified, named, and investigated the spirochete of the genus *Treponema (T. pallidum)* that causes syphilis in humans, and his discovery of a specific antigen for it led to his development of a complement-fixation test for syphilis. He also described the entoptic symptoms of digitalis intoxication and wrote an important monograph on the use of vaccines.

re·ject \ri-'jekt\ vt **1** : to rebuff, repel, refuse to hear, or withhold love from; esp : to communicate negative feelings toward and a wish to be free of ⟨parents who ~ their children⟩ **2** : to subject to immunological rejection ⟨~ed a heart transplant⟩ — **re·jec·tive** \ri-'jek-tiv\ adj

re·jec·tion \ri-'jek-shən\ n **1** : the action of rejecting or the state of being rejected ⟨feelings of ~⟩ ⟨~ of the atypical child by the . . . group —G. S. Speer⟩ **2** : an immune response in which foreign tissue (as of a skin graft or transplanted organ) is attacked by immune system components (as antibodies, T cells, and macrophages) of the recipient organism

re·ju·ve·nate \ri-'jü-və-‚nāt\ vb **-nat·ed; -nat·ing** vt : to make young or youthful again; specif : to restore sexual vigor in (as by hormones or an operation) ~ vi : to cause or undergo a renewal of youthfulness — **re·ju·ve·na·tion** \ri-‚jü-və-'nā-shən, ‚rē-\ n — **re·ju·ve·na·tor** \ri-'jü-və-‚nāt-ər\ n

¹re·lapse \ri-'laps, 'rē-\ n : a recurrence of illness; esp : a recurrence of symptoms of a disease after a period of improvement ⟨a ~ after an 18-month remission —M. T. Fosburg et al⟩ — compare RECRUDESCENCE

²re·lapse \ri-'laps\ vi **re·lapsed; re·laps·ing** : to slip or fall back into a former worse state (as of illness) after a change for the better ⟨the patient *relapsed* twice in four years⟩

relapsing febrile nodular non·sup·pu·ra·tive panniculi·tis \-ˌnän-ˈsəp-yə-rət-iv-, -ˌrāt-\ *n* : PANNICULITIS 2

relapsing fever *n* : any of several forms of an acute epidemic infectious disease marked by sudden recurring paroxysms of high fever lasting from five to seven days, articular and muscular pains, and a sudden crisis and caused by a spirochete of the genus *Borrelia* transmitted by the bites of lice and ticks and found in the circulating blood — see MIANEH FEVER

relapsing polychondritis *n* : a connective tissue disease esp. of cartilage that is characterized usu. by recurrent progressively destructive episodes of tissue inflammation (as of the ears, nose, larynx, trachea, eyes, joints, kidney, or heart) and that is inferred to have an autoimmune etiology from its frequent association with autoimmune diseases (as rheumatoid arthritis or systemic lupus erythematosus)

re·late \ri-ˈlāt\ *vi* **re·lat·ed; re·lat·ing** : to have meaningful social relationships : interact realistically ⟨an inability to ~ emotionally to others —Willow Lawson⟩

re·la·tion \ri-ˈlā-shən\ *n* **1** : an aspect or quality (as resemblance or causality) that connects two or more things or parts as being or belonging or working together, as being of the same kind, or as being logically connected ⟨the strong ~ between genotype and phenotype —Anne M. Glazier *et al*⟩ **2** : the attitude or stance which two or more persons or groups assume toward one another ⟨race ~s⟩ **3 a** : the state of being mutually or reciprocally interested (as in social matters) **b relations** *pl* : SEXUAL INTERCOURSE ⟨testified that ~s had occurred —*Newsweek*⟩ — **re·la·tion·al** \-əl\ *adj*

re·la·tion·ship \-shən-ˌship\ *n* **1** : the state of being related or interrelated ⟨research into the ~ between diet, blood, cholesterol levels, and coronary heart disease —*Current Biog.*⟩ **2 a** : a state of affairs existing between those having relations or dealings ⟨called on to assume the role of personal advisor in the doctor-patient ~ —*Jour. Amer. Med. Assoc.*⟩ **b** : an emotional attachment between individuals ⟨a meaningful ~⟩

rel·a·tive biological effectiveness \ˈrel-ət-iv-\ *n* : the relative capacity of a particular ionizing radiation to produce a response in a biological system — abbr. *RBE*

relative humidity *n* : the ratio of the amount of water vapor actually present in the air to the greatest amount possible at the same temperature — compare ABSOLUTE HUMIDITY

relative refractory period *n* : the period shortly after the firing of a nerve fiber when partial repolarization has occurred and a greater than normal stimulus can stimulate a second response — called also *relative refractory phase;* compare ABSOLUTE REFRACTORY PERIOD

re·lax \ri-ˈlaks\ *vt* **1** : to slacken or make less tense or rigid ⟨alternately contracting and ~ing their muscles⟩ **2** : to relieve from nervous tension **3** : to relieve from constipation ⟨medications to ~ the bowels⟩ ~ *vi* **1** *of a muscle or muscle fiber* : to return to an inactive or resting state; *esp* : to become inactive and lengthen **2** : to cast off social restraint, nervous tension, or anxiety ⟨couldn't ~ in crowds⟩

¹**re·lax·ant** \ri-ˈlak-sənt\ *adj* : of, relating to, or producing relaxation ⟨an anesthetic and ~ agent⟩

²**relaxant** *n* : a substance (as a drug) that relaxes; *specif* : one that relieves muscular tension

re·lax·ation \ˌrē-ˌlak-ˈsā-shən, ri-ˌlak-, *esp Brit* ˌrel-ək-\ *n* **1** : the act of relaxing or state of being relaxed ⟨maximal abdominal ~ was not evident until at least five minutes after the injection —*Lancet*⟩ **2** : the reduction of contractile force in a muscle or muscle fiber; *esp* : the lengthening that typically characterizes inactive muscles or muscle fibers

re·lax·in \ri-ˈlak-sən\ *n* : a polypeptide sex hormone of the corpus luteum that facilitates birth by causing relaxation of the pelvic ligaments

re·learn \ˈrē-ˈlərn\ *vt* : to learn again (what has been forgotten) — **re·learn·ing** *n*

re·leas·er \ri-ˈlē-sər\ *n* : a stimulus that serves as the initiator of complex reflex behavior

re·leas·ing factor \ri-ˈlēs-iŋ-\ *n* : HYPOTHALAMIC RELEASING FACTOR

re·li·abil·i·ty \ri-ˌlī-ə-ˈbil-ət-ē\ *n, pl* **-ties** : the extent to which an experiment, test, or measuring procedure yields the same results on repeated trials

re·li·able \ri-ˈlī-ə-bəl\ *adj* : giving the same result on successive trials ⟨a ~ psychological test⟩

re·lief \ri-ˈlēf\ *n* : removal or lightening of something oppressive or distressing ⟨~ of pain⟩ ⟨symptomatic ~⟩

re·lieve \ri-ˈlēv\ *vt* **re·lieved; re·liev·ing 1** : to bring about the removal or alleviation of (pain or discomfort) **2** : to discharge the bladder or bowels of (oneself) — **re·liev·er** *n*

rem \ˈrem\ *n* : the dosage of an ionizing radiation that will cause the same biological effect as one roentgen of X-ray or gamma-ray dosage — compare REP

REM \ˈrem\ *n* : RAPID EYE MOVEMENT

Re·mak's fiber \ˈrā-ˌmäks-\ *n* : an unmyelinated nerve fiber — called also *fiber of Remak*

Remak, Robert (1815–1865), German neurologist and embryologist. Remak published his first studies on the fine structure of nerve tissue in 1836 and published his dissertation on the subject two years later. He studied the function of the sympathetic nervous system, coming to the conclusion that the function of these nerves was concerned with all involuntary muscle movement, with secretion, and possibly with the skin. In 1843 and 1844 he demonstrated the presence of extremely thin fibrils in the axis cylinder, the central core of nerve fibers. As an embryologist Remak conducted research on chicken embryos. In 1842 he discovered the three germ layers of the embryo: the ectoderm, the mesoderm, and the endoderm.

re·me·di·a·ble \ri-ˈmēd-ē-ə-bəl\ *adj* : capable of being remedied ⟨~ speech defects⟩

re·me·di·al \ri-ˈmēd-ē-əl\ *adj* : affording a remedy : intended as a remedy ⟨~ surgery⟩ — **re·me·di·al·ly** \-ē\ *adv*

re·me·di·a·tion \ri-ˌmēd-ē-ˈā-shən\ *n* : the act or process of remedying ⟨~ of learning disabilities⟩

rem·e·dy \ˈrem-əd-ē\ *n, pl* **-dies** : a medicine, application, or treatment that relieves or cures a disease — **remedy** *vt* **-died; -dy·ing**

re·min·er·al·iza·tion *also Brit* **re·min·er·al·isa·tion** \ˌrē-ˌmin-(ə)-rə-lə-ˈzā-shən\ *n* : the restoring of minerals to demineralized structures or substances ⟨~ of bone⟩ — **re·min·er·al·ize** \(ˈ)rē-ˈmin-(ə)-rə-ˌlīz\ *vb* **-ized; -iz·ing**

re·mis·sion \ri-ˈmish-ən\ *n* : a state or period during which the symptoms of a disease are abated ⟨cancer in ~ after treatment⟩ — compare ARREST, CURE 1, INTERMISSION

re·mit \ri-ˈmit\ *vi* **re·mit·ted; re·mit·ting** : to abate symptoms for a period : go into or be in remission ⟨her leukemia *remitted* for a year⟩

re·mit·tent \ri-ˈmit-ᵊnt\ *adj* : marked by alternating periods of abatement and increase of symptoms ⟨~ fever⟩

REM latency *n* : the time span between the start of sleeping and the start of REM sleep

re·mod·el·ing \(ˌ)rē-ˈmäd-ᵊl-iŋ\ *n* : the process of bone resorption and formation that involves the activity of osteoclasts and osteoblasts ⟨osteoporosis results when the dynamic, constant process of bone ~ becomes unbalanced —Larry Deblinger⟩ — **re·mod·el** \-ˈmäd-ᵊl\ *vt*

REM sleep *n* : a state of sleep that recurs cyclically several times during a normal period of sleep and that is characterized by increased neuronal activity of the forebrain and midbrain, by depressed muscle tone, and esp. in humans by dreaming, rapid eye movements, and vascular congestion of the sex organs — called also *desynchronized sleep, paradoxical sleep, rapid eye movement sleep;* compare SLOW-WAVE SLEEP

re·nal \ˈrēn-ᵊl\ *adj* : relating to, involving, affecting, or located in the region of the kidneys : NEPHRIC ⟨~ function⟩

renal artery *n* : either of two branches of the abdominal aorta of which each supplies one of the kidneys, arises immedi-

\ə\ abut \ᵊ\ kitten \ər\ further \a\ ash \ā\ ace \ä\ cot, cart
\au̇\ out \ch\ chin \e\ bet \ē\ easy \g\ go \i\ hit \ī\ ice \j\ job
\ŋ\ sing \ō\ go \ȯ\ law \ȯi\ boy \th\ thin \t͟h\ the \ü\ loot
\u̇\ foot \y\ yet \zh\ vision *See also* Pronunciation Symbols page

Q
R

ately below the origin of the corresponding superior mesenteric artery, divides into four or five branches which enter the hilum of the kidney, and gives off smaller branches to the ureter, adrenal gland, and adjoining structures

renal calculus *n* : KIDNEY STONE

renal cast *n* : a cast of a renal tubule consisting of granular, hyaline, albuminoid, or other material formed in and discharged from the kidney in renal disease

renal clearance *n* : CLEARANCE

renal colic *n* : the severe pain produced by the passage of a calculus from the kidney through the ureter

renal column *n* : any of the masses of cortical tissue extending between the sides of the renal pyramids of the kidney as far as the renal pelvis — called also *Bertin's column, column of Bertin*

renal corpuscle *n* : the part of a nephron that consists of Bowman's capsule with its included glomerulus — called also *Malpighian body, Malpighian corpuscle*

renal diabetes *n* : RENAL GLYCOSURIA

renal glycosuria *n* : excretion of glucose associated with increased permeability of the kidneys without increased sugar concentration in the blood — called also *renal diabetes*

renal hypertension *n* : hypertension that is associated with disease of the kidneys and is caused by kidney damage or malfunctioning

renal osteodystrophy *n* : a painful rachitic condition of abnormal bone growth that is associated with chronic acidosis, hypocalcemia, hyperplasia of the parathyroid glands, and hyperphosphatemia caused by chronic renal insufficiency — called also *renal rickets*

renal papilla *n* : the apex of a renal pyramid which projects into the lumen of a calyx of the kidney and through which collecting tubules discharge urine

renal pelvis *n* : a funnel-shaped structure in each kidney that is formed at one end by the expanded upper portion of the ureter lying in the renal sinus and at the other end by the union of the calyxes of the kidney

renal plexus *n* : a plexus of the autonomic nervous system that arises esp. from the celiac plexus, surrounds the renal artery, and accompanies it into the kidney which it innervates

renal pyramid *n* : any of the conical masses that form the medullary substance of the kidney, project as the renal papillae into the renal pelvis, and are made up of bundles of straight uriniferous tubules opening at the apex of the conical mass — called also *Malpighian pyramid*

renal rickets *n* : RENAL OSTEODYSTROPHY

renal sinus *n* : the main cavity of the kidney that is an expansion behind the hilum and contains the renal pelvis, calyxes, and the major renal vessels

renal syndrome — see HEMORRHAGIC FEVER WITH RENAL SYNDROME

renal threshold *n* : the concentration level up to which a substance (as glucose) in the blood is prevented from passing through the kidneys into the urine

renal tubular acidosis *n* : decreased ability of the kidneys to excrete hydrogen ions that is associated with a defect in the renal tubules without a defect in the glomeruli and that results in the production of urine deficient in acidity

renal tubule *n* : the part of a nephron that leads away from a glomerulus, that is made up of a proximal convoluted tubule, loop of Henle, and distal convoluted tubule, and that empties into a collecting tubule

renal vein *n* : a short thick vein that is formed in each kidney by the convergence of the interlobar veins, leaves the kidney through the hilum, and empties into the inferior vena cava

re·na·tur·a·tion \ˌrē-ˌnā-chə-'rā-shən\ *n* : the process of renaturing ⟨denaturation and ∼ of proteins⟩

re·na·ture \(')rē-'nā-chər\ *vt* **-tured; -tur·ing** \-'nāch-(ə-)riŋ\ : to restore (as a denatured protein) to an original or normal condition

Ren·du–Os·ler–Web·er disease \ˌrän-ˌd(y)ü-'äs-lər-'web-ər-\ *n* : HEREDITARY HEMORRHAGIC TELANGIECTASIA

  Ren·du \rän-dūe\, **Henry–Jules–Louis–Marie** (1844–

1902), French physician. Rendu was the leading French clinician of his day. His major writings include monographs on dysfunctions of the heart and liver and on chronic nephritis. In 1888 he described a form of hysterical tremor that is precipitated or aggravated by volitional movements. Eight years later he published a report of a single case of hereditary hemorrhagic telangiectasia. Additional cases and information were supplied by Sir William Osler in 1901 and by Frederick Parkes Weber in 1907.

  Osler, Sir William (1849–1919), American physician. Osler was the greatest clinician and arguably the most famous and revered physician of his time. He held successive professorships in medicine at McGill University in Montreal, at the University of Pennsylvania in Philadelphia, and, most importantly, at Johns Hopkins University in Baltimore. During his 16 years there he became enormously skillful and celebrated as a teacher of medicine. He modeled the clinical and tutorial practice after European schools and did much to establish Hopkins as the premier medical school in the U.S. Osler did research on cardiovascular diseases and anatomy, blood platelets, typhoid fever, malaria, pneumonia, amebiasis, tuberculosis, and gallstones. In 1892 he published a text on the principles and practice of medicine that dominated the field for the next 30 years. The book is credited with inspiring the founding of the Rockefeller Institute for Medical Research and the Rockefeller Foundation. After his tenure at Hopkins he accepted a professorship at Oxford University. He was among the founders of the Royal Society of Medicine in 1907, and he was widely known as a medical historian.

  F. P. Weber — see WEBER-CHRISTIAN DISEASE

Ren·ese \'ren-ˌēz\ *trademark* — used for a preparation of polythiazide

re·ni·form \'rē-nə-ˌfȯrm, 'ren-ə-\ *adj* : suggesting a kidney in outline

re·nin \'rē-nən *also* 'ren-ən\ *n* : a proteolytic enzyme of the blood that is produced and secreted by the juxtaglomerular cells of the kidney and hydrolyzes angiotensinogen to angiotensin I

ren·net \'ren-ət\ *n* **1 a** : the contents of the stomach of an unweaned animal and esp. a calf   **b** : the lining membrane of a stomach or one of its compartments (as the fourth of a ruminant) used for curdling milk; *also* : a preparation of the stomach of animals used for this purpose   **2 a** : RENNIN   **b** : a substitute for rennin

ren·nin \'ren-ən\ *n* : a crystallizable enzyme that coagulates milk, that occurs esp. with pepsin in the gastric juice of young animals and is obtained as a yellowish powder, grains, or scales usu. by extraction of the mucous membrane of the fourth stomach of calves, and that is used chiefly in making cheese and casein for plastics — called also *chymosin*

re·no·gram \'rē-nə-ˌgram\ *n* : a photographic depiction of the course of renal excretion of a radiolabeled substance —

re·no·graph·ic \ˌrē-nə-'graf-ik\ *adj* — **re·nog·ra·phy** \rē-'näg-rə-fē\ *n, pl* **-phies**

re·no·pri·val \ˌrē-nō-'prī-vəl\ *adj* : of, relating to, resulting from, or characterized by the loss of the kidneys or of renal function ⟨∼ patients⟩ ⟨∼ hypertension⟩

re·no·re·nal reflex \ˌrē-nō-ˌrēn-ᵊl-\ *n* : pain or dysfunction in a healthy kidney occurring in association with disease or injury of the contralateral kidney

re·no·tro·pic \ˌrē-nə-'trō-pik, -'träp-ik\ *or* **re·no·tro·phic** \-'trō-fik\ *adj* : tending to induce enlargement of the kidney

re·no·vas·cu·lar \ˌrē-nō-'vas-kyə-lər\ *adj* : of, relating to, or involving the blood vessels of the kidneys ⟨∼ hypertension⟩

Ren·shaw cell \'ren-ˌshȯ-\ *n* : an inhibitory interneuron in the ventral horn of gray matter of the spinal cord that is held to be reciprocally innervated with a motor neuron so that nerve impulses received by way of processes of the motor neuron stimulate inhibitory impulses back to the motor neuron along an axon of the internuncial cell

  Renshaw, Birdsey (1911–1948), American neurologist. Renshaw is credited with investigating the nerve cells of the spinal cord that bear his name.

re·oc·clu·sion \ˌrē-ə-ˈklü-zhən\ n : the reoccurrence of occlusion in an artery after it has been treated (as by balloon angioplasty) with apparent success — **re·oc·clude** \-ə-ˈklüd\ vb **-clud·ed; -clud·ing**

re·op·er·a·tion \ˌrē-ˌäp-ə-ˈrā-shən\ n : an operation to correct a condition not corrected by a previous operation or to correct the complications of a previous operation — **re·op·er·ate** \-ˈäp-ə-ˌrāt\ vb **-at·ed; -at·ing**

Reo·Pro \ˈrē-ō-ˌprō\ trademark — used for a preparation of abciximab

Reo·vi·ri·dae \ˌrē-ō-ˈvir-ə-ˌdē\ n pl : a family of double-stranded RNA viruses that have a virion with icosahedral structural symmetry but may appear spherical, that have a capsid with one to three concentric protein layers, and that comprise many pathogens of plants and animals including the causative agents of bluetongue and Colorado tick fever — see ORBIVIRUS, ROTAVIRUS

reo·vi·rus \ˌrē-ō-ˈvī-rəs\ n : any of the family Reoviridae of double-stranded RNA viruses — **reo·vi·ral** \-rəl\ adj

rep \ˈrep\ n, pl **rep** or **reps** : the dosage of an ionizing radiation that will develop the same amount of energy upon absorption in human tissues as one roentgen of X-ray or gamma-ray exposure — compare REM

rep abbr [Latin repetatur] let it be repeated — used in writing prescriptions

¹re·pair \ri-ˈpa(ə)r, -ˈpe(ə)r\ vt : to restore to a sound or healthy state ⟨a surgical procedure to ~ damaged tissue⟩

²repair n **1 a** : the act or process of repairing ⟨surgical ~ of a detached retina⟩ **b** : an instance or result of repairing **2** : the replacement of destroyed cells or tissues by new formations

re·pand \ri-ˈpand\ adj : having a slightly undulating margin ⟨a ~ colony of bacteria⟩

re·par·a·tive \ri-ˈpar-ət-iv\ adj : of, relating to, or effecting repair ⟨~ dentistry⟩

re·peat \ri-ˈpēt, ˈrē-\ n : genetic duplication in which the duplicated parts are adjacent to each other along the chromosome

¹re·pel·lent also **re·pel·lant** \ri-ˈpel-ənt\ adj : serving or tending to drive away or ward off — often used in combination ⟨a mosquito-repellent spray⟩

²repellent also **repellant** n : something that repels; esp : a substance used to prevent insect attacks

re·per·fu·sion \ˌrē-pər-ˈfyü-zhən\ n : restoration of the flow of blood to a previously ischemic tissue or organ (as the heart or brain) ⟨~ following heart attack⟩ — **re·per·fuse** \-ˈfyüz\ vt **-fused; -fus·ing**

rep·e·ti·tion compulsion \ˌrep-ə-ˈtish-ən-\ n : an irresistible tendency to repeat an emotional experience or to return to a previous psychological state

re·pet·i·tive strain injury \ri-ˈpet-ət-iv-\ n : any of various musculoskeletal disorders (as carpal tunnel syndrome or tendinitis) that are caused by cumulative damage to muscles, tendons, ligaments, nerves, or joints (as of the hand, wrist, arm, or shoulder) from highly repetitive movements and that are characterized chiefly by pain, weakness, and loss of feeling — called also cumulative trauma disorder, repetitive motion injury, repetitive stress injury, repetitive stress syndrome, RSI

re·place·ment therapy \ri-ˈplā-smənt-\ n : therapy involving the supplying of something (as nutrients or blood) lacking from or lost to the system — see ESTROGEN REPLACEMENT THERAPY, HORMONE REPLACEMENT THERAPY

re·plant \(ˈ)rē-ˈplant\ vt : to subject to replantation ⟨~ an avulsed tooth⟩

re·plan·ta·tion \ˌrē-(ˌ)plan-ˈtā-shən\ n : reattachment or reinsertion of a bodily part (as a limb or tooth) after separation from the body

re·ple·tion \ri-ˈplē-shən\ n : the act or process of replenishing or state of being replenished following depletion (as of a constituent of the blood) ⟨sodium ~⟩

rep·li·ca·ble \ˈrep-li-kə-bəl\ adj : capable of replication ⟨~ experimental results⟩

rep·li·case \ˈrep-li-ˌkās, -ˌkāz\ n : a polymerase that pro-

motes synthesis of a particular RNA in the presence of a template of RNA — called also RNA replicase, RNA synthetase

¹rep·li·cate \ˈrep-lə-ˌkāt\ vb **-cat·ed; -cat·ing** vt : to repeat or duplicate (as an experiment) ~ vi : to undergo replication : produce a replica of itself ⟨virus particles replicating in cells⟩

²rep·li·cate \-li-kət\ n **1** : one of several identical experiments, procedures, or samples **2** : something (as a gene, DNA, or a cell) produced by replication

rep·li·ca·tion \ˌrep-lə-ˈkā-shən\ n **1** : the action or process of reproducing or duplicating ⟨~ of DNA⟩ **2** : performance of an experiment or procedure more than once

rep·li·ca·tive \ˈrep-li-ˌkāt-iv\ adj : of, relating to, involved in, or characterized by replication ⟨conversion of single stranded . . . DNA to a double stranded ~ form —Nature⟩

rep·li·con \ˈrep-li-ˌkän\ n : a linear or circular section of DNA or RNA which replicates sequentially as a unit

re·po·lar·iza·tion also Brit **re·po·lar·isa·tion** \ˌrē-ˌpō-lə-rə-ˈzā-shən\ n : restoration of the difference in charge between the inside and outside of the plasma membrane of a muscle fiber or cell following depolarization — **re·po·lar·ize** also Brit **re·po·lar·ise** \(ˈ)rē-ˈpō-lə-ˌrīz\ vb **-ized** also Brit **-ised; -iz·ing** also Brit **-is·ing**

re·port·able \ri-ˈpōrt-ə-bəl, -ˈpȯrt-\ adj : required by law to be reported ⟨~ diseases⟩

re·port·er gene \ri-ˈpōrt-ər-, -ˈpȯrt-\ n : a gene often of prokaryotic origin that produces a product easily detected in eukaryotic cells and that is used as a marker to determine the activity of another gene with which its DNA has been closely linked or combined — called also reporter

re·po·si·tion \ˌrē-pə-ˈzish-ən\ vt : to return to or place in a normal or proper position ⟨~ a dislocated shoulder⟩

re·pos·i·to·ry \ri-ˈpäz-ə-ˌtōr-ē\ adj, of a drug : designed to act over a prolonged period ⟨~ penicillin⟩

re·pre·cip·i·tate \ˌrē-pri-ˈsip-ə-ˌtāt\ vb **-tat·ed; -tat·ing** : to precipitate again

re·press \ri-ˈpres\ vt **1** : to exclude from consciousness ⟨~ conflicts⟩ **2** : to inactivate (a gene or formation of a gene product) by allosteric combination at a DNA binding site

re·pressed \ri-ˈprest\ adj : subjected to or marked by repression ⟨a ~ child⟩ ⟨~ anger⟩

re·press·ible \ri-ˈpres-ə-bəl\ adj : capable of being repressed ⟨~ enzymes controlled by their end products⟩ — **re·press·ibil·i·ty** \-ˌpres-ə-ˈbil-ət-ē\ n, pl **-ties**

re·pres·sion \ri-ˈpresh-ən\ n **1** : the action or process of repressing ⟨gene ~⟩ **2 a** : a process by which unacceptable desires or impulses are excluded from consciousness and left to operate in the unconscious — compare SUPPRESSION c **b** : an item so excluded

re·pres·sive \ri-ˈpres-iv\ adj : tending to repress or to cause repression ⟨~ psychological defenses⟩

re·pres·sor \ri-ˈpres-ər\ n : one that represses; esp : a protein that is determined by a regulatory gene, binds to a genetic operator, and inhibits the initiation of transcription of messenger RNA

re·pro·duce \ˌrē-prə-ˈd(y)üs\ vb **-duced; -duc·ing** vt **1** : to produce (new individuals of the same kind) by a sexual or asexual process **2** : to achieve (an original result or score) again or anew by repeating an experiment or test ~ vi **1** : to undergo reproduction **2** : to produce offspring

re·pro·duc·tion \ˌrē-prə-ˈdək-shən\ n : the act or process of reproducing; specif : the process by which plants and animals give rise to offspring and which fundamentally consists of the segregation of a portion of the parental body by a sexual or an asexual process and its subsequent growth and differentiation into a new individual

re·pro·duc·tive \ˌrē-prə-ˈdək-tiv\ adj : of, relating to, func-

---

\ə\ abut \ˈə, ˌə\ kitten \ər\ further \a\ ash \ā\ ace \ä\ cot, cart
\aú\ out \ch\ chin \e\ bet \ē\ easy \g\ go \i\ hit \ī\ ice \j\ job
\ŋ\ sing \ō\ go \ȯ\ law \ȯi\ boy \th\ thin \t̲h̲\ the \ü\ loot
\ú\ foot \y\ yet \zh\ vision   See also Pronunciation Symbols page

Q
R

tioning in, or capable of reproduction ⟨∼ organs⟩ — **re·pro·duc·tive·ly** *adv*

reproductive system *n* : the system of organs and parts which function in reproduction consisting in the male esp. of the testes, penis, seminal vesicles, prostate, and urethra and in the female esp. of the ovaries, fallopian tubes, uterus, vagina, and vulva

re·pul·sion \ri-'pəl-shən\ *n* : the tendency of some linked genetic characters to be inherited separately because a dominant allele for each character occurs on the same chromosome as a recessive allele of the other — compare COUPLING 2

re·ra·di·ate \(')rē-'rād-ē-ˌāt\ *vt* **-at·ed; -at·ing** : to radiate again or anew; *esp* : to emit (energy) in the form of radiation after absorbing incident radiation — **re·ra·di·a·tion** \(ˌ)rē-ˌrād-ē-'ā-shən\ *n*

RES *abbr* reticuloendothelial system

res·azur·in \rez-'azh-ə-rən\ *n* : a blue crystalline dye $C_{12}H_7NO_4$ used chiefly as an oxidation-reduction indicator in the resazurin test for bacteria

resazurin test *n* : a test of the keeping quality of milk based on the speed with which a standard quantity of the dye resazurin is reduced by a sample of milk

res·cin·na·mine \re-'sin-ə-ˌmēn, -mən\ *n* : an antihypertensive, tranquilizing, and sedative drug $C_{35}H_{42}N_2O_9$

re·sect \ri-'sekt\ *vt* : to perform resection on ⟨∼ an ulcer⟩

re·sect·able \ri-'sek-tə-bəl\ *adj* : capable of being resected : suitable for resection ⟨∼ cancer⟩ — **re·sect·abil·i·ty** \ri-ˌsek-tə-'bil-ət-ē\ *n, pl* **-ties**

re·sec·tion \ri-'sek-shən\ *n* : the surgical removal of part of an organ or structure ⟨pancreatic ∼⟩ ⟨∼ of the lower bowel⟩ ⟨∼ of a tumor⟩ — see ABDOMINOPERINEAL RESECTION, MIKULICZ RESECTION, SEGMENTAL RESECTION, WEDGE RESECTION

re·sec·to·scope \ri-'sek-tə-ˌskōp\ *n* : an instrument consisting of a tubular fenestrated sheath with a sliding knife within it that is used for surgery within cavities (as of the prostate through the urethra)

re·ser·pine \ri-'sər-ˌpēn *also* 'res-ər-pən\ *n* : an alkaloid $C_{33}H_{40}N_2O_9$ extracted esp. from the root of rauwolfias and used in the treatment of hypertension, mental disorders, and tensions states — see RAUDIXIN, SANDRIL, SERPASIL

re·ser·pin·ized *also Brit* **re·ser·pin·ised** \ri-'sər-pə-ˌnīzd\ *adj* : treated or medicated with reserpine or a reserpine derivative — **re·ser·pin·iza·tion** *also Brit* **re·ser·pin·isa·tion** \ri-ˌsər-pə-nə-'zā-shən\ *n*

reservatus — see COITUS RESERVATUS

¹**re·serve** \ri-'zərv\ *n* **1** : something stored or kept available for future use or need ⟨oxygen ∼⟩ — see CARDIAC RESERVE **2** : the capacity of a solution to neutralize alkali or acid when its reaction is shifted from one hydrogen-ion concentration to another; *esp* : the capacity of blood or bacteriological media to react with acid or alkali within predetermined and usu. physiological limits of hydrogen-ion concentration — compare BUFFER, BUFFER SOLUTION

²**reserve** *adj* : constituting or having the form or function of a reserve ⟨a ∼ supply⟩ ⟨∼ strength⟩

reserve air *n* : SUPPLEMENTAL AIR

res·er·voir \'rez-ə(r)v-ˌwär, -ə(r)v-ˌ(w)òr\ *n* **1** : a space (as an enlargement of a vessel or the cavity of a glandular acinus) in which a body fluid is stored **2** : an organism in which a parasite that is pathogenic for some other species lives and multiplies without damaging its host; *also* : a noneconomic organism within which a pathogen of economic or medical importance flourishes without regard to its pathogenicity for the reservoir ⟨rats are ∼s of plague⟩ — compare CARRIER 1a

reservoir host *n* : RESERVOIR 2

res·i·den·cy \'rez-əd-ən-sē\ *n, pl* **-cies** : a period of advanced medical training and education that normally follows graduation from medical school and licensing to practice medicine and that consists of supervised practice of a specialty in a hospital and in its outpatient department and instruction from specialists on the hospital staff

res·i·dent \'rez-əd-ənt, 'rez-dənt\ *n* : a physician serving a residency

res·i·den·tial \ˌrez-(ə)-'den-chəl\ *adj* : provided to patients residing in a facility ⟨∼ drug treatment⟩

residua *pl of* RESIDUUM

¹**re·sid·u·al** \ri-'zij-(ə-)wəl, -'zij-əl\ *adj* **1** : of, relating to, or being something that remains: as **a** : remaining after a disease or operation ⟨∼ paralysis⟩ **b** : remaining in a body cavity after maximum normal expulsion has occurred ⟨∼ urine⟩ — see RESIDUAL VOLUME **2 a** : leaving a residue that remains effective for some time after application ⟨∼ insecticides⟩ **b** : of or relating to a residual insecticide ⟨a ∼ spray⟩

²**residual** *n* **1** : an internal aftereffect of experience or activity that influences later behavior **2** : a residual abnormality (as a scar or limp)

residual air *n* : RESIDUAL VOLUME

residual body *n* **1** : a cytoplasmic vacuole containing the leftover products of digestion after fusion with the contents of a lysosome **2** : any of the small cytoplasmic masses that are shed from the developing sperms in spermiogenesis and that lack a nucleus but contain lipids, ribosomes, mitochondria, and cytoplasmic membranes

residual volume *n* : the volume of air still remaining in the lungs after the most forcible expiration possible and amounting usu. to 60 to 100 cubic inches (980 to 1640 cubic centimeters) — called also *residual air;* compare SUPPLEMENTAL AIR

res·i·due \'rez-ə-ˌd(y)ü\ *n* : something that remains after a part is taken, separated, or designated; *specif* : a constituent structural unit (as a group or monomer) of a usu. complex molecule ⟨amino acid ∼s in a protein⟩

re·sid·u·um \ri-'zij-ə-wəm\ *n, pl* **re·sid·ua** \-ə-wə\ *also* **residuums** : something that remains; *esp* : RESIDUAL 2

re·sil·ience \ri-'zil-yən(t)s\ *n* **1** : the capability of a strained body to recover its size and shape after deformation caused esp. by compressive stress **2** : an ability to recover from or adjust easily to misfortune or change ⟨emotional ∼⟩

re·sil·ien·cy \ri-'zil-yən-sē\ *n, pl* **-cies** : RESILIENCE

re·sil·ient \-yənt\ *adj* : characterized or marked by resilience

res·in \'rez-ᵊn\ *n* **1 a** : any of various solid or semisolid amorphous fusible flammable natural organic substances that are usu. transparent or translucent and yellowish to brown, are formed esp. in plant secretions, are soluble in organic solvents (as ether) but not in water, and are electrical nonconductors **b** : ROSIN **c** : a solid pharmaceutical preparation consisting chiefly of the resinous principles of a drug or drugs usu. extracted by solvents ⟨∼ of jalap⟩ **2 a** : any of a large class of synthetic products that have some of the physical properties of natural resins but are different chemically and are used chiefly in plastics **b** : any of various products made from a natural resin or a natural polymer

res·in·oid \'rez-ᵊn-ˌòid\ *n* **1** : a thermosetting synthetic resin **2 a** : any of a class of resinous preparations made by pouring a concentrated alcoholic extract of a drug into cold water and separating and drying the precipitate formed **b** : GUM RESIN

res·in·ous \'rez-nəs, -ᵊn-əs\ *adj* : of, relating to, resembling, containing, or derived from resin

re·sis·tance \ri-'zis-tən(t)s\ *n* **1 a** : power or capacity to resist; *esp* : the inherent ability of an organism to resist harmful influences (as disease, toxic agents, or infection) **b** : the capacity of a species or strain of microorganism to survive exposure to a toxic agent (as a drug) formerly effective against it due to genetic mutation and selection for and accumulation of genes conferring protection from the agent esp. as a result of overuse of the agent which selectively destroys individual microorganisms lacking the protective genes **2 a** : the opposition offered by a body to the passage through it of a steady electric current **b** : opposition or impediment to the flow of a fluid (as blood or respiratory gases) through one or more passages — see VASCULAR RESISTANCE **3** : a psychological defense mechanism wherein a psychoanalysis patient rejects, denies, or otherwise opposes therapeutic efforts by the analyst

re·sis·tant *also* **re·sis·tent** \-tənt\ *adj* : giving, capable of, or exhibiting resistance — often used in combination ⟨a drug= *resistant* strain of virus⟩

re·sis·tiv·i·ty \ri-ˌzis-'tiv-ət-ē, ˌrē-\ *n, pl* **-ties** : the longitudinal electrical resistance of a uniform rod of unit length and unit cross-sectional area : the reciprocal of conductivity

re·so·cial·iza·tion *also Brit* **re·so·cial·isa·tion** \ˌrē-ˌsōsh-(ə-)lə-'zā-shən\ *n* : readjustment of an individual (as a mentally or physically disabled person) to life in society

res·o·lu·tion \ˌrez-ə-'lü-shən\ *n* 1 : the separating of a chemical compound or mixture into its constituents 2 : the process or capability of making distinguishable the individual parts of an object, closely adjacent optical images, or sources of light 3 : the subsidence of a pathological state (as inflammation)

re·solve \ri-'zälv, -'zolv *also* -'zäv *or* -'zov\ *vb* **re·solved; re·solv·ing** *vt* 1 : to separate (a racemic compound or mixture) into the two components 2 : to cause resolution of (as inflammation) 3 : to distinguish between or make independently visible adjacent parts of ∼ *vi* 1 : to become separated into component parts; *also* : to become reduced by dissolving or analysis 2 : to undergo resolution — used esp. of disease or inflammation — **re·solv·able** \-'zäl-və-bəl, -'zol-*also* -'zäv-ə- *or* -'zov-ə-\ *adj*

¹**re·sol·vent** \ri-'zäl-vənt, -'zol-\ *adj* : having power to resolve ⟨a ∼ drug⟩

²**resolvent** *n* : an agent capable of dispersing or absorbing inflammatory products

resolving power *n* : the ability of an optical system to form distinguishable images of objects separated by small angular distances

res·o·nance \'rez-ᵊn-ən(t)s, 'rez-nən(t)s\ *n* 1 : a quality imparted to voiced sounds by vibration in anatomical resonating chambers or cavities (as the mouth or the nasal cavity) 2 : the sound elicited on percussion of the chest 3 : the conceptual alternation of a chemical species (as a molecule or ion) between two or more equivalent allowed structural representations differing only in the placement of electrons that aids in understanding the actual state of the species as an amalgamation of its possible structures and the usu. higher= than-expected stability of the species 4 a : the enhancement of an atomic, nuclear, or particle reaction or a scattering event by excitation of internal motion in the system b : MAGNETIC RESONANCE — see ELECTRON SPIN RESONANCE

resonance theory *n* 1 : a theory of hearing: different sections of the basilar membrane of the organ of Corti are tuned to different vibration rates and set up sympathetic vibrations that stimulate sensory nerve endings when the cochlear endolymph is vibrating at a corresponding frequency 2 : a theory in physiology: different forms of excitation arise in the central nervous system, are transmitted diffusely to the end organs, but are individually capable of effectively stimulating only those muscles or other motor organs that are responsive to their particular frequency

res·o·nant \'rez-ᵊn-ənt, 'rez-nənt\ *adj* 1 : capable of inducing resonance 2 : relating to or exhibiting resonance

re·sorb \(')rē-'sȯ(ə)rb, -'zȯ(ə)rb\ *vt* : to break down and assimilate (something previously differentiated) ⟨∼ed bone⟩ ∼ *vi* : to undergo resorption ⟨the injected protein ∼s after some days⟩ — **re·sorb·a·ble** \-'sȯ(ə)r-bə-bəl, -'zȯ(ə)r-\ *adj*

res·or·cin \rə-'zȯrs-ᵊn\ *n* : RESORCINOL

res·or·cin·ol \-ˌȯl, -ˌōl\ *n* : a crystalline phenol $C_6H_6O_2$ obtained from various resins or artificially and used in medicine as a fungicidal, bactericidal, and keratolytic agent

resorcinol mono·ac·e·tate \-ˌmän-ō-'as-ə-ˌtāt\ *n* : a thick yellow liquid compound $C_8H_8O_3$ that slowly liberates resorcinol and that is used esp. to treat diseases of the scalp

re·sorp·tion \(')rē-'sȯrp-shən, -'zȯrp-\ *n* : the action or process of resorbing something ⟨age-related bone loss . . . is caused by a slight but persistent elevation in the rate of bone ∼ over the rate of bone formation —P. S. Millard *et al*⟩

re·sorp·tive \-tiv\ *adj* : of, relating to, or characterized by resorption ⟨∼ processes⟩

re·source–based rel·a·tive val·ue scale \'rē-ˌsō(ə)rs-'bāst-'rel-ət-iv-'val-(ˌ)yü-\ *n* : a system of payments to physicians for treating Medicare patients that takes into account the work done by the physicians, malpractice insurance, and practice expenses including staff salaries, overhead, supplies, and equipment — abbr. *RBRVS*

re·spi·ra·ble \'res-p(ə-)rə-bəl, ri-'spī-rə-\ *adj* 1 : fit for breathing ⟨∼ air⟩ 2 : capable of being taken in by breathing ⟨∼ particles of ash⟩

res·pi·ra·tion \ˌres-pə-'rā-shən\ *n* 1 a : the movement of respiratory gases (as oxygen and carbon dioxide) into and out of the lungs b : a single complete act of breathing ⟨30 ∼s per minute⟩ 2 : the physical and chemical processes (as breathing and diffusion) by which an organism supplies its cells and tissues with the oxygen needed for metabolism and relieves them of the carbon dioxide formed in energy= producing reactions 3 : CELLULAR RESPIRATION

res·pi·ra·tor \'res-pə-ˌrāt-ər\ *n* 1 : a device (as a gas mask) worn over the mouth and nose to protect the respiratory system by filtering out dangerous substances (as dust or fumes) from inhaled air 2 : a device for maintaining artificial respiration ⟨a mechanical ∼⟩ — called also *ventilator*

res·pi·ra·to·ry \'res-p(ə-)rə-ˌtōr-ē, ri-'spī-rə-, -ˌtȯr-\ *adj* 1 : of or relating to respiration ⟨∼ function⟩ ⟨∼ diseases⟩ 2 : serving for or functioning in respiration ⟨∼ organs⟩

respiratory acidosis *n* : acidosis that is caused by excessive retention of carbon dioxide due to a respiratory abnormality (as obstructive lung disease)

respiratory alkalosis *n* : alkalosis that is caused by excessive elimination of carbon dioxide due to a respiratory abnormality (as hyperventilation)

respiratory center *n* : a region in the medulla oblongata that regulates respiratory movements

respiratory chain *n* : the metabolic pathway along which electron transport occurs in cellular respiration; *also* : the series of respiratory enzymes involved in this pathway

respiratory distress syndrome *n* : a respiratory disorder that occurs in newborn premature infants and is characterized by deficiency of the surfactant coating the inner surface of the lungs, by failure of the lungs to expand and contract properly during breathing with resulting collapse, and by the accumulation of a protein-containing film lining the alveoli and their ducts — abbr. *RDS;* called also *hyaline membrane disease;* see ADULT RESPIRATORY DISTRESS SYNDROME

respiratory enzyme *n* : an enzyme (as an oxidase, dehydrogenase, or catalase) associated with the processes of cellular respiration

respiratory pigment *n* : any of various permanently or intermittently colored conjugated proteins and esp. hemoglobin that function in the transfer of oxygen in cellular respiration

respiratory quotient *n* : the ratio of the volume of carbon dioxide given off in respiration to that of the oxygen consumed that has a value near 1 when the organism is burning chiefly carbohydrates, near 0.7 when chiefly fats, and near 0.8 when chiefly proteins but sometimes exceeding 1 when carbohydrates are being changed to fats for storage — abbr. *RQ*

respiratory syncytial virus *n* : a paramyxovirus (species *Human respiratory syncytial virus* of the genus *Pneumovirus*) that has three strains, forms syncytia in tissue culture, and is responsible for severe respiratory diseases (as bronchopneumonia and bronchiolitis) in children and esp. in infants — abbr. *RSV*

respiratory system *n* : a system of organs functioning in respiration and consisting esp. of the nose, nasal passages, nasopharynx, larynx, trachea, bronchi, and lungs — called

Q
R

also *respiratory tract;* see LOWER RESPIRATORY TRACT, UP-
PER RESPIRATORY TRACT

respiratory therapist *n* : a specialist in respiratory therapy

respiratory therapy *n* : therapy that is concerned with the
maintenance or improvement of respiratory functioning (as
in patients with pulmonary disease)

respiratory tract *n* : RESPIRATORY SYSTEM

respiratory tree *n* : the trachea, bronchi, and bronchioles

re·spire \ri-'spī(ə)r\ *vb* **re·spired; re·spir·ing** *vi* 1
: BREATHE; *specif* : to inhale and exhale air successively 2 *of
a cell or tissue* : to take up oxygen and produce carbon dioxide through oxidation ~ *vt* : BREATHE

res·pi·rom·e·ter \ˌres-pə-'räm-ət-ər\ *n* : an instrument for
studying the character and extent of respiration

res·pi·ro·met·ric \ˌres-pə-rō-'me-trik\ *adj* : of or relating to
respirometry or to the use of a respirometer ⟨~ studies⟩

res·pi·rom·e·try \ˌres-pə-'räm-ə-trē\ *n, pl* **-tries** : the study
of respiration (as cellular respiration) by means of a respirometer

re·spond \ri-'spänd\ *vi* 1 : to react in response 2 : to show
favorable reaction ⟨~ to surgery⟩

¹**re·spon·dent** \ri-'spän-dənt\ *n* : a reflex that occurs in response to a specific external stimulus ⟨the knee jerk is a typical ~⟩

²**respondent** *adj* : relating to or being behavior or responses to
a stimulus that are followed by a reward ⟨~ conditioning⟩
— compare OPERANT

re·spond·er \ri-'spän-dər\ *n* : one that responds (as to treatment or to an antigen)

re·sponse \ri-'spän(t)s\ *n* : the activity or inhibition of previous activity of an organism or any of its parts resulting from
stimulation ⟨a conditioned ~⟩

re·spon·sive \ri-'spän(t)-siv\ *adj* : making a response; *esp*
: responding to treatment ⟨pain ~ to opioids⟩

re·spon·sive·ness *n* : the quality or state of being responsive

res·sen·ti·ment \rə-säⁿ-tē-'mäⁿ\ *n* : deep-seated resentment,
frustration, and hostility accompanied by a sense of being
powerless to express these feelings directly

¹**rest** \'rest\ *n* 1 : a state of repose or sleep — see BED REST 2
: cessation or temporary interruption of motion, exertion, or
labor ⟨~ from hard physical effort⟩ ⟨a ten-minute ~ peri-
od⟩ 3 : a bodily state (as that attained by a fasting individual lying supine) characterized by minimal functional and
metabolic activities ⟨the patient must have complete ~⟩ 4
: the part of a partial denture that rests on an abutment
tooth, distributes stresses, and holds the clasp in position 5
: a firm but moldable cushion used to raise or support a portion of the body during surgery ⟨a kidney ~⟩

²**rest** *vi* 1 : to get rest by lying down; *esp* : SLEEP 2 : to cease
from action or motion : refrain from labor or exertion ~ *vt*
: to give rest to ⟨~ your eyes⟩

³**rest** *n* : a mass of surviving embryonic cells or of cells misplaced in development ⟨most tumors derived from embryonic ~s are benign —Shields Warren⟩

rest cure *n* : treatment of disease (as tuberculosis) by rest
and isolation in a good hygienic environment

re·ste·no·sis \ˌres-tə-'nō-səs, ˌrē-stə-\ *n, pl* **-no·ses** \-ˌsēz\ : the
reoccurrence of stenosis in a blood vessel or heart valve after
it has been treated (as by balloon angioplasty or valvuloplas-
ty) with apparent success

rest home *n* : an establishment that provides housing and
general care for the aged or the convalescent — compare
NURSING HOME

res·ti·form body \'res-tə-ˌfȯrm-\ *n* : CEREBELLAR PEDUN-
CLE c

re·stim·u·late \(ˈ)rē-'stim-yə-ˌlāt\ *vt* **-lat·ed; -lat·ing** : to re-
activate by stimulation

rest·ing *adj* 1 : not physiologically active ⟨red blood cells in
a ~ state⟩ 2 : occurring in or performed on a subject at
rest ⟨a ~ EEG⟩ ⟨a ~ tremor⟩

resting cell *n* : a living cell with a resting nucleus

resting nucleus *n* : a cell nucleus when not undergoing the
process of division (as by mitosis)

resting potential *n* : the membrane potential of a cell that is

not exhibiting the activity resulting from a stimulus — compare ACTION POTENTIAL, POTENTIAL DIFFERENCE

resting spore *n* : a spore that remains dormant for a period
before germination

resting stage *n* : INTERPHASE

resting wandering cell *n* : a fixed macrophage of the loose
connective tissue of the body

rest·less \'rest-ləs\ *adj* 1 : deprived of rest or sleep ⟨the patient was ~ from pain⟩ 2 : providing no rest ⟨a ~ night⟩

restless legs syndrome *n* : a neurological disorder of uncertain pathophysiology that is characterized by aching, burning, crawling, or creeping sensations of the legs that occur
esp. at night usu. when lying down (as before sleep) and
cause a compelling urge to move the legs and that is often
accompanied by difficulty in falling or staying asleep and by
involuntary twitching of the legs during sleep — called also
restless legs

res·to·ra·tion \ˌres-tə-'rā-shən\ *n* : the act of restoring or the
condition of being restored: as **a** : a returning to a normal
or healthy condition **b** : the replacing of missing teeth or
crowns; *also* : a dental replacement (as a denture) used for
restoration

¹**re·stor·ative** \ri-'stȯr-ət-iv, -'stȯr-\ *adj* : of, relating to, or
providing restoration ⟨~ treatment⟩ ⟨~ dentistry⟩

²**restorative** *n* : something (as a medicine) that serves to restore to consciousness, vigor, or health

re·store \ri-'stō(ə)r, -'stȯ(ə)r\ *vt* **re·stored; re·stor·ing** : to
bring back to or put back into a former or original state ⟨a
tooth *restored* with an inlay⟩

Res·to·ril \'res-tə-ˌril\ *trademark* — used for a preparation of
temazepam

re·straint \ri-'strānt\ *n* : a device that restricts movement
⟨~s such as straitjackets for violent patients⟩

re·stric·tion \ri-'strik-shən\ *n, often attrib* : the breaking of
double-stranded DNA into fragments by restriction enzymes
⟨~ sites⟩

restriction endonuclease *n* : RESTRICTION ENZYME

restriction enzyme *n* : any of various enzymes that cleave
DNA into fragments at specific sites in the interior of the
molecule and are often used as tools in molecular analysis

restriction fragment *n* : a segment of DNA produced by the
action of a restriction enzyme on a molecule of DNA

restriction fragment length polymorphism *n* : variation
in the length of a restriction fragment produced by a specific
restriction enzyme acting on DNA from different individuals
that usu. results from a genetic mutation (as an insertion or
deletion) and that may be used as a genetic marker — called
also *RFLP*

rest seat *n* : an area on the surface of a tooth that is specially
prepared (as by grinding) for the attachment of a dental rest

res·ur·rec·tion·ist \ˌrez-ə-'rek-sh(ə-)nəst\ *n* : BODY SNATCH-
ER

res·ur·rec·tion man \ˌrez-ə-'rek-shən-\ *n* : BODY SNATCHER

re·sus·ci·tate \ri-'səs-ə-ˌtāt\ *vt* **-tat·ed; -tat·ing** : to revive
from apparent death or from unconsciousness ⟨~ a nearly
drowned person by artificial respiration⟩

re·sus·ci·ta·tion \ri-ˌsəs-ə-'tā-shən, rē-\ *n* : an act of resusci-
tating or the state of being resuscitated ⟨~ by means of artificial respiration or cardiac massage⟩ — see CARDIOPULMO-
NARY RESUSCITATION

re·sus·ci·ta·tive \ri-'səs-ə-ˌtāt-iv\ *adj* : of or relating to resuscitation ⟨~ methods⟩

re·sus·ci·ta·tor \ri-'səs-ə-ˌtāt-ər\ *n* : one that resuscitates;
specif : an apparatus used to restore respiration (as of a partially asphyxiated person)

res·ver·a·trol \rez-'vir-ə-ˌtrȯl, -ˌträl, -ˌtrōl\ *n* : a compound
$C_{14}H_{12}O_3$ that is a trihydroxy trans form of stilbene found in
some plants, fruits (as the mulberry), and seeds (as the peanut) and esp. in the skin of grapes and certain grape-derived
products (as red wine) and that has been linked to a reduced
risk of coronary artery disease and cancer

re·syn·the·sis \(ˌ)rē-'sin(t)-thə-səs\ *n, pl* **-the·ses** \-ˌsēz\ : the
action or process of resynthesizing something ⟨~ of a dam-
aged section of DNA⟩

re·syn·the·size *also Brit* **re·syn·the·sise** \-,sīz\ *vt* **-sized** *also Brit* **-sised; -siz·ing** *also Brit* **-sis·ing** : to synthesize again

re·tain \ri-'tān\ *vt* **1** : to hold or keep in ⟨∼ fluids⟩ **2** : to keep in mind or memory

re·tain·er \ri-'tān-ər\ *n* **1** : the part of a dental replacement (as a bridge) by which it is made fast to adjacent natural teeth **2** : a dental appliance used to hold teeth in their correct position esp. following orthodontic treatment

re·tard \ri-'tärd\ *vt* : to slow up esp. by preventing or hindering advance or development ⟨∼ spoilage⟩ ⟨∼ hair loss⟩

re·tar·date \ri-'tärd-,āt, -ət\ *n, often offensive* : a mentally retarded individual

re·tar·da·tion \,rē-,tär-'dā-shən, ri-\ *n* **1** : an abnormal slowness of thought or action; *esp* : MENTAL RETARDATION **2** : slowness in development or progress

re·tard·ed \ri-'tärd-əd\ *adj, sometimes offensive* : slow or limited in intellectual or emotional development : characterized by mental retardation

retch \'rech, *esp Brit* 'rēch\ *vi* : to make an effort to vomit ∼ *vt* : VOMIT — **retch** *n*

re·te \'rēt-ē, 'rāt-\ *n, pl* **re·tia** \'rēt-ē-ə, 'rāt-\ **1** : a network esp. of blood vessels or nerves : PLEXUS **2** : an anatomical part resembling or including a network

rete cord *n* : any of the strands of cells that grow from the region of the mesonephros into the developing gonad of the vertebrate embryo

re·ten·tion \ri-'ten-chən\ *n* **1** : the act of retaining: as **a** : abnormal retaining of a fluid or secretion in a body cavity ⟨∼ of urine⟩ ⟨∼ of bile⟩ **b** : the holding in place of a tooth or dental replacement by means of a retainer **2** : a preservation of the aftereffects of experience and learning that makes recall or recognition possible

re·ten·tive \ri-'ten-tiv\ *adj* : tending to retain: as **a** : retaining knowledge : having a good memory ⟨a ∼ mind⟩ **b** : of, relating to, or being a dental retainer

rete peg *n* : any of the inwardly directed prolongations of the Malpighian layer of the epidermis that intermesh with the dermal papillae of the skin

rete testis *n, pl* **retia tes·ti·um** \-'tes-tē-əm\ : the network of tubules in the mediastinum testis

retia *pl of* RETE

reticula *pl of* RETICULUM

re·tic·u·lar \ri-'tik-yə-lər\ *adj* : of, relating to, or forming a network ⟨∼ layers in the adrenal cortex⟩

reticular activating system *n* : a part of the reticular formation that extends from the brain stem to the midbrain and thalamus with connections distributed throughout the cerebral cortex and that controls the degree of activity of the central nervous system (as in maintaining sleep and wakefulness and in making transitions between the two states)

reticular cell *n* : RETICULUM CELL; *esp* : RETICULOCYTE

reticular fiber *n* : any of the thin branching fibers of connective tissue that form an intricate interstitial network ramifying through other tissues and organs

reticular formation *n* : a mass of nerve cells and fibers situated primarily in the brain stem and functioning upon stimulation esp. in arousal of the organism — called also *reticular substance*

reticularis — see LIVEDO RETICULARIS, ZONA RETICULARIS

reticular lamina *n* : a thin extracellular layer that sometimes lies below the basal lamina, is composed chiefly of collagenous fibers, and serves to anchor the basal lamina to underlying connective tissue

reticular layer *n* : the deeper layer of the dermis formed of interlacing fasciculi of white fibrous tissue

reticular substance *n* : RETICULAR FORMATION

reticular tissue *n* : RETICULUM 2a

reticulata — see PARS RETICULATA

re·tic·u·late body \ri-'tik-yə-lət-\ *n* : a chlamydial cell of a spherical intracellular form that is larger than an elementary body and reproduces by binary fission

re·tic·u·lat·ed \ri-'tik-yə-,lāt-əd\ *or* **re·tic·u·late** \-lət, -,lāt\ *adj* : resembling a net ⟨the lesions formed a ∼ pattern⟩ — **re·tic·u·la·tion** \ri-,tik-yə-'lā-shən\ *n*

re·tic·u·lin \ri-'tik-yə-lən\ *n* : a protein substance similar to collagen that is a constituent of reticular tissue

re·tic·u·li·tis \ri-,tik-yə-'līt-əs\ *n* : inflammation of the reticulum of a ruminant

re·tic·u·lo·cyte \ri-'tik-yə-lō-,sīt\ *n* : an immature red blood cell that appears esp. during regeneration of lost blood and that has a fine basophilic reticulum formed of the remains of ribosomes — **re·tic·u·lo·cyt·ic** \ri-,tik-yə-lō-'sit-ik\ *adj*

re·tic·u·lo·cy·to·pe·nia \ri-,tik-yə-lō-,sīt-ə-'pē-nē-ə\ *n* : an abnormal decrease in the number of reticulocytes in the blood

re·tic·u·lo·cy·to·sis \-,sī-'tō-səs\ *n, pl* **-to·ses** \-,sēz\ : an increase in the number of reticulocytes in the blood typically following hemorrhage or accompanying hemolytic anemia

re·tic·u·lo·en·do·the·li·al \ri-'tik-yə-lō-,en-də-'thē-lē-əl\ *adj* : of, relating to, or being the reticuloendothelial system ⟨∼ tissue⟩ ⟨∼ cells⟩

reticuloendothelial system *n* : a diffuse system of cells of varying lineage that include esp. the macrophages and the phagocytic endothelial cells lining blood sinuses and that were orig. grouped together because of their supposed phagocytic properties based on their ability to take up the vital dye trypan blue — called also *lymphoreticular system;* compare MONONUCLEAR PHAGOCYTE SYSTEM

re·tic·u·lo·en·do·the·li·o·sis \-,thē-lē-'ō-səs\ *n, pl* **-o·ses** \-,sēz\ : any of several disorders characterized by proliferation of reticuloendothelial cells or their derivatives — called also *reticulosis*

re·tic·u·lo·en·do·the·li·um \-,en-də-'thē-lē-əm\ *n, pl* **-lia** \-lē-ə\ : the cells of the reticuloendothelial system regarded as a tissue

re·tic·u·lo·sar·co·ma \-sär-'kō-mə\ *n, pl* **-mas** *also* **-ma·ta** \-mət-ə\ : RETICULUM CELL SARCOMA

re·tic·u·lo·sis \ri-,tik-yə-'lō-səs\ *n, pl* **-lo·ses** \-,sēz\ : RETICULOENDOTHELIOSIS

re·tic·u·lo·spi·nal tract \ri-,tik-yə-lō-,spī-n'l-\ *n* : a tract of nerve fibers that originates in the reticular formation of the pons and medulla oblongata and descends to the spinal cord

re·tic·u·lum \ri-'tik-yə-ləm\ *n, pl* **-la** \-lə\ **1** : the second compartment of the stomach of a ruminant in which folds of the mucous membrane form hexagonal cells — called also *honeycomb;* compare ABOMASUM, OMASUM, RUMEN **2** : a reticular structure : NETWORK: as **a** : the network of interstitial tissue composed of reticular fibers — called also *reticular tissue* **b** : the network often visible in fixed protoplasm both of the cell body and the nucleus of many cells

reticulum cell *n* : any of the branched anastomosing reticuloendothelial cells that form the reticular fibers

reticulum cell sarcoma *n* : a malignant lymphoma arising from reticulum cells — called also *reticulosarcoma*

ret·i·na \'ret-ᵊn-ə, 'ret-nə\ *n, pl* **retinas** *or* **ret·i·nae** \-ᵊn-,ē\ : the sensory membrane that lines most of the large posterior chamber of the vertebrate eye, is composed of several layers including one containing the rods and cones, and functions as the immediate instrument of vision by receiving the image formed by the lens and converting it into chemical and nervous signals which reach the brain by way of the optic nerve

Ret·in-A \,ret-ᵊn-'ā\ *trademark* — used for a preparation of tretinoin

ret·i·nac·u·lar \,ret-ᵊn-'ak-yə-lər\ *adj* : of, relating to, or being a retinaculum ⟨∼ tissue⟩ ⟨a ∼ repair⟩

ret·i·nac·u·lum \-ləm\ *n, pl* **-la** \-lə\ : a connecting or retaining band esp. of fibrous tissue — see EXTENSOR RETINACULUM, FLEXOR RETINACULUM, INFERIOR EXTENSOR RETINACULUM, INFERIOR PERONEAL RETINACULUM, PERONEAL RETINACULUM, SUPERIOR EXTENSOR RETINACULUM, SUPERIOR PERONEAL RETINACULUM

¹**ret·i·nal** \'ret-ᵊn-əl, 'ret-nəl\ *adj* : of, relating to, involving, or being a retina ⟨a ∼ examination⟩ ⟨∼ rods⟩

\ə\ abut \ᵊ\ kitten \ər\ further \a\ ash \ā\ ace \ä\ cot, cart \aú\ out \ch\ chin \e\ bet \ē\ easy \g\ go \i\ hit \ī\ ice \j\ job \ŋ\ sing \ō\ go \ò\ law \òi\ boy \th\ thin \t͟h\ the \ü\ loot \ù\ foot \y\ yet \zh\ vision *See also* Pronunciation Symbols page

Q
R

²**ret·i·nal** \'ret-ᵊn-ₐal, -ₐȯl\ *n* : a yellowish to orange aldehyde $C_{20}H_{28}O$ derived from vitamin A that in combination with proteins forms the visual pigments of the retinal rods and cones — called also *retinene, retinene₁, vitamin A aldehyde*

retinal artery — see CENTRAL RETINAL ARTERY

retinal detachment *n* : a condition of the eye in which the retina has separated from the choroid — called also *detached retina, detachment of the retina*

retinal disparity *n* : the slight difference in the two retinal images due to the angle from which each eye views an object

retinal rivalry *n* : the oscillating perception of first one then the other of two visual stimuli which differ radically in color or form when they are presented simultaneously to congruent areas of both eyes

retinal vein — see CENTRAL RETINAL VEIN

ret·i·nene \'ret-ᵊn-ₐēn\ *n* : either of two aldehydes derived from vitamin A: **a** : RETINAL   **b** : an orange-red crystalline compound $C_{20}H_{26}O$ related to vitamin A₂ and formed from porphyropsin by the action of light

retinene₁ \-'wən\ *n* : RETINAL

retinene₂ \-'tü\ *n* : RETINENE b

ret·i·ni·tis \ₐret-ᵊn-'īt-əs\ *n, pl* **-nit·i·des** \-'it-ə-ₐdēz\ : inflammation of the retina

retinitis pig·men·to·sa \-ₐpig-mən-'tō-sə, -(ₐ)men-, -zə\ *n* : any of several hereditary progressive degenerative diseases of the eye marked by night blindness in the early stages, atrophy and pigment changes in the retina, constriction of the visual field, and eventual blindness — abbr. *RP;* called also *pigmentary retinopathy*

retinitis pro·lif·er·ans \-prə-'lif-ə-ₐranz\ *n* : neovascularization of the retina associated esp. with diabetic retinopathy

ret·i·no·blas·to·ma \ₐret-ᵊn-ō-ₐblas-'tō-mə\ *n, pl* **-mas** *also* **-ma·ta** \-mət-ə\ : a hereditary malignant tumor of the retina that develops during childhood, is derived from retinal germ cells, and is associated with a chromosomal abnormality

ret·i·no·cho·roid·i·tis \-ₐkȯr-ₐȯid-'īt-əs\ *n* : inflammation of the retina and the choroid

ret·i·no·ic acid \ₐret-ᵊn-ₐō-ik-\ *n* : either of two isomers of an acid $C_{20}H_{28}O_2$ derived from vitamin A and used esp. in the treatment of acne: **a** *or* **all–trans–retinoic acid** : TRETINOIN   **b** *or* **13–cis–retinoic acid** : ISOTRETINOIN

ret·i·noid \'ret-ᵊn-ₐȯid\ *n* : any of various synthetic or naturally occurring analogs of vitamin A — **retinoid** *adj*

ret·i·nol \'ret-ᵊn-ₐȯl, -ₐōl\ *n* : VITAMIN A a

retinol palmitate *n* : RETINYL PALMITATE

ret·i·nop·a·thy \ₐret-ᵊn-'äp-ə-thē\ *n, pl* **-thies** : any of various noninflammatory disorders of the retina including some that cause blindness ⟨diabetic ~⟩

retinopathy of prematurity *n* : an ocular disorder of premature infants that occurs when the incompletely vascularized retina of such an infant completes an abnormal pattern of vascularization and that is characterized by the presence of an opaque fibrous membrane behind the lens of each eye — abbr. *ROP;* called also *retrolental fibroplasia*

ret·i·nos·chi·sis \ₐret-ᵊn-'äs-kə-səs\ *n, pl* **-chi·ses** \-ₐsēz\ *also* **-chi·sis·es** : degenerative splitting of the retina into separate layers

ret·i·no·scope \'ret-ᵊn-ə-ₐskōp\ *n* : an apparatus used in retinoscopy

ret·i·nos·co·py \ₐret-ᵊn-'äs-kə-pē\ *n, pl* **-pies** : a method of determining the state of refraction of the eye by illuminating the retina with a mirror and observing the direction of movement of the retinal illumination and adjacent shadow when the mirror is turned — **ret·i·no·scop·ic** \ₐret-ᵊn-ə-'skäp-ik\ *adj*

ret·i·no·tec·tal \ₐret-ᵊn-ō-'tek-təl\ *adj* : of, relating to, or being the nerve fibers connecting the retina and the tectum of the midbrain ⟨~ pathways⟩

ret·i·nyl palmitate \'ret-ᵊn-əl-\ *n* : a light yellow to red oil $C_{36}H_{60}O_2$ that is a derivative of vitamin A and is about half as potent — called also *retinol palmitate*

re·tort \ri-'tȯ(ə)rt, 'rē-ₐ\ *n* : a vessel or chamber in which substances are distilled or decomposed by heat

re·tract \ri-'trakt\ *vt* : to draw back or in ⟨~ the lower jaw⟩

— compare PROTRACT ~ *vi* : to draw something (as tissue) back or in; *also* : to use a retractor

re·trac·tile \ri-'trak-tᵊl, -ₐtīl\ *adj* : capable of being drawn back or in

re·trac·tion \ri-'trak-shən\ *n* : an act or instance of retracting; *specif* : backward or inward movement of an organ or part ⟨~ of the nipple or skin overlying the tumor —*Jour. Amer. Med. Assoc.*⟩

re·trac·tor \ri-'trak-tər\ *n* : one that retracts: as **a** : any of various surgical instruments for holding tissues away from the field of operation **b** : a muscle that draws in an organ or part — compare PROTRACTOR

ret·ro·ac·tive \ₐre-trō-'ak-tiv\ *adj* : having relation or reference to or efficacy in a prior time; *specif* : relating to, caused by, or being obliteration of the results of learning by immediately subsequent activity ⟨~ inhibition⟩

ret·ro·bul·bar \-'bəl-bər, -ₐbär\ *adj* : situated, occurring, or administered behind the eyeball ⟨a ~ injection⟩

retrobulbar neuritis *n* : inflammation of the part of the optic nerve lying immediately behind the eyeball

ret·ro·ca·val \-'kā-vəl\ *adj* : situated or occurring behind the vena cava

ret·ro·ces·sion \-'sesh-ən\ *n* : abnormal backward displacement ⟨~ of the uterus⟩

ret·ro·cli·na·tion \-klə-'nā-shən\ *n* : the condition of being inclined backward ⟨~ of the lower incisors⟩

ret·ro·col·ic \-'kō-lik, -'käl-ik\ *adj* : situated or occurring behind the colon

ret·ro·fec·tion \ₐre-trə-'fek-shən\ *n* : infection with pinworms in which the eggs hatch on the anal skin and mucosa and the larvae migrate up the bowel to the cecum where they mature

ret·ro·flex·ion \ₐre-trə-'flek-shən\ *n* : the state of being bent back; *specif* : the bending back of the body of the uterus upon the cervix — compare RETROVERSION

ret·ro·gnath·ia \-'nath-ē-ə\ *n* : RETROGNATHISM

ret·ro·gnath·ic \-'nath-ik\ *adj* : relating to or characterized by retrognathism

ret·ro·gnath·ism \ₐre-trō-'nath-ₐiz-əm\ *n* : a condition characterized by recession of one or both of the jaws ⟨mandibular ~⟩

ret·ro·grade \'re-trə-ₐgrād\ *adj* **1** : characterized by retrogression **2** : affecting a period immediately prior to a precipitating cause ⟨~ amnesia⟩ **3** : occurring or performed in a direction opposite to the normal or forward direction of conduction or flow: as **a** : occurring along nerve cell processes toward the cell body ⟨~ axonal transport⟩ ⟨~ degeneration of nerve fibers⟩ **b** : occurring opposite to the normal direction or path of blood circulation ⟨apply bandaging to the lower extremities to produce pressure to reduce ~ blood flow in veins with incompetent valves⟩ — compare ANTEROGRADE 2 — **ret·ro·grade·ly** *adv*

retrograde pyelogram *n* : a radiograph of the kidney made by retrograde pyelography

retrograde pyelography *n* : pyelography performed by injection of radiopaque material through the ureter

ret·ro·gres·sion \ₐre-trə-'gresh-ən\ *n* : a reversal in development or condition: as **a** : return to a former and less complex level of development or organization **b** : subsidence or decline of symptoms or manifestations of a disease

ret·ro·gres·sive \-'gres-iv\ *adj* : characterized by retrogression: as **a** : declining from a better to a worse state ⟨a ~ disease⟩ **b** : passing from a higher to a lower level of organization ⟨~ evolution⟩

ret·ro·len·tal \ₐre-trō-'lent-ᵊl\ *adj* : situated or occurring behind the lens of the eye

retrolental fibroplasia *n* : RETINOPATHY OF PREMATURITY

ret·ro·len·tic·u·lar \ₐre-trō-len-'tik-yə-lər\ *adj* : RETROLENTAL

ret·ro·lin·gual \-'liŋ-g(yə-)wəl\ *adj* : situated or occurring behind or near the base of the tongue ⟨~ salivary glands⟩

ret·ro·mam·ma·ry \-'mam-ə-rē\ *adj* : situated or occurring behind the mammae

ret·ro·man·dib·u·lar \-man-'dib-yə-lər\ *adj* : situated or occurring behind the lower jaw

ret·ro·mo·lar \-'mō-lər\ *adj* : situated or occurring behind the last molar 〈~ tissue〉

ret·ro·oc·u·lar \ˌre-trō-'äk-yə-lər\ *adj* : situated or occurring behind the eye : RETROBULBAR 〈~ pain〉

ret·ro·or·bit·al \-'ȯr-bət-ᵊl\ *adj* : situated or occurring behind the orbit of the eye

ret·ro·per·i·to·ne·al \-ˌper-ət-ᵊn-'ē-əl\ *adj* : situated or occurring behind the peritoneum 〈~ bleeding〉 〈a ~ tumor〉 — **ret·ro·per·i·to·ne·al·ly** \-ə-lē\ *adv*

retroperitoneal fibrosis *n* : proliferation of fibrous tissue behind the peritoneum often leading to blockage of the ureters — called also *Ormond's disease*

retroperitoneal space *n* : RETROPERITONEUM

ret·ro·per·i·to·ne·um \-ˌper-ət-ᵊn-'ē-əm\ *n, pl* **-ne·ums** *or* **-nea** \-'ē-ə\ : the space between the peritoneum and the posterior abdominal wall that contains esp. the kidneys and associated structures, the pancreas, and part of the aorta and inferior vena cava

ret·ro·pha·ryn·geal \-ˌfar-ən-'jē-əl, -fə-'rin-j(ē-)əl\ *adj* : situated or occurring behind the pharynx 〈a ~ abscess〉

ret·ro·pla·cen·tal \-plə-'sent-ᵊl\ *adj* : situated, occurring, or obtained from behind the placenta 〈~ blood〉

ret·ro·po·son \-'pō-ˌzän\ *n* : RETROTRANSPOSON

ret·ro·pu·bic \ˌre-trō-'pyü-bik\ *adj* **1** : situated or occurring behind the pubis **2** : performed by way of the retropubic space 〈~ prostatectomy〉

retropubic space *n* : the potential space occurring between the pubic symphysis and the urinary bladder — called also *space of Retzius*

ret·ro·pul·sion \-'pəl-shən\ *n* : a disorder of locomotion associated esp. with Parkinson's disease that is marked by a tendency to walk backwards

ret·ro·rec·tal \-'rek-tᵊl\ *adj* : situated or occurring behind the rectum 〈a ~ abscess〉

ret·ro·spec·tive \-'spek-tiv\ *adj* **1 a** : of, relating to, or given to introspection **b** : relating to or being a study (as of a disease) that starts with the present condition of a population of individuals and collects data about their past history to explain their present condition — compare PROSPECTIVE 2 : based on memory — **ret·ro·spec·tive·ly** *adv*

ret·ro·stal·sis \ˌre-trō-'stȯl-səs, -'stäl-, -'stal-\ *n, pl* **-stal·ses** \-ˌsēz\ : backward motion of the intestines : reversed peristalsis — **ret·ro·stal·tic** \-tik\ *adj*

ret·ro·ster·nal \-'stər-nəl\ *adj* : situated or occurring behind the sternum 〈~ pain〉

ret·ro·tar·sal \-'tär-səl\ *adj* : situated or occurring behind the tarsal plate of the eyelid

ret·ro·trans·po·son \-ˌtran(t)s-'pō-ˌzän\ *n* : a transposable element that undergoes transposition from one place to another in the genome of a cell by forming an intermediate RNA transcript from which a copy of the DNA of the transposable element is made using a reverse transcriptase and inserted into the genome at a new location — called also *retroposon*

ret·ro·ver·sion \-'vər-zhən *also* -shən\ *n* : the bending backward of the uterus and cervix out of the normal axis so that the fundus points toward the sacrum and the cervix toward the pubic symphysis — compare RETROFLEXION

Ret·ro·vir \'re-trō-ˌvir\ *trademark* — used for a preparation of AZT

Ret·ro·vi·ri·dae \ˌre-trō-'vir-ə-ˌdē\ *n pl* : a family of single-stranded RNA viruses that produce reverse transcriptase by means of which DNA is synthesized using their RNA as a template and incorporated into the genome of infected cells, that are often tumorigenic, and that include the foamy viruses, HIV, HTLV-I, Rous sarcoma virus, SIV, and the causative agents of avian leukosis, equine infectious anemia, ovine progressive pneumonia, and jaagsiekte — see LENTIVIRUS

ret·ro·vi·rol·o·gy \ˌre-trō-vī-'räl-ə-jē\ *n, pl* **-gies** : a branch of virology concerned with the study of retroviruses — **ret·ro·vi·rol·o·gist** \-jəst\ *n*

ret·ro·vi·rus \'re-trō-ˌvī-rəs\ *n* : any of the family *Retroviri-*

dae of single-stranded RNA viruses — called also *RNA tumor virus* — **ret·ro·vi·ral** \-rəl\ *adj* — **ret·ro·vi·ral·ly** \-ē\ *adv*

re·trude \ri-'trüd\ *vt* **re·trud·ed; re·trud·ing** : to move backward : displace posteriorly 〈~ the mandible〉

re·tru·sion \ri-'trü-zhən\ *n* : backward displacement; *specif* : a condition in which a tooth or the jaw is posterior to its proper occlusal position

re·tru·sive \-siv\ *adj* : marked by retrusion 〈a ~ chin〉

Rett's syndrome *or* **Rett syndrome** \'ret(s)-\ *n* : a familial disorder that affects females usu. during infancy, that results from arrested brain development, and that is characterized by cognitive and psychomotor deterioration, dementia, stunted head growth, stereotyped hand movements, and mild hyperammonemia

Rett, Andreas (*fl* 1966–1968), Austrian physician. Rett published his first description of Rett's syndrome in 1966, supplementing it with another report in 1968.

reuniens — see DUCTUS REUNIENS

re·up·take \(')rē-'əp-ˌtāk\ *n* : the reabsorption by a neuron of a neurotransmitter following the transmission of a nerve impulse across a synapse 〈antidepressants which block the ~ of norepinephrine〉

re·vac·ci·na·tion \'rē-ˌvak-sə-'nā-shən\ *n* : vaccination administered some period after an initial vaccination esp. to strengthen or renew immunity — **re·vac·ci·nate** \(')rē-'vak-sə-ˌnāt\ *vt* **-nat·ed; -nat·ing**

re·vas·cu·lar·iza·tion \'rē-ˌvas-kyə-lə-rə-'zā-shən\ *n* : a surgical procedure for the provision of a new, augmented, or restored blood supply to a body part or organ 〈myocardial ~〉

re·ver·sal \ri-'vər-səl\ *n* : an act or the process of reversing

re·verse \ri-'vərs\ *vt* **re·versed; re·vers·ing** : to change drastically or completely the course or effect of: as **a** : to initiate recovery from 〈~ a disease〉 **b** : to make of no effect or as if not done 〈~ a surgical procedure〉

reverse genetics *n pl but sing in constr* : genetics that is concerned with genetic material whose nucleotide sequence is known and that analyzes its contribution to the phenotype of the organism by varying the nucleotide sequence and observing the results of such variation in the living organism, in living cells, or in vitro on macromolecules — **reverse–genetic** *adj*

reverse transcriptase *n* : a polymerase esp. of retroviruses that catalyzes the formation of DNA using RNA as a template

reverse transcriptase inhibitor *n* : an agent that inhibits the activity of a reverse transcriptase; *esp* : a drug (as AZT) that acts by inhibiting retroviral reverse transcription

reverse transcription *n* : the process of synthesizing DNA using RNA as a template and reverse transcriptase as a catalyst — **reverse–transcribe** *vt* **-scribed; -scrib·ing**

re·vers·ible \ri-'vər-sə-bəl\ *adj* **1** : capable of going through a series of actions (as changes) either backward or forward 〈the chemical reaction was not ~〉 **2** : capable of being corrected or undone : not permanent or irrevocable 〈~ hypertension〉 〈a ~ vasectomy〉 — **re·vers·ibil·i·ty** \-ˌvər-sə-'bil-ət-ē\ *n, pl* **-ties** — **re·vers·ibly** \-'vər-sə-blē\ *adv*

reversible colloid *n* : a colloid that can be precipitated as a gel and then again dispersed as a sol

re·ver·sion \ri-'vər-zhən, -shən\ *n* **1 a** : an act or the process of returning (as to a former condition) **b** : a return toward an ancestral type or condition : reappearance of an ancestral character **2** : a product of reversion; *specif* : an organism with an atavistic character

re·vert \ri-'vərt\ *vi* : to undergo reversion — **re·vert·ible** \-'vərt-ə-bəl\ *adj*

re·ver·tant \ri-'vərt-ᵊnt\ *n* : a mutant gene, individual, or strain that regains a former capability (as the production of a

---

\ə\ abut \ᵊ\ kitten \ər\ further \a\ ash \ā\ ace \ä\ cot, cart
\au̇\ out \ch\ chin \e\ bet \ē\ easy \g\ go \i\ hit \ī\ ice \j\ job
\ŋ\ sing \ō\ go \ȯ\ law \ȯi\ boy \th\ thin \t͟h\ the \ü\ loot
\u̇\ foot \y\ yet \zh\ vision *See also* Pronunciation Symbols page

Q
R

particular protein) by undergoing further mutation ⟨yeast ∼s⟩ — **revertant** *adj*

re·vi·sion surgery \ri-'vizh-ən-\ *n* : surgery performed to replace or compensate for a failed implant (as a hip replacement) or to correct undesirable sequelae (as scars or scar tissue) of previous surgery

re·vi·tal·ize *also Brit* **re·vi·tal·ise** \(')rē-'vīt-ᵊl-ͺīz\ *vt* **-ized** *also Brit* **-ised; -iz·ing** *also Brit* **-is·ing** : to impart new life or vigor or to : restore to an active or fresh condition — **re·vi·tal·iza·tion** *also Brit* **re·vi·tal·isa·tion** \(ͺ)rē-ͺvīt-ᵊl-ə-'zā-shən\ *n*

re·vive \ri-'vīv\ *vb* **re·vived; re·viv·ing** *vi* : to return to consciousness or life ∼ *vt* **1** : to restore to consciousness or life **2** : to restore from a depressed, inactive, or unused state — **re·viv·able** \-'vī-və-bəl\ *adj*

re·viv·i·fi·ca·tion \'rē-ͺviv-ə-fə-'kā-shən\ *n* : renewal or restoration of life

re·vul·sion \ri-'vəl-shən\ *n* : alleviation of a localized disease by treatment (as with counterirritants) of an adjacent region

¹re·ward \ri-'wȯ(ə)rd\ *vt* : to give a reward to or for

²reward *n* : a stimulus (as food) that serves to reinforce a desired response

Reye's syndrome \'rīz- *also* 'rāz-\ *also* **Reye syndrome** \'rī- *also* 'rā-\ *n* : an often fatal encephalopathy esp. of childhood characterized by fever, vomiting, fatty infiltration of the liver, and swelling of the kidneys and brain

   Reye \'rī\, **Ralph Douglas Kenneth (1912–1977)**, Australian pathologist. Reye held the post of director of pathology at a hospital for children in Sydney, Australia. From 1951 to 1962 he studied 21 cases of Reye's syndrome. He presented his findings in an article published in 1963.

Rf *symbol* rutherfordium

RF *abbr* rheumatic fever

R factor \'är-\ *n* : a group of genes present in some bacteria that provide a basis for resistance to antibiotics and can be transferred from cell to cell by conjugation

RFLP \ͺär-(ͺ)ef-(ͺ)el-'pē\ *n* : RESTRICTION FRAGMENT LENGTH POLYMORPHISM

Rh \'är-'āch\ *adj* : of, relating to, or being an Rh factor ⟨∼ antigens⟩ ⟨∼ sensitization in pregnancy⟩

Rh *symbol* rhodium

RH *abbr* relative humidity

rhab·dit·i·form \rab-'dit-ə-ͺfȯrm\ *adj* : RHABDITOID

Rhab·di·tis \rab-'dīt-əs *also* -'dēt-\ *n* : a genus (the type of the family Rhabditidae) of minute nematode worms that have the esophagus clearly divided into three regions, live in soil and organic debris, and occas. occur as facultative parasites in mammalian tissues including those of humans

rhab·di·toid \'rab-di-ͺtȯid\ *adj, of a larval nematode* : having the esophagus functional and with an enlarged pharyngeal bulb

rhab·do·my·ol·y·sis \ͺrab-dō-mī-'äl-ə-səs\ *n, pl* **-y·ses** \-ͺsēz\ : the destruction or degeneration of skeletal muscle tissue (as from traumatic injury, excessive exertion, or stroke) that is accompanied by the release of muscle cell contents (as myoglobin and potassium) into the bloodstream resulting in hypovolemia, hyperkalemia, and sometimes acute renal failure

rhab·do·my·o·ma \ͺrab-dō-mī-'ō-mə\ *n, pl* **-mas** *also* **-ma·ta** \-mət-ə\ : a benign tumor composed of striated muscle fibers ⟨a cardiac ∼⟩

rhab·do·myo·sar·co·ma \'rab-(ͺ)dō-ͺmī-ə-sär-'kō-mə\ *n, pl* **-mas** *also* **-ma·ta** \-mət-ə\ : a malignant tumor composed of striated muscle fibers

Rhab·do·vi·ri·dae \ͺrab-(ͺ)dō-'vir-ə-ͺdē\ *n pl* : a family of single-stranded RNA viruses that are rod- or bullet-shaped, are found in plants and animals, and include the causative agents of rabies and vesicular stomatitis

rhab·do·vi·rus \'rab-(ͺ)dō-ͺvī-rəs\ *n* : any of the family *Rhabdoviridae* of single-stranded RNA viruses

rhachitis *var of* RACHITIS

rhag·a·des \'rag-ə-ͺdēz\ *n pl* : linear cracks or fissures in the skin occurring esp. at the angles of the mouth or about the anus

rha·gad·i·form \rə-'gad-ə-ͺfȯrm\ *adj* : having or characterized by cracks or fissures ⟨∼ eczema⟩

rham·nose \'ram-ͺnōs, -ͺnōz\ *n* : a crystalline sugar $C_6H_{12}O_5$ that occurs combined in many plants and is obtained in the common dextrorotatory L-form

rham·no·side \'ram-nə-ͺsīd\ *n* : a glycoside that yields rhamnose on hydrolysis

Rham·nus \'ram-nəs\ *n* : a genus (family Rhamnaceae) of trees and shrubs that have small flowers and a fruit which is a drupe and that comprise the buckthorns (as cascara buckthorn, *R. purshiana*) of which some yield pigments or purgatives (as cascara sagrada)

rhaphe *var of* RAPHE

rha·pon·tic \rə-'pän-tik\ *n* : a rhubarb (*Rheum rhaponticum*); *also* : the root of this plant used esp. formerly in pharmacy

rhat·a·ny \'rat-ᵊn-ē\ *n, pl* **-nies** : KRAMERIA 2

Rh disease *n* : ERYTHROBLASTOSIS FETALIS

rhe·ni·um \'rē-nē-əm\ *n* : a rare heavy metallic element that resembles manganese, is obtained either as a powder or as a silver-white hard metal, and is used in catalysts for dehydrogenation and in thermocouples — symbol *Re*; see ELEMENT table

rheo·base \'rē-ō-ͺbās\ *n* : the minimal electric current required to excite a tissue (as nerve or muscle) given an indefinitely long time during which the current is applied — compare CHRONAXIE — **rheo·ba·sic** \-ͺbā-sik, -zik\ *adj*

rheo·car·di·og·ra·phy \ͺrē-ō-ͺkärd-ē-'äg-rə-fē\ *n, pl* **-phies** : the recording of the changes in the body's electrical conductivity that are synchronous with the beating of the heart

rheo·log·i·cal \ͺrē-ə-'läj-i-kəl\ *also* **rheo·log·ic** \-ik\ *adj* : of or relating to rheology or to the phenomena of flowing matter — **rheo·log·i·cal·ly** \-i-k(ə-)lē\ *adv*

rhe·ol·o·gy \rē-'äl-ə-jē\ *n, pl* **-gies** : a science dealing with the deformation and flow of matter

rhe·om·e·ter \rē-'äm-ət-ər\ *n* : an instrument for measuring flow (as of viscous substances)

rheo·stat \'rē-ə-ͺstat\ *n* : a resistor for regulating a current by means of variable resistances — **rheo·stat·ic** \ͺrē-ə-'stat-ik\ *adj*

rheo·tac·tic \ͺrē-ə-'tak-tik\ *adj* : relating to or exhibiting rheotaxis ⟨∼ response⟩

rheo·tax·is \ͺrē-ə-'tak-səs\ *n, pl* **-tax·es** \-ͺsēz\ : a taxis in which mechanical stimulation by a stream of fluid (as water) is the directive factor

rhe·ot·ro·pism \rē-'ä-trə-ͺpiz-əm\ *n* : a tropism in which mechanical stimulation by a stream of fluid (as water) is the orienting factor

rhe·sus \'rē-səs\ *n* : RHESUS MONKEY

rhesus factor *n* : RH FACTOR

rhesus monkey *n* : a pale brown Asian monkey of the genus *Macaca* (*M. mulatta*) often used in medical research

rheum \'rüm\ *n* : a watery discharge from the mucous membranes esp. of the eyes or nose; *also* : a condition (as a cold) marked by such discharge — **rheumy** \-ē\ *adj*

Rhe·um \'rē-əm\ *n* : a genus of Asian herbs (family Polygonaceae) that have large leaves, small flowers, and a 3-winged fruit and that include the rhubarbs (as the Chinese rhubarb, *R. officinale*, and rhapontic, *R. rhaponticum*)

¹rheu·mat·ic \rù-'mat-ik\ *adj* : of, relating to, characteristic of, or affected with rheumatism ⟨∼ pain⟩ ⟨a ∼ joint⟩

²rheumatic *n* : an individual affected with rheumatism

rheumatica — see POLYMYALGIA RHEUMATICA, PURPURA RHEUMATICA

rheumatic disease *n* : any of several diseases (as rheumatic fever or fibrositis) characterized by inflammation and pain in muscles or joints : RHEUMATISM

rheumatic fever *n* : an acute often recurrent disease occurring chiefly in children and young adults and characterized by fever, inflammation, pain, and swelling in and around the joints, inflammatory involvement of the pericardium and valves of the heart, and often the formation of small nodules chiefly in the subcutaneous tissues and the heart

rheumatic heart disease *n* : active or inactive disease of the heart that results from rheumatic fever and that is characterized by reduced functional capacity of the heart caused by inflammatory changes in the myocardium or scarring of the valves

rheu·ma·tism \'rü-mə-ˌtiz-əm, 'rùm-ə-\ *n* **1** : any of various conditions characterized by inflammation or pain in muscles, joints, or fibrous tissue ⟨muscular ∼⟩ **2** : RHEUMATOID ARTHRITIS

rheu·ma·toid \-ˌtóid\ *adj* : characteristic of or affected with rheumatoid arthritis

rheumatoid arthritis *n* : a usu. chronic disease that is considered an autoimmune disease and is characterized esp. by pain, stiffness, inflammation, swelling, and sometimes destruction of joints — abbr. *RA;* called also *atrophic arthritis;* compare OSTEOARTHRITIS

rheumatoid factor *n* : an autoantibody of high molecular weight that reacts against immunoglobulins of the class IgG and is often present in rheumatoid arthritis

rheumatoid spondylitis *n* : ANKYLOSING SPONDYLITIS

rheu·ma·tol·o·gist \ˌrü-mə-'täl-ə-jəst, ˌrùm-ə-\ *n* : a specialist in rheumatology

rheu·ma·tol·o·gy \ˌrü-mə-'täl-ə-jē, ˌrùm-ə-\ *n, pl* **-gies** : a medical science dealing with rheumatic diseases — **rheu·ma·to·log·ic** \-tə-'läj-ik\ *or* **rheu·ma·to·log·i·cal** \-i-kəl\ *adj*

rhex·is \'rek-səs\ *n, pl* **rhex·es** \-ˌsēz\ : RUPTURE 1 ⟨∼ of a blood vessel⟩ ⟨∼ of an organ⟩

Rh factor \'är-'āch-\ *n* : a genetically determined protein on the red blood cells of some people that is one of the substances used to classify human blood as to compatibility for transfusion and that when present in a fetus but not in the mother causes a serious immunogenic reaction in which the mother produces antibodies that cross the placenta and attack the red blood cells of the fetus — called also *rhesus factor*

rhi·nal \'rīn-ᵊl\ *adj* : of or relating to the nose : NASAL

rhin·en·ceph·a·lon \ˌrī-(ˌ)nen-'sef-ə-ˌlän, -lən\ *n, pl* **-la** \-lə\ : the anterior inferior part of the forebrain that is chiefly concerned with olfaction and that is considered to include the olfactory bulb together with the forebrain olfactory structures receiving fibers directly from it and often esp. formerly the limbic system which is now known to be concerned with emotional states and affect — called also *smell brain* — **rhin·en·ce·phal·ic** \ˌrī-nen-sə-'fal-ik\ *adj*

rhi·ni·tis \rī-'nīt-əs\ *n, pl* **-nit·i·des** \-'nit-ə-ˌdēz\ : inflammation of the mucous membrane of the nose marked esp. by rhinorrhea, nasal congestion and itching, and sneezing; *also* : of various conditions characterized by rhinitis — see ALLERGIC RHINITIS, RHINITIS MEDICAMENTOSA, RHINITIS SICCA, VASOMOTOR RHINITIS

rhinitis me·dic·a·men·to·sa \-mə-ˌdik-ə-men-'tō-sə\ *n* : an increase in the severity or duration of rhinitis that results from prolonged use of decongestant nasal spray

rhinitis sic·ca \-'sik-ə\ *n* : a form of rhinitis in which the mucous membrane of the nose is abnormally dry

rhi·no·gen·ic \ˌrī-nə-'jen-ik\ *adj* : originating in or transmitted by way of the nose ⟨∼ meningitis⟩

rhi·no·la·lia \ˌrī-nə-'lā-lē-ə\ *n* : nasal tone in speech esp. when caused by excessive closure or openness of the posterior nares

rhi·no·lar·yn·gol·o·gy \'rī-nō-ˌlar-ən-'gäl-ə-jē\ *n, pl* **-gies** : a branch of medical science dealing with the nose and larynx

rhi·no·lith \'rī-nə-ˌlith\ *n* : a concretion formed within the cavities of the nose

rhi·no·li·thi·a·sis \ˌrī-nō-li-'thī-ə-səs\ *n, pl* **-a·ses** \-ˌsēz\ : the formation or presence of rhinoliths

rhi·no·log·ic \ˌrī-nə-'läj-ik\ *or* **rhi·no·log·i·cal** \-i-kəl\ *adj* : of or relating to the nose ⟨∼ disease⟩

rhi·nol·o·gist \rī-'näl-ə-jəst\ *n* : a physician who specializes in rhinology

rhi·nol·o·gy \-jē\ *n, pl* **-gies** : a branch of medicine that deals with the nose and its diseases

rhi·no·pha·ryn·geal \ˌrī-nō-ˌfar-ən-'jē-əl, -fə-'rin-j(ē-)əl\ *adj* : NASOPHARYNGEAL ⟨∼ cancer⟩

rhi·no·phar·yn·gi·tis \-ˌfar-ən-'jīt-əs\ *n, pl* **-git·i·des** \-'jit-ə-

ˌdēz\ : inflammation of the mucous membrane of the nose and pharynx

rhi·no·phar·ynx \-'far-iŋ(k)s\ *n, pl* **-pha·ryn·ges** \-fə-'rin-(ˌ)jēz\ *also* **-phar·ynx·es** : NASOPHARYNX

rhi·no·phy·ma \-'fī-mə\ *n, pl* **-mas** *or* **-ma·ta** \-mət-ə\ : a nodular swelling and congestion of the nose in an advanced stage of rosacea

rhi·no·plas·tic \-'plas-tik\ *adj* : of, relating to, or being rhinoplasty ⟨∼ surgery⟩

rhi·no·plas·ty \'rī-nō-ˌplas-tē\ *n, pl* **-ties** : plastic surgery on the nose usu. for cosmetic purposes — called also *nose job*

rhi·no·pneu·mo·ni·tis \ˌrī-nō-ˌn(y)ü-mə-'nīt-əs\ *n* : an acute febrile respiratory disease of horses that is caused by two herpesviruses of the genus *Varicellovirus* (species *Equid herpesvirus 1* and *Equid herpesvirus 4*), that is characterized esp. by rhinopharyngitis and tracheobronchitis, and that sometimes causes abortion in pregnant mares

rhi·nor·rha·gia \ˌrī-nə-'rā-j(ē-)ə\ *n* : NOSEBLEED

rhi·nor·rhea *or chiefly Brit* **rhi·nor·rhoea** \ˌrī-nə-'rē-ə\ *n* : excessive mucous secretion from the nose

rhi·no·scle·ro·ma \ˌrī-nō-sklə-'rō-mə\ *n, pl* **-ma·ta** \-mət-ə\ : a chronic inflammatory disease of the nasopharyngeal mucosa that is characterized by the formation of granulomas and by dense induration of the tissues and nodular deformity

rhi·no·scope \'rī-nə-ˌskōp\ *n* : an instrument (as an endoscope) for examining the cavities and passages of the nose — called also *nasoscope*

rhi·nos·co·py \rī-'näs-kə-pē\ *n, pl* **-pies** : examination of the nasal passages — **rhi·no·scop·ic** \ˌrī-nə-'skäp-ik\ *adj*

rhi·no·spo·rid·i·o·sis \ˌrī-nō-spə-ˌrid-ē-'ō-səs\ *n, pl* **-o·ses** \-ˌsēz\ : a fungal disease of the external mucous membranes (as of the nose) that is characterized by the formation of pinkish red, friable, sessile, or pedunculated polyps and is caused by an ascomycetous fungus of the genus *Rhinosporidium* (*R. seeberi*)

rhi·no·spo·rid·i·um \ˌrī-nō-spə-'rid-ē-əm\ *n* **1** *cap* : a genus of ascomycetous fungi that include the causative agent (*R. seeberi*) of rhinosporidiosis **2** *pl* **-ia** \-ē-ə\ : any fungus of the genus *Rhinosporidium*

rhi·not·o·my \rī-'nät-ə-mē\ *n, pl* **-mies** : surgical incision of the nose

rhi·no·tra·che·itis \ˌrī-nō-ˌtrā-kē-'īt-əs\ *n* : inflammation of the nasal cavities and trachea; *esp* : a disease of the upper respiratory system in cats and esp. young kittens that is characterized by sneezing, conjunctivitis with discharge, and nasal discharges — see INFECTIOUS BOVINE RHINOTRACHEITIS

rhi·no·vi·rus \ˌrī-nō-'vī-rəs\ *n* : any of a genus (*Rhinovirus*) of single-stranded RNA viruses of the family *Picornaviridae* including two species (*Human rhinovirus A* and *Human rhinovirus B*) and numerous serotypes currently unassigned to species that affect humans causing respiratory infections including the common cold

Rhipi·ceph·a·lus \ˌrip-ə-'sef-ə-ləs\ *n* : a large and widely distributed genus of ixodid ticks that are parasitic on many mammals and some birds and include vectors of serious diseases (as babesiosis of canines and east coast fever)

rhi·zo·bi·um \rī-'zō-bē-əm\ *n* **1** *cap* : a genus (family Rhizobiaceae) of small heterotrophic soil bacteria capable of forming symbiotic nodules on the roots of leguminous plants where they fix atmospheric nitrogen **2** *pl* **-bia** \-bē-ə\ : any bacterium of the genus *Rhizobium*

rhi·zoid \'rī-ˌzóid\ *n* : a rootlike structure — **rhi·zoi·dal** \rī-'zóid-ᵊl\ *adj*

rhi·zo·ma·tous \rī-'zō-mət-əs\ *adj* : having or resembling a rhizome ⟨a drug from a ∼ root⟩

rhi·zome \'rī-ˌzōm\ *n* : a usu. horizontal subterranean plant stem that is distinguished from a true root in possessing buds, nodes, and usu. scalelike leaves

---

\ə\ **abut** \ᵊ\ **kitten** \ər\ **further** \a\ **ash** \ā\ **ace** \ä\ **cot, cart**
\aù\ **out** \ch\ **chin** \e\ **bet** \ē\ **easy** \g\ **go** \i\ **hit** \ī\ **ice** \j\ **job**
\ŋ\ **sing** \ō\ **go** \ò\ **law** \òi\ **boy** \th\ **thin** \th̲\ **the** \ü\ **loot**
\ù\ **foot** \y\ **yet** \zh\ **vision** *See also* Pronunciation Symbols page

rhi·zo·me·lic \ˌrī-zə-'mē-lik\ *adj* : of or relating to the hip and shoulder joints

rhi·zo·plast \'rī-zə-ˌplast\ *n* : a fibril that connects the blepharoplast with the nucleus in flagellated cells or organisms

rhi·zo·pod \'rī-zə-ˌpäd\ *n* : any protozoan of the subclass Rhizopoda

¹Rhi·zop·o·da \rī-'zäp-ə-də\ *n pl* : a subclass of the class Sarcodina comprising usu. creeping protozoans (as an ameba or a foraminifer) having lobate or rootlike pseudopodia

²Rhizopoda *n pl, syn of* SARCODINA

rhi·zo·pus \'rī-zə-pəs\ *n* **1** *cap* : a genus of fungi of the family Mucoraceae that have columellate hemispherical aerial sporangia formed in fascicles anchored to the substrate and tufts of rhizoids or root hyphae connected by stolons and that include a common bread mold (*R. nigricans*) and several forms found in phycomycoses of some mammals including humans **2** : any fungus of the genus *Rhizopus*

rhi·zot·o·my \rī-'zät-ə-mē\ *n, pl* **-mies** : the operation of cutting the anterior or posterior spinal nerve roots

Rh–neg·a·tive \ˌär-ˌāch-'neg-ət-iv\ *adj* : lacking Rh factor in the blood

rho·da·mine \'rōd-ə-ˌmēn\ *n* : any of a group of yellowish red to blue fluorescent dyes; *esp* : RHODAMINE B

rhodamine B \-'bē\ *n* : a brilliant bluish red dye made by fusing an amine derivative of phenol with phthalic anhydride and used esp. in coloring paper and as a biological stain

rho·da·nese \'rōd-ə-ˌnēz, -ˌnēs\ *n* : a crystallizable enzyme that catalyzes the conversion of cyanide and thiosulfate to thiocyanate and sulfite and that occurs in animal tissues and bacteria

rho·da·nine \'rōd-ə-ˌnēn\ *n* : a pale yellow crystalline acid $C_3H_3NOS_2$ that is derived from thiazole and is used in the synthesis of phenylalanine

rho·di·um \'rōd-ē-əm\ *n* : a white hard ductile metallic element that is resistant to attack by acids, occurs in platinum ores, and is used in alloys with platinum — symbol *Rh*; see ELEMENT table

Rhod·ni·us \'räd-nē-əs\ *n* : a genus of reduviid bugs including some that are intermediate hosts of the trypanosome causing Chagas' disease

rho·dop·sin \rō-'däp-sən\ *n* : a red photosensitive pigment in the retinal rods of marine fishes and most higher vertebrates that is important in vision in dim light, is quickly bleached by light to a mixture of opsin and retinal, and is regenerated in the dark — called also *visual purple*

Rho·do·tor·u·la \ˌrōd-ə-'tor-yə-lə\ *n* : a genus of yeasts (family Cryptococcaceae) including one (*R. rubra* syn. *R. mucilaginosa*) sometimes present in the blood or involved in endocarditis prob. as a secondary infection

rhomb·en·ceph·a·lon \ˌräm-(ˌ)ben-'sef-ə-ˌlän, -lən\ *n, pl* **-la** \-lə\ : HINDBRAIN — **rhomb·en·ce·phal·ic** \-sə-'fal-ik\ *adj*

rhomboidalis — see SINUS RHOMBOIDALIS

rhom·boi·de·us \räm-'boid-ē-əs\ *n, pl* **-dei** \-ē-ˌī\ : either of two muscles that lie beneath the trapezius muscle and connect the spinous processes of various vertebrae with the medial border of the scapula: **a** : RHOMBOIDEUS MINOR **b** : RHOMBOIDEUS MAJOR

rhomboideus major *n* : a muscle arising from the spinous processes of the second through fifth thoracic vertebrae, inserted into the vertebral border of the scapula, and acting to adduct and laterally rotate the scapula — called also *rhomboid major*

rhomboideus minor *n* : a muscle arising from the inferior part of the ligamentum nuchae and from the spinous processes of the seventh cervical and first thoracic vertebrae, inserted into the vertebral border of the scapula at the base of the bony process terminating in the acromion, and acting to adduct and laterally rotate the scapula — called also *rhomboid minor*

rhomboid fossa *n* : the floor of the fourth ventricle of the brain formed by the dorsal surfaces of the pons and medulla oblongata

rhomboid major *n* : RHOMBOIDEUS MAJOR

rhomboid minor *n* : RHOMBOIDEUS MINOR

rhon·chus \'räŋ-kəs\ *n, pl* **rhon·chi** \'räŋ-ˌkī\ : a whistling or snoring sound heard on auscultation of the chest when the air channels are partly obstructed — compare RALE, RATTLE 2

rho·ta·cism \'rōt-ə-ˌsiz-əm\ *n* : a defective pronunciation of *r; esp* : substitution of some other sound for that of *r*

Rh–pos·i·tive \ˌär-ˌāch-'päz-ət-iv, -'päz-tiv\ *adj* : containing Rh factor in the red blood cells

rhu·barb \'rü-ˌbärb\ *n* **1** : any of several plants of the genus *Rheum* having large leaves with thick succulent petioles often used as food **2** : the dried rhizome and roots of any of several rhubarbs (esp. *Rheum officinale* and *R. palmatum*) grown in China and Tibet and used as a purgative and stomachic

rhus \'rüs\ *n* **1** *cap* : a genus of shrubs and trees of the cashew family (Anacardiaceae) that are native to temperate and warm regions, have compound trifoliolate or pinnate leaves, and include some (as poison ivy, poison oak, and poison sumac) producing irritating oils that cause dermatitis — see SUMAC, TOXICODENDRON **2** *pl* **rhuses** *or* **rhus** : any shrub or tree of the genus *Rhus*

rhus dermatitis *n* : dermatitis caused by contact with various plants of the genus *Rhus* and esp. with the common poison ivy (*R. radicans*)

rhythm \'rith-əm\ *n* **1** : a regularly recurrent quantitative change in a variable biological process: as **a** : the pattern of recurrence of the cardiac cycle ⟨an irregular ∼⟩ **b** : the recurring pattern of physical and functional changes associated with the mammalian and esp. human sexual cycle **2** : RHYTHM METHOD

rhyth·mic \'rith-mik\ *or* **rhyth·mi·cal** \-mi-kəl\ *adj* **1** : of, relating to, or involving rhythm **2** : marked by or moving in pronounced rhythm ⟨∼ contractions⟩ — **rhyth·mi·cal·ly** \-mi-k(ə-)lē\ *adv*

rhyth·mic·i·ty \rith-'mis-ət-ē\ *n, pl* **-ties** : the state of being rhythmic or responding rhythmically ⟨the ∼ of the heart⟩

rhythm method *n* : a method of birth control involving continence during the period of the sexual cycle in which ovulation is most likely to occur

rhyt·i·dec·to·my \ˌrit-ə-'dek-tə-mē\ *n, pl* **-mies** : FACE-LIFT

RIA *abbr* radioimmunoassay

rib \'rib\ *n* : any of the paired curved bony or partly cartilaginous rods that stiffen the lateral walls of the body of most vertebrates and protect the viscera, that occur in mammals exclusively or almost exclusively in the thoracic region, and that in humans normally include 12 pairs of which all are articulated with the spinal column at the dorsal end and the first 10 are connected also at the ventral end with the sternum by costal cartilages — see FALSE RIB, FLOATING RIB, TRUE RIB

ri·ba·vi·rin \ˌrī-bə-'vī-rən\ *n* : a synthetic broad-spectrum antiviral drug $C_8H_{12}N_4O_5$ that is a nucleoside resembling guanosine

rib cage *n* : the bony enclosing wall of the chest consisting chiefly of the ribs and the structures connecting them — called also *thoracic cage*

ri·bi·tol \'rī-bə-ˌtol, -ˌtōl\ *n* : ADONITOL

ri·bo·fla·vin \ˌrī-bə-'flā-vən, 'rī-bə-ˌ\ *also* **ri·bo·fla·vine** \-ˌvēn\ *n* : a yellow crystalline compound $C_{17}H_{20}N_4O_6$ that is a growth-promoting member of the vitamin B complex and occurs both free (as in milk) and combined (as in liver) — called also *lactoflavin, ovoflavin, vitamin B_2*

riboflavin phosphate *or* **riboflavin 5′–phosphate** \-'fiv-'prīm-\ *n* : FMN

ri·bo·nu·cle·ase \ˌrī-bō-'n(y)ü-klē-ˌās, -ˌāz\ *n* : an enzyme that catalyzes the hydrolysis of RNA — called also *RNase*

ri·bo·nu·cle·ic acid \ˌrī-bō-n(y)ü-ˌklē-ik-, -ˌklā-\ *n* : RNA

ri·bo·nu·cleo·pro·tein \-ˌn(y)ü-klē-ō-'prō-ˌtēn, -'prōt-ē-ən\ *n* : a nucleoprotein that contains RNA

ri·bo·nu·cle·o·side \-'n(y)ü-klē-ə-ˌsīd\ *n* : a nucleoside that contains ribose

ri·bo·nu·cle·o·tide \-ˌtīd\ n : a nucleotide that contains ribose and occurs esp. as a constituent of RNA

ri·bose \ˈrī-ˌbōs, -ˌbōz\ n : a pentose $C_5H_{10}O_5$ found esp. in the levorotatory D-form as a constituent of a number of nucleosides (as adenosine, cytidine, and guanosine) esp. in RNA

ri·bo·side \ˈrī-bə-ˌsīd\ n : a glycoside that yields ribose on hydrolysis

ribosomal RNA n : RNA that is a fundamental structural element of ribosomes — called also *rRNA*

ri·bo·some \ˈrī-bə-ˌsōm\ n : any of the RNA- and protein‑rich cytoplasmic granules that are sites of protein synthesis — **ri·bo·som·al** \ˌrī-bə-ˈsō-məl\ adj

ri·bo·zyme \ˈrī-bə-ˌzīm\ n : a molecule of RNA that functions as an enzyme (as by catalyzing the cleavage of other RNA molecules)

ri·bu·lose \ˈrib-yə-ˌlōs also -ˌlōz\ n : a ketose $C_5H_{10}O_5$ that plays a role in carbohydrate metabolism

Ric·co's law \ˈrik-ōz-\ n : a statement in physiology: when a light source of a given size and intensity is just capable of producing visual sensation, reduction of either size or intensity will make it invisible

    Ric·cò \rēk-ˈkō\, **Annibale (1844–1919)**, Italian astrophysicist. A professor of astrophysics, Riccò founded an astronomical and meteorological station on Mt. Etna. For over forty years, he conducted a regular series of direct and spectroscopic observations of the sun, accumulating data on the frequency, position, and development of sunspots and clouds of solar gases and on their influence on terrestrial phenomena. Also interested in geodesy and geophysics, he made measurements in Sicily of the local values of the earth's gravitational and magnetic fields.

RICE abbr rest, ice, compression, elevation — used esp. for the initial treatment of many usu. minor sports-related injuries (as sprains)

rice body n : any of the smooth glistening ovoid particles resembling grains of rice that occur in joints and the sheaths of tendons and bursae as a result of chronic inflammation

rice pol·ish \-ˌpäl-ish\ n : RICE POLISHINGS

rice polishings n pl : the inner bran layer of rice rubbed off in milling and used as a source of thiamin, riboflavin, and niacin — called also *tikitiki*

rice–water stool n : a watery stool containing white flecks of mucus, epithelial cells, and bacteria and discharged from the bowels in severe forms of diarrhea (as in Asiatic cholera)

ri·cin \ˈrīs-ᵊn, ˈris-\ n : a poisonous protein in the castor bean

ri·cin·ole·ic acid \ˌrīs-ᵊn-ō-ˌlē-ik-, ˌris-, -ˌlā-\ n : an oily unsaturated hydroxy fatty acid $C_{18}H_{34}O_3$ that occurs in castor oil as a glyceride

ric·i·nus \ˈris-ᵊn-əs\ n **1** cap : a genus of plants of the spurge family (Euphorbiaceae) that have large palmate leaves and flowers with numerous stamens and include the castor-oil plant (*R. communis*) **2** : any plant of the genus *Ricinus*

rick·ets \ˈrik-əts\ n pl but sing in constr : a deficiency disease that affects the young during the period of skeletal growth, is characterized esp. by soft and deformed bones, and is caused by failure to assimilate and use calcium and phosphorus normally due to inadequate sunlight or vitamin D — called also *rachitis*

rick·etts·emia or chiefly Brit **rick·etts·ae·mia** \ˌrik-ət-ˈsē-mē-ə\ n : the abnormal presence of rickettsiae in the blood

    Rick·etts \ˈrik-əts\, **Howard Taylor (1871–1910)**, American pathologist. Ricketts is remembered for his discovery of the causative organisms and mode of transmission of Rocky Mountain spotted fever and typhus. He began studying Rocky Mountain spotted fever in 1906. He showed that the disease could be transmitted to a healthy animal by the bite of a certain tick. Two years later he described the causative microorganism. He had discovered it in the blood of the infected animals as well as in the ticks and their eggs. In 1909 he went to Mexico to study typhus. He found that the kind of typhus he was studying was transmitted by the body louse, and he was able to locate the disease-causing organism in the blood of the victim and in the lice. He went on to

demonstrate that the disease could be transmitted to monkeys, who, after they had recovered, would develop immunity to the disease. His work on immunity and sera became the basis for further advancement in vaccines.

rick·ett·sia \ri-ˈket-sē-ə\ n **1** cap : the type genus of the family Rickettsiaceae comprising rod-shaped, coccoid, or diplococcus-shaped often pleomorphic bacteria that live intracellularly in biting arthropods (as lice or ticks) and when transmitted to humans by the bite of an arthropod host cause a number of serious diseases (as Rocky Mountain spotted fever and typhus) **2** pl **-si·ae** \-ˌē\ also **-sias** or **-sia** : any bacterium of the order Rickettsiales and esp. of the family Rickettsiaceae

Rick·ett·si·a·ce·ae \ri-ˌket-sē-ˈā-sē-ˌē\ n pl : a family of bacteria of the order Rickettsiales that are typically inhabitants of arthropod tissues, are capable in some cases of causing serious disease when transmitted to vertebrates including humans, and include esp. the genera *Rickettsia* and *Cowdria*

rick·ett·si·al \ri-ˈket-sē-əl\ adj : of, relating to, or caused by rickettsiae ⟨a ∼ disease⟩ ⟨∼ vaccines⟩

Rick·ett·si·a·les \ri-ˌket-sē-ˈā-(ˌ)lēz\ n pl : an order of small pleomorphic gram-negative bacteria that are obligate parasites living in vertebrates or in arthropods which often serve as vectors of those parasitic in vertebrates and are placed in the families Anaplasmataceae, Bartonellaceae, and Rickettsiaceae

rick·ett·si·al·pox \ri-ˌket-sē-əl-ˈpäks\ n : a disease characterized by fever, chills, headache, backache, and a spotty rash and caused by a bacterium of the genus *Rickettsia* (*R. akari*) transmitted to humans by the bite of a mite of the genus *Allodermanyssus* (*A. sanguineus*) living on rodents (as the house mouse)

rick·ett·si·ol·o·gy \ri-ˌket-sē-ˈäl-ə-jē\ n, pl **-gies** : a branch of science that deals with the rickettsiae

rick·ett·si·o·sis \ri-ˌket-sē-ˈō-səs\ n, pl **-o·ses** \-ˌsēz\ : infection with or disease caused by a rickettsia ⟨a mild ∼⟩

rick·ett·sio·stat·ic \ri-ˌket-sē-ə-ˈstat-ik\ adj : inhibiting the growth of rickettsiae ⟨the ∼ effect of chloramphenicol⟩

rick·ety \ˈrik-ət-ē\ adj : affected with rickets : RACHITIC

Ri·de·al–Walk·er test \ri-ˈdē(ə)l-ˈwȯ-kər-\ n : a test for determining the phenol coefficient esp. of a disinfectant

    Rideal, Samuel (1863–1929), and **Walker, J. T. Ainslie (1868–1930)**, British chemists. Rideal taught chemistry and was an expert on the purification of water and sewage. He wrote extensively on food preservation, disinfection and disinfectants, and public water supplies. Rideal and Walker introduced their method for testing disinfectants in 1903.

rid·er embolus \ˈrīd-ər-\ n : SADDLE EMBOLUS

ridge \ˈrij\ n : a raised or elevated part and esp. a body part: as **a** : the projecting or elevated part of the back along the line of the backbone **b** : an elevated body part projecting from a surface

ridg·el \ˈrij-əl\ n : RIDGELING

ridge·ling or **ridg·ling** \ˈrij-liŋ\ n **1** : a partially castrated male animal **2** : a male animal having one or both testes retained in the inguinal canal

Rie·del's disease \ˈrēd-ᵊlz-\ n : chronic thyroiditis in which the thyroid gland becomes hard and stony and firmly attached to surrounding tissues

    Riedel, Bernhard Moritz Karl Ludwig (1846–1916), German surgeon. Riedel was a professor of surgery at Jena, Germany. He performed the first surgical operation for hip luxation. He published classic descriptions of a tongue-shaped part of the liver attached to its right lobe (1888), a tumor found in chronic pancreatitis (1896), and a type of chronic inflammation of the thyroid (1896).

Riedel's struma n : RIEDEL'S DISEASE

rif·a·bu·tin \ˈrif-ə-ˌbyüt-ᵊn\ n : a semisynthetic antibacterial drug $C_{46}H_{62}N_4O_{11}$ used esp. to prevent infection with bacte-

---

\ə\ abut \ᵊ\ kitten \ər\ further \a\ ash \ā\ ace \ä\ cot, cart \au̇\ out \ch\ chin \e\ bet \ē\ easy \g\ go \i\ hit \ī\ ice \j\ job \ŋ\ sing \ō\ go \ȯ\ law \ȯi\ boy \th\ thin \th\ the \ü\ loot \u̇\ foot \y\ yet \zh\ vision See also Pronunciation Symbols page

ria of the Mycobacterium avium complex in individuals affected with AIDS

ri·fam·pin \rī-'fam-pən\ *or* **ri·fam·pi·cin** \rī-'fam-pə-sən\ *n* : a semisynthetic antibiotic $C_{43}H_{58}N_4O_{12}$ that is used esp. in the treatment of tuberculosis and to treat asymptomatic carriers of meningococci

rif·a·my·cin \rif-ə-'mīs-ᵊn\ *n* : any of several antibiotics that are derived from a bacterium of the genus *Streptomyces* (*S. mediterranei*)

Rift Val·ley fever \'rift-val-ē-\ *n* : an acute usu. epizootic mosquito-borne disease of domestic animals (as sheep and cattle) chiefly of eastern and southern Africa that is caused by a bunyavirus of the genus *Phlebovirus* (species *Rift Valley fever virus*), is marked esp. by fever, abortion, death of newborns, diarrhea, and jaundice, and is sometimes transmitted to humans usu. in a milder form marked by flulike symptoms

Riggs' disease \'rigz-\ *n* : PYORRHEA 2

Riggs, John Mankey (1810–1885), American dentist. Riggs is remembered for his description and treatment of the advanced form of periodontal disease known as pyorrhea or pyorrhea alveolaris. His method of treatment consisted of removing from the teeth, with scrapers that he had designed, the salivary and serumal deposits and necrosed bone. A tincture prepared from powdered myrrh was then applied as a protective, and the teeth were polished. He first demonstrated his method in 1865. He published a description of pyorrhea alveolaris (or Riggs' disease, as it is sometimes called) and his treatment for it in 1876. His other notable accomplishment was extracting a tooth in 1844 using nitrous oxide gas to produce anesthesia.

right \'rīt\ *adj* : of, relating to, or being the side of the body which is away from the heart and on which the hand is stronger in most people ⟨her ∼ foot⟩; *also* : located nearer to this side than to the left — **right** *adv*

right atrioventricular valve *n* : TRICUSPID VALVE

right brain *n* : the right cerebral hemisphere of the human brain esp. when viewed in terms of its predominant thought processes (as creativity and intuitive thinking) — **right–brained** \-'brānd\ *adj*

right colic artery *n* : COLIC ARTERY a

right colic flexure *n* : HEPATIC FLEXURE

right–eyed *adj* : using the right eye in preference (as in using a camera or a monocular microscope)

right gastric artery *n* : an artery that arises from the hepatic artery, passes to the left along the lesser curvature of the stomach while giving off a number of branches, and eventually joins a branch of the left gastric artery

right gastroepiploic artery *n* : GASTROEPIPLOIC ARTERY a

right–hand \'rīt-hand\ *adj* **1** : situated on the right **2** : RIGHT-HANDED

right hand *n* **1** : the hand on a person's right side **2** : the right side

right–hand·ed \-'han-dəd\ *adj* **1** : using the right hand habitually or more easily than the left **2** : relating to, designed for, or done with the right hand **3** : having the same direction or course as the movement of the hands of a watch viewed from in front **4** : DEXTROROTATORY — **right–handed** *adv*

right–hand·ed·ness \-nəs\ *n* : the quality or state of being right-handed

right heart *n* : the right atrium and ventricle : the half of the heart that receives blood from the systemic circulation and passes it into the pulmonary arteries

right lymphatic duct *n* : a short vessel that receives lymph from the right side of the head, neck, and thorax, the right arm, right lung, right side of the heart, and convex surface of the liver and that discharges it into the right subclavian vein at its junction with the right internal jugular vein

right pulmonary artery *n* : PULMONARY ARTERY b

right subcostal vein *n* : SUBCOSTAL VEIN a

right–to–life *adj* : ANTIABORTION

right–to–lif·er \rīt-tə-'lī-fər\ *n* : ANTIABORTIONIST

rig·id \'rij-əd\ *adj* : deficient in or devoid of flexibility : characterized by stiffness ⟨∼ muscles⟩

ri·gid·i·ty \rə-'jid-ət-ē\ *n, pl* **-ties** : the quality or state of being rigid: as **a** : abnormal stiffness of muscle ⟨muscle ∼ symptomatic of Parkinson's disease —Diane Gershon⟩ **b** : emotional inflexibility and resistance to change

rigidus — see HALLUX RIGIDUS

rig·or \'rig-ər, *Brit also* 'rī-gör\ *n* **1 a** : CHILL 1 **b** : a tremor caused by a chill **2 a** : rigidity or torpor of organs or tissue that prevents response to stimuli **b** : RIGOR MORTIS

rig·or mor·tis \rig-ər-'mört-əs *also chiefly Brit* rī-gö(ə)r-\ *n* : temporary rigidity of muscles occurring after death

Ri·ley–Day syndrome \'rī-lē-'dā-\ *n* : FAMILIAL DYSAUTONOMIA

Riley, Conrad Milton (*b* 1913), American pediatrician. Riley served for several years as professor of pediatrics at Columbia University's College of Physicians and Surgeons before assuming the permanent position of professor of pediatrics and preventive medicine at the University of Colorado's School of Medicine. He and R. L. Day published their description of familial dysautonomia in a 1949 issue of *Pediatrics*. Other topics of Riley's research included nephrosis and osseous diseases in children.

Day, Richard Lawrence (1905–1989), American pediatrician. Day held successive positions as instructor or professor of pediatrics at the medical schools of Columbia University, Cornell University, the State University of New York, the University of Pittsburgh, and New York City's Mt. Sinai School of Medicine. His varied topics of research included neonatology, the Heimlich maneuver, and acupuncture.

ri·ma \'rī-mə\ *n, pl* **ri·mae** \-mē\ : an anatomical fissure or cleft

rima glot·ti·dis \-'glät-əd-əs\ *n* : the passage in the glottis between the true vocal cords

ri·man·ta·dine \rə-'man-tə-dēn, -dīn\ *n* : a synthetic antiviral drug that is chemically related to amantadine and is administered orally in the form of its hydrochloride $C_{12}H_{21}N \cdot HCl$ in the prevention and treatment of influenza A

rima pal·pe·bra·rum \-pal-pē-'brer-əm\ *n* : PALPEBRAL FISSURE

rima pu·den·di \-pyü-'den-dī\ *n* : PUDENDAL CLEFT

rin·der·pest \'rin-dər-pest\ *n* : an acute infectious usu. fatal disease of ruminant animals (as cattle) that is caused by a paramyxovirus of the genus *Morbillivirus* (species *Rinderpest virus*) and is marked by fever, diarrhea, and inflammation of mucous membranes — called also *cattle plague*

¹ring \'rin\ *n* **1 a** : a circular band **b** : an anatomical structure having a circular opening : ANNULUS **2** : an arrangement of atoms represented in formulas or models in a cyclic manner as a closed chain — called also *cycle*

²ring *vi* **rang** \'ran\; **rung** \'rən\; **ring·ing** \'rin-in\ : to have the sensation of being filled with a humming sound ⟨his ears *rang*⟩

ring·bone \-bōn\ *n* : a bony outgrowth on the phalangeal bones of a horse's foot that usu. produces lameness

Ring·er's fluid \'rin-ərz-\ *n* : RINGER'S SOLUTION

Ringer, Sidney (1835–1910), British physiologist. Ringer spent his entire career as a member of the faculty of a university hospital. He was known as the author of a popular handbook on therapeutics that was a practical treatise summarizing the actions and effects of drugs. Having a lifelong interest in pharmacology, he contributed papers on the actions of various substances, including digitalis, atropine, muscarine, and pilocarpine. From 1882 to 1885 in a series of classic experiments on frog hearts, Ringer developed a balanced solution for keeping isolated organs functional for long periods of time. The solution is now called Ringer's solution.

Ringer's lactate *or* **Ringer's lactate solution** *n* : LACTATED RINGER'S SOLUTION

Ringer's solution *also* **Ring·er solution** \'rin-ər-\ *n* : a sterile aqueous solution of calcium chloride, sodium chloride, and potassium chloride that provides a medium essentially isotonic to many animal tissues and that is used esp. to replenish fluids and electrolytes by intravenous infusion or to irrigate tissues by topical application — compare LACTATED RINGER'S SOLUTION

ring·hals \'riŋ-ˌhals\ *n* : a venomous African elapid snake (*Haemachates haemachatus*) that is closely related to the true cobras but has carinate scales and that seldom strikes but spits or sprays its venom aiming at the eyes of its victim where the poison causes intense pain and possible blindness

ring test *n* : a test for antigens or antibodies in which a layer of diluted material suspected of containing antigen is placed over a column of known antiserum in a small test tube or a layer of diluted known antigen is placed over serum suspected of containing antibodies and is then examined for a positive reaction signaled by formation of a thin plane or ring of precipitate

ring·worm \'riŋ-ˌwərm\ *n* : any of several contagious diseases of the skin, hair, or nails of humans and domestic animals caused by fungi (as of the genus *Trichophyton*) and characterized by ring-shaped discolored patches on the skin that are covered with vesicles and scales — called also *tinea*

Rin·ne's test \'rin-əz-\ *or* **Rin·ne test** \'rin-ə-\ *n* : a test for determining a subject's ability to hear a vibrating tuning fork when it is held next to the ear and when it is placed on the mastoid process with diminished hearing acuity through air and somewhat heightened hearing acuity through bone being symptomatic of conduction deafness

   Rinne, Heinrich Adolf R. (1819–1868), German otologist. Rinne engaged in private medical practice before accepting a position at a public asylum. He published a notable work on the vocal organs and the development of speech in 1850. In 1855 in a treatise on the physiology of the human ear he introduced Rinne's test for hearing loss.

ris·ed·ro·nate \ri-'sed-rə-ˌnāt\ *n* : a sodium bisphosphonate salt $C_7H_{10}NNaO_7P_2$ used esp. to prevent or treat osteoporosis in postmenopausal women

risk \'risk\ *n* **1** : possibility of loss, injury, disease, or death ⟨hypertension increases the ∼ of stroke⟩ **2** : a person considered in terms of the possible bad effects of a particular course of treatment ⟨a poor surgical ∼⟩ — **at risk** : characterized by high risk or susceptibility (as to disease) ⟨patients *at risk* of developing infections⟩

risk factor *n* : something which increases risk or susceptibility ⟨a fatty diet is a *risk factor* for heart disease⟩

ri·so·ri·us \ri-'sōr-ē-əs, -'zòr-\ *n, pl* **-rii** \-ē-ˌī\ : a narrow band of muscle fibers arising from the fascia over the masseter muscle, inserted into the tissues at the corner of the mouth, and acting to retract the angle of the mouth

Ris·per·dal \'ris-pər-ˌdal\ *trademark* — used for a preparation of risperidone

ris·per·i·done \ri-'sper-ə-ˌdōn\ *n* : an antipsychotic drug $C_{23}H_{27}FN_4O_2$ noted for its affinity for certain serotonin, dopamine, alpha-adrenergic, and histamine receptors in the brain — see RISPERDAL

ris·to·ce·tin \ˌris-tə-'sēt-ᵊn\ *n* : either of two antibiotics or a mixture of both produced by an actinomycete of the genus *Nocardia* (*N. lurida*)

ri·sus sar·do·ni·cus \'rī-səs-ˌsär-'dän-i-kəs, 'rē-\ *n* : a facial expression characterized by raised eyebrows and grinning distortion of the face resulting from spasm of facial muscles esp. in tetanus

Rit·a·lin \'rit-ə-lən\ *trademark* — used for a preparation of the hydrochloride of methylphenidate

rit·o·drine \'rit-ə-ˌdrēn, -drən\ *n* : a drug administered intravenously in the form of its hydrochloride $C_{17}H_{21}NO_3 \cdot HCl$ as a smooth muscle relaxant esp. to inhibit premature labor

ri·to·na·vir \ˌrī-'tō-nə-ˌvir, -'tän-ə-, ri-\ *n* : an antiviral protease inhibitor $C_{37}H_{48}N_6O_5S_2$ administered orally to treat HIV infection and AIDS — see NORVIR

Rit·ter's disease \'rit-ərz-\ *n* : STAPHYLOCOCCAL SCALDED SKIN SYNDROME

   Ritter von Rittershain \'rit-ər-fòn-'rit-ərz-ˌhīn\, **Gottfried (1820–1883)**, German physician. Ritter first described

staphylococcal scalded skin syndrome in brief in 1870, publishing a full description in 1878.

rit·u·al \'rich-(ə-)wəl\ *n* : any act or practice regularly repeated in a set precise manner for relief of anxiety ⟨obsessive-compulsive ∼s⟩

ri·val·ry \'rī-vəl-rē\ *n, pl* **-ries** **1** : a competitive or antagonistic state or condition **2** : RETINAL RIVALRY

riv·er blindness \'riv-ər-\ *n* : ONCHOCERCIASIS

RK *abbr* radial keratotomy

RLF *abbr* retrolental fibroplasia

RLQ *abbr* right lower quadrant (abdomen)

RLS *abbr* restless legs syndrome

Rn *symbol* radon

RN \'är-'en\ *n* : REGISTERED NURSE

RNA \ˌär-ˌen-'ā\ *n* : any of various nucleic acids that contain ribose and uracil as structural components and are associated with the control of cellular chemical activities — called also *ribonucleic acid;* see MESSENGER RNA, RIBOSOMAL RNA, TRANSFER RNA

RNAi \ˌär-ˌen-ˌā-'ī\ *n* : RNA INTERFERENCE

RNA interference *n* : a posttranscriptional genetic mechanism of various eukaryotes (as plants, fungi, nematodes, and mammals) which suppresses gene expression and in which double-stranded RNA cleaved into small fragments initiates the degradation of a complementary messenger RNA; *also* : a technique (as the introduction of double-stranded RNA into an organism) that artificially induces RNA interference and is used for studying or regulating gene expression

RNA polymerase *n* : any of a group of enzymes that promote the synthesis of RNA using DNA or RNA as a template

RNA replicase *n* : REPLICASE

RN·ase *or* **RNA·ase** \ˌär-ˌen-'ā-ˌās, -'ā-ˌāz\ *n* : RIBONUCLE-ASE

RNA syn·the·tase \-'sin-thə-ˌtās, -ˌtāz\ *n* : REPLICASE

RNA tumor virus *n* : RETROVIRUS

RNA virus *n* : a virus (as a paramyxovirus or a retrovirus) whose genome consists of RNA

roach \'rōch\ *n* : COCKROACH

roar·er \'rōr-ər, 'ròr-\ *n* : a horse subject to roaring

roar·ing \-iŋ\ *n* : noisy inhalation in a horse esp. upon exercising that is caused by paralysis and muscular atrophy of part of the larynx — compare GRUNTING, THICK WIND

Rob·ert·so·ni·an \ˌräb-ərt-'sō-nē-ən\ *adj* : relating to or being a reciprocal translocation that takes place between two acrocentric chromosomes and that yields one nonfunctional chromosome having two short arms and one functional chromosome having two long arms of which one arm is derived from each parent chromosome

   Rob·ert·son \'räb-ərt-sən\, **William Rees Brebner (1881–1941)**, American biologist. Robertson held a series of academic posts as an instructor in anatomy, histology, and embryology. He first described Robertsonian translocations in 1916.

Ro·bi·nul \'rō-bi-ˌnùl\ *trademark* — used for a preparation of glycopyrrolate

Rob·i·son ester \'räb-ə-sən-\ *n* : GLUCOSE-6-PHOSPHATE

   Robison, Robert (1883–1941), British biochemist. Robison was appointed to the staff of the Lister Institute of Preventive Medicine in London in 1913. He began research in the products of yeast fermentation. Within a short time he successfully isolated glucose-6-phosphate, which came to be known also as the Robison ester. In 1923 he announced the discovery of the enzyme phosphatase in aqueous extracts of bones of young, rapidly growing animals. He published a volume on the significance of phosphoric esters in metabolism in 1932.

rob·o·rant \'räb-ə-rənt, 'rōb-\ *n* : an invigorating drug : TONIC

Q
R

\ə\ **abut** \ᵊ\ **kitten** \ər\ **further** \a\ **ash** \ā\ **ace** \ä\ **cot, cart**
\aù\ **out** \ch\ **chin** \e\ **bet** \ē\ **easy** \g\ **go** \i\ **hit** \ī\ **ice** \j\ **job**
\ŋ\ **sing** \ō\ **go** \ò\ **law** \òi\ **boy** \th\ **thin** \t̲h̲\ **the** \ü\ **loot**
\ù\ **foot** \y\ **yet** \zh\ **vision** *See also* Pronunciation Symbols page

Ro·cha·li·maea \‚rō-kə-li-'mē-ə, ‚rō-shə-, ‚rash-ə-; ‚rō-chə-'lī-mā-ə\ *n, syn of* BARTONELLA

Ro·chelle salt \rō-'shel-\ *n* : a crystalline salt $C_4H_4KNaO_6 \cdot 4H_2O$ that is a mild purgative — called also *potassium sodium tartrate, Seignette salt, sodium potassium tartrate*

rock \'räk\ *n* **1** : a small crystallized mass of crack cocaine **2** : CRACK — called also *rock cocaine*

Rocky Moun·tain spotted fever \'räk-ē-'maůnt-ᵊn-\ *n* : an acute bacterial disease that is characterized by chills, fever, prostration, pains in muscles and joints, and a red purple eruption and that is caused by a bacterium of the genus *Rickettsia* (*R. rickettsii*) usu. transmitted by ixodid ticks and esp. by the American dog tick and Rocky Mountain wood tick

Rocky Mountain wood tick *n* : a widely distributed wood tick of the genus *Dermacentor* (*D. andersoni*) of western No. America that is a vector of Rocky Mountain spotted fever and sometimes causes tick paralysis

rod \'räd\ *n* **1** : a straight slender pole or bar **2** : any of the long rod-shaped photosensitive receptors in the retina responsive to faint light — compare CONE 2a **3** : a bacterium shaped like a rod

ro·dent \'rōd-ᵊnt\ *n* : any mammal (as a mouse or rat) of the order Rodentia — **rodent** *adj*

Ro·den·tia \rō-'den-chə, -'dent-ē-ə\ *n pl* : an order of the division Eutheria comprising relatively small gnawing mammals having a single pair of incisors in each jaw that grow from persistent pulps and bear enamel chiefly in front to produce a chisel-shaped edge

ro·den·ti·ci·dal \rō-‚dent-ə-'sīd-ᵊl\ *adj* : of, relating to, or being a rodenticide ⟨a ∼ agent⟩

ro·den·ti·cide \rō-'dent-ə-‚sīd\ *n* : an agent that kills, repels, or controls rodents

rodent ulcer *n* : a chronic persistent ulcer of the exposed skin and esp. of the face that is destructive locally, spreads slowly, and is usu. a carcinoma derived from basal cells

rod·like \'räd-‚līk\ *adj* : resembling a rod ⟨∼ bacteria⟩

rod of Cor·ti \-'kórt-ē\ *n* : any of the minute modified epithelial elements that rise from the basilar membrane of the organ of Corti in two spirally arranged rows so that the free ends of the members incline toward and interlock with corresponding members of the opposite row and enclose the tunnel of Corti

A. G. G. Corti — see ORGAN OF CORTI

¹roent·gen *also* **rönt·gen** \'rent-gən, 'rənt-, -jən; 'ren-chən, 'rən-\ *adj* : of, relating to, or using X-rays : X-RAY ⟨∼ examinations⟩ ⟨∼ therapy⟩

Rönt·gen *or* **Roent·gen** \'roent-gən\, **Wilhelm Conrad (1845–1923)**, German physicist. Röntgen is famous for his discovery of X-rays in 1895. He made the discovery while experimenting with electric current flow in a cathode-ray tube. He observed that a nearby piece of the platinocyanide of barium gave off light when the tube was in operation. He attributed the fluorescence of the chemical to some unknown form of radiation. Because of the uncertain nature of the radiation he called the phenomenon X radiation. For his discovery of X-rays he was awarded the Nobel Prize for Physics in 1901. His discovery had a great impact on both physics and medicine.

²roentgen *also* **röntgen** *n* : the international unit of x-radiation or gamma radiation equal to the amount of radiation that produces in one cubic centimeter of dry air at 0°C (32°F) and standard atmospheric pressure ionization of either sign equal to one electrostatic unit of charge

roent·gen·o·gram \-ə-‚gram\ *n* : RADIOGRAPH

roent·gen·o·graph \-ə-‚graf\ *n* : RADIOGRAPH

roent·gen·og·ra·phy \‚rent-gən-'äg-rə-fē, ‚rənt-, -jən-; ‚ren-chən-, ‚rən-\ *n, pl* **-phies** : RADIOGRAPHY — **roent·gen·o·graph·ic** \-ə-'graf-ik\ *adj* — **roent·gen·o·graph·i·cal·ly** \-i-k(ə-)lē\ *adv*

roent·gen·ol·o·gist \-'äl-ə-jəst\ *n* : RADIOLOGIST

roent·gen·ol·o·gy \-'äl-ə-jē\ *n, pl* **-gies** : RADIOLOGY 2 —

roent·gen·o·log·ic \-ə-'läj-ik\ *or* **roent·gen·o·log·i·cal** \-i-kəl\ *adj* — **roent·gen·o·log·i·cal·ly** \-i-k(ə-)lē\ *adv*

roent·gen·om·e·ter \-'äm-ət-ər\ *n* : a radiometer for measuring the intensity of X-rays or gamma radiation

roent·gen·os·co·py \‚rent-gən-'äs-kə-pē, ‚rənt-, -jən-; ‚ren-chən-, ‚rən-\ *n, pl* **-pies** : observation or examination by means of a fluoroscope : FLUOROSCOPY — **roent·gen·o·scop·ic** \-ə-'skäp-ik\ *adj*

roent·gen·o·ther·a·py \‚rent-gən-ə-'ther-ə-pē, ‚rənt-, -jən-; ‚ren-chən-, ‚rən-\ *n, pl* **-pies** : X-RAY THERAPY

roentgen ray *n* : X-RAY 1

ro·fe·cox·ib \‚rō-fe-'käk-sib\ *n* : a COX-2 inhibitor $C_{17}H_{14}O_4S$ used to relieve the signs and symptoms of osteoarthritis and rheumatoid arthritis, to manage acute pain in adults, and to treat primary dysmenorrhea but withdrawn from sale by the manufacturer because of its link to cardiovascular events (as heart attack and stroke) — see VIOXX

Ro·gaine \'rō-‚gān\ *trademark* — used for a preparation of minoxidil

Rog·er·ian \rä-'jer-ē-ən\ *adj* : of or relating to the system of therapy or the theory of personality of Carl Rogers — **Rogerian** *n*

Rog·ers \'räj-ərz\, **Carl Ransom (1902–1987),** American psychologist. Rogers originated an approach to psychotherapy emphasizing a person-to-person relationship between the therapist and the client. The client determines the course, speed, and duration of treatment. He first presented his views on psychotherapy in an article in 1940, and two years later he elaborated on his concepts in *Counseling and Psychotherapy*. Rogers proposed that a client could find the means to restructure his or her life by establishing a relationship with an understanding therapist. He went on to establish a counseling center at the University of Chicago where he put his theories into practice. In 1951 and 1954 he published two more volumes that presented his theories on psychotherapy and his clinical findings.

Ro·hyp·nol \rō-'hip-‚nól, -‚nöl\ *n* : a preparation of flunitrazepam — formerly a U.S. registered trademark

Ro·lan·dic \rō-'lan-dik\ *adj* : of, relating to, or discovered by Luigi Rolando

L. Rolando — see FISSURE OF ROLANDO

Rolandic area *n* : the motor area of the cerebral cortex lying just anterior to the central sulcus and comprising part of the precentral gyrus

L. Rolando — see FISSURE OF ROLANDO

Rolandic fissure *n* : CENTRAL SULCUS

role *also* **rôle** \'rōl\ *n* : a socially prescribed pattern of behavior usu. determined by an individual's status in a particular society

role model *n* : a person whose behavior in a particular role is imitated by others ⟨watching our parents and other *role models* deal with conflict —Melody Beattie⟩

role–play \'rōl-‚plā\ *vt* : ACT OUT ∼ *vi* : to play a role

rolf \'rólf *also* 'rōf\ *vt, often cap* : to practice Rolfing on — **rolf·er** \'ról-fər *also* 'rō-\ *n, often cap*

Rolf \'rólf\, **Ida P. (1896–1979),** American biochemist and physiotherapist. Rolf received a doctorate in biochemistry and physiology. After working 12 years as a biochemist, she devoted 40 years to developing a new kind of physical therapy involving vigorous manipulation of the body's underlying musculature. The muscular manipulation was held to correct the body's structure so that it would be in alignment with the earth's gravitational field. Rolfing became an object of considerable popular interest in the 1970s.

Rolf·ing \'rólf-iŋ *also* 'róf-\ *service mark* — used for a system of deep muscle massage intended to serve as both physical and emotional therapy

ro·li·tet·ra·cy·cline \‚rō-li-‚te-trə-'sī-‚klēn\ *n* : a semisynthetic broad-spectrum tetracycline antibiotic $C_{27}H_{33}N_3O_8$ used esp. for parenteral administration in cases requiring high concentrations or when oral administration is impractical

roller — see TONGUE ROLLER

roll·er bandage \'rō-lər-\ *n* : a long rolled bandage

Ro·ma·now·sky stain *or* **Ro·ma·now·sky's stain** *also* **Ro-**

ma·nov·sky stain *or* **Ro·ma·nov·sky's stain** \ˌrō-mə-ˈnȯf-skē(z)-\ *n* : a stain made from water-soluble eosin, methylene blue, and absolute methanol and used in parasitology
 Romanowsky, Dimitri Leonidovich (1861–1921), Russian physician. Romanowsky made important studies of the malaria parasite. In an 1891 monograph on the parasitology and treatment of malaria, he introduced the original eosin= methylene blue stain for blood smears and malaria parasites.

Rom·berg's sign *or* **Rom·berg sign** \ˈräm-ˌbərg(z)-\ *n* : a diagnostic sign of tabes dorsalis and other diseases of the nervous system consisting of a swaying of the body when the feet are placed close together and the eyes are closed
 Rom·berg \ˈróm-berk\, **Moritz Heinrich (1795–1873),** German pathologist. A professor of medicine at Berlin, Romberg wrote the first formal treatise on diseases of the nervous system. Published 1840 to 1846, it was the first attempt to organize scattered data and to systematize methods of treatment. The manual was notable for emphasizing the significance of physiological principles in interpreting neurological function and for its precise clinical illustrations. The treatise contains descriptions of the pathognomonic symptom of tabes dorsalis, now known as Romberg's sign, and of neuralgia affecting the eye, brow, or temple. Romberg is also remembered for his classic description of achondroplasia in 1817.

Romberg's test *or* **Romberg test** *n* : a test for the presence of Romberg's sign by placing the feet close together and closing the eyes

¹ron·geur \rō⁻ˈzhər\ *n* : a heavy-duty forceps for removing small pieces of bone or tough tissue

²rongeur *vt* : to remove (bone or other tissue) with a rongeur

ron·nel \ˈrän-ᵊl\ *n* : an organophosphate $C_8H_8Cl_3O_3PS$ used esp. as a systemic insecticide to protect cattle from pests

röntgen *var of* ROENTGEN

roof \ˈrüf, ˈrúf\ *n, pl* **roofs** \ˈrüfs, ˈrúfs *also* ˈrüvz, ˈrúvz\ **1** : the vaulted upper boundary of the mouth supported largely by the palatine bones and limited anteriorly by the dental lamina and posteriorly by the uvula and upper part of the fauces **2** : a covering structure of any of various parts of the body other than the mouth ⟨∼ of the skull⟩ ⟨∼ of the dental pulp chamber⟩

roof·ie \ˈrü-fē\ *n, pl* **roof·ies** *slang* : a tablet of flunitrazepam used illicitly

roof nucleus *n* : FASTIGIAL NUCLEUS

roof rat *n* : a grayish brown rat that belongs to a variety (*Rattus rattus alexandrinus*) of the black rat, is common in warm regions, and often nests in trees or the upper parts of buildings

room \ˈrüm, ˈrùm\ *n* : a partitioned part of the inside of a hospital; *esp* : a space for lodging patients

room·ing–in \ˈrüm-iŋ-ˈin, ˈrùm-\ *n* : an arrangement in a hospital whereby a newborn infant is kept in the mother's hospital room instead of in a nursery

room temperature *n* : a temperature of from 59° to 77°F (15° to 25°C) which is suitable for human occupancy and at which laboratory experiments are usu. performed

root \ˈrüt, ˈrút\ *n* **1 a** : the usu. underground part of a seed plant body that functions as an organ of absorption, aeration, and food storage or as a means of anchorage and support and that differs from a stem esp. in lacking nodes, buds, and leaves **b** : any subterranean plant part (as a true root or a bulb, tuber, rootstock, or other modified stem) esp. when fleshy and edible **2 a (1)** : the part of a tooth within the socket **(2)** : any of the processes into which the root of a tooth is often divided **b** : the enlarged basal part of a hair within the skin — called also *hair root* **c** : the proximal end of a nerve; *esp* : one or more bundles of nerve fibers joining the cranial and spinal nerves with their respective nuclei and columns of gray matter — see DORSAL ROOT, VENTRAL ROOT **d** : the part of an organ or physical structure by which it is attached to the body ⟨the ∼ of the tongue⟩ — **root·less** \-ləs\ *adj*

root canal *n* **1** : the part of the pulp cavity lying in the root

of a tooth — called also *pulp canal* **2** : a dental operation to save a tooth by removing the contents of its root canal and filling the cavity with a protective substance (as gutta= percha)

root·ed \ˈrüt-əd, ˈrút-\ *adj* **1** : having such or so many roots ⟨single-*rooted* molars⟩ **2** : having a contracted root nearly closing the pulp cavity and preventing further growth

root·let \-lət\ *n* : a small root; *also* : one of the ultimate divisions of a nerve root

root plan·ing \-ˌplā-niŋ\ *n* : the scraping of a bacteria= impregnated layer of cementum from the surface of a tooth root to prevent or treat periodontitis

root sheath *n* : the epidermal lining of a hair follicle

ROP *abbr* retinopathy of prematurity

ropy *also* **rop·ey** \ˈrō-pē\ *adj* **rop·i·er; -est 1** : capable of being drawn into a thread : VISCOUS; *also* : tending to adhere in stringy masses **2** : having a gelatinous or slimy quality from bacterial or fungal contamination ⟨∼ milk⟩ — **rop·i·ness** *n*

Ror·schach \ˈrȯ(ə)r-ˌshäk\ *adj* : of, relating to, used in connection with, or resulting from the Rorschach test

Rorschach test *n* : a projective psychological test that uses a subject's interpretation of 10 standard black or colored inkblot designs to assess personality traits and emotional tendencies — called also *Rorschach, Rorschach inkblot test*
 Ror·schach \ˈrȯr-ˌshäk\, **Hermann (1884–1922),** Swiss psychiatrist. Rorschach was an early supporter of psychoanalytic theory. In 1921 he published his major work on psychodiagnosis in which he introduced his famous inkblot test. He based his findings on the testing of 300 mentally ill patients and 100 average people over a 14-year period. His work included a systematic analysis of his subjects' attention to the wholes or details of the symmetrical figures used in his test. Although controversial, his inkblot test has since been widely used for the clinical diagnosing of psychopathology.

ro·sa·cea \rō-ˈzā-sh(ē-)ə\ *n* : a chronic inflammatory disorder involving esp. the skin of the nose, forehead, and cheeks that is characterized by congestion, flushing, telangiectasia, and marked nodular swelling of tissues esp. of the nose — called also *acne rosacea*

ros·an·i·line \rō-ˈzan-ᵊl-ən\ *n* **1** : a white crystalline compound $C_{20}H_{21}N_3O$ that is the parent of many dyes **2** : FUCHSIN

ro·sa·ry \ˈrōz-(ə-)rē\ *n, pl* **-ries** : BEADING

rosary pea *n* **1** : a tropical leguminous twining herb of the genus *Abrus* (*A. precatorius*) that bears jequirity beans and has a root used as a substitute for licorice — called also *jequirity bean* **2** : JEQUIRITY BEAN 1

rose \ˈrōz\ *n* **1 a** : any of a genus (*Rosa* of the family Rosaceae, the rose family) of usu. prickly shrubs with pinnate leaves and showy flowers of which some are sources of rose oil **b** : the flower of a rose **2** : ERYSIPELAS

rosea — see PITYRIASIS ROSEA

rose ben·gal \-ben-ˈgȯl, -beŋ-\ *n* : either of two bluish red acid dyes that are iodinated and chlorinated derivatives of fluorescein

rose bengal test *n* : a test of liver function by determining the time taken for an injected quantity of rose bengal to be absorbed from the bloodstream

rose cold *n* : ROSE FEVER

rose fever *n* : hay fever occurring in the spring or early summer

rose·mary \ˈrōz-ˌmer-ē\ *n, pl* **-mar·ies** : a fragrant shrubby mint (*Rosmarinus officinalis*) of southern Europe and Asia Minor that is the source of rosemary oil and was formerly used medicinally as a stimulant and carminative

rosemary oil *n* : a pungent essential oil obtained from the flowering tops of rosemary and used chiefly in soaps, colognes, hair lotions, and pharmaceutical preparations

---

\ə\ abut \ᵊ\ kitten \ər\ further \a\ ash \ā\ ace \ä\ cot, cart \aú\ out \ch\ chin \e\ bet \ē\ easy \g\ go \i\ hit \ī\ ice \j\ job \ŋ\ sing \ō\ go \ȯ\ law \ȯi\ boy \th\ thin \t͟h\ the \ü\ loot \ú\ foot \y\ yet \zh\ vision *See also* Pronunciation Symbols page

Q
R

rose oil *n* : a fragrant essential oil obtained from roses and used chiefly in perfumery and in flavoring; *esp* : ATTAR OF ROSES

ro·se·o·la \ˌrō-zē-ˈō-lə, rō-ˈzē-ə-lə\ *n* : a rose-colored eruption in spots or a disease marked by such an eruption; *esp* : ROSEOLA INFANTUM — **ro·se·o·lar** \-lər\ *adj*

roseola in·fan·tum \-in-ˈfant-əm\ *n* : a mild virus disease of infants and children that is characterized by fever lasting three days followed by an eruption of rose-colored spots and is caused by a herpesvirus (species *Human herpesvirus 6* of the genus *Roseolovirus*) — called also *exanthema subitum, exanthem subitum*

ro·sette \rō-ˈzet\ *n* : a rose-shaped cluster of cells

ro·si·glit·a·zone \ˌrō-sə-ˈglit-ə-ˌzōn\ *n* : a thiazolidine derivative administered in the form of its maleate $C_{18}H_{19}N_3O_3S\cdot C_4H_4O_4$ to treat type 2 diabetes by decreasing insulin resistance — see AVANDIA

ros·in \ˈräz-ᵊn, ˈröz-\ *n* : a translucent amber-colored to almost black brittle friable resin that is obtained from the oleoresin or dead wood of pine trees or from tall oil and is used in pharmacology as an adhesive constituent in plasters, cerates, and ointments — called also *colophony*

ro·sol·ic acid \rō-ˌzäl-ik-\ *n* : AURIN

ros·tel·lum \rä-ˈstel-əm\ *n* : an anterior prolongation of the head of a tapeworm often bearing hooks

ros·trad \ˈräs-ˌtrad\ *adv* : toward a rostrum : in a rostral direction ⟨the dorsal layer of this fascia ... projects ∼ —*Science*⟩

ros·tral \ˈräs-trəl *also* ˈrös-\ *adj* **1** : of or relating to a rostrum **2** : situated toward the oral or nasal region: as **a** *of a part of the spinal cord* : SUPERIOR 1 **b** *of a part of the brain* : anterior or ventral ⟨the ∼ pons⟩ — **ros·tral·ly** \-ē\ *adv*

ros·trum \ˈräs-trəm *also* ˈrös-\ *n, pl* **rostrums** *or* **ros·tra** \-trə\ : a bodily part or process suggesting a bird's bill: as **a** : the reflected anterior portion of the corpus callosum below the genu **b** : the interior median spine of the body of the basisphenoid bone articulating with the vomer

rosy periwinkle \ˈrō-zē-\ *n* : a commonly cultivated shrub (*Catharanthus roseus* syn. *Vinca rosea*) of the dogbane family (Apocynaceae) that is native to the Old World tropics and is the source of several antineoplastic drugs (as vinblastine and vincristine) — called also *Madagascar periwinkle, periwinkle*

¹rot \ˈrät\ *vi* **rot·ted; rot·ting** : to undergo decomposition from the action of bacteria or fungi

²rot *n* **1** : the process of rotting : the state of being rotten **2** : any of several parasitic diseases esp. of sheep marked by necrosis and wasting

ro·ta·me·ter \ˈrōt-ə-ˌmēt-ər, rō-ˈtam-ət-\ *n* : a gauge that consists of a graduated glass tube containing a free float for measuring the flow of a liquid or gas

ro·tate \ˈrō-ˌtāt, *esp Brit* rō-ˈ\ *vb* **ro·tat·ed; ro·tat·ing** *vi* : to turn about an axis or a center ∼ *vt* : to cause to turn about an axis or a center ⟨∼ the head⟩

ro·ta·tion \rō-ˈtā-shən\ *n* : the action or process of rotating on or as if on an axis or center; *specif* : the turning of a body part about its long axis as if on a pivot ⟨∼ of the head to look over the shoulder⟩ — **ro·ta·tion·al** \-shnəl, -shən-ᵊl\ *adj*

rotation flap *n* : a pedicle flap that is rotated on its base to graft an adjacent area

ro·ta·tor \ˈrō-ˌtāt-ər *also* rō-ˈ\ *n, pl* **rotators** *or* **ro·ta·to·res** \ˌrōt-ə-ˈtōr-ēz\ : a muscle that partially rotates a part on its axis; *specif* : any of several small muscles in the dorsal region of the spine arising from the upper and back part of a transverse process and inserted into the lamina of the vertebra above

rotator cuff \-ˌkəf\ *n* : a supporting and strengthening structure of the shoulder joint that is made up of part of its capsule blended with tendons of the subscapularis, infraspinatus, supraspinatus, and teres minor muscles as they pass to the capsule or across it to insert on the humerus — called also *musculotendinous cuff*

ro·ta·to·ry \ˈrōt-ə-ˌtōr-ē, -ˌtōr-, *Brit* -t(ə-)rē *also* rō-ˈtā-tə-rē\ *adj* : of, relating to, or producing rotation

ro·ta·vi·rus \ˈrōt-ə-ˌvī-rəs\ *n* : any of a genus (*Rotavirus*) of double-stranded RNA viruses of the family *Reoviridae* that have a capsid composed of two layers and cause diarrhea esp. in young vertebrates including human infants and young children — **ro·ta·vi·ral** \-rəl\ *adj*

ro·te·none \ˈrōt-ᵊn-ˌōn\ *n* : a crystalline insecticide $C_{23}H_{22}O_6$ that is of low toxicity for warm-blooded animals and is used esp. in home gardens

ro·ti·fer \ˈrōt-ə-fər\ *n* : any member of the class Rotifera

Ro·tif·era \rō-ˈtif-ə-rə\ *n pl* : a class of minute usu. microscopic but many-celled aquatic invertebrate animals of the phylum Aschelminthes

rott·ler·in \ˈrät-lə-rən\ *n* : a salmon-colored crystalline phenolic ketone $C_{30}H_{28}O_8$ that is the active principle of kamala

rotunda — see FENESTRA ROTUNDA

rotundum — see FORAMEN ROTUNDUM

Rou·get cell \rü-ˈzhā-\ *n* : any of numerous branching cells adhering to the endothelium of capillaries and regarded as a contractile element in the capillary wall

Rou·get \rü-zhā\, **Charles–Marie–Benjamin** (1824–1904), French physiologist and anatomist. Rouget's early researches dealt with the anatomy and physiology of the reproductive organs. He made his best contributions in correlating physiology with microscopic structure. Using special photographic techniques, he was able to examine the muscle fibers of vertebrates under high magnification. He made noteworthy observations in three areas: contractile tissue, nerve endings, and the eye. For his study of capillary contractility he examined the capillaries of the hyaloid membrane of the eye of a frog. He presented his first findings in 1874, and five years later he made another report on the contractility of blood capillaries. He described certain contractile cells, now called Rouget cells, on the walls of capillaries. His research on nerve endings produced two reports on the sensory receptors in the skin. His later research dealt with the termination of sensory nerve fibers in skeletal muscle and with end plates in particular. Rouget's most important contribution to the study of the eye dealt with accommodation of the lens.

rough \ˈrəf\ *adj* : having a broken, uneven, or bumpy surface; *specif* : forming or being rough colonies usu. made up of organisms that form chains or filaments and tend to marked decrease in capsule formation and virulence — used of dissociated strains of bacteria; compare SMOOTH

rough·age \ˈrəf-ij\ *n* : FIBER 2; *also* : food (as bran) containing much indigestible material acting as fiber

rough endoplasmic reticulum *n* : endoplasmic reticulum that is studded with ribosomes

rou·leau \rü-ˈlō\ *n, pl* **rou·leaux** \-ˈlō(z)\ *or* **rouleaus** : a group of red blood corpuscles resembling a stack of coins

round \ˈraund\ *vi* : to go on rounds

round cell *n* : a small lymphocyte or a closely related cell esp. occurring in an area of chronic infection or as the typical cell of some sarcomas

round ligament *n* **1** : a fibrous cord resulting from the obliteration of the umbilical vein of the fetus and passing from the navel to the notch in the anterior border of the liver and along the undersurface of that organ **2** : either of a pair of rounded cords arising from each side of the uterus and traceable through the inguinal canal to the tissue of the labia majora into which they merge

rounds *n pl* : a series of professional calls on hospital patients made by a doctor or nurse — see GRAND ROUNDS

round–shoul·dered \ˈraun(d)-ˈshōl-dərd\ *adj* : having the shoulders stooping or rounded

round window *n* : a round opening between the middle ear and the cochlea that is closed over by a membrane — called also *fenestra cochleae, fenestra rotunda*

round·worm \ˈraun-ˌdwərm\ *n* : NEMATODE; *also* : a related round-bodied unsegmented worm (as an acanthocephalan) as distinguished from a flatworm

roup \ˈrüp, ˈraup\ *n* : any of various respiratory disorders of poultry; *esp* : TRICHOMONIASIS c

Rous sarcoma \ˈraus-\ *n* : a readily transplantable malignant fibrosarcoma of chickens that is caused by the Rous sarcoma virus

Rous, Francis Peyton (1879–1970), American pathologist. Rous spent almost all of his career as a researcher at the Rockefeller Institute of Medical Research. In a series of classic experiments involving hens he was able to transplant, by means of a cell-free filtrate, a sarcoma from one hen to another and to show that the cancer was of viral origin. He published an initial report of his findings in 1910. After further experimentation in 1911 in which he multiplied the number of transplanted tumors, he published in 1912 the first evidence that a virus was etiologically related to a malignant tumor. Because his findings contradicted prevailing medical opinion, his work was dismissed, and he had to wait decades before being vindicated. In 1915 and 1916 he studied the physiology of the blood and helped to develop a solution for preserving whole blood, an achievement which made possible the creation of the first blood banks. In the 1940s and 1950s he introduced new techniques that advanced the science of virology. In 1966 he was awarded the Nobel Prize for Physiology or Medicine.

Rous sarcoma virus *n* : a single-stranded RNA virus of the family *Retroviridae* (species *Rous sarcoma virus* of the genus *Alpharetrovirus*) that contains an oncogene causing Rous sarcoma

route \'rüt, 'raùt\ *n* : a method of transmitting a disease or of administering a remedy ⟨the airborne ∼ of . . . infection —M. L. Furculow⟩

Roux–en–Y gastric bypass \ˌrü-ˌen-'wī-, ˌrü-ˌän-ˌē-'grek-\ *n* : a gastric bypass surgical procedure in the treatment of severe obesity that involves partitioning off part of the upper stomach (as by stapling and separation from the lower stomach) to form a small pouch, dividing the jejunum into upper and lower parts, and forming a Y-shaped anastomosis by attaching the free end of the lower part of the jejunum to a new outlet on the upper stomach pouch and attaching the free end of what was the upper jejunum to a new opening on the small intestine — called also *Roux-en-Y*

Roux \'rü\, **César (1857–1934),** Swiss surgeon. Roux served as chief of surgery at the University of Lausanne's medical school. In 1892 he began using the technique of the Y-shaped loop in gastrointestinal surgeries involving antral or pyloric obstruction. Although he subsequently abandoned the procedure, on account of the frequency of late peptic ulcerations in the loop, the concept of the Y-shaped loop was eventually adapted for hepatic, biliary, and pancreatic surgeries, as well as for other gastrointestinal procedures.

RP *abbr* retinitis pigmentosa

RPh *abbr* registered pharmacist

rpm *abbr* revolutions per minute

RPR card test \ˌär-ˌpē-ˌär-'kärd-\ *n* : RAPID PLASMA REAGIN TEST

RPT *abbr* registered physical therapist

RQ *abbr* respiratory quotient

RR *abbr* recovery room

RRA *abbr* registered records administrator

RRL *abbr* registered records librarian

rRNA \ˌär-ˌär-ˌen-ˌā\ *n* : RIBOSOMAL RNA

RRT *abbr* registered respiratory therapist

RSD *abbr* reflex sympathetic dystrophy

RSI \ˌär-(ˌ)es-'ī\ *n* : REPETITIVE STRAIN INJURY

RS–T segment \ˌär-ˌes-'tē-\ *n* : ST SEGMENT

RSV *abbr* **1** respiratory syncytial virus **2** Rous sarcoma virus

RT *abbr* **1** reaction time **2** recreational therapy **3** respiratory therapist

Ru *symbol* ruthenium

RU *abbr* rat unit

rub \'rəb\ *n* **1** : the application of friction with pressure ⟨an alcohol ∼⟩ **2** : a sound heard in auscultation that is produced by the friction of one structure moving against another

rub·ber \'rəb-ər\ *n* **1** : an elastic substance that is obtained

by coagulating the milky juice of any of various tropical plants (as of the genera *Hevea* and *Ficus*), is essentially a polymer of isoprene, and is prepared as sheets and then dried — called also *caoutchouc, india rubber* **2** : CONDOM 1

rubber dam *n* : a thin sheet of rubber that is stretched around a tooth to keep it dry during dental work or is used in strips to provide drainage in surgical wounds

rub·bing alcohol \'rəb-iŋ-ˌ\ *n* : a cooling and soothing liquid for external application that contains approximately 70 percent denatured ethanol or isopropyl alcohol

ru·be·an·ic acid \ˌrü-bē-ˌan-ik-\ *n* : an intensely colored weak acid $(CSNH_2)_2$ that is used as a reagent for copper, cobalt, and nickel

¹ru·be·fa·cient \ˌrü-bə-'fā-shənt\ *adj* : causing redness of the skin ⟨a ∼ cream⟩

²rubefacient *n* : a substance (as capsaicin) for external application that produces redness of the skin

ru·be·fac·tion \-'fak-shən\ *n* **1** : the act or process of causing redness **2** : redness due to a rubefacient

ru·bel·la \rü-'bel-ə\ *n* : GERMAN MEASLES — see MATERNAL RUBELLA

ru·be·o·la \ˌrü-bē-'ō-lə, rü-'bē-ə-lə\ *n* : MEASLES 1a — **ru·be·o·lar** \-lər\ *adj*

ru·be·o·sis \ˌrü-bē-'ō-səs\ *n, pl* **-o·ses** \-'ō-ˌsēz\ *or* **-osises** : a condition characterized by abnormal redness; *esp* : RUBEOSIS IRIDIS

rubeosis iri·dis \-'ī-rəd-əs\ *n* : abnormal redness of the iris resulting from neovascularization and often associated with diabetes

ru·bid·i·um \rü-'bid-ē-əm\ *n* : a soft silvery metallic element that decomposes water with violence and bursts into flame spontaneously in air — symbol *Rb*; see ELEMENT table

Ru·bin test \'rü-bən-\ *n* : a test to determine the patency or occlusion of the fallopian tubes by insufflating them with carbon dioxide by transuterine injection

Rubin, Isidor Clinton (1883–1958), American gynecologist. Rubin's early researches dealt with the pathology of cancer of the cervix of the uterus. He turned toward the study of sterility, and after several years he successfully developed the first test for determining the patency of the fallopian tubes. The test, now known as the Rubin test, was first performed in 1919, and a report was published in 1920. The author of three major gynecological texts and over 132 articles, Rubin was widely regarded as the foremost researcher of fertility in the 20th century.

ru·bor \'rü-ˌbòr\ *n* : redness of the skin (as from inflammation)

rubra — see PITYRIASIS RUBRA PILARIS

ru·bri·blast \'rü-bri-ˌblast\ *n* : PRONORMOBLAST

ru·bri·cyte \'rü-bri-ˌsīt\ *n* : an immature red blood cell that has a nucleus, is about half the size of developing red blood cells in preceding stages, and has cytoplasm that stains erratically blue, purplish, and gray due to the presence of hemoglobin : polychromatic normoblast

ru·bro·spi·nal \ˌrü-brō-'spī-n²l\ *adj* **1** : of, relating to, or connecting the red nucleus and the spinal cord **2** : of, relating to, or constituting a tract of crossed nerve fibers passing from the red nucleus to the spinal cord and relaying impulses from the cerebellum and corpora striata to the motor neurons of the spinal cord

rubrum — see PRONTOSIL RUBRUM

Ru·bu·la·vi·rus \ˌrü-byə-lə-'vī-rəs\ *n* : a genus of single-stranded RNA viruses of the family *Paramyxoviridae* that includes several parainfluenza viruses and the causative agents of mumps and Newcastle disease

rud·dy \'rəd-ē\ *adj* **rud·di·er; -est** : having a healthy reddish color ⟨a ∼ complexion⟩

ru·di·ment \'rüd-ə-mənt\ *n* : an incompletely developed or-

\ə\ **abut** \ᵊ\ **kitten** \ər\ **further** \a\ **ash** \ā\ **ace** \ä\ **cot, cart**
\aù\ **out** \ch\ **chin** \e\ **bet** \ē\ **easy** \g\ **go** \i\ **hit** \ī\ **ice** \j\ **job**
\ŋ\ **sing** \ō\ **go** \ò\ **law** \òi\ **boy** \th\ **thin** \th̲\ **the** \ü\ **loot**
\ù\ **foot** \y\ **yet** \zh\ **vision** *See also* Pronunciation Symbols page

Q
R

gan or part; *esp* : an organ or part just beginning to develop : ANLAGE

ru·di·men·ta·ry \ˌrüd-ə-ˈment-ə-rē, -ˈmen-trē\ *adj* : very imperfectly developed or represented only by a vestige

rue \ˈrü\ *n* : a strong-scented perennial woody herb (*Ruta graveolens* of the family Rutaceae, the rue family) that has bitter leaves used in medicine

Ruf·fi·ni's corpuscle \rü-ˈfē-nēz-\ *or* **Ruf·fi·ni corpuscle** \-nē-\ *n* : any of numerous oval sensory end organs occurring in the subcutaneous tissue of the fingers — called also *Ruffini's brush, Ruffini's end organ*

> **Ruf·fi·ni** \rüf-ˈfē-nē\, **Angelo (1864–1929)**, Italian histologist and embryologist. Ruffini served as director of a small hospital in Lucignano, Italy, where he set up his own laboratory for histological research. Concurrently, at the University of Siena he was instructor of histology and later professor of embryology. From 1912 until his death he held the post of professor of histology and general physiology at the University of Bologna. From 1890 to 1906 Ruffini worked on proprioceptive sensibility. In 1888 he had begun research on nerve receptors. In 1891 he discovered a new form of human sensory nerve ending now known as Ruffini's corpuscle; he published his discovery in 1894.

RU–486 \ˌär-(ˌ)yü-ˌfō(ə)r-ˌāt-ē-ˈsiks\ *n* : a drug $C_{29}H_{35}NO_2$ taken orally to induce abortion esp. early in pregnancy by blocking the body's use of progesterone — called also *mifepristone*

ru·ga \ˈrü-gə\ *n, pl* **ru·gae** \-ˌgī, -ˌgē, -ˌjē\ : an anatomical fold or wrinkle esp. of the viscera — usu. used in pl. ⟨the *rugae* of an empty stomach⟩

ru·gose \ˈrü-ˌgōs\ *adj* : having many wrinkles ⟨∼ skin⟩

ru·gos·i·ty \rü-ˈgäs-ət-ē\ *n, pl* **-ties** : the quality or state of being rugose; *also* : WRINKLE

ru·men \ˈrü-mən\ *n, pl* **ru·mi·na** \-mə-nə\ *or* **rumens** : the large first compartment of the stomach of a ruminant from which food is regurgitated for rumination and in which cellulose is broken down by the action of symbiotic microorganisms — called also *paunch;* compare ABOMASUM, OMASUM, RETICULUM

ru·men·ot·o·my \ˌrü-mə-ˈnät-ə-mē\ *n, pl* **-mies** : surgical incision into the rumen

Ru·mex \ˈrü-ˌmeks\ *n* : a genus of herbs and shrubs of the buckwheat family (Polygonaceae) that are mainly native to temperate regions of the northern hemisphere and used as potherbs and in folk medicine

ru·mi·nal \ˈrü-mə-n³l\ *adj* : of, relating to, or occurring in the rumen ⟨a ∼ ulcer⟩

¹ru·mi·nant \ˈrü-mə-nənt\ *n* : a ruminant mammal

²ruminant *adj* : of or relating to two suborders (Ruminantia and Tylopoda) of even-toed hoofed mammals (as sheep, oxen, deer, and camels) that chew the cud and have a complex 3- or 4-chambered stomach

ru·mi·nate \ˈrü-mə-ˌnāt\ *vi* **-nat·ed; -nat·ing** **1** : to chew again what has been chewed slightly and swallowed : chew the cud **2** : to engage in contemplation

ru·mi·na·tion \ˌrü-mə-ˈnā-shən\ *n* : the act or process of ruminating: **a** : the act or process of regurgitating and chewing again previously swallowed food **b** : obsessive or abnormal reflection upon an idea or deliberation over a choice

ru·mi·na·tive \ˈrü-mə-ˌnāt-iv\ *adj* : inclined to or engaged in rumination

rump \ˈrəmp\ *n* **1** : the upper rounded part of the hindquarters of a quadruped mammal **2** : the seat of the body : BUTTOCKS

Rum·pel–Leede test \ˈrùm-pel-ˈlēd-\ *n* : a test in which the increased bleeding tendency characteristic of various disorders (as scarlet fever and thrombocytopenia) is indicated by the formation of multiple petechiae on the forearm following application of a tourniquet to the upper arm

> **Rumpel, Theodor (1862–1923)**, German physician. Rumpel was the first to discover that in a patient with scarlet fever petechiae appear when the arm is constricted. He recorded his observation in 1909.
>
> **Leede, Carl Stockbridge (1882–1964)**, American physi-

cian. Leede published independently a description of the Rumpel-Leede test in 1911.

run \ˈrən\ *vi* **ran** \ˈran\; **run; run·ning** : to discharge fluid (as pus or serum) ⟨a *running* sore⟩ — **run a fever** *or* **run a temperature** : to have a fever

run·around \ˈrən-ə-ˌraùnd\ *n* : a whitlow encircling a fingernail or toenail

rung *past part of* RING

run·ner's high \ˈrən-ərz-\ *n* : a feeling of euphoria that is experienced by some individuals engaged in strenuous running and that is held to be associated with the release of endorphins by the brain

runner's knee *n* : pain in the region of the knee esp. when related to running that may have a simple anatomical basis (as tightness of a muscle) or may be a symptom of iliotibial band friction syndrome or may be an indication of chondromalacia patellae

run·ny \ˈrən-ē\ *adj* : secreting a thin flow of mucus ⟨a ∼ nose⟩

run·round \ˈrən-ˌraùnd\ *n* : RUNAROUND

runs \ˈrənz\ *n pl but sing or pl in constr* : DIARRHEA — used with *the*

runt disease \ˈrənt-\ *n* : graft-versus-host disease produced experimentally in laboratory animals that is characterized esp. by severely retarded growth and is often fatal

ru·pia \ˈrü-pē-ə\ *n* : an eruption occurring esp. in tertiary syphilis consisting of vesicles having an inflamed base and filled with serous purulent or bloody fluid which dries up and forms large blackish conical crusts — **ru·pi·al** \-əl\ *adj*

¹rup·ture \ˈrəp-chər\ *n* **1** : the tearing apart of a tissue ⟨∼ of heart muscle⟩ ⟨∼ of an intervertebral disk⟩ **2** : HERNIA

²rupture *vb* **rup·tured; rup·tur·ing** \-chə-riŋ, -shriŋ\ *vt* : to produce a rupture in ⟨∼ an eardrum⟩ ∼ *vi* : to have or undergo a rupture

RUQ *abbr* right upper quadrant (abdomen)

rush \ˈrəsh\ *n* **1** : a rapid and extensive wave of peristalsis along the walls of the intestine ⟨peristaltic ∼⟩ **2** : the immediate pleasurable feeling produced by a drug (as heroin or amphetamine) — called also *flash*

Rus·sell's viper \ˌrəs-əlz-\ *n* : a strikingly marked highly venomous snake of the genus *Vipera* (*V. russellii*) occurring in southeastern Asia — called also *tic-polonga*

> **Russell, Patrick (1727–1805)**, British physician and naturalist. For the first part of his career Russell was a physician in Aleppo, Syria, where he studied plague and other diseases. In the 1780s he traveled to India, and while employed as a naturalist for the East India Company, he made large collections of specimens and drawings of the plants, fishes, and reptiles of the country. From 1796 to 1809 the East India Company published his multivolume, illustrated work on the snakes of the Coromandel coast. In 1797 the naturalist George Shaw named Russell's viper in his honor.

Rus·sian spring–sum·mer encephalitis \ˈrəsh-ən-ˌspriŋ-ˈsəm-ər-\ *n* : a tick-borne encephalitis of Europe and Asia that is transmitted by ticks of the genus *Ixodes* — see LOUPING ILL

rust \ˈrəst\ *n* **1** : the reddish brittle coating formed on iron esp. when chemically attacked by moist air and composed essentially of hydrated ferric oxide **2** : any of numerous destructive diseases of plants produced by fungi (order Uredinales) and characterized by reddish brown pustular lesions; *also* : a fungus causing this

¹rut \ˈrət\ *n* **1** : an annually recurrent state of sexual excitement in the male deer; *broadly* : sexual excitement in a mammal (as estrus in the female) esp. when periodic **2** : the period during which rut normally occurs — often used with *the*

²rut *vi* **rut·ted; rut·ting** : to be in or enter into a state of rut

ru·the·ni·um \rü-ˈthē-nē-əm\ *n* : a hard brittle grayish polyvalent rare metallic element occurring in platinum ores and used in hardening platinum alloys — symbol *Ru*; see ELEMENT table

ruth·er·ford \ˈrəth-ə(r)-fərd, ˈrəth-\ *n* : a unit strength of a radioactive source corresponding to one million disintegrations per second — abbr. *rd*

Rutherford, Ernest (Baron Rutherford of Nelson) (1871–1937), British physicist. Rutherford is ranked with Isaac Newton and Michael Faraday for his fundamental contributions to physics and his lasting influence on scientific thought. He developed the basis for nuclear physics by investigating radioactivity, discovering the alpha particle, and developing the concept of the nuclear atom. In 1902 with Frederick Soddy he developed the theory of radioactive decay. A year later he demonstrated that alpha particles can be deflected by electric and magnetic fields, the direction of the deflection proving that the rays are particles of positive charge. In 1904 he identified the alpha particle as a helium atom. He produced in 1919 the first nuclear reaction by bombarding atoms of nitrogen with alpha particles, thus demonstrating that the atom is not the ultimate building block of the physical universe. His research opened up the whole new field of nuclear energy. In 1908 he was awarded the Nobel Prize for Chemistry.

ruth·er·ford·ium \ˌrəth-ə(r)-ˈfȯ(ə)rd-ē-əm\ *n* : a short-lived radioactive element that is artificially produced — symbol *Rf*; see ELEMENT table

ru·tin \ˈrüt-ᵊn\ *n* : a yellow crystalline flavonol glycoside $C_{27}H_{30}O_{16}$ that occurs in various plants (as rue, tobacco, and buckwheat), that yields quercetin and rutinose on hydrolysis, and that is used chiefly for strengthening capillary blood vessels (as in cases of hypertension and radiation injury)

ru·tin·ose \ˈrüt-ᵊn-ˌōs\ *n* : a hygroscopic reducing disaccharide sugar $C_{12}H_{22}O_{10}$ that is obtained from rutin and yields D-glucose and L-rhamnose on hydrolysis

R wave \ˈär-ˌwāv\ *n* : the positive upward deflection in the QRS complex of an electrocardiogram that follows the Q wave

Rx \ˈär-ˈeks\ *n* : a medical prescription

rye \ˈrī\ *n* **1** : a hardy annual grass (*Secale cereale*) that is widely grown for grain and as a cover crop **2** : the seeds of rye used for bread flour, whiskey manufacture, feed for farm animals (as poultry), and esp. formerly in the roasted state as a coffee substitute

S

S *abbr* **1** sacral — used esp. with a number from 1 to 5 to indicate a vertebra or segment of the spinal cord in the sacral region ⟨the relative length of cord segments *S1* to *S5*⟩ **2** signa — used to introduce the signature in writing a prescription **3** smooth — used of bacterial colonies **4** subject **5** svedberg

S *symbol* sulfur

sa *abbr* [Latin *secundum artem*] according to art — used in writing prescriptions

S–A *abbr* sinoatrial

sab·a·dil·la \ˌsab-ə-ˈdil-ə, -ˈdē-(y)ə\ *n* : a Mexican plant (*Schoenocaulon officinalis*) of the lily family (Liliaceae); *also* : its seeds that are used as a source of veratrine and in insecticides and formerly in a preparation against external parasites (as head lice)

sa·bal \ˈsā-ˌbal\ *n* : SAW PALMETTO 2

sa·ber shin \ˈsā-bər-\ *n* : a tibia that has a pronounced anterior convexity resembling the curve of a saber and caused by congenital syphilis

sa·bi·na \sə-ˈbī-nə, -ˈbē-\ *n* : SAVIN

Sa·bin vaccine \ˈsā-bin-\ *n* : a polio vaccine that is taken by mouth and contains the three serotypes of poliovirus in a weakened live state — called also *Sabin oral vaccine;* compare SALK VACCINE

Sabin, Albert Bruce (1906–1993), American immunologist. Beginning in the 1930s Sabin embarked upon a research project that was to occupy his time for the next 25 years: the development of a vaccine for the prevention of poliomyelitis. From 1939 he was a professor of pediatrics at the University of Cincinnati College of Medicine. During World War II, as a member of the army medical corps, he developed vaccines effective against dengue fever and Japanese B encephalitis. Although Jonas Salk had perfected a vaccine using virus inactivated by treatment with formaldehyde by 1954, Sabin worked on the development of a vaccine prepared from live virus that had been attenuated. In 1956 he released his vaccine for use by other researchers. A year later the World Health Organization began using the Sabin vaccine on a worldwide basis. It had several advantages over the type prepared by using virus treated with formaldehyde: it was cheaply produced, it provided lifelong immunity, and it could be given orally.

sab·u·lous \ˈsab-yə-ləs\ *adj* : being sandy or gritty

sac \ˈsak\ *n* : a soft-walled anatomical cavity usu. having a

narrow opening or none at all and often containing a special fluid ⟨a synovial ∼⟩ — see AIR SAC, AMNIOTIC SAC, DENTAL SAC, LACRIMAL SAC

sac·cade \sa-ˈkäd\ *n* : a small rapid jerky movement of the eye esp. as it jumps from fixation on one point to another (as in reading) — **sac·cad·ic** \-ˈkäd-ik\ *adj*

sac·cate \ˈsak-ˌāt\ *adj* : having the form of a sac or pouch

sac·cha·rase \ˈsak-ə-ˌrās, -ˌrāz\ *n* : INVERTASE

sac·cha·rate \ˈsak-ə-ˌrāt, -rət\ *n* **1** : a salt or ester of saccharic acid **2** : a metallic derivative of a sugar usu. with a bivalent metal (as calcium or barium); *esp* : SUCRATE

sac·cha·rat·ed \-ˌrāt-əd\ *adj* : mixed or combined with sucrose

sac·char·ic acid \sə-ˌkar-ik-\ *n* : a dicarboxylic acid $C_6H_{10}O_8$ derived from glucose or its derivatives by oxidation with nitric acid

sac·cha·ride \ˈsak-ə-ˌrīd *also* -rəd\ *n* : a simple sugar, combination of sugars, or polymerized sugar — see DISACCHARIDE, MONOSACCHARIDE, OLIGOSACCHARIDE, POLYSACCHARIDE, TRISACCHARIDE

sac·cha·rif·er·ous \ˌsak-ə-ˈrif-(ə-)rəs\ *adj* : producing or containing sugar

sac·char·i·fi·ca·tion \sə-ˌkar-ə-fə-ˈkā-shən\ *n* : the process of breaking a complex carbohydrate (as starch) into simple sugars — **sac·char·i·fy** \sə-ˈkar-ə-ˌfī, sa-\ *vt* **-fied; -fy·ing**

sac·cha·rim·e·ter \ˌsak-ə-ˈrim-ət-ər\ *n* : a device for measuring the amount of sugar in a solution; *esp* : a polarimeter so used — **sac·char·i·met·ric** \sə-ˌkar-ə-ˈme-trik\ *adj* — **sac·cha·rim·e·try** \ˌsak-ə-ˈrim-ə-trē\ *n, pl* **-tries**

sac·cha·rin \ˈsak-(ə-)rən\ *n* : a crystalline cyclic imide $C_7H_5NO_3S$ that is unrelated to the carbohydrates, is several hundred times sweeter than sucrose, and is used as a calorie-free sweetener — called also *benzosulfimide, gluside*

sac·cha·rine \ˈsak-(ə-)rən *also* -ə-ˌrēn *or* -ə-ˌrīn\ *adj* **1 a** : of, relating to, or resembling that of sugar ⟨∼ taste⟩ **b** : yielding or containing sugar ⟨a ∼ fluid⟩ **2** : overly or sickeningly sweet ⟨∼ flavor⟩

sac·cha·ro·gen·ic \ˌsak-ə-rō-ˈjen-ik\ *adj* : producing sugar ⟨∼ enzymatic activity⟩ — compare DEXTRINOGENIC

sac·cha·ro·lyt·ic \ˌsak-ə-rō-ˈlit-ik\ *adj* : breaking down sug-

---

\ə\ **abut** \ᵊ\ **kitten** \ər\ **further** \a\ **ash** \ā\ **ace** \ä\ **cot, cart**
\au̇\ **out** \ch\ **chin** \e\ **bet** \ē\ **easy** \g\ **go** \i\ **hit** \ī\ **ice** \j\ **job**
\ŋ\ **sing** \ō\ **go** \ȯ\ **law** \ȯi\ **boy** \th\ **thin** \th̲\ **the** \ü\ **loot**
\u̇\ **foot** \y\ **yet** \zh\ **vision** *See also* Pronunciation Symbols page

S
T

ars in metabolism with the production of energy ⟨∼ enzymes⟩ ⟨∼ microorganisms⟩

sac·cha·rom·e·ter \ˌsak-ə-'räm-ət-ər\ *n* : SACCHARIMETER; *esp* : a hydrometer with a special scale

sac·cha·ro·my·ces \ˌsak-ə-rō-'mī-(ˌ)sēz\ *n* **1** *cap* : a genus of unicellular yeasts (as a brewer's yeast) of the family Saccharomycetaceae that are distinguished by their sparse or absent mycelium and by their facility in reproducing asexually by budding **2** *pl* **saccharomyces** : any yeast of the genus *Saccharomyces*

Sac·cha·ro·my·ce·ta·ce·ae \ˌsak-ə-rō-ˌmī-sə-'tā-sē-ˌē\ *n pl* : a family of ascomycetous fungi (order Endomycetales) comprising the typical yeasts that form asci or reproduce by budding and that typically produce alcoholic fermentations in carbohydrate substrates

sac·cha·rose \'sak-ə-ˌrōs, -ˌrōz\ *n* : SUCROSE; *broadly* : DISACCHARIDE

sacci *pl of* SACCUS

sac·ci·form \'sak-(s)ə-ˌfȯrm\ *adj* : SACCULAR ⟨∼ lesions⟩

sac·cu·lar \'sak-yə-lər\ *adj* : resembling a sac ⟨a ∼ aneurysm⟩

sac·cu·lat·ed \-ˌlāt-əd\ *also* **sac·cu·late** \-ˌlāt, -lət\ *adj* : having or formed of a series of saccular expansions

sac·cu·la·tion \ˌsak-yə-'lā-shən\ *n* **1** : the quality or state of being sacculated **2** : the process of developing or segmenting into sacculated structures **3** : a sac or sacculated structure; *esp* : one of a linear series of such structures ⟨the ∼s of the colon⟩

sac·cule \'sak-(ˌ)yü(ə)l\ *n* : a little sac; *specif* : the smaller chamber of the membranous labyrinth of the ear

sacculi — see MACULA SACCULI

sac·cu·lus \'sak-yə-ləs\ *n, pl* **-li** \-ˌlī, -ˌlē\ : SACCULE

sac·cus \'sak-əs\ *n, pl* **sac·ci** \'sa-ˌkī\ : SAC

sac·like \'sak-ˌlīk\ *adj* : having the form of or suggesting a sac ⟨the gallbladder is a ∼ structure⟩

sacra *pl of* SACRUM

¹**sa·cral** \'sak-rəl, 'sā-krəl\ *adj* : of, relating to, or lying near the sacrum ⟨the ∼ region of the spinal cord⟩

²**sacral** *n* : a sacral vertebra or sacral nerve

sacral artery — see LATERAL SACRAL ARTERY, MIDDLE SACRAL ARTERY

sacral canal *n* : the part of the vertebral canal lying in the sacrum

sacral cornu *n* : a rounded process on each side of the fifth sacral vertebra that projects downward and represents an inferior articular process of the vertebra

sacral crest *n* : any of several crests or tubercles on the sacrum: as **a** : one on the midline of the dorsal surface — called also *median sacral crest* **b** : any of a series of tubercles on each side of the dorsal surface lateral to the sacral foramina that represent the transverse processes of the sacral vertebrae and serve as attachments for ligaments — called also *lateral crest, lateral sacral crest*

sacral foramen *n* : any of 16 openings in the sacrum of which there are four on each side of the dorsal surface giving passage to the posterior branches of the sacral nerves and four on each side of the pelvic surface giving passage to the anterior branches of the sacral nerves

sacral hiatus *n* : the opening into the vertebral canal in the midline of the dorsal surface of the sacrum between the laminae of the fifth sacral vertebra

sacral index *n* : the ratio of the breadth of the sacrum to its length multiplied by 100

sa·cral·iza·tion \ˌsā-krə-lə-'zā-shən\ *also Brit* **sa·cral·isa·tion** \-ˌlī-'zā-\ *n* : incorporation (as of the last lumbar vertebra or any of its parts) into the sacrum; *specif* : a congenital anomaly in which the fifth lumbar vertebra is fused to the sacrum in varying degrees

sacral nerve *n* : any of the spinal nerves of the sacral region of which there are five pairs and which have anterior and posterior branches passing out through the sacral foramina

sacral plexus *n* : a nerve plexus that lies against the posterior and lateral walls of the pelvis, is formed by the union of the lumbosacral trunk and the first, second, and third sacral nerves, and continues into the thigh as the sciatic nerve

sacral promontory *n* : the inwardly projecting anterior part of the body of the first sacral vertebra

sacral vein — see LATERAL SACRAL VEIN, MEDIAN SACRAL VEIN

sacral vertebra *n* : any of the five fused vertebrae that make up the sacrum

sa·cro·coc·cy·geal \ˌsā-krō-käk-'sij(-ē)-əl, ˌsak-rō-\ *adj* : of, relating to, affecting, or performed by way of the region of the sacrum and coccyx ⟨a ∼ teratoma⟩

sa·cro·coc·cy·geus dor·sa·lis \-käk-'sij-ē-əs-ˌdȯr-'sā-ləs\ *n* : an inconstant muscle that sometimes extends from the dorsal part of the sacrum to the coccyx — called also *posterior sacrococcygeal muscle*

sacrococcygeus ven·tra·lis \-ven-'trā-ləs\ *n* : an inconstant muscle that sometimes extends from the ventral surface of the lower sacral vertebrae to the coccyx — called also *anterior sacrococcygeal muscle*

¹**sa·cro·il·i·ac** \ˌsak-rō-'il-ē-ˌak, ˌsā-krō-\ *adj* : of, relating to, affecting, or being the region of the joint between the sacrum and the ilium ⟨∼ distress⟩

²**sacroiliac** *n* : SACROILIAC JOINT

sacroiliac joint *n* : the joint or articulation between the sacrum and ilium — called also *sacroiliac, sacroiliac articulation*

sa·cro·il·i·i·tis \ˌsā-krō-ˌil-ē-'īt-əs, ˌsak-rō-\ *n* : inflammation of the sacroiliac joint or region

sa·cro·spi·na·lis \ˌsā-krō-spī-'nā-ləs, ˌsak-rō-spī-'nal-əs\ *n* : a muscle that extends the length of the back and neck, that arises from the iliac crest, the sacrum, and the lumbar and two lower thoracic vertebrae, and that splits in the upper lumbar region into three divisions of which the lateral is made up of the three iliocostalis muscles, the intermediate is made up of the three longissimus muscles, and the medial is made up of the three spinalis muscles — called also *erector spinae*

sa·cro·spi·nous ligament \ˌsā-krō-ˌspī-nəs-, ˌsak-rō-\ *n* : a ligament on each side of the body that is attached by a broad base to the lateral margins of the sacrum and coccyx and passes to the ischial spine and that closes off the greater sciatic notch to form the greater sciatic foramen and with the sacrotuberous ligament closes off the lesser sciatic notch to form the lesser sciatic foramen

sa·cro·tu·ber·ous ligament \ˌsā-krō-ˌt(y)ü-b(ə-)rəs-, ˌsak-rō-\ *n* : a thin fan-shaped ligament on each side of the body that is attached above to the posterior superior and posterior inferior iliac spines and to the sacrum and coccyx, that passes obliquely downward to insert into the inner margin of the ischial tuberosity, and that with the sacrospinous ligament closes off the lesser sciatic notch to form the lesser sciatic foramen

sa·cro·uter·ine ligament \-ˌyüt-ə-ˌrīn-, -rən-\ *n* : UTEROSACRAL LIGAMENT

sa·crum \'sak-rəm, 'sā-krəm\ *n, pl* **sa·cra** \'sak-rə, 'sā-krə\ : the part of the spinal column that is directly connected with or forms a part of the pelvis by articulation with the ilia and that in humans forms the dorsal wall of the pelvis and consists of five fused vertebrae diminishing in size to the apex at the lower end which bears the coccyx

SAD *abbr* seasonal affective disorder

sad·dle \'sad-əl\ *n* : the part of a partial denture that carries an artificial tooth and has connectors for adjacent teeth attached to its ends

sad·dle·bag \'sad-əl-ˌbag\ *n* : a bulge of lumpy fat in the outer area of the upper thighs

saddle block anesthesia *n* : spinal anesthesia confined to the perineum, the buttocks, and the inner aspect of the thighs — called also *saddle block*

saddle embolus *n* : an embolus that straddles the branching of an artery blocking both branches — called also *rider embolus*

saddle joint *n* : a joint (as the carpometacarpal joint of the thumb) with saddle-shaped articular surfaces that are convex in one direction and concave in another and that permit movements in all directions except axial rotation

sad·dle·nose \'sad-ᵊl-ˌnōz\ *n* : a nose marked by depression of the bridge resulting from injury or disease

sa·dism \'sā-ˌdiz-əm, 'sad-ˌiz-\ *n* : a sexual perversion in which gratification is obtained by the infliction of physical or mental pain on others (as on a love object) — compare ALGOLAGNIA, MASOCHISM — **sa·dis·tic** \sə-'dis-tik *also* sā- *or* sa-\ *adj* — **sa·dis·ti·cal·ly** \-ti-k(ə-)lē\ *adv*

Sade \säd\, **Marquis de (Comte Donatien–Alphonse–François) (1740–1814),** French soldier and writer. From the time that he was a young nobleman Sade consorted with prostitutes and developed a taste for sexual perversions. He was imprisoned on several occasions for his harsh abuse of prostitutes and gross licentiousness. After arriving at the Bastille in 1784 he began writing erotic novels in which he gave full expression to his sexual fantasies. His most famous novel was *The Adversities of Virtue* (1787). His works are known for their graphic descriptions of sexual perversions. His last years were spent in an insane asylum at Charenton, where he wrote plays for his fellow inmates to perform. His compulsion for physically and sexually abusing others gave rise to the concept of *sadism.*

sa·dist \'säd-əst, 'sad-\ *n* : an individual who practices sadism

sa·do·mas·och·ism \ˌsäd-(ˌ)ō-'mas-ə-ˌkiz-əm, ˌsad-, -'maz-\ *n* : the derivation of pleasure from the infliction of physical or mental pain either on others or on oneself

L. von Sacher–Masoch — see MASOCHISM

sa·do·mas·och·ist \-kəst\ *n* : an individual who practices sadomasochism

sa·do·mas·och·ist·ic \-ˌmas-ə-'kist-ik\ *also* **sadomasochist** *adj* : of, relating to, involving, or exhibiting sadomasochism

safe \'sāf\ *adj* **saf·er; saf·est** : not causing harm or injury; *esp* : having a low incidence of adverse reactions and significant side effects when adequate instructions for use are given and having a low potential for harm under conditions of widespread availability ⟨a list of drugs generally regarded as ∼⟩ ⟨∼ use in pregnancy has not been established —*Emergency Medicine*⟩ — **safe·ty** \'sāf-tē\ *n, pl* **-ties**

safe period *n* : a portion of the menstrual cycle of the human female during which conception is least likely to occur and which usu. includes several days immediately before and after the menstrual period and the period itself

safe sex *n* : sexual activity and esp. sexual intercourse in which various measures (as the use of latex condoms or the practice of monogamy) are taken to avoid disease (as AIDS) transmitted by sexual contact — called also *safer sex*

saf·flow·er \'saf-ˌlaů(-ə)r\ *n* **1** : a widely grown Old World composite herb (*Carthamus tinctorius*) that has large orange or red flower heads from which a red dyestuff is prepared and seeds rich in oil **2** : a drug consisting of the dried florets of the safflower that has been used in medicine in place of saffron — called also *carthamus*

safflower oil *n* : an edible drying oil that is low in saturated fatty acids and is obtained from the seeds of the safflower

saf·fron \'saf-rän, -rən\ *n* **1** : the deep orange aromatic pungent dried stigmas of a purple-flowered crocus used to color and flavor foods and formerly as a dyestuff and as a stimulant antispasmodic emmenagogue in medicine **2** : a purple-flowered crocus (*Crocus sativa*) that is the source of saffron — called also *saffron crocus*

saf·ra·nine \'saf-rə-ˌnēn, -nən\ *or* **saf·ra·nin** \-nən\ *n* **1** : any of various usu. red synthetic dyes that are amino derivatives of bases **2** : any of various mixtures of safranine salts used in dyeing and as biological stains

saf·role \'saf-ˌrōl\ *also* **saf·rol** \-ˌrōl, -ˌrȯl\ *n* : a poisonous oily cyclic carcinogenic ether $C_{10}H_{10}O_2$ that is the principal component of sassafras oil and occurs also in other essential oils (as camphor oil) and that is used chiefly in perfumery

sage \'sāj\ *n* : a perennial mint of the genus *Salvia* (*S. officinalis*) having grayish green pungent and aromatic leaves that are much used in flavoring foods and as a mild tonic and astringent; *broadly* : any plant of the genus *Salvia*

sag·it·tal \'saj-ət-ᵊl\ *adj* **1** : of, relating to, or being the sagit-

tal suture of the skull **2** : of, relating to, situated in, or being the median plane of the body or any plane parallel to it ⟨a ∼ section dividing the body into unequal right and left parts⟩ — **sag·it·tal·ly** *adv*

sagittal crest *n* : an elevated bony ridge along the sagittal suture of many mammalian skulls including those of some extinct hominids

sagittal plane *n* : MIDSAGITTAL PLANE; *also* : any plane parallel to a midsagittal plane : a parasagittal plane

sagittal sinus *n* : either of two venous sinuses of the dura mater: **a** : one passing backward in the convex attached superior margin of the falx cerebri and ending at the internal occipital protuberance by fusion with the transverse sinus — called also *superior sagittal sinus* **b** : one lying in the posterior two thirds of the concave free inferior margin of the falx cerebri and ending posteriorly by joining the great cerebral vein to form the straight sinus — called also *inferior sagittal sinus*

sagittal suture *n* : the deeply serrated articulation between the two parietal bones in the median plane of the top of the head

sa·go \'sā-(ˌ)gō\ *n, pl* **sagos** : a dry granulated or powdered starch prepared from the pith of a sago palm and used in foods and as textile stiffening

sago palm *n* : a plant that yields sago; *esp* : any of various lofty pinnate-leaved Malaysian palms (genus *Metroxylon*)

sago spleen *n* : a spleen which is affected with amyloid degeneration and in which the amyloid is deposited in the Malpighian corpuscles which appear in cross section as gray translucent bodies resembling grains of sago

sagrada — see CASCARA SAGRADA

sail·or's skin \'sā-lərz-\ *n* : skin of exposed portions of the body marked by warty thickening, pigmentation, and presenile keratosis and often considered to be precancerous and to lead to formation of epitheliomas

Saint An·tho·ny's fire \ˌsānt-ˌan(t)-thə-nēz-, *chiefly Brit* -ˌan-tə-\ *n* : any of several inflammatory or gangrenous conditions (as erysipelas or ergotism) of the skin

Anthony, Saint (*ca* 250–350), Egyptian monk. St. Anthony is regarded as the founder of Christian monasticism. From the age of 20 he practiced an ascetic life, living in absolute solitude on mountains or in the desert. He occasionally emerged from his seclusion in order to instruct and organize the monastic life of other hermits who had imitated him or to preach against heresies. He is the patron saint of swineherds, and in the art of the Middle Ages he is shown with a small pig at his side. Since pork fat was used to dress the wounds of skin diseases, he became the saint of those who care for the sick, and skin diseases such as erysipelas and ergotism became known as Saint Anthony's fire.

Saint–Ig·na·tius's–bean \-ig-'nā-sh(ē-)əs-\ *n* : the greenish straw-colored seed of a Philippine woody vine of the genus *Strychnos* (*S. ignatii*) that is like nux vomica in its action and uses — called also *Ignatius bean*

Aze·ve·do \ə-zə-'vā-thü\, **Blessed Ignacio de (1527–1570),** Portuguese missionary. Azevedo became a Jesuit in 1548 and subsequently served as rector of religious colleges in Lisbon and Braga, Portugal. In 1566 he journeyed to Brazil to serve the Jesuit missions there. While on a trip to Europe to recruit new missionaries, he and 39 other Jesuits were attacked by Huguenot privateers, who brutally slaughtered them. Azevedo and the other martyrs were beatified in 1854.

Saint–John's–wort \-'jänz-ˌwərt, -ˌwȯ(ə)rt\ *n* **1** : any of a genus (*Hypericum* of the family Guttiferae, the Saint-John's-wort family) of herbs and shrubs with showy yellow flowers; *esp* : one (*H. perforatum*) of dry soil, roadsides, pastures, and ranges that contains a photodynamic pigment causing dermatitis due to photosensitization in sheep, cattle, horses, and

---

\ə\ **abut** \ᵊ\ **kitten** \ər\ **further** \a\ **ash** \ā\ **ace** \ä\ **cot, cart** \aů\ **out** \ch\ **chin** \e\ **bet** \ē\ **easy** \g\ **go** \i\ **hit** \ī\ **ice** \j\ **job** \ŋ\ **sing** \ō\ **go** \ȯ\ **law** \ȯi\ **boy** \th\ **thin** \t̲h̲\ **the** \ü\ **loot** \ů\ **foot** \y\ **yet** \zh\ **vision** *See also* Pronunciation Symbols page

S
T

goats when ingested — see HYPERICISM **2** *usu* **Saint John's wort** : the dried aerial parts of a Saint-John's-wort (*Hypericum perforatum*) that are held to relieve depression and are used in herbal remedies and dietary supplements

John the Bap·tist \-'bap-təst\, **Saint** (*fl* **1st century** AD) Jewish prophet. John lived approximately at the same time as Jesus Christ. He is considered by Christians the last of the Jewish prophets and the forerunner of Christ. John preached the imminence of God's Final Judgment and the Messiah. He baptized his followers as a token of repentance, and Jesus himself received his rite of baptism. He was executed by Herod Antipas for publicly opposing the latter's marriage to Herodias. Saint-John's-wort derives its name from the fact that it was traditionally gathered on the eve of his feast day (June 24) and used to ward off evil spirits and as a medicinal herb.

Saint Lou·is encephalitis \-,lü-əs-\ *n* : a No. American encephalitis that is caused by a single-stranded RNA virus of the genus *Flavivirus* (species *St. Louis encephalitis virus*) transmitted by several mosquitoes of the genus *Culex*

Saint Vi·tus' dance also **Saint Vitus's dance** \-,vīt-əs(-əz)-\ *n* : CHOREA; *esp* : SYDENHAM'S CHOREA

Vitus, Saint (*d ca* 300), Italian martyr. Saint Vitus is believed by some to have lived during the reign of the Roman emperor Diocletian. According to legend, while still a child he delivered the emperor's daughter of an evil spirit. Because he was a Christian, however, he was subjected to various tortures, including being thrown into a cauldron filled with pitch and molten lead. He survived the torture intact, but he and his Christian nurse were ultimately put to death. People suffering from chorea have traditionally invoked his name for relief.

sal \'sal\ *n* : SALT — see SAL AMMONIAC

sal·abra·sion \,sal-ə-'brā-zhən\ *n* : a method of removing tattoos from skin in which moist gauze pads saturated with sodium chloride are used to abrade the tattooed area by rubbing

sal am·mo·ni·ac \,sal-ə-'mō-nē-,ak\ *n* : AMMONIUM CHLORIDE

sal·bu·ta·mol \sal-'byüt-ə-,mȯl, -,mōl\ *n* : ALBUTEROL

sa·lep \'sal-əp, sə-'lep\ *n* : the starchy or mucilaginous dried tubers of various orchids (genus *Orchis* or *Eulophia*) used for food or in medicine

sal·i·cin \'sal-i-sin\ *n* : a bitter white crystalline glucoside $C_{13}H_{18}O_7$ found in the bark and leaves of several willows and poplars, yielding saligenin and glucose on hydrolysis, and formerly used in medicine as an antipyretic, antirheumatic, and tonic

sal·i·cyl al·co·hol \'sal-i-sil-\ *n* : SALIGENIN

sal·i·cyl·al·de·hyde \-'al-də-,hīd\ *n* : an oily liquid phenolic aldehyde $C_7H_6O_2$ that has a bitter almond odor and is used chiefly in perfumery and in making coumarin — called also *salicylic aldehyde*

sal·i·cyl·amide \,sal-ə-'sil-ə-,mīd\ *n* : the crystalline amide $C_7H_7NO_2$ of salicylic acid that is used chiefly as an analgesic, antipyretic, and antirheumatic

sal·i·cyl·an·il·ide \,sal-ə-sə-'lan-ᵊl-īd\ *n* : a crystalline compound $C_{13}H_{11}NO_2$ that is used as a fungicidal agent esp. in the external treatment of tinea capitis caused by a fungus of the genus *Microsporum* (*M. audouini*)

sa·lic·y·late \sə-'lis-ə-,lāt\ *n* : a salt or ester of salicylic acid; *also* : SALICYLIC ACID

sa·lic·y·lat·ed \-,lāt-əd\ *adj* : treated with salicylic acid

sal·i·cyl·azo·sul·fa·pyr·i·dine *or chiefly Brit* **sal·i·cyl·azo·sul·pha·pyr·i·dine** \,sal-ə-sil-,ā-zō-,səl-fə-'pir-ə-,dēn\ *n* : SULFASALAZINE

sal·i·cyl·ic acid \,sal-ə-,sil-ik-\ *n* : a crystalline phenolic acid $C_7H_6O_3$ that is the ortho form of hydroxybenzoic acid and is used esp. in making pharmaceuticals and dyes, as an antiseptic and disinfectant esp. in treating skin diseases, as a keratolytic agent for skin exfoliation, and in the form of salts and other derivatives as an analgesic and antipyretic and in the treatment of rheumatism — see ASPIRIN

salicylic aldehyde *n* : SALICYLALDEHYDE

sal·i·cyl·ism \'sal-ə-sil-,iz-əm\ *n* : a toxic condition produced by the excessive intake of salicylic acid or salicylates and marked by ringing in the ears, nausea, and vomiting

sal·i·cyl·iza·tion *or chiefly Brit* **sal·i·cyl·isa·tion** \,sal-ə-,sil-ə-'zā-shən\ *n* **1** : the act or process of administering salicylates until physiological effects are produced in the patient **2** : the condition produced by salicylization

sal·i·cyl·ize *or chiefly Brit* **sal·i·cyl·ise** \'sal-ə-sil-,īz\ *vt* **-cyl·ized** *or chiefly Brit* **-cyl·ised; -cyl·iz·ing** *or chiefly Brit* **-cyl·is·ing** : to treat (a patient) with salicylic acid or its compounds until physiological effects are produced

sal·i·cyl·uric acid \,sal-ə-sil-,(y)ùr-ik-\ *n* : a crystalline acid $C_9H_9NO_4$ found in the urine after the administration of salicylic acid or one of its derivatives

sal·i·gen·in \,sal-ə-'jen-ən, sə-'lij-ə-nən\ *n* : a crystalline phenolic alcohol $C_7H_8O_2$ that is obtained usu. by hydrolysis of salicin and that acts as a local anesthetic — called also *salicyl alcohol*

sa·lim·e·ter \sā-'lim-ət-ər, sə-\ *n* : SALOMETER

¹sa·line \'sā-,lēn, -,līn\ *adj* **1** : consisting of or containing salt ⟨a ~ solution⟩ **2** : of, relating to, or resembling salt : SALTY ⟨a ~ taste⟩ **3** : consisting of or relating to the salts esp. of lithium, sodium, and magnesium ⟨a ~ cathartic⟩ **4** : relating to or being abortion induced by the injection of a highly concentrated saline solution into the amniotic sac ⟨~ amniocentesis⟩

²saline *n* **1 a** : a metallic salt; *esp* : a salt of potassium, sodium, or magnesium with a cathartic action **b** : an aqueous solution of one or more such salts **2** : a saline solution used in physiology; *esp* : PHYSIOLOGICAL SALINE

sa·lin·i·ty \sā-'lin-ət-ē, sə-\ *n, pl* **-ties** **1** : the quality or state of being saline **2** : a concentration (as in a solution) of salt

sa·li·nom·e·ter \,sal-ə-'näm-ət-ər, ,sā-lə-\ *n* : an instrument (as a hydrometer) for measuring the amount of salt in a solution

sa·li·va \sə-'lī-və\ *n* : a slightly alkaline secretion of water, mucin, protein, salts, and often a starch-splitting enzyme (as ptyalin) that is secreted into the mouth by salivary glands, lubricates ingested food, and often begins the breakdown of starches

saliva ejector *n* : a narrow tubular device providing suction to draw saliva, blood, and debris from the mouth of a dental patient in order to maintain a clear operative field

sal·i·vary \'sal-ə-,ver-ē\ *adj* : of or relating to saliva or the glands that secrete it; *esp* : producing or carrying saliva

salivary corpuscles *n pl* : degenerating lymphocytes originating in the tonsils and passing into the saliva in the mouth

salivary gland *n* : any of various glands that discharge a fluid secretion and esp. saliva into the mouth cavity and that in humans comprise large compound racemose glands including the parotid glands, the sublingual glands, and the submandibular glands

sal·i·vate \'sal-ə-,vāt\ *vb* **-vat·ed; -vat·ing** *vt* : to produce an abnormal flow of saliva in (as by the use of mercury) ~ *vi* : to have a flow of saliva esp. in excess

sal·i·va·tion \,sal-ə-'vā-shən\ *n* : the act or process of salivating; *esp* : excessive secretion of saliva often accompanied by soreness of the mouth and gums

sal·i·va·to·ry \'sal-ə-və-,tōr-ē, *Brit usu* ,sal-ə-'vā-trē\ *adj* : inducing salivation

Salk vaccine \'sȯ(l)k-\ *n* : a polio vaccine consisting of the three serotypes of poliovirus grown on embryonated eggs and inactivated by treatment with formaldehyde — compare SABIN VACCINE

Salk, Jonas Edward (1914–1995), American immunologist. In 1942 while on a fellowship in epidemiology, Salk began studies of the influenza virus with the purpose of producing vaccines in commercial quantities. In 1947 he became the director of the virus research laboratory at the University of Pittsburgh, and two years later he changed his interest to developing a serum against poliomyelitis. A problem was presented by the fact that poliomyelitis is caused by three strains of virus and a single effective vaccine was needed that could neutralize all of the strains. In

1953 he announced the successful development of a vaccine prepared from virus inactivated by treatment with formaldehyde. In the next two years mass inoculation of school children with the Salk vaccine was undertaken. 1953 was also the year in which he published the results of experimental inoculations of 20,000 people with a flu vaccine which had produced immunity for as long as two years. That vaccine also went into wide use.

sal·met·er·ol \sal-ˈmet-ə-ˌròl, -ˌrōl, -ˈmē-tə-\ *n* : a bronchodilator administered by oral inhalation in the form of a salt C₂₅H₃₇NO₄·C₁₁H₈O₃ to treat asthma and bronchospasm — see ADVAIR DISKUS

sal·mine \ˈsal-ˌmēn\ *n* : a protamine obtained from the sperm of salmon and used chiefly in the form of its sulfate to reverse the anticoagulant effect of heparin or as the protamine component of protamine zinc insulin

sal·mo·nel·la \ˌsal-mə-ˈnel-ə\ *n* **1** *cap* : a genus of aerobic gram-negative rod-shaped nonspore-forming usu. motile bacteria of the family Enterobacteriaceae that grow well on artificial media and form acid and gas on many carbohydrates but not on lactose, sucrose, or salicin, that are pathogenic for humans and other warm-blooded animals, and that cause food poisoning, acute gastrointestinal inflammation, typhoid fever, and septicemia **2** *pl* **-nel·lae** \-ˈnel-ē\ *or* **-nellas** *or* **-nella** : any bacterium of the genus *Salmonella*

Salm·on \ˈsam-ən\, **Daniel Elmer (1850–1914)**, American veterinarian. For the greater part of his career Salmon was associated with the U.S. Department of Agriculture, having joined the department to investigate diseases of domestic animals, especially Texas fever. He later founded and became chief of the Bureau of Animal Industry. In 1900 the genus *Salmonella* of bacteria was named after him.

sal·mo·nel·lal \-ˈnel-əl\ *adj* : of, relating to, being, or caused by salmonellae ⟨∼ food poisoning⟩

sal·mo·nel·lo·sis \ˌsal-mə-ˌne-ˈlō-səs\ *n, pl* **-lo·ses** \-ˌsēz\ : infection with or disease caused by bacteria of the genus *Salmonella* typically marked by gastroenteritis but often complicated by septicemia, meningitis, endocarditis, and various focal lesions (as in the kidneys)

salmon poisoning *n* : a highly fatal febrile disease of fish-eating dogs and other canine mammals that resembles canine distemper and is caused by a rickettsial bacterium (*Neorickettsia helminthoeca*) transmitted by encysted larvae of a fluke (*Nanophyetus salmincola*) ingested with the raw flesh of infested salmon, trout, or salamanders

sal·ol \ˈsal-ˌòl, -ˌōl\ *n* : PHENYL SALICYLATE

sa·lom·e·ter \sā-ˈläm-ət-ər, sə-\ *n* : a hydrometer for indicating the percentage of salt in a solution — called also *salimeter*

sal·pin·gec·to·my \ˌsal-pən-ˈjek-tə-mē\ *n, pl* **-mies** : surgical excision of a fallopian tube

sal·pin·gi·tis \ˌsal-pən-ˈjīt-əs\ *n, pl* **-git·i·des** \-ˈjit-ə-ˌdēz\ : inflammation of a fallopian or eustachian tube

salpingitis isth·mi·ca no·do·sa \-ˈis-mə-kə-nə-ˈdō-sə\ *n* : salpingitis of the fallopian tubes marked by nodular thickening of the muscular coat esp. of the tubal portion adjacent to the uterus

sal·pin·go·gram \sal-ˈpiŋ-gə-ˌgram\ *n* : a radiograph produced by salpingography

sal·pin·gog·ra·phy \ˌsal-piŋ-ˈgäg-rə-fē\ *n, pl* **-phies** : visualization of a fallopian tube by radiography following injection of an opaque medium

sal·pin·gol·y·sis \ˌsal-piŋ-ˈgäl-ə-səs\ *n, pl* **-y·ses** : surgical correction of adhesions in a fallopian tube

sal·pin·go-oo·pho·rec·to·my \sal-ˌpiŋ-gō-ˌō-ə-fə-ˈrek-tə-mē\ *n, pl* **-mies** : surgical excision of a fallopian tube and an ovary

sal·pin·go-oo·pho·ri·tis \-ˌō-ə-fə-ˈrīt-əs\ *n* : inflammation of a fallopian tube and an ovary

sal·pin·go·pha·ryn·ge·us \-fə-ˈrin-jē-əs\ *n* : a muscle of the pharynx that arises from the inferior part of the eustachian tube near its opening and passes downward to join the posterior part of the palatopharyngeus

sal·pin·go·plas·ty \sal-ˈpiŋ-gə-ˌplas-tē\ *n, pl* **-ties** : plastic surgery of a fallopian tube

sal·pin·gos·to·my \ˌsal-piŋ-ˈgäs-tə-mē\ *n, pl* **-mies** : a surgical opening of a fallopian tube (as to establish patency)

sal soda \ˈsal-ˌsòd-ə\ *n* : WASHING SODA

¹salt \ˈsòlt\ *n* **1 a** : a crystalline compound NaCl that is the chloride of sodium, is abundant in nature, and is used esp. to season or preserve food or in industry — called also *common salt, sodium chloride* **b** : a substance (as Glauber's salt) resembling common salt **c** : any of numerous compounds that result from replacement of part or all of the acid hydrogen of an acid by a metal or a group acting like a metal : an ionic crystalline compound **2 salts** *pl* **a** : a mineral or saline mixture (as Epsom salts) used as an aperient or cathartic **b** : SMELLING SALTS

²salt *adj* **1** : SALINE, SALTY **2** : being or inducing the one of the four basic taste sensations that is suggestive of seawater — compare BITTER, SOUR, SWEET

sal·ta·tion \sal-ˈtā-shən, sòl-\ *n* **1** : the origin of a new species or a higher taxon in essentially a single evolutionary step that in some esp. former theories is held to be due to macromutation **2** : MUTATION — used esp. of bacteria and fungi

sal·ta·to·ry \ˈsal-tə-ˌtōr-ē, ˈsòl-, -ˌtòr-\ *adj* : proceeding by leaps rather than by gradual transitions ⟨∼ conduction of impulses in myelinated nerve fibers⟩

salt out *vt* : to precipitate, coagulate, or separate (as a dissolved substance or lyophilic sol) esp. from a solution by the addition of salt ∼ *vi* : to become salted out

salt·pe·ter *or chiefly Brit* **salt·pe·tre** \ˈsòlt-ˈpēt-ər\ *n* **1** : POTASSIUM NITRATE **2** : SODIUM NITRATE

salty \ˈsòl-tē\ *adj* **salt·i·er; -est** : of, seasoned with, or containing salt — **salt·i·ness** \-tē-nəs\ *n*

sa·lu·bri·ous \sə-ˈlü-brē-əs\ *adj* : favorable to or promoting health or well-being ⟨a ∼ climate⟩ — **sa·lu·bri·ous·ness** *n* — **sa·lu·bri·ty** \-brət-ē\ *n, pl* **-ties**

¹sal·uret·ic \ˌsal-tə-ˈret-ik\ *adj* : facilitating the urinary excretion of salt and esp. of sodium ion ⟨a ∼ drug⟩ ⟨∼ therapy⟩ — **sal·uret·i·cal·ly** \-i-k(ə-)lē\ *adv*

²saluretic *n* : a saluretic agent (as a drug)

Sal·u·ron \ˈsal-(y)ə-ˌrän\ *n* : a preparation of hydroflumethiazide — formerly a U.S. registered trademark

sal·u·tary \ˈsal-yə-ˌter-ē\ *adj* : promoting health : CURATIVE

¹sal·vage \ˈsal-vij\ *n* : the act or an instance of salvaging ⟨thrombolytic therapy has permitted ∼ of some limbs —Richard Lennihan *et al*⟩

²salvage *vt* **sal·vaged; sal·vag·ing** : to save (an organ, tissue, or patient) by preventive or therapeutic measures ⟨a *salvaged* cancer patient⟩ ⟨*salvaged* lung tissue⟩

sal·vage·able \ˈsal-vij-ə-bəl\ *adj* : capable of being salvaged ⟨∼ patients⟩ — **sal·vage·abil·i·ty** *n, pl* **-ties**

sal·var·san \ˈsal-vər-ˌsan\ *n* : ARSPHENAMINE

salve \ˈsav, ˈsäv, ˈsàv, ˈsalv, ˈsälv\ *n* : an unctuous adhesive substance for application to wounds or sores

sal·via \ˈsal-vē-ə\ *n* **1** *cap* : a genus of widely distributed herbs or shrubs of the mint family (Labiatae) including the sage (*S. officinalis*) **2** : any herb or shrub of the genus *Salvia*

sal vo·la·ti·le \ˌsal-və-ˈlat-ᵊl-ē\ *n* **1** : AMMONIUM CARBONATE **2** : SMELLING SALTS

sa·mar·i·um \sə-ˈmer-ē-əm, -ˈmar-\ *n* : a pale gray lustrous metallic element used esp. in alloys that form permanent magnets — symbol *Sm*; see ELEMENT table

sam·bu·cus \sam-ˈb(y)ü-kəs\ *n* **1** *cap* : a genus of trees or shrubs of the honeysuckle family (Caprifoliaceae) that bear flat clusters of small white or pink flowers and that include the elderberries **2** : the dried flowers of either of two elderberries (*Sambucus canadensis* or *S. nigra*) formerly used esp. in the form of an infusion as a mild stimulant, carminative, and diaphoretic but of little medicinal effect

SAMe \ˈsam-ē\ *n* : *S*-adenosylmethionine esp. when used as

\ə\ abut \ᵊ\ kitten \ər\ further \a\ ash \ā\ ace \ä\ cot, cart \aù\ out \ch\ chin \e\ bet \ē\ easy \g\ go \i\ hit \ī\ ice \j\ job \ŋ\ sing \ō\ go \ò\ law \òi\ boy \th\ thin \t͟h\ the \ü\ loot \ù\ foot \y\ yet \zh\ vision *See also* Pronunciation Symbols page

a dietary supplement with the intention of relieving depression or arthritic pain and inflammation

sam·ple \'sam-pəl\ *n* **1 :** a representative part or a single item from a larger whole or group esp. when presented for inspection or shown as evidence of quality : SPECIMEN ⟨a blood ∼⟩ **2 :** a finite part of a statistical population whose properties are studied to gain information about the whole

sam·pling \'sam-pliŋ\ *n* **1 :** the act, process, or technique of selecting a suitable sample; *specif* : the act, process, or technique of selecting a representative part of a population for the purpose of determining parameters or characteristics of the whole population **2 :** SAMPLE ⟨obtain a ∼ of urine⟩

san·a·tive \'san-ət-iv\ *adj* : having the power to cure or heal : CURATIVE

san·a·to·ri·um \ˌsan-ə-'tōr-ē-əm, -'tȯr-\ *n, pl* **-ri·ums** *or* **-ria** \-ē-ə\ **1 :** an establishment that provides therapy combined with a regimen (as of diet and exercise) for treatment or rehabilitation **2 a :** an institution for rest and recuperation (as of convalescents) **b :** an establishment for the treatment of the chronically ill ⟨a tuberculosis ∼⟩

sand \'sand\ *n* : gritty particles in various body tissues or fluids — see BRAIN SAND

san·dal·wood oil \'san-dᵊl-ˌwu̇d-\ *n* : a pale yellow somewhat viscous aromatic liquid essential oil obtained from a sandalwood (*Santalum album*) and used chiefly in perfumes and soaps and esp. formerly in medicine — called also *santal oil*

san·da·rac \'san-də-ˌrak\ *n* : a brittle aromatic translucent resin obtained from a large northern African tree (*Callitris articulata*) of the cypress family (Cupressaceae) and used chiefly in making varnish and as incense; *also* : a similar resin obtained from any of several related Australian trees

sand bath *n* : a bath of sand in which laboratory vessels to be heated are partly immersed; *also* : a pan for holding the sand

sand crack *n* : a fissure in the wall of a horse's hoof often causing lameness

sand flea *n* : CHIGOE 1

sand fly *n* : any of various small biting dipteran flies (families Psychodidae, Simuliidae, and Ceratopogonidae); *esp* : any fly of the genus *Phlebotomus*

sand-fly fever \ˌsan(d)-ˌflī-\ *n* : a virus disease of brief duration that is characterized by fever, headache, pain in the eyes, malaise, and leukopenia and is caused by either of two bunyaviruses of the genus *Phlebovirus* transmitted by the bite of a sand fly of the genus *Phlebotomus* (esp. *P. papatasii*) — called also *pappataci fever, phlebotomus fever*

Sand·hoff–Jatz·ke·witz disease \-'jats-kə-ˌvits\ *n* : SANDHOFF'S DISEASE

Sand·hoff's disease \'sand-ˌhȯfs-\ *or* **Sand·hoff disease** \-ˌhȯf-\ *n* : a hereditary disorder of lipid metabolism that is closely related to or a variant of Tay-Sachs disease, that typically affects individuals of non-Jewish ancestry, and that is characterized by great reduction in or absence of both hexosaminidase A and hexosaminidase B

  Sandhoff, K., An·dreae \än-'drā-ə\, U., and Jatz·ke·witz \'yäts-kə-ˌvits\, H., German medical scientists. Sandhoff, Andreae, and Jatzkewitz jointly published a description of a variant form of Tay-Sachs disease in 1968. They based their report on three typical cases of Tay-Sachs, one exceptional case, and seven controls.

San·dril \'san-ˌdril\ *n* : a preparation of reserpine — formerly a U.S. registered trademark

sandy blight \'sand-ē-\ *n* : BLIGHT

sane \'sān\ *adj* **san·er; san·est** **1 :** free from hurt or disease : HEALTHY **2 :** mentally sound; *esp* : able to anticipate and appraise the effect of one's actions **3 :** proceeding from a sound mind ⟨∼ behavior⟩ — **sane·ly** *adv*

san·gui·fi·ca·tion \ˌsaŋ-gwə-fə-'kā-shən\ *n* : formation of blood : HEMATOPOIESIS

san·gui·nar·ia \ˌsaŋ-gwə-'ner-ē-ə, -'nar-\ *n* : the rhizome and roots of the bloodroot formerly used as an expectorant and emetic

san·guin·a·rine \saŋ-'gwin-ə-ˌrēn, -rən\ *n* : a poisonous bit-

ter crystalline alkaloid $C_{20}H_{15}NO_5$ obtained esp. from the bloodroot

san·guine \'saŋ-gwən\ *adj* **1 a :** consisting of or relating to blood **b** *of the complexion* : RUDDY **2 :** having blood as the predominating bodily humor; *also* : having the bodily conformation and temperament held characteristic of such predominance and marked by sturdiness, high color, and cheerfulness

san·guin·e·ous \saŋ-'gwin-ē-əs, san-\ *adj* **1 :** of, relating to, or containing blood **2 :** SANGUINE 2 ⟨a ∼ temperament⟩

san·guin·o·lent \-'gwin-ᵊl-ənt\ *adj* : of, containing, or tinged with blood ⟨∼ sputum⟩

san·gui·no·pu·ru·lent \ˌsaŋ-gwə-nō-'pyu̇r-(y)ə-lənt\ *adj* : containing blood and pus ⟨∼ discharge⟩

san·guin·ous \saŋ-'gwə-nəs\ *adj* : SANGUINEOUS ⟨slightly ∼, frothy material was slowly exuding from her nose and mouth —*Jour. Amer. Med. Assoc.*⟩

sa·ni·es \'sā-nē-ˌēz\ *n, pl* **sanies** : a thin blood-tinged seropurulent discharge from ulcers or infected wounds — compare ICHOR

sa·ni·ous \'sā-nē-əs\ *adj* : consisting of a thin mixture of serum and pus with a slightly bloody tinge ⟨a ∼ discharge⟩

san·i·tar·i·an \ˌsan-ə-'ter-ē-ən\ *n* : a specialist in sanitary science and public health ⟨a milk ∼⟩

san·i·tar·i·um \ˌsan-ə-'ter-ē-əm\ *n, pl* **-i·ums** *or* **-ia** \-ē-ə\ : SANATORIUM

san·i·tary \'san-ə-ˌter-ē\ *adj* **1 :** of or relating to health ⟨∼ measures⟩ **2 :** of, relating to, or used in the disposal esp. of domestic waterborne waste ⟨∼ sewage⟩ **3 :** characterized by or readily kept in cleanliness ⟨∼ food handling⟩ — **san·i·tari·ly** \ˌsan-ə-'ter-ə-lē\ *adv*

sanitary napkin *n* : a disposable absorbent pad used (as during menstruation) to absorb the flow from the uterus

san·i·tate \'san-ə-ˌtāt\ *vt* **-tat·ed; -tat·ing** : to make sanitary esp. by providing with sanitary appliances or facilities ⟨epidemics which occurred in areas which had not been *sanitated*⟩

san·i·ta·tion \ˌsan-ə-'tā-shən\ *n* **1 :** the act or process of making sanitary **2 :** the promotion of hygiene and prevention of disease by maintenance of sanitary conditions ⟨mouth ∼⟩

san·i·tize *also Brit* **san·i·tise** \'san-ə-ˌtīz\ *vt* **-tized** *also Brit* **-tised; -tiz·ing** *also Brit* **-tis·ing** : to make sanitary (as by cleaning or sterilizing) ⟨∼ all surfaces with a solution of bleach and water⟩ — **san·i·ti·za·tion** *also Brit* **san·i·ti·sa·tion** \ˌsan-ət-ə-'zā-shən\ *n*

san·i·to·ri·um \ˌsan-ə-'tōr-ē-əm, -'tȯr-\ *n, pl* **-ri·ums** *or* **-ria** \-ē-ə\ : SANATORIUM

san·i·ty \'san-ət-ē\ *n, pl* **-ties** : the quality or state of being sane; *esp* : soundness or health of mind

San Joa·quin fever \ˌsan-wä-'kēn-\ *n* : COCCIDIOIDOMYCOSIS

San Joaquin valley fever *n* : COCCIDIOIDOMYCOSIS

S–A node \ˌes-'ā-\ *n* : SINOATRIAL NODE

santa — see YERBA SANTA

san·tal oil \'sant-ᵊl-\ *n* : SANDALWOOD OIL

san·ta·lol \'san-tə-ˌlȯl, -ˌlōl\ *n* : a mixture of two liquid isomeric alcohols $C_{15}H_{23}OH$ that is the chief constituent of sandalwood oil; *also* : either of these alcohols

san·ton·i·ca \san-'tän-i-kə\ *n* : the unopened dried flower heads of Levant wormseed or of another plant of the genus *Artemisia* (esp. *A. maritima*) used as an anthelmintic; *also* : one of these plants

san·to·nin \'sant-ᵊn-ən, san-'tän-ən\ *n* : a poisonous slightly bitter crystalline compound $C_{15}H_{18}O_3$ found esp. in the unopened flower heads of santonicas and used esp. formerly as an anthelmintic

San·to·ri·ni's duct \ˌsant-ə-'rē-nēz-, ˌsänt-\ *n* : ACCESSORY PANCREATIC DUCT

sap — see CELL SAP, NUCLEAR SAP

sa·phe·na \sə-'fē-nə\ *n, often attrib* : SAPHENOUS VEIN

sa·phe·no·fem·o·ral \sə-ˌfē-nō-'fem-(ə-)rəl\ *adj* : of or relating to the saphenous and the femoral veins ⟨the ∼ junction⟩

sa·phe·nous \sə-'fē-nəs, 'saf-ə-nəs\ *adj* : of, relating to, associated with, or being either of the saphenous veins

saphenous nerve *n* : a nerve that is the largest and longest branch of the femoral nerve and supplies the skin over the medial side of the leg

saphenous opening *n* : a passage for the great saphenous vein in the fascia lata of the thigh — called also *fossa ovalis*

saphenous vein *n* : either of two chief superficial veins of the leg : **a** : one originating in the foot and passing up the medial side of the leg and through the saphenous opening to join the femoral vein — called also *great saphenous vein, long saphenous vein* **b** : one originating similarly and passing up the back of the leg to join the popliteal vein at the knee — called also *short saphenous vein, small saphenous vein*

sap·id \'sap-əd\ *adj* : affecting the organs of taste : possessing flavor and esp. a strong agreeable flavor

sapiens — see HOMO SAPIENS

sa·po \'sā-ˌpō\ *n, pl* **sa·pos** : SOAP 1

sa·po·ge·nin \ˌsap-ə-'jen-ən, sə-'päj-ə-nən\ *n* : a nonsugar portion of a saponin that is typically obtained by hydrolysis, has either a complex terpenoid or a steroid structure and in the latter case forms a practicable starting point in the synthesis of steroid hormones

sap·o·na·ceous \ˌsap-ə-'nā-shəs\ *adj* : resembling or having the qualities of soap ⟨a ∼ preparation⟩

sap·o·nat·ed \'sap-ə-ˌnāt-əd\ *adj* : treated or combined with a soap ⟨∼ cresol solution⟩

sa·pon·i·fi·able \sə-ˌpän-ə-'fī-ə-bəl\ *adj* : capable of being saponified

sa·pon·i·fi·ca·tion \sə-ˌpän-ə-fə-'kā-shən\ *n* **1** : the hydrolysis of a fat by an alkali with the formation of a soap and glycerol **2** : the hydrolysis esp. by an alkali of an ester into the corresponding alcohol and acid; *broadly* : HYDROLYSIS

saponification number *n* : a measure of the total free and combined acids esp. in a fat, wax, or resin expressed as the number of milligrams of potassium hydroxide required for the complete saponification of one gram of substance — called also *saponification value*

sa·pon·i·fy \sə-'pän-ə-ˌfī\ *vb* **-fied; -fy·ing** *vt* : to convert (as a fat or fatty acid) into soap : subject to saponification ∼ *vi* : to undergo saponification

sa·po·nin \'sap-ə-nən, sə-'pō-\ *n* : any of various mostly toxic glucosides that occur in plants (as soapbark) and are characterized by the property of producing a soapy lather; *esp* : a hygroscopic amorphous saponin mixture used esp. as a foaming and emulsifying agent and detergent

sap·o·tox·in \ˌsap-ə-'täk-sən\ *n* : any of various highly poisonous saponins

sap·phic \'saf-ik\ *adj or n* : LESBIAN

Sap·pho \'saf-(ˌ)ō\ (*fl ca* **610** BC–*ca* **580** BC), Greek lyric poet. Sappho was the leading spirit of a coterie of female poets on the Aegean isle of Lesbos. Because of the homosexual themes in her poetry, she herself has traditionally been regarded as homosexual.

sap·phism \'saf-ˌiz-əm\ *n* : LESBIANISM

sap·phist \-əst\ *n* : LESBIAN

sa·pre·mia *or chiefly Brit* **sa·prae·mia** \sə-'prē-mē-ə\ *n* : a toxic state resulting from the presence in the blood of toxic products of putrefactive bacteria and often accompanying gangrene of a part of the body

sap·robe \'sap-ˌrōb\ *n* : a saprobic organism — called also *saprobiont*

sa·pro·bic \sə-'prō-bik\ *adj* : SAPROPHYTIC; *also* : living in or being an environment rich in organic matter and relatively free from oxygen — **sa·pro·bi·cal·ly** \-bi-k(ə-)lē\ *adv*

sap·ro·bi·ont \ˌsap-rō-'bī-ˌänt, sə-'prō-bē-ˌänt\ *n* : SAPROBE

sap·ro·gen \'sap-rə-jən, -ˌjen\ *n* : an organism (as a fungus) living upon and causing decay of nonliving organic matter

sap·ro·gen·ic \ˌsap-rə-'jen-ik\ *also* **sa·prog·e·nous** \sa-'präj-ə-nəs\ *adj* : of, causing, or resulting from putrefaction ⟨∼ bacteria⟩ — **sap·ro·ge·nic·i·ty** \-rō-jə-'nis-ət-ē\ *n, pl* **-ties**

sa·proph·a·gous \sa-'präf-ə-gəs\ *adj* : feeding on decaying matter ⟨∼ insects⟩

sa·proph·i·lous \sa-'präf-ə-ləs\ *adj* : SAPROPHYTIC; *specif* : thriving in decaying matter ⟨∼ bacteria⟩

sap·ro·phyte \'sap-rə-ˌfīt\ *n* : a saprophytic organism; *esp* : a plant living on dead or decaying organic matter

sap·ro·phyt·ic \ˌsap-rə-'fit-ik\ *adj* : obtaining food by absorbing dissolved organic material; *esp* : obtaining nourishment osmotically from the products of organic breakdown and decay ⟨∼ fungi⟩ — **sap·ro·phyt·i·cal·ly** \-i-k(ə-)lē\ *adv*

sap·ro·phyt·ism \'sap-rə-ˌfīt-ˌiz-əm\ *n* : the condition of feeding saprophytically

sap·ro·zo·ic \ˌsap-rə-'zō-ik\ *adj* : SAPROPHYTIC — used of animals (as protozoans)

sa·quin·a·vir \sə-'kwin-ə-ˌvir\ *n* : a protease inhibitor $C_{38}H_{50}N_6O_5$ or its mesylate $C_{38}H_{50}N_6O_5 \cdot CH_4O_3S$ administered orally often in combination with other antiretroviral drugs to treat HIV infection

sar·al·a·sin \sä-'ral-ə-sən\ *n* : an antihypertensive polypeptide composed of eight amino acid residues that is used esp. in the form of its hydrated acetate $C_{42}H_{65}N_{13}O_{10} \cdot nC_2H_4O_2 \cdot nH_2O$ in the treatment and diagnosis of hypertension

sar·ci·na \'sär-si-nə\ *n* **1** *cap* : a genus of bacteria (family Peptococcaceae) that are gram-positive cocci, are mostly harmless saprophytes but include a few serious brewery pests, and have cells which under favorable conditions divide in three directions into cubical masses **2** *pl* **-nas** *or* **-nae** \-nē\ : any bacterium of the genus *Sarcina*

sar·co·blast \'sär-kə-ˌblast\ *n* : MYOBLAST

sar·co·cele \'sär-kə-ˌsēl\ *n* : a fleshy swelling of the testicle resembling a tumor

sar·co·cyst \'sär-kə-ˌsist\ *n* : SARCOCYSTIS 2; *specif* : the large intramuscular cyst of a protozoan of the genus *Sarcocystis*

sar·co·cys·tis \ˌsär-kə-'sis-təs\ *n* **1** *cap* : a genus of sporozoan protozoans of the order Sarcosporidia that form cysts in vertebrate muscle **2** *pl* **-tis** *or* **-tis·es** : any sporozoan protozoan of the genus *Sarcocystis*; *broadly* : any of the order Sarcosporidia

sar·co·cys·to·sis \-sis-'tō-səs\ *n* : infestation with or disease caused by sporozoan protozoans of the genus *Sarcocystis* — called also *sarcosporidiosis*

sar·code \'sär-ˌkōd\ *n* : PROTOPLASM 1

Sar·co·di·na \ˌsär-kə-'dī-nə, -'dē-\ *n, pl* : a subphylum of protozoans of the phylum Sarcomastigophora that includes protozoans forming pseudopodia which ordinarily serve as organs for locomotion and taking food — see RHIZOPODA — **sar·co·din·i·an** \-'din-ē-ən\ *n*

¹sar·coid \'sär-ˌkȯid\ *adj* : of, relating to, resembling, or being sarcoid or sarcoidosis ⟨∼ fibroblastic tissue⟩

²sarcoid *n* **1** : any of various diseases characterized esp. by the formation of nodules in the skin **2** : a nodule characteristic of sarcoid or of sarcoidosis

sar·coid·o·sis \ˌsär-ˌkȯid-'ō-səs\ *n, pl* **-o·ses** \-ˌsēz\ : a chronic disease of unknown cause that is characterized by the formation of nodules resembling true tubercles esp. in the lymph nodes, lungs, bones, and skin — called also *Boeck's disease, Boeck's sarcoid, lupus pernio*

sar·co·lac·tic acid \ˌsär-kə-ˌlak-tik-\ *n* : the dextrorotatory L-form of lactic acid occurring in muscle

sar·co·lem·ma \ˌsär-kə-'lem-ə\ *n* : the thin transparent homogeneous sheath enclosing a striated muscle fiber — **sar·co·lem·mal** \-əl\ *adj*

sar·co·ly·sin \ˌsär-kə-'līs-ᵊn\ *or* **sar·co·ly·sine** \-ˌsēn\ *also* **L–sar·co·ly·sin** \'el-\ *or* **L–sar·co·ly·sine** *n* : MELPHALAN

sar·col·y·sis \sär-'käl-ə-səs\ *n, pl* **-y·ses** \-ˌsēz\ : lysis of muscular tissue

sar·co·ma \sär-'kō-mə\ *n, pl* **-mas** *also* **-ma·ta** \-mət-ə\ : a malignant tumor arising in tissue of mesodermal origin (as connective tissue, bone, cartilage, or striated muscle) that spreads by extension into neighboring tissue or by way of the bloodstream — compare CARCINOMA

\ə\ abut \ᵊ\ kitten \ər\ further \a\ ash \ā\ ace \ä\ cot, cart \au̇\ out \ch\ chin \e\ bet \ē\ easy \g\ go \i\ hit \ī\ ice \j\ job \ŋ\ sing \ō\ go \ȯ\ law \ȯi\ boy \th\ thin \t͟h\ the \ü\ loot \u̇\ foot \y\ yet \zh\ vision *See also* Pronunciation Symbols page

S
T

sarcoma bot·ry·oi·des \-ˌbä-trē-ˈoid-ˌēz\ *n* : a malignant tumor of striated muscle that resembles a bunch of grapes and occurs esp. in the urogenital tract of young children

sar·co·ma·gen·ic \ˌsär-ˌkō-mə-ˈjen-ik\ *adj* : producing sarcoma ⟨shown to be highly ∼ in mice⟩

Sar·co·mas·ti·goph·o·ra \ˌsär-(ˌ)kō-ˌmas-tə-ˈgäf-ə-rə\ *n pl* : a phylum of protozoans that includes forms moving by flagella, pseudopodia, or both and that is divided into the subphyla Mastigophora and Sarcodina — compare CILIOPHORA

sar·co·ma·toid \sär-ˈkō-mə-ˌtoid\ *adj* : resembling a sarcoma

sar·co·ma·to·sis \(ˌ)sär-ˌkō-mə-ˈtō-səs\ *n, pl* **-to·ses** \-ˌsēz\ : a disease characterized by the presence and spread of sarcomas

sar·co·ma·tous \sär-ˈkō-mət-əs\ *adj* : of, relating to, or resembling sarcoma

sar·co·mere \ˈsär-kə-ˌmi(ə)r\ *n* : any of the repeating structural units of striated muscle fibrils — **sar·co·mer·ic** \ˌsär-kə-ˈmer-ik\ *adj*

Sar·coph·a·ga \sär-ˈkäf-ə-gə\ *n* : the type genus of the family Sarcophagidae comprising typical flesh flies

¹**sar·coph·a·gid** \sär-ˈkäf-ə-jid\ *adj* : of or relating to the family Sarcophagidae

²**sarcophagid** *n* : any dipteran fly of the family Sarcophagidae

Sar·co·phag·i·dae \ˌsär-kə-ˈfaj-ə-ˌdē\ *n pl* : a family of dipteran flies of the superfamily Muscoidea that include flesh flies, some that cause myiases, and others that develop in organic materials (as manure)

sar·co·plasm \ˈsär-kə-ˌplaz-əm\ *n* : the cytoplasm of a striated muscle fiber — compare MYOPLASM

sar·co·plas·mic \ˌsär-kə-ˈplaz-mik\ *also* **sar·co·plas·mat·ic** \-ˌplaz-ˈmat-ik\ *adj* : of or relating to the sarcoplasm ⟨∼ proteins⟩

sarcoplasmic reticulum *n* : the endoplasmic reticulum of cardiac muscle and skeletal striated muscle that functions esp. as a storage and release area for calcium

Sar·cop·tes \sär-ˈkäp-(ˌ)tēz\ *n* : a genus of whitish itch mites that is the type genus of the family Sarcoptidae

sar·cop·tic \sär-ˈkäp-tik\ *adj* : of, relating to, caused by, or being itch mites of the family Sarcoptidae and esp. the genus *Sarcoptes* ⟨∼ infection⟩ ⟨∼ mites⟩

sar·cop·ti·cide \sär-ˈkäp-tə-ˌsīd\ *n* : an agent used for killing itch mites

sarcoptic mange *n* : a mange caused by mites of the genus *Sarcoptes* that burrow in the skin esp. of the head and face — compare CHORIOPTIC MANGE, DEMODECTIC MANGE

Sar·cop·ti·dae \sär-ˈkäp-tə-ˌdē\ *n pl* : a family of small whitish itch mites that attack the skin of humans and other mammals

sar·cop·toid \sär-ˈkäp-ˌtoid\ *adj* : of, relating to, or having the characteristics of the superfamily Sarcoptoidea or the family Sarcoptidae

Sar·cop·toi·dea \ˌsär-ˌkäp-ˈtoid-ē-ə\ *n pl, in some classifications* : a superfamily of mites containing the family Sarcoptidae and related families

sar·co·sine \ˈsär-kə-ˌsēn, -sən\ *n* : a sweetish crystalline amino acid $C_3H_7NO_2$ formed by the decomposition of creatine or made synthetically

sar·co·some \ˈsär-kə-ˌsōm\ *n* : a mitochondrion of a striated muscle fiber — **sar·co·som·al** \ˌsär-kə-ˈsō-məl\ *adj*

Sar·co·spo·rid·ia \ˌsär-kō-spə-ˈrid-ē-ə\ *n pl* : an order of a subclass (Acnidosporidia) of sporozoans that comprises imperfectly known parasites of the muscles of vertebrates and includes the genus *Sarcocystis* — **sar·co·spo·rid·ian** \-ē-ən\ *adj or n*

sar·co·spo·rid·i·o·sis \-spə-ˌrid-ē-ˈō-səs\ *n, pl* **-o·ses** \-ˌsēz\ : SARCOCYSTOSIS

sar·co·tu·bu·lar \-ˈt(y)ü-byə-lər\ *adj* : relating to or being the system of membranes, vesicles, and tubules in the sarcoplasm of a striated muscle fiber that make up the sarcoplasmic reticulum and the T tubules

sar·don·ic laugh \sär-ˌdän-ik-\ *n* : RISUS SARDONICUS

sardonicus — see RISUS SARDONICUS

sar·gram·o·stim \sär-ˈgram-əs-təm\ *n* : a granulocyte-macrophage colony-stimulating factor produced by recombinant DNA technology that is used esp. following autologous bone marrow transplantation (as that used to treat non-Hodgkin's lymphoma, acute lymphoblastic leukemia, or Hodgkin's disease) to accelerate the division and differentiation of the transplanted bone marrow cells

sa·rin \ˈsär-ən, zä-ˈrēn\ *n* : an extremely toxic chemical warfare agent $C_4H_{10}FO_2P$ that is a powerful cholinesterase inhibitor — called also *GB*

sar·men·to·cy·ma·rin \sär-ˌmen-tō-ˈsī-mə-rən\ *n* : a crystalline steroid cardiac glycoside $C_{30}H_{46}O_8$ found in the seeds of several plants of the genus *Strophanthus* (as *S. sarmentosus*)

sar·men·to·gen·in \sär-ˌmen-tə-ˈjen-ən, ˌsär-mən-ˈtäj-ə-nən\ *n* : a crystalline steroid lactone $C_{23}H_{34}O_5$ closely related to digitoxigenin, found in several plants of the genus *Strophanthus,* obtained esp. by hydrolysis of sarmentocymarin, and used in a synthesis of cortisone

sar·men·tose \ˈsär-mən-ˌtōs\ *n* : a sugar $C_7H_{14}O_4$ that is obtained from sarmentocymarin by hydrolysis and that is stereoisomeric with cymarose and closely related to digitalose

SARS \ˈsärz\ *n* : a severe respiratory illness that is transmitted esp. by contact with infectious material (as respiratory droplets or body fluids), is caused by a single-stranded RNA virus of the genus *Coronavirus*, is characterized by fever, headache, body aches, a dry cough, and hypoxia and usu. by pneumonia — called also *severe acute respiratory syndrome*

sar·sa·pa·ril·la \ˌsas-(ə-)pə-ˈril-ə, ˌsärs-, -ˈrel-\ *n* **1 a** : any of various tropical American plants of the genus *Smilax* **b** : any of various plants (as wild sarsaparilla, *Aralia nudicaulis*) that resemble or are used as a substitute for the sarsaparillas **2 a** : the dried roots of any of several sarsaparillas of the genus *Smilax* (esp. *S. aristolochiaefolia, S. febrifuga,* and *S. regelii*) used now esp. as a flavoring and formerly for the diaphoretic, expectorant, and laxative effects of the saponins found in them and without curative effect in the treatment of syphilis **b** : the roots of wild sarsaparilla (*Aralia nudicaulis*) used similarly

sar·sa·sap·o·gen·in \ˌsär-sə-ˌsap-ə-ˈjen-ən, ˌsas-ə-, -sə-ˈpäj-ə-nən\ *n* : a crystalline steroid sapogenin $C_{27}H_{44}O_3$ obtained esp. by hydrolysis of sarsasaponin

sar·sa·sap·o·nin \-ˈsap-ə-nən, -sə-ˈpō-\ *also* **sar·sap·o·nin** \ˌsär-\ *n* : a saponin $C_{45}H_{74}O_{17}$ obtained from sarsaparilla root

sar·to·ri·us \sär-ˈtōr-ē-əs\ *n, pl* **-rii** \-ē-ˌī\ : a muscle that arises from the anterior superior iliac spine, crosses the front of the thigh obliquely to insert on the upper part of the inner surface of the tibia, is the longest muscle in the human body, and acts to flex, abduct, and rotate the thigh laterally at the hip joint and to flex the leg at the knee joint and to rotate it medially in a way that enables one to sit with the heel of one leg on the knee of the opposite leg

sas·sa·fras \ˈsas-ə-ˌfras\ *n* **1** : a tall eastern No. American tree (*Sassafras albidum*) of the laurel family (Lauraceae) with mucilaginous twigs and leaves **2** : the dried root bark of the sassafras formerly used as a diaphoretic and flavoring agent but now prohibited for use as a flavoring or food additive because of its carcinogenic properties

sassafras oil *n* : a yellow or reddish yellow aromatic essential oil obtained from the roots and stumps of the sassafras and used chiefly in perfuming and as a disinfectant

sas·sy bark \ˈsas-ē-\ *n* : the poisonous bark of a western African tree (*Erythrophloeum guineënse*) that contains erythrophleine

sat *abbr* saturated

sat·el·lite \ˈsat-ºl-ˌīt\ *n* **1** : a short segment separated from the main body of a chromosome by a constriction — called also *trabant* **2** : the secondary or later member of a chain of gregarines **3** : a bodily structure lying near or associated with another (as a vein accompanying an artery) **4** : a smaller lesion accompanying a main one and situated nearby **5** : a spectral line of low intensity having a frequency close to that of another stronger line to which it is closely related (as by having a common energy level) — **satellite** *adj*

satellite cell *n* **1** : a cell surrounding a ganglion cell **2** : a stem cell that lies adjacent to a skeletal muscle fiber and plays a role in muscle growth, repair, and regeneration

sat·el·lit·ed \-ˌīt-əd\ *adj* : having a satellite ⟨a ∼ chromosome⟩

satellite DNA *n* : a fraction of a eukaryotic organism's DNA that differs in density from most of its DNA as determined by centrifugation, that consists of short repetitive nucleotide sequences, that does not undergo transcription, and that is often found in centromeric regions

sat·el·lit·ism \ˈsat-ᵊl-ˌit-ˌiz-əm\ *n* : the growth of bacteria of one type in culture about colonies of another type that supply needed micronutrients or growth factors

sat·el·lit·o·sis \ˌsat-ᵊl-ī-ˈtō-səs\ *n, pl* **-o·ses** \-ˌsēz\ : the usu. abnormal clustering of one type of cell around another; *esp* : the clustering of glial cells around neurons in the brain that is associated with certain pathological states (as oligodendroglioma)

sa·ti·ety \sə-ˈtī-ət-ē *also* ˈsā-sh(ē-)ət-\ *n, pl* **-eties** : the quality or state of being fed or gratified to or beyond capacity

sat·u·ra·ble \ˈsach-(ə-)rə-bəl\ *adj* : capable of being saturated

¹sat·u·rate \ˈsach-ə-ˌrāt\ *vt* **-rat·ed; -rat·ing 1** : to treat, furnish, or charge with something to the point where no more can be absorbed, dissolved, or retained ⟨water *saturated* with salt⟩ ⟨a bandage *saturated* with blood⟩ **2** : to cause to combine till there is no further tendency to combine

²sat·u·rate \-rət\ *n* : a saturated chemical compound

sat·u·rat·ed \ˈsach-ə-ˌrāt-əd\ *adj* **1** : being a solution that is unable to absorb or dissolve any more of a solute at a given temperature and pressure **2** : being an organic compound having no double or triple bonds between carbon atoms

sat·u·ra·tion \ˌsach-ə-ˈrā-shən\ *n* **1** : the act of saturating : the state of being saturated **2** : conversion of an unsaturated to a saturated chemical compound (as by hydrogenation) **3** : a state of maximum impregnation; *esp* : the presence in air of the most water possible under existent pressure and temperature **4 a** : the one of the three psychological dimensions of color perception that is related to the purity of the color and that decreases as the amount of white present in the stimulus increases — called also *intensity;* compare BRIGHTNESS, HUE **b** (1) : degree of difference from the gray having the same lightness — used of an object color (2) : degree of difference from the achromatic light-source color or of the same brightness — used of a light-source color

sat·ur·nine \ˈsat-ər-ˌnīn\ *adj* **1** : of or relating to lead **2** : of, relating to, or produced by the absorption of lead into the system ⟨∼ poisoning⟩ ⟨∼ gout⟩

Sat·urn \ˈsat-ərn\, Roman mythological character. A god of agriculture in Roman mythology, Saturn taught humans how to till the fields and enjoy the fruits of civilization. His festival was called the Saturnalia and took place in late December. Lasting a week, it was the merriest and most popular of the Roman festivals. The planet Saturn, named after the god, was believed by the ancients to be made of lead.

sat·urn·ism \ˈsat-ər-ˌniz-əm\ *n* : LEAD POISONING

sa·ty·ri·a·sis \ˌsāt-ə-ˈrī-ə-səs, ˌsat-\ *n, pl* **-a·ses** \-ˌsēz\ : excessive or abnormal sexual desire in the male — compare NYMPHOMANIA

sau·cer·iza·tion *also Brit* **sau·cer·isa·tion** \ˌsȯ-sər-ə-ˈzā-shən\ *n* : the operation of saucerizing something (as a bone or the gingiva)

sau·cer·ize *also Brit* **sau·cer·ise** \ˈsȯ-sər-ˌīz\ *vt* **-ized** *also Brit* **-ised; -iz·ing** *also Brit* **-is·ing** : to form a shallow depression by excavation of tissue to promote granulation and healing of (a wound)

sau·na \ˈsaů-nə, ˈsȯ-nə\ *n* **1** : a Finnish steam bath in which the steam is provided by water thrown on hot stones; *also* : a bathhouse or room used for such a bath **2** : a dry heat bath; *also* : a room or cabinet used for such a bath

sa·vant \sa-ˈvänt, sə-, ˈsav-ˌvant\ *n* : IDIOT SAVANT

sav·in \ˈsav-ən\ *n* : a mostly prostrate Eurasian evergreen juniper (*Juniperus sabina*) with dark foliage and small berries having a glaucous bloom and with bitter acrid tops that are

sometimes used in folk medicine (as for amenorrhea or as an abortifacient) — called also *sabina*

savin oil *n* : a pungent essential oil from the tops of a savin (*Juniperus sabina*) that causes inflammation of the skin and mucous membranes

¹saw *past of* SEE

²saw \ˈsȯ\ *n* : a hand or power tool used to cut hard material (as bone) and equipped usu. with a toothed blade or disk

saw pal·met·to \-pal-ˈmet-(ˌ)ō\ *n* **1** : any of several shrubby palms chiefly of the southern U.S. and West Indies with spiny-toothed leafstalks; *esp* : a common palm (*Serenoa repens*) of the southeastern U.S. with a usu. creeping stem **2** : a preparation derived from the berrylike fruit of a saw palmetto (*Serenoa repens*) that is held to have a therapeutic effect on the prostate gland and is used in herbal remedies and dietary supplements — called also *sabal*

saxi·tox·in \ˌsak-sə-ˈtäk-sən\ *n* : a potent nonprotein neurotoxin $C_{10}H_{17}N_7O_4$·2HCl that originates in dinoflagellates of the genus *Gonyaulax* found in red tides and that sometimes occurs in and renders toxic normally edible mollusks which feed on them

Sb *symbol* [Latin *stibium*] antimony

SBS *abbr* sick building syndrome

Sc *symbol* scandium

SCA *abbr* **1** sickle-cell anemia **2** spinocerebellar ataxia **3** sudden cardiac arrest

¹scab \ˈskab\ *n* **1** : scabies of domestic animals **2** : a hardened covering of dried secretions (as blood, plasma, or pus) that forms over a wound — called also *crust* — **scab·by** \-ē\ *adj* **scab·bi·er; -est**

²scab *vi* **scabbed; scab·bing** : to become covered with a scab ⟨the wound *scabbed* over⟩

scabby mouth *n* : SORE MOUTH 1

sca·bi·ci·dal \ˌskā-bə-ˈsīd-ᵊl\ *adj* : destroying the itch mite causing scabies

sca·bi·cide \ˈskā-bə-ˌsīd\ *n* : a drug that destroys the itch mite causing scabies

sca·bies \ˈskā-bēz\ *n, pl* **scabies** : contagious itch or mange esp. with exudative crusts that is caused by parasitic mites and esp. by a mite of the genus *Sarcoptes* (*S. scabiei*)

sca·bi·et·ic \ˌskā-bē-ˈet-ik\ *also* **sca·bet·ic** \skə-ˈbet-ik\ *adj* : of, relating to, or affected with scabies ⟨a ∼ infection⟩

sca·bi·et·i·cide \ˌskā-bē-ˈet-ə-ˌsīd\ *n* : SCABICIDE

sca·bi·ous \ˈskā-bē-əs\ *adj* **1** : relating to or characterized by scabs **2** : of, relating to, or resembling scabies ⟨∼ eruptions⟩

scab mite *n* : any of several small mites that cause mange, scabies, or scab; *esp* : one of the genus *Psoroptes*

sca·la \ˈskā-lə\ *n, pl* **sca·lae** \-ˌlē\ : any of the three spirally arranged canals into which the bony canal of the cochlea is partitioned by the vestibular and basilar membranes and which comprise the scala media, scala tympani, and scala vestibuli

scala me·dia \-ˈmēd-ē-ə\ *n, pl* **scalae me·di·ae** \-ē-ˌē\ : the spirally arranged canal in the bony canal of the cochlea that contains the organ of Corti, is triangular in cross section, and is bounded by the vestibular membrane above, by the periosteum-lined wall of the cochlea laterally, and by the basilar membrane below — called also *cochlear canal, cochlear duct, ductus cochlearis*

scala tym·pa·ni \-ˈtim-pə-ˌnī, -ˌnē\ *n, pl* **scalae tym·pa·no·rum** \-ˌtim-pə-ˈnōr-əm, -ˈnȯr-əm\ : the lymph-filled spirally arranged canal in the bony canal of the cochlea that is separated from the scala media by the basilar membrane, communicates at its upper end with the scala vestibuli, and abuts at its lower end upon the membrane that separates the round window from the middle ear

scala ves·tib·u·li \-ve-ˈstib-yə-ˌlī\ *n, pl* **scalae ves·tib·u·lo·rum** \-ve-ˌstib-yə-ˈlō-rəm\ : the lymph-filled spirally ar-

S
T

ranged canal in the bony canal of the cochlea that is separated from the scala media below by the vestibular membrane, is connected with the oval window, and receives vibrations from the stapes

¹**scald** \'skȯld\ *vt* : to burn with hot liquid or steam

²**scald** *n* : an injury to the body caused by scalding

scald·ed–skin syndrome \'skȯld-əd-\ *n* : TOXIC EPIDERMAL NECROLYSIS — see STAPHYLOCOCCAL SCALDED SKIN SYNDROME

¹**scale** \'skā(ə)l\ *n* **1 a** : either pan or tray of a balance **b** : a beam that is supported freely in the center and has two pans of equal weight suspended from its ends — usu. used in pl. **2** : an instrument or machine for weighing

²**scale** *vb* **scaled; scal·ing** *vt* : to weigh in scales ∼ *vi* : to have a specified weight on scales

³**scale** *n* **1** : a small thin dry lamina shed (as in many skin diseases) from the skin **2** : a film of tartar encrusting the teeth

⁴**scale** *vb* **scaled; scal·ing** *vt* : to take off in thin layers or scales ⟨∼ tartar from the teeth⟩ ∼ *vi* **1** : to separate or come off in thin layers or laminae **2** : to shed scales or fragmentary surface matter : EXFOLIATE ⟨*scaling* skin⟩

⁵**scale** *n* **1** : a series of marks or points at known intervals used to measure distances (as the height of the mercury in a thermometer) **2** : a graduated series or scheme of rank or order **3** : a graded series of tests or of performances used in rating individual intelligence or achievement

¹**sca·lene** \'skā-ˌlēn, skā-'\ *adj* : of, relating to, or being a scalenus muscle

²**scalene** *n* : SCALENUS — called also *scalene muscle*

scalene tubercle *n* : a tubercle on the upper surface of the first rib that serves for insertion of the scalenus anterior

sca·le·not·o·my \ˌskā-lə-'nät-ə-mē\ *also* **sca·le·ni·ot·o·my** \ˌskā-lē-nē-'ät-\ *n, pl* **-mies** : surgical severing of one or more scalenus muscles near their insertion on the ribs

sca·le·nus \skā-'lē-nəs\ *n, pl* **sca·le·ni** \-ˌnī\ : any of usu. three deeply situated muscles on each side of the neck of which each extends from the transverse processes of two or more cervical vertebrae to the first or second rib: **a** : one arising from the transverse processes of the third to sixth cervical vertebrae, inserting on the scalene tubercle of the first rib, and functioning to bend the neck forward and laterally and to rotate it to the side — called also *anterior scalene, scalenus anterior, scalenus anticus* **b** : one arising from the transverse processes of the lower six cervical vertebrae, inserting on the upper surface of the first rib, and functioning similarly to the scalenus anterior — called also *middle scalene, scalenus medius* **c** : one arising from the transverse processes of the fourth to sixth cervical vertebrae, inserting on the outer surface of the second rib, and functioning to raise the second rib and to bend and slightly rotate the neck — called also *posterior scalene, scalenus posterior*

scalenus anterior *n* : SCALENUS a

scalenus an·ti·cus \-an-'tī-kəs\ *n* : SCALENUS a

scalenus anticus syndrome *n* : a complex of symptoms including pain and numbness in the region of the shoulder, arm, and neck that is caused by compression of the brachial plexus or subclavian artery or both by the scalenus anticus muscle

scalenus me·di·us \-'mēd-ē-əs\ *n* : SCALENUS b

scalenus posterior *n* : SCALENUS c

scal·er \'skā-lər\ *n* : any of various dental instruments for removing tartar from teeth

scalp \'skalp\ *n* : the part of the integument of the head usu. covered with hair in both sexes

scal·pel \'skal-pəl *also* skal-'pel\ *n* : a small straight thin=bladed knife used esp. in surgery

scalp ringworm *n* : TINEA CAPITIS

scaly \'skā-lē\ *adj* **scal·i·er; -est** : covered with or composed of scale or scales ⟨dry ∼ skin⟩ — **scal·i·ness** *n*

scaly leg *also* **scaly legs** *n* : a disease of poultry that is transmitted by a mite of the genus *Knemidokoptes* (*K. mutans*) and that produces an abnormal rough hard scaliness on the featherless parts of the legs

scam·mo·ny \'skam-ə-nē\ *n, pl* **-nies** **1** : a twining plant of the genus *Convolvulus* (*C. scammonia*) of Asia Minor with a large thick root **2 a** : the dried root of scammony **b** : a cathartic resin obtained from scammony

¹**scan** \'skan\ *vb* **scanned; scan·ning** *vt* **1 a** : to examine esp. systematically with a sensing device (as a photometer or a beam of radiation) **b** : to pass an electron beam over and convert (an image) into variations of electrical properties (as voltage) that convey information electronically **2** : to make a scan of (as the human body) in order to detect the presence or localization of radioactive material ∼ *vi* : to make a scan of the body or of an organ or part

²**scan** *n* **1** : the act or process of scanning **2 a** : a depiction (as a photograph) of the distribution of a radioactive material in something (as a bodily organ) **b** : an image of a bodily part produced (as by computer) by combining ultrasonographic or radiographic data obtained from several angles or sections

scan·di·um \'skan-dē-əm\ *n* : a white trivalent metallic element found in association with rare earth elements — symbol *Sc*; see ELEMENT table

scan·ner \'skan-ər\ *n* : a device (as a CAT scanner) for making scans of the human body

scanning electron micrograph *n* : a micrograph made by scanning electron microscopy

scanning electron microscope *n* : an electron microscope in which a beam of focused electrons moves across the object with the secondary electrons produced by the object and the electrons scattered by the object being collected to form a three-dimensional image on a cathode-ray tube — called also *scanning microscope;* compare TRANSMISSION ELECTRON MICROSCOPE — **scanning electron microscopy** *n*

scanning speech *n* : speech characterized by regularly recurring pauses between words or syllables

Scan·zo·ni maneuver *also* **Scan·zo·ni's maneuver** \skän-'tsō-nē(z)-\ *n* : rotation of an abnormally positioned fetus by means of forceps with subsequent reapplication of forceps for delivery

Scanzoni, Friedrich Wilhelm (1821–1891), German obstetrician. In 1849 Scanzoni announced his development of a procedure for changing a presentation in which the occiput is presented first into an anterior presentation. The procedure called for the use of forceps twice in the birth process and has since been identified with his name.

sca·pha \'skaf-ə\ *n* : an elongated depression of the ear that separates the helix and antihelix

scaph·o·ceph·a·ly \ˌskaf-ə-'sef-ə-lē\ *n, pl* **-lies** : a congenital deformity of the skull in which the vault is narrow, elongated, and boat-shaped because of premature ossification of the sagittal suture

¹**scaph·oid** \'skaf-ˌȯid\ *adj* **1** : shaped like a boat : NAVICULAR **2** : characterized by concavity ⟨the abdomen was soft and ∼ without tenderness —Nancy M. Heiss *et al*⟩

²**scaphoid** *n* **1** : NAVICULAR a **2** : the largest carpal bone of the proximal row of the wrist that occupies the most lateral position on the thumb side — called also *navicular*

scaphoid bone *n* : SCAPHOID

scaphoid fossa *n* : a shallow oval depression that is situated above the pterygoid fossa on the pterygoid process of the sphenoid bone and that provides attachment for the origin of the tensor veli palatini muscle

scap·u·la \'skap-yə-lə\ *n, pl* **-lae** \-ˌlē, -ˌlī\ *or* **-las** : either of a pair of large essentially flat and triangular bones lying one in each dorsolateral part of the thorax, being the principal bone of the corresponding half of the pectoral girdle, divided on the posterior surface into the supraspinous and infraspinous fossae by an oblique transverse bony process or spine terminating in the acromion, having a hook-shaped bony coracoid process on the anterior surface of the superior border of the bone, providing articulation for the humerus, and articulating with the corresponding clavicle — called also *shoulder blade*

scapulae — see LEVATOR SCAPULAE

scap·u·lar \'skap-yə-lər\ *adj* : of, relating to, or affecting the shoulder or scapula ⟨a ∼ fracture⟩

scapular notch *n* : a semicircular notch on the superior border of the scapula next to the coracoid process that gives passage to the suprascapular nerve and is converted to a foramen by the suprascapular ligament

scap·u·lo·hu·mer·al \ˌskap-yə-lō-ˈhyüm-(ə-)rəl\ *adj* : of or relating to the scapula and the humerus ⟨∼ movement⟩

scap·u·lo·pexy \ˈskap-yə-lōˌpek-sē\ *n, pl* **-pex·ies** : a surgical procedure in which the scapula is attached (as by a wire) to a rib or vertebra

scap·u·lo·tho·rac·ic \ˌskap-yə-lō-thə-ˈras-ik\ *adj* : of or relating to the scapula and the thorax ⟨∼ pain⟩

¹**scar** \ˈskär\ *n* **1** : a mark left (as in the skin) by the healing of injured tissue **2** : a lasting emotional injury ⟨psychological ∼s⟩

²**scar** *vb* **scarred; scar·ring** *vt* : to mark with a scar ⟨scarred heart valves⟩ ∼ *vi* **1** : to form a scar **2** : to become scarred

scarf·skin \ˈskärfˌskin\ *n* : EPIDERMIS; *esp* : that forming the cuticle of a nail

scar·i·fi·ca·tion \ˌskar-ə-fə-ˈkā-shən, ˌsker-\ *n* **1** : the act or process of scarifying ⟨vaccination by ∼⟩ **2** : a mark or marks made by scarifying

scar·i·fy \ˈskar-əˌfī, ˈsker-\ *vt* **-fied; -fy·ing** : to make scratches or small cuts in (as the skin) ⟨∼ an area for vaccination⟩

scar·la·ti·na \ˌskär-lə-ˈtē-nə\ *n* : SCARLET FEVER — **scar·la·ti·nal** \-ˈtēn-ᵊl\ *adj*

scar·la·ti·ni·form \-ˈtē-nəˌförm\ *adj* : resembling the rash of scarlet fever ⟨a ∼ eruption⟩

scar·la·ti·no·gen·ic \-ˌtē-nə-ˈjen-ik\ *adj* : causing scarlet fever ⟨a ∼ streptococcus⟩

scar·let fever \ˈskär-lət-\ *n* : an acute contagious febrile disease caused by Group A bacteria of the genus *Streptococcus* (esp. various strains of *S. pyogenes*) and characterized by inflammation of the nose, throat, and mouth, generalized toxemia, and a red rash — called also *scarlatina*

scarlet red *n* : SUDAN IV

Scar·pa's fascia \ˈskär-pəz-\ *n* : the deep layer of the superficial fascia of the anterior abdominal wall that is composed mostly of yellow elastic fibers with little adipose tissue

Scar·pa \ˈskär-pä\, **Antonio (1752–1832),** Italian anatomist and surgeon. Scarpa was one of the preeminent anatomists and surgeons of his time. He wrote classic descriptions of several anatomical features that have since been associated with his name: Scarpa's fascia (1809), Scarpa's foramen (1799), and Scarpa's triangle (1809).

Scarpa's foramen *n* : either of two canals opening into the incisive foramen in the median plane behind the upper incisors and transmitting the nasopalatine nerves

Scarpa's triangle *n* : FEMORAL TRIANGLE

scar tissue *n* : the connective tissue forming a scar and composed chiefly of fibroblasts in recent scars and largely of dense collagenous fibers in old scars

scat·o·log·i·cal \ˌskat-ᵊl-ˈäj-i-kəl\ *also* **scat·o·log·ic** \-ˈäj-ik\ *adj* **1** : of or relating to the study of excrement ⟨∼ data⟩ **2** : marked by an interest in excrement or obscenity **3** : of or relating to excrement or excremental functions ⟨∼ terms⟩

scat·ol·o·gy \ska-ˈtäl-ə-jē, skə-\ *n, pl* **-gies 1** : interest in or treatment of obscene matters esp. in literature **2** : the biologically oriented study of excrement (as for taxonomic purposes or for the determination of diet)

sca·to·ma \skə-ˈtō-mə\ *n, pl* **-mas** *or* **-ma·ta** \-mət-ə\ : a fecal mass in the colon or rectum that gives the impression of a tumor on palpation

sca·toph·a·gy \-fə-jē\ *n, pl* **-gies** : the practice of eating excrement or other filth esp. as a pathological obsession

¹**scat·ter** \ˈskat-ər\ *vt* : to cause (a beam of radiation) to diffuse or disperse

²**scatter** *n* **1** : the act of scattering **2** : the state or extent of being scattered; *esp* : SCATTERING

scat·ter·ing *n* : the random change in direction of the particles constituting a beam or wave front due to collision with particles of the medium traversed

ScD *abbr* doctor of science

scene — see PRIMAL SCENE

Scha·fer method *or* **Schae·fer method** *also* **Scha·fer's method** \ˈshā-fər(z)-\ *n* : PRONE PRESSURE METHOD

Shar·pey–Scha·fer \ˌshär-pē-ˈshā-fər\, **Sir Edward Albert (1850–1935),** British physiologist. Schafer held positions as professor of physiology at several British universities, his longest tenure being at the university in Edinburgh. He introduced the Schafer method of artificial respiration in a paper published in 1903. His method came into wide use as a means of reviving apparent drowning victims.

Scham·berg's disease \ˈsham-bərgz-\ *n* : a progressive purpuric disorder of the skin esp. of the legs characterized by petechiae and patches of orange to brown pigmentation

Schamberg, Jay Frank (1870–1934), American dermatologist. Schamberg held a number of positions with several medical schools in Philadelphia. He described the progressive pigmentary skin disease since known as Schamberg's disease in 1901.

Schar·ding·er dextrin \ˈshär-diŋ-ər-\ *n* : any of several nonreducing water-soluble low-molecular-weight polysaccharides formed by cultivation of a bacterium of the genus *Bacillus* (*B. macerans*) upon starch solutions

Schardinger, Franz (fl 1902), Austrian biochemist. Schardinger discovered xanthine oxidase in 1902.

Schardinger enzyme *n* : XANTHINE OXIDASE

Schatz·ki ring \ˈshats-kē-\ *or* **Schatz·ki's ring** \-kēz-\ *n* : a local narrowing in the lower part of the esophagus that may cause dysphagia

Schatzki, Richard (1901–1992), American radiologist. Schatzki held positions in radiology at several Boston hospitals.

¹**sched·ule** \ˈskej-(ˌ)ü(ə)l, ˈskej-əl, *Canad also* ˈshej-, *Brit usu* ˈshed-(ˌ)yü(ə)l\ *n* **1** : a program or plan that indicates the sequence of each step or procedure ⟨reinforcement ∼s used in conditioning experiments⟩; *esp* : REGIMEN ⟨antibiotic ∼s for treating Lyme disease⟩ **2** *often cap* : an official list of drugs that are subject to the same legal controls and restrictions — usu. used with a Roman numeral from I to V indicating decreasing potential for abuse or addiction ⟨the Drug Enforcement Administration classifies heroin as a ∼ I drug while the tranquilizer chlordiazepoxide is on ∼ IV⟩

²**schedule** *vt* **sched·uled; sched·ul·ing** : to place in a schedule ⟨methadone and phenobarbital are *scheduled* substances⟩

scheduled disease *n, Brit* : a notifiable disease

Schee·le's green \ˈshā-ləz-, -lēz-\ *n* : a poisonous yellowish green pigment consisting essentially of a copper arsenite and used esp. as an insecticide

Schee·le \ˈshā-lə\, **Carl Wilhelm (1742–1786),** Swedish chemist. Scheele is most famous as the chemist who is now credited with discovering oxygen at least two years before Joseph Priestley. (Priestley had long been accepted as the original discoverer.) Scheele spent his life as an apothecary, working in his small chemical laboratory in his spare time. He first described Scheele's green in an article on arsenic published in 1775.

Scheie syndrome \ˈshī-\ *n* : an autosomal recessive mucopolysaccharidosis similar to Hurler's syndrome but less severe that is characterized by clouding of the cornea, slight deformity of the extremities, and disease of the aorta but not by mental retardation or early death

Scheie, Harold Glendon (1909–1990), American ophthalmologist. Throughout his medical career Scheie was associated with the hospital and medical school of the University of Pennsylvania in Philadelphia. He described Scheie syndrome in 1962.

sche·ma \ˈskē-mə\ *n, pl* **sche·ma·ta** \-mət-ə\ *also* **schemas 1** : a nonconscious adjustment of the brain to the afferent impulses indicative of bodily posture that is a prerequisite of appropriate bodily movement and of spatial perception **2**

\ə\ **abut** \ᵊ\ **kitten** \ər\ **further** \a\ **ash** \ā\ **ace** \ä\ **cot, cart**
\au̇\ **out** \ch\ **chin** \e\ **bet** \ē\ **easy** \g\ **go** \i\ **hit** \ī\ **ice** \j\ **job**
\ŋ\ **sing** \ō\ **go** \ȯ\ **law** \ȯi\ **boy** \th\ **thin** \t͟h\ **the** \ü\ **loot**
\u̇\ **foot** \y\ **yet** \zh\ **vision** *See also* Pronunciation Symbols page

: the organization of experience in the mind or brain that includes a particular organized way of perceiving cognitively and responding to a complex situation or set of stimuli

sche·mat·ic \ski-'mat-ik\ *adj* : of or relating to a scheme or schema — **sche·mat·i·cal·ly** \-i-k(ə-)lē\ *adv*

scheme \'skēm\ *n* : SCHEMA

Scheuer·mann's disease \'shòi-ər-ˌmänz-\ *n* : osteochondrosis of the vertebrae associated with the active state with pain and kyphosis

  Scheuermann, Holger Werfel (1877–1960), Danish orthopedist. Scheuermann practiced radiology in Copenhagen. He described osteochondrosis of the vertebrae in 1920.

Schick test \'shik-\ *n* : a serological test for susceptibility to diphtheria by cutaneous injection of a diluted diphtheria toxin that causes an area of reddening and induration in susceptible individuals

  Schick, Béla (1877–1967), American pediatrician. In 1913 Schick announced his development of the Schick test for susceptibility to diphtheria. The test was a safe, reliable method of detection that eliminated the unnecessary use of sera with serious side effects.

Schiff base \'shif-\ *also* **Schiff's base** *n* : any of a class of bases of the general formula RR′C=NR″ that are obtained typically by condensation of an aldehyde or ketone with a primary amine (as aniline) with elimination of water, that usu. polymerize readily if made from aliphatic aldehydes, and that are used chiefly as intermediates in organic synthesis and in some cases as dyes

  Schiff, Hugo Josef (1834–1915), German chemist. In 1864 Schiff discovered the condensation products of aldehydes and amines; the products are now known as Schiff bases. Two years later he introduced a test for aldehydes, in which decolorized fuchsin regains its color in the presence of aldehydes.

Schiff reaction *n* : a reaction that is used as a test for aldehydes and consists in the formation by them of a reddish violet color with a solution of fuchsin decolorized with sulfurous acid

Schiff's reagent \ˌshifs-\ *or* **Schiff reagent** \ˌshif-\ *n* : a solution of fuchsin decolorized by treatment with sulfur dioxide that gives a useful test for aldehydes because they restore the reddish violet color of the dye — compare FEULGEN REACTION

Schil·der's disease \'shil-dərz-\ *n* : ADRENOLEUKODYSTROPHY

  Schilder, Paul Ferdinand (1886–1940), Austrian psychiatrist. In 1912 Schilder described encephalitis periaxialis diffusa, which is now usually called adrenoleukodystrophy or Schilder's disease.

Schilder's encephalitis *n* : ADRENOLEUKODYSTROPHY

Schil·ler's test \'shil-ərz-\ *n* : a preliminary test for cancer of the uterine cervix in which the cervix is painted with an aqueous solution of iodine and potassium iodide and which shows up healthy tissue by staining it brown and possibly cancerous tissue as white or yellow due to its failure to take up the stain because of a deficiency of glycogen in the cells

  Schiller, Walter (1887–1960), American pathologist. In 1933 Schiller introduced the test for cancer of the cervix that is now known as Schiller's test.

Schil·ling index \'shil-iŋ-\ *n* : an age classification of blood neutrophils which is based on increasing irregularity or lobulation of the nucleus and in which the classes are myelocytes, metamyelocytes, band forms, and mature neutrophils having nuclei with two or more lobes — compare ARNETH INDEX

  Schilling, Victor Theodor Adolf Georg (1883–1960), German hematologist. Schilling introduced in 1924 a differential count of white blood cells, dividing the neutrophil cells into four groups.

Schilling test *n* : a test for gastrointestinal absorption of vitamin B₁₂ in which a dose of the radioactive vitamin is taken orally, a dose of the nonradioactive vitamin is given by injection to impede uptake of the absorbed radioactive dose by the liver, and the proportion of the radioactive dose absorbed is determined by measuring the radioactivity of the urine

  Schilling, Robert Frederick (b 1919), American hematologist. Schilling undertook research on the absorption and utilization of vitamin B₁₂, the mechanisms involved in the causation of anemia, and on the gastrointestinal absorption of nutrients. He introduced the Schilling test in 1953.

Schim·mel·busch's disease \'shim-ᵊl-ˌbùsh-əz-\ *n* : a benign disease affecting one or both breasts of the female and characterized by the formation of numerous small cysts due to dilation and hyperplasia of the epithelial lining of the ducts of the mammary glands

  Schimmelbusch, Curt (1860–1895), German surgeon. Schimmelbusch published a description of Schimmelbusch's disease in 1892.

schin·dy·le·sis \ˌskin-də-'lē-səs\ *n, pl* **-le·ses** \-ˌsēz\ : an articulation in which one bone is received into a groove or slit in another

Schiotz tonometer \'shyœts-, 'shyərts-\ *n* : a tonometer used to measure intraocular pressure in millimeters of mercury

  Schiøtz, Hjalmar (1850–1927), Norwegian physician. With the French ophthalmologist Louis-Emile Javal (1839–1907), Schiøtz invented a tonometer for measuring intraocular pressure. They introduced their tonometer in an article published in 1881.

schis·to·cor·mus \ˌshis-tə-'kòr-məs, ˌskis-\ *n, pl* **-mi** \-ˌmī\ : an individual with a congenital cleft of the thorax, neck, or abdominal wall

schis·to·cyte \'shis-tə-ˌsīt, 'skis-\ *n* : a hemoglobin-containing fragment of a red blood cell

schis·to·cy·to·sis \ˌshis-tə-sī-'tō-səs, ˌskis-\ *n* : the presence of an abnormal number of schistocytes in the blood

schis·tor·rha·chis \shis-'tòr-ə-kəs, skis-\ *n* : SPINA BIFIDA

schis·to·so·ma \ˌshis-tə-'sō-mə, ˌskis-\ **1** *cap* : a genus that is the type genus of the family Schistosomatidae and that includes elongated digenetic trematode worms parasitizing the blood vessels of birds and mammals and several forms (as *S. haematobium, S. japonicum,* and *S. mansoni*) causing human schistosomiasis **2** : any digenetic trematode worm of the genus *Schistosoma* : SCHISTOSOME

Schis·to·so·mat·i·dae \ˌshis-tə-sō-'mat-ə-ˌdē, ˌskis-\ *n pl* : a family of slender elongated digenetic trematodes of the superfamily Schistosomatoidea in which the sexes are separate and in which marked sexual dimorphism is usu. present

Schis·to·so·ma·toi·dea \ˌshis-tə-sō-mə-'tòid-ē-ə, ˌskis-\ *n pl* : a superfamily of digenetic trematodes that lack a metacercaria and have instead a furcocercous cercaria that actively penetrates the skin of a definitive host

schis·to·some \'shis-tə-ˌsōm, 'skis-\ *n* : any trematode worm of the genus *Schistosoma* or of the family Schistosomatidae — called also *blood fluke* — **schis·to·so·mal** \ˌshis-tə-'sō-məl, ˌskis-\ *adj*

schistosome dermatitis *n* : SWIMMER'S ITCH

schis·to·so·mi·a·sis \ˌshis-tə-sō-'mī-ə-səs, ˌskis-\ *n, pl* **-a·ses** \-ˌsēz\ : infestation with or disease caused by schistosomes; *specif* : a severe endemic disease of humans in much of Africa and parts of Asia and So. America that is caused by any of three trematode worms of the genus *Schistosoma* (*S. haematobium, S. mansoni,* and *S. japonicum*) which multiply in snail intermediate hosts and are disseminated into freshwaters as furcocercous cercariae that bore into the body when it is in contact with infested water, migrate through the tissues to the visceral venous plexuses (as of the bladder or intestine) where they attain maturity, and cause much of their injury through hemorrhage and damage to tissues resulting from the passage of the usu. spiny eggs to the intestine and bladder whence they pass out to start a new cycle of infection in snail hosts — called also *bilharzia, bilharziasis, snail fever;* compare SWIMMER'S ITCH

schistosomiasis hae·ma·to·bi·um \-ˌhē-mə-'tō-bē-əm\ *n* : schistosomiasis caused by a schistosome (*Schistosoma haematobium*) occurring over most of Africa and in Asia Minor and predominantly involving infestation of the veins of the urinary bladder

schis·to·so·mi·a·sis ja·pon·i·ca \-jə-'pän-i-kə\ *n* : schistosomiasis caused by a schistosome (*Schistosoma japonicum*) occurring chiefly in eastern Asia and the Pacific islands and predominantly involving infestation of the portal and mesenteric veins — see KATAYAMA SYNDROME

schistosomiasis man·so·ni \-'man(t)-sə-ˌnī\ *n* : schistosomiasis caused by a schistosome (*Schistosoma mansoni*) occurring chiefly in central Africa and eastern So. America and predominantly involving infestation of the mesenteric and portal veins — called also *Manson's disease*

   P. Manson — see MANSONELLA

schis·to·so·mi·cid·al \ˌshis-tə-ˌsō-mə-'sīd-ᵊl, ˌskis-\ *adj* : destructive to schistosomes ⟨a ~ agent⟩ ⟨~ activity⟩

Schis·to·so·moph·o·ra \ˌshis-tə-sə-'mäf-ə-rə, ˌskis-\ *n* : a genus of Asian freshwater snails (family Bulimidae) including important intermediate hosts of a trematode worm of the genus *Schistosoma* (*S. japonicum*) esp. in the Philippines

schis·to·som·u·lum \ˌshis-tə-'säm-yə-ləm, ˌskis-\ *n, pl* **-la** \-lə\ : an immature schistosome in the body of the definitive host

schis·to·tho·rax \ˌshis-tə-'thōr-ˌaks, ˌskis-\ *n, pl* **-tho·rax·es** *or* **-tho·ra·ces** \-'thōr-ə-ˌsēz\ : congenital fissure of the chest or sternum

schizo \'skit-(ˌ)sō\ *n, pl* **schiz·os** : SCHIZOPHRENIC

schizo·af·fec·tive \-a-'fek-tiv\ *adj* : relating to, characterized by, or exhibiting symptoms of both schizophrenia and bipolar disorder ⟨~ disorders⟩ ⟨~ patients⟩

schizo·gon·ic \ˌskit-sə-'gän-ik\ *or* **schi·zog·o·nous** \ski-'zäg-ə-nəs, skit-'säg-\ *adj* : of, relating to, or reproducing by schizogony ⟨the ~ cycle of the malaria parasite⟩

schi·zog·o·ny \ski-'zäg-ə-nē, skit-'säg-\ *n, pl* **-nies** : asexual reproduction by multiple segmentation characteristic of sporozoans (as the malaria parasite)

¹schiz·oid \'skit-ˌsȯid\ *adj* : characterized by, resulting from, tending toward, or suggestive of schizophrenia ⟨~ behavior⟩

²schizoid *n* : a schizoid individual

schiz·oid·ism \'skit-sȯi-ˌdiz-əm\ *n* : the state of being split off (as in schizoid personality and schizophrenia) from one's social and vital environment

schizoid personality *n* **1** : a personality disorder characterized by shyness, withdrawal, inhibition of emotional expression, and apparent diminution of affect — called also *schizoid personality disorder* **2** : an individual with a schizoid personality

Schizo·my·ce·tes \-mī-'sēt-ˌēz\ *n pl, in former classifications* : a class of unicellular or noncellular microorganisms that lack true chlorophyll and are now usu. grouped with the cyanobacteria

schiz·ont \'skiz-ˌänt, 'skit-ˌsänt\ *n* : a multinucleate sporozoan (as a malaria parasite) that reproduces by schizogony — called also *agamont, segmenter*

schi·zon·ti·ci·dal \ski-ˌzän-tə-'sīd-ᵊl, skit-ˌsän-\ *adj* : of or relating to a schizonticide

schi·zon·ti·cide \ski-'zän-tə-ˌsīd, skit-'sän-\ *n* : an agent selectively destructive of the schizont of a sporozoan parasite

schizo·pha·sia \ˌskit-sō-'fā-zh(ē-)ə\ *n* : the disorganized speech characteristic of schizophrenia

schizo·phrene \'skit-sə-ˌfrēn\ *n* : SCHIZOPHRENIC

schizo·phre·nia \ˌskit-sə-'frē-nē-ə\ *n* : a psychotic disorder characterized by loss of contact with the environment, by noticeable deterioration in the level of functioning in everyday life, and by disintegration of personality expressed as disorder of feeling, thought (as in delusions), perception (as in hallucinations), and behavior — called also *dementia praecox;* see PARANOID SCHIZOPHRENIA

¹schizo·phren·ic \-'fren-ik\ *adj* : relating to, characteristic of, or affected with schizophrenia ⟨~ behavior⟩ ⟨~ patients⟩

²schizophrenic *n* : an individual affected with schizophrenia

schizophrenic reaction *n* : SCHIZOPHRENIA

schiz·o·phren·i·form \ˌskit-sə-'fren-ə-ˌfȯrm\ *adj* : being similar to schizophrenia in appearance or manifestations but

tending to last usu. more than two weeks and less than six months ⟨~ disorder⟩

schiz·o·phreno·gen·ic \ˌskit-sə-ˌfren-ə-'jen-ik\ *adj* : tending to produce schizophrenia ⟨~ factors⟩

schizos *pl of* SCHIZO

schizo·thy·mic \ˌskit-sə-'thī-mik\ *adj* : tending toward an introverted temperament that while remaining within the bounds of normality somewhat resembles schizophrenia

Schizo·tryp·a·num \ˌskiz-ə-'trip-ə-nəm\ *n, in some classifications* : a genus of flagellates including the trypanosome (*S. cruzi*) of Chagas' disease — used when the organism is viewed as generically distinct from the genus *Trypanosoma*

schizo·ty·pal \ˌskit-sə-'tī-pəl\ *adj* : characterized by, exhibiting, or being patterns of thought, perception, communication, and behavior suggestive of schizophrenia but not of sufficient severity to warrant a diagnosis of schizophrenia ⟨~ personality⟩

Schlemm's canal \'shlemz-\ *n* : CANAL OF SCHLEMM

Schmorl's node \'shmȯrlz-\ *n* : a spinal defect characterized by protrusion of the nucleus pulposus into the spongiosa of a vertebra

   Schmorl, Christian Georg (1861–1932), German pathologist. Schmorl described the spinal defect now known as Schmorl's node in 1926.

Schnei·de·ri·an membrane \shnī-ˌdir-ē-ən-\ *n* : modified mucous membrane forming the epithelial part of the olfactory organ

   Schnei·der \'shnīd-ər\, **Conrad Victor (1614–1680),** German anatomist. Schneider was professor of medicine at Wittenberg. In 1660 he published a work on catarrh in which he described the nasal mucous membrane, now known as the Schneiderian membrane.

Schnei·der index \'shnīd-ər-\ *n* : a measure of comparative circulatory efficiency based on determination of pulse rates under several test conditions (as reclining, standing, or after exercise), time required for rate to alter with change of state, and accompanying variations in systolic blood pressure

   Schneider, Edward Christian (1874–1954), American biologist. Schneider published several studies on the influence of high altitudes and low oxygen on humans, aviation physiology, and the effects of physical exercise and training. He introduced in 1920 a cardiovascular rating as a measure of physical fatigue and efficiency; the rating is now known as the Schneider index.

Schön·lein–Hen·och \ˌshœn-līn-'hen-ək\ *adj* : being a form of purpura that is characterized by swelling and pain of the joints in association with gastrointestinal bleeding and pain ⟨the ~ syndrome⟩ ⟨~ disease⟩

   Schönlein, Johann Lucas (1793–1864), German physician. Schönlein was one of the leading clinicians of his time. The early part of his career was spent at the university in Würzburg, Germany, where he lectured in pathological anatomy and eventually became director of the medical clinic there. His later appointments were as professor of medicine at Zurich, Switzerland, and Berlin, Germany. In 1837 he described a form of purpura often associated with pains in the joints.

   Henoch, Eduard Heinrich (1820–1910), German pediatrician. Henoch was one of Johann Schönlein's outstanding students at the University of Berlin. He described purpura associated with joint disease in two papers delivered before the Berlin Medical Society. His reports were published in 1868 and 1874. Henoch's descriptions expanded upon the observations made earlier by Schönlein.

Schönlein's disease *n* : Schönlein-Henoch purpura that is characterized esp. by swelling and pain of the joints — called also *purpura rheumatica;* compare HENOCH'S PURPURA

schra·dan \'shrä-ˌdan\ *n* : OCTAMETHYLPYROPHOSPHORAMIDE

S
T

\ə\ **abut** \ᵊ\ **kitten** \ər\ **further** \a\ **ash** \ā\ **ace** \ä\ **cot, cart** \aú\ **out** \ch\ **chin** \e\ **bet** \ē\ **easy** \g\ **go** \i\ **hit** \ī\ **ice** \j\ **job** \ŋ\ **sing** \ō\ **go** \ȯ\ **law** \ȯi\ **boy** \th\ **thin** \t̲h̲\ **the** \ü\ **loot** \ú\ **foot** \y\ **yet** \zh\ **vision** *See also* Pronunciation Symbols page

Schra·der \'shräd-ər\, **Gerhard (1903–1990),** German chemist. Schrader developed schradan in 1941 as part of the German research on poison gases for use in World War II.

Schuff·ner's dots \'shuf-nərz-\ *n pl* : punctate granulations present in red blood cells invaded by the tertian malaria parasite — compare MAURER'S DOTS

Schüff·ner \'shuef-nər\, **Wilhelm August Paul (1867–1949),** German pathologist. In 1904 Schüffner described small round granules appearing in the red blood cells of malarial patients; they are now known as Schuffner's dots.

Schüller–Christian disease *n* : HAND-SCHÜLLER= CHRISTIAN DISEASE

Schultz–Dale reaction \'shultz-'dāl-\ *n* : a reaction of anaphylaxis carried out in vitro with isolated tissues

Schultz, Werner (1878–1947), German internist. Schultz is best known for his classic description of agranulocytosis in 1922. He did his research on anaphylaxis independently of Dale and carried out his in vitro testing using the intestinal muscles of guinea pigs.

Dale, Sir Henry Hallet (1875–1968), British physiologist and pharmacologist. Dale was one of the outstanding physiologists and pharmacologists of the first half of the 20th century. His early research work centered on the physiological actions of ergot. His work with isolated guinea pig uteri established that the anaphylactic antibodies are attached to cells. He reported on the results of his research on anaphylaxis in 1919. For their discoveries in the chemical transmission of nerve impulses, he and the German pharmacologist Otto Loewi were awarded the Nobel Prize for Physiology or Medicine in 1936.

Schwann cell \'shwän-\ *n* : a cell that forms spiral layers around a myelinated nerve fiber between two nodes of Ranvier and forms the myelin sheath consisting of the inner spiral layers from which the protoplasm has been squeezed out

Schwann \'shvän\, **Theodor Ambrose Hubert (1810–1882),** German anatomist and physiologist. Schwann is regarded as the founder of modern histology. He is best known for his conception of the structure and function of cells: he defined the cell as the basic unit of human anatomy. Investigating the digestive processes in 1836, he isolated a substance responsible for digestion in the stomach. He named this first enzyme prepared from animal tissue *pepsin.* Schwann is also regarded as a founder of the germ theory of putrefaction and fermentation. He was the first to investigate the laws of muscular contraction by physical and mathematical methods and to demonstrate that the tension of a contracting muscle varies with its length. In 1838 he published his description of the myelin sheath covering peripheral axons. He also formulated a basic principle of embryology by observing that the egg is a single cell that eventually develops into a complete organism.

schwan·no·ma \shwä-'nō-mə\ *n, pl* **-mas** *also* **-ma·ta** \-mət-ə\ : NEURILEMMOMA

Schwann's sheath *n* : NEURILEMMA

sci·at·ic \sī-'at-ik\ *adj* **1** : of, relating to, or situated near the hip **2** : of, relating to, or caused by sciatica ⟨∼ pains⟩

sci·at·i·ca \sī-'at-i-kə\ *n* : pain along the course of a sciatic nerve esp. in the back of the thigh caused by compression, inflammation, or reflex mechanisms; *broadly* : pain in the lower back, buttocks, hips, or adjacent parts

sciatic foramen *n* : either of two foramina on each side of the pelvis that are formed by the hip bone, the sacrospinous ligament, and the sacrotuberous ligament and that form a passage from the pelvis to the gluteal and peroneal regions: **a** : one giving passage to the piriformis muscle and to the sciatic, superior and inferior gluteal, and pudendal nerves together with their associated arteries and veins — called also *greater sciatic foramen* **b** : one giving passage to the tendon of the obturator internus muscle and its nerve, to the internal pudendal artery and veins, and to the pudendal nerve — called also *lesser sciatic foramen*

sciatic nerve *n* : either of the pair of largest nerves in the body that arise one on each side from the sacral plexus and that pass out of the pelvis through the greater sciatic fora-

men and down the back of the thigh to its lower third where division into the tibial and common peroneal nerves occurs

sciatic notch *n* : either of two notches on the dorsal border of the hip bone on each side that when closed off by ligaments form the corresponding sciatic foramina: **a** : a relatively large notch just above the ischial spine that is converted into the greater sciatic foramen by the sacrospinous ligament — called also *greater sciatic notch* **b** : a smaller notch just below the ischial spine that is converted to the lesser sciatic foramen by the sacrospinous ligament and the sacrotuberous ligament — called also *lesser sciatic notch*

SCID *abbr* severe combined immunodeficiency

sci·ence \'sī-ən(t)s\ *n* : knowledge or a system of knowledge covering general truths or the operation of general laws esp. as obtained and tested through the scientific method and concerned with the physical world and its phenomena

sci·en·tif·ic \,sī-ən-'tif-ik\ *adj* : of, relating to, or exhibiting the methods or principles of science — **sci·en·tif·i·cal·ly** \-i-k(ə-)lē\ *adv*

scientific method *n* : principles and procedures for the systematic pursuit of knowledge involving the recognition and formulation of a problem, the collection of data through observation and experiment, and the formulation and testing of hypotheses

sci·en·tist \'sī-ənt-əst\ *n* : a person learned in science and esp. natural science : a scientific investigator

scil·li·ro·side \'sil-ə-rə-,sīd\ *n* : a crystalline steroid cardiac glucoside $C_{32}H_{44}O_{12}$ obtained from red squill

scin·ti·gram \'sin-tə-,gram\ *n* : a picture produced by scintigraphy

scin·tig·ra·phy \sin-'tig-rə-fē\ *n, pl* **-phies** : a diagnostic technique in which a two-dimensional picture of internal body tissue is produced through the detection of radiation emitted by a radioactive substance administered into the body ⟨myocardial ∼⟩ — **scin·ti·graph·ic** \,sint-ə-'graf-ik\ *adj*

scin·til·late \'sint-ºl-,āt\ *vi* **-lat·ed; -lat·ing** : to produce scintillation

scintillating scotoma *n* : a blind spot in the visual field that is bordered by shimmering or flashing light and that is often a premonitory symptom of migraine attack

scin·til·la·tion \,sint-ºl-'ā-shən\ *n, often attrib* : a flash of light produced in a phosphor by an ionizing event

scintillation camera *n* : a camera that records scintillations

scintillation counter *n* : a device for detecting and registering individual scintillations (as in radioactive emission) — called also *scintillometer*

scin·til·la·tor \'sint-ºl-,āt-ər\ *n* **1** : a phosphor in which scintillations occur (as in a scintillation counter) **2** : a device for sending out scintillations of light **3** : SCINTILLATION COUNTER

scin·til·lom·e·ter \,sint-ºl-'äm-ət-ər\ *n* : SCINTILLATION COUNTER

scin·ti·scan \'sint-i-,skan\ *n* : a two-dimensional representation of radioisotope radiation from a bodily organ (as the spleen or kidney)

scin·ti·scan·ner \-,skan-ər\ *n* : a device for producing a scintiscan

scin·ti·scan·ning \-,skan-iŋ\ *n* : the action or process of making a scintiscan

scir·rhoid \'s(k)i-,ròid\ *adj* : resembling a scirrhous carcinoma

scir·rhous \'s(k)ir-əs\ *adj* : of, relating to, or being a scirrhous carcinoma ⟨∼ infiltration⟩

scirrhous carcinoma *n* : a hard slow-growing malignant tumor having a preponderance of fibrous tissue

scir·rhus \'s(k)ir-əs\ *n, pl* **scir·rhi** \'s(k)i(ə)r-,ī, 's(k)i(ə)r-,ē\ : SCIRRHOUS CARCINOMA

scis·sile \'sis-əl, -,īl\ *adj* : capable of being cut smoothly or split easily ⟨a ∼ peptide bond⟩

scis·sion \'sizh-ən\ *n* : an action or process of cutting, dividing, or splitting : the state of being cut, divided, or split ⟨single strand ∼s in DNA⟩

scis·sors \'siz-ərz\ *n pl but sing or pl in constr* : a cutting instrument having two blades whose cutting edges slide past each other

sclera \\'skler-ə\\ *n* : the dense fibrous opaque white outer coat enclosing the eyeball except the part covered by the cornea — called also *sclerotic, sclerotic coat*

sclerae — see SINUS VENOSUS SCLERAE

scler·al \\'skler-əl\\ *adj* : of or relating to the sclera ⟨∼ tissue⟩ ⟨∼ contact lenses⟩

scle·rec·to·my \\sklə-'rek-tə-mē\\ *n, pl* **-mies** : surgical removal of a part of the sclera

scle·re·ma neo·na·to·rum \\sklə-'rē-mə-,nē-ə-nə-'tōr-əm\\ *n* : hardening of the cutaneous and subcutaneous tissues in newborn infants

scle·ri·tis \\sklə-'rīt-əs\\ *n* : inflammation of the sclera

sclero·cor·nea \\,skler-ō-'kȯr-nē-ə\\ *n* : a congenital condition in which the cornea is opaque like the sclera

sclero·cor·ne·al \\-nē-əl\\ *adj* : of or involving both sclera and cornea ⟨the ∼ junction⟩

sclero·dac·tyl·ia \\,skler-ō-dak-'til-ē-ə\\ *or* **sclero·dac·ty·ly** \\-'dak-tə-lē\\ *n, pl* **-ias** *or* **-lies** : scleroderma of the fingers and toes

sclero·der·ma \\,skler-ə-'dər-mə\\ *n, pl* **-mas** *or* **-ma·ta** \\-mət-ə\\ : a usu. slowly progressive disease marked by the deposition of fibrous connective tissue in the skin and often in internal organs and structures, by hand and foot pain upon exposure to cold, and by tightening and thickening of the skin — called also *dermatosclerosis*

sclero·der·ma·tous \\-'dər-mət-əs\\ *adj* : of, relating to, or affected with scleroderma ⟨∼ changes over the shins, forearms, knees, hands, and feet —*Lancet*⟩

sclero·ker·a·ti·tis \\,skler-ō-,ker-ə-'tīt-əs\\ *n, pl* **-tit·i·des** \\-'tit-ə-,dēz\\ : inflammation of the sclera and cornea

scle·ro·ma \\sklə-'rō-mə\\ *n, pl* **-mas** *or* **-ma·ta** \\-mət-ə\\ : hardening of tissues; *specif* : RHINOSCLEROMA

sclero·pro·tein \\,skler-ō-'prō-,tēn, -'prōt-ē-ən\\ *n* : any of various proteins (as collagen and keratin) that occur esp. in connective and skeletal tissues, are usu. insoluble in aqueous solvents, and are resistant to chemical reagents — called also *albuminoid*

scle·rose \\sklə-'rōs, -'rōz\\ *vb* **-rosed; -ros·ing** *vt* : to cause sclerosis in ⟨chronic infections may ∼ kidneys⟩ ∼ *vi* : to undergo or become affected with sclerosis : become sclerotic ⟨arteries of older people often tend to ∼⟩

scle·ros·ing \\sklə-'rō-siŋ, -ziŋ\\ *adj* : causing or characterized by sclerosis ⟨a ∼ agent that induces an inflammatory response leading to a fibrotic process —Lisette R. Teixeira *et al*⟩ — see SUBACUTE SCLEROSING PANENCEPHALITIS

scle·ro·sis \\sklə-'rō-səs\\ *n, pl* **-ro·ses** \\-,sēz\\ **1** : a pathological condition in which a tissue has become hard and which is produced by overgrowth of fibrous tissue and other changes (as in arteriosclerosis) or by increase in interstitial tissue and other changes (as in multiple sclerosis) — called also *hardening* **2** : any of various diseases characterized by sclerosis — usu. used in combination; see ARTERIOSCLEROSIS, MULTIPLE SCLEROSIS, MYELOSCLEROSIS

scle·ro·stome \\'skler-ə-,stōm\\ *n* : STRONGYLE

sclerosus — see LICHEN SCLEROSUS ET ATROPHICUS

sclero·ther·a·py \\,skler-ō-'ther-ə-pē\\ *n, pl* **-pies** : the injection of a sclerosing agent (as morrhuate sodium) into a varicose vein to produce inflammation and scarring which closes the lumen and is followed by shrinkage; *also* : PROLOTHERAPY

scle·ro·thrix \\'skler-ə-,thriks, 'sklir-\\ *n, pl* **scle·rot·ri·ches** \\sklə-'rä-trə-,kēz\\ *or* **scle·ro·thrix·es** : abnormal hardness of the hair

scle·ro·tial \\sklə-'rō-shəl\\ *adj* : of or relating to a sclerotium : bearing sclerotia

¹scle·rot·ic \\sklə-'rät-ik\\ *adj* **1** : being or relating to the sclera ⟨the ∼ layer of the eye⟩ **2** : of, relating to, or affected with sclerosis ⟨a ∼ blood vessel⟩

²sclerotic *n* : SCLERA

sclerotic coat *n* : SCLERA

scle·ro·tium \\sklə-'rō-sh(ē-)əm\\ *n, pl* **-tia** \\-sh(ē-)ə\\ : a compact mass of hardened mycelium (as in an ergot) stored with

reserve food material that in some higher fungi becomes detached and remains dormant until a favorable opportunity for growth occurs

sclero·tome \\'skler-ə-,tōm\\ *n* : the ventral and mesial portion of a somite that proliferates mesenchyme which migrates about the notochord to form the axial skeleton and ribs — **sclero·tom·ic** \\,skler-ə-'tō-mik, -'tä-mik\\ *adj*

scle·rot·o·my \\sklə-'rät-ə-mē\\ *n, pl* **-mies** : surgical cutting of the sclera

sclerotriches *pl of* SCLEROTHRIX

sclero·trich·ia \\,skler-ə-'trik-ē-ə\\ *n* : SCLEROTHRIX

ScM *abbr or n* master of science

SCM *abbr* state certified midwife

SCN *abbr* suprachiasmatic nucleus

sco·lex \\'skō-,leks\\ *n, pl* **sco·li·ces** \\'skō-lə-,sēz\\ *also* **sco·le·ces** \\'skäl-ə-,sēz, 'skōl-\\ *or* **scolexes** : the head of a tapeworm either in the larva or adult stage from which the proglottids are produced by budding

sco·li·o·sis \\,skō-lē-'ō-səs\\ *n, pl* **-o·ses** \\-,sēz\\ : a lateral curvature of the spine — compare KYPHOSIS, LORDOSIS — **sco·li·ot·ic** \\-'ät-ik\\ *adj*

scom·broid \\'skäm-,brȯid\\ *n* : any of a suborder (Scombroidea) of marine bony fishes (as mackerels, tunas, albacores, bonitos, and swordfishes) which are of great economic importance as food fishes and are sometimes a source of poisoning due to heat-stable toxins produced by bacterial action on fish with dark meat — **scombroid** *adj*

scoop \\'sküp\\ *n* : a spoon-shaped surgical instrument used in extracting various materials (as pus or foreign bodies)

sco·par·i·us \\skō-'par-ē-əs\\ *n* : the dried tops of the Scotch broom (*Cytisus scoparius*) containing the alkaloid sparteine and formerly used as a diuretic

scope \\'skōp\\ *n* : any of various instruments (as an endoscope or microscope) for viewing or observing

sco·po·la \\'skō-pə-lə\\ *also* **sco·po·lia** \\skə-'pō-lē-ə\\ *n* : the dried rhizome of an herb (*Scopolia carniolica*) of the family Solanaceae that contains the alkaloids scopolamine, atropine, and hyoscyamine and is used as a hypnotic and analgesic

sco·pol·amine \\skō-'päl-ə-,mēn, -mən\\ *n* : a poisonous alkaloid $C_{17}H_{21}NO_4$ similar to atropine that is found in various solanaceous plants (as jimsonweed) and is used chiefly in the form of its hydrated hydrobromide $C_{17}H_{21}NO_4 \cdot HBr \cdot 3H_2O$ for its anticholinergic effects (as preventing nausea in motion sickness and inducing mydriasis) — called also *hyoscine*

sco·po·le·tin \\,skō-pə-'lēt-ᵊn, skə-'päl-ət-ən\\ *n* : a crystalline lactone $C_{10}H_8O$ that is found in various solanaceous plants (as members of the genus *Scopolia* or belladonna)

sco·po·phil·ia \\,skō-pə-'fil-ē-ə\\ *or* **scop·to·phil·ia** \\,skäp-tə-'fil-ē-ə\\ *n* : a desire to look at sexually stimulating scenes esp. as a substitute for actual sexual participation — **sco·po·phil·ic** *or* **scop·to·phil·ic** \\-'fil-ik\\ *adj*

sco·po·phil·i·ac *or* **scop·to·phil·i·ac** \\-'fil-ē-,ak\\ *n* : an individual affected with scopophilia — **scopophiliac** *or* **scoptophiliac** *adj*

scor·bu·tic \\skȯr-'byüt-ik\\ *adj* : of, relating to, producing, or affected with scurvy ⟨a ∼ diet⟩

scor·bu·ti·gen·ic \\skȯr-,byüt-ə-'jen-ik\\ *adj* : causing scurvy ⟨a ∼ diet⟩

scor·bu·tus \\skȯr-'byüt-əs\\ *n* : SCURVY

scor·pi·on \\'skȯr-pē-ən\\ *n* : any of an order (Scorpionida) of arachnids that have an elongated body and a narrow segmented tail bearing a venomous stinger at the tip

scorpion fish *n* : any of a family (Scorpaenidae) of marine spiny-finned fishes; *esp* : one having a venomous spine or spines on its dorsal fin

Scotch broom \\'skäch-\\ *n* : a deciduous broom (*Cytisus scoparius*) of western Europe that contains the alkaloid sparte-

S
T

\\ə\\ **abut** \\ᵊ\\ **kitten** \\ər\\ **further** \\a\\ **ash** \\ā\\ **ace** \\ä\\ **cot, cart**
\\au̇\\ **out** \\ch\\ **chin** \\e\\ **bet** \\ē\\ **easy** \\g\\ **go** \\i\\ **hit** \\ī\\ **ice** \\j\\ **job**
\\ŋ\\ **sing** \\ō\\ **go** \\ȯ\\ **law** \\ȯi\\ **boy** \\th\\ **thin** \\th̲\\ **the** \\ü\\ **loot**
\\u̇\\ **foot** \\y\\ **yet** \\zh\\ **vision** *See also* Pronunciation Symbols page

ine, is the source of scoparius, and is widely cultivated for its bright yellow or partly red flowers

sco·to·ma \skə-'tō-mə\ *n, pl* **-mas** *or* **-ma·ta** \-mət-ə\ : a spot in the visual field in which vision is absent or deficient

sco·top·ic \skə-'tō-pik, -'täp-ik\ *adj* : of, relating to, being, or suitable for scotopic vision ⟨rods functioning under ∼ conditions⟩ ⟨∼ sensitivity⟩

scotopic vision *n* : vision in dim light with dark-adapted eyes that involves only the retinal rods as light receptors — called also *twilight vision*

sco·top·sin \skə-'täp-sən\ *n* : a protein in the retinal rods that combines with retinal to form rhodopsin

¹**scour** \'skau̇(ə)r\ *vi, of a domestic animal* : to suffer from diarrhea or dysentery ⟨a diet causing cattle to ∼⟩

²**scour** *n* : diarrhea or dysentery occurring esp. in young domestic animals — usu. used in pl. but sing. or pl. in constr.

scra·pie \'skrā-pē\ *n* : a usu. fatal spongiform encephalopathy esp. of sheep that is caused by a prion and is characterized by twitching, excitability, intense itching, excessive thirst, emaciation, weakness, and finally paralysis

scrap·ing \'skrā-piŋ\ *n* : material scraped esp. from diseased tissue (as infected skin) for microscopic examination

scratch test *n* : a test for allergic susceptibility made by rubbing an extract of an allergy-producing substance into small breaks or scratches in the skin — compare INTRADERMAL TEST, PATCH TEST, PRICK TEST

screen \'skrēn\ *vt* : to test or examine for the presence of something (as a disease) ⟨∼ patients for prostate cancer⟩ ⟨a test to ∼ donor blood for HIV and hepatitis C —Penni Crabtree⟩

screen — see INTENSIFYING SCREEN, SUNSCREEN, TRIPLE SCREEN

screen memory *n* : a recollection of early childhood that may be falsely recalled or magnified in importance and that masks another memory of deep emotional significance

screw \'skrü\ *n* : a threaded device used in bone surgery for fixation of parts (as fragments of fractured bones)

screw·fly \'skrü-ˌflī\ *n, pl* **-flies** : SCREWWORM FLY

screw·worm \'skrü-ˌwərm\ *n* **1** : either of two dipteran flies of the genus *Cochliomyia*: **a** : one (*C. hominivorax*) of the warmer parts of America whose larva develops in sores or wounds or in the nostrils of mammals including humans with serious or sometimes fatal results; *esp* : its larva **b** : SECONDARY SCREWWORM **2** : a dipteran fly of the genus *Chrysomyia* (*C. bezziana*) that causes myiasis in the Old World

screwworm fly *n* : the adult of a screwworm — called also *screwfly*

scrip \'skrip\ *n* : PRESCRIPTION 1

script \'skript\ *n* : PRESCRIPTION 1

scrof·u·la \'skrȯf-yə-lə, 'skräf-\ *n* : tuberculosis of lymph nodes esp. in the neck — called also *king's evil*

scrof·u·lo·der·ma \ˌskrȯf-yə-lō-'dər-mə, ˌskräf-\ *n* : a disease of the skin of tuberculous origin (as an inflammation of the neck from draining tuberculous lymph nodes) — **scrof·u·lo·der·mic** \-mik\ *adj*

scrof·u·lous \'skrȯf-yə-ləs, 'skräf-\ *adj* : of, relating to, or affected with scrofula ⟨∼ ulcers⟩

scro·tal \'skrōt-ᵊl\ *adj* **1** : of or relating to the scrotum ⟨∼ skin⟩ **2** : lying in or having descended into the scrotum ⟨∼ testes⟩

scro·to·cele \'skrōt-ə-ˌsēl\ *n* : a scrotal hernia

scro·to·plas·ty \'skrōt-ə-ˌplas-tē\ *n, pl* **-ties** : plastic surgery performed on the scrotum

scro·tum \'skrōt-əm\ *n, pl* **scro·ta** \-ə\ *or* **scrotums** : the external sac that in most mammals contains the testes

¹**scrub** \'skrəb\ *vb* **scrubbed; scrub·bing** *vt* : to clean and disinfect (the hands and forearms) before participating in surgery ∼ *vi* : to prepare for surgery by scrubbing oneself

²**scrub** *n* **1** : an act or instance of scrubbing ⟨a surgical ∼⟩ **2** *pl* : loose-fitting clothing worn by hospital staff ⟨surgical ∼s⟩

scrub nurse *n* : a nurse who assists the surgeon in an operating room

scrub typhus *n* : TSUTSUGAMUSHI DISEASE

scru·ple \'skrü-pəl\ *n* : a unit of apothecaries' weight equal to 20 grains or ⅓ dram or 1.296 grams

scurf \'skərf\ *n* : thin dry scales detached from the epidermis esp. in an abnormal skin condition; *specif* : DANDRUFF — **scurfy** \'skər-vē\ *adj*

scur·vy \'skər-vē\ *n, pl* **scur·vies** : a disease caused by a lack of vitamin C and characterized by spongy gums, loosening of the teeth, and bleeding into the skin and mucous membranes — called also *scorbutus*

scurvy grass *n* : a cress (as *Cochlearia officinalis*) formerly believed useful in preventing or treating scurvy

scu·tel·lar·ia \ˌsk(y)üt-ə-'lar-ē-ə\ *n* **1** *cap* : a very large widely distributed genus of herbs of the mint family (Labiatae) **2** : the dried aboveground portion of a plant of the genus *Scutellaria* (*S. lateriflora*) used esp. formerly as a bitter tonic, antispasmodic, and stomachic

scu·tu·lum \'skü-chə-ləm\ *n, pl* **scu·tu·la** \-lə\ : one of the yellow cup-shaped crusts occurring over hair follicles in favus

scyb·a·lous \'sib-ə-ləs\ *adj* : formed of hardened feces ⟨a ∼ mass⟩

scyb·a·lum \-ləm\ *n, pl* **scyb·a·la** \-lə\ : a hardened fecal mass

Scyph·o·zoa \ˌskif-ə-'zō-ə\ *n pl* : a class of coelenterates that includes jellyfishes (as the sea wasps) having gastric tentacles and no true polyp stage — **scyph·o·zo·an** \-'zō-ən\ *adj or n*

SDA *abbr* specific dynamic action

Se *symbol* selenium

sea·bath·er's eruption \'sē-ˌbā-ˌthərz-\ *n* : acute pruritic dermatitis that occurs on parts of the body covered by a bathing suit within 24 hours after exposure to seawater containing certain tiny coelenterate larvae (as of jellyfishes, sea anemones, or corals) and that is caused by nematocysts fired by the larvae caught in the mesh of the bathing suit or compressed between the bathing suit and the skin — see THIMBLE JELLYFISH

sea·borg·i·um \sē-'bȯr-gē-əm\ *n* : a short-lived radioactive element that is artificially produced — symbol *Sg*; see ELEMENT table

sea hol·ly \'sē-ˌhäl-ē\ *n* : a European coastal herb of the genus *Eryngium* (*E. maritimum*) that has spiny leaves and pale blue flowers and was formerly used as an aphrodisiac

seal \'sēl\ *vt* : to apply dental sealant to ⟨the teeth to be ∼ed are surrounded by cotton rolls and dried thoroughly —J. W. Friedman⟩

seal·ant \'sē-lənt\ *n* : a plastic material that is applied to parts of teeth (as the occlusal surfaces of molars and premolars) with imperfections (as pits and fissures) usu. to prevent dental decay

seal finger *n* : a finger rendered swollen and painful by erysipeloid or a similar infection and occurring esp. in individuals handling seals or sealskins — called also *blubber finger*

sea lice *n pl* : tiny coelenterate larvae (as of the thimble jellyfish) that cause seabather's eruption; *also* : SEABATHER'S ERUPTION

sea on·ion \-ˌən-yən\ *n* : SQUILL 1a

sea·sick \-ˌsik\ *adj* : affected with seasickness

sea·sick·ness \-nəs\ *n* : motion sickness experienced on the water — called also *mal de mer*

sea snake *n* : any of a family (Hydrophidae) of numerous venomous snakes inhabiting the tropical parts of the Pacific and Indian oceans

sea·son·al affective disorder \ˌsēz-ᵊn-əl-\ *n* : depression that tends to recur as the days grow shorter during the fall and winter — abbr. *SAD*

¹**seat** \'sēt\ *n* : a part or surface esp. in dentistry on or in which another part or surface rests — see REST SEAT

²**seat** *vt* : to provide with or position on a dental seat ∼ *vi* : to fit correctly on a dental seat

seat·worm \-ˌwərm\ *n* : a pinworm of the genus *Enterobius* (*E. vermicularis*) that is parasitic in humans

sea wasp *n* : any of various scyphozoan jellyfishes (order or suborder Cubomedusae) that sting virulently and sometimes fatally

se·ba·ceous \si-'bā-shəs\ *adj* **1** : secreting sebum **2** : of, relating to, or being fatty material ⟨a ∼ exudate⟩

sebaceous cyst *n* : a cyst filled with sebaceous matter and formed by distension of a sebaceous gland as a result of obstruction of its excretory duct — called also *wen*

sebaceous gland *n* : any of the small sacculated glands lodged in the substance of the derma, usu. opening into the hair follicles, and secreting an oily or greasy material composed in great part of fat which softens and lubricates the hair and skin

sebaceum — see MOLLUSCUM SEBACEUM

seb·or·rhea *or Brit* **seb·or·rhoea** \ˌseb-ə-'rē-ə\ *n* : abnormally increased secretion and discharge of sebum producing an oily appearance of the skin and the formation of greasy scales

seb·or·rhe·al *or Brit* **seb·or·rhoe·al** \ˌseb-ə-'rē-əl\ *adj* : SEBORRHEIC

seb·or·rhe·ic *or Brit* **seb·or·rhoe·ic** \-'rē-ik\ *adj* : of, relating to, marked by, or characteristic of seborrhea ⟨∼ lesions⟩

seborrheic dermatitis *n* : a red, scaly, itchy dermatitis chiefly affecting areas (as of the face, scalp, or chest) with many large sebaceous glands

seborrheic keratosis *n* : a benign hyperkeratotic tumor that occurs singly or in clusters on the surface of the skin, is usu. light to dark brown or black in color, and typically has a warty texture often with a waxy appearance

se·bum \'sē-bəm\ *n* : fatty lubricant matter secreted by sebaceous glands of the skin

seco·bar·bi·tal \ˌsek-ō-'bär-bə-ˌtȯl\ *n* : a barbiturate that is used chiefly in the form of its bitter hygroscopic sodium salt $C_{12}H_{17}N_2NaO_3$ as a hypnotic and sedative — called also *quinalbarbitone;* see SECONAL

Sec·o·nal \'sek-ə-ˌnȯl, -ˌnal, -ən-ᵊl\ *trademark* — used for a preparation of the sodium salt of secobarbital

sec·ond·ar·ies *n pl* : the lesions characteristic of secondary syphilis

sec·ond·ary \'sek-ən-ˌder-ē\ *adj* **1** : not first in order of occurrence or development: as **a** : dependent or consequent on another disease ⟨∼ diabetes⟩ ⟨Bright's disease is often ∼ to scarlet fever⟩ **b** : occurring or being in the second stage ⟨∼ symptoms of syphilis⟩ **c** : occurring some time after the original injury ⟨a ∼ hemorrhage⟩ **2** : characterized by or resulting from the substitution of two atoms or groups in a molecule ⟨a ∼ salt⟩; *esp* : being, characterized by, or attached to a carbon atom having bonds to two other carbon atoms **3** : relating to or being the three-dimensional coiling of the polypeptide chain of a protein esp. in the form of an alpha-helix — compare PRIMARY 4, TERTIARY 2c — **sec·ond·ari·ly** \ˌsek-ən-'der-ə-lē\ *adv*

secondary amenorrhea *n* : the temporary or permanent cessation of menstruation in a woman who has previously experienced normal menses

secondary amine *n* : an amine (as piperidine) having two organic groups attached to the nitrogen in place of two hydrogen atoms

secondary care *n* : medical care provided by a specialist or facility upon referral by a primary care physician that requires more specialized knowledge, skill, or equipment than the primary care physician has — compare PRIMARY CARE, TERTIARY CARE

secondary color *n* : a color formed by mixing primary colors in equal or equivalent quantities

secondary dentin *n* : dentin formed following the loss (as by erosion, abrasion, or disease) of original dentin

secondary emission *n* : the emission of electrons from a surface that is bombarded by particles (as electrons or ions) from a primary source

secondary gain *n* : a benefit (as sympathetic attention) associated with a mental illness

secondary hypertension *n* : hypertension that results from an underlying identifiable cause (as aldosteronism, thyroid dysfunction, or coarctation of the aorta)

secondary infection *n* : infection occurring at the site of a preexisting infection

secondary oocyte *n* : an oocyte that is produced by division of a primary oocyte in the first meiotic division

secondary screwworm *n* : a screwworm of the genus *Cochliomyia* (*C. macellaria*)

secondary sex characteristic *n* : a physical characteristic (as the breasts of a female mammal or the nuptial plumage of a male bird) that appears in members of one sex at puberty or in seasonal breeders at the breeding season and is not directly concerned with reproduction — called also *secondary sex character, secondary sexual characteristic*

secondary spermatocyte *n* : a spermatocyte that is produced by division of a primary spermatocyte in the first meiotic division, that has a haploid number of chromosomes in forms (as the human male) having a single centromere, and that divides in the second meiotic division to give spermatids

secondary syphilis *n* : the second stage of syphilis that appears from 2 to 6 months after primary infection, that is marked by lesions esp. in the skin but also in organs and tissues, and that lasts from 3 to 12 weeks

secondary tympanic membrane *n* : a membrane closing the round window and separating the scala tympani from the middle ear

sec·ond childhood \ˌsek-ᵊnd-\ *n* : DOTAGE

second cranial nerve *n* : OPTIC NERVE

second–degree burn *n* : a burn marked by pain, blistering, and superficial destruction of dermis with edema and hyperemia of the tissues beneath the burn

second filial generation *n* : F_2 GENERATION

second generation hybrid *n* : F_2 HYBRID

sec·ond·hand smoke \ˌsek-ᵊn(d)-ˌhan(d)-\ *n* : tobacco smoke that is exhaled by a smoker or is given off by burning tobacco (as of a cigarette) and is inhaled by persons nearby — called also *passive smoke*

second in·ten·tion \-in-'ten-chən\ *n* : the healing of an incised wound by granulations that bridge the gap between skin edges — compare FIRST INTENTION

second law of thermodynamics *n* : LAW OF THERMODYNAMICS 2

sec·ond–line \ˌsek-ᵊn(d)-ˌlīn\ *adj* : being or using a drug that is not the usual or preferred choice — compare FIRST-LINE

second messenger *n* : an intracellular substance (as cyclic AMP) that mediates cell activity by relaying a signal from an extracellular molecule (as of a hormone or neurotransmitter) bound to the cell's surface — compare FIRST MESSENGER

second polar body *n* : POLAR BODY b

second wind *n* : recovered full power of respiration after the first exhaustion during exertion due to improved heart action

se·cre·ta·gogue *also* **se·cre·to·gogue** \si-'krēt-ə-ˌgäg\ *n* : a substance that stimulates secretion (as by the stomach or pancreas)

se·cre·tase \si-'krē-ˌtās\ *n* : any of several transmembrane proteases that are capable of cleaving amyloid precursor protein and include two forms that function in the generation of beta-amyloid

se·crete \si-'krēt\ *vt* **se·cret·ed; se·cret·ing** : to form and give off (a secretion) ⟨cells *secreting* mucus⟩

se·cre·tin \si-'krēt-ᵊn\ *n* : an intestinal proteinaceous hormone capable of stimulating secretion by the pancreas and liver

se·cre·tion \si-'krē-shən\ *n* **1** : the process of segregating, elaborating, and releasing some material either functionally specialized (as saliva) or isolated for excretion (as urine) **2** : a product of secretion formed by an animal or plant; *esp* : one performing a specific useful function in the organism

se·cre·tor \si-'krēt-ər\ *n* : an individual of blood group A, B,

S
T

\ə\ **abut** \ᵊ\ **kitten** \ər\ **further** \a\ **ash** \ā\ **ace** \ä\ **cot, cart**
\aú\ **out** \ch\ **chin** \e\ **bet** \ē\ **easy** \g\ **go** \i\ **hit** \ī\ **ice** \j\ **job**
\ŋ\ **sing** \ō\ **go** \ȯ\ **law** \ȯi\ **boy** \th\ **thin** \t̲h̲\ **the** \ü\ **loot**
\ú\ **foot** \y\ **yet** \zh\ **vision** *See also* Pronunciation Symbols page

or AB who secretes the antigens characteristic of these blood groups in bodily fluids (as saliva)

se·cre·to·ry \'sē-krə-ˌtór-ē, *esp Brit* si-'krēt-(ə-)rē\ *adj* : of, relating to, or promoting secretion; *also* : produced by secretion

secretory otitis media *n* : SEROUS OTITIS MEDIA

¹sec·tion \'sek-shən\ *n* **1** : the action or an instance of cutting or separating by cutting; *esp* : the action of dividing (as tissues) surgically ⟨nerve ∼⟩ ⟨abdominal ∼⟩ — see CESAREAN SECTION **2** : a natural subdivision of a taxonomic group **3** : a very thin slice (as of tissue) suitable for microscopic examination

²section *vt* **sec·tioned; sec·tion·ing** \-sh(ə-)niŋ\ **1** : to divide (a body part or organ) surgically ⟨∼ a nerve⟩ **2** : to cut (fixed tissue) into thin slices for microscopic examination

se·cun·di·grav·id \si-ˌkənd-ē-'grav-əd\ *adj* : pregnant for the second time

se·cun·di·grav·i·da \-'grav-id-ə\ *n, pl* **-dae** \-ˌdē, -ˌdī\ *also* **-das** : a woman in her second pregnancy

sec·un·dines \'sek-ən-ˌdēnz, -ˌdīnz; se-'kən-dənz\ *n pl* : AFTERBIRTH

sec·un·dip·a·ra \ˌsek-ən-'dip-ə-rə\ *n, pl* **-ras** *or* **-rae** \-ˌrē, -ˌrī\ : a woman who has borne children in two separate pregnancies

secundum — see OSTIUM SECUNDUM

se·cu·ri·ty \si-'kyùr-ət-ē\ *n, pl* **-ties** : freedom from fear or anxiety ⟨need for ∼ dates back into infancy —K. C. Garrison⟩

security blanket *n* : a blanket carried by a child as a protection against anxiety

SED *abbr* skin erythema dose

se·date \si-'dāt\ *vt* **se·dat·ed; se·dat·ing** : to dose with sedatives ⟨the patient was *sedated* before the procedure⟩

se·da·tion \si-'dā-shən\ *n* **1** : the inducing of a relaxed easy state esp. by the use of sedatives **2** : a state resulting from sedation — see CONSCIOUS SEDATION, DEEP SEDATION

¹sed·a·tive \'sed-ət-iv\ *adj* : tending to calm, moderate, or tranquilize nervousness or excitement ⟨∼ effects of anesthetics and analgesics —Linda C. Haynes *et al*⟩

²sedative *n* : a sedative agent or drug

sed·en·tary \'sed-ºn-ˌter-ē\ *adj* : doing or requiring much sitting : characterized by a lack of physical activity ⟨increased risk of heart disease for those with ∼ jobs⟩

¹sed·i·ment \'sed-ə-mənt\ *n* : the matter that settles to the bottom of a liquid

²sed·i·ment \-ˌment\ *vt* : to deposit as sediment ⟨the synaptosomes were ∼*ed* by centrifugation⟩ ∼ *vi* **1** : to settle to the bottom in a liquid ⟨let the red blood cells ∼ for 30 minutes⟩ **2** : to deposit sediment

sed·i·ment·able \ˌsed-ə-'ment-ə-bəl\ *adj* : capable of being sedimented by centrifugation ⟨∼ ribosomal particles⟩

sed·i·men·ta·tion \ˌsed-ə-(ˌ)men-'tā-shən\ *n* **1** : the action or process of depositing sediment **2** : the depositing esp. by mechanical means of matter suspended in a liquid

sedimentation coefficient *n* : a measure of the rate at which a molecule (as a protein) suspended in a colloidal solution sediments in an ultracentrifuge usu. expressed in svedbergs

sedimentation rate *n* : the speed at which red blood cells settle to the bottom of a column of citrated blood measured in millimeters deposited per hour and which is used esp. in diagnosing the progress of various abnormal conditions (as chronic infections)

sedis — see INCERTAE SEDIS

se·do·hep·tose \ˌsēd-ō-'hep-ˌtōs, -ˌtōz\ *n* : SEDOHEPTULOSE

se·do·hep·tu·lose \ˌsēd-ō-'hep-tyə-ˌlōs, -ˌlōz\ *n* : an amorphous ketose sugar $C_7H_{14}O_7$ that plays a role in carbohydrate metabolism but is not fermented by yeast and that is a laboratory source of D-altrose and D-ribose

sed rate \'sed-\ *n* : SEDIMENTATION RATE

see \'sē\ *vb* **saw** \'sò\; **seen** \'sēn\; **see·ing** \'sē-iŋ\ *vt* : to perceive by the eye ∼ *vi* **1** : to have the power of sight **2** : to apprehend objects by sight

¹seed \'sēd\ *n, pl* **seed** *or* **seeds** **1 a** : the fertilized ripened ovule of a flowering plant containing an embryo and capable normally of germination to produce a new plant; *broadly* : a propagative plant structure (as a spore or small dry fruit) **b** : a propagative animal structure: (1) : MILT, SEMEN (2) : a small egg (as of an insect) (3) : a developmental form of a lower animal — see SEED TICK **2** : a small usu. glass and gold or platinum capsule used as a container for a radioactive substance (as radium or radon) to be applied usu. interstitially in the treatment of cancer ⟨implantation of radon ∼s for bladder cancer⟩

²seed *vi* : to bear or shed seed ∼ *vt* **1** : to furnish with something that causes or stimulates growth or development **2** : INOCULATE **3** : to supply with nuclei (as of crystallization or condensation)

³seed *adj* **1** : selected or used to produce a new crop or stock ⟨∼ virus⟩ **2** : left or saved for breeding ⟨a ∼ population⟩

seed tick *n* : the 6-legged larva of a tick

Seeing Eye *trademark* — used for a guide dog trained to lead the blind

¹seg·ment \'seg-mənt\ *n* : one of the constituent parts into which a body, entity, or quantity is divided or marked off by or as if by natural boundaries ⟨bronchopulmonary ∼s⟩ ⟨the affected ∼ of the colon was resected⟩

²seg·ment \'seg-ˌment\ *vt* **1** : to cause to undergo segmentation by division or multiplication of cells **2** : to separate into segments

seg·men·tal \seg-'ment-ºl\ *adj* **1 a** : of, relating to, or having the form of a segment **b** : situated in, affecting, or performed on a segment ⟨a ∼ pancreas transplant using only the lower third of the organ⟩ ⟨∼ versus total mastectomy⟩ **2** : of, relating to, or composed of somites or metameres : METAMERIC **3** : divided into segments **4** : resulting from segmentation

segmental in·ter·change \-'int-ər-ˌchānj\ *n* : RECIPROCAL TRANSLOCATION

seg·men·tal·ly \-ºl-ē\ *adv* : in a segmental manner ⟨∼ arranged organs⟩

segmental resection *n* : excision of a segment of an organ; *specif* : excision of a portion of a lobe of a lung — called also *segmentectomy;* compare PNEUMONECTOMY

seg·men·ta·tion \ˌseg-(ˌ)men-'tā-shən\ *n* **1** : the act or process of dividing into segments; *esp* : the formation of many cells from a single cell (as in a developing egg) **2** : annular contraction of smooth muscle (as of the intestine) that seems to cut the part affected into segments — compare PERISTALSIS

segmentation cavity *n* : BLASTOCOEL

seg·men·tec·to·my \ˌseg-mən-'tek-tə-mē\ *n, pl* **-mies** : SEGMENTAL RESECTION

seg·ment·ed \'seg-ˌment-əd, seg-'\ *adj* **1** : having or made up of segments **2** : being a cell in which the nucleus is divided into lobes connected by a fine filament ⟨∼ neutrophils⟩

seg·ment·er \'seg-ˌment-ər\ *n* : SCHIZONT

Seg·men·ti·na \ˌseg-mən-'tī-nə\ *n* : a genus of Asian freshwater snails of the family Planorbidae that are of medical importance as intermediate hosts of an intestinal fluke of the genus *Fasciolopsis* (*F. buski*)

seg·re·gant \'seg-ri-gənt\ *n* : SEGREGATE

¹seg·re·gate \'seg-ri-ˌgāt\ *vi* **-gat·ed; -gat·ing** : to undergo genetic segregation

²seg·re·gate \-gət\ *n* : an individual or class of individuals differing in one or more genetic characters from the parental line usu. because of segregation of genes

seg·re·ga·tion \ˌseg-ri-'gā-shən\ *n* : the separation of allelic genes that occurs typically during meiosis

seg·re·ga·tor \'seg-ri-ˌgāt-ər\ *n* : an instrument for collecting the urine from each kidney separately

Seid·litz powders \'sed-ləts-\ *n pl* : effervescing salts that consist of two separate powders with one made up of 40 grains of sodium bicarbonate mixed with 2 drams of Rochelle salt and the other of 35 grains of tartaric acid and that are mixed in water and drunk while effervescing as a mild cathartic

Sei·gnette salt *or* **Seignette's salt** \sen-'yet(s)-\ *n* : RO-CHELLE SALT

Sei·gnette \se-n^yet\, **Pierre (1660–1719)**, French pharmacist. Seignette first prepared potassium sodium tartrates in 1672. Ten years later he introduced Seignette salt as a laxative.

sei·zure \'sē-zhər\ *n* **1** : a sudden attack (as of disease); *esp* : the physical manifestations (as convulsions, sensory disturbances, or loss of consciousness) resulting from abnormal electrical discharges in the brain (as in epilepsy) **2** : an abnormal electrical discharge in the brain

sel·a·chyl alcohol \'sel-ə-ˌkil-\ *n* : a liquid unsaturated alcohol $C_{20}H_{40}O_2$ found in the portion of fish oils (as shark-liver oil) that is not saponifiable

Sel·dane \'sel-ˌdān\ *n* : a preparation of terfenadine — formerly a U.S. registered trademark

se·lect \sə-'lekt\ *vi* : to cause a specified gene, trait, or organism to become more frequent or less frequent — usu. used with *for* or *against* ⟨animal breeders need to ∼ simultaneously for improved conformity to breed characteristics and against defective genes causing disease⟩

se·lec·tin \sə-'lek-tin\ *n* : any of a family of sugar-binding lectins that are found on the surface of cells (as endothelial cells and white blood cells) and that promote their adhesion to other cells and mediate their migration to sites of inflammation

se·lec·tion \sə-'lek-shən\ *n* : a natural or artificial process that results or tends to result in the survival and propagation of some individuals or organisms but not of others with the result that the inherited traits of the survivors are perpetuated — compare DARWINISM, NATURAL SELECTION

selection coefficient *n* : a measure of the disadvantage of a given gene or mutation that is usu. the frequency of individuals having the gene or mutation which fail to leave fertile offspring

se·lec·tion·ist \sə-'lek-sh(ə-)nəst\ *n* : a person who considers natural selection a fundamental factor in evolution

selection pressure *n* : the effect of selection on the relative frequency of one or more genes within a population

se·lec·tive \sə-'lek-tiv\ *adj* **1** : of, relating to, or characterized by selection : selecting or tending to select **2** : highly specific in activity or effect ⟨∼ pesticides⟩ ⟨∼ permeability of a plasma membrane⟩ — **se·lec·tive·ly** *adv*

selective estrogen receptor modulator *n* : any of a class of drugs (as raloxifene or tamoxifen) that bind with estrogen receptors and act as estrogen agonists in some tissues and estrogen antagonists in other tissues — abbr. *SERM*

selective reduction *n* : abortion of one or more but not all embryos in a pregnancy with multiple embryos — called also *selective termination*

selective serotonin reuptake inhibitor *n* : SSRI

selective termination *n* : SELECTIVE REDUCTION

se·lec·tiv·i·ty \sə-ˌlek-'tiv-ət-ē, ˌsē-\ *n, pl* **-ties** : the quality, state, or degree of being selective ⟨porous materials . . . fixed in both pore size and ∼ —Elizabeth Wilson⟩

se·leg·i·line \si-'lej-ə-ˌlēn\ *n* : the levorotatory form of the monoamine oxidase inhibitor deprenyl that is administered in the form of its hydrochloride $C_{13}H_{17}N \cdot HCl$ as an adjuvant to therapy using the combination of L-dopa and carbidopa in the treatment of Parkinson's disease and is sometimes used alone to treat endogenous depression or to treat dementia associated with Alzheimer's disease

sel·e·nif·er·ous \ˌsel-ə-'nif-(ə-)rəs\ *adj* : containing or yielding selenium ⟨∼ vegetation⟩

se·le·ni·ous acid \sə-ˌlē-nē-əs-\ *n* : a poisonous hygroscopic crystalline acid H_2SeO_3 that is a weaker acid than sulfurous acid and is an oxidizing agent yielding selenium as it is reduced

se·le·ni·um \sə-'lē-nē-əm\ *n* : a nonmetallic element that resembles sulfur and tellurium chemically, causes poisoning in range animals when ingested by eating some plants growing in soils in which it occurs in quantity, and occurs in allotropic forms of which a gray stable form varies in electrical con-

ductivity with the intensity of its illumination and is used in electronic devices — symbol *Se*; see ELEMENT table

selenium sulfide *n* : the disulfide SeS_2 of selenium usu. in the form of an orange powder that is used in preparations for treating dandruff and seborrheic dermatitis of the scalp

sel·e·no·cys·teine \ˌsel-ə-nō-'sis-tə-ˌēn\ *n* : a cysteine analog $C_3H_7NO_2Se$ in which one atom of sulfur has been replaced with one atom of selenium

se·len·odont \sə-'lē-nə-ˌdänt, sə-'len-ə-\ *adj* : of, relating to, characteristic of, or being molar teeth with crescentic ridges on the crown ⟨the ∼ teeth of sheep⟩

sel·e·no·me·thi·o·nine \-mə-'thī-ə-ˌnēn\ *n* : a selenium analog $C_5H_{11}NO_2Se$ of methionine in which sulfur is replaced by selenium and that is used as a diagnostic aid in scintigraphy esp. of the pancreas and as a dietary supplement

sel·e·no·sis \ˌsel-ə-'nō-səs\ *n* : poisoning of livestock by selenium due to ingestion of plants grown in seleniferous soils that is characterized in the acute phase by diffuse necrosis and hemorrhage resulting from capillary damage and in chronic poisoning by degenerative and fibrotic changes esp. of the liver and of the skin and its derivatives — called also *alkali disease;* see BLIND STAGGERS

self \'self\ *n, pl* **selves** \'selvz\ **1** : the union of elements (as body, emotions, thoughts, and sensations) that constitute the individuality and identity of a person **2** : material that is part of an individual organism ⟨ability of the immune system to distinguish ∼ from nonself⟩

self–abuse \ˌself-ə-'byüs\ *n* : MASTURBATION

self–ac·tu·al·ize *also Brit* **self–ac·tu·al·ise** \'self-'ak-ch(ə-w)ə-ˌlīz\ *vi* **-ized** *also Brit* **-ised; -iz·ing** *also Brit* **-is·ing** : to realize fully one's potential — **self–ac·tu·al·iza·tion** *also Brit* **self–ac·tu·al·isa·tion** \-ˌak-ch(ə-w)ə-lə-'zā-shən\ *n*

self–ad·min·i·ster \-əd-'mi-nə-stər\ *vt* : to administer (as a drug) to oneself ⟨∼ed an analgesic⟩ — **self–ad·min·i·stra·tion** \-ˌmin-ə-'strā-shən\ *n*

self–administered *adj* : administered by oneself ⟨∼ analgesia⟩

self–anal·y·sis \-ə-'nal-ə-səs\ *n, pl* **-y·ses** \-ˌsēz\ : a systematic attempt by an individual to understand his or her own personality without the aid of another person — **self–an·a·lyt·i·cal** \-ˌan-ə-'lit-i-kəl\ *or* **self–an·a·lyt·ic** \-ik\ *adj*

self–an·ti·gen \-'ant-i-jən\ *n* : any molecule or chemical group of an organism which acts as an antigen in inducing antibody formation in another organism but to which the healthy immune system of the parent organism is tolerant

self–as·sem·bly \-ə-'sem-blē\ *n, pl* **-blies** : the process by which a complex macromolecule (as collagen) or a supramolecular system (as a virus) spontaneously assembles itself from its components — **self–as·sem·ble** \-bəl\ *vi*

self–aware \-ə-'we(ə)r\ *adj* : characterized by self-awareness

self–aware·ness *n* : an awareness of one's own personality or individuality

self–care \-'ke(ə)r\ *n* : care for oneself : SELF-TREATMENT

self–con·cept \'self-'kän-ˌsept\ *n* : the mental image one has of oneself

self–de·struc·tion \-di-'strək-shən\ *n* : destruction of oneself; *esp* : SUICIDE

self–de·struc·tive \-'strək-tiv\ *adj* : acting or tending to harm or destroy oneself ⟨∼ behavior⟩; *also* : SUICIDAL — **self–de·struc·tive·ly** *adv* — **self–de·struc·tive·ness** *n*

self–dif·fer·en·ti·a·tion \-ˌdif-ə-ˌren-chē-'ā-shən\ *n* : differentiation of a structure or tissue due to factors existent in itself and essentially independent of other parts of the developing organism

self–di·ges·tion \ˌself-(ˌ)dī-'jes(h)-chən, -də-\ *n* : AUTOLYSIS

self–ex·am·i·na·tion \-ig-ˌzam-ə-'nā-shən\ *n* : examination of one's body esp. for evidence of disease ⟨regular ∼ for early detection of breast cancer⟩

self–fer·til·iza·tion \ˌself-ˌfərt-ᵊl-ə-'zā-shən\ *n* : fertilization

\ə\ abut \ᵊ\ kitten \ər\ further \a\ ash \ā\ ace \ä\ cot, cart \au̇\ out \ch\ chin \e\ bet \ē\ easy \g\ go \i\ hit \ī\ ice \j\ job \ŋ\ sing \ō\ go \ȯ\ law \ȯi\ boy \th\ thin \ṯẖ\ the \ü\ loot \u̇\ foot \y\ yet \zh\ vision   *See also* Pronunciation Symbols page

S
T

effected by union of ova with pollen or sperm from the same individual

self–fer·til·ized \'self-'fərt-ᵊl-ˌīzd\ *adj* : fertilized by one's own pollen or sperm

self–hyp·no·sis \ˌself-(h)ip-'nō-səs\ *n, pl* **-no·ses** \-ˌsēz\ : hypnosis of oneself : AUTOHYPNOSIS

self–im·age \-'im-ij\ *n* : one's conception of oneself or of one's role

self–in·duced \-in-'d(y)üst\ *adj* : induced by oneself ⟨∼ vomiting⟩

self–in·duc·tance \-in-'dək-tən(t)s\ *n* : inductance that induces an electromotive force in the same circuit as the one in which the current varies

self–in·flict·ed \-in-'flik-təd\ *adj* : inflicted by oneself ⟨a ∼ wound⟩

self–in·ject·able \-in-'jek-tə-bəl\ *adj* : suitable for self= injection ⟨a ∼ prescription drug⟩

self–in·jec·tion \-in-'jek-shən\ *n* : an act of injecting oneself with a drug or other substance

self·ish \'sel-fish\ *adj* : being an actively replicating repetitive sequence of nucleic acid that serves no known function ⟨∼ DNA⟩; *also* : being genetic material solely concerned with its own replication ⟨∼ genes⟩

self–lim·it·ed \-'lim-ət-əd\ *adj* : limited by one's or its own nature; *specif* : running a definite and limited course ⟨the disease is ∼, and the prognosis is good —*Science*⟩

self–lim·it·ing \-ət-iŋ\ *adj* : SELF-LIMITED ⟨a ∼ disease⟩

self–med·i·cate \-'med-ə-ˌkāt\ *vb* **-cat·ed; -cat·ing** *vt* : to treat by self-medication ⟨the patient had attempted to ∼ depression⟩ ∼ *vi* : to treat oneself by self-medication ⟨patients with dental pain often ∼ with analgesics⟩

self–med·i·ca·tion \-ˌmed-ə-'kā-shən\ *n* : medication of oneself esp. without the advice of a physician : SELF= TREATMENT ⟨∼ with nonprescription drugs⟩

self–mu·ti·la·tion \-ˌmyüt-ə-'lā-shən\ *n* : injury or disfigurement of oneself ⟨∼ associated with the Lesch-Nyhan syndrome⟩

self–pun·ish·ment \-'pən-ish-mənt\ *n* : punishment of oneself ⟨masochistic ∼⟩

self–re·ac·tive \-rē-'ak-tiv\ *adj* : capable of participating in an autoimmune response ⟨∼ T cells⟩

self–rec·og·ni·tion \-ˌrek-əg-'nish-ən\ *n* : the process by which the immune system of an organism distinguishes between the body's own chemicals, cells, and tissues and those of foreign organisms or agents — compare SELF= TOLERANCE

self–re·fer·ral \-ri-'fər-əl\ *n* : the referral of a patient to a specialized medical facility (as a medical imaging center) in which the referring physician has a financial interest — **self– re·fer** \-ri-'fər\ *vt* **-re·ferred; -re·fer·ring**

self–rep·li·cat·ing \-'rep-lə-ˌkāt-iŋ\ *adj* : reproducing itself autonomously ⟨DNA is a ∼ molecule⟩ — **self–rep·li·ca· tion** \-ˌrep-lə-'kā-shən\ *n*

self–stim·u·la·tion \'self-ˌstim-yə-'lā-shən\ *n* : stimulation of oneself as a result of one's own activity or behavior ⟨electrical ∼ of the brain in rats⟩; *esp* : MASTURBATION — **self– stim·u·la·to·ry** \'self-'stim-yə-lə-ˌtōr-ē, -ˌtȯr-\ *adj*

self–tan·ner \-'tan-ər\ *n* : a cosmetic product (as one containing dihydroxyacetone) that when applied to the skin reacts chemically with its surface layer to give the appearance of a tan

self–tol·er·ance \'self-'täl(-ə)-rən(t)s\ *n* : the physiological state that exists in a developing organism when its immune system has proceeded far enough in the process of self= recognition to lose the capacity to attack and destroy its own bodily constituents — called also *horror autotoxicus*

self–treat·ment \'self-'trēt-mənt\ *n* : medication of oneself or treatment of one's own disease without medical supervision or prescription

sel·la \'se-lə\ *n, pl* **sellas** *or* **sel·lae** \-lē\ : SELLA TURCICA

sel·lar \'sel-ər, -ˌär\ *adj* : of, relating to, or involving the sella turcica ⟨the ∼ region⟩

sella tur·ci·ca \-'tər-ki-kə, -si-\ *n, pl* **sellae tur·ci·cae** \-ki-ˌkī,

-si-ˌsē\ : a depression in the middle line of the upper surface of the sphenoid bone in which the pituitary gland is lodged

selves *pl of* SELF

SEM *abbr* scanning electron microscope; scanning electron microscopy

se·man·tic aphasia \si-ˌman-tik-\ : aphasia characterized by the loss of recognition of the meaning of words and phrases

se·man·tics \si-'mant-iks\ *n pl but sing or pl in constr* : the study of meanings: **a** : the historical and psychological study and the classification of changes in the signification of words or forms viewed as factors in linguistic development **b** (1) : SEMIOTIC (2) : a branch of semiotic dealing with the relations between signs and what they refer to and including theories of denotation, extension, naming, and truth

semeiology *var of* SEMIOLOGY

se·mei·ot·ic \ˌsem-ē-'ät-ik, ˌsē-mī-\ *adj* : of or relating to symptoms of disease

se·men \'sē-mən\ *n* : a viscid whitish fluid of the male reproductive tract consisting of spermatozoa suspended in secretions of accessory glands (as of the prostate and Cowper's glands)

semi·car·ba·zide \ˌsem-i-'kär-bə-ˌzīd\ *n* : a crystalline compound CH_5N_3O that is used chiefly as a reagent for aldehydes and ketones

semi·car·ba·zone \-'kär-bə-ˌzōn\ *n* : any of a class of usu. well-crystallized compounds having the general formula $RR'C{=}NNHCONH_2$ and formed by the action of semicarbazide on an aldehyde or ketone

semi·car·ti·lag·i·nous \-ˌkärt-ᵊl-'aj-ə-nəs\ *adj* : consisting partly of cartilaginous tissue

semi·cir·cu·lar canal \-ˌsər-kyə-lər-\ *n* : any of the loop= shaped tubular parts of the labyrinth of the ear that together constitute a sensory organ associated with the maintenance of bodily equilibrium, that consist of an inner membranous canal of the membranous labyrinth and a corresponding outer bony canal of the bony labyrinth, and that in all vertebrates above cyclostomes form a group of three in each ear usu. in planes nearly at right angles to each other — see SEMICIRCULAR DUCT

semicircular duct *n* : any of the three loop-shaped membranous inner tubular parts of the semicircular canals that are about one-fourth the diameter of the corresponding outer bony canals, that communicate at each end with the utricle, and that have near one end an expanded ampulla containing an area of sensory epithelium — called also *membranous semicircular canal*

semi·co·ma \-'kō-mə\ *n* : a semicomatose state from which a person can be aroused

semi·co·ma·tose \-'kō-mə-ˌtōs\ *adj* : lethargic and disoriented but not completely comatose ⟨a ∼ patient⟩

semi·con·duc·tor \-kən-'dək-tər\ *n* : any of a class of solids (as germanium or silicon) whose electrical conductivity is between that of a conductor and that of an insulator in being nearly as great as that of a metal at high temperatures and nearly absent at low temperatures

semi·con·scious \-'kän-chəs\ *adj* : incompletely conscious : imperfectly aware or responsive — **semi·con·scious·ness** *n*

semi·con·ser·va·tive \-kən-'sər-vət-iv\ *adj* : relating to or being genetic replication in which a double-stranded molecule of nucleic acid separates into two single strands each of which serves as a template for the formation of a complementary strand that together with the template forms a complete molecule — **semi·con·ser·va·tive·ly** *adv*

semi·dom·i·nant \-'däm-(ə-)nənt\ *adj* : producing an intermediate phenotype in the heterozygous condition ⟨a ∼ mutant gene⟩

semi·dry·ing \-'drī-iŋ\ *adj* : that dries imperfectly or slowly — used of some oils (as rapeseed oil)

semi·flu·id \-'flü-əd\ *adj* : having the qualities of both a fluid and a solid : VISCOUS — **semifluid** *n*

semi·le·thal \-'lē-thəl\ *n* : a mutation that in the homozygous condition produces more than 50 percent mortality but not complete mortality — **semilethal** *adj*

semi·lu·nar \-'lü-nər\ *adj* : shaped like a crescent

semilunar bone *n* : LUNATE BONE

semilunar cartilage *n* : MENISCUS 2a

semilunar cusp *n* : any of the crescentic cusps making up the semilunar valves

semilunares — see LINEA SEMILUNARIS, PLICA SEMILUNARIS

semilunar fibrocartilage *n* : MENISCUS 2a

semilunar fold *n* : a small fold of membrane in the inner corner of the eye that is a vestige of a nictitating membrane

semilunar ganglion *n* : TRIGEMINAL GANGLION

semilunaris — see HIATUS SEMILUNARIS, LINEA SEMILUNARIS, PLICA SEMILUNARIS

semilunar line *n* : LINEA SEMILUNARIS

semilunar lobule *n* : either of a pair of crescent-shaped lobules situated one on each side in the posterior and ventral part of the cerebellum

semilunar notch *n* : TROCHLEAR NOTCH

semilunar valve *n* **1** : either of two valves of which one is situated at the opening between the heart and the aorta and the other at the opening between the heart and the pulmonary artery, which prevent regurgitation of blood into the ventricles, and each of which is made up of three crescent-shaped cusps that are forced apart by pressure in the ventricles exerted during systole and are pushed together by pressure in the arteries exerted during diastole **2** : SEMILUNAR CUSP

semi·mem·bra·no·sus \ˌsem-ē-ˌmem-brə-'nō-səs\ *n, pl* **-no·si** \-ˌsī\ : a large muscle of the inner part and back of the thigh that arises by a thick tendon from the back part of the tuberosity of the ischium, is inserted into the medial condyle of the tibia, and acts to flex the leg and rotate it medially and to extend the thigh

sem·i·nal \'sem-ən-ᵊl\ *adj* : of, relating to, or consisting of seed or semen ⟨~ discharge⟩

seminal duct *n* : a tube or passage serving esp. or exclusively as an efferent duct of the testis and in humans being made up of the tubules of the epididymis, the vas deferens, and the ejaculatory duct

seminal fluid *n* **1** : SEMEN **2** : the part of the semen that is produced by various accessory glands (as the prostate gland and seminal vesicles) : semen excepting the spermatozoa

seminal vesicle *n* : either of a pair of glandular pouches that lie one on either side of the male reproductive tract and that in human males secrete a sugar- and protein-containing fluid into the ejaculatory duct

sem·i·nate \'sem-ə-ˌnāt\ *vt* **-nat·ed; -nat·ing** : INSEMINATE — **sem·i·na·tion** \ˌsem-ə-'nā-shən\ *n*

sem·i·nif·er·ous \ˌsem-ə-'nif-(ə-)rəs\ *adj* : producing or bearing seed or semen ⟨the ~ epithelium of the testis⟩

seminiferous tubule *n* : any of the coiled threadlike tubules that make up the bulk of the testis and are lined with a layer of epithelial cells from which the spermatozoa are produced

sem·i·no·ma \ˌsem-i-'nō-mə\ *n, pl* **-mas** *also* **-ma·ta** \-mət-ə\ : a germinoma of the testis

se·mi·ol·o·gy *or* **se·mei·ol·o·gy** \ˌsem-ē-'äl-ə-jē, ˌsē-mē-\ *n, pl* **-gies** : the study of signs: as **a** : SYMPTOMATOLOGY 2 **b** : SEMIOTIC

se·mi·ot·ic \-'ät-ik\ *or* **se·mi·ot·ics** \-iks\ *n, pl* **semiotics** : a general philosophical theory of signs and symbols that deals esp. with their function in both artificially constructed and natural languages and comprises syntactics, semantics, and pragmatics — **semiotic** *adj*

semi·per·me·able \ˌsem-i-'pər-mē-ə-bəl, ˌsem-ˌī-\ *adj* : partially but not freely or wholly permeable; *specif* : permeable to some usu. small molecules but not to other usu. larger particles ⟨a ~ membrane⟩ — **semi·per·me·abil·i·ty** \-ˌpər-mē-ə-'bil-ət-ē\ *n, pl* **-ties**

semi·pri·vate \-'prī-vət\ *adj* : of, receiving, or associated with hospital service giving a patient more privileges than a ward patient but fewer than a private patient ⟨a ~ room⟩

semi·quan·ti·ta·tive \-'kwän(t)-ə-ˌtāt-iv\ *adj* : constituting or involving less than quantitative precision ⟨~ analysis⟩ — **semi·quan·ti·ta·tive·ly** *adv*

semi·sol·id \-'säl-əd\ *adj* : having the qualities of both a solid and a liquid : highly viscous ⟨~ waste⟩

semi·spi·na·lis \-ˌspī-'nā-ləs\ *n, pl* **-les** \-ˌlēz\ : any of three muscles of the cervical and thoracic parts of the spinal column that arise from transverse processes of the vertebrae and pass to spinous processes higher up and that help to form a layer underneath the sacrospinalis muscle: **a** : SEMISPINALIS THORACIS **b** : SEMISPINALIS CERVICIS **c** : SEMISPINALIS CAPITIS

semispinalis cap·i·tis \-'kap-ət-əs\ *n* : a deep longitudinal muscle of the back that arises esp. from the transverse processes of the upper six or seven thoracic and the seventh cervical vertebrae, is inserted on the outer surface of the occipital bone between two ridges behind the foramen magnum, and acts to extend and rotate the head — called also *complexus*

semispinalis cer·vi·cis \-'sər-və-səs\ *n* : a deep longitudinal muscle of the back that arises from the transverse processes of the upper five or six thoracic vertebrae, is inserted into the cervical spinous processes from the axis to the fifth cervical vertebra, and with the semispinalis thoracis acts to extend the spinal column and rotate it toward the opposite side

semispinalis tho·ra·cis \-thə-'rā-səs\ *n* : a deep longitudinal muscle of the back that arises from the transverse processes of the lower five thoracic vertebrae, is inserted into the spinous processes of the upper four thoracic and lower two cervical vertebrae, and with the semispinalis cervicis acts to extend the spinal column and rotate it toward the opposite side

semi·syn·thet·ic \-sin-'thet-ik\ *adj* **1** : produced by chemical alteration of a natural starting material ⟨~ penicillins⟩ **2** : containing both chemically identified and complex natural ingredients ⟨a ~ diet⟩ — **semi·syn·thet·i·cal·ly** \-i-k(ə-)lē\ *adv*

sem·i·ten·di·no·sus \ˌsem-ē-ˌten-də-'nō-səs\ *n, pl* **-no·si** \-ˌsī\ : a fusiform muscle of the posterior and inner part of the thigh that arises from the ischial tuberosity along with the biceps femoris, that is inserted by a long round tendon which forms part of the inner hamstring into the inner surface of the upper part of the shaft of the tibia, and that acts to flex the leg and rotate it medially and to extend the thigh

Sem·li·ki Forest virus \'sem-lē-kē-'fôr-əst-\ *n* : a togavirus of the genus *Alphavirus* that was isolated from mosquitoes in a Ugandan forest and is capable of infecting humans and laboratory animals

Sen·dai virus \'sen-ˌdī-\ *n* : a parainfluenza virus (species *Sendai virus* of the genus *Respirovirus*) first reported from Japan that infects swine, mice, and humans

sen·e·ca snakeroot \'sen-i-kə-\ *n* : a No. American plant of the genus *Polygala* (*P. senega*) whose dried root was formerly used as an expectorant

se·ne·cio \si-'nē-sh(ē-)ō\ *n* **1** *cap* : a genus of widely distributed plants (family Compositae) including some containing various alkaloids which are poisonous to livestock **2** *pl* **-cios** : any plant of the genus *Senecio*

se·ne·ci·o·sis \si-ˌnē-sē-'ō-səs\ *n, pl* **-o·ses** \-ˌsēz\ : a frequently fatal intoxication esp. of livestock feeding on plants of the genus *Senecio* that is marked by intense acute or chronic necrosis and cirrhosis of the liver

sen·e·ga \'sen-i-gə\ *n* : the dried root of seneca snakeroot that contains an irritating saponin and was formerly used as an expectorant

senega root *n* **1** : SENECA SNAKEROOT **2** : SENEGA

senega snakeroot *n* : SENECA SNAKEROOT

se·nes·cence \si-'nes-ᵊn(t)s\ *n* : the state of being old : the process of becoming old

se·nes·cent \si-'nes-ᵊnt\ *adj* : relating to, characterized by, or associated with senescence ⟨~ persons⟩ ⟨~ arthritis⟩

se·nile \'sēn-ˌīl *also* 'sen-\ *adj* **1** : of, relating to, exhibiting, or characteristic of old age ⟨~ weakness⟩; *esp* : exhibiting a

---

S

T

loss of mental faculties associated with old age   **2** : being a cell that cannot undergo mitosis and is in the stage of declining functional capacities prior to the time of death ⟨∼ red blood cells⟩

senile cataract *n* : a cataract of a type that occurs in the aged and is characterized by an initial opacity in the lens, subsequent swelling of the lens, and final shrinkage with complete loss of transparency

senile dementia *n* : a mental disorder of old age esp. of the degenerative type associated with Alzheimer's disease — called also *senile psychosis*

senile gangrene *n* : gangrene due to lack of blood supply resulting from sclerosis of blood vessels

senile plaque *n* : PLAQUE 1d

senile psychosis *n* : SENILE DEMENTIA

senilis — see ARCUS SENILIS, LENTIGO SENILIS, MORBUS COXAE SENILIS

se·nil·i·ty \si-'nil-ət-ē *also* se-\ *n, pl* **-ties** : the quality or state of being senile; *specif* : the physical and mental infirmity of old age

se·ni·um \'sē-nē-əm\ *n* : the final period in the normal life span ⟨from birth to the ∼⟩

sen·na \'sen-ə\ *n* **1** : any plant of the genus *Cassia*; *esp* : one used medicinally   **2** : the dried leaflets or pods of various sennas (esp. *Cassia acutifolia* and *C. angustifolia*) used as a purgative

sen·no·side \'sen-ə-ˌsīd\ *n* : either of two cathartic glucosides obtained from senna

sen·sa·tion \sen-'sā-shən, sən-\ *n* **1 a** : a mental process (as seeing, hearing, or smelling) due to immediate bodily stimulation often as distinguished from awareness of the process — compare PERCEPTION   **b** : awareness (as of heat or pain) due to stimulation of a sense organ   **c** : a state of consciousness of a kind usu. due to physical objects or internal bodily changes ⟨a burning ∼ in his chest⟩   **2** : something (as a physical object, sense-datum, pain, or afterimage) that causes or is the object of sensation

¹sense \'sen(t)s\ *n* **1 a** : the faculty of perceiving by means of sense organs   **b** : a specialized animal function or mechanism (as sight, hearing, smell, taste, or touch) basically involving a stimulus and a sense organ   **c** : the sensory mechanisms constituting a unit distinct from other functions (as movement or thought)   **2** : a particular sensation or kind or quality of sensation ⟨a good ∼ of balance⟩

²sense *vt* **sensed; sens·ing** : to perceive by the senses

sense–da·tum \-ˌdāt-əm, -ˌdat-, -ˌdät-\ *n, pl* **sense–da·ta** \-ə\ : the immediate private perceived object of sensation as distinguished from the objective material object itself

sense impression *n* : a psychic and physiological effect resulting directly from the excitation of a sense organ : SENSATION

sense organ *n* : a bodily structure that receives a stimulus (as heat or sound waves) and is affected in such a manner as to initiate a wave of excitation in associated sensory nerve fibers which convey specific impulses to the central nervous system where they are interpreted as corresponding sensations : RECEPTOR

sen·si·bil·i·ty \ˌsen(t)-sə-'bil-ət-ē\ *n, pl* **-ties** **1** : ability to receive sensations ⟨∼ to pain⟩   **2** : awareness of and responsiveness toward something (as emotion in another)

sen·si·ble \'sen(t)-sə-bəl\ *adj* : perceptible to the senses or to reason or understanding ⟨felt a ∼ chill⟩   **2** : capable of receiving sensory impressions ⟨∼ to pain⟩

sen·si·tive \'sen(t)-sət-iv, 'sen(t)-stiv\ *adj* **1** : SENSORY 2 ⟨∼ nerves⟩   **2 a** : receptive to sense impressions   **b** : capable of being stimulated or excited by external agents (as light, gravity, or contact) ⟨a photographic emulsion ∼ to red light⟩ ⟨∼ protoplasm⟩   **3** : highly responsive or susceptible: as   **a** : easily hurt or damaged ⟨∼ skin⟩; *esp* : easily hurt emotionally   **b** : excessively or abnormally susceptible : HYPERSENSITIVE ⟨∼ to egg protein⟩   **c** : capable of indicating minute differences ⟨∼ scales⟩   **d** : readily affected or changed by various agents (as light or mechanical shock) ⟨a ∼ colloid⟩ — **sen·si·tive·ness** *n*

sen·si·tiv·i·ty \ˌsen(t)-sə-'tiv-ət-ē\ *n, pl* **-ties** : the quality or state of being sensitive: as   **a** : the capacity of an organism or sense organ to respond to stimulation : IRRITABILITY   **b** : the quality or state of being hypersensitive

sensitivity training *n* : training in a small interacting group that is designed to increase each individual's awareness of his or her own feelings and the feelings of others and to enhance interpersonal relations through the exploration of the behavior, needs, and responses of the individuals making up the group

sen·si·ti·za·tion *also Brit* **sen·si·ti·sa·tion** \ˌsen(t)-sət-ə-'zā-shən, ˌsen(t)-stə-'zā-\ *n* **1** : the action or process of making sensitive or hypersensitive ⟨allergic ∼ of the skin⟩   **2** : the process of becoming sensitive or hypersensitive (as to an antigen); *also* : the resulting state   **3** : a form of nonassociative learning characterized by an increase in responsiveness upon repeated exposure to a stimulus — compare HABITUATION 3

sen·si·tize *also Brit* **sen·si·tise** \'sen(t)-sə-ˌtīz\ *vt* **-tized** *also Brit* **-tised; -tiz·ing** *also Brit* **-tis·ing** : to make sensitive or hypersensitive ⟨the patient was *sensitized* to the drug⟩

sen·si·tiz·er *also Brit* **sen·si·tis·er** \-ər\ *n* : one that sensitizes: as   **a** : AMBOCEPTOR   **b** : a substance that sensitizes the skin on first contact so that subsequent contact causes inflammation

sen·sor \'sen-ˌsȯ(ə)r, 'sen(t)-sər\ *n* : a device that responds to a physical stimulus (as heat, light, sound, pressure, magnetism, or a particular motion) and transmits a resulting impulse (as for measurement or operating a control); *also* : SENSE ORGAN

sen·so·ri·al \sen-'sōr-ē-əl, -'sȯr-\ *adj* : SENSORY

sen·so·ri·mo·tor \ˌsen(t)s-(ə-)rē-'mōt-ər\ *adj* : of, relating to, or functioning in both sensory and motor aspects of bodily activity ⟨∼ disturbances⟩ ⟨∼ skills⟩

sen·so·ri·neu·ral \-'n(y)ùr-əl\ *adj* : of, relating to, or involving the aspects of sense perception mediated by nerves ⟨∼ hearing loss⟩

sen·so·ri·um \sen-'sōr-ē-əm, -'sȯr-\ *n, pl* **-ri·ums** *or* **-ria** \-ē-ə\ **1** : the parts of the brain or the mind concerned with the reception and interpretation of sensory stimuli; *broadly* : the entire sensory apparatus   **2 a** : ability of the brain to receive and interpret sensory stimuli ⟨decreasing ∼⟩   **b** : the state of consciousness judged in terms of this ability ⟨a clouded ∼⟩ ⟨the ∼ remained clear⟩

sen·so·ry \'sen(t)s-(ə-)rē\ *adj* **1** : of or relating to sensation or the senses ⟨∼ stimulation⟩ ⟨∼ data⟩   **2** : conveying nerve impulses from the sense organs to the nerve centers : AFFERENT ⟨∼ nerve fibers⟩

sensory aphasia *n* : inability to understand spoken, written, or tactile speech symbols that results from damage (as by a brain lesion) to an area of the brain (as Wernicke's area) concerned with language — called also *receptive aphasia, Wernicke's aphasia*

sensory area *n* : an area of the cerebral cortex that receives afferent nerve fibers from lower sensory or motor areas

sensory cell *n* **1** : a peripheral nerve cell (as an olfactory cell) located at a sensory receiving surface and being the primary receptor of a sensory impulse   **2** : a nerve cell (as a spinal ganglion cell) transmitting sensory impulses

sensory neuron *n* : a neuron that transmits nerve impulses from a sense organ towards the central nervous system — compare INTERNEURON, MOTOR NEURON

sensory root *n* : a nerve root containing only sensory fibers; *specif* : DORSAL ROOT — compare MOTOR ROOT

sen·su·al \'sench-(ə-)wəl, 'sen-shəl\ *adj* **1** : SENSORY 1   **2** : relating to or consisting in the gratification of the senses or the indulgence of appetite   **3** : devoted to or preoccupied with the senses or appetites

sen·su·al·ism \'sench-(ə-)wə-ˌliz-əm, 'sen-shə-ˌliz-\ *n* : persistent or excessive pursuit of sensual pleasures and interests — **sen·su·al·ist** \-ləst\ *n*

sen·su·al·i·ty \ˌsen-chə-'wal-ət-ē\ *n, pl* **-ities** : the quality or state of being sensual

sen·tient \'sen-ch(ē-)ənt, 'sent-ē-ənt\ *adj* : responsive to or conscious of sense impressions — **sen·tient·ly** *adv*

sen·ti·ment \'sent-ə-mənt\ *n* **1** : an attitude, thought, or judgment colored or prompted by feeling or emotion **2** : EMOTION 2, FEELING 2

sen·ti·nel \'sent-ᵊn-əl\ *adj* : being an individual or part of a population potentially susceptible to an infection or infestation that is being monitored for the appearance or recurrence of the causative pathogen or parasite

sentinel node *n* : the first lymph node to receive lymphatic drainage from the site of a primary tumor ⟨studies concluded that *sentinel node* biopsy can predict whether axillary node metastasis is present —Lecia M. Apantaku⟩ ⟨the use of *sentinel nodes* for pathologic staging of bladder cancer —Anne Scheck⟩ — called also *sentinel lymph node*

sep·a·rate \'sep-(ə-)ˌrāt\ *vb* **-rat·ed; -rat·ing** *vt* **1** : to isolate from a mixture : EXTRACT **2** : DISLOCATE ⟨*separated* his right shoulder⟩ ∼ *vi* : to become isolated from a mixture

sep·a·ra·tion \ˌsep-ə-'rā-shən\ *n* **1** : the process of isolating or extracting from or of becoming isolated from a mixture; *also* : the resulting state **2** : DISLOCATION — see SHOULDER SEPARATION

separation anxiety *n* : a form of anxiety that is caused by separation from a significant nurturant figure and typically a parent or from familiar surroundings and that has an onset during childhood or sometimes adolescence

sep·a·ra·tor \'sep-(ə-)ˌrāt-ər\ *n* : one that separates: as **a** : a device for separating liquids of different specific gravities (as cream from milk) or liquids from solids **b** : a dental appliance for separating adjoining teeth to give access to their surfaces

se·pia \'sē-pē-ə\ *n* **1** *cap* : a genus (the type of the family Sepiidae) of oval-bodied cephalopods that comprise the cuttlefishes and have a saclike organ containing a dark fluid and an internal shell mostly of calcium carbonate which has been used as an antacid and in tooth and polishing powders **2** : the inky secretion of a cuttlefish or a brown pigment from it

sep·sis \'sep-səs\ *n, pl* **sep·ses** \'sep-ˌsēz\ : a systemic response typically to a serious usu. localized infection (as of the abdomen or lungs) esp. of bacterial origin that is usu. marked by abnormal body temperature and white blood cell count, tachycardia, and tachypnea; *specif* : systemic inflammatory response syndrome induced by a documented infection — see MULTIPLE ORGAN DYSFUNCTION SYNDROME, SEPTIC SHOCK

septa *pl of* SEPTUM

sep·tal \'sep-tᵊl\ *adj* : of or relating to a septum ⟨∼ defects⟩

septal cartilage *n* : the cartilage of the nasal septum

septal cell *n* : a small macrophage characteristic of the lung

septa pellucida *pl of* SEPTUM PELLUCIDUM

sep·tate \'sep-ˌtāt\ *adj* : divided by or having a septum

sep·ta·tion \sep-'tā-shən\ *n* **1** : division into parts by a septum : the condition of being septate **2** : SEPTUM

septa transversa *pl of* SEPTUM TRANSVERSUM

sep·tec·to·my \sep-'tek-tə-mē\ *n, pl* **-mies** : surgical excision of a septum

septi — see DEPRESSOR SEPTI

sep·tic \'sep-tik\ *adj* **1** : PUTREFACTIVE **2** : relating to, involving, caused by, or affected with sepsis ⟨∼ complications⟩ ⟨∼ arthritis⟩ ⟨∼ patients⟩

septic abortion *n* : spontaneous or induced abortion associated with bacterial infection (as by E. coli, beta-hemolytic streptococci, or *Clostridium perfringens*)

sep·ti·ce·mia *or chiefly Brit* **sep·ti·cae·mia** \ˌsep-tə-'sē-mē-ə\ *n* : invasion of the bloodstream by virulent microorganisms (as bacteria, viruses, or fungi) from a focus of infection that is accompanied by acute systemic illness — called also *blood poisoning;* see PYEMIA; compare SEPSIS — **sep·ti·ce·mic** *or chiefly Brit* **sep·ti·cae·mic** \-'sē-mik\ *adj*

sep·ti·co·py·emia *or Brit* **sep·ti·co·py·ae·mia** \ˌsep-ti-(ˌ)kō-pī-'ē-mē-ə\ *n* : PYEMIA — **sep·ti·co·py·emic** *or Brit* **sep·ti·co·py·ae·mic** \-'ē-mik\ *adj*

septic shock *n* : a life-threatening severe form of sepsis that usu. results from the presence of bacteria and their toxins in the bloodstream and is characterized esp. by persistent hy-

potension with reduced blood flow to organs and tissues and often organ dysfunction

septic sore throat *n* : STREP THROAT

sep·to·mar·gin·al \ˌsep-tō-'märj-ən-ᵊl, -'märj-nəl\ *adj* : of or relating to the margin of a septum

sep·to·na·sal \-'nā-zəl\ *adj* : of, relating to, or situated in the region of the nasal septum

sep·to·plas·ty \'sep-tə-ˌplas-tē\ *n, pl* **-ties** : surgical repair of the nasal septum

sep·tos·to·my \sep-'täs-tə-mē\ *n, pl* **-mies** : the surgical creation of an opening through the interatrial septum

Sep·tra \'sep-trə\ *trademark* — used for a preparation of sulfamethoxazole and trimethoprim

sep·tum \'sep-təm\ *n, pl* **sep·ta** \-tə\ : a dividing wall or membrane esp. between bodily spaces or masses of soft tissue: as **a** : NASAL SEPTUM **b** : CRURAL SEPTUM

septum pel·lu·ci·dum \-pə-'lü-sə-dəm\ *n, pl* **septa pel·lu·ci·da** \-də\ : the thin double partition extending vertically from the lower surface of the corpus callosum to the fornix and neighboring parts, separating the lateral ventricles of the brain, and enclosing the fifth ventricle

septum trans·ver·sum \-tranz-'vər-səm\ *n, pl* **septa trans·ver·sa** \-sə\ : the diaphragm or the embryonic structure from which it in part develops

sep·tup·let \sep-'təp-lət, -'t(y)üp-lət *also* 'sep-təp-\ *n* **1** : one of seven offspring born at one birth **2 septuplets** *pl* : a group of seven such offspring

se·quel \'sē-kwəl *also* -ˌkwel\ *n* : SEQUELA ⟨gangrene is . . . a ∼ of wounds —Robert Chawner⟩

se·quela \si-'kwe-lə\ *n, pl* **se·quel·ae** \-(ˌ)lē\ : a negative aftereffect ⟨prevention of the post-phlebitic *sequelae* —A. G. Sharf⟩ ⟨the emotional *sequelae* of early parental death —Sheila Ballantyne⟩

¹se·quence \'sē-kwən(t)s, -ˌkwen(t)s\ *n* **1** : a continuous or connected series; *specif* : the exact order of bases in a nucleic acid or of amino acids in a protein **2** : a consequence, result, or subsequent development (as of a disease)

²sequence *vt* **se·quenced; se·quenc·ing** : to determine the sequence of chemical constituents (as amino acid residues in a protein or bases in a strand of DNA) in ⟨*sequenced* the DNA of the entire genome of an organism⟩

se·quenc·er \'sē-kwən-sər, -ˌkwen(t)-sər\ *n* : one that sequences; *esp* : a device for determining the order of occurrence of amino acids in a protein or of bases in a nucleic acid

¹se·quen·tial \si-'kwen-chəl\ *adj* **1** : occurring as a sequela of disease or injury **2** : of, relating to, forming, or taken in a sequence ⟨∼ pills for contraception⟩

²sequential *n* : a birth control pill of which those taken during approximately the first three weeks contain only estrogen and those taken during the rest of the cycle contain both estrogen and progestogen

¹se·ques·ter \si-'kwes-tər\ *vt* : to hold (as a metallic ion) in solution esp. for the purpose of suppressing undesired chemical or biological activity

²sequester *n* : SEQUESTRUM

se·ques·trant \-trənt\ *n* : a sequestering agent (as citric acid)

se·ques·tra·tion \ˌsēk-wəs-'trā-shən, ˌsek-, si-ˌkwes-\ *n* **1** : the formation of a sequestrum **2** : the process of sequestering or result of being sequestered

se·ques·trec·to·my \ˌsē-kwe-'strek-tə-mē\ *n, pl* **-mies** : the surgical removal of a sequestrum

se·ques·trum \si-'kwes-trəm\ *n, pl* **-trums** *also* **-tra** \-trə\ : a fragment of dead bone detached from adjoining sound bone

Ser *abbr* serine; seryl

sera *pl of* SERUM

ser·e·noa \ˌser-ə-'nō-ə, si-'rē-nō-ə\ *n* : SAW PALMETTO 2

se·ri·al·o·graph \ˌsir-ē-'al-ə-ˌgraf\ *or* **se·rio·graph** \'sir-ē-ə-ˌ\ *n* : a device for making a number of radiographs in rapid sequence

---

\ə\ abut \ᵊ\ kitten \ər\ further \a\ ash \ā\ ace \ä\ cot, cart \au̇\ out \ch\ chin \e\ bet \ē\ easy \g\ go \i\ hit \ī\ ice \j\ job \ŋ\ sing \ō\ go \ȯ\ law \ȯi\ boy \th\ thin \t̲h̲\ the \ü\ loot \u̇\ foot \y\ yet \zh\ vision   *See also* Pronunciation Symbols page

S
T

se·ri·al·og·ra·phy \,sir-ē-ə-'läg-rə-fē\ n, pl **-phies** : SERIAL RADIOGRAPHY

se·ri·al radiography \'sir-ē-əl-\ n : the technique of making radiographs in rapid sequence for the study of high-speed phenomena (as the flow of blood through an artery)

serial section n : any of a series of sections cut in sequence by a microtome from a prepared specimen (as of tissue) — **serially sectioned** adj — **serial sectioning** n

se·ries \'si(ə)r-(,)ēz\ n, pl **series** **1** : a number of things or events of the same class coming one after another in spatial or temporal succession ⟨described a new ~ of cases⟩ **2** : a group of specimens or types progressively differing from each other in some morphological or physiological attribute ⟨a ~ of antitoxins⟩ **3** : a group of chemical compounds related in composition and structure

ser·ine \'se(ə)r-,ēn\ n : a nonessential amino acid $C_3H_7NO_3$ that occurs esp. as a structural part of many proteins and phosphatidylethanolamines and is a precursor of glycine — abbr. *Ser*

seriograph var of SERIALOGRAPH

se·ri·ous \'sir-ē-əs\ adj : having important or dangerous possible consequences ⟨a ~ injury⟩

SERM abbr selective estrogen receptor modulator

se·ro·con·ver·sion \,sir-ō-kən-'vər-zhən, ,ser-ō-\ n : the production of antibodies in response to an antigen — **se·ro·con·vert** \-'vərt\ vi

se·ro·con·vert·er \-kən-'vərt-ər\ n : one that is undergoing or has undergone seroconversion

se·ro·di·ag·no·sis \'sir-ō-,dī-ig-'nō-səs\ n, pl **-no·ses** \-,sēz\ : diagnosis by the use of serum (as in the Wassermann test) — **se·ro·di·ag·nos·tic** \-'näs-tik\ adj

se·ro·ep·i·de·mi·o·log·ic \-,ep-ə-,dē-mē-ə-'läj-ik\ or **se·ro·ep·i·de·mi·o·log·i·cal** \-i-kəl\ adj : of, relating to, or being epidemiological investigations involving the identification of antibodies to specific antigens in populations of individuals — **se·ro·ep·i·de·mi·ol·o·gy** \-mē-'äl-ə-jē\ n, pl **-gies**

se·ro·fi·brin·ous \-'fī-brin-əs\ adj : composed of or characterized by serum and fibrin ⟨a ~ exudate⟩ ⟨~ pleurisy⟩

se·ro·group \'sir-ō-,grüp\ n : a group of serotypes having one or more antigens in common

se·ro·log·i·cal \,sir-ə-'läj-i-kəl\ or **se·ro·log·ic** \-ik\ adj : of, relating to, or employing the methods of serology ⟨a ~ test⟩ — **se·ro·log·i·cal·ly** \-i-k(ə-)lē\ adv

se·rol·o·gist \si-'räl-ə-jəst\ n : a specialist in serology

se·rol·o·gy \si-'räl-ə-jē\ n, pl **-gies** : a medical science dealing with blood sera and esp. their immunological reactions and properties

se·ro·mu·coid \,sir-ō-'myü-,kȯid, ,ser-ō-\ n : a glycoprotein of serum that is not coagulated by heat

se·ro·mu·cous \-'myü-kəs\ adj : containing or consisting of a mixture of serum and mucus

se·ro·mus·cu·lar \-'məs-kyə-lər\ adj : relating to or consisting of the serous and muscular layer of an organ

se·ro·neg·a·tive \-'neg-ə-tiv\ adj : having or being a negative serum reaction esp. in a test for the presence of an antibody ⟨early ~ syphilis⟩ ⟨a ~ patient⟩

se·ro·neg·a·tiv·i·ty \-,neg-ə-'tiv-ət-ē\ n, pl **-ties** : the state of being seronegative often used as a criterion of the elimination of an infection

se·ro·pos·i·tive \-'päz-ət-iv, -'päz-tiv\ adj : having or being a positive serum reaction esp. in a test for the presence of an antibody ⟨a ~ donor⟩

se·ro·pos·i·tiv·i·ty \-,päz-ə-'tiv-ət-ē\ n, pl **-ties** : the state of being seropositive

se·ro·prev·a·lence \-'prev-(ə-)lən(t)s\ n : the frequency of individuals in a population that have a particular element (as antibodies to HIV) in their blood serum

se·ro·pu·ru·lent \,sir-ō-'pyur-(y)ə-lənt, ,ser-\ adj : consisting of a mixture of serum and pus ⟨a ~ exudate⟩

se·ro·pus \'sir-ō-,pəs\ n : a seropurulent exudate

se·ro·re·ac·tion \,sir-ō-rē-'ak-shən, ,ser-\ n : a serological reaction ⟨a positive ~ for syphilis⟩

se·ro·re·ac·tiv·i·ty \-(,)rē-,ak-'tiv-ət-ē\ n, pl **-ties** : reactivity

of blood serum ⟨~ to the human papillomavirus⟩ — **se·ro·re·ac·tive** \-rē-'ak-tiv\ adj

se·ro·re·sis·tance \-ri-'zis-tən(t)s\ n : failure to attain seronegativity after intensive or prolonged treatment that results in subsidence of clinical symptoms — used chiefly of advanced or congenital syphilis — **se·ro·re·sis·tant** \-tənt\ adj

se·ro·sa \sə-'rō-zə\ n, pl **-sas** also **-sae** \-zē\ : a usu. enclosing serous membrane ⟨the peritoneal ~⟩

se·ro·sal \-zəl\ adj : of, relating to, or consisting of serosa ⟨the ~ surface of the bowel⟩ ⟨a ~ cyst on the ovary⟩

se·ro·san·guin·e·ous \,sir-ō-san-'gwin-ē-əs, ,ser-ō-, -saŋ-\ or **se·ro·san·guin·ous** \-'saŋ-gwə-nəs\ adj : containing or consisting of both blood and serous fluid ⟨a ~ discharge⟩

se·ro·si·tis \,sir-ō-'sīt-əs, ,ser-\ n, pl **-tis·es** : inflammation of one or more serous membranes ⟨peritoneal ~⟩

se·ro·sta·tus \'sir-ə-,stāt-əs, 'ser-, -,stat-\ n : status with respect to being seropositive or seronegative for a particular antibody ⟨HIV ~⟩

se·ro·sur·vey \-,sər-(,)vā\ n : a test of blood serum from a group of individuals to determine seroprevalence (as of antibodies to HIV)

se·ro·ther·a·py \,sir-ō-'ther-ə-pē, ,ser-\ n, pl **-pies** : the treatment of a disease with specific immune serum — called also *serum therapy*

serotina — see DECIDUA SEROTINA

se·ro·to·ner·gic \,sir-ə-tə-'nər-jik\ or **se·ro·to·nin·er·gic** \,sir-ə-,tō-nə-'nər-jik\ adj : liberating, activated by, or involving serotonin in the transmission of nerve impulses

se·ro·to·nin \,sir-ə-'tō-nən, ,ser-\ n : a phenolic amine neurotransmitter $C_{10}H_{12}N_2O$ that is a powerful vasoconstrictor and is found esp. in the brain, blood serum, and gastric mucous membrane of mammals — called also *5-HT, 5-hydroxytryptamine*

¹se·ro·type \'sir-ə-,tīp, 'ser-\ n **1** : a group of intimately related microorganisms distinguished by a common set of antigens **2** : the set of antigens characteristic of a serotype — **se·ro·typ·ic** \,sir-ə-'tip-ik\ adj — **se·ro·typ·i·cal·ly** \-i-k(ə-)lē\ adv

²serotype vt **-typed; -typ·ing** : to determine the serotype of ⟨~ streptococci⟩ ⟨*serotyped* isolates from 100 patients⟩

se·rous \'sir-əs\ adj : of, relating to, producing, or resembling serum; esp : having a thin watery constitution ⟨a ~ exudate⟩

serous cavity n : a cavity (as the peritoneal cavity, pleural cavity, or pericardial cavity) that is lined with a serous membrane

serous cell n : a cell (as of the parotid gland) that secretes a serous fluid

serous gland n : a gland secreting a serous fluid

serous membrane n : any of various thin membranes (as the peritoneum, pericardium, or pleurae) that consist of a single layer of thin flat mesothelial cells resting on a connective-tissue stroma, secrete a serous fluid, and usu. line bodily cavities or enclose the organs contained in such cavities — compare MUCOUS MEMBRANE

serous otitis media n : a form of otitis media that is characterized by the accumulation of serous exudate in the middle ear and that typically results from an unresolved attack of acute otitis media — called also *secretory otitis media*

ser·o·var \'sir-ə-,vär, -,ve(ə)r, -,va(ə)r, 'ser-\ n : SEROTYPE 1

Ser·pa·sil \'sər-pə-,sil\ n : a preparation of reserpine — formerly a U.S. registered trademark

ser·pen·tar·ia \,sər-pən-'tar-ē-ə\ n : the dried rhizome and roots of the Virginia snakeroot or the Texas snakeroot used in pharmacology esp. as a bitter tonic

ser·pig·i·nous \(,)sər-'pij-ə-nəs\ adj : slowly spreading; esp : healing or worn in one portion while continuing to advance in another ⟨~ ulcer⟩

ser·pin \'sir-pən, 'ser-\ n [*serine* *p*roteinase *in*hibitor] : any of a group of structurally related proteins that typically are serine protease inhibitors (as antithrombin and antitrypsin) whose inhibiting activity is conferred by an active site in a highly variable and mobile peptide loop and that include some (as ovalbumin and angiotensinogen) which have apparently lost the inhibitory action due to mutation in the course of evolutionary change

serrata — see ORA SERRATA

ser·rat·ed \'se(ə)r-ˌāt-əd, sə-'rāt-əd\ *or* **ser·rate** \'se(ə)r-ˌāt, sə-'rāt\ *adj* : notched or toothed on the edge

Ser·ra·tia \se-'rā-sh(ē-)ə\ *n* : a genus of aerobic saprophytic flagellated rod-shaped bacteria of the family Enterobacteriaceae that occur as rods, commonly produce a bright red pigment, and are now usu. considered serotypes of a single species (*S. marcescens*) which has been implicated in some human opportunistic infections

Ser·ra·ti \se-'rä-tē\, **Serafino**, Italian boatman. The genus *Serratia* was so named in 1823 by Bartolomeo Bizio, a bacteriologist at the University of Padua, Italy, in honor of Serrati, who was engaged in operating a steamboat on the Arno River.

ser·ra·tus \se-'rāt-əs\ *n, pl* **ser·ra·ti** \-'rā-ˌtī\ : any of three muscles of the thorax that have complex origins but arise chiefly from the ribs or vertebrae: **a** : SERRATUS ANTERIOR **b** : SERRATUS POSTERIOR INFERIOR **c** : SERRATUS POSTERIOR SUPERIOR

serratus anterior *n* : a thin muscular sheet of the thorax that arises from the first eight or nine ribs and from the intercostal muscles between them, is inserted into the ventral side of the medial margin of the scapula, and acts to stabilize the scapula by holding it against the chest wall and to rotate it in raising the arm

serratus mag·nus \-'mag-nəs\ *n* : SERRATUS ANTERIOR

serratus posterior inferior *n* : a thin quadrilateral muscle at the junction of the thoracic and lumbar regions that arises chiefly from the spinous processes of the lowest two thoracic and first two or three lumbar vertebrae, is inserted into the lowest four ribs, and acts to counteract the pull of the diaphragm on the ribs to which it is attached

serratus posterior superior *n* : a thin quadrilateral muscle of the upper and dorsal part of the thorax that arises chiefly from the spinous processes of the lowest cervical and the first two or three thoracic vertebrae, is inserted into the second to fifth ribs, and acts to elevate the upper ribs

serre·fine \ˌser-'fēn\ *n* : a small forceps for clamping a blood vessel

Ser·to·li cell \'sert-ə-lē-, ser-'tō-lē-\ *also* **Ser·to·li's cell** \-lēz-\ *n* : any of the elongated striated cells in the seminiferous tubules of the testis to which the spermatids become attached and from which they apparently derive nourishment

Ser·to·li \ser-'tō-lē\, **Enrico (1842–1910)**, Italian physiologist. In 1865 Sertoli identified and described the branched cells in the seminiferous tubules of the human testicle; the cells are now known as Sertoli cells. He went on to study the anatomy of the testicle and spermatogenesis.

ser·tra·line \'sər-trə-ˌlēn\ *n* : an antidepressant drug that functions as an SSRI and is administered orally in the form of its hydrochloride $C_{17}H_{17}NCl_2 \cdot HCl$ — see ZOLOFT

¹se·rum \'sir-əm\ *n, pl* **se·ra** \-ə\ *or* **serums** : the watery portion of an animal fluid remaining after coagulation: **a** (1) : the clear yellowish fluid that remains from blood plasma after fibrinogen, prothrombin, and other clotting factors have been removed by clot formation — called also *blood serum* (2) : ANTISERUM **b** : a normal or pathological serous fluid (as in a blister)

²serum *adj* : occurring or found in the serum of the blood ⟨~ cholesterol⟩ ⟨~ glutamic-oxaloacetic transaminase⟩

se·rum·al \'sir-əm-əl\ *adj* : relating to or derived from serum or serous exudations ⟨a ~ calculus at the root of a tooth⟩

serum albumin *n* : a crystallizable albumin or mixture of albumins that normally constitutes more than half of the protein in blood serum, that serves to maintain the osmotic pressure of the blood, and that is used in transfusions esp. for the treatment of shock

serum disease *n* : SERUM SICKNESS

serum globulin *n* : a globulin or mixture of globulins occurring in blood serum and containing most of the antibodies of the blood

serum hepatitis *n* : HEPATITIS B

serum prothrombin conversion accelerator *n* : FACTOR VII

serum sickness *n* : an allergic reaction to the injection of foreign serum manifested by hives, swelling, eruption, arthritis, and fever — called also *serum disease*

serum therapy *n* : SEROTHERAPY

ser·vice \'sər-vəs\ *n* : a branch of a hospital medical staff devoted to a particular specialty ⟨pediatric ~⟩

service mark *n* : a mark or device used to identify a service (as transportation or insurance) offered to customers — compare TRADEMARK

se·ryl \'sir-əl, 'ser-\ *n* : the amino acid radical or residue $HOCH_2CH(NH_2)CO–$ of serine — abbr. *Ser*

ses·a·me \'ses-ə-mē *also* 'sez-\ *n* : a widely cultivated annual erect herb (*Sesamum indicum* syn. *S. orientale* of the family Pedaliaceae); *also* : its small somewhat flat seeds used as a source of sesame oil and a flavoring agent

sesame oil *n* : a pale yellow bland semidrying fatty oil obtained from sesame seeds and used chiefly as an edible oil, as a vehicle for various pharmaceuticals, and in cosmetics and soaps — called also *benne oil, teel oil*

¹ses·a·moid \'ses-ə-ˌmȯid\ *adj* : of, relating to, or being a nodular mass of bone or cartilage in a tendon esp. at a joint or bony prominence ⟨the patella is the largest ~ bone in the human body⟩

²sesamoid *n* : a sesamoid bone or cartilage

ses·a·moid·itis \ˌses-ə-ˌmȯi-'dīt-əs\ *n* : inflammation of the navicular bone and adjacent structures in the horse

ses·qui·ox·ide \ˌses-kwē-'äk-ˌsīd\ *n* : an oxide containing three atoms of oxygen combined with two of the other constituent in the molecule

ses·qui·ter·pene \ˌses-kwi-'tər-ˌpēn\ *n* : any of a class of terpenes $C_{15}H_{24}$ containing half again as many atoms in each molecule as monoterpenes; *also* : a derivative of such a terpene

ses·sile \'ses-īl, -əl\ *adj* **1** : attached directly by a broad base : not pedunculated ⟨a ~ tumor⟩ **2** : firmly attached (as to a cell) : not free to move about ⟨~ antibodies⟩

¹set \'set\ *vb* **set; set·ting** *vt* : to restore to normal position or connection when dislocated or fractured ⟨~ a broken bone⟩ ~ *vi* **1** : to become solid or thickened by chemical or physical alteration **2** *of a bone* : to become whole by knitting

²set *n* : a state of psychological preparedness usu. of limited duration for action in response to an anticipated stimulus or situation ⟨the influence of mental ~ on problem solving⟩

se·ta \'sēt-ə\ *n, pl* **se·tae** \'sē-ˌtē\ : a slender usu. rigid or bristly and springy organ or part of an animal or plant

Se·tar·ia \se-'tar-ē-ə\ *n* : a genus of filarial worms parasitic as adults in the body cavity of various ungulate mammals (as cattle and deer) and producing larvae that wander in the tissues and occas. invade the eye

set·fast \'set-ˌfast\ *n* : SITFAST

se·ton \'sēt-ᵊn\ *n* : one or more threads or horsehairs or a strip of linen introduced beneath the skin by a knife or needle to provide drainage or formerly to produce or prolong inflammation

set point *n* : the level or point at which a variable physiological state (as body temperature or weight) tends to stabilize

set·tle \'set-ᵊl\ *vb* **set·tled; set·tling** *vt, of an animal* : IMPREGNATE 1a ~ *vi, of an animal* : CONCEIVE

sev·enth cranial nerve \'sev-ən(t)th-\ *n* : FACIAL NERVE

seventh nerve *n* : FACIAL NERVE

severe acute respiratory syndrome *n* : SARS

severe combined immunodeficiency *n* : a rare congenital disorder of the immune system that is characterized by inability to produce a normal complement of antibodies and T cells and that results usu. in early death — abbr. *SCID*;

\ə\ abut \ᵊ\ kitten \ər\ further \a\ ash \ā\ ace \ä\ cot, cart \au̇\ out \ch\ chin \e\ bet \ē\ easy \g\ go \i\ hit \ī\ ice \j\ job \ŋ\ sing \ō\ go \ȯ\ law \ȯi\ boy \th\ thin \t̲h̲\ the \ü\ loot \u̇\ foot \y\ yet \zh\ vision *See also* Pronunciation Symbols page

S
T

called also *severe combined immune deficiency, severe combined immunodeficiency disease;* see ADENOSINE DEAMINASE

Sev·in \'sev-ən\ *trademark* — used for an insecticide consisting of a preparation of carbaryl

sew·age \'sü-ij\ *n* : refuse liquids or waste matter carried off by sewers

¹sex \'seks\ *n* **1** : either of the two major forms of individuals that occur in many species and that are distinguished respectively as male or female **2** : the sum of the structural, functional, and behavioral characteristics of living things that are involved in reproduction by two interacting parents and that distinguish males and females **3 a** : sexually motivated phenomena or behavior **b** : SEXUAL INTERCOURSE

²sex *vt* : to identify the sex of ⟨techniques for ~ing human embryos⟩

sex cell *n* : GAMETE; *also* : its cellular precursor

sex chromatin *n* : BARR BODY

sex chromosome *n* : a chromosome (as the X chromosome or the Y chromosome in humans) of a sexually reproducing eukaryotic organism that is directly concerned with the inheritance of sex, that contains the genes governing the inheritance of various sex-linked and sex-limited characters, and that is represented differently in the two sexes either by being present in one and not the other or by being present a different number of times in one sex compared to the other — called also *heterochromosome*

sex determination *n* : the process by which sex and the characteristics distinctive of a sex are imparted to a developing organism

sex·dig·i·tal \(')seks-'dij-ət-³l\ *or* **sex·dig·i·tate** \-'dij-ə-,tāt\ *adj* : having six fingers on one hand or six toes on one foot

sex gland *n* : GONAD

sex hormone *n* : a steroid hormone (as estradiol, progesterone, androstenedione, or testosterone) that is produced esp. by the ovaries, testes, or adrenal cortex and that exerts estrogenic, progestational, or androgenic activity on the growth or function of the reproductive organs or on the development of secondary sex characteristics

sexi·va·lent \,sek-sə-'vā-lənt\ *adj* : HEXAVALENT

sex–lim·it·ed \'seks-,lim-ət-əd\ *adj* : expressed in the phenotype of only one sex ⟨a ~ character⟩

sex–link·age \-,liŋk-ij\ *n* : the quality or state of being sex=linked

sex–linked *adj* **1** : located in a sex chromosome ⟨a ~ gene⟩ **2** : mediated by a sex-linked gene ⟨a ~ character⟩

sex object *n* : a person regarded esp. exclusively as an object of sexual interest

sex·ol·o·gist \,sek-'säl-ə-jəst\ *n* : a specialist in sexology

sex·ol·o·gy \sek-'säl-ə-jē\ *n, pl* **-gies** : the study of sex or of the interaction of the sexes esp. among human beings — **sex·o·log·i·cal** \,sek-sə-'läj-i-kəl\ *adj*

sex ratio *n* : the proportion of males to females in a population as expressed by the number of males per hundred females

sex·ti·grav·i·da \,sek-stə-'grav-əd-ə\ *n* : a woman who is pregnant for the sixth time

sex·tu·plet \sek-'stəp-lət, -'st(y)üp-; 'sek-st(y)əp-\ *n* **1** : any of six offspring born at one birth **2 sextuplets** *pl* : a group of six offspring born at one birth

sex·u·al \'seksh-(ə-)wəl, 'sek-shəl\ *adj* **1** : of, relating to, or associated with sex or the sexes ⟨~ differentiation⟩ ⟨~ conflict⟩ **2** : having or involving sex ⟨~ reproduction⟩ — **sex·u·al·ly** \'seksh-(ə-)wə-lē, 'seksh-ə-)lē\ *adv*

sexual as·sault \-ə-'sȯlt\ *n* : illegal sexual contact that usu. involves force upon a person without consent or is inflicted upon a person who is incapable of giving consent (as because of age or physical or mental incapacity) or who places the assailant (as a family friend) in a position of trust or authority

sexual cell *n* : GAMETE

sexual cord *n* : any of the cords of mesothelial cells that contain the primitive sexual cells in the developing ovaries and

testes of vertebrate embryos and that in the male develop into the seminiferous tubules

sexual cycle *n* : a cycle of bodily functional and structural changes associated with sex: as **a** : ESTROUS CYCLE **b** : MENSTRUAL CYCLE

sexual intercourse *n* **1** : heterosexual intercourse involving penetration of the vagina by the penis : COITUS **2** : intercourse (as anal or oral intercourse) that does not involve penetration of the vagina by the penis

sex·u·al·i·ty \,seksh-shə-'wal-ət-ē\ *n, pl* **-ties** : the quality or state of being sexual: **a** : the condition of having sex **b** : sexual activity **c** : expression of sexual receptivity or interest esp. when excessive

sex·u·al·ize *also Brit* **sex·u·al·ise** \'seksh-(ə-)wə-,līz, 'sek-shə-,līz\ *vt* **-ized** *also Brit* **-ised; -iz·ing** *also Brit* **-is·ing** : to make sexual : endow with a sexual character or quality — **sex·u·al·iza·tion** *also Brit* **sex·u·al·isa·tion** \,seksh-(ə-)wə-lə-'zā-shən\ *n*

sexually transmitted disease *n* : any of various diseases or infections that can be transmitted by direct sexual contact including some (as syphilis, gonorrhea, chlamydia, and genital herpes) chiefly spread by sexual means and others (as hepatitis B and AIDS) often contracted by nonsexual means — called also *STD*

sexual orientation *n* : the inclination of an individual with respect to heterosexual, homosexual, and bisexual behavior

sexual pref·er·ence \-'pref-(ə-)rens\ *n* : SEXUAL ORIENTATION

sexual relations *n pl* : COITUS

sexual selection *n* : natural selection for characters that confer success in competition for a mate as distinguished from competition with other species; *also* : the choice of a mate based on a preference for certain characteristics (as color or bird song)

Se·za·ry cell \sā-zä-'rē-\ *n* : any of the large mononuclear T cells with irregularly shaped nuclei that are characteristic of the Sezary syndrome

Sé·za·ry \sā-zà-rē\, **Albert (1880–1956),** French physician. Sézary was associated with clinics and research laboratories in Paris. He specialized in venereal disease and diseases of the skin but also did research within neurology and endocrinology. His publications covered such topics as disorders of the adrenal glands, tuberculin therapy, and antituberculous serotherapy. He was the author of a number of works on syphilis and its treatment and a dermatology text.

Sezary syndrome *or* **Se·za·ry's syndrome** \,sā-zä-'rēz-\ *n* : mycosis fungoides of a variant form that is characterized by exfoliative dermatitis with intense itching and by the presence in the blood and in the skin of numerous large atypical mononuclear T cells with irregularly shaped nuclei

SFA \,es-(,)ef-'ā\ *n* : a saturated fatty acid

sg *abbr* specific gravity

Sg *symbol* seaborgium

SGOT *abbr* serum glutamic-oxaloacetic transaminase

SGPT *abbr* serum glutamic pyruvic transaminase

SH *abbr* serum hepatitis

¹shad·ow \'shad-(,)ō, -ə(-w)\ *n* **1 a** : partial darkness or obscurity within a part of space from which rays from a source of light are cut off by an interposed opaque body **b** : a dark outline or image on an X-ray photograph where the X-rays have been blocked by a radiopaque mass (as a tumor) **2** : a colorless or scantily pigmented or stained body (as a degenerate cell or empty membrane) only faintly visible under the microscope

²shadow *vt* : to perform shadow-casting on ⟨freeze-dried and ~ed myosin molecules⟩

shadow–casting *n* : the production of exaggerated contrast in electron microscopy by irradiating the specimen obliquely with a beam esp. of gold atoms which makes opaque films on the slide in exact imitation of shadows

shaft \'shaft\ *n, pl* **shafts** \'shaf(t)s\ : a long slender cylindrical body or part: as **a** : the cylindrical part of a long bone between the enlarged ends **b** : HAIR SHAFT

shaft louse *n* : a biting louse of the genus *Menopon* (*M. gallinae*) that commonly infests domestic fowls

shak·en baby syndrome \'shā-kən-\ *n* : one or more of a group of symptoms (as limb paralysis, epilepsy, vision loss, or mental retardation) that tend to occur in an infant which has been severely shaken but that may also result from other actions (as tossing) causing internal trauma (as hemorrhage, hematoma, or contusions) esp. to the brain region, and that may ultimately result in the death of the infant — called also *shaken infant syndrome;* compare BATTERED CHILD SYNDROME

shakes \'shāks\ *n pl but sing or pl in constr* **1** : a condition of trembling; *specif* : DELIRIUM TREMENS **2** : MALARIA 1

shak·ing palsy \'shā-kiŋ-\ *n* : PARKINSON'S DISEASE

shal·low \'shal-(ˌ)ō, -ə(-w)\ *adj* : displacing comparatively little air ⟨~ breathing⟩

sham \'sham\ *adj* : being a treatment or procedure that is performed as a control and that is similar to but omits a key therapeutic element of the treatment or procedure under investigation ⟨~ surgery, in which doctors make an incision in a patient's knee and manipulate the joint, but don't clean out fluid, debris, and torn cartilage —Liz Kowalczyk⟩ ⟨a ~ injection of saline solution⟩

shank \'shaŋk\ *n* : the part of the leg between the knee and the ankle in humans or a corresponding part in other vertebrates

shape \'shāp\ *vt* **shaped; shap·ing** : to modify (behavior) by rewarding changes that tend toward a desired response

shark–liver oil \'shärk-ˌliv-ər-\ *n* : a yellow to red-brown fatty oil obtained from the livers of various sharks and used as a source of vitamin A

sharp \'shärp\ *n* : a medical instrument (as a scalpel, hypodermic needle, or breakable culture dish) that is sharp or may produce sharp pieces by shattering ⟨stuck by a ~ left in the workplace⟩ — usu. used in pl. ⟨a container for ~s⟩

Shar·pey's fiber \'shär-pēz-\ *n* : any of the thready processes of the periosteum that penetrate the tissue of the superficial lamellae of bones

Sharpey, William (1802–1880), British anatomist and physiologist. Sharpey was one of the founders of modern physiology in Great Britain and the first to occupy a chair of physiology in a British medical school. Joseph Lister was one of his pupils. In 1830 he wrote an early important work on cilia and ciliary motion. Renowned also as an anatomist, he furnished the description of the fibers that now bear his name for the 1848 edition of Jones Quain's *Anatomy.*

sheath \'shēth\ *n, pl* **sheaths** \'shēthz, 'shēths\ **1** : an investing cover or case of a plant or animal body or body part: as **a** : the tubular fold of skin into which the penis of many mammals is retracted **b** : the connective tissue of an organ or part that binds together its component elements and holds it in place **2** : CONDOM 1 — **sheathed** *adj*

sheath of Hen·le \-'hen-lē\ *n* : ENDONEURIUM

F. G. J. Henle — see HENLE'S LAYER

sheath of Hert·wig \-'hert-ˌvig\ *n* : a two-layered epithelial wall that covers the developing root of a tooth, is derived from cells of the enamel organ, and later breaks up during the process of cement deposition — called also *Hertwig's sheath*

Hert·wig \'hert-ˌvik\, **Wilhelm August Oskar (1849–1922),** German embryologist and cytologist. Hertwig's important investigations concerned the nuclear transmission of hereditary characteristics, biogenetic theory, and the effect of radium rays on somatic and germ cells. He is most famous for being the first to recognize that the fusion of the nuclei of the sperm and ovum is the central event in fertilization. He also made the important observation that only one spermatozoan is required to fertilize one egg. With his brother, Richard von Hertwig, he studied the formation of the coelom and the theory of the germ layer.

sheath of Schwann \-'shwän\ *n* : NEURILEMMA

T. A. H. Schwann — see SCHWANN CELL

shed \'shed\ *vt* **shed; shed·ding** : to give off or out: as **a** : to lose as part of a natural process ⟨~ the deciduous teeth⟩ **b**

: to discharge usu. gradually from the body ⟨exposed persons may ~ virus from the oropharynx —D. R. Franz *et al*⟩

Shee·han's syndrome \'shē-ənz-\ *also* **Shee·han syndrome** \-ən-\ *n* : necrosis of the pituitary gland with associated hypopituitarism resulting from postpartum hemorrhage

Sheehan, Harold Leeming (1900–1988), British pathologist. As a professor of pathology, Sheehan served at various times on the faculties of universities in Liverpool and Manchester, England, and in Glasgow, Scotland. From 1935 to 1946 he was director of research at Glasgow Royal Maternity Hospital. His published research included papers on pathology, endocrinology, and renal physiology.

sheep botfly \'shēp-\ *n* : a dipteran fly of the genus *Oestrus* (*O. ovis*) whose larvae parasitize sheep and lodge esp. in the nasal passages, frontal sinuses, and throat

sheep–dip \-ˌdip\ *n* : a liquid preparation of usu. toxic chemicals into which sheep are plunged esp. to destroy parasitic arthropods

sheep ked *n* : a wingless bloodsucking hippoboscid fly of the genus *Melophagus* (*M. ovinus*) that feeds chiefly on sheep and is a vector of sheep trypanosomiasis — called also *ked, sheep tick*

sheep pox *n* : a disease of sheep that is caused by a poxvirus (species *Sheeppox virus* of the genus *Capripoxvirus*), was formerly epizootic in warmer Old World areas, is marked by formation of vesicles or pocks esp. on the bare or thinly wooled areas of the body, and is frequently complicated by a secondary septic infection

sheep tick *n* **1** : SHEEP KED **2** : CASTOR-BEAN TICK

sheet \'shēt\ *n* **1** : a broad piece of cloth; *esp* : an oblong of usu. cotton or linen cloth used as an article of bedding **2** : a portion of something that is thin in comparison to its length and breadth ⟨a ~ of connective tissue⟩

shelf life \'shelf-ˌ\ *n* : the period of time during which a material (as a food or drug) may be stored and remain suitable for use

shellfish poisoning — see PARALYTIC SHELLFISH POISONING

shell shock *n* : COMBAT FATIGUE

shell–shocked \'shel-ˌshäkt\ *adj* : affected with combat fatigue

shi·at·su *also* **shi·at·zu** \shē-'ät-sü\ *n, often cap* : acupressure esp. of a form that originated in Japan

shield \'shēld\ *n* : a structure, device, or part that serves as a protective cover or barrier ⟨a lead ~ to protect against X-rays⟩

shift \'shift\ *n* : a change in place, position, or frequency: as **a** : a change in frequency resulting in a change in position of a spectral line or band — compare DOPPLER EFFECT **b** : a removal or transfer from one thing or place to another — see CHLORIDE SHIFT

shift to the left *n* : alteration of an Arneth index by an increase of immature neutrophils in the circulating blood

shift to the right *n* : alteration of an Arneth index by an increase in mature or overage neutrophils in the circulating blood

Shi·ga bacillus \'shē-gə-\ *n* : a widely distributed but chiefly tropical bacterium of the genus *Shigella* (*S. dysenteriae*) that causes dysentery in humans and monkeys

Shi·ga \shē-gä\, **Kiyoshi (1870–1957),** Japanese bacteriologist. Shiga is best known for the discovery in 1897 of a bacillus that causes dysentery. Originally the bacterium was classified in the genus *Bacillus,* but in 1919 along with several other species it was placed in a new genus, *Shigella,* which was named in honor of Shiga.

shi·gel·la \shi-'gel-ə\ *n* **1** *cap* : a genus of nonmotile aerobic bacteria of the family Enterobacteriaceae that form acid but no gas on many carbohydrates and that cause dysenteries in

S
T

\ə\ abut \ʹ\ kitten \ər\ further \a\ ash \ā\ ace \ä\ cot, cart
\aů\ out \ch\ chin \e\ bet \ē\ easy \g\ go \i\ hit \ī\ ice \j\ job
\ŋ\ sing \ō\ go \ô\ law \ôi\ boy \th\ thin \t͟h\ the \ü\ loot
\ů\ foot \y\ yet \zh\ vision *See also* Pronunciation Symbols page

animals and esp. humans **2** *pl* **-gel·lae** \-ˌē\ *also* **-gellas** : any bacterium of the genus *Shigella* **3** : SHIGELLOSIS

shig·el·lo·sis \ˌshig-ə-'lō-səs\ *n, pl* **-lo·ses** \-'lō-ˌsēz\ : infection with or dysentery caused by bacteria of the genus *Shigella*

shi·kim·ic acid \shi-ˌkim-ik-\ *n* : a crystalline acid $C_7H_{10}O_5$ that is formed as a precursor in the biosynthesis of aromatic amino acids and of lignin

shin \'shin\ *n* : the front part of the leg below the knee

shin·bone \'shin-ˌbōn, -ˌbōn\ *n* : TIBIA

shin·er \'shī-nər\ *n* : BLACK EYE

shin·gles \'shiŋ-gəlz\ *n pl but sing in constr* : an acute viral inflammation of the sensory ganglia of spinal and cranial nerves associated with a vesicular eruption and neuralgic pain and caused by reactivation of the herpesvirus causing chicken pox — called also *herpes zoster, zona, zoster*

shin splints *n pl but sing or pl in constr* : painful injury to and inflammation of the tibial and toe extensor muscles or their fasciae that is caused by repeated minimal traumas (as by running on a hard surface)

ship fever \'ship-\ *n* : TYPHUS a

ship·ping fever *n* : an often fatal febrile disease esp. of young cattle and sheep that occurs under highly stressful conditions (as shipment over long distances and crowding in feedlots), is marked by high fever and pneumonia, and is caused by bacteria (esp. *Pasteurella haemolytica*) usu. in association with a virus

ship rat *n* : a rat (as the brown rat or roof rat) that frequently infests ships

¹shiv·er \'shiv-ər\ *vi* : to undergo trembling : experience rapid involuntary muscular twitching esp. in response to cold

²shiver *n* : an instance of shivering

shivering *n* **1** : an act or action of one that shivers **2** : a constant abnormal twitching of various muscles in the horse that is prob. due to sensory nerve derangement

¹shock \'shäk\ *n* **1** : a sudden or violent disturbance in the mental or emotional faculties **2** : a state of profound depression of the vital processes of the body that is characterized by pallor, rapid but weak pulse, rapid and shallow respiration, reduced total blood volume, and low blood pressure and that is caused usu. by severe esp. crushing injuries, hemorrhage, burns, or major surgery **3** : sudden stimulation of the nerves or convulsive contraction of the muscles that is caused by the discharge through the animal body of electricity from a charged source — compare ELECTROCONVULSIVE THERAPY

²shock *vt* **1** : to cause to undergo a physical or nervous shock **2** : to subject to the action of an electrical discharge

shock lung *n* : a condition of severe pulmonary edema associated with shock

shock organ *n* : an organ or part that is the principal site of an allergic reaction

shock therapy *n* : the treatment of mental disorder by the artificial induction of coma or convulsions through use of drugs or electric current — called also *convulsive therapy;* see ELECTROCONVULSIVE THERAPY

shock treatment *n* : SHOCK THERAPY

shoe boil \'shü-\ *n* : a soft swelling on the elbow of a horse caused by irritation (as from bruising in lying down)

shoot \'shüt\ *vt* shot \'shät\; **shoot·ing** **1** : to give an injection to **2** : to take or administer (as a drug) by hypodermic needle

shoot·ing *adj* : characterized by sudden sharp piercing sensations ⟨~ pains⟩

Shope papilloma \'shōp-\ *also* **Shope's papilloma** \'shōps-\ *n* : a transmissible fibroma of cottontail rabbits that occurs esp. on the legs, feet, and ears, is caused by a poxvirus (species *Rabbit fibroma virus* of the genus *Leporipoxvirus*), and has under certain circumstances been transmitted to domestic rabbits

Shope, Richard Edwin (1901–1966), American pathologist. Shope was the first to isolate an influenza virus, the first to establish the feasibility of animal immunization against influenza, and the first to explain the cause of the

pandemic of Spanish influenza following World War I. During the 1920s and 1930s he demonstrated that pseudorabies is caused by a virus for which pigs act as intermediate hosts. In 1933, while studying tumors in cottontail rabbits, he discovered a virus causing similar growths in domestic rabbits that can eventually become malignant. This discovery marked the first time that a potentially cancerous tumor was shown to be caused by a virus.

short bone \'shòrt-\ *n* : a bone (as of the tarsus or carpus) that is of approximately equal length in all dimensions

short bowel syndrome *n* : malabsorption from the small intestine that is marked by diarrhea, malnutrition, and steatorrhea and that results from resection of the small intestine

short ciliary nerve *n* : any of 6 to 10 delicate nerve filaments of parasympathetic, sympathetic, and general sensory function that arise in the ciliary ganglion and innervate the smooth muscles and tunics of the eye — compare LONG CILIARY NERVE

short gut syndrome *n* : SHORT BOWEL SYNDROME

shortness of breath *n* : difficulty in drawing sufficient breath : labored breathing

short–nosed cattle louse *n* : a large bluish broad-bodied and short-headed louse of the genus *Haematopinus* (*H. eurysternus*) that attacks domestic cattle

short posterior ciliary artery *n* : any of 6 to 10 arteries that arise from the ophthalmic artery or its branches, pass to the posterior part of the eyeball while surrounding the optic nerve, and enter or divide into branches entering the sclera to supply the choroid and the ciliary processes — compare LONG POSTERIOR CILIARY ARTERY

short saphenous vein *n* : SAPHENOUS VEIN b

short sight *n* : MYOPIA

short·sight·ed \'shòrt-'sīt-əd\ *adj* : NEARSIGHTED

short·sight·ed·ness *n* : MYOPIA

short–term memory *n* : memory that involves recall of information for a relatively short time (as a few seconds) ⟨*short-term memory* is involved when a phone number is remembered just long enough to dial it⟩ — abbr. *STM*

short·wave \'shòrt-'wāv\ *n* **1** : a radio wave having a wavelength between 10 and 100 meters **2** : electromagnetic radiation having a wavelength equal to or less than that of visible light

shortwave diathermy *n* : diathermy in which wavelengths of about 11 meters are employed

shortwave therapy *n* : SHORTWAVE DIATHERMY

short–wind·ed \-'win-dəd\ *adj* : affected with or characterized by shortness of breath

¹shot \'shät\ *n* : an injection of a drug, immunizing substance, nutrient, or medicament ⟨a flu ~⟩

²shot *past and past part of* SHOOT

shoul·der \'shōl-dər\ *n* **1** : the laterally projecting part of the human body formed of the bones and joints with their covering tissue by which the arm is connected with the trunk **2** : the two shoulders and the upper part of the back — usu. used in pl.

shoulder blade *n* : SCAPULA

shoulder girdle *n* : PECTORAL GIRDLE

shoulder–hand syndrome *n* : reflex sympathetic dystrophy affecting the upper extremities and characterized by pain in and stiffening of the shoulder followed by swelling and stiffening of the hand and fingers

shoulder joint *n* : the ball-and-socket joint of the humerus and the scapula

shoulder separation *n* : a dislocation of the shoulder at the acromioclavicular joint

show \'shō\ *n* **1** : a discharge of mucus streaked with blood from the vagina at the onset of labor **2** : the first appearance of blood in a menstrual period

Shrap·nell's membrane \'shrap-nəlz-\ *n* : a triangular flaccid part of the tympanic membrane of the ear

Shrapnell, Henry Jones (1761–1841), British anatomist. Shrapnell published the first description of the flaccid portion of the tympanic membrane in 1832.

shrink \\'shriŋk\\ *n* : a clinical psychiatrist or psychologist — called also *headshrinker*

shud·der \\'shəd-ər\\ *vi* **shud·dered; shud·der·ing** : to tremble convulsively : SHIVER — **shudder** *n*

¹shunt \\'shənt\\ *vt* : to divert by or as if by a shunt; *esp* : to divert (blood) from one part to another by a surgical shunt

²shunt *n* **1** : a passage by which a bodily fluid (as blood) is diverted from one channel, circulatory path, or part to another; *esp* : such a passage established by surgery or occurring as an abnormality ⟨an arteriovenous ∼⟩ **2 a** : a surgical procedure for the establishment of an artificial shunt — see PORTACAVAL SHUNT **b** : a device (as a narrow tube) used to establish an artificial shunt ⟨plastic ∼s have been used to bypass temporarily sections of major arteries —Johnson McGuire & Arnold Iglauer⟩

¹shut–in \\'shət-ˌin\\ *n* : a person who is confined to home, a room, or bed because of illness or incapacity

²shut–in \\'shət-ˌin\\ *adj* **1** : confined to one's home or an institution by illness or incapacity **2** : tending to avoid social contact : WITHDRAWN ⟨diagnostic and prognostic significance of the ∼ personality type —S. K. Weinberg⟩

Shwartz·man reaction \\'shwȯrts-mən-, 'shwärts-\\ *n* : either of two reactions resulting from administration of endotoxin to experimental animals and esp. rabbits: **a** : a generalized reaction following two intravenous injections of endotoxin given 24 hours apart and marked by widespread hemorrhage, reduced numbers of white blood cells and platelets, renal necrosis, and death of the animal — called also *generalized Shwartzman reaction* **b** : a localized cutaneous reaction following subcutaneous injection of endotoxin followed 24 hours later by intravenous injection of endotoxin and marked by hemorrhage, necrosis, and white blood cell infiltration at the site of first injection — called also *Shwartzman phenomenon*

Shwartzman, Gregory (1896–1965), American bacteriologist. Born in Odessa, Russia, Shwartzman received his medical degree in Brussels and later worked as a researcher at London's Lister Institute before coming to the U.S. in 1923. In 1926 he became head of the department of bacteriology at New York's Mount Sinai Hospital, where he spent the bulk of his career. Concurrently he held a professorship at Columbia University. His areas of research included immunological reactions in tissue cultures and the effects of vitamins on bacterial growth. In 1928 he published an article on the phenomenon of local skin reactivity to bacterial filtrates in which he described what is now known as the Shwartzman reaction or Shwartzman phenomenon.

Shy–Dra·ger syndrome \\'shī-'drā-gər-\\ *n* : an uncommon degenerative disease of unknown cause that affects the autonomic nervous system, that typically occurs in late middle age or old age, and that is characterized by orthostatic hypotension, muscular wasting and atrophy, rigidity, tremors, urinary and fecal incontinence, impotence, anhidrosis, and atrophy of the iris — called also *Shy-Drager disease*

Shy, George Milton (1919–1967), and **Drager, Glenn Albert (1917–1967),** American neurologists. Shy's major positions included those of clinical director of the National Institute of Neurological Diseases and Blindness at the National Institutes of Health and professor at Columbia University's New York Neurological Institute. His areas of research included nuclear medicine and neuromuscular disease; he was one of the coauthors of *Atlas of Muscle* (1957). In 1960 he and G. A. Drager published their description of the disease that bears their names.

Si *symbol* silicon

SI *abbr* [French *Système International d'Unités*] International System of Units

si·al·ad·e·ni·tis \\ˌsī-əl-ˌad-ᵊn-'īt-əs\\ *also* **si·alo·ad·e·ni·tis** \\ˌsī-ə-lō-\\ *n* : inflammation of a salivary gland

si·al·a·gogue \\sī-'al-ə-ˌgäg\\ *n* : an agent that promotes the flow of saliva — called also *sialogogue*

si·al·ec·ta·sis \\ˌsī-əl-'ek-tə-səs\\ *n* : abnormal dilation of the ducts of a salivary gland

si·al·ic acid \\(ˌ)sī-ˌal-ik-\\ *n* : any of a group of reducing amido acids that are essentially carbohydrates and are found esp. as components of blood glycoproteins and mucoproteins

si·alo·ad·e·nec·to·my \\ˌsī-ə-lō-ˌad-ᵊn-'ek-tə-mē\\ *n, pl* **-mies** : surgical excision of a salivary gland

sialoadenitis *var of* SIALADENITIS

si·alo·do·cho·plas·ty \\ˌsī-ə-lō-'dō-kə-ˌplas-tē\\ *n, pl* **-ties** : plastic surgery performed on a duct of a salivary gland

si·alo·gly·co·pro·tein \\-ˌglī-kō-'prō-ˌtēn, -'prōt-ē-ən\\ *n* : a glycoprotein (as of blood) having sialic acid as a component

si·al·o·gogue \\sī-'al-ə-ˌgäg\\ *n* : SIALAGOGUE

si·al·o·gram \\sī-'al-ə-ˌgram\\ *n* : a radiograph of the salivary tract made by sialography

si·a·log·ra·phy \\ˌsī-ə-'läg-rə-fē\\ *n, pl* **-phies** : radiography of the salivary tract after injection of a radiopaque substance

si·al·o·lith \\sī-'al-ə-ˌlith\\ *n* : a calculus occurring in a salivary gland

si·al·o·li·thi·a·sis \\ˌsī-ə-lō-li-'thī-ə-səs\\ *n, pl* **-a·ses** \\-ˌsēz\\ : the formation or presence of a calculus or calculi in a salivary gland

si·alo·li·thot·o·my \\-li-'thät-ə-mē\\ *n, pl* **-mies** : surgical incision of a salivary gland for removal of a calculus

si·al·or·rhea *or chiefly Brit* **si·al·or·rhoea** \\ˌsī-ə-lə-'rē-ə\\ *n* : excessive salivation

Si·a·mese twin \\'sī-ə-ˌmēz-, -ˌmēs-\\ *n* : either of a pair of conjoined twins

sib \\'sib\\ *n* : a brother or sister considered irrespective of sex; *broadly* : any plant or animal of a group sharing a degree of genetic relationship corresponding to that of human sibs

¹sib·i·lant \\'sib-ə-lənt\\ *adj* : having, containing, or producing the sound of or a sound resembling that of the *s* or *sh* in *sash* ⟨a ∼ speech sound⟩ ⟨∼ breathing⟩ ⟨∼ rales⟩

²sibilant *n* : a sibilant speech sound (as English \\s\\, \\z\\, \\sh\\, \\zh\\, \\ch(=t + sh)\\, or \\j(=d + zh)\\)

sib·ling \\'sib-liŋ\\ *n* : SIB; *also* : one of two or more individuals having one common parent

sibling rivalry *n* : competition between siblings esp. for the attention, affection, and approval of their parents

sib·ship \\'sib-ˌship\\ *n* : a group of sibs ⟨a small ∼⟩

si·bu·tra·mine \\sə-'byü-trə-ˌmēn, -mən\\ *n* : an appetite suppressant that is administered orally in the form of its hydrated hydrochloride $C_{17}H_{26}ClN·HCl·H_2O$ in the treatment of obesity and that exerts its therapeutic effect by inhibiting the reuptake of norepinephrine, serotonin, and dopamine

sicca — see KERATOCONJUNCTIVITIS SICCA, RHINITIS SICCA

sic·ca syndrome \\'sik-ə-\\ *n* : SJÖGREN'S SYNDROME

sick \\'sik\\ *adj* **1 a** : affected with disease or ill health **b** : of, relating to, or intended for use in sickness ⟨a ∼ ward⟩ **c** : affected with nausea : inclined to vomit or being in the act of vomiting ⟨∼ to one's stomach⟩ ⟨was ∼ in the car⟩ **2** : mentally or emotionally unsound or disordered

sick bay *n* : a compartment in a ship used as a dispensary and hospital; *broadly* : a place for the care of the sick or injured

sick·bed \\'sik-ˌbed\\ *n* : the bed upon which one lies sick

sick build·ing syndrome \\-'bil-diŋ-\\ *n* : a set of symptoms (as headache, fatigue, eye irritation, and breathing difficulties) that typically affect workers in modern airtight office buildings, that are believed to be caused by indoor pollutants (as formaldehyde fumes, particulate matter, or microorganisms), and that tend to disappear when affected individuals leave the building — *abbr.* SBS; compare BUILDING-RELATED ILLNESS

sick call *n* : a scheduled time at which individuals (as soldiers) may report as sick to a medical officer

sick·en \\'sik-ən\\ *vt* : to make sick ∼ *vi* : to become sick

sick·en·ing \\'sik-(ə-)niŋ\\ *adj* : causing sickness or nausea

sick headache *n* : MIGRAINE

sicklaemia *chiefly Brit var of* SICKLEMIA

\\ə\\ abut \\ᵊ\\ kitten \\ər\\ further \\a\\ ash \\ā\\ ace \\ä\\ cot, cart \\au̇\\ out \\ch\\ chin \\e\\ bet \\ē\\ easy \\g\\ go \\i\\ hit \\ī\\ ice \\j\\ job \\ŋ\\ sing \\ō\\ go \\ȯ\\ law \\ȯi\\ boy \\th\\ thin \\t̲h̲\\ the \\ü\\ loot \\u̇\\ foot \\y\\ yet \\zh\\ vision   *See also* Pronunciation Symbols page

¹**sick·le** \'sik-əl\ *n* : a dental scaler with a curved 3-sided point

²**sickle** *adj* : of, relating to, or characteristic of sickle-cell anemia or sickle-cell trait ⟨~ hemoglobin⟩

³**sickle** *vb* **sick·led; sick·ling** \'sik-(ə-)liŋ\ *vt* : to change (a red blood cell) into a sickle cell ~ *vi* : to undergo change into a sickle cell ⟨the ability of red blood cells to ~⟩

sick leave *n* **1** : an absence from work permitted because of illness **2** : the number of days per year for which an employer agrees to pay employees who are sick

sickle cell *n* **1** : an abnormal red blood cell of crescent shape **2** : a condition characterized by sickle cells : SICKLE-CELL ANEMIA, SICKLE-CELL TRAIT

sickle–cell anemia *n* : a chronic anemia that occurs in individuals (as those of African or Mediterranean descent) who are homozygous for the gene controlling hemoglobin S and that is characterized by destruction of red blood cells and by episodic blocking of blood vessels by the adherence of sickle cells to the vascular endothelium which causes the serious complications of the disease (as organ failure)

sickle–cell disease *n* : SICKLE-CELL ANEMIA

sickle–cell trait *n* : a usu. asymptomatic blood condition in which some red blood cells tend to sickle but usu. not enough to produce anemia and which occurs in individuals (as those of African or Mediterranean descent) who are heterozygous for the gene controlling hemoglobin S

sick·le·mia *or chiefly Brit* **sick·lae·mia** \si-'klē-mē-ə\ *n* : SICKLE-CELL TRAIT — **sick·le·mic** *or chiefly Brit* **sick·lae·mic** \-mik\ *adj*

sick·ler \'sik-lər\ *n* : an individual with sickle-cell trait or sickle-cell anemia

sick·ly \'sik-lē\ *adj* **1** : somewhat unwell; *also* : habitually ailing ⟨a ~ child⟩ **2** : produced by or associated with sickness ⟨a ~ complexion⟩ **3** : producing or tending to produce disease ⟨a ~ climate⟩ **4** : tending to produce nausea ⟨a ~ odor⟩

sick·ness \'sik-nəs\ *n* **1** : the condition of being ill : ill health **2** : a specific disease **3** : NAUSEA

sick·room \'sik-ˌrüm, -ˌrüm\ *n* : a room in which a person is confined by sickness

sick sinus syndrome *n* : a cardiac disorder typically characterized by alternating tachycardia and bradycardia

side \'sīd\ *n* **1** : the right or left part of the wall or trunk of the body ⟨a pain in the ~⟩ **2** : one of the halves of the animal body on either side of the midsagittal plane **3** : a lateral half or part of an organ or structure ⟨burned on the right ~ of one leg⟩

side·bone \-ˌbōn\ *n* **1** *or* sidebones *pl but sing in constr* : abnormal ossification of the cartilages in the lateral posterior part of a horse's hoof (as of a forefoot) often causing lameness **2** : one of the bony structures characteristic of sidebone

side chain *n* : a branched chain of atoms attached to the principal chain or to a ring in a molecule

side effect *n* : a secondary and usu. adverse effect (as of a drug) ⟨toxic *side effects*⟩ ⟨a *side effect* of drowsiness caused by antihistamines⟩ — called also *side reaction*

side reaction *n* **1** : a less important reaction of two or more chemical reactions occurring at the same time ⟨undesirable complex *side reactions*⟩ **2** : SIDE EFFECT

sid·ero·blast \'sid-ə-rə-ˌblast\ *n* : an erythroblast containing cytoplasmic iron granules

sid·ero·blas·tic \ˌsid-ə-rə-'blas-tik\ *adj* : of, relating to, or characterized by the presence of sideroblasts ⟨~ anemia⟩

sid·ero·cyte \'sid-ə-rə-ˌsīt\ *n* : an atypical red blood cell containing iron not bound in hemoglobin

sid·ero·fi·bro·sis \ˌsid-ə-rō-fī-'brō-səs\ *n, pl* **-bro·ses** \-'brō-ˌsēz\ : fibrosis esp. of the spleen associated with deposits containing iron

sid·ero·pe·nia \ˌsid-ə-rə-'pē-nē-ə\ *n* : iron deficiency in the blood serum — **sid·ero·pe·nic** \-'pē-nik\ *adj*

sid·er·oph·i·lin \ˌsid-ə-'räf-ə-lən\ *n* : TRANSFERRIN

sid·ero·phore \'sid-ə-rə-ˌfō(ə)r\ *n* : any of a group of low molecular weight compounds produced esp. by various microorganisms that bind ferric iron extracellularly to form a stable chelate for transport into the cell

sid·er·o·sis \ˌsid-ə-'rō-səs\ *n, pl* **-o·ses** \-ˌsēz\ *also* **-o·sis·es** **1** : pneumoconiosis occurring in iron workers from inhalation of particles of iron **2** : deposit of iron pigment in a bodily tissue

sid·er·ot·ic \ˌsid-ə-'rät-ik\ *adj* : of or relating to siderosis

side·stream \'sīd-ˌstrēm\ *adj* : relating to or being tobacco smoke that is emitted from the lit end of a cigarette or cigar — compare MAINSTREAM

side·wind·er \'sīd-ˌwīnd-ər\ *n* : a small pale-colored rattlesnake of the genus *Crotalus* (*C. cerastes*) of the southwestern U.S. that moves by thrusting its body diagonally forward in a series of S-shaped curves — called also *horned rattlesnake*

SIDS *abbr* sudden infant death syndrome

sie·mens \'sē-mənz, 'zē-\ *n, pl* **siemens** : a unit of conductance in the mks system equivalent to one ampere per volt

sie·vert \'sē-vərt\ *n* : an SI unit for the dosage of ionizing radiation equal to 100 rems — abbr. *Sv*

> **Sievert, Rolf Maximilian (1896–1966),** Swedish physicist. Sievert was a pioneer in radiation physics and protection from radiation. He served as head of the physics laboratory at Sweden's Radiumhemmet from 1924 to 1937, when he became head of the department of radiation physics at the Karolinska Institute. He played a pioneering role in the measurement of doses of radiation especially in its use in the diagnosis and treatment of cancer. In later years he focused his research on the biological effects of repeated exposure to low doses of radiation. In 1964 he founded the International Radiation Protection Association, serving for a time as its chairman. He also chaired the United Nations Scientific Committee on the Effects of Atomic Radiation. In 1979 a scientific conference named a unit for the dosage of ionizing radiation in his honor.

Sig *abbr* signa — used to introduce the signature in writing a prescription

sight \'sīt\ *n* **1** : something that is seen **2** : the process, power, or function of seeing; *specif* : the one of the five basic physical senses by which light stimuli received by the eye are interpreted by the brain and constructed into a representation of the position, shape, brightness, and usu. color of objects in space **3 a** : a perception of an object by the eye **b** : the range of vision

sight·ed \'sīt-əd\ *adj* : having sight : not blind

sight·less \'sīt-ləs\ *adj* : lacking sight : BLIND — **sight·less·ness** *n*

sig·ma factor \'sig-mə-\ *n* : a detachable polypeptide subunit of RNA polymerase that facilitates the initiation of transcription by recognizing specific DNA promoter sites

sig·ma·tism \'sig-mə-ˌtiz-əm\ *n* : faulty articulation of sibilants

¹**sig·moid** \'sig-ˌmȯid\ *adj* **1 a** : curved like the letter C **b** : curved in two directions like the letter S **2** : of, relating to, or being the sigmoid colon of the intestine ⟨~ lesions⟩

²**sigmoid** *n* : SIGMOID COLON

sigmoid artery *n* : any of several branches of the inferior mesenteric artery that supply the sigmoid colon

sigmoid colon *n* : the contracted and crooked part of the colon immediately above the rectum — called also *pelvic colon, sigmoid flexure*

sig·moid·ec·to·my \ˌsig-mȯi-'dek-tə-mē\ *n, pl* **-mies** : surgical excision of part of the sigmoid colon

sigmoid flexure *n* : SIGMOID COLON

sig·moid·itis \ˌsig-mȯi-'dīt-əs\ *n* : inflammation of the sigmoid colon

sigmoid notch \-'näch\ *n* **1** : MANDIBULAR NOTCH **2** : TROCHLEAR NOTCH

sig·moid·o·pexy \sig-'mȯid-ə-ˌpek-sē\ *n, pl* **-pex·ies** : surgical attachment of the sigmoid colon to the wall of the abdomen for relief of rectal prolapse

sig·moid·o·scope \sig-'mȯid-ə-ˌskōp\ *n* : an endoscope designed to be passed through the anus in order to permit inspection, diagnosis, treatment, and photography esp. of the sigmoid colon — called also *proctosigmoidoscope*

sig·moid·os·co·py \ˌsig-ˌmȯi-'däs-kə-pē\ *n, pl* **-pies** : the process of using a sigmoidoscope — called also *proctosigmoidoscopy* — **sig·moid·o·scop·ic** \-də-'skäp-ik\ *adj*

sig·moid·os·to·my \ˌsig-ˌmȯi-'däs-tə-mē\ *n, pl* **-mies** : surgical creation of an artificial anus in the sigmoid colon

sigmoid sinus *n* : a sinus on each side of the brain that is a continuation of the transverse sinus on the same side, follows an S-shaped course to the jugular foramen, and empties into the internal jugular vein

sigmoid vein *n* : any of several veins that drain the sigmoid colon and empty into the superior rectal vein

sign \'sīn\ *n* **1** : one of a set of gestures used to represent language **2** : an objective evidence of disease esp. as observed and interpreted by the physician rather than by the patient or lay observer 〈narrow retinal vessels are a ∼ of arteriosclerosis〉 — see BRUDZINSKI SIGN, CHVOSTEK'S SIGN, HOMANS' SIGN, KERNIG SIGN, PHYSICAL SIGN, PLACENTAL SIGN, ROMBERG'S SIGN, TINEL'S SIGN, VITAL SIGNS, VON GRAEFE'S SIGN; compare SYMPTOM

sig·na \'sig-nə\ *vb imper* : write on label — used to introduce the signature in writing a prescription; abbr. *S, Sig*

sig·nal node \'sig-nəl-\ *n* : a supraclavicular lymph node which when tumorous is often a secondary sign of gastrointestinal cancer — called also *Virchow's node*

sig·na·ture \'sig-nə-ˌchu̇(ə)r, -chər, -ˌt(y)u̇(ə)r\ *n* **1** : a feature in the appearance or qualities of a natural object formerly held to indicate its utility in medicine either because of a fancied resemblance to a body part (as a heart-shaped leaf indicating utility in heart disease) or because of a presumed relation to some phase of a disease (as the prickly nature of thistle indicating utility in case of a stitch in the side) **2** : the part of a medical prescription which contains the directions to the patient

sig·net cell \'sig-nət-\ *n* : SIGNET RING CELL

signet ring *n* : a malaria parasite in an intracellular developmental stage in which the nucleus is peripheral and the cytoplasm somewhat attenuated and annular

signet ring cell *n* : a cell that has its nucleus shifted to one side by a large cytoplasmic vacuole and that occurs esp. in mucin-producing adenocarcinomas esp. of the stomach

sig·nif·i·cant \sig-'nif-i-kənt\ *adj* : probably caused by something other than mere chance 〈a statistically ∼ correlation between diet and disease〉 — **sig·nif·i·cant·ly** *adv*

significant oth·er \-'əth̶-ər\ *n* : a person who is important to one's well-being; *esp* : a spouse or one in a similar relationship

sign language *n* : a formal language employing a system of hand gestures for communication (as by the deaf) — compare FINGER SPELLING

Si·las·tic \si-'las-tik\ *trademark* — used for a silicone material resembling rubber

sil·den·a·fil \sil-'den-ə-ˌfil\ *n* : a drug that is used in the form of its citrate $C_{22}H_{30}N_6O_4S \cdot C_6H_8O_7$ to treat erectile dysfunction in males, that by suppressing a phosphodiesterase enzyme also suppresses the enzyme's inhibitory effect on the hormone cyclic GMP, and that enables the cyclic GMP produced during sexual arousal to initiate the muscular and vascular changes which produce an erection — see VIAGRA

si·lence \'sī-lən(t)s\ *vt* **si·lenced; si·lenc·ing** : to block the genetic expression of : SUPPRESS 〈the gene was *silenced* using the technique of RNA interference〉

si·lent \'sī-lənt\ *adj* **1** : not exhibiting the usual signs or symptoms of presence 〈a ∼ infection〉 〈∼ gallstones〉 〈∼ tuberculosis〉 〈∼ ischemia〉 **2** : yielding no detectable response to stimulation — used esp. of an association area of the brain 〈∼ cortex〉 **3** : having no detectable function or effect 〈∼ DNA〉 〈∼ genes〉 — **si·lent·ly** *adv*

si·lex \'sī-ˌleks\ *n* : silica or a siliceous material esp. for use as a filler in paints or wood or as a dental material

sil·i·ca \'sil-i-kə\ *n* : the dioxide of silicon SiO_2 that is used as an ingredient of simethicone and that occurs naturally in crystalline, amorphous, and impure forms (as in quartz, opal, and sand respectively) — called also *silicon dioxide*

silica gel *n* : colloidal silica resembling coarse white sand in

appearance but possessing many fine pores and therefore extremely adsorbent

sil·i·cate \'sil-ə-ˌkāt, 'sil-i-kət\ *n* : a salt or ester derived from a silicic acid; *esp* : any of numerous insoluble often complex metal salts that contain silicon and oxygen in the anion and constitute the largest class of minerals

silicate cement *n* : a dental cement used in restorations

si·li·ceous *also* **si·li·cious** \sə-'lish-əs\ *adj* : of, relating to, or containing silica or a silicate 〈a ∼ cement used in dentistry〉

si·lic·ic \sə-'lis-ik\ *adj* : of, relating to, or derived from silica or silicon

silicic acid *n* : any of various weakly acid substances obtained as gelatinous masses by treating silicates with acids

sil·i·co·flu·o·ride \ˌsil-i-kō-'flu̇(-ə)r-ˌīd\ *n* : FLUOSILICATE — see SODIUM FLUOSILICATE

sil·i·con \'sil-i-kən, 'sil-ə-ˌkän\ *n* : a tetravalent nonmetallic element that occurs combined as the most abundant element next to oxygen in the earth's crust and is used esp. in alloys — symbol *Si*; see ELEMENT table

silicon carbide *n* : a very hard dark crystalline compound SiC of silicon and carbon that is used as an abrasive in dentistry

silicon dioxide *n* : SILICA

sil·i·cone \'sil-ə-ˌkōn\ *n* : any of various polymeric organic silicon compounds which are obtained as oils, greases, or plastics and some of which have been used as surgical implants

sil·i·con·ize \-ˌīz\ *vt* **-ized; -iz·ing** : to provide with a silicone surface 〈∼ hypodermic needles to reduce friction〉

sil·i·co·sis \ˌsil-ə-'kō-səs\ *n, pl* **-co·ses** \-ˌsēz\ : pneumoconiosis characterized by massive fibrosis of the lungs resulting in shortness of breath and caused by prolonged inhalation of silica dusts — compare BLACK LUNG, PNEUMOCONIOSIS

¹sil·i·cot·ic \ˌsil-ə-'kät-ik\ *adj* : relating to, caused by, or affected with silicosis 〈∼ patients〉 〈∼ lungs〉

²silicotic *n* : an individual affected with silicosis

sil·i·co·tu·ber·cu·lo·sis \ˌsil-i-kō-t(y)u̇-ˌbər-kyə-'lō-səs\ *n, pl* **-lo·ses** \-ˌsēz\ : silicosis and tuberculosis in the same lung

silk \'silk\ *n* **1** : a fine continuous protein fiber produced by various insect larvae usu. for cocoons; *esp* : a lustrous tough elastic fiber produced by silkworms and used for textiles **2** : strands of silk thread of various thicknesses used as suture material in surgery 〈surgical ∼〉

silk vine *n* : a Eurasian woody nearly evergreen vine of the genus *Periploca* (*P. graeca*) with silky seeds that is a source of the glycosides periplocin and periplocymarin

sil·ver \'sil-vər\ *n* : a white metallic element that is sonorous, ductile, very malleable, capable of a high degree of polish, and chiefly monovalent in compounds, and that has the highest thermal and electric conductivity of any substance — symbol *Ag*; see ELEMENT table

silver iodide *n* : a compound AgI that darkens on exposure to light and is used in medicine as a local antiseptic

silver nitrate *n* : an irritant compound $AgNO_3$ that in contact with organic matter turns black and is used as a chemical reagent, in photography, and in medicine esp. as an antiseptic and caustic

silver protein *n* : any of several colloidal light-sensitive preparations of silver and protein used in aqueous solution on mucous membranes as antiseptics and classified by their efficacy and irritant properties: as **a** : a preparation containing 19 to 23 percent of silver and consisting of dark brown or almost black shining scales or granules — called also *mild silver protein* **b** : a more irritant preparation containing 7.5 to 8.5 percent of silver and consisting of a pale yellowish orange to brownish black powder — called also *strong silver protein*

Sil·ves·ter method \sil-'ves-tər-\ *n* : a method of artificial respiration in which the subject is laid on his or her back and

\ə\ abut \ᵊ\ kitten \ər\ further \a\ ash \ā\ ace \ä\ cot, cart \au̇\ out \ch\ chin \e\ bet \ē\ easy \g\ go \i\ hit \ī\ ice \j\ job \ŋ\ sing \ō\ go \ȯ\ law \ȯi\ boy \th\ thin \t̶h\ the \ü\ loot \u̇\ foot \y\ yet \zh\ vision   *See also* Pronunciation Symbols page

air is expelled from the lungs by pressing the arms over the chest and fresh air drawn in by pulling them above the head

Silvester, Henry Robert (1828–1908), British physician. Silvester introduced his method of artificial respiration in 1858.

sil·y·mar·in \ˌsil-i-ˈmar-ən\ *n* : an antioxidant flavonoid $C_{25}H_{22}O_{10}$ consisting of a mixture of three isomers isolated from seeds of the milk thistle, held to have properties protecting the liver from or clearing it of toxins, and used in dietary supplements and herbal remedies

Sim·a·rou·ba \ˌsim-ə-ˈrü-bə\ *n* : a genus (the type of the family Simaroubaceae) of tropical American shrubs and trees having bitter bark sometimes used medicinally — compare QUASSIA 1

si·meth·i·cone \si-ˈmeth-i-ˌkōn, sī-\ *n* : a mixture of dimethylpolysiloxanes and silica in liquid or tablet form that is used as an antiflatulent — see MYLICON

sim·i·an crease \ˈsim-ē-ən-\ *n* : a deep crease extending across the palm that results from the fusion of the two normally occurring horizontal palmar creases and is found esp. in individuals with Down syndrome

simian immunodeficiency virus *n* : SIV

simian virus 40 \-ˈfȯrt-ē\ *n* : a double-stranded DNA virus of the genus *Polyomavirus* (species *Simian virus 40*) that infects monkeys and has been shown experimentally to cause tumors in laboratory animals (as newborn hamsters) — called also *SV40*

Sim·monds' disease \ˈsim-ən(d)z-\ *n* : a disease that is characterized by extreme and progressive emaciation with atrophy of internal organs, loss of body hair, and evidences of premature aging resulting from atrophy or destruction of the anterior lobe of the pituitary gland

Sim·monds \ˈzim-ȯnts\, **Morris (1855–1925)**, German physician. Simmonds described a disease caused by atrophy of the anterior lobe of the pituitary gland in 1914.

¹sim·ple \ˈsim-pəl\ *adj* **sim·pler** \-p(ə-)lər\; **sim·plest** \-p(ə-)ləst\ **1** : free from complexity or difficulty: as **a** : easily treated or cured ⟨a ~ vitamin deficiency⟩ **b** : controlled by a single gene ⟨~ inherited characters⟩ **2** : of, relating to, or being an epithelium in which the cells are arranged in a single layer

²simple *n* **1** : a medicinal plant **2** : a vegetable drug having only one ingredient

simple fracture *n* : a bone fracture that does not form an open wound in the skin — compare COMPOUND FRACTURE

simple mastectomy *n* : a mastectomy in which the breast tissue, associated skin, nipple, and areola are removed — called also *total mastectomy*

simple ointment *n* : WHITE OINTMENT

simple sugar *n* : MONOSACCHARIDE

simplex — see EPIDERMOLYSIS BULLOSA SIMPLEX, GENITAL HERPES SIMPLEX, HERPES SIMPLEX, ICHTHYOSIS SIMPLEX, LICHEN SIMPLEX CHRONICUS, PERIODONTITIS SIMPLEX

Sim·plex·vi·rus \ˈsim-ˌpleks-ˌvī-rəs\ *n* : a genus of double-stranded DNA viruses of the family *Herpesviridae* that usu. infect primates including two (HSV-1 and HSV-2) specific for humans and that tend to persist in the host as latent infections in neurons

sim·u·late \ˈsim-yə-ˌlāt\ *vt* **-lat·ed; -lat·ing** : to have or produce a symptomatic resemblance to ⟨lesions *simulating* leprosy⟩ — **sim·u·la·tion** \ˌsim-yə-ˈlā-shən\ *n*

sim·u·la·tor \ˈsim-yə-ˌlāt-ər\ *n* : a device that enables the operator to reproduce or represent under test conditions phenomena likely to occur in actual performance ⟨a driving ~ used to study behavior in highway emergencies⟩

Sim·u·li·i·dae \ˌsim-yə-ˈlī-ə-ˌdē\ *n pl* : a family of small biting dipteran flies including the blackflies and related pests and having larvae that usu. live in rapidly flowing water

Si·mu·li·um \si-ˈmyü-lē-əm\ *n* : the type genus of the family Simuliidae comprising dark-colored bloodsucking dipteran flies of which some are vectors of onchocerciasis or of protozoan diseases of birds — see BLACKFLY

sim·va·stat·in \ˈsim-və-ˌstat-ᵊn, ˌsim-və-ˈstat-\ *n* : a semisynthetic lipid-lowering drug $C_{25}H_{38}O_5$ derived from a compound produced by a mold of the genus *Aspergillus* (*A. terreus*) and administered orally to lower a high cholesterol level in the blood by inhibiting the action of an enzyme catalyzing the synthesis of cholesterol — see VYTORIN, ZOCOR

si·nal \ˈsī-nᵊl\ *adj* : of, relating to, or coming from a sinus ⟨a ~ discharge⟩

sin·a·pism \ˈsin-ə-ˌpiz-əm\ *n* : MUSTARD PLASTER

sin·cip·i·tal \sin-ˈsip-ət-ᵊl\ *adj* : of or relating to the sinciput

sin·ci·put \ˈsin(t)-sə-(ˌ)pət\ *n, pl* **sinciputs** *or* **sin·cip·i·ta** \sin-ˈsip-ət-ə\ **1** : FOREHEAD **2** : the upper half of the skull

Sind·bis virus \ˈsind-bis-\ *n* : a togavirus of the genus *Alphavirus* (species *Sindbis virus*) that is transmitted by mosquitoes and causes a febrile disease marked by joint pain, a rash, and malaise in parts of Africa, the Middle East, Europe, Asia, and Australia

Sin·e·met \ˈsin-ə-ˌmet\ *trademark* — used for a preparation containing carbidopa and L-dopa

Sin·e·quan \ˈsin-ə-ˌkwan\ *trademark* — used for a preparation of the hydrochloride of doxepin

sin·ew \ˈsin-(ˌ)yü, -yə(-w) *also* ˈsin-(ˌ)ü\ *n* : TENDON

sin·gle–blind \ˌsiŋ-gəl-ˈblīnd\ *adj* : of, relating to, or being an experimental procedure in which the experimenters but not the subjects know the makeup of the test and control groups during the actual course of the experiments — compare DOUBLE-BLIND, OPEN-LABEL

single bond *n* : a chemical bond consisting of one covalent bond between two atoms in a molecule esp. when the atoms can have more than one bond

single nucleotide polymorphism *n* : SNP

single photon absorptiometry *n* : a scanning technique using photons of a single energy to measure the density of a material and esp. bone

single photon emission computed tomography *n* : a medical imaging technique that is used esp. for mapping brain function and that is similar to positron-emission tomography in using the photons emitted by the agency of a radioactive tracer to create an image but that differs in being able to detect only a single photon for each nuclear disintegration and in generating a lower-quality image — abbr. *SPECT*

sin·gle·ton \ˈsiŋ-gəl-tən\ *n* : an offspring born singly

Sin·gu·lair \ˌsiŋ-gyə-ˈler\ *trademark* — used for a preparation of the sodium salt of montelukast

sin·gul·tus \siŋ-ˈgəl-təs\ *n* : HICCUP

sin·i·grin \ˈsin-i-grin\ *n* : a crystalline glucoside $C_{10}H_{16}KNO_9S_2$ found in the seeds of black mustard (*Brassica nigra*) from which allyl isothiocyanate is obtained — compare MUSTARD OIL 1

sinistra — see COLICA SINISTRA

¹si·nis·tral \ˈsin-əs-trəl, sə-ˈnis-\ *adj* : of, relating to, or inclined to the left; *esp* : LEFT-HANDED

²sinistral *n* : a person exhibiting dominance of the left hand and eye : a left-handed person

sin·is·tral·i·ty \ˌsin-ə-ˈstral-ət-ē\ *n, pl* **-ties** : the quality or state of having the left side or one or more of its parts (as the hand or eye) different from and usu. more efficient than the right or its corresponding parts; *also* : LEFT-HANDEDNESS

sin·is·troc·u·lar \ˌsin-ə-ˈsträk-yə-lər\ *adj* : using the left eye habitually or more effectively than the right

si·no·atri·al \ˌsī-nō-ˈā-trē-əl\ *also* **si·nu·atri·al** \ˌsī-n(y)ü-\ *adj* : of, involving, or being the sinoatrial node ⟨~ block⟩

sinoatrial node *n* : a small mass of tissue that is made up of Purkinje fibers, ganglion cells, and nerve fibers, that is embedded in the musculature of the right atrium of higher vertebrates, and that originates the impulses stimulating the heartbeat — called also *S-A node, sinus node*

si·no·au·ric·u·lar \-ȯ-ˈrik-yə-lər\ *adj* : SINOATRIAL

si·no·gram \ˈsī-nə-ˌgram\ *n* : a radiograph of a sinus following the injection of a radiopaque medium

si·nog·ra·phy \sī-ˈnäg-rə-fē\ *n, pl* **-phies** : radiography of a sinus following the injection of a radiopaque medium

si·no·pul·mo·nary \ˌsī-nō-ˈpùl-mə-ˌner-ē, -ˈpəl-\ *adj* : of, relating to, involving, or affecting the paranasal sinuses and the airway of the lungs ⟨∼ infections⟩ ⟨the ∼ tract⟩

si·no·res·pi·ra·to·ry \ˌsī-nō-ˈres-p(ə-)rə-ˌtōr-ē, -ri-ˈspī-rə-, -ˌtȯr-ē\ *adj* : of, relating to, or affecting both the sinuses and the respiratory tract ⟨∼ infection⟩

sin·se·mil·la \ˌsin-sə-ˈmē-yə, -ˈmēl-, -ˈmil-; -ˈmēl-ə, -ˈmil-\ *n* : highly potent marijuana from female plants that are specially tended and kept seedless by preventing pollination in order to induce a high resin content; *also* : a female hemp plant grown to produce sinsemilla

sin·ter \ˈsint-ər\ *vt* : to cause to become a coherent mass by heating without melting ⟨the binding of ∼ed hydroxyapatite with bone⟩

sinuatrial *var of* SINOATRIAL

si·nus \ˈsī-nəs\ *n* : a cavity or hollow in the body: as **a** : a narrow elongated tract extending from a focus of suppuration and serving for the discharge of pus ⟨a tuberculous ∼⟩ **b** (1) : a cavity in the substance of a bone of the skull that usu. communicates with the nostrils and contains air (2) : a channel for venous blood (3) : a dilatation in a bodily canal or vessel

sinus bradycardia *n* : abnormally slow sinus rhythm; *specif* : sinus rhythm at a rate lower than 60 beats per minute

si·nus·itis \ˌsī-n(y)ə-ˈsīt-əs\ *n* : inflammation of a sinus of the skull

sinus node *n* : SINOATRIAL NODE

sinus of Mor·ga·gni \-ˌmȯr-ˈgän-yē\ *n* : a space at the upper back part of each side of the pharynx where the walls are deficient in muscular fibers between the upper border of the superior constrictor and the base of the skull and closed only by the aponeurosis of the pharynx

G. B. Morgagni — see CRYPT OF MORGAGNI

sinus of the dura mater *n* : any of numerous venous channels (as the sagittal sinuses, straight sinus, and transverse sinuses) that are situated between the two layers of the dura mater, that have no valves, and that drain blood from the brain and the bones forming the cranium and empty it into the internal jugular vein — called also *dural sinus*

sinus of Val·sal·va \-ˌväl-ˈsäl-və\ *n* : any one of the pouches of the aorta and pulmonary artery which are located behind the flaps of the semilunar valves and into which the blood in its regurgitation toward the heart enters and thereby closes the valves — called also *aortic sinus*

Valsalva, Antonio Maria (1666–1723), Italian anatomist. In 1704 Valsalva published a major treatise on the anatomy and physiology of the human ear. Among other things this work is notable for its outstanding illustrations. For the middle ear he gave clear illustrations of the hammer and the tube, calling the latter the eustachian tube. He described the morphology of the pharyngeal musculature and the muscle fasciae controlling the eustachian tube. In his treatise on the ear he introduced the Valsalva maneuver. The maneuver was originally designed as a method of removing foreign bodies from the ear. As a surgeon Valsalva did work in ophthalmology and rhinology and performed vasal and tumor surgery.

si·nu·soid \ˈsī-n(y)ə-ˌsȯid\ *n* : a minute endothelium-lined space or passage for blood in the tissues of an organ (as the liver) — **si·nu·soi·dal** \ˌsī-n(y)ə-ˈsȯid-ᵊl\ *adj* — **si·nu·soi·dal·ly** \-ᵊl-ē\ *adv*

si·nus·ot·o·my \ˌsī-n(y)ə-ˈsät-ə-mē\ *n, pl* **-mies** : surgical incision into a sinus of the skull

sinus rhom·boi·da·lis \-ˌräm-ˌbȯid-ˈā-ləs\ *n* : the posterior expanded and for a long time incompletely closed part of the neural groove of vertebrate embryos; *also* : an expansion of the central canal in the sacral region derived from it

sinus rhythm *n* : the rhythm of the heart produced by impulses from the sinoatrial node

sinus tachycardia *n* : abnormally rapid sinus rhythm; *specif* : sinus rhythm at a rate greater than 100 beats per minute

sinus ter·mi·na·lis \-ˌtər-mi-ˈnā-ləs\ *n* : a circular blood sinus bordering the area vasculosa of the vertebrate embryo

si·nus ve·no·sus \ˌsī-nəs-vi-ˈnō-səs\ *n* : an enlarged pouch that adjoins the heart, is formed by the union of the large systemic veins, and is the passage through which venous blood enters the heart in lower vertebrates and in embryos of higher forms

sinus venosus scle·rae \-ˈsklē-rē\ *n* : CANAL OF SCHLEMM

sinuum — see CONFLUENS SINUUM

Si·phon·ap·tera \ˌsī-fən-ˈap-tə-rə\ *n pl* : an order of insects consisting of the fleas

si·pho·no·phore \sī-ˈfän-ə-ˌfō(ə)r, ˈsī-fə-nə-, -ˌfȯ(ə)r\ *n* : any of an order (Siphonophora) of compound free-swimming or floating pelagic hydrozoans — see PORTUGUESE MAN-OF-WAR

Si·phun·cu·li·na \(ˌ)sī-ˌfən-kyə-ˈlē-nə\ *n* : a genus of dipteran flies of the family Chloropidae that includes an eye gnat (*S. funicola*) responsible for spreading conjunctivitis in southeastern Asia

Sip·py diet \ˈsip-ē-\ *n* : a bland diet for the treatment of peptic ulcer consisting mainly of measured amounts of milk and cream, farina, and egg taken at regular hourly intervals for a specified period of time

Sippy, Bertram Welton (1866–1924), American physician. Sippy was a professor of medicine at Rush Medical College in Chicago. In 1915 he published a description of his special diet for the treatment of peptic ulcer.

¹sire \ˈsī(ə)r\ *n* : the male parent of an animal and esp. of a domestic animal

²sire *vt* **sired; sir·ing** : to procreate as the male parent of

si·re·no·me·lia \ˌsī-rə-nō-ˈmē-lē-ə\ *n* : a congenital malformation in which the lower limbs are fused

si·re·nom·e·lus \ˌsī-rə-ˈnäm-ə-ləs\ *n, pl* **-li** \-ˌlī\ : an individual exhibiting sirenomelia

si·ri·a·sis \si-ˈrī-ə-səs\ *n, pl* **-a·ses** \-ˌsēz\ : SUNSTROKE

SIRS *abbr* systemic inflammatory response syndrome

sirup, sirupy *var of* SYRUP, SYRUPY

sis·ter \ˈsis-tər\ *n, chiefly Brit* : a head nurse in a hospital ward or clinic; *broadly* : NURSE

sister chromatid *n* : any of the chromatids formed by replication of one chromosome during interphase of the cell cycle esp. while they are still joined by a centromere

Sis·tru·rus \si-ˈstrūr-əs\ *n* : a genus of small rattlesnakes (as a massasauga) having the top of the head covered with scales

site \ˈsīt\ *n* : the place, scene, or point of something ⟨the ∼ of inflammation⟩ — see ACTIVE SITE

sit·fast \ˈsit-ˌfast\ *n* : a callosity with inflamed edges formed on a horse's back by the chafing of the saddle — called also *setfast*

si·to·sta·nol \ˌsī-tō-ˈstan-ᵊl, sə-ˈtäs-tə-ˌnȯl\ *n* : a plant sterol $C_{29}H_{52}O$ that is derived from sitosterol and has been shown to significantly reduce serum cholesterol by inhibiting cholesterol absorption when made part of the human diet

si·tos·ter·ol \sī-ˈtäs-tə-ˌrȯl, sə-, -ˌrōl\ *n* : any of several sterols that are widespread esp. in plant products (as wheat germ or soybean oil) and are used as starting materials for the synthesis of steroid hormones

situ — see IN SITU

sit·u·a·tion \ˌsich-ə-ˈwā-shən\ *n* **1** : the way in which something is placed in relation to its surroundings **2** : the total set of physical, social, and psychocultural factors that act upon an individual in orienting and conditioning his or her behavior **3** : relative position or combination of circumstances at a particular moment

sit·u·a·tion·al \-shnəl, -shən-ᵊl\ *adj* : of, relating to, or occurring in a particular set of circumstances ⟨∼ impotence⟩ ⟨∼ hypertension⟩ — **sit·u·a·tion·al·ly** \-ē\ *adv*

si·tus \ˈsīt-əs\ *n* : the place where something exists or originates : SITE ⟨∼ of an inflammation⟩

situs in·ver·sus \-in-ˈvər-səs\ *n* : a congenital abnormality characterized by lateral transposition of the viscera (as of the heart or the liver)

sitz bath \ˈsits-\ *n* **1** : a tub in which one bathes in a sitting

\ə\ abut \ᵊ\ kitten \ər\ further \a\ ash \ā\ ace \ä\ cot, cart \aù\ out \ch\ chin \e\ bet \ē\ easy \g\ go \i\ hit \ī\ ice \j\ job \ŋ\ sing \ō\ go \ȯ\ law \ȯi\ boy \th\ thin \th\ the \ü\ loot \ù\ foot \y\ yet \zh\ vision *See also* Pronunciation Symbols page

posture **2** : a bath in which the hips and buttocks are immersed in hot water for the therapeutic effect of moist heat in the perineal and anal regions

SIV \,es-,ī-'vē\ *n* : a retrovirus of the genus *Lentivirus* (species *Simian immunodeficiency virus*) that causes a disease in monkeys similar to AIDS and that is closely related to HIV-2 of humans — called also *simian immunodeficiency virus*

six–o–six *or* **606** \,sik-,sō-'siks\ *n* : ARSPHENAMINE

sixth cranial nerve \'siks(th)-\ *n* : ABDUCENS NERVE

six–year molar \,siks-,yi(ə)r-\ *n* : one of the first permanent molar teeth of which there are four including one on each side of the upper and lower jaws and which erupt at about six years of age — called also *sixth-year molar;* compare TWELVE-YEAR MOLAR

Sjö·gren's syndrome *also* **Sjögren syndrome** \'shȫ-,gren(z)-\ *n* : a chronic inflammatory autoimmune disease that affects esp. older women, that is characterized by dryness of mucous membranes esp. of the eyes and mouth and by infiltration of the affected tissues by lymphocytes, and that is often associated with rheumatoid arthritis — called also *sicca syndrome, Sjögren's, Sjögren's disease*

Sjögren, Henrik Samuel Conrad (1899–1986), Swedish ophthalmologist. Sjögren served as a professor of medicine at Lund, Sweden, and eventually held the position of chief physician at the hospital there. He invented ophthalmological instruments. He first described Sjögren's syndrome in 1933.

SK *abbr* streptokinase

ska·tole \'skat-,ōl, 'skāt-\ *also* **ska·tol** \-,ōl, -,ōl\ *n* : a foul-smelling compound C_9H_9N found in the intestines and feces, in civet, and in several plants or made synthetically and used in perfumes as a fixative

skel·e·tal \'skel-ət-ºl, *Brit sometimes* ske-'lēt-ºl\ *adj* : of, relating to, forming, attached to, or resembling a skeleton ⟨∼ structures⟩ ⟨the ∼ system⟩

skeletal muscle *n* : striated muscle that is usu. attached to the skeleton and is usu. under voluntary control; *also* : a muscle composed of skeletal muscle

skel·e·tog·e·nous \,skel-ə-'täj-ə-nəs\ *adj* : forming skeletal tissue : OSTEOGENIC

skel·e·to·mus·cu·lar \,skel-ə-tō-'məs-kyə-lər\ *adj* : constituting, belonging to, or dependent upon the skeleton and the muscles that move it ⟨the ∼ system⟩

skel·e·ton \'skel-ət-ºn\ *n* **1** : a usu. rigid supportive or protective structure or framework of an organism; *esp* : the bony or more or less cartilaginous framework supporting the soft tissues and protecting the internal organs of a vertebrate **2** : the straight or branched chain or ring of atoms that forms the basic structure of an organic molecule

skene·i·tis *also* **sken·i·tis** \skē-'nīt-əs\ *n* : inflammation of the paraurethral glands

Skene's gland \'skēnz-\ *n* : PARAURETHRAL GLAND

Skene, Alexander Johnston Chalmers (1838–1900), American gynecologist. Skene was a pioneer in the field of gynecology and the author of over a hundred medical papers. In 1878 he published a monograph on the diseases of the bladder and urethra in women. Two years later he reported on his discovery of the paraurethral glands, now also known as Skene's glands. He is also credited with devising 31 surgical instruments.

skia·gram \'skī-ə-,gram\ *n* : RADIOGRAPH

skia·graph \-,graf\ *n* : RADIOGRAPH

skia·scope \'skī-ə-,skōp\ *n* : a device for determining the refractive state of the eye from the movement of retinal lights and shadows

ski·as·co·py \skī-'as-kə-pē\ *n, pl* **-pies** : RETINOSCOPY

skilled nursing facility \,skild-\ *n* : a health-care institution that meets federal criteria for Medicaid and Medicare reimbursement for nursing care including esp. the supervision of the care of every patient by a physician, the employment full-time of at least one registered nurse, the maintenance of records concerning the care and condition of every patient, the availability of nursing care 24 hours a day, the presence of facilities for storing and dispensing drugs, the implemen-

tation of a utilization review plan, and overall financial planning including an annual operating budget and a 3-year capital expenditures program

skim milk \,skim-\ *n* : milk from which the cream has been taken — called also *skimmed milk*

¹**skin** \'skin\ *n* : the 2-layered covering of the body consisting of an outer ectodermal epidermis that is more or less cornified and penetrated by the openings of sweat and sebaceous glands and an inner mesodermal dermis that is composed largely of connective tissue and is richly supplied with blood vessels and nerves

²**skin** *vt* **skinned; skin·ning** : to cut or scrape the skin of ⟨fell and *skinned* his knee⟩

skin erythema dose *n* : the minimal dose of radiation required to cause perceptible reddening of the skin — abbr. *SED*

skin·fold \'skin-,fōld\ *n, often attrib* : a fold of skin formed by pinching or compressing the skin and subcutaneous layers esp. in order to estimate the amount of body fat

skinfold caliper *n* : a pair of calipers used to form and measure the thickness of skinfolds in order to estimate the amount of body fat — usu. used in pl.

skin graft *n* : a piece of skin that is surgically removed from a donor area to replace skin in a defective or denuded area (as one that has been burned); *also* : the procedure by which such a piece of skin is removed and transferred to a new area

skin grafting *n* : the action or process of making a skin graft

skinned \'skind\ *adj* : having skin esp. of a specified kind — usu. used in combination ⟨dark-*skinned*⟩

Skin·ner box \'skin-ər-,bäks\ *n* : a laboratory apparatus in which an animal is caged for experiments in operant conditioning and which typically contains a lever that must be pressed by the animal to gain reward or avoid punishment

Skinner, Burrhus Frederic (1904–1990), American psychologist. Skinner made a major contribution to 20th-century psychology. He is famous as a major proponent of behaviorism, a philosophy that studies human behavior in terms of physiological responses to the environment and believes that human nature can be revealed through the controlled scientific study of these responses. Skinner conducted innovative experiments in animal learning, training laboratory animals to perform a number of complex actions. To carry out some of his experiments he designed the Skinner box, an apparatus later adopted by pharmaceutical research for observing the effects of drugs on animal behavior. His work with research animals led to his development of the principles of programmed learning. His revolutionary innovations in educational method included the invention of teaching machines. Central to his methods was the concept of reinforcement, or reward.

¹**Skin·ner·ian** \ski-'nir-ē-ən, -'ner-\ *adj* : of, relating to, or suggestive of the behavioristic theories of B. F. Skinner

²**Skinnerian** *n* : an advocate of the behavioristic theories of B. F. Skinner

skin patch *n* : PATCH 1b

skin tag \-,tag\ *n* : a small soft pendulous growth on the skin esp. around the eyes or on the neck, armpits, or groin — called also *acrochordon*

skin test *n* : a test (as a scratch test or a tuberculin test) for an allergic or immune response to a substance that is performed by administering the substance to or through the skin and is used esp. in detecting allergic hypersensitivity

skin testing *n* : the process of administering and interpreting skin tests

skull \'skəl\ *n* : the skeleton of the head forming a bony case that encloses and protects the brain and chief sense organs and supports the jaws

skull·cap \'skəl-,kap\ *n* : the upper portion of the skull : CALVARIUM

slant \'slant\ *n* : a culture medium solidified obliquely in a tube so as to increase the surface area ⟨a blood-agar ∼⟩ — compare STAB 2a

slant culture *n* : a culture (as of bacteria) made by inoculating the surface of a slant

¹sla·ver \'slav-ər, 'slāv-, 'släv-\ *vi* **sla·vered; sla·ver·ing** \-(ə-)riŋ\ : DROOL

²slaver *n* : saliva dribbling from the mouth

SLE *abbr* systemic lupus erythematosus

¹sleep \'slēp\ *n* **1** : the natural periodic suspension of consciousness during which the powers of the body are restored — compare REM SLEEP, SLOW-WAVE SLEEP **2** : a state resembling sleep: as **a** : DEATH 1 ⟨put a pet cat to ∼⟩ **b** : a state marked by a diminution of feeling followed by tingling ⟨her foot went to ∼⟩

²sleep *vi* **slept** \'slept\; **sleep·ing** : to rest in a state of sleep

sleep apnea *n* : brief periods of recurrent cessation of breathing during sleep that is caused esp. by obstruction of the airway or a disturbance in the brain's respiratory center and is associated esp. with excessive daytime sleepiness

sleeping pill *n* : a drug and esp. a barbiturate that is taken as a tablet or capsule to induce sleep — called also *sleeping tablet*

sleeping sickness *n* **1** : a serious disease that is prevalent in much of tropical Africa, is marked by fever, headache, protracted lethargy, confusion, sleep disturbances, tremors, and loss of weight, is caused by either of two trypanosomes (*Trypanosoma brucei gambiense* and *T. b. rhodesiense*), and is transmitted by tsetse flies — called also *African sleeping sickness* **2** : any of various viral encephalitides or encephalomyelitides of which lethargy or somnolence is a prominent feature; *esp* : EQUINE ENCEPHALOMYELITIS

sleeping tablet *n, chiefly Brit* : SLEEPING PILL

sleep–learn·ing \-ˌlərn-iŋ\ *n* : HYPNOPEDIA

sleep·less \'slē-pləs\ *adj* : not able to sleep : INSOMNIAC — **sleep·less·ness** *n*

sleep paralysis *n* : a complete temporary paralysis occurring in connection with sleep and esp. upon waking

sleep spindle *n* : a burst of synchronous alpha waves that occurs during light sleep

sleep–teach·ing \-ˌtēch-iŋ\ *n* : HYPNOPEDIA

sleep·walk·er \'slēp-ˌwȯ-kər\ *n* : one who is subject to somnambulism : one who walks while sleeping — called also *somnambulist* — **sleep·walk** \-ˌwȯk\ *vi*

sleepy \'slē-pē\ *adj* **sleep·i·er; -est** : ready to fall asleep — **sleep·i·ness** \-pē-nəs\ *n*

sleepy sickness *n, Brit* : ENCEPHALITIS LETHARGICA

slept *past and past part of* SLEEP

slide \'slīd\ *n* : a flat piece of glass or plastic on which an object is mounted for microscopic examination

slid·ing filament hypothesis \'slīd-iŋ-\ *n* : a theory in physiology holding that muscle contraction occurs when the actin filaments next to the Z line at each end of a sarcomere are drawn toward each other between the thicker myosin filaments more centrally located in the sarcomere by the projecting globular heads of myosin molecules that form temporary attachments to the actin filaments and become detached when the actin filaments move in the opposite directions toward the ends of the sarcomere — called also *sliding filament theory;* see CROSSBRIDGE

sliding microtome *n* : a microtome in which the object to be cut is fixed and the knife is carried obliquely across it

slim disease \'slim-\ *n* : AIDS; *also* : severe wasting of the body in the later stages of AIDS

slime bacterium \'slīm-\ *n* : MYXOBACTERIUM

slime mold *n* : any organism of the group Myxomycetes — called also *myxomycete*

sling \'sliŋ\ *n* **1** : a hanging bandage suspended from the neck to support an arm or hand **2** : a harness esp. constructed for supporting a sick animal in a standing position

slipped disk \ˌslipt-\ *n* : a protrusion of an intervertebral disk and its nucleus pulposus that produces pressure upon spinal nerves resulting in low-back pain and often sciatic pain

slipped tendon *n* : PEROSIS

slit lamp \'slit-ˌlamp\ *n* : a lamp for projecting a narrow beam of intense light that is used in conjunction with a biomicroscope for examining the anterior parts (as the conjunctiva or cornea) of an eye; *also* : a unit consisting of both the lamp and biomicroscope

¹slough \'sləf\ *n* : dead tissue separating from living tissue; *esp* : a mass of dead tissue separating from an ulcer

²slough *vi* : to separate in the form of dead tissue from living tissue ⟨dermal ∼*ing*⟩ ∼ *vt* : to cast off ⟨∼ dead tissue⟩ ⟨the uterine lining is ∼*ed*⟩

slow infection \'slō-\ *n* : a degenerative disease (as scrapie or Creutzfeldt-Jakob disease) caused by a slow virus

slow–reacting substance *n* : SLOW-REACTING SUBSTANCE OF ANAPHYLAXIS — *abbr. SRS*

slow–reacting substance of anaphylaxis *n* : a mixture of three leukotrienes produced in anaphylaxis that causes contraction of smooth muscle after minutes in contrast to histamine which acts in seconds and that is prob. responsible for the bronchoconstriction occurring in anaphylaxis — *abbr. SRS-A*

slow–re·lease \ˌslō-ri-ˌlēs\ *adj* : SUSTAINED-RELEASE

slow–twitch \ˌslō-ˌtwich\ *adj* : of, relating to, or being muscle fiber that contracts slowly esp. during sustained physical activity requiring endurance — compare FAST-TWITCH

slow virus *n* : any of various viruses or prions having a long incubation period between infection and the clinical appearance of the slowly progressive serious or fatal disease (as scrapie or Creutzfeldt-Jakob disease) associated with it

slow wave *n* : DELTA WAVE

slow–wave sleep *n* : a state of deep usu. dreamless sleep that occurs regularly during a normal period of sleep with intervening periods of REM sleep and that is characterized by delta waves and a low level of autonomic physiological activity — called also *non-REM sleep, NREM sleep, orthodox sleep, S sleep, synchronized sleep*

¹sludge \'sləj\ *n* : a semisolid precipitated mass or deposit ⟨biliary ∼⟩; *esp* : SLUDGED BLOOD

²sludge *vi* **sludged; sludg·ing** : to form sludge ⟨positions that cause blood to ∼ —L. K. Altman⟩

sludged blood *n* : blood in which the red blood cells become massed along the walls of the blood vessels and reduce the lumen of the vessels and the rate of blood flow

slug·gish \'sləg-ish\ *adj* : markedly slow in movement, progression, or response ⟨∼ healing⟩ — **slug·gish·ly** *adv* — **slug·gish·ness** *n*

slur·ry \'slər-ē, 'slə-rē\ *n, pl* **slur·ries** : a watery mixture of insoluble matter

Sm *symbol* samarium

small bowel \'smȯl-\ *n* : SMALL INTESTINE

small calorie *n* : CALORIE 1a

small cardiac vein *n* : CARDIAC VEIN c

small–cell lung cancer *n* : cancer of a highly malignant form that affects the lungs, tends to metastasize to other parts of the body, and is characterized by small round or oval cells resembling oat grains and having a high ratio of nuclear protoplasm to cytoplasm — called also *oat-cell cancer, oat-cell carcinoma, small-cell carcinoma, small-cell lung carcinoma*

small intestine *n* : the part of the intestine that lies between the stomach and colon, consists of duodenum, jejunum, and ileum, secretes digestive enzymes, and is the chief site of the absorption of digested nutrients — called also *small bowel*

small·pox \'smȯl-ˌpäks\ *n* : an acute contagious febrile disease of humans that is caused by a poxvirus of the genus *Orthopoxvirus* (species *Variola virus*), is characterized by skin eruption with pustules, sloughing, and scar formation, and is believed to have been eradicated globally by widespread vaccination — called also *variola;* see VARIOLA MAJOR, VARIOLA MINOR

small saphenous vein *n* : SAPHENOUS VEIN b

smart \'smärt\ *vi* : to cause or be the cause or seat of a sharp poignant pain ⟨rapid fatigue with burning and ∼*ing* of the conjunctiva —H. G. Armstrong⟩; *also* : to feel or have such a pain

---

\ə\ abut \ᵊ\ kitten \ər\ **further** \a\ **ash** \ā\ **ace** \ä\ **cot, cart**
\au̇\ **out** \ch\ **chin** \e\ **bet** \ē\ **easy** \g\ **go** \i\ **hit** \ī\ **ice** \j\ **job**
\ŋ\ **sing** \ō\ **go** \ȯ\ **law** \ȯi\ **boy** \th\ **thin** \t͟h\ **the** \ü\ **loot**
\u̇\ **foot** \y\ **yet** \zh\ **vision** *See also* Pronunciation Symbols page

S
T

smart drug *n* : NOOTROPIC

¹**smear** \'smi(ə)r\ *n* : material spread on a surface (as of a microscopic slide); *also* : a preparation made by spreading material on a surface — see PAP SMEAR, VAGINAL SMEAR

²**smear** *vt* : to prepare as a smear for microscopic examination : make a smear of

¹**smec·tic** \'smek-tik\ *adj* : of, relating to, or being the phase of a liquid crystal characterized by the arrangement of the molecules in layers with the long axes of the molecules in a given layer being parallel to one another and perpendicular to the plane of the layer ⟨a ~ phase of cholesterol esters in denatured LDL⟩ — compare MESOMORPHIC 1, NEMATIC

²**smectic** *n* : a liquid crystal in its smectic phase

smeg·ma \'smeg-mə\ *n* : the secretion of a sebaceous gland; *specif* : the cheesy sebaceous matter that collects between the glans penis and the foreskin or around the clitoris and labia minora

smegma bacillus *n* : an acid-fast bacterium of the genus *Mycobacterium* (*M. smegmatis*) found in smegma

¹**smell** \'smel\ *vb* **smelled** \'smeld\ *or* **smelt** \'smelt\; **smell·ing** *vt* : to perceive the odor or scent of through stimuli affecting the olfactory nerves : get the odor or scent of with the nose ~ *vi* : to exercise the sense of smell

²**smell** *n* **1** : the property of a thing that affects the olfactory organs : ODOR **2** : the special sense concerned with the perception of odor

smell brain *n* : RHINENCEPHALON

smelling salts *n pl but sing or pl in constr* : a usu. scented aromatic preparation of ammonium carbonate and ammonia water used as a stimulant and restorative

Smi·lax \'smī-ˌlaks\ *n* : a large widely distributed genus of plants of the lily family (Liliaceae) which includes the sarsaparillas

Smith fracture \'smith-\ *or* **Smith's fracture** \'smiths-\ *n* : a fracture of the lower portion of the radius with forward displacement of the lower fragment — compare COLLES' FRACTURE

Smith, Robert William (1807–1873), British surgeon. Smith is best known for his description of generalized neurofibromatosis, which was included in his 1849 treatise on the pathology, diagnosis, and treatment of neuroma. He described the Smith fracture in 1847 in a treatise on fractures and dislocations.

Smith–Pe·ter·sen nail \'smith-'pēt-ər-sən-\ *n* : a flanged metal nail used to fix the femoral head in fractures of the neck of the femur

Smith–Petersen, Marius Nygaard (1886–1953), American orthopedic surgeon. Smith-Petersen practiced orthopedic surgery in Boston. He had long-term associations with Massachusetts General Hospital and Harvard Medical School. In 1925 he introduced a three-flanged steel nail for insertion across the fracture site in hip fractures. This innovation reduced considerably the death rate from hip fracture and brought about successful unions of fragments in a greater percentage of the cases. To further improve hip disabilities he developed an operative procedure which involved placing a Vitallium alloy cup or mold between surgically reshaped joint surfaces. The operation was widely adopted from 1938 on.

smog \'smäg *also* 'smȯg\ *n* : a fog made heavier and darker by smoke and chemical fumes; *also* : a photochemical haze caused by the action of solar ultraviolet radiation on atmosphere polluted with hydrocarbons and oxides of nitrogen esp. from automobile exhaust

smoke \'smōk\ *vb* **smoked; smok·ing** *vi* : to inhale and exhale the fumes of burning plant material and esp. tobacco; *esp* : to smoke tobacco habitually ~ *vt* : to inhale and exhale the smoke of ⟨*smoked* 30 cigarettes a day⟩

smok·er \'smō-kər\ *n* : a person who smokes habitually

smooth \'smüth\ *adj* : forming or being a colony with a flat shiny surface usu. made up of organisms that form no chains or filaments, show characteristic internal changes, and tend toward marked increase in capsule formation and virulence — used of dissociated strains of bacteria; compare ROUGH

smooth muscle *n* : muscle tissue that lacks cross striations, that is made up of elongated spindle-shaped cells having a central nucleus, and that is found esp. in vertebrate hollow organs and structures (as the small intestine and bladder) as thin sheets performing functions not subject to direct voluntary control and in all or most of the musculature of invertebrates other than arthropods — called also *nonstriated muscle, unstriated muscle;* compare CARDIAC MUSCLE, STRIATED MUSCLE

smut \'smət\ *n* : any of various destructive diseases esp. of cereal grasses caused by parasitic fungi (order Ustilaginales); *also* : a fungus causing a smut

Sn *symbol* tin

snail \'snā(ə)l\ *n* : any of various gastropod mollusks and esp. those having an external enclosing spiral shell including some which are important in medicine as intermediate hosts of trematodes

snail fever *n* : SCHISTOSOMIASIS

snake \'snāk\ *n* : any of numerous limbless scaled reptiles (suborder Serpentes syn. Ophidia) with a long tapering body and with salivary glands often modified to produce venom which is injected through grooved or tubular fangs

snake·bite \-ˌbīt\ *n* : the bite of a snake; *also* : the condition resulting from the bite of a venomous snake and characterized by variable symptoms (as pain and swelling at the puncture site, blurred vision, difficulty in breathing, or internal bleeding)

snake oil *n* : any of various substances or mixtures sold (as by a traveling medicine show) as medicine usu. without having had the claims of their medical worth or properties substantiated by scientific tests

snake·root \-ˌrüt, -ˌru̇t\ *n* : any of numerous plants most of which have roots sometimes believed to cure snakebites; *also* : the root of such a plant — see SENECA SNAKEROOT

snare \'sna(ə)r, 'sne(ə)r\ *n* : a surgical instrument consisting usu. of a wire loop constricted by a mechanism in the handle and used for removing tissue masses (as tonsils or polyps)

¹**sneeze** \'snēz\ *vi* **sneezed; sneez·ing** : to make a sudden violent spasmodic audible expiration of breath through the nose and mouth esp. as a reflex act following irritation of the nasal mucous membrane

²**sneeze** *n* : an act or instance of sneezing

sneezing gas *n* : a gaseous sternutator created for chemical warfare

Snel·len chart \'snel-ən-\ *n* : the chart used in the Snellen test with black letters of various sizes against a white background

Snellen, Hermann (1834–1908), Dutch ophthalmologist. Snellen was director of an eye clinic at Utrecht. In 1862 he introduced a test for measuring the acuteness of vision which consisted of printed letters or words in type of various sizes. He also introduced operations for entropion and ectropion and for ptosis, the latter operation being performed by shortening the aponeurosis of the levator palpebrae superioris of the upper eyelid. Snellen is additionally famous for constructing an artificial eye consisting of two concavo-convex plates with intervening empty space.

Snellen test *n* : a test for visual acuity presenting letters of graduated sizes to determine the smallest size that can be read at a standard distance

SNF *abbr* skilled nursing facility

snif·fles \'snif-əlz\ *n pl* **1** : a head cold marked by nasal discharge ⟨a case of the ~⟩ **2** *usu sing in constr* : BULLNOSE

¹**snore** \'snō(ə)r, 'snȯ(ə)r\ *vi* **snored; snor·ing** : to breathe during sleep with a rough hoarse noise due to vibration of the soft palate

²**snore** *n* **1** : an act of snoring **2** : a noise of snoring

snor·er *n* : one who snores ⟨a chronic ~⟩

snort \'snȯ(ə)rt\ *vi* : to take in a drug by inhalation ~ *vt* : to inhale (a narcotic drug in powdered form) through the nostrils ⟨~ cocaine⟩

snout \'snau̇t\ *n* : a long projecting nose (as of a swine)

snow \'snō\ *n* **1** : any of various congealed or crystallized substances resembling snow in appearance ⟨carbon dioxide ∼⟩ **2** *slang* **a** : COCAINE **b** : HEROIN

snow–blind \-ˌblīnd\ *or* **snow–blind·ed** \-ˌblīn-dəd\ *adj* : affected with snow blindness

snow blindness *n* : inflammation and photophobia caused by exposure of the eyes to ultraviolet rays reflected from snow or ice

SNP \ˈsnip\ *n* : a variant DNA sequence in which the purine or pyrimidine base (as cytosine) of a single nucleotide has been replaced by another such base (as thymine) — called also *single nucleotide polymorphism*

snuff \ˈsnəf\ *n* : a preparation of pulverized tobacco to be inhaled through the nostrils, chewed, or placed against the gums; *also* : a preparation of a powdered drug to be inhaled through the nostrils

snuf·fles \ˈsnəf-əlz\ *n pl* **1** : SNIFFLES 1 **2** *usu sing in constr* : a respiratory disorder in animals marked esp. by catarrhal inflammation and sniffling: as **a** : a disease of the upper respiratory tract of rabbits that is often a precursor of pneumonia **b** : BULLNOSE

soak \ˈsōk\ *n* : an often hot medicated solution with which a body part is soaked usu. long or repeatedly esp. to promote healing, relieve pain, or stimulate local circulation

soap \ˈsōp\ *n* **1** : a cleansing and emulsifying agent made usu. by action of alkali on fat or fatty acids and consisting essentially of sodium or potassium salts of such acids **2** : a salt of a fatty acid and a metal

soap·bark \ˈsōp-ˌbärk\ *n* **1** : a Chilean tree of the genus *Quillaja* (*Q. saponaria*) with shiny leaves and white flowers **2** : the saponin-rich bark of the soapbark tree used in cleaning and in emulsifying oil — called also *quillaja*

SOB *abbr* short of breath

so·cial \ˈsō-shəl\ *adj* **1 a** : tending to form cooperative and interdependent relationships with others of one's kind **b** : living and breeding in more or less organized communities ⟨∼ insects⟩ **2** : of or relating to human society, the interaction of the individual and the group, or the welfare of human beings as members of society ⟨immature ∼ behavior⟩ — **so·cial·ly** \-ē\ *adv*

social disease *n* **1** : VENEREAL DISEASE **2** : a disease (as tuberculosis) whose incidence is directly related to social and economic factors

so·cial·iza·tion *also Brit* **so·cial·isa·tion** \ˌsōsh-(ə-)lə-ˈzā-shən\ *n* : the process by which a human being beginning at infancy acquires the habits, beliefs, and accumulated knowledge of society through education and training for adult status

so·cial·ize *also Brit* **so·cial·ise** \ˈsō-shə-ˌlīz\ *vt* **-ized** *also Brit* **-ised; -iz·ing** *also Brit* **-is·ing** : to make social; *esp* : to fit or train for society or a social environment ⟨children are *socialized* according to a given cultural pattern —H. A. Murray & C. K. Kluckhohn⟩

socialized medicine *n* : medical and hospital services for the members of a class or population administered by an organized group (as a state agency) and paid for from funds obtained usu. by assessments, philanthropy, or taxation

social psychiatry *n* **1** : a branch of psychiatry that deals in collaboration with related specialties (as sociology and anthropology) with the influence of social and cultural factors on the causation, course, and outcome of mental disorder **2** : the application of psychodynamic principles to the solution of social problems

social psychologist *n* : a specialist in social psychology

social psychology *n* : the study of the manner in which the personality, attitudes, motivations, and behavior of the individual influence and are influenced by social groups

social recovery *n* : an improvement in a psychiatric patient's clinical status that is not a total recovery but is sufficient to permit the patient's return to his or her former social milieu

social science *n* **1** : a branch of science that deals with the institutions and functioning of human society and with the interpersonal relationships of individuals as members of so-

ciety **2** : a science (as anthropology or social psychology) dealing with a particular phase or aspect of human society

social scientist *n* : a specialist in the social sciences

social wel·fare \-ˈwel-ˌfa(ə)r, -ˌfe(ə)r\ *n* : organized public or private social services for the assistance of disadvantaged groups; *specif* : SOCIAL WORK

social work *n* : any of various professional services, activities, or methods concretely concerned with the investigation, treatment, and material aid of the economically, physically, mentally, or socially disadvantaged

social work·er \-ˈwər-kər\ *n* : a person engaged in social work

so·cio·bi·ol·o·gist \ˌsō-sē-ō-bī-ˈäl-ə-jəst, ˌsō-shē-\ *n* : an expert in sociobiology : a person who professes or supports the theories of sociobiology

so·cio·bi·ol·o·gy \ˌsō-sē-ō-bī-ˈäl-ə-jē, ˌsō-shē-\ *n, pl* **-gies** : the comparative study of the biological basis of social organization and behavior in animals and humans esp. with regard to their genetic basis and evolutionary history — **so·cio·bio·log·i·cal** \-ˌbī-ə-ˈläj-i-kəl\ *adj* — **so·cio·bio·log·i·cal·ly** \-k(ə-)lē\ *adv*

so·cio·cul·tur·al \ˌsō-sē-ō-ˈkəlch-(ə-)rəl, ˌsō-shē-\ *adj* : of, relating to, or involving a combination of social and cultural factors — **so·cio·cul·tur·al·ly** \-rə-lē\ *adv*

so·cio·dra·ma \ˈsō-sē-ō-ˌdräm-ə, ˈsō-shē-, -ˌdram-ə\ *n* : a dramatic play in which several individuals act out assigned roles for the purpose of studying and remedying problems in group or collective relationships — **so·cio·dra·mat·ic** \-drə-ˈmat-ik\ *adj*

so·cio·gram \ˈsō-sē-ə-ˌgram, ˈsō-shē-\ *n* : a sociometric chart plotting the structure of interpersonal relations in a group situation

so·cio·log·i·cal \ˌsō-sē-ə-ˈläj-i-kəl, ˌsō-sh(ē-)ə-\ *also* **so·cio·log·ic** \-ik\ *adj* : of or relating to sociology or to the methodological approach of sociology — **so·cio·log·i·cal·ly** \-i-k(ə-)lē\ *adv*

so·ci·ol·o·gist \ˌsō-sē-ˈäl-ə-jəst, ˌsō-shē-\ *n* : a specialist in sociology

so·ci·ol·o·gy \ˌsō-sē-ˈäl-ə-jē, ˌsō-shē-\ *n, pl* **-gies** : the science of society, social institutions, and social relationships; *specif* : the systematic study of the development, structure, interaction, and collective behavior of organized groups of human beings

so·cio·med·i·cal \ˌsō-sē-ō-ˈmed-i-kəl, ˌsō-shē-\ *adj* : of or relating to the interrelations of medicine and social welfare

so·ci·om·e·try \ˌsō-sē-ˈäm-ə-trē, ˌsō-shē-\ *n, pl* **-tries** : the study and measurement of interpersonal relationships in a group of people — **so·cio·met·ric** \ˌsō-sē-ə-ˈme-trik, ˌsō-shē-\ *adj*

so·cio·path \ˈsō-sē-ə-ˌpath, ˈsō-sh(ē-)ə-\ *n* : a sociopathic individual : PSYCHOPATH

so·cio·path·ic \ˌsō-sē-ə-ˈpath-ik, ˌsō-sh(ē-)ə-\ *adj* : of, relating to, or characterized by asocial or antisocial behavior or an antisocial personality

so·ci·op·a·thy \ˌsō-sē-ˈäp-ə-thē, ˌsō-shē-\ *n, pl* **-thies** : the condition of being sociopathic

so·cio·psy·cho·log·i·cal \ˌsō-sē-ō-ˌsī-kə-ˈläj-i-kəl, ˌsō-shē-\ *adj* **1** : of, relating to, or involving a combination of social and psychological factors **2** : of or relating to social psychology

so·cio·sex·u·al \-ˈseksh-(ə-)wəl, -ˈsek-shəl\ *adj* : of or relating to the interpersonal aspects of sexuality ⟨∼ behavior⟩

sock·et \ˈsäk-ət\ *n* : an opening or hollow that forms a holder for something: as **a** : any of various hollows in body structures in which some other part normally lodges ⟨the bony ∼ of the eye⟩ ⟨an inflamed tooth ∼⟩; *esp* : the depression in a bone with which the rounded head of another bone fits in a ball-and-socket joint **b** : a cavity terminating an artificial

---

\ə\ abut \ᵊ\ kitten \ər\ further \a\ ash \ā\ ace \ä\ cot, cart
\au̇\ out \ch\ chin \e\ bet \ē\ easy \g\ go \i\ hit \ī\ ice \j\ job
\ŋ\ sing \ō\ go \ȯ\ law \ȯi\ boy \th\ thin \th\ the \ü\ loot
\u̇\ foot \y\ yet \zh\ vision *See also* Pronunciation Symbols page

S
T

limb into which the bodily stump fits — see SUCTION SOCK-ET

SOD *abbr* superoxide dismutase

so·da \'sōd-ə\ *n* : SODIUM CARBONATE; *also* : SODIUM BICARBONATE

soda lime *n* : a granular mixture of calcium hydroxide with sodium hydroxide or potassium hydroxide or both used to absorb moisture and acid gases and esp. carbon dioxide (as in gas masks, in the rebreathing technique of inhalation anesthesia, and in oxygen therapy)

sod disease \'säd-\ *n* : VESICULAR DERMATITIS

so·di·um \'sōd-ē-əm\ *n* : a silver white soft waxy ductile element of the alkali metal group that occurs abundantly in nature in combined form and is very active chemically — symbol *Na*; see ELEMENT table

sodium acetate *n* : the hygroscopic crystalline sodium salt $C_2H_3NaO_2$ of acetic acid used chiefly in organic synthesis and photography and as a mordant or as an analytical reagent

sodium acid carbonate *n* : SODIUM BICARBONATE

sodium acid phosphate *n* : SODIUM PHOSPHATE 1

sodium acid pyrophosphate *n* : SODIUM PYROPHOSPHATE

sodium alginate *n* : ALGIN b

sodium ascorbate *n* : the sodium salt $C_6H_7NaO_6$ of vitamin C

sodium au·ro·thio·sul·fate \-ˌȯr-ō-ˌthī-ō-'səl-ˌfāt\ *n* : GOLD SODIUM THIOSULFATE

sodium benzoate *n* : a crystalline or granular salt $C_7H_5O_2Na$ used chiefly as a food preservative

sodium bicarbonate *n* : a white crystalline weakly alkaline salt $NaHCO_3$ used in baking powders and in medicine esp. as an antacid — called also *baking soda, bicarb, bicarbonate of soda, sodium acid carbonate*

sodium borate *n* : a sodium salt of a boric acid; *esp* : BORAX

sodium bromide *n* : a crystalline salt $NaBr$ having a biting saline taste that is used in medicine as a sedative, hypnotic, and anticonvulsant

sodium cacodylate *n* : a poisonous arsenic-containing salt $C_2H_6AsNaO_2\cdot 3H_2O$ formerly used in medicine to treat skin diseases and leukemia

sodium caprylate *n* : the sodium salt $C_8H_{15}O_2Na$ of caprylic acid used esp. in the topical treatment of fungal infections

sodium carbonate *n* : a sodium salt of carbonic acid used esp. in making soaps and chemicals, in water softening, in cleaning and bleaching, and in photography: as **a** : a hygroscopic crystalline anhydrous strongly alkaline salt Na_2CO_3 **b** : WASHING SODA

sodium chloride *n* : an ionic crystalline chemical compound consisting of equal numbers of sodium and chlorine atoms : SALT 1a

sodium citrate *n* : a crystalline salt $C_6H_5Na_3O_7$ used chiefly as an expectorant, a systemic and urinary alkalizer, a chelator to increase urinary excretion of calcium in hypercalcemia and lead in lead poisoning, and in combination as an anticoagulant (as in stored blood)

sodium cro·mo·gly·cate \-ˌkrō-mō-'glī-ˌkāt\ *n* : CROMOLYN SODIUM

sodium di·hy·dro·gen phosphate \-ˌdī-'hī-drə-jən-\ *n* : SODIUM PHOSPHATE 1

sodium do·dec·yl sulfate \-dō-'des-il-\ *n* : SODIUM LAURYL SULFATE

sodium fluoride *n* : a poisonous crystalline salt NaF that is used in trace amounts in the fluoridation of drinking water, toothpastes, and oral rinses and in metallurgy, as a flux, as an antiseptic, and as a pesticide — see LURIDE

sodium flu·o·ro·ace·tate \-ˌflü(-ə)r-ō-'as-ə-ˌtāt\ *n* : a poisonous powdery compound $C_2H_2FNaO_2$

sodium fluosilicate *n* : a crystalline salt Na_2SiF_6 used as an insecticide — called also *sodium silicofluoride*

sodium glutamate *n* : MONOSODIUM GLUTAMATE

sodium hydroxide *n* : a white brittle deliquescent solid $NaOH$ that dissolves readily in water to form a strongly alkaline and caustic solution and that is used in pharmacy as an alkalizing agent — called also *caustic soda*

sodium hypochlorite *n* : an unstable salt $NaOCl$ produced usu. in aqueous solution and used as a bleaching and disinfecting agent

sodium hy·po·sul·fite \-ˌhī-pō-'səl-ˌfīt\ *n* : SODIUM THIOSULFATE

sodium iodide *n* : a crystalline salt NaI used as an iodine supplement and expectorant

sodium iodohippurate *n* : HIPPURAN

sodium lactate *n* : a hygroscopic syrupy salt $C_3H_5NaO_3$ used chiefly as an antacid in medicine and as a substitute for glycerol

sodium lauryl sulfate *n* : the crystalline sodium salt $C_{12}H_{25}NaO_4S$ of sulfated lauryl alcohol; *also* : a mixture of sulfates of sodium consisting principally of this salt and used as a detergent, wetting, and emulsifying agent (as in toothpastes, ointments, and shampoos)

sodium meta·bi·sul·fite \-ˌmet-ə-ˌbī-'səl-ˌfīt\ *n* : a compound $Na_2S_2O_5$ used as an antioxidant in pharmaceutical preparations

sodium morrhuate *n* : MORRHUATE SODIUM

sodium nitrate *n* : a deliquescent crystalline salt $NaNO_3$ used as a fertilizer and an oxidizing agent and in curing meat — called also *saltpeter;* see CHILE SALTPETER

sodium nitrite *n* : a colorless or yellowish deliquescent salt $NaNO_2$ that is used as a meat preservative and in medicine as a vasodilator and an antidote for cyanide poisoning

sodium ni·tro·prus·side \-ˌnī-trō-'prəs-ˌīd\ *n* : a red crystalline salt $C_5FeN_6Na_2O$ administered intravenously as a vasodilator esp. in hypertensive emergencies — see NIPRIDE

sodium oleate *n* : the sodium salt $C_{18}H_{33}NaO_2$ of oleic acid that has been used in the treatment of cholelithiasis

sodium oxalate *n* : a poisonous crystalline salt $Na_2C_2O_4$ having anticoagulant properties

sodium pentobarbital *n* : the sodium salt of pentobarbital

sodium pentobarbitone *n, Brit* : SODIUM PENTOBARBITAL

sodium perborate *n* : a white crystalline hydrated powder $NaBO_3\cdot 4H_2O$ used as an oral antiseptic

sodium peroxide *n* : a pale-yellow hygroscopic granular compound Na_2O_2 that is used chiefly as an oxidizing and bleaching agent

sodium phosphate *n* **1** : a phosphate NaH_2PO_4 of sodium containing one sodium atom per molecule that with the phosphate containing two sodium atoms per molecule constitutes the principal buffer system of the urine — called also *monobasic sodium phosphate, sodium acid phosphate, sodium dihydrogen phosphate* **2** : a phosphate Na_2HPO_4 of sodium containing two sodium atoms per molecule that is used in medicine as a laxative and antacid — called also *dibasic sodium phosphate* **3** : a phosphate Na_3PO_4 of sodium containing three sodium atoms per molecule that is used chiefly in cleaning compositions and in water treatment

sodium potassium tartrate *n* : ROCHELLE SALT

sodium propionate *n* : a deliquescent crystalline salt $C_3H_5NaO_2$ used as a fungicide (as in retarding the growth of mold in the baking and dairy industries)

sodium pump *n* **1** : a molecular mechanism by which sodium ions are actively transported across a cell membrane; *esp* : one by which a high concentration of potassium ions and a low concentration of sodium ions are maintained within a cell and that is controlled by a specialized plasma membrane protein linking the hydrolysis of ATP to the active transport of intracellular sodium ions out of the cell and extracellular potassium ions into the cell to create an electrical and chemical gradient across the plasma membrane necessary for vital cell functions (as nerve cell excitation and cell volume regulation) **2** : the specialized plasma membrane protein that controls the sodium pump mechanism

sodium pyrophosphate *n* : a crystalline acid salt $Na_2H_2P_2O_7$ of pyrophosphoric acid that has been added to hot dogs to give them color — called also *sodium acid pyrophosphate*

sodium salicylate *n* : a crystalline salt $NaC_7H_5O_3$ that has a sweetish saline taste and is used chiefly as an analgesic, antipyretic, and antirheumatic

sodium secobarbital *n* : the sodium salt $C_{12}H_{17}N_2NaO_3$ of secobarbital

sodium silicofluoride *n* : SODIUM FLUOSILICATE

sodium stearate *n* : a white powdery salt $C_{17}H_{35}COONa$ that is soluble in water, is the chief constituent of some laundry soaps, and is used esp. in glycerin suppositories, cosmetics, and some toothpastes

sodium succinate *n* : a compound $C_4H_4Na_2O_4$ that has been used as a respiratory stimulant, analeptic, diuretic, and laxative

sodium sulfate *n* : a bitter salt Na_2SO_4 used esp. in detergents, in the manufacture of wood pulp and rayon, in dyeing and finishing textiles, and in its hydrated form as a cathartic — see GLAUBER'S SALT

sodium tetraborate *n* : BORAX

sodium thiosulfate *n* : a hygroscopic crystalline salt $Na_2O_3S_2$ that is used as a fixing agent in photography, as a reducing agent and bleaching agent, in chemical analysis for the titration of iodine, and in medicine as an antidote in poisoning esp. by cyanides and as an antifungal agent — called also *hypo, sodium hyposulfite*

sodium valproate *n* : the sodium salt $C_8H_{15}NaO_2$ of valproic acid used as an anticonvulsant — called also *valproate sodium*

so·do·ku \'sōd-ə-ˌkü\ *n* : RAT-BITE FEVER b

sod·om·ist \'säd-ə-məst\ *n* : SODOMITE

sod·om·ite \-ˌmīt\ *n* : one who practices sodomy

sod·om·ize \-ˌmīz\ *vt* **-ized; -iz·ing** : to perform sodomy on

sod·omy \'säd-ə-mē\ *n, pl* **-om·ies** : anal or oral copulation with a member of the same or opposite sex; *also* : copulation with an animal — **sod·om·it·ic** \ˌsäd-ə-'mit-ik\ *or* **sod·om·it·i·cal** \-i-kəl\ *adj*

soft \'sóft\ *adj* **1** : yielding to physical pressure **2** : deficient in or free from substances (as calcium and magnesium salts) that prevent lathering of soap ⟨~ water⟩ **3** : having relatively low energy ⟨~ X-rays⟩ **4** : BIODEGRADABLE ⟨~ pesticides⟩ **5** *of a drug* : considered less detrimental than a hard narcotic ⟨marijuana is usually regarded as a ~ drug⟩ **6** : easily polarized — used of acids and bases **7 a** : being or based on interpretive or speculative data ⟨~ evidence⟩ **b** : utilizing or based on soft data ⟨~ science⟩

soft chancre *n* : CHANCROID

soft contact lens *n* : a contact lens made of soft water-absorbing plastic that adheres closely and with minimal discomfort to the eye

soft·gel \'sóft-ˌjel\ *n* : a pliable soft gelatin capsule containing a liquid preparation (as a medicine)

soft lens *n* : SOFT CONTACT LENS

soft palate *n* : the membranous and muscular fold suspended from the posterior margin of the hard palate and partially separating the mouth cavity from the pharynx

soft soap *n* : soap of a semifluid consistency made principally with potash and having various medical uses (as in the treatment of skin diseases); *specif* : GREEN SOAP

soft spot *n* : a fontanel of a fetal or young skull

sol \'säl, 'sól\ *n* : a fluid colloidal system; *esp* : one in which the dispersion medium is a liquid

So·la·na·ce·ae \ˌsō-lə-'nā-sē-ˌē\ *n pl* : a large family of widely distributed often strongly scented herbs, shrubs, and trees (order Polemoniales) that include the tomato, potato, jimsonweed, and belladonna

so·la·na·ceous \ˌsō-lə-'nā-shəs\ *adj* : relating to, derived from, or being plants of the family Solanaceae ⟨~ drugs⟩

so·la·nine *or* **so·la·nin** \'sō-lə-ˌnēn, -nən\ *n* : a bitter poisonous crystalline alkaloid $C_{45}H_{72}NO_{15}$ from several plants (as some potatoes or tomatoes) of the family Solanaceae

so·la·num \sə-'lān-əm, -'län-, -'lan-\ *n* **1** *cap* : the type genus of the family Solanaceae comprising often spiny herbs, shrubs, and trees that have white, purple, or yellow flowers and a fruit that is a berry **2** : any plant of the genus *Solanum* : NIGHTSHADE

solare — see ERYTHEMA SOLARE

so·lar·i·um \sō-'lar-ē-əm, sə-, -'ler-\ *n, pl* **-ia** \-ē-ə\ *also* **-ums** : a room (as in a hospital) used esp. for sunbathing or therapeutic exposure to light

so·lar plexus \'sō-lər-\ *n* **1** : CELIAC PLEXUS **2** : the part of the abdomen including the stomach and celiac plexus that is particularly vulnerable to the effects of a blow to the body wall in front of it — not used technically

sol·ate \'säl-ˌāt, 'sól-\ *vt* **sol·at·ed; sol·at·ing** : to change to a sol — **sol·ation** \sä-'lā-shən, sō-\ *n*

sol·dier's heart \'sōl-jərz-\ *n* : NEUROCIRCULATORY ASTHENIA

sole \'sōl\ *n* **1** : the undersurface of a foot **2** : the somewhat concave plate of moderately dense horn that covers the lower surface of the coffin bone of the horse, partly surrounds the frog, and is bounded externally by the wall

So·le·nog·ly·pha \ˌsō-lə-'näg-lə-fə\ *n pl, in some classifications* : a group of venomous snakes with tubular erectile fangs comprising the families Viperidae and Crotalidae

So·le·nop·sis \ˌsō-lə-'näp-səs\ *n* : a genus of small stinging ants including several abundant tropical and subtropical forms (as the imported fire ants)

sole·plate \'sōl-ˌplāt\ *n* : a flattened nucleated mass of soft granular protoplasm surrounding the end of a motor nerve in a striated muscle fiber

sole·print \-ˌprint\ *n* : a print of the sole of the foot; *esp* : one made in the manner of a fingerprint and used for the identification of an infant

so·le·us \'sō-lē-əs\ *n, pl* **so·lei** \-lē-ˌī\ *also* **soleuses** : a broad flat muscle of the calf of the leg that lies deep to the gastrocnemius, arises from the back and upper part of the tibia and fibula and from a tendinous arch between them, inserts by a tendon that unites with that of the gastrocnemius to form the Achilles tendon, and acts to flex the foot

¹sol·id \'säl-əd\ *adj* **1** : being without an internal cavity : not hollow ⟨~ tumors⟩ **2** : possessing or characterized by the properties of a solid : neither gaseous nor liquid **3** *of immunity* : capable of resisting severe challenge — **sol·id·ly** *adv*

²solid *n* **1** : a substance that does not flow perceptibly under moderate stress, has a definite capacity for resisting forces (as compression or tension) which tend to deform it, and under ordinary conditions retains a definite size and shape **2** : the part of a solution or suspension that when freed from solvent or suspending medium has the qualities of a solid — usu. used in pl. ⟨milk ~s⟩

sol·i·da·go \ˌsäl-ə-'dā-(ˌ)gō, -'däg-(ˌ)ō\ *n* **1** *cap* : a genus of chiefly No. American composite herbs including the typical goldenrods **2** *pl* **-gos** : any plant of the genus *Solidago*

solitarius — see TRACTUS SOLITARIUS

sol·i·tary \'säl-ə-ˌter-ē\ *adj* : occurring singly and not as part of a group ⟨a ~ lesion⟩

sol·u·bil·i·ty \ˌsäl-yə-'bil-ət-ē\ *n, pl* **-ties** **1** : the quality or state of being soluble **2** : the amount of a substance that will dissolve in a given amount of another substance and is typically expressed as the number of parts by weight dissolved by 100 parts of solvent at a specified temperature and pressure or as percent by weight or by volume

sol·u·bi·lize *also Brit* **sol·u·bi·lise** \'säl-yə-bə-ˌlīz\ *vt* **-lized** *also Brit* **-lised; -liz·ing** *also Brit* **-lis·ing** : to make soluble or increase the solubility of — **sol·u·bi·li·za·tion** *also Brit* **sol·u·bi·li·sa·tion** \ˌsäl-yə-bə-lə-'zā-shən\ *n*

sol·u·bi·liz·er *also Brit* **sol·u·bi·lis·er** \-ˌlīz-ər\ *n* : an agent that increases the solubility of a substance

sol·u·ble \'säl-yə-bəl\ *adj* **1** : susceptible of being dissolved in or as if in a fluid **2** : capable of being emulsified ⟨a ~ oil⟩

soluble RNA *n* : TRANSFER RNA

sol·ute \'säl-ˌyüt\ *n* : a dissolved substance; *esp* : a component of a solution present in smaller amount than the solvent

so·lu·tion \sə-'lü-shən\ *n* **1 a** : an act or the process by which a solid, liquid, or gaseous substance is homogeneously

S
T

mixed with a liquid or sometimes a gas or solid — called also *dissolution* **2 a :** a liquid containing a dissolved substance ⟨an aqueous ∼⟩ **b :** a liquid and usu. aqueous medicinal preparation with the solid ingredients soluble **c :** the condition of being dissolved ⟨a substance in ∼⟩

solution pressure *n* : the pressure by which the particles of a dissolved substance are driven into solution and which when equal to the osmotic pressure establishes equilibrium so that the concentration of the solution becomes constant

¹**sol·vate** \'säl-ˌvāt, 'sȯl-\ *n* : an aggregate that consists of a solute ion or molecule with one or more solvent molecules; *also* : a substance (as a hydrate) containing such ions

²**solvate** *vt* **sol·vat·ed; sol·vat·ing :** to make part of a solvate

sol·va·tion \säl-'vā-shən, sȯl-\ *n* : the formation of a solvate; *also* : the state or degree of being solvated

¹**sol·vent** \'säl-vənt, 'sȯl-\ *adj* : that dissolves or can dissolve ⟨∼ fluids⟩ ⟨∼ action of water⟩

²**solvent** *n* : a substance capable of or used in dissolving or dispersing one or more other substances; *esp* : a liquid component of a solution present in greater amount than the solute

sol·vol·y·sis \säl-'väl-ə-səs, sȯl-\ *n, pl* **-y·ses** \-ˌsēz\ : a chemical reaction (as hydrolysis) of a solvent and solute that results in the formation of new compounds

sol·vo·lyt·ic \ˌsäl-və-'lit-ik, ˌsȯl-\ *adj* : of, relating to, or involving solvolysis

so·ma \'sō-mə\ *n, pl* **so·ma·ta** \'sō-mət-ə\ *or* **somas** **1 :** the body of an organism **2 :** all of an organism except the germ cells **3 :** CELL BODY

somaesthesis, somaesthetic *chiefly Brit var of* SOMESTHESIS, SOMESTHETIC

So·man \'sō-mən\ *n* : a poisonous gas $C_7H_{16}FO_2P$ with potent anticholinesterase activity created for use in chemical warfare

so·mat·ic \sō-'mat-ik, sə-\ *adj* **1 a :** of, relating to, or affecting the body esp. as distinguished from the germ plasm or psyche : PHYSICAL **b :** of, relating to, supplying, or involving skeletal muscles ⟨the ∼ nervous system⟩ ⟨a ∼ reflex⟩ **2 :** of or relating to the wall of the body as distinguished from the viscera : PARIETAL — **so·mat·i·cal·ly** \-i-k(ə-)lē\ *adv*

somatic antigen *n* : O ANTIGEN

somatic cell *n* : any of the cells of the body that compose the tissues, organs, and parts of that individual other than the germ cells

somatic mutation *n* : a mutation occurring in a somatic cell and inducing a chimera

so·ma·ti·za·tion \ˌsō-mət-ə-'zā-shən\ *or chiefly Brit* **so·ma·ti·sa·tion** \-mə-ˌtī-'-\ *n* : conversion of a mental state (as depression or anxiety) into physical symptoms; *also* : the existence of physical bodily complaints in the absence of a known medical condition

somatization disorder *n* : a somatoform disorder characterized by multiple and recurring physical complaints for which the patient has sought medical treatment over several years without any organic or physiological basis for the symptoms being found

so·ma·tize *or chiefly Brit* **so·ma·tise** \'sō-mə-ˌtīz\ *vb* **-tized** *or chiefly Brit* **-tised; -tiz·ing** *or chiefly Brit* **-tis·ing** *vt* : to express (as psychological conflicts) through somatic symptoms ⟨*somatized* anxieties⟩ ∼ *vi* : to express psychological conflicts through somatic symptoms ⟨some people ∼ — they have all kinds of body aches and pains that their doctors can't explain —Roger Callahan *et al*⟩

so·ma·tiz·er \-ˌtī-zər\ *n* : a patient with frequent physical complaints for which no organic basis is found

so·ma·to·form disorder \'sō-mət-ə-ˌfȯrm-, sə-'mat-ə-\ *n* : any of a group of psychological disorders (as body dysmorphic disorder or hypochondriasis) marked by physical complaints for which no organic or physiological explanation is found and for which there is a strong likelihood that psychological factors are involved

so·ma·to·gen·ic \ˌsō-mət-ə-'jen-ik, sō-ˌmat-ə-\ *adj* : originat-

ing in, affecting, or acting through the body ⟨a ∼ disorder⟩ — compare PSYCHOGENIC

so·ma·tol·o·gy \ˌsō-mə-'täl-ə-jē\ *n, pl* **-gies :** PHYSICAL ANTHROPOLOGY — **so·ma·to·log·i·cal** \ˌsō-mət-ə-'läj-i-kəl\ *adj*

so·ma·to·mam·mo·tro·pin \ˌsō-mət-ə-ˌmam-ə-'trōp-ⁿn, sə-ˌmat-ə-\ *n* : any of several hormones (as growth hormone and prolactin) having lactogenic and somatotropic properties; *esp* : PLACENTAL LACTOGEN

so·ma·to·me·din \sō-ˌmat-ə-'mēd-ⁿn, ˌsō-mət-ə-\ *n* : any of several endogenous peptides produced esp. in the liver that are dependent on and prob. mediate growth hormone activity (as in sulfate uptake by epiphyseal cartilage)

so·ma·tom·e·try \ˌsō-mə-'täm-ə-trē\ *n, pl* **-tries :** a branch of anthropometry that is concerned with measurement of parts of the body other than the head — **so·ma·to·met·ric** \ˌsō-ˌmat-ə-'me-trik, ˌsō-mət-ə-\ *adj*

so·ma·to·pause \sō-'mat-ə-ˌpȯz, 'sō-mət-ə-\ *n* : a gradual and progressive decrease in growth hormone secretion that occurs normally with increasing age during adult life and is associated with an increase in adipose tissue and LDL levels and a decrease in lean body mass

so·ma·to·plasm \sō-'mat-ə-ˌplaz-əm, 'sō-mət-ə-\ *n* **1 :** protoplasm of somatic cells as distinguished from that of germ cells **2 :** somatic cells as distinguished from germ cells

so·ma·to·pleure \sō-'mat-ə-ˌplü(ə)r, 'sō-mət-ə-\ *n* : a complex fold of tissue in the embryo of craniate vertebrates that consists of an outer layer of mesoderm together with the ectoderm ensheathing it and that gives rise to the amnion and chorion — compare SPLANCHNOPLEURE — **so·ma·to·pleu·ric** \sō-ˌmat-ə-'plür-ik, ˌsō-mət-ə-\ *adj*

so·ma·to·psy·chic \sō-ˌmat-ə-'sī-kik, ˌsō-mət-ə-\ *adj* : of or relating to the body and the mind; *esp* : of, relating to, or concerned with mental symptoms caused by bodily illness

so·ma·to·sen·so·ry \sō-ˌmat-ə-'sen(t)s-(ə-)rē, ˌsō-mət-ə-\ *adj* : of, relating to, or being sensory activity having its origin elsewhere than in the special sense organs (as eyes and ears) and conveying information about the state of the body proper and its immediate environment ⟨∼ pathways⟩

somatosensory cortex *n* : either of two regions in the postcentral gyrus that receive and process somatosensory stimuli — called also *somatosensory area, somesthetic area*

so·ma·to·stat·in \sō-ˌmat-ə-'stat-ⁿn\ *n* : a polypeptide neurohormone that is found esp. in the hypothalamus, is composed of a chain of 14 amino acid residues, and inhibits the secretion of several other hormones (as growth hormone, insulin, and gastrin)

so·ma·to·ther·a·py \ˌsō-mət-ə-'ther-ə-pē, sō-ˌmat-ə-\ *n, pl* **-pies :** therapy for psychological problems that uses physiological intervention (as by drugs or surgery) to modify behavior — **so·ma·to·ther·a·peu·tic** \-ˌther-ə-'pyüt-ik\ *adj*

so·ma·to·to·nia \ˌsō-mət-ə-'tō-nē-ə, sō-ˌmat-ə-\ *n* : a pattern of temperament that is marked by predominance of physical over social or intellectual factors, aggressiveness, love of physical activity, vigor, and alertness — compare CEREBROTONIA, VISCEROTONIA

so·ma·to·ton·ic \-'tän-ik\ *adj* : relating to or characterized by somatotonia

so·ma·to·top·ic \-'täp-ik\ *adj* : of, relating to, or mediating the orderly and specific relation between particular body regions (as a hand or the tongue) and corresponding motor areas of the brain ⟨the ∼ arrangement within the thalamus⟩ — **so·ma·to·top·i·cal·ly** \-i-k(ə-)lē\ *adv*

so·ma·to·trope \sō-'mat-ə-ˌtrōp, 'sō-mət-ə-\ *n* : SOMATOTROPH

so·ma·to·troph \-ˌtrōf, -ˌträf\ *n* : any of various cells of the adenohypophysis of the pituitary gland that secrete growth hormone — called also *somatotrope*

so·ma·to·trop·ic \ˌsō-mət-ə-'trō-pik, sə-ˌmat-ə-, -'träp-ik\ *or* **so·ma·to·tro·phic** \-'trō-fik\ *adj* : promoting growth ⟨∼ activity⟩

somatotropic hormone *n* : GROWTH HORMONE

so·ma·to·tro·pin \-'trō-pən\ *also* **so·ma·to·tro·phin** \-fən\ *n* : GROWTH HORMONE

¹**so·ma·to·type** \'sō-mət-ə-ˌtīp, sō-'mat-ə-\ *n* : a body type or

physique esp. in a system of classification based on the relative development of ectomorphic, endomorphic, and mesomorphic components — **so·ma·to·typ·ic** \-₁tip-ik\ *adj* — **so·ma·to·typ·i·cal·ly** \-i-k(ə-)lē\ *adv*

²**somatotype** *vt* **-typed; -typ·ing** : to determine the somatotype of (as a human body) : classify according to physique

so·ma·tro·pin \sō-ˈmat-rə-pən, ₁sō-mə-ˈtrō-\ *n* : HUMAN GROWTH HORMONE; *esp* : a recombinant version of human growth hormone

som·es·the·sis *or chiefly Brit* **som·aes·the·sis** \₁sōm-es-ˈthē-səs\ *n, pl* **-sis·es** : body sensibility including the cutaneous and kinesthetic senses

som·es·thet·ic *or chiefly Brit* **som·aes·thet·ic** \-es-ˈthet-ik\ *adj* : of, relating to, or concerned with bodily sensations ⟨a ~ image of the body created by the brain from sensory inputs of touch, pressure, cold, heat, and pain⟩

somesthetic area *n* : SOMATOSENSORY CORTEX

so·mite \ˈsō-₁mīt\ *n* : one of the longitudinal series of segments into which the body of many animals (as articulate animals and vertebrates) is divided : METAMERE — **so·mit·ic** \sō-ˈmit-ik\ *adj*

som·nam·bu·lance \säm-ˈnam-byə-lən(t)s\ *n* : SOMNAMBULISM

som·nam·bu·lant \säm-ˈnam-byə-lənt\ *adj* : walking or tending to walk while asleep

som·nam·bu·late \-₁lāt\ *vi* **-lat·ed; -lat·ing** : to walk while asleep — **som·nam·bu·la·tion** \-₁nam-byə-ˈlā-shən\ *n*

som·nam·bu·lism \säm-ˈnam-byə-₁liz-əm\ *n* **1** : an abnormal condition of sleep in which motor acts (as walking) are performed **2** : actions characteristic of somnambulism — **som·nam·bu·lis·tic** \(₁)säm-₁nam-byə-ˈlis-tik\ *adj*

som·nam·bu·list \-ləst\ *n* : SLEEPWALKER

¹**som·ni·fa·cient** \₁säm-nə-ˈfā-shənt\ *adj* : inducing sleep : HYPNOTIC 1 ⟨a ~ drug⟩

²**somnifacient** *n* : a somnifacient agent (as a drug) : HYPNOTIC 1

som·nif·er·ous \säm-ˈnif-(ə-)rəs\ *adj* : SOPORIFIC

som·nil·o·quism \säm-ˈnil-ə-₁kwiz-əm\ *n* : SOMNILOQUY

som·nil·o·quy \-kwē\ *n, pl* **-quies** : the action or habit of talking in one's sleep

som·no·lence \ˈsäm-nə-lən(t)s\ *n* : the quality or state of being drowsy

som·no·lent \-lənt\ *adj* : inclined to or heavy with sleep : DROWSY

So·mo·gyi effect \ˈsō-mō-jē-\ *n* : hyperglycemia following an episode of hypoglycemia; *esp* : hyperglycemia that occurs after breakfast following nocturnal hypoglycemia and that may occur in type 1 diabetes esp. when too much insulin has been taken the day before — called also *Somogyi phenomenon*; compare DAWN PHENOMENON

Somogyi, Michael (1883–1971), American biochemist. Somogyi was head chemist in Budapest's municipal laboratories before immigrating to the U.S. and becoming an instructor of biochemistry at Washington University's medical school and a biochemist at the Jewish Hospital of St. Louis. In 1926 he introduced a method for determining reducing sugars in human blood. In 1940 he developed a method for the determination of serum amylase in healthy and diabetic individuals. He is also credited with devising a test for acute pancreatitis.

Somogyi unit *n* : a unit that is a measure of the hydrolyzing action of serum amylase on starch and that is equivalent to the amount of enzyme in 100 milliliters of blood serum required to produce 1 milligram of glucose when acting on a standard starch solution under defined conditions

sone \ˈsōn\ *n* : a subjective unit of loudness for an average listener equal to the loudness of a 1000-hertz sound that has an intensity 40 decibels above the listener's own threshold of hearing

son·ic \ˈsän-ik\ *adj* **1** : having a frequency within the audibility range of the human ear — used of waves and vibrations **2** : utilizing, produced by, or relating to sound waves ⟨a ~ device used to rupture cell walls⟩ — **son·i·cal·ly** \-i-k(ə-)lē\ *adv*

¹**son·i·cate** \ˈsän-ə-₁kāt\ *vt* **-cat·ed; -cat·ing** : to disrupt (as bacterial cells) by exposure to high-frequency sound waves — **son·i·ca·tion** \₁sän-ə-ˈkā-shən\ *n*

²**son·i·cate** \-kət\ *n* : a product of sonication ⟨a bacterial ~⟩

sono·gram \ˈsän-ə-₁gram\ *n* : an image produced by ultrasound — called also *echogram, ultrasonogram*

so·nog·ra·pher \sō-ˈnäg-rə-fər\ *n* : a specialist in the use of ultrasound — called also *ultrasonographer*

so·nog·ra·phy \sō-ˈnäg-rə-fē\ *n, pl* **-phies** : ULTRASOUND 2 — **sono·graph·ic** \₁sän-ə-ˈgraf-ik\ *adj* — **sono·graph·i·cal·ly** \-i-k(ə-)lē\ *adv*

sono·lu·cent \₁sän-ō-ˈlü-sənt\ *adj* : allowing passage of ultrasonic waves without production of echoes that are due to reflection of some of the waves ⟨a ~ mass⟩

so·phis·ti·cate \sə-ˈfis-tə-₁kāt\ *vt* **-cat·ed; -cat·ing** : to make impure : ADULTERATE ⟨a *sophisticated* oil⟩

so·phis·ti·ca·tion \sə-₁fis-tə-ˈkā-shən\ *n* : the process or result of making impure or weak : ADULTERATION ⟨~ of a drug⟩

soph·o·rine \ˈsäf-ə-₁rēn\ *n* : CYTISINE

so·por \ˈsō-pər, -₁pȯ(ə)r\ *n* : profound or lethargic sleep

so·po·rif·er·ous \₁säp-ə-ˈrif-(ə-)rəs, ₁sō-pə-\ *adj* : SOPORIFIC

¹**so·po·rif·ic** \-ˈrif-ik\ *adj* : causing or tending to cause sleep

²**soporific** *n* : a soporific agent (as a drug)

sorb \ˈsȯrb\ *vt* : to take up and hold by either adsorption or absorption

sor·bate \ˈsȯr-₁bāt\ *n* : a salt or ester of sorbic acid

sor·bent \ˈsȯr-bənt\ *n* : a substance that sorbs

sor·bic acid \₁sȯr-bik-\ *n* : a crystalline acid $C_6H_8O_2$ obtained from the unripe fruits of the mountain ash (genus *Sorbus*) or synthesized and used esp. as a fungicide and food preservative

sor·bi·nil \ˈsȯr-bə-₁nil\ *n* : a drug $C_{11}H_{19}FN_2O_3$ that inhibits the activity of a reductase which catalyzes the conversion of glucose to sorbitol and that has been used experimentally in the treatment of diabetic neuropathy

sor·bi·tan \ˈsȯr-bə-₁tan\ *n* : an anhydride $C_6H_{12}O_5$ of sorbitol from which various fatty acid esters are derived for use as surfactants and emulsifying agents

sor·bi·tol \ˈsȯr-bə-₁tȯl, -₁tōl\ *n* : a faintly sweet alcohol $C_6H_{14}O_6$ that occurs esp. in fruits of the mountain ash (genus *Sorbus*), is made synthetically, and is used esp. as a humectant, a softener, and a sweetener and in making ascorbic acid

sor·bose \ˈsȯr-₁bōs, -₁bōz\ *n* : a sweet crystalline levorotatory ketohexose sugar $C_6H_{12}O_6$ that is derived from sorbitol

sor·des \ˈsȯr-(₁)dēz\ *n, pl* **sordes** : the crusts that collect on the teeth and lips in debilitating diseases with protracted low fever

¹**sore** \ˈsō(ə)r, ˈsȯ(ə)r\ *adj* **sor·er; sor·est** : causing, characterized by, or affected with pain : PAINFUL ⟨~ muscles⟩ ⟨a ~ wound⟩ — **sore·ly** *adv* — **sore·ness** *n*

²**sore** *n* : a localized sore spot on the body; *esp* : one (as an ulcer) with the tissues ruptured or abraded and usu. with infection

sore·head \-₁hed\ *n* : FOWL POX a

sore mouth *n* **1** : a highly contagious virus disease of sheep and goats that is caused by a poxvirus (species *Orf virus* of the genus *Parapoxvirus*), occurs esp. in young animals, is characterized by extensive vesiculation and subsequent ulceration about the lips, gums, and tongue, and rarely ends fatally but interferes with nutrition and may be complicated by secondary bacterial infection — called also *orf, scabby mouth* **2** : necrobacillosis affecting the mouth; *esp* : CALF DIPHTHERIA

sore·muz·zle \-₁məz-ᵊl\ *n* : BLUETONGUE

sore throat *n* : painful throat due to inflammation of the fauces and pharynx

\ə\ abut \ᵊ\ kitten \ər\ further \a\ ash \ā\ ace \ä\ cot, cart \aú\ out \ch\ chin \e\ bet \ē\ easy \g\ go \i\ hit \ī\ ice \j\ job \ŋ\ sing \ō\ go \ȯ\ law \ȯi\ boy \th\ thin \th\ the \ü\ loot \ú\ foot \y\ yet \zh\ vision See also Pronunciation Symbols page

sorp·tion \'sȯrp-shən\ n : the process of sorbing : the state of being sorbed ⟨selective ∼ of the components of a mixture⟩

SOS abbr [Latin si opus sit] if occasion require; if necessary — used in writing prescriptions

so·ta·lol \'sōt-ə-ˌlȯl, -ˌlōl\ n : a beta-adrenergic blocking agent administered in the form of its hydrochloride $C_{12}H_{20}N_2O_3S·HCl$ to treat ventricular arrhythmias

souf·fle \'sü-fəl\ n : a blowing sound heard on auscultation ⟨the uterine ∼ heard in pregnancy⟩

¹**sound** \'saùnd\ adj **1** : free from injury or disease : exhibiting normal health **2** : deep and undisturbed ⟨a ∼ sleep⟩ — **sound·ness** n

²**sound** n **1** : a particular auditory impression ⟨heart ∼s heard by auscultation⟩ **2** : the sensation perceived by the sense of hearing **3** : mechanical radiant energy that is transmitted by longitudinal pressure waves in a material medium (as air) and is the objective cause of hearing

³**sound** vt : to explore or examine (a body cavity) with a sound

⁴**sound** n : an elongated instrument for exploring or examining body cavities ⟨a uterine ∼⟩

sound pollution n : NOISE POLLUTION

sound wave n **1** : SOUND 1 **2 sound waves** pl : longitudinal pressure waves esp. when transmitting audible sound

¹**sour** \'saù(ə)r\ adj : causing, characterized by, or being the one of the four basic taste sensations that is produced chiefly by acids — compare BITTER, SALT 2, SWEET — **sour·ness** n

²**sour** n : the primary taste sensation produced by acid stimuli

South American blastomycosis \'saùth-\ n : blastomycosis caused by a fungus of the genus *Paracoccidioides* (*P. brasiliensis* syn. *Blastomyces brasiliensis*) and characterized by formation of ulcers on the mucosal surfaces of the mouth that spread to lips, nose, and cheeks, by great enlargement of lymph nodes esp. of the throat and chest, and by involvement of the gastrointestinal tract — called also *paracoccidioidomycosis*

South·ern blot \'səth-ərn-\ n : a blot consisting of a sheet of cellulose nitrate or nylon that contains spots of DNA for identification by a suitable molecular probe — compare NORTHERN BLOT, WESTERN BLOT — **Southern blot·ting** \-'blät-iŋ\ n

Southern, Edwin M. (fl 1975), British molecular biologist. In 1975 Southern delineated a method for identifying specific DNA sequences that had been previously separated by gel electrophoresis.

sov·er·eign \'säv-(ə-)rən\ adj : having generalized curative powers ⟨a ∼ remedy⟩

soya \'sȯi-(y)ə\ n : SOYBEAN

soy·bean \'sȯi-ˌbēn\ also **soya bean** n : a hairy annual Asian legume (*Glycine max*) grown for its oil-rich proteinaceous seeds and for forage and soil improvement; also : its seed

soybean oil also **soya–bean oil** n : a pale yellow drying or semidrying oil that is obtained from soybeans and is used chiefly as a food, in paints, varnishes, linoleum, printing ink, and soap, and as a source of phospholipids, fatty acids, and sterols

sp abbr species (sing) — compare SPP

spa \'spä, 'spȯ\ n **1 a** : a mineral spring **b** : a resort with mineral springs **2** : a commercial establishment with facilities for exercising and bathing; esp : HEALTH SPA

space \'spās\ n **1** : a period of time; also : its duration **2** : a limited extent in one, two, or three dimensions **3** : a particular area or cavity within the body

space lattice n : LATTICE a

space main·tain·er \-mān-ˌtā-nər\ n : a temporary orthodontic appliance used following the loss or extraction of a tooth (as a milk tooth) to prevent the shifting of adjacent teeth into the resulting space — called also *space retainer*

space medicine n : a branch of medicine concerned with the physiological and biological effects on the human body of spaceflight

space of Fon·tana \-ˌfän-'tän-ə\ n : any of the spaces between trabeculae of Descemet's membrane through which the anterior chamber of the eye communicates with the canal of Schlemm

Fon·ta·na \ˌfōn-'tä-nä\, **Felice (1730–1805)**, Italian neurologist and physiologist. Fontana lectured in physics at the University of Pisa, Italy. He is remembered for developing a museum of natural history in Florence that was known for its collection of wax models of anatomical parts. In 1765 he published his observations on the movements of the iris. He observed that the reflex response to light in the pupil of one eye occurs also in the other eye, even if the latter is not exposed to light. In this study he described the spaces between the fibers of the posterior elastic lamina of the cornea which serve as passages between the canal of Schlemm and the anterior chamber of the eye; these spaces are now known as the spaces of Fontana.

space of Nu·el \-'n(y)ü-əl, -nǖ-'el\ n : NUEL'S SPACE

space of Ret·zi·us \-'ret-sē-əs\ n : RETROPUBIC SPACE

Retzius, Anders Adolf (1796–1860), Swedish anatomist and anthropologist. A professor of anatomy and physiology in Stockholm, Retzius conducted his early research in comparative anatomy, of which he was a pioneer in Sweden. An early discovery was an organ of elasmobranch fishes homologous with the adrenal cortex of higher animals. His investigations of the chordate amphioxus were very important in the development of comparative anatomy and embryology. Retzius is best known for his pioneering studies in craniometry, however. In 1842 he devised the cranial index, which is based upon the ratio of the skull's width to its height and serves as a preliminary indicator of racial identity for human fossils.

space perception n : the perception of the properties and relationships of objects in space esp. with respect to direction, size, distance, and orientation

spac·er \'spā-sər\ n : a region of chromosomal DNA between genes that is not transcribed into messenger RNA and is of uncertain function

space retainer n : SPACE MAINTAINER

space·sick \-ˌsik\ adj : affected with space sickness

space sickness n : sickness and esp. nausea and dizziness that occurs under the conditions of sustained spaceflight

span \'span\ n **1** : an extent of distance or of time; esp : LIFE SPAN **2** : MEMORY SPAN

Span·ish flu \'span-ish-\ n : influenza that is caused by a subtype (H1N1) of the orthomyxovirus causing influenza A and that was responsible for about 500,000 deaths in the U.S. in the influenza pandemic of 1918–1919 — called also *Spanish influenza*; compare ASIAN FLU, HONG KONG FLU

Spanish fly n **1** : a green blister beetle (*Lytta vesicatoria* of the family Meloidae) of southern Europe that is the source of cantharides **2** : CANTHARIS 2

spar·er \'sper-ər\ n : a substance that reduces the body's need for or consumption of something ⟨carbohydrates are protein ∼s⟩

spar·ga·no·sis \ˌspär-gə-'nō-səs\ n, pl **-no·ses** \-ˌsēz\ : the condition of being infected with sparganum

spar·ga·num \'spär-gə-nəm\ n, pl **-na** \-nə\ also **-nums** : an intramuscular or subcutaneous vermiform parasite of various vertebrates including humans that is the plerocercoid larva of a tapeworm — sometimes used as though a generic name when describing such a larva ⟨*Sparganum mansoni* is the larva of *Spirometra mansoni*⟩

Spar·ine \'spär-ˌēn\ n : a preparation of the hydrochloride of promazine — formerly a U.S. registered trademark

spar·te·ine \'spärt-ē-ən, 'spär-ˌtēn\ n : a liquid alkaloid extracted from the Scotch broom that has been used esp. formerly in medicine in the form of its hydrated sulfate $C_{15}H_{26}N_2·H_2SO_4·5H_2O$

spasm \'spaz-əm\ n **1** : an involuntary and abnormal contraction of muscle or muscle fibers or of a hollow organ (as an artery, the colon, or the esophagus) that consists largely of involuntary muscle fibers **2** : the state or condition of a muscle or organ affected with spasms ⟨the renal artery went into ∼⟩

spas·mod·ic \spaz-'mäd-ik\ adj : of, relating to, characterized by, or resulting from spasm ⟨a ∼ twitching⟩ ⟨a ∼ cough⟩ — **spas·mod·i·cal·ly** \-i-k(ə-)lē\ adv

spasmodic dysmenorrhea *n* : dysmenorrhea associated with painful contractions of the uterus

spas·mo·gen·ic \ˌspaz-mə-ˈjen-ik\ *adj* : inducing spasm

spas·mol·y·sis \spaz-ˈmäl-ə-səs\ *n, pl* **-y·ses** \-ˌsēz\ : the relaxation of spasm

¹**spas·mo·lyt·ic** \ˌspaz-mə-ˈlit-ik\ *adj* : tending or having the power to relieve spasms or convulsions ⟨∼ drugs⟩ — **spas·mo·lyt·i·cal·ly** \-i-k(ə)lē\ *adv*

²**spasmolytic** *n* : a spasmolytic agent

spas·mo·phe·mia \ˌspaz-mə-ˈfē-mē-ə\ *n* : STUTTERING 2

spas·mo·phil·ia \ˌspaz-mə-ˈfil-ē-ə\ *n* : an abnormal tendency to convulsions, tetany, or spasms from even slight mechanical or electrical stimulation ⟨∼ associated with rickets⟩ — **spas·mo·phile** \ˈspaz-mə-ˌfīl\ *or* **spas·mo·phil·ic** \ˌspaz-mə-ˈfil-ik\ *adj*

¹**spas·tic** \ˈspas-tik\ *adj* **1** : of, relating to, or characterized by spasm **2** : affected with or marked by spasticity or spastic paralysis ⟨a ∼ patient⟩ ⟨∼ hemiplegia⟩ — **spas·ti·cal·ly** \-ti-k(ə)lē\ *adv*

²**spastic** *n* : an individual affected with spastic paralysis

spastic cerebral palsy *n* : the most common form of cerebral palsy marked by hypertonic muscles and stiff and jerky movements

spastic colon *n* : IRRITABLE BOWEL SYNDROME

spas·tic·i·ty \spa-ˈstis-ət-ē\ *n, pl* **-ties** : a spastic state or condition; *esp* : muscular hypertonicity with increased tendon reflexes

spastic paralysis *n* : paralysis with tonic spasm of the affected muscles and with increased tendon reflexes

spastic paraplegia *n* : spastic paralysis of the legs

spat *past and past part of* SPIT

spa·tial \ˈspā-shəl\ *adj* **1** : relating to, occupying, or having the character of space ⟨affected with ∼ disorientation⟩ **2** : of or relating to facility in perceiving relations (as of objects) in space ⟨tests of ∼ ability⟩ — **spa·tial·ly** \ˈspāsh-(ə-)lē\ *adv*

spatial summation *n* : sensory summation that involves stimulation of several spatially separated neurons at the same time

spa·tia zon·u·lar·ia \ˈspā-sh(ē-)ə-ˌzän-yə-ˈlar-ē-ə\ *n* : a sacculated canal that is situated behind the suspensory ligament of the eye and circles the lens at its equator

spat·u·la \ˈspach-(ə-)lə\ *n* : a flat thin instrument for spreading or mixing soft substances, scooping, lifting, or scraping

¹**spat·u·late** \-lət\ *adj* : shaped like a spatula or a spoon

²**spat·u·late** \ˈspach-ə-ˌlāt\ *vt* **-lat·ed; -lat·ing** : to mix or treat with a spatula ⟨after the powder has been incorporated in the water, the mass is *spatulated* thoroughly —M. G. Swenson⟩

spat·u·la·tion \ˌspach-ə-ˈlā-shən\ *n* : the act or process of spatulating

spav·in \ˈspav-ən\ *n* : a bony enlargement of the hock of a horse associated with strain — **spav·ined** \-ənd\ *adj*

spay \ˈspā\ *vt* **spayed; spay·ing** : to remove the ovaries and uterus of (a female animal)

SPCA *abbr* **1** serum prothrombin conversion accelerator **2** Society for the Prevention of Cruelty to Animals

spear·mint \ˈspi(ə)r-ˌmint, -mənt\ *n* : a common herb of the genus *Mentha* (*M. spicata*) cultivated for use as a flavoring agent and esp. for its aromatic oil

spearmint oil *n* : an aromatic essential oil obtained from spearmint and used in pharmacology as a flavoring agent

spe·cial·ist \ˈspesh-(ə-)ləst\ *n* : a medical practitioner whose practice is limited to a particular class of patients (as children) or of diseases (as skin diseases) or of technique (as surgery); *esp* : a physician who is qualified by advanced training and certification by a specialty examining board to so limit his or her practice

spe·cial·iza·tion \ˌspesh-(ə-)lə-ˈzā-shən\ *also Brit* **spe·cial·isa·tion** \ˌspesh-ə-ˌlī-\ *n* **1** : a making or becoming specialized ⟨∼ in pediatrics⟩ **2 a** : structural adaptation of a body part to a particular function or of an organism for life in a particular environment **b** : a body part or an organism adapted by specialization

spe·cial·ize *also Brit* **spe·cial·ise** \ˈspesh-ə-ˌlīz\ *vi* **-ized** *also Brit* **-ised; -iz·ing** *also Brit* **-is·ing** **1** : to concentrate one's efforts in a special activity or field : become or be a specialist ⟨∼ in anesthesiology⟩ **2** : to undergo evolutionary specialization

Spe·cial K \ˈspesh-əl-ˈkā\ *n, slang* : the anesthetic ketamine used illicitly usu. by being inhaled in powdered form esp. for the dreamlike or hallucinogenic state it produces

spe·cial sense \ˈspesh-əl-\ *n* : any of the senses of sight, hearing, equilibrium, smell, taste, or touch

spe·cial·ty \ˈspesh-əl-tē\ *n, pl* **-ties** : something (as a branch of medicine) in which one specializes

spe·ci·ate \ˈspē-sē-ˌāt, -shē-\ *vi* **-at·ed; -at·ing** : to differentiate into new biological species — **spe·ci·a·tion** \ˌspē-s(h)ē-ˈā-shən\ *n* — **spe·ci·a·tion·al** \-shnəl, -shən-ᵊl\ *adj*

spe·cies \ˈspē-(ˌ)shēz, -(ˌ)sēz\ *n, pl* **species** **1 a** : a category of biological classification ranking immediately below the genus or subgenus, comprising related organisms or populations potentially capable of interbreeding, and being designated by a binomial that consists of the name of the genus followed by a Latin or latinized uncapitalized noun or adjective agreeing grammatically with the genus name **b** : an individual or kind belonging to a biological species **2** : a particular kind of atomic nucleus, atom, molecule, or ion ⟨production of DNA damage by active oxygen ∼⟩

species–spe·cif·ic \-spi-ˈsif-ik\ *adj* : relating to or being a substance (as an antigen or drug) that is limited in action or effect to a particular species and esp. to the species from which it is derived ⟨interferon is a ∼ substance⟩

¹**spe·cif·ic** \spi-ˈsif-ik\ *adj* **1 a** : restricted by nature to a particular individual, situation, relation, or effect ⟨a disease ∼ to horses⟩ **b** : exerting a distinctive influence (as on a body part or a disease) ⟨∼ antibodies⟩ **2** : of, relating to, or constituting a species and esp. a biological species

²**specific** *n* : a drug or remedy having a specific mitigating effect on a disease

specific dynamic action *n* : the effect of ingestion and assimilation of food and esp. of protein in increasing the production of heat in the body — abbr. *SDA*

specific epithet *n* : the Latin or latinized noun or adjective that follows the genus name in a taxonomic binomial

specific gravity *n* : the ratio of the density of a substance to the density of some substance (as pure water) taken as a standard when both densities are obtained by weighing in air

specific heat *n* **1** : the ratio of the quantity of heat required to raise the temperature of a body one degree to that required to raise the temperature of an equal mass of water one degree **2** : the heat in calories required to raise the temperature of one gram of a substance one degree Celsius

spec·i·fic·i·ty \ˌspes-ə-ˈfis-ət-ē\ *n, pl* **-ties** : the quality or condition of being specific: as **a** : the condition of being peculiar to a particular individual or group of organisms ⟨host ∼ of a parasite⟩ **b** : the condition of participating in or catalyzing only one or a few chemical reactions ⟨the ∼ of an enzyme⟩

spec·i·men \ˈspes-(ə-)mən\ *n* **1** : an individual, item, or part typical of a group, class, or whole **2** : a portion or quantity of material for use in testing, examination, or study ⟨a urine ∼⟩

SPECT *abbr* single photon emission computed tomography

spec·ta·cles \ˈspek-ti-kəlz\ *n pl* : GLASS 2b

spec·ti·no·my·cin \ˌspek-tə-nō-ˈmīs-ᵊn\ *n* : a white crystalline broad-spectrum antibiotic derived from a bacterium of the genus *Streptomyces* (*S. spectabilis*) that is used clinically esp. in the form of its hydrated dihydrochloride $C_{14}H_{24}N_2O_7 \cdot 2HCl \cdot 5H_2O$ to treat gonorrhea — called also *actinospectacin;* see TROBICIN

spectra *pl of* SPECTRUM

S

T

spec·tral \'spek-trəl\ *adj* : of, relating to, or made by a spectrum — **spec·tral·ly** *adv*

spectral line *n* : one of a series of linear images of the narrow slit of a spectrograph or similar instrument corresponding to a component of the spectrum of the radiation emitted by a particular source

spec·trin \'spek-trən\ *n* : a large cytoskeletal protein that is found on the inner cell membrane of red blood cells and that functions esp. in maintaining cell shape

spec·tro·chem·i·cal \ˌspek-trō-'kem-i-kəl\ *adj* : of, relating to, or applying the methods of spectrochemistry ⟨∼ analysis of a toxin⟩

spec·tro·chem·is·try \-'kem-ə-strē\ *n, pl* **-tries** : a branch of chemistry based on a study of the spectra of substances

spec·tro·flu·o·rom·e·ter \'spek-(ˌ)trō-ˌflü(-ə)r-'äm-ət-ər\ *also* **spec·tro·flu·o·rim·e·ter** \-'im-\ *n* : a device for measuring and recording fluorescence spectra — **spec·tro·flu·o·ro·met·ric** \-ˌflü(-ə)r-ə-'me-trik\ *adj* — **spec·tro·flu·o·rom·e·try** \-ˌflü(-ə)r-'äm-ə-trē\ *n, pl* **-tries**

spec·tro·gram \'spek-t(r)ə-ˌgram\ *n* : a photograph or diagram of a spectrum

spec·tro·graph \-ˌgraf\ *n* : an instrument for dispersing radiation (as electromagnetic radiation or sound waves) into a spectrum and photographing or mapping the spectrum — **spec·tro·graph·ic** \ˌspek-t(r)ə-'graf-ik\ *adj* — **spec·tro·graph·i·cal·ly** \-i-k(ə-)lē\ *adv* — **spec·trog·ra·phy** \spek-'träg-rə-fē\ *n, pl* **-phies**

spec·trom·e·ter \spek-'träm-ət-ər\ *n* **1** : an instrument used for measuring wavelengths of light spectra **2** : any of various analytical instruments in which an emission (as of particles or radiation) is dispersed according to some property (as mass or energy) of the emission and the amount of dispersion is measured ⟨nuclear magnetic resonance ∼⟩ — **spec·tro·met·ric** \ˌspek-trə-'me-trik\ *adj* — **spec·trom·e·try** \spek-'träm-ə-trē\ *n, pl* **-tries**

spec·tro·pho·tom·e·ter \ˌspek-trō-fə-'täm-ət-ər\ *n* : a photometer for measuring the relative intensities of the light in different parts of a spectrum — **spec·tro·pho·to·met·ric** \-trə-ˌfōt-ə-'me-trik\ *adj* — **spec·tro·pho·to·met·ri·cal·ly** \-tri-k(ə-)lē\ *adv* — **spec·tro·pho·tom·e·try** \ˌspek-(ˌ)trō-fə-'täm-ə-trē\ *n, pl* **-tries**

spec·tro·po·lar·im·e·ter \-ˌpō-lə-'rim-ət-ər\ *n* : a combined spectroscope and polarimeter that is used for the determination of the rotatory power of solutions at different wavelengths

spec·tro·scope \'spek-trə-ˌskōp\ *n* : an instrument for forming and examining optical spectra — **spec·tro·scop·ic** \ˌspek-trə-'skäp-ik\ *adj* — **spec·tro·scop·i·cal·ly** \-i-k(ə-)lē\ *adv*

spec·tros·co·pist \spek-'träs-kə-pəst\ *n* : a person trained in or specializing in spectroscopy

spec·tros·co·py \spek-'träs-kə-pē\ *n, pl* **-pies** **1 a** : the production and investigation of spectra **b** : the process or technique of using a spectroscope or spectrometer **2** : physics that deals with the theory and interpretation of interactions between matter and radiation (as electromagnetic radiation)

spec·trum \'spek-trəm\ *n, pl* **spec·tra** \-trə\ *or* **spectrums** **1 a** : a continuum of color formed when a beam of white light is dispersed (as by passage through a prism) so that its component wavelengths are arranged in order **b** : any of various continua that resemble a spectrum in consisting of an ordered arrangement by a particular characteristic (as frequency or energy): as **(1)** : ELECTROMAGNETIC SPECTRUM **(2)** : MASS SPECTRUM **c** : the representation (as a plot) of a spectrum **2** : a continuous sequence or range; *specif* : a range of effectiveness against pathogenic organisms ⟨an antibiotic with a broad ∼⟩

spec·u·lar \'spek-yə-lər\ *adj* : conducted with the aid of a speculum ⟨a ∼ examination⟩

spec·u·lum \'spek-yə-ləm\ *n, pl* **-la** \-lə\ *also* **-lums** : any of various instruments for insertion into a body passage to facilitate visual inspection or medication ⟨a vaginal ∼⟩

speech \'spēch\ *n* : the communication or expression of thoughts in spoken words

speech center *n* : a brain center exerting control over speech : BROCA'S AREA

speech therapist *n* : a person specially trained in speech therapy

speech therapy *n* : therapeutic treatment of speech defects (as lisping and stuttering)

speed \'spēd\ *n* : METHAMPHETAMINE; *also* : a related stimulant drug and esp. an amphetamine

speed freak \-'frēk\ *n* : one who habitually misuses amphetamines and esp. methamphetamine

spell \'spel\ *n* : a period of bodily or mental distress or disorder ⟨a ∼ of coughing⟩ ⟨fainting ∼s⟩

sperm \'spərm\ *n, pl* **sperm** *or* **sperms** **1** : the male impregnating fluid : SEMEN **2** : a male gamete; *esp* : SPERMATOZOON

sper·ma·ce·ti \ˌspər-mə-'sēt-ē, -'set-\ *n* : a waxy solid obtained from the oil of cetaceans and esp. sperm whales and used esp. formerly in pharmacology as a constituent of ointments

sper·mat·ic \(ˌ)spər-'mat-ik\ *adj* : relating to, resembling, carrying, or full of sperm

spermatic artery — see INTERNAL SPERMATIC ARTERY

spermatic canal *n* : INGUINAL CANAL a

spermatic cord *n* : a cord that suspends the testis within the scrotum, contains the vas deferens and vessels and nerves of the testis, and extends from the deep inguinal ring through the inguinal canal and superficial inguinal ring downward into the scrotum

spermatic duct *n* : VAS DEFERENS

spermatic fluid *n* : SEMEN

spermatic plexus *n* : a nerve plexus that receives fibers from the renal plexus and a plexus associated with the aorta and that passes with the testicular artery to the testis

spermatic vein *n* : TESTICULAR VEIN

sper·ma·tid \'spər-mət-əd\ *n* : one of the haploid cells that are formed by the second meiotic division of a spermatocyte and that differentiate into spermatozoa — compare OOTID

sper·mato·cele \(ˌ)spər-'mat-ə-ˌsēl\ *n* : a cystic swelling of the ducts in the epididymis or in the rete testis usu. containing spermatozoa

sper·mato·cide \(ˌ)spər-'mat-ə-ˌsīd\ *n* : SPERMICIDE — **sper·mato·cid·al** \(ˌ)spər-ˌmat-ə-'sīd-ᵊl\ *adj*

sper·mato·cyte \(ˌ)spər-'mat-ə-ˌsīt\ *n* : a cell giving rise to sperm; *esp* : a cell that is derived from a spermatogonium and ultimately gives rise to four haploid spermatids

sper·mato·gen·e·sis \(ˌ)spər-ˌmat-ə-'jen-ə-səs\ *n, pl* **-e·ses** \-ˌsēz\ : the process of male gamete formation including formation of a primary spermatocyte from a spermatogonium, meiotic division of the spermatocyte, and transformation of the four resulting spermatids into spermatozoa

sper·mato·gen·ic \-'jen-ik\ *adj* : of, relating to, or constituting spermatogenesis

sper·mato·go·ni·um \-'gō-nē-əm\ *n, pl* **-nia** \-nē-ə\ : a primitive male germ cell that gives rise to primary spermatocytes in spermatogenesis — **sper·mato·go·ni·al** \-nē-əl\ *adj*

sper·ma·tor·rhea *or chiefly Brit* **sper·ma·tor·rhoea** \ˌspər-mət-ə-'rē-ə, (ˌ)spər-ˌmat-\ *n* : abnormally frequent or excessive emission of semen without orgasm

sper·ma·tox·in \'spər-mə-ˌtäk-sən\ *n* : a substance (as an antibody) poisonous to spermatozoa or derived from spermatozoa and tending to prevent conception

sper·ma·to·zo·al \ˌspər-mət-ə-'zō-əl, (ˌ)spər-ˌmat-\ *adj* : of or relating to spermatozoa

sper·ma·to·zo·an \(ˌ)spər-ˌmat-ə-'zō-ən, ˌspər-mət-\ *n* : SPERMATOZOON — **spermatozoan** *adj*

sper·ma·to·zo·id \-'zō-əd\ *n* : a male gamete of a plant motile by anterior cilia

sper·ma·to·zo·on \-'zō-ˌän, -'zō-ən\ *n, pl* **-zoa** \-'zō-ə\ : a motile male gamete of an animal usu. with rounded or elongate head and a long posterior flagellum

sper·ma·tu·ria \ˌspər-mə-'t(y)ùr-ē-ə\ *n* : discharge of semen in the urine

sperm cell *n* : SPERM 2

sperm duct *n* : VAS DEFERENS

sper·mi·a·tion \ˌspər-mē-ˈā-shən\ *n* : the discharge of spermatozoa from the testis

sper·mi·cid·al \ˌspər-mə-ˈsīd-ᵊl\ *adj* : killing sperm ⟨∼ jelly⟩ — **sper·mi·cid·al·ly** \-ē\ *adv*

sper·mi·cide \ˈspər-mə-ˌsīd\ *n* : a preparation or substance (as nonoxynol-9) used to kill sperm — called also *spermatocide*

sper·mi·dine \ˈspər-mə-ˌdēn\ *n* : a crystalline aliphatic amine $C_7H_{19}N_3$ which is found esp. in semen

sperm·ine \ˈspər-ˌmēn, -mən\ *n* : a deliquescent crystalline aliphatic tetramine $C_{10}H_{26}N_4$ found in semen in combination with phosphoric acid, in blood serum and body tissues, and in yeast

sper·mio·gen·e·sis \ˌspər-mē-ō-ˈjen-ə-səs\ *n, pl* **-e·ses** \-ˌsēz\ **1** : SPERMATOGENESIS **2** : transformation of a spermatid into a spermatozoon

sper·mo·tox·in \ˈspər-mə-ˌtäk-sən\ *n* : SPERMATOXIN

spes phthis·i·ca \ˈspās-ˈtiz-i-kə\ *n* : a state of euphoria occurring in patients with pulmonary tuberculosis

SPF \ˌes-ˌpē-ˈef\ *n* : a number assigned to a sunscreen that is the factor by which the time required for unprotected skin to become sunburned is increased when the sunscreen is used — called also *sun protection factor*

sp gr *abbr* specific gravity

sphac·e·late \ˈsfas-ə-ˌlāt\ *vb* **-lat·ed; -lat·ing** *vi* : to become gangrenous ∼ *vt* : to cause to become gangrenous — **sphac·e·la·tion** \ˌsfas-ə-ˈlā-shən\ *n*

sphac·e·lus \ˈsfas-ə-ləs\ *n* : GANGRENE; *also* : a gangrenous or necrosed part or mass : SLOUGH

sphag·num \ˈsfag-nəm\ *n* **1** : any of an order (Sphagnales, containing a single genus *Sphagnum*) of atypical mosses that grow only in wet acid areas where their remains become compacted with other plant debris to form peat **2** : a mass of dehydrated sphagnum plants used as a surgical dressing esp. during World War I

S phase *n* : the period in the cell cycle during which DNA replication takes place — compare G_1 PHASE, G_2 PHASE, M PHASE

sphe·no·eth·moid recess \ˌsfē-nō-ˌeth-ˌmȯid-\ *or* **sphe·no·eth·moi·dal recess** \-ˌmȯid-ᵊl-\ *n* : a small space between the sphenoid bone and the superior nasal concha into which the sphenoid sinus opens

sphe·no·fron·tal suture \ˌsfē-nō-ˌfrənt-ᵊl-\ *n* : the suture occurring between the greater wing of the sphenoid and the frontal bone

¹**sphe·noid** \ˈsfē-ˌnȯid\ *or* **sphe·noi·dal** \sfē-ˈnȯid-ᵊl\ *adj* : of, relating to, or being a compound bone of the base of the cranium of various vertebrates formed by the fusion of several bony elements with the basisphenoid and in humans consisting of a median body from whose sides extend a pair of broad curved winglike expansions in front of which is another pair of much smaller triangular lateral processes while ventrally two large deeply cleft processes extend downward — see GREATER WING, LESSER WING

²**sphenoid** *n* : a sphenoid bone

sphenoidal fissure *n* : a fissure between the greater and lesser wing of the sphenoid bone

sphenoidal process *n* **1** : a process on the superior border of the vertical plate of the palatine bone articulating with the sphenoid **2** : a backward prolongation of the cartilage of the nasal septum between the vomer and the perpendicular plate of the ethmoid

sphe·noid·itis \ˌsfē-ˌnȯi-ˈdīt-əs\ *n* : inflammation of the sphenoid sinuses

sphenoid sinus *or* **sphenoidal sinus** *n* : either of two irregular cavities in the body of the sphenoid bone that communicate with the nasal cavities

sphe·no·man·dib·u·lar ligament \ˌsfē-nō-man-ˌdib-yə-lər-\ *n* : a flat thin band of fibrous tissue derived from Meckel's cartilage which extends downward from the sphenoid bone to the lingula of the mandibular foramen

sphe·no·max·il·lary fissure \ˌsfē-nō-ˈmak-sə-ˌler-ē-, *chiefly Brit* -mak-ˈsil-ə-rē-\ *n* : ORBITAL FISSURE b

sphenomaxillary fossa *n* : PTERYGOPALATINE FOSSA

sphe·no–oc·cip·i·tal synchondrosis \ˌsfē-nō-äk-ˈsip-ət-ᵊl-\ *n* : the cartilaginous junction between the basisphenoid and basioccipital bones of the mammalian skull that in humans is usu. closed by the age of 25

¹**sphe·no·pal·a·tine** \ˌsfē-nō-ˈpal-ə-ˌtīn\ *adj* : of, relating to, lying in, or distributed to the vicinity of the sphenoid and palatine bones

²**sphenopalatine** *n* : a sphenopalatine part; *specif* : PTERYGOPALATINE GANGLION

sphenopalatine foramen *n* : a foramen between the sphenoidal and orbital parts of the vertical plate of the palatine bone; *also* : a deep notch between these parts that by articulation with the sphenoid bone is converted into a foramen

sphenopalatine ganglion *n* : PTERYGOPALATINE GANGLION

sphe·no·pa·ri·etal sinus \ˌsfē-nō-pə-ˈrī-ət-ᵊl-\ *n* : a venous sinus of the dura mater on each side of the cranium arising at a meningeal vein near the apex of the lesser wing of the sphenoid bone and draining into the anterior part of the cavernous sinus

sphenoparietal suture *n* : the suture occurring between the greater wing of the sphenoid bone and the parietal bone

sphe·no·squa·mo·sal suture \ˌsfē-nō-skwə-ˌmō-səl-\ *n* : the suture occurring between the greater wing of the sphenoid bone and the squamous portion of the temporal bone

sphe·no·zy·go·mat·ic suture \ˌsfē-nō-ˌzī-gə-ˌmat-ik-\ *n* : the suture occurring between the greater wing of the sphenoid bone and the zygomatic bone

spher·i·cal aberration \ˈsfir-i-kəl-, ˈsfer-\ *n* : aberration that is caused by the spherical form of a lens or mirror and that gives different foci for central and marginal rays

sphe·ro·cyte \ˈsfir-ə-ˌsīt, ˈsfer-\ *n* : a more or less globular red blood cell that is characteristic of some hemolytic anemias

sphe·ro·cyt·ic \ˌsfir-ə-ˈsit-ik, ˌsfer-\ *adj* : of, relating to, or characterized by spherocytes ⟨∼ anemia⟩

sphe·ro·cy·to·sis \ˌsfir-ō-sī-ˈtō-səs, ˌsfer-\ *n* : the presence of spherocytes in the blood; *esp* : HEREDITARY SPHEROCYTOSIS

sphe·roi·dal \sfir-ˈȯid-ᵊl\ *also* **spher·oid** \ˈsfi(ə)r-ˌȯid, ˈsfe(ə)r-\ *adj* : having the shape of a sphere

sphe·rom·e·ter \sfir-ˈäm-ət-ər\ *n* : an instrument for measuring the curvature of a surface

sphe·ro·pha·kia \ˌsfir-ə-ˈfā-kē-ə, ˌsfer-\ *n* : a congenital vision defect characterized by lenses which are abnormally small and spherical

sphe·ro·plast \ˈsfir-ə-ˌplast, ˈsfer-\ *n* : a bacterium or yeast cell that has been modified by nutritional or environmental factors or by artificial means (as by the use of a lysozyme) and that is characterized by partial loss of the cell wall and by increased osmotic sensitivity

spher·u·lin \ˈsfir-yə-lən, ˈsfer-\ *n* : an antigen that is derived from a fungus of the genus *Coccidioides* (*C. immitis*) while in its endospore-producing phase and that is used similarly to coccidioidin

spher·u·lite \ˈsfir-yə-ˌlīt, ˈsfer-\ *n* : a usu. spherical crystalline body of radiating crystal fibers — **spher·u·lit·ic** \ˌsfir-yə-ˈlit-ik, ˌsfer-\ *adj*

sphinc·ter \ˈsfiŋ(k)-tər\ *n* : an annular muscle surrounding and able to contract or close a bodily opening — see ANAL SPHINCTER, CARDIAC SPHINCTER, PRECAPILLARY SPHINCTER, PYLORIC SPHINCTER — **sphinc·ter·al** \-t(ə-)rəl\ *adj*

sphincter ani ex·ter·nus \-ˈā-ˌnī-ik-ˈstər-nəs\ *n* : ANAL SPHINCTER a

sphincter ani in·ter·nus \-in-ˈtər-nəs\ *n* : ANAL SPHINCTER b

sphinc·ter·ec·to·my \ˌsfiŋk-tər-ˈek-tə-mē\ *n, pl* **-mies** : surgical excision of a sphincter

sphinc·ter·ic \sfiŋ(k)-ˈter-ik\ *adj* : of, relating to, or being a sphincter ⟨∼ control⟩ ⟨a ∼ muscle⟩

\ə\ abut \ᵊ\ kitten \ər\ further \a\ ash \ā\ ace \ä\ cot, cart
\aú\ out \ch\ chin \e\ bet \ē\ easy \g\ go \i\ hit \ī\ ice \j\ job
\ŋ\ sing \ō\ go \ȯ\ law \ȯi\ boy \th\ thin \t͟h\ the \ü\ loot
\ú\ foot \y\ yet \zh\ vision *See also* Pronunciation Symbols page

S
T

sphincter of Od·di \-'äd-ē\ *n* : a complex sphincter closing the duodenal orifice of the common bile duct

Od·di \'ȯd-dē\, **Ruggero (1864–1913)**, Italian physician. While studying in vivo the action of the bile on digestion, Oddi discovered the sphincter of the common bile duct. He later measured the tone of the sphincter by perfecting an experimental device very similar to the device now used for the intraoperative manometry of the bile ducts.

sphinc·tero·plas·ty \'sfiŋk-tər-ə-ˌplas-tē\ *n, pl* **-ties** : plastic surgery of a sphincter ⟨anal ∼⟩

sphinc·ter·ot·o·my \ˌsfiŋk-tər-'ät-ə-mē\ *n, pl* **-mies** : surgical incision of a sphincter

sphincter pu·pil·lae \-pyü-'pil-ē\ *n* : a broad flat band of smooth muscle in the iris that surrounds the pupil of the eye

sphincter ure·thrae \-yu̇-'rē-thrē\ *n* : a muscle composed of fibers that arise from the inferior ramus of the ischium and that interdigitate with those from the opposite side of the body to form in the male a narrow ring of muscle around the urethra just distal to the apex of the prostate gland and in the female a ring of muscle more generally distributed around the urethra — called also *urethral sphincter*

sphincter va·gi·nae \-və-'jī-nē\ *n* : the bulbocavernosus of the female

sphin·go·lip·id \ˌsfin-gō-'lip-əd\ *n* : any of a group of lipids (as sphingomyelins and cerebrosides) that yield sphingosine or one of its derivatives as one product of hydrolysis

sphin·go·lip·i·do·sis \-ˌlip-ə-'dō-səs\ *n, pl* **-do·ses** \-ˌsēz\ : any of various usu. hereditary disorders (as Gaucher's disease and Tay-Sachs disease) characterized by abnormal metabolism and storage of sphingolipids

sphin·go·my·elin \ˌsfin-gō-'mī-ə-lən\ *n* : any of a group of crystalline phosphatides that are obtained esp. from nerve tissue and that on hydrolysis yield a fatty acid (as lignoceric acid), sphingosine, choline, and phosphoric acid

sphin·go·my·elin·ase \-'mī-ə-lə-ˌnās, -ˌnāz\ *n* : any of several enzymes that catalyze the hydrolysis of sphingomyelin and are lacking in some metabolic deficiency diseases (as Niemann-Pick disease) in which sphingomyelin accumulates in bodily organs (as the spleen and liver)

sphin·go·sine \'sfin-gə-ˌsēn, -sən\ *n* : an unsaturated amino diol $C_{18}H_{37}NO_2$ obtained by hydrolysis of various sphingomyelins, cerebrosides, and gangliosides

sphyg·mic \'sfig-mik\ *adj* : of or relating to the circulatory pulse

sphyg·mo·gram \'sfig-mə-ˌgram\ *n* : a tracing made by a sphygmograph and consisting of a series of curves that correspond to the beats of the heart

sphyg·mo·graph \'sfig-mə-ˌgraf\ *n* : an instrument that records graphically the movements or character of the pulse — **sphyg·mo·graph·ic** \ˌsfig-mə-'graf-ik\ *adj*

sphyg·mo·ma·nom·e·ter \ˌsfig-mō-mə-'näm-ət-ər\ *n* : an instrument for measuring blood pressure and esp. arterial blood pressure

sphyg·mo·mano·met·ric \-ˌman-ə-'me-trik\ *adj* **1** : obtained with a sphygmomanometer ⟨∼ readings⟩ **2** : of, relating to, or used for sphygmomanometry ⟨an ambulatory ∼ device⟩ — **sphyg·mo·mano·met·ri·cal·ly** \-tri-k(ə-)lē\ *adv*

sphyg·mo·ma·nom·e·try \-mə-'näm-ə-trē\ *n, pl* **-tries** : measurement of blood pressure by means of the sphygmomanometer

sphyg·mom·e·ter \sfig-'mäm-ət-ər\ *n* : an instrument for measuring the strength of the pulse beat

spi·ca \'spī-kə\ *n, pl* **spi·cae** \-ˌkē\ *or* **spicas** : a bandage that is applied in successive V-shaped crossings and is used to immobilize a limb esp. at a joint; *also* : such a bandage impregnated with plaster of paris ⟨a ∼ cast applied at the hip⟩

spic·ule \'spik-(ˌ)yü(ə)l\ *n* : a minute slender pointed usu. hard body (as of bone)

spi·der \'spīd-ər\ *n* **1** : any of an order (Araneae syn. Araneida) of arachnids having a body with two main divisions, four pairs of walking legs, and two or more pairs of abdominal spinnerets for spinning threads of silk used esp. in making webs for catching prey **2** : SPIDER NEVUS ⟨an arterial

∼⟩ **3** : an obstruction in the teat of a cow; *esp* : a small irregular horny growth resulting from irritation or bruising

spider nevus *n* : a pigmented area on the skin formed of dilated capillaries or arterioles radiating from a central point like the legs of a spider — called also *spider angioma*

spider vein *n* : a telangiectasia (as on the legs or face) often appearing as a central area with outward radiations resembling the legs of a spider

Spiel·mey·er–Vogt disease \'shpēl-ˌmī-ər-'fōkt-\ *n* : BATTEN DISEASE

Spielmeyer, Walter (1879–1935), German neurologist. Spielmeyer is known for his descriptions of a method of microscopic examination of myelin sheaths of the nervous system (1911) and of a fatal form of lipofuscinosis (1908).

Vogt, Heinrich (1875–1957), German neurologist. After psychiatric posts at the universities of Göttingen and Frankfurt, Vogt became director of a neurological sanatorium at Wiesbaden. Following a major change in his area of interest in the 1920s, he commenced a practice in medical hydrology at a health spa and later founded an institute for research in balneology at Breslau (now Wrocław, Poland). He published his own description of what is now known as Batten disease in 1905.

spi·ge·lia \spī-'jē-l(ē-)yə\ *n* **1** *cap* : a large genus of American herbs (family Loganiaceae) with showy flowers **2** : PINKROOT

Spie·ghel \'spē-gəl\, **Adriaan van den (1578–1625)**, Flemish anatomist. Spieghel was for many years professor of anatomy at Padua, Italy. He published a major treatise on human anatomy in 1627. He is also remembered for an introductory text on botany (1606). The genus *Spigelia* of herbs was named in his honor by Linnaeus in 1753.

spi·ge·lian hernia \spī-'jē-l(ē-)yən-\ *n, often cap S* : a hernia occurring along the linea semilunaris

spigelian lobe *n, often cap S* : CAUDATE LOBE

¹spike \'spīk\ *n* : a change (as in voltage) involving a sharp increase and fall or a recording of this: as **a** : the pointed element in the wave tracing in an electroencephalogram **b** : a sharp increase in body temperature followed by a rapid fall ⟨a fever with ∼s to 103°⟩ **c (1)** : the sharp increase and fall in the recorded action potential of a stimulated nerve cell that during the increasing phase corresponds to an inrush of sodium ions to the interior of the cell and during the decreasing phase corresponds to a slowing of the influx of sodium ions and to an increasing efflux of potassium ions to the exterior **(2)** : ACTION POTENTIAL

²spike *vt* **spiked; spik·ing** : to undergo a sudden sharp increase in (temperature or fever) usu. up to an indicated level ⟨infected patients *spiked* fevers as high as 105°F⟩

spike·nard \'spīk-ˌnärd\ *n* **1 a** : a fragrant ointment of the ancients **b** : a Himalayan aromatic plant (*Nardostachys jatamansi*) from which spikenard is believed to have been derived **2** : an American herb of the genus *Aralia* (*A. racemosa*) whose dried rhizome and roots have been used as a diaphoretic and aromatic

spike potential *n* **1** : SPIKE c(1) **2** : ACTION POTENTIAL

spik·ing *adj* : characterized by recurrent sharp rises in body temperature ⟨a ∼ fever⟩; *also* : resulting from a sharp rise in body temperature ⟨a ∼ temperature of 105°⟩

spin \'spin\ *n* **1** : a quantum characteristic of an elementary particle that is visualized as the rotation of the particle on its axis and that is responsible for measurable angular momentum and magnetic moment **2** : the angular momentum which is associated with spin, whose magnitude is quantized, and which may assume either of two possible directions; *also* : the angular momentum of a system of elementary particles derived from their spins and orbital motions — see SPIN ECHO, SPIN LABEL

spi·na \'spī-nə\ *n, pl* **spi·nae** \-ˌnē\ : an anatomical spine or spinelike process

spina bi·fi·da \-'bif-ə-də *also* -'bīf-\ *n* : a neural tube defect marked by congenital cleft of the spinal column usu. with hernial protrusion of the meninges and sometimes the spinal cord — see MENINGOCELE, MYELOCELE, MYELOMENINGO-CELE

spina bifida oc·cul·ta \-ə-ˈkəl-tə\ *n* : a mild often asymptomatic form of spina bifida in which there is no hernial protrusion of the meninges or spinal cord

spinae — see ERECTOR SPINAE

¹spi·nal \ˈspīn-ᵊl\ *adj* **1** : of, relating to, or situated near the spinal column **2 a** : of, relating to, or affecting the spinal cord ⟨∼ reflexes⟩ **b** : having the spinal cord functionally isolated (as by surgical section) from the brain ⟨experiments on ∼ animals⟩ **c** : used for spinal anesthesia ⟨a ∼ anesthetic⟩ **3** : made for or fitted to the spinal column ⟨a ∼ brace⟩ — **spi·nal·ly** \-ē\ *adv*

²spinal *n* : a spinal anesthetic

spinal accessory nerve *n* : ACCESSORY NERVE

spinal and bulbar muscular atrophy *n* : KENNEDY'S DISEASE

spinal anesthesia *n* : anesthesia produced by injection of an anesthetic into the subarachnoid space of the spine

spinal artery *n* : any of three arteries that supply the spinal cord and its membranes and adjacent structures: **a** : a single unpaired artery that is formed by the anastomosis of a branch of the vertebral artery on each side and that descends in the anterior median fissure of the spinal cord — called also *anterior spinal artery* **b** : either of two arteries of which one arises from a vertebral artery on each side below the level at which the corresponding branch of the anterior spinal artery arises and which descend on the posterior lateral surface of the spinal cord along a line passing close to the entrance of the dorsal roots to the spinal cord — called also *posterior spinal artery*

spinal canal *n* : VERTEBRAL CANAL

spinal column *n* : the articulated series of vertebrae connected by ligaments and separated by more or less elastic intervertebral fibrocartilages that in nearly all vertebrates forms the supporting axis of the body and a protection for the spinal cord and that extends from the hind end of the skull through the median dorsal part of the body to the coccyx or end of the tail — called also *backbone, spine, vertebral column*

spinal cord *n* : the thick longitudinal cord of nervous tissue that in vertebrates extends along the back dorsal to the bodies of the vertebrae and is enclosed in the vertebral canal formed by their neural arches, is continuous anteriorly with the medulla oblongata, gives off at intervals pairs of spinal nerves to the various parts of the trunk and limbs, serves not only as a pathway for nervous impulses to and from the brain but as a center for carrying out and coordinating many reflex actions independently of the brain, and is composed largely of white matter arranged in columns and tracts of longitudinal fibers about a large central core of gray matter somewhat H-shaped in cross section and pierced centrally by a small longitudinal canal continuous with the ventricles of the brain — called also *medulla spinalis*

spinal fluid *n* : CEREBROSPINAL FLUID

spinal fusion *n* : surgical fusion of two or more vertebrae for remedial immobilization of the spine

spinal ganglion *n* : a ganglion on the dorsal root of each spinal nerve that is one of a series of ganglia containing cell bodies of sensory neurons — called also *dorsal root ganglion*

spi·na·lis \spī-ˈnā-ləs, spi-ˈna-lis\ *n, pl* **spi·na·les** \-(ˌ)lēz\ : the most medial division of the sacrospinalis situated next to the spinal column and acting to extend it or any of the three muscles making up this division: **a** : SPINALIS THORACIS **b** : SPINALIS CERVICIS **c** : SPINALIS CAPITIS

spinalis — see MEDULLA SPINALIS

spinalis cap·i·tis \-ˈkap-ət-əs\ *n* : a muscle that arises with, inserts with, and is intimately associated with the semispinalis capitis

spinalis cer·vi·cis \-ˈsər-və-səs\ *n* : an inconstant muscle that arises esp. from the spinous processes of the lower cervical and upper thoracic vertebrae and inserts esp. into the spinous process of the axis

spinalis tho·ra·cis \-thə-ˈrā-səs\ *n* : an upward continuation

of the sacrospinalis that is situated medially to and blends with the longissimus thoracis, arises from the spinous processes of the first two lumbar and last two thoracic vertebrae, and inserts into the spinous processes of the upper thoracic vertebrae

spinal meningitis *n* : inflammation of the meninges of the spinal cord; *also* : CEREBROSPINAL MENINGITIS

spinal muscular atrophy *n* : any of several inherited disorders (as Kugelberg-Welander disease) that are characterized by the degeneration of motor neurons in the spinal cord resulting in muscular weakness and atrophy and that in some forms (as Werdnig-Hoffmann disease) are fatal

spinal nerve *n* : any of the paired nerves which leave the spinal cord of a craniate vertebrate, supply muscles of the trunk and limbs, and connect with the nerves of the sympathetic nervous system, which arise by a short motor ventral root and a short sensory dorsal root, and of which there are 31 pairs in humans classified according to the part of the spinal cord from which they arise into 8 pairs of cervical nerves, 12 pairs of thoracic nerves, 5 pairs of lumbar nerves, 5 pairs of sacral nerves, and one pair of coccygeal nerves

spinal puncture *n* : LUMBAR PUNCTURE

spinal seg·ment \-ˈseg-mənt\ *n* : a segment of the spinal cord including a single pair of spinal nerves and representing the spinal innervation of a single primitive metamere

spinal shock *n* : a temporary condition following transection of the spinal cord that is characterized by muscular flaccidity and loss of motor reflexes in all parts of the body below the point of transection

spinal stenosis *n* : narrowing of the lumbar spinal column that produces pressure on the nerve roots resulting in sciatica and a condition resembling intermittent claudication and that usu. occurs in middle or old age

spinal tap *n* : LUMBAR PUNCTURE

spin·dle \ˈspin-dᵊl\ *n* **1** : something shaped like a round stick or pin with tapered ends: as **a** : a network of chiefly microtubular fibers along which the chromosomes are distributed during mitosis and meiosis **b** : MUSCLE SPINDLE **2** : SLEEP SPINDLE

spindle cell *n* : a spindle-shaped cell (as in some tumors)

spindle–cell sarcoma *n* : a sarcoma (as a fibrosarcoma) composed chiefly or entirely of spindle cells

spindle fiber *n* : any of the apparent filaments constituting a mitotic spindle

spine \ˈspīn\ *n* **1** : SPINAL COLUMN **2** : a pointed prominence or process (as on a bone)

spin echo *n* : a signal that is detected in a nuclear magnetic resonance spectrometer, that is an echo-like replication of a free induction decay produced by a planned series of radio=frequency pulses, and that can be used to extract more information from a test sample or subject than conventional nuclear magnetic resonance spectroscopy — usu. used attributively ⟨*spin-echo* magnetic resonance imaging of the cervical spine⟩; compare GRADIENT ECHO

spine of the scapula *n* : a projecting triangular bony process on the dorsal surface of the scapula that divides it obliquely into the area of origin of parts of the supraspinatus and infraspinatus muscles and that terminates in the acromion

spin label *n* : a chemical species (as a free radical or metal complex) that has an unpaired electron and that is introduced into a molecule so that the molecule can be investigated using electron spin resonance — **spin–la·beled** *or* **spin–la·belled** *adj* — **spin la·bel·ing** *or* **spin la·bel·ling** *n*

spinn·bar·keit \ˈspin-ˌbär-ˌkīt, ˈshpin-\ *n* : the elastic quality that is characteristic of mucus of the uterine cervix esp. shortly before ovulation

spi·no·cer·e·bel·lar \ˌspī-nō-ˌser-ə-ˈbel-ər\ *adj* : of or relating to the spinal cord and cerebellum ⟨∼ degeneration⟩

spinocerebellar ataxia *n* : any of a group of inherited neu-

S

T

\ə\ **abut** \ᵊ\ **kitten** \ər\ **further** \a\ **ash** \ā\ **ace** \ä\ **cot, cart** \aů\ **out** \ch\ **chin** \e\ **bet** \ē\ **easy** \g\ **go** \i\ **hit** \ī\ **ice** \j\ **job** \ŋ\ **sing** \ō\ **go** \ȯ\ **law** \ȯi\ **boy** \th\ **thin** \ṯẖ\ **the** \ü\ **loot** \ů\ **foot** \y\ **yet** \zh\ **vision** *See also* Pronunciation Symbols page

rodegenerative disorders that are characterized by cerebellar dysfunction manifested esp. by progressive ataxia

spinocerebellar tract *n* : any of four nerve tracts which pass from the spinal cord to the cerebellum and of which two are situated on each side external to the crossed corticospinal tracts: **a** : a posterior tract on each side that arises from cells in the nucleus dorsalis esp. on the same side and passes to the inferior cerebellar peduncle and vermis of the cerebellum — called also *dorsal spinocerebellar tract, posterior spinocerebellar tract* **b** : an anterior tract on each side that arises from cells mostly in the dorsal column of gray matter on the same or opposite side and passes through the medulla oblongata and pons to the superior cerebellar peduncle and vermis — called also *anterior spinocerebellar tract, Gowers's tract, tract of Gowers, ventral spinocerebellar tract*

spi·no·ol·i·vary \-'äl-ə-ˌver-ē\ *adj* : connecting the spinal cord with the olivary nuclei ⟨∼ fibers⟩ ⟨the ∼ tract⟩

spi·nose ear tick \'spī-ˌnōs-\ *n* : an ear tick of the genus *Otobius* (*O. megnini*) of the southwestern U.S. and Mexico that is a serious pest of cattle, horses, sheep, and goats

spinosum — see FORAMEN SPINOSUM, STRATUM SPINOSUM

spi·no·tec·tal tract \ˌspī-nō-ˌtek-t⁸l-\ *n* : an ascending tract of nerve fibers in each lateral funiculus of white matter of the spinal cord that passes upward and terminates in the superior colliculus of the opposite side

spi·no·tha·lam·ic \ˌspī-nō-thə-'lam-ik\ *adj* : of, relating to, comprising, or associated with the spinothalamic tracts ⟨the ∼ system⟩

spinothalamic tract *n* : any of four tracts of nerve fibers of the spinal cord that are arranged in pairs with one member of a pair on each side and that ascend to the thalamus by way of the brain stem: **a** : one on each side of the anterior median fissure that carries nerve impulses relating to the sense of touch — called also *anterior spinothalamic tract, ventral spinothalamic tract* **b** : one on each lateral part of the spinal cord that carries nerve impulses relating to the senses of touch, pain, and temperature — called also *lateral spinothalamic tract*

spi·nous \'spī-nəs\ *adj* : slender and pointed like a spine

spinous process *n* : SPINE 2; *specif* : the median spinelike or platelike dorsal process of the neural arch of a vertebra

spin resonance — see ELECTRON SPIN RESONANCE

spinulosus — see LICHEN SPINULOSUS

spiny–head·ed worm \ˌspī-nē-ˌhed-əd-\ *n* : ACANTHOCEPHALAN

¹spi·ral \'spī-rəl\ *adj* **1 a** : winding around a center or pole and gradually receding from or approaching it **b** : HELICAL ⟨the ∼ structure of DNA⟩ **2** : being a fracture in which the break is produced by twisting apart the bone ⟨a double ∼ break⟩ — **spi·ral·ly** \-rə-lē\ *adv*

²spiral *n* **1** : the path of a point in a plane moving around a central point while continuously receding from or approaching it **2** : a three-dimensional curve (as a helix) with one or more turns about an axis ⟨the double ∼ of DNA⟩

spiral ganglion *n* : a mass of bipolar cell bodies occurring in the modiolus of the organ of Corti and giving off axons which comprise the cochlear nerve

spiralis — see LAMINA SPIRALIS

spiral lamina *n* : a twisting shelf of bone which projects from the modiolus into the canal of the cochlea as it coils around the modiolus and to which the inner margin of the basilar membrane is attached — called also *lamina spiralis*

spiral ligament *n* : the thick periosteum that forms the outer wall of the scala media and that gives attachment to the outer edge of the basilar membrane

spiral organ *n* : ORGAN OF CORTI

spiral valve *n* : a series of crescentic folds of mucous membrane somewhat spirally arranged on the interior of the gallbladder and continuing into the cystic duct — called also *valve of Heister*

spi·ra·my·cin \ˌspī-rə-'mīs-⁸n\ *n* : a mixture of macrolide antibiotics produced by a soil bacterium of the genus *Streptomyces* (*S. ambofaciens*) and having antibacterial activity

spi·reme \'spī-ˌrēm\ *n* : a continuous thread observed in fixed preparations of the prophase of mitosis that appears to be a strand of chromatin but is generally held to be an artifact

Spi·ril·la·ce·ae \ˌspī-rə-'lā-sē-ˌē\ *n pl, in former classifications* : a family of phylogenetically heterogeneous bacteria including *Spirillum, Campylobacter, Bdellovibrio,* and associated genera, and comprising rigid more or less spirally curved elongate forms

spi·ril·li·ci·dal \spī-ˌril-ə-'sīd-⁸l\ *adj* : destroying spirilla ⟨a drug's ∼ action⟩

spi·ril·lo·sis \ˌspī-rə-'lō-səs\ *n, pl* **-lo·ses** \-ˌsēz\ *or* **-lo·sis·es** : infection with or disease caused by spirilla

spi·ril·lum \spī-'ril-əm\ *n* **1** *cap* : a genus of gram-negative bacteria comprising elongated forms having tufts of flagella at both poles and usu. living in stagnant water rich in organic matter — see RAT-BITE FEVER b **2** *pl* **-ril·la** \-'ril-ə\ : any bacterium of the genus *Spirillum*

spir·it \'spir-ət\ *n* **1 a** : DISTILLATE; *esp* : the liquid containing ethyl alcohol and water that is distilled from an alcoholic liquid or mash — often used in pl. **b** : a usu. volatile organic solvent (as an alcohol, ester, or hydrocarbon) **2** : an alcoholic solution of a volatile substance ⟨∼ of camphor⟩

spirit of harts·horn *or* **spirits of harts·horn** \-'härts-ˌhȯ(ə)rn\ *n* : AMMONIA WATER

spirits of wine *or* **spirit of wine** *n* : rectified spirit : ETHANOL, ALCOHOL 1a

spir·i·tu·ous \'spir-ich-(ə-)wəs, -ich-əs, 'spir-ət-əs\ *adj* : containing or impregnated with alcohol obtained by distillation

Spi·ro·cer·ca \ˌspī-rō-'sər-kə\ *n* : a genus of red filarial worms of the family Thelaziidae forming nodules in the walls of the digestive tract and sometimes the aorta of canines esp. in warm regions

Spi·ro·chae·ta \ˌspī-rə-'kēt-ə\ *n* : a genus (the type of the family Spirochaetaceae) of spirochetes distinguished by a flexible undulating body with the protoplasm wound spirally around an elastic axis filament and comprising as now restricted various chiefly aquatic forms or formerly these together with important pathogens now placed in the genera *Treponema, Borrelia,* and *Leptospira*

Spi·ro·chae·ta·ce·ae \ˌspī-rə-kē-'tā-sē-ˌē\ *n pl* : a family comprising large coarsely spiral bacteria of the order Spirochaetales that are free-living in fresh or salt water or associated with animal or human hosts

Spi·ro·chae·ta·les \ˌspī-rə-kē-'tā-(ˌ)lēz\ *n pl* : an order of higher bacteria comprising slender elongated flexuous spiral forms in which the body makes up at least one complete turn of the spiral

spi·ro·chet·al *or chiefly Brit* **spi·ro·chaet·al** \ˌspī-rə-'kēt-⁸l\ *adj* : relating to or caused by spirochetes ⟨∼ infection⟩

spi·ro·chete *or chiefly Brit* **spi·ro·chaete** \'spī-rə-ˌkēt\ *n* : any bacterium of the order Spirochaetales including those causing syphilis and relapsing fever

spi·ro·chet·emia *or chiefly Brit* **spi·ro·chaet·ae·mia** \ˌspī-rə-ˌkē-'tē-mē-ə\ *n* : the abnormal presence of spirochetes in the circulating blood

spi·ro·che·ti·ci·dal *or chiefly Brit* **spi·ro·chae·ti·ci·dal** \ˌspī-rə-ˌkēt-ə-'sīd-⁸l\ *adj* : destructive to spirochetes esp. within the body of an animal host ⟨a ∼ drug⟩

spi·ro·che·ti·cide *or chiefly Brit* **spi·ro·chae·ti·cide** \ˌspī-rə-'kēt-ə-ˌsīd\ *n* : an agent (as a drug) capable of killing spirochetes esp. within the human or animal body

spi·ro·chet·ol·y·sis *or chiefly Brit* **spi·ro·chaet·ol·y·sis** \ˌspī-rə-ˌkē-'täl-ə-səs\ *n, pl* **-y·ses** \-ˌsēz\ : destruction of spirochetes

spi·ro·chet·osis *or chiefly Brit* **spi·ro·chaet·osis** \ˌspī-rə-ˌkēt-'ō-səs\ *n, pl* **-oses** \-ˌsēz\ : infection with or a disease caused by spirochetes

spi·ro·gram \'spī-rə-ˌgram\ *n* : a graphic record of respiratory movements traced on a revolving drum

spi·ro·graph \'spī-rə-ˌgraf\ *n* : an instrument for recording respiratory movements — **spi·ro·graph·ic** \ˌspī-rə-'graf-ik\ *adj*

spi·rog·ra·phy \spī-'räg-rə-fē\ *n, pl* **-phies** : the recording of respiratory movements by means of a spirograph

spi·rom·e·ter \spi-'räm-ət-ər\ *n* : an instrument for measuring the air entering and leaving the lungs — **spi·ro·met·ric** \ˌspī-rə-'me-trik\ *adj*

Spi·rom·e·tra \spī-'räm-ə-trə, spi-\ *n* : a genus of tapeworms of the order Pseudophyllidea that include several (as *S. mansoni* of Asia and *S. mansonoides* of the southern U.S.) which sometimes cause sparganosis in humans

spi·rom·e·try \-ə-trē\ *n, pl* **-tries** : measurement by means of a spirometer of the air entering and leaving the lungs

spi·ro·no·lac·tone \ˌspī-rə-nō-'lak-ˌtōn, spi-ˌrō-nə-\ *n* : an aldosterone antagonist $C_{24}H_{32}O_4S$ that promotes diuresis and sodium excretion and is used to treat essential hypertension, edema with congestive heart failure, hepatic cirrhosis with ascites, nephrotic syndrome, and idiopathic edema

Spi·ru·ri·da \spī-'rur-ə-də\ *n pl* : an order of parasitic nematodes of the subclass Aphasmidia that are characterized by an esophagus divided into two cylinder-shaped regions and having six lips and no buccal stylet and that include various parasites (as the filarial worms) of vertebrates having complex life cycles requiring an invertebrate intermediate host

Spi·rur·i·dae \-ˌdē\ *n pl* : a family of nematode worms that have the adults parasitic in vertebrates, that have the larval stages parasitic in insects, and that with related forms constitute a distinct superfamily of the order Spirurida

spi·rur·oid \'spī-rə-ˌroid\ *adj* : resembling or related to the family Spiruridae ⟨a ~ nematode⟩

¹**spit** \'spit\ *vb* **spit** *or* **spat** \'spat\; **spit·ting** *vt* : to eject (as saliva) from the mouth ~ *vi* : to eject saliva from the mouth

²**spit** *n* : SALIVA

spitting cobra *n* : BLACK-NECKED COBRA; *also* : an African cobra (*Hemachatus hemachatus*) that in defense typically ejects its venom toward the victim without striking

spit·tle \'spit-ᵊl\ *n* : SALIVA

splanch·nic \'splaŋk-nik\ *adj* : of or relating to the viscera : VISCERAL ⟨~ circulation⟩

splanch·ni·cec·to·my \ˌsplaŋk-nə-'sek-tə-mē\ *n, pl* **-mies** : surgical excision of a segment of one or more splanchnic nerves to relieve hypertension

splanchnic ganglion *n* : a small ganglion on the greater splanchnic nerve that is usu. located near the eleventh or twelfth thoracic vertebra

splanchnic nerve *n* : any of three important nerves situated on each side of the body and formed by the union of branches from the six or seven lower thoracic and first lumbar ganglia of the sympathetic system: **a** : a superior one ending in the celiac ganglion — called also *greater splanchnic nerve* **b** : a middle one ending in a detached ganglionic mass of the celiac ganglion at the origin of the renal artery — called also *lesser splanchnic nerve* **c** : an inferior one ending in the renal plexus — called also *least splanchnic nerve, lowest splanchnic nerve*

splanch·ni·cot·o·my \ˌsplaŋk-nə-'kät-ə-mē\ *n, pl* **-mies** : surgical division of one or more splanchnic nerves

splanch·no·cra·ni·um \ˌsplaŋk-nō-'krā-nē-əm\ *n, pl* **-ni·ums** *or* **-nia** \-nē-ə\ : the portion of the skull that arises from the first three branchial arches and forms the supporting structure of the jaws

splanch·nol·o·gy \splaŋk-'näl-ə-jē\ *n, pl* **-gies** : a branch of anatomy concerned with the viscera

splanch·no·meg·a·ly \ˌsplaŋk-nō-'meg-ə-lē\ *n, pl* **-lies** : ORGANOMEGALY

splanch·no·mi·cria \-'mī-krē-ə\ *n* : abnormal smallness of the viscera

splanch·no·pleure \'splaŋk-nə-ˌplu̇(ə)r\ *n* : a layer of tissue that consists of the inner of the two layers into which the unsegmented sheet of mesoderm splits in the embryo of a craniate vertebrate together with the endoderm internal to it and that forms most of the walls and substance of the visceral organs — compare SOMATOPLEURE — **splanch·no·pleu·ric** \ˌsplaŋk-nə-'plu̇r-ik\ *adj*

splanch·nop·to·sis \ˌsplaŋk-ˌnäp-'tō-səs\ *n, pl* **-to·ses** \-ˌsēz\ : VISCEROPTOSIS

splay·foot \'splā-ˌfu̇t, -'fu̇t\ *n* : a foot abnormally flattened

and spread out; *specif* : FLATFOOT — **splay·foot·ed** \-'fu̇t-əd\ *adj*

spleen \'splēn\ *n* : a highly vascular ductless abdominal organ of vertebrates that resembles a gland in organization but is closely associated with the circulatory system, that plays a role in the final destruction of red blood cells, filtration and storage of blood, and production of lymphocytes, and that in humans is a dark purplish flattened oblong object of a soft fragile consistency lying near the cardiac end of the stomach and consisting largely of blood and lymphoid tissue enclosed in a fibroelastic capsule from which trabeculae ramify through the tissue of the organ which is divisible into a loose friable red pulp in intimate connection with the blood supply and with red blood cells free in its interstices and a denser white pulp chiefly of lymphoid tissue condensed in masses about the small arteries

sple·nec·to·mize *or chiefly Brit* **sple·nec·to·mise** \spli-'nek-tə-ˌmīz\ *vt* **-mized** *or chiefly Brit* **-mised; -miz·ing** *or chiefly Brit* **-mis·ing** : to excise the spleen of

sple·nec·to·my \spli-'nek-tə-mē\ *n, pl* **-mies** : surgical excision of the spleen

splenia *pl of* SPLENIUM

splen·ic \'splen-ik\ *adj* : of, relating to, or located in the spleen ⟨~ blood flow⟩

splenic artery *n* : the branch of the celiac artery that carries blood to the spleen and sends branches also to the pancreas and the cardiac end of the stomach

splenic fever *n* **1** : ANTHRAX **2** : TEXAS FEVER

splenic flexure *n* : the sharp bend of the colon under the spleen where the transverse colon joins the descending colon — called also *left colic flexure*

splenic flexure syndrome *n* : pain in the upper left quadrant of the abdomen that may radiate upward to the left shoulder and inner aspect of the left arm and that sometimes mimics angina pectoris but is caused by bloating and gas in the colon

splenic pulp *n* : the characteristic tissue of the spleen

splenic vein *n* : the vein that carries blood away from the spleen, that is formed by five or six large branches which unite a short distance from the spleen, and that joins the superior mesenteric vein to form the portal vein — called also *lienal vein*

sple·ni·tis \splē-'nīt-əs\ *n* : inflammation of the spleen

sple·ni·um \'splē-nē-əm\ *n, pl* **-nia** \-nē-ə\ : the thick rounded fold that forms the posterior border of the corpus callosum and is continuous by its undersurface with the fornix

sple·ni·us \-nē-əs\ *n, pl* **-nii** \-nē-ˌī\ : either of two flat oblique muscles on each side of the back of the neck and upper thoracic region: **a** : SPLENIUS CAPITIS **b** : SPLENIUS CERVICIS

splenius cap·i·tis \-'kap-ət-əs\ *n* : a flat muscle on each side of the back of the neck and the upper thoracic region that arises from the caudal half of the ligamentum nuchae and the spinous processes of the seventh cervical and the first three or four thoracic vertebrae, that is inserted into the occipital bone and the mastoid process of the temporal bone, and that rotates the head to the side on which it is located and with the help of the muscle on the opposite side extends it

splenius cer·vi·cis \-'sər-və-səs\ *n* : a flat narrow muscle on each side of the back of the neck and the upper thoracic region that arises from the spinous processes of the third to sixth thoracic vertebrae, is inserted into the transverse processes of the first two or three cervical vertebrae, and acts to rotate the head to the side on which it is located and with the help of the muscle on the opposite side to extend and arch the neck

sple·no·cyte \'splē-nə-ˌsīt, 'splen-ə-\ *n* : a macrophage of the spleen

spleno·he·pa·to·meg·a·ly \ˌsplen-ō-ˌhep-ət-ō-'meg-ə-lē, -hi-

\ə\ abut \ᵊ\ kitten \ər\ further \a\ ash \ā\ ace \ä\ cot, cart
\au̇\ out \ch\ chin \e\ bet \ē\ easy \g\ go \i\ hit \ī\ ice \j\ job
\ŋ\ sing \ō\ go \ȯ\ law \ȯi\ boy \th\ thin \t͟h\ the \ü\ loot
\u̇\ foot \y\ yet \zh\ vision *See also* Pronunciation Symbols page

ˌpat-ō-\ *n, pl* **-lies** : abnormal enlargement of the spleen and the liver

spleno·meg·a·ly \ˌsplen-ō-ˈmeg-ə-lē\ *n, pl* **-lies** : abnormal enlargement of the spleen

sple·nop·a·thy \splē-ˈnäp-ə-thē\ *n, pl* **-thies** : disease of the spleen

spleno·por·to·gram \ˌsplen-ō-ˈpȯrt-ə-ˌgram\ *n* : a radiograph produced by splenoportography

spleno·por·tog·ra·phy \-pȯr-ˈtäg-rə-fē\ *n, pl* **-phies** : radiography of the splenic and portal veins following the injection of a radiopaque medium

spleno·re·nal \splen-ō-ˈrēn-ᵊl\ *adj* : of, relating to, or joining the splenic and renal veins or arteries ⟨a ∼ shunt⟩

splenorenal shunt *n* : an anastomosis between the splenic vein and the renal vein of the left kidney made esp. for the relief of portal hypertension

sple·no·sis \splē-ˈnō-səs\ *n, pl* **-no·ses** \-ˌsēz\ *or* **-no·sis·es** : a rare condition in which fragments of tissue from a ruptured spleen become implanted throughout the peritoneal cavity and often undergo regeneration and vascularization

splice \ˈsplīs\ *vt* **spliced; splic·ing** : to combine or insert (as genes) by genetic engineering ⟨*spliced* a human gene for insulin into a bacterium⟩ — see GENE-SPLICING

spli·ce·o·some \ˈsplī-sē-ə-ˌsōm\ *n* : a ribonucleoprotein complex that is the site in the cell nucleus where introns are excised from precursor messenger RNA and exons are joined together to form functional messenger RNA — **spli·ce·o·som·al** \ˌsplī-sē-ə-ˈsō-məl\ *adj*

splicing *n* : the process that occurs chiefly in eukaryotic nuclei by which introns in an RNA transcript are removed and exons are joined to form functional messenger RNA; *also* : GENE-SPLICING

¹**splint** \ˈsplint\ *n* **1** : material or a device used to protect and immobilize a body part ⟨a plaster ∼ for a fractured leg⟩ ⟨a dental ∼⟩ **2** : a bony enlargement on the upper part of the cannon bone of a horse usu. on the inside of the leg

²**splint** *vt* **1** : to support and immobilize (as a broken bone) with a splint **2** : to protect against pain by reducing the motion of ⟨the patient ∼*ed* his chest by a fixed position and shallow breathing⟩

splint·age \ˈsplint-ij\ *n* : the application of splints

splint bone *n* : one of the slender rudimentary metacarpal or metatarsal bones on either side of the cannon bone in the limbs of the horse and related animals

splin·ter \ˈsplint-ər\ *n* : a thin piece (as of wood) split or broken off lengthwise; *esp* : such a piece embedded in the skin ⟨used tweezers to remove a ∼⟩ — **splinter** *vt* **splin·tered; splin·ter·ing** \ˈsplint-ə-riŋ, ˈsplin-triŋ\

split \ˈsplit\ *vt* **split; split·ting** : to divide or break down (a chemical compound) into constituents ⟨∼ a fat into glycerol and fatty acids⟩; *also* : to remove by such separation

split–brain \ˌsplit-ˌbrān\ *adj* : of, relating to, concerned with, or having undergone separation of the two cerebral hemispheres by surgical division of the optic chiasma and corpus callosum ⟨∼ research⟩ ⟨∼ patients⟩

split personality *n* **1** : SCHIZOPHRENIA — not used technically **2** : MULTIPLE PERSONALITY DISORDER — not used technically

sp nov *abbr* [Latin *species nova*] new species — used following a taxonomic binomial proposed as new

spon·dyl·ar·thri·tis \ˌspän-dil-är-ˈthrīt-əs\ *n, pl* **-thrit·i·des** \-ˈthrit-ə-ˌdēz\ : arthritis of the spine

spon·dy·lit·ic \ˌspän-də-ˈlit-ik\ *adj* : of, relating to, or affected with spondylitis

spon·dy·li·tis \ˌspän-də-ˈlīt-əs\ *n* : inflammation of the vertebrae ⟨tuberculous ∼⟩ — see ANKYLOSING SPONDYLITIS

spon·dy·lo·ar·throp·a·thy \ˌspän-də-lō-är-ˈthräp-ə-thē\ *also* **spon·dyl·ar·throp·a·thy** \ˌspän-dil-är-ˈthräp-\ *n, pl* **-thies** : any of several diseases (as ankylosing spondylitis) affecting the joints of the spine

spon·dy·lo·lis·the·sis \ˌspän-də-lō-lis-ˈthē-səs\ *n* : forward displacement of a lumbar vertebra on the one below it and esp. of the fifth lumbar vertebra on the sacrum producing pain by compression of nerve roots

spon·dy·lol·y·sis \ˌspän-də-ˈläl-ə-səs\ *n, pl* **-y·ses** \-ˌsēz\ : disintegration or dissolution of a vertebra

spon·dy·lop·a·thy \ˌspän-də-ˈläp-ə-thē\ *n, pl* **-thies** : any disease or disorder of the vertebrae

spon·dy·lo·sis \ˌspän-də-ˈlō-səs\ *n, pl* **-lo·ses** \-ˌsēz\ *or* **-lo·sis·es** : any of various degenerative diseases of the spine

¹**sponge** \ˈspənj\ *n* **1** : an elastic porous mass of interlacing horny fibers that forms the internal skeleton of various marine animals (phylum Porifera) and is able when wetted to absorb liquid **2 a** : a small pad made of multiple folds of gauze or of cotton and gauze used to mop blood from a surgical incision, to carry inhalant medicaments to the nose, or to cover a superficial wound as a dressing **b** : a porous dressing (as of fibrin or gelatin) applied to promote wound healing **c** : a plastic prosthesis used in chest cavities following lung surgery **3** : an absorbent contraceptive device impregnated with spermicide that is inserted into the vagina before sexual intercourse to cover the cervix and act as a barrier to sperm

²**sponge** *vt* **sponged; spong·ing** : to cleanse, wipe, or moisten with or as if with a sponge ⟨∼ the patient's back⟩

sponge bath *n* : a bath in which water is applied to the body without actual immersion

sponge biopsy *n* : biopsy performed on matter collected with a sponge from a lesion

spon·gi·form \ˈspən-ji-ˌfȯrm\ *adj* : of, relating to, or being a degenerative disease which causes the brain tissue to have a porous structure like that of a sponge ⟨∼ lesions⟩

spongiform encephalopathy *n* : any of a group of degenerative diseases of the brain characterized by the development of spongiform lesions and by deterioration in neurological functioning — see BOVINE SPONGIFORM ENCEPHALOPATHY, TRANSMISSIBLE SPONGIFORM ENCEPHALOPATHY

spon·gin \ˈspən-jən\ *n* : a scleroprotein that is the chief constituent of flexible fibers in sponge skeletons

spon·gi·o·blast \ˈspən-jē-ō-ˌblast, ˈspän-\ *n* : any of the ectodermal cells of the embryonic spinal cord or other nerve center that are at first columnar but become branched at one end and that give rise to the glial cells

spon·gi·o·blas·to·ma \ˌspən-jē-ō-(ˌ)bla-ˈstō-mə, ˌspän-\ *n, pl* **-mas** *also* **-ma·ta** \-mət-ə\ : GLIOBLASTOMA

spon·gi·o·cyte \ˈspən-jē-ō-ˌsīt, ˈspän-\ *n* : any of the cells of the adrenal cortex that have a spongy appearance due to lipid vacuoles the contents of which have been dissolved out in the process of cytological or histological preparation

spon·gi·o·sa \ˌspən-jē-ˈō-sə, ˌspän-\ *n* : the part of a bone (as much of the epiphyseal area of long bones) made up of spongy cancellous bone

spon·gi·o·sis \ˌspän-jē-ˈō-səs, ˌspän-\ *n* : swelling localized in the epidermis and often occurring in eczema

spongiosum — see CORPUS SPONGIOSUM, STRATUM SPONGIOSUM

spongy \ˈspən-jē\ *adj* **spong·i·er; -est** : resembling a sponge; *esp* : full of cavities : CANCELLOUS ⟨∼ bone⟩ — **spong·i·ness** *n*

spon·ta·ne·ous \spän-ˈtā-nē-əs\ *adj* **1** : proceeding from natural feeling or native tendency without external constraint **2** : developing without apparent external influence, force, cause, or treatment ⟨a ∼ nosebleed⟩ — **spon·ta·ne·ous·ly** *adv*

spontaneous abortion *n* : naturally occurring expulsion of a nonviable fetus

spontaneous generation *n* : ABIOGENESIS

spontaneous recovery *n* : reappearance of an extinguished conditioned response without positive reinforcement

spoon nails \ˈspün-\ *n pl but sing in constr* : KOILONYCHIA

spo·rad·ic \spə-ˈrad-ik\ *adj* : occurring occasionally, singly, or in scattered instances ⟨∼ diseases⟩ — compare ENDEMIC, EPIDEMIC 1 — **spo·rad·i·cal·ly** \-i-k(ə-)lē\ *adv*

spo·ran·gio·phore \spə-ˈran-jē-ə-ˌfō(ə)r, -ˌfȯ(ə)r\ *n* : a stalk or similar structure bearing sporangia

spo·ran·gio·spore \-ˌspō(ə)r\ *n* : a spore that develops in a sporangium

spo·ran·gi·um \spə-ˈran-jē-əm\ *n, pl* **-gia** \-jē-ə\ : a structure (as of an alga or fungus) within which spores are produced — **spo·ran·gial** \-j(ē-)əl\ *adj*

Spor·a·nox \'spōr-ə-ˌnäks, 'spór-\ *trademark* — used for a preparation of itraconazole

¹**spore** \'spō(ə)r, 'spó(ə)r\ *n* : a primitive usu. unicellular often environmentally resistant dormant or reproductive body produced by plants, fungi, and some microorganisms and capable of developing into a new individual either directly or after fusion with another spore

²**spore** *vi* **spored; spor·ing** : to produce or reproduce by spores

spo·ri·cid·al \ˌspōr-ə-'sīd-ᵊl, ˌspór-\ *adj* : tending to kill spores

spo·ri·cide \'spōr-ə-ˌsīd, 'spór-\ *n* : an agent that kills spores

spo·rid·i·al \spór-'id-ē-əl\ *adj* : of, relating to, or producing sporidia : developing from a sporidium

spo·rid·i·um \spór-'id-ē-əm\ *n, pl* **-rid·ia** \-ē-ə\ : a small spore (as in various smuts and rusts)

spo·ro·blast \'spō-rə-ˌblast\ *n* : a cell of a sporozoan resulting from sexual reproduction and producing spores and sporozoites

spo·ro·cyst \-ˌsist\ *n* **1** : a case or cyst secreted by some sporozoans preliminary to sporogony; *also* : a sporozoan encysted in such a case **2** : a saccular body that is the first asexual reproductive form of a digenetic trematode, develops from a miracidium, and buds off cells from its inner surface which develop into rediae

spo·ro·gen·e·sis \ˌspōr-ə-'jen-ə-səs, ˌspór-\ *n, pl* **-e·ses** \-ˌsēz\ **1** : reproduction by spores **2** : spore formation

spo·rog·e·nous \spə-'räj-ə-nəs, spó-\ *also* **spo·ro·gen·ic** \ˌspōr-ə-'jen-ik, ˌspór-\ *adj* : of, relating to, involving, or reproducing by sporogenesis

spo·ro·gon·ic \ˌspōr-ə-'gän-ik\ *also* **spo·rog·o·nous** \spə-'räg-ə-nəs\ *adj* : of, relating to, involving, or produced by sporogony

spo·rog·o·ny \spə-'räg-ə-nē, spó-\ *n, pl* **-nies** : reproduction by spores; *specif* : formation of spores containing sporozoites that is characteristic of some sporozoans and that results from the encystment and subsequent division of a zygote

spo·ront \'spōr-ˌänt\ *n* : a sporozoan that engages in sporogony

spo·ro·phore \'spōr-ə-ˌfō(ə)r, 'spór-ə-ˌfó(ə)r\ *n* : the spore-producing organ esp. of a fungus

spo·ro·phyte \-ˌfīt\ *n* : an individual or generation of a plant exhibiting alternation of generations that bears asexual spores, is usu. not clearly differentiated in algae and fungi, and in vascular plants is the conspicuous form ordinarily seen — compare GAMETOPHYTE — **spo·ro·phyt·ic** \ˌspōr-ə-'fit-ik, ˌspór-\ *adj*

spo·ro·thrix \-ˌthriks\ *n* **1** *cap* : a genus of imperfect fungi of the family Moniliaceae that includes the causative agent (*S. schenckii*) of sporotrichosis **2** : any fungus of the genus *Sporothrix*

spo·ro·tri·cho·sis \spə-ˌrä-trik-'ō-səs, ˌspōr-ə-trik-, ˌspór-\ *n, pl* **-cho·ses** \-ˌsēz\ : infection with or disease caused by a fungus of the genus *Sporothrix* (*S. schenckii* syn. *Sporotrichum schenckii*) that is characterized by often ulcerating or suppurating nodules in the skin, subcutaneous tissues, and nearby lymph nodes, that occurs esp. in humans and horses, and that is usu. transmitted by entry of the fungus through a skin abrasion or wound

spo·ro·tri·chot·ic \spə-ˌrä-tri-'kät-ik\ *adj* : of or relating to sporotrichosis ⟨∼ lesions⟩

spo·rot·ri·chum \spə-'rä-tri-kəm\ *n* **1** *cap* : a genus of saprophytic or parasitic imperfect fungi of the family Moniliaceae that formerly included the causative agent (*Sporothrix schenckii*) of sporotrichosis **2** *pl* **-cha** \-kə\ : any fungus of the genus *Sporotrichum*

spo·ro·zoa \ˌspōr-ə-'zō-ə, ˌspór-\ *n pl* **1** *cap* : a large class of strictly parasitic protozoans that pass through a complicated life cycle usu. involving alternation of a sexual with an asexual generation, that often require two or more dissimilar hosts to complete their life cycle, that are typically immobile and usu. intracellular parasites, and that include many seri-

ous pathogens (as the malaria parasites, coccidia, and babesias **2** : protozoans of the class Sporozoa

spo·ro·zo·an \ˌspōr-ə-'zō-ən, ˌspór-\ *n* : any protozoan of the class Sporozoa — **sporozoan** *adj*

spo·ro·zo·ite \-'zō-ˌīt\ *n* : a usu. motile infective form of some sporozoans (as the malaria parasite) that is a product of sporogony and initiates an asexual cycle in the new host

spo·ro·zo·it·i·cide \ˌspōr-ə-zō-'it-ə-ˌsīd\ *n* : an agent selectively destructive of the sporozoite form of a sporozoan parasite

sport \'spō(ə)rt, 'spó(ə)rt\ *n* : an individual exhibiting a sudden deviation from type beyond the normal limits of individual variation usu. as a result of mutation esp. of somatic tissue

sports medicine \'spō(ə)rts-, 'spó(ə)rts-\ *n* : a medical specialty concerned with the prevention and treatment of injuries and disorders that are related to participation in sports

spor·u·late \'spōr-(y)ə-ˌlāt, 'spór-\ *vi* **-lat·ed; -lat·ing** : to undergo sporulation

spor·u·la·tion \ˌspōr-(y)ə-'lā-shən, ˌspór-\ *n* : the formation of spores; *esp* : division into many small spores (as after encystment)

¹**spot** \'spät\ *n* : a circumscribed mark or area: as **a** : a circumscribed surface lesion of disease (as measles) **b** : a circumscribed abnormality in an organ seen by means of X-rays or an instrument ⟨X-rays revealed a ∼ on the lung⟩

²**spot** *vi* **spot·ted; spot·ting** : to experience abnormal and sporadic bleeding in small amounts from the uterus

spot film *n* : a radiograph of a restricted area in the body

spotted cow·bane \-'kaú-ˌbān\ *n* : a tall biennial No. American herb of the genus *Cicuta* (*C. maculata*) chiefly of wetlands of northeastern No. America with clusters of tuberous roots that resemble small sweet potatoes and are extremely poisonous — called also *spotted hemlock;* compare WATER HEMLOCK

spotted fever *n* : any of various eruptive fevers: as **a** : TYPHUS a **b** : ROCKY MOUNTAIN SPOTTED FEVER

spotted hemlock *n* : SPOTTED COWBANE

spp *abbr* species (*pl*) — compare SP

¹**sprain** \'sprān\ *n* : a sudden or violent twist or wrench of a joint causing the stretching or tearing of ligaments and often rupture of blood vessels with hemorrhage into the tissues; *also* : the condition resulting from a sprain that is usu. marked by swelling, inflammation, hemorrhage, and discoloration — compare ³STRAIN b

²**sprain** *vt* : to weaken (a joint or ligament) by sudden and violent twisting or wrenching : stretch (ligaments) injuriously without dislocation of the joint

sprain fracture *n* : AVULSION FRACTURE

¹**spray** \'sprā\ *n* : a jet of vapor or finely divided liquid; *specif* : a jet of fine medicated vapor used as an application to a diseased part or to charge the air of a room with a disinfectant or deodorant

²**spray** *vi* : to emit a stream or spray of urine ⟨a cat may ∼ to mark its territory⟩

spread·ing factor \'spred-iŋ-\ *n* : HYALURONIDASE

Spren·gel's deformity \'shpreŋ-əlz-\ *n* : a congenital elevation of the scapula

Sprengel, Otto Gerhard Karl (1852–1915), German surgeon. Sprengel described a congenital elevation of the scapula in 1891.

spring \'spriŋ\ *n* : any of various elastic orthodontic devices used esp. to apply constant pressure to misaligned teeth

spring·halt \-ˌhólt\ *n* : STRINGHALT

spring ligament *n* : PLANTAR CALCANEONAVICULAR LIGAMENT

¹**sprout** \'spraút\ *vi* : to send out new growth : produce sprouts ⟨vascular endothelial growth factor . . . has been shown to spur blood vessels to ∼ —Greg Miller⟩

\ə\ **abut** \ᵊ\ **kitten** \ər\ **further** \a\ **ash** \ā\ **ace** \ä\ **cot, cart**
\aú\ **out** \ch\ **chin** \e\ **bet** \ē\ **easy** \g\ **go** \i\ **hit** \ī\ **ice** \j\ **job**
\ŋ\ **sing** \ō\ **go** \ó\ **law** \ói\ **boy** \th\ **thin** \th̲\ **the** \ü\ **loot**
\ú\ **foot** \y\ **yet** \zh\ **vision** *See also* Pronunciation Symbols page

²**sprout** *n* : a new outgrowth (as of nerve tissue) resembling the young shoot of a plant ⟨segments of the axon above the injury . . . produce new ~s —J. L. Marx⟩

sprue \'sprü\ *n* **1** : CELIAC DISEASE **2** : a disease of tropical regions that is of unknown cause and is characterized by fatty diarrhea and malabsorption of nutrients — called also *tropical sprue*

spud \'spəd\ *n* : any of various small surgical instruments with a shape resembling that of a spade ⟨use of a ~ to remove a foreign object from the eye⟩

spu·ma·vi·rus \'spü-mə-ˌvī-rəs\ *n* : FOAMY VIRUS

spur \'spər\ *n* : a sharp and esp. bony outgrowth (as on the heel of the foot) — **spurred** \'spərd\ *adj*

spurge \'spərj\ *n* : any of various mostly shrubby plants (family Euphorbiaceae, the spurge family, and esp. genus *Euphorbia*) that have a bitter milky juice and that include several which have been used medicinally — see IPECAC SPURGE

spu·ri·ous \'spyùr-ē-əs\ *adj* : simulating a symptom or condition without being pathologically or morphologically genuine ⟨~ labor pains⟩ ⟨~ polycythemia⟩

spu·tum \'sp(y)üt-əm\ *n, pl* **spu·ta** \-ə\ : the matter discharged from the air passages in diseases of the lungs, bronchi, or upper respiratory tract that contains mucus and often pus, blood, fibrin, or bacterial products

squa·la·mine \'skwä-lə-ˌmēn, ˌskwäl-'am-ˌēn\ *n* : any of a group of steroid antimicrobials that were orig. discovered in the blood of sharks and that have a broad spectrum of activity against bacteria, protozoans, and fungi

squa·lene \'skwä-ˌlēn\ *n* : an acyclic hydrocarbon $C_{30}H_{50}$ that is widely distributed in nature (as a major component of sebum and in shark-liver oils) and is a precursor of sterols (as cholesterol)

squa·ma \'skwä-mə, 'skwā-\ *n, pl* **squa·mae** \'skwä-ˌmē, 'skwā-ˌmī\ : a structure resembling a scale or plate: as **a** : the curved platelike posterior portion of the occipital bone **b** : the vertical portion of the frontal bone that forms the forehead **c** : the thin anterior upper portion of the temporal bone

squame \'skwām\ *n* : a scale or flake (as of skin)

squa·mo·co·lum·nar junction \ˌskwä-mō-kə-ˌləm-nər-\ *n* : the region in the uterine cervix in which the squamous lining of the vagina is replaced by the columnar epithelium typical of the body of the uterus and which is a common site of neoplastic change

¹**squa·mo·sal** \skwä-'mō-səl, skwə-\ *n* : a squamosal bone

²**squamosal** *adj* **1** : SQUAMOUS 2 **2** : of, relating to, or being a bone in the skull of many vertebrates that corresponds to the squamous portion of the temporal bone in humans

squa·mous \'skwä-məs\ *adj* **1 a** : covered with or consisting of scales **b** : of, relating to, or being a stratified epithelium that consists at least in its outer layers of small scalelike cells **2** : resembling a scale or plate; *esp* : of, relating to, or being the thin anterior upper portion of the temporal bone

squamous carcinoma *n* : SQUAMOUS CELL CARCINOMA

squamous cell *n* : a cell of or derived from squamous epithelium

squamous cell carcinoma *n* : a carcinoma that is made up of or arises from squamous cells and usu. occurs in areas of the body exposed to strong sunlight over a period of many years

square \'skwa(ə)r, 'skwe(ə)r\ *adj* : being or converted to a unit of area equal in measure to a square each side of which measures one unit of a specified unit of length ⟨a ~ foot⟩

squash \'skwäsh, 'skwòsh\ *n* : a bit of tissue crushed between a slide and cover glass and stained in situ esp. for cytological study of chromosomes

squash bite *n* : an impression of the teeth and mouth made by closing the teeth on modeling composition or wax

squill \'skwil\ *n* **1 a** : a Mediterranean bulbous herb of the genus *Urginea* (*U. maritima*) of the lily family — called also *sea onion* **b** : any of several other plants of the genus *Urginea* **c** : the bulbs of a squill (esp. *U. maritima*) **2 a** : the dried sliced bulb of the white-bulbed form of the squill (*Urginea*

maritima) of the Mediterranean region or the dried sliced bulb of a related Asian plant (*U. indica*) that contains one or more physically active cardiac glycosides and was formerly used as an expectorant, cardiac stimulant, and diuretic — see URGINEA 2a; compare WHITE SQUILL **b** : RED SQUILL 2

¹**squint** \'skwint\ *vi* **1** : to be cross-eyed **2** : to look or peer with eyes partly closed

²**squint** *n* **1** : STRABISMUS **2** : an instance or habit of squinting

squir·rel corn \'skwər(-ə)l-, *chiefly Brit* 'skwir-əl-\ *n* : a poisonous No. American herb (*Dicentra canadensis* of the family Fumariaceae) from which bulbocapnine is obtained

Sr *symbol* strontium

SR *abbr* slow-release; sustained-release

S–R *abbr* stimulus-response

sRNA \ˌes-ˌär-ˌen-'ā\ *n* : TRANSFER RNA

SRS *abbr* slow-reacting substance

SRS–A *abbr* slow-reacting substance of anaphylaxis

ss *abbr* [Latin *semis*] one half — used in writing prescriptions

S sleep *n* : SLOW-WAVE SLEEP

SSPE *abbr* subacute sclerosing panencephalitis

SSRI \ˌes-ˌ(ˌ)es-ˌ(ˌ)är-'ī\ *n* : any of a class of antidepressants (as fluoxetine or sertraline) that inhibit the inactivation of serotonin by blocking its reuptake by presynaptic nerve cell endings — called also *selective serotonin reuptake inhibitor*

SSSS *abbr* staphylococcal scalded skin syndrome

ST \ˌes-'tē\ *n* : ST SEGMENT

¹**stab** \'stab\ *n* **1** : a wound produced by a pointed object or weapon **2 a** : a culture medium solidified in an upright column in a tube to reduce the surface to a minimum — compare SLANT **b** : STAB CULTURE

²**stab** *vt* **stabbed; stab·bing** : to wound or pierce by the thrust of a pointed object or weapon

stabbing *adj* : having a sharp piercing quality ⟨~ pain⟩

stab cell *n* : BAND FORM

stab culture *n* : a culture (as of bacteria) made by inoculating deep into a stab

stab form *n* : BAND FORM

sta·bi·late \'stā-bə-ˌlāt\ *n* : a population of microbes maintained or preserved (as by freezing) in a stable and viable condition

sta·bile \'stā-ˌbīl, -ˌbil\ *adj* **1** : STABLE 1 **2** : resistant to chemical change ⟨native proteins are never ~ —Otto Rahn⟩

sta·bil·i·ty \stə-'bil-ət-ē\ *n, pl* **-ties** : the quality, state, or degree of being stable ⟨emotional ~⟩ ⟨chemical ~⟩

sta·bi·lize *also Brit* **sta·bi·lise** \'stā-bə-ˌlīz\ *vb* **-lized** *also Brit* **-lised; -liz·ing** *also Brit* **-lis·ing** *vt* : to make stable ⟨~ a patient's condition⟩ ~ *vi* : to become stable ⟨when pulse and blood pressure respond and ~ —*Jour. Amer. Med. Assoc.*⟩ — **sta·bi·li·za·tion** *also Brit* **sta·bi·li·sa·tion** \ˌstā-bə-lə-'zā-shən\ *n*

sta·bi·liz·er *also Brit* **sta·bi·lis·er** \'stā-bə-ˌlī-zər\ *n* : one that stabilizes something; *esp* : a substance added to another substance or to a system (as an emulsion) to prevent or retard an unwanted alteration of physical state

stab incision *n* : STAB WOUND

sta·ble \'stā-bəl\ *adj* **sta·bler** \-b(ə-)lər\; **sta·blest** \-b(ə-)ləst\ **1** : not changing or fluctuating ⟨the patient's condition was listed as ~⟩ **2** : not subject to insecurity or emotional illness ⟨a ~ personality⟩ **3** : not readily altering in chemical makeup or physical state ⟨~ emulsions⟩ **b** : not spontaneously radioactive ⟨a ~ isotope⟩

stable factor *n* : FACTOR VII

stable fly *n* : a biting dipteran fly of the genus *Stomoxys* (*S. calcitrans*) that is abundant about stables and often enters dwellings esp. in autumn

stab wound *n* : a small surgical incision (as for drainage) made by a thrust with a sharp instrument — called also *stab incision*

stachy·bot·ryo·tox·i·co·sis \ˌstak-i-ˌbä-trē-ō-ˌtäk-sə-'kō-səs\ *n, pl* **-co·ses** \-ˌsēz\ : a serious and sometimes fatal intoxication chiefly affecting domestic animals (as horses) that is due to ingestion of a toxic substance elaborated by a mold (*Stachybotrys alternans*)

stach·y·drine \'stak-i-₁drēn, -drən\ *n* : a crystalline alkaloid $C_7H_{13}NO_2$ found in various plants (as alfalfa)

stach·y·ose \'stak-ē-₁ōs\ *n* : a sweet crystalline tetrasaccharide sugar $C_{24}H_{42}O_{21}$ that yields glucose, fructose, and galactose on hydrolysis

Sta·der splint \'stā-dər-\ *n* : a splinting device consisting of two stainless steel pins inserted in the bone above and below a fracture and a bar joining the pins for drawing and holding the broken ends together

Stader, Otto (1894–1962), American veterinary surgeon. Stader devised the Stader splint in 1931. He developed this type of splint because his canine patients gnawed off plaster casts fitted on their legs. After several years of use on animals, the splint was adopted for treating fractures in human patients.

sta·di·om·e·ter \₁stād-ē-'äm-ət-ər\ *n* : a device for measuring height that typically consists of a vertical ruler with a sliding horizontal rod or paddle which is adjusted to rest on the top of the head

Sta·dol \'stā-₁dȯl\ *trademark* — used for a preparation of the tartrate of butorphanol

staff \'staf\ *n* : the doctors and surgeons regularly attached to a hospital and helping to determine its policies and guide its activities

staff cell *n* : BAND FORM

staff nurse *n* : a registered nurse employed by a medical facility who does not assist in surgery

staff of Aes·cu·la·pi·us \₁es-kyə-'lā-pē-əs\ *n* : a conventionalized representation of a staff branched at the top with a single snake twined around it that is used as a symbol of medicine and as the official insignia of the American Medical Association — called also *Aesculapian staff;* compare CADUCEUS a

Aesculapius *or* **As·cle·pi·us** \as-'klē-pē-əs\, mythological character. Aesculapius was the god of medicine in Greek and Roman mythology. Snakes were the god's sacred emblems, and the god was believed to be incarnate in them. According to myth, the chief god Zeus struck him with a lightning bolt for daring to bring the dead back to life.

¹stage \'stāj\ *n* **1** : a period or step in a process, activity, or development: as **a** : one of the distinguishable periods of growth and development of a plant or animal ⟨the larval ∼ of an insect⟩ **b** : a period or phase in the course of a disease ⟨the rash ∼ of Lyme disease —R. H. Boyle⟩; *also* : the degree of involvement or severity of a disease ⟨advanced ∼ II or III disease (more than 10 positive lymph nodes found after axillary dissection) —M. S. Anscher *et al*⟩ **c** : one of two or more operations performed at different times but constituting a single procedure ⟨a two-*stage* thoracoplasty⟩ **d** : any of the four degrees indicating depth of general anesthesia **2** : the small platform of a microscope on which an object is placed for examination

²stage *vt* **staged; stag·ing** : to determine the phase or severity of (a disease) based on a classification of established symptomatic criteria; *also* : to evaluate (a patient) to determine the phase, severity, or progression of a disease

stage micrometer *n* : a finely divided scale ruled on a microscope slide and used to calibrate the filar micrometer

stag·gers \'stag-ərz\ *n pl* **1** *sing or pl in constr* : any of various abnormal conditions of domestic mammals and birds associated with damage to the central nervous system and marked by incoordination and a reeling unsteady gait — see BLIND STAGGERS; compare GRASS TETANY **2** : vertigo occurring as a symptom of decompression sickness; *also* : DECOMPRESSION SICKNESS

stag·horn calculus \'stag-₁hȯ(ə)rn-\ *n* : a large renal calculus with multiple irregular branches

staging *n* : the classification of the severity of a disease in distinct stages on the basis of established symptomatic criteria

¹stain \'stān\ *vt* **1** : to cause discoloration of ⟨smoking ∼s teeth⟩ **2** : to color by processes affecting chemically or oth-

erwise the material itself ⟨∼ bacteria with a fluorescent dye⟩ ∼ *vi* : to receive a stain

²stain *n* **1** : a discolored spot or area (as on the skin or teeth) — see PORT-WINE STAIN **2** : a preparation (as of dye or pigment) used in staining something; *esp* : a dye or mixture of dyes used in microscopy to make minute and transparent structures visible, to differentiate tissue elements, or to produce specific chemical reactions

stain·abil·i·ty \₁stā-nə-'bil-ət-ē\ *n, pl* **-ties** : the capacity of cells and cell parts to stain specifically and consistently with particular dyes and stains — **stain·able** \'stā-nə-bəl\ *adj*

stair·case effect \'sta(ə)r-₁kās-\ *n* : TREPPE

staircase phenomenon *n* : TREPPE

stal·ag·mom·e·ter \₁stal-ag-'mäm-ət-ər\ *n* : a device for determining the number of drops in a given volume of liquid esp. for use in calculating the surface tension (as of blood or serum) — **sta·lag·mo·met·ric** \stə-₁lag-mə-'me-trik\ *adj*

stalk \'stȯk\ *n* : a slender supporting or connecting part : PEDUNCLE ⟨the pituitary ∼⟩ — **stalked** \'stȯkt\ *adj* — **stalk·less** *adj*

stam·i·na \'stam-ə-nə\ *n* : the strength or vigor of bodily constitution : capacity for standing fatigue or resisting disease ⟨restoration of weight, strength and ∼ following recovery from major surgery —*Jour. Amer. Med. Assoc.*⟩

¹stam·mer \'stam-ər\ *vi* **stam·mered; stam·mer·ing** \-(ə-)riŋ\ : to make involuntary stops and repetitions in speaking

²stammer *n* **1** : an act or instance of stammering **2** : the condition of habitually speaking with stammers ⟨a severe ∼⟩

stam·mer·er \'stam-ər-ər\ *n* : one who stammers

stammering *n* **1** : the act of one who stammers **2** : a disorder of speech characterized by involuntary stops and repetitions or blocking of utterance

stanch *also* **staunch** \'stȯnch, 'stänch\ *vt* : to check or stop the flowing of ⟨∼ bleeding⟩; *also* : to stop the flow of blood from ⟨∼ a wound⟩

¹stan·dard \'stan-dərd\ *n* : something set up or established by an authority as a rule for the measure of quantity, weight, extent, value, or quality

²standard *adj* : constituting or conforming to a standard esp. as established by law or custom ⟨∼ weight⟩

stan·dard·ize *also Brit* **stan·dard·ise** \'stan-dərd-₁īz\ *vt* **-ized** *also Brit* **-ised; -iz·ing** *also Brit* **-is·ing** **1** : to reduce to or compare with a standard ⟨∼ a solution⟩ **2** : to bring into conformity with a standard **3** : to arrange or order the component items of a test (as of intelligence or personality) so that the probability of their eliciting a designated class of response varies with some quantifiable psychological or behavioral attribute, function, or characteristic — **stan·dard·iza·tion** *also Brit* **stan·dard·isa·tion** \₁stan-dərd-ə-'zā-shən\ *n*

standard solution *n* : a solution having a standard or accurately known strength that is used as a reagent in chemical analysis

stand·still \'stand-₁stil\ *n* : a state characterized by absence of motion or of progress : ARREST ⟨cardiac ∼⟩

Stan·ford–Bi·net test \₁stan-fərd-bi-'nā-\ *n* : an intelligence test prepared at Stanford University as a revision of the Binet-Simon scale and commonly employed with children — called also *Stanford-Binet*

A. Binet — see BINET AGE

stan·nic \'stan-ik\ *adj* : of, relating to, or containing tin esp. with a valence of four

stan·nous \'stan-əs\ *adj* : of, relating to, or containing tin esp. with a valence of two

stannous fluoride *n* : a white compound SnF_2 of tin and fluorine used in toothpastes and oral rinses to prevent tooth decay

stan·num \'stan-əm\ *n* : TIN

\ə\ **abut** \ᵊ\ **kitten** \ər\ **further** \a\ **ash** \ā\ **ace** \ä\ **cot, cart**
\aú\ **out** \ch\ **chin** \e\ **bet** \ē\ **easy** \g\ **go** \i\ **hit** \ī\ **ice** \j\ **job**
\ŋ\ **sing** \ō\ **go** \ȯ\ **law** \ȯi\ **boy** \th\ **thin** \t͟h\ **the** \ü\ **loot**
\ú\ **foot** \y\ **yet** \zh\ **vision** *See also* Pronunciation Symbols page

S T

sta·nol \'stan-ˌȯl, 'stā-ˌnȯl\ *n* : any of the fully saturated phytosterols — see SISTOSTANOL

stan·o·lone \'stan-ə-ˌlōn\ *n* : a semisynthetic dihydrotestosterone derivative $C_{19}H_{30}O_2$ used esp. in the treatment of breast cancer

stan·o·zo·lol \'stan-ə-zō-ˌlȯl\ *n* : an anabolic steroid $C_{21}H_{32}N_2O$

sta·pe·dec·to·mized \ˌstā-pi-'dek-tə-ˌmīzd\ *adj* : having undergone a stapedectomy

sta·pe·dec·to·my \ˌstā-pi-'dek-tə-mē\ *n, pl* **-mies** : surgical removal and prosthetic replacement of part or all of the stapes to relieve deafness

sta·pe·di·al \stā-'pēd-ē-əl, stə-\ *adj* : of, relating to, or located near the stapes ⟨~ surgery⟩

sta·pe·di·us \stə-'pē-dē-əs\ *n, pl* **-dii** \-dē-ˌī\ : a small muscle of the middle ear that arises from the wall of the tympanum, is inserted into the neck of the stapes by a tendon that sometimes contains a slender spine of bone, and serves to check and dampen vibration of the stapes — called also *stapedius muscle*

sta·pes \'stā-(ˌ)pēz\ *n, pl* **stapes** or **sta·pe·des** \stə-'pē-ˌdēz\ : the innermost of the chain of three ossicles in the middle ear of a mammal having the form of a stirrup, a base occupying the oval window of the tympanum, and a head connected with the incus — called also *stirrup*

staph \'staf\ *n* : STAPHYLOCOCCUS 2; *also* : an infection with staphylococci

staph·i·sa·gria \ˌstaf-ə-'sā-grē-ə\ *n* : STAVESACRE 2

staph·y·lec·to·my \ˌstaf-i-'lek-tə-mē\ *n, pl* **-mies** : surgical excision of the uvula

staph·y·lo·co·ag·u·lase \'staf-ə-(ˌ)lō-kō-'ag-yə-ˌlās, -ˌlāz\ *n* : a coagulase produced by pathogenic staphylococci

staph·y·lo·coc·cal \ˌstaf-(ə)lō-'käk-əl\ *also* **staph·y·lo·coc·cic** \-'käk-(s)ik\ *adj* : of, relating to, caused by, or being a staphylococcus ⟨~ infection⟩ ⟨a ~ organism⟩

staphylococcal scalded skin syndrome *n* : an acute skin disorder esp. of infants and immunocompromised individuals that is characterized by widespread erythema, peeling, and necrosis of the skin, that is caused by a toxin produced by a bacterium of the genus *Staphylococcus* (*S. aureus*), and that exposes the affected individual to serious infections but is rarely fatal if diagnosed and treated promptly — abbr. *SSSS*; compare TOXIC EPIDERMAL NECROLYSIS

staph·y·lo·coc·ce·mia *or chiefly Brit* **staph·y·lo·coc·cae·mia** \ˌstaf-ə-lō-käk-'sē-mē-ə\ *n* : the presence of staphylococci in the circulating blood — **staph·y·lo·coc·ce·mic** *or chiefly Brit* **staph·y·lo·coc·cae·mic** \-'sē-mik\ *adj*

staph·y·lo·coc·co·sis \ˌstaf-ə-lō-kä-'kō-səs\ *n* : infection with or disease caused by staphylococci

staph·y·lo·coc·cus \ˌstaf-ə-lō-'käk-əs\ *n* **1** *cap* : a genus of nonmotile gram-positive spherical bacteria of the family Micrococcaceae that occur singly, in pairs or tetrads, or in irregular clusters and include causative agents of various diseases and disorders (as food poisoning, skin infections, and endocarditis) **2** *pl* **-coc·ci** \-'käk-ˌ(s)ī\ : any bacterium of the genus *Staphylococcus*; *broadly* : MICROCOCCUS 2

staph·y·lo·ki·nase \-'kī-ˌnās, -ˌnāz\ *n* : a protease from some pathogenic staphylococci that converts plasminogen to plasmin but does not activate the plasminogen of the ox as urokinase does

staph·y·lol·y·sin \ˌstaf-i-'läl-ə-sən\ *n* : a hemolysin produced by staphylococci

staph·y·lo·ma \ˌstaf-ə-'lō-mə\ *n* : a protrusion of the cornea or sclera of the eye

staph·y·lo·tox·in \ˌstaf-ə-lō-'täk-sən\ *n* : a toxin produced by staphylococci

sta·ple \'stā-pəl\ *n* : a usu. U-shaped and typically metal surgical fastener used to hold layers of tissue together (as in the closure of an incision) — **staple** *vt* **sta·pled; sta·pling** — **sta·pler** \-plər\ *n*

star anise oil \'stär-\ *n* : a fragrant essential oil obtained from the dried fruit of a tree of the genus *Illicium* (*I. verum*) and used chiefly as a flavoring agent, expectorant, and carminative — called also *anise oil*

starch \'stärch\ *n* : a white odorless tasteless granular or powdery complex carbohydrate $(C_6H_{10}O_5)_x$ that is the chief storage form of carbohydrate in plants, is an important foodstuff, has demulcent and absorbent properties, and is used in pharmacy esp. as a dusting powder and as a constituent of ointments and pastes

starchy \'stär-chē\ *adj* **starch·i·er; -est** : containing, consisting of, or resembling starch ⟨~ foods⟩

Star·ling's hypothesis \'stär-liŋz-\ *also* **Starling hypothesis** \-liŋ-\ *n* : a hypothesis in physiology: the flow of fluids across capillary walls depends on the balance between the force of blood pressure on the walls which tends to force fluids out and the osmotic pressure across the walls which tends to force them in due to the greater concentration of dissolved substances in the blood so that the declining gradient in blood pressure from the arterial to the venous end of the capillary results in an outflow of fluids at its arterial end with an increasing inflow toward its venous end

E. H. Starling — see FRANK-STARLING LAW

Starling's law of the heart *n* : a statement in physiology: the strength of the heart's systolic contraction is directly proportional to its diastolic expansion with the result that under normal physiological conditions the heart pumps out of the right atrium all the blood returned to it without letting any back up in the veins — called also *Frank-Starling law, Frank=Starling law of the heart, Starling's law*

star·va·tion \stär-'vā-shən\ *n* **1** : the act or an instance of starving **2** : the state of being starved

starve \'stärv\ *vb* **starved; starv·ing** *vi* **1** : to perish from lack of food **2** : to suffer extreme hunger ~ *vt* **1** : to kill with hunger **2** : to deprive of nourishment

sta·sis \'stā-səs, 'stas-əs\ *n, pl* **sta·ses** \'stā-ˌsēz, 'stas-ˌēz\ : a slowing or stoppage of the normal flow of a bodily fluid or semifluid ⟨biliary ~⟩: as **a** : slowing of the current of circulating blood **b** : reduced motility of the intestines with retention of feces

stasis dermatitis *n* : inflammation of skin caused by slowing or stoppage of blood flow to the affected area

stasis ulcer *n* : an ulcer (as on the lower leg) caused by localized slowing or stoppage of blood flow

stat \'stat\ *adv* : STATIM

stat·am·pere \'stat-ˌam-pi(ə)r\ *n* : the cgs electrostatic unit of current equal to about 3.3×10^{-10} ampere

stat·cou·lomb \'stat-ˌkü-ˌläm\ *n* : the cgs electrostatic unit of charge equal to about 3.3×10^{-10} coulomb

state \'stāt\ *n* : mode or condition of being: as **a** : condition of mind or temperament ⟨a manic ~⟩ **b** : a condition or stage in the physical being of something ⟨the gaseous ~ of water⟩

state hospital *n* : a hospital for the mentally ill that is run by a state

state medicine *n* : administration and control by the national government of medical and hospital services provided to the whole population and paid for out of funds raised by taxation

stat·ic \'stat-ik\ *adj* **1** : characterized by a lack of movement or change ⟨a ~ condition⟩ **2** : ELECTROSTATIC — **stat·i·cal·ly** \-i-k(ə-)lē\ *adv*

stat·im \'stat-im\ *adv* : immediately or without delay

stat·in \'stat-ᵊn\ *n* : any of a group of drugs (as lovastatin and simvastatin) that inhibit the synthesis of cholesterol and promote the production of LDL-binding receptors in the liver resulting in a usu. marked decrease in the level of LDL and a modest increase in the level of HDL circulating in blood plasma

sta·tion \'stā-shən\ *n* **1** : the place at which someone is positioned or is assigned to remain ⟨the nurse's ~ on a hospital ward⟩ **2** : the act or manner of standing : POSTURE ⟨~ was unsteady with the eyes open or closed —*Diseases of the Nervous System*⟩ **3** : a place established to provide a service — see AID STATION

sta·tion·ary \'stā-shə-ˌner-ē\ *adj* **1** : fixed in position : not moving **2** : characterized by a lack of change ⟨the patient's condition remained ~⟩

stato·co·nia \ˌstat-ə-'kō-nē-ə\ *n pl* : OTOCONIA

stato·ki·net·ic \ˌstat-ō-kə-'net-ik\ *adj* : of, relating to, or constituting a kinetic postural reflex that is initiated by stimulation of the semicircular canals through movements of the head and involves compensatory movements of the limbs and eyes ⟨the effect of ∼ stimuli on pilots during training flights⟩ — compare STATOTONIC

stato·lith \'stat-ᵊl-ˌith\ *n* : OTOLITH

stato·ton·ic \ˌstat-ə-'tän-ik\ *adj* : of, relating to, or being a tonic reflex that serves to establish or maintain the posture of an individual against the force of gravity and that is initiated by stimulation of the utricle of the labyrinth through position of the head or movements of the neck muscles and involves alteration of skeletal muscle tone ⟨∼ reflexes⟩ — compare STATOKINETIC

stat·ure \'stach-ər\ *n* : natural height (as of a person) in an upright position

sta·tus \'stāt-əs, 'stat-\ *n, pl* **sta·tus·es** : a particular state or condition ⟨a patient's neurological ∼⟩

status asth·mat·i·cus \-az-'mat-i-kəs\ *n* : a prolonged severe attack of asthma that is unresponsive to initial standard therapy, is characterized esp. by dyspnea, dry cough, wheezing, and hypoxemia, and that may lead to respiratory failure

status ep·i·lep·ti·cus \-ˌep-ə-'lep-ti-kəs\ *n* : a single prolonged seizure or a series of seizures without intervening full recovery of consciousness

status lym·phat·i·cus \-(ˌ)lim-'fat-i-kəs\ *n* : hyperplasia of the lymphatic tissue formerly believed to be a cause of sudden death in infancy and childhood but now no longer recognized as a genuine pathological entity — called also *lymphatism*

status thy·mi·co·lym·phat·i·cus \-'thī-mi-kō-(ˌ)lim-'fat-i-kəs\ *n* : status lymphaticus with enlargement of the thymus

stat·u·to·ry rape \ˌstach-ə-ˌtōr-ē-\ *n* : sexual intercourse with a person who is below the age of consent as defined by law

staunch *var of* STANCH

staves·acre \'stāv-ˌzā-kər\ *n* **1** : a Eurasian plant of the genus *Delphinium* (*D. staphisagria*) having purple flowers **2** : the ripe seeds of the stavesacre that contain delphinine, are violently emetic and cathartic, and have been used to kill head lice — called also *staphisagria*

stav·u·dine \'stav-yü-ˌdēn\ *n* : D4T

STD \ˌes-ˌtē-'dē\ *n* : SEXUALLY TRANSMITTED DISEASE

steady state *n* **1** : a state or condition of a system or process (as one of the energy states of an atom) that does not change in time **2** : a state of physiological equilibrium esp. in connection with a specified metabolic relation or activity

steal \'stēl\ *n* : abnormal circulation characterized by deviation (as through collateral vessels or by backward flow) of blood to tissues where the normal flow of blood has been cut off by occlusion of an artery ⟨subclavian ∼⟩ ⟨coronary ∼⟩

ste·ap·sin \stē-'ap-sən\ *n* : the lipase in pancreatic juice

stea·rate \'stē-ə-ˌrāt, 'sti(ə)r-ˌāt\ *n* : a salt or ester of stearic acid

stea·ric acid \stē-'ar-ik-, ˌsti(ə)r-ik-\ *n* : a white crystalline fatty acid $C_{18}H_{36}O_2$ obtained by saponifying tallow or other hard fats containing stearin; *also* : a commercial mixture of stearic and palmitic acids

stea·rin \'stē-ə-rən, 'sti(ə)r-ən\ *n* **1** : an ester of glycerol and stearic acid $C_3H_5(C_{18}H_{35}O_2)_3$ that is a predominant constituent of many hard fats **2** *also* **stea·rine** *same or* 'stē-ə-ˌrēn, 'sti(ə)r-ˌēn\ : the solid portion of a fat

stea·rop·tene \ˌstē-ə-'räp-ˌtēn, sti-'räp-\ *n* : the portion of a natural essential oil that separates as a solid on cooling or long standing — compare ELEOPTENE

stea·ryl alcohol \'stē-ə-ˌril-, 'sti-ˌril-\ *n* : an unctuous solid alcohol $C_{18}H_{38}O$ that has uses similar to those of cetyl alcohol

ste·a·ti·tis \ˌstē-ə-'tīt-əs\ *n* : inflammation of fatty tissue; *esp* : YELLOW FAT DISEASE

steatoides — see PITYRIASIS STEATOIDES

ste·a·to·ma \ˌstē-ə-'tō-mə\ *n, pl* **-mas** *or* **-ma·ta** \-mət-ə\ : SEBACEOUS CYST

ste·a·to·py·gia \ˌstē-at-ə-'pij-ē-ə *also* stē-ˌat-ō-, -'pī-j(ē-)ə\ *n*

: an accumulation of a large amount of fat on the buttocks — **ste·a·to·py·gous** \-'pī-gəs\ *or* **ste·a·to·py·gic** \-'pij-ik *also* -'pī-jik\ *adj*

ste·at·or·rhea *or chiefly Brit* **ste·at·or·rhoea** \(ˌ)stē-ˌat-ə-'rē-ə\ *n* : an excess of fat in the stools ⟨idiopathic ∼⟩

ste·a·to·sis \ˌstē-ə-'tō-səs\ *n, pl* **-to·ses** \-ˌsēz\ : FATTY DEGENERATION ⟨∼ of the liver⟩

stego·my·ia \ˌsteg-ə-'mī-ə\ *n* **1** *cap, in some classifications* : a genus of mosquitoes including the yellow-fever mosquito (*Aedes aegypti*) and several related mosquitoes **2** : any mosquito of the genus *Stegomyia*; *specif* : YELLOW-FEVER MOSQUITO

Stei·nert's disease \'stī-nərts-\ *n* : MYOTONIC DYSTROPHY

Stei·nert \'shtī-nərt\, **Hans Gustav Wilhelm (1875–1911)**, German physician. Steinert published his description of myotonic dystrophy in 1909. In that same year the disease was described independently by British physician Frederic Eustace Batten, and consequently in the past his name was attached to it as well.

Stein–Lev·en·thal syndrome \'stīn-'lev-ᵊn-ˌthäl-\ *n* : POLYCYSTIC OVARY SYNDROME

Stein, Irving Freiler (1887–1976), and **Leventhal, Michael Leo (1901–1971)**, American gynecologists. Stein and Leventhal published the first description of polycystic ovary syndrome in 1935.

Stein·mann pin \'stīn-mən-\ *n* : a stainless steel spike used for the internal fixation of fractures of long bones

Stein·mann \'shtīn-ˌmän\, **Fritz (1872–1932)**, Swiss surgeon. Steinmann invented for insertion into the distal end of a fractured bone a surgical pin that provided a hold for skeletal traction. He published a report of his invention in 1907.

Stel·a·zine \'stel-ə-ˌzēn\ *trademark* — used for a preparation of trifluoperazine

stel·late \'ste-ˌlāt\ *adj* : shaped like a star ⟨a ∼ ulcer⟩

stellate cell *n* : a cell (as a Kupffer cell) with radiating cytoplasmic processes

stellate ganglion *n* : a composite ganglion formed by fusion of the inferior cervical ganglion and the first thoracic ganglion of the sympathetic chain of a vertebrate animal

stellate ligament *n* : RADIATE LIGAMENT

stellate reticulum *n* : a loosely connected mass of stellate epithelial cells that in early developmental stages makes up a large portion of the enamel organ

stel·lec·to·my \stə-'lek-tə-mē\ *n, pl* **-mies** : surgical excision of the stellate ganglion

stem cell \'stem-\ *n* : an unspecialized cell that gives rise to differentiated cells ⟨hematopoietic *stem cells* in bone marrow⟩

Sten·der dish \'sten-dər-\ *n* : a small circular glass dish with vertical walls and loosely fitting cover used in laboratories usu. to hold stains, culture media, or specimens

Sten·der \'shten-dər\, **Wilhelm P.**, German manufacturer. Stender was a manufacturer of scientific apparatus in Leipzig in the 19th century.

steno·car·dia \ˌsten-ə-'kärd-ē-ə\ *n* : ANGINA PECTORIS

ste·nosed \ste-'nōst, -'nōzd\ *adj* : affected with stenosis : abnormally constricted ⟨a ∼ eustachian tube⟩

ste·nos·ing \ste-'nō-siŋ, -ziŋ\ *adj* : causing or characterized by stenosis (as of a tendon sheath) ⟨∼ tenosynovitis⟩

ste·no·sis \stə-'nō-səs\ *n, pl* **-no·ses** \-ˌsēz\ : a narrowing or constriction of the diameter of a bodily passage or orifice ⟨esophageal ∼⟩ — see AORTIC STENOSIS, MITRAL STENOSIS, PULMONARY STENOSIS, SPINAL STENOSIS, SUBAORTIC STENOSIS

ste·not·ic \stə-'nät-ik\ *adj* : of, relating to, characterized by, or causing stenosis ⟨∼ lesions⟩

Sten·sen's duct *also* **Sten·son's duct** \'sten-sənz-\ *n* : PAROTID DUCT

S
T

\ə\ abut \ᵊ\ kitten \ər\ further \a\ ash \ā\ ace \ä\ cot, cart \aů\ out \ch\ chin \e\ bet \ē\ easy \g\ go \i\ hit \ī\ ice \j\ job \ŋ\ sing \ō\ go \ȯ\ law \ȯi\ boy \th\ thin \t̲h̲\ the \ü\ loot \ů\ foot \y\ yet \zh\ vision *See also* Pronunciation Symbols page

Sten·sen *or* **Steen·sen** \'stän-sən\, **Niels** (*Latin* **Nicolaus Steno**) **(1638–1686),** Danish anatomist and geologist. Although Stensen had prepared to become a physician and eventually became a Catholic priest, his importance in science rests with his anatomical and geological researches. An early discovery was the duct of the parotid gland in 1660. In 1669 he published his geological observations in a work that was seminal to the development of geology. He put forth the revolutionary concept that fossils are the remains of ancient living organisms. He was the first to realize that the earth's crust contains a chronological history of geologic events and that the earth's history could be reconstructed by a careful analysis of the strata and fossils.

stent \'stent\ *also* **stint** \'stint\ *n* **1 :** a mold formed from a resinous compound and used for holding a surgical graft in place; *also* : something (as a pad of gauze immobilized by sutures) used like a stent **2 :** a short narrow metal or plastic tube often in the form of a mesh that is inserted into the lumen of an anatomical vessel (as an artery or bile duct) esp. to keep a previously blocked passageway open

Stent, Charles Thomas (1807–1885), British dentist. In the mid 19th century Stent developed a dental-impression compound containing gutta-percha, stearine, and talc, which he produced and sold with the aid of his sons Charles Robert (1845–1901) and Arthur Howard (1859–1900), who also became dentists. In 1899 the compound was trademarked under the name *Stents*. During World War I the Dutch plastic surgeon J. F. S. Esser discovered that Stent's compound could also be used to form molds for holding skin grafts in place, and in a 1917 publication he referred to such molds as "stents molds." Over the next several decades the singular form *stent* became a generally used term in plastic and oral surgery. The meaning of *stent* continued to be expanded to include other types of artificial supports for human tissue. In 1954 the American surgeon William ReMine applied the term *stent* to a polyethylene tube used to support an anastomosis in an experimental biliary reconstruction. By 1966 *stent* (or sometimes *stint*) had been used for tubular supports in cardiovascular surgery, and by 1972 the term was also being used for urological supports.

stent·ing \'sten-tiŋ\ *n* : a surgical procedure or operation for inserting a stent into an anatomical vessel — **stent** *vt*

Steph·a·no·fi·lar·ia \,stef-ə-,nō-fi-'lar-ē-ə\ *n* : a genus of filarial worms parasitic in the skin and subcutaneous tissues of ruminants and horses where they may cause dermatitis and extensive degenerative lesions — see HUMP SORE

steph·a·no·fil·a·ri·a·sis \-,fil-ə-'rī-ə-səs\ *n, pl* **-a·ses** \-,sēz\ : infestation with or disease caused by worms of the genus *Stephanofilaria*

Steph·a·nu·rus \,stef-ə-'n(y)ùr-əs\ *n* : a genus of nematode worms of the family Strongylidae that includes the kidney worm (*S. dentatus*) of swine

step·page gait \'step-ij-\ *n* : an abnormal gait that is characterized by high lifting of the legs with the toes pointing downward and that is associated with neurological disorders which prevent normal flexion of the feet

ste·ra·di·an \sti-'rād-ē-ən\ *n* : a unit of measure of solid angles that is expressed as the solid angle subtended at the center of the sphere by a portion of the surface whose area is equal to the square of the radius of the sphere

ster·co·bi·lin \,stər-kō-'bī-lin\ *n* : UROBILIN; *esp* : a brown levorotatory pigment $C_{33}H_{46}N_4O_6$ found in feces and urine

ster·co·bi·lin·o·gen \-bī-'lin-ə-jən\ *n* : UROBILINOGEN

ster·co·ra·ceous \,stər-kə-'rā-shəs\ *adj* : of, relating to, containing, produced by, or being feces : FECAL

ster·co·ral \'stər-kə-rəl\ *adj* : STERCORACEOUS

Ster·cu·lia \stər-'k(y)ül-yə\ *n* : a genus of tropical trees (family Sterculiaceae) including several from which karaya gum is obtained

sterculia gum *n* : KARAYA GUM

ste·reo·acui·ty \,ster-ē-ō-ə-'kyü-ət-ē, ,stir-\ *n, pl* **-ties** : the ability to detect differences in distance using stereoscopic cues that is measured by the smallest difference in the images presented to the two eyes that can be detected reliably — compare GRATING ACUITY, HYPERACUITY, VERNIER ACUITY

ste·reo·cam·pim·e·ter \-kam-'pim-ət-ər\ *n* : a campimeter equipped for the simultaneous testing of both eyes

ste·reo·chem·i·cal \-'kem-i-kəl\ *adj* : of or relating to stereochemistry — **ste·reo·chem·i·cal·ly** \-i-k(ə-)lē\ *adv*

ste·reo·chem·is·try \,ster-ē-ō-'kem-ə-strē, ,stir-\ *n, pl* **-tries** **1 :** a branch of chemistry that deals with the spatial arrangement of atoms and groups in molecules **2 :** the spatial arrangement of atoms and groups in a compound and its relation to the properties of the compound

ste·reo·cil·i·um \-'sil-ē-əm\ *n, pl* **-cil·ia** \-ē-ə\ : a specialized microvillus that superficially resembles a cilium and projects from the surface of certain cells (as the auditory hair cells and the superficial epithelial cells of the epididymis) — see KINOCILIUM

ste·re·og·no·sis \,ster-ē-äg-'nō-səs, ,stir-\ *n* : ability to perceive or the perception of material qualities (as shape) of an object by handling or lifting it : tactile recognition

ste·re·og·nos·tic \-'näs-tik\ *adj* : of, relating to, or involving stereognosis ⟨∼ abilities⟩

ste·reo·gram \'ster-ē-ə-,gram, 'stir-\ *n* **1 :** a diagram or picture representing objects with an impression of solidity or relief **2 :** STEREOGRAPH

ste·reo·graph \-,graf\ *n* : a pair of stereoscopic pictures or a picture composed of two superposed stereoscopic images that gives a three-dimensional effect when viewed with a stereoscope or special glasses

ste·reo·iso·mer \,ster-ē-ō-'ī-sə-mər, ,stir-\ *n* : any of a group of isomers in which atoms are linked in the same order but differ in their spatial arrangement — **ste·reo·iso·mer·ic** \-,ī-sə-'mer-ik\ *adj* — **ste·reo·isom·er·ism** \-ī-'säm-ə-,riz-əm\ *n*

ste·re·ol·o·gy \,ster-ē-'äl-ə-jē, ,stir-\ *n, pl* **-gies** : a branch of science concerned with inferring the three-dimensional properties of objects or matter ordinarily observed two≈ dimensionally — **ste·reo·log·i·cal** \-ē-ə-'läj-i-kəl\ *also* **ste·reo·log·ic** \-'läj-ik\ *adj* — **ste·reo·log·i·cal·ly** \-i-k(ə-)lē\ *adv*

ste·reo·mi·cro·scope \,ster-ē-ō-'mī-krə-,skōp\ *n* : a microscope having a set of optics for each eye to make an object appear in three dimensions — **ste·reo·mi·cro·scop·ic** \-,mī-krə-'skäp-ik\ *adj* — **ste·reo·mi·cro·scop·i·cal·ly** \-i-k(ə-)lē\ *adv*

ste·reo·pho·to·mi·cro·graph \,ster-ē-ō-,fōt-ō-'mī-krə-,graf, ,stir-\ *n* : a stereoscopic photograph made through a microscope

ste·re·op·sis \,ster-ē-'äp-səs, ,stir-\ *n* : stereoscopic vision

ste·reo·ra·dio·graph \,ster-ē-ō-'rād-ē-ə-,graf, ,stir-\ *n* : a stereoscopic radiograph — **ste·reo·ra·dio·graph·ic** \-,rād-ē-ə-'graf-ik\ *adj*

ste·reo·ra·di·og·ra·phy \-,rād-ē-'äg-rə-fē\ *n, pl* **-phies** : the production or use of stereoradiographs

ste·reo·scope \'ster-ē-ə-,skōp, 'stir-\ *n* : an optical instrument with two eyepieces for helping the observer to combine the images of two pictures taken from points of view a little way apart and thus to get the effect of solidity or depth

ste·reo·scop·ic \,ster-ē-ə-'skäp-ik, ,stir-\ *adj* **1 :** of or relating to stereoscopy or the stereoscope **2 :** characterized by stereoscopy ⟨∼ vision⟩ — **ste·reo·scop·i·cal·ly** \-i-k(ə-)lē\ *adv*

ste·re·os·co·py \,ster-ē-'äs-kə-pē, ,stir-; 'ster-ē-ə-,skō-pē, 'stir-\ *n, pl* **-pies** **1 :** a science that deals with stereoscopic effects and methods **2 :** the seeing of objects in three dimensions

ste·reo·se·lec·tive \,ster-ē-ō-sə-'lek-tiv, ,stir-\ *adj* : relating to or being a reaction or process producing a stereoisomer having one particular configuration regardless of the stereoisomeric configuration of the reactant

ste·reo·se·lec·tiv·i·ty \-sə-,lek-'tiv-ət-ē, -,sē-\ *n, pl* **-ties** : the state or condition of being stereoselective

ste·reo·spe·cif·ic \-spə-'sif-ik\ *adj* : relating to, being, or effecting a reaction or process in which different stereoisomeric starting materials produce different stereoisomeric products ⟨∼ polymerization⟩ ⟨∼ catalysts⟩ — **ste·reo·spe·cif·i·cal·ly** \-i-k(ə-)lē\ *adv*

ste·reo·spec·i·fic·i·ty \-,spes-ə-'fis-ət-ē\ *n, pl* **-ties** : the state or condition of being stereospecific

ste·reo·tac·tic \,ster-ē-ə-'tak-tik, ,stir-\ *adj* : involving, being, utilizing, or used in a surgical technique for precisely directing the tip of a delicate instrument (as a needle) or beam of radiation in three planes using coordinates provided by medical imaging (as computed tomography) in order to reach a specific locus in the body (as a tumor in the brain or breast) ⟨a ∼ biopsy⟩ ⟨a ∼ surgical probe⟩ — **ste·reo·tac·ti·cal·ly** \-ti-k(ə-)lē\ *adv*

stereotactic radiosurgery *n* : a surgical technique involving the use of narrow beams of radiation (as gamma rays) that are precisely targeted by stereotactic methods to destroy tumors or lesions esp. of the brain

ste·reo·tax·ic \,ster-ē-ə-'tak-sik, ,stir-\ *adj* : STEREOTACTIC — **ste·reo·tax·i·cal·ly** \-si-k(ə-)lē\ *adv*

ste·reo·tax·is \-'tak-səs\ *n, pl* **-tax·es** \-,sēz\ : a stereotactic technique or procedure

¹**ste·reo·type** \'ster-ē-ə-,tīp, 'stir-\ *vt* **-typed; -typ·ing** **1** : to repeat without variation ⟨*stereotyped* behavior⟩ **2** : to develop a mental stereotype about

²**stereotype** *n* : something conforming to a fixed or general pattern; *esp* : an often oversimplified or biased mental picture held to characterize the typical individual of a group — **ste·reo·typ·i·cal** \,ster-ē-ə-'tip-i-kəl\ *also* **ste·reo·typ·ic** \-ik\ *adj*

ste·reo·ty·py \'ster-ē-ə-,tī-pē, 'stir-\ *n, pl* **-pies** : frequent almost mechanical repetition of the same posture, movement, or form of speech (as in schizophrenia)

ste·ric \'ster-ik, 'stir-\ *adj* : relating to or involving the arrangement of atoms in space — **ste·ri·cal·ly** \-i-k(ə-)lē\ *adv*

ste·rig·ma \stə-'rig-mə\ *n, pl* **-ma·ta** \-mət-ə\ *also* **-mas** : any of the slender stalks at the top of the basidium of some fungi from the tips of which the basidiospores are produced; *broadly* : a stalk or filament that bears conidia or spermatia

ste·rig·ma·to·cys·tin \stə-,rig-mət-ō-'sis-tin\ *n* : a mycotoxin produced by an ascomycete of the genus *Aspergillus* (*A. versicolor*)

ster·il·ant \'ster-ə-lənt\ *n* : a sterilizing agent

ster·ile \'ster-əl, *chiefly Brit* -,īl\ *adj* **1** : failing to produce or incapable of producing offspring ⟨a ∼ hybrid⟩ — compare INFERTILE **2** : free from living organisms and esp. microorganisms ⟨a ∼ syringe⟩ ⟨a ∼ cyst⟩ — **ster·ile·ly** \-əl-(l)ē\ *adv* — **ste·ril·i·ty** \stə-'ril-ət-ē\ *n, pl* **-ties**

sterilisans — see THERAPIA STERILISANS MAGNA

ster·il·ize *also Brit* **ster·il·ise** \'ster-ə-,līz\ *vt* **-ized** *also Brit* **-ised; -iz·ing** *also Brit* **-is·ing** : to make sterile: **a** : to deprive of the power of reproducing **b** : to free from living microorganisms (as by the use of physical or chemical agents) ⟨∼ a surgical instrument⟩ — **ster·il·iza·tion** \,ster-ə-lə-'zā-shən\ *also Brit* **ster·il·isa·tion** \-,lī-'\ *n*

ster·il·iz·er *also Brit* **ster·il·is·er** \'ster-ə-,lī-zər\ *n* : an apparatus for sterilizing (as by the agency of steam, ultraviolet radiation, or chemicals)

sterna *pl of* STERNUM

ster·nal \'stərn-ᵊl\ *adj* : of or relating to the sternum

sternal angle *n* : the angle formed by the joining of the manubrium to the gladiolus of the sternum

ster·na·lis \stər-'nā-ləs\ *n, pl* **ster·na·les** \-(,)lēz\ : a muscle that sometimes occurs on the surface of the pectoralis major at its sternal end and that has its fibers running parallel to the sternum and perpendicular to the pectoralis major

Stern·berg cell \'stərn-bərg-\ *n* : REED-STERNBERG CELL

Sternberg–Reed cell *n* : REED-STERNBERG CELL

ster·ne·bra \'ster-nə-brə\ *n, pl* **-brae** \-,brē, -,brī\ : any of the four segments into which the body of the sternum is divided in childhood and which fuse to form the gladiolus

sterni — see MANUBRIUM STERNI

ster·no·cla·vic·u·lar \,stər-nō-kla-'vik-yə-lər\ *adj* : of, relating to, or being articulation of the sternum and the clavicle ⟨the ∼ joint⟩ ⟨∼ dislocation⟩

¹**ster·no·clei·do·mas·toid** \,stər-nō-,klīd-ə-'mas-,tóid\ *n* : a thick superficial muscle on each side that arises by one head from the first segment of the sternum and by a second from

the inner part of the clavicle, that inserts into the mastoid process and occipital bone, and that acts esp. to bend, rotate, flex, and extend the head

²**sternocleidomastoid** *adj* : of, relating to, supplying, or being a sternocleidomastoid ⟨the ∼ artery⟩

ster·no·clei·do·mas·toi·de·us \-,mas-'tóid-ē-əs\ *n, pl* **-dei** \-ē-,ī\ : STERNOCLEIDOMASTOID

ster·no·cos·tal \,stər-nō-'käs-tᵊl\ *adj* : of, relating to, or situated between the sternum and ribs ⟨∼ articulations⟩

ster·no·hy·oid \,stər-nō-'hī-,óid\ *n* : an infrahyoid muscle on each side of the midline that arises from the medial end of the clavicle and the first segment of the sternum, inserts into the body of the hyoid bone, and acts to depress the hyoid bone and the larynx — **sternohyoid** *adj*

ster·no·hy·oi·de·us \-hī-'ói-dē-əs\ *n, pl* **-dei** \-dē-,ī\ : STERNOHYOID

ster·no·mas·toid muscle \-'mas-,tóid-\ *n* : STERNOCLEIDOMASTOID

ster·no·thy·roid \,stər-nō-'thī-,róid\ *n* : an infrahyoid muscle on each side of the body below the sternohyoid that arises from the sternum and from the cartilage of the first and sometimes of the second ribs, inserts into the thyroid cartilage, and acts to draw the larynx downward by depressing the thyroid cartilage — **sternothyroid** *adj*

ster·no·thy·roi·de·us \-thī-'rói-dē-əs\ *n, pl* **-dei** \-dē-,ī\ : STERNOTHYROID

ster·not·o·my \stər-'nät-ə-mē\ *n, pl* **-mies** : surgical incision through the sternum

ster·num \'stər-nəm\ *n, pl* **-nums** *or* **-na** \-nə\ : a compound ventral bone or cartilage that lies in the median central part of the body of most vertebrates above fishes and that in humans is about seven inches (18 centimeters) long, consists in the adult of three parts, and connects with the clavicles and the cartilages of the upper seven pairs of ribs — called also *breastbone*

ster·nu·ta·tion \,stər-nyə-'tā-shən\ *n* : the act, fact, or noise of sneezing

ster·nu·ta·tor \'stər-nyə-,tāt-ər\ *n* : an agent that induces sneezing and often lacrimation and vomiting

¹**ster·nu·ta·to·ry** \,stər-'nyüt-ə-,tō-rē\ *adj* : inducing sneezing

²**sternutatory** *n, pl* **-ries** : STERNUTATOR

ste·roid \'sti(ə)r-,óid *also* 'ste(ə)r-\ *n* : any of numerous natural or synthetic compounds containing a 17-carbon 4-ring system and including the sterols and various hormones and glycosides — see ANABOLIC STEROID — **steroid** *or* **ste·roi·dal** \stə-'róid-ᵊl\ *adj*

steroid hormone *n* : any of numerous hormones (as estrogen, testosterone, cortisone, and aldosterone) having the characteristic ring structure of steroids and formed in the body from cholesterol

ste·roido·gen·e·sis \stə-,róid-ə-'jen-ə-səs; ,stir-,óid- *also* ,ster-\ *n, pl* **-e·ses** \-,sēz\ : synthesis of steroids ⟨adrenal ∼⟩

ste·roido·gen·ic \-'jen-ik\ *adj* : of, relating to, or involved in steroidogenesis ⟨∼ cells⟩ ⟨∼ response of ovarian tissue⟩

ste·rol \'sti(ə)r-,ól, 'ste(ə)r-, -,ōl\ *n* : any of various solid steroid alcohols (as cholesterol) widely distributed in animal and plant lipids

ster·tor \'stərt-ər, 'stər-,tó(ə)r\ *n* : the act or fact of snoring : stertorous breathing

ster·to·rous \'stərt-ə-rəs\ *adj* : characterized by a harsh snoring or gasping sound — **ster·to·rous·ly** *adv*

stetho·graph \'steth-ə-,graf\ *n* : an instrument that records graphically the heart sounds heard through a stethoscope — **stetho·graph·ic** \,steth-ə-'graf-ik\ *adj*

stetho·scope \'steth-ə-,skōp *also* 'steth-\ *n* : an instrument used to detect and study sounds produced in the body that are conveyed to the ears of the listener through rubber tubing connected with a usu. cup-shaped piece placed upon the

\ə\ abut \ᵊ\ kitten \ər\ further \a\ ash \ā\ ace \ä\ cot, cart \aú\ out \ch\ chin \e\ bet \ē\ easy \g\ go \i\ hit \ī\ ice \j\ job \ŋ\ sing \ō\ go \ó\ law \ói\ boy \th\ thin \t̲h̲\ the \ü\ loot \ú\ foot \y\ yet \zh\ vision *See also* Pronunciation Symbols page

area to be examined — **stetho·scop·ic** \ˌsteth-ə-ˈskäp-ik *also* ˌsteth-\ *adj* — **stetho·scop·i·cal·ly** \-i-k(ə-)lē\ *adv*

Ste·vens–John·son syndrome \ˌstē-vənz-ˈjän(t)-sən-\ *n* : a severe and sometimes fatal form of erythema multiforme that is characterized esp. by purulent conjunctivitis, Vincent's angina, and ulceration of the genitals and anus and that often results in blindness

 Stevens, Albert Mason (1884–1945), and **Johnson, Frank Chambliss (1894–1934),** American pediatricians. Stevens and Johnson jointly published a description of Stevens-Johnson syndrome in 1922. They based their report upon two cases found in children.

ste·via \ˈstē-vē-ə\ *n* : a So. American perennial shrub (*Stevia rebaudiana*) of the composite family; *also* : a very sweet non-caloric glycoside-containing substance that is obtained from the leaves of the stevia and is approved in the U.S. as a dietary supplement

STH *abbr* somatotropic hormone

sthen·ic \ˈsthen-ik\ *adj* **1** : notably or excessively vigorous or active ⟨∼ fever⟩ ⟨∼ emotions⟩ **2** : PYKNIC

stib·amine glucoside \ˈstib-ə-ˌmēn-\ *n* : an amorphous powder $C_{36}H_{49}N_3NaO_{22}Sb_3$ formerly used in the treatment of various tropical diseases (as leishmaniasis)

stib·o·phen \ˈstib-ə-ˌfen\ *n* : a crystalline antimony derivative $C_{12}H_4Na_5O_{16}S_4Sb\cdot7H_2O$ of pyrocatechol used in the treatment of various tropical diseases

stick·ing plaster \ˈstik-iŋ-ˌ\ *n* : an adhesive plaster esp. for closing superficial wounds

Stick·ler syndrome \ˈstik-lər-\ *n* : a variable disorder of connective tissue involving the skeleton, face, and eyes that is characterized by myopia, retinal detachment, cleft palate, micrognathia, flat facies, premature arthritis, hip deformity, and hyperextensibility of the large joints and that is inherited as an autosomal dominant trait

 Stickler, Gunnar B. (*fl* 1965–67), American pediatrician. Stickler published his first description of the syndrome identified by his name in 1965 and then followed it up with another report in 1967. The earliest known description of the disorder, however, is one published in 1953 by German physician B. David.

stick·tight flea \ˈstik-ˈtīt-\ *n* : a flea of the genus *Echidnophaga* (*E. gallinacea*) that is parasitic esp. on the heads of chickens and is a pest in the southern U.S.

sties *pl of* STY

stiff \ˈstif\ *adj* : lacking in suppleness ⟨∼ muscles⟩ — **stiffness** *n*

stiff–lamb disease \ˈstif-ˈlam-\ *n* : white muscle disease occurring in lambs

stiff–man syndrome *n* : a chronic progressive disorder of uncertain etiology that is characterized by painful spasms and increasing stiffness of the muscles

sti·fle \ˈstī-fəl\ *n* : the joint next above the hock in the hind leg of a quadruped (as a horse) corresponding to the knee in humans

stig·ma \ˈstig-mə\ *n, pl* **stig·ma·ta** \stig-ˈmät-ə, ˈstig-mət-ə\ *or* **stigmas 1** : an identifying mark or characteristic; *specif* : a specific diagnostic sign of a disease ⟨the *stigmata* of syphilis⟩ **2** : PETECHIA **3** : a small spot, scar, or opening on a plant or animal

stig·mas·ter·ol \stig-ˈmas-tə-ˌròl, -ˌrōl\ *n* : a crystalline sterol $C_{29}H_{48}O$ obtained esp. from soybean oil

stig·mat·ic \stig-ˈmat-ik\ *adj* : ANASTIGMATIC — used esp. of a bundle of light rays intersecting at a single point — **stig·mat·i·cal·ly** \-i-k(ə-)lē\ *adv*

stil·bam·i·dine \(ˈ)stil-ˈbam-ə-ˌdēn\ *n* : a diamidine $C_{16}H_{16}N_4$ derived from stilbene and used chiefly in the form of its crystalline isethionate salt $C_{20}H_{28}N_4O_8S_2$ in treating various fungal infections

stil·bene \ˈstil-ˌbēn\ *n* **1** : an aromatic hydrocarbon $C_{14}H_{12}$ used as a phosphor and in making dyes **2** : a compound derived from stilbene

stil·bes·trol \stil-ˈbes-ˌtròl, -ˌtrōl\ *or chiefly Brit* **stil·boes·trol** \-ˈbēs-\ *n* : DIETHYLSTILBESTROL

Stiles–Craw·ford effect \ˌstīlz-ˈkrò-fərd-\ *n* : an optical phenomenon in which light passing through the center of the pupil is perceived as more intense than light passing through the periphery of the pupil

 Stiles, Walter Stanley (1901–1985), and **Crawford, Brian Hewson (1906–1991),** British physicists. Stiles spent almost all of his career as a research scientist at the National Physical Laboratory in Great Britain. He was the author of numerous papers on illuminating engineering and physiological optics. He published book-length studies on thermionic emission (1932), the science of color (1967), and the mechanisms of color vision (1978). The Stiles-Crawford effect honors their names.

sti·let \ˈstī-lət\ *or* **sti·lette** \sti-ˈlet\ *n* : STYLET 1 — **sti·let·ted** *adj*

stili *pl of* STYLUS

still·birth \ˈstil-ˌbərth, -ˈbərth\ *n* : the birth of a dead fetus — compare LIVE BIRTH

still·born \-ˈbò(ə)rn\ *adj* : dead at birth — compare LIVE=BORN — **still·born** \-ˌbò(ə)rn\ *n*

stil·lin·gia \sti-ˈlin-j(ē-)ə\ *n* **1** *cap* : a genus of widely distributed herbs and shrubs (family Euphorbiaceae) **2** : the dried root of a plant of the genus *Stillingia* (*S. sylvatica*) formerly used as a sialagogue, diuretic, and laxative

 Stil·ling·fleet \ˈstil-iŋ-flēt\, **Benjamin (1702–1771),** British botanist. Stillingfleet is famous for helping to establish the Linnaean system of botany in England. One of Linnaeus's earliest defenders, he published in 1759 the first fundamental treatise in English on the principles of Linnaeus. The genus name *Stilingia* was introduced in 1767.

Still's disease \ˈstilz-\ *n* : rheumatoid arthritis esp. in children

 Still, Sir George Frederic (1868–1941), British pediatrician. Still was associated for many years with London's King's College Hospital, which was the first hospital with a medical school to establish a special department for the diseases of children. In 1897 he published a description of chronic rheumatoid arthritis found in children; it is now known as Still's disease.

stilus *var of* STYLUS

stim·u·lant \ˈstim-yə-lənt\ *n* **1** : an agent (as a drug) that produces a temporary increase of the functional activity or efficiency of an organism or any of its parts **2** : STIMULUS 2

stim·u·late \-ˌlāt\ *vt* **-lat·ed; -lat·ing 1** : to excite to activity or growth or to greater activity **2 a** : to function as a physiological stimulus to (as a nerve or muscle) **b** : to arouse or affect by a stimulant (as a drug) — **stim·u·la·tive** \ˈstim-yə-ˌlāt-iv\ *adj* — **stim·u·la·to·ry** \-lə-ˌtōr-ē, -ˌtòr-\ *adj*

stim·u·la·tion \ˌstim-yə-ˈlā-shən\ *n* **1** : the act or process of stimulating **2** : the stimulating action of various agents on muscles, nerves, or a sensory end organ by which activity is evoked; *esp* : the reaction produced in a sensory end organ by a stimulus that initiates a nerve impulse and results in functional activity of an effector (as a muscle or gland) ⟨gastric secretion induced by ∼ of the sense of smell⟩

stim·u·la·tor \ˈstim-yə-ˌlāt-ər\ *n* : one that stimulates or provides a stimulus ⟨an electronic nerve ∼⟩ ⟨immune system ∼s⟩ ⟨interdental ∼s⟩

stim·u·lus \ˈstim-yə-ləs\ *n, pl* **-li** \-ˌlī, -ˌlē\ **1** : STIMULANT 1 **2** : an agent (as an environmental change) that directly influences the activity of living protoplasm (as by exciting a sensory organ or evoking muscular contraction or glandular secretion) ⟨a visual ∼⟩

stimulus–object *n* : the physical source of a stimulus

stimulus–response *adj* : of, relating to, or being a reaction to a stimulus; *also* : representing the activity of an organism as composed of such reactions ⟨∼ psychology⟩

¹sting \ˈstiŋ\ *vb* **stung** \ˈstəŋ\; **sting·ing** \ˈstiŋ-iŋ\ *vt* : to prick painfully: as **a** : to pierce or wound with a poisonous or irritating process **b** : to affect with sharp quick pain ∼ *vi* : to feel or cause a keen burning pain or smart ⟨the injection *stung*⟩

²sting *n* **1 a** : the act of stinging; *specif* : the thrust of a stinger into the flesh **b** : a wound or pain caused by or as if by stinging **2** : STINGER 1

sting·er \'stiŋ-ər\ *n* **1** : a sharp organ (as of a wasp, bee, scorpion, or stingray) that is usu. connected with a poison gland or otherwise adapted to wound by piercing and injecting a poison **2** : a usu. sports-related injury of the brachial plexus marked by a painful burning sensation that radiates from the neck down the arm and is often accompanied by weakness or numbness of the affected area — called also *burner*

stinging cell *also* **sting cell** *n* : NEMATOCYST

stinging nettle *n* : NETTLE 1; *esp* : a perennial Eurasian nettle (*Urtica dioica*) established in No. America and having broad coarsely toothed leaves with stinging hairs

sting·ray \'stiŋ-ˌrā *also* -rē\ *n* : any of numerous large flat cartilaginous fishes (order Rajiformes and esp. family Dasyatidae) with one or more large sharp barbed dorsal spines near the base of the whiplike tail capable of inflicting severe wounds

stint *var of* STENT

stip·pling \'stip-liŋ\ *n* : the appearance of spots : a spotted condition (as in basophilic red blood cells, X-rays of the lungs, or bones) — **stip·pled** \-əld\ *adj*

stir·rup \'stər-əp *also* 'stir-əp *or* 'stə-rəp\ *n* **1** : STAPES **2** : an attachment to an examining or operating table designed to raise and spread the legs of a patient

¹**stitch** \'stich\ *n* **1** : a local sharp and sudden pain esp. in the side **2 a** : one in-and-out movement of a threaded needle in suturing **b** : a portion of a suture left in the tissue after one stitch ⟨removal of ∼*es*⟩

²**stitch** *vt* : to fasten, join, or close with stitches ⟨∼ a wound⟩

STM *abbr* short-term memory

sto·chas·tic \stə-'kas-tik, stō-\ *adj* **1** : involving a random variable ⟨a ∼ process⟩ **2** : involving chance or probability ⟨a ∼ model of radiation-induced mutation⟩ — **sto·chas·ti·cal·ly** \-ti-k(ə)lē\ *adv*

stock \'stäk\ *n* : a population, colony, or culture of organisms used for scientific research or medical purposes ⟨smallpox virus ∼*s* retained for research into new vaccines and treatments against smallpox⟩

Stock·holm syndrome \'stäk-ˌhō(l)m-\ *n* : the psychological tendency of a hostage to bond with, identify with, or sympathize with his or her captor

stock·i·nette *or* **stock·i·net** \ˌstäk-ə-'net\ *n* : a soft elastic usu. cotton fabric used esp. for bandages

stock·ing \'stäk-iŋ\ *n* : a usu. knit close-fitting covering for the foot and leg — see ELASTIC STOCKING

stoi·chi·om·e·try \ˌstȯi-kē-'äm-ə-trē\ *n, pl* **-tries** **1** : a branch of chemistry that deals with the application of the laws of definite proportions and of the conservation of mass and energy to chemical activity **2 a** : the quantitative relationship between constituents in a chemical substance **b** : the quantitative relationship between two or more substances esp. in processes involving physical or chemical change — **stoi·chi·o·met·ric** \-kē-ə-'me-trik\ *adj*

stoke \'stōk\ *n* : the cgs unit of kinematic viscosity being that of a fluid which has a viscosity of one poise and a density of one gram per cubic centimeter

Stokes \'stōks\, **Sir George Gabriel (1819–1903),** British mathematician and physicist. Stokes enjoyed a long and illustrious association with Cambridge University. He is noted for his studies of the behavior of viscous fluids and for a theorem which is fundamental to vector analysis. The stoke unit honors his name.

Stokes–Ad·ams syndrome \ˌstōks-'ad-əmz-\ *n* : fainting and convulsions induced by complete heart block with a pulse rate of 40 beats per minute or less — called also *Adams-Stokes attack, Adams-Stokes disease, Adams-Stokes syndrome, Stokes-Adams attack, Stokes-Adams disease*

W. Stokes — see CHEYNE-STOKES RESPIRATION

Adams, Robert (1791–1875), British physician. Adams enjoyed a high reputation as a surgeon and specialist in pathological anatomy. He practiced medicine at several Dublin hospitals. His most important scientific contributions were made in cardiology and the autopsies of patients suffering from various cardiac disorders. He associated cerebral symptoms and slowing of the pulse with cardiac disease.

This phenomenon had been noted earlier by Morgagni and would be confirmed later by William Stokes. Adams published his monograph on diseases of the heart in 1827.

sto·ma \'stō-mə\ *n, pl* **-mas** **1** : any of various small simple bodily openings esp. in a lower animal **2** : an artificial permanent opening esp. in the abdominal wall made in surgical procedures ⟨a colostomy ∼⟩

stom·ach \'stəm-ək, -ik\ *n* **1 a** : a saclike expansion of the alimentary canal of a vertebrate communicating anteriorly with the esophagus and posteriorly with the duodenum and being typically a simple often curved sac with an outer serous coat, a strong complex muscular wall that contracts rhythmically, and a mucous lining membrane that contains gastric glands **b** : one of the compartments of a ruminant stomach ⟨the abomasum is the fourth ∼ of a ruminant⟩ **2** : a cavity in an invertebrate animal that is analogous to a stomach **3** : the part of the body that contains the stomach : BELLY, ABDOMEN

stom·ach·ache \-ˌāk\ *n* : pain in or in the region of the stomach

stom·ach·al \'stəm-ə-kəl\ *adj* : STOMACHIC

¹**sto·mach·ic** \stə-'mak-ik\ *adj* : of or relating to the stomach ⟨∼ vessels⟩

²**stomachic** *n* : a stimulant or tonic for the stomach

stomach pump *n* : a suction pump with a flexible tube for removing the contents of the stomach

stomach tooth *n* : a lower canine esp. of the first dentition

stomach tube *n* : a flexible rubber tube to be passed through the esophagus into the stomach for introduction of material or removal of gastric contents

stomach worm *n* : any of various nematode worms parasitic in the stomach of mammals or birds — see BARBER'S POLE WORM, HYOSTRONGYLUS

sto·mal \'stō-məl\ *adj* : of, relating to, or situated near a surgical stoma ⟨a ∼ ulcer⟩

sto·ma·ti·tis \ˌstō-mə-'tīt-əs\ *n, pl* **-tit·i·des** \-'tit-ə-ˌdēz\ *or* **-ti·tis·es** \-'tīt-ə-səz\ : any of numerous inflammatory diseases of the mouth having various causes (as mechanical trauma, allergy, vitamin deficiency, or infection) ⟨erosive ∼⟩

sto·ma·to·de·um *or chiefly Brit* **sto·ma·to·dae·um** \ˌstō-mət-ə-'dē-əm\ *n, pl* **-dea** *or chiefly Brit* **-daea** \-'dē-ə\ : STOMODEUM

sto·ma·to·gnath·ic \ˌstō-mə-(ˌ)tō(g)-'nath-ik\ *adj* : of or relating to the jaws and the mouth

sto·ma·tol·o·gist \ˌstō-mə-'täl-ə-jəst\ *n* : a specialist in stomatology

sto·ma·tol·o·gy \ˌstō-mə-'täl-ə-jē\ *n, pl* **-gies** : a branch of medical science dealing with the mouth and its disorders — **sto·ma·to·log·i·cal** \ˌstō-mət-ᵊl-'äj-i-kəl\ *also* **sto·ma·to·log·ic** \-ik\ *adj*

sto·ma·to·scope \stə-'mat-ə-ˌskōp, 'stō-mət-ə-\ *n* : an instrument used for examination of the mouth

sto·mo·de·um *or* **sto·mo·dae·um** \ˌstō-mə-'dē-əm\ *n, pl* **-dea** \-'dē-ə\ *or* **-daea** \-'dē-ə\ *also* **-deums** *or* **-daeums** : the embryonic anterior ectodermal part of the alimentary canal or tract — **sto·mo·de·al** *or* **sto·mo·dae·al** \-'dē-əl\ *adj*

Sto·mox·ys \stə-'mäk-səs\ *n* : a genus of bloodsucking dipteran flies of the family Muscidae that includes the stable fly (*S. calcitrans*)

stone \'stōn\ *n* **1** : CALCULUS 1 **2** *pl usu* **stone** : any of various units of weight; *esp* : an official British unit equal to 14 pounds (6.3 kilograms)

stone–blind \'stōn-'blīnd\ *adj* : totally blind

stoned \'stōnd\ *adj* : being drunk or under the influence of a drug (as marijuana) taken esp. for pleasure : HIGH

stone–deaf \-'def\ *adj* : totally deaf

stool \'stül\ *n* : a discharge of fecal matter

stop codon \'stäp-\ *n* : a genetic codon in messenger RNA

\ə\ abut \ᵊ\ kitten \ər\ further \a\ ash \ā\ ace \ä\ cot, cart
\au̇\ out \ch\ chin \e\ bet \ē\ easy \g\ go \i\ hit \ī\ ice \j\ job
\ŋ\ sing \ō\ go \ȯ\ law \ȯi\ boy \th\ thin \th̲\ the \ü\ loot
\u̇\ foot \y\ yet \zh\ vision *See also* Pronunciation Symbols page

S
T

that signals the termination of protein synthesis during translation

stop·ping \\'stäp-iŋ\ *n* : FILLING 1

stor·age disease \\'stȯr-ij-\ *n* : the abnormal accumulation in the body of one or more specific substances and esp. metabolic substances (as cerebrosides in Gaucher's disease) — called also *thesaurosis;* see GLYCOGEN STORAGE DISEASE

sto·rax \\'stō(ə)r-ˌaks, 'stȯ(ə)r-\ *n* 1 : a fragrant balsam obtained from the bark of an Asian tree of the genus *Liquidambar* (*L. orientalis*) that is used as an expectorant and sometimes in perfumery — called also *Levant storax, liquid storax* 2 : a balsam from the sweet gum (*Liquidambar styraciflua*) that is similar to storax — called also *American storax, liquidambar*

stor·es·in \\'stȯr-ez-ᵊn\ *n* : a resin that is an alcohol, exists in two forms, and is the chief constituent of storax

sto·ri·form \\'stȯr-i-ˌfȯrm\ *adj* : having a spiral appearance ⟨xanthomatous . . . pseudotumor of the lung . . . may show a striking ∼ pattern —W. A. D. Anderson & J. M. Kissane⟩

storm \\'stȯ(ə)rm\ *n* : a crisis or sudden increase in the symptoms of a disease — see THYROID STORM

stormy \\'stȯr-mē\ *adj* **storm·i·er; -est** : having alternating exacerbations and remissions of symptoms

STP \ˌes-ˌtē-ˈpē\ *n* : a hallucinogenic drug chemically related to mescaline and amphetamine — called also *DOM*

STP *abbr* standard temperature and pressure

stra·bis·mic \strə-ˈbiz-mik\ *adj* : of, relating to, or affected with strabismus

stra·bis·mus \strə-ˈbiz-məs\ *n* : inability of one eye to attain binocular vision with the other because of imbalance of the muscles of the eyeball — called also *heterotropia, squint;* compare CROSS-EYE

straight chain \\'strāt-\ *n* : an open chain of atoms having no side chains

straightjacket *var of* STRAITJACKET

straight sinus *n* : a venous sinus of the brain that is located along the line of junction of the falx cerebri and tentorium cerebelli, is formed by the junction of the great cerebral vein and the inferior sagittal sinus, and passes posteriorly to terminate in the confluence of sinuses

¹strain \\'strān\ *n* : a group of presumed common ancestry with clear-cut physiological but usu. not morphological distinctions ⟨a highly virulent ∼ of bacteria⟩

²strain *vt* **1 a** : to exert (as oneself) to the utmost **b** : to injure by overuse, misuse, or excessive pressure ⟨∼ed his heart by overwork⟩ **c** : to cause a change of form or size in (a body) by application of external force **2** : to cause to pass through a strainer ∼ *vi* : to contract the muscles forcefully in attempting to defecate — often used in the phrase *strain at stool*

³strain *n* : an act of straining or the condition of being strained: as **a** : excessive physical or mental tension; *also* : a force, influence, or factor causing such tension **b** : bodily injury from excessive tension, effort, or use ⟨heart ∼⟩; *esp* : one resulting from a wrench or twist and involving undue stretching of muscles or ligaments ⟨back ∼⟩ — compare SPRAIN **c** : deformation of a material body under the action of applied forces

strain·er \\'strā-nər\ *n* : a device (as a sieve) to retain solid pieces while a liquid passes through

strain gauge *n* : EXTENSOMETER

strait·jack·et *or* **straight·jack·et** \\'strāt-ˌjak-ət\ *n* : a cover or garment of strong material (as canvas) used to bind the body and esp. the arms closely in restraining a violent prisoner or patient

stra·mo·ni·um \strə-ˈmō-nē-əm\ *n* 1 : the dried leaves of the jimsonweed (*Datura stramonium*) or of a related plant of the genus *Datura* containing the anticholinergic and antispasmodic alkaloids atropine, hyoscyamine, and scopolamine and used esp. formerly in the treatment of asthma and parkinsonism 2 : JIMSONWEED

strand \\'strand\ *n* : something (as a molecular chain) resembling a thread ⟨a ∼ of DNA⟩

strand·ed \\'stran-dəd\ *adj* : having a strand or strands esp. of

a specified kind or number — usu. used in combination ⟨the double-*stranded* molecule of DNA⟩ — **strand·ed·ness** *n*

stran·gle \\'straŋ-gəl\ *vb* **stran·gled; stran·gling** \-g(ə-)liŋ\ *vt* **1** : to choke to death by compressing the throat with something (as a hand or rope) **2** : to obstruct seriously or fatally the normal breathing of ⟨the bone wedged in his throat and *strangled* him⟩ ∼ *vi* **1** : to become strangled : undergo a severe interference with breathing **2** : to die from interference with breathing

stran·gles \-gəlz\ *n pl but sing or pl in constr* : an infectious febrile disease of horses and other equines that is caused by a bacterium of the genus *Streptococcus* (*S. equi*), is characterized by inflammation and congestion of mucous membranes and a tendency to swelling and suppuration of the intermaxillary and cervical lymph nodes, usu. affects young animals, has a low mortality rate, and confers subsequent immunity after one attack

stran·gu·late \\'straŋ-gyə-ˌlāt\ *vb* **-lat·ed; -lat·ing** *vt* : STRANGLE ∼ *vi* : to become constricted so as to stop circulation ⟨the hernia will ∼ and become necrotic⟩

strangulated hernia *n* : a hernia in which the blood supply of the herniated viscus is so constricted by swelling and congestion as to arrest its circulation

stran·gu·la·tion \ˌstraŋ-gyə-ˈlā-shən\ *n* **1** : the action or process of strangling or strangulating **2** : the state of being strangled or strangulated; *esp* : excessive or pathological constriction or compression of a bodily tube (as a blood vessel or a loop of intestine) that interrupts its ability to act as a passage

stran·gu·ry \\'straŋ-gyə-rē, -ˌgyu̇r-ē\ *n, pl* **-ries** : a slow and painful discharge of urine drop by drop produced by spasmodic muscular contraction of the urethra and bladder

¹strap \\'strap\ *n* : a flexible band or strip

²strap *vt* **strapped; strap·ping** **1** : to secure with or attach by means of a strap **2** : to support (as a sprained joint) with overlapping strips of adhesive plaster

strapping *n* : the application of adhesive plaster in overlapping strips upon or around a part (as a sprained ankle or the chest in pleurisy) to serve as a splint to reduce motion or to hold surgical dressings in place upon a surgical wound; *also* : material so used

strata *pl of* STRATUM

strat·e·gy \\'strat-ə-jē\ *n, pl* **-gies** : an adaptation or complex of adaptations (as of behavior, metabolism, or structure) that serves or appears to serve an important function in achieving evolutionary success

strat·i·fi·ca·tion \ˌstrat-ə-fə-ˈkā-shən\ *n* : arrangement or formation in layers or strata ⟨∼ of epithelial cells⟩

strat·i·fied \\'strat-ə-ˌfīd\ *adj* : arranged in layers; *esp* : of, relating to, or being an epithelium consisting of more than one layer of cells

stra·tig·ra·phy \strə-ˈtig-rə-fē\ *n, pl* **-phies** : TOMOGRAPHY

stra·tum \\'strāt-əm, 'strat-\ *n, pl* **stra·ta** \\'strāt-ə, 'strat-\ **1** : a layer of tissue ⟨a deep ∼ of the skin⟩ **2** : a statistical subpopulation

stratum ba·sa·le \-bā-ˈsā-lē\ *n, pl* **strata ba·sa·lia** \-lē-ə\ **1** : the basal layer of the epidermis consisting of a single row of columnar or cuboidal epithelial cells that continually divide and replace the rest of the epidermis as it wears away — called also *stratum germinativum;* see MALPIGHIAN LAYER **2** : the deep layer of the endometrium that is between the stratum spongiosum and the myometrium and that is retained during menstruation

stratum com·pac·tum \-kəm-ˈpakt-əm\ *n, pl* **strata com·pac·ta** \-ˈpakt-ə\ : the relatively dense superficial layer of the endometrium

stratum corneum *n, pl* **strata cornea** : the outer more or less horny part of the epidermis consisting chiefly of layers of dead flattened nonnucleated cells filled with keratin

stratum ger·mi·na·ti·vum \-ˌjər-mə-nə-ˈtī-vəm\ *n, pl* **strata ger·mi·na·ti·va** \-və\ : STRATUM BASALE 1

stratum gran·u·lo·sum \-ˌgran-yə-ˈlō-səm\ *n, pl* **strata gran·u·lo·sa** \-sə\ : a layer of granular nondividing cells lying immediately above the stratum basale in most parts of the epidermis

stratum in·ter·me·di·um \-₁in-tər-'mē-dē-əm\ *n, pl* **strata in·ter·me·dia** \-dē-ə\ : the cell layer of the enamel organ next to the layer of ameloblasts

stratum lu·ci·dum \-'lü-sə-dəm\ *n, pl* **strata lu·ci·da** \-də\ : a thin somewhat translucent layer of cells lying superficial to the stratum granulosum and under the stratum corneum esp. in thickened parts of the epidermis (as of the palms or the soles of the feet)

stratum spi·no·sum \-spi-'nō-səm\ *n, pl* **strata spi·no·sa** \-sə\ : the layers of prickle cells over the layer of the stratum basale capable of undergoing mitosis — called also *prickle cell layer;* see MALPIGHIAN LAYER

stratum spon·gi·o·sum \-₁spən-jē-'ō-səm\ *n, pl* **strata spon·gi·o·sa** \-sə\ : the middle layer of the endometrium between the stratum basale and stratum compactum that contains dilated and tortuous portions of the uterine glands

straw·ber·ry gallbladder \'strò-₁ber-ē-, -brē-\ *n* : an abnormal condition characterized by the deposition of cholesterol in the lining of the gallbladder in a pattern resembling the surface of a strawberry

strawberry mark *n* : a tumor of the skin filled with small blood vessels and appearing usu. as a red and elevated birthmark

strawberry tongue *n* : a tongue that is red from swollen congested papillae and that occurs esp. in scarlet fever and Kawasaki disease

¹**streak** \'strēk\ *n* **1** : a usu. irregular line or stripe — see PRIMITIVE STREAK **2** : inoculum implanted (as with a needle drawn across the surface) in a line on a solid medium

²**streak** *vt* : to implant (inoculum) in a line on a solid medium

stream \'strēm\ *n* : an unbroken current or flow (as of water, a bodily fluid, or a gas) — see BLOODSTREAM, MIDSTREAM

stream·ing \'strē-miŋ\ *n* : an act or instance of flowing; *specif* : CYCLOSIS

stream of consciousness *n* : the continuous unedited flow of conscious experience through the mind

street virus \'strēt-\ *n* : a naturally occurring rabies virus as distinguished from virus attenuated in the laboratory

strength \'streŋ(k)th, 'stren(t)th\ *n, pl* **strengths** \'streŋ(k)ths, 'stren(t)ths, 'streŋks\ **1** : the quality or state of being strong : capacity for exertion or endurance **2** : degree of potency of effect or of concentration **3** : degree of ionization of a solution — used of acids and bases

strep \'strep\ *n, often attrib* : STREPTOCOCCUS ⟨a ~ infection⟩

strepho·sym·bo·lia \₁stref-ō-sim-'bō-lē-ə\ *n* : a learning disorder in which symbols and esp. phrases, words, or letters appear to be reversed or transposed in reading — **strepho·sym·bol·ic** \-'bäl-ik\ *adj*

strepo·gen·in \₁strep-ə-'jen-ən\ *n* : a biologically active principle, characteristic chemical structure, or amino acid content attributed esp. formerly to various proteins, peptides, or mixtures of them to account for their ability to stimulate growth of various microorganisms and esp. one of the genus *Lactobacillus* (*L. casei*)

strep sore throat *n* : STREP THROAT

strep·ta·mine \'strep-tə-₁mēn, -mən\ *n* : a cyclic diamino alcohol $C_6H_{14}N_2O_4$ obtained by alkaline hydrolysis of streptomycin or streptidine

strep·ta·vi·din \₁strep-'tav-əd-ən, -tə-'vīd-ᵊn\ *n* : a protein similar to avidin that is produced by a bacterium of the genus *Streptomyces* (*S. avidinii*), has four identical subunits that each bind tightly to a molecule of biotin, and is used esp. in the detection of molecules (as nucleic acids or antibodies) linked to a biotin label

strep throat *n* : an inflammatory sore throat caused by hemolytic streptococci and marked by fever, prostration, and toxemia — called also *septic sore throat, strep sore throat*

strep·ti·dine \'strep-tə-₁dēn, -dən\ *n* : a cyclic basic alcohol $C_8H_{18}N_6O_4$ that is obtained from streptomycin by acid hydrolysis

strep·to·ba·cil·la·ry \₁strep-tō-'bas-ə-₁ler-ē, -bə-'sil-ə-rē\ *adj* : caused by a streptobacillus ⟨~ fever⟩

strep·to·ba·cil·lus \-bə-'sil-əs\ *n* **1** *cap* : a genus of facultatively anaerobic gram-negative rod bacteria of uncertain family affiliation that includes one (*S. moniliformis*) that is the causative agent of one form of rat-bite fever **2** *pl* **-li** \-₁lī\ : any of various nonmotile gram-negative bacilli in which the individual cells are joined in a chain; *esp* : one of the genus *Streptobacillus*

strep·to·bi·o·sa·mine \-bī-'ō-sə-₁mēn, -mən\ *n* : a glycosidic compound $C_{13}H_{23}NO_9$ that is obtained along with streptidine from streptomycin by hydrolysis

strep·to·coc·cal \₁strep-tə-'käk-əl\ *also* **strep·to·coc·cic** \-'käk-(s)ik\ *adj* : of, relating to, caused by, or being streptococci ⟨a ~ sore throat⟩ ⟨~ organisms⟩ ⟨~ gingivitis⟩

strep·to·coc·co·sis \-kä-'kō-səs\ *n* : infection with or disease caused by hemolytic streptococci

strep·to·coc·cus \-'käk-əs\ *n* **1** *cap* : a genus of spherical or ovoid chiefly nonmotile and parasitic gram-positive bacteria (family Streptococcaceae) that divide only in one plane, occur in pairs or chains, and include important pathogens of humans and domestic animals **2** *pl* **-coc·ci** \-'käk-₁(s)ī\ : any bacterium of the genus *Streptococcus*; *broadly* : a coccus occurring in chains

strep·to·dor·nase \₁strep-tō-'dòr-₁nās, -₁nāz\ *n* : a deoxyribonuclease from hemolytic streptococci that causes hydrolysis of DNA and deoxyribonucleoprotein outside of living cells or in the nuclei of degenerating cells and dissolves pus and that is usu. administered in a mixture with streptokinase — see VARIDASE

strep·to·gram·in \₁strep-tō-'gram-ən\ *n* : an antibiotic complex produced by a bacterium of the genus *Streptomyces* (*S. graminofaciens*)

strep·to·ki·nase \₁strep-tō-'kī-₁nās, -₁nāz\ *n* : a proteolytic enzyme produced by hemolytic streptococci that promotes the dissolution of blood clots by activating plasminogen to produce plasmin — see VARIDASE

strep·to·ly·sin \₁strep-tə-'līs-ᵊn\ *n* : any of various antigenic hemolysins produced by streptococci

strep·to·my·ces \-'mī-₁sēz\ *n* **1** *cap* : the type genus of the family Streptomycetaceae comprising mostly soil actinomycetes including some that form antibiotics as by-products of their metabolism **2** *pl* **streptomyces** : any bacterium of the genus *Streptomyces*

Strep·to·my·ce·ta·ce·ae \₁strep-tō-₁mī-sə-'tā-sē-₁ē\ *n pl* : a family of higher bacteria (order Actinomycetales) that form vegetative mycelia which rarely break up into bacillary forms, have conidia borne on sporophores, and are typically aerobic soil saprophytes but include a few parasites of plants and animals

strep·to·my·cete \-'mī-₁sēt, -₁mī-'sēt\ *n* : any actinomycete (as a streptomyces) of the family Streptomycetaceae

strep·to·my·cin \-'mīs-ᵊn\ *n* : an antibiotic organic base $C_{21}H_{39}N_7O_{12}$ that is produced by a soil actinomycete of the genus *Streptomyces* (*S. griseus*), is active against bacteria, and is used esp. in the treatment of infections (as tuberculosis) by gram-negative bacteria

strep·to·ni·grin \-'nī-grən\ *n* : a toxic antibiotic $C_{25}H_{22}N_4O_8$ from an actinomycete of the genus *Streptomyces* (*S. flocculus*) that interferes with DNA metabolism and is used as an antineoplastic agent

strep·to·thri·cin \₁strep-tō-'thrīs-ᵊn, -'thris-\ *n* : a basic antibiotic $C_{19}H_{34}N_8O_8$ that is produced by a soil actinomycete of the genus *Streptomyces* (*S. lavendulae*) and is active esp. against bacteria; *also* : any of several related antibiotics

strep·to·thrix \'strep-tə-₁thriks\ *n* **1** *cap, in some classifications* : a genus of higher bacteria that somewhat resemble molds, have branched filaments, and comprise forms now usu. placed in *Actinomyces* or in *Leptothrix* **2** *pl* **strep·to-**

\ə\ abut \ᵊ\ kitten \ər\ further \a\ ash \ā\ ace \ä\ cot, cart \au̇\ out \ch\ chin \e\ bet \ē\ easy \g\ go \i\ hit \ī\ ice \j\ job \ŋ\ sing \ō\ go \ȯ\ law \ȯi\ boy \th\ thin \t͟h\ the \ü\ loot \u̇\ foot \y\ yet \zh\ vision *See also* Pronunciation Symbols page

thri·ces \ˌstrep-tə-ˈthrī-ˌsēz\ : any bacterium of the genus *Streptothrix*

strep·to·tri·cho·sis \ˌstrep-tō-ˌtrī-ˈkō-səs\ *also* **strep·to·thri·cho·sis** \-ˌthrī-\ *n* : infection with or disease caused by actinomycetes of the genus *Streptothrix*

strep·to·var·i·cin \ˌstrep-tō-ˈvar-ə-sən\ *n* : any of a group of antibiotics isolated from a bacterium of the genus *Streptomyces* (*S. spectabilis*)

strep·to·zo·cin \ˌstrep-tə-ˈzō-sən\ *n* : STREPTOZOTOCIN

strep·to·zot·o·cin \ˌstrep-tə-ˈzät-ə-sən\ *n* : a broad-spectrum antibiotic $C_8H_{15}N_3O_7$ with antineoplastic and diabetogenic properties that has been isolated from a bacterium of the genus *Streptomyces* (*S. achromogenes*)

¹stress \ˈstres\ *n*   **1 a** : a force exerted when one body or body part presses on, pulls on, pushes against, or tends to compress or twist another body or body part; *esp* : the intensity of this mutual force commonly expressed in pounds per square inch   **b** : the deformation caused in a body by such a force   **2 a** : a physical, chemical, or emotional factor that causes bodily or mental tension and may be a factor in disease causation   **b** : a state of bodily or mental tension resulting from factors that tend to alter an existent equilibrium   **3** : the force exerted between teeth of the upper and lower jaws during mastication

²stress *vt* : to subject to stress ⟨a patient ~ed by surgery⟩

stress breaker *n* : a flexible dental device used to lessen the occlusal forces exerted on teeth to which a partial denture is attached

stress fracture *n* : a usu. hairline fracture of a bone (as of the foot or lower leg) that has been subjected to repeated stress ⟨occurrence of *stress fractures* among joggers⟩

stress·ful \ˈstres-fəl\ *adj* : full of or subject to stress ⟨~ situations⟩ — **stress·ful·ly** \-fə-lē\ *adv*

stress incontinence *n* : involuntary leakage of urine from the bladder accompanying physical activity (as in laughing, coughing, sneezing, or physical exercise) which places increased pressure on the abdomen — compare URGE INCONTINENCE

stress·or \ˈstres-ər, -ˌȯ(ə)r\ *n* : a stimulus that causes stress ⟨psychological ~s⟩

stress test *n* : an electrocardiographic test of heart function before, during, and after a controlled period of increasingly strenuous exercise (as on a treadmill)

¹stretch \ˈstrech\ *vt*   **1** : to extend in length ⟨was told to ~ the leg muscles before running⟩   **2** : to enlarge or distend esp. by force ~ *vi*   **1** : to become extended in length or breadth   **2** : to extend one's body or limbs

²stretch *n* : the act of stretching : the state of being stretched ⟨a muscle or group of muscles in ~ —C. R. Houck⟩

stretch·er \ˈstrech-ər\ *n* : a device for carrying a sick, injured, or dead person

stretch·er–bear·er \-ˌbar-ər, -ˌber-\ *n* : a person who carries one end of a stretcher

stretch marks *n pl* : striae on the skin (as of the hips, abdomen, and breasts) from excessive stretching and rupture of elastic fibers esp. due to pregnancy or obesity

stretch receptor *n* : MUSCLE SPINDLE

stretch reflex *n* : a spinal reflex involving reflex contraction of a muscle in response to stretching — called also *myotatic reflex*

stria \ˈstrī-ə\ *n, pl* **stri·ae** \ˈstrī-ˌē\   **1** : STRIATION 2   **2** : a narrow structural band esp. of nerve fibers   **3** : a stripe or line (as in the skin) distinguished from surrounding tissue by color, texture, or elevation — see STRETCH MARKS

stria longitudinalis *n, pl* **striae lon·gi·tu·di·na·les** \-ˌlän-jə-ˌt(y)üd-ə-ˈnā-ˌlēz\ : NERVE OF LANCISI

striata *pl of* STRIATUM

stri·a·tal \strī-ˈāt-ᵊl\ *adj* : of or relating to the corpus striatum ⟨~ neurons⟩

stri·ate \ˈstrī-ət, -ˌāt\ *adj* : STRIATED

striate cortex *n* : an area of the brain that receives visual impulses, contains a conspicuous band of myelinated fibers, and is located mostly in the walls and along the edges of the

calcarine sulcus of the occipital lobe — called also *visual projection area*

stri·at·ed \ˈstrī-ˌāt-əd\ *adj*   **1** : marked with striae   **2** : of, relating to, or being striated muscle

striated muscle *n* : muscle tissue that is marked by transverse dark and light bands, that is made up of elongated fibers, and that includes skeletal and usu. cardiac muscle of vertebrates and most muscle of arthropods — compare SMOOTH MUSCLE, VOLUNTARY MUSCLE

stria ter·mi·na·lis \-ˌtər-mə-ˈnā-ləs\ *n* : a bundle of nerve fibers that passes from the amygdala along the demarcation between the thalamus and caudate nucleus mostly to the anterior part of the hypothalamus with a few fibers crossing the anterior commissure to the amygdala on the opposite side

stri·a·tion \strī-ˈā-shən\ *n*   **1** : the fact or state of being striated   **2** : a minute groove, scratch, or channel esp. when one of a parallel series   **3** : any of the alternate dark and light cross bands of a myofibril of striated muscle

stri·a·to·ni·gral \strī-ˌāt-ə-ˈnī-grəl\ *adj* : connecting the corpus striatum and substantia nigra ⟨~ axons⟩

stri·a·tum \strī-ˈāt-əm\ *n, pl* **stri·a·ta** \-ˈāt-ə\   **1** : CORPUS STRIATUM   **2** : NEOSTRIATUM

stria vas·cu·la·ris \-ˌvas-kyə-ˈler-əs\ *n* : the upper part of the spiral ligament of the scala media that contains numerous small blood vessels

stric·ture \ˈstrik-chər\ *n* : an abnormal narrowing of a bodily passage (as from inflammation, cancer, or the formation of scar tissue) ⟨esophageal ~⟩; *also* : the narrowed part

stri·dor \ˈstrīd-ər, ˈstrī-ˌdȯ(ə)r\ *n* : a harsh vibrating sound heard during respiration in cases of obstruction of the air passages ⟨laryngeal ~⟩

strid·u·lous \ˈstrij-ə-ləs\ *adj* : characterized by stridor ⟨~ breathing⟩

stridulus \ˈ\ — see LARYNGISMUS STRIDULUS

strike \ˈstrīk\ *n* : cutaneous myiasis (as of sheep) ⟨body ~⟩ ⟨blowfly ~⟩

string galvanometer *n* : a galvanometer for measuring oscillating currents by the lateral motions of a silver-plated quartz fiber traversed by the current and stretched under adjustable tension perpendicular to the field of an electromagnet

string·halt \ˈstriŋ-ˌhȯlt\ *n* : a condition of lameness in the hind legs of a horse caused by muscular spasms — called also *springhalt* — **string·halt·ed** \-ˌhȯl-təd\ *adj*

strip \ˈstrip\ *vt* **stripped** \ˈstript\; **strip·ping** : to remove (a vein) by means of a stripper ⟨*stripping* a varicose saphenous vein⟩

strip–chart re·cord·er \ˈstrip-ˌchärt-ri-ˈkȯrd-ər\ *n* : a device used for the continuous graphic recording of time-dependent data — **strip–chart re·cord·ing** \-ri-ˈkȯrd-iŋ\ *n*

strip·per \ˈstrip-ər\ *n* : a surgical instrument used for removal of a vein

stro·bi·la \strō-ˈbī-lə, ˈstrō-bə-\ *n, pl* **-lae** \-(ˌ)lē\ : a linear series of similar animal structures (as the segmented body of a tapeworm) produced by budding — **stro·bi·lar** \-ˈbī-lər; -bə-lər, -ˌlär\ *adj*

stro·bi·late \ˈstrō-bə-ˌlāt\ *vi* **-lat·ed; -lat·ing** : to become a strobila : undergo strobilation ⟨a *strobilating* tapeworm⟩

stro·bi·la·tion \ˌstrō-bə-ˈlā-shən\ *n* : asexual reproduction by transverse division of the body into segments which develop into separate individuals, zooids, or proglottids in many coelenterates and worms

strob·i·lo·cer·cus \ˌsträb-ə-lō-ˈsər-kəs\ *n, pl* **-ci** \-ˌsī\ : a larval tapeworm that has undergone strobilation and eversion from its bladder while still in the intermediate host

stroke \ˈstrōk\ *n* : sudden diminution or loss of consciousness, sensation, and voluntary motion caused by rupture or obstruction (as by a clot) of a blood vessel of the brain — called also *apoplexy, brain attack, cerebral accident, cerebrovascular accident;* see HEMORRHAGIC STROKE, ISCHEMIC STROKE, LITTLE STROKE

stroke volume *n* : the volume of blood pumped from a ventricle of the heart in one beat

stro·ma \'strō-mə\ *n, pl* **stro·ma·ta** \-mət-ə\ **1** : the supporting framework of an animal organ typically consisting of connective tissue **2** : the spongy protoplasmic framework of some cells (as a red blood cell) — **stro·mal** \-məl\ *adj*

stro·ma·tin \'strō-mət-ən\ *n* : a protein in some respects comparable to keratin that is present in the stroma of some cells (as red blood cells)

strom·uhr \'strō-ˌmù(ə)r\ *n* : a rheometer designed to measure the amount and speed of blood flow through an artery

strong silver protein \'stroŋ-\ *n* : SILVER PROTEIN b

stron·gyle \'strän-ˌjīl\ *n* : STRONGYLID; *esp* : a worm of the genus *Strongylus* or closely related genera that is parasitic esp. in the intestines and tissues of the horse and may induce severe diarrhea and debility

stron·gy·lid \'strän-jə-ləd\ *n* : any nematode worm of the family Strongylidae — **strongylid** *adj*

Stron·gyl·i·dae \strän-'jil-ə-ˌdē\ *n pl* : a large family of nematode worms of the suborder Strongylina that are parasites of vertebrates and have a globular to cylindrical buccal capsule and a circlet of laminar processes about the mouth

stron·gy·li·do·sis \ˌsträn-jə-lə-'dō-səs\ *n* : STRONGYLOSIS

Stron·gy·li·na \ˌsträn-jə-'lī-nə\ *n pl* : a suborder (order Rhabditida) that comprises nematode worms parasitic as adults in vertebrates often with a complex life cycle involving an invertebrate larval host and that includes important parasites (as the strongyles and the hookworms) of humans and domestic animals

¹**stron·gy·loid** \'strän-jə-ˌlòid\ *adj* : of or relating to the superfamily Strongyloidea

²**strongyloid** *n* : a worm of the superfamily Strongyloidea

Stron·gy·loi·dea \ˌsträn-jə-'lòid-ē-ə\ *n pl* : a superfamily of parasitic nematode worms (order Rhabditida) comprising the hookworms, strongyles, and related forms

Stron·gy·loi·des \ˌsträn-jə-'lòi-ˌdēz\ *n* : a genus (the type of the family Strongyloididae) of nematode worms having both free-living males and females and parthenogenetic females parasitic in the intestine of various vertebrates and including some medically and economically important pests of humans

stron·gy·loi·di·a·sis \-ˌlòi-'dī-ə-səs\ *n, pl* **-a·ses** \-ə-ˌsēz\ : infestation with or disease caused by nematodes of the genus *Strongyloides*

stron·gy·loi·do·sis \-ˌlòi-'dō-səs\ *n* : STRONGYLOIDIASIS

stron·gy·lo·sis \ˌsträn-jə-'lō-səs\ *n* : infestation with or disease caused by strongyles — called also *strongylidosis*

Stron·gy·lus \'strän-jə-ləs\ *n* : the type genus of the family Strongylidae of parasitic nematode worms comprising worms with a pair of elongated buccal glands and including gastrointestinal parasites of the horse

stron·tium \'strän-ch(ē-)əm, 'stränt-ē-əm\ *n* : a soft malleable ductile bivalent metallic element of the alkaline-earth group occurring only in combination — symbol *Sr*; see ELEMENT table

strontium 90 *n* : a heavy radioactive isotope of strontium having the mass number 90 that is present in the fallout from nuclear explosions and is hazardous because like calcium it can be assimilated in biological processes and deposited in the bones of human beings and animals — called also *radiostrontium*

stro·phan·thi·din \strō-'fan(t)-thə-dən\ *n* : a very toxic crystalline steroidal gamma-lactone $C_{23}H_{32}O_6$ obtained by hydrolysis of strophanthin, cymarin, and various other glycosides

stro·phan·thin \strō-'fan(t)-thən\ *n* : any of several glycosides (as ouabain) or mixtures of glycosides from African plants of the genera *Strophanthus* and *Acocanthera*; *esp* : a bitter toxic glycoside $C_{36}H_{54}O_{14}$ from a woody vine of the genus *Strophanthus* (*S. kombé*) used similarly to digitalis

stro·phan·thus \-thəs\ *n* **1** *cap* : a genus of tropical Asian and African trees, shrubs, and woody vines of the dogbane family (Apocynaceae) that include several African forms with poisonous seeds as well as forms (as *S. kombé*) that furnish strophanthin **2** : the dried cleaned ripe seeds of any of several plants of the genus *Strophanthus* (as *S. kombé* and *S.*

hispidus) that are in moderate doses a cardiac stimulant like digitalis but in larger doses a violent poison and that have strophanthin as their most active constituent

struck \'strək\ *n* : enterotoxemia esp. of adult sheep

struc·tur·al \'strək-chə-rəl, 'strək-shrəl\ *adj* **1** : of or relating to the physical makeup of a plant or animal body ⟨∼ defects of the heart⟩ — compare FUNCTIONAL 1a **2** : of, relating to, or affecting structure ⟨∼ stability⟩ — **struc·tur·al·ly** \-ē\ *adv*

structural formula *n* : an expanded molecular formula (as H-O-H for water) showing the arrangement within the molecule of atoms and of bonds

structural gene *n* : a gene that codes for the amino acid sequence of a protein (as an enzyme) or for a ribosomal RNA or transfer RNA

struc·tur·al·ism \'strək-chə-rə-ˌliz-əm, 'strək-shrə-\ *n* : psychology concerned esp. with resolution of the mind into structural elements

structural isomer *n* : one of two or more compounds that contain the same number and kinds of atoms but that differ significantly in their geometric arrangement — **structural isomerism** *n*

struc·ture \'strək-chər\ *n* **1** : something (as an anatomical part) arranged in a definite pattern of organization **2 a** : the arrangement of particles or parts in a substance or body ⟨molecular ∼⟩ **b** : organization of parts as dominated by the general character of the whole ⟨personality ∼⟩ **3** : the aggregate of elements of an entity in their relationships to each other

struc·ture·less \'strək-chər-ləs\ *adj* : lacking structure; *esp* : devoid of cells ⟨a ∼ membrane⟩ — **struc·ture·less·ness** *n*

stru·ma \'strü-mə\ *n, pl* **-mae** \-(ˌ)mē\ *or* **-mas** : GOITER

struma lym·pho·ma·to·sa \-lim-ˌfō-mə-'tō-sə\ *n* : HASHIMOTO'S THYROIDITIS

stru·vite \'strü-ˌvīt\ *n* : a hydrated magnesium-containing mineral $Mg(NH_4)(PO_4)\cdot 6H_2O$ which is found in kidney stones associated with bacteria that cleave urea

strych·nine \'strik-ˌnīn, -nən, -ˌnēn\ *n* : a bitter poisonous alkaloid $C_{21}H_{22}N_2O_2$ that is obtained from nux vomica and related plants of the genus *Strychnos* and is used as a poison (as for rodents) and medicinally as a stimulant of the central nervous system

Strych·nos \'strik-nəs, -ˌnäs\ *n* : a large genus of tropical trees and woody vines (family Loganiaceae) — see CURARE, NUX VOMICA, STRYCHNINE

STS *abbr* serologic test for syphilis

ST segment *or* **S–T segment** \ˌes-'tē-\ *n* : the part of an electrocardiogram between the QRS complex and the T wave

Stu·art–Prow·er factor \'st(y)ü-ərt-'praú-ər-\ *n* : FACTOR X
  Stuart and **Prower**, 20th-century hospital patients in whom factor X deficiency was first found.

stuff \'stəf\ *vt* : to choke or block up (as nasal passages) ⟨a ∼ed up nose⟩

stuffy \'stəf-ē\ *adj* **stuff·i·er; -est** : affected with congestion ⟨a ∼ nose⟩ — **stuff·i·ness** \'stəf-ē-nəs\ *n*

stump \'stəmp\ *n* **1** : the basal portion of a bodily part (as a limb) remaining after the rest is removed **2** : a rudimentary or vestigial bodily part

stump sock *n* : a special sock worn over an amputation stump with various types of prostheses

stun \'stən\ *vt* **stunned; stun·ning** : to make senseless, groggy, or dizzy by or as if by a blow

stung *past and past part of* STING

stunt \'stənt\ *vt* : to hinder the normal growth, development, or progress of ⟨an emotionally ∼ed child⟩

stupe \'st(y)üp\ *n* : a hot wet often medicated cloth applied externally (as to stimulate circulation) ⟨a turpentine ∼⟩

stu·pe·fac·tion \ˌst(y)ü-pə-'fak-shən\ *n* : the act of stupefying or the state of being stupefied

---

\ə\ **abut** \ˀ\ **kitten** \ər\ **further** \a\ **ash** \ā\ **ace** \ä\ **cot, cart** \aú\ **out** \ch\ **chin** \e\ **bet** \ē\ **easy** \g\ **go** \i\ **hit** \ī\ **ice** \j\ **job** \ŋ\ **sing** \ō\ **go** \ò\ **law** \òi\ **boy** \th\ **thin** \th\ **the** \ü\ **loot** \ù\ **foot** \y\ **yet** \zh\ **vision** *See also* Pronunciation Symbols page

S T

stu·pe·fy \'st(y)ü-pə-ˌfī\ vt **-fied; -fy·ing** : to make stupid, groggy, or insensible ⟨*stupefied* by anesthesia⟩

stu·por \'st(y)ü-pər\ n : a condition of greatly dulled or completely suspended sense or sensibility ⟨a drunken ∼⟩; *specif* : a chiefly mental condition marked by absence of spontaneous movement, greatly diminished responsiveness to stimulation, and usu. impaired consciousness

stu·por·ose \'st(y)ü-pə-ˌrōs\ adj : STUPOROUS ⟨if so much drug is given that the patient becomes ∼ —*Lancet*⟩

stu·por·ous \'st(y)ü-p(ə-)rəs\ adj : marked or affected by stupor ⟨was found in her home in a ∼ and unresponsive state —Irving Robinson *et al*⟩ ⟨a ∼ patient⟩

stur·dy \'stərd-ē\ n, pl **sturdies** : GID

Sturge–Web·er syndrome \'stərj-'web-ər-\ n : a rare congenital condition that is characterized by a port-wine stain affecting the facial skin on one side in the area innervated by the first branch of the trigeminal nerve and by malformed blood vessels in the brain that may cause progressive mental retardation, epilepsy, and glaucoma in the eye on the affected side — called also *Sturge-Weber disease*

> **Sturge, William Allen (1850–1919),** British physician. Sturge served as physician to the Royal Free Hospital and the Hospital for Epilepsy and Paralysis, both in London. In later years he was in private practice at Nice. Sturge-Weber syndrome was described by him in 1879 and by F. P. Weber in 1922.
>
> **F. P. Weber** — see WEBER-CHRISTIAN DISEASE

¹**stut·ter** \'stət-ər\ vi : to speak with involuntary disruption or blocking of speech (as by spasmodic repetition or prolongation of vocal sounds) ∼ vt : to say, speak, or sound with or as if with a stutter

²**stutter** n **1** : an act or instance of stuttering **2** : a speech disorder involving stuttering

stut·ter·er \'stət-ər-ər\ n : an individual who stutters

stuttering n **1** : the act of one who stutters **2** : a disorder of vocal communication marked by involuntary disruption or blocking of speech (as by spasmodic repetition or prolongation of vocal sounds), by fear and anxiety, and by a struggle to avoid speech errors

Stutt·gart disease \'stüt-ˌgärt-, 'shtüt-\ n : canine leptospirosis; *esp* : a severe highly contagious form of canicola fever marked by predominantly renal infection with nephritis and uremia, intense calf diphtheria, and bloody vomit and diarrhea and commonly leading to collapse and death

sty or **stye** \'stī\ n, pl **sties** or **styes** : an inflamed swelling of a sebaceous gland at the margin of an eyelid — called also *hordeolum*

sty·let \stī-'let, 'stī-lət\ n **1** also **sty·lette** \stī-'let\ **a** : a slender surgical probe **b** : a thin wire inserted into a catheter to maintain rigidity or into a hollow needle to maintain patency **2** : a relatively rigid elongated organ or appendage (as a piercing mouthpart) of an animal

styli pl of STYLUS

sty·lo·glos·sus \ˌstī-lō-'gläs-əs, -'glòs-\ n, pl **-glos·si** \-'gläs-ˌī, -'glòs-\ : a muscle that arises from the styloid process of the temporal bone, inserts along the side and underpart of the tongue, and functions to draw the tongue upwards

sty·lo·hy·oid \ˌstī-lō-'hī-ˌòid\ n : STYLOHYOID MUSCLE

sty·lo·hy·oi·de·us \-hī-'òid-ē-əs\ n, pl **-dei** \-ē-ˌī\ : STYLOHYOID MUSCLE

stylohyoid ligament n : a band of fibrous tissue connecting the tip of the styloid process of the temporal bone to the ceratohyal of the hyoid bone

stylohyoid muscle n : a slender muscle that arises from the posterior surface of the styloid process of the temporal bone, inserts into the body of the hyoid bone, and acts to elevate and retract the hyoid bone resulting in elongation of the floor of the mouth — called also *stylohyoid, stylohyoideus*

sty·loid \'stī(ə)l-ˌòid\ adj : having a slender pointed shape

styloid process n : any of several long slender pointed bony processes: as **a** : a sharp spine that projects downward and forward from the inferior surface of the temporal bone just in front of the stylomastoid foramen and that is derived from cartilage of the second visceral arch **b** : an eminence on the

distal extremity of the ulna projecting from the medial and posterior part of the bone and giving attachment to a ligament of the wrist joint **c** : a conical prolongation of the lateral surface of the distal extremity of the radius that gives attachment to several tendons and ligaments

sty·lo·man·dib·u·lar ligament \ˌstī-lō-man-'dib-yə-lər-\ : a band of deep fascia that connects the styloid process of the temporal bone to the gonial angle

sty·lo·mas·toid foramen \-'mas-ˌtòid-\ n : a foramen that occurs on the lower surface of the temporal bone between the styloid and mastoid processes and that forms the termination of the facial canal

sty·lo·pha·ryn·ge·us \ˌstī-lō-fə-'rin-jē-əs, -ˌfar-ən-'jē-əs\ n, pl **-gei** \-jē-ˌī\ : a slender muscle that arises from the base of the styloid process of the temporal bone, inserts into the side of the pharynx, and acts with the contralateral muscle in swallowing to increase the transverse diameter of the pharynx by drawing its sides upward and laterally

sty·lus also **sti·lus** \'stī-ləs\ n, pl **sty·li** \'stī(ə)l-ˌī\ also **sty·lus·es** \'stī-lə-səz\ or **sti·li** or **sti·lus·es** : an instrument for writing, marking, or incising: as **a** : a hard-pointed instrument for punching the dots in writing braille with a braille slate **b** : a device that traces a recording (as of an electrocardiograph) on paper

¹**styp·tic** \'stip-tik\ adj : tending to check bleeding ⟨the ∼ effect of cold⟩; *esp* : having the property of arresting oozing of blood (as from a shallow surface injury) when applied to a bleeding part ⟨∼ agent⟩

²**styptic** n : an agent (as a drug) having a styptic effect

styptic cotton n : cotton that is prepared by impregnating with a styptic agent and drying and that is applied to minor wounds to stop bleeding

styptic pencil n : a cylindrical stick of a medicated styptic substance used esp. in shaving to stop the bleeding from small cuts

sty·rax \'stī-ˌraks\ n **1** : STORAX **2** cap : a large genus (the type genus of the family Styracaceae) of shrubs and trees including forms yielding commercially important resins (as benzoin)

sty·rene \'stī-ˌrēn\ n : a fragrant liquid unsaturated hydrocarbon C_8H_8 used chiefly in making synthetic rubber, resins, and plastics and in improving drying oils; *also* : any of various synthetic plastics made from styrene by polymerization or copolymerization

sty·rol \'stī-ˌròl, -ˌrōl\ n : STYRENE

sub·acro·mi·al \ˌsəb-ə-'krō-mē-əl\ adj : of, relating to, or affecting the subacromial bursa ⟨∼ bursitis⟩

subacromial bursa n : a bursa lying between the acromion and the capsule of the shoulder joint

sub·acute \ˌsəb-ə-'kyüt\ adj **1** : falling between acute and chronic in character esp. when closer to acute ⟨∼ endocarditis⟩ **2** : less marked in severity or duration than a corresponding acute state ⟨∼ pain⟩ — **sub·acute·ly** adv

subacute sclerosing panencephalitis n : a usu. fatal neurological disease of children and young adults that is caused by infection of the brain by a previously latent morbillivirus causing measles and that is marked esp. by behavioral changes, myoclonic seizures, progressive deterioration of motor and mental functioning, and coma — abbr. *SSPE*

sub·aor·tic stenosis \ˌsəb-ā-ˌòrt-ik-\ n : aortic stenosis produced by an obstruction in the left ventricle below the aortic valve

sub·api·cal \ˌsəb-'ā-pi-kəl also -'ap-i-\ adj : situated below or near an apex

sub·apo·neu·rot·ic \ˌsəb-ˌap-ə-n(y)ù-'rät-ik\ adj : lying beneath an aponeurosis

sub·arach·noid \ˌsəb-ə-'rak-ˌnòid\ also **sub·arach·noid·al** \-rak-'nòid-ᵊl\ adj **1** : situated or occurring under the arachnoid membrane ⟨∼ hemorrhage⟩ **2** : of, relating to, or involving the subarachnoid space and the fluid within it ⟨∼ meningitis⟩

subarachnoid space n : the space between the arachnoid and the pia mater through which the cerebrospinal fluid circulates and across which extend delicate trabeculae of connective tissue

sub·at·mo·spher·ic \ˌsəb-ˌat-mə-ˈsfir-ik, -ˈsfer-\ *adj* : less or lower than that of the atmosphere ⟨∼ pressure⟩

sub·atom·ic \ˌsəb-ə-ˈtäm-ik\ *adj* **1** : of or relating to the inside of the atom **2** : of, relating to, or being particles smaller than atoms

sub·cal·lo·sal \ˌsəb-ka-ˈlō-səl\ *adj* : situated below the corpus callosum ⟨the ∼ cortex⟩

subcallosal area *n* : a small area of cortex in each cerebral hemisphere below the genu of the corpus callosum — called also *parolfactory area*

sub·cap·su·lar \ˌsəb-ˈkap-sə-lər\ *adj* : situated or occurring beneath or within a capsule ⟨∼ cataracts⟩

subcarbonate — see BISMUTH SUBCARBONATE

sub·car·ci·no·gen·ic \ˌsəb-ˌkärs-ᵊn-ō-ˈjen-ik\ *adj* : relating to or being a dose of a carcinogen that is smaller than that required to produce or incite cancer

sub·car·di·nal vein \-ˈkärd-nəl-, -ᵊn-əl-\ *n* : a vein in the mammalian embryo or the adult of some lower vertebrates that is located on each side of the abdominal region ventromedial to the mesonephros and that in mammals participates in the formation of the inferior vena cava and the renal vein

sub·cel·lu·lar \ˌsəb-ˈsel-yə-lər\ *adj* **1** : of less than cellular scope or level of organization ⟨∼ organelles⟩ ⟨∼ studies using synaptosomes⟩; *also* : containing or composed of subcellular elements ⟨recovered ∼ fractions by centrifuging homogenized cells⟩ **2** : relating to or being a local or restricted area within a cell ⟨a ∼ site of hormonal activity⟩

sub·chon·dral \-ˈkän-drəl\ *adj* : situated beneath cartilage ⟨∼ bone⟩

sub·cho·roi·dal \ˌsəb-kə-ˈrȯid-ᵊl\ *adj* : situated or occurring between the choroid and the retina ⟨∼ fluid⟩

sub·class \ˈsəb-ˌklas\ *n* : a category in biological classification ranking below a class and above an order

subclavia — see ANSA SUBCLAVIA

¹sub·cla·vi·an \ˌsəb-ˈklā-vē-ən\ *adj* : of, relating to, being, performed on, or inserted into a part (as an artery or vein) located under the clavicle ⟨a ∼ catheter⟩

²subclavian *n* : a subclavian part (as a subclavian artery or vein)

subclavian artery *n* : the proximal part of the main artery of the arm that arises on the right side from the brachiocephalic artery and on the left side from the arch of the aorta, that extends from its point of origin to the outer border of the first rib where it becomes the axillary artery and passes through the axilla and into the arm to become the brachial artery, and that supplies or gives off branches supplying the brain, neck, anterior wall of the thorax, and shoulder

subclavian trunk *n* : a large lymphatic vessel on each side of the body that receives lymph from the axilla and arms and that on the right side empties into the right lymphatic duct and on the left side into the thoracic duct

subclavian vein *n* : the proximal part of the main vein of the arm that is a continuation of the axillary vein and extends from the level of the first rib to the sternal end of the clavicle where it unites with the internal jugular vein to form the brachiocephalic vein

sub·cla·vi·us \ˌsəb-ˈklā-vē-əs\ *n, pl* **-vii** \-vē-ˌī\ : a small muscle on each side of the body that arises from the junction of the first rib and its cartilage, inserts into the inferior surface of the clavicle, and acts to stabilize the clavicle by depressing and drawing forward its lateral end during movements of the shoulder joint

sub·clin·i·cal \-ˈklin-i-kəl\ *adj* : not detectable or producing effects that are not detectable by the usual clinical tests ⟨a ∼ infection⟩ ⟨∼ cancer⟩ — **sub·clin·i·cal·ly** \-k(ə-)lē\ *adv*

sub·clone \ˈsəb-ˌklōn\ *n* : a clone selected from a clone esp. after a mutation occurs ⟨clones and ∼*s* of human-mouse somatic cell hybrids were selected —T. B. Shows *et al*⟩

sub·co·ma \ˌsəb-ˈkō-mə\ *adj* : relating to, used in, or being psychiatric therapy in which insulin is administered in doses too small to produce coma ⟨∼ insulin therapy⟩

sub·com·mis·sur·al organ \ˌsəb-ˌkäm-ə-ˌshùr-əl-\ *n* : an aggregation of columnar cells situated between the posterior commissure and the third ventricle of the brain

sub·con·junc·ti·val \ˌsəb-ˌkän-ˌjəŋ(k)-ˈtī-vəl\ *adj* : situated or occurring beneath the conjunctiva ⟨∼ hemorrhage⟩ — **sub·con·junc·ti·val·ly** \-ē\ *adv*

¹sub·con·scious \ˌsəb-ˈkän-chəs, ˈsəb-\ *adj* **1** : existing in the mind but not immediately available to consciousness : affecting thought, feeling, and behavior without entering awareness ⟨∼ motives⟩ ⟨a ∼ reflex⟩ **2** : imperfectly conscious : partially but not fully aware ⟨the persistence of ∼ dream activity for several minutes after waking —*Psychological Abstracts*⟩ — **sub·con·scious·ly** *adv* — **sub·con·scious·ness** *n*

²subconscious *n* : the mental activities just below the threshold of consciousness; *also* : the aspect of the mind concerned with such activities — compare UNCONSCIOUS

sub·con·vul·sive \ˌsəb-kən-ˈvəl-siv\ *adj* **1** : inadequate to produce convulsions ⟨∼ doses of insulin⟩ **2** : approaching the convulsive in character ⟨a ∼ reaction to noise⟩

sub·cor·a·coid \-ˈkȯr-ə-ˌkȯid, -ˈkȯr-\ *adj* : situated or occurring under the coracoid process of the scapula ⟨a ∼ dislocation of the humerus⟩

sub·cor·tex \ˌsəb-ˈkȯr-ˌteks, ˈsəb-\ *n* : the parts of the brain immediately beneath the cerebral cortex

sub·cor·ti·cal \-ˈkȯrt-i-kəl\ *adj* : of, relating to, involving, or being nerve centers below the cerebral cortex ⟨∼ lesions⟩ ⟨∼ sensation⟩ — **sub·cor·ti·cal·ly** \-i-k(ə-)lē\ *adv*

¹sub·cos·tal \-ˈkäs-təl\ *adj* : situated or performed below a rib ⟨a left ∼ incision⟩

²subcostal *n* : a subcostal part (as a muscle)

subcostal artery *n* : either of a pair of arteries that are the most posterior branches of the thoracic aorta and follow a course beneath the last pair of ribs

sub·cos·ta·lis \ˌsəb-käs-ˈtā-ləs\ *n, pl* **-ta·les** \-ˌlēz\ : any of a variable number of small muscles that arise on the inner surface of a rib, are inserted into the inner surface of the second or third rib below, and prob. function to draw adjacent ribs together

subcostal muscle *n* : SUBCOSTALIS

subcostal vein *n* : either of two veins: **a** : one that arises on the right side of the anterior abdominal wall, follows a course along the lower margin of the twelfth rib, and joins in the formation of the azygos vein — called also *right subcostal vein* **b** : one on the left side of the body that usu. empties into the hemiazygos vein — called also *left subcostal vein*

sub·crep·i·tant \-ˈkrep-ət-ənt\ *adj* : partially crepitant : faintly crepitant ⟨∼ rales⟩

¹sub·cul·ture \ˈsəb-ˌkəl-chər\ *n* **1** : a culture (as of bacteria) derived from another culture **2** : an act or instance of producing a subculture — **sub·cul·tur·al** \-ˈkəlch-(ə-)rəl\ *adj* — **sub·cul·tur·al·ly** \-ē\ *adv*

²subculture *vt* **-tured; -tur·ing** : to culture (as bacteria) anew on a fresh medium by inoculation from an older culture

sub·cu·ra·tive \ˌsəb-ˈkyùr-ət-iv\ *adj* : relating to or being a dose that is too small to produce a cure ⟨∼ amounts of one drug may become curative when given with another⟩

subcutanea — see TELA SUBCUTANEA

sub·cu·ta·ne·ous \ˌsəb-kyù-ˈtā-nē-əs\ *adj* : being, living, used, or made under the skin ⟨∼ parasites⟩ — **sub·cu·ta·ne·ous·ly** *adv*

subcutaneous bursa *n* : a bursa lying between the skin and a bony process (as the olecranon of the elbow) or a ligament

subcutaneous emphysema *n* : the presence of a gas and esp. air in the subcutaneous tissue

sub·cu·tic·u·lar \-kyù-ˈtik-yə-lər\ *adj* : situated or occurring beneath a cuticle ⟨∼ sutures⟩ ⟨∼ tissues⟩

sub·cu·tis \ˌsəb-ˈkyüt-əs, ˈsəb-\ *n* : the deeper part of the dermis

S
T

sub·del·toid \ˌsəb-ˈdel-ˌtȯid\ *adj* : situated underneath or inferior to the deltoid muscle ⟨~ calcareous deposits⟩

subdeltoid bursa *n* : the bursa that lies beneath the deltoid muscle and separates it from the capsule of the shoulder joint

sub·der·mal \-ˈdər-məl\ *adj* : SUBCUTANEOUS ⟨a ~ injection⟩ — **sub·der·mal·ly** \-ē\ *adv*

sub·di·a·phrag·mat·ic \ˌsəb-ˌdī-ə-frə(g)-ˈmat-ik, -ˌfrag-\ *adj* : situated, occurring, or performed below the diaphragm ⟨a ~ vagotomy⟩

sub·di·vi·sion \ˈsəb-də-ˌvi-zhən\ *n* : a category in botanical classification ranking below a division and above a class

sub·du·ral \ˌsəb-ˈd(y)ùr-əl\ *adj* : situated, occurring, or performed under the dura mater or between the dura mater and the arachnoid ⟨~ hematoma⟩ — **sub·du·ral·ly** \-ē\ *adv*

subdural hematoma *n* : a hematoma that occurs between the dura mater and arachnoid in the subdural space and that may apply neurologically significant pressure to the cerebral cortex

subdural space *n* : a fluid-filled space or potential space between the dura mater and the arachnoid

sub·en·do·car·di·al \ˌsəb-ˌen-dō-ˈkärd-ē-əl\ *adj* : situated or occurring beneath the endocardium or between the endocardium and myocardium ⟨~ blood loss⟩

sub·en·do·the·li·al \-ˌen-dō-ˈthē-lē-əl\ *adj* : situated under an endothelium ⟨~ tissues⟩

sub·ep·en·dy·mal \-e-ˈpend-ə-məl\ *adj* : situated under the ependyma ⟨~ lesions⟩

sub·epi·car·di·al \-ˌep-i-ˈkärd-ē-əl\ *adj* : situated or occurring beneath the epicardium or between the epicardium and myocardium ⟨~ hemorrhages⟩

sub·epi·der·mal \ˌsəb-ˌep-ə-ˈdər-məl\ *adj* : lying beneath or constituting the innermost part of the epidermis

sub·epi·the·li·al \-ˌep-ə-ˈthē-lē-əl\ *adj* : situated or occurring beneath an epithelial layer; *also* : SUBCUTANEOUS

su·ber·in \ˈsü-bə-rən\ *n* : a complex fatty substance that is found in the cells of cork

sub·fam·i·ly \ˈsəb-ˌfam-(ə-)lē\ *n* : a category in biological classification ranking below a family and above a genus

sub·fas·cial \-ˈfash-(ē-)əl\ *adj* : situated, occurring, or performed below a fascia ⟨a ~ tumor⟩ ⟨~ suturing⟩

sub·fe·brile \-ˈfeb-ˌrīl *also* -ˈfēb-\ *adj* : of, relating to, or constituting a body temperature very slightly above normal but not febrile ⟨a ~ rise in temperature⟩

sub·fe·cun·di·ty \-fi-ˈkən-dət-ē\ *n, pl* **-ties** : SUBFERTILITY

sub·fer·til·i·ty \-fər-ˈtil-ət-ē\ *n, pl* **-ties** : the condition of being less than normally fertile though still capable of effecting fertilization — **sub·fer·tile** \-ˈfərt-ᵊl\ *adj*

sub·gal·late \-ˈgal-ˌāt\ *n* : a basic gallate ⟨bismuth ~⟩

sub·ge·nus \ˈsəb-ˌjē-nəs\ *n, pl* **-gen·e·ra** \-ˌjen-ər-ə\ : a category in biological classification ranking below a genus and above a species

sub·gin·gi·val \ˌsəb-ˈjin-jə-vəl\ *adj* : situated, performed, or occurring beneath the gums and esp. between the gums and the basal part of the crowns of the teeth ⟨~ calculus⟩ ⟨~ curettage⟩ — **sub·gin·gi·val·ly** \-ē\ *adv*

sub·glot·tic \-ˈglät-ik\ *adj* : situated or occurring below the glottis

sub·he·pat·ic \-hi-ˈpat-ik\ *adj* : situated or occurring under the liver

sub·hu·man \ˌsəb-ˈhyü-mən, ˈsəb-, -ˈyü-\ *adj* : less than human; *esp* : of or relating to an infrahuman taxonomic group ⟨the ~ primates⟩ — **subhuman** *n*

sub·ic·ter·ic \ˌsəb-ik-ˈter-ik\ *adj* : very slightly jaundiced ⟨a ~ tint in the skin⟩

su·bic·u·lar \sə-ˈbik-yə-lər\ *adj* : of, relating to, or constituting the subiculum ⟨~ recording electrodes⟩

su·bic·u·lum \-ləm\ *n, pl* **-la** \-lə\ : a part of the parahippocampal gyrus that is a ventral continuation of the hippocampus and is situated ventrally and medially to the dentate gyrus; *also* : a section of this that borders the hippocampal sulcus

sub·in·ci·sion \ˌsəb-in-ˈsizh-ən\ *n* : a ritual operation performed as a part of puberty rites among some Australasian peoples that involves slitting the underside of the penis with permanent opening of the urethra

sub·in·oc·u·late \-in-ˈäk-yə-ˌlāt\ *vt* **-lat·ed; -lat·ing** : to introduce (infective material) from a laboratory strain into a potential host — **sub·in·oc·u·la·tion** \-in-ˌäk-yə-ˈlā-shən\ *n*

sub·in·tern \-ˈin-ˌtərn\ *n* : a medical student in the last year of medical school who performs work supervised by interns and residents in a hospital

sub·in·ti·mal \-ˈint-ə-məl\ *adj* : situated beneath an intima and esp. between the intima and media of an artery ⟨~ hemorrhages⟩

sub·in·vo·lu·tion \-ˌin-və-ˈlü-shən\ *n* : partial or incomplete involution ⟨~ of the uterus⟩

subitum — see EXANTHEMA SUBITUM

sub·ja·cent \ˌsəb-ˈjās-ᵊnt\ *adj* : lying immediately under or below ⟨~ tissue⟩ ⟨severe bone loss ~ to gingival inflammation⟩

sub·ject \ˈsəb-jikt\ *n* **1** : an individual whose reactions or responses are studied **2** : a dead body for anatomical study and dissection

sub·jec·tive \(ˌ)səb-ˈjek-tiv\ *adj* **1 a** : relating to or determined by the mind as the subject of experience ⟨~ reality⟩ **b** : characteristic of or belonging to reality as perceived rather than as independent of mind **c** : relating to or being experience or knowledge as conditioned by personal mental characteristics or states **2 a** : arising from conditions within the brain or sense organs and not directly caused by external stimuli ⟨~ sensations⟩ **b** : arising out of or identified by means of one's perception of one's own states and processes and not observable by an examiner ⟨a ~ symptom of disease⟩ ⟨caused objective or ~ clinical improvement or both —*Jour. Amer. Med. Assoc.*⟩ — compare OBJECTIVE 2 — **sub·jec·tive·ly** *adv*

subjective vertigo *n* : vertigo characterized by a sensation that one's body is revolving in space — compare OBJECTIVE VERTIGO

sub·jec·tiv·i·ty \ˌsəb-jek-ˈtiv-ət-ē\ *n, pl* **-ties** **1** : subjective character, quality, state, or nature **2** : the personal qualities of an investigator that affect the outcome of scientific or medical research (as by unconsciously communicating a bias to the subject of the experiment)

sub·king·dom \ˈsəb-ˌkiŋ-dəm\ *n* : a category in biological classification ranking below a kingdom and above a phylum

sub·le·thal \ˌsəb-ˈlē-thəl, ˈsəb-\ *adj* : less than but usu. only slightly less than lethal ⟨a ~ dose⟩ — **sub·le·thal·ly** \-thə-lē\ *adv*

sub·leu·ke·mic *or chiefly Brit* **sub·leu·kae·mic** \-lü-ˈkē-mik\ *adj* : not marked by the presence of excessive numbers of white blood cells in the circulating blood ⟨~ leukemia⟩

¹sub·li·mate \ˈsəb-lə-ˌmāt, -mət\ *n* **1** : MERCURIC CHLORIDE **2** : a chemical product obtained by sublimation

²sub·li·mate \ˈsəb-lə-ˌmāt\ *vt* **-mat·ed; -mat·ing** **1** : SUBLIME **2** : to divert the expression of (an instinctual desire or impulse) from its unacceptable form to one that is considered more socially or culturally acceptable

sub·li·ma·tion \ˌsəb-lə-ˈmā-shən\ *n* **1** : the act, process, or an instance of subliming a chemical **2** : the process of converting and expressing a primitive instinctual desire or impulse to a form that is socially or culturally acceptable

sub·lime \sə-ˈblīm\ *vb* **sub·limed; sub·lim·ing** *vt* : to cause to pass from the solid to the vapor state by heating and to condense back to solid form ~ *vi* : to pass directly from the solid to the vapor state

sub·lim·i·nal \(ˌ)səb-ˈlim-ən-ᵊl, ˈsəb-\ *adj* **1** : inadequate to produce a sensation or a perception **2** : existing or functioning below the threshold of consciousness ⟨the ~ mind⟩ ⟨~ advertising⟩ — **sub·lim·i·nal·ly** \-ē\ *adv*

subliminal self *n* : the portion of an individual's personality that lies below or beyond the reach of his or her personal awareness

sub·line \ˈsəb-ˌlīn\ *n* : an inbred or selectively cultured line (as of cells) within a strain

¹sub·lin·gual \ˌsəb-ˈliŋ-g(yə-)wəl, ˈsəb-\ *adj* **1** : situated or administered under the tongue ⟨∼ tablets⟩ **2** : of or relating to the sublingual glands — **sub·lin·gual·ly** \-ē\ *adv*

²**sublingual** *n* : SUBLINGUAL GLAND

sublingual gland *n* : a small salivary gland on each side of the mouth lying beneath the mucous membrane in a fossa in the mandible near the symphysis — called also *sublingual salivary gland*

sublingualis — see PLICA SUBLINGUALIS

sub·lob·u·lar \-ˈläb-yə-lər\ *adj* : situated at the bases of the lobules of the liver

sublobular vein *n* : one of several veins in the liver into which the central veins empty and which in turn empty into the hepatic veins

sub·lux·at·ed \-ˈlək-ˌsāt-əd\ *adj* : partially dislocated ⟨a ∼ vertebra⟩

sub·lux·a·tion \ˌsəb-ˌlək-ˈsā-shən\ *n* : partial dislocation (as of one of the bones in a joint)

¹**sub·man·dib·u·lar** \ˌsəb-man-ˈdib-yə-lər\ *adj* **1** : of, relating to, situated, or performed in the region below the lower jaw ⟨a ∼ lymph node⟩ **2** : of, relating to, or associated with the submandibular glands

²**submandibular** *n* : a submandibular part (as an artery or bone)

submandibular ganglion *n* : an autonomic ganglion that is situated on the hyoglossus muscle above the deep part of the submandibular gland, receives preganglionic fibers from the facial nerve by way of the chorda tympani, and sends postganglionic fibers to the submandibular and sublingual glands — called also *submaxillary ganglion*

submandibular gland *n* : a salivary gland inside of and near the lower edge of the mandible on each side and discharging by Wharton's duct into the mouth under the tongue — called also *mandibular gland, submandibular salivary gland, submaxillary gland, submaxillary salivary gland*

sub·mar·gin·al \ˌsəb-ˈmärj-nəl, ˈsəb-, -ən-ᵊl\ *adj* **1** : adjacent to a margin or a marginal part or structure ⟨∼ areas of the gingiva⟩ **2** : falling below a necessary minimum ⟨∼ diets⟩

¹**sub·max·il·lary** \ˌsəb-ˈmak-sə-ˌler-ē, ˈsəb-, *chiefly Brit* ˌsəb-mak-ˈsil-ə-rē\ *adj* : SUBMANDIBULAR

²**submaxillary** *n, pl* **-lar·ies** : SUBMANDIBULAR

submaxillary ganglion *n* : SUBMANDIBULAR GANGLION

submaxillary gland *n* : SUBMANDIBULAR GLAND

submaxillary salivary gland *n* : SUBMANDIBULAR GLAND

sub·max·i·mal \ˌsəb-ˈmak-s(ə-)məl\ *adj* : being less than the maximum of which an individual is capable ⟨∼ exercise⟩

sub·men·tal \-ˈment-ᵊl\ *adj* : located in, affecting, or performed on the area under the chin

submental artery *n* : a branch of the facial artery that branches off near the submandibular gland and is distributed to the muscles of the jaw

¹**sub·meta·cen·tric** \ˌsəb-ˌmet-ə-ˈsen-trik\ *adj* : having the centromere situated so that one chromosome arm is somewhat shorter than the other

²**submetacentric** *n* : a submetacentric chromosome

sub·mi·cron \-ˈmī-ˌkrän\ *adj* **1** : being less than a micron in a (specified) measurement and esp. in diameter ⟨a ∼ particle⟩ **2** : having or consisting of submicron particles ⟨∼ aerosols⟩

sub·mi·cro·scop·ic \ˌsəb-ˌmī-krə-ˈskäp-ik\ *adj* : too small to be seen in an ordinary light microscope ⟨∼ particles⟩ ⟨∼ organization of a bacterium⟩ — compare MACROSCOPIC, MICROSCOPIC 2, ULTRAMICROSCOPIC 1 — **sub·mi·cro·scop·i·cal·ly** \-i-k(ə-)lē\ *adv*

sub·min·i·mal \-ˈmin-ə-məl\ *adj* : smaller than the minimum that is required for a particular result ⟨a ∼ stimulus⟩

sub·mis·sion \səb-ˈmish-ən\ *n* : the condition of being submissive

sub·mis·sive \səb-ˈmis-iv\ *adj* : characterized by tendencies to yield to the will or authority of others ⟨bullying usually involves a stronger, more dominant personality coercing a weaker, more ∼ personality —S. W. Twemlow *et al*⟩ — **sub·mis·sive·ness** *n*

sub·mi·to·chon·dri·al \ˌsəb-ˌmīt-ə-ˈkän-drē-əl\ *adj* : relating to, composed of, or being parts and esp. fragments of mitochondria ⟨∼ membranes⟩ ⟨∼ particles⟩

sub·mu·co·sa \ˌsəb-myü-ˈkō-sə\ *n* : a supporting layer of loose connective tissue directly under a mucous membrane — called also *tela submucosa* — **sub·mu·co·sal** \-zəl\ *adj* — **sub·mu·co·sal·ly** \-zə-lē\ *adv*

sub·mu·cous \ˌsəb-ˈmyü-kəs, ˈsəb-\ *adj* : lying under or involving the tissues under a mucous membrane ⟨∼ layers⟩ ⟨a ∼ resection⟩ — **sub·mu·cous·ly** *adv*

sub·nar·co·tic \-när-ˈkät-ik\ *adj* : somewhat narcotic; *esp* : insufficient to produce deep sleep ⟨barbiturates in ∼ amounts⟩

sub·na·sale \ˌsəb-nā-ˈzā-lē\ *n* : a point on the living body where the nasal septum and the upper lip meet in the midsagittal plane

sub·ni·trate \-ˈnī-ˌtrāt\ *n* : a basic nitrate — see BISMUTH SUBNITRATE

sub·nor·mal \ˌsəb-ˈnȯr-məl\ *adj* **1** : lower or smaller than normal ⟨a ∼ temperature⟩ **2** : having less of something and esp. of intelligence than is normal — **sub·nor·mal·i·ty** \ˌsəb-nȯr-ˈmal-ət-ē\ *n, pl* **-ties**

sub·nu·tri·tion \-n(y)ü-ˈtrish-ən\ *n* : inadequate nutrition

sub·oc·cip·i·tal \-äk-ˈsip-ət-ᵊl\ *adj* **1** : situated or performed below the occipital bone **2** : situated or performed below the occipital lobe of the brain

suboccipital nerve *n* : the first cervical nerve that supplies muscles around the suboccipital triangle including the rectus capitis posterior major, obliquus capitis superior, and obliquus capitis inferior and that sends branches to the rectus capitis posterior minor and semispinalis capitis

suboccipital triangle *n* : a space of the suboccipital region on each side of the dorsal cervical region that is bounded superiorly and medially by a muscle arising by a tendon from a spinous process of the axis and inserting into the inferior nuchal line and the adjacent inferior region of the occipital bone, that is bounded superiorly and laterally by the obliquus capitis superior, and that is bounded inferiorly and laterally by the obliquus capitis inferior

sub·op·ti·mal \ˌsəb-ˈäp-tə-məl\ *adj* : less than optimal ⟨a ∼ diet⟩ ⟨a ∼ dose of a drug⟩

sub·op·ti·mum \-məm\ *adj* : SUBOPTIMAL

sub·or·bit·al \ˌsəb-ˈȯr-bət-ᵊl\ *adj* : situated or occurring beneath the eye or the orbit of the eye ⟨∼ fat⟩

sub·or·der \ˈsəb-ˌȯrd-ər\ *n* : a category in biological classification ranking below an order and above a family

sub·ox·ide \ˌsəb-ˈäk-ˌsīd\ *n* : an oxide containing a relatively small proportion of oxygen

sub·peri·os·te·al \-ˌper-ē-ˈäs-tē-əl\ *adj* : situated or occurring beneath the periosteum ⟨∼ bone deposition⟩ ⟨a ∼ fibroma⟩ — **sub·peri·os·te·al·ly** \-ē\ *adv*

sub·phren·ic \ˌsəb-ˈfren-ik\ *adj* : situated or occurring below the diaphragm ⟨a ∼ abscess⟩

subphrenic space *n* : a space on each side of the falciform ligament between the underside of the diaphragm and the upper side of the liver

sub·phy·lum \ˈsəb-ˌfī-ləm\ *n, pl* **-la** \-lə\ : a category in biological classification ranking below a phylum and above a class

sub·pi·al \-ˈpī-əl, -ˈpē-\ *adj* : situated or occurring beneath the pia mater ⟨∼ tissue⟩

sub·platy·hi·er·ic \ˌsəb-ˌplat-i-hī-ˈer-ik\ *adj* : having a sacrum of moderate length and breadth with a cranial index of 100 to 105.9 — compare DOLICHOHIERIC, PLATYHIERIC

sub·pleu·ral \-ˈplu̇r-əl\ *adj* : situated or occurring between the pleura and the body wall — **sub·pleu·ral·ly** \-ē\ *adv*

sub·pop·u·la·tion \ˈsəb-ˌpäp-yə-ˈlā-shən\ *n* : an identifiable fraction or subdivision of a population

sub·po·tent \ˌsəb-ˈpōt-ᵊnt-, ˈsəb-\ *adj* : less potent than normal ⟨∼ drugs⟩ — **sub·po·ten·cy** \-ˈpōt-ᵊn-sē\ *n, pl* **-cies**

\ə\ abut \ᵊ\ kitten \ər\ further \a\ ash \ā\ ace \ä\ cot, cart \au̇\ out \ch\ chin \e\ bet \ē\ easy \g\ go \i\ hit \ī\ ice \j\ job \ŋ\ sing \ō\ go \ȯ\ law \ȯi\ boy \th\ thin \t͟h\ the \ü\ loot \u̇\ foot \y\ yet \zh\ vision *See also* Pronunciation Symbols page

S
T

sub·pu·bic angle \ˌsəb-'pyü-bik-\ *n* : the angle that is formed just below the pubic symphysis by the meeting of the inferior or ramus of the pubis on one side with the corresponding part on the other side and that is usu. less than 90° in the male and usu. more than 90° in the female

sub·rect·an·gu·lar \-rek-'taŋ-gyə-lər\ *adj* : approximately rectangular ⟨∼ cells⟩

sub·ret·i·nal \-'ret-ᵊn-əl\ *adj* : situated or occurring beneath the retina ⟨∼ fluid⟩

sub·sa·lic·y·late \-sə-'lis-ə-ˌlāt\ *n* : a basic salicylate (as bismuth subsalicylate)

sub·sar·co·lem·mal \-ˌsär-kə-'lem-əl\ *adj* : situated or occurring beneath a sarcolemma ⟨∼ mitochondria⟩

sub·scap·u·lar \ˌsəb-'skap-yə-lər\ *adj* : situated under the scapula; *esp* : of or relating to the ventral or in humans the anterior surface of the scapula

subscapular artery *n* : an artery that is usu. the largest branch of the axillary artery, that arises opposite the lower border of the subscapularis muscle, and that passes down and back to the lower part of the scapula where it forms branches and anastomoses with arteries in that region

subscapular fascia *n* : a thin sheet of fascia fixed to the circumference of the subscapular fossa

subscapular fossa *n* : the concave depression of the anterior surface of the scapula

sub·scap·u·lar·is \ˌsəb-ˌskap-yə-'lar-əs\ *n* : a large triangular muscle that fills up the subscapular fossa, that arises from the surface of the scapula, that is inserted into the lesser tubercle of the humerus, and that stabilizes the shoulder joint as part of the rotator cuff and rotates the humerus medially when the arm is held by the side of the body

sub·scrip·tion \səb-'skrip-shən\ *n* : a part of a prescription that contains directions to the pharmacist

sub·se·ro·sa \ˌsəb-sə-'rō-zə\ *n* : subserous tissue

sub·se·rous \ˌsəb-'sir-əs\ *or* **sub·se·ro·sal** \-sə-'rō-zəl\ *adj* : situated or occurring under a serous membrane ⟨a ∼ uterine fibroid⟩ ⟨∼ fat⟩

sub·side \səb-'sīd\ *vi* **sub·sid·ed; sub·sid·ing** : to lessen in severity : become diminished ⟨the fever *subsided*⟩ — **sub·si·dence** \səb-'sīd-ᵊn(t)s, 'səb-səd-ən(t)s\ *n*

sub·specialist \ˌsəb-'spesh-(ə-)ləst\ *n* : a physician having a subspecialty

sub·spe·cial·ty \ˌsəb-'spesh-əl-tē, 'səb-ˌ\ *n, pl* **-ties** : a subordinate field of specialization ⟨child psychiatry is a ∼ of general psychiatry —Bruno Bettelheim *et al*⟩

sub·spe·cies \'səb-ˌspē-shēz, -sēz\ *n* : a subdivision of a species: as **a** : a category in biological classification that ranks immediately below a species and designates a population of a particular geographical region genetically distinguishable from other such populations of the same species and capable of interbreeding successfully with them where its range overlaps theirs **b** : a named subdivision (as a race or variety) of a species — **sub·spe·cif·ic** \ˌsəb-spi-'sif-ik\ *adj*

sub·stage \'səb-ˌstāj\ *n* : an attachment to a microscope by means of which accessories (as mirrors, diaphragms, or condensers) are held in place beneath the stage of the instrument

sub·stance \'səb-stən(t)s\ *n* **1** : physical material from which something is made or which has discrete existence ⟨the ∼ of nerve tissue⟩ **2** : matter of particular or definite chemical constitution **3** : something (as alcohol, methamphetamine, or marijuana) deemed harmful and usu. subject to legal restriction ⟨heroin is a controlled ∼⟩ ⟨∼ abuse⟩

substance P *n* : a neuropeptide that consists of 11 amino acid residues, that is widely distributed in the brain, spinal cord, and peripheral nervous system, and that acts across nerve synapses to produce prolonged postsynaptic excitation

sub·stan·tia \səb-'stan-ch(ē-)ə\ *n, pl* **-ti·ae** \-chē-ˌē\ : anatomical material, substance, or tissue

substantia gel·a·ti·no·sa \-ˌjel-ət-ᵊn-'ō-sə\ *n* : a mass of gelatinous gray matter that lies on the dorsal surface of the dorsal column and extends the entire length of the spinal cord into the medulla oblongata and that functions in the transmission of painful sensory information

substantia in·nom·i·na·ta \-i(n)-ˌnäm-ə-'nāt-ə\ *n* : a band of large cells of indeterminate function that lie just under the surface of the globus pallidus

sub·stan·tia ni·gra \səb-ˌstan-chē-ə-'nī-grə, -'nig-rə\ *n, pl* **sub·stan·ti·ae ni·grae** \-chē-ˌē-'nī-(ˌ)grē, -'nig-(ˌ)rē\ : a layer of deeply pigmented gray matter situated in the midbrain and containing the cell bodies of a tract of dopamine-producing nerve cells whose secretion tends to be deficient in Parkinson's disease

substantia pro·pria \-'prō-prē-ə\ *n, pl* **substantiae pro·pri·ae** \-prē-ˌē\ : the layer of lamellated transparent fibrous connective tissue that makes up the bulk of the cornea of the eye

sub·ster·nal \ˌsəb-'stər-nəl\ *adj* : situated or perceived behind or below the sternum ⟨∼ pain⟩

sub·stit·u·ent \səb-'stich-(ə-)wənt\ *n* : an atom or group that replaces another atom or group in a molecule — **substituent** *adj*

¹**sub·sti·tute** \'səb-stə-ˌt(y)üt\ *n* : a person or thing that takes the place or function of another ⟨father and mother ∼s⟩ — **substitute** *adj*

²**substitute** *vt* **-tut·ed; -tut·ing** : to put or use in the place of another: as **a** : to introduce (an atom or group) as a substituent **b** : to alter (as a compound) by introduction of a substituent

sub·sti·tu·tion \ˌsəb-stə-'t(y)ü-shən\ *n* **1** : a chemical reaction in which one or more atoms or groups in a molecule are replaced by equivalent atoms or groups to form at least two products; *esp* : the replacement of hydrogen in an organic compound by another element or group **2 a** : the turning from an obstructed desire to another desire whose gratification is socially acceptable **b** : the turning from an obstructed form of behavior to a different and often more primitive expression of the same tendency ⟨a ∼ neurosis⟩ **c** : the reacting to each of a set of stimuli by a response prescribed in a key ⟨a ∼ test for speed of learning new responses⟩

sub·sti·tu·tive \'səb-stə-ˌt(y)üt-iv\ *adj* : serving or suitable as a substitute ⟨∼ behavior⟩ — **sub·sti·tu·tive·ly** *adv*

sub·strate \'səb-ˌstrāt\ *n* **1** : SUBSTRATUM 1 **2** : the base on which an organism lives **3** : a substance acted upon (as by an enzyme)

sub·stra·tum \'səb-ˌstrāt-əm, -ˌstrat-, 'səb-'\ *n, pl* **-stra·ta** \-ə\ **1** : the material of which something is made and from which it derives its special qualities **2** : SUBSTRATE 2

sub·struc·ture \'səb-ˌstrək-chər\ *n* : an underlying or supporting structure — **sub·struc·tur·al** \-chə-rəl, -shrəl\ *adj*

sub·syn·dro·mal \ˌsəb-sin-'drō-məl\ *adj* : characterized by or exhibiting symptoms that are not severe enough for diagnosis as a clinically recognized syndrome ⟨∼ seasonal affective disorder⟩ ⟨a ∼ patient⟩

sub·ta·lar \ˌsəb-'tā-lər\ *adj* : situated or occurring beneath the talus; *specif* : of, relating to, or being the articulation formed between the posterior facet of the inferior surface of the talus and the posterior facet of the superior surface of the calcaneus ⟨the ∼ joint⟩ ⟨∼ arthrodesis⟩

sub·tem·po·ral decompression \ˌsəb-'tem-p(ə-)rəl-\ *n* : relief of intracranial pressure by excision of a portion of the temporal bone

sub·ter·tian malaria \-'tər-shən-\ *n* : FALCIPARUM MALARIA

sub·te·tan·ic \ˌsəb-te-'tan-ik\ *adj* : approaching tetany or tetanus esp. in form or degree of contraction ⟨∼ contractions of the duodenum⟩ ⟨a ∼ convulsion⟩

sub·tha·lam·ic \ˌsəb-thə-'lam-ik\ *adj* : of or relating to the subthalamus

subthalamic nucleus *n* : an oval mass of gray matter that is located in the caudal part of the subthalamus along the medial part of the internal capsule, receives fibers from the lateral part of the globus pallidus, sends fibers through the internal capsule to the medial part of the globus pallidus, and when affected with lesions is associated with hemiballismus of the contralateral side of the body

sub·thal·a·mus \ˌsəb-'thal-ə-məs\ *n, pl* **-mi** \-ˌmī\ : the ventral part of the thalamus

sub·ther·a·peu·tic \-,ther-ə-'pyüt-ik\ *adj* : not producing a therapeutic effect ⟨∼ doses of penicillin⟩

sub·thresh·old \,səb-'thresh-,(h)ōld, 'səb-\ *adj* : inadequate to produce a response ⟨∼ dosages⟩ ⟨a ∼ stimulus⟩

sub·ti·lin \'səb-tə-lən\ *n* : a polypeptide antibiotic or mixture of antibiotics that is similar to bacitracin and is produced by a soil bacterium of the genus *Bacillus* (*B. subtilis*)

sub·til·i·sin \,səb-'til-ə-sən\ *n* : an extracellular protease that is secreted by a soil bacterium of the genus *Bacillus* (*B. amyloliquefaciens*) and has various commercial uses (as in laundry detergents)

sub·to·tal \,səb-'tōt-ᵊl\ *adj* : somewhat less than complete : nearly total ⟨∼ thyroidectomy⟩ — **sub·to·tal·ly** \-ᵊl-ē\ *adv*

sub·tro·chan·ter·ic \,səb-,trō-kən-'ter-ik, -,kan-\ *adj* : situated or occurring below a trochanter

¹sub·type \'səb-,tīp\ *n* : a type that is subordinate to or included in another type ⟨the blood group ∼s⟩ ⟨∼s of a disease⟩

²subtype *vt* **sub·typed; sub·typ·ing** : to classify according to subtype ⟨schizophrenic patients *subtyped* as paranoid or catatonic⟩

sub·un·gual \,səb-'əŋ-gwəl, -'ən-\ *adj* : situated or occurring under a fingernail or toenail ⟨a ∼ abscess⟩

sub·unit \'səb-,yü-nət\ *n* : a unit that forms a discrete part of a more comprehensive unit ⟨∼s of a protein⟩

sub·val·vu·lar \,səb-'val-vyə-lər\ *adj* : situated or occurring below a valve (as a semilunar valve) ⟨∼ stenosis⟩

sub·vi·ral \,səb-'vī-rəl\ *adj* : relating to, being, or caused by a piece or a structural part (as a protein) of a virus ⟨∼ infection⟩

sub·vo·cal \-'vō-kəl\ *adj* : characterized by the occurrence in the mind of words in speech order with or without inaudible articulation of the speech organs — **sub·vo·cal·ly** \-kə-lē\ *adv*

sub·vo·cal·iza·tion *also Brit* **sub·vo·cal·isa·tion** \-,vō-kə-lə-'zā-shən\ *n* : the act or process of inaudibly articulating speech with speech organs — **sub·vo·cal·ize** *also Brit* **sub·vo·cal·ise** \-'vō-kə-,līz\ *vb* **-ized** *also Brit* **-ised; -iz·ing** *also Brit* **-is·ing**

sub·xi·phoid \,səb-'zī-,fòid, -'zif-,òid\ *adj* : situated, occurring, or performed below the xiphoid process ⟨a ∼ incision⟩

suc·ce·da·ne·ous tooth \,sək-sə-'dā-nē-əs-\ *n* : SUCCESSIONAL TOOTH

succedaneum — see CAPUT SUCCEDANEUM

suc·cen·tu·ri·ate \,sək-,sen-'t(y)ur-ē-ət\ *adj* : ACCESSORY 1b ⟨a ∼ lobe of a placenta⟩

suc·ces·sion·al tooth \sək-'sesh-nəl-, -ən-ᵊl-\ *n* : any permanent tooth that grows in the place of a milk tooth — called also *succedaneous tooth*

suc·ci·nate \'sək-sə-,nāt\ *n* : a salt or ester of succinic acid

succinate dehydrogenase *n* : an iron-containing flavoprotein enzyme that catalyzes often reversibly the dehydrogenation of succinic acid to fumaric acid in the presence of a hydrogen acceptor and that is widely distributed esp. in animal tissues, bacteria, and yeast — called also *succinic dehydrogenase*

suc·cin·ic acid \(,)sək-'sin-ik-\ *n* : a crystalline dicarboxylic acid $C_4H_6O_4$ that is found widely in nature, that is formed in the Krebs cycle and in various fermentation processes, and that is used chiefly as an intermediate in synthesis (as of pharmaceuticals and synthetic resins)

succinic dehydrogenase *n* : SUCCINATE DEHYDROGENASE

suc·cin·i·mide \,sək-sin-'im-əd; sək-'sin-ə-,mīd, -məd\ *n* : a crystalline cyclic imide $C_4H_5NO_2$ obtained from succinic acid or succinic anhydride

suc·cin·ox·i·dase \,sək-sən-'äk-sə-,dās, -,dāz\ *n* : the entire complex system containing succinate dehydrogenase and cytochromes that catalyzes the reaction between a succinate ion and molecular oxygen with the formation of a fumarate ion

suc·ci·nyl \'sək-sən-ᵊl, -sə-,nil\ *n* : either of two groups of succinic acid: **a** : a bivalent group $OCCH_2CH_2CO$ **b** : a monovalent group $HOOCCH_2CH_2CO$

suc·ci·nyl·cho·line \,sək-sən-ᵊl-'kō-,lēn, -sə-,nil-\ *n* : a basic compound that acts similarly to curare and is used intrave-

nously chiefly in the form of its chloride salt $C_{14}H_{30}Cl_2N_2O_4$ as a short-acting relaxant of skeletal muscle in surgery — called also *suxamethonium;* see ANECTINE

suc·ci·nyl·sul·fa·thi·a·zole *or chiefly Brit* **suc·ci·nyl·sul·pha·thi·a·zole** \,sək-sən-ᵊl-,səl-fə-'thī-ə-,zōl, -sə-,nil-\ *n* : a crystalline sulfa drug $C_{13}H_{13}N_3O_5S_2$ used esp. for treating gastrointestinal infections

suc·cu·bus \'sək-yə-bəs\ *n, pl* **-bi** \-,bī, -,bē\ : an imaginary demon assuming female form and formerly held to have sexual intercourse with men in their sleep — compare INCUBUS 1

suc·cus en·ter·i·cus \,sək-əs-en-'ter-i-kəs\ *n* : INTESTINAL JUICE

suc·cus·sion \sə-'kəsh-ən\ *n* : the action or process of shaking or the condition of being shaken esp. with violence: **a** : a shaking of the body to ascertain if fluid is present in a cavity and esp. in the thorax **b** : the splashing sound made by succussion

suck \'sək\ *vt* **1** : to draw (as liquid) into the mouth through a suction force produced by movements of the lips and tongue ⟨∼ed milk from her mother's breast⟩ **2** : to draw out by suction ∼ *vi* : to draw something in by or as if by exerting a suction force; *esp* : to draw milk from a breast or udder with the mouth

suck·er \'sək-ər\ *n* **1** : an organ in various animals (as a trematode or tapeworm) used for adhering or holding **2** : a mouth (as of a leech) adapted for sucking or adhering

sucking louse *n* : any of an order (Anoplura) of wingless insects comprising the true lice with mouthparts adapted for sucking body fluids

sucking wound *n* : a perforating wound of the chest through which air enters and leaves during respiration

suck·le \'sək-əl\ *vt* **suck·led; suck·ling** \-(ə-)liŋ\ **1** : to give milk to from the breast or udder ⟨a mother *suckling* her child⟩ **2** : to draw milk from the breast or udder of

su·cral·fate \sü-'kral-,fāt\ *n* : an aluminum complex $C_{12}H_mAl_{16}O_nS_8$ where *m* and *n* are approximately 54 and 75 that is used in the treatment of duodenal ulcers — see CARAFATE

su·cra·lose \'sü-krə-,lōs\ *n* : a white crystalline powder $C_{12}H_{19}Cl_3O_8$ that is derived from sucrose by the chemical substitution of three chlorine atoms for three hydroxyl groups and that is used as a low-calorie sweetener having a sweetness of much greater intensity than sucrose

su·crase \'sü-,krās, -,krāz\ *n* : INVERTASE

su·crate \'sü-,krāt\ *n* : a metallic derivative of sucrose

su·crose \'sü-,krōs, -,krōz\ *n* : a sweet crystalline dextrorotatory nonreducing disaccharide sugar $C_{12}H_{22}O_{11}$ that occurs naturally in most plants and is obtained commercially esp. from sugarcane or sugar beets

¹suc·tion \'sək-shən\ *n* **1** : the act or process of sucking **2 a** : the act or process of exerting a force upon a solid, liquid, or gaseous body by reason of reduced air pressure over part of its surface **b** : force so exerted **3** : the act or process of removing secretions or fluids from hollow or tubular organs or cavities by means of a tube and a device (as a suction pump) that operates on negative pressure

²suction *vt* : to remove from a body cavity or passage by suction

suction cup *n* : a cup of glass or of a flexible material (as rubber) in which a partial vacuum is produced when applied to a surface and which is used variously (as to bring blood to the surface of the skin)

suction lipectomy *n* : LIPOSUCTION

suction pump *n* : a common pump in which the liquid to be raised is pushed by atmospheric pressure into the partial vacuum under a retreating valved piston on the upstroke and reflux is prevented by a valve in the pipe that permits flow in only one direction — see STOMACH PUMP

S
T

\ə\ abut \ᵊ\ kitten \ər\ further \a\ ash \ā\ ace \ä\ cot, cart \aù\ out \ch\ chin \e\ bet \ē\ easy \g\ go \i\ hit \ī\ ice \j\ job \ŋ\ sing \ō\ go \ò\ law \òi\ boy \th\ thin \th\ the \ü\ loot \ù\ foot \y\ yet \zh\ vision *See also* Pronunciation Symbols page

suction socket *n* : a socket on an artificial leg that is held to the stump by the suction of negative pressure maintained within the socket

Suc·to·ria \ˌsək-ˈtōr-ē-ə\ *n pl* : a class of complex protozoans (subphylum Ciliophora) which in the mature form are fixed to the substrate, lack locomotor organelles or a mouth, and obtain food through specialized suctorial tentacles

suc·to·ri·an \-ē-ən\ *n* : any protozoan of the class Suctoria

su·dam·i·na \sü-ˈdam-ə-nə\ *n pl* : a transient eruption of minute translucent vesicles caused by retention of sweat in the sweat glands and in the corneous layer of the skin and occurring after profuse perspiration — called also *miliaria crystallina*

su·dam·i·nal \sü-ˈdam-ən-ᵊl\ *adj* : of or relating to sudamina ⟨∼ eruptions⟩

Su·dan \sü-ˈdan\ *n* : any of several azo solvent dyes including some which have a specific affinity for fatty substances and are used as biological stains

Sudan IV \-ˈfō(ə)r\ *n* : a red disazo solvent dye used chiefly as a biological stain and in ointments for promoting the growth of epithelium (as in the treatment of burns, wounds, or ulcers) — called also *scarlet red*

su·dan·o·phil·ia \sü-ˌdan-ə-ˈfil-ē-ə\ *n* : the quality or state of being sudanophilic

su·dan·o·phil·ic \ˌsü-ˌdan-ə-ˈfil-ik\ *also* **su·dan·o·phil** \sü-ˈdan-ə-ˌfil\ *adj* : staining selectively with Sudan dyes; *also* : containing lipids

su·da·tion \sü-ˈdā-shən\ *n* : the action or process of sweating

sud·den cardiac arrest \ˈsəd-ᵊn-\ *n* : CARDIAC ARREST

sudden cardiac death *n* : death occurring within minutes or hours following onset of acute symptoms of cardiac arrest resulting esp. from an arrhythmia

sudden death *n* : unexpected death that is instantaneous or occurs within minutes or hours from any cause other than violence ⟨*sudden death* following coronary occlusion⟩; *esp* : SUDDEN CARDIAC DEATH

sudden infant death syndrome *n* : death of an apparently healthy infant usu. before one year of age that is of unknown cause and occurs esp. during sleep — abbr. *SIDS;* called also *cot death, crib death*

su·do·mo·tor \ˈsüd-ə-ˌmōt-ər\ *adj* : of, relating to, or being nerve fibers controlling the activity of sweat glands ⟨∼ activity⟩

su·do·rif·er·ous gland \ˌsüd-ə-ˈrif-(ə-)rəs-\ *n* : SWEAT GLAND

¹**su·do·rif·ic** \-ˈrif-ik\ *adj* : causing or inducing sweat : DIAPHORETIC 1 ⟨∼ herbs⟩

²**sudorific** *n* : a sudorific agent or medicine

su·do·rip·a·rous gland \ˌsüd-ə-ˈrip-ə-rəs-\ *n* : SWEAT GLAND

su·et \ˈsü-ət\ *n* : the hard fat about the kidneys and loins in beef and mutton that yields tallow and that in prepared form is used in some pharmaceutical ointments

su·fen·ta·nil \sü-ˈfen-tə-ˌnil\ *n* : an opioid analgesic that is administered intravenously in the form of its citrate $C_{22}H_{30}N_2O_2S \cdot C_6H_8O_7$ as an anesthetic or an anesthetic adjuvant

suf·fo·cate \ˈsəf-ə-ˌkāt\ *vb* **-cat·ed; -cat·ing** *vt* **1** : to stop the respiration of (as by strangling or asphyxiation) **2** : to deprive of oxygen ∼ *vi* : to die from being unable to breathe — **suf·fo·ca·tive** \-ˌkāt-iv\ *adj*

suf·fo·ca·tion \ˌsəf-ə-ˈkā-shən\ *n* : the act of suffocating or state of being suffocated : stoppage of breathing — compare ASPHYXIA

suf·frag·i·nis \sə-ˈfraj-ə-nəs\ *n* : the long bone of the pastern that is a common site of fracture in racehorses

suf·fuse \sə-ˈfyüz\ *vt* **suf·fused; suf·fus·ing** : to flush or spread over or through in the manner of a fluid and esp. blood

suf·fu·sion \sə-ˈfyü-zhən\ *n* **1** : the act or process of suffusing or state of being suffused with something; *specif* : the spreading of a fluid of the body into the surrounding tissues ⟨a ∼ of blood⟩ **2** : a coloring spread over a surface (as the face)

sug·ar \ˈshüg-ər\ *n* **1** : a sweet crystallizable substance that consists chiefly of sucrose, is colorless or white when pure and tending to brown when less refined, is obtained commercially from sugarcane or sugar beet and less extensively from sorghum, maples, and palms, and is important as a source of dietary carbohydrate and as a sweetener and preservative for other foods and for drugs and in the chemical industry as an intermediate **2** : any of various water-soluble compounds that vary widely in sweetness and comprise the oligosaccharides including sucrose

sugar diabetes *n* : DIABETES MELLITUS

sugar of lead *n* : LEAD ACETATE

sugar pill *n* : a pharmacologically inert pill : PLACEBO

sug·gest·ibil·i·ty \sə(g)-ˌjes-tə-ˈbil-ət-ē\ *n, pl* **-ties** : the quality or state of being suggestible : susceptibility to suggestion

sug·gest·ible \sə(g)-ˈjes-tə-bəl\ *adj* : easily influenced by suggestion ⟨a ∼ hypnotic subject⟩

sug·ges·tion \sə(g)-ˈjes-chən, -ˈjesh-\ *n* **1 a** : the act or process of impressing something (as an idea, attitude, or desired action) upon the mind of another ⟨∼ in response to propaganda —*Psychological Abstracts*⟩ **b** : the process by which a physical or mental state is influenced by a thought or idea ⟨the power of ∼⟩ **2** : something impressed upon the mind by suggestion ⟨the posthypnotic carrying out of ∼s held in the unconscious —G. S. Blum⟩

sug·ges·tive \sə(g)-ˈjes-tiv\ *adj* **1** : serving to indicate ⟨a butterfly-shaped red rash . . . is highly ∼ of the disease —S. E. Goldfinger *et al*⟩ **2** : tending to act like or have the effect of suggestion

sug·gil·la·tion \ˌsə(g)-jə-ˈlā-shən\ *n* : ECCHYMOSIS, BRUISE; *esp* : one that develops post-mortem

sui·cid·al \ˌsü-ə-ˈsīd-ᵊl\ *adj* **1** : of, relating to, or tending to cause suicide ⟨∼ tendencies⟩ **2** : marked by an impulse to commit suicide ⟨∼ patients⟩ — **sui·cid·al·ly** \-ᵊl-ē\ *adv*

¹**sui·cide** \ˈsü-ə-ˌsīd\ *n* **1** : the act or an instance of taking one's own life voluntarily and intentionally **2** : a person who commits or attempts suicide

²**suicide** *vb* **sui·cid·ed; sui·cid·ing** *vi* : to commit suicide ∼ *vt* : to put (oneself) to death

sui·cid·ol·o·gy \ˌsü-ə-ˌsī-ˈdäl-ə-jē\ *n, pl* **-gies** : the study of suicide and suicide prevention — **sui·cid·ol·o·gist** \-jəst\ *n*

suit — see G SUIT, PRESSURE SUIT

suite \ˈswēt\ *n* : a group of rooms in a medical facility dedicated to a specified function or specialty ⟨a surgical ∼⟩

sul·bac·tam \səl-ˈbak-ˌtam, -təm\ *n* : a beta-lactamase inhibitor that is usu. administered in the form of its sodium salt $C_8H_{10}NNaO_5S$ in combination with a beta-lactam antibiotic (as ampicillin)

sul·cal \ˈsəl-kəl\ *adj* : of or relating to a sulcus

sul·cu·lus \ˈsəl-kyə-ləs\ *n, pl* **-cu·li** \-kyə-ˌlī\ : a small sulcus — **sul·cu·lar** \-lər\ *adj*

sul·cus \ˈsəl-kəs\ *n, pl* **sul·ci** \-ˌkī, -ˌsī\ : FURROW, GROOVE; *esp* : a shallow furrow on the surface of the brain separating adjacent convolutions — compare FISSURE 1c

sulcus lu·na·tus \-lü-ˈnāt-əs\ *n, pl* **sulci lu·na·ti** \-ˈnā-ˌtī\ : LUNATE SULCUS

sulcus ter·mi·na·lis \-ˌtər-mə-ˈnā-ləs\ *n, pl* **sulci ter·mi·na·les** \-ˌlēz\ **1** : a V-shaped groove separating the anterior two thirds of the tongue from the posterior third and containing the circumvallate papillae **2** : a shallow groove on the outside of the right atrium of the heart

¹**sul·fa** *or chiefly Brit* **sul·pha** \ˈsəl-fə\ *adj* **1** : related chemically to sulfanilamide **2** : of, relating to, employing, or containing sulfa drugs ⟨∼ therapy⟩

²**sulfa** *or chiefly Brit* **sulpha** *n* : SULFA DRUG

sul·fa·cet·a·mide *also* **sul·fa·cet·i·mide** *or chiefly Brit* **sul·pha·cet·a·mide** *also* **sul·pha·cet·i·mide** \ˌsəl-fə-ˈset-ə-ˌmīd, -məd\ *n* : a sulfa drug $C_8H_{10}N_2O_3S$ that is used chiefly for treating infections of the urinary tract and in the form of its sodium salt $C_8H_9N_2NaO_3S$ to treat infections of the eye and acne vulgaris

sul·fa·di·a·zine *or chiefly Brit* **sul·pha·di·a·zine** \ˌsəl-fə-ˈdī-ə-ˌzēn\ *n* : a sulfa drug $C_{10}H_{10}N_4O_2S$ that is used esp. in the treatment of toxoplasmosis

sulfa drug *n* : any of various synthetic organic bacteria-inhibiting drugs that are sulfonamides closely related chemically to sulfanilamide — called also *sulfa*

sul·fa·gua·ni·dine *or chiefly Brit* **sul·pha·gua·ni·dine** \ˌsəl-fə-ˈgwän-ə-ˌdēn\ *n* : a sulfa drug $C_7H_{10}N_4O_2S$ used esp. in veterinary medicine — called also *sulfanilylguanidine*

sul·fa·mate *or chiefly Brit* **sul·pha·mate** \ˈsəl-fə-ˌmāt\ *n* : a salt or ester of sulfamic acid

sul·fa·mer·a·zine *or chiefly Brit* **sul·pha·mer·a·zine** \ˌsəl-fə-ˈmer-ə-ˌzēn\ *n* : a sulfa drug $C_{11}H_{12}N_4O_2S$ that is a derivative of sulfadiazine having one methyl group replacing a hydrogen and is used similarly

sul·fa·meth·a·zine *or chiefly Brit* **sul·pha·meth·a·zine** \-ˈmeth-ə-ˌzēn\ *n* : a sulfa drug $C_{12}H_{14}N_4O_2S$ that is a dimethyl derivative of sulfadiazine and is used similarly

sul·fa·meth·ox·a·zole *or chiefly Brit* **sul·pha·meth·ox·a·zole** \-ˌmeth-ˈäk-sə-ˌzōl\ *n* : an antibacterial sulfonamide $C_{10}H_{11}N_3O_3S$ used alone (as in the treatment of urinary tract infections or prophylaxis against meningococcal meningitis) or in combination with trimethoprim (as in the treatment of Pneumocystis carinii pneumonia, shigellosis, acute otitis media, or urinary tract infections) — see BACTRIM, SEPTRA

sul·fa·mez·a·thine *or chiefly Brit* **sul·pha·mez·a·thine** \-ˈmez-ə-ˌthēn\ *n* : SULFAMETHAZINE

sul·fam·ic acid *or chiefly Brit* **sul·pham·ic acid** \səl-ˈfam-ik-\ *n* : a strong crystalline acid H_3NSO_3 made usu. by reaction of sulfuric acid, sulfur trioxide, and urea

Sul·fa·my·lon \ˌsəl-fə-ˈmī-ˌlän\ *trademark* — used for a preparation of the acetate of mafenide

sul·fa·nil·amide *or chiefly Brit* **sul·pha·nil·amide** \ˌsəl-fə-ˈnil-ə-ˌmīd, -məd\ *n* : a crystalline sulfonamide $C_6H_8N_2O_3S$ that is the amide of sulfanilic acid and the parent compound of most of the sulfa drugs

sul·fa·nil·ic acid *or chiefly Brit* **sul·pha·nil·ic acid** \ˌsəl-fə-ˌnil-ik-\ *n* : a crystalline acid $C_6H_7NO_3S$ obtained from aniline and used esp. in making dyes and as a reagent

sul·fan·i·lyl·gua·ni·dine *or chiefly Brit* **sul·phan·i·lyl·gua·ni·dine** \səl-ˈfan-i-lil-ˈgwän-ə-ˌdēn\ *n* : SULFAGUANIDINE

sul·fa·pyr·i·dine *or chiefly Brit* **sul·pha·pyr·i·dine** \ˌsəl-fə-ˈpir-ə-ˌdēn\ *n* : a sulfa drug $C_{11}H_{11}N_3O_2S$ that is derived from pyridine and sulfanilamide and is used in small doses in the treatment of dermatitis herpetiformis and esp. formerly against pneumococcal and gonococcal infections

sul·fa·qui·nox·a·line *or chiefly Brit* **sul·pha·qui·nox·a·line** \-kwi-ˈnäk-sə-ˌlēn\ *n* : a sulfa drug $C_{14}H_{12}N_4O_2S$ used esp. in veterinary medicine

sulf·ars·phen·a·mine *or chiefly Brit* **sulph·ars·phen·a·mine** \ˌsəl-ˌfärs-ˈfen-ə-ˌmēn, -mən\ *n* : an orange-yellow powder $C_{14}H_{14}As_2N_2Na_2O_8S_2$ formerly used to treat syphilis

sul·fa·sal·a·zine *or chiefly Brit* **sul·pha·sal·a·zine** \ˌsəl-fə-ˈsal-ə-ˌzēn\ *n* : a sulfonamide $C_{18}H_{14}N_4O_5S$ used in the treatment of chronic ulcerative colitis — called also *salicylazosulfapyridine*

sul·fa·tase *or chiefly Brit* **sul·pha·tase** \ˈsəl-fə-ˌtās, -ˌtāz\ *n* : any of various esterases that accelerate the hydrolysis of sulfuric esters and that are found in animal tissues and in microorganisms

¹sul·fate *or chiefly Brit* **sul·phate** \ˈsəl-ˌfāt\ *n* **1** : a salt or ester of sulfuric acid **2** : a bivalent group or anion SO_4 characteristic of sulfuric acid and the sulfates

²sulfate *or chiefly Brit* **sulphate** *vt* **sul·fat·ed** *or chiefly Brit* **sul·phat·ed; sul·fat·ing** *or chiefly Brit* **sul·phat·ing** : to treat or combine with sulfuric acid or a sulfate

sul·fa·thi·a·zole *or chiefly Brit* **sul·pha·thi·a·zole** \ˌsəl-fə-ˈthī-ə-ˌzōl\ *n* : a sulfa drug $C_9H_9N_3O_2S_2$ derived from thiazole and sulfanilamide that is seldom prescribed because of its toxicity but was formerly used esp. in the treatment of pneumococcus and staphylococcus infections

sul·fa·tide *or chiefly Brit* **sul·pha·tide** \ˈsəl-fə-ˌtīd\ *n* : any of the sulfates of cerebrosides that often accumulate in the central nervous systems of individuals affected with metachromatic leukodystrophy

sulf·he·mo·glo·bin \ˌsəlf-ˈhē-mə-ˌglō-bən\ *or chiefly Brit* **sul·phae·mo·glo·bin** \-ˌhē-mə-ˈglō-bən\ *n* : a green pigment formed by the reaction of hemoglobin with a sulfide in the

presence of oxygen or hydrogen peroxide and found in putrefied organs and cadavers

sulf·he·mo·glo·bi·ne·mia *or chiefly Brit* **sul·phae·mo·glo·bi·nae·mia** \ˌsəlf-ˌhē-mə-ˌglō-bə-ˈnē-mē-ə\ *n* : the presence of sulfhemoglobin in the blood

sulf·hy·dryl *or chiefly Brit* **sul·phy·dryl** \ˌsəlf-ˈ(h)ī-drəl\ *n* : THIOL 2 — used chiefly in molecular biology

sul·fide *or chiefly Brit* **sul·phide** \ˈsəl-ˌfīd\ *n* **1** : any of various organic compounds characterized by a sulfur atom attached to two carbon atoms **2** : a binary compound (as CuS) of sulfur usu. with a more electropositive element or group : a salt of hydrogen sulfide

sul·fin·ic acid *or chiefly Brit* **sul·phin·ic acid** \səl-ˌfin-ik-\ *n* : any of a series of monobasic organic acids of sulfur having the general formula RSO_2H

sul·fin·py·ra·zone *or chiefly Brit* **sul·phin·py·ra·zone** \ˌsəl-fən-ˈpī-rə-ˌzōn\ *n* : a uricosuric drug $C_{23}H_{20}N_2O_3S$ used in the long-term treatment of chronic gout

sul·fi·nyl *or chiefly Brit* **sul·phi·nyl** \ˈsəl-fə-ˌnil\ *n* : the bivalent group SO

sul·fi·sox·a·zole *or chiefly Brit* **sul·phi·sox·a·zole** \ˌsəl-fə-ˈsäk-sə-ˌzōl\ *n* : a sulfa drug $C_{11}H_{13}N_3O_3S$ that is derived from sulfanilamide and isoxazole, is used similarly to other sulfanilamide derivatives, but is less likely to produce renal damage because of its greater solubility

sul·fite *or chiefly Brit* **sul·phite** \ˈsəl-ˌfit\ *n* : a salt or ester of sulfurous acid

sul·fo·bro·mo·phtha·lein *or chiefly Brit* **sul·pho·bro·mo·phtha·lein** \ˌsəl-fə-ˌbrō-mō-ˈthal-ē-ən, -ˈthal-ˌēn, -ˈthāl-\ *n* : a diagnostic material used in the form of its disodium salt $C_{20}H_8Br_4Na_2O_{10}S_2$ in a liver function test

sul·fon·amide *or chiefly Brit* **sul·phon·amide** \ˌsəl-ˈfän-ə-ˌmīd, -məd; -ˈfō-nə-ˌmīd\ *n* : any of various amides (as sulfanilamide) of a sulfonic acid; *also* : SULFA DRUG

¹sul·fo·nate *or chiefly Brit* **sul·pho·nate** \ˈsəl-fə-ˌnāt\ *n* : a salt or ester of a sulfonic acid

²sulfonate *or chiefly Brit* **sulphonate** *vt* **sul·fo·nat·ed** *or chiefly Brit* **sul·pho·nat·ed; sul·fo·nat·ing** *or chiefly Brit* **sul·pho·nat·ing** : to introduce the SO_3H group into; *broadly* : to treat (an organic substance) with sulfuric acid — **sul·fo·na·tion** *or chiefly Brit* **sul·pho·na·tion** \ˌsəl-fə-ˈnā-shən\ *n*

sul·fone *or chiefly Brit* **sul·phone** \ˈsəl-ˌfōn\ *n* : any of various compounds containing the sulfonyl group with its sulfur atom having two bonds with carbon

sul·fon·eth·yl·meth·ane \ˌsəl-ˌfōn-eth-əl-ˈmeth-ˌān\ *or chiefly Brit* **sul·phon·eth·yl·me·thane** \-ˈmē-ˌthān\ *n* : a crystalline hypnotic sulfone $C_8H_{18}O_4S_2$ that is an ethyl analog of sulfonmethane

sul·fon·ic *or chiefly Brit* **sul·phon·ic** \ˌsəl-ˈfän-ik, -ˈfōn-\ *adj* : of, relating to, being, or derived from the monovalent acid group SO_3H

sulfonic acid *n* : any of numerous acids that contain the SO_3H group and may be derived from sulfuric acid by replacement of a hydroxyl group by either an inorganic anion or a monovalent organic group

sul·fo·ni·um *or chiefly Brit* **sul·pho·ni·um** \ˌsəl-ˈfō-nē-əm\ *n* : a monovalent group or cation SH_3 or derivative SR_3

sul·fon·meth·ane \ˌsəl-ˌfōn-ˈmeth-ˌān\ *or chiefly Brit* **sul·phon·me·thane** \-ˈmē-ˌthān\ *n* : a crystalline hypnotic sulfone $C_5H_{10}O_4S_2$

sul·fo·nyl *or chiefly Brit* **sul·pho·nyl** \ˈsəl-fə-ˌnil\ *n* : the bivalent group SO_2

sul·fo·nyl·urea *or chiefly Brit* **sul·pho·nyl·urea** \ˌsəl-fə-ˌnil-ˈ(y)ùr-ē-ə\ *n* : any of several hypoglycemic compounds (as glipizide and tolbutamide) related to the sulfonamides and used in the oral treatment of type 2 diabetes

sul·fo·raph·ane *or chiefly Brit* **sul·pho·raph·ane** \ˌsəl-fō-ˈraf-ˌān, -ˈrāf-\ *n* : an anticarcinogenic isothiocyanate $C_6H_{11}NOS_2$ found in cruciferous vegetables (as broccoli and cauliflower)

S
T

that is thought to function by stimulating the production of enzymes in the body that detoxify cancer-causing substances

sul·fo·sal·i·cyl·ic acid *or chiefly Brit* **sul·pho·sal·i·cyl·ic acid** \ˌsəl-fō-ˌsal-ə-ˌsil-ik-\ *n* : a sulfonic acid derivative $C_7H_6O_6S_3$ used esp. to detect and precipitate proteins (as albumin) from urine

sulf·ox·ide *or chiefly Brit* **sulph·ox·ide** \ˌsəl-ˈfäk-ˌsīd\ *n* : any of a class of organic compounds characterized by a sulfinyl group with its sulfur atom having two bonds with carbon

sulf·ox·one sodium *or chiefly Brit* **sulph·ox·one sodium** \ˌsəl-ˈfäk-ˌsōn-\ *n* : a crystalline salt $C_{14}H_{14}N_2Na_2O_6S_3$ used in the treatment of leprosy

¹sul·fur *or chiefly Brit* **sul·phur** \ˈsəl-fər\ *n* : a nonmetallic element that occurs either free or combined esp. in sulfides and sulfates, is a constituent of proteins, exists in several allotropic forms including yellow orthorhombic crystals, resembles oxygen chemically but is less active and more acidic, and is used esp. in the chemical and paper industries, in rubber vulcanization, and in medicine for treating skin diseases — symbol *S*; see ELEMENT table

²sulfur *or chiefly Brit* **sulphur** *adj* : of, relating to, or resembling sulfur : containing or impregnated with sulfur

sul·fu·rate *or chiefly Brit* **sul·phu·rate** \ˈsəl-f(y)ə-ˌrāt\ *vt* **-rat·ed; -rat·ing** : to combine or treat with sulfur : SULFURIZE

sulfurated lime solution *n* : an orange-colored solution containing sulfides of calcium made by boiling a mixture of hydrated lime and sublimed sulfur in water and applied externally as a topical antiseptic and scabicide — called also *Vleminckx' lotion, Vleminckx' solution*

sulfurated potash *n* : a mixture composed principally of sulfurated potassium compounds that is used in treating skin diseases — called also *liver of sulfur*

sulfur bacterium *n* : any of various bacteria capable of reducing sulfur compounds; *esp* : one of the genus *Thiobacillus*

sulfur dioxide *n* : a heavy pungent toxic gas SO_2 that is easily condensed to a colorless liquid, is used esp. in making sulfuric acid, in bleaching, as a preservative, and as a refrigerant, and is a major air pollutant esp. in industrial areas

sul·fu·ret *or chiefly Brit* **sul·phu·ret** \ˈsəl-f(y)ə-ˌret\ *vt* **-ret·ed** *or* **-ret·ted; -ret·ing** *or* **-ret·ting** : to combine or impregnate with sulfur

sulfur granule *n* : any of the small yellow bodies found in the pus of actinomycotic abscesses and consisting of clumps of the causative actinomycete

sul·fu·ric *or chiefly Brit* **sul·phu·ric** \ˌsəl-ˈfyu̇(ə)r-ik\ *adj* : of, relating to, or containing sulfur esp. with a higher valence than sulfurous compounds ⟨~ esters⟩

sulfuric acid *n* : a heavy corrosive oily dibasic strong acid H_2SO_4 that is colorless when pure and is a vigorous oxidizing and dehydrating agent — see OIL OF VITRIOL

sul·fur·ize *or chiefly Brit* **sul·phur·ize** *also* **sul·phur·ise** \ˈsəl-f(y)ə-ˌrīz\ *vt* **sul·fur·ized** *or chiefly Brit* **sul·phur·ized** *also* **sul·phur·ised; sul·fur·iz·ing** *or chiefly Brit* **sul·phur·iz·ing** *also* **sul·phur·is·ing** : to treat with sulfur or a sulfur compound — **sul·fur·iza·tion** *or chiefly Brit* **sul·phur·iza·tion** *also* **sul·phur·isa·tion** \ˌsəl-f(y)ə-rə-ˈzā-shən\ *n*

sulfur mustard *n* : MUSTARD GAS

sul·fu·rous *or chiefly Brit* **sul·phu·rous** \ˈsəl-f(y)ə-rəs, *also esp for 1* ˌsəl-ˈfyu̇r-əs\ *adj* **1** : of, relating to, or containing sulfur esp. with a lower valence than sulfuric compounds ⟨~ esters⟩ **2** : resembling or emanating from sulfur and esp. burning sulfur

sulfurous acid *n* : a weak unstable dibasic acid H_2SO_3 known in solution and through its salts and used as a reducing and bleaching agent and in medicine as an antiseptic

sul·fu·ryl *or chiefly Brit* **sul·phu·ryl** \ˈsəl-f(y)ə-ˌril\ *n* : SULFONYL — used esp. in names of inorganic compounds

su·lin·dac \sə-ˈlin-ˌdak\ *n* : a nonsteroidal anti-inflammatory drug $C_{20}H_{17}FO_3S$ used esp. in the treatment of rheumatoid arthritis

sul·i·so·ben·zone \ˌsəl-i-sō-ˈben-ˌzōn\ *n* : a sunscreening agent $C_{14}H_{12}O_6S$

sul·lage \ˈsəl-ij\ *n* : SEWAGE

Each boldface word in the list below is a chiefly British variant of the word to its right in small capitals.

sulpha	SULFA
sulphaceta-mide	SULFACETA-MIDE
sulphaceti-mide	SULFACETA-MIDE
sulphadiazine	SULFADIAZINE
sulphaemo-globin	SULFHEMO-GLOBIN
sulphaemo-globinemia	SULFHEMO-GLOBINEMIA
sulphaguani-dine	SULFAGUANI-DINE
sulphamate	SULFAMATE
sulphamera-zine	SULFAMERA-ZINE
sulphametha-zine	SULFAMETHA-ZINE
sulphamethox-azole	SULFAMETHOX-AZOLE
sulphameza-thine	SULFAMEZA-THINE
sulphamic acid	SULFAMIC ACID
sulphanil-amide	SULFANIL-AMIDE
sulphanilic acid	SULFANILIC ACID
sulphanilyl-guanidine	SULFANILYL-GUANIDINE
sulphapyri-dine	SULFAPYRI-DINE
sulphaquinox-aline	SULFAQUINOX-ALINE
sulpharsphen-amine	SULFARSPHEN-AMINE
sulphasalazine	SULFASALAZINE
sulphatase	SULFATASE
sulphate	SULFATE
sulphathia-zole	SULFATHIA-ZOLE

sulphatide	SULFATIDE
sulphide	SULFIDE
sulphinic acid	SULFINIC ACID
sulphinpyra-zone	SULFINPYRA-ZONE
sulphinyl	SULFINYL
sulphisoxazole	SULFISOXA-ZOLE
sulphite	SULFITE
sulphobromo-phthalein	SULFOBROMO-PHTHALEIN
sulphonamide	SULFONAMIDE
sulphonate	SULFONATE
sulphonation	SULFONATION
sulphone	SULFONE
sulphonethyl-methane	SULFONETHYL-METHANE
sulphonic	SULFONIC
sulphonium	SULFONIUM
sulphonme-thane	SULFONME-THANE
sulphonyl	SULFONYL
sulphonylurea	SULFONYLUREA
sulphoraphane	SULFORAPHANE
sulphosalicylic acid	SULFOSALICYL-IC ACID
sulphoxide	SULFOXIDE
sulphoxone sodium	SULFOXONE SODIUM
sulphur	SULFUR
sulphurate	SULFURATE
sulphuret	SULFURET
sulphuric	SULFURIC
sulphurisation	SULFURIZATION
sulphurise	SULFURIZE
sulphurization	SULFURIZATION
sulphurize	SULFURIZE
sulphurous	SULFUROUS
sulphuryl	SULFURYL
sulphydryl	SULFHYDRYL

sul·pir·ide \ˈsəl-(ˌ)pir-ˌīd\ *n* : an antidepressant and antiemetic drug $C_{15}H_{23}N_3O_4S$

sul·tone \ˈsəl-ˌtōn\ *n* : any of a class of esters of hydroxy sulfonic acids having the sulfonyl-oxy group –OSO₂– in a ring and analogous to lactones

su·mac *also* **su·mach** \ˈsü-ˌmak, ˈshü-\ *n* : any of various plants of the genus *Rhus* including several (as poison sumac) having foliage poisonous to the touch — compare POISON IVY, POISON OAK

su·ma·trip·tan \ˌsü-mə-ˈtrip-ˌtan, -tən\ *n* : a triptan $C_{14}H_{21}N_3O_2S$ that is administered as a nasal spray or in the form of its succinate $C_{14}H_{21}N_3O_2S \cdot C_4H_6O_4$ either as an oral tablet or by injection and that is used in the treatment of migraine attacks

sum·bul \ˈsəm-ˌbu̇l\ *n* : the root of a plant of the genus *Ferula* (*F. sumbul*) formerly used as a tonic and antispasmodic

sum·mate \ˈsəm-ˌāt\ *vb* **sum·mat·ed; sum·mat·ing** *vt* : to add together or sum up ⟨impulses . . . are *summated* with the subliminal impulses arriving over the sensory neuron —L. L. Langley *et al*⟩ ~ *vi* : to form a sum or cumulative effect

sum·ma·tion \(ˌ)sə-ˈmā-shən\ *n* : cumulative action or effect; *esp* : the process by which a sequence of stimuli that are individually inadequate to produce a response are cumulatively able to induce a nerve impulse — see SPATIAL SUMMATION, TEMPORAL SUMMATION

sum·mer complaint \ˈsəm-ər-\ *n* : SUMMER DIARRHEA

summer diarrhea *n* : diarrhea esp. of children that is prevalent in hot weather and is usu. caused by ingestion of food contaminated by various microorganisms responsible for gastrointestinal infections

summer mastitis *n* : bovine mastitis that occurs sporadically esp. in cattle on summer pasture and is caused by a pus-forming bacterium of the genus *Corynebacterium* (*C. pyogenes*)

summer sores *n pl but sing or pl in constr* : a skin disease of the horse caused by larval roundworms of the genus *Habronema* deposited by flies in skin wounds or abrasions where they cause intense inflammation with exudate and local necrosis

sun·block \ˈsən-ˌbläk\ *n* : a preparation (as a lotion) applied to the skin to prevent sunburn (as by physically blocking out ultraviolet radiation); *also* : its active ingredient (as titanium dioxide) — compare SUNSCREEN

¹**sun·burn** \-ˌbərn\ *vt* **sun·burned** \-ˌbərnd\ *or* **sun·burnt** \-ˌbərnt\; **sun·burn·ing** : to affect with sunburn ⟨~*ed* skin⟩

²**sunburn** *n* : inflammation of the skin caused by overexposure to ultraviolet radiation esp. from sunlight — called also *erythema solare*

sun·down·ing \'sən-ˌdaun-iŋ\ *n* : a state of increased agitation, confusion, disorientation, and anxiety that typically occurs in the late afternoon or evening in some individuals affected with dementia

sun·glass·es \-ˌglas-əs\ *n pl* : glasses used to protect the eyes from the sun

sun·lamp \'sən-ˌlamp\ *n* : an electric lamp designed to emit radiation of wavelengths from ultraviolet to infrared and used esp. for therapeutic purposes or for producing a tan artificially

sun protection factor *n* : SPF

sun·screen \-ˌskrēn\ *n* : a preparation (as a lotion) applied to the skin to prevent sunburn (as by chemically absorbing ultraviolet radiation); *also* : its active ingredient (as benzophenone) — compare SUNBLOCK — **sun·screen·ing** *adj*

sun·shine vitamin \-ˌshīn-\ *n* : VITAMIN D

sun·stroke \-ˌstrōk\ *n* : heatstroke caused by direct exposure to the sun

sun·tan \-ˌtan\ *n* : a browning of the skin from exposure to the rays of the sun — **sun·tanned** \-ˌtand\ *adj*

su·per·al·i·men·ta·tion \ˌsü-pər-ˌal-ə-mən-'tā-shən\ *n* : the action or process of overfeeding — called also *hypernutrition*

su·per·an·ti·gen \-'ant-i-jən\ *n* : a substance (as an enterotoxin) that acts as an antigen capable of stimulating much larger numbers of T cells than an ordinary antigen — **su·per·an·ti·gen·ic** \-ˌant-i-'jen-ik\ *adj*

su·per·cil·i·ary \ˌsü-pər-'sil-ē-ˌer-ē\ *adj* : of, relating to, or adjoining the eyebrow : SUPRAORBITAL

superciliary arch *n* : SUPERCILIARY RIDGE

superciliary ridge *n* : a prominence of the frontal bone above the eye caused by the projection of the frontal sinuses — called also *browridge, supraorbital ridge*

su·per·coil \'sü-pər-ˌkòi(ə)l\ *n* : a double helix (as of DNA) that has undergone additional twisting in the same direction as or in the opposite direction from the turns in the original helix — called also *superhelix* — **supercoil** *vb*

su·per·ego \ˌsü-pər-'ē-(ˌ)gō *also* 'sü-pər-ˌ, -'eg-(ˌ)ō\ *n* : the one of the three divisions of the psyche in psychoanalytic theory that is only partly conscious, represents internalization of parental conscience and the rules of society, and functions to reward and punish through a system of moral attitudes, conscience, and a sense of guilt — compare EGO, ¹ID

su·per·fam·i·ly \'sü-pər-ˌfam-(ə-)lē\ *n, pl* **-lies** **1** : a category of taxonomic classification between a family and an order or a suborder **2** : a large group of closely related molecules or chemical compounds usu. possessing a similar function

su·per·fat·ted \'sü-pər-ˌfat-əd\ *adj* : containing extra oil or fat ⟨~ soap⟩

su·per·fe·cun·da·tion \ˌsü-pər-ˌfek-ən-'dā-shən, -ˌfē-kən-\ *n* **1** : successive fertilization of two or more ova from the same ovulation esp. by different sires **2** : fertilization at one time of a number of ova excessive for the species

su·per·fe·ta·tion *or chiefly Brit* **su·per·foe·ta·tion** \ˌsü-pər-fē-'tā-shən\ *n* : successive fertilization of two or more ova of different ovulations resulting in the presence of embryos of unlike ages in the same uterus

su·per·fi·cial \ˌsü-pər-'fish-əl\ *adj* **1** : of, relating to, or located near the surface ⟨~ blood vessels⟩ **2** : lying on, not penetrating below, or affecting only the surface ⟨~ wounds⟩ — **su·per·fi·cial·ly** \-ē\ *adv*

superficial cleavage *n* : meroblastic cleavage in which a layer of cells is produced about a central mass of yolk (as in many arthropod eggs)

superficial epigastric artery *n* : EPIGASTRIC ARTERY c

superficial external pudendal artery *n* : EXTERNAL PUDENDAL ARTERY a

superficial fascia *n* : the thin layer of loose fatty connective tissue underlying the skin and binding it to the parts beneath — called also *hypodermis, tela subcutanea;* compare DEEP FASCIA

superficial inguinal ring *n* : the inguinal ring that is the external opening of the inguinal canal — called also *external inguinal ring;* compare DEEP INGUINAL RING

superficialis — see FLEXOR DIGITORUM SUPERFICIALIS, TRANSVERSUS PERINEI SUPERFICIALIS

superficial origin *n* : a site on the surface of the brain where the nerve fibers of a cranial nerve enter or leave the brain — compare NUCLEUS OF ORIGIN

superficial palmar arch *n* : PALMAR ARCH b

superficial peroneal nerve *n* : a nerve that arises as a branch of the common peroneal nerve where it forks between the fibula and the peroneus longus and that innervates or supplies branches innervating the muscles of the anterior part of the leg and the skin on the lower anterior part of the leg, on the dorsum of the foot, on the lateral and medial sides of the foot, and between the toes — called also *musculocutaneous nerve;* compare DEEP PERONEAL NERVE

superficial temporal artery *n* : the one of the two terminal branches of each external carotid artery that arises in the substance of the parotid gland, passes upward over the zygomatic process of the temporal bone, and is distributed by way of branches esp. to the more superficial parts of the side of the face and head

superficial temporal vein *n* : TEMPORAL VEIN a(1)

superficial transverse metacarpal ligament *n* : a transverse ligamentous band across the palm of the hand in the superficial fascia at the base of the fingers — called also *superficial transverse ligament*

superficial transverse perineal muscle *n* : TRANSVERSUS PERINEI SUPERFICIALIS

superfoetation *chiefly Brit var of* SUPERFETATION

su·per·fu·sate \ˌsü-pər-'fyü-ˌzāt, -zət\ *n* : a fluid that is used to superfuse an organ or tissue

su·per·fuse \ˌsü-pər-'fyüz\ *vt* **-fused; -fus·ing** : to maintain the metabolic or physiological activity of (as an isolated organ) by submitting it to a continuous flow of a sustaining medium over the outside ⟨the artificial cerebrospinal fluid ... that *superfused* the isolated cortical tissue —C. D. Richards *et al*⟩ — **su·per·fu·sion** \-'fyü-zhən\ *n*

su·per·gene \'sü-pər-ˌjēn\ *n* : a group of linked genes acting as an allelic unit esp. when due to the suppression of crossing-over

su·per·glue \'sü-pər-ˌglü\ *n* : a very strong glue; *specif* : a glue whose chief ingredient is cyanoacrylate that becomes adhesive through polymerization rather than evaporation of a solvent

su·per·he·lix \'sü-pər-ˌhē-liks\ *n* : SUPERCOIL — **su·per·he·li·cal** \ˌsü-pər-'hel-i-kəl, ˌsü-, -'hē-li-\ *adj* — **su·per·he·lic·i·ty** \-hi-'lis-ət-ē\ *n, pl* **-ties**

su·per·in·duce \ˌsü-pər-in-'d(y)üs\ *vt* **-duced; -duc·ing** : to increase the rate of formation of (as an enzyme) above the normal — **su·per·in·duc·tion** \-'dək-shən\ *n*

su·per·in·fect \-in-'fekt\ *vt* : to cause or produce superinfection of ⟨~*ed* cells⟩

su·per·in·fec·tion \-in-'fek-shən\ *n* : a second infection superimposed on an earlier one esp. by a different microbial agent of exogenous or endogenous origin that is resistant to the treatment used against the first infection

su·pe·ri·or \sù-'pir-ē-ər\ *adj* **1** : situated toward the head and further away from the feet than another and esp. another similar part of an upright body esp. of a human being ⟨the ~ medial edge of the patient's right scapula —J. M. Lewis⟩ — compare INFERIOR 1 **2** : situated in a more anterior or dorsal position in the body of a quadruped — compare INFERIOR 2

\ə\ abut \ᵊ\ kitten \ər\ further \a\ ash \ā\ ace \ä\ cot, cart \aù\ out \ch\ chin \e\ bet \ē\ easy \g\ go \i\ hit \ī\ ice \j\ job \ŋ\ sing \ō\ go \ò\ law \òi\ boy \th\ thin \th\ the \ü\ loot \ù\ foot \y\ yet \zh\ vision *See also* Pronunciation Symbols page

superior alveolar nerve *n* : any of the branches of the maxillary nerve or of the infraorbital nerve that supply the teeth and gums of the upper jaw

superior articular process *n* : ARTICULAR PROCESS a

superior cardiac nerve *n* : CARDIAC NERVE c

superior carotid triangle *n* : a space in each lateral half of the neck that is bounded in back by the sternocleidomastoid muscle, below by the omohyoid muscle, and above by the stylohyoid and digastric muscles — called also *carotid triangle*

superior cerebellar artery *n* : an artery that arises from the basilar artery just before it divides to form the posterior cerebral arteries and supplies or gives off branches supplying the superior part of the cerebellum, midbrain, pineal gland, and choroid plexus of the third ventricle

superior cerebellar peduncle *n* : CEREBELLAR PEDUNCLE a

superior cervical ganglion *n* : CERVICAL GANGLION a

superior cervical sympathetic ganglion *n* : CERVICAL GANGLION a

superior colliculus *n* : either member of the anterior and higher pair of corpora quadrigemina that together constitute a primitive center for vision — called also *optic lobe, optic tectum;* compare INFERIOR COLLICULUS

superior concha *n* : NASAL CONCHA c

superior constrictor *n* : a 4-sided muscle of the pharynx that arises from the posterior and medial parts of the pterygoid plate, from the pterygomandibular raphe, from the alveolar process above the end of the mylohyoid line, and from the side of the tongue, that inserts into the median line at the back of the pharynx, and that acts to constrict part of the pharynx in swallowing — called also *constrictor pharyngis superior, superior pharyngeal constrictor muscle;* compare INFERIOR CONSTRICTOR, MIDDLE CONSTRICTOR

superior epigastric artery *n* : EPIGASTRIC ARTERY a

superior extensor retinaculum *n* : EXTENSOR RETINACULUM 1b

superior ganglion *n* **1** : the upper and smaller of the two sensory ganglia of the glossopharyngeal nerve that may be absent but when present is situated in a groove in which the nerve passes through the jugular foramen — called also *jugular ganglion;* compare INFERIOR GANGLION 1 **2** : the upper of the two ganglia of the vagus nerve that is situated at the point where it exits through the jugular foramen — called also *jugular ganglion, superior vagal ganglion;* compare INFERIOR GANGLION 2

superior gluteal artery *n* : GLUTEAL ARTERY a

superior gluteal nerve *n* : GLUTEAL NERVE a

superior gluteal vein *n* : any of several veins that accompany the superior gluteal artery and empty into the internal iliac vein either individually or as a single united vein

superior hemorrhoidal artery *n* : RECTAL ARTERY c

superior hemorrhoidal vein *n* : RECTAL VEIN c

superior intercostal vein *n* : a vein on each side formed by the union of the veins draining the first two or three intercostal spaces of which the one on the right usu. empties into the azygos vein but sometimes into the right brachiocephalic vein and the one on the left empties into the left brachiocephalic vein after crossing the arch of the aorta

superioris — see LEVATOR LABII SUPERIORIS, LEVATOR LABII SUPERIORIS ALAEQUE NASI, LEVATOR PALPEBRAE SUPERIORIS, QUADRATUS LABII SUPERIORIS

superiority complex *n* : an excessive striving for or pretense of superiority to compensate for supposed inferiority

superior laryngeal *n* : SUPERIOR LARYNGEAL NERVE

superior laryngeal artery *n* : LARYNGEAL ARTERY b

superior laryngeal nerve *n* : LARYNGEAL NERVE a — called also *superior laryngeal*

superior longitudinal fasciculus *n* : a large bundle of association fibers in the white matter of each cerebral hemisphere that extends above the insula from the frontal lobe to the occipital lobe where it curves downward and forward into the temporal lobe

su·pe·ri·or·ly \sū-ˈpir-ē-ər-lē\ *adv* : in or to a more superior

position or direction ⟨those branches of the aorta which are ∼ oriented —H. T. Karsner⟩

superior maxillary nerve *n* : MAXILLARY NERVE

superior meatus *n* : a curved relatively short anteroposterior passage on each side of the nose that occupies the middle third of the lateral wall of a nasal cavity between the superior and middle nasal conchae — compare INFERIOR MEATUS, MIDDLE MEATUS

superior mesenteric artery *n* : MESENTERIC ARTERY b

superior mesenteric ganglion *n* : MESENTERIC GANGLION b

superior mesenteric plexus *n* : MESENTERIC PLEXUS b

superior mesenteric vein *n* : MESENTERIC VEIN b

superior nasal concha *n* : NASAL CONCHA c

superior nuchal line *n* : NUCHAL LINE a

superior oblique *n* : OBLIQUE b(1)

superior olive *n* : a small gray nucleus situated on the dorsolateral aspect of the trapezoid body — called also *superior olivary nucleus;* compare INFERIOR OLIVE

superior ophthalmic vein *n* : OPHTHALMIC VEIN a

superior orbital fissure *n* : ORBITAL FISSURE a

superior pancreaticoduodenal artery *n* : PANCREATICODUODENAL ARTERY b

superior pectoral nerve *n* : PECTORAL NERVE a

superior peroneal retinaculum *n* : PERONEAL RETINACULUM a

superior petrosal sinus *n* : PETROSAL SINUS a

superior pharyngeal constrictor muscle *n* : SUPERIOR CONSTRICTOR

superior phrenic artery *n* : PHRENIC ARTERY a

superior phrenic vein *n* : PHRENIC VEIN a

superior radioulnar joint *n* : PROXIMAL RADIOULNAR JOINT

superior ramus *n* : RAMUS b(1)

superior rectal artery *n* : RECTAL ARTERY c

superior rectal vein *n* : RECTAL VEIN c

superior rectus *n* : RECTUS 2a

superior sagittal sinus *n* : SAGITTAL SINUS a

superior temporal gyrus *n* : TEMPORAL GYRUS a

superior thyroid artery *n* : THYROID ARTERY a

superior thyroid vein *n* : THYROID VEIN a

superior transverse scapular ligament *n* : SUPRASCAPULAR LIGAMENT

superior turbinate *n* : NASAL CONCHA c

superior turbinate bone *also* **superior tur·bi·nat·ed bone** \-ˈtər-bə-ˌnāt-əd-\ *n* : NASAL CONCHA c

superior ulnar collateral artery *n* : a long slender artery that arises from the brachial artery or one of its branches just below the middle of the upper arm, descends to the elbow following the course of the ulnar nerve, and terminates under the flexor carpi ulnaris by anastomosing with two other arteries — compare INFERIOR ULNAR COLLATERAL ARTERY

superior vagal ganglion *n* : SUPERIOR GANGLION 2

superior vena cava *n* : a vein that is the second largest vein in the human body, is formed by the union of the two brachiocephalic veins at the level of the space between the first two ribs, and returns blood to the right atrium of the heart from the upper half of the body

superior vena cava syndrome *n* : a condition characterized by elevated venous pressure of the upper extremities with accompanying distension of the affected veins and swelling of the face and neck and caused by blockage (as by a thrombus or an aneurysm) or compression (as by a tumor) of the superior vena cava

superior vermis *n* : VERMIS 1a

superior vesical *n* : VESICAL ARTERY a

superior vesical artery *n* : VESICAL ARTERY a

superior vestibular nucleus *n* : the one of the four vestibular nuclei on each side of the medulla oblongata that is situated dorsal to the lateral vestibular nucleus at the junction of the floor and lateral wall of the fourth ventricle and that sends ascending fibers to the oculomotor and trochlear nuclei in the cerebrum on the same side of the brain — called also *Bekhterev's nucleus*

superior vocal cords *n pl* : FALSE VOCAL CORDS

su·per·na·tant \ˌsü-pər-ˈnāt-ᵊnt\ *n* : the usu. clear liquid overlying material deposited by settling, precipitation, or centrifugation — **supernatant** *adj*

su·per·nate \ˈsü-pər-ˌnāt\ *n* : SUPERNATANT

su·per·nor·mal \ˌsü-pər-ˈnȯr-məl\ *adj* **1** : exceeding the normal or average **2** : being beyond normal human powers : PARANORMAL — **su·per·nor·mal·i·ty** \-ˌnȯr-ˈmal-ət-ē\ *n, pl* **-ties** — **su·per·nor·mal·ly** \-ˈnȯr-mə-lē\ *adv*

su·per·nu·mer·ary \ˌsü-pər-ˈn(y)ü-mə-ˌrer-ē, -ˈn(y)üm-(ə-)rē\ *adj* : exceeding the usual or normal number ⟨~ teeth⟩ ⟨a ~ rib⟩

su·pero·lat·er·al \ˌsü-pə-rō-ˈlat-ə-rəl\ *adj* : situated above and toward the side

su·pero·me·di·al \-ˈmēd-ē-əl\ *adj* : situated above and at or toward the midline — **su·pero·me·di·al·ly** \-ə-lē\ *adv*

su·per·or·der \ˈsü-pər-ˌȯrd-ər\ *n* : a category of taxonomic classification between an order and a class or a subclass

su·per·ovu·late \ˌsü-pər-ˈäv-yə-ˌlāt\ *vt* **-lat·ed; -lat·ing** : to induce excessive ovulation in (as by administration of hormones)

su·per·ovu·la·tion \-ˌäv-yə-ˈlā-shən\ *n* : ovulation marked by the production of more than the normal number of mature eggs at one time ⟨infertility treatment including the use of gonadotropins to induce ~⟩

su·per·ox·ide \-ˈäk-ˌsīd\ *n* : any of various toxic oxygen-containing free radicals; *esp* : the monovalent anion O_2^- or a compound containing it ⟨potassium ~ KO_2⟩

superoxide dis·mu·tase \-ˈdis-myü-ˌtās\ *n* : a metal-containing antioxidant enzyme that reduces potentially harmful free radicals of oxygen formed during normal metabolic cell processes to oxygen and hydrogen peroxide — abbr. *SOD*

su·per·po·tent \ˌsü-pər-ˈpōt-ᵊnt\ *adj* : of greater than normal or acceptable potency ⟨~ topical corticosteroids⟩ — **su·per·po·ten·cy** \-ᵊn(t)-sē\ *n, pl* **-cies**

su·per·sat·u·rate \ˌsü-pər-ˈsach-ə-ˌrāt\ *vt* **-rat·ed; -rat·ing** : to add to beyond saturation — **su·per·sat·u·ra·tion** \-ˌsach-ə-ˈrā-shən\ *n*

su·per·scrip·tion \ˌsü-pər-ˈskrip-shən\ *n* : the part of a pharmaceutical prescription which contains or consists of the Latin word *recipe* or the sign ℞

su·per·sen·si·tive \-ˈsen(t)-sət-iv, -ˈsen(t)-stiv\ *adj* : HYPERSENSITIVE — **su·per·sen·si·tiv·i·ty** \-ˌsen(t)-sə-ˈtiv-ət-ē\ *n, pl* **-ties**

¹su·per·son·ic \-ˈsän-ik\ *adj* **1** : ULTRASONIC 1 **2** : of, being, or relating to speeds from one to five times the speed of sound in air — compare SONIC **3** : moving, capable of moving, or utilizing air currents moving at supersonic speed **4** : relating to supersonic airplanes or missiles ⟨the ~ age⟩ — **su·per·son·i·cal·ly** \-i-k(ə-)lē\ *adv*

²supersonic *n* **1** : a supersonic wave or frequency **2** : a supersonic airplane

su·per·vene \ˌsü-pər-ˈvēn\ *vi* **-vened; -ven·ing** : to follow or result as an additional, adventitious, or unlooked-for development (as in the course of a disease) ⟨the majority of patients die once this complication ~s —*Scientific Amer. Medicine*⟩

su·per·volt·age \ˈsü-pər-ˌvōl-tij\ *adj* : of, relating to, or employing very high X-ray voltage ⟨~ radiation therapy⟩

su·pi·nate \ˈsü-pə-ˌnāt\ *vb* **-nat·ed; -nat·ing** *vt* : to cause to undergo supination ⟨~ the hand⟩ ~ *vi* : to undergo supination

su·pi·na·tion \ˌsü-pə-ˈnā-shən\ *n* **1** : rotation of the forearm and hand so that the palm faces forward or upward and the radius lies parallel to the ulna; *also* : a corresponding movement of the foot and leg in which the foot rolls outward with an elevated arch so that in walking the foot tends to come down on its outer edge **2** : the position resulting from supination

su·pi·na·tor \ˈsü-pə-ˌnāt-ər\ *n* : a muscle that produces the motion of supination; *specif* : a deeply situated muscle of the forearm that arises in two layers from the lateral epicondyle of the humerus and adjacent parts of the ligaments and bones of the elbow and that passes over the head of the radius to insert into its neck and the lateral surface of its shaft

supinator crest *n* : a bony ridge on the upper lateral surface of the shaft of the ulna that is the origin for part of the supinator muscle

su·pine \su̇-ˈpīn, ˈsü-ˌpīn\ *adj* **1** : lying on the back or with the face upward **2** : marked by supination

¹sup·ple·ment \ˈsəp-lə-mənt\ *n* : something that completes or makes an addition ⟨dietary ~s⟩

²sup·ple·ment \ˈsəp-lə-ˌment\ *vt* : to add a supplement to : serve as a supplement for ⟨utilizes . . . surgery to ~ the traditional treatment —*Therapeutic Notes*⟩ — **sup·ple·men·ta·tion** \ˌsəp-lə-ˌmen-ˈtā-shən, -mən-\ *n*

sup·ple·men·tal \ˌsəp-lə-ˈment-ᵊl\ *adj* : serving to supplement : SUPPLEMENTARY

supplemental air *n* : the air that can still be expelled from the lungs after an ordinary expiration — compare RESIDUAL VOLUME

sup·ple·men·ta·ry \ˌsəp-lə-ˈment-ə-rē, -ˈmen-trē\ *adj* : added or serving as a supplement ⟨~ vitamins⟩

sup·ply \sə-ˈplī\ *vt* **sup·plied; sup·ply·ing** : to furnish (organs, tissues, or cells) with a vital element (as blood or nerve fibers) — used of nerves and blood vessels ⟨the mandibular foramen transmits blood vessels and nerves *supplying* the lower teeth⟩

¹sup·port \sə-ˈpō(ə)rt, -ˈpȯ(ə)rt\ *vt* **1** : to hold up or serve as a foundation or prop for **2** : to maintain in condition, action, or existence ⟨~ respiration⟩ ⟨~ life⟩

²support *n* **1** : the act or process of supporting : the condition of being supported ⟨respiratory ~⟩ **2** : SUPPORTER

sup·port·er *n* : a woven or knitted band or elastic device supporting a part; *esp* : ATHLETIC SUPPORTER

support group *n* : a group of people with common experiences and concerns who provide emotional and moral support for one another

support hose *n* : stockings (as elastic stockings) worn to supply mild compression to assist the veins of the legs — usu. pl. in constr.; called also *support hosiery*

sup·port·ive \-ˈpȯrt-iv, -ˈpȯrt-\ *adj* : furnishing support; *specif* : serving to sustain the strength and condition of a patient ⟨administration of fluids, glucose, and proteins is ~ against liver failure⟩ ⟨~ care⟩

support system *n* : a network of people who provide an individual with practical or emotional support

sup·pos·i·to·ry \sə-ˈpäz-ə-ˌtōr-ē, -ˌtȯr-\ *n, pl* **-ries** : a solid but readily meltable cone or cylinder of usu. medicated material for insertion into a bodily passage or cavity (as the rectum, vagina, or urethra)

sup·press \sə-ˈpres\ *vt* **1** : to exclude from consciousness ⟨~ed anxiety⟩ **2** : to restrain from a usual course or action ⟨~ a cough⟩ **3** : INHIBIT 2 ⟨~es the human immune response —Josie Glausiusz⟩; *esp* : to inhibit the genetic expression of ⟨~ a mutation⟩ — **sup·press·ibil·i·ty** \-ˌpres-ə-ˈbil-ət-ē\ *n, pl* **-ties** — **sup·press·ible** \-ˈpres-ə-bəl\ *adj*

¹sup·press·ant \sə-ˈpres-ᵊnt\ *adj* : SUPPRESSIVE

²suppressant *n* : an agent (as a drug) that tends to suppress or reduce in intensity rather than eliminate something ⟨a cough ~⟩

sup·pres·sion \sə-ˈpresh-ən\ *n* : an act or instance of suppressing: as **a** : stoppage of a bodily function or a symptom ⟨~ of urine secretion⟩ ⟨~ of a cough⟩ **b** : the failure of development of a bodily part or organ **c** : the conscious intentional exclusion from consciousness of a thought or feeling — compare REPRESSION 2a

sup·pres·sive \-ˈpres-iv\ *adj* : tending or serving to suppress something (as the symptoms of a disease) ⟨~ drugs⟩ — **sup·pres·sive·ness** *n*

\ə\ **abut** \ᵊ\ **kitten** \ər\ **further** \a\ **ash** \ā\ **ace** \ä\ **cot, cart** \au̇\ **out** \ch\ **chin** \e\ **bet** \ē\ **easy** \g\ **go** \i\ **hit** \ī\ **ice** \j\ **job** \ŋ\ **sing** \ō\ **go** \ȯ\ **law** \ȯi\ **boy** \th\ **thin** \t͟h\ **the** \ü\ **loot** \u̇\ **foot** \y\ **yet** \zh\ **vision** *See also* Pronunciation Symbols page

S
T

sup·pres·sor \-'pres-ər\ *n* : one that suppresses; *esp* : a mutant gene that suppresses the expression of another nonallelic mutant gene when both are present

suppressor T cell *n* : a T cell that suppresses the immune response of B cells and other T cells to an antigen resulting in tolerance for the antigen by the organism containing the T cell — called also *suppressor cell, suppressor lymphocyte, suppressor T lymphocyte, T suppressor cell;* compare CYTOTOXIC T CELL, HELPER T CELL

sup·pu·rate \'səp-yə-ˌrāt\ *vi* **-rat·ed; -rat·ing** : to form or discharge pus ⟨a *suppurating* wound⟩

sup·pu·ra·tion \ˌsəp-yə-'rā-shən\ *n* : the formation of, conversion into, or process of discharging pus ⟨an abscess is a localized area of ∼⟩ ⟨∼ in a wound⟩

suppurativa — see HIDRADENITIS SUPPURATIVA

sup·pu·ra·tive \'səp-yə-ˌrāt-iv\ *adj* : of, relating to, or characterized by suppuration ⟨∼ arthritis⟩ ⟨∼ lesions⟩

su·pra·car·di·nal vein \ˌsü-prə-'kärd-nəl-, -ˌprä-, -'kard-ᵊn-əl\ *n* : either of two veins in the mammalian embryo and various adult lower vertebrate forms located in the thoracic and abdominal regions dorsolateral to and on either side of the descending aorta and giving rise to the azygous and hemiazygous veins and a part of the inferior vena cava

su·pra·cer·vi·cal hysterectomy \-'sər-vi-kəl-\ *n* : a hysterectomy in which the uterine cervix is not removed

su·pra·chi·as·mat·ic \-ˌkī-əz-'mat-ik\ *adj* : SUPRAOPTIC

suprachiasmatic nucleus *n* : either of a pair of neuron clusters in the hypothalamus situated directly above the optic chiasma that receive photic input from the retina via the optic nerve and that regulate the body's circadian rhythms — abbr. SCN

su·pra·cho·roi·dal \-kə-'ròid-ᵊl\ *adj* : of, relating to, or being the layer of loose connective tissue situated between the choroid and sclerotic coats of the eyeball

su·pra·cil·i·ary \-'sil-ē-ˌer-ē\ *adj* : SUPERCILIARY

su·pra·cla·vic·u·lar \-kla-'vik-yə-lər, -klə-\ *adj* : situated or occurring above the clavicle ⟨∼ lymph nodes⟩

supraclavicular nerve *n* : any of three nerves that are descending branches of the cervical plexus arising from the third and fourth cervical nerves and that supply the skin over the upper chest and shoulder

su·pra·clu·sion \ˌsü-prə-'klü-zhən\ *n* : SUPRAOCCLUSION

su·pra·con·dy·lar \ˌsü-prə-'kän-də-lər, -ˌprä-\ *adj* : of, relating to, affecting, or being the part of a bone situated above a condyle ⟨∼ osteotomy⟩ ⟨a ∼ fracture of the humerus⟩

supracondylar ridge *n* : either of two ridges above the condyle of the humerus of which one is situated laterally and the other medially and which give attachment to muscles

su·pra·di·a·phrag·mat·ic \ˌsü-prə-ˌdī-ə-ˌfrag-'mat-ik, -frə(g)-\ *adj* : situated or performed from above the diaphragm ⟨∼ vagotomy⟩ — **su·pra·di·a·phrag·mat·i·cal·ly** \-i-k(ə-)lē\ *adv*

su·pra·gin·gi·val \-'jin-jə-vəl\ *adj* : located on the part of the surface of a tooth that is not surrounded by gingiva ⟨∼ calculus⟩

su·pra·gle·noid \-'glen-ˌòid, -'glēn-\ *adj* : situated or occurring superior to the glenoid cavity

su·pra·glot·tic \-'glät-ik\ *also* **su·pra·glot·tal** \-'glät-ᵊl\ *adj* : situated or occurring above the glottis ⟨∼ cancers⟩

su·pra·glot·ti·tis \-(ˌ)glä-'tīt-əs\ *n* : epiglottitis that is not confined to the epiglottis but that extends to other structures (as the pharynx, uvula, base of the tongue, aryepiglottic folds, or false vocal cords)

su·pra·he·pat·ic \-hi-'pat-ik\ *adj* : situated superior to or on the surface of the liver ⟨a ∼ abscess⟩

su·pra·hy·oid \-'hī-ˌòid\ *adj* : situated or occurring superior to the hyoid bone ⟨∼ lymphadenectomy⟩

suprahyoid muscle *n* : any of several muscles (as the mylohyoid and geniohyoid) passing upward to the jaw and face from the hyoid bone

su·pra·le·thal \-'lē-thəl\ *adj* : of, relating to, or being a dose above the lethal level ⟨∼ radiation⟩

su·pra·lim·i·nal \ˌsü-prə-'lim-ən-ᵊl, -ˌprä-\ *adj* **1** : existing

above the threshold of consciousness **2** : adequate to evoke a response or induce a sensation ⟨a ∼ stimulus⟩

su·pra·mar·gi·nal gyrus \-ˌmärj-ən-ᵊl-, -ˌmärj-nəl-\ *n* : a gyrus of the inferior part of the parietal lobe that is continuous in front with the postcentral gyrus and posteriorly and inferiorly with the superior temporal gyrus

su·pra·max·i·mal \-'mak-si-məl\ *adj* : higher or greater than a corresponding maximal ⟨a ∼ stimulus⟩ — **su·pra·max·i·mal·ly** \-ē\ *adv*

su·pra·mo·lec·u·lar \-mə-'lek-yə-lər\ *adj* : more complex than a molecule; *also* : composed of many molecules

su·pra·na·sal \-'nā-zəl\ *adj* : situated superior to the nose or a nasal part

su·pra·nu·cle·ar \-'n(y)ü-klē-ər\ *adj* : situated, occurring, or produced by a lesion superior or cortical to a nucleus esp. of the brain

supranuclear palsy *n* : PROGRESSIVE SUPRANUCLEAR PALSY

su·pra·oc·cip·i·tal \-äk-'sip-ət-ᵊl\ *adj* : situated or performed over or in the upper part of the occiput ⟨∼ craniotomy⟩

su·pra·oc·clu·sion \-ə-'klü-zhən\ *n* : the projection of a tooth beyond the plane of occlusion

su·pra·op·tic \-'äp-tik\ *adj* : situated or occurring above the optic chiasma

supraoptic nucleus *n* : a small nucleus of closely packed neurons that overlies the optic chiasma and is intimately connected with the neurohypophysis

su·pra·op·ti·mal \-'äp-tə-məl\ *adj* : greater than optimal ⟨∼ temperatures⟩

su·pra·or·bit·al \-'òr-bət-ᵊl\ *adj* : situated or occurring above the orbit of the eye

supraorbital artery *n* : a branch of the ophthalmic artery supplying the orbit and parts of the forehead

supraorbital fissure *n* : ORBITAL FISSURE a

supraorbital foramen *n* : SUPRAORBITAL NOTCH

supraorbital nerve *n* : a branch of the frontal nerve supplying the forehead, scalp, cranial periosteum, and adjacent parts

supraorbital notch *n* : a notch or foramen in the bony border of the upper inner part of the orbit serving for the passage of the supraorbital nerve, artery, and vein

supraorbital ridge *n* : SUPERCILIARY RIDGE

supraorbital vein *n* : a vein that drains the supraorbital region and unites with the frontal vein to form the angular vein

su·pra·phys·i·o·log·i·cal \-ˌfiz-ē-ə-'läj-i-kəl\ *also* **su·pra·phys·i·o·log·ic** \-'läj-ik\ *adj* : greater than normally present in the body ⟨estrogens were delivered in ∼ concentrations⟩

su·pra·pu·bic \-'p(y)ü-bik\ *adj* : situated, occurring, or performed from above the pubis ⟨∼ prostatectomy⟩ — **su·pra·pu·bi·cal·ly** \-bi-k(ə-)lē\ *or* **su·pra·pu·bic·ly** *adv*

¹**su·pra·re·nal** \-'rēn-ᵊl\ *adj* : situated above or anterior to the kidneys; *specif* : ADRENAL

²**suprarenal** *n* : a suprarenal part; *esp* : ADRENAL GLAND

suprarenal artery *n* : any of three arteries on each side of the body that supply the adrenal gland located on the same side and that arise from the inferior phrenic artery, the abdominal aorta, or the renal artery

suprarenal body *n* : ADRENAL GLAND

su·pra·re·nal·ec·to·my \ˌsü-prə-ˌrē-nᵊl-'ek-tə-mē\ *n, pl* **-mies** : ADRENALECTOMY

suprarenal gland *n* : ADRENAL GLAND

suprarenal vein *n* : either of two veins of which one arises from the right adrenal gland and empties directly into the inferior vena cava while the other arises from the left adrenal gland, passes behind the pancreas, and empties into the renal vein on the left side

su·pra·scap·u·lar \ˌsü-prə-'skap-yə-lər, -ˌprä-\ *adj* : situated or occurring superior to the scapula

suprascapular artery *n* : a branch of the thyrocervical trunk that passes obliquely from within outward and over the suprascapular ligament to the back of the scapula

suprascapular ligament *n* : a thin flat ligament that is attached at one end to the coracoid process, bridges over the suprascapular notch converting it into a foramen, and is attached at the other end to the upper margin of the scapula on its dorsal surface — called also *superior transverse scapular ligament*

suprascapular nerve *n* : a branch of the brachial plexus that supplies the supraspinatus and infraspinatus muscles

suprascapular notch *n* : a deep notch in the upper border of the scapula at the base of the coracoid process giving passage to the suprascapular nerve

su·pra·sel·lar \-'sel-ər\ *adj* : situated or rising above the sella turcica — used chiefly of tumors of the hypophysis

su·pra·spi·nal \-'spī-nəl\ *adj* : situated or occurring above a spine; *esp* : situated above the spine of the scapula

supraspinal ligament *n* : a fibrous cord that joins the tips of the spinous processes of the vertebrae from the seventh cervical vertebra to the sacrum and that continues forward to the skull as the ligamentum nuchae — called also *supraspinous ligament*

su·pra·spi·na·tus \-,spī-'nāt-əs\ *n* : a muscle of the back of the shoulder that arises from the supraspinous fossa of the scapula, that inserts into the top of the greater tubercle of the humerus, that is one of the muscles making up the rotator cuff of the shoulder, and that rotates the humerus laterally and helps to abduct the arm

su·pra·spi·nous \-'spī-nəs\ *adj* : SUPRASPINAL

supraspinous fossa *n* : a smooth concavity above the spine on the dorsal surface of the scapula that gives origin to the supraspinatus muscle

supraspinous ligament *n* : SUPRASPINAL LIGAMENT

su·pra·ster·nal \-'stərn-ᵊl\ *adj* : situated above or measured from the top of the sternum ⟨~ height⟩

suprasternal notch *n* : the depression in the top of the sternum between its articulations with the two clavicles — called also *jugular notch*

suprasternal space *n* : a long narrow space in the lower part of the deep fascia of the cervical region containing areolar tissue, the sternal part of the sternocleidomastoid muscles, and the lower part of the anterior jugular veins

su·pra·syl·vi·an \-'sil-vē-ən\ *adj* : situated or occurring superior to the sylvian fissure

su·pra·ten·to·ri·al \-ten-'tōr-ē-əl\ *adj* : relating to, occurring in, affecting, or being the tissues overlying the tentorium cerebelli ⟨a ~ glioma⟩ — **su·pra·ten·to·ri·al·ly** \-ē\ *adv*

su·pra·thresh·old \-'thresh-,(h)ōld\ *adj* : of sufficient strength or quantity to produce a perceptible physiological effect ⟨~ stimuli⟩

su·pra·troch·le·ar artery \-,träk-lē-ər-\ *n* : one of the terminal branches of the ophthalmic artery that ascends upon the forehead from the inner angle of the orbit — called also *frontal artery*

supratrochlear nerve *n* : a branch of the frontal nerve supplying the skin of the forehead and the upper eyelid

su·pra·vag·i·nal \-'vaj-ən-ᵊl\ *adj* : situated or occurring above the vagina

su·pra·val·vu·lar \-'valv-yə-lər\ *adj* : situated or occurring above a valve ⟨~ aortic stenosis⟩

su·pra·ven·tric·u·lar \-ven-'trik-yə-lər\ *adj* : relating to or being a rhythmic abnormality of the heart caused by impulses originating above the ventricles (as in the atrioventricular node) ⟨~ tachycardia⟩

su·pra·vi·tal \-'vīt-ᵊl\ *adj* : constituting or relating to the staining of living tissues or cells surviving after removal from a living body by dyes that penetrate living substance but induce more or less rapid degenerative changes — compare INTRAVITAL 2 — **su·pra·vi·tal·ly** \-ᵊl-ē\ *adv*

su·preme thoracic artery \sə-'prēm-, sü-\ *n* : THORACIC ARTERY a

surae — see TRICEPS SURAE

su·ral \'sur-əl\ *adj* : of, relating to, or being a sural nerve or branches of the popliteal artery or vein that ramify in the area of the calf of the leg

sural nerve *n* : any of several nerves in the region of the calf of the leg; *esp* : one formed by the union of a branch of the tibial nerve with a branch of the common peroneal nerve

that supplies branches to the skin of the back of the leg and sends a continuation to the little toe by way of the lateral side of the foot

sur·a·min \'sur-ə-mən\ *n* : a trypanocidal drug $C_{51}H_{34}N_6Na_6O_{23}S_6$ obtained as a white powder and administered intravenously in the early stages of African sleeping sickness — called also *germanin, suramin sodium*

sur·face \'sər-fəs\ *n* : the exterior or upper boundary of an object or body ⟨the mesial and distal ~s of a tooth⟩

surface–active *adj* : altering the properties and esp. lowering the tension at the surface of contact between phases ⟨soaps and wetting agents are typical ~ substances⟩

surface tension *n* : the attractive force exerted upon the surface molecules of a liquid by the molecules beneath that tends to draw the surface molecules into the bulk of the liquid and makes the liquid assume the shape having the least surface area

sur·fac·tant \(,)sər-'fak-tənt, 'sər-,\ *n* : a surface-active substance; *specif* : a surface-active lipoprotein mixture which coats the alveoli and which prevents collapse of the lungs by reducing the surface tension of pulmonary fluids — **surfactant** *adj*

surf·er's knot \'sər-fərz-\ *n* : a knobby lump just below a surfer's knee or on the upper surface of the foot caused by friction and pressure between surfboard and skin — called also *surfer's knob, surfer's lump, surfer's nodule*

surg *abbr* **1** surgeon **2** surgery **3** surgical

sur·geon \'sər-jən\ *n* **1** : a medical specialist who performs surgery : a physician qualified to treat those diseases that are amenable to or require surgery — compare INTERNIST **2** : the senior medical officer of a military unit

surgeon general *n, pl* **surgeons general** : the chief medical officer of a branch of the armed services or of a public health service

surgeon–in–chief *n* : the surgeon in charge of the surgical service of a hospital and esp. a teaching hospital

surgeon's knot *n* : any of several knots used in tying ligatures or surgical stitches; *esp* : a square knot in which the first knot has two turns

sur·gery \'sərj-(ə-)rē\ *n, pl* **-ger·ies 1** : a branch of medicine concerned with diseases and conditions requiring or amenable to operative or manual procedures **2 a** *Brit* : a physician's or dentist's office **b** : a room or area where surgery is performed **3 a** : the work done by a surgeon **b** : OPERATION

sur·gi·cal \'sər-ji-kəl\ *adj* **1** : of, relating to, or concerned with surgeons or surgery ⟨~ skill⟩ **2** : requiring surgical treatment ⟨a ~ appendix⟩ **3** : used in or in connection with surgery ⟨~ gauze⟩ **4** : following or resulting from surgery ⟨~ fevers⟩

surgical diathermy *n* : surgery by electrocoagulation

sur·gi·cal·ly \'sər-ji-k(ə-)lē\ *adv* : by means of surgery

surgical neck *n* : a slightly narrowed part of the humerus below the greater and lesser tubercles that is frequently the site of fractures

surgical needle *n* : a needle designed to carry sutures when sewing tissues

sur·gi·cen·ter \'sər-jə-,sent-ər\ *n* : a medical facility that performs minor surgery on an outpatient basis

sur·ra \'sur-ə\ *n* : a severe tropical or subtropical disease of domestic animals that is caused by a protozoan of the genus *Trypanosoma* (*T. evansi*), is transmitted by biting flies, and is marked esp. by fever, anemia, edema, emaciation, and petechiae

sur·ro·ga·cy \'sər-ə-gə-sē, 'sə-rə-\ *n, pl* **-cies** : the practice of serving as a surrogate mother

sur·ro·gate \-gət, -,gāt\ *n* : one that serves as a substitute: as **a** : a representation of a person substituted through symbolizing (as in a dream) for conscious recognition of the person

---

\ə\ **abut** \ᵊ\ **kitten** \ər\ **further** \a\ **ash** \ā\ **ace** \ä\ **cot, cart** \au̇\ **out** \ch\ **chin** \e\ **bet** \ē\ **easy** \g\ **go** \i\ **hit** \ī\ **ice** \j\ **job** \ŋ\ **sing** \ō\ **go** \ȯ\ **law** \ȯi\ **boy** \th\ **thin** \t̲h̲\ **the** \ü\ **loot** \u̇\ **foot** \y\ **yet** \zh\ **vision** *See also* Pronunciation Symbols page

S
T

b : a drug substituted for another drug   **c** : SURROGATE MOTHER

surrogate mother *n* : a woman who becomes pregnant usu. by artificial insemination or surgical implantation of a fertilized egg for the purpose of carrying the fetus to term for another woman — **surrogate motherhood** *n*

su·ru·cu·cu \ˌsùr-ə-kü-ˈkü\ *n* : BUSHMASTER

sur·veil·lance \sər-ˈvā-lən(t)s *also* -ˈvāl-yən(t)s *or* -ˈvā-ən(t)s\ *n* : close and continuous observation or testing ⟨serological ∼⟩ — see IMMUNOLOGICAL SURVEILLANCE

sur·viv·al of the fittest \sər-ˈvī-vəl-\ *n* : NATURAL SELECTION

sur·vive \sər-ˈvīv\ *vb* **sur·vived; sur·viv·ing** *vi* : to remain alive or in existence : live on ∼ *vt* **1** : to remain alive after the death of ⟨his son *survived* him⟩ **2** : to continue to exist or live after ⟨*survived* the stroke⟩ — **sur·vi·val** \-ˈvī-vəl\ *n* — **sur·vi·vor** \-ˈvī-vər\ *n*

sur·vi·vor·ship \-ˈvī-vər-ˌship\ *n* **1** : the state of being a survivor ⟨quality of life in long-term ∼ (five years or longer) of patients who have experienced breast cancer⟩ **2** : the probability of surviving to a particular age; *also* : the number or proportion of survivors (as of an age group)

sus·cep·ti·bil·i·ty \sə-ˌsep-tə-ˈbil-ət-ē\ *n, pl* **-ties 1** : the quality or state of being susceptible : the state of being predisposed to, sensitive to, or of lacking the ability to resist something (as a pathogen, familial disease, or a drug) : SENSITIVITY **2 a** : the ratio of the magnetization in a substance to the corresponding magnetizing force — see PARAMAGNETIC **b** : the ratio of the electric polarization to the electric intensity in a polarized dielectric

¹sus·cep·ti·ble \sə-ˈsep-tə-bəl\ *adj* **1** : having little resistance to a specific infectious disease : capable of being infected **2** : predisposed to develop a noninfectious disease ⟨∼ to diabetes⟩ **3** : abnormally reactive to various drugs

²susceptible *n* : one that is susceptible (as to a disease) ⟨vaccinate all ∼s in each region where outbreaks appeared —A. J. Bollet⟩

sus·pend·ed animation \sə-ˈspend-əd-\ *n* : temporary suspension of the vital functions (as in persons nearly drowned)

sus·pen·sion \sə-ˈspen-chən\ *n* **1 a** : the state of a substance when its particles are mixed with but undissolved in a fluid or solid **b** : a substance in this state — see ORAL SUSPENSION **2** : a system consisting of a solid dispersed in a solid, liquid, or gas usu. in particles of larger than colloidal size

sus·pen·soid \sə-ˈspen(t)-ˌsòid\ *n* **1** : a colloidal system in which the dispersed particles are solid **2** : a lyophobic sol

¹sus·pen·so·ry \sə-ˈspen(t)s-(ə-)rē\ *adj* : serving to suspend : providing support ⟨the ∼ nature of the periodontal membrane —John Osborne *et al*⟩

²suspensory *n, pl* **-ries** : something that suspends or holds up; *esp* : a fabric supporter for the scrotum

suspensory ligament *n* : a ligament or fibrous membrane suspending an organ or part: as **a** : a ringlike fibrous membrane connecting the ciliary body and the lens of the eye and holding the lens in place **b** : FALCIFORM LIGAMENT

suspensory ligament of the ovary *n* : a fold of peritoneum that consists of a part of the broad ligament that is attached to the ovary near the end joining the fallopian tube and that contains blood and lymph vessels passing to and from the ovary — called also *infundibulopelvic ligament;* compare LIGAMENT OF THE OVARY

sus·tained–re·lease \səs-ˌtānd-ri-ˌlēs\ *adj* : designed to slowly release a drug in the body over an extended period of time ⟨∼ capsules⟩ ⟨a ∼ drug delivery system⟩ — compare TIMED-RELEASE

sus·ten·tac·u·lar \ˌsəs-tən-ˈtak-yə-lər, -ˌten-\ *adj* : serving to support or sustain ⟨∼ bone⟩

sustentacular cell *n* : a supporting epithelial cell (as a Sertoli cell or a cell of the olfactory epithelium) that lacks a specialized function (as nerve-impulse conduction)

sustentacular fiber of Müller *n* : FIBER OF MÜLLER

sus·ten·tac·u·lum \ˌsəs-tən-ˈtak-yə-ləm\ *n, pl* **-la** \-lə\ : a body part that supports or suspends another organ or part

sustentaculum ta·li \-ˈtā-ˌlī\ *n* : a medial process of the calcaneus supporting part of the talus

su·tur·al \ˈsü-chə-rəl\ *adj* : of, relating to, or occurring in a suture

sutural bone *n* : WORMIAN BONE

¹su·ture \ˈsü-chər\ *n* **1 a** : a stitch made with a suture **b** : a strand or fiber used to sew parts of the living body **c** : the act or process of sewing with sutures **2 a** : the line of union in an immovable articulation (as between the bones of the skull); *also* : such an articulation **b** : a furrow at the junction of adjacent bodily parts

²suture *vt* **su·tured; su·tur·ing** \ˈsüch-(ə-)riŋ\ : to unite, close, or secure with sutures ⟨∼ a wound⟩

suture needle *n* : SURGICAL NEEDLE

suxa·me·tho·ni·um \ˌsùk-sə-mə-ˈthō-nē-əm\ *n, chiefly Brit* : SUCCINYLCHOLINE

Sv *abbr* sievert

sved·berg \ˈsfed-ˌbərg, -ˌber-ē\ *n* : a unit of time amounting to 10⁻¹³ second that is used to measure the sedimentation velocity of a colloidal solution (as of a protein) in an ultracentrifuge and to determine molecular weight by substitution in an equation — called also *svedberg unit*

Sved·berg \ˈsved-ˌber-ē\, **Theodor (1884–1971),** Swedish chemist. Svedberg was associated with the University of Uppsala for virtually all of his research career. In 1924 he developed the ultracentrifuge to facilitate the separation of colloids and large molecules. His ultracentrifuge helped determine the presence of substances contaminating protein molecules. In 1926 he was awarded the Nobel Prize for Chemistry for his development of the ultracentrifuge.

SV40 \ˌes-ˌvē-ˈfòrt-ē\ *n* : SIMIAN VIRUS 40

SVT *abbr* supraventricular tachycardia

¹swab \ˈswäb\ *n* **1** : a wad of absorbent material usu. wound around one end of a small stick and used for applying medication or for removing material from an area **2** : a specimen taken with a swab ⟨a throat ∼⟩

²swab *vt* **swabbed; swab·bing** : to apply medication to with a swab ⟨*swabbed* the wound with iodine⟩

swabbing *n* : the material removed from tissue (as of a lesion) by means of a swab — usu. used in pl.

swage \ˈswāj, ˈswej\ *vt* **swaged; swag·ing** : to fuse (a strand of suture) onto the end of a surgical needle

¹swal·low \ˈswäl-(ˌ)ō\ *vt* : to take through the mouth and esophagus into the stomach ∼ *vi* : to receive something into the body through the mouth and esophagus

²swallow *n* **1** : an act of swallowing **2** : an amount that can be swallowed at one time

swamp fever \ˈswämp-, ˈswòmp-\ *n* **1** : LEPTOSPIROSIS **2** : EQUINE INFECTIOUS ANEMIA

Swan–Ganz catheter \ˈswän-ˈganz-\ *n* : a soft catheter with an expandable balloon tip that is used for measuring blood pressure in the pulmonary artery

Swan, Harold James Charles (*b* 1922), and **Ganz, William (*b* 1919),** American cardiologists. From the 1960s Swan served as director of cardiology at a Los Angeles medical center and as professor of medicine at the University of California. In 1970 he introduced a catheter with an expandable balloon tip for use in measuring blood pressure in the pulmonary artery. Swan was greatly assisted in the development of the balloon catheter by Ganz. Together Swan and Ganz also developed a multipurpose catheter that incorporates a number of electrodes in its shaft.

swarm·ing \ˈswòr-miŋ\ *n* : movement or spreading in a swarm ⟨∼ of bacteria in a culture medium⟩

swarm spore *n* : any of various minute motile sexual or asexual spores; *esp* : ZOOSPORE

S wave \ˈes-ˌ\ *n* : the negative downward deflection in the QRS complex of an electrocardiogram that follows the R wave

sway·back \ˈswā-ˌbak, -ˈbak\ *n* **1** : an abnormally hollow condition or sagging of the back found esp. in horses; *also* : a back so shaped **2** : LORDOSIS **3** : a copper-deficiency disease of young or newborn lambs that is marked by demyelination of the brain resulting in weakness, staggering gait, and collapse and is almost universally fatal but is readily preventable by copper supplementation of the diet of the pregnant ewe — **sway·backed** \-ˌbakt\ *adj*

¹sweat \ˈswet\ *vi* **sweat** *or* **sweat·ed; sweat·ing** : to excrete moisture in visible quantities through the opening of the sweat glands : PERSPIRE

²sweat *n* **1** : the fluid excreted from the sweat glands of the skin : PERSPIRATION **2** : abnormally profuse sweating — often used in pl. ⟨soaking ∼*s*⟩ — **sweaty** \-ē\ *adj* **sweat·i·er; -est**

sweat duct *n* : the part of a sweat gland which extends through the dermis to the surface of the skin

sweat gland *n* : a simple tubular gland of the skin that secretes perspiration, in humans is widely distributed in nearly all parts of the skin, and consists typically of an epithelial tube extending spirally from a minute pore on the surface of the skin into the dermis or subcutaneous tissues where it ends in a convoluted tuft — called also *sudoriferous gland, sudoriparous gland*

sweating sickness *n* : an epidemic febrile disease esp. of young cows that occurs chiefly in Africa, is characterized by profuse sweating and early high mortality, and is caused by a toxin produced and transmitted by a tick of the genus *Hyalomma* (*H. truncatum*)

sweat test *n* : a test for cystic fibrosis that involves measuring the subject's sweat for abnormally high sodium chloride content

swee·ny *also* **swee·ney** \ˈswē-nē\ *or* **swin·ney** \ˈswin-ē\ *n, pl* **sweenies** *also* **sweeneys** *or* **swinneys** : an atrophy of the shoulder muscles of a horse; *broadly* : any muscular atrophy of a horse

¹sweet \ˈswēt\ *adj* : being or inducing the one of the four basic taste sensations that is typically induced by disaccharides and is mediated esp. by receptors in taste buds at the front of the tongue — compare BITTER, SALT 2, SOUR — **sweet·ness** *n*

²sweet *n* **1** : something that is sweet to the taste; *esp* : a food (as a candy or preserve) having a high sugar content ⟨don't fill up on ∼*s*⟩ **2** : a sweet taste sensation

sweet almond *n* : an almond that produces sweet edible seeds and forms a distinct variety (*Prunus amygdalus dulcis*) of the common almond; *also* : the edible seed of this tree

sweet almond oil *n* : ALMOND OIL 1a

sweet birch *n* : a common birch (*Betula lenta*) of the eastern U.S. with spicy brown bark that yields birch oil

sweet–birch oil *n* : BIRCH OIL

sweet clover disease *n* : a hemorrhagic diathesis of sheep and cattle feeding on improperly cured sweet clover (genus *Melilotus* of the family Leguminosae) containing excess quantities of dicumarol

sweet flag \-ˈflag\ *n* : a perennial marsh herb (*Acorus calamus*) of the arum family (Araceae) having long leaves and a pungent rootstock and used esp. formerly as a flavoring agent and in folk medicine but now largely abandoned because of demonstrated carcinogenicity and toxicity in laboratory animals — see CALAMUS

sweet gum *n* : a No. American tree of the genus *Liquidambar* (*L. styraciflua*) with a round spiny brown fruit cluster and an inner bark that is the source of American storax

sweet marjoram *n* : an aromatic European herb (*Majorana hortensis*) with dense spikelike flower clusters formerly used as a mild stimulant and carminative

sweet orange oil *n* : ORANGE OIL a

Sweet's syndrome \ˈswēts-\ *n* : a disease that occurs esp. in middle-aged women, that is characterized by red raised often painful patches on the skin, fever, and neutrophilia in the peripheral blood, that responds to treatment with corticosteroids but not antibiotics, and that is of unknown cause but is sometimes associated with an underlying malignant disorder — called also *acute febrile neutrophilic dermatosis*
 Sweet, Robert Douglas (*fl* **1964),** British dermatologist. Sweet published his description of acute febrile neutrophilic dermatosis in 1964.

swell \ˈswel\ *vi* **swelled; swelled** *or* **swol·len** \ˈswō-lən\;

swell·ing : to become distended or puffed up ⟨her ankle ∼*ed*⟩

swelled head *n* : BIGHEAD

swell·ing \ˈswel-iŋ\ *n* : an abnormal bodily protuberance or localized enlargement ⟨an inflammatory ∼⟩

Swift's disease \ˈswifts-\ *n* : ACRODYNIA
 Swift, H. (*fl* **1918),** Australian physician. Swift described acrodynia about 1918. His description was not the first, for the German pediatrician Paul Selter had described it in 1903. Later, other physicians would offer more detailed descriptions of the disease.

swim·mer's ear \ˈswim-ərz-\ *n* : inflammation of the canal in the outer ear that is characterized by itching, redness, swelling, pain, discharge, and sometimes hearing loss and that typically occurs when water trapped in the outer ear during swimming becomes infected with a bacterium (as *Pseudomonas aeruginosa* or *Staphylococcus aureus*) or rarely with a fungus

swimmer's itch *n* : an itching inflammation that is a reaction to the invasion of the skin by schistosomes that are not normally parasites of humans — called also *schistosome dermatitis*

swine \ˈswīn\ *n* : any of various stout-bodied short-legged mammals (family Suidae) with a thick bristly skin and a long mobile snout; *esp* : a domesticated member of a species (*Sus scrofa*) that occurs wild in the Old World

swine dysentery *n* : an acute infectious hemorrhagic dysentery of swine

swine erysipelas *n* : a destructive contagious disease of various mammals and birds that is caused by a bacterium of the genus *Erysipelothrix* (*E. rhusiopathiae*), that may occur in an acute highly fatal septicemic form or take a chronic course marked by endocarditis, arthritis, or hives, and that is of esp. economic importance in swine and domesticated turkeys — called also *erysipelas*

swine fever *n* **1** : HOG CHOLERA **2** : AFRICAN SWINE FEVER

swine flu *n* : SWINE INFLUENZA

swine·herd's disease \ˈswīn-ˌhərdz-\ *n* : a form of leptospirosis contracted from swine — called also *swineherder's disease*

swine influenza *n* : an acute contagious febrile disease of swine that is marked by severe coughing and inflammation of the upper respiratory tract, that sometimes develops into bronchopneumonia but is rarely fatal, that is caused by infection with a subtype (H1N1 or sometimes H3N2) of the orthomyxovirus causing influenza A, and that is often complicated by infection with another microorganism (as the pseudorabies virus or a pneumonia-causing bacterium) — called also *swine flu*

swine plague *n* : hemorrhagic septicemia of swine with symptoms resembling those of hog cholera but commonly complicated by pneumonia

swine pox *n* : a mild virus disease of young pigs that is marked by fever, loss of appetite, relative indifference to normal stimuli, and skin lesions suggestive of those of smallpox and that is caused by a poxvirus (species *Swinepox virus* of the genus *Suipoxvirus*) transmitted by the hog louse

swinny *var of* SWEENY

swol·len *adj* : protuberant or abnormally distended (as by injury or disease) ⟨a ∼ finger⟩

sy·co·sis \sī-ˈkō-səs\ *n, pl* **sy·co·ses** \-ˌsēz\ : a chronic inflammatory disease involving the hair follicles esp. of the bearded part of the face and marked by papules, pustules, and tubercles perforated by hairs with crusting

sycosis bar·bae \-ˈbär-bē\ *n* : sycosis of the bearded part of the face

sycosis par·a·sit·i·ca \-ˌpar-ə-ˈsit-i-kə\ *n* : BARBER'S ITCH

\ə\ abut \ᵊ\ kitten \ər\ further \a\ ash \ā\ ace \ä\ cot, cart
\au̇\ out \ch\ chin \e\ bet \ē\ easy \g\ go \i\ hit \ī\ ice \j\ job
\ŋ\ sing \ō\ go \ȯ\ law \ȯi\ boy \th\ thin \t̲h̲\ the \ü\ loot
\u̇\ foot \y\ yet \zh\ vision   *See also* Pronunciation Symbols page

Syd·en·ham's chorea \'sid-ᵊn-əmz-\ *n* : chorea following infection (as rheumatic fever) and occurring usu. in children and adolescents — called also *Saint Vitus' dance*

Sydenham, Thomas (1624–1689), British physician. Sydenham has been called the founder of epidemiology and the English Hippocrates for his reliance on close personal observation of patients and clinical experience to treat disease. He introduced the use of opium into medical practice and helped to popularize the use of quinine for the treatment of malaria. He is also known for his classic descriptions of arthritis due to gout (1683) and Sydenham's chorea (1686).

syl·vat·ic \sil-'vat-ik\ *adj* : occurring in, affecting, or transmitted by wild animals ⟨∼ diseases⟩ ⟨∼ yellow fever⟩

sylvatic plague *n* : a form of plague of which wild rodents and their fleas are the reservoirs and vectors and which is widely distributed in western No. and So. America though rarely affecting humans

syl·vi·an \'sil-vē-ən\ *adj, often cap S* : of or relating to the sylvian fissure

sylvian aqueduct *n, often cap S* : AQUEDUCT OF SYLVIUS

sylvian fissure *n, often cap 1st S* : a deep fissure of the lateral aspect of each cerebral hemisphere that divides the temporal from the parietal and frontal lobes — called also *fissure of Sylvius, lateral fissure, lateral sulcus*

Du·bois \dǖ-'bȯ-ä\ *or* **De Le Boë** \,dā-lā-'bō-ä\, **François** *or* **Franz** (*Latin* **Franciscus Sylvius**) **(1614–1672)**, Dutch anatomist, physician, and chemist. As a professor of medicine at Leiden, Dubois was one of Europe's most celebrated teachers. He is considered by many the founder of the 17th=century school of iatrochemical medicine, a school that held that all the phenomena of life and disease are based on chemical action. This school sought to apply rationally the universal laws of chemistry and physics to medicine. He extensively investigated the anatomy of the brain, and in 1641 he discovered the deep cleft separating the temporal, frontal, and parietal lobes of the brain. This cleft is now known as the sylvian fissure. He published his collected medical works in 1671.

sylvian fossa *n, often cap 1st S* : a depression that forms in the lateral surface of each embryonic cerebral hemisphere during the third month of development and contains the insula at its bottom which is later covered by the operculum whose edges form the border of the sylvian fissure

sym·bal·lo·phone \sim-'bȯl-ə-ˌfōn\ *n* : a double stethoscope having two chest pieces for comparing and determining the location of sounds in the body

sym·bi·ont \'sim-ˌbī-ˌänt, -bē-\ *n* : an organism living in symbiosis; *esp* : the smaller member of a symbiotic pair — called also *symbiote* — **sym·bi·on·tic** \,sim-ˌbī-'änt-ik, -bē-\ *adj*

sym·bi·o·sis \,sim-ˌbī-'ō-səs, -bē-\ *n, pl* **-bi·o·ses** \-ˌsēz\ **1** : the living together of two dissimilar organisms in more or less intimate association or close union **2** : the intimate living together of two dissimilar organisms in a mutually beneficial relationship; *esp* : MUTUALISM

sym·bi·ote \'sim-ˌbī-ˌōt, -bē-\ *n* : SYMBIONT

sym·bi·ot·ic \,sim-ˌbī-'ät-ik, -bē-\ *also* **sym·bi·ot·i·cal** \-i-kəl\ *adj* : relating to, characterized by, living in, or resulting from a state of symbiosis — **sym·bi·ot·i·cal·ly** \-i-k(ə-)lē\ *adv*

sym·bleph·a·ron \sim-'blef-ə-ˌrän\ *n* : adhesion between an eyelid and the eyeball

sym·bol \'sim-bəl\ *n* : something that stands for or suggests something else: as **a** : an arbitrary or conventional sign used in writing or printing relating to a particular field to represent operations, quantities, elements, relations, or qualities **b** : an object or act representing something in the unconscious mind that has been repressed ⟨phallic ∼s⟩ — **sym·bol·ic** \sim-'bäl-ik\ *adj* — **sym·bol·i·cal·ly** \-i-k(ə-)lē\ *adv*

sym·bol·ism \'sim-bə-ˌliz-əm\ *n* : the art or practice of using symbols esp. by investing things with a symbolic meaning or by expressing the invisible or intangible by means of visible or sensuous representations

sym·bol·iza·tion *also Brit* **sym·bol·isa·tion** \,sim-bə-lə-'zā-shən, -ˌlī-\ *n* : the act or process of symbolizing; *specif* : symbolic representation of a repressed complex (as in dreams)

sym·bol·ize *also Brit* **sym·bol·ise** \'sim-bə-ˌlīz\ *vt* **-ized** *also Brit* **-ised; -iz·ing** *also Brit* **-is·ing** **1** : to serve as a symbol of **2** : to represent, express, or identify by a symbol

Syme's amputation \'sīmz-\ *or* **Syme amputation** \'sīm-\ *n* : amputation of the foot through the articulation of the ankle with removal of the malleoli of the tibia and fibula — compare PIROGOFF'S AMPUTATION

Syme, James (1799–1870), British surgeon. Syme was generally recognized as one of the leading surgical authorities of his time. During his lifetime he held the positions of surgeon to the queen in Scotland, senior attending surgeon at the Royal Infirmary, and professor of clinical surgery at the University of Edinburgh, Scotland. He performed his first amputation at the ankle on a patient suffering from osteomyelitis of the foot. He described the operation in an 1843 medical communication.

sym·me·lus \'sim-ə-ləs\ *n, pl* **-li** \-ˌlī\ : SIRENOMELUS

Sym·met·rel \'sim-ə-ˌtrel\ *trademark* — used for a preparation of the hydrochloride of amantadine

sym·met·ri·cal \sə-'me-tri-kəl\ *or* **sym·met·ric** \-trik\ *adj* : having, involving, or exhibiting symmetry: as **a** : affecting corresponding parts simultaneously and similarly ⟨a ∼ rash⟩ **b** : exhibiting symmetry in a structural formula; *esp* : being a derivative with groups substituted symmetrically in the molecule — **sym·met·ri·cal·ly** \-tri-k(ə-)lē\ *adv*

sym·me·try \'sim-ə-trē\ *n, pl* **-tries** **1** : correspondence in size, shape, and relative position of parts on opposite sides of a dividing line or median plane or about a center or axis — see BILATERAL SYMMETRY, RADIAL SYMMETRY **2** : the property of remaining invariant under certain changes (as of orientation in space, of the sign of the electric charge, of parity, or of the direction of time flow) — used of physical phenomena and of equations describing them

sym·pa·thec·to·my \,sim-pə-'thek-tə-mē\ *n, pl* **-mies** : surgical interruption of sympathetic nerve pathways — **sym·pa·thec·to·mized** *or chiefly Brit* **-mised** \-ˌmīzd\ *adj*

¹sym·pa·thet·ic \,sim-pə-'thet-ik\ *adj* **1** : of or relating to the sympathetic nervous system **2** : mediated by or acting on the sympathetic nerves — **sym·pa·thet·i·cal·ly** \-i-k(ə-)lē\ *adv*

²sympathetic *n* : a sympathetic structure; *esp* : SYMPATHETIC NERVOUS SYSTEM

sympathetic chain *n* : either of the pair of ganglionated longitudinal cords of the sympathetic nervous system of which one is situated on each side of the spinal column — called also *sympathetic trunk;* compare VERTEBRAL GANGLION

sympathetic nerve *n* : a nerve of the sympathetic nervous system

sympathetic nervous system *n* : the part of the autonomic nervous system that is concerned esp. with preparing the body to react to situations of stress or emergency, that contains chiefly adrenergic fibers and tends to depress secretion, decrease the tone and contractility of smooth muscle, increase heart rate, and that consists essentially of preganglionic fibers arising in the thoracic and upper lumbar parts of the spinal cord and passing through delicate white rami communicantes to ganglia located in a pair of sympathetic chains situated one on each side of the spinal column or to more peripheral ganglia or ganglionated plexuses and postganglionic fibers passing typically through gray rami communicantes to spinal nerves with which they are distributed to various end organs — called also *sympathetic system;* compare PARASYMPATHETIC NERVOUS SYSTEM

sym·pa·thet·i·co·ad·re·nal \,sim-pə-'thet-i-(ˌ)kō-ə-'drēn-ᵊl\ *adj* : of, relating to, or made up of sympathetic nervous and adrenal elements ⟨the ∼ system⟩

sym·pa·thet·i·co·lyt·ic \-'lit-ik\ *adj* : SYMPATHOLYTIC

¹sym·pa·thet·i·co·mi·met·ic \-mə-'met-ik\ *adj* : SYMPATHOMIMETIC

²sympatheticomimetic *n* : SYMPATHOMIMETIC

sympathetic ophthalmia *n* : inflammation in an uninjured eye as a result of injury and inflammation of the other

sym·pa·thet·i·co·to·nia \,sim-pə-,thet-i-kə-'tō-nē-ə\ n : SYMPATHICOTONIA — **sym·pa·thet·i·co·ton·ic** \-'tän-ik\ adj

sympathetic system n : SYMPATHETIC NERVOUS SYSTEM

sympathetic trunk n : SYMPATHETIC CHAIN

sym·path·i·co·blast \sim-'path-i-kō-,blast\ n : a cell that is a precursor of a sympathetic neuron

¹**sym·path·i·co·lyt·ic** \sim-,path-i-kō-'lit-ik\ adj : SYMPATHOLYTIC

²**sympathicolytic** n : SYMPATHOLYTIC

sym·path·i·co·mi·met·ic \-mə-'met-ik, -mī-\ adj or n : SYMPATHOMIMETIC

sym·path·i·co·to·nia \sim-,path-i-kō-'tō-nē-ə\ n : a condition produced by relatively great activity or stimulation of the sympathetic nervous system and characterized by goose bumps, vascular spasm, and abnormally high blood pressure — called also *sympatheticotonia;* compare VAGOTONIA — **sym·path·i·co·ton·ic** \-'tän-ik\ adj

sym·path·i·co·trop·ic cell \-'träp-ik-\ n : any of various large epithelioid cells found in intimate association with unmyelinated nerve fibers in the hilum of the ovary

sym·pa·thin \'sim-pə-thən\ n : a substance (as norepinephrine) that is secreted by sympathetic nerve endings and acts as a chemical mediator

sym·pa·tho·ad·re·nal \,sim-pə-thō-ə-'drēn-ᵊl\ adj : relating to or involving the sympathetic nervous system and the adrenal medulla ⟨the ∼ system⟩ ⟨∼ pathways⟩

sym·pa·tho·blast \'sim-pə-thō-,blast\ n : SYMPATHICOBLAST

sym·pa·tho·go·nia \,sim-pə-thō-'gō-nē-ə\ n : precursor cells of the sympathetic nervous system

sym·pa·tho·go·ni·o·ma \-,gō-nē-'ō-mə\ n, pl **-ma·ta** \-mət-ə\ or **-mas** : a tumor derived from sympathogonia; also : NEUROBLASTOMA

¹**sym·pa·tho·lyt·ic** \,sim-pə-thō-'lit-ik\ adj : tending to oppose the physiological results of sympathetic nervous activity or of sympathomimetic drugs — compare PARASYMPATHOLYTIC

²**sympatholytic** n : a sympatholytic agent

¹**sym·pa·tho·mi·met·ic** \-mə-'met-ik, -(,)mī-\ adj : simulating sympathetic nervous action in physiological effect — compare PARASYMPATHOMIMETIC, SYMPATHOLYTIC

²**sympathomimetic** n : a sympathomimetic agent

sym·pa·thy \'sim-pə-thē\ n, pl **-thies** **1 a** : an affinity, association, or relationship between persons or things wherein whatever affects one similarly affects the other **b** : mutual or parallel susceptibility or a condition brought about by it **2 a** : the act or capacity of entering into or sharing the feelings or interests of another **b** : the feeling or mental state brought about by such sensitivity

sym·phal·an·gism \(,)sim-'fal-ən-,jiz-əm\ n : ankylosis of the joints of one or more digits

sym·phy·se·al \,sim(p)-fə-'sē-əl\ also **sym·phys·i·al** \sim-'fiz-ē-əl\ adj : of, relating to, or constituting a symphysis

symphyseal height n : the distance from the gnathion to a point between the two middle incisors of the lower jaw

sym·phys·i·on \sim-'fiz-ē-,än\ n **1** : the upper end of the symphysis of the jaw at the outer surface **2** : the middle point in the upper border of the pubic arch

sym·phy·si·ot·o·my \,sim(p)-fə-zē-'ät-ə-mē, sim-,fiz-ē-\ n, pl **-mies** : the operation of dividing the pubic symphysis (as to facilitate childbirth)

sym·phy·sis \'sim(p)-fə-səs\ n, pl **-phy·ses** \-,sēz\ **1** : an immovable or more or less movable articulation of various bones in the median plane of the body — see PUBIC SYMPHYSIS **2** : an articulation (as between the bodies of vertebrae) in which the bony surfaces are connected by pads of fibrous cartilage without a synovial membrane

symphysis men·ti \-'men-,tī\ n : the median articulation of the two bones of the lower jaw

symphysis pubis n : PUBIC SYMPHYSIS

sym·plasm \'sim-,plaz-əm\ n **1** : COENOCYTE 1a **2** : an amorphous mass made up of numerous intimately fused bacteria — **sym·plas·mic** \(,)sim-'plaz-mik\ adj

symp·tom \'sim(p)-təm\ n : subjective evidence of disease or physical disturbance observed by the patient ⟨headache is a

∼ of many diseases⟩ ⟨visual disturbances may be a ∼ of retinal arteriosclerosis⟩; *broadly* : something that indicates the presence of a physical disorder — compare SIGN 2

symp·tom·at·ic \,sim(p)-tə-'mat-ik\ adj **1 a** : being a symptom of a disease ⟨gummas ∼ of syphilis⟩ **b** : having the characteristics of a particular disease but arising from another cause ⟨∼ epilepsy resulting from brain damage⟩ **2** : concerned with or affecting symptoms ⟨∼ treatment⟩ **3** : having symptoms ⟨a ∼ patient⟩ — **symp·tom·at·i·cal·ly** \-i-k(ə-)lē\ adv

symptomatic anthrax n : BLACKLEG

symp·tom·atol·o·gy \,sim(p)-tə-mə-'täl-ə-jē\ n, pl **-gies 1** : SYMPTOM COMPLEX **2** : a branch of medical science concerned with symptoms of diseases — **symp·tom·at·o·log·i·cal** \-,mat-ᵊl-'äj-i-kəl\ or **symp·tom·at·o·log·ic** \-'äj-ik\ adj — **symp·tom·at·o·log·i·cal·ly** \-i-k(ə-)lē\ adv

symptom complex n : a group of symptoms occurring together and characterizing a particular disease ⟨the *symptom complex* of epilepsy⟩

symp·tom·less \'sim(p)-təm-ləs\ adj : exhibiting no symptoms ⟨a ∼ infection⟩

symp·to·mol·o·gy \,sim(p)-tə-'mäl-ə-jē\ n, pl **-gies** : SYMPTOMATOLOGY

sym·pus di·pus \'sim-pùs-'dī-pùs\ n : a sirenomelus in which the feet are partly or wholly distinct

synaeresis var of SYNERESIS

synaesthesia, synaesthetic chiefly Brit var of SYNESTHESIA, SYNESTHETIC

syn·anas·to·mo·sis \,sin-ə-,nas-tə-'mō-səs\ n, pl **-mo·ses** \-,sēz\ : an anastomosis involving several vessels

syn·an·throp·ic \,sin-ən-'thräp-ik\ adj : ecologically associated with humans ⟨∼ flies⟩ — **syn·an·thro·py** \sin-'an(t)-thrə-pē\ n, pl **-pies**

¹**syn·apse** \'sin-,aps also sə-'naps, chiefly Brit 'sī-,naps\ n **1** : the place at which a nervous impulse passes from one neuron to another **2** : SYNAPSIS

²**synapse** vi **syn·apsed; syn·aps·ing** : to form a synapse or come together in synapsis

syn·ap·sis \sə-'nap-səs\ n, pl **-ap·ses** \-,sēz\ : the association of homologous chromosomes with chiasma formation that is characteristic of the first meiotic prophase and is held to be the mechanism for genetic crossing-over

syn·ap·tic \si-'nap-tik, Brit also sī-\ adj **1** : of, relating to, or participating in synapsis ⟨∼ chromosomes⟩ **2** : of or relating to a synapse ⟨∼ transmission⟩ — **syn·ap·ti·cal·ly** \-ti-k(ə-)lē\ adv

synaptic cleft n : the space between neurons at a nerve synapse across which a nerve impulse is transmitted by a neurotransmitter — called also *synaptic gap*

synaptic vesicle n : a small secretory vesicle that contains a neurotransmitter, is found inside an axon near the presynaptic membrane, and releases its contents into the synaptic cleft after fusing with the membrane

syn·ap·to·gen·e·sis \sə-,nap-tə-'jen-ə-səs\ n, pl **-e·ses** \-,sēz\ : the formation of nerve synapses

syn·ap·tol·o·gy \,sin-ap-'täl-ə-jē\ n, pl **-gies** : the scientific study of nerve synapses

syn·ap·to·ne·mal complex \sə-,nap-tə-,nē-məl-\ or **syn·ap·ti·ne·mal complex** \same\ n : a complex triparite protein structure that spans the region between synapsed chromosomes in meiotic prophase

syn·ap·to·some \sə-'nap-tə-,sōm\ n : a nerve ending that is isolated from homogenized nerve tissue (as of the brain) — **syn·ap·to·som·al** \-,nap-tə-'sō-məl\ adj

syn·ar·thro·di·al \,sin-är-'thrōd-ē-əl\ adj : of, relating to, or being a synarthrosis

syn·ar·thro·sis \-'thrō-səs\ n, pl **-thro·ses** \-,sēz\ : an immovable articulation in which the bones are united by intervening fibrous connective tissues

---

\ə\ abut \ᵊ\ kitten \ər\ further \a\ ash \ā\ ace \ä\ cot, cart \aù\ out \ch\ chin \e\ bet \ē\ easy \g\ go \i\ hit \ī\ ice \j\ job \ŋ\ sing \ō\ go \ò\ law \òi\ boy \th\ thin \th\ the \ü\ loot \ù\ foot \y\ yet \zh\ vision *See also* Pronunciation Symbols page

syn·car·yon *var of* SYNKARYON

syn·ceph·a·lus \sin-'sef-ə-ləs\ *n, pl* **-li** \-ˌlī\ : a teratological twin fetus having the two heads fused

syn·chon·dro·sis \ˌsin-ˌkän-'drō-səs\ *n, pl* **-dro·ses** \-ˌsēz\ : an immovable skeletal articulation in which the union is cartilaginous

syn·cho·ri·al \ˌsin-'kōr-ē-əl, ˌsin-, -'kȯr-\ *adj* : having a common placenta — used of multiple fetuses ⟨fraternal twins showing ∼ fusion⟩

syn·chro·nic·i·ty \ˌsiŋ-krə-'nis-ət-ē, ˌsin-\ *n, pl* **-ties** : the co-incidental occurrence of events and esp. psychic events (as similar thoughts in widely separated persons or a mental image of an unexpected event before it happens) that seem related but are not explained by conventional mechanisms of causality — used esp. in the psychology of C. G. Jung

syn·chro·nized sleep \'siŋ-krə-ˌnīzd-, 'sin-\ *n* : SLOW-WAVE SLEEP

syn·chro·nous \'siŋ-krə-nəs, 'sin-\ *adj* **1** : happening, existing, or arising at precisely the same time **2** : recurring or operating at exactly the same periods **3** : having the same period; *also* : having the same period and phase — **syn·chro·nous·ly** *adv*

syn·chro·ny \'siŋ-krə-nē, 'sin-\ *n, pl* **-nies** : synchronous occurrence, arrangement, or treatment ⟨cells dividing in ∼⟩

syn·chro·tron \'siŋ-krə-ˌträn, 'sin-\ *n* : an apparatus for imparting very high speeds to charged particles by means of a combination of a high-frequency electric field and a low-frequency magnetic field

syn·co·pal \'siŋ-kə-pəl, 'sin-\ *adj* : of, relating to, or characterized by syncope ⟨experienced ∼ episodes on awakening⟩

syn·co·pe \'siŋ-kə-pē, 'sin-\ *n* : loss of consciousness resulting from insufficient blood flow to the brain : FAINT

syn·cy·tial \sin-'sish-(ē-)əl\ *adj* : of, relating to, or constituting syncytium ⟨∼ tissue⟩

syn·cy·tio·tro·pho·blast \sin-ˌsish-ē-ō-'trō-fə-ˌblast\ *n* : the outer syncytial layer of the trophoblast that actively invades the uterine wall forming the outermost fetal component of the placenta — called also *syntrophoblast;* compare CYTO-TROPHOBLAST

syn·cy·tium \sin-'sish-(ē-)əm\ *n, pl* **-tia** \-(ē-)ə\ **1** : a multinucleate mass of cytoplasm resulting from fusion of cells **2** : COENOCYTE 1

syn·dac·tyl \ˌsin-'dak-tᵊl\ *adj* : having two or more digits wholly or partly united

syn·dac·tyl·ia \ˌsin-ˌdak-'til-ē-ə\ *n* : SYNDACTYLY

syn·dac·ty·lism \(')sin-'dak-tə-ˌliz-əm\ *n* : SYNDACTYLY

syn·dac·ty·lous \(')sin-'dak-tə-ləs\ *adj* : SYNDACTYL

syn·dac·ty·ly \-lē\ *n, pl* **-lies** : a union of two or more digits that is normal in many birds (as kingfishers) and in some lower mammals (as the kangaroos) and that occurs in humans often as a hereditary disorder marked by the joining or webbing of two or more fingers or toes

syn·de·sis \'sin-də-səs\ *n* : SYNAPSIS

syn·des·mo·cho·ri·al \ˌsin-ˌdez-mə-'kō-rē-əl\ *adj, of a placenta* : having fetal epithelium in contact with maternal submucosa (as in ruminants)

syn·des·mo·sis \ˌsin-ˌdez-'mō-səs, -ˌdes-\ *n, pl* **-mo·ses** \-ˌsēz\ : an articulation in which the contiguous surfaces of the bones are rough and are bound together by a ligament

syn·drome \'sin-ˌdrōm *also* -drəm\ *n* : a group of signs and symptoms that occur together and characterize a particular abnormality

syndrome X \-'eks\ *n* **1** : angina pectoris of a usu. benign form in which the coronary arteriogram is normal **2** : METABOLIC SYNDROME

syn·drom·ic \sin-'drō-mik, -'dräm-ik\ *adj* : occurring as a syndrome or part of a syndrome ⟨∼ deafness has obvious other symptoms associated with it⟩

syn·e·chia \si-'nek-ē-ə, -'nēk-\ *n, pl* **-chi·ae** \-ē-ˌē, -ˌī\ : an adhesion of parts and esp. one involving the iris of the eye: as **a** : adhesion of the iris to the cornea — called also *anterior synechia* **b** : adhesion of the iris to the crystalline lens — called also *posterior synechia*

syn·eph·rine \sē-'nef-rən\ *n* : a crystalline sympathomimetic amine $C_9H_{13}NO_2$ isomeric with phenylephrine

syn·ere·sis *also* **syn·ae·re·sis** \ˌsin-ə-'rē-səs, sə-'ner-ə-səs\ *n* : the separation of liquid from a gel caused by contraction

syn·er·get·ic \ˌsin-ər-'jet-ik\ *adj* : SYNERGIC

syn·er·gic \sin-'ər-jik\ *adj* : working together ⟨∼ muscle contraction⟩ — **syn·er·gi·cal·ly** \-ji-k(ə-)lē\ *adv*

syn·er·gism \'sin-ər-ˌjiz-əm\ *n* : interaction of discrete agents (as drugs) such that the total effect is greater than the sum of the individual effects — called also *synergy;* compare ANTAGONISM b

syn·er·gist \-jəst\ *n* **1** : an agent that increases the effectiveness of another agent when combined with it; *esp* : a drug that acts in synergism with another **2** : an organ (as a muscle) that acts in concert with another to enhance its effect — compare AGONIST 1, ANTAGONIST a

syn·er·gis·tic \ˌsin-ər-'jis-tik\ *adj* **1** : having the capacity to act in synergism ⟨∼ drugs⟩ ⟨∼ muscles⟩ **2** : of, relating to, or resembling synergism ⟨a ∼ reaction⟩ ⟨a ∼ effect⟩ — **syn·er·gis·ti·cal·ly** \-ti-k(ə-)lē\ *adv*

syn·er·gize \'sin-ər-ˌjīz\ *vb* **-gized; -giz·ing** *vi* : to act as synergists : exhibit synergism ∼ *vt* : to increase the activity of (a substance)

syn·er·gy \'sin-ər-jē\ *n, pl* **-gies** : SYNERGISM

syn·er·ize \'sin-ə-ˌrīz\ *vi* **-ized; -iz·ing** : to undergo syneresis

syn·es·the·sia *or chiefly Brit* **syn·aes·the·sia** \ˌsin-əs-'thē-zh(ē-)ə\ *n* : a concomitant sensation and esp. a subjective sensation or image of a sense (as of color) other than the one (as of sound) being stimulated; *also* : the condition marked by the experience of such sensations — **syn·es·thet·ic** *or chiefly Brit* **syn·aes·thet·ic** \-'thet-ik\ *adj*

syn·es·thete \'sin-əs-ˌthēt\ *n* : one who experiences synesthesia ⟨for a ∼, a voice can spark color or taste as well as sound —*Psychology Today*⟩

syn·ga·mo·sis \ˌsiŋ-gə-'mō-səs\ *n, pl* **-mo·ses** \-ˌsēz\ : infestation with or disease caused by roundworms of the genus *Syngamus* : GAPES

Syn·ga·mus \'siŋ-gə-məs\ *n* : a genus of strongyloid nematode worms (family Syngamidae) that are parasitic in the trachea or esophagus of various birds and mammals and include the gapeworm (*S. trachea*)

syn·ga·my \'siŋ-gə-mē\ *n, pl* **-mies** : sexual reproduction by union of gametes

syn·ge·ne·ic \ˌsin-jə-'nē-ik\ *adj* : genetically identical esp. with respect to antigens or immunological reactions ⟨∼ tumor cells⟩ ⟨grafts between ∼ mice⟩ — compare ALLOGENEIC, XENOGENEIC

syn·ge·ne·sio·trans·plan·ta·tion \ˌsin-jə-ˌnē-zē-ō-ˌtran(t)s-ˌplan-'tā-shən\ *n* : a graft of material or tissue between closely related individuals of the same species

syn·kary·on *also* **syn·cary·on** \sin-'kar-ē-ˌän, -ē-ən\ *n* : a cell nucleus formed by the fusion of two preexisting nuclei

syn·ki·ne·sia \ˌsin-kə-'nē-zh(ē-)ə, -ˌkī-\ *n* : SYNKINESIS

syn·ki·ne·sis \-'nē-səs\ *n, pl* **-ne·ses** \-ˌsēz\ : involuntary movement in one part when another part is moved : an associated movement

syn·ki·net·ic \-'net-ik\ *adj* : relating to or involving synkinesis ⟨∼ movements⟩

syn·onym \'sin-ə-ˌnim\ *n* : a taxonomic name rejected as being incorrectly applied or incorrect in form — **syn·onym·i·ty** \ˌsin-ə-'nim-ət-ē\ *n, pl* **-ties**

syn·on·y·mize *also Brit* **syn·on·y·mise** \sə-'nän-ə-ˌmīz\ *vt* **-mized** *also Brit* **-mised; -miz·ing** *also Brit* **-mis·ing** : to demonstrate (a taxonomic name) to be a synonym

syn·on·y·my \-mē\ *n, pl* **-mies** : the scientific names that have been used in different publications to designate a taxonomic group (as a species); *also* : a list of these

syn·op·to·phore \sin-'äp-tə-ˌfō(ə)r\ *n* : an instrument for diagnosing imbalance of eye muscles and treating them by orthoptic methods

syn·or·chi·dism \sin-'ȯr-kə-ˌdiz-əm\ *n* : partial or complete fusion of the testes

syn·os·to·sis \ˌsin-ˌäs-'tō-səs\ *n, pl* **-to·ses** \-ˌsēz\ : union of two or more separate bones to form a single bone; *also* : the union so formed (as at an epiphyseal line) — **syn·os·tot·ic** \-ˈtät-ik\ *adj* — **syn·os·tot·i·cal·ly** \-i-k(ə-)lē\ *adv*

syn·o·vec·to·my \ˌsin-ə-ˈvek-tə-mē\ *n, pl* **-mies** : surgical removal of a synovial membrane

sy·no·via \sə-ˈnō-vē-ə, sī-\ *n* : SYNOVIAL FLUID

sy·no·vi·al \-vē-əl\ *adj* : of, relating to, or secreting synovial fluid ⟨∼ effusion⟩; *also* : lined with synovial membrane ⟨a ∼ bursa⟩ ⟨∼ tendon sheaths⟩

synovial cyst *n* : a cyst (as a Baker's cyst) containing synovial fluid

synovial fluid *n* : a transparent viscid lubricating fluid secreted by a membrane of an articulation, bursa, or tendon sheath — called also *joint fluid, synovia*

synovial joint *n* : DIARTHROSIS

synovial membrane *n* : the dense connective-tissue membrane that secretes synovial fluid and that lines the ligamentous surfaces of joint capsules, tendon sheaths where free movement is necessary, and bursae

syn·ovi·o·ma \si-ˌnō-vē-ˈō-mə\ *n, pl* **-mas** *also* **-ma·ta** \-mət-ə\ : a tumor of a synovial membrane

sy·no·vi·tis \ˌsī-nə-ˈvīt-əs\ *n* : inflammation of a synovial membrane usu. with pain and swelling of the joint

sy·no·vi·um \sə-ˈnō-vē-əm, si-\ *n* : SYNOVIAL MEMBRANE

syn·tac·tic \sin-ˈtak-tik\ *or* **syn·tac·ti·cal** \-ti-kəl\ *adj* : of or relating to syntactics — **syn·tac·ti·cal·ly** \-ti-k(ə-)lē\ *adv*

syntactical aphasia *n* : the loss of power to form grammatical constructions

syn·tac·tics \-tiks\ *n pl but sing or pl in constr* : a branch of semiotic that deals with the formal relations between signs or expressions in abstraction from their signification and their interpreters

syn·ten·ic \sin-ˈten-ik\ *adj* : located on the same chromosome ⟨two ∼ genes⟩ — **syn·te·ny** \ˈsin-tə-nē\ *n, pl* **-nies**

syn·thase \ˈsin-ˌthās, -ˌthāz\ *n* : any of various enzymes that catalyze the synthesis of a substance without involving the breaking of a high-energy phosphate bond (as in ATP)

syn·the·sis \ˈsin(t)-thə-səs\ *n, pl* **-the·ses** \-ˌsēz\ **1** : the composition or combination of parts or elements so as to form a whole **2** : the production of a substance by the union of chemical elements, groups, or simpler compounds or by the degradation of a complex compound ⟨protein ∼⟩

syn·the·size *also Brit* **syn·the·sise** \-ˌsīz\ *vt* **-sized** *also Brit* **-sised**; **-siz·ing** *also Brit* **-sis·ing** : to combine or produce by synthesis ⟨∼ penicillin⟩

syn·the·tase \ˈsin-thə-ˌtās, -ˌtāz\ *n* : an enzyme that catalyzes the linking together of two molecules esp. by using the energy derived from the concurrent splitting off of a pyrophosphate group from a triphosphate (as ATP) — called also *ligase*

¹**syn·thet·ic** \sin-ˈthet-ik\ *adj* : of, relating to, or produced by chemical or biochemical synthesis; *esp* : produced artificially ⟨∼ drugs⟩ ⟨∼ dyes⟩ — **syn·thet·i·cal·ly** \-i-k(ə-)lē\ *adv*

²**synthetic** *n* : a product (as a drug) of chemical synthesis

synthetic resin *n* : RESIN 2a

Syn·throid \ˈsin-ˌthróid\ *trademark* — used for a preparation of the sodium salt of levothyroxine

syn·ton·ic \sin-ˈtän-ik\ *adj* : normally responsive and adaptive to the social or interpersonal environment ⟨a ∼ personality⟩

syn·tro·phism \ˈsin-trə-ˌfiz-əm\ *n* : mutual dependence (as of different strains of bacteria) for the satisfaction of nutritional needs

syn·tro·pho·blast \(ˈ)sin-ˈtrō-fə-ˌblast\ *n* : SYNCYTIOTROPHOBLAST

Sy·pha·cia \sī-ˈfā-shē-ə\ *n* : a genus of nematode worms of the family Oxyuridae that includes one (*S. obvelata*) normally parasitic in the cecum and colon of rodents and rarely in humans

syph·i·lid \ˈsif-ə-lid\ *n* : a skin eruption caused by syphilis — called also *syphiloderm*

syph·i·lis \ˈsif-(ə-)ləs\ *n* : a chronic contagious usu. venereal and often congenital disease that is caused by a spirochete of the genus *Treponema* (*T. pallidum*) and if left untreated produces chancres, rashes, and systemic lesions in a clinical course with three stages continued over many years — called also *lues;* see PRIMARY SYPHILIS, SECONDARY SYPHILIS, TERTIARY SYPHILIS

Syph·i·lus \ˈsif-ə-ləs\, literary character. Syphilus is the hero of the 1530 Latin poem "Syphilis or the French Disease," which was written by the Italian physician and poet Girolamo Fracastoro. Syphilus is a swineherd who blasphemes a sun god and as a punishment is afflicted with a disease.

¹**syph·i·lit·ic** \ˌsif-ə-ˈlit-ik\ *adj* : of, relating to, or infected with syphilis — **syph·i·lit·i·cal·ly** \-i-k(ə-)lē\ *adv*

²**syphilitic** *n* : an individual infected with syphilis

syph·i·lo·derm \ˈsif-ə-lō-ˌdərm\ *n* : SYPHILID

syph·i·loid \ˈsif-ə-ˌlóid\ *adj* : resembling syphilis ⟨a ∼ disease⟩

syph·i·lol·o·gist \ˌsif-ə-ˈläl-ə-jəst\ *n* : a physician who specializes in syphilology

syph·i·lol·o·gy \-jē\ *n, pl* **-gies** : a branch of medicine that deals with the diagnosis and treatment of syphilis — **syph·i·lo·log·ic** \ˌsif-ə-lə-ˈläj-ik\ *adj*

syph·i·lo·ma \ˌsif-ə-ˈlō-mə\ *n, pl* **-mas** *or* **-ma·ta** \-mət-ə\ : a syphilitic tumor : GUMMA ⟨a testicular ∼⟩

syph·i·lo·pho·bia \ˌsif-ə-lō-ˈfō-bē-ə\ *n* : abnormal dread of syphilis or fear of being infected with it

syph·i·lo·ther·a·py \-ˈther-ə-pē\ *n, pl* **-pies** : the treatment of syphilis ⟨∼ with penicillin⟩

Syr·a·cuse watch glass \ˈsir-ə-ˌkyüs-, -ˌkyüz-\ *n* : a small circular flat-bottomed dish of thick glass with a shallow depression used in biology (as for staining, culturing, and various phases of microtechnique) — called also *Syracuse dish*

sy·rette \sə-ˈret\ *n, often cap* : a small collapsible tube fitted with a hypodermic needle for injecting a single dose of a medicinal agent

syr·ing·ad·e·no·ma \ˌsir-iŋ-ˌ(g)ad-ᵊn-ˈō-mə\ *n, pl* **-mas** *also* **-ma·ta** \-mət-ə\ : adenoma of a sweat gland

sy·ringe \sə-ˈrinj *also* ˈsir-inj\ *n* : a device used to inject fluids into or withdraw them from something (as the body or its cavities): as **a** : a device that consists of a nozzle of varying length and a compressible rubber bulb and is used for injection or irrigation ⟨an ear ∼⟩ **b** : an instrument (as for the injection of medicine or the withdrawal of bodily fluids) that consists of a hollow barrel fitted with a plunger and a hollow needle **c** : a gravity device consisting of a reservoir fitted with a long rubber tube ending with an exchangeable nozzle that is used for irrigation of the vagina or bowel — **syringe** *vt* **sy·ringed; sy·ring·ing**

sy·rin·go·bul·bia \sə-ˌriŋ-gō-ˈbəl-bē-ə\ *n* : the presence of abnormal cavities in the medulla oblongata

sy·rin·go·cyst·ad·e·no·ma \sə-ˌriŋ-gō-ˌsist-ˌad-ᵊn-ˈō-mə\ *n, pl* **-mas** *also* **-ma·ta** \-mət-ə\ : SYRINGADENOMA

syr·in·go·ma \ˌsir-iŋ-ˈgō-mə\ *n, pl* **-mas** *also* **-ma·ta** \-mət-ə\ : SYRINGADENOMA

sy·rin·go·my·elia \sə-ˌriŋ-gō-mī-ˈē-lē-ə\ *n* : a chronic progressive disease of the spinal cord associated with sensory disturbances, muscle atrophy, and spasticity — **sy·rin·go·my·el·ic** \-ˈel-ik\ *adj*

syr·inx \ˈsir-iŋ(k)s\ *n, pl* **sy·rin·ges** \sə-ˈriŋ-ˌgēz, -ˈrin-ˌjēz\ *or* **syr·inx·es** **1** : the vocal organ of birds that is a special modification of the lower part of the trachea or of the bronchi or of both **2** : a pathological cavity in the brain or spinal cord esp. in syringomyelia

syr·o·sin·go·pine \ˌsir-ō-ˈsiŋ-gə-ˌpēn, -ˌpīn\ *n* : a white crystalline powder $C_{35}H_{42}N_2O_{11}$ that is closely related to reserpine and is used as an antihypertensive drug

syr·up *also* **sir·up** \ˈsər-əp, ˈsir-əp\ *n* : a thick sticky liquid consisting of a concentrated solution of sugar and water with or without the addition of a flavoring agent or medicinal substance ⟨∼ of codeine⟩ — **syr·upy** *or* **sir·upy** \-ē\ *adj*

syrup of ipecac *n* : IPECAC SYRUP

\ə\ **abut** \ᵊ\ **kitten** \ər\ **further** \a\ **ash** \ā\ **ace** \ä\ **cot, cart** \aú\ **out** \ch\ **chin** \e\ **bet** \ē\ **easy** \g\ **go** \i\ **hit** \ī\ **ice** \j\ **job** \ŋ\ **sing** \ō\ **go** \ó\ **law** \ói\ **boy** \th\ **thin** \t̲h̲\ **the** \ü\ **loot** \ú\ **foot** \y\ **yet** \zh\ **vision** *See also* Pronunciation Symbols page

S
T

sys·tem \'sis-təm\ *n* **1 a** : a group of body organs or structures that together perform one or more vital functions — see CIRCULATORY SYSTEM, DIGESTIVE SYSTEM, ENDOCRINE SYSTEM, LIMBIC SYSTEM, NERVOUS SYSTEM, REPRODUCTIVE SYSTEM, RESPIRATORY SYSTEM **b** : the body considered as a functional unit **2** : a manner of classifying, symbolizing, or schematizing ⟨a taxonomic ∼⟩

sys·tem·at·ic \ˌsis-tə-'mat-ik\ *adj* : of, relating to, or concerned with classification; *specif* : TAXONOMIC — **sys·tem·at·i·cal·ly** \-i-k(ə-)lē\ *adv*

sys·tem·at·ics \ˌsis-tə-'mat-iks\ *n pl but sing in constr* **1** : the science of classification **2 a** : a system of classification **b** : the classification and study of organisms with regard to their natural relationships : TAXONOMY

sys·tem·a·tist \'sis-tə-mət-əst\ *n* : a classifying scientist : TAXONOMIST

sys·tem·atize *also Brit* **sys·tem·atise** \'sis-tə-mə-ˌtīz\ *vt* **-atized** *also Brit* **-atised; -atiz·ing** *also Brit* **-atis·ing** : to arrange in accord with a definite plan or scheme : order systematically ⟨a patient with *systematized* delusions⟩ — **sys·tem·ati·za·tion** *also Brit* **sys·tem·ati·sa·tion** \ˌsis-tə-mət-ə-'zā-shən, sis-ˌtem-ət-\ *n*

¹sys·tem·ic \sis-'tem-ik\ *adj* : of, relating to, or common to a system: as **a** : affecting the body generally — compare LOCAL **b** : supplying those parts of the body that receive blood through the aorta rather than through the pulmonary artery **c** : being a pesticide that as used is harmless to a higher animal or a plant but when absorbed into the bloodstream or the sap makes the whole organism toxic to pests (as cattle grubs, mites, or aphids) — **sys·tem·i·cal·ly** \-i-k(ə-)lē\ *adv*

²systemic *n* : a systemic pesticide

systemic circulation *n* : the passage of arterial blood from the left atrium of the heart through the left ventricle, the systemic arteries, and the capillaries to the organs and tissues that receive much of its oxygen in exchange for carbon dioxide and the return of the carbon-dioxide carrying blood via the systemic veins to enter the right atrium of the heart and to participate in the pulmonary circulation

systemic heart *n* : the part of the heart propelling blood through the systemic circulation; *specif* : the left atrium and ventricle of higher vertebrates

systemic inflammatory response syndrome *n* : a severe systemic response to a condition (as trauma, an infection, or a burn) that provokes an acute inflammatory reaction indicated by the presence of two or more of a group of symptoms including abnormally increased or decreased body temperature, heart rate greater than 90 beats per minute, respiratory rate greater than 20 breaths per minute or a reduced concentration of carbon dioxide in the arterial blood, and the white blood cell count greatly decreased or increased or consisting of more than ten percent immature neutrophils — abbr. *SIRS*; see SEPSIS

systemic lupus er·y·the·ma·to·sus \-ˌer-ə-ˌthē-mə-'tō-səs\ *n* : an inflammatory connective tissue disease of unknown cause that occurs chiefly in women and that is characterized esp. by fever, skin rash, and arthritis, often by acute hemolytic anemia, by small hemorrhages in the skin and mucous membranes, by inflammation of the pericardium, and in serious cases by involvement of the kidneys and central nervous system — called also *systemic lupus*

systemic necrotizing vasculitis *n* : NECROTIZING VASCULITIS

sys·to·le \'sis-tə-(ˌ)lē\ *n* : the contraction of the heart by which the blood is forced onward and the circulation kept up — compare DIASTOLE 1 — **sys·tol·ic** \sis-'täl-ik\ *adj*

systolic blood pressure *n* : the highest arterial blood pressure of a cardiac cycle occurring immediately after systole of the left ventricle of the heart — called also *systolic pressure;* compare DIASTOLIC BLOOD PRESSURE

T

T *abbr* **1** tesla **2** thoracic — used with a number from 1 to 12 to indicate a vertebra or segment of the spinal cord ⟨multiple injuries with a fracture of *T-12*⟩ **3** thymine

T *symbol* **1** absolute temperature **2** tritium

2,4,5–T — see entry alphabetized as TWO,FOUR,FIVE-T

Ta *symbol* tantalum

TA *abbr* transactional analysis

tab \'tab\ *n* : TABLET

¹tab·a·nid \'tab-ə-nid, tə-'ban-id\ *adj* : of or relating to the family Tabanidae

²tabanid *n* : any fly (as a horsefly) of the family Tabanidae

Ta·ban·i·dae \tə-'ban-ə-ˌdē\ *n pl* : a very large family of the order Diptera comprising the horseflies and deerflies whose females suck blood and sometimes transmit disease (as loaiasis) to human beings

Ta·ba·nus \tə-'bā-nəs, -'ba-\ *n* : the type genus of the family Tabanidae comprising various horseflies

ta·bar·dil·lo \ˌtä-bär-'dē-yō\ *n* : murine typhus occurring esp. in Mexico

ta·bel·la \tə-'bel-ə\ *n, pl* **-lae** \-ˌlē\ : a medicated lozenge or tablet

ta·bes \'tā-(ˌ)bēz\ *n, pl* **tabes 1** : wasting accompanying a chronic disease **2** : TABES DORSALIS

tabes dor·sa·lis \-dȯr-'sā-ləs, -'sal-əs\ *n* : a syphilitic disorder that involves the dorsal horns of the spinal cord and the sensory nerve trunks and that is marked by wasting, pain, lack of coordination of voluntary movements and reflexes, and disorders of sensation, nutrition, and vision — called also *locomotor ataxia*

¹ta·bet·ic \tə-'bet-ik\ *adj* : of, relating to, or affected with tabes and esp. tabes dorsalis ⟨∼ pains⟩ ⟨a ∼ joint⟩

²tabetic *n* : an individual affected with tabes dorsalis

tab·id \'tab-əd\ *adj* : TABETIC

ta·ble \'tā-bəl\ *n* **1** : a piece of furniture consisting of a smooth flat slab fixed on legs; *esp* : one used for examining or operating **2** : either of the two layers of compact bone of the skull which are separated by cancellous diploe

table salt *n* : salt and esp. sodium chloride refined for use at the table and in cooking

ta·ble·spoon \'tā-bəl-ˌspün\ *n* : a unit of measure equal to 4 fluid drams or ½ fluid ounce or 15 milliliters

ta·ble·spoon·ful \ˌtā-bəl-'spün-ˌfůl, 'tā-bəl-ˌ\ *n, pl* **ta·ble·spoon·fuls** \-ˌfůlz\ *also* **ta·ble·spoons·ful** \-'spünz-ˌfůl, -ˌspünz-\ : TABLESPOON

tab·let \'tab-lət\ *n* : a small mass of medicated material (as in the shape of a disk) ⟨an aspirin ∼⟩

tablet triturate *n* : a small tablet made by molding fine moistened powder containing a medicinal and a diluent

¹ta·boo *also* **ta·bu** \tə-'bü, ta-\ *n, pl* **taboos** *also* **tabus 1** : a prohibition in some cultures against touching, saying, or doing something for fear of immediate harm from a mysterious superhuman force **2** : a prohibition imposed by social custom or as a protective measure ⟨the view that incest, not cannibalism, was the world's first ∼ —Phyllis Grosskurth⟩ **3** : belief in taboos — **taboo** *also* **tabu** *adj*

²taboo *also* **tabu** *vt* : to avoid or ban as taboo

ta·bo·pa·ral·y·sis \ˌtä-bō-pə-'ral-ə-səs\ *n, pl* **-y·ses** \-ˌsēz\ : TABOPARESIS

ta·bo·pa·re·sis \-pə-'rē-səs, -'par-ə-səs\ *n, pl* **-re·ses** \-ˌsēz\ : paresis occurring with tabes and esp. with tabes dorsalis

tab·u·lar \'tab-yə-lər\ *adj* : having the form of a thin plate or scale ⟨a ∼ crystal⟩

ta·bun \'tä-ˌbùn\ *n* : a liquid organic phosphorus ester $C_5H_{11}N_2O_2P$ that acts as a nerve gas

tache noire \'täsh-'nwär\ *n, pl* **taches noires** \'täsh-'nwär(z)\ : a small dark-centered ulcer that appears at the site of a tick bite and is the primary lesion of boutonneuse fever

ta·chis·to·scope \tə-'kis-tə-ˌskōp-, ta-\ *n* : an apparatus for the brief exposure of visual stimuli that is used in the study of learning, attention, and perception — **ta·chis·to·scop·ic** \-ˌkis-tə-'skäp-ik\ *adj* — **ta·chis·to·scop·i·cal·ly** \-i-k(ə-)lē\ *adv*

tachy·ar·rhyth·mia \ˌtak-ē-ā-'rith-mē-ə\ *n* : arrhythmia characterized by a rapid irregular heartbeat

tachy·car·dia \ˌtak-i-'kärd-ē-ə\ *n* : relatively rapid heart action whether physiological (as after exercise) or pathological — see JUNCTIONAL TACHYCARDIA, PAROXYSMAL TACHYCARDIA, SINUS TACHYCARDIA, VENTRICULAR TACHYCARDIA; compare BRADYCARDIA

tachy·car·di·ac \-ē-ˌak\ *adj* : relating to or affected with tachycardia

tachy·phy·lac·tic \-fi-'lak-tik\ *adj* : of or relating to tachyphylaxis

tachy·phy·lax·is \ˌtak-i-fi-'lak-səs\ *n, pl* **-lax·es** \-ˌsēz\ : diminished response to later increments in a sequence of applications of a physiologically active substance (as the diminished pressor response that follows repeated injections of renin)

tachy·pnea *or chiefly Brit* **tachy·pnoea** \ˌtak-i(p)-'nē-ə\ *n* : increased rate of respiration — **tachy·pne·ic** *or chiefly Brit* **tachy·pnoe·ic** \-'nē-ik\ *adj*

tachy·rhyth·mia \ˌtak-i-'rith-mē-ə\ *n* : TACHYCARDIA

ta·chys·ter·ol \ta-'kist-ə-ˌról, -ˌrōl\ *n* : an oily liquid alcohol $C_{28}H_{43}OH$ isomeric with ergosterol that is formed by ultraviolet irradiation of ergosterol or lumisterol and that on further irradiation yields vitamin D_2 — see DIHYDROTACHYSTEROL

tac·rine \'tak-ˌrēn, -ˌrīn\ *n* : an anticholinesterase that is administered in the form of its hydrochloride $C_{13}H_{14}N_2 \cdot HCl$ and is used esp. in the palliative treatment of cognitive deficits in learning, memory, and mood associated with Alzheimer's disease — called also *tetrahydroaminoacridine, THA;* see COGNEX

tac·tic \'tak-tik\ *adj* **1** : regular in structure of repeating units in a polymer **2** : of, relating to, or showing biological taxis

tac·tic·i·ty \tak-'tis-ət-ē\ *n, pl* **-ties** : the quality or state of being stereochemically tactic

¹tac·tile \'tak-t⁰l, -ˌtīl\ *adj* **1** : of, relating to, mediated by, or affecting the sense of touch ⟨~ sensations⟩ ⟨~ stimuli⟩ ⟨~ anesthesia⟩ **2** : having or being organs or receptors for the sense of touch — **tac·tile·ly** \-ē\ *adv*

²tactile *n* : a person whose prevailing mental imagery is tactile rather than visual, auditory, or motor — compare AUDILE, MOTILE, VISUALIZER

tactile cell *n* : one of the oval nucleated cells (as in a Meissner's corpuscle) that are in close contact with the expanded ends of nerve fibers in the deeper layers of the epidermis and dermis of some parts of the body and prob. serve a tactile function

tactile corpuscle *n* : one of the numerous minute bodies (as a Meissner's corpuscle) in the skin and some mucous membranes that usu. consist of a group of cells enclosed in a capsule, contain nerve terminations, and are held to be end organs of touch — called also *touch corpuscle*

tactile receptor *n* : an end organ (as a Meissner's corpuscle or a Pacinian corpuscle) that responds to light touch

tac·toid \'tak-ˌtóid\ *n* : an elongated particle (as in a sickle cell, myosin, or fibrin) that appears as a spindle-shaped body under a polarizing microscope

tac·tu·al \'tak-chə-wəl\ *adj* : of or relating to the sense or the organs of touch : derived from or producing the sensation of touch : TACTILE ⟨~ stimuli⟩ — **tac·tu·al·ly** \-ē\ *adv*

ta·dal·a·fil \tə-'dal-ə-ˌfil\ *n* : a drug $C_{22}H_{19}N_3O_4$ that is used to treat erectile dysfunction and has a mechanism of action similar to that of sildenafil — see CIALIS

tae·di·um vi·tae \ˌtēd-ē-əm-'vī-ˌtē, ˌtīd-ē-əm-'wē-ˌtī\ *n* : weariness or loathing of life

tae·nia \'tē-nē-ə\ *n* **1 a** *also* **te·nia** \'tē-nē-ə\ *pl* **taenias** *also* **tenias** : TAPEWORM **b** *cap* : a genus of cyclophyllidean tapeworms that is the type of the family Taeniidae, that comprises forms usu. occurring as adults in the intestines of carnivores and as larvae in various ruminants, and that includes the beef tapeworm (*T. saginata*) and the pork tapeworm (*T. solium*) of humans **2** *or* **tenia** *pl* **tae·ni·ae** \-nē-ˌē, -ˌī\ *or* **tae·nias** *or* **te·ni·ae** *or* **tenias** : a band of nervous tissue or of muscle

tae·nia·cide *also* **te·nia·cide** \'tē-nē-ə-ˌsīd\ *n* : an agent that destroys tapeworms — **tae·nia·cid·al** *also* **te·nia·cid·al** \ˌtē-nē-ə-'sīd-⁰l\ *adj*

taenia co·li *or* **tenia coli** \-'kō-ˌlī\ *n, pl* **taeniae coli** *or* **teniae coli** : any of three external longitudinal muscle bands of the large intestine

tae·nia·fuge *also* **te·nia·fuge** \'tē-nē-ə-ˌfyüj\ *n* : an agent that expels tapeworms

Tae·nia·rhyn·chus \ˌtē-nē-ə-'riŋ-kəs\ *n, in some classifications* : a genus of tapeworms comprising the beef tapeworm of humans that is now usu. placed in the genus *Taenia*

tae·ni·a·sis *or* **te·ni·a·sis** \tē-'nī-ə-səs\ *n* : infestation with or disease caused by tapeworms

tae·ni·id \'tē-nē-əd\ *n* : any tapeworm of the family Taeniidae — **taeniid** *adj*

Tae·ni·idae \tē-'nī-ə-ˌdē\ *n pl* : a large family of tapeworms of the order Cyclophyllidea that includes numerous forms of medical or veterinary importance

tae·ni·oid \'tē-nē-ˌóid\ *adj* : resembling or related to the family Taeniidae

¹tag \'tag\ *n* **1 a** : a shred of flesh or muscle **b** : a small abnormal projecting piece of tissue esp. when potentially or actually neoplastic in character **2** : LABEL

²tag *vt* **tagged; tag·ging** : LABEL ⟨*tagged* antibodies⟩

Tag·a·met \'tag-ə-mət, -ˌmet\ *trademark* — used for a preparation of cimetidine

tag·a·tose \'tag-ə-ˌtōs *also* -ˌtōz\ *n* : a crystalline ketohexose sugar $C_6H_{12}O_6$ found naturally in the D-form (as in gum from a West African tree *Sterculia setigera* and in various dairy products) and also obtainable from galactose by treatment with dilute alkali that is nearly as sweet as sucrose and is used as a low-calorie sweetener

tai chi *also* **t'ai chi** \'tī-'jē, -'chē\ *n, often cap T&C* : an ancient Chinese discipline involving a continuous series of controlled usu. slow movements designed to improve physical and mental well-being — called also *t'ai chi ch'uan, tai chi chuan* \-chü-'än\

tail \'tā(ə)l\ *n, often attrib* **1** : the rear end or a process or prolongation of the rear end of the body of an animal **2** : one end of a molecule regarded as opposite to the head; *esp* : the end of a lipid molecule that consists of a nonpolar hydrocarbon chain and is opposite to the polar group ⟨most surface-active agents have a long hydrophobic ~ attached to a polar head —R. E. Kirk & D. F. Othmer⟩ **3** : any of various parts of bodily structures that are terminal: as **a** : the distal tendon of a muscle **b** : the slender left end of the human pancreas **c** : the common convoluted tube that forms the lower part of the epididymis **4** : the motile part of a sperm that extends from the middle piece to the end and comprises the flagellum **5** : a thin protein tube which forms part of the coat of some bacteriophages and through which DNA is injected into a cell — **tailed** \'tā(ə)ld\ *adj* — **tail·less** \'tā(ə)l-les\ *adj*

tail·bone \-'bōn, -ˌbōn\ *n* **1** : a caudal vertebra **2** : COCCYX

tail bud *n* : a knob of embryonic tissue not divided into germ layers that arises at the primitive knot and contributes to the formation of the posterior part of the vertebrate body — called also *end bud*

S
T

tai·lor's muscle *or* **tai·lor muscle** \'tā-lər(z)-\ *n* : SARTORIUS

Taka–Di·a·stase \'tä-kə-'dī-ə-ˌstās\ *trademark* — used for an enzyme preparation obtained from a mold of the genus *Aspergillus* (*A. oryzae*) and used chiefly as a starch digestant

Ta·ka·ya·su's arteritis \ˌtä-kə-'yä-süz-\ *n* : a chronic inflammatory disease esp. of the aorta and its major branches (as the brachiocephalic artery and left common carotid artery) that results in progressive stenosis, occlusion, and aneurysm formation and is marked esp. by diminution or loss of the pulse (as in the arm) and by ischemic symptoms (as pain or weakness of the extremities, fainting, visual disturbances, or renovascular hypertension) — called also *pulseless disease, Takayasu's disease*

Ta·ka·ya·su \tä-kä-yä-sü\, **Michishige** (1872–1938), Japanese physician.

¹**take** \'tāk\ *vi* **took** \'túk\; **tak·en** \'tā-kən\; **tak·ing 1** : to establish a take esp. by uniting or growing ⟨with an experienced surgeon some 90 percent of the grafts ∼ —*Lancet*⟩ **2** *of a vaccine or vaccination* : to produce a take

²**take** *n* **1** : a local or systemic reaction indicative of successful vaccination **2** : a successful union (as of a graft)

take up *vt* : to absorb or incorporate into itself ⟨the rate at which the cells *took up* glucose⟩ — **take–up** *n*

talc \'talk\ *n* : a very soft mineral $Mg_3Si_4O_{10}(OH)_2$ that is a basic silicate of magnesium, has a soapy feel, and is used esp. in making talcum powder

tal·cum \'tal-kəm\ *n* : TALC

talcum powder *n* **1** : powdered talc **2** : a toilet powder composed of perfumed talc or talc and some mild antiseptic

tali *pl of* TALUS

tali — see SUSTENTACULUM TALI

tali·pes \'tal-ə-ˌpēz\ *n* : CLUBFOOT 1

talipes equi·no·var·us \-ˌek-wi-nō-'var-əs\ *n* : a congenital deformity of the foot in which both talipes equinus and talipes varus occur so that walking is done on the toes and outer side of the foot

talipes equi·nus \-'ek-wi-nəs\ *n* : a congenital deformity of the foot in which the sole is permanently flexed so that walking is done on the toes without touching the heel to the ground

talipes valgus *n* : a congenital deformity of the foot in which it is rotated inward so that walking is done on the inner side of the sole

talipes varus *n* : a congenital deformity of the foot in which it is rotated outward so that walking is done on the outer side of the sole

talk therapy \'tók-\ *n* : psychotherapy emphasizing conversation between therapist and patient

tall fescue \'tól-\ *n* : a European fescue (*Festuca elatior* syn. *F. arundinacea*) with erect smooth stems 3 to 4 feet (about 1 meter) high that has been introduced into No. America — called also *tall fescue grass;* see FESCUE FOOT

tal·low \'tal-(ˌ)ō, -ə-(w)\ *n* : the white nearly tasteless solid rendered fat of cattle and sheep which is used chiefly in soap, margarine, candles, and lubricants and of which the form obtained from domestic sheep (*Ovis aries*) is used in pharmacy in ointments and cerates

ta·lo·cal·ca·ne·al \ˌtä-lō-kal-'kä-nē-əl\ *adj* **1** : of or relating to the talus and the calcaneus **2** : relating to or being the articulation of the talus and the calcaneus

ta·lo·cru·ral \-'krúr-əl\ *adj* : relating to or being the ankle joint ⟨the ∼ articulation⟩

tal·on \'tal-ən\ *n* : the crushing region of the crown of an upper molar

ta·lo·na·vic·u·lar \ˌtä-lō-nə-'vik-yə-lər\ *adj* : of or relating to the talus and the navicular of the tarsus

tal·on·id \'tal-ə-nəd\ *n* : the crushing region of a lower molar tooth usu. better developed than the corresponding talon

tal·ose \'tal-ˌōs\ *n* : a rare aldohexose sugar $C_6H_{12}O_6$ obtained indirectly from galactose

ta·lo·tib·i·al \ˌtä-lō-'tib-ē-əl\ *adj* : of or relating to the talus and the tibia ⟨performed a ∼ capsulotomy⟩

ta·lus \'tā-ləs\ *n, pl* **ta·li** \'tā-ˌlī\ **1** : the human astragalus that bears the weight of the body and together with the tibia and fibula forms the ankle joint — called also *anklebone* **2** : the entire ankle

Tal·win \'tal-ˌwin\ *trademark* — used for a preparation of pentazocine

tam·a·rind \'tam-ə-rənd, -ˌrind\ *n* **1** : a tropical leguminous tree (*Tamarindus indica*) with hard yellowish wood and a fruit with an acid pulp **2** : the pulp of the partially dried ripe fruit of a tamarind used in herbal medicine esp. for its laxative properties

tam·bour \'tam-ˌbú(ə)r, tam-'\ *n* : a shallow metallic cup or drum with a thin elastic membrane supporting a writing lever used to transmit and register slight motions (as arterial pulsations and peristaltic contractions)

ta·mox·i·fen \ta-'mäk-si-ˌfen\ *n* : a selective estrogen receptor modulator that acts as an estrogen antagonist in breast tissue and is administered orally in the form of its citrate $C_{26}H_{29}NO·C_6H_8O_7$ esp. to treat breast cancer — see NOLVADEX

tam·pan \'tam-ˌpan\ *n* : any of various ticks of the family Argasidae; *esp* : FOWL TICK

Tam·pi·co jalap \tam-'pē-kō-\ *n* : the dried root of a Mexican morning glory of the genus *Ipomoea* (*I. simulans*) or the powdered drug containing a resin prepared from it

¹**tam·pon** \'tam-ˌpän\ *n* : a wad of absorbent material (as cotton) introduced into a body cavity or canal usu. to absorb secretions (as from menstruation) or to arrest hemorrhaging

²**tampon** *vt* : to place or insert a tampon into

tam·pon·ade \ˌtam-pə-'nād\ *also* **tam·pon·age** \'tam-pə-nij\ *n* **1** : the closure or blockage (as of a wound or body cavity) by or as if by a tampon esp. to stop bleeding **2** : CARDIAC TAMPONADE

tam·su·lo·sin \tam-'sü-lə-sən\ *n* : an alpha-adrenergic blocking agent administered orally in the form of its hydrochloride $C_{20}H_{28}N_2O_5S·HCl$ to treat benign prostatic hyperplasia — see FLOMAX

¹**tan** \'tan\ *vb* **tanned**; **tan·ning** *vt* : to make (skin) tan esp. by exposure to the sun ∼ *vi* : to get or become tanned

²**tan** *n* : a brown color imparted to the skin by exposure to the sun or wind

T and A *abbr* tonsillectomy and adenoidectomy

tan·dem repeat \'tan-dəm-\ *n* : any of several identical DNA segments lying one after the other in a sequence — compare LONG TERMINAL REPEAT

tan·gle \'taŋ-gəl\ *n* : NEUROFIBRILLARY TANGLE

tan·nate \'tan-ˌāt\ *n* : a compound of a tannin

tan·nic acid \ˌtan-ik-\ *n* **1** : a tannin occurring esp. in extracts from nutgalls and yielding gallic acid on hydrolysis — called also *digallic acid, gallotannic acid, gallotannin* **2** : TANNIN 1

tan·nin \'tan-ən\ *n* **1** : any of various soluble astringent complex phenolic substances of plant origin used in tanning, dyeing, the making of ink, and in medicine as astringents and formerly in the treatment of burns **2** : a substance that has a tanning effect

tan·ning \'tan-iŋ\ *n* : a browning of the skin by exposure to the sun

tan·ta·lum \'tant-ᵊl-əm\ *n* : a hard ductile gray-white acid‑resisting metallic element of the vanadium family found combined in rare minerals and sometimes used in surgical implants and sutures — symbol *Ta*; see ELEMENT table

T antigen \'tē-\ *n* : any of several proteins that are produced by some tumorigenic DNA viruses (as simian virus 40) when they infect cells and that function in the transformation of normal cells into tumor cells or into tumor-forming cells and in the unwinding and replication of the DNA of the virus

tan·trum \'tan-trəm\ *n* : a fit of bad temper

¹**tap** \'tap\ *n* : the procedure of removing fluid (as from a body cavity) — see LUMBAR PUNCTURE

²**tap** *vt* **tapped**; **tap·ping** : to pierce so as to let out or draw off a fluid ⟨∼ the spine for a specimen of cerebrospinal fluid⟩

³**tap** *vt* **tapped**; **tap·ping** : to strike lightly esp. with a slight sound

⁴**tap** *n* : a light usu. audible blow; *also* : its sound

¹tape \'tāp\ *n* : a narrow band of woven fabric; *esp* : ADHESIVE TAPE

²tape *vt* **taped; tap·ing** : to fasten, tie, bind, cover, or support with tape and esp. adhesive tape

ta·pe·tal \tə-'pēt-ᵊl\ *adj* : of or relating to a tapetum

ta·pe·to·ret·i·nal \tə-ˌpēt-ō-'ret-ᵊn-əl\ *adj* : of, relating to, or involving both tapetum and retina ⟨∼ degeneration⟩

ta·pe·tum \tə-'pēt-əm\ *n, pl* **ta·pe·ta** \-'pēt-ə\ **1** : any of various membranous layers or areas esp. of the choroid and retina of the eye; *specif* : TAPETUM LUCIDUM **2** : a layer of nerve fibers derived from the corpus callosum and forming part of the roof of each lateral ventricle of the brain

tapetum lu·ci·dum \-'lü-si-dəm\ *n* : a layer in the choroid chiefly of nocturnal mammals that reflects light causing the eyes to glow when light strikes them at night and that is made up of several layers of flattened cells covered by a zone of doubly refracting crystals

tape·worm \'tāp-ˌwərm\ *n* : any of the class Cestoda of flatworms that are parasitic as adults in the alimentary tract of vertebrates including humans and as larvae in a great variety of vertebrates and invertebrates, that typically consist of an attachment organ usu. with suckers, grooves, hooks, or other devices for adhering to the host's intestine followed by an undifferentiated growth region from which buds off a chain of segments of which the anterior members are little more than blocks of tissue, the median members have fully developed organs of both sexes, and the posterior members are degenerated to egg-filled sacs, that have no digestive system and absorb food through the body wall, and that have a nervous system consisting of ganglia and commissures in the scolex and longitudinal cords extending the length of the strobila — called also *cestode;* see BEEF TAPEWORM, CAT TAPEWORM, DOG TAPEWORM, FISH TAPEWORM, FRINGED TAPEWORM, PORK TAPEWORM

ta·pote·ment \tə-'pōt-mənt\ *n* : PERCUSSION 2

tar \'tär\ *n* **1** : any of various dark brown or black bituminous usu. odorous viscous liquids obtained by destructive distillation of organic material (as wood, coal, or peat); *esp* : one used medicinally (as to treat skin diseases) — see COAL TAR, JUNIPER TAR, PINE TAR **2** : a substance in some respects resembling tar; *esp* : a condensable residue present in smoke from burning tobacco that contains combustion by-products (as resins, acids, phenols, and essential oils)

tar·an·tism \'tar-ən-ˌtiz-əm\ *n* : a dancing mania or malady of late medieval Europe popularly regarded as being caused by the bite of the European tarantula (*Lycosa tarentula*)

ta·ran·tu·la \tə-'ranch-(ə-)lə, -'rant-ᵊl-ə\ *n, pl* **-las** *also* **-lae** \-'ran-chə-ˌlē, -'rant-ᵊl-ˌē\ **1** : a European spider (*Lycosa tarentula* of the family Lycosidae) popularly held to be the cause of tarantism **2** : any of a family (Theraphosidae) of large hairy American spiders that are typically rather sluggish and capable of biting sharply though most forms are not significantly poisonous to humans

ta·rax·a·cum \tə-'rak-sə-kəm\ *n* **1** *cap* : a genus of chiefly weedy perennial composite herbs which includes the dandelions **2** : the dried rhizome and roots of a dandelion (*T. officinale*) used as a diuretic, a tonic, and an aperient

ta·rax·e·in \tə-'rak-sē-ən\ *n* : a substance orig. reported to have been isolated from the blood of schizophrenics and to cause schizophrenic behavior but not chemically characterized or confirmed by later workers attempting to replicate the results

tarda — see OSTEOGENESIS IMPERFECTA TARDA

tar·dive \'tär-div\ *adj* : tending to or characterized by lateness esp. in development or maturity ⟨∼ syphilis develops after the second year —E. R. Pund⟩

tardive dyskinesia *n* : a neurological disorder characterized by involuntary uncontrollable movements esp. of the mouth, tongue, trunk, and limbs and occurring esp. as a side effect of prolonged use of antipsychotic drugs (as phenothiazine) — abbr. *TD*

¹tare \'ta(ə)r, 'te(ə)r\ *n* **1** : a deduction from the gross weight of a substance and its container made in allowance for the weight of the container **2** : an empty vessel that is similar in physical properties to a weighing container and that is used as a counterbalance to compensate for changes in the weight of the weighing container due to changes in environmental conditions (as temperature or moisture)

²tare *vt* **tared; tar·ing** : to ascertain or mark the tare of; *esp* : to weigh so as to determine the tare

tar·get \'tär-gət\ *n* **1** : something to be affected by an action or development; *specif* : an organ, part, or tissue that is affected by the action of a hormone **2 a** : the metallic surface usu. of platinum or tungsten upon which the stream of electrons within an X-ray tube is focused and from which the X-rays are emitted **b** : a body, surface, or material bombarded with nuclear particles or electrons **3** : the thought or object that is to be recognized (as by telepathy) or affected (as by psychokinesis) in a parapsychological experiment

target cell *n* : a cell that is acted on selectively by a specific agent (as a virus, drug, or hormone) ⟨the receptor that HIV binds to in entering its *target cells* —Michael Balter⟩

target gland *n* : an endocrine organ of which the functional activity is controlled by tropic hormones secreted by the pituitary gland

tar·ry stool \'tär-ē-\ *n* : an evacuation from the bowels having the color of tar caused esp. by hemorrhage in the stomach or small intestine

¹tar·sal \'tär-səl\ *adj* **1** : of or relating to the tarsus **2** : being or relating to plates of dense connective tissue that serve to stiffen the eyelids

²tarsal *n* : a tarsal part (as a bone or cartilage)

tarsal gland *n* : MEIBOMIAN GLAND

tarsal plate *n* : the plate of strong dense fibrous connective tissue that forms the supporting structure of the eyelid

tar·so·meta·tar·sal \ˌtär-sō-ˌmet-ə-'tär-səl\ *adj* : of or relating to the tarsus and metatarsus ⟨∼ articulations⟩

tar·sor·rha·phy \tär-'sòr-ə-fē\ *n, pl* **-phies** : the operation of suturing the eyelids together entirely or in part

tar·sus \'tär-səs\ *n, pl* **tar·si** \-ˌsī, -ˌsē\ **1** : the part of the foot of a vertebrate between the metatarsus and the leg; *also* : the small bones supporting this part of the limb that include the three cuneiform bones and the cuboid in a distal row and the navicular, calcaneus, and talus in a proximal row **2** : TARSAL PLATE

tar·tar \'tärt-ər\ *n* : an incrustation on the teeth consisting of plaque that has become hardened by the deposition of mineral salts (as calcium carbonate)

tartar emetic *n* : a poisonous efflorescent crystalline salt $KSbOC_4H_4O_6 \cdot \frac{1}{2}H_2O$ of sweetish metallic taste that is used in dyeing as a mordant and esp. formerly in medicine as an expectorant, anthelmintic, and emetic — called also *antimony potassium tartrate, potassium antimonyltartrate, tartrated antimony*

tar·tar·ic acid \(ˌ)tär-ˌtar-ik-\ *n* : a strong dicarboxylic acid $C_4H_6O_6$ of plant origin that occurs in three optically isomeric crystalline forms; *esp* : a dextrorotatory L-form of tartaric acid that is widely distributed in plants and esp. in fruits (as grapes) both free and combined as salts and that is used chiefly in effervescent beverages and pharmaceutical preparations, in desserts and candies, in photography, in making salts and esters, and as a sequestering agent

tar·trate \'tär-ˌtrāt\ *n* : a salt or ester of tartaric acid

tartrated antimony *n* : TARTAR EMETIC

tar·tra·zine \'tär-trə-ˌzēn, -zən\ *n* : a yellow azo dye that is used in making organic pigments and in coloring foods and drugs and that sometimes causes bronchoconstriction in individuals with asthma

task \'task\ *n* : the performance that is required of the subject in a psychological experiment or test and that is usu. communicated to a human subject by verbal instructions

¹taste \'tāst\ *vb* **tast·ed; tast·ing** *vt* : to ascertain the flavor of

\ə\ abut \ᵊ\ kitten \ər\ further \a\ ash \ā\ ace \ä\ cot, cart
\aù\ out \ch\ chin \e\ bet \ē\ easy \g\ go \i\ hit \ī\ ice \j\ job
\ŋ\ sing \ō\ go \ò\ law \òi\ boy \th\ thin \ṯh\ the \ü\ loot
\ù\ foot \y\ yet \zh\ vision *See also* Pronunciation Symbols page

S
T

by taking a little into the mouth ~ *vi* : to have a specific flavor 〈the milk ~*s* sour〉

²**taste** *n*   **1** : the one of the special senses that is concerned with distinguishing the sweet, sour, bitter, or salty quality of a dissolved substance and is mediated by taste buds on the tongue   **2** : the objective sweet, sour, bitter, or salty quality of a dissolved substance as perceived by the sense of taste   **3** : a sensation obtained from a substance in the mouth that is typically produced by the stimulation of the sense of taste combined with those of touch and smell : FLAVOR

taste bud *n* : an end organ that mediates the sensation of taste, lies chiefly in the epithelium of the tongue and esp. in the walls of the circumvallate papillae, and consists of a conical or flask-shaped mass made up partly of supporting cells and partly of neuroepithelial sensory cells terminating peripherally in short hairlike processes which project into the pore in the overlying epithelium and by which communication with the mouth cavity is effected

taste cell *n* : a neuroepithelial cell that is located in a taste bud and is the actual receptor of the sensation of taste — called also *gustatory cell*

taste hair *n* : the hairlike free end of a neuroepithelial cell in a taste bud

tast·er \'tā-stər\ *n* : a person able to taste the chemical phenylthiocarbamide

tat \'tat\ *n, often cap*   **1** : a small protein produced by a lentivirus (as HIV) within infected cells that greatly increases the rate of viral transcription and replication and that is also secreted extracellularly where it plays a role in increasing viral replication in newly infected cells and in enhancing the susceptibility of T cells to infection — called also *tat protein*   **2** : the viral gene that codes for the tat protein

TAT *abbr* thematic apperception test

¹**tat·too** \ta-'tü\ *vt* : to mark or color (the skin) with tattoos

²**tattoo** *n, pl* **tattoos** : an indelible mark or figure fixed upon the body by insertion of pigment under the skin or by production of scars

tau \'taù, 'tò\ *n* : a protein that binds to and regulates the assembly and stability of neuronal microtubules and that is found in an abnormal form as the major component of neurofibrillary tangles — called also *tau protein*

tau·rine \'tò-ˌrēn\ *n* : a colorless crystalline acid $C_2H_7NO_3S$ that is synthesized in the body from cysteine and methionine, is similar to amino acids but is not a component of proteins, and is involved in various physiological functions (as bile acid conjugation and cell membrane stabilization)

tau·ro·cho·late \ˌtòr-ə-'kō-lāt\ *n* : a salt or ester of taurocholic acid

tau·ro·cho·lic acid \ˌtòr-ə-ˌkō-lik-, -ˌkäl-ik-\ *n* : a deliquescent acid occurring in the form of its sodium salt $C_{26}H_{44}NNaO_7S$ in the bile of humans, the ox, and various carnivores

tau·ro·dont \'tòr-ə-ˌdänt\ *adj* : having the pulp cavities of the teeth very large and the roots reduced 〈a ~ tooth〉

tau·ro·dont·ism \ˌtòr-ə-'dän-ˌtiz-əm\ *n* : a dental condition marked by the enlargement of the pulp cavities and the reduction of the roots

tau·to·mer \'tòt-ə-mər\ *n* : any of the forms of a tautomeric compound

tau·to·mer·ic \ˌtòt-ə-'mer-ik\ *adj* : of, relating to, or marked by tautomerism

tau·tom·er·ism \tò-'täm-ə-ˌriz-əm\ *n* : isomerism in which the isomers change into one another with great ease so that they ordinarily exist together in equilibrium

tau·tom·er·iza·tion *or chiefly Brit* **tau·tom·er·isa·tion** \tò-ˌtäm-ə-rə-'zā-shən\ *n* : the process of changing into a tautomeric form — **tau·tom·er·ize** *or chiefly Brit* **tau·tom·er·ise** \tò-'täm-ə-ˌrīz\ *vb* **-ized** *or chiefly Brit* **-ised; -iz·ing** *or chiefly Brit* **-is·ing**

tax·is \'tak-səs\ *n, pl* **tax·es** \-ˌsēz\   **1** : the manual restoration of a displaced body part; *specif* : the reduction of a hernia manually   **2 a** : reflex translational or orientational movement by a freely motile and usu. simple organism in relation

to a source of stimulation (as a light or a temperature or chemical gradient)   **b** : a reflex reaction involving a taxis

Tax·ol \'tak-ˌsòl\ *trademark* — used for a preparation of paclitaxel

tax·on \'tak-ˌsän\ *n, pl* **taxa** \-sə\ *also* **tax·ons**   **1** : a taxonomic group or entity   **2** : the name applied to a taxonomic group in a formal system of nomenclature

tax·on·o·mist \tak-'sän-ə-məst\ *n* : a specialist in taxonomy

tax·on·o·my \tak-'sän-ə-mē\ *n, pl* **-mies**   **1** : the study of the general principles of scientific classification : SYSTEMATICS   **2** : orderly classification of plants and animals according to their presumed natural relationships — **tax·o·nom·ic** \ˌtak-sə-'näm-ik\ *adj* : of, relating to, or having the character of taxonomy — **tax·o·nom·i·cal·ly** \-i-k(ə-)lē\ *adv*

Tax·o·tere \'tak-sə-ˌter, -ˌtir\ *trademark* — used for a preparation of docetaxel

Tay–Sachs disease \'tā-'saks-\ *n* : a hereditary disorder of lipid metabolism that typically affects individuals of eastern European Jewish ancestry, that is marked by the accumulation of lipids esp. in nervous tissue due to a deficiency of hexosaminidase A, that is characterized by weakness, macrocephaly, red retinal spots, hyperacusis, retarded development, blindness, convulsions, paralysis, and death in early childhood, and that is inherited as an autosomal recessive trait — called also *infantile amaurotic idiocy, Tay-Sachs;* see SANDHOFF'S DISEASE; compare GAUCHER'S DISEASE, NIEMANN-PICK DISEASE

Tay, Warren (1843–1927), British physician. Tay specialized in ophthalmology, dermatology, and pediatrics. In 1881 he described a degenerative condition of the choroid found in a genetic disorder of lipid metabolism.

Sachs, Bernard (1858–1944), American neurologist. Sachs was a neurologist associated with several New York City hospitals. In 1887 he published a comprehensive description of a genetic disorder of lipid metabolism. His observations were made independently of Tay. The condition is known as Tay-Sachs disease as an acknowledgment of Sachs' later but more comprehensive account.

Tb *symbol* terbium

TB \('')tē-'bē\ *n* : TUBERCULOSIS

TB *abbr* tubercle bacillus

TBG *abbr* thyroid-binding globulin; thyroxine-binding globulin

TBI *abbr* traumatic brain injury

Tc *symbol* technetium

TCA *abbr* tricyclic antidepressant

TCDD \ˌtē-ˌsē-ˌdē-'dē\ *n* : a carcinogenic dioxin $C_{12}H_4O_2Cl_4$ found esp. as a contaminant in 2,4,5-T — called also *2,3,7,8=tetrachlorodibenzo-para-dioxin, 2,3,7,8-tetrachlorodibenzo-p=dioxin*

TCE *abbr* trichloroethylene

T cell *n* : any of several lymphocytes (as a helper T cell) that differentiate in the thymus, possess highly specific cell=surface antigen receptors, and include some that control the initiation or suppression of cell-mediated and humoral immunity (as by the regulation of T and B cell maturation and proliferation) and others that lyse antigen-bearing cells — called also *T lymphocyte;* see CYTOTOXIC T CELL, HELPER T CELL, SUPPRESSOR T CELL, T4 CELL

T–cell leukemia — see ADULT T-CELL LEUKEMIA

TCR *abbr* T cell (antigen) receptor — used for the receptor on an immunoreactive T cell that enables it to bind and react with a specific antigen

Td *abbr* tetanus diphtheria — used for a vaccine containing toxoids of the bacteria causing tetanus and diphtheria

TD *abbr* tardive dyskinesia

tds *abbr* [Latin *ter die sumendum*] to be taken three times a day — used in writing prescriptions

Te *symbol* tellurium

tea \'tē\ *n*   **1 a** : a shrub (*Camellia sinensis* of the family Theaceae, the tea family) cultivated esp. in China, Japan, and the East Indies   **b** : the prepared and cured leaves, leaf buds, and internodes of the tea plant   **2** : a mildly stimulating aromatic beverage prepared from tea leaves by infusion with boiling water **3** : any of various plants resembling tea in properties; *also* : an infusion of their leaves used medicinally or as a beverage

TEA *abbr* tetraethylammonium

teach·ing hospital \'tē-chiŋ-\ *n* : a hospital that is affiliated with a medical school and provides the means for medical education to students, interns, residents, and sometimes postgraduates

¹tear \'ti(ə)r\ *n* **1 a** : a drop of clear saline fluid secreted by the lacrimal gland and diffused between the eye and eyelids to moisten the parts and facilitate their motion **b tears** *pl* : a secretion of profuse tears that overflow the eyelids and dampen the face **2** : a transparent drop of fluid or hardened fluid matter (as resin)

²tear *vi* : to fill with tears : shed tears ⟨my eyes sting and ∼⟩

³tear \'ta(ə)r, 'te(ə)r\ *vt* **tore** \'tō(ə)r, 'tȯ(ə)r\; **torn** \'tō(ə)rn, 'tȯ(ə)rn\; **tear·ing** : to wound by or as if by pulling apart by force ⟨∼ the skin⟩

⁴tear *n* : a wound made by tearing a bodily part ⟨a muscle ∼⟩

tear duct *n* : LACRIMAL DUCT

tear gas *n* : a solid, liquid, or gaseous substance that on dispersion in the atmosphere blinds the eyes with tears and is used chiefly in dispelling mobs

tear gland *n* : LACRIMAL GLAND

tease \'tēz\ *vt* **teased; teas·ing** : to tear in pieces; *esp* : to shred (a tissue or specimen) for microscopic examination

teasing needle *n* : a tapering needle mounted in a handle and used for teasing tissues for microscopic examination

tea·spoon \'tē-ˌspün, -ˌspün\ *n* : a unit of measure equal to ⅙ fluid ounce or ⅓ tablespoon or 5 milliliters

tea·spoon·ful \-ˌfúl\ *n, pl* **tea·spoon·fuls** \-ˌfúlz\ *also* **tea·spoons·ful** \-ˌspünz-ˌfúl, -ˈspünz-\ : TEASPOON

teat \'tit, 'tēt\ *n* : the protuberance through which milk is drawn from an udder or breast : NIPPLE

tech *abbr* technician

tech·ne·tium \tek-ˈnē-sh(ē-)əm\ *n* : a metallic element that is obtained by bombarding molybdenum with deuterons or neutrons and in the fission of uranium and that is used in medicine in the preparation of radiopharmaceuticals — symbol *Tc*; see PERTECHNETATE; ELEMENT table

tech·nic \'tek-nik\ *n* : TECHNIQUE

tech·ni·cal \'tek-ni-kəl\ *adj* **1 a** : marked by or characteristic of specialization **b** : of or relating to a special field or subject **2** : of or relating to technique ⟨a surgeon with great ∼ skill⟩ **3** : of, relating to, or produced by ordinary commercial processes without being subjected to special purification ⟨∼ sulfuric acid⟩ — **tech·ni·cal·ly** \-k(ə-)lē\ *adv*

tech·ni·cian \tek-ˈnish-ən\ *n* : a specialist in the technical details of a subject or occupation ⟨a medical ∼⟩

tech·nique \tek-ˈnēk\ *n* : a method or body of methods for accomplishing a desired end ⟨new surgical ∼s⟩

tech·nol·o·gist \tek-ˈnäl-ə-jəst\ *n* : a specialist in technology

tech·nol·o·gy \-jē\ *n, pl* **-gies** **1** : the science of the application of knowledge to practical purposes : applied science **2** : a scientific method of achieving a practical purpose — **tech·no·log·i·cal** \ˌtek-nə-ˈläj-i-kəl\ *also* **tech·no·log·ic** \-ik\ *adj*

tec·tal \'tek-təl\ *adj* : of or relating to a tectum; *esp* : of or relating to the tectum mesencephali ⟨∼ lesions⟩

tec·to·bul·bar \ˌtek-tō-ˈbəl-bər\ *adj* : of, relating to, or being a tract of nerve fibers that originate in the superior colliculus, descend with the tectospinal tract, and terminate in a fasciculus at the level of the medulla oblongata

tec·to·ri·al membrane \tek-ˈtōr-ē-əl-\ *n* : a membrane having the consistency of jelly that covers the surface of the organ of Corti

tec·to·spi·nal \ˌtek-tō-ˈspīn-ᵊl\ *adj* : of, relating to, or being a tract of myelinated nerve fibers that mediate various visual and auditory reflexes and that originate in the superior colliculus, cross to the opposite side, and descend in the anterior funiculus of the spinal cord to terminate in the ventral horn of gray matter in the cervical region of the spinal cord ⟨∼ pathways⟩

tec·tum \'tek-təm\ *n, pl* **tec·ta** \-tə\ **1** : a bodily structure resembling or serving as a roof **2** : the dorsal part of the midbrain including the corpora quadrigemina — called also *tectum mesencephali*

tectum mes·en·ceph·a·li \-ˌmez-ˌen-ˈsef-ə-ˌlī\ *n* : TECTUM 2

teel oil \'tēl-\ *n* : SESAME OIL

teeth *pl of* TOOTH

teethe \'tēth\ *vi* **teethed; teeth·ing** : to cut one's teeth : grow teeth

teeth·ing \'tē-thiŋ\ *n* **1** : the first growth of teeth **2** : the phenomena accompanying the growth of teeth through the gums

Tef·lon \'tef-ˌlän\ *trademark* — used for polytetrafluoroethylene used esp. for molding articles and for coatings to prevent sticking (as of food in cookware)

teg·men \'teg-mən\ *n, pl* **teg·mi·na** \-mə-nə\ : an anatomical layer or cover; *specif* : TEGMEN TYMPANI

teg·men·tal \teg-ˈment-ᵊl\ *adj* : of, relating to, or associated with a tegmentum esp. of the brain

teg·men·tum \teg-ˈment-əm\ *n, pl* **-men·ta** \-ˈment-ə\ : an anatomical covering : TEGMEN; *esp* : the part of the ventral midbrain above the substantia nigra formed of longitudinal white fibers with arched transverse fibers and gray matter

tegmen tym·pa·ni \-ˈtim-pə-ˌnī\ *n* : a thin plate of bone that covers the middle ear and separates it from the cranial cavity

Teg·o·pen \'teg-ə-ˌpen\ *trademark* — used for a preparation of cloxacillin

Teg·re·tol \'teg-rə-ˌtȯl\ *trademark* — used for a preparation of carbamazepine

teg·u·ment \'teg-yə-mənt\ *n* : INTEGUMENT — **teg·u·men·tal** \ˌteg-yə-ˈment-ᵊl\ *adj*

teg·u·men·ta·ry \ˌteg-yə-ˈment-ə-rē\ *adj* : of, relating to, or consisting of an integument : serving as a covering

Teich·mann's crystal \'tīk-mənz-\ *n* : a crystal of hemin obtainable from hemoglobin that is used in a test for the detection of blood (as in a stain)

Teich·mann \'tīk-ˌmän\, **Ludwik Karol (1823–1895),** Polish anatomist. Teichmann attended medical school in Göttingen, Germany, and after graduation remained there as prosector of anatomy. In an 1853 paper on the crystallization of certain organic compounds of the blood, he described the preparation of microscopic crystals of hemin. The simple, specific test developed by Teichmann for the presence of blood in suspect stains on clothes and other items became widely used in forensic medicine.

tei·cho·ic acid \tī-ˌkō-ik-\ *n* : any of a class of strongly acidic polymers found in the cell walls, capsules, and membranes of all gram-positive bacteria and containing residues of the phosphates of glycerol and adonitol

te·la \'tē-lə\ *n, pl* **te·lae** \-ˌlē\ : an anatomical tissue or layer of tissue

tela cho·roi·dea \-kō-ˈrȯid-ē-ə\ *also* **tela cho·ri·oi·dea** \-ˌkōr-ē-ˈȯid-ē-ə\ *n* : a fold of pia mater roofing a ventricle of the brain

telaesthesia, telaesthetic *chiefly Brit var of* TELESTHESIA, TELESTHETIC

tel·an·gi·ec·ta·sia \ˌtel-ˌan-jē-ˌek-ˈtā-zh(ē-)ə, ˌtēl-, təl-\ *or* **tel·an·gi·ec·ta·sis** \-ˈek-tə-səs\ *n, pl* **-ta·sias** *or* **-ta·ses** \-tə-ˌsēz\ **1** : an abnormal dilation of red, blue, or purple superficial capillaries, arterioles, or venules typically located just below the skin's surface (as on the face) — see SPIDER VEIN **2** : HEREDITARY HEMORRHAGIC TELANGIECTASIA — **tel·an·gi·ec·tat·ic** \-ˌek-ˈtat-ik\ *adj*

te·la sub·cu·ta·nea \'tē-lə-ˌsəb-kyü-ˈtā-nē-ə\ *n* : SUPERFICIAL FASCIA

tela submucosa *n* : SUBMUCOSA

tele·bin·oc·u·lar \ˌtel-ə-bī-ˈnäk-yə-lər\ *n* : a stereoscopic instrument for determining various eye defects, measuring vi-

S
T

sual acuity or fusion of images, and conducting orthoptic training

teledendron *var of* TELODENDRON

tele·di·ag·no·sis \ˌtel-ə-ˌdī-əg-'nō-səs\ *n, pl* **-no·ses** \-ˌsēz\ : medical diagnosis made by means of telemedicine

tele·ki·ne·sis \ˌtel-ə-kə-'nē-səs, -kī-\ *n, pl* **-ne·ses** \-ˌsēz\ : the apparent production of motion in objects (as by a spiritualistic medium) without contact or other physical means — compare PRECOGNITION, PSYCHOKINESIS — **tele·ki·net·ic** \-'net-ik\ *adj* — **tele·ki·net·i·cal·ly** \-i-k(ə-)lē\ *adv*

tele·med·i·cine \-'med-ə-sən, -'med-sən\ *n* : the practice of medicine when the doctor and patient are widely separated using two-way voice and visual communication (as by satellite, computer, or closed-circuit television) — **tele·med·i·cal** \-'med-i-kəl\ *adj*

¹tele·me·ter \'tel-ə-ˌmēt-ər\ *n* : an electrical apparatus for measuring a quantity (as pressure, speed, or temperature), transmitting the result esp. by radio to a distant station, and there indicating or recording the quantity measured

²telemeter *vt* : to transmit by telemeter

te·lem·e·try \tə-'lem-ə-trē\ *n, pl* **-tries** **1** : the science or process of telemetering data **2** : data transmitted by telemetry **3** : BIOTELEMETRY — **tele·met·ric** \ˌtel-ə-'me-trik\ *adj* — **tele·met·ri·cal·ly** \-tri-k(ə-)lē\ *adv*

tel·en·ce·phal·ic \ˌtel-ˌen-sə-'fal-ik\ *adj* : of or relating to the telencephalon

tel·en·ceph·a·lon \ˌtel-en-'sef-ə-ˌlän, -lən\ *n, pl* **-la** \-lə\ *or* **-lons** : the anterior subdivision of the embryonic forebrain or the corresponding part of the adult forebrain that includes the cerebral hemispheres and associated structures

te·le·o·log·i·cal \ˌtel-ē-ə-'läj-i-kəl, ˌtēl-\ *also* **te·le·o·log·ic** \-'läj-ik\ *adj* : exhibiting or relating to design or purpose esp. in nature — **te·le·o·log·i·cal·ly** \-i-k(ə-)lē\ *adv*

te·le·ol·o·gy \ˌtel-ē-'äl-ə-jē, ˌtēl-\ *n, pl* **-gies** **1 a** : the study of evidences of design in nature **b** : a doctrine (as in vitalism) that ends are immanent in nature **c** : a doctrine explaining phenomena by final causes **2** : the fact or character attributed to nature or natural processes of being directed toward an end or shaped by a purpose **3** : the use of design or purpose as an explanation of natural phenomena

te·le·on·o·my \ˌtel-ē-'än-ə-mē, ˌtēl-\ *n, pl* **-mies** : the quality of apparent purposefulness of structure or function in living organisms that derives from their evolutionary adaptation — **te·le·o·nom·ic** \ˌtel-ē-ə-'näm-ik, ˌtēl-\ *adj*

te·lep·a·thy \tə-'lep-ə-thē\ *n, pl* **-thies** : apparent communication from one mind to another by extrasensory means — **tele·path·ic** \ˌtel-ə-'path-ik\ *adj* — **tele·path·i·cal·ly** \-i-k(ə-)lē\ *adv*

tele·phone theory \'tel-ə-ˌfōn-\ *n* : a theory in physiology: the perception of pitch depends on the frequency of the nerve impulses induced by sounds of different pitch — compare PLACE THEORY

tele·ra·di·ol·o·gy \ˌtel-ə-ˌrād-ē-'äl-ə-jē\ *n, pl* **-gies** : radiology concerned with the transmission of digitized medical images (as X-rays, CAT scans, and sonograms) over electronic networks and with the interpretation of the transmitted images for diagnostic purposes

tel·es·the·sia *or chiefly Brit* **tel·aes·the·sia** \ˌtel-əs-'thē-zh(ē-)ə\ *n* : an impression supposedly received at a distance without the normal operation of the organs of sense — **tel·es·thet·ic** *or chiefly Brit* **tel·aes·thet·ic** \-'thet-ik\ *adj*

tele·ther·a·py \ˌtel-ə-'ther-ə-pē\ *n, pl* **-pies** : the treatment of diseased tissue with high-intensity radiation (as gamma rays from radioactive cobalt)

tel·lu·ri·um \tə-'lùr-ē-əm, te-\ *n* : a semimetallic element related to selenium and sulfur that occurs in a silvery white brittle crystalline form of metallic luster, in a dark amorphous form, or combined with metals and that is used esp. in alloys — symbol *Te*; see ELEMENT table

¹telo·cen·tric \ˌtel-ō-'sen-trik, ˌtēl-\ *adj* : having the centromere terminally situated so that there is only one chromosomal arm ⟨∼ chromosomes⟩ — compare ACROCENTRIC, METACENTRIC

²telocentric *n* : a telocentric chromosome

telo·den·dri·on \ˌtel-ə-'den-drē-ən\ *also* **tele·den·dron** *or* **telo·den·dron** \-'den-drən\ *n, pl* **telo·den·dria** \-drē-ə\ *also* **tele·den·dra** *or* **telo·den·dra** \-drə\ : the terminal arborization of a nerve fiber — used orig. of dendrites but now esp. of the main arborization of an axon

te·lo·gen \'tē-lə-ˌjen\ *n* : the resting phase of the hair growth cycle following anagen and preceding shedding

telo·lec·i·thal \ˌtel-ō-'les-ə-thəl, ˌtēl-\ *adj, of an egg* : having the yolk large in amount and concentrated at one pole — compare CENTROLECITHAL, ISOLECITHAL

tel·o·mer·ase \te-'lō-mə-ˌrās, -ˌrāz\ *n* : a DNA polymerase that is a ribonucleoprotein catalyzing the elongation of chromosomal telomeres in eukaryotic cell division and is particularly active in cancer cells

telo·mere \'tel-ə-ˌmi(ə)r, 'tēl-\ *n* : the natural end of a eukaryotic chromosome composed of a usu. repetitive DNA sequence and serving to stabilize the chromosome — **telo·mer·ic** \ˌtel-ə-'mer-ik\ *adj*

telo·phase \'tel-ə-ˌfāz, 'tēl-\ *n* **1** : the final stage of mitosis and of the second division of meiosis in which the spindle disappears and the nucleus reforms around each set of chromosomes **2** : the final stage in the first division of meiosis that may be missing in some organisms and that is characterized by the gathering at opposite poles of the cell of half the original number of chromosomes including one from each homologous pair

telo·phrag·ma \ˌtel-ə-'frag-mə, ˌtēl-\ *n, pl* **-ma·ta** \-mət-ə\ : KRAUSE'S MEMBRANE

Telo·spo·rid·ia \ˌtel-ə-spə-'rid-ē-ə, ˌtēl-\ *n pl* : a subclass of the class Sporozoa comprising parasitic protozoans that form spores or filaments which contain one or more infective sporozoites and including the orders Gregarinida, Coccidia, and Haemosporidia — **telo·spo·rid·i·an** \-ē-ən\ *adj*

telo·syn·ap·sis \-sə-'nap-səs\ *n, pl* **-ap·ses** \-ˌsēz\ : synapsis of chromosomes by end-to-end union that is now known to be an observational artifact — **telo·syn·ap·tic** \-sə-'nap-tik\ *adj*

telo·tax·is \ˌtel-ə-'tak-səs, ˌtēl-\ *n, pl* **-tax·es** \-ˌsēz\ : a taxis in which an organism orients itself in respect to a stimulus (as a light source) as though that were the only stimulus acting on it

tel·son \'tel-sən\ *n* : the terminal segment of the body of an arthropod or segmented worm

TEM \'tē-'ē-'em\ *n* : TRIETHYLENEMELAMINE

TEM *abbr* transmission electron microscope; transmission electron microscopy

Tem·a·ril \'tem-ə-ˌril\ *trademark* — used for a preparation of the tartrate of trimeprazine

te·maz·e·pam \tə-'maz-ə-ˌpam\ *n* : a benzodiazepine $C_{16}H_{13}ClN_2O_2$ used for its sedative and tranquilizing effects in the treatment of insomnia — see RESTORIL

temp \'temp\ *n* : TEMPERATURE ⟨spike a ∼⟩

tem·per·a·ment \'tem-p(ə-)rə-mənt, -pər-mənt\ *n* **1** : the peculiar or distinguishing mental or physical character determined by the relative proportions of the humors according to medieval physiology **2** : characteristic or habitual inclination or mode of emotional response ⟨a nervous ∼⟩

tem·per·ance \'tem-p(ə-)rən(t)s, -pərn(t)s\ *n* : habitual moderation in the indulgence of the appetites or passions; *specif* : moderation in or abstinence from the use of alcoholic beverages

tem·per·ate \'tem-p(ə-)rət\ *adj* **1** : marked by moderation; *esp* : moderate in the use of intoxicating liquors **2** : existing as a prophage in infected cells and rarely causing lysis ⟨∼ bacteriophages⟩ — **tem·per·ate·ly** *adv*

tem·per·a·ture \'tem-pə(r)-ˌchủ(ə)r, -p(ə-)rə-, -chər, -ˌt(y)ủ(ə)r\ *n* **1** : degree of hotness or coldness measured on a definite scale — see THERMOMETER **2 a** : the degree of heat that is natural to a living body ⟨a normal oral ∼ of about 98.6°F⟩ **b** : a condition of abnormally high body heat ⟨was running a ∼⟩

tem·plate \'tem-plət\ *n* **1** *also* **tem·plet** : a gauge, pattern, or mold used as a guide to the form of a piece being made **2** : a molecule (as of DNA) that serves as a pattern for the synthesis of another macromolecule (as messenger RNA)

tem·ple \'tem-pəl\ *n* **1** : the flattened space on each side of the forehead of some mammals (as humans) **2** : one of the side supports of a pair of glasses jointed to the bows and passing on each side of the head

¹tem·po·ral \'tem-p(ə-)rəl\ *adj* : of or relating to time as distinguished from space; *also* : of or relating to the sequence of time or to a particular time — **tem·po·ral·ly** \-ē\ *adv*

²temporal *n* : a temporal part (as a bone or muscle)

³temporal *adj* : of or relating to the temples or the sides of the skull behind the orbits

temporal arteritis *n* : GIANT CELL ARTERITIS

temporal artery *n* **1** : either of two branches of the maxillary artery that supply the temporalis and anastomose with the middle temporal artery — called also *deep temporal artery* **2 a** : SUPERFICIAL TEMPORAL ARTERY **b** : a branch of the superficial temporal artery that arises just above the zygomatic arch, sends branches to the temporalis, and forms anastomoses with the deep temporal artery — called also *middle temporal artery* **3** : any of three branches of the middle cerebral artery: **a** : one that supplies the anterior parts of the superior, middle, and inferior temporal gyri — called also *anterior temporal artery* **b** : one that supplies the middle parts of the superior and middle temporal gyri — called also *intermediate temporal artery* **c** : one that supplies the middle and posterior parts of the superior temporal gyrus and the posterior parts of the middle and inferior temporal gyri — called also *posterior temporal artery*

temporal bone *n* : a compound bone of the side of the skull that has four principal parts including the squamous, petrous, and tympanic portions and the mastoid process

temporal fascia *n* : a broad fascia covering the temporalis and attached below to the zygomatic arch

temporal fossa *n* : a broad fossa on the side of the skull of higher vertebrates behind the orbit that contains muscles for raising the lower jaw and that in humans is occupied by the temporalis muscle, is separated from the orbit by the zygomatic bone, is bounded laterally by the zygomatic arch, and lies above the infratemporal crest of the greater wing of the sphenoid bone

temporal gyrus *n* : any of three major convolutions of the external surface of the temporal lobe of a cerebral hemisphere that are arranged approximately horizontally with one above the other: **a** : the one that is uppermost and borders the sylvian fissure — called also *superior temporal gyrus* **b** : one lying in the middle between the other two — called also *middle temporal gyrus* **c** : the lowest of the three — called also *inferior temporal gyrus*

tem·po·ral·is \ˌtem-pə-'rā-ləs\ *n* : a large muscle in the temporal fossa that serves to raise the lower jaw and is composed of fibers that arise from the surface of the temporal fossa and converge to an aponeurosis which contracts into a thick flat tendon inserted into the coronoid process of the mandible — called also *temporalis muscle, temporal muscle*

temporal line *n* : either of two nearly parallel ridges or lines on each side of the skull that begin as a single ridge on the temporal bone, run upward and backward from the zygomatic process above the temporal fossa, divide into upper and lower lines, and continue on the parietal bone

temporal lobe *n* : a large lobe of each cerebral hemisphere that is situated in front of the occipital lobe and contains a sensory area associated with the organ of hearing

temporal lobe epilepsy *n* : epilepsy characterized by partial rather than generalized seizures that typically originate in the temporal lobe and are marked by impairment of consciousness, automatisms, unusual changes in behavior, and hallucinations (as of odors) — abbr. *TLE;* called also *psychomotor epilepsy*

temporal muscle *n* : TEMPORALIS

temporal nerve — see AURICULOTEMPORAL NERVE, DEEP TEMPORAL NERVE

temporal process *n* : a process of the zygomatic bone that with the zygomatic process of the temporal bone with which it articulates laterally forms part of the zygomatic arch

temporal summation *n* : sensory summation that involves the addition of single stimuli over a short period of time

temporal vein *n* : any of several veins draining the temporal region: as **a** (1) : a large vein on each side of the head that is formed by anterior and posterior tributaries from the scalp and adjacent parts, receives the middle temporal vein, and unites with the maxillary vein to form a vein that contributes to the formation of the external jugular vein — called also *superficial temporal vein* (2) : a vein that drains the lateral orbital region and empties into the superficial temporal vein just above the zygomatic arch — called also *middle temporal vein* **b** : any of several veins arising from behind the temporalis and emptying into the pterygoid plexus — called also *deep temporal vein*

tem·po·ro·man·dib·u·lar \ˌtem-pə-rō-man-'dib-yə-lər\ *adj* : of, relating to, or affecting the temporomandibular joint ⟨~ pain and dysfunction —George Dimitroulis⟩

temporomandibular disorder *n* : TEMPOROMANDIBULAR JOINT SYNDROME — abbr. *TMD*

temporomandibular joint *n* : the diarthrosis between the temporal bone and mandible that includes the condyloid process below separated by an articular disk from the glenoid fossa above and that allows for the opening, closing, protrusion, retraction, and lateral movement of the mandible — abbr. *TMJ*

temporomandibular joint syndrome *n* : a group of symptoms that may include pain or tenderness in the temporomandibular joint or surrounding muscles, headache, earache, neck, back, or shoulder pain, limited jaw movement, or a clicking or popping sound in the jaw and that are caused either by dysfunction of the temporomandibular joint (as derangement of the articular disk) or another problem (as spasm or tension of the masticatory muscles) affecting the region of the temporomandibular joint — called also *temporomandibular disorder, temporomandibular joint disorder, temporomandibular joint dysfunction, TMJ syndrome*

tem·po·ro–oc·cip·i·tal \-äk-'sip-ət-ᵊl\ *adj* : of or relating to the temporal and occipital regions

tem·po·ro·pa·ri·etal \-pə-'rī-ət-ᵊl\ *adj* : of or relating to the temporal and parietal bones or lobes ⟨the ~ region⟩

te·na·cious \tə-'nā-shəs\ *adj* : tending to adhere or cling esp. to another substance : VISCOUS ⟨coughed up 150 cc. of thick ~ sputum —*Jour. Amer. Med. Assoc.*⟩

te·nac·u·lum \tə-'nak-yə-ləm\ *n, pl* **-la** \-ˌlə\ *or* **-lums** : a slender sharp-pointed hook attached to a handle and used mainly in surgery for seizing and holding parts (as arteries)

ten·der \'ten-dər\ *adj* : sensitive to touch or palpation ⟨~ skin⟩ ⟨a ~ palpable kidney⟩ — **ten·der·ness** \-nəs\ *n*

tendinea — see CHORDA TENDINEA

tendinis — see VAGINA TENDINIS

ten·di·ni·tis *or* **ten·don·itis** \ˌten-də-'nīt-əs\ *n* : inflammation of a tendon

ten·di·nous *also* **ten·do·nous** \'ten-də-nəs\ *adj* **1** : consisting of tendons ⟨~ tissue⟩ **2** : of, relating to, or resembling a tendon

tendinous arch *n* : a thickened arch of fascia which gives origin to muscles or ligaments or through which pass vessels or nerves; *esp* : a thickening in the pelvic fascia that gives attachment to supporting ligaments

ten·do cal·ca·ne·us \'ten-dō-kal-'kā-nē-əs\ *n* : ACHILLES TENDON

ten·don \'ten-dən\ *n* : a tough cord or band of dense white fibrous connective tissue that unites a muscle with some other part, transmits the force which the muscle exerts, and is continuous with the connective-tissue epimysium and perimysium of the muscle and when inserted into a bone with the periosteum of the bone

tendonitis *var of* TENDINITIS

tendon of Achil·les \-ə-'kil-ēz\ *n* : ACHILLES TENDON

\ə\ **abut** \ᵊ\ **kitten** \ər\ **further** \a\ **ash** \ā\ **ace** \ä\ **cot, cart** \aú\ **out** \ch\ **chin** \e\ **bet** \ē\ **easy** \g\ **go** \i\ **hit** \ī\ **ice** \j\ **job** \ŋ\ **sing** \ō\ **go** \ó\ **law** \ói\ **boy** \th\ **thin** \th̲\ **the** \ü\ **loot** \ú\ **foot** \y\ **yet** \zh\ **vision** *See also* Pronunciation Symbols page

S
T

tendon of Zinn \-ˈtsin\ *n* : LIGAMENT OF ZINN

tendon organ *n* : GOLGI TENDON ORGAN

tendonous *var of* TENDINOUS

tendon reflex *n* : a reflex act (as a knee jerk) in which a muscle is made to contract by a blow upon its tendon

tendon sheath *n* : a synovial sheath covering a tendon (as in the hand or foot)

tendon spindle *n* : GOLGI TENDON ORGAN

ten·do·vag·i·ni·tis \ˌten-dō-ˌvaj-ə-ˈnīt-əs\ *n* : TENOSYNOVITIS

tenens, tenentes — see LOCUM TENENS

te·nes·mus \tə-ˈnez-məs\ *n* : a distressing but ineffectual urge to evacuate the rectum or urinary bladder

tenia, teniacidal, teniacide, tenia coli, teniafuge, teniasis *var of* TAENIA, TAENIACIDAL, TAENIACIDE, TAENIA COLI, TAENIAFUGE, TAENIASIS

te·nip·o·side \tə-ˈnip-ə-ˌsīd\ *n* : an antineoplastic agent $C_{32}H_{32}O_{13}S$ that is a semisynthetic derivative of podophyllotoxin

ten·nis elbow \ˈten-əs-\ *n* : inflammation and pain over the outer side of the elbow involving the lateral epicondyle of the humerus and usu. resulting from excessive strain on and twisting of the forearm — called also *lateral humeral epicondylitis;* compare LITTLE LEAGUE ELBOW

te·no·de·sis \ˌten-ə-ˈdē-səs\ *n, pl* **-de·ses** \-ˌsēz\ : the operation of suturing the end of a tendon to a bone

te·nol·y·sis \te-ˈnäl-ə-səs\ *n, pl* **-y·ses** \-ə-ˌsēz\ : a surgical procedure to free a tendon from surrounding adhesions

teno·my·ot·o·my \ˌten-ō-mī-ˈät-ə-mē\ *n, pl* **-mies** : surgical excision of a portion of a tendon and muscle

Te·non's capsule \tə-ˈnōⁿz-, ˈten-ənz-\ *n* : a thin connective-tissue membrane ensheathing the eyeball behind the conjunctiva

   Te·non \tə-nōⁿ\, **Jacques René (1724–1816),** French surgeon. Tenon was an army surgeon who later became a professor of surgery and specialized in ophthalmology. In 1806 in a work on the anatomy of the eye, he described the space between the eyeball and the fibrous capsule of the eye. He also described the fibrous capsule itself which covers the posterior two-thirds of the eyeball and serves as a synovial sac. The capsule and the space have been named Tenon's capsule and Tenon's space in his honor.

Tenon's space *n* : a space between Tenon's capsule and the sclerotic coat of the eye that is traversed by strands of reticular tissue and by the optic nerve and ocular muscles

teno·plas·ty \ˈten-ə-ˌplas-tē\ *n, pl* **-ties** : plastic surgery performed on a tendon

Ten·or·min \ˈten-ər-ˌmin\ *trademark* — used for a preparation of atenolol

te·nor·rha·phy \te-ˈnȯr-ə-fē\ *n, pl* **-phies** : surgical suture of a divided tendon

teno·syn·o·vec·to·my \ˈten-ō-ˌsin-ə-ˈvek-tə-mē\ *n, pl* **-mies** : surgical excision of a tendon sheath

teno·syn·o·vi·tis \ˌten-ō-ˌsin-ə-ˈvīt-əs\ *n* : inflammation of a tendon sheath — called also *tendovaginitis, tenovaginitis*

ten·o·tome \ˈten-ə-ˌtōm\ *n* : a slender narrow-bladed surgical instrument mounted on a handle

te·not·o·mize *or Brit* **te·not·o·mise** \te-ˈnät-ə-ˌmīz\ *vt* **-mized** *or Brit* **-mised; -miz·ing** *or Brit* **-mis·ing** : to perform a tenotomy on

te·not·o·my \te-ˈnät-ə-mē\ *n, pl* **-mies** : surgical division of a tendon

teno·vag·i·ni·tis \ˌten-ō-ˌvaj-ə-ˈnīt-əs\ *n* : TENOSYNOVITIS

TENS *abbr* transcutaneous electrical nerve stimulation; transcutaneous electrical nerve stimulator

¹**tense** \ˈten(t)s\ *adj* **tens·er; tens·est** **1** : stretched tight : made taut or rigid ⟨the skeletal musculature involuntarily becomes ∼ —H. G. Armstrong⟩ **2** : feeling or showing nervous tension ⟨was ∼ and irritable⟩ — **tense·ness** *n*

²**tense** *vb* **tensed; tens·ing** *vt* : to make tense ⟨∼ a muscle⟩ ∼ *vi* : to become tense

Ten·si·lon \ˈten-si-ˌlän\ *trademark* — used for a preparation of edrophonium

ten·si·om·e·ter \ˌten(t)-sē-ˈäm-ət-ər\ *n* **1** : a device for mea-

suring tension **2** : an instrument for measuring the surface tension of liquids

ten·sion \ˈten-chən\ *n* **1 a** : the act or action of stretching or the condition or degree of being stretched to stiffness ⟨muscular ∼⟩ **b** : STRESS 1b **2 a** : either of two balancing forces causing or tending to cause extension **b** : the stress resulting from the elongation of an elastic body **3** : inner striving, unrest, or imbalance often with physiological indication of emotion **4** : PARTIAL PRESSURE — **ten·sion·al** \ˈtench-nəl, -ən-ᵊl\ *adj* — **ten·sion·less** \ˈten-chən-ləs\ *adj*

tension headache *n* : headache marked by mild to moderate pain of variable duration that affects both sides of the head and is typically accompanied by contraction of neck and scalp muscles

tension pneumothorax *n* : pneumothorax resulting from a wound in the chest wall which acts as a valve that permits air to enter the pleural cavity but prevents its escape

tension–time index *n* : a measure of ventricular work and oxygen demand that is found by multiplying the average pressure in the ventricle during the period in which it ejects blood by the time it takes to do this

ten·sor \ˈten(t)-sər, ˈten-ˌsȯ(ə)r\ *n* : a muscle that stretches a part or makes it tense — called also *tensor muscle*

tensor fas·ci·ae la·tae \-ˈfash-ē-ē-ˈlā-tē\ *or* **tensor fas·cia la·ta** \-ˈfash-ē-ə-ˈlā-tə\ *n* : a muscle that arises esp. from the anterior part of the iliac crest and from the anterior superior iliac spine, is inserted into the iliotibial band of the fascia lata about one third of the way down the thigh, and acts to flex and abduct the thigh

tensor pa·la·ti \-ˈpal-ə-ˌtī\ *n* : TENSOR VELI PALATINI

tensor tym·pa·ni \-ˈtim-pə-ˌnī\ *n* : a small muscle of the middle ear that is located in the bony canal just above the bony part of the eustachian tube, that arises from the canal containing it, from the cartilaginous portion of the eustachian tube, and from the adjacent greater wing of the sphenoid bone, that is inserted by a long tendon into the manubrium of the malleus near its base, and that serves to adjust the tension of the tympanic membrane — called also *tensor tympani muscle*

tensor ve·li pa·la·ti·ni \-ˈvē-ˌlī-ˌpal-ə-ˈtī-ˌnī\ *n* : a ribbonlike muscle of the palate that arises from the scaphoid fossa, from the spine of the sphenoid bone, and from the lateral cartilaginous wall of the eustachian tube, that is attached by a tendon which hooks around the pterygoid plate of the sphenoid bone to insert esp. into the soft palate, and that acts esp. to tense the soft palate

tent \ˈtent\ *n* : a canopy or enclosure placed over the head and shoulders to retain vapors or oxygen during medical administration

ten·ta·cle \ˈtent-i-kəl\ *n* : any of various elongate flexible usu. tactile or prehensile processes borne by animals chiefly on the head or about the mouth; *esp* : one of the threadlike processes bearing nematocysts that hang down from the margin of the umbrella of many jellyfishes

tenth cranial nerve \ˈten(t)th-\ *n* : VAGUS NERVE

ten·to·ri·al \ten-ˈtōr-ē-əl\ *adj* : of, relating to, or involving the tentorium cerebelli ⟨a ∼ meningioma⟩

tentorial notch *n* : an oval opening that is bounded by the anterior border of the tentorium cerebelli, that surrounds the midbrain, and that gives passage to the posterior cerebral arteries — called also *tentorial incisure*

ten·to·ri·um \-ē-əm\ *n, pl* **-ria** \-ē-ə\ : TENTORIUM CEREBELLI

tentorium ce·re·bel·li \-ˌser-ə-ˈbe-ˌlī\ *n* : an arched fold of dura mater that covers the upper surface of the cerebellum, supports the occipital lobes of the cerebrum, and has its posterior and lateral border attached to the skull and its anterior border free

Ten·u·ate \ˈten-yə-ˌwāt\ *trademark* — used for a preparation of the hydrochloride of diethylpropion

te·pa \ˈtē-pə\ *n* : a soluble crystalline compound $C_6H_{12}N_3OP$ that is used esp. as a chemical sterilizing agent of insects, a palliative in some kinds of cancer, and in finishing and flameproofing textiles — see THIOTEPA

TEPP \ˌtē-ˌē-ˌpē-'pē\ *n* : a mobile hygroscopic corrosive liquid organophosphate $C_8H_{20}O_7P_2$ that is a powerful anticholinesterase and is used as an insecticide and parasympathomimetic agent — called also *tetraethyl pyrophosphate*

ter·as \'ter-əs\ *n, pl* **ter·a·ta** \'ter-ət-ə\ : an organism (as a fetus) that is grossly abnormal in structure due to genetic or developmental causes

ter·a·tism \'ter-ə-ˌtiz-əm\ *n* : anomaly of organic form and structure : MONSTROSITY 1a

te·rato·car·ci·no·ma \ˌter-ət-ō-ˌkärs-ᵊn-'ō-mə\ *n, pl* **-mas** *also* **-ma·ta** \-mət-ə\ : a malignant teratoma; *esp* : one involving germinal cells of the testis or ovary

te·rato·gen \tə-'rat-ə-jən\ *n* : a teratogenic agent (as a drug or virus)

ter·a·to·gen·e·sis \ˌter-ə-tə-'jen-ə-səs\ *n, pl* **-e·ses** \-ˌsēz\ : production of developmental malformations

ter·a·to·ge·net·ic \-jə-'net-ik\ *adj* : TERATOGENIC

ter·a·to·gen·ic \-'jen-ik\ *adj* : of, relating to, or causing developmental malformations ⟨∼ substances⟩ ⟨∼ effects⟩ — **ter·a·to·ge·nic·i·ty** \-jə-'nis-ət-ē\ *n, pl* **-ties**

ter·a·toid \'ter-ə-ˌtoid\ *adj* : of, resembling, or being a teratoma ⟨a ∼ tumor⟩

ter·a·to·log·i·cal \ˌter-ət-ᵊl-'äj-i-kəl\ *or* **ter·a·to·log·ic** \-ik\ *adj* **1** : abnormal in growth or structure **2** : of or relating to teratology

ter·a·tol·o·gist \ˌter-ə-'täl-ə-jəst\ *n* : a specialist in teratology

ter·a·tol·o·gy \ˌter-ə-'täl-ə-jē\ *n, pl* **-gies** : the study of malformations or serious deviations from the normal type in organisms

ter·a·to·ma \ˌter-ə-'tō-mə\ *n, pl* **-mas** *also* **-ma·ta** \-mət-ə\ : a tumor derived from more than one embryonic layer and made up of a heterogeneous mixture of tissues (as epithelium, bone, cartilage, or muscle) — **ter·a·to·ma·tous** \-mət-əs\ *adj*

ter·a·to·sis \ˌter-ə-'tō-səs\ *n, pl* **-to·ses** \-ˌsēz\ : TERATISM

te·ra·zo·sin \tə-'rā-zə-ˌsin\ *n* : an alpha-adrenergic blocking agent administered orally in the form of its hydrated hydrochloride $C_{19}H_{25}N_5O_4\cdot HCl\cdot 2H_2O$ esp. in the treatment of benign prostatic hyperplasia and hypertension — see HYTRIN

ter·bin·a·fine \(ˌ)tər-'bin-ə-ˌfēn\ *n* : a synthetic derivative of allylamine that is used in the form of its hydrochloride $C_{21}H_{25}N\cdot HCl$ as an antifungal agent for topical dermatologic use (as in the treatment of athlete's foot and tinea cruris)

ter·bi·um \'tər-bē-əm\ *n* : a usu. trivalent metallic element of the rare-earth group — symbol *Tb*; see ELEMENT table

ter·bu·ta·line \tər-'byüt-ə-ˌlēn\ *n* : a bronchodilator used esp. in the form of its sulfate $(C_{12}H_{19}NO_3)_2\cdot H_2SO_4$

ter·e·bene \'ter-ə-ˌbēn\ *n* : a mixture of terpenes from oil of turpentine that has been used as an expectorant

teres — see LIGAMENTUM TERES, PRONATOR TERES

te·res major \'ter-ēz-, 'tir-\ *n* : a thick somewhat flattened muscle that arises chiefly from the lower third of the axillary border of the scapula, passes in front of the long head of the triceps to insert on the medial border of the bicipital groove of the humerus, and functions in opposition to the muscles comprising the rotator cuff by extending the arm when it is in the flexed position and by rotating it medially

teres minor *n* : a long cylindrical muscle that arises from the upper two-thirds of the axillary border of the scapula, passes behind the long head of the triceps to insert chiefly on the greater tubercle of the humerus, contributes to the formation of the rotator cuff of the shoulder, and acts to rotate the arm laterally and draw the humerus toward the glenoid fossa

ter·fen·a·dine \(ˌ)tər-'fen-ə-ˌdēn\ *n* : a drug $C_{32}H_{41}NO_2$ formerly used as a nonsedating antihistamine but now withdrawn from U.S. markets because of its link to cardiac arrhythmias — see SELDANE

tergo — see VIS A TERGO

ter·gum \'tər-gəm\ *n, pl* **ter·ga** \-gə\ : the dorsal part or plate of a segment of an arthropod — **ter·gal** \-gəl\ *adj*

¹term \'tərm\ *n* : the time at which a pregnancy of normal length terminates ⟨had her baby at full ∼⟩

²term *adj* : carried to, occurring at, or associated with full term ⟨a ∼ infant⟩ ⟨∼ births⟩

¹ter·mi·nal \'tərm-nəl, -ən-ᵊl\ *adj* **1** : of, relating to, or being at an end, extremity, boundary, or terminus ⟨the ∼ phalanx of a finger⟩ **2 a** : leading ultimately to death : FATAL ⟨∼ cancer⟩ **b** : approaching or close to death : being in the final stages of a fatal disease ⟨a ∼ patient⟩ **c** : of or relating to patients with a terminal illness ⟨∼ care⟩ **3** : being at or near the end of a chain of atoms making up a molecule ⟨the ∼ carbon⟩ — **ter·mi·nal·ly** \-ē\ *adv*

²terminal *n* : a part that forms an end; *esp* : NERVE ENDING ⟨synthesis of a neurotransmitter in the presynaptic ∼ of a neuron —R. J. Wurtman⟩

terminale — see FILUM TERMINALE

terminal ganglion *n* : a usu. parasympathetic ganglion situated on or close to an innervated organ and being the site where preganglionic nerve fibers terminate

terminalis — see LAMINA TERMINALIS, NERVUS TERMINALIS, SINUS TERMINALIS, STRIA TERMINALIS, SULCUS TERMINALIS

terminal nerve *n* : NERVUS TERMINALIS

ter·mi·na·tion \ˌtər-mə-'nā-shən\ *n* : an end or ending of something; *esp* : a distal end of an anatomical part

ter·mi·na·tor \'tər-mə-ˌnāt-ər\ *n* : a codon that stops protein synthesis since it does not code for a transfer RNA — called also *termination codon, terminator codon*; compare INITIATION CODON

ter·mi·nus \'tər-mə-nəs\ *n, pl* **-ni** \-ˌnī, -ˌnē\ *also* **-nus·es** : an end or ending esp. of a molecular chain, a chromosome, or a process of a nerve cell

ter·na·ry \'tər-nə-rē\ *adj* **1** : having three elements, parts, or divisions **2 a** : being or consisting of an alloy of three elements **b** : of, relating to, or containing three different elements, atoms, radicals, or groups ⟨a ∼ acid⟩

Ter·ni·dens \'tər-nə-ˌdenz\ *n* : a genus of nematode worms of the family Strongylidae parasitic in the intestine of various African apes and monkeys and sometimes in humans

ter·pene \'tər-ˌpēn\ *n* : any of various isomeric hydrocarbons $C_{10}H_{16}$ found present in essential oils (as from conifers) and used esp. as solvents and in organic synthesis; *broadly* : any of numerous hydrocarbons $(C_5H_8)_n$ found esp. in essential oils, resins, and balsams — **ter·pene·less** \-ləs\ *adj* — **ter·pe·nic** \ˌtər-'pē-nik, -'pen-ik\ *adj*

¹ter·pe·noid \'tər-pə-ˌnoid\ *adj* : resembling a terpene in molecular structure

²terpenoid *n* : any of a class of compounds that are characterized by an isoprenoid structure like that of the terpene hydrocarbons

ter·pin \'tər-pin\ *n* : a crystalline saturated terpenoid glycol $C_{10}H_{18}(OH)_2$ that is known in cis and trans forms and is obtained readily in the form of terpin hydrate

ter·pin·e·ol \ˌtər-'pin-ē-ˌól, -ˌōl\ *n* : any of three fragrant isomeric alcohols $C_{10}H_{17}OH$ or a mixture of them found in essential oils or made artificially and used esp. formerly as an antiseptic

terpin hydrate *n* : an efflorescent crystalline or powdery compound $C_{10}H_{18}(OH)_2\cdot H_2O$ used as an expectorant for coughs

Ter·ra·my·cin \ˌter-ə-'mīs-ᵊn\ *trademark* — used for a preparation of oxytetracycline

¹ter·tian \'tər-shən\ *adj* : recurring at approximately 48-hour intervals — used chiefly of vivax malaria; compare QUARTAN

²tertian *n* : a tertian fever; *specif* : VIVAX MALARIA

¹ter·tia·ry \'tər-shē-ˌer-ē, 'tər-shə-rē\ *n, pl* **-ries** **1** : TERTIARY COLOR **2** : a lesion of tertiary syphilis

²tertiary *adj* **1** : of third rank, importance, or value **2 a** : involving or resulting from the substitution of three atoms or groups ⟨a ∼ salt⟩ **b** : being or containing a carbon atom having bonds to three other carbon atoms ⟨an acid containing a ∼ carbon⟩ **c** : of, relating to, or being the normal

S
T

folded structure of the coiled chain of a protein or of a DNA or RNA — compare PRIMARY 4, SECONDARY 3 **3** : occurring in or being a third stage ⟨∼ lesions of syphilis⟩ **4** : providing tertiary care ⟨a ∼ medical center⟩

tertiary alcohol *n* : an alcohol characterized by the group ≡COH consisting of a carbon atom holding the hydroxyl group and attached by its other three valences to other carbon atoms in a chain or ring

tertiary amine *n* : an amine (as trimethylamine or nicotine) having three organic groups attached to the nitrogen in place of three hydrogen atoms

tertiary care *n* : highly specialized medical care usu. over an extended period of time that involves advanced and complex procedures and treatments performed by medical specialists in state-of-the-art facilities — compare PRIMARY CARE, SECONDARY CARE

tertiary color *n* : a color produced by mixing two secondary colors

tertiary syphilis *n* : the third stage of syphilis that develops after the disappearance of the secondary symptoms and is marked by ulcers in and gummas under the skin and commonly by involvement of the skeletal, cardiovascular, and nervous systems

ter·tip·a·ra \ˌtər-ˈtip-ə-rə\ *n, pl* **-ras** *or* **-rae** \-ˌrē\ : a woman who has given birth three times

tertius — see PERONEUS TERTIUS

Tesch·en disease \ˈte-shən-\ *n* : a now uncommon mild to severe encephalomyelitis of swine that is caused by picornaviruses of several serogroups belonging to the genus *Enterovirus*, that is marked by lesions of the central nervous system and by varying degrees of systemic paralysis, and that is considered analogous to human poliomyelitis

tes·la \ˈtes-lə\ *n* : a unit of magnetic flux density in the mks system equivalent to one weber per square meter

Tesla, Nikola (1856–1943), American electrical engineer and inventor. Tesla was a prolific genius who claimed more than 700 inventions. The tesla, a unit of magnetic induction, was named in his honor.

¹test \ˈtest\ *n* **1** : a critical examination, observation, evaluation, or trial; *specif* : the procedure of submitting a statement to such conditions or operations as will lead to its proof or disproof or to its acceptance or rejection ⟨a ∼ of a statistical hypothesis⟩ **2** : a means of testing: as **a** (1) : a procedure or reaction used to identify or characterize a substance or constituent ⟨a ∼ for starch using iodine⟩ (2) : a reagent used in such a test **b** : a diagnostic procedure for determining the presence or nature of a condition or disease or for revealing a change in function ⟨∼ : something (as a series of questions or exercises) for measuring the skill, knowledge, intelligence, capacities, or aptitudes of an individual or group **3** : a result or value determined by testing

²test *vt* : to subject to a test ∼ *vi* **1** : to undergo a test **2** : to apply a test as a means of analysis or diagnosis — used with *for* ⟨∼ for the presence of starch⟩

³test *adj* **1** : of, relating to, or constituting a test ⟨the ∼ environment affected the scores⟩ **2** : subjected to, used for, or revealed by testing ⟨∼ substances⟩

test·cross \ˈtes(t)-ˌkròs\ *n* : a genetic cross between a homozygous recessive individual and a corresponding suspected heterozygote to determine the genotype of the latter — **test·cross** *vt*

tested *adj* : subjected to test; *esp* : pronounced free of disease as a result of testing ⟨tuberculin-*tested* cattle⟩

testes *pl of* TESTIS

tes·ti·cle \ˈtes-ti-kəl\ *n* : TESTIS; *esp* : one with its enclosing structures

tes·tic·u·lar \tes-ˈtik-yə-lər\ *adj* : of, relating to, or derived from the testes ⟨∼ hormones⟩

testicular artery *n* : either of a pair of arteries which supply blood to the testes and of which one arises on each side from the front of the aorta a little below the corresponding renal artery and passes downward to the spermatic cord of the same side and along it to the testis — called also *internal spermatic artery*

testicular feminization *n* : a genetic defect characterized by the presence in a phenotypically female individual of the normal X and Y chromosomes of a male, undeveloped and undescended testes, and functional sterility — called also *testicular feminization syndrome*

testicular vein *n* : any of the veins leading from the testes, forming with tributaries from the epididymis the pampiniform plexus in the spermatic cord, and thence accompanying the testicular artery and eventually uniting to form a single trunk which on the right side opens into the vena cava and on the left into the renal vein — called also *spermatic vein*

tes·tis \ˈtes-təs\ *n, pl* **tes·tes** \ˈtes-ˌtēz\ : a typically paired male reproductive gland that usu. consists largely of seminiferous tubules from the epithelium of which spermatozoa develop, that contains androgen-secreting Leydig cells in the interstitial tissue, that corresponds to the ovary of the female and in craniate vertebrates develops from the genital ridges of the embryo, and that in most mammals descends into the scrotum before the attainment of sexual maturity and in many cases before birth

tes·tos·ter·one \te-ˈstäs-tə-ˌrōn\ *n* : a male hormone that is a crystalline hydroxy steroid ketone $C_{19}H_{28}O_2$ produced primarily by the testes or made synthetically and that is the main androgen responsible for inducing and maintaining male secondary sex characteristics

testosterone enan·thate \-ē-ˈnan-ˌthāt\ *n* : a white or whitish crystalline ester $C_{26}H_{40}O_3$ of testosterone that is used esp. in the treatment of eunuchism, eunuchoidism, androgen deficiency after castration, symptoms of andropause, and oligospermia

testosterone propionate *n* : a white or whitish crystalline ester $C_{22}H_{32}O_3$ of testosterone that is used esp. in the treatment of postpubertal cryptorchidism and symptoms of andropause, in palliation of inoperable breast cancer, and in the prevention of postpartum pain and breast engorgement, that is usu. administered intramuscularly, and that has a half-life of about four hours

test paper *n* : paper (as litmus paper) cut usu. in strips and saturated with a reagent and esp. an indicator that changes color in testing for various substances

test–tube *adj* **1** : IN VITRO ⟨∼ experiments⟩ **2** : produced by in vitro fertilization ⟨∼ babies⟩

test tube *n* : a plain or lipped tube usu. of thin glass closed at one end and used esp. in chemistry and biology

tet·a·nal \ˈtet-ᵊn-əl\ *adj* : of, relating to, or derived from tetanus ⟨∼ toxin⟩

te·tan·ic \te-ˈtan-ik\ *adj* : of, relating to, being, or tending to produce tetany or tetanus ⟨a ∼ condition⟩ ⟨∼ contractions⟩ — **te·tan·i·cal·ly** \-i-k(ə-)lē\ *adv*

tet·a·nize *also Brit* **tet·a·nise** \ˈtet-ᵊn-ˌīz\ *vt* **-nized** *also Brit* **-nised; -niz·ing** *also Brit* **-nis·ing** : to induce tetanus in ⟨∼ a muscle⟩ — **tet·a·ni·za·tion** *also Brit* **tet·a·ni·sa·tion** \ˌtet-ᵊn-ə-ˈzā-shən, ˌtet-nə-\ *n*

tet·a·noid \ˈtet-ᵊn-ˌòid\ *adj* : resembling tetanus or tetany ⟨∼ spasms⟩

tet·a·no·ly·sin \ˌtet-ə-ˈnäl-ə-sən, ˌtet-ᵊn-ō-ˈlīs-ᵊn\ *n* : a hemolytic toxin produced by the tetanus bacillus (*Clostridium tetani*)

tet·a·no·spas·min \ˌtet-ᵊn-ō-ˈspaz-mən\ *n* : a crystalline unstable neurotoxin produced by the tetanus bacillus and held to be the cause of the tetanic convulsions of tetanus — called also *tetanus toxin*

tet·a·nus \ˈtet-ᵊn-əs, ˈtet-nəs\ *n* **1 a** : an acute infectious disease characterized by tonic spasm of voluntary muscles and esp. of the muscles of the jaw and caused by the specific toxin produced by a bacterium of the genus *Clostridium* (*C. tetani*) which is usu. introduced through a wound — compare LOCKJAW **b** : TETANUS BACILLUS **2** : prolonged contraction of a muscle resulting from a series of motor impulses following one another too rapidly to permit intervening relaxation of the muscle

tetanus bacillus *n* : the bacterium of the genus *Clostridium* (*C. tetani*) that causes tetanus

tetanus toxin *n* : TETANOSPASMIN

tet·a·ny \'tet-ᵊn-ē, 'tet-nē\ *n, pl* **-nies** : a condition of physiological calcium imbalance that is marked by intermittent tonic spasm of the voluntary muscles and is associated with deficiencies of parathyroid secretion or other disturbances (as vitamin D deficiency)

te·tar·ta·no·pia \te-ˌtär-tə-'nō-pē-ə\ *n* : dichromatism in which the spectrum is seen in tones of red and green with blue and yellow replaced by gray

tet·ra·ac·e·tate \ˌte-trə-'as-ə-ˌtāt\ *n* : an acetate containing four acetate groups

tet·ra·ben·a·zine \-'ben-ə-ˌzēn\ *n* : a serotonin antagonist $C_{19}H_{27}NO_3$ that is used esp. in the treatment of psychosis and anxiety

tet·ra·bo·rate \-'bō(ə)r-ˌāt\ *n* : a salt or ester of tetraboric acid — see SODIUM TETRABORATE

tet·ra·bo·ric acid \-ˌbō-rik-\ *n* : a dibasic acid $H_2B_4O_7$ containing four atoms of boron in a molecule, formed by heating ordinary boric acid, and known esp. in the form of its salts (as borax)

tet·ra·caine \'te-trə-ˌkān\ *n* : a crystalline basic ester that is closely related chemically to procaine and is used chiefly in the form of its hydrochloride $C_{15}H_{24}N_2O_2$·HCl as a local anesthetic — called also *amethocaine, pantocaine;* see PONTOCAINE

tet·ra·chlo·ride \ˌte-trə-'klō(ə)r-ˌīd, -'klō(ə)r-\ *n* : a chloride containing four atoms of chlorine

2,3,7,8–tet·ra·chlo·ro·di·ben·zo–para–di·ox·in \ˌtü-ˌthrē-ˌsev-ən-ˌāt-ˌte-trə-ˌklō-rō-(ˌ)dī-ˌben-zō-ˌpar-ə-dī-'äk-sən\ *n* : TCDD

2,3,7,8–tet·ra·chlo·ro·di·ben·zo–p–di·ox·in \-'pē-dī-'äk-sən\ *n* : TCDD

tet·ra·chlo·ro·eth·yl·ene \ˌte-trə-ˌklō-rō-'eth-ə-ˌlēn\ *n* : PERCHLOROETHYLENE

tet·ra·chlo·ro·meth·ane \-'meth-ˌān, *Brit usu* -'mē-ˌthän\ *n* : CARBON TETRACHLORIDE

tet·ra·cy·clic \-'sī-klik, -'sik-lik\ *adj* : containing four usu. fused rings in the molecule structure

tet·ra·cy·cline \ˌte-trə-'sī-ˌklēn, -klən\ *n* : a yellow crystalline broad-spectrum antibiotic that is produced by a soil actinomycete of the genus *Streptomyces* (*S. viridifaciens*) or made synthetically and that is administered chiefly in the form of its hydrochloride $C_{22}H_{24}N_2O_8$·HCl; *also* : any of several chemically related antibiotics (as doxycycline)

tet·rad \'te-ˌtrad\ *n* : a group or arrangement of four: as **a** : a tetravalent element, atom, or radical **b** : a group of four cells arranged usu. in the form of a tetrahedron and produced by the successive divisions of a mother cell ⟨a ∼ of spores⟩ **c** : a group of four synapsed chromatids that become visibly evident in the pachytene stage of meiotic prophase and are produced by the longitudinal splitting of each of two paired homologous chromosomes

tet·ra·deca·no·ic acid \ˌte-trə-ˌdek-ə-ˌnō-ik-\ *n* : MYRISTIC ACID

tet·ra·deca·pep·tide \ˌte-trə-ˌdek-ə-'pep-ˌtīd\ *n* : a polypeptide (as somatostatin) that contains 14 amino acids

tet·ra·eth·yl·am·mo·ni·um \ˌte-trə-ˌeth- əl-ə-'mō-nē-əm\ *n* : the quaternary ammonium ion $(C_2H_5)_4N^+$ containing four ethyl groups; *also* : a salt of this ion (as the deliquescent crystalline chloride used as a ganglionic blocking agent) — abbr. *TEA*

tet·ra·eth·yl lead \ˌte-trə-ˌeth-əl-'led\ *n* : a heavy oily poisonous liquid $Pb(C_2H_5)_4$ used as an antiknock agent in gasoline — called also *lead tetraethyl*

tetraethyl pyrophosphate *n* : TEPP

tet·ra·eth·yl·thi·u·ram disulfide \ˌte-trə-ˌeth-əl-'thī-yu-ˌram-\ *n* : DISULFIRAM

tet·ra·flu·or·o·eth·yl·ene \ˌte-trə-ˌflu(-ə)r-ō-'eth-ə-ˌlēn\ *n* : a flammable gaseous fluorocarbon $CF_2=CF_2$ used in making polytetrafluoroethylene resins

tet·ra·hy·drate \-'hī-ˌdrāt\ *n* : a chemical compound with four molecules of water — **tet·ra·hy·drat·ed** *adj*

tet·ra·hy·dro·ami·no·ac·ri·dine \ˌte-trə-ˌhī-drə-ə-ˌmē-nō-'ak-rə-ˌdēn\ *n* : TACRINE

tet·ra·hy·dro·can·nab·i·nol \-kə-'nab-ə-ˌnȯl, -ˌnōl\ *n* : THC; *esp* : THC a

Δ⁹–tetrahydrocannabinol *var of* DELTA-9-TETRAHYDROCANNABINOL

tet·ra·hy·dro·fo·late \-'fō-ˌlāt\ *n* : a salt or ester of tetrahydrofolic acid

tet·ra·hy·dro·fo·lic acid \-ˌfō-lik-\ *n* : a metabolically active reduced form $C_{19}H_{23}N_7O_6$ of folic acid that acts as a coenzyme in the transfer of groups (as a methyl group) containing a single carbon atom in metabolic synthesis (as of purines)

tet·ra·hy·me·na \-'hī-mə-nə\ *n* **1** *cap* : a genus of free-living ciliate protozoans much used for genetic and biochemical research **2** : any ciliate protozoan of the genus *Tetrahymena*

tet·ra·iodo·phe·nol·phtha·lein \ˌte-trə-ī-ˌō-dō-ˌfēn-ᵊl-'thal-ē-ən, -'thal-ˌēn, -'thāl-\ *n* : IODOPHTHALEIN

te·tral·o·gy of Fal·lot \te-'tral-ə-jē-əv-fä-'lō\ *n* : a congenital abnormality of the heart characterized by pulmonary stenosis, an opening in the interventricular septum, malposition of the aorta over both ventricles, and hypertrophy of the right ventricle

Fal·lot \fä-lō\, **Étienne–Louis–Arthur (1850–1911)**, French physician. Fallot published in 1888 an article on cardiac anomalies in which he described the form of congenital heart disease producing cyanosis that now bears his name. His description was not the first but an improvement that analyzed and correlated the clinical with postmortem observations and gave all four of the identifying characteristics.

tet·ra·mer \'te-trə-mər\ *n* : a molecule (as an enzyme or a polymer) that consists of four structural subunits (as peptide chains or condensed monomers) — **tet·ra·mer·ic** \ˌte-trə-'mer-ik\ *adj*

tet·ra·meth·yl·am·mo·ni·um \ˌte-trə-ˌmeth-əl-ə-'mō-nē-əm\ *n* : the quaternary ammonium ion $(CH_3)_4N^+$ containing four methyl groups

tet·ra·mine \'te-trə-ˌmēn\ *n* **1** : a compound (as methenamine) containing four amino groups **2** : a strong toxic unstable base $C_4H_{13}NO$ obtained from sea anemones or made synthetically

tetranitrate — see ERYTHRITYL TETRANITRATE, PENTAERYTHRITOL TETRANITRATE

tet·ra·nu·cle·o·tide \ˌte-trə-'n(y)ü-klē-ə-ˌtīd\ *n* : a nucleotide consisting of a chain of four mononucleotides

tet·ra·pa·ren·tal \-pə-'rent-ᵊl\ *adj* : produced from a mosaic cellular mass composed of cells integrated from two genetically different embryos

tet·ra·pa·re·sis \-pə-'rē-səs, -'par-ə-\ *n, pl* **-re·ses** \-ˌsēz\ : muscle weakness affecting all four limbs — called also *quadriparesis*

tet·ra·pa·ret·ic \-pə-'ret-ik\ *adj* : of, relating to, or affected with tetraparesis ⟨a ∼ patient⟩

tet·ra·pep·tide \-'pep-ˌtīd\ *n* : a peptide consisting of four amino acid residues

tetraphosphate — see HEXAETHYL TETRAPHOSPHATE

Tet·ra·phyl·lid·ea \ˌte-trə-fi-'lid-ē-ə\ *n pl* : an order of the class Cestoda comprising tapeworms parasitic in elasmobranch fishes and distinguished by a scolex having four bothridia and sometimes also hooks or suckers for attachment to the host

tet·ra·ple·gia \ˌte-trə-'plē-j(ē-)ə\ *n* : QUADRIPLEGIA

tet·ra·ple·gic \-'plē-jik\ *adj or n* : QUADRIPLEGIC

¹tet·ra·ploid \'te-trə-ˌplȯid\ *adj* : having or being a chromosome number four times the monoploid number ⟨a ∼ cell⟩ — **tet·ra·ploi·dy** \-ˌplȯid-ē\ *n, pl* **-dies**

²tetraploid *n* : a tetraploid individual

tet·ra·pyr·role *also* **tet·ra·pyr·rol** \ˌte-trə-'pi(ə)r-ˌōl\ *n* : a chemical group consisting of four pyrrole rings joined either

---

\ə\ **abut** \ᵊ\ **kitten** \ər\ **further** \a\ **ash** \ā\ **ace** \ä\ **cot, cart**
\au̇\ **out** \ch\ **chin** \e\ **bet** \ē\ **easy** \g\ **go** \i\ **hit** \ī\ **ice** \j\ **job**
\ŋ\ **sing** \ō\ **go** \ȯ\ **law** \ȯi\ **boy** \th\ **thin** \th̲\ **the** \ü\ **loot**
\u̇\ **foot** \y\ **yet** \zh\ **vision** *See also* Pronunciation Symbols page

S
T

in a straight chain (as in phycobilins) or in a ring (as in chlorophyll)

tet·ra·sac·cha·ride \-'sak-ə-ˌrīd\ *n* : any of a class of carbohydrates (as stachyose) that yield on complete hydrolysis four monosaccharide molecules

tet·ra·so·mic \ˌte-trə-'sō-mik\ *adj* : having one or a few chromosomes tetraploid in otherwise diploid nuclei due to nondisjunction

tet·ra·va·lent \ˌte-trə-'vā-lənt\ *adj* : having a chemical valence of four ⟨∼ carbon⟩

tet·ra·zole \'te-trə-ˌzōl\ *n* : a crystalline acidic compound CH_2N_4 containing a five-membered ring composed of one carbon and four nitrogen atoms; *also* : any of various derivatives of this compound

tet·ra·zo·li·um \ˌte-trə-'zō-lē-əm\ *n* : a monovalent cation or group CH_3N_4 that is analogous to ammonium; *also* : any of several of its derivatives used esp. as electron acceptors to test for metabolic activity in living cells

te·tro·do·tox·in \te-ˌtrōd-ə-'täk-sən\ *n* : a neurotoxin $C_{11}H_{17}N_3O_8$ that is found esp. in pufferfishes and that blocks nerve conduction by suppressing permeability of the nerve fiber to sodium ions

tet·rose \'te-ˌtrōs\ *n* : any of a class of monosaccharides $C_4H_8O_4$ (as erythrose) containing four carbon atoms

te·trox·ide \te-'träk-ˌsīd\ *n* : a compound of an element or group with four atoms of oxygen — see OSMIUM TETROXIDE

Tex·as fever \'tek-səs-\ *n* : an infectious disease of cattle transmitted by the cattle tick and caused by a sporozoan of the genus *Babesia* (*B. bigemina*) that multiplies in the blood and destroys red blood cells — called also *cattle-tick fever, Texas cattle fever*

Texas fever tick *n* : a cattle tick of the genus *Boophilus* (*B. annulatus*)

Texas snakeroot *n* : a plant of the genus *Aristolochia* (*A. reticulata*) that occurs in the southwestern U.S. and resembles the Virginia snakeroot in its medicinal properties — see SERPENTARIA

T4 *or* **T₄** \'tē-'fō(ə)r\ *n* : THYROXINE

T4 cell \ˌtē-'fō(ə)r-\ *n* : any of the T cells (as a helper T cell) that display the CD4 molecule on their surface and become severely depleted in AIDS — called also *helper-inducer T cell, T4 lymphocyte*

TGF *abbr* transforming growth factor

T–group \'tē-ˌgrüp\ *n* : a group of people under the leadership of a trainer who seek to develop self-awareness and sensitivity to others by verbalizing feelings uninhibitedly at group sessions — compare ENCOUNTER GROUP

Th *symbol* thorium

THA \ˌtē-(ˌ)āch-'ā\ *n* : TACRINE

tha·lam·ic \thə-'lam-ik\ *adj* : of, relating to, or involving the thalamus ⟨bilateral medial ∼ lesions —L. R. Squire⟩

thalamic radiation *n* : any of several large bundles of nerve fibers connecting the thalamus with the cerebral cortex by way of the internal capsule

thal·a·mo·cor·ti·cal \ˌthal-ə-mō-'kȯrt-i-kəl\ *adj* : of, relating to, or connecting the thalamus and the cerebral cortex ⟨∼ axons⟩ ⟨∼ activity⟩

thal·a·mot·o·my \ˌthal-ə-'mät-ə-mē\ *n, pl* **-mies** : a surgical operation involving electrocoagulation of areas of the thalamus to interrupt pathways of nervous transmission through the thalamus for relief of certain mental and psychomotor disorders

thal·a·mus \'thal-ə-məs\ *n, pl* **-mi** \-ˌmī, -ˌmē\ : the largest subdivision of the diencephalon that consists chiefly of an ovoid mass of nuclei in each lateral wall of the third ventricle and serves to relay impulses and esp. sensory impulses to and from the cerebral cortex

thal·as·sa·ne·mia *or Brit* **thal·as·sa·nae·mia** \ˌthal-ə-sə-'nē-mē-ə\ *n* : THALASSEMIA

thal·as·se·mia *or Brit* **thal·as·sae·mia** \ˌthal-ə-'sē-mē-ə\ *n* : any of a group of inherited hypochromic anemias esp. Cooley's anemia controlled by a series of allelic genes that cause reduction in or failure of synthesis of one of the globin chains making up hemoglobin and that tend to occur esp. in individuals of Mediterranean, African, or southeastern Asian ancestry — sometimes used with a prefix (as alpha-, beta-, or delta-) to indicate the hemoglobin chain affected; called also *Mediterranean anemia;* see BETA-THALASSEMIA

thalassemia major *n* : COOLEY'S ANEMIA

thalassemia minor *n* : a mild form of thalassemia associated with the heterozygous condition for the gene involved

¹thal·as·se·mic *or Brit* **thal·as·sae·mic** \ˌthal-ə-'sē-mik\ *adj* : of, relating to, or affected with thalassemia

²thalassemic *or Brit* **thalassaemic** *n* : an individual affected with thalassemia

tha·las·so·ther·a·py \thə-ˌlas-ō-'ther-ə-pē\ *n, pl* **-pies** : exposure to seawater (as in a hot tub) or application of sea products (as seaweed or sea salt) to the body for health or beauty benefits

tha·lid·o·mide \thə-'lid-ə-ˌmīd, -məd\ *n* : a sedative, hypnotic, and antiemetic drug $C_{13}H_{10}N_2O_4$ that was used chiefly in Europe during the late 1950s and early 1960s esp. to treat morning sickness but was soon withdrawn after being shown to cause serious malformations (as missing or severely shortened arms and legs) in infants born to mothers using it during the first trimester of pregnancy and has now been reintroduced for use as a treatment for the cutaneous complications of leprosy and is being investigated for use as an immunomodulatory, anti-inflammatory, and antiangiogenic agent in the treatment of various diseases

thalli *pl of* THALLUS

thal·li·um \'thal-ē-əm\ *n* : a sparsely but widely distributed poisonous metallic element that resembles lead in physical properties and is used chiefly in the form of compounds in photoelectric cells or as a pesticide — symbol *Tl;* see ELEMENT table

thallium sulfate *n* : a poisonous crystalline salt Tl_2SO_4 used chiefly as a rodenticide and insecticide — called also *thallous sulfate*

thal·lo·spore \'thal-ə-ˌspō(ə)r, -ˌspȯ(ə)r\ *n* : a spore (as a blastospore) developing by septation or budding of hyphal cells

thal·lous sulfate \'thal-əs-\ *n* : THALLIUM SULFATE

thal·lus \'thal-əs\ *n, pl* **thal·li** \'thal-ˌī, -ˌē\ *or* **thal·lus·es** : a plant or plantlike body (as of an alga, fungus, or moss) that lacks differentiation into distinct members (as stem, leaves, and roots) and does not grow from an apical point

than·a·tol·o·gist \ˌthan-ə-'täl-ə-jəst\ *n* : a person who specializes in thanatology

than·a·tol·o·gy \ˌthan-ə-'täl-ə-jē\ *n, pl* **-gies** : the description or study of the phenomena of death and of psychological mechanisms for coping with them — **than·a·to·log·i·cal** \ˌthan-ət-ᵊl-'äj-i-kəl\ *adj*

than·a·to·pho·bia \ˌthan-ət-ə-'fō-bē-ə\ *n* : fear of death

than·a·to·pho·ric \ˌthan-ət-ə-'fȯr-ik\ *adj* : relating to, affected with, or being a severe form of congenital dwarfism which results in early death

Than·a·tos \'than-ə-ˌtäs\ *n* : DEATH INSTINCT

THC \ˌtē-ˌāch-'sē\ *n* : either of two physiologically active isomers $C_{21}H_{30}O_2$ that occur naturally in hemp plant resin or are synthetically prepared: **a** : one that is the chief intoxicant in marijuana and is used medicinally — called also *delta-9-tetrahydrocannabinol, delta-9-THC;* see DRONABINOL **b** : one that is present in marijuana only in minute quantities

Δ⁹–THC *var of* DELTA-9-THC

the·ater *or* **the·atre** \'thē-ət-ər\ *n* **1** : a room often with rising tiers of seats for assemblies (as for lectures or surgical demonstrations) **2** *usu theatre, Brit* : a hospital operating room

the·ba·ine \thə-'bā-ˌēn\ *n* : a poisonous crystalline alkaloid $C_{19}H_{21}NO_3$ found in opium in small quantities, related chemically to morphine and codeine, and possessing a sharp astringent taste and a tetanic action like strychnine

The·be·sian vein \thə-'bē-zhən-\ *n* : any of the minute veins of the heart wall that drain directly into the cavity of the heart — called also *Thebesian vessel*

The·be·si·us \te-'bā-zē-əs\, **Adam Christian (1686–1732),** German anatomist. Thebesius was the first to examine the details of the circulation of the blood in the heart. He described the valve at the orifice of the coronary sinus, now known as the coronary valve or the valve of Thebesius, and the small veins by which the blood passes from the walls of the heart to the right atrium.

the·ca \'thē-kə\ *n, pl* **the·cae** \'thē-ˌsē, -ˌkē\ : an enveloping case or sheath (as the theca folliculi) of an anatomical part

theca cell *n* **1** : THECA LUTEIN CELL **2** : a cell of the columnar epithelium lining the gastric pits of the stomach

theca ex·ter·na \-ek-'stər-nə\ *n* : the outer layer of the theca folliculi that is composed of fibrous and muscular tissue

theca fol·lic·u·li \-fə-'lik-yə-ˌlī\ *n* : the outer covering of a graafian follicle that is made up of the theca externa and theca interna

theca in·ter·na \-in-'tər-nə\ *n* : the inner layer of the theca folliculi that is highly vascular and that contributes theca lutein cells to the formation of the corpus luteum

the·cal \'thē-kəl\ *adj* : of or relating to a theca

theca lutein cell *n* : any of the relatively deeply staining cells of the corpus luteum that are derived from cells of the theca interna, lack microvilli on the surface, and secrete estrone and estradiol as well as progesterone — called also *theca cell;* compare GRANULOSA LUTEIN CELL

Thee·lin \'thē-(ə)-lən\ *n* : a preparation of estrone — formerly a U.S. registered trademark

thei·le·ria \thī-'lir-ē-ə\ *n* **1** *cap* : a genus of sporozoan protozoans (family Theileriidae) that includes a parasite (*T. parva*) causing east coast fever of cattle **2** *pl* **-ri·ae** \-ē-ˌē\ *also* **-rias** : any organism of the genus *Theileria* — **thei·le·ri·al** \-ē-əl\ *adj*

Thei·ler \'tī-lər\, **Sir Arnold (1867–1936),** South African veterinary bacteriologist.

thei·le·ri·a·sis \ˌthī-lə-'rī-ə-səs\ *n, pl* **-a·ses** \-ˌsēz\ : THEILERIOSIS

thei·le·ri·o·sis \thī-ˌlir-ē-'ō-səs\ *n, pl* **-o·ses** \-ˌsēz\ *or* **-o·sis·es** : infection with or disease caused by a protozoan of the genus *Theileria; esp* : EAST COAST FEVER

the·lar·che \thē-'lär-kē\ *n* : the beginning of breast development at the onset of puberty ⟨premature ∼⟩

The·la·zia \thə-'lā-zē-ə\ *n* : a genus of nematode worms that is the type of the family Thelaziidae and includes various eye worms

thel·a·zi·a·sis \ˌthel-ə-'zī-ə-səs\ *n, pl* **-a·ses** \-ˌsēz\ : infestation with or disease caused by roundworms of the genus *Thelazia*

Thel·a·zi·idae \ˌthel-ə-'zī-ə-ˌdē\ *n pl* : a family of spiruroid nematode worms containing various forms of medical and veterinary importance — see THELAZIA

T–help·er cell \(')tē-'hel-pər-\ *n* : HELPER T CELL

T–helper lymphocyte *n* : HELPER T CELL

the·lyt·o·ky \thə-'lit-ə-kē\ *n, pl* **-kies** : parthenogenesis in which only female offspring are produced — compare ARRHENOTOKY, DEUTEROTOKY

the·mat·ic apperception test \thi-'mat-ik-\ *n* : a projective psychological test that is used in clinical psychology to make personality, psychodynamic, and diagnostic assessments based on the subject's verbal responses to a series of black and white pictures — abbr. *TAT*

the·nar \'thē-ˌnär, -nər\ *adj* : of, relating to, involving, or constituting the thenar eminence or the thenar muscles

thenar eminence *n* : the ball of the thumb

thenar muscle *n* : any of the muscles that comprise the intrinsic musculature of the thumb and include the abductor pollicis brevis, adductor pollicis, flexor pollicis brevis, and opponens pollicis

The·o·bro·ma \ˌthē-ə-'brō-mə\ *n* : a genus of tropical American trees (family Sterculiaceae) which includes the cacao (*T. cacao*)

theobroma oil *n* : COCOA BUTTER — used esp. in pharmacy

theo·bro·mine \ˌthē-ə-'brō-ˌmēn, -mən\ *n* : a bitter alkaloid $C_7H_8N_4O_2$ closely related to caffeine that occurs esp. in cacao beans and is used as a diuretic, myocardial stimulant, and vasodilator

the·oph·yl·line \thē-'äf-ə-lən\ *n* : a feebly basic bitter crystalline compound $C_7H_8N_4O_2$ that is present in small amounts in tea but is prepared chiefly by synthesis, that is isomeric with theobromine, and that is used in medicine often in the form of derivatives or in combination with other drugs esp. as a bronchodilator to relieve or prevent symptoms of asthma and bronchospasm associated with chronic bronchitis and emphysema

theophylline ethylenediamine *n* : AMINOPHYLLINE

the·o·ry \'thē-ə-rē, 'thi(-ə)r-ē\ *n, pl* **-ries** **1** : the general or abstract principles of a body of fact, a science, or an art ⟨the ∼ and practice of medicine⟩ **2** : a plausible or scientifically acceptable general principle or body of principles offered to explain natural phenomena ⟨a ∼ of organic evolution⟩ — see ATOMIC THEORY, CELL THEORY, GERM THEORY **3** : a working hypothesis that is considered probable based on experimental evidence or factual or conceptual analysis and is accepted as a basis for experimentation — **the·o·ret·i·cal** \ˌthē-ə-'ret-i-kəl, ˌthi(ə)r-'et-\ *also* **the·o·ret·ic** \-ik\ *adj* — **the·o·ret·i·cal·ly** \-i-k(ə-)lē\ *adv*

theory of epigenesis *n* : a theory in biology: development involves differentiation of an initially undifferentiated entity

ther·a·peu·sis \ˌther-ə-'pyü-səs\ *n, pl* **-peu·ses** \-ˌsēz\ : THERAPEUTICS

ther·a·peu·tic \-'pyüt-ik\ *adj* **1** : of or relating to the treatment of disease or disorders by remedial agents or methods ⟨a ∼ rather than a diagnostic specialty⟩ **2** : CURATIVE, MEDICINAL ⟨∼ activity of a drug⟩ ⟨∼ diets⟩ — **ther·a·peu·ti·cal·ly** \-i-k(ə-)lē\ *adv*

therapeutic abortion *n* : abortion induced when pregnancy constitutes a threat to the physical or mental health of the mother

therapeutic index *n* : a measure of the relative desirability of a drug for the attaining of a particular medical end that is usu. expressed as the ratio of the largest dose producing no toxic symptoms to the smallest dose routinely producing cures

therapeutic nihilism *n* : skepticism regarding the worth of therapeutic agents esp. in a particular disease

ther·a·peu·tics \ˌther-ə-'pyüt-iks\ *n pl but sing or pl in constr* : a branch of medical science dealing with the application of remedies to diseases ⟨cancer ∼⟩ — called also *therapeusis*

therapeutic touch *n* : a technique often included in alternative medicine in which the practitioner passes his or her hands over the body of the person being treated and that is held to induce relaxation, reduce pain, and promote healing

therapeutic window *n* **1** : the range of dosage of a drug or of its concentration in a bodily system that provides safe effective therapy ⟨the narrow *therapeutic window* . . . the effect may go from therapeutic to toxic with an increase of just 10 micrograms per milliliter [in] blood concentration —Lisa Davis⟩ **2** : a usu. short time interval (as after a precipitating event) during which a particular therapy can be given safely and effectively ⟨has a narrow *therapeutic window*: the drug must be given within three hours of a stroke in order to be effective —*Genesis Report-RX*⟩

ther·a·peu·tist \-'pyüt-əst\ *n* : a person skilled in therapeutics

the·ra·pia ste·ri·li·sans mag·na \the-'rā-pē-ə-ˌster-ə-'lī-ˌzanz-'mag-nə\ *n* : treatment of infectious disease by the administration of large doses of a specific remedy for the destruction of the infectious agent in the body without doing serious harm to the patient

ther·a·pist \'ther-ə-pəst\ *n* : a person specializing in therapy; *esp* : one trained in methods of treatment and rehabilitation other than the use of drugs or surgery

ther·a·py \'ther-ə-pē\ *n, pl* **-pies** : therapeutic treatment: as **a** : remedial treatment of mental or bodily disorder **b** : an agency (as treatment) designed or serving to bring about re-

\ə\ abut \ᵊ\ kitten \ər\ further \a\ ash \ā\ ace \ä\ cot, cart
\aú\ out \ch\ chin \e\ bet \ē\ easy \g\ go \i\ hit \ī\ ice \j\ job
\ŋ\ sing \ō\ go \ò\ law \òi\ boy \th\ thin \t̲h̲\ the \ü\ loot
\ú\ foot \y\ yet \zh\ vision   *See also* Pronunciation Symbols page

S
T

habilitation or social adjustment — see OCCUPATIONAL THERAPY, RECREATIONAL THERAPY

the·ri·ac \'thir-ē-ˌak\ n : THERIACA

the·ri·a·ca \thi-'rī-ə-kə\ n : an antidote to poison consisting typically of about 70 drugs pulverized and reduced with honey to an electuary — called also *Venice treacle*

theriaca An·drom·a·chi \-an-'dräm-ə-ˌkī\ n : THERIACA

An·drom·a·chus \an-'dräm-ə-kəs\ (*fl* 1st century AD), Greek physician. Andromachus was physician to the Roman emperor Nero. He is credited with the invention of the famous antidote for poison now known as theriaca Andromachi.

Ther·i·di·idae \ˌther-ə-'dī-ə-ˌdē\ n pl : a family of spiders that includes the genus *Latrodectus* and comprises those (as the black widow) which spin netlike webs and have usu. a small globose body and slender legs

the·rio·ge·nol·o·gist \ˌthir-ē-ō-jə-'näl-ə-jəst\ n : a veterinarian who specializes in theriogenology

the·rio·ge·nol·o·gy \ˌthir-ē-ō-jə-'näl-ə-jē\ n, pl **-gies** : a branch of veterinary medicine concerned with veterinary obstetrics and with the diseases and physiology of animal reproductive systems — **the·rio·gen·o·log·i·cal** \ˌthir-ē-ō-ˌjen-ə-'läj-i-kəl\ adj

the·rio·mor·phism \ˌthir-ē-ō-'mȯr-ˌfiz-əm\ n : the ascription of animal characteristics to humans — compare ANTHROPOMORPHISM

therm \'thərm\ n : any of several units of quantity of heat: as **a** : 1000 kilogram calories **b** : 100,000 British thermal units

ther·mal \'thər-məl\ adj **1** : of, relating to, or caused by heat ⟨tactile and ~ senses⟩ **2** : being or involving a state of matter dependent upon temperature ⟨~ agitation of molecular structure⟩ — **ther·mal·ly** \-mə-lē\ adv

thermal capacity n : HEAT CAPACITY

thermal death point n : the temperature at which all organisms of a culture will be killed by heat either instantaneously or within an arbitrary brief finite period

therm·ion·ic emission \ˌthər-(ˌ)mī-'än-ik-\ n : emission of particles (as electrons) from materials at high temperature due to the heat energy imparted to them

therm·is·tor \'thər-ˌmis-tər\ n : an electrical resistor making use of a semiconductor whose resistance varies sharply in a known manner with the temperature

ther·mo·cau·ter·iza·tion or chiefly Brit **ther·mo·cau·ter·isa·tion** \ˌthər-mō-ˌkȯt-ə-rə-'zā-shən\ n : cautery by the application of heat

ther·mo·cau·tery \-'kȯt-ə-rē\ n, pl **-ter·ies** **1** : THERMOCAUTERIZATION **2** : ACTUAL CAUTERY

ther·mo·chem·is·try \ˌthər-mō-'kem-ə-strē\ n, pl **-tries** : a branch of chemistry that deals with the interrelation of heat with chemical reaction or physical change of state — **ther·mo·chem·i·cal** \-'kem-i-kəl\ adj

ther·mo·co·ag·u·la·tion \ˌthər-mō-kō-ˌag-yə-'lā-shən\ n : surgical coagulation of tissue by the application of heat

ther·mo·cou·ple \'thər-mə-ˌkəp-əl\ n : a device for measuring temperature in which a pair of wires of dissimilar metals (as copper and iron) are joined and the free ends of the wires are connected to an instrument (as a voltmeter) that measures the difference in potential created at the junction of the two metals

ther·mo·di·lu·tion \ˌthər-mō-dī-'lü-shən\ adj : relating to or being a method of determining cardiac output by measurement of the change in temperature in the bloodstream after injecting a measured amount of cool fluid (as saline)

ther·mo·du·ric \ˌthər-mō-'d(y)u̇(ə)r-ik\ adj : THERMOTOLERANT ⟨~ bacteria⟩

ther·mo·dy·nam·ic \ˌthər-mō-dī-'nam-ik, -də-\ also **ther·mo·dy·nam·i·cal** \-i-kəl\ adj **1** : of or relating to thermodynamics **2** : being or relating to a system of atoms, molecules, colloidal particles, or larger bodies considered as an isolated group in the study of thermodynamic processes — **ther·mo·dy·nam·i·cal·ly** \-i-k(ə)lē\ adv

ther·mo·dy·nam·ics \-iks\ n pl but sing or pl in constr **1** : physics that deals with the mechanical action or relations of heat **2** : thermodynamic processes and phenomena

ther·mo·elec·tric \ˌthər-mō-i-'lek-trik\ adj : of, relating to, or dependent on phenomena that involve relations between the temperature and the electrical condition in a metal or in contacting metals

ther·mo·gen·e·sis \ˌthər-mō-'jen-ə-səs\ n, pl **-e·ses** \-ˌsēz\ : the production of heat esp. in the body (as by oxidation)

ther·mo·gen·ic \ˌthər-mə-'jen-ik\ adj : of or relating to the production of heat : producing heat

ther·mo·gram \'thər-mə-ˌgram\ n **1** : the record made by a thermograph **2** : a photographic record made by thermography

ther·mo·graph \-ˌgraf\ n **1** : THERMOGRAM **2** : the apparatus used in thermography **3** : a thermometer that produces an automatic record

ther·mog·ra·phy \(ˌ)thər-'mäg-rə-fē\ n, pl **-phies** : a technique for detecting and measuring variations in the heat emitted by various regions of the body and transforming them into visible signals that can be recorded photographically (as for diagnosing abnormal or diseased underlying conditions) — **ther·mo·graph·ic** \ˌthər-mə-'graf-ik\ adj — **ther·mo·graph·i·cal·ly** \-i-k(ə)lē\ adv

ther·mo·la·bile \ˌthər-mō-'lā-ˌbīl, -bəl\ adj : unstable when heated; specif : subject to loss of characteristic properties on being heated to or above 55°C ⟨~ enzymes and vitamins⟩ — **ther·mo·la·bil·i·ty** \-lā-'bil-ət-ē\ n, pl **-ties**

ther·mol·y·sin \thər-'mäl-ə-sən\ n : a zinc-containing microbial enzyme that is used to catalyze the hydrolysis of proteins esp. when it is desired to keep the disulfide bonds intact

ther·mol·y·sis \(ˌ)thər-'mäl-ə-səs\ n, pl **-y·ses** \-ˌsēz\ **1** : the dissipation of heat from the living body **2** : decomposition by heat — **ther·mo·lyt·ic** \ˌthər-mə-'lit-ik\ adj

ther·mom·e·ter \thə(r)-'mäm-ət-ər\ n : an instrument for determining temperature that usu. consists either of a device providing a digital readout or of a glass bulb attached to a fine tube of glass with a numbered scale and containing a liquid (as mercury or colored alcohol) that is sealed in and rises and falls with changes of temperature

ther·mo·met·ric \ˌthər-mə-'me-trik\ adj : of or relating to a thermometer or to thermometry

ther·mom·e·try \thə(r)-'mäm-ə-trē\ n, pl **-tries** : the measurement of temperature

ther·mo·phile \'thər-mə-ˌfīl\ n : a thermophilic organism — compare MESOPHILE, PSYCHROPHILE

ther·mo·phil·ic \ˌthər-mə-'fil-ik\ adj also **ther·moph·i·lous** \(ˌ)thər-'mäf-ə-ləs\ adj : of, relating to, or being an organism living at a high temperature ⟨~ bacteria⟩

¹ther·mo·plas·tic \ˌthər-mə-'plas-tik\ adj : capable of softening or fusing when heated and of hardening again when cooled ⟨~ synthetic resins⟩ — **ther·mo·plas·tic·i·ty** \-ˌplas-'tis-ət-ē\ n, pl **-ties**

²thermoplastic n : a thermoplastic material

ther·mo·re·cep·tor \ˌthər-mō-ri-'sep-tər\ n : a sensory end organ that is stimulated by heat or cold

ther·mo·reg·u·la·tion \-ˌreg-yə-'lā-shən\ n : the maintenance or regulation of temperature; specif : the maintenance of a particular temperature of the living body — **ther·mo·reg·u·late** \-'reg-yə-ˌlāt\ vb **-lat·ed; -lat·ing**

ther·mo·reg·u·la·tor \-'reg-yə-ˌlāt-ər\ n : a device (as a thermostat) for the regulation of temperature

ther·mo·reg·u·la·to·ry \-'reg-yə-lə-ˌtōr-ē, -ˌtȯr-\ adj : tending to maintain a body at a particular temperature whatever its environmental temperature ⟨~ adjustments⟩

ther·mo·scope \'thər-mə-ˌskōp\ n : an instrument for indicating changes of temperature by accompanying changes in volume (as of a gas)

ther·mo·set·ting \-ˌset-iŋ\ adj : capable of becoming permanently rigid when heated or cured ⟨a ~ resin⟩

ther·mo·sta·ble \ˌthər-mō-'stā-bəl\ adj : stable when heated; specif : retaining characteristic properties on being moderately heated ⟨a ~ bacterial protease⟩ — **ther·mo·sta·bil·i·ty** \-stə-'bil-ət-ē\ n, pl **-ties**

¹ther·mo·stat \'thər-mə-ˌstat\ n **1** : an automatic device for regulating temperature (as by controlling the supply of gas or electricity to a heating apparatus) **2** : a piece of apparatus (as a constant-temperature chamber) regulated by a thermostat — **ther·mo·stat·ic** \ˌthər-mə-ˈstat-ik\ *adj* — **ther·mo·stat·i·cal·ly** \-i-k(ə-)lē\ *adv*

²**thermostat** *vt* **-stat·ed** \-ˌstat-əd\ *or* **-stat·ted; -stat·ing** *or* **-stat·ting** : to provide with or control the temperature of by a thermostat ⟨a *thermostated* centrifuge⟩

ther·mo·strom·uhr \ˌthər-mō-ˈstrō-ˌmù(ə)r\ *n* : a stromuhr that measures the rate of blood flow in an intact blood vessel by determining the amount of heating of the blood as indicated by a sensitive galvanometer when a radio-frequency current is passed through the vessel between thermocouples so that the amount of heating is inversely proportional to the rate of flow

ther·mo·tac·tic \ˌthər-mə-ˈtak-tik\ *adj* : of, relating to, or exhibiting thermotaxis

ther·mo·tax·is \-ˈtak-səs\ *n, pl* **-tax·es** \-ˌsēz\ **1** : a taxis in which a temperature gradient constitutes the directive factor **2** : the regulation of body temperature

ther·mo·ther·a·py \-ˈther-ə-pē\ *n, pl* **-pies** : treatment of disease by heat (as by hot air, hot baths, or diathermy)

ther·mo·tol·er·ant \-ˈtäl-(ə-)rənt\ *adj* : able to survive high temperatures; *specif* : able to survive pasteurization — used of microorganisms ⟨~ bacteria⟩ ⟨~ yeast⟩

ther·mo·trop·ic \-ˈträp-ik\ *adj* : of, relating to, or exhibiting thermotropism

ther·mot·ro·pism \ˌ(ˌ)thər-ˈmä-trə-ˌpiz-əm\ *n* : a tropism in which a temperature gradient determines the orientation

the·sau·ro·sis \ˌthē-sȯ-ˈrō-səs\ *n, pl* **-ro·ses** \-ˌsēz\ *or* **-ro·sis·es** : STORAGE DISEASE

the·ta rhythm \ˈthāt-ə-, *Brit usu* ˈthēt-ə-\ *n* : a relatively high amplitude brain wave pattern between approximately 4 and 9 hertz that is characteristic esp. of the hippocampus but occurs in many regions of the brain including the cortex — called also *theta, theta wave*

the·ve·tin \thə-ˈvēt-ⁿn, ˈthev-ət-ən\ *n* : a poisonous crystalline cardiac glycoside $C_{42}H_{66}O_{18}$ obtained esp. from the seeds of a West Indian shrub or small tree (*Thevetia nereifolia*) of the dogbane family (Apocynaceae) that yields glucose, digitalose, and a sterol on hydrolysis

thia·ben·da·zole \ˌthī-ə-ˈben-də-ˌzōl\ *n* : a drug $C_{10}H_7N_3S$ used in the control of parasitic nematodes and in the treatment of fungus infections and as an agricultural fungicide

thi·acet·azone \ˌthī-ə-ˈset-ə-ˌzōn\ *n* : a bitter pale yellow crystalline tuberculostatic drug $C_{10}H_{12}N_4OS$

thi·ami·nase \thī-ˈam-ə-ˌnās, ˈthī-ə-mə-, -ˌnāz\ *n* : an enzyme that catalyzes the breakdown of thiamine

thi·a·mine \ˈthī-ə-mən, -ˌmēn\ *also* **thi·a·min** \-mən\ *n* : a vitamin $C_{12}H_{17}N_4OSCl$ of the B complex that is an amino hydroxy quaternary ammonium water-soluble salt containing a thiazole ring and a pyrimidine ring, that occurs widely both free (as in the germs of cereals and hulls of grain) and combined (as in yeast and in animal tissues like liver, kidneys, and heart) but is usu. synthesized commercially, that functions in the body as a cocarboxylase and is essential for carbohydrate metabolism and for normal functioning of the nervous system, and that is used in nutrition (as in vitamin preparations and in enriching flour and bread) and in medicine — called also *vitamin B₁*

thiamine pyrophosphate *n* : COCARBOXYLASE

Thi·ara \thī-ˈar-ə\ *n* : a genus of freshwater snails (the type genus of the family Thiaridae) that includes several forms (as *T. granifera* of eastern Asia and the western Pacific islands) which are intermediate hosts of medically important trematodes

thi·a·zide \ˈthī-ə-ˌzīd, -zəd\ *n* : any of a group of drugs used as oral diuretics esp. in the control of high blood pressure

thi·a·zine \ˈthī-ə-ˌzēn\ *n* : any of various compounds that are characterized by a ring composed of four carbon atoms, one sulfur atom, and one nitrogen atom and include some that are important as dyes and others that are important as tranquilizers — see PHENOTHIAZINE

thi·a·zole \ˈthī-ə-ˌzōl\ *n* **1** : a colorless basic liquid C_3H_3NS consisting of a 5-membered ring and having an odor like pyridine **2** : any of various thiazole derivatives including

some that are used in medicine and others that are important as chemical accelerators

thi·a·zol·i·dine \ˌthī-ə-ˈzō-lə-ˌdēn\ *n* : a basic liquid saturated heterocyclic compound C_3H_7NS whose ring is present in the structure of penicillin

thi·a·zol·i·dine·di·one \ˌthī-ə-ˌzō-lə-ˌdēn-ˈdī-ˌōn\ *n* : any of a class of drugs (as pioglitazone and rosiglitazone) that are thiazolidine derivatives used to reduce insulin resistance in the treatment of type 2 diabetes

thick filament *n* : a myofilament of one of the two types making up myofibrils that is 10 to 12 nanometers (100 to 120 angstroms) in width and is composed of the protein myosin — compare THIN FILAMENT

thick wind \ˈthik-ˌwind\ *n* : a chronic defect of respiration in the horse due to obstruction of the respiratory passages (as by nasal polyps or deformed bones) — compare ROARING — **thick–wind·ed** \-ˈwind-əd\ *adj*

Thiersch graft \ˈtirsh-\ *n* : a skin graft that consists of thin strips or sheets of epithelium with the tops of the dermal papillae and that is split off with a sharp knife

   Thiersch, Carl (1822–1895), German surgeon. Thiersch is famous for introducing epidermal grafting in plastic surgery and for his monographs on epithelial cancer of the skin and the healing of wounds. He introduced the Thiersch graft in 1874.

thigh \ˈthī\ *n* **1** : the proximal segment of the vertebrate hind or lower limb extending from the hip to the knee and supported by a single large bone — compare FEMUR 1 **2** : the segment of the leg immediately distal to the thigh in a bird or in a quadruped in which the true thigh is obscured **3** : the femur of an insect

thigh bone \ˈthī-ˌbōn, -ˌbōn\ *n* : FEMUR 1

thig·mo·tac·tic \ˌthig-mə-ˈtak-tik\ *adj* : of, relating to, or involving a thigmotaxis

thig·mo·tax·is \ˌthig-mə-ˈtak-səs\ *n, pl* **-tax·es** \-ˌsēz\ : a taxis in which contact esp. with a solid body is the directive factor

thig·mo·trop·ic \ˌthig-mə-ˈträp-ik\ *adj* : of, relating to, or exhibiting thigmotropism

thig·mot·ro·pism \thig-ˈmä-trə-ˌpiz-əm\ *n* : a tropism in which physical contact esp. with a solid or a rigid surface is the factor causing orientation of the whole organism

thim·ble jellyfish \ˈthim-bəl-\ *n* : a small scyphozoan jellyfish (*Linuche unguiculata*) whose tiny larvae cause seabather's eruption esp. in coastal waters of southern Florida and the Caribbean

thi·mer·o·sal \thī-ˈmer-ə-ˌsal\ *n* : a crystalline organic mercurial antiseptic $C_9H_9HgNaO_2S$ used esp. for its antifungal and bacteriostatic properties — see MERTHIOLATE

thin filament *n* : a myofilament of the one of the two types making up myofibrils that is about 5 nanometers (50 angstroms) in width and is composed chiefly of the protein actin — compare THICK FILAMENT

thin–layer chromatography \ˈthin-ˌlā-ər-\ *n* : chromatography in which the solution containing the substances to be separated migrates by capillarity through a thin layer of the adsorbent medium (as silica gel, alumina, or cellulose) arranged on a rigid support — abbr. *TLC*; compare COLUMN CHROMATOGRAPHY, GAS CHROMATOGRAPHY, PAPER CHROMATOGRAPHY — **thin–layer chromatogram** *n* — **thin–layer chromatographic** *adj*

thio \ˈthī-ō\ *adj* : relating to or containing sulfur esp. in place of oxygen

thio acid *n* : an acid in which oxygen is partly or wholly replaced by sulfur

thio·al·co·hol \ˌthī-ō-ˈal-kə-ˌhȯl\ *n* : a thiol with the general formula RSH in which the R group is an alkyl or a cyclic alkyl

thio·al·de·hyde \-ˈal-də-ˌhīd\ *n* : a compound having the

\ə\ **abut** \ˌ,ˌ\ **kitten** \ər\ **further** \a\ **ash** \ā\ **ace** \ä\ **cot, cart**
\aù\ **out** \ch\ **chin** \e\ **bet** \ē\ **easy** \g\ **go** \i\ **hit** \ī\ **ice** \j\ **job**
\ŋ\ **sing** \ō\ **go** \ȯ\ **law** \ȯi\ **boy** \th\ **thin** \t̲h̲\ **the** \ü\ **loot**
\ù\ **foot** \y\ **yet** \zh\ **vision** *See also* Pronunciation Symbols page

S
T

general formula RCHS that is an aldehyde in which oxygen is replaced by sulfur

thio·amide \-'am-,īd, -əd\ *n* : an amide of a thio acid; *esp* : an amide having the general formula RCSNH₂

thio·ba·cil·lus \-bə-'sil-əs\ *n* **1** *cap* : a genus of small rod-shaped bacteria (family Thiobacteriaceae) that live in water, sewage, and soils, derive energy from oxidation of sulfides, thiosulfates, or elemental sulfur, and obtain carbon from carbon dioxide, bicarbonates, or carbonates in solution **2** *pl* **-li** \-,lī\ : any bacterium (as some sulfur bacteria) of the genus *Thiobacillus*

thio·bar·bi·tu·ric acid \-,bär-bə-,t(y)ùr-ik-\ *n* : a barbituric acid derivative $C_6H_4N_2O_2S$ that is used to form a series of thio analogs of the barbiturates

thio·car·ba·mide \,thī-ō-'kär-bə-,mīd, -kär-'bam-,īd\ *n* : THIOUREA

thio·chrome \'thī-ə-,krōm\ *n* : a yellow crystalline tricyclic alcohol $C_{12}H_{14}N_4OS$ found in yeast, formed by oxidation of thiamine, and giving a blue fluorescence under ultraviolet light that serves as the basis of a method of determining thiamine

thi·oc·tic acid *also* **6,8-thi·oc·tic acid** \(,siks-,āt-)thī-,äk-tik-\ *n* : a lipoic acid $C_8H_{14}O_2S_2$ that has been reported to ameliorate the effects of poisoning by mushrooms (as the death cap) of the genus *Amanita*

thio·cy·a·nate \,thī-ō-'sī-ə-,nāt, -nət\ *n* : a compound that consists of the chemical group SCN bonded by the sulfur atom to a group or an atom other than a hydrogen atom

thio·cy·an·ic \-sī-'an-ik\ *adj* : of, relating to, or being a colorless unstable liquid acid HSCN of strong odor

thiocyanoacetate — see ISOBORNYL THIOCYANOACETATE

thio·di·phe·nyl·amine \-,dī-,fen-ᵊl-'am-,ēn, -,fēn-ᵊl-, -ə-'mēn\ *n* : PHENOTHIAZINE 1

thio·es·ter \,thī-ō-'es-tər\ *n* : an ester formed by uniting a carboxyl group of one compound (as acetic acid) with a sulfhydryl group of another (as coenzyme A)

thio·ether \-'ē-thər\ *n* : a compound analogous to ether in which the oxygen has been replaced by sulfur

thio·fla·vine \-'flā-,vēn\ *also* **thio·fla·vin** \-'flā-vən\ *n* : either of two yellow thiazole dyes used as biological stains as well as in dyeing or making organic pigments

thioglucose — see GOLD THIOGLUCOSE

thio·gly·co·late *also* **thio·gly·col·late** \,thī-ō-'glī-kə-,lāt\ *n* : a salt or ester of thioglycolic acid

thio·gly·col·ic acid *also* **thio·gly·col·lic acid** \-glī-,käl-ik-\ *n* : an ill-smelling liquid mercapto acid $C_2H_4O_2S$ that is used as a reagent for ferric iron and esp. in the form of its calcium salt as a depilatory

thio·gua·nine \-'gwän-,ēn\ *n* : a crystalline compound $C_5H_5N_5S$ that is an antimetabolite and has been used in the treatment of leukemia

thi·ol \'thī-,ȯl, -,ōl\ *n* **1** : any of a class of compounds that are analogous to alcohols and phenols but contain sulfur in place of oxygen with the general formula RSH and in the case of those of low molecular weight have very disagreeable odors — called also *mercaptan* **2** : the functional group –SH characteristic of thiols — **thi·o·lic** \thī-'ō-lik\ *adj*

thiol group *n* : THIOL 2

thiomalate — see GOLD SODIUM THIOMALATE

thio·ne·ine \,thī-ə-'nē-ən, -ēn\ *n* : ERGOTHIONEINE

thi·on·ic acid \thī-'än-ik-\ *n* : any of a series of unstable acids of the general formula $H_2S_nO_6$ in which the number of atoms of sulfur in the molecule varies from 2 to 6

thi·o·nine \'thī-ə-,nēn, -nən\ *n* : a dark crystalline basic thiazine dye that is used chiefly as a biological stain

thi·o·nyl chloride \'thī-ə-,nil-\ *n* : a volatile corrosive liquid compound $SOCl_2$ used chiefly in making acyl chlorides from carboxylic acids

thio·pen·tal \,thī-ō-'pen-,tal, -,tȯl\ *n* : a barbiturate used in the form of its sodium salt $C_{11}H_{17}N_2NaO_2S$ esp. as an intravenous anesthetic — see PENTOTHAL

thio·pen·tone \-,tōn\ *n, Brit* : THIOPENTAL

thio·phene \'thī-ə-,fēn\ *also* **thio·phen** \-,fen\ *n* : a heterocyclic liquid C_4H_4S from coal tar that resembles benzene and is used chiefly in organic synthesis

thio·phos·phate \,thī-ō-'fäs-,fāt\ *n* : a salt or ester of an acid derived from a phosphoric acid by replacement of one or more atoms of oxygen with sulfur

thio·rid·a·zine \,thī-ə-'rid-ə-,zēn, -zən\ *n* : a phenothiazine tranquilizer used in the form of its hydrochloride $C_{21}H_{26}N_2S_2\cdot HCl$ for relief of anxiety states and in the treatment of psychotic disorders and severe childhood behavioral problems — see MELLARIL

thio·semi·car·ba·zide \,thī-ō-,sem-i-'kär-bə-,zīd\ *n* : a crystalline compound CH_5N_3S that is the analog of semicarbazide in which oxygen is replaced by sulfur

thio·semi·car·ba·zone \-'kär-bə-,zōn\ *n* : any of a class of compounds analogous to semicarbazones and formed by the action of thiosemicarbazide on an aldehyde or ketone

thio·sin·amine \,thī-ō-'sin-ə-,mēn\ *n* : ALLYLTHIOUREA

thio·sul·fate *or chiefly Brit* **thio·sul·phate** \-'səl-,fāt\ *n* : a salt or ester of thiosulfuric acid

thio·sul·fu·ric *or chiefly Brit* **thio·sul·phu·ric** \-,səl-'fyù(ə)r-ik\ *adj* : of, relating to, or being an unstable acid $H_2S_2O_3$ derived from sulfuric acid by replacement of one oxygen atom by sulfur and known only in solution or in salts and esters

thio·te·pa \,thī-ə-'tē-pə\ *n* : a sulfur analog of tepa $C_6H_{12}N_3PS$ that is used esp. as an antineoplastic agent and is less toxic than tepa

thio·thix·ene \,thī-ō-'thik-,sēn\ *n* : an antipsychotic drug $C_{23}H_{29}N_3O_2S_2$ used esp. in the treatment of schizophrenia — see NAVANE

thio·ura·cil \,thī-ō-'yùr-ə-,sil\ *n* : a bitter crystalline compound $C_4H_4N_2OS$ that depresses the function of the thyroid gland

thio·urea \-yù-'rē-ə\ *n* : a colorless bitter crystalline compound $CS(NH_2)_2$ analogous to and resembling urea that is used esp. as a reagent and in medicine as an antithyroid drug — called also *thiocarbamide*

thio·xan·thene \,thī-ō-'zan-,thēn\ *n* : a compound $C_{13}H_{10}S$ that is the parent compound of various antipsychotic drugs (as thiothixene); *also* : a derivative of thioxanthene

thi·ram \'thī-,ram\ *n* : a compound $C_6H_{12}N_2S_4$ used as a fungicide

third cranial nerve *n* : OCULOMOTOR NERVE

third–de·gree burn \'thərd-di-,grē-\ *n* : a severe burn characterized by destruction of the skin through the depth of the dermis and possibly into underlying tissues, loss of fluid, and sometimes shock

third eyelid *n* : NICTITATING MEMBRANE

third law of thermodynamics *n* : LAW OF THERMODYNAMICS 3

third ventricle *n* : the median unpaired ventricle of the brain bounded by parts of the telencephalon and diencephalon

thirst \'thərst\ *n* : a sensation of dryness in the mouth and throat associated with a desire for liquids; *also* : the bodily condition (as of dehydration) that induces this sensation

thirsty \'thər-stē\ *adj* **thirst·i·er; -est** : feeling thirst

thix·ot·ro·py \thik-'sä-trə-pē\ *n, pl* **-pies** : the property of various gels of becoming fluid when disturbed (as by shaking) — **thixo·tro·pic** \,thik-sə-'trō-pik, -'träp-ik\ *adj*

THM *abbr* trihalomethane

Thom·as splint \'täm-əs-\ *n* : a metal splint for fractures of the arm or leg that consists of a ring at one end to fit around the upper arm or leg and two metal shafts extending down the sides of the limb in a long U with a crosspiece at the bottom where traction is applied

Thomas, Hugh Owen (1834–1891), British orthopedic surgeon. Thomas is considered by many the founder of modern orthopedics in Great Britain. He introduced a splint for immobilization of the hip, a knee splint for immobilization of the knee, and a caliper splint for ambulatory patients.

Thom·sen's disease \'tȯm-sənz-\ *n* : MYOTONIA CONGENITA

Thomsen, Asmus Julius Thomas (1815–1896), Danish physician. In 1876 Thomsen gave the first full description of a congenital disease marked by tonic spasm of some of the muscles. He himself suffered from this condition, which is now known as myotonia congenita or Thomsen's disease.

thon·zyl·a·mine \thän-'zil-ə-ˌmēn, -mən\ *n* : an antihistamine derived from pyrimidine and used in the form of its crystalline hydrochloride $C_{16}H_{22}N_4O\cdot HCl$

tho·ra·cen·te·sis \ˌthō-rə-sen-'tē-səs\ *n, pl* **-te·ses** \-ˌsēz\ : aspiration of fluid from the chest (as in empyema) — called also *thoracocentesis*

thoraces *pl of* THORAX

tho·rac·ic \thə-'ras-ik\ *adj* : of, relating to, located within, or involving the thorax ⟨~ trauma⟩ ⟨~ surgery⟩ — **tho·rac·i·cal·ly** \-i-k(ə-)lē\ *adv*

thoracic aorta *n* : the part of the aorta that lies in the thorax and extends from the arch to the diaphragm

thoracic artery *n* : either of two arteries that branch from the axillary artery or from one of its branches: **a** : a small artery that usu. arises from the axillary artery below the clavicle and that supplies or sends branches to the two pectoralis muscles and the walls of the chest — called also *supreme thoracic artery* **b** : an artery that often arises from the thoracoacromial artery or from the subscapular artery rather than the axillary artery and that supplies both pectoralis muscles and the serratus anterior and sends branches to the lymph nodes of the axilla and to the subscapularis muscle — called also *lateral thoracic artery*; compare INTERNAL THORACIC ARTERY

thoracic cage *n* : RIB CAGE

thoracic cavity *n* : the division of the body cavity that lies above the diaphragm, is bounded peripherally by the wall of the chest, and contains the heart and lungs

thoracic duct *n* : the main trunk of the system of lymphatic vessels that lies along the front of the spinal column, extends from a dilatation behind the aorta and opposite the second lumbar vertebra up through the thorax where it turns to the left and opens into the left subclavian vein, and receives chyle from the intestine and lymph from the abdomen, the lower limbs, and the entire left side of the body — called also *left lymphatic duct*

thoracic ganglion *n* : any of the ganglia of the sympathetic chain in the thoracic region that occur in 12 or fewer pairs

thoracic nerve *n* : any of the spinal nerves of the thoracic region that consist of 12 pairs of which one pair emerges just below each thoracic vertebra

thoracic vertebra *n* : any of the 12 vertebrae dorsal to the thoracic region and characterized by articulation with the ribs — called also *dorsal vertebra*

thoracis — see ILIOCOSTALIS THORACIS, LONGISSIMUS THORACIS, SEMISPINALIS THORACIS, SPINALIS THORACIS, TRANSVERSUS THORACIS

tho·ra·co·ab·dom·i·nal \ˌthō-rə-ˌkō-ab-'däm-ən-ᵊl\ *also* **tho·rac·i·co·ab·dom·i·nal** \thə-ˌras-i-ˌkō-\ *adj* : of, relating to, involving, or affecting the thorax and the abdomen ⟨a ~ incision⟩ ⟨a ~ tumor⟩

tho·ra·co·acro·mi·al artery \ˌthō-rə-ˌkō-ə-'krō-mē-əl-\ *n* : a short branch of the axillary artery that divides into four branches supplying the region of the pectoralis muscles, deltoid, subclavius, and sternoclavicular joint

tho·ra·co·cen·te·sis \-sen-'tē-səs\ *n, pl* **-te·ses** \-ˌsēz\ : THORACENTESIS

tho·ra·co·dor·sal artery \ˌthō-rə-kō-ˌdor-səl-\ *n* : an artery that is continuous with the axillary artery, accompanies the thoracodorsal nerve, and supplies or gives off branches supplying the subscapularis muscle, latissimus dorsi, serratus anterior, and the intercostal muscles

thoracodorsal nerve *n* : a branch of the posterior cord of the brachial plexus that supplies the latissimus dorsi

tho·ra·co·gas·tros·chi·sis \ˌthō-rə-ˌkō-gas-'träs-kə-səs\ *n, pl* **-chi·ses** \-ˌsēz\ *or* **-chi·sis·es** : a congenital developmental defect in which the body wall fails to close properly along the midline of the front of the thorax and abdomen allowing protrusion of the viscera

tho·ra·co·lum·bar \-'ləm-bər, -ˌbär\ *adj* **1** : of, relating to,

arising in, or involving the thoracic and lumbar regions **2** : SYMPATHETIC 1 ⟨~ nerve fibers⟩

tho·ra·cop·a·gus \ˌthor-ə-'käp-ə-gəs, ˌthor-\ *n, pl* **-gi** \-ˌjī\ : conjoined twins that are united at the thorax

tho·ra·co·plas·ty \'thor-ə-kō-ˌplas-tē, 'thor-\ *n, pl* **-ties** : the surgical operation of removing or resecting one or more ribs so as to obliterate the pleural cavity and collapse a diseased lung

tho·ra·co·scope \thə-'rāk-ə-ˌskōp, -'rak-\ *n* : an endoscope that is inserted through a puncture in the chest wall in an intercostal space (as for the visual examination of the chest cavity) — **tho·ra·co·scop·ic** \thə-ˌrak-ə-'skäp-ik, -ˌrak-\ *adj*

tho·ra·cos·co·py \ˌthor-ə-'käs-kə-pē, ˌthor-\ *n, pl* **-pies** : examination of the chest and esp. the pleural cavity by means of a thoracoscope

tho·ra·cos·to·my \ˌthor-ə-'käs-tə-mē, ˌthor-\ *n, pl* **-mies** : surgical opening of the chest (as for drainage)

tho·ra·cot·o·my \ˌthor-ə-'kät-ə-mē, ˌthor-\ *n, pl* **-mies** : surgical incision of the chest wall

tho·rax \'thō(ə)r-ˌaks, 'thò(ə)r-\ *n, pl* **tho·rax·es** *or* **tho·ra·ces** \'thor-ə-ˌsēz, 'thor-\ **1** : the part of the mammalian body that is situated between the neck and the abdomen and supported by the ribs, costal cartilages, and sternum; *also* : THORACIC CAVITY **2** : the middle of the three chief divisions of the body of an insect; *also* : the corresponding part of a crustacean or an arachnid

Tho·ra·zine \'thor-ə-ˌzēn, 'thor-\ *trademark* — used for a preparation of the hydrochloride of chlorpromazine

tho·ri·um \'thor-ē-əm, 'thor-\ *n* : a radioactive metallic element that occurs combined in minerals and is usu. associated with rare earths — symbol *Th*; see ELEMENT table

thorium dioxide *n* : a refractory crystalline compound obtained usu. as a dense white powder and formerly used as a contrast medium in radiography — called also *thorium oxide, thorotrast*

thorn apple \'thor(ə)rn-\ *n* : JIMSONWEED; *also* : any plant of the genus *Datura*

thorn–head·ed worm *or* **thorny–head·ed worm** \'thorn(-ē)-ˌhed-əd-\ *n* : any worm of the group Acanthocephala

tho·ron \'thō(ə)r-ˌän, 'thò(ə)r-\ *n* : a heavy radioactive isotope of radon of mass number 220 that is formed as a decay product of thorium, decays by emission of an alpha particle, and has a half-life of less than a minute

tho·ro·trast \'thor-ə-ˌtrast\ *n* : THORIUM DIOXIDE

thor·ough·pin \'thər-ə-ˌpin, 'thə-rə-\ *n* : a synovial swelling just above the hock of a horse on both sides of the leg and slightly anterior to the hamstring tendon that is often associated with lameness

thought \'thot\ *n* **1 a** : the action or process of thinking **b** : serious consideration **2 a** : reasoning power **b** : the power to imagine : CONCEPTION **3** : something that is thought: as **a** : an individual act or product of thinking **b** : a developed intention or plan ⟨he had no ~ of leaving home⟩ **c** : something (as an opinion or belief) in the mind ⟨she spoke her ~s freely⟩ **d** : the intellectual product or the organized views and principles of a period, place, group, or individual

Thr *abbr* threonine; threonyl

thread lungworm \'thred-\ *n* : a slender widely distributed nematode worm of the genus *Dictyocaulus* (*D. filaria*) that parasitizes the air passages of the lungs of sheep

thread·worm \'thred-ˌwərm\ *n* : any long slender nematode worm (as a pinworm or strongyle)

thready \-ē\ *adj* **1** : resembling a thread **2** : of, relating to, or being a thready pulse

thready pulse *n* : a scarcely perceptible and commonly rapid pulse that feels like a fine mobile thread under a palpating finger

three–day fever \'thrē-ˌdā-\ *n* : a fever or febrile state lasting three days: as **a** : SANDFLY FEVER **b** : EPHEMERAL FEVER

\ə\ abut \ᵊ\ kitten \ər\ further \a\ ash \ā\ ace \ä\ cot, cart
\aù\ out \ch\ chin \e\ bet \ē\ easy \g\ go \i\ hit \ī\ ice \j\ job
\ŋ\ sing \ō\ go \ò\ law \òi\ boy \th\ thin \th\ the \ü\ loot
\ù\ foot \y\ yet \zh\ vision *See also* Pronunciation Symbols page

S
T

3TC \ˌthrē-(ˌ)tē-ˈsē\ *trademark* — used for a preparation of lamivudine

thre·o·nine \ˈthrē-ə-ˌnēn\ *n* : a colorless crystalline essential amino acid $C_4H_9NO_3$ that is found in various proteins — abbr. *Thr*

thre·o·nyl \-ˌnil\ *n* : the amino acid radical or residue $CH_3CH(OH)CH(NH_3)COO-$ of threonine — abbr. *Thr*

thre·ose \ˈthrē-ˌōs\ *n* : a syrupy synthetic sugar $C_4H_8O_4$ that is the epimer of erythrose and that occurs as two optical isomers

thresh·old \ˈthresh-ˌ(h)ōld\ *n* : the point at which a physiological or psychological effect begins to be produced (as the degree of stimulation of a nerve which just produces a response or the concentration of sugar in the blood at which sugar just begins to pass the barrier of the kidneys and enter the urine) ⟨below the ∼ of consciousness⟩ ⟨the ∼ of pain⟩ ⟨a high renal clearance ∼⟩ — called also *limen*

thrill \ˈthril\ *n* : an abnormal fine tremor or vibration in the respiratory or circulatory systems felt on palpation ⟨a continuous systolic and diastolic murmur, frequently associated with a ∼ —R. L. Cecil & R. F. Loeb⟩

throat \ˈthrōt\ *n* **1** : the part of the neck in front of the spinal column **2** : the passage through the throat to the stomach and lungs containing the pharynx and upper part of the esophagus, the larynx, and the trachea

throat botfly *n* : a rusty reddish hairy botfly of the genus *Gasterophilus* (*G. nasalis*) that lays its eggs on the hairs about the mouth of the horse from where the larvae migrate on hatching and attach themselves to the walls of the stomach and intestine — called also *chin fly, throat fly*

¹throb \ˈthräb\ *vi* **throbbed; throb·bing** : to pulsate or pound esp. with abnormal force or rapidity ⟨a finger *throbbing* from an infected cut⟩

²throb *n* : a single pulse of a pulsating movement or sensation ⟨a sudden ∼ of pain⟩

throe \ˈthrō\ *n* : PANG, SPASM — usu. used in pl. ⟨death ∼s⟩ ⟨∼s of childbirth⟩

throm·base \ˈthräm-ˌbās\ *n* : THROMBIN

throm·bas·the·nia \ˌthräm-bəs-ˈthē-nē-ə\ *n* : an inherited abnormality of the blood platelets characterized esp. by defective clot retraction and often by prolonged bleeding time

throm·bec·to·my \thräm-ˈbek-tə-mē\ *n, pl* **-mies** : surgical excision of a thrombus

thrombi *pl of* THROMBUS

throm·bin \ˈthräm-bən\ *n* : a proteolytic enzyme formed from prothrombin that facilitates the clotting of blood by catalyzing conversion of fibrinogen to fibrin and that is used in the form of a powder as a topical hemostatic — called also *thrombase*

throm·ban·gi·i·tis \ˌthräm-bō-ˌan-jē-ˈīt-əs\ *n, pl* **-it·i·des** \-ˈit-ə-ˌdēz\ : inflammation of the lining of a blood vessel with thrombus formation

thromboangiitis ob·lit·er·ans \-ə-ˈblit-ə-ˌranz\ *n* : BUERGER'S DISEASE

throm·bo·ar·ter·i·tis \ˌthräm-bō-ˌärt-ə-ˈrīt-əs\ *n* : inflammation of an artery with thrombus formation

throm·bo·blast \ˈthräm-bə-ˌblast\ *n* : an immature blood platelet

throm·bo·cyte \-bə-ˌsīt\ *n* : PLATELET — **throm·bo·cyt·ic** \ˌthräm-bə-ˈsit-ik\ *adj*

throm·bo·cy·the·mia *or chiefly Brit* **throm·bo·cy·thae·mia** \ˌthräm-bō-ˌsī-ˈthē-mē-ə\ *n* : THROMBOCYTOSIS

throm·bo·cy·top·a·thy \ˌthräm-bə-ˌsī-ˈtäp-ə-thē\ *n, pl* **-thies** : any of various functional disorders of the blood platelets

throm·bo·cy·to·pe·nia \ˌthräm-bə-ˌsīt-ə-ˈpē-nē-ə, -nyə\ *n* : persistent decrease in the number of blood platelets that is often associated with hemorrhagic conditions — called also *thrombopenia* — **throm·bo·cy·to·pe·nic** \-ˈpē-nik\ *adj*

thrombocytopenic purpura *n* : purpura that is characterized by bleeding into the skin with the production of petechiae or ecchymoses and by hemorrhages into mucous membranes and that is associated with a reduction in circulating blood platelets and prolonged bleeding time ⟨idiopath-

ic *thrombocytopenic purpura*⟩ — called also *purpura hemorrhagica, Werlhof's disease*

throm·bo·cy·to·poi·e·sis \ˌthräm-bə-ˌsīt-ə-ˌpȯi-ˈē-səs\ *n, pl* **-e·ses** \-ˌsēz\ : the production of blood platelets from megakaryocytes typically in the bone marrow

throm·bo·cy·to·sis \ˌthräm-bə-ˌsī-ˈtō-səs\ *n, pl* **-to·ses** \-ˈtō-sēz\ : increase and esp. abnormal increase in the number of blood platelets — called also *thrombocythemia*

throm·bo·em·bol·ic \ˌthräm-bō-em-ˈbäl-ik\ *adj* : marked by or associated with thromboembolism ⟨∼ disease⟩

throm·bo·em·bo·lism \ˌthräm-bō-ˈem-bə-ˌliz-əm\ *n* : the blocking of a blood vessel by a particle that has broken away from a blood clot at its site of formation

throm·bo·end·ar·te·rec·to·my \ˌthräm-bō-ˌen-ˌdär-tə-ˈrek-tə-mē\ *n, pl* **-mies** : surgical excision of a thrombus and the adjacent arterial lining

throm·bo·gen·e·sis \-ˈjen-ə-səs\ *n, pl* **-e·ses** \-ˌsēz\ : the formation of a thrombus

throm·bo·gen·ic \ˌthräm-bə-ˈjen-ik\ *adj* : tending to produce a thrombus ⟨a ∼ diet⟩ — **throm·bo·ge·nic·i·ty** \-jə-ˈnis-ət-ē\ *n, pl* **-ties**

throm·bo·ki·nase \ˌthräm-bō-ˈkī-ˌnās, -ˌnāz\ *n* : THROMBOPLASTIN

¹throm·bo·lyt·ic \ˌthräm-bə-ˈlit-ik\ *adj* : destroying or breaking up a thrombus ⟨a ∼ agent⟩ ⟨∼ therapy⟩ — **throm·bol·y·sis** \ˌthräm-ˈbäl-ə-səs\ *n, pl* **-y·ses** \-ˌsēz\

²thrombolytic *n* : a thrombolytic drug (as streptokinase or urokinase) : CLOT-BUSTER

throm·bop·a·thy \ˌthräm-ˈbäp-ə-thē\ *n, pl* **-thies** : any disease affecting the functioning of blood platelets

throm·bo·pe·nia \ˌthräm-bə-ˈpē-nē-ə\ *n* : THROMBOCYTOPENIA — **throm·bo·pe·nic** \-ˈpē-nik\ *adj*

throm·bo·phil·ia \-ˈfil-ē-ə\ *n* : a hereditary or acquired predisposition to thrombosis

throm·bo·phle·bi·tis \-fli-ˈbīt-əs\ *n, pl* **-bit·i·des** \-ˈbit-ə-ˌdēz\ : inflammation of a vein with formation of a thrombus — compare PHLEBOTHROMBOSIS

throm·bo·plas·tic \ˌthräm-bō-ˈplas-tik\ *adj* : initiating or accelerating the clotting of blood ⟨a ∼ substance⟩ — **throm·bo·plas·ti·cal·ly** \-ti-k(ə-)lē\ *adv*

throm·bo·plas·tin \ˌthräm-bō-ˈplas-tən\ *n* : a complex enzyme that is found in brain, lung, and other tissues and esp. in blood platelets and that functions in the conversion of prothrombin to thrombin in the clotting of blood — called also *thrombokinase*

throm·bo·plas·tin·o·gen \-plas-ˈtin-ə-jən\ *n* : FACTOR VIII

throm·bo·poi·e·tin \-ˈpȯi-ət-ən\ *n* : a hormone that regulates blood platelet production by promoting the proliferation and maturation of megakaryocyte progenitor cells and the development of megakaryocytes into blood platelets

throm·bose \ˈthräm-ˌbōs, -ˌbōz\ *vb* **-bosed; -bos·ing** *vt* : to affect with thrombosis ⟨a *thrombosed* blood vessel⟩ ∼ *vi* : to undergo thrombosis

throm·bo·sis \thräm-ˈbō-səs, thrəm-\ *n, pl* **-bo·ses** \-ˌsēz\ : the formation or presence of a blood clot within a blood vessel — see CORONARY THROMBOSIS, DEEP VEIN THROMBOSIS

throm·bo·sthe·nin \ˌthräm-bō-ˈsthē-nən\ *n* : a complex of contractile proteins occurring in blood platelets

throm·bo·test \ˈthräm-bō-ˌtest\ *n* : a test for the functional intactness of the prothrombin complex that is used in controlling the amount of anticoagulant used in preventing thrombosis

throm·bot·ic \thräm-ˈbät-ik\ *adj* : of, relating to, or affected with thrombosis ⟨a ∼ disorder⟩ ⟨a ∼ patient⟩

thrombotic thrombocytopenic purpura *n* : hemolytic uremic syndrome that primarily affects adult females, is typically distinguished by only mild renal dysfunction but significant neurological deficits, and is marked by the presence of large aggregates of von Willebrand factor and a deficiency in or absence of a protease that cleaves von Willebrand factor — called also *TTP*

throm·box·ane \thräm-ˈbäk-ˌsān\ *n* : any of several substances that are produced esp. by platelets, are formed from endoperoxides, cause constriction of vascular and bronchial smooth muscle, and promote blood clotting

throm·bus \'thräm-bəs\ *n, pl* **throm·bi** \-ˌbī, -ˌbē\ : a clot of blood formed within a blood vessel and remaining attached to its place of origin — compare EMBOLUS

throw·back \'thrō-ˌbak\ *n* **1** : reversion to an earlier type or phase : ATAVISM **2** : an instance or product of atavistic reversion

throw up \ˌthrō-'əp\ *vi* : VOMIT

thrush \'thrəsh\ *n* **1** : a disease that is caused by a fungus of the genus *Candida* (*C. albicans*), occurs esp. in infants and children, and is marked by white patches in the oral cavity; *broadly* : CANDIDIASIS ⟨vaginal ∼⟩ **2** : a suppurative disorder of the feet in various animals (as the horse)

thu·jone \'thü-ˌjōn\ *n* : a fragrant oily ketone $C_{10}H_{16}O$ occurring in various essential oils — called also *absinthol*

thu·li·um \'th(y)ü-lē-əm\ *n* : a trivalent metallic element of the rare-earth group — symbol *Tm*; see ELEMENT table

thumb \'thəm\ *n* : the short and thick first or most preaxial digit of the human hand that differs from the other fingers in having only two phalanges, in having greater freedom of movement, and in being opposable to the other fingers

thumb–suck·er \'thəm-ˌsək-ər\ *n* : an infant or young child that habitually sucks a thumb

thumb–suck·ing \-ˌsək-iŋ\ *n* : the habit of sucking a thumb beyond the period of physiological need

thumps \'thəmps\ *n pl but sing in constr* : a dyspneic breathing that is marked by throbbing movements of the sides of the chest due to spasmodic contractions of the diaphragm analogous to those of hiccups in humans, is esp. common in young pigs, and is associated with nutritional anemia or the passage of larval ascarid worms through the lungs; *also* : a disease (as a nutritional anemia or verminous pneumonia) of young pigs of which thumps is a symptom

thy·la·ken·trin \ˌthī-lə-'ken-trən\ *n* : FOLLICLE-STIMULATING HORMONE

thyme \'tīm *also* 'thīm\ *n* : any of a genus (*Thymus*) of mints with small pungent aromatic leaves; *esp* : a garden herb (*T. vulgaris*) used in seasoning and formerly in medicine esp. as a stimulant and carminative

thy·mec·to·mize *also Brit* **thy·mec·to·mise** \thī-'mek-tə-ˌmīz\ *vt* **-mized** *also Brit* **-mised; -miz·ing** *also Brit* **-mis·ing** : to subject to thymectomy ⟨rats *thymectomized* at birth⟩

thy·mec·to·my \thī-'mek-tə-mē\ *n, pl* **-mies** : surgical excision of the thymus

thyme oil *n* : a fragrant essential oil containing thymol and carvacrol that is obtained from various thymes and is used chiefly as an antiseptic in pharmaceutical and dental preparations and as a flavor in foods

thymi *pl of* THYMUS

thy·mic \'thī-mik\ *adj* : of or relating to the thymus ⟨a ∼ tumor⟩

thymic corpuscle *n* : HASSALL'S CORPUSCLE

thy·mi·co·lym·phat·ic \ˌthī-mi-(ˌ)kō-lim-'fat-ik\ *adj* : of, relating to, or affecting both the thymus and the lymphatic system ⟨∼ involution⟩

thymicolymphaticus — see STATUS THYMICOLYMPHATICUS

thy·mi·dine \'thī-mə-ˌdēn\ *n* : a nucleoside $C_{10}H_{14}N_2O_5$ that is composed of thymine and deoxyribose and occurs as a structural part of DNA

thymidine kinase *n* : an enzyme that catalyzes the phosphorylation of thymidine in a pathway leading to DNA synthesis, that is active esp. in tissues undergoing growth or regeneration, and that is the key enzyme mediating replication in certain viruses (as the herpesvirus causing herpes simplex)

thy·mi·dyl·ate \ˌthī-mə-'dil-ˌāt\ *n* : a salt or ester of thymidylic acid

thy·mi·dyl·ic acid \ˌthī-mə-ˌdil-ik-\ *n* : either of two isomeric crystalline nucleotides $C_{10}H_{15}N_2O_8P$ obtained by partial hydrolysis of DNA

thy·mine \'thī-ˌmēn\ *n* : a pyrimidine base $C_5H_6N_2O_2$ that is one of the four bases coding genetic information in the polynucleotide chain of DNA — compare ADENINE, CYTOSINE, GUANINE, URACIL

thy·mo·cyte \'thī-mə-ˌsīt\ *n* : a cell of the thymus; *esp* : a thymic lymphocyte

thy·mol \'thī-ˌmól, -ˌmōl\ *n* : a crystalline phenol $C_{10}H_{14}O$ of aromatic odor and antiseptic properties found esp. in thyme oil or made synthetically and used chiefly as a fungicide and preservative

thymol blue *n* : a greenish crystalline compound $C_{27}H_{30}O_5S$ derived from thymol and used as an acid-base indicator

thy·mol·phtha·lein \-'thal-ˌēn, -'thā-ˌlēn, -'thal-ē-ən\ *n* : a crystalline compound $C_{28}H_{30}O_4$ analogous to phenolphthalein and likewise used as an acid-base indicator

thy·mo·lyt·ic \ˌthī-mə-'lit-ik\ *adj* : causing destruction of thymic tissue ⟨a ∼ disease⟩

thy·mo·ma \thī-'mō-mə\ *n, pl* **-mas** *also* **-ma·ta** \-mət-ə\ : a tumor that arises from the tissue elements of the thymus

thy·mo·nu·cle·ic acid \ˌthī-mō-n(y)ù-ˌklā-ik-, -ˌklē-\ *n* : DNA

thy·mo·poi·et·in \-'pói-ət-ən\ *n* : either of two heat-stable polypeptide hormones obtained from extracts of the thymus

thy·mo·sin \'thī-mə-sən\ *n* : a mixture of polypeptides isolated from the thymus; *also* : any of these polypeptides

thy·mus \'thī-məs\ *n, pl* **thy·mus·es** *also* **thy·mi** \-ˌmī\ : a glandular structure of largely lymphoid tissue that functions in cell-mediated immunity by being the site where T cells develop, that is present in the young of most vertebrates typically in the upper anterior chest or at the base of the neck, that arises from the epithelium of one or more embryonic branchial clefts, and that tends to disappear or become rudimentary in the adult — called also *thymus gland*

thy·ro·ac·tive \ˌthī-rō-'ak-tiv\ *adj* **1** : capable of entering into the thyroid metabolism and of being incorporated into the thyroid hormone ⟨∼ iodine⟩ **2** : simulating the action of the thyroid hormone ⟨∼ iodinated casein⟩

thy·ro·ar·y·te·noid \-ˌar-ə-'tē-ˌnóid, -ə-'rit-ᵊn-ˌóid\ *n* : a broad thin muscle that arises esp. from the thyroid cartilage, inserts into the arytenoid cartilage, and functions to relax and shorten the vocal cords by drawing the arytenoid cartilage forward and to narrow the rima glottidis by rotating the arytenoid cartilage inward causing the vocal cords to approach each other — called also *thyroarytenoid muscle, thyroarytenoideus;* see INFERIOR THYROARYTENOID LIGAMENT

thy·ro·ar·y·te·noi·de·us \-ˌar-ət-ə-'nóid-ē-əs\ *n* : THYROARYTENOID

thyroarytenoid muscle *n* : THYROARYTENOID

thy·ro·cal·ci·to·nin \ˌthī-rō-ˌkal-sə-'tō-nən\ *n* : CALCITONIN

thy·ro·cer·vi·cal \-'sər-vi-kəl\ *adj* : of, relating to, or being the thyrocervical trunk ⟨the ∼ artery⟩

thyrocervical trunk *n* : a short thick branch of the subclavian artery that divides into the inferior thyroid, suprascapular, and transverse cervical arteries

thy·ro·epi·glot·tic ligament \ˌthī-rō-ˌep-ə-ˌglät-ik-\ *n* : a long narrow ligamentous cord connecting the thyroid cartilage and epiglottis

thy·ro·gen·ic \ˌthī-rə-'jen-ik\ *adj* : originating in or caused by activity of the thyroid ⟨a drug containing ∼ substances⟩

thy·ro·glob·u·lin \ˌthī-rō-'gläb-yə-lən\ *n* : an iodine-containing protein of the thyroid gland that on proteolysis yields thyroxine and triiodothyronine

thy·ro·glos·sal \ˌthī-rō-'gläs-əl\ *adj* : of, relating to, or originating in the thyroglossal duct ⟨∼ cysts⟩

thyroglossal duct *n* : a temporary duct connecting the embryonic thyroid gland and the tongue

thy·ro·hy·al \ˌthī-rō-'hī-əl\ *n* : the larger and more lateral of the two lateral projections on each side of the human hyoid bone — called also *greater cornu;* compare CERATOHYAL

¹**thy·ro·hy·oid** \-'hī-ˌóid\ *adj* : of, relating to, or supplying the thyrohyoid muscle ⟨the ∼ branch of the hypoglossal nerve⟩

²**thyrohyoid** *n* : a thyrohyoid part; *esp* : THYROHYOID MUSCLE

thyrohyoid membrane *n* : a broad fibroelastic sheet that

S
T

\ə\ abut \ᵊ\ kitten \ər\ further \a\ ash \ā\ ace \ä\ cot, cart
\aù\ out \ch\ chin \e\ bet \ē\ easy \g\ go \i\ hit \ī\ ice \j\ job
\ŋ\ sing \ō\ go \ò\ law \ói\ boy \th\ thin \th\ the \ü\ loot
\ù\ foot \y\ yet \zh\ vision   See also Pronunciation Symbols page

connects the upper margin of the thyroid cartilage and the upper margin of the back of the hyoid bone

thyrohyoid muscle *n* : a small quadrilateral muscle that arises from the thyroid cartilage, inserts into the thyrohyal of the hyoid bone, and functions to depress the hyoid bone and to elevate the thyroid cartilage — called also *thyrohyoid*

¹**thy·roid** \'thī-ˌrȯid\ *also* **thy·roi·dal** \thī-'rȯid-ᵊl\ *adj* **1 a** : of, relating to, affecting, or being the thyroid gland ⟨∼ disorders⟩ **2** : of, relating to, or being the thyroid cartilage

²**thyroid** *n* **1** : a large bilobed endocrine gland of craniate vertebrates that arises as a median ventral outgrowth of the pharynx, lies in the anterior base of the neck or anterior ventral part of the thorax, is often accompanied by lateral accessory glands sometimes more or less fused with the main mass, and produces esp. the hormones thyroxine and triiodothyronine — called also *thyroid gland* **2** : a preparation of the thyroid gland of various domesticated food animals (as pigs) containing approximately ¹/₁₀ percent of iodine combined in thyroxine and used in treating thyroid disorders — called also *thyroid extract*

thyroid artery *n* : either of two arteries supplying the thyroid gland and nearby structures at the front of the neck: **a** : one that branches from the external carotid artery or sometimes from the common carotid artery at the level of the thyrohyal of the hyoid bone and that gives off branches to nearby muscles and to the thyroid gland — called also *superior thyroid artery* **b** : one that branches from the thyrocervical trunk and that divides to form branches supplying the inferior portion of the thyroid gland and anastomosing with the superior thyroid artery or with a corresponding branch from the opposite side — called also *inferior thyroid artery*

thyroid–binding globulin *n* : THYROXINE-BINDING GLOBULIN

thyroid cartilage *n* : the chief cartilage of the larynx that consists of two broad lamellae joined at an angle and that forms the Adam's apple

thy·roid·ec·to·mize *also Brit* **thy·roid·ec·to·mise** \ˌthī-ˌrȯid-'ek-tə-ˌmīz\ *vt* **-mized** *also Brit* **-mised; -miz·ing** *also Brit* **-mis·ing** : to subject to thyroidectomy

thy·roid·ec·to·my \ˌthī-ˌrȯid-'ek-tə-mē, -rəd-\ *n, pl* **-mies** : surgical excision of thyroid gland tissue

thyroid extract *n* : THYROID 2

thyroid ganglion *n* : a ganglion that is a variant of the middle cervical ganglion and is found in some dissections in close association with the inferior thyroid artery

thyroid gland *n* : THYROID 1

thyroid hormone *n* : any of several closely related metabolically active compounds (as triiodothyronine) that are stored in the thyroid gland in the form of thyroglobulin or circulate in the blood usu. bound to plasma proteins; *esp* : THYROXINE

thy·roid·itis \ˌthī-ˌrȯid-'īt-əs, -rəd-\ *n* : inflammation of the thyroid gland

thy·roid·ol·o·gist \ˌthī-ˌrȯi-'däl-ə-jəst\ *n* : an expert in thyroidology

thy·roid·ol·o·gy \-jē\ *n, pl* **-gies** : the study of the thyroid gland

thyroid–stimulating hormone *n* : a hormone secreted by the adenohypophysis of the pituitary gland that regulates the formation and secretion of thyroid hormone — called also *thyrotropic hormone, thyrotropin, TSH*

thyroid storm *n* : a sudden life-threatening exacerbation of the symptoms (as high fever, tachycardia, weakness, or extreme restlessness) of hyperthyroidism that is brought on by various causes (as infection, surgery, or stress)

thyroid vein *n* : any of several small veins draining blood from the thyroid gland and nearby structures in the front of the neck: **a** : a vein on each side that drains the upper part of the thyroid and empties into the internal jugular vein — called also *superior thyroid vein* **b** : a vein on each side that drains the lateral part of the thyroid and empties into the internal jugular vein — called also *middle thyroid vein* **c** : any of two to four veins on each side that drain the thyroid gland

and unite to empty into the brachiocephalic vein on the same side or that unite with the veins on the opposite side to form a common trunk emptying into the left brachiocephalic vein — called also *inferior thyroid vein*

thy·ro·nine \'thī-rə-ˌnēn, -nən\ *n* : a phenolic amino acid $C_{15}H_{15}NO_4$ of which thyroxine is a derivative; *also* : any of various derivatives of this

thy·ro·para·thy·roid·ec·to·my \ˌthī-rō-ˌpar-ə-ˌthī-ˌrȯid-'ek-tə-mē\ *n, pl* **-mies** : excision of both the thyroid and parathyroid glands — **thy·ro·para·thy·roid·ec·to·mized** *also Brit* **thy·ro·para·thy·roid·ec·to·mised** \-tə-ˌmīzd\ *adj*

thy·ro·pro·tein \ˌthī-rō-'prō-ˌtēn, -'prōt-ē-ən\ *n* : any of various preparations made by iodinating proteins and having physiological activity similar to that of thyroxine and related iodinated protein constituents from the thyroid gland; *esp* : IODINATED CASEIN — compare IODOPROTEIN

thy·rot·o·my \thī-'rät-ə-mē\ *n, pl* **-mies** : surgical incision or division of the thyroid cartilage

thy·ro·tox·ic \ˌthī-rō-'täk-sik\ *adj* : of, relating to, induced by, or affected with hyperthyroidism ⟨∼ heart failure⟩ ⟨∼ patients⟩ — **thy·ro·tox·ic·i·ty** \-täk-'sis-ət-ē\ *n, pl* **-ties**

thy·ro·tox·i·co·sis \'thī-rō-ˌtäk-sə-'kō-səs\ *n, pl* **-co·ses** \-ˌsēz\ : HYPERTHYROIDISM

thy·ro·tro·pic \ˌthī-rə-'trō-pik, -'träp-ik\ *also* **thy·ro·tro·phic** \-'trō-fik\ *adj* : exerting or characterized by a direct influence on the secretory activity of the thyroid gland

thyrotropic hormone *also* **thyrotrophic hormone** *n* : THYROID-STIMULATING HORMONE

thy·ro·tro·pin \ˌthī-rə-'trō-pən\ *also* **thy·ro·tro·phin** \-fən\ *n* **1** : THYROID-STIMULATING HORMONE **2** : a recombinant form of thyroid-stimulating hormone used esp. as a diagnostic agent (as in the detection of thyroid cancer) — called also *thyrotropin alfa*

thyrotropin–releasing hormone *n* : a tripeptide hormone synthesized in the hypothalamus that stimulates secretion of thyroid-stimulating hormone by the anterior lobe of the pituitary gland — abbr. *TRH;* called also *protirelin, thyrotropin-releasing factor*

thy·rox·ine *or* **thy·rox·in** \thī-'räk-ˌsēn, -sən\ *n* : an iodine containing hormone $C_{15}H_{11}I_4NO_4$ that is an amino acid produced by the thyroid gland as a product of the cleavage of thyroglobulin, increases the metabolic rate, and is used to treat thyroid disorders — called also *T4*

thyroxine–binding globulin *n* : a blood serum glycoprotein that is synthesized in the liver and that binds tightly to thyroxine and less firmly to triiodothyronine preventing their removal from the blood by the kidneys and releasing them as needed at sites of activity — abbr. *TBG;* called also *thyroid-binding globulin*

Thysa·no·so·ma \ˌthis-ə-nō-'sō-mə, ˌthīs-\ *n* : a genus of tapeworms (family Anoplocephalidae) including the common fringed tapeworm of ruminants

Ti *symbol* titanium

TIA *abbr* transient ischemic attack

tib·ia \'tib-ē-ə\ *n, pl* **-i·ae** \-ē-ˌē, -ē-ˌī\ *also* **-i·as** : the inner and usu. larger of the two bones of the leg between the knee and ankle that articulates above with the femur and below with the talus — called also *shinbone*

tib·i·al \'tib-ē-əl\ *adj* : of, relating to, or located near a tibia ⟨a ∼ fracture⟩

tibial artery *n* : either of the two arteries of the lower leg formed by the bifurcation of the popliteal artery: **a** : a larger posterior artery that divides between the medial malleolus and heel into the lateral and medial plantar arteries — called also *posterior tibial artery* **b** : a smaller anterior artery that passes between the tibia and fibula, descends in the anterior portion of the leg, and continues beyond the ankle joint into the foot as the dorsalis pedis artery — called also *anterior tibial artery*

tibial collateral ligament *n* : MEDIAL COLLATERAL LIGAMENT

tib·i·a·le \ˌtib-ē-'ā-lē\ *n, pl* **-a·lia** \-'ā-lē-ə\ : the upper margin and edge of the interior prominence of the head of the tibia

tib·i·a·lis \ˌtib-ē-'ā-ləs\ *n, pl* **tib·i·a·les** \-(ˌ)lēz\ : either of two muscles of the calf of the leg: **a** : a muscle arising chiefly from the lateral condyle and part of the shaft of the tibia, inserting by a long tendon into the first cuneiform and first metatarsal bones, and acting to flex the foot dorsally and to invert it — called also *tibialis anterior, tibialis anticus* **b** : a deeply situated muscle that arises from the tibia and fibula, interosseous membrane, and intermuscular septa, that is inserted by a tendon passing under the medial malleolus into the navicular and first cuneiform bones, and that flexes the foot in the direction of the sole and tends to invert it — called also *tibialis posterior, tibialis posticus*

tibialis anterior *n* : TIBIALIS a

tibialis an·ti·cus \-an-'tī-kəs\ *n* : TIBIALIS a

tibialis posterior *n* : TIBIALIS b

tibialis pos·ti·cus \-pōs-'tī-kəs\ *n* : TIBIALIS b

tibial nerve *n* : the large nerve in the back of the leg that is a continuation of the sciatic nerve and terminates at the medial malleolus in the lateral and medial plantar nerves — called also *medial popliteal nerve*

tibial plateau *n* : the smooth bony surface of either the lateral condyle or the medial condyle of the tibia that articulates with the corresponding condylar surface of the femur

tibial vein *n* : any of several veins that accompany the corresponding tibial arteries and that unite to form the popliteal vein: **a** : one accompanying the posterior tibial artery — called also *posterior tibial vein* **b** : one accompanying the anterior tibial artery — called also *anterior tibial vein*

tib·io·fem·o·ral \,tib-ē-ō-'fem-(ə-)rəl\ *adj* : relating to or being the articulation occurring between the tibia and the femur ⟨the ~ joint⟩

tib·io·fib·u·lar \-'fib-yə-lər\ *adj* : of, relating to, or connecting the tibia and fibula ⟨~ fusion⟩ ⟨the proximal ~ joint⟩

tib·io·ta·lar \,tib-ē-ō-'tā-lər\ *adj* : of or relating to the tibia and the talus ⟨noninflammatory effusion in the ~ joint —S. B. Baker *et al*⟩

tib·io·tar·sal \,tib-ē-ō-'tar-səl\ *adj* : of, relating to, or affecting the tibia and the tarsus ⟨~ abnormalities⟩

ti·bric acid \,tī-brik-\ *n* : an antihyperlipidemic drug $C_{14}H_{18}ClNO_4S$

tic \'tik\ *n* **1** : local and habitual spasmodic motion of particular muscles esp. of the face : TWITCHING **2** : a habitual usu. unconscious quirk of behavior or speech

ti·car·cil·lin \,tī-kär-'sil-ən\ *n* : a semisynthetic antibiotic used esp. in the form of its disodium salt $C_{15}H_{14}N_2Na_2O_6S_2$

tic dou·lou·reux \'tik-,dü-lə-'rü, -'rə(r)\ *n* : TRIGEMINAL NEURALGIA

tick \'tik\ *n* **1** : any of numerous bloodsucking arachnids that constitute the acarine superfamily Ixodoidea, are much larger than the closely related mites, attach themselves to warm-blooded vertebrates to feed, include important vectors of various infectious diseases of humans and lower animals, and although the immature larva has but six legs, may be readily distinguished from an insect by the complete lack of external segmentation **2** : any of various usu. wingless parasitic dipteran flies (as the sheep ked)

tick–bite fever *n* : boutonneuse fever esp. as it occurs in South Africa

tick–borne \'tik-,bō(ə)rn, -,bȯ(ə)rn\ *adj* : capable of being transmitted by the bites of ticks ⟨~ encephalitis⟩

tick–borne fever *n* : a usu. mild rickettsial disease of ruminant animals (as sheep and cattle) esp. in Europe that is caused by a bacterium of the genus *Ehrlichia* (*E. phagocytophilia* syn. *Rickettsia phagocytophilia*) which is transmitted by a tick of the genus *Ixodes,* and that is marked by fever, listlessness, and anorexia

tick fever *n* **1** : TEXAS FEVER **2** : a febrile disease (as Rocky Mountain spotted fever or relapsing fever) transmitted by the bites of ticks

tick·icide \'tik-ə-,sīd\ *n* : an agent used to kill ticks — **tick·icid·al** \,tik-ə-'sīd-ᵊl\ *adj*

¹tick·le \'tik-əl\ *vb* **tick·led; tick·ling** \-(ə-)liŋ\ *vi* **1** : to have a tingling or prickling sensation ⟨my back ~s⟩ **2** : to excite the surface nerves to prickle ~ *vt* : to touch (as a body part)

lightly so as to excite the surface nerves and cause uneasiness, laughter, or spasmodic movements

²tickle *n* **1** : the act of tickling **2** : a tickling sensation ⟨a cough is a reflex to a ~ in the throat —Karl Menninger⟩ **3** : something that tickles

tick paralysis *n* : a progressive spinal paralysis that moves upward toward the brain in humans or lower animals and that is caused by a neurotoxin secreted by some ticks (as *Dermacentor andersoni*) and injected into the host during feeding

tick typhus *n* : any of various tick-borne rickettsial spotted fevers (as Rocky Mountain spotted fever or boutonneuse fever)

tick–wor·ry \'tik-,wər-ē\ *n* : a generalized state of unease and irritability of cattle severely infested with ticks often leading to serious loss of energy and weight

tic–po·lon·ga \,tik-pə-'lȯŋ-gə\ *n* : RUSSELL'S VIPER

ti·cryn·a·fen \tī-'krin-ə-,fen\ *n* : a diuretic, uricosuric, and antihypertensive agent $C_{13}H_8Cl_2O_4S$ withdrawn from use because of its link to hepatic disorders

tid *abbr* [Latin *ter in die*] three times a day — used in writing prescriptions

tid·al \'tīd-ᵊl\ *adj* : of, relating to, or constituting tidal air ⟨interference with the normal ~ exchange of the lungs —F. R. Mautz & R. M. Hosler⟩

tidal air *n* : the air that passes in and out of the lungs in an ordinary breath and averages 500 cubic centimeters in a normal adult human male

tidal volume *n* : the volume of the tidal air

tide \'tīd\ *n* : a temporary increase or decrease in a specified substance or quality in the body or one of its systems ⟨a postprandial alkaline ~, the typical rise in urinary pH associated with gastric acid secretion —E. J. Jacobson & Gerhard Fuchs⟩

tie off \'tī-'ȯf\ *vt* **tied off; ty·ing off** *or* **tie·ing off** : to close by means of an encircling or enveloping ligature ⟨*tie off* a bleeding vessel⟩

Tie·tze's syndrome \'tēt-səz-\ *n* : a condition of unknown origin that is characterized by inflammation of costochondral cartilage — called also *costochondritis, Tietze's disease*

ti·ger mosquito \'tī-gər-\ *n* **1** : YELLOW-FEVER MOSQUITO **2** : ASIAN TIGER MOSQUITO

tiger rattlesnake *n* : a rather small yellow or tawny rattlesnake of the genus *Crotalus* (*C. tigris*) that is narrowly striped with black and occurs in mountainous deserts of western No. America

tiger snake *n* : a widely distributed extremely venomous elapid snake (*Notechis scutatus*) of Australia and Tasmania that is predominantly brown with dark crossbars

tig·lic acid \,tig-lik-\ *n* : a vesicant crystalline unsaturated acid $C_5H_8O_2$ with a spicy odor that is the stable stereoisomer of angelic acid and occurs in the form of esters esp. in chamomile oil from a European chamomile (*Chamaemelum nobile*) and in croton oil

ti·gog·e·nin \ti-'gäj-ə-nən\ *n* : a crystalline steroid sapogenin $C_{27}H_{44}O_3$ obtained esp. by hydrolysis of tigonin

ti·go·nin \'tig-ə-nən\ *n* : a steroid saponin obtained esp. from the leaves of either of two foxgloves (*Digitalis purpurea* and *D. lanata*)

ti·groid \'tī-,grȯid\ *adj* **1** : having a striped or spotted appearance ⟨pathological changes in the eye resulted in a ~ fundus⟩ **2** : being or consisting of Nissl substance

tigroid substance *n* : NISSL BODIES

ti·grol·y·sis \tī-'gräl-ə-səs\ *n, pl* **-y·ses** \-,sēz\ : loss of Nissl bodies or Nissl substance that accompanies degenerative changes in nerve tissue

ti·ki·ti·ki \,tē-kē-'tē-kē\ *n* : RICE POLISHINGS

TIL \,tē-(,)ī-'el\ *n* : TUMOR-INFILTRATING LYMPHOCYTE

tilt table \'tilt-\ *n* : an apparatus that is used to rotate a per-

---

\ə\ **abut** \ᵊ\ **kitten** \ər\ **further** \a\ **ash** \ā\ **ace** \ä\ **cot, cart** \aú\ **out** \ch\ **chin** \e\ **bet** \ē\ **easy** \g\ **go** \i\ **hit** \ī\ **ice** \j\ **job** \ŋ\ **sing** \ō\ **go** \ȯ\ **law** \ȯi\ **boy** \th\ **thin** \th\ **the** \ü\ **loot** \ú\ **foot** \y\ **yet** \zh\ **vision** *See also* Pronunciation Symbols page

S
T

son from a horizontal to a vertical or oblique position in order to test perception of bodily position and to assist in teaching a person affected with paralysis to stand — called also *tiltboard*

tim·ber rattlesnake \'tim-bər-\ *n* : a moderate-sized rattlesnake of the genus *Crotalus* (*C. horridus*) that is widely distributed through the eastern half of the U.S. and feeds largely on mice and other rodents

tim·bre *also* **tim·ber** \'tam-bər, 'tim-; 'tam(br²)\ *n* : the quality given to a sound by its overtones: as **a** : the resonance by which the ear recognizes and identifies a voiced speech sound **b** : the quality of tone distinctive of a particular singing voice or musical instrument — **tim·bral** \'tam-brəl, 'tim-\ *adj*

time \'tīm\ *n* **1 a** : the measured or measurable period during which an action, process, or condition exists or continues — see BLEEDING TIME, COAGULATION TIME, PROTHROMBIN TIME, REACTION TIME **b** : a continuum which lacks spatial dimensions and in which events succeed one another from past through present to future **2** : the point or period when something occurs **3** : a moment, hour, day, or year as indicated by a clock or calendar ⟨what ∼ is it⟩

timed–re·lease *or* **time–release** \'tīm(d)-ri-'lēs\ *adj* : consisting of or containing a drug that is released in small amounts over time (as by dissolution of a coating) usu. in the gastrointestinal tract ⟨∼ capsules⟩ — compare SUSTAINED≈ RELEASE

time–of–flight \,tīm-ə(v)-,flīt\ *adj* : of, relating to, being, or done with an instrument (as a mass spectrometer) that separates particles (as ions) according to the time required for them to traverse a tube of a certain length ⟨a ∼ imaging system⟩ ⟨∼ magnetic resonance angiography⟩ — abbr. *TOF*

ti·mo·lol \'tī-mə-,lōl, -,lȯl\ *n* : a beta-blocker used esp. in the form of its maleate C₁₃H₂₄N₄O₃S·C₄H₄O₄ to treat hypertension, to reduce the risk of reinfarction, and to lower intraocular pressure associated with open-angle glaucoma and ocular hypertension

Ti·mop·tic \tə-'mäp-tik\ *trademark* — used for a preparation of the maleate of timolol

tin \'tin\ *n* : a soft faintly bluish white lustrous low-melting crystalline metallic element that is malleable and ductile at ordinary temperatures and that is used as a protective coating, in tinfoil, and in soft solders and alloys — symbol *Sn*; see ELEMENT table

Ti·nac·tin \ti-'nak-tən\ *trademark* — used for a preparation of tolnaftate

tinct *abbr* tincture

tinc·to·ri·al \tiŋk-'tōr-ē-əl\ *adj* : of or relating to dyeing or staining ⟨the ∼ reaction of eosin⟩ — **tinc·to·ri·al·ly** \-ē\ *adv*

tinc·tu·ra \tiŋk-'t(y)ü-rə\ *n, pl* **-rae** \-rē\ : TINCTURE

tinc·ture \'tiŋ(k)-chər\ *n* : a solution of a medicinal substance in an alcoholic or hydroalcoholic menstruum — compare LIQUOR b

tin·ea \'tin-ē-ə\ *n* : any of several fungal diseases of the skin; *esp* : RINGWORM

tinea bar·bae \-'bär-bē\ *n* : BARBER'S ITCH

tinea cap·i·tis \-'kap-ət-əs\ *n* : an infection of the scalp caused by fungi of the genera *Trichophyton* and *Microsporum* and characterized by scaly patches penetrated by a few dry brittle hairs

tinea cor·po·ris \-'kȯr-pə-rəs\ *n* : a fungal infection involving parts of the body not covered with hair — called also *body ringworm*

tinea cru·ris \-'krùr-əs\ *n* : a fungal infection involving esp. the groin and perineum

tinea pe·dis \-'ped-əs\ *n* : ATHLETE'S FOOT

tinea ver·si·col·or \-'vər-si-,kəl-ər\ *n* : a chronic noninflammatory infection of the skin esp. of the trunk that is caused by a lipophilic fungus (*Pityrosporum orbiculare* syn. *Melassezia furfur*) and is marked by the formation of irregular macular patches that often appear lighter than the surrounding area if the skin is tanned and may appear darker than the surrounding skin if the skin is not tanned or black — called also *pityriasis versicolor*

Ti·nel's sign \ti-'nelz-\ *n* : a tingling sensation felt in the distal portion of a limb upon percussion of the skin over a regenerating nerve in the limb

   Ti·nel \tē-nel\, **Jules (1879–1952),** French neurologist. In 1916 Tinel published a study of the effect of gunshot wounds on nerves. The work included a discussion of Tinel's sign.

tine test \'tīn-\ *n* : a tuberculin test in which the tuberculin is introduced intradermally by means of four tines on a stainless steel disk

tin·gle \'tiŋ-gəl\ *vi* **tin·gled; tin·gling** \-g(ə-)liŋ\ : to feel a stinging or prickling sensation — **tingle** *n*

Tin·ne·vel·ly senna \,tin-ə-'vel-ē-\ *n* : senna obtained from a cassia (*Cassia angustifolia*) esp. in southern India

tin·ni·tus \'tin-ət-əs, ti-'nīt-əs\ *n* : a sensation of noise (as a ringing or roaring) that is caused by a bodily condition (as a disturbance of the auditory nerve or wax in the ear) and typically is of the subjective form which can only be heard by the one affected

ti·queur \tē-'kər\ *n* : one affected with a tic

tire \'tī(ə)r\ *vb* **tired; tir·ing** *vi* : to become weary ∼ *vt* : to exhaust or greatly decrease the physical strength of : FATIGUE

tired \'tī(ə)rd\ *adj* : drained of strength and energy : fatigued often to the point of exhaustion

ti·sane \ti-'zan, -'zän\ *n* : an infusion (as of dried herbs) used as a beverage or for medicinal effects

Ti·se·li·us apparatus \ti-'sā-lē-əs-\ *n* : an apparatus used for electrophoresis esp. of proteins in a biological system (as blood plasma) — called also *Tiselius cell*

   Ti·se·li·us \te-'sā-lē-ùs\, **Arne Wilhelm Kaurin (1902–1971),** Swedish biochemist. Tiselius developed the use of electrophoresis in the 1920s for the separation of proteins in suspension on the basis of their electrical charge. In 1937 he introduced the radically improved apparatus that is now known as the Tiselius apparatus. He was awarded the Nobel Prize for Chemistry in 1948.

tis·sue \'tish-(,)ü, 'tish-ə-(w), *chiefly Brit* 'tis-(,)yü\ *n* : an aggregate of cells usu. of a particular kind together with their intercellular substance that form one of the structural materials of a plant or an animal and that in animals include connective tissue, epithelium, muscle tissue, and nerve tissue

tissue culture *n* : the process or technique of making body tissue grow in a culture medium outside the organism; *also* : a culture of tissue (as epithelium)

tissue fluid *n* : a fluid that permeates the spaces between individual cells, that is in osmotic contact with the blood and lymph, and that serves in interstitial transport of nutrients and waste

tissue plasminogen activator *n* : a clot-dissolving enzyme that has an affinity for fibrin, that catalyzes the conversion of plasminogen to plasmin, that is produced naturally in blood vessel linings, and that is used in a genetically engineered form to prevent damage to heart muscle following a heart attack and to reduce neurological damage following ischemic stroke — abbr. *tPA*

tissue space *n* : an intercellular space

tissue typing *n* : the determination of the degree of compatibility of tissues or organs from different individuals based on the similarity of histocompatibility antigens esp. on lymphocytes and used esp. as a measure of potential rejection in an organ transplant procedure

tis·su·lar \'tish-(y)ə-lər\ *adj* : of, relating to, or affecting organismal tissue ⟨∼ grafts⟩ ⟨∼ lesions⟩

titanate — see BARIUM TITANATE

ti·ta·ni·um \tī-'tān-ē-əm, tə- *also* -'tan-\ *n* : a silvery gray light strong metallic element found combined in ilmenite and rutile and used esp. in alloys (as steel) and combined in refractory materials and in coatings — symbol *Ti*; see ELEMENT table

titanium dioxide *n* : an oxide TiO₂ of titanium that is used esp. as a pigment and in sunblocks

ti·ter \'tīt-ər\ *or chiefly Brit* **ti·tre** \'tī-tər *also* 'tē-\ *n* **1 a** : the strength of a solution or the concentration of a substance in solution as determined by titration   **b** : the dilution of a serum containing a specific antibody at which the solution just retains a specific activity (as neutralizing or precipitating an antigen) which it loses at any greater dilution ⟨a test for toxoplasmosis antibodies yielded a ∼ of 1:1024⟩   **2** : the solidifying point of the fatty acids liberated from a fat that is determined by melting the acids in a tube and noting the temperature at which they solidify again on cooling — **ti‧tered** \-ərd\ *adj*

ti‧trant \'tī-trənt\ *n* : a substance (as a reagent solution of precisely known concentration) that is added in titration

ti‧trat‧able \'tī-ˌtrāt-ə-bəl\ *adj* : capable of being determined by titration ⟨∼ acidity⟩

ti‧trate \'tī-ˌtrāt\ *vb* **ti‧trat‧ed; ti‧trat‧ing** *vt* : to subject to titration — *vi* : to perform titration — **ti‧tra‧tor** \-ˌtrāt-ər\ *n*

ti‧tra‧tion \tī-'trā-shən\ *n* : a method or the process of determining the concentration of a dissolved substance in terms of the smallest amount of a reagent of known concentration required to bring about a given effect in reaction with a known volume of the test solution; *esp* : the analytical process of successively adding from a burette measured amounts of a reagent to a known volume of a sample in solution or a known weight of a sample until a desired end point (as a color change) is reached

titre *chiefly Brit var of* TITER

ti‧trim‧e‧try \tī-'trim-ə-trē\ *n, pl* **-tries** : measurement or analysis by titration — **ti‧tri‧met‧ric** \ˌtī-trə-'me-trik\ *adj* — **ti‧tri‧met‧ri‧cal‧ly** \-tri-k(ə-)lē\ *adv*

tit‧u‧ba‧tion \ˌtich-ə-'bā-shən\ *n* : a staggering gait observed in some nervous disturbances

Tl *symbol* thallium

TLC *abbr* **1** tender loving care   **2** thin-layer chromatography

TLE *abbr* temporal lobe epilepsy

T lymphocyte \'tē-\ *n* : T CELL

Tm *symbol* thulium

TM \'tē-'em\ *service mark* — used for a Transcendental Meditation technique

T–maze \'tē-ˌmāz\ *n* : a maze for the study of learning usu. consisting of a wood or metal structure shaped like the letter T in which the experimental subject (as a rat or mouse) must at a given point make a choice between a left or right turn with one choice usu. involving a reward

TMD *abbr* temporomandibular disorder

TMJ *abbr* temporomandibular joint; temporomandibular joint syndrome

TMJ syndrome \ˌtē-(ˌ)em-'jā-\ *n* : TEMPOROMANDIBULAR JOINT SYNDROME

TNF *abbr* tumor necrosis factor

TNT \ˌtē-ˌen-'tē\ *n* : TRINITROTOLUENE

toad skin \'tōd-\ *n* : PHRYNODERMA

toad‧stool \-ˌstül\ *n* : a fungus having an umbrella-shaped pileus : MUSHROOM; *esp* : a poisonous or inedible one as distinguished from an edible mushroom

to‧bac‧co \tə-'bak-(ˌ)ō\ *n, pl* **-cos**   **1** : any plant of the genus *Nicotiana*; *esp* : an annual So. American herb (*N. tabacum*) cultivated for its leaves   **2** : the leaves of cultivated tobacco prepared for use in smoking or chewing or as snuff   **3** : manufactured products of tobacco; *also* : the use of tobacco as a practice

tobacco heart *n* : a functional disorder of the heart marked by irregularity of action and caused by excessive use of tobacco

to‧bra‧my‧cin \ˌtō-brə-'mīs-ᵊn\ *n* : a colorless water-soluble antibiotic $C_{18}H_{37}N_5O_9$ isolated from a soil bacterium of the genus *Streptomyces* (*S. tenebrarius*) and effective esp. against gram-negative bacteria

tocodynamometer *var of* TOKODYNAMOMETER

tocology *var of* TOKOLOGY

to‧col‧y‧sis \tō-'käl-ə-səs\ *n, pl* **-y‧ses** \-ˌsēz\ : inhibition of uterine contractions

¹to‧co‧lyt‧ic \ˌtō-kə-'lit-ik\ *adj* : inhibiting uterine contractions ⟨a ∼ drug⟩ — **to‧co‧lyt‧i‧cal‧ly** \-i-k(ə-)lē\ *adv*

²tocolytic *n* : a tocolytic drug

to‧coph‧er‧ol \tō-'käf-ə-ˌról, -ˌról\ *n* : any of several fat‑soluble oily phenolic compounds with varying degrees of antioxidant vitamin E activity; *esp* : ALPHA-TOCOPHEROL

to‧co‧tri‧en‧ol \ˌtō-kō-'trī-ə-ˌnól, -ˌnól\ *n* : any of several compounds that are similar to the tocopherols but in which the isoprenoid units of the side chain are unsaturated

Todd's paralysis \'tädz-\ *n* : temporary weakness or paralysis of one limb or one side of the body that occurs following a seizure

> **Todd, Robert Bentley (1809–1860),** British physician. Born and educated in Ireland, Todd served as professor of physiology and general and morbid anatomy at London's King's College from 1836 to 1853. He is credited with contributing to the founding of King's College Hospital and to the establishment of a program for the training of nurses. As coeditor, he contributed important articles on the heart, brain, and nervous system to *The Cyclopedia of Anatomy and Physiology* (1835–59). This multivolume reference was credited with doing more than any previous work to advance the study of physiology and of comparative and microscopic anatomy. The condition now known as Todd's paralysis was described by him in 1856 in *Clinical Lectures on Paralysis and Certain Diseases of the Brain*.

toe \'tō\ *n* : one of the terminal members of a vertebrate's foot

toed \'tōd\ *adj* : having a toe or toes esp. of a specified kind or number — usu. used in combination ⟨five-*toed*⟩

toe‧nail \'tō-ˌnāl, -'nā(ə)l\ *n* : a nail of a toe

TOF *abbr* time-of-flight

To‧fra‧nil \tō-'frā-nil\ *trademark* — used for a preparation of imipramine

To‧ga‧vi‧ri‧dae \ˌto-gə-'vir-ə-ˌdē\ *n pl* : a family of single‑stranded RNA viruses that have a spherical virion about 70 nanometers in diameter and that include the causative agents of German measles and the three equine encephalomyelitides — see ALPHAVIRUS

to‧ga‧vi‧rus \'tō-gə-ˌvī-rəs\ *n* : any of the family *Togaviridae* of single-stranded RNA viruses

toi‧let \'tói-lət\ *n* : cleansing in preparation for or in association with a medical or surgical procedure ⟨a pharyngeal ∼⟩

toilet train‧ing \-ˌtrān-iŋ\ *n* : the process of training a child to control bladder and bowel movements and to use the toilet — **toilet train** \-ˌtrān\ *vt*

to‧ken economy \'tō-kən-\ *n* : a system of operant conditioning used for behavior modification that involves rewarding desirable behaviors with tokens which can be exchanged for items or privileges (as food or free time) and punishing undesirable behaviors (as destruction or violence) by taking away tokens

to‧ko‧dy‧na‧mom‧e‧ter *or* **to‧co‧dy‧na‧mom‧e‧ter** \ˌtō-kō-ˌdī-nə-'mäm-ə-tər\ *n* : an instrument by means of which the force of uterine puerperal contractions can be measured

to‧kol‧o‧gy *or* **to‧col‧o‧gy** \tō-'käl-ə-jē\ *n, pl* **-gies** : OBSTETRICS

to‧laz‧amide \tō-'laz-ə-ˌmīd\ *n* : a sulfonylurea $C_{14}H_{21}N_3O_3S$ used orally to lower blood sugar in the treatment of type 2 diabetes — see TOLINASE

to‧laz‧o‧line \tō-'laz-ə-ˌlēn\ *n* : a weak alpha-adrenergic blocking agent used in the form of its hydrochloride $C_{10}H_{12}N_2 \cdot HCl$ to produce peripheral vasodilation

tol‧bu‧ta‧mide \täl-'byüt-ə-ˌmīd\ *n* : a sulfonylurea $C_{12}H_{18}N_2O_3S$ used orally to lower blood sugar in the treatment of type 2 diabetes

Tol‧ec‧tin \'täl-ek-tin\ *trademark* — used for a preparation of the hydrated sodium salt of tolmetin

tol‧er‧ance \'täl-(ə)-rən(t)s\ *n*   **1** : the capacity of the body to endure or become less responsive to a substance (as a drug) or a physiological insult esp. with repeated use or exposure

---

\ə\ abut   \ᵊ\ kitten   \ər\ further   \a\ ash   \ā\ ace   \ä\ cot, cart
\aú\ out   \ch\ chin   \e\ bet   \ē\ easy   \g\ go   \i\ hit   \ī\ ice   \j\ job
\ŋ\ sing   \ō\ go   \ó\ law   \ói\ boy   \th\ thin   \th\ the   \ü\ loot
\ú\ foot   \y\ yet   \zh\ vision   *See also* Pronunciation Symbols page

⟨developed a ～ to painkillers⟩ **2** : the immunological state marked by unresponsiveness to a specific antigen

tol·er·ant \-rənt\ *adj* : exhibiting tolerance (as for a drug or physiological insult) ⟨lactose ～⟩

tol·er·ate \'täl-ə-ˌrāt\ *vt* **-at·ed; -at·ing** : to endure or resist the action of (as a drug or food) without serious side effects or discomfort : exhibit physiological tolerance for ⟨a premature baby . . . does not ～ fats very well —H. R. Litchfield & L. H. Dembo⟩

tol·er·a·tion \ˌtäl-ə-'rā-shən\ *n* : TOLERANCE

tol·ero·gen \'täl-ə-rə-jən\ *n* : a tolerogenic antigen

tol·ero·gen·ic \ˌtäl-ə-rə-'jen-ik\ *adj* : capable of producing immunological tolerance ⟨～ antigens⟩

To·li·nase \'tō-lə-ˌnās, 'täl-ə-ˌnāz\ *n* : a preparation of tolazamide — formerly a U.S. registered trademark

tol·met·in \'täl-mət-ən\ *n* : an anti-inflammatory drug administered esp. in the form of its hydrated sodium salt $C_{15}H_{14}NNaO_3·2H_2O$ — see TOLECTIN

tol·naf·tate \täl-'naf-ˌtāt\ *n* : a topical antifungal drug $C_{19}H_{17}NOS$ — see TINACTIN

to·lo·ni·um chloride \tə-'lō-nē-əm-\ *n* : TOLUIDINE BLUE

tol·ter·o·dine \ˌtäl-'ter-ə-ˌdēn\ *n* : an anticholinergic drug administered in the form of its tartrate $C_{22}H_{31}NO·C_4H_6O_6$ to treat urge incontinence, frequent urination, and urinary urgency associated with an overactive bladder

to·lu \tə-'lü, tō-\ *n* : BALSAM OF TOLU

tolu balsam *n* : BALSAM OF TOLU

tol·u·ene \'täl-yə-ˌwēn\ *n* : a liquid aromatic hydrocarbon C_7H_8 that resembles benzene but is less volatile, flammable, and toxic and is used as a solvent, in organic synthesis, and as an antiknock agent for gasoline — called also *methylbenzene*

tol·u·ene·sul·fon·ic acid *or Brit* **tol·u·ene·sul·phon·ic acid** \ˌtäl-yə-ˌwēn-səl-ˌfän-ik-\ *n* : any of three isomeric crystalline oily liquid strong acids $CH_3C_6H_4SO_3H$ of which the para isomer has important use in organic synthesis (as of dyes)

tol·u·ene·sul·fo·nyl *or Brit* **tol·u·ene·sul·pho·nyl** \-'səl-fə-ˌnil\ *n* : any of three radicals $CH_3C_6H_4SO_2-$ derived from the toluenesulfonic acids

to·lu·ic \tə-'lü-ik\ *adj* : of, relating to, or being any of four isomeric acids $C_8H_8O_2$ derived from toluene

to·lu·idine \tə-'lü-ə-ˌdēn\ *n* : any of three isomeric amino derivatives of toluene C_7H_9N that are analogous to aniline and are used as dye intermediates

toluidine blue *n* : a basic thiazine dye that is related to methylene blue and is used as a biological stain and esp. formerly as an antihemorrhagic drug — called also *tolonium chloride*

toluidine blue O *n* : TOLUIDINE BLUE

tol·u·ol \'täl-yə-ˌwól, -ˌwōl\ *n* : toluene esp. of commercial grade

tol·yl \'täl-il\ *n* : any of three monovalent radicals $CH_3C_6H_4$ derived from toluene

tom·a·tine \'täm-ə-ˌtēn\ *or* **tom·a·tin** \-ˌtin\ *n* : a crystalline antibiotic glycosidic alkaloid $C_{50}H_{83}NO_{21}$ that is obtained esp. from the juice of the stems and leaves of tomato plants resistant to wilt, that is active against fungi including some causing disease in humans, and that is used as a precipitating agent for steroids

Tomes' fiber \'tōmz-\ *n* : any of the fibers extending from the odontoblasts into the alveolar canals : a dentinal fiber — called also *Tomes' process*

Tomes, Sir John (1815–1895), British dental surgeon. Tomes did much during his career to upgrade the practice of dentistry, working to establish it as a profession and to ensure the proper education and registration of its practitioners. Between 1849 and 1856 he wrote a series of important papers on bone and dental tissues, and in 1850 he described Tomes' fibers.

Tom·my John surgery \ˌtäm-ē-'jän-\ *n* : ULNAR COLLATERAL LIGAMENT RECONSTRUCTION

John, Thomas Edward (b 1943), American baseball player. As a left-handed pitcher, John enjoyed a 26-year career in the major leagues, most notably with the Chicago White Sox, Los Angeles Dodgers, and the New York Yankees.

During the 1974 season he permanently damaged the ulnar collateral ligament in his pitching arm. In a revolutionary surgical procedure, the elbow tendon in his left arm was replaced with a tendon from his right wrist. Despite predictions that he would never pitch again, he made a full recovery and returned to baseball in 1976. From that point until his retirement in 1989, he pitched a total of 164 winning games.

to·mo·gram \'tō-mə-ˌgram\ *n* : a radiograph made by tomography

to·mo·graph \-ˌgraf\ *n* : an X-ray machine used for tomography

to·mog·ra·phy \tō-'mäg-rə-fē\ *n, pl* **-phies** : a method of producing a three-dimensional image of the internal structures of a solid object (as the human body) by the observation and recording of the differences in the effects on the passage of waves of energy impinging on those structures — called also *stratigraphy;* see COMPUTED TOMOGRAPHY, POSITRON= EMISSION TOMOGRAPHY — **to·mo·graph·ic** \ˌtō-mə-'graf-ik\ *adj*

¹tone \'tōn\ *n* **1** : a sound of definite pitch and vibration **2 a** : the state of a living body or of any of its organs or parts in which the functions are healthy and performed with due vigor or **b** : normal tension or responsiveness to stimuli; *specif* : TONUS 2

²tone *vt* **toned; ton·ing** : to impart tone to ⟨～ the muscles⟩

tone–deaf \'tōn-ˌdef\ *adj* : relatively insensitive to differences in musical pitch — **tone deafness** *n*

ton·er \'tō-nər\ *n* : one that tones ⟨a muscle ～⟩; *esp* : a liquid cosmetic for cleansing the skin and contracting the pores ⟨facial ～s⟩

tongue \'təŋ\ *n* : a process of the floor of the mouth that is attached basally to the hyoid bone, that consists essentially of a mass of extrinsic muscle attaching its base to other parts, intrinsic muscle by which parts of the structure move in relation to each other, and an epithelial covering rich in sensory end organs and small glands, and that functions esp. in taking and swallowing food and as a speech organ

tongue blade *n* : TONGUE DEPRESSOR

tongue depressor *n* : a thin wooden blade rounded at both ends that is used to depress the tongue to allow for inspection of the mouth and throat

tongue roll·er \-ˌrō-lər\ *n* : a person who carries a dominant gene which confers the capacity to roll the tongue into the shape of a U

tongue thrust \-ˌthrəst\ *n* : the thrusting of the tongue against or between the incisors during the act of swallowing which if persistent in early childhood can lead to various dental abnormalities

tongue–tie *n* : a congenital defect characterized by limited mobility of the tongue due to shortness of its frenulum

tongue–tied \'təŋ-ˌtīd\ *adj* : characteristic of or affected with tongue-tie

tongue worm *n* : any of a phylum or arthropod class (Pentastomida) of parasitic invertebrates that live as adults in the respiratory passages of reptiles, birds, or mammals — see HALZOUN

¹ton·ic \'tän-ik\ *adj* **1 a** : characterized by tonus ⟨～ contraction of muscle⟩; *also* : marked by or being prolonged muscular contraction ⟨～ convulsions⟩ **b** : producing or adapted to produce healthy muscular condition and reaction of organs (as muscles) **2 a** : increasing or restoring physical or mental tone **b** : yielding a tonic substance — **ton·i·cal·ly** \'tän-i-k(ə-)lē\ *adv*

²tonic *n* : an agent (as a drug) that increases body tone

ton·ic–clon·ic \'tän-i(k)-'klä-nik\ *adj* : relating to, marked by, or being a generalized seizure that is initially tonic and then becomes clonic and is characterized by the abrupt loss of consciousness ⟨～ epilepsy⟩ ⟨～ seizures⟩

to·nic·i·ty \tō-'nis-ət-ē\ *n, pl* **-ties** **1** : the property of possessing tone; *esp* : healthy vigor of body or mind **2** : TONUS 2 **3** : the osmotic pressure of a solution ⟨the cells swell and shrink with changing ～ of the environment⟩

ton·i·co·clon·ic \ˌtän-i-kō-'klän-ik\ *adj* : TONIC-CLONIC

ton·ka bean \ˈtäŋ-kə-\ *n* : the seed of any of several leguminous trees of the genus *Dipteryx* that contains coumarin and is used in perfumes and as a flavoring; *also* : a tree bearing tonka beans

tono·clon·ic \ˌtän-ō-ˈklän-ik\ *adj* : TONIC-CLONIC

tono·fi·bril \-ˈfīb-rəl, -ˈfib-\ *n* : a thin fibril made up of tonofilaments

tono·fil·a·ment \-ˈfil-ə-mənt\ *n* : a slender cytoplasmic organelle found esp. in some epithelial cells

to·nog·ra·phy \tō-ˈnäg-rə-fē\ *n, pl* **-phies** : the procedure of recording measurements (as of intraocular pressure) with a tonometer — **to·no·graph·ic** \ˌtō-nə-ˈgraf-ik, ˌtän-ə-\ *adj*

to·nom·e·ter \tō-ˈnäm-ət-ər\ *n* : an instrument for measuring tension or pressure and esp. intraocular pressure — **to·no·met·ric** \ˌtō-nə-ˈme-trik, ˌtän-ə-\ *adj* — **to·nom·e·try** \tō-ˈnäm-ə-trē\ *n, pl* **-tries**

to·no·top·ic \ˌtō-nə-ˈtäp-ik\ *adj* : relating to or being the anatomic organization by which specific sound frequencies are received by specific receptors in the inner ear with nerve impulses traveling along selected pathways to specific sites in the brain

ton·sil \ˈtän(t)-səl\ *n* **1 a** : either of a pair of prominent masses of lymphoid tissue that lie one on each side of the throat between the anterior and posterior pillars of the fauces and are composed of lymph follicles grouped around one or more deep crypts and except for the exposed surface which is covered only by epithelium are surrounded by diffuse lymphoid tissue in a fibrous capsule — called also *palatine tonsil* **b** : PHARYNGEAL TONSIL **c** : LINGUAL TONSIL **2** : a rounded prominence situated medially on the lower surface of each lateral hemisphere of the cerebellum

ton·sil·lar \ˈtän(t)-sə-lər\ *adj* : of, relating to, or affecting the tonsils ⟨~ tissue⟩

tonsillar crypt *n* : any of the deep invaginations occurring on the surface of the palatine and pharyngeal tonsils

ton·sil·lec·tome \ˈtän(t)-sə-ˈlek-ˌtōm\ *n* : a surgical instrument for excising the tonsils

ton·sil·lec·to·my \ˌtän(t)-sə-ˈlek-tə-mē\ *n, pl* **-mies** : surgical excision of the tonsils

ton·sil·li·tis \ˌtän(t)-sə-ˈlīt-əs\ *n* : inflammation of the tonsils and esp. the palatine tonsils typically due to viral or bacterial infection and marked by red enlarged tonsils usu. with sore throat, fever, difficult swallowing, hoarseness or loss of voice, and tender or swollen lymph nodes

ton·sil·lo·phar·yn·geal \ˌtän(t)-sə-lō-ˌfar-ən-ˈjē-əl, -fə-ˈrin-j(ē-)əl\ *adj* : of, relating to, or involving the tonsils and pharynx ⟨the ~ area⟩

ton·sil·lo·phar·yn·gi·tis \-ˌfar-ən-ˈjīt-əs\ *n, pl* **-git·i·des** \-ˈjit-ə-ˌdēz\ : inflammation of the tonsils and pharynx

ton·sil·lo·tome \ˈtän-ˈsil-ə-ˌtōm\ *n* : a surgical instrument for partial or complete excision of the tonsils

to·nus \ˈtō-nəs\ *n* **1** : TONE 2a **2** : a state of partial contraction that is characteristic of normal muscle, is maintained at least in part by a continuous bombardment of motor impulses originating reflexly, and serves to maintain body posture — called also *muscle tone;* compare CLONUS

took *past of* TAKE

tooth \ˈtüth\ *n, pl* **teeth** \ˈtēth\ : any of the hard bony appendages that are borne on the jaws and serve esp. for the prehension and mastication of food — see MILK TOOTH, PERMANENT TOOTH

tooth·ache \ˈtüth-ˌāk\ *n* : pain in or about a tooth — called also *odontalgia*

tooth·brush \-ˌbrəsh\ *n* : a brush for cleaning the teeth

tooth·brush·ing \-ˌbrəsh-iŋ\ *n* : the action of using a toothbrush to clean the teeth

tooth bud *n* : a mass of tissue having the potentiality of differentiating into a tooth

toothed \ˈtütht also ˈtü-thəd\ *adj* **1** : having teeth esp. of an indicated kind or number ⟨small-*toothed* individuals⟩ **2** : having pointed projections on the margin or surface

tooth germ *n* : TOOTH BUD

tooth·less \ˈtüth-ləs\ *adj* : having no teeth

tooth·paste \-ˌpāst\ *n* : a paste for cleaning the teeth

tooth·pick \-ˌpik\ *n* : a pointed instrument (as a slender tapering piece of wood) used for removing food particles lodged between the teeth

tooth powder *n* : a powder for cleaning the teeth

tooth sac *n* : DENTAL SAC

to·pec·to·my \tə-ˈpek-tə-mē\ *n, pl* **-mies** : surgical excision of selected portions of the frontal cortex of the brain esp. for the relief of medically intractable epilepsy

to·pha·ceous \tə-ˈfā-shəs\ *adj* : relating to, being, or characterized by the occurrence of tophi ⟨~ deposits⟩ ⟨~ gout⟩

to·phus \ˈtō-fəs\ *n, pl* **to·phi** \ˈtō-ˌfī, -ˌfē\ : a deposit of urates in tissues (as cartilage) characteristic of gout

top·i·cal \ˈtäp-i-kəl\ *adj* : designed for or involving application to or action on the surface of a part of the body ⟨applied a ~ anesthetic to numb the skin⟩ ⟨eyedrops used in the ~ treatment of glaucoma⟩ — **top·i·cal·ly** \-k(ə-)lē\ *adv*

top·og·no·sia \ˌtäp-ˌäg-ˈnō-zh(ē-)ə, ˌtōp-\ *n* : recognition of the location of a stimulus on the skin or elsewhere in the body

topo·graph·i·cal \ˌtäp-ə-ˈgraf-i-kəl\ *or* **topo·graph·ic** \-ik\ *adj* **1** : of, relating to, or concerned with topography ⟨~ correspondences between the skin and the cortex —F. A. Geldard⟩ **2** : of or relating to a mind made up of different strata and esp. of the conscious, preconscious, and unconscious — **topo·graph·i·cal·ly** \-i-k(ə-)lē\ *adv*

topographic anatomy *n* : REGIONAL ANATOMY

to·pog·ra·phy \tə-ˈpäg-rə-fē\ *n, pl* **-phies** **1** : the physical or natural features of an object or entity and their structural relationships ⟨the ~ of the abdomen⟩ ⟨the ~ (size and fluorescent staining intensity) of human chromosomes —*Science News*⟩ **2** : REGIONAL ANATOMY

topo·isom·er·ase \ˌtō-pō-ī-ˈsäm-ə-ˌrās, -ˌrāz\ *n* : any of a class of enzymes that reduce supercoiling in DNA by breaking and rejoining one or both strands of the DNA molecule

to·pol·o·gy \tə-ˈpäl-ə-jē, tä-\ *n, pl* **-gies** **1** : REGIONAL ANATOMY **2** : CONFIGURATION 1 ⟨the ~ of a molecule⟩ — **topo·log·i·cal** \ˌtäp-ə-ˈläj-i-kəl\ *also* **topo·log·ic** \-ik\ *adj*

Top·rol \ˈtäp-ˌról\ *trademark* — used for a preparation of the succinate of metoprolol

TORCH \ˈtórch\ *n* [*t*oxoplasma, *r*ubella virus, *c*ytomegalovirus, *h*erpes simplex virus] : a group of pathological agents that cause similar symptoms in newborns and that include esp. a toxoplasma (*Toxoplasma gonii*), cytomegalovirus, herpes simplex virus, and the togavirus causing German measles

TORCH infection *n* : a group of symptoms esp. of newborn infants that include hepatosplenomegaly, jaundice, and thrombocytopenia and are caused by infection with one or more of the TORCH agents — called also *TORCH syndrome*

tor·cu·lar He·roph·i·li \ˈtór-kyə-lər-he-ˈräf-ə-ˌlī\ *n* : CONFLUENCE OF SINUSES

He·roph·i·lus \he-ˈräf-ə-ləs\ (335 BC?–280 BC?), Greek physician. Herophilus is often called the father of anatomy because of his advocacy of dissection and especially human dissection as an essential means to an understanding of human anatomy. He investigated the brain's cavities and followed the sinuses of the dura mater to their meeting point. He likened the junction of the sinuses to a winepress, and accordingly the junction has since been known as the torcular Herophili, *torcular* being the Latin word meaning "winepress." None of his original works have survived; he is known only through Galen and other later writers.

tore *past of* TEAR

tori *pl of* TORUS

to·ric \ˈtór-ik, ˈtòr-\ *adj* : of, relating to, or shaped like a torus or segment of a torus; *specif* : being a simple lens having for one of its surfaces a segment of an equilateral zone of a torus and consequently having different refracting power in different meridians

\ə\ abut \ˈə\ kitten \ər\ further \a\ ash \ā\ ace \ä\ cot, cart \aú\ out \ch\ chin \e\ bet \ē\ easy \g\ go \i\ hit \ī\ ice \j\ job \ŋ\ sing \ō\ go \ò\ law \ói\ boy \th\ thin \th\ the \ü\ loot \ù\ foot \y\ yet \zh\ vision *See also* Pronunciation Symbols page

torn *past part of* TEAR

tor·pid \'tor-pəd\ *adj* : sluggish in functioning or acting : characterized by torpor — **tor·pid·i·ty** \tor-'pid-ət-ē\ *n, pl* -ties

tor·por \'tor-pər\ *n* : a state of mental and motor inactivity with partial or total insensibility : extreme sluggishness or stagnation of function

¹**torque** \'tork\ *n* : a force that produces or tends to produce rotation or torsion; *also* : a measure of the effectiveness of such a force that consists of the product of the force and the perpendicular distance from the line of action of the force to the axis of rotation

²**torque** *vt* **torqued; torqu·ing** : to impart torque to : cause to twist (as a shaft about its long axis)

torr \'to(ə)r\ *n, pl* **torr** : a unit of pressure equal to ¹⁄₇₆₀ of an atmosphere or about 0.019 pounds per square inch or about 133.3 pascals

tor·sades de pointes \tor-ˌsäd(z)-də-'pwant\ *or* **tor·sade de pointes** \-ˌsäd-\ *n* : ventricular tachycardia that is characterized by fluctuation of the QRS complexes around the electrocardiographic baseline and is typically caused by a long QT interval

tor·sion \'tor-shən\ *n* **1** : the twisting of a bodily organ or part on its own axis ⟨intestinal ∼⟩ **2** : the twisting or wrenching of a body by the exertion of forces tending to turn one end or part about a longitudinal axis while the other is held fast or turned in the opposite direction; *also* : the state of being twisted — **tor·sion·al** \'tor-shnəl, -shən-ᵊl\ *adj*

torsion dystonia *n* : DYSTONIA MUSCULORUM DEFORMANS

tor·si·ver·sion \ˌtor-sə-'vər-zhən\ *n* : malposition of a tooth that is turned on its long axis

tor·so \'tor-(ˌ)sō\ *n, pl* **torsos** *or* **tor·si** \'tor-ˌsē\ : the human trunk

tort·ed \'tort-əd\ *adj, chiefly Brit* : marked by torsion ⟨tenderness over the ∼ appendix —J. A. Fracchia *et al*⟩

tor·ti·col·lis \ˌtort-ə-'käl-əs\ *n* : a twisting of the neck to one side that results in abnormal carriage of the head and is usu. caused by muscle spasms — called also *wryneck*

tor·tu·ous \'torch-(ə-)wəs\ *adj* : marked by repeated twists, bends, or turns ⟨a ∼ blood vessel⟩ — **tor·tu·os·i·ty** \ˌtor-chə-'wäs-ət-ē\ *n, pl* -ties — **tor·tu·rous·ly** *adv*

tor·u·la \'tor-yə-lə, 'tär-\ *n* **1** *pl* **-lae** \-ˌlē, -ˌlī\ *also* **-las** **a** : any of various yeasts or fungi resembling yeasts that lack sexual spores, do not produce alcoholic fermentations, and are typically acid formers **b** : CRYPTOCOCCUS **2** *cap* **a** : a genus of usu. dark colored chiefly saprophytic imperfect fungi (family Dematiaceae) **b** *in some classifications* : a genus of yeasts including pathogens (as *T. histolytica* syn. *Cryptococcus neoformans* that causes cryptococcosis) usu. placed in the genus *Cryptococcus*

Tor·u·lop·sis \ˌtor-yə-'läp-səs, ˌtär-\ *n* : a genus of round, oval, or cylindrical yeasts that form no spores and no pellicle when growing in a liquid culture medium and that include forms which in other classifications are placed in *Torula* or *Cryptococcus*

tor·u·lo·sis \ˌtor-yə-'lō-səs, ˌtär-\ *n* : CRYPTOCOCCOSIS

to·rus \'tor-əs, 'tor-\ *n, pl* **to·ri** \'tō(ə)r-ˌī, 'tó(ə)r-, -ˌē\ **1** : a doughnut-shaped surface generated by a circle rotated about an axis in its plane that does not intersect the circle **2** : a smooth rounded anatomical protuberance (as a bony ridge on the skull) ⟨a supraorbital ∼⟩

torus tu·ba·ri·us \-t(y)ü-'ber-ē-əs\ *n* : a protrusion on the lateral wall of the nasopharynx marking the pharyngeal end of the cartilaginous part of the eustachian tube

torus ure·ter·i·cus \-ˌyùr-ə-'ter-i-kəs\ *n* : a band of smooth muscle joining the orifices of the ureter and forming the base of the trigone of the bladder — called also *Mercier's bar*

tos·yl·ate \'täs-ə-ˌlāt\ *n* : an ester of the para isomer of toluenesulfonic acid

to·tal hysterectomy \'tōt-ᵊl-\ *n* : PANHYSTERECTOMY

total mastectomy *n* : SIMPLE MASTECTOMY

to·ta·quine \'tōt-ə-ˌkwēn\ *also* **to·ta·qui·na** \ˌtōt-ə-'kē-nə\ *n* : an antimalarial drug that is obtained as a yellowish brown powder by extraction of cinchona bark and that contains quinine and other alkaloids but is less effective than quinine

to·ti·po·ten·cy \ˌtōt-ə-'pōt-ᵊn-sē\ *n, pl* -cies : ability of a cell or bodily part to generate or regenerate the whole organism

to·ti·po·tent \tō-'tip-ət-ənt\ *adj* : capable of developing into a complete organism or differentiating into any of its cells or tissues ⟨∼ blastomeres⟩

to·ti·po·ten·tial \ˌtōt-ə-pə-'ten-chəl\ *adj* : TOTIPOTENT

to·ti·po·ten·ti·al·i·ty \-pə-ˌten-chē-'al-ət-ē\ *n, pl* -ties : the quality or state of being totipotential

¹**touch** \'təch\ *vt* : to bring a bodily part into contact with esp. so as to perceive through the tactile sense : handle or feel gently usu. with the intent to understand or appreciate ∼ *vi* : to feel something with a body part (as the hand or foot)

²**touch** *n* **1** : the special sense by which pressure or traction exerted on the skin or mucous membrane is perceived **2** : a light attack ⟨a ∼ of fever⟩

touch corpuscle *n* : TACTILE CORPUSCLE

Tou·rette's \tùr-'et(s)\ *or* **Tou·rette** \-'et\ *n* : TOURETTE'S SYNDROME

Tourette's syndrome *or* **Tourette syndrome** *n* : a familial neuropsychiatric disorder of variable expression that is characterized by multiple recurrent involuntary tics involving body movements (as eye blinks, grimaces, or knee bends) and vocalizations (as grunts, snorts, or utterance of inappropriate words), that often has one or more associated behavioral or psychiatric conditions (as attention deficit disorder or obsessive-compulsive behavior), that is more common in males than females, and that usu. has an onset in childhood and often stabilizes or ameliorates in adulthood — abbr. *TS;* called also *Gilles de la Tourette syndrome, Tourette's disease, Tourette's disorder*

   Gilles de la Tourette \zhēl-də-lä-tür-et\, **Georges (1857–1904),** French physician. Gilles de la Tourette first described Tourette's syndrome in 1884. He is also remembered for his clinical studies, published in 1891, in which he expounded the ideas of the French neurologist Jean-Martin Charcot about hysteria and hystero-epilepsy.

tour·ni·quet \'tùr-ni-kət, 'tər-\ *n* : a device (as a bandage twisted tight with a stick) to check bleeding or blood flow

tow·el \'taù(-ə)l\ *n* **1** : an absorbent cloth or paper for wiping or drying **2** *Brit* : SANITARY NAPKIN

tow·er head \'taù(-ə)r-\ *n* : OXYCEPHALY

tower skull *n* : OXYCEPHALY

toxaemia, toxaemic *chiefly Brit var of* TOXEMIA, TOXEMIC

tox·al·bu·min \ˌtäks-al-'byü-mən\ *n* : any of a class of toxic substances of protein nature

tox·a·phene \'täk-sə-ˌfēn\ *n* : an insecticide with the approximate empirical formula $C_{10}H_{10}Cl_8$ that is a complex mixture of chlorinated compounds and has been shown to have carcinogenic properties in experiments with laboratory animals

Tox·as·ca·ris \täks-'as-kə-rəs\ *n* : a cosmopolitan genus of ascarid roundworms that infest the small intestine of the dog and cat and related wild animals

tox·e·mia *or chiefly Brit* **tox·ae·mia** \täk-'sē-mē-ə\ *n* : an abnormal condition associated with the presence of toxic substances in the blood: as **a** : a generalized intoxication due to absorption and systemic dissemination of bacterial toxins from a focus of infection **b** : intoxication due to dissemination of toxic substances (as some by-products of protein metabolism) that cause functional or organic disturbances (as in the kidneys) — **tox·e·mic** *or chiefly Brit* **tox·ae·mic** \-mik\ *adj*

toxemia of pregnancy *n* : a disorder of unknown cause that is peculiar to pregnancy, is usu. of sudden onset, is marked by hypertension, albuminuria, edema, headache, and visual disturbances, and may or may not be accompanied by convulsions — compare ECLAMPSIA a, PREECLAMPSIA

¹**tox·ic** \'täk-sik\ *adj* **1** : of, relating to, or caused by a poison or toxin ⟨a ∼ effect⟩ **2 a** : affected by a poison or toxin **b** : affected with toxemia of pregnancy ⟨∼ pregnant women⟩ **3** : POISONOUS ⟨∼ drugs⟩

²**toxic** *n* : a toxic substance

tox·i·cant \'täk-si-kənt\ *n* : a toxic agent; *esp* : one for insect control that kills rather than repels

toxic epidermal necrolysis *n* : a skin disorder characterized by widespread erythema and the formation of flaccid bullae and later by skin that is scalded in appearance and separates from the body in large sheets — called also *epidermal necrolysis, Lyell's syndrome, scalded-skin syndrome*; compare STAPHYLOCOCCAL SCALDED SKIN SYNDROME

tox·ic·i·ty \täk-'sis-ət-ē\ *n, pl* **-ties** : the quality, state, or relative degree of being toxic or poisonous

tox·i·co·den·drol \,täk-si-kō-'den-,dról\ *n* : a nonvolatile irritant oil that is the active constituent of various plants (as poison ivy) of the genus *Rhus*

Tox·i·co·den·dron \,täk-si-kō-'den-,drän\ *n* : a genus of shrubs and trees of the cashew family (Anacardiaceae) that includes poison ivy and related plants when they are split off from the genus *Rhus*

tox·i·co·der·ma \,täk-si-kō-'dər-mə\ *n* : a disease of the skin caused by a toxic agent

tox·i·co·der·ma·ti·tis \-,dər-mə-'tīt-əs\ *n, pl* **-ti·tis·es** *or* **-tit·i·des** \-'tit-ə-,dēz\ : an inflammation of the skin caused by a toxic substance

tox·i·co·gen·ic \,täk-si-kō-'jen-ik\ *adj* : producing toxins or poisons 〈∼ bacteria〉

tox·i·co·log·i·cal \-kə-'läj-i-kəl\ *or* **tox·i·co·log·ic** \-ik\ *adj* : of or relating to toxicology or toxins 〈a ∼ examination〉 — **tox·i·co·log·i·cal·ly** \-i-k(ə-)lē\ *adv*

tox·i·col·o·gist \,täk-si-'käl-ə-jəst\ *n* : a specialist in toxicology

tox·i·col·o·gy \-'käl-ə-jē\ *n, pl* **-gies** : a science that deals with poisons and their effect and with the problems involved (as clinical, industrial, or legal)

tox·i·co·ma·nia \,täk-si-kō-'mā-nē-ə, -nyə\ *n* : addiction to a drug (as opium or cocaine)

tox·i·co·sis \,täk-sə-'kō-səs\ *n, pl* **-co·ses** \-,sēz\ : a pathological condition caused by the action of a poison or toxin

toxic shock *n* : TOXIC SHOCK SYNDROME

toxic shock syndrome *n* : an acute and sometimes fatal disease that is characterized by fever, nausea, diarrhea, diffuse erythema, and shock, that is associated esp. with the presence of a bacterium of the genus *Staphylococcus* (*S. aureus*), and that occurs esp. in menstruating females using tampons — called also *toxic shock*

toxi·gen·ic \,täk-sə-'jen-ik\ *adj* : producing toxin 〈∼ bacteria and fungi〉 — **toxi·ge·nic·i·ty** \,täk-si-jə-'nis-ət-ē\ *n, pl* **-ties**

tox·in \'täk-sən\ *n* : a colloidal proteinaceous poisonous substance that is a specific product of the metabolic activities of a living organism and is usu. very unstable, notably toxic when introduced into the tissues, and typically capable of inducing antibody formation

toxin–antitoxin *n* : a mixture of toxin and antitoxin used esp. formerly in immunizing against a disease (as diphtheria) for which they are specific

toxi·pho·bia \,täk-sə-'fō-bē-ə\ *n* : abnormal fear of poisons or of being poisoned

Tox·o·cara \,täk-sə-'kar-ə\ *n* : a genus of nematode worms of the family Ascaridae including the common ascarids (*T. canis* and *T. cati*) of the dog and cat

tox·o·ca·ri·a·sis \,täk-sə-kə-'rī-ə-səs\ *n, pl* **-a·ses** \-ə-,sēz\ : infection with or disease caused by nematode worms of the genus *Toxocara*

tox·oid \'täk-,sóid\ *n* : a toxin of a pathogenic organism treated so as to destroy its toxicity but leave it capable of inducing the formation of antibodies on injection 〈diphtheria ∼〉 — called also *anatoxin*

toxo·phore \'täk-sə-,fó(ə)r\ *n* : a chemical group that produces the toxic effect in a toxin molecule — **toxo·phor·ic** \,täk-sə-'fór-ik\ *or* **tox·oph·o·rous** \täk-'säf-ə-rəs\ *adj*

toxo·plasm \'täk-sə-,plaz-əm\ *n* : TOXOPLASMA

toxo·plas·ma \,täk-sə-'plaz-mə\ *n* **1** *cap* : a genus of sporozoans that are typically serious pathogens of vertebrates **2** *pl* **-mas** *or* **-ma·ta** \-mət-ə\ *also* **-ma** : any microorganism of the genus *Toxoplasma* — **toxo·plas·mic** \-mik\ *adj*

toxo·plas·mo·sis \-,plaz-'mō-səs\ *n, pl* **-mo·ses** \-,sēz\ : infection with or disease caused by a sporozoan of the genus *Toxoplasma* (*T. gondii*) that invades the tissues and may seriously damage the central nervous system esp. of infants

tPA *abbr* tissue plasminogen activator

TPI *abbr* Treponema pallidum immobilization (test)

TPN \'tē-'pē-'en\ *n* : NADP

TPN *abbr* total parenteral nutrition

TPP *abbr* thiamine pyrophosphate

TPR *abbr* temperature, pulse, respiration

tra·bant \trə-'bänt\ *n* : SATELLITE 1

tra·bec·u·la \trə-'bek-yə-lə\ *n, pl* **-lae** \-,lē\ *also* **-las** **1** : a small bar, rod, bundle of fibers, or septal membrane in the framework of a bodily organ or part (as the spleen) **2** : one of a pair of longitudinally directed more or less curved cartilaginous rods in the developing skull of a vertebrate that develop under the anterior part of the brain on each side of the pituitary gland and subsequently fuse with each other and with the parachordal cartilages to form the base of the cartilaginous cranium **3** : any of the intersecting osseous bars occurring in cancellous bone

tra·bec·u·lar \-lər\ *adj* : of, relating to, consisting of, or being trabeculae 〈∼ tissue〉

trabecular meshwork *n* : trabecular tissue that separates the angle of the anterior chamber from the canal of Schlemm and that contains the spaces of Fontana through which aqueous humor normally drains from the anterior chamber into the canal of Schlemm

tra·bec·u·la·tion \trə-,bek-yə-'lā-shən\ *n* : the formation or presence of trabeculae 〈∼ of the spleen〉

tra·bec·u·lec·to·my \trə-,bek-yə-'lek-tə-mē\ *n, pl* **-mies** : surgical excision of a small portion of the trabecular tissue lying between the anterior chamber of the eye and the canal of Schlemm in order to facilitate drainage of aqueous humor for the relief of glaucoma

tra·bec·u·lo·plas·ty \trə-'bek-yə-lō-,plas-tē\ *n, pl* **-ties** : plastic surgery of a trabecula; *specif* : laser surgery to create small openings in the trabecular meshwork of the eye from which the aqueous humor can drain to reduce intraocular pressure caused by open-angle glaucoma

trace \'trās\ *n* **1** : the marking made by a recording instrument (as a kymograph) **2** : an amount of a chemical constituent not always quantitatively determinable because of minuteness **3** : ENGRAM — **trace** *vt* — **trace·able** \-ə-bəl\ *adj*

trace element *n* : a chemical element present in minute quantities; *esp* : one used by organisms and held essential to their physiology — compare MICRONUTRIENT 2

trac·er \'trā-sər\ *n* : a substance used to trace the course of a process; *specif* : a labeled element or atom that can be traced throughout chemical or biological processes by its radioactivity or its unusual isotopic mass

tra·chea \'trā-kē-ə, *Brit also* trə-'kē-ə\ *n, pl* **tra·che·ae** \-kē-,ē\ *also* **tra·che·as** : the main trunk of the system of tubes by which air passes to and from the lungs that is about four inches (10 centimeters) long and somewhat less than an inch (2.5 centimeters) in diameter, extends down the front of the neck from the larynx, divides in two to form the bronchi, has walls of fibrous and muscular tissue stiffened by incomplete cartilaginous rings which keep it from collapsing, and is lined with mucous membrane whose epithelium is composed of columnar ciliated mucus-secreting cells — called also *windpipe*

tra·che·al \-əl\ *adj* : of, relating to, or functioning in the manner of a trachea : resembling a trachea

tra·che·a·lis \,trā-kē-'ā-ləs, -'al-əs\ *n, pl* **-a·les** \-'ā-(,)lēz, -'al-(,)ēz\ : a muscle associated with the trachea that in humans

---

S
T

\ə\ **abut** \ᵊ\ **kitten** \ər\ **further** \a\ **ash** \ā\ **ace** \ä\ **cot, cart** \aú\ **out** \ch\ **chin** \e\ **bet** \ē\ **easy** \g\ **go** \i\ **hit** \ī\ **ice** \j\ **job** \ŋ\ **sing** \ō\ **go** \ó\ **law** \ói\ **boy** \th\ **thin** \t̲h̲\ **the** \ü\ **loot** \ú\ **foot** \y\ **yet** \zh\ **vision** *See also* Pronunciation Symbols page

consists of smooth muscle fibers extending transversely between the ends of the tracheal rings and the intervals between them at the back of the trachea

tracheal node *n* : any of a group of lymph nodes arranged along each side of the thoracic part of the trachea

tracheal ring *n* : any of the 16 to 20 C-shaped bands of highly elastic cartilage which are found as incomplete rings in the anterior two-thirds of the tracheal wall and of which there are usu. 6 to 8 in the right bronchus and 9 to 12 in the left

tracheal tug \-'təg\ *n* : a downward pull of the trachea and larynx observed in aneurysm of the aorta — called also *tracheal tugging*

tra·che·itis \ˌtrā-kē-'īt-əs\ *n* : inflammation of the trachea

trach·e·lec·to·my \ˌtrak-ə-'lek-tə-mē\ *n, pl* **-mies** : CERVICECTOMY

trach·e·lo·mas·toid muscle \ˌtrak-ə-lō-'mas-ˌtȯid-\ *n* : LONGISSIMUS CAPITIS — called also *trachelomastoid*

trach·e·lo·plas·ty \'trak-ə-lō-ˌplas-tē\ *n, pl* **-ties** : a plastic operation on the neck of the uterus

trach·e·lor·rha·phy \ˌtrak-ə-'lȯr-ə-fē\ *n, pl* **-phies** : the operation of sewing up a laceration of the uterine cervix

tra·cheo·bron·chi·al \ˌtrā-kē-ō-'bräŋ-kē-əl\ *adj* : of, relating to, affecting, or produced in the trachea and bronchi ⟨∼ secretion⟩ ⟨∼ lesions⟩

tracheobronchial node *n* : any of the lymph nodes arranged in four or five groups along the trachea and bronchi — called also *tracheobronchial lymph node*

tracheobronchial tree *n* : the trachea and bronchial tree considered together

tra·cheo·bron·chi·tis \ˌtrā-kē-ō-bräŋ-'kīt-əs\ *n, pl* **-chit·i·des** \-'kit-ə-ˌdēz\ : inflammation of the trachea and bronchi

tra·cheo·esoph·a·ge·al *or chiefly Brit* **tra·cheo·oe·soph·a·ge·al** \-i-ˌsäf-ə-'jē-əl\ *adj* : relating to or connecting the trachea and the esophagus ⟨a ∼ fistula⟩

tra·cheo·plas·ty \'trā-kē-ə-ˌplas-tē\ *n, pl* **-ties** : plastic surgery on the trachea

tra·che·os·co·py \ˌtrā-kē-'äs-kə-pē\ *n, pl* **-pies** : inspection of the interior of the trachea (as by a bronchoscope or through an established tracheostomy)

tra·cheo·sto·ma \ˌtrā-kē-ə-'stō-mə\ *n* : an opening into the trachea created by tracheostomy

tra·che·os·to·my \ˌtrā-kē-'äst-ə-mē\ *n, pl* **-mies** : the surgical formation of an opening into the trachea through the neck esp. to allow the passage of air; *also* : the opening itself

tra·che·ot·o·my \ˌtrā-kē-'ät-ə-mē\ *n, pl* **-mies** **1** : the surgical operation of cutting into the trachea esp. through the skin **2** : the opening created by a tracheotomy

tra·cho·ma \trə-'kō-mə\ *n* : a chronic contagious conjunctivitis marked by inflammatory granulations on the conjunctival surfaces, caused by a bacterium of the genus *Chlamydia* (*C. trachomatis*), and commonly resulting in blindness if left untreated — **tra·cho·ma·tous** \trə-'kō-mət-əs, -'käm-ət-əs\ *adj*

trac·ing \'trā-siŋ\ *n* : a graphic record made by an instrument (as an electrocardiograph) that registers some movement

tract \'trakt\ *n* **1** : a system of body parts or organs that act together to perform some function ⟨the digestive ∼⟩ — see GASTROINTESTINAL TRACT, LOWER RESPIRATORY TRACT, UPPER RESPIRATORY TRACT **2** : a bundle of nerve fibers having a common origin, termination, and function and esp. one within the spinal cord or brain — called also *fiber tract*; see CORTICOSPINAL TRACT, OLFACTORY TRACT, OPTIC TRACT, SPINOTHALAMIC TRACT; compare FASCICULUS b

trac·tion \'trak-shən\ *n* **1** : the pulling of or tension established in one body part by another **2** : a pulling force exerted on a skeletal structure (as in a fracture) by means of a special device or apparatus ⟨a ∼ splint⟩; *also* : a state of tension created by such a pulling force ⟨a leg in ∼⟩

traction fiber *n* : a spindle fiber of a dividing cell that extends from a pole to the chromosomal centromere and along which a daughter chromosome moves to the pole of the spindle

tract of Burdach *n* : FASCICULUS CUNEATUS
  K. F. Burdach — see COLUMN OF BURDACH

tract of Gowers *n* : SPINOCEREBELLAR TRACT b
  W. R. Gowers — see GOWERS'S TRACT

tract of Lissauer *n* : DORSOLATERAL TRACT
  H. Lissauer — see LISSAUER'S TRACT

trac·tor \'trak-tər\ *n* : an instrument used to exert traction on a body part or tissue (as in surgical procedures) ⟨a urethral ∼⟩

trac·tot·o·my \trak-'tät-ə-mē\ *n, pl* **-mies** : surgical division of a nerve tract

trac·tus \'trak-təs\ *n, pl* **tractus** : TRACT 2

tractus sol·i·ta·ri·us \-ˌsäl-i-'tar-ē-əs\ *n* : a descending tract of nerve fibers that is situated near the dorsal surface of the medulla oblongata, mediates esp. the sense of taste, and includes fibers from the facial, glossopharyngeal, and vagus nerves

trade·mark \'trād-ˌmärk\ *n* : a device (as a word or mark) that points distinctly to the origin or ownership of merchandise to which it is applied and that is legally reserved for the exclusive use of the owner — compare SERVICE MARK

trag·a·canth \'traj-ə-ˌkan(t)th, 'trag-, -kən(t)th; *also* 'trag-ə-ˌsan(t)th\ *n* : a gum obtained from various Asian or East European leguminous plants (genus *Astragalus* and esp. *A. gummifer*) that swells in water and is used as an emulsifying, suspending, and thickening agent and as a demulcent — called also *gum tragacanth, hog gum*

trag·a·can·thin \ˌtrag-ə-'kan(t)-thən, ˌtraj-; *also* -'san(t)-\ *n* : a substance obtained from tragacanth that is soluble in water forming a hydrosol — compare BASSORIN

trag·i·on \'traj-ē-ˌän\ *n* : an anthropometric point situated in the notch just above the tragus of the ear

tra·gus \'trā-gəs\ *n, pl* **tra·gi** \-ˌgī, -ˌjī\ : a small projection in front of the external opening of the ear

train·able \'trā-nə-bəl\ *adj* : affected with moderate mental retardation and capable of being trained in self-care and in simple social and work skills in a sheltered environment — compare EDUCABLE

trained nurse \ˌtrānd-\ *n* : GRADUATE NURSE

trait \'trāt, *Brit usu* 'trā\ *n* : an inherited characteristic

tram·a·dol \'tram-ə-ˌdȯl\ *n* : a synthetic opioid analgesic administered orally in the form of its hydrochloride $C_{16}H_{25}NO_2 \cdot HCl$ to treat moderate to severe pain — see ULTRAM

trance \'tran(t)s\ *n* **1** : a sleeplike altered state of consciousness (as of deep hypnosis) usu. characterized by partly suspended animation with diminished or absent sensory and motor activity and subsequent lack of recall **2** : a state of profound abstraction or absorption — **trance·like** \-ˌlīk\ *adj*

tran·ex·am·ic acid \ˌtran-eks-ˌam-ik-\ *n* : an antifibrinolytic drug $C_8H_{15}NO_2$

tran·quil·ize *or chiefly Brit* **tran·quil·lize** *or* **tran·quil·lise** \'traŋ-kwə-ˌlīz, 'tran-\ *vt* **-ized** *or chiefly Brit* **-lized** *or* **-lised**; **-iz·ing** *or chiefly Brit* **-liz·ing** *or* **-lis·ing** : to make tranquil or calm; *esp* : to relieve of mental tension and anxiety by means of drugs — **tran·quil·iza·tion** *or chiefly Brit* **tran·quil·li·za·tion** *or* **tran·quil·li·sa·tion** \ˌtraŋ-kwə-lə-'zā-shən, ˌtran-\ *n*

tran·quil·iz·er *or chiefly Brit* **tran·quil·liz·er** *or* **tran·quil·lis·er** \-ˌlī-zər\ *n* : a drug used to reduce mental disturbance (as anxiety and tension) — see ANTIPSYCHOTIC

trans \'tran(t)s, 'tranz\ *adj* **1** : characterized by or having certain groups of atoms on opposite sides of the longitudinal axis of a double bond or of the plane of a ring in a molecule — see ALL-TRANS **2** : relating to or being an arrangement of two very closely linked genes in the heterozygous condition in which one mutant allele and one wild-type allele are on each of the two homologous chromosomes — compare CIS 2

trans·ab·dom·i·nal \ˌtran(t)s-ab-'dam-ən-ᵊl, ˌtranz-əb-'dam-nᵊl\ *adj* : passing through or performed by passing through the abdomen or the abdominal wall ⟨∼ amniocentesis⟩

trans·acet·y·lase \-ə-'set-ᵊl-ˌās\ *n* : ACETYLTRANSFERASE

trans·ac·tion·al analysis \-ˌak-shnəl-, -shən-ᵊl-\ *n* : a system of psychotherapy involving analysis of individual episodes of social interaction for insight that will aid communication — abbr. *TA*

trans·am·i·nase \tran(t)s-'am-ə-ˌnās, tranz-, -ˌnāz\ *n* : an enzyme-promoting transamination — called also *amino-transferase*

trans·am·i·nate \-ˌnāt\ *vb* **-nat·ed; -nat·ing** *vi* : to induce or catalyze a transamination ~ *vt* : to induce or catalyze the transamination of

trans·am·i·na·tion \ˌtran(t)s-ˌam-ə-ˈnā-shən, ˌtranz-\ *n* : a reversible oxidation-reduction reaction in which an amino group is transferred typically from an alpha-amino acid to the carbonyl carbon atom of an alpha-keto acid

trans·bron·chi·al \tran(t)s-ˈbräŋ-kē-əl, tranz-\ *adj* : occurring or performed by way of a bronchus; *specif* : involving the passage of a bronchoscope through the lumen of a bronchus ⟨a ~ lung biopsy⟩

trans·cal·lo·sal \-ka-ˈlō-səl\ *adj* : passing through the corpus callosum ⟨~ pathways⟩

trans·cap·il·lary \-ˈkap-ə-ˌler-ē, *Brit usu* -kə-ˈpil-ə-rē\ *adj* : existing or taking place across the capillary walls ⟨~ absorption of extravascular fluids⟩

trans·car·ba·myl·ase \-ˌkär-bə-ˈmil-ˌās\ *n* : any of several enzymes that catalyze the addition of a carbamyl radical to a molecule — see ORNITHINE TRANSCARBAMYLASE

trans·cath·e·ter \-ˈkath-(ə-)tər\ *adj* : performed through the lumen of a catheter ⟨~ embolization⟩

Tran·scen·den·tal Meditation \ˌtran(t)s-ˌen-ˈdent-ᵊl-, -ən-\ *service mark* — used for a meditation technique

trans·cer·vi·cal \tran(t)s-ˈsər-vi-kəl, tranz-, *Brit usu* -sər-ˈvī-kəl\ *adj* : performed by way of the uterine cervix ⟨~ chorionic villus sampling⟩ — **trans·cer·vi·cal·ly** \-k(ə-)lē\ *adv*

trans·con·dy·lar \-ˈkän-də-lər\ *adj* : passing through a pair of condyles ⟨a ~ fracture of the humerus⟩

trans·cor·ti·cal \-ˈkȯrt-i-kəl\ *adj* : crossing the cortex of the brain; *esp* : passing from the cortex of one hemisphere to that of the other ⟨~ stimulation⟩

trans·cor·tin \-ˈkȯrt-ᵊn\ *n* : an alpha globulin produced in the liver that binds with and transports cortisol in the blood

trans·cra·ni·al \-ˈkrā-nē-əl\ *adj* : passing or performed through the skull ⟨~ Doppler ultrasound⟩

tran·scribe \tran(t)s-ˈkrīb\ *vt* **tran·scribed; tran·scrib·ing** : to cause (as DNA) to undergo genetic transcription

tran·script \ˈtran(t)s-ˌkript\ *n* : a sequence of RNA produced by transcription from a DNA template

tran·scrip·tase \tran-ˈskrip-ˌtās, -ˌtāz\ *n* : RNA POLYMERASE; *also* : REVERSE TRANSCRIPTASE

tran·scrip·tion \tran(t)s-ˈkrip-shən\ *n* : the process of constructing a messenger RNA molecule using a DNA molecule as a template with resulting transfer of genetic information to the messenger RNA — compare REVERSE TRANSCRIPTION, TRANSLATION — **tran·scrip·tion·al** \-shnəl, -shən-ᵊl\ *adj* — **tran·scrip·tion·al·ly** \-ē\ *adv*

transcription factor *n* : any of various proteins that bind to DNA and play a role in the regulation of gene expression by promoting transcription

tran·scrip·tion·ist \-shə-nəst\ *n* : one that transcribes; *esp* : MEDICAL TRANSCRIPTIONIST

trans·cu·ta·ne·ous \ˌtran(t)s-kyü-ˈtā-nē-əs\ *adj* : passing, entering, or made by penetration through the skin ⟨~ infection⟩

transcutaneous electrical nerve stimulation *n* : electrical stimulation of the skin to relieve pain by interfering with the neural transmission of signals from underlying pain receptors — abbr. *TENS;* called also *transcutaneous nerve stimulation* — **transcutaneous electrical nerve stimulator** *n*

trans·der·mal \ˌtran(t)s-ˈdər-məl, ˌtranz-\ *adj* : relating to, being, or supplying a medication in a form for absorption through the skin into the bloodstream ⟨~ drug delivery⟩ ⟨a ~ nicotine patch⟩ — **trans·der·mal·ly** \-ē\ *adv*

trans·dia·phrag·mat·ic \-ˌdī-ə-frə(g)-ˈmat-ik, -ˌfrag-\ *adj* : occurring, passing, or performed through the diaphragm ⟨~ hernia⟩ ⟨~ pressure⟩

trans·duce \tran(t)s-ˈd(y)üs, tranz-\ *vt* **trans·duced; trans·duc·ing** **1** : to convert (as energy or a message) into another form ⟨essentially sense organs ~ physical energy into a nervous signal⟩ **2** : to cause (genetic material) to undergo transduction; *also* : to introduce genetic material into (a cell) by transduction

trans·duc·er \-ˈd(y)ü-sər\ *n* : a device that is actuated by power from one system and supplies power usu. in another form to a second system

trans·duc·tant \-ˈdek-tənt\ *n* : a cell or organism (as a bacterium) that has undergone transduction

trans·duc·tion \-ˈdek-shən\ *n* **1** : the action or process of converting something and esp. energy or a message into another form **2** : the transfer of genetic material from one organism (as a bacterium) to another by a genetic vector and esp. a bacteriophage — compare TRANSFORMATION 2 — **trans·duc·tion·al** \-shnəl, -shən-ᵊl\ *adj*

trans·du·o·de·nal \-ˌd(y)ü-ə-ˈdē-nəl, -d(y)u-ˈäd-ᵊn-əl\ *adj* : performed by cutting across or through the duodenum

tran·sect \tran-ˈsekt\ *vt* : to cut transversely

tran·sec·tion \-ˈsek-shən\ *n* : an act or instance of transecting ⟨therapeutic ~ of sensory nerves —E. R. Kandel *et al*⟩

trans·epi·the·li·al \-ˌep-ə-ˈthē-lē-əl\ *adj* : existing or taking place across an epithelium ⟨~ sodium transport⟩

tran·sep·tal \tran-ˈsep-təl\ *adj* **1** : passing across a septum ⟨~ fibers between teeth⟩ **2** : passing or performed through a septum ⟨~ cardiac catheterization⟩

trans·esoph·a·ge·al \-ˌsäf-ə-ˈjē-əl\ *adj* : passing through or performed by way of the esophagus ⟨~ echocardiography⟩

trans·es·ter·i·fi·ca·tion \ˌtran(t)s-e-ˌster-ə-fə-ˈkā-shən, tranz-\ *n* : a reversible reaction in which one ester is converted into another (as by interchange of ester groups with an alcohol in the presence of a base)

transexual, transexualism, transexuality *var of* TRANSSEXUAL, TRANSSEXUALISM, TRANSSEXUALITY

trans fat *n* : a fat containing trans-fatty acids

trans–fatty acid \ˈtran(t)s-ˈfat-ē-, ˈtranz-\ *n* : any of various unsaturated fatty acids that are characterized by a trans arrangement of alkyl chains, that are formed esp. during the hydrogenation of vegetable oils, and that have been linked to an increase in blood cholesterol

trans·fec·tant \tran(t)s-ˈfek-tənt\ *n* : a cell that has incorporated foreign nucleic acid and esp. DNA through a process of transfection

trans·fec·tion \tran(t)s-ˈfek-shən\ *n* : infection of a cell with isolated viral nucleic acid followed by production of the complete virus in the cell; *also* : the incorporation of exogenous DNA into a cell — **trans·fect** \-ˈfekt\ *vt*

trans·fem·o·ral \-ˈfem-(ə-)rəl\ *adj* **1** : passing through or performed by way of the femoral artery ⟨~ angiography⟩ **2 a** : occurring across or involving the femur ⟨~ amputation⟩ **b** : having undergone transfemoral amputation ⟨a ~ amputee⟩; *also* : suitable for use following transfemoral amputation ⟨~ prostheses⟩

trans·fer \ˈtran(t)s-ˌfər\ *n* **1** : TRANSFERENCE **2** : the carryover or generalization of learned responses from one type of situation to another — see NEGATIVE TRANSFER

trans·fer·ase \ˈtran(t)s-(ˌ)fər-ˌās, -ˌāz\ *n* : an enzyme that promotes transfer of a group from one molecule to another

trans·fer·ence \tran(t)s-ˈfər-ən(t)s, ˈtran(t)s-(ˌ)\ *n* : the redirection of feelings and desires and esp. of those unconsciously retained from childhood toward a new object (as a psychoanalyst conducting therapy)

transference neurosis *n* : a neurosis developed in the course of psychoanalytic treatment and manifested by the reliving of infantile experiences in the presence of the analyst

transfer factor *n* : a substance that is produced and secreted by a lymphocyte functioning in cell-mediated immunity and that upon incorporation into a lymphocyte which has not been sensitized confers on it the same immunological specificity as the sensitized cell

trans·fer·rin \tran(t)s-ˈfer-ən\ *n* : a beta globulin in blood

---

\ə\ abut \ᵊ\ kitten \ər\ further \a\ ash \ā\ ace \ä\ cot, cart \au̇\ out \ch\ chin \e\ bet \ē\ easy \g\ go \i\ hit \ī\ ice \j\ job \ŋ\ sing \ō\ go \ȯ\ law \ȯi\ boy \th\ thin \t͟h\ the \ü\ loot \u̇\ foot \y\ yet \zh\ vision *See also* Pronunciation Symbols page

plasma capable of combining with ferric ions and transporting iron in the body — called also *siderophilin*

transfer RNA *n* : a relatively small RNA that transfers a particular amino acid to a growing polypeptide chain at the ribosomal site of protein synthesis during translation — called also *adapter RNA, soluble RNA, tRNA;* compare MESSENGER RNA

trans·fix·ion \tran(t)s-'fik-shən\ *n* : a piercing of a part of the body (as by a suture, nail, or other device) in order to fix it in position — **trans·fix** \-'fiks\ *vt*

trans·form \tran(t)s-'fȯ(ə)rm\ *vt* : to cause to change: as **a** : to change (a current) in potential (as from high voltage to low) or in type (as from alternating to direct) **b** : to cause (a cell) to undergo genetic transformation ~ *vi* : to become transformed

trans·for·mant \-'fȯr-mənt\ *n* : an individual (as a bacterium) that has undergone genetic transformation

trans·for·ma·tion \ˌtran(t)s-fər-'mā-shən, -fȯr-\ **1** : an act, process, or instance of transforming or being transformed — see MALIGNANT TRANSFORMATION **2 a** : genetic modification of a bacterium by incorporation of free DNA from another ruptured bacterial cell — compare TRANSDUCTION 2 **b** : genetic modification of a cell by the uptake and incorporation of exogenous DNA

transforming growth factor *n* : any of a group of polypeptides that are secreted by a variety of cells (as monocytes, T cells, or blood platelets) and have diverse effects (as inducing angiogenesis, stimulating fibroblast proliferation, or inhibiting T cell proliferation) on the division and activity of cells — abbr. *TGF*

transforming principle *n* : DNA that is transferred from one individual to another in genetic transformation

trans·fus·able *or* **trans·fus·ible** \tran(t)s-'fyü-zə-bəl\ *adj* : capable of being transfused ⟨~ blood⟩

trans·fuse \tran(t)s-'fyüz\ *vt* **trans·fused; trans·fus·ing 1** : to transfer (as blood) into a vein or artery of a human being or an animal **2** : to subject (a patient) to transfusion

trans·fu·sion \tran(t)s-'fyü-zhən\ *n* **1** : the process of transfusing fluid into a vein or artery **2** : something transfused

trans·fu·sion·al \-zhən-ᵊl\ *adj* : of, relating to, or caused by transfusion ⟨~ shock⟩ ⟨~ reactions⟩

trans·fu·sion·ist \-zhə-nəst\ *n* : one skilled in performing transfusions

trans·gen·der \tran(t)s-'jen-dər\ *or* **trans·gen·dered** \-dərd\ *adj* : of, relating to, or being a person (as a transsexual or a transvestite) who identifies with or expresses a gender identity that differs from the one which corresponds to the person's sex at birth — **trans·gen·der·ism** \-də-ˌriz-əm\ *n*

trans·gene \'tran(t)s-ˌjēn, 'tranz-\ *n* : a gene that is taken from the genome of one organism and introduced into the genome of another organism by artificial techniques

¹trans·gen·ic \ˌtran(t)s-'jen-ik, ˌtranz-\ *adj* : being or used to produce an organism or cell of one species into which one or more genes of other species have been incorporated ⟨~ mice⟩ ⟨~ corn plants⟩ ⟨~ techniques⟩; *also* : produced by or composed of transgenic plants or animals ⟨~ foods⟩

²transgenic *n* **1** : a transgenic plant or animal **2 transgenics** *pl but sing in constr* : a branch of biotechnology concerned with the production of transgenic plants, animals, and foods

trans·glu·co·syl·ase \-'glü-kə-ˌsil-ˌās, -ˌglü-kə-'sil-ˌāz\ *n* : GLUCOSYLTRANSFERASE

trans·glu·ta·min·ase \-'glüt-ə-mə-ˌnās, -glü-'tam-ə-ˌnāz\ *n* : a clotting factor that is a variant of factor XIII and that promotes the formation of cross-links between strands of fibrin

trans·he·pat·ic \-hi-'pat-ik\ *adj* : passing through or performed by way of the bile ducts; *specif* : involving direct injection (as of a radiopaque medium) into the bile ducts ⟨~ cholangiography⟩ — **trans·he·pat·i·cal·ly** \-i-k(ə-)lē\ *adv*

tran·sient \'tran-zē-ənt, 'tranch-ənt\ *adj* : passing away in time : existing temporarily ⟨~ symptoms⟩

transient global amnesia *n* : temporary amnesia of short duration (as several hours) that is marked by sudden onset, by loss of past memories, and by an inability to form new memories, and that is believed to result from a transient

ischemic attack affecting the posteromedial thalamus or hippocampus on both sides of the brain

transient ischemic attack *n* : a brief episode of cerebral ischemia that is usu. characterized by temporary blurring of vision, slurring of speech, numbness, paralysis, or syncope and that is often predictive of a serious stroke — abbr. *TIA;* called also *mini-stroke*

trans·il·lu·mi·nate \ˌtran(t)s-ə-'lü-mə-ˌnāt, ˌtranz-\ *vt* **-nat·ed; -nat·ing** : to cause light to pass through; *esp* : to pass light through (a body part) for medical examination

trans·il·lu·mi·na·tion \-ə-ˌlü-mə-'nā-shən\ *n* : the act, process, or an instance of transilluminating

tran·sis·tor \tranz-'is-tər, tran(t)s-\ *n* : a solid-state electronic device that is used to control the flow of electricity in electronic equipment and consists of a small block of a semiconductor (as germanium) with at least three electrodes

tran·si·tion \tran(t)s-'ish-ən, tranz-, *chiefly Brit* tran(t)s-'izh-\ *n* **1** : passage from one state or stage to another; *esp* : an abrupt change in energy state or level (as of an atomic nucleus or a molecule) usu. accompanied by loss or gain of a single quantum of energy **2** : a genetic mutation in RNA or DNA that results from the substitution of one purine base for the other or of one pyrimidine base for the other

tran·si·tion·al \-'ish-nəl, -'izh-ən-ᵊl\ *adj* **1** : of, relating to, or characterized by transition **2** : of, relating to, or being epithelium (as in the urinary bladder) that consists of several layers of soft cuboidal cells which become flattened when stretched (as when the bladder is distended)

trans·ke·tol·ase \ˌtran(t)s-'kēt-ȯl-ˌās, -ˌāz\ *n* : an enzyme that catalyzes the transfer of the ketonic residue $HOCH_2CO-$ from the phosphate of xylulose to that of ribose to form the phosphate of sedoheptulose

trans·late \tran(t)s-'lāt, tranz-\ *vt* **trans·lat·ed; trans·lat·ing** : to subject (as genetic information) to translation in protein synthesis

trans·la·tion \tran(t)s-'lā-shən, tranz-\ *n* : the process of forming a protein molecule at a ribosomal site of protein synthesis from information contained in messenger RNA — compare TRANSCRIPTION — **trans·la·tion·al** \-shnəl, -shən-ᵊl\ *adj*

trans·la·to·ry \'tran(t)s-lə-ˌtōr-ē, 'tranz-, -ˌtȯr-; tran(t)s-'lāt-ə-rē, tranz-\ *adj* : of, relating to, involving, or being uniform motion in one direction ⟨receptor organs for rotatory and ~ motion in the inner ear —*Scientific American*⟩

trans·lo·ca·tion \ˌtran(t)s-lō-'kā-shən, ˌtranz-\ *n* **1** : transfer of part of a chromosome to a different position esp. on a nonhomologous chromosome; *esp* : the exchange of parts between nonhomologous chromosomes **2** : a chromosome or part of a chromosome that has undergone translocation — **trans·lo·cate** \-'lō-ˌkāt\ *vb* **-cat·ed; -cat·ing**

trans·lu·cence \tran(t)s-'lüs-ᵊn(t)s, tranz-\ *n* : the quality or state of being translucent

trans·lu·cen·cy \-ᵊn-sē\ *n, pl* **-cies** : TRANSLUCENCE

trans·lu·cent \-ᵊnt\ *adj* : permitting the passage of light; *esp* : transmitting and diffusing light so that objects beyond cannot be seen clearly

trans·lum·bar \ˌtran(t)s-'ləm-bər, ˌtranz-, -'ləm-ˌbär\ *adj* : passing through or performed by way of the lumbar region; *specif* : involving the injection of a radiopaque medium through the lumbar region ⟨~ aortography⟩

trans·lu·mi·nal \-'lü-mə-nəl\ *adj* : passing across or performed by way of a lumen; *specif* : involving the passage of an inflatable catheter along the lumen of a blood vessel ⟨~ angioplasty⟩

trans·mem·brane \(ˈ)tran(t)s-'mem-ˌbrān, (ˈ)tranz-\ *adj* : taking place, existing, or arranged from one side to the other of a membrane ⟨a ~ potential⟩ ⟨~ proteins⟩

trans·meth·yl·a·tion \-ˌmeth-ə-'lā-shən\ *n* : a chemical reaction in which a methyl group is transferred from one compound to another

trans·mis·si·ble \tran(t)s-'mis-ə-bəl, tranz-\ *adj* : capable of being transmitted (as from one person to another) ⟨~ diseases⟩ — **trans·mis·si·bil·i·ty** \(ˌ)tran(t)s-ˌmis-ə-'bil-ət-ē, (ˌ)tranz-\ *n, pl* **-ties**

transmissible mink encephalopathy \-'miŋk-\ *n* : a transmissible spongiform encephalopathy of mink that resembles scrapie and that has been transmitted experimentally to mink by injecting or feeding them with infected tissue from sheep

transmissible spongiform encephalopathy *n* : any of a group of spongiform encephalopathies (as Creutzfeldt-Jakob disease, kuru, and scrapie) that are now usu. considered to be caused and transmitted by prions

trans·mis·sion \tran(t)s-'mish-ən, tranz-\ *n* : an act, process, or instance of transmitting ⟨~ of HIV⟩ ⟨synaptic ~⟩

transmission deafness *n* : CONDUCTION DEAFNESS

transmission electron microscope *n* : a conventional electron microscope which produces an image of a cross-sectional slice of a specimen all points of which are illuminated by the electron beam at the same time — compare SCANNING ELECTRON MICROSCOPE — **transmission electron microscopy** *n*

trans·mit \tran(t)s-'mit, tranz-\ *vt* **trans·mit·ted; trans·mit·ting** : to pass, transfer, or convey from one person or place to another: as **a** : to pass or convey by heredity ⟨~ a genetic abnormality⟩ **b** : to convey (infection) abroad or to another ⟨mosquitoes ~ malaria⟩ **c** : to cause (energy) to be conveyed through space or a medium ⟨substances that ~ nerve impulses⟩

trans·mit·ta·ble \-'mit-ə-bəl\ *adj* : TRANSMISSIBLE

trans·mit·tance \-'mit-ᵊn(t)s\ *n* **1** : TRANSMISSION **2** : the fraction of radiant energy that having entered a layer of absorbing matter reaches its farther boundary

trans·mit·ter \-'mit-ər\ *n* : one that transmits; *specif* : NEUROTRANSMITTER

trans·mu·ral \tran(t)s-'myur-əl, tranz-\ *adj* : passing or administered through an anatomical wall ⟨~ stimulation of the ileum⟩; *also* : involving the whole thickness of a wall ⟨~ myocardial infarction⟩ — **trans·mu·ral·ly** \-ē\ *adv*

trans·mu·ta·tion \tran(t)s-myü-'tā-shən, tranz-\ *n* : an act or instance of changing: as **a** : the evolutionary change of one species into another **b** : the conversion of one element or nuclide into another either naturally or artificially

trans·neu·ro·nal \tran(t)s-n(y)ù-'rōn-ᵊl, tranz-, -'n(y)ùr-ən-ᵊl\ *adj* : TRANSSYNAPTIC ⟨~ cell atrophy⟩

trans·or·bit·al \-'ór-bət-ᵊl\ *adj* : passing through or performed by way of the eye socket

trans·ovar·i·al \-ō-'var-ē-əl, -'ver-\ *adj* : relating to or being transmission of a pathogen from an organism (as a tick) to its offspring by infection of eggs in its ovary — **trans·ovar·i·al·ly** \-ē\ *adv*

trans·ovar·i·an \-ē-ən\ *adj* : TRANSOVARIAL — **trans·ovar·i·an·ly** *adv*

trans·par·en·cy \tran(t)s-'par-ən-sē\ *n, pl* **-cies** : the quality or state of being transparent

trans·par·ent \-ənt\ *adj* **1** : having the property of transmitting light without appreciable scattering so that bodies lying beyond are seen clearly **2** : allowing the passage of a specified form of radiation (as X-rays or ultraviolet light)

trans·pep·ti·dase \-'pep-tə-ˌdās, -ˌdāz\ *n* : an enzyme that catalyzes the transfer of an amino acid residue or a peptide residue from one amino compound to another

trans·pep·ti·da·tion \-ˌpep-tə-'dā-shən\ *n* : a chemical reaction (as the reversible conversion of one peptide to another by a protease) in which an amino acid residue or a peptide residue is transferred from one amino compound to another

trans·peri·to·ne·al \-ˌper-ət-ᵊn-'ē-əl\ *adj* : passing or performed through the peritoneum

trans·per·son·al \-'pərs-nəl, -ᵊn-əl\ *adj* : of, relating to, or being psychology or psychotherapy concerned esp. with esoteric mental experience (as mysticism and altered states of consciousness) beyond the usual limits of ego and personality

trans·phos·phor·y·lase \-fäs-'fór-ə-ˌlās, -ˌlāz\ *n* : any of a group of enzymes that promote transphosphorylation processes

trans·phos·phor·y·la·tion \-ˌfäs-ˌfór-ə-'lā-shən\ *n* : phos-

phorylation in which an organic phosphate group is transferred from one molecule to another

tran·spi·ra·tion \tran(t)s-pə-'rā-shən\ *n* : the passage of water vapor from a living body through a membrane or pores — **tran·spi·ra·tion·al** \-shnəl, -shən-ᵊl\ *adj*

trans·pla·cen·tal \tran(t)s-plə-'sent-ᵊl\ *adj* : relating to, involving, or being passage (as of an antibody) between mother and fetus through the placenta ⟨~ immunization⟩ — **trans·pla·cen·tal·ly** \-ᵊl-ē\ *adv*

¹trans·plant \tran(t)s-'plant\ *vt* : to transfer from one place to another; *esp* : to transfer (an organ or tissue) from one part or individual to another

²trans·plant \'tran(t)s-ˌplant\ *n* **1** : something (as an organ or part) that is transplanted **2** : the act or process of transplanting : TRANSPLANTATION ⟨performed a kidney ~⟩

trans·plant·able \-'plant-ə-bəl\ *adj* : capable of being transplanted ⟨~ tumors⟩ — **trans·plant·abil·i·ty** \-ˌplant-ə-'bil-ət-ē\ *n, pl* **-ties**

trans·plan·ta·tion \ˌtran(t)s-ˌplan-'tā-shən\ *n* : an act, process, or instance of transplanting; *esp* : the removal of tissue from one part of the body or from one individual and its implantation or insertion in another esp. by surgery ⟨corneal ~⟩ ⟨the ~ of lung tissue⟩

trans·pleu·ral \-'plùr-əl\ *adj* : passing through or requiring passage through the pleura ⟨a ~ surgical procedure⟩

¹trans·port \tran(t)s-'pō(ə)rt, -'pó(ə)rt, 'tran(t)s-ˌ\ *vt* : to transfer or convey from one place to another ⟨mechanisms of ~ing ions across a living membrane⟩

²trans·port \'tran(t)s-ˌpō(ə)rt, -ˌpó(ə)rt\ *n* : an act or process of transporting; *specif* : ACTIVE TRANSPORT

transposable element *n* : a segment of genetic material that is capable of changing its location in the genome or that in some bacteria is capable of undergoing transfer between an extrachromosomal plasmid and a chromosome — called also *transposable genetic element*

trans·pos·ase \ˌtran(t)s-'pō-ˌzās\ *n* : an enzyme that catalyzes the transposition of a transposon

trans·pose \tran(t)s-'pōz\ *vb* **trans·posed; trans·pos·ing** *vt* : to transfer from one place or period to another; *specif* : to subject to genetic transposition ~ *vi* : to undergo genetic transposition — **trans·pos·able** \-'pō-zə-bəl\ *adj*

trans·po·si·tion \ˌtran(t)s-pə-'zish-ən\ *n* : an act, process, or instance of transposing or being transposed: as **a** : the displacement of a viscus to a side opposite from that which it normally occupies ⟨~ of the heart⟩ **b** : the transfer of a segment of DNA from one site to another in the genome either between chromosomal sites or between an extrachromosomal site (as on a plasmid) and a chromosome — **trans·po·si·tion·al** \-'zish-nəl\ *adj*

trans·po·son \ˌtran(t)s-'pō-ˌzän\ *n* : a transposable element esp. when it contains genetic material controlling functions other than those related to its relocation

trans·py·lor·ic \-pī-'lór-ik\ *adj* : relating to or being the transverse plane or the line marking its intersection with the surface of the abdomen that passes below the rib cage cutting the pylorus of the stomach and the first lumbar vertebra and that is one of the four planes marking off the nine abdominal regions

trans·rec·tal \-'rek-tᵊl\ *adj* : passing through or performed by way of the rectum ⟨~ prostatic biopsy⟩

trans·sep·tal \-'sep-tᵊl\ *adj* : passing through a septum

trans·sex·u·al *also* **tran·sex·u·al** \(')tran(t)s-'sek-sh(ə)-wəl, -'sek-shəl\ *n* : a person who psychologically identifies with the opposite sex and may seek to live as a member of this sex esp. by undergoing surgery and hormone therapy to obtain the necessary physical appearance (as by changing the external sex organs) — **transsexual** *also* **transexual** *adj* — **trans·sex·u·al·ism** *also* **tran·sex·u·al·ism** \-wə-ˌliz-əm, -shə-ˌliz-\ *n*

\ə\ **abut** \ᵊ\ **kitten** \ər\ **further** \a\ **ash** \ā\ **ace** \ä\ **cot, cart**
\aù\ **out** \ch\ **chin** \e\ **bet** \ē\ **easy** \g\ **go** \i\ **hit** \ī\ **ice** \j\ **job**
\ŋ\ **sing** \ō\ **go** \ó\ **law** \ói\ **boy** \th\ **thin** \th\ **the** \ü\ **loot**
\ù\ **foot** \y\ **yet** \zh\ **vision** *See also* Pronunciation Symbols page

S
T

— **trans·sex·u·al·i·ty** *also* **tran·sex·u·al·i·ty** \-ˌsek-shə-ˈwal-ət-ē\ *n, pl* **-ties**

trans·sphe·noi·dal \-sfi-ˈnȯid-ᵊl\ *adj* : performed by entry through the sphenoid bone ⟨~ hypophysectomy⟩

trans·syn·ap·tic \-sə-ˈnap-tik\ *adj* : occurring or taking place across nerve synapses ⟨~ degeneration⟩

trans·tho·rac·ic \-thə-ˈras-ik\ *adj* **1** : performed or made by way of the thoracic cavity **2** : crossing or having connections that cross the thoracic cavity ⟨a ~ pacemaker⟩ — **trans·tho·rac·i·cal·ly** \-i-k(ə-)lē\ *adv*

trans·thy·re·tin \-ˈthī-rət-ən\ *n* : a protein component of blood serum that functions esp. in the transport of thyroxine — called also *prealbumin*

trans·tib·i·al \tran(t)s-ˈtib-ē-əl\ *adj* **1** : occurring across or involving the tibia ⟨~ amputation⟩ **2** : having undergone transtibial amputation ⟨~ amputees⟩; *also* : suitable for use following transtibial amputation ⟨a ~ prosthesis⟩

trans·tra·che·al \-ˈtrā-kē-əl\ *adj* : passing through or administered by way of the trachea ⟨~ anesthesia⟩

tran·su·date \ˌtran(t)s-ˈ(y)üd-ət, ˌtranz-, -ˌāt; ˈtran(t)s-(y)ù-ˌdāt, ˈtranz-\ *n* : a transuded substance

tran·su·da·tion \ˌtran(t)s-(y)ü-ˈdā-shən, ˌtranz-\ *n* **1** : the act or process of transuding or being transuded **2** : TRANSUDATE

tran·su·da·tive \tran(t)s-ˈ(y)üd-ət-iv, tranz-\ *adj* : of, relating to, or constituting transudation or a transudate ⟨a ~ synovial fluid⟩

tran·sude \tran(t)s-ˈ(y)üd, tranz-\ *vb* **tran·sud·ed; tran·sud·ing** *vi* : to pass through a membrane or permeable substance ~ *vt* : to permit passage of

trans·ure·tero·ure·ter·os·to·my \ˌtran(t)s-yù-ˌrēt-ə-ˌrō-yù-ˌrēt-ə-ˈräs-tə-mē, ˌtranz-\ *n, pl* **-mies** : anastomosis of a ureter to the contralateral ureter

trans·ure·thral \-yù-ˈrē-thrəl\ *adj* : passing through or performed by way of the urethra ⟨~ prostatectomy⟩

trans·vag·i·nal \-ˈvaj-ən-ᵊl\ *adj* : passing through or performed by way of the vagina ⟨~ laparoscopy⟩

trans·ve·nous \-ˈvē-nəs\ *adj* : relating to or involving the use of an intravenous catheter containing an electrode carrying electrical impulses from an extracorporeal source to the heart ⟨~ pacing of the heart⟩

trans·ven·tric·u·lar \-ven-ˈtrik-yə-lər, -vən-\ *adj* : passing through or performed by way of a ventricle ⟨a ~ valvulotomy⟩

transversalis — see PLICA TRANSVERSALIS RECTI

trans·ver·sa·lis cer·vi·cis \ˌtran(t)s-vər-ˈsā-ləs-ˈsər-və-səs\ *n* : LONGISSIMUS CERVICIS

transversalis fascia *n* : the whole deep layer of fascia lining the abdominal wall; *also* : the part of this covering the inner surface of the transversus abdominis and separating it from the peritoneum

trans·verse \tran(t)s-ˈvərs, tranz-, ˈtran(t)s-ˌ, ˈtranz-ˌ\ *adj* **1** : acting, lying, or being across : set crosswise **2** : made at right angles to the long axis of the body ⟨a ~ section⟩ — **trans·verse·ly** *adv*

transverse carpal ligament *n* : FLEXOR RETINACULUM 2

transverse cervical artery *n* : an inconstant branch of the thyrocervical trunk or of the subclavian artery that when present supplies or divides into branches supplying the region at the base of the neck and the muscles of the scapula

transverse colon *n* : the part of the large intestine that extends across the abdominal cavity joining the ascending colon to the descending colon

transverse crural ligament *n* : EXTENSOR RETINACULUM 1b

transverse facial artery *n* : a large branch of the superficial temporal artery that arises in the parotid gland and supplies or gives off branches supplying the parotid gland, masseter muscle, and adjacent parts

transverse fissure *n* : PORTA HEPATIS

transverse foramen *n* : a foramen in each transverse process of a cervical vertebra through which the vertebral artery and vertebral vein pass in each cervical vertebra except the seventh

transverse ligament *n* : any of various ligaments situated transversely with respect to a bodily axis or part: as **a** : the transverse part of the cruciate ligament of the atlas **b** : one in the anterior part of the knee connecting the anterior margins of the lateral and medial menisci

transverse process *n* : a process that projects on the dorsolateral aspect of each side of the neural arch of a vertebra

transverse sinus *n* : either of two large venous sinuses of the cranium that begin at the bony protuberance on the middle of the inner surface of the occipital bone at the intersection of its bony ridges and that terminate at the jugular foramen on either side to become the internal jugular vein — called also *lateral sinus*

transverse thoracic muscle *n* : TRANSVERSUS THORACIS

transverse tubule *n* : T TUBULE

trans·ver·sion \tran(t)s-ˈvər-zhən, tranz-\ *n* **1** : the eruption of a tooth in an abnormal position on the jaw **2** : a genetic mutation in RNA or DNA that results from the substitution of a purine base for a pyrimidine base or of a pyrimidine base for a purine base

transversum — see SEPTUM TRANSVERSUM

trans·ver·sus ab·dom·i·nis \tran(t)s-ˈvər-səs-əb-ˈdäm-ə-nəs\ *n* : a flat muscle with transverse fibers that forms the innermost layer of the anterolateral wall of the abdomen and ends in a broad aponeurosis which joins that of the opposite side at the linea alba with its upper three fourths passing behind the rectus abdominis muscle and the lower fourth in front of it and that acts to constrict the abdominal viscera and assist in expulsion of the contents of various abdominal organs (as in defecation, vomiting, and parturition)

transversus pe·rin·ei su·per·fi·ci·a·lis \-pe-ˈrin-ē-ˌī-ˌsü-pər-ˌfish-ē-ˈā-ləs\ *n* : a small band of muscle of the urogenital region of the perineum that arises from the ischial tuberosity and that with the contralateral muscle inserts into and acts to stabilize the mass of tissue in the midline between the anus and the penis or vagina — called also *superficial transverse perineal muscle*

transversus tho·ra·cis \-thə-ˈrā-səs\ *n* : a thin flat sheet of muscle and tendon fibers of the anterior wall of the chest that arises esp. from the xiphoid process and lower third of the sternum, inserts into the costal cartilages of the second to sixth ribs, and acts to draw the ribs downward — called also *transverse thoracic muscle*

trans·ves·i·cal \tran(t)s-ˈves-i-kəl, tranz-\ *adj* : passing through or performed by way of the urinary bladder

trans·ves·tism \tran(t)s-ˈves-ˌtiz-əm, tranz-\ *also* **trans·ves·tit·ism** \-ˈves-ˌtit-ˌiz-əm\ *n* : adoption of the dress and often the behavior of the opposite sex — called also *eonism*

trans·ves·tite \tran(t)s-ˈves-ˌtīt, tranz-\ *n* : a person and esp. a male who adopts the dress and often the behavior typical of the opposite sex esp. for purposes of emotional or sexual gratification — **transvestite** *adj*

Tran·xene \ˈtran-ˌzēn\ *trademark* — used for a preparation of clorazepate

tran·yl·cy·pro·mine \ˌtran-ᵊl-ˈsī-prə-ˌmēn\ *n* : an antidepressant drug that is an inhibitor of monoamine oxidase and is administered in the form of its sulfate $(C_9H_{11}N)_2 \cdot H_2SO_4$

tra·pe·zi·um \trə-ˈpē-zē-əm, tra-\ *n, pl* **-zi·ums** *or* **-zia** \-zē-ə\ : a bone in the distal row of the carpus at the base of the thumb — called also *greater multangular*

tra·pe·zi·us \trə-ˈpē-zē-əs, tra-\ *n, pl* **-zii** \-zē-ˌī\ *also* **-zi·us·es** : a large flat triangular superficial muscle of each side of the upper back that arises from the occipital bone, the ligamentum nuchae, and the spinous processes of the last cervical and all the thoracic vertebrae, is inserted into the outer part of the clavicle, the acromion, and the spine of the scapula, and serves chiefly to rotate the scapula so as to present the glenoid cavity upward

trap·e·zoid \ˈtrap-ə-ˌzȯid\ *n* : a bone in the distal row of the carpus at the base of the index finger — called also *lesser multangular, trapezoid bone, trapezoideum*

trapezoid body *n* : a bundle of transverse fibers in the dorsal part of the pons

trapezoid bone *n* : TRAPEZOID

trap·e·zoi·de·um \,trap-ə-'zȯid-ē-əm\ *n* : TRAPEZOID

tras·en·tine \'tras-ən-,tēn\ *n, often cap* : a preparation of the hydrochloride of adiphenine — formerly a U.S. registered trademark

tras·tu·zu·mab \,tras-'tü-zü-,mab\ *n* : a genetically engineered monoclonal antibody that is administered by injection to slow or inhibit tumor growth in some advanced breast cancers by blocking a cell membrane receptor which receives signals promoting cancer cell growth — see HERCEPTIN

Tras·y·lol \'tras-ə-,lȯl\ *trademark* — used for a preparation of aprotinin

trau·ma \'trȯ-mə, 'traȯ-\ *n, pl* **traumas** *also* **trau·ma·ta** \-mət-ə\ **1 a** : an injury (as a wound) to living tissue caused by an extrinsic agent ⟨surgical ∼⟩ ⟨the intra-abdominal organs at greatest risk to athletic ∼ are the spleen, pancreas, and kidney —M. R. Eichelberger⟩ — see BLUNT TRAUMA **b** : a disordered psychic or behavioral state resulting from mental or emotional stress or physical injury **2** : an agent, force, or mechanism that causes trauma

trauma center *n* : a hospital unit specializing in the treatment of patients with acute and esp. life-threatening traumatic injuries

trau·mat·ic \trə-'mat-ik, trȯ-, traȯ-\ *adj* : of, relating to, resulting from, or causing a trauma ⟨cases of ∼ rupture —*Jour. Amer. Med. Assoc.*⟩ ⟨a ∼ experience⟩ — **trau·mat·i·cal·ly** \-i-k(ə-)lē\ *adv*

trau·ma·tism \'trȯ-mə-,tiz-əm, 'traȯ-\ *n* : the development or occurrence of trauma ⟨periodontal ∼⟩; *also* : TRAUMA

trau·ma·tize *also Brit* **trau·ma·tise** \-,tīz\ *vt* **-tized** *also Brit* **-tised; -tiz·ing** *also Brit* **-tis·ing** : to inflict a trauma upon ⟨*traumatized* tissues⟩ — **trau·ma·ti·za·tion** *also Brit* **trau·ma·ti·sa·tion** \,trȯ-mət-ə-'zā-shən, ,traȯ-\ *n*

trau·ma·tol·o·gist \,trȯ-mə-'täl-ə-jəst, ,traȯ-\ *n* : a surgeon who practices traumatology or who is on duty at a trauma center

trau·ma·tol·o·gy \-jē\ *n, pl* **-gies** : the surgical treatment of wounds ⟨pediatric ∼⟩

trau·ma·to·pho·bia \,trȯ-mət-ə-'fō-bē-ə, ,traȯ-\ *n* : excessive or disabling fear of war or physical injury usu. resulting from experiences in combat

tra·vail \trə-'vā(ə)l, 'trav-,āl\ *n* : LABOR, PARTURITION

trav·el·er's diarrhea \'trav-(ə-)lərz-\ *n* : intestinal sickness and diarrhea affecting a traveler and typically caused by ingestion of pathogenic microorganisms (as some E. coli) — compare MONTEZUMA'S REVENGE

trav·el sickness \'trav-əl-\ *n* : MOTION SICKNESS

tray \'trā\ *n* : an appliance consisting of a flanged body and a handle for use in holding plastic material against the gums or teeth in making negative impressions for dentures

traz·o·done \'traz-ə-,dōn\ *n* : an antidepressant drug that is administered in the form of its hydrochloride $C_{19}H_{22}ClN_5O\cdot HCl$ and inhibits the uptake of serotonin by the brain

Trea·cher Col·lins syndrome \'trē-chər-'käl-ənz-\ *n* : MANDIBULOFACIAL DYSOSTOSIS

Collins, Edward Treacher (1862–1932), British ophthalmologist. Collins was on the staff of the Royal London Ophthalmic Hospital and a visiting ophthalmic surgeon to several schools of ophthalmology. He published works on the anatomy and pathology of the eye (1896), on the bacteriology and pathology of the eye (1911), and on the evolution of the eye (1922).

trea·cle \'trē-kəl\ *n* : a medicinal compound formerly in wide use as a remedy against poison

tread·mill \'tred-,mil\ *n* : a device having an endless belt on which an individual walks or runs in place that is used for exercise and in tests of physiological functions — see STRESS TEST

treat \'trēt\ *vt* : to care for or deal with medically or surgically : deal with by medical or surgical means ⟨∼*ed* their diseases⟩ ⟨∼*s* a patient⟩

treat·able \'trēt-ə-bəl\ *adj* : capable of being treated : yielding or responsive to treatment ⟨a ∼ disease⟩ — **treat·abil·i·ty** \,trēt-ə-'bil-ət-ē\ *n, pl* **-ties**

treat·ment \'trēt-mənt\ *n* **1** : the action or manner of treating a patient medically or surgically ⟨∼ of tuberculosis⟩ **2** : an instance of treating ⟨the cure required many ∼*s*⟩

tree \'trē\ *n* : an anatomical system or structure having many branches ⟨the vascular ∼⟩ — see BILIARY TREE, BRONCHIAL TREE, TRACHEOBRONCHIAL TREE

tree of heav·en \-'hev-ən\ *n* : an Asian tree of the genus *Ailanthus* (*A. glandulosa*) widely grown as a shade and ornamental tree and having bark that has been used as a tonic, purgative, and anthelmintic

tre·ha·lase \tri-'häl-,ās, -,āz\ *n* : an enzyme that accelerates the hydrolysis of trehalose and is found in yeasts and molds

tre·ha·lose \-'häl-,ōs, -,ōz\ *n* : a crystalline disaccharide $C_{12}H_{22}O_{11}$ stored instead of starch by many fungi and found in the blood of many insects

Trem·a·to·da \,trem-ə-'tōd-ə\ *n pl* : a class of the phylum Platyhelminthes including the flukes and related parasitic flatworms that usu. have no cellular epidermis or cilia but have a chitinous cuticle covering the body, suckers for adhesion, and a well-developed alimentary canal — **trem·a·to·dan** \-'tōd-ᵊn\ *or* **trem·a·to·de·an** \-'tōd-ē-ən\ *adj*

trem·a·tode \'trem-ə-,tōd\ *n* : any parasitic flatworm (as a liver fluke) of the class Trematoda — **trematode** *adj*

trem·bles \'trem-bəlz\ *n pl but sing in constr* : severe poisoning of livestock and esp. cattle by a toxic alcohol present in a snakeroot (*Eupatorium rugosum*) and several rayless goldenrods (esp. *Haplopappus heterophyllus*) that is characterized by muscular tremors, weakness, and constipation

tremens — see DELIRIUM TREMENS

trem·e·tol \'trem-ə-,tȯl, -,tōl\ *n* : an unsaturated alcohol obtained as an oil of aromatic odor from a snakeroot (*Eupatorium rugosum*) and several rayless goldenrods (esp. *Haplopappus heterophyllus*) that causes trembles in animals and milk sickness in humans

trem·or \'trem-ər\ *n* : a trembling or shaking usu. from physical weakness, emotional stress, or disease ⟨∼*s* of the hands⟩

trem·or·ine \'trem-ə-,rēn\ *n* : a compound $C_{12}H_{20}N_2$ from which oxotremorine is derived and which has effects and uses like those of oxotremorine

trem·oro·gen·ic \,trem-ər-ə-'jen-ik\ *adj* : inducing tremors

trem·u·lous \'trem-yə-ləs\ *adj* : characterized by or affected with trembling or tremors — **trem·u·lous·ness** *n*

trench fever \'trench-\ *n* : a disease that is usu. marked by fever and pain in muscles, bones, and joints and that is caused by a bacterium (*Bartonella quintana* syn. *Rochalimaea quintana*) transmitted by the human body louse (*Pediculus humanus humanus*)

trench foot *n* : a painful foot disorder resembling frostbite and resulting from exposure to cold and wet

trench mouth *n* : ACUTE NECROTIZING ULCERATIVE GINGIVITIS; *also* : VINCENT'S ANGINA

Tren·de·len·burg position \'tren-dᵊl-ən-,bərg-\ *n* : a position of the body for medical examination or operation in which the patient is placed head down on a table inclined at about 45 degrees from the floor with the knees uppermost and the legs hanging over the end of the table

Tren·de·len·burg \'tren-də-lən-,bu̇rk\, **Friedrich (1844–1924),** German surgeon. A professor of surgery, Trendelenburg was the author of numerous articles. It was in an 1890 paper on vesicovaginal fistula that he presented the advantages of an elevated pelvic position for operations within the abdominal cavity.

Tren·tal \'tren-,tal\ *trademark* — used for a preparation of pentoxifylline

trep·a·na·tion \,trep-ə-'nā-shən\ *n* **1** : TREPHINATION **2** : a hole in the skull produced surgically

\ə\ **abut** \ᵊ\ **kitten** \ər\ **further** \a\ **ash** \ā\ **ace** \ä\ **cot, cart** \au̇\ **out** \ch\ **chin** \e\ **bet** \ē\ **easy** \g\ **go** \i\ **hit** \ī\ **ice** \j\ **job** \ŋ\ **sing** \ō\ **go** \ȯ\ **law** \ȯi\ **boy** \th\ **thin** \th\ **the** \ü\ **loot** \u̇\ **foot** \y\ **yet** \zh\ **vision** *See also* Pronunciation Symbols page

S

T

treph·i·na·tion \ˌtref-ə-'nā-shən\ n : an act or instance of using a trephine (as to perforate the skull)

¹**tre·phine** \'trē-ˌfīn\ n : a surgical instrument for cutting out circular sections (as of bone or corneal tissue)

²**tre·phine** \'trē-ˌfīn, tri-'\ vt **tre·phined; tre·phin·ing** : to operate on with or extract by means of a trephine

trep·o·ne·ma \ˌtrep-ə-'nē-mə\ n **1** cap : a genus of the family Spirochaetaceae comprising anaerobic spirochetes that are pathogenic in humans and other warm-blooded animals and include one (*T. pallidum*) causing syphilis and another (*T. pertenue*) causing yaws **2** pl **-ma·ta** \-mət-ə\ or **-mas** : any spirochete of the genus *Treponema*

trep·o·ne·mal \-'nē-məl\ adj : of, relating to, or caused by spirochetes of the genus *Treponema* ⟨a ∼ disease⟩

Treponema pal·li·dum immobilization test \-'pal-əd-əm-\ n : a serological test for syphilis in which a solution containing the living causative spirochete (*Treponema pallidum*) is combined with serum in the presence of complement with immobilization of the active spirochetes indicating a positive result — abbr. *TPI*

Trep·o·ne·ma·ta·ce·ae \ˌtrep-ə-ˌnē-mə-'tā-sē-ˌē\ n pl, in former classifications : a family of the order Spirochaetales comprising small variable spirochetes without obvious structural differentiation and including a number of important pathogens

trepo·ne·ma·to·sis \-ˌnē-mə-'tō-səs, -ˌnem-ə-\ n, pl **-to·ses** \-ˌsēz\ : infection with or disease caused by spirochetes of the genus *Treponema*

trepo·neme \'trep-ə-ˌnēm\ n : TREPONEMA 2

trep·o·ne·mi·ci·dal \ˌtrep-ə-ˌnē-mə-'sīd-ᵊl\ adj : destroying spirochetes of the genus *Treponema*

trep·pe \'trep-ə\ n : the graduated series of increasingly vigorous contractions that results when a corresponding series of identical stimuli is applied to a rested muscle — called also *staircase effect, staircase phenomenon*

tre·tin·o·in \trə-'tin-ə-wən\ n : the all-trans isomer of retinoic acid that is applied topically to the skin to treat acne vulgaris and to reduce facial wrinkles, roughness, and pigmented spots and that is administered orally to induce remission of acute myelogenous leukemia in which more than half the cells are malignant promyelocytes — called also *all-trans-retinoic acid, retinoic acid, vitamin A acid*; see ISOTRETINOIN, RETIN-A

TRF abbr thyrotropin-releasing factor

TRH abbr thyrotropin-releasing hormone

tri·ac·e·tate \(ˈ)trī-'as-ə-ˌtāt\ n : an acetate containing three CH₃COO groups

tri·ac·e·tin \(ˈ)trī-'as-ət-ən\ n : ACETIN c

tri·ac·e·tyl·ole·an·do·my·cin \(ˌ)trī-ˌas-ət-ᵊl-ˌō-lē-ˌan-dō-'mīs-ᵊn\ n : TROLEANDOMYCIN

tri·ad \'trī-ˌad also -əd\ n **1** : a union or group of three ⟨a ∼ of symptoms⟩ **2** : a trivalent element, atom, or radical — **tri·ad·ic** \trī-'ad-ik\ adj

tri·age \trē-'äzh, 'trē-ˌ\ n **1** : the sorting of and allocation of treatment to patients and esp. battle and disaster victims according to a system of priorities designed to maximize the number of survivors **2** : the sorting of patients (as in an emergency room) according to the urgency of their need for care — **triage** vt

tri·al \'trī-(ə)l\ n **1** : a tryout or experiment to test quality, value, or usefulness — see CLINICAL TRIAL **2** : one of a number of repetitions of an experiment

tri·am·cin·o·lone \ˌtrī-am-'sin-ᵊl-ˌōn\ n : a glucocorticoid drug C₂₁H₂₇FO₆ that is administered esp. in the form of its acetal and acetate derivatives for its anti-inflammatory and immunosuppressant effects and that is used chiefly in the treatment of skin disorders, asthma, and allergic rhinitis — see AZMACORT, KENACORT, NASACORT

tri·am·ter·ene \trī-'am-tər-ˌēn\ n : a diuretic drug C₁₂H₁₁N₇ that promotes potassium retention — see DYAZIDE

tri·an·gle \'trī-ˌaŋ-gəl\ n : a three-sided region or space and esp. an anatomical one — see ANTERIOR TRIANGLE, POSTERIOR TRIANGLE, SCARPA'S TRIANGLE, SUBOCCIPITAL TRIANGLE, SUPERIOR CAROTID TRIANGLE

triangle of Hes·sel·bach \-'hes-əl-ˌbäk\ n : an area of the abdominal wall bounded laterally by the inferior epigastric artery, medially by the margin of the rectus muscle, and below by the inguinal ligament — called also *Hesselbach's triangle*

Hes·sel·bach \'hes-əl-ˌbäk\, **Franz Kaspar (1759–1816)**, German surgeon and anatomist. Hesselbach served as professor of anatomy and surgery at Würzburg, Germany. In 1806 he published an anatomical-surgical treatise on the origin of hernias which included a description of the triangle of Hesselbach.

tri·an·gu·lar \trī-'aŋ-gyə-lər\ n : TRIQUETRAL BONE

triangular bone n : TRIQUETRAL BONE

triangular fossa n : a shallow depression in the anterior part of the top of the ear's auricle between the two crura into which the antihelix divides

tri·an·gu·la·ris \trī-ˌaŋ-gyə-'lar-əs\ n, pl **-la·res** \-'lar-ˌēz\ **1** : a flat triangular muscle that extends from the base of the mandible to the angle formed by the joining of the upper and lower lips and that acts to depress this angle **2** : TRIQUETRAL BONE

triangular ridge n : a triangular surface that slopes downward from the tip of a cusp of a molar or premolar toward the center of its occlusal surface

tri·at·o·ma \trī-'at-ə-mə\ n **1** cap : a genus of large blood-sucking bugs that are usu. placed in the family Reduviidae but sometimes assigned to a separate family and that feed on mammals and sometimes transmit Chagas' disease to their hosts — see CONENOSE **2** : any bug of the genus *Triatoma*

tri·atom·ic \ˌtrī-ə-'täm-ik\ adj : having three atoms in the molecule ⟨ozone is ∼ oxygen⟩

¹**tri·at·o·mid** \trī-'at-ə-mid\ adj : belonging to the genus *Triatoma*

²**triatomid** n : a triatomid bug : TRIATOMA 2

tri·az·i·quone \trī-'az-ə-ˌkwōn\ n : an antineoplastic drug C₁₂H₁₃N₃O₂

tri·azo·lam \trī-'ā-zə-ˌlam\ n : a benzodiazepine C₁₇H₁₂Cl₂N₄ used as a sleep-inducing agent in the short-term treatment of insomnia — see HALCION

tri·azole \'trī-ə-ˌzōl\ n : any of a group of compounds that are characterized by a ring composed of two carbon atoms and three nitrogen atoms and that include a number of antifungal agents (as fluconazole)

trib·ade \'trib-əd, tri-'bäd\ n : a woman who practices tribadism — **tri·bad·ic** \tri-'bad-ik\ adj

trib·a·dism \'trib-ə-ˌdiz-əm\ n : a homosexual practice among women in which the external genitalia are rubbed together

tri·ba·sic \(ˈ)trī-'bā-sik\ adj **1** : having three replaceable hydrogen atoms — used of acids **2** : containing three atoms of a monovalent metal or their equivalent

tribe \'trīb\ n : a category of taxonomic classification sometimes equivalent to or ranking just below a suborder but more commonly ranking below a subfamily

tri·bol·o·gy \trī-'bäl-ə-jē, trib-'äl-\ n, pl **-gies** : a branch of mechanical engineering that deals with the design, friction, wear, and lubrication of interacting surfaces (as bodily joints) in relative motion — **tri·bo·log·i·cal** \ˌtrī-bə-'läj-i-kəl, ˌtrib-ə-\ adj

tri·bo·lu·mi·nes·cence \'trī-bō-ˌlü-mə-'nes-ᵊn(t)s, 'trib-ō-\ n : luminescence due to friction — **tri·bo·lu·mi·nes·cent** \-ᵊnt\ adj

tri·bro·mo·eth·a·nol \ˌtrī-ˌbrō-mō-'eth-ə-ˌnȯl, -ˌnōl\ n : a crystalline bromine derivative C₂H₃Br₃O of ethyl alcohol used as a basal anesthetic

tri·bro·mo·eth·yl alcohol \-ˌeth-əl-\ n : TRIBROMOETHANOL

trib·u·tary \'trib-yə-ˌter-ē\ n, pl **-tar·ies** : a vein that empties into a larger vein

tri·bu·tyr·in \trī-'byüt-ə-rən\ n : the bitter oily liquid triglyceride C₁₅H₂₆O₆ of butyric acid used as a plasticizer — called also *butyrin*

tri·car·box·yl·ic acid cycle \ˌtrī-ˌkär-ˌbäk-ˌsil-ik-\ n : KREBS CYCLE

tri·ceps \'trī-ˌseps\ *n, pl* **triceps** *also* **tri·ceps·es** : a muscle that arises from three heads: **a** : the large extensor muscle that is situated along the back of the upper arm, arises by the long head from the infraglenoid tubercle of the scapula and by two heads from the shaft of the humerus, is inserted into the olecranon at the elbow, and extends the forearm at the elbow joint — called also *triceps brachii* **b** : the gastrocnemius and soleus muscles viewed as constituting together one muscle — called also *triceps surae*

triceps bra·chii \-ˈbrā-kē-ˌī\ *n* : TRICEPS a

triceps su·rae \-ˈsu̇r-ē\ *n* : TRICEPS b

tri·chi·a·sis \trik-ˈī-ə-səs\ *n* : a turning inward of the eyelashes often causing irritation of the eyeball

tri·chi·na \tri-ˈkī-nə\ *n, pl* **-nae** \-(ˌ)nē\ *also* **-nas** : a small slender nematode worm of the genus *Trichinella* (*T. spiralis*) that as an adult is a short-lived parasite of the intestines of a flesh-eating mammal (as a human being, rat, or pig) where it produces immense numbers of larvae which migrate to the striated muscles either directly or through the blood, establish themselves in or between the muscle fibers where they become encysted and may persist for years, and if consumed by a new host in raw or insufficiently cooked meat are liberated by the digestive processes and rapidly become adult to initiate a new parasitic cycle — see TRICHINOSIS

Trichina *n, syn of* TRICHINELLA

trich·i·nel·la \ˌtrik-ə-ˈnel-ə\ *n* **1** *cap* : a genus (coextensive with the family Trichinellidae of the order Enoplida) of nematode worms comprising the trichinae and being often isolated in a distinct superfamily **2** *pl* **-lae** \-ˌlē\ : TRICHINA

trich·i·nel·li·a·sis \ˌtrik-ə-nə-ˈlī-ə-səs\ *n, pl* **-a·ses** \-ˌsēz\ : TRICHINOSIS

trich·i·ni·a·sis \ˌtrik-ə-ˈnī-ə-səs\ *n, pl* **-a·ses** \-ˌsēz\ : TRICHINOSIS

trich·i·nize *also Brit* **trich·i·nise** \'trik-ə-ˌnīz\ *vt* **-nized** *also Brit* **-nised; -niz·ing** *also Brit* **-nis·ing** : to infest with trichinae ⟨*trichinized* pork⟩

trich·i·nosed \'trik-ə-ˌnōst\ *adj* : TRICHINOUS

trich·i·no·sis \ˌtrik-ə-ˈnō-səs\ *n, pl* **-no·ses** \-ˌsēz\ : infestation with or disease caused by trichinae contracted by eating raw or insufficiently cooked infested food and esp. pork and marked initially by colicky pains, nausea, and diarrhea and later by muscular pain, dyspnea, fever, and edema — called also *trichinelliasis, trichiniasis*

tri·chi·nous \'trik-ə-nəs, trik-ˈī-\ *adj* **1** : infested with trichinae ⟨~ meat⟩ **2** : of, relating to, or involving trichinae or trichinosis ⟨~ infection⟩

tri·chlor·fon *also* **tri·chlor·phon** \(ˈ)trī-ˈklō(ə)r-ˌfän, -ˈklȯ(ə)r-\ *n* : an organophosphate $C_4H_8Cl_3O_4P$ used as a parasiticide in veterinary medicine

tri·chlor·me·thi·a·zide \ˌtrī-ˌklȯr-me-ˈthī-ə-ˌzīd\ *n* : a diuretic and antihypertensive drug $C_8H_8Cl_3N_3O_4S_2$ — see METAHYDRIN, NAQUA

tri·chlo·ro·ace·tic acid \ˌtrī-ˌklȯr-ō-ə-ˌsēt-ik-, -ˌklȯr-\ *also* **tri·chlor·ace·tic acid** \-ˌklȯr-ə-ˌsēt-ik-\ *n* : a strong vesicant pungent acid $C_2Cl_3HO_2$ made usu. by chlorinating acetic acid or by oxidizing chloral and used in medicine as a caustic and astringent — compare MONOCHLOROACETIC ACID

tri·chlo·ro·eth·ane \-ˈeth-ˌān\ *n* : either of two nonflammable irritating liquid isomeric compounds $C_2H_3Cl_3$: **a** *or* **1,1,1–trichloroethane** \'wən-ˌwən-ˈwən-\ : the isomer CH_3CCl_3 that is the parent compound of various insecticides (as DDT) — called also *methyl chloroform* **b** *or* **1,1,2–trichloroethane** \-ˈtü-\ : the isomer $CH_2ClCHCl_2$ that is used chiefly as a solvent

tri·chlo·ro·eth·y·lene *also* **tri·chlor·eth·y·lene** \-ˈeth-ə-ˌlēn\ *n* : a nonflammable liquid C_2HCl_3 used as a solvent and in medicine as an anesthetic and analgesic — abbr. TCE

tri·chlo·ro·meth·ane \-ˈmeth-ˌān, *Brit usu* -ˈmē-ˌthān\ *n* : CHLOROFORM

tri·chlo·ro·phe·nol \-ˈfē-ˌnȯl, -ˌnȯl, -fi-ˈ\ *n* : a bactericide and fungicide $C_6H_3Cl_3O$ that is a major constituent of hexachlorophene

tri·chlo·ro·phen·oxy·ace·tic acid \(ˈ)trī-ˈklȯr-ō-fə-ˌnäk-sē-ə-ˌsēt-ik-, -ˌklȯr-\ *n* : 2,4,5-T

trichlorphon *var of* TRICHLORFON

tricho·be·zoar \ˌtrik-ō-ˈbē-ˌzō(ə)r, -ˌzȯ(ə)r\ *n* : HAIR BALL

Tricho·bil·har·zia \ˌtrik-ō-bil-ˈhär-zē-ə, -ˈhärt-sē-ə\ *n* : a genus of digenetic trematode worms of the family Schistosomatidae including forms that normally parasitize aquatic birds and are leading causes of swimmer's itch in humans

tricho·ceph·a·li·a·sis \-ˌsef-ə-ˈlī-ə-səs\ *n, pl* **-a·ses** \-ˌsēz\ : TRICHURIASIS

Tricho·ceph·a·lus \-ˈsef-ə-ləs\ *n, syn of* TRICHURIS

tricho·cyst \'trik-ə-ˌsist\ *n* : any of the minute projectile organs that release adhesive threads when discharged and that occur on the body of protozoans and esp. of many ciliates

Tricho·dec·tes \ˌtrik-ə-ˈdek-ˌtēz\ *n* : the type genus of the family Trichodectidae including various biting lice of domesticated mammals

Tricho·dec·ti·dae \ˌtrik-ə-ˈdek-ti-ˌdē\ *n pl* : a widespread family of biting lice that have a single simple tarsal claw and include economically important parasites of mammals — see CAT LOUSE

Tricho·der·ma \ˌtrik-ə-ˈdər-mə\ *n* : a form genus of imperfect fungi of the family Moniliaceae having nonseptate conidia borne in heads on 2-branched or 3-branched conidiophores

tricho·epi·the·li·o·ma \ˌtrik-ō-ˌep-ə-ˌthē-lē-ˈō-mə\ *n, pl* **-mas** *also* **-ma·ta** \-mət-ə\ : a benign epithelial tumor developing from the hair follicles esp. on the face

tri·chol·o·gy \tri-ˈkäl-ə-jē\ *n, pl* **-gies** **1** : scientific study of hair and its diseases **2** : the occupation of hairdressing

tri·chome \'trik-ˌōm, 'trī-ˌkōm\ *n* : a strand or chain of cells (as in a filamentous colony of bacteria or algae)

tricho·mo·na·cide \ˌtrik-ə-ˈmō-nə-ˌsīd\ *n* : an agent used to destroy trichomonads — **tricho·mo·na·cid·al** \-ˌmō-nə-ˈsīd-ᵊl\ *adj*

¹tricho·mo·nad \ˌtrik-ə-ˈmō-ˌnad, -nəd\ *n* : any protozoan of the genus *Trichomonas*

²trichomonad *adj* : TRICHOMONAL

tricho·mo·nal \ˌtrik-ə-ˈmō-nəl\ *adj* : of, relating to, or caused by flagellated protozoans of the genus *Trichomonas* ⟨~ infections⟩

trich·o·mo·nas \ˌtrik-ə-ˈmō-nəs\ *n* **1** *cap* : a genus (the type of the family Trichomonadidae) of polymastigote parasitic flagellated protozoans that have four anterior flagella and another at the margin of an undulating membrane or in some classifications also include forms with three or four anterior flagella and that are parasites of the alimentary or genitourinary tracts of numerous vertebrate and invertebrate hosts including one (*T. vaginalis*) causing human vaginitis **2** : a protozoan of the genus *Trichomonas*

tricho·mo·ni·a·sis \ˌtrik-ə-mə-ˈnī-ə-səs\ *n, pl* **-a·ses** \-ˌsēz\ : infection with or disease caused by trichomonads: as **a** : a human sexually transmitted disease occurring esp. as vaginitis with a persistent discharge and caused by a trichomonad (*Trichomonas vaginalis*) that may also invade the male urethra and bladder **b** : a venereal disease of domestic cattle caused by a trichomonad (*T. foetus*) and marked by abortion and sterility **c** : one or more diseases of various birds caused by trichomonads (esp. *T. gallinae*) and resembling blackhead — called also *roup*

tricho·my·co·sis \-ˌmī-ˈkō-səs\ *n, pl* **-co·ses** \-ˌsēz\ : a disease of the hair caused by fungi — called also *lepothrix*

tricho·phy·tid \ˌtrik-ə-ˈfīt-əd, tri-ˈkäf-ət-əd\ *n* : a skin eruption accompanying infection by fungi of the genus *Trichophyton*

tricho·phy·tin \ˌtrik-ə-ˈfīt-ᵊn, tri-ˈkäf-ət-ᵊn\ *n* : an antigenic extract from cultures of fungi of the genus *Trichophyton* used esp. formerly in a test for trichophytosis

tricho·phy·ton \ˌtrik-ə-ˈfī-ˌtän, tri-ˈkäf-ə-ˌtän\ *n* **1** *cap* : a genus of ringworm fungi of the family Moniliaceae that have hyaline single-celled spores and are parasitic in the skin and

\ə\ abut \ᵊ\ kitten \ər\ further \a\ ash \ā\ ace \ä\ cot, cart \au̇\ out \ch\ chin \e\ bet \ē\ easy \g\ go \i\ hit \ī\ ice \j\ job \ŋ\ sing \ō\ go \ȯ\ law \ȯi\ boy \th\ thin \th̲\ the \ü\ loot \u̇\ foot \y\ yet \zh\ vision   *See also* Pronunciation Symbols page

hair follicles of humans and lower mammals — see EPIDER-
MOPHYTON **2** : any fungus of the genus *Trichophyton*

tricho·phy·to·sis \ˌtrik-ə-ˌfī-'tō-səs\ *n, pl* **-to·ses** \-ˌsēz\ : a
disease of the skin, nails, or hair caused by fungi of the genus
Trichophyton

Tricho·spo·ron \ˌtrik-ə-'spōr-ˌän, tri-'käs-pə-ˌrän\ *n* : a genus
of parasitic imperfect fungi of the order Moniliales that includes the causative agent (*T. beigelii*) of white piedra

tricho·spo·ro·sis \ˌtrik-ə-spōr-'ō-səs\ *n, pl* **-ro·ses** \-ˌsēz\ *or*
-ro·sis·es : PIEDRA

tricho·stron·gyle \ˌtrik-ə-'strän-ˌjīl\ *n* : any worm of the genus *Trichostrongylus*

Tricho·stron·gyl·i·dae \ˌtrik-ō-strän-'jil-ə-ˌdē\ *n pl* : a family of nematode worms of the suborder Strongylina that have
a reduced buccal capsule with three or fewer basal teeth and
parasitize the alimentary tract of vertebrates — **tricho·
stron·gy·lid** \-'strän-jə-ləd\ *adj or n*

tricho·stron·gy·lo·sis \ˌtrik-ō-ˌsträn-jə-'lō-səs\ *n* : infestation with or disease caused by roundworms of the genus
Trichostrongylus chiefly in young sheep and cattle where it is
commonly marked by diarrhea, inappetence, and loss of
weight

Tricho·stron·gy·lus \ˌtrik-ō-'strän-jə-ləs\ *n* : the type genus
of the family Trichostrongylidae containing nematode
worms that are parasites of birds and of mammals including
humans and comprising forms formerly placed in the genus
Strongylus

tricho·the·cene \ˌtrik-ə-'thē-ˌsēn, tri-'käth-ə-ˌsēn\ *n* : any of
several mycotoxins that are produced by various fungi (as of
the genera *Fusarium* and *Trichothecium*) and that include
some contaminants of livestock feed and some held to be
found in yellow rain

tricho·til·lo·ma·nia \-ˌtil-ə-'mā-nē-ə\ *n* : abnormal desire to
pull out one's hair — called also *hairpulling* — **tricho·til·lo·
man·ic** \-'man-ik\ *adj*

tri·chro·ism \'trī-ˌkrō-ˌiz-əm\ *n* : pleochroism in which the
colors are unlike when a crystal is viewed in the direction of
three different axes

tri·chro·mat \'trī-krō-ˌmat, (')trī-'\ *n* : an individual with
normal color vision requiring that three primary colors be
mixed in order to match the perceived spectrum

tri·chro·mat·ic \ˌtrī-krō-'mat-ik\ *adj* **1** : of, relating to, or
consisting of three colors ⟨~ light⟩ **2 a** : relating to or being the theory that human color vision involves three types
of retinal sensory receptors **b** : characterized by trichromatism ⟨~ vision⟩

tri·chro·ma·tism \(')trī-'krō-mə-ˌtiz-əm\ *n* **1** : the quality or
state of being trichromatic **2** : color vision based on the
perception of three primary colors and esp. red, green and
blue — compare DEUTERANOMALY, PROTANOMALY

tri·chrome \'trī-ˌkrōm\ *adj* : coloring tissue elements differentially in three colors ⟨a ~ biological stain⟩

trich·u·ri·a·sis \ˌtrik-yə-'rī-ə-səs\ *n, pl* **-a·ses** \-ˌsēz\ : infestation with or disease caused by nematode worms of the genus
Trichuris — called also *trichocephaliasis*

Trich·u·ri·dae \ˌtrik-'yùr-ə-ˌdē\ *n pl* : a family of nematode
worms (order Enoplida) that are parasitic in the intestines of
vertebrates and have a slender body sometimes with a thickened posterior end and a tubular capillary esophagus

Trich·u·ris \ˌtrik-'yùr-əs\ *n* : the type genus of the family
Trichuridae of nematode worms comprising the whipworms

Tri·clad·i·da \ˌtrī-'klad-əd-ə\ *n pl* : an order of small turbellarian worms (as the planarians) including marine, freshwater, and terrestrial forms

tri·clo·car·ban \ˌtrī-ˌklō-'kär-ˌban\ *n* : an antiseptic
$C_{13}H_9Cl_3N_2O$ used esp. in soaps

tri·clo·san \ˌtrī-'klō-ˌsan\ *n* : a whitish crystalline powder
$C_{12}H_7Cl_3O_2$ used esp. as a broad-spectrum antibacterial
agent (as in soaps, deodorants, and mouthwash)

Tri·Cor \'trī-ˌkȯr\ *trademark* — used for a preparation of
fenofibrate

tri·cre·sol \(')trī-'krē-ˌsȯl, -ˌsōl\ *n* : CRESOL 2

¹tri·cus·pid \(')trī-'kəs-pəd\ *adj* **1** : having three cusps ⟨~

molars⟩ **2** : of, relating to, or involving the tricuspid valve
of the heart ⟨~ disease⟩

²tricuspid *n* : a tricuspid anatomical structure; *esp* : a tooth
having three cusps

tricuspid valve *n* : a valve that is situated at the opening of
the right atrium of the heart into the right ventricle and that
resembles the mitral valve in structure but consists of three
triangular membranous flaps — called also *right atrioventricular valve*

¹tri·cy·clic \(')trī-'sī-klik, -'sik-lik\ *adj* : being a chemical with
three usu. fused rings in the molecular structure and esp. a
tricyclic antidepressant

²tricyclic *n* : TRICYCLIC ANTIDEPRESSANT

tricyclic antidepressant *n* : any of a group of antidepressant drugs (as imipramine, amitriptyline, desipramine, and
nortriptyline) that contain three fused benzene rings, that
potentiate the action of catecholamines (as norepinephrine
and serotonin) by inhibiting their uptake by nerve endings,
and that do not inhibit the action of monoamine oxidase

tri·di·hex·eth·yl chloride \ˌtrī-ˌdī-ˌheks-'eth-ᵊl-\ *n* : a quaternary ammonium compound $C_{21}H_{36}ClNO$ used as an anticholinergic drug — see PATHILON

Tri·di·one \ˌtrī-'dī-ˌōn\ *trademark* — used for a preparation
of trimethadione

tri–es·ter \(')trī-'es-tər\ *n* : a compound containing three es-
ter groups

tri·eth·a·nol·amine \(')trī-ˌeth-ə-'näl-ə-ˌmēn, -'nōl-\ *n* : a sol-
uble hygroscopic basic amino alcohol $C_6H_{15}NO_3$ that is used
as a reducing agent, a corrosion inhibitor in aqueous solution, and in making fatty acid soaps

triethiodide — see GALLAMINE TRIETHIODIDE

tri·eth·yl·amine \(')trī-ˌeth-ᵊl-ə-'mēn, -'am-ˌēn\ *n* : a water-
soluble flammable liquid tertiary amine $(C_2H_5)_3N$ that is
used chiefly in synthesis (as of quaternary ammonium compounds)

tri·eth·yl·ene glycol \-'eth-ə-ˌlēn-\ *n* : a hygroscopic liquid
alcohol $C_6H_{14}O_4$ that is used chiefly as a solvent and in medicine as an air disinfectant

tri·eth·yl·ene·mel·amine \(')trī-ˌeth-ə-ˌlēn-'mel-ə-ˌmēn,
-mən\ *n* : a cytotoxic crystalline compound $C_9H_{12}N_6$ used as
an antineoplastic drug — called also *TEM*

tri·fa·cial nerve \ˌtrī-'fā-shəl-\ *n* : TRIGEMINAL NERVE

trifacial neuralgia *n* : TRIGEMINAL NEURALGIA

tri·fluo·per·a·zine \ˌtrī-ˌflü-ō-'per-ə-ˌzēn, -zən\ *n* : a phenothiazine tranquilizer $C_{21}H_{24}F_3N_3S$ used esp. to treat psychotic conditions and esp. schizophrenia — see STELAZINE

tri·flu·pro·ma·zine \ˌtrī-ˌflü-'prō-mə-ˌzēn, -zən\ *n* : a phenothiazine tranquilizer used in the form of its hydrochloride
$C_{18}H_{19}F_3N_2S\cdot HCl$ esp. in the treatment of psychotic disorders and as an antiemetic — see VESPRIN

¹tri·fo·cal \(')trī-'fō-kəl\ *adj* **1** : having three focal lengths **2**
of an eyeglass lens : having one part that corrects for near vision, one for intermediate vision (as at arm's length), and one
for distant vision

²trifocal *n* **1** : a trifocal glass or lens **2 trifocals** *pl* : eyeglasses with trifocal lenses

tri·fo·li·o·sis \ˌtrī-ˌfō-lē-'ō-səs\ *n, pl* **-o·ses** \-'ō-ˌsēz\ : CLOVER
DISEASE

tri·func·tion·al \ˌtrī-'fəŋk-shən-ᵊl\ *adj* : of, relating to, or being a compound with three sites in the molecule that are
highly reactive (as in polymerization) ⟨a ~ amino acid⟩

tri·fur·ca·tion \ˌtrī-fər-'kā-shən\ *n* : division into three
branches ⟨~ of a blood vessel⟩

¹tri·gem·i·nal \trī-'jem-ən-ᵊl\ *adj* : of or relating to the trigeminal nerve

²trigeminal *n* : TRIGEMINAL NERVE

trigeminal ganglion *n* : the large flattened sensory root ganglion of the trigeminal nerve that lies within the skull and behind the orbit — called also *gasserian ganglion, semilunar
ganglion*

trigeminal nerve *n* : either of the fifth pair of cranial nerves
that are mixed nerves and in humans are the largest of the
cranial nerves and that arise by a small motor root and a
larger sensory root which both emerge from the side of the

pons with the sensory root bearing the trigeminal ganglion and dividing into ophthalmic, maxillary, and mandibular nerves and the motor root supplying fibers to the mandibular nerve and through this to the muscles of mastication — called also *fifth cranial nerve, trifacial nerve, trigeminus*

trigeminal neuralgia *n* : an intense paroxysmal neuralgia involving one or more branches of the trigeminal nerve — called also *tic douloureux*

trig·ger area \'trig-ər-\ *n* : TRIGGER POINT

trigger finger *n* : an abnormal condition in which flexion or extension of a finger may be momentarily obstructed by spasm followed by a snapping into place

trigger mechanism *n* : something (as a specific act or stimulus) that in interaction with the body constitutes a physiological trigger; *esp* : one by which an attack (as of disease or referred pain) is precipitated

trigger point *n* : a sensitive area of the body which when stimulated gives rise to a reaction elsewhere in the body; *esp* : a localized usu. tender or painful area of the body and esp. of a muscle that when stimulated gives rise to pain elsewhere in the body — called also *trigger area, trigger zone*

tri·glyc·er·ide \(')trī-'glis-ə-ˌrīd\ *n* : any of a group of lipids that are esters formed from one molecule of glycerol and three molecules of one or more fatty acids, are widespread in adipose tissue, and commonly circulate in the blood in the form of lipoproteins — called also *neutral fat*

trigona *pl of* TRIGONUM

tri·gone \'trī-ˌgōn\ *also* **tri·gon** \-ˌgän\ *n* : a triangular body part; *specif* : a smooth triangular area on the inner surface of the bladder limited by the apertures of the ureters and urethra

trig·o·nel·line \ˌtrig-ə-'nel-ˌēn, -ən\ *n* : a crystalline alkaloid $C_7H_7NO_2$ obtained esp. from the seeds of fenugreek and found in the urine (as after ingestion of nicotinic acid)

tri·go·nid \'trī-gə-ˌnid\ *n* : the first three cusps of a lower molar

tri·go·ni·tis \ˌtrī-gə-'nīt-əs\ *n* : inflammation of the trigone of the bladder

tri·go·no·ceph·a·ly \ˌtrig-ə-nə-'sef-ə-lē, ˌtrī-ˌgō-nō-\ *n, pl* **-lies** : a congenital deformity in which the head is somewhat triangular and flat

tri·go·num \trī-'gō-nəm\ *n, pl* **-nums** *or* **-na** \-nə\ : a triangular anatomical part : TRIGONE

trigonum ha·ben·u·lae \-hə-'ben-yə-ˌlē\ *n* : a triangular area on the dorsomedial surface of the lateral geniculate body rostral to the pineal gland

trigonum ves·i·cae \-'ves-i-kē\ *n* : the trigone of the urinary bladder

tri·halo·meth·ane \(ˌ)trī-ˌhā-lə-'meth-ˌān, *Brit usu* -'mē-ˌthān\ *n* : any of various derivatives CHX_3 of methane (as chloroform) that have three halogen atoms per molecule and are formed esp. during the chlorination of drinking water — abbr. THM

tri·hy·brid \-'hī-brəd\ *n* : an individual or strain that is heterozygous for three pairs of genes — **trihybrid** *adj*

tri·hy·drate \ˌtrī-'hī-ˌdrāt\ *n* : a chemical compound with three molecules of water

tri·hy·dric \-'hī-drik\ *adj* : TRIHYDROXY

tri·hy·droxy \ˌtrī-hī-'dräk-sē\ *adj* : containing three hydroxyl groups in a molecule

tri·io·dide \ˌtrī-'ī-ə-ˌdīd\ *n* : a binary compound containing three atoms of iodine combined with an element or radical

tri·io·do·thy·ro·nine \ˌtrī-ˌī-əd-ō-'thī-rə-ˌnēn\ *n* : a crystalline iodine-containing hormone $C_{15}H_{12}I_3NO_4$ that is an amino acid derived from thyroxine and is used esp. in the form of its soluble sodium salt $C_{15}H_{11}I_3NNaO_4$ in the treatment of hypothyroidism and metabolic insufficiency — called also *liothyronine, T3*

tri·lam·i·nar \(')trī-'lam-ə-nər\ *adj* : having or built up of three layers

tri·lobed \'trī-ˌlōbd\ *adj* : having three lobes

tri·mep·ra·zine \trī-'mep-rə-ˌzēn\ *n* : a phenothiazine used esp. in the form of its tartrate $(C_{18}H_{22}N_2S)_2 \cdot C_4H_6O_6$ as an antipruritic — see TEMARIL

tri·mer \'trī-mər\ *n* : a polymer formed from three molecules of a monomer — **tri·mer·ic** \trī-'mer-ik\ *adj*

Trim·er·e·su·rus \ˌtrim-ə-rə-'sùr-əs\ *n* : a genus of usu. green prehensile-tailed arboreal Asian pit vipers that includes the habu — see LACHESIS

tri·mer·iza·tion *also Brit* **tri·mer·isa·tion** \ˌtrī-mə-rə-'zā-shən\ *n* : polymerization resulting in a trimer

tri·mes·ter \(')trī-'mes-tər, 'trī-ˌ\ *n* : a period of three or about three months; *esp* : any of three periods of approximately three months each into which a human pregnancy is divided

tri·metha·di·one \ˌtrī-ˌmeth-ə-'dī-ˌōn\ *n* : a crystalline anticonvulsant $C_6H_9NO_3$ used chiefly in the treatment of absence seizures — see TRIDIONE

tri·meth·a·phan \trī-'meth-ə-ˌfan\ *n* : a ganglionic blocking agent used as a salt $C_{32}H_{40}N_2O_5S_2$ to lower blood pressure esp. in hypertensive emergencies

tri·metho·ben·za·mide \ˌtrī-ˌmeth-ə-'ben-zə-ˌmīd\ *n* : an antiemetic drug used esp. in the form of its hydrochloride salt $C_{21}H_{28}N_2O_5 \cdot HCl$

tri·meth·o·prim \trī-'meth-ə-ˌprim\ *n* : a synthetic antibacterial drug $C_{14}H_{18}N_4O_3$ used alone esp. to treat urinary tract infections and Pneumocystis carinii pneumonia and in combination with sulfamethoxazole to treat these as well as other infections (as shigellosis or acute otitis media) — see BACTRIM

tri·meth·yl \(')trī-'meth-ᵊl, *Brit also* -'mē-ˌthīl\ *adj* : containing three methyl groups in a molecule

tri·meth·yl·amine \ˌtrī-ˌmeth-ᵊl-'am-ˌēn, -ə-'mēn\ *n* : an irritating gaseous or volatile liquid tertiary amine $(CH_3)_3N$ that has a fishy odor, is only slightly more basic than ammonia, is flammable and forms explosive mixtures with air, is formed as a degradation product of many nitrogenous animal and plant substances, and is used chiefly in making quaternary ammonium compounds (as choline)

tri·meth·y·lene \(')trī-'meth-ə-ˌlēn, -lən\ *n* : CYCLOPROPANE

tri·me·trex·ate \ˌtrī-mi-'trek-ˌsāt\ *n* : a toxic drug structurally related to methotrexate that is administered in the form of its glucuronate $C_{19}H_{23}N_5O_3 \cdot C_6H_{10}O_7$ with concomitant administration of leucovorin to reduce toxicity and is used esp. in the treatment of Pneumocystis carinii pneumonia and certain carcinomas

tri·mo·lec·u·lar \-mə-'lek-yə-lər\ *adj* : relating to or formed from three molecules

tri·mor·phic \(')trī-'mòr-fik\ *or* **tri·mor·phous** \-fəs\ *adj* : occurring in or having three distinct forms — **tri·mor·phism** \-ˌfiz-əm\ *n*

Tri·mox \'trī-ˌmäks\ *trademark* — used for a preparation of amoxicillin

tri·ni·trate \(')trī-'nī-ˌtrāt, -trət\ *n* : a nitrate containing three nitrate groups in a molecule

tri·ni·trin \-'nī-trən\ *n* : NITROGLYCERIN

tri·ni·tro·glyc·er·in \ˌtrī-ˌnī-trə-'glis-(ə-)rən\ *n* : NITROGLYCERIN

tri·ni·tro·phe·nol \-'fē-ˌnòl, -ˌnòl, -fi-'nōl\ *or* **2,4,6–trinitrophenol** \ˌtü-'fòr-ˌsiks-\ *n* : PICRIC ACID

tri·ni·tro·tol·u·ene \ˌtrī-ˌnī-trō-'täl-yə-ˌwēn\ *n* : a flammable toxic compound $C_7H_5N_3O_6$ obtained by nitrating toluene and used as a high explosive and in chemical synthesis — called also *TNT*

trin·oc·u·lar \(')trī-'näk-yə-lər\ *adj* : relating to or being a binocular microscope equipped with a lens for photographic recording during direct visual observation

¹tri·no·mi·al \trī-'nō-mē-əl\ *n* : a trinomial name

²trinomial *adj* **1** : being a name belonging to botanical or zoological nomenclature composed of a first term designating the genus, a second term designating the species, and a third term designating the subspecies or variety to which an

---

S
T

organism belongs   **2** : of or relating to trinomials ⟨~ nomenclature⟩

tri·nu·cle·ate \(')trī-'n(y)ü-klē-ət\ *adj* : having three nuclei

tri·nu·cle·o·tide \(')trī-'n(y)ü-klē-ə-ˌtīd\ *n* : a nucleotide consisting of three mononucleotides in combination : CODON

tri·ole·in \-'ō-lē-ən\ *n* : OLEIN

tri·or·tho·cre·syl phosphate \ˌtrī-ˌòr-thō-ˌkres-əl-, -ˌkrēs-\ *n* : a usu. colorless, odorless, tasteless neurotoxic organophosphate $C_{21}H_{21}O_4P$ that sometimes is the cause of poisoning of workers handling it in industry

tri·ose \'trī-ˌōs, -ˌōz\ *n* : either of two simple sugars $C_3H_6O_3$ containing three carbon atoms

triose phosphate *n* : a phosphoric ester or acylal of a triose; *esp* : either of two monophosphates $C_3H_7O_6P$ or an equilibrium mixture of them formed as intermediates in carbohydrate metabolism

tri·ox·ide \(')trī-'äk-ˌsīd\ *n* : an oxide containing three atoms of oxygen

tri·ox·sa·len \ˌtrī-'äk-sə-lən\ *n* : a synthetic psoralen $C_{14}H_{12}O_3$ that promotes tanning of the skin

tri·pal·mi·tin \(')trī-'pal-mət-ən, -'pä(l)m-ət-ən\ *n* : PALMITIN

trip·a·ra \'trip-ə-rə\ *n* : a woman who has borne three children

tri·par·a·nol \trī-'par-ə-ˌnòl, -ˌnōl\ *n* : a drug $C_{27}H_{32}ClNO_2$ that inhibits the formation of cholesterol but that has numerous toxic side effects

tri·pel·en·na·mine \ˌtrī-pe-'len-ə-ˌmēn, -mən\ *n* : an antihistamine drug derived from pyridine and ethylenediamine and used in the form of its crystalline citrate $C_{16}H_{21}N_3 \cdot C_6H_8O_7$ or hydrochloride $C_{16}H_{21}N_3 \cdot HCl$ — see PYRIBENZAMINE

tri·pep·tide \(')trī-'pep-ˌtīd\ *n* : a peptide that yields three amino acid residues on hydrolysis

tri·pha·sic \(')trī-'fā-zik\ *adj* : having or occurring in three phases

tri·phe·nyl·meth·ane \ˌtrī-ˌfen-ᵊl-'meth-ˌān, -ˌfēn-\ *n* : a crystalline hydrocarbon $CH(C_6H_5)_3$ that is the parent compound of many dyes

triphenylmethane dye *n* : any of a group of dyes (as pararosaniline) derived from triphenylmethane and used esp. as organic pigments and biological stains

tri·phos·pha·tase \(')trī-'fäs-fə-ˌtās, -ˌtāz\ *n* : an enzyme that catalyzes hydrolysis of a triphosphate — see ATPASE

tri·phos·phate \(')trī-'fäs-ˌfāt\ *n* : a salt or acid that contains three phosphate groups — see ATP, GTP

tri·phos·pho·pyr·i·dine nucleotide \'trī-ˌfäs-fō-'pir-ə-ˌdēn-\ *n* : NADP

tri·ple bond \'trip-əl-\ *n* : a chemical bond in which three pairs of electrons are shared by two atoms in a molecule — compare DOUBLE BOND, UNSATURATED b

triple dye *n* : an antiseptic consisting of the aniline dyes gentian violet, brilliant green, and acriflavine that was orig. used in the treatment of burns and later as a general bactericide

tri·ple·gia \(')trī-'plē-j(ē-)ə\ *n* : hemiplegia plus paralysis of a limb on the opposite side

triple point *n* : the condition of temperature and pressure under which the gaseous, liquid, and solid phases of a substance (as water) can exist in equilibrium

triple screen *n* : a blood test for pregnant women for alpha-fetoprotein, human chorionic gonadotropin, and estriol in order to assess the risk of fetal abnormality (as Down syndrome, anencephaly, and spina bifida) — called also *triple test*

trip·let \'trip-lət\ *n*   **1 a** : a combination, set, or group of three   **b** : an atom or molecule with an even number of electrons that have a net magnetic moment   **c** : CODON   **2 a** : one of three children or offspring born at one birth   **b triplets** *pl* : a group of three offspring born at one birth   **3** : a combination of three lenses

triple test *n* : TRIPLE SCREEN

trip·lo·blas·tic \ˌtrip-lō-'blas-tik\ *adj* : having three primary germ layers ⟨human beings are ~ organisms⟩

¹trip·loid \'trip-ˌlòid\ *adj* : having or being a chromosome number three times the monoploid number — **trip·loi·dy** \-ˌlòid-ē\ *n, pl* **-dies**

²triploid *n* : a triploid individual

tri·pod \'trī-ˌpäd\ *n* : a bone having three processes

trip·tan \'trip-ˌtan, -tən\ *n* : any of a class of drugs (as sumatriptan) that bind to and are agonists of serotonin receptors, that are used to treat migraine attacks, and that are thought to function by producing vasoconstriction of cranial blood vessels, by inhibiting secretion of inflammatory neuropeptides, and by blocking neurotransmission of pain

tri·que·tral bone \trī-'kwē-trel-\ *n* : the bone in the proximal row of the carpus that is third counting from the thumb side of the wrist, has a pyramidal shape, and is situated between the lunate and pisiform bones — called also *triangular, triangular bone, triangularis, triquetral, triquetrum*

tri·que·trum \trī-'kwē-trəm\ *n, pl* **tri·que·tra** \-trə\ : TRIQUETRAL BONE

tri·ra·di·us \-'rād-ē-əs\ *n, pl* **-dii** \-ē-ˌī\ *also* **-di·us·es** : a group of ridges forming a Y at the base of each finger on the palm of the hand

tris \'tris\ *n, often cap* : a white crystalline powder $C_4H_{11}NO_3$ used as a buffer (as in the treatment of acidosis) — called also *tris buffer, tromethamine*

Tris *n* : a phosphoric acid ester $C_9H_{15}Br_6O_4P$ formerly used to flameproof clothes and esp. children's nightclothes until it was found to cause cancer in animals

tri·sac·cha·ride \(')trī-'sak-ə-ˌrīd\ *n* : a sugar that yields on complete hydrolysis three monosaccharide molecules

tris buffer *n* : TRIS

tris·kai·deka·pho·bia \ˌtris-ˌkī-ˌdek-ə-'fō-bē-ə, ˌtris-kə-\ *n* : fear of the number 13

tris·mus \'triz-məs\ *n* : spasm of the muscles of mastication resulting from any of various abnormal conditions or diseases (as tetanus)

¹tri·so·mic \(')trī-'sō-mik\ *adj* : relating to, caused by, or characterized by trisomy ⟨~ cells⟩

²trisomic *n* : a trisomic individual

tri·so·my \'trī-ˌsō-mē\ *n, pl* **-mies** : the condition (as in Down syndrome) of having one or a few chromosomes triploid in an otherwise diploid set

trisomy 18 \-'ā(t)-'tēn\ *n* : a congenital condition that is characterized esp. by mental retardation and by craniofacial, cardiac, gastrointestinal, and genitourinary abnormalities, is caused by trisomy of the human chromosome numbered 18, and is typically fatal esp. within the first year of life — called also *Edwards syndrome*

trisomy 13 \-'thər(t)-'tēn\ *n* : a congenital condition that is characterized esp. by usu. severe mental retardation and by craniofacial, cardiac, ocular, and cerebral abnormalities, is caused by trisomy of the human chromosome numbered 13, and is typically fatal esp. within the first six months of life — called also *Patau syndrome*

trisomy 21 \-ˌtwent-ē-'wən\ *n* : DOWN SYNDROME

tri·stea·rin \(')trī-'stē-ə-rən, -'sti(ə)r-ən\ *n* : the crystallizable triglyceride $C_{57}H_{110}O_6$ of stearic acid that is found esp. in hard fats

tri·sub·sti·tut·ed \'trī-'səb-stə-ˌt(y)üt-əd\ *adj* : having three substituent atoms or groups in the molecule ⟨a ~ amine⟩

trit·an·ope \'trīt-ᵊn-ˌōp, 'trit-\ *n* : an individual affected with tritanopia

trit·an·opia \ˌtrīt-ᵊn-'ō-pē-ə, ˌtrit-\ *n* : dichromatism in which the spectrum is seen in tones of red and green

trit·an·opic \ˌtrīt-ᵊn-'ō-pik, ˌtrit-ᵊn-'äp-ik\ *adj* : characterized by or affected by tritanopia ⟨~ vision⟩ ⟨a ~ person⟩

tri·ter·pene \(')trī-'tər-ˌpēn\ *n* : any of a class of terpenes $C_{30}H_{48}$ (as squalene) containing three times as many atoms in the molecule as monoterpenes; *also* : a derivative of such a terpene

tri·ter·pe·nic \ˌtrī-ˌtər-'pē-nik\ *adj* : relating to or being a triterpene

¹tri·ter·pe·noid \(')trī-'tər-pə-ˌnòid\ *adj* : resembling or derived from a triterpene ⟨~ sapogenins⟩

²triterpenoid *n* : a triterpene or triterpene derivative

tri·ti·at·ed \'trit-ē-ˌāt-əd, 'trish-ē-\ *adj* : containing and esp. labeled with tritium ⟨~ water⟩

trit·i·cum \'trit-i-kəm\ *n*   **1** *cap* : a genus of cereal grasses including the wheats **2** : the dried rhizome of the quack grass used esp. formerly as a diuretic and to treat cystitis

tri·ti·um \'trit-ē-əm, 'trish-ē-\ *n* : a radioactive isotope of hydrogen with atoms of three times the mass of ordinary light hydrogen atoms — symbol *T*

tri·tu·ber·cu·lar \,trī-t(y)ù-'bər-kyə-lər\ *adj* : having three cusps : TRICUSPID ⟨a ∼ molar⟩

¹trit·u·rate \'trich-ə-,rāt\ *vt* **-rat·ed; -rat·ing** : to pulverize and comminute thoroughly by rubbing or grinding ⟨*triturated* the drug with a diluent⟩

²trit·u·rate \-rət\ *n* : a triturated substance : TRITURATION 2

trit·u·ra·tion \,trich-ə-'rā-shən\ *n* **1** : the act or process of triturating : the state of being triturated **2** : a triturated medicinal powder made by triturating a substance with a diluent

trit·u·ra·tor \'trich-ə-,rāt-ər\ *n* : an apparatus used for trituration

¹tri·va·lent \(')trī-'vā-lənt\ *adj* **1** : having a chemical valence of three **2** : conferring immunity to three different pathogenic strains or species ⟨a ∼ influenza vaccine⟩

²trivalent *n* : a group of three synapsed homologous chromosomes in meiosis

triv·i·al name \'triv-ē-əl-\ *n* **1** : SPECIFIC EPITHET **2** : a common or vernacular name of an organism or chemical

tri·zy·got·ic \,trī-zī-'gät-ik\ *adj* : produced from three zygotes ⟨∼ triplets⟩

tRNA \,tē-,är-,en-'ā, 'tē-,är-,en-,ā\ *n* : TRANSFER RNA

Tro·bi·cin \trō-'bīs-³n\ *trademark* — used for a preparation of the hydrated dihydrochloride of spectinomycin

tro·car *also* **tro·char** \'trō-,kär\ *n* : a sharp-pointed surgical instrument fitted with a cannula and used esp. to insert the cannula into a body cavity as a drainage outlet

tro·chan·ter \trō-'kant-ər\ *n* : a rough prominence or process at the upper part of the femur of many vertebrates serving usu. for the attachment of muscles and being usu. two on each femur in mammals including humans: **a** : a larger one situated on the outer part of the upper end of the shaft at its junction with the neck — called also *greater trochanter* **b** : a smaller one situated at the lower back part of the junction of the shaft and neck — called also *lesser trochanter* — **tro·chan·ter·ic** \,trō-kən-'tcr-ik, -,kan-\ *adj*

trochanteric fossa *n* : a depression at the base of the internal surface of the greater trochanter of the femur for the attachment of the tendon of the obturator externus

trochar *var of* TROCAR

tro·che \'trō-kē, *Brit usu* 'trōsh\ *n* : LOZENGE

troch·lea \'träk-lē-ə\ *n* : an anatomical structure resembling a pulley: as **a** : the articular surface on the medial condyle of the humerus that articulates with the ulna **b** : the fibrous ring in the inner upper part of the orbit through which the tendon of the superior oblique muscle of the eye passes

troch·le·ar \-ər\ *adj* **1** : of, relating to, or being a trochlea **2** : of, relating to, or being a trochlear nerve ⟨∼ fibers⟩

trochlear fovea *n* : a depression that is located in the anteromedial aspect of the orbital surface of each bony plate of the frontal bone making up the superior part of one of the orbits and that forms a point of attachment for the corresponding superior oblique muscle of the eye

troch·le·ar·is \,träk-lē-'ar-əs\ *n* : TROCHLEAR NERVE

trochlear nerve *n* : either of the fourth pair of cranial nerves that arise from the dorsal aspect of the brain stem just below the inferior colliculus and supply the superior oblique muscle of the eye with motor fibers

trochlear notch *n* : the deep depression in the proximal end of the ulna by which the ulna articulates with the trochlea of the humerus at the elbow — called also *semilunar notch, sigmoid notch*

trochlear nucleus *n* : a nucleus situated behind the oculomotor nucleus on the dorsal surface of a medial longitudinal fasciculus near the midline that is the source of the motor fibers of the trochlear nerve

tro·choid \'trō-,kóid\ *n* : PIVOT JOINT

tro·glit·a·zone \trō-'glit-ə-,zōn\ *n* : a thiazolidine derivative $C_{24}H_{27}NO_5S$ formerly used to treat type 2 diabetes but now withdrawn from use because of its link to serious hepatic reactions

Trog·lo·tre·ma \,träg-lə-'trē-mə\ *n* : a genus that is the type genus of the family Troglotrematidae and includes small spiny egg-shaped digenetic trematodes including one (*T. salmincola*) that transmits the causative agent of salmon poisoning

Trog·lo·tre·mat·i·dae \,träg-lə-trə-'mat-ə-,dē\ *n pl* : a small family of trematode worms that are parasitic chiefly in mammals — see PARAGONIMUS, TROGLOTREMA

tro·land \'trō-lənd\ *n* : PHOTON 1

Troland, Leonard Thompson (1889–1932), American psychologist and physicist. Troland was a university instructor of psychology and a practical engineer. He devised most of the photographic and mechanical apparatus for color motion pictures. In 1922 he wrote a monograph summarizing the current state of visual science. In 1929 and 1930 he published a major two-volume treatise on the principles of psychophysiology.

tro·le·an·do·my·cin \,trō-lē-,an-də-'mīs-³n\ *n* : an orally administered antibacterial drug $C_{41}H_{67}NO_{15}$ that is the triacetate ester derivative of oleandomycin used chiefly against bacteria of the genus *Streptococcus* (esp. *S. pneumoniae* and *S. pyogenes*) — called also *triacetyloleandomycin*

trol·ley *also* **trol·ly** \'träl-ē\ *n, pl* **trolleys** *also* **trollies** *Brit* : GURNEY

trol·ni·trate \,träl-'nī-,trāt\ *n* : an organic nitrate with vasodilator activity that is used in the form of its diphosphate salt $C_6H_{12}N_4O_9\cdot2H_3PO_4$ to prevent or ameliorate attacks of angina pectoris

Trom·bic·u·la \träm-'bik-yə-lə\ *n* : a genus of mites that is the type genus of the family Trombiculidae and that contains some forms which transmit tsutsugamushi disease in Asia

Trom·bi·cu·li·dae \,träm-bə-'kyü-lə-,dē\ *n pl* : a large and widely distributed family of mites whose nymphs and adults feed on early stages of small arthropods but whose larvae include the chiggers and are parasites on terrestrial vertebrates including humans — **trom·bic·u·lid** \träm-'bik-yə-ləd\ *adj or n*

Trom·bi·di·idae \,träm-bə-'dī-ə-,dē\ *n pl* : a family of mites that now includes only forms that feed in all stages on other arthropods but formerly included mites whose larvae are chiggers and which are now included in the family Trombiculidae — **trom·bid·i·id** \-'bid-ē-əd\ *adj or n*

Trom·bid·i·um \träm-'bid-ē-əm\ *n* : a genus of mites that is the type genus of the family Trombidiidae and formerly included mites whose larvae are chiggers and which are now included in the family Trombiculidae

tro·meth·a·mine \trō-'meth-ə-,mēn\ *n* : TRIS

tro·pa·co·caine \,trō-pə-kō-'kān\ *n* : a crystalline alkaloid $C_{15}H_{19}NO_2$ that is obtained from coca leaves grown esp. in Java or made synthetically, that is the ester of pseudotropine and benzoic acid, and that acts like cocaine but is about one-half as toxic

tro·pane \'trō-,pān\ *n* : a bicyclic tertiary amine $C_8H_{15}N$ that is the parent compound of atropine, cocaine, and related alkaloids

tropane alkaloid *n* : any of a large group of alkaloids (as cocaine, atropine, hyoscyamine, and scopolamine) that can be derived from ornithine

tro·pate \'trō-,pāt\ *n* : a salt or ester of tropic acid

tro·pe·ine \'trō-pē-,ēn, -ən\ *n* : any of a series of crystalline basic esters of tropine; *esp* : such an ester made synthetically

troph·ec·to·derm \,trōf-'ek-tə-,dərm\ *n* : TROPHOBLAST; *esp* : the outer layer of the mammalian blastocyst after differentiation of the ectoderm, mesoderm, and endoderm when the outer layer is continuous with the ectoderm of the embryo

troph·ede·ma *or chiefly Brit* **troph·oe·de·ma** \,trōf-i-'dē-mə\

n, pl **-mas** *also* **-ma·ta** \-mət-ə\ : chronic edema of the legs and feet caused by inadequate or faulty nutrition

tro·phic \'trō-fik\ *adj* **1** : of or relating to nutrition : NUTRI-TIONAL ⟨∼ disorders⟩ **2** : TROPIC **3** : promoting cellular growth, differentiation, and survival ⟨nerve growth factor is a ∼ agent⟩ — **tro·phi·cal·ly** \-fi-k(ə-)lē\ *adv*

trophic ulcer *n* : an ulcer (as a bedsore) caused by faulty nutrition in the affected part

tro·pho·blast \'trō-fə-ˌblast\ *n* : the outer layer of the mammalian blastocyst that supplies nutrition to the embryo, facilitates implantation by eroding away the tissues of the uterus with which it comes in contact allowing the blastocyst to sink into the cavity formed in the uterine wall, and differentiates into the extraembryonic membranes surrounding the embryo — called also *trophoderm* — **tro·pho·blas·tic** \ˌtrō-fə-'blas-tik\ *adj*

tro·pho·chro·ma·tin \ˌtrō-fō-'krō-mət-ən\ *n* : chromatin in some protozoans that is held to be concerned with vegetative functions only

troph·o·derm \'trō-fə-ˌdərm\ *n* : TROPHOBLAST

trophoedema *chiefly Brit var of* TROPHEDEMA

tro·phol·o·gy \trō-'fäl-ə-jē\ *n, pl* **-gies** : a branch of science dealing with nutrition

tro·pho·neu·ro·sis \ˌtrō-fō-n(y)ù-'rō-səs\ *n, pl* **-ro·ses** \-ˌsēz\ : a functional disease of a part due to failure of nutrition from defective nerve action in the parts involved

tro·pho·neu·rot·ic \-n(y)ù-'rät-ik\ *adj* : of, relating to, constituting, or affected by a trophoneurosis ⟨∼ blisters⟩

tro·pho·nu·cle·us \ˌtrō-fō-'n(y)ü-klē-əs\ *n* : MACRONUCLE-US

tro·pho·plasm \'trō-fə-ˌplaz-əm\ *n* : apparently relatively undifferentiated protoplasm once held to be nutritive in function — **tro·pho·plas·mic** \ˌtrō-fə-'plaz-mik\ *adj*

tro·pho·zo·ite \ˌtrō-fə-'zō-ˌīt\ *n* : a protozoan of a vegetative form as distinguished from one of a reproductive or resting form

tro·pia \'trō-pē-ə\ *n* : deviation of an eye from the normal position with respect to the line of vision when the eyes are open : STRABISMUS — see ESOTROPIA, HYPERTROPIA

tro·pic \'trō-pik\ *adj* **1** : of, relating to, or characteristic of tropism or of a tropism **2** *of a hormone* : influencing the activity of a specified gland

trop·ic acid \ˌträp-ik-\ *n* : a crystalline acid $C_9H_{10}O_3$ obtained by hydrolysis of atropine

trop·i·cal disease \'träp-i-kəl-\ *n* : a disease that is indigenous to and may be endemic in a tropical area but may also occur in sporadic or epidemic form in areas that are not tropical

tropical horse tick *n* : an ixodid tick (*Anocenter nitens* syn. *Dermacentor nitens*) that is common in the American tropics, has been found in southern Texas and in Florida, and transmits a causative agent (*Babesia caballi*) of equine babesiosis

tropical medicine *n* : a branch of medicine dealing with tropical diseases and other medical problems of tropical regions

tropical oil *n* : any of several oils (as coconut oil and palm oil) of tropical origin that are high in saturated fatty acids and are used esp. in commercially prepared baked goods, snack products, and confections

tropical rat mite *n* : a widely distributed mite (*Ornithonyssus bacoti* of the family Macronyssidae) that is primarily a parasite of rodents but sometimes bites humans causing painful itching and irritation and that has been implicated as a vector or potential vector of various diseases

tropical sprue *n* : SPRUE 2

tropical ulcer *n* : a chronic sloughing sore of unknown cause occurring usu. on the legs and prevalent in wet tropical regions

tro·pic·amide \trə-'pik-ə-ˌmīd\ *n* : a synthetic anticholinergic $C_{17}H_{20}N_2O_2$ used esp. to dilate pupils in ophthalmological examinations — see MYDRIACYL

tropicus — see LICHEN TROPICUS

tro·pine \'trō-ˌpēn\ *n* : a poisonous hygroscopic crystalline

heterocyclic amino alcohol $C_8H_{15}NO$ derived from tropane and obtained by hydrolysis of atropine and other solanaceous alkaloids or by synthesis

tro·pism \'trō-ˌpiz-əm\ *n* : involuntary orientation by an organism or one of its parts that involves turning or curving by movement or by differential growth and is a positive or negative response to a source of stimulation; *also* : a reflex reaction involving a tropism — **tro·pis·tic** \trō-'pis-tik\ *adj*

tro·po·col·la·gen \ˌträp-ə-'käl-ə-jən, ˌtrōp-\ *n* : a subunit of collagen fibrils consisting of three polypeptide strands arranged in a helix

tro·po·my·o·sin \ˌträp-ə-'mī-ə-sən, ˌtrōp-\ *n* : a protein of muscle that forms a complex with troponin regulating the interaction of actin and myosin in muscular contraction

tro·po·nin \'trōp-ə-nən, 'träp-, -ˌnin\ *n* : a protein of muscle that together with tropomyosin forms a regulatory protein complex controlling the interaction of actin and myosin and that when combined with calcium ions permits muscular contraction

trough — see GINGIVAL TROUGH

troy \'tròi\ *adj* : expressed in troy weight ⟨a ∼ ounce⟩

troy pound *n* : POUND a

troy weight *n* : a series of units of weight based on a pound of 12 ounces and an ounce of 480 grains or 31.103 grams

Trp *abbr* tryptophan; tryptophanyl

true bug \'trü-\ *n* : BUG 1c

true conjugate *n* : CONJUGATE DIAMETER

true fly *n* : FLY 2a

true pelvis *n* : the lower more contracted part of the pelvic cavity — called also *true pelvic cavity;* compare FALSE PELVIS

true rib *n* : any of the ribs having costal cartilages connected directly with the sternum and in humans constituting the first seven pairs — called also *vertebrosternal rib*

true vocal cords *n pl* : the lower pair of vocal cords each of which encloses a vocal ligament, extends from the inner surface of one side of the thyroid cartilage near the median line to a process of the corresponding arytenoid cartilage on the same side of the larynx, and when drawn taut, approximated to the contralateral member of the pair, and subjected to a flow of breath produces the voice — called also *inferior vocal cords, vocal folds*

trun·cal \'trən-kəl\ *adj* : of or relating to the trunk of the body or of a bodily part (as a nerve) ⟨∼ obesity⟩

trun·cus \'trən-kəs\ *n* : TRUNK 2

truncus ar·te·ri·o·sus \-ˌär-ˌtir-ē-'ō-səs\ *n* : the part of the embryonic arterial system which develops into the ascending aorta and the pulmonary trunk

truncus bra·chio·ce·phal·i·cus \-ˌbrā-kē-(ˌ)ō-se-'fal-i-kəs\ *n* : BRACHIOCEPHALIC ARTERY

truncus ce·li·a·cus \-se-'lī-ə-kəs\ *n* : CELIAC ARTERY

trunk \'trəŋk\ *n* **1** : the human body apart from the head and appendages : TORSO **2** : the main body of an anatomical part (as a nerve or blood vessel) that divides into branches

truss \'trəs\ *n* : a device worn to reduce a hernia by pressure

truth drug \'trüth-\ *n* : TRUTH SERUM

truth serum *n* : a hypnotic or anesthetic (as thiopental) held to induce a subject under questioning to talk freely

Try *abbr* tryptophan

tryp·an blue \'trip-ən-\ *n* : a teratogenic disazo dye $C_{34}H_{24}N_6Na_4O_{14}S_4$ used as an intravital stain and esp. formerly as a trypanocide

try·pano·ci·dal \tri-ˌpan-ə-'sīd-ᵊl\ *adj* : destroying trypanosomes ⟨∼ antibodies⟩ ⟨a ∼ drug⟩

try·pano·cide \tri-'pan-ə-ˌsīd\ *n* : a trypanocidal agent

try·pano·so·ma \tri-ˌpan-ə-'sō-mə\ *n* **1** *cap* : the type genus of the family Trypanosomatidae comprising kinetoplastid flagellates that as adults are elongated and somewhat spindle-shaped, have a posteriorly arising flagellum which passes forward at the margin of an undulating membrane and emerges near the anterior end of the body as a short free flagellum, and are parasitic in the blood or rarely the tissues of vertebrates, that following development in the digestive tract of a blood-sucking invertebrate and usu. an insect pass ultimately to the mouthparts or salivary structures where they may be transmitted into a new vertebrate host bitten by the invertebrate host, and that are responsible for various serious diseases (as Chagas' disease, dourine, nagana, sleeping sickness, and surra) of humans and domestic animals **2** pl **-mas** or **-ma·ta** \-mət-ə\ : TRYPANOSOME

try·pano·so·mal \-məl\ adj : of, relating to, caused by, or being flagellates of the genus Trypanosoma ⟨a ∼ infection⟩

Try·pano·so·mat·i·dae \tri-ˌpan-ə-sō-ˈmat-ə-ˌdē\ n pl : a family of strictly parasitic more or less slender and elongated uniflagellate protozoans of the order Kinetoplastida that includes serious pathogens of humans and domestic animals

try·pano·some \tri-ˈpan-ə-ˌsōm\ n : any flagellate of the genus Trypanosoma

try·pano·so·mi·a·sis \tri-ˌpan-ə-sə-ˈmī-ə-səs\ n, pl **-a·ses** \-ˌsēz\ : infection with or disease (as African sleeping sickness or Chagas' disease) caused by flagellates of the genus Trypanosoma

trypan red n : a disazo dye $C_{32}H_{19}N_6Na_5O_{15}S_5$ formerly used in the treatment of trypanosomiasis

tryp·ars·amide \trip-ˈär-sə-ˌmīd\ n : an organic arsenical $C_8H_{10}AsN_2O_4Na·½H_2O$ used in the treatment of African sleeping sickness and syphilis

trypo·mas·ti·gote \ˌtrip-ə-ˈmas-ti-ˌgōt\ n : any flagellate of the family Trypanosomatidae that has the typical form of a mature blood trypanosome

tryp·sin \ˈtrip-sən\ n **1** : a crystallizable proteolytic enzyme that differs from pepsin in several ways (as in being most active in a slightly alkaline medium and in hydrolyzing esters as well as amides) and that is produced and secreted in the pancreatic juice in the form of inactive trypsinogen and activated in the intestine — compare CHYMOTRYPSIN **2** : a preparation from the pancreatic juice differing from pancreatin in containing principally proteolytic enzymes and used chiefly as a digestive and lytic agent

tryp·sin·ize or Brit **tryp·sin·ise** \ˈtrip-sə-ˌnīz\ vt **-ized** or Brit **-ised; -iz·ing** or Brit **-is·ing** : to subject to the action of trypsin ⟨trypsinized tissue cells⟩ — **tryp·sin·iza·tion** or Brit **tryp·sin·isa·tion** \ˌtrip-sə-nə-ˈzā-shən\ n

tryp·sin·o·gen \trip-ˈsin-ə-jən\ n : the inactive substance released by the pancreas into the duodenum to form trypsin

tryp·amine \ˈtrip-tə-ˌmēn\ n : a crystalline amine $C_{10}H_{12}N_2$ derived from tryptophan; also : any of various substituted derivatives of this amine of which some are significantly hallucinogenic or neurotoxic

tryp·tase \ˈtrip-ˌtās, -ˌtāz\ n : a protease of human mast cells that has been implicated as a pathological mediator of numerous allergic and inflammatory conditions (as asthma, rhinitis, and conjunctivitis)

tryp·tic \ˈtrip-tik\ adj : of, relating to, or produced by trypsin or its action ⟨∼ digestion⟩

tryp·to·phan \ˈtrip-tə-ˌfan\ also **tryp·to·phane** \-ˌfān\ n : a crystalline essential amino acid $C_{11}H_{12}N_2O_2$ that is widely distributed in proteins — abbr. Trp

L–tryptophan — see entry alphabetized in the letter l

tryp·to·pha·nase \ˈtrip-tə-fə-ˌnās, trip-ˈtäf-ə-, -ˌnāz\ n : an enzyme that catalyzes the decomposition of tryptophan into indole, pyruvic acid, and ammonia

tryp·to·pha·nyl \ˌtrip-tə-ˈfān-ᵊl\ n : the amino acid radical or residue $(C_8H_6N)CH_2CH(NH_2)CO-$ of tryptophan — abbr. Trp

TS abbr Tourette's syndrome; Tourette syndrome

TSA abbr Tourette Syndrome Association

TSE abbr transmissible spongiform encephalopathy

tset·se \ˈt(s)et-sē, ˈt(s)ēt-, ˈset-, ˈsēt-\ n, pl **tsetse** or **tset·ses** : TSETSE FLY

tsetse fly n : any of several dipteran flies of the genus Glossina that occur in sub-Saharan Africa and include vectors of human and animal trypanosomes (as those causing sleeping sickness and nagana) — called also tsetse

TSH \ˌtē-ˌes-ˈāch\ n : THYROID-STIMULATING HORMONE

TSS abbr toxic shock syndrome

T suppressor cell n : SUPPRESSOR T CELL

tsu·tsu·ga·mu·shi disease \ˌ(t)süt-sə-gə-ˈmü-shē-, ˌtüt-, -ˈgäm-ù-shē-\ n : an acute febrile bacterial disease that is caused by a rickettsial bacterium (Rickettsia tsutsugamushi) transmitted by mite larvae, resembles louse-borne typhus, and is widespread in the western Pacific area — called also scrub typhus, tsutsugamushi

T system \ˈtē-\ n : the system of T tubules in striated muscle

T3 or **T₃** \ˌtē-ˈthrē\ n : TRIIODOTHYRONINE

TTP \ˌtē-ˌtē-ˈpē\ n : THROMBOTIC THROMBOCYTOPENIC PURPURA

T–tube \ˈtē-\ n : a narrow flexible tube in the form of a T that is used for drainage esp. of the common bile duct

T tubule n : any of the small tubules which run transversely through a striated muscle fiber and through which electrical impulses are transmitted from the sarcoplasm to the fiber's interior

tub·al \ˈt(y)ü-bəl\ adj : of, relating to, or involving a tube and esp. a fallopian tube ⟨∼ lumens⟩ ⟨a ∼ infection⟩

tubal abortion n : an aborted tubal pregnancy

tubal ligation n : ligation of the fallopian tubes that by preventing passage of ova from the ovaries to the uterus serves as a method of female sterilization

tubal pregnancy n : ectopic pregnancy in a fallopian tube

tubarius — see TORUS TUBARIUS

¹tube \ˈt(y)üb\ n **1** : a slender channel within a plant or animal body : DUCT — see BRONCHIAL TUBE, EUSTACHIAN TUBE, FALLOPIAN TUBE **2 a** : an often complex piece of laboratory or technical apparatus usu. of glass and commonly serving to isolate or convey a product of reaction ⟨a distillation ∼⟩ **b** : TEST TUBE **3** : a soft tubular container whose contents (as toothpaste) can be dispensed by squeezing **4** : a hollow cylindrical device (as a cannula) used for insertion into bodily passages or hollow organs for removal or injection of materials

²tube vt **tubed; tub·ing** : to furnish with, enclose in, or pass through a tube ⟨the patient is then anesthetized . . . and tubed —Anesthesia Digest⟩

tu·bec·to·my \t(y)ü-ˈbek-tə-mē\ n, pl **-mies** : surgical excision of a fallopian tube

tube curare n : curare from a So. American vine (Chondrodendron tomentosum of the family Menispermaceae) that is a source of tubocurarine

tubed adj : having the sides sewn together so as to form a tube ⟨a ∼ pedicle flap⟩

tu·ber \ˈt(y)ü-bər\ n : an anatomical prominence : TUBEROSITY

tuberalis — see PARS TUBERALIS

tuber ci·ne·re·um \-si-ˈnir-ē-əm\ n : an eminence of gray matter which lies on the lower surface of the brain between the optic tracts and in front of the mammillary bodies and of which the upper surface forms part of the floor of the third ventricle and the lower surface bears the infundibulum to which the pituitary gland is attached

tu·ber·cle \ˈt(y)ü-bər-kəl\ n **1** : a small knobby prominence or excrescence: as **a** : a prominence on the crown of a molar tooth **b** : a small rough prominence (as the greater tubercle or adductor tubercle) on a bone usu. being smaller than a tuberosity and serving for the attachment of one or more muscles or ligaments **c** : an eminence near the head of a rib that articulates with the transverse process of a vertebra **d** : any of several prominences (as the acoustic tubercle) in the central nervous system that mark the nuclei of various nerves **2** : a small discrete lump in the substance of an organ or in the skin; esp : the specific lesion of tuberculosis consisting of a packed mass of epithelioid cells, giant cells, disintegration products of white blood cells and bacilli, and usu. a necrotic center

tubercle bacillus n : a bacterium of the genus Mycobacterium (M. tuberculosis) that causes tuberculosis in humans; also

\ə\ abut \ᵊ\ kitten \ər\ further \a\ ash \ā\ ace \ä\ cot, cart \aù\ out \ch\ chin \e\ bet \ē\ easy \g\ go \i\ hit \ī\ ice \j\ job \ŋ\ sing \ō\ go \ò\ law \òi\ boy \th\ thin \t̲h̲\ the \ü\ loot \ù\ foot \y\ yet \zh\ vision See also Pronunciation Symbols page

S
T

: a related mycobacterium (*M. bovis*) that causes tuberculosis in cattle and sometimes humans esp. in underdeveloped countries

tubercle of Ca·ra·bel·li \-ˌkä-rä-ˈbel-ē\ *n* : a fifth cusp sometimes found on the lingual surface of the upper second deciduous molars and the upper first permanent molars
  Carabelli, Georg (1787–1842), Hungarian dentist. Carabelli was a professor of dental surgery in Vienna. The tubercle of Carabelli was first illustrated in his text of oral anatomy, published in 1842, and was first described in writing in his handbook of dentistry, published posthumously in 1844.

tubercle of Ro·lan·do \-rō-ˈlän-(ˌ)dō\ *n* : TUBER CINEREUM
  L. Rolando — see FISSURE OF ROLANDO

tubercula *pl of* TUBERCULUM

¹tu·ber·cu·lar \t(y)ù-ˈbər-kyə-lər\ *adj* **1 a** : of, relating to, or affected with tuberculosis : TUBERCULOUS **b** : caused by the tubercle bacillus ⟨∼ meningitis⟩ **2** : characterized by lesions that are or resemble tubercles **3** : relating to, resembling, or constituting a tubercle : TUBERCULATED

²tubercular *n* : an individual affected with tuberculosis

tu·ber·cu·lat·ed \t(y)ù-ˈbər-kyə-ˌlāt-əd\ *also* **tu·ber·cu·late** \-lət\ *adj* : having tubercles : characterized by or beset with tubercles

tu·ber·cu·la·tion \t(y)ù-ˌbər-kyə-ˈlā-shən\ *n* : formation of or affection with tubercles

tu·ber·cu·lid \t(y)ù-ˈbər-kyə-ləd\ *also* **tu·ber·cu·lide** \-kyə-ˌlīd\ *n* : a tuberculous lesion of the skin; *esp* : one that is an id

tu·ber·cu·lin \t(y)ù-ˈbər-kyə-lən\ *n* : a sterile solution containing the growth products of or specific substances extracted from the tubercle bacillus and used in the diagnosis of tuberculosis — see OLD TUBERCULIN, PURIFIED PROTEIN DERIVATIVE

tuberculin reaction *n* : a skin reaction that occurs at the site of a tuberculin test ⟨an induration measuring 10 mm or more is considered a positive *tuberculin reaction* for all individuals⟩

tuberculin test *n* : a test (as the Mantoux test or tine test) for hypersensitivity to tuberculin in which tuberculin is introduced (as by injection or puncture) usu. into the skin of the individual tested and the appearance of inflammation or induration at the site of introduction is construed as indicating past or present tubercular infection — called also *tuberculin skin test*

tu·ber·cu·lo·cid·al \t(y)ù-ˌbər-kyə-lō-ˈsīd-ᵊl\ *adj* : destroying tubercle bacilli

tu·ber·cu·lo·derm \t(y)ù-ˈbər-kyə-lə-ˌdərm\ *n* : a tuberculous lesion of the skin

tu·ber·cu·loid \t(y)ù-ˈbər-kyə-ˌlȯid\ *adj* **1** : resembling tuberculosis and esp. the tubercles characteristic of it **2** : of, relating to, characterized by, or affected with tuberculoid leprosy

tuberculoid leprosy *n* : the one of the two major forms of leprosy that is characterized by the presence of few or no Hansen's bacilli in the lesions, by the loss of sensation in affected areas of the skin, and by a positive skin reaction to lepromin and that is usu. not infectious to others — compare LEPROMATOUS LEPROSY

tu·ber·cu·lo·ma \t(y)ù-ˌbər-kyə-ˈlō-mə\ *n, pl* **-mas** *also* **-ma·ta** \-mət-ə\ : a large solitary caseous tubercle of tuberculous character occurring esp. in the brain

tu·ber·cu·lo·pro·tein \t(y)ù-ˌbər-kyə-lō-ˈprō-ˌtēn, -ˈprōt-ē-ən\ *n* : protein occurring in or obtained from the tubercle bacillus

tu·ber·cu·lo·sis \t(y)ù-ˌbər-kyə-ˈlō-səs\ *n, pl* **-lo·ses** \-ˌsēz\ : a usu. chronic highly variable disease that is caused by a bacterium of the genus *Mycobacterium* (*M. tuberculosis*) and rarely in the U.S. by a related mycobacterium (*M. bovis*), is usu. communicated by inhalation of the airborne causative agent, affects esp. the lungs but may spread to other areas (as the kidney or spinal column) from local lesions or by way of the lymph or blood vessels, and is characterized by fever, cough, difficulty in breathing, inflammatory infiltrations, formation of tubercles, caseation, pleural effusion, and fibrosis — called also *TB*

¹tu·ber·cu·lo·stat·ic \t(y)ù-ˌbər-kyə-lō-ˈstat-ik\ *adj* : inhibiting the growth of the tubercle bacillus ⟨a ∼ drug⟩

²tuberculostatic *n* : a tuberculostatic agent

tu·ber·cu·lo·stea·ric acid \t(y)ù-ˌbər-kyə-(ˌ)lō-stē-ˌär-ik-, -ˌsti(ə)r-ik-\ *n* : a fatty acid $C_{19}H_{38}O_2$ obtained from the wax of tubercle bacilli

tu·ber·cu·lous \t(y)ù-ˈbər-kyə-ləs\ *adj* **1** : constituting or affected with tuberculosis ⟨a ∼ process⟩ ⟨a ∼ patient⟩ **2** : caused by or resulting from the presence or products of the tubercle bacillus ⟨∼ peritonitis⟩

tu·ber·cu·lum \t(y)ù-ˈbər-kyə-ləm\ *n, pl* **-la** \-lə\ : TUBERCLE

tuberculum im·par \-ˈim-ˌpär\ *n* : an embryonic swelling that is situated in the midline of the floor of the pharynx between the ventral ends of the two sides of the mandibular arch and of the second branchial arch and that prob. contributes to the formation of the anterior part of the tongue

tu·ber·os·i·ty \ˌt(y)ü-bə-ˈräs-ət-ē\ *n, pl* **-ties** : a rounded prominence; *esp* : a large prominence on a bone usu. serving for the attachment of muscles or ligaments

tu·ber·ous \ˈt(y)ü-b(ə-)rəs\ *adj* : characterized by or being knobby or nodular lesions ⟨∼ xanthomas on the knees⟩

tuberous sclerosis *n* : an inherited disorder of the skin and nervous system that is characterized typically by epilepsy and mental retardation, by a rash of the face resembling acne, and by multiple noncancerous tumors of the brain, kidney, retina, and heart and that is controlled by an autosomal dominant gene maintained in human populations by a high mutation rate — called also *epiloia*

tu·bo·cu·ra·rine \ˌt(y)ü-bō-kyù-ˈrär-ən, -ˌēn\ *n* : a toxic alkaloid that is obtained chiefly from the bark and stems of a So. American vine (*Chondrodendron tomentosum* of the family Menispermaceae), that in its dextrorotatory form constitutes the chief active constituent of curare, and that is used in the form of its hydrated hydrochloride $C_{37}H_{41}ClN_2O_6 \cdot HCl \cdot 5H_2O$ esp. as a skeletal muscle relaxant

tu·bo–ovar·i·an \ˌt(y)ü-bō-ō-ˈvar-ē-ən, -ˈver-\ *adj* : of, relating to, or affecting a fallopian tube and ovary ⟨a ∼ abscess⟩

tu·bo·uter·ine \ˌt(y)ü-bō-ˈyüt-ə-ˌrīn, -rən\ *n* : of or relating to the uterus and a fallopian tube

tu·bu·lar \ˈt(y)ü-byə-lər\ *adj* **1** : having the form of or consisting of a tube **2** : of, relating to, or sounding as if produced through a tube or tubule ⟨∼ rales⟩

tu·bule \ˈt(y)ü-(ˌ)byü(ə)l\ *n* : a small tube; *esp* : a slender elongated anatomical channel

tu·bu·lin \ˈt(y)ü-byə-lən\ *n* : a globular protein that polymerizes to form microtubules

tu·bu·lo·ac·i·nar \ˌt(y)ü-byə-lō-ˈas-ə-nər\ *or* **tu·bu·lo·ac·i·nous** \-nəs\ *adj* : TUBULOALVEOLAR

tu·bu·lo·al·ve·o·lar \ˌt(y)ü-byə-lō-al-ˈvē-ə-lər\ *adj* : of, relating to, or being a gland having branching tubules which end in secretory alveoli ⟨Cowper's gland is ∼⟩

tu·bu·lo·in·ter·stit·ial \-ˌint-ər-ˈstish-əl\ *adj* : affecting or involving the tubules and interstitial tissue of the kidney

tu·bu·lus \ˈt(y)ü-byə-ləs\ *n, pl* **tu·bu·li** \-yə-ˌlī\ : TUBULE

tuck \ˈtək\ *n* : a cosmetic surgical operation for the removal of excess skin or fat from a body part — see TUMMY TUCK

tuft \ˈtəft\ *n* **1** : a small cluster of elongated flexible outgrowths or parts attached or close together at the base and free at the opposite ends; *esp* : a small bunch of hairs on the body **2** : a branching anatomical structure that resembles a tuft

tug — see TRACHEAL TUG

Tu·i·nal \ˈtü-i-ˌnäl\ *trademark* — used for a preparation of amobarbital and secobarbital

tu·la·re·mia *or chiefly Brit* **tu·la·rae·mia** \ˌt(y)ü-lə-ˈrē-mē-ə\ *n* : an infectious disease esp. of wild rabbits, rodents, humans, and some domestic animals that is caused by a bacterium (*Francisella tularensis*), is transmitted esp. by the bites of insects, and in humans is marked by symptoms (as fever) of toxemia — called also *rabbit fever* — **tu·la·re·mic** *or chiefly Brit* **tu·la·rae·mic** \-mik\ *adj*

tulle gras \ˌtül-ˈgrä\ *n* : fine-meshed gauze impregnated with a fatty substance (as vegetable oil or soft paraffin) and used in medicine as an application to raw surfaces

tum·bu fly \\'tùm-ˌbü-\ *n* : an African fly (*Cordylobia anthropophaga*) of the family Calliphoridae whose larvae are subcutaneous parasites in various mammals and sometimes in humans

tu·me·fa·cient \ˌt(y)ü-mə-'fā-shənt\ *adj* : producing swelling

tu·me·fac·tion \-'fak-shən\ *n* **1** : an action or process of swelling or becoming tumorous **2** : SWELLING ⟨benign ∼s⟩

tu·me·fac·tive \-'fak-tiv\ *adj* : producing swelling

tumeric *var of* TURMERIC

tu·mes·cence \t(y)ü-'mes-ᵊn(t)s\ *n* : the quality or state of being tumescent; *esp* : readiness for sexual activity marked esp. by vascular congestion of the sex organs

tu·mes·cent \-'mes-ᵊnt\ *adj* : somewhat swollen ⟨∼ tissue⟩

tu·mid \'t(y)ü-məd\ *adj* : marked by swelling : SWOLLEN ⟨an infected ∼ leg⟩ — **tu·mid·i·ty** \t(y)ü-'mid-ət-ē\ *n, pl* **-ties**

tum·my tuck \'təm-ē-\ *n* : ABDOMINOPLASTY

tu·mor *or chiefly Brit* **tu·mour** \'t(y)ü-mər\ *n* : an abnormal benign or malignant new growth of tissue that possesses no physiological function and arises from uncontrolled usu. rapid cellular proliferation — see CANCER 1, CARCINOMA, SARCOMA — **tu·mor·like** \-ˌlīk\ *adj*

tu·mor·al \'t(y)ü-mə-rəl\ *adj* : of, relating to, or constituting a tumor ⟨a ∼ mass⟩ ⟨a ∼ syndrome⟩

tu·mor·i·cid·al \ˌt(y)ü-mə-rə-'sīd-ᵊl\ *adj* : destroying tumor cells ⟨∼ activity⟩ ⟨∼ macrophages⟩

tu·mor·i·gen·e·sis \-'jen-ə-səs\ *n, pl* **-e·ses** \-ˌsēz\ : the formation of tumors

tu·mor·i·gen·ic \-'jen-ik\ *adj* : producing or tending to produce tumors; *also* : CARCINOGENIC — **tu·mor·i·ge·nic·i·ty** \-jə-'nis-ət-ē\ *n, pl* **-ties**

tumor–infiltrating lymphocyte *n* : a T cell that is isolated from a malignant tumor, cultured with interleukin-2, and injected back into the patient as a tumor-killing cell and that has greater cytotoxicity than lymphokine-activated killer cells — called also *TIL*

tumor necrosis factor *n* : a protein that is produced chiefly by monocytes and macrophages in response esp. to endotoxins, that mediates inflammation, and that induces the destruction of some tumor cells and the activation of white blood cells — abbr. *TNF*

tu·mor·ous \'t(y)üm-(ə-)rəs\ *adj* : of, relating to, or resembling a tumor ⟨a ∼ disease⟩

tumor suppressor gene *n* : any of a class of genes (as p53) that act in normal cells to inhibit unrestrained cell division and that when inactivated (as by mutation) place the cell at increased risk for malignant proliferation — called also *antioncogene*

tumor virus *n* : a virus (as Rous sarcoma virus) that causes neoplastic or cancerous growth

tumour *chiefly Brit var of* TUMOR

Tums \'təmz\ *trademark* — used for an antacid tablet containing calcium carbonate

Tun·ga \'təŋ-gə\ *n* : a genus of fleas (family Tungidae) that have conspicuous mouthparts, that lack or have very small setae on the head, and that include the chigoe (*T. penetrans*)

tung·sten \'təŋ-stən\ *n* : a gray-white heavy high-melting ductile hard polyvalent metallic element that resembles chromium and molybdenum in many of its properties and is used esp. for electrical purposes and in hardening alloys (as steel) — symbol *W*; called also *wolfram*; see ELEMENT table

tung·stic acid \ˌtəŋ-stik-\ *n* : a yellow crystalline powder WO_3 that is the trioxide of tungsten; *also* : an acid (as H_2WO_4) derived from this trioxide

tu·nic \'t(y)ü-nik\ *n* : an enclosing or covering membrane or tissue : TUNICA ⟨the ∼s of the eye⟩

tu·ni·ca \'t(y)ü-ni-kə\ *n, pl* **tu·ni·cae** \-nə-ˌkē, -ˌkī, -ˌsē\ : an enveloping membrane or layer of body tissue

tunica adventitia *n* : ADVENTITIA

tunica albuginea *n, pl* **tunicae albugineae** : a white fibrous capsule esp. of the testis

tunica ex·ter·na \-ek-'stər-nə\ *n* : ADVENTITIA

tunica fi·bro·sa \-fī-'brō-sə\ *n* : a fibrous or connective tissue capsule or coat (as of the kidney)

tunica intima *n* : INTIMA

tunica media *n* : MEDIA

tunica mucosa *n* : mucous membrane and esp. that lining the digestive tract

tunica muscularis *n* : MUSCULAR COAT

tunica pro·pria \-'prō-prē-ə\ *n* : LAMINA PROPRIA

tunica va·gi·na·lis \-ˌvaj-ə-'nā-ləs, -'nal-əs\ *n, pl* **tunicae va·gi·na·les** \-'nā-(ˌ)lez, -'nal-(ˌ)ēz\ : a pouch of serous membrane covering the testis and derived from the peritoneum

tun·ing fork \'t(y)ün-iŋ-\ *n* : a 2-pronged metal implement that gives a fixed tone when struck

tun·nel \'tən-ᵊl\ *n* : a bodily channel — see CARPAL TUNNEL

tunnel of Cor·ti \-'kȯrt-ē\ *n* : a spiral passage in the organ of Corti

tunnel vision *n* : constriction of the visual field resulting in loss of peripheral vision

tu·ran·ose \'t(y)ù-rə-ˌnōs\ *n* : a crystalline reducing disaccharide sugar $C_{12}H_{22}O_{11}$ obtained by the partial hydrolysis of melezitose

Tur·ba·trix \ˌtər-'bā-triks\ *n* : a genus of small slender nematode worms (family Cephalobidae) including the vinegar eel

Tur·bel·lar·ia \ˌtər-bə-'ler-ē-ə, -'lar-\ *n pl* : a class of the phylum Platyhelminthes comprising flatworms that are mostly aquatic and free-living but occas. live on land or as parasites

tur·bel·lar·i·an \-'ler-ē-ən, -'lar-\ *n* : any flatworm of the class Turbellaria — **turbellarian** *adj*

tur·bid \'tər-bəd\ *adj* : thick or opaque with matter in suspension : cloudy or muddy in appearance ⟨∼ urine⟩

tur·bi·dim·e·ter \ˌtər-bə-'dim-ət-ər\ *n* **1** : an instrument for measuring and comparing the turbidity of liquids by viewing light through them and determining how much light is transmitted **2** : NEPHELOMETER — **tur·bi·di·met·ric** \ˌtər-bəd-ə-'me-trik, ˌtər-ˌbid-ə-\ *adj* — **tur·bi·di·met·ri·cal·ly** \-tri-k(ə-)lē\ *adv*

tur·bi·dim·e·try \-'dim-ə-trē\ *n, pl* **-tries** : the determination and measurement of the concentration of suspended matter in a liquid by use of a turbidimeter

tur·bid·i·ty \ˌtər-'bid-ət-ē\ *n, pl* **-ties** : the quality or state of being turbid

tur·bi·nal \'tər-bən-ᵊl\ *n* : NASAL CONCHA

¹tur·bi·nate \'tər-bə-nət, -ˌnāt\ *adj* : of, relating to, or being a nasal concha

²turbinate *n* : NASAL CONCHA

turbinate bone *also* **tur·bi·nat·ed bone** \'tər-bə-ˌnāt-əd-\ *n* : NASAL CONCHA

tur·bi·nec·to·my \ˌtər-bə-'nek-tə-mē\ *n, pl* **-mies** : surgical excision of a nasal concha

turcica — see SELLA TURCICA

turf toe \'tərf-\ *n* : a minor but painful usu. sports-related injury involving hyperextension of the big toe that results in spraining or tearing of the ligament of the metatarsophalangeal joint

tur·ges·cence \ˌtər-'jes-ᵊn(t)s\ *n* : the quality or state of being turgescent

tur·ges·cent \-'jes-ᵊnt\ *adj* : becoming turgid, distended, or swollen

tur·gid \'tər-jəd\ *adj* : being in a normal or abnormal state of distension : SWOLLEN, TUMID ⟨∼ limbs⟩ ⟨∼ living cells⟩

tur·gid·i·ty \ˌtər-'jid-ət-ē\ *n, pl* **-ties** : the quality or state of being turgid : condition of being swollen ⟨breast ∼⟩

tur·gor \'tər-gər, -ˌgȯ(ə)r\ *n* : the normal state of turgidity and tension in living cells; *esp* : the rigidity of a plant that is due to the pressure of the cell contents against the cell walls and that is lost or greatly diminished in wilting

tu·ris·ta \tù-'rē-stə\ *n* : TRAVELER'S DIARRHEA

tur·mer·ic \'tər-mə-rik\ *also* **tu·mer·ic** \'t(y)ü-mə-\ *n* **1** : an Indian perennial herb (*Curcuma longa*) of the ginger family with a large aromatic yellow rhizome **2** : the cleaned, boiled, dried, and usu. ground rhizome of the turmeric plant

---

\ə\ **abut** \ᵊ\ **kitten** \ər\ **further** \a\ **ash** \ā\ **ace** \ä\ **cot, cart**
\aù\ **out** \ch\ **chin** \e\ **bet** \ē\ **easy** \g\ **go** \i\ **hit** \ī\ **ice** \j\ **job**
\ŋ\ **sing** \ō\ **go** \ȯ\ **law** \ȯi\ **boy** \th\ **thin** \th̲\ **the** \ü\ **loot**
\ù\ **foot** \y\ **yet** \zh\ **vision**   *See also* Pronunciation Symbols page

used as a coloring agent, a condiment, or a stimulant **3** : a yellow to reddish brown dyestuff obtained from turmeric

turn \'tərn\ *vt* : to injure by twisting or wrenching ⟨∼ed his ankle⟩

Tur·ner's syndrome \'tər-nərz-\ *or* **Tur·ner syndrome** \-nər-\ *n* : a genetically determined condition that is typically associated with the presence of only one complete X chromosome and no Y chromosome and with characteristics including a female phenotype, underdeveloped and usu. infertile ovaries, absence of menstrual onset, short stature, excess skin about the neck, cubitus valgus, aortic coarctation, and a low hairline on the back of the neck

    Turner, Henry Hubert (1892–1970), American endocrinologist. Turner practiced internal medicine privately and served as a consulting endocrinologist and chief of a metabolic clinic at a university hospital in Oklahoma. He described Turner's syndrome in 1938.

turn·over \'tər-ˌnō-vər\ *n* : the continuous process of loss and replacement of a constituent (as a neurotransmitter, cell, or tissue) of a living system ⟨protein ∼ in various pathological states —J. C. Waterlow⟩ ⟨hyperthyroidism accelerates bone ∼ and shortens the normal bone remodeling cycle —Richard Sadovsky⟩

turn–sick \'tərn-ˌsik\ *n* : GID

TURP *abbr* transurethral resection of the prostate

tur·pen·tine \'tər-pən-ˌtīn, 'tərp-ᵊm-\ *n* **1 a** : a yellow to brown semifluid oleoresin obtained as an exudate from the terebinth (*Pistacia terebinthus*) of the sumac family **b** : an oleoresin obtained from various conifers (as some pines and firs) **2 a** : an essential oil obtained from turpentines by distillation and used esp. as a solvent and thinner — called also *oil of turpentine* **b** : a similar oil obtained by distillation or carbonization of pinewood — called also *wood turpentine*

tur·ri·ceph·a·ly \ˌtər-ə-'sef-ə-lē, ˌtə-rə-\ *n, pl* **-lies** : OXYCEPHALY

tur·tle \'tərt-ᵊl\ *n, pl* **turtles** *also* **turtle** *often attrib* : any of an order (Testudines) of terrestrial, freshwater, and marine reptiles that have a toothless horny beak and a shell of bony dermal plates usu. covered with horny shields enclosing the trunk and into which the head, limbs, and tail usu. may be withdrawn — called also *chelonian*

tusk \'təsk\ *n* : an elongated greatly enlarged tooth that projects when the mouth is closed and serves for digging food or as a weapon; *broadly* : a long protruding tooth

tus·sal \'təs-əl\ *adj* : of, relating to, or manifested by a cough or coughing ⟨a ∼ attack⟩

tus·sic \'təs-ik\ *adj* : TUSSAL

tus·sis \'təs-əs\ *n* : COUGH

tus·sive \'təs-iv\ *adj* : of, relating to, or involved in coughing

T wave \'tē-ˌwāv\ *n* : the deflection in an electrocardiogram that represents the electrical activity produced by ventricular repolarization — compare P WAVE, QRS COMPLEX

Tween \'twēn\ *trademark* — used for any of several preparations of polysorbates

tween–brain \'twēn-ˌbrān\ *n* : DIENCEPHALON

twee·zers \'twē-zərz\ *n pl but sing or pl in constr* : any of various small metal instruments that are usu. held between the thumb and index finger, are used for plucking, holding, or manipulating, and consist of two legs joined at one end

twelfth cranial nerve \'twelf(t)th-\ *n* : HYPOGLOSSAL NERVE

12–step \'twelv-ˌstep\ *adj* : of, relating to, or characteristic of a program that is designed esp. to help an individual overcome an addiction, compulsion, serious shortcoming, or traumatic experience by adherence to 12 tenets emphasizing personal growth and dependence on a higher spiritual being

twelve–year molar \ˌtwelv-ˌyi(ə)r-\ *n* : any of the second permanent molar teeth which erupt at about 12 years of age and include four of which one is located on each side of the upper and lower jaws — compare SIX-YEAR MOLAR

twen·ty–twen·ty *or* **20/20** \ˌtwent-ē-'twent-ē\ *adj* : having the normal visual acuity of the human eye that according to one common scale can distinguish at a distance of 20 feet characters one-third inch in diameter ⟨∼ vision⟩

twig \'twig\ *n* : a minute branch of a nerve or artery ⟨∼s of sensory nerves in the skin —Lynda Charters⟩

twi·light sleep \'twī-ˌlīt-\ *n* : a state in which awareness of pain is dulled and memory of pain is dimmed or effaced and which is produced by hypodermic injection of morphine and scopolamine and used esp. formerly chiefly in childbirth

twilight state *n* : a dreamy state lacking touch with present reality, occurring in epilepsy, hysteria, and schizophrenia, and sometimes induced with narcotics

twilight vision *n* : SCOTOPIC VISION

¹twin \'twin\ *adj* : born with one other or as a pair at one birth ⟨a ∼ brother⟩ ⟨∼ girls⟩

²twin *n* **1** : either of two offspring produced at a birth **2 twins** *pl* : a group of two offspring born at one birth — **twin·ship** \-ˌship\ *n*

twin disease *n* : PREGNANCY DISEASE

twinge \'twinj\ *n* : a sudden sharp stab of pain

twin–lamb disease \'twin-ˌlam-\ *n* : PREGNANCY DISEASE

twin·ning \'twin-iŋ\ *n* : the bearing of twins

¹twitch \'twich\ *vi* : to undergo a brief spasmodic muscular contraction ⟨the muscle ∼ed⟩

²twitch *n* : a brief spasmodic contraction of muscle fibers; *also* : a slight jerk of a body part caused by such a contraction

³twitch *n* : QUACK GRASS

two–egg \'tü-ˌeg\ *adj* : DIZYGOTIC ⟨∼ twins⟩

2,4–D \ˌtü-ˌfōr-'dē, -ˌfȯr-\ *n* : a white crystalline irritant compound $C_8H_6Cl_2O_3$ used as a weed killer — called also *2,4=dichlorophenoxyacetic acid;* see AGENT ORANGE

2,4,5–T \-ˌfiv-'tē\ *n* : an irritant compound $C_8H_5Cl_3O_3$ used esp. as an herbicide and defoliant — called also *trichlorophenoxyacetic acid;* see AGENT ORANGE

two–winged fly \ˌtü-ˌwiŋ(d)-\ *n* : FLY 2a

Tx *abbr* treatment

ty·ba·mate \'tī-bə-ˌmāt\ *n* : a tranquilizing drug $C_{13}H_{26}N_2O_4$

ty·lec·to·my \tī-'lek-tə-mē\ *n, pl* **-mies** : LUMPECTOMY

Ty·le·nol \'tī-lə-ˌnȯl\ *trademark* — used for a preparation of acetaminophen

ty·lo·sin \'tī-lə-sən\ *n* : an antibacterial antibiotic $C_{45}H_{77}NO_{17}$ from an actinomycete of the genus *Streptomyces* (*S. fradiae*) used in veterinary medicine and as a feed additive

ty·lo·sis \tī-'lō-səs\ *n, pl* **ty·lo·ses** \-'lō-sēz\ : a thickening and hardening of the skin : CALLOSITY

tympani — see CHORDA TYMPANI, SCALA TYMPANI, TEGMEN TYMPANI, TENSOR TYMPANI

tym·pan·ic \tim-'pan-ik\ *adj* : of, relating to, or being a tympanum

tympanic antrum *n* : a large air-containing cavity in the mastoid process communicating with the tympanum and often being the location of dangerous inflammation — called also *mastoid antrum*

tympanic canal *n* : SCALA TYMPANI

tympanic cavity *n* : MIDDLE EAR

tympanic membrane *n* : a thin membrane separating the middle ear from the inner part of the external auditory canal that vibrates in response to sound energy and transmits the resulting mechanical vibrations to the structures of the middle ear — called also *eardrum, tympanum*

tympanic nerve *n* : a branch of the glossopharyngeal nerve arising from the petrosal ganglion and entering the middle ear where it takes part in forming the tympanic plexus — called also *Jacobson's nerve*

tympanic plate *n* : a curved platelike bone that is part of the temporal bone and forms the floor and anterior wall of the external auditory canal

tympanic plexus *n* : a nerve plexus of the middle ear that is formed by the tympanic nerve and two or three filaments from the carotid plexus, sends fibers to the mucous membranes of the middle ear, the eustachian tube, and the mastoid cells, and gives off the lesser petrosal nerve to the otic ganglion

tym·pa·ni·tes \ˌtim-pə-'nīt-ēz\ *n* : a distension of the abdomen caused by accumulation of gas in the intestinal tract or peritoneal cavity

tym·pa·nit·ic \ˌtim-pə-ˈnit-ik\ *adj* **1** : of, relating to, or affected with tympanites ⟨a ∼ abdomen⟩ **2** : resonant on percussion : hollow-sounding

tym·pa·no·plas·ty \ˈtim-pə-nō-ˌplas-tē\ *n, pl* **-ties** : a reparative surgical operation performed on the middle ear

tym·pa·nos·to·my \ˌtim-pə-ˈnäs-tə-mē\ *n, pl* **-mies** MYRINGOTOMY

tym·pa·no·sym·pa·thec·to·my \ˌtim-pə-nō-ˌsim-pə-ˈthek-tə-mē\ *n, pl* **-mies** : surgical excision of the tympanic plexus for relief of tinnitus

tym·pa·not·o·my \ˌtim-pə-ˈnät-ə-mē\ *n, pl* **-mies** : MYRINGOTOMY

tym·pa·num \ˈtim-pə-nəm\ *n, pl* **-na** \-nə\ *also* **-nums** **1** : TYMPANIC MEMBRANE **2** : MIDDLE EAR

tym·pa·ny \-nē\ *n, pl* **-nies** **1** : TYMPANITES **2** : a resonant sound heard in percussion (as of the abdomen)

Tyn·dall beam \ˈtind-ᵊl-\ *n* : the luminous path formed in the Tyndall effect by the breaking up of the entering light by the suspended particles — called also *Tyndall cone*

    Tyndall, John (1820–1893), British physicist. Tyndall was appointed professor of natural philosophy at the Royal Institution in London. He studied the diffusion of light by large molecules and dust. Basing his experiments on the fact that blue light more than any other light color tends to scatter, he demonstrated that the sky's blue color results from the scattering of the sun's rays by dust.

Tyndall effect *n* : the scattering of a beam of light when passed through a medium containing small suspended particles (as smoky or mist-laden air or colloidal solutions) — called also *Tyndall phenomenon*

¹type \ˈtīp\ *n* **1** : a lower taxonomic category selected as a standard of reference for a higher category; *also* : a specimen or series of specimens on which a taxonomic species or subspecies is actually based **2** : the morphological, physiological, or ecological characters by which relationship between organisms may be recognized **3** : a particular kind, class, or group ⟨cell ∼s⟩; *specif* : a group distinguishable on physiological or serological bases ⟨salmonella ∼s⟩

²type *vt* **typed; typ·ing** : to determine the type of (as a sample of blood or a culture of bacteria)

¹type A *adj* : relating to, characteristic of, having, or being a personality that is marked by impatience, aggressiveness, and competitiveness and that has been implicated by some studies as a factor increasing the risk of cardiovascular disease ⟨*type A* behavior⟩

²type A *n* : an individual with a type A personality

¹type B *adj* : relating to, characteristic of, having, or being a personality that is marked by a lack of excessive aggressiveness and tension and that has been implicated by some studies as a factor reducing the risk of cardiovascular disease ⟨*type B* behavior⟩

²type B *n* : an individual with a type B personality

type genus *n* : the genus of a taxonomic family or subfamily from which the name of the family or subfamily is formed

type 1 diabetes \ˌtīp-ˈwən-\ *n* : diabetes of a form that usu. develops during childhood or adolescence and is characterized by a severe deficiency of insulin secretion resulting from atrophy of the islets of Langerhans and causing hyperglycemia and a marked tendency toward ketoacidosis — called also *insulin-dependent diabetes, insulin-dependent diabetes mellitus, juvenile diabetes, juvenile-onset diabetes, type 1 diabetes mellitus*

type species *n* : the species of a genus with which the generic name is permanently associated

type 2 diabetes \-ˈtü-\ *n* : diabetes mellitus of a common form that develops esp. in adults and most often in obese individuals and that is characterized by hyperglycemia resulting from impaired insulin utilization coupled with the body's inability to compensate with increased insulin production — called also *adult-onset diabetes, late-onset diabetes, maturity-onset diabetes, non-insulin-dependent diabetes, non-insulin-dependent diabetes mellitus, type 2 diabetes mellitus*

typh·li·tis \tif-ˈlīt-əs\ *n* : inflammation of the cecum

¹ty·phoid \ˈtī-ˌfȯid, (ˈ)tī-ˈ\ *adj* **1** : of, relating to, or suggestive of typhus **2** : of, relating to, affected with, or constituting typhoid fever

²typhoid *n* **1** : TYPHOID FEVER **2** : any of several diseases of domestic animals resembling human typhus or typhoid fever

ty·phoi·dal \tī-ˈfȯid-ᵊl\ *adj* : of, relating to, or resembling typhoid fever ⟨a ∼ infection⟩

typhoid fever *n* : a communicable disease marked by fever, diarrhea, prostration, headache, splenomegaly, eruption of rose-colored spots, leukopenia, and intestinal inflammation and caused by a bacterium of the genus *Salmonella* (*S. typhi*)

ty·phus \ˈtī-fəs\ *n* : any of various bacterial diseases caused by rickettsial bacteria: as **a** : a severe human febrile disease that is caused by one (*Rickettsia prowazekii*) transmitted esp. by body lice and is marked by high fever, stupor alternating with delirium, intense headache, and a dark red rash — called also *louse-borne typhus* **b** : MURINE TYPHUS **c** : TSUTSUGAMUSHI DISEASE

typhus fever *n* : TYPHUS

typ·i·cal \ˈtip-i-kəl\ *adj* : conforming to a type ⟨a ∼ specimen⟩ ⟨∼ symptoms of a disease⟩

ty·pol·o·gy \tī-ˈpäl-ə-jē\ *n, pl* **-gies** : study of or study based on types; *esp* : classification (as of personality, human physique, or bacterial strains) based on the comparative study of types — **ty·po·log·i·cal** \ˌtī-pə-ˈläj-i-kəl\ *adj*

Tyr *abbr* tyrosine; tyrosyl

ty·ra·mine \ˈtī-rə-ˌmēn\ *n* : a phenolic amine $C_8H_{11}NO$ that is found in various foods and beverages (as cheese and red wine), has a sympathomimetic action, and is derived from tyrosine

ty·ro·ci·dine *also* **ty·ro·ci·din** \ˌtī-rə-ˈsīd-ᵊn\ *n* : a basic polypeptide antibiotic produced by a soil bacterium of the genus *Bacillus* (*B. brevis*) and constituting the major component of tyrothricin

Ty·rode solution *or* **Ty·rode's solution** \ˈtī-ˌrōd(z)-\ *n* : physiological saline containing sodium chloride 0.8, potassium chloride 0.02, calcium chloride 0.02, magnesium chloride 0.01, sodium bicarbonate 0.1, and sodium dihydrogen phosphate 0.005 percent

    Tyrode, Maurice Vejux (1878–1930), American pharmacologist. An instructor of pharmacology at Harvard Medical School, Tyrode specialized in therapeutics.

Ty·ro·glyph·i·dae \ˌtī-rə-ˈglif-ə-ˌdē\ *n pl, syn of* ACARIDAE

Ty·rog·ly·phus \tī-ˈräg-lə-fəs, ˌtī-rə-ˈglif-əs\ *n, syn of* ACARUS

ty·ros·i·nase \tə-ˈräs-ə-ˌnās, tī-, -ˌnāz\ *n* : an enzyme that promotes the oxidation of phenols (as tyrosine) and is widespread in plants and animals

ty·ro·sine \ˈtī-rə-ˌsēn\ *n* : a phenolic amino acid $C_9H_{11}NO_3$ that is a precursor of several important substances (as epinephrine and melanin) — abbr. *Tyr*

tyrosine hydroxylase *n* : an enzyme that catalyzes the first step in the biosynthesis of catecholamines (as dopamine and norepinephrine)

ty·ro·sin·emia *or Brit* **ty·ro·sin·ae·mia** \ˌtī-rō-si-ˈnē-mē-ə\ *n* : a rare inherited disorder of tyrosine metabolism that is characterized by abnormally high concentrations of tyrosine in the blood and urine with associated abnormalities esp. of the liver and kidneys

ty·ro·sin·osis \ˌtī-rō-si-ˈnō-səs\ *n* : a condition of faulty metabolism of tyrosine marked by the excretion of unusual amounts of tyrosine in the urine

ty·ro·sin·uria \ˌtī-rō-si-ˈn(y)ùr-ē-ə\ *n* : the excretion of tyrosine in the urine

ty·ro·syl \ˈtī-rə-ˌsil\ *n* : the amino acid radical or residue $HOC_6H_4CH_2CH(NH_2)CO-$ of tyrosine — abbr. *Tyr*

ty·ro·thri·cin \ˌtī-rə-ˈthrīs-ᵊn\ *n* : an antibiotic mixture that consists chiefly of tyrocidine and gramicidin, is obtained from a soil bacterium of the genus *Bacillus* (*B. brevis*), and is used in the topical treatment of infections esp. of the skin and mouth caused by gram-positive bacteria

---

\ə\ abut \ᵊ\ kitten \ər\ further \a\ ash \ā\ ace \ä\ cot, cart
\aù\ out \ch\ chin \e\ bet \ē\ easy \g\ go \i\ hit \ī\ ice \j\ job
\ŋ\ sing \ō\ go \ò\ law \òi\ boy \th\ thin \th̲\ the \ü\ loot
\ù\ foot \y\ yet \zh\ vision *See also* Pronunciation Symbols page

U

U *abbr* uracil

U *symbol* uranium

ubi·qui·none \yü-'bik-wə-ˌnōn, ˌyü-bi-kwi-'nōn\ *n* : any of a group of lipid-soluble quinones that contain a long isoprenoid side chain and that function in the part of cellular respiration comprising oxidative phosphorylation as electron-carrying coenzymes in the transport of electrons from organic substrates to oxygen esp. along the chain of reactions leading from the Krebs cycle; *esp* : COENZYME Q10

ubiq·ui·tin \yü-'bik-wət-ən\ *n* : a chiefly eukaryotic protein that when covalently bound to other cellular proteins marks them for proteolytic degradation

UCL \ˌyü-ˌsē-'el\ *n* : ULNAR COLLATERAL LIGAMENT

ud·der \'əd-ər\ *n* : a large pendulous organ in various mammals and esp. a female domestic bovine consisting of two or more mammary glands enclosed in a common envelope and each provided with a single nipple

UDP \'yü-ˌdē-'pē\ *n* : a diphosphate of uridine $C_9H_{14}N_2O_{12}P_2$ that functions esp. as a glycosyl carrier in the synthesis of glycogen and starch and is used to form polyuridylic acid — called also *uridine diphosphate*

¹ul·cer \'əl-sər\ *n* : a break in skin or mucous membrane with loss of surface tissue, disintegration and necrosis of epithelial tissue, and often pus ⟨a stomach ∼⟩

²ulcer *vb* **ul·cered; ul·cer·ing** \'əls-(ə-)riŋ\ : ULCERATE

ul·cer·ate \'əl-sə-ˌrāt\ *vb* **-at·ed; -at·ing** *vi* : to become affected with or as if with an ulcer ∼ *vt* : to affect with or as if with an ulcer ⟨an *ulcerated* stomach⟩

ul·cer·ation \ˌəl-sə-'rā-shən\ *n* : the process of becoming ulcerated : the state of being ulcerated

ul·cer·a·tive \'əl-sə-ˌrāt-iv, 'əls-(ə-)rət-iv\ *adj* : of, relating to, or characterized by an ulcer or by ulceration ⟨∼ gingivitis⟩

ulcerative colitis *n* : a chronic inflammatory disease of the colon that is of unknown cause and is characterized by diarrhea with discharge of mucus and blood, cramping abdominal pain, and inflammation and edema of the mucous membrane with patches of ulceration

ul·cero·gen·ic \ˌəl-sə-rō-'jen-ik\ *adj* : tending to produce or develop into ulcers or ulceration ⟨an ∼ drug⟩

ul·cero·glan·du·lar \ˌəl-sə-rō-'glan-jə-lər\ *adj* : being a type of tularemia in which the place of infection is the skin where a papule and then an ulcer develops with enlargement of the lymph nodes in the associated region

ul·cer·ous \'əls-(ə-)rəs\ *adj* **1** : characterized or caused by ulceration ⟨∼ lesions⟩ **2** : affected with an ulcer

ul·cus \'əl-kəs\ *n, pl* **ul·cera** \'əl-sə-rə\ : ULCER

ule·gy·ria \ˌyü-lə-'jī-rē-ə\ *n* : a condition in which the convolutions of the cerebral cortex are abnormally narrow and misshapen due to scarring following the production of lesions in fetal or postnatal life

ul·mus \'əl-məs\ *n* : the dried inner bark of the slippery elm (*Ulmus rubra* syn. *U. fulva*) of No. America used esp. formerly as a demulcent and an emollient

ul·na \'əl-nə\ *n, pl* **ul·nae** \-nē\ *or* **ul·nas** : the bone on the little-finger side of the human forearm that forms with the humerus the elbow joint and serves as a pivot in rotation of the hand

¹ul·nar \'əl-nər\ *adj* **1** : of or relating to the ulna **2** : located on the same side of the forearm as the ulna

²ulnar *n* : an ulnar anatomical part (as the ulnar nerve or the ulnar artery)

ulnar artery *n* : an artery that is the larger of the two terminal branches of the brachial artery, runs along the ulnar side of the forearm, and gives off near its origin the anterior and posterior ulnar recurrent arteries

ulnar collateral artery — see INFERIOR ULNAR COLLATERAL ARTERY, SUPERIOR ULNAR COLLATERAL ARTERY

ulnar collateral ligament *n* : a triangular ligament of the elbow that connects the medial epicondyle with the medial edge of the coronoid process and the olecranon, that helps to stabilize the elbow joint, and that is often injured in sports (as baseball) which involve repeated overhand throwing — called also *medial collateral ligament, UCL;* compare RADIAL COLLATERAL LIGAMENT

ulnar collateral ligament reconstruction *n* : a surgical procedure in which a torn ulnar collateral ligament is replaced with a tendon graft typically obtained from the palmaris longus — called also *Tommy John surgery*

ulnaris — see EXTENSOR CARPI ULNARIS, FLEXOR CARPI ULNARIS

ulnar nerve *n* : a large superficial nerve of the arm that is a continuation of the medial cord of the brachial plexus, passes around the elbow superficially in a groove between the olecranon and the medial epicondyle of the humerus, and continues down the inner side of the forearm to supply the skin and muscles of the little-finger side of the forearm and hand — see FUNNY BONE

ulnar notch \-'näch\ *n* : the narrow medial concave surface on the lower end of the radius that articulates with the ulna

ulnar recurrent artery *n* : either of the two small branches of the ulnar artery arising from its medial side: **a** : one that arises just below the elbow and supplies the brachialis muscle and the pronator teres — called also *anterior ulnar recurrent artery* **b** : one that is larger, arises lower on the arm, and supplies the elbow and associated muscles — called also *posterior ulnar recurrent artery*

ulnar vein *n* : any of several deep veins of the forearm that accompany the ulnar artery and unite at the elbow with the radial veins to form the brachial veins

ul·ti·mo·bran·chi·al \ˌəl-tə-mō-'braŋ-kē-əl\ *adj* : being, relating to, produced by, or derived from the ultimobranchial bodies

ultimobranchial body *n* : a hollow vesicle that is formed from the fourth pharyngeal pouch, may represent a fifth pharyngeal pouch, and gives rise to cells that produce calcitonin and later become incorporated into the thyroid gland in higher vertebrates or persist as distinct organs in birds and lower vertebrates — called also *postbranchial body*

ul·tra·cen·trif·u·gal \ˌəl-trə-ˌsen-'trif-yə-gəl, -'trif-i-gəl\ *adj* : of, relating to, or obtained by means of an ultracentrifuge ⟨∼ analysis⟩ — **ul·tra·cen·trif·u·gal·ly** \-gə-lē\ *adv*

ul·tra·cen·tri·fu·ga·tion \-ˌsen-trə-fyü-'gā-shən\ *n* : the process of using an ultracentrifuge

¹ul·tra·cen·tri·fuge \-'sen-trə-ˌfyüj\ *n* : a high-speed centrifuge able to sediment colloidal and other small particles and used esp. in determining sizes of such particles and molecular weights of large molecules

²ultracentrifuge *vt* **-fuged; -fug·ing** : to subject to centrifugal action in an ultracentrifuge ⟨∼ blood plasma⟩

ul·tra·di·an \ˌəl-'trād-ē-ən\ *adj* : being, characterized by, or occurring in periods or cycles (as of biological activity) that are repeated frequently (as every 90 to 100 minutes) throughout a 24-hour period ⟨∼ rhythms⟩ — compare CIRCADIAN, INFRADIAN

ul·tra·fil·ter \'əl-trə-ˌfil-tər\ *n* : a dense filter used for the filtration of a colloidal solution that holds back the dispersed particles but not the liquid

ul·tra·fil·tra·ble \ˌəl-trə-'fil-trə-bəl\ *adj* : capable of passing through the pores of an ultrafilter

ul·tra·fil·trate \-'fil-ˌtrāt\ *n* : material that has passed through an ultrafilter in the process of ultrafiltration

ul·tra·fil·tra·tion \ˌəl-trə-fil-'trā-shən\ *n* : filtration through a medium (as a semipermeable capillary wall) which allows small molecules (as of water) to pass but holds back larger ones (as of protein)

Ul·tram \'əl-ˌtram\ *trademark* — used for a preparation of the hydrochloride of tramadol

ul·tra·mi·cro·scope \ˌəl-trə-'mī-krə-ˌskōp\ *n* : an apparatus for making visible by scattered light particles too small to be perceived by the ordinary microscope — called also *dark= field microscope* — **ul·tra·mi·cros·co·py** \-mī-'kräs-kə-pē\ *n, pl* **-pies**

ul·tra·mi·cro·scop·ic \-,mī-krə-'skäp-ik\ *also* **ul·tra·mi·cro·scop·i·cal** \-i-kəl\ *adj* **1 :** too small to be seen with an ordinary microscope — compare MACROSCOPIC, MICROSCOPIC 2, SUBMICROSCOPIC **2 :** of or relating to an ultramicroscope — **ul·tra·mi·cro·scop·i·cal·ly** \-i-k(ə-)lē\ *adv*

ul·tra·mi·cro·tome \-'mī-krə-,tōm\ *n* : a microtome for cutting extremely thin sections for electron microscopy — **ul·tra·mi·crot·o·my** \-mī-'krät-ə-mē\ *n, pl* **-mies**

ul·tra·son·ic \-'sän-ik\ *adj* **1 a :** having a frequency above the human ear's audibility limit of about 20,000 hertz — used of waves and vibrations **b :** utilizing, produced by, or relating to ultrasonic waves or vibrations ⟨removal of tartar with an ∼ scaler⟩ **2 :** ULTRASOUND — **ul·tra·son·i·cal·ly** \-i-k(ə-)lē\ *adv*

ul·tra·son·ics \,əl-trə-'sän-iks\ *n pl but sing in constr* **1 :** the science or technology of ultrasonic phenomena **2 :** ULTRASOUND 2

ul·tra·sono·gram \-'sän-ə-,gram\ *n* : SONOGRAM

ul·tra·so·nog·ra·pher \,əl-trə-sə-'näg-rə-fər\ *n* : SONOGRAPHER

ul·tra·so·nog·ra·phy \-fē\ *n, pl* **-phies** : ULTRASOUND 2 — **ul·tra·so·no·graph·ic** \-,sän-ə-'graf-ik, -,sō-nə-\ *adj*

¹**ul·tra·sound** \'əl-trə-,saúnd\ *n* **1 :** vibrations of the same physical nature as sound but with frequencies above the range of human hearing — compare INFRASOUND **2 :** the diagnostic or therapeutic use of ultrasound and esp. a noninvasive technique involving the formation of a two-dimensional image used for the examination and measurement of internal body structures and the detection of bodily abnormalities — called also *echography, sonography, ultrasonography* **3 :** a diagnostic examination using ultrasound

²**ultrasound** *adj* : of, relating to, performed by, using, or specializing in ultrasound ⟨an ∼ technician⟩ ⟨∼ imaging⟩

ul·tra·struc·ture \'əl-trə-,strək-chər\ *n* : biological structure and esp. fine structure (as of a cell) not visible through a light microscope — **ul·tra·struc·tur·al** \,əl-trə-'strək-chə-rəl, -'strək-shrəl\ *adj* — **ul·tra·struc·tur·al·ly** \-ē\ *adv*

ul·tra·thin \,əl-trə-'thin\ *adj* : exceedingly thin ⟨∼ sections for use in electron microscopy⟩

¹**ul·tra·vi·o·let** \,əl-trə-'vī-(ə-)lət\ *adj* **1 :** situated beyond the visible spectrum at its violet end — used of radiation having a wavelength shorter than wavelengths of visible light and longer than those of X-rays **2 :** relating to, producing, or employing ultraviolet radiation

²**ultraviolet** *n* : ultraviolet radiation

ultraviolet A \-'ā\ *n* : UVA

ultraviolet B \-'bē\ *n* : UVB

ultraviolet light *n* : ultraviolet radiation

ultraviolet microscope *n* : a microscope equipped to irradiate material under examination with ultraviolet radiation in order to detect or study fluorescent components — called also *fluorescence microscope*

ul·tra·vi·rus \'əl-trə-,vī-rəs\ *n* : VIRUS 1b

uma·mi \ü-'mä-mē\ *n* : a taste sensation that is meaty or savory and is produced by several amino acids and nucleotides (as aspartate, inosinate, and glutamate) — **umami** *adj*

Um·bel·lif·er·ae \,əm-bə-'lif-ə-,rē\ *n pl* : a large family of often fragrant or aromatic plants (order Umbellales) that have small flowers borne in umbels and include numerous economically important plants (as the carrot, anise, caraway, dill, and parsley) — **um·bel·li·fer** \əm-'bel-ə-fər\ *n*

um·bel·lif·er·one \-,rōn\ *n* : a crystalline phenolic lactone $C_9H_6O_3$ obtained by the distillation of resins (as galbanum or asafetida) from various plants of the family Umbelliferae

um·bi·lec·to·my \,əm-bi-'lek-tə-mē\ *n, pl* **-mies** : OMPHALECTOMY

um·bil·i·cal \,əm-'bil-i-kəl *also* ,əm-bə-'lī-kəl\ *adj* **1 :** of, relating to, or used at the navel ⟨∼ infection⟩ **2 :** of or relating to the central abdominal region that is situated between the right and left lumbar regions and between the epigastric region above and the hypogastric region below ⟨∼ pain⟩

umbilical artery *n* : either of a pair of arteries that arise from the hypogastric arteries of the mammalian fetus and pass through the umbilical cord to the placenta to which they carry the deoxygenated blood from the fetus

umbilical cord *n* : a cord arising from the navel that connects the fetus with the placenta and contains the two umbilical arteries and the umbilical vein

umbilical hernia *n* : a hernia of abdominal viscera at the navel — called also *exomphalos*

umbilical ligament — see MEDIAL UMBILICAL LIGAMENT, MEDIAN UMBILICAL LIGAMENT

umbilical vein *n* : a vein that passes through the umbilical cord to the fetus and returns the oxygenated and nutrient blood from the placenta to the fetus

umbilical vesicle *n* : the yolk sac of a mammalian embryo usu. having the form of a fluid-filled pouch, corresponding to the yolk sac of an oviparous vertebrate, and having a transitory connection with the alimentary canal by way of the omphalomesenteric duct

um·bil·i·cat·ed \,əm-'bil-ə-,kāt-əd\ *or* **um·bil·i·cate** \-kət\ *adj* : having a small depression that resembles a navel ⟨∼ vesicles⟩ — **um·bil·i·cate** \-,kāt\ *vi* **-cat·ed; -cat·ing**

um·bil·i·ca·tion \,əm-,bil-ə-'kā-shən\ *n* : a depression resembling a navel ⟨an ∼ in the center of a lesion⟩; *also* : the state or condition of having such depressions ⟨a tendency to ∼⟩

um·bi·li·cus \,əm-'bil-i-kəs, ,əm-bə-'lī-\ *n, pl* **um·bi·li·ci** \,əm-'bil-ə-,kī, -,kē; ,əm-bə-'lī-,kī, -,sī\ *or* **um·bi·li·cus·es** : NAVEL

um·bo \'əm-(,)bō\ *n, pl* **um·bo·nes** \,əm-'bō-(,)nēz\ *or* **umbos** : an elevation in the tympanic membrane of the ear

UMP \,yü-,em-'pē\ *n* : URIDYLIC ACID

un·anes·the·tized *or chiefly Brit* **un·anaes·the·tized** *also* **un·anaes·the·tised** \,ən-ə-'nes-thə-,tīzd\ *adj* : not having been subjected to an anesthetic ⟨an ∼ patient⟩

un·armed \,ən-'ärmd\ *adj* : having no arms or armlike projections ⟨an ∼ tapeworm⟩

un·bal·anced \,ən-'bal-ən(t)st\ *adj* : mentally disordered or disturbed ⟨an ∼ mind⟩

un·ban·dage \-'ban-dij\ *vt* **-daged; -dag·ing** : to remove a bandage from

un·blind·ed \-'blīnd-əd\ *adj* : made or done with knowledge of significant facts by the participants : not blind ⟨an ∼ study of a drug's effectiveness⟩

un·born \-'bȯ(ə)rn\ *adj* : not yet born : existing in utero ⟨∼ children⟩

un·branched \-'brancht\ *adj* **1 :** having no branches ⟨∼ filaments⟩ **2 :** having a straight chain of atoms in a molecule : NORMAL 4d

un·bro·ken \-'brō-kən\ *adj* : not broken ⟨∼ skin⟩

un·cal \'ən-kəl\ *adj* : of or relating to the uncus ⟨the ∼ region⟩

un·cal·ci·fied \,ən-'kal-sə-,fīd\ *adj* : not calcified ⟨∼ osteoid tissue⟩

uncal herniation *n* : downward displacement of the uncus and adjacent structures into the tentorial notch

un·charged \-'chärjd\ *adj* : not charged; *specif* : having no electric charge ⟨an ∼ atom⟩

unci *pl of* UNCUS

¹**un·ci·form** \'ən(t)-sə-,fȯrm\ *adj* : hook-shaped : UNCINATE

²**unciform** *n* : HAMATE

unciform bone *n* : HAMATE

Un·ci·nar·ia \,ən(t)-sə-'nar-ē-ə\ *n* : a genus of hookworms of the family Ancylostomatidae now usu. restricted to a few parasites of carnivorous mammals but formerly often including most of the common hookworms

un·ci·na·ri·a·sis \,ən-,sin-ə-'rī-ə-səs\ *n, pl* **-a·ses** \-,sēz\ : ANCYLOSTOMIASIS

un·ci·nate \'ən(t)-sə-,nāt\ *adj* **1 :** bent at the tip like a hook

\ə\ **abut** \ᵊ\ **kitten** \ər\ **further** \a\ **ash** \ā\ **ace** \ä\ **cot, cart** \aú\ **out** \ch\ **chin** \e\ **bet** \ē\ **easy** \g\ **go** \i\ **hit** \ī\ **ice** \j\ **job** \ŋ\ **sing** \ō\ **go** \ȯ\ **law** \ȯi\ **boy** \th\ **thin** \th\ **the** \ü\ **loot** \ú\ **foot** \y\ **yet** \zh\ **vision** *See also* Pronunciation Symbols page

U Z

2 a : of, relating to, affecting, or involving the uncus ⟨the ∼ area of the parahippocampal gyrus⟩ **b** : relating to, characterized by, or being an uncinate fit ⟨∼ epilepsy⟩ ⟨an ∼ seizure⟩

uncinate fasciculus *n* : a hook-shaped bundle of long association fibers connecting the frontal lobe with the anterior portion of the temporal lobe

uncinate fit *n* : a seizure of a form of temporal lobe epilepsy that originates in the region of the uncus and is characterized by hallucinations of taste and odor and disturbances of consciousness

uncinate process *n* : a hooklike body part: as **a** : an irregular downwardly and backwardly directed process of each lateral mass of the ethmoid bone that articulates with the inferior nasal conchae **b** : a bony upward projection arising from each side of the upper surface of any of the cervical vertebrae numbered three to seven and forming a raised lateral margin **c** : the portion of the pancreas that wraps behind the superior mesenteric artery and superior mesenteric vein

un·cir·cum·cised \ˌən-ˈsər-kəm-ˌsīzd, ˈən-ˌ\ *adj* : not circumcised

un·cloned \-ˈklōnd\ *adj* : not produced or reproduced by cloning ⟨an ∼ virus⟩ ⟨∼ DNA⟩

un·com·pen·sat·ed \-ˈkäm-pən-ˌsāt-əd, -ˌpen-\ *adj* **1** : accompanied by a change in the pH of the blood ⟨∼ acidosis⟩ ⟨∼ alkalosis⟩ — compare COMPENSATED **2** : not corrected or affected by physiological compensation ⟨∼ congestive heart failure⟩

un·com·pli·cat·ed \ˌən-ˈkäm-plə-ˌkāt-əd\ *adj* : not involving or marked by complications ⟨∼ peptic ulcer⟩ ⟨the clinical course is usually benign and ∼ —M. A. Baumann *et al*⟩

un·con·di·tion·al \ˌən-kən-ˈdish-nəl, -ˈdish-ən-ᵊl\ *adj* : UNCONDITIONED 2

un·con·di·tioned \-ˈdish-ənd\ *adj* **1** : not dependent on or subjected to conditioning or learning ⟨∼ responses⟩ **2** : producing an unconditioned response ⟨∼ stimuli⟩

un·con·ju·gat·ed \-ˈkän-jə-ˌgāt-əd\ *adj* : not chemically conjugated ⟨∼ bilirubin⟩

¹un·con·scious \ˌən-ˈkän-chəs\ *adj* **1** : not marked by conscious thought, sensation, or feeling ⟨∼ motivation⟩ **2** : of or relating to the unconscious **3** : having lost consciousness ⟨was ∼ for three days⟩ — **un·con·scious·ly** *adv* — **un·con·scious·ness** *n*

²unconscious *n* : the part of mental life that is not ordinarily integrated or available to consciousness yet may be manifested as a motive force in overt behavior (as in neurosis) and is often revealed (as through dreams, slips of the tongue, or dissociated acts) — compare SUBCONSCIOUS

un·con·trolled \ˌən-kən-ˈtrōld\ *adj* **1** : not being under control ⟨∼ hypertension⟩ **2** : not incorporating suitable experimental controls ⟨∼ drug trials⟩

un·co·or·di·nat·ed \-kō-ˈȯrd-ᵊn-ˌāt-əd\ *adj* : not coordinated : lacking proper or effective coordination ⟨∼ muscles⟩

un·cor·rect·ed \-kə-ˈrek-təd\ *adj* : not corrected ⟨∼ vision⟩

un·cou·pler \ˈən-ˈkəp-(ə-)lər\ *n* : an agent that dissociates two integrated series of chemical reactions; *esp* : one that prevents the formation of ATP in oxidative phosphorylation in mitochondria by dissociating the reactions of phosphorylation from those concerned with electron transport and oxidation

un·crossed \-ˈkròst\ *adj* : not forming a decussation ⟨an ∼ tract of nerve fibers⟩

unc·tion \ˈəŋ(k)-shən\ *n* **1** : the application of a soothing or lubricating oil or ointment **2** : something that is used for anointing : OINTMENT

unc·tu·ous \ˈəŋ(k)-chə(-wə)s, ˈəŋ(k)sh-wəs\ *adj* : rich in oil or fat ⟨an ∼ pharmaceutical preparation⟩

un·cur·able \ˌən-ˈkyùr-ə-bəl\ *adj* : INCURABLE

un·cus \ˈəŋ-kəs\ *n, pl* **un·ci** \ˈən-ˌsī\ : a hooked anatomical part or process; *specif* : the anterior curved end of the parahippocampal gyrus

un·deca·pep·tide \ˌən-ˌdek-ə-ˈpep-ˌtīd\ *n* : a peptide (as substance P) composed of a chain of 11 amino acid residues

un·dec·e·no·ic acid \ˌən-ˌdes-ə-ˌnō-ik-\ *n* : any of several isomeric straight-chain unsaturated acids $C_{11}H_{20}O_2$ (as undecylenic acid)

un·dec·y·len·ate \ˌən-ˌdes-ə-ˈlen-ˌāt\ *n* : a salt or ester of undecylenic acid

un·dec·y·le·nic acid \ˌən-ˌdes-ə-ˌlen-ik-, -ˌlēn-\ *n* : an acid $C_{11}H_{20}O_2$ found in perspiration, obtained commercially from castor oil, and used in the treatment of fungus infections (as ringworm) of the skin

¹un·der \ˈən-dər\ *adv* : in or into a condition of unconsciousness ⟨put the patient ∼ prior to surgery⟩

²under *prep* : receiving or using the action or application of ⟨an operation performed ∼ local anesthesia⟩

³under *adj* : being in an induced state of unconsciousness ⟨given intravenously when the patient is ∼ —C. A. Birch⟩

un·der·achiev·er \ˌən-dər-ə-ˈchē-vər\ *n* : a person (as a student) who fails to achieve his or her potential or does not do as well as expected — **un·der·achieve** \-ˈchēv\ *vi* **-achieved; -achiev·ing** — **un·der·achieve·ment** \-mənt\ *n*

un·der·ac·tive \-ˈak-tiv\ *adj* : characterized by an abnormally low level of activity ⟨an ∼ thyroid gland⟩ — **un·der·ac·tiv·i·ty** \-ak-ˈtiv-ət-ē\ *n, pl* **-ties**

un·der·arm \ˈən-dər-ˌärm\ *n* : ARMPIT

un·der·cut \ˈən-dər-ˌkət\ *n* : the part of a tooth lying between the gum and the points of maximum outward bulge on the tooth's surfaces

un·der·de·vel·oped \ˌən-dər-di-ˈvel-əpt\ *adj* : not normally or adequately developed ⟨∼ muscles⟩ ⟨∼ lungs⟩

un·der·de·vel·op·ment \-əp-mənt\ *n* : lack of adequate development ⟨∼ of the jaw⟩

un·der·di·ag·nose \ˌən-dər-ˈdī-ig-ˌnōs, -ˌnōz; -ˌdī-ig-ˈ, -əg-\ *vt* **-nosed; -nos·ing** : to diagnose (a condition or disease) less often than it is actually present ⟨a tendency to ∼ degenerative joint disease⟩

un·der·di·ag·no·sis \-ˌdī-ig-ˈnō-səs, -əg-\ *n, pl* **-no·ses** \-ˌsēz\ : failure to recognize or correctly diagnose a disease or condition esp. in a significant proportion of patients

un·der·dos·age \-ˈdō-sij\ *n* : the administration or taking of an underdose ⟨∼ of a drug⟩

¹un·der·dose \-ˈdōs\ *vb* **-dosed; -dos·ing** *vi* : to take or administer an insufficient dose ⟨noncompliant patients may tend to ∼⟩ ∼ *vt* : to administer an insufficient dose of or to ⟨antidepressants are *underdosed* in the study group of elderly patients⟩ ⟨a tendency to ∼ some patients⟩

²un·der·dose \-ˈdōs\ *n* : an insufficient dose ⟨received an ∼ of radiation for chest cancer⟩

un·der·feed \ˌən-dər-ˈfēd\ *vb* **-fed** \-ˈfed\; **-feed·ing** *vt* : to feed with too little food ⟨an *underfed* woman has a higher probability of a miscarriage and of a stillbirth —Rose E. Frisch⟩ ∼ *vi* : to eat too little food

un·der·ly·ing \-ˌlī-iŋ\ *adj* : serving as a basis or cause (as of secondary symptoms) ⟨the ∼ brain malformation that caused the hydrocephalus —R. M. Henig⟩

un·der·nour·ished \ˌən-dər-ˈnər-isht, -ˈnə-risht\ *adj* : supplied with less than the minimum amount of the foods essential for sound health and growth — **un·der·nour·ish·ment** \-ˈnər-ish-mənt, -ˈnə-rish-\ *n*

un·der·nu·tri·tion \-n(y)ù-ˈtrish-ən\ *n* : deficient bodily nutrition due to inadequate food intake or faulty assimilation — called also *hyponutrition* — **un·der·nu·tri·tion·al** \-əl\ *adj*

un·der·sexed \-ˈsekst\ *adj* : deficient in sexual desire

un·der·shot \ˈən-dər-ˌshät\ *adj* : having the lower incisor teeth or lower jaw projecting beyond the upper when the mouth is closed — used chiefly of animals

un·der·tak·er \ˈən-dər-ˌtā-kər\ *n* : an individual whose business is to prepare the dead for burial and to arrange and manage funerals — called also *mortician*

un·der·treat \-ˈtrēt\ *vt* : to treat inadequately or inappropriately ⟨∼ a disease⟩ ⟨evidence shows that hospitalized patients are ∼*ed* for pain —*Harvard Med. School Health Letter*⟩ — **un·der·treat·ment** \-mənt\ *n*

un·der·vac·ci·na·tion \-ˌvak-sə-ˈnā-shən\ *n* : a vaccination of significantly less than the proportion of a population that should be vaccinated

un·der·ven·ti·la·tion \ˌən-dər-ˌven-ti-ˈlā-shən\ *n* : HYPOVEN-TILATION

un·der·weight \-ˈwāt\ *adj* : weighing less than the normal amount for one's age, height, and build ⟨~ children⟩ ⟨~ adults typically have a body mass index of less than 18.5⟩

un·de·scend·ed \ˌən-di-ˈsen-dəd\ *adj* : retained within the iliac region rather than descending into the scrotum ⟨an ~ testis⟩

un·de·vel·oped \ˌən-di-ˈvel-əpt\ *adj* : lacking in development : not developed ⟨physiologically ~⟩

un·di·ag·nos·able \-ˌdī-ig-ˈnō-sə-bəl\ *adj* : not capable of being diagnosed ⟨an ~ complaint⟩

un·di·ag·nosed \-ˈnōst\ *adj* : not diagnosed : eluding diagnosis ⟨~ disease⟩

un·dif·fer·en·ti·at·ed \-ˌdif-ə-ˈren-chē-ˌāt-əd\ *adj* : not differentiated ⟨an ~ sarcoma⟩

un·di·gest·ed \ˌən-dī-ˈjest-əd\ *adj* : not digested ⟨~ food⟩

un·di·gest·ible \-dī-ˈjes-tə-bəl\ *adj* : not capable of being digested

un·dine \ˈən-ˌdēn, ˌən-ˈdēn\ *n* : a small glass container used for irrigating the eyes

un·dis·so·ci·at·ed \ˌən-dis-ˈō-sē-ˌāt-əd, -shē-\ *adj* : not electrolytically dissociated

un·du·lant fever \ˈən-jə-lənt-, ˈən-d(y)ə-\ *n* : BRUCELLOSIS a

un·du·late \ˈən-jə-lət, ˈən-d(y)ə-, -ˌlāt\ *adj* : having a wavy surface, edge, or markings ⟨an ~ cell⟩

un·du·lat·ing membrane \ˈən-jə-ˌlāt-iŋ-, ˈən-d(y)ə-\ *n* : a vibratile cytoplasmic membrane: **a** : a lateral expansion of the plasma membrane in some flagellates that is usu. associated with a flagellum **b** : a row of laterally fused long cilia associated in many ciliates with the oral structures

un·du·la·to·ry theory \ˈən-jə-lə-ˌtōr-ē-, ˈən-d(y)ə-lə-, -ˌtȯr-ē-\ *n* : WAVE THEORY

un·erupt·ed \ˌən-i-ˈrəp-təd\ *adj, of a tooth* : not yet having emerged through the gum

un·es·ter·i·fied \ˌən-e-ˈster-ə-ˌfīd\ *adj* : not esterified ⟨~ cholesterol⟩

un·fer·til·ized \-ˈfərt-ᵊl-ˌīzd\ *adj* : not fertilized ⟨an ~ egg⟩

un·frac·tion·at·ed \-ˈfrak-shə-ˌnāt-əd\ *adj* : not fractionated ⟨~ DNA⟩

ung *abbr* [Latin *unguentum*] ointment — used in writing prescriptions

un·gual \ˈəŋ-gwəl, ˈən-\ *adj* : of or relating to a fingernail or toenail

un·guent \ˈəŋ-gwənt *also* ˈən-jənt\ *n* : a soothing or healing salve : OINTMENT

un·guis \ˈəŋ-gwəs, ˈən-\ *n, pl* **un·gues** \-ˌgwēz\ : a fingernail or toenail

unguis in·car·na·tus \-ˌin-ˌkär-ˈnāt-əs\ *n* : an ingrown fingernail or toenail

¹**un·gu·late** \ˈəŋ-gyə-lət, ˈən-, -ˌlāt\ *adj* **1** : having hooves **2** : of or relating to the ungulates

²**ungulate** *n* : a hoofed typically herbivorous quadruped mammal (as a pig, camel, hippopotamus, horse, tapir, rhinoceros, or elephant) of a polyphyletic group formerly considered a major mammalian taxon (Ungulata)

un·gu·li·grade \ˈəŋ-gyə-lə-ˌgrād, ˈən-\ *adj* : walking on hooves ⟨horses are ~ animals⟩

Unh *symbol* unnilhexium

un·healed \ˌən-ˈhēld\ *adj* : not healed ⟨~ wounds⟩

un·health·ful \-ˈhelth-fəl\ *adj* : detrimental to good health ⟨~ working conditions⟩ — **un·health·ful·ness** *n*

un·healthy \-ˈhel-thē\ *adj* **un·health·i·er; -est** **1** : not conducive to health ⟨an ~ climate⟩ **2** : not in good health : SICKLY — **un·health·i·ness** *n*

un·hy·gi·en·ic \ˌən-ˌhī-jē-ˈen-ik, -ˈjen-, -ˈjēn-\ *adj* : not healthful or sanitary ⟨~ conditions⟩ ⟨~ habits⟩ — **un·hy·gi·en·i·cal·ly** \-i-k(ə-)lē\ *adv*

uni·cel·lu·lar \ˌyü-ni-ˈsel-yə-lər\ *adj* : having or consisting of a single cell ⟨~ microorganisms⟩ — **uni·cel·lu·lar·i·ty** \-ˌsel-yə-ˈlar-ət-ē\ *n, pl* **-ties**

uni·corn \ˈyü-nə-ˌkȯ(ə)rn\ *adj* : having a single horn or hornlike process ⟨a ~ uterus⟩

uni·cus·pid \ˌyü-ni-ˈkəs-pəd\ *adj* : having a single cusp ⟨canines and other ~ teeth⟩

uni·di·rec·tion·al \ˌyü-ni-də-ˈrek-shnəl, -dī-, -shən-ᵊl\ *adj* : involving, functioning, moving, or responsive in a single direction — **uni·di·rec·tion·al·ly** \-ē\ *adv*

uni·fac·to·ri·al \ˌyü-ni-fak-ˈtōr-ē-əl, -ˈtȯr-\ *adj* **1** : having or being characters or a mode of inheritance dependent on genes at a single genetic locus **2** : having, involving, concerned with, or produced by a single element or cause ⟨a ~ versus multifactorial analysis of mortality⟩

uni·fla·gel·late \ˌyü-ni-ˈflaj-ə-lət, -flə-ˈjel-ət\ *adj* : having a single flagellum ⟨a ~ spore⟩

uni·fo·cal \ˌyü-ni-ˈfō-kəl\ *adj* : arising from or occurring in a single focus or location ⟨~ infection⟩

uni·la·mel·lar \ˌyü-ni-lə-ˈmel-ər\ *adj* : having only one lamella or layer ⟨a ~ liposome⟩

uni·lat·er·al \ˌyü-ni-ˈlat-ə-rəl, -ˈla-trəl\ *adj* : occurring on, performed on, or affecting one side of the body or one of its parts ⟨~ exophthalmos⟩ — **uni·lat·er·al·ly** \-ē\ *adv*

uni·loc·u·lar \ˌyü-ni-ˈläk-yə-lər\ *adj* : containing a single cavity ⟨a ~ blister⟩

un·im·mu·nized *or chiefly Brit* **un·im·mu·nised** \(ˈ)ən-ˈim-yə-ˌnīzd\ *adj* : not immunized ⟨~ children⟩

uni·ne·phrec·to·my \ˌyü-ni-nə-ˈfrek-tə-mē\ *n, pl* **-mies** : surgical excision of one kidney — **uni·ne·phrec·to·mized** *or chiefly Brit* **uni·ne·phrec·to·mised** \-tə-ˌmīzd\ *adj*

un·in·fect·ed \ˌən-in-ˈfek-təd\ *adj* : free from infection ⟨an ~ infant⟩ ⟨~ cells⟩

uni·nu·cle·ate \ˌyü-ni-ˈn(y)ü-klē-ət\ *also* **uni·nu·cle·at·ed** \-ˌāt-əd\ *adj* : having a single nucleus : MONONUCLEAR

uni·oc·u·lar \ˌyü-nē-ˈäk-yə-lər\ *adj* : MONOCULAR ⟨~ blindness⟩

union \ˈyü-nyən\ *n* : an act or instance of uniting or joining two or more things into one: as **a** : the growing together of severed parts ⟨~ of a fractured bone⟩ **b** : a chemical combination : BOND **c** : the joining of two germ cells in the process of fertilization

uni·ovu·lar \ˌyü-nē-ˈäv-yə-lər\ *adj* : MONOZYGOTIC ⟨~ twins⟩

unip·a·ra \yü-ˈnip-ə-rə\ *n, pl* **-ras** *or* **-rae** \-ˌrē\ : a woman who has borne one child

uni·pa·ren·tal \ˌyü-ni-pə-ˈrent-ᵊl\ *adj* : having, involving, or derived from a single parent; *specif* : involving or being inheritance in which an offspring's complete genotype or all copies of one or more genes, chromosome parts, or whole chromosomes are derived from a single parent ⟨~ disomy⟩ — **uni·pa·ren·tal·ly** \-ᵊl-ē\ *adv*

unip·a·rous \yü-ˈnip-ə-rəs\ *adj* **1** : producing but one egg or offspring at a time **2** : having produced but one offspring

uni·pen·nate \ˌyü-ni-ˈpen-ˌāt\ *adj* : having the fibers arranged obliquely and inserting into a tendon only on one side in the manner of a feather barbed on one side ⟨a ~ muscle⟩

uni·po·lar \ˌyü-ni-ˈpō-lər\ *adj* **1** : having but one process ⟨a ~ neuron⟩ **2** : relating to or being a manic-depressive disorder in which there is a depressive phase only ⟨~ depression⟩ — compare BIPOLAR 3 **3** : involving or being electrodes or leads recording electrical potentials between the scalp and the ground or a distant bodily site

unip·o·tent \yü-ˈnip-ət-ənt\ *adj* : having power in one way only; *esp* : capable of developing only in one direction or to one end product ⟨~ cells⟩

un·ir·ra·di·at·ed \ˌən-ir-ˈād-ē-ˌāt-əd\ *adj* : not having been exposed to radiation ⟨~ lymphocytes⟩

unit \ˈyü-nət\ *n* **1** : an amount of a biologically active agent (as a drug or antigen) required to produce a specific result under strictly controlled conditions ⟨a ~ of penicillin⟩ — see INTERNATIONAL UNIT **2** : a small molecule esp. when combined in a larger molecule ⟨repeating ~s of a polymer⟩

\ə\ abut \ᵊ\ kitten \ər\ further \a\ ash \ā\ ace \ä\ cot, cart
\au̇\ out \ch\ chin \e\ bet \ē\ easy \g\ go \i\ hit \ī\ ice \j\ job
\ŋ\ sing \ō\ go \ȯ\ law \ȯi\ boy \th\ thin \t͟h\ the \ü\ loot
\u̇\ foot \y\ yet \zh\ vision *See also* Pronunciation Symbols page

U
Z

3 : an area in a medical facility and esp. a hospital that is specially staffed and equipped to provide a particular type of care ⟨an intensive care ∼⟩

unit·age \\'yü-nət-ij\ *n* **1** : specification of the amount constituting a unit (as of a vitamin) **2** : amount in units ⟨a ∼ of 50,000 per capsule⟩

unit character *n* : a natural character inherited on an all-or-none basis; *esp* : one dependent on the presence or absence of a single gene

unit membrane *n* : the limiting membrane of cells and various organelles viewed formerly as a 3-layered structure with an inner lipid layer and two outer protein layers and currently as a fluid phospholipid bilayer with intercalated proteins

¹**uni·va·lent** \\,yü-ni-'vā-lənt\ *n* : a chromosome that lacks a synaptic mate

²**univalent** *adj* **1** : MONOVALENT 1 **2** : being a chromosomal univalent **3** *of an antibody* : capable of agglutinating or precipitating but not both : having only one combining group

uni·ver·sal antidote \\,yü-ni-,vər-səl-\ *n* : an antidote for ingested poisons having activated charcoal as its principal ingredient

universal donor *n* **1** : a person who has Rh-negative blood of the blood group O and whose blood can be donated to any recipient; *broadly* : a person with blood group O blood **2** : the blood or blood group of a universal donor

universal recipient *n* **1** : a person who has Rh-positive blood of the blood group AB and who can receive blood from any donor; *broadly* : a person with blood group AB blood **2** : the blood or blood group of a universal recipient

universal serologic reaction *n* : the Kahn test used to detect serological changes characteristic of various diseases (as tuberculosis, malaria, and leprosy)

un·la·beled *or* **un·la·belled** \\,ən-'lā-bəld\ *adj* : not labeled esp. with an isotopic label ⟨∼ DNA⟩

un·la·bored \-'lā-bərd\ *adj* : produced without exertion, pain, or undue effort ⟨∼ breathing⟩

un·li·censed *or chiefly Brit* **un·li·cenced** \-'līs-ᵊn(t)st\ *adj* : not licensed; *esp, of a drug* : not approved for use by the appropriate regulating authority (as the Food and Drug Administration in the U.S.)

un·linked \-'liŋ(k)t\ *adj* : not belonging to the same genetic linkage group ⟨∼ genes⟩

un·med·ul·lat·ed \-'med-ᵊl-,āt-əd, -'mej-ə-,lāt-\ *adj* : UNMYELINATED ⟨∼ nerve fiber⟩

un·my·elin·at·ed \-'mī-ə-lə-,nāt-əd\ *adj* : lacking a myelin sheath ⟨∼ axons⟩

Un·na's boot *or* **Un·na boot** \'ü-nə(z)-\ *n* : a compression dressing for varicose veins or ulcers consisting of a paste made of zinc oxide, gelatin, glycerin, and water that is applied to the lower leg, covered with a bandage, and then applied to the outside of the bandage

Un·na \'ú-nä\, **Paul Gerson (1850–1929),** German dermatologist. Unna was one of the leading dermatologists of his time. Near Hamburg, Germany, he founded a private clinic for skin diseases, and in 1882 he founded his own journal of practical dermatology. Unna introduced into medicine hard and soft zinc oxide pastes, including the paste used in Unna's boot.

Unna's paste boot *n* : UNNA'S BOOT

un·nil·hex·i·um \\,yün-ᵊl-'hek-sē-əm\ *n* : SEABORGIUM — symbol *Unh*

un·nil·pen·ti·um \\,yün-ᵊl-'pent-ē-əm\ *n* : DUBNIUM — symbol *Unp*

un·nil·qua·di·um \\,yün-ᵊl-'kwäd-ē-əm\ *n* : RUTHERFORDIUM — symbol *Unq*

un·of·fi·cial \\,ən-ə-'fish-əl\ *adj* : not official; *specif* : of, relating to, or being a drug not described in the *U.S. Pharmacopeia* and *National Formulary* — compare NONOFFICIAL, OFFICIAL

un·op·posed \-ə-'pōzd\ *adj* : being or relating to estrogen replacement therapy in which a progestin (as medroxyprogesterone acetate) is not coadministered to reduce the side effects (as endometrial cancer) of estrogen

un·or·ga·nized *also Brit* **un·or·ga·nised** \-'or-gə-,nīzd\ *adj* : not organized : lacking order or coherence ⟨∼ delusions⟩

un·os·si·fied \-'äs-ə-,fīd\ *adj* : not ossified

un·ox·y·gen·at·ed \-'äk-si-jə-,nāt-əd, -äk-'sij-ə-\ *adj* : not oxygenated ⟨∼ blood⟩

Unp *symbol* unnilpentium

un·paired \,ən-'pa(ə)rd, -'pe(ə)rd\ *adj* **1 a** : not paired; *esp* : not matched or mated **b** : characterized by the absence of pairing ⟨electrons in the ∼ state⟩ **2** : situated in the median plane of the body ⟨an ∼ anatomical part⟩; *also* : not matched by a corresponding part on the opposite side

un·pas·teur·ized *also Brit* **un·pas·teur·ised** \-'pas-chə-,rīzd\ *adj* : not pasteurized ⟨∼ milk⟩

un·phys·i·o·log·i·cal \-,fiz-ē-ə-'läj-i-kəl\ *or* **un·phys·i·o·log·ic** \-ik\ *adj* : not characteristic of or appropriate to an organism's normal functioning ⟨∼ conditions⟩

un·pig·ment·ed \-'pig-mənt-əd\ *adj* : not pigmented : having no pigment

un·pro·tect·ed \-prə-'tek-təd\ *adj* : not protected; *esp* : performed without measures to prevent pregnancy or sexually transmitted disease ⟨∼ sexual intercourse⟩

Unq *symbol* unnilquadium

un·re·ac·tive \-rē-'ak-tiv\ *adj* : not reactive ⟨pupils ∼ to light⟩ ⟨an ∼ gas⟩

un·re·sect·able \-ri-'sek-tə-bəl\ *adj* : not capable of being resected ⟨an ∼ tumor⟩

un·re·solved \-ri-'zälvd, -'zolvd\ *adj* : not resolved : not having undergone resolution ⟨∼ pneumonia⟩

un·re·spon·sive \,ən-ri-'spän(t)-siv\ *adj* : not responsive (as to a stimulus or treatment) ⟨an ∼ ulcer⟩ — **un·re·spon·sive·ness** *n*

un·san·i·tary \-'san-ə-,ter-ē\ *adj* : not sanitary : INSANITARY ⟨∼ conditions⟩

un·sa·pon·i·fi·able \-sə-,pän-ə-'fī-ə-bəl\ *adj* : incapable of being saponified — used esp. of the portion of oils and fats other than the glycerides ⟨∼ fractions such as steroids or vitamin A⟩

un·sat·u·rate \-'sach-ə-rət\ *n* : an unsaturated chemical compound (as an alkene)

un·sat·u·rat·ed \-'sach-ə-,rāt-əd\ *adj* : not saturated: as **a** : capable of absorbing or dissolving more of something ⟨an ∼ solution⟩ **b** : able to form products by chemical addition; *esp* : containing double or triple bonds between carbon atoms ⟨∼ fats⟩

un·sat·u·ra·tion \-,sach-ə-'rā-shən\ *n* : the quality or state of being unsaturated

un·seg·ment·ed \-'seg-,ment-əd\ *adj* : not divided into or made up of segments

un·sex \-'seks\ *vt* : to deprive of sexual qualities or characteristics; *esp* : CASTRATE 1a

un·sound \-'saùnd\ *adj* : not sound: as **a** : not healthy or whole ⟨an ∼ limb⟩ ⟨an ∼ horse⟩ **b** : not mentally normal : not wholly sane ⟨of ∼ mind⟩ **c** : not fit to be eaten ⟨∼ food⟩ — **un·sound·ness** *n*

un·sta·ble \-'stā-bəl\ *adj* : not stable: as **a** : characterized by frequent or unpredictable changes ⟨a patient in ∼ condition⟩ **b** : readily changing (as by decomposing) in chemical composition or biological activity ⟨∼ compounds⟩ **c** : characterized by lack of emotional control or stability

unstable angina *n* : angina pectoris characterized by sudden changes (as an increase in the severity or length of anginal attacks or a decrease in the exertion required to precipitate an attack) esp. when symptoms were previously stable

un·stri·at·ed \,ən-'strī-,āt-əd\ *adj* : not striated : not marked by striae

unstriated muscle *n* : SMOOTH MUSCLE

un·struc·tured \,ən-'strək-chərd\ *adj* : lacking structure : not formally organized ⟨∼ psychological tests⟩

un·trans·formed \-tran(t)s-'förmd\ *adj* : not transformed; *specif* : not having undergone genetic transformation ⟨∼ cells⟩

un·trans·lat·ed \-'tran(t)s-,lāt-əd\ *adj* : not subjected to genetic translation ⟨∼ polynucleotide chains⟩

un·trau·ma·tized *also Brit* **un·trau·ma·tised** \-'trȯ-mə-ˌtīzd, -'traȯ-\ *adj* : not subjected to trauma ⟨~ skin⟩

un·treat·able \-'trēt-ə-bəl\ *adj* : not susceptible to medical treatment ⟨~ patients⟩ ⟨an ~ disease⟩

un·treat·ed \-'trēt-əd\ *adj* : not subjected to treatment ⟨an ~ disease⟩

un·vac·ci·nat·ed \-'vak-sə-ˌnāt-əd\ *adj* : not vaccinated ⟨~ children⟩

un·well \-'wel\ *adj* **1** : being in poor health : SICK **2** : undergoing menstruation

up·grade \'əp-ˌgrād, ˌəp-'\ *vt* **-grad·ed; -grad·ing 1** : to assign a less serious status to ⟨*upgraded* the patient's condition from fair to good⟩ **2** : to reclassify (as a cancer, concussion, or bone fracture) to a more serious grade when the grades are numbered from least to most serious

¹up·per \'əp-ər\ *n* : an upper tooth or denture

²upper *n* : a stimulant drug; *esp* : AMPHETAMINE

upper airway *n* : any or all of the air-conducting passages of the respiratory system that extend to the larynx from the two external openings of the nose and from the lips through the mouth

upper facial index *n* : the ratio of the distance between the nasion and prosthion to the bizygomatic breadth multiplied by 100

upper gastrointestinal series *n* : UPPER GI SERIES

upper GI series *n* : fluoroscopic and radiographic examination (as for the detection of gastroesophageal reflux, hiatal hernia, or ulcers) of the esophagus, stomach, and duodenum during and following oral ingestion of a solution of barium sulfate — called also *upper gastrointestinal series*

upper jaw *n* : JAW 1a

upper respiratory *adj* : of, relating to, or affecting the upper respiratory tract ⟨*upper respiratory* infection⟩

upper respiratory tract *n* : the part of the respiratory system including the nose, nasal passages, and nasopharynx — compare LOWER RESPIRATORY TRACT

up·reg·u·la·tion \'əp-ˌreg-yə-'lā-shən, -ˌreg-ə-'lā-\ *n* : the process of increasing the response to a stimulus; *specif* : increase in a cellular response to a molecular stimulus due to increase in the number of receptors on the cell surface — **up·reg·u·late** \-'reg-yə-ˌlāt\ *vt* **-lat·ed; -lat·ing**

¹up·set \(ˌ)əp-'set\ *vt* **-set; -set·ting 1** : to trouble mentally or emotionally ⟨the news ~ me⟩ **2** : to cause a physical disorder in; *specif* : to make somewhat ill ⟨greasy food ~s my stomach⟩

²up·set \'əp-ˌset\ *n* **1** : a minor physical disorder ⟨a stomach ~⟩ **2** : an emotional disturbance

³up·set \(ˌ)əp-'set\ *adj* **1** : affected with a minor physical disturbance ⟨an ~ stomach⟩ **2** : emotionally disturbed or agitated ⟨was too ~ to speak⟩

up·stream \'əp-'strēm\ *adv or adj* : in a direction along a molecule of DNA or RNA opposite to that in which transcription and translation take place and toward the end having a phosphate group attached to the position labeled 5′ in the terminal nucleotide ⟨a small coding sequence is located just ~ from each . . . gene —J. N. Goldman *et al*⟩ — compare DOWNSTREAM

up·take \'əp-ˌtāk\ *n* : an act or instance of absorbing and incorporating something esp. into a living organism, tissue, or cell ⟨oxygen ~⟩ ⟨thyroid function should be determined by radioiodine ~ studies —*Jour. Amer. Med. Assoc.*⟩

ura·chal \'yùr-ə-kəl\ *adj* : of or relating to the urachus ⟨a ~ cyst⟩

ura·chus \-kəs\ *n* : a cord of fibrous tissue extending from the bladder to the navel and constituting the functionless remnant of a part of the duct of the allantois of the embryo

ura·cil \'yùr-ə-ˌsil, -səl\ *n* : a pyrimidine base $C_4H_4N_2O_2$ that is one of the four bases coding genetic information in the polynucleotide chain of RNA — compare ADENINE, CYTOSINE, GUANINE, THYMINE

uraemia, uraemic *chiefly Brit var of* UREMIA, UREMIC

ura·mil \'yùr-ə-ˌmil\ *n* : a nitrogenous cyclic compound $C_4H_5N_3O_3$ obtained from derivatives of uric acid or urea in colorless crystals that redden on exposure

ura·nin \'yùr-ə-nən\ *n* : the sodium salt of fluorescein

ura·ni·nite \yù-'rā-nə-ˌnīt\ *n* : a mineral that is basically a black octahedral or cubic oxide of uranium containing lead, thorium, and rare earth elements and that is the chief ore of uranium

ura·nism \'yùr-ə-ˌniz-əm\ *n* : HOMOSEXUALITY

ura·nist \-nəst\ *n* : HOMOSEXUAL

ura·ni·um \yù-'rā-nē-əm\ *n* : a silvery heavy radioactive polyvalent metallic element that is found esp. in pitchblende and uraninite and exists naturally as a mixture of three isotopes of mass number 234, 235, and 238 in the proportions of 0.006 percent, 0.71 percent, and 99.28 percent respectively — symbol *U*; see ELEMENT table

uranium 235 *n* : a light isotope of uranium of mass number 235 that when bombarded with slow neutrons undergoes rapid fission into smaller atoms with the release of neutrons and atomic energy

ura·no·plas·ty \'yùr-ə-nō-ˌplas-tē\ *n, pl* **-ties** : PALATOPLASTY

ura·nos·chi·sis \ˌyùr-ə-'näs-kə-səs\ *n, pl* **-chi·ses** \-ˌsēz\ *also* **-chi·sis·es** : CLEFT PALATE

ura·no·staph·y·lo·plas·ty \ˌyùr-ə-nō-'staf-ə-lə-ˌplas-tē\ *n, pl* **-ties** : PALATOPLASTY

ura·nyl acetate \'yùr-ə-ˌnil-, yù-'rān-ᵊl-\ *n* : a yellow crystalline uranium salt $C_4H_6O_6U$ used as a reagent and esp. as a biological stain

urate \'yù(ə)r-ˌāt\ *n* : a salt of uric acid ⟨deposits of ~s in the joints⟩

urat·ic \yù-'rat-ik\ *adj* : of, relating to, or containing urates ⟨~ deposits⟩

urea \yù-'rē-ə\ *n* : a soluble weakly basic nitrogenous compound CH_4N_2O that is the chief solid component of mammalian urine and an end product of protein decomposition and that is administered intravenously as a diuretic drug — called also *carbamide*

urea peroxide *n* : a crystalline compound $CH_4N_2O·H_2O_2$ of urea and hydrogen peroxide used as a disinfectant

urea·plas·ma \yù-'rē-ə-ˌplaz-mə\ *n* **1** *cap* : a genus of mycoplasmas of the family Mycoplasmataceae that are able to hydrolyze urea with the formation of ammonia and that include one (*U. urealyticum*) found in the human genitourinary tract, oropharynx, and anal canal **2** : a mycoplasma of the genus *Ureaplasma*

ure·ase \'yùr-ē-ˌās, -ˌāz\ *n* : a crystallizable enzyme that catalyzes the hydrolysis of urea into ammonia and carbon dioxide, is present in the alkaline fermentation of urine, and is produced by many bacteria and found in various seeds

Ure·cho·line \ˌyùr-ə-'kō-ˌlēn\ *trademark* — used for a preparation of the chloride of bethanechol

ure·ide \'yùr-ē-ˌīd\ *n* : an acyl derivative of urea

ure·mia *or chiefly Brit* **urae·mia** \yù-'rē-mē-ə\ *n* **1** : accumulation in the blood of constituents normally eliminated in the urine that produces a severe toxic condition and usu. occurs in severe kidney disease **2** : the toxic bodily condition associated with uremia ⟨the patient was in ~⟩ — **ure·mic** *or chiefly Brit* **urae·mic** \-mik\ *adj*

ure·mi·gen·ic \yù-ˌrē-mə-'jen-ik\ *adj* : caused by uremia ⟨~ cholangitis⟩

ure·om·e·ter \ˌyùr-ē-'äm-ət-ər\ *n* : an apparatus for the detection and measurement of urea (as in blood or urine)

ureo·se·cre·to·ry \yù-ˌrē-ə-si-'krēt-ə-rē, ˌyùr-ē-ō-\ *adj* : of or relating to the secretion of urea

ureo·tel·ic \yù-ˌrē-ə-'tel-ik, ˌyùr-ē-ō-\ *adj* : excreting nitrogen mostly in the form of urea ⟨~ mammals⟩ — **ureo·te·lism** \-'tel-ˌiz-əm, ˌyùr-ē-'ät-ᵊl-ˌiz-əm\ *n*

ure·ter \'yùr-ət-ər, yù-'rēt-ər\ *n* : either of the paired ducts that carry away urine from a kidney to the bladder or cloaca and that in humans are slender membranous epithelium-lined flat tubes about sixteen inches (41 centimeters) long

---

\ə\ abut \ᵊ\ kitten \ər\ further \a\ ash \ā\ ace \ä\ cot, cart \aù\ out \ch\ chin \e\ bet \ē\ easy \g\ go \i\ hit \ī\ ice \j\ job \ŋ\ sing \ō\ go \ȯ\ law \ȯi\ boy \th\ thin \t̶h̶\ the \ü\ loot \ù\ foot \y\ yet \zh\ vision *See also* Pronunciation Symbols page

U
Z

which open above into the pelvis of a kidney and below into the back part of the same side of the bladder at a very oblique angle

ure·ter·al \yu̇-ˈrēt-ə-rəl\ *or* **ure·ter·ic** \ˌyu̇r-ə-ˈter-ik\ *adj* : of or relating to a ureter ⟨∼ occlusion⟩

ure·ter·ec·ta·sis \ˌyu̇r-ət-ər-ˈek-tə-səs, yu̇-ˌrēt-ər-\ *n, pl* **-ta·ses** \-ˌsēz\ : dilation of a ureter

ure·ter·ec·to·my \ˌyu̇r-ət-ər-ˈek-tə-mē, yu̇-ˌrēt-ər-\ *n, pl* **-mies** : surgical excision of all or part of a ureter

uretericus — see TORUS URETERICUS

ure·ter·itis \ˌyu̇r-ət-ər-ˈīt-əs, yu̇-ˌrēt-ər-\ *n* : inflammation of a ureter

ure·ter·o·cele \yu̇-ˈrēt-ə-rə-ˌsēl\ *n* : cystic dilation of the lower part of a ureter into the bladder

ure·ter·o·col·ic \yu̇-ˌrēt-ə-rō-ˈkō-lik, -ˈkäl-ik\ *adj* : relating to or joining the colon and a ureter ⟨a ∼ anastomosis⟩

ure·ter·o·co·los·to·my \yu̇-ˌrēt-ə-rō-kə-ˈläs-tə-mē\ *n, pl* **-mies** : surgical implantation of a ureter into the colon

ure·ter·o·en·ter·os·to·my \-ˌen-tə-ˈräs-tə-mē\ *n, pl* **-mies** : surgical formation of an artificial opening between a ureter and the intestine

ure·ter·o·gram \yu̇-ˈrēt-ə-rə-ˌgram\ *n* : an X-ray photograph of the ureters after injection of a radiopaque substance

ure·ter·og·ra·phy \yu̇-ˌrēt-ə-ˈräg-rə-fē, ˌyu̇r-ət-ə-\ *n, pl* **-phies** : the making of ureterograms

ure·ter·o·il·e·al \yu̇-ˌrēt-ə-rō-ˈil-ē-əl\ *adj* : relating to or connecting a ureter and the ileum

ure·ter·o·in·tes·ti·nal \yu̇-ˌrēt-ə-rō-in-ˈtes-tən-ᵊl, Brit often -ˌin-(ˌ)tes-ˈtīn-ᵊl\ *adj* : of, relating to, or connecting the intestine and a ureter ⟨∼ anastomosis⟩

ure·ter·o·li·thot·o·my \yu̇-ˌrēt-ə-rō-li-ˈthät-ə-mē\ *n, pl* **-mies** : removal of a calculus by incision of a ureter

ure·ter·ol·y·sis \ˌyu̇r-ət-ər-ˈäl-ə-səs, yu̇-ˌrēt-ər-\ *n, pl* **-y·ses** \-ˌsēz\ : a surgical procedure to free a ureter from abnormal adhesions or surrounding tissue (as in retroperitoneal fibrosis)

ure·ter·o·neo·cys·tos·to·my \yu̇-ˌrēt-ər-ō-ˌnē-ō-sis-ˈtäs-tə-mē\ *n, pl* **-mies** : surgical reimplantation of a ureter into the bladder

ure·ter·o·ne·phrec·to·my \yu̇-ˌrēt-ə-rō-ni-ˈfrek-tə-mē\ *n, pl* **-mies** : surgical excision of a kidney with its ureter

ure·ter·o·pel·vic \-ˈpel-vik\ *adj* : of, relating to, or involving a ureter and the adjoining renal pelvis ⟨∼ obstruction⟩

ure·ter·o·pel·vio·plas·ty \yu̇-ˌrēt-ə-rō-ˈpel-vē-ə-ˌplas-tē\ *n, pl* **-ties** : plastic surgery for the repair of a ureter and its adjacent renal pelvis

ure·ter·o·plas·ty \yu̇-ˈrēt-ə-rə-ˌplas-tē\ *n, pl* **-ties** : plastic surgery performed on a ureter

ure·ter·o·py·elog·ra·phy \yu̇-ˌrēt-ə-rō-ˌpī-ə-ˈläg-rə-fē\ *n, pl* **-phies** : X-ray photography of a renal pelvis and a ureter following the injection of a radiopaque medium

ure·ter·o·py·elo·ne·os·to·my \yu̇-ˌrēt-ə-rō-ˌpī-(ə)lō-nē-ˈäs-tə-mē\ *n, pl* **-mies** : surgical creation of a new channel joining a renal pelvis to a ureter

ure·ter·o·py·e·los·to·my \-ˌpī-(ə)-ˈläs-tə-mē\ *n, pl* **-mies** : URETEROPYELONEOSTOMY

ure·ter·or·rha·phy \ˌyu̇-ˌrēt-ə-ˈrȯr-ə-fē, ˌyu̇r-ət-ə-\ *n, pl* **-phies** : the surgical operation of suturing a ureter

ure·ter·o·scope \yu̇-ˈrēt-ə-rō-ˌskōp\ *n* : an endoscope for visually examining and passing instruments into the interior of the ureter

ure·ter·os·co·py \yu̇-ˌrēt-ə-ˈräs-kə-pē, ˌyu̇r-ət-ə-\ *n, pl* **-pies** : examination of the interior of a ureter by means of a ureteroscope

ure·ter·o·sig·moid·os·to·my \yu̇-ˌrēt-ə-rō-ˌsig-ˌmȯid-ˈäs-tə-mē\ *n, pl* **-mies** : surgical implantation of a ureter in the sigmoid colon

ure·ter·o·ste·no·sis \yu̇-ˌrēt-ə-rō-stə-ˈnō-səs\ *n, pl* **-no·ses** \-ˌsēz\ : stricture of a ureter

ure·ter·os·to·my \ˌyu̇r-ət-ər-ˈäs-tə-mē, yu̇-ˌrēt-ər-\ *n, pl* **-mies** : surgical creation of an opening on the surface of the body for the ureters

ure·ter·ot·o·my \ˌyu̇r-ət-ər-ˈät-ə-mē, yu̇-ˌrēt-ər-\ *n, pl* **-mies** : the operation of cutting into a ureter

ure·tero·ure·ter·os·to·my \yu̇-ˌrēt-ə-rō-yu̇-ˌrēt-ər-ˈäs-tə-mē\ *n, pl* **-mies** : surgical establishment of an artificial communication between two ureters or between different parts of the same ureter

ure·tero·ves·i·cal \yu̇-ˌrēt-ə-rō-ˈves-i-kəl\ *adj* : of or relating to the ureters and the urinary bladder

ure·thane \ˈyu̇r-ə-ˌthān\ *or* **ure·than** \-ˌthan\ *n* **1** : a crystalline compound $C_3H_7NO_2$ that is the ethyl ester of carbamic acid and is used esp. as a solvent and in anesthetizing laboratory animals — called also *ethyl carbamate* **2** : an ester of carbamic acid other than the ethyl ester

ure·thra \yu̇-ˈrē-thrə\ *n, pl* **-thras** *or* **-thrae** \-(ˌ)thrē\ : the canal that in most mammals carries off the urine from the bladder and in the male serves also as a passageway for semen — **ure·thral** \-thrəl\ *adj*

urethrae — see SPHINCTER URETHRAE

urethral crest *n* : a narrow longitudinal fold or ridge along the posterior wall or floor of the female urethra or the prostatic portion of the male urethra

urethral gland *n* : any of the small mucous glands in the wall of the male or female urethra — see GLAND OF LITTRÉ

urethral sphincter *n* : SPHINCTER URETHRAE

urethral syndrome *n* : a group of symptoms (as urinary frequency and urgency, pain and discomfort in the lower abdominal region, and dysuria) that resemble those of a urinary tract infection but for which no significant bacteriuria exists

ure·threc·to·my \ˌyu̇r-i-ˈthrek-tə-mē\ *n, pl* **-mies** : total or partial surgical excision of the urethra

ure·thri·tis \ˌyu̇r-i-ˈthrīt-əs\ *n* : inflammation of the urethra

ure·thro·cele \yə-ˈrēth-rə-ˌsēl\ *n* : a pouched protrusion of urethral mucous membrane in the female

ure·thro·cu·ta·ne·ous \yu̇-ˌrē-thrō-kyu̇-ˈtā-nē-əs\ *adj* : of, relating to, or joining the urethra and the skin ⟨a ∼ fistula⟩

ure·thro·cys·tog·ra·phy \yu̇-ˌrē-thrō-sis-ˈtäg-rə-fē\ *n, pl* **-phies** : radiography of the urethra and bladder that utilizes a radiopaque substance

ure·thro·gram \yu̇-ˈrē-thrə-ˌgram\ *n* : a radiograph of the urethra made after injection of a radiopaque substance

ure·throg·ra·phy \ˌyu̇r-i-ˈthräg-rə-fē\ *n, pl* **-phies** : radiography of the urethra after injection of a radiopaque substance

ure·thro·pexy \yu̇-ˈrē-thrə-ˌpek-sē\ *n, pl* **-pex·ies** : surgical fixation to nearby tissue of a displaced urethra that is causing incontinence by placing stress on the opening from the bladder

ure·thro·plas·ty \yu̇-ˈrē-thrə-ˌplas-tē\ *n, pl* **-ties** : plastic surgery of the urethra

ure·thro·rec·tal \yu̇-ˌrē-thrō-ˈrek-tᵊl\ *adj* : of, relating to, or joining the urethra and the rectum ⟨a ∼ fistula⟩

ure·thror·rha·phy \ˌyu̇r-ə-ˈthrȯr-ə-fē\ *n, pl* **-phies** : suture of the urethra for an injury or fistula

ure·thro·scope \yu̇-ˈrē-thrə-ˌskōp\ *n* : an endoscope for viewing the interior of the urethra — **ure·thro·scop·ic** \yu̇-ˌrē-thrə-ˈskäp-ik\ *adj*

ure·thros·co·py \ˌyu̇r-ə-ˈthräs-kə-pē\ *n, pl* **-pies** : examination of the urethra by means of a urethroscope

ure·thros·to·my \ˌyu̇r-ə-ˈthräs-tə-mē\ *n, pl* **-mies** : the creation of a surgical opening between the perineum and the urethra

ure·thro·tome \yu̇-ˈrēth-rə-ˌtōm\ *n* : a surgical instrument for cutting a urethral stricture

ure·throt·o·my \ˌyu̇r-ə-ˈthrät-ə-mē\ *n, pl* **-mies** : surgical incision into the urethra esp. for the relief of stricture

ure·thro·vag·i·nal \yu̇-ˌrē-thrō-ˈvaj-ən-ᵊl\ *adj* : of, relating to, or joining the urethra and the vagina ⟨a ∼ fistula⟩

urge incontinence \ˈərj-\ *n* : involuntary leakage of urine from the bladder when a sudden strong need to urinate is felt — compare STRESS INCONTINENCE

ur·gen·cy \ˈər-jən-sē\ *n, pl* **-cies** : a sudden compelling need to urinate or defecate

ur·gin·ea \ər-ˈjin-ē-ə\ *n* **1** *cap* : a genus of bulbous herbs of the lily family native to the Old World and esp. to the Mediterranean region — see SQUILL 1a **2 a** *often cap* : squill for medicinal use composed of the sliced young bulbs of the squill (*Urginea indica*) of the Orient — used in the British Pharmacopoeia; called also *Indian squill;* compare WHITE SQUILL   **b :** any plant of the genus *Urginea*

URI *abbr* upper respiratory infection

uric \'yu̇r-ik\ *adj* : of, relating to, or found in urine

uric acid *n* : a white odorless nearly insoluble weak acid $C_5H_4N_4O_3$ that is present in small quantity in mammalian urine as an end product of purine metabolism, is present abundantly in the form of urates in the excreta of most lower vertebrates and invertebrates as the chief nitrogenous waste, and occurs pathologically in renal calculi and the tophi of gout

uric·ac·i·de·mia *or chiefly Brit* **uric·ac·i·dae·mia** \,yu̇r-ik-,as-ə-'dē-mē-ə\ *n* : HYPERURICEMIA

uric·ac·id·uria \,yu̇r-ik-,as-ə-'d(y)u̇r-ē-ə\ *n* : the presence of excess uric acid in the urine

uri·case \'yu̇r-ə-,kās, -,kāz\ *n* : an enzyme that promotes oxidation of uric acid to allantoin, carbon dioxide, and other products and that is found esp. in the liver, kidney, and brains of most animals other than primates

uri·ce·mia *or chiefly Brit* **uri·cae·mia** \,yu̇r-ə-'sē-mē-ə\ *n* : HYPERURICEMIA — **uri·ce·mic** *or chiefly Brit* **uri·cae·mic** \-mik\ *adj*

uri·col·y·sis \,yu̇r-i-'käl-ə-səs\ *n, pl* **-y·ses** \-,sēz\ : breakdown of uric acid esp. in the body

uri·co·lyt·ic \,yu̇r-i-kō-'lit-ik\ *adj* : of, relating to, or functioning in uricolysis ⟨a ~ enzyme⟩

uri·co·su·ria \-'su̇r-ē-ə, -'shu̇r-\ *n* : the excretion of uric acid in the urine esp. in excessive amounts

¹**uri·co·su·ric** \-'su̇r-ik, -'shu̇r-\ *adj* : relating to or promoting uricosuria ⟨~ drugs⟩

²**uricosuric** *n* : a uricosuric agent (as probenecid)

uri·co·tel·ic \,yu̇r-i-kō-'tel-ik\ *adj* : excreting nitrogen mostly in the form of uric acid ⟨birds are typical ~ animals⟩ — **uri·co·tel·ism** \-'tel-,iz-əm, -'kät-ᵊl-,iz-əm\ *n*

uri·dine \'yu̇r-ə-,dēn\ *n* : a crystalline pyrimidine nucleoside $C_9H_{12}N_2O_6$ that is composed of uracil attached to ribose, that is derived by hydrolysis from nucleic acids, and that in the form of phosphate derivatives plays an important role in carbohydrate metabolism

uridine diphosphate *also* **uridine 5′–diphosphate** \-'fīv-'prīm-\ *n* : UDP

uridine diphosphate glucose *n* : a coenzyme $C_{15}H_{24}N_2O_{17}P_2$ that reversibly catalyzes the formation of glucose-1-phosphate from the corresponding phosphate of galactose and that acts as a donor of glucose residues in the biosynthesis of glycogen

uridine di·phos·pho·glu·cose \-,dī-,fäs-fō-'glü-,kōs\ *n* : URIDINE DIPHOSPHATE GLUCOSE

uridine triphosphate *also* **uridine 5′–triphosphate** \-'fīv-'prīm-\ *n* : UTP

urid·y·late \yu̇-'rid-ə-,lāt, -lət\ *n* : a salt or ester of uridylic acid

uri·dyl·ic acid \,yu̇r-ə-,dil-ik-\ *n* : a nucleotide $C_9H_{13}N_2O_9P$ known in three isomeric forms obtained by hydrolysis of RNA — called also *UMP*

urinae — see ARDOR URINAE, DETRUSOR URINAE

uri·nal \'yu̇r-ən-ᵊl\ *n* **1 :** a vessel so constructed that it can be used for urination by a bedridden patient   **2 :** a container worn by a person with urinary incontinence

uri·nal·y·sis \,yu̇r-ə-'nal-ə-səs\ *n, pl* **-y·ses** \-,sēz\ : chemical analysis of urine

urinaria — see VESICA URINARIA

uri·nary \'yu̇r-ə-,ner-ē\ *adj* **1 :** relating to, occurring in, or constituting the organs concerned with the formation and discharge of urine   **2 :** of, relating to, or for urine   **3 :** excreted as or in urine ⟨~ sugar⟩

urinary bladder *n* : a distensible membranous sac that serves for the temporary retention of the urine, is situated in the pelvis in front of the rectum, receives the urine from the two ureters and discharges it at intervals into the urethra through an orifice closed by a sphincter, is lined with transitional hypoblastic epithelium, and develops from the proximal part of the allantois of the embryo

urinary calculus *n* : a calculus occurring in any portion of the urinary tract and esp. in the pelvis of the kidney — called also *urinary stone, urolith*

urinary system *n* : the organs of the urinary tract comprising the kidneys, ureters, urinary bladder, and urethra

urinary tract *n* : the tract through which urine passes and which consists of the renal tubules and renal pelvis of the kidney, the ureters, the bladder, and the urethra

uri·nate \'yu̇r-ə-,nāt\ *vi* **-nat·ed; -nat·ing :** to discharge urine : MICTURATE

uri·na·tion \,yu̇r-ə-'nā-shən\ *n* : the act of urinating — called also *micturition*

urine \'yu̇r-ən\ *n* : waste material that is secreted by the kidney, is rich in end products (as urea, uric acid, and creatinine) of protein metabolism together with salts and pigments, and forms a clear amber and usu. slightly acid fluid

uri·nif·er·ous tubule \,yu̇r-ə-'nif-(ə-)rəs-\ *n* : a tubule (as a convoluted tubule) of the kidney that collects or conducts urine

uri·no·gen·i·tal \,yu̇r-ə-nō-'jen-ə-tᵊl\ *adj* : UROGENITAL

uri·no·ma \,yu̇r-ə-'nō-mə\ *n, pl* **-mas** *also* **-ma·ta** \-mət-ə\ : a cyst that contains urine

uri·nom·e·ter \,yu̇r-ə-'näm-ət-ər\ *n* : a small hydrometer for determining the specific gravity of urine

uri·nous \'yu̇r-ə-nəs\ *adj* : of, relating to, like, or having the qualities or odor of urine

ur·ning \'u̇r-niŋ\ *n* : HOMOSEXUAL

uro·bi·lin \,yu̇r-ə-'bī-lən\ *n* : any of several brown bile pigments formed from urobilinogens and found in normal feces, in normal urine in small amounts, and in pathological urines in larger amounts

uro·bi·lin·o·gen \,yu̇r-ə-bī-'lin-ə-jən, -,jen\ *n* : any of several chromogens that are reduction products of bilirubin and yield urobilins on oxidation — called also *stercobilinogen*

uro·bi·lin·o·gen·uria \-,lin-ə-jə-'n(y)u̇r-ē-ə\ *n* : the presence of urobilinogen in the urine esp. in excess

uro·ca·nic acid \,yu̇r-ə-,kā-nik-, -,kan-ik-\ *n* : a crystalline acid $C_6H_6N_2O_2$ normally present in human skin that is held to act as a screening agent for ultraviolet radiation

uro·chlo·ral·ic acid \,yu̇r-ə-klō-,ral-ik-\ *n* : a crystalline glycoside $C_8H_{11}Cl_3O_7$ found in the urine after chloral hydrate is administered

uro·chrome \'yu̇r-ə-,krōm\ *n* : a yellow pigment to which the color of normal urine is principally due

uro·dy·nam·ics \,yu̇r-ə-dī-'nam-iks\ *n pl but sing in constr* : the hydrodynamics of the urinary tract — **uro·dy·nam·ic** \-ik\ *adj* — **uro·dy·nam·i·cal·ly** \-i-k(ə-)lē\ *adv*

uro·ep·i·the·li·al \,yu̇r-ō-,ep-ə-'thē-lē-əl\ *adj* : of or affecting the epithelium of the urinary tract ⟨~ cells⟩ ⟨~ cancers⟩ — **uro·ep·i·the·li·um** \-əm\ *n*

uro·er·y·thrin \,yu̇r-ō-'er-ə-thrən\ *n* : a pink or reddish pigment found in many pathological urines and also frequently in normal urine in very small quantity

uro·gas·trone \,yu̇r-ə-'gas-,trōn\ *n* : a polypeptide that has been isolated from urine and inhibits gastric secretion — compare ENTEROGASTRONE

uro·gen·i·tal \,yu̇r-ō-'jen-ə-tᵊl\ *adj* : of, relating to, affecting, treating, or being the organs or functions of excretion and reproduction : GENITOURINARY

urogenital diaphragm *n* : a double layer of pelvic fascia with its included muscle that is situated between the ischial and pubic rami, supports the prostate in the male, is traversed by the vagina in the female, gives passage to the membranous part of the urethra, and encloses the sphincter urethrae

urogenital ridge *n* : a pair of dorsolateral mesodermal ridges in the vertebrate embryo out of which the urogenital organs are developed

urogenital sinus *n* : the ventral part of the embryonic mam-

---

\ə\ abut \ᵊ\ kitten \ər\ further \a\ ash \ā\ ace \ä\ cot, cart
\au̇\ out \ch\ chin \e\ bet \ē\ easy \g\ go \i\ hit \ī\ ice \j\ job
\ŋ\ sing \ō\ go \ȯ\ law \ȯi\ boy \th\ thin \t̲h\ the \ü\ loot
\u̇\ foot \y\ yet \zh\ vision   *See also* Pronunciation Symbols page

U Z

malian cloaca that is formed by the growth of a fold dividing the cloaca where the gut and allantois meet and that eventually forms the neck of the bladder and some of the more distal portions of the genitourinary tract

urogenital system *n* : GENITOURINARY TRACT

urogenital tract *n* : GENITOURINARY TRACT

uro·gram \\'yu̇r-ə-ˌgram\\ *n* : a radiograph made by urography

uro·graph·ic \\ˌyu̇r-ə-'graf-ik\\ *adj* : of or relating to urography ⟨∼ findings⟩

urog·ra·phy \\yu̇-'räg-rə-fē\\ *n, pl* **-phies** : radiography of a part of the urinary tract (as a kidney or ureter) after injection of a radiopaque substance

uro·gy·ne·col·o·gist *or chiefly Brit* **uro·gy·nae·col·o·gist** \\ˌyu̇r-ō-ˌgīn-ə-'käl-ə-jəst, -ˌjin-\\ *n* : a specialist in urogynecology

uro·gy·ne·col·o·gy *or chiefly Brit* **uro·gy·nae·col·o·gy** \\-'käl-ə-jē\\ *n, pl* **-gies** : a branch of medicine concerned with the urological problems (as urinary incontinence) of women — **uro·gy·ne·co·log·ic** \\-ˌgīn-ə-kə-'läj-ik, -ˌjin-\\ *or* **uro·gy·ne·co·log·i·cal** \\-i-kəl\\ *or chiefly Brit* **uro·gy·nae·co·log·ic** *or* **uro·gy·nae·co·log·i·cal** *adj*

uro·ki·nase \\ˌyu̇r-ō-'kī-ˌnās, -ˌnāz\\ *n* : an enzyme that is produced by the kidney and is found in human urine, that activates plasminogen, and that is used therapeutically to dissolve blood clots (as in the heart)

uro·lag·nia \\ˌyu̇r-ō-'lag-nē-ə\\ *n* : sexual excitement associated with urine or with urination

uro·lith \\'yu̇r-ə-ˌlith\\ *n* : URINARY CALCULUS

uro·lith·ia·sis \\ˌyu̇r-ə-lith-'ī-ə-səs\\ *n, pl* **-ia·ses** \\-ˌsēz\\ : a condition that is characterized by the formation or presence of calculi in the urinary tract

uro·log·i·cal \\ˌyu̇r-ə-'läj-i-kəl\\ *also* **uro·log·ic** \\-'läj-ik\\ *adj* : of or relating to the urinary tract or to urology ⟨a ∼ examination⟩ ⟨∼ infections⟩

urol·o·gist \\yu̇-'räl-ə-jəst\\ *n* : a physician who specializes in urology

urol·o·gy \\-jē\\ *n, pl* **-gies** : a branch of medicine dealing with the urinary or urogenital organs

uron·ic acid \\yu̇-ˌrän-ik-\\ *n* : any of a class of acidic compounds of the general formula HOOC(CHOH)$_n$CHO that contain both carboxylic and aldehydic groups, are oxidation products of sugars, and occur combined in many polysaccharides and in urine

uro·patho·gen·ic \\ˌyu̇r-ō-ˌpath-ə-'jen-ik\\ *adj* : of, relating to, or being a pathogen (as some strains of E. coli) of the urinary tract — **uro·patho·gen** \\-'path-ə-jən\\ *n*

urop·a·thy \\yu̇-'räp-ə-thē\\ *n, pl* **-thies** : a disease of the urinary or urogenital organs — **uro·path·ic** \\ˌyu̇r-ə-'path-ik\\ *adj*

uro·pep·sin \\ˌyu̇r-ō-'pep-sən\\ *n* : a proteolytic hormone found in urine esp. in cases of peptic ulcers and other disorders of the digestive tract

uro·por·phy·rin \\ˌyu̇r-ō-'pȯr-fə-rən\\ *n* : any of four isomeric porphyrins $C_{40}H_{38}N_4O_{16}$ which contain acetic acid and propionic acid groups on the porphin nucleus and are closely related to the coproporphyrins

uro·por·phy·rin·ogen \\ˌyu̇r-ō-ˌpȯr-fə-'rin-ə-jən\\ *n* : any of several porphyrins that can be converted to uroporphyrins or to a precursor of coproporphyrins

uro·ra·di·ol·o·gy \\ˌyu̇r-ō-ˌrād-ē-'äl-ə-jē\\ *n, pl* **-gies** : radiology of the urinary tract — **uro·ra·dio·log·ic** \\-ˌrād-ē-ə-'läj-ik\\ *adj*

uros·co·py \\yu̇-'äs-kə-pē\\ *n, pl* **-pies** : examination or analysis of the urine (as for the purpose of medical diagnosis)

uro·sep·sis \\ˌyu̇r-ō-'sep-səs\\ *n, pl* **-sep·ses** \\-ˌsēz\\ : a toxic condition caused by the extravasation of urine into bodily tissues

uros·to·my \\yu̇-'räs-tə-mē\\ *n, pl* **-mies** : an ostomy for the elimination of urine from the body

ur·so·de·oxy·cho·lic acid \\ˌər-sō-dē-ˌäk-sē-ˌkō-lik-\\ *n* : URSODIOL

ur·so·di·ol \\ˌər-sō-'dī-ˌȯl, -ˌōl\\ *n* : a bile acid $C_{24}H_{40}O_4$ stereoisomeric with chenodeoxycholic acid that is used to dissolve uncalcified radiolucent gallstones — called also *ursodeoxycholic acid*

ur·ti·ca \\'ərt-i-kə\\ *n*   **1** *cap* : a genus (the type of the family Urticaceae) of widely distributed plants comprising the nettles and having leaves with stinging hairs and small greenish flowers   **2** : NETTLE 1

ur·ti·car·ia \\ˌərt-ə-'kar-ē-ə, -'ker-\\ *n* : HIVES — **ur·ti·car·i·al** \\-ē-əl\\ *adj*

ur·ti·car·io·gen·ic \\ˌərt-ə-ˌkar-ē-ə-'jen-ik\\ *adj* : being an agent or substance that induces or predisposes to urticarial lesions (as wheals on the skin)

urticata — see ACNE URTICATA

ur·ti·cate \\'ərt-ə-ˌkāt\\ *vi* **-cat·ed; -cat·ing** : to produce wheals or itching; *esp* : to induce hives — **ur·ti·ca·tion** \\ˌərt-ə-'kā-shən\\ *n*

uru·shi·ol \\(y)u̇-'rü-shē-ˌȯl, -ˌōl\\ *n* : a mixture of pyrocatechol derivatives with saturated or unsaturated side chains of 15 or 17 carbon atoms that is an oily toxic irritant principle present in poison ivy and some related plants of the genus *Rhus*

USAN *abbr* United States Adopted Names — used to designate officially recognized nonproprietary names of drugs as established by a joint committee of medical and pharmaceutical professionals

Ush·er's syndrome \\'əsh-ərz-\\ *also* **Ush·er syndrome** \\-ər-\\ *n* : an inherited disease that is characterized by congenital deafness or progressive hearing loss during childhood and by retinitis pigmentosa and that is inherited chiefly as an autosomal recessive trait

  Usher, Charles Howard (1865–1942), British ophthalmologist. Usher published his description of Usher's syndrome in a 1914 article reporting on some cases of inherited retinitis pigmentosa.

Us·nea \\'əs-nē-ə\\ *n* : a genus of widely distributed lichens (family Usneaceae) including old-man's beard from which usnic acid is obtained

us·nic acid \\ˌəs-nik-\\ *n* : a yellow crystalline antibiotic $C_{18}H_{16}O_7$ that is obtained from various lichens (as old-man's beard)

USP *abbr* United States Pharmacopeia

USPSTF *abbr* U.S. Preventive Services Task Force

us·ti·lag·i·nism \\ˌəs-tə-'laj-ə-ˌniz-əm\\ *n* : a toxic condition caused by eating corn infested with a parasitic fungus of the genus *Ustilago* (*U. maydis*)

Us·ti·la·go \\ˌəs-tə-'lā-gō\\ *n* : a genus (the type of the family Ustilaginaceae) of parasitic fungi that cause various destructive plant diseases esp. of cereal grasses

uta \\'üt-ə\\ *n* : a leishmaniasis of the skin occurring in Peru : ESPUNDIA

ut dict *abbr* [Latin *ut dictum*] as directed — used in writing prescriptions

uter·ec·to·my \\ˌyüt-ə-'rek-tə-mē\\ *n, pl* **-mies** : HYSTERECTOMY

uteri *pl of* UTERUS

uteri — see CERVIX UTERI, CORPUS UTERI

uter·ine \\'yüt-ə-ˌrīn, -rən\\ *adj* : of, relating to, occurring in, or affecting the uterus ⟨∼ tissue⟩ ⟨∼ cancer⟩

uterine artery *n* : an artery that arises from the internal iliac artery and after following a course between the layers of the broad ligament reaches the uterus at the cervix and supplies the uterus and adjacent parts and during pregnancy the placenta

uterine gland *n* : any of the branched tubular glands in the mucous membrane of the uterus

uterine milk *n* : a nutritive secretion that is produced by uterine glands esp. during the early phases of mammalian gestation and that nourishes the young mammalian embryo prior to implantation

uterine plexus *n* : a plexus of veins tributary to the internal iliac vein by which blood is returned from the uterus

uterine tube *n* : FALLOPIAN TUBE

uterine vein *n* : any of the veins that make up the uterine plexus

utero·ges·ta·tion \ˌyüt-ə-(ˌ)rō-jes-ˈtā-shən\ *n* : normal gestation within the uterus

uter·o·gram \ˈyüt-ə-rə-ˌgram\ *n* : HYSTEROGRAM

uter·og·ra·phy \ˌyüt-ə-ˈräg-rə-fē\ *n, pl* **-phies** : HYSTEROGRAPHY

utero·ma·nia \ˌyüt-ə-rə-ˈmā-nē-ə\ *n* : NYMPHOMANIA

utero·ovar·ian \ˌyüt-ə-(ˌ)rō-ō-ˈvar-ē-ən\ *adj* : of or relating to the uterus and the ovary ⟨∼ blood flow⟩

utero·pla·cen·tal \-plə-ˈsent-ᵊl\ *adj* : of or relating to the uterus and the placenta ⟨∼ circulation⟩

utero·sa·cral ligament \ˌyüt-ə-rō-ˈsak-rəl-, -ˌsāk-\ *n* : a fibrous fascial band on each side of the uterus that passes along the lateral wall of the pelvis from the uterine cervix to the sacrum and that serves to support the uterus and hold it in place — called also *sacrouterine ligament*

utero·sal·pin·gog·ra·phy \-ˌsal-ˌpiŋ-ˈgäg-rə-fē\ *n, pl* **-phies** : HYSTEROSALPINGOGRAPHY

utero·ton·ic \ˌyüt-ə-rō-ˈtän-ik\ *adj* : stimulating muscular tone in the uterus ⟨a ∼ substance⟩

utero·tub·al \-ˈt(y)ü-bəl\ *adj* : of or relating to the uterus and fallopian tubes ⟨the ∼ junction⟩

utero·vag·i·nal \-ˈvaj-ən-ᵊl\ *adj* : of or relating to the uterus and the vagina ⟨∼ prolapse⟩

utero·ves·i·cal pouch \-ˈves-i-kəl-\ *n* : a pouch formed by the peritoneum between the uterus and the bladder

uter·us \ˈyüt-ə-rəs\ *n, pl* **uteri** \-ˌrī\ *also* **uter·us·es** : an organ in female mammals for containing and usu. for nourishing the young during development prior to birth that consists of a greatly modified and enlarged section of an oviduct (as in rodents and marsupials) or of the two oviducts united (as in the higher primates including humans), that has thick walls consisting of an outer serous layer, a very thick middle layer of smooth muscle, and an inner mucous layer containing numerous glands, and that during pregnancy undergoes great increase in size and change in the condition of its walls — called also *womb;* see CERVIX 2a, CORPUS UTERI, ENDOMETRIUM, FUNDUS c, MYOMETRIUM, PERIMETRIUM

UTI \ˌyü-(ˌ)tē-ˈī\ *n* : a urinary tract infection

uti·li·za·tion re·view \ˌyüt-ᵊl-ə-ˈzā-shən-ri-ˈvyü\ *n* : the critical examination (as by a physician or nurse) of health-care services provided to patients esp. for the purpose of controlling costs (as by identifying unnecessary medical procedures) and monitoring the quality of care

UTP \ˈyü-ˈtē-ˈpē\ *n* : a phosphorylated nucleoside $C_9H_{15}N_2O_{15}P_3$ of uridine that is formed by the phosphorylation of uridylic acid and that reacts with glucose-1-phosphate to yield uridine diphosphate glucose in the biosynthetic pathway of glycogen — called also *uridine triphosphate*

utri·cle \ˈyü-tri-kəl\ *n* : a small anatomical pouch: as **a** : the part of the membranous labyrinth of the ear into which the semicircular canals open — called also *utriculus* **b** : PROSTATIC UTRICLE — **utric·u·lar** \yu̇-ˈtrik-yə-lər\ *adj*

utriculi — see MACULA UTRICULI

utric·u·lo·sac·cu·lar duct \yu̇-ˌtrik-yə-lō-ˌsak-yə-lər-\ *n* : a narrow tube connecting the utricle to the saccule in the membranous labyrinth of the ear

utric·u·lus \yu̇-ˈtrik-yə-ləs\ *n, pl* **-li** \-ˌlī\ : UTRICLE a

UV \(ˈ)yü-ˈvē\ *abbr* ultraviolet

UVA \-ˈā\ *n* : radiation that is in the region of the ultraviolet spectrum which is nearest to visible light and extends from 320 to 400 nm in wavelength and that causes tanning and contributes to aging of the skin

uva·ur·si \ˌyü-və-ˈər-sē\ *n* : the dried leaves of the bearberry used esp. formerly as an astringent and diuretic

UVB \-ˈbē\ *n* : radiation that is in the region of the ultraviolet spectrum which extends from 280 to 320 nm in wavelength and that is primarily responsible for sunburn, aging of the skin, and the development of skin cancer

UVC \-ˈsē\ *n* : radiation that is in the region of the ultraviolet spectrum which extends from about 200 to 280 nm in wavelength and that is more hazardous than UVB but is mostly absorbed by the earth's upper atmosphere

uvea \ˈyü-vē-ə\ *n* : the middle layer of the eye consisting of the iris and ciliary body together with the choroid coat — called also *vascular tunic*

uve·al \ˈyü-vē-əl\ *adj* : of, relating to, affecting, or being the uvea ⟨∼ tissue⟩

uve·itis \ˌyü-vē-ˈīt-əs\ *n, pl* **uve·it·i·des** \-ˈit-ə-ˌdēz\ : inflammation of the uvea

uveo·pa·rot·id fever \ˌyü-vē-ō-pə-ˈrät-əd-\ *n* : chronic inflammation of the parotid gland and uvea marked by low-grade fever, lassitude, and bilateral iridocyclitis and sometimes associated with sarcoidosis — called also *Heerfordt's syndrome, uveoparotitis*

uveo·par·oti·tis \-ˌpar-ō-ˈtīt-əs\ *n* : UVEOPAROTID FEVER

UV index *n* : a number on a scale which extends indefinitely upward from a baseline of 0 and whose values express the intensity of solar ultraviolet radiation at noon on a given day for a particular location with 0 indicating negligible ultraviolet exposure and values over 10 indicating very high ultraviolet exposure

uvu·la \ˈyü-vyə-lə\ *n, pl* **-las** \-ləz\ *or* **-lae** \-ˌlē\ **1** : the pendent fleshy lobe in the middle of the posterior border of the soft palate **2** : a lobe of the inferior vermis of the cerebellum located in front of the pyramid — **uvu·lar** \-lər\ *adj*

uvula ves·i·cae \-ˈves-ə-ˌkē\ *n* : an elevation of the mucous membrane lining the lower anterior part of the bladder

uvu·lec·to·my \ˌyü-vyə-ˈlek-tə-mē\ *n, pl* **-mies** : surgical excision of the uvula

U wave \ˈyü-ˌ\ *n* : a positive wave following the T wave on an electrocardiogram

V

V *abbr* volt

V *symbol* vanadium

vac·cen·ic acid \vak-ˈsen-ik-\ *n* : a crystalline unsaturated acid $C_{18}H_{34}O_2$ that is isomeric with elaidic acid and oleic acid and that is obtained esp. from animal fats

vac·ci·nal \ˈvak-sən-ᵊl, vak-ˈsēn-\ *adj* : of or relating to vaccine or vaccination ⟨a ∼ allergy⟩ ⟨∼ control of a disease⟩

¹vac·ci·nate \ˈvak-sə-ˌnāt\ *vb* **-nat·ed; -nat·ing** *vt* **1** : to inoculate (a person) with cowpox virus in order to produce immunity to smallpox **2** : to administer a vaccine to usu. by injection ∼ *vi* : to perform or practice vaccination

²vac·ci·nate \ˈvak-sə-ˌnāt, -nət\ *n* : a vaccinated individual

vac·ci·na·tion \ˌvak-sə-ˈnā-shən\ *n* **1** : the introduction into humans or domestic animals of microorganisms that have previously been treated to make them harmless for the purpose of inducing the development of immunity ⟨oral ∼⟩ ⟨∼ against smallpox⟩ ⟨∼ for whooping cough⟩ **2** : the scar left by vaccinating

vac·ci·na·tor \ˈvak-sə-ˌnāt-ər\ *n* : one that vaccinates

vac·cine \vak-ˈsēn, ˈvak-ˌ\ *n* **1** : matter or a preparation containing the virus of cowpox used to vaccinate a person against smallpox **2** : a preparation of killed microorganisms, living attenuated organisms, or living fully virulent organisms that is administered to produce or artificially increase immunity to a particular disease ⟨chicken pox ∼⟩;

\ə\ abut \ᵊ\ kitten \ər\ further \a\ ash \ā\ ace \ä\ cot, cart
\au̇\ out \ch\ chin \e\ bet \ē\ easy \g\ go \i\ hit \ī\ ice \j\ job
\ŋ\ sing \ō\ go \ȯ\ law \ȯi\ boy \th\ thin \th\ the \ü\ loot
\u̇\ foot \y\ yet \zh\ vision   *See also* Pronunciation Symbols page

U
Z

also : a mixture of several such vaccines ⟨measles-mumps‑rubella ∼⟩

vac·ci·nee \ˌvak-sə-ˈnē\ *n* : a vaccinated individual

vac·cin·ia \vak-ˈsin-ē-ə\ *n* **1 a** : COWPOX **b** : a reaction to smallpox vaccine prepared from live vaccinia virus that may involve a rash, fever, headache, and body pain **2** : a poxvirus of the genus *Orthopoxvirus* (species *Vaccinia virus*) that differs from but is closely related to the viruses causing smallpox and cowpox and that includes a strain of uncertain natural origin used in making vaccines against smallpox — called also *vaccinia virus* — **vac·cin·i·al** \-ē-əl\ *adj*

vac·ci·noid \ˈvak-sə-ˌnȯid\ *adj* : resembling vaccinia

vac·ci·no·style \ˈvak-sə-nō-ˌstīl\ *n* : a small pointed instrument formerly used in vaccination

vac·ci·no·ther·a·py \ˌvak-sə-nō-ˈther-ə-pē\ *n, pl* **-pies** : the use of vaccines as therapy

vacua *pl of* VACUUM

vacuo — see IN VACUO

vac·u·o·lar \ˌvak-yə-ˈwō-lər, -ˌlär\ *adj* : of or relating to a vacuole ⟨∼ contents⟩

vac·u·o·late \ˈvak-yə-(ˌ)wō-ˌlāt\ *or* **vac·u·o·lat·ed** \-ˌlāt-əd\ *adj* : containing one or more vacuoles ⟨*vacuolated* cells⟩

vac·u·o·la·tion \ˌvak-yə-(ˌ)wō-ˈlā-shən\ *n* : the development or formation of vacuoles ⟨neuronal ∼⟩

vac·u·ole \ˈvak-yə-ˌwōl\ *n* **1** : a small cavity or space in the tissues of an organism containing air or fluid **2** : a cavity or vesicle in the cytoplasm of a cell containing fluid

vac·u·ol·iza·tion *also Brit* **vac·u·ol·isa·tion** \ˌvak-yə-ˌwō-lə-ˈzā-shən\ *n* : VACUOLATION ⟨∼ of erythroid cells⟩

¹vac·u·um \ˈvak-(ˌ)yüm, -yü-əm, -yəm\ *n, pl* **vac·u·ums** *or* **vac·ua** \-yə-wə\ **1** : emptiness of space **2 a** : a space absolutely devoid of matter **b** : a space partially exhausted (as to the highest degree possible) by artificial means (as an air pump) **c** : a degree of rarefaction below atmospheric pressure — see NEGATIVE PRESSURE

²vacuum *adj* **1** : of, containing, producing, or utilizing a partial vacuum ⟨separated by means of ∼ distillation⟩ **2** : of or relating to a vacuum device or system

vacuum aspiration *n* : a method of abortion performed in the later half of the first trimester of pregnancy by aspiration of the contents of the uterus through a narrow tube

vacuum aspirator *n* : an aspirator used to perform vacuum aspiration

vacuum tube *n* : an electronic device in which conduction by electrons takes place through a vacuum within a sealed glass or metal container and which has various uses based on the controlled flow of electrons

VAD \ˈvē-ˌā-ˈdē\ *n* : an artificial device that is implanted in the chest to assist a damaged or weakened heart in pumping blood — called also *ventricular assist device*

vag·a·bond's disease \ˈvag-ə-ˌbändz-\ *n* : a condition of pigmentation of the skin caused by long continued exposure, uncleanliness, and esp. by scratch marks and other lesions due to the presence of body lice

va·gal \ˈvā-gəl\ *adj* : of, relating to, mediated by, or being the vagus nerve ⟨∼ stimulation⟩ — **va·gal·ly** \-gə-lē\ *adv*

vagal escape *n* : resumption of the heartbeat after stimulation of the vagus nerve has caused it to stop that occurs despite continuation of such stimulation

vagal tone *n* : impulses from the vagus nerve producing inhibition of the heartbeat

vagi *pl of* VAGUS

va·gi·na \və-ˈjī-nə\ *n, pl* **-nae** \-(ˌ)nē\ *or* **-nas** : a canal in a female mammal that leads from the uterus to the external orifice opening into the vestibule between the labia minora

vaginae — see SPHINCTER VAGINAE

¹va·gi·nal \ˈvaj-ən-ᵊl, *sometimes* və-ˈjī-nᵊl\ *adj* **1** : of, relating to, or resembling a vagina : THECAL ⟨a ∼ synovial membrane surrounding a tendon⟩ **2 a** : of, relating to, or affecting the genital vagina ⟨∼ discharge⟩ ⟨∼ infection⟩ **b** : occurring through the birth canal ⟨a ∼ delivery⟩ ⟨a ∼ birth⟩ — **va·gi·nal·ly** \-ē\ *adv*

²vaginal *n* : a vaginal anatomical part (as a muscle)

vaginal artery *n* : any of the several arteries that supply the vagina and that usu. arise from the internal iliac artery or the uterine artery

vaginal hysterectomy *n* : a hysterectomy performed through the vagina

vaginalis — see PROCESSUS VAGINALIS, TUNICA VAGINALIS

vaginal process *n* **1** : a projecting lamina of bone on the inferior surface of the petrous portion of the temporal bone that is continuous with the tympanic plate and surrounds the root of the styloid process **2** : either of a pair of projecting laminae on the inferior surface of the sphenoid that articulate with the alae of the vomer

vaginal smear *n* : a smear taken from the vaginal mucosa for cytological diagnosis

vaginal thrush *n* : candidiasis of the vagina or vulva

vagina ten·di·nis \-ˈten-də-nəs\ *n* : the synovial sheath of a tendon esp. of the hand or foot

vag·i·nec·to·my \ˌvaj-ə-ˈnek-tə-mē\ *n, pl* **-mies** : COLPECTOMY

vag·i·nis·mus \ˌvaj-ə-ˈniz-məs\ *n* : a painful spasmodic contraction of the vagina

vag·i·ni·tis \ˌvaj-ə-ˈnīt-əs\ *n, pl* **-nit·i·des** \-ˈnit-ə-ˌdēz\ **1** : inflammation (as from bacterial or fungal infection, allergic reaction, or hormone deficiency) of the vagina that may be marked by irritation and vaginal discharge — see ATROPHIC VAGINITIS, BACTERIAL VAGINOSIS, TRICHOMONIASIS **2** : inflammation of a sheath (as a tendon sheath)

vag·i·no·plas·ty \ˈvaj-ə-nə-ˌplas-tē\ *n, pl* **-ties** : plastic surgery of the vagina — called also *colpoplasty*

vag·i·no·scope \ˈvaj-ə-nə-ˌskōp\ *n* : an instrument and esp. a speculum used to examine the vagina

vag·i·no·sis \ˌvaj-ə-ˈnō-səs\ *n, pl* **-no·ses** \-ˌsēz\ : an abnormal or diseased condition of the vagina; *specif* : BACTERIAL VAGINOSIS

va·go·de·pres·sor \ˌvā-gō-di-ˈpres-ər\ *adj* : depressing activity of the vagus nerve ⟨a ∼ reaction⟩

va·go·lyt·ic \ˌvā-gō-ˈlit-ik\ *adj* : PARASYMPATHOLYTIC

va·got·o·mize *or chiefly Brit* **va·got·o·mise** \vā-ˈgät-ə-ˌmīz\ *vt* **-mized** *or chiefly Brit* **-mised; -miz·ing** *or chiefly Brit* **-mis·ing** : to perform a vagotomy on

va·got·o·my \vā-ˈgät-ə-mē\ *n, pl* **-mies** : surgical division of the vagus nerve

va·go·to·nia \ˌvā-gə-ˈtō-nē-ə\ *n* : excessive excitability of the vagus nerve resulting typically in vasomotor instability, constipation, and sweating — compare SYMPATHICOTONIA — **va·go·ton·ic** \-ˈtän-ik\ *adj*

va·go·tro·pic \-ˈtrō-pik\ *adj* : acting selectively upon the vagus nerve ⟨∼ drugs⟩

va·go–va·gal \ˌvā-gō-ˈvā-gəl\ *adj* : relating to or arising from both afferent and efferent impulses of the vagus nerve ⟨a ∼ reflex⟩

va·grant \ˈvā-grənt\ *adj* : having no fixed course : moving from place to place ⟨a ∼ infection⟩

va·gus \ˈvā-gəs\ *n, pl* **va·gi** \ˈvā-ˌgī, -ˌjī\ : VAGUS NERVE

vagus nerve *n* : either of the tenth pair of cranial nerves that arise from the medulla and supply chiefly the viscera esp. with autonomic sensory and motor fibers — called also *pneumogastric nerve, tenth cranial nerve, vagus*

Val *abbr* valine; valyl

val·a·cy·clo·vir \ˌval-ə-ˈsī-klō-ˌvir\ *n* : a prodrug of acyclovir that is administered orally in the form of its hydrochloride $C_{13}H_{20}N_6O_4 \cdot HCl$ to treat shingles, genital herpes, and cold sores — see VALTREX

val·de·cox·ib \ˌval-də-ˈkäk-sib\ *n* : an NSAID $C_{16}H_{14}N_2O_3S$ that is a COX-2 inhibitor administered orally esp. to treat osteoarthritis, rheumatoid arthritis, and primary dysmenorrhea but withdrawn from sale by the manufacturer because of its link to cardiovascular events (as heart attacks) and severe skin rashes — see BEXTRA

va·lence \ˈvā-lən(t)s\ *n* **1 a** : the degree of combining power of an element or radical as shown by the number of atomic weights of a monovalent element (as hydrogen) with which the atomic weight of the element or the partial molecular weight of the radical will combine or for which it can be substituted or with which it can be compared **b** : a unit of valence ⟨the four ∼s of carbon⟩ **2 a :** relative capacity to unite, react, or interact (as with antigens or a biological substrate) **b :** the degree of attractiveness an individual, activity, or object possesses as a behavioral goal ⟨the relative potency of the ∼s of success and failure —Leon Festinger⟩

valence electron *n* : a single electron or one of two or more electrons in the outer shell of an atom that is responsible for the chemical properties of the atom

va·len·cy \'vā-lən-sē\ *n, pl* **-cies** : VALENCE

va·lent \'vā-lənt\ *adj* : having valence — usu. used in combination ⟨bi*valent*⟩ ⟨multi*valent*⟩

val·er·ate \'val-ə-ˌrāt\ *n* : a salt or ester of valeric acid

va·le·ri·an \və-'lir-ē-ən\ *n* **1 :** any of a genus (*Valeriana* of the family Valerianaceae, the valerian family) of perennial herbs many of which possess medicinal properties **2 :** a preparation of the dried rhizome and roots of the garden heliotrope (*Valeriana officinalis*) that is used as an herbal remedy and is held to be beneficial in treating nervousness and insomnia — called also *valerian root*

va·le·ric acid \və-ˌlir-ik-\ *also* **va·le·ri·an·ic acid** \və-ˌlir-ē-ˌan-ik-\ *n* : any of four isomeric fatty acids $C_5H_{10}O_2$ or a mixture of two or more of them: **a :** a liquid normal acid that has a disagreeable odor and that is used in organic synthesis — called also *pentanoic acid* **b :** ISOVALERIC ACID **c :** a liquid acid existing in three optically isomeric forms and occurring usu. in the dextrorotatory form in a few essential oils **d :** PIVALIC ACID

¹val·e·tu·di·nar·i·an \ˌval-ə-ˌt(y)üd-ᵊn-'er-ē-ən\ *n* : a person of a weak or sickly constitution; *esp* : one whose chief concern is his or her ill health

²valetudinarian *adj* : of, relating to, or being a valetudinarian : SICKLY

valgum — see GENU VALGUM

val·gus \'val-gəs\ *adj* **1 :** turned outward; *esp* : of, relating to, or being a deformity in which an anatomical part is turned outward away from the midline of the body to an abnormal degree ⟨a ∼ heel⟩ ⟨∼ deformity of the big toe⟩ — see CUBITUS VALGUS, HALLUX VALGUS, TALIPES VALGUS; compare GENU VALGUM, GENU VARUM **2 :** VARUS 1 — used esp. in orthopedics of the knee ⟨changes spontaneously from the initial varus (bowing) to a ∼ position (knock-knee) at about age 2 to 3 —Joan M. Walker⟩ — **valgus** *n*

va·line \'vā-ˌlēn, 'va-ˌlēn\ *n* : a crystalline essential amino acid $C_5H_{11}NO_2$ that occurs esp. in fibrous proteins — abbr. *Val*

val·in·o·my·cin \ˌval-ə-nō-'mīs-ᵊn\ *n* : an antibiotic $C_{54}H_{90}N_6O_{18}$ produced by a bacterium of the genus *Streptomyces* (*S. fulvissimus*)

Val·ium \'val-ē-əm, 'val-yəm\ *trademark* — used for a preparation of diazepam

val·late \'val-ˌāt\ *adj* : having a raised edge surrounding a depression

vallate papilla *n* : CIRCUMVALLATE PAPILLA

val·lec·u·la \va-'lek-yə-lə\ *n, pl* **-lae** \-ˌlē\ : an anatomical groove, channel, or depression: as **a :** a groove between the base of the tongue and the epiglottis **b :** a fossa on the underside of the cerebellum separating the hemispheres and including the inferior vermis — **val·lec·u·lar** \-yə-lər\ *adj*

val·ley fever \'val-ē-\ *n* : COCCIDIOIDOMYCOSIS

val·lum \'va-ləm\ *n, pl* **val·la** \-lə\ *or* **val·lums** : an anatomical wall

val·pro·ate \val-'prō-ˌāt\ *n* : a salt or ester of valproic acid; *esp* : SODIUM VALPROATE

valproate sodium *n* : SODIUM VALPROATE

val·pro·ic acid \val-ˌprō-ik-\ *n* : a valeric-acid derivative $C_8H_{16}O_2$ used as an anticonvulsant often in the form of its sodium salt $C_8H_{15}NaO_2$ — see DEPAKENE; SODIUM VALPROATE

Val·sal·va maneuver *also* **Val·sal·va's maneuver** \val-'sal-və(z)-\ *n* : a forceful attempt at expiration when the airway is closed at some point; *esp* : a conscious effort made while holding the nostrils closed and keeping the mouth shut esp. for the purpose of testing the patency of the eustachian tubes, adjusting middle ear pressure, or aborting tachycardia — called also *Valsalva*

A. M. Valsalva — see SINUS OF VALSALVA

val·sar·tan \val-'sär-ˌtan\ *n* : an antihypertensive drug $C_{24}H_{29}N_5O_3$ that blocks the action of angiotensin II — see DIOVAN

Val·trex \'val-ˌtreks\ *trademark* — used for a preparation of the hydrochloride of valacyclovir

val·va \'val-və\ *n, pl* **val·vae** \-ˌvē\ : VALVE

val·val \'val-vəl\ *adj* : VALVULAR ⟨∼ calcification⟩

valve \'valv\ *n* **1 :** a bodily structure (as the mitral valve) that closes temporarily a passage or orifice or permits movement of fluid in one direction only **2 :** any of various mechanical devices by which the flow of liquid (as blood) may be started, stopped, or regulated by a movable part that opens, shuts, or partially obstructs one or more ports or passageways; *also* : the movable part of such a device

valve of Has·ner \-'häs-nər\ *n* : PLICA LACRIMALIS

Hasner, Joseph Ritter von Artha (1819–1892), Bohemian ophthalmologist. Hasner was a professor of ophthalmology at Prague. In 1850 he published a monograph on the physiology and pathology of the nasolacrimal duct in which he described a fold of mucous membrane that is now sometimes called the valve of Hasner.

valve of Hei·ster \-'hī-stər\ *n* : SPIRAL VALVE

Heister, Lorenz (1683–1758), German anatomist and surgeon. Heister was one of the founders of scientific surgery. His works on medicine, anatomy, and surgery were widely read for several generations. His main work, a general treatise on surgery, was originally published in 1718 and eventually translated into seven languages. Another major work was an illustrated compendium of anatomical structures first published in 1717. It includes the description of the spiral valve sometimes known as the valve of Heister.

valves of Kerck·ring *or* **valves of Kerck·ring** \-'ker-kriŋ\ *n pl* : PLICAE CIRCULARES

Kerckring, Theodor (1640–1693), Dutch anatomist. Kerckring was an anatomist and physician practicing in Amsterdam. In 1670 he described the permanent transverse folds of the luminal surface of the small intestine. Although they were previously described by Gabriele Falloppio, they are now sometimes called the valves of Kerckring.

valve of The·be·si·us \-te-'bā-zē-əs\ *n* : CORONARY VALVE

A. C. Thebesius — see THEBESIAN VEIN

val·vot·o·my \val-'vät-ə-mē\ *n, pl* **-mies** : VALVULOTOMY

val·vu·la \'val-vyə-lə\ *n, pl* **-lae** \-ˌlē *also* -ˌlī\ : a small valve or fold

valvula co·li \-'kō-ˌlī\ *n* : ILEOCECAL VALVE

valvulae con·ni·ven·tes \-ˌkän-ə-'ven-ˌtēz\ *n pl* : PLICAE CIRCULARES

val·vu·lar \'val-vyə-lər\ *adj* **1 :** resembling or functioning as a valve ⟨established a ∼ connection to the esophagus⟩ **2 :** of, relating to, or affecting a valve esp. of the heart ⟨∼ heart disease⟩

val·vu·li·tis \ˌval-vyə-'līt-əs\ *n* : inflammation of a valve esp. of the heart ⟨rheumatic ∼⟩

val·vu·lo·plas·ty \'val-vyə-lō-ˌplas-tē\ *n, pl* **-ties** : plastic surgery performed on a heart valve

val·vu·lo·tome \'val-vyə-lō-ˌtōm\ *n* : a surgical blade designed for valvulotomy or commissurotomy

val·vu·lot·o·my \ˌval-vyə-'lät-ə-mē\ *n, pl* **-mies** : surgical incision of a valve; *specif* : the operation of enlarging a narrowed heart valve by cutting through the mitral commissures with a knife or by a finger thrust to relieve the symptoms of mitral stenosis

va·lyl \'vā-ˌlil, 'va-\ *n* : the amino acid radical or residue $(CH_3)_2CHCH(NH_2)CO-$ of valine — abbr. *Val*

vam·pire \'vam-ˌpī(ə)r\ *n* : VAMPIRE BAT

vampire bat *n* : any of several Central and So. American bats (*Desmodus rotundus, Diaemus youngi,* and *Diphylla ecaudata*) that feed on the blood of birds and mammals and esp. domestic animals and that are sometimes vectors of disease and esp. of rabies; *also* : any of several other bats that do not feed on blood but are sometimes reputed to do so

vam·pir·ism \-ˌpī(ə)r-ˌiz-əm\ *n* : a sexual perversion in which gratification is obtained by the drawing of blood

van·a·date \ˈvan-ə-ˌdāt\ *n* : a salt derived from the pentoxide of vanadium and containing pentavalent vanadium

va·na·di·um \və-ˈnād-ē-əm\ *n* : a grayish malleable ductile polyvalent metallic element found combined in minerals and used esp. to form alloys (as vanadium steel) — symbol *V*; see ELEMENT table

Van·co·cin \ˈvan-kə-ˌsin\ *trademark* — used for a preparation of the hydrochloride of vancomycin

van·co·my·cin \ˌvaŋ-kə-ˈmīs-ᵊn\ *n* : an antibiotic $C_{66}H_{75}Cl_2N_9O_{24}$ derived from an actinomycete (*Amycolatopsis orientalis* syn. *Streptomyces orientalis* syn. *Nocardia orientalis*) that is effective against gram-positive bacteria and is used chiefly in the form of its hydrochloride $C_{66}H_{75}Cl_2N_9O_{24}\cdot HCl$ esp. against staphylococci resistant to methicillin — see VANCOCIN

Van de Graaff generator \ˈvan-də-ˌgraf-\ *n* : an apparatus for the production of electrical discharges at high voltage commonly consisting of an insulated hollow conducting sphere that accumulates in its interior the charge continuously conveyed from a source of direct current by an endless belt of flexible nonconducting material — called also *electrostatic generator*

Van de Graaff, Robert Jenison (1901–1967), American physicist. Van de Graaff developed his generator as a device for producing the very high voltages necessary to accelerate particles to energies high enough to create new elements heavier than uranium. He built his first machine in the early 1930s, and in 1946 he cofounded a company to manufacture particle accelerators incorporating the Van de Graaff generator. These particle accelerators have found widespread use in medicine and industry as well as in high-energy physics research.

van den Bergh reaction \ˈvan-dən-ˌbərg-\ *n* : the chemical reaction that takes place in the van den Bergh test when bilirubin is present in the blood

Van den Bergh, Albert Abraham Hijmans (1869–1943), Dutch physician. Van den Bergh introduced in 1913 a test for the presence of bilirubin in the blood.

van den Bergh test *also* **van den Bergh's test** \ˈvan-dən-ˌbərgz-\ *n* : a test indicating presence of bilirubin in the blood when a diazotizing reagent added to blood serum turns it red (as in jaundice)

van der Waals forces \ˈvan-dər-ˌwȯlz-\ *n pl* : the relatively weak attractive forces that are operative between neutral atoms and molecules and that arise because of the electric polarization induced in each of the particles by the presence of other particles

Waals \ˈwäls\, **Johannes Diederik van der (1837–1923),** Dutch physicist. Van der Waals was a professor of physics at the University of Amsterdam. In 1873 he first postulated the van der Waals forces in support of his theoretical treatment of real as distinguished from ideal gases. In 1910 he was awarded the Nobel Prize for Physics for his research on the mathematical equations describing the gaseous and liquid states of matter.

va·nil·la \və-ˈnil-ə, -ˈnel-\ *n* **1 a** : VANILLA BEAN **b** : a commercially important extract of the vanilla bean that is prepared by soaking comminuted vanilla beans in water and ethyl alcohol and that is used esp. as a flavoring (as in pharmaceutical preparations) **2** : any of a genus (*Vanilla*) of tropical American climbing orchids

vanilla bean *n* : the long capsular fruit of a vanilla (esp. *Vanilla planifolia*) that is an important article of commerce

va·nil·late \və-ˈnil-ət, -ˌāt; ˈvan-ᵊl-ˌāt\ *n* : a salt or ester of vanillic acid

va·nil·lic acid \və-ˌnil-ik-\ *n* : an odorless crystalline phenolic acid $C_8H_8O_4$ found in some varieties of vanilla, formed by oxidation of vanillin, and used chiefly in the form of esters as food preservatives

van·il·lin \ˈvan-ᵊl-ən\ *n* : a crystalline phenolic aldehyde $C_8H_8O_3$ that is prepared synthetically or is obtained as the chief fragrant component of vanilla extracted from vanilla beans and that is used esp. in flavoring and in perfumery

va·nil·lism \və-ˈnil-ˌiz-əm, ˈvan-ᵊl-ˌiz-əm\ *n* : a grocer's itch caused by a grain mite of the genus *Acarus* (*A. siro*) commonly infesting vanilla pods

van·il·lyl·man·de·lic acid \ˌvan-ə-ˌlil-man-ˌdē-lik-\ *n* : a principal catecholamine metabolite $C_9H_{10}O_5$ whose presence in excess in the urine is used as a test for pheochromocytoma — abbr. *VMA*

van·il·man·de·lic acid \ˌvan-ᵊl-man-ˌdē-lik-\ *n* : VANILLYLMANDELIC ACID

Van Slyke method \van-ˈslīk-\ *n* : any of several analytical methods; *esp* : the determination of free amino groups (as in amino acids or proteins) by measuring the volume or pressure of nitrogen gas formed by reaction with nitrous acid

Van Slyke, Donald Dexter (1883–1971), American biochemist. Van Slyke served as a research biochemist first at the Rockefeller Institute for Medical Research (1907–49) and then at the Brookhaven National Laboratory (1949–71). He conducted extensive research in the application of chemistry to clinical and investigative medicine and in so doing made major discoveries in chemistry, medicine, and physiology which brought about the development of new analytical methods and apparatuses.

van't Hoff's law \vant-ˈhȯfs-\ *n* : a statement in physical chemistry: the effect of a change in temperature on a system in equilibrium is to shift the equilibrium in the direction that acts to nullify the temperature change ⟨according to *van't Hoff's law,* an increase in temperature will cause an increase in the rate of an endothermic reaction⟩

Van't Hoff, Jacobus Henricus (1852–1911), Dutch physical chemist. Van't Hoff is considered the father of physical chemistry. As a professor of chemistry he taught first at the University of Amsterdam and later at the Prussian Academy of Science at Berlin. In 1886 he demonstrated a similarity between the behavior of dilute solutions and gases. He also introduced the modern concept of chemical affinity. Van't Hoff was awarded the first Nobel Prize for Chemistry in 1901 for his work on rates of reaction, chemical equilibrium, and osmotic pressure.

va·por *or chiefly Brit* **va·pour** \ˈvā-pər\ *n* **1 a** : a substance in the gaseous state as distinguished from the liquid or solid state **b** : a substance (as alcohol or benzoin) vaporized for industrial, therapeutic, or military uses **2 vapors** *or chiefly Brit* **vapours** *pl* **a** : exhalations of bodily organs (as the stomach) formerly held to affect the physical or mental condition **b** : a depressed or hysterical nervous condition

va·por·ish *or chiefly Brit* **va·pour·ish** \ˈvāp-ər-ish\ *adj* : affected by the vapors : given to fits of depression or hysteria — **va·por·ish·ness** *or chiefly Brit* **va·pour·ish·ness** *n*

va·por·iza·tion *also Brit* **va·por·isa·tion** \ˌvā-p(ə-)rə-ˈzā-shən\ *n* : the action or process of vaporizing : the state of being vaporized

va·por·ize *also Brit* **va·por·ise** \ˈvā-pə-ˌrīz\ *vb* **-ized** *also Brit* **-ised; -iz·ing** *also Brit* **-is·ing** *vt* : to convert from a liquid or solid into a vapor ⟨*vaporized* plaque in an artery with laser treatment⟩ ~ *vi* : to become vaporized — **va·por·iz·able** *also Brit* **va·por·is·able** \-ˌrī-zə-bəl\ *adj*

va·por·iz·er *also Brit* **va·por·is·er** \-ˌrī-zər\ *n* : one that vaporizes: as **a** : ATOMIZER **b** : a device for converting water or a medicated liquid into a vapor for inhalation

Va·quez's disease \vä-ˈkez-əz-\ *n* : POLYCYTHEMIA VERA

Va·quez \vä-kez\, **Louis Henri (1860–1936),** French physician. Vaquez developed an interest in the diseases of the heart and circulation early in his career and eventually became a leading clinical cardiologist of his time. He is famous for describing polycythemia vera in 1892. (An equally famous description of this entity was written later by Sir William Osler in 1903.)

Var \ˈvär\ *n* : a vaccine that protects against chicken pox — see VARIVAX

var·den·a·fil \vär-ˈden-ə-ˌfil\ *n* : a drug that is administered in the form of its hydrated hydrochloride $C_{23}H_{32}N_6O_4S$·HCl·3H$_2$O to treat erectile dysfunction and has a mechanism of action similar to sildenafil — see LEVITRA

¹vari·able \'ver-ē-ə-bəl, 'var-\ *adj* **1** : able or apt to vary : subject to variation or changes ⟨allergy is perhaps the most ~ of all diseases —H. G. Rapaport & Shirley Linde⟩ **2** : characterized by variations **3** : not true to type : ABERRANT — used of a biological group or character — **vari·abil·i·ty** \,ver-ē-ə-'bil-ət-ē, ,var-\ *n, pl* **-ties**

²variable *n* : something that is variable

variable region *n* : the part of the polypeptide chain of a light or heavy chain of an antibody that ends in a free amino group –NH₂, that varies greatly in its sequence of amino acid residues from one antibody to another, and that prob. determines the conformation of the combining site which confers the specificity of the antibody for a particular antigen — called also *variable domain;* compare CONSTANT REGION

¹vari·ant \'ver-ē-ənt, 'var-\ *adj* : manifesting variety or deviation : exhibiting variation ⟨~ forms of the disease⟩

²variant *n* : one that exhibits variation from a type, norm, or wild type : MUTATION; *also* : one whose behavior is at variance with the norms of society

variant Creutzfeldt–Jakob disease *n* : a fatal spongiform encephalopathy that is held to be a variant of Creutzfeldt-Jakob disease caused by the prion associated with bovine spongiform encephalopathy and contracted by consuming infected beef or beef products — abbr. *v*CJD; called also *new variant Creutzfeldt-Jakob disease, variant CJD*

var·i·a·tion \,ver-ē-'ā-shən, ,var-\ *n* **1** : divergence in one or more characteristics of an organism or biotype from those typical of or usual for its group **2** : something (as an individual or group) that exhibits variation — **var·i·a·tion·al** \-shnəl, -shən-³l\ *adj*

var·i·ce·al \,var-ə-'sē-əl, və-'ris-ē-əl\ *adj* : of, relating to, or caused by varices ⟨~ hemorrhage⟩

var·i·cel·la \,var-ə-'sel-ə\ *n* : CHICKEN POX

varicella zoster *n* : a herpesvirus that causes chicken pox and shingles — called also *varicella-zoster virus*

var·i·cel·li·form \,var-ə-'sel-ə-,förm\ *adj* : resembling chicken pox ⟨a ~ eruption⟩

Var·i·cel·lo·vi·rus \,var-ə-'sel-ə-,vī-rəs\ *n* : a genus of double-stranded DNA viruses of the family *Herpesviridae* that include the causative agents of chicken pox, infectious bovine rhinotracheitis, pseudorabies, rhinopneumonitis, and shingles

varices *pl of* VARIX

var·i·co·cele \'var-i-kō-,sēl\ *n* : a varicose enlargement of the veins of the spermatic cord producing a soft compressible tumor mass in the scrotum

var·i·co·cel·ec·to·my \,var-i-kō-sēl-'ek-tə-mē\ *n, pl* **-mies** : surgical treatment of varicocele by excision of the affected veins often with removal of part of the scrotum

var·i·cog·ra·phy \,var-i-'käg-rə-fē\ *n, pl* **-phies** : radiographic visualization of varicose veins after injection of a radiopaque substance

var·i·cose \'var-ə-,kōs\ *also* **var·i·cosed** \-,kōst\ *adj* **1** : abnormally swollen or dilated ⟨~ lymph vessels⟩ **2** : affected with varicose veins ⟨a patient with ~ legs⟩

varicose vein *n* : an abnormal swelling and tortuosity esp. of a superficial vein of the legs — usu. used in pl.

var·i·co·sis \,var-ə-'kō-səs\ *n, pl* **-co·ses** \-,sēz\ : the condition of being varicose or of having varicose vessels

var·i·cos·i·ty \,var-ə-'käs-ət-ē\ *n, pl* **-ties** **1** : the quality or state of being abnormally or markedly swollen or dilated **2** : VARIX

Var·i·dase \'var-ə-,dās\ *n* : a preparation containing a mixture of streptodornase and streptokinase — formerly a U.S. registered trademark

va·ri·e·ty \və-'rī-ət-ē\ *n, pl* **-ties** : any of various groups of plants or animals ranking below a species : SUBSPECIES

va·ri·o·la \və-'rī-ə-lə\ *n* : SMALLPOX; *also* : the poxvirus of the genus *Orthopoxvirus* (species *Variola virus*) that is the causative agent of smallpox

variola major *n* : a severe form of smallpox characterized historically by a death rate up to 40 percent or more

variola minor *n* : a mild form of smallpox of low mortality — called also *alastrim, amaas*

var·i·o·late \'var-ē-ə-,lāt\ *vt* **-lat·ed; -lat·ing** : to subject to variolation

var·i·o·la·tion \,var-ē-ə-'lā-shən\ *n* : the deliberate inoculation of an uninfected person with the smallpox virus (as by contact with pustular matter) that was widely practiced before the era of vaccination as prophylaxis against the severe form of smallpox

variola vac·cin·ia \-vak-'sin-ē-ə\ *n* : COWPOX

var·i·ol·i·form \,var-ē-'ō-lə-,förm\ *adj* : resembling smallpox

varioliformis — see PITYRIASIS LICHENOIDES ET VARIOLIFORMIS ACUTA

va·ri·o·loid \'var-ē-ə-,lóid, və-'rī-ə-,lóid\ *n* : a modified mild form of smallpox occurring in persons who have been vaccinated or who have had smallpox

va·ri·o·lous \və-'rī-ə-ləs\ *adj* : of or relating to smallpox ⟨inoculated with ~ matter⟩

Var·i·vax \'var-ə-,vaks\ *trademark* — used for a vaccine against chicken pox composed of live attenuated varicella-zoster virus

var·ix \'var-iks\ *n, pl* **var·i·ces** \'var-ə-,sēz\ : an abnormally dilated and lengthened vein, artery, or lymph vessel; *esp* : VARICOSE VEIN

var·nish \'vär-nish\ *n* : any of various liquid preparations that when spread and allowed to dry on a surface form a hard lustrous typically transparent coating and that include some used in dentistry to line deep cavities in order to protect the pulp of a tooth — **varnish** *vt*

Va·ro·li·an \və-'rō-lē-ən\ *adj* : of or relating to the pons Varolii

C. Varolio — see PONS VAROLII

varum — see GENU VARUM

var·us \'var-əs, 'ver-\ *adj* **1** : of, relating to, or being a deformity in which an anatomical part is turned inward toward the midline of the body to an abnormal degree ⟨a ~ heel⟩ ⟨~ angulation of the little toe⟩ — see CUBITUS VARUS, TALIPES VARUS; compare GENU VALGUM, GENU VARUM **2** : VALGUS 1 — used esp. in orthopedics of the knee ⟨changes spontaneously from the initial ~ (bowing) to a valgus position (knock-knee) at about age 2 to 3 —Joan M. Walker⟩ — **varus** *n*

vary \'ver-ē, 'var-ē\ *vi* **var·ied; vary·ing** : to exhibit divergence in structural or physiological characters from the typical form

vas \'vas\ *n, pl* **va·sa** \'vā-zə\ : an anatomical vessel : DUCT

VAS *abbr* visual analog scale

vasa ab·er·ran·tia \-,ab-ə-'ran-ch(ē-)ə\ *n pl* : slender arteries that are only occas. present and that connect the axillary or brachial artery with an artery (as the radial artery) of the forearm or with its branches

vas ab·er·rans of Hal·ler \-'ab-ə-,ranz-əv-'häl-ər\ *n, pl* **vasa ab·er·ran·tia of Haller** \-,ab-ə-'ran-ch(ē-)ə-\ : a blind tube that is occas. present parallel to the first part of the vas deferens and that may communicate with the vas deferens or with the epididymis — called also *ductulus aberrans*

Haller, Albrecht von (1708–1777), Swiss biologist. Haller made important contributions to physiology, anatomy, botany, embryology, scientific bibliography, and even poetry. One of his preeminent publications was his eight-volume work on the physiology of the human body. Published between 1757 and 1766, it constitutes a landmark in medical history. He also published works summarizing the anatomy of the genitals, the brain, and the cardiovascular system. His discoveries in nerve and muscle action laid the foundations for the advent of modern neurology.

vasa bre·via \-'brē-vē-ə\ *n pl* : short branches of the splenic

\ə\ abut \ᵊ\ kitten \ər\ further \a\ ash \ā\ ace \ä\ cot, cart \au̇\ out \ch\ chin \e\ bet \ē\ easy \g\ go \i\ hit \ī\ ice \j\ job \ŋ\ sing \ō\ go \ȯ\ law \ȯi\ boy \th\ thin \t͟h\ the \ü\ loot \u̇\ foot \y\ yet \zh\ vision *See also* Pronunciation Symbols page

U Z

artery and vein that run to the greater curvature of the stomach

vasa deferentia *pl of* VAS DEFERENS

vasa ef·fer·en·tia \-ˌef-ə-ˈren-ch(ē-)ə\ *n pl* : the 12 to 20 ductiles that lead from the rete testis to the vas deferens and except near their commencement are greatly convoluted and form the compact head of the epididymis

va·sal \ˈvā-zəl\ *adj* : of, relating to, or constituting an anatomical vessel ⟨a ∼ obstruction⟩

vasa rec·ta \-ˈrek-tə\ *n pl* **1** : numerous small vessels that arise from the terminal branches of arteries supplying the intestine, encircle the intestine, and divide into more branches between its layers **2** : hairpin-shaped vessels that arise from the arteriole leading away from a renal glomerulus, descend into the renal pyramids, reunite as they ascend, and play a role in the concentration of urine

vasa va·so·rum \-vā-ˈsōr-əm\ *n pl* : small blood vessels that supply or drain the walls of the larger arteries and veins and connect with a branch of the same vessel or a neighboring vessel

vas·cu·lar \ˈvas-kyə-lər\ *adj* **1** : of, relating to, constituting, or affecting a tube or a system of tubes for the conveyance of a body fluid (as blood or lymph) ⟨∼ disease⟩ ⟨∼ surgical techniques⟩ **2** : supplied with or containing ducts and esp. blood vessels ⟨a ∼ tumor⟩ ⟨the ∼ layer of the skin⟩

vascular bed *n* : an intricate network of minute blood vessels that ramifies through the tissues of the body or of one of its parts

vascular dementia *n* : dementia (as multi-infarct dementia) of abrupt or gradual onset that is caused by cerebrovascular disease

vascular endothelial growth factor *n* : a protein that is a major factor in promoting the growth of new blood vessels — abbr. *VEGF*

vascularis — see STRIA VASCULARIS

vas·cu·lar·i·ty \ˌvas-kyə-ˈlar-ət-ē\ *n, pl* **-ties** : the quality or state of being vascular ⟨tumor ∼⟩

vas·cu·lar·iza·tion *also Brit* **vas·cu·lar·isa·tion** \ˌvas-kyə-lə-rə-ˈzā-shən\ *n* : the process of becoming vascular; *also* : abnormal or excessive formation of blood vessels (as in the retina or on the cornea)

vas·cu·lar·ize *also Brit* **vas·cu·lar·ise** \ˈvas-kyə-lə-ˌrīz\ *vt* **-ized** *also Brit* **-ised; -iz·ing** *also Brit* **-is·ing** : to make vascular ⟨*vascularized* allografts⟩

vascular resistance *n* : resistance to blood flow through blood vessels and esp. arterioles ⟨internal vessel diameter is inversely proportional to pulmonary and systemic *vascular resistance*⟩ — see PERIPHERAL VASCULAR RESISTANCE

vascular tunic *n* : UVEA

vas·cu·la·ture \ˈvas-kyə-lə-ˌchù(ə)r, -ˌt(y)ù(ə)r\ *n* : the disposition or arrangement of blood vessels in an organ or part ⟨vasoconstriction of the renal ∼ —Mary Jo Holechek⟩

vas·cu·li·tis \ˌvas-kyə-ˈlīt-əs\ *n, pl* **-lit·i·des** \-ˈlit-ə-ˌdēz\ : inflammation of a blood or lymph vessel — called also *angiitis* — **vas·cu·lit·ic** \ˌvas-kyə-ˈlit-ik\ *adj*

vas·cu·lo·gen·e·sis \ˌvas-kyə-lō-ˈjen-ə-səs\ *n, pl* **-e·ses** \-ˌsēz\ : embryonic formation and differentiation of the vascular system

vas·cu·lo·gen·ic \ˌvas-kyə-lō-ˈje-nik\ *adj* : caused by disorder or dysfunction of the blood vessels ⟨∼ impotence⟩

vasculosa — see AREA VASCULOSA

vas·cu·lo·tox·ic \ˌvas-kyə-lō-ˈtäk-sik\ *adj* : destructive to blood vessels or the vascular system ⟨∼ agents⟩

vas def·er·ens \-ˈdef-ə-rənz, -ˌrenz\ *n, pl* **vasa def·er·en·tia** \-ˌdef-ə-ˈren-ch(ē-)ə\ : a sperm-carrying duct esp. of a higher vertebrate that in humans is a small but thick-walled tube about two feet (0.6 meter) long formed by the union of the vasa efferentia, is greatly convoluted in its proximal portion, begins at and is continuous with the tail of the epididymis, runs in the spermatic cord through the inguinal canal, and descends into the pelvis where it joins the duct of the seminal vesicle to form the ejaculatory duct — called also *ductus deferens, spermatic duct*

va·sec·to·mist \və-ˈsek-tə-məst, vā-ˈzek-\ *n* : a physician who performs vasectomies

va·sec·to·mize *or chiefly Brit* **va·sec·to·mise** \və-ˈsek-tə-ˌmīz, vā-ˈzek-\ *vt* **-mized** *or chiefly Brit* **-mised; -miz·ing** *or chiefly Brit* **-mis·ing** : to perform a vasectomy on

va·sec·to·my \-tə-mē\ *n, pl* **-mies** : surgical division or resection of all or part of the vas deferens usu. to induce sterility

Vaseline *trademark* — used for a preparation of petrolatum

va·so·ac·tive \ˌvā-zō-ˈak-tiv\ *adj* : affecting the blood vessels esp. in respect to the degree of their relaxation or contraction — **va·so·ac·tiv·i·ty** \-ak-ˈtiv-ət-ē\ *n, pl* **-ties**

vasoactive intestinal polypeptide *n* : a protein hormone that consists of a chain of 28 amino acid residues, was first isolated from the gut of the pig, has been implicated as a neurotransmitter, and has a wide range of physiological activities (as stimulation of secretion by the pancreas and small intestine, vasodilation, and inhibition of gastric juice production) — abbr. *VIP*; called also *vasoactive intestinal peptide*

va·so·con·strict·ing \ˌvā-zō-kən-ˈstrikt-iŋ\ *adj* : VASOCONSTRICTIVE ⟨∼ drugs⟩

va·so·con·stric·tion \-kən-ˈstrik-shən\ *n* : narrowing of the lumen of blood vessels esp. as a result of vasomotor action

va·so·con·stric·tive \-ˈstrik-tiv\ *adj* : inducing vasoconstriction ⟨a ∼ agent⟩

va·so·con·stric·tor \ˌvā-zō-kən-ˈstrik-tər\ *n* : an agent (as a sympathetic nerve fiber or a drug) that induces or initiates vasoconstriction — **vasoconstrictor** *adj*

va·so·den·tin \ˌvā-zō-ˈdent-ⁿn\ *or* **va·so·den·tine** \-ˈden-ˌtēn\ *n* : a modified dentin permeated by blood capillaries and common in the teeth of the lower vertebrates

va·so·de·pres·sor \ˌvā-zō-di-ˈpres-ər\ *adj* : causing or characterized by vasomotor depression resulting in lowering of the blood pressure ⟨∼ agents⟩ ⟨∼ fainting⟩

vasodepressor syncope *n* : VASOVAGAL SYNCOPE

va·so·di·la·tin \ˌvā-zō-ˈdī-lət-ən\ *n* : a substance (as acetylcholine) that induces vasodilation

va·so·di·lat·ing \-ˈdī-ˌlāt-iŋ, -dī-ˈlāt-\ *adj* : inducing or initiating vasodilation ⟨a ∼ drug⟩

va·so·di·la·tion \ˌvā-zo-dī-ˈlā-shən\ *or* **va·so·di·la·ta·tion** \-ˌdil-ə-ˈtā-shən, -ˌdī-lə-\ *n* : widening of the lumen of blood vessels

¹**va·so·di·la·tor** \ˌvā-zō-ˈdī-ˌlāt-ər\ *n* : an agent (as a parasympathetic nerve fiber or a drug) that induces or initiates vasodilation

²**vasodilator** *also* **va·so·di·la·to·ry** \-ˈdil-ə-ˌtōr-ē, -ˈdī-lə-, -ˌtòr-\ *adj* : relating to, inducing, or initiating vasodilation ⟨a drug with a ∼ effect⟩

va·so·ex·ci·tor \-ik-ˈsīt-ər\ *adj* : VASOPRESSOR

va·so·for·ma·tive \ˌvā-zō-ˈfòr-mət-iv\ *adj* : functioning in the development and formation of vessels and esp. blood vessels ⟨∼ cells⟩

va·sog·ra·phy \vā-ˈzäg-rə-fē\ *n, pl* **-phies** : radiography of blood vessels

va·so·li·ga·tion \ˌvā-zō-lī-ˈgā-shən\ *n* : surgical ligation of a vessel and esp. of the vas deferens

va·so·mo·tion \ˌvā-zō-ˈmō-shən\ *n* : alteration in the caliber of blood vessels

va·so·mo·tor \ˌvā-zō-ˈmōt-ər\ *adj* : of, relating to, affecting, or being those nerves or the centers (as in the medulla and spinal cord) from which they arise that supply the muscle fibers of the walls of blood vessels, include sympathetic vasoconstrictors and parasympathetic vasodilators, and by their effect on vascular diameter regulate the amount of blood passing to a particular body part or organ

vasomotor rhinitis *n* : chronic rhinitis that is not attributable to allergy or infection and is thought to be a hypersensitive reaction to various potentially irritating stimuli (as strong odors, air pollution, or sudden temperature changes)

va·so·neu·ro·sis \ˌvā-zō-n(y)ù-ˈrō-səs\ *n, pl* **-ro·ses** \-ˌsēz\ : a disorder of blood vessels (as a vascular spasm) that is of basically neural origin

va·so·neu·rot·ic \-n(y)ù-ˈrät-ik\ *adj* : of, relating to, or affected with a vasoneurosis

va·so·oc·clu·sive \-ə-ˈklü-siv\ *adj* : relating to, resulting from, or caused by occlusion of a blood vessel ⟨~ retinopathy⟩ ⟨a ~ crisis characteristic of sickle-cell anemia⟩

va·so·pres·sin \ˌvā-zō-ˈpres-ᵊn\ *n* : a polypeptide hormone that is secreted together with oxytocin by the posterior lobe of the pituitary gland, is also obtained synthetically, and increases blood pressure and exerts an antidiuretic effect — called also *antidiuretic hormone, beta-hypophamine;* see ARGININE VASOPRESSIN, LYSINE VASOPRESSIN, PITRESSIN

¹**va·so·pres·sor** \-ˈpres-ər\ *adj* : causing a rise in blood pressure by exerting a vasoconstrictor effect ⟨~ drugs⟩

²**vasopressor** *n* : a vasopressor agent (as a drug)

va·so·re·flex \-ˈrē-ˌfleks\ *n* : a reflex reaction of a blood vessel

¹**va·so·re·lax·ant** \-ri-ˈlak-sənt\ *adj* : relating to or producing vasorelaxation

²**vasorelaxant** *n* : a vasorelaxant agent

va·so·re·lax·ation \ˌvā-zō-ˌrē-ˌlak-ˈsā-shən, *esp Brit* -ˌrel-ak-\ *n* : reduction of vascular tension

vasorum — see VASA VASORUM

va·so·spasm \ˈvā-zō-ˌspaz-əm\ *n* : sharp and often persistent contraction of a blood vessel reducing its caliber and blood flow

va·so·spas·tic \ˌvā-zō-ˈspas-tik\ *adj* : of, relating to, inducing, or characterized by vasospasm ⟨~ disorders⟩

Va·so·tec \ˈvā-zō-ˌtek\ *trademark* — used for a preparation of enalaprilat or the maleate of enalapril

va·so·to·cin \ˌvā-zə-ˈtōs-ᵊn\ *n* : a polypeptide pituitary hormone of most lower vertebrates that is held to have an antidiuretic function

va·sot·o·my \vā-ˈzät-ə-mē\ *n, pl* **-mies** : surgical incision of the vas deferens

va·so·ton·ic \ˌvā-zō-ˈtän-ik\ *adj* : of, relating to, or promoting tone of blood vessel walls

va·so·va·gal \ˌvā-zō-ˈvā-gəl\ *adj* : of, relating to, or involving both vascular and vagal factors ⟨a ~ reaction⟩

vasovagal syncope *n* : a usu. transitory condition that is marked esp. by fainting associated with hypotension, peripheral vasodilation, and bradycardia resulting from increased stimulation of the vagus nerve — called also *neurocardiogenic syncope, vasodepressor syncope*

va·so·va·sos·to·my \ˌvā-zō-vā-ˈzäs-tə-mē\ *n, pl* **-mies** : surgical anastomosis of a divided vas deferens to reverse a previous vasectomy

Va·sox·yl \vā-ˈzäk-səl\ *n* : a preparation of the hydrochloride of methoxamine — formerly a U.S. registered trademark

vas·tus ex·ter·nus \ˈvas-təs-ek-ˈstər-nəs\ *n* : VASTUS LATERALIS

vastus in·ter·me·di·us \-ˌin-tər-ˈmēd-ē-əs\ *n* : the division of the quadriceps muscle that arises from and covers the front of the shaft of the femur

vastus in·ter·nus \-in-ˈtər-nəs\ *n* : VASTUS MEDIALIS

vastus lat·er·a·lis \-ˌlat-ər-ˈā-ləs, -ˈal-əs\ *n* : the division of the quadriceps muscle that covers the outer aspect of the femur, arises chiefly from the femur, and inserts into the outer border of the patella by a flat tendon which blends with that of the other divisions of the muscle and sends an expansion to the capsule of the knee — called also *vastus externus*

vastus me·di·a·lis \-ˌmēd-ē-ˈā-ləs, -ˈal-əs\ *n* : the division of the quadriceps muscle that covers the inner anterior aspect of the femur, arises chiefly from the femur and the adjacent intermuscular septum, inserts into the inner border of the patella and into the tendon of the other divisions of the muscle, sends also a tendinous expansion to the capsule of the knee joint, and is closely and in the upper part often inseparably united with the vastus intermedius — called also *vastus internus*

vault \ˈvȯlt, *chiefly Brit* ˈvält\ *n* : an arched or dome-shaped anatomical structure: as **a** : SKULLCAP, CALVARIUM ⟨the cranial ~⟩ **b** : FORNIX d

VBAC \ˈvē-ˌbak\ *n* [*v*aginal *b*irth *a*fter *c*esarean] : delivery through the birth canal in a pregnancy subsequent to one in which delivery was by cesarean section

VCG *abbr* vectorcardiogram

vCJD *abbr* variant Creutzfeldt-Jakob disease

VD *abbr* venereal disease

VDRL \ˈvē-ˌdē-ˌär-ˈel\ *n* : VDRL TEST

VDRL *abbr* venereal disease research laboratory

VDRL slide test *n* : VDRL TEST

VDRL test *n* : a flocculation test for syphilis employing cardiolipin in combination with lecithin and cholesterol

¹**vec·tor** \ˈvek-tər\ *n* **1** : a quantity that has magnitude and direction and that is usu. represented by part of a straight line with the given direction and with a length representing the magnitude **2** : an organism (as an insect) that transmits a pathogen from one organism or source to another ⟨fleas are ~s of plague⟩ — compare CARRIER 1a **3** : an agent (as a plasmid or virus) that contains or carries modified genetic material (as recombinant DNA) and can be used to introduce exogenous genes into the genome of an organism — **vec·to·ri·al** \vek-ˈtōr-ē-əl, -ˈtȯr-\ *adj*

²**vector** *vt* **vec·tored; vec·tor·ing** \-t(ə-)riŋ\ : to transmit (a pathogen or disease) from one organism to another : act as a vector for ⟨a disease ~ed by flies⟩

vec·tor·car·dio·gram \ˌvek-tər-ˈkärd-ē-ə-ˌgram\ *n* : a graphic record made by vectorcardiography

vec·tor·car·di·og·ra·phy \-ˌkärd-ē-ˈäg-rə-fē\ *n, pl* **-phies** : a method of recording the direction and magnitude of the electrical forces of the heart by means of a continuous series of vectors that form a curving line around a center — **vec·tor·car·dio·graph·ic** \-ē-ə-ˈgraf-ik\ *adj*

veg·an \ˈvē-gən; ˈvej-ən, -ˌan\ *n* : a strict vegetarian who consumes no animal food or dairy products — **vegan** *adj* — **veg·an·ism** \ˈvē-gə-ˌniz-əm, ˈvej-ə-\ *n*

¹**veg·e·ta·ble** \ˈvej-tə-bəl, ˈvej-ət-ə-\ *adj* **1 a** : of, relating to, constituting, or growing like plants **b** : consisting of plants **2** : made or obtained from plants or plant products

²**vegetable** *n* **1** : a usu. herbaceous plant (as the cabbage, bean, or potato) grown for an edible part; *also* : such an edible part **2** : a person whose mental and physical functioning is severely impaired and esp. who requires supportive measures (as intravenous feeding or mechanical ventilation) to survive

vegetable mercury *n* : MANACA ROOT

vegetable oil *n* : an oil of plant origin; *esp* : a fatty oil from seeds or fruits

veg·e·tal \ˈvej-ət-ᵊl\ *adj* **1** : VEGETABLE **2** : of or relating to the vegetal pole of an egg or to that part of an egg from which the endoderm normally develops ⟨~ blastomeres⟩

vegetal pole *n* : the point on the surface of an egg that is diametrically opposite to the animal pole and usu. marks the center of the protoplasm containing more yolk, dividing more slowly and into larger blastomeres than that about the animal pole, and giving rise to the hypoblast of the embryo

¹**veg·e·tar·i·an** \ˌvej-ə-ˈter-ē-ən\ *n* : an individual who believes in or practices vegetarianism

²**vegetarian** *adj* **1** : of or relating to vegetarians **2** : consisting wholly of vegetables, fruits, grains, nuts, and sometimes eggs or dairy products ⟨a ~ diet⟩

veg·e·tar·i·an·ism \-ē-ə-ˌniz-əm\ *n* : the theory or practice of living on a vegetarian diet

veg·e·ta·tion \ˌvej-ə-ˈtā-shən\ *n* : an abnormal outgrowth upon a body part; *specif* : any of the warty excrescences on the valves of the heart that are composed of various tissue elements including fibrin and collagen and that are typical of endocarditis

veg·e·ta·tive \ˈvej-ə-ˌtāt-iv\ *adj* **1 a** (1) : growing or having the power of growing (2) : of, relating to, or engaged in nutritive and growth functions as contrasted with reproductive functions ⟨a ~ nucleus⟩ **b** : of, relating to, or involving propagation by nonsexual processes or methods **2** : of or relating to the division of nature comprising the plant kingdom **3** : affecting, arising from, or relating to involuntary

---

\ə\ abut \ᵊ\ kitten \ər\ further \a\ ash \ā\ ace \ä\ cot, cart
\aù\ out \ch\ chin \e\ bet \ē\ easy \g\ go \i\ hit \ī\ ice \j\ job
\ŋ\ sing \ō\ go \ȯ\ law \ȯi\ boy \th\ thin \ṭh\ the \ü\ loot
\ù\ foot \y\ yet \zh\ vision *See also* Pronunciation Symbols page

U
Z

bodily functions   **4** : characterized by, resulting from, or being a state in which there is total loss of cognitive functioning typically indicated by a lack of awareness of oneself and one's environment and in which only involuntary bodily functions (as breathing or blinking of the eyes) are sustained ⟨entered a ∼ state following a serious head injury⟩ — **veg·e·ta·tive·ly** *adv*

vegetative nervous system *n* : AUTONOMIC NERVOUS SYSTEM

vegetative pole *n* : VEGETAL POLE

VEGF *abbr* vascular endothelial growth factor

ve·hi·cle \'vē-ₚ(h)ik-əl, 'vē-ə-kəl\ *n* **1** : an inert medium in which a medicinally active agent is administered **2** : an agent of transmission ⟨a ∼ of infection⟩

veil \'vā(ə)l\ *n* : a covering body part or membrane; *esp* : CAUL 2

vein \'vān\ *n* : any of the tubular branching vessels that carry blood from the capillaries toward the heart and have thinner walls than the arteries and often valves at intervals to prevent reflux of the blood which flows in a steady stream and is in most cases dark-colored due to the presence of reduced hemoglobin

vein of Galen *n* : GALEN'S VEIN

vein·ous \'vā-nəs\ *adj* **1** : having veins that are esp. prominent ⟨∼ hands⟩ **2** : VENOUS ⟨less evidence of a ∼ stasis —*Diseases of the Nervous System*⟩

veiny \'vā-nē\ *adj* : full of veins : marked by conspicuous veins ⟨∼ legs⟩

vela *pl of* VELUM

ve·la·men·tous insertion \ₚvel-ə-'men-təs-, ₚvēl-\ *n* : attachment of the umbilical cord to the chorion beyond the margin of the placenta

ve·lar \'vē-lər\ *adj* : of, forming, or relating to a velum and esp. the soft palate

veli — see LEVATOR VELI PALATINI, TENSOR VELI PALATINI

ve·lo·pha·ryn·geal \ₚvē-lō-ₚfar-ən-'jē-əl, -fə-'rin-j(ē-)əl\ *adj* : of or relating to the soft palate and the pharynx ⟨∼ structures⟩

Vel·peau bandage *or* **Vel·peau's bandage** \vel-'pō(z)-\ *n* : a bandage used to support and immobilize the arm when the clavicle is fractured

 Vel·peau \vel-pō\, **Alfred–Armand–Louis–Marie (1795–1867),** French surgeon. Velpeau was the leading French surgeon in the first half of the 19th century. In 1839 he introduced a bandage designed to support the arm in dislocation or fracture of the clavicle.

ve·lum \'vē-ləm\ *n, pl* **ve·la** \-lə\ : a membrane or membranous part resembling a veil or curtain: as **a** : SOFT PALATE **b** : SEMILUNAR CUSP

ve·na ca·va \ₚvē-nə-'kā-və\ *n, pl* **ve·nae ca·vae** \-ni-'kā-(ₚ)vē\ : either of two large veins by which the blood is returned to the right atrium of the heart: **a** : INFERIOR VENA CAVA **b** : SUPERIOR VENA CAVA — **vena ca·val** \-vəl\ *adj*

vena co·mi·tans \-'kō-mə-ₚtanz\ *n, pl* **venae co·mi·tan·tes** \-ₚkō-mə-'tan-ₚtēz\ : a vein accompanying an artery

venae cor·dis min·i·mae \-'kȯr-dəs-'min-ə-ₚmē\ *n pl* : minute veins in the wall of the heart that empty into the atria or ventricles

vena vor·ti·co·sa \-ₚvȯrt-ə-'kō-sə\ *n, pl* **venae vor·ti·co·sae** \-(ₚ)sē\ : any of the veins of the outer layer of the choroid of the eye — called also *vorticose vein*

ve·neer \və-'ni(ə)r\ *n* : a plastic or porcelain coating bonded to the surface of a cosmetically imperfect tooth

ven·e·na·tion \ₚven-ə-'nā-shən\ *n* : the condition or process of being poisoned esp. by a venom of animal origin — **ven·e·nate** \'ven-ə-ₚnāt\ *vb* **-nat·ed; -nat·ing**

ven·e·nif·er·ous \ₚven-ə-'nif-(ə-)rəs\ *adj* : bearing or transmitting poison and esp. a natural venom

venepuncture *var of* VENIPUNCTURE

ve·ne·re·al \və-'nir-ē-əl\ *adj* **1** : of or relating to sexual pleasure or indulgence **2 a** : resulting from or contracted during sexual intercourse ⟨∼ infections⟩ **b** : of, relating to, or affected with venereal disease ⟨a high ∼ rate⟩ **c** : involving the genital organs ⟨∼ sarcoma⟩ — **ve·ne·re·al·ly** \-ē\ *adv*

venereal disease *n* : a contagious disease (as gonorrhea or syphilis) that is typically acquired in sexual intercourse — abbr. *VD*; compare SEXUALLY TRANSMITTED DISEASE

venereal wart *n* : GENITAL WART

ve·ne·re·ol·o·gist \və-ₚnir-ē-'äl-ə-jəst\ *n* : a physician specializing in venereal diseases

ve·ne·re·ol·o·gy \və-ₚnir-ē-'äl-ə-jē\ *also* **ven·er·ol·o·gy** \ₚven-ə-'räl-ə-jē\ *n, pl* **-gies** : a branch of medical science concerned with venereal diseases — **ve·ne·re·o·log·i·cal** \və-ₚnir-ē-ə-'läj-i-kəl\ *adj*

venereum — see GRANULOMA VENEREUM, LYMPHOGRANULOMA VENEREUM, LYMPHOPATHIA VENEREUM

veneris — see MONS VENERIS

ven·ery \'ven-ə-rē\ *n, pl* **ven·er·ies** **1** : the pursuit of or indulgence in sexual pleasure **2** : SEXUAL INTERCOURSE

vene·sec·tion *also* **veni·sec·tion** \'ven-ə-ₚsek-shən, 'vēn-\ *n* : PHLEBOTOMY

Ven·e·zu·e·lan equine encephalitis \ₚven-əz(-ə)-'wā-lən-\ *n* : EQUINE ENCEPHALOMYELITIS C

Venezuelan equine encephalomyelitis *n* : EQUINE ENCEPHALOMYELITIS C

Ven·ice treacle \'ven-əs-\ *n* : THERIACA

ve·ni·punc·ture *also* **ve·ne·punc·ture** \'vēn-ə-ₚpəŋ(k)-chər, 'ven-ə-\ *n* : surgical puncture of a vein esp. for the withdrawal of blood or for administration of intravenous fluids or drugs

venisection *var of* VENESECTION

ven·la·fax·ine \ₚven-lə-'fak-ₚsēn\ *n* : an antidepressant drug that is used in the form of its hydrochloride $C_{17}H_{27}NO_2$·HCl and acts by inhibiting the reuptake of serotonin and norepinephrine by neurons — see EFFEXOR

ve·no·ar·te·ri·al \ₚvē-nō-är-'tir-ē-əl\ *adj* : relating to or involving an artery and vein

ve·noc·ly·sis \vē-'näk-lə-səs\ *n, pl* **-ly·ses** \-ₚsēz\ : clysis into a vein

ve·no·con·stric·tion \ₚvē-nō-kən-'strik-shən\ *n* : constriction of a vein

ve·no·fi·bro·sis \ₚvē-nō-fī-'brō-səs\ *n, pl* **-bro·ses** \-ₚsēz\ : PHLEBOSCLEROSIS

ve·no·gram \'vē-nə-ₚgram\ *n* : a radiograph after the injection of an opaque substance into a vein

ve·no·graph·ic \ₚvē-nə-'graf-ik\ *adj* : of, relating to, or involving venography or a venogram ⟨a ∼ assessment⟩

ve·nog·ra·phy \vi-'näg-rə-fē, vā-\ *n, pl* **-phies** : radiography of a vein after injection of an opaque substance

ven·om \'ven-əm\ *n* : poisonous matter normally secreted by some animals (as snakes, scorpions, or bees) and transmitted to prey or an enemy chiefly by biting or stinging

ven·om·ous \'ven-ə-məs\ *adj* **1** : POISONOUS **2** : having a venom-producing gland and able to inflict a poisoned wound ⟨the vipers, pit vipers, and coral snakes are ∼⟩

ve·no·oc·clu·sive \ₚvē-nō-ə-'klü-siv\ *adj* : marked by occlusion or compression of small veins ⟨∼ disease⟩

ve·no·pres·sor \ₚvē-nə-'pres-ₚȯr, -ər\ *adj* : of, relating to, or controlling venous blood pressure

ve·nos·i·ty \vi-'näs-ət-ē\ *n, pl* **-ties** : the quality or state of being venous

ve·nos·ta·sis \vi-'näs-tə-səs\ *n, pl* **-ta·ses** \-ₚsēz\ : an abnormal slowing or stoppage of the flow of blood in a vein

venosum — see LIGAMENTUM VENOSUM

venosus — see DUCTUS VENOSUS, SINUS VENOSUS, SINUS VENOSUS SCLERAE

ve·not·o·my \vi-'nät-ə-mē\ *n, pl* **-mies** : PHLEBOTOMY

ve·nous \'vē-nəs\ *adj* **1 a** : full of or characterized by veins **b** : made up of or carried on by veins ⟨the ∼ circulation⟩ **2** : of, relating to, or performing the functions of a vein ⟨a ∼ inflammation⟩ ⟨∼ arteries⟩ **3** *of blood* : having passed through the capillaries and given up oxygen for the tissues and become charged with carbon dioxide and ready to pass through the respiratory organs to release its carbon dioxide and renew its oxygen supply : dark red from reduced hemoglobin — compare ARTERIAL 2

venous hum *n* : a humming sound sometimes heard during auscultation of the veins of the neck esp. in anemia

venous re·turn \-ri-'tərn\ *n* : the flow of blood from the venous system into the right atrium of the heart

venous sinus *n* **1** : a large vein or passage (as the canal of Schlemm) for venous blood **2** : SINUS VENOSUS

vent \'vent\ *n* : an opening for the escape of a gas or liquid or for the relief of pressure; *esp* : the external opening of the rectum or cloaca : ANUS

ven·ter \'vent-ər\ *n* : an anatomical structure that is protuberant and often hollow: as **a** : ABDOMEN; *also* : a large bodily cavity (as in the head, thorax, or abdomen) containing organs **b** : BELLY 2

vent gleet *n* : CLOACITIS

ven·ti·late \'vent-ᵊl-ˌāt\ *vt* **-lat·ed; -lat·ing** **1** : to expose to air and esp. to a current of fresh air for purifying or refreshing **2 a** : OXYGENATE, AERATE ⟨∼ blood in the lungs⟩ **b** : to subject the lungs of (an individual) to ventilation ⟨artificially ∼ a patient in respiratory distress⟩ **3** : to give verbal expression to (as mental or emotional conflicts)

ven·ti·la·tion \ˌvent-ᵊl-'ā-shən\ *n* **1** : the act or process of ventilating **2** : the circulation and exchange of gases in the lungs or gills that is basic to respiration

ven·ti·la·tor \'vent-ᵊl-ˌāt-ər\ *n* : RESPIRATOR 2

ven·ti·la·to·ry \'vent-ᵊl-ə-ˌtōr-ē, -ˌtȯr-\ *adj* : of, relating to, or provided with ventilation ⟨∼ support⟩ ⟨no further decrement in ∼ function —A. R. Morton⟩

Ven·to·lin \'vent-ᵊl-ən\ *trademark* — used for a preparation of albuterol

ven·tral \'ven-trəl\ *adj* **1** : of or relating to the belly : ABDOMINAL **2 a** : being or located near, on, or toward the lower surface of an animal (as a quadruped) opposite the back or dorsal surface **b** : being or located near, on, or toward the front or anterior part of the human body

ventral column *n* : VENTRAL HORN

ventral corticospinal tract *n* : a band of nerve fibers that descends in the ventrolateral part of the spinal cord and consists of fibers arising in the motor cortex of the brain on the same side of the body and not crossing over in the decussation of pyramids — called also *anterior corticospinal tract, direct pyramidal tract*

ventral funiculus *n* : ANTERIOR FUNICULUS

ventral gray column *n* : VENTRAL HORN

ventral horn *n* : a longitudinal subdivision of gray matter in the anterior part of each lateral half of the spinal cord that contains neurons giving rise to motor fibers of the ventral roots of the spinal nerves — called also *anterior column, anterior gray column, anterior horn, ventral column, ventral gray column;* compare DORSAL HORN, LATERAL COLUMN 1

ventralis — see SACROCOCCYGEUS VENTRALIS

ven·tral·ly \'ven-trə-lē\ *adv* : in a ventral direction or position ⟨attached ∼ to the mesentery⟩

ventral median fissure *n* : ANTERIOR MEDIAN FISSURE

ventral mesogastrium *n* : MESOGASTRIUM 1

ventral root *n* : the one of the two roots of a spinal nerve that passes anteriorly from the spinal cord separating the anterior and lateral funiculi and that consists of motor fibers — called also *anterior root;* compare DORSAL ROOT

ventral spinocerebellar tract *n* : SPINOCEREBELLAR TRACT b

ventral spinothalamic tract *n* : SPINOTHALAMIC TRACT a

ven·tri·cle \'ven-tri-kəl\ *n* : a cavity of a bodily part or organ: as **a** : a chamber of the heart which receives blood from a corresponding atrium and from which blood is forced into the arteries **b** : one of the system of communicating cavities in the brain that are continuous with the central canal of the spinal cord, that like it are derived from the medullary canal of the embryo, that are lined with an epithelial ependyma, and that contain a serous fluid — see LATERAL VENTRICLE, THIRD VENTRICLE, FOURTH VENTRICLE **c** : a fossa or pouch on each side of the larynx between the false vocal cords above and the true vocal cords below

ven·tri·cor·nu \ˌven-tri-'kȯr-ˌn(y)ü\ *n* : VENTRAL HORN

ven·tric·u·lar \ven-'trik-yə-lər, vən-\ *adj* : of, relating to, or being a ventricle esp. of the heart or brain

ventricular as·sist device \-ə-'sist-\ *n* : VAD

ventricular fibrillation *n* : very rapid uncoordinated fluttering contractions of the ventricles of the heart resulting in loss of synchronization between heartbeat and pulse beat — abbr. *VF, V-fib*

ventricular folds *n pl* : FALSE VOCAL CORDS

ven·tric·u·lar·is \ven-ˌtrik-yə-'lar-əs\ *n* : a small bundle of fibers of the thyroarytenoid that extends along the wall of the ventricle from the arytenoid cartilage to the epiglottis

ventricular septal defect *n* : a congenital defect in the interventricular septum — abbr. *VSD*

ventricular tachycardia *n* : tachycardia that is associated with the generation of electrical impulses within the ventricles and is characterized by an electrocardiogram having a broad QRS complex — abbr. *VT, V-tach*

ven·tric·u·li·tis \ven-ˌtrik-yə-'līt-əs\ *n* : inflammation of the ventricles of the brain

ven·tric·u·lo·atri·al \ven-ˌtrik-yə-lō-'ā-trē-əl\ *adj* **1** : of, relating to, or being an artificial shunt between a ventricle of the brain and an atrium of the heart esp. to drain cerebrospinal fluid (as in hydrocephalus) **2** : of, relating to, or being conduction from the ventricle to the atrium of the heart

ven·tric·u·lo·atri·os·to·my \-ˌā-trē-'äs-tə-mē\ *n, pl* **-mies** : surgical establishment of a shunt to drain cerebrospinal fluid (as in hydrocephalus) from a ventricle of the brain to the right atrium

ven·tric·u·lo·cis·ter·nos·to·my \-ˌsis-tər-'näs-tə-mē\ *n, pl* **-mies** : the surgical establishment of a communication between a ventricle of the brain and the subarachnoid space and esp. the cisterna magna to drain cerebrospinal fluid esp. in hydrocephalus

ven·tric·u·lo·gram \ven-'trik-yə-lə-ˌgram\ *n* : an X-ray photograph made by ventriculography

ven·tric·u·log·ra·phy \ven-ˌtrik-yə-'läg-rə-fē\ *n, pl* **-phies** **1** : the act or process of making an X-ray photograph of the ventricles of the brain after withdrawing fluid from the ventricles and replacing it with air or a radiopaque substance **2** : the act or process of making an X-ray photograph of a ventricle of the heart after injecting a radiopaque substance — **ven·tric·u·lo·graph·ic** \-yə-lō-'graf-ik\ *adj*

ven·tric·u·lo·peri·to·ne·al \ven-ˌtrik-yə-lō-ˌper-ət-ᵊn-'ē-əl\ *adj* : relating to or serving to communicate between a ventricle of the brain and the peritoneal cavity ⟨a ∼ shunt⟩

ven·tric·u·los·to·my \ven-ˌtrik-yə-'läs-tə-mē\ *n, pl* **-mies** : the surgical establishment of an opening in a ventricle of the brain to drain cerebrospinal fluid esp. in hydrocephalus

ven·tric·u·lot·o·my \ven-ˌtrik-yə-'lät-ə-mē\ *n, pl* **-mies** : surgical incision of a ventricle (as of the heart)

ven·tric·u·lus \ven-'trik-yə-ləs, vən-\ *n, pl* **-li** \-ˌlī\ : a digestive cavity (as the stomach or gizzard)

ven·tro·lat·er·al \ˌven-trō-'lat-ə-rəl, -'la-trəl\ *adj* : ventral and lateral — **ven·tro·lat·er·al·ly** \-ē\ *adv*

ven·tro·me·di·al \-'mēd-ē-əl\ *adj* : ventral and medial — **ven·tro·me·di·al·ly** \-ē\ *adv*

ventromedial nucleus *n* : a medially located nucleus of the hypothalamus that is situated between the lateral wall of the third ventricle and the fornix and that is held to suppress the urge to eat when satiety is reached

ven·u·lar \'ven-yə-lər\ *adj* : of, relating to, or involving venules ⟨∼ disorders⟩

ve·nule \'vēn-(ˌ)yü(ə)l, 'ven-\ *n* : a small vein; *esp* : any of the minute veins connecting the capillaries with the larger systemic veins

Ve·nus·hair \'vē-nəs-ˌha(ə)r, -ˌhe(ə)r\ *n* : a delicate maidenhair fern (*Adiantum capillus-veneris*) that has been used in the preparation of expectorants and demulcents

vera — see ALOE VERA, CUTIS VERA, DECIDUA VERA, POLYCYTHEMIA VERA

ve·rap·am·il \və-'rap-ə-ˌmil\ *n* : a calcium channel blocker that is administered in the form of its hydrochloride

$C_{27}H_{38}N_2O_4 \cdot HCl$ esp. to treat hypertension and angina pectoris — see CALAN

ve·rat·ri·dine \və-'ra-trə-ˌdēn\ *n* : a poisonous amorphous alkaloid $C_{36}H_{51}NO_{11}$ occurring esp. in sabadilla seeds

ver·a·trine \'ver-ə-ˌtrēn\ *n* : a mixture of alkaloids that is obtained as a white or grayish powder from sabadilla seeds, that is an intense local irritant and a powerful muscle and nerve poison, and that has been used as a counterirritant in neuralgia and arthritis

ve·ra·trum \və-'rā-trəm\ *n* **1 a** *cap* : a genus of coarse herbs of the lily family (Liliaceae) having short poisonous rootstocks **b** : any hellebore of the genus *Veratrum* **2** : HELLEBORE 2b

ver·big·er·a·tion \(ˌ)vər-ˌbij-ə-'rā-shən\ *n* : continual repetition of stereotyped phrases (as in some forms of mental disorder)

ver·di·gris \'vərd-ə-ˌgrēs, -ˌgris, -grəs *also* -ˌgrē\ *n* : a green or greenish blue poisonous pigment resulting from the action of acetic acid on copper, consisting of one or more basic copper acetates, and formerly used in medicine

ver·do·glo·bin \'vər-də-ˌglō-bən\ *n* : any of several green compounds derived from hemoglobin or related compounds by cleavage of the porphyrin ring

ver·do·per·ox·i·dase \ˌvər-dō-pə-'räk-sə-ˌdās, -ˌdāz\ *n* : a green-colored peroxidase obtained from white blood cells that is responsible for the peroxidase activity of pus

verge — see ANAL VERGE

ver·gence \'vər-jən(t)s\ *n* : a movement of one eye in relation to the other

Ver·hoeff's stain \'vər-ˌhófs-\ *n* : a stain containing hematoxylin, ferric chloride, and iodine that is used to demonstrate the presence of elastin

    Verhoeff, Frederick Herman (1874–1968), American ophthalmologist. Verhoeff was an ophthalmic surgeon and pathologist at a Boston eye and ear infirmary and had a parallel career as a professor of ophthalmology at Harvard Medical School. He introduced Verhoeff's stain in 1908.

vermes *pl of* VERMIS

Ver·mes \'vər-(ˌ)mēz\ *n pl* : any of several major divisions of the animal kingdom: as **a** *in former classifications* : a taxon containing all invertebrates with the exception of the arthropods **b** *in some esp former classifications* : a taxon comprising the typically soft-bodied and more or less vermiform invertebrates including the flatworms, roundworms, annelid worms, and minor forms, and usu. held to be a purely artificial grouping

ver·mi·an \'vər-mē-ən\ *adj* **1** : of, relating to, or resembling worms **2** : of or relating to the vermis of the cerebellum

ver·mi·ci·dal \ˌvər-mə-'sīd-ᵊl\ *adj* : destroying worms

ver·mi·cide \'vər-mə-ˌsīd\ *n* : an agent that destroys worms; *esp* : ANTHELMINTIC

ver·mi·form \'vər-mə-ˌfórm\ *adj* : resembling a worm in shape

vermiform appendix *n* : a narrow blind tube usu. about three or four inches (7.6 to 10.2 centimeters) long that extends from the cecum in the lower right-hand part of the abdomen, has much lymphoid wall tissue, normally communicates with the cavity of the cecum, and represents an atrophied terminal part of the cecum

vermiform process *n* : VERMIFORM APPENDIX

ver·mif·u·gal \vər-'mif-yə-gəl, ˌvər-mə-'fyü-gəl\ *adj* : serving to destroy or expel parasitic worms : ANTHELMINTIC

ver·mi·fuge \'vər-mə-ˌfyüj\ *n* : a vermifugal agent : ANTHELMINTIC

ver·mil·ion border \vər-'mil-yən-\ *n* : the exposed pink or reddish margin of a lip

ver·mil·ion·ec·to·my \vər-ˌmil-yən-'ek-tə-mē\ *n, pl* **-mies** : surgical excision of the vermilion border

ver·min \'vər-mən\ *n, pl* **vermin** : small common harmful or objectionable animals (as lice or fleas) that are difficult to control

ver·min·osis \ˌvər-mə-'nō-səs\ *n, pl* **-oses** \-ˌsēz\ : infestation with or disease caused by parasitic worms

ver·min·ous \'vər-mə-nəs\ *adj* **1** : consisting of, infested with, or being vermin **2** : caused by parasitic worms ⟨~ gastritis⟩

ver·mis \'vər-mis\ *n, pl* **ver·mes** \-ˌmēz\ **1** : either of two parts of the median lobe of the cerebellum: **a** : one slightly prominent on the upper surface — called also *superior vermis* **b** : one on the lower surface sunk in the vallecula — called also *inferior vermis* **2** : the median lobe or part of the cerebellum

ver·nal catarrh \'vərn-ᵊl-\ *n* : VERNAL CONJUNCTIVITIS

vernal conjunctivitis *n* : conjunctivitis occurring in warm seasons as a result of exposure to allergens

Ver·ner–Mor·ri·son syndrome \'vər-nər-'mór-ə-sən-, -'mär-\ *n* : a syndrome characterized esp. by severe watery diarrhea and hypokalemia that is often due to an excessive secretion of vasoactive intestinal peptide from a vipoma esp. of the pancreas — called also *pancreatic cholera, WDHA syndrome*

    Verner, John Victor (b 1927), American internist, and **Morrison, Ashton Byrom (b 1922),** American pathologist. Verner and Morrison published their description of Verner–Morrison syndrome in 1958. A brief report on the same syndrome had been published a year earlier by British physicians W. M. Priest and M. K. Alexander. In addition to pancreatic cholera, Morrison's areas of research included chronic renal insufficiency and nephropathies. Morrison held a series of professorships at the medical schools for Duke University, the University of Pennsylvania, and the University of Rochester before settling at Rutgers University Medical School, first as professor of pathology and eventually as dean.

ver·ni·er acuity \'vər-nē-ər-\ *n* : the aspect of visual acuity that involves the ability to detect the alignment or lack of alignment of the two parts of a broken line (as in reading a vernier scale) — compare GRATING ACUITY, HYPERACUITY, STEREOACUITY

ver·nix \'vər-niks\ *n* : VERNIX CASEOSA

vernix ca·se·o·sa \-ˌkas-ē-'ō-sə\ *n* : a pasty covering chiefly of dead cells and sebaceous secretions that protects the skin of the fetus

ver·o·nal \'ver-ə-ˌnól, -ən-ᵊl\ *n, often cap* : a preparation of the sodium salt $C_8H_{11}N_2NaO_3$ of barbital formerly used in medicine as a sedative and hypnotic

ver·ru·ca \və-'rü-kə\ *n, pl* **-cae** \-(ˌ)kē\ : a wart or warty skin lesion

verruca acu·mi·na·ta \-ə-ˌkyü-mə-'nāt-ə\ *n* : GENITAL WART

verruca pla·na \-'plā-nə\ *n* : FLAT WART

verruca plan·ta·ris \-ˌplan-'tar-əs, -'ter-\ *n* : PLANTAR WART

verruca vul·ga·ris \-ˌvəl-'gar-əs, -'ger-\ *n* : WART 1; *esp* : one occurring on the back of the fingers and hands

ver·ru·cose \və-'rü-ˌkōs\ *adj* **1** : covered with warty elevations ⟨a ~ surface⟩ **2** : having the form of a wart ⟨a ~ nevus⟩

ver·ru·cous \və-'rü-kəs\ *adj* **1** : VERRUCOSE ⟨~ vegetations⟩ **2** : characterized by the formation of warty lesions ⟨~ dermatitis⟩

verrucous endocarditis *n* : endocarditis marked by the formation or presence of warty nodules of fibrin on the lips of the heart valves

ver·ru·ga \və-'rü-gə\ *n* **1** : VERRUCA **2** : VERRUGA PERUANA

verruga per·u·a·na \-ˌper-ə-'wä-nə\ *also* **verruga pe·ru·vi·ana** \-pə-ˌrü-vē-'an-ə\ *n* : the second stage of bartonellosis characterized by warty nodules tending to ulcerate and bleed

versicolor — see PITYRIASIS VERSICOLOR, TINEA VERSICOLOR

ver·sion \'vər-zhən, -shən\ *n* **1** : a condition in which an organ and esp. the uterus is turned from its normal position **2** : manual turning of a fetus in the uterus to aid delivery

ver·te·bra \'vərt-ə-brə\ *n, pl* **-brae** \-ˌbrā, -(ˌ)brē\ *or* **-bras** : any of the bony or cartilaginous segments that make up the spinal column and that have a short more or less cylindrical body whose ends articulate by pads of elastic or cartilaginous tissue with those of adjacent vertebrae and a bony arch that encloses the spinal cord

¹**ver·te·bral** \\(ˌ)vər-'tē-brəl, 'vərt-ə-\ *adj* **1** : of, relating to, or being vertebrae or the spinal column : SPINAL **2** : composed of or having vertebrae

²**vertebral** *n* : a vertebral part or element (as an artery)

vertebral arch *n* : NEURAL ARCH

vertebral artery *n* : a large branch of the subclavian artery that ascends through the foramina in the transverse processes of each of the cervical vertebrae except the last one or two, enters the cranium through the foramen magnum, and unites with the corresponding artery of the opposite side to form the basilar artery

vertebral body *n* : the main anterior bony part of a vertebra that consists of the centrum, the ossified posterolateral joints linking the centrum and each half of the neural arch, and part of the neural arch

vertebral canal *n* : a canal that contains the spinal cord and is delimited by the neural arches on the dorsal side of the vertebrae — called also *spinal canal*

vertebral column *n* : SPINAL COLUMN

vertebral foramen *n* : the opening formed by a neural arch through which the spinal cord passes

vertebral ganglion *n* : any of a group of sympathetic ganglia which form two chains extending from the base of the skull to the coccyx along the sides of the spinal column — compare SYMPATHETIC CHAIN

vertebral notch *n* : either of two concave constrictions of which one occurs on the inferior surface and one on the superior surface of the pedicle on each side of a vertebra and which are arranged so that the superior notches of one vertebra and the corresponding inferior notches of a contiguous vertebra combine to form an intervertebral foramen on each side

vertebral plexus *n* : a plexus of veins associated with the spinal column

vertebral vein *n* : a tributary of the brachiocephalic vein that is formed by the union of branches originating in the occipital region and forming a plexus about the vertebral artery in its passage through the foramina of the cervical vertebrae and that receives various branches which join it near its termination

vertebra pro·mi·nens \-'prä-mi-ˌnenz\ *n* : the seventh cervical vertebra characterized by a prominent spinous process which can be felt at the base of the neck

Ver·te·bra·ta \ˌvər-tə-'brät-ə, -'brāt-\ *n pl* : a subphylum of chordates comprising animals (as mammals, birds, reptiles, amphibians, and fishes) with a segmented spinal column together with a few primitive forms in which the backbone is represented by a notochord

¹**ver·te·brate** \'vərt-ə-brət, -ˌbrāt\ *adj* **1** : having a spinal column **2** : of or relating to the subphylum Vertebrata

²**vertebrate** *n* : an animal of the subphylum Vertebrata

ver·te·bro·ba·si·lar \ˌvər-tə-brō-'bā-sə-lər\ *adj* : of, relating to, or being the vertebral and basilar arteries ⟨~ injuries⟩

ver·te·bro·chon·dral rib \ˌvər-tə-brō-ˌkän-drəl-\ *n* : any of the three false ribs that are located above the floating ribs and that are attached to each other by costal cartilages

ver·te·bro·plas·ty \'vər-tə-brō-ˌplas-tē\ *n, pl* **-ties** : a medical procedure for reducing pain caused by a vertebral compression fracture (as that associated with osteoporosis) that involves injection of an acrylic cement (as methyl methacrylate) into the body of the fractured vertebra for stabilization — compare KYPHOPLASTY

ver·te·bro·ster·nal rib \ˌvər-tə-brō-ˌstər-nəl-\ *n* : TRUE RIB

ver·tex \'vər-ˌteks\ *n, pl* **ver·ti·ces** \'vərt-ə-ˌsēz\ *also* **ver·tex·es** **1** : the top of the head **2** : the highest point of the skull

vertex presentation *n* : normal obstetric presentation in which the fetal occiput lies at the opening of the uterus

ver·ti·cal \'vərt-i-kəl\ *adj* : relating to or being transmission (as of a disease) by genetic inheritance or by a congenital or perinatal route ⟨~ transmission of the hepatitis B virus from mother to infant⟩ — compare HORIZONTAL 2 — **ver·ti·cal·ly** \'vərt-i-k(ə-)lē\ *adv*

vertical dimension *n* : the distance between two arbitrarily chosen points on the face above and below the mouth when the teeth are in occlusion

vertical nystagmus *n* : nystagmus characterized by up-and-down movement of the eyes

ver·tig·i·nous \(ˌ)vər-'tij-ə-nəs\ *adj* : of, relating to, characterized by, or affected with vertigo or dizziness

ver·ti·go \'vərt-i-ˌgō\ *n, pl* **-goes** *or* **-gos** **1** : a disordered state which is associated with various disorders (as of the inner ear) and in which the individual or the individual's surroundings seem to whirl dizzily — see OBJECTIVE VERTIGO, SUBJECTIVE VERTIGO; compare DIZZINESS **2** : disordered vertiginous movement as a symptom of disease in lower animals; *also* : a disease (as gid) causing this

ver·u·mon·ta·ni·tis \ˌvər-ə-ˌmän-tə-'nīt-əs\ *n* : inflammation of the verumontanum

ver·u·mon·ta·num \ˌvər-ə-ˌmän-'tā-nəm\ *n* : an elevation in the floor of the prostatic portion of the urethra where the seminal ducts enter

ver·vain \'vər-ˌvān\ *n* : any of a genus (*Verbena* of the family Verbenaceae, the vervain family) of plants including several (as *V. hastata*) formerly used as medicinal herbs

ver·vet monkey \ˌvər-vət-\ *n* : GREEN MONKEY — called also *vervet*

very–low–density lipoprotein \'ver-ē-\ *n* : VLDL

vesicae — see TRIGONUM VESICAE, UVULA VESICAE

ves·i·ca fel·lea \'ves-i-kə-'fel-ē-ə\ *n* : GALLBLADDER

¹**ves·i·cal** \'ves-i-kəl\ *adj* : of or relating to a bladder and esp. to the urinary bladder ⟨~ burning⟩

²**vesical** *n* : VESICAL ARTERY

vesical artery *n* : any of several arteries that arise from the internal iliac artery or one of its branches and that supply the urinary bladder and adjacent parts: as **a** : any of several arteries that arise from the umbilical artery and supply the upper part of the bladder — called also *superior vesical, superior vesical artery* **b** : one that arises from the internal iliac artery or the internal pudendal artery and that supplies the bladder, prostate, and seminal vesicles — called also *inferior vesical, inferior vesical artery*

vesical plexus *n* : a plexus of nerves that comprises preganglionic fibers derived chiefly from the hypogastric plexus and postganglionic neurons whose fibers are distributed to the bladder and adjacent parts

vesical venous plexus *n* : a plexus of veins surrounding the neck of the bladder and the base of the prostate gland and draining eventually into the internal iliac vein

¹**ves·i·cant** \'ves-i-kənt\ *n* : an agent (as a drug or a war gas) that induces blistering — called also *blister gas*

²**vesicant** *adj* : producing or tending to produce blisters ⟨a ~ substance⟩

ves·i·ca·tion \ˌves-ə-'kā-shən\ *n* **1** : BLISTER **2** : an instance or the process of blistering

vesica uri·nar·ia \-ˌyùr-i-'nar-ē-ə\ *n* : URINARY BLADDER

ves·i·cle \'ves-i-kəl\ *n* **1 a** : a membranous and usu. fluid-filled pouch (as a cyst, vacuole, or cell) in a plant or animal **b** : SYNAPTIC VESICLE **2** : a small abnormal elevation of the outer layer of skin enclosing a watery liquid : BLISTER **3** : a pocket of embryonic tissue that is the beginning of an organ — see AUDITORY VESICLE, BRAIN VESICLE, OPTIC VESICLE

ves·i·co·en·ter·ic \ˌves-i-kō-en-'ter-ik\ *adj* : of, relating to, or connecting the urinary bladder and the intestinal tract ⟨a ~ fistula⟩

ves·i·cos·to·my \ˌves-i-'käs-tə-mē\ *n, pl* **-mies** : CYSTOSTOMY

ves·i·co·ure·ter·al reflux \ˌves-i-kō-yù-'rēt-ə-rəl\ *n* : reflux of urine from the bladder into a ureter

ves·i·co·ure·ter·ic reflux \-'rēt-ə-rik-\ *n* : VESICOURETERAL REFLUX

ves·i·co·ure·thral \ˌves-i-kō-yù-'rē-thrəl\ *adj* : of, relating to,

\ə\ **abut** \ə\ **kitten** \ər\ **further** \a\ **ash** \ā\ **ace** \ä\ **cot, cart** \aù\ **out** \ch\ **chin** \e\ **bet** \ē\ **easy** \g\ **go** \i\ **hit** \ī\ **ice** \j\ **job** \ŋ\ **sing** \ō\ **go** \ò\ **law** \ói\ **boy** \th\ **thin** \th\ **the** \ü\ **loot** \ù\ **foot** \y\ **yet** \zh\ **vision** *See also* Pronunciation Symbols page

U
Z

or connecting the urinary bladder and the urethra ⟨the ~ junction⟩

ves·i·co·uter·ine \ˌves-i-kō-ˈyüt-ə-ˌrīn, -rən\ *adj* : of, relating to, or connecting the urinary bladder and the uterus ⟨a ~ fistula⟩

ves·i·co·vag·i·nal \ˌves-i-kō-ˈvaj-ən-ᵊl\ *adj* : of, relating to, or connecting the urinary bladder and vagina ⟨a ~ fistula⟩

ve·sic·u·lar \və-ˈsik-yə-lər, ve-\ *adj* **1** : characterized by the presence or formation of vesicles ⟨a ~ rash⟩ **2** : having the form of a vesicle ⟨a ~ lesion⟩

vesicular breathing *n* : normal breathing that is soft and low-pitched when heard in auscultation

vesicular dermatitis *n* : a severe dermatitis esp. of young chickens and turkeys ranging on sod that is characterized by vesicle and scab formation on the feet and frequent sloughing of toes — called also *sod disease*

vesicular exanthema *n* : an acute virus disease primarily of swine that is caused by a single-stranded RNA virus of the family *Caliciviridae* (species *Vesicular exanthema of swine virus* of the genus *Vesivirus*), that closely resembles foot-and-mouth disease, and that occurred in the U.S. in an epidemic of the 1950s

vesicular ovarian follicle *n* : GRAAFIAN FOLLICLE

vesicular rickettsiosis *n* : RICKETTSIALPOX

vesicular stomatitis *n* : an acute virus disease esp. of various domesticated animals (as horses and cows) that resembles foot-and-mouth disease, that is marked by erosive blisters in and about the mouth, and that is caused by any of three single-stranded RNA viruses of the family *Rhabdoviridae* (genus *Vesiculovirus*) which sometimes infect humans producing symptoms resembling influenza

ve·sic·u·la·tion \və-ˌsik-yə-ˈlā-shən\ *n* **1** : the presence or formation of vesicles **2** : the process of becoming vesicular ⟨~ of a papule⟩

ve·sic·u·lec·to·my \və-ˌsik-yə-ˈlek-tə-mē\ *n, pl* **-mies** : surgical excision of a seminal vesicle

ve·sic·u·li·tis \və-ˌsik-yə-ˈlīt-əs\ *n* : inflammation of a vesicle and esp. a seminal vesicle

ve·sic·u·lo·bul·lous \və-ˌsik-yə-lō-ˈbùl-əs\ *adj* : of, relating to, or being both vesicles and bullae ⟨a ~ rash⟩

ve·sic·u·lo·gram \və-ˈsik-yə-lə-ˌgram\ *n* : a radiograph produced by vesiculography

ve·sic·u·log·ra·phy \və-ˌsik-yə-ˈläg-rə-fē\ *n, pl* **-phies** : radiography of the seminal vesicles following the injection of a radiopaque medium

ve·sic·u·lo·pap·u·lar \və-ˌsik-yə-lō-ˈpap-yə-lər\ *adj* : marked by both vesicles and papules ⟨a ~ skin eruption⟩

ve·sic·u·lo·pus·tu·lar \və-ˌsik-yə-lō-ˈpəs-chə-lər\ *adj* : of, relating to, or marked by both vesicles and pustules ⟨a ~ eruption⟩

ve·sic·u·lot·o·my \və-ˌsik-yə-ˈlät-ə-mē\ *n, pl* **-mies** : surgical incision of a seminal vesicle

Ves·prin \ˈves-prən\ *trademark* — used for a preparation of triflupromazine

ves·sel \ˈves-əl\ *n* : a tube or canal (as an artery, vein, or lymphatic) in which a body fluid (as blood or lymph) is contained and conveyed or circulated

vestibula *pl of* VESTIBULUM

ves·tib·u·lar \ve-ˈstib-yə-lər\ *adj* **1** : of or relating to the vestibule of the inner ear, the vestibular system, the vestibular nerve, or the labyrinthine sense ⟨~ impulses⟩ **2** : lying within or facing the vestibule of the mouth ⟨the ~ surface of a tooth⟩ — **ves·tib·u·lar·ly** *adv*

vestibular apparatus *n* : VESTIBULAR SYSTEM

vestibular canal *n* : SCALA VESTIBULI

vestibular folds *n pl* : FALSE VOCAL CORDS

vestibular ganglion *n* : a sensory ganglion in the trunk of the vestibular nerve in the internal auditory canal that contains cell bodies supplying nerve fibers comprising the vestibular nerve

vestibular gland *n* : any of the glands (as Bartholin's glands) that open into the vestibule of the vagina

vestibular ligament *n* : the narrow band of fibrous tissue

contained in each of the false vocal cords and stretching between the thyroid and arytenoid cartilages

vestibular membrane *n* : a thin cellular membrane separating the scala media and scala vestibuli — called also *Reissner's membrane*

vestibular nerve *n* : a branch of the auditory nerve that consists of bipolar neurons with cell bodies collected in the vestibular ganglion, with peripheral processes passing to the semicircular canals, utricle, and saccule, and with central processes passing to the vestibular nuclei of the medulla oblongata

vestibular neuronitis *n* : a disorder of uncertain etiology that is characterized by transitory attacks of severe vertigo

vestibular nucleus *n* : any of four nuclei in the medulla oblongata on each side of the floor of the fourth ventricle of the brain in which fibers of the vestibular nerve terminate — see INFERIOR VESTIBULAR NUCLEUS, LATERAL VESTIBULAR NUCLEUS, MEDIAL VESTIBULAR NUCLEUS, SUPERIOR VESTIBULAR NUCLEUS

vestibular system *n* : the vestibule of the inner ear together with the end organs and nerve fibers that function in mediating the labyrinthine sense — called also *vestibular apparatus*

ves·ti·bule \ˈves-tə-ˌbyül\ *n* : any of various bodily cavities esp. when serving as or resembling an entrance to some other cavity or space: as **a** (1) : the central cavity of the bony labyrinth of the ear (2) : the parts of the membranous labyrinth comprising the utricle and the saccule and contained in the cavity of the bony labyrinth **b** : the space between the labia minora containing the orifice of the urethra **c** : the part of the left ventricle of the heart immediately below the aortic orifice **d** : the part of the mouth cavity outside the teeth and gums

vestibuli — see FENESTRA VESTIBULI, SCALA VESTIBULI

ves·tib·u·lo·co·chle·ar nerve \ve-ˌstib-yə-lō-ˌkō-klē-ər-, -ˌkäk-lē-\ *n* : AUDITORY NERVE

ves·tib·u·lo·plas·ty \ve-ˈstib-yə-lō-ˌplas-tē\ *n, pl* **-ties** : plastic surgery of the vestibular region of the mouth

ves·tib·u·lo·spi·nal \ve-ˌstib-yə-lō-ˈspī-nᵊl\ *adj* : of, relating to, or being the vestibulospinal tracts

vestibulospinal tract *n* : a nerve tract on each side of the central nervous system containing nerve fibers that arise from cell bodies in the lateral vestibular nucleus on one side of the medulla oblongata and that descend on the same side in the lateral and anterior funiculi of the spinal cord to synapse with motor neurons in the ventral roots

ves·tib·u·lum \ve-ˈstib-yə-ləm\ *n, pl* **-la** \-lə\ : VESTIBULE

ves·tige \ˈves-tij\ *n* : a bodily part or organ that is small and degenerate or imperfectly developed in comparison to one more fully developed in an earlier stage of the individual, in a past generation, or in closely related forms

ves·tig·ial \ve-ˈstij-(ē-)əl\ *adj* : of, relating to, or being a vestige ⟨a ~ structure⟩ — **ves·tig·ial·ly** \-ē\ *adv*

vestigial fold of Mar·shall \-ˈmär-shəl\ *n* : a fold of endocardium that extends from the left pulmonary artery to the left superior pulmonary vein

J. Marshall — see OBLIQUE VEIN OF MARSHALL

¹vet \ˈvet\ *n* : VETERINARIAN

²vet *vt* **vet·ted; vet·ting 1** : to provide veterinary care for (an animal) or medical care for (a person) **2** : to subject (a person or animal) to a physical examination or checkup

ve·ta \ˈvāt-ə\ *n* : MOUNTAIN SICKNESS

vet·er·i·nar·i·an \ˌvet-ə-rən-ˈer-ē-ən, ˌve-trən-, ˌvet-ᵊn-\ *n* : a person qualified and authorized to practice veterinary medicine

¹vet·er·i·nary \ˈvet-ə-rən-ˌer-ē, ˈve-trən-, ˈvet-ᵊn-\ *adj* : of, relating to, or being veterinary medicine

²veterinary *n, pl* **-nar·ies** : VETERINARIAN

veterinary medicine *n* : the science and art that deals with the maintenance of health in and the prevention, alleviation, and cure of disease and injury in animals and esp. domestic animals

veterinary surgeon *n, Brit* : VETERINARIAN

VF *abbr* ventricular fibrillation

V–fib *abbr* ventricular fibrillation

V gene \\'vē-\\ *n* : a gene that codes genetic information for the variable region of an immunoglobulin — compare C GENE

Vi *abbr* virulent

vi·a·bil·i·ty \\ˌvī-ə-'bil-ət-ē\\ *n, pl* **-ties** : the quality or state of being viable : the ability to live, grow, and develop

vi·a·ble \\'vī-ə-bəl\\ *adj* **1** : capable of living ⟨the skin graft was ∼⟩ ⟨∼ cancer cells⟩; *esp* : having attained such form and development as to be normally capable of living outside the uterus — often used of a human fetus at seven months but may be interpreted according to the state of the art of medicine ⟨a ∼ fetus is one sufficiently developed for extrauterine survival —*Words & Phrases*⟩ ⟨the fetus is considered ∼ when it weighs 500 grams or more and the pregnancy is over 20 weeks in duration —S. W. Jacob & C. A. Francone⟩ **2** : capable of growing or developing ⟨∼ eggs⟩

Vi·ag·ra \\vī-'ag-rə\\ *trademark* — used for a preparation of the citrate of sildenafil

vi·al \\'vī(-ə)l\\ *n* : a small closed or closable vessel esp. for liquids — called also *phial*

Vi antigen \\'vē-ˌ ī-\\ *n* : a heat-labile somatic antigen thought to be associated with virulence in some bacteria (as of the genus *Salmonella*) and esp. in the typhoid fever bacterium and used to detect typhoid carriers through the presence in their serum of agglutinins against this antigen

vi·at·i·cal \\vī-'at-i-kəl\\ *adj* : of, concerned with, or dealing in viatical settlements ⟨adding provisions to the state's ∼ law to better protect consumers —J. T. Fakler⟩

viatical set·tle·ment \\-'set-ᵊl-mənt\\ *n* : an agreement by which the owner of a life insurance policy that covers a person (as the owner) who has a catastrophic or life-threatening illness receives compensation for less than the expected death benefit of the policy in return for a turning over (as by sale or bequest) of the death benefit or ownership of the policy to the other party (as a company specializing in such transactions) — called also *viatical*

vi·at·i·cate \\vī-'at-i-ˌkāt\\ *vb* **-cat·ed; -cat·ing** *vt* : to sell or assign (a life insurance policy) in a viatical settlement ∼ *vi* : to sell or assign a life insurance policy in a viatical settlement — **vi·at·i·ca·tion** \\vī-ˌat-i-'kā-shən\\ *n*

vi·a·tor \\vī-'āt-ər\\ *n* : a person with a catastrophic or life-threatening illness who has a life insurance policy and sells or intends to sell it in a viatical settlement; *broadly* : one who owns and assigns a life insurance policy in a viatical settlement

Vi·bra·my·cin \\ˌvī-brə-'mīs-ᵊn\\ *trademark* — used for a preparation of doxycycline

vi·bra·tile \\'vī-brət-ᵊl, -brə-ˌtīl\\ *adj* : characterized by vibration ⟨∼ motion⟩

vi·bra·tion \\vī-'brā-shən\\ *n* **1 a** : a periodic motion of the particles of an elastic body or medium in alternately opposite directions from the position of equilibrium when that equilibrium has been disturbed (as when particles of air transmit sounds to the ear) **b** : the action of vibrating : the state of being vibrated or in vibratory motion **2** : an instance of vibration — **vi·brate** \\'vī-ˌbrāt\\ *vb* **vi·brat·ed; vi·brat·ing** — **vi·bra·tion·al** \\-shnəl, -shən-ᵊl\\ *adj*

vibration white finger *n, chiefly Brit* : Raynaud's disease esp. when caused by severe vibration (as in prolonged and repeated use of a chain saw)

vi·bra·tor \\'vī-ˌbrāt-ər\\ *n* : a vibrating electrical apparatus used in massage or for sexual stimulation

vi·bra·to·ry \\'vī-brə-ˌtōr-ē, -ˌtòr-\\ *adj* **1** : of, consisting in, capable of, or causing vibration or oscillation ⟨cutaneous ∼ sensation⟩ **2** : characterized by vibration

vib·rio \\'vib-rē-ō\\ *n* **1** *cap* : a genus of short rigid motile bacteria of the family Vibrionaceae that are straight or curved rods, have one or sometimes two or three polar flagella enclosed in a sheath, and include various saprophytes and a few pathogens (as *V. cholerae*, the cause of cholera in humans) **2** : any bacterium of the genus *Vibrio*; *broadly* : a curved rod-shaped bacterium

vib·ri·on \\'vib-rē-ˌän\\ *n* : VIBRIO 2; *also* : a motile bacterium

Vib·rio·na·ce·ae \\ˌvib-rē-ō-'nā-sē-ˌē\\ *n pl* : a family of facultatively anaerobic gram-negative rod bacteria that are motile by means of polar flagella

vib·ri·on·ic \\ˌvib-rē-'än-ik\\ *adj* : caused by a bacterium of the genus *Vibrio* ⟨∼ enteritis⟩

vibrionic abortion *n* : abortion in sheep and cattle associated with vibriosis

vib·ri·o·sis \\ˌvib-rē-'ō-səs\\ *n, pl* **-o·ses** \\-ˌsēz\\ **1** : an infectious disease of sheep and cattle caused by a bacterium of the genus *Campylobacter* (*C. fetus* syn. *Vibrio fetus*) and marked esp. by by infertility and abortion **2** : infection with or disease caused by a bacterium of the genus *Vibrio*: as **a** : an infectious disease of fish that is caused by a vibrio (*V. anguillarum*) and is marked esp. by hemorrhages and ulcerations of the skin **b** : a gastrointestinal illness of humans that is caused by consuming raw or undercooked fish or shellfish contaminated with a vibrio (as *V. parahaemolyticus* or *V. vulnificus*)

vi·bris·sa \\vī-'bris-ə, və-\\ *n, pl* **vi·bris·sae** \\vī-'bris-(ˌ)ē; və-'bris-(ˌ)ē, -ˌī\\ **1** : any of the stiff hairs that are located esp. about the nostrils or on other parts of the face in many mammals and that often serve as tactile organs **2** : any of the stiff hairs growing within the nostrils that serve to impede the inhalation of foreign substances — **vi·bris·sal** \\-əl\\ *adj*

vi·bur·num \\vī-'bər-nəm\\ *n* **1** *cap* : a large genus of widely distributed shrubs or trees of the honeysuckle family (Caprifoliaceae) including several species whose dried bark has been used in folk medicine **2** : any plant of the genus *Viburnum*

vi·car·i·ous \\vī-'ker-ē-əs, və-, -'kar-\\ *adj* : occurring in an unexpected or abnormal part of the body instead of the usual one ⟨bleeding from the gums sometimes occurs in the absence of the normal discharge from the uterus in ∼ menstruation⟩

vice \\'vīs\\ *n* : an abnormal behavior pattern in a domestic animal detrimental to its health or usefulness

vi·ci·a·nose \\'vis-ē-ə-ˌnōs\\ *n* : a crystalline disaccharide sugar $C_{11}H_{20}O_{10}$ that yields arabinose and glucose on hydrolysis

vi·cious \\'vish-əs\\ *adj* **1** : dangerously aggressive ⟨a ∼ dog⟩ **2** : of, relating to, or being perverse or abnormal behavior in a domestic animal

Vi·co·din \\'vī-kō-dən\\ *trademark* — used for a preparation of acetaminophen and the bitartrate of hydrocodone

Vic·to·ria blue \\vik-'tōr-ē-ə-, -'tòr-\\ *n* : any of several basic blue dyes that are used as biological stains and organic pigments

vid·ar·a·bine \\vid-'är-ə-ˌbēn\\ *n* : an antiviral agent $C_{10}H_{13}N_5O_4 \cdot H_2O$ derived from adenine and arabinoside and used esp. to treat keratitis and encephalitis caused by the herpes simplex virus — called also *adenine arabinoside, ara-A*

Vi·dex \\'vī-ˌdeks\\ *trademark* — used for a preparation of ddI

Vid·i·an artery \\'vid-ē-ən-\\ *n* : a branch of the maxillary artery passing through the pterygoid canal of the sphenoid bone

Gui·di \\'gwēd-ē\\, **Guido** (*Latin* **Vidus Vidius**) **(1508–1569)**, Italian anatomist and surgeon. Guidi practiced medicine in Rome and Florence before going to Paris to serve as royal physician and as the first professor of medicine at the College Royal. He eventually became professor of philosophy and medicine at Pisa. In his writings he allied himself with classical Galenism, but about 1560 he began to record his own anatomical observations in manuscript form. He is remembered for his descriptions of the maxillary artery (the Vidian artery is one of its branches), the pterygoid canal (the Vidian canal), and the nerve of the pterygoid canal (the Vidian nerve).

Vidian canal *n* : PTERYGOID CANAL

Vidian nerve *n* : a nerve formed by the union of the greater petrosal and the deep petrosal nerves that passes forward through the pterygoid canal in the sphenoid bone and joins the pterygopalatine ganglion

view \\'vyü\ *n* : a radiographic image of the body or a body part often taken with the body or part oriented in a standardized way in relation to the imaging beam of radiation — called also *projection;* see WATERS' VIEW

vi·gab·a·trin \vī-'gab-ə-trən\ *n* : an anticonvulsant drug $C_6H_{11}NO_2$ that inhibits enzymatic degradation of gamma-aminobutyric acid

vig·i·lance \\'vij-ə-lən(t)s\ *n* : the quality or state of being wakeful and alert : degree of wakefulness or responsiveness to stimuli — **vig·i·lant** \-lənt\ *adj*

vigor *or chiefly Brit* **vigour** — see HYBRID VIGOR

vil·li·form \\'vil-ə-ˌfórm\ *adj* : having the form or appearance of villi ⟨∼ polyps in the distal large bowel —H. E. Mulcahy *et al*⟩

vil·li·ki·nin \ˌvil-ə-'kī-nən\ *n* : a hormone postulated to exist in order to explain the activity of intestinal extracts in stimulating the intestinal villi

vil·lo·nod·u·lar \ˌvil-ō-'näj-ə-lər\ *adj* : characterized by villous and nodular thickening (as of a synovial membrane) ⟨∼ synovitis⟩

vil·lous \\'vil-əs\ *adj* : covered or furnished with or as if with villi — **vil·lous·ly** *adv*

vil·lus \\'vil-əs\ *n, pl* **vil·li** \-ˌī\ : a small slender vascular process: as **a** : one of the minute fingerlike processes which more or less thickly cover and give a velvety appearance to the surface of the mucous membrane of the small intestine and serve in the absorption of nutriment and of which each has a central blindly ending lacteal surrounded by blood capillaries and covered with epithelium **b** : one of the branching processes of the surface of the chorion of the developing embryo of most mammals that are restricted to particular areas or diffusely arranged and over parts of the surface become vascular and help to form the placenta

vin·blas·tine \(')vin-'blas-ˌtēn\ *n* : an alkaloid that is obtained from the rosy periwinkle and that is used esp. in the form of its sulfate $C_{46}H_{58}N_4O_9 \cdot H_2SO_4$ to treat human neoplastic diseases (as Hodgkin's disease and testicular carcinoma) — called also *vincaleukoblastine*

vin·ca \\'viŋ-kə\ *n* : PERIWINKLE

vinca alkaloid *n* : any of several alkaloids (as vinblastine and vincristine) obtained esp. from the rosy periwinkle

vin·ca·leu·ko·blas·tine \ˌviŋ-kə-ˌlü-kə-'blas-ˌtēn\ *n* : VINBLASTINE

Vin·cent's angina \ˌvin(t)-sən(t)s-, (ˌ)vaⁿ-ˌsänz-\ *n* : acute necrotizing ulcerative gingivitis in which the ulceration has spread to surrounding tissues (as of the pharynx and tonsils) — called also *trench mouth*

  Vin·cent \vaⁿ-saⁿ\, **Jean Hyacinthe (1862–1950),** French bacteriologist. Vincent was a researcher and later director at various French laboratories engaged in bacteriological and epidemiological research. In 1896 he described a fusiform bacillus and a spirochete which in association are the cause of hospital gangrene. These bacteria are called Vincent's organisms. Two years later he demonstrated that these two microorganisms are present in necrotizing ulcerative infections of the gums, tonsils, and throat; two forms of these infections are now known as Vincent's angina and acute necrotizing ulcerative gingivitis or Vincent's infection.

Vincent's infection *n* : ACUTE NECROTIZING ULCERATIVE GINGIVITIS

Vincent's organisms *n pl* : a bacterium of the genus *Fusobacterium* (*F. nucleatum* syn. *F. fusiforme*) and a spirochete of the genus *Treponema* (*T. vincentii* syn. *Borrelia vincentii*) that are part of the normal oral flora and undergo a great increase in numbers in the mucous membrane of the mouth and adjacent parts in acute necrotizing ulcerative gingivitis and Vincent's angina

vin·cris·tine \(')vin-'kris-ˌtēn\ *n* : an alkaloid that is obtained from the rosy periwinkle and that is used esp. in the form of its sulfate $C_{46}H_{56}N_4O_{10} \cdot H_2SO_4$ to treat some human neoplas-

tic diseases (as acute leukemia) — called also *leurocristine;* see ONCOVIN

Vine·berg procedure \\'vīn-ˌbərg-\ *n* : surgical implantation of an internal thoracic artery into the myocardium

  Vineberg, Arthur Martin (1903–1988), Canadian surgeon. Vineberg served as director of cardiothoracic surgery at one Montreal hospital and as a consultant in cardiac surgery at several others. In 1945 he began research on the revascularization of the myocardium for the treatment of coronary insufficiency.

vin·e·gar \\'vin-i-gər\ *n* **1** : a sour liquid used as a condiment or a preservative that is obtained by acetic fermentation of dilute alcoholic liquids (as fermented cider, malt beer, or wine) or of dilute distilled alcohol **2** : a pharmaceutical solution of the active principles of drugs in dilute acetic acid usu. prepared by maceration ⟨aromatic ∼⟩

vinegar eel \-ˈēl\ *n* : a minute free-living nematode worm of the genus *Turbatrix* (*T. aceti*) often found in great numbers in acidic vegetable or vegetable-derived fermenting matter (as unpasteurized vinegar)

vinegar fly *n* : DROSOPHILA 2

vi·nyl \\'vīn-ᵊl\ *n* **1** : a monovalent radical $CH_2=CH$ derived from ethylene by removal of one hydrogen atom **2** : a polymer of a vinyl compound or a product (as a resin or a textile fiber) made from one — **vi·nyl·ic** \vī-'nil-ik\ *adj*

vi·nyl·ben·zene \\'vīn-ᵊl-'ben-ˌzēn\ *n* : STYRENE

vinyl chloride *n* : a flammable gaseous carcinogenic compound C_2H_3Cl that is used esp. to make vinyl resins

vinyl ether *n* : a volatile flammable liquid unsaturated ether C_4H_6O formerly used as an inhalation anesthetic

vi·o·la·ceous \ˌvī-ə-'lā-shəs\ *adj* : of the color violet

vi·o·my·cin \ˌvī-ə-'mīs-ᵊn\ *n* : a basic polypeptide antibiotic that is produced by several soil actinomycetes of the genus *Streptomyces* (as *S. puniceus*) and is administered intramuscularly in the form of its sulfate $C_{25}H_{43}N_{13}O_{10} \cdot xH_2SO_4$ in the treatment of tuberculosis esp. in combination with other antituberculous drugs

vi·os·ter·ol \vī-'äs-tə-ˌról, -ˌrōl\ *n* : CALCIFEROL

Vi·oxx \\'vī-ˌäks\ *trademark* — used for a preparation of rofecoxib

VIP *abbr* vasoactive intestinal peptide; vasoactive intestinal polypeptide

vi·per \\'vī-pər\ *n* **1** : a common Eurasian venomous snake of the genus *Vipera* (*V. berus*) that attains a length of about two feet (0.6 meter), varies in color from red, brown, or gray with dark markings to black, and whose bite is usu. not fatal to humans; *broadly* : any snake of an Old World subfamily (Viperinae) of the family Viperidae **2** : PIT VIPER **3** : a venomous or reputedly venomous snake

Vi·pera \\'vī-pə-rə\ *n* : a genus of Old World venomous snakes of the family Viperidae

Vi·per·i·dae \vī-'per-ə-ˌdē\ *n pl* : a widely distributed family comprising heavy-bodied venomous snakes that include Old World snakes (subfamily Viperinae) and the pit vipers (subfamily Crotalinae) and that are characterized by large tubular venom-conducting fangs erected by rotation of the movable premaxillae — compare CROTALIDAE — **vi·per·id** \\'vī-pə-ˌrid\ *adj*

vi·per·ine \\'vī-pə-ˌrīn\ *adj* : of, relating to, or resembling a viper : VENOMOUS ⟨∼ snakes⟩

vi·po·ma \vī-'pō-mə, vi-\ *n* : a tumor of endocrine tissue esp. in the pancreas that secretes vasoactive intestinal polypeptide

Vi·ra·cept \\'vī-rə-ˌsept\ *trademark* — used for a preparation of nelfinavir

viraemia *chiefly Brit var of* VIREMIA

vi·ral \\'vī-rəl\ *adj* : of, relating to, or caused by a virus ⟨∼ infections⟩ — **vi·ral·ly** \-rə-lē\ *adv*

viral hepatitis *n* : hepatitis (as hepatitis A) caused by a virus

Vir·chow–Ro·bin space \\'fir-ˌkō-rō-'baⁿ-\ *n* : any of the spaces that surround blood vessels as they enter the brain and that communicate with the subarachnoid space

  Virchow, Rudolf Ludwig Karl (1821–1902), German pathologist, anthropologist, and statesman. Virchow was the leading German physician of the 19th century. He sought to make medicine the paramount science. His long influential career coincided with the effective adoption by the medical world of the scientific method.

Ro·bin \rō-baⁿ\, **Charles–Philippe (1821–1885)**, French anatomist and histologist. Robin held professorships at the Faculty of Medicine of Paris, first in natural history and later in histology. In 1864 he founded a journal of comparative anatomy, and in 1873 he also assumed directorship of a marine zoology laboratory. In 1868 he described small spaces in the external coat of arteries communicating with the lymphatic system. In 1872 Virchow described similar spaces in the vessels of the brain.

Virchow's node *n* : SIGNAL NODE

vi·re·mia *or chiefly Brit* **vi·rae·mia** \vī-ˈrē-mē-ə\ *n* : the presence of viruses in the blood — **vi·re·mic** *or chiefly Brit* **vi·rae·mic** \-mik\ *adj*

vires a tergo *pl of* VIS A TERGO

¹**vir·gin** \ˈvər-jən\ *n* : one who has not had sexual intercourse

²**virgin** *adj* : not affected or altered by previous use or exposure (as to an antigen) : NAIVE ⟨∼ B cells⟩

vir·gin·al \ˈvər-jən-ᵊl, ˈvərj-nəl\ *adj* : of, relating to, or characteristic of a virgin or virginity

Vir·gin·ia snakeroot \vər-ˌjin-yə-, -ˌjin-ē-ə-\ *n* : a plant of the genus *Aristolochia* (*A. serpentaria*) of the eastern U.S. with oblong leaves cordate at the base and a solitary basal brownish purple flower — see SERPENTARIA

vir·gin·i·ty \(ˌ)vər-ˈjin-ət-ē\ *n, pl* **-ties** : the quality or state of being a virgin

vi·ri·ci·dal \ˌvī-rə-ˈsīd-ᵊl\ *adj* : VIRUCIDAL

vi·ri·cide \ˈvī-rə-ˌsīd\ *n* : VIRUCIDE

vir·i·dans \ˈvir-ə-ˌdanz\ *adj* : producing alpha hemolysis ⟨∼ streptococci⟩

vir·i·din \ˈvir-əd-ən\ *n* : a crystalline fungistatic antibiotic C₁₉H₁₆O₆ isolated from a fungus of the genus *Trichoderma* (*T. viride*) and one of the genus *Gliocladium* (*G. virens*)

vir·ile \ˈvir-əl, ˈvi(ə)r-ˌīl, *Brit also* ˈvī(ə)r-ˌīl\ *adj* **1** : having the nature, properties, or qualities of an adult male; *specif* : capable of functioning as a male in copulation **2** : characteristic of or associated with men : MASCULINE

vir·il·ism \ˈvir-ə-ˌliz-əm\ *n* **1** : precocious development of secondary sex characteristics in the male **2** : the appearance of secondary sex characteristics of the male in a female

vi·ril·i·ty \və-ˈril-ət-ē, vī-\ *n, pl* **-ties** : the quality or state of being virile: as **a** : the period of developed manhood **b** : the capacity to function as a male in copulation

vir·il·iza·tion *also Brit* **vir·il·isa·tion** \ˌvir-ə-lə-ˈzā-shən\ *n* : the condition of being or process of becoming virilized

vir·il·ize *also Brit* **vir·il·ise** \ˈvir-ə-ˌlīz\ *vt* **-ized** *also Brit* **-ised**; **-iz·ing** *also Brit* **-is·ing** : to make virile; *esp* : to cause or produce virilism in

vi·ri·on \ˈvī-rē-ˌän, ˈvir-ē-\ *n* : a complete virus particle that consists of an RNA or DNA core with a protein coat sometimes with external envelopes and that is the extracellular infective form of a virus

¹**vi·roid** \ˈvī-ˌròid\ *n* **1** : a hypothetical symbiont resembling a virus that was formerly held to be present in cells, to be favorable to the host, and to tend to mutate to a virus **2** : any of two families (*Pospiviroidae* and *Avsunviroidae*) of subviral particles that consist of a small single-stranded RNA arranged in a closed loop without a protein shell and that replicate in their host plants where they may or may not be pathogenic

²**viroid** *adj* **1** : caused by a virus ⟨∼ pneumonia⟩ **2** : of or relating to viroids

vi·ro·log·i·cal \ˌvī-rə-ˈläj-i-kəl\ *or* **vi·ro·log·ic** \-ik\ *adj* : of or relating to virology ⟨∼ studies⟩ — **vi·ro·log·i·cal·ly** \-i-k(ə)lē\ *adv*

vi·rol·o·gist \vī-ˈräl-ə-jəst\ *n* : a specialist in virology

vi·rol·o·gy \vī-ˈräl-ə-jē\ *n, pl* **-gies** : a branch of science that deals with viruses

vi·ro·pause \ˈvī-rə-ˌpóz\ *n* : ANDROPAUSE

vi·ro·some \ˈvī-rə-ˌsōm\ *n* : a liposome that has protein or lipid from the envelope of a virus (as the influenza virus) at-

tached to its membrane and that possesses the antigenic properties of the virus

vi·ro·stat·ic \ˌvī-rə-ˈstat-ik\ *adj* : tending to check the growth of viruses ⟨a ∼ agent⟩

vir·tu·al dead space \ˈvərch-(ə-)wəl-\ *n* : PHYSIOLOGICAL DEAD SPACE

virtual focus *n* : a point from which divergent rays (as of light) seem to emanate but do not actually do so (as in the image of a point source seen in a plane mirror)

virtual image *n* : an image (as seen in a plane mirror) formed of virtual foci

vi·ru·cid·al \ˌvī-rə-ˈsīd-ᵊl\ *adj* : having the capacity to or tending to destroy or inactivate viruses ⟨∼ activity⟩

vi·ru·cide \ˈvī-rə-ˌsīd\ *n* : an agent having the capacity to destroy or inactivate viruses — called also *viricide*

vir·u·lence \ˈvir-(y)ə-lən(t)s\ *n* : the quality or state of being virulent: as **a** : relative severity and malignancy ⟨ameliorate the ∼ of a disease⟩ **b** : the relative capacity of a pathogen to overcome body defenses — compare INFECTIVITY

vir·u·len·cy \-lən-sē\ *n, pl* **-cies** : VIRULENCE

vir·u·lent \-lənt\ *adj* **1 a** : marked by a rapid, severe, and malignant course ⟨a ∼ infection⟩ **b** : able to overcome bodily defense mechanisms ⟨a ∼ pathogen⟩ **2** : extremely poisonous or venomous : NOXIOUS

vir·u·lif·er·ous \ˌvir-(y)ə-ˈlif-(ə-)rəs\ *adj* : containing, producing, or conveying an agent of infection ⟨∼ insects⟩

vi·rus \ˈvī-rəs\ *n* **1 a** : the causative agent of an infectious disease **b** : any of a large group of submicroscopic infective agents that are regarded either as extremely simple microorganisms or as extremely complex molecules, that typically contain a protein coat surrounding an RNA or DNA core of genetic material but no semipermeable membrane, that are capable of growth and multiplication only in living cells, and that cause various important diseases in humans, animals, or plants; *also* : FILTERABLE VIRUS **c** : a disease caused by a virus **2** : an antigenic but not infective material (as vaccine lymph) obtainable from a case of an infectious disease

vi·rus·ci·dal \ˌvī-rə-ˈsīd-ᵊl\ *adj* : VIRUCIDAL

virus disease *n* : a disease caused by a virus (sense 1b)

virus hepatitis *n* : VIRAL HEPATITIS

vi·rus·like \ˈvī-rəs-ˌlīk\ *adj* : resembling a virus ⟨a ∼ agent⟩

virus pneumonia *n* : pneumonia caused or thought to be caused by a virus; *esp* : PRIMARY ATYPICAL PNEUMONIA

vi·ru·stat·ic \ˌvī-rə-ˈstat-ik\ *adj* : VIROSTATIC

vi·sam·min \vi-ˈsam-ən\ *n* : KHELLIN

vis a ter·go \vis-ə-ˈtər-(ˌ)gō\ *n, pl* **vi·res a tergo** \ˌvī-rēz-\ : a force acting from behind ⟨the *vis a tergo* imparted by the heart and transmitted through the arteries —*Science*⟩

viscera *pl of* VISCUS

vis·cer·al \ˈvis-ə-rəl\ *adj* : of, relating to, or located on or among the viscera ⟨∼ organs⟩ — compare PARIETAL 1 — **vis·cer·al·ly** \-rə-lē\ *adv*

visceral arch *n* : BRANCHIAL ARCH

visceral cleft *n* : BRANCHIAL CLEFT

visceral leishmaniasis *n* : KALA-AZAR

visceral muscle *n* : smooth muscle esp. in visceral structures

visceral pericardium *n* : EPICARDIUM

visceral peritoneum *n* : the part of the peritoneum that lines the abdominal viscera — compare PARIETAL PERITONEUM

visceral reflex *n* : a reflex mediated by autonomic nerves and initiated in the viscera

vis·cero·cra·ni·um \ˌvis-ə-rō-ˈkrā-nē-əm\ *n* : SPLANCHNOCRANIUM

vis·cero·gen·ic \ˌvis-ə-rə-ˈjen-ik\ *adj* : arising within the body ⟨∼ needs⟩

vis·cero·in·hib·i·to·ry \ˌvis-ə-(ˌ)rō-in-ˈhib-ə-ˌtōr-ē, -ˌtòr-\ *adj* : inhibiting functional activity of the viscera ⟨∼ nerves⟩

\ə\ abut \ᵊ\ kitten \ər\ further \a\ ash \ā\ ace \ä\ cot, cart
\aú\ out \ch\ chin \e\ bet \ē\ easy \g\ go \i\ hit \ī\ ice \j\ job
\ŋ\ sing \ō\ go \ò\ law \ói\ boy \th\ thin \t̲h̲\ the \ü\ loot
\ú\ foot \y\ yet \zh\ vision   *See also* Pronunciation Symbols page

vis·cero·meg·a·ly \ˌvis-ə-rō-ˈmeg-ə-lē\ *n, pl* **-lies** : ORGANO-MEGALY

vis·cero·mo·tor \-ˈmōt-ər\ *adj* : causing or concerned with the functional activity of the viscera ⟨~ nerves⟩

vis·cer·op·to·sis \ˌvis-ər-äp-ˈtō-səs\ *n, pl* **-to·ses** \-ˌsēz\ : downward displacement of the abdominal viscera

vis·cer·op·tot·ic \-äp-ˈtät-ik\ *adj* : of, relating to, or affected with visceroptosis ⟨~ patients⟩

vis·cero·sen·so·ry \ˌvis-ə-rō-ˈsen(t)s-(ə-)rē\ *adj* : of, relating to, or mediated by the sensory innervation of the viscera ⟨~ pain⟩

vis·cero·tome \ˈvis-ə-rə-ˌtōm\ *n* : an instrument used to obtain a liver tissue sample from a cadaver

vis·cer·o·to·nia \ˌvis-ə-rə-ˈtō-nē-ə\ *n* : a pattern of temperament that is marked by predominance of social over intellectual or physical factors and exhibits conviviality, tolerance, complacency, and love of food — compare CEREBROTONIA, SOMATOTONIA

¹vis·cer·o·ton·ic \ˌvis-ə-rə-ˈtän-ik\ *adj* : of, relating to, or characterized by viscerotonia

²viscerotonic *n* : a viscerotonic individual

vis·cer·o·trop·ic \ˌvis-ə-rə-ˈträp-ik\ *adj* : tending to affect or having an affinity for the viscera ⟨~ leishmaniasis⟩

vis·cer·ot·ro·pism \ˌvis-ə-ˈrä-trə-ˌpiz-əm\ *n* : the quality or state of being viscerotropic ⟨~ of the flavivirus causing yellow fever⟩

vis·cid \ˈvis-əd\ *adj* **1** : having an adhesive quality **2** : having a glutinous consistency : VISCOUS

vis·cid·i·ty \vis-ˈid-ət-ē\ *n, pl* **-ties** : the quality or state of being viscid ⟨increased ~ of the blood —F. G. Slaughter⟩

vis·co·elas·tic \ˌvis-kō-ə-ˈlas-tik\ *adj* : having appreciable and conjoint viscous and elastic properties; *also* : constituting or relating to the state of viscoelastic materials ⟨~ properties⟩ — **vis·co·elas·tic·i·ty** \-ˌlas-ˈtis-ət-ē, -ˈtis-tē\ *n, pl* **-ties**

vis·com·e·ter \vis-ˈkäm-ət-ər\ *n* : an instrument used to measure viscosity ⟨a blood ~⟩ — called also *viscosimeter*

vis·co·met·ric \ˌvis-kə-ˈme-trik\ *adj* : of, relating to, or determined by a viscometer or viscometry ⟨~ readings⟩ — **vis·co·met·ri·cal·ly** \-tri-k(ə-)lē\ *adv*

vis·com·e·try \vis-ˈkäm-ə-trē\ *n, pl* **-tries** : measurement of viscosity — called also *viscosimetry*

vis·co·sim·e·ter \ˌvis-kə-ˈsim-ət-ər\ *n* : VISCOMETER

vis·co·si·met·ric \vis-ˌkäs-ə-ˈme-trik\ *adj* : VISCOMETRIC

vis·co·sim·e·try \ˌvis-kə-ˈsim-ə-trē\ *n, pl* **-tries** : VISCOMETRY

vis·cos·i·ty \vis-ˈkäs-ət-ē\ *n, pl* **-ties** **1** : the quality of being viscous; *esp* : the property of resistance to flow in a fluid or semifluid **2** : the ratio of the tangential frictional force per unit area to the velocity gradient perpendicular to the direction of flow of a liquid — called also *coefficient of viscosity*

vis·cous \ˈvis-kəs\ *adj* **1** : having a glutinous consistency and the quality of sticking or adhering : VISCID **2** : having or characterized by viscosity ⟨a ~ flow⟩

vis·cus \ˈvis-kəs\ *n, pl* **vis·cera** \ˈvis-ə-rə\ : an internal organ of the body; *esp* : one (as the heart, liver, or intestine) located in the large cavity of the trunk

vis·i·bil·i·ty \ˌviz-ə-ˈbil-ət-ē\ *n, pl* **-ties** **1** : the quality or state of being visible **2** : a measure of the ability of radiant energy to evoke visual sensation

vis·i·ble \ˈviz-ə-bəl\ *adj* **1** : capable of being seen : perceptible to vision ⟨particulates ~ to the naked eye⟩ **2** : situated in the visible spectrum ⟨~ light⟩

visible spectrum *n* : the part of the electromagnetic spectrum to which the human eye is sensitive extending from a wavelength of about 400 nm for violet light to about 700 nm for red light

vi·sion \ˈvizh-ən\ *n* **1** : the act or power of seeing : SIGHT **2** : the special sense by which the qualities of an object (as color, luminosity, shape, and size) constituting its appearance are perceived through a process in which light rays entering the eye are transformed by the retina into electrical signals that are transmitted to the brain via the optic nerve

¹vis·it \ˈviz-ət\ *vt* **vis·it·ed** \ˈviz-ət-əd, ˈviz-təd\; **vis·it·ing** \ˈviz-

ət-iŋ, ˈviz-tiŋ\ **1** : to go to attend (a patient) **2** : to go to see (as a physician or dentist) for professional service

²visit *n* **1** : a professional call (as by a physician to treat a patient) **2** : a call upon a professional person (as a physician or dentist) for consultation or treatment ⟨make regular ~s to your dentist⟩

visiting nurse *n* : a nurse employed (as by a hospital or social-service agency) to perform public health services and esp. to visit and provide care for sick persons in a community — called also *public health nurse*

vis·na \ˈvis-nə\ *n* : ovine progressive pneumonia of a chronic encephalitic form that is characterized typically by demyelination in the central nervous system and that leads eventually to paralysis — see MAEDI

Vis·ta·ril \ˈvis-tə-ˌril\ *trademark* — used for a preparation of hydroxyzine

vi·su·al \ˈvizh-(ə-)wəl, ˈvizh-əl\ *adj* **1** : of, relating to, or used in vision ⟨~ organs⟩ **2** : attained or maintained by sight ⟨~ impressions⟩ — **vi·su·al·ly** \ˈvizh-(ə-)wə-lē, ˈvizh-(ə-)lē\ *adv*

visual acuity *n* : the relative ability of the visual organ to resolve detail that is usu. expressed as the reciprocal of the minimum angular separation in minutes of two lines just resolvable as separate and that forms in the average human eye an angle of one minute — compare MINIMUM SEPARABLE, MINIMUM VISIBLE

visual agnosia *n* : a form of agnosia characterized by inability to recognize familiar objects observed by the sense of sight — compare PROSOPAGNOSIA

visual analog scale *n* : a testing technique for measuring subjective or behavioral phenomena (as pain or dietary consumption) in which a subject selects from a gradient of alternatives (as from "no pain" to "worst imaginable pain" or from "every day" to "never") arranged in linear fashion — abbr. *VAS*

visual angle *n* : the angle formed by two rays of light or two straight lines drawn from the extreme points of a viewed object to the nodal point of the eye

visual area *n* : a sensory area of the occipital lobe of the cerebral cortex receiving afferent projection fibers concerned with the sense of sight — called also *visual cortex*

visual axis *n* : LINE OF VISION

visual cortex *n* : VISUAL AREA

visual field *n* : the entire expanse of space visible at a given instant without moving the eyes — called also *field of vision*

vi·su·al·i·za·tion *also Brit* **vi·su·al·i·sa·tion** \ˌvizh-(ə-)wə-lə-ˈzā-shən, ˌvizh-ə-lə-\ *n* **1** : formation of mental visual images **2** : the process of making an internal organ or part visible by the introduction (as by swallowing, by an injection, or by an enema) of a radiopaque substance followed by radiography

vi·su·al·ize *also Brit* **vi·su·al·ise** \ˈvizh-(ə-)wə-ˌlīz, ˈvizh-ə-ˌlīz\ *vt* **-ized** *also Brit* **-ised**; **-iz·ing** *also Brit* **-is·ing** : to make visible: as **a** : to see or form a mental image of **b** : to make (an organ) visible by radiographic visualization ⟨~ the gallbladder⟩ **c** : to prepare (as an organism or tissue) for microscopic examination esp. by staining

vi·su·al·iz·er *also Brit* **vi·su·al·is·er** \-ˌlī-zər\ *n* : one that visualizes; *esp* : one whose mental imagery is prevailingly visual — compare AUDILE, MOTILE, TACTILE

visual projection area *n* : STRIATE CORTEX

visual purple *n* : RHODOPSIN

vi·suo·mo·tor \ˌvizh-ə-wō-ˈmōt-ər\ *adj* : of or relating to vision and muscular movement ⟨~ coordination⟩

vi·suo·psy·chic \-ˈsī-kik\ *adj* : of, relating to, or being the portion of the cerebral cortex that functions in the evaluation of visual impressions

vi·suo·sen·so·ry \-ˈsen(t)-sə-rē\ *adj* : of, relating to, or being the portion of the cerebral cortex that functions in the perception of visual stimuli

vi·suo·spa·tial \-ˈspā-shəl\ *adj* : of, relating to, or being thought processes that involve visual and spatial awareness ⟨~ problem solving⟩

vitae — see AQUA VITAE, LIGNUM VITAE, TAEDIUM VITAE

vi·tal \ˈvīt-ᵊl\ *adj* **1 a** : existing as a manifestation of life **b**

: concerned with or necessary to the maintenance of life ⟨∼ organs⟩ ⟨blood and other ∼ fluids⟩ **2** : characteristic of life or living beings ⟨∼ activities⟩ **3** : recording data relating to lives ⟨∼ records⟩ **4** : of, relating to, or constituting the staining of living tissues — **vi·tal·ly** \-ᵊl-ē\ *adv*

vital capacity *n* : the breathing capacity of the lungs expressed as the number of cubic inches or cubic centimeters of air that can be forcibly exhaled after a full inspiration

vital dye *n* : a dye or stain capable of penetrating living cells or tissues and not inducing immediate evident degenerative changes — called also *vital stain*

vital function *n* : a function of the body (as respiration or the circulation of the blood) on which life is directly dependent

vital index *n* : the ratio of births to deaths in a human population at any given time

vi·tal·ism \'vīt-ᵊl-ˌiz-əm\ *n* **1** : a doctrine that the functions of a living organism are due to a vital principle distinct from physicochemical forces **2** : a doctrine that the processes of life are not explicable by the laws of physics and chemistry alone and that life is in some part self-determining

¹vi·tal·ist \'vīt-ᵊl-əst\ *adj* : VITALISTIC

²vitalist *n* : one who believes in vitalism

vi·tal·is·tic \ˌvīt-ᵊl-'ist-ik\ *adj* : of, relating to, or characteristic of vitalism or vitalists

vi·tal·i·ty \vī-'tal-ət-ē\ *n, pl* **-ties** **1** : the peculiarity distinguishing the living from the nonliving **2** : capacity to live and develop; *also* : physical or mental vigor esp. when highly developed

Vi·tal·li·um \vī-'tal-ē-əm\ *trademark* — used for a cobalt-chromium alloy of platinum-white color used esp. for cast dentures and prostheses

vital red *n* : a disazo acid dye used as a biological stain and in the determination of the volume of blood in the body

vi·tals \'vīt-ᵊlz\ *n pl* : vital organs (as the heart, liver, lungs, and brain)

vital signs *n pl* : signs of life; *specif* : the pulse rate, respiratory rate, body temperature, and often blood pressure of a person

vital stain *n* : VITAL DYE

vital sta·tis·tics \-stə-'tis-tiks\ *n pl* : statistics relating to births, deaths, marriages, health, and disease

vi·ta·mer \'vīt-ə-mər\ *n* : any of two or more compounds that relieve a particular vitamin deficiency; *also* : a structural analog of a vitamin — **vi·ta·mer·ic** \ˌvīt-ə-'mer-ik\ *adj*

vi·ta·min *also* **vi·ta·mine** \'vīt-ə-mən, *Brit also* 'vit-\ *n* : any of various organic substances that are essential in minute quantities to the nutrition of most animals and some plants, act esp. as coenzymes and precursors of coenzymes in the regulation of metabolic processes but do not provide energy or serve as building units, and are present in natural foodstuffs or are sometimes produced within the body

vitamin A *n* : any of several fat-soluble vitamins or a mixture of two or more of them whose lack in the animal body causes keratinization of epithelial tissues (as in the eye with resulting night blindness and xerophthalmia): as **a** : a pale yellow crystalline highly unsaturated alicyclic alcohol $C_{20}H_{29}OH$ that is found in animal products (as egg yolk, milk, and butter) and esp. in marine fish-liver oils (as of cod, halibut, and shark) and that is used in various forms in medicine and nutrition — called also *retinol, vitamin A₁* **b** : a yellow viscous liquid alicyclic alcohol $C_{20}H_{27}OH$ that contains one more double bond in a molecule than vitamin A₁ and is less active biologically in mammals and that occurs esp. in the liver oil of freshwater fish — called also *vitamin A₂*

vitamin A acid *n* : TRETINOIN

vitamin A aldehyde *n* : RETINAL

vitamin A₁ \-'ā-'wən\ *n* : VITAMIN A a

vitamin A palmitate *n* : an ester $C_{36}H_{60}O_2$ of vitamin A

vitamin A₂ \-'ā-'tü\ *n* : VITAMIN A b

vitamin B *n* **1** : VITAMIN B COMPLEX **2** : any of numerous members of the vitamin B complex; *esp* : THIAMINE

vitamin Bₑ \-'bē-'sē\ *n* : FOLIC ACID

vitamin B complex *n* : a group of water-soluble vitamins found esp. in yeast, seed germs, eggs, liver and flesh, and vegetables that have varied metabolic functions and include coenzymes and growth factors — called also *B complex;* see BIOTIN, NIACIN, PANTOTHENIC ACID

vitamin B₁ \-'bē-ˌwən\ *n* : THIAMINE

vitamin B₁₇ \-ˌbē-ˌsev-ən-'tēn\ *n* : LAETRILE

vitamin B₆ \-'bē-'siks\ *n* : pyridoxine or a closely related compound found widely in combined form and considered essential to vertebrate nutrition

vitamin B_T \-'bē-'tē\ *n* : CARNITINE

vitamin B₃ \-'bē-'thrē\ *n* : NIACIN

vitamin B₁₂ \-'bē-'twelv\ *n* **1** : a complex cobalt-containing compound $C_{63}H_{88}CoN_{14}O_{14}P$ that occurs esp. in liver, is essential to normal blood formation, neural function, and growth, and is used esp. in treating pernicious and related anemias and in animal feed as a growth factor — called also *cyanocobalamin* **2** : any of several compounds similar to vitamin B₁₂ in action but having different chemistry

vitamin B₂ \-'bē-'tü\ *n* : RIBOFLAVIN

vitamin C *n* : a water-soluble vitamin $C_6H_8O_6$ found in plants and esp. in fruits and leafy vegetables or made synthetically and used in the prevention and treatment of scurvy and as an antioxidant for foods — called also *ascorbic acid*

vitamin D *n* : any or all of several fat-soluble vitamins chemically related to steroids, essential for normal bone and tooth structure, and found esp. in fish-liver oils, egg yolk, and milk or produced by activation (as by ultraviolet irradiation) of sterols: as **a** : CALCIFEROL **b** : CHOLECALCIFEROL — called also *sunshine vitamin*

vitamin D milk *n* : milk enriched (as by irradiation) with added vitamin D

vitamin D₃ \-'dē-'thrē\ *n* : CHOLECALCIFEROL

vitamin D₂ \-'dē-'tü\ *n* : CALCIFEROL

vitamin E *n* : any of several fat-soluble vitamins that are chemically tocopherols or tocotrienols, are essential in the nutrition of various vertebrates in which their absence is associated with infertility, degenerative changes in muscle, or vascular abnormalities, are found esp. in wheat germ, vegetable oils, egg yolk, and green leafy vegetables or are made synthetically, and are used chiefly in animal feeds and as antioxidants; *esp* : ALPHA-TOCOPHEROL

vitamin G *n* : RIBOFLAVIN

vitamin H *n* : BIOTIN

vi·ta·min·iza·tion \ˌvīt-ə-mə-nə-'zā-shən\ *also Brit* **vi·ta·min·isa·tion** \ˌvit-ə-min-ˌī-'zā-shən\ *n* : the action or process of vitaminizing

vi·ta·min·ize \'vīt-ə-mə-ˌnīz\ *also Brit* **vi·ta·min·ise** \'vit-\ *vt* **-ized** *also Brit* **-ised; -iz·ing** *also Brit* **-is·ing** : to provide or supplement with vitamins ⟨*vitaminized* margarine⟩

vitamin K *n* **1** : either of two naturally occurring fat-soluble vitamins that are essential for the clotting of blood because of their role in the production of prothrombin in the liver and that are used in preventing and treating hypoprothrombinemia and hemorrhage: **a** : a yellow oily naphthoquinone $C_{31}H_{46}O_2$ that is obtained esp. from alfalfa or made synthetically and that has a fast, potent, and prolonged biological effect, is effective orally, and is useful esp. in treating hypoprothrombinemia induced by anticoagulant drugs — called also *phylloquinone, phytonadione, vitamin K₁;* see MEPHYTON **b** : a pale yellow crystalline naphthoquinone $C_{41}H_{56}O_2$ that is obtained esp. from putrefied fish meal and is synthesized by various bacteria (as in the intestines of humans and higher animals) and that is much more unsaturated than vitamin K₁ and slightly less active biologically — called also *menaquinone, vitamin K₂* **2** : any of several synthetic compounds that are closely related chemically to vitamins K₁ and K₂ but are

\ə\ abut \ᵊ\ kitten \ər\ further \a\ ash \ā\ ace \ä\ cot, cart \aù\ out \ch\ chin \e\ bet \ē\ easy \g\ go \i\ hit \ī\ ice \j\ job \ŋ\ sing \ō\ go \ò\ law \òi\ boy \th\ thin \th̲\ the \ü\ loot \ù\ foot \y\ yet \zh\ vision   *See also* Pronunciation Symbols page

U
Z

simpler in structure and that have similar biological activity; *esp* : MENADIONE

vitamin K₁ \-ˈkā-ˌwən\ *n* : VITAMIN K 1a

vitamin K₃ \-ˈkā-ˌthrē\ *n* : MENADIONE

vitamin K₂ \-ˈkā-ˌtü\ *n* : VITAMIN K 1b

vitamin M *n* : FOLIC ACID

vi·ta·min·ol·o·gy \ˌvīt-ə-mə-ˈnäl-ə-jē\ *n, pl* **-gies** : a branch of knowledge dealing with vitamins, their nature, action, and use

vitamin P *n* : a substance or mixture of substances obtained from various plant sources, identified as any of a number of substances (as citrin or a mixture of bioflavonoids), and formerly held to be useful in reducing the extent of hemorrhage but never precisely characterized chemically or proved to have the effects claimed for it

vitamin PP \-ˈpē-ˈpē\ *n* : NIACIN

vi·tel·lar·i·um \ˌvīt-ᵊl-ˈar-ē-əm\ *n, pl* **-lar·ia** \-ē-ə\ : a modified part of the ovary that in many flatworms and rotifers produces yolk-filled cells serving to nourish the true eggs

vi·tel·lin \vī-ˈtel-ən, və-\ *n* : a phosphoprotein in egg yolk — called also *ovovitellin*

vi·tel·line \-ˈtel-ən, -ˌēn, -ˌīn\ *adj* : of, relating to, or producing yolk

vitelline artery *n* : OMPHALOMESENTERIC ARTERY

vitelline duct *n* : OMPHALOMESENTERIC DUCT

vitelline membrane *n* : a membrane enclosing the egg proper and corresponding to the plasma membrane of an ordinary cell

vitelline vein *n* : OMPHALOMESENTERIC VEIN

vi·tel·lo·gen·e·sis \vī-ˌtel-ō-ˈjen-ə-səs, və-\ *n, pl* **-e·ses** \-ˌsēz\ : yolk formation — **vi·tel·lo·gen·ic** \-ˈjen-ik\ *adj*

vi·tel·lo·in·tes·ti·nal duct \vī-ˌtel-ō-in-ˈtes-tən-əl-, *Brit often* -ˌin-(ˌ)tes-ˈtīn-ᵊl-\ *n* : OMPHALOMESENTERIC DUCT

vi·tel·lus \-ˈtel-əs\ *n* : the egg cell proper including the yolk but excluding any albuminous or membranous envelopes; *also* : YOLK

vit·i·lig·i·nous \ˌvit-ᵊl-ˈij-ə-nəs\ *adj* : of, relating to, or characterized by vitiligo ⟨~ skin⟩

vit·i·li·go \ˌvit-ᵊl-ˈī-(ˌ)gō *also* -ˈē-(ˌ)\ *n* : a skin disorder manifested by smooth white spots on various parts of the body — compare LEUKODERMA

vit·i·li·goid \-ˌgȯid\ *adj* : resembling vitiligo ⟨~ patches⟩

vit·rec·to·my \və-ˈtrek-tə-mē\ *n, pl* **-mies** : surgical removal of all or part of the vitreous body

vit·reo·ret·i·nal \ˌvi-trē-ō-ˈret-ᵊn-əl\ *adj* : of or relating to the vitreous body and the retina ⟨~ research⟩

¹vit·re·ous \ˈvi-trē-əs\ *adj* : of, relating to, constituting, or affecting the vitreous body ⟨~ hemorrhages⟩

²vitreous *n* : VITREOUS BODY

vitreous body *n* : the clear colorless transparent jelly that fills the eyeball posterior to the lens, is enclosed by a delicate hyaloid membrane, and in the adult is nearly homogeneous but in the fetus is pervaded by fibers with minute nuclei at their points of junction

vitreous chamber *n* : the space in the eyeball between the lens and the retina that is occupied by the vitreous body

vitreous detachment *n* : separation of the posterior part of the vitreous body from the retina due to contraction of the vitreous that occurs as part of the process of aging and may occur sooner in serious cases of myopia, that is usu. accompanied by the presence of floaters often seen as spots or structures resembling cobwebs, and that may result in a torn retina or in retinal detachment — called also *posterior vitreous detachment*

vitreous humor *n* : VITREOUS BODY

vitreous silica *n* : a chemically stable and refractory glass made from silica alone — see QUARTZ GLASS

vit·ri·ol \ˈvi-trē-əl\ *n* **1** : a sulfate of any of various metals (as copper, iron, or zinc) **2** : OIL OF VITRIOL

vitro — see IN VITRO

vit·ro·nec·tin \ˌvi-trō-ˈnek-tən\ *n* : a glycoprotein of blood plasma that promotes cell adhesion and migration and is similar to fibronectin

Vi·vac·til \vī-ˈvak-til\ *trademark* — used for a preparation of protriptyline

vi·var·i·um \vī-ˈvar-ē-əm, -ˈver-\ *n, pl* **-ia** \-ē-ə\ *or* **-i·ums** : an enclosure for keeping or raising and observing animals esp. for laboratory research

¹vi·vax \ˈvī-ˌvaks\ *n* : the malaria parasite (*Plasmodium vivax*) that causes vivax malaria

²vivax *adj* : of, relating to, caused by, or being vivax or vivax malaria ⟨malaria of the ~ type⟩ ⟨treated 20 ~ cases⟩

vivax malaria *n* : malaria caused by a plasmodium (*Plasmodium vivax*) that induces paroxysms at 48-hour intervals — compare FALCIPARUM MALARIA

vivi·dif·fu·sion \ˌviv-ə-di-ˈfyü-zhən\ *n* : dialysis performed by passing the blood through celloidin tubes immersed in an isotonic solution into which diffusible substances from the blood diffuse before the blood returns to the circulatory system

vi·vi·par·i·ty \ˌvī-və-ˈpar-ət-ē, ˌviv-ə-\ *n, pl* **-ties** : the quality or state of being viviparous

vi·vip·a·rous \vī-ˈvip-(ə-)rəs, və-\ *adj* : producing living young instead of eggs from within the body in the manner of nearly all mammals, many reptiles, and a few fishes — compare LARVIPAROUS, OVIPAROUS, OVOVIVIPAROUS — **vi·vip·a·rous·ly** *adv*

vivi·sec·tion \ˌviv-ə-ˈsek-shən, ˈviv-ə-ˌ\ *n* : the cutting of or operation on a living animal usu. for physiological or pathological investigation; *broadly* : animal experimentation esp. if considered to cause distress or result in injury or death to the subject — **vivi·sect** \-ˈsekt\ *vb* — **vivi·sec·tion·al** \ˌviv-ə-ˈsek-shnəl, -shən-ᵊl\ *adj*

vivi·sec·tion·ist \ˌviv-ə-ˈsek-sh(ə-)nəst\ *n* : a practitioner or advocate of vivisection : VIVISECTOR

vivi·sec·tor \ˌviv-ə-ˈsek-tər\ *n* : one who performs vivisection

vivo — see IN VIVO

VLDL \ˈvē-ˌel-ˈdē-ˈel\ *n* : a plasma lipoprotein that is produced primarily by the liver with lesser amounts contributed by the intestine, that contains relatively large amounts of triglycerides compared to protein, and that leaves a residue of cholesterol in the tissues during the process of conversion to LDL — called also *very-low-density lipoprotein;* compare HDL, LDL

Vlem·inckx' lotion \ˈvlem-iŋks-\ *n* : SULFURATED LIME SOLUTION

Vleminckx, Jean–François (1800–1876), Belgian physician. Vleminckx practiced medicine in Brussels. He was the author of several papers on ophthalmia and one on whooping cough. His major concerns were public health care and the health of the army. He contributed to a number of medical journals and was coeditor of the Belgian Archives of Medicine.

Vleminckx' solution *n* : SULFURATED LIME SOLUTION

VMA *abbr* vanillylmandelic acid

VMD *abbr* doctor of veterinary medicine

VNA *abbr* Visiting Nurse Association

VNTR \ˌvē-(ˌ)en-(ˌ)tē-ˈär\ *n, often attrib* : a segment of DNA that consists of repetitions of a fixed sequence of consecutive DNA base pairs a constant number of times in any one individual and that is widely used for identification purposes in forensic medicine because the number of repetitions of the fixed sequence within the segment varies from individual to individual

VOC \ˌvē-(ˌ)ō-ˈsē\ *n* : any of various organic chemical compounds (as formaldehyde or gasoline) that evaporate quickly esp. from solvents, adhesives, fuels, or industrial wastes and that contribute to photochemical smog in the atmosphere

vo·cal \ˈvō-kəl\ *adj* **1** : uttered by the voice : ORAL **2** : having or exercising the power of producing voice, speech, or sound **3** : of, relating to, or resembling the voice ⟨~ dysfunction due to throat infection⟩ — **vo·cal·i·ty** \vō-ˈkal-ət-ē\ *n, pl* **-ties** — **vo·cal·ly** \ˈvō-kə-lē\ *adv*

vocal cord *n* **1 vocal cords** *pl* : either of two pairs of folds of mucous membrane of which each member of each pair stretches from the thyroid cartilage in front to the arytenoid cartilage in back, contains a band of fibrous or elastic tissue, and has a free edge projecting into the cavity of the larynx toward the contralateral member of the same pair forming a cleft which can be opened or closed: **a** : FALSE VOCAL CORDS **b** : TRUE VOCAL CORDS **2** : VOCAL LIGAMENT

vocal folds *n pl* : TRUE VOCAL CORDS

vo·ca·lis \vō-'kā-ləs\ *n* : a small muscle that is the medial part of the thyroarytenoid, originates in the lamina of the thyroid cartilage, inserts in the vocal process of the arytenoid cartilage, and modulates the tension of the true vocal cords

vo·cal·i·za·tion *also Brit* **vo·cal·i·sa·tion** \ˌvō-kə-lə-'zā-shən\ *n* : the act or process of producing sounds with the voice; *also* : a sound thus produced — **vo·cal·ize** *also Brit* **vo·cal·ise** *vb* **-ized** *also Brit* **-ised; -iz·ing** *also Brit* **-is·ing**

vocal ligament *n* : the band of yellow elastic tissue contained in each true vocal cord and stretching between the thyroid and arytenoid cartilages — called also *inferior thyroarytenoid ligament*

vocal process *n* : the anterior angle of the arytenoid cartilage on each side of the larynx to which the vocal ligament of the corresponding side is attached

Vo·ges–Pros·kau·er reaction \'fō-gəs-'präs-ˌkaù-ər-\ *n* : a method for detecting the presence of acetoin in a bacterial broth culture in which the addition of a concentrated solution of sodium hydroxide produces a red color in the presence of the substance

Voges, Daniel Wilhelm Otto (*b* 1867), and Pros·kau·er \'pros-ˌkaù-ər\, Bernhard (1851–1915), German bacteriologists. In 1898 at the Institute for Infectious Diseases, Proskauer and Voges developed the Voges-Proskauer reaction.

Voges–Proskauer test *n* : VOGES-PROSKAUER REACTION

voice \'vóis\ *n* **1** : sound produced by vertebrates by means of lungs, larynx, or syrinx; *esp* : sound so produced by human beings **2** : the faculty of utterance : SPEECH — **voice** *vt* **voiced; voic·ing**

voice box *n* : LARYNX

void \'vóid\ *vt* : to discharge or emit ⟨∼ urine⟩ ∼ *vi* : to eliminate solid or liquid waste from the body ⟨frequent ∼*ing*⟩

vol *abbr* volume

vo·lar \'vō-lər, -ˌlär\ *adj* : relating to the palm of the hand or the sole of the foot; *specif* : located on the same side as the palm of the hand ⟨the ∼ part of the forearm⟩

¹vol·a·tile \'väl-ət-ᵊl, *esp Brit* -ə-ˌtīl\ *n* : a volatile substance

²volatile *adj* : readily vaporizable at a relatively low temperature — **vol·a·til·i·ty** \ˌväl-ə-'til-ət-ē\ *n, pl* **-ties**

volatile oil *n* : an oil that vaporizes readily; *esp* : ESSENTIAL OIL — compare FATTY OIL

vol·a·til·ize *also Brit* **vol·a·til·ise** \'väl-ət-ᵊl-ˌīz, *Brit also* və-'lat-\ *vb* **-ized** *also Brit* **-ised; -iz·ing** *also Brit* **-is·ing** *vt* : to make volatile; *esp* : to cause to pass off in vapor ∼ *vi* : to pass off in vapor — **vol·a·til·iz·able** *also Brit* **vol·a·til·is·able** \-ˌī-zə-bəl\ *adj* — **vol·a·til·iza·tion** *also Brit* **vol·a·til·isa·tion** \ˌväl-ət-ᵊl-ə-'zā-shən, *Brit also* və-ˌlat-ᵊl-ī-'\ *n*

vole \'vōl\ *n* : any of various small rodents (family Cricetidae and esp. genus *Microtus*) that typically have a stout body, rather blunt nose, and short ears, that inhabit both moist meadows and dry uplands and do much damage to crops, and that are closely related to muskrats and lemmings but in general resemble stocky mice or rats

vole bacillus *n* : a bacterium of the genus *Mycobacterium* (*M. microti*) that is closely related to the tubercle bacillus (*M. tuberculosis*), was first isolated from a wild European vole of the genus *Microtus* (*M. agrestis*), and has been used in vaccines against tuberculosis

volitantes — see MUSCAE VOLITANTES

vo·li·tion \vō-'lish-ən, və-\ *n* **1** : an act of making a choice or decision; *also* : a choice or decision made **2** : the power of choosing or determining

vo·li·tion·al \-'lish-nəl, -ən-ᵊl\ *adj* : of, relating to, or produced by volition ⟨∼ movements⟩ — **vo·li·tion·al·ly** \-ē\ *adv*

Volk·mann's canal \'fō(l)k-mənz-\ *n* : any of the small channels in bone that transmit blood vessels from the perios-

teum into the bone and that lie perpendicular to and communicate with the haversian canals

Volk·mann \'fólk-ˌmän\, **Alfred Wilhelm (1800–1877),** German physiologist. Volkmann held a succession of academic posts in Germany, serving variously as professor of zoology, physiology, pathology, and anatomy. His description of the canals in compact bone which transmit blood vessels from the periosteum was published in 1863; the canals are now known as Volkmann's canals.

Volkmann's contracture *or* **Volkmann contracture** *n* : ischemic contracture of an extremity and esp. of a hand

Volkmann's paralysis *n* : paralysis (as of the muscles of the hand) associated with Volkmann's contracture

vol·ley \'väl-ē\ *n, pl* **volleys** : a burst of simultaneous or immediately sequential nerve impulses passing to an end organ, synapse, or center

vol·sel·la \väl-'sel-ə\ *n* : VULSELLUM

volt \'vōlt\ *n* **1** : the practical mks unit of electrical potential difference and electromotive force equal to the difference of potential between two points in a conducting wire carrying a constant current of one ampere when the power dissipated between these two points is equal to one watt and equivalent to the potential difference across a resistance of one ohm when one ampere is flowing through it **2** : a unit of electrical potential difference and electromotive force equal to 1.00034 volts and formerly taken as the standard in the U.S.

Vol·ta \'vòl-tä\, **Alessandro Giuseppe Antonio Anastasio (1745–1827),** Italian physicist. Volta served as professor of physics at the University of Pavia, Italy, from 1779 to 1804. From 1815 he was director of the philosophical faculty at the University of Padua, Italy. His interest in electricity led him to invent in 1775 a device used to generate static electricity. In 1800 he demonstrated his electric battery for the first time. The volt, a unit of potential difference that drives current, was named in his honor.

volt·age \'vōl-tij\ *n* : electrical potential or potential difference expressed in volts

voltage clamp *n* : stabilization of a membrane potential by depolarization and maintenance at a given potential by means of an electric current from a source outside the living system esp. in order to study the flow of potassium and sodium ions independently of the effects of changes in the membrane potential — **voltage clamp** *vt*

voltage–gat·ed \-ˌgā-təd\ *adj* : permitting or blocking passage through a cell membrane in response to an electrical stimulus (as a potential difference between the two sides of the membrane)

vol·tam·me·try \ˌvōl-'tam-ə-trē\ *n, pl* **-ries** : the detection of minute quantities of chemicals (as metals) by measuring the currents generated in electrolytic solutions when known voltages are applied — **vol·tam·me·tric** \ˌvōlt-ə-'me-trik\ *adj*

volt–am·pere \'vōlt-'am-ˌpi(ə)r *also* -ˌpe(ə)r\ *n* : a unit of electric measurement equal to the product of a volt and an ampere that for direct current constitutes a measure of power equivalent to a watt

Vol·ta·ren \'vòl-tə-rən\ *trademark* — used for a preparation of the sodium salt of diclofenac

volt·me·ter \'vōlt-ˌmēt-ər\ *n* : an instrument (as a galvanometer) for measuring in volts the differences of potential between different points of an electrical circuit

vol·ume \'väl-yəm, -(ˌ)yüm\ *n* **1** : the amount of space occupied by a three-dimensional figure as measured in cubic units (as inches, quarts, or centimeters) : cubic capacity **2** : the amount of a substance occupying a particular volume

vol·u·me·nom·e·ter \ˌväl-yə-me-'näm-ət-ər\ *n* : an instrument for measuring the volume and indirectly the specific gravity of a body (as a solid) by means of the difference in

\ə\ abut \ᵊ\ kitten \ər\ further \a\ ash \ā\ ace \ä\ cot, cart
\aú\ out \ch\ chin \e\ bet \ē\ easy \g\ go \i\ hit \ī\ ice \j\ job
\ŋ\ sing \ō\ go \ò\ law \òi\ boy \th\ thin \th̲\ the \ü\ loot
\ù\ foot \y\ yet \zh\ vision *See also* Pronunciation Symbols page

U
Z

pressure caused by its presence and absence in a closed air space

vol·u·met·ric \ˌväl-yû-'me-trik\ *adj* : of, relating to, or involving the measurement of volume — **vol·u·met·ri·cal·ly** \-tri-k(ə-)lē\ *adv*

volumetric analysis *n* **1** : quantitative analysis by the use of definite volumes of standard solutions of reagents **2** : analysis of gases by volume

volumetric flask *n* : a flask for use in volumetric analysis that contains a specific volume when filled to an indicated level

volumetric solution *n* : a standard solution for use in volumetric analysis

vol·un·tary \'väl-ən-ˌter-ē\ *adj* **1** : proceeding from the will or from one's own choice or consent **2** : of, relating to, subject to, or regulated by the will ⟨∼ behavior⟩ — **vol·un·tari·ly** *adv*

voluntary hospital *n* : a private nonprofit hospital that is operated under individual, partnership, or corporate control

voluntary muscle *n* : muscle (as most striated muscle) under voluntary control

vo·lu·tin \'väl-yə-ˌtin, və-'lüt-ᵊn\ *n* : a granular basophilic substance containing nucleic acids that is found esp. in cells of microorganisms (as bacteria, yeast, and protozoans) and is believed to function as a phosphate reserve — called also *metachromatin*

vol·vu·lus \'väl-vyə-ləs\ *n* : a twisting of the intestine upon itself that causes obstruction — compare ILEUS

vo·mer \'vō-mər\ *n* : a bone of the skull of most vertebrates that is situated below the ethmoid region, that develops from lateral halves which remain separate in some animals, and that in humans forms the posterior and inferior part of the nasal septum comprising a vertical plate pointed in front and expanding at the upper back part into lateral wings

vo·mer·ine \'vō-mə-ˌrīn\ *adj* : of or relating to the vomer

vom·ero·na·sal \ˌväm-ə-rō-'nā-zəl, ˌvōm-\ *adj* : of or relating to the vomer and the nasal region and esp. to the vomeronasal organ or the vomeronasal cartilage

vomeronasal cartilage *n* : a narrow process of cartilage between the vomer and the cartilage of the nasal septum — called also *Jacobson's cartilage*

vomeronasal nerve *n* : a nerve that exists in the human fetus but disappears before birth, that originates in the olfactory epithelial cells of the vomeronasal organ, and that passes through the submucous tissue of the nasal septum and the cribriform plate of the ethmoid bone to the olfactory bulb

vomeronasal organ *n* : either of a pair of small blind pouches or tubes in many vertebrates that are situated one on either side of the nasal septum or in the buccal cavity and that are reduced to rudimentary pits in adult humans but are developed in reptiles, amphibians, and some mammals as chemoreceptors — called also *Jacobson's organ, organ of Jacobson*

vomica — see NUX VOMICA

¹**vom·it** \'väm-ət\ *n* **1** : VOMITING **2** : stomach contents disgorged through the mouth — called also *vomitus*

²**vomit** *vi* : to disgorge the stomach contents ∼ *vt* : to disgorge (the contents of the stomach) through the mouth

vom·it·ing \-iŋ\ *n* : an act or instance of disgorging the contents of the stomach through the mouth — called also *emesis*

vomiting center *n* : a nerve center in the medulla oblongata which when stimulated initiates the act of vomiting

vomiting gas *n* : chloropicrin in aerosol form for use esp. as a war gas or crowd-control agent

vo·mi·tion \vō-'mish-ən\ *n* : VOMITING

vom·i·tive \'väm-ət-iv\ *n* : EMETIC

vom·i·to·ry \'väm-ə-ˌtōr-ē, -ˌtòr-\ *adj* : EMETIC

vom·i·tu·ri·tion \ˌväm-ə-chə-'rish-ən, -ə-tü-'\ *n* : repeated ineffectual attempts at vomiting

vom·i·tus \'väm-ət-əs\ *n* : VOMIT 2

von Gier·ke disease \vän-'gir-kə-\ *or* **von Gier·ke's disease** \-kəz-\ *n* : a glycogen storage disease that is caused by a deficiency of glucose-6-phosphate and has a clinical onset at birth or during infancy, that is characterized esp. by enlargement of the liver and kidney, hypoglycemia, hyperlipidemia, hyperuricemia, acidosis, adiposity, xanthomas, and nosebleeds, and is inherited as an autosomal recessive trait

Gierke, Edgar Otto Konrad von (1877–1945), German pathologist. Von Gierke's chief academic position was a professorship of bacteriology at Karlsruhe's Technical University. During World War I he served first as a field doctor and then as a military pathologist. In 1911 he published a textbook of pathological anatomy. He described the type of glycogen storage disease identified with his name in 1929. Other areas of his research included thyroid gland structure, bone tumors, and metabolic diseases.

von Grae·fe's sign \vän-'grā-fəz-\ *n* : the failure of the upper eyelid to follow promptly and smoothly the downward movement of the eyeball that is seen in Graves' disease

von Grae·fe \fòn-'gre-fə\, **Albrecht Friedrich Wilhelm Ernst (1828–1870),** German ophthalmologist. Von Graefe is generally regarded as the founder of modern ophthalmology. In 1850 he founded what was to become one of Europe's leading eye clinics. He described von Graefe's sign for Graves' disease in 1864. His comprehensive seven-volume manual of ophthalmology was published posthumously (1874–1880).

von Hip·pel–Lin·dau disease \vän-'hip-əl-'lin-ˌdaù-\ *n* : a rare genetically determined disease that is characterized by angiomatosis of the retina and cerebellum and often by cysts or tumors of the liver, pancreas, and kidneys — called also *Lindau's disease*

von Hip·pel \fòn-'hip-əl\, **Eugen (1867–1939),** German ophthalmologist. Von Hippel held professorships at a succession of German universities and became head of the eye clinic at Halle, Germany. In 1895 he published the original description of von Hippel-Lindau disease.

Lindau, Arvid Vilhelm (1892–1958), Swedish pathologist. Lindau published his own description of von Hippel-Lindau disease in 1926. His report of the disease is important for its histological findings.

von Korff fiber \vän-'kòrf-\ *n* : KORFF'S FIBER

von Reck·ling·hau·sen's disease \-'rek-liŋ-ˌhaù-zənz-\ *n* : NEUROFIBROMATOSIS

F. D. von Recklinghausen — see RECKLINGHAUSEN'S DISEASE

von Wil·le·brand factor \vän-'vil-ə-ˌbränt-\ *n* : a protein secreted esp. by endothelial cells that circulates in blood plasma as a large variable aggregation consisting usu. of repeating dimers, that mediates platelet adhesion to collagen in subendothelial tissue at injury sites, that is often found complexed to factor VIII in plasma where it serves to protect it from degradation, and that is deficient or defective in individuals affected with von Willebrand's disease — called also *VW factor*

Willebrand, Erik Adolf von (1870–1949), Finnish physician. He described von Willebrand's disease first in 1926 and again in 1931 in a follow-up article.

von Wil·le·brand's disease \-ˌbränts-\ *n* : a genetic disorder that is caused by deficient or defective von Willebrand factor, is characterized by mucosal and petechial bleeding due to abnormal blood vessels, and is inherited chiefly as an autosomal dominant trait

vor·tex \'vò(ə)r-ˌteks\ *vt* : to mix (as the contents of a test tube) by means of a rapid whirling or circular motion ⟨∼ air into a solution⟩ — **vor·tex·ing** *n*

vorticosa — see VENA VORTICOSA

vor·ti·cose vein \ˌvòrt-ə-ˌkōs-\ *n* : VENA VORTICOSA

VO₂ max \ˌvē-ō-'tü-ˌmaks\ *n* : the maximum amount of oxygen the body can use during a specified period of usu. intense exercise that depends on body weight and the strength of the lungs — called also *maximal oxygen consumption, maximal oxygen uptake, max VO₂*

voy·eur \vwä-'yər, vòi-'ər\ *n* : one obtaining sexual gratification from observing unsuspecting individuals who are partly undressed, naked, or engaged in sexual acts; *broadly*

: one who habitually seeks sexual stimulation by visual means

voy·eur·ism \-ˌiz-əm\ *n* : the tendencies or behavior of a voyeur

voy·eur·is·tic \ˌvwä-(ˌ)yər-ˈis-tik, ˌvȯi-ər-\ *adj* : of, relating to, or having the characteristics of a voyeur ⟨~ drives⟩ — **voy·eur·is·ti·cal·ly** \-ti-k(ə-)lē\ *adv*

VRE \ˌvē-ˌär-ˈē\ *n* [*vancomycin-resistant enterococcus*] : any of various bacterial strains of the genus *Enterococcus* (as *E. faecium* and *E. faecalis*) that are resistant to the antibiotic-vancomycin, occur as part of the normal flora esp. of the gastrointestinal tract, and may cause serious infections (as of the urinary tract, blood, or surgical wounds) typically in immunocompromised individuals in a hospital setting

VS *abbr* vesicular stomatitis

VSD *abbr* ventricular septal defect

VT *abbr* ventricular tachycardia

V–tach *abbr* ventricular tachycardia

vulgaris — see ACNE VULGARIS, ICHTHYOSIS VULGARIS, LUPUS VULGARIS, PEMPHIGUS VULGARIS, VERRUCA VULGARIS

vul·ner·a·ble \ˈvəln-(ə-)rə-bəl, ˈvəl-nər-bəl\ *adj* : capable of being hurt : susceptible to injury or disease ⟨the liver is itself ~ to nutritional impairment —*Jour. Amer. Med. Assoc.*⟩ — **vul·ner·a·bil·i·ty** \ˌvəln-(ə-)rə-ˈbil-ət-ē\ *n, pl* **-ties**

¹**vul·ner·ary** \ˈvəl-nə-ˌrer-ē\ *adj* : used for or useful in healing wounds ⟨~ plants⟩

²**vulnerary** *n, pl* **-ar·ies** : a vulnerary remedy

vul·sel·lum \vəl-ˈsel-əm\ *n, pl* **-sel·la** \-ˈsel-ə\ : a surgical forceps with serrated, clawed, or hooked blades

vul·va \ˈvəl-və\ *n, pl* **vul·vae** \-ˌvē, -ˌvī\ : the external parts of the female genital organs comprising the mons pubis, labia majora, labia minora, clitoris, vestibule of the vagina, bulb of the vestibule, and Bartholin's glands

vulvae — see KRAUROSIS VULVAE, PRURITUS VULVAE

vul·val \ˈvəl-vəl\ *or* **vul·var** \-vər\ *adj* : of or relating to the vulva ⟨~ infection⟩

vul·vec·to·my \ˌvəl-ˈvek-tə-mē\ *n, pl* **-mies** : surgical excision of the vulva

vul·vi·tis \ˌvəl-ˈvīt-əs\ *n* : inflammation of the vulva

vul·vo·dyn·ia \ˌvəl-vō-ˈdin-ē-ə\ *n* : chronic discomfort of the vulva of uncertain cause that is experienced as burning, stinging, or irritation

vul·vo·vag·i·nal \ˌvəl-vō-ˈvaj-ən-ᵊl\ *adj* : of or relating to the vulva and the vagina ⟨~ hematoma⟩ ⟨~ thrush⟩

vul·vo·vag·i·ni·tis \ˌvəl-vō-ˌvaj-ə-ˈnīt-əs\ *n, pl* **-nit·i·des** \-ˈnit-ə-ˌdēz\ : coincident inflammation of the vulva and vagina

v/v *abbr* volume per volume

VW factor \ˌvē-ˈdəb-ə(l)-(ˌ)yü-\ *n* : VON WILLEBRAND FACTOR

VX \ˈvē-ˈeks\ *n* : a cholinesterase inhibitor $C_{11}H_{26}NO_2PS$ prepared and stockpiled for use in chemical warfare as a nerve gas

Vy·tor·in \vī-ˈtȯr-ən\ *trademark* — used for a preparation of ezetimibe and simvastatin

W

W *symbol* [German *wolfram*] tungsten

Waar·den·burg's syndrome \ˈvärd-ᵊn-ˌbərgz-\ *n* : a highly variable genetic disorder inherited as an autosomal dominant trait and accompanied by all, any, or none of deafness, a white forelock, widely spaced eyes, and heterochromia of the irises

Waar·den·burg \ˈvärd-ᵊn-ˌbůrk\, **Petrus Johannes (1886–1979)**, Dutch ophthalmologist. Waardenburg published his description of Waardenburg's syndrome in 1951. The same syndrome had been reported on by J. van der Hoeve in 1916 and D. Klein in 1950.

Wa·da test \ˈwä-də-\ *n* : a test that is used to determine whether the right or left cerebral hemisphere is dominant for speech and that involves injection of amobarbital into the internal carotid artery first on one side and then on the other so that transient aphasia results when the injection is made into the artery on the dominant side

Wada, Juhn Atsushi (*b* 1924), Canadian (Japanese-born) neurologist. Wada held the concurrent positions of professor of neurology at the University of British Columbia and attending neurologist at Vancouver General Hospital. His areas of research included epilepsy and the brain mechanisms of human behavior. He introduced the Wada test for determining which side of the brain is dominant for speech in 1960.

wad·ding \ˈwäd-iŋ\ *n* : a soft absorbent sheet of cotton, wool, or cellulose used esp. in hospitals for surgical dressings

wa·fer \ˈwā-fər\ *n* : CACHET

wafer capsule *n* : CACHET

wa·hoo \ˈwä-ˌhü\ *n, pl* **wahoos** : a shrubby No. American tree of the genus *Euonymus* (*E. atropurpureus*) having a root bark with cathartic properties — compare EUONYMUS 2

WAIS *abbr* Wechsler Adult Intelligence Scale

waist \ˈwāst\ *n* : the typically narrowed part of the body between the thorax and hips

waist·line \ˈwāst-ˌlīn\ *n* : body circumference at the waist

wake·ful \ˈwāk-fəl\ *adj* : not sleeping or able to sleep : SLEEPLESS — **wake·ful·ness** *n*

Wal·den·ström's macroglobulinemia \ˈväl-dən-ˌstremz-, -ˌstrœmz-\ *n* : a rare progressive syndrome associated with a high serum concentration of a monoclonal antibody of the class IgM and characterized by adenopathy, hepatomegaly, splenomegaly, anemia, and lymphocytosis and plasmacytosis of the bone marrow

Wal·den·ström \ˈväl-dən-ˌstrœm\, **Jan Gosta (1906–1996)**, Swedish physician. Waldenström held positions as professor of internal medicine at the University of Lund and as head of the department of medicine at the hospital in Malmö, Sweden. He was the author of numerous articles and textbook chapters on metabolism and hematology. He undertook research on diseases in which the function of red blood pigment is disturbed and on the treatment of malignant diseases of blood and bone marrow. In 1968 he published a study of monoclonal and polyclonal hypergammaglobulinemia.

Wal·dey·er's ring \ˈväl-ˌdī-ərz-\ *n* : a ring of lymphatic tissue formed by the two palatine tonsils, the pharyngeal tonsil, the lingual tonsil, and intervening lymphoid tissue

Wal·dey·er–Hartz \ˈväl-ˌdī-ər-ˈhärts\, **Heinrich Wilhelm Gottfried von (1836–1921)**, German anatomist. Waldeyer held successively the positions of professor of pathology at the University of Breslau, Germany; professor of anatomy at the University of Strasbourg, France; and professor of anatomy at the University of Berlin. As director of the department of anatomy at Berlin for more than 33 years, he gained a wide reputation as an outstanding teacher of anatomy and histology. He coined the word *neuron* and helped to lay the foundation upon which the neuron doctrine was established. He also coined the term *chromosome* to describe the bodies in the nucleus of cells. He described Waldeyer's tonsillar ring in 1884.

\ə\ **abut** \ᵊ\ **kitten** \ər\ **further** \a\ **ash** \ā\ **ace** \ä\ **cot, cart** \aů\ **out** \ch\ **chin** \e\ **bet** \ē\ **easy** \g\ **go** \i\ **hit** \ī\ **ice** \j\ **job** \ŋ\ **sing** \ō\ **go** \ȯ\ **law** \ȯi\ **boy** \th\ **thin** \t̲h̲\ **the** \ü\ **loot** \ů\ **foot** \y\ **yet** \zh\ **vision** *See also* Pronunciation Symbols page

U Z

walk·about disease \'wȯk-ə-ˌbau̇t-\ *n* : a disease of horses marked by cirrhosis of the liver, severe nervous symptoms, and continuous aimless walking and usu. believed to be caused by eating poisonous vegetation esp. of leguminous plants of the genus *Crotalaria* — called also *walking disease;* compare CROTALISM

walk·er \'wȯ-kər\ *n* : a framework designed to support an infant learning to walk or an infirm or physically disabled person

¹walk–in \'wȯk-ˌin\ *adj* : providing medical services to ambulatory patients without an appointment ⟨a ∼ clinic⟩; *also* : being an individual who uses such services

²walk–in *n* : a walk-in patient

walk·ing \'wȯ-kiŋ\ *adj* : able to walk : AMBULATORY

walking cast *n* : a cast that is worn on a patient's leg and has a stirrup with a heel or other supporting device embedded in the plaster to facilitate walking

walking disease *n* : WALKABOUT DISEASE

walking pneumonia *n* : a usu. mild pneumonia caused by a microorganism of the genus *Mycoplasma* (*M. pneumoniae*) and characterized by malaise, cough, and often fever

wall \'wȯl\ *n* : a structural layer surrounding a cavity, hollow organ, or mass of material ⟨molecules small enough to be absorbed through the intestinal ∼ —Josie Glausiusz⟩ ⟨muscles of the abdominal ∼⟩ — **walled** \'wȯld\ *adj*

Wal·le·ri·an degeneration \wä-'lir-ē-ən-\ *n* : degeneration of nerve fibers that occurs following injury or disease and that progresses from the place of injury along the axon away from the cell body while the part between the place of injury and the cell body remains intact

Wal·ler \'wäl-ər\, **Augustus Volney (1816–1870),** British physiologist. Waller began in private practice, but after several years he decided to devote full time to research, first in Bonn and then in Paris. For a time he was professor of physiology in Birmingham, England. He is best known for pioneering a major technique for unraveling the complex structure of the nervous system using the type of nerve degeneration that is now associated with his name. By cutting the nerves in the frog's tongue, Waller discovered in 1849 that degeneration occurred throughout the axon's distal segment, and he concluded from this that the nerve cell body is the axon's source of nutriment. The method became a major means of tracing the origin and course of nerve fibers and tracts.

wall·eye \'wȯ-ˌlī\ *n* **1 a** : an eye with a bluish white iris **b** : an eye with an opaque white cornea **2 a** : strabismus in which the eye turns outward away from the nose — called also *exotropia;* compare CROSS-EYE 1 **b wall·eyes** \-ˌlīz\ *pl* : eyes affected with divergent strabismus

wall·eyed \-'līd\ *adj* : having walleyes or affected with wall-eye

¹wan·der·ing \'wän-də-riŋ\ *adj* : FLOATING ⟨a ∼ spleen⟩

²wandering *n* : movement of a tooth out of its normal position esp. as a result of periodontal disease

wandering cell *n* : any of various ameboid phagocytic tissue cells

wandering pacemaker *n* : a back-and-forth shift in the location of cardiac pacemaking esp. from the sinoatrial node to or near the atrioventricular node

Wan·gen·steen apparatus \'waŋ-(g)ən-ˌstēn-\ *n* : the apparatus used in Wangensteen suction — called also *Wangensteen appliance*

Wangensteen, Owen Harding (1898–1981), American surgeon. Wangensteen enjoyed a career-long association with the University of Minnesota medical school and hospital. From 1937 to 1970 he was also coeditor of the medical journal *Surgery.* He did research on bowel obstruction, appendicitis, the genesis of peptic ulcers and their surgical management, and on the etiology of gallstones. In 1956 he published a study of cancer of the esophagus and stomach. He devised the Wangensteen apparatus in 1932 for the relief of distension in cases of intestinal obstruction.

Wangensteen suction *n* : a method of draining fluid or se-cretions from body cavities (as the stomach) by means of an apparatus that operates on negative pressure

war·ble \'wȯr-bəl\ *n* **1** : a swelling under the hide esp. of the back of cattle, horses, and wild mammals caused by the maggot of a botfly or warble fly **2** : the maggot of a warble fly — **war·bled** \-bəld\ *adj*

warble fly *n* : any of various dipteran flies of the genus *Hypoderma* that are parasites of cattle and other mammals and lay eggs on their feet and legs which are licked off and hatch in the mouth or esophagus and burrow as larvae through the tissues to the skin and beneath it to the back of the animal where they live until ready to pupate and cause warbles

War·burg apparatus \'wȯr-ˌbərg-, 'vär-ˌbu̇rk-\ *n* : an analytic apparatus that employs a manometer to determine changes in the amount of gas produced or absorbed by a test sample kept at constant temperature in a flask of constant gas volume and is used esp. in the study of cellular respiration and metabolism and of some enzymatic reactions (as fermentation)

War·burg \'vär-ˌbu̇rk\, **Otto Heinrich (1883–1970),** German biochemist. Warburg is considered by some the most accomplished biochemist of all time. He received doctorates in both medicine and chemistry. After World War I he began investigating the process by which oxygen is consumed in the cells of living organisms. He introduced the use of manometry as a means of studying the rates at which slices of living tissue take up oxygen. His research led to the identification of the role of the cytochromes. In 1931 Warburg was awarded the Nobel Prize for Physiology or Medicine for his research on respiratory enzymes. He also investigated photosynthesis and was the first to observe that the growth of malignant cells requires markedly smaller amounts of oxygen than that of normal cells.

Warburg respirometer *n* : WARBURG APPARATUS

ward \'wȯrd\ *n* : a division in a hospital; *esp* : a large room in a hospital where a number of patients often requiring similar treatment are accommodated ⟨a diabetic ∼⟩

war·fa·rin \'wȯr-fə-rən\ *n* : a crystalline anticoagulant coumarin derivative $C_{19}H_{16}O_4$ related to dicumarol that inhibits the production of prothrombin by vitamin K and is used as a rodent poison and in medicine; *also* : its sodium salt $C_{19}H_{15}NaO_4$ used esp. in the prevention or treatment of thromboembolic disease — see COUMADIN

war gas \'wȯr-\ *n* : a gas for use in warfare — compare LACRIMATOR, NERVE GAS, STERNUTATOR, VESICANT

warm–blood·ed \'wȯrm-'bləd-əd\ *adj* : having warm blood; *specif* : having a relatively high and constant body temperature relatively independent of the surroundings — **warm–blood·ed·ness** *n*

warm–up \'wȯr-ˌməp\ *n* : the act or an instance of warming up; *also* : a procedure (as a set of exercises) used in warming up

warm up \(')wȯr-'məp\ *vi* : to engage in preliminary exercise (as to stretch the muscles) ⟨important to *warm up* properly before running⟩

war neurosis *n* : COMBAT FATIGUE

wart \'wȯ(ə)rt\ *n* **1** : a horny projection on the skin usu. of the extremities produced by proliferation of the skin papillae and caused by any of numerous genotypes of the human papillomavirus — see FLAT WART, GENITAL WART, PLANTAR WART, VERRUCA VULGARIS **2** : any of numerous warty skin lesions not caused by human papillomaviruses

War·thin–Star·ry stain \'wȯr-thən-'stär-ē-\ *n* : a silver nitrate stain used to show the presence of bacilli

Warthin, Aldred Scott (1866–1931), and **Starry, Allen Chronister (b 1890),** American pathologists. Warthin served for many years as professor and director of the department of pathology at the University of Michigan. He was the author of several textbooks of pathology. He did research on tuberculosis of the placenta, the hemolymph nodes, lipemia, mustard gas poisoning, the aging process, and especially syphilis. In 1920 Warthin and Starry introduced a silver nitrate stain as a method for demonstrating spirochetes in tissues.

warty \'wȯrt-ē\ *adj* **wart·i·er; wart·i·est 1** : characterized by warts **2** : of the nature of or resembling a wart ⟨~ cutaneous nodules⟩

¹**wash** \'wȯsh, 'wäsh\ *vt* **1** : to cleanse by or as if by the action of liquid (as water) **2** : to flush or moisten (a bodily part or injury) with a liquid ⟨~ the wound with saline solution⟩ **3** : to pass through a liquid to carry off impurities or soluble components ~ *vi* **1** : to wash oneself or a part of one's body **2** : to clean something by rubbing or dipping in water

²**wash** *n* : a liquid medicinal preparation used esp. for cleansing or antisepsis — see EYEWASH, MOUTHWASH

wash·able \'wȯsh-ə-bəl\ *adj* **1** : capable of being washed without damage **2** : soluble in water ⟨~ ointment bases⟩

wash bottle *n* : a bottle or flask with a bent tube through its cap or stopper that is used to direct a stream of water (as by squeezing the bottle if it is flexible) onto something to be washed or rinsed

washings *n pl* : material collected by the washing of a bodily cavity ⟨sinus ~⟩ ⟨throat ~⟩

washing soda *n* : a transparent crystalline hydrated sodium carbonate — called also *sal soda*

wash·out \'wȯsh-ˌaút, 'wäsh-\ *n* : the action or process of progressively reducing the concentration of a substance (as a dye injected into the left ventricle of the heart)

wasp \'wäsp, 'wȯsp\ *n* : any of numerous social or solitary winged insects (esp. families Sphecidae and Vespidae) of the order Hymenoptera that usu. have a slender smooth body with the abdomen attached by a narrow stalk, well-developed wings, biting mouthparts, and in the females and workers an often formidable sting

Was·ser·mann \'wäs-ər-mən, 'väs-\ *n* : WASSERMANN TEST

Was·ser·mann \'väs-ər-ˌmän\, **August Paul von (1866–1925),** German bacteriologist. Wassermann is famous for discovering a universal blood-serum test for syphilis that helped to extend the basic tenets of immunology to diagnosis. His early research dealt with cholera immunity and diphtheria antitoxin. He established a relationship between the presence of diphtheria in an individual's serum and an ability to resist diphtheria infection. In 1906 he and the German dermatologist Albert Neisser developed a test for the antibody produced by persons infected with the causative agent of syphilis. The Wassermann reaction, in combination with other diagnostic procedures, is still used to test for the disease.

Wassermann reaction *n* : the complement-fixing reaction that occurs in a positive complement-fixation test for syphilis using the serum of an infected individual

Wassermann test *n* : a test for the detection of syphilitic infection using the Wassermann reaction — called also *Wassermann*

¹**waste** \'wāst\ *n* **1** : loss through breaking down of bodily tissue **2 wastes** *pl* : bodily waste materials : EXCREMENT

²**waste** *vb* **wast·ed; wast·ing** *vt* : to cause to shrink in physical bulk or strength : EMACIATE ~ *vi* : to lose weight, strength, or vitality — often used with *away*

³**waste** *adj* : excreted from or stored in inert form in a living body as a by-product of vital activity ⟨~ products⟩

¹**wast·ing** \'wā-stiŋ\ *adj* : undergoing or causing decay or loss of strength ⟨~ diseases such as tuberculosis⟩

²**wasting** *n* : unintended loss of weight and lean body tissue characteristic of many diseases (as cancer, tuberculosis, and AIDS) : gradual loss of strength or substance : ATROPHY

¹**wa·ter** \'wȯt-ər, 'wät-\ *n* **1** : the liquid that descends from the clouds as rain, forms streams, lakes, and seas, and is a major constituent of all living matter and that is an odorless, tasteless, very slightly compressible liquid oxide of hydrogen H_2O which appears bluish in thick layers, freezes at 0°C (32°F) and boils at 100°C (212°F), has a maximum density at 4°C (39°F) and a high specific heat, is feebly ionized to hydrogen and hydroxyl ions, and is a poor conductor of electricity and a good solvent **2** : liquid containing or resembling water: as **a** (1) : a pharmaceutical or cosmetic preparation made with water (2) : a watery solution of a gaseous or readily volatile substance — see AMMONIA WATER **b** : a watery fluid (as

tears or urine) formed or circulating in a living body **c** : AMNIOTIC FLUID — often used in pl.; *also* : BAG OF WATERS

²**water** *vi* : to form or secrete water or watery matter (as tears or saliva)

water bag *n* : BAG OF WATERS — used esp. of domestic animals

water balance *n* : the ratio between the water assimilated into the body and that lost from the body; *also* : the condition of the body when this ratio approximates unity

water bath *n* **1** : a bath composed of or using water **2** : a vessel containing usu. heated water over or in which something in a separate container is processed

water bed *n* : a bed whose mattress is a plastic bag filled with water — called also *hydrostatic bed*

water blister *n* : a blister with a clear watery content that is not purulent or sanguineous

wa·ter·borne \'wȯt-ər-ˌbō(ə)rn, 'wät-, -ˌbȯ(ə)rn\ *adj* : carried or transmitted by water and esp. by drinking water ⟨~ diseases⟩

water brash *n* : regurgitation of an excessive accumulation of saliva from the lower part of the esophagus often with some acid material from the stomach — compare HEARTBURN

water cure *n* : HYDROPATHY, HYDROTHERAPY

water–hammer pulse *n* : CORRIGAN'S PULSE

water hemlock *n* : a tall poisonous Eurasian perennial herb of the genus *Cicuta* (*C. virosa*) that is locally abundant in marshy areas or along streams; *also* : any of several poisonous No. American plants of the genus *Cicuta* (as spotted cowbane)

Wa·ter·house–Frid·er·ich·sen syndrome \'wȯt-ər-ˌhaús-'frid-(ə-)rik-sən-\ *n* : acute and severe meningococcemia with hemorrhage into the adrenal glands

Waterhouse, Rupert (1873–1958), British physician, and **Friderichsen, Carl (1886–1979),** Danish physician. Waterhouse described in 1911 a syndrome of acute collapse associated with hemorrhages in the adrenal glands, usually observed in severe cases of meningitis caused by the meningococcus. Friderichsen published his own independent description of the syndrome in 1918.

wa·ter·logged \-ˌlägd\ *adj* : EDEMATOUS ⟨the scrotum and abdominal wall become ~ —R. L. Cecil & R. F. Loeb⟩

water moc·ca·sin \-ˌmäk-ə-sən\ *n* : a venomous semiaquatic pit viper (*Agkistrodon piscivorus*) of the southern U.S. closely related to the copperhead — called also *cottonmouth, cottonmouth moccasin*

water of constitution *n* : water so combined into a molecule that it cannot be removed without disrupting the entire molecule

water of crystallization *n* : water of hydration present in many crystallized substances that is usu. essential for maintenance of a particular crystal structure

water of hydration *n* : water that is chemically combined with a substance to form a hydrate and can be expelled (as by heating) without essentially altering the composition of the substance

water on the brain *n* : HYDROCEPHALUS

water on the knee *n* : an accumulation of synovial fluid in the knee joint (as from injury or disease) marked esp. by swelling

water pick \-ˌpik\ *n* : a tooth-cleaning device that cleans by directing a stream of water over and between teeth

water pill *n* : a diuretic pill

water–soluble *adj* : soluble in water ⟨~ vitamin B⟩

Wa·ters' view \'wȯt-ərz-\ *n* : a radiographic image obtained by passing a beam of X-rays through the chin at an angle and used esp. to obtain diagnostic information in a single X-ray image about the bony structures of the front of the head and esp. the maxillary sinuses and frontal sinuses

\ə\ **abut** \ˀ\ **kitten** \ər\ **further** \a\ **ash** \ā\ **ace** \ä\ **cot, cart** \aú\ **out** \ch\ **chin** \e\ **bet** \ē\ **easy** \g\ **go** \i\ **hit** \ī\ **ice** \j\ **job** \ŋ\ **sing** \ō\ **go** \ȯ\ **law** \ȯi\ **boy** \th\ **thin** \th\ **the** \ü\ **loot** \ú\ **foot** \y\ **yet** \zh\ **vision** *See also* Pronunciation Symbols page

Waters, Charles Alexander (1888–1961), American radiologist. For the bulk of his career Waters was associated with Johns Hopkins University and Hospital. His specialties included urological radiology and injuries and diseases of the bones and joints.

water vapor *n* : water in a vaporous form esp. when below boiling temperature and diffused (as in the atmosphere)

wa·tery \\'wȯt-ə-rē, 'wät-\\ *adj* **1** : consisting of or filled with water **2** : containing, sodden with, or yielding water or a thin liquid ⟨a ∼ solution⟩ ⟨∼ stools⟩

Wat·son–Crick \\,wät-sən-'krik\\ *adj* : of or relating to the Watson-Crick model ⟨the *Watson-Crick* helix⟩

Watson, James Dewey (*b* 1928), American molecular biologist. Watson is famous for his major role in the discovery of the molecular structure of DNA. In 1951 he began working with Francis Crick at Cambridge, England, learning X-ray diffraction techniques and studying the problem of DNA structure. In 1953 he realized that the essential DNA components—four organic bases—must be linked in definite pairs. This discovery was the key factor that enabled Watson and Crick to formulate a molecular model for DNA in which the organic base pairs are linked by hydrogen bonds to form the rungs of a flexible ladder spiraling in the form of a helix. In this model, DNA replicates itself by splitting lengthwise and reconstructing a double strand of DNA from each of the single strands. This was a major stepping-stone in understanding the process by which genetic material replicates.

Crick, Francis Harry Compton (1916–2004), British molecular biologist. Crick had a major role in the determination of the molecular structure of DNA, a discovery which is widely regarded as one of the most important of 20th-century biology. He joined the research staff at Cavendish Laboratories in Cambridge, England. By 1961 Crick demonstrated that each group of three bases on a single DNA strand designates the position of a specific amino acid on the polypeptide chain of a protein molecule. He also helped to determine the base triplets that code for each of the 20 amino acids normally found in proteins. Watson, Crick, and Maurice Wilkins were awarded the Nobel Prize for Physiology or Medicine in 1962.

Watson–Crick model *n* : a model of DNA structure in which the molecule is a cross-linked double-stranded helix, each strand is composed of alternating links of phosphate and deoxyribose, and the strands are cross-linked by pairs of purine and pyrimidine bases projecting inward from the deoxyribose sugars and joined by hydrogen bonds with adenine paired with thymine and with cytosine paired with guanine — compare DOUBLE HELIX

Wat·so·ni·an \\wät-'sō-nē-ən\\ *adj* : of or relating to the behavioristic theories of the psychologist John B. Watson

Watson, John Broadus (1878–1958), American psychologist. Watson popularized the theories of behaviorism in the U.S. During the 1920s and 1930s Watsonian behaviorism was the dominant school of psychology in the U.S., where it still has an enduring influence. Before joining the advertising business in 1921, Watson served as professor of psychology at Johns Hopkins University, where he established a laboratory of comparative psychology. In 1913 he published a manifesto for behaviorist psychology, asserting that psychology, like other sciences, is to be studied under exacting laboratory conditions. In 1919 he published a major work on behaviorist psychology in which he sought to extend the principles and methods of comparative psychology to the study of human beings. His other writings include a book on behaviorism intended for the general reader (1925) and a guide for the psychological care of infants and children (1928).

Wat·so·ni·us \\wät-'sō-nē-əs\\ *n* : a genus of conical amphistome digenetic trematodes that is related to the genus *Paramphistomum* and includes parasites infesting the intestine of African primates and rarely humans

Watson, Sir Malcom (1873–1955), British physician. In 1900 Watson entered the medical service in Malaya, the site of frequent epidemics of malaria. He quickly embarked upon a vigorous program of mosquito control. Malaria and its prevention were to become his lifelong interests. In 1928 he left Malaya to serve at the Ross Institute of Tropical Hygiene in London. He later served as the director of the Institute and of the branches he established in India and West Africa.

watt \\'wät\\ *n* : the absolute mks unit of power equal to the work done at the rate of one joule per second or to the power produced by a current of one ampere across a potential difference of one volt : $\frac{1}{746}$ horsepower

Watt, James (1736–1819), British engineer and inventor. Watt's steam engine played a major role in the coming of the Industrial Revolution and came to be used in paper mills, flour mills, cotton mills, iron mills, distilleries, canals, and waterworks. At the end of the 19th century the International Electrical Congress named the watt, the unit of electrical power, in his honor.

watt·age \\'wät-ij\\ *n* : amount of power expressed in watts

wat·tle \\'wät-ᵊl\\ *n* : a fleshy process that hangs usu. from the head or neck (as of a bird) — **wat·tled** \-ᵊld\ *adj*

watt·me·ter \\'wät-,mēt-ər\\ *n* : an instrument for measuring electric power in watts

wave \\'wāv\\ *n* **1 a** : a disturbance or variation that transfers energy progressively from point to point in a medium and that may take the form of an elastic deformation or of a variation of pressure, electrical or magnetic intensity, electrical potential, or temperature **b** : one complete cycle of such a disturbance **2** : an undulating or jagged line constituting a graphic representation of an action ⟨an electroencephalographic ∼⟩

wave·form \\'wāv-,fȯrm\\ *n* : a usu. graphic representation of the shape of a wave that indicates its characteristics (as frequency and amplitude) — called also *waveshape*

wave front *n* : a surface composed at any instant of all the points just reached by a vibrational disturbance in its propagation through a medium

wave·guide \\'wāv-,gīd\\ *n* : a device (as a glass fiber) designed to confine and direct the propagation of electromagnetic waves (as light) ⟨use of ∼s for visual examination of the stomach⟩

wave·length \-,len(k)th\ *n* : the distance in the line of advance of a wave from any one point to the next point of corresponding phase — symbol λ

wave mechanics *n* : QUANTUM MECHANICS

wave·shape \-,shāp\ *n* : WAVEFORM

wave theory *n* : a theory in physics: light is transmitted from luminous bodies to the eye and other objects by an undulatory movement — called also *undulatory theory*

wave train *n* : a succession of similar waves at equal intervals

wax \\'waks\\ *n* **1** : a substance that is secreted by bees and is used by them for constructing the honeycomb, that is a dull yellow solid plastic when warm, and that is composed of a mixture of esters, cerotic acid, and hydrocarbons — called also *beeswax* **2** : any of various substances resembling beeswax: as **a** : any of numerous substances of plant or animal origin that differ from fats in being less greasy, harder, and more brittle and in containing principally compounds of high molecular weight (as fatty acids, alcohols, and saturated hydrocarbons) **b** : a pliable or liquid composition used esp. in uniting surfaces, excluding air, making patterns or impressions, or producing a polished surface ⟨dental ∼es⟩ **3** : a waxy secretion; *esp* : EARWAX

wax·ing *n* : the process of removing body hair with a depilatory wax

waxy \\'wak-sē\\ *adj* **wax·i·er; -est 1** : made of, abounding in, or covered with wax ⟨a ∼ surface⟩ **2** : resembling wax ⟨a ∼ complexion⟩ ⟨∼ secretions⟩

waxy degeneration *n* : ZENKER'S DEGENERATION

waxy flexibility *n* : a condition in which a patient's limbs retain any position into which they are manipulated by another person and which occurs esp. in catatonic schizophrenia — compare CATALEPSY

WBC *abbr* white blood cell

WDHA syndrome \dəb-ə(l)-(ˌ)yü-(ˌ)dē-(ˌ)āch-ˈā-\ *n* [watery *d*iarrhea, *h*ypokalemia, and *a*chlorhydria] : VERNER-MORRISON SYNDROME

weal \ˈwē(ə)l\ *n* : WELT

wean \ˈwēn\ *vt* **1** : to accustom (as a child) to take food otherwise than by nursing **2** : to detach usu. gradually from a cause of dependence or form of treatment

wean·ling \ˈwēn-liŋ\ *n* : a child or animal newly weaned — **weanling** *adj*

wea·sand \ˈwēz-ᵊnd, ˈwiz-ᵊn(d)\ *n* : THROAT, GULLET; *also* : WINDPIPE

weav·ing \ˈwē-viŋ\ *n* : a debilitating vice of stabled horses consisting of rhythmic swaying back and forth while shifting the weight from one side to the other

web \ˈweb\ *n* : a tissue or membrane of an animal or plant; *esp* : that uniting fingers or toes either at their bases (as in humans) or for a greater part of their length (as in many waterbirds) — **webbed** \ˈwebd\ *adj*

we·ber \ˈweb-ər, ˈvā-bər\ *n* : the practical mks unit of magnetic flux equal to that flux which in linking a circuit of one turn produces in it an electromotive force of one volt as the flux is reduced to zero at a uniform rate in one second : 10^8 maxwells

> **We·ber** \ˈvā-bər\, **Wilhelm Eduard (1804–1891)**, German physicist. Weber, who was a professor at Göttingen, Germany, was notable for his researches in magnetism and electricity. With Carl Friedrich Gauss he investigated terrestrial magnetism. Weber introduced the absolute system of electrical units patterned after Gauss's system of magnetic units. The term *weber* was officially introduced for the practical unit of magnetic flux in 1935.

Web·er–Chris·tian disease *also* **Web·er–Chris·tian's disease** \ˈweb-ər-ˈkris(h)-chən(z)-\ *n* : PANNICULITIS 2

> **Weber, Frederick Parkes (1863–1962)**, British physician. Weber was on the staff of an English hospital for patients with tuberculosis. He is best known for his studies of the therapeutic benefits of climate and mineral waters. In 1925 he published a description of a disease which was described independently by Christian in 1928; it is now identified with both their names.
>
> **H. A. Christian** — see HAND-SCHÜLLER-CHRISTIAN DISEASE

We·ber–Fech·ner law \ˈweb-ər-ˈfek-nər-, ˈvā-bər-ˈfek-nər-\ *n* : an approximately accurate generalization in psychology: the intensity of a sensation is proportional to the logarithm of the intensity of the stimulus causing it — called also *Fechner's law*

> **We·ber** \ˈvā-bər\, **Ernst Heinrich (1795–1878)**, German anatomist and physiologist. Weber undertook studies of the sense of touch that are important to both psychology and sensory physiology. He introduced the concept of the just noticeable difference between two similar stimuli. In 1851 he published an expanded report on his experimental findings on the sense of touch. Some consider this work to mark the founding of experimental psychology. Weber's empirical observations were expressed mathematically by Gustav Fechner.
>
> **Fech·ner** \ˈfek̲-nər\, **Gustav Theodor (1801–1887)**, German physicist and psychologist. Fechner was one of the founders of the science of psychophysics. He brought out a fundamental work in this field in 1860 which established his lasting importance in psychology. Fechner also developed experimental procedures for measuring sensations in relation to the physical magnitude of stimuli. In particular he formulated an equation to express Weber's theory of the just noticeable difference. Subsequent research has revealed that the equation is applicable within the middle range of stimulus intensity and then is only approximately true.

We·ber's law \ˈweb-ərz-, ˈvā-bərz-\ *n* : an approximately accurate generalization in psychology: the smallest change in the intensity of a stimulus capable of being perceived is proportional to the intensity of the original stimulus

E. H. Weber — see WEBER-FECHNER LAW

We·ber test *or* **We·ber's test** \ˈweb-ər(z)-, ˈvā-bər(z)-\ *n* : a test to determine the nature of unilateral hearing loss in which a vibrating tuning fork is held against the forehead at the midline and conduction deafness is indicated if the sound is heard more loudly in the affected ear and nerve deafness is indicated if it is heard more loudly in the normal ear

> **We·ber–Liel** \ˈvā-bər-ˈlēl\, **Friedrich Eugen (1832–1891)**, German otologist. Weber-Liel taught otology at the universities of Berlin and Jena. He is remembered for a surgical operation consisting of a tenotomy of the tensor tympani. This operation was used in the treatment of certain forms of partial deafness, subjective aural sensations, and the vertiginous feelings associated with these.

Wechs·ler Adult Intelligence Scale \ˈweks-lər-\ *n* : an updated version of the Wechsler-Bellevue test having the same structure but standardized against a different population to more accurately reflect the general population — abbr. *WAIS*

> **Wechsler, David (1896–1981)**, American psychologist. Wechsler enjoyed a long association with New York City's Bellevue Hospital, serving as chief psychologist from 1932 to 1967. He is known as the inventor of several widely used intelligence tests for adults and children, including the Wechsler-Bellevue Intelligence Scale (1939), the Wechsler Intelligence Scale for Children (1949), and the Wechsler Adult Intelligence Scale (1955).

Wechs·ler–Belle·vue test \-ˈbel-ˌvyü-\ *n* : a test of general intelligence and coordination in adults that involves both verbal and performance tests and is now superseded by the Wechsler Adult Intelligence Scale — called also *Wechsler= Bellevue scale*

Wechsler Intelligence Scale for Children *n* : an intelligence test for children of elementary- and secondary-school age that tests knowledge and abilities of a verbal nature (as vocabulary, comprehension, and verbal mathematical reasoning) and the application of knowledge and various skills to the performance of specified tasks (as the arrangement of a series of pictures into a meaningful sequence and the assembly of an object given its parts) — abbr. *WISC*

wedge biopsy \ˈwej-\ *n* : a biopsy in which a wedge-shaped sample of tissue is obtained; *also* : the tissue sample itself

wedge pressure *n* : intravascular pressure that is measured by means of a catheter wedged into the pulmonary artery so as to block the flow of blood and that is equivalent to the pressure in the left atrium — called also *pulmonary capillary wedge pressure, pulmonary wedge pressure*

wedge resection *n* : any of several surgical procedures for removal of a wedge-shaped mass of tissue (as from the ovary or a lung)

WEE *abbr* western equine encephalomyelitis

weep \ˈwēp\ *vb* **wept** \ˈwept\; **weep·ing** *vt* **1** : to pour forth (tears) from the eyes **2** : to exude (a fluid) slowly ~ *vi* **1** : to shed tears **2** : to exude a serous fluid ⟨a ~*ing* burn⟩

Weg·e·ner's granulomatosis \ˈveg-ə-nərz-\ *n* : an uncommon disease of unknown cause that is characterized esp. by vasculitis of small vessels, by granuloma formation in the respiratory tract, and by glomerulonephritis

> **Wegener, Friedrich (1907–1990)**, German pathologist. Wegener first described Wegener's granulomatosis in 1936, issuing another report in 1939. The disease was actually first described by German pathologist Heinz Karl Ernst Klinger in 1931.

weigh \ˈwā\ *vt* **1** : to ascertain the heaviness of by or as if by a balance **2** : to measure or apportion (a definite quantity) on or as if on a scale ~ *vi* : to have a certain amount of heaviness : experience a specific force due to gravity

---

\ə\ **abut** \ᵊ\ **kitten** \ər\ **further** \a\ **ash** \ā\ **ace** \ä\ **cot, cart** \aů\ **out** \ch\ **chin** \e\ **bet** \ē\ **easy** \g\ **go** \i\ **hit** \ī\ **ice** \j\ **job** \ŋ\ **sing** \ō\ **go** \ȯ\ **law** \ȯi\ **boy** \th\ **thin** \th̲\ **the** \ü\ **loot** \ů\ **foot** \y\ **yet** \zh\ **vision** *See also* Pronunciation Symbols page

U
Z

weight \'wāt\ *n* **1** : the amount that a thing weighs **2** : a unit of weight or mass

weight·less·ness \'wāt-ləs-nəs\ *n* : the state or condition of having little or no weight due to lack of apparent gravitational pull — **weight·less** *adj*

Weil–Fe·lix reaction \'vī(ə)l-'fā-liks-\ *n* : an agglutination test for various rickettsial infections (as typhus and tsutsugamushi disease) using particular strains of bacteria of the genus *Proteus* that have antigens in common with the rickettsiae to be identified

> **Weil, Edmund (1880–1922),** and **Felix, Arthur (1887–1956),** Austrian bacteriologists. During World War I Felix served as a bacteriologist charged with the diagnosing of typhus in the Austrian army. As a result of his work he and Weil developed an agglutination test for typhus in 1916.

Weil–Felix test *n* : WEIL-FELIX REACTION

Weil's disease \'vī(ə)lz-, 'wī(ə)lz-\ *n* : a leptospirosis that is characterized by chills, fever, muscle pain, and hepatitis manifested by more or less severe jaundice and that is caused by a spirochete of the genus *Leptospira* (*L. interrogans,* esp. serotype icterohaemorrhagiae) — called also *leptospiral jaundice*

> **Weil** \'vī(ə)l\, **Adolf (1848–1916),** German physician. Weil held professorships in Berlin and later in Tartu, Estonia. In 1886 he published a classic description of a type of leptospirosis characterized by jaundice, nephritis, muscular pain, fever, and enlargement of the spleen and liver. The disease had been described originally by an English physician some 23 years before.

Weis·mann·ism \'wī-smə-ˌniz-əm, 'vī-\ *n* : the theories of heredity proposed by August Weismann stressing particularly the continuity of the germ plasm and the separateness of the germ cells and soma

> **Weis·mann** \'vīs-ˌmän\, **August Friedrich Leopold (1834–1914),** German biologist. Weismann ranks as one of the founders of the science of genetics. In his later years he established himself as one of the leading biologists of his time. In 1863 he joined the faculty of the University of Freiburg, where he remained until his retirement. He introduced his theory of the germ plasm in a book published in 1886. Its essence was the notion that all living things contain a special hereditary substance. His theory was the forerunner of the DNA theory. In addition he predicted that there must be a form of nuclear division in which each daughter nucleus receives only half the ancestral germ plasm contained in the original nucleus. He was an early and ardent supporter of Darwinism. Weismann firmly opposed the idea of the inheritance of acquired traits, however. In later life he became famous as a lecturer on heredity and evolution.

Welch bacillus \'welch-\ *n* : a clostridium (*Clostridium perfringens* syn. *C. welchii*) that causes gas gangrene

> **Welch, William Henry (1850–1934),** American pathologist and bacteriologist. Welch played a major role in the introduction of modern medical practice and education in the U.S. As dean of the Johns Hopkins Medical School he demanded of his students a rigorous study of the physical sciences and an active involvement in clinical duties and laboratory work. Under his direction Johns Hopkins became a model for American medical schools. In his own investigations he is remembered for his demonstration of the pathological effects of diphtheria toxin and for his discovery in 1892 of the bacterium of the genus *Clostridium* (*C. perfringens* syn. *C. welchii*) that causes gas gangrene.

well \'wel\ *adj* **1** : free or recovered from infirmity or disease : HEALTHY ⟨a ∼ person⟩ **2** : completely cured or healed ⟨the wound is nearly ∼⟩

well–ad·just·ed \(')wel-ə-'jəs-təd\ *adj* : WELL-BALANCED 2

well–ba·lanced \-'bal-ən(t)st\ *adj* **1** : nicely or evenly balanced, arranged, or regulated ⟨a ∼ diet⟩ **2** : emotionally or psychologically untroubled

Well·bu·trin \ˌwel-'byü-trin\ *trademark* — used for a preparation of the hydrochloride of bupropion

well·ness *n* : the quality or state of being in good health esp. as an actively sought goal ⟨lifestyles that promote ∼⟩

welt \'welt\ *n* : a ridge or lump raised on the body usu. by a blow

wen \'wen\ *n* : SEBACEOUS CYST; *broadly* : an abnormal growth or a cyst protruding from a surface esp. of the skin

Wencke·bach period \'weŋ-kə-ˌbäk-\ *n* : WENCKEBACH PHENOMENON

> **Wencke·bach** \'veŋ-kə-ˌbäk\, **Karel Frederik (1864–1940),** Dutch internist. Wenckebach held professorships in internal medicine at Groningen, Netherlands, at Strasbourg, and at Vienna. His areas of research included embryological problems and the pathology of heart diseases and the circulation of the blood. In 1914 he published classic descriptions of various forms of cardiac arrhythmia. He was the first to demonstrate the value of quinine in the treatment of paroxysmal fibrillation. In 1928 he established a mechanical theory of cardiac pain in coronary occlusion.

Wenckebach phenomenon *n* : heart block in which a pulse from the atrium periodically does not reach the ventricle and which is characterized by progressive prolongation of the P-R interval until a pulse is skipped

Werd·nig–Hoff·mann disease \'vert-nik-'hof-ˌmän-\ *n* : atrophy of muscles that is caused by degeneration of the ventral horn cells of the spinal cord, is inherited as an autosomal recessive trait, becomes symptomatic during early infancy, is characterized by hypotonia and flaccid paralysis, and is often fatal during childhood — called also *Werdnig-Hoffmann syndrome;* compare KUGELBERG-WELANDER DISEASE

> **Werd·nig** \'vert-nik\, **Guido (1844–1919),** Austrian neurologist, and **Hoffmann, Johann (1857–1919),** German neurologist. Independently of each other, Werdnig and Hoffmann published descriptions of Werdnig-Hoffmann disease in 1891. Hoffmann is also remembered for his 1897 descriptions of peroneal muscular atrophy and myopathy associated with hypothyroidism.

Werl·hof's disease \'ver(-ə)l-ˌhōfs-\ *n* : THROMBOCYTOPENIC PURPURA

> **Werlhof, Paul Gottlieb (1699–1767),** German physician. Werlhof served as the court physician at Hannover, Germany. In 1735 he published a classic description of thrombocytopenic purpura, now also known as Werlhof's disease.

Wer·ner's syndrome \'ver-nərz\ *n* : a rare hereditary disorder characterized by premature aging with associated abnormalities (as dwarfism, cataracts, osteoporosis, and hypogonadism) — called also *Werner syndrome*

> **Werner, Otto (1879–1936),** German physician.

Wer·nicke's aphasia \'ver-nə-kəz-, -kēz-\ *n* : SENSORY APHASIA; *specif* : sensory aphasia in which the affected individual speaks words fluently but without meaningful content

> **Wer·nicke** \'ver-nə-kə\, **Carl (1848–1905),** German neurologist. Wernicke is important for his work in relating nerve diseases to specific areas of the brain. The last two decades of his life were spent as professor of neurology and psychiatry first at Breslau and then at Halle, Germany. Wernicke belonged to a 19th-century school of German neuropsychiatry that made no distinction between disorders of the mind and disorders of the brain. He is best known for his studies of aphasia.

Wernicke's area *n* : an area located in the posterior part of the superior temporal gyrus that plays an important role in the comprehension of language

Wernicke's encephalopathy *n* : an inflammatory hemorrhagic encephalopathy that is caused by thiamine deficiency, affects esp. chronic alcoholics, and is characterized by nystagmus, diplopia, ataxia, and degenerative mental disorders (as Korsakoff's psychosis)

Wert·heim operation \'vert-ˌhīm-\ *or* **Wert·heim's operation** \-ˌhīmz-\ *n* : radical hysterectomy performed by way of an abdominal incision

> **Wertheim, Ernst (1864–1920),** Austrian gynecologist. Wertheim held a series of surgical positions at women's clinics in Vienna. As a gynecologist he devoted much time to research and is remembered for his fundamental research on gonorrhea in the female genital tract. Wertheim is

best known for his development of a radical abdominal operation for cervical cancer. He first performed the operation in 1898 and published a full account of it in 1911. He also developed an operation for prolapse of the uterus, presenting a written account of it in 1919.

Wes·ter·gren erythrocyte sedimentation rate \\'ves-tər-grən-\ *n* : sedimentation rate of red blood cells determined by the Westergren method — called also *Westergren sedimentation rate*

Westergren, Alf Vilhelm (1891–1968), Swedish physician. In 1921 in an article on blood in pulmonary tuberculosis, Westergren introduced his method for measuring the sedimentation rate of red blood cells.

Westergren method *n* : a method for estimating the sedimentation rate of red blood cells in fluid blood by observing the level to which the cells fall in one hour in a tube of 2 or 2.5 mm bore that is 300 mm long and is graduated downward in millimeters from 0 to 200 when 4.5 ml of venous blood is mixed with 0.5 ml of 3.8 percent aqueous solution of sodium citrate

Westergren sedimentation rate *n* : WESTERGREN ERYTHROCYTE SEDIMENTATION RATE

wes·tern black–legged tick \\'wes-tərn-'blak-ˌlegd-\ *n* : a tick of the genus *Ixodes* (*I. pacificus*) that is a vector of Lyme disease and is found esp. in some parts of the Pacific coastal states of the U.S.

West·ern blot \\ˌwes-tərn-'blät\ *n* : a blot consisting of a sheet of cellulose nitrate or nylon that contains spots of protein for identification by a suitable molecular probe and is used esp. for the detection of antibodies — compare NORTHERN BLOT, SOUTHERN BLOT — **Western blot·ting** \-'blät-iŋ\ *n*

western equine encephalomyelitis *n* : EQUINE ENCEPHALOMYELITIS b

West Nile encephalitis \\'west-'nīl-\ *n* : severe West Nile fever marked by encephalitis

West Nile fever *n* : illness caused by the West Nile virus

West Nile virus *n* : a single-stranded RNA virus of the genus *Flavivirus* (species *West Nile virus*) that causes an illness marked by fever, headache, muscle ache, skin rash, and sometimes encephalitis or meningitis, that is spread chiefly by mosquitoes, and that is closely related to the viruses causing Japanese B encephalitis and Saint Louis encephalitis; *also* : WEST NILE FEVER

wet \\'wet\ *adj* : marked by the presence or abundance of fluid (as secretions or effusions) ⟨the ∼ form of age-related macular degeneration⟩

wet–and–dry–bulb thermometer *n* : PSYCHROMETER

wet dream *n* : an erotic dream culminating in orgasm and in the male accompanied by seminal emission — compare NOCTURNAL EMISSION

wet lab *n* : a laboratory equipped with appropriate plumbing, ventilation, and equipment to allow for hands-on scientific research and experimentation — called also *wet laboratory;* compare DRY LAB

wet mount *n* : a glass slide holding a specimen suspended in a drop of liquid (as water) for microscopic examination; *also* : a specimen mounted in this way — **wet–mount** *adj*

wet nurse *n* : a woman who cares for and suckles young not her own

wet pleurisy *n* : pleurisy with effusion of exudate into the pleural cavity

wetting agent *n* : a substance that promotes the spreading of a liquid on a surface or the penetration of a liquid into a material esp. by becoming adsorbed in such a way that the liquid is no longer repelled

Whar·ton's duct \\'(h)wȯrt-ᵊnz-\ *n* : the duct of the submandibular gland that opens into the mouth on a papilla at the side of the frenulum of the tongue

Wharton, Thomas (1614–1673), British anatomist. Wharton was a physician attached to St. Thomas's Hospital and is remembered as one of the very few physicians to remain on duty while London was ravaged by the great plague of 1665. A noted anatomist, he provided the most complete description of the glands up to that time. In 1650 he described the

soft connective tissue that forms the matrix of the umbilical cord and is now known as Wharton's jelly. In 1656 he published a work describing many glands of the body, including the submandibular gland for the conveyance of saliva. He is credited with discovering the gland's duct.

Wharton's jelly *n* : a soft connective tissue that occurs in the umbilical cord and consists of large stellate fibroblasts and a few wandering cells and macrophages embedded in a homogeneous jellylike intercellular substance

wheal \\'hwē(ə)l, 'wē(ə)l\ *n* : a suddenly formed elevation of the skin surface: as **a** : WELT **b** : the transient lump occurring at the site of injection of a solution before the solution is normally dispersed **c** : a flat burning or itching eminence on the skin ⟨urticarial ∼s⟩

whealing *n* : the presence or development of wheals

wheat germ \\'hwēt-, 'wēt-\ *n* : the embryo of the wheat kernel separated in milling and used esp. as a source of vitamins and protein

wheat–germ oil *n* : a yellow unsaturated fatty oil obtained from wheat germ and containing vitamin E

Wheat·stone bridge \\ˌhwēt-ˌstōn-, ˌwēt-, *chiefly Brit* -stən-\ *n* : a bridge for measuring electrical resistances that consists of a conductor joining two branches of a circuit

Wheatstone, Sir Charles (1802–1875), British physicist. Wheatstone was professor of experimental philosophy at King's College, London. He is remembered for his researches in electricity, sound, and light. In 1834 he devised a revolving mirror for an experiment to measure the speed of electricity in a conductor. In 1843 he constructed the Wheatstone bridge and began to popularize its use. He initiated the use of electromagnets in electric generators, and in 1837 he and Sir William Fothergill Cooke patented an early telegraph.

wheel·chair \\'hwē(ə)l-ˌche(ə)r, 'wē(ə)l-, -ˌcha(ə)r\ *n* : a chair mounted on wheels esp. for the use of disabled individuals

¹wheeze \\'hwēz, 'wēz\ *vi* **wheezed; wheez·ing** : to breathe with difficulty usu. with a whistling sound

²wheeze *n* : a sibilant whistling sound caused by difficult or obstructed respiration

¹whelp \\'hwelp, 'welp\ *n* : one of the young of various carnivorous mammals and esp. of the dog

²whelp *vt* : to give birth to — used of various carnivores and esp. the dog ∼ *vi* : to bring forth young

whey \\'hwā, 'wā\ *n* : the serum or watery part of milk that is separated from the coagulable part or curd esp. in the process of making cheese and that is rich in lactose, minerals, and vitamins and contains lactalbumin and traces of fat

whip·lash \\'hwip-ˌlash, 'wip-\ *n* : injury resulting from a sudden sharp whipping movement of the neck and head (as of a person in a vehicle that is struck head-on or from the rear by another vehicle)

Whip·ple operation \\'(h)wip-əl-\ *or* **Whip·ple's operation** \-əlz-\ *n* : WHIPPLE PROCEDURE

Whipple procedure *or* **Whipple's procedure** *n* : PANCREATICODUODENECTOMY; *esp* : one in which there is complete excision of the pancreas and partial excision of the duodenum

Whipple, Allen Oldfather (1881–1963), American surgeon. Whipple's chief medical positions were with the surgical faculty of Columbia University's College of Physicians and Surgeons and the surgical staff of New York City's Presbyterian Hospital. After his retirement from Columbia University, he reformed the medical training programs at Memorial Hospital in New York City and American University in Beirut, Lebanon. A leader in abdominal, spleen, and gallbladder surgery, he was credited with the creation of the spleen clinic in the surgery department at the College of Physicians and Surgeons, which was responsible for many important advances, including prosthetic materials for aor-

---

\ə\ abut \ᵊ\ kitten \ər\ further \a\ ash \ā\ ace \ä\ cot, cart
\aù\ out \ch\ chin \e\ bet \ē\ easy \g\ go \i\ hit \ī\ ice \j\ job
\ŋ\ sing \ō\ go \ȯ\ law \ȯi\ boy \th\ thin \ṯh\ the \ü\ loot
\ù\ foot \y\ yet \zh\ vision   *See also* Pronunciation Symbols page

U
Z

tic grafting and the measurement and treatment of portal hypertension. Whipple is best known for his triad of criteria for hyperinsulinism with tumors of the islets of Langerhans and for his operation for carcinoma of the pancreas, the latter having been introduced in 1938.

Whipple's disease *also* **Whipple disease** *n* : a rare malabsorption syndrome that is caused by an actinomycetous fungus (*Tropheryma whippelli*) in the mucous membrane of the intestine, that affects primarily the small intestine but becomes more generalized affecting esp. the joints, brain, liver, and heart, that is marked by the accumulation of lipid deposits in the intestinal lymphatic tissues, weight loss, joint pain, mental confusion, and generalized lymphadenopathy, and that is diagnosed by the presence of macrophages in the lamina propria of the small intestine which give a positive reaction to a periodic acid-Schiff test — called also *intestinal lipodystrophy*

Whipple, George Hoyt (1878–1976), American pathologist. For more than 30 years Whipple served as dean of the Rochester (New York) School of Medicine and Dentistry, an institution which he developed into a medical center of the first rank. He is best known for his studies of the role of dietary iron. He initially conceived the idea of using a liver diet to treat pernicious anemia. For his work he shared the Nobel Prize for Physiology or Medicine in 1934. Whipple also did significant research on tuberculosis, pancreatitis, regeneration of plasma protein, chloroform poisoning in animals, and blackwater fever. He described intestinal lipodystrophy in 1907.

whip·worm \-ˌwərm\ *n* : a parasitic nematode worm of the family Trichuridae with a body that is thickened posteriorly and that is very long and slender anteriorly; *esp* : one of the genus *Trichuris* (*T. trichiura*) that parasitizes the human intestine

whirl·ing disease \ˈhwər(-ə)l-iŋ-, ˈwər(-ə)l-\ *n* : an infectious often fatal disease of salmonid fish (as trout and salmon) that is caused by a protozoan (*Myxobolus cerebralis* syn. *Myxosoma cerebralis*) of the order Myxosporidia which attacks cartilage of the head and spinal cord esp. of young fish and that causes the fish to swim in circles and is marked by skeletal deformities

whirl·pool \ˈhwər(-ə)l-ˌpül, ˈwər(-ə)l-\ *n* : WHIRLPOOL BATH

whirlpool bath *n* : a therapeutic bath in which all or part of the body is exposed to forceful whirling currents of hot water

whis·key *or* **whis·ky** \ˈhwis-kē, ˈwis-\ *n, pl* **whiskeys** *or* **whiskies** : a liquor that is distilled from the fermented mash of grain (as rye, corn, or barley) and was formerly used medicinally as a sedative and vasodilator

white agaric \ˈ(h)wīt-\ *n* : PURGING AGARIC

white arsenic *n* : ARSENIC TRIOXIDE

white blood cell *n* : any of the blood cells that are colorless, lack hemoglobin, contain a nucleus, and include the lymphocytes, monocytes, neutrophils, eosinophils, and basophils — called also *leukocyte, white blood corpuscle, white cell, white corpuscle;* compare RED BLOOD CELL

white coat hypertension *n* : a temporary elevation in a patient's blood pressure that occurs when measured in a medical setting (as a physician's office) and that is usu. due to anxiety on the part of the patient — called also *white coat effect*

white comb *n* : favus of fowls that is marked by proliferation of grayish white crumbly crusts about the comb, earlobes, and wattles

white corpuscle *n* : WHITE BLOOD CELL

white count *n* : the count or the total number of white blood cells in the blood usu. stated as the number in one cubic millimeter — compare DIFFERENTIAL BLOOD COUNT

white fat *n* : normal fat tissue that replaces brown fat in infants during the first year of life

white fibrous tissue *n* : typical connective tissue in which white inelastic fibers predominate as distinguished from elastic tissue

white–foot·ed mouse \ˌ(h)wīt-ˌfüt-əd-\ *n* : a common wood-

land mouse (*Peromyscus leucopus*) that has whitish feet and underparts and that is a reservoir for the spirochete of the genus *Borrelia* (*B. burgdorferi*) causing Lyme disease

white·head \-ˌhed\ *n* : MILIUM

white hellebore *n* : FALSE HELLEBORE; *also* : HELLEBORE 2b

white horehound *n* : HOREHOUND 1

white lead *n* : any of several white lead-containing pigments; *esp* : a heavy poisonous basic carbonate of lead of variable composition used esp. formerly in paints

white light *n* : light that is composed of a wide range of electromagnetic frequencies and that appears colorless to the eye

white lotion *n* : a preparation made of sulfurated potash and zinc sulfate that is applied topically in the treatment of various skin disorders

white matter *n* : neural tissue esp. of the brain and spinal cord that consists largely of myelinated nerve fibers bundled into tracts, has a whitish color, and typically underlies the gray matter

white mineral oil *n* : MINERAL OIL 2

white muscle disease *n* : a disease of young domestic animals (as lambs and calves) that is characterized by muscular degeneration and is associated esp. with inadequate intake of vitamin E — see STIFF-LAMB DISEASE

white mustard *n* : a Eurasian mustard (*Brassica hirta*) with pale yellow seeds that yield mustard and mustard oil

white noise *n* : a heterogeneous mixture of sound waves extending over a wide frequency range that has been used to mask out unwanted noise interfering with sleep — called also *white sound*

white ointment *n* : an ointment consisting of 5 percent white wax and 95 percent white petrolatum — called also *simple ointment*

white pepper *n* : a condiment that consists of the fruit of an Indian plant of the genus *Piper* (*P. nigrum*) ground after the black husk has been removed

white petrolatum *n* : PETROLATUM b

white petroleum jelly *n* : PETROLATUM b

white piedra *n* : a form of piedra that affects esp. the facial hairs and is caused by a fungus of the genus *Trichosporan* (*T. beigelii*)

white plague *n* : TUBERCULOSIS

white pulp *n* : a parenchymatous tissue of the spleen that consists of compact masses of lymphatic cells and that forms the Malpighian corpuscles — compare RED PULP

white quebracho *n* : QUEBRACHO 1

white ramus *n* : RAMUS COMMUNICANS a

white ramus communicans *n* : RAMUS COMMUNICANS a

white rat *n* : a rat of an albino strain of the brown rat that is used extensively as a laboratory animal in biological experimentation

whites *n pl* : LEUKORRHEA

white shark *n* : GREAT WHITE SHARK

white snakeroot *n* : a poisonous No. American herb of the genus *Eupatorium* (*E. rugosum*) that is a cause of trembles and milk sickness

white sound *n* : WHITE NOISE

white squill *n* : squill for medicinal use composed of the sliced bulbs of the white-bulbed form of the squill (*Urginea maritima*) of the Mediterranean region — compare RED SQUILL 1, URGINEA 2a

white vitriol *n* : ZINC SULFATE

white wax *n* : bleached yellow wax used esp. in cosmetics, ointments, and cerates — called also *beeswax, cera alba*

Whit·field's ointment \ˈ(h)wit-ˌfēldz-\ *also* **Whit·field ointment** \-ˌfēld-\ *n* : an ointment that contains benzoic acid and salicylic acid and is used for its keratolytic effect in treating fungal skin diseases (as ringworm)

Whitfield, Arthur (1868–1947), British dermatologist. Whitfield was a London professor of dermatology and the author of numerous articles on skin diseases. In 1907 he published a handbook of skin diseases and their treatment. The handbook introduced an antiseptic ointment composed of benzoic and salicylic acids and petrolatum and used for the treatment of fungus infections.

whit·low \'hwit-(,)lō, 'wit-\ n : a deep usu. suppurative inflammation of the finger or toe esp. near the end or around the nail — called also *felon;* compare PARONYCHIA

WHO *abbr* World Health Organization

whole \'hōl\ *adj* : containing all its natural constituents, components, or elements : deprived of nothing by refining, processing, or separation ⟨~ milk⟩

whole blood n : blood with all its components intact that has been withdrawn from a donor into an anticoagulant solution for use to restore blood volume esp. after traumatic blood loss

whole–body *adj* : of, relating to, or affecting the entire body ⟨~ radiation⟩ ⟨~ hyperthermia⟩

whole food n : a natural food and esp. an unprocessed one (as a vegetable or fruit)

¹**whoop** \'hüp, 'hu̇p\ vi : to make the characteristic whoop of whooping cough

²**whoop** n : the crowing intake of breath following a paroxysm in whooping cough

whooping cough n : an infectious disease esp. of children caused by a bacterium of the genus *Bordetella* (*B. pertussis*) and marked by a convulsive spasmodic cough sometimes followed by a crowing intake of breath — called also *pertussis*

whorl \'hwȯr(-ə)l, 'wȯr(-ə)l, '(h)wər(-ə)l\ n : a fingerprint in which the central papillary ridges turn through at least one complete turn

¹**wick** \'wik\ n : a strip of material (as gauze) placed in a wound to serve as a drain

²**wick** vt : to absorb or drain (as fluid or moisture) like a wick — often used with *away* ⟨a dry gauze dressing was used to ~ exudate away from the wound⟩

Wi·dal reaction *also* **Wi·dal's reaction** \vē-'däl(z)-\ n : a specific reaction consisting in agglutination of typhoid bacilli or other salmonellas when mixed with serum from a patient having typhoid fever or other salmonella infection and constituting a test for the disease

Wi·dal \vē-däl\, **Georges–Fernand–Isidore (1862–1929),** French physician and bacteriologist. Widal held a professorship of pathology and internal medicine at the University of Paris. In 1896 he developed the Widal reaction, a procedure for diagnosing typhoid fever based on the fact that antibodies in the blood of an infected individual cause the bacteria to bind together into clumps. In 1906 he recognized that the retention of sodium chloride was a feature found in cases of nephritis and cardiac edema, and he recommended salt deprivation as part of the treatment for both diseases.

Widal test *also* **Widal's test** n : a test for detecting typhoid fever and other salmonella infections using the Widal reaction — compare AGGLUTINATION TEST

wide–spec·trum \'wīd-'spek-trəm\ *adj* : BROAD-SPECTRUM

wild cherry \'wīld-\ n : the dried bark of a tree of the genus *Prunus* (*P. serotina*) that is used in pharmacology as a flavoring agent

wild ginger n : a No. American perennial herb of the genus *Asarum* (*A. canadense*) whose dried rhizome is used in pharmacology — see ASARUM 2

wild type n : a phenotype, genotype, or gene that predominates in a natural population of organisms or strain of organisms in contrast to that of natural or laboratory mutant forms; *also* : an organism or strain displaying the wild type — **wild–type** *adj*

Wil·liams syndrome \'wil-yəmz-\ n : a rare genetic disorder characterized esp. by hypercalcemia of infants, heart defects (as supravalvular aortic stenosis), characteristic facial features (as an upturned nose, long philtrum, wide mouth, full lips, and pointed chin), a sociable personality, and a high verbal aptitude, but with mild to moderate mental retardation

Williams, J. C. P. (*fl* 1961), New Zealand cardiologist. Williams was the principal author on a 1961 article on su-

pravalvular aortic stenosis, with B. G. Barratt-Boyes and J. B. Lowe listed as secondary authors.

Wilms' tumor *also* **Wilms's tumor** \'vilmz-(əz-)\ n : a malignant tumor of the kidney that primarily affects children and is made up of embryonic elements — called also *nephroblastoma*

Wilms, Max (1867–1918), German surgeon. Wilms held professorships at Basel, Switzerland, and at Leipzig and Heidelberg, Germany. He developed several operations, including resection of the ribs to produce depression of the chest and compression of the lungs (1911) and benign stricture of the common bile duct (1912). He described Wilms' tumor in 1899.

Wil·son's disease \'wil-sənz-\ n : a hereditary disease that is characterized by the accumulation of copper in the body (as in the liver, brain, or cornea) due to abnormal copper metabolism associated with ceruloplasmin deficiency, that is determined by an autosomal recessive gene, and that is marked esp. by liver dysfunction and disease and neurologic or psychiatric symptoms (as tremors, slowness of speech, inappropriate behaviors, or personality changes) — called also *hepatolenticular degeneration;* see KAYSER-FLEISCHER RING

Wilson, Samuel Alexander Kinnier (1877–1937), British neurologist. Wilson enjoyed long-term associations with King's College Hospital and the National Hospital for the Paralyzed and Epileptic, both in London. His neurological studies covered such diverse topics as epilepsy, narcolepsy, speech disorders, apraxia, and pathological laughing and crying. In 1912 he published a monograph on progressive lenticular degeneration, which is now known as Wilson's disease. He was the first to detect the relationship between liver disease and putaminous destruction.

wind–bro·ken \'win(d)-,brō-kən\ *adj, of a horse* : affected with pulmonary emphysema or with heaves

wind·burn \-,bərn\ n : irritation of the skin caused by wind — **wind·burned** \-,bərnd\ *adj*

wind·chill \'win(d)-,chil\ n : a still-air temperature that would have the same cooling effect on exposed human flesh as a given combination of temperature and wind speed — called also *chill factor, windchill factor, windchill index*

wind colic n : BLOAT 1

wind·gall \-,gȯl\ n : a soft tumor or synovial swelling on a horse's leg in the region of the fetlock joint

win·dow \'win-(,)dō, -də(-w)\ n **1** : FENESTRA 1 **2** : a small surgically created opening : FENESTRA 2a **3** : a usu. narrow interval of time or range of values for which a certain condition or an opportunity exists ⟨coma and multiorgan failure can occur within hours and there may be a very narrow ~ of opportunity for transplantation —J. P. A. Lodge⟩ — see THERAPEUTIC WINDOW

wind·pipe \'win(d)-,pīp\ n : TRACHEA

wind puff \-,pəf\ n : WINDGALL

wind sucking n : a vice of horses that is related to and often associated with cribbing and that is characterized by repeated swallowing of air

wine \'wīn\ n **1** : fermented grape juice containing varying percentages of alcohol together with ethers and esters that give it bouquet and flavor **2** : a pharmaceutical preparation using wine as a vehicle

wing \'wiŋ\ n **1** : one of the movable feathered or membranous paired appendages by means of which a bird, bat, or insect is able to fly **2** : a winglike anatomical part or process : ALA; *esp* : any of the four winglike processes of the sphenoid bone — see GREATER WING, LESSER WING — **winged** \'wiŋd, 'wiŋ-əd\ *adj*

¹**wink** \'wiŋk\ vi : to close and open the eyelids quickly

²**wink** n : a quick closing and opening of the eyelids : BLINK

win·ter·green \'wint-ər-,grēn\ n **1** : any plant of the genus *Gaultheria;* esp : a low evergreen plant (*G. procumbens*) with

U Z

white flowers and spicy red berries **2** : OIL OF WINTER-GREEN

wintergreen oil *n* : OIL OF WINTERGREEN

win·ter itch \'wint-ər-\ *n* : an itching disorder caused by prolonged exposure to cold dry air

winter tick *n* : an ixodid tick of the genus *Dermacentor* (*D. albipictus*) that is actively parasitic during the winter months on domestic and big-game animals in parts of Canada and the northern and western U.S.

Win·ton disease \'wint-ən-\ *n* : cirrhosis of the liver in horses and cattle resulting from the chronic poisoning by toxic constituents of ragwort and other noxious plants eaten in the pasturage

wire \'wī(ə)r\ *n* : metal thread or a rod used in surgery to suture soft tissue or transfix fractured bone and in orthodontic dentistry to position teeth — **wire** *vt* **wired; wir·ing**

Wir·sung's duct \'vir-ˌsùnz-\ *n* : PANCREATIC DUCT a J. G. Wirsung — see DUCT OF WIRSUNG

WISC *abbr* Wechsler Intelligence Scale for Children

wis·dom tooth \'wiz-dəm-\ *n* : the third molar that is the last tooth to erupt on each side of the upper and lower human jaw

wish–ful·fill·ing \'wish-fù(l)-ˌfil-iŋ\ *adj* : relating to or serving the function of wish fulfillment ⟨a ~ fantasy⟩

wish ful·fill·ment \-mənt\ *n* : the gratification of a desire esp. symbolically (as in dreams or fantasies)

Wis·kott–Al·drich syndrome \'vis-ˌkät-'ȯl-ˌdrich-\ *n* : an inherited usu. fatal childhood immunodeficiency disease characterized esp. by thrombocytopenia, leukopenia, recurrent infections, eczema, and abnormal bleeding

Wis·kott \'vis-ˌkòt\, **Alfred (1898–1978),** German pediatrician. A professor of pediatrics in Munich, Wiskott wrote on diseases of the respiratory system and on the pathogenesis, clinical treatment, and classification of pneumonias in early childhood.

Aldrich, Robert Anderson (1917–1998), American pediatrician. Aldrich held professorships in pediatrics at the medical schools of the University of Oregon and the University of Washington. Later he was professor of preventive medicine and comprehensive health care at the University of Colorado. His areas of research included the biochemistry of bilirubin and porphyrins, the mechanism of heme synthesis, and inborn errors of metabolism.

Wis·tar rat \'wist-ər-\ *n* : an albino rat widely used in biological and medical research

witch·grass \'wich-ˌgras\ *n* : QUACK GRASS

witch ha·zel \'wich-ˌhā-zəl\ *n* **1** : any small tree or shrub of the genus *Hamamelis*; *esp* : one (*Hamamelis virginiana*) of eastern No. America that blooms in the fall **2** : an alcoholic solution of a distillate of the bark of a witch hazel (*Hamamelis virginiana*) used as a soothing and mildly astringent lotion

with·draw \with-'drȯ, with-\ *vb* **-drew** \-'drü\; **-drawn** \-'drȯn\; **-draw·ing** \-'drȯ(-)iŋ\ *vt* : to discontinue use or administration of ⟨~ a drug⟩ ~ *vi* : to become socially or emotionally detached

with·draw·al \-'drȯ(ə)l\ *n* **1 a** : a pathological retreat from objective reality (as in some schizophrenic states) **b** : social or emotional detachment **2 a** : the discontinuance of administration or use of a drug **b** : the syndrome of often painful physical and psychological symptoms that follows discontinuance of an addicting substance ⟨a heroin addict going through ~⟩ **3** : COITUS INTERRUPTUS

withdrawal symptom *n* : one of a group of symptoms (as nausea, sweating, or depression) produced in a person by deprivation of an addicting drug

with·drawn \with-'drȯn\ *adj* : socially detached and unresponsive : exhibiting withdrawal : INTROVERTED

with·ers \'with-ərz\ *n pl* **1** : the ridge between the shoulder bones of a horse **2** : a part corresponding to the withers in a quadruped other than a horse

Wit·zel·sucht \'vit-səl-ˌzükt\ *n* : excessive facetiousness and inappropriate or pointless humor esp. when considered as part of an abnormal condition

wob·bles \'wäb-əlz\ *n pl but usu sing in constr* : a disease of

horses that is marked by degenerative changes in the spinal cord and nerves resulting in ataxia chiefly of the hind legs

wohl·fahr·tia \ˌvōl-'färt-ē-ə\ *n* **1** *cap* : a genus of larviparous dipteran flies of the family Sarcophagidae that commonly deposit their larvae in wounds or on the intact skin of humans and domestic animals causing severe cutaneous myiasis **2** : any fly of the genus *Wohlfahrtia*

Wol·fart \'vōl-ˌfärt\, **Peter (1675–1726),** German physician. Wolfart was a practicing physician in Hanau, Germany, as well as a professor of medicine and anatomy, first at the secondary school and later at the college there.

Wolff·ian body \ˌwùl-fē-ən-\ *n* : MESONEPHROS

Wolff \'vȯlf\, **Caspar Friedrich (1734–1794),** German anatomist and embryologist. Wolff spent most of his career as a lecturer on anatomy at the Academy of Sciences at St. Petersburg, Russia. His primary achievement was his refutation of the theory of preformation, the theory which held that the development of an organism was simply the expansion of a fully formed embryo. In his studies of the chick embryo he followed the development of the mesonephros and discovered the embryonic kidneys that become the final metanephros and are now known as Wolffian bodies.

Wolffian duct *n* : the duct of the mesonephros that persists in the female chiefly as part of the epoophoron and in the male as the duct system leaving the testis and including the epididymis, vas deferens, seminal vesicle, and ejaculatory duct — called also *Leydig's duct, mesonephric duct*

Wolff–Par·kin·son–White syndrome \'wùlf-'pär-kən-sən-'(h)wīt-\ *n* : an abnormal heart condition characterized by preexcitation of the ventricle and an electrocardiographic tracing with a shortened P-R interval and a widened QRS complex — called also *WPW syndrome*

Wolff, Louis (1898–1972), American cardiologist. Wolff, Parkinson, and White described the syndrome that bears their names in an article published in 1930.

Parkinson, Sir John (1885–1976), British cardiologist. Parkinson served as a cardiologist at the London and National Heart Hospitals and as a consulting cardiologist with the Royal Air Force.

White, Paul Dudley (1886–1973), American cardiologist. White was an international authority on heart disease who gained national celebrity status when he became cardiologist to President Dwight Eisenhower. White maintained lifelong associations with Massachusetts General Hospital and Harvard Medical School. He was among the first to employ electrocardiograms for the diagnosis of heart disease. He used some 21,000 as the basis for *Heart Diseases,* a classic text that he published in 1931. He also helped to found the American Heart Association and the International Society of Cardiology. White was an advocate of physical exercise, and in later years he would be credited with helping to plant the seeds for the ensuing increased interest in fitness.

wol·fram \'wùl-frəm\ *n* : TUNGSTEN

Wol·fram syndrome \'wùl-frəm-\ *or* **Wolfram's syndrome** *n* : a rare hereditary disorder that is characterized esp. by type 1 diabetes, diabetes insipidus, optic atrophy, sensorineural deafness, and bladder dysfunction and that is inherited as an autosomal recessive trait

Wolfram, D. J. (fl 1938), American physician. Wolfram published a report on four cases of Wolfram syndrome in 1938.

wolfs·bane \'wùlfs-ˌbān\ *n* : a plant of the genus *Aconitum*; *esp* : a monkshood (*A. napellus*) that is the source of the drug aconite

womb \'wüm\ *n* : UTERUS

won·der drug \'wənd-ər-\ *n* : MIRACLE DRUG

wood alcohol \'wùd-\ *n* : METHANOL

wood·en tongue \'wùd-ən-\ *n* : actinobacillosis or actinomycosis of cattle esp. when chiefly affecting the tongue

Wood's lamp \'wùdz-\ *also* **Wood lamp** \'wùd-\ *n* : a lamp for producing ultraviolet radiation in which a filter made of nickel-containing glass is used to block all light having a wavelength above 365 nanometers and which is used esp. to detect various skin conditions (as some fungus infections) by the fluorescence induced in the affected areas by ultraviolet radiation

Wood, Robert Williams (1868–1955), American physicist. Wood spent the bulk of his scientific career at Johns Hopkins University, first as professor and later as research professor of experimental physics. His greatest contributions were in optics, especially spectroscopy, in which he obtained experimental results of prime importance for the advancement of atomic physics. A recognized authority on the optical properties of gases and vapors, especially sodium vapor, he did fundamental work on fluorescence in vapors. Equally important was his research on the effect of electric and magnetic fields on spectral lines. With his improvements in the diffraction grating he greatly stimulated research in spectroscopy by other scientists. Other areas of Wood's research included color photography, the photographing of sound waves, the properties of ultrasonic vibrations, and criminalistics. During World War II he served as a consultant for the Manhattan project. He also had numerous inventions to his credit. In 1903 he first used a filter of nickel-containing glass to remove visible light from a beam of radiation, producing a beam consisting only of ultraviolet light. Lamps incorporating such filters have since been named after him.

Wood's light *also* **Wood light** *n* : WOOD'S LAMP; *also* : ultraviolet radiation produced by a Wood's lamp

wood sugar *n* : XYLOSE

wood tick *n* : any of several ixodid ticks: as **a** : ROCKY MOUNTAIN WOOD TICK **b** : AMERICAN DOG TICK

wood turpentine *n* : TURPENTINE 2b

woody tongue \'wùd-ē-\ *n* : WOODEN TONGUE

wool fat \'wùl-\ *n* : wool grease esp. after refining : LANOLIN

wool grease *n* : a fatty slightly sticky wax coating the surface of the fibers of sheep's wool that is used as a source of lanolin — compare WOOL FAT

wool maggot *n* : the larva of a blowfly that causes strike in sheep

wool·sort·er's disease \'wùl-ˌsȯrt-ərz-\ *n* : pulmonary anthrax resulting esp. from inhalation of bacterial spores from contaminated wool or hair

word–association test \'wərd-\ *n* : a test of personality and mental function in which the subject is required to respond to each of a series of words with the first word that comes to mind or with a word of a specified class of words (as antonyms)

word blindness *n* : ALEXIA — **word–blind** *adj*

word deafness *n* : AUDITORY APHASIA — **word–deaf** *adj*

word sal·ad \-ˌsal-əd\ *n* : a jumble of extremely incoherent speech as sometimes observed in schizophrenia

work·a·hol·ic \ˌwər-kə-'hȯl-ik, -'häl-\ *n* : a compulsive worker

work·a·hol·ism \'wər-kə-ˌhȯl-ˌiz-əm, -ˌhäl-\ *n* : an obsessive need to work

work–related musculoskeletal disorder \'wərk-ri-ˌlāt-əd-\ *n* : REPETITIVE STRAIN INJURY

work·up \'wər-ˌkəp\ *n* : an intensive diagnostic study ⟨a gastrointestinal ∼⟩ ⟨a psychiatric ∼⟩

work up \wər-'kəp, 'wər-\ *vt* : to perform a diagnostic work-up upon ⟨*work up* a patient⟩

¹**worm** \'wərm\ *n* **1** : any of various relatively small elongated usu. naked and soft-bodied parasitic animals (as of the phylum Platyhelminthes) **2** : HELMINTHIASIS — usu. used in pl. ⟨a dog with ∼s⟩ — **worm·like** \-ˌlīk\ *adj*

²**worm** *vt* : to treat (an animal) with a drug to destroy or expel parasitic worms

worm·er \'wər-mər\ *n* : an agent used in veterinary medicine to destroy or expel parasitic worms

Wor·mi·an bone \'wȯr-mē-ən-\ *n* : a small irregular inconstant plate of bone interposed in a suture between large cranial bones — called also *sutural bone*

Worm \'vȯrm\, **Ole** (*Latin* **Olaus Wormius**) (1588–1654), Danish physician. Worm was a professor of medicine at the University of Copenhagen and personal physician to King

Christian V as well. In 1634 he described the small bones that occasionally occur along the lambdoid suture of the human skull.

worm·seed \'wərm-ˌsēd\ *n* **1** : any of various plants whose seeds possess anthelmintic properties: as **a** : any of several artemisias **b** : MEXICAN TEA **2 a** : the fruit of the Mexican tea **b** : SANTONICA; *also* : LEVANT WORMSEED

wormseed oil *n* : CHENOPODIUM OIL

worm·wood \'wərm-ˌwùd\ *n* : ARTEMISIA 2; *esp* : a European plant (*Artemisia absinthium*) yielding a bitter slightly aromatic dark green oil used in absinthe

worse *comparative of* ILL

worst *superlative of* ILL

Woulff bottle \'wùlf-\ *n* : a bottle or jar with two or three necks used in washing or absorbing gases

Woulfe, Peter (1727–1803), British chemist. The Woulff bottle had been known to chemists before Woulfe's time, but the association of the bottle with Woulfe apparently derives from his use of a vessel with two outlets in a series of experiments described in 1767.

¹**wound** \'wünd\ *n* **1 a** : a physical injury to the body consisting of a laceration or breaking of the skin or mucous membrane ⟨has a deep festering knife ∼ across the palm⟩ ⟨a gunshot ∼⟩ **b** : an opening made in the skin or a membrane of the body incidental to a surgical operation or procedure **2** : a mental or emotional hurt or blow

²**wound** *vt* : to cause a wound to or in

wounded *n pl* : wounded persons

WPW syndrome \ˌdəb-ə(l)-(ˌ)yü-ˌpē-'dəb-ə(l)-(ˌ)yü-\ *n* : WOLFF-PARKINSON-WHITE SYNDROME

¹**wrench** \'rench\ *vt* : to injure or disable by a violent twisting or straining ⟨slipped and ∼ed her back⟩

²**wrench** *n* : a sharp twist or sudden jerk straining muscles or ligaments; *also* : the resultant injury (as of a joint)

Wright's stain \'rīts-\ *n* : a stain that is a modification of the Romanowsky stain and is used in staining blood and parasites living in blood

Wright, James Homer (1869–1928), American pathologist. Wright was a professor of pathology at Harvard Medical School and on the staff of Massachusetts General Hospital. He devised several stains for blood cells, among them the well-known Wright's stain (1902).

¹**wrin·kle** \'riŋ-kəl\ *n* : a small ridge or furrow in the skin esp. when due to age, care, or fatigue

²**wrinkle** *vb* **wrin·kled; wrin·kling** \-k(ə-)liŋ\ *vi* : to become marked with or contracted into wrinkles ∼ *vt* : to contract into wrinkles ⟨*wrinkled* skin⟩

Wris·berg's ganglion \'riz-ˌbərgz-, 'vris-ˌberks-\ *n* : a small ganglion that sometimes occurs in the superficial part of the cardiac plexus at the right side of the ligamentum arteriosum

H. A. Wrisberg — see CARTILAGE OF WRISBERG

wrist \'rist\ *n* : the joint or the region of the joint between the human hand and the arm or a corresponding part on a lower animal

wrist·bone \-ˌbōn\ *n* **1** : a carpal bone **2** : the styloid process of the human radius that forms a prominence on the outer side of the wrist above the thumb

wrist–drop \-ˌdräp\ *n* : paralysis of the extensor muscles of the hand causing the hand to hang down at the wrist

wrist joint *n* : the articulation at the wrist

wri·ter's block \'rīt-ərz-\ *n* : a psychological inhibition preventing a writer from proceeding with a piece of writing

writer's cramp *n* : a painful spasmodic cramp of muscles of the hand or fingers brought on by excessive writing — called also *graphospasm*

wry·neck \'rī-ˌnek\ *n* : TORTICOLLIS

ws *abbr* water-soluble

\ə\ abut \ᵊ\ kitten \ər\ further \a\ ash \ā\ ace \ä\ cot, cart
\aù\ out \ch\ chin \e\ bet \ē\ easy \g\ go \i\ hit \ī\ ice \j\ job
\ŋ\ sing \ō\ go \ȯ\ law \ȯi\ boy \th\ thin \th̲\ the \ü\ loot
\ù\ foot \y\ yet \zh\ vision   *See also* Pronunciation Symbols page

U Z

wt *abbr* weight

Wuch·er·e·ria \ˌwük-ə-ˈrir-ē-ə\ *n* : a genus of filarial worms of the family Dipetalonematidae including a parasite (*W. bancrofti*) that causes elephantiasis

Wu·cher·er \ˈvük̲-ər-ər\, **Otto Eduard Heinrich (1820–1873)**, German physician. Wucherer practiced medicine in London, Lisbon, and in several cities in Brazil. In 1866 he discovered hookworms in Brazil. That same year he discov-

ered filarial worms of the genus *Wuchereria* (*W. bancrofti*) in chylous urine.

w/v *abbr* weight in volume — used to indicate that a particular weight of a solid is contained in a particular volume of solution

w/w *abbr* weight in weight — used esp. to indicate that a particular weight of a gas is contained in a particular weight of liquid solution

X

x \ˈeks\ *n, pl* **x's** *or* **xs** *or* **x'es** *or* **xes** \ˈek-səz\ : the basic or monoploid number of chromosomes of a polyploid series : the number contained in a single genome — compare N 1

x *symbol* **1** *cap* halogen atom — used in general formulas (as of trihalomethane CHX₃) **2** power of magnification

Xal·a·tan \ˈzal-ə-ˌtan\ *trademark* — used for a preparation of latanoprost

Xan·ax \ˈzan-ˌaks\ *trademark* — used for a preparation of alprazolam

xan·than gum \ˈzan-thən-\ *n* : a polysaccharide that is produced by fermentation of carbohydrates by a bacterium (*Xanthomonas campestris*) and is a thickening and suspending agent used esp. in pharmaceuticals and prepared foods — called also *xanthan*

xan·thate \ˈzan-ˌthāt\ *n* : a salt or ester of any of various thio acids and esp. $C_3H_6OS_2$

xan·the·las·ma \ˌzan-thə-ˈlaz-mə\ *n* : a xanthoma of the eyelid

xanthelasma pal·pe·bra·rum \-ˌpal-ˌpē-ˈbrer-əm\ *n* : XANTHELASMA

xan·thene \ˈzan-ˌthēn\ *n* **1** : a white crystalline heterocyclic compound $C_{13}H_{10}O$; *also* : an isomer of this that is the parent of the colored forms of the xanthene dyes **2** : any of various derivatives of xanthene

xanthene dye *n* : any of various brilliant fluorescent yellow to pink to bluish red dyes that are characterized by the presence of the xanthene nucleus

xan·thine \ˈzan-ˌthēn\ *n* : a feebly basic compound $C_5H_4N_4O_2$ that occurs esp. in animal or plant tissue, is derived from guanine and hypoxanthine, and yields uric acid on oxidation; *also* : any of various derivatives of this

xanthine oxidase *n* : a crystallizable flavoprotein enzyme containing iron and molybdenum that promotes the oxidation esp. of hypoxanthine and xanthine to uric acid and of many aldehydes to acids — called also *Schardinger enzyme*

xan·tho·chro·mia \ˌzan-thə-ˈkrō-mē-ə\ *n* : xanthochromic discoloration

xan·tho·chro·mic \-ˈkrō-mik\ *adj* : having a yellowish discoloration ⟨~ cerebrospinal fluid⟩

xan·tho·der·ma \ˌzan-thə-ˈdər-mə\ *n* : yellow color of the skin

xan·tho·ma \zan-ˈthō-mə\ *n, pl* **-mas** *also* **-ma·ta** \-mət-ə\ : a fatty irregular yellow patch or nodule containing lipid-filled foam cells that occurs on the skin (as of the eyelids, neck, or back) or in internal tissue and is associated esp. with disturbances of lipid metabolism

xan·tho·ma·to·sis \ˌ(ˌ)zan-ˌthō-mə-ˈtō-səs\ *n, pl* **-to·ses** \-ˌsēz\ : a condition marked by the presence of multiple xanthomas

xan·tho·ma·tous \zan-ˈthō-mət-əs\ *adj* : of, relating to, marked by, or characteristic of a xanthoma or xanthomatosis ⟨~ lesions⟩

xan·thone \ˈzan-ˌthōn\ *n* : a ketone $C_{13}H_8O_2$ that is the parent of several natural yellow pigments

xan·tho·phyll \ˈzan-thə-ˌfil\ *n* : any of several neutral yellow

to orange carotenoid pigments that are oxygen derivatives of carotenes; *esp* : LUTEIN

xan·tho·pro·te·ic test \ˌzan-thə-prō-ˈtē-ik-\ *n* : a test for the detection of proteins in which concentrated nitric acid reacts with the proteins to form a yellow color that is intensified to orange-yellow by the addition of alkali — called also *xanthoproteic reaction*

xan·thop·sia \zan-ˈthäp-sē-ə\ *n* : a visual disturbance in which objects appear yellow

xan·thop·ter·in \zan-ˈthäp-tə-rən\ *n* : a yellow crystalline amphoteric pigment $C_6H_5N_5O_2$ that occurs esp. in the wings of yellow butterflies and also in the urine of mammals and that is convertible into folic acid by the action of various microorganisms

xan·tho·sine \ˈzan-thə-ˌsēn\ *n* : a crystalline nucleoside $C_{10}H_{12}N_4O_6$ that yields xanthine and ribose on hydrolysis

xan·tho·tox·in \ˈzan-thə-ˌtäk-sən\ *n* : METHOXSALEN

xanth·uren·ic acid \ˌzanth-yə-ˌren-ik-\ *n* : a yellow crystalline phenolic acid $C_{10}H_7NO_4$ closely related to kynurenic acid and excreted in the urine when tryptophan is added to the diet of experimental animals deficient in pyridoxine

xan·thy·drol \zan-ˈthī-ˌdrol, -ˌdröl\ *n* : a crystalline secondary alcohol $C_{13}H_{10}O_2$ that is used esp. for the detection of urea with which it forms an insoluble product

X chromosome *n* : a sex chromosome that usu. occurs paired in each female cell and single in each male cell in species in which the male typically has two unlike sex chromosomes — compare Y CHROMOSOME

X–disease *n* : any of various usu. virus diseases of obscure etiology and relationships: as **a** : MURRAY VALLEY ENCEPHALITIS **b** : HYPERKERATOSIS 2b

Xe *symbol* xenon

Xen·i·cal \ˈzen-i-ˌkal\ *trademark* — used for a preparation of orlistat

xe·no·bi·ot·ic \ˌzen-ō-bī-ˈät-ik, ˌzēn-, -bē-\ *n* : a chemical compound (as a drug, pesticide, or carcinogen) that is foreign to a living organism — **xenobiotic** *adj*

xe·no·di·ag·no·sis \ˌzen-ō-ˌdī-ig-ˈnō-səs, ˌzēn-\ *n, pl* **-no·ses** \-ˌsēz\ : the detection of a parasite (as of humans) by feeding supposedly infected material (as blood) to a suitable intermediate host (as an insect) and later examining the intermediate host for the parasite — **xe·no·di·ag·nos·tic** \-ˈnäs-tik\ *adj*

xe·no·ge·ne·ic \ˌzen-ō-jə-ˈnē-ik, ˌzēn-\ *also* **xe·no·gen·ic** \-ˈjen-ik\ *adj* : derived from, originating in, or being a member of another species ⟨~ tissue⟩ — compare ALLOGENEIC, SYNGENEIC

xe·no·graft \ˈzen-ə-ˌgraft, ˈzēn-\ *n* : a graft of tissue taken from a donor of one species and grafted into a recipient of another species — called also *heterograft, heterotransplant, xenotransplant;* compare HOMOGRAFT — **xenograft** *vt*

xe·non \ˈzē-ˌnän, ˈzen-ˌän\ *n* : a heavy, colorless, and relatively inert gaseous element that occurs in air as about one part in 20 million by volume — symbol *Xe*; see ELEMENT table

xe·no·phobe \'zen-ə-ˌfōb, 'zēn-\ *n* : one unduly fearful of what is foreign and esp. of people of foreign origin — **xe·no·pho·bic** \ˌzen-ə-'fō-bik, ˌzēn-\ *adj*

xe·no·pho·bia \ˌzen-ə-'fō-bē-ə, ˌzēn-\ *n* : fear and hatred of strangers or foreigners or of anything that is strange or foreign

xe·no·plas·tic \ˌzen-ə-'plas-tik, ˌzēn-\ *adj* : involving or occurring between distantly related individuals

Xen·op·syl·la \ˌzen-äp-'sil-ə\ *n* : a genus of fleas of the family Pulicidae including several (as the oriental rat flea) that are important as vectors of plague

Xen·o·pus \'zen-ə-pəs\ *n* : a genus of African aquatic frogs including one (*X. laevis*) formerly used in a test for pregnancy

xe·no·trans·plant \ˌzen-ə-'tran(t)s-ˌplant, ˌzēn-\ *n* : XENOGRAFT — **xe·no·trans·plant** \-'tran(t)s-ˌplant\ *vt*

xe·no·trans·plan·ta·tion \-ˌtran(t)s-ˌplan-'tā-shən\ *n* : transplantation of an organ, tissue, or cells between two different species (as a human and a domestic swine)

xe·no·tro·pic \-'träp-ik, -'trō-pik\ *adj* : replicating or reproducing only in cells other than those of the host species ⟨∼ viruses⟩

xe·ro·der·ma \ˌzir-ə-'dər-mə\ *n* : a disease of the skin characterized by dryness and roughness and a fine scaly desquamation

xeroderma pig·men·to·sum \-ˌpig-mən-'tō-səm, -ˌmen-\ *n* : a genetic condition inherited as a recessive autosomal trait that is caused by a defect in mechanisms that repair DNA mutations (as those caused by ultraviolet light) and is characterized by the development of pigment abnormalities and multiple skin cancers in body areas exposed to the sun — abbr. XP

xe·rog·ra·phy \zə-'räg-rə-fē, zir-'äg-\ *n, pl* **-phies 1** : a process for copying graphic matter by the action of light on an electrically charged photoconductive insulating surface in which the latent image is developed with a resinous powder **2** : XERORADIOGRAPHY — **xe·ro·graph·ic** \ˌzir-ə-'graf-ik\ *adj* — **xe·ro·graph·i·cal·ly** \-i-k(ə-)lē\ *adv*

xe·ro·mam·mog·ra·phy \ˌzir-ō-ma-'mäg-rə-fē\ *n, pl* **-phies** : xeroradiography of the breast — **xe·ro·mam·mo·gram** \-'mam-ə-ˌgram\ *n*

xe·roph·thal·mia \ˌzir-ˌäf-'thal-mē-ə, -ˌäp-'thal-\ *n* : a dry thickened lusterless condition of the eyeball resulting esp. from a severe systemic deficiency of vitamin A — compare KERATOMALACIA — **xe·roph·thal·mic** \-mik\ *adj*

xe·ro·ra·dio·graph \ˌzir-ō-'räd-ē-ō-ˌgraf\ *n* : a radiograph produced by xeroradiography

xe·ro·ra·di·og·ra·phy \ˌzir-ō-ˌräd-ē-'äg-rə-fē\ *n, pl* **-phies** : radiography used esp. in mammographic screening for breast cancer that produces an image using X-rays in a manner similar to the way an image is produced by light in xerography — **xe·ro·ra·dio·graph·ic** \-ˌräd-ē-ō-'graf-ik\ *adj*

xe·ro·sis \zi-'rō-səs\ *n, pl* **xe·ro·ses** \-ˌsēz\ : abnormal dryness of a body part or tissue (as the skin or conjunctiva)

xe·ro·sto·mia \ˌzir-ə-'stō-mē-ə\ *n* : abnormal dryness of the mouth due to insufficient secretions — called also *dry mouth*

xi·phi·ster·num \ˌzī-fə-'stər-nəm, ˌzif-ə-\ *n, pl* **-na** \-nə\ : XIPHOID PROCESS

xi·pho·cos·tal \ˌzī-fə-'käs-t°l, ˌzif-ə-\ *adj* : of, relating to, or connecting the xiphoid process and the ribs

xi·phoid \'zī-ˌfòid, 'zif-ˌòid\ *n* : XIPHOID PROCESS — **xiphoid** *adj*

xiphoid cartilage *n* : XIPHOID PROCESS

xiphoid process *n* : the smallest and lowest division of the human sternum that is cartilaginous early in life but becomes more or less ossified during adulthood — called also *ensiform cartilage, ensiform process*

xi·phop·a·gus \zī-'fäp-ə-gəs\ *n* : congenitally joined twins united at the xiphoid process

x-ir·ra·di·a·tion \'eks-\ *n, often cap X* : X-RADIATION 1 — **x-ir·ra·di·ate** *vt* **-at·ed; -at·ing** *often cap X*

X–linked *adj* : located on an X chromosome ⟨an ∼ gene⟩; *also* : transmitted by an X-linked gene ⟨an ∼ disease⟩

XP *abbr* xeroderma pigmentosum

x-ra·di·a·tion *n, often cap X* **1** : exposure to X-rays **2** : radiation composed of X-rays

x-radiograph *n* : X-RAY 2

x-ra·di·og·ra·phy *n, pl* **-phies** *often cap X* : radiography by means of X-rays

x-ray \'eks-ˌrā\ *vt, often cap X* : to examine, treat, or photograph with X-rays

X–ray *n* **1** : any of the electromagnetic radiations of the same nature as visible radiation but of an extremely short wavelength less than 100 angstroms that is produced by bombarding a metallic target with fast electrons in vacuum or by transition of atoms to lower energy states and that has the properties of ionizing a gas upon passage through it, of penetrating various thicknesses of all solids, of producing secondary radiations by impinging on material bodies, of acting on photographic films and plates as light does, and of causing fluorescent screens to emit light — called also *roentgen ray* **2** : a photograph obtained by use of X-rays ⟨a chest X-ray⟩ — **X–ray** *adj*

X–ray crystallography *n* : an analytical technique in which X-ray diffraction is used to obtain information about the identity or structure of a crystalline substance

X–ray diffraction *n* : a scattering of X-rays by the atoms of a crystal that produces an interference effect so that the diffraction pattern gives information on the structure of the crystal or the identity of a crystalline substance

X–ray microscope *n* : an instrument in which X-ray diffraction patterns of crystals are translated into pictures showing the relative positions of the atoms in a crystal as if in a photomicrograph of very high magnification

X–ray therapy *n* : medical treatment (as of cancer) by controlled application of X-rays

X–ray tube *n* : a vacuum tube in which a concentrated stream of electrons from a cathode strikes a metal target and produces X-rays from the side of the tube at right angles in a quantity and intensity that is controlled by the cathode temperature and with a wavelength and hardness that depends upon the voltage applied to the tube terminals

XTC \'ek-stə-sē\ *n* : ECSTASY 2

XX disease \'eks-'eks-\ *n* : HYPERKERATOSIS 2b

xy·lan \'zī-ˌlan\ *n* : a yellow gummy pentosan that yields xylose on hydrolysis and is abundantly present in plant cell walls and woody tissue

xy·la·zine \'zī-lə-ˌzēn\ *n* : a veterinary sedative, analgesic, and muscle relaxant administered in the form of its hydrochloride $C_{12}H_{16}N_2S\cdot HCl$

xy·lene \'zī-ˌlēn\ *n* : any of three toxic flammable oily isomeric aromatic hydrocarbons C_8H_{10} that are dimethyl homologues of benzene and are usu. obtained from petroleum or natural gas distillates; *also* : a commercial mixture of xylenes used chiefly as a solvent

xy·le·nol \'zī-lə-ˌnól, -ˌnōl\ *n* : any of six crystalline isomeric phenols $C_8H_{10}O$ or a mixture of them derived from the xylenes, found in coal tar, and used chiefly as disinfectants and in making phenolic resins — compare CHLOROXYLENOL

xy·li·dine \'zī-lə-ˌdēn\ *n* : any of six toxic liquid or low-melting crystalline compounds $C_8H_{11}N$ that are amino derivatives of the xylenes and are used chiefly as intermediates for azo dyes and in organic synthesis

xy·li·tol \'zī-lə-ˌtòl, -ˌtōl\ *n* : a crystalline alcohol $C_5H_{12}O_5$ that is a derivative of xylose, is obtained esp. from birch bark, and is used as a sweetener

Xy·lo·caine \'zī-lə-ˌkān\ *trademark* — used for a preparation of lidocaine

xy·lol \'zī-ˌlòl, -ˌlōl\ *n* : XYLENE

\ə\ **abut** \ᵊ\ **kitten** \ər\ **further** \a\ **ash** \ā\ **ace** \ä\ **cot, cart**
\aú\ **out** \ch\ **chin** \e\ **bet** \ē\ **easy** \g\ **go** \i\ **hit** \ī\ **ice** \j\ **job**
\ŋ\ **sing** \ō\ **go** \ò\ **law** \òi\ **boy** \th\ **thin** \t͟h\ **the** \ü\ **loot**
\ú\ **foot** \y\ **yet** \zh\ **vision**   *See also* Pronunciation Symbols page

U Z

xy·lo·met·a·zo·line \ˌzī-lə-ˌmet-ə-'zō-ˌlēn\ *n* : a sympathomimetic agent with vasoconstrictive activity that is used in the form of its hydrochloride $C_{16}H_{24}N_2 \cdot HCl$ esp. as a topical nasal decongestant

xy·lose \'zī-ˌlōs, -ˌlōz\ *n* : a crystalline aldose sugar $C_5H_{10}O_5$ that is not fermentable with ordinary yeasts and occurs esp. as a constituent of xylans from which it is obtained by hydrolysis

xy·lo·side \'zī-lə-ˌsīd\ *n* : a glycoside that yields xylose on hydrolysis

xy·lu·lose \'zīl-(y)ə-ˌlōs *also* -ˌlōz\ *n* : a ketose sugar $C_5H_{10}O_5$ of the pentose class that plays a role in carbohydrate metabolism and is found in the urine in cases of pentosuria

xy·lyl \'zī-lil\ *n* : any of several isomeric monovalent radicals C_8H_9 derived from the three xylenes by removal of a hydrogen atom; *esp* : a radical of the formula $(CH_3)_2C_6H_3$

Y

Y *symbol* yttrium

YAC *abbr* yeast artificial chromosome

ya·ge *or* **ya·gé** *or* **ya·je** *or* **ya·jé** \'yä-ˌhā\ *n* : a powerful hallucinogenic beverage prepared from any of several tropical plants (genus *Banisteriopsis* of the family Malpighiaceae)

yaw \'yò\ *n* : one of the lesions characteristic of yaws — see MOTHER YAW

¹**yawn** \'yòn, 'yän\ *vi* : to open the mouth wide and take a deep breath usu. as an involuntary reaction to fatigue or boredom

²**yawn** *n* : an opening of the mouth wide while taking a deep breath often as an involuntary reaction to fatigue or boredom

yaws \'yòz\ *n pl but sing or pl in constr* : an infectious contagious tropical disease that is caused by a spirochete of the genus *Treponema* (*T. pertenue*) and that is characterized by a primary ulcerating lesion on the skin followed by a secondary stage in which ulcers develop all over the body and by a third stage in which the bones are involved — called also *frambesia, pian*

Yb *symbol* ytterbium

Y chromosome \'wī-\ *n* : a sex chromosome that is characteristic of male cells in species in which the male typically has two unlike sex chromosomes — compare X CHROMOSOME

yeast \'yēst\ *n* **1** : a unicellular chiefly ascomycetous fungus (as of the family Saccharomycetaceae) that has usu. little or no mycelium, that typically reproduces asexually by budding, and that includes forms (as *Saccharomyces cerevisiae*) which cause alcoholic fermentation and are used esp. in the making of alcoholic beverages and leavened bread **2** : a yellowish surface froth or sediment that occurs esp. in sugary fermenting liquids (as fruit juices) and consists chiefly of yeast cells and carbon dioxide **3** : a commercial product containing yeast cells in a moist or dry medium — **yeast·like** \-ˌlīk\ *adj*

yeast artificial chromosome *n* : a chromosome that is used esp. to clone DNA segments longer than those capable of being cloned in bacteria, that is introduced for cloning into a yeast of the genus *Saccharomyces* (*S. cerevisiae*), that contains a centromere, a telomere, and a replication initiation site suitable for use in the yeast, and into which a segment of foreign DNA up to about a million base pairs in length has been spliced for cloning — abbr. *YAC*

yeast infection *n* : an infection of the vagina with an overgrowth of a yeastlike fungus of the genus *Candida* (*C. albicans*) normally present in the vaginal flora and characterized by vaginal discharge and vulvovaginitis; *broadly* : an infection (as thrush or tinea versicolor) caused by a yeast or yeastlike fungus

yeast nucleic acid *n* : RNA

yel·low bile \'yel-ō-\ *n* : the one of the four humors of ancient and medieval physiology that was believed to be secreted by the liver and to cause irascibility

yellow body *n* : CORPUS LUTEUM

yellow cinchona *n* : CALISAYA BARK

yellow enzyme *n* : any of several yellow flavoprotein respiratory enzymes

yellow fat disease *n* : a disease esp. of swine, cats, and ranch-raised mink that is associated with a deficiency of vi-

tamin E and is marked by inflammation of the fatty tissue, subcutaneous edema, and varied visceral lesions — called also *steatitis, yellow fat*

yellow fever *n* : an acute infectious disease of warm regions (as sub-Saharan Africa and tropical South America) marked by sudden onset, prostration, fever, and headache and sometimes albuminuria, jaundice, and hemorrhage and caused by a single-stranded RNA virus of the genus *Flavivirus* (species *Yellow fever virus*) transmitted esp. by the yellow-fever mosquito — called also *yellow jack*

yellow–fever mosquito *n* : a small dark-colored mosquito of the genus *Aedes* (*A. aegypti*) that is the usual vector of yellow fever — called also *tiger mosquito*

yellow flag \-'flag\ *n* : QUARANTINE FLAG

yellow jack *n* **1** : YELLOW FEVER **2** : QUARANTINE FLAG

yellow jacket *n* **1** : any of various yellow-marked social wasps (esp. genus *Vespula* of the family Vespidae) that usu. nest in the ground, aggressively defend their nests, and can sting repeatedly and painfully **2** *slang* : pentobarbital esp. in a yellow capsule — usu. used in pl.

yellow jes·sa·mine \-'jes-(ə-)mən\ *n* : a twining evergreen shrub of the genus *Gelsemium* (*G. sempervirens*) with fragrant yellow flowers and a root formerly used in medicine — called also *yellow jasmine;* see GELSEMIUM 2

yellow marrow *n* : BONE MARROW a

yellow petrolatum *n* : PETROLATUM a

yellow precipitate *n* : yellow mercuric oxide used esp. formerly in ophthalmic ointments

yellow rain \-'rān\ *n* : a yellow substance that has occurred in southeastern Asia as a mist or as spots on rocks and vegetation and has been held to be a biological warfare agent used in the Vietnam War but appears upon scientific examination to be identical to the pollen-laden feces of bees

yel·lows \'yel-(ˌ)ōz\ *n pl but sing or pl in constr* : any of several diseases of domestic animals (as sheep) that are characterized by jaundice

yellow spot *n* : MACULA LUTEA

yellow wax *n* : a wax obtained as a yellow to brown solid by melting a honeycomb with boiling water, straining, and cooling and used esp. in polishes, modeling, ointments, and making patterns — called also *beeswax, cera flava*

yer·ba ma·té \ˌyer-bə-'mä-ˌtā, ˌyər-\ *n* : MATÉ

yerba san·ta \-'sän-tə, -'san-\ *n* : an evergreen shrub of the genus *Eriodictyon* (*E. californicum*) of California whose aromatic dried leaves are used as an expectorant and to mask the bitter taste of various drugs; *also* : ERIODICTYON 2

yer·sin·ia \yər-'sin-ē-ə\ *n* **1** *cap* : a genus of gram-negative bacteria of the family Enterobacteriaceae that includes several important pathogens (as the plague bacterium, *Y. pestis*) affecting animals and humans and formerly included in the genus *Pasteurella* — see PLAGUE 2 **2** : any bacterium of the genus *Yersinia*

    Yer·sin \yer-saⁿ\, **Alexandre–Émile–John (1863–1943),** French bacteriologist. Yersin studied bacteriology under Émile Roux in Paris and Robert Koch in Berlin. Later, in Hong Kong, he and Kitasato Shibasaburo independently discovered the plague bacillus at about the same time. In 1944 the genus *Yersinia* containing the plague bacillus (*Y. pestis*) was named after Yersin.

yer·sin·i·o·sis \yər-ˌsin-ē-ˈō-səs\ n : infection with or disease caused by a bacterium of the genus *Yersinia* (as *Y. pseudotuberculosis*); *esp* : an infectious disease that is caused by a yersinia (*Y. enterocolitica*) transmitted chiefly in contaminated water and food or raw or undercooked pork products and that is marked esp. by fever, abdominal pain, and diarrhea

yew \ˈyü\ n : any of a genus (*Taxus* of the family Taxaceae, the yew family) of evergreen trees and shrubs with stiff linear leaves and seeds surrounded by a fleshy red aril; *esp* : one (*T. brevifolia*) of the Pacific coast of the U.S. and Canada whose bark yields the antineoplastic drug paclitaxel

Y ligament n : ILIOFEMORAL LIGAMENT

yo·ga \ˈyō-gə\ n **1** *cap* : a Hindu theistic philosophy teaching the suppression of all activity of body, mind, and will in order that the self may realize its distinction from them and attain liberation **2** : a system of physical postures, breathing techniques, and meditation derived from Yoga but often practiced independently esp. in Western cultures to promote bodily or mental control and well-being — see HATHA YOGA — **yo·gic** \-gik\ adj

yo·gurt *also* **yo·ghurt** \ˈyō-gərt\ n : a fermented slightly acid often flavored semisolid food made of milk and milk solids to which cultures of bacteria of the genus *Lactobacillus* (*L. bulgarius*) and *Streptococcus* (*S. thermophilus*) have been added

yo·him·be \yō-ˈhim-bā, yə-, -bē\ n : a tropical African tree (*Pausinystalia yohimbe* syn. *Corynanthe yohimbe*) of the madder family whose bark yields the alkaloid yohimbine; *also* : a preparation of the bark that is used esp. as an aphrodisiac

yo·him·bine \yō-ˈhim-ˌbēn, -bən\ n : an alkaloid obtained from the bark of yohimbe that is a weak blocker of alpha-adrenergic receptors and has been used in the form of its hydrochloride $C_{21}H_{26}N_2O_3 \cdot HCl$ as a mydriatic and aphrodisiac and to treat male impotence — called also *quebrachine*

yoked \ˈyōkt\ adj : relating to or being a control organism or group that is subjected to stimuli at the same time or on the same schedule as the subject of an experiment

yolk \ˈyōk\ n : material stored in an ovum that supplies food to the developing embryo and consists chiefly of proteins, lecithin, and cholesterol

yolk plug n : a mass of yolk cells found in the blastopore of the embryos of some vertebrates

yolk sac n : a membranous sac of most vertebrates that is attached to an embryo and encloses the yolk, that is continuous in most forms including humans through the omphalomesenteric duct with the intestinal cavity of the embryo, that is abundantly supplied with blood vessels which transport nutritive yolk products to the developing embryo, and that in placental mammals is nearly vestigial and functions chiefly prior to the formation of the placenta

yolk stalk n : OMPHALOMESENTERIC DUCT

young \ˈyəŋ\ n, pl **young** **1** : immature offspring — used esp. of animals **2** : a single recently born or hatched animal — **with young** : PREGNANT — used of a female animal

Young–Helm·holtz theory \ˈyəŋ-ˈhelm-ˌhōlts-\ n : a theory in color vision: the eye has three separate elements each of which is stimulated by a different primary color

Young, Thomas (1773–1829), British physician, physicist, and Egyptologist. Young is remembered for his efforts to win broad acceptance for the undulatory theory of light. His research led him to the discovery of accommodation, the means by which the lens of the eye changes shape to focus on objects at differing distances, and to the discovery in 1801 of the cause of astigmatism. He also studied the problem of color perception and proposed that the eye does not have or need a separate mechanism for every individual color but only for three: blue, green, and red. Young's modulus was first defined by him in a lecture on passive strength and friction that appeared in print in 1807. Young is equally famous for being one of the first to translate Egyptian hieroglyphics. He began studying the Rosetta Stone in 1814, and after obtaining additional hieroglyphic writings from other sources, he produced a nearly accurate translation within a few years. His work was a major contribution to the deciphering of the ancient Egyptian language.

Helmholtz, Hermann Ludwig Ferdinand von (1821–1894), German physicist and physiologist. Helmholtz made fundamental contributions to physiology, optics, electrodynamics, and meteorology. He is best known for his statement of the conservation of energy, which he presented in 1847. He invented the ophthalmoscope in 1851, and he determined the mechanisms of focusing in the eye and of the motion of the eyeballs to give single vision. In 1852 he revived the theory of color vision that Young had first postulated in 1801—only to refute it. In 1858 he reversed his position, amending Young's original theory and becoming its foremost advocate. He also examined the structure and function of the organs and bones of the ear and developed the theory that harmonics are determinants of musical tone.

Young's modulus \ˈyəŋz-\ n : the ratio of the tensile stress in a material to the corresponding tensile strain

yo-yo di·et·ing \ˈyō-(ˌ)yō-ˈdī-ət-in\ n : the practice of repeatedly losing weight by dieting and subsequently regaining it

yper·ite \ˈē-pə-ˌrīt\ n : MUSTARD GAS

yt·ter·bi·um \i-ˈtər-bē-əm\ n : a bivalent or trivalent metallic element of the rare-earth group that resembles yttrium and occurs with it and related elements in several minerals — symbol *Yb*; see ELEMENT table

yt·tri·um \ˈi-trē-əm\ n : a trivalent metallic element usu. included among the rare earth elements which it resembles chemically and with which it occurs in minerals — symbol *Y*; see ELEMENT table

yup·pie flu \ˈyəp-ē-\ n : CHRONIC FATIGUE SYNDROME

Z

Z *symbol* **1** atomic number **2** impedance

za·fir·lu·kast \zə-ˈfir-lü-ˌkast, ˌza-fir-ˈlü\ n : an anti-asthma drug $C_{31}H_{33}N_3O_6S$ that is administered orally and tends to inhibit bronchoconstriction caused by certain allergenic substances

zal·cit·a·bine \zal-ˈsit-ə-ˌbēn, -ˌbin\ n : DDC

zal·e·plon \ˈzal-ə-ˌplän\ n : a sedative and hypnotic drug $C_{17}H_{15}N_5O$ used in the treatment of insomnia

za·nam·i·vir \zə-ˈnam-ə-ˌvir\ n : an antiviral drug $C_{12}H_{20}N_4O_7$ administered by oral inhalation in the treatment of influenza A and B

Zan·tac \ˈzan-ˌtak\ *trademark* — used for a preparation of the hydrochloride of ranitidine

Z–DNA \ˈzē-\ n : the left-handed uncommon form of double helix DNA in which the chains twist up and to the left around the front of the axis of the helix and which has 12 base pairs in each helical turn and one groove on the external surface — compare B-DNA

ZDV \ˌzē-(ˌ)dē-ˈvē\ n : AZT

ze·a·tin \ˈzē-ət-ən\ n : a cytokinin first isolated from the endosperm of Indian corn

ze·a·xan·thin \ˌzē-ə-ˈzan-thən\ n : a yellow crystalline carot-

\ə\ **abut**	\ᵊ\ **kitten**	\ər\ **further**	\a\ **ash**	\ā\ **ace**	\ä\ **cot, cart**
\aů\ **out**	\ch\ **chin**	\e\ **bet**	\ē\ **easy**	\g\ **go**	\i\ **hit**	\ī\ **ice**	\j\ **job**
\ŋ\ **sing**	\ō\ **go**	\ȯ\ **law**	\ȯi\ **boy**	\th\ **thin**	\t͟h\ **the**	\ü\ **loot**
\ů\ **foot**	\y\ **yet**	\zh\ **vision**	*See also* Pronunciation Symbols page

U
Z

enoid alcohol $C_{40}H_{56}O_2$ that is isomeric with lutein and occurs widely with it and that is the chief pigment of yellow Indian corn

zed·o·ary \\'zed-ə-ˌwer-ē\ *n, pl* **-ar·ies** : the dried rhizome of an Indian plant (*Curcuma zedoaria*) of the ginger family that has a bitter taste and is used medicinally esp. as an intestinal stimulant and carminative

Zei·gar·nik effect \zī-'gär-nik-\ *n* : the psychological tendency to remember an uncompleted task rather than a completed one

> **Zeigarnik, Bluma (1900–1988)**, Russian psychologist. Zeigarnik first described the Zeigarnik effect in her 1927 doctoral thesis.

ze·in \\'zē-ən\ *n* : a protein from Indian corn that lacks lysine and tryptophan

zeit·ge·ber \\'tsīt-ˌgā-bər, 'zīt-\ *n* : an environmental agent or event (as the occurrence of light or dark) that provides the stimulus setting or resetting a biological clock of an organism

Zen·ker's degeneration \\'tseŋ-kərz-, 'zeŋ-\ *n* : hyaline degeneration of voluntary muscles associated with severe infectious diseases (as typhoid fever) — called also *waxy degeneration*

> **Zen·ker** \\'tseŋ-kər\, **Friedrich Albert von (1825–1898)**, German pathologist and anatomist. Zenker held professorships at Dresden and Erlengen, Germany. He introduced Zenker's fluid in 1894.

Zenker's diverticulum *n* : an abnormal pouch in the upper part of the esophagus in which food may become trapped causing bad breath, irritation, difficulty in swallowing, and regurgitation — called also *pharyngoesophageal diverticulum;* compare PULSION DIVERTICULUM

Zenker's fluid *n* : a fixing fluid used in histological technique that is composed of potassium dichromate, mercuric chloride, sodium sulfate, glacial acetic acid, and water

Zenker's necrosis *n* : ZENKER'S DEGENERATION

ze·o·lite \\'zē-ə-ˌlīt\ *n* : any of various hydrous silicates that can act as ion exchangers; *also* : any of various natural or synthesized silicates of similar structure used in water softening and as adsorbents — **ze·o·lit·ic** \ˌzē-ə-'lit-ik\ *adj*

Zeph·i·ran \\'zef-ə-ˌran\ *trademark* — used for a preparation of benzalkonium chloride

ze·ro \\'zē-(ˌ)rō, 'zi(ə)r-(ˌ)ō\ *n, pl* **zeros** *also* **zeroes** **1** : the arithmetical symbol 0 or Ø denoting the absence of all magnitude or quantity **2 a** : the point of departure in reckoning; *specif* : the point from which the graduation of a scale (as of a thermometer) begins **b** : the temperature represented by the zero mark on a thermometer

Zes·tril \\'zes-tril\ *trademark* — used for a preparation of lisinopril

Zet·ia \\'zet-ē-ə\ *trademark* — used for a preparation of ezetimibe

zi·con·o·tide \zī-'kän-ō-ˌtīd\ *n* : a calcium channel blocker $C_{102}H_{172}N_{36}O_{32}S_7$ with analgesic and neuroprotective effects that has been used to relieve chronic intractable pain and is a synthetic analog of a constituent of the venom of a tropical marine snail of the genus *Conus* (*C. magus*)

zi·do·vu·dine \zī-'dō-v(y)ü-ˌdēn\ *n* : AZT

Ziehl–Neel·sen stain \\'tsēl-'nāl-sən-\ *n* : a carbolfuchsin stain used esp. for detecting the tubercle bacillus

> **Ziehl, Franz (1857–1926)**, German bacteriologist. A professor in Lübeck, Ziehl introduced the carbolfuchsin stain for the tubercle bacillus in 1882.
>
> **Neelsen, Friedrich Carl Adolf (1854–1894)**, German pathologist. Neelsen published a handbook of staining methods in 1892.

ZIFT *abbr* zygote intrafallopian transfer

zi·leu·ton \zī-'lüt-ᵊn\ *n* : an anti-asthma drug $C_{11}H_{12}N_2O_2S$ that is administered orally and acts by inhibiting the lipoxygenase catalyzing the formation of leukotrienes

zi·mel·i·dine \zi-'mel-ə-ˌdēn\ *n* : a bicyclic antidepressant drug $C_{16}H_{17}BrN_2$

zinc \\'ziŋk\ *n* : a bluish white crystalline bivalent metallic element of low to intermediate hardness that is an essential mi

cronutrient for both plants and animals — symbol *Zn*; see ELEMENT table

zinc carbonate *n* : a crystalline salt $ZnCO_3$ having astringent and antiseptic properties

zinc chloride *n* : a poisonous caustic deliquescent readily soluble salt $ZnCl_2$ that is used as a catalyst in organic synthesis and as a disinfectant and astringent

zinc finger *n* : any of a class of proteins that typically possess tandem repeats of fingerlike loops of amino acids with each loop containing a zinc-binding site at its base consisting of two molecules of cysteine and two molecules of histidine and that regulates transcription by binding to specific regions of a gene's DNA; *also* : one of the fingerlike amino acid loops of such a protein

zinc ointment *n* : ZINC OXIDE OINTMENT

zinc oxide *n* : a white solid ZnO used in pharmaceutical and cosmetic preparations (as ointments and powders)

zinc oxide ointment *n* : an ointment that contains about 20 percent zinc oxide and is used in treating skin disorders

zinc peroxide *n* : any of various white to yellowish white powders that have the peroxide ZnO_2 of zinc as their chief ingredient and are used chiefly as disinfectants, astringents, and deodorants

zinc phosphide *n* : a dark gray powdery compound Zn_3P_2 having an odor resembling that of garlic and used as a rodenticide

zinc picolinate *n* : a biologically active zinc salt $C_{12}H_8N_2O_4Zn$ containing two picolinic acid ligands that is used as a dietary supplement

zinc pyr·i·thi·one \-ˌpir-i-'thī-ˌōn\ *n* : an antibacterial and antifungal compound $C_{10}H_8N_2O_2S_2Zn$ that is nearly insoluble in water, possesses cytostatic activity against epidermal cells, and is the active ingredient in various shampoos used to control dandruff and seborrheic dermatitis — called also *pyrithione zinc*

zinc stearate *n* : an insoluble salt usu. of commercial stearic acid and usu. containing some zinc oxide that has astringent and antiseptic properties and is used as a constituent of ointments and powders

zinc sulfate *n* : a crystalline salt $ZnSO_4$ used in medicine as an astringent, emetic, and weak antiseptic

zinc undecylenate *n* : a fine white powder $C_{22}H_{38}O_4Zn$ that is used as a fungistatic agent in powders, ointments, and aerosols

zinc white *n* : ZINC OXIDE

zir·co·ni·um \(ˌ)zər-'kō-nē-əm\ *n* : a steel-gray strong ductile chiefly tetravalent metallic element with a high melting point — symbol *Zr*; see ELEMENT table

zit \\'zit\ *n, slang* : PIMPLE 1

Zith·ro·max \\'zith-rō-ˌmaks\ *trademark* — used for a preparation of azithromycin

Z line *n* : any of the dark bands across a striated muscle fiber that mark the junction of actin filaments in adjacent sarcomeres

Zn *symbol* zinc

Zo·cor \\'zō-ˌkȯr\ *trademark* — used for a preparation of simvastatin

Zo·fran \\'zō-ˌfran\ *trademark* — used for a preparation of the hydrated hydrochloride of ondansetron

Zol·ling·er–El·li·son syndrome \\'zäl-iŋ-ər-'el-i-sən-\ *n* : a syndrome consisting of fulminant intractable peptic ulcers, gastric hypersecretion and hyperacidity, and the occurrence of gastrinomas of the pancreatic cells of the islets of Langerhans

> **Zollinger, Robert Milton (1903–1992)**, American surgeon. Zollinger served for many years as professor and chief of surgical services at the medical school of Ohio State University. He was also editor in chief of the *American Journal of Surgery*.
>
> **Ellison, Edwin Homer (1918–1970)**, American surgeon. Ellison was a professor of surgery at Marquette University's medical school. His fields of research included blood volume studies in surgical patients, hormones of the pancreas, pathogenesis of ulcers, and nutrition in surgical patients.

zol·mi·trip·tan \ˌzōl-mi-'trip-ˌtan\ *n* : a triptan $C_{16}H_{21}N_3O_2$ administered orally to treat migraine headaches

Zo·loft \'zō-ˌlȯft\ *trademark* — used for a preparation of the hydrochloride of sertraline

zol·pi·dem \'zōl-pə-ˌdem\ *n* : a sedative and hypnotic drug administered orally in the form of its tartrate $(C_{19}H_{21}N_3O)_2 \cdot C_4H_6O_6$ in the short-term treatment of insomnia — see AMBIEN

Zo·max \'zō-ˌmaks\ *n* : a preparation of zomepirac — formerly a U.S. registered trademark

zo·me·pir·ac \ˌzō-mə-'pir-ˌak\ *n* : a compound $C_{15}H_{13}ClNNaO_3 \cdot 2H_2O$ formerly used as an anti-inflammatory and analgesic agent but now withdrawn from use because of its link to life-threatening anaphylactic reactions — see ZOMAX

zo·na \'zō-nə\ *n, pl* **zo·nae** \-ˌnē *also* -ˌnī\ *or* **zonas** **1** : an anatomical zone or layer; *esp* : ZONA PELLUCIDA **2** : SHINGLES

zona fas·cic·u·la·ta \-fa-ˌsik-yə-'lāt-ə\ *n* : the middle of the three layers of the adrenal cortex that consists of radially arranged columnar epithelial cells

zona glo·mer·u·lo·sa \-ˌglō-ˌmer-yə-'lō-sə\ *n* : the outermost of the three layers of the adrenal cortex that consists of round masses of granular epithelial cells that stain deeply — called also *glomerulosa*

zona in·cer·ta \-in-'sərt-ə\ *n* : a flat thin layer of gray matter located in the dorsal part of the subthalamus

zon·al \'zōn-ᵊl\ *adj* : of, relating to, affecting, or having the form of a zone ⟨a ∼ boundary⟩

zona pel·lu·ci·da \-pə-'lü-sə-də\ *n* : the transparent more or less elastic noncellular glycoprotein outer layer or envelope of a mammalian ovum often traversed by numerous radiating striae

zona re·tic·u·lar·is \-re-ˌtik-yə-'lar-əs\ *n* : the innermost of the three layers of the adrenal cortex that consists of irregularly arranged cylindrical masses of epithelial cells

zone \'zōn\ *n* **1** : an encircling anatomical structure **2** : a region or area set off as distinct

zo·nu·la \'zōn-yə-lə\ *n, pl* **-lae** \-ˌlē\ *or* **-las** : ZONULE OF ZINN

zonula cil·i·ar·is \-ˌsil-ē-'ar-əs\ *n* : ZONULE OF ZINN

zo·nu·lar \'zōn-yə-lər\ *adj* **1** : of, relating to, or affecting an anatomical zone **2** : of or relating to the zonule of Zinn ⟨∼ attachments⟩

zonularia — see SPATIA ZONULARIA

zon·ule \'zōn-ˌyül\ *n* : ZONULE OF ZINN

zonule of Zinn \-'tsin\ *n* : the suspensory ligament of the crystalline lens of the eye — called also *ciliary zonule, zonula, zonula ciliaris*

J. G. Zinn — see LIGAMENT OF ZINN

zo·nu·ly·sis \ˌzōn-yə-'lī-səs\ *n, pl* **-ly·ses** \-ˌsēz\ : the use of enzymes to dissolve the zonule of Zinn in order to facilitate cataract removal

zoo·eras·tia \ˌzō-ə-ē-'ras-tē-ə\ *n* : BESTIALITY

zoo·eras·ty \'zō-(ə-)ē-ˌras-tē\ *n, pl* **-ties** : BESTIALITY

zoo·ge·og·ra·pher \ˌzō-ə-jē-'äg-rə-fər\ *n* : a person who specializes in zoogeography

zoo·ge·og·ra·phy \ˌzō-ə-jē-'äg-rə-fē\ *n, pl* **-phies** : a branch of biogeography concerned with the geographical distribution of animals and esp. with the determination of the areas characterized by special groups of animals and the study of the causes and significance of such groups — **zoo·geo·graph·ic** \-ˌjē-ə-'graf-ik\ *or* **zoo·geo·graph·i·cal** \-i-kəl\ *adj* — **zoo·geo·graph·i·cal·ly** \-i-k(ə-)lē\ *adv*

zo·o·glea *or chiefly Brit* **zo·o·gloea** \ˌzō-ə-'glē-ə\ *n, pl* **-gle·as** *or* **-gle·ae** *or chiefly Brit* **-gloe·as** *or* **-gloe·ae** \-'glē-ˌē\ : a gelatinous or mucilaginous mass that is characteristic of the growth of various bacteria when growing in fluid media rich in organic material and is made up of the bodies of the bacteria embedded in a matrix of swollen confluent capsule substance — **zo·o·gle·al** *or chiefly Brit* **zo·o·gloe·al** \-'glē-əl\ *adj*

zoo·graft·ing \'zō-ə-ˌgraft-iŋ\ *n* : the use of animal tissue in surgical grafting

zo·oid \'zō-ˌȯid\ *n* : one of the asexually produced individuals of a compound organism (as a coral colony)

zoo·log·i·cal \ˌzō-ə-'läj-i-kəl\ *also* **zoo·log·ic** \-ik\ *adj* **1** : of, relating to, or occupied with zoology **2** : of, relating to, or affecting lower animals often as distinguished from humans ⟨∼ infections⟩

zo·ol·o·gist \zō-'äl-ə-jəst\ *n* : a specialist in zoology

zo·ol·o·gy \zō-'äl-ə-jē\ *n, pl* **-gies** **1** : a branch of biology that deals with the classification and the properties and vital phenomena of animals **2** : the properties and vital phenomena exhibited by an animal, animal type, or group

zoo·no·sis \ˌzō-ə-'nō-səs, zō-'än-ə-səs\ *n, pl* **-no·ses** \-ˌsēz\ : a disease communicable from animals to humans under natural conditions — **zoo·not·ic** \ˌzō-ə-'nät-ik\ *adj*

zoo·par·a·site \ˌzō-ə-'par-ə-ˌsīt\ *n* : a parasitic animal — **zoo·par·a·sit·ic** \-ˌpar-ə-'sit-ik\ *adj*

zo·oph·a·gous \zō-'äf-ə-gəs\ *adj* : feeding on animals : CARNIVOROUS

zoo·phil·ia \ˌzō-ə-'fil-ē-ə\ *n* : an erotic fixation on animals that may result in sexual excitement through real or fancied contact

zoo·phil·ic \ˌzō-ə-'fil-ik\ *adj* : having an attraction to or preference for animals: as **a** : affected with zoophilia **b** *of an insect* : preferring lower animals to humans as a source of food ⟨∼ mosquitoes⟩

zo·oph·i·lism \zō-'äf-ə-ˌliz-əm\ *n* : attraction to or preference for animals: as **a** : ZOOPHILIA **b** : preference by an insect of lower animals to humans as a source of food

zo·oph·i·lous \zō-'äf-ə-ləs\ *adj* : ZOOPHILIC ⟨a ∼ mosquito⟩

zo·oph·i·ly \zō-'äf-ə-lē\ *n, pl* **-lies** : ZOOPHILIA

zoo·pho·bia \ˌzō-ə-'fō-bē-ə\ *n* : abnormal fear of animals

zoo·phyte \'zō-ə-ˌfīt\ *n* : an invertebrate animal (as a coral or sponge) more or less resembling a plant in appearance or mode of growth

zoo·spo·ran·gi·um \ˌzō-ə-spə-'ran-jē-əm\ *n, pl* **-gia** \-jē-ə\ : a sporangium bearing zoospores

zoo·spore \'zō-ə-ˌspō(ə)r, -ˌspȯ(ə)r\ *n* : an independently motile spore; *esp* : a motile usu. naked and flagellated asexual spore esp. of an alga or lower fungus — **zoo·spor·ic** \ˌzō-ə-'spȯr-ik, -'spȯr-\ *adj*

zo·os·ter·ol \zō-'äs-tə-ˌrȯl, -ˌrōl\ *n* : any of a group of sterols (as cholesterol or coprostanol) of animal origin — compare PHYTOSTEROL

zoo·tech·ni·cal \ˌzō-ə-'tek-ni-kəl\ *also* **zoo·tech·nic** \-nik\ *adj* : of or relating to zootechnics

zo·o·tech·ni·cian \-tek-'nish-ən\ *n* : a specialist in zootechnics

zoo·tech·nics \ˌzō-ə-'tek-niks\ *n pl but sing or pl in constr* : the scientific art of maintaining and improving animals under domestication that includes breeding, genetics, nutrition, and housing : the technology of animal husbandry

zo·ot·omy \zō-'ät-ə-mē\ *n, pl* **-mies** : animal anatomy esp. as studied on a comparative basis

zoo·tro·phic \ˌzō-ə-'trō-fik\ *adj* : HETEROTROPHIC

zos·ter \'zäs-tər\ *n* : SHINGLES

zos·ter·i·form \zäs-'ter-ə-ˌfȯrm\ *adj* : resembling shingles ⟨a ∼ rash⟩

Zos·trix *trademark* — used for a preparation containing capsaicin

Zo·vi·rax \zō-'vī-ˌraks\ *trademark* — used for a preparation of acyclovir

zox·a·zol·amine \ˌzäk-sə-'zäl-ə-ˌmēn\ *n* : a drug $C_7H_5ClN_2O$ used esp. formerly as a skeletal muscle relaxant and uricosuric agent

ZPG *abbr* zero population growth

Z–plas·ty \'zē-ˌplas-tē\ *n, pl* **-ties** : a surgical procedure for the repair of constricted scar tissue in which a Z-shaped incision is made in the skin and the two resulting flaps are interposed

Zr *symbol* zirconium

\ə\ abut \ᵊ\ kitten \ər\ further \a\ ash \ā\ ace \ä\ cot, cart \au̇\ out \ch\ chin \e\ bet \ē\ easy \g\ go \i\ hit \ī\ ice \j\ job \ŋ\ sing \ō\ go \ȯ\ law \ȯi\ boy \th\ thin \t͟h\ the \ü\ loot \u̇\ foot \y\ yet \zh\ vision *See also* Pronunciation Symbols page

zwit·ter·ion \'tsvit-ər-ˌī-ˌän also 'zwit-\ n : a dipolar ion — **zwit·ter·ion·ic** \ˌtsvit-ər-ī-'än-ik\ adj

Zy·ban \'zī-ˌban\ trademark — used for a preparation of the hydrochloride of bupropion

zyg·a·de·nine \ˌzig-ə-'dē-ˌnēn\ n : a crystalline alkaloid $C_{27}H_{43}NO_7$ that is obtained from plants of a genus (*Zigadenus*) of the lily family (Liliaceae)

zyg·apoph·y·sis \ˌzī-gə-'päf-ə-səs\ n, pl **-y·ses** \-ˌsēz\ : any of the articular processes of the neural arch of a vertebra of which there are usu. two anterior and two posterior

zyg·i·on \'zig-ē-ˌän, 'zij-\ n, pl **zyg·ia** \-ē-ə\ also **zygions** : a craniometric point at either end of the bizygomatic diameter

zy·goc·i·ty \zī-'gäs-ət-ē\ n, pl **-ties** : the number of ova from which a pair of twins are derived : the condition of being monozygotic or dizygotic

zy·go·dac·tyl \ˌzī-gə-'dak-t³l\ adj : SYNDACTYL

zy·go·dac·ty·ly \-'dak-tə-lē\ n, pl **-lies** : SYNDACTYLY

zy·go·gen·e·sis \ˌzī-gō-'jen-ə-səs\ n, pl **-e·ses** \-ˌsēz\ : reproduction by means of specialized germ cells or gametes : sexual and biparental reproduction

zy·goid \'zī-ˌgoid\ adj : DIPLOID

zy·go·ma \zī-'gō-mə\ n, pl **-ma·ta** \-mət-ə\ also **-mas** 1 : ZYGOMATIC ARCH 2 : ZYGOMATIC BONE

¹zy·go·mat·ic \ˌzī-gə-'mat-ik\ adj : of, relating to, constituting, or situated in the region of the zygomatic bone and the zygomatic arch ⟨a ∼ reconstruction involving multiple bone grafts⟩

²zygomatic n : ZYGOMATIC BONE

zygomatic arch n : the arch of bone that extends along the front or side of the skull beneath the orbit and that is formed by the union of the temporal process of the zygomatic bone in front with the zygomatic process of the temporal bone behind

zygomatic bone n : a bone of the side of the face below the eye that in mammals forms part of the zygomatic arch and part of the orbit and articulates with the temporal, sphenoid, and frontal bones and with the maxilla of the upper jaw — called also *cheekbone, jugal, malar bone, zygoma*

zygomatic nerve n : a branch of the maxillary nerve that divides into a facial branch supplying the skin of the prominent part of the cheek and a temporal branch supplying the skin of the anterior temporal region

zy·go·mat·i·co·fa·cial \ˌzī-gə-ˌmat-i-kō-'fā-shəl\ adj 1 : of, relating to, or being the branch of the zygomatic nerve that supplies the skin of the prominent part of the cheek 2 : of, relating to, or being a foramen in the zygomatic bone that gives passage to the zygomaticofacial branch of the zygomatic nerve

zy·go·mat·i·co·max·il·lary \-'mak-sə-ˌler-ē, chiefly Brit -mak-'sil-ə-rē\ adj : of, relating to, or uniting the zygomatic bone and the maxilla of the upper jaw ⟨the ∼ suture⟩

zy·go·mat·i·co·tem·po·ral \-'tem-p(ə-)rəl\ adj 1 : of, relating to, or uniting the zygomatic arch and the temporal bone ⟨the ∼ suture⟩ 2 a : of, relating to, or being the branch of the zygomatic nerve that supplies the skin of the anterior temporal region ⟨the zygomatic nerve divides into ∼ and zygomaticofacial branches⟩ b : of, relating to, or being a foramen in the zygomatic bone that gives passage to the zygomaticotemporal branch of the zygomatic nerve

zygomatic process n : any of several bony processes that articulate with the zygomatic bone: as a : a long slender process of the temporal bone helping to form the zygomatic arch b : a narrow process of the frontal bone articulating with the zygomatic bone c : a rough triangular eminence of the maxilla of the upper jaw articulating with the zygomatic bone

zy·go·mat·i·cus \ˌzī-gə-'mat-i-kəs\ n 1 : ZYGOMATICUS MAJOR 2 : ZYGOMATICUS MINOR

zygomaticus major n : a slender band of muscle on each side of the face that arises from the zygomatic bone, inserts into the orbicularis oris and skin at the corner of the mouth, and acts to pull the corner of the mouth upward and backward when smiling or laughing

zygomaticus minor n : a slender band of muscle on each side of the face that arises from the zygomatic bone, inserts into the upper lip between the zygomaticus major and the levator labii superioris, and acts to raise the upper lip upward and laterally

Zy·go·my·ce·tes \ˌzī-gō-mī-'sēt-ēz\ n pl : a subclass of fungi of the class Phycomycetes characterized by gametangia that are morphologically alike and by sexually produced zygospores — **zy·go·my·ce·tous** \-'sēt-əs\ adj

zy·gos·i·ty \zī-'gäs-ət-ē\ n, pl **-ties** : the makeup or characteristics of a particular zygote

zy·go·spore \'zī-gə-ˌspō(ə)r, -ˌspo(ə)r\ n : a plant spore that is formed by union of two similar sexual cells, usu. serves as a resting spore, and produces the sporophytic phase of the plant

zy·go·style \'zī-gə-ˌstīl\ n : the terminal caudal vertebra

zy·gote \'zī-ˌgōt\ n : a cell formed by the union of two gametes; broadly : the developing individual produced from such a cell

zygote in·tra·fal·lo·pi·an transfer \-ˌin-trə-fə-'lō-pē-ən\ n : a method of assisting reproduction in cases of infertility in which eggs are obtained from an ovary and fertilized with sperm in vitro and the resulting fertilized eggs are inserted into a fallopian tube by a laparoscope — abbr. *ZIFT*; compare GAMETE INTRAFALLOPIAN TRANSFER

zy·go·tene \'zī-gə-ˌtēn\ n : the stage of meiotic prophase which immediately follows the leptotene and during which synapsis of homologous chromosomes occurs — **zygotene** adj

zy·got·ic \zī-'gät-ik\ adj : of, relating to, or existing as a zygote — **zy·got·i·cal·ly** \-i-k(ə-)lē\ adv

zy·go·zoo·spore \ˌzī-gō-'zō-ə-ˌspō(ə)r, -ˌspo(ə)r\ n : a motile zygospore

zy·mase \'zī-ˌmās, -ˌmāz\ n : an enzyme or enzyme complex that promotes glycolysis

zy·min \'zī-mən\ n : FERMENT 1

zy·mo·gen \'zī-mə-jən\ n : an inactive protein precursor of an enzyme secreted by living cells and converted (as by a kinase or an acid) into an active form — called also *proenzyme*

zy·mog·e·nous \zī-'mäj-ə-nəs\ adj : producing fermentation ⟨∼ organisms⟩

zy·mo·gram \'zī-mə-ˌgram\ n : an electrophoretic strip (as of starch gel) or a representation of it exhibiting the pattern of separated enzymes and esp. isoenzymes after electrophoresis

zy·mol·o·gy \zī-'mäl-ə-jē\ n : a science that deals with fermentation

zy·mo·plas·tic \ˌzī-mō-'plas-tik\ adj : participating in the formation of enzymes ⟨∼ substances⟩

zy·mo·san \'zī-mə-ˌsan\ n : an insoluble largely polysaccharide fraction of yeast cell walls

zy·mos·ter·ol \zī-'mäs-tə-ˌrol, -ˌrōl\ n : a crystalline unsaturated sterol $C_{27}H_{43}OH$ occurring with ergosterol in yeast fat, resembling ergosterol chemically, and yielding cholestanol on hydrogenation

zy·mos·then·ic \ˌzī-məs-'then-ik\ adj : strengthening the activity of an enzyme

zy·mot·ic \zī-'mät-ik\ adj 1 : of, relating to, causing, or caused by fermentation 2 : relating to or being an infectious or contagious disease

Zy·prexa \zī-'prek-sə\ trademark — used for a preparation of olanzapine

Zyr·tec \'zər-ˌtek\ trademark — used for a preparation of the dihydrochloride of cetirizine

Signs and Symbols

Biology

○	an individual, specif., a female — used chiefly in inheritance charts
☐	an individual, specif., a male — used chiefly in inheritance charts
♀	female

♂ or ⚦	male
+	wild type
×	crossed with; hybrid

Chemistry and Physics

(for element symbols see ELEMENT table)

α alpha particle

β beta particle, beta ray

λ wavelength

+   signifies "plus," "and," "together with" — used between the symbols of substances brought together for, or produced by, a reaction;

signifies a unit charge of positive electricity when placed to the right of a symbol as a superscript: Ca^{2+} or Ca^{++} denotes the ion of calcium, which carries two positive charges;

signifies a dextrorotatory compound when preceding in parentheses a compound name [as in (+)-tartaric acid]

−   signifies removal or loss of a part from a compound during a reaction (as in $-CO_2$);

signifies a unit charge of negative electricity when placed to the right of a symbol as a superscript: Cl^- denotes a chlorine ion carrying a negative charge;

signifies a levorotatory compound when preceding in parentheses a compound name [as in (−)-quinine]

−   signifies a single bond — used between the symbols of elements or groups which unite to form a compound (as in H–Cl for HCl and H–O–H for H_2O)

>   signifies separate single bonds from an atom to two other atoms or groups (as in the group >C=NNHR characteristic of hydrazone)

·   used to separate parts of a compound regarded as loosely joined (as in $CuSO_4 \cdot 5H_2O$);

also used to denote the presence of a single unpaired electron (as in H·)

=   indicates a double bond;

signifies two unit charges of negative electricity when placed to the right of a symbol as a superscript (as in $SO_4^=$, the negative ion of sulfuric acid)

≡   signifies a triple bond or a triple negative charge

:   signifies a pair of electrons belonging to an atom that are not shared with another atom (as in :NH_3);

sometimes signifies a double bond (as in CH_2:CH_2)

( )   marks groups within a compound [as in $C_6H_4(CH_3)_2$, the formula for xylene which contains two methyl groups (CH_3)]

⌐ or ⌐   joins attached atoms or groups in structural formulas for cyclic compounds, as that for glucose

$$\overline{\qquad O \qquad}$$
$$CH_2OHCH(CHOH)_3CHOH$$

1-, 2-, etc.   used in names to indicate the positions of substituting groups, attached to the first, second, etc., of the numbered atoms of the parent compound (as in 5-fluorouracil or glucose-6-phosphate)

x, m, n used as subscripts following an atom or group in a chemical formula to indicate that the number of times the atom or group occurs is indefinite [as in $(C_6H_{10}O_5)$ for glycogen] or approximate [as in $C_{12}H_mAl_{16}O_nS_8$ for sucralfate where m and n are approximately 54 and 75]

R   group—used esp. of an organic group

′   used to distinguish between different substituents of the same kind (as R′, R″, R‴ to indicate different organic groups)

Medicine

℞ take — used on prescriptions; prescription; treatment

☠ poison

☣ biohazard, biohazardous materials

☢ *or* ☢ radiation, radioactivity, radioactive materials

☢ fallout shelter

APOTHECARIES' MEASURES

℥ ounce

ƒ℥ fluid ounce

ƒ ʒ fluid dram

min *or* ℞ minim

APOTHECARIES' WEIGHTS

℔ pound

℥ ounce: as

℥ i *or* ℥ j, one ounce;

℥ ss, half an ounce;

℥ iss *or* ℥ jss, one ounce and a half;

℥ ij, two ounces

ʒ dram

℈ scruple

A Handbook of Style

Punctuation

Punctuation is used to separate groups of words for meaning and emphasis; to convey an idea of the variations of pitch, volume, pause, and intonation of speech; and to help avoid ambiguity. Punctuation marks, together with general rules and examples of their use, follow.

Apostrophe

1. Indicates the possessive of nouns and indefinite pronouns.

> Dr. Donohue's office
>
> anyone's guess
>
> the boy's mother
>
> the boys' mothers
>
> the AMA's convention
>
> 2001's Nobel Prize winners
>
> the Browns' house

2. Marks omissions in contracted words.

> didn't
>
> o'clock

3. Often forms plurals of letters, figures, abbreviations, and words referred to as words.

> cross your *t*'s
>
> three 8's *or* three 8s
>
> two Ph.D.'s *or* two PhDs
>
> used &'s instead of *and*'s

Brackets

1. Enclose editorial comments, corrections, and clarifications inserted into quoted matter.

> Surely that should have peaked [sic] the curiosity of a serious researcher.

2. Function as parentheses within parentheses.

> A tranquilizer (such as chlorpromazine [Thorazine]) should be prescribed.

3. Sometimes indicate that the charge on an ionic complex belongs to the whole complex rather than to an individual atom.

> $[Fe(CN)_5NO]^{--}$

4. Sometimes indicate the site of attachment of a substituent in a molecule.

> benzo[*a*]pyrene

Colon

1. Introduces a clause or phrase that explains, illustrates, amplifies, or restates what has gone before.

> The medication appeared to be working: the patient was regaining lost weight and was no longer disoriented.

2. Directs attention to an appositive.

> He had only one pleasure: eating.

3. Introduces a series.

> The patient presented the following medical problems: diabetes mellitus, chronic bronchitis, and emphysema.

4. Introduces lengthy quoted material set off from the rest of a text by indentation but not by quotation marks.

> I quote from part I of the study:

5. Separates data in bibliographical references (such as the volume number from a page number or a publisher's location from the name of the publisher).

> *JAMA* 2001;285:2987
>
> New York: Random House

6. Follows the salutation in formal correspondence.

> Ladies and Gentlemen:
>
> Dear Dr. McCarthy:

Comma

1. Separates main clauses joined by a coordinating conjunction (such as *and, but, or, nor,* or *so*) and very short clauses not joined by a conjunction.

> Seven out of ten patients claimed that the drug relieved their symptoms, and three said that it completely eliminated them.
>
> I came, I saw, I conquered.

2. Sets off an adverbial clause or long phrase that precedes the main clause.

> When she found that the tests were positive, she called the doctor.

3. Sets off transitional words and expressions (such as *on the contrary, on the other hand*), conjunctive adverbs (such as *consequently, however*), and expressions that introduce an illustration or example (such as *namely, for example*).

> Your second question, on the other hand, remains unanswered.
>
> They are eager to begin construction of the clinic; however, the necessary materials have not yet arrived.
>
> She expects to evaluate two drugs, namely, propranolol and fluoxetine.

4. Separates words, phrases, or clauses in a series.

> Men, women, and children crowded aboard the train.
>
> Her job required her to pack quickly, to travel often, and to have no personal life.

5. Separates coordinate adjectives modifying a noun.

> It is a safe, effective, reliable drug.

6. Sets off parenthetical elements such as nonrestrictive modifiers and appositives.

> These programs, all of which should be under a physician's supervision, are not recommended for patients with high blood pressure.
>
> The nursing supervisor, Sally Dowd, attended the meeting.

7. Introduces a direct quotation, terminates a direct quotation that is neither a question nor an exclamation, and sets off split quotations.

> The nurse said, "I am leaving."
>
> "I am leaving,"the nurse said.
>
> "I am leaving,"the nurse said in a friendly way, "but I'll come back soon."

8. Sets off words in direct address, absolute phrases, and mild interjections.

> We would like to discuss your account, Mr. Baker.
>
> I fear the encounter, her temper being what it is.
>
> Ah, that's my idea of a sensible procedure.

9. Indicates the omission of a word or phrase used in a parallel construction earlier in a sentence.

> Some medical transcriptionists work for single-physician practices; others, for group practices.

10. Is used to avoid ambiguity that might arise from adjacent words.

> To John, Marshall was someone special.
>
> Whatever will be, will be.

11. Is used to group numbers into units of three to separate thousands, millions, and so on; however, it is not used in page numbers, street numbers, or numbers within dates.

> 2,000 case histories
>
> a population of 1,350,000
>
> > *but*
>
> page 1411
>
> 4507 Chestnut Street
>
> the year 2000

12. Punctuates an inverted name.

> Salk, Jonas E.

13. Separates a surname from a following academic degree or honorary, governmental, or military title.

> Amelia P. Artandi, D.V.M.
>
> Robert Menard, M.A., Ph.D.
>
> Sandra Cobb, Vice President

14. Sets off geographical names (such as state or country from city), items in dates, and addresses.

> Houston, Texas, is the site of a large Air Force medical center.
>
> On July 18, 2001, the patient was examined.
>
> Mail your check to South Suburban Hospital, 5600 Swarthmore Street, Evans, MO 56789.

15. Follows the salutation in informal correspondence and follows the complimentary close of a letter.

> Dear Rachel,
>
> Warm regards,
>
> Very truly yours,

Dash

1. Marks an abrupt change or break in the structure of a sentence.

> The students seemed happy with the change, but the alumni—there was the problem.

> If I had kept my notes—and I really wish that I had—I would be able to tell you the exact date of the visit.

2. Introduces a summary statement that follows a series of words or phrases.

> Cancer, heart attacks, and strokes—these are the health problems that people seem to fear most.

3. Often precedes the attribution of a quotation.

> What wound did ever heal but by degrees—
> William Shakespeare

Ellipsis Points

1. Indicate the omission of one or more words within a quoted sentence.

> Now we are engaged in a great civil war testing whether that nation . . . can long endure.

2. Indicate the omission of one or more sentences within a quoted passage or the omission of words up to, including, or following the end of a sentence by using four dots, the first of which represents the period. Alternatively, the period may be dropped and all omissions may be indicated simply by three ellipsis points.

> Now we are engaged in a great civil war. . . . We are met on a great battlefield of that war.

> From these honored dead we take increased devotion to that cause for which they gave the last full measure of devotion. . . .

3. Indicate halting speech or an unfinished sentence in dialogue.

> "I'd like to . . . that is . . . if you don't mind . . . "

Exclamation Point

1. Ends an emphatic sentence or phrase.

> Get out of here!

> And now our competition—get this!—wants to start sharing secrets.

2. Ends an emphatic interjection.

> Stat!

Hyphen

1. Is used to link elements in compound words.

> secretary-treasurer
> cost-effective
> fund-raiser
> spin-off

2. Is usually used between elements of a compound modifier preceding the word it modifies. However, foreign phrases and names of diseases and chemical compounds are not hyphenated even when they serve as preceding compound modifiers.

> low-level radiation
> first-degree burns
> *but*
> cri du chat syndrome
> in vivo examination
> diabetes mellitus complications
> carbon monoxide poisoning

3. Is often used with prefixes to separate two identical adjoining vowels. However, there are many exceptions, including most words beginning with *pre-* and *re-*.

> anti-inflation
> de-escalate
> intra-arterial
> *but*
> preeclampsia
> reeducation

4. Is used with prefixes attached to numerals or capitalized base words.

> pre-2000 projections
> non-20th-century ideas
> neo-Freudian
> post-Victorian architecture

5. Suspends the first part of a hyphenated compound when used with another hyphenated compound.

> a 4- to 8-mg dose
> *but*
> a dose of 4 to 8 mg

6. Is used in writing out compound numbers between 21 and 99.

> thirty-four
> one hundred twenty-eight

7. Marks an end-of-line division of a word.

> Smallpox, formerly a great scourge, was declared totally eradicated by the World Health Organization.

8. Serves as an equivalent to the phrase "(up) to and including" when used between numbers and dates; in typeset material, it is replaced by an en dash.

> pages 40–98
>
> the years 2002–2005

9. Serves as the equivalent of *to, and,* or *versus* in indicating linkage or opposition. (In typeset material the longer en dash is used.)

> the New York–Paris flight
>
> the Hardy–Weinberg law
>
> Hand–Schüller–Christian disease
>
> The final score was 7–2.

Parentheses

1. Enclose supplementary, parenthetical, or explanatory material.

> A large number of patients (44.8%) required two calls before follow-up could be obtained.
>
> as shown in the graph (Figure 1)

2. Enclose numerals that confirm a written number in a business or legal context.

> Delivery will be made in thirty (30) days.

3. Enclose a bibliographic reference given in running text.

> A similar view was noted by Watson (*Science* 1990;248:45).

4. Enclose numbers or letters indicating individual elements or items in a series.

> We must set forth (1) our long-term goals, (2) our immediate objectives, and (3) the means at our disposal.

5. Enclose abbreviations that follow their spelled-out forms.

> the presence of benign prostatic hyperplasia (BPH)

6. Enclose proprietary names of drugs when they follow generic names in running text, and sometimes vice versa.

> administration of lisinopril (Zestril) to lower blood pressure
>
> U.S. embassies were instructed to stock up on the antibiotic Cipro (ciprofloxacin) in case of a bioterrorist anthrax attack.

Period

1. Ends a sentence or sentence fragment that is neither interrogative nor exclamatory.

> She answered all of the questions on the form.
>
> She asked whether he had answered all the questions on the form.
>
> Not bad.

2. Punctuates some abbreviations.

> Dr.
>
> No. 2 pencils
>
> Fig. 15
>
> etc.
>
> e.g.
>
> A.D.
>
> b.i.d.

Question Mark

1. Ends a direct question.

> Who authorized the procedure?
>
> "Who signed the memo?" she asked.

2. Punctuates each element of an interrogative series that is neither numbered nor lettered; however, only one such mark punctuates a numbered or lettered interrogative series.

> Has the patient completed the needed insurance forms? Checked the data? Signed the forms where indicated?
>
> Has the patient (1) completed the needed insurance forms, (2) checked the data, (3) signed the forms where indicated?

3. Indicates that a piece of information is unknown or uncertain.

> Jean Nicot (1530?–1600), French diplomat who introduced tobacco to France and for whom *nicotine* is named.

Quotation Marks

1. Enclose direct quotations but not indirect quotations.

> He said, "I am leaving."
>
> *but*
>
> He said he was leaving.

2. Enclose words or phrases borrowed from others, words used in a special way, and often a word of marked informality when introduced into formal writing.

> Be sure to send a copy of your résumé—or as some folks would say, your "biodata summary."

They were afraid the patient had "stroked out"—had had a stroke.

3. Enclose titles of reports, short poems, short stories, articles, lectures, chapters of books, short musical compositions, and radio and television program episodes.

> the report "Smoking and Health"
>
> Robert Frost's "The Death of the Hired Man"
>
> O'Conner's story "Good Country People"
>
> an article on doctors' compensation, "Differences in Earnings between Male and Female Physicians," in *The New England Journal of Medicine*
>
> the chapter entitled "Medical Ethics"
>
> "America the Beautiful"
>
> Ravel's "Bolero"
>
> M*A*S*H's final episode, "Goodbye, Farewell and Amen"

4. Are used with other punctuation marks in the following ways:
The period and the comma fall *within* the quotation marks.

> "The doctor will see you," she said.
>
> The bandage was described as "waterproof," but a better description would have been "moisture-resistant."

The semicolon and colon fall *outside* the quotation marks.

> They spoke of their "little cottage in the country"; they might better have called it a mansion.

The question mark and exclamation point fall *within* the quotation marks when they refer to the quoted matter only; they fall *outside* when they refer to the whole sentence.

> He asked, "When did the doctor arrive?"
>
> What is the meaning of "greenstick fracture"?
>
> She shouted, "Stop right there!"
>
> Save us from his "mercy"!

5. Are not used with *yes* or *no* except in direct discourse.

> We said yes to all their proposals.

6. Are not used with lengthy quotations set off from the rest of the text.

> John Dirckx begins his essay with a general description of medical English:
>
> > The language of modern medicine, a vigorous, versatile idiom of vast range and formidable intricacy, expands constantly to meet the needs of a complex and rapidly evolving discipline. Medical English in its broadest sense includes not only the official nomenclatures of the basic medical sciences (such as anatomy, biochemistry, pathology, and immunology) and the clinical specialties (such as pediatrics, dermatology, thoracic surgery, and psychiatry) but also a large body of less formal expressions, a sort of

trade jargon used by physicians and their professional associates in speech, correspondence, and record-keeping.

7. Are replaced by single quotation marks when enclosing a quotation within a quotation.

> The witness said, "I distinctly heard him say, 'Don't be late,' and then I heard the door close."

8. Are often replaced by single quotation marks in British usage.

> The witness said, 'I distinctly heard him say, "Don't be late," and then I heard the door close.'

Semicolon

1. Separates main clauses joined without a coordinating conjunction.

> Some people have the ability to handle sick people effectively; others do not.

2. Separates main clauses joined by a conjunctive adverb (such as *consequently, furthermore, however*).

> It won't be easy to sort out the facts of this confusing situation; however, a decision must be made.

3. Separates phrases and clauses that themselves contain commas often even when such clauses are joined by a coordinating conjunction.

> Send copies to my colleagues in Portland, Maine; Savannah, Georgia; and Springfield, Illinois.
>
> We fear that this situation may, in fact, occur; but for the time being, we don't know when.

Slash

1. Represents the words *per* or *to* when used between units of measure or the terms of a ratio.

> 40,000 tons/year
>
> 29 mi/gal
>
> cost/benefit analysis　*or*　cost-benefit analysis
>
> 20/20 vision

2. Separates alternatives, usually representing the words *or* or *and/or*.

> alumni/ae
>
> his/her

3. Replaces the word *and* in some compound terms.

> the May/June issue　*or*　the May–June issue
>
> 2001/02　*or*　2001–02
>
> travel/study trip　*or*　travel-study trip

4. Is sometimes used to replace certain prepositions such as *at, versus,* and *for.*

U.C./Berkeley *or* U.C.–Berkeley

parent/child issues *or* parent-child issues

5. Punctuates a few abbreviations.

w/o [*for* without]

c/o [*for* care of]

d/b/a [*for* doing business as]

o/a [*for* on or about]

Capitalization

Capital letters are used for two broad purposes: they mark a beginning (as of a sentence), and they signal a proper noun or adjective. The following principles, each with examples, describe the most common uses of capital letters.

1. The first word of a sentence or sentence fragment is capitalized.

> The meeting was postponed.
>
> No! I cannot.
>
> How are you feeling?
>
> Bravo!

2. The first word of a sentence within parentheses is capitalized; however, if the sentence occurs within another sentence, the first word is not capitalized.

> The meeting ended. (The results were not revealed.)
>
> She studied medicine with Dr. Heller (he wrote this text, you know) at the university.

3. The first word of a direct quotation is capitalized, but the first word of the continuation of a split quotation is not capitalized unless it begins a new sentence. However, when a quotation is tightly bound to the rest of the sentence, its first word is not capitalized.

> The medical director said, "We have rejected this report entirely."
>
> "We have rejected this report entirely," the medical director said, "and we will not comment on it further."
>
> The medical director made it clear that "there is no room for compromise."

4. The first word of a direct question within a sentence is capitalized.

> The question is, Who is responsible for keeping track of instruments in the operating room?

5. The first word following a colon may be lowercased or capitalized if it introduces a complete sentence. While the former is the more usual styling, the latter is common especially when the sentence introduced by the colon is fairly long and distinctly separate from the preceding clause.

> The advantage of this particular system is clear: it's inexpensive.
>
> The situation is critical: This hospital cannot hope to recoup the fourth-quarter losses that were sustained this fiscal year.

6. The first word of the salutation of a letter and the first word of the complimentary close are capitalized.

> Dear Mary,
>
> Ladies and Gentlemen:
>
> Sincerely yours,

7. Words in titles of printed matter are capitalized except for internal conjunctions and prepositions (especially those having fewer than four letters) and for articles. (For the capitalization of titles in medical references see the section on References that follows.)

> *Writing and Communicating in Medicine*
>
> "A Logical Basis for Medical Mythology"

8. The names of persons and places, of organizations and their members, of congresses and councils, and of historical periods and events are capitalized.

> Joseph Lister
>
> Rome
>
> Texas
>
> England
>
> American Medical Association
>
> Baptists
>
> the United Methodist Church
>
> the Food and Drug Administration
>
> the Yalta Conference
>
> the Middle Ages
>
> World War II

9. Words designating peoples and their languages are capitalized.

> Canadians
>
> Turks
>
> Swedish
>
> Welsh
>
> Iroquois
>
> Ibo
>
> Vietnamese

10. Derivatives of proper names are capitalized when used in their primary sense; consult a dictionary when in doubt about styling.

>Adlerian therapy
>
>Asiatic cholera
>
>Skinnerian theory
>
>>*but*
>
>pasteurize
>
>cesarean section

11. Words of family relationship preceding the name of a person are capitalized when they are treated as part of the name; otherwise they are lowercased.

>Aunt Mona and Uncle George came to see us.
>
>It's good to see you, Cousin Julia.
>
>>*but*
>
>Have you met my uncle George?

12. Titles preceding the name of a person and epithets used instead of a name are capitalized whether spelled out in full or abbreviated.

>President Roosevelt
>
>Professor Harris
>
>Dr. Collins
>
>Old Hickory
>
>the Iron Chancellor
>
>>*but*
>
>the doctor's assistant

13. Days of the week, months of the year, holidays, and holy days are capitalized.

>Tuesday
>
>July
>
>Independence Day
>
>Easter
>
>Good Friday
>
>Yom Kippur

14. Names of specific courts of law are capitalized.

>the United States Court of Appeals for the Second Circuit

15. Brand names, trademarks, and service marks are capitalized.

>Breathalyzer
>
>Viagra
>
>Planned Parenthood
>
>Rolfing
>
>Kleenex
>
>Band-Aid

16. Geologic eras, periods, epochs, strata, and names of prehistoric divisions are capitalized.

>Silurian period

>Pleistocene epoch
>
>Neolithic age

17. Planets, constellations, asteroids, stars, and groups of stars are capitalized; however, *sun, earth,* and *moon* are usually not capitalized unless they are listed with other astronomical names.

>Venus
>
>Big Dipper
>
>Sirius
>
>Pleiades
>
>a trip to the moon
>
>the effect of solar radiation on Mercury, Venus, and Earth

18. New Latin names of genera in binomial nomenclature in zoology, botany, and bacteriology are capitalized; names of species in zoology and bacteriology are not. Although the *International Code of Botanical Nomenclature* recommends that all species names start with a lowercase letter, it allows capitalization in certain cases (as a species name derived from the name of a person) at the discretion of the author of the species

>the rhesus monkey (*Macaca mulatta*)
>
>a bacterium (*Chlamydia trachomatis*)

19. New Latin names of all groups above genera (as families, orders, classes, and phyla) in zoology, botany, and bacteriology are capitalized; however, their derivative adjectives and nouns are not.

>the family Tabanidae
>
>the order Diptera
>
>the class Insecta
>
>the phylum Arthropoda
>
>>*but*
>
>arthropod evolution
>
>arthropods
>
>insect pests
>
>insects
>
>dipteran flies
>
>dipterans

20. Proper names forming essential elements of terms designating diseases, syndromes, and tests are capitalized.

>Parkinson's disease
>
>Down syndrome
>
>Rorschach test

21. Proper names forming essential elements of scientific laws, theorems, and principles are capitalized.

>Weber–Fechner law
>
>Bell's law
>
>Planck's constant

Italicization

The following are usually italicized in print and underlined in manuscript and typescript.

1. Titles of books, journals, published theses, magazines, newspapers, plays, movies, works of art, and long musical compositions.

> Fishbein's *Medical Writing*
>
> the magazine *Drug Topics*
>
> a thesis entitled *Recent Trends in Lung Cancer Mortality among Coal Miners*
>
> Shakespeare's *Othello*
>
> the movie *Arachnophobia*
>
> Norman Rockwell's *Doctor and Doll*
>
> Mozart's *Don Giovanni*

2. Names of ships and airplanes and often spacecraft.

> M.V. *West Star*
>
> Lindbergh's *Spirit of St. Louis*
>
> *Apollo 11*

3. Words, letters, and figures when referred to as such.

> The word *receive* is often misspelled.
>
> The *g* in *align* is silent.
>
> The first *2* and the last *0* are barely legible.

4. Foreign words and phrases that have not been naturalized in English.

> *ad manus medici*
>
> *modo prescriptio*
>
> *oculus dexter*
>
> *quater in die*
>
> > *but*
>
> in vitro
>
> in vivo

5. New Latin scientific names of genera, species, subspecies, and varieties (but not groups of high rank, as phyla, classes, or orders) in botanical or zoological names.

> a spirochete of the genus *Treponema*
>
> poison sumac (*Rhus vernix*)
>
> > *but*
>
> the phylum Arthropoda
>
> the order Diptera

6. Case titles in legal citations, both in full and shortened form ("v." for "versus" is set roman or italic).

> *Jones* v. *Massachusetts*
>
> the *Jones* case
>
> *Jones*

References

Writers give credit to other authors' published work by the use of references within the text that are keyed to a list at the end of the article, chapter, or book. The references in the list are either numbered and listed in the order cited in the text or are listed in alphabetical order with or without numbers and by date for references to several works by the same author. References in journals are usually listed in the order cited while those in books and comprehensive monographs are more often ordered alphabetically. When the date is used to order references to publications by the same author, the publication date of every reference usually follows the list of authors. In a list given in the order cited in the text the publication date is usually placed near the end of the reference. Typical examples of the two systems are given below. The first is from a journal and the second from a book:

> 11. Cregler LL, Mark H. Medical complications of cocaine abuse. N Engl J Med 1986;315:1495–500.
>
> Pullman W E, Bodmer W F 1992 Cloning and characterization of a gene that regulates cell adhesion. Nature 356: 529–532

Within the text, the references to the bibliographic list may appear as small superscript numerals or in parentheses on the line of text as numbers or as last names and dates. Journals tend to use numbers while longer monographs and books with a comprehensive bibliography tend to mention the author and date. Examples are given below:

Superscript reference to a numbered list — Two weeks later, serologic data from case patients suggested that a new *Hantavirus* was associated with these cases.[5,7]

Unfortunately, the increasing widespread emergence of acquired resistance to antibiotics over the past 40 years now constitutes a serious threat to global public health[1–3]. . . .

Parenthetical reference to a numbered list   A large part of the problem is that all cancer risk assessments are derived from studies of cohorts exposed to very high levels of insult (*1, 2*).

The chemical and physical properties of atomic-level surface defects play a crucial role in governing the outcome of many important interfacial processes such as chemical catalysis (*1–4*) and crystal growth (*5–8*).

Parenthetical reference to an alphabetical list   In contrast there is evidence, anatomical (Hoff & Hoff 1934, Kupyers 1960, Liu & Chambers 1964) and physiological (Bernhard et al 1953, Preston & Whitlock 1961, Landgren et al 1962), that in monkeys some corticospinal fibres end. . . .

In a journal, the principal features of the reference entry are these: (1) the author or list of authors is placed first; (2) the names of no more than usually three or six authors are listed, and "et al." is used to indicate that a list of authors has been truncated; (3) initials are used for an author's first and middle names and increasingly are closed up without any punctuation and follow an author's name without being set off by a comma; (4) words in titles are lowercased except for the first word, the first word of any subtitle, and proper nouns and adjectives; (5) titles of books and articles are not enclosed in quotation marks and depending on the style of the source may or may not be italicized; and (6) the date follows the title and for journal articles is followed by a semicolon, the volume number (which is sometimes in boldface), a colon, and the page numbers. As indicated above, in books or publications with a comprehensive bibliography where the date is used to order references by the same author (or authors), it is placed immediately after the author's name.

In preparing a manuscript for publication, the author should look carefully for subtleties in styling the list of references. The first example below is a reference from the *Journal of the American Medical Association* (*JAMA*) to an article in *The New England Journal of Medicine* (*N Eng J Med*), and the second is a reference in an article in *The New England Journal of Medicine* to one in *JAMA*:

27. Croog SH, Levine S, Testa MA, et al. The effects of antihypertensive therapy on the quality of life. *N Eng J Med.* 1986;314:1657–1664.

10. Reinhardt UE. Wanted: a clearly articulated social ethic for American health care. JAMA 1997;278:1446–7.

The reader will note the use of boldface in the reference number, lack of indentation on the second and succeeding lines of the reference, the presence or absence of italics in the journal name, the presence or absence of a period following the journal name, and the use of full page numbers or a cutback for the final page of the article. Both journals permit lists of up to six authors but cut them back to three when "et al."(styled in roman type and terminated by a period) is used.

In the following three pairs of bibliographic citations for a book, government document or publication, and newspaper, the first of each pair is from *JAMA* and the second is from *The New England Journal of Medicine:*

Book   **20.** Fuchs VR. *Who Shall Live: Health, Economics, and Social Choice.* New York, NY: Basic Books Inc Publishers; 1974.

4. Daniel WW. Biostatistics: a foundation for analysis in the health sciences. 7th ed. New York: John Wiley, 1999.

Government publication   **62.** *Effects of Managed Care: An Update.* Washington, DC: Congressional Budget Office; 1994.

1. Centers for Disease Control and Prevention. Tuberculosis statistics in the United States, 1991. Atlanta: Department of Health and Human Services, 1993.

Newspaper   **82.** Henneberger M. Managed care changing practice of psychotherapy. *New York Times.* October 9, 1994:A1, A50.

5. Kolata G. Boom in Ritalin sales raises ethical issues. New York Times. May 15, 1996:C8.

Several of the references above have been restyled below as they might appear in an alphabetical list in a monograph or book:

Center for Disease Control and Prevention. 1993. Tuberculosis statistics in the United States, 1991. Atlanta: Department of Health and Human Services.

Daniel WW. 1999. Biostatistics: a foundation for analysis in the health sciences, 7th ed. New York, NY: John Wiley & Sons, Inc.

Croog SH, Levine S, Testa MA, et al. 1986. The effects of antihypertensive therapy on the quality of life. N Eng J Med. 314:1657–1664.

Henneberger M. 1994. Managed care changing practice of psychotherapy. New York Times. October 9: A1, A50.

Many authors use more capitals in titles and more punctuation and italics than are shown above, but the current trend is toward a bare-bones approach to reference lists.

The styling of references to journal articles in two leading British medical publications, the *British Medical Journal* (*BMJ*) and *The Lancet,* is very similar to that in *JAMA* and *The New England Journal of Medicine* except for the unpunctuated lightface reference numbers, the boldface volume numbers in *The Lancet*, the even sparser punctuation in both journals, and the listing of six authors with "et al." in *BMJ*. The first example below is from *BMJ* and the second from *The Lancet:*

17 Friel JK, Andrews WL, Matthew JD, Long DR, Cornel AM, Cox M, et al. Iron status of very-low-birth-weight infants during the first 15 months of infancy. *Can Med Assoc J* 1990;143:733–36.

18 Jendrossek V, Peters AMJ, Buth S, et al. Improvement of superoxide production in monocytes from patients with chronic granulomatous disease by recombinant cyto-kines. *Blood* 1993; **81**: 211–36.

Two of the world's leading interdisciplinary scientific journals published in English, the American publication *Science* and the British journal *Nature,* eliminate the titles of articles in references to journals but not in references to books. Their styles of punctuation are somewhat more conservative than in the examples given above. Volume numbers are in boldface, and *Science* permits several references to be grouped following one number in the reference list. Reference 13 below is from *Science* and 31 and 38 from *Nature:*

13. M. J. Thirman, D. A. Levitan, H. Kobayashi, M. C. Simon, J. D. Rowley, *Proc. Natl. Acad. Sci. U.S.A.* **91**, 12110 (1994); K. Mitani *et al., Blood* **85**, 2017 (1995).

31. Halachmi, S. *et al. Science* **264**, 1455–1458 (1994).

38. Saha, S., Brickman, J. M., Lehming, N. & Ptashne, M. *Nature* **363**, 648–652 (1993).

Science cites only the beginning page number of an article, and lists of authors in both *Science* and *Nature* are cut back to a single name when *et al.* (in italics) is used. Other differences can be found by comparing the styles of these two journals between themselves and with those of others mentioned above.

It is hoped that the examples given here will show an editor or author what to look for in preparing a list of references for an established journal and will help in selecting an individual style for a comprehensive list of references in a monograph or book. For more extensive treatment on the styling of references than can be provided here, consult *Merriam-Webster's Manual for Writers and Editors, The Chicago Manual of Style,* or *The American Medical Association Manual of Style: A Guide for Authors and Editors.*